# Modern Surgical Pathology

**Noel Weidner, M.D.**

*Professor and Director of Anatomic Pathology*
*University of California, San Diego*
*School of Medicine*
*San Diego, California*

**Richard J. Cote, M.D.**

*Professor of Pathology and Urology*
*University of Southern California*
*Keck School of Medicine*
*Director, Genitourinary Cancer Program*
*USC Norris Comprehensive Cancer Center*
*Los Angeles, California*

**Saul Suster, M.D.**

*Professor and Vice Chair of Pathology*
*Director of Anatomic Pathology*
*The Ohio State University Medical Center*
*Columbus, Ohio*

**Lawrence M. Weiss, M.D.**

*Chair, Division of Pathology*
*Director, Surgical Pathology*
*City of Hope National Medical Center*
*Duarte, California*

SAUNDERS
An Imprint of Elsevier Science
Philadelphia  London  New York  St. Louis  Sydney  Tokyo

**SAUNDERS**
An Imprint of Elsevier Science

The Curtis Center
Independence Square West
Philadelphia, PA 19106

ISBN Volume 1 0-7216-7254-X
Volume 2 0-7216-7255-8
2 Volume Set 0-7216-7253-1

Modern Surgical Pathology

---

**Notice**

Medicine is an ever-changing field. Standard safety precautions must be followed, but as new research and clinical experience broaden our knowledge, changes in treatment and drug therapy become necessary or appropriate. Readers are advised to check the product information currently provided by the manufacturer of each drug to be administered to verify the recommended dose, the method and duration of administration, and the contraindications. It is the responsibility of the treating physician, relying on experience and knowledge of the patient, to determine dosages and the best treatment for the patient. Neither the publisher nor the editor assumes any responsibility for any injury and/or damage to persons or property.

The Publisher

---

**Library of Congress Cataloging-in-Publication Data**
Modern surgical pathology/[edited by] Noel Weidner . . . [et al.].—1st ed.
    p.;cm.
     ISBN 0-7216-7253-1(set)
    1. Pathology, Surgical.   I. Weidner, Noel.
    [DNLM: 1. Pathology, Surgical. WO 142 M689 2003]
  RD57.M59 2003
  617'.07—dc21                               2002029405

All material in Chapter 11 is in the public domain, with the exception of any borrowed figures or tables. Figures 24–2 through 24–5, 24–7, 24–8, 24–10, 24–11, 24–17, and 24–28 are also in the public domain.

*Acquisitions Editor:* Allan Ross
*Developmental Editor:* Ann Ruzycka
*Project Manager:* Peter Faber
*Indexer:* Julie Shawvan

PI/PAR

Printed in Hong Kong

Last digit is the print number:  9  8  7  6  5  4  3  2  1

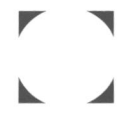

# Contributors

**Mahul B. Amin, MD**
Associate Professor of Pathology and Urology
Emory University School of Medicine
Director of Surgical Pathology
Emory University Hospital
Atlanta, Georgia
*Bladder and Urethra; Penis and Scrotum; Testis and Paratestis Including Spermatic Cord*

**Daniel A. Arber, MD**
Professor of Pathology
Director of Clinical Hematology and
Associate Director of Molecular Pathology
Stanford University Medical Center
Stanford, California
*Lymph Nodes; Spleen; Bone Marrow*

**Sylvia L. Asa, MD, PhD**
Professor, Department of Laboratory Medicine and
Pathobiology
University of Toronto Faculty of Medicine
Pathologist-in-Chief
University Health Network and Toronto Medical
Laboratories
Toronto, Ontario, Canada
*Pituitary*

**James B. Atkinson, MD, PhD**
Associate Professor of Pathology
Vanderbilt University School of Medicine
Attending Pathologist
Vanderbilt University Hospital
Nashville, Tennessee
*Muscle and Nerve Biopsy*

**Paul L. Auclair, DMD, MS**
Attending Pathologist
Department of Pathology
Maine Medical Center
Portland, Maine
*Pathology of the Salivary Glands*

**Michael J. Becich, MD, PhD**
Associate Professor of Pathology
University of Pittsburgh School of Medicine, and
Associate Professor of Information Science and
Telecommunications
University of Pittsburgh School of Information
Science

Director of Pathology Informatics and Director of
Urologic Pathobiology Laboratory
UPMC Health System
Pittsburgh, Pennsylvania
*Anatomic Pathology Laboratory Information Systems*

**David G. Bostwick, MD, MBA**
Clinical Professor of Pathology
University of Virginia School of Medicine
Charlottesville
Medical Director
Bostwick Laboratories
Richmond, Virginia
*Surgical Pathology of the Prostate*

**Allen Burke, MD**
Adjunct Professor
Georgetown University
Staff Pathologist, Cardiovascular Pathology
Armed Forces Institute of Pathology
Washington, District of Columbia
*Heart and Blood Vessels*

**R. Tucker Burks, MD**
Assistant Professor
Department of Pathology
Virginia Commonwealth University School of
Medicine
Richmond, Virgina
*Vulva and Vagina*

**Norman J. Carr, MBBS, FRCPath**
Head of Histopathology and Consultant Pathologist
Department of Cellular Pathology
Southampton General Hospital
Head of Histopathology and Consultant Pathologist
Pathology Department
Royal Hospital Haslar
Southampton, Hampshire, United Kingdom
*Appendix*

**John K. C. Chan, MBBS, FRCPath, FRCPA**
(DR) Consultant Pathologist
Department of Pathology
Queen Elizabeth Hospital
Hong Kong
*Thyroid and Parathyroid*

**Karen L. Chang, MD**
Staff Pathologist
Department of Pathology
City of Hope National Medical Center
Duarte, California
*Lymph Nodes*


**Richard J. Cote, MD, FRCPath**
Professor of Pathology and Urology
University of Southern California
Keck School of Medicine
Director, Genitourinary Cancer Program
USC Norris Comprehensive Cancer Center
Los Angeles, California
*Immunohistochemistry; Bladder and Urethra*


**Antonio L. Cubilla, MD**
Professor of Pathology
Facultad de Cíencías Medicas
Universidad Nacional
Director, Instituto de Pathologia e Investigacion
Asuncion, Paraguay
*Penis and Scrotum*


**Moacyr M. Da Silva, MD**
Medical Director, Western Division
IMPATH Inc.
Assistant Professor of Pathology
New York University
Adjunct Assistant Professor of Pathology
Cornell Medical College
New York, New York
*The Surgical Pathology Report*


**Stephen J. DeArmond, BS, MS, MD, PhD**
Professor of Neuropathology
University of California
San Francisco School of Medicine
Neuropathology Consultant
San Francisco General Hospital
San Francisco, California
*The Molecular and Genetic Basis of Neurodegenerative Diseases*


**John N. Eble, MD, MBA**
Nordschow Professor of Laboratory Medicine
Professor of Pathology and Laboratory Medicine,
and Chairman, Department of Pathology and
Laboratory Medicine
Indiana University School of Medicine
Chief Pathologist
Clarian Health Partners (Methodist–IU–Riley)
Indianapolis, Indiana
*Renal Neoplasia*


**Gary L. Ellis, DDS**
Director, Oral and Maxillofacial Pathology
ARUP Laboratories, Inc.
Salt Lake City, Utah
*Pathology of the Salivary Glands*


**Robert A. Erlandson, MS, PhD**
Associate Professor of Pathology
Weill Medical College of Cornell University
Attending Electron Microscopist and
Head, Diagnostic Electron Microscopy Laboratory
Memorial Sloan-Kettering Cancer Center
New York, New York
*Role of Electron Microscopy in Modern Diagnostic Surgical Pathology*


**Juan C. Felix, MD**
Professor of Pathology and
Obstetrics and Gynecology
University of Southern California Keck School of
Medicine
Chief of Surgical Pathology
Los Angeles County Women's and Children's
Hospital
Director of Obstetrical and Gynecological Pathology
Los Angeles County–University of Southern
California Medical Center
Los Angeles, California
*Vulva and Vagina; Cervix*


**Linda D. Ferrell, MD**
Professor of Pathology
University of California
San Francisco, School of Medicine
Vice-Chair of Clinical Affairs
UC Stanford Health Care–North Campus
San Francisco, California
*Liver; Gallbladder and Extrahepatic Bile Ducts*


**David A. Gaskin, MD, BMSc, BSc**
Clinical Instructor (Neuropathology)
Department of Pathology
University of California
San Francisco, School of Medicine
UCSF Medical Center
San Francisco, California
*The Molecular and Genetic Basis of Neurodegenerative Diseases*


**John R. Gilbertson, MD**
Adjunct Assistant Professor of Pathology
University of Pittsburgh School of Medicine
Pittsburgh, Pennsylvania
*Anatomic Pathology Laboratory Information Systems*

**Scott R. Granter, MD**
Assistant Professor of Pathology
Harvard Medical School
Associate Pathologist
Department of Pathology
Brigham and Women's Hospital
Consultant Pathologist
Children's Hospital
Boston, Massachusetts
*Inflammatory Skin Conditions*

**William C. Gross**
LIS Manager, Information Services Division
UPMC Health System
Pittsburgh, Pennsylvania
*Anatomic Pathology Laboratory Information Systems*

**Noam Harpaz, MD, PhD**
Associate Professor
Department of Pathology
Director, Gastrointestinal Pathology
Mount Sinai Medical Center
New York, New York
*Large Intestine*

**James H. Harrison, Jr., MD, PhD**
Associate Professor of Pathology
University of Pittsburgh School of Medicine
Pittsburgh, Pennsylvania
*Anatomic Pathology Laboratory Information Systems*

**Debra Hawes, MD**
Assistant Professor of Clinical Pathology
University of Southern California Keck School of Medicine
Los Angeles, California
*Immunohistochemistry*

**David R. Hinton, MD, FRCPC**
Professor of Pathology, Neurological Surgery, and Ophthalmology
Gavin S. Herbert Professor of Retinal Research
University of Southern California Keck School of Medicine
Director of Neuropathology
USC University Hospital
Los Angeles, California
*Pituitary*

**Bruce C. Horten, MD**
Medical Director, East Coast
IMPATH, Inc.
Consultant, Lenox Hill Hospital
New York, New York
*Central Nervous System Tumors*

**Lester O. Hosten, MD**
Fellow
Department of Ophthalmic Pathology
Armed Forces Institute of Pathology
Washington, DC
*The Eye and Ocular Adnexa*

**Ralph H. Hruban, MD**
Professor of Pathology and Oncology
Johns Hopkins University School of Medicine
Pathologist, Johns Hopkins Hospital
Baltimore, Maryland
*Pancreas*

**Mahlon D. Johnson, MD, PhD**
Associate Professor of Pathology
Vanderbilt University School of Medicine
Attending Pathologist
Vanderbilt University Hospital
Nashville, Tennessee
*Muscle and Nerve Biopsy*

**Cynthia G. Kaplan, MD**
Associate Professor of Pathology
State University of New York at Stony Brook School of Medicine
Pediatric Pathologist
University Hospital
Stony Brook, New York
*Gestational Pathology*

**Steve A. Kargas, MD, PhD**
Surgical Pathologist
IMPATH Inc.
Los Angeles, California
*The Surgical Pathology Report*

**Michael N. Koss, MD**
Professor
Department of Pathology
University of Southern California
Keck School of Medicine
Los Angeles, California
*The Non-neoplastic Kidney*

**Michael Kyriakos, MD**
Professor of Surgical Pathology
Washington University School of Medicine
St. Louis, Missouri
*Bone and Joint Pathology*

**W. Dwayne Lawrence, MD**
Professor and Vice Chair
Department of Pathology and Laboratory Medicine
Brown University Medical School
Chief, Department of Pathology and Laboratory Medicine
Women and Infants Hospital of Rhode Island
Providence, Rhode Island
*Uterus; Fallopian Tubes and Broad Ligament*

**David N. Lewin, MD**
Associate Professor
Department of Pathology and Laboratory Medicine
Medical University of South Carolina
Section of Surgical Pathology
Charleston, South Carolina
*Stomach; Small Intestine*

**Klaus J. Lewin, MD, FRCPath**
Professor of Pathology and Medicine
Department of Pathology
Division of Surgical Pathology
University of California, Los Angeles
UCLA School of Medicine
Los Angeles, California
*Stomach; Small Intestine*

**M. Beatriz S. Lopes, MD**
Associate Professor of Pathology–Neuropathology
University of Virginia School of Medicine
Director of Autopsy Services
University of Virginia Health Systems
Charlottesville, Virginia
*Central Nervous System Tumors*

**Ian W. McLean, MD**
Department of Ophthalmic Pathology
Armed Forces Institute of Pathology
Washington, District of Columbia
*The Eye and Ocular Adnexa*

**Martin C. Mihm, Jr., MD**
Professor of Pathology
Harvard Medical School
Consultant in Dermatopathology
Dermatopathology Unit
Massachusetts General Hospital
Boston, Massachusetts
*Inflammatory Skin Conditions; Tumors of the Skin*

**Thomas J. Montine, MD, PhD**
Assistant Professor of Pathology and Pharmacology
Vanderbilt University School of Medicine
Attending Pathologist
Vanderbilt University Hospital
Nashville, Tennessee
*Muscle and Nerve Biopsy*

**Cesar Moran, MD**
Professor of Pathology
University of Texas
M.D. Anderson Cancer Center
Houston, Texas
*The Lung; The Mediastinum*

**Christopher Moskaluk, MD, PhD**
Assistant Professor of Pathology and Biochemistry
Division of Surgical Pathology and Cytopathology
Department of Pathology
University of Virginia School of Medicine
Charlottesville, Virginia
*Esophagus*

**Lucien E. Nochomovitz, MD**
Clinical Professor of Pathology
State University of New York (S.U.N.Y.)
Stony Brook School of Medicine
Stony Brook
Chief of Anatomic Pathology
Department of Pathology
Winthrop University Hospital
Mineola, New York
*Gross Room and Specimen Handling*

**Debra Budwit Novotny, MD**
Associate Professor of Pathology and Laboratory
Medicine
University of North Carolina
Chapel Hill School of Medicine
Chapel Hill, North Carolina
*Ovaries*

**David A. Owen, MB, BCh, FRCPC, FRCPath**
Professor of Pathology
University of British Columbia Facility of Medicine
Consultant Pathologist
Vancouver General Hospital
Vancouver, British Columbia
*Anus*

**Zdena Pavlova, MD**
Associate Professor
Departments of Pathology and Pediatrics
University of Southern California
Keck School of Medicine
Los Angeles, California
*The Non-neoplastic Kidney*

**Nilsa C. Ramirez, MD**
Associate Professor–Clinical
Department of Pathology
Ohio State University College of Medicine
Attending Pathologist
Division of Anatomic Pathology
Department of Pathology
Ohio State University Medical Center
Columbus, Ohio
*Uterus; Fallopian Tubes and Broad Ligament*

**Mahendra Ranchod, MB, ChB, MMed(Path)**
Clinical Professor of Pathology
Stanford University School of Medicine, Stanford
Director of Anatomic Pathology
Department of Pathology
Good Samaritan Hospital
San Jose, California
*Intraoperative Consultations in Surgical Pathology*


**Joseph A. Regezi, DDS, MS**
Professor of Oral Pathology
University of California
San Francisco, Schools of Dentistry
Professor of Pathology
University of California
San Francisco, School of Medicine
Oral Pathologist
Department of Dentistry
UCSF Medical Center
San Francisco, California
*Oral Cavity and Jaws*


**Robert R. Rickert, MD**
Clinical Professor of Pathology
University of Medicine and Dentistry of New
Jersey–New Jersey Medical School
Newark
Co-Chairman, Department of Pathology
Saint Barnabas Medical Center
Livingston, New Jersey
*Essential Quality Improvement and Educational
Programs in Surgical Pathology*


**Capt. William B. Ross, MD**
Department of Scientific Laboratories
Armed Forces Institute of Pathology
Washington, District of Columbia
*The Non-neoplastic Kidney*


**Sharda G. Sabnis, MD**
Chief, Division of Nephropathology
Armed Forces Institute of Pathology
Washington, District of Columbia
*The Non-neoplastic Kidney*


**Eric D. Schubert, MD**
Staff Pathologist
Memorial Hospital
Chattanooga, Tennessee
*Anatomic Pathology Laboratory Information Systems*

**Jeffry P. Simko, PhD, MD, BSc**
Clinical Fellow
Department of Pathology
University of California
San Francisco, School of Medicine
Clinical Fellow
Department of Pathology
UCSF Medical Center
San Francisco, California
*The Molecular and Genetic Basis of Neurodegenerative
Diseases*


**Leslie H. Sobin, MD, FRCPath**
Chief, Division of Gastrointestinal Pathology
Department of Hepatic and Gastrointestinal
Pathology
Armed Forces Institute of Pathology
Washington, District of Columbia
*Appendix*


**Rashida A. Soni, MD**
Assistant Professor of Pathology
University of Southern California
Keck School of Medicine
Associate Attending
USC/Norris Comprehensive Cancer Center
Los Angeles, California
*Bladder and Urethra*


**Saul Suster, MD**
Professor and Vice-Chair
Department of Pathology
Ohio State University School of Medicine
Director of Anatomic Pathology
Department of Pathology
Ohio State University Medical Center
Columbus, Ohio
*The Lung; The Mediastinum; Tumors of the Skin*


**Pheroze Tamboli, MD**
Assistant Professor
Department of Pathology
University of Texas
M.D. Anderson Cancer Center
Houston, Texas
*Penis and Scrotum; Testis and Paratestis Including
Spermatic Cord*


**Clive R. Taylor, MD, PhD**
Professor and Chair
Department of Pathology
Senior Associate Dean for Educational Affairs
University of Southern California
Keck School of Medicine
Director of Laboratories
LAC–USC Healthcare Network General Hospital
Los Angeles, California
*Immunohistochemistry*

**Lester D. R. Thompson, MD**
Clinical Instructor of Pathology
Uniformed Services University of the Health Sciences
Assistant Chairman
Department of Otolaryngologic Pathology
Armed Forces Institute of Pathology
Washington, District of Columbia
*Larynx Pathology*

**Satish K. Tickoo, MD**
Assistant Professor of Pathology
Weill Medical College of Cornell University
Assistant Attending Pathologist
New York Presbyterian Hospital
New York, New York
*Testis and Paratestis Including Spermatic Cord*

**David B. Troxel, MD**
Clinical Professor
Health and Medical Sciences
University of California, Berkeley
School of Public Health
Berkeley, California
Pathology Consultant and Governor
The Doctors Company
Napa, California
Pathologist
Mt. Diablo Medical Center
Concord, California
*Medicolegal Issues in Surgical Pathology*

**Renu Virmani, MD**
Clinical Professor of Pathology
Vanderbilt University School of Medicine
Nashville, Tennessee
Chair, Department of Cardiovascular Pathology
Armed Forces Institute of Pathology
Washington, District of Columbia
*Heart and Blood Vessels*

**Nancy E. Warner, MD**
Hastings Professor of Pathology Emeritus
University of Southern California
Keck School of Medicine
Los Angeles, California
*Testis and Paratestis Including Spermatic Cord*

**Noel Weidner, MD**
Professor and Director of Anatomic Pathology
Department of Pathology
University of California
San Diego, School of Medicine,
San Diego, California
*Breast; Bone and Joint Pathology*

**Lawrence M. Weiss, MD**
Chair, Division of Pathology
Director, Surgical Pathology
City of Hope National Medical Center
Duarte, California
*Serosal Membranes; Lymph Nodes; Adrenal Gland; Soft Tissues*

**Bruce M. Wenig, MD**
Professor of Pathology
Albert Einstein College of Medicine
Vice Chairman, Anatomic Pathology
Department of Pathology
Beth Israel Medical Center
New York, New York
*Nasal Cavity, Paranasal Sinuses, and Nasopharynx; The Ear*

**William O. Whetsell, Jr., MD**
Professor of Pathology and Psychiatry
Vanderbilt University School of Medicine
Attending Pathologist
Vanderbilt University Hospital
Nashville, Tennessee
*Muscle and Nerve Biopsy*

**Sharon P. Wilczynski, MD, PhD**
Staff Pathologist and Director of Cytology
City of Hope National Medical Center
Duarte, California
*Molecular Biology*

**Robb E. Wilentz, MD**
Chief Resident, Department of Pathology
Johns Hopkins University Hospital
Baltimore, Maryland
*Pancreas*

**Tai-Yuen Wong, MB, ChB, FCAP**
Chairman, Pathology Consultants and Diagnostic Pathology System
Hockessin, Delaware
*Inflammatory Skin Conditions; Tumors of the Skin*

**Thomas C. Wright, MD**
Associate Professor of Pathology
Director of Obstetrical and Gynecological Pathology
Columbia University
College of Physicians and Surgeons
New York, New York
*Cervix*

# Preface

Creating a new (modern) comprehensive textbook of general surgical pathology was a daunting task. Our goal was to produce a text that fully integrates the latest concepts and techniques in surgical pathology in a way that not only would be useful today but would also indicate the future direction of the field. The Editors of the current volume see this as a vital part of our practice and teaching, and this focus has informed the overall objectives and content of the text. As Editors, we are looking not only to the present time but also to the future. Hence, we asked the contributors to emphasize new developments in immunohistochemistry and molecular biology that have had a significant impact in their areas of expertise, and to integrate these developments in their respective chapters.

Although advanced techniques have had a major impact on the practice of surgical pathology, in current daily practice the major core for all diagnostic surgical pathology remains the gross and microscopic examinations. Thus, we continue to stress the importance of having in-depth knowledge of both gross and microscopic pathology. Indeed, the book is illustrated with numerous color gross and microscopic photographs. A textbook can never have enough illustrative examples of pathologic entities, despite the fact that in practice, often subtle morphologic differences can have a major diagnostic impact. Recognizing this, we have taken advantage of readily available computer technology to greatly expand the collection of figures and photomicrographs through the inclusion of a companion CD-ROM. Importantly, the CD-ROM figures are directly referred to and integrated in the text and thus can be placed in the context of the overall discussion. In addition, summaries of important staging parameters and the necessary components of the final surgical pathology report are also provided. We have coupled this traditional approach with descriptions of many of the startling recent advances in immunohistochemistry and molecular biology, which are slowly but surely changing our overall approach to diagnostic pathology. We believe that the final product can serve as a comprehensive working companion or consultative source for all those interested in diagnostic pathology. We have worked to produce a book that will be useful to all surgical pathologists, both in training and in practice.

The Editors chose the authors for the various chapters on the basis of their recognized expertise as well as their writing skills. We thank them heartily and sincerely appreciate the high quality of their individual contributions. We believe that each contribution is authoritative and comprehensive. Without these hard-working and dedicated contributors, this text would not exist. We thank all of our colleagues who allowed us to use in this book many of their unique and superb examples of pathologic entities; their contributions are acknowledged throughout the text. Finally, we want to thank our family, friends, and colleagues, who have been a constant source of inspiration to all those involved in this undertaking. Their patience and their understanding of our workaholic natures are deeply appreciated.

The initial launch of a textbook project such as this one is a tremendous undertaking and could not have been accomplished without the support, guidance, and direction (and prodding) of a large number of people. We would thus like to thank the staff at Elsevier Science/W.B. Saunders, in particular Allan Ross, Ann Ruzycka, Delores Meloni, and Peter Faber, for their efforts on our behalf and for their great patience.

We hope that you enjoy and learn from this book, which is intended as an evolving work to be continually improved. We believe that in its initial presentation, it is a much-needed text on modern surgical pathology that reflects the growing intimacy between traditional diagnostic pathology and new molecular approaches.

*Noel Weidner, M.D.*
*Richard J. Cote, M.D.*
*Saul Suster, M.D.*
*Lawrence M. Weiss, M.D.*

# Contents

PART **XII**
# Nervous System .................................................................2021

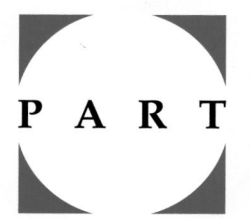

# PART VI

# Urinary Tract and Male Genital System

# 29

# *The Non-Neoplastic Kidney*

Sharda G. Sabnis    W.B. Ross
Zdena Pavlova    Michael N. Koss

## KIDNEY: DEVELOPMENTAL ABNORMALITIES

The kidney and lower urinary tract are commonly affected by congenital anomalies. In our experience at Los Angeles County General Hospital, the incidence of major renal malformations is 11% to 12% of perinatal autopsies (Table 29–1). The most common renal congenital anomalies are renal agenesis; renal dysgenesis; abnormalities in position, size, and

**TABLE 29–1.** Lethal Congenital Malformations in 223 Perinatal Autopsies*

| Malformation | No. | % |
|---|---|---|
| CNS | 73 | 33 |
| MCA | 57 | 26 |
| Chromosomal abnormalities | 23 | 10 |
| Renal | 24 | 11 |
| Cardiac | 20 | 9 |
| GI | 17 | 8 |
| Musculoskeletal | 13 | 6 |
| Pulmonary | 3 | 1 |

*Lethal congenital malformations by organ system affected at autopsy, Los Angeles County–University of Southern California Medical Center, 5-year experience.
CNS, central nervous system; GI, gastrointestinal; MCA, multiple congenital abnormalities.

number of the kidneys; and congenital hydronephrosis. Furthermore, the anomalies can be limited to the kidney or they can occur as a component of multiorgan syndromes. Of the anomalies, bilateral renal agenesis and some forms of dysgenesis are invariably fatal in early postnatal life. After an initial discussion of renal development, we review the more common developmental disorders.

## Development

The embryology of the kidney is considered only briefly. The urogenital ridge, which is derived from mesoderm, gives rise to two nonfunctioning systems, pronephros and mesonephros. The mesonephric, or wolffian duct, develops from the mesonephros and ultimately forms the vas deferens, epididymis, efferent ductules, and rete testis in men, whereas it mostly degenerates in women.

The definitive kidney is formed from the metanephros, which develops caudally to the mesonephros. The ureter is formed from the lower mesonephric duct, and grows cephalad to extend into the metanephric mesenchyme. The proximal end undergoes a series of branchings, forming initially the renal pelvis and calyces and subsequently the collecting ducts of the kidney. The distal portions of these branches, or ampullae, induce formation of nephrons from the metanephric blastema. Glomerulogenesis begins in the seventh gestational week, with the final 8 to 12 generations of nephrons formed by 32 to 36 weeks of gestation, at which time nephrogenesis is completed. The development is initiated by S-shaped renal vesicles, which become invaginated by capillaries to form a glomerulus.

Excretion of fetal urine is detectable radiographically by the end of the 16th week. Many severe renal disorders can be detected during fetal life by the finding of oligohydramnios or by radiologic or ultrasonographic imaging.

## Renal Agenesis

Bilateral renal agenesis is not uncommon, occurring in 1 in 4000 births at Los Angeles County Medical Center. This relatively high incidence may be due to both improved clinical diagnostic accuracy and a relatively high autopsy rate. The cause of renal agenesis is unknown. Clinically, oligohydramnios is invariably present. The infants are frequently small for gestational age and they have a remarkably similar dehydrated appearance and bowing of the legs. They also exhibit characteristic Potter's facies with prominent infraorbital and nasolabial creases, beaked noses, and variably dysmorphic, enlarged, posteriorly rotated ears (Fig. 29–1). Although this appearance is classic for renal agenesis, it is also seen in severe oligohydramnios due to other etiologic factors, for example, bilateral renal dysgenesis. All of the infants in our experience are liveborn, but none survive beyond 1 day. The immediate cause of death is respiratory distress due to pulmonary hypoplasia, the latter being invariably present. The Rokitansky anomaly (incomplete to atretic vagina and rudimentary to bicornuate uterus) is occasionally associated with renal agenesis.

Unilateral renal agenesis is more common than bilateral agenesis, but because the contralateral kidney is usually normal, unilateral disease typically remains asymptomatic. Anomalies associated with unilateral agenesis include ipsilateral absence or malformation of the fallopian tube, ovary, and

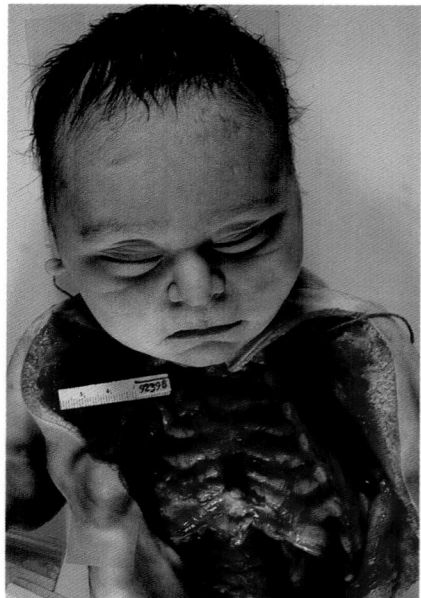

**FIGURE 29–1.** The gross appearance of Potter's facies. Note the prominent infraorbital and nasolabial creases, beaked nose, and enlarged, posteriorly rotated ears. In this case, there is also hypoplasia of the thoracic cavity.

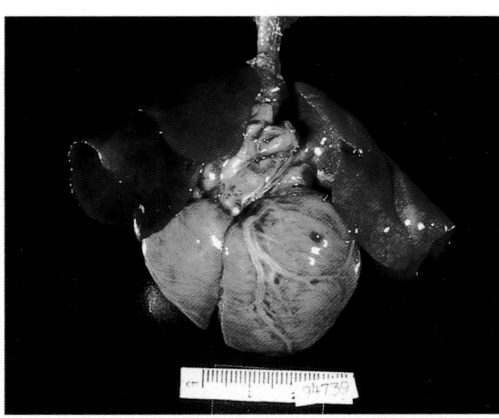

**FIGURE 29-2.** Pulmonary hypoplasia is a frequent cause of death in infants with renal dysgenesis, Potter type I. This photograph shows the typical gross appearance of pulmonary hypoplasia. The small lungs are dwarfed by the enlarged heart, which has been partially opened.

uterus in women, and of the testis, seminal vesicles, and vas deferens in men.

## Renal Dysgenesis

### RENAL DYSGENESIS (SYNONYMS: RENAL DYSPLASIA, POLYCYSTIC KIDNEY DISEASE, AND MULTICYSTIC KIDNEY DISEASE)

The nomenclature of cystic disorders of diverse etiologies is confusing and complex. The Potter classification of cystic or dysgenetic diseases of the kidney is based on anatomic microdissection of renal tubules, but it also appears to have clinical relevance. Renal dysgenesis, whether occurring as an isolated malformation or as part of various malformation syndromes (e.g., Meckel-Gruber, Zellweger's, Ivemark's, or Jeune's syndrome or trisomy 13), is the most frequent malformation of the kidney in perinatal as well as pediatric age groups. Moreover, polycystic kidney disease is one of the most common hereditary disorders in the United States.

### RENAL DYSGENESIS, POTTER TYPE I (SPONGE KIDNEY, HAMARTOMA, AUTOSOMAL RECESSIVE POLYCYSTIC KIDNEY, INFANTILE POLYCYSTIC KIDNEY)

CLINICAL CONSIDERATIONS. This form of dysgenesis is an autosomal recessive disorder reported to be present in 1 per 6000 to 14,000 live births. The disorder presents clinically in the newborn period. Pulmonary hypoplasia of varying degree is usually present, and it is the most common cause of death (Fig. 29-2). The patients who survive generally have lesser degrees of lung hypoplasia, but they then develop renal failure within the first decade of life. Liver abnormalities due to hepatic fibrosis, including portal hypertension and varices, may also occur

later in life. A gene present on chromosome 6 has been implicated in the disease.

DIAGNOSTIC CONSIDERATIONS. Grossly, the kidneys are bilaterally symmetric and massively enlarged, but their normal reniform shape is preserved (Fig. 29-3). The cut surface of the kidneys reveals a spongiform surface with radial orientation of the cysts, which are often most pronounced in the medulla. The renal pelves, ureters, and urinary bladder show no evidence of dilatation. Histologically, there is diffuse enlargement of the collecting ducts, which are lined by simple flat to cuboidal epithelium (Fig. 29-4A and B). The distal tubules are sometimes involved. Occasional small glomerular cysts are present.

There is always congenital hepatic fibrosis in association with the kidney disease, and fibrotic expansion of the portal triads can usually be appreciated grossly (Fig. 29-5A). Occasionally liver cysts are also present. Microscopically, the hepatic bile ducts show cystic dilatation (biliary dysgenesis) associated with portal fibrosis (Fig. 29-5B).

### RENAL DYSGENESIS, POTTER TYPE II (MULTICYSTIC KIDNEY DISEASE)

CLINICAL CONSIDERATIONS. The disease can involve either one kidney, or it can present as bilateral renal involvement. There is no evidence of genetic inheritance, although a familial incidence has been reported occasionally.

DIAGNOSTIC CONSIDERATIONS. Grossly, the kidneys can be of small, normal, or large size (Fig. 29-6A). The reniform contour is lost and the parenchyma is replaced by cysts of variable size. The ureters and urinary bladder are usually hypoplastic.

Microscopically, the cysts are surrounded by increased connective tissue (Fig. 29-6B). Incomplete glomeruli and rare tubules are frequently present. Islands of metaplastic cartilage are reported to occur in 50% of cases, and large nerve trunks are common.

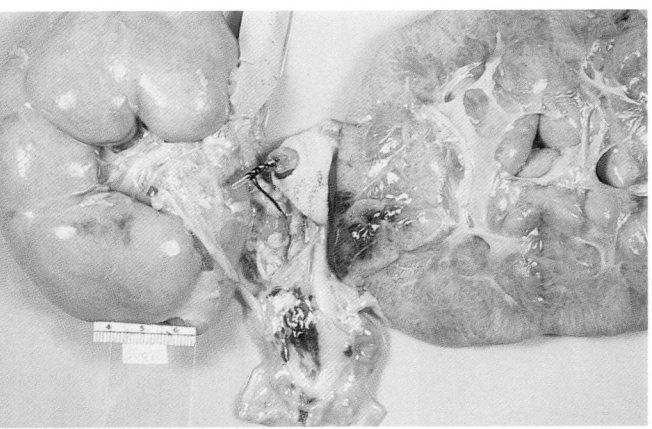

**FIGURE 29-3.** Renal dysgenesis, Potter type I, gross appearance. The kidneys are markedly enlarged but retain the usual lobular architecture.

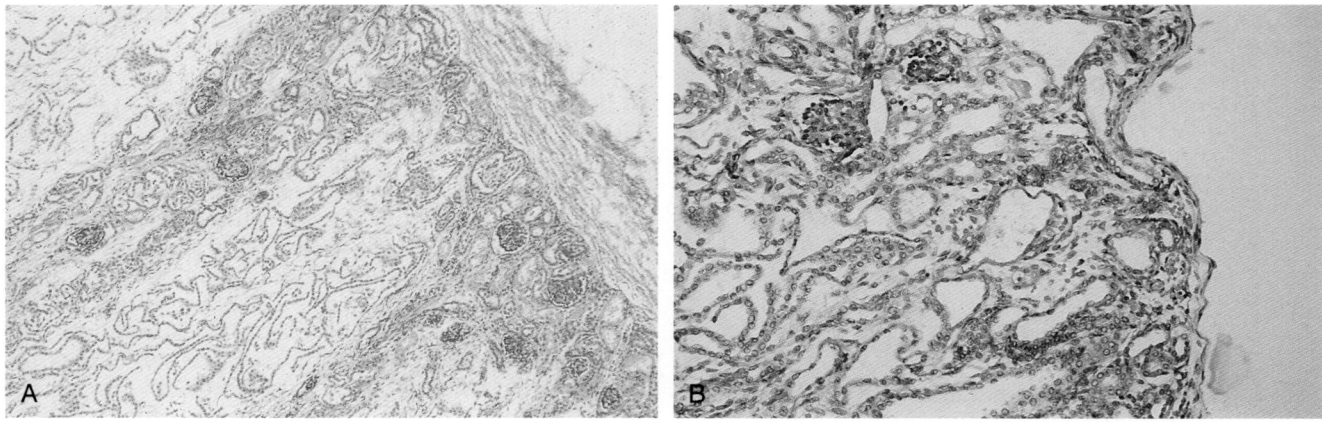

**FIGURE 29–4.** *A.* Renal dysgenesis, Potter type I, low-power microscopic view. Cystic dilatation of tubules is readily seen. *B.* Renal dysgenesis, Potter type I, high-power microscopic view. Dilated distal tubules and collecting ducts are lined by flattened epithelium.

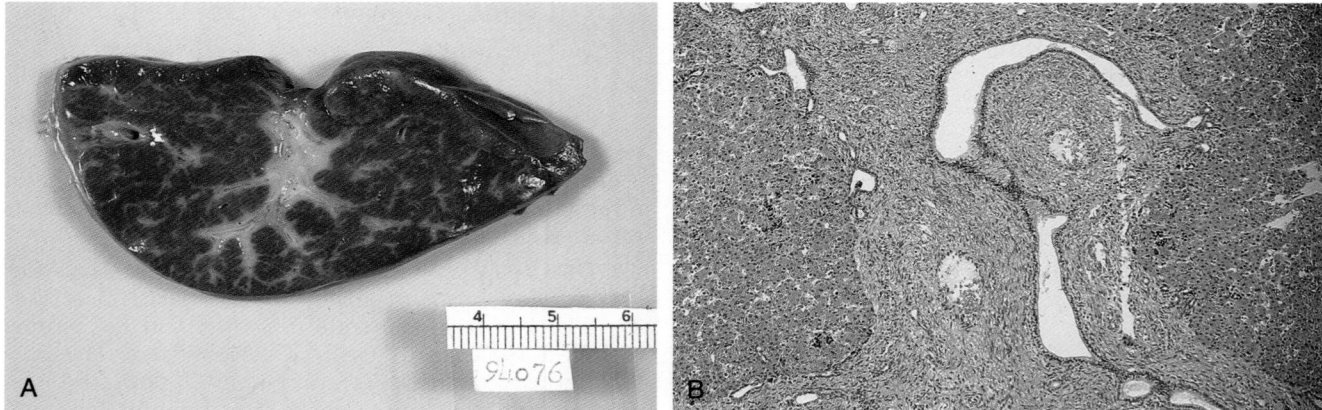

**FIGURE 29–5.** *A.* Gross appearance of liver showing fibrosis in an arborizing pattern in a patient with renal dysgenesis, Potter type I. *B.* Microscopic appearance of liver in the same case. Note the marked fibrotic expansion of the portal zone with mild dilatation of bile ducts.

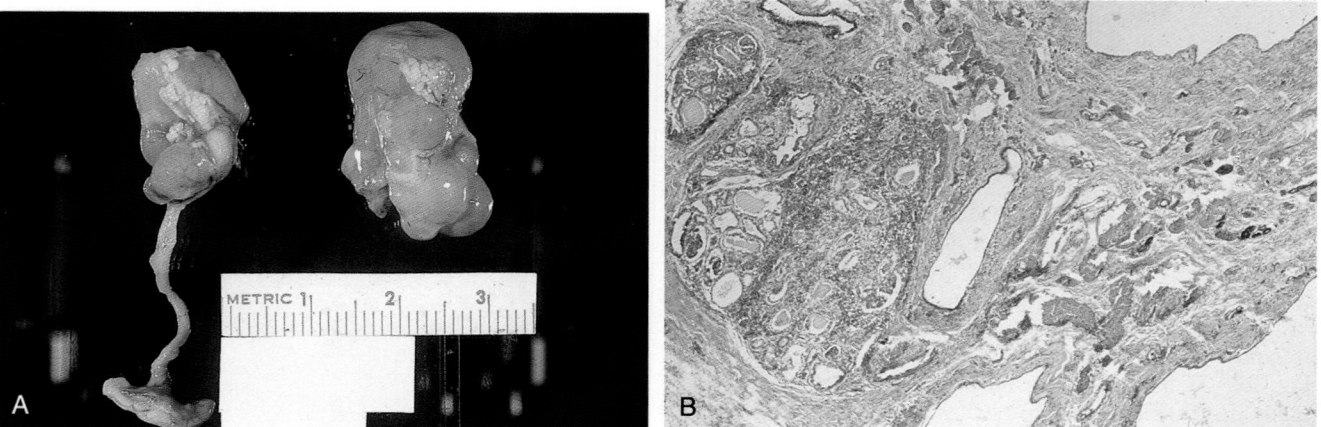

**FIGURE 29–6.** *A.* Renal dysgenesis, Potter type II. The normal gross appearance of the kidney is distorted by numerous cysts of varying size. *B.* Renal dysgenesis, Potter type II. Microscopic view showing large cysts that are bordered by broad bands of fibrous tissue. Glomeruli and rare tubules are also present.

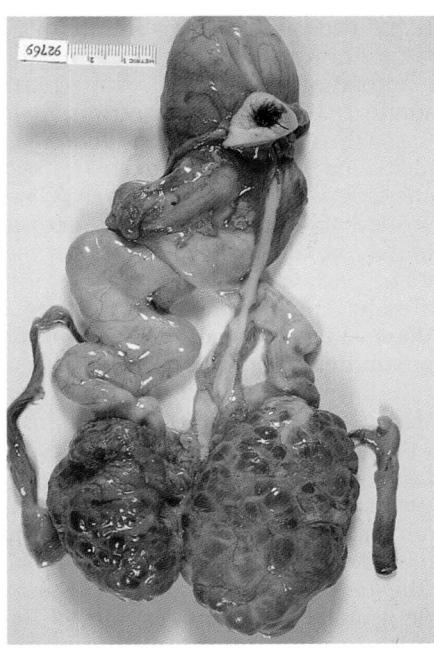

**FIGURE 29–7.** Renal dysgenesis, Potter type IV. The gross appearance is that of numerous renal cysts in conjunction with ureteral dilatation.

## RENAL DYSGENESIS, POTTER TYPE III (POLYCYSTIC KIDNEY DISEASE, AUTOSOMAL DOMINANT POLYCYSTIC KIDNEY, ADULT POLYCYSTIC KIDNEY)

CLINICAL CONSIDERATIONS. The incidence of this disease in the general population is 1 in 1000, making it one of the most common heritable single gene disorders.[1, 2] Although much remains to be explained in the pathogenesis of this disease, the gene *PKD1*, located on the short arm of chromosome 16, appears to be present in at least 90% of the 500,000 adult patients with polycystic disease in the United States and it is likely the cause of the disease.[3] More recently, the *PKD2* gene has been reported on chromosome 4.[4] Because this form of renal dysgenesis generally presents in adulthood, only rare cases are reported in neonates. The disease usually affects 30- to 40-year-old individuals of either sex, whose symptoms include flank pain, hypertension, hematuria, and renal stones. There is usually bilateral renal involvement. Cysts can develop in other sites, such as liver, pancreas, and lungs. So-called berry aneurysms may be present in the cerebral arteries, and coronary artery aneurysms are also reported to occur.

DIAGNOSTIC CONSIDERATIONS. The kidneys are usually enlarged by myriads of cysts of varying, but often large, size. Histologically, normal and abnormal nephrons can be intermixed, but in later stages of disease, only small amounts of normal renal parenchyma are present. The cysts can involve any part of the nephron, but they occur most commonly in the cortex. They are lined by cuboidal to flattened epithelium. Renal adenomas occur in one fifth of patients.

## RENAL DYSGENESIS, POTTER TYPE IV

The disease is secondary to partial or intermittent urethral obstruction. The changes in the renal parenchyma occur later than in type II disease, after sufficient urine has been produced and retrograde pressure within the urinary collecting system causes damage to the developing nephrons. As expected, associated abnormalities include urinary bladder muscle hypertrophy and dilatation, massive dilatation of the ureters, and hydronephrosis (Fig. 29–7). The changes are more severe when the urethral obstruction occurs early. Massive urinary bladder dilatation can result in the so-called prune-belly syndrome (Fig. 29–8). Malformations of extrarenal organs are rare. There is no evidence of an inherited predisposition.

## Juvenile Nephronophthisis– Medullary Cystic Disease

CLINICAL CONSIDERATIONS. This set of diseases is believed to be the cause of up to one quarter of childhood cases of chronic renal insufficiency. Probably several diseases of tubules are involved. When the disease occurs in childhood and is heritable as an autosomal recessive, it is termed juvenile nephronophthisis. Patients are children who present with symptoms related to failure of the tubules to concentrate (polyuria and polydipsia) and growth retardation. They usually proceed over a period of about 10 years to chronic renal failure. Medullary cystic

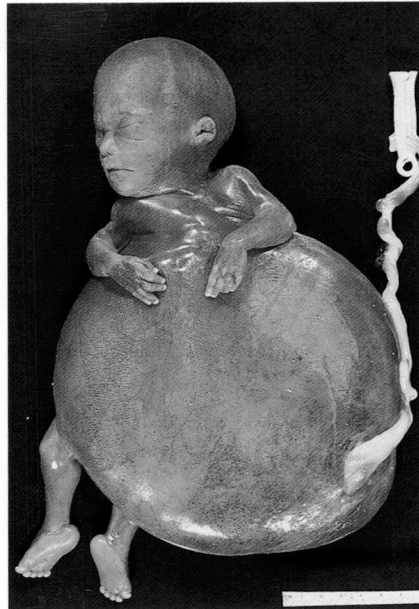

**FIGURE 29–8.** Typical example of prune-belly syndrome due to massive enlargement of the bladder.

disease usually presents in patients who are 20 to 30 years of age. It is inherited as an autosomal dominant. Patients show many of the clinical features noted above.

DIAGNOSTIC CONSIDERATIONS. The kidney may not be greatly enlarged, but on cut section it shows numerous cortical and medullary cysts measuring up to 2 cm. The cysts have a flattened lining, with variable amounts of fibrosis and chronic inflammation in the adjacent interstitium. They appear to arise from the distal tubules and collecting ducts.

## Horseshoe Kidney

Fusion of the kidneys occurs most commonly at the lower poles, producing a horseshoe-shaped appearance. When this occurs, the kidney is often situated lower in the abdomen than is normal. This abnormality is seen in approximately 1 in 600 radiographic examinations of the abdomen. The renal pelves are anterior and superior, and the ureters take an anterior course over the fused kidney. Often, hydronephrosis results from kinking of the ureters, and secondary renal calculi and infection frequently supervene. Horseshoe kidney is more common in men than in women. It is frequently seen in Turner's syndrome and in trisomy 18.

## INTERPRETATION OF THE RENAL BIOPSY

Evaluation of kidney biopsies is an essential and integral part in the assessment of kidney diseases because it allows the pathologist and clinician to study the type, extent, site, and nature of renal involvement by a disease; plan treatment; and estimate outcome. The remainder of this chapter includes the most common renal lesions encountered in the routine practice of nephropathology. In particular, it is intended to familiarize the reader with the various lesions associated with medical renal diseases.

Proper evaluation of a renal biopsy requires close attention to the processing of renal tissue. For light microscopy, the tissue is fixed immediately in 10% neutral buffered formalin and then processed in the conventional manner. Paraffin sections are cut at 2 $\mu$m and they are routinely stained with hematoxylin and eosin (H&E), periodic acid–Schiff (PAS), Masson trichrome, and Jones methenamine silver or periodic acid–methenamine silver (PAMS) stains. In addition, Congo red stain is used where indicated.

Tissue for electron microscopy is fixed in a glutaraldehyde-based electron microscopy fixative, postfixed with osmium tetroxide, dehydrated through graded alcohols, and embedded in plastic resin. Following sectioning with an ultramicrotome and staining with lead citrate and uranyl acetate, the tissue is examined in a transmission electron microscope.

Tissue for direct or indirect immunofluorescence microscopy is immediately snap-frozen in a cryomatrix or is immersed in a transport medium containing ammonium sulfate.[5] After sectioning in a cryostat, the sections are routinely stained for the immunoglobulins IgG, IgA, and IgM; for $\kappa$ and $\lambda$ light chains; complement components (C3 and C1q); fibrinogen; and for albumin. If indicated, additional antibodies may be applied.

As noted earlier, kidney biopsies are routinely evaluated using H&E and a variety of special stains. Among these stains, Masson trichrome is useful in estimating tubulointerstitial changes, such as edema, fibrosis, tubular atrophy, and vascular sclerosis. The stain is also useful for demonstrating proteinaceous deposits, such as immune complex deposits and fibrinoid necrosis. PAMS stain is particularly useful for demonstrating basement membrane spikes, or honeycomb patterns and double contour lesions, as well as basement membrane changes in all components of the nephron. Similarly, PAS stain is useful for basement membrane changes and to demonstrate the presence of inflammatory cells.

For objective evaluation, sections for light, electron, and immunofluorescence microscopy are examined separately without knowledge of clinical history. Each component of the renal biopsy is evaluated for changes in glomeruli, tubules, interstitium, and vessels. Final diagnosis is rendered by correlating the histologic findings with clinical history.

Glomeruli (Fig. 29–9) are evaluated for

1. Pattern of involvement: (a) Diffuse or generalized when all glomeruli are involved and each glomerulus is totally involved, or (b) focal and segmental where only some glomeruli and segments of each individual glomerulus are involved.
2. Cellularity: Glomeruli may show an increase in one or several components, including endocapillary cells (mesangial and endothelial cells), epithelial cell hypertrophy, epithelial crescents, and inflammatory cell infiltration.

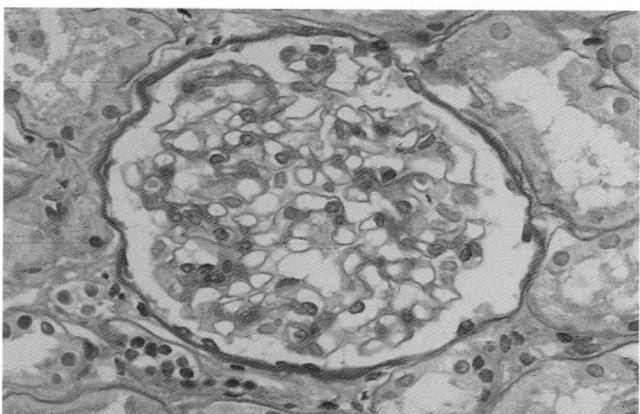

**FIGURE 29–9.** Normal glomerulus: Glomerulus showing normal cellularity, thin capillary walls, and normal mesangium. (PAS stain.)

3. Changes in capillary walls, including thickening, attenuation (thinning), splintering, spikes, reduplication of basement membranes resulting in a tram-track pattern, and breaks in glomerular basement membrane.
4. Changes in the mesangial matrix, which may be increased with a generalized diffuse pattern or irregular or nodular pattern.
5. The glomerular capillary tufts can show segmental or global solidification (sclerosis), fibrinoid necrosis, intracapillary thrombi, hyaline thrombi, and karyorrhexis, nuclear pyknosis, and hematoxylin bodies (in vivo lupus erythematosus [LE] cells).
6. Inclusions in the cellular components may be seen in certain metabolic or familial diseases.

The tubules are evaluated for

1. Atrophy and tubular dropout. With advanced atrophy, the tubules are often dilated with changes described as thyroidization.
2. Changes in lining epithelium showing degeneration and regeneration (acute tubular necrosis [ATN]).
3. Lymphocytic or neutrophilic infiltration of the epithelium (tubulitis).
4. Thickening of tubular basement membranes associated with tubular atrophy, or due to deposition of extracellular material (e.g., amyloid or light chains).

The interstitium is evaluated for edema, inflammatory cell infiltration by mononuclear cells (lymphocytes, plasma cells, macrophages), neutrophils and eosinophils, giant cells with granuloma, foam cells or lipid-laden cells, and chronic changes such as fibrosis.

Evaluation of vessels includes searching for thickening of walls by subintimal fibrosis; medial, intimal, or adventitial hyperplasia; hyaline deposition; reduplication of elastica; onion peel pattern; deposition of extracellular material; and other changes such as fibrinoid necrosis, thrombi, inflammatory cell infiltration (by neutrophils and/or mononuclear cells) of vessel walls, and extravasation of red blood cells into the vessel walls.

Immunofluorescence microscopic evaluation of the renal biopsy centers mainly on the glomeruli, with determination of pattern and type of immune complex or other deposits (e.g., light chains). A panel of antibodies, including IgG, IgA, IgM, C3, C1q, fibrinogen, κ and λ light chains, and albumin (as a control), is performed, and the presence and combinations of the various antibodies, their patterns (granular or linear), their distribution, and the strength or intensity of staining (1+ to 3+) are used in the report and diagnosis. Deposits (immune complexes) may be mesangial, peripheral along capillary walls, or both. They may be coarse or finely granular or they may appear linear. Fibrinogen is usually seen in epithelial cell crescents and in areas of necrosis. Tubular basement membranes often demonstrate granular staining with immune-complex deposition and linear staining with light chain deposition (κ or λ). The vessels may show granular staining with immunoglobulins and with complement. In certain diseases, such as Goodpasture's syndrome, IgA nephropathy, and IgM nephropathy, immunohistochemistry is absolutely essential, whereas in other diseases it serves as an additional tool to confirm the diagnosis.

Electron microscopic examination is an absolutely essential part of renal biopsy interpretation (Fig. 29–10). In addition to the demonstration of immune-complex deposits, which usually appear as granular electron-dense deposits, electron microscopy also enables the examiner to evaluate ultrastructural changes in glomerular basement membranes and mesangium, and to demonstrate various inclusions and changes in the cellular components, especially in the epithelial and endothelial cells, as well as in other components of the nephron. Certain diseases, such as thin basement membrane syndrome and Alport's syndrome, are strongly suggested by the thickness of the glomerular basement membrane. Capillary basement membranes are evaluated primarily for electron-dense deposits in subepithelial, intramembranous, and subendothelial regions. The location of these deposits may provide a clue to diagnosis. For example, postinfectious glomerulonephritis shows characteristic moth-eaten subepithelial humplike deposits, membranous glomerulopathy demonstrates smaller but often numerous subepithelial deposits with spikelike projections of basement membranes between the deposits, mesangiocapillary glomerulonephritis shows either characteristic mesangial interpositioning and duplication of capillary basement membranes (in type I disease) or wormlike dense deposits within the lamina densa of the glomerular basement membranes (in type II disease), whereas IgA nephropathy and lupus nephritis typically show a mesangial and subendothelial pattern of deposits. The epithelial podocytes are

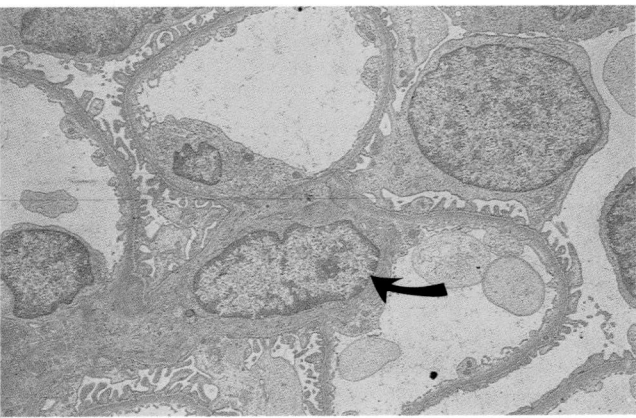

**FIGURE 29–10.** Normal glomerulus: Electron micrograph of glomerulus showing mesangium with mesangial cell (*arrow*), basement membrane, and visceral epithelial cell with foot processes and endothelial cell.

evaluated for effacement or fusion and for intracellular inclusions, typical features of proteinuric states. The mesangial areas are evaluated for an increase in matrix (a typical feature of diabetes) and for deposits. Deposition of distinctive extracellular material in the mesangium and along capillary basement membranes, such as in amyloidosis, cryoglobulinemia, light chain disease, and immunotactoid glomerulonephropathy can be strongly suggestive of a specific diagnosis. Intracellular inclusions seen in metabolic or familial diseases are looked for in all cellular elements, and tubuloreticular structures (TRSs) (mistakenly termed myxovirus-like particles), which are abundant in lupus nephritis and in the setting of human immunodeficiency virus (HIV) infection, are sought in the endothelial cells.

## CLASSIFICATION OF GLOMERULONEPHRITIS: CLINICAL SYMPTOMS

Glomerulonephritis is a type of disease characterized by intraglomerular inflammation and cellular proliferation, typically associated with hematuria. Patterns of glomerular injury help in understanding a variety of lesions and may have an association with a particular glomerular disease.[6] Classification of glomerulonephritis constitutes a major problem, because often there is overlap of diseases in more than one category.[7] There is no one satisfactory classification, although it is useful to divide lesions associated with glomerulonephritis into two subgroups: primary and associated with systemic diseases.

Glomerulonephritis can be also classified by clinical manifestations. For example, renal diseases may be associated with nephrotic syndrome, nephritic syndrome, asymptomatic hematuria, acute renal failure, and chronic renal failure. Still, this classification also poses problems, because a given disease may present with more than one type of clinical manifestation.

## PRIMARY GLOMERULAR DISEASES

### Minimal Change Disease (Synonyms: Lipoid Nephrosis, Visceral Epithelial Cell Disease, Foot Process Disease, Nil Disease, Minimal Change Glomerulopathy)

NOMENCLATURE. Munk[8] introduced the term *lipoid nephrosis* to describe a group of patients with heavy proteinuria but without glomerular changes by light microscopy. Perhaps the most prominent finding by light microscopy was the presence of lipid droplets in proximal tubular epithelium; hence, the disease was called lipoid nephrosis. Because of the normal appearance of glomeruli or minimal

mesangial cellularity, the term minimal change disease is used commonly.

CLINICAL CONSIDERATIONS. This lesion accounts for about 80% of cases of nephrotic syndrome in children and 20% of cases in adults.[9] In children, the average age is 3 years, and there is a male preponderance.[10, 11] Although the overwhelming majority of cases are idiopathic, minimal change disease can occur secondary to specific causes, such as lymphoma, including Hodgkin's disease,[12, 13] drugs such as nonsteroidal anti-inflammatory drugs (NSAIDs),[14] and HIV infection. Viral upper respiratory tract infection is a common antecedent feature, and a history of allergy, atopy, or recent immunization[15, 16] may be found. Patients typically present with nephrotic-range proteinuria (more than 3.0 to 3.5 g per 24 hours). The proteinuria is often selective (mainly albuminuria), and it is usually associated with hypoalbuminemia, lipiduria, and hyperlipidemia. Occasionally, renal insufficiency can be associated with the nephrotic syndrome, particularly in patients with accompanying tubular damage or interstitial nephritis. The disease typically responds to corticosteroids, although one or a few relapses can occur on cessation of treatment. Still, the prognosis is excellent.

DIAGNOSTIC CONSIDERATIONS. All glomeruli are similar and are either normocellular or show a slight increase in endocapillary cells (minimal changes) (Fig. 29–11). The glomerular capillary walls are unremarkable, and the capillary lumina are widely patent. There is usually prominence or swelling of visceral epithelial cells and there is often edema in the renal interstitium. Tubules may contain hyaline (protein reabsorption) droplets or lipid droplets. Blood vessels are usually normal.

By electron microscopy, there is visceral epithelial cell swelling, with diffuse or extensive effacement of epithelial cell foot processes and formation of villi on the external surface of the epithelial cells (so-called villous transformation) (Fig. 29–12). The glomerular capillary basement membranes are usu-

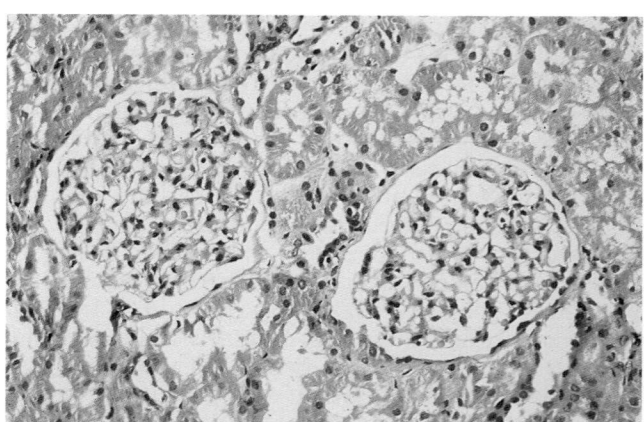

**FIGURE 29–11.** Minimal change disease: Glomerulus shows slight increase in cells and widely open capillary lumina.

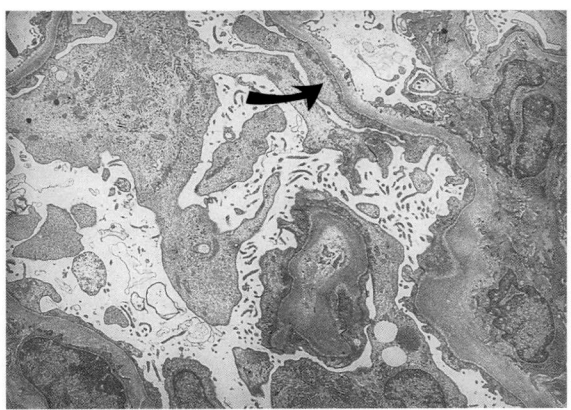

**FIGURE 29–12.** Minimal change disease: Electron micrograph of a portion of a glomerulus shows effacement of foot processes (foot process fusion) (*arrow*) and villous transformation of visceral epithelial cells.

ally of normal thickness. Electron microscopy is essential for the diagnosis of minimal change disease.

Immunofluorescence microscopy is negative for immunoglobulins, complement components, and fibrin.

## Mesangial Proliferative Glomerulopathy (Synonyms: Diffuse Mesangial Proliferation, IgM Nephropathy)

CLINICAL CONSIDERATIONS. The dominant clinical feature in mesangial proliferative glomerulonephritis is the insidious onset of heavy proteinuria. Individuals of any age may be affected, but usually the patients are older children and young adults.[17-20] Unlike minimal change disease, hematuria is present in the majority of cases, and there can be mild hypertension in about 30% of cases. Patients usually respond to corticosteroid therapy, but they are often corticosteroid dependent, with repeated recurrence of proteinuria following tapering or discontinuation of corticosteroids.

DIAGNOSTIC CONSIDERATIONS. By light microscopy, the glomeruli show mild to moderate increase in endocapillary cells and widening of the mesangium. Interstitial, tubular, and blood vessel changes are usually minimal or may be similar to those seen with minimal change disease.

By electron microscopy, the mesangial regions are widened, with increase in cells and matrix. Occasionally, mesangial electron-dense deposits are seen. There is diffuse effacement or fusion of foot processes and villous transformation. By immunofluorescence microscopy, deposits of IgM are seen in the mesangium. They are essential for diagnosis and are often associated with C3. Rarely, mesangial deposits of IgG or IgA may be present, but their intensity is lower than that of IgM and deposits are minimal.

## Focal Segmental Glomerulosclerosis (Synonym: Focal Segmental Glomerulosclerosis and Hyalinosis)

NOMENCLATURE. Rich[21] first described this lesion in 1957 as a new pathologic finding in the autopsy kidneys of 20 patients who, on clinical grounds, were considered to have minimal change disease. However, these kidneys showed focal and segmental glomerular scars, hence the name. This change also seemed to affect earliest the glomeruli in the deep cortex (juxtamedullary glomeruli). Later, a number of other authors[22-24] pointed out the frequency of this lesion in idiopathic nephrotic syndrome in children and adults. The poor response to corticosteroid and other immunosuppressive therapy and the progressive loss of renal function found in association with focal segmental glomerulosclerosis have been repeatedly emphasized.[25] Some investigators regard this lesion as a nonspecific feature superimposed on the basic lesions of minimal change disease and mesangial proliferative glomerulopathy (IgM nephropathy). Still others consider minimal change disease, diffuse mesangial proliferation, and focal segmental glomerulosclerosis to be separate entities.[26] However, over the years it has become apparent that there is definite clinical overlap among these different morphologic expressions and, furthermore, it is known that the initial morphologic changes of recurrent focal segmental glomerulosclerosis in kidney transplants are those of minimal change disease or diffuse mesangial proliferation, suggesting a continuum of disease from mild damage (minimal changes) to severe disease (focal glomerulosclerosis).

CLINICAL CONSIDERATIONS. Patients commonly present with nephrotic-range proteinuria and nephrotic syndrome. The proteinuria is typically nonselective, with loss of large-molecular-weight immunoglobulins as well as the lower molecular weight albumin. Hypertension and microscopic hematuria are commonly present. Renal insufficiency at clinical presentation is common in adults. There is a higher incidence in blacks.

Although focal segmental glomerulosclerosis is an idiopathic glomerular disease, it can be associated with a variety of conditions (secondary form). In particular, the lesion is often seen in intravenous drug abusers (heroin nephropathy) and in patients with acquired immunodeficiency syndrome (AIDS-associated or HIV-associated nephropathy).[27] Here, the disease may be rapidly progressive, leading to renal failure in a matter of months, rather than the years that are often required in idiopathic disease (see later). Additional conditions associated with focal segmental glomerulosclerosis are reflux nephropathy, morbid obesity, renal dysplasia, and, sometimes, sickle cell disease.

DIAGNOSTIC CONSIDERATIONS. Solidification or scarring of a portion or segment (hence the term segmental) of the tuft of some glomeruli (hence the term focal) by light microscopy is the basis for this diagnosis (Fig. 29–13).[28, 29] Depending on the stage of disease, varying numbers of glomeruli show focal or segmental widening of their mesangia, with solidification or sclerosis of glomerular lobules. These areas are often adherent to Bowman's capsule, without alteration in the parietal epithelium. Sometimes in the solidifying areas, the capillary lumen is filled with proteinaceous material—a phenomenon referred to as hyalinosis (see Fig. 29–13).[28–30] Prominent visceral epithelial cells can fill the urinary space or surround a collapsed or sclerotic lobule, a finding referred to as the cellular lesion or as collapsing glomerulopathy, and one which is more common in heroin nephropathy or AIDS-associated nephropathy.[28–31] Glomeruli can also be completely solidified (global sclerosis). Most often, the sclerotic areas are seen at the hilus of the glomerulus (hilar focal and segmental glomerulosclerosis) but they can also be adjacent to the proximal tubule end (glomerular tip lesion).[32] Depending on the type of lesion, a subclassification of focal segmental glomerulosclerosis can be made, but the clinical significance of this subclassification is not clear, and its relation to prognosis is controversial.[29] Glomeruli that do not have sclerotic lesions usually show minimal change disease or diffuse mesangial proliferation. Tubulointerstitial and vascular changes usually correlate with the degree of glomerular changes.

By electron microscopy, the glomerular capillary basement membranes are of normal thickness (Fig. 29–14). In areas of sclerosis, there is an increase in mesangial matrix and the surrounding capillary basement membranes are thickened, wrinkled, and collapsed. There may be capillary loops containing homogeneous, proteinaceous, electron-dense material, often with lipid droplets, corresponding to the hyalinotic lesions (see Fig. 29–14). The mesangial regions are widened by an increase in matrix or mesangial cells. Mesangial regions can contain electron-dense deposits. As noted earlier, the nonsclerotic glomeruli also typically show variable mesangial widening. All glomeruli, whether sclerotic or

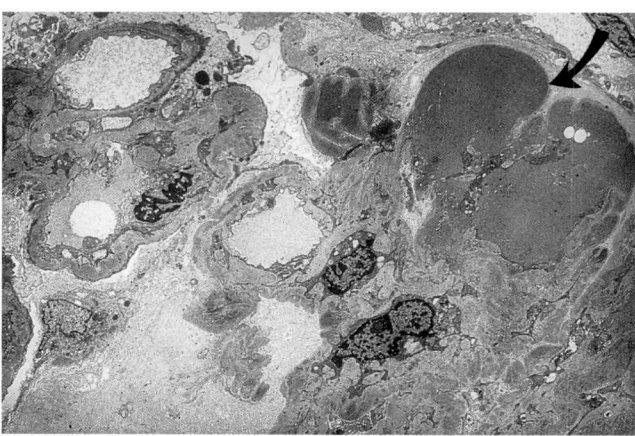

**FIGURE 29–14.** Focal segmental glomerulosclerosis: Electron micrograph of a portion of a glomerulus confirms changes seen by light microscopy in Figure 29–13. There is diffuse effacement of foot processes. The capillary lumen is filled with electron-dense material (hyalinosis) (*arrow*). Around this area, the epithelial cell is detached and fibrillary material fills the intervening space.

not, show diffuse effacement or fusion of visceral epithelial cell foot processes, which is associated with villous transformation (see Fig. 29–14). This change by itself is also seen in minimal change disease and mesangial proliferative glomerulonephritis, but as a sign of more severe injury, there can be focal detachment of visceral epithelial cells from the basement membrane.

By immunofluorescence microscopy, deposits of IgM are seen in the mesangium in a focal distribution and in areas corresponding to hyalinosis, with or without accompanying deposits of C3 (Fig. 29–15). They are not due to immune-complex deposits, but rather, they are considered to be secondary to trapping of large-molecular-weight proteins within the scarred glomeruli. The same trapping mechanism is believed to account for the presence of lipoproteins in the hyalinotic lesions.

The renal changes of focal and segmental glomerulosclerosis in intravenous drug abusers can dif-

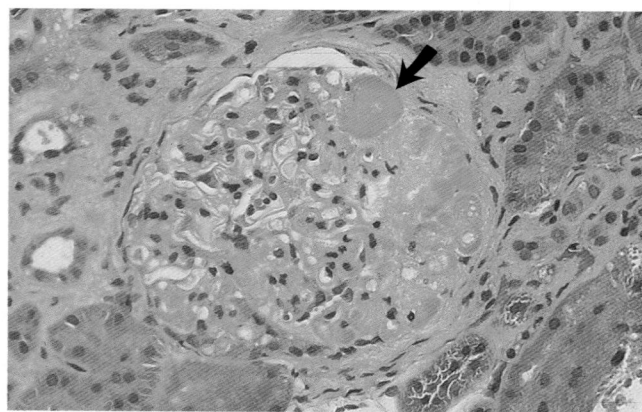

**FIGURE 29–13.** Focal segmental glomerulosclerosis: Portion of a glomerulus shows increase in matrix material with solidification (sclerosis) and adhesion to Bowman's capsule. Intracapillary eosinophilic hyaline material (hyalinosis) is seen in this area (*arrow*).

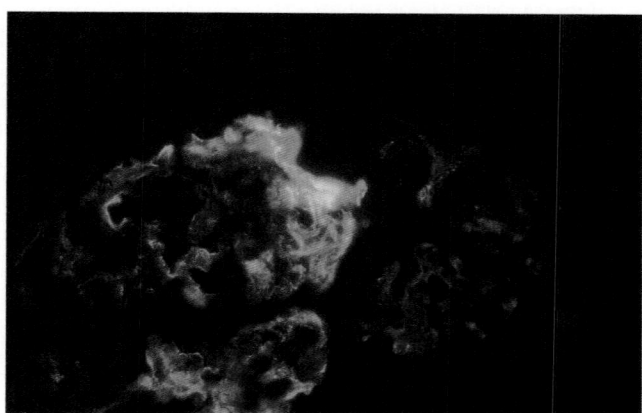

**FIGURE 29–15.** Focal segmental glomerulosclerosis: Immunofluorescence microscopy reveals irregular distribution of IgM in sclerotic areas and in the mesangium.

fer from those in idiopathic focal segmental glomerulosclerosis (Fig. 29–16). The glomeruli by light microscopy are cellular, there is often extensive chronic tubulointerstitial changes with marked interstitial mononuclear cell infiltration, and vascular sclerosis is often present (see Fig. 29–16). These histologic changes are important prognostic markers that point to accelerated development of end-stage renal disease. Patients with HIV-associated nephropathy can show collapsing glomerulopathy, which is characterized by prominent glomerular capillary collapse with large, hypertrophied visceral epithelial cells and cystic dilatation of Bowman's capsule. In addition, there can be cystic dilatation of tubules, which are filled with protein casts due to the rapid leakage of protein through the glomeruli, extensive interstitial edema, fibrosis, and a moderate interstitial chronic inflammatory cellular infiltrate (see Fig. 29–16). Finding these changes is also indicative of an ominous prognosis.

By electron microscopy, in addition to the glomerular changes of focal segmental glomerulosclerosis, heroin abusers and HIV-infected patients show visceral epithelial cells that have vacuolar and degenerative changes. Tubuloreticular structures (myxovirus-like particles) are seen in the endothelial cell cytoplasm of glomerular capillaries, interstitial capillaries, and vessels. In HIV-infected patients, Cohen and colleagues[33] reported viral nucleic acid in tubular and visceral epithelial cells, whereas Kimmel and associates[34] demonstrated the presence of HIV nucleic acid in renal tubular epithelial cells using polymerase chain reaction. However, there are conflicting opinions regarding the need for the presence of virus for the development of HIV-associated focal segmental glomerulosclerosis.

PATHOGENESIS. Various theories have been proposed for the pathogenesis of the group of lesions encompassing minimal changes, mesangial proliferative disease, and focal segmental glomerulosclerosis.[35–38] The reason for the increased permeability of the glomerular capillary wall to macromolecules in these diseases is not apparent. Although some decrease of glomerular polyanion has been demonstrated, the cause for this loss is not known. An experimental model of minimal change disease has been developed by administration of the aminoglycoside puromycin, an agent specifically toxic to the glomerular epithelial cells, which synthesize the negatively charged sialoproteins and proteoglycans so abundant in the glomerular basement membrane. Thus, it is believed that injury to the glomerular visceral epithelial cells results in reduction of glomerular polyanions, which, in turn, leads to a loss of the anionic charge barrier considered necessary to preventing anionic intravascular proteins, particularly albumin, from leaking across the glomerular basement membrane. Another hypothesis of pathogenesis is based on the association of minimal change disease with allergies, abnormal T-cell function, and abnormal cellular immunity, suggesting that a circulating lymphokine or vasculotoxic substance produced by an aberrant clone of lymphocytes causes the disease. The rapid recurrence of focal segmental glomerulosclerosis in transplant patients indicates that the idiopathic nephrotic syndrome is probably not a disease of the kidneys, but that it is related to an as yet unknown circulating factor that increases glomerular permeability.

## Membranous Glomerulopathy (Primary, Idiopathic) (Synonyms: Epimembranous Glomerulopathy, Membranous Glomerulonephritis, and Extramembranous Glomerulopathy)

CLINICAL CONSIDERATIONS. Membranous glomerulopathy is an immune-complex glomerulopathy.[39–43] It is one of the common causes of nephrotic syndrome in adults (20% to 30% of cases) and although rare in children, it accounts for 1% to 9% of patients with nephrotic syndrome in this age group as well. The disease is common in men, with a peak incidence between the fourth and fifth decades. Most patients present with nephrotic range proteinuria that is usually nonselective, that is, it contains large-molecular-weight proteins such as immunoglobulins as well as low-molecular-weight proteins such as albumin. Microscopic hematuria is present at some time during the course of the disease. Idiopathic membranous glomerulopathy typically produces recurrent episodes of nephrotic syndrome. About 20% to 25% of untreated patients progress to end-stage renal disease.[39, 44, 45] Renal vein thrombosis may supervene. Transplanted patients can show recurrence of their initial membranous glomerulopathy or can develop de novo membranous disease. In general, recurrence is less common than de novo lesions.

In about one third of cases, membranous glomerulopathy is associated with a secondary cause (specific antigen), and the antigen can be demonstrated in the deposits. It is of great importance to differentiate a secondary membranous glomerulopa-

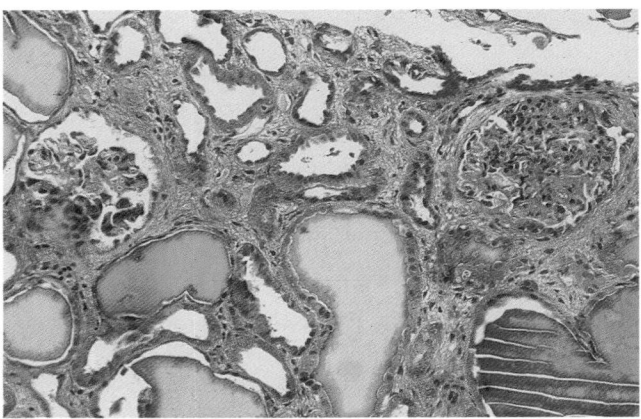

FIGURE 29–16. HIV-associated nephropathy: Glomeruli show lesions of focal segmental glomerulosclerosis. The tubules are cystically dilated, and there is chronic tubulointerstitial change. (Masson trichrome stain.)

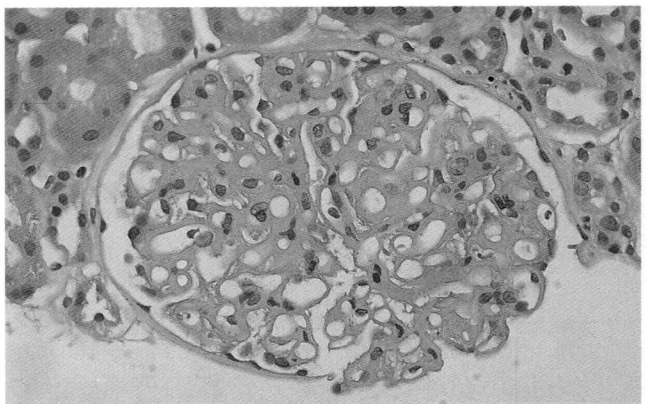

**FIGURE 29–17.** Membranous glomerulopathy: The glomerulus is normocellular. The capillary walls show diffuse uniform thickening.

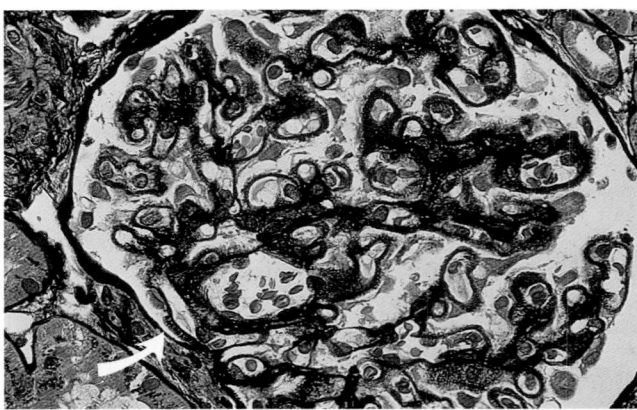

**FIGURE 29–19.** Membranous glomerulopathy: Spikes (*arrow*) and honeycomb patterns are seen along glomerular capillary walls. (Periodic acid-methenamine silver stain.)

thy from idiopathic (primary) membranous glomerulopathy, because elimination of a causative agent combined with appropriate treatment may change the prognosis or even lead to complete restoration of renal function and normal morphology. In secondary membranous glomerulopathy, the causes (antigens) include infections (hepatitis B, syphilis),[46–48] autoimmune disease (systemic lupus erythematosus [SLE]),[49, 50] drugs (e.g., gold, penicillamine, or mercury),[51] and solid tumors (e.g., colon or lung).[52, 53] It is a clinical axiom that if membranous glomerulopathy occurs in a patient older than 60 years of age, he or she should be investigated for a lung or gastrointestinal tract carcinoma. About 10% to 20% of cases of lupus nephritis present with membranous glomerulopathy. Occasionally, the patient may not have extrarenal manifestations of SLE. Membranous glomerulopathy is also associated with congenital and secondary syphilis.[46, 47] Treatment with penicillin can lead to complete recovery from the renal disease within several weeks, particularly in secondary syphilis.

DIAGNOSTIC CONSIDERATIONS. By light microscopy, all glomeruli are affected. They are normocellular and, depending on the stage, show mild, moderate, or marked thickening of peripheral capillary walls (Fig. 29–17). With Masson trichrome stain, magenta red deposits of protein (corresponding to immune deposits) are seen along the outer surface of the glomerular capillary walls (Fig. 29–18). Basement membrane spikes are seen with the PAMS silver stain (Fig. 29–19).[54] Mild interstitial edema and tubular degeneration may be present in the early stage of disease, and interstitial fibrosis with varying degrees of tubular atrophy as well as vascular sclerosis appear in advanced disease. Severe interstitial edema associated with inflammatory cell infiltration of glomerular capillaries (leukocytic margination) is often associated with renal vein thrombosis.[55]

By electron microscopy, all capillaries contain subepithelial or intramembranous electron-dense deposits (Fig. 29–20). The glomerular capillary wall changes are subdivided into stages I to IV.[56] The glomerular capillary basement membranes are thick-

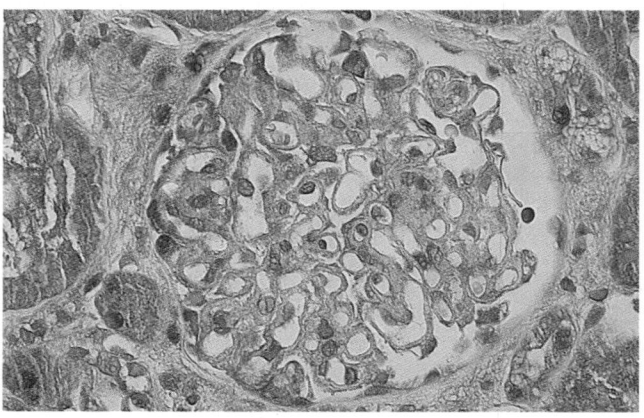

**FIGURE 29–18.** Membranous glomerulopathy: Magenta red granules (deposits) are present along the thickened glomerular capillary walls. (Masson trichrome stain.)

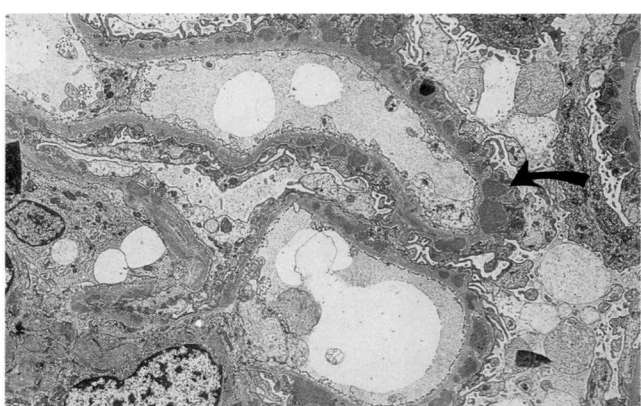

**FIGURE 29–20.** Membranous glomerulopathy. Electron micrograph of stage II disease, in which subepithelial electron-dense deposits (*arrow*) are bordered by spikelike projections of glomerular basement membrane.

ened initially (stage I) by subepithelial and later by intramembranous (stages II to III) electron-dense deposits along with spikes of basement membrane between the deposits. There is diffuse foot process fusion and villous transformation, a rather nonspecific finding indicative of heavy proteinuria. In advanced stages (stages III to IV), the capillary walls are markedly thickened and consist of masses of dense and fading deposits, old and newly laid down basement membrane material, and cytoplasmic fragments (i.e., stage IV—membranous transformation).

By immunofluorescence microscopy, the predominant finding is diffuse granular deposits of IgG of high intensity along the glomerular capillary walls (Fig. 29–21). In 50% of cases, less intense deposits of complement (C3 component) are also present in a similar location.[57, 58] Crescents are not a common feature of membranous glomerulopathy, but there have been case reports of crescentic glomerulonephritis with antecedent membranous glomerulopathy,[59–61] and some of these cases show antiglomerular basement membrane (anti-GBM) antibodies.[60]

The morphologic expression of secondary membranous glomerulopathy differs slightly from the idiopathic form of disease. By light microscopy, the glomeruli often show a mild to moderate increase in mesangial cellularity. By electron and immunofluorescence microscopy, in addition to subepithelial deposits, mesangial, perimesangial, and rarely, subendothelial deposits are present.[62]

In gold-induced membranous nephropathy, the primary site of gold deposition is the mitochondria of proximal convoluted tubules. Accumulation of gold in the mitochondria results in their disruption and the consequent degeneration and necrosis of the lining epithelium. By electron microscopy, in addition to subepithelial electron-dense deposits in glomeruli, granules of gold (aurosomes) may be found in proximal tubular epithelium and rarely in glomerular visceral epithelial cells.

In membranous glomerulopathy associated with neoplasia, several studies have identified tumor-associated antigens, such as carcinoembryonic antigen, in renal biopsy specimens in individual cases.[52, 53] Finally, treponemal antigen has been demonstrated in glomeruli of cases of both congenital and secondary syphilis.

Recently, we have discovered that CD30 (Ki-1) is a possible new antigen in a subgroup of cases of membranous glomerulopathy.[63] The pilot study has shown that in some cases of secondary membranous glomerulopathy, the glomerular deposits stain with antibody to CD30 (Ki-1), and that some of these patients have lesions of the gastrointestinal tract, such as a recent or past history of gastrointestinal tumors or irritable bowel syndrome.[63]

PATHOGENESIS. Until the 1980s, it was universally believed that membranous glomerulopathy resulted from deposition of circulating immune complexes. However, it now appears that the subepithelial immune-complex deposits actually form by interaction of an in situ antigen (intrinsic or structural antigen) or extrarenal planted antigen with antibody.[64] In most cases of idiopathic membranous glomerulopathy, circulating immune complexes are not detected, and when they are detected, attempts to establish an antigen responsible for the membranous glomerulopathy have failed.[39,65]

# DIFFUSE PROLIFERATIVE GLOMERULONEPHRITIS

## Acute Postinfectious (Post-Streptococcal) Glomerulonephritis

CLINICAL CONSIDERATIONS. Poststreptococcal glomerulonephritis usually results from throat or skin infection with nephritogenic strains of group A $\beta$-hemolytic streptococci. The principal serotypes implicated are streptococci of group M types 1, 2, 12, 49, 55, 57, and 60. The overall risk of developing nephritis after a nephritogenic streptococcus infection is estimated at 15%. The disease commonly occurs in children, but no age group is exempt. Patients present with an abrupt onset of renal disease within 21 days of the appearance of infection. Streptococcal infection is accepted as the cause of the glomerulonephritis; however, demonstration of streptococcal antigen or antibody in glomeruli is controversial.[66, 67] The disease is characterized by generalized edema, hematuria with smoky-colored urine, a nephritic urine sediment containing red blood cells and red blood cell casts, hypertension, and mild proteinuria. The antistreptolysin O titer usually rises, and levels of the C3 component of complement decrease early in the course of the nephritis (within the first month), only to rise to normal levels later. Complete resolution of nephritis is the rule. Progressive renal failure can occur, but it is more common in adults and it is usually accompanied by severe hypertension.[68–71]

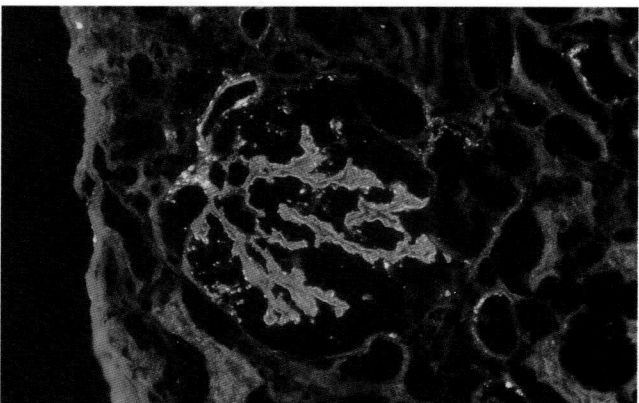

**FIGURE 29–21.** Membranous glomerulopathy: Immunofluorescence showing finely granular deposits along glomerular capillary walls with antibodies to IgG.

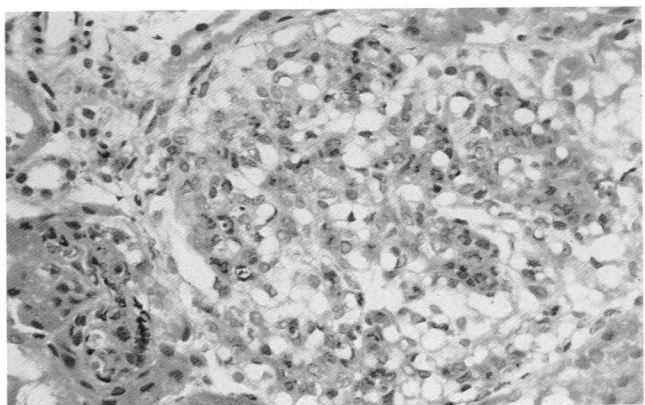

**FIGURE 29–22.** Acute postinfectious glomerulonephritis: The glomerulus is hypercellular with increase in intrinsic cells and inflammatory cell (neutrophil) infiltration.

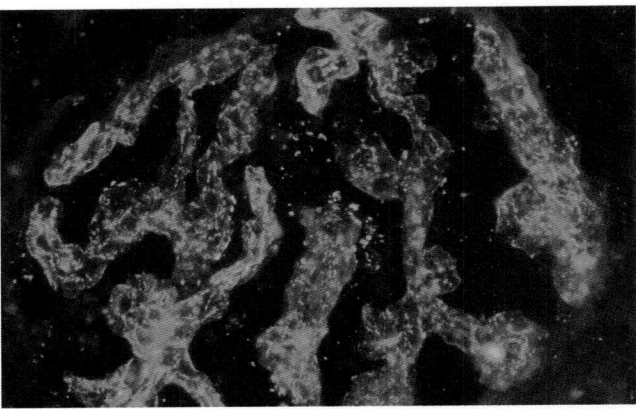

**FIGURE 29–24.** Postinfectious glomerulonephritis: Immunofluorescence microscopy shows granular deposits along capillary walls with antibodies to IgG.

DIAGNOSTIC CONSIDERATIONS. By light microscopy, all glomeruli are large, similarly involved, and hypercellular, with an increase in endocapillary cells and with inflammatory cell (neutrophil) infiltration (Fig. 29–22).[72] The glomerular capillary walls are normal in appearance. There is usually interstitial edema, and periglomerular inflammatory cell infiltration can be seen. Tubules may contain red blood cell casts. The blood vessels are unremarkable.

By electron microscopy, the glomerular capillary basement membranes are normal in thickness. Widely spaced, large, dome-shaped or humplike subepithelial deposits resting on an intact basement membrane is the characteristic lesion (Fig. 25–23). They are seen only within the first few weeks following the onset of nephritis. In addition, mesangial and occasional subendothelial deposits may be present. In general, the epithelial cell foot processes are slender. Depending on the stage and severity of the disease, the glomerular capillary lumina contain a variable number of leukocytes.

By immunofluorescence microscopy, coarse and fine granular deposits of IgG, and to a lesser extent of C3, are seen along the glomerular capillary walls and sometimes in the mesangium (Fig. 29–24).[73]

Although poststreptococcal glomerulonephritis has become synonymous with postinfectious glomerulonephritis, the disease also occurs with other organisms, such as *Staphylococcus, Meningococcus, Pneumococcus, Klebsiella, Salmonella, Enterococcus, Brucellae, Leptospira,* and mycobacteria. The list of organisms causing glomerulonephritis is ever expanding. The aforementioned organisms cause a diffuse proliferative glomerulonephritis; however, some infectious agents cause lesions other than a diffuse proliferative glomerulonephritis. Some important organisms and their associated lesions are shown in Table 29–2.[74]

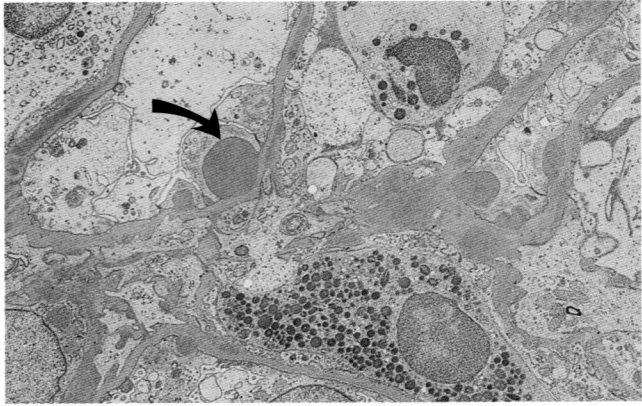

**FIGURE 29–23.** Postinfectious glomerulonephritis: Electron micrograph showing subepithelial humplike deposits along capillary basement membranes (*arrow*). Small intramembranous/subendothelial deposits are present. The capillary lumen is filled with inflammatory cells.

**TABLE 29–2.** Renal Glomerular Abnormalities Secondary to Infectious Agents[74]

| Agent | Glomerular Disease |
|---|---|
| Viral: | |
|   Hepatitis B | Membranous glomerulopathy or mesangiocapillary glomerulonephritis |
|   Hepatitis C | Mesangiocapillary glomerulonephritis[157, 158] |
|   Human immunodeficiency virus | Focal segmental glomerulosclerosis[27] |
| Bacterial: | Shunt nephritis[369]; chronic deep tissue abscesses; focal (common) and, less commonly, diffuse glomerulonephritis[366] |
| Secondary syphilis | Membranous glomerulopathy |
| Parasitic diseases: | |
|   Schistosomiasis, filariasis, hydatidosis | Membranous glomerulopathy |
|   Schistosomiasis, malaria | Mesangiocapillary glomerulonephritis[74] |

## Mesangiocapillary Glomerulonephritis, Types I, II, and III

On the basis of morphology, mesangiocapillary glomerulonephritis is divided into types I to III. The clinical presentation in the three types is similar, but their appearance is distinctive by electron microscopy.[75]

## Mesangiocapillary Glomerulonephritis, Type I (Synonyms: Membranoproliferative Glomerulonephritis Type I, Lobular Glomerulonephritis, Hypocomplementemic Glomerulonephritis)

CLINICAL CONSIDERATIONS. In type I mesangiocapillary glomerulonephritis, usually children or young adults are affected. Both sexes are equally affected. Patients present with overt nephrotic syndrome, asymptomatic proteinuria, or hematuria. Some present with nephritic syndrome, and a combination of nephrotic and nephritic syndromes is often present. Some patients also have a previous history of an upper respiratory tract infection that can cause clinical confusion with acute postinfectious glomerulonephritis. The two diseases do share some morphologic features by light microscopy, but the prognosis is quite different. In most, but not all, cases of type I membranoproliferative glomerulonephritis (MPGN), the C3 component of complement is decreased (hypocomplementemic glomerulonephritis).[76] The disease is chronic, with periods of clinical remission in some individuals. It progresses to end-stage renal disease within 10 to 15 years and recurs in about 30% to 40% of renal transplant recipients.

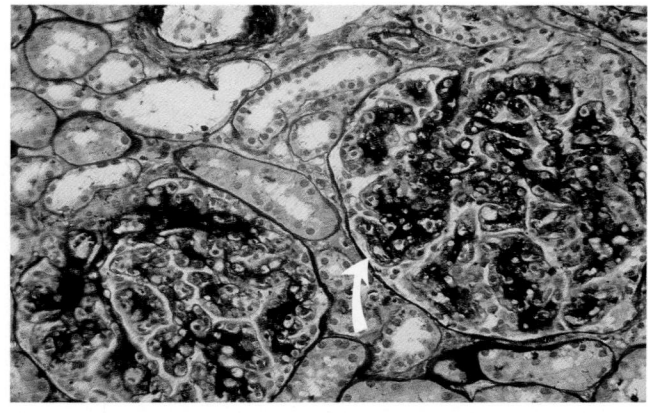

FIGURE 29–26. Mesangiocapillary glomerulonephritis, type I: Glomerulus displays double contours or tram-track pattern (reduplication) along capillary walls (*arrow*). The inherent lobularity of the glomerulus is accentuated.

DIAGNOSTIC CONSIDERATIONS. By light microscopy, all glomeruli are uniformly involved. They are large, hypercellular, with an increase in endocapillary cells and with leukocytic infiltration that obliterates glomerular capillary lumina and that leads to simplification of the glomerular tufts, producing a lobular pattern (Fig. 29–25). In PAS- and methenamine silver-stained sections, a double contour or tram-track pattern of the glomerular capillary wall is recognized (mesangiocapillary pattern) (Fig. 29–26).[77] Both lobular and double contour patterns can be present together and represent morphologic variants of the lesion. Crescents may be present.

By electron microscopy, the glomerular capillary basement membranes proper are of normal thickness and they show subendothelial mesangial extension (the double contour seen by light microscopy) or when the lobular pattern is pronounced, they can show obliteration of capillary lumina by intraluminal expansion of proliferating mesangial cells and matrix (Fig. 29–27). In addition, mostly discrete sub-

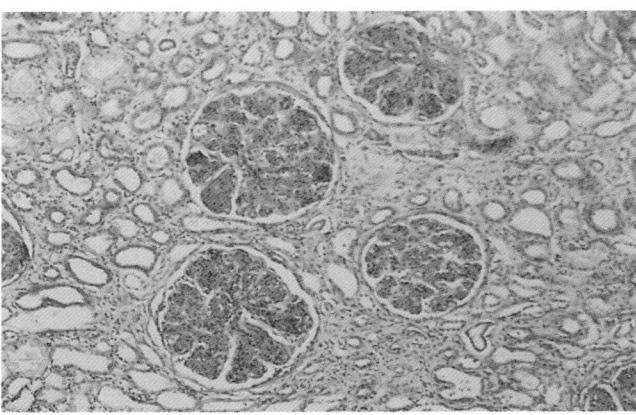

FIGURE 29–25. Mesangiocapillary glomerulonephritis, type I: The glomeruli are similar in appearance. They are hypercellular and they show lobular simplification with obliteration of capillary lumina and thickening of capillary walls.

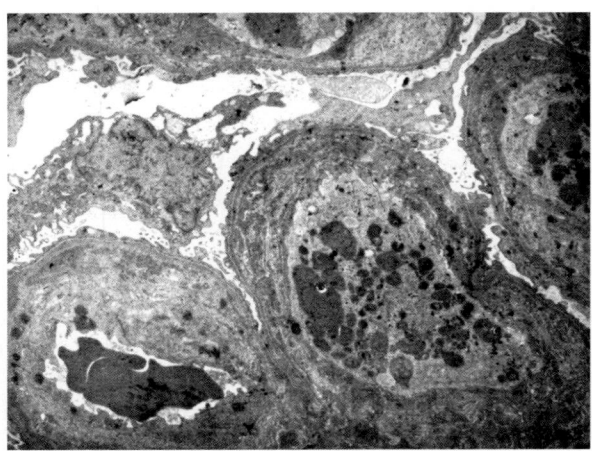

FIGURE 29–27. Mesangiocapillary glomerulonephritis, type I: Electron micrograph reveals subendothelial mesangial extension and subendothelial deposits. There is diffuse effacement of epithelial cell foot processes.

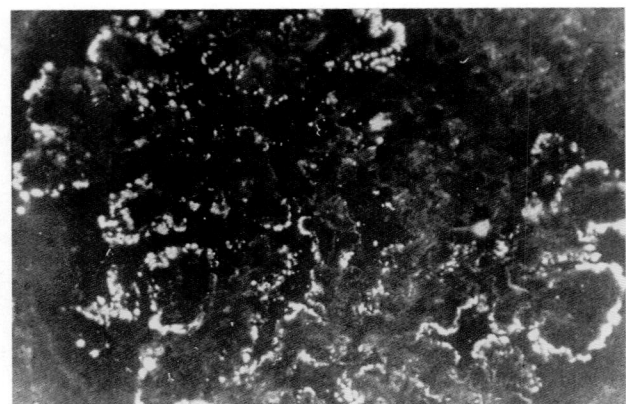

**FIGURE 29–28.** Mesangiocapillary glomerulonephritis, type I: Immunofluorescence microscopy shows granular deposits of C3 along capillary walls at the periphery of the accentuated glomerular lobules.

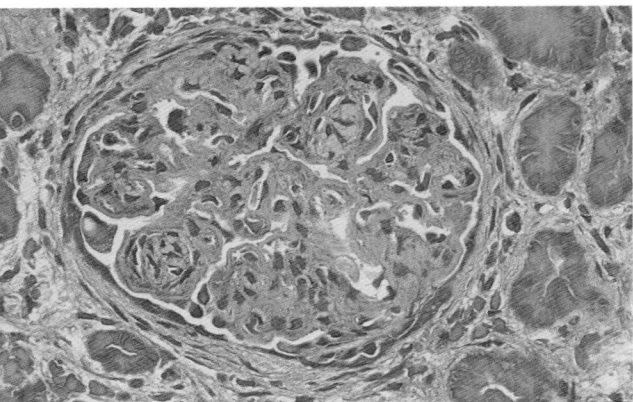

**FIGURE 29–29.** Dense deposit disease (MPGN type II): Glomerulus shows increase in cellularity, lobular simplification, obliteration of lumina, and thickening of capillary walls. (Masson trichrome stain.)

endothelial and mesangial electron-dense deposits are seen. There is diffuse effacement of epithelial foot processes.

By immunofluorescence microscopy, the glomerular capillary walls contain predominantly deposits of C3, which outline the lobules and are rarely associated with deposits of IgG (Fig. 29–28). Other immunoglobulins are usually absent.

## Mesangiocapillary Glomerulonephritis Type III (Synonym: Membranoproliferative Glomerulonephritis, Type III)

A morphologic variant of MPGN type I was introduced in the 1980s.[78, 79] In this subtype, subepithelial, often humplike deposits are seen in addition to the subendothelial and mesangial deposits. Clinically, the disease appears to be similar to MPGN type I and the lesion is referred to as a variant of type I MPGN.

## Dense Deposit Disease; Mesangiocapillary Glomerulonephritis, Type II (Synonym: Membranoproliferative Glomerulonephritis, Type II)

CLINICAL CONSIDERATIONS. The clinical presentation of patients with type II MPGN is similar to those with type I MPGN, but the serum levels of C3 are more often depressed and remain depressed for longer periods of time than in patients with type I MPGN.[71, 80–84] More than 60% of the patients exhibit a complement-activating antibody called C3 nephritic factor. This factor, an IgG autoantibody, binds to the alternate pathway convertase called C3b,Bb. The C3 nephritic factor stabilizes and pro-

longs the activity of the enzyme by interfering with normal factors controlling the enzyme convertase activity, with resultant sustained activation and depletion of serum C3 levels.[71] Some patients also have partial lipodystrophy.[85]

In our experience, type III MPGN is common in patients from Iran, possibly suggesting a relationship with socioeconomic standards that may lead to higher incidences of infection.

DIAGNOSTIC CONSIDERATIONS. By light microscopy, the changes are similar to those seen in type I MPGN (Fig. 29–29). Often there is irregular, bright pink, refractile thickening of capillary walls, best seen with the PAS stain. This change can also be seen in plastic sections stained with toluidine blue, and it can be appreciated sometimes in extraglomerular locations, such as along tubular and vascular basement membranes.

Electron microscopy is essential to establish the diagnosis of dense deposit disease. Ribbon-like electron-dense deposits of uniform density are seen

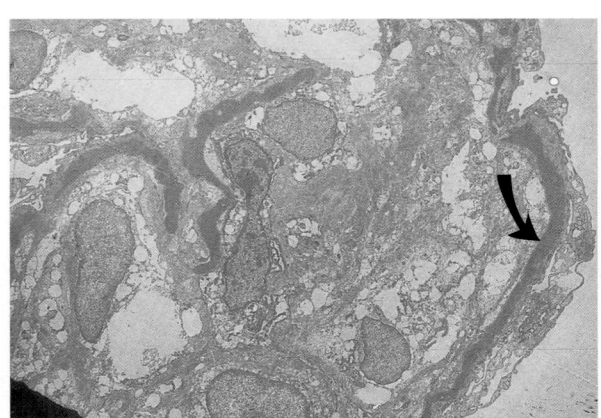

**FIGURE 29–30.** Dense deposit disease (MPGN type II): Electron micrograph showing intramembranous ribbon-like deposits occupying the lamina densa (*arrow*). There is effacement of epithelial cell foot processes.

within the lamina densa of glomerular capillary basement membranes and in the mesangium (Fig. 29–30). In addition, deposits can be seen in Bowman's capsule and tubular or vascular basement membranes. In early stages, deposits are interrupted and occupy only portions of the basement membranes, but in later phases of disease, they occupy the entire length of capillaries.

By immunohistochemistry, wide, bandlike or interrupted pseudolinear deposits of C3 are seen along the glomerular capillary walls, outlining the lobules, as well as within the mesangium.[86]

In all three types of MPGN, depending on the stage of the disease, a variety of chronic changes, such as glomerular and vascular sclerosis, interstitial fibrosis, and tubular atrophy, can be seen.

## IgA Nephropathy (Synonyms: IgA–IgG Nephropathy, Berger's Disease)

This disease was originally described by Berger and Hinglais[87] in 1968, and it is characterized by mesangial cell proliferation with mesangial deposits by electron microscopy and mesangial IgA deposits by immunohistochemistry.[74, 87–89]

CLINICAL CONSIDERATIONS. IgA nephropathy is common worldwide, but it varies in frequency from country to country. The disease can affect any age, but it is most common in young adults in the second to third decades of life. Men are affected three to six times more often than women; however this may vary. The clinical presentation in most cases is microhematuria with episodic gross hematuria, often associated with upper respiratory tract infection. Proteinuria, if present, is non-nephrotic; only about 10% of patients develop nephrotic syndrome. The disease originally was considered benign; however, 25% to 40% of patients develop end-stage renal disease. The recurrence rate in renal transplants is 50%.

DIAGNOSTIC CONSIDERATIONS. By light microscopy, the glomeruli usually show similar changes,

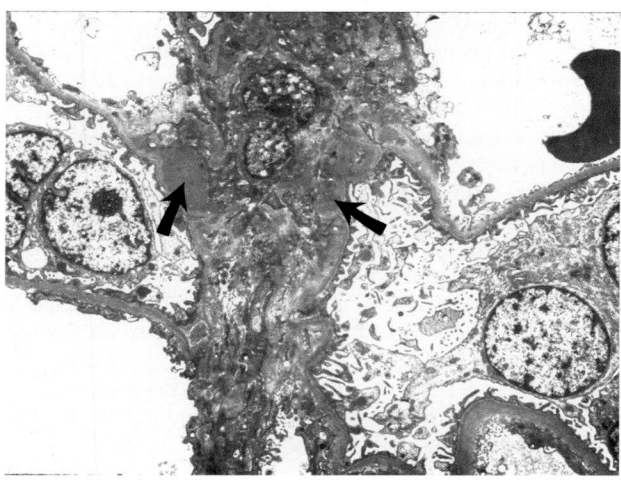

**FIGURE 29–32.** IgA nephropathy: Electron micrograph shows mesangial widening with deposits (*arrow*).

with minor variation. They most often have a moderate increase in mesangial cells and matrix (Fig. 29–31). In a smaller percentage of biopsies with progressive lesions, focal or even diffuse endocapillary proliferation and/or crescents are seen.

By electron microscopy, the mesangial deposits are often large, and they are present in most mesangial areas (Fig. 29–32). Occasionally, perimesangial or rare subendothelial deposits can also be seen.

By immunofluorescence microscopy, mesangial IgA is necessary to make the diagnosis (Fig. 29–33). It is associated with C3 in most patients. IgG and IgM have been reported in more than 50% of cases, but early complement components C1q and C4 are not commonly found. Fibrinogen may be present, but it is often inconspicuous; in contrast, Henoch-Schönlein purpura (HSP) has prominent deposits of fibrinogen.

PATHOGENESIS. IgA nephropathy is an immune-complex disease with high levels of circulating IgA immune complexes found in some patients. Plasma cells in the gastrointestinal tract and possibly in the respiratory tract are believed to be the source of the antibody. The nature of the antigen in serum

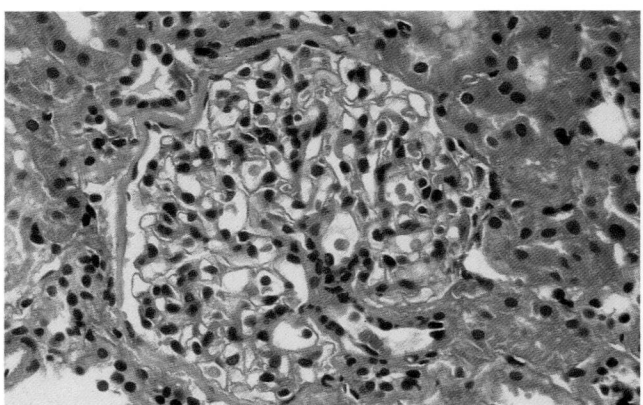

**FIGURE 29–31.** IgA nephropathy: Glomerulus shows a mild increase in mesangial cells and matrix.

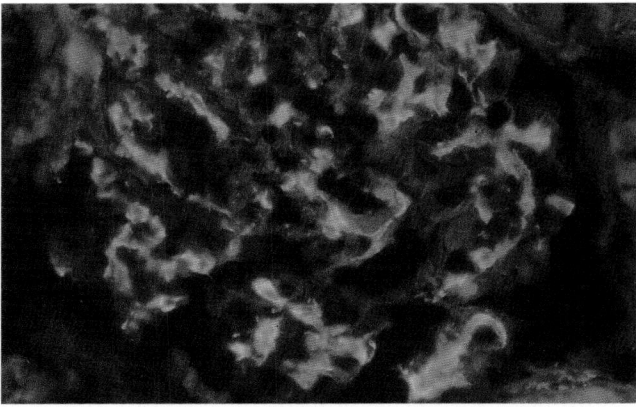

**FIGURE 29–33.** IgA nephropathy: Immunofluorescence microscopy shows a mesangial distribution of IgA.

immune complexes and in the mesangial deposits remains unknown; it may be food, viral, or microbial antigens.[74, 89] This disease is now considered by many to be one manifestation of a clinicopathologic syndrome that includes IgA nephropathy and HSP. The two diseases share many common factors, such as similar circulating immune complexes and histologic changes, the presence of mesangial IgA, and similar histologic changes in transplanted kidneys. Because of the often overlapping histologic findings, differentiation between IgA nephropathy and HSP is still based solely on clinical features. IgA nephropathy can also be associated with other systemic diseases—the secondary form includes diseases such as alcoholic liver disease,[89] celiac disease, dermatitis herpetiformis, and HIV infection.

## Crescentic Glomerulonephritis (Synonyms: Rapidly Progressive Glomerulonephritis, Subacute Glomerulonephritis, Extracapillary Glomerulonephritis, Malignant Glomerulonephritis)

DEFINITION. Crescentic glomerulonephritis is a histopathologic term for a pattern of diseases characterized morphologically by extensive crescent formation in the glomeruli and clinically by rapid deterioration of renal function with progression to end-stage renal failure within weeks or months. The main histologic feature is the presence of crescents in most glomeruli without an underlying disease.[74, 90-92] It has been suggested that crescents represent an inflammatory response (principally macrophagic) to the presence of fibrin and formed elements of the blood within Bowman's space, arising from breaks in the glomerular basement membrane.

On the basis mainly of immunohistochemical findings, crescentic glomerulonephritis can be subdivided into several subtypes (Table 29–3). Still, regardless of the underlying mechanism, light microscopy reveals similar findings, that is, crescents.

CLINICAL CONSIDERATIONS. This pattern of disease is found in approximately 10% of renal biopsies. It affects adults, and it is more common in men than in women. The presenting symptoms can be vague and can include nausea, tiredness, weakness, and fatigue. Most patients present with rapid deterioration of renal function and oliguria or anuria, occasionally associated with hematuria. Hypertension is uncommon. In patients with anti-glomerular basement membrane (anti-GBM) antibody-associated crescentic glomerulonephritis, pulmonary hemorrhage can occur with onset of renal disease or later in the course. The triad of crescentic glomerulonephritis, pulmonary hemorrhage, and circulating anti-GBM antibodies is known as Goodpasture's disease. The autoantibody reacts with the NC-1 domain of type IV collagen of the GBM, which is therefore known as the Goodpasture antigen. This type of crescentic glomerulonephritis is more common in patients with HLA-DR2 immunophenotype. Serum complement is typically normal in these patients.

In crescentic glomerulonephritis associated with immune complexes, there can be an occult or overt source of infection. In the authors' experience, this subtype is common in elderly patients. The source of the immune complexes is often unknown.

In the nonimmune or pauci-immune type of crescentic glomerulonephritis, no known etiologic agent is demonstrable and serum complement values are again typically normal. However, antineutrophil cytoplasmic antibody (ANCA) is often present, and therefore this disease is believed by many to be a renal-limited variant of microscopic polyangiitis (see the discussion of that disease later).

DIAGNOSTIC CONSIDERATIONS. By light microscopy, the hallmark of this pattern of glomerulonephritis is the crescent, a collection of cells in Bowman's space that, in filling the space, produces a configuration resembling a crescent moon (Fig. 29–34). Although crescents are often present in 80% to 90% of glomeruli in crescentic glomerulonephritis, there is no agreement on the percentage of glomeruli that need to be involved, and crescentic disease can range from 50% to 90% of glomeruli. The crescents are usually circumferential and compress the

**TABLE 29–3.** Subtypes of Crescentic Glomerulonephritis[92]

Glomerulonephritis associated with antibodies to glomerular basement membrane antigens (antiglomerular basement membrane glomerulonephritis)
Glomerulonephritis associated with immune-complex deposition in the glomeruli
Nonimmune or pauci-immune glomerulonephritis, without association with antigen-antibody complexes, or anti-glomerular basement membrane antibodies.
　ANCA-positive crescentic glomerulonephritis
　ANCA-negative crescentic glomerulonephritis

ANCA, antineutrophil-associated cytoplasmic antibody.

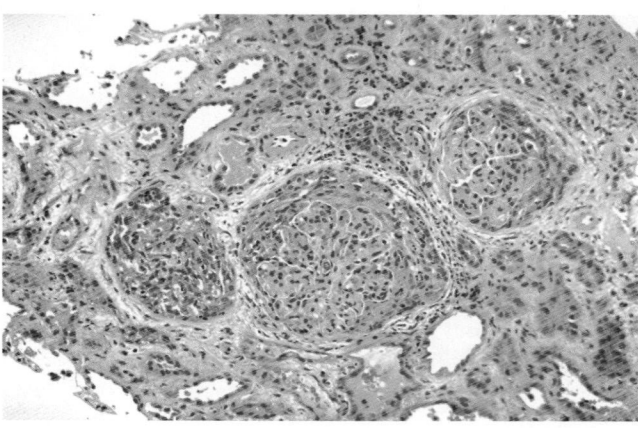

**FIGURE 29–34.** Crescentic glomerulonephritis: The glomeruli are compressed by epithelial crescents. The tubules are dilated.

glomerular tufts. The glomerular tufts proper usually do not show any changes, but they may appear hypercellular due to inflammatory cell infiltration. Glomeruli that are uninvolved by crescents usually fail to show tuft abnormalities. Crescents are made up of proliferating epithelial cells, fibrin, and inflammatory cells, including monocyte-type cells. Depending on the time of biopsy, fibroepithelial or purely fibrous crescents can be seen. There are usually associated tubulointerstitial changes, including tubular necrosis and dilatation, red blood cell casts, interstitial edema, and rarely, interstitial fibrosis. Blood vessels do not reveal changes of vasculitis, but they may show arteriosclerosis.

By electron microscopy, glomerular capillary basement membranes are usually compressed by the crescent and they are thickened, collapsed, and show a widening of the lamina rara interna, with loss of normal appearance of the lamina densa. Breaks in the basement membranes are common. Usually, electron-dense deposits or immune complexes are not seen, but occasionally (approximately 40% of cases) they can be present.

By immunohistochemistry several patterns are possible. In anti-GBM–associated glomerulonephritis, a continuous fine linear pattern of IgG is present along glomerular capillary basement membranes (Fig. 29–35). These deposits also have been described along Bowman's capsule and tubular basement membranes, but they are less common in these locations. The deposits can be associated with linear or semilinear deposits of the C3 fraction of complement, but often immunoglobulins and complement components are absent. A linear immunofluorescence pattern, usually thicker than that seen with anti-GBM glomerulonephritis, can also be present in patients with diabetes; however, albumin and, less commonly, other immunoglobulins are also co-expressed in a linear pattern in diabetics, which helps in differentiating the two entities.

In 40% of crescentic glomerulonephritides, granular deposits of IgG and C3 and, less commonly, of other immunoglobulins are seen. In these cases, the IgG, C3, and, rarely, IgA are present along glomerular capillary walls, and they are seen in the mesangium. In most of the cases, a convincing underlying cause for the immune-complex deposits is not found.

In all three groups of crescentic glomerulonephritis, deposits of fibrin are present both within the glomerular tufts and within Bowman's spaces or the crescents themselves.

Finally, in about 40% of cases of crescentic glomerulonephritis, immunofluorescence microscopy is negative for immunoglobulins and complement components (pauci-immune crescentic glomerulonephritis).

## GLOMERULAR INVOLVEMENT WITH SYSTEMIC DISEASES

Renal involvement occurs in a variety of systemic diseases. The glomerular involvement is basically focal (some glomeruli) and segmental (portions of glomeruli), a feature that separates the primary glomerular diseases from those associated with systemic disease, also called secondary.

### Lupus Nephritis

CLINICAL CONSIDERATIONS. SLE is an autoimmune disease that commonly affects young adults. Ten times as many woman are affected as men. Laboratory criteria formulated by the American College of Rheumatology (ACR) are often used for the diagnosis of SLE.

Renal involvement occurs in as many as 80% of patients with SLE. Nephritis is a major cause of morbidity and mortality. Patients present with diverse clinical findings. In particular, symptomatic hematuria or proteinuria, nephrotic or nephritic syndromes, hypertension, azotemia, nephritic urinary sediment with hematuria, red blood cell and cellular casts (telescope urine), hypocomplementemia, and high anti-DNA titers can be present.[93]

DIAGNOSTIC CONSIDERATIONS. On light microscopy, lupus nephritis can mimic almost any other renal disease. The most characteristic feature of the renal lesion is its great morphologic variability.[94–96] Through the years, numerous attempts to classify lupus nephritis on clinical and histologic bases have been made. The latest, now widely used, classification is that of the World Health Organization (WHO), which is essentially based on light microscopic features. It is recognized, however, that a more precise definition of renal biopsy findings can only be made by light microscopy in combination with electron and immunofluorescence microscopy. The WHO classification divides the lesions into six subgroups (I to VI) (Table 29–4). Further subclassification of each group includes additional findings.[97]

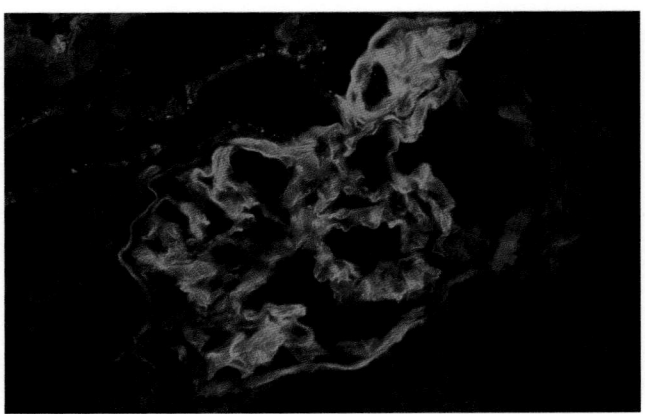

**FIGURE 29–35.** Crescentic glomerulonephritis (anti-GBM antibody-associated glomerulonephritis): Immunofluorescence microscopy shows linear deposits when stained with antibody against IgG.

**TABLE 29–4.** WHO Classification of Lupus Nephritis

| WHO I | Normal | Normal by all parameters |
|---|---|---|
| WHO II | Mesangial lupus nephritis | Mesangial hypercellularity and/or sclerosis. (Mesangial electron-dense and immune deposits seen) |
| WHO III | Focal proliferative lupus nephritis | Mesangial hypercellularity diffusely present; endocapillary proliferative lesions in less than 50% of glomeruli. (Mesangial and subendothelial electron-dense and immune-complex deposits) |
| WHO IV | Diffuse proliferative lupus nephritis | Mesangial hypercellularity diffusely present; endocapillary proliferative lesions in more than 50% of glomeruli. (Mesangial and subendothelial electron-dense and immune-complex deposits) |
| WHO V | Membranous lupus nephritis | Mesangial hypercellularity and diffuse thickening of glomerular capillary basement membranes. (Mesangial and subepithelial electron-dense and immune-complex deposits) |
| WHO VI | Sclerosing lupus nephritis | Glomerular sclerosis, sometimes associated with fibrous crescents, and interstitial fibrosis, tubular atrophy, and vascular sclerosis. |

The details of the WHO classification are as follows:

1. Normal (WHO I): There are no abnormalities by light, electron, or immunofluorescence microscopy.
2. Mesangial lupus nephritis (WHO II): By light microscopy, the mesangial regions show a variable but usually mild to moderate increase in cells and matrix (Fig. 29–36). By electron microscopy, the widened mesangia contain electron-dense deposits that extend into the perimesangial areas in some cases (Fig. 29–37). Tubuloreticular structures (TRSs) or myxovirus-like particles (a misnomer, because no viral nucleic acid has ever been demonstrated within them) are seen in endothelial cells (Fig. 29–37). The glomerular capillary basement membranes are normal, without deposits. Epithelial cells are also unremarkable, and the epithelial foot processes are slender.

   By immunofluorescence microscopy, deposits of IgG and C3 and at times other immunoglobulins (IgA, IgM) and C1q are seen in the mesangium.

3. Proliferative lupus nephritis (WHO III and IV): The difference between types III (focal) and IV (diffuse) proliferative nephritis is based on the percentage of glomeruli involved. Although the glomerular lesions seen in the two groups are often similar, they are typically less severe in type III than in type IV disease. By light microscopy, the glomerular involvement varies in degree and extent. Most but not necessarily all of the following glomerular changes are present: an increase in cellularity, leukocyte infiltration, fibrinoid necrosis, karyorrhexis, nuclear pyknosis, focal eosinophilic thickening of peripheral capillary walls or "wire loop" lesions (due to massive subendothelial immune-complex deposits), hyaline eosinophilic intracapillary thrombi, and crescents (Fig. 29–38). At times, glomeruli exhibit a mesangiocapillary pattern similar to, but not identical with, that of mesangiocapillary glomerulonephri-

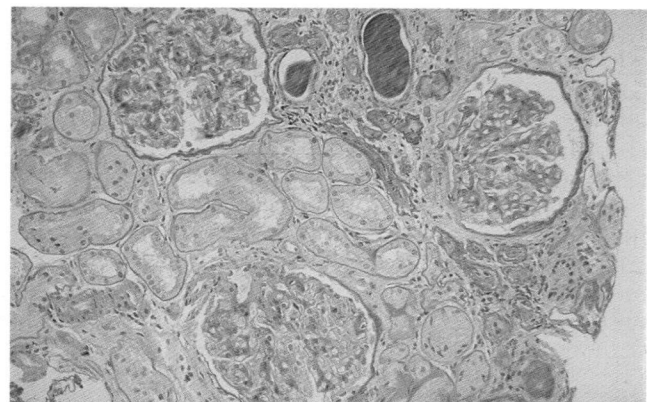

**FIGURE 29–36.** Lupus nephritis, mesangial: The glomeruli show moderate increase in mesangial cells and matrix. (PAS stain.)

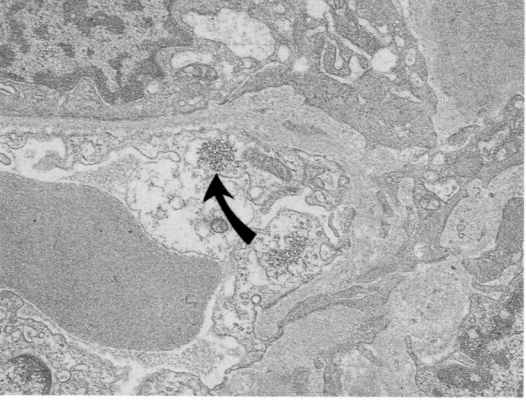

**FIGURE 29–37.** Lupus nephritis, mesangial: Electron micrograph shows a mesangial deposit and tubuloreticular structures (*arrow*) in an endothelial cell.

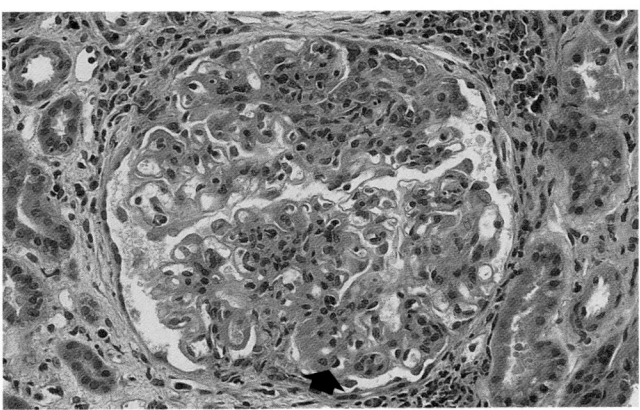

**FIGURE 29–38.** Lupus nephritis, proliferative: Glomerulus shows segmental hypercellularity, inflammatory cell infiltration, and irregular thickening of capillary walls. Some thickened walls show wire loop lesion (*arrow*).

tis, type I. Intraglomerular hematoxyphil bodies, a pathognomonic marker for SLE, are rare. The tubulointerstitial changes include interstitial infiltrates made up predominantly of plasma cells, lymphocytes, and mononuclear cells. The degree of interstitial inflammation usually increases with the severity of the glomerular lesions. Vascular sclerosis with hyaline change and fibrinoid necrosis or thrombosis of arteries may be present.

By electron microscopy, electron-dense deposits are present in mesangial, perimesangial, subendothelial, subepithelial, and intramembranous locations (Fig. 29–39). Massive subendothelial deposits correspond to the "wire loop" lesion seen by light microscopy. Large deposits in the capillary lumen may, in cross-section, appear as free intraluminal masses; they correspond to the "hyaline" thrombi seen by light microscopy. At times, lupus nephritis can be complicated by cryoglobulinemia and it can be associated with electron-dense deposits that reveal a curvilinear substructure resembling fingerprints. Intracapillary cryoglobulin

"thrombi" that appear bright pink by light microscopy also have a crystalline or fibrillar substructure by electron microscopy. True intraluminal thrombi with fibrin and platelets are rarely present in lupus nephritis. Deposits are often present in extraglomerular sites, such as the wall of vessels, tubular basement membranes, and in the interstitium.

TRSs are present within the endothelial cell cytoplasm of glomerular and intratubular capillaries.[94, 98] They are present in almost every case of lupus nephritis. Originally thought to be diagnostic for lupus nephritis, these structures are now known to be present in renal biopsies of patients with AIDS and occasionally in cases of hepatitis-associated nephritis. They may be correlated with a high interferon level.

By immunofluorescence microscopy, granular or lumpy deposits of immunoglobulins IgG, IgA, IgM, complement components C3 and C1q, and often fibrin/fibrinogen (the so-called full-house staining pattern) are seen with an irregular, focal or diffuse glomerular distribution (Fig. 29–40). Extraglomerular deposits are often present. In occasional cases, the extraglomerular deposits are numerous in comparison to the glomerular deposits and are associated with heavy interstitial inflammatory cell infiltration.

4. Membranous lupus nephritis (WHO V): The changes are those of a secondary membranous glomerulopathy with a mild to moderate increase in mesangial cellularity and with subepithelial or intramembranous and mesangial deposits by electron microscopy and immunofluorescence microscopy (Figs. 29–41 and 29–42). TRSs are present in endothelial cells (Fig. 29–42).

5. Sclerosing lupus nephritis (WHO VI): In sclerosing lupus nephritis, varying degrees of glomerular sclerosis, sometimes associated with fibrous crescents, and interstitial fibrosis, tubular atrophy, and vascular sclerosis are present. By electron microscopy, irregular thickening and collapse of capillary basement membranes, increase in mes-

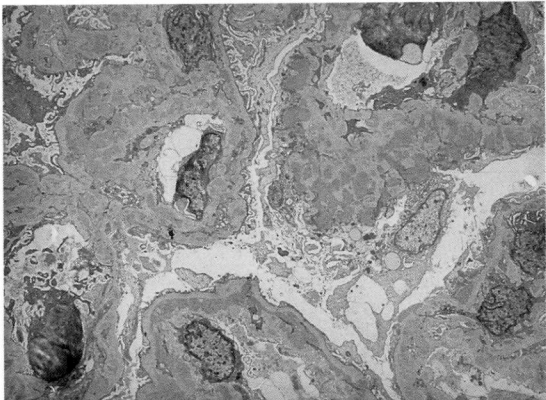

**FIGURE 29–39.** Lupus nephritis, proliferative: Electron micrograph shows thickened capillary basement membranes due to subepithelial, subendothelial, and mesangial deposits.

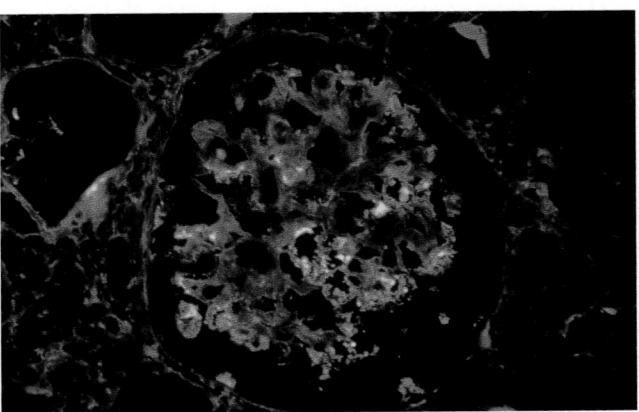

**FIGURE 29–40.** Lupus nephritis, proliferative: Immunofluorescence microscopy shows variable but diffuse distribution of granular deposits of IgG.

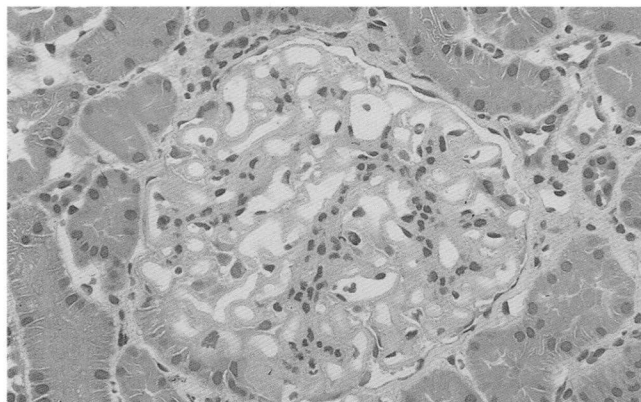

**FIGURE 29–41.** Lupus nephritis, membranous: The glomerulus shows thickening of capillary walls and increase in endocapillary cells.

angial matrix, and varying amounts of electron-dense or variably lucent intramembranous or intraluminal deposits are seen. TRSs may not be found.

It is well known that lupus nephritis is not a static disease. The renal disease can change from a given WHO class to another during the clinical course in 15% to 40% of patients.[96, 99] This change can occur spontaneously or following treatment. Usually with a change in WHO class, there is a corresponding change in clinical signs and symptoms; thus, rebiopsies may be performed to decide the current WHO type and treatment. A new WHO subgroup, consisting of a combination of membranous and proliferative lupus nephritis with a membranous pattern by light microscopy and subepithelial, mesangial, and subendothelial deposits by electron microscopy, has been reported by some; however, its impact on treatment and outcome needs to be studied.

In addition to the WHO classification system, investigators at the National Institutes of Health (NIH) have developed a scoring methodology that produces morphologic indices of activity and chronicity of renal disease.[100, 101] The system is based on the idea that patients with significant scarring in the glomerular or tubulointerstitial compartments can be and ought to be separated from those who have more active lesions, such as cellular crescents or necrotizing glomerular lesions, in deciding whether to use aggressive immunosuppressive therapy, and that these findings may also be useful to predict renal prognosis over time. Although considered controversial by some and not routinely used by others, in our view, it remains a useful measure to quantify renal damage, separate acute from chronic renal disease, and to decide treatment.

VASCULAR LESIONS IN LUPUS NEPHRITIS. The most common vascular lesions in lupus nephritis are arteriosclerosis and arteriolosclerosis. They are similar to those seen in benign hypertension. These vas-

cular lesions are common in patients with chronic lupus nephritis and in those on long-term corticosteroid treatment. Another lesion known as lupus vasculopathy[96, 102] is associated with proliferative lupus nephritis and affects primarily arterioles. It is a noninflammatory lesion that shows eosinophilic granular material in the media and intima of arteries, narrowing the lumen. By immunofluorescence microscopy, immunoglobulins, complement, and fibrin are observed, and electron microscopy reveals electron-dense deposits in the subendothelial region and between the myointimal cells. The presence of these deposits is usually associated with proliferative lupus nephritis with a high activity index (see NIH scoring, which is discussed earlier), and it is associated with hypertension and with poor outcome. Thrombotic vasculopathy is seen in a small number of patients who clinically develop a hemolytic-uremic syndrome or thrombotic thrombocytopenic purpura–like syndrome. The lesions affect glomerular capillaries, arterioles, and small arteries, and are similar to the lesions of hemolytic-uremic syndrome or thrombotic thrombocytopenia purpura. Vascular lesions associated with antiphospholipid antibodies usually affect the arterioles and small arteries, and show organizing and often recanalized thrombi occluding the lumen.[103] These changes are not associated with an inflammatory response. Vascular lesions with necrotizing inflammation of vessel walls similar to those seen in polyarteritis nodosa (PAN) are rare and, when present, they may represent an overlap lesion.[96] Lupus-like syndromes are encountered from time to time; they include drug-induced lupus and lupus anticoagulant syndrome, and these conditions can occur in HIV infection.

DIFFERENTIAL DIAGNOSIS. With the variety of morphologic lesions seen in lupus nephritis, there is a wide differential diagnosis with non–lupus glomerulopathies. For example, mesangial lupus nephritis requires differentiation from IgA nephropathy, IgM

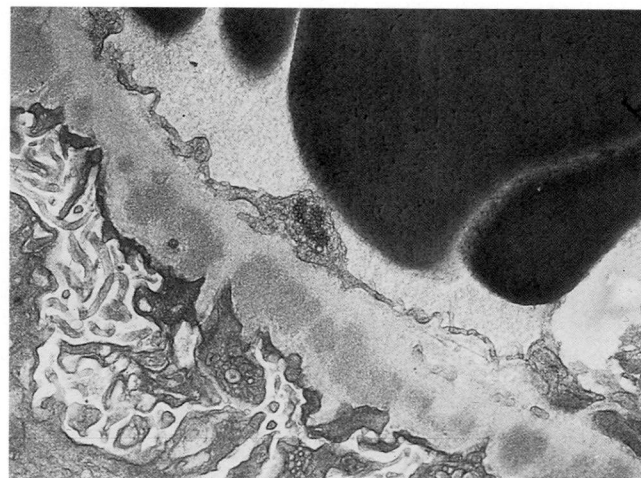

**FIGURE 29–42.** Lupus nephritis, membranous: Electron micrograph shows intramembranous deposits, basement membrane spikes, and a tubuloreticular structure in the endothelial cell.

nephropathy, and subsiding postinfectious glomerulonephritis. Membranous lupus nephritis requires distinction from other forms of secondary membranous glomerulopathies.[95] Finally, proliferative lupus nephritis needs to be distinguished from other proliferative glomerulonephritides, such as HSP, mesangiocapillary glomerulonephritis, cryoglobulinemic glomerulonephritis, and crescentic glomerulonephritis. Thus, correlation with clinical and laboratory findings and certain subtle histologic changes become very important in establishing the diagnosis of lupus nephritis.

## Henoch-Schönlein Purpura

TERMINOLOGY. HSP is a systemic disease caused by immune-complex deposits of IgA. Most patients have circulating IgA; some have IgA-cytoplasmic-antineutrophil cytoplasmic antibodies.[104]

CLINICAL CONSIDERATIONS. The disease commonly affects children,[105–107] and it is rare in adults.[108, 109] The clinical symptoms include skin rash (leukocytoclastic vasculitis), joint pains, abdominal pain and melena (produced by gastrointestinal vasculitis), and renal symptoms. Renal involvement occurs in 70% of patients. The kidney findings range from mild hematuria or proteinuria with normal renal function to nephrotic syndrome and severe renal insufficiency. The disease undergoes remission in some patients, but often it progresses to end-stage renal disease within 5 to 10 years, and it can recur in transplanted patients.

DIAGNOSTIC CONSIDERATIONS. By light microscopy, there is diffuse mesangial accentuation produced by an increase in mesangial cells. In addition, focal or diffuse proliferative glomerulonephritis, fibrinoid necrosis, epithelial crescents, and focal sclerosis with segmental fibrous crescents can be present. The blood vessels appear normal.

By electron microscopy, mesangial, sometimes subendothelial, and rarely subepithelial electron-dense deposits are seen. Immunofluorescence microscopy is necessary for diagnosis; it reveals mesangial deposits of IgA. Deposits of IgG, IgM, C3, properdin, and fibrin of lesser intensity and amount can also be present. Skin biopsies contain granular deposits of IgA and C3 within dermal vascular walls. The renal disease is often difficult to differentiate from a progressive IgA nephropathy (Berger's disease),[106] and it can only be separated by the clinical symptoms.

## Glomerulonephritis Associated with Bacterial Endocarditis

Glomerular involvement in bacterial endocarditis can occur as an acute or subacute form.[110–113] In both forms, the pathogenesis revolves around deposition of immune complexes in the glomeruli. Cardiac valvular lesions secondary to infection are the usual cause of the disease. The valvular lesions develop in patients who have undergone vascular or cardiac surgery; however, a high incidence is also encountered in drug abusers.[111] *Streptococcus viridans* is most commonly implicated, but endocarditis can also be associated with *Staphylococcus*. In acute bacterial endocarditis, the systemic symptoms often overshadow the renal symptoms, which can show minimal proteinuria and few casts, but rarely there is renal failure. In contrast, in subacute bacterial endocarditis, hematuria, red blood cell casts, proteinuria, and renal insufficiency are common, and some patients also develop nephrotic syndrome. In addition, extrarenal signs are also present.

In both types of bacterial endocarditis, clinical correlation, positive blood cultures, and renal involvement are necessary for diagnosis. If treated in time, the prognosis in both types is excellent.

DIAGNOSTIC CONSIDERATIONS. In acute bacterial endocarditis, the glomerular involvement is diffuse and often resembles postinfectious glomerulonephritis; however, neutrophil infiltration is much less intense than in postinfectious glomerulonephritis.

Electron microscopy reveals scant subepithelial and mesangial deposits and by immunofluorescence microscopy, IgG, IgM, and C3 may be seen as scattered granules along capillary walls and in the mesangium.

In subacute bacterial endocarditis,[112–114] a variable number of glomeruli commonly show focal acute or healing lesions involving a few capillaries or lobules. Occasionally, there can be diffuse glomerular involvement similar to that seen in acute bacterial endocarditis. In the acute lesions, small foci of fibrinoid necrosis or intracapillary fibrin thrombi associated with endocapillary cell proliferation and mononuclear cell and neutrophil infiltration are seen. These lesions are usually adherent to Bowman's capsule, with or without crescents. The healing lesions show focal and segmental solidification of the glomerular tuft, usually associated with fibrous crescents. The vessels and tubules show no specific changes. The interstitium has patchy infiltrates composed of mononuclear cells and plasma cells.

By electron microscopy, mesangial and focal subendothelial deposits are seen, but they are scant. By immunofluorescence microscopy, granular deposits of IgG and C3, at times associated with other immunoglobulins, C1q, and fibrinogen, have been reported within the mesangia and along capillary walls. Occasionally no immunoreactants are present.

## Diabetic Nephropathy

TERMINOLOGY. Diabetes mellitus is a systemic disease that affects many organs. The basic lesion is a microangiopathy resulting from an increase in vascular basement membrane material.

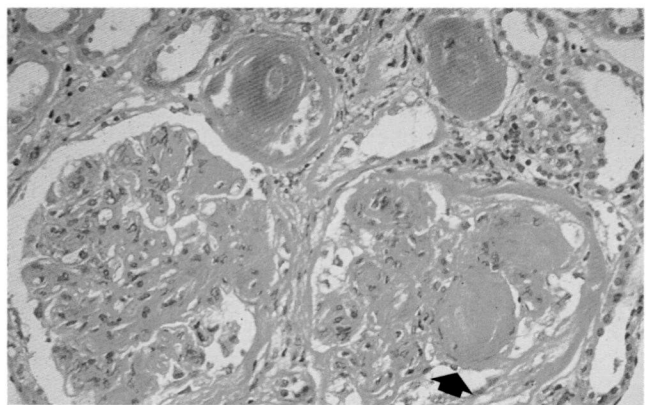

**FIGURE 29–43.** Diabetic glomerulosclerosis: Glomeruli show mesangial expansion. In one glomerulus, there is an acellular nodule (Kimmelstiel-Wilson nodule) (*arrow*). The capillary walls are thick, and the arterioles show hyaline sclerosis.

CLINICAL CONSIDERATIONS. Diabetes mellitus clinically can be subdivided into insulin-dependent diabetes mellitus, non–insulin-dependent diabetes mellitus, chemical diabetes (e.g., associated with corticosteroids, FK506, cyclosporine), and gestational diabetes mellitus, which is transient. Thirty to forty percent of insulin-dependent and 10% to 15% of non–insulin-dependent diabetics develop nephropathy, and about 30% of all diabetics develop chronic renal failure. Proteinuria is the most consistent and common abnormality. Microalbuminuria at the level of 20 to 200 $\mu$g/min (30 to 300 mg/day)[115] is a sign of early renal involvement and has a sensitivity of 95%, but it cannot be detected by routine urinalysis such as dipstick examination. Most patients who develop diabetic nephropathy have had diabetes for at least 8 to 10 years, and they usually present with nephrotic range proteinuria.

PATHOLOGIC CONSIDERATIONS. Two types of glomerular lesions are seen in diabetic nephropathy: nodular glomerulosclerosis, first described by Kimmelstiel and Wilson in l936,[116] and diffuse glomerular sclerosis, described by Spuhler and Zollinger.[117] By light microscopy, diffuse diabetic glomerulosclerosis shows mild to moderate diffuse mesangial widening due to an increase in mesangial matrix. This finding may be associated with a mild increase in mesangial cells, with or without thickening of peripheral glomerular capillary walls.

In nodular diabetic glomerulosclerosis, there are both changes of diffuse diabetic glomerulosclerosis and marked, focal expansion of the mesangial matrix, forming nodules (Kimmelstiel-Wilson nodules) of varying sizes that displace mesangial cells toward their periphery (Fig. 29–43). A well-developed diabetic nodule is acellular, stains positively with PAS stain, blue (or green) with trichrome stains, and often has a laminated appearance with silver stain (PAMS).

Additional frequent but nonspecific lesions include fibrin or hyaline caps and capsular drops.

These insudative lesions are made up of a variety of serum proteins and lipid. The fibrin cap lesion occludes peripheral capillary lumina, whereas capsular drop lesions project from Bowman's capsule into the urinary space. In contrast to the mesangial nodules, they stain bright red with trichrome stains. The changes of diabetic glomerulosclerosis are always associated with hyaline arteriolar sclerosis, often involving both afferent and efferent arterioles. Simultaneous afferent and efferent hyaline arteriolosclerosis is the only histologic feature pathognomonic for diabetic glomerulosclerosis. There is initially patchy, and later extensive, tubular atrophy with marked thickening of the tubular basement membranes, which stain similar to the glomerular nodules. The thickening of glomerular and tubular basement membranes is associated with moderate to marked interstitial fibrosis and varying degrees of interstitial inflammatory cell infiltration. The glomerular changes, along with tubulointerstitial changes, are collectively called diabetic nephropathy.

By electron microscopy, early diabetic nephropathy shows mild to moderate diffuse thickening of glomerular basement membranes and an increase in mesangial matrix. In advanced disease, the basement membrane, and in particular its lamina densa, may be approximately 10 times thicker than normal (Fig. 29–44). The diabetic (or Kimmelstiel-Wilson) nodule is composed of an acellular nodule of mesangial matrix. The mesangial cellular elements are typically displaced to the periphery of the nodule. Other cellular elements are usually unremarkable, and in particular, epithelial cell foot processes are often slender despite nephrotic range proteinuria. Sometimes, diffuse or focal thickening of basement membranes similar to that seen in diabetic glomerulosclerosis is noted without evidence of clinical diabetes. Although aging and hypertension do cause thickening of glomerular basement membranes, diffuse thickening of this type without clinical evidence of diabetes

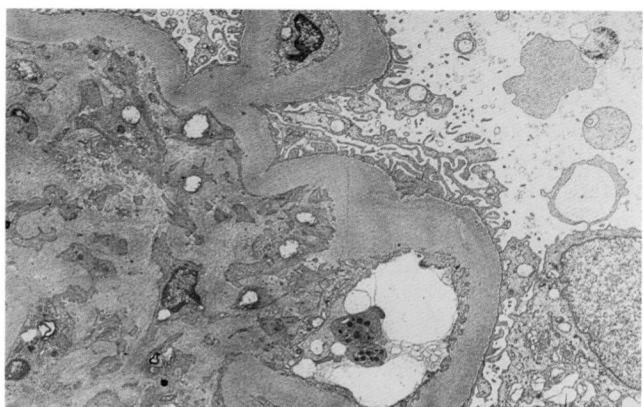

**FIGURE 29–44.** Diabetic glomerulosclerosis: Electron micrograph shows that the glomerular capillary basement membrane is markedly thickened. The mesangium is widened by an increase in matrix that compresses the mesangial cells. The epithelial cell foot processes are slender.

may still be the earliest histologic evidence of renal involvement by the disease.

By immunofluorescence microscopy, bandlike linear deposits of IgG and albumin are often present along glomerular capillary walls. They are sometimes accompanied by other immunoglobulins, and they are therefore believed to represent nonspecific trapping or leakage, rather than immune binding. Deposits of IgM, corresponding to fibrin caps, are often, but not always, seen in the mesangium and in capillary lumina.

PATHOGENESIS. The pathophysiology of the initiation and progression of diabetic nephropathy has not been completely established, but the pathogenetic mechanisms appear to be multifactorial. They include (1) renal hemodynamic abnormalities with elevated glomerular filtration rate (GFR) and capillary hydraulic pressure that precede structural changes, and (2) persistent hyperglycemia that itself can cause an increase in GFR, induce biochemical abnormalities in the polyol pathway,[118] and participate in formation of nonenzymatic glycosylation. The products of glycosylation bind to a wide variety of proteins, which results in a reduction in their turnover and interference with their function. These proteins are lipoproteins affecting cholesterol metabolism and extracellular matrix proteins, including collagen, mesangium, vascular walls, and glomerular and tubular basement membranes. The result is increased synthesis and accumulation of basement membranes, with disruption of architecture and microvascular complications.[119]

## Renal Diseases Associated with Plasma Cell Dyscrasias

TERMINOLOGY. Plasma cell dyscrasias are defined as an excessive proliferation of a single clone of cells producing either entire immunoglobulins (Ig), immunoglobulin fragments, heavy chains, or light chains. The list of these dyscrasias includes multiple myeloma (MM) with a monoclonal spike of IgG, IgA, or light chains; Waldenström's macroglobulinemia with an excess of IgM; heavy-chain diseases; and benign monoclonal gammopathies. Cryoglobulinemias types I and II are often included in plasma cell dyscrasias because they contain monoclonal immunoglobulin components. Amyloid is also included in this section, because it is often produced by overproduction of one of the light chains. Fibrillary glomerulopathy, although not a plasma cell dyscrasia, is included owing to its similarities with amyloid. Only the most commonly encountered lesions are discussed.

CLINICAL CONSIDERATIONS. The clinical presentations vary according to the lesion. Most frequently there is proteinuria; it is often very heavy, and frequently in the nephrotic range. Hematuria is less common. Renal insufficiency or failure may be the only presenting symptom in some patients, or it

may be associated with proteinuria in others. Monoclonal immunoglobulin is usually detectable in the serum and urine of most of these patients, but it may be absent in 10% to 15% of cases, particularly in patients with pure light-chain disease. The renal biopsy often provides the first clue to the diagnosis of plasma cell dyscrasia.

## The Kidney in Multiple Myeloma

CLINICAL CONSIDERATIONS. Among the plasma cell dyscrasias, MM is the most frequent cause of renal disease. The incidence is 3:100,000 persons among the 50- to 70-year-old age group. There is a slight male predominance. Although patients with MM have fatigue, bone pain, and infections, many of them present with only renal findings, such as proteinuria, with or without renal failure, and less commonly hematuria.

PATHOLOGIC CONSIDERATIONS. The renal involvement includes manifestations presumably related to the pathologic immunoglobulin itself, or to the toxic effect of the light chain synthesized in excess. In addition, secondary metabolic disturbances play an increasingly important role. Finally, renal manifestations may be related to adverse effects of either diagnostic procedures or treatment. It is obvious that the concomitance of multiple factors is responsible for the so-called myeloma kidney. These manifestations are shown in Table 29-5.

## Multiple Myeloma

GLOMERULI. Glomerulosclerosis was reported in several cases of MM as early as the 1970s; however, glomerular lesions remained unexplained until

**TABLE 29-5.** Renal Abnormalities Occurring in Patients with Multiple Myeloma

*Renal Abnormalities Directly Related to Multiple Myeloma*
Light-chain proteinuria (light-chain nephropathy)
Renal acidosis
Fanconi's syndrome with tubular degeneration
Salt-losing nephropathy
Renal insufficiency
Tubular cast formation (myeloma cast nephropathy)
Interstitial plasmacytic infiltration
Amyloidosis
Glomerulosclerosis

*Renal Abnormalities Due to Metabolic Disturbances*
Hypercalcemia
Hyperuricemia

*Acute Renal Failure Following Intravenous Pyelography*
Dehydration
Toxic effect of contrast media

*Infectious Complications*
Pyelonephritis
Infectious interstitial nephritis

renal tissue was studied by immunofluorescence microscopy. This technique showed deposition of light chains in the kidneys of these patients, so-called light-chain disease.[120, 121] Electron microscopy further defined the nature of these deposits.[122]

By light microscopy, the lesion resembles the Kimmelstiel-Wilson nodule of diabetic glomerulosclerosis (Fig. 29–45). It is characterized by the presence of dense mesangial nodules of varying sizes. The deposits are PAS positive. With Masson trichrome stain, the nodules sometimes stain magenta red or exhibit a metachromatic staining pattern; they are not strongly argyrophilic in silver stains. The peripheral capillary walls are usually not thickened. Hyaline arteriolosclerotic changes are either absent or uncommon, which helps distinguish myelomatous glomerular nodules from diabetic nodular glomerulosclerosis.

The diagnosis of light-chain disease can be made only by immunohistochemical methods using antisera specific for light chains. $\kappa$ Light chains are found in most cases, but $\lambda$-chains are seen in some. The pattern of deposits by immunofluorescence microscopy presents certain common characteristics. The outer part of the basal lamina of most distal and a few proximal tubules are sharply stained by the antisera with a linear pattern (Fig. 29–46). The tubular basement membrane deposits are characteristic enough to be considered a diagnostic morphologic feature. When found in the glomeruli, these immunoglobulin components tend to accumulate in nodules, but the glomerular basement membranes may also exhibit a linear pattern. Often, the glomerular deposits are less impressive than the tubular basement membrane deposits; however, this depends on the degree of involvement of various parts of the nephron. Granular deposits of C3 have been noted in the mesangium.

By electron microscopy, finely granular electron-dense deposits are located in the widened mesangium, including within the mesangial nodules, in the subendothelial aspects of the glomerular basement membranes with an irregular distribution, and

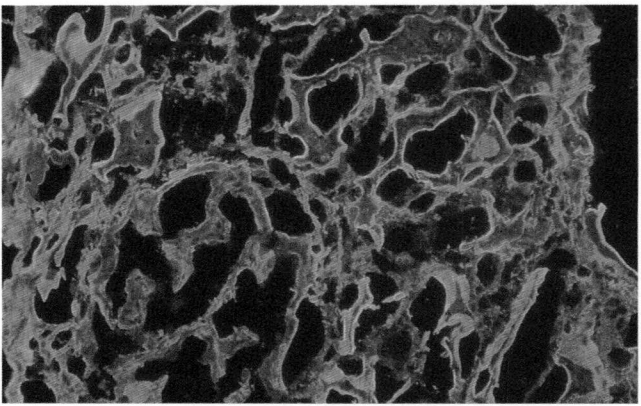

**FIGURE 29–46.** Light-chain nephropathy: Immunofluorescence microscopy reveals pseudolinear and finely granular deposits with antibodies to $\kappa$ light chain.

in the tubular basement membranes (Fig. 29–47). These electron microscopic deposits are diagnostic of the disease.[122]

TUBULES. The most conspicuous tubular lesion is the presence of tubular casts, known as cast nephropathy. Immunoglobulin light chains, or Bence Jones proteins, are filtered through the glomerulus and reabsorbed by the proximal tubules.[122, 123] The overproduction causes accumulation of these proteins in the tubules, with resultant cast nephropathy. The casts are characteristic, and they are commonly located in the distal convoluted and collecting tubules, which are dilated. The casts are strongly eosinophilic or polychromatic, and they are PAS positive. They are of varying size, appear solid, and often have a multilamellar, fragmented or fractured appearance. The casts are surrounded by mononuclear and multinucleated giant cells, most of which are of monocytic origin and some of which may be tubular cells, a cellular response which is regarded as the most characteristic lesion of myeloma kidney (Fig. 29–48).[124–126] Similar casts can be seen rarely in other conditions but never in significant numbers.

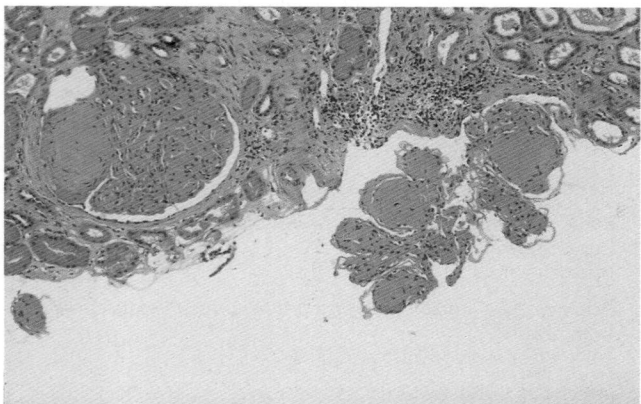

**FIGURE 29–45.** Light-chain nephropathy: Glomeruli show acellular nodules identical to diabetic nodules.

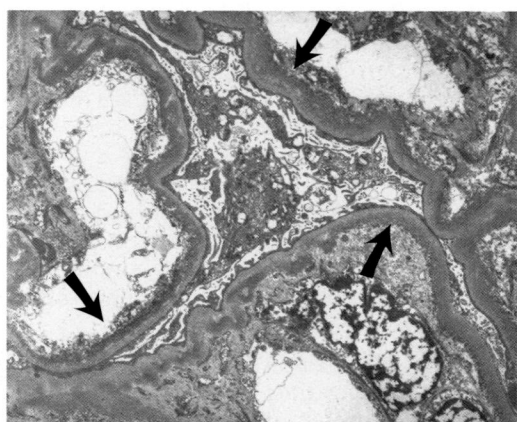

**FIGURE 29–47.** Light-chain nephropathy: Electron micrograph reveals fine granular electron-dense deposits (*arrow*) within and along the endothelial side of the basement membrane.

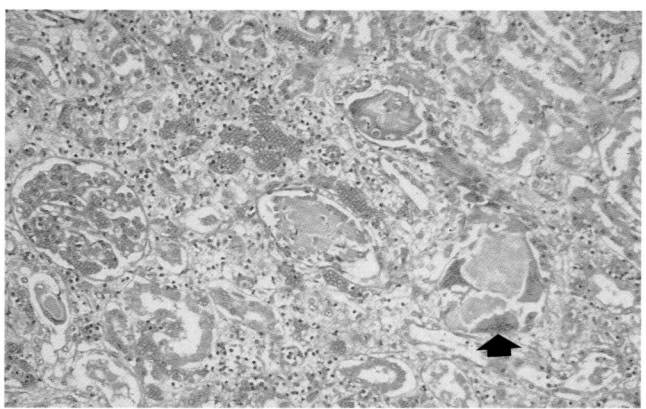

**FIGURE 29–48.** Myeloma casts: Intratubular protein casts with giant cell reaction (*arrow*) around some of the casts.

Cytoplasmic and nuclear debris, calcium deposits, and in a number of cases, amyloid are also detectable, especially at the periphery of the casts. These changes are often associated with interstitial lymphocytic infiltration. In some instances, long crystals, probably related to precipitation of the abnormal light chain, are present within the casts or within the tubular epithelial cells. Plasma cells are often present in close contact with these crystals.[127, 128] Usually, the glomeruli do not show any changes in cast nephopathy unless involved by amyloid or by light-chain disease. Of interest, concomitant presence of light-chain disease or amyloidosis with cast nephropathy is rare.

By immunofluorescence microscopy, the casts stain commonly with antibodies to $\kappa$ or sometimes $\lambda$ light chain.[121] A clear relationship between the pathologic circulating protein and the composition of the casts is often not present. Apart from the myeloma casts, extensive tubular atrophy and dedifferentiation of tubular cells is frequently seen. In patients with acute renal failure, changes of ATN are present.

INTERSTITIUM. Neoplastic plasma cell infiltration of the interstitium is rare. Most often, there are mixed inflammatory cells and foci of interstitial fibrosis that parallel the degree of tubular damage. Neutrophilic infiltration is frequent. In cases of MM associated with amyloidosis, deposits of amyloid can be seen.

VESSELS. Arterial and arteriolar changes vary from hypertensive sclerosis with hyaline deposition to light-chain or amyloid fibril deposition in vessel walls.

## Renal Amyloidosis

TERMINOLOGY AND PATHOGENESIS. Amyloidosis refers to the accumulation of peculiar extracellular deposits that exhibit a fibrillar structure by ultrastructural examination and a $\beta$-pleated sheet structure by x-ray diffraction studies. It was described as a $\beta$-fibrillosis by Glenner.[129] The amyloid deposits are derived from various precursors; they can have different chemical structures, but they all have in common the same tertiary structure with the $\beta$-pleated configuration that produces the tinctorial and optical properties of staining with cotton dyes, such as Congo red, and apple green birefringence under polarization.[130]

A number of types of amyloid can involve the kidney (Table 29–6). However, two major species of amyloid, AA and AL, are recognized.[131] AL amyloid fibrils are derived from light chains, usually $\lambda$ light chains. Patients with AL amyloidosis have either overt or silent myeloma, suggesting underlying plasma cell dyscrasias, or they may present as primary disease. Amyloidosis is common in patients with IgD-type myeloma; it is also encountered in 10% of patients with MM.

The precursor for AA amyloid is a plasma protein known as serum amyloid A protein. It is a high-density lipoprotein that is synthesized by liver, and levels are increased in chronic inflammatory and infectious diseases, some tumors,[132] and patients with familial Mediterranean fever.[133]

CLINICAL CONSIDERATIONS. Regardless of type of amyloid, patients commonly present with proteinuria in the nephrotic range. Often, proteinuria is massive and it is unaccompanied by hematuria or hypertension. Abnormal renal function is present in advanced stages of the disease. The age range of patients is variable; however, AA amyloid often affects younger patients, because it is associated with a variety of underlying diseases. In contrast, patients with AL amyloid are usually older because of the association with plasma cell dyscrasias, which typically occur in older individuals.

PATHOLOGIC CONSIDERATIONS. Renal amyloid deposits commonly occur in glomeruli, with varying degrees of involvement of blood vessels, interstitium, and tubular basement membranes. Renal involvement is similar regardless of the type of amyloid. By light microscopy, in early stages there is only minimal widening of the mesangium by amyloid that can be easily missed. Later, the mesangial amyloid appears as irregular masses or nodules of varying size that extend into the adjacent capillary

**TABLE 29–6.** Classification of Renal Amyloidosis

| Disease | Amyloid Type |
| --- | --- |
| Primary amyloidosis | AL |
| Amyloidosis associated with multiple myeloma | AL |
| Secondary amyloidosis with coexisting disease | AA |
| Familial amyloidosis (in familial Mediterranean fever) | AA |
| Dialysis-associated amyloidosis (does not involve kidney)[370, 371] | $\beta_2$-microglobulin |

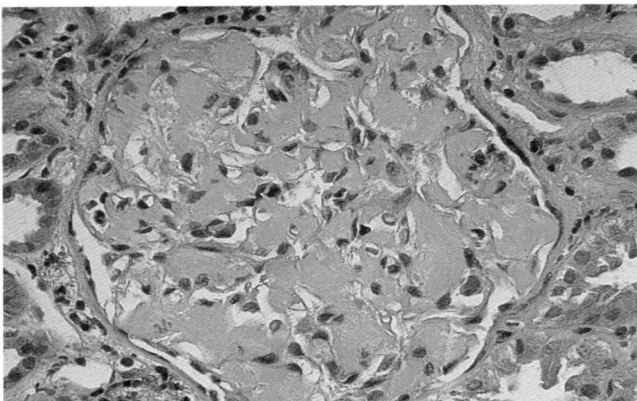

**FIGURE 29–49.** Renal amyloidosis: Glomerulus reveals pale eosinophilic nodular expansion of the mesangium and thickening of some capillary walls.

walls (Fig. 29–49). Therefore, they can be confused with Kimmelstiel-Wilson nodules of diabetic glomerulosclerosis. The deposits have a pale eosinophilic appearance, and they often have a ground-glass–like appearance (Fig. 29–49). With PAS stain, they appear pale pink and they show pale blue staining with Masson trichrome stain. With PAMS stain, spikes larger than the spikes seen in membranous glomerulonephritis are seen along the mesangium and capillary walls.[134, 135]

The Congo red stain is the gold standard for the diagnosis of amyloid.[136] It stains amyloid deposits orange; under polarized light, these stained deposits exhibit a brilliant apple green birefringence (Fig. 29–50). This staining should not be confused with the yellow, pale green birefringence of collagen. Other less specific stains that may be used to demonstrate amyloid are thioflavine B/T and crystal violet. With thioflavine, amyloid stains bright green in fluorescence microscopy. Crystal violet stains amyloid pink (metachromasia). A histochemical method using pretreatment of paraffin sections with potassium permanganate can also be used to distinguish between AA and AL amyloid. Permanganate-pretreated sec-

tions of AL amyloid retain their Congo red affinity, whereas sections of AA amyloid lose their Congo red staining.[137] However, more specific immunohistochemical methods for AA amyloid and for AL amyloid have replaced this method for identifying the two subgroups.[138]

Involvement of tubules, interstitium, and blood vessels is variable. It occurs in about 50% of cases, and it parallels the severity of renal involvement. Concomitant involvement of large blood vessels may indicate primary amyloidosis.

By electron microscopy, amyloid, regardless of its origin, is made up of characteristic fibrils that measure 8 to 12 nm in diameter (Fig. 29–51). These extracellular fibrils are of varying lengths, appear rigid, and are arranged in a haphazard or crisscross pattern. The fibrils are commonly seen in the mesangium. The capillary basement membranes, when involved, are widened by fibrils that occupy the entire thickness of the basement membrane. The fibrils often form spicules that project perpendicular to the glomerular basement membrane, corresponding to the spicules seen with PAMS stain (Fig. 29–51).

By immunofluorescence microscopy, antibodies to $\kappa$ or $\lambda$ light chains often stain glomeruli, tubules, interstitium, and vessels.[139] The glomerular deposits are often smudgy. In contrast to the specific staining of light chains in AL amyloidosis, other components such as immunoglobulin heavy chains and complement may show staining in AA amyloidosis. Although the findings are confusing at times, this more diverse staining may help in differentiating AA amyloid from the AL type.

## Fibrillary Glomerulopathy and Immunotactoid Glomerulopathy

TERMINOLOGY. These terms were first used to describe renal disease characterized by Congo red–negative, extracellular immunoglobulin–containing fibrillary deposits.[140] The deposits may have either a

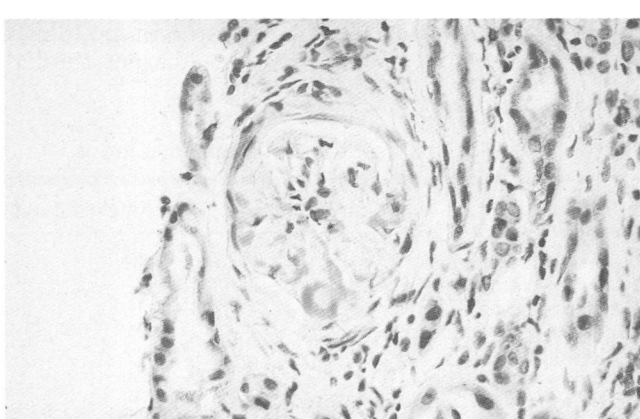
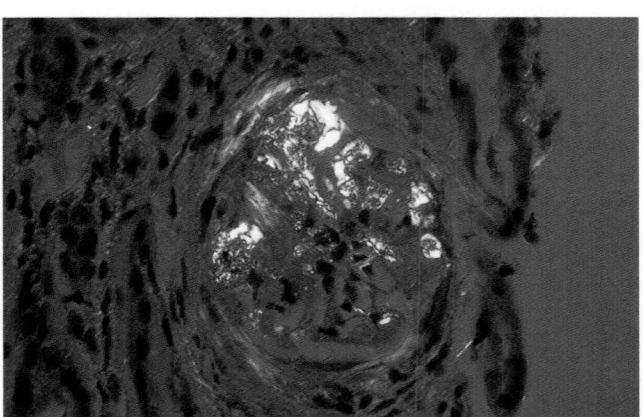

**FIGURE 29–50.** Renal amyloidosis: Congo red stain without polarization (*left*). On polarization (*right*), the Congo red stain shows apple green birefringence. (Congo red stain.)

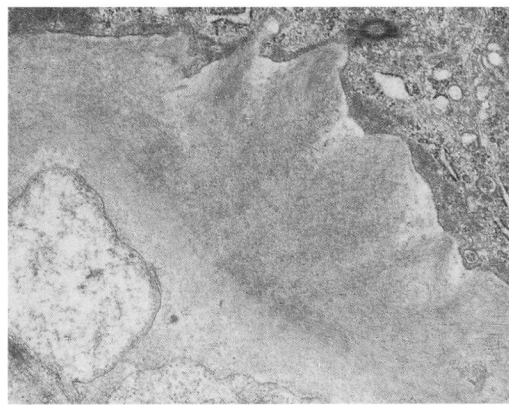

**FIGURE 29–51.** Renal amyloidosis: Electron micrograph reveals fine fibrils of amyloid in the glomerular basement membrane, destroying the lamina densa and forming spikes between the epithelial cells.

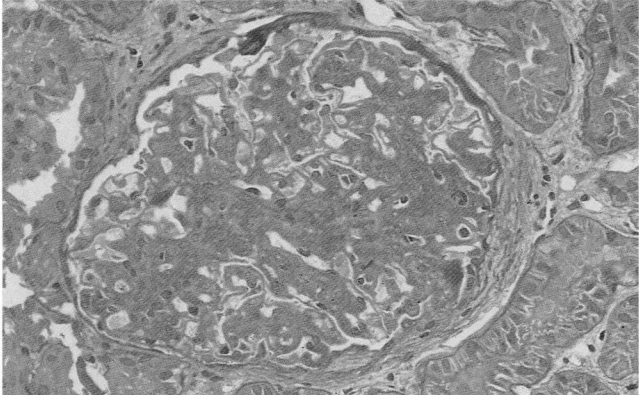

**FIGURE 29–52.** Immunotactoid/fibrillary glomerulopathy: Glomerulus shows variable widening of the mesangium and thickening of some capillary walls. (PAS stain.)

microtubular substructure (termed immunotactoid glomerulopathy) or randomly organized fibrils (termed fibrillary glomerulopathy).[141, 142] Characteristically, these fibrils are larger in diameter than amyloid fibrils (8 to 10 nm),[141–147] measuring 16 to 24 nm in fibrillary glomerulopathy and 30 nm or larger in immunotactoid glomerulopathy.[148]

CLINICAL CONSIDERATIONS. The disease occurs in adults, most commonly in the fifth decade of life, but the age range of patients can be wide. They usually present with proteinuria in the nephrotic range, hematuria, and hypertension, with renal insufficiency in some. Fibrillary glomerulopathy and immunotactoid glomerulopathy often progress to renal failure. Currently, serologic diagnostic tests for the disease are not available, nor do patients usually respond to therapy. The disease can recur in patients transplanted. It has been proposed that the disease should be separated into two lesions (fibrillary glomerulopathy or immunotactoid glomerulopathy) based on fibril diameter, as noted earlier.[148] The distinction may be clinically important to study the natural history, outcome, response to therapy, and pathogenesis of these lesions; however, this proposal requires further confirmation with additional studies. For example, one caveat is that there may be changes in the size of deposited fibrils with the method of tissue processing.[149]

DIAGNOSTIC CONSIDERATIONS. By light microscopy, the glomeruli commonly show widening of mesangial regions and irregular thickening of capillary walls with a membranous pattern (Fig. 29–52); however, mesangiocapillary-like and nodular patterns have been described as well. Lack of staining with PAMS stain of some capillary walls should raise the suspicion of replacement or destruction of the glomerular basement membrane by deposits of extracellular material.

By electron microscopy, fibrils are present in capillary walls and mesangium (Fig. 29–53). There is a predilection for fibril deposition in the glomeru-

lus and occasionally within vascular walls; only rarely are fibrils seen in tubular basement membranes. Taking into consideration the size of the fibrils by electron microscopy (see Terminology, earlier), the diseases are subdivided into two groups: immunotactoid glomerulonephritis and fibrillary glomerulonephritis. In cases of immunotactoid glomerulonephritis with a tubular distribution, underlying lesions such as cryoglobulinemia and macroglobulinemia should be excluded.

By immunofluorescence microscopy, deposits of IgG and C3 are present in a capillary and mesangial distribution in all cases. In some biopsies, deposits of IgM, IgA, or C1q may be present.

Exclusion of other systemic diseases, particularly cryoglobulinemia and amyloidosis, is essential to the diagnosis of immunotactoid and fibrillary glomerulonephritis. Of interest, patients with rheumatoid arthritis and mixed connective tissue and concomitant fibrillary and immunotactoid disease have been described.

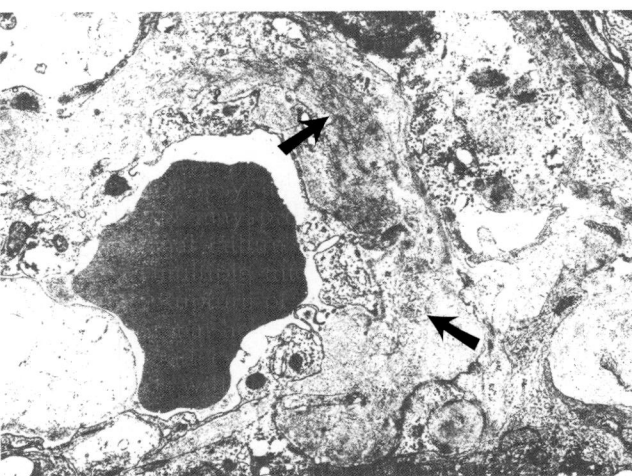

**FIGURE 29–53.** Immunotactoid/fibrillary glomerulopathy: Electron micrograph shows thickening of capillary basement membrane and widening of mesangium by fibrils larger than amyloid fibrils (*arrows*).

## Renal Changes in Sickle Cell Anemia

CLINICAL CONSIDERATIONS. Three major renal complications are known to be associated with, or related to, sickle cell disease: hematuria, hyposthenuria, and nephrotic syndrome.

Hematuria is the most common renal manifestation of the sickling disorders.[150] It occurs not only in homozygous SS individuals but also in AS and SC genotypes. It is seen in early adult life, it is more common in men, and it is often unilateral, arising from the left kidney. The hematuria is typically gross, painless, and occurs spontaneously. There may be renal colic. When unilateral severe hematuria occurs, nephrectomy may be required for relief of pain.

Hyposthenuria is manifested as a defect in ability to concentrate the urine. Patients with nephrotic syndrome show the typical features of this condition, with heavy proteinuria, edema, and hypercholesterolemia.

DIAGNOSTIC CONSIDERATIONS. Hematuria occurs owing to intense stasis, dilatation, and congestion of the vasa recta and capillaries. The resultant small foci of papillary necrosis contribute to the bleeding. In patients with hematuria, light microscopy shows patchy glomerular and arterial stasis of red blood cells and striking dilatation and congestion of peritubular capillaries and vasa recta. Peritubular edema, extravasation of red blood cells, focal tubular degeneration (particularly in the medulla), iron pigment within tubular epithelial and interstitial cells, foci of recent and old hemorrhage and scarring, and papillary necrosis can be seen.

In patients with hyposthenuria, light microscopy also shows peritubular capillary stasis, interstitial fibrosis, deposits of iron pigment in tubular epithelium and tubular atrophy. The defect in concentrating ability is probably related to changes in the papillae. The red blood cells containing the SA hemoglobin become sickled when they enter the hypertonic and hypoxic areas of the renal medulla, thereby increasing blood viscosity and restricting blood flow. Congestion and dilatation of the vasa recta and capillaries together produce papillary necrosis. The defect in concentration of the urine can be explained as a result of decreased medullary blood flow, which, in turn, limits the production of a high concentration of sodium in the interstitium, thereby interfering with the concentrating mechanism.

The morphologic lesions associated with nephrotic syndrome include minimal change disease, MPGN, focal segmental glomerulosclerosis, and renal vein thrombosis.[151–153] It is often difficult to determine whether these are merely chance associations; however, a form of MPGN has been described on several occasions[153, 154] and the association between it and sickle cell disease has been suggested as real. By light microscopy, the glomeruli show many features of MPGN, with an increase in mesangial cells and matrix and enhanced lobularity.

By electron microscopy, focal subendothelial mesangial extension, rare mesangial and subendothelial electron-dense deposits, and visceral epithelial cell foot process fusion are seen. The red blood cells may show paracrystalline structures. By immunofluorescence microscopy, IgG and C3 have been described along the capillary walls and tubular antigen has been demonstrated in the glomerular deposits.

## Renal Involvement in Hepatitis B and C

Both hepatitis B and C infection can produce kidney disease. The renal lesions associated with hepatitis B antigenemia are membranous glomerulopathy,[155] MPGN, and PAN. Of these, membranous glomerulopathy is by far the commonest. In fact, a high percentage of children with membranous glomerulopathy have hepatitis B antigenemia.

Clinical presentation varies with the type of renal lesion, but proteinuria is almost always present. Histologic changes by light and electron microscopy correspond to the underlying lesion. In membranous glomerulopathy, the morphologic and ultrastructural changes correspond to those of a "secondary" membranous glomerulopathy. By immunofluorescence microscopy, IgG and C3 and sometimes IgA and IgM, are present along glomerular capillary walls.

In the lesion resembling MPGN, the glomerular involvement is more uneven than in idiopathic mesangiocapillary glomerulonephritis. Electron microscopy shows type I and sometimes type III mesangiocapillary patterns. By immunofluorescence microscopy, IgG and C3 are present in equal strength and amount. Hepatitis B antigens have been demonstrated in the glomerular deposits (immune complexes).[156] In children, the prognosis is better, resolution of proteinuria is common, and progression to end-stage disease is uncommon; in contrast, the outcome in adults is less favorable.[157]

In hepatitis C, the renal lesion is that of mesangiocapillary glomerulonephritis,[158] and in some cases, it is associated with cryoglobulinemia. Patients commonly present with proteinuria sometimes in the nephrotic range, which may be associated with hematuria. The light, electron, and immunofluorescence microscopic findings are those of type I mesangiocapillary glomerulonephritis; however, hepatitis C antigen has not been demonstrated in the glomerular deposits.

## Renal Involvement in Human Immunodeficiency Virus Infection

In HIV infection, manifestations affect almost every organ in the body, susceptibility to even the most innocuous infectious agents is increased, and there is an increased tendency to certain malignancies. HIV infection is acquired mainly through the parenteral route or through mucosal sites and through breast-feeding (mother to child). Although intravenous drug abuse and homosexual contact were the most important factors in the 1980s, heterosexual transmission of the disease has gained importance in the 1990s. Autopsy and biopsy studies have shown significant renal complications occurring in patients with asymptomatic HIV infection as well as in those with fully developed AIDS. The renal involvement ranges from tubular functional abnormalities, such as fluid, electrolyte, and acid-base imbalances,[159, 160] to structural changes of ATN, to interstitial nephritis secondary to the toxicity of antiviral or antifungal drugs and aminoglycosides. In addition, lesions associated with opportunistic infections and malignancies are also encountered. Glomerular lesions associated with HIV infection include focal segmental glomerulosclerosis and its variant collapsing glomerulopathy, minimal change disease, IgA nephropathy, amyloidosis, and lesions associated with thrombotic angiopathy.[161] Based on autopsy series, the incidence of HIV-associated nephropathy varies from 3% to 8% of patients. Most cases of HIV-associated nephropathy develop early in the course of HIV infection (asymptomatic carriers), but the disease can occur at any stage. HIV-associated nephropathy is particularly prevalent among intravenous drug abusers, which is considered a major risk factor for nephropathy. In both HIV-associated nephropathy and heroin-associated nephropathy, the principal glomerular lesion is that of focal segmental glomerulosclerosis and it often becomes difficult to separate the two entities. However, absence of drug abuse in many HIV-associated nephropathy patients, presence of TRSs in HIV-associated nephropathy, rapid progression to end-stage renal disease in HIV-associated nephropathy, and demonstration of genome for HIV in renal cells[33] help in differentiating the two entities.

CLINICAL CONSIDERATIONS. The clinical presentation of HIV-associated nephropathy and other renal complications varies with the underlying lesion. It includes proteinuria to severe nephrotic syndrome, hematuria with or without varying degrees of renal insufficiency, acute renal failure, chronic renal failure, and, rarely, autoimmune (lupus-like) manifestations.[162] Ultrasonographic studies show highly echogenic large kidneys. Renal manifestations may be the primary presentation in a small proportion of cases.

The prognosis of renal disease is generally poor, particularly in African Americans and in those with an advanced stage of HIV infection, nephrotic-range proteinuria, and higher creatinine levels at the time of their initial presentation. These patients rapidly reach end-stage renal disease within 6 months to 3 years.

PATHOLOGIC CONSIDERATIONS. At autopsy, the kidneys generally appear normal or enlarged in size, with a smooth outer surface and an edematous cortex. In more advanced cases of HIV-associated nephropathy, a patchy or diffuse microcystic change is present on the cut surface, particularly in the cortex.

By light microscopy, the glomerular and tubulointerstitial features, although nonspecific, are sufficient to make a diagnosis of HIV-associated nephropathy. Focal segmental glomerulosclerosis is the most common lesion associated with HIV-associated nephropathy. It is noted in about 75% to 80% of adult patients with HIV-associated renal disease.[27, 163, 164] The glomerular change is characterized by a severe form of focal segmental and global glomerulosclerosis that often correlates with a rapid decline in renal function. The changes include focal or global capillary wall wrinkling, thickening, and collapse; varying degrees of segmental or global mesangial hypercellularity; glomerular sclerosis and hyalinosis, surrounded by large visceral epithelial cells containing abundant hyaline droplets; and dilated Bowman's spaces often containing protein precipitates (see Fig. 29–16). In late stages, progressive segmental and global sclerosis with loss of cellularity ensues, accompanied by severe tubulointerstitial and vascular changes. Other milder glomerular lesions of mesangial hypercellularity or minimal change disease can be associated with considerable proteinuria.

Tubulointerstitial changes such as tubular cell degeneration, luminal dilatation leading to microcystic changes with protein casts, interstitial edema or fibrosis, and moderate to marked active or chronic interstitial inflammation consisting of predominantly CD8-bearing lymphocytes are recognized in HIV-associated nephropathy (see Fig. 29–16).

Immunofluorescence microscopy reveals deposits of IgM, C3, and sometimes C1q in the glomerular mesangium, corresponding to electron-dense mesangial deposits seen by electron microscopy. The presence of frequent TRSs in the glomerular endothelial cells and of TRSs and confronting cylindrical cisternae in interstitial lymphocytes[165] is thought to be the result of elevated cytokine interferon-$\alpha$ levels elaborated by activated T cells. In addition, nuclear bodies and granular transformation of nuclear chromatin, particularly of the nuclei of tubular and interstitial cells, may be seen. In those cases co-infected with hepatitis B or C virus, some biopsies may show immune-complex glomerulonephritis with or without cryoglobulinemia.[166] On occasion, lupus or lupus-like syndromes expressed in HIV patients may induce glomerulonephritis similar to lupus nephritis.[167]

HIV-infected children also develop the glomerular and tubulointerstitial lesions of HIV-associated nephropathy, although the disease tends to be milder. IgA nephropathy and other forms of immune-complex glomerulopathies have also been identified in children.

PATHOGENESIS. The pathogenesis of HIV-associated nephropathy is not completely known.[33, 34, 168–172] Several explanations have been offered following controlled studies and experimental models. They include

1. A direct injury caused by HIV infecting the glomerular and tubular epithelial cells.[171]
2. The presence of factors or triggering mechanisms in African-American individuals that predispose them to develop glomerulosclerosis.
3. Dose of the virus.
4. Immunologic (cell-mediated) factors.
5. Other virus-host interactions necessary for the development of renal disease.
6. That there may be a role for immune complexes isolated from the circulation and renal tissue that contain p24 or gpl20 HIV in the pathogenesis of glomerular disease in HIV-infected patients, and even more so in those with IgA nephropathy.
7. That HIV-1 gp/60 protein can modulate mesangial cell proliferation, possibly through cytokine tumor necrosis factor (TNF)-$\alpha$ and that the latter at higher concentrations can even lead to mesangial cell apoptosis.[172]
8. That indirectly, viral gene products, cytokines, and growth factors elaborated by monocytes and lymphocytes can induce altered glomerular basement membrane permeability and glomerular and tubular epithelial cell injury, initiating glomerulosclerosis.[34] However, some investigators have found that certain host cells, namely glomerular epithelial and mesangial cells, are relatively resistant when exposed to HIV.[173] Still, investigation of a murine model of HIV-associated nephropathy has shown that HIV transgene expression in renal epithelium causes altered podocyte proliferation.

## Tuberculosis of the Kidney

With increasing numbers of cases of HIV infection, the incidence of tuberculosis has also increased. The main renal symptoms are frequent micturition, painless hematuria, loin pain, weight loss, and fever associated with the presence of tuberculous bacilli in the urine.

The renal lesions occur in two forms: miliary and ulcerative.[174] In the miliary type, the renal involvement is overshadowed by a serious generalized infection. The kidney shows numerous white, hard, pinhead-sized nodules scattered throughout the parenchyma but present predominantly in the cortex.

The caseous or ulcerative type of tuberculous infection in the kidneys is an important form of renal infection, because it may cause severe destruction of the parenchyma and necessitate removal of the kidney. In autopsy series, there is a high incidence of bilateral involvement. The pathologic changes vary greatly in extent, but the process is essentially one of destruction of the renal parenchyma by the tuberculous process. The lesions usually begin in the medulla, causing ulceration and deformity of the peripelvic system. Histologically,

there are typical necrotizing and non-necrotizing tuberculous granulomas in which acid-fast bacilli can be demonstrated.

## RENAL VASCULAR DISEASES

### Renal Vasculitis—Introduction

Vasculitis affecting the kidney is not rare; in fact, vasculitis is a common cause of crescentic glomerulonephritis in some centers. For example, in one series, 8% of all glomerular disease diagnosed by renal biopsy was ANCA-associated crescentic glomerulonephritis.[175] In Great Britain, the overall incidence of systemic vasculitides is about 40 per 1 million adults.[176]

There are two recent classifications of the vasculitides: the Chapel Hill Consensus Conference on the Nomenclature of Systemic Vasculitis (Tables 29–7 and 29–8)[92, 177] and that of the American College of Rheumatology (ACR) (Table 29–9).[178, 179] The ACR classification provides selected clinicopathologic criteria for the diagnosis (see Table 29–9), whereas the Chapel Hill criteria rely chiefly on pathologic (histologic) criteria (see Table 29–8). In the latter schema, large vessel vasculitis affects the aorta and the largest arterial branches directed toward major body regions; medium-sized vessel vasculitis affects the main visceral arteries and their branches; and small vessel vasculitis affects arterioles, venules, and capillaries, although arteries, especially small arteries, can also be affected (see Table 29–7). Classic PAN is an example of medium-sized vessel vasculitis. By contrast, Wegener's granulomatosis, microscopic polyangiitis, and Churg-Strauss syndrome are all variants of ANCA-associated small vessel vasculitides.

**TABLE 29–7.** Chapel Hill Consensus Conference Classification of Systemic Vasculitides[92, 177]

*Large Vessel Vasculitis*
Giant cell (temporal) arteritis
Takayasu's arteritis

*Medium-size Vessel Vasculitis*
Classic polyarteritis nodosa
Kawasaki disease

*Small Vessel Vasculitis*
ANCA-associated (see Table 29–8)
  Wegener's granulomatosis
  Microscopic polyangiitis
  Churg-Strauss syndrome (allergic granulomatosis)
  Drug-induced ANCA-associated vasculitis
Immune-complex small vessel vasculitis
  Henoch-Schönlein purpura
  Anti-GBM disease
  Lupus vasculitis
  Rheumatoid vasculitis
  Essential cryoglobulinemic vasculitis
Paraneoplastic small vessel vasculitis

**TABLE 29–8.** Definitions of Vasculitis Suggested by the Chapel Hill Consensus Conference on the Nomenclature of Systemic Vasculitis[92, 177]

**Wegener's Granulomatosis**
Granulomatous inflammation of respiratory tract, and necrotizing vasculitis affecting small to medium-sized vessels, for example, capillaries, venules, arterioles, and arteries. Necrotizing glomerulonephritis is common.

**Polyarteritis Nodosa (PAN)**
Necrotizing inflammation of medium-sized or small arteries without glomerulonephritis or vasculitis in arterioles, capillaries, or venules.

**Microscopic Polyangiitis**
Necrotizing vasculitis with few or no immune deposits affecting small vessels, that is, capillaries, venules, or arterioles. Necrotizing arteritis of small and medium-sized arteries may be present. Necrotizing glomerulonephritis is very common. Pulmonary capillaritis often occurs.

**Churg-Strauss Syndrome (CSS)**
Eosinophil-rich and granulomatous inflammation involving the respiratory tract and necrotizing vasculitis affecting small to medium-sized vessels and associated with asthma and blood eosinophilia.

**TABLE 29–9.** 1990 ACR Criteria for Diagnosis of Wegener's Granulomatosis, Churg-Strauss Syndrome, and Polyarteritis Nodosa[178, 179, 375, 376]

**Wegener's Granulomatosis** (requires at least two of the following)
Nasal or oral inflammation
Abnormal chest radiograph
Abnormal urinary sediment (microhematuria with more than 5 red blood cells/high power field or red cell casts)
Granulomatous inflammation on biopsy (histologic changes showing inflammation within the wall of an artery or in the perivascular or extravascular area (artery or arteriole)

**Churg-Strauss Syndrome** (requires at least 4 of the following)
Asthma
Blood eosinophilia greater than 10%
Mononeuropathy or polyneuropathy
Pulmonary infiltrates, nonfixed
Paranasal sinus abnormality
Extravascular eosinophils (biopsy including artery, arteriole, or venule showing accumulations of eosinophils in extravascular areas)

**Polyarteritis Nodosa** (requires at least 3 of the following)
Weight loss of more than 4 kg
Livedo reticularis
Testicular pain and tenderness
Myalgia, weakness, or leg tenderness
Mononeuropathy or polyneuropathy
Diastolic BP >90 mm Hg
Elevated BUN (>40 mg/dL) or creatinine (>1.5 mg/dL)
Hepatitis B virus
Arteriographic abnormality (aneurysms or occlusions of visceral arteries not due to arteriosclerosis or other noninflammatory causes)
Biopsy of small or medium-sized artery containing neutrophils in artery wall

A recent critical analysis of these two classification systems has found significant discordances between them.[180] In particular, the ACR system overestimates the frequency of Wegener's granulomatosis by including cases of microscopic polyangiitis, which was not defined by the ACR, whereas the Chapel Hill system's definitions, which are largely biopsy dependent, are sometimes not easily used in routine clinical practice, particularly because vasculitides may develop in a staged fashion.[180] Finally, morphologic and clinical overlap of diseases continues to cause difficulties in classification. For example, the Chapel Hill system emphasizes the involvement of small vessels in microscopic polyangiitis, whereas only larger muscular arteries are supposed to be affected in classic PAN, but a recent study showed that small-sized arteries can be affected by classic polyarteritis; that is, that vessel size alone is not sufficient to diagnose microscopic polyangiitis.[181] In fact, in one recent series, 9 of 24 patients with vasculitis remained unclassifiable in the Chapel Hill System. Use of additional clinical criteria, such as ANCA status, promises to facilitate classification (see later).[181]

## Pathogenetic Mechanisms of Vasculitis

Several principal pathogenetic mechanisms have been proposed for vasculitis. These include infection, immune-complex mediated, autoimmune antibody mediated, pauci-immune, and cell mediated. There are also diseases of unknown etiology. Immune-complex and cell-mediated diseases are covered in other portions of this chapter. For the pauci-immune vasculitides, which include Wegener's granulomatosis, microscopic polyangiitis, and Churg-Strauss syndrome, ANCAs have been suggested to play a key pathogenic role. All three diseases share the presence of these antibodies in the serum in most patients, and there is a correlation between disease activity and ANCA titers. Also, no evidence for an alternative pathogenic mechanism has been produced. It has been suggested that ANCA may interact with neutrophils that have been previously primed by cytokines and which may express small amounts of ANCA antigens on their cell surface as a result.[182] The interaction with ANCA causes the partially activated neutrophils to release their enzymatic contents prematurely when they initially adhere to the endothelium, rather than at the site of the inflammatory stimulus.[183]

## Wegener's Granulomatosis

NOMENCLATURE. In 1936 and 1939, Friedrich Wegener described a form of PAN characterized by peculiar destructive granulomatous lesions that occurred initially in the nasopharyngeal region and later progressed to involve lung and kidney.[184] Later, a detailed clinicopathologic description of the disease was given by Godman and Churg.[185] As described by these authors, so-called classic Wegener's granulomatosis shows

1. Necrotizing extravascular granulomas of undetermined etiology, most frequently involving upper and lower respiratory tracts
2. Glomerulonephritis
3. Systemic granulomatous vasculitis

A limited form of the disease lacking renal involvement was later reported.[186] More recently, the ACR and the Chapel Hill Consensus conference have offered definitions and diagnostic criteria based on these earlier findings (see Tables 29–8 and 29–9).

CLINICAL CONSIDERATIONS. The disease is uncommon: Its prevalence is estimated at approximately 3 per 100,000,[187] but this figure may be an underestimate, because the use of ANCA has shown that there are milder forms of the disease not previously recognized. The mean age of patients is approximately 41 years, but there is a wide age range.[188, 189] The male-to-female ratio is 3:2.

Renal involvement is frequent. When assessed by an abnormal urinalysis or by the finding of pathologic changes on renal biopsy, it appears to occur in 11% to 18% of patients at clinical onset of disease and in 77% to 85% of patients at some time during the clinical course. Patients can show hematuria, red and white cell casts, or mild proteinuria. The finding of red blood cell casts is nearly 100% predictive of glomerulonephritis.[187] There can be a rapid (and irreversible) rise in the blood urea nitrogen levels within days or weeks.

The last 10 years have seen striking advances in the diagnosis of Wegener's granulomatosis through the use of ANCA tests. Cytoplasmic ANCA (c-ANCA), and particularly the antiproteinase 3 (anti-PR3) form of c-ANCA, shows variable sensitivity depending on the extent and activity of disease, with the highest levels (84% to 99%) occurring in generalized active disease and lower frequencies found in limited and treated forms.[190, 191] The overall sensitivity of c-(anti-PR3)-ANCA for Wegener's granulomatosis is approximately 75%.[192] The specificity of proteinase-3 for Wegener's granulomatosis is also good, although proteinase 3 identifies some patients with microscopic polyangiitis.[192, 193] A homogeneous c-ANCA has been seen rarely in several infectious diseases, such as symptomatic HIV infection, endocarditis, cystic fibrosis associated with chronic infection, and tuberculosis, but it is unclear whether any of these cases are due to anti-PR3.

Untreated Wegener's granulomatosis has a 2-year survival rate of 10%. Before the use of cytotoxic therapy, renal failure was the cause of 50% of deaths. The development of renal insufficiency is still an ominous prognostic sign; treatment must begin immediately with cyclophosphamide, usually

with corticosteroids. It usually produces prolonged remissions in 70% to 90% of patients, with 5-year survival rates of at least 80%.[187, 194] Still, disease relapse is seen in approximately 50% of patients.[191] Patients who receive kidney transplants have a good outcome, with little evidence of recurrent disease, even when there is circulating ANCA.[195]

DIAGNOSTIC CONSIDERATIONS. The kidney is involved by a focal and segmental necrotizing glomerulonephritis with crescents in about 75% of cases at some time during the clinical course (Fig. 29–54).[189] The disease rapidly progresses to diffuse crescentic glomerulonephritis, so that anywhere between 2% and 100% of glomeruli may be involved in the renal biopsy.[189, 194, 196] Fibrinoid necrosis of a portion of the glomerular tuft is most common; as more glomeruli are affected, the disease more frequently affects the whole tuft. The fibrinoid necrosis is characterized by brightly eosinophilic material. Neutrophils, macrophages, and T cells may infiltrate these portions of the tuft, but the glomeruli usually lack hypercellularity and fail to show endocapillary proliferation.[197–199] The necrotic portion of the tuft shows vascular cell adhesion molecule-1, which is a macrophage, lymphocyte, and eosinophil attractant, and it also shows intercellular adhesion molecule-1. These adhesion molecules may play a role in the recruitment and retention of glomerular inflammatory cells.[199, 200] Furthermore, serum levels of soluble endothelial leukocyte adhesion molecule-1 are also elevated in ANCA-positive vasculitis.[201] The damaging role of neutrophils in development of the necrotic lesions is suggested by the presence of neutrophil elastase within glomeruli.[202]

Crescents are usually present over the area of tuft necrosis and thrombosis. Extensive crescents or sclerotic glomeruli are common in patients with irreversible renal failure.[189, 194] A granulomatous glomerulonephritis caused by epithelioid histiocytes and lymphocytes lined up along Bowman's space can occur (see Fig. 29–54).[199, 203, 204] It is in no way specific for Wegener's granulomatosis; it can also be

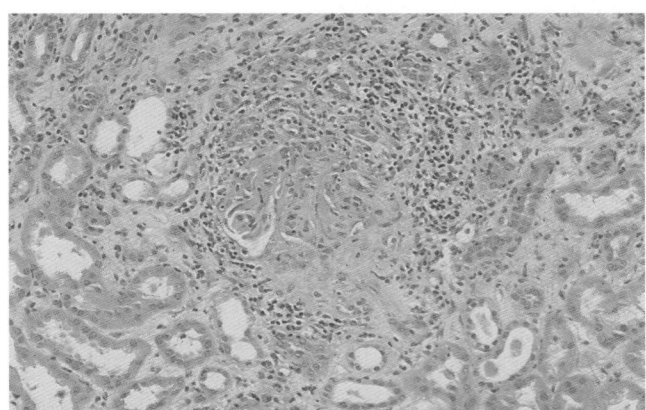

**FIGURE 29–54.** Wegener's granulomatosis: The glomerular tufts are compressed by crescents and are surrounded and infiltrated by inflammatory cells, forming a so-called granuloma.

seen in microscopic polyangiitis and occasionally in anti-GBM disease.

Vasculitis is uncommon in renal biopsies, occurring in 3% to 12% of biopsies.[189, 205–207] The vasculitis most often affects interlobular muscular arteries. There is infiltration of the vessel wall by neutrophils, lymphocytes, or macrophages with subintimal fibrin and endothelial cell swelling and detachment. Occasionally, granulomatous arteritis occurs.

Immunofluorescence microscopy either fails to show immunoglobulins or complement or shows small granular deposits of them (staining of less than 1+ intensity), that is, pauci-immune features.[203, 208, 209] Fibrin is typically seen, particularly when crescentic lesions are present.[197] Monocytes and T cells can be found within the crescents and in the interstitium of patients with crescentic glomerulonephritis, including Wegener's granulomatosis.[210]

By electron microscopy, there are glomerular intracapillary and subendothelial fibrin and platelet aggregates, suggesting that endothelial cell damage and intracapillary thrombosis are major factors in pathogenesis of the disease. Glomerular basement membrane breaks may be present, with fibrin deposits within Bowman's space. Traditional electron-dense deposits are infrequent and small, as expected in a pauci-immune type of glomerulonephritis. Vasculitic lesions show swelling of endothelial cells, subendothelial fibrin, platelets, electron-dense deposits that can be insudated plasma, and infiltrating lymphocytes and neutrophils.

DIFFERENTIAL DIAGNOSIS. In clinically ambiguous cases, renal biopsy is a necessary procedure to exclude lupus nephritis, anti-GBM disease, IgA nephropathy, and HSP, none of which are pauci-immune diseases, but the chief differential diagnosis in Wegener's glomerulonephritis is microscopic polyangiitis. The finding of granulomatous vasculitis somewhat favors Wegener's granulomatosis over microscopic polyangiitis, but because granulomatous glomerulonephritis can be seen in both diseases, it may be difficult to distinguish them and clinical correlation as well as type of ANCA may be necessary to establish the diagnosis.

## Churg-Strauss Syndrome (Allergic Granulomatosis)

NOMENCLATURE. Churg-Strauss syndrome is a clinicopathologic syndrome characterized by the presence of asthma, prominent tissue and blood eosinophilia, systemic vasculitis, and pulmonary and systemic necrotizing allergic granulomas. The Chapel Hill Consensus Conference offered a largely pathologic definition, namely eosinophil-rich and granulomatous inflammation involving the respiratory tract, necrotizing vasculitis affecting small to medium-sized vessels, and associated asthma and blood eosinophilia (see Table 29–8). The definition

has gradually shifted from pathologic findings to clinical parameters because the typical pathologic findings are not seen in all cases and can be induced by other diseases, such as parasitic infections and drug hypersensitivity. The ACR definition offers this view (see Table 29–9).

CLINICAL CONSIDERATIONS. Churg-Strauss syndrome is rare, representing only 2% of consultations for vasculitis in one series.[211] Still, in France, the disease is considered to represent 20% of cases of PAN.[212] The male-to-female ratio varies between 1:1 and 3:1. Children as young as 7 years and adults as old as 69 years can acquire the disease.

Certain organs are often targeted by the disease, and certain symptoms are characteristic. Patients initially show a prodrome of allergic rhinitis and nasal polyps, leading to prominent tissue and blood eosinophilia associated with Löffler's syndrome, chronic eosinophilic pneumonia, or eosinophilic gastroenteritis.[213] In the last phase, systemic vasculitis emerges, usually following the asthmatic symptoms by 2 to 3 years.

Kidney disease is variable, occurring in 16% to 49% of patients, but it is not generally as prominent or severe clinically as in Wegener's granulomatosis or microscopic polyangiitis, although exceptions occur.[213–216] Microscopic hematuria or mild proteinuria (often less than 500 mg/24 hours) are typically present.

There is an elevated eosinophil count (greater than $1000/mm^3$) in most cases and markedly elevated IgE levels that may reach 1000 mg/dL. Serum ANCA can be present; elevated titers have been reported in 38% to 85% of patients.[216–219] Most of these ANCAs are p-ANCAs, more specifically myeloperoxidase (MPO)–ANCA, although in one series c-ANCA predominated.[217, 218]

The untreated 5-year survival rate is 5%; treated patients have a 5-year survival rate of about 60% to 75%. The disease responds to corticosteroids, but patients may be steroid dependent and some require cytotoxic therapy.

DIAGNOSTIC CONSIDERATIONS. Glomerular changes range from none to very severe glomerulonephritis. Most commonly, the renal involvement is a focal segmental glomerulonephritis, sometimes necrotizing and sometimes associated with crescents.[213, 215, 220, 221] Mild mesangial hypercellularity may occur, but it is inconstant. In sum, the histologic appearance of the glomerulonephritis itself is similar to that which can be seen in Wegener's granulomatosis and microscopic polyangiitis, only milder.

Vasculitis occurs in more than 50% of renal biopsies.[220] It is often granulomatous, involving small to intermediate arteries and occasionally veins. It differs little from the vasculitis of Wegener's granulomatosis and microscopic polyangiitis, except that there are abundant perivascular and intra-arterial eosinophils. There may also be distinctive extravascular necrotizing or non-necrotizing granulomas with numerous central eosinophils (so-called eosinophilic abscesses), but the granulomas are inconstant.[211, 220, 222] Also, granulomatous crescents have not been reported.

By immunofluorescence microscopy, IgM, C3, and fibrinogen are the most constant findings,[213, 223] but their significance is unclear, particularly since by electron microscopy no electron-dense deposits have been reported within glomeruli or arteries.[221, 223]

DIFFERENTIAL DIAGNOSIS. As far as the kidney is concerned, the differential diagnosis is very much the same as in Wegener's granulomatosis and microscopic polyangiitis, namely that of focal segmental glomerulonephritis. Anti-GBM disease and the varieties of immune-complex–induced glomerulonephritis, including lupus nephritis, IgA nephropathy, HSP, and endocarditis-associated glomerulonephritis need to be considered, but are usually readily excluded when attention is paid to immunofluorescence and electron microscopic findings. The distinction from other pauci-immune glomerulonephritides, such as Wegener's granulomatosis and microscopic polyangiitis, is made easier when abundant vascular, perivascular, and interstitial eosinophils are seen; this finding should strongly raise the diagnosis of Churg-Strauss syndrome.

Diagnosis of Churg-Strauss syndrome can be made on clinicopathologic grounds with high specificity and sensitivity by demonstrating that a patient has at least four of the ACR criteria (see Table 29–9).

## Microscopic Polyangiitis (Synonym: Microscopic Polyarteritis Nodosa)

NOMENCLATURE. Microscopic polyangiitis, formerly termed microscopic PAN, is a systemic necrotizing vasculitis that affects small vessels, varying from small arteries, arterioles, and capillaries to venules, including pulmonary and glomerular capillaries (where it produces focal segmental necrotizing glomerulonephritis) (see Table 29–8).[177, 211] The Chapel Hill Consensus Conference favored the term microscopic polyangiitis over microscopic PAN because the disease is not restricted to arteries.

CLINICAL CONSIDERATIONS. The average age of patients is 50 years, but there is a wide age range, from 3 to 80 years. The clinical course before presentation may be prolonged, varying from several months to several years before development of the full syndrome.[224] The principal organs of involvement are lungs in the form of pulmonary hemorrhage, kidneys in the form of rapidly progressive renal failure, and skin in the form of purpuric lesions.

Clinically, most patients have reduced renal function on presentation; untreated disease rapidly progresses to azotemia.[224] Dialysis is needed in 25% to 45% of cases.[225, 226]

Relapses occur in about 35% of cases, with a median time of 2 years. They can occur during or after cessation of treatment. The survival rate at 5 years is 65%, with most deaths caused by active vasculitis, renal failure, or lung hemorrhage. Renal transplantation can be performed; in the era of cyclosporine treatment, relapse of ANCA-associated disease is uncommon.[195]

Serum ANCA, most often p-ANCA, can be seen in 75% to 82% of cases.[192, 227]

DIAGNOSTIC CONSIDERATIONS. Grossly, the kidney capsular surface is smooth and lacks infarcts, as opposed to the coarse granularity of classic PAN.

Microscopically, the kidney most often shows focal to diffuse segmental necrotizing glomerulonephritis, as in Wegener's granulomatosis. There are segmental areas of fibrinoid necrosis and thrombosis of the glomerular tufts with rupture of the glomerular basement membranes, best seen in silver-stained sections. Fibrin and red blood cells escape from the damaged glomerular capillaries into Bowman's space, leading to at first cellular and later fibrous crescents, very much as in Wegener's granulomatosis (Fig. 29–55). Both macrophages and, to a lesser extent, T cells can be present in the glomerular capillary loops.[199] As in Wegener's granulomatosis, palisaded granulomas may also occur around Bowman's capsule, leading to destruction of the glomerular tufts.

Although microscopic polyangiitis affects glomerular capillaries routinely in the form of a glomerulonephritis, it produces a vasculitis involving arterioles and arteries in only 25% or less of renal biopsies, suggesting the importance of sampling.[224, 228–230] Typically, the affected vessels show fibrinoid necrosis with infiltrating macrophages, lymphocytes, and neutrophils, but eosinophils can also be present in perivascular areas (see Fig. 29–55). A granulomatous vasculitis also can occur, as in Wegener's granulomatosis. In healing phases of the disease, there may be arterial wall fibrosis.

There is a pauci-immune pattern of immunofluorescent staining; that is, there is either no staining

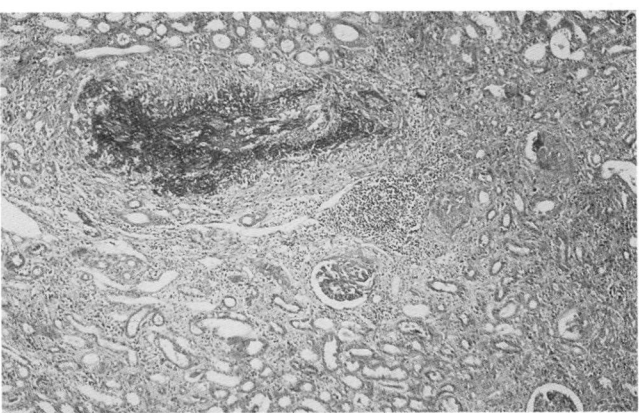

**FIGURE 29–55.** Polyarteritis nodosa: The artery shows fibrinoid necrosis and perivascular inflammatory cell infiltration. Two glomeruli are involved and show in part fibrous crescents. (Masson trichrome stain.)

or weak (<1 to 2+) focal staining for C3 and, to a lesser extent, immunoglobulins, most often in necrotic areas of the glomerular tuft.[229, 231] Fibrinogen, by contrast, is fairly frequent, being present in approximately 60% of cases, as expected in the setting of crescentic glomerular disease. It is seen in the glomerular tuft and within Bowman's space. Fibrinogen is also the most frequent immunoreactant in arteries, followed by complement and, in a few cases, immunoglobulins.

Electron microscopy shows swelling and loss of glomerular capillary endothelial cells. The capillary lumina are filled with fibrin and platelet aggregates, and fibrin may be seen within Bowman's space. In necrotizing lesions, breaks may be present within glomerular basement membranes. There are either no or very scant electron-dense deposits.[229] Arteries show endothelial cell swelling and intravascular and subendothelial fibrin.

DIFFERENTIAL DIAGNOSIS. Microscopic polyangiitis may be difficult to distinguish from classic PAN. Absence of aneurysms by angiography, presence of glomerulonephritis, small (<200 $\mu$m) vessel vasculitis, and serum ANCA suggest microscopic polyangiitis over classic PAN. Indeed, it has been suggested that finding ANCA is an exclusion criterion for classic PAN.[181] However, microscopic polyangiitis can occasionally show saccular and sausage-shaped aneurysms of arteries up to 300 $\mu$m in diameter.[232] Also, inflammation of arteries smaller than 200 $\mu$m in diameter can occur in cases of classic PAN, showing radiographic evidence of strictures.[181]

There may also be significant overlap in the clinical and microscopic features of Wegener's granulomatosis and microscopic polyangiitis.[180] p-ANCA is far more common in microscopic polyangiitis, whereas c-ANCA is typical of Wegener's granulomatosis. The finding of granulomatous arteritis also favors Wegener's granulomatosis. Necrotizing granulomas in the upper respiratory tract support Wegener's granulomatosis.

Unfortunately, the specificity of p-ANCA for microscopic polyangiitis or its renal-limited variant, idiopathic crescentic glomerulonephritis, is only moderate. Myeloperoxidase-ANCA can be seen in other vasculitides, such as Churg-Strauss syndrome, giant cell arteritis, and Wegener's granulomatosis. Elevated p-ANCA titers can also be seen in lupus nephritis, anti-GBM disease, postinfectious glomerulonephritis, sarcoidosis, idiopathic colitis, and bacterial pneumonia.[190, 193, 233]

## Classic Polyarteritis Nodosa

NOMENCLATURE. Classic PAN or macroscopic arteritis is less common than microscopic polyangiitis. It was initially described by Kussmaul and Maier in 1866.[234] The Chapel Hill Consensus Conference defined it as a necrotizing vasculitis that affects medium and small muscular arteries, rather than elastic arteries, without evidence of glomerulonephritis (see Table 29–8).[92] The disease typically involves bifurcations of arteries with formation of aneurysms, thrombosis, and infarction of organs. There is dispute about whether arterioles and even glomeruli can be affected. The Chapel Hill Consensus Conference definition excludes cases showing glomerulonephritis, arteriolitis, or venulitis (see Table 29–8),[177] whereas others suggest that arteries less than 200 $\mu$m in diameter, arterioles, and venules may be affected rarely.[181, 211] The clinicopathologic definition given by the ACR in 1990 (see Table 29–9) does not distinguish between classic PAN and microscopic polyangiitis (microscopic PAN) and is therefore somewhat outdated. Recent clinicopathologic studies have suggested that an abnormal angiogram supports the diagnosis of classical PAN whereas ANCA in the blood helps exclude it.[181]

CLINICAL CONSIDERATIONS. Evaluation of clinical and demographic features of classic PAN is difficult because cases of microscopic polyangiitis are admixed. Estimates using biopsy-proven cases suggest an overall annual incidence of only 0.7 per 100,000 to 6.3 per 100,000,[235] but two recent series that strictly distinguished microscopic polyangiitis from classic PAN showed classic PAN in 0% to 4% of patients with systemic vasculitis.[176, 186, 236] Most patients are between 40 and 60 years old.[212]

The frequency of hepatitis B virus (HBV)–associated PAN varies from 7% to 36% of cases, but was reported as less than 10% in a recent study. Clinical evidence of renal involvement is moderately frequent (about 35% of patients), but at autopsy, the kidney is the organ most often involved by the disease. There may be proteinuria, a mildly active urinary sediment, and evolving azotemia.[224] In HBV–related PAN, renal insufficiency occurs in about 25% of cases and nephrotic syndrome in 5%. ANCAs are infrequent in classic PAN: Only 10% of patients with HBV-associated PAN show them. The pattern may be either p- or c-ANCA.[212] Angiographic evidence of aneurysms in kidneys, liver, or mesentery are not pathognomonic, but they are frequently found in the disease. The aneurysms range in size from 1 to 5 mm, and they often involve the kidney. Therefore, performance of angiography is of some importance before renal biopsy to minimize the possibility of bleeding. PAN may produce multiple renal infarcts leading to renal failure. In these cases, arteriograms often show multiple microaneurysms with or without infarcts. Rupture of microaneurysms can lead to renal or perirenal hematomas. Treatment is with corticosteroids and cyclophosphamide. Poor prognosis is associated with proteinuria of greater than 1 g/day, renal insufficiency, cardiomyopathy, and gastrointestinal tract or central nervous system involvement.[212] Patients with HBV-associated disease are treated initially with corticosteroids followed by antiviral agents and plasma exchanges, with a 10-year survival rate of 83%.[212, 237, 238]

DIAGNOSTIC CONSIDERATIONS. Grossly, the kidney in classic PAN shows zones of fresh red hemorrhagic cortical infarcts in early cases and low flat scars, representing healed infarcts, in older cases. The arcuate and smaller muscular arteries may be prominent, owing to aneurysmal dilatation. Perirenal hematomas due to rupture of vascular aneurysms can occur.

The histologic hallmark is necrotizing vasculitis, but diagnosis is dependent on the finding of arteries, particularly arcuate to interlobular arteries, in the renal biopsy. Thus, a normal needle biopsy of kidney does not exclude the diagnosis.[228] The affected vessels are muscular arteries or occasionally arterioles as well.[211] They show inflammation, with or without fibrinoid necrosis. The vasculitis is typically segmental, affecting portions of the vascular wall, rather than the whole circumference. The lesions may be of varying ages. Early or acute lesions show a mixed inflammatory infiltrate affecting the intima and media as well as adventitia of the artery. The predominant cells in the arterial walls are a mixture of CD4-positive lymphocytes and macrophages,[211] but neutrophils and occasional eosinophils can be present. Sometimes, the appearance is that of a granulomatous arteritis. There is fibrinoid necrosis of intimal areas of the arteries, with intensely eosinophilic amorphous deposits that stain for fibrin in the subintima; fibrin thrombi can be present within the vascular lumina. Elastic stains usually show disruption of the elastic lamina. Microaneurysms, the classic arteriographic finding, are usually seen only at autopsy or in large specimens and not in needle biopsies. Older lesions show endarteritic fibrosis and eccentric narrowing or even occlusion of the affected vessels.

A striking feature is cortical infarcts, either recent or healed. Glomeruli are either normal or show ischemic contraction of their tufts.

DIFFERENTIAL DIAGNOSIS. The principal differential diagnosis is between classic PAN, microscopic polyangiitis, and Wegener's granulomatosis. Microscopically, the presence of glomerulonephritis makes a diagnosis of classic PAN unlikely, and leads to the alternate consideration of microscopic polyangiitis and Wegener's granulomatosis. Still, on occasion there may be cases that are difficult to classify, that is, appear to be overlap disease.[224] These cases may show involvement of larger arteries, but they also may have a focal glomerulonephritis.

The differential diagnosis is made considerably easier if attention is paid to clinical as well as pathologic features. Recent studies suggest that ANCA is usually, although not always, absent in classic PAN, whereas it is present in most cases of microscopic polyangiitis and Wegener's granulomatosis. Radiographic evidence of aneurysms is common in classic PAN and supports the diagnosis; indeed, angiographic evidence of aneurysms should be viewed as exclusionary of microscopic polyangiitis.

## Miscellaneous Vasculitides

There are two forms of large vessel vasculitis that can affect the kidney, but they are very rare and are discussed only briefly.

Giant cell or temporal arteritis is a vasculitis in which granulomatous inflammation and, in particular, multinucleated giant cells affect the media or the whole vessel wall.[239] Patients most often have polymyalgia rheumatica and are older than 40 years of age. Although the disease usually affects the carotid arteries and their branches, large arteries elsewhere in the body, including the main renal artery and its branches, may occasionally be involved.

Histologically, large arteries show a mixture of multinucleated giant cells that are typically arrayed around fragmented elastica of the artery, mononuclear cells, and occasional eosinophils. In healing phases of the disease, subintimal, intimal, and medial sclerosis can occur.

In the kidney, the disease is most often found in postmortem tissues. In these cases, it affects arteries, sometimes extending to smaller arteries, without evidence of glomerulonephritis.[239, 240]

Takayasu's arteritis is a large vessel vasculitis that most frequently involves the aorta and its branches. It occurs in a somewhat younger age group than does giant cell arteritis. The renal artery can show radiographic abnormalities in the form of stenosis or occlusion, resembling renal artery stenosis and producing renovascular hypertension.[239]

Histologically, the large arteries show multinucleated giant cells and mononuclear cells in early stages of disease, and medial and subintimal fibrosis in later stages. The disease is typically patchy. Mesangioproliferative glomerulonephritis has rarely been reported in association with the vasculitis.[241]

Kawasaki disease (mucocutaneous lymph node syndrome) is a disease of medium-size (main visceral) arteries. It is characterized by mucosal and skin inflammation, lymphadenopathy, fever, and arteritis, and it occurs most typically in children.[242] Iliac and axillary arteries are most commonly involved, but the main renal arteries are affected in 25% of cases.

Histologically, neutrophils and macrophages are present in the arterial walls, sometimes with small amounts of fibrinoid necrosis.[239] Healing lesions produce arterial fibroplasia and stenosis. Glomerulonephritis does not occur.

## Pauci-immune Crescentic Glomerulonephritis

NOMENCLATURE. An idiopathic form of crescentic glomerulonephritis typically lacks significant deposits within glomeruli and most often is associated with ANCA. The disease is sometimes called renal-limited vasculitis or ANCA-associated crescentic glomerulonephritis.

CLINICAL CONSIDERATIONS. The disease is associated with the presence of serum ANCA in 80% to 90% of cases, most often p-(myeloperoxidase or MPO)-ANCA.[243–245] Some patients eventually do develop a full-fledged vasculitis, such as Wegener's granulomatosis, months to years after clinical presentation.[246] Cases can be associated with the use of drugs, including penicillamine[247] and hydralazine, and the disease may rarely occur in relapsing polychondritis. Some patients with crescentic glomerulonephritis and serum ANCA also have antiglomerular basement membrane disease; in fact, about one third of patients with anti-GBM disease have concomitant serum ANCA. These patients should be considered to have anti-GBM disease, rather than pauci-immune glomerulonephritis. Pauci-immune glomerulonephritis is treated with corticosteroids, with or without cyclophosphamide. There does not appear to be a significant difference in kidney survival rates between those with renal-limited pauci-immune glomerulonephritis (75% renal survival at 2 years) and those who have pauci-immune glomerulonephritis in the setting of vasculitis.

DIAGNOSTIC CONSIDERATIONS. The classic early finding is segmental fibrinoid necrosis of glomerular tufts, followed by the formation of epithelial crescents. Endocapillary proliferation is typically absent. In glomeruli with crescents, basement membranes show segmental rupture, which is well demonstrated with such basement membrane stains as PAS and Jones silver. Bowman's capsules can show necrosis, and granulomatous reaction may be present around the glomeruli. The light microscopic appearance of the glomeruli is identical to that seen in anti-GBM disease, microscopic polyangiitis, or Wegener's granulomatosis. Because of this, a careful evaluation for vasculitis must be done in each case. The crescents and glomeruli undergo progressive fibrosis.

Immunofluorescence microscopy can show fibrinogen within the areas of segmental tuft necrosis and within Bowman's spaces of glomeruli with crescents, but immunoglobulins are either absent or present in low intensity. The level of staining is controversial but most have less than 1+ intensity for immunoglobulins. Electron microscopic appearance of the glomeruli is virtually identical to that seen in other ANCA-positive vasculitic diseases. Electron-dense deposits are usually absent, but occasionally, there can be small amounts of electron-dense material.

## Cryoglobulinemia

NOMENCLATURE. Cryoglobulins are immunoglobulins in the blood that are reversibly precipitable by a drop in temperature. Three types exist. Type I is composed of monoclonal immunoglobulins and occurs in the setting of hematologic malignancies, particularly B-cell lymphomas and leukemias and plasma cell neoplasms. Types II and III are mixed cryoglobulins containing at least two types of immunoglobulin, one of which (most often but not always an IgM) is directed against the Fc fragment of polyclonal IgG. In type II disease, this antiglobulin is monoclonal, whereas in type III, it is polyclonal. These mixed cryoglobulins are pathogenic because of their ability to fix complement, thereby acting as immune complexes, and by their capacity to deposit in many sites, particularly vessels and glomeruli, where they produce disease.

CLINICAL CONSIDERATIONS. As noted earlier, most cases of type I disease occur in patients with immunoglobulin-producing malignancies, such as B-cell lymphomas, chronic lymphocytic leukemias, and plasma cell dyscrasias or MM. The frequency of type I disease is hard to assess, but it is most likely less common than type II or III disease. Types II and III disease cause 60% to 75% of all cases of cryoglobulinemia, and they are most often seen in chronic liver disease, autoimmune diseases, infections, lymphoproliferative disorders, and in the setting of some immune-complex diseases. Before the 1990s, the etiology of many cases of types II and III cryoglobulinemia was undetermined and therefore the clinical disease in these cases was termed essential cryoglobulinemia. It is now known that most of these cases are due to hepatitis C viral infection. The cryoglobulins often contain hepatitis C viral RNA; curiously, they also usually contain a monoclonal IgM.

Clinically, patients with cryoglobulinemia often present with a syndrome of purpura of the lower extremities, weakness, joint pains, and nephrotic or nephritic syndrome, or proteinuria. A characteristic finding is hypocomplementemia in which early complement components (C1, C4) and CH50 are depressed, whereas C3 may be normal. The cryoglobulin level in the blood (cryocrit) varies between 2% to 70%, but the level does not correlate with the activity of the renal disease. Work-up for a cause, as well as evaluation of the type of cryoglobulin, is of value in the clinical management of the disease, because it may point to a specific etiology.

DIAGNOSTIC CONSIDERATIONS. The usual glomerular lesion of essential cryoglobulinemia and hepatitis C viral infections is mesangiocapillary glomerulonephritis.[248–253] There is hyperlobulation of the glomeruli owing to mesangial cell and matrix increase and prominent mesangial cell interpositioning producing characteristic tram-tracks (Fig. 29–56). Numerous monocytes are present within capillaries, and these monocytes may contain PAS-positive cytoplasmic droplets. A frequent helpful finding is the presence of PAS-positive intracapillary thrombi, which begin as subendothelial globules (see Fig. 29–56). These globules can resemble hyaline thrombi of the type seen in lupus nephritis. Rarely, a membranous rather than mesangiocapillary pattern is seen.

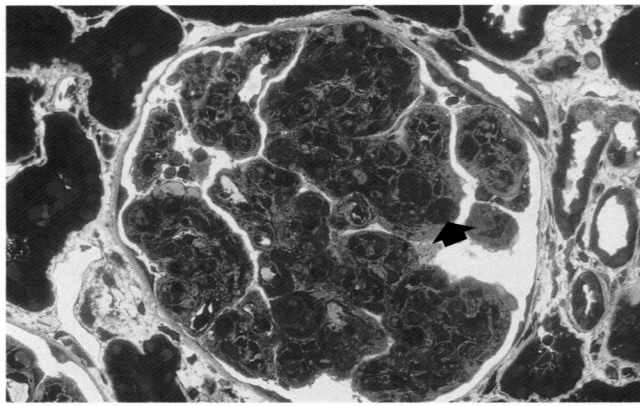

**FIGURE 29–56.** Cryoglobulinemic glomerulonephritis: The glomerulus is hypercellular, shows lobular simplification, and some capillary lumina are filled with protein-like material ("thrombi") (*arrow*). (Toluidine blue.)

Vasculitis with necrotizing, neutrophilic, or cicatricial features can also be seen.

Electron microscopy shows subendothelial electron-dense deposits; occasionally mesangial and subepithelial deposits can be seen as well (Fig. 29–57). Mesangial cell interpositioning can be seen (see Fig. 29–57). The deposits often have an organized, typically microtubular substructure, with the tubules measuring 250 to 300 angstroms in diameter. Paracrystalline arrays and patterns resembling fingerprints can also be seen.[249, 251] These organized arrays can also be seen in other related diseases, such as benign monoclonal gammopathy, Waldenström's macroglobulinemia, MM, and lupus nephritis. The capillary lumina are filled with macrophages that show large, membrane-bound, electron-dense inclusions, presumably derived from the cryoglobulin.

Immunofluorescence microscopy shows granular or globular deposits, most commonly IgG, IgM, and C3, in the capillary loops, corresponding to the composition of the circulating cryoglobulin.[252, 253] The capillary thrombi seen by light microscopy stain intensely for these immunoglobulins, but not for C3. Arteries show the same deposits.

## Benign Nephrosclerosis

CLINICAL CONSIDERATIONS. The kidney is a major end organ affected by hypertension. The rate of damage depends on the degree of hypertension. Benign nephrosclerosis occurs with mild to moderate hypertension, and it results in slow decline in glomerular filtration rate. In the early stages, it is not associated with symptoms and may be unsuspected during routine evaluation. The urinary sediment is benign and proteinuria, when present, is in the non-nephrotic range.

DIAGNOSTIC CONSIDERATIONS. With long-standing hypertension, the kidney is reduced in size, its surface is granular, it often contains V-shaped scars, and its cortex is thinned.[254] In the early stages, only small numbers of glomeruli in the outer cortex or subcapsular area are involved, but as the disease progresses, a greater proportion of deeper glomeruli show changes. These changes include collapse of the tufts with accumulation of collagen internal to Bowman's capsule and focally hyalinotic lesions.[255–257]

The vascular lesions associated with benign nephrosclerosis involve vessels of all sizes. In the small arteries and arterioles, there is hyperplasia of myointimal cells, a common and early lesion representing direct response to hypertension. Another well-recognized lesion is hyaline thickening, which appears to be initiated by the deposition of inactive C3b nonspecifically binding to the hyaluronic acid of the vessel wall.[258] Hypertension apparently accelerates this process by enhancing the permeability of the vessel wall to macromolecules. By light microscopy, arteriolar walls are thickened by deposition of homogenous eosinophilic material with accompanying atrophy of muscle cells (Fig. 29–58). This change is marked in afferent arterioles and vessels lacking internal elastic lamina.[255] Hyaline arteriolosclerosis is also seen with advanced age, but it is milder when compared with the hyaline changes seen in hypertensive or diabetic patients.

By electron microscopy, electron-dense, finely granular material, often of variable density, is deposited in the arteriolar wall, displacing or compressing the myointimal cells (Fig. 29–59). By immunofluorescence microscopy, C3 and IgM are often seen in the vessels. In larger arteries approximately the size of arcuate arteries, subintimal fibrosis and narrowing of the lumen are present.[255, 259] All of these changes also can occur with aging in the absence of hypertension, in which case they may result from the reduction in glomerular filtration rate that is normally seen in aging individuals.[258]

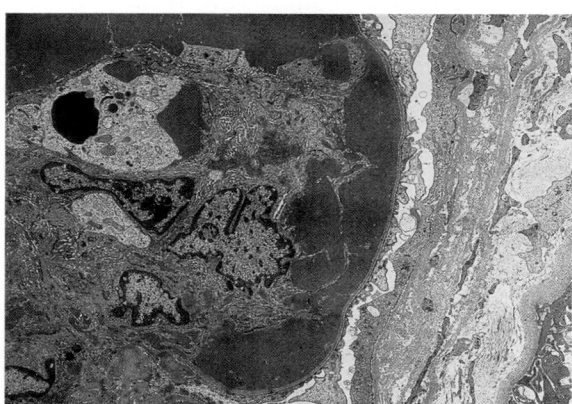

**FIGURE 29–57.** Cryoglobulinemic glomerulonephritis: Electron micrograph reveals intracapillary electron-dense granular material and focal mesangial extension.

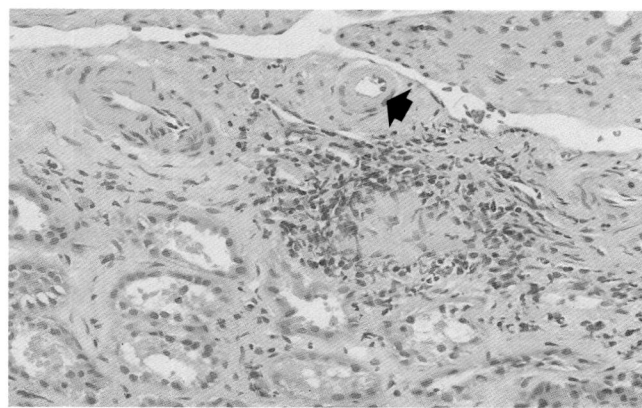

**FIGURE 29–58.** Benign hypertension, hyaline arteriolosclerosis: The arterioles (*arrow*) are thickened and show hyaline changes.

## Malignant Nephrosclerosis

CLINICAL CONSIDERATIONS. As in benign hypertension, the kidney is a major target organ for malignant hypertension. Malignant hypertension is usually preceded by a benign phase[260, 261]; however, some patients may develop malignant hypertension without a benign phase.

Patients with malignant nephrosclerosis typically present with the clinical findings of malignant hypertension, including headaches, blurred vision, dizziness, confusion, and hypertensive encephalopathy. On physical examination, retinal hemorrhages, exudates, and papilledema are common findings. The renal findings include elevated creatinine levels, hematuria with red blood cell casts, and non-nephrotic–range proteinuria. Anemia and thrombocytopenia can be present.

DIAGNOSTIC CONSIDERATIONS. On gross examination, the size of the kidney varies with the length of the clinical course. It is often large with a smooth surface, particularly if there is no prior history of benign nephrosclerosis, but later in the clinical course the kidneys are often small with a granular surface. The cut surface is mottled red and yellow with evident petechial hemorrhages.

Microscopically, both glomeruli and blood vessels are involved. The glomeruli are often collapsed, with shrunken lobules, and they may show areas of fibrinoid necrosis. Crescents may be present in severe cases. The vascular changes are commonly seen in interlobular arteries and arterioles. The arteries show a laminated onionskin intimal hyperplasia, red blood cell extravasation, and marked luminal narrowing or occasionally even thrombosis (Fig. 29–60).[255, 262] The arterioles demonstrate subintimal mucoid change and fibrinoid necrosis of their walls.

By electron microscopy, the glomerular capillaries are collapsed and may show subendothelial widening containing electron-lucent, granular, acellular material. With fibrinoid necrosis, electron-dense granular material and fibrin or platelets can be seen in the vessel walls.[263, 264]

By immunofluorescence microscopy, in more than half of the cases, fibrinogen, complement, and immunoglobulins (most commonly IgM) are seen in the small arteries and arterioles. IgM and complement can also be seen in the glomerular mesangium.[264] Similar vascular changes are seen in kidneys of patients with scleroderma and hemolytic-uremic syndrome. In scleroderma, the lesions are mainly confined to the interlobular arteries, whereas in hemolytic-uremic syndrome, in contrast to malignant hypertension, the vascular lesions are focal and more acute.

PATHOGENESIS. The pathogenesis of malignant nephrosclerosis is believed to be damage to the endothelium and vascular wall, with increased permeability and resultant insudation of plasma proteins and fibrin into the wall, leading to vascular necrosis and damage to the wall.[263, 264]

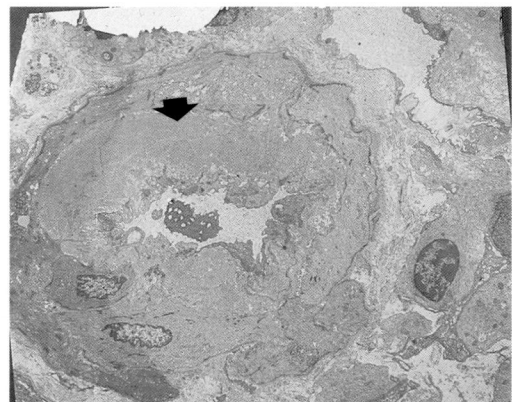

**FIGURE 29–59.** Benign hypertension, hyaline arteriolosclerosis: Electron micrograph reveals a thickened arteriole with subendothelial electron-dense granular material (*arrow*) (hyaline changes).

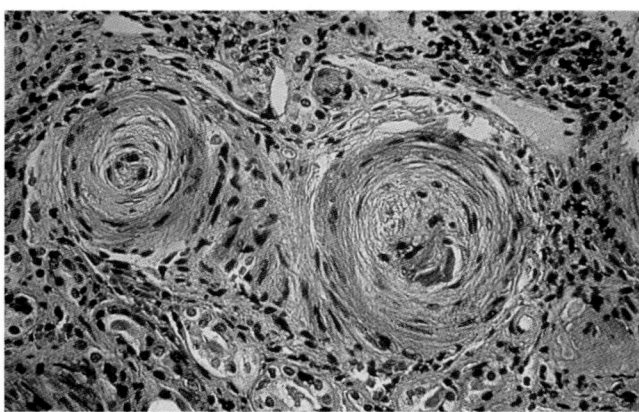

**FIGURE 29–60.** Malignant hypertension: The arterioles show an onion-peel pattern, with marked narrowing of the lumen.

## Renal Artery Stenosis

Stenosis of the main renal artery can cause secondary hypertension.[265–270] One of the principal causes of narrowing of the artery is atherosclerosis. Atheromas of the renal artery usually form a localized plaque, destroying the intima and internal elastic membrane and reducing or almost completely obstructing the vascular lumen. Thrombosis of the renal artery can be superimposed on renal artery atherosclerosis or can occur in abdominal aortic atherosclerotic aneurysms, and it rarely complicates PAN. It may also result from extension of a thrombus from the ascending aorta or trauma to the renal pedicle.

Atheromatous involvement of the aorta can also lead to atheromatous emboli lodging in the smaller (arcuate or interlobular) renal arteries. The occluded arteries contain needle-shaped cholesterol crystals, which appear as slits that can be surrounded by intimal fibrous tissue or show an inflammatory and sometimes giant cell reaction around them.[266] Patients commonly present with deterioration of renal function, frequently following arteriography that causes fragments of the plaques to break off into the blood stream.

The second group of conditions that leads to stenosis of the renal artery is known as renal artery dysplasia.[265–268] Typically, these lesions occur in the distal portion of the renal artery. They are bilateral in approximately 50% of cases, and they can involve other systemic arteries as well. The result is usually severe hypertension that is not responsive to therapy. Renal artery dysplasias can be divided into several subtypes (Table 29–10).

Medial fibroplasia is the most common form, representing 60% to 85% of cases. It is predominantly seen in young women between the ages of 20 and 50 years. It affects the distal two thirds of the main artery, it is usually bilateral, and the changes may extend into the first branches of the renal artery. Microscopically, thickened fibromuscular ridges due to medial fibrosis alternate with aneurysmally dilated, thinned areas of the arterial wall due to atrophy of muscle cells and loss of the internal elastica. The result is a characteristic sausage-string or string-of-beads appearance on arteriography. Extrarenal sites of involvement may include the carotid, coronary, mesenteric, hepatic, and iliac arteries.

Perimedial fibroplasia is the second most common lesion, with an incidence of 10% to 25% of cases. It affects the right artery more than the left artery, but it is often bilateral. This form of disease is seen in women younger than 30 years of age. Microscopically, the outer half of the media is replaced by a variably thick layer of collagen, but the media, elastica, and intima maintain their architecture. Extrarenal vascular lesions are not seen.

Medial hyperplasia affects only short segments of the renal artery with uniform circumferential thickening of the smooth muscle of its media and resultant narrowing of the lumen. It occurs in adolescence and in late middle age, and it affects both sexes equally. Extrarenal involvement is not seen.

Intimal fibroplasia is uncommon, with an incidence of 1% to 5% of cases. It occurs most often in women of childbearing age. It is characterized by hyperplasia of the intima. Microscopically, there is circumferential accumulation of loose ground substance, collagen fibers, and myointimal cells in the subintimal area of the renal artery, markedly reducing the lumen. Intimal fibroplasia can resemble atherosclerotic changes, but lipid accumulation is absent. The architecture of the elastica and media is preserved. Extrarenal involvement can occur in cerebral, mesenteric, and extremity arteries.

Periarterial fibroplasia is the rarest of all fibroplasias, with an incidence of less than 1%. There is no sex predilection. It occurs in patients between the ages of 15 and 30 years. There is fibrosis of the adventitia that extends into the perivascular connective tissue, constricting the vessel wall from its external surface.

Dissecting renal artery aneurysms are seen in 5% to 10% of cases of renal artery stenosis. They can be seen with renal artery dysplasias, especially in the intimal and perimedial fibroplasias. Medial dissection usually occurs, with the new channel in the outer third of the media. Other lesions of the main renal artery, such as inflammatory involvement (vasculitis), are discussed elsewhere in this chapter.

**TABLE 29–10.** Types of Renal Artery Dysplasia

**Medial fibroplasia:** Bands of fibrous tissue in the arterial media alternate with marked thinning of the arterial wall due to atrophy of muscle cells, loss of the internal elastica, and aneurysmal dilatation, producing a characteristic sausage-string or string of beads.

**Perimedial fibroplasia:** Fibrosis of the outer half of the arterial media; the media, elastica, and intima maintain their architecture.

**Medial hyperplasia:** Uniform circumferential thickening of the smooth muscle of the media of the artery.

**Intimal fibroplasia:** Subintimal circumferential accumulation of stroma and myointimal cells.

**Periarterial fibroplasia:** Adventitial and perivascular fibrosis, externally constricting the artery.

## Renal Vein Thrombosis

CLINICAL CONSIDERATIONS. Renal vein thrombosis is most commonly associated with three conditions: dehydration in infants resulting from severe diarrhea; nephrotic syndrome, most commonly due to membranous glomerulopathy and amyloidosis; and compression trauma to the kidney.[271–273] Often the patients are asymptomatic, but in its acute stage, renal vein thrombosis can present with flank pain, hematuria, and acute renal failure.

Radiographic findings in renal vein thrombosis depend on the acuteness and completeness of the venous occlusion. With complete, acute occlusion, there is nonvisualization of the kidney. When the occlusion is partial or accompanied by adequate collateral formation, the kidney is large and smooth, but some degree of contrast material excretion can be demonstrated. The collecting system has a normal distribution, but it is attenuated by surrounding interstitial edema. The nephrogram may continue to increase in density with time, or it may show striations of alternating radiolucent and radiopaque stripes. Ureteral notching may be a manifestation of collateral circulation. Occasionally, filling defects within the renal pelvis mimicking ureteritis cystica is identified. If thrombosis is insidious and adequate collaterals have developed, the urogram will be normal. In all cases, venography, ultrasonography, or computed tomography is required to confirm the diagnosis.

DIAGNOSTIC CONSIDERATIONS. Histologic changes are nonspecific, because venous thrombi are not usually seen in needle biopsy of the kidney. There is typically interstitial edema or fibrosis that is out of proportion to the glomerular disease. The most common glomerular diseases associated with renal vein thrombosis are membranous glomerulopathy and renal amyloidosis. When neutrophils are present in glomerular capillary lumina, known as leukocytic margination, the suspicion of renal vein thrombosis should be raised.[272, 273]

PATHOGENESIS. Renal vein thrombosis is now accepted as the result, rather than the cause, of the nephrotic syndrome. In particular, nephrotic syndrome can cause hypercoagulability, owing to urinary loss of the anticoagulant antithrombin III.[271] Elevated fibrinogen levels, enhanced platelet aggregation, and increased inhibition of fibrinolysis probably all contribute to the clotting tendency. Involvement of extrarenal arteries occurs, and deep vein thrombosis with pulmonary thromboembolism can cause death.

## Renal Infarction

Renal artery embolism is usually a complication of heart disease, such as mitral stenosis with atrial fibrillation, myocardial infarction with mural thrombosis, or bacterial endocarditis. Emboli usually lodge in secondary arterial branches in the kidney; they often involve both kidneys. Rarely, they can occlude the main renal artery, at which point surgical intervention is indicated. Arterial occlusion results in ischemic infarction. Small infarcts may also result from cholesterol emboli that are derived from atheromatous lesions of the abdominal aorta (see Renal Artery Stenosis), from severe narrowing of small intrarenal branches in scleroderma or malignant hypertension, and from sickling of red blood cells in small vessels in sickle cell anemia. Radiographic features vary with the age and extent of the infarct. Within the first week of an infarct, there may be a nephrographic defect in the area of infarction. This defect is triangular, with the base situated on the outer margin of the kidney. The calyx and infundibulum may be attenuated and incompletely filled due to adjacent edema. After approximately 4 weeks, a wide-based depression in the renal contour develops at the site of the infarct. The underlying papilla remains normal. When the entire kidney is infarcted, intravenous urography demonstrates nonfunction.

## Thrombotic Microangiopathies

NOMENCLATURE. Thrombotic microangiopathies encompass many clinical and pathologic features, including microangiopathic hemolytic anemia, the presence of schistocytes in the peripheral blood smear, thrombocytopenia, elevated serum lactate dehydrogenase levels, and renal failure. Two basic abnormalities include damage to the endothelium and coagulation. Two main diseases that come under the thrombotic microangiopathies are hemolytic-uremic syndrome (HUS) and thrombotic thrombocytopenic purpura (TTP). Besides these two major entities, other diseases such as scleroderma, malignant hypertension, primary anti-phospholipid syndrome, SLE, and pregnancy (eclampsia/preeclampsia), as well as contraceptive drugs, cyclosporine, transplantation (bone marrow and kidney), and cancer and chemotherapy are associated with thrombotic microangiopathy. There are many overlapping clinical and histologic features between HUS and TTP; therefore, some consider the two diseases to be different expressions of the same disease.[274] In spite of similarities, there are certain features that tend to separate these two diseases. Therefore, these are described separately below.

### HEMOLYTIC-UREMIC SYNDROME

CLINICAL CONSIDERATIONS. The triad that describes HUS includes microangiopathic hemolytic anemia, thrombocytopenia, and acute renal failure. The lesion of HUS was originally described in infants and children; however, cases in older patients are now known to occur.[275] Drummond[276] subdivided HUS into six categories (Table 29–11). The renal manifestations include oliguria, anuria, hematuria, proteinuria, and renal failure.

**TABLE 29–11.** Subtypes of Hemolytic-Uremic Syndrome[276, 372–374]

Classic form
Associated with infection (*Shigella dysenteriae, Salmonella typhi, Streptococcus pneumoniae,* and verotoxin-producing *E. coli*)
Hereditary and recurrent forms
Associated with abnormalities of complement system
Associated with systemic disease (scleroderma, SLE, malignant hypertension)
Miscellaneous form (pregnancy related, contraceptive use, radiation of kidney, transplantation, use of cyclosporine, mitomycin)

DIAGNOSTIC CONSIDERATIONS. By light microscopy, the glomeruli appear bloodless and show obliteration of capillary lumina due to endothelial swelling. Occasionally, double contours are seen with PAS or PAMS stains. Focal tuft necrosis can be present; it is usually associated with afferent arteriolar thrombosis and necrosis. There is also basophilic mucoid widening of the intima that develops over weeks. Extravasation of red blood cells into the vessel wall may be present. Occasionally, glomerular crescents are present. There is usually interstitial edema but chronic tubulointerstitial changes can be present, depending on a variety of factors.

Electron microscopy reveals the most characteristic glomerular lesion. The lamina rara interna of the glomerular basement membrane is widened and electron lucent due to finely granular or fibrillar material in which entrapped red blood cells may occasionally be seen (Fig. 29–61). The endothelium is swollen and may be detached, and the capillary lumen is often completely or almost completely obliterated by the swollen cells. Capillary lumina may contain thrombi made up of platelets and fibrin.[277] There is often diffuse effacement of epithelial cell foot processes. The arterioles and small arteries also show similar changes, with mucoid intimal widening, endothelial swelling, and narrowing of lumina. In addition, an onion-peel pattern, fibrinoid necrosis of the wall, and extravasation of red blood cells in the wall may be seen.

Immune-complex–type deposits are absent. Fibrinogen is present along glomerular capillary walls and along blood vessels. IgM and C3 are often associated with the fibrinogen. In secondary forms of the disease, the changes are similar, but alterations associated with the underlying disease also accompany the lesions of HUS.

PATHOGENESIS. The pathogenesis of HUS is by no means fully understood, but the disease is believed to result from damage to vascular endothelium with resultant platelet adhesion, leading to intravascular thrombus formation.[278]

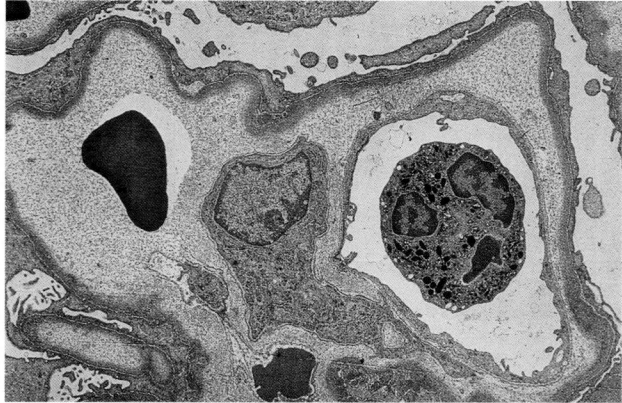

**FIGURE 29–61.** Hemolytic-uremic syndrome: Electron micrograph showing marked widening of lamina rara interna with an electron-lucent zone containing a red blood cell.

## Thrombotic Thrombocytopenic Purpura

CLINICAL CONSIDERATIONS. This disease, first described by Moschcowitz, has five features: fever, hemolytic anemia, thrombocytopenia, neurologic involvement, and renal manifestations.[279] Women are more commonly affected than men, and patients are most often in the second to fifth decades of life. The anemia is of the microangiopathic hemolytic type, and it produces petechiae and ecchymoses. The neurologic manifestations include headache, coma, paresis, aphasia, syncope, seizures, and visual and mental changes. TTP is a fatal disease with rapid course; only 10% of patients survive. Renal involvement occurs in 70% to 76% of patients.[280, 281] The renal presentation includes hematuria, proteinuria, urinary casts, and elevation in blood urea nitrogen and serum creatinine. However, renal manifestations are less frequent and less acute than in HUS.

DIAGNOSTIC CONSIDERATIONS. The light microscopic changes are usually similar to those seen in HUS. The most conspicuous feature is the presence of granular eosinophilic thrombi in the arterioles and interlobular arteries. The thrombotic material is often well organized and endothelialized, and the lumen is rarely completely obliterated but rather appears slitlike. This lesion is often referred to as the glomera or glomeruloid structure.[282]

By electron microscopy, the thrombi contain fragments of basement membrane–like and proteinaceous material along with cellular and platelet fragments. The organizing thrombi are covered by endothelium. Immune-complex–type deposits are absent and immunofluorescence microscopy reveals deposits of fibrinogen, without immunoglobulins or complement.

## Scleroderma and Progressive Systemic Sclerosis

CLINICAL CONSIDERATIONS. Progressive systemic sclerosis is an uncommon systemic disease that produces prominent changes in the skin, along with multisystem involvement of such organs as gastrointestinal tract, lungs, heart, and kidney. It is classified into generalized and limited forms. The limited form consists of Raynaud's phenomenon and sclerosis of the skin of hands, face, fingers, and forearms; it rarely affects the kidney. In the generalized form, there is fibrosis of the skin of the face, trunk, and extremities. In addition, sclerosis of the esophagus, interstitial fibrosis in the lungs, cardiac involvement, or kidney disease is present.

Renal involvement is particularly important for prognostication because, if the condition is left untreated, it leads to rapid progression to end-stage renal disease and is a major cause of death. Patients are usually women between the second and fifth decades of life, but any age and either sex can be affected. The clinical signs and symptoms affecting various organs are secondary to vascular sclerosis, increased deposition of collagen in various organs, and smooth muscle atrophy. The most common symptoms are dermal changes, particularly thickening of skin and Raynaud's phenomenon (95% of cases), and dysphagia due to decreased esophageal motility (50% to 70% of cases). Lung, heart, and renal symptoms are present in approximately 50% of cases. Kidney disease accounts for 40% of deaths. Approximately 20% of patients with renal involvement present with renal crisis, characterized by abrupt onset of rapidly progressive renal failure and hypertension. The course is variable and no form of treatment alters the extrarenal disease.

DIAGNOSTIC CONSIDERATIONS. In the kidney, the major microscopic abnormality is in the vessels. Interlobular arteries show concentric onion-skin thickening, deposition of mucoid substance in their intima, and perivascular collagen deposition. Glomerular and vascular changes are similar to those seen in malignant hypertension.[283, 284] The tubulointerstitial changes are variable. They range from necrosis of tubules in early and acute phases to scarring in later stages. In a scleroderma crisis, areas of infarction are commonly seen. Immunohistochemical findings commonly include IgM and C3 in vessel walls and fibrin in areas of necrosis.

PATHOGENESIS. The pathogenesis of scleroderma is unknown. Three theories have been proposed: (1) abnormal collagen metabolism; (2) impaired control of vascular microcirculation; and (3) autoimmune vascular damage.[285-288]

## Renal Diseases Associated with Pregnancy

Disease associated with pregnancy can be divided into two categories: (1) underlying diseases exacerbated by pregnancy; and (2) disease initiated or caused by pregnancy. The most common diseases exacerbated by pregnancy are hypertension, SLE, and focal segmental glomerulosclerosis. The diseases initiated by pregnancy are preeclampsia and eclampsia and postpartum acute renal failure; these diseases are described in this section.

### PREECLAMPSIA AND ECLAMPSIA (SYNONYM: TOXEMIA OF PREGNANCY)

CLINICAL CONSIDERATIONS. Preeclampsia develops in 5% to 7% of primiparas, it is six to eight times more common in primiparas than multiparas, and it tends to occur at extremes of reproductive age. In multiparas, it is often associated with multifetal pregnancy, fetal hydrops, and hypertension.

Patients present with hypertension, proteinuria, and edema. Nephrotic syndrome is rare. Recovery is usually rapid after delivery. Rarely, the course can be complicated by a decline in glomerular function and by signs and symptoms of HUS and TTP. When the disease progresses to a convulsive stage, it is referred to as eclampsia. With better clinical management, the need for kidney biopsies has become rare.

DIAGNOSTIC CONSIDERATIONS. The primary site of injury is the glomerulus. Both endothelial and mesangial cells are involved.[74, 289-293] These cells are swollen, which results in narrowing of the glomerular capillary lumina. The glomeruli therefore appear bloodless and they are normocellular.

By electron microscopy, a variety of vacuoles are seen in the endothelial cell cytoplasm, which is swollen; sometimes, the vacuoles contain membrane-bound myelin-like figures. The lamina rara interna of the glomerular basement membranes are often widened. Electron-dense deposits of immune-complex type are not seen.

By immunofluorescence microscopy, fibrinogen is present in the capillaries. Crescent formation is rare.

PATHOGENESIS. The disease is common in the third trimester. The etiology is unclear; however, it is thought to be multifactorial. Pregnancy predisposes to intravascular coagulation and to the effects of endotoxins. Ischemia of the uterus and placenta possibly triggers release of thromboplastic substances, and immunologic reactivity to fetal products may be implicated. These factors cause spasm of arterioles and they trigger endothelial damage.[74]

### POSTPARTUM ACUTE RENAL FAILURE

In this disease, the clinical and histologic changes are again similar to those of HUS and TTP. In particular, there is microangiopathic hemolytic anemia, thrombocytopenia, and sudden development of acute renal failure soon after a normal delivery or within the first 3 months after delivery. Blood pressure is usually normal but rises with progression of disease. The mortality rate is over 50%.

## TUBULOINTERSTITIAL DISEASE

Tubulointerstitial disease (TID) affects primarily the tubules and interstitium of the kidney; it is therefore separated from conditions that primarily affect the glomeruli and blood vessels. It can also be referred to as the tubulointerstitial nephropathies or interstitial nephritis. TID can be classified according to its pathogenesis, pathologic features, or clinical presentation, but broadly it is most often classified as acute or chronic and by etiology, if known.[294, 295]

## Acute Tubulointerstitial Disease Associated with Drugs

CLINICAL CONSIDERATIONS. Acute TID is characterized by an abrupt clinical onset and is associated with infiltration of the renal parenchyma by inflammatory cells. The three major causes of acute TID are drugs, infections, and idiopathic.[294]

**TABLE 29–12.** Selected Effects of Drugs on the Kidney*

| Disease | Drugs |
| --- | --- |
| Tubulointerstitial nephritis | Penicillins, cephalosporins sulfonamides, rifampin, NSAIDs |
| Membranous glomerulopathy | Gold, penicillamine |
| Minimal change disease | NSAIDs, diuretics |
| Acute TID and minimal change disease | NSAIDs |
| Necrotizing crescentic glomerulonephritis | Allopurinol |
| Acute tubular necrosis | NSAIDs |
| Interstitial fibrosis | CCNU |
| Vascular lesions | Cyclosporine, FK506, corticosteroids |

* Only selected diseases and the drugs that cause them are listed in this table.
NSAIDs, nonsteroidal anti-inflammatory agents; TID, tubulointerstitial disease.

Drugs often cause a clinically recognized TID that is due to hypersensitivity reaction. It is associated with fever, rash, eosinophilia, nonoliguric renal insufficiency, sterile pyuria, eosinophiluria, mild proteinuria, and hematuria. The kidney is one of the major routes of drug elimination, and its unique anatomic configuration and complex physiologic function renders it particularly prone to adverse drug reactions. A detailed list of drugs associated with TID is available in many textbooks. The most common drugs causing acute disease are the $\beta$-lactam antibiotics, such as the penicillins and cephalosporins. Other drugs that may cause it include sulfonamides, rifampin, nonsteroidal anti-inflammatory drugs, and diuretics.

Drugs also cause other renal lesions besides TID (Table 29–12). Drugs affect the kidney via a variety of mechanisms. These include direct effect on the nephron, production of fluid and electrolyte imbalances, hemodynamic disturbances, vascular involvement, hypersensitivity,[296] and exacerbation of underlying renal disease. With the variety of renal lesions associated with drugs, a high level of suspicion and detailed clinical information is critical for diagnosis.

DIAGNOSTIC CONSIDERATIONS. The histologic changes in the kidney in drug-induced acute tubulointerstitial nephritis are interstitial edema and irregular, patchy interstitial inflammation (Fig. 29–62). The infiltrates are composed predominantly of lymphocytes, macrophages, and a variable number of plasma cells (Fig. 29–63). Eosinophils may be present in large numbers or may be absent; they are not necessary to make a diagnosis of drug-induced TID (Fig. 29–63). Despite the name "acute" given to the disease, neutrophils, the classic acute inflammatory cells, are only occasionally seen and when present are usually sparse. The inflammatory cells line the tubular basement membranes and often invade the tubular epithelium (so-called tubulitis) (Fig.

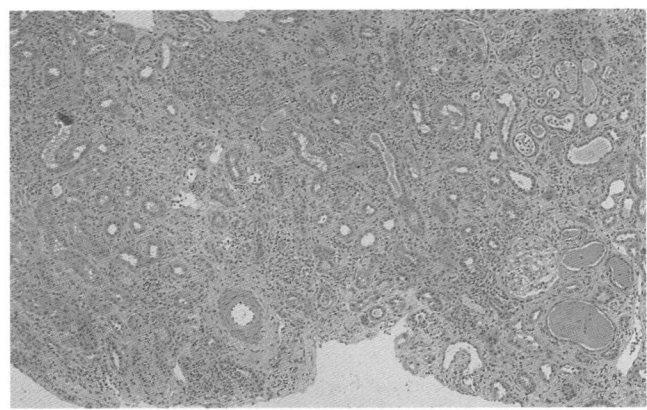

**FIGURE 29–62.** Acute tubulointerstitial disease: At low magnification, the parenchyma shows edema and is infiltrated by inflammatory cells. The glomeruli are unremarkable.

29–63). Epithelioid granulomas may be seen rarely with penicillin-associated acute TID.[294–297]

## Acute Tubulointerstitial Disease Associated with Infections (Synonym: Acute Pyelonephritis)

CLINICAL CONSIDERATIONS. Acute TID associated with systemic infections was first described at the end of the 19th century by Councilman[298] in autopsy kidneys of children dying of diptheria and scarlet fever, prior to the era of antibiotics. Other organisms associated with acute TID are listed in Table 29–13. The TID produced by acute infection is often termed acute pyelonephritis.

While systemic infection may seed the kidney and cause acute pyelonephritis, pyelonephritis is most often caused by vesicoureteric reflux and ascending infection from the bladder. Gram-negative organisms, such as *E. coli*, are the typical agents. Acute pyelonephritis has a sudden onset with chills,

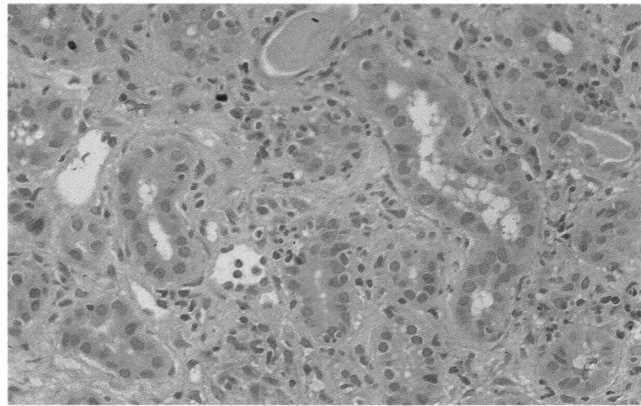

**FIGURE 29–63.** Acute tubulointerstitial disease: At high magnification, the tubular epithelium is infiltrated by inflammatory cells (tubulitis). Occasional eosinophils can be recognized.

**TABLE 29–13.** Systemic Infections Producing Acute Tubulointerstitial Disease

Systemic streptococcal infection
Leptospirosis
Toxoplasmosis
Infectious mononucleosis
Measles
Brucellosis
Syphilis
*Mycoplasma* pneumonia
Rocky mountain spotted fever
Legionnaire's disease

**TABLE 29–14.** Selected Causes of Chronic Tubulointerstitial Disease

*Bacterial Infections*
Either alone (chronic pyelonephritis) or associated with vesicoureteral reflux, xanthogranulomatous pyelonephritis, urinary tract obstruction, renal tuberculosis, or malakoplakia.

*Drugs*
Analgesics, lithium, CCNU

*Heavy Metals*
Lead, mercury, cadmium

*Metabolic Disorders*
Sickle cell disease, calcium disturbances, cystinosis, and oxalosis
Glomerulonephritis: a secondary component of the inflammatory reaction
Nonglomerular immunologic diseases, malignancies, and hereditary diseases

fever, back pain, tenderness, and pain and frequency of micturition. Renal function may be abnormal, but acute renal failure is rare. Urinalysis reveals bacteriuria with more than 100,000 organisms/mL and pyuria with white blood cells and white blood cell casts. Red blood cell casts may also be present. Proteinuria is usually absent.

In animal models, bacterial antigens have been demonstrated in the renal interstitium.[294, 299] With the advent of antibiotics, it may be difficult to differentiate between drug-induced acute TID and acute TID secondary to infection, because patients with infection often receive antibiotics before biopsy.

DIAGNOSTIC CONSIDERATIONS. Microscopic examination of the kidney reveals interstitial inflammatory cells that are predominantly neutrophils and to a lesser extent mononuclear cells. Parenchymal abscesses may be present. The tubules show epithelial degeneration and contain neutrophil casts.

## Idiopathic Acute Tubulointerstitial Disease

The term *idiopathic acute TID* refers to acute TID not associated with any documented cause such as hypersensitivity to drugs or infections. Patients can present with findings varying from minimal nonspecific symptoms to renal failure. Urinalysis reveals leukocytes, erythrocytes, rare casts, and minimal proteinuria. Some patients show features of hypersensitivity, such as blood eosinophilia, increased serum IgE levels, and granular or linear immune deposits of IgG and C3 along tubular basement membranes.[300, 301] The kidney biopsy shows infiltration by mononuclear cells and occasionally eosinophils. The etiology in most patients is unknown, and the prognosis is usually favorable with treatment.

## Chronic Tubulointerstitial Disease

This manifestation of TID results from a variety of chronic underlying conditions (Table 29–14).[294] The histologic hallmark is interstitial fibrosis of varying extent, along with tubular atrophy and patchy but heavy interstitial infiltration by mononuclear cells,

lymphocytes, and plasma cells. Sometimes, there can be superimposed acute TID, and eosinophils can be present on occasion. Vascular sclerosis and glomerular scarring occur secondary to the tubulointerstitial inflammation and fibrosis, but in advanced cases, it may be difficult to distinguish where the primary area of disease lies, because all three zones of the kidney (i.e., glomeruli, arteries, and tubulointerstitium) often show extensive damage.

## Radiation Nephropathy

CLINICAL CONSIDERATIONS. Improved radiation delivery systems and better localization of kidney and target organs have reduced the incidence of radiation nephropathy. Over time, it has become evident that more than 2300 rad delivered over a period of 5 weeks to the kidney often leads to renal failure.[302-304] The pathologic lesions associated with radiation depend on dose, time of exposure, age of the patient, preexisting renal disease, and concomitant use of chemotherapeutic agents.[302, 303, 305]

Acute radiation nephritis usually occurs 6 to 12 months after exposure to radiation, but it can occur earlier. Clinically, there is edema, hypertension, dyspnea on exertion, pleural and peritoneal effusions, anemia, headaches, proteinuria, renal insufficiency, and urinary casts. About half of the patients develop renal failure with chronic renal impairment. In patients who also develop malignant hypertension, the mortality rate is high.

Chronic radiation nephritis occurs either after an episode of acute radiation nephritis or secondary to long-standing chronic exposure to radiation, with insidious development of symptoms of hypertension, isolated proteinuria, and renal insufficiency.

DIAGNOSTIC CONSIDERATIONS. The histologic changes vary greatly, depending on the severity and stage of the disease.[302, 305-307] In acute radiation nephritis, the glomerular changes include fibrinoid necrosis, thickening of capillary walls, double contours or tram tracks along the capillary walls, occasional crescents, and segmental scarring. By electron microscopy, the subendothelial areas of the capillary walls are widened by electron-lucent, fluffy material. This material appears to be fibrinogen or fibrin by immunohistochemistry. In chronic disease, there is partial or complete glomerular sclerosis.

The vascular changes include fibrinoid necrosis of arterioles and small arteries without inflammatory cell reaction. Intimal proliferation in arterioles and interlobular arteries is a common finding. Foam cells may narrow arterial lumina, particularly in chronic disease; this is a characteristic lesion of radiation vasculopathy.

Tubular changes include vacuolization, necrosis, and sloughing of lining epithelium, predominantly in the proximal tubules. This change occurs even before vascular and glomerular abnormalities are observed. The interstitial abnormalities reflect the glomerular, vascular, and tubular disease. There can be interstitial edema and fibrosis with rare mononuclear cell infiltration.

## Acute Tubular Necrosis

Acute tubular necrosis (ATN) is defined as renal tubular injury associated with clinical evidence of renal failure.[308-310] The common underlying causes for ATN include either ischemia (e.g., shock, sepsis, or burns) or toxins such as antibiotics, hemoglobin, myoglobin, and chemical toxins. Patients present with either oliguric or nonoliguric renal failure. ATN involves primarily and often exclusively proximal tubules. Depending on the stage, the morphologic changes include minimal swelling, dilatation of the lumen and flattening of lining epithelium (Fig. 29–64), or marked necrosis and sloughing of epithelium. These changes are often associated with intratubular granular and cellular casts; however, inflammatory cell casts are not common. In the regenerative stage, the lining epithelium shows a ba-

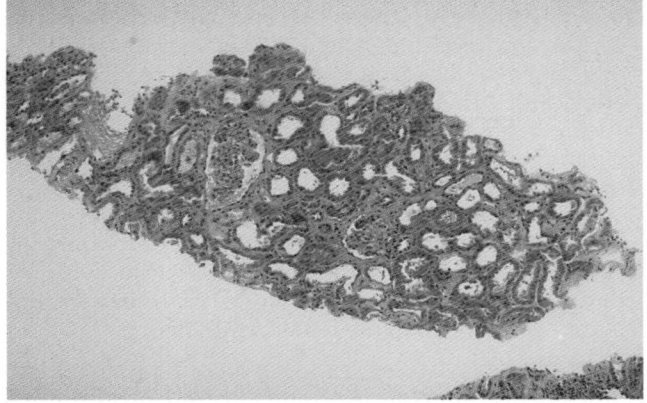

**FIGURE 29–64.** Acute tubular necrosis. The proximal tubules are dilated and lined by flattened epithelium.

sophilic cytoplasm and hyperchromatic nuclei. The tubular changes are associated with interstitial edema and minimal inflammatory cell infiltration. There is a distinct lack of tubulitis, which helps in the diagnosis of ATN. When tubular changes are associated with heavy inflammatory cell infiltration, the lesion is more often that of acute interstitial nephritis, rather than ATN, or a combination of the two lesions. The glomeruli and blood vessels do not show any significant changes. Immunofluorescence and electron microscopy do not contribute toward the diagnosis but help in excluding glomerular lesions.

## HEREDITARY NEPHROPATHIES

### Congenital Nephrotic Syndrome

CLINICAL CONSIDERATIONS. The appearance of nephrotic syndrome at birth or shortly thereafter is unusual; however, when it occurs, it is known as congenital nephrotic syndrome. Two types of congenital nephrotic syndrome are recognized: the Finnish type and the mesangial sclerosis type.

Finnish-type congenital nephrotic syndrome, also known as microcystic disease, is transmitted as an autosomal recessive disease. It has an incidence of 1:8000 in newborns of Finnish extraction. The pathogenesis is not clear, but there appears to be a chromosomal defect linked to 19q12-13.1. Hoyer and associates[311] suggested a possible genetic metabolic defect, and chemical analysis of the glomerular basement membrane in these patients has shown increased numbers of hydroxylysine, 3- and 4-hydroxyproline and glucosyl-galactosyl hydroxylysine units.[312] Still, immunohistochemical studies have shown that staining for collagen type IV, laminin, and fibronectin is the same as in the normal glomerulus.[311, 313, 314] The disease is limited to the kidneys. Nephrotic syndrome occurs in these infants from the early postnatal period up to 6 months of age.

The diffuse mesangial sclerosis–type of congenital nephrotic syndrome is differentiated from the Finnish type by its later age at onset and slower progression to renal failure and death.[315, 316]

DIAGNOSTIC CONSIDERATIONS. Pathologic changes in the early stages of the Finnish type of disease include cystic dilatation of proximal and distal tubules, predominantly in the corticomedullary junction area. Glomeruli show absent or minimal changes in the form of mesangial widening. The glomeruli appear immature and cellular, and are often surrounded by prominent epithelial cells. Later, glomerulosclerosis, both segmental and global, and chronic tubulointerstitial changes accompany vascular changes. Because infection is a common complication, it is sometimes difficult to determine whether the glomerular and tubulointerstitial changes are part of the disease or whether they are secondary to infection. By electron microscopy, the glomerular basement membranes are thin and show focal splitting. The mesangial areas are widened due to increase in matrix. The visceral epithelial cells are hypertrophic, and there is diffuse effacement of foot processes. Immune-complex–type deposits are not present.

By light microscopy, the diffuse mesangial sclerosis–type of congenital nephrotic syndrome reveals the presence of fetal glomeruli and focal or extensive mesangial sclerosis, with or without increase in cellularity. Prominent epithelial cells surround the collapsed glomeruli, a change often interpreted as crescents. The deeper glomeruli are less affected, and there can be dilatation of tubules, but this is minor in comparison to the Finnish variety of congenital nephrotic syndrome. By electron microscopy, the glomerular basement membrane is split and wavy, and there is epithelial cell foot process fusion, reflecting the nephrotic range proteinuria. By immunofluorescence microscopy, IgM and C3 are present in the mesangium of less affected glomeruli. This variety of congenital nephrotic syndrome is associated with Drash syndrome.[317]

## Nail-Patella Syndrome (Synonyms: Osteo-onychodysplasia, Turner-Keiser Syndrome)

CLINICAL CONSIDERATIONS. The disease is very uncommon. It is transmitted as an autosomal dominant trait with a gene frequency of 2/100,000. A strong linkage is recognized to the locus 9q34, containing the ABO blood group and adenylate kinase gene, on chromosome 9.[318] Although abnormalities of COL5A1 have so far not been identified, a linkage between the COL5A1 gene and the 9q34.2-9q34.3 region of chromosome 9 has been suggested recently, because the nail-patella locus is also localized on 9q34.[74] Patients with this disease present with hematuria and proteinuria. Nephrotic syndrome is rare, but it can occur with progression to renal failure. The renal symptoms may be the first presentation of the disease, and renal involvement is seen in approximately 40% of cases. Other characteristic features include hypoplasia or absence of the patella, dysplasia of fingernails, iliac horns, and subluxation of the radial heads. The disease does not recur in renal transplants.[319–321]

DIAGNOSTIC CONSIDERATIONS. By light microscopy, the renal tissue may be normal or it may show progressive glomerulosclerosis and chronic TID. The glomerular capillary walls may be focally thickened. Electron microscopy is essential for the diagnosis.[319, 322] It demonstrates a thickened glomerular basement membrane that contains fibrils with cross striations resembling interstitial collagen. The distribution of the fibrils is irregular, with involvement of some, but not all, capillaries. Depending on the amount of proteinuria, there is variable effacement of epithelial cell foot processes. Electron-dense deposits (immune-complex type) are absent. Deposits are also absent on routine immunohistochemistry.

## Fabry's Disease (Synonym: Angiokeratoma Corporis Diffusum Universale)

CLINICAL CONSIDERATIONS. Fabry's disease is an X-linked inborn error of metabolism caused by deficiency of $\alpha$-galactosidase A, a lysozymal enzyme present in all tissues. A defective gene is located on the long arm of the X chromosome, and it has been specifically linked to Xq22.[323] The disease is encountered in hemizygous men. Female carriers, being heterozygous, are mildly affected. As a consequence of the deficiency, neutral glycosphingolipids, predominantly ceramide trihexoside and cerebroside dihexoside, accumulate in many organs, including the kidney. These glycosphingolipids aggregate in the lysosomes, causing a clinical syndrome with punctate skin lesions, renal disease, and shooting pain in the lower extremities. Systemic manifestations result from accumulation of glycosphingolipids in blood vessels, heart, kidney, and other organs. Renal involvement manifests itself by hematuria and proteinuria, usually developing in the second decade, with gradual decrease in renal function by the third or fourth decade.[324] Death occurs around the fifth decade of life due to renal, cardiac, and cerebrovascular involvement. It was initially thought that kidney transplantation might provide the missing enzyme, but this procedure produces no significant release of the enzyme, and there is continued progression of the disease.[325]

DIAGNOSTIC CONSIDERATIONS. Glycosphingolipid accumulation is seen in all affected tissues but primarily in vascular endothelium, smooth muscles and perithelium, glomerular and tubular epithelium, corneal epithelium, myocardium, reticuloendothelial system of bone marrow, spleen, liver, and bronchial and synovial lining. In the kidney by light microscopy, the glomerular cellular elements, especially the epithelial cells, are enlarged and appear vacuolated; these features are best seen with the PAS stain (Fig. 29–65). The mesangium may show an increase in matrix. Progression of the disease is manifested by sclerotic changes. Vacuoles can be seen in the tubular epithelium, vascular endothelium, and vascular smooth muscle.

The disease is most readily diagnosed by electron microscopy, which shows whorled, laminated inclusion bodies that measure approximately 5 $\mu$m in diameter. These inclusions are ovoid or round in shape. They consist of concentric, myelin-like structures with parallel layers, forming so-called zebra bodies (Fig. 29–66). These structures are easily visualized in plastic-embedded tissue stained with toluidine blue (Fig. 29–67). By electron microscopy, zebra bodies are common in both visceral and parietal

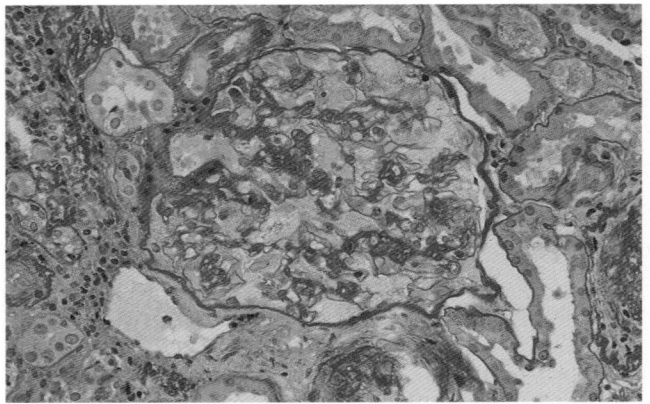

**FIGURE 29–65.** Fabry's disease: The glomerulus shows marked swelling of epithelial cells (pale areas) that have a foamy appearance. (PAS stain.)

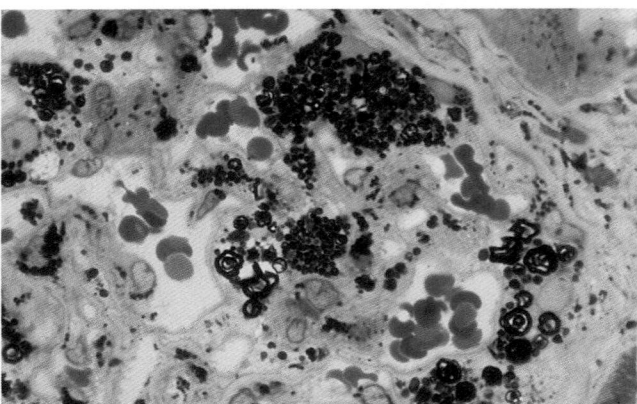

**FIGURE 29–67.** Fabry's disease: Intracytoplasmic inclusions are present in all cellular elements. (Toluidine blue stain.)

glomerular epithelial cells; they are less frequent in endothelial and mesangial cells (see Fig. 29–66). The inclusions are also seen in vascular endothelium and muscle cells and in the tubular epithelium, especially of the distal tubules.[326] Immunofluorescence microscopy is negative for immunoreactants.

## Alport's Syndrome (Synonym: Hereditary Nephritis)

CLINICAL CONSIDERATIONS. Alport[327] in 1927 described a clinical syndrome of familial renal disease associated in most cases with deafness. It is known to represent a disorder of basement membrane synthesis affecting collagen type IV; in addition, basement membranes in a number of organs are involved.[328–331] The disease affects men more often than women. It occurs in children and young adults.

The major clinical symptom involving the kidney is hematuria, which can be present at birth or commence within the first few months or years of life. The hematuria can be either continuous or recurrent, and it can be either microscopic or gross. Proteinuria is absent in the early stages of disease, but with progression of the disease, it can reach nephrotic range in 30% to 40% of patients. The renal disease commonly progresses to end stage in men and in some women. Two clinical variants are recognized: a juvenile form, in which end-stage renal disease occurs before the age of 31 years, and an adult form, in which the disease occurs in patients older than 31 years of age.[328] In the juvenile group, the course is similar in most patients, but in the adult group, the prognosis is less predictable.[328] Neural deafness occurs in 50% of patients; it is bilateral and sensorineural, and it primarily affects high-tone hearing. Ocular defects include anterior lenticonus, cataracts, and whitish perimacular lesions in the retina. Other less common lesions include peripheral neuropathy, retinitis pigmentosa, and platelet dysfunction.[327, 328, 332] The disease does not recur in renal transplants, but patients can develop antiglomerular basement membrane disease in the transplant owing to the presence of normal, hence antigenically different, glomerular basement membrane in the graft.[333, 334]

GENETICS OF ALPORT'S SYNDROME. There are two principal modes of inheritance of Alport's syndrome: (1) genetically heterogeneous—including an X-linked dominant form and an autosomal dominant type (which explains the male to male transmission); and (2) an autosomal dominant form with variable penetrance and expression and reduced penetrance in men who receive the mutant gene from their father.

What is the site of mutation in this disease? Human basement membranes are composed of a number of glycoproteins, including type IV collagen. Type IV collagen consists of a family of proteins comprising six isomeric chains, designated as a1 through a6. The human a1 and a2 type IV collagens are encoded on chromosome 13, a3 and a4 are encoded on chromosome 2, and a5 and a6 are encoded

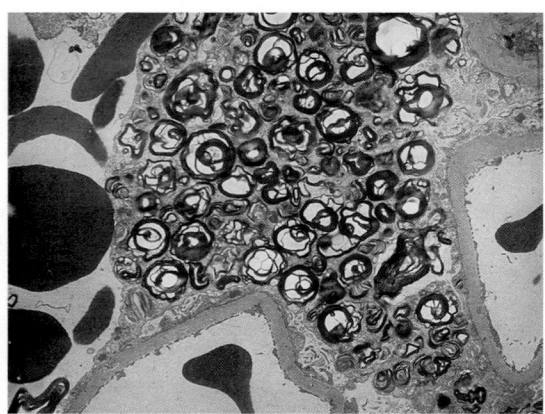

**FIGURE 29–66.** Fabry's disease: In the electron micrograph, a visceral epithelial cell contains whorled laminated zebra bodies.

on the X chromosome. Polypeptides containing an epitope in the NC1 domain of collagen IV (and recognized by the antiglomerular basement membrane antibody of Goodpasture's disease) are absent in the glomerular basement membrane in Alport's syndrome. The defective gene has been mapped to the Xq22 locus, where mutations have been noted in the a5 locus in the collagen IV gene. The X-linked dominant form of Alport's syndrome arises from mutation in the collagen a5 locus, whereas the autosomal recessive form arises as a result of mutation at the a3 or a4 locus. The X-linked form of Alport's syndrome is seen in approximately 80% of patients; however, mutation of a5 has been noted in only 50% of patients believed to have X-linked Alport's syndrome. Autosomal-recessive Alport's syndrome was identified as a mutation of a3 in two children and a4 in two other kindreds. Several more cases have since been reported.[335]

DIAGNOSTIC CONSIDERATIONS. Light microscopic changes are nonspecific.[327, 328, 332, 336, 337] The glomeruli can appear normal, show mild to moderate increase in mesangial cells and matrix, or demonstrate partial or complete glomerulosclerosis. Similarly, the tubulointerstitial changes are nonspecific, and a variable amount of chronic TID may be present. Often foam cells are present in the interstitium,[333] and their presence without proteinuria should raise the suspicion of Alport's syndrome. Although they are considered to be nonspecific, some suggest that they occur as a consequence of altered lipid metabolism in the tubules.[336]

The diagnosis of Alport's syndrome can be made only by electron microscopy. In the early stages, the glomerular basement membrane is extremely thin and has a poorly formed, reticulated lamina densa that shows splitting and splintering (Fig. 29–68). These areas often contain electron-dense granules or small amounts of fragmented cytoplasmic-like material. With progression of disease, the basement membrane becomes thick and often has an irregular epithelial surface.[331, 337, 338]

Routine immunofluorescence microscopy is negative, but in sclerotic glomeruli, IgM and C3 may be present. Of interest, the serum from a patient with anti-GBM antibody disease (Goodpasture's disease), when applied to the kidney of a patient with Alport's syndrome, does not show linear immunofluorescence because the antigen associated with anti-GBM antibody disease is absent in the native kidneys of Alport's syndrome patients.[333, 334] This may serve as an additional tool in the diagnosis of Alport's syndrome.

## Benign Familial Hematuria and Thin Basement Membrane Disease

These conditions include a heterogeneous group of patients with overlapping clinical and morphologic findings. To date, studies of type IV collagen in the glomerular basement membrane in these patients have failed to uncover any consistent abnormality in the distribution of any of the six collagen subchains. However, one study reported a defect in the a4 chain of collagen IV.[339] This finding suggests the possibility of a partial penetrance or expression of the gene for Alport's syndrome, with incomplete morphologic expression.[335]

In recent years, the term thin basement membrane disease has been preferred to benign familial hematuria by some authors. The patients present with gross or microscopic hematuria that may be intermittent or continuous. In most, the mode of inheritance is autosomal dominant; indeed, many patients have relatives with hematuria. Autosomal recessive inheritance is also suggested in some individuals. Some cases of IgA nephropathy have been reported in association with this lesion.[340] The prognosis is excellent, unless the lesion is associated with other renal disease.

By light microscopy, glomerular changes may be minimal, or there may be mesangial expansion. By electron microscopy, the glomerular basement membranes are thin, but they have a well-developed lamina densa.[341]

## PATHOLOGY OF RENAL TRANSPLANTATION

Over the last 40 years, better monitoring and treatment of renal transplant patients have resulted in increasingly successful use of this procedure with long-term survival times. Transplant rejection in its many manifestations still remains the most important issue in the management and survival of renal allografts; both clinical and pathologic findings are important in the evaluation of transplant biopsies. The morphologic changes in a renal transplant biopsy usually correlate with the clinical findings, although histologic changes without overt clinical symptoms of rejection have been observed.[342–345]

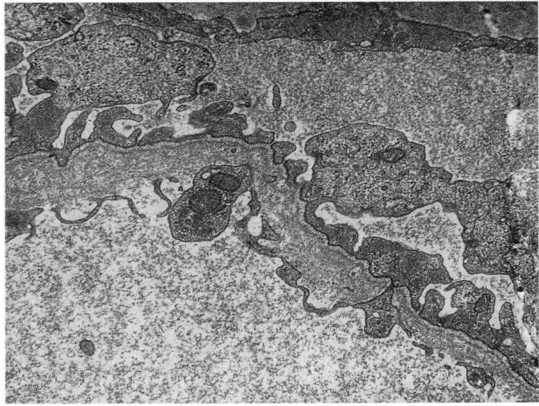

**FIGURE 29–68.** Hereditary nephropathy (Alport's syndrome): Electron micrograph shows thickening of glomerular basement membrane with fibrillar/reticulated appearance.

**TABLE 29–15.** Pathologic Alterations in Renal Transplants

Preservation injury
Hyperacute rejection
Imminent rejection
Acute rejection
    Acute cellular rejection
    Acute vascular rejection
Chronic rejection
    Chronic transplant glomerulopathy
Cyclosporine/FK506 toxicity
Recurrent and de novo diseases

Knowledge of the histologic appearance of the donor kidney is important to compare with changes seen in the transplant; however, baseline (1 hour post anastomosis) biopsies are no longer routinely performed in many centers.

The histologic changes of the renal transplant biopsy are broadly subdivided as listed in Table 29–15.[346] Although the morphologic patterns in each subgroup have characteristic features with specific lesions, overlap between two or more categories is often present.[347]

## Preservation Injury

Preservation injury is seen in the biopsy of donor kidneys before anastomosis into the recipient. Whether it occurs depends primarily on the methods of preservation and on ischemia time. The light microscopic changes are mainly confined to the tubules. The tubular lining epithelial cells show necrosis, leading to sloughing of lining epithelium. The tubular lumen often contains detached epithelial cellular fragments. There is often loss of the proximal tubular brush border, which is best seen in sections stained with PAS. Later in the course, as the tubular epithelium regenerates, a flattened or piled up tubular epithelium containing occasional mitoses can be seen. The interstitium is usually edematous and may contain a few scattered inflammatory cells.

The electron microscopic findings include marked lysosomal and mitochondrial swelling, increased cytoplasmic protein droplets, and widening of the basal infoldings of tubular lining cells. The glomeruli usually are unremarkable, although they can reveal swelling of all cellular elements and focal effacement of epithelial cell foot processes. Blood vessels are usually unremarkable, or they may show endothelial hypertrophy. Immunofluorescence microscopy fails to show significant abnormalities.

## Hyperacute Rejection

Hyperacute rejection usually occurs within minutes or hours following renal transplantation. It occurs in recipients who have high titers of preformed antibodies against ABO antigens or against antigens expressed on the donor lymphocytes or endothelium of the transplanted kidney. Hyperacute rejection causes irreversible damage to the transplant. The antibodies in the majority of these patients are of IgG class; they are directed against human leukocyte antigen class I antigens on both T and B lymphocytes.[343, 348]

The light microscopic changes result from widespread vascular thromboses, which are best seen in the muscular arteries. They include fibrin and platelet thrombi and occasional fibrinoid necrosis of vessel walls, resulting in infarction and necrosis of renal parenchyma. The glomeruli appear congested. Glomerular capillaries may be filled with sludged red blood cells, clumps of platelets, and inflammatory cells (neutrophils), and there is necrosis of cellular elements. There is also interstitial edema, hemorrhage, and interstitial infiltration by mainly neutrophils. Mononuclear cell infiltrates are a later event, if the transplant remains for more than 4 to 6 days.[349] The changes are focal in early stages and become extensive with time.

By electron microscopy, the glomeruli reveal intracapillary platelets and fibrin thrombi, and degeneration of all cellular elements, mainly endothelial cells. Electron-dense deposits (immune complexes) are not present.

By immunofluorescence microscopy, there are linear deposits of IgG along glomerular and interstitial capillaries. Staining for C3 is discontinuous in the glomerular capillaries, but it is widespread in peritubular capillaries. Deposits of fibrin are seen in the glomerular capillaries and in blood vessels. With the passage of time, immunoglobulin and complement either diminish or disappear.[343, 347]

## Imminent Rejection

Glomerular and interstitial cellular infiltrates and occasionally glomerular intracapillary thrombi can occur in immediate or 1-hour post-transplant biopsies.[349–351] Their precise meaning still remains controversial, because they may be secondary to preservation injury, preformed antibodies, or a combination of the two. In our experience, the presence of histologic abnormalities in 1-hour post-anastomosis biopsies probably correlates with early post-transplant graft loss, and this finding is a useful indicator of early rejection.[350] These light microscopic changes include the presence of mononuclear and polymorphonuclear cells in the interstitial and glomerular capillaries, which may be associated with glomerular intracapillary thrombi. By electron microscopy, except for the changes described by light microscopy, no other additional features are seen. Immunofluorescence microscopy is either negative or it reveals deposits of fibrinogen in the glomerular thrombi.

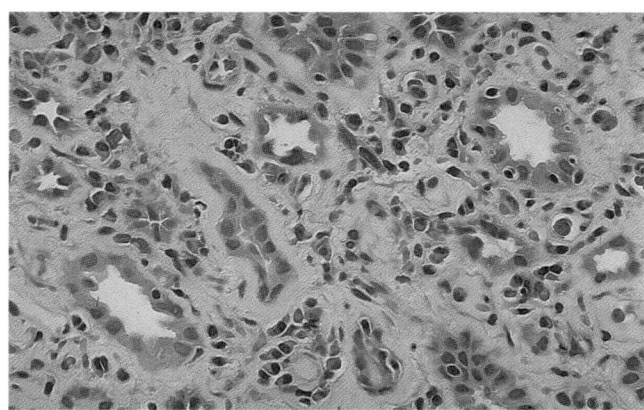

**FIGURE 29–69.** Renal transplant, acute cellular rejection: The interstitium is infiltrated mainly by mononuclear cells. In many tubules, inflammatory cells infiltrate the epithelium (tubulitis).

## Acute Rejection

Acute rejection usually occurs within the first few weeks after transplantation, but it can also occur months or years after transplantation, superimposed on chronic rejection. Both cellular and humoral immune mechanisms play a role. Two types of acute rejection are recognized—acute cellular rejection and vascular (humoral) rejection.

ACUTE CELLULAR REJECTION. In this type of rejection, there is either diffuse or focal, but extensive, inflammatory cell infiltration of the interstitium (Fig. 29–69). The infiltrates are composed of small and large (activated) lymphocytes, monocytes, and plasma cells; to a lesser degree, polymorphonuclear leukocytes and eosinophils are also present.[343, 347, 351–353] Invasion of the tubular lining epithelium by the inflammatory cells resulting in so-called tubulitis occurs, denoting recent damage (see Fig. 29–69).[345, 352] Both tubulitis and interstitial cellular infiltrates are important in the diagnosis and grading of cellular rejection.[354] The interstitium is often edematous. Interstitial fibrosis and vascular changes may be present, depending on the age of the transplant; however, a variety of other factors also play a role. The glomeruli are normal.

The electron microscopic findings are noncontributory. Immunohistochemical staining shows the majority (60% to 80%) of the infiltrating cells to be suppressor or cytotoxic (CD8$^+$) cells. The remaining cells are a combination of helper (CD4$^+$) T cells, plasma cells, and monocytes.[343, 352] Routine immunofluorescence microscopy for immunoglobulins and complement is negative.

ACUTE VASCULAR (HUMORAL) REJECTION. This type of rejection includes both vessel (vasculopathy) and glomerular (glomerulopathy) involvement. The blood vessels are always involved but often in a patchy manner (Fig. 29–70). The involved arteries and arterioles show marked subendothelial swelling due to edema, with accumulation of mucoid material, which can be demonstrated as acid mucosubstances by Alcian blue staining.[353] The endothelial cells are hypertrophic, with resultant narrowing of the vascular lumina. They may show focal necrosis and detachment (see Fig. 29–70). There is widening and infiltration of the subendothelial space by small and large lymphocytes, monocytes, foam cells, and rare plasma cells. Arterial media may show degenerative changes and fibrin may be seen between muscle cells. Breaks in the elastica, focal medial necrosis, and rarely, inflammatory cell infiltration of the necrotic vessel wall may be seen.

The glomeruli show endothelial hypertrophy, diffuse effacement of epithelial cell foot processes, and villous transformation (glomerulopathy). More severely affected glomeruli show cellular detachment from the basement membrane, platelet aggregates and strands of fibrin in the vascular and urinary spaces. At times, breaks in the capillary basement membranes may be seen. These changes are associated with extensive tubulointerstitial changes, including interstitial cellular infiltrates, tubular dilatation with necrosis of lining epithelium, red blood cell casts, interstitial edema, hemorrhages, and dilatation of peritubular capillaries.

Electron microscopy is noncontributory. Immunofluorescence microscopy often reveals linear deposits of immunoglobulin (IgG, IgM) and granular deposits of complement components (C1q and C3) and fibrin in the walls of glomerular and interstitial vessels.[340, 355] The cellular infiltrates are similar to those seen in acute cellular rejection and contain both CD4$^+$ and CD8$^+$ cells; however, in severe lesions, there is predominance of CD8$^+$ cells.

## Chronic Rejection

Chronic rejection is a slow and progressive loss of renal function and parenchyma over months or

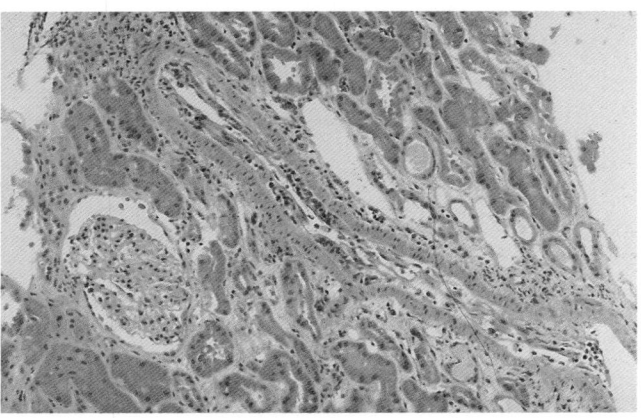

**FIGURE 29–70.** Renal transplant, acute vascular rejection: The arterial endothelium is sloughed off and inflammatory cells and edema are present in the subendothelial area. Edema and cellular infiltrates are seen in the renal interstitium. The glomerulus is normal.

years, and usually occurs as the end result of clinically apparent or silent repeated episodes of rejection affecting the nephron, interstitium, and vasculature.[343, 356] The histologic changes are often subdivided into chronic vascular rejection and chronic transplant glomerulopathy; however, these two entities may be seen together and there is often an overlap of histologic findings.

In chronic rejection, the glomeruli are either normocellular and unremarkable or they show focal or diffuse thickening or collapse of capillary walls. Some glomeruli may be completely sclerosed. The mesangium demonstrates a variable increase in matrix, resulting in focal areas of sclerosis. These changes may be associated with periglomerular fibrosis. Immunofluorescence microscopy reveals granular deposits of IgM and C3 along the capillary walls or in areas of sclerosis.[343, 352] IgG is found less frequently; it is often associated with the presence of albumin.

CHRONIC TRANSPLANT GLOMERULOPATHY. Transplant glomerulopathy can occur as early as the first few months after transplantation.[355, 356] It is associated with proteinuria, which can be progressive and which can reach nephrotic range.[343, 353, 355, 356]

The glomeruli are enlarged, they may appear hypercellular, and they commonly show thickening of their walls or lobular simplification of their tufts (Fig. 29–71). The glomerular capillary walls often demonstrate diffuse or focal double contours or tram tracks in silver stains (Fig. 29–72). These glomerular changes can easily be misinterpreted as membranous or mesangiocapillary glomerulonephritis, and they often lead to consideration of recurrent or de novo glomerulonephritis in the differential diagnosis.

By electron microscopy, the thickening of the glomerular capillary walls is due to widening of the subendothelial zone by granular or filamentous electron-dense material or membrane-bound structures, suggestive of cytoplasmic fragments and cellular debris (Fig. 29–73). Extensive electron-dense deposits

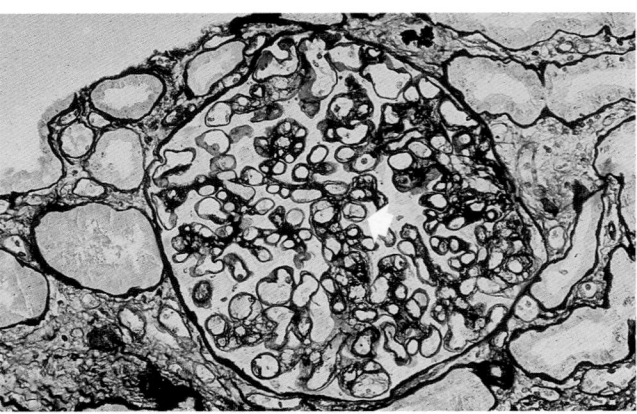

FIGURE 29–72. Renal transplant, chronic transplant glomerulopathy: Glomerulus shows thickening and double contours (*arrow*) along some capillary walls (PAMS).

(immune-complex type) are not seen; if present, they should raise the possibility of recurrent or de novo glomerulonephritis. The double contour lesion appears as partial or circumferential subendothelial interposition of mesangial cells and matrix. It does not contain substantial numbers of subendothelial deposits.

By immunofluorescence microscopy, granular deposits of IgM are seen in the mesangium and occasionally along glomerular capillary walls. Deposits of C3 are seen in the vessel walls and occasionally in the mesangium as well. In rare instances, IgG may be seen in the mesangium or capillary wall.[343, 355]

CHRONIC VASCULAR REJECTION. The vascular changes are those of a progressive obliterative arteriopathy (Fig. 29–74). The arteries are thickened due to a combination of intimal widening, subintimal fibrosis, reduplication of elastica, and hyaline changes. The arterioles are thickened and they often show hyaline changes. These glomerular and vascular changes are associated with interstitial fibrosis of

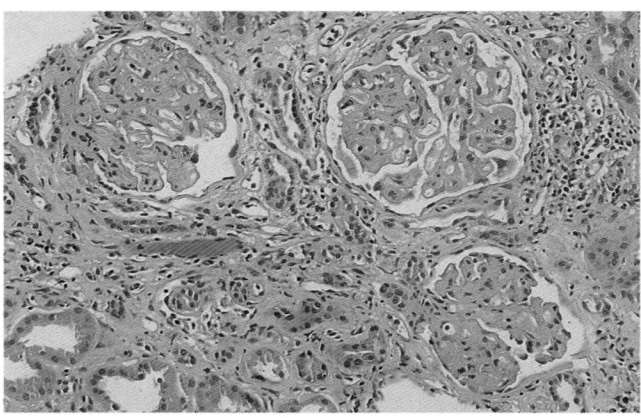

FIGURE 29–71. Renal transplant, chronic transplant glomerulopathy: The glomeruli show thickening of capillary walls.

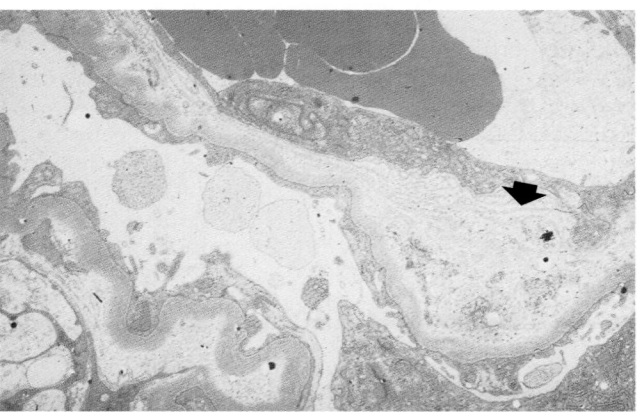

FIGURE 29–73. Renal transplant, chronic transplant glomerulopathy: In this electron micrograph, the capillary basement membranes show subendothelial widening containing fibrillar material (*arrow*).

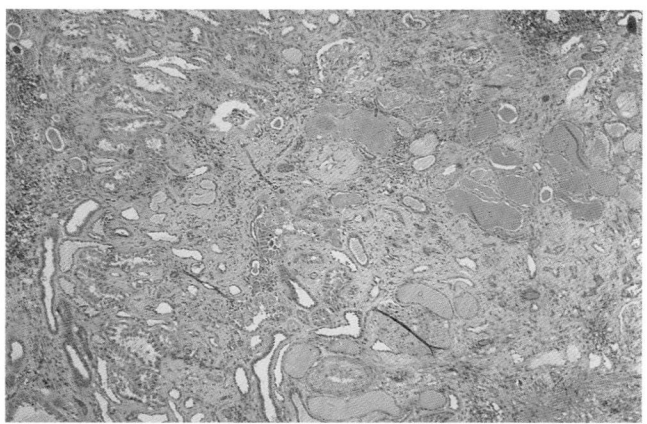

**FIGURE 29–74.** Renal transplant, chronic rejection: There is extensive interstitial fibrosis, tubular loss, and glomerular and vascular sclerosis associated with interstitial inflammatory cell infiltrates.

variable extent, tubular atrophy, and interstitial infiltration of lymphocytes and plasma cells.

## Drug Toxicity

A number of drugs used in immunosuppression of renal transplants can cause toxicity to the kidney as well.

### CYCLOSPORINE

Since the 1980s, cyclosporine, a lymphokine synthesis inhibitor, has been routinely used as an immunosuppressive agent in organ transplantation. There have been a number of studies to evaluate the toxic effects of the drug, especially on the kidney.[357–360]

The morphologic changes predominantly involve the vascular and tubulointerstitial components of the kidney. The vascular changes commonly affect arterioles and small arteries. The endothelium is hypertrophied with a picket fence appearance. There may be subintimal edema or mucoid change narrowing the lumen or subintimal eosinophilic granular material widening the vessel wall (Fig. 29–75). Hyaline arteriolar change, when present, is similar to the hyaline arteriolosclerosis associated with hypertension. Another abnormality that can occur is circular deposition of hyaline-type granular material in muscle cells, forming a beaded appearance.[357] This finding can also be seen in patients with hypertension who are not receiving cyclosporine.

Tubular changes are generally patchy and include isometric tubular vacuolization, microcalcification, and tubular epithelial cell inclusions (see Fig. 29–75). The isometric vacuolization is composed of intracytoplasmic vacuoles of uniform size, devoid of lipid, and probably occurring as a result of dilatation of smooth endoplasmic reticulum. These intracytoplasmic inclusions are commonly seen in the proximal convoluted tubules. Electron microscopy reveals giant mitochondria and phagolysosomes that are often as large as the nuclei of the tubular epithelial cells. With improved management of cyclosporine dosage, tubular lesions have become less frequent.

Microcalcification may be seen throughout the parenchyma, but it is infrequent. Another finding of interest is striped fibrosis, zones of interstitial fibrosis alternating with areas of relatively normal parenchyma. These scarred areas correspond to zones fed by thickened blood vessels.

Glomerular abnormalities resembling those of HUS, as well as arterial thrombi, have been described in cases of cyclosporine toxicity, but they are infrequent.[357, 361]

Overall, the changes associated with cyclosporine toxicity or effect are nonspecific, being similar to those seen in a variety of conditions affecting the kidney. Therefore, in a renal transplant biopsy with histologic alterations due to rejection, a conclusive diagnosis of cyclosporine toxicity is often difficult to make without clinical correlation.

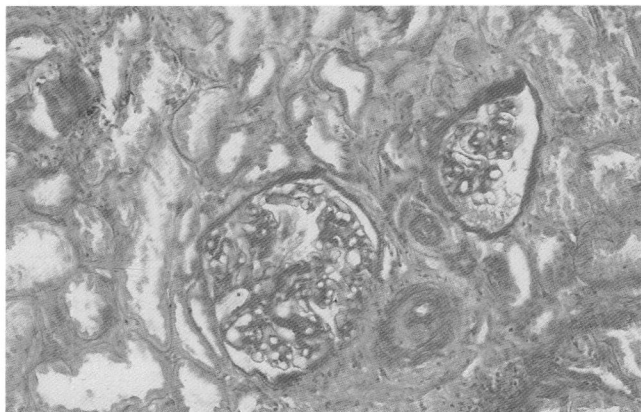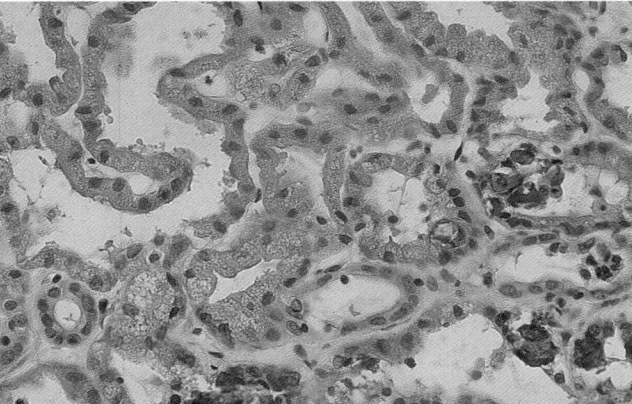

**FIGURE 29–75.** Renal transplant, cyclosporine effect: The arterioles are thickened by granular and mucoid change, with marked narrowing of the lumina (PAS stain, *left*). Tubules show isometric vacuolization and calcification (H&E, *right*).

## TACROLIMUS (FK506)

FK506 is a macrolide immunosuppressant that inhibits cytokine gene transcription in a manner identical to cyclosporine. The side effects of FK506 are similar to those of cyclosporine, but the drugs are structurally unrelated compounds. The parallelism observed in their nephrotoxicity suggests that the interactions of these drugs with renal tissue involve different initial mechanisms that ultimately activate the same final metabolic pathway.[362]

Acute adverse side effects of tacrolimus include headache, nausea, vomiting, diarrhea, pruritus, tremor, abdominal pain, and impairment of renal function.[363-365] The renal toxic effects are similar to those of cyclosporine, with tubular vacuolization, myocyte vacuolization, hyaline arteriolar sclerosis, chronic tubulointerstitial changes with striped interstitial fibrosis, and reduction in the glomerular filtration rate. HUS and necrotizing arteriopathy are also associated with both drugs.[366]

Development of diabetes mellitus in nondiabetic patients is an important side effect with both cyclosporine and FK506; however, it is more pronounced with FK506.[363, 367] FK506 can induce early changes of diabetic glomerulosclerosis, occasionally with development of nodular lesions within a year of transplantation.

## Recurrent and De Novo Diseases

A variety of diseases affecting the kidney recur in transplanted kidneys, and they may or may not be associated with clinical symptoms. Similar to the native kidney, any disease can affect a functioning renal transplant.[343, 351, 353, 361] The true rate of recurrence of renal diseases in transplants is unknown because (1) in many patients, the original disease is unknown; (2) transplant biopsy is often not performed because symptoms are construed to be secondary to rejection; (3) biopsy of the donor kidney (post-anastomosis biopsy) to establish the absence of glomerular disease is often not performed; and (4) on many occasions, the transplant biopsy is performed at an advanced stage of disease when other histologic lesions secondary to rejection or drugs overlap and obscure the histologic changes of recurrent disease.[343, 351, 353, 361] Some diseases, such as dense deposit disease or mesangiocapillary glomerulonephritis type 2 (MPGN type II) and diabetes, have a high incidence of recurrence in renal allografts, but they do not cause major clinical symptoms. By contrast, other diseases, such as mesangiocapillary glomerulonephritis type 1 (MPGN type I) and focal segmental glomerulosclerosis, have a lower incidence of recurrence, but they cause distinct clinical symptoms in the early post-transplant period, producing significant problems in the management and survival of transplants.

The histologic changes of recurrent diseases may or may not be associated with changes of rejection. De novo glomerulonephritis in the transplant is less common than recurrent glomerulonephritis and acute and chronic transplant glomerulopathies. Any disease that can affect the native kidney can also occur as a de novo disease in the transplant, but membranous glomerulopathy is by far the most common glomerulopathy to recur. The diagnosis of de novo disease in a transplant can be made only when the transplant disease is histologically different from the original renal disease and when the transplant disease is not due to acute or chronic rejection.[343, 351, 353, 361] Detailed accounts of various diseases recurrent or de novo in the transplanted kidney are available elsewhere.[343, 351, 353, 361] Study of sequential biopsies of the recurrent disease allows evaluation of histologic progression, and it can help to gain insight into the earliest histologic changes of a lesion and possibly into the pathogenesis of renal diseases.

## Banff Classification

In 1993, the Banff working classification of the pathology of kidney transplants was published.[345] It established a schema to grade and standardize the nomenclature describing the histologic changes in renal transplants. Two histologic changes, tubulitis and intimal arteritis, were established as the diagnostic criteria for acute rejection. Interstitial inflammatory cell infiltration, a common finding in rejection, which had been used previously for grading the severity of rejection, was not considered a useful marker due to the likelihood of sampling error. Similarly, the Banff classification did not incorporate glomerulitis as a definite feature of rejection.

A revision of the Banff classification was proposed in 1996 (Table 29-16).[354] It included interstitial inflammation as an additional criterion, with changes made to make the classification compatible with the simplified system used in the National Institutes of Health–sponsored collaborative clinical trial (CCTT).[344, 354] The CCTT schema divides rejection into three types: (1) tubulointerstitial; (2) vascular with intimal arteritis; and (3) vascular with fibrinoid necrosis or transmural arteritis.[368] Although this classification may bring uniformity to the nomenclature of renal transplant pathology, many factors need to

**TABLE 29-16.** Revised (1997) Banff Classification for Acute Renal Allograft Rejection[354]

| Grade | Finding |
| --- | --- |
| Suspicious | 10% of cortex has tubulointerstitial inflammation with tubulitis |
| Type I (a and b) | >25% of cortex shows tubulointerstitial inflammation with tubulitis |
| Type II (a and b) | Endarteritis (arterial mononuclear endothelial inflammation) |
| Type III | Fibrinoid necrosis/transmural inflammation |

be considered in the interpretation of renal transplant biopsies. These factors include (1) the focal nature of the lesions (sampling error); (2) the presence of histologic changes without clinical signs of rejection; (3) the changing or dynamic nature of histologic findings during the life of a transplant; (4) the use of various therapeutic agents and their effect on the transplant; (5) infections; (6) the presence of recurrent or de novo disease; and (7) the frequent lack of a baseline post-anastomosis biopsy. These factors play a role in establishing the overall final diagnosis, and they often prevent objective classification, requiring evaluation of transplant biopsies on an individual case basis.

In conclusion, kidney transplant biopsy still remains an important tool to diagnose rejection, but evaluation of transplant biopsy has become more complex due to a variety of factors that affect and alter renal morphology.

### Acknowledgments

*We thank Mr. Joseph Rosamont for the excellent electron micrographs, Dr. Sam Michaels for assistance in references, and the Department of Scientific Illustrations for their assistance in photography.*

## REFERENCES

1. Glassberg KI, Stephens FD, Lebowitz RI, et al: Renal dysgenesis and cystic diseases of the kidney: A report of the Committee of Terminology, Nomenclature and Classification, Section on Urology, American Academy of Pediatrics. J Urol 139:1085–1092, 1987.
2. Gabow PA: Autosomal dominant polycystic kidney disease. N Engl J Med 329:332–342, 1993.
3. Grantham JJ: Polycystic kidney disease: hereditary and acquired. Adv Intern Med 38:409–420, 1993.
4. Kimberling WJ, Kumar S, Gabow PA, et al: Autosomal dominant polycystic kidney disease: localization of the second gene to chromosome 4q13-q23. Genomics 18:467–472, 1993.
5. Michel B, Milner Y, David K: Preservation of tissue-fixed immunoglobulins in skin biopsies of patients with lupus erythematosus and bullous diseases—preliminary report. J Invest Dermatol 59:449–452, 1972
6. Mostofi FK, Antonovych TT, Limas E: Patterns of glomerular reaction to injury. Hum Pathol 2:233–252, 1971.
7. Hricik DE, Chung-Park M, Cedor JR: Medical progress: glomerulonephritis. N Engl J Med 339:888–899, 1998.
8. Munk F: Die Nephrosen. Med Klin 12:1019, 1946.
9. Korbet SM, Schwartz MM, Lewis EJ: Minimal change glomerulopathy of adulthood. Am J Nephrol 8:291–297, 1988.
10. Churg J, Habib R, White R: Pathology of the nephrotic syndrome in children: a report of the International Study of Kidney Disease in Children. Lancet 760:1299–1302, 1970.
11. Primary nephrotic syndrome in children: clinical significance of histopathologic variants of minimal change and diffuse mesangial hypercellularity. A report of the International Study of Kidney Disease in Children. Kidney Int 20:765–771, 1981.
12. Ghosh L, Muehrcke RC: The nephrotic syndrome: a prodrome to lymphoma. Ann Intern Med 72:379–382, 1970.
13. Hyman LR, Burkholder PM, Joo PA, et al: Malignant lymphoma and nephrotic syndrome: A clinicopathologic analysis with light, immunofluorescence, and electron microscopy of the renal lesions. J Pediatr 82:207–212, 1973.
14. Warren GV, Korbet SM, Schwartz MM, et al: Minimal change glomerulopathy associated with nonsteroidal anti-inflammatory drugs. Am J Kidney Dis 13:129–130, 1989.
15. Sabbah DM, Bonneau JC, Le Sellin J: Renal complications due to desensitization. Allerg Immunol (Paris) 18:17–19, 1986.
16. Cuoghi D, Venturi P, Cheli E: Bee sting and relapse of nephrotic syndrome. Child Nephrol Urol 9:82–83, 1988–89.
17. Cohen AH, Border W, Glassock RJ: Nephrotic syndrome with glomerular mesangial IgM deposits. Lab Invest 38:610–619, 1978.
18. Saha H, Mustonen J, Pasternak A, et al: Clinical follow up of 564 patients with IgM nephropathy. Am J Nephrol 9:124–128, 1989.
19. Murphy WM, Jukkola AF, Roy S: Nephrotic syndrome with mesangial cell proliferation in children—a distinct entity. Am J Clin Pathol 72:42–47, 1979.
20. Waldherr R, Gubler MC, Levy M, et al: The significance of pure diffuse mesangial proliferation in idiopathic nephrotic syndrome. Clin Nephrol 10:171–179, 1978.
21. Rich, AR: A hitherto undescribed vulnerability of the juxtamedullary glomeruli in lipoid nephrosis. Bull Johns Hopkins Hosp 100:173–186, 1957.
22. Habib R, Gubler MC: Les lesions glomerulaires focales des syndromes nephrotiques idiopathiques de l'enfant. Apropos de 49 observations. Nephron 8:382–401, 1971.
23. Habib R: Focal glomerular sclerosis. Kidney Int 4:355–361, 1973.
24. McGovern VJ: Persistant nephrotic syndrome: a renal biopsy study. Australasia Ann Med 13:306–312, 1964.
25. Beaufils H, Alphonse JC, Guedon J, et al: Focal glomerulosclerosis: natural history and treatment. A report of 70 cases. Nephron 21:75–85, 1978.
26. Border WA: Distinguishing minimal-change disease from mesangial disorders. Kidney Int 18:419–434, 1988.
27. Rao TK, Filippone EJ, Nicastri AD, et al: Associated focal and segmental glomerulosclerosis in the acquired immunodeficiency syndrome. N Engl J Med 310:669–673, 1984.
28. Schwartz MM, Korbet SM: Primary focal segmental glomerulosclerosis: pathology, histologic variants, and pathogenesis. Am J Kidney Dis 22:874–883, 1993.
29. Schwartz MM: Nephrotic syndrome and proteinuria. In Silva FG, D'Agati VD, Nadasdy T (eds): Renal Biopsy Interpretation. New York, Churchill Livingstone, 1996, pp 115–146.
30. Bariety J, Nochy D, Jacquot C, et al: Diversity and unity of focal segmental glomerular sclerosis. In Grunfeld JP, Bach JF, Kreis H, Maxwell MH (eds): Advances in Nephrology. St. Louis, Mosby, 1998.
31. Nagata M, Hattori M, Hamano Y, et al: Origin and phenotypic features of hyperplastic epithelial cells in collapsing glomerulopathy. Am J Kidney Dis 32:962–969, 1998.
32. Howie A, Brewer D: Further studies on the glomerular tip lesion: early and late stages and life table analysis. J Pathol 147:245–255, 1985.
33. Cohen AH, Sun NC, Shapshak P, et al: Demonstration of human immunodeficiency virus in renal epithelium in HIV-associated nephropathy. Mod Pathol 2:125–128, 1989.
34. Kimmel PL, Ferreira-Centeno A, Farkas-Szallasi T, et al: Viral DNA in microdissected renal biopsy tissue from HIV-infected patients with nephrotic syndrome. Kidney Int 43:1347–1352, 1993.
35. Mallick NP: The pathogenesis of minimal change nephropathy. Clin Nephrol 7:87–95, 1977.
36. Michael AF, Blau E, Vernier RL, et al: Glomerular polyanion. Alteration in aminonucleoside nephrosis. Lab Invest 23:649–657, 1970.
37. Michael AF: Immunologic mechanism in renal disease. In Robinson RR (ed): Nephrology I. Proceedings of the IX International Congress of Nephrology. New York, Springer-Verlag, 1984, pp 485–503.
38. Farquar MG, Lemkin MC, Jennifer JL: Role of proteoglycans in glomerular function and pathology. In Robinson RR (ed): Nephrology I. Proceedings of the IX International Congress of Nephrology. New York, Springer-Verlag, 1984, pp 580–600.
39. Ordonez NG, Rosai J: Urinary Tract. In Rosai J (ed): Ackerman's Surgical Pathology. 8th ed. St. Louis, Mosby, pp 1059–1184.
40. Gluck MC, Gallo G, Lowenstein J, et al: Membranous glomerulonephritis; evolution of clinical and pathologic features. Ann Intern Med 78:1–11, 1973.

41. Berger J, Michielsen P, Galle P: Les syndrome nephrotiques avec depots intermembranou-epitheliaux. J Urol Nephrol (Paris) 67:52–57, 1961.
42. Tornroth T: Membranous glomerulonephritis. *In* Rosen S (ed): Pathology of Glomerular Disease. New York, Churchill Livingstone, 1983, pp 125–150.
43. Rosen S: Membranous glomerulonephritis: current status. Hum Pathol 2:209–231, 171.
44. Donadio JV, Torres VE, Velosa JA, et al: Idiopathic membranous nephropathy. The natural history of untreated patients. Kidney Int 33:708–715, 1988.
45. Schieppati A, Mosconi, L, Perna A, et al: Prognosis of untreated patients with idiopathic membranous nephropathy. N Engl J Med 329:85–89, 1993.
46. Bhorade MS, Carag HG, Lee HJ, et al: Nephropathy of secondary syphilis: a clinical and pathological spectrum. JAMA 216:1159–1166, l971.
47. Hill LL, Singer DB, Falletta J, et al: The nephrotic syndrome in congenital syphilis: an immunopathy. Pediatrics 49:260–266, 1972.
48. Guerra IL, Abraham AA, Kimmel PL, et al: Nephrotic syndrome associated with chronic persistent hepatitis B in an HIV antibody positive patient. Am J Kidney Dis 10:335–388, 1987.
49. Gonzalez-Dettoni H, Tron J: Membranous glomerulopathy in sytemic lupus erythematosus. Adv Nephrol Necker Hosp 14:347–364, 1985.
50. Schwartz MM, Kawala K, Roberts JL, et al: Clinical and pathological features of membranous glomerulonephritis of systemic lupus erythematosus. Am J Nephrol 4:301–311, 1984
51. Antonovych TT: Gold nephropathy. Ann Clin Lab Sci 11:386–391, 1981.
52. Eagen JW, Lewis EJ: Editorial review: glomerulopathies of neoplasia. Kidney Int 11:297–306, 1977.
53. Morel-Moroger Striker L, Striker GE: Glomerular lesions in malignancies. Contrib Nephrol 48:111–124, 1985.
54. Jones DB: Nephrotic glomerulonephritis. Am J Pathol 33:313–330, 1957.
55. Llach F, Arieff AI, Massry SG: Renal vein thrombosis and the nephrotic syndrome. A prospective study of 36 adult patients. Ann Intern Med 83:8–14, 1975.
56. Ehrenreich T, Churg J: Pathology of membranous nephropathy. *In* Sommers S (ed): Pathology Annual. New York, Appleton-Century-Croft, 1968, pp 145–186.
57. Davies DR, Tighe JR, Wing AJ, et al: Immunoglobulin deposition in membranous glomerulonephritis: immunofluorescence and immunoelectron microscopy findings. Histopathology 1:39–52, 1977.
58. Germuth FGJ, Rodriquez E: Immunopathology of the Renal Glomerulus. Boston, Little, Brown, 1973.
59. Moorthy AV, Zimmerman SW, Burkholder PM, et al: Association of crescentic glomerulonephritis with membranous glomerulonephropathy: a report of three cases. Clin Nephrol 6:319–325, 1976.
60. Klassen J, Elwood C, Grossberg AL, et al: Evolution of membranous nephropathy into anti-glomerular-basement-membrane glomerulonephritis. N Engl J Med 290:1340–1344, 1974.
61. Cheong IK, Chong SM, Singh N, et al: Extensive crescent formation in idiopathic membranous glomerulonephritis. A case report. Med J Malasia 36:8–10, 1981.
62. Honig C, Mouradian JA, Montoliu J, et al: Mesangial electron-dense deposits in membranous nephropathy. Lab Invest 42:427–432, 1980.
63. Sabnis SG, Ross WB, Bratthauer GL: Presence of CD30 (Ki-1) antibodies in membranous glomerulopathy (MG): a useful marker? (Abstract). Lab Invest 76:179A, 1997.
64. Cameron JS: Pathogenesis and treatment of membranous nephropathy. Kidney Int 15:88–103, 1979.
65. Abrass CK, Hall CL, Border WA, et al: Circulating immune complexes in adults with idiopathic nephrotic syndrome. Collaborative study of the adult nephrotic syndrome. Kidney Int 17:545–553, 1980
66. Friedman J, Van de Rijn I, Ohkuni H, et al: Immunological studies of post-streptococcal sequelae. Evidence for presence of streptococcal antigens in circulating immune complexes. J Clin Invest 74:1027–1034, 1984.
67. Treser G, Ehrenreich T, Ores R, et al: Antigenic streptococcal components in acute glomerulonephritis. Science 163:676–677, 1969.
68. Baldwin DS, Gluck MC, Schacht RG, et al: The long term course of poststreptococcal glomerulonephritis. Ann Intern Med 80:342–358, 1974.
69. Cameron JS: Bright's disease today. The pathogenesis and treatment of glomerulonephritis I. Br Med J 4:87–90, 1972.
70. Cameron JS: Bright's disease today. The pathogenesis and treatment of glomerulonephritis II. Br Med J 4:160–163, 1972.
71. Balow J, Austin H, Boumpas D: Immunologic renal diseases. *In* Rich R (ed): Clinical Immunology: Principles and Practice. Boston, Mosby, 1996, pp 1444–1462.
72. Dunn JS: The fundamental lesion in acute diffuse intracapillary glomerulonephritis. J Pathol Bacteriol 51:169–188, 1940.
73. McClusky RT, Vassalli P, Gallo G, et al: An immunofluorescent study of pathogenetic mechanisms in glomerular diseases. N Engl J Med 274:695–701, 1966.
74. Striker G, Striker LJ, D'Agati V: The Renal Biopsy: Major Problems in Pathology. Philadelphia, WB Saunders, 1997.
75. Watson AR, Poucell S, Thorner P, et al: Membranoproliferative glomerulonephritis type I in children: correlation of clinical features with pathologic subtypes. Am J Kidney Dis 4:141–146, 1984.
76. Cameron JS, Glasgow EF, Ogg CS, et al: Membranoproliferative glomerulonephritis and persistent hypocomplementemia. Br Med J 4:7–14, 1970.
77. Mandalenakis N, Mendoza N, Pirani CL, et al: Lobular glomerulonephritis and membranoproliferative glomerulonephritis. Medicine 50:319–355, 1971.
78. Strife CE, Jackson EC, McAdams AJ: Type III membranoproliferative glomerulonephritis: long-term clinical and morphologic evaluation. Clin Nephrol 21:323–334, 1984.
79. Anders, D: Membranoproliferative glomerulonephritis (MPGN): morphogenesis of the type III lesion. (Abstract). Kidney Int 28:259, 1985
80. Lamb V, Tisher CC, McCly RC: Membranoproliferative glomerulonephritis with dense intramembranous alterations (a clinico-pathologic study). Lab Invest 36:607–617, 1977.
81. Antoine B, Faye C: The clinical course associated with dense deposits in the kidney basement membrane. Kidney Int 1:420–427, 1972
82. Scully RE: Case records of the Massachusetts General Hospital. N Engl J Med 297:713–720, 1976
83. Habib R, Gubler MC, Loriat C: Dense deposit disease: A variant of membranoproliferative glomerulonephritis. Kidney Int 7:204–215, 1975
84. Donadio JV, Slack TK, Holley KE: Idiopathic membranoproliferative (mesangiocapillary) glomerulonephritis: a clinico-pathologic study. Mayo Clin Proc 54:141–150, 1979.
85. Eisinger AJ, Shorter JR, Moorhead PJ: Renal disease in partial lipodystrophy. Q J Med 41:343–354, 1972.
86. Sibley RK, Kim Y: Dense intramembranous deposit disease: new pathologic features. Kidney Int 25:660–670, 1984.
87. Berger J, Hinglais N: Les depots intercapillaries d'IgA-IgG. J Urol Nephrol 74:694–695, 1968.
88. Emancipator SN: IgA nephropathy: morphologic expression and pathogenesis. Current concepts in renal pathology. Am J Kidney Dis 23:451–462, 1994.
89. Clarkson AR, Woodroffe AJ, Bannister KM, et al: The syndrome of IgA nephropathy. Clin Nephrol 21:7–14, 1984.
90. Rose BD, Jacobs JB: Nephrotic syndrome and glomerulonephritis. *In* Rose BD (ed): Pathophysiology of Renal Disease. 2nd ed. New York, McGraw-Hill, 1987, pp 179–296.
91. Couser WG: Idiopathic rapidly progressive glomerulonephritis. Am J Kidney Dis 2:57–69, 1982.
92. Jennette JC, Falk RJ, Andrassy K, et al: Nomenclature of systemic vasculitides. Proposal of an international consensus conference. Arthritis Rheum 37:187–192, 1994.
93. Cameron JS: Lupus nephritis. J Am Soc Nephrol 10:413–424, 1999.

94. Pollack VE, Pirani CL: Renal histologic findings in systemic lupus erythematosus. Mayo Clin Proc 44:630–644, 1969.

95. Jennette JC, Iskandar SS, Daldorf FG: Pathologic differentiation between lupus and nonlupus membranous glomerulopathy. Kidney Int 24:337–385, 1983.

96. D'Agati, VD: Systemic lupus erythematosus. In Silva FG, D'Agati VD, Nadasdy T (eds): Renal Biposy Interpretation. New York, Churchill Livingstone, 1997, pp 181–220.

97. Churg J, Sobin LH: Renal Disease: Classification and Atlas of Glomerular Diseases. Tokyo, Ikagu-Shoin, 1982.

98. Burkholder PM, Hyman LR, Barber TA: Extracellular clusters of spherical microparticles in glomeruli in human renal glomerular diseases. Lab Invest 28:415–425, 1973.

99. Mahajan SK, Ordonez NG, Spargo BH, et al: Changing histopathology patterns in lupus nephropathy. Clin Nephrol 10:1–8, 1978.

100. Austin HA, Muenz LR, Joyce KM, et al: Prognostic factors in lupus nephritis. Contribution of renal histologic data. Am J Med 75:382–391, 1983.

101. Austin HA, Boumpas DT, Vaughan EM, et al: Predicting renal outcome in severe lupus nephritis: contributions of clinical histologic data. Kidney Int 45:544–550, 1994.

102. Bhathena DB, Sobel BJ, Migdal SD: Non-inflammatory renal microangiopathy of systemic lupus erythematosus ("lupus vasculitis"). Am J Nephrol 1:144–159, 1981.

103. Love PE, Santoro SA: Antiphospholipid antibodies: anticardiolipin and the lupus anticoagulant in SLE and in non-SLE disorders. Ann Intern Med 112:682–698, 1990.

104. Li L, Liu Z, Zhang J: Circulating antibodies to neutrophil cytoplasmic antigens in patients with Henoch-Schönlein purpura and IgA nephropathy. J Am Soc Nephrol 3:599–604, 1991.

105. Goldstein AR, White RH, Akuse R, et al: Long-term follow-up of childhood Henoch-Schönlein nephritis. Lancet 339:280–282, 1992.

106. Niaudet P, Murcia I, Beaufils H, et al: Primary IgA nephropathies in children: prognosis and treatment. Adv Nephrol Necker Hosp 22:121–140, 1993.

107. Glasgow EF: Renal changes in Henoch-Schönlein purpura. Arch Dis Child 45:151, 1970.

108. Meadows SR, Glasgow EF, White RHR, et al: Schönlein-Henoch nephritis. Q J Med 41:241–258, 1972.

109. Ballard HS, Eisinger RP, Gallo G: Renal manifestations of the Henoch-Schönlein syndrome in adults. Am J Med 49:328–335, 1970.

110. Montseny JJ, Meyrier A, Kleinknecht D, et al: The current spectrum of infectious glomerulonephritis. Experience with 76 patients and review of literature. Medicine 74:63–73, 1995.

111. Beaufils M, Gibert C, Morel-Maroger L, et al: Glomerulonephritis in severe bacterial infections with and without endocarditis. Adv Nephrol Necker Hosp 7:217–234, 1977.

112. Morel-Maroger L, Sraer JD, Herreman G, et al: Kidney in subacute bacterial endocarditis: pathological and immunofluorescent findings. Arch Pathol 94:205–213, 1972.

113. Neugarten J, Gallo GR, Baldwin DS: Glomerulonephritis in bacterial endocarditis. Am J Kidney Dis 3:371–379, 1984.

114. Neugarten J, Baldwin DS: Glomerulonephritis in bacterial endocarditis. Am J Med 77:297–304, 1984.

115. Bennett PH, Haffner S, Kasiske BL, et al: Screening and management of microalbuminuria in patients with diabetes mellitus: Recommendations to the Scientific Advisory Board of the National Kidney Foundation from an Ad Hoc Committee of the Council on Diabetes Mellitus of the National Kidney Foundation. Am J Kidney Dis 25:107–112, 1995.

116. Kimmelstiel P, Wilson C: Intercapillary lesions in the glomeruli of the kidney. Am J Pathol 12:83–98, 1936.

117. Spuhler O: Die diabetische glomerulosklerose. Helvet Med Acta 11:27–30, 1944.

118. Beyer-Mears A: The polyol pathway, sorbinil and renal dysfunction. Metabolism 35 (4 suppl 1):46–54, 1986.

119. Vlassara H, Bucala R, Striker L: Biology of disease. Pathogenic effects of advanced glycosylation: biochemical, biologic, and clinical implications of diabetes and aging. Lab Invest 70:138–151, 1994.

120. Levi DF, Willams RC, Lindstrom FD: Immunofluorescent studies of the myeloma kidney with special reference to light chain disease. Am J Med 44:922–933, 1968.

121. Cohen AH, Border WA: Myeloma kidney: an immunomorphogenetic study of renal biopsies. Lab Invest 42:248–256, 1980.

122. Pirani CL, Silva FG, D'Agati V, et al: Renal lesions in plasma cell dyscrasias: ultrastructural observations. Am J Kidney Dis 10:208–221, 1987.

123. Koss MN, Pirani CL, Osserman EF: Experimental Bence Jones cast nephropathy. Lab Invest 34:579–591, 1976.

124. Papadimitriou JM, Matz LR: Origin of multinucleated giant cells in myeloma kidney from mononuclear phagocytes: an ultrastructural study. Pathology 11:583–593, 1979.

125. Sandres PW, Herreras GA, Kirk KA, et al: Spectrum of glomerular and tubulointerstitial renal lesions associated with monotypical immunoglobulin light chain deposition. Lab Invest 64:527–537, 1991.

126. Factor SM, Winn RM, Biempica L: The histocytic origin of multinucleated giant cells in myeloma kidney. Hum Pathol 9:114–120, 1978.

127. Neumann V: Multiple plasma cell myeloma with crystalline deposits in the tumor cells and in the kidney. J Pathol Bacteriol 61:165–169, 1949.

128. Sickel GW: Crystalline glomerular deposits in multiple myeloma. Am J Med 27:354–356, 1959.

129. Glenner GG: Amyloid deposits and amyloidosis: the beta-fibrilloses (second of two parts). N Engl J Med 302:1333–1344, 1980.

130. Watanabe T, Saniter T: Morphological and clinical features of renal amyloidosis. Virchows Arch A Pathol Anat Histopathol 366:125–135, 1975.

131. Isobe T, Osserman EF: Patterns of amyloidosis and their association with plasma cell dyscrasias, monoclonal immunoglobulins and Bence Jones proteins. N Engl J Med 290:473–477, 1974.

132. Browning MJ, Banks RA, Tribe CR, et al: Ten years' experience of an amyloid clinic—a clinicopathologic survey. Q J Med 215:213–227, 1985.

133. Sohar E, Gafni J, Pras M, et al: Familial Mediterranean fever. A survey of 470 cases and a review of literature. Am J Med 43:227–253, 1967.

134. Nolting SF, Campbell WG: Subepithelial argyrophilic spicular structures in renal amyloidosis: an aid in diagnosis. Hum Pathol 12:724–734, 1981.

135. Gallo G, Kumar A: Hematopoietic disorders. In Silva FG, D'Agati VD, Nadasdy T (eds): Renal Biopsy Interpretation. New York, Churchill Livingstone, 1996, pp 259–282.

136. Puchtler H, Sweat F, Levine M: On the binding of Congo red by amyloid. J Histochem Cytochem 10:355–364, 1962.

137. Wright JR, Calkin, E, Humphrey RL: Potassium permanganate reaction in amyloidosis. Lab Invest 36:274–281, 1977.

138. Noel LH, Droz GD: Immunohistochemical characterization of renal amyloidosis. Am J Clin Pathol 87:756–761, 1987.

139. Gallo GR, Feiner HD, Chuba JV, et al: Characterization of tissue amyloid by immunofluorescence microscopy. Clin Immunol Immunopathol 39:479–490, 1986.

140. Rosenmann E, Eliakim M: Nephrotic syndrome associated with amyloid-like glomerular deposits. Nephron 18:301–308, 1977.

141. Alpers CE, Renke GH, Hopper J: Fibrillary glomerulonephritis: an entity with unusual immunofluorescence features. Kidney Int 31:781–789, 1987.

142. Schwartz MM: Immunotactoid glomerulopathy: the case for Occam's razor. Am J Kid Dis 22:446–447, 1993.

143. Devaney K, Sabnis SG, Antonovych TT: Nonamyloidotic fibrillary glomerulopathy, immunotactoid glomerulopathy, and differential diagnosis of filamentous glomerulopathies. Mod Pathol 4:34–45, 1991.

144. Korbet SM, Schwartz MM, Lewis EJ: Immunotactoid glomerulopathy. Am J Kidney Dis 17:247–257, 1991.

145. Korbet SM, Schwartz MM, Rosenberg BF, et al: Immunotactoid glomerulopathy. Medicine (Baltimore) 64:228–243, 1985.

146. Neill J, Rubin J: Nonamyloidotic fibrillary glomerulopathy. Arch Pathol Lab Med 113:553–555, 1989.

147. Sturgill BC, Bolton WK, Griffith KM: Congo red negative amyloidosis-like glomerulopathy. Hum Pathol 16:220–224, 1985.

148. Fogo A, Qureshi N, Horn RG: Morphologic and clinical features of fibrillary glomerulonephritis versus immunotactoid glomerulopathy. Am J Kid Dis 22:367–377, 1993.

149. Yang GCH, Nieto R: Ultrastructural immunochemical localization of polyclonal IgG, C3 and amyloid P component on the Congo red negative amyloid-like fibrils of fibrillary glomerulopathy. Am J Pathol 141:409–419, 1992.

150. Redman JF, Mobley JE: Hematuria associated with sickle cell disease. J Ark Med Sci 65:110–111, 1968.

151. Strom T, Muehrcke RC, Smith RD: Sickle cell anemia with the nephrotic syndrome and renal vein obstruction. Arch Intern Med 129:104–108, 1972.

152. McCoy RC: Ultrastructural alterations in the kidney of patients with sickle cell disease and nephrotic syndrome. Lab Invest 21:85–95, 1969.

153. Elfenbein IB, Patchefsky A, Schwartz W: Pathology of the glomerulus in sickle cell anemia with and without nephrotic syndrome. Am J Pathol 77:357–374, 1974.

154. Pardo V, Strauss J, Kramer H, et al: Nephropathy associated with sickle cell anemia: an autologous immune complex nephritis. II. Clinicopathologic study of seven patients. Am J Med 59:650–659, 1975.

155. Yoshikawa N, Ito H, Yamada Y, et al: Membranous glomerulonephritis associated with hepatitis B antigen in children: a comparison with idiopathic membranous glomerulonephritis. Clin Nephrol 23:28–34, 1985.

156. Collins AB, Bhan AK, Dienstag JL, et al: Hepatitis B immune complex glomerulonephritis: simultaneous glomerular deposition of hepatitis B surface and e antigens. Clin Immunol Immunopathol 26:137–153, 1983.

157. Johnson RJ, Couser WG: Hepatitis B infection and renal disease: clinical immunopathogenetic and therapeutic considerations. Kidney Int 37:663–676, 1990.

158. Johnson RJ, Gretch DR, Yamabe H, et al: Membranoproliferative glomerulonephritis associated with hepatitis C viral infection. N Engl J Med 328:465–470, 1993.

159. Seney FD, Burns DK, Silva FG: Acquired immunodeficiency syndrome and the kidney. Am J Kidney Dis 16:1–13, 1990.

160. Glassock RJ, Cohen AH, Danovitch G, et al: Human immunodeficiency virus (HIV) infection and the kidney. Ann Intern Med 112:35–49, 1990.

161. Maslo C, Peraldi MN, Desenclos JC, et al: Thrombotic microangiopathy and cytomegalovirus disease in patients infected with human immunodeficiency virus. Clin Infect Dis 24:350–355, 1997.

162. Oritz-Butcher C: The spectrum of kidney diseases in patients with human immunodeficiency virus infection. Curr Opin Nephrol Hypertens 2:355–364, 1993.

163. Gardenswartz MH, Lerner CW, Seligson GR, et al: Renal disease in patients with AIDS. Clin Nephrol 21:197–204, 1984.

164. Pardo V, Aldana M, Colton RM, et al: Glomerular lesions in the acquired immunodeficiency syndrome. Ann Intern Med 101:429–434, 1984.

165. Luu JY, Bockus D, Remington F, et al: Tubuloreticular structures and cylindrical confronting cisternae: a review. Hum Pathol 20:617–627, 1989.

166. Stokes MB, Chawla H, Brody RI, et al: Immune complex glomerulonephritis in patients coinfected with human immunodeficiency virus and hepatitis C virus. Am J Kid Dis 29:514–525, 1997.

167. Contreras G, Green DF, Pardo V, et al: Systemic lupus erythematosus in two adults with human immunodeficiency virus infection. Am J Kid Dis 28:292–295, 1996.

168. Bourgoignie JJ, Ortiz-Interian C, Green DF, et al: A co-factor in HIV-1 associated nephropathy. Transplant Proc 21:3899–3901, 1989.

169. Kopp JB, Ray PF, Adler SA, et al: Nephropathy in HIV-transgenic mice. Contrib Nephrol 107:194–204, 1994.

170. Rappaport J, Kopp JB, Klotman PE: Host-virus interactions and the molecular regulation of HIV-1: Role in the pathogenesis of HIV-associated nephropathy. Kidney Int 46:16–27, 1994.

171. Ray PE, Liu XH, Henry,D, et al: Infection of human primary renal epithelial cells with HIV-1 from children with HIV-associated nephropathy. Kidney Int 53:1217–1229, 1998.

172. Singhal PC, Sharma P, Reddy K, et al: HIV-1 gp 160 envelope protein modulates proliferation and apoptosis in mesangial cells. Nephron 76:284–295, 1997.

173. Alpers C, McClure J, Bursten SL: Human mesangial cells are resistant to productive infection by multiple strains of human immunodeficiency virus types 1 and 2. Am J Kidney Dis 19:126–130, 1992.

174. Christensen WI: Genitourinary tuberculosis; review of 102 cases. Medicine (Baltimore) 53:377–390, 1974.

175. D'Agati, VD, Appel, GB: Polyarteritis nodosa, Wegener's granulomatosis, Churg-Strauss syndrome, temporal arteritis, Takayasu arteritis, and lymphomatoid granulomatosis. *In* Tisher C, Brenner BM (eds): Renal Pathology: With Clinical and Functional Correlations. Philadelphia, JB Lippincott, 1994, pp 1087–1153.

176. Watts RA, Scott DG: Classification and epidemiology of the vasculitides. Baillieres Clin Rheumatol 11:191–217, 1997.

177. Jennette JC, Falk RJ: Small vessel vasculitis. N Engl J Med 337:1512–1523, 1997.

178. Fries JF, Hunder GG, Black DA, et al: The American College of Rheumatology criteria for the classification of vasculitis. Summary. Arthritis Rheum 33:1135–1136, 1990.

179. Lightfoot RW, Michel BA, Bloch, DA, et al: The American College of Rheumatology 1990 criteria for the classification of polyarteritis nodosa. Arthritis Rheum 33:1088–1093, 1990

180. Bruce IN, Bell AN: A comparison of two nomenclature systems for primary systemic vasculitis. Br J Rheumatol 36:453–458, 1997

181. Guillevin L, Lhote F, Amouroux J, et al: Antineutrophil cytoplasmic antibodies, abnormal angiograms and pathological findings in polyarteritis nodosa and Churg-Strauss syndrome: indications for the classification of vasculitides of the polyarteritis nodosa group. Br J Rheumatol 35:958–964, 1996.

182. Falk RJ, Terrell RS, Charles LA, et al: Anti-neutrophil cytoplasmic auto-antibodies induce neutrophils to degranulate and produce oxygen radicals in vitro. Proc Natl Acad Sci U S A 87:4115–4119, 1990.

183. Jennette JC: Renal involvement in systemic vasculitis. *In* Jennette JC, Olson JL, Schwartz MM, Silva FG (eds): Heptinstall's Pathology of the Kidney. 5th ed. Philadelphia, Lippincott-Raven, 1998, pp 1059–1095.

184. Wegener F: Uber generalisierte, septische Gefasserkrankungen. Verh Dtsch Ges Pathol 29:202–210, 1936.

185. Godman G, Churg J: Wegener's granulomatosis: Pathology and review of the literature. Arch Pathol Lab Med 58:533–553, 1954.

186. Carrington CB, Liebow AA: Limited forms of angiitis and granulomatosis of Wegener's type. Am J Med 41:497–527, 1966.

187. Duna GF, Galperin C, Hoffman GS: Wegener's granulomatosis. Rheum Dis Clin North Am 21:949–986, 1995.

188. Halstead LA, Karmody CS, Wolff SM: Presentation of Wegener's granulomatosis in young patients. Otol Head Neck Surg 94:368–371, 1986.

189. Hoffman GS, Kerr GS, Leavitt RY, et al: Wegener's granulomatosis: an analysis of 158 patients. Ann Intern Med 116:488–498, 1992.

190. Gross WL: Antineutrophil cytoplasmic autoantibody testing in vasculitides. Rheum Dis Clin North Am 21:987–1011, 1995.

191. Schmitt WH, Gross WL: Vasculitis in the seriously ill patient: diagnostic approaches and therapeutic options in ANCA-associated vasculitis. Kidney Int 64:S39–44, 1998.

192. Hagen EC, Daha MR, Hermans J, et al: Diagnostic value of standardized assays for anti-neutrophil cytoplasmic antibodies in idiopathic systemic vasculitis. EC/BCR Project for ANCA assay standardization. Kidney Int 53:743–753, 1998.

193. Franssen C, Gans R, Kallenber C, et al: Disease spectrum of patients with antineutrophil cytoplasmic autoantibodies of defined specificity: distinct differences between anti-protein-

ase and anti-myeloperoxidase autoantibodies. J Intern Med 244:209–216, 1998.

194. Fauci AS, Hayes BF, Katz P, et al: Wegener's granulomatosis: prospective clinical and therapeutic experience with 85 patients for 21 years. Ann Intern Med 98:76–85, 1983.

195. Rostaing L, Modesto A, Oksman F, et al: Outcome of patients with antineutrophil cystoplasmic autoantibody-associated vasculitis following cadaveric kidney transplantation. Am J Kidney Dis 29:96–102, 1997.

196. Wolff SM, Fauci AS, Horn RG, et al: Wegener's granulomatosis. Ann Intern Med 81:513–525, 1974.

197. Weiss MA, Crissman JD: Renal biopsy findings in Wegener's granulomatosis: segmental necrotizing glomerulonephritis with glomerular thrombosis. Hum Pathol 1984:943–956, 1984.

198. Weiss MA, Crissman JD: Segmental necrotizing glomerulonephritis: diagnostic, prognostic and therapeutic significance. Am J Kidney Dis 6:199–211, 1985.

199. Rastaldi MP, Ferrario F, Tunesi S, et al: Intraglomerular and interstitial leukocyte infiltration, adhesion molecules, and interleukin-1 alpha expression in 15 cases of antineutrophil cytoplasmic autoantibody–associated renal vasculitis. Am J Kidney Dis 27:48–57, 1996.

200. Pall AA, Howie AJ, Adu D, et al: Glomerular vascular cell adhesion molecule-1 expression in renal vasculitis. J Clin Pathol 49:238–242, 1996.

201. Yaqoob M, West DC, McDicken I, et al: Monitoring of endothelial leucocyte adhesion molecule-1 in anti-neutrophil-cytoplasmic-antibody-positive vasculitis. Am J Nephrol 16:106–113, 1996.

202. Hotta O, Oda, T, Taguma Y, et al: Role of neutrophil elastase in the development of renal necrotizing vasculitis. Clin Nephrol 45:211–216, 1996.

203. Ronco P, Verroust P, Mignon F, et al: Immunopathological studies of polyarteritis nodosa and Wegener's granulomatosis: a report of 43 patients with 51 renal biopsies. Q J Med 206:212–223, 1983.

204. Yoshikawa Y, Watanabe T: Granulomatous glomerulonephritis in Wegener's granulomatosis. Virchows Arch A Pathol Anat Histopathol 402:361–372, 1984.

205. Appel GB, Gee B, Kashgarian M, et al: Wegener's granulomatosis: clinico-pathologic correlations and long-term course. Am J Kidney Dis 1:27–37, 1981.

206. Grotz W, Wanner C, Keller E, et al: Crescentic glomerulonephritis in Wegener's granulomatosis: morphology, therapy, outcome. Clin Nephrol 35:243–251, 1991

207. Watanabe T, Yoshikawa Y: Morphological and clinical features of the kidney in Wegener's granulomatosis. Jpn J Nephrol 32:921–930, 1981

208. Fauci AS, Wolff SM: Wegener's granulomatosis: studies in eighteen patients and a review of the literature. 1973. [classic article.] Medicine (Baltimore) 73:315–324, 1994.

209. Andrassy K, Erb A, Koderisch J, et al: Wegener's granulomatosis with renal involvement: patient survival and correlations between initial renal function, renal histology, therapy, and renal outcome. Clin Nephrol 35:139–147, 1991.

210. Boucher A, Droz D, Adafer E, et al: Relationship between the integrity of Bowman's capsule and the composition of cellular crescents in human crescentic glomerulonephritis. Lab Invest 56:526–533, 1987.

211. Lie JT: Histopathologic specificity of systemic vasculitis. Rheum Dis Clin North Am 21:883–908, 1995.

212. Lhote F, Guillevin L: Polyarteritis nodosa, microscopic polyangiitis, and Churg-Strauss syndrome. Rheum Dis Clin North Am 21:911–946, 1995.

213. Lanham JG, Elkon, KB, Pusey CD, et al: Systemic vasculitis with asthma and eosinophilia: a clinical approach to the Churg-Strauss syndrome. Medicine 63:65–80, 1984.

214. Chumbley LC, Harrison EGJ, DeRemee RA: Allergic granulomatosis and angiitis (Churg-Strauss syndrome). Report and analysis of 30 cases. Mayo Clin Proc 52:477–484, 1977.

215. Clutterbuck EJ, Evans DJ, Pusey CD: Renal involvement in Churg-Strauss syndrome. Nephrol Dial Transplant 5:161–167, 1990.

216. Gaskin G, Clutterbuck EJ, Pusey CD: Renal disease in Churg-Strauss syndrome. Diagnosis, management and outcome. Contrib Nephrol 94:58–65, 1991.

217. Cohen Tervaert JW, Kallenberg CM: Neurologic manifestations of systemic vasculitides. Rheum Dis Clin North Am 19:913–940, 1990.

218. Gross WL, Schmitt WH, Csernok E: Antineutrophil cytoplasmic autoantibody-associated diseases: a rheumatologist's perspective. Am J Kidney Dis 18:175–179, 1991.

219. Guillevin L, Visser H, Noel LH, et al: Antineutrophil cytoplasmic antibodies in systemic polyarteritis nodosa with and without hepatitis B virus infection and Churg-Strauss syndrome—62 patients. J Rheumatol 20:1345–1349, 1993.

220. Churg J, Strauss L: Allergic granulomatosis, allergic angiitis and periarteritis nodosa. Am J Pathol 27:277–301, 1951.

221. Koss MN, Antonovych T, Hochholzer L: Allergic granulomatosis (Churg-Strauss syndrome). Pulmonary and renal morphologic findings. Am J Surg Pathol 5:21–28, 1981.

222. Jessurum J, Azevedo M, Saldana MJ: Allergic angiitis and granulomatosis (Churg-Strauss syndrome). Hum Pathol 17:637–639, 1986.

223. Antiga G, Volpi A, Battini G, et al: Acute renal failure in a patient affected with Churg and Strauss syndrome. Nephron 57:113–114, 1991.

224. Balow JE: Renal vasculitis (nephrology forum). Kidney Int 27:954–964, 1985.

225. Savage CO, Winearls CG, Evans DJ, et al: Microscopic polyarteritis: presentation, pathology and prognosis. Q J Med 56:467–483, 1985.

226. Adu D, Howie AJ, Scott DG, et al: Polyarteritis and the kidney. Q J Med 62:221–237, 1987.

227. Hauschild S, Schmit W, Csernok E: ANCA in systemic vasculitides, collagen vascular disorders, and inflammatory bowel diseases. In Gross WL (ed): ANCA-Associated Vasculitis. New York, Plenum, 1993, pp 245.

228. Kirkland GS, Savige J, Wilson D, et al: Classical polyarteritis nodosa and microscopic polyarteritis with medium vessel involvement—a comparison of the clinical and laboratory features. Clin Nephrol 47:176–180, 1997.

229. Jennette JC, Falk RJ: Antineutrophil cytoplasmic autoantibodies and associated diseases: a review. Am J Kidney Dis 15:517–529, 1990.

230. Guillevin L, Jaronesse B, Lok C, et al: Long-term follow-up after treatment of polyarteritis nodosa and Churg-Strauss angiitis with comparison of steroids, plasma exchange: a prospective randomized trial of 71 patients. J Rheumatol 18:567–574, 1991.

231. D'Agati V, Chander P, Nash M, et al: Idiopathic microscopic polyarteritis nodosa: ultrastructural observations on the renal vascular and glomerular lesions. Am J Kidney Dis 7:95–110, 1986.

232. Inoue M, Akikusa B, Masuda Y, et al: Demonstration of microaneurysms at the interlobular arteries of the kidneys in microscopic polyangiitis: a three-dimensional study. Hum Pathol 29:223–227, 1998.

233. Velosa JA, Homburger HA, Holley KE: Prospective study of anti-neutrophil cytoplasmic autoantibody tests in the diagnosis of idiopathic necrotizing-crescentic glomerulonephritis and renal vasculitis. Mayo Clin Proc 68:561–565, 1993.

234. Kussmaul A, Maier R: Ueber eine bisher micht beshriebene eigenthumliche Arterienerkrankung (periartereritis nodosa) die mit Morbus Brightu und rapid fortschreitender allgemeiner Muskellahmung einhergeht. Dtsch Arch Klin Med 1:484–518, 1866.

235. Conn DL: Polyarteritis. Rheum Dis Clin North Am 16:341–362, 1990.

236. Watts RA, Jolliffe VA, Carruthers DM, et al: Effect of classification on the incidence of polyarteritis nodosa and microscopic polyangiitis. Arthritis Rheum 39:1208–1212, 1996.

237. Guillevin L, Lhote F, Sauvaget F, et al: Treatment of polyarteritis nodosa related to hepatitis B virus with interferon-alpha and plasma exchanges. Ann Rheum Dis 53:334–337, 1994.

238. Guillevin L, Lhote F, Jarrousse, B et al: Treatment of polyarteritis nodosa and Churg-Strauss syndrome. A meta-analysis

of 3 prospective controlled trials including 182 patients over 12 years. Ann Med Interne (Paris) 143:405–416, 1992.

239. Jennette JC, Falk RJ: The pathology of vasculitis involving the kidney. Am J Kidney Dis 24:130–141, 1994.

240. Sonnenblick M, Nasher G, Rosin A: Nonclassical organ involvement in temporal arteritis. Semin Arthritis Rheum 19:183–190, 1989.

241. Lai KN, Chan KW, Ho CP: Glomerulonephritis associated with Takayasu's arteritis: report of three cases and review of literature. Am J Kidney Dis 7:197–204, 1986.

242. Gribetz D, Landing BH, Larson EJ: Mucocutaneous lymph node syndrome (MCLS). *In* Churg A, Churg J (eds): Systemic Vasculitides. New York, Igaku-Shoin, 1991, pp 257–272.

243. Andrassy K, Kuster S, Waldherr R, et al: Rapidly progressive glomerulonephritis: analysis or prevalence and clinical course. Nephron 59:206–212, 1991.

244. Bindi P, Mougenot B, Mentre F, et al: Necrotizing crescentic glomerulonephritis without significant immune deposits: a clinical and serological study. Q J Med 86:55–68, 1993.

245. Falk RJ, Jennette JC: Anti-neutrophil cytoplasmic autoantibodies with specificity for myeloperoxidase in patients with systemic vasculitis and idiopathic necrotizing and crescentic glomerulonephritis. N Engl J Med 318:1651–1657, 1988.

246. Woodworth TG, Abuelo JG, Austin HA, et al: Severe glomerulonephritis with late emergence of classic Wegener's granulomatosis. Report of 4 cases and review of the literature. Medicine (Baltimore) 66:181–191, 1987.

247. Mathieson PW, Peat DS, Short A, et al: Coexistent membranous nephropathy and ANCA-positive crescentic glomerulonephritis in association with penicillamine. Nephrol Dial Transplant 11:863–866, 1996.

248. Tarantino A, De Vecchi A, Montagnino G, et al: Renal disease in essential mixed cryoglobulinemia: long-term follow-up of 44 patients. Q J Med 50:1–30, 1981.

249. D'Amico G, Colasanti G, Ferrario F, et al: Renal involvement in essential mixed cryoglobulinemia. Kidney Int 35:1004–1014, 1989.

250. Johnson RJ, Gretch DR, Yamabe H, et al: Membranoproliferative glomerulonephritis associated with hepatitis C virus infection. N Engl J Med 328:465–470, 1993.

251. Feiner H: Pathology of dysproteinemia: light chain amyloidosis, non-amyloid immunoglobulin deposition disease, cryoglobulinemia syndromes, and macroglobulinemia of Waldenström. Hum Pathol 19:1255–1272, 1988.

252. Druet P, Letonturier P, Contet A, et al: Cryoglobulinaemia in human renal disease. A study of seventy-six cases. Clin Exp Immunol 15:483–496, 1973.

253. Faraggiana T, Parolini C, Previato G, et al: Light and electron microscopic findings in five cases of cryoglobulinemic glomerulonephritis. Virchows Arch A Pathol Anat Histopathol 384:29–44, 1979.

254. Tracy RE: Blood pressure related separately to parenchymal fibrosis and vasculopathy of the kidney. Am J Kidney Dis 20:124–131, 1992.

255. Heptinstall RH: Hypertension I: Essential hypertension. *In* Heptinstall RH (ed): Pathology of the Kidney. 4th ed. Boston, Little Brown, 1992, pp 951–1028.

256. McManus JFA, Lupton CH Jr: Ischemic obsolescence of renal glomeruli. The natural history of the lesions and their relation to hypertension. Lab Invest 9:413–434, 1960.

257. Sommers SC, Melamed J: Renal pathology of essential hypertension. Am J Hypertens 3:583–587, 1990.

258. Gamble CN: The pathogenesis of hyaline arteriolosclerosis. Am J Pathol 122:410–420, 1986.

259. Valenzuela R, Gogate PA, Deodhar SD, et al: Hyaline arteriolar nephrosclerosis. Immunofluorescent findings in the vascular lesion. Lab Invest 43:530–534, 1980.

260. Kinkaid-Smith P, McMichael J, Murphy FA: The clinical course and pathology of hypertension with papilloedema (malignant hypertension). Q J Med 105:117–163, 1958.

261. Klemperer P, Otani S: Malignant nephrosclerosis. Arch Pathol 11:60–117, 1931.

262. Hsu H, Churg J: The ultrastructure of mucoid "onionskin" intimal lesions in malignant nephrosclerosis. Am J Pathol 99:67–80, 1980.

263. Jones DB: Arterial and glomerular lesions associated with severe hypertension. Lab Invest 31:303–313, 1974.

264. Bohle A, Helmchen U, Grund RE, et al: Malignant nephrosclerosis in patients with hemolytic uremic syndrome (primary malignant nephrosclerosis). Curr Top Pathol 65:81–113, 1977.

265. Goldblatt PJ, Gohara AF, Khan NH, et al: Benign and malignant nephrosclerosis and renovascular hypertension. *In* Tisher CC, Brenner BM (eds): Renal Pathology with Clinical and Functional Correlations. New York, JB Lippincott, 1989, pp 1131–1162.

266. Hughson MD, Lajoie G: Vascular Diseases. *In* Silva FG, D'Agati VD, Nadasdy T (eds): Renal Biospy Interpretation. New York, Churchill Livingstone, 1996, pp 333–355.

267. Luscher TF, Keller HM, Imhof HG, et al: Fibromuscular hyperplasia: extension of the disease and therapeutic outcome. Results of the University Hospital Zurich Cooperative Study on Fibromuscular Hyperplasia. Nephron 44 (suppl 1):S109–114, 1986.

268. Luscher TF, Lie JT, Stanson AW, et al: Arterial fibromuscular dysplasia. Mayo Clin Proc 62:931–952, 1987.

269. Treadway KK, Slater EE: Renovascular hypertension. Annu Rev Med 35:665–692, 1984.

270. Perloff D, Schambelan M: Renovascular hypertension. Clin Endocrinol Metab 10:513–535, 1981.

271. Llach F, Papper S, Massry, SG: The clinical spectrum of renal vein thrombosis: acute and chronic. Am J Med 69:819–829, 1980.

272. Pollack VE, Kark RM, Pirani CL, et al: Renal vein thrombosis and the nephrotic syndrome. Am J Med 21:496–520, 1956.

273. Wagoner RD, Stanson AW, Holley KE, et al: Renal vein thrombosis in idiopathic membranous glomerulopathy and nephrotic syndrome: incidence and significance. Kidney Int 23:368–374, 1983.

274. Remmuzi G: HUS and TTP: variable expression of a single entity. Kidney Int 32:292–308, 1987.

275. Churg J, Goldstein MH, Bernstein J: Thrombotic microangiopathy. *In* Tisher CC, Brenner BM (eds): Renal Pathology with Clinical and Functional Correlations. Philadelphia, JB Lippincott, 1989, pp 1081–1113.

276. Drummond KN: Hemolytic uremic syndrome: then and now. N Engl J Med 312:116–118, 1985.

277. John HD, Thoenes W: The glomerular lesions in endotheliotropic hemolytic nephroangiopathy (hemolytic uremic syndrome, malignant nephrosclerosis, post partum renal insufficiency). Pathol Res Pract 173:236–259, 1982.

278. Remuzzi G, Ruggententi P: The hemolytic uremic syndrome. Kidney Int 48:2–19, 1995.

279. Moschcowitz, E: An acute febrile pleiochromic anemia with hyaline thrombosis of the terminal arterioles and capillaries: an undescribed disease. Arch Intern Med 36:89–93, 1925.

280. Ridolfi RL, Bell WR: Thrombotic thrombocytopenic purpura: report of 25 cases and review of the literature. Medicine (Baltimore) 60:413–428, 1981.

281. Eknoyan G, Riggs SA: Renal involvement in patients with thrombotic thrombocytopenic purpura. Am J Nephrol 6:117–131, 1986.

282. Umlas J: Glomeruloid structures in thrombohemolytic thrombocytopenic purpura, glomerulonephritis, and disseminated intravascular coagulation. Hum Pathol 3:437–441, 1972.

283. McCoy RC, Tisher CC, Pepe PF, et al: The kidney in progressive systemic sclerosis: immunohistochemical and antibody elution studies. Lab Invest 35:124–131, 1976.

284. Kovalchik MT, Guggenheim SJ, Silverman MH, et al: The kidney in progressive systemic sclerosis: a prospective study. Ann Intern Med 89:881–887, 1978.

285. D'Agati VD, Cannon PJ: Scleroderma (progressive systemic sclerosis). *In* Tisher CC, Brenner BM (eds): Renal Pathology with Clinical and Functional Correlations. Philadelphia, JB Lippincott, 1989, pp 994–1020.

286. Lee EB, Anhalt GJ, Voorhees JJ, et al: Pathogenesis of scleroderma. Current concepts. Int J Dermatol 23:85–89, 1984.

287. Fries JF: The microvasculature pathogenesis of scleroderma: a hypothesis. Ann Intern Med 91:788–789, 1979.

288. Jimenez SA: Cellular immune dysfunction and the pathogen-

esis of scleroderma. Semin Arthritis Rheum 13 (suppl 1):104–113, 1983.

289. Spargo B, McCartney CP, Winemiller R: Glomerular capillary endotheliosis in toxemia of pregnancy. Arch Pathol 68:593, 1959.

290. Roberts, JM, Taylor, RN, Goldfine A, et al: Clinical and biochemical evidence of endothelial cell dysfunction in the pregnancy syndrome preeclampsia. An endothelial disorder. Hypertension 4:700–708, 1991.

291. Gaber LW, Spargo BH, Lindheimer MD: Renal pathology in pre-eclampsia. Baillieres Clin Obstet Gynaecol 8:443–468, 1994.

292. Pollack VE, Nettles JB: The kidney in toxemia of pregnancy: a clinical and pathological study based on renal biopsies. Medicine 39:469–526, 1960.

293. Sheehan HL: Renal morphology in preeclampsia. Kidney Int 18:241–252, 1980.

294. Cogan MG: Classification and patterns of renal dysfunction. In Cotran RS, Brenner BM, Stein JH (eds): Contemporary Issues in Nephrology: Tubulo-Interstitial Nephropathies. New York, Churchill Livingstone, 1983, pp 35–48.

295. Apple GB, Kunis CL: Acute tubulo-interstitial nephritis. In Cotran RS, Brenner BM, Stein JH (eds): Contemporary Issues in Nephrology: Tubulo-Interstitial Nephropathies. New York, Churchill Livingstone, 1983, pp 151–185.

296. Mills RM Jr: Severe hypersensitivity reaction associated with allopurinol. J Am Med Assoc 216:799–802, 1971.

297. Appel GB, Neu HC: The nephrotoxicity of antimicrobial agents. N Engl J Med 296:784–787, l977.

298. Councilman WT: Acute interstitial nephritis. J Exp Med 3:393–420, 1898.

299. Morrison WI, Wright NG: Canine leptospirosis: an immunopathological study of interstitial nephritis due to Leptospira canicola. J Pathol 120:83–89, 1976.

300. Cotran RS, Galvanek E: Immunopathology of human tubulo-interstitial diseases: localization of immunoglobulins, complement and Tamm-Horsfall protein. Contrib Nephrol 16:126–131, 1979.

301. Bergstein J, Litman N: Interstitial nephritis with anti-tubular basement membrane antibody. N Engl J Med 292:875–878, 1975.

302. Crosson JT, Keane WF, Anderson WR: Radiation nephropathy. In Tisher CC, Brenner BM (eds): Renal Pathology with Clinical and Functional Correlations. Philadelphia, JB Lippincott, 1989, pp 866–876.

303. Kunkler PB, Farr RF, Luxton RW: Limit of renal tolerance of x-ray: investigation into renal damage occurring following treatment of tumors of testis by abdominal bath. Br J Radiol 25:190–205, 1952.

304. Krochak RJ, Baker DG: Radiation nephritis: clinical manifestations and pathophysiologic mechanisms. Urology 27:389–393, 1986.

305. Madrazo A, Churg J: Radiation nephritis: chronic changes following moderate doses of radiation. Lab Invest 34:283–290, 1976.

306. Mostofi FK, Pani CK, Ericsson J: Effects of radiation on canine kidney. Am J Pathol 44:707–725, 1964.

307. Mostofi FK, Berdjis CC: The kidney. In Berdjis CC (eds): Pathology of Radiation. Baltimore, Williams & Wilkins, 1971, pp 597–635.

308. Striker G, Striker LJ, D'Agati VD: Tubular and Interstitial Lesions in the Renal Biopsy: Major Problems in Pathology. Philadelphia, WB Saunders 1997, pp 269–290.

309. Racusen LC, Fivush BA, Li YL, et al: Dissociation of tubular cell detachment and tubular cell death in clinical and experimental acute tubular necrosis. Lab Invest 64: 546–556, 1991.

310. Kashgarian M: Acute tubular necrosis and ischemic renal injury. In Jennette JC, Olsen JL, Schwartz MM, Silva FG (eds): Heptinstall's Pathology of the Kidney. Philadelphia, Lippincott-Raven, 1998, pp 863–889.

311. Hoyer JR, Michael AF, Good RA, et al: The nephrotic syndrome of infancy: clinical, morphologic, and immunologic studies of four infants. Pediatrics 40:233–246, 1967.

312. Mahieu P, Monnens L, Van Haelst U: Chemical properties of

glomerular basement membrane in congenital nephrotic syndrome. Clin Nephrol 5:135–139, 1976.

313. Rapola J, Sariola H, Ekbolm P: Pathology of fetal congenital nephrosis: immunohistochemical and ultrastructural studies. Kidney Int 25:701–707, 1984.

314. Autio-Harmainen H, Rapola, J: Renal pathology of fetuses with congenital nephrotic syndrome of the Finnish type. Nephron 29:158–163, 1981.

315. Naruse T, Hirokawa N, Maekawa T, et al: Familial nephrotic syndrome with focal glomerular sclerosis. Am J Med Sci 280:109–113, 1980.

316. Olson JL: The nephrotic syndrome. In Heptinstall RH (ed): Pathology of the Kidney. 4th ed. Boston, Little Brown, 1992, pp 779–869.

317. Eddy AA, Mauer SM: Pseudohermaphroditism, glomerulopathy and Wilm's tumor (Drash syndrome): frequency in end stage renal failure. J Pediatr 106:584–587, 1985.

318. Schleutermann DA, Bias WB, Murdoch JL, et al: Linkage of the loci for the nail-patella syndrome and adenylate kinase. Am J Hum Genet 21:606–630, 1969.

319. Ben-Bassat M, Cohen L, Rosenfeld J: The glomerular basement membrane in nail-patella syndrome. Arch Pathol 92:350–355, 1971.

320. Hoyer JR, Michael AF, Vernier RL: Renal disease in nail-patella syndrome: clinical and morphologic studies. Kidney Int 2:231–238, 1972.

321. Bennett WM, Musgrave JE, Campbell RA, et al: The nephropathy of the nail-patella syndrome: clinicopathologic analysis of 11 kindreds. Am J Med 54:304–319, 1973.

322. Sabnis SG, Antonovych TT, Argy WP, et al: Nail-patella syndrome. Clin Nephrol 14:148–153, 1980.

323. Desnick RJ, Astrin KH, Bishop DF: Fabry's disease. Molecular genetics of the inherited nephropathy. Adv Nephrol 18:113–128, 1989.

324. Sheth KJ, Roth DA, Adams MB: Early renal failure in Fabry's disease. Am J Kidney Dis 2:651–654, 1983.

325. Kramer W, Thronman J, Mueller K, et al: Progressive cardiac involvement by Fabry's disease despite successful renal allotransplantation. Int J Cardiol 7:72–75, 1985.

326. Faraggiana T, Churg J, Grishman E, et al: Light- and electron-microscopic histochemistry of Fabry's disease. Am J Pathol l03:247–262, 1981.

327. Alport AC: Hereditary familial congenital haemorrhagic nephritis. Br Med J 1:504–506, 1927.

328. Gregory MC, Atkin CL: Alport syndrome. In Schrier RW, Gottschalk CW (eds): Diseases of the Kidney. Boston, Little Brown, 1993, pp 571–591.

329. Throner P, Janse B, Baumal R, et al: Samoyed hereditary glomerulopathy. Immunohistochemical staining of basement membranes of kidney for laminin, collagen type IV, fibronectin, and Goodpasture antigen, and correlation with electron microscopy of glomerular capillary basement membranes. Lab Invest 56:435–443, 1987.

330. Yoshioka K, Michael AF, Velso J, et al: Detection of hidden nephritogenic antigen determinants in human renal and nonrenal basement membranes. Am J Pathol 121:156–165, 1985.

331. Bernstein J: The glomerular basement membrane abnormality in Alport's syndrome. Am J Kidney Dis 10:222–229, 1987.

332. Gubler M, Levy M, Brolyer M, et al: Alport's syndrome. A report of 58 cases and a review of the literature. Am J Med 70:493–505, 1981.

333. Shah B, First MR, Mendoza NC, et al: Alport's syndrome: risk of glomerulonephritis induced by antiglomerular-basement-membrane antibody after renal transplantation. Nephron 50:34–38, 1988.

334. Savage CO, Pusey CD, Kershaw MJ, et al: The Goodpasture antigen in Alport's syndrome: Studies with a monoclonal antibody. Kidney Int 30:107–112, 1986.

335. Kashtan CE: Alport syndrome and thin basement membrane disease. J Am Soc Nephrol 9:1736–1750, 1998

336. Kees-Folts D, Sadow JL, Schreiner GF: Tubular catabolism of albumin is associated with the release of an inflammatory lipid. Kidney Int 45:1697–1709, 1994.

337. Antonovych TT, Deasy PF, Tina LU, et al: Hereditary ne-

phritis. Early clinical, functional, and morphological studies. Pediatr Res 6:545–556, 1969.

338. Spear SG, Slusser RJ: Alport's Syndrome, emphasizing electron microscopic studies of the glomerulus. Am J Pathol 59:213–220, 1972.

339. Lemmink HH, Nillesen WN, Mochizuki T, et al: Benign familial hematuria due to mutation of type IV collagen a4 gene. J Clin Invest 98:1114–1118, 1996.

340. Cosio FG, Falkenhain ME, Sedmak DD: Association of thin glomerular basement membrane with other glomerulopathies. Kidney Int 46:471–474, 1994.

341. Piel CF, Biava CG, Goodman JR: Glomerular basement membrane attenuation in familial nephritis and "benign" hematuria. J Pediatr 101:358–365, 1982.

342. Burdick JF, Beschorner WE, Smith WJ, et al: Characteristics of early routine renal allograft biopsies. Transplantation 38:679–684, 1984.

343. Porter, K: Renal transplantation. *In* Heptinstall RH (ed): Pathology of the Kidney. 4th ed. Boston, Little Brown, 1992, pp 1799–1988.

344. Colvin BR: The renal allograft biopsy. Kidney Int 50:1069–1082, 1996.

345. Solez K, Axelsen RA, Benediktsson H, et al: International standardization of criteria for the histologic diagnosis of renal allograft rejection: the Banff working classification of kidney transplant pathology. Kidney Int 44:411–422, 1993

346. Sabnis SG: Histopathologic diagnosis of kidney transplant rejection. *In* Lieberman R, Mukherjee A (eds): Principles of Drug Development in Transplantation and Autoimmunity. New York, Chapman & Hall, 1995, pp 521–528.

347. Ratner LE, Hadley GA, Hanto DW, et al: Immunology of renal allograft rejection. Arch Pathol Lab Med 115:283–287, 1991.

348. Ito S, Camussi G, Tetta C, et al: Hyperacute renal allograft rejection in the rabbit: the role of platelet-activating factor and of cationic proteins derived from polymorphonuclear leukocytes and from platelets. Lab Invest 51:148–161, 1984.

349. Kinkaid-Smith P, Morris PJ, Saker BM, et al: Immediate renal-graft biopsy and subsequent rejection. Lancet 5:748–749, 1968.

350. Sabnis SG, Antonovych TT, Alijani MR: The value of one-hour post-anastomosis biopsy in renal allograft transplantation. Transplant India 1:30–38, 1997.

351. Crocker BP, Salomon DR: Pathology of the renal allograft. *In* Tisher CC, Brenner BM (eds): Renal Pathology. Philadelphia, JB Lippincott, 1989, pp 1518–1554.

352. Olsen S: Pathology of renal allograft rejection. In Churg J, Spargo BH, Mostofi FK, et al (eds): Kidney Disease: Present Status. International Academy of Pathology Monograph. Baltimore, Williams & Wilkins, 1979, pp 327–355.

353. Zollinger HU, Mihatsch MJ: Renal Pathology in Biopsy. New York, Springer-Verlag, 1978.

354. Solez K, Benediktsson H, Cavallo T, et al: Report of the third Banff conference on classification and lesion scoring in allograft pathology. Transplant Proc 28:441–444, 1996.

355. Maryniak R, First MR, Weiss MA: Transplant glomerulopathy: evolution of morphologically distinct changes. Kidney Int 27:799–780, 1985.

356. Monaco AP, Burke JF, Ferguson RM, et al: Current thinking on chronic allograft rection: issues, concerns, and recommendations from a 1997 roundtable discussion. Am J Kidney Dis 33:150–160, 1999.

357. Mihatsch MJ, Ryffel B, Gudat F, et al: Cyclosporine nephropathy. In Tisher CC, Brenner BM (eds): Renal Pathology. Philadelphia, JB Lippincott, 1989, pp 1555–1586.

358. Antonovych TT, Sabnis SG, Austin HA, et al: Cyclosporine A–induced arteriolopathy. Transplant Proc 20 (suppl):951–958, 1988.

359. Palestine AG, Austin HA, Balow JE, et al: Renal histopathologic alterations in patients treated with cyclosporine in uveitis. N Engl J Med 314:1293–1298, 1986.

360. Austin HA, Palestine AG, Sabnis SG, et al: Evolution of cyclosporin nephropathy in patients treated for autoimmune uveitis. Am J Nephrol 9:392–402, 1989.

361. Mathew TH: Recurrence of disease following renal transplantation. Am J Kidney Dis 12:85–96, 1988.

362. Randhawa PS, Shapiro R, Jordan ML, et al: The histopathologic changes associated with allograft rejection and drug toxicity in renal transplant recipients maintained on FK506. Clinical significance and comparison with cyclosporine. Am J Surg Pathol 17:60–68, 1993.

363. Katari SR, Magnone M, Shapiro R, et al: Clinical features of acute reversible tacrolimus (FK506) nephrotoxicity in kidney transplant patients. Clin Transplant 11:237–242, 1997.

364. Ciancio G, Burke GW, Roth D, et al: Tacrolimus and mycophenolate mofetil as primary immunosuppression for renal allograft recipients. *In* Racusen LC, Solez K, Burdick JF (eds): Kidney Transplant Rejection: Diagnosis and Treatment. New York, Marcel Dekker, 1998, pp 519–529.

365. McKee M, Segev D, Wise B, et al: Initial experience with FK 506 (tacrolimus) in pediatric renal transplant recipients. J Pediatr Surg 32:688–690, 1997.

366. Porayko MK, Textor SC, Krom RA, et al: Nephrotoxic effects of primary immunosuppression with FK506 and cyclosporine regimens after liver transplantation. Mayo Clin Proc 69:105–111, 1994.

367. Shapiro R, Jordan M, Scantlebury VP, et al: Renal transplantation at the University of Pittsburgh: the impact of FK506. Clin Transplant 12:229–236, 1994.

368. Racusen LC, Solez K, Olsen S: Pathology of kidney transplantation. *In* Racusen LC, Solez K, Burdick JF (eds): Kidney Transplant Rejection: Diagnosis and Tratment. New York, Marcel Dekker, 1998, pp 383–387.

369. Beaufils M, Morel-Maroger L, Sraer JD, et al: Acute renal failure of glomerular origin during visceral abscesses. N Engl J Med 295:185–189, 1976.

370. Miyata T, Jadaul M, Kurokawa K, et al: Beta-2 microglobulin in renal disease. J Am Soc Nephrol 9:1722–1735, 1998.

371. Alfrey AC: Beta-2 microglobulins amyloidosis (letter). AKF Nephrology 6:27–33, 1989.

372. Murgo AJ: Thrombotic microangiopathy in the cancer patient including those induced by chemotherapeutic agents. Semin Hematol 24:161–177, 1987.

373. Kaplan BS, Chesney RW, Drummond KN: Hemolytic uremic syndrome in families. N Engl J Med 292:1090–1093, 1975.

374. Sammaritano LR, Gharavi AE: Antiphospholipid antibody syndrome. Clin Lab Med 12:41–54, 1992.

375. Leavitt RY, Fauci AS, Bloch DA, et al: The American College of Rheumatology 1990 criteria for the classification of Wegener's granulomatosis. Arthritis Rheum 33:1101–1107, 1990.

376. Masi AT, Hunder GG, Lie JT, et al: The American College of Rheumatology 1990 criteria for the classification of Churg-Strauss syndrome (allergic granulomatosis and angiitis). Arthritis Rheum 33:1094–1100, 1990.

# 30

# *Renal Neoplasia*

John N. Eble

Since the time when the two diagnoses of Wilms' tumor and renal cell carcinoma encompassed almost all renal neoplasms three decades ago, the classification of renal neoplasia has grown more complex. In the following sections on neoplasms of children, epithelial neoplasms, and mesenchymal neoplasms, the diagnostic and prognostic aspects of renal neoplasia are presented with emphasis on the gross pathology and histologic examination, including recently recognized and rare entities. Tumors of the renal pelvis and ureter are discussed in their own section following those of the renal parenchyma.

## RENAL NEOPLASIA IN CHILDREN

Primary renal neoplasms are uncommon in children; approximately 500 new cases are diagnosed annually in the United States. On the other hand, they make up the fifth most common group of pediatric cancers and are the second most frequent abdominal malignancy of children. Although these tumors are not very numerous in absolute terms, progress in the treatment of Wilms' tumor and the recognition of two highly malignant neoplasms as specific entities distinct from Wilms' tumor make the correct diagnosis and staging of pediatric renal neoplasms important.[1–3] The variable and overlapping appearances of the tumors and their rarity make them an especially challenging group of lesions for the surgical pathologist.

The most common tumor in this group is Wilms' tumor (nephroblastoma). Clear cell sarcoma and rhabdoid tumor are important because of their poor response to therapy and consequent morbidity and mortality. Mesoblastic nephroma is the most common renal neoplasm in children younger than 3 months of age, and the tumor usually is cured surgically. Renal cell carcinoma, lymphoma, sarcomas, neuroendocrine tumors, and angiomyolipoma are usually found in the kidneys of adults and occur rarely in children. The pathology of these tumors is essentially the same in children as it is in adults.

Much of what we know today about the pathology of renal neoplasia in childhood is the result of the work of the National Wilms' Tumor Study (NWTS) and its pathology center under the direction of Bruce Beckwith.

## Wilms' Tumor

More than 80% of renal tumors of childhood are Wilms' tumors.[4] A synonym for Wilms' tumor is nephroblastoma. Most often, these tumors occur in children 2 to 4 years old (median ages for boys and girls, respectively, are 37 and 43 months[5]) and Wilms' tumors are relatively uncommon in the first 6 months of life and after 6 years of age.[6, 7] The incidence of Wilms' tumors is about the same throughout the world.[8] They are slightly more common in girls.[5] The tumors are bilateral in approximately 5% of cases.[9] Patients with bilateral Wilms' tumors average more than a year younger than patients with unilateral tumors.[5] Associations with congenital anomalies, such as cryptorchidism, hypospadias, other genital anomalies, hemihypertrophy, and aniridia, are well recognized.[10] As many as 5% of patients with Beckwith-Wiedemann syndrome develop Wilms' tumors.[11] Patients with the Drash syndrome also have an increased risk of developing Wilms' tumors.[12] A variety of other malformations are less frequently associated with Wilms' tumors.[7, 13] It is uncommon for Wilms' tumors to have a familial association.[5] Wilms' tumors are rare in adults, and the stage at presentation and frequency of anaplasia are higher than in children and response to therapy is less.[14, 15]

### PATHOGENESIS

Aggregates of cells resembling blastema have been found in autopsies of young children and in kidneys resected from patients with Wilms' tumors. These nephrogenic rests are now believed to be the source of Wilms' tumors. Beckwith and associates[16] have classified these based on the extensive case material of the NWTS, and the following discussion is based on that work.

Nephrogenic rests are foci of nephrogenic cells resembling those of the developing kidney (Fig. 30–1). There are two types: perilobar nephrogenic rests, which occur at the periphery of the renal lobes, and intralobar nephrogenic rests, which occur in the cortex or medulla within the renal lobe. In addition to their location, perilobar nephrogenic rests differ from intralobar nephrogenic rests in having well-defined smooth borders and predominance of blastema, are often multiple, and rarely may be diffuse. Intralobar nephrogenic rests usually are single and mingle irregularly with renal parenchyma; stroma is usually the predominant element. Nephrogenic rests are subclassified according to their histologic ap-

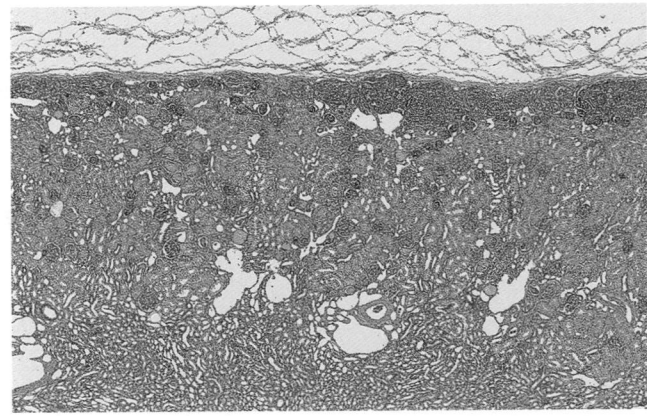

**Figure 30–1.** Perilobar nephrogenic rest consisting of blastemal cells at the periphery of the renal lobe, beneath the renal capsule.

pearance as dormant or nascent; maturing, sclerosing, and obsolescent; hyperplastic; and neoplastic. The first are usually composed of blastema, are of microscopic size, and exhibit rare mitotic figures. In the maturing, sclerosing and obsolescent types, there are differentiating stromal and epithelial cells with hyalinization of stroma. Hyperplastic rests are macroscopically visible and may contain blastemal, embryonic, or sclerosing areas. Uncommonly, hyperplastic rests may diffusely replace much of the renal parenchyma. Neoplastic rests are divided into adenomatous and nephroblastomatous types, based on cellular crowding and the prevalence of mitotic figures. In adenomatous rests, mitotic figures are uncommon, whereas in nephroblastomatous rests (incipient Wilms' tumors), mitotic figures are common. Typically, neoplastic rests are expansile nodules arising within and compressing a rest. Nephroblastomatosis is defined as the diffuse or multifocal presence of nephrogenic rests, or multicentric or bilateral Wilms' tumors.

Autopsy studies have shown that perilobar nephrogenic rests are present in approximately 1% of infants younger than 3 months,[17] a frequency much greater than that of Wilms' tumor (1 per 10,000). Intralobar nephrogenic rests are rare except in kidneys with Wilms' tumor. Nephrogenic rests are almost never found in adults.[18] In patients with unilateral Wilms' tumor, the NWTS has found that perilobar and intralobar nephrogenic rests occur approximately equally frequently and are present in 41% of cases. The situation differs in patients with synchronous or metachronous bilateral tumors in whom nephrogenic rests are present in more than 95% of cases. Thus, careful examination of the grossly uninvolved kidney is important because the presence of nephrogenic rests indicates a greater probability of bilaterality.

### MACROSCOPIC FINDINGS

Wilms' tumors are usually large compared with the kidneys in which they have arisen, often more than 5 cm in diameter and a third or more are larger

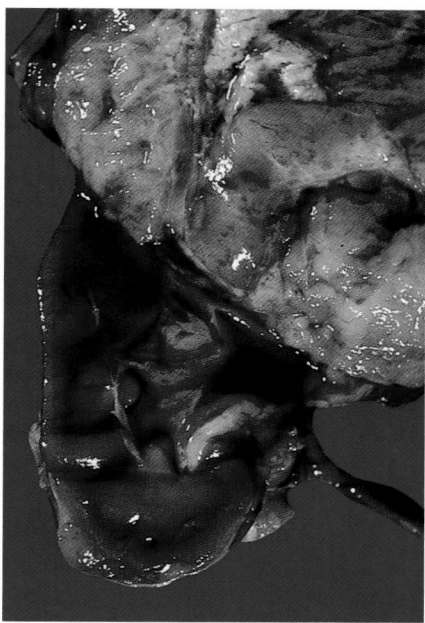

**Figure 30–2.** Wilms' tumor with gelatinous gray parenchyma sharply circumscribed from the non-neoplastic kidney.

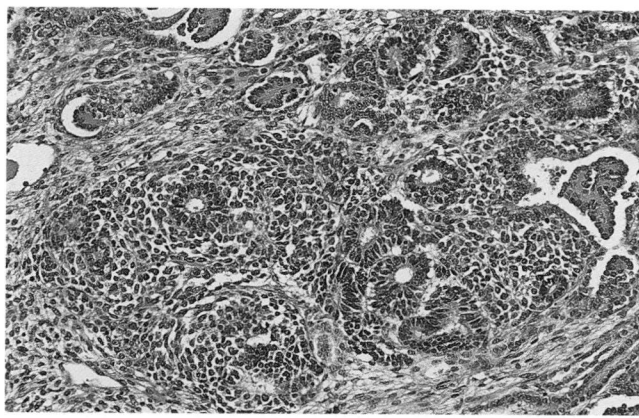

**Figure 30–4.** Wilms' tumor with epithelial differentiation forming tubules and blunt papillae.

than 10 cm.[7] The cut surfaces are typically solid, soft, and grayish or pinkish resembling fresh brain tissue (Fig. 30–2). Hemorrhage and necrosis are common, as are cysts. Occasionally, the cysts are extensive. Wilms' tumors usually are enclosed by a pseudocapsule composed of compressed renal and perirenal tissues, giving an appearance of encapsulation.

## MICROSCOPIC FINDINGS

Wilms' tumors are typically composed of variable proportions of blastema, epithelium, and stroma, although in some tumors, only two and occasionally only one component is present. Blastema consists of randomly arranged, densely packed small cells with darkly staining nuclei, frequent mitotic figures, and inconspicuous cytoplasm. Blastema is commonly arranged in three patterns—serpentine, nodular, and diffuse. Serpentine and nodular are most diagnostically helpful. They consist of anastomosing serpiginous or spheroidal aggregates of blastema sharply circumscribed from the surrounding stromal elements (Fig. 30–3).

The epithelial component usually consists of small tubules or cysts lined by primitive columnar or cuboidal cells (Fig. 30–4). The nuclei of the epithelium are often elongate and wedge shaped. The epithelium of Wilms' tumor may also form structures resembling glomeruli or may differentiate in extrarenal directions: mucinous, squamous, neural,[19] or endocrine.[20–22] Predominantly cystic Wilms' tumors contain blastema and other Wilms' tumor tissues in their septa and have been called cystic partially differentiated nephroblastoma.[23]

The stroma of Wilms' tumors' may differentiate along the lines of almost any type of soft tissue. Although loose myxoid and fibroblastic spindle cell stroma are most common (Fig. 30–5), smooth mus-

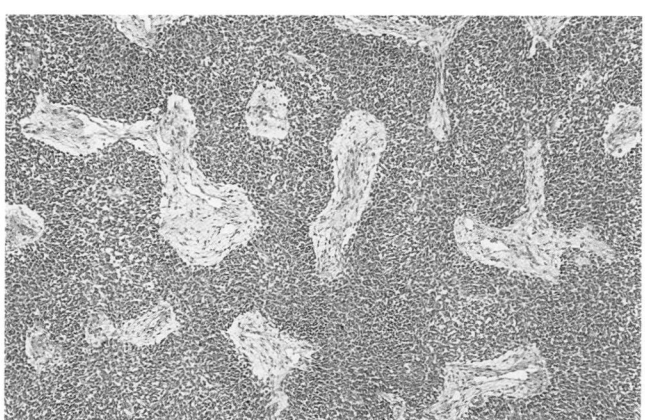

**Figure 30–3.** Wilms' tumor with predominance of blastema, which forms serpentine cords.

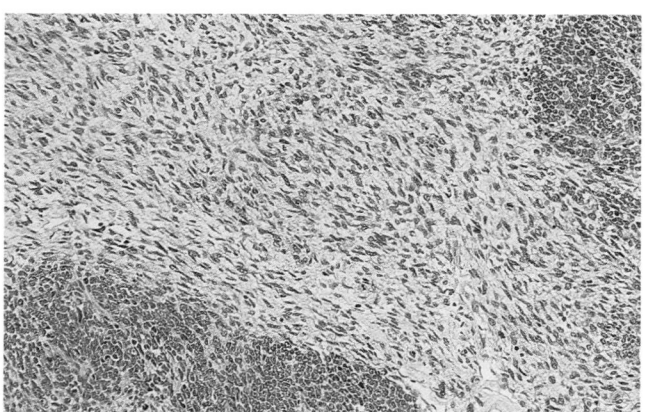

**Figure 30–5.** Wilms' tumor stroma consisting of a sheet of undifferentiated spindle cells with a sharp border with islands of blastema.

cle, skeletal muscle, fat, cartilage, bone, and neural components also occur.[22] Uncommonly, the differentiation toward more mature soft tissue types is diffuse and predominant, and such tumors have sometimes been given special names, such as fetal rhabdomyomatous nephroblastoma.[24] Sometimes tumors with complex combinations of differentiated epithelium and stroma have been called teratoid Wilms' tumor.[25, 26]

## DIFFERENTIAL DIAGNOSIS

Some Wilms' tumors have a monomorphous epithelial appearance and can pose difficult diagnostic problems, especially in adolescents and adults, in their distinction from renal cell carcinoma. Recognition of the nuclear characteristics typical of Wilms' tumor epithelium is usually helpful in distinguishing these Wilms' tumors from renal cell carcinoma. The epithelial nuclei in Wilms' tumor are often elongate or ovoid with molded, sometimes wedge-shaped, contours, a feature helpful in distinguishing monophasic tubular Wilms' tumor from renal cell carcinomas in which the nuclei usually are roughly spherical.

Cystic, partially differentiated nephroblastomas grossly resemble cystic nephroma, and because the elements typical of Wilms' tumor may be inconspicuous, cystic renal tumors in children should be sampled extensively to identify blastema or other elements of Wilms' tumor.

Because it has a favorable prognosis, fetal rhabdomyomatous nephroblastoma must not be misinterpreted as a rhabdomyosarcoma. It contains extensive areas of relatively mature skeletal muscle but lacks the malignant small cells and rhabdomyoblasts found in rhabdomyosarcoma.

The distinction of Wilms' tumor from rhabdoid tumor and clear cell sarcoma is discussed later.

## GRADING, STAGING, AND PROGNOSTIC FACTORS IN WILMS' TUMORS

Based on the results of the NWTS, Wilms' tumors are divided into two categories—favorable and unfavorable histology, based on the absence or presence of anaplasia. Anaplasia is found in approximately 6% of Wilms' tumors. More than 80% of patients with anaplasia are older than 24 months of age; it is rare in patients younger than 12 months.[27] The presence of anaplasia was recognized to carry a greatly increased risk of treatment failure and death early in the NWTS.[28] Thus, it is important to sample Wilms' tumor specimens extensively.

Anaplasia has been defined by the NWTS as the combination of cells with very large hyperchromatic nuclei and multipolar mitotic figures. Correct recognition of anaplasia demands good histologic preparations. The enlarged nuclei must be at least three times as large as typical blastemal nuclei in both axes and their hyperchromasia must be obvious (Fig. 30–6). In addition to the enlarged nuclei, hyperdiploid mitotic figures must be present. However, enlarged nuclei in skeletal muscle fibers in the

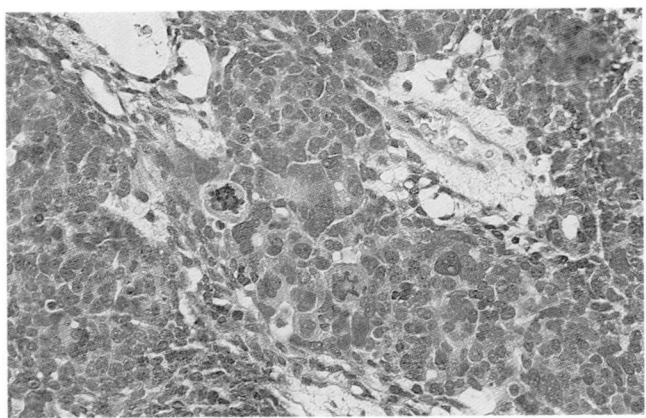

**Figure 30–6.** Anaplasia in Wilms' tumor with giant hyperchromatic nuclei.

stroma of Wilms' tumors are not evidence of anaplasia. The criteria for abnormal hyperdiploid mitotic figures demand not only structural abnormalities but also enlargement of the mitotic figure as evidence of hyperploidy. When anaplasia is present only focally, surgical cure remains likely.[29]

The NWTS has established a staging scheme for Wilms' tumor and other pediatric renal malignancies (Table 30–1). The tabular presentation, however, does not do justice to the challenges that staging presents to the surgical pathologist. Stage I and Stage II require assessment of the renal sinus and capsule. The renal sinus is the space within the kid-

**TABLE 30–1.** National Wilms' Tumor Study System for Staging Pediatric Renal Tumors

| | |
|---|---|
| Stage I | Tumor confined to kidney and completely resected |
| | *Specific Criteria:* |
| | The renal capsule is not penetrated by the tumor |
| | Renal sinus veins and lymphatics not invaded |
| | There is no lymph node or hematogenous spread |
| Stage II | Tumor extends locally outside the kidney but is completely resected |
| | *Specific Criteria:* |
| | The renal capsule is penetrated by tumor |
| | Renal sinus veins or lymphatics invaded |
| | The renal vein contains tumor |
| | Local spillage or biopsy involves only the flank |
| | Specimen margins are free of tumor and no residual tumor remains after surgery |
| | No metastases |
| Stage III | There is residual tumor confined to the abdomen without hematogenous spread |
| | *Specific Criteria:* |
| | Grossly visible residual tumor in abdomen |
| | There are tumor implants on the peritoneal surface |
| | The specimen margins contain tumor |
| | Abdominal lymph nodes contain tumor |
| Stage IV | There are blood-borne metastases or spread beyond abdomen |
| Stage V | Tumors are present in both kidneys |

ney extending from the plane defined by the medial-most limits of the cortex laterally to the limits of the space between the medullary pyramids and contains the major branches of the renal artery and vein and the bulk of the renal pelvis. In NWTS 5, vascular invasion in the renal sinus was adopted as evidence of extension requiring upstaging to stage II. Invasion of the soft tissue of the renal sinus is acceptable in stage I unless it involves the margin, in which case stage III is the appropriate assignment. Stage I also requires evaluation of the renal capsule, but this is often difficult because as a renal neoplasm grows, it sequentially is surrounded by an intrarenal pseudocapsule, the renal capsule, a pseudocapsule external to the kidney, Gerota's fascia, and the ultimate limits of the specimen. These layers frequently fuse, confusing the identification of the true renal capsule. In fact, when Wilms' tumor invades perirenal fat, it may destroy the fat cells and a fibrous response may give the appearance of stage I limitation by renal capsule. If the renal capsule can be identified, it is the structure that must be used for staging. When the renal capsule is joined to the soft tissue of Gerota's fascia, this layer must be used for staging. The presence of an inflammatory pseudocapsule beyond the renal capsule is at present not sufficient justification for assigning stage II but has been shown to be associated with an increase in the rate of relapse.[30] Stages II and IV are more straightforward, as shown in Table 30-1. For stage V, the most advanced individual tumor should be assigned a substage according to the stage it would be assigned if it had occurred alone, for example stage V, substage I.

## Clear Cell Sarcoma of Kidney

### CLINICAL CONSIDERATIONS

Clear cell sarcoma was recognized in 1978 approximately simultaneously by Morgan and Kidd,[31] Marsden and Lawler,[32] and Beckwith and Palmer.[33] Marsden and colleagues originally called this tumor bone-metastasizing renal tumor of childhood,[32] but the name clear cell sarcoma[33] has prevailed. Clear cell sarcoma is highly malignant and resistant to conventional therapy for Wilms' tumor but is often responsive to doxorubicin. Thus, it is important that clear cell sarcoma is distinguished from other tumors. Clear cell sarcomas make up approximately 4% of renal tumors in children.[34] Most patients are between 12 and 36 months old.[35] Approximately 66% of the patients are boys. Clear cell sarcoma is approximately 10 times more likely to metastasize to bone than are other pediatric renal cancers. The origin of clear cell sarcoma is unknown.

### MACROSCOPIC FINDINGS

The appearance of the cut surfaces of these tumors is variable: They may be homogeneous, grayish and lobular or variegated, including firm grayish

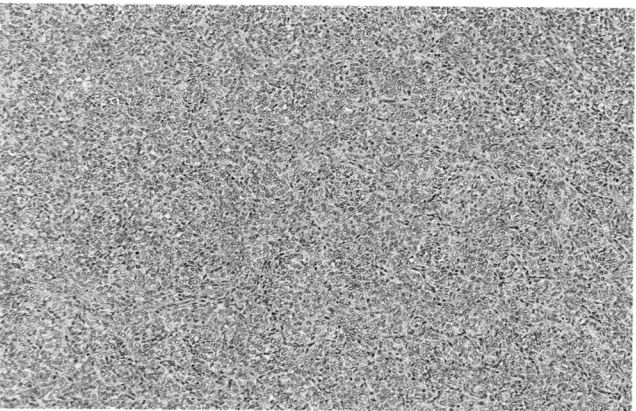

**Figure 30–7.** Clear cell sarcoma of kidney; low magnification shows a monotonous pale gray array.

whorled tissues and light pink soft areas.[36] Occasionally the tumor may produce abundant mucin, which gives a slimy glistening appearance. Most appear to be well circumscribed. Approximately 33% contain cysts ranging from a few millimeters to centimeters in diameter.[36] Bilaterality has not been reported.[4]

### MICROSCOPIC FINDINGS

Most clear cell sarcomas of kidney consist of a monotonous array of cells with pale staining or vacuolated cytoplasm and indistinct borders (Fig. 30–7). The nuclei contain fine chromatin and the nucleoli are small (Fig. 30–8). These nuclear characteristics are helpful in distinguishing clear cell sarcomas from rhabdoid tumors. In the classic pattern, the cells are arranged in cords supplied with a distinctive branching array of small blood vessels, which form septa between the cords (see Fig. 30–8).[37] Another characteristic feature is the infiltrative border between the clear cell sarcoma and the surrounding renal parenchyma; residual renal tubules are fre-

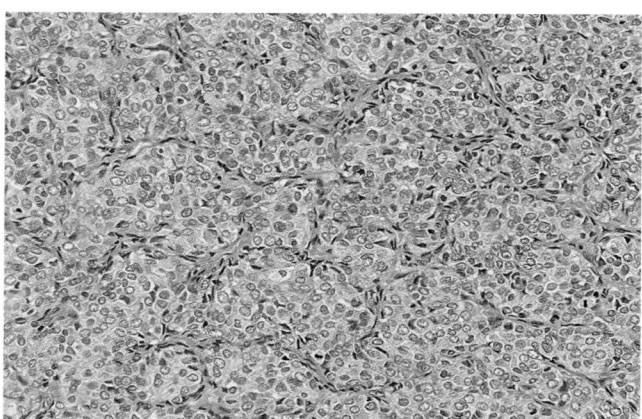

**Figure 30–8.** Clear cell sarcoma of kidney; high magnification shows the architecture of cords and septa and the characteristic pale nuclei.

quently seen surrounded by the sarcoma.[36] The cytoplasm of most clear cell sarcomas is much less clear than that of clear cell renal cell carcinoma. Confusing variations on the classic appearance occur, including spindle cell proliferation, cystic change, hyaline sclerosis, and palisading.[22] Generous sampling may help the clinician find areas in which the vascular pattern and finely dispersed chromatin and small nucleoli in the nuclei indicate the correct diagnosis.

### DIFFERENTIAL DIAGNOSIS

In distinguishing clear cell sarcoma of kidney from Wilms' tumor, some negatives are important: blastema is not found in clear cell sarcoma, heterologous elements such as cartilage or muscle are not found in clear cell sarcomas, clear cell sarcomas are unilateral and unicentric, and sclerotic stroma is uncommon in Wilms' tumors before therapy. The vascular pattern typical of clear cell sarcoma is often helpful in distinguishing it from Wilms' tumor. The border with the kidney is usually infiltrative, whereas the border of Wilms' tumor is typically pushing. Exceptionally, a clear cell sarcoma of kidney may contain foci in which the cells have prominent nucleoli, similar to those of rhabdoid tumor of kidney; examination of other areas with patterns typical of clear cell sarcoma usually will clarify the diagnosis.

## Rhabdoid Tumor of Kidney

### CLINICAL CONSIDERATIONS

The most malignant of the renal neoplasms of childhood, the rhabdoid tumor usually metastasizes widely and causes the death of the patient within 12 months of diagnosis.[38] Most patients are very young at the time of diagnosis (median age 11 months and rare after 3 years in the NWTS population). There is a 1.5:1 predominance of boys.[39] Associations with embryonal tumors of the central nervous system[40] and paraneoplastic hypercalcemia[41, 42] have been reported. The origin of rhabdoid tumor is unknown

### MACROSCOPIC FINDINGS

Rhabdoid tumors lack the appearance of encapsulation commonly seen in cases of Wilms' tumor or clear cell sarcoma. The tumors usually are located medially in the kidney,[39] and the renal sinus and pelvis are almost always infiltrated. They are typically yellow-gray or light tan crumbly tumors with indistinct borders. Necrosis and hemorrhage are common.

### MICROSCOPIC FINDINGS

Microscopically, the classic pattern of rhabdoid tumor of kidney is a diffuse and monotonous array of medium or large polygonal cells with abundant eosinophilic cytoplasm and spheroidal nuclei with thick nuclear membranes and large nucleoli (Fig. 30–9). It is the resemblance of the cytoplasm of

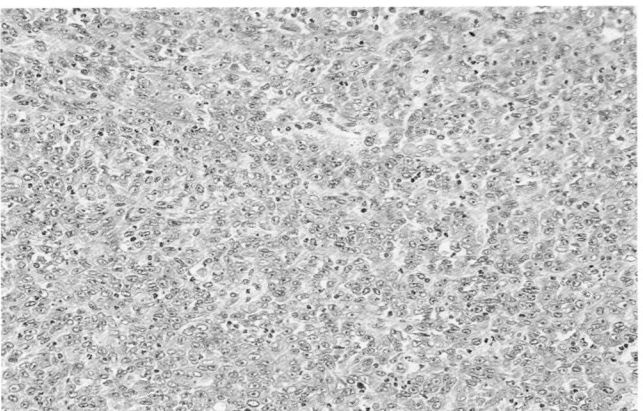

**Figure 30–9.** Rhabdoid tumor of kidney forming a diffuse sheet of cells; nucleoli are visible even at low magnification.

these cells to differentiating rhabdomyoblasts that gave the tumor its name.[33] Often, the cytoplasm contains a large eosinophilic globular inclusion that displaces the nucleus (Fig. 30–10). Electron microscopy has shown that the inclusions consist of aggregates of whorled filaments.[43] As more cases have accrued to the NWTS, a wide range of patterns has been appreciated, including sclerosing, epithelioid, spindled, lymphomatoid, vascular, pseudopapillary, and cystic.[39] These patterns are usually mixed with the classic pattern and with each other. The characteristic nuclear features of large centrally placed nucleoli and thick nuclear membranes are usually retained.

### DIFFERENTIAL DIAGNOSIS

An important problem in the diagnosis of rhabdoid tumor of kidney is the fact that a wide variety of renal and extrarenal tumors may mimic it in routine sections. The NWTS has been referred cases of Wilms' tumor, mesoblastic nephroma, renal cell carcinoma, urothelial carcinoma, collecting duct carcinoma, oncocytoma, rhabdomyosarcoma, neuroendocrine carcinoma, and lymphoma that have been

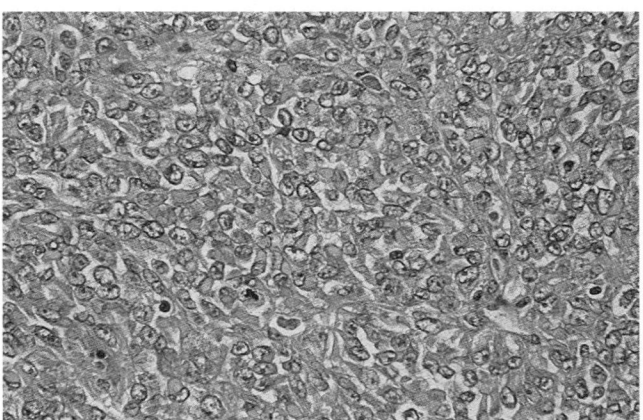

**Figure 30–10.** Rhabdoid tumor of kidney with eosinophilic cytoplasmic inclusions.

confused with rhabdoid tumor of kidney.[44] Filamentous cytoplasmic inclusions or conspicuous macronucleoli have been the misleading features in most cases. Although examination of routine sections was able to clarify most cases, electron microscopy and immunohistochemistry were sometimes necessary to exclude rhabdoid tumor. Although blastemal cells rarely contain inclusions suggestive of rhabdoid tumor, the presence of characteristic aggregates of blastema, such as nodules or serpentine groupings, clarifies the diagnosis.

## Mesoblastic Nephroma

### CLINICAL CONSIDERATIONS

Mesoblastic nephroma makes up less than 3% of primary renal tumors in children, but it predominates in the first 3 months of life.[4, 6] After 6 months, it is uncommon. Polyhydramnios and prematurity have been associated with these tumors.[46, 47] An abdominal mass is the usual presentation. Mesoblastic nephroma was first recognized in 1966,[48] and subsequent studies[49] have shown it to have a good prognosis. Almost all patients are cured by surgical resection.[50–52] A few recurrences and adverse outcomes have been recorded, principally in patients older than 3 months of age at presentation.[53, 54] Characteristically, mesoblastic nephromas have infiltrative borders and the surgical pathologist must study these carefully because the risk of recurrence appears related to incomplete resection.[55, 56] These tumors are very rare in adults.[57, 58] Cellular mesoblastic nephroma is characterized by the same genetic lesion as infantile fibrosarcoma but classic mesoblastic nephroma does not share that genetic lesion.[59]

### MACROSCOPIC FINDINGS

Most mesoblastic nephromas are large relative to the kidney in which they have arisen. Externally, the surface of the tumor and kidney is smooth and the

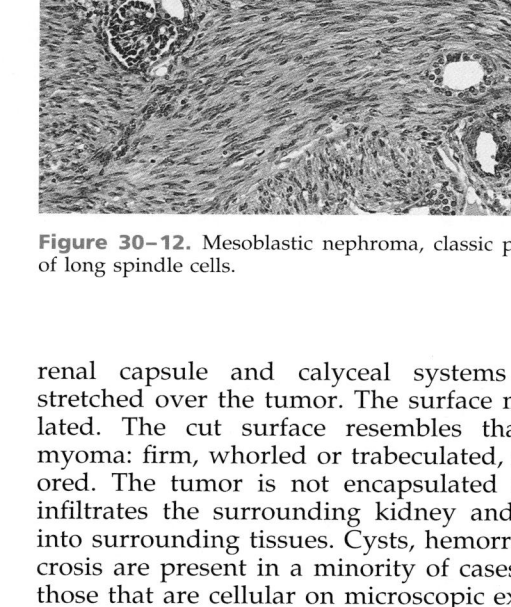

**Figure 30–12.** Mesoblastic nephroma, classic pattern composed of long spindle cells.

renal capsule and calyceal systems are usually stretched over the tumor. The surface may be bosselated. The cut surface resembles that of a leiomyoma: firm, whorled or trabeculated, and light colored. The tumor is not encapsulated and typically infiltrates the surrounding kidney and may extend into surrounding tissues. Cysts, hemorrhage, and necrosis are present in a minority of cases, particularly those that are cellular on microscopic examination.[60]

### MICROSCOPIC FINDINGS

The pattern described by Bolande[49] was a moderately cellular proliferation of thick interlacing bundles of spindle cells with elongated nuclei and a marked proclivity for infiltration of renal and perirenal tissues (Figs. 30–11 and 30-12). Entrapment of glomeruli and renal tubules is common. Another more common pattern was recognized later that consists of a more densely cellular proliferation of polygonal cells (Fig. 30–13) with easy-to-find mitotic figures and often has pushing borders. This pattern has been called cellular mesoblastic nephroma. In

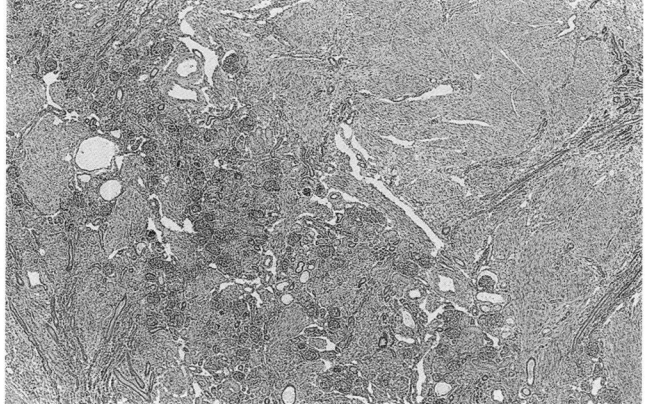

**Figure 30–11.** Mesoblastic nephroma, classic pattern with an infiltrative border with the kidney.

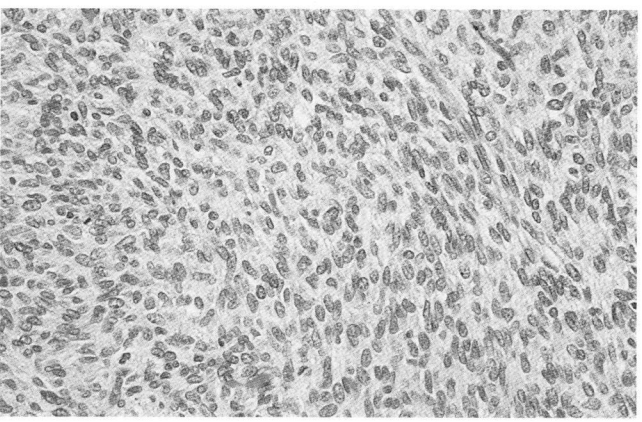

**Figure 30–13.** Mesoblastic nephroma, cellular pattern composed of densely packed short spindle cells.

view of the generally favorable outcome for patients with mesoblastic nephroma and the predominance of lesions containing the cellular pattern, the histologic pattern should not be a primary indication for therapy beyond adequate surgical resection.

### DIFFERENTIAL DIAGNOSIS

Mesoblastic nephroma usually is easily diagnosed when the microscopic appearance and patient's age are considered. Wilms' tumors with stromal predominance may be confused with mesoblastic nephroma, particularly in the case of Wilms' tumors treated preoperatively. This problem can usually be solved by remembering that blastema is not found in mesoblastic nephroma and that Wilms' tumors usually have sharply circumscribed borders, whereas those of mesoblastic nephromas are infiltrative. Age assists in making the correct diagnosis and bilaterality favors Wilms' tumor. Although both occur in the same age group, mesoblastic nephroma, even the cellular variant, and rhabdoid tumor are usually easily distinguished.

# EPITHELIAL TUMORS OF THE KIDNEY

## Papillary Adenoma

### CLINICAL CONSIDERATIONS

Notwithstanding the historical problems and success of surgery, it is our view that the data support the definition of a set of criteria within which the diagnosis of papillary adenoma is safe and justified (Table 30–2). The first criterion indicates that the microscopic morphology of papillary adenoma resembles that of papillary renal cell carcinoma, including lesions with both type 1 and type 2 characteristics.[61] The second criterion defines a group of tumors which appear to be limited in growth potential. This includes more than 95% of all papillary neoplasms of the renal tubules.[62, 63] Larger ones are more worrisome because they have demonstrated a greater capacity for growth and may have the potential for metastasis.[64] The third criterion reflects the fact that there is no convincing evidence that very small tumors of those other cell types are not small carcinomas. As early as 1938, Bell[65] recognized that the distinction between papillary neoplasms and those histologically resembling clinically apparent clear cell renal cell carcinoma was important and that among those resembling clear cell renal carci-

noma, "the size of the tumor is not a certain criterion as to its malignancy." Subsequent investigations and case reports of small clear cell renal cell carcinomas with metastases have reinforced this conclusion.[66, 67] Similar criteria for papillary adenoma were accepted at consensus conferences in Heidelberg, Germany, and Rochester, Minnesota.[68]

The frequency of small epithelial tumors in the cortices of kidneys is approximately 37% in autopsy patients, depending on the patient population and study methods.[69] The frequency of small papillary tumors increases with age to approximately 40% of the population over age 65. Similar lesions frequently develop in patients on long-term hemodialysis and have been reported in approximately 33% of patients with acquired renal cystic disease.[70] The association between arteriosclerotic renal vascular disease and papillary adenomas has long been recognized.[65, 71] Budin and McDonnell[72] studied autopsy material and found that the prevalence of papillary adenomas not only was much increased in kidneys with arteriosclerotic renal vascular disease but that this was independent of age. Xipell[73] found a strong correlation between tobacco smoking and the presence of papillary adenomas; this also was observed by Bennington.[74]

That kidneys bearing renal cell carcinoma or oncocytoma are more likely to contain papillary adenomas than normal kidneys has long been recognized.[75] Occasionally, more than one adenoma will be present adjacent to the carcinoma or oncocytoma, as if some local factor were promoting the development of the adenomas.

### MACROSCOPIC FINDINGS

Papillary adenomas appear to the naked eye as well-circumscribed, yellow to grayish white nodules in the renal cortex. Most occur just below the renal capsule, but those that are invisible from the cortical surface are fairly common. The smallest ones usually are spherical, but larger ones sometimes are roughly conical with a wedge-shaped appearance in sections cut at right angles to the cortical surface. An association with scars in the renal cortex has been asserted but is controversial.[72, 76] In most patients, adenomas are solitary,[76] but occasionally, papillary adenomas are multiple and bilateral, rarely miliary; this condition has been called renal adenomatosis,[77–80] analogous to renal oncocytomatosis.[81, 82]

### MICROSCOPIC FINDINGS

Papillary adenomas have tubular, papillary, or tubulopapillary architectures (Fig. 30–14), often corresponding closely to the chromophil-basophil cell type described by Thoenes and associates.[83] Some are surrounded by thin fibrous pseudocapsules, whereas others have none.[62] The cells have round to oval nuclei with chromatin that ranges from stippled to clumped, and inconspicuous nucleoli. Nuclear grooves may be present. Mitotic figures usually are absent.[62] In most papillary adenomas, the cytoplasm is scant and pale, and amphophilic to basophilic. Occasionally, it is slightly more voluminous and ap-

**TABLE 30–2.** Diagnostic Criteria for Papillary Adenoma of the Kidney

Papillary or tubulopapillary architecture
Diameter less than or equal to 5 mm
Does not histologically resemble clear cell, chromophobe, or collecting duct renal cell carcinoma

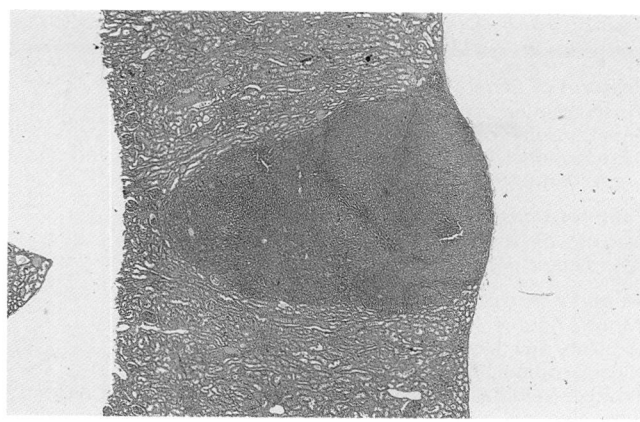

**Figure 30–14.** Papillary adenoma, compact endophytic growth forming a wedge-shaped profile.

pears clear or filled with minute vacuoles.[62] Less frequently, the cytoplasm is voluminous and eosinophilic, resembling type 2 papillary renal cell carcinoma.[61] Psammoma bodies often are present, as are foamy macrophages.[62]

## IMMUNOHISTOCHEMISTRY, ULTRASTRUCTURE, AND SPECIAL STUDIES

Cohen and coworkers[84] found that almost all papillary adenomas react with antibodies to epithelial membrane antigen and low-molecular-weight cytokeratin, whereas a majority react with antibody to high-molecular-weight cytokeratin. Neuron-specific enolase and $\alpha_1$-antitrypsin occasionally were present, and carcinoembryonic antigen could not be detected.[84] Hiasa and associates[85] studied 65 adenomas ranging from 1 to 5 mm in diameter and found 52 to be positive for peanut agglutinin and epithelial membrane antigen and negative for both Leu M1 and *Lotus tetragonolobus* lectin, a pattern similar to that in the normal distal tubule. Thirteen had the opposite pattern and were similar to the lining cells of the normal proximal tubule.[85]

## Renal Oncocytoma

### CLINICAL CONSIDERATIONS

Renal oncocytomas are neoplasms of the renal cortex that often are discovered incidentally by radiologic examinations of the kidneys for other reasons but may also present as a palpable mass or with hematuria.[86] In 1976, Klein and Valensi[87] drew attention to renal oncocytoma as a renal tumor previously classified as renal cell carcinoma but distinguishable from it by its pathologic features and benign course. There is a 2:1 male-to-female ratio, and almost all cases have occurred in adults, mostly from age 50 to 80 years. Resection of the tumor is curative. A striking spoke-and-wheel appearance on radiography was at first thought to be diagnostic of oncocytoma, but greater experience has indicated that this is not specific because renal cell carcinomas

may have similar appearances.[88] The tumor cannot reliably be distinguished preoperatively from renal cell carcinoma by imaging or biopsy. Thus, radical nephrectomy is the usual operation. However, a number of patients have had multicentric or bilateral tumors,[89] and conservative operations[90] have been successful when they are performed for these reasons.

### MACROSCOPIC FINDINGS

The most characteristic feature of renal oncocytoma is its mahogany brown color (Fig. 30–15), which contrasts with the bright yellow color typical of clear cell renal cell carcinomas. Many oncocytomas have central zones of whitish stroma that may connect with the periphery, giving the subcapsular surface a bosselated contour. Occasional tumors exhibit foci of hemorrhage, but necrosis is rare and often can be related to extrinsic factors.[86] Generally, the presence of gross necrosis or hemorrhage suggests extra caution is called for in making the diagnosis of oncocytoma. Bilaterality or unilateral multicentricity occurs in approximately 4% of cases and is more frequent than with renal cell carcinoma. Rarely, there may be large numbers of small oncocytomas in the cortices of both kidneys, a condition that has been termed oncocytomatosis.[81]

### MICROSCOPIC FINDINGS

The cells usually are arranged either in diffuse sheets (Fig. 30–16) or as cellular islands in a background of loose edematous connective tissue (Fig. 30–17). Tubules, often mildly dilated, also are common. Rarely, the groups of cells contain hyaline deposits of type IV collagen, giving a cylindromatous appearance.[91] In sections stained with hematoxylin and eosin, the cytoplasm is intensely eosinophilic and finely granular. Although the cytoplasmic volume ranges from moderate to abundant, its staining qualities are the same. The nuclei are mainly round with small clumps of chromatin and nucleoli, which may be visible with a 10× microscope objective.[92] Occasional bizarre, enlarged nuclei, sometimes con-

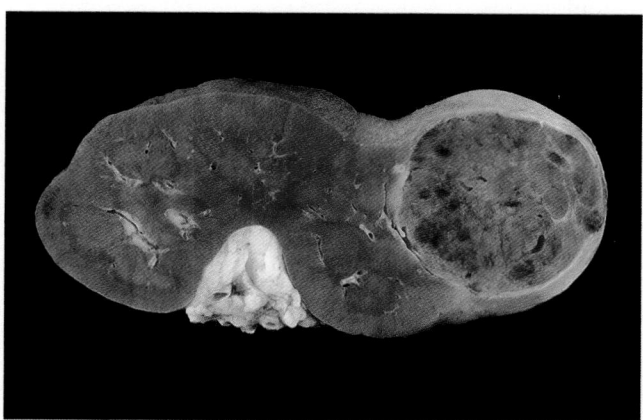

**Figure 30–15.** Oncocytoma forming a well-circumscribed globular mass with brown parenchyma.

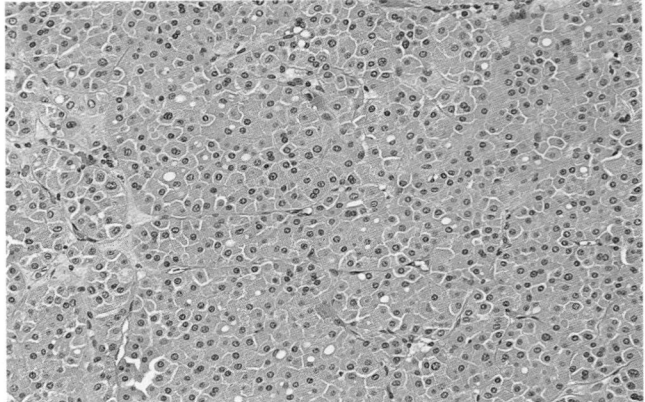

**Figure 30–16.** Oncocytoma growing in sheets of cells with abundant eosinophilic cytoplasm and inconspicuous vasculature.

**TABLE 30–3.** Diagnostic Features of Renal Oncocytoma

***Features of Renal Oncocytoma***
Finely granular, strongly eosinophilic cytoplasm
Sheet, insular, or tubulocystic architectural patterns
Mitochondria filling cytoplasm with other organelles and
    sparse microvilli

***Features Unusual in Renal Oncocytoma***
Microscopic vascular invasion
Microscopic extension into perirenal fat

***Features Rare or Impermissible in Renal Oncocytoma***
Mitotic figures
Papillary architecture
Clear or spindle cells
Positive colloidal iron stain or chromophobe-type vesicles seen
    by electron microscopy
Gross vascular invasion
Gross extension into perirenal fat

taining cytoplasmic invaginations, may be present. Mitotic figures are absent or very rare in oncocytomas. Because they are benign, oncocytomas are not graded. By electron microscopy, the cytoplasm is seen to be filled with mitochondria and other organelles are scant. Microvilli are sparse, and completely formed brush borders usually are not present.[93]

Extension into small veins is seen microscopically in a little more than 5% of cases and appears to have no adverse prognostic significance.[86] Small extensions into perirenal fat are seen in almost 10% of cases and also appear to have no adverse effect.[86]

### DIFFERENTIAL DIAGNOSIS

The principal consideration is the eosinophilic variant of chromophobe renal cell carcinoma. In most cases, strict adherence to the criteria listed in Table 30–3 will enable this distinction. Immunohistochemistry can be helpful because oncocytomas do not express vimentin[94] and often have a characteristic punctate pattern of staining for cytokeratin.[95]

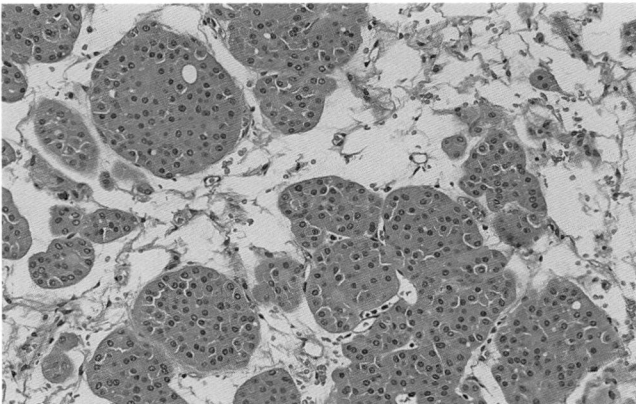

**Figure 30–17.** Oncocytoma growing as archipelagoes of oncocytic cells in an edematous stroma.

## Metanephric Adenoma and Metanephric Adenofibroma

### CLINICAL CONSIDERATIONS

In 1980, Pagès and Granier[96] drew attention to a previously unrecognized renal neoplasm that they called néphrome néphronogèn" (nephronogenic nephroma) and considered to be a purely epithelial neoplasm arising from persistent blastema. Since that time, almost 100 cases have been described individually or in aggregated studies and the name metanephric adenoma has become accepted.[69]

In 1992, Hennigar and Beckwith[97] described five cases of a composite neoplasm in which an epithelial component identical to metanephric adenoma was combined with a proliferation of spindle cells; they proposed the name nephrogenic adenofibroma for this tumor. However, Beckwith now favors the name metanephric adenofibroma for these tumors to emphasize their close relationship with metanephric adenoma.

Metanephric adenoma occurs at all ages, most commonly in the fifth and sixth decades, and there is a 2:1 female-to-male ratio.[98] Approximately 50% are incidental findings, with others presenting with polycythemia, abdominal or flank pain, mass, or hematuria. Often, the polycythemia has resolved after the tumor was removed. Cases reported to date have neither recurred nor metastasized. Four of the 50 patients reported by Davis and associates[98] also had renal cell carcinoma.

Patients with metanephric adenofibroma have ranged from 3.5 to 36 years (mean = 16 years). Although the number of cases is small, there does not appear to be any gender predominance. More than 50% of the patients have had polycythemia. Other symptoms of metanephric adenofibroma have included hematuria[97, 99] and hypertension.[97] Some have been incidental findings. Three of the five cases reported by Hennigar and Beckwith had separate small papillary epithelial tumors near the renal pelvis, which they considered to be low-grade collecting duct carcinomas.

## MACROSCOPIC FINDINGS

Metanephric adenomas have ranged widely in size, with the largest being 150 mm in diameter; most have been 30 to 60 mm in diameter.[98] Davis and associates[98] found no instance of bilaterality and only two instances of unilateral multifocality in 50 patients. The tumors are typically well circumscribed, but in most instances, they are not encapsulated. A thin and discontinuous pseudocapsule is more common than a substantial one. The cut surfaces vary from gray to tan to yellow and may be soft or firm. Calcification is present in approximately 20% and a few are densely calcified. Small cysts are present in about 10% of tumors, and a unique example was entirely cystic.[98] Foci of hemorrhage and necrosis are common.[98, 100] Metanephric adenofibromas are typically solitary firm bosselated masses without capsules and with indistinct borders.[97] The cut surfaces range from gray to tan to yellow and solid with only occasional cysts in some of the tumors.

## MICROSCOPIC FINDINGS

Histologically, metanephric adenoma is typically a highly cellular tumor composed of tightly packed small, uniform, round acini (Fig. 30–18). Because the acini and their lumens are so small, at low magnification, this pattern may be mistaken for a solid sheet of cells. Long branching and angulated tubular structures are also common. The stroma ranges from inconspicuous to a loose paucicellular edematous stroma. Hyalinized scar or focal osseous metaplasia of the stroma are present in 10% to 20% of tumors.[98] Approximately 50% of tumors contain papillary structures (Fig. 30–19), usually consisting of minute cysts into which have grown short blunt papillae reminiscent of immature glomeruli. In most of these, no blood vessel is visible. Psammoma bodies are common and may be numerous. The junction with

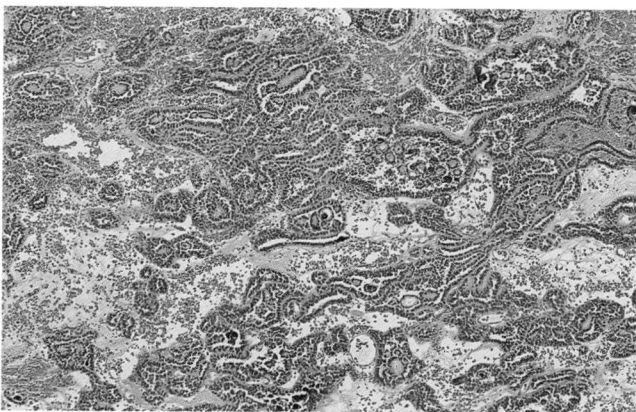

**Figure 30–19.** Metanephric adenoma forming papillae and psammoma bodies.

the kidney is usually abrupt and lacking a pseudo-capsule.

The cells of metanephric adenoma have small, uniform nuclei with absent or inconspicuous nucleoli. The nuclei are only slightly larger than lymphocytes and are round or oval and have delicate chromatin. The cytoplasm is scant and pale or light pink. Mitotic figures are absent or rare.

Metanephric adenofibroma is a composite tumor in which nodules of epithelium identical to metanephric adenoma are embedded in sheets of moderately cellular spindle cells. The spindle cell component consists of fibroblast-like cells.[97] Their cytoplasm is eosinophilic but pale and the nuclei are oval or fusiform. Nucleoli are inconspicuous and mitotic figures are absent or rare. Variable amounts of hyalinization and myxoid change are present. The relative amounts of the spindle cell and epithelial components vary from predominance of spindle cells to a minor component of spindle cells. The border of the tumor with the kidney is typically irregular and the spindle cell component may entrap renal structures as it advances. The epithelial component consists of small acini, tubules, and papillary structures, as described earlier in metanephric adenoma. Psammoma bodies are common and may be numerous. Neither metanephric adenoma nor metanephric adenofibroma contains blastema, nor is either associated with nephrogenic rests.

Immunohistochemistry and lectin histochemistry have given varied results in different laboratories and consequently do not play a large role in the differential diagnosis of metanephric adenoma.[69] Metanephric neoplasms composed exclusively of stromal elements have been called metanephric stromal tumors.[101]

## DIFFERENTIAL DIAGNOSIS

At first inspection, metanephric adenoma brings Wilms' tumor to mind because of the dense array of small blue cells and epithelial differentiation. However, the nuclei of metanephric adenoma are smaller

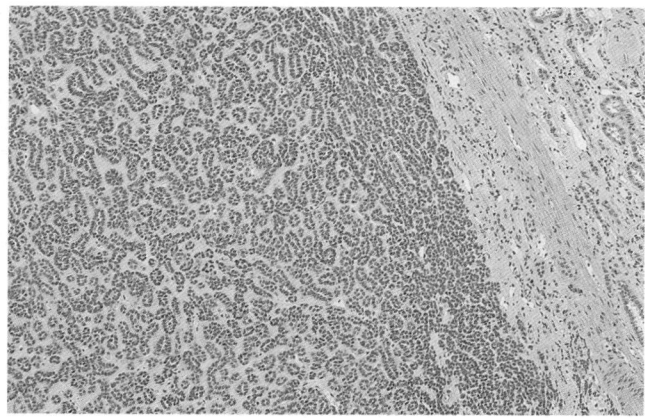

**Figure 30–18.** Metanephric adenoma forming small tubules and a sharp border with the kidney.

and lack the elongation and tapered ends often present in the nuclei of epithelial cells in Wilms' tumor. Furthermore, mitotic figures are rare in metanephric adenoma and blastema is not present. The fibromatous component of metanephric adenofibroma could be mistaken for the stroma of Wilms' tumor, but cytologically, it is benign and its lacks the variety of differentiation often seen in the stroma of Wilms' tumor.

The other major consideration is papillary renal cell carcinoma, type 1. The small cytoplasmic volume, papillary structures, and psammoma bodies bring this to mind. However, most metanephric adenomas are composed mainly of arrays of fairly uniform structures resembling renal tubules in cross section. This architecture is not typical of papillary renal cell carcinoma. Additionally, metanephric adenomas often have long pointed, branching channels lined by epithelial cells. These are not found in papillary renal cell carcinoma, nor in Wilms' tumor. The edema of papillary cores and collections of stromal foam cells that are common in papillary renal cell carcinoma are not typical of metanephric adenoma.

Metanephric stromal tumors may be difficult to distinguish from mesoblastic nephromas.

## RENAL CELL CARCINOMA

At present, renal cell carcinoma is recognized to be a family of carcinomas that arise from the epithelium of the renal tubules. The carcinomas have distinct morphologic features and arise through different constellations of genetic lesions.[68, 102, 103] The classification of renal cell carcinoma is presented in Table 30–4.

Since the recognition that renal cell carcinoma is a family of diseases that arise through different genetic lesions is recent, almost all of the clinical and epidemiologic information available comes from studies in which all types of renal cell carcinoma

**TABLE 30–4.** Classification of Renal Cell Neoplasms

Benign
  Papillary adenoma
  Oncocytoma
  Metanephric adenoma
Malignant
  Clear cell renal cell carcinoma
  Papillary renal cell carcinoma
    Type 1
    Type 2
  Chromophobe renal cell carcinoma
    Classic
    Eosinophilic
  Collecting duct carcinoma
    Medullary carcinoma
  Renal cell carcinoma, unclassified
  Neuroendocrine neoplasms
    Carcinoid
    Small cell carcinoma

were aggregated. This is the source of the following generalizations. Renal cell carcinoma is almost exclusively a cancer of adults, and approximately 28,000 new cases are diagnosed each year in the United States. Its incidence increases with each decade of life until the 6th decade, and it is two to three times more common in men than in women.[104] Renal cell carcinoma is rare in the first 2 decades of life, and makes up approximately 2% of pediatric renal tumors.[105] Obesity,[106] smoking,[107] and exposure to industrial chemicals[108] are risk factors for renal cell carcinomas, but in most cases, there is no clear carcinogenic influence. Although from 33% to 50% of patients with von Hippel–Lindau disease develop renal cell carcinoma, they make up only a minute fraction of the overall population with renal cell carcinoma.[109, 110] Renal cell carcinoma is also associated with tuberous sclerosis[111, 112] and autosomal dominant polycystic kidney disease.[113–115] Acquired renal cystic disease arising in patients with chronic renal failure is strongly associated with renal cell carcinoma.[116–118] Hematuria, pain, and a mass in the flank are the classic triad of presenting symptoms, but many patients lack any of these symptoms and present with systemic ones[119] such as fever, malaise, or anemia.[120, 121] Paraneoplastic syndromes of hypercalcemia,[122] erythrocytosis,[123] hypertension,[124] and amyloidosis[125] have occasionally been associated with renal cell carcinoma.[123, 126, 127] Renal cell carcinoma is also notorious for presenting as metastatic carcinoma of unknown primary, sometimes in unusual sites. Multicentricity occurs within the same kidney in from 7% to 13% of cases[128] and tumors are present in both kidneys in approximately 1% of patients.[17]

The clinical course of renal cell carcinoma is unpredictable, and there are well-documented cases of spontaneous regression of metastases.[129–132] Recurrences 10 years or more after nephrectomy occur in more than 10% of patients who survive that long.[133] There is some evidence that resection of solitary metastases improves survival,[134] while the presence of multiple metastases indicates a worse prognosis.[135] However, the resistance of renal cell carcinoma to radiation and chemotherapy gives most patients with remote metastases extremely poor prognoses.[136, 137] Metastases to bone occur frequently, and the scapula is an unusually frequent site.[138]

## Staging and Grading Renal Cell Carcinoma

The extent of spread of renal cell carcinoma is the dominant factor in prognosis.[139] Two staging systems are presently widely used for renal cell carcinoma. The system proposed by Robson and associates[140, 141] is compared with the tumor, nodes, metastases (TNM) system[142, 143] in Table 30–5. These schemes are roughly parallel, and comparable groupings have been set off by horizontal alignment.

**TABLE 30–5.** Staging of Renal Cell Carcinoma

| Robson System | TNM System |
| --- | --- |
| Stage 1<br>  Confined within the renal capsule<br>Stage 2<br>  Confined by Gerota's fascia<br>Stage 3<br>  A grossly visible extension into renal vein or vena cava<br>  B Lymphatic metastasis<br><br>  C Both vascular extension and metastasis to nodes<br>Stage 4<br>  Invasion of adjacent organs (except adrenal)<br>  Hematogenous metastases | T1 Confined by renal capsule & ≤70 mm<br>T2 Confined by renal capsule & >70 mm<br>T3a Invasion of adrenal or fat within Gerota's fascia<br><br>T3b Gross extension into veins or cava below diaphragm<br>T3c Intravascular extension above diaphragm<br>N1 Single regional node<br>N2 More than one regional node<br><br>T4 Extension beyond Gerota's fascia<br>M1 |

Surgery is the principal therapy for renal cell carcinoma, and for this reason, both systems include tumors confined within the renal capsule in the most favorable category. The TNM system takes into account the correlation between size and survival by dividing this group according to size. Invasion of the perinephric fat within Gerota's fascia indicates the next stage in both systems. The next group is more complicated and controversial; renal cell carcinoma frequently invades the renal venous system and this is the criterion for stage 3A. The prognostic significance of venous invasion has been difficult to establish because many tumors with venous invasion have other features of high stage disease, such as metastases. Medeiros and associates[144, 145] compared stage 1 tumors with stage 3 tumors, which would have been stage 1 but for venous invasion, and found that it was an independent prognostic factor among high-grade tumors but did not affect prognosis in low-grade tumors. Invasion of small veins within the main tumor is not sufficient reason to assign stage 3; rather, the invasion must be macroscopically visible or microscopically must occur in large veins with smooth muscle in their walls and must be at the edge or outside of the main tumor. Metastasis to regional lymph nodes without distant metastasis occurs in approximately 10% to 15% of cases[146, 147] but more than 50% of patients with enlarged regional lymph nodes have only inflammatory or hyperplastic changes.[148] Radical nephrectomy with regional lymph node dissection has been the standard operation for renal cell carcinoma for more than 3 decades,[140] but the therapeutic contribution of the lymph node dissection remains controversial.[149] Occasionally, metastasis occurs via paraureteral veins or lymphatics,[150] and for this reason, the end of the ureter and its adventitial tissues constitute a relevant surgical margin and should be examined histologically in radical nephrectomy specimens.

Since Hand and Broders[151] introduced grading of renal cell carcinomas in 1932, several different systems have been proposed, with variable success. In addition to nuclear characteristics, cytoplasmic and architectural features have been incorporated, leading to a long controversy and considerable frustration for practicing surgical pathologists. In 1971, Skinner and coworkers[152] redirected attention to the correlation between nuclear features and survival. These observations were confirmed and refined into a system of practically applicable criteria by Fuhrman and associates.[153] The Fuhrman system consists of four grades based on the size, contour, and conspicuousness of nucleoli (Table 30–6). Medeiros and colleagues[144] showed that the Fuhrman system correlated well with survival in a large population of patients with renal cell carcinoma and in a smaller population of patients with stage I tumors. Survival ranged from 86% for patients with grade 1 tumors to 24% for those with grade 4 tumors. The grade assigned is that of the highest grade found, regardless of extent.[154] Green and coworkers[155] studied 55 patients with stage I renal cell carcinoma and found a significant decrease in 5-year survival of patients with grade 4 tumors. The importance of nucleolar morphology also has been confirmed by Helpap and associates.[156] Mitotic figures are not a part of this system but typically are rare in grade 1 and 2 tumors, and the finding of more than one mitotic figure per 10 high power fields has adverse prognostic significance.[154] Störkel and associates have proposed reducing the nuclear grades to three to improve the discriminatory power of the grades.[157]

**TABLE 30–6.** Nuclear Grading of Renal Cell Carcinoma

| | |
| --- | --- |
| Grade 1 | Round, uniform nuclei approximately 10 μm in diameter with minute or absent nucleoli |
| Grade 2 | Slightly irregular nuclear contours and diameters of approximately 15 μm with nucleoli visible at ×400 |
| Grade 3 | Moderately to markedly irregular nuclear contours and diameters of approximately 20 μm with large nucleoli visible at ×100 |
| Grade 4 | Nuclei similar to those of Grade 3 but also multilobular or multiple nuclei or bizarre nuclei and heavy clumps of chromatin |

# Clear Cell Renal Cell Carcinoma

## CLINICAL CONSIDERATIONS

Approximately two thirds to three quarters of all renal cell carcinomas are clear cell renal cell carcinomas. This name is given to these tumors because most of them are composed wholly or partially of cells with abundant clear cytoplasm. However, clear cell renal cell carcinoma is merely a name, and many of these carcinomas have extensive areas in which the cytoplasm is eosinophilic, and rare examples are composed entirely of cells with eosinophilic cytoplasm. Recently, there has been some interest in changing this name to conventional renal cell carcinoma, but it remains unclear whether or not this change will take hold.[68] Some geneticists have proposed that these carcinomas be called nonpapillary renal cell carcinoma, but this terminology is ambiguous because it could include several types of renal cell carcinoma, so it should be avoided.

Clear cell renal cell carcinomas are characterized by loss of genetic material in 3p. The loss ranges from loss of whole chromosomes to loss of function through hypermethylation.[158–160] Other genetic abnormalities are common and there is some evidence that loss of heterozygosity on chromosome 14 is associated with a worse prognosis.[161]

Clear cell renal cell carcinoma is resistant to present regimens of chemotherapy and radiation therapy. Immunotherapy has also been disappointing. Since surgery is the main treatment, stage is the principal determinant of prognosis.[162] Within stage groups, grade adds to the prognostic predictive power. Grading is discussed later.

## MACROSCOPIC FINDINGS

Clear cell renal cell carcinomas are typically globular masses that may arise anywhere in the renal cortex and often protrude beyond the normal contour of the kidney. However, they occasionally grow inward or are diffusely infiltrative. The cut surface is usually variegated (Fig. 30–20), composed of soft bright yellow parenchyma with areas of grayish edematous stroma, hemorrhage, necrosis, and cysts. The cysts are filled with clear straw-colored fluid or with hemorrhage. Clear cell renal cell carcinoma may invade the renal venous system, occasionally filling the renal vein and extending into the vena cava or even the right atrium. Approximately 5% of clear cell renal cell carcinomas have areas of sarcomatoid change. These tend to appear grossly as firm solid whitish tissue.

Rarely, cystic masses grossly resembling cystic nephroma and meeting the criteria listed in Table 30–7 contain aggregates of clear epithelial cells within their septa.[23] These cells almost always have small dark-staining nuclei and are histologically identical to nuclear grade 1 clear cell renal cell carcinoma. Although there is little or no evidence of malignant behavior by such tumors, they should be diagnosed as multilocular cystic clear cell renal cell carcinoma.

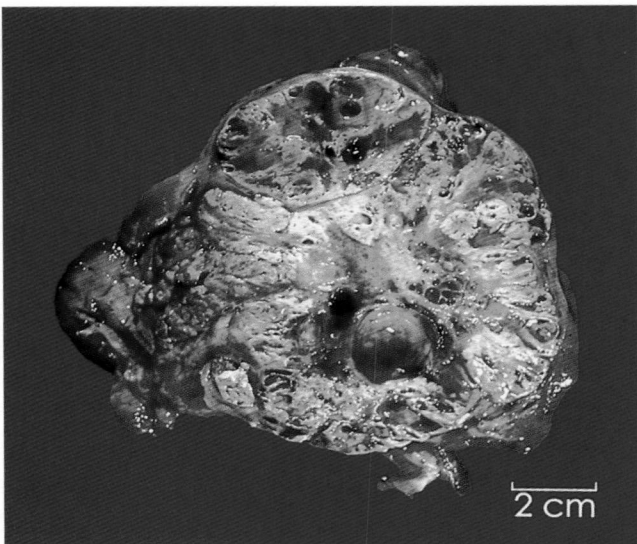

**Figure 30–20.** Clear cell renal cell carcinoma consisting of yellow parenchyma with cysts and hemorrhage.

## MICROSCOPIC FINDINGS

Clear cell renal cell carcinomas typically have a network of small blood vessels that invest alveolar clusters of carcinoma cells (Fig. 30–21). These blood vessels are very delicate and of a uniform small caliber. This vascular pattern is of great help in diagnosis because it is particular to clear cell renal cell carcinoma and not found in other types of renal cell carcinoma.

Although a solid sheet of alveoli is a common pattern of growth, the alveoli often have small central lumens that contain freshly extravasated erythrocytes. Commonly, some of the lumens are larger, forming microscopic cysts of variable size (Fig. 30–22). Among renal cell carcinomas, clear cell renal cell carcinoma is the one most prone to the formation of small and large cysts and this is a helpful diagnostic clue.

The cytoplasmic volume of clear cell renal cell carcinoma is variable over a range from moderate to voluminous (Fig. 30–23). However, it is typical that the cells in one area of a tumor are similar in size. This zonal pattern of cellular sizes contrasts with the

**TABLE 30–7.** Diagnostic Criteria of Eble and Bonsib for Multilocular Cystic Renal Cell Carcinoma

Expansile mass surrounded by fibrous pseudocapsule
Interior of tumor entirely composed of cysts and septa with no expansile solid nodules
Septa contain aggregates of epithelial cells with clear cytoplasm

Eble JN, Bonsib SM: Extensively cystic renal neoplasms: Cystic nephroma, cystic partially differentiated nephroblastoma, multilocular cystic renal cell carcinoma, and cystic hamartoma of renal pelvis. Semin Diagn Pathol 15:2–20, 1998.

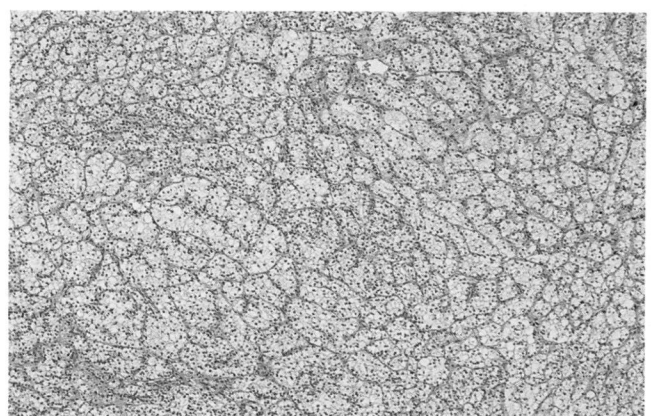

**Figure 30–21.** Clear cell renal cell carcinoma growing in a pattern of alveoli invested by delicate blood vessels.

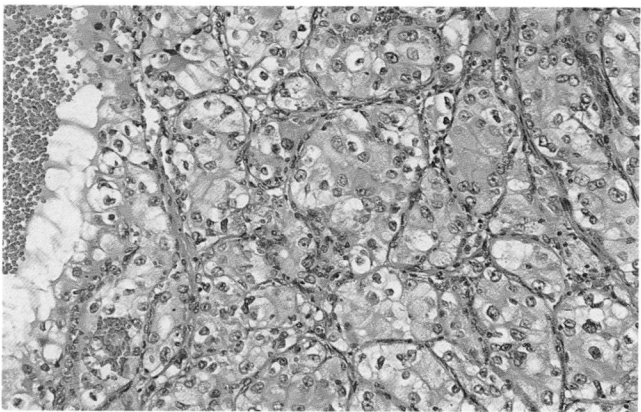

**Figure 30–23.** Clear cell renal cell carcinoma. Although there is a mixture of cells with eosinophilic and clear cytoplasm, the vascular pattern and microscopic cysts are guides to the correct diagnosis.

mosaic pattern characteristic of chromophobe renal cell carcinoma. The clarity of the cytoplasm is caused by the abundant lipid and glycogen that dissolve in tissue processing.

In clear cell renal cell carcinoma, papillary architecture is exceptional and, to some extent, controversial. One should think twice before diagnosing a tumor with obvious papillary architecture as clear cell renal cell carcinoma. Psammoma bodies and foamy macrophages, which are common in papillary renal cell carcinoma, are rare in clear cell renal cell carcinoma. Mucin is at most rare in clear cell renal cell carcinoma, and some would categorize tumors containing mucin as renal cell carcinoma, unclassified.

## DIFFERENTIAL DIAGNOSIS

The diagnosis of the typical clear cell renal cell carcinoma is usually straightforward. Sarcomatoid change may cause difficulty because it may very closely mimic a sarcoma. This problem is well known, however, and because of the rarity of renal sarcomas, they should be diagnosed with caution.

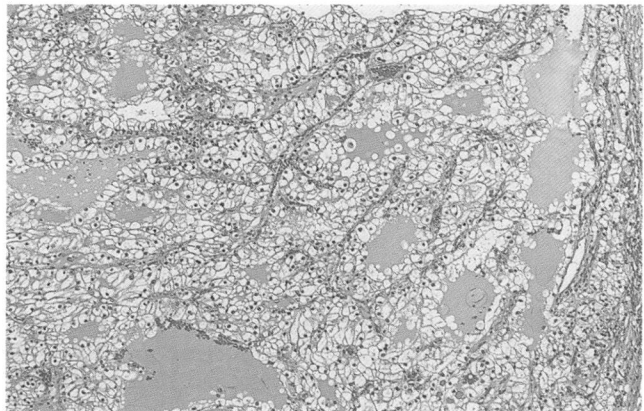

**Figure 30–22.** Clear cell renal cell carcinoma forming microscopic cysts.

Extensive sampling may be helpful because these tumors frequently have foci, albeit sometimes small, of typical renal cell carcinoma that make the correct diagnosis obvious. Ultrastructural examination[163, 164] and immunohistochemistry[165] may demonstrate epithelial features in cells that appear to be sarcomatous in sections stained with hematoxylin and eosin.

In adults, urothelial carcinomas of the renal pelvis may be confused with renal cell carcinomas, especially when the tumors are large and extensively infiltrate the kidney. Microscopically, the diagnosis may be difficult, particularly when the pelvic tumor is predominantly sarcomatoid, as has been described recently.[166] Extensive sampling may be necessary in order to find small areas of typical urothelial carcinoma, even in situ, or renal cell carcinoma. Immunohistochemical demonstration of high-molecular-weight cytokeratin or carcinoembryonic antigen indicate that such a tumor is of urothelial origin.[167]

Xanthogranulomatous pyelonephritis is an unusual inflammatory disorder that can clinically and pathologically be confused with renal cell carcinoma.[168, 169] The presenting symptoms overlap with those of renal cell carcinoma, because most of the patients present with various symptoms from the constellation of flank pain, fever, malaise, weight loss, and hematuria.[170, 171] The preoperative diagnosis is confused further by the frequent finding of a flank mass. The gross appearance also is confusing because the inflammation may produce a tumor-like mass of yellow tissue and infiltrate the perinephric fat (Fig. 30–24). The renal outflow is almost always obstructed, usually by a calculus, but sometimes by deformity of the ureteropelvic junction.[172] Xanthogranulomatous pyelonephritis may also be confusing microscopically because an infiltrate of foamy histiocytes that may be misconstrued as the clear cells of renal cell carcinoma is usually the predominant element[173] (Fig. 30–25). Close attention to the cytoplasm reveals its foamy character, unlike that of clear cell renal cell carcinoma. There is also a lack of

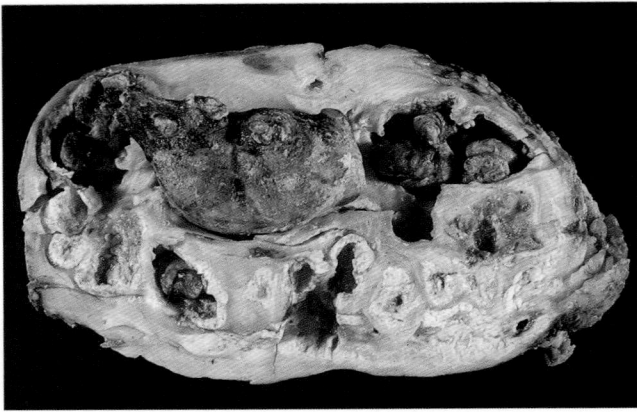

**Figure 30–24.** Xanthogranulomatous pyelonephritis in which masses of yellow tissue permeate the kidney. Note the stones in the hydronephrotic renal pelvis.

the vascular pattern typical of clear cell renal cell carcinomas, and the other inflammatory cells, principally lymphocytes and plasma cells, should assist further in its recognition. Malakoplakia is another inflammatory process that may resemble a primary renal tumor.[174]

Clinically occult renal cell carcinomas presenting at distant sites with unknown primaries or recurring years after an apparently successful radical nephrectomy may pose special diagnostic problems. The coexpression of cytokeratin and vimentin, which occurs in a majority of clear cell renal cell carcinomas,[175] is unusual among carcinomas and is suggestive of a renal primary when found in a metastasis of unknown origin.[167] Ultrastructurally, dense arrays of microvilli at intercellular areas or on luminal surfaces and prominence of glycogen in the cytoplasm are suggestive of renal cell carcinoma.[176] Solitary metastasis to the contralateral adrenal gland can resemble primary adrenal cortical carcinoma.[177] In such cases, immunohistochemical staining for epi-

thelial membrane antigen and cytokeratins can be helpful because renal cell carcinomas almost always stain for epithelial membrane antigen or cytokeratin, or both, whereas adrenal cortical carcinomas do not contain epithelial membrane antigen[178] and stain for cytokeratin only weakly and after a strong protease digestion procedure.[167] Metastasis to the thyroid can mimic clear cell carcinoma of the thyroid[179]; thyroglobulin immunohistochemistry and ultrastructural detection of intracytoplasmic glycogen (which is not found in clear cell carcinomas primary in the thyroid) can be helpful in making the distinction. Metastases to the ovary can be confused with primary ovarian clear cell adenocarcinoma.[180] Capillary hemangioblastoma of the central nervous system may closely resemble clear cell renal cell carcinoma in sections stained with hematoxylin and eosin, and it poses a particular problem because both neoplasms are associated with von Hippel–Lindau disease. This problem can usually be resolved by staining for epithelial membrane antigen because capillary hemangioblastomas fail to stain,[181] whereas renal cell carcinomas usually do.

## Papillary Renal Cell Carcinoma

### CLINICAL CONSIDERATIONS

Approximately 10% to 15% of renal cell carcinomas in surgical series are papillary renal cell carcinomas.[102, 182–187] Men predominate in a male-to-female ratio of approximately 2:1. Ages range from early adulthood to old age, with the mean between 50 and 55 years. These carcinomas have a mortality rate of at least 16% at 10 years[187] and sometimes present with metastases.[188]

Papillary renal cell carcinoma has a characteristic pattern of genetic abnormalities that differs from those of other renal cell neoplasms. The pattern of lesions is one of chromosomal gains. Most commonly, these are trisomy or tetrasomy of 7 and 17.[189, 190] Most papillary renal cell carcinomas in men lose the Y chromosome.[190] These results have been confirmed by several laboratories.[159, 191–194] Gains limited to chromosomes 7 and 17 may correlate with low grade and development of further trisomy correlates with progression.[190]

### MACROSCOPIC FINDINGS

Papillary renal cell carcinomas usually are well-circumscribed, globular tumors with pale tan or brown parenchyma (Fig. 30–26). In about two thirds of cases, hemorrhage and necrosis are prominent, which may cause the tumor to appear hypovascular radiographically.[182, 183] Many of these carcinomas are large. Often, the cut surface is friable or granular, a reflection of the papillae seen microscopically. The larger tumors are often surrounded by a rim of dense fibrous tissue.[195, 196] In about one third of cases, there are calcifications.[182, 183]

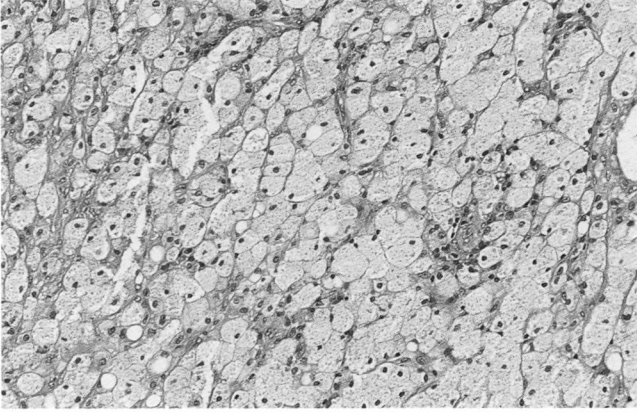

**Figure 30–25.** Xanthogranulomatous pyelonephritis. Cluster of pale-staining foamy histiocytes resemble clear cell renal cell carcinoma.

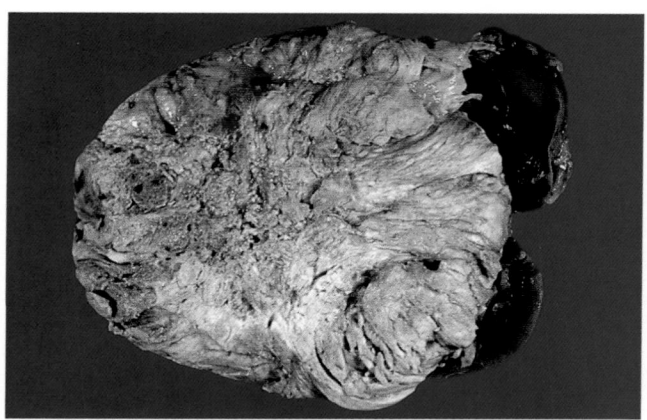

**Figure 30–26.** Papillary renal cell carcinoma forming a large globular mass of fronds.

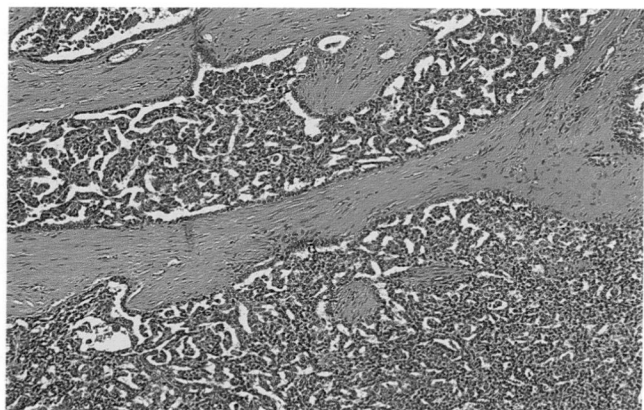

**Figure 30–28.** Papillary renal cell carcinoma type 1 with a tubulopapillary growth pattern.

## MICROSCOPIC FINDINGS

The architecture is predominantly papillary or tubulopapillary (Figs. 30–27 and 30–28) in more than 90% of papillary renal cell carcinomas.[102] Tight packing of papillae imparts the appearance of a solid growth pattern in some tumors. The papillae usually have delicate fibrovascular cores covered by a single layer of cells. The form of the papillae varies, ranging from complex branching to long parallel arrays.[186] The cores are sometimes expanded by foamy macrophages (Fig. 30–29) or edema fluid. Psammoma bodies occasionally are present.[197] Rarely, the papillary cores are wide and collagenous.[186] The tubular architecture consists of small tubules lined by a single layer of cells identical to those covering papillae.

There are two types of papillary renal cell carcinoma that Delahunt and Eble have designated type 1 and type 2.[61] Type 1 is more common than type 2. In type 1, the cells usually are small, with inconspicuous pale cytoplasm (see Fig. 30–27). The nuclei are typically uniform, nearly spherical, and small, with nucleoli that are small or invisible. In type 2, the cells are usually larger and often have abundant eosinophilic cytoplasm. The nuclei are arranged in a pseudostratified pattern, are large and spherical, and often have prominent nucleoli (Fig. 30–30).

In a series of 39 cases, nuclear morphology correlated with stage and outcome.[188] Thus, the nuclear grading system is recommended.[153]

## DIFFERENTIAL DIAGNOSIS

In children and adolescents, papillary renal cell carcinomas must be distinguished from Wilms' tumors with epithelial predominance. Beckwith[22] has emphasized the similarity of some Wilms' tumors to typical renal cell carcinoma. Thorough sampling of such tumors usually reveals blastema or differentiated stroma (e.g., skeletal muscle) and the diagnosis of Wilms' tumor is made with relative ease. The appearance of the nuclei, elongated with tapered ends in the epithelium of Wilms' tumor and roughly spherical in renal cell carcinoma, also may be helpful. The diagnosis of papillary renal cell carcinoma

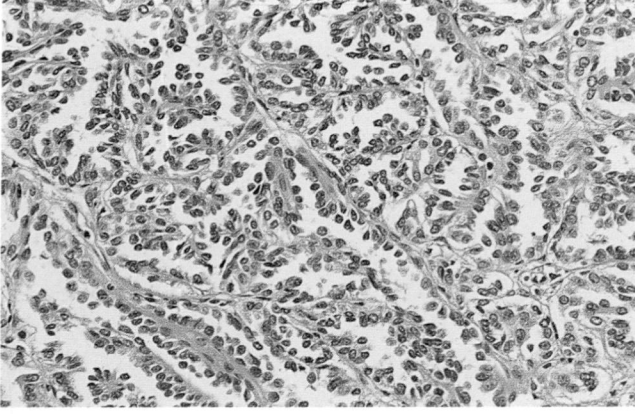

**Figure 30–27.** Papillary renal cell carcinoma type 1, consisting of complex branching papillae covered by a single layer of small cells.

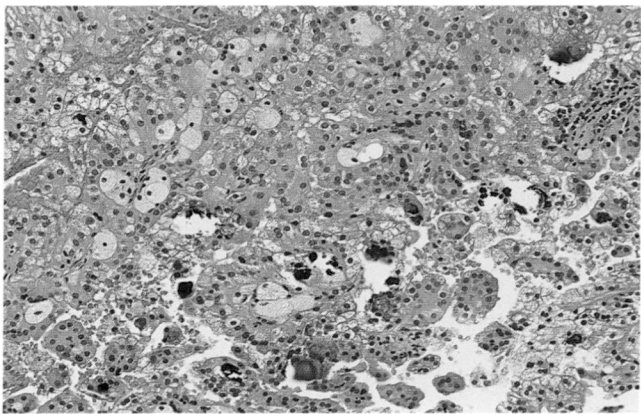

**Figure 30–29.** Papillary renal cell carcinoma type 1 with foamy histiocytes in the papillary cores and with psammoma bodies.

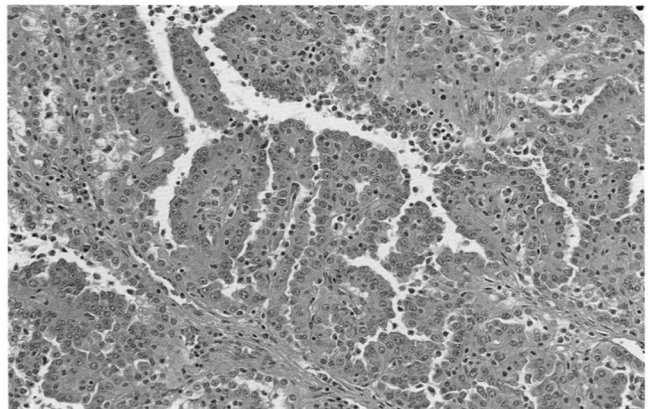

**Figure 30–30.** Papillary renal cell carcinoma type 2 consisting of papillae covered by cells with a pseudostratified appearance and abundant eosinophilic cytoplasm.

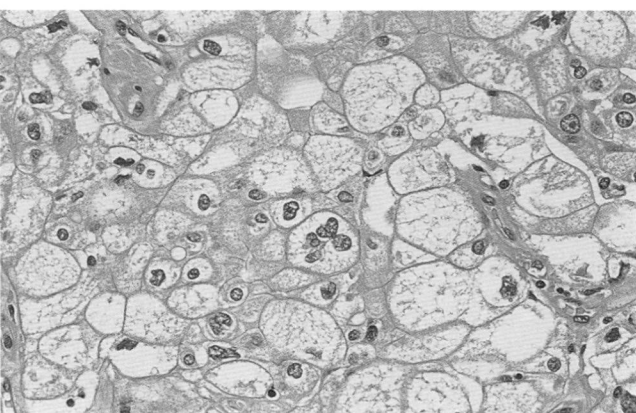

**Figure 30–32.** Chromophobe renal cell carcinoma consisting of a mosaic of cells with variable cytoplasmic volume.

in a young person should be made only after epithelial predominant Wilms' tumor has been excluded.

## Chromophobe Renal Cell Carcinoma

### CLINICAL CONSIDERATIONS

In 1985, Thoenes and colleagues[198] first described and named chromophobe renal cell carcinoma. Since then, it has become apparent that approximately 5% of renal cell carcinomas are chromophobe renal cell carcinomas.[199–201] The genetic hallmark of chromophobe renal cell carcinoma is the loss of multiple chromosomes.[202]

Although several deaths have been recorded from chromophobe renal cell carcinoma, it appears that this neoplasm is the least aggressive of the renal cell carcinomas. Sarcomatoid change occurs in chromophobe renal cell carcinoma at about the same frequency as in the other types of renal cell carcinoma but appears to account for a substantial fraction of the deaths.[203]

### MACROSCOPIC FINDINGS

Chromophobe renal cell carcinomas are usually well-circumscribed globular solid tan or brown tumors. Formalin fixation may change their color to a pale off white. Macroscopically visible cysts are not typical of chromophobe renal cell carcinoma.

### MICROSCOPIC FINDINGS

Chromophobe renal cell carcinoma is characterized by the presence of cells with large numbers of minute intracytoplasmic vesicles that impart a pale, reticular or flocculent appearance to the cytoplasm in preparations stained with hematoxylin and eosin (Figs. 30–31 and 30–32). The vesicles are demonstrable by electron microscopy. The Hale's colloidal iron stain colors the cytoplasm blue (Fig. 30–33).[199] The initial descriptions[198] emphasized the well-defined thick cytoplasmic membranes and lightly staining flocculent cytoplasm of what is now called the typical variant of chromophobe renal cell carcinoma. The typical variant also has thick-walled blood vessels. The cells range widely in size, and

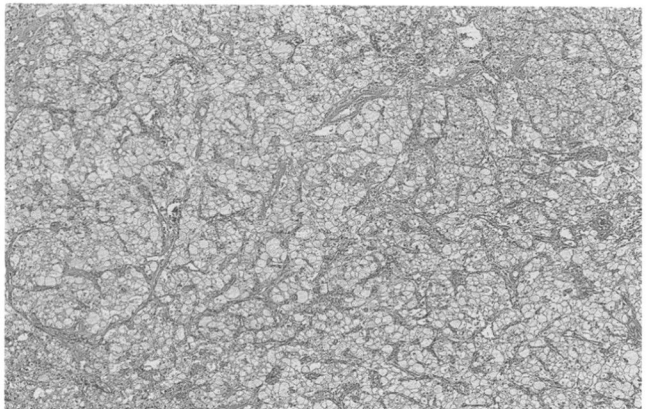

**Figure 30–31.** Chromophobe renal cell carcinoma consisting of cells with pale cytoplasm and an irregular vascular pattern with considerable variability in the thickness of the vessels' walls.

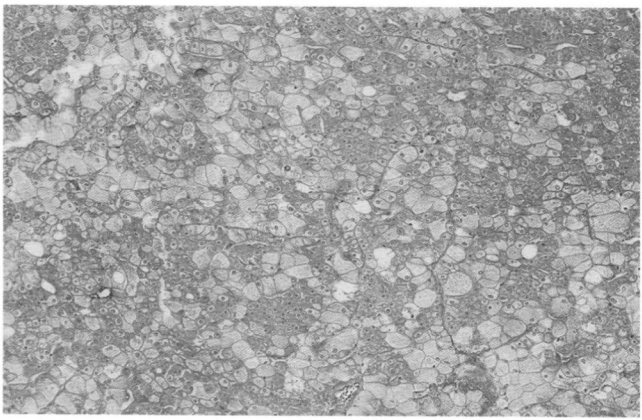

**Figure 30–33.** Chromophobe renal cell carcinoma in which the Hale's colloidal iron stain colors the cytoplasm blue.

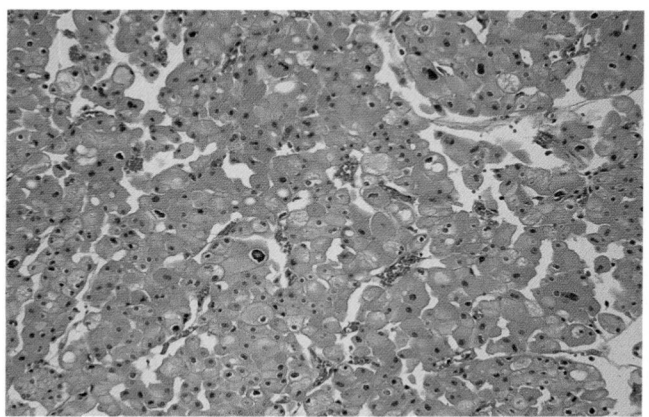

**Figure 30–34.** Chromophobe renal cell carcinoma, the eosinophilic variant. Note the perinuclear haloes.

small and large cells are mixed together in a mosaic pattern. Later, the eosinophilic variant of chromophobe cell renal cell carcinoma was recognized.[199] This variant shares the ultrastructural and colloidal iron–staining features of the typical variant, but in hematoxylin and eosin-stained slides, it often closely resembles renal oncocytoma (Fig. 30–34[204]). For this reason, it is worthwhile to collect specimens routinely for electron microscopy from renal tumors, especially those that do not have the yellow color characteristic of clear cell renal cell carcinoma. It is prudent to perform a colloidal iron stain on any tumor in which the differential diagnosis includes renal oncocytoma and chromophobe cell renal cell carcinoma.

### DIFFERENTIAL DIAGNOSIS

The vasculature, mosaic pattern of variability of cell size, and cytoplasmic characteristics make the classic form of chromophobe renal cell carcinoma distinctive, and the diagnosis can usually be easily achieved in routine sections. The eosinophilic variant is more problematic because of its close resemblance to oncocytoma. In sections stained with hematoxylin and eosin, perinuclear haloes, wrinkled irregular nuclei, and microcystic architecture lend support to the diagnosis of the eosinophilic variant of chromophobe renal cell carcinoma. However, histochemical staining for the Hale's colloidal iron reaction can be helpful and a diffuse cytoplasmic positive reaction is diagnostic of chromophobe renal cell carcinoma, whereas a diffusely negative reaction supports oncocytoma.

## Collecting Duct Carcinoma

### CLINICAL CONSIDERATIONS

The collecting ducts begin in the renal cortex and descend through the medulla to the renal papillae; the short segments just above the papillary orifices are called the ducts of Bellini.[205] There is evidence

that the intercalated cells of the collecting duct may be the source of renal oncocytomas[206] and chromophobe renal cell carcinomas.[207] Rumpelt and colleagues,[208] Fleming and Lewi,[209] Aizawa and coworkers,[210] and Kennedy and associates[211] have recently described a different group of tumors to which they attribute collecting duct origin. The criteria for this diagnosis are presently evolving.[212]

In general, the prognosis for collecting duct carcinomas is poor.[212] A variant of collecting duct carcinoma that occurs in young patients with sickle cell trait has recently been described and given the name medullary carcinoma of the kidney.[213] The prognosis for these patients has been exceptionally bad.

### MACROSCOPIC FINDINGS

Although the collecting ducts are present in the cortex and the medulla, the gross pathologic finding of a tumor arising in the inner medulla, where most other parts of the renal tubular system are absent, is an important aid to the diagnosis.[210] Unfortunately, precise localization to the medulla is only possible with small tumors, and many tumors are too large at the time of resection for the specific site of origin within the kidney to be recognizable. The tumors are usually centered in the medulla, often with extensions into the cortex or hilar tissues.[209, 211] Infiltrative borders and white or gray cut surfaces with central necrosis are typical.[208] A connection with the renal pelvis is common.

### MICROSCOPIC FINDINGS

Characteristically, these are histopathologically distinctive carcinomas with features of adenocarcinoma and urothelial carcinoma.[208, 214–216] Microscopic examination shows highly irregular duct-like structures, nests, and cords of cells in an abundant loose, slightly basophilic stroma (Fig. 30–35). The carcinoma cells lining the lumens have small or moderate amounts of cytoplasm and nuclei which are pleomorphic and have thick nuclear membranes. An especially useful feature, rarely found in renal cell

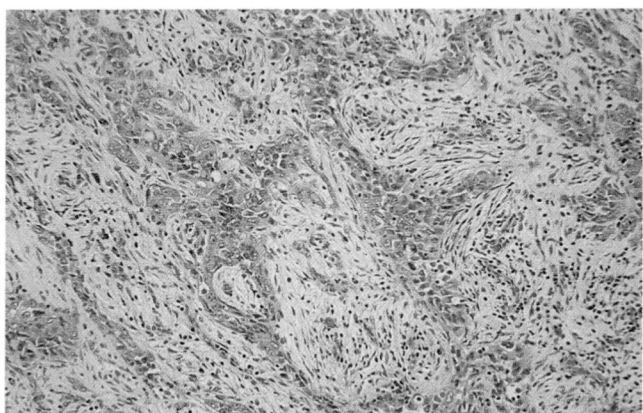

**Figure 30–35.** Collecting duct carcinoma forming irregular channels in an inflamed desmoplastic stroma.

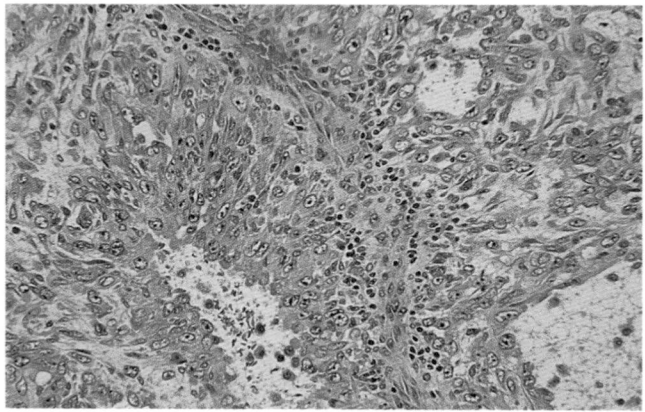

**Figure 30–36.** Collecting duct carcinoma; high magnification shows marked nuclear atypia and scattered hobnail cells.

carcinoma and not found in urothelial carcinoma, is the hobnail appearance sometimes seen in the cells lining duct lumens (Fig. 30–36). Some of the reported cases have a different pattern, consisting of papillary fronds covered by cells with small amounts of cytoplasm, similar to papillary renal cell carcinoma.[210, 211] Atypical epithelium in the medullary tubules adjacent to the carcinoma has been seen in some cases.[182, 211]

A lower grade neoplasm composed of many small cysts lined by epithelium with eosinophilic or amphophilic cytoplasm has been proposed as a low-grade collecting duct carcinoma.[217] The evidence for its origin in the distal collecting ducts is not as strong as the evidence for the more typical type.

### DIFFERENTIAL DIAGNOSIS

Awareness of collecting duct carcinoma and appreciation of the differences between microscopic features described earlier and those of other renal cancers should establish the diagnosis in most cases. Rumpelt and coworkers[208] found immunohistochemical differences in cytokeratin patterns and lectin binding between six collecting duct carcinomas and similar

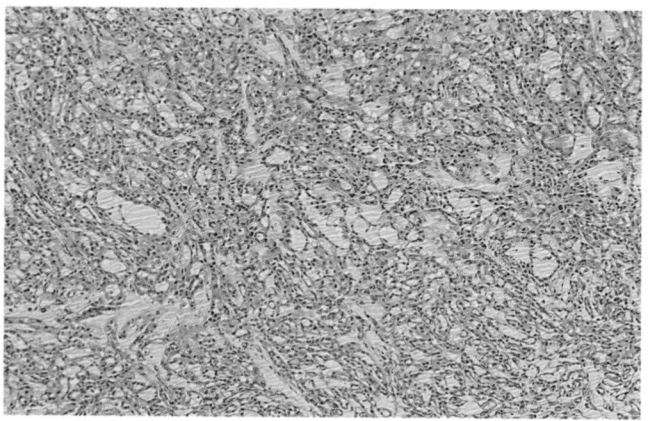

**Figure 30–37.** Renal cell carcinoma, unclassified. In this example, small glands are filled with basophilic mucinous material.

numbers of urothelial carcinomas and renal cell carcinomas. Collecting duct carcinomas stained strongly positively for cytokeratin 19 and *Ulex europaeus* lectin, and moderately for vimentin, but failed to stain for cytokeratin 13. The urothelial carcinomas uniformly failed to stain for vimentin, and the renal cell carcinomas failed to stain for *U. europaeus* lectin. If these differences prove consistent in larger series, immunohistochemistry will make valuable contributions to the diagnosis of collecting duct carcinoma. Until this is better understood, it is better to restrict the diagnosis of collecting duct carcinoma to those tumors for which the gross pathologic findings indicate this origin or that have the characteristic histopathologic appearance described earlier. Borderline cases should be diagnosed as renal cell carcinoma, unclassified.

## Renal Cell Carcinoma, Unclassified

Renal cell carcinoma, unclassified is a diagnostic category to which renal carcinomas should be assigned when they do not fit readily into one of the other categories.[68] In some surgical series, this group has amounted to approximately 4% and 5% of cases. Because this category must contain tumors with variety of appearances and genetic lesions, it cannot be precisely defined. Features that should prompt assignment of a carcinoma to this category include apparent composites of recognized types, sarcomatoid carcinoma without recognizable epithelial elements, production of mucin (Fig. 30–37), mixtures of epithelial and stromal elements, and unrecognizable cell types.

## NEUROENDOCRINE NEOPLASMS OF THE KIDNEY

More than two dozen neuroendocrine neoplasms in the spectrum from carcinoid to small cell carcinoma have been described in the kidney.[216] Arising equally frequently in men and women, the patients' ages have ranged from adolescence to the ninth decade of life, with a mean age of approximately 50 years. A variety of endocrine manifestations have been reported, including cases of the carcinoid syndrome[218] and excess secretion of glucagon.[219] Metastases have been common, even among the cases of carcinoid carcinoma.[220, 221]

Although pheochromocytomas arising in the renal sinus and compressing the renal artery appear to be more common than pheochromocytomas within the renal capsule,[222–224] intrarenal pheochromocytomas also occur[225–229] and are associated with hypertension. Neuroblastoma rarely arises in the kidneys of adults.[230]

## Macroscopic Appearances

The carcinoids often are well circumscribed[220, 231, 232] and consist of red-tan tissue with areas of hemorrhage[233] and necrosis.[234] Two cases have been de-

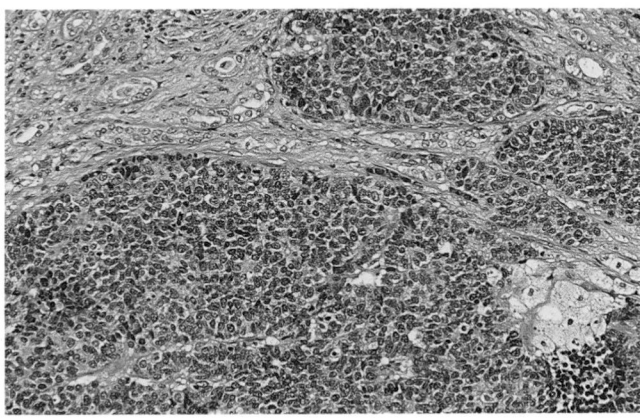

**Figure 30–38.** Small cell carcinoma of the kidney is histologically similar to small cell carcinoma of other sites.

scribed in which dysplastic teratoid elements have been associated with renal carcinoid.[235, 236] Renal small cell carcinomas often are large and infiltrate retroperitoneal soft tissues; regional lymph node metastases are common.[237, 238] Renal neuroblastomas are often large, firm tumors with yellowish red cut surfaces with areas of hemorrhage.[230] Intrarenal pheochromocytomas range in size from 2.5 to 9 cm in diameter[225, 227] and consist of yellow-brown or brownish tissue, often containing cysts.[226, 227]

## Histologic Appearances

Histopathologically, the tumors fill the spectrum from carcinoid to small cell carcinoma. The carcinoids consist of cords or nests of cells with the cytologic features characteristic of carcinoid tumors. At the other end of the spectrum of differentiation, the small cell carcinomas consist of sheets of poorly differentiated cells with darkly staining nuclei and inconspicuous cytoplasm (Fig. 30–38). Necrosis is common, and two studies[237, 238] noted the Azzopardi phenomenon (deposition of DNA in the walls of blood vessels). Neuroblastoma is diagnosed using the same criteria applied in the adrenal gland; the presence of neuropil or Homer-Wright rosettes is helpful in distinguishing it from small cell carcinoma and neuron-specific enolase is usually demonstrable by immunohistochemistry.[230] Intrarenal pheochromocytomas resemble their adrenal counterparts histologically.

## MESENCHYMAL TUMORS OF THE KIDNEY

### Angiomyolipoma

These benign neoplasms of the kidney are composed of fat, smooth muscle, and thick-walled blood vessels in varying proportions.[239] In surgical series, approximately half are associated with tuberous sclero-

sis and half occur sporadically. In patients with tuberous sclerosis, they are usually asymptomatic, multiple, bilateral, and small, whereas in the general population, they are usually symptomatic, single, and large (Fig. 30–39).[240] They are uncommon in the general population, but more than 50% of patients with tuberous sclerosis develop them.[111] Local invasion has been reported occasionally and has exceptionally been lethal[241]; however, in only rare instances have well-documented sarcomas arisen from an angiomyolipoma.[242]

### MACROSCOPIC APPEARANCES

Ranging from less than a centimeter to 20 cm or more in diameter. The likelihood of symptoms increases above 4 cm and symptomatic tumors average about 9 cm. These tumors are typically golden yellow, but the color varies according to the proportions of smooth muscle and blood vessels. They are not encapsulated, and although they are generally well demarcated, they may be locally infiltrative. The appearance of the cut surface of the tumor may resemble that of a lipoma.

### HISTOLOGIC APPEARANCES

The histology of these tumors varies according to the relative proportions of fat, smooth muscle, and blood vessels (Fig. 30–40). The smooth muscle component is also variable in appearance. A frequent finding is radial arrays of smooth muscle fibers about blood vessels, but smooth muscle also is found in bundles and scattered as individual fibers. The smooth muscle cells are typically spindle shaped, but occasionally they are epithelioid and have abundant eosinophilic cytoplasm. The blood vessels are often abnormal, with thick walls resembling those of arteries but with eccentrically placed or very small lumens. Nuclear pleomorphism may be pronounced, and mitotic figures may be present. These findings have no adverse prognostic significance in most cases. In some cases, angiomyolipomatous tissue has been found in regional lymph

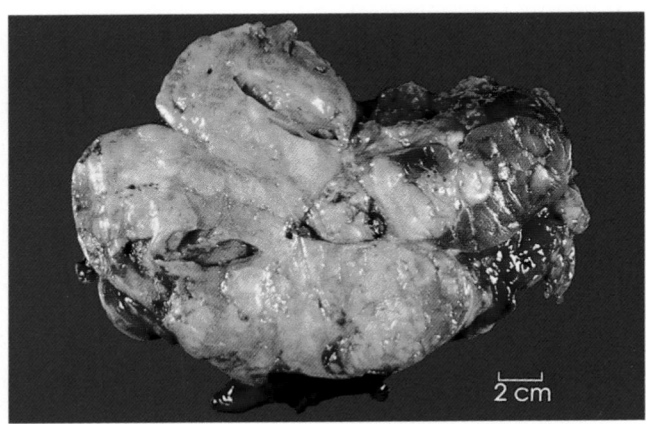

**Figure 30–39.** Angiomyolipoma forms a large irregular yellow mass.

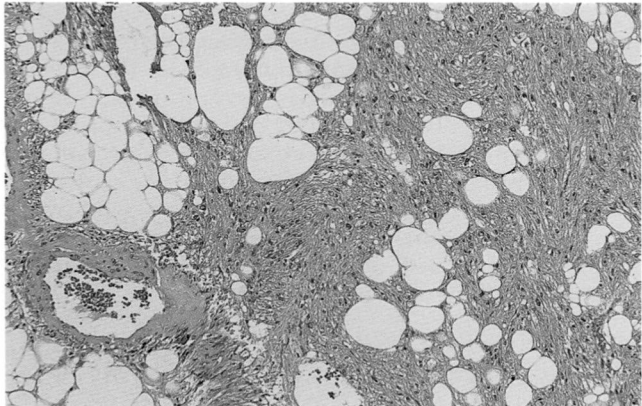

**Figure 30–40.** Angiomyolipoma composed of thick-walled blood vessels, smooth muscle, and fat.

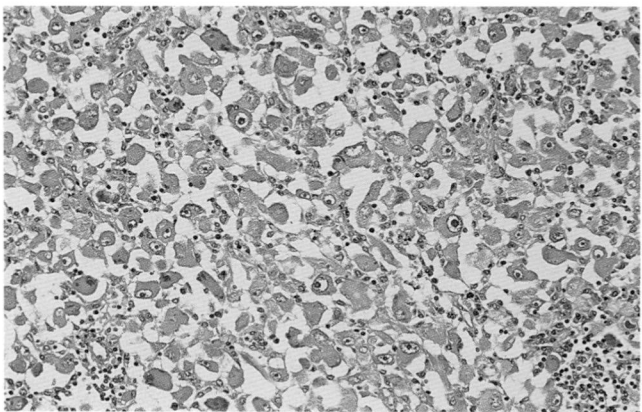

**Figure 30–42.** Epithelioid angiomyolipoma with many large round cells with eccentrically located nuclei with prominent nucleoli, reminiscent of ganglion cells.

nodes[243–245] (Fig. 30–41) and spleen.[246] This appearance should not be misinterpreted as metastatic sarcoma. Occasionally, angiomyolipoma invades the renal vein or vena cava; all of these patients have been cured surgically, so this lesion does not indicate malignancy.[239]

A variant of angiomyolipoma that can be mistaken for carcinoma has recently been recognized and categorized as epithelioid angiomyolipoma.[247–249] The tumors are composed of a mixture of large polygonal cells with abundant eosinophilic cytoplasm (Fig. 30–42), some of which superficially resemble ganglion cells, and short spindle cells. Often, there is extensive hemorrhage and edema in the tumors. Immunohistochemistry shows the presence of actin and HMB-45 and the absence of epithelial markers. The diagnosis is clinically important because a substantial fraction of these tumors have progressed and been lethal.

### DIFFERENTIAL DIAGNOSIS

In cases with an extreme predominance of fat, angiomyolipoma can be confused with lipoma; extensive sampling may be necessary to identify the vascular and smooth muscle components of the tumor. Tumors with scant fat may be confused with other mesenchymal tumors, such as leiomyoma. Tumors with epithelioid features may mimic epithelial tumors of the kidney and the possibility should be considered when examining an epithelial-like renal tumor that is hard to classify, particularly if the patient has tuberous sclerosis.

Epithelioid angiomyolipoma is often incorrectly diagnosed as carcinoma at frozen section, in fine-needle aspirations or in permanent sections. It should be considered when confronted by any unusual renal neoplasm composed of poorly cohesive polygonal cells with eosinophilic cytoplasm.

## Hemangioma

Hemangiomas of the kidney have been found mainly in adults and occur equally in men and women.[250, 251] Solitary lesions are the most frequent, but more than 10% are multiple and bilaterality has been reported. Rarely, they may be associated with the Klippel-Trenaunay and Sturge-Weber syndromes.[252] Many are asymptomatic and found only at autopsy. In symptomatic patients, recurrent hematuria is the usual complaint, frequently associated with anemia.[253]

### MACROSCOPIC APPEARANCES

Most are less than 1 cm in diameter and unimpressive to the naked eye. Larger lesions, approximately 18 cm in diameter, occur and have a spongy reddish appearance. Although hemangiomas may arise anywhere in the kidney, the medulla and papilla are the sites of the majority of symptomatic lesions.[253]

### HISTOLOGIC APPEARANCES

Microscopically, these lesions are composed of vascular spaces of variable size, some of which may have smooth muscle and elastic tissue in their walls. Thrombosis and organization are common. Although they often have irregular borders and merge

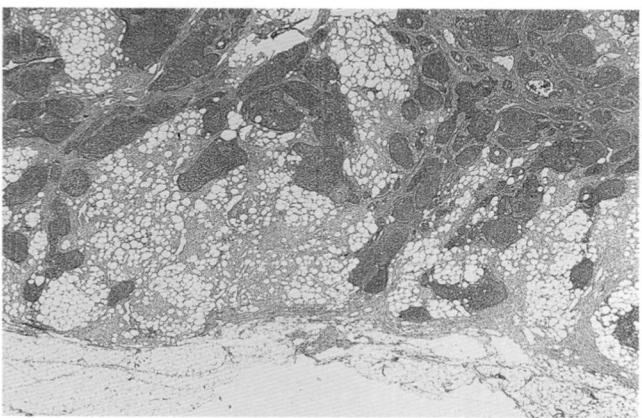

**Figure 30–41.** Angiomyolipoma in para-aortic node from a patient with renal angiomyolipoma.

with the surrounding renal parenchyma, the lack of nuclear atypia and mitotic figures should make recognition of their benign nature easy in most cases. They are distinguished from angiosarcomas using the same criteria applied in soft tissue; this also pertains to the other benign mesenchymal tumors discussed here.

## Lymphangioma

Renal lymphangiomas are much less common than renal hemangiomas. A few dozen cases have been described in patients ranging in age from infancy[254] to old age, about a third in children and two thirds in adults.[255, 256] Grossly, most have been solitary encapsulated masses composed of small cysts containing clear fluid. Microscopic examination shows spaces lined by benign endothelial cells with septa that are generally fibrous but may contain smooth muscle. Lesions in the renal sinus may infiltrate the renal medulla,[254] obstructing the flow of urine.

## Leiomyoma

Symptomatic renal leiomyomas are rare,[257] but they rarely are large masses as great as 37 kg;[258] small ones are usually found incidentally at autopsy. Most occur in adults.[259] Grossly, they are well-circumscribed solid rubbery masses with whorled cut surfaces. As in the uterus, they consist of bundles of smooth muscle fibers that may focally calcify and show other degenerative changes. The finding of necrosis, nuclear atypia, or more than rare mitotic figures strongly suggests that the tumor is a leiomyosarcoma.

## Lipoma

Symptomatic renal lipomas are rare.[260] The patients usually present with abdominal or flank pain. They occur almost exclusively in middle-aged women. Unlike angiomyolipomas, these tumors are not associated with tuberous sclerosis. Grossly, these are yellow lobulated and encapsulated masses, and histopathologically, they consist entirely of mature fat. Generous sampling is indicated because, as noted earlier, angiomyolipomas may consist predominantly of fat and thorough sectioning may be necessary to find the smooth muscle and vascular elements which distinguish them from lipomas. Rarely, renal sinus fat around the renal pelvis may proliferate excessively, mimicking a neoplasm.[261]

## Leiomyosarcoma

This is the most common primary renal sarcoma, more than 100 cases having been reported.[262] Although the patients' ages have ranged from childhood to older than 80 years of age, most have oc-

curred in patients older than 40, with a peak in the fifth and sixth decades. There have been approximately twice as many women as men. Mass and flank pain are the most common presentation.

### MACROSCOPIC APPEARANCES

The gross appearance of the tumors often resembles that of leiomyomas: firm, solid tumors with well-circumscribed margins and whorled cut surfaces, but necrosis and hemorrhage are more common.[263] Leiomyosarcomas may also arise from the renal capsule,[263] and renal vein and the bulk of the tumor may be in the renal sinus.[264] Renal and perirenal infiltration are frequent.

### HISTOLOGIC APPEARANCES

Microscopically, they are composed of fascicles of spindle-shaped cells with features resembling smooth muscle. A myxoid variant has been described.[265] The degree of nuclear pleomorphism and the prevalence of mitotic figures vary over a wide range and no clear minimum criteria of malignancy have been established.[266] Necrosis, nuclear pleomorphism, or more than rare mitotic figures should be taken as indications that a renal smooth muscle tumor is probably a leiomyosarcoma. Especially in large smooth muscle tumors, suspicion of leiomyosarcoma should be high because metastasis and death have occasionally been caused by tumors with very low mitotic counts.[267]

## Liposarcoma

Liposarcoma is common in the retroperitoneal soft tissues but rare in the kidney.[268, 269] Careful gross examination is important to establish the intrarenal origin of the tumors because liposarcomas of the retroperitoneal soft tissues invading or compressing the kidney are more common than renal liposarcomas invading the retroperitoneal soft tissues.[263] In cases in which the origin is unclear (the larger and more infiltrative ones), the presumption should be in favor of a primary in retroperitoneal soft tissue. Some of the reported cases have, in retrospect, been large solitary angiomyolipomas, giving renal liposarcoma a reputation for a more favorable prognosis than is warranted. Grossly, the tumors are relatively well circumscribed yellow lobulated masses. Histopathologically, renal liposarcomas have shown the usual variety of patterns found elsewhere; 80% of the tumors described by Farrow and colleagues[263] were myxoid.

## Malignant Fibrous Histiocytoma

Malignant fibrous histiocytomas may arise from the renal parenchyma or from the renal capsule.[270, 271] Because the retroperitoneal soft tissues are a common site for malignant fibrous histiocytoma, the recommendations made earlier for the attribution of primary site for liposarcomas involving the kidney also apply here. Clinically, renal malignant fibrous histiocytomas have mainly occurred in adults and there has been a strong male predominance. For the most part, they have been large infiltrative lesions and histopathologically of the storiform-pleomorphic and inflammatory types. The former may be difficult to distinguish from sarcomatoid renal cell carcinoma, and sarcomatoid renal cell carcinoma may resemble xanthogranulomatous pyelonephritis.

## Rhabdomyosarcoma

Rhabdomyosarcomas of the kidney are rare[272–274]; Grignon and associates[275] reviewed the literature and found only eight convincing cases, evenly divided between the genders and occurring in patients from 36 to 70 years old. Four died of the sarcoma within 14 months, and the other four were reported with less than 12 months of follow-up. Most renal tumors with appearances suggesting rhabdomyosarcoma are something else, so the diagnosis of rhabdomyosarcoma should be made reluctantly. In children, Wilms' tumors may contain elements of skeletal muscle and the existence of rhabdomyosarcoma distinct from Wilms' tumor in children is questionable. Rhabdoid tumor of kidney may also mimic rhabdomyosarcoma, as may sarcomatoid renal cell carcinoma.

## Other Sarcomas

A hemangiopericytoma primary in the kidney is rare[276, 277] and subject to the confusion between intrarenal and extrarenal origin discussed in the section on liposarcoma.[263, 278] The tumors usually are large and cysts and foci of hemorrhage are common.[277] Osteogenic sarcomas arise rarely from the renal parenchyma or pelvis[279, 280] and a few chondrosarcomas,[281, 282] angiosarcomas,[283–285] and malignant mesenchymomas[286] have been reported. Histologically, they show the typical features seen elsewhere.

## Juxtaglomerular Cell Tumor

Juxtaglomerular cell tumors, also known as reninomas, were recognized independently in 1967 by Robertson and associates and Kihara and associates. More than 50 examples have been reported.[216, 287] Although all of the patients have been hypertensive, Corvol and associates[288] found only seven tumors in 30,000 new hypertensive patients. Elevation of plasma renin levels is typical of these patients, and selective catheterization of the renal veins has been an important guide to the resection of small tumors.[289] Most of the patients have been young adults and adolescents, averaging 27 years old at the time of resection.[216] However, many of the patients have been hypertensive for years before resection. The average age of onset of hypertension is only 22

years. The incidence of the tumor in women exceeds that in men by almost 2:1. Resection has cured the hypertension in most cases, and conservative resection has been effective in several cases. No instance of metastasis, local invasion or recurrence, multifocality, or bilaterality has been reported.

### MACROSCOPIC APPEARANCES

Most juxtaglomerular cell tumors have been smaller than 3 cm, and some have not been visible when the renal capsule was stripped. Thus, when a juxtaglomerular cell tumor is suspected, the specimen must be carefully dissected and any abnormal foci submitted for histopathologic examination. The masses are sharply circumscribed and composed of rubbery off-white tissue, sometimes containing small cystlike smooth-walled cavities.

### HISTOLOGIC APPEARANCES

The histopathology of these lesions is varied. A common pattern is one of irregular trabeculae of polygonal cells in a loose myxoid stroma (Fig. 30–43). Tubules and cysts often are present. There is frequently prominent vascularity and a lymphocytic infiltrate may be conspicuous. Modified Bowie's stain may reveal intracytoplasmic granules and immunohistochemistry may demonstrate intracytoplasmic renin.[290, 291] Electron microscopy is helpful in demonstrating the typical rhomboid granules of juxtaglomerular cell tumors.[292]

### DIFFERENTIAL DIAGNOSIS

Because it is almost invariably discovered in the investigation of hypertension, the nature of the tumor is often suspected preoperatively. The gross finding of a small light-colored rubbery tumor narrows the differential diagnosis, and the histopathologic appearance is distinctive. However, because immunoreactive renin has been found in renal cell carcinomas and Wilms' tumors,[293–295] some of which have caused hypertension, these may rarely cause diagnostic confusion.

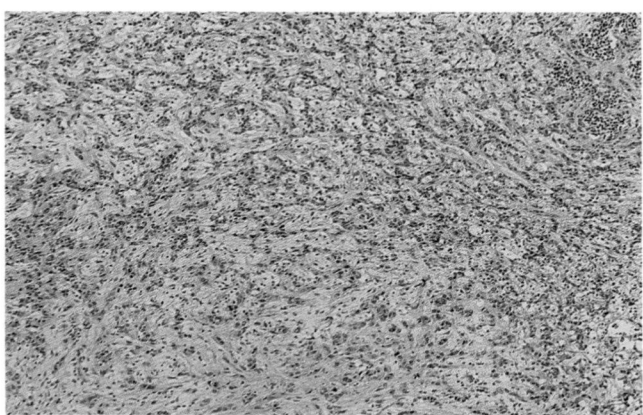

**Figure 30–43.** Juxtaglomerular cell tumor consisting of cords of cells in a loose edematous background scattered with lymphocytes.

## Renomedullary Interstitial Cell Tumor

These small tumors of the renal medulla are frequent findings at autopsy. Ultrastructural and other studies have shown that these lesions are composed of the renomedullary interstitial cells, which contain vasoactive substances that are important in the regulation of blood pressure. Whether these are neoplasms or hyperplastic nodules that arise in response to hypertension remains controversial. They are rare in patients younger than 20 years, but in a large series of carefully dissected autopsy kidneys, almost half of the patients older than 20 years of age had at least one lesion and 57% of the patients with renomedullary interstitial cell tumors had more than one.[296]

Because most of these tumors are small, they rarely cause symptoms or diagnostic difficulty in surgical specimens. Most problems have arisen when one is an unexpected finding in a kidney resected for other reasons, such as transplantation. The few symptomatic tumors have usually been pedunculated masses in the renal pelvis, and the early reports called them renal pelvic fibromas.[216]

### MACROSCOPIC APPEARANCES

These tumors are white nodules that can occur anywhere in the renal medulla (Fig. 30–44). They are well circumscribed and usually spheroidal, and most are smaller than 5 mm in diameter.

### HISTOLOGIC APPEARANCES

Microscopically, small stellate cells lie in a faintly basophilic loose stroma, reminiscent of the stroma of the renal medulla. Bundles of loose fibers arranged in an interlacing pattern frequently are present (Fig. 30–45). The stromal matrix often entraps medullary tubules at the periphery of the nodules. The name fibroma is a misnomer because most of these lesions contain little collagen. Some do contain amyloid,[297] which may be deposited in irregular clumps (see

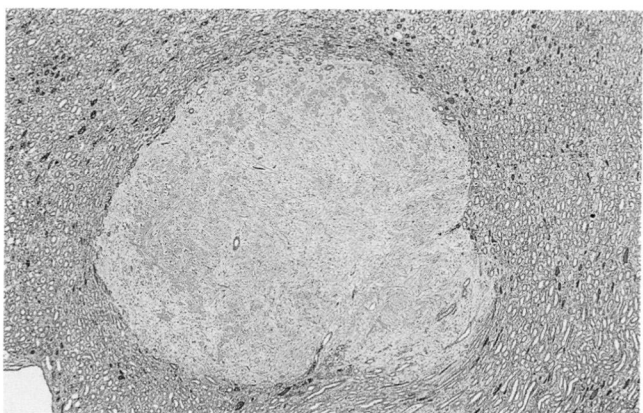

**Figure 30–45.** Renomedullary interstitial cell tumor forming a well-circumscribed nodule composed of stellate and spindle cells. Pink-staining amyloid is present. Renal tubules are entrapped mainly at the periphery.

Fig. 30–45), obscuring the characteristic delicate stroma.

## Cystic Nephroma

Cystic nephroma, which has also been called multilocular cyst[298] and multilocular cystic nephroma,[299] is an uncommon benign renal neoplasm that occurs in adults.[23, 300] Women predominate over men in a ratio of approximately 7:1. In a few patients, sarcoma has arisen in cystic nephroma.[23] Conservative surgery is generally curative, but in one case, cystic nephroma recurred after incomplete excision.[23, 301] The diagnostic criteria for cystic nephroma are listed in Table 30–8.

### MACROSCOPIC APPEARANCES

These lesions are well-circumscribed globular masses surrounded by a fibrous capsule. They are composed of multiple noncommunicating cystic locules with smooth inner surfaces. The cysts are filled with clear yellowish fluid (Fig. 30–46). Solid areas are

**TABLE 30–8.** Diagnostic Criteria of Eble and Bonsib for Cystic Nephroma

---

Adult patient
Expansile mass surrounded by fibrous pseudocapsule
Interior entirely composed of cysts and septa with no expansile solid nodules
Cysts lined by flattened, hobnail, or cuboidal epithelium
Septa may contain epithelial structures resembling mature renal tubules
Septa may not contain epithelial cells with clear cytoplasm
Septa may not contain skeletal muscle fibers

---

Eble JN, Bonsib SM: Extensively cystic renal neoplasms: Cystic nephroma, cystic partially differentiated nephroblastoma, multilocular cystic renal cell carcinoma, and cystic hamartoma of renal pelvis. Semin Diagn Pathol 15:2–20, 1998.

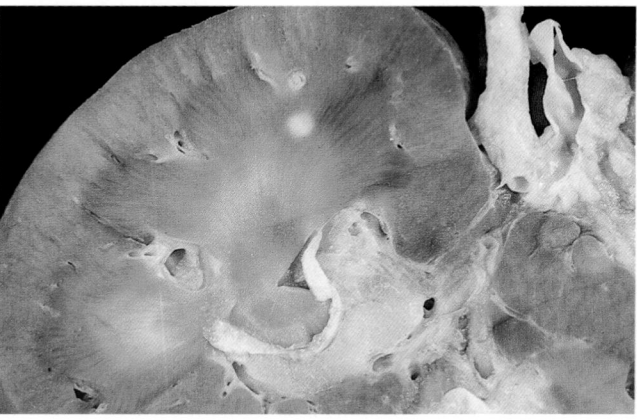

**Figure 30–44.** Renomedullary interstitial cell tumor, a 2-mm white nodule in the medullary pyramid.

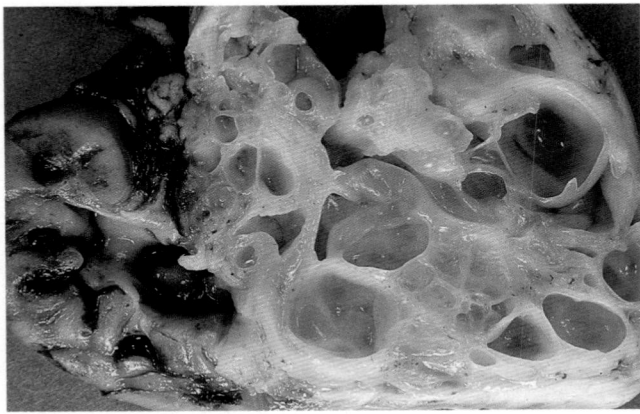

**Figure 30–46.** Cystic nephroma forms a well-circumscribed mass of cysts of variable size.

absent, and the septa range from paper thin to a few millimeters thick. Grossly, cystic nephroma is indistinguishable from multilocular cystic renal cell carcinoma and from cystic partially differentiated nephroblastoma.

### HISTOLOGIC APPEARANCES

Microscopically, the septa are composed of fibrous tissue (Fig. 30–47), which may contain foci of calcification. The septa may contain structures resembling differentiated renal tubules (as opposed to tubules with the morphology characteristic of Wilms' tumor), inflammatory cells, and reactive fibroblasts.[302] The cellularity of the septa ranges from sparsely cellular hyalinized tissue to highly cellular spindle cell stroma superficially resembling ovarian stroma. The cysts are usually lined by flattened or low cuboidal epithelium with small amounts of cytoplasm; occasionally the lining cells have a hobnail configuration. The cytoplasm ranges from eosinophilic to clear.

### DIFFERENTIAL DIAGNOSIS

Cystic Wilms' tumor and cystic renal cell carcinoma are the principal differential diagnostic considerations, clinically, radiographically, and pathologically. The criteria set out in Table 30–8 distinguish cystic nephroma from these tumors. Of critical importance is the absence of blastema and other elements of Wilms' tumor and the lack of collections of epithelial cells with clear cytoplasm within the septa.

## Mixed Epithelial and Stromal Tumor of the Kidney

A rare and distinctive renal neoplasm apparently composed of a complex mixture of neoplastic stroma and epithelium has been recognized in recent years.[23] A variety of names have been applied to these tumors,[303–305] but the one that most accurately describes them is mixed epithelial and stromal tumor.[306] To date, these patients have been cured surgically and there is no report of malignant behavior.

Grossly, the tumors typically contain small and large cysts mixed with solid areas (Fig. 30–48A).[307] A few have been extensively cystic and have resembled cystic nephroma. They appear to arise from the renal parenchyma, probably the medulla, and a majority have extended into the renal pelvis.

Microscopically, they consist of stroma ranging from hyalinized fibrous tissue to smooth muscle.[307] Fat has been present in some. The stroma contains complex epithelial elements forming cysts and tubules (Fig. 30–48B). The tubules range from small ones resembling nephrogenic adenoma to long branching tubules. The lining epithelium may be cuboidal, columnar, flattened, or urothelial. Immunohistochemistry often confirms smooth muscle differentiation. HMB45 is absent.

## Lymphoma

Secondary involvement of the kidney in cases of disseminated malignant lymphoma occurs in as many as 50% of cases. However, whether or not lymphomas occur as primary tumors in the kidney is controversial.[308, 309] Small numbers of cases of lymphoma that have appeared to be renal masses have been reported but in most, extrarenal lymphoma has been discovered shortly thereafter. The symptoms resemble those of renal cell carcinoma.[310]

### MACROSCOPIC APPEARANCES

The gross appearance of lymphoma in the kidney is variable. Frequently, the mass is parenchymal and well circumscribed; less frequently, it is diffuse.[311] In the former case, the lesions consist of whitish nodules in the kidney, typically visible on the cortical surface. In the latter case, the renal volume is ex-

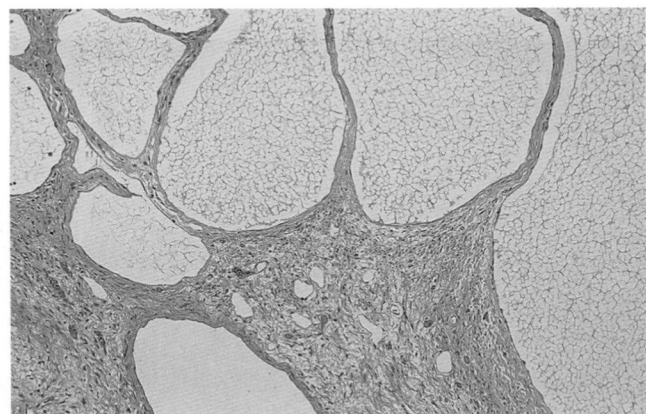

**Figure 30–47.** Cystic nephroma with thin fibrous septa delimiting cysts lined by flattened epithelium.

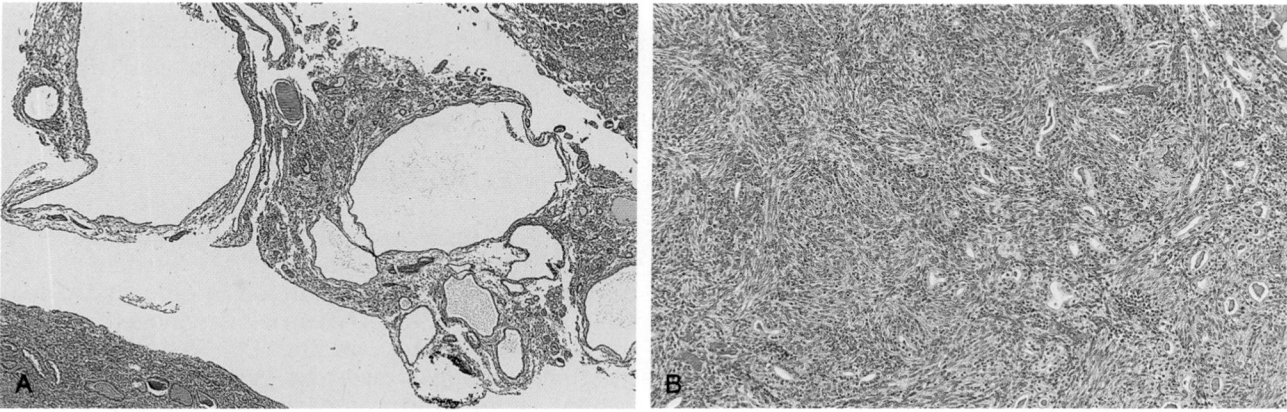

**Figure 30–48.** *A,* Mixed epithelial and stromal tumor with cystic and solid areas. *B,* Mixed epithelial and stromal tumor; complex tubular structures lined by cuboidal cells and embedded in spindle cell stroma.

panded and the cortex and medulla are pale and their junctions are obscured by the infiltrate. Lymphoma presenting as a renal mass often arises in the renal sinus, surrounding and invading the hilar structures.[311]

### HISTOLOGIC APPEARANCES

The microscopic appearance varies according to the gross appearance and type of lymphoma. In cases in which the lymphoma consists of circumscribed nodules, the lesions consist almost entirely of lymphoma cells microscopically. In examples in which there is diffuse infiltration, the renal interstitium is infiltrated by a monomorphous population of atypical lymphoid cells; there may be sparing of the glomeruli and tubules. Among those presenting as renal primaries, large cell lymphomas are more common than small cell lymphomas[310, 311] and Hodgkin's disease is unusual.[311] Plasmacytomas also occur in the kidney.[312, 313]

## SECONDARY NEOPLASMS OF THE KIDNEY

In a study of 11,328 autopsies of cancer patients, Bracken and associates[314] found that 7.2% of patients had metastases to the kidneys. These findings are supported by other studies.[315–318] Bronchogenic carcinomas are the most frequent sources of metastatic carcinoma.[314, 317] Metastases more rarely present as primary renal tumors and may be treated surgically for that mistaken diagnosis.[316] Although solitary metastases may closely mimic primary renal neoplasms grossly, microscopic examination usually clarifies the case when the typical features of a nonrenal primary are found. Occasionally, carcinoma metastatic to the kidney is found only as widespread microscopic metastases to the glomeruli[319] or diffusely to renal lymphatics.[320]

## Germ Cell Neoplasms

Renal teratomas are rare and controversial lesions that may be difficult to distinguish from Wilms' tumors because they can contain areas of immature renal tissue with primitive glomerulogenesis and tubule formation.[321] The presence of a wide variety of tissue types representing all three germ cell layers is important in the diagnosis. Structures not ordinarily found in Wilms' tumors, such as lymph node or gut-like structures combining epithelium with smooth muscle[322] or hair follicle and sweat glands,[323] are most helpful.[322] However, most renal tumors consisting of a variety of epithelial and mesenchymal elements are Wilms' tumors.

Choriocarcinoma has been reported to arise in the kidney.[324] Because differentiation toward choriocarcinoma is seen in some high-grade urothelial carcinomas,[325] a thorough search for recognizable urothelial carcinoma should be made in all such cases.

## TUMORS OF THE RENAL PELVIS AND URETER

Given the similarities of the anatomic structures and exposure to urine-borne carcinogens of the renal pelvis, ureter, and urinary bladder, it is not surprising that most of the kinds of tumors that are found in the urinary bladder have also occurred in the segments of the urinary tract above it. The following discussion focuses mainly on those aspects which are particular to the upper urinary tract. For a more general and detailed discussion, the reader should look to the sections addressing the same tumors as they occur in the urinary bladder.

Primary tumors of ureters are uncommon, and in a comprehensive review, Abeshouse[326] found that carcinomas were more common than benign tumors.

# BENIGN TUMORS AND TUMOR-LIKE LESIONS

## Nephrogenic Adenoma

These lesions also are known as nephrogenic metaplasia. They are rare in the ureter and much more common in the urinary bladder. Nephrogenic adenomas are exophytic lesions which grossly mimic urothelial carcinoma and microscopically are characterized by benign papillary and tubular proliferations lined by cuboidal or hobnail epithelium.[327, 328]

## Inverted Papilloma

Inverted papillomas are benign urothelial tumors that occur less commonly in the renal pelvis and ureter than in the urinary bladder.[329, 330] They are almost twice as common in the ureter as in the renal pelvis.[331] Men predominate, and the mean age of presentation is in the mid-60s.[331] In the upper tract, these tumors are found incidentally by intravenous pyelography[330] or cause hematuria.[332, 333] These tumors may be multiple and associated with urothelial carcinoma at other sites.[334] Grossly, they are broad-based domed lesions. The tumors consist of trabeculae of histologically typical urothelial epithelium, which in some cases, forms small glandular structures lined by metaplastic mucinous epithelium.[335] The histologic features of these tumors are discussed in more detail in connection with their occurrence in the urinary bladder. Rarely, urothelial carcinoma may arise within an inverted papilloma of the ureter.[336, 337]

## Fibroepithelial Polyp

This is an uncommon benign mesenchymal tumor of the renal pelvis[338] and ureter.[339] Most are found in adults of young or middle age, but pediatric[340, 341] and geriatric[342] cases have occurred. Macksood and colleagues concluded that these are the most frequent benign polypoid lesions of the ureters in children.[341] Most (70%) of the patients are male.[343] Colicky flank pain and hematuria are the most common symptoms. Grossly, these tumors consist of single or multiple smooth-surfaced slender fronds arising close together from the mucosa. The most common locations are the ureteropelvic junction and upper ureter.[344] The etiology is uncertain.[344] Histopathologically, they consist of a vascular loose edematous stromal core with a variable inflammatory infiltrate, covered by essentially normal urothelium, which may show foci of squamous metaplasia or ulceration.

## Hemangioma

Hemangiomas of the ureter and renal pelvis are uncommon polypoid tumors consisting of hypervascular fibrous stroma covered by normal urothelial epithelium.[345, 346] They occur in children and adults, and these lesions may be multiple and frequently cause obstruction.

# UROTHELIAL CARCINOMA

Urothelial carcinomas of the upper tract have epidemiology similar to those of the bladder[347]: male predominance,[348] most common in older individuals, and tobacco[349] and industrial carcinogen exposure risk factors. Phenacetin abuse[350, 351] is the most important etiologic factor in some populations, accounting for nearly a quarter of renal pelvic tumors and more than 10% of ureteral tumors. Balkan nephropathy and exposure to thorium-containing radiologic contrast material[352, 353] are risk factors for upper tract carcinomas but not for urinary bladder tumors. Tumors of the renal pelvis and calyces are approximately twice as common as tumors of the ureters.[348] Hematuria is the principal symptom, but flank pain also is frequent.[354] Multifocality is a significant problem for patients with upper tract tumors.[348, 355] Nearly 50% of them have histories of urothelial carcinoma of the bladder or ureters or later develop additional urothelial carcinomas.[356] In the ureter, the most common location is the distal segment.[357] Grade and stage are the most important prognostic factors in urothelial carcinomas of the upper tract, whereas multiplicity of tumors also has an effect.[355] Approximately 75% of cases are classified as low grade and stage 1.[358] The grading scheme is identical to that applied in the bladder, and the staging system is similar to that used in the bladder. The AJCC staging system is shown in Table 30–9.[359] Tumors that are grade 1 and stage 1 at the time of resection have little effect on survival.[360] Muscle invasion is a critical point in the progression of these tumors, and survival decreases markedly when it is present. The lung is the most common site of metastasis.[361] Owing to the high rate of recur-

**TABLE 30–9.** Staging System for Urothelial Carcinomas of the Renal Pelvis and Ureter

| | |
|---|---|
| Ta | Noninvasive papillary carcinoma |
| Tis | Urothelial carcinoma in situ |
| T1 | Invasion of lamina propria |
| T2 | Invasion of muscularis propria |
| T3 (renal pelvis) | Extension into peripelvic fat or renal parenchyma |
| T3 (ureter) | Extension into periureteric fat |
| T4 | Invasion of adjacent organs or extension through kidney into perirenal fat |
| N1 | Metastasis in single node, <20 mm |
| N2 | Metastasis in single node, >20 mm & <50 mm or multiple nodes each <50 mm |
| N3 | Metastasis >50 mm |
| M1 | Distant metastasis |

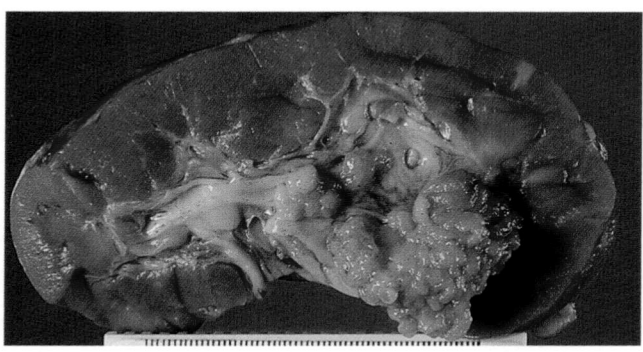

**Figure 30–49.** Papillary urothelial carcinoma of the renal pelvis.

rence (more than 15%) in the ureter distal to the resected tumor, nephroureterectomy with resection of a cuff of urinary bladder is the operation of choice.[362]

### MACROSCOPIC APPEARANCES

The gross appearance of the tumors is similar to that seen in the bladder, except that large papillary tumors frequently fill the pelvic cavity or ureter (Fig. 30–49) and cause obstruction resulting in hydronephrosis. Large tumors of the pelvis may invade the renal parenchyma extensively in an ill-defined infiltrative manner, even extending into the paracortical fat and may be very scirrhous. Sometimes, in such tumors, little evidence remains of a mucosal origin in the pelvis and extensive histologic sampling is necessary to demonstrate it.

### HISTOLOGIC APPEARANCES

The histopathology of upper tract tumors has the same spectrum as do urothelial carcinomas of the urinary bladder, including squamous and glandular[363] differentiation and the sarcomatoid (Fig. 30–50[166, 364, 365]) and small cell[366] variants. Rare variants, such as trophoblastic differentiation and osteoclast-type giant cells,[367, 368] have been reported. When the sarcomatoid elements obscure the clearly carcinomatous elements, immunohistochemical studies[166, 364] or ultrastructural examination[363] may be of diagnostic help. Mapping studies have shown that virtually all urothelial carcinomas of the renal pelvis and ureter are associated with changes ranging from hyperplasia to carcinoma in situ in the mucosa elsewhere in the specimen.[369] Thickening of basement membranes around capillaries in the lamina propria of the renal pelvis and ureter has been found to be a histologic marker for analgesic abuse and termed capillarosclerosis.[350]

## Adenocarcinoma

Primary adenocarcinomas of the upper tract are rare, and the reports consist mainly of single cases or small series.[370–375] Most patients are adult, but pediatric cases occur.[376] Calculi and chronic inflammation and infection appear to be predisposing conditions. Glandular metaplasia[377, 378] may be a precursor lesion, and noninvasive carcinoma is sometimes found in the mucosa adjacent to the tumors. A papillary architecture and resemblance to mucinous adenocarcinoma of the colon are common. One tumor had hepatoid areas and contained bile pigment.[374]

## Squamous Cell Carcinoma

Approximately 10% of renal pelvic tumors are squamous cell carcinomas,[379] and the percentage of ureteral carcinomas is even smaller. Calculi and chronic infection often are associated with squamous cell carcinoma. The relationship with squamous metaplasia is more controversial, with series of tumors finding strong association,[380, 381] whereas some studies of squamous metaplasia have found little association.[382] This disagreement may be the result of the rarity of squamous cell carcinoma of the upper urinary tract. Prognostically, high stage is common,[383] and the results are unfavorable.[381] The histopathology of these tumors is similar to that of their counterparts in the urinary bladder. Extensive infiltration of the renal parenchyma is very common, and survival for 5 years is rare.[381] These tumors should be distinguished from metastatic squamous cell carcinomas, which usually is straightforward when clinical and pathologic features are considered. An exceptional case of adenosquamous carcinoma of the renal pelvis, without urothelial carcinoma, has been described in association with staghorn calculi.[384]

## Other Tumors

Smooth muscle neoplasms are the most common mesenchymal tumors of the renal pelvis and ureter; both leiomyomas[385, 386] and leiomyosarcomas[387–389]

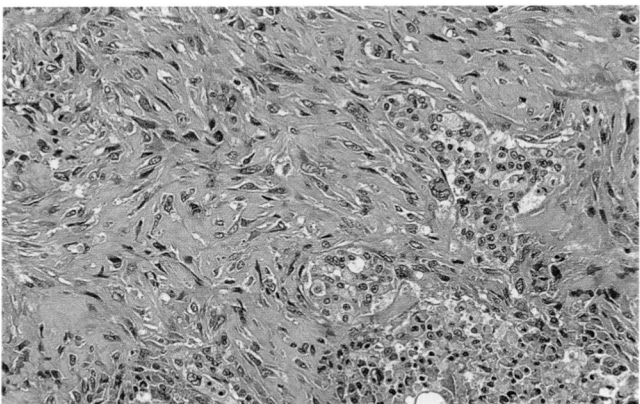

**Figure 30–50.** Sarcomatoid urothelial carcinoma of the renal pelvis. Both ordinary high-grade urothelial carcinoma and sarcomatoid urothelial carcinoma are present.

have been reported. Other sarcomas, such as osteogenic sarcoma[279] and malignant schwannoma[390] are extremely rare. Malignant melanoma has arisen in the mucosa of the renal pelvis.[391] Carcinosarcomas combining squamous or urothelial carcinoma with heterologous sarcomas such as osteogenic sarcoma, chondrosarcoma, or rhabdomyosarcoma, are extremely rare.[392, 393] A pure choriocarcinoma of the renal pelvis has been reported.[394] Obstruction caused by secondary infiltration by malignant lymphoma occurs in approximately 16% of cases of disseminated lymphoma.[395]

## REFERENCES

1. Beckwith JB: Wilms' tumor and other renal tumors of childhood. *In* Finegold M (ed): Pathology of Neoplasia in Children and Adolescents. Philadelphia, WB Saunders, 1986, pp 313–332.
2. Mierau GW, Beckwith JB, Weeks DA: Ultrastructure and histogenesis of the renal tumors of childhood: An overview. Ultrastruct Pathol 11:313–333, 1987.
3. Webber BL, Parham DM, Drake LG, Wilimas JA: Renal tumors in childhood. Pathol Annu 27 Pt 1:191–232, 1992.
4. Sotelo-Avila C: Nephroblastoma and other pediatric renal cancers. *In* Eble JN (ed): Tumors and Tumor-like Conditions of the Kidneys and Ureters. New York, Churchill Livingstone, 1990, pp 71–121.
5. Breslow N, Beckwith JB, Ciol M, Sharples K: Age distribution of Wilms' tumor: Report from the National Wilms' Tumor Study. Cancer Res 48:1653–1657, 1988.
6. Hrabovsky EE, Othersen HB Jr, deLorimier A, et al: Wilms' tumor in the neonate: A report from the National Wilms' Tumor Study. J Pediatr Surg 21:385–387, 1986.
7. Lemerle J, Tournade M-F, Gerard-Marchant R, et al: Wilms' tumor: Natural history and prognostic factors, a retrospective study of 248 cases treated at the Institut Gustave-Roussy 1952–1967. Cancer 37:2557–2566, 1976.
8. Innis MD: Nephroblastoma: Index cancer of childhood. Med J Aust 2:322–323, 1973.
9. Blute ML, Kelalis PP, Offord KP, et al: Bilateral Wilms' tumor. J Urol 138:968–973, 1987.
10. Breslow NE, Beckwith JB: Epidemiological features of Wilms' tumor: Results of the National Wilms' Tumor Study. J Natl Cancer Inst 68:429–436, 1982.
11. Sotelo-Avila C, Gonzalez-Crussi F, Fowler JW: Complete and incomplete forms of Beckwith-Wiedemann syndrome: Their oncogenic potential. J Pediatr 96:47–50, 1980.
12. Heppe RK, Koyle MA, Beckwith JB: Nephrogenic rests in Wilms tumor patients with Drash syndrome. J Urol 145:1225–1228, 1991.
13. Miller RW, Fraumeni JF Jr, Manning MD: Association of Wilms's tumor with aniridia, hemihypertrophy and other congenital malformations. N Engl J Med 270:922–927, 1964.
14. Huser J, Grignon DJ, Ro JY, et al: Adult Wilms' tumor: A clinicopathologic study of 11 cases. Mod Pathol 3:321–326, 1990.
15. Arrigo S, Beckwith JB, Sharples K, et al: Better survival after combined modality care for adults with Wilms' tumor, a report from the National Wilms' Tumor Study. Cancer 66:827–830, 1990.
16. Beckwith JB, Kiviat NB, Bonadio JF: Nephrogenic rests, nephroblastomatosis, and the pathogenesis of Wilms' tumor. Pediatr Pathol 10:1–36, 1990.
17. Bennington JL, Beckwith JB: Atlas of Tumor Pathology, Second Series, Fascicle 12, Tumors of the Kidney, Renal Pelvis, and Ureter. Bethesda, Armed Forces Institute of Pathology, 1975, p 1.
18. Scharfenberg JC, Beckman EN: Persistent renal blastema in an adult. Hum Pathol 15:791–793, 1984.
19. Grimes MM, Wolff M, Wolff JA, et al: Ganglion cells in metastatic Wilms' tumor, review of a histogenetic controversy. Am J Surg Pathol 6:565–571, 1982.
20. Fetissof F, Dubois MP, Robert M, Jobard P: Néphroblastome avec cellules endocrines, Étude immunohistochimique. Ann Pathol 5:279–281, 1985.
21. Cummins GE, Cohen D: Cushing's syndrome secondary to ACTH-secreting Wilms' tumor. J Pediatr Surg 9:535–539, 1974.
22. Beckwith JB: Wilms' tumor and other renal tumors of childhood: A selective review from the National Wilms' Tumor Study Pathology Center. Hum Pathol 14:481–492, 1983.
23. Eble JN, Bonsib SM: Extensively cystic renal neoplasms: Cystic nephroma, cystic partially differentiated nephroblastoma, multilocular cystic renal cell carcinoma, and cystic hamartoma of renal pelvis. Semin Diagn Pathol 15:2–20, 1998.
24. Wigger HJ: Fetal rhabdomyomatous nephroblastoma—a variant of Wilms' tumor. Hum Pathol 7:613–623, 1976.
25. Fernandes ET, Parham DM, Ribeiro RC, et al: Teratoid Wilms' tumor: The St. Jude experience. J Pediatr Surg 23:1131–1134, 1988.
26. Variend S, Spicer RD, MacKinnon AE: Teratoid Wilms' tumor. Cancer 53:1936–1942, 1984.
27. Bonadio JF, Storer B, Norkool P, et al: Anaplastic Wilms' tumor: Clinical and pathologic studies. J Clin Oncol 3:513–520, 1985.
28. Breslow NE, Palmer NF, Hill LR, et al: Wilms' tumor: Prognostic factors for patients without metastases at diagnosis, results of the National Wilms' Tumor Study. Cancer 41:1577–1589, 1978.
29. Faria P, Beckwith JB, Mishra K, et al: Focal versus diffuse anaplasia in Wilms tumor—new definitions with prognostic significance, a report from the National Wilms Tumor Study Group. Am J Surg Pathol 20:909–920, 1996.
30. Weeks DA, Beckwith JB, Luckey DW: Relapse-associated variables in stage I favorable histology Wilms' tumor, a report of the National Wilms' Tumor Study. Cancer 60:1204–1212, 1987.
31. Morgan E, Kidd JM: Undifferentiated sarcoma of the kidney, a tumor of childhood with histopathologic and clinical characteristics distinct from Wilms' tumor. Cancer 42:1916–1921, 1978.
32. Marsden HB, Lawler W: Bone-metastasizing renal tumour of childhood. Br J Cancer 38:437–441, 1978.
33. Beckwith JB, Palmer NF: Histopathology and prognosis of Wilms tumor, results from the First National Wilms' Tumor Study. Cancer 41:1937–1948, 1978.
34. Mierau GW, Weeks DA, Beckwith JB: Anaplastic Wilms' tumor and other clinically aggressive childhood renal neoplasms: Ultrastructural and immunocytochemical features. Ultrastruct Pathol 13:225–248, 1989.
35. Argani P, Perlman EJ, Breslow NE, et al: Clear cell sarcoma of the kidney, a review of 351 cases from the National Wilms Tumor Study Group Pathology Center. Am J Surg Pathol 24:4–18, 2000.
36. Sotelo-Avila C, Gonzalez-Crussi F, Sadowinski S, et al: Clear cell sarcoma of the kidney: A clinicopathologic study of 21 patients with long-term follow-up evaluation. Hum Pathol 16:1219–1230, 1986.
37. Marsden HB, Lawler W: Bone metastasizing renal tumour of childhood, histopathological and clinical review of 38 cases. Virchows Arch [A] 387:341–351, 1980.
38. Palmer NF, Sutow W: Clinical aspects of the rhabdoid tumor of the kidney: A report of the National Wilms' Tumor Study Group. Med Pediatr Oncol 11:242–245, 1983.
39. Weeks DA, Beckwith JB, Mierau GW, Luckey DW: Rhabdoid tumor of kidney, a report of 111 cases from the National Wilms' Tumor Study Pathology Center. Am J Surg Pathol 13:439–458, 1989.
40. Bonnin JM, Rubinstein LJ, Palmer NF, Beckwith JB: The association of embryonal tumors originating in the kidney and in the brain, a report of seven cases. Cancer 54:2137–2146, 1984.
41. Rousseau-Merck MF, Boccon-Gibod L, Nogues C, et al: An original hypercalcemic infantile renal tumor without bone metastasis: Heterotransplantation to nude mice, report of two cases. Cancer 50:85–93, 1982.
42. Mayes LC, Kasselberg AG, Roloff JS, Lukens JN: Hypercal-

cemia associated with immunoreactive parathyroid hormone in a malignant rhabdoid tumor of the kidney (rhabdoid Wilms' tumor). Cancer 54:882–884, 1984.

43. Haas JE, Palmer NF, Weinberg AG, Beckwith JB: Ultrastructure of malignant rhabdoid tumor of the kidney, a distinctive renal tumor of children. Hum Pathol 12:646–657, 1981.
44. Weeks DA, Beckwith JB, Mierau GW, Zuppan CW: Renal neoplasms mimicking rhabdoid tumor of kidney, a report from the National Wilms' Tumor Study Pathology Center. Am J Surg Pathol 15:1042–1054, 1991.
45. Marsden HB, Lawler W: Primary renal tumours in the first year of life. A population based review. Virchows Arch [A] 399:1–9, 1983.
46. Blank E, Neerhout RC, Burry KA: Congenital mesoblastic nephroma and polyhydramnios. JAMA 240:1504–1505, 1978.
47. Favara BE, Johnson W, Ito J: Renal tumors in the neonatal period. Cancer 22:845–855, 1968.
48. Kay S, Pratt CB, Salzberg AM: Hamartoma (leiomyomatous type) of the kidney. Cancer 19:1825–1832, 1966.
49. Bolande RP: Congenital mesoblastic nephroma of infancy. Perspect Pediatr Pathol 1:227–250, 1973.
50. Howell CG, Othersen HB, Kiviat NE, et al: Therapy and outcome in 51 children with mesoblastic nephroma: A report of the National Wilms' Tumor Study. J Pediatr Surg 17:826–831, 1982.
51. Chan HSL, Cheng M-Y, Mancer K, et al: Congenital mesoblastic nephroma: A clinicoradiologic study of 17 cases representing the pathologic spectrum of the disease. J Pediatr 111:64–70, 1987.
52. Sandstedt B, Delemarre JFM, Krul EJ, Tournade MF: Mesoblastic nephromas: A study of 29 tumours from the SIOP nephroblastoma file. Histopathology 9:741–750, 1985.
53. Joshi VV, Kasznica J, Walters TR: Atypical mesoblastic nephroma. Arch Pathol Lab Med 110:100–106, 1986.
54. Gonzalez-Crussi F, Sotelo-Avila C, Kidd JM: Malignant mesenchymal nephroma of infancy, report of a case with pulmonary metastases. Am J Surg Pathol 4:185–190, 1980.
55. Beckwith JB, Weeks DA: Congenital mesoblastic nephroma, when should we worry? Arch Pathol Lab Med 110:98–99, 1986.
56. Gormley TS, Skoog SJ, Jones RV, Maybee D: Cellular congenital mesoblastic nephroma: What are the options. J Urol 142:479–483, 1989.
57. Trillo AA: Adult variant of congenital mesoblastic nephroma. Arch Pathol Lab Med 114:533–535, 1990.
58. Van Velden DJJ, Schneider JW, Allen FJ: A case of adult mesoblastic nephroma: Ultrastructure and discussion of histogenesis. J Urol 143:1216–1219, 1990.
59. Rubin BP, Chen C-J, Morgan TW, et al: Congenital mesoblastic nephroma t(12;15) is associated with ETV6-NTRK3 gene fusion; cytogenetic and molecular relationship to congenital (infantile) fibrosarcoma. Am J Pathol 153:1451–1458, 1998.
60. Pettinato G, Manivel JC, Wick MR, Dehner LP: Classical and cellular (atypical) congenital mesoblastic nephroma: A clinicopathologic, ultrastructural, immunohistochemical, and flow cytometric study. Hum Pathol 20:682–690, 1989.
61. Delahunt B, Eble JN: Papillary renal cell carcinoma: A clinicopathologic and immunohistochemical study of 105 tumors. Mod Pathol 10:537–544, 1997.
62. Reese AJM, Winstanley DPL: The small tumor-like lesions of the kidney. Br J Cancer 12:507–516, 1958.
63. Eble JN, Warfel K: Early human renal cortical epithelial neoplasia. Mod Pathol 4:45A (Abstract) 1991.
64. Evins SC, Varner W: Renal adenoma—a misnomer. Urology 13:85–86, 1979.
65. Bell ET: A classification of renal tumors with observations on the frequency of the various types. J Urol 39:238–243, 1938.
66. Talamo TS, Shonnard JW: Small renal adenocarcinoma with metastases. J Urol 124:132–134, 1980.
67. Eschwege P, Saussine C, Steichen G, et al: Radical nephrectomy for renal cell carcinoma 30 mm. or less: Long-term followup results. J Urol 155:1196–1199, 1996.
68. Störkel S, Eble JN, Adlakha K, et al: Classification of renal cell carcinoma, workgroup 1. Cancer 80:987–989, 1997.
69. Grignon DJ, Eble JN: Papillary and metanephric adenomas of the kidney. Semin Diagn Pathol 15:41–53, 1998.

70. Hughson MD, Buchwald D, Fox M: Renal neoplasia and acquired cystic kidney disease in patients receiving long-term dialysis. Arch Pathol Lab Med 110:592–601, 1986.
71. Cabot H, Middleton AW: The relation of so-called adenoma of the kidney to carcinoma of the kidney. Trans Am Assoc Genitourin Surg 31:91–109, 1938.
72. Budin RE, McDonnell PJ: Renal cell neoplasms, their relationship to arteriolonephrosclerosis. Arch Pathol Lab Med 108:138–140, 1984.
73. Xipell JM: The incidence of benign renal nodules (a clinicopathologic study). J Urol 106:503–506, 1971.
74. Bennington JL: Cancer of the kidney—etiology, epidemiology, and pathology. Cancer 32:1017–1029, 1973.
75. Cristol DS, McDonald JR, Emmett JL: Renal adenomas in hypernephromatous kidneys: A study of their incidence, nature and relationship. J Urol 55:18–27, 1946.
76. Reis M, Faria V, Lindoro J, Adolfo A: The small cystic and noncystic noninflammatory renal nodules: A postmortem study. J Urol 140:721–724, 1988.
77. Turley LA, Steel J: Multiple miliary adenomas of the kidney cortex, with special reference to histogenesis. JAMA 82:857–859, 1924.
78. Corwin WC: Multiple adenomas of the kidneys, report of a case. J Urol 43:249–252, 1940.
79. Syrjänen KJ: Renal adenomatosis, report of an autopsy case. Scand J Urol Nephrol 13:329–334, 1979.
80. Ullrich R, Susani M, Schuster FX, et al: Multiple Adenome bei der Nieren—"renale Adenomatose?." Pathologe 11:120–124, 1990.
81. Warfel KA, Eble JN: Renal oncocytomatosis. J Urol 127:1179–1180, 1982.
82. Katz DS, Gharagozloo AM, Peebles TR, Oliphant M: Renal oncocytomatosis. Am J Kidney Dis 27:579–582, 1996.
83. Thoenes W, Störkel S, Rumpelt H-J: Histopathology and classification of renal cell tumors (adenomas, oncocytomas and carcinomas). The basic cytological and histopathological elements and their use for diagnostics. Pathol Res Pract 181:125–143, 1986.
84. Cohen C, McCue PA, DeRose PB: Immunohistochemistry of renal adenomas and carcinomas. J Urol Pathol 3:61–71, 1995.
85. Hiasa Y, Kitamura M, Nakaoka S, et al: Antigen immunohistochemistry of renal cell adenomas in autopsy cases: Relevance to histogenesis. Oncology 52:97–105, 1995.
86. Davis CJ Jr, Mostofi FK, Sesterhenn IA, Ho CK: Renal oncocytoma, clinicopathological study of 166 patients. J Urogenital Pathol 1:41–52, 1991.
87. Klein MJ, Valensi QJ: Proximal tubular adenomas of kidney with so-called oncocytic features, a clinicopathologic study of 13 cases of a rarely reported neoplasm. Cancer 38:909–914, 1976.
88. Defossez SM, Yoder IC, Papanicolaou N, et al: Nonspecific magnetic resonance appearance of renal oncocytomas: Report of 3 cases and review of the literature. J Urol 145:552–554, 1991.
89. Mead GO, Thomas LR Jr, Jackson JG: Renal oncocytoma: Report of a case with bilateral multifocal oncocytomas. Clin Imaging 14:231–234, 1990.
90. Takai K, Kakizoe T, Tobisu K, et al: Renal oncocytoma treated by partial nephrectomy, a case report. Nippon Hinyokika Gakkai Zasshi 78:935–938, 1987.
91. Kragel PJ, Williams J, Emory TS, Merino MJ: Renal oncocytoma with cylindromatous changes: Pathologic features and histogenetic significance. Mod Pathol 3:277–281, 1990.
92. Tickoo SK, Amin MB: Discriminant nuclear features of renal oncocytoma and chromophobe renal cell carcinoma: Analysis of their potential utility in the differential diagnosis. Am J Clin Pathol 110:782–787, 1998.
93. Eble JN, Hull MT: Morphologic features of renal oncocytoma: A light and electron microscopic study. Hum Pathol 15:1054–1061, 1984.
94. Pitz S, Moll R, Störkel S, Thoenes W: Expression of intermediate filament proteins in subtypes of renal cell carcinomas and in renal oncocytomas, distinction of two classes of renal cell tumors. Lab Invest 56:642–653, 1987.

95. Bonsib SM, Bromley C, Lager DJ: Renal oncocytoma: Diagnostic utility of cytokeratin-containing globular filamentous bodies. Mod Pathol 4:16–23, 1991.

96. Pagès A, Granier M: Le néphrome néphronogène. Arch Anat Cytol Pathol 28:99–103, 1980.

97. Hennigar RA, Beckwith JB: Nephrogenic adenofibroma, a novel kidney tumor of young people. Am J Surg Pathol 16:325–334, 1992.

98. Davis CJ Jr, Barton JH, Sesterhenn IA, Mostofi FK: Metanephric adenoma, clinicopathological study of fifty patients. Am J Surg Pathol 19:1101–1114, 1995.

99. Bigg SW, Bari WA: Nephrogenic adenofibroma: An unusual renal tumor. J Urol 157:1835–1836, 1997.

100. Jones EC, Pins M, Dickersin GR, Young RH: Metanephric adenoma of the kidney, a clinicopathological, immunohistochemical, flow cytometric, cytogenetic, and electron microscopic study of seven cases. Am J Surg Pathol 19:615–626, 1995.

101. Beckwith JB: Metanephric stromal tumor (MST): A new renal neoplasm resembling mesoblastic nephroma (MN) but related to metanephric adenofibroma (MAF) (Abstract). Mod Pathol 11:p 1P 1998.

102. Thoenes W, Störkel S, Rumpelt HJ, Moll R: Cytomorphological typing of renal cell carcinoma—a new approach. Eur Urol 18(suppl):6–9, 1990.

103. Kovacs G, Akhtar M, Beckwith JB, et al: The Heidelberg classification of renal cell tumours. J Pathol 183:131–133, 1997.

104. Dayal HH, Wilkinson GS: Epidemiology of renal cell cancer. Semin Urol 7:139–143, 1989.

105. Leuschner I, Harms D, Schmidt D: Renal cell carcinoma in children: Histology, immunohistochemistry, and follow-up of 10 cases. Med Pediatr Oncol 19:33–41, 1991.

106. Maclure M, Willett W: A case-control study of diet and risk of renal adenocarcinoma. Epidemiol 1:430–440, 1990.

107. La Vecchia C, Negri E, D'Avanzo B, Franceschi S: Smoking and renal cell carcinoma. Cancer Res 50:5231–5233, 1990.

108. Sharpe CR, Rochon JE, Adam JM, Suissa S: Case-control study of hydrocarbon exposures in patients with renal cell carcinoma. Can Med Assoc J 140:1309–1318, 1989.

109. Solomon D, Schwartz A: Renal pathology in von Hippel-Lindau disease. Hum Pathol 19:1072–1079, 1988.

110. Maher ER, Yates JRW, Harries R, et al: Clinical features and natural history of von Hippel-Lindau disease. Q J Med 77:1151–1163, 1990.

111. Bernstein J, Robbins TO: Renal involvement in tuberous sclerosis. Ann N Y Acad Sci 615:36–49, 1991.

112. Washecka R, Hanna M: Malignant renal tumors in tuberous sclerosis. Urology 37:340–343, 1991.

113. Gregoire JR, Torres VE, Holley KE, Farrow GM: Renal epithelial hyperplastic and neoplastic proliferation in autosomal dominant polycystic kidney disease. Am J Kidney Dis 9:27–38, 1987.

114. Bernstein J, Evan AP, Gardner KD Jr: Epithelial hyperplasia in human polycystic kidney diseases, its role in pathogenesis and risk of neoplasia. Am J Pathol 129:92–101, 1987.

115. Bonacina R, Di Natale G, Zois G, et al: Adenocarcinoma renale associato a rene policistico (presentazione di un caso e revisone della literatura). Chir Ital 38:406–411, 1986.

116. Fallon B, Williams RD: Renal cancer associated with acquired cystic disease of the kidney and chronic renal failure. Semin Urol 7:228–236, 1989.

117. Matson MA, Cohen EP: Acquired cystic kidney disease: occurrence, prevalence and renal cancers. Medicine 69:217–226, 1990.

118. Ishikawa I: Development of adenocarcinoma and acquired cystic disease of the kidney in hemodialysis patients. Int Symp Princess Takamatsu Cancer Res Fund 18:77–86, 1987.

119. Gibbons RP, Montie JE, Correa RJ Jr, Mason JT: Manifestations of renal cell carcinoma. Urology 8:201–206, 1976.

120. Cronin RE, Kaehny WD, Miller PD, et al: Renal cell carcinoma: Unusual systemic manifestations. Medicine 555:291–311, 1976.

121. Kiely JM: Hypernephroma—the internist's tumor. Med Clin North Am 50:1067–1083, 1966.

122. Fahn H-J, Lee Y-H, Chen M-T, et al: The incidence and prognostic significance of humoral hypercalcemia in renal cell carcinoma. J Urol 145:248–250, 1991.

123. Sufrin G, Chasan S, Golio A, Murphy GP: Paraneoplastic and serologic syndromes of renal adenocarcinoma. Semin Urol 7:158–171, 1989.

124. Moran A: Malignant hypertension due to renal carcinoma. Br J Urol 65:299, 1990.

125. Somer TP, Törnroth TS: Renal adenocarcinoma and systemic amyloidosis, immunohistochemical and histochemical studies. Arch Pathol Lab Med 109:571–574, 1985.

126. Althaffer LF III, Chenault OW, Jr: Paraneoplastic endocrinopathies associated with renal tumors. J Urol 122:573–577, 1979.

127. Rosenblum SL: Paraneoplastic syndromes associated with renal cell carcinoma. J S C Med Assoc 83:375–378, 1987.

128. Cheng WS, Farrow GM, Zincke H: The incidence of multicentricity in renal cell carcinoma. J Urol 146:1221–1223, 1991.

129. Katz SE, Schapira HE: Spontaneous regression of genitourinary cancer—an update. J Urol 128:1–4, 1982.

130. Kavoussi LR, Levine SR, Kadmon D, Fair WR: Regression of metastatic renal cell carcinoma: A case report and literature review. J Urol 135:1005–1007, 1986.

131. De Riese W, Goldenberg K, Allhoff E, et al: Metastatic renal cell carcinoma (RCC): Spontaneous regression, long-term survival and late recurrence. Int Urol Nephrol 23:13–25, 1991.

132. Rodier JF, Rodier D, Janser JC, et al: Régression spontanée de métastases pulmonaires de cancer du rein. J Chir 125:341–345, 1988.

133. McNichols DW, Segura JW, DeWeerd JH: Renal cell carcinoma: Long-term survival and late recurrence. J Urol 126:17–23, 1981.

134. Hienert G, Latal D, Rummelhardt S: Urological aspects of surgical management for metastatic renal cell cancer. Semin Surg Oncol 4:137–138, 1988.

135. Neves RJ, Zincke H, Taylor WF: Metastatic renal cell cancer and radical nephrectomy: Identification of prognostic factors and patient survival. J Urol 139:1173–1176, 1988.

136. Elson PJ, Witte RS, Trump DL: Prognostic factors for survival in patients with recurrent or metastatic renal cell carcinoma. Cancer Res 48:7310–7313, 1988.

137. Tobisu K-I, Kakizoe T, Takai K, Tanaka Y: Prognosis in renal cell carcinoma: Analysis of clinical course following nephrectomy. Jpn J Clin Oncol 19:142–148, 1989.

138. Gurney H, Larcos G, McKay M, et al: Bone metastases in hypernephroma, frequency of scapular involvement. Cancer 64:1429–1431, 1989.

139. Schouman M, Warter A, Roos M, Bollack C: Renal cell carcinoma: Statistical study of survival based on pathological criteria. World J Urol 2:109–113, 1984.

140. Robson CJ: Radical nephrectomy for renal cell carcinoma. J Urol 89:37–42, 1963.

141. Robson CJ, Churchill BM, Anderson W: The results of radical nephrectomy for renal cell carcinoma. J Urol 101:297–301, 1969.

142. International Union Against Cancer: Kidney. In Sobin LH, Wittekind C (eds): TNM Classification of Malignant Tumours. New York, Wiley-Liss, 1997, pp 180–182

143. American Joint Committee on Cancer: Kidney (sarcomas and adenomas are not included). AJCC Cancer Staging Manual. Philadelphia, Lippincott-Raven, 1997, pp 231–234.

144. Medeiros LJ, Gelb AB, Weiss LM: Renal cell carcinoma, prognostic significance of morphologic parameters in 121 cases. Cancer 61:1639–1651, 1988.

145. Medeiros LJ, Gelb AB, Weiss LM: Low-grade renal cell carcinoma, a clinicopathologic study of 53 cases. Am J Surg Pathol 11:633–642, 1987.

146. Giuliani L, Giberti C, Martorana G, Rovida S: Radical extensive surgery for renal cell carcinoma: Long-term results and prognostic factors. J Urol 143:468–474, 1990.

147. Herrlinger A, Schrott KM, Sigel A, Giedl J: Results of 381 transabdominal radical nephrectomies for renal cell carcinoma with partial and complete en-bloc lymph-node dissection. World J Urol 2:114–121, 1984.

148. Studer UE, Scherz S, Scheidegger J, et al: Enlargement of regional lymph nodes in renal cell carcinoma is often not due to metastases. J Urol 144:243–245, 1990.

149. Ramon J, Goldwasser B, Raviv G, et al: Long-term results of simple and radical nephrectomy for renal cell carcinoma. Cancer 67:2506–2511, 1991.

150. Mitty HA, Droller MJ, Dikman SH: Ureteral and renal pelvic metastases from renal cell carcinoma. Urol Radiol 9:16–20, 1987.

151. Hand JR, Broders AC: Carcinoma of the kidney: The degree of malignancy in relation to factors bearing on prognosis. J Urol 28:199–216, 1932.

152. Skinner DG, Colvin RB, Vermillion CD, et al: Diagnosis and management of renal cell carcinoma, a clinical and pathological study of 309 cases. Cancer 28:1165–1177, 1971.

153. Fuhrman SA, Lasky LC, Limas C: Prognostic significance of morphologic parameters in renal cell carcinoma. Am J Surg Pathol 6:655–663, 1982.

154. Grignon DJ, Ayala AG, El-Naggar A, et al: Renal cell carcinoma, a clinicopathologic and DNA flow cytometric analysis of 103 cases. Cancer 64:2133–2140, 1989.

155. Green LK, Ayala AG, Ro JY, et al: Role of nuclear grading in stage I renal cell carcinoma. Urology 34:310–315, 1989.

156. Helpap B, Knüpffer J, Essmann S: Nucleolar grading of renal cancer, correlation of frequency and localization of nucleoli to histologic and cytologic grading and stage of renal cell carcinomas. Mod Pathol 3:671–678, 1990.

157. Störkel S, Thoenes W, Jacobi GH, Lippold R: Prognostic parameters in renal cell carcinoma—a new approach. Eur Urol 16:416–422, 1989.

158. Gnarra JR, Duan DR, Weng Y, et al: Molecular cloning of the von Hippel-Lindau tumor suppressor gene and its role in renal carcinoma. Biochim Biophys Acta 1242:201–210, 1996.

159. van der Hout AH, van den Berg E, van der Vlies P, et al: Loss of heterozygosity at the short arm of chromosome 3 in renal-cell cancer correlates with the cytological tumour type. Int J Cancer 53:353–357, 1993.

160. Zbar B, Lerman M: Inherited carcinomas of the kidney: Histology. Adv Cancer Res 75:164–201, 1998.

161. Schullerus D, Herbers J, Chudek J, et al: Loss of heterozygosity at chromosomes 8p, 9p, and 14q is associated with stage and grade of nonpapillary renal cell carcinomas. J Pathol 183:151–155, 1997.

162. Delahunt B: Histopathologic prognostic indicators for renal cell carcinoma. Semin Diagn Pathol 15:68–76, 1998.

163. Deitchman B, Sidhu GS: Ultrastructural study of a sarcomatoid variant of renal cell carcinoma. Cancer 46:1152–1157, 1980.

164. Bonsib SM, Fischer J, Plattner S, Fallon B: Sarcomatoid renal tumors, clinicopathologic correlation of three cases. Cancer 59:527–532, 1987.

165. Lanzafame S: Carcinoma <<sarcomatode>> del rene, distribuzione dei filamenti intermedi di citocheratine e di vimentina nelle cellule carcinomatose e sarcomatose. Pathologica 79:323–337, 1987.

166. Wick MR, Perrone TL, Burke BA: Sarcomatoid transitional cell carcinoma of the renal pelvis, an ultrastructural and immunohistochemical study. Arch Pathol Lab Med 109:55–58, 1985.

167. Wick MR, Cherwitz DL, Manivel JC, Sibley R: Immunohistochemical findings in tumors of the kidney. *In* Eble JN (ed): Tumors and Tumor-like Conditions of the Kidneys and Ureters. New York, Churchill Livingstone, 1990, pp 207–247.

168. Kimura I, Takahashi N, Okumura R, et al: Perinephric xanthogranulomatous pyelonephritis simulating a renal or retroperitoneal tumor on x-ray CT and angiography. Radiat Med 7:111–117, 1989.

169. Malek RS, Greene LF, DeWeerd JH, Farrow GM: Xanthogranulomatous pyelonephritis. Br J Urol 44:296–308, 1972.

170. Goodman M, Curry T, Russell T: Xanthogranulomatous pyelonephritis (XGP): A local disease with systemic manifestations, report of 23 patients and review of the literature. Medicine 58:171–181, 1979.

171. Rosi P, Selli C, Carini M, et al: Xanthogranulomatous pyelonephritis: Clinical experience with 62 cases. Eur Urol 12:96–100, 1986.

172. Chuang C-K, Lai M-K, Chang P-L, et al: Xanthogranulomatous pyelonephritis: Experience in 36 cases. J Urol 147:333–336, 1992.

173. Parsons MA, Harris SC, Longstaff AJ, Grainger RG: Xanthogranulomatous pyelonephritis: A pathological, clinical and aetiological analysis of 87 cases. Diagn Histopathol 6:203–219, 1983.

174. Esparza AR, McKay DB, Cronan JJ, Chazan JA: Renal parenchymal malakoplakia, histologic spectrum and its relationship to megalocytic interstitial nephritis and xanthogranulomatous pyelonephritis. Am J Surg Pathol 13:225–236, 1989.

175. Waldherr R, Schwechheimer K: Co-expression of cytokeratin and vimentin intermediate-sized filaments in renal cell carcinoma, a comparative study of the intermediate-sized filaments in renal cell carcinoma and normal human kidney. Virchows Arch 408:15–27, 1985.

176. Taxy JB: Renal adenocarcinoma presenting as a solitary metastasis: Contribution of electron microscopy to diagnosis. Cancer 48:2056–2062, 1981.

177. Lemmers M, Ward K, Hatch T, Stenzel P: Renal adenocarcinoma with solitary metastasis to the contralateral adrenal gland: Report of 2 cases and review of the literature. J Urol 141:1177–1180, 1989.

178. Wick MR, Cherwitz DL, McGlennen RC, Dehner LP: Adrenocortical carcinoma, an immunohistochemical comparison with renal cell carcinoma. Am J Pathol 122:343–352, 1986.

179. Green LK, Ro JY, Mackay B, et al: Renal cell carcinoma metastatic to the thyroid. Cancer 63:1810–1815, 1989.

180. Young RH, Hart WR: Renal cell carcinoma metastatic to the ovary: A report of three cases emphasizing possible confusion with ovarian clear cell carcinoma. Int J Gynecol Pathol 11:96–104, 1992.

181. Hufnagel TJ, Kim JH, True LD, Manuelidis EE: Immunohistochemistry of capillary hemangioblastoma, immunoperoxidase-labeled antibody staining resolves the differential diagnosis with metastatic renal cell carcinoma, but does not explain the histogenesis of the capillary hemangioblastoma. Am J Surg Pathol 13:207–216, 1989.

182. Mancilla-Jimenez R, Stanley RJ, Blath RA: Papillary renal cell carcinoma, a clinical, radiologic, and pathologic study of 34 cases. Cancer 38:2469–2480, 1976.

183. Bard RH, Lord B, Fromowitz F: Papillary adenocarcinoma of kidney, II. Radiographic and biologic characteristics. Urology 19:16–20, 1982.

184. Gutíerrez Baños JL, Martín García B, Hernández Rodríguez R, et al: Adenocarcinoma papilar de riñon. Aportacion de 12 casos y puesta al dia. Actas Urol Esp 15:437–441, 1991.

185. El-Naggar AK, Ro JY, Ensign LG: Papillary renal cell carcinoma: Clinical implication of DNA content analysis. Hum Pathol 24:316–321, 1993.

186. Renshaw AA, Corless CL: Papillary renal cell carcinoma, histology and immunohistochemistry. Am J Surg Pathol 19:842–849, 1995.

187. Thoenes W, Störkel S: Die Pathologie der benignen und malignen Nierenzelltumoren. Urologe [A] 30:W41–W50, 1991.

188. Lager DJ, Huston BJ, Timmerman TG, Bonsib SM: Papillary renal tumors, morphologic, cytochemical, and genotypic features. Cancer 76:669–673, 1995.

189. Kovacs G: Papillary renal cell carcinoma, a morphologic and cytogenetic study of 11 cases. Am J Pathol 134:27–34, 1989.

190. Kovacs G, Fuzesi L, Emanuel A, Kung H-F: Cytogenetics of papillary renal cell tumors. Genes Chromosom Cancer 3:249–255, 1991.

191. Presti JC Jr, Rao PH, Chen Q, et al: Histopathological, cytogenetic, and molecular characterization of renal cortical tumors. Cancer Res 51:1544–1552, 1991.

192. Fournet JC, Béroud C, Austruy E, Léonard C: Aspects génétiques des tumeurs rénales de l'adulte. Arch Anat Cytol Pathol 40:301–306, 1992.

193. Henn W, Zwergel T, Wullich B, et al: Bilateral multicentric papillary renal tumors with heteroclonal origin based on tissue-specific karyotype instability. Cancer 72:1315–1318, 1993.

194. van den Berg E, van der Hout AH, Oosterhuis JW, et al: Cytogenetic analysis of epithelial renal-cell tumors: Relationship with a new histopathological classification. Int J Cancer 55:223–227, 1993.

195. Reznicek SB, Narayana AS, Culp DA: Cystadenocarcinoma of the kidney: A profile of 13 cases. J Urol 134:256–259, 1985.

196. Landier JF, Deslignières S, Debré B, et al: Les cystadénocarcinomes papillaires du rein. Ann Urol 14:205–208, 1980.

197. Orain I, Buzelin F, Ferry N: Les tumeurs tubulo-papillaires du rein, à propos de 20 nouveaux et d'une revue de la littérature. J Urol (Paris) 93:1–9, 1987.

198. Thoenes W, Störkel S, Rumpelt H-J: Human chromophobe cell renal carcinoma. Virchows Arch [B] 48:207–217, 1985.

199. Thoenes W, Störkel S, Rumpelt H-J, et al: Chromophobe cell renal carcinoma and its variants—a report on 32 cases. J Pathol 155:277–287, 1988.

200. Crotty TB, Farrow GM, Lieber MM: Chromophobe renal cell carcinoma: clinicopathologic features of 50 cases. J Urol 154:964–967, 1995.

201. Durham JR, Keohane M, Amin MB: Chromophobe renal cell carcinoma. Adv Anat Pathol 3:336–342, 1996.

202. Bugert P, Gaul C, Weber K, et al: Specific genetic changes of diagnostic importance in chromophobe renal cell carcinoma. Lab Invest 76:203–208, 1997.

203. Akhtar M, Tulbah A, Kardar AH, Ali MA: Sarcomatoid renal cell carcinoma: The chromophobe connection. Am J Surg Pathol 21:1188–1195, 1997.

204. Bonsib SM, Lager DJ: Chromophobe cell carcinoma: Analysis of five cases. Am J Surg Pathol 14:260–267, 1990.

205. Kriz W, Bankir L: A standard nomenclature for structures of the kidney. Kidney Int 33:1–7, 1988.

206. Störkel S, Pannen B, Thoenes W, et al: Intercalated cells as a probable source for the development of renal oncocytoma. Virchows Arch [B] 56:185–189, 1988.

207. Störkel S, Steart PV, Drenckhahn D, Thoenes W: The human chromophobe cell renal carcinoma: Its probable relation to intercalated cells of the collecting duct. Virchows Arch [B] 56:237–245, 1989.

208. Rumpelt HJ, Störkel S, Moll R, et al: Bellini duct carcinoma: Further evidence for this rare variant of renal cell carcinoma. Histopathology 18:115–122, 1991.

209. Fleming S, Lewi HJE: Collecting duct carcinoma of the kidney. Histopathology 10:1131–1141, 1986.

210. Aizawa S, Kikuchi Y, Suzuki M, Furusato M: Renal cell carcinoma of lower nephron origin. Acta Pathol Jpn 37:567–574, 1987.

211. Kennedy SM, Merino MJ, Linehan WM, et al: Collecting duct carcinoma of the kidney. Hum Pathol 21:449–456, 1990.

212. Srigley JR, Eble JN: Collecting duct carcinoma of kidney. Semin Diagn Pathol 15:54–67, 1998.

213. Davis CJ Jr, Mostofi FK, Sesterhenn IA: Renal medullary carcinoma: The seventh sickle cell nephropathy. Am J Surg Pathol 19:1–11, 1995.

214. Hai MA, Diaz-Perez R: Atypical carcinoma of kidney originating from collecting duct epithelium. Urology 19:89–92, 1982.

215. Cromie WJ, Davis CJ Jr: Atypical carcinoma of kidney possibly originating from collecting duct epithelium. Urology 13:315–317, 1979.

216. Eble JN: Unusual renal tumors and tumor-like conditions. In Eble JN (ed): Tumors and Tumor-like Conditions of the Kidneys and Ureters. New York, Churchill Livingstone, 1990, pp 145–176.

217. MacLennan GT, Farrow GM, Bostwick DG: Low-grade collecting duct carcinoma of the kidney: Report of 13 cases of low-grade mucinous tubulocystic renal carcinoma of possible collecting duct origin. Urology 50:679–684, 1997.

218. Resnick ME, Unterberger H, McLoughlin PT: Renal carcinoid producing the carcinoid syndrome. Med Times 94:895–896, 1966.

219. Gleeson MH, Bloom SR, Polak JM, et al: Endocrine tumour in kidney affecting small bowel structure, motility, and absorptive function. Gut 12:773–782, 1971.

220. Ghazi MR, Brown JS, Warner RS: Carcinoid tumor of kidney. Urology 14:610–612, 1979.

221. Stahl RE, Sidhu GS: Primary carcinoid of the kidney, light and electron microscopic study. Cancer 44:1345–1349, 1979.

222. Raghavaiah NV, Singh SM: Extra-adrenal pheochromocytoma producing renal artery stenosis. J Urol 116:243–245, 1976.

223. Naidich TP, Sprayregen S, Goldman AG, Siegelman SS: Renal artery alterations associated with pheochromocytoma. Angiology 23:488–499, 1972.

224. Van Way CW III, Michelakis AM, Alper BJ, et al: Renal vein renin studies in a patient with renal hilar pheochromocytoma and renal artery stenosis. Ann Surg 172:212–217, 1970.

225. Pengelly CDR: Phaeochromocytoma within the renal capsule. Br Med J 2:477–478, 1959.

226. Preger L, Gardner RE, Kawala BO, Steinbach HL: Intrarenal pheochromocytoma, preoperative angiographic diagnosis. Urology 8:194–196, 1976.

227. Simon H, Carlson DH, Hanelin J, et al: Intrarenal pheochromocytoma: Report of a case. J Urol 121:805–807, 1979.

228. Bezirdjian DR, Tegtmeyer CJ, Leef JL: Intrarenal pheochromocytoma and renal artery stenosis. Urol Radiol 3:121–122, 1981.

229. Rothwell DL, Vorstman B, Patton I, Allan JS: Intrarenal pheochromocytoma. Urology 21:175–177, 1983.

230. Gohji K, Nakanishi T, Hara I, et al: Two cases of primary neuroblastoma of the kidney in adults. J Urol 137:966–968, 1987.

231. Zak FG, Jindrak K, Capozzi F: Carcinoidal tumor of the kidney. Ultrastruct Pathol 4:51–59, 1983.

232. Acconcia A, Miracco C, Mattei FM, et al: Primary carcinoid tumor of kidney, light and electron microscopy, and immunohistochemical study. Urology 31:517–520, 1988.

233. Cauley JE, Almagro UA, Jacobs SC: Primary renal carcinoid tumor. Urology 32:564–566, 1988.

234. Huettner PC, Bird DJ, Chang YC, Seiler M: Carcinoid tumor of the kidney with morphologic and immunohistochemical profile of a hindgut endocrine tumor: Report of a case. Ultrastruct Pathol 15:655–661, 1991.

235. Kojiro M, Ohishi H, Isobe H: Carcinoid tumor occurring in cystic teratoma of the kidney, a case report. Cancer 38:1636–1640, 1976.

236. Fetissof F, Benatre A, Dubois MP, et al: Carcinoid tumor occurring in a teratoid malformation of the kidney, an immunohistochemical study. Cancer 54:2305–2308, 1984.

237. Capella C, Eusebi V, Rosai J: Primary oat cell carcinoma of the kidney. Am J Surg Pathol 8:855–861, 1984.

238. Têtu B, Ro JY, Ayala AG, et al: Small cell carcinoma of the kidney, a clinicopathologic, immunohistochemical, and ultrastructural study. Cancer 60:1809–1814, 1987.

239. Eble JN: Angiomyolipoma of kidney. Semin Diagn Pathol 15:21–40, 1998.

240. Klapproth HJ, Poutasse EF, Hazard JB: Renal angiomyolipomas, report of four cases. Arch Pathol 67:400–411, 1959.

241. Kragel PJ, Toker C: Infiltrating recurrent renal angiomyolipoma with fatal outcome. J Urol 133:90–91, 1985.

242. Ferry JA, Malt RA, Young RH: Renal angiomyolipoma with sarcomatous transformation and pulmonary metastases. Am J Surg Pathol 15:1083–1088, 1991.

243. Taylor RS, Joseph DB, Kohaut EC, et al: Renal angiomyolipoma associated with lymph node involvement and renal cell carcinoma in patients with tuberous sclerosis. J Urol 141:930–932, 1989.

244. McIntosh GS, Hamilton Dutoit S, Chronos NV, Kaisary AV: Multiple unilateral renal angiomyolipomas with regional lymphangioleiomyomatosis. J Urol 142:1305–1307, 1989.

245. Ro JY, Ayala AG, El-Naggar A, et al: Angiomyolipoma of kidney with lymph node involvement, DNA flow cytometric analysis. Arch Pathol Lab Med 114:65–67, 1990.

246. Hulbert JC, Graf R: Involvement of the spleen by renal angiomyolipoma: Metastasis or multicentricity. J Urol 130:328–329, 1983.

247. Mai KT, Perkins DG, Collins JP: Epithelioid variant of renal angiomyolipoma. Histopathology 28:277–280, 1996.

248. Eble JN, Amin MB, Young RH: Epithelioid angiomyolipoma of the kidney, a report of five cases with a prominent and diagnostically confusing epithelioid smooth muscle component. Am J Surg Pathol 21:1123–1130, 1997.

249. Pea M, Bonetti F, Martignoni G, et al: Apparent renal cell carcinomas in tuberous sclerosis are heterogeneous: The identification of malignant epithelioid angiomyolipoma. Am J Surg Pathol 22:180–187, 1998.

250. Peterson NE, Thompson HT: Renal hemangioma. J Urol 105:27–31, 1971.

251. Edward HG, DeWeerd JH, Woolner LB: Renal hemangiomas. Mayo Clin Proc 37:545–566, 1962.

252. Schofield D, Zaatari GS, Gay BB: Klippel-Trenaunay and Sturge-Weber syndromes with renal hemangioma and double inferior vena cava. J Urol 136:442–445, 1986.

253. Moros Garcia M, Martinez Tello D, Ramon y Cajal Junquera S, et al: Multiple cavernous hemangioma of the kidney. Eur Urol 14:90–92, 1988.

254. Pickering SP, Fletcher BD, Bryan PJ, Abramowsky CR: Renal lymphangioma: A cause of neonatal nephromegaly. Pediatr Radiol 14:445–448, 1984.

255. Singer DRJ, Miller JDB, Smith G: Lymphangioma of kidney. Scott Med J 28:293–294, 1983.

256. Joost J, Schäfer R, Altwein JE: Renal lymphangioma. J Urol 118:22–24, 1977.

257. Di Palma S, Giardini R: Leiomyoma of the kidney. Tumori 74:489–493, 1988.

258. Clinton-Thomas CL: A giant leiomyoma of the kidney. Br J Surg 43:497–501, 1956.

259. Zollikofer C, Castaneda-Zuniga W, et al: The angiographic appearance of intrarenal leiomyoma. Radiology 136:47–49, 1980.

260. Dineen MK, Venable DD, Misra RP: Pure intrarenal lipoma—report of a case and review of the literature. J Urol 132:104–107, 1984.

261. Hurwitz RS, Benjamin JA, Cooper JF: Excessive proliferation of peripelvic fat of the kidney. Urology 11:448–456, 1978.

262. Grignon DJ, Ro JY, Ayala AG: Mesenchymal tumors of the kidney. In Eble JN (ed): Tumors and Tumor-like Conditions of the Kidneys and Ureters. New York, Churchill Livingstone, 1990, pp 123–144.

263. Farrow GM, Harrison EG Jr, Utz DC, ReMine WH: Sarcomas and sarcomatoid and mixed malignant tumors of the kidney in adults—part I. Cancer 22:545–550, 1968.

264. Herman C, Morales P: Leiomyosarcoma of renal vein. Urology 18:395–398, 1981.

265. Yokose T, Fukuda H, Ogiwara A, et al: Myxoid leiomyosarcoma of the kidney accompanying ipsilateral ureteral transitional cell carcinoma. A case report with cytological, immunohistochemical and ultrastructural study. Acta Pathol Jpn 41:694–700, 1991.

266. Krech RH, Loy V, Dieckmann K-P, et al: Leiomyosarcoma of the kidney: Immunohistological and ultrastructural findings with special emphasis on the growth fraction. Br J Urol 63:132–134, 1989.

267. Grignon DJ, Ayala AG, Ro JY, et al: Primary sarcomas of the kidney, a clinicopathologic and DNA flow cytometric study of 17 cases. Cancer 65:1611–1618, 1990.

268. Mayes DC, Fechner RE, Gillenwater JY: Renal liposarcoma. Am J Surg Pathol 14:268–273, 1990.

269. Cano JY, D'Altorio RA: Renal liposarcoma: Case report. J Urol 115:747–749, 1976.

270. Takashi M, Murase T, Kato K, et al: Malignant fibrous histiocytoma arising from the renal capsule: Report of a case. Urol Int 42:227–230, 1987.

271. Joseph TJ, Becker DI, Turton AF: Renal malignant fibrous histiocytoma. Urology 37:483–489, 1991.

272. Srinivas V, Sogani PC, Hajdu SI, Whitmore WF Jr: Sarcomas of the kidney. J Urol 132:13–16, 1984.

273. Penchansky L, Gallo G: Rhabdomyosarcoma of the kidney in children. Cancer 44:285–292, 1979.

274. Gonzalez-Crussi F, Baum ES: Renal sarcomas of childhood, a clinicopathologic and ultrastructural study. Cancer 51:898–912, 1983.

275. Grignon DJ, McIsaac GP, Armstrong RF, Wyatt JK: Primary rhabdomyosarcoma of the kidney, a light microscopic, immunohistochemical, and electron microscopic study. Cancer 62:2027–2032, 1988.

276. Ordóñez NG, Bracken RB, Stroehlein KB: Hemangiopericytoma of kidney. Urology 20:191–195, 1982.

277. Siniluoto TMJ, Päivänsalo M, Hellström PA, et al: Hemangiopericytoma of the kidney: A case with preoperative ethanol embolization. J Urol 140:137–138, 1988.

278. Weiss JP, Pollack HM, McCormick JF, et al: Renal hemangiopericytoma: Surgical, radiological and pathological implications. J Urol 132:337–339, 1984.

279. Eble JN, Young RH, Störkel S, Thoenes W: Primary osteosarcoma of the kidney: A report of three cases. J Urogenital Pathol 1:83–88, 1991.

280. O'Malley FP, Grignon DJ, Shepherd RR, Harker LA: Primary osteosarcoma of the kidney, report of a case studied by immunohistochemistry, electron microscopy, and DNA flow cytometry. Arch Pathol Lab Med 115:1262–1265, 1991.

281. Malhotra CM, Doolittle CH, Rodil JV, Vezeridis MP: Mesenchymal chondrosarcoma of the kidney. Cancer 54:2495–2499, 1984.

282. Nativ O, Horowitz A, Lindner A, Many M: Primary chondrosarcoma of the kidney. J Urol 134:120–121, 1985.

283. Cason JD, Waisman J, Plaine L: Angiosarcoma of kidney. Urology 30:281–283, 1987.

284. Desai MB, Chess Q, Naidich JB, Weiner R: Primary renal angiosarcoma mimicking a renal cell carcinoma. Urol Radiol 11:30–32, 1989.

285. Terris D, Plaine L, Steinfeld A: Renal angiosarcoma. Am J Kidney Dis 8:131–133, 1986.

286. Mead JH, Herrera GA, Kaufman MF, Herz JH: Case report of a primary cystic sarcoma of the kidney, demonstrating fibrohistiocytic, osteoid, and cartilaginous components (malignant mesenchymoma). Cancer 50:2211–2214, 1982.

287. Remynse LC, Begun FP, Jacobs SC, Lawson RK: Juxtaglomerular cell tumor with elevation of serum erythropoietin. J Urol 142:1560–1562, 1989.

288. Corvol P, Pinet F, Galen FX, et al: Seven lessons from seven renin secreting tumors. Kidney Int Suppl 34(Suppl 25):S-38–S-44, 1988.

289. Valdés G, Lopez JM, Martinez P, et al: Renin-secreting tumor, case report. Hypertension 2:714–718, 1980.

290. Tetu B, Totovic V, Bechtelsheimer H, Smend J: Tumeur rénale à sécrétion de rénine, à propos d'un cas avec étude ultrastructurale et immunohistochimique. Ann Pathol 4:55–59, 1984.

291. Camilleri J-P, Hinglais N, Bruneval P, et al: Renin storage and cell differentiation in juxtaglomerular cell tumors: An immunohistochemical and ultrastructural study of three cases. Hum Pathol 15:1069–1079, 1984.

292. Lindop GBM, Stewart JA, Downie TT: The immunocytochemical demonstration of renin in a juxtaglomerular cell tumour by light and electron microscopy. Histopathology 7:421–431, 1983.

293. Lindop GBM, Fleming S: Renin in renal cell carcinoma—an immunocytochemical study using an antibody to pure human renin. J Clin Pathol 37:27–31, 1984.

294. Steffens J, Bock R, Braedel HU, et al: Renin-producing renal cell carcinoma. Eur Urol 18:56–60, 1990.

295. Lindop GBM, Fleming S, Gibson AAM: Immunocytochemical localisation of renin in nephroblastoma. J Clin Pathol 37:738–742, 1984.

296. Warfel KA, Eble JN: Renomedullary interstitial cell tumors. Am J Clin Pathol 83:262, 1985.

297. Zimmermann A, Luscieti P, Flury B, et al: Amyloid-containing renal interstitial cell nodules (RICNs) associated with chronic arterial hypertension in older age groups. Am J Pathol 105:288–294, 1981.

298. Taxy JB, Marshall FF: Multilocular renal cysts in adults, possible relationship to renal adenocarcinoma. Arch Pathol Lab Med 107:633–637, 1983.

299. Boggs LK, Kimmelstiel P: Benign multilocular cystic nephroma: Report of two cases of so-called multilocular cyst of the kidney. J Urol 76:530–541, 1956.

300. Kanomata N, Halling K, Eble JN: Non-random X chromosome inactivation in cystic nephroma demonstrates its neoplastic nature. J Urol Pathol 7:81–87, 1997.

301. Castillo OA, Boyle ET Jr, Kramer SA: Multilocular cysts of kidney, a study of 29 patients and review of the literature. Urology 37:156–162, 1991.

302. Joshi VV, Beckwith JB: Multilocular cyst of the kidney (cystic nephroma) and cystic, partially differentiated nephroblastoma. Terminology and criteria for diagnosis. Cancer 64:466–479, 1989.
303. Pawade J, Soosay GN, Delprado W, et al: Cystic hamartoma of the renal pelvis. Am J Surg Pathol 17:1169–1175, 1993.
304. Truong LD, Williams R, Ngo T, et al: Adult mesoblastic nephroma. Am J Surg Pathol 22:827–839, 1998.
305. Durham JR, Bostwick DG, Farrow GM, Ohorodnik JM: Mesoblastic nephroma of adulthood, report of three cases. Am J Surg Pathol 17:1029–1038, 1993.
306. Michal M, Syrucek M: Benign mixed epithelial and stromal tumor of the kidney. Pathol Res Pract 194:445–448, 1998.
307. Adsay NV, Eble JN, Srigley JR, et al: Mixed epithelial and stromal tumor of the kidney. Am J Surg Pathol 24:958–970, 2000.
308. Ferry JA, Harris NL, Papanicolaou N, Young RH: Lymphoma of the kidney, a report of 11 cases. Am J Surg Pathol 19:134–144, 1995.
309. Ferry JA, Young RH: Malignant lymphoma of the genitourinary tract. Curr Diagn Pathol 4:145–169, 1997.
310. Osborne BM, Brenner M, Weitzner S, Butler JJ: Malignant lymphoma presenting as a renal mass: Four cases. Am J Surg Pathol 11:375–382, 1987.
311. Farrow GM, Harrison EG Jr, Utz DC: Sarcomas and sarcomatoid and mixed malignant tumors of the kidney in adults—part II. Cancer 22:551–555, 1968.
312. Jaspan T, Gregson R: Extra-medullary plasmacytoma of the kidney. Br J Radiol 57:95–97, 1984.
313. Igel TC, Engen DE, Banks PM, Keeney GL: Renal plasmacytoma: Mayo Clinic experience and review of the literature. Urology 37:385–389, 1991.
314. Bracken RB, Chica G, Johnson DE, Luna M: Secondary renal neoplasms: An autopsy study. South Med J 72:806–807, 1979.
315. Klinger ME: Secondary tumors of the genito-urinary tract. J Urol 65:144–153, 1951.
316. Payne RA: Metastatic renal tumours. Br J Surg 48:310–315, 1960.
317. Wagle DG, Moore RH, Murphy GP: Secondary carcinomas of the kidney. J Urol 114:30–32, 1975.
318. Pascal RR: Renal manifestations of extrarenal neoplasms. Hum Pathol 11:7–17, 1980.
319. Melato M, Laurino L, Bianchi P, Faccini L: Intraglomerular metastases. A possibly maldiagnosed entity. Zentralbl Allg Pathol 137:90–92, 1991.
320. Naryshkin S, Tomaszewski JE: Acute renal failure secondary to carcinomatous lymphatic metastases to kidneys. J Urol 146:1610–1612, 1991.
321. Dehner LP: Intrarenal teratoma occurring in infancy: Report of a case with discussion of extragonadal germ cell tumors in infancy. J Pediatr Surg 8:369–378, 1973.
322. Aubert J, Casamayou J, Denis P, et al: Intrarenal teratoma in a newborn child. Eur Urol 4:306–308, 1978.
323. Aaronson IA, Sinclair-Smith C: Multiple cystic teratomas of the kidney. Arch Pathol Lab Med 104:614, 1980.
324. Mihatsch MJ, Bleisch A, Six P, Heitz P: Primary choriocarcinoma of the kidney in a 49-year-old woman. J Urol 108:537–539, 1972.
325. Young RH, Eble JN: Unusual forms of carcinoma of the urinary bladder. Hum Pathol 22:948–965, 1991.
326. Abeshouse BS: Primary benign and malignant tumors of the ureter, a review of the literature and report of one benign and twelve malignant tumors. Am J Surg 91:237–271, 1956.
327. Satodate R, Koike H, Sasou S, et al: Nephrogenic adenoma of the ureter. J Urol 131:332–334, 1984.
328. Lugo M, Petersen RO, Elfenbein IB, et al: Nephrogenic metaplasia of the ureter. Am J Clin Pathol 80:92–97, 1983.
329. Naito S, Minoda M, Hirata H: Inverted papilloma of ureter. Urology 22:290–291, 1983.
330. Lausten GS, Anagnostaki L, Thomsen OF: Inverted papilloma of the upper urinary tract. Eur Urol 10:67–70, 1984.
331. Kyriakos M, Royce RK: Multiple simultaneous inverted papillomas of the upper urinary tract. A case report with a review of ureteral and renal pelvic inverted papillomas. Cancer 63:368–380, 1989.
332. Embon OM, Saghi N, Bechar L: Inverted papilloma of ureter. Eur Urol 10:139–140, 1984.
333. Arrufat JM, Vera-Román JM, Casas V, et al: Papiloma invertido de uréter. Actas Urol Esp 7:225–228, 1983.
334. Palvio DHB: Inverted papillomas of the urinary tract, a case of multiple, recurring inverted papillomas of the renal pelvis, ureter and bladder associated with malignant change. Scand J Urol Nephrol 19:299–302, 1985.
335. Kunze E, Schauer A, Schmitt M: Histology and histogenesis of two different types of inverted urothelial papillomas. Cancer 51:348–358, 1983.
336. Kimura G, Tsuboi N, Nakajima H, et al: Inverted papilloma of the ureter with malignant transformation: A case report and review of the literature. Urol Int 42:30–36, 1987.
337. Grainger R, Gikas PW, Grossman HB: Urothelial carcinoma occurring within an inverted papilloma of the ureter. J Urol 143:802–804, 1990.
338. Wolgel CD, Parris AC, Mitty HA, Schapira HE: Fibroepithelial polyp of renal pelvis. Urology 19:436–439, 1982.
339. Goldman SM, Bohlman ME, Gatewood OMB: Neoplasms of the renal collecting system. Semin Roentgenol 22:284–291, 1987.
340. Bartone FF, Johansson SL, Markin RJ, Imray TJ: Bilateral fibroepithelial polyps of ureter in a child. Urology 35:519–522, 1990.
341. Macksood MJ, Roth DR, Chang C-H, Perlmutter AD: Benign fibroepithelial polyps as a cause of intermittent ureteropelvic junction obstruction in a child: A case report and review of the literature. J Urol 134:951–952, 1985.
342. van Poppel H, Nuttin B, Oyen R, et al: Fibroepithelial polyps of the ureter, etiology, diagnosis, treatment and pathology. Eur Urol 12:174–179, 1986.
343. Williams PR, Feggeter J, Miller RA, Wickham JEA: The diagnosis and management of benign fibrous ureteric polyps. Br J Urol 52:253–256, 1980.
344. Stuppler SA, Kandzari SJ: Fibroepithelial polyps of ureter, a benign ureteral tumor. Urology 5:553–558, 1975.
345. Uhlí K: Hemangioma of the ureter. J Urol 110:647–649, 1973.
346. Jansen TTH, van deWeyer FPH, deVries HR: Angiomatous ureteral polyp. Urology 20:426–427, 1982.
347. Kvist E, Lauritzen AF, Bredesen J, et al: A comparative study of transitional cell tumors of the bladder and upper urinary tract. Cancer 61:2109–2112, 1988.
348. Mazeman E: Tumours of the upper urinary tract calyces, renal pelvis and ureter. Eur Urol 2:120–128, 1976.
349. McLaughlin JK, Blot WJ, Mandel JS, et al: Etiology of cancer of the renal pelvis. J Natl Cancer Inst 71:287–291, 1983.
350. Palvio DHB, Andersen JC, Falk E: Transitional cell tumors of the renal pelvis and ureter associated with capillarosclerosis indicating analgesic abuse. Cancer 59:972–976, 1987.
351. Steffens J, Nagel R: Tumours of the renal pelvis and ureter, observations in 170 patients. Br J Urol 61:277–283, 1988.
352. Christensen P, Rørbæk Madsen M, Myhre Jensen O: Latency of thorotrast-induced renal tumors. Scand J Urol Nephrol 17:127–130, 1983.
353. Verhaak RLOM, Harmsen AE, van Unnik AJM: On the frequency of tumor induction in a thorotrast kidney. Cancer 34:2061–2068, 1974.
354. Nielsen K, Ostri P: Primary tumors of the renal pelvis: Evaluation of clinical and pathological features in a consecutive series of 10 years. J Urol 140:19–21, 1988.
355. Corrado F, Ferri C, Mannini D, et al: Transitional cell carcinoma of the upper urinary tract: Evaluation of prognostic factors by histopathology and flow cytometric analysis. J Urol 145:1159–1163, 1991.
356. Bonsib SM: Pathology of the renal pelvis and ureter. In Eble JN (ed): Tumors and Tumor-like Conditions of the Kidneys and Ureters. New York, Churchill Livingstone, 1990, pp 177–205.
357. Anderström C, Johansson SL, Pettersson S, Wahlqvist L: Carcinoma of the ureter: A clinicopathologic study of 49 cases. J Urol 142:280–283, 1989.
358. Blute ML, Tsushima K, Farrow GM, et al: Transitional cell carcinoma of the renal pelvis: Nuclear deoxyribonucleic acid ploidy studied by flow cytometry. J Urol 140:944–949, 1988.

359. American Joint Committee on Cancer: Renal pelvis and ureter. AJCC Cancer Staging Manual. Philadelphia, Lippincott-Raven, 1997, pp 235–239.
360. Murphy DM, Zincke H, Furlow WL: Primary grade 1 transitional cell carcinoma of the renal pelvis and ureter. J Urol 123:629–631, 1980.
361. Huben RP, Mounzer AM, Murphy GP: Tumor grade and stage as prognostic variables in upper tract urothelial tumors. Cancer 62:2016–2020, 1988.
362. Nocks BN, Heney NM, Daly JJ, et al: Transitional cell carcinoma of renal pelvis. Urology 19:472–477, 1982.
363. Tajima Y, Aizawa M: Unusual renal pelvic tumor containing transitional cell carcinoma, adenocarcinoma and sarcomatoid elements (so-called sarcomatoid carcinoma of the renal pelvis), a case report and review of the literature. Acta Pathol Jpn 38:805–814, 1988.
364. Piscioli F, Bondi A, Scappini P, Luciani L: 'True' sarcomatoid carcinoma of the renal pelvis. Eur Urol 10:350–355, 1984.
365. Rao SS, Rao NN, Venkataratnam G: Carcino-sarcoma of renal pelvis in a child, a case report. Indian J Pathol Microbiol 29:313–316, 1986.
366. Essenfeld H, Manivel JC, Benedetto P, Albores-Saavedra J: Small cell carcinoma of the renal pelvis: A clinicopathological, morphological and immunohistochemical study of 2 cases. J Urol 144:344–347, 1990.
367. Kenney RM, Prat J, Tabernero M: Giant-cell tumor-like proliferation associated with a papillary transitional cell carcinoma of the renal pelvis. Am J Surg Pathol 8:139–144, 1984.
368. Tarry WF, Morabito RA, Belis JA: Carcinosarcoma of the renal pelvis with extension into the renal vein and vena cava. J Urol 128:582–585, 1982.
369. Mahadevia PS, Karwa GL, Koss LG: Mapping of urothelium in carcinomas of the renal pelvis and ureter. Cancer 51:890–897, 1983.
370. Martínez García R, Boronat Tormo F, Domínguez Hinarejos C, et al: Adenocarcinoma de pelvis renal. Actas Urol Esp 13:470–472, 1989.
371. Takezawa Y, Saruki K, Jinbo S, Yamanaka H: A case of adenocarcinoma of the renal pelvis. Acta Urol Jpn 36:841–845, 1990.
372. Stein A, Sova Y, Lurie M, Lurie A: Adenocarcinoma of the renal pelvis, report of two cases, one with simultaneous transitional cell carcinoma of the bladder. Urol Int 43:299–301, 1988.
373. Kim YI, Yoon DH, Lee SW, Lee C: Multicentric papillary adenocarcinoma of the renal pelvis and ureter: Report of a case with ultrastructural study. Cancer 62:2402–2407, 1988.
374. Ishikura H, Ishiguro T, Enatsu C, et al: Hepatoid adenocarcinoma of the renal pelvis producing alpha-fetoprotein of hepatic type and bile pigment. Cancer 67:3051–3056, 1991.
375. Brawer MK, Waisman J: Papillary adenocarcinoma of ureter. Urology 19:205–209, 1982.
376. Moncino MD, Friedman HS, Kurtzberg J, Pizzo SV: Papillary adenocarcinoma of the renal pelvis in a child: Case report and brief review of the literature. Med Pediatr Oncol 18:81–86, 1990.
377. Bullock PS, Thoni DE, Murphy WM: The significance of colonic mucosa (intestinal metaplasia) involving the urinary tract. Cancer 59:2086–2090, 1987.
378. Gordon A: Intestinal metaplasia of the urinary tract epithelium. J Pathol Bacteriol 85:441–444, 1963.
379. Utz DC, McDonald JR: Squamous cell carcinoma of the kidney. J Urol 78:540–552, 1957.
380. Vyas MCR, Joshi KR, Mathur DR, Bais CS: Primary squamous cell carcinoma of the renal pelvis, a report of four cases with review of literature. Indian J Pathol Microbiol 25:151–155, 1982.
381. Blacher EJ, Johnson DE, Abdul-Karim FW, Ayala AG: Squamous cell carcinoma of renal pelvis. Urology 25:124–125, 1985.
382. Hertle L, Androulakakis P: Keratinizing desquamative squamous metaplasia of the upper urinary tract: Leukoplakia-cholesteatoma. J Urol 127:631–635, 1982.
383. Strobel SL, Jasper WS, Gogate SA, Sharma HM: Primary carcinoma of the renal pelvis and ureter, evaluation of clinical and pathologic features. Arch Pathol Lab Med 108:697–700, 1984.
384. Howat AJ, Scott E, Mackie B, Pinkerton JR: Adenosquamous carcinoma of the renal pelvis. Am J Clin Pathol 79:731–733, 1983.
385. Kao VCT, Graff PW, Rappaport H: Leiomyoma of the ureter, a histologically problematic rare tumor confirmed by immunohistochemical studies. Cancer 24:535–542, 1969.
386. Zaitoon MM: Leiomyoma of ureter. Urology 28:50–51, 1986.
387. Gislason T, Arnarson OO: Primary ureteral leiomyosarcoma. Scand J Urol Nephrol 18:253–254, 1984.
388. Tolia BM, Hajdu SI, Whitmore WF Jr: Leiomyosarcoma of the renal pelvis. J Urol 109:974–976, 1973.
389. Rushton HG, Sens MA, Garvin AJ, Turner WR Jr: Primary leiomyosarcoma of the ureter: A case report with electron microscopy. J Urol 129:1045–1046, 1983.
390. Fein RL, Hamm FC: Malignant schwannoma of the renal pelvis: A review of the literature and a case report. J Urol 94:356–361, 1965.
391. Frasier BL, Wachs BH, Watson LR, Tomasulo JP: Malignant melanoma of the renal pelvis presenting as a primary tumor. J Urol 140:812–813, 1988.
392. Chen KTK, Workman RD, Flam MS, DeKlotz RJ: Carcinosarcoma of renal pelvis. Urology 22:429–431, 1983.
393. Yano S, Arita M, Ueno F, et al: Carcinosarcoma of the ureter. Eur Urol 10:71, 1984.
394. Vahlensieck W, Riede U, Wimmer B, Ihling C: Beta-human chorionic gonadotropin-positive extragonadal germ cell neoplasia of the renal pelvis. Cancer 67:3051–3056, 1991.
395. Scharifker D, Chalasani A: Ureteral involvement by malignant lymphoma, ten years' experience. Arch Pathol Lab Med 102:541–542, 1978.

# 31

# *Bladder and Urethra*

Richard J. Cote   Rashida A. Soni   Mahul B. Amin

## BLADDER

### Anatomy of the Urinary Bladder

The urinary bladder varies in size, shape, position, and relations, according to the fluid it contains. When empty, it is entirely in the lesser pelvis, but as it becomes distended, it extends into the abdominal cavity.[1] The bladder lies relatively free within the fibrofatty tissue of the pelvis to expand freely when filled except in the area of the bladder neck, where it is secured firmly by the pubovesical ligaments in the female and puboprostatic ligaments in the male.[2, 3] The superior surface of the bladder is covered by the pelvic parietal peritoneum. The base of the bladder faces posteriorly and inferiorly. It is separated from the rectum by the uterine cervix and the proximal portions of the vagina in the female and by the seminal vesicles and the ampulla of the vasa deferentia in the male. Posterior anatomic relations are important. The two inferolateral surfaces face laterally, inferiorly, and anteriorly and are in contact with the fascia of the levator and other muscles. The most anterosuperior point of the bladder is known as the *apex,* which marks the point of insertion of the median umbilical ligament and is the area where urachal carcinomas are located. The trigone is a complex anatomic structure located at the base of the bladder, extending to the posterior bladder neck. In the proximal and lateral aspects of the trigone, the ureters enter into the bladder obliquely. Distally the portion of the bladder where the posterior and inferolateral walls converge and open into the urethra is called the *bladder neck.* In the male, the blad-der neck merges with the prostate gland, where prostatic ducts can be seen occasionally.

The lymphatic vessels of the bladder take their origin in three plexuses—mucosal, intramuscular, and extramuscular. Most of the collecting vessels end in the external iliac lymph nodes; however, one of these vessels may go to the internal or common iliac lymph nodes. The lymphatic vessels, derived from the prostatic and membranous part of the urethra in the male and from the entire urethra in the female, pass mainly to the internal iliac lymph nodes. The principal vascular supply to the bladder is the superior and the inferior vesical arteries, derived from the anterior trunk of the internal iliac artery. The obturator and inferior gluteal arteries also send branches to it, and in the female, additional branches are derived from the uterine and vaginal branches. The veins form a complicated plexus on the inferolateral surfaces near the prostate and end in the internal iliac veins.

The bladder wall consists of epithelium, lamina propria, muscularis mucosae, muscularis propria, subserosa, and serosa (Fig. 31–1). The epithelium of the urinary bladder is lined by transitional cells and is known also as *urothelium.* It is derived endodermally from the cranial portion of the urogenital sinus, which is in continuity with the allantois. Lamina propria and muscularis propria and the adventitia develop from the adjacent splanchnic mesenchyme. The urothelium is usually six to seven cells thick in the contracted state and is composed of three regions: superficial umbrella cells, intermediate cells, and basal cells. The intermediate cells may be five cells thick in contracted bladder. They have oval

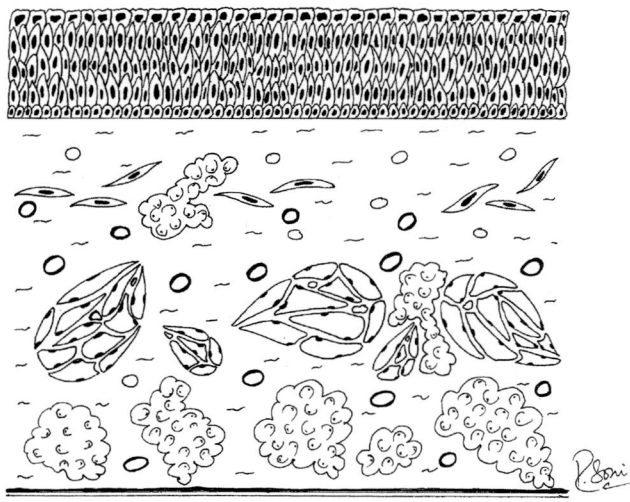

**FIGURE 31–1.** Schematic cross-section of bladder wall. The muscularis mucosae is discontinuous. Where it is found, the portion of the nonmuscular bladder wall deep to it is considered the submucosa and contains larger thick-walled blood vessels. Note also the presence of fat, which can be seen (occasionally in substantial deposits) in lamina propria and muscularis propria. Muscularis mucosae and fat in the bladder wall represent potential pitfalls in staging of bladder cancer, particularly in biopsy specimens.

nuclei with finely stippled chromatin and ample cytoplasm, which sometimes can be vacuolated, and are arranged in pseudostratified orientation, in vertical cellular polarity. The basal cells are cuboidal and are seen clearly only in contracted bladder. The luminal cells are called *umbrella cells* and are larger with irregular cytoplasmic membrane and abundant eosinophilic cytoplasm. The lamina propria contains delicate blood vessels, nerves, and loose connective tissue with delicate wisps of smooth muscle fibers, sometimes referred to as *muscularis mucosae*,[4, 5] which has considerable relevance in bladder cancer staging (discussed later). The muscularis mucosae is considered by some to separate the lamina propria from the submucosa. The submucosa generally shows larger, thick-walled blood vessels compared to the lamina propria. The lamina propria and muscularis propria also contain fat, which is important in assessing the bladder biopsy specimens because the presence of fat sometimes can pose difficulty in assessing extent of invasion.[6, 7]

Urothelium may show divergent differentiation on histologic evaluation. Glandular features within benign lesions, such as cystitis glandularis and nephrogenic adenoma, and in malignant lesions, such as adenocarcinoma, are not due to mesodermal or müllerian rests within the trigone but constitute urothelial metaplasia. Normally the lining of the urachus is composed of transitional epithelium, but it frequently undergoes metaplastic change, mostly glandular.

Muscularis propria, which constitutes a detrusor muscle, consists of three layers of nonstriated myocytes: an external and an internal layer consisting of longitudinal fibers and a middle layer consisting of circular fibers. The serosa is composed mainly of peritoneal covering. In the male, the superior surface is covered completely with peritoneum, which extends slightly to the base and is continued behind into the rectovesical pouch. In the female, the superior surface is covered almost entirely with peritoneum, but posteriorly the serosa is reflected onto the uterus to form the vesicouterine pouch.

## Bladder Cancer

### EPIDEMIOLOGY

Bladder cancer is a common malignancy, with more than 50,000 new cases diagnosed annually. The incidence of bladder cancer is higher in the United States and Europe than the rest of the world. In the United States, bladder cancer is the fourth most common malignancy[8] and fifth most common cause of cancer deaths. The disease is three times more common in men than women, and whites are affected more commonly than blacks.

The high incidence of bladder cancer in men may be explained by environmental and dietary exposures, innate sexual characteristics (e.g., anatomic differences), urination habits, or hormonal factors.[9] Most bladder cancers occur in adults over 50 years of age. Cases also can occur in younger individuals, however, and even in children.[10–12] The mortality rate for bladder cancer has declined in the last 50 years. This situation is due in part to improvements in diagnosis and treatment.

Many factors have been linked to the development of bladder cancer, including cigarette smoke, chemical exposure, analgesic and artificial sweetener use, certain urinary infections, and radiation. These factors may induce changes in the genome of the transitional cells that line the urinary tract and initiate carcinogenesis.

Bladder cancer incidence has increased with industrialization and was one of the first cancers to be investigated epidemiologically. Initial evidence found a risk in workers who manufactured aniline dyes used for coloring fabrics. Aniline dyes are part of a class of chemicals known as *arylamines*, which include naphthylamine and aminobiphenyl. Occupational exposure to arylamines such as benzidine, 2-naphthylamine, and 4-aminobiphenyl is associated with a greatly elevated risk of bladder cancer (≥100-fold).[13, 14] In one cohort study,[15] the incidence of bladder cancer increased with the duration of work in industries that exposed workers to aromatic amines, with an average latency period of more than 20 years.

Besides textile industries, exposure to arylamines is seen in the aluminum industry. Arylamines are found in tobacco smoke, which may explain the increased incidence of bladder cancer in smokers.[16] Epidemiologic analyses of timing of exposure in workers occupationally exposed to arylamines suggest that arylamines exert an early-stage and a late-stage activity, compatible with a two-mutation the-

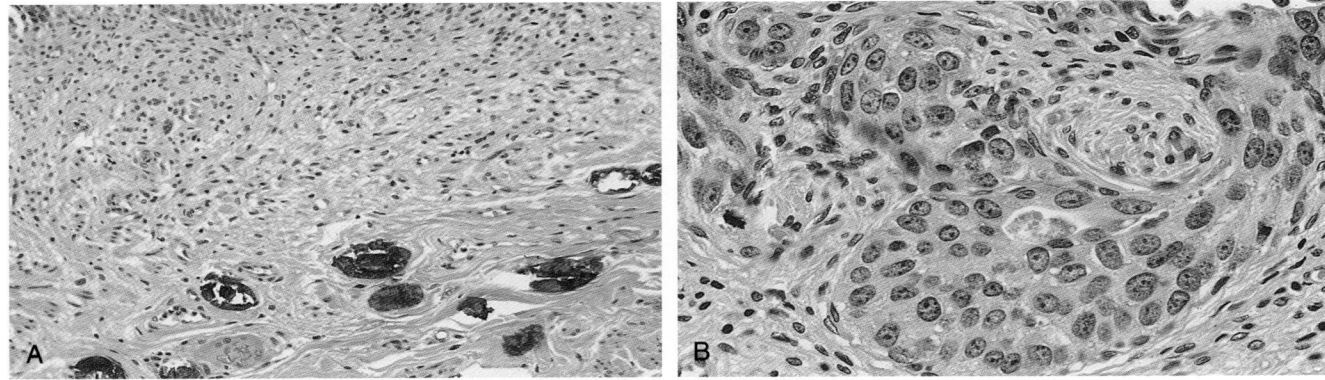

**FIGURE 31–2.** Section of bladder wall from an Egyptian man. *A,* Note the presence of *Schistosoma* eggs, associated with pronounced inflammation. *B,* A section from the same bladder, showing squamous carcinoma.

ory of bladder carcinogenesis.[17] Approximately one quarter of U.S. men with bladder cancer have a history of occupational exposure to the compounds commonly implicated in bladder cancer risk.

In the United States, the most important risk factor for bladder cancer is cigarette smoking. There is a dose-response relationship in men and women, with a threshold limit of 15 to 20 cigarettes per day, after which no increased risk is observed. A study has shown, however, that risk of bladder cancer in women who smoke is higher than that in men who smoke a comparable number of cigarettes.[18] Studies have shown a linear increasing risk of bladder cancer with increasing duration of smoking.[18, 19] The risk for bladder cancer seems much lower in pipe and cigar smokers. The mechanism of carcinogenicity of smoking seems to be related to chemicals in the smoke, especially aromatic amines.[20]

Certain drugs are implicated in causing bladder cancer. Cyclophosphamide chemotherapy produces a 5% risk of bladder cancer in humans. This risk is dose related and has a latency period of 20 years. Radiation to the pelvis is an additional risk factor for bladder cancer. This risk factor is important diagnostically in a patient with a radiated pelvis who presents with gross or microscopic hematuria. Phenacetin-containing analgesics are associated with urinary tract tumors, especially in the renal pelvis and ureter. Evidence suggests, however, that nonsteroidal analgesics may reduce the risk of bladder cancer.[21] Although saccharin was implicated previously in bladder carcinogenesis in rats, more recent evidence suggests that the compound does not play a significant role in bladder cancer causation. Some studies have shown an increased risk of bladder cancer among daily coffee drinkers.[22] The data on tea consumption are largely negative.[23] Chlorinated water consumption is linked weakly to bladder cancer development,[24] and use of permanent hair dyes has been linked to bladder cancer.[25]

Chronic bladder inflammation secondary to urinary tract infection or an indwelling foreign body, such as a stone or a catheter, is related to the development of squamous cell carcinoma of the bladder.

This relationship is seen especially in patients with spinal cord injury, in elderly patients with an indwelling catheter, or patients in parts of the world where bladder infections with schistosomiasis are endemic.[26]

Approximately 90% of the tumors of the urinary bladder in the United States are transitional cell type, 7% are squamous, 2% are glandular, and 1% are undifferentiated.[27] This distribution is in contrast to *Schistosoma haematobium*–endemic areas, such as Egypt and parts of the Middle East, where squamous cell carcinoma is the most common form of bladder cancer (Fig. 31–2). In *S. haematobium* infection, the toxins produced by the organism itself or through secondary bacterial infection induce damage to urothelium, which can lead to squamous metaplasia and subsequently to squamous cell carcinoma. The patients usually present at a younger age[28] and with advanced stage.

## GENETIC ALTERATIONS IN BLADDER CANCER

Bladder cancer is known to be a disease that results from molecular alterations, many of which have been defined over the past several years. Cytogenetic and molecular genetic analyses of bladder cancer have identified alterations in many chromosomes that seem to be involved in the development and progression of the disease. The earliest cytogenetic studies in bladder cancer showed evidence of alterations in chromosomes 9q, 11p, and 17p,[29–34] the most common defects being allelic losses, loss of heterozygosity, and microsatellite alterations. In general, amplification of regions within chromosomes reflects the identification of possible oncogene loci, and allelic losses or loss of heterozygosity reflects the possible presence of tumor-suppressor genes. From early studies, it was evident that tumor-suppressor genes probably play an important role in bladder tumorigenesis.

The role of tumor-suppressor genes on chromosome 9 became more clear when repeated reports showed allelic losses and loss of heterozygosity of more than one marker on chromosome 9.[33, 35, 36] Alle-

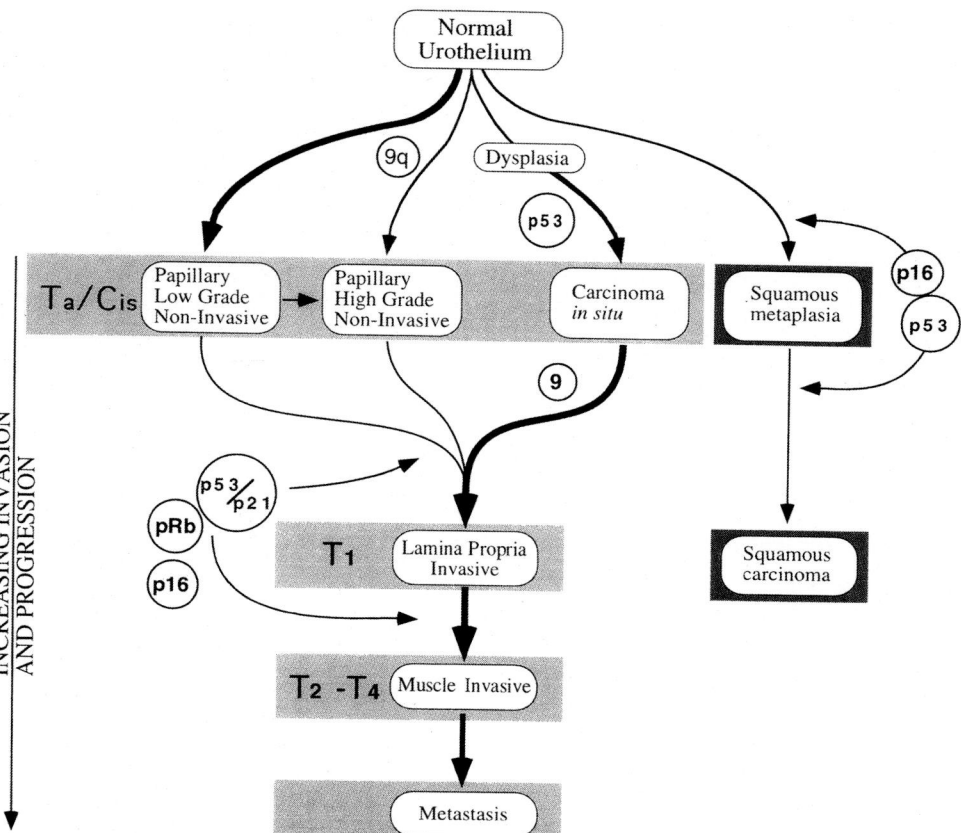

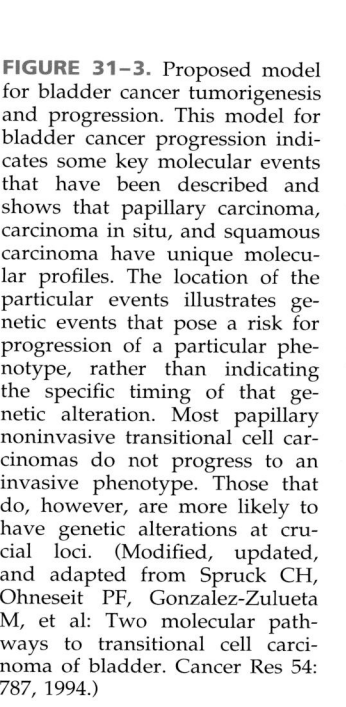

**FIGURE 31–3.** Proposed model for bladder cancer tumorigenesis and progression. This model for bladder cancer progression indicates some key molecular events that have been described and shows that papillary carcinoma, carcinoma in situ, and squamous carcinoma have unique molecular profiles. The location of the particular events illustrates genetic events that pose a risk for progression of a particular phenotype, rather than indicating the specific timing of that genetic alteration. Most papillary noninvasive transitional cell carcinomas do not progress to an invasive phenotype. Those that do, however, are more likely to have genetic alterations at crucial loci. (Modified, updated, and adapted from Spruck CH, Ohneseit PF, Gonzalez-Zulueta M, et al: Two molecular pathways to transitional cell carcinoma of bladder. Cancer Res 54: 787, 1994.)

lic losses were seen in 9p and 9q; the regions of deletions were between 9p12 and 9q34.[33] Subsequently the genes encoding cyclin-dependent kinase inhibitors p16[INK4a] and p15[INK4b] were found to reside on chromosome band 9p2[37, 38]; p16[INK4a] may play an important role in bladder tumorigenesis. Chromosome 17p, which harbors the *p53* tumor-suppressor gene, also shows allelic losses in bladder cancer[30–32]; *p53* is important in the pathogenesis of bladder cancer. The other tumor-suppressor gene found altered in many bladder cancers is the retinoblastoma susceptibility gene *Rb*, located on chromosome 13q. The tumor-suppressor genes *p53*, *Rb*, and *p16* all are involved in cell cycle control, and it has become clear that regulators of the cell cycle machinery are crucial in bladder cancer progression.

On the basis of consistent and frequent genetic defects in bladder tumors and increasing understanding of cell cycle regulation and its role in tumor behavior, studies from many groups have led to the description of a detailed and sophisticated model of important molecular events in bladder cancer[31, 32, 36, 39–47] (Fig. 31–3). These studies have shown that lesions long recognized as being morphologically and biologically distinct (papillary tumors versus flat and invasive tumors) are characterized by distinct molecular alterations. It seems that alteration in cell cycle regulation is a key event in determining the biologic behavior of bladder cancer. It is becom-

ing increasingly clear that these regulatory events are linked through specific pathways. It is now evident that a crucial event in bladder cancer progression involves the *p53* gene, not only through its role in cell cycle regulatory pathways, but also through other pathways.

Classic methods, particularly histologic grade and pathologic stage, are the mainstays of bladder cancer assessment. As knowledge of molecular pathways improves and the relationship between molecular alterations and bladder cancer tumorigenesis, progression, and response to therapy is elucidated further, there is no doubt that molecular assessment will become crucial in the evaluation of bladder cancer. We discuss in detail the issues regarding the standard diagnosis and staging of bladder cancer and point out where molecular evaluation already has had an impact.

## CLASSIFICATION OF MALIGNANT NEOPLASMS OF THE BLADDER

Most bladder tumors are epithelial, with 90% classified as *urothelial (transitional cell carcinoma)* (Table 31–1). The terms *transitional cell carcinoma* and *urothelial carcinoma* are interchangeable, and we use both terms to denote the primary neoplasms of the bladder. The most important subtypes of epithelial carcinomas of the bladder are adenocarcinomas and squamous cell carcinomas. Most epithelial neo-

**TABLE 31–1.** Classification of Malignant Neoplasms of the Bladder

Urothelial (transitional cell carcinoma)
  Papillary
  Flat carcinoma in situ
  Invasive, with or without mixed epithelial components
Distinctive histologic variants
  Micropapillary
  Sarcomatoid/carcinosarcoma
  Lymphoepithelial-like
  Small cell/neuroendocrine
  Giant cell
  Clear cell features
  Urothelial carcinoma with trophoblasts
  Plasmacytoid variant
Deceptively bland features
  Tubular
  Microcystic
  Nested
  Endophytic
Adenocarcinoma
  Intestinal type (enteric)
  Mucinous
  Signet ring cell
  Clear cell
  Hepatoid
Squamous cell carcinoma
  Verrucous
  Basaloid
  Sarcomatoid
Urachal carcinoma
  Mucinous
  Enteric
  Signet ring
Mesenchymal neoplasms (malignant)
  Leiomyosarcoma
  Rhabdomyosarcoma
  Malignant fibrous histiocytoma
  Osteosarcoma, liposarcoma, angiosarcoma, hemangiopericytoma
Other
  Melanoma
  Hematologic
  Carcinoid
  Pheochromocytoma

plasms involving the bladder are believed to be of urothelial origin, arising from metaplastic urothelium.

The terms *transitional cell carcinoma* and *urothelial carcinoma* are used for tumors that have recognizable areas of urothelial differentiation, including tumors that have as a major component areas of glandular, squamous, or other type of differentiation, including small cell and neuroendocrine features. We reserve the terms *adenocarcinoma* and *squamous carcinoma* for tumors that show essentially pure patterns of that designation. The presence of other components is noted, however, and we often comment on their relative proportion.

## GRADING PAPILLARY TUMORS

Papillary neoplasms are the most common tumors of the bladder, comprising 70% to 80% of all bladder tumors. Papillary tumors tend to recur locally and they infrequently become invasive and metastasize. It was recognized by Virchow[48] that papillary tumors of the bladder can exist for many years "and yet no trace of any cancerous infiltration of the base of the growth . . . existed, but the tumor was quite simply a papillary one, a benignant formation. . . ." It also was recognized, however, that some bladder tumors acted in an aggressive fashion and that one of the correlates of behavior was the microscopic appearance of the tumor. This recognition has led to classification schemes based on the histologic appearance of a tumor (or, more elegantly stated, the degree of differentiation of a tumor). The goal of these schemes is to predict the behavior of tumors.[49]

In the case of urothelial carcinomas, grading systems are applied to papillary neoplasms. Although all are not restricted to noninvasive neoplasms, it is in the superficial noninvasive tumors that grading schemes have the greatest utility. The first widely used grading scheme was developed by Broders in 1922.[50] This system was based on the degree of differentiation present in the lesion, and to some extent all other systems are related to it. Many systems and variations on systems have been proposed since[50–57] (Table 31–2); all have as their goal predicting behavior, in particular the risk for development of invasive disease. Although an attempt has been made here to compare the different grading systems directly, it is recognized that the overlap is by no means complete. For example, based on high nuclear grade, some tumors classified as grade 2 in the World Health Organization (WHO) system may be classified as high grade in the WHO/International Society of Urologic Pathologists (ISUP) system.

In general, four main grades of papillary neoplasm can be defined, as distinguished by their histologic characteristics (Table 31–3; Fig. 31–4 and CD

**TABLE 31–2.** Grading Systems for Papillary Urothelial Neoplasms

| Broders[50] | Ash[51] | Bergkvist[52] | Koss[53] | WHO 1973[54] | Murphy[55] | WHO/ISUP[56] | WHO 1999[57] |
|---|---|---|---|---|---|---|---|
|  | I | 0 | Papilloma | Papilloma | Papilloma | Papilloma | Papilloma |
| Grade 1 | II | Grade 1 | Grade 1 | Grade 1 |  | LMP | LMP |
|  |  |  |  |  | Low grade |  | Grade 1 |
| Grade 2 | III | Grade 2 | Grade 2 | Grade 2 |  | Low grade | Grade 2 |
| Grade 3, 4 | IV | Grade 3, 4 | Grade 3 | Grade 3 | High grade | High grade | Grade 3 |

LMP, Low malignant potential.

**TABLE 31–3.** Histologic Features of Papillary Urothelial Neoplasms

| Grade | Features |
|---|---|
| Papilloma | Normal urothelial cytology<br>Cellular polarity maintained<br>No/rare mitoses<br>Intact umbrella cell layer<br>7 to 8 cell layers |
| Grade 1/LMP | Normal urothelial cytology<br>Cellular polarity maintained<br>No/rare mitoses<br>± umbrella cell layer<br>Increased cellular density<br>>8 cell layers |
| Grade 2/low grade | Mild to moderate urothelial atypia<br>Increased nuclear-to-cytoplasmic ratio<br>Mild to moderate nuclear pleomorphism<br>Loss of cellular polarity<br>Infrequent mitoses<br>Variable loss of umbrella cell layer<br>Variable cell layer thickness |
| Grade 3, 4/high grade | Moderate to marked urothelial atypia<br>Increased nuclear-to-cytoplasmic ratio<br>Moderate to marked nuclear pleomorphism<br>Loss of cellular polarity<br>Mitoses easily seen, particularly in upper layers<br>Loss of umbrella cell layer<br>Variable cell layer thickness<br>Discohesion<br>Presence of necrosis |

LMP, Low malignant potential.

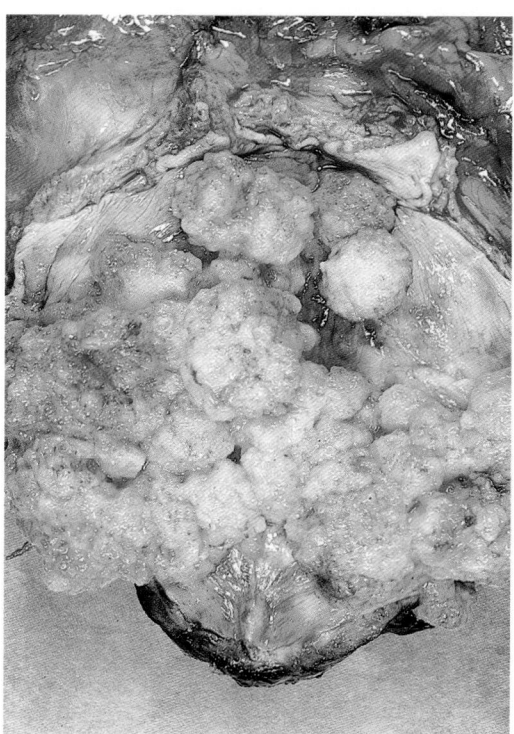

**FIGURE 31–4.** Papillary carcinoma of the bladder, gross specimen. These tumors can fill the bladder. These are unlikely to invade and metastasize, however, despite their exuberant appearance.

Fig. 31–1; see Table 31–2). *Papillomas* are composed of normal-appearing urothelium having an umbrella cell layer, with no more than seven or eight cell layers.[51, 53] These cells are arranged in delicate papillary fronds with a central fibrovascular core (Fig. 31–5). These tumors are rare and are considered benign.[58] *Grade 1/low malignant potential (LMP)* tumors are composed of essentially normal-appearing urothelium but with a thickness greater than seven or eight cell layers (Fig. 31–6 and CD Fig. 31–2). These tumors are called grade 1 carcinomas in many grading schemes, but it now is recognized that although they may recur, they only rarely progress to invasive or higher grade lesions.[52, 55, 56, 59] Invasion virtually always is preceded by evidence of increasing grade (or carcinoma in situ [CIS]).[49] Recognizing the low propensity of these tumors to progress (either in grade or stage), the ISUP has suggested the term *papillary neoplasms of LMP.*[56]

*Grade 2/low-grade* tumors have clear evidence of cytologic atypia, including increased nuclear-to-cytoplasmic ratio, loss of cellular polarity, and infrequent mitoses (Fig. 31–7). *Grade 3, 4/high-grade* tumors are clearly cytologically atypical, with features approaching or similar to CIS, including increased nuclear-to-cytoplasmic ratio, loss of normal architectural orientation, and moderate-to-frequent mitoses (Fig. 31–8). These tumors have a definite propensity for invasion, may have concurrent CIS, and must be followed closely and aggressively.[49, 53, 60, 61]

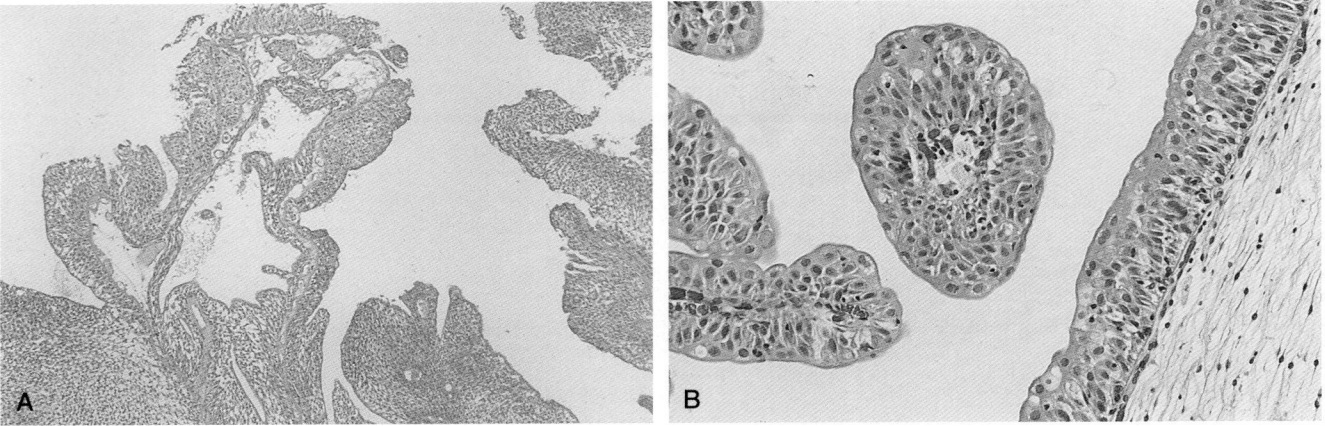

**FIGURE 31–5.** Papilloma of the bladder. *A,* Low-power view. *B,* High-power view. Note the delicate fibrovascular core. On cytologic evaluation, the cells are orderly and arranged in a pseudocolumnar arrangement, with round, regular, nonpleomorphic nuclei. A pronounced umbrella cell layer is noted. The thickness of the urothelial lining of a papilloma is generally seven to eight cell layers, although this can seem to be greater because of tangential sectioning. The urothelial lining is virtually indistinguishable from normal urothelium.

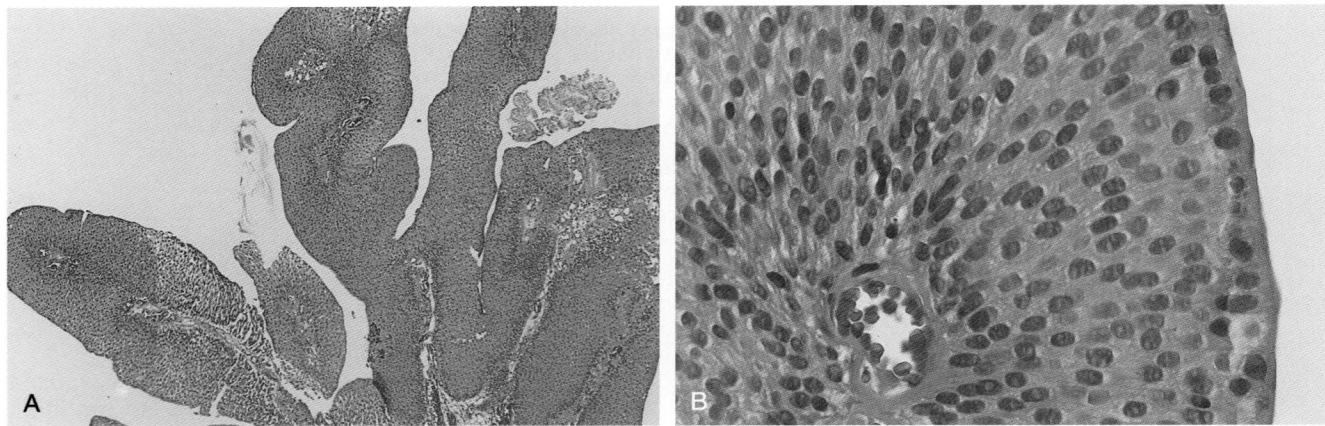

**FIGURE 31–6.** Grade 1 papillary carcinoma, papillary neoplasm of low malignant potential. *A,* Low-power view. *B,* High-power view. These tumors have a delicate fibrovascular core. They are lined by essentially normal-appearing urothelium but with a thickness greater than seven or eight cell layers. In addition, the density of the cells is increased. Cellular polarity is largely maintained, and an umbrella cell layer often can be appreciated. These tumors rarely progress.

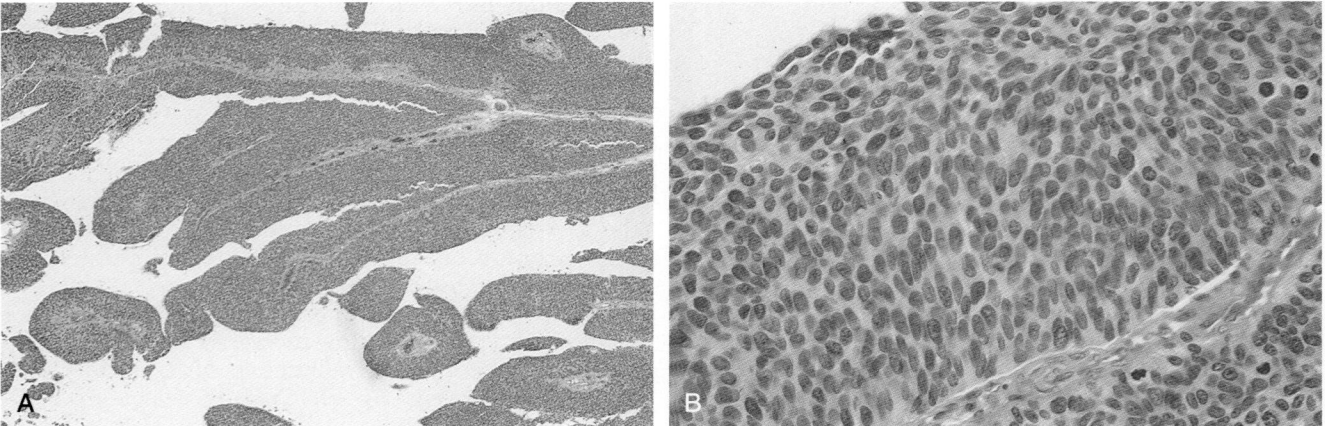

**FIGURE 31–7.** Grade 2, low-grade papillary carcinoma. *A,* Low-power view. *B,* High-power view. The fibrovascular core is not as delicate as for papillomas or grade 1 papillary carcinomas. In this example, the urothelial cell lining is composed of multiple cell layers, although this can be variable. The high-power view shows loss of cellular polarity. Mild-to-moderate nuclear pleomorphism can be appreciated, although individually the nuclei are not far deviated from normal. Mitoses usually can be appreciated but are relatively infrequent. The risk for local recurrence in these tumors is substantial. (Courtesy of Dr. Peter W. Nichols.)

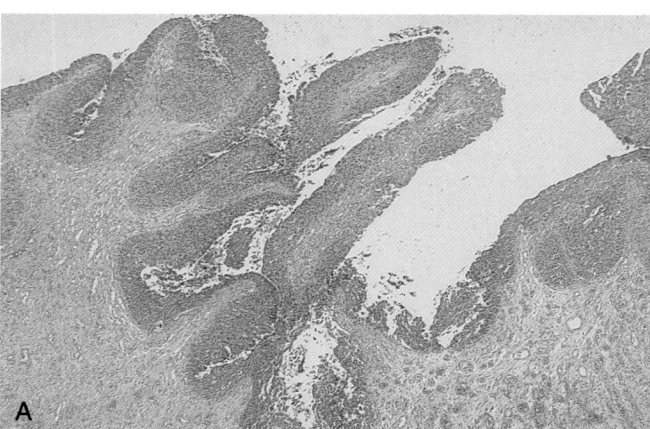
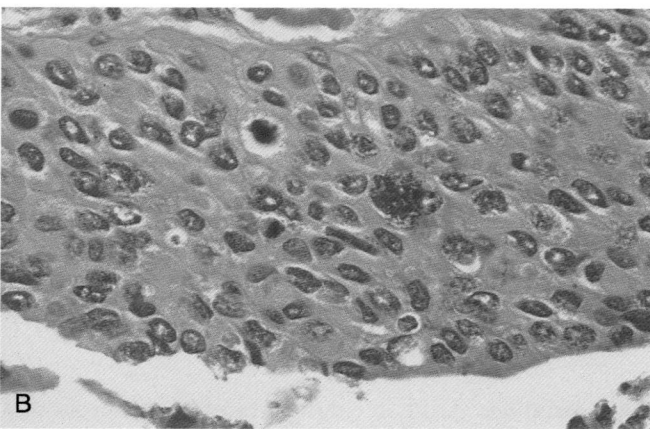

**FIGURE 31-8.** Grade 3 and 4, high-grade papillary carcinomas. *A*, Low-power view. *B*, High-power view. Although the tumor has a papillary configuration, the fibrovascular cores are thickened. The urothelial lining can be of variable thickness. On cytologic evaluation, these tumors have lost cellular polarity. They show moderate-to-marked nuclear pleomorphism, and mitoses are easily appreciated, including in the upper cell layers. The presence of discohesion or necrosis (not shown in this example) is diagnostic of high-grade tumors. The cytologic appearance of a high-grade papillary urothelial carcinoma is similar to that of flat carcinoma in situ. These tumors are aggressive and have a high propensity to recur and to progress to invasion.

Histologic grading is by its nature subjective. This subjectivity, combined with the numerous proposed grading systems, has resulted in significant interobserver variability.[62-65] This variability is important to recognize because grading of noninvasive papillary neoplasms is the basis for treatment and management decisions. In our opinion, however, this variability is mitigated substantially by the fact that the primary distinction that must be made is between tumors with low propensities for invasion (papilloma and grade 1/LMP) versus tumors with moderate-to-high risk for invasion (grade 2/low grade and grade 3, 4/high grade). This distinction is relatively straightforward because the former are composed of urothelium that looks normal (although thicker in the case of grade 1/LMP neoplasms), whereas the latter have urothelium with varying degrees of cytologic atypia and recognizable mitoses. The next most important distinction is between grade 2/low-grade tumors and grade 3, 4/high-grade tumors. This distinction is considerably more difficult. Cytologic criteria must be observed; more than moderate pleomorphism should be classified as high grade (see Fig. 31-8). Necrosis and cellular discohesion indicate the presence of a high-grade lesion. In addition, in our experience, mitotic activity can be useful; the presence of more than infrequent mitoses, particularly in the upper layers of the urothelium, should be cause to consider classification as high grade, even in the presence of mild-to-moderate cytologic atypia.

This discussion illustrates the difficulty inherent in the histologic grading of papillary urothelial neoplasms. Grade must be reported in all cases of noninvasive papillary tumors, however. Although less important for invasive tumors, it is still common practice to report grade. The choice of a grading system should be made in conjunction with the urologist and oncologist and should be consistent within an institution. It is helpful to specify which grading system is being used or at least to indicate the denominator. When reporting grade, the pathologist should list the range of grades seen or the highest grade because management is based on the highest grade of the tumor. The most commonly used grading systems are WHO[54] and Bergkvist,[52] although the WHO/ISUP classification is gaining popularity.[56]

The most important use of grading in the management of bladder cancer is for noninvasive papillary lesions. The risk of local recurrence for LMP tumors is approximately 30%, whereas it is greater than 60% for low-grade carcinomas (WHO grade 2, WHO/ISUP low grade).[58, 66, 67] The risk of progression (either grade or stage progression) for LMP tumors and low-grade carcinomas is low and increases with higher grade tumors.[49, 58, 66-68] When a tumor has invaded the bladder wall, however, stage of disease, including depth of invasion, extension to adjacent structures, and lymph node involvement, are the most important classic prognostic parameters.[60, 69] Although some studies have shown that grade remains an important prognostic feature of invasive tumors,[70] more recent studies have shown that grade is not an independent predictor of long-term outcome.[71] In our experience, when a tumor has invaded, it almost always is high grade, making grading virtually moot for invasive tumors.

The impact of specific genetic alterations on the behavior of bladder tumors in general and papillary noninvasive tumors in particular is becoming increasingly clear[41] (see Fig. 31-3). The presence of *p53* or *Rb* alterations now is known to be a risk factor for progression to invasive disease.[72-76] Studies show that superficial (Ta/T1) papillary tumors that show alterations in *p53* or *Rb* tumor-suppressor

**TABLE 31–4.** Progression-Free Survival in Patients with Superficial (Ta/T1) Bladder Cancer Based on *p53* and pRb Tumor-Suppressor Status*

| | | 5-year Progression-Free Survival | | | |
| --- | --- | --- | --- | --- | --- |
| Study | No. Patients | *Wild-Type* p53 *and pRb* | *Altered* p53 *or pRb* | *Altered* p53 *and pRb* | P Value |
| Grossman et al[76] | 45 | 100% | 70% | 53% | .005 |
| Cordon-Cardo et al[73] | 59 | 95% | 57% | 45% | .0001 |

\* *p53* and pRb status determined by immunohistochemistry.
pRb, *Rb* protein.

gene products have a higher rate of progression than tumors with no detectable alterations in either *p53* or *Rb*. Tumors with alterations in both gene products have the highest rate of progression (Table 31–4). Future grading systems no doubt will combine morphology with molecular assessment. This combination will greatly facilitate reproducibility and specific management decisions for patients with papillary neoplasms.

## CARCINOMA IN SITU

CIS is a high-grade lesion with severe cytologic abnormalities, similar to those seen in high-grade papillary carcinoma. CIS usually refers to a flat (nonpapillary) lesion, although CIS can be described within a papillary tumor and often is associated with papillary tumors. As its name implies, CIS is a noninvasive lesion, and, as with papillary tumors, the recognition of early invasion is important (described further subsequently).

First described by Melicow[77] as highly atypical epithelium adjacent to invasive bladder cancer, CIS has long been recognized as a dangerous and aggressive form of noninvasive urothelial carcinoma; Melamed and colleagues[78] first recognized that CIS has a high propensity to progress to invasive cancer, and this has been confirmed by many subsequent studies.[79–84] Although CIS may occur in the absence of other urothelial tumors (papillary or invasive tumors), it is seen most commonly in association with high-grade papillary tumors or with invasive urothelial carcinomas.[79, 85, 86]

Clinically, patients with pure CIS either have no symptoms or present with symptoms that resemble cystitis.[87] The cystoscopic and gross appearance of CIS is subtle, but it is well recognized by urologists and pathologists. Bladder mucosa involved with CIS shows a hyperemic, velvety appearance. This appearance reflects the high degree of angiogenesis observed in response to these tumors and their mucosal friability (Fig. 31–9).

An important feature of CIS is its multifocality; involvement of the bladder can be extensive,[78, 88] and CIS often can be seen involving urethra, prostatic ducts, and ureters.[89–94] Skinner and coworkers[94] recognized that in bladders where it occurred, CIS was noted at the ureter and urethral margins in a substantial proportion of cases. The multifocality, involvement of urethra (including prostatic urethra and ducts), and involvement of ureteral and urethral margins have led some investigators to propose aggressive management for patients with CIS (see later).

The most common microscopic presentation of CIS is full-thickness replacement of the urothelium by cytologically atypical cells (see Fig. 31–9). The cells have a high nuclear-to-cytoplasmic ratio, moderate-to-severe nuclear pleomorphism, and an irregular or stippled chromatin pattern. An important feature is the recognition of mitoses in the mid to upper urothelium. Architecturally, there is loss of normal urothelial orientation, similar to that seen in high-grade papillary carcinoma. The number of cell layers, or the thickness of the mucosa, can be variable, ranging from hyperplastic to attenuated to fully denuded. This last situation reflects the friability of CIS involving the mucosa and must be recognized as a potential diagnostic pitfall in its presentation.[84] This friability also leads to abundant material for examination in urine by cytology, however. The general features of CIS are similar to those seen in high-grade papillary tumors (see Table 31–3). Several patterns of CIS have been recognized and are well summarized by McKenney and associates,[95] including large cell CIS, small cell CIS, and CIS with pagetoid spread (Table 31–5; Fig. 31–10; and CD Figs. 31–3 to 31–7).

Although CIS usually is characterized by full-thickness replacement of the mucosa, it now is recognized that cytologic abnormalities can exist without such full-thickness replacement and that the diagnosis of CIS should be based on the presence of cytologic atypia.[55] It also is recognized, however, that urothelium with less than high-grade cytologic atypia can be seen, and terms such as *dysplasia* and *atypia* have been used to describe these types of change.[59, 96–98] Grading systems similar to those used in papillary carcinomas have been proposed for lower grade epithelial atypias,[99, 100] but these have suffered from lack of reproducibility.[64, 101] In our practice, we report only the high-grade lesions. The usual situation is in the case of a high-grade lesion that does not involve the full thickness of the mucosa. We manage these cases as if they represent full-blown CIS.

An important and well-recognized diagnostic di-

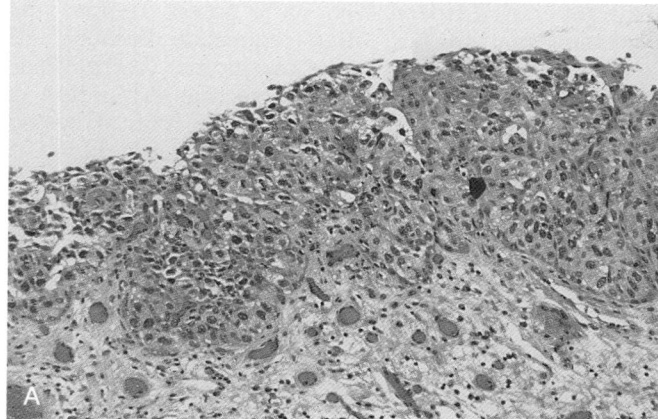

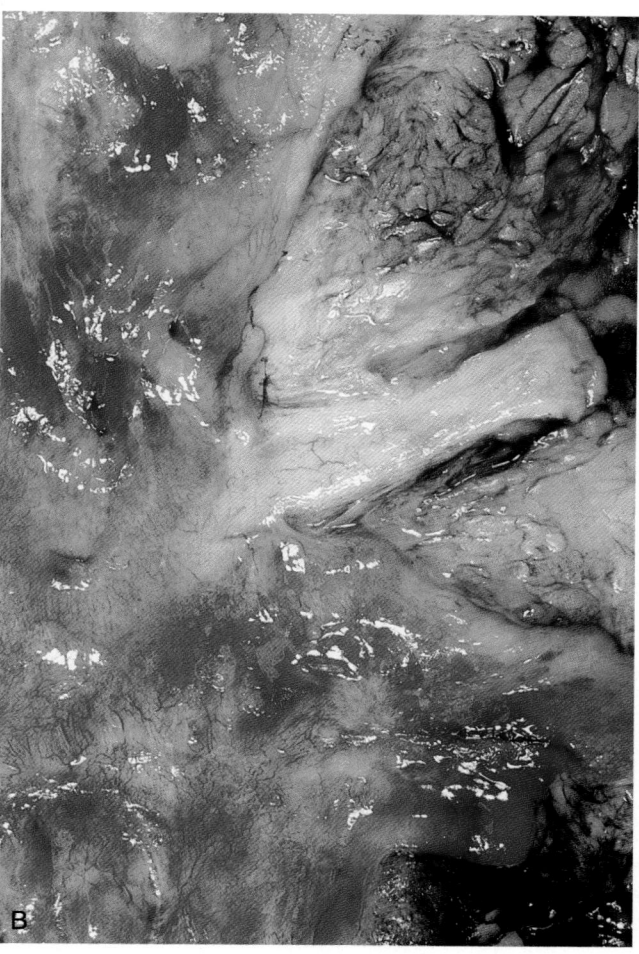

**FIGURE 31–9.** Flat urothelial carcinoma in situ (CIS). *A,* Microscopic appearance. Note loss of cellular polarity, marked cellular and nuclear pleomorphism, and easily identifiable mitoses, including in the upper cell layers. This example shows cellular discohesion, another important feature in the recognition of CIS. Many blood vessels are seen in the upper layers of the lamina propria, extending into the mucosa (neovascularity). This represents increased angiogenesis, a characteristic feature seen in CIS. *B,* This increased angiogenesis is used by pathologists and urologists. It is recognized as increased vascularity in the mucosa and can direct not only the urologist in performing biopsies but also the pathologist in gross evaluation of a specimen. Note the increased vascularity in the ureter from this radical cystectomy specimen. This patient had multifocal CIS, extending up the ureter and involving the ureter margins of resection.

lemma, particularly at the time of intraoperative frozen section, is the differentiation between CIS and reactive urothelial atypia. Reactive atypia can occur for a variety of reasons and is seen commonly in response to inflammation induced as a result of surgical manipulation or intravesicular treatment. In reactive atypia, nuclear enlargement can be prominent, and mitoses may be recognized. The nuclear enlargement is generally not accompanied by pleomor-

phism, however, and the chromatin pattern is more open than that seen in CIS. The nuclear enlargement in atypia often is accompanied by increased cellular size so that the nuclear-to-cytoplasmic ratio is not as high as in CIS. Although mitoses are seen com-

**TABLE 31–5.** Patterns of Carcinoma In Situ

Large cell CIS with pleomorphism
Large cell CIS without pleomorphism
Small cell CIS*
Clinging CIS
Cancerization of normal urothelium
  Pagetoid
  Undermining or overriding

* The term *small cell* is a morphologic description referring to the size of the cells and is not meant to imply neuroendocrine differentiation.
CIS, Carcinoma in situ.
From McKenney JK, Gomez JA, Desai S, et al: Morphologic expressions of urothelial carcinoma in situ. A detailed evaluation of its histologic patterns with emphasis on carcinoma in situ with microinvasion. Am J Surg 25: 357, 2001.

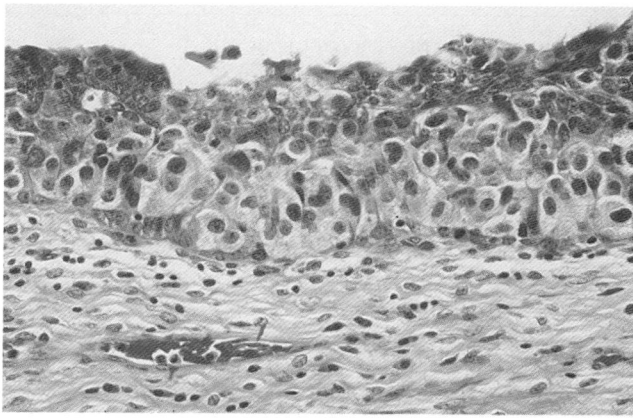

**FIGURE 31–10.** Pagetoid spread of carcinoma in situ. The upper layers of urothelium are cytologically normal, whereas the lower layers have been replaced by cytologically abnormal cells. This should not be mistaken for urothelial dysplasia.

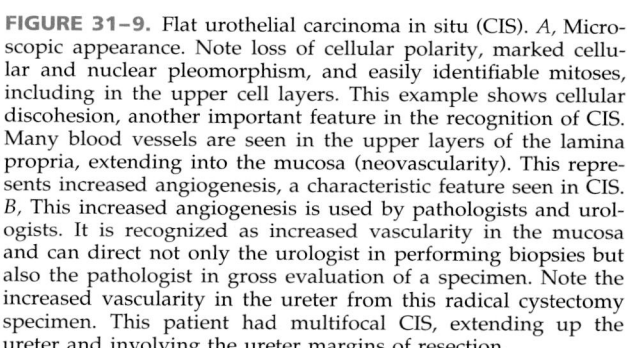

monly in atypia, generally they are located toward the base of the mucosa and not in the upper levels, as is seen in CIS. Nucleoli can be prominent in reactive atypia. Finally, reactive atypia often is accompanied by visible and pronounced inflammation. When evaluating urothelium, particularly at frozen section for surgical margins, it is important to note the presence of inflammation. A diagnosis of CIS in the presence of significant inflammation should be made with great care.

CIS is clinically and morphologically distinct from papillary carcinomas, and it now is recognized that it is distinct at the molecular level. Most CIS lesions have *p53* abnormalities, whereas few papillary carcinomas show *p53* alterations.[41] Loss of heterozygosity of chromosome 9 is observed commonly in papillary tumors and observed only infrequently in CIS.[41] It seems that papillary carcinoma and CIS, long recognized to be pathologically and clinically distinct, evolve through two distinct genetic pathways[31, 32, 42–47] (see Fig. 31–3), reflecting their morphologic and biologic differences.

For patients with CIS and no evidence of invasion, intravesical therapy with bacille Calmette-Guérin (BCG) or other agents is usually the first course of therapy.[83, 102–104] A significant proportion of patients with CIS progress to invasive disease, however. It also is recognized that a high proportion of patients with the diagnosis of CIS and no invasion in the biopsy can have microinvasion on cystectomy and even muscle-invasive disease.[87, 105] As mentioned previously, CIS is recognized as being multifocal, commonly involving urethra and ureters.[94] For this reason, several investigators have advocated early cystectomy in the treatment of CIS.[94, 105, 106] When radical cystectomy is performed in the presence of CIS (with or without invasion),

intraoperative frozen sections to assess urethral and ureteral margins are often requested. Because CIS often accompanies invasive carcinoma, we routinely perform intraoperative frozen section evaluation of ureteral and urethral margins at the time of cystectomy for bladder cancer, even in cases in which CIS was not appreciated on diagnostic biopsy.

In women with bladder cancer, it previously was believed that orthotopic reconstruction with continent urinary diversion to urethra could not be performed because of the short length of the female urethra and its possible involvement with CIS. We now have shown that continent orthotopic urinary diversions can be performed reliably in women.[107, 108] We routinely perform intraoperative frozen sections to evaluate margins in these cases. We also have observed that when CIS involves the female urethra, it almost always is seen in the bladder neck.[107] Biopsy of the bladder neck should be performed routinely by transurethral resection in women with bladder cancer who are candidates for cystectomy.

## STAGING BLADDER CANCER

When a tumor has invaded the bladder wall, the most important classic prognostic factor is pathologic stage. Staging systems are based on depth of invasion and assessment of regional and systemic spread of tumor and for bladder cancer are based on the depth of invasion of the tumor to involve specific anatomic areas of the bladder wall, as first proposed by Jewett and Strong[109, 110] and later modified by Marshall[111] and the basis for the tumor/nodes/metastasis (TNM) system proposed by the American Joint Committee on Cancer[112] (Table 31–6). The power of these staging systems is the ability to define outcome for populations of patients with invasive bladder cancer. Many studies have

**TABLE 31–6.** Staging of Bladder Cancer

| Jewett-Strong[109] Marshall[111] | | AJCC[112] | T1 Substage (proposed) | |
|---|---|---|---|---|
| | No residual tumor | T0 | | |
| 0 | Papillary noninvasive | Ta | | |
| 0 | Carcinoma in situ | Tis | T1a[120] | Superficial to muscularis mucosae |
| | | | T1b | To muscularis mucosae |
| A | Invades lamina propria | T1 | T1c | Through muscularis mucosae |
| | | | T1a[121, 122] | Superficial to muscularis mucosae |
| | | | T1b | Involving muscularis mucosae |
| B | Invades muscularis propria | T2 | | |
| B1 | Superficial (<50%) | T2a | | |
| B2 | Deep (>50%) | T2b | | |
| C | Invades perivesicle fat | T3 | <1.5 mm[123] | Depth of lamina propria invasion |
| | Microscopic | T3a | >1.5 mm | |
| | Macroscopic | T3b | | |
| D | Direct extension | T4 | | |
| | Prostate, uterus, vagina | T4a | | |
| | Pelvic/abdominal wall | T4b | | |

T, Depth of invasion of primary tumor (TNM system).

**TABLE 31–7.** Recurrence and Survival for 1054 Patients with Bladder Cancer Based on Stage of Disease

| Pathologic Stage* | No. Patients | 5-Year Recurrence-Free Survival (%) | 5-Year Overall Survival (%) |
|---|---|---|---|
| pT0, pTa, pTis† | 208 | 89 | 85 |
| pT1 N0 | 194 | 83 | 76 |
| pT2a N0 | 94 | 89 | 77 |
| pT2b N0 | 98 | 78 | 64 |
| pT3 N0 | 135 | 62 | 49 |
| pT4 N0 | 79 | 50 | 44 |
| N+ | 246 | 35 | 31 |

Based on Stein JP, Lieskovsky G, Cote RJ, et al: Radical cystectomy in the treatment of invasive bladder cancer. Long-term results in 1,054 patients. J Clin Oncol 19:666–675, 2001.
NOTE. All patients were treated by radical cystectomy.
\* Pathologic stage at time of cystectomy, based on 1997 TNM.[112]
† Includes patients with invasive disease at the time of biopsy.

shown that depth of invasion and regional and systemic spread of tumor can distinguish distinct prognostic groups.[69, 98, 113–116] In one of the largest and more recent studies, investigators at the University of Southern California showed that stage of disease is related directly to recurrence and survival[69] (Table 31–7). This study is noteworthy in that all patients were treated by radical cystectomy so that the variation in treatment found in several other series was not a variable in outcome. For node-negative disease, the greatest distinctions were between patients with organ-confined disease (pT1, pT2) and patients with extravesicular extension of tumor (pT3, pT4). Patients showing regional spread of tumor (node-positive) had the poorest prognosis. We have used the designation *pT* to indicate depth of invasion on cystectomy specimens and *T* to indicate depth of invasion on transurethral biopsy specimens.

### Prostate Stromal Invasion

Invasion of tumor into the prostate represents advanced (pT4) disease and has a poor prognosis. It now is recognized, however, that urothelial carcinoma can invade the prostate through two distinct routes. The first is through direct extension of tumor through the entire thickness of the bladder wall. The second is through extension of CIS down the prostatic urethra and its prostatic ducts, where stromal invasion of the prostate through the basement membrane of the urethra or ducts can occur. This stromal invasion often can be focal and microscopic and is distinct from that seen in tumor involving prostate through direct extension through bladder wall.[117] When prostate stromal invasion through extension of CIS in the prostate urethra and ducts occurs, it can be associated with early-stage invasive disease in the bladder. It was shown that although prostatic stromal invasion through extension of CIS along the prostatic urethra and ducts predicts a higher rate of recurrence on a stage-adjusted basis, these patients do better than those with prostate involvement through direct extension through the bladder wall (Table 31–8).[118] In particular, patients with lamina

propria invasive (pT1) disease in the bladder, with prostate stromal invasion through extension of CIS along prostatic urethra and ducts, have a favorable long-term outcome (see Table 31–8). It was recommended that patients with organ-confined (pT1/pT2) tumors and prostate stromal invasion through prostatic urethra and ducts be distinguished from other patients with pT4a disease and given the designation *Pstr*. Although this is not yet standard nomenclature, we recommend that this distinction be communicated in the surgical pathology report.

### Superficial Versus Invasive Bladder Cancer

Although invasion is an ominous sign, it is common practice at some institutions and in some countries to distinguish between *superficial* and *muscularis propria* invasive cancer, with the superficial group including patients with noninvasive disease and patients with lamina propria invasion (T1). T1 lesions are regarded as being amenable to local therapy (transurethral resection with intravesicular BCG therapy or chemotherapy). We believe it is most appropriate to distinguish noninvasive lesions from

**TABLE 31–8.** Urothelial Carcinoma Involving Prostate via Prostatic Ducts Versus Extravesical Extension of Tumor

| Stage | No. Patients | 5-Year Recurrence Free Survival (%) |
|---|---|---|
| pT1str* | 23 | 76 |
| pT2str* | 13 | 39 |
| pT3str* | 22 | 27 |
| pT4a† | 19 | 25 |

\* str Indicates tumor involving prostate stroma via the prostatic ducts. The depth of invasion in the bladder is designated according to the TNM system.
† Transitional cell carcinoma invading through the entire thickness of the bladder wall and extending into the prostate.
Based on Esrig D, Freeman JA, Elamjian DA, et al: Transitional cell carcinoma involving the prostate with a proposed staging classification for stromal invasion, J Urol 153:1071–1076, 1996.

those that show evidence of invasion[69, 119] because patients with any invasive disease have a substantially worse long-term outcome than patients with noninvasive disease.

### Substaging T1 Disease

Because of the controversy regarding the management of patients with superficially invasive (T1) tumors, several groups have used depth of invasion into lamina propria to subclassify T1 tumors[120-123] (see Table 31–6). These attempts have focused primarily on the use of the muscularis mucosae to define the depth of invasion and have indicated that patients with tumors invading to or beyond the muscularis mucosae have poorer outcomes than patients with more superficially invasive tumors. These subclassification schemes are attractive because they fit well in classic staging systems and are consistent with the current concept of the natural history of bladder cancer. The main problem with these schemes is that the muscularis mucosae is discontinuous and is not a consistent finding in bladder biopsy specimens or in sections from cystectomy specimens. One way investigators have attempted to deal with this problem is by using the large vessels present in the lamina propria/submucosa as a secondary anatomic landmark.[122] Others have recognized, however, that muscularis mucosae is seen in only a few biopsy specimens and that the use of blood vessels as a secondary landmark may not provide prognostic information.[124] As a result, the actual measurement of depth of invasion has been proposed; patients with tumors invading to a depth of less than 1.5 mm had a better outcome than patients with tumors invading to greater than 1.5 mm[123] (see Table 31–6). This method obviates the need to identify specific anatomic landmarks in the resected material.

The depth of lamina propria invasion seems to define prognostic groups and is an attractive concept overall. When possible, we recommend that some assessment of depth of lamina propria invasion be expressed in the surgical pathology report. Because of the limitations described, however, and the limited data, T1 substaging has not been adopted as routine at this time and is not recommended by the WHO/ISUP system.[56]

### Assessing Invasion: Problems and Pitfalls

The assessment of invasion in radical cystectomy specimens is generally straightforward, but this is not always the case in transurethral biopsy specimens, in which there can be substantial interobserver variability, particularly in the case of superficially invasive disease.[63, 125, 126] The distinction between noninvasive and superficially invasive disease is important because it may make a dramatic difference in management. Noninvasive disease generally is treated conservatively, with transurethral resection and intravesicular therapy, whereas in some centers in the United States the presence of early invasion can lead to radical cystectomy.[127] Distinguishing invasive from noninvasive disease can sometimes be difficult in biopsy material for several reasons.[125] Transurethral resections of bladder tumors produce fragmented and poorly oriented specimens; tangential sectioning can give the appearance of tumor cell nests in lamina propria. Thermal injury or cautery artifact can produce severe cellular distortion, occasionally to the degree that definitive assessment of invasion cannot be made (this should be stated in the pathology report). Similarly an intense inflammatory response (as a reaction to the tumor or to intravesicular therapy) may obscure tumor cells in the lamina propria. Involvement of Brunn's nests by CIS may mimic superficial invasion, and invasion can be difficult to identify for certain types of tumors, such as microcystic carcinoma, the nested variant of urothelial carcinoma, or carcinoma with an endophytic growth pattern.[125] In all of these cases, strict criteria should be applied in the assessment of invasion (see later).

Even when there is unequivocal evidence for invasion, there are other potential pitfalls in staging, particularly in biopsy specimens. The distinction between lamina propria versus muscularis propria invasion (T1 versus T2) is important because management can be quite different. It now is well recognized that the bladder has a muscularis mucosae.[128] These muscle fibers are typically small and wispy and do not form the large bundles characteristic of the muscularis propria. Overstaging can occur, however, if the presence of tumor in muscle fibers is interpreted as muscularis propria invasion[129, 130] (Fig. 31–11). It no longer is acceptable to describe tumor as simply "involving muscle" in the surgical pathology report; a specific distinction should be between muscularis mucosae and muscularis propria. Occasionally, it may be difficult or impossible for the pathologist to determine whether the muscle fibers seen in a biopsy specimen belong

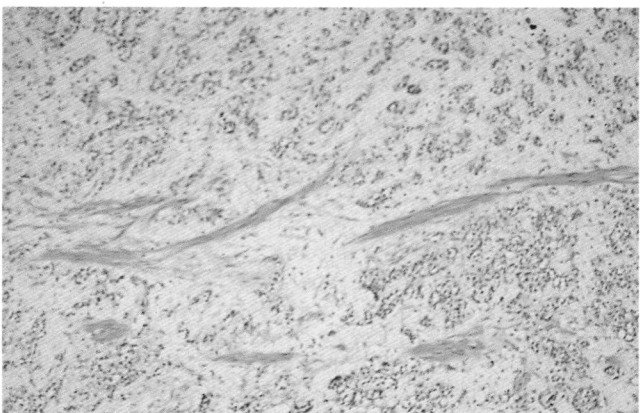

**FIGURE 31–11.** Urothelial carcinoma involving muscularis mucosae. Involvement of this wispy, discontinuous layer of muscle should not be mistaken for involvement of muscularis propria. Involvement of muscularis mucosae has been used to substage patients with urothelial carcinoma invading into lamina propria.

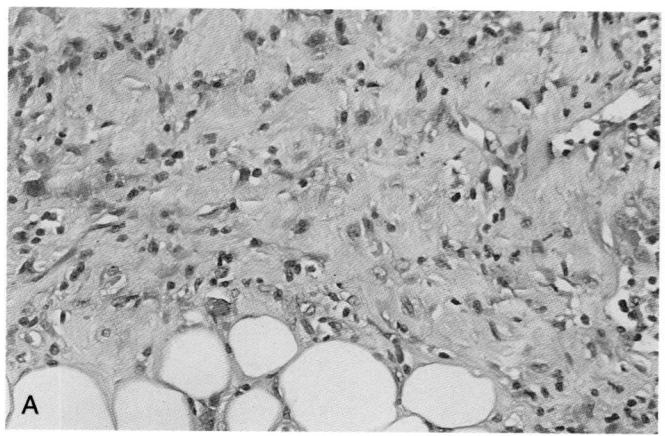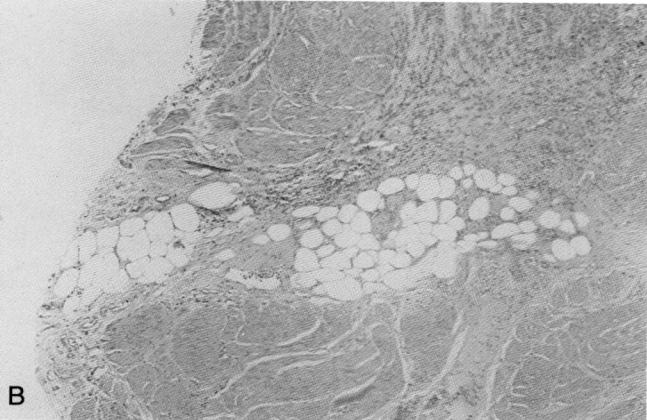

**FIGURE 31–12.** *A,* Urothelial carcinoma involving fatty tissue. *B,* Low-power view of the same area. This deposit of fat is in the muscularis propria. Involvement of fat by tumor in biopsy specimens should not be mistaken for invasion through the bladder wall into perivesical soft tissues.

to muscularis propria or muscularis mucosa. In these situations, we recommend that this uncertainty be stated in the pathology report.

It has been recognized that fat can be present in the lamina propria and muscularis propria, occasionally in substantial deposits (Fig. 31–12), and that its presence can represent another potential source of error in staging.[7, 131] It is important to recognize that fat can exist in the bladder wall and that the presence of tumor in fat in a biopsy specimen does not represent extravesicular extension of tumor into perivascular fat.

### Patterns of Invasion

As discussed, the diagnosis of lamina propria invasion is a particularly challenging problem because the pathologist often is faced with distorted, tangentially sectioned, and cauterized specimens. Strict criteria must be used to diagnose lamina propria invasion (Table 31–9). While evaluating tumors

**TABLE 31–9.** Criteria for Diagnosis of Invasion into Lamina Propria by Urothelial Carcinoma

**Histologic grade**
  Invasion seen much more frequently in high-grade lesions
**Invading epithelium**
  Irregularly shaped nests
  Single cell infiltration
  Irregular or absent basement membrane
  Tentacular finger-like projections
  Invasive component with higher nuclear grade and/or more cytoplasm than overlying noninvasive component
**Stromal response**
  Desmoplasia or sclerosis
  Retraction artifact
  Inflammation
  Myxoid stroma
  Pseudosarcomatous stroma
  Absent stromal response

From Jimenez RE, Keane TE, Hardy HT, Amin MB: pT1 urothelial carcinoma of the bladder: Criteria for diagnosis, pitfalls, and clinical implications. Adv Anat Pathol 7:16, 2000.

for invasion, it is important to focus on 1) histologic grade, 2) characteristics of the invading epithelium, 3) stromal response, 4) histologic pattern of invasion, and 5) possible pitfalls.

Invasion is much more likely to be encountered in a high-grade tumor compared with a low-grade tumor, and there should be a high index of suspicion for lamina propria invasion in all high-grade papillary tumors. Most tumors that show invasion are high grade.[70, 98]

The invasive front of the neoplasm may show one of several features: single cells or irregularly shaped nests of tumor within the stroma; architectural complexity not conforming to the usual regularity of papillary neoplasms; or an irregular, disrupted, or absent basement membrane. Sometimes tentacular or finger-like extensions can be seen arising from the base of the papillary tumor. Frequently the invading nests appear morphologically different from the cells at the base of the noninvasive component of the tumor, with more abundant cytoplasm and often with a higher degree of pleomorphism (Fig. 31–13 and CD Fig. 31–8), as is seen in early invasion of squamous carcinomas of the uterine cervix.

There are several ways the lamina propria can show a response to invasion. The most common include desmoplastic or sclerotic stromal response, retraction artifact, and inflamed stroma. In our experience, retraction artifact is one of the earliest signs of invasion and often is focal and characterized by single cells or small clusters of cells present at the base of papillae, mimicking vascular invasion (CD Fig. 31–9; see Fig. 31–13). Invasion may elicit a brisk inflammatory response in which numerous inflammatory cells that may obscure the interface between epithelium and stroma infiltrate the lamina propria heavily. The stroma less commonly may be myxoid, loose, and hypocellular or may be exuberant and cellular, resembling a sarcoma. The juxtaposition of invasive carcinoma and the reactive spindle cell

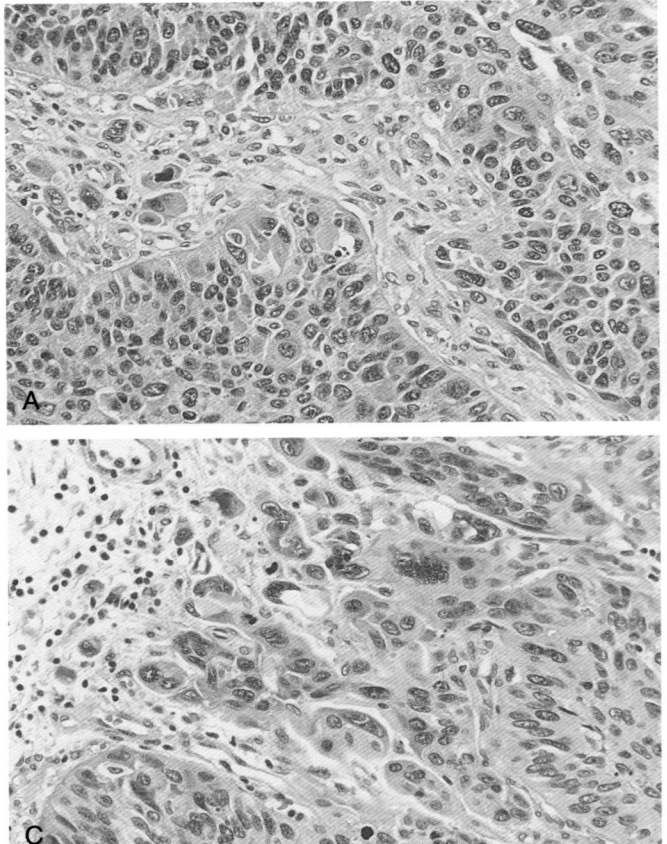
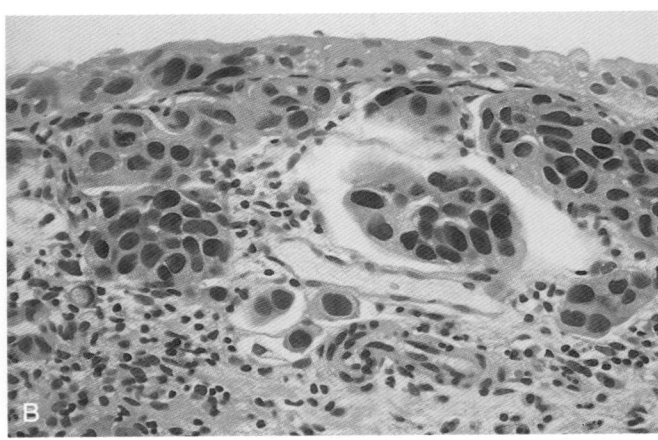

**FIGURE 31-13.** Patterns of early invasion of urothelial carcinoma. *A,* Papillary carcinoma showing single cell invasion. Note the morphologic change associated with the invasive cells, including increased cellular size. *B,* Carcinoma in situ showing single cell invasion and a small invasive nest of cells showing retraction artifact. Retraction artifact sometimes can be the first evidence of early invasion. *C,* Papillary carcinoma showing early invasion. The cells show finger-like projections with loss of the rounded regular borders of the noninvasive component. Note also the morphologic change associated with the invasive component.

component should not be mistaken for a biphasic sarcomatoid urothelial cancer. The proliferating stroma is usually nonexpansile, being limited to areas around the neoplasm, and it is composed cytologically of cells that have a degenerate or smudged appearance. A stromal response to an invading carcinoma may be absent. In these cases, as mentioned previously, diagnosis of invasion should rely on the characteristics of the invading epithelium.

Lamina propria invasion may be classified morphologically according to several patterns (Table 31-10 and CD Fig. 31-10). Awareness of these patterns may be important to the surgical pathologist to focus on particular areas of the tumor while assessing for invasion, facilitating its recognition, even when it is extremely focal. Not all patterns are associated with a known clinical significance.

Microinvasion by CIS (Fig. 31-14) was defined by Farrow and Utz[132] as an invasive component measuring less than 5 mm in depth. In that study, microinvasion was found in 34% of a series of entirely submitted bladders harboring CIS, and in 5.8% of these cases metastatic disease developed. These data suggest that microinvasion confers the ability to metastasize and cause death in a few cases. Amin and colleagues[133] have proposed that the 5-mm criterion may be liberal and suggested a 2-mm cutoff for this diagnosis. Using this criterion, McKenney and coworkers[95] reported 13 cases in which the invasive

component was accompanied by retraction artifact in 10 cases; nests, cords, and single cells in 1 case; and absent stromal response in 12 cases.

Microinvasion by papillary tumors (Fig. 31-15) can be defined similarly as in cases with CIS and should be mentioned in the diagnosis to document minimal, focal, or early invasion. Papillary urothelial carcinomas rarely invade the stalk of a tumor (CD Fig. 31-11). Appreciation of this pattern requires

**TABLE 31-10.** Histologic Patterns of Invasion into Lamina Propria by Urothelial Carcinoma

Carcinoma in situ with microinvasion
Papillary urothelial carcinoma with microinvasion
Papillary urothelial carcinoma with invasion into stalk
Well-established invasion into lamina propria
   Invasion up to muscularis mucosae
   Invasion beyond muscularis mucosae
   Lamina propria invasion not further specified (no muscularis mucosae present)
Urothelial carcinoma with endophytic or broad-front growth pattern with destructive stromal invasion
Urothelial carcinoma with deceptively bland patterns of invasion

Modified from Amin MB, Gomez JA, Young RH: Urothelial transitional cell carcinoma with endophytic growth patterns. A discussion of patterns of invasion and problems associated with assessment of invasion in 18 cases. Am J Surg Pathol 21:1057-1068, 1997.

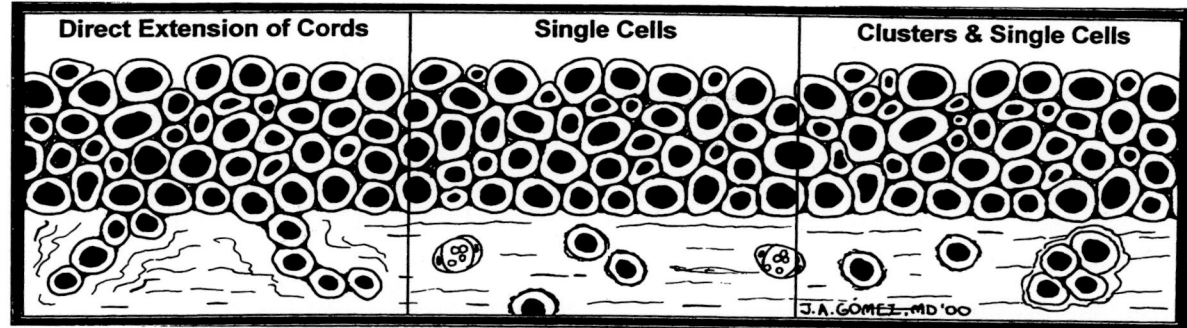

**FIGURE 31–14.** Schematic representation of patterns of invasion (microinvasion) associated with carcinoma in situ. (From McKenney JK, Gomez JA, Desai S, et al: Morphologic expressions of urothelial carcinoma in situ. Am J Surg Pathol 25:361, 2001.)

optimal orientation of the entire papillary tumor, which may not always be the case, especially in transurethral resection bladder tumor specimens. In most cases, invasion is seen at the base of the papillary neoplasm (CD Fig. 31–12).

Urothelial carcinomas with an endophytic growth pattern may be associated with two separate although sometimes overlapping problems. In tumors with trabeculae and cords growing within the lamina propria, distinction from inverted papilloma sometimes is difficult[133] and requires attention to architectural and cytologic features of the lesion. Urothelial carcinoma with an inverted growth pattern has thicker columns, with irregularity in the width of the columns, and transition of cords and columns into more solid areas (Fig. 31–16). The characteristic orderly maturation, spindling, and pe-

ripheral palisading seen in inverted papilloma are generally absent or inconspicuous in urothelial carcinoma with an inverted growth pattern. Unequivocal invasion into the lamina propria or muscularis propria rules out the diagnosis of inverted papilloma. Cytologic atypia, including nuclear pleomorphism, irregularities of nuclear borders and chromatin distribution, prominent nucleoli, and appreciable mitotic rate, is an important feature for the diagnosis of carcinoma because only focal and minor degrees of cytologic atypia are acceptable in inverted papilloma.

The second and more common histologic appearance of urothelial carcinoma with an endophytic growth pattern is the pushing broad-front extension into the lamina propria, akin to cutaneous and mucosal verrucous carcinoma (CD Fig. 31–13). In some

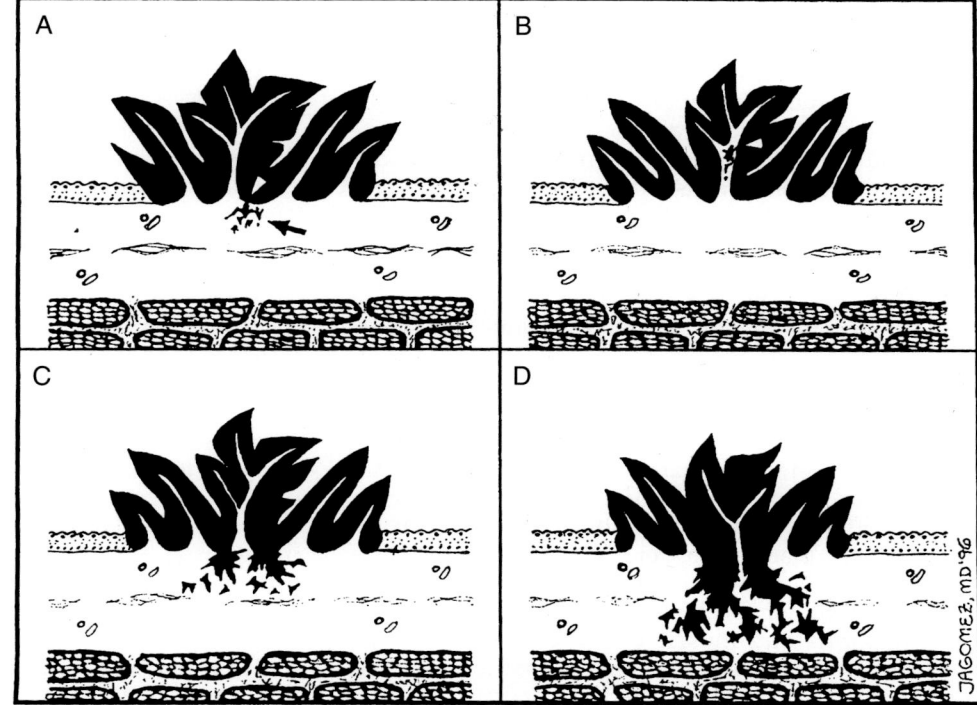

**FIGURE 31–15.** Patterns of invasion of papillary urothelial carcinoma. *A,* Microinvasion at the base. *B,* Invasion into the stalk. *C,* Invasion into lamina propria to the level of the muscularis mucosae. *D,* Invasion into lamina propria beyond muscularis mucosae. (From Amin MB, Gomez JA, Young RH: Urothelial transitional cell carcinoma with endophytic growth patterns. Am J Surg Pathol 21:1067, 1997.

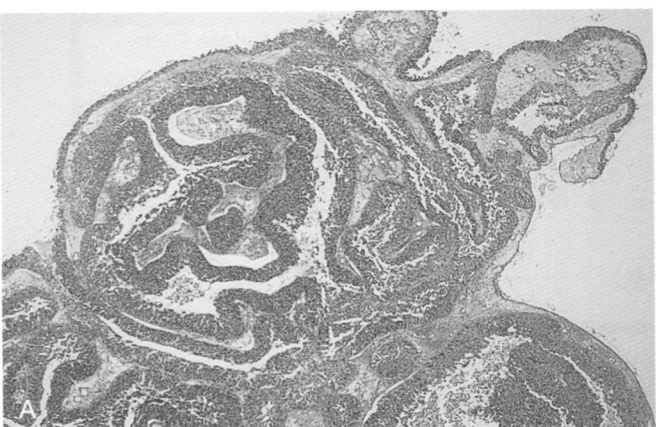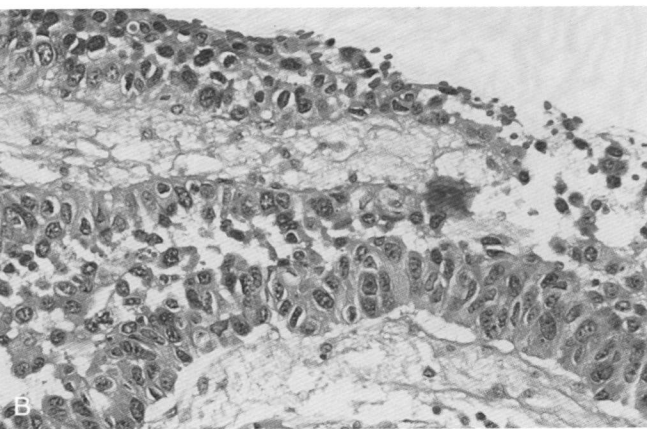

**FIGURE 31–16.** Urothelial carcinoma with endophytic growth pattern resembling inverted papilloma. *A,* Low-power view shows normal overlying urothelium. *B,* High-power view shows pronounced cytologic atypia of the endophytic component; this distinguishes this lesion from a benign inverted papilloma.

examples, this downward projection is so pronounced that the base of the tumor lies on the muscularis propria. The mere depth of this extension into the bladder wall may be enough to merit diagnosis as invasion in a strict sense; however, unless this pattern is accompanied by true destructive stromal invasion, the likelihood of metastasis is small because the basement membrane is not truly breached.

When limited to the lamina propria, deceptively bland patterns of invasive urothelial carcinoma may make the recognition of invasive pT1 disease extremely difficult. Microcystic urothelial carcinoma[134, 135] can mimic cystitis cystica easily, and the relatively recently described *nested* pattern may be confused with Brunn's nests, particularly in limited superficial biopsy specimens.[136] Attention should be paid to general features useful in assessing invasion, such as cytologic atypia, infiltrative architecture, desmoplasia, and architectural complexity, especially because they may be subtle in superficial biopsy specimens.

Invasive urothelial carcinoma can produce unusual and pronounced stromal reactions.[137] Pseudosarcomatous stroma, consisting of atypical proliferations of mesenchymal cells, has been described. The stromal response also can include osseous or cartilaginous metaplasia and the formation of osteoclast-like giant cells. The importance is recognizing that these types of unusual stromal reactions can occur and should not be mistaken for sarcomatous proliferations.

### Vascular and Lymphatic Invasion

Vascular and lymphatic vessel invasion by tumor is considered an important prognostic factor for several different types of tumors and has been investigated in bladder cancer.[138–141] The diagnosis of vessel invasion may be difficult, however, because of the well-known problems of retraction artifact in lamina propria and muscle (CD Fig. 31–14). Several investigators have used endothelial markers, such as *Ulex europaeus* and factor VIII, to confirm the presence of vessel invasion and have shown that only a few cases initially reported as having vascular and lymphatic invasion were confirmed by the special studies.[142, 143] The prognostic value of vessel invasion has not been shown by all studies, particularly when endothelial markers are used to confirm its presence.[138, 142] The documented or presumed presence of vessel invasion can lead to errors in staging. We have seen cases staged as superficial muscularis propria invasion (pT2a) even though tumor was present in deep muscle because the deep muscle involvement was interpreted as vessel invasion. In this case, the presence of tumor in deep muscle, whatever its source, is the basis for a pT2b stage assessment. Vascular and lymphatic invasion should be documented only when it is unequivocal and should not be used as a primary prognostic factor.

### Cystectomy and Lymph Node Evaluation

For patients with invasive bladder cancer, particularly patients with muscle-invasive disease, the standard treatment in the United States is radical cystectomy. (In some parts of the world, radiation therapy may be a primary form of treatment for invasive bladder cancer.) Other indications for radical cystectomy include intractable CIS and multifocal recurrent papillary tumors that do not respond to transurethral resection and intravesicular therapy. In some instances, when the tumor is small and not deeply invasive, a partial cystectomy may be performed to spare the bladder. The advent of modern surgical techniques has mitigated to a large extent one of the most undesirable postoperative consequences of the radical cystectomy—the necessity to drain urine to skin and into a bag. The use of orthotopic bladder reconstruction allows for the construction of a neobladder using a short segment of intestine. The neobladder is connected directly to the urethra, and drainage of urine takes place by normal routes.[69, 144]

When cystectomy is performed, the tumor type, growth pattern (papillary versus nonpapillary), location, presence of multifocality, presence and location of in situ disease, presence of unequivocal vascular and lymphatic invasion, and status of the margins of resection all must be evaluated and documented. Margin status includes bilateral ureters, urethra, perivesicular soft tissues including peritoneum, and any adjacent structures that may be removed, such as prostate, vagina, or rectum. Invasion into adjacent organs is an important staging parameter and must be evaluated. As mentioned earlier, the route of invasion into the prostate also should be documented (i.e., through extension along prostatic urothelial ducts versus through bladder wall). Adjacent organs must be evaluated not only for bladder cancer but also for other conditions. It is common to find incidental prostate cancer in men undergoing radical cystoprostatectomy for bladder cancer. Because of this common occurrence, we routinely evaluate the prostate as if it has primary tumor (i.e., margins, extent, and seminal vesicle status). This evaluation allows staging of the prostate cancer if it is found.

It is highly recommended that staging by bilateral pelvic lymph node dissection be performed as part of the overall surgical procedure.[145–148] The rate of lymph node metastasis increases with increasing depth of invasion. A small but substantial proportion of patients with pT1 disease have regional lymph node metastases, however.[60] All lymph nodes submitted by the surgeon should be submitted for microscopic examination and documented as to site. On histologic evaluation, the number of lymph nodes at each site and the total number of lymph nodes should be documented because this is one measure of the adequacy of the surgical procedure.[60, 69] As with other tumor types, the number of lymph nodes containing tumor should be documented. Other factors that should be included in the surgical pathology report include size of the largest metastasis and the presence of extranodal extension by tumor. There is some evidence that pelvic lymph node dissection is more than a staging procedure and may have therapeutic benefit.[146–148] This evidence includes data from the University of Southern California, where the 5-year recurrence-free survival rate was 35% for 246 patients with node-positive bladder cancer[69] who underwent a complete pelvic lymph node dissection (see Table 31–7).

## MOLECULAR STAGING OF BLADDER CANCER

Standard methods of bladder cancer assessment are based on histologic grade and stage of the tumor. There has been active modification and refinement of these parameters, but they have remained, in principal, basically intact for more than 50 years. This fact attests to the power of classic histopathologic classification and staging parameters. Although these criteria can provide reliable and reproducible information about populations of patients, however, they are unable to specify risk for progression or response to treatment for the individual patient with bladder cancer.

There have been enormous advances in understanding of the molecular basis for bladder cancer tumorigenesis and progression. Bladder cancer now is understood as a disease characterized by specific molecular defects (see Fig. 31–3), and this information is being translated to develop methods to assess cancer at the cellular and molecular level in ways previously inconceivable. The increased understanding of the molecular basis for bladder cancer is leading to the development of a new wave of therapeutic intervention targeted at specific disease mechanisms.

It is now clear that genes and proteins that exert regulatory control on the cell cycle have an important role in the progression of bladder (and other) cancers.[149] Attention has focused on genes and proteins that belong to the class of so-called tumor suppressors, in particular $p53$ and $Rb$. Alterations in $p53$ and $Rb$ are among the most common genetic defects in human tumors.[150–153] One of the primary features of cancer is uncontrolled cellular proliferation, and $p53$ and $Rb$ play an important role in cell cycle regulation, specifically by inhibiting cellular proliferation at the $G_1/S$ transition.[149] Several studies have shown that $p53$ alteration, as determined by immunohistochemical techniques, is an important predictor of bladder cancer progression[72, 154–156] (Fig. 31–17). Increased $p53$ immunoreactivity has been found in higher grade and higher stage bladder cancers and is associated with disease progression and decreased survival. Our group showed that $p53$ nuclear accumulation was associated with an increased risk of recurrence in 243 patients with invasive bladder cancer.[154] This association was most pronounced in patients with organ-confined tumors (Table 31–11), in which $p53$ nuclear accumulation was found to be the only independent predictor of disease progression when compared with tumor stage and grade. Similar results have been reported by other groups.[72, 76, 155, 156] On the basis of evidence from

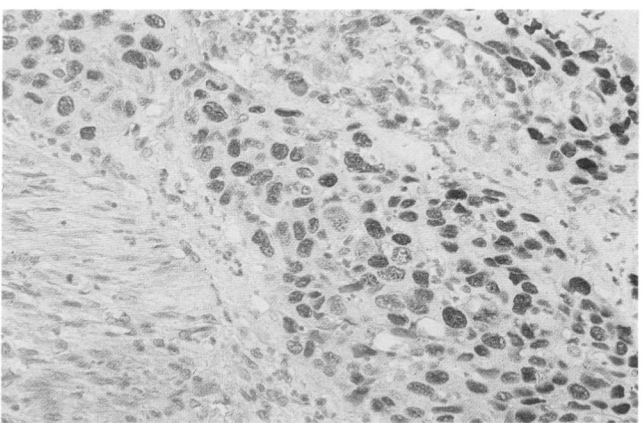

**FIGURE 31–17.** Invasive urothelial carcinoma showing nuclear immunoreactivity for the p53 protein, using monoclonal antibody clone 1801. This is indicative of alterations in the *p53* gene.

**TABLE 31–11.** Estimated 5-Year Recurrence Rate on Patients with Bladder Cancer Based on *p53* Tumor-Suppressor Status*

| Stage | No. of Patients | Rate of Recurrence (%) | | P Value |
|---|---|---|---|---|
| | | *p53* Wild-Type | *p53* Altered | |
| Lymph node negative | | | | |
| pTa/pTis | 15 | 18 | 33 | .48 |
| pT1 | 39 | 7 | 62 | .002 |
| pT2a | 29 | 12 | 56 | .003 |
| pT2b | 20 | 11 | 80 | .01 |
| pT3 | 36 | 59 | 73 | .23 |
| pT4 | 7 | 43 | 100 | .20 |
| Lymph node positive | 42 | 69 | 91 | .05 |

* *p53* status based on immunohistochemical reactivity; tumors considered *p53* wild-type had less than 10% positive tumor cell nuclei, whereas tumors considered *p53* altered had greater than 10% positive tumor cell nuclei. *p53* Antibody clone 1801 used.

Based on Esrig D, Elmajian D, Groshen S, et al: Accumulation of nuclear *p53* and tumor progression in bladder cancer. N Engl J Med 331:1259–1264, 1994.

many independent studies, *p53* assessment seems to be a reliable and consistent prognostic marker for bladder cancer progression. The specificity and reliability by which *p53* status can predict tumor progression strongly suggests it can be used in the management of bladder cancer.

The retinoblastoma gene, *Rb*, is the prototype tumor suppressor gene. The protein product of the *Rb* gene, pRb, interacts with multiple cell cycle regulatory proteins involved in control of cell growth. Alterations in pRb expression, as determined by immunohistochemistry, have been shown to be a significant predictor of outcome in patients with bladder cancer; patients with loss of pRb expression (usually indicative of mutations and deletions in the *Rb* gene) have a higher rate of disease progression than patients with normal pRb expression.[74, 157, 158] The evaluation of bladder tumors for *p53* and pRb alterations seems to provide particularly useful information, which stratifies patients into distinct prognostic groups; patients with tumors altered in *p53* and pRb have significantly increased rates of recurrence compared with patients with no alterations in either *p53* or pRb, whereas patients with alternations in only one of these proteins have intermediate rates of recurrence and survival.[73, 76, 158] As noted previously in the discussion on grading of papillary tumors, the combination of *p53* and pRb evaluation may be particularly useful in determining risk of progression for patients with superficial papillary tumors[73, 76] (see Table 31–4). There is evidence that the status of other cell cycle regulatory genes and proteins, such as *p21 (WAF1/CIP1)* and the *INK4A* locus, may be important predictors of bladder cancer progression.[149, 159]

Another pathway that is likely to have important prognostic and therapeutic implications is angiogenesis. The ability to induce new blood vessel growth is a tightly regulated process in normal tissues. Disregulation of this process is a key feature of tumors.[160] The prognostic significance of tumor angiogenesis, as determined by microvessel density, has been investigated in a variety of tumor systems, in-

cluding bladder cancer (CD Fig. 31–15).[6, 161, 162] The expression of factors that regulate angiogenesis may be important prognostically and therapeutically (CD Fig. 31–16).[163–169]

Other molecular features of bladder tumors have been studied and are important because they not only may have prognostic value, but also may be targets for therapy. Blood group antigens are highly expressed on normal urothelium, and changes in their structure have been investigated for their potential prognostic value.[75, 170–172] The examination of antigens associated with normal and malignant urothelium using mouse monoclonal antibody technology has led to the identification of a series of antigens that seem to be associated with urothelial transformation and progression.[173] One clear and exciting use of tumor-associated antigens is in the evaluation of urine cytologies,[174] in which the use of tumor markers has been shown to be significantly more sensitive than urine cytology in identifying bladder tumors, in particular recurrences of low-grade papillary tumors.[175–177] The use of in situ hybridization markers also has shown promise in detecting tumor recurrences in bladder wash specimens.[178, 179] Increased proliferation has been associated with disease progression for many cancers, including bladder cancer.[180] Microsatellite analysis has been used to detect tumor in urine and bladder wash specimens, with promising results.[108, 181] Telomerase activity has been studied as a potential method to detect bladder cancer in cytologic preparations; however, results are mixed because there are many false-positive results.[182, 183] Several oncogenes have been identified in bladder cancer, including *H-ras*, *c-myc*, and *mdm2*.[184, 185] The proto-oncogene *c-erbB-2* (also known as *Her2-neu*) may have particular relevance in bladder cancer. It has been shown to be important in several tumors[186] and may be a prognostic factor in bladder cancer, although results are mixed.[187, 188] Even if *c-erbB-2* is not a prognostic factor in bladder cancer, however, it may be a potential therapeutic target. The epidermal growth factor receptor is found in a substantial proportion of bladder cancers and may have relevance as a prognostic factor and as a therapeutic target.[189, 190] Other molecular factors that may have relevance in invasion, metastasis, and progression include peptide growth factors and cellular adhesion molecules, such as E-cadherin and integrins.[191, 192]

As alluded to earlier, the increased understanding of molecular pathways is leading to the development of new therapeutic strategies. These have focused on many pathways, including angiogenesis, cell cycle regulation, oncogenes, and growth factor receptors.[149, 191] One of the more exciting areas, which has relevance in the near term, is the role of p53 alterations in the development of resistance and response to standard chemotherapeutic agents. A body of clinical studies provides support for the view that p53 alterations confer a chemoresistant phenotype in patients with a variety of cancers.[75, 193–195] A series of studies now suggest, however, that p53 alterations may promote selective tumor chemosensitivity, at least to certain types of agents,[196] in particular those that induce DNA damage (e.g., cisplatin),[197, 198] disrupt the microtubule apparatus (e.g., paclitaxel),[199] or inhibit $G_2/M$ phase checkpoint regulation.[197, 200] Our group has shown that bladder tumors that have p53 alterations may be particularly sensitive to chemotherapeutic regimens that contain cisplatin.[201] The evaluation of bladder tumors for p53 alterations not only may have prognostic significance but also may help to specify the type of treatment that would most benefit a particular patient.

Bladder cancer tumorigenesis and progression is a process involving multiple genetic defects and pathways. Knowledge of the status of multiple pathways is important in assessing the prognosis of patients with bladder cancer and for evaluating the expression of potential therapeutic targets.

The ultimate goal of studying molecular determinants of bladder cancer outcome is to define risk and response for the individual patient. Bladder cancer is a model of modern cancer management, in which advances in pathology, surgery, oncology, and basic science have converged to produce the possibility of a more rational, biologically based approach.[202] Understanding of molecular pathways is leading to the development of an increasing array of nontraditional treatment possibilities. The evaluation and integration of pathologic and molecular parameters that have a direct bearing on the management of individual patients is clearly the purview of the surgical pathologist.

## IMMUNOHISTOCHEMISTRY

Immunohistochemical methods can be used to distinguish primary urothelial carcinoma from other epithelial malignancies. Primary urothelial carcinomas are known to express certain epithelial markers, including most cytokeratins. Low-molecular-weight cytokeratins appear early in development and predominate in tumors derived from simple nonstratified epithelia, whereas high-molecular-weight cytokeratins appear in complex stratified epithelia and predominate in tumors derived from stratified epithelia. Normal urothelium expresses low-molecular-weight and high-molecular-weight cytokeratins, as do many primary urothelial carcinomas. As urothelial carcinomas become less differentiated (i.e., higher grade), the expression of high-molecular-weight cytokeratins decreases, whereas the low-molecular-weight cytokeratins continue to be expressed. Of particular value in differentiating urothelial carcinomas from other forms of cancer is the assessment of the CK 7 and CK 20 cytokeratin subtypes. Urothelial carcinomas usually express CK 7 and CK 20,[203] whereas primary colon tumors express CK 20 but do not express CK 7, and primary prostate tumors do not express either subtype.[203–206]

Thrombomodulin and uroplakins have been shown to be of value in differentiating urothelial carcinoma from other tumors. Thrombomodulin is a surface glycoprotein commonly expressed in normal and neoplastic urothelium and is not generally expressed by tumors of other primary sites.[207] Uroplakins, a family of transmembrane proteins, have been found to be expressed only in urothelial mucosa.[208] It has been shown that uroplakin antibodies on paraffin-embedded tissue were positive in 66% of metastatic urothelial carcinoma cases and were negative in all breast, ovarian, lung, and gastrointestinal carcinomas tested.[208] Immunohistochemical markers specific for other tumor types may be used in differentiating urothelial carcinomas from other tumor types. Prostate-specific antigen (PSA) and prostate-specific acid phosphatase (PSAP) are especially useful in identifying tumors of prostate origin, although it must be remembered that high-grade prostate tumors may be PSA and PSAP negative.[205] Urothelial carcinomas, particularly those that are high-grade, also may express carcinoembryonic antigen (CEA), cathepsin-D, CA 19-9 and Leu-M1. Pleomorphic areas may show immunoreactivity with human chorionic gonadotropin and human placental lactogen (CD Fig. 31–17), even in the absence of trophoblastic differentiation.

## BLADDER CANCER SUBTYPES

### Micropapillary Transitional Cell Carcinoma

A recently described histologic variant of urothelial carcinoma is termed *micropapillary transitional cell carcinoma*.[209] These tumors have a characteristic architecture resembling papillary serous carcinoma of the ovary. The micropapillary pattern may be focal or extensive and in some cases is the only pattern seen. In the original series by Amin and colleagues,[209] it also was described as part of the surface component of the tumor (Fig. 31–18). The invasive component has well-formed papillary clusters, which can show retraction artifact that mimics vascular invasion (CD Figs. 31–18 and 31–19; see Fig. 31–18). This architectural pattern is retained in metastases from these tumors (see Fig. 31–18).

These tumors can have a deceptively low-grade appearance, with relatively low nuclear-to-cytoplasmic ratio and nuclei that show minimal-to-moderate pleomorphism. In contrast to the histologic appear-

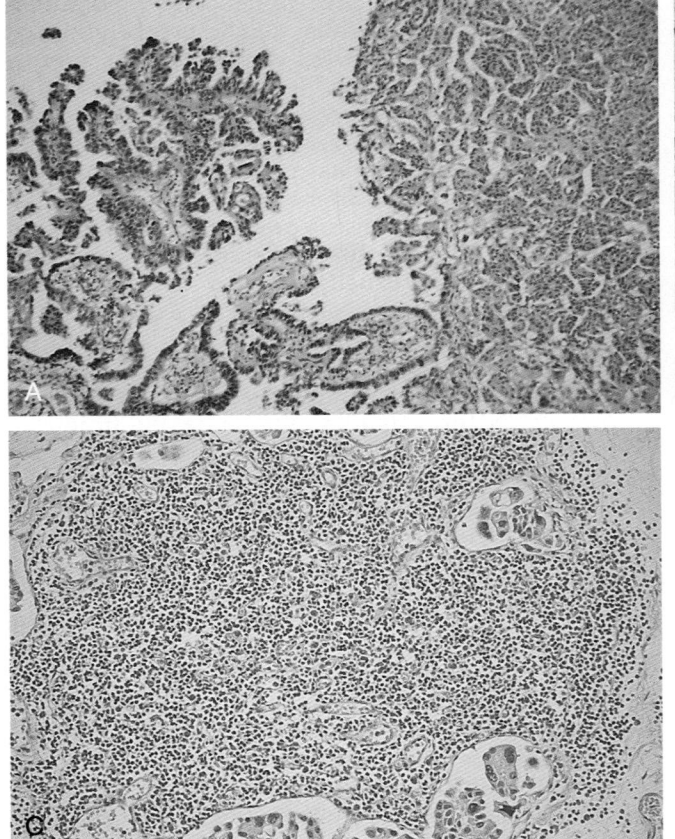

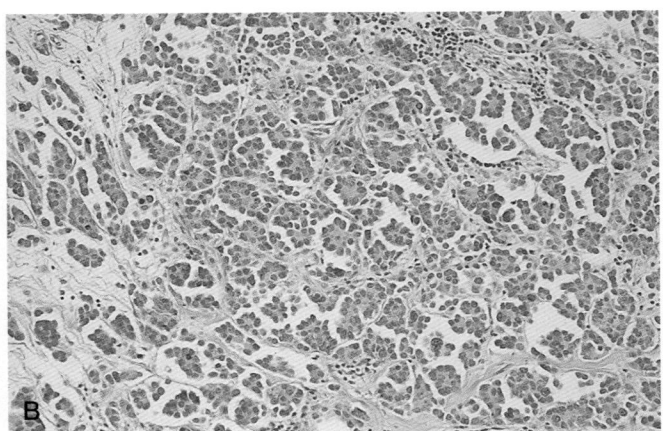

FIGURE 31-18. Micropapillary transitional cell carcinoma. *A*, Micropapillary features can be seen as part of the surface component of the tumor. *B*, The invasive component shows well-formed papillary clusters. A prominent feature is retraction artifact that mimics vascular invasion. *C*, The micropapillary features are retained in lymph metastases.

ance, this tumor tends to be aggressive, with most patients presenting with disease invading the muscularis propria and many showing evidence of metastatic disease at the time of presentation.[209] Although this variant is considered to be relatively rare, this may be due largely to its more recent description; our personal review of cases at the University of Southern California indicates that this variant can be seen either in its pure form or as a component of urothelial carcinoma in a substantial minority of cases previously diagnosed as urothelial carcinoma, and when it is seen, it portends a particularly poor prognosis (PW Nichols and RJ Cote, personal communication). We believe this is an important histologic feature to identify in urothelial carcinomas.

### Carcinosarcoma and Sarcomatoid Carcinoma

Sarcomatoid carcinoma is a variant of typical urothelial carcinoma. It is more common than primary sarcomas of the bladder. These tumors have been given a variety of names, including metaplastic carcinoma, spindle cell carcinoma, carcinosarcoma, sarcomatoid carcinoma, and myxoid sarcomatoid carcinoma. The tumors often are associated with urothelial CIS and with elements of more typical urothelial carcinoma or its variants.

The tumors frequently present as large polypoid masses (CD Fig. 31-20). Microscopically, the tumors show undifferentiated malignant spindle cells, which is often the most prominent feature (Fig. 31-19). They can show prominent myxoid features and can be associated with heterologous elements, showing muscular, cartilaginous, or osseous differentiation.[210, 211] These heterologous elements have no particular prognostic significance.

The primary differential diagnosis for these tumors is sarcoma, either primary or metastatic to the bladder. Because sarcomas of the bladder are rare (see later), spindle cell neoplasms generally are sarcomatoid carcinomas. A history of prior urothelial carcinoma and the presence of recognizable urothelial differentiation or CIS are helpful in distinguishing sarcomatoid carcinomas from sarcomas. The most common form of bladder sarcoma is leiomyosarcoma, which is usually readily recognizable. Sarcomatoid carcinomas should be distinguished from reactive processes, such as pseudosarcoma, postoperative spindle cell nodules, or a pseudosarcomatous stromal response to urothelial carcinoma. These distinctions are generally not difficult because sarcomatoid carcinomas are high-grade pleomorphic tumors. The tumors can show prominent myxoid features and can be associated with a pronounced inflammatory response (CD Figs. 31-21 and 31-22). The spindle cells of sarcomatoid carcinoma show expression of cytokeratin in virtually all cases,[212] demonstrating their epithelial origin (see Fig. 31-19), and lack expression of muscle antigens. The presence of

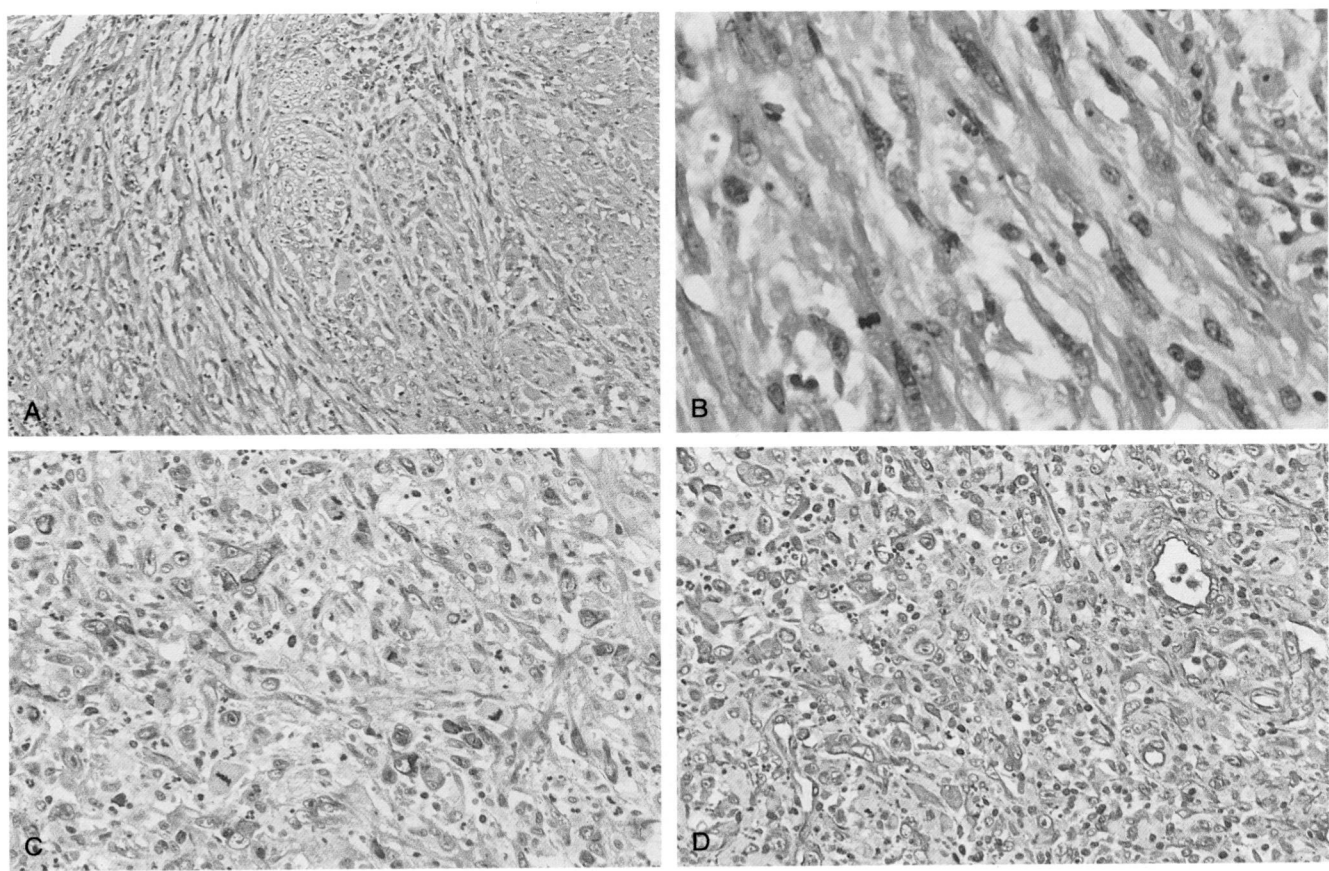

**FIGURE 31-19.** Sarcomatoid urothelial carcinoma. *A,* Low-power view shows spindle cells infiltrating through muscularis propria. *B,* High-power view shows prominent nuclear pleomorphism and mitotic activity. *C,* The spindle cells show immunoreactivity with antibodies to cytokeratin. *D,* The spindle cells show prominent immunoreactivity with antibody to vimentin.

cytokeratin immunoreactivity distinguishes sarcomatoid carcinomas from mesenchymal neoplasms and reactive spindle cell proliferations, although myofibroblasts may occasionally be cytokeratin positive. This distinction is discussed further later in the chapter. These tumors generally have a poor prognosis because of their advanced stage at presentation; however, compared stage for stage with typical urothelial carcinomas, the survival rate is similar.[213] The primary treatment for tumors that do not show systemic metastases is surgery, just as for typical urothelial carcinoma.

### Lymphoepithelioma

A distinct form of bladder carcinoma that seems to be morphologically and clinically distinct from urothelial carcinoma is lymphoepithelioma-like carcinoma of the bladder. It has a histologic appearance similar to lymphoepitheliomas of the nasopharynx, showing diffuse sheets of malignant cells having indistinct cytoplasmic borders, large vesicular nuclei with prominent nucleoli, and an associated extensive lymphocytic infiltrate[214] (Fig. 31-20). In contrast to its nasopharyngeal counterpart, lymphoepitheliomas of the bladder are not associated with the Epstein-Barr virus.[215] These tumors are seen either in their pure form or in association with more typical

urothelial carcinoma.[214] The differential diagnosis includes lymphoma. Lymphoepitheliomas can be distinguished from lymphomas by their strong expression of cytokeratin (see Fig. 31-20). Also included in the differential diagnosis is small cell carcinoma, either primary from the urinary bladder or metastatic. In general, histologic criteria and the characteristic lymphoid infiltrate can help to make this distinction. The distinction of lymphoepithelioma-like lesions from lymphoma or from other forms of bladder carcinoma is important because prognosis and therapy may differ. Lymphoepitheliomas seem to respond well to chemotherapy, and there is evidence that they have a better outcome than typical urothelial carcinomas.[214, 216]

### Small Cell and Neuroendocrine Cell Carcinoma

Small cell carcinoma is a rare form of bladder tumor that is being increasingly described.[217, 218] These tumors have a similar histologic and immunohistochemical appearance as small cell carcinomas seen in the lung and are classified similarly (carcinoid tumors, small cell carcinoma, large cell neuroendocrine carcinoma). By electron microscopy, they show dense core granules and express neuron-specific enolase, chromogranin, and synaptophysin, con-

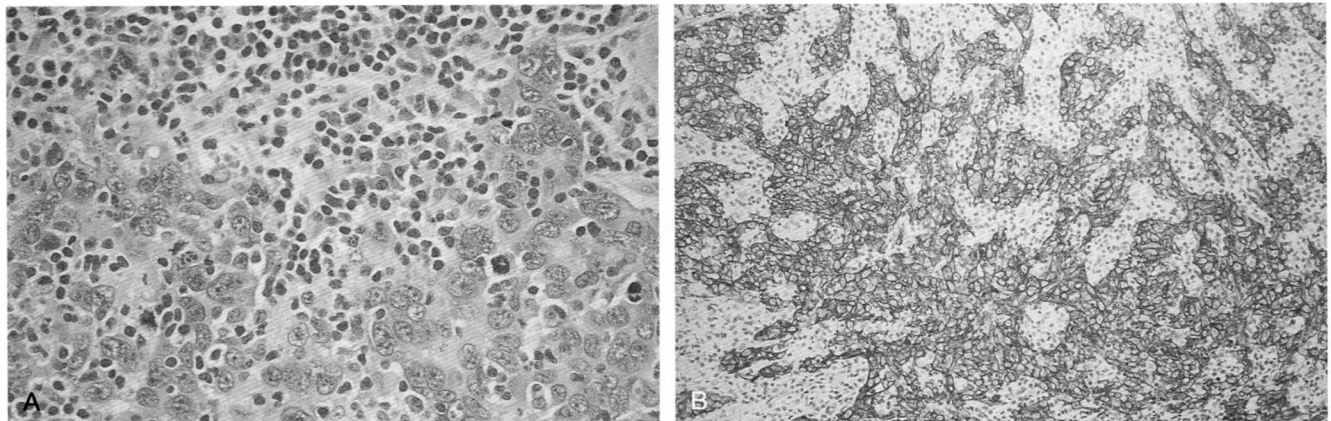

**FIGURE 31–20.** *A,* Lymphoepithelioma of the bladder. Note the sheets of large cytologically atypical cells, associated with a prominent lymphocytic infiltrate. *B,* The cytologically atypical cells show strong immunoreactivity to cytokeratin antigens. The lymphocytic population does not react with antibodies to cytokeratin.

firming their neuroendocrine differentiation. They are thought to arise from multipotential stem cells in the urothelium,[217] and their frequent association with typical urothelial carcinoma and other variants supports this.[219]

The tumors are composed of small uniform cells with scant cytoplasm and a high nuclear-to-cytoplasmic ratio. Similar to the small cell carcinomas of the lung, the nuclear chromatin is finely dispersed, and nucleoli are absent or inconspicuous (Fig. 31–21; CD

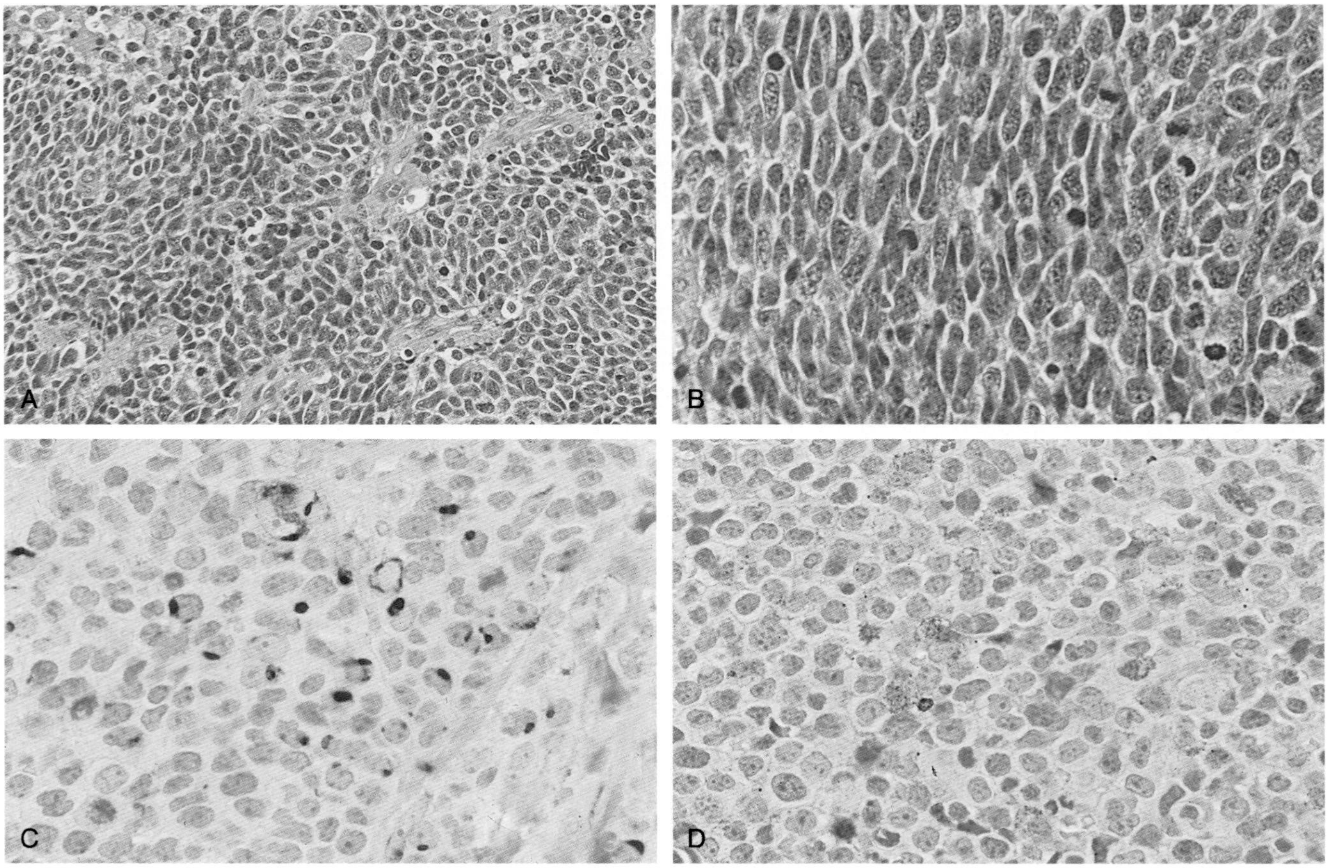

**FIGURE 31–21.** Small cell/neuroendocrine carcinoma of the bladder. *A,* Low-power view shows high cellular density and angiotropism. *B,* High-power view shows cellular molding, prominent mitotic activity, and apoptosis. *C,* The tumor cells show characteristic perinuclear punctate immunoreactivity with antibodies to cytokeratin. *D,* The tumor cells also show focal immunoreactivity with antibody to chromogranin, showing the neuroendocrine nature of this tumor.

Figs. 31–23 and 31–24). There is brisk mitotic activity. By immunohistochemistry, the tumors show the typical dotlike perinuclear pattern of cytokeratin expression (see Fig. 31–21), also characteristic of these tumors from the lung. A case of large cell neuroendocrine carcinoma has been reported,[220] but this tumor is extremely rare. Small cell carcinoma of the bladder is an aggressive tumor and usually presents at an advanced stage. Most patients die of disease in a short period,[217, 218] although long-term survivors have been reported. This tumor is particularly sensitive to chemotherapy (similar to that for small cell tumors of the lung), however, with greatly improved survival times for patients receiving adjuvant chemotherapy.[221] This fact makes recognition of this tumor crucial.

The primary differential diagnosis for small cell carcinomas of the bladder are metastasis from another site and malignant lymphoma. Metastases rarely may arise from the lung but more commonly arise from the prostate, where small cell carcinoma generally is seen in association with typical prostatic adenocarcinoma. In these cases, the small cell component is often negative for PSA and prostatic acid phosphastase; immunohistochemistry for PSA and prostatic acid phosphastase should be performed but when negative does not rule out a prostate primary.[222] The presence of a urothelial component, in particular urothelial CIS, strongly supports a bladder origin. Distinction from malignant lymphoma is important because of differences in prognosis and therapy. This differentiation can be achieved through immunohistochemical analysis for cytokeratin and leukocyte common antigen (CD45).

### Deceptively Bland Variants of Urothelial Carcinoma

It has been recognized that urothelial carcinomas have variants that mimic non-neoplastic conditions, such as cystitis cystica, Brunn's nests, nephrogenic adenoma, and inverted papilloma. It is important to be aware of these variants to avoid underdiagnosis, which can be a particular problem in cystoscopic biopsy specimens. Although these variants are not common, they can pursue an aggressive biologic course.[223, 224] Four such variants have been described.

*Transitional cell carcinomas with tubules* consist of small nests of cells and tubules, which mimic nephrogenic adenoma[224] (Fig. 31–22). A feature that dis-

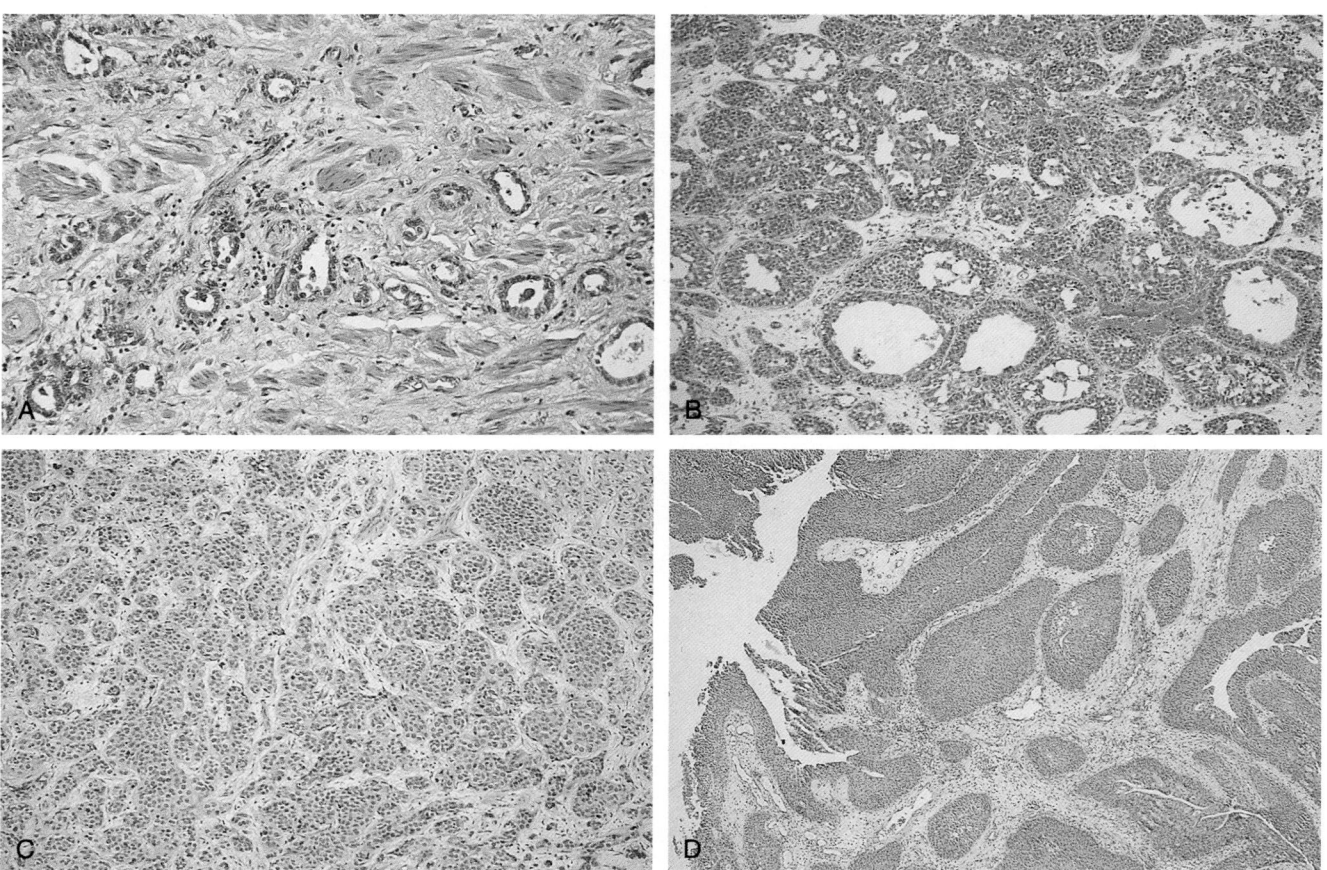

**FIGURE 31–22.** Deceptively bland variants of urothelial carcinoma. *A,* Transitional cell carcinoma with tubules. Note involvement of muscle bundles. *B,* Microcystic transitional cell carcinoma. Note similarities to cystitis glandularis. This photomicrograph shows the extensive nature of the lesion and solid areas characteristic of this subtype. *C,* Nested variant of transitional cell carcinoma. Note similarities to Brunn's nests. *D,* Transitional cell carcinoma with an endophytic growth pattern. This photomicrograph shows the verrucous form of this lesion.

tinguishes these tumors from nephrogenic adenoma is that some of the tubules may be lined by urothelium. *Microcystic transitional cell carcinoma* consists of variably sized cysts within nests of invasive urothelial carcinoma (CD Fig. 31–25; see Fig. 31–22). These may be confused with cystitis cystica, particularly in superficial biopsy specimens in which the invasive nature may not be readily recognized.[134, 135, 225] Variation in the shape and size of the cysts and the identification of nuclear atypia may be helpful in distinguishing microcystic carcinoma from cystitis cystica in superficial biopsy specimens. The presence of muscularis propria invasion is particularly helpful. *Nested transitional cell carcinoma* consists of a packed arrangement of small nests of tumor cells that closely resemble Brunn's nests (see Fig. 31–22).[224, 226] These tumors show bland cytologic features, which may make distinction from Brunn's nests particularly difficult, especially on superficial biopsy specimens. Distinguishing features include the presence of larger sized nests that are irregularly shaped, focal nuclear atypia, stromal reaction, and muscularis propria invasion. This variant is reported to behave in an aggressive fashion despite its bland appearance.[224, 226] *Transitional cell carcinoma with an endophytic growth pattern* shows broad pushing borders extending into the lamina propria, similar to that seen in verrucous carcinoma (see Fig. 31–22). The downward projections have regular contours, but more invasive finger-like extensions also may be seen. Another pattern consists of cords and nests of cells involving the lamina propria (CD Fig. 31–26; see Fig. 31–16). This pattern closely resembles inverted papilloma.[135, 227] Nests vary in size and shape and occasionally show microcystic and macrocystic areas.[133] The inverted papilloma-like and broad-front patterns may coexist. When the broad-front pattern is present, the tumor should be considered noninvasive if the basement membrane is intact by light microscopy because the likelihood of metastases is small.[133] It is important to recognize invasion, however, because this increases the risk for metastasis.[133] The identification of invasion can be complicated by sectioning, crush, or cautery artifact. The recognition of invasion was discussed in earlier sections.

### Adenocarcinoma

Pure adenocarcinomas of the bladder are relatively rare, constituting about 1% to 2% of primary bladder tumors.[228, 229] Most cases seem to arise from metaplasia of the urothelium, most commonly cystitis glandularis with intestinal metaplasia.[229, 230] Exstrophy of the bladder is also a risk factor for adenocarcinoma.[231] We have observed adenocarcinoma of the bladder arising in association with glandular metaplasia seen in the surface urothelium (Fig. 31–23; CD Figs. 31–27 and 31–28). Glandular differentiation also can be seen in cases of recognizable urothelial carcinoma; however, these are classified as urothelial carcinomas with glandular differentiation.[229, 232] Adenocarcinoma arising in the bladder also can be of urachal origin (see later).

Many histologic variants of adenocarcinoma of the urinary bladder have been described, including adenocarcinoma of no specific type, enteric variants in which the cancer is composed of pseudostratified columnar cells resembling colonic adenocarcinoma, mucinous or colloid carcinoma, signet ring cell carcinoma (further described subsequently), clear cell variants, and mixed types in which two or more patterns are found (CD Figs. 31–29 and 31–30).[232] A hepatoid variant has been described; this tumor morphologically resembles and has molecular characteristics similar to hepatocellular carcinoma, including expression of alpha-fetoprotein, $\alpha_1$-antitrypsin, and albumin.[233, 234]

Although adenocarcinomas tend to have a poorer prognosis overall than typical urothelial carcinomas, this is due to the fact that they generally are found at higher stages at diagnosis. Staging for

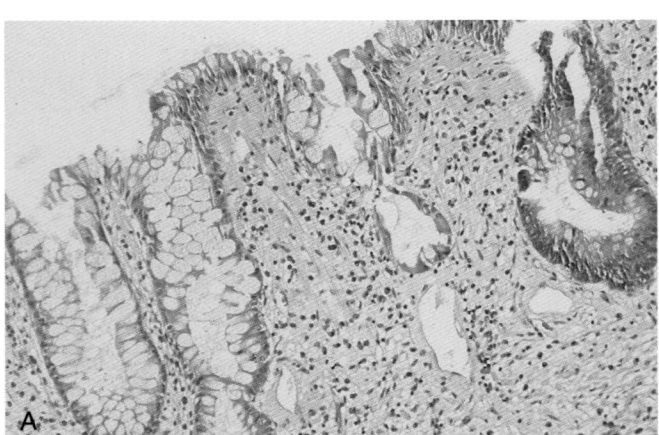
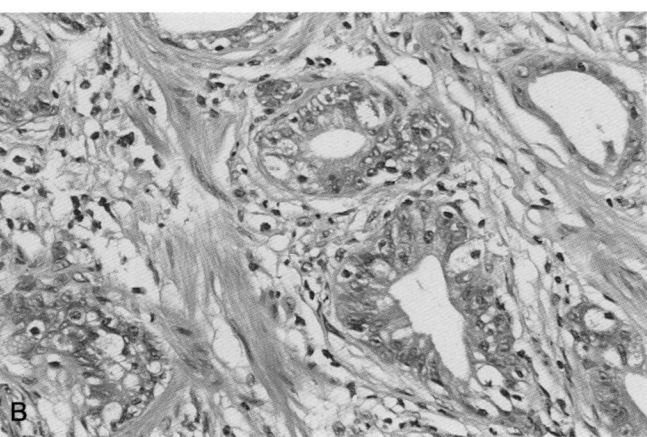

**FIGURE 31–23.** Adenocarcinoma of the bladder arising in association with urothelial intestinal metaplasia and dysplasia. *A,* Surface urothelial and glandular metaplasia of intestinal type is shown. Transition to intestinal dysplasia is noted. The dysplastic cells show cellular basophilia, increased nuclear-to-cytoplasmic ratio, nuclear pleomorphism, and increased mitotic activity. *B,* Invasive adenocarcinoma seen in the same case.

adenocarcinoma is the same as for typical urothelial carcinomas. The primary differential diagnosis for adenocarcinoma of the bladder includes typical urothelial carcinoma with extensive glandular differentiation. More importantly, primary adenocarcinoma must be distinguished from benign conditions, including cystitis cystica and cystitis glandularis. Nephrogenic adenoma can be a particularly difficult diagnostic distinction. Nephrogenic adenomas can infiltrate the muscularis propria, so this feature alone should not be used to distinguish this entity from adenocarcinoma. Nephrogenic adenomas lack cytologic atypia, are typically small, and lack solid areas, which are common features of adenocarcinoma (see later).[235, 236] Also nephrogenic adenomas commonly are associated with a history of trauma or instrumentation. Endometriosis and endocervicosis occasionally are seen in the bladder wall and should be distinguished from adenocarcinoma. Pure adenocarcinomas of the bladder must be distinguished from metastatic adenocarcinoma or from direct extension of adenocarcinoma from other sites, such as the rectum. The presence of intestinal metaplasia in the surface urothelium can be particularly helpful in defining origin in the bladder.

### Signet Ring Cell Carcinoma

Signet ring cell carcinoma, first reported in the 1950s,[237, 238] is a rare variant of adenocarcinoma. It is seen most commonly in association with well-differentiated forms of adenocarcinoma and in association with more typical urothelial carcinoma (Fig. 31–24 and CD Fig. 31–31). The pure form of signet ring carcinoma is uncommon[239]; it tends to present with diffuse involvement of the bladder wall, which results in induration and thickening similar to the linitis plastica seen in signet ring cell carcinomas of the stomach. These tumors have a particularly poor prognosis, primarily as a result of advanced stage at presentation. They must be distinguished from metastases and from direct extension of signet ring

carcinomas from adjacent sites, in particular, rectum, urethra, and prostate. Metastatic lobular carcinoma of the breast also may resemble signet ring cell carcinoma involving the bladder. It is important to distinguish the mixed form of signet ring carcinoma from its pure form because the prognosis is significantly worse for the pure form. These tumors rarely may have their origin in the urachus.

### Squamous Cell Carcinoma

In certain parts of the world, particularly where schistosomiasis (S. haematobium) is prevalent, squamous cell carcinoma is the major form of bladder cancer.[240] This type of bladder cancer is seen in the Nile River Valley, and schistosome eggs can be identified in most cases (see Fig. 31–2). In other areas, such as the United States, squamous cell carcinoma composes 3% to 6% of bladder malignancies.[241] In these areas, squamous cell carcinoma often is associated with a history of bladder irritation, such as chronic infection, stones, or the long-term presence of indwelling catheters. Paraplegic patients with indwelling catheters are at risk for the development of squamous cell carcinoma.[242] Tumors arising from bladder diverticula are often squamous cell carcinomas.[242, 243] Rarely, bladder exstrophy can give rise to squamous cell carcinoma.[244]

As with adenocarcinoma, squamous cell carcinoma of the bladder is thought to arise from squamous metaplasia of the urothelium, which often is seen in association with squamous carcinoma of the bladder. Squamous carcinomas commonly are associated with loss of expression of the cyclin-dependent kinase inhibitor *p16* through mutation, deletion, or methylation of the *p16* promoter.[245] Another possible cause, which has been described only rarely, is infection with human papillomavirus, which can give rise to bladder condylomata and subsequently squamous cell carcinomas, particularly of the verrucous type[246] (Fig. 31–25 and CD Fig. 31–32). Squamous cell carcinomas should be distinguished from

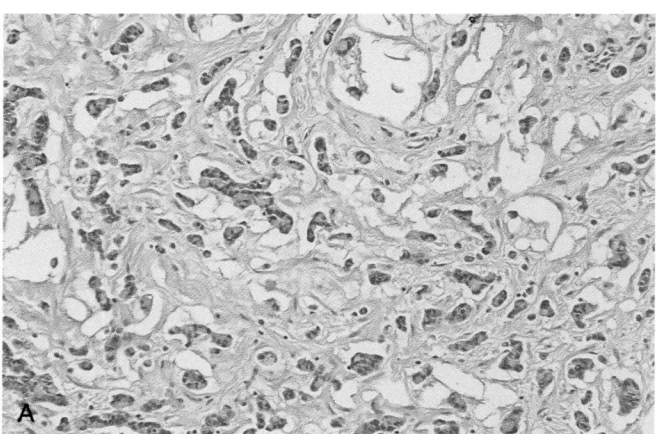
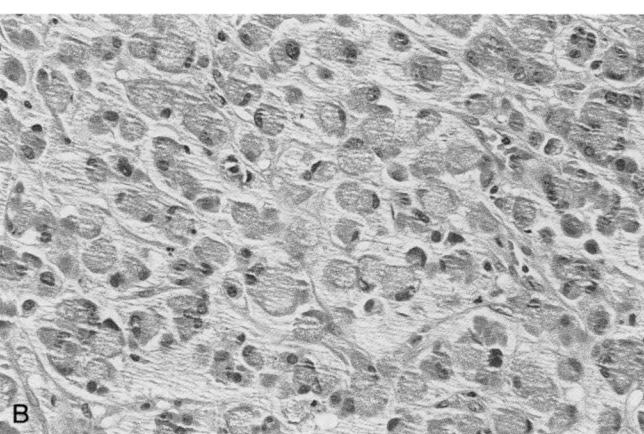

**FIGURE 31–24.** *A*, Adenocarcinoma of the bladder with mucinous features. *B*, An area from the same case shows prominent signet ring cell features. Signet ring cells often are seen in association with more well-differentiated forms of adenocarcinoma.

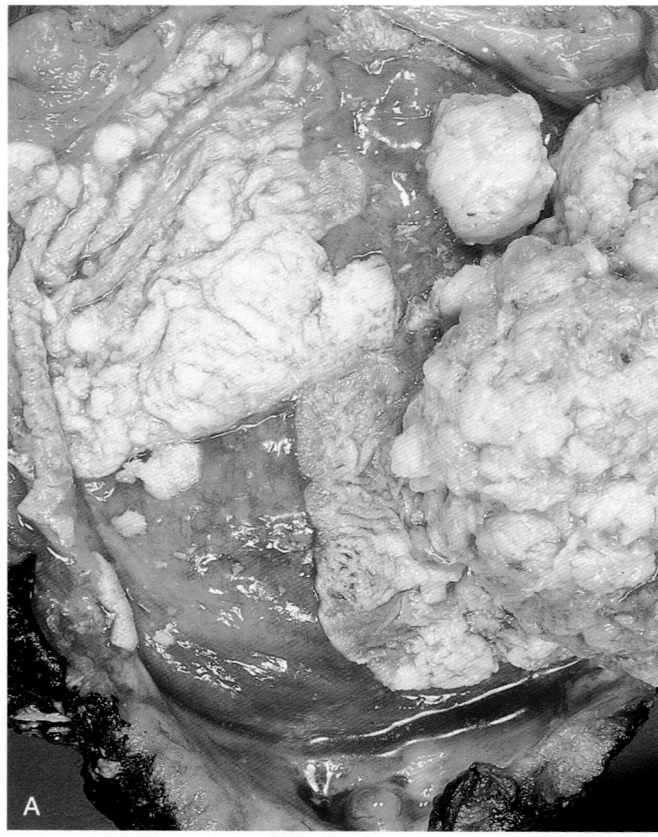

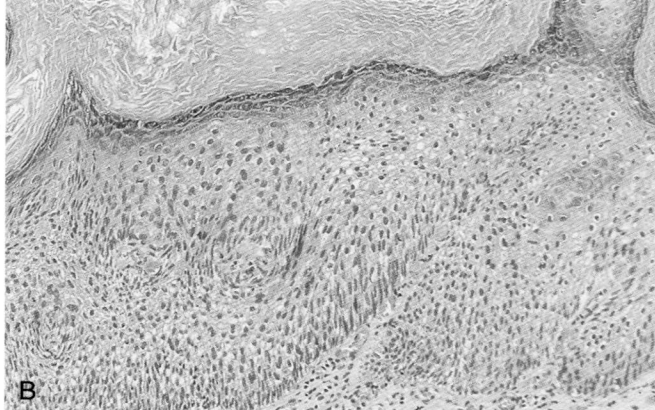

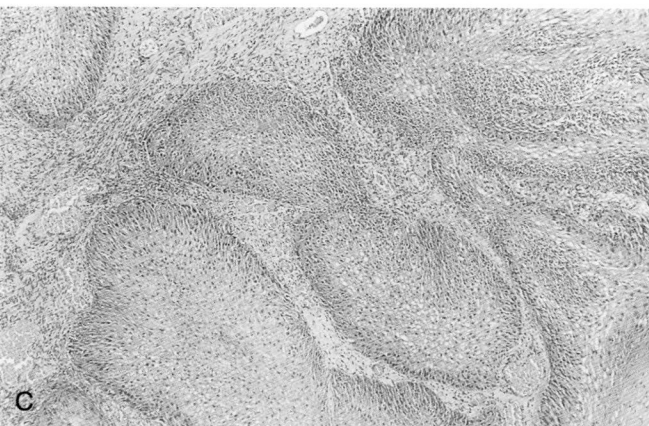

**FIGURE 31–25.** Verrucous carcinoma arising in human papillomavirus–associated condyloma. *A,* Gross photograph shows the flat and slightly raised areas of squamous metaplasia and condyloma. In the upper part of the photograph, the large verrucous carcinoma is identified. *B,* Condylomatous area with koilocytotic changes identified. *C,* Verrucous carcinoma. Note the broad pushing borders.

typical urothelial carcinomas with areas with squamous differentiation, which can be seen in a substantial proportion of urothelial carcinomas. When areas of squamous differentiation are seen, the urothelial carcinoma is considered high grade. If an identifiable urothelial element is seen, in particular urothelial CIS, the tumor should be classified as a urothelial carcinoma with squamous differentiation. Squamous cell carcinomas of the bladder often are associated with a poor prognosis, but this is due to their generally advanced stage at presentation. Stage for stage, the prognosis for squamous cell carcinoma is similar to that for typical urothelial carcinoma.[247]

Squamous carcinomas are classified as typical or conventional (not otherwise specified), verrucous type, basaloid type, and sarcomatoid (CD Figs. 31–33 to 31–36). The last-mentioned variant has spindle cell features. The tumors show squamous cells with keratinization. Intracellular bridges often are seen, particularly with well-differentiated forms. The verrucous type usually is well differentiated and shows broad pushing borders, whereas the basaloid type is similar in appearance to basal cell carcinomas of the skin, with smaller, more basophilic cells. The tumors can be graded based on their degree of keratinization and histologic differentiation, although this has not always been associated with outcome.[247, 248] Tumors are staged by the standard staging

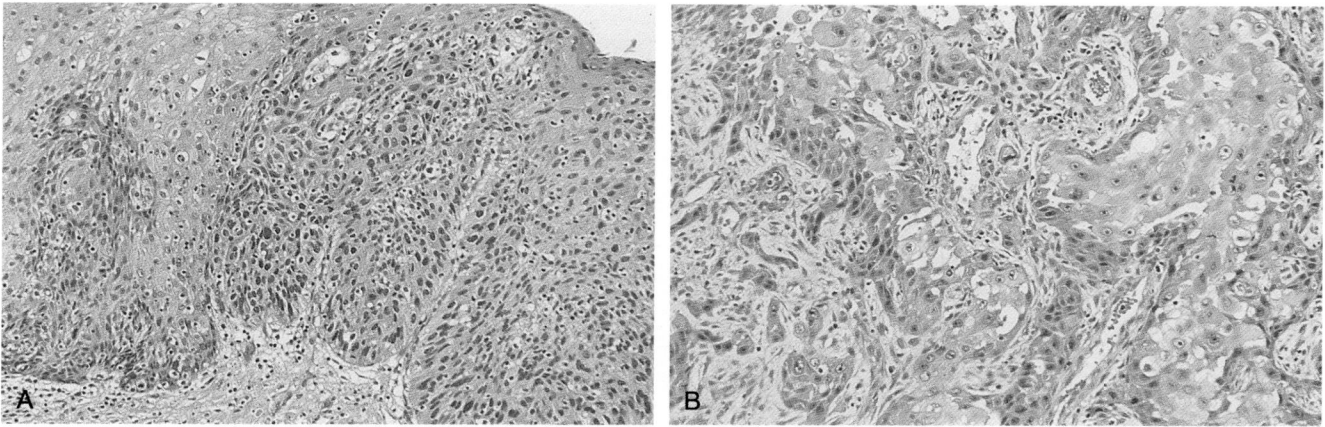

FIGURE 31–26. *A,* Squamous cell carcinoma in situ of the bladder. *B,* Invasive squamous cell carcinoma from the same case. The presence of the squamous cell carcinoma in situ is helpful in differentiating high-grade transitional cell carcinoma with prominent squamous features from pure squamous cell carcinoma of the bladder.

systems, and depth of invasion is the most important prognostic factor for squamous cell carcinoma.[247]

The primary differential diagnosis for pure squamous cell carcinoma is typical urothelial carcinoma with squamous differentiation. The presence of identifiable urothelial elements, in particular urothelial CIS or a history of CIS in the upper or lower urinary tracts, favors a diagnosis of urothelial carcinoma with squamous differentiation. The finding of squamous metaplasia and dysplasia, with a history of bladder irritation, favors a diagnosis of squamous cell carcinoma (Fig. 31–26). Extension of squamous cell carcinoma from adjacent sites, in particular the cervix and anal canal, and metastatic squamous cell carcinoma should be considered in the differential diagnosis. In these cases, the presence of squamous metaplasia and dysplasia involving surface urothelium is helpful in making the distinction.

## Urachal Carcinoma

Carcinomas arising in the urachus or urachal remnants are generally adenocarcinomas, although they occasionally can show squamous and transitional cell features. Although most adenocarcinomas primary to the bladder arise from urothelium, 20% are of urachal origin.[238] The identification of adenocarcinomas of urachal origin is based on several clinical and pathologic features, the most important of which are location of the tumor in the dome of the bladder, location centered in the muscular wall of the bladder rather than in the mucosa, and the absence of intestinal metaplasia or CIS in the surface urothelium. Also helpful are the identification of urachal remnants (Fig. 31–27 and CD Fig. 31–37), a sharp demarcation between tumor and normal urothelium, and the exclusion of metastatic adenocarcinoma from other sites.[230, 238, 249] Most cases occur in individuals in their 40s and 50s, with a mean age of

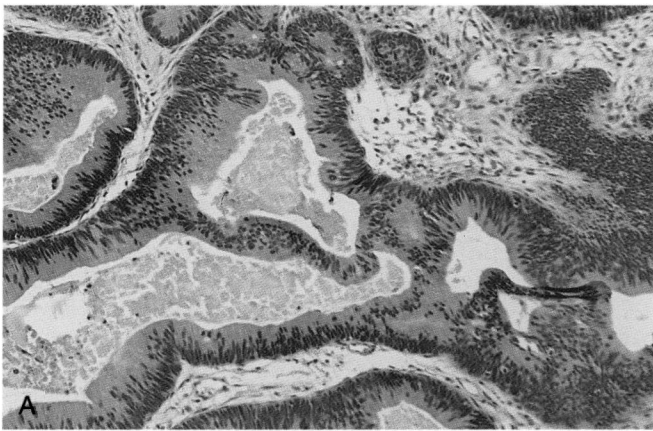
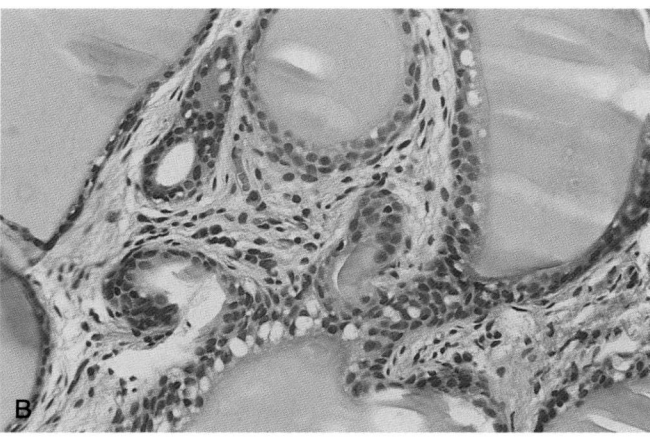

FIGURE 31–27. *A,* Enteric-type urachal carcinoma arising in the dome of the bladder. *B,* The presence of urachal remnants in the same case helps to identify the tumor as of urachal origin.

occurrence approximately 10 years younger than for carcinoma arising in urothelium.[232]

The most common form of urachal adenocarcinoma is the mucinous type. The next most frequent pattern is the enteric type; these tumors closely resemble colonic adenocarcinoma, and tumors with enteric morphology must be distinguished from adenocarcinomas of colonic origin involving the bladder wall through direct extension or by metastatic spread (CD Figs. 31–38 to 31–40). A rare subtype of adenocarcinoma of the urachus shows a signet ring pattern.[232, 239, 250]

Staging for urachal adenocarcinomas is the same as for urothelial carcinomas.[232, 251] Because these cancers arise in the muscular wall of the bladder, however, and by definition are invading into muscularis propria, a separate staging system has been proposed that evaluates extent of invasion into the urachus.[252]

The importance of distinguishing adenocarcinomas of urachal versus urothelial origin is based on the surgical approach to the tumor. The location of an adenocarcinoma in the dome of the bladder should suggest the possibility of urachal origin, and the urologist should proceed accordingly. Partial or total cystectomy with en bloc resection of urachus and umbilicus is performed for tumors originating in the urachus[251] (CD Fig. 31–41). This procedure is done because urachal tumors occasionally may extend along the urachal tract and involve the abdominal wall. It has been suggested that urachal adenocarcinomas may be resistant to radiation therapy.[252]

## BENIGN MESENCHYMAL NEOPLASMS

Benign mesenchymal tumors of the bladder are rare. The most common subtypes are leiomyoma, hemangioma, and neurofibroma,[253] with rare examples including granular cell tumor, lymphangioma, and ganglioneuroma.[254–257] Leiomyoma[258] usually presents as a submucosal mass protruding into the bladder lumen. The tumors are generally small (1 to 4 cm), although larger tumors have been described.[259] On gross examination, cut surfaces of these lesions resemble leiomyoma seen in the uterus, with a circumscribed border. The features are typical for leiomyoma seen elsewhere, including fascicles of spindle-shaped cells that show minimal atypia and rare-to-absent mitotic figures. A distinction must be made between leiomyoma and leiomyosarcoma. Because the criteria used to determine malignant potential for smooth muscle tumors varies depending on the site of origin, Mills and coworkers[260] proposed that the presence of an infiltrating border should give rise to the diagnosis of low-grade leiomyosarcoma. These authors recognize, however, that smooth muscle tumors that show minimal mitotic activity and pleomorphism rarely metastasize, even when they have infiltrating borders. The primary consideration in distinguishing leiomyoma from leiomyosarcoma is based on the surgical approach. For smooth muscle tumors that are sharply circumscribed and show minimal pleomorphism and mi-

totic activity, local resection is generally curative. For tumors with similar histologic characteristics but with an infiltrating border, a wider resection is recommended. Malignant degeneration of leiomyomas has not been described.

## SARCOMAS

Sarcomas of the bladder are rare and constitute fewer than 1% of neoplasms arising at that site,[261, 262] although they are the most common malignant tumors involving the bladder in children. Bladder sarcomas show a distinct age distribution: Rhabdomyosarcomas are seen almost exclusively in children, whereas leiomyosarcomas are the most common soft tissue malignancy seen in adults.[261, 263, 264] In children, rhabdomyosarcomas are most commonly of the embryonal type and show the typical histologic features of small round blue cells with scant cytoplasm. Gross examination shows polypoid masses extending into the bladder lumen, or the so-called botryoid appearance. Rhabdoid or strap cells may be seen, but this is not necessary for the diagnosis. Generally, immunohistochemical analysis should be performed on these cases, in particular to distinguish them from lymphomas and other tumors. Rhabdomyosarcomas typically express desmin and MyoD1, at least focally, and the embryonal type occasionally expresses the p30/32[MIC-2] oncoprotein.[265, 266] When they occur in adults, rhabdomyosarcomas may show alveolar, pleomorphic, or rarely embryonal patterns.[267] Rhabdomyosarcomas of the bladder traditionally have had a poor prognosis, although in children combination therapy including surgery, radiation, and chemotherapy has shown dramatic results.[268]

Leiomyosarcomas are the most common sarcoma of the bladder in adults. The tumors often protrude into the lumen and may be ulcerated (CD Fig. 31–42). Although they are generally small (2 to 5 cm), larger tumors have been described.[261, 269–271] The tumors have the histologic appearance of leiomyosarcomas at other sites, with interwoven fascicles of spindle-shaped cells. The degree of cellular pleomorphism and mitotic activity is variable. Necrosis may be present, and the tumors may show myxoid areas.[260] Although the gross tumors can appear well circumscribed, the microscopic tumors always show infiltrating borders, most commonly into the surrounding smooth muscle of the bladder wall. This feature is crucial in distinguishing leiomyosarcomas from leiomyomas.[260] By immunohistochemistry, the tumors nearly always express muscle-specific actin and commonly express desmin. Cytokeratin and epithelial membrane antigen reactivity has not been observed.[260] The behavior of these tumors seems to be related to the level of mitotic activity; tumors with 5 or more mitoses per 10 high-power fields have a higher rate of metastasis than tumors with lower mitotic activity, although even in cases with elevated mitotic rates, the development of metastases is relatively uncommon.[260]

Distinguishing leiomyosarcomas from other spindle cell lesions of the bladder is crucial.[272] Most spindle cell tumors of the bladder that are clearly malignant are epithelial (sarcomatoid carcinomas) and not sarcomas. These cases can be distinguished by immunohistochemistry; sarcomatoid carcinomas express keratin at least focally but lack expression of muscle antigens. Differentiating leiomyosarcomas from spindle cell carcinomas is important because sarcomatoid carcinomas have a much worse prognosis.[213, 260] As mentioned previously, the distinction from leiomyoma may be difficult. Although mitotic activity can be helpful, smooth muscle tumors that show little pleomorphism and rare mitoses should be considered leiomyosarcomas if they have infiltrating borders.[260] Non-neoplastic spindle cell proliferations may be confused with leiomyosarcoma, in particular postoperative spindle cell nodules and inflammatory pseudotumor.[272-280] These lesions can show many features of sarcomas, including relatively high mitotic activity and infiltrating borders. Features that can help distinguish these non-neoplastic proliferations from leiomyosarcoma include a history of prior manipulation of the bladder (for postoperative spindle cell nodules). Mitoses can be seen, but the non-neoplastic spindle cell proliferation should show an absence of atypical mitotic figures and a lack of nuclear and cellular pleomorphism. These distinctions are not absolute, however, and may be particularly difficult, especially on biopsy specimens. The diagnosis may not be clear until the definitive resection specimen is obtained. Immunohistochemical analysis is of little value in these cases because the non-neoplastic spindle cell proliferations can show reactivity for muscle antigens. The distinction between spindle cell proliferations is discussed more fully later.

Treatment of leiomyosarcomas is generally surgical, by either partial or radical cystectomy.[281] Although these tumors can be locally aggressive, the outcome is generally favorable, with most patients cured by surgery.

A wide variety of malignant mesenchymal neoplasms have been reported arising in the bladder, including malignant fibrous histiocytoma, osteosarcoma, liposarcoma, angiosarcoma, and hemangiopericytoma.[282-285] These are all rare and must be distinguished from metastases to the bladder, which are much more common.

## MISCELLANEOUS TUMORS

Malignant melanoma arising in the bladder is rare.[286-289] When it occurs, it has an appearance typical of melanoma at other sites. The tumors express S-100 and HMB-45.[288, 289] Metastatic melanoma involving the bladder is much more common than primary melanoma arising in the bladder. Criteria have been proposed that should be met to make a diagnosis of primary melanoma of the bladder.[286, 289] Patients should have no history of melanoma involving the skin or other sites, such as the eye, and they should undergo a thorough examination to rule out other sources of melanoma. Most importantly, atypical melanocytes should be identified in adjacent bladder mucosa.

Malignant lymphoma occasionally can arise in the bladder but much more commonly involves the bladder secondary to systemic lymphoma.[290] Lymphoma generally presents as a solid mass, which is submucosal on cystoscopic examination and can be multifocal. Lymphomas primary in the bladder have been classified most commonly as large cell diffuse and small lymphocytic; other classifications reported are follicular, plasmacytoid, mantle zone, and monocytoid lymphoma.[291] Most cases have been of B-cell origin.[291] Lymphomas of the bladder must be distinguished from florid cystitis and bladder carcinomas, in particular small cell carcinoma and lymphoepithelial-like carcinoma. Immunohistochemical analysis can be crucial in distinguishing epithelial lesions from primary lymphomas; lymphomas are cytokeratin negative and express lymphoid-associated antigens, in particular CD45 and B-cell markers. Immunohistochemical and molecular analysis can be useful in establishing the monoclonality of a lymphoid infiltrate. As with lymphomas primary to other visceral sites (e.g., the stomach), lymphomas primary to the bladder can be treated surgically. Other treatment is similar to that for lymphomas at other sites, including radiation therapy for local control and systemic chemotherapy.

Many other tumors have been described arising in the bladder, including carcinoid tumors[292-294] and paragangliomas. In the case of paragangliomas (pheochromocytomas), patients often present with symptoms of catecholamine hypersecretion, including paroxysmal hypertension. The carcinoid tumors and paragangliomas have histologic appearances similar to those found at other sites. Both show immunohistochemical expression of neuroendocrine markers. It is important to establish the diagnosis of paraganglioma because these tumors almost always behave in a benign fashion, although paragangliomas with more aggressive behavior have been described.[295]

## SIGNOUT AND FINAL REPORT

The final surgical pathology report should summarize all of the features observed by the pathologist and all of the relevant information obtained, including the status of special studies (Table 31–12). Several different types of specimens can be generated in the evaluation of bladder cancer, the most common being transurethral biopsy specimens and cystectomies (partial or radical). Cystectomies often include other structures, including the prostate, uterus, vagina, and colon. The status of these structures, along with any intrinsic disease they may have, must be commented on.

In the case of transurethral specimens, it is crucial to note the presence and type of tumor, the pattern (papillary versus nonpapillary), the tumor grade, the presence or absence of invasion, and the level of invasion. Invasion into muscularis propria

**TABLE 31–12.** Signout and Final Report for Bladder Cancer

*Transurethral Biopsy*
Gross description
  Number of chips, total size, weight (optional)
  Proportion embedded (often all submitted for microscopic examination)
Microscopic description
  Presence or absence of tumor
  Tumor type (papillary, CIS)
  Tumor grade
  Invasion, including depth and pattern of invasion
    Presence and involvement of muscularis mucosae
  Lymphovascular invasion (optional and only if unequivocal)
Molecular marker status
  *p53, Rb*, others

*Cystectomy*
Gross description
  Dimensions
  Location, size, and number of tumors
  Gross depth of infiltration
  Urethra, ureters, and adjacent structures (e.g., prostate, vagina, uterus, colon)
  Lymph nodes, with location noted
Microscopic description
  All points described under transurethral biopsy
  Status of mucosa, especially at ureter-vesicle junction, trigone, and bladder neck
  Margins (urethra, ureters, radial, adjacent structures)
  Status of tumor involvement of adjacent structures, including type of prostatic involvement (CIS, stromal invasion via prostatic urethra or via extension through bladder wall)
  Status of adjacent structures, including presence of primary tumor (in particular, prostate carcinoma)
  Lymph nodes
    Location, number, number involved, extent of involvement including extranodal extension, and size of largest involved lymph node
Pathologic stage (TNM)
Molecular marker status
  *p53, Rb*, others

CIS, Carcinoma in situ.

should be identified specifically and distinguished from invasion into muscularis mucosae. The presence of muscularis propria in a biopsy specimen is worth noting; if it is not present, the depth of invasion of a tumor cannot be assessed accurately. These features are the primary basis for future treatment decisions. As discussed, the presence of vascular and lymphatic invasion should be noted only when it is unequivocal. The status of invasion sometimes is equivocal, and if this is the case, it must be so stated. It is important to recognize the pitfalls in evaluating biopsy specimens, as outlined previously.

In the case of cystectomy specimens, all of the features noted in the biopsy specimen are relevant to the cystectomy specimen as well. The status of margins and adjacent structures also is relevant in cystectomy specimens. As noted previously, the way adjacent structures are involved can be important (as it is with the prostate). A thorough evaluation for lymph nodes must be performed as part of the gross dissection, and the lymph node status needs to be reported fully, including number and location

of lymph nodes, number and location of involved lymph nodes, extent of involvement, and size of the largest involved lymph node. All of these gross and histologic features are used to generate a pathologic stage for the patient.

The status of molecular markers, including *p53, Rb,* and growth factor receptors, is increasingly important in the evaluation of bladder cancer. In particular, *p53* and *Rb* status may be important in the management of patients with superficial and organ-confined bladder cancer. There is an increasing emphasis on target-directed therapy, including therapy based on *p53* status and growth factor receptor status. The status of the molecular markers and the way these markers were evaluated should be reported when marker status and evaluation would affect management.

An excellent review of the general features of the surgical pathology report is provided in Chapter 3, and there are excellent published and on-line resources available that outline the features to be considered for inclusion in the surgical pathology report.[296, 297] These should be considered guidelines; the final format of the report should be designed in conjunction with the urologists and oncologists and with the needs and practices of the particular institution in mind. An increasingly popular option is the synoptic report, which is basically a checklist that includes all possible important features. This provides a complete report, although it is cumbersome and may not be suitable for all practices.

The pathologist plays a crucial and central role in the management of patients with bladder cancer; this is communicated through the surgical pathology report, not only by way of the traditional methods of gross and microscopic evaluation but also increasingly by way of the evaluation of the molecular status of the tumor. Far from reducing the pathologist's role, new technologies are making the evaluation of bladder cancer by the pathologist even more crucial and specific for the management of patients. We do not expect the pathologist's role to be diminished any time soon.

## Benign Conditions of the Bladder

### TUMOR-LIKE CONDITIONS

Many benign variants of metaplastic change can form tumor-like growths, which can be indistinguishable clinically and grossly from the true neoplasms. The following tumor-like lesions generally occur as a result of either reactive or metaplastic change.

#### Inverted Papilloma

Inverted papilloma of the urinary bladder is rare and can occur anywhere in the genitourinary tract but is most common in the bladder. On cystoscopic examination, it can mimic urothelial carcinoma. Clinically the lesions show a male predominance,[298]

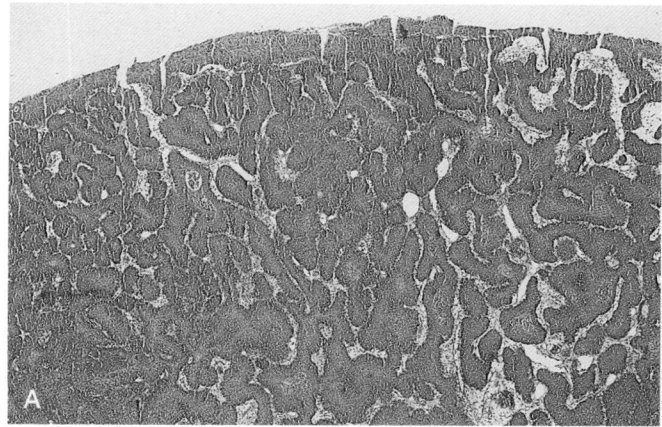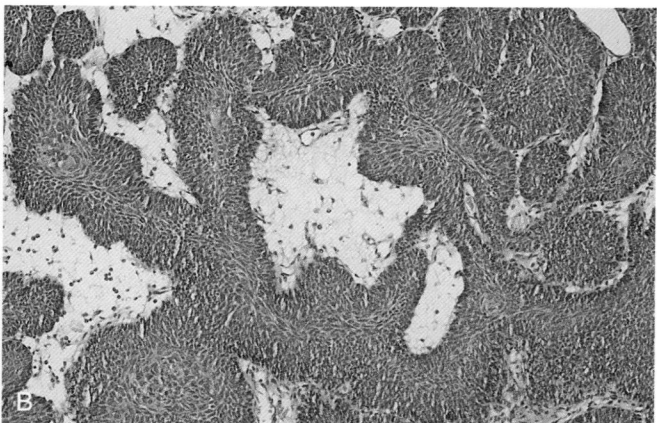

FIGURE 31-28. Inverted papilloma of the bladder. *A,* Low-power view. *B,* High-power view shows architectural organization and maturation in this lesion.

and patients present with hematuria. Inverted papillomas generally are believed to be a reactive proliferative process secondary to irritative stimuli. The gross lesions are polypoid in appearance with a smooth mucosal surface. The surface urothelium is unremarkable; however, the lamina propria is invaginated by nests and cords of oval or spindle-shaped transitional cells that show normal maturation and minimal or no cytologic atypia (Fig. 31-28). Mitotic figures can be seen, but they are rare[299] and usually are limited to the basal layer. Epithelial nests may become centrally cystic, dilated, and lined by cuboidal epithelium. The lesion shows smooth pushing borders that are not invasive. This endophytic invagination of the transitional mucosa in inverted papilloma should be differentiated from invasive transitional cell carcinoma by the absence of stromal reaction and surface epithelial abnormalities in the former. When inverted papilloma becomes fragmented during transurethral resection, it appears pseudopapillary and can be particularly difficult to differentiate from papillary transitional carcinoma. Inverted papillomas generally are considered to be benign lesions by histologic examination.[300] Some reports suggest association with transitional cell carcinoma,[301-304] but the evidence is not strong. According to some studies, the two lesions may be related, but in general inverted papilloma is not considered a risk factor for transitional cell carcinoma.[305] Inverted papilloma is included in the benign conditions in the WHO/ISUP classification.[56] They can be treated successfully by transurethral resection and fulguration of the tumor bed.[303]

### Condylomata Acuminata

Condylomata acuminata, caused by human papillomavirus, are common lesions of the genital tract, and sometimes they can extend into the urethra or more rarely can involve ureters and bladder.[306] Condylomata acuminata are described in detail in the section on urethra.

### Nephrogenic Adenoma

Nephrogenic adenoma is a relatively uncommon benign metaplastic lesion occurring in the urothelium, usually as a response to chronic irritation, trauma, or immunosuppression.[307] It has been associated with urinary tract infections, BCG treatment for transitional cell carcinoma,[308] polytetrafluoroethylene (Teflon) injections for vesicoureteric reflux,[309] and hemodialysis.[310] It is more common in males.[311] The most frequent site is the trigone of the bladder followed by ureter and urethra.[311] Nephrogenic adenoma can mimic papillary carcinoma on cystoscopy, and the diagnosis is essentially histologic[312] (CD Fig. 31-43).

Microscopic characteristics include a papillary proliferation of tubules and cysts lined by cuboidal-to-low columnar cells without cytologic atypia and with occasional clear cell change (Fig. 31-29; CD Figs. 31-44 to 31-47). The differential diagnosis includes clear cell adenocarcinoma of the bladder and prostatic carcinoma. There is no evidence that clear cell carcinomas arise from the malignant transformation of nephrogenic adenoma.[313] Immunohistochemical studies show that clear cell carcinoma and nephrogenic adenoma are strongly positive for AE1, AE3, and CAM 5.2, and both are negative for high molecular weight cytokeratin, PSA, and PSAP. PSA and PSAP help in distinguishing nephrogenic adenoma from prostate cancer. Features that favor clear cell carcinoma over nephrogenic adenoma include overt infiltrative growth, severe cytologic atypia, high mitotic rate, necrosis, high MIB-1 positivity, and strong staining for $p53$[314] (Table 31-13). Recognition of nephrogenic adenoma is important because it can be cured by conservative resection, and generally no additional therapy is required.[307] The clinical course is benign.

### Villous Adenoma

Villous adenoma of the bladder is an extremely rare tumor-like condition that is histologically iden-

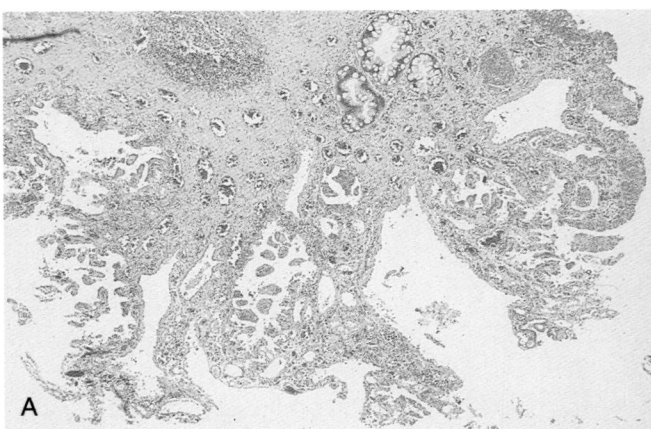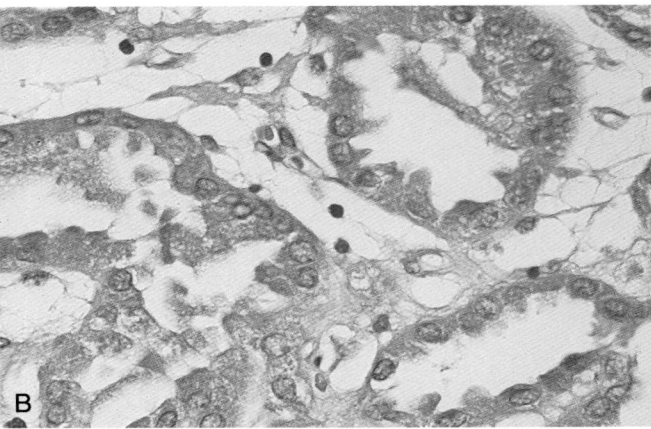

**FIGURE 31–29.** *A,* Nephrogenic adenoma, surface component. The surface component can show papillary-like projections. *B,* High-power view shows tubules lined by cuboidal cells showing minimal cytologic atypia. (Courtesy of Dr. Andy E. Sherrod.)

tical to villous adenomas of the colon.[315] These lesions appear as exophytic masses, and the gross lesions mimic papillary tumors. Microscopic characteristics include complex branching papillary fronds lined by pseudostratified columnar epithelium with goblet cells. These lesions are biologically benign and do not show invasion into the lamina propria. Extravasation of mucin into the stroma can mimic invasion, however. Similar lesions can occur in the patent urachus.[316]

### Endometriosis and Endocervicosis

Endometriosis uncommonly affects the urinary bladder and usually is seen in premenopausal women. It is rare in postmenopausal women, unless hormone replacement therapy is administered. Clinically, patients are either asymptomatic or can present with dysuria during menstruation and intermittent gross hematuria, urgency, and pain, symptoms that can mimic interstitial cystitis.[317] Frequently, there is an apparent mass, which is palpable or is discovered on cystoscopy. Ureteric involvement can occur with silent obstructive uropathy.

**TABLE 31–13.** Differential Diagnosis: Nephrogenic Adenoma Versus Clear Cell Carcinoma of Bladder Versus Prostatic Adenocarcinoma

| Features | Nephrogenic Adenoma | Clear Cell Carcinoma | Prostatic Carcinoma |
|---|---|---|---|
| Clear cell change | Focal | Predominant | Variable |
| Nuclear atypia | Mild to absent | Moderate to severe | Mild to severe |
| Mitotic activity | Absent | Increased | Slightly increased |
| Cytokeratin | ++ | ++ | ++ |
| PSA and PSAP | – | – | ++ |

PSA, Prostate-specific antigen; PSAP, Prostate-specific acid phosphatase.

In most cases, endometriosis is found on the serosal surface of the urinary bladder or the ureter (CD Fig. 31–48). The kidneys and urethra are involved much less commonly.[318] Gross examination typically reveals a solitary blue, red, or brown multicystic mass that thickens the wall and projects into the lumen, causing a filling defect on urography. Because of the intramuscular or serosal location of the lesion, a simple mucosal biopsy may not provide the diagnosis. The mucosal surface is usually intact but can ulcerate and bleed, especially during menses. Serosal foci of endometriosis are characterized by endometrial-type glands and stroma with surrounding fibrosis and proliferation of the muscularis. The endometrial glands are often cystically dilated and are associated with hemosiderin-filled macrophages. Complications include fibrotic obstruction of both ureteric orifices, vesicocolic fistula, and rarely malignant transformation.[318] Endometriosis also has been described in men with prostate carcinoma who are receiving estrogen therapy, which most likely represents activation of müllerian nests.[319]

Another müllerian lesion of the bladder has been described, termed *endocervicosis* (CD Fig. 31–49). Endocervicosis is a benign lesion in which endocervical-type glands typically are seen in the posterior wall or posterior dome of the urinary bladder.[320, 321] This lesion also can show transmural involvement of the bladder.[322] Glands rupture and can cause mucin extravasation, which can be confused with mucinous adenocarcinoma. Recognition of this entity may prevent a faulty diagnosis of adenocarcinoma. Local treatment is satisfactory for this lesion.[323]

### Pseudosarcoma, Inflammatory Pseudotumor, and Postoperative Spindle Cell Nodule

Pseudosarcomas of the urinary bladder are unusual benign proliferative lesions[324] with histologic features mimicking malignant spindle cell neoplasms.

Pseudosarcomatous spindle cell proliferations have been reported in other sites, such as lung. These lesions have a spindle cell morphology and are described by variety of names, including pseudosarcoma, inflammatory pseudotumor, pseudosarcomatous fibromyxoid tumor, inflammatory myofibroblastic tumor, and plasma cell granuloma. These lesions arise de novo, with no prior history of surgery or injury. Similar histologic lesions seen arising after surgery, most commonly after transurethral resection of prostate or bladder, are termed *postoperative spindle cell nodules*.[276] All of these lesions can grossly mimic papillary tumors. The lesions are characterized by a cellular spindle cell proliferation that infiltrates the bladder wall and can focally invade and destroy the muscle. The spindle cells are plump fibroblasts and myofibroblasts, which are traversed by a delicate network of small blood vessels, in a chronically inflamed myxoid stroma. The myxoid stroma is more pronounced in pseudosarcomatous fibromyxoid tumor. In plasma cell granuloma, the plasma cells are so abundant that they can resemble plasmacytoid lymphoma or myeloma. Postoperative spindle cell nodules generally lack the nuclear pleomorphism that is seen with pseudosarcomas.

The differential diagnosis usually includes leiomyosarcoma and spindle cell carcinoma. The histologic characteristics of pseudosarcoma and malignant spindle cell neoplasms overlap to a considerable degree so that definite distinction frequently cannot be made on histologic grounds alone. Histologic features, such as nuclear pleomorphism, can be helpful but can be pronounced in pseudosarcomatous fibromyxoid tumor. Mitotic figures are often present in the benign pseudosarcomatous lesions, but atypical forms are generally lacking. Although immunohistochemistry can be helpful, its use is limited (Table 31–14). Vimentin can be positive in all three types of lesions. Keratin immunoreactivity can help distinguish a spindle cell carcinoma; however, spindle cell carcinomas are high-grade pleomorphic tumors and are unlikely to be mistaken for a benign entity. Smooth muscle actin, generally positive in leiomyosarcoma, also can show reactivity in pseudosarcoma and postoperative spindle cell nodule. In the case of plasma cell granuloma, the plasma cell component is so abundant that the differential diag-

nosis may include a plasmacytoid lymphoma[325] and myeloma. Immunohistochemical analysis for $\kappa$ and $\lambda$ light chains can distinguish the polyclonal plasma cells of the plasma cell granuloma from the monoclonal proliferation seen in lymphoma and myeloma. Morphologic features, clinical presentation, and immunohistochemistry all can be used in conjunction to make a precise diagnosis. The distinction of benign pseudosarcomatous lesions from malignant spindle cell neoplasms is extremely important clinically because management of the benign spindle cell lesions is conservative and consists of a simple transurethral resection or partial cystectomy.

## Reactive Epithelial Changes

### BRUNN'S NEST, CYSTITIS CYSTICA, AND CYSTITIS GLANDULARIS

Brunn's nests are a common finding and are considered a hyperplastic epithelial alteration resulting from invagination of the surface urothelium into the underlying lamina propria. Chronic insult with inflammation or physical stimulation causes the urothelium to form an inflammatory crypt. This crypt is an immature cyst, and Brunn's nests represent a cut surface of the immature cyst.[326] When these nests are filled with debris or mucin, as a result of inflammatory stimulation, they gradually grow into a complete cyst[326]; they then are termed *cystitis cystica* and are lined by flattened transitional epithelium. In some cases, the lining epithelium undergoes glandular metaplasia, however, with cells transforming into cuboidal-to-columnar type with goblet cell metaplasia. This condition is called *cystitis glandularis* (CD Fig. 31–50). It is not clear if the aforementioned changes represent normal histologic variants or the residual effect of inflammatory processes.[327, 328]

### METAPLASIA

Urothelium frequently undergoes metaplastic changes, either squamous or glandular metaplasia, most likely as a response to chronic inflammatory stimuli, such as urinary tract infections, calculi, diverticuli, or frequent catheterizations.[329, 330] *Squamous metaplasia*, especially in the area of the trigone, is common in women (CD Fig. 31–51); it is thought to

**TABLE 31–14.** Differential Diagnosis: Pseudosarcoma/Postoperative Spindle Cell Nodule Versus Spindle Cell Malignancies of the Bladder

| Features | Pseudosarcoma/Postoperative Spindle Cell Nodule | Leiomyosarcoma | Spindle Cell Carcinoma |
|---|---|---|---|
| Nuclear pleomorphism | Mild to moderate | Moderate to marked | Moderate to marked |
| Mitotic activity | Present but no atypical mitotic figures | Atypical mitosis present | Atypical mitosis present |
| Vimentin | + + | + + | + + |
| Keratin | −/+ | − | + + |
| Actin | −/+ | + + | − |
| Electron microscopy | Fibroblast and myofibroblast | Smooth muscle cells | Epithelial |

occur in response to estrogen and is not considered preneoplastic. In the setting of repeated chronic inflammation, such as schistosomal infection or bladder diverticula, squamous cell carcinoma occasionally may arise from squamous metaplasia.[331] Metaplastic squamous cells are histologically similar to cervicovaginal mucosa with intercellular bridges and surface keratin. *Glandular metaplasia* most commonly occurs in the form of cystitis glandularis described earlier. Surface metaplasia can be seen and can be extensive (CD Figs. 31–52 and 31–53; see Fig. 31–23). This common finding is important to recognize because when the intestinal type of mucinous epithelium is seen, it can be associated with prominent mucin extravasation into the stroma, a finding that should not lead to the misdiagnosis of adenocarcinoma.[332]

## Cystitis

### MALAKOPLAKIA

Malakoplakia is an unusual reaction to infection, characterized by granulomatous inflammation of the urinary tract that can affect any age group but usually occurs in middle-aged individuals. Although malakoplakia usually involves the urinary tract, it also can occur in the genital tract, gastrointestinal tract,[333] and retroperitoneum, where it can be associated with considerable morbidity. Urinary tract malakoplakia often is associated with coliform infection. Although there remains much uncertainty regarding the specific cause of malakoplakia, it seems to be associated with a defect in intracellular killing of ingested microorganisms by macrophages.[334] There seems to be an association with immunosuppression.[335, 336]

Clinically, malakoplakia can present as hematuria, fever of unknown origin, or mass lesion. The clinical and radiologic features often mimic carcinoma. In the gross specimen, yellow-brown or pink-brown nodular plaques with central ulceration usually are seen at the trigone and can simulate bladder carcinoma (CD Fig. 31–54). On microscopic examination, the lamina propria is infiltrated by dense clusters of mononuclear histiocytes with eosinophilic cytoplasmic granules. The granules stain strongly with periodic acid–Schiff and show ultrastructural features of autophagic vacuoles. Some of these histiocytes contain the characteristic Michaelis-Gutmann bodies, which are concentrically laminated basophilic structures, resembling corpora amylacea. The calcium-containing Michaelis-Gutmann bodies stain positive with von Kossa's stain[337] and can stain positive with periodic acid–Schiff and iron stain.

Generally, upper urinary tract involvement requires surgical intervention, whereas most cases of lower tract involvement can be managed with antibiotics and endoscopic resection.[336] The differential diagnosis includes xanthogranulomatous cystitis, which also shows mononucleated and multinucleated histiocytes but without the calcified bodies. Similar histiocytic infiltrates can be seen in dissemi-

nated *Mycobacterium avium* infection, such as in patients infected by human immunodeficiency virus; these infections can be excluded by acid-fast stain.

### EOSINOPHILIC CYSTITIS

Eosinophilic cystitis is encountered more commonly in children and women and often is associated with allergic disorders and peripheral blood eosinophilia. It also may affect elderly men, in whom it is often associated with trauma, in particular with transurethral resection of the prostate or bladder. On cystoscopic examination, mucosal edema, erythema, friability, and ulceration are present or can produce polypoid masses that mimic a neoplasm. On microscopic examination, submucosal and intramural eosinophilic infiltration with fibrosis is seen. The disorder is self-limited and generally resolves without treatment.[338]

### INTERSTITIAL CYSTITIS

Interstitial cystitis is a sterile inflammation of the bladder occurring primarily in women. The cause and pathogenesis are undetermined.[339] Clinically, it is characterized by frequency, nocturia, and suprapubic pain. The symptoms are exacerbated during ovulation and stress, implicating neurohormonal processes.[340] Studies suggest that interstitial cystitis is a clinicopathologic syndrome with neural, immune, and endocrine components, in which activated mast cells play a central role.[340] Interstitial cystitis has been described in patients with chronic urticaria and angioedema.[341]

The microscopic changes are variable. The early stages show mucosal microhemorrhages. Ulcers may also be seen. The ulcer bed usually is covered by fibrin and necrotic material, and the underlying lamina propria shows varying degrees of edema and vascular congestion. The inflammatory infiltrate is composed predominantly of lymphocytes, with lesser numbers of plasma cells, histiocytes, neutrophils, and occasionally eosinophils.[342] There is usually diffuse involvement of the bladder wall with activated mast cells, especially surrounding vessels, in submucosa and in the muscularis propria. The mast cells can be identified using toluidine blue, Leder stain, or Giemsa stain. Human bladder mast cells also express estrogen receptors, which may explain worsening of the condition during ovulation.[340]

### TREATMENT (BACILLE CALMETTE-GUÉRIN)–ASSOCIATED CYSTITIS

Intravesicle administration of BCG is used frequently for the treatment of CIS and can lead to marked chronic granulomatous inflammation of the mucosa and the lamina propria. Epithelioid histiocytes, small mature lymphocytes, fibrosis, and multinucleated giant cells characterize the inflammation. The granulomas usually are noncaseating, and a history of BCG therapy usually is helpful in differentiating it from other causes of granulomatous inflammation. The giant cells in BCG cystitis may contain

**TABLE 31–15.** Differential Diagnosis: Radiation-Induced Changes Versus Malignancy

| Features | Radiation Damage | Urothelial Malignancy |
|---|---|---|
| Nuclear-to-cytoplasmic ratio | Not increased | Increased |
| Nuclear irregularity | Absent to minimal | Present |
| Chromatin | Karyorrhectic to finely dispersed | Coarse |
| Binucleation and multinucleation | Frequently present | Can be present |
| Cytoplasmic vacuolation | Frequently present | Absent except in adenocarcinoma |

crystalloid material, which may represent the product of the vaccine.

## RADIATION CYSTITIS

Radiation cystitis is a frequent complication of radiation therapy administered for urologic[343] and nonurologic malignancies. Patients receiving greater than 7000 rads to the pelvis are at highest risk of developing radiation cystitis. Chronic radiation cystitis occasionally can result in massive bleeding. On cystoscopy, acutely irradiated mucosa is red and edematous, with abnormal telangiectasia and focal ulceration (CD Fig. 31–55). The epithelium is atrophic with dilated vessels and inflammatory cells in the lamina propria.[344] Radiation damage primarily affects the basal epithelium and the lamina propria. Urothelial atypia can be marked, and the differentiation from malignancy, particularly CIS, can be difficult. Radiated cells frequently show significant nuclear pleomorphism, multinucleation, and significant hyperchromasia, but the nuclear-to-cytoplasmic ratio is generally low compared with malignant cells. The nuclear chromatin in irradiated cells is more indistinct and blurred, whereas malignant nuclei show coarse chromatin. The cytoplasm generally is wispy in irradiated cells, with streaming morphology and degenerative vacuoles, which should be distinguished from the vacuoles of adenocarcinoma; a mucicarmine stain can be helpful in difficult cases. Vacuoles can be seen in the nuclei of irradiated cells (Table 31–15). The lamina propria shows bizarre fibroblasts that sometimes can mimic sarcomatous proliferation. Clinical history of prior radiation is crucial for the diagnosis.

## HEMORRHAGIC CYSTITIS

Cyclophosphamide is a common chemotherapeutic agent used for a variety of malignancies. It is a significant cause of hemorrhagic cystitis, which can develop after short-term, high-dose therapy with this alkylating agent. The drug's metabolite, acrolein, seems to be the causative agent. Busulfan is a rare cause of hemorrhagic cystitis.[345] Clinically, patients present with a variety of urinary problems, including incontinence, hematuria, and vesicoureteral reflux.[346] On cystoscopic examination, the mucosa is edematous and reddened with multiple telangiectatic vessels. On microscopic examination, the mucosa may be focally to extensively denuded, with atypical urothelial cells, similar to those seen in radiation injury. The lamina propria shows varying degrees of edema, fibroblastic proliferation, vascular dilation, or intimal proliferation with sclerosis. A variant of acute hemorrhagic cystitis in children is associated with viral infection. Drug-related lesions tend to resolve several weeks after the cessation of therapy.

## POLYPOID CYSTITIS

Polypoid cystitis is a variant of simple cystitis that frequently results as a complication of radiation therapy, long-term indwelling catheters, or after any inflammatory insult to the urothelial mucosa. Two thirds of the cases are related to indwelling catheters with an average time interval of 2.3 months.[347] In polypoid cystitis, the edema in the lamina propria is so pronounced that the mucosa is projected into the lumen, producing a polypoid mass that can mimic papillary transitional cell carcinoma grossly and cystoscopically.[348] When the edema is pronounced enough to cause bulbous projections with attenuated mucosa, the histologic diagnosis is usually straightforward (Fig. 31–30 and CD Fig. 31–56). The difficulty arises when mucosal projections are thin and show branching, resembling papillary transitional cell carcinoma. The fronds in polypoid cystitis are generally composed of edematous, capillary-rich fi-

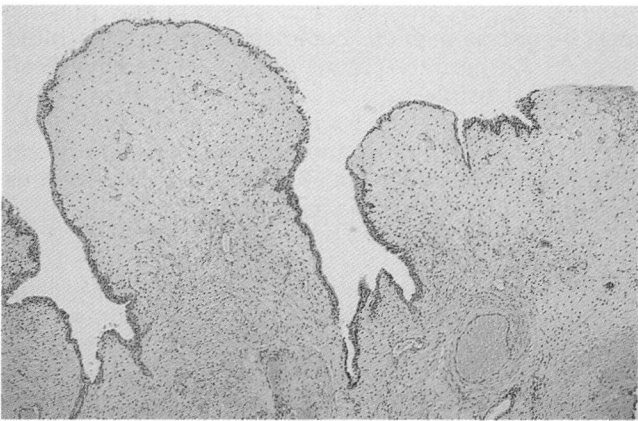

**FIGURE 31–30.** Polypoid cystitis showing edema of lamina propria with papillary projections into the bladder lumen. On gross examination, this lesion can mimic papillary carcinoma. The overlying urothelium is benign.

brovascular cores, which contain inflammatory cells and show absent or minimal branching into smaller papillae, whereas papillary transitional cell carcinomas usually have thin fibrovascular cores, which lack prominent edema and inflammation and frequently branch.[349] The urothelium in polypoid cystitis can show reactive cellular changes and contains fewer layers than papillary carcinomas. Polypoid cystitis usually resolves after the removal of the inflammatory insult.

## Amyloidosis

Although the kidney is the most common site of urinary tract amyloidosis, isolated cases of amyloidosis can occur rarely in the bladder, ureters, or urethra. The urinary tract can be involved in secondary amyloidosis. Bladder amyloidosis usually manifests with hematuria. It does not have any typical cystoscopic features; however, a localized amyloid tumor can mimic a neoplastic mass lesion. On microscopic examination, as with any other site, amyloidosis is characterized by deposition of amorphous eosinophilic material in the interstitium of lamina propria and around the blood vessels (CD Fig. 31–57). Inflammation is usually minimal or absent. Amyloid stains positive with Congo red and shows apple-green birefringence by polarized microscopy.

## Congenital Abnormalities

### URACHAL MALDEVELOPMENT AND PATENT URACHUS

Urachal maldevelopment is a common congenital abnormality of the urinary tract, with a male predominance. The urachal tract links the dome of the bladder to the allantois, which atrophies during caudad descent of the bladder. Urachal vestiges, which are present as microcysts in the bladder wall, are common in the general population (CD Fig. 31–58; see Fig. 31–27 and CD Fig. 31–37). The urachus may persist as a microscopic sinus or a gross blind sinus.[350] An entirely patent urachus forming a vesicoumbilical fistula can occur as an isolated anomaly, or it may be associated with prune-belly syndrome. These sinuses, cysts, and fistulas are prone to trauma and infection, which can result in squamous and glandular metaplasia and carcinoma.

### EXSTROPHY

Bladder exstrophy is rare but one of the most challenging congenital urinary tract abnormalities.[351] It occurs in about 1 in every 40,000 births and is more common in boys. The severity ranges from a small cutaneous fistula to complete exposure of the bladder on the abdominal wall. This anomaly is the result of failure of mesoderm to cause cephalic extension of the cloacal membrane. The consequences of the untreated bladder exstrophy is total urinary incontinence and increased incidence of bladder cancer, usually adenocarcinoma. Apart from the open bladder, there are other abnormalities, including urogenital, musculoskeletal, and anorectal defects.

### CONGENITAL BLADDER DIVERTICULA

Most bladder diverticula are acquired. Congenital bladder diverticula occur at the ureterovesical junction and are associated with vesicoureteral reflux. These are commonly associated with distal urethral obstruction or neurogenic bladder dysfunction and can lead to severe kidney damage.[352]

## Acquired Bladder Diverticula

Most acquired bladder diverticula occur in middle-aged to elderly men with bladder outlet obstruction secondary to prostatic hyperplasia. Increased intravesicle pressure causes mucosal invagination into the bladder wall. They are more common near the ureteric orifices and usually communicate with the bladder lumen. Bladder diverticula are susceptible to repeated infection resulting from stasis and stone formation. Infection and obstruction lead to squamous metaplasia of the epithelium, which carries a small but significant risk of developing squamous cell carcinoma in the wall of the diverticula and transitional cell carcinoma.[353] When carcinoma does occur, it has a poor prognosis, owing to delay in early detection and ease of invasion secondary to the thin diverticular wall.

## URETHRA

## Urethral Carcinoma

Urethral involvement by urothelial carcinoma warrants serious consideration when cystectomy is necessary and reconstruction of the urinary tract is indicated. In male patients, it has been reported that 4% to 18% of patients develop recurrent carcinoma in the remnant urethra after cystectomy. Urethral recurrences can occur with an average interval of 3 years after cystectomy. Urethral recurrences generally are associated with multifocal cancers in the bladder, concurrent upper urinary tract cancers, diffuse CIS, involvement by cancer of the bladder neck or trigone, involvement of the prostatic urethra or prostatic ducts or prostatic tissue, and positive urethral margin on intraoperative frozen section.[107]

Primary urethral carcinomas are rare and relatively more common in women. Most are urothelial carcinomas. Rarely, melanomas[286] or periurethral sarcomas can occur. The prognosis of urethral cancer depends on its anatomic location and the depth of invasion. Superficial tumors located in the anterior urethra of the female and male are generally curable; deeply invasive lesions and lesions located in the posterior urethra are rarely curable. Prognosis is determined by the anatomic location of the neo-

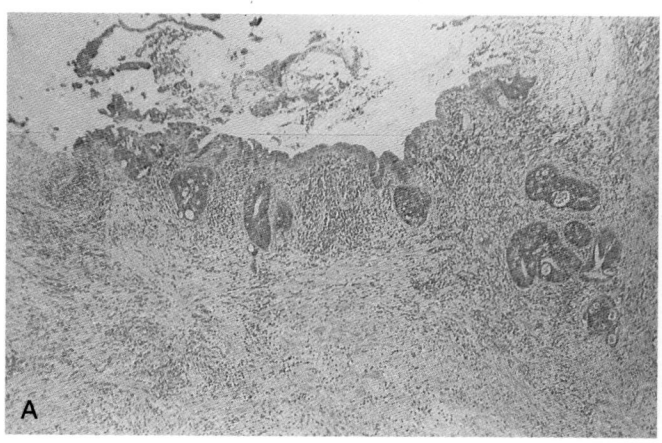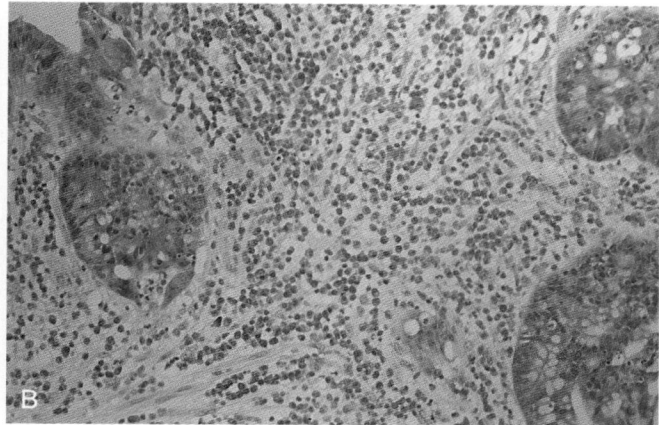

**FIGURE 31–31.** Adenocarcinoma arising in the urethra. *A,* Low-power view. *B,* High-power view shows infiltrating glands. (Courtesy of Dr. Peter W. Nichols.)

plasm, the size, and the depth of invasion of the primary tumor. The histology of the primary tumor is less important in determining response to therapy and survival.[354]

The female urethra is lined by transitional cell mucosa proximally and stratified squamous cells distally. Transitional cell carcinoma is most common in the proximal urethra, and squamous cell carcinoma predominates in the distal urethra (CD Fig. 31–59). Adenocarcinoma is found in both locations and arises from metaplasia of the numerous periurethral glands (Fig. 31–31).

The male urethra is lined by transitional cells in its prostatic and membranous portion and stratified columnar epithelium–to–stratified squamous epithelium in the bulbous and penile portions. The submucosa of the urethra contains numerous glands. Urethral cancer in men can manifest the histologic characteristics of transitional cell carcinoma, squamous cell carcinoma, or adenocarcinoma. Except for the prostatic urethra, where transitional cell carcinoma is most common, squamous cell carcinoma is the predominant histology of male urethral neoplasms.

## Benign Conditions of the Urethra

### TUMOR-LIKE CONDITIONS

#### Fibroepithelial Polyps

Fibroepithelial polyps are benign lesions that usually occur in children and are regarded as possibly congenital.[355] They usually occur in the prostatic urethra close to the verumontanum.[356, 357] They also have been reported in adults. Microscopic examination shows they are composed of a fibrous stalk lined by either transitional or squamous epithelium.

#### Urethral Pseudotumors and Postoperative Spindle Cell Nodules

When the urethra is examined shortly after a transurethral procedure, pseudosarcomatous lesions, similar to postoperative spindle cell nodules of the bladder, are encountered frequently.[278] These lesions are described in detail in the section on the bladder.

### Condylomata Acuminata

Condylomata acuminata, caused by human papillomavirus, are common lesions of the genital tract and sometimes can extend into the urethra or more rarely can involve ureters and bladder.[306] Intraurethral spread of venereal warts is a serious complication and clinically manifests with severe irritative symptoms. It is more common in men. Recurrence is frequent, and the condition is difficult to treat. The usual subtypes of human papillomavirus are 6, 11, 16, and 18. Most lesions are confined to the fossa navicularis (which is the distal dilated end of the urethra). Some lesions can be extensive, however. On cystoscopic and gross examinations, the lesions appear as polypoid or papillary excrescences on the mucosal surface. Sometimes there can be diffuse involvement, giving a velvety granular appearance to the mucosa. The lesions show a papillary growth pattern lined by metaplastic squamous urothelium. The epithelial cells show koilocytic change, characterized by perinuclear clearing, nuclear hyperchromasia, and nuclear membrane irregularities (Fig. 31–32 and CD Fig. 31–60). Condylomata acuminata have a potential for malignant transformation, but it is rare.[358] Immunohistochemical or in situ hybridization studies for human papillomavirus can be helpful in some cases (see Fig. 31–32).

### INFLAMMATORY CONDITIONS OF THE URETHRA

Lower urinary tract infections can affect the urethra and generally include *Neisseria gonorrhoeae, Chlamydia,* and *Mycoplasma.* Infection with *Mycobacterium tuberculosis* can cause strictures and fistulas. Urethral stones are more common in men and generally are formed in the bladder, then become lodged in the posterior urethra. In women, stones can be formed in urethral diverticula.[350]

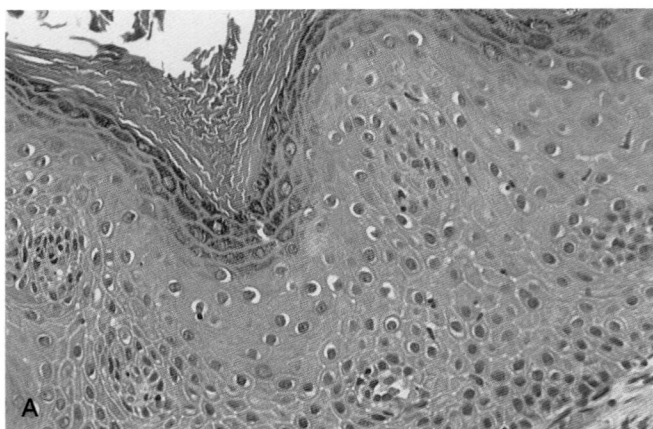 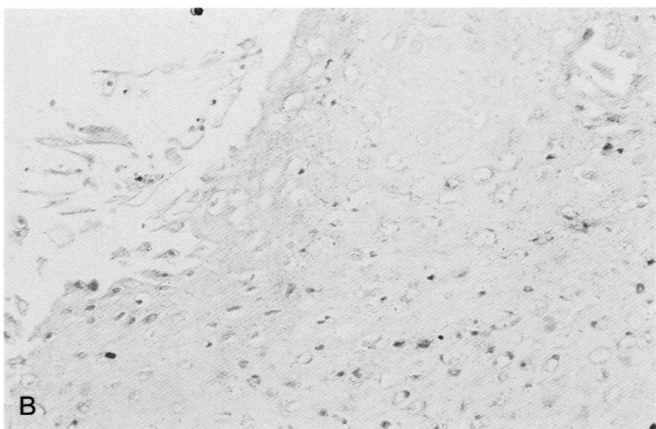

**FIGURE 31–32.** *A,* Urethral condyloma. Note the squamous metaplasia and hyperkeratosis. Koilocytotic changes are identified. *B,* In situ hybridization for human papillomavirus (HPV) subtypes 6 and 11 show presence of HPV transcripts (as demonstrated by the dark blue nuclear stain).

## REFERENCES

1. Gray H, Lewis WH: Anatomy of the Human Body. 20th ed. Philadelphia, Lea & Febiger, 1918. Available at Bartleby.com, www.bartleby.com/107/.
2. Carroll PH, Dixon CM: Surgical anatomy of male and female urethra. Urol Clin North Am 19:339–340, 1992.
3. Tanagho E: Anatomy of the lower urinary tract. *In* Walsh PC, Retik AB, Starney TA, et al (eds): Campbell's Urology, 6th ed. Philadelphia, WB Saunders, 1992.
4. Vera-Sempere FJ, Jaen Martinez J, Vera Donoso CD, Jimenez Cruz JF: Assessment of the tunica muscularis mucosae of the bladder wall. Necropsy study [in Spanish]. Acta Urol Espan 22:726–734, 1998.
5. Sanchez-Chapado M, Angulo Cuesta J: The presence of muscularis mucosae in the urinary bladder of samples from transurethral resection [in Spanish]. Arch Espan Urol 48:117–122, 1995.
6. Bochner BH, Cote RJ, Weidner N, et al: Angiogenesis in bladder cancer. Relationship between microvessel density and tumor prognosis. J Natl Cancer Inst 87:1603–1612, 1995.
7. Philip AT, Amin MB, Tamboli P, et al: Intravesical adipose tissue. Am J Surg Pathol 24:1286–1290, 2000.
8. Lamm DL: Efficacy and safety of bacille Calmette-Guérin immunotherapy in superficial bladder cancer. Clin Infect Dis 31(suppl 3):S86–90, 2000.
9. Hartge P, Harvey EB, Linehan WM, et al: Unexplained excess risk of bladder cancer in men. J Natl Cancer Inst 82:1636–1640, 1990.
10. Khasidy LR, Khashu B, Mallett EC, et al: Transitional cell carcinoma of bladder in children. Urology 35:142–144, 1990.
11. Yanase M, Tsukamoto T, Kumamoto Y, et al: Transitional cell carcinoma of the bladder or renal pelvis in children. Eur Urol 19:312–314, 1991.
12. Keetch DW, Manley CB, Catalona WJ: Transitional cell carcinoma of bladder in children and adolescents. Urology 42:447–449, 1993.
13. Zenser TV, Lakshmi VM, Davis BB: N-glucuronidation of benzidine and its metabolites. Role in bladder cancer. Drug Metab Dispos 26:856–859, 1998.
14. Carel R, Levitas-Langman A, Kordysh E, et al: Case-referent study on occupational risk factors for bladder cancer in southern Israel. Int Arch Occup Environ Health 72:304–308, 1999.
15. Schulte PA, Ringen K, Hemstreet GP, et al: Risk assessment of a cohort exposed to aromatic amines. Initial results. J Occupat Med 27:115–121, 1985.
16. Hoffmann D, Patrianakos C, Brunnemann KD, Gori GB: Chromatographic determination of vinyl chloride in tobacco smoke. Anal Chem 48:47–50, 1976.
17. Vineis P: Epidemiology of cancer from exposure to arylamines. Environ Health Perspect 102(suppl 6):7–10, 1994.
18. Castelao JE, Yuan JM, Skipper PL, et al: Gender- and smoking-related bladder cancer risk. J Natl Cancer Inst 93:538–545, 2001.
19. Brennan P, Bogillot O, Cordier S, et al: Cigarette smoking and bladder cancer in men. A pooled analysis of 11 case-control studies. Int J Cancer 86:289–294, 2000.
20. Vineis P, Pirastu R: Aromatic amines and cancer. Cancer Causes Control 8:346–355, 1997.
21. Castelao JE, Yuan JM, Gago-Dominguez M, et al: Non-steroidal anti-inflammatory drugs and bladder cancer prevention. Br J Cancer 82:1364–1369, 2000.
22. D'Avanzo B, La Vecchia C, Franceschi S, et al: Coffee consumption and bladder cancer risk. Eur J Cancer 28:1480–1484, 1992.
23. Yu MC, Ross RK, Skinner DG: Epidemiology of bladder cancer. *In* Petrovich Z, Baert L, Brady LW (eds): Carcinoma of the Bladder. Innovations in Management. Berlin, Springer-Verlag, 1998, pp 1–13.
24. Cantor KP, Lynch CF, Hildesheim ME, et al: Drinking water source and chlorination byproducts. I. Risk of bladder cancer. Epidemiology 9:21–28, 1998.
25. Gago-Dominguez M, Castelao JE, Yuan JM, et al: Use of permanent hair dyes and bladder-cancer risk. Int J Cancer 91:575–579, 2001.
26. Bedwani R, Renganathan E, El Kwhsky F, et al: Schistosomiasis and the risk of bladder cancer in Alexandria, Egypt. Br J Cancer 77:1186–1189, 1998.
27. Mostofi FK, Davis CJ, Sesterhenn IA: Diagnosis and management of genitourinary cancer. *In* Skinner DG, Lieskovsky G (eds): Diagnosis and Management of Genitourinary Cancer. Philadelphia, WB Saunders, 1988, pp 83–117.
28. Tawfik HN: Carcinoma of the urinary bladder associated with shistosomiasis in Egypt. The possible causal relationship. *In* Princess Takamatsu Symposia, Baltimore: University Park Press, Princeton, NJ: Princeton Scientific Publishing, 1987.
29. Fearon ER, Feinberg AP, Hamilton SH, Vogelstein B: Loss of genes on the short arm of chromosome 11 in bladder cancer. Nature 318:377–380, 1985.
30. Olumi AF, Tsai YC, Nichols PW, et al: Allelic loss of chromosome 17p distinguishes high grade from low grade transitional cell carcinomas of the bladder. Cancer Res 50:7081–7083, 1990.
31. Presti JCJ, Reuter VE, Galan T, et al: Molecular genetic alterations in superficial and locally advanced human bladder cancer. Cancer Res 51:5405–5409, 1991.
32. Sidransky D, Frost P, Von Eschenbach A, et al: Clonal origin bladder cancer. N Engl J Med 326:737–740, 1992.

33. Miyao N, Tsai YC, Lerner SP, et al: Role of chromosome 9 in human bladder cancer. Cancer Res 53:4066–4070, 1993.
34. Gonzalez-Zulueta M, Ruppert JM, Tokino K, et al: Microsatellite instability in bladder cancer. Cancer Res 53:5620–5623, 1993.
35. Ruppert JM, Tokino K, Sidransky D: Evidence of two bladder cancer suppressor loci on human chromosome 9. Cancer Res 53:5093–5095, 1993.
36. Orlow I, Lianes P, Lacombe L, et al: Chromosome 9 allelic losses and microsatellite alterations in human bladder tumors. Cancer Res 54:2848–2851, 1994.
37. Kamb A, Gruis NA, Weaver-Feldhaus J, et al: A cell cycle regulator potentially involved in genesis of many tumor types. Science 264:436–440, 1994.
38. Nobori T, Miura K, Wu DJ, et al: Deletions of the cyclin-dependent kinase-4 inhibitor gene in multiple human cancers. Nature 368:753–756, 1994.
39. Reznikoff CA, Belair CD, Yeager TR, et al: A molecular genetic model of human bladder cancer pathogenesis. Semin Oncol 23:571–584, 1996.
40. Knowles MA, Elder PA, Williamson M, et al: Allelotype of human bladder cancer. Cancer Res 54:531–538, 1994.
41. Spruck CHI, Ohneseit PF, Gonzalez-Zulueta M, et al: Two molecular pathways to transitional cell carcinoma of the bladder. Cancer Res 54:784–788, 1994.
42. Dalbagni G, Presti J, Reuter V, et al: Genetic alterations in bladder cancer. Lancet 342:469–471, 1993.
43. Reznikoff CA, Kao CH, Messing EM, et al: A molecular-genetic model of human bladder carcinogenesis. Semin Cancer Biol 4:143–152, 1993.
44. Reznikoff CA, Loretz LJ, Christian BJ, et al: Neoplastic transformation of SV40 immortalized human urinary tract epithelial cells by in vitro exposure to 3-methylcholanthrene. Carcinogens (Lond) 9:1427–1436, 1988.
45. Sidransky D, Von Eschenbach A, Tsai YC, et al: Identification of *p53* gene mutations in bladder cancers and urine samples. Science (Washington DC) 252:706–709, 1991.
46. Spruck CHI, Rideout III WM, Olumi AF, et al: Distinct pattern of *p53* mutations in bladder cancer. Relationship to tobacco usage. Cancer Res 53:1162–1166, 1993.
47. Cairns P, Proctor AJ, Knowles MA: Loss of heterozygosity at the RB locus is frequent and correlates with muscle invasion in bladder carcinoma. Oncogene 6:2305–2309, 1991.
48. Virchow R: Cellular Pathology as Based Upon Physiological and Pathological Histology. Translated from the second edition of the original by F Chance, 1860. *In* Bogdonoff MD, Good RA, McGovern JP, et al (eds): The Classics of Medicine Library, Special Edition, 1978. Birmingham, UK, The Classics of Medicine Library, Division of Gryphon Editions, 1978, p 468.
49. Busch C, Hawes D, Johansson SL, Cote RJ: Pathologic assessment of bladder cancer and pitfalls in staging. In: Bladder: Current Diagnosis and Treatment, ed. M.J. Droller. 2001, Totwa, NJ: Humana Press.
50. Broders AC: Epithelioma of the genitourinary organs. Ann Surg 75:574–604, 1922.
51. Ash JE: Epithelial tumors of the bladder. J Urol 44:135–145, 1940.
52. Bergkvist A, Lungqvist A, Moberger G: Classification of bladder tumours based on the cellular pattern. Acta Chir Scand 130:371–378, 1961.
53. Koss LG: Tumors of the urinary bladder. In: Atlas of Tumor Pathology, American Registry of Pathology. Second Series, Fascicle II. Washington, DC, Armed Forces Institute of Pathology, 1975.
54. Mostofi FK, Sobin HL, Torlini H: Histologic Typing of Urinary Bladder Tumors. Geneva, World Health Organization, 1973.
55. Murphy WM, Beckwith JB, Farrow GM: Tumors of the kidney, bladder and related urinary structures. In: Atlas of Tumor Pathology, American Registry of Pathology. Third Series, Fascicle 14. Washington, DC, Armed Forces Institute of Pathology, 1994, pp 198–233.
56. Epstein JI, Amin MB, Reuter VR, Mostofi FK: The World Health Organization/International Society of Urological Pathology consensus classification of urothelial (transitional cell) neoplasms of the urinary bladder. Bladder Consensus Conference Committee. Am J Surg Pathol 22:1435–1448, 1998.
57. Mostofi FK, Davis CJ, Sesterhenn IA, et al: Histology Typing of Urinary Tumors. 2nd ed. Bladder Tumours (International Histological Classification of Tumors) Springer Verlag, 2nd edition, NY, 1999.
58. Cheng L, Darson M, Cheville JC, et al: Urothelial papilloma of the bladder. Clinical and biologic implications. Cancer 86:2098–2101, 1999.
59. Busch C, Engberg A, Norlen BJ, Stenkvist B: Malignancy grading of epithelial bladder tumours. Scand J Urol Nephrol 11:143–148, 1977.
60. Skinner DG: Current perspectives in the management of high-grade invasive bladder cancer. Cancer 45(7 suppl):1866–1874, 1980.
61. Marshall VF: Current clinical problems regarding bladder tumors. Cancer 9:543, 1956.
62. Ooms ECM, Anderson WAD, Alons CL, et al: Analysis of the performance of pathologists in the grading of bladder tumors. Hum Pathol 14:140–143, 1983.
63. Abel PD, Henderson D, Bennett MK, et al: Differing interpretations by pathologists of the pT category and grade of transitional cell cancer of the bladder. Br J Urol 62:339–342, 1988.
64. Robertson AJ, Beck J, Burnett MK, et al: Observer variability in histopathological reporting of transitional cell carcinoma and epithelial dysplasia in bladders. J Clin Pathol 43:17–21, 1990.
65. Amin MB, Grignon DJ, Eble J, et al: Intraepithelial lesions of the urothelium. An interobserver reproducibility study study with proposed terminology and histologic criteria (abstract). Mod Pathol 10:69A, 1997.
66. Holmang S, Hedelin H, Anderstom C, et al: Recurrence and progression in low grade papillary urothelial tumors. J Urol 162:702–707, 1999.
67. Desai S, Lim SD, Jimenez RE, et al: Relationship of cytokeratin 20 and CD44 protein expression with WHO/ISUP grade in pTa and pT1 papillary urothelial neoplasia. Mod Pathol 13:1315–1323, 2000.
68. Gilbert HA, Logan JL, Kagan AR, et al: The natural history of papillary transitional cell carcinoma of the bladder and its treatment in an unselected population on the basis of histologic grading. J Urol 119:488–492, 1978.
69. Stein JP, Lieskovsky G, Cote RJ, et al: Radical cystectomy in the treatment of invasive bladder cancer. Long-term results in 1,054 patients. J Clin Oncol 19:666–675, 2001.
70. Jordan AM, Weingarten J, Murphy WM: Transitional cell neoplasms of the bladder. Can biologic potential be predicted from histologic grading? Cancer 60:2766–2774, 1987.
71. Jimenez RE, Gheiler E, Oskanian P, et al: Grading the invasive component of urothelial carcinoma of the bladder and its relationship with progression-free survival. Am J Surg Pathol 24:980–987, 2000.
72. Sarkis AS, Zhang Z, Cordon-Cardo C: *p53* nuclear overexpression and disease progression in Ta bladder cancer. Int J Oncol 3:355–360, 1993.
73. Cordon-Cardo C, Zhang ZF, Dalbagni G, et al: Cooperative effects of *p53* and *pRb* alterations in primary superficial bladder tumors. Cancer Res 57:1217–1221, 1997.
74. Logothetis CJ, Xu H-J, Ro JY, et al: Altered expression of retinoblastoma protein and known prognostic variables in locally advanced bladder cancer. J Natl Cancer Inst 84:1256–1261, 1992.
75. Sarkis AS, Bajorin DF, Reuter VE, et al: Prognostic value of *p53* nuclear overexpression in patients with invasive bladder cancer treated with neoadjuvant MVAC. J Clin Oncol 13:1384–1390, 1995.
76. Grossman HB, Liebert M, Dinney AM, et al: *p53* and *Rb* expression predict progression in T1 bladder cancer. Clin Cancer Res 4:829–834, 1998.
77. Melicow MM: Histological study of vesical urothelium intervening between gross neoplasms in total cystectomy. J Urol 68:261–279, 1952.

78. Melamed MR, Voutsa NG, Grabstald H: Natural history and clinical behavior of in situ carcinoma of the human urinary bladder. Cancer 17:1533–1545, 1964.

79. Farrow GM, Utz DC, Rife CC: Morphological and clinical observations of patients with early bladder cancer treated with total cystectomy. Cancer Res 36:2495–2501, 1976.

80. Utz DC, Hanash KA, Farrow GM: The plight of the patient with carcinoma in situ of the bladder. J Urol 103:160–164, 1970.

81. Yates-Bell AJ: Carcinoma in situ of the bladder. Br J Surg 58:359–364, 1971.

82. Barlebo H, Sorensen BL, Soeborg OA: Carcinoma in situ of the urinary bladder. Scand J Urol Nephrol 6:213–223, 1972.

83. Farrow GM, Utz DC, Rife CC, Greene LF: Clinical observations on sixty-nine cases of in situ carcinoma of the urinary bladder. Cancer Res 37(8 pt 2):2794–2798, 1977.

84. Elliott GB, Moloney PJ, Anderson GH: "Denuding cystitis" and in situ urothelial carcinoma. Arch Pathol 96:91–94, 1973.

85. Dona ST, Flamm J: The significance of bladder quadrant biopsies in patients with primary superficial bladder carcinoma. Eur Urol 16:81–85, 1989.

86. Mufti GR, Singh M: Value of random mucosal biopsies in the management of superficial bladder cancer. Eur Urol 22:288–293, 1992.

87. Zincke H, Utz DC, Farrow GM: Review of Mayo Clinic experience with carcinoma in situ. Urology 26(suppl):39–46, 1985.

88. Koss LG: Mapping of the urinary bladder. Its impact on the concepts of bladder cancer. Hum Pathol 10:533–549, 1979.

89. Richie JP, Skinner DG: Carcinoma in situ of the urethra associated with bladder carcinoma. The role of urethrectomy. J Urol 119:80–81, 1978.

90. Schellhammer PF, Whitmore Jr WF: Transitional cell carcinoma of the urethra in men having cystectomy for bladder cancer. J Urol 115:56–60, 1976.

91. Culp OSU, Utz DC, Harrison Jr EG: Experiences with ureteral carcinomas in situ detected during operations for vesical neoplasm. J Urol 97:679–682, 1967.

92. Sharma TC, Melamed MR, Whitmore Jr WF: Carcinoma in situ of the ureter in patients with bladder carcinoma treated by cystectomy. Cancer 26:583–587, 1970.

93. Schade ROK, Tubingen MD, Serck-Hanssen A, Swinney J: Morphological changes in the ureter in cases of bladder carcinoma. Cancer 27:1267–1272, 1971.

94. Skinner DG, Richie JP, Cooper PH, et al: The clinical significance of carcinoma in situ of the bladder and its association with overt carcinoma. J Urol 112:68–71, 1974.

95. McKenney JK, Gomez JA, Desai S, et al: Morphologic expressions of urothelial carcinoma in situ. A detailed evaluation of its histologic patterns with emphasis on carcinoma in situ with microinvasion. Am J Surg Pathol 25:356–362, 2001.

96. Boon ME, Ooms ECM: Carcinoma in situ of transitional cell epithelium. Clinical and pathological considerations. Prog Surg Pathol 8:153–168, 1988.

97. Murphy WM, Soloway MS: Urothelial dysplasia. J Urol 127:p. 849–854, 1982.

98. Malmstrom P-U, Busch C, Norlen BJ: Recurrence, progression and survival in bladder cancer. Scand J Urol Nephrol 21:185–195, 1987.

99. Mostofi FK, Setherhenn IA, Davis Jr CJ: Dysplasia versus atypia versus carcinoma in situ of bladder. In McCullough DL (ed): Difficult Diagnoses in Urology. New York, Churchill Livingstone, 1988.

100. Nagy GK, Friedell GHY: Urinary bladder. In Henson DE, Albores-Saavedra J (eds): Pathology of Incipient Neoplasia. 2nd ed. Philadelphia, WB Saunders, 1993.

101. Droller MJ: A rose is a rose, or is it? J Urol 136:1057–1058, 1986.

102. Prout GRJ, Griffin PP, Daly JJ: The outcome of conservative treatment of carcinoma in situ of the bladder. J Urol 138:766–770, 1987.

103. Stanisic TH, Donovan JM, Lebouton J, Graham AR: 5-year experience with intravesical therapy of carcinoma in situ. An inquiry into the risks of "conservative" management. J Urol 138:1158–1161, 1987.

104. Bretton PR, Herr HW, Whitmore Jr WF, et al: Intravesical bacillus Calmette-Guerin therapy for in situ transitional cell carcinoma involving the prostatic urethra. J Urol 141:853–856, 1989.

105. Amling CL, Thrasher JB, Dodge RK, et al: Radical cystectomy for stages Ta, Tis and T1 transitional cell carcinoma of the bladder. J Urol 151:31–35, 1994.

106. Malkowicz SB, Nichols P, Lieskovsky G, et al: The role of radical cystectomy in the management of high grade superficial bladder cancer (PA, P1, PIS and P2). J Urol 144:641–645, 1990.

107. Stein JP, Cote RJ, Freeman JA, et al: Indications for lower urinary tract reconstruction in women after cystectomy for bladder cancer. A pathological review of female cystectomy specimens. J Urol 154:1329–1333, 1995.

108. Stein JP, Grossfeld GD, Freeman JA, et al: Orthotopic lower urinary tract reconstruction in women using the Kock ileal neobladder. Updated experience in 34 patients. J Urol 158:400–405, 1997.

109. Jewett HJ, Strong GH: Infiltrating carcinoma of the bladder. Relation of the depth of penetration of the bladder wall to incidence of local extension and metastasis. J Urol 55:336–372, 1946.

110. Jewett HJ: Carcinoma of the bladder. Influence of depth infiltration on the 5-year results following complete extirpation of the primary growth. J Urol 67:672–676, 1952.

111. Marshall VF: The relation of the preoperative estimate of the pathologic demonstration of the extent of vesical neoplasms. J Urol 68:714–723, 1952.

112. Fleming ID, Cooper JS, Henson DE, et al: Urinary bladder. In: AJCC Cancer Staging Manual. Fleming, Irving D. Philadelphia, Lippincott-Raven, 1997, pp 241–243.

113. Smith JA, Batata M, Grabstald H: Preoperative irradiation and cystectomy for bladder cancer. Cancer 49:869–873, 1982.

114. Pagano F, Bassi P, Galetti TP: Results of contemporary radical cystectomy for invasive bladder cancer. A clinicopathological study with an emphasis on the inadequacy of the tumor, nodes, and metastases classification. J Urol 145:45–50, 1991.

115. Richie JP, Skinner DG, Kaufman JJ: Radical cystectomy for carcinoma of the bladder: 16 years experience. J Urol 113:186–189, 1975.

116. Abel PD: Prognostic indices in transitional cell carcinoma of the bladder. Br J Urol 62:103–109, 1988.

117. Hardman SW, Soloway MS: Transitional cell carcinoma of the prostate. Diagnosis, staging and management. World J Urol 8:170, 1988.

118. Esrig D, Freeman JA, Elamjian DA, et al: Transitional cell carcinoma involving the prostate with a proposed staging classification for stromal invasion. J Urol 156:1071–1076, 1996.

119. Abel PD, Hall RR, Williams G: Should pT1 transitional cell cancers of the bladder still be classified as superficial? Br J Urol 62:235–239, 1988.

120. Younes M, Sussman J, True LD: The usefulness of the level of the muscularis mucosae in the staging of invasive transitional cell carcinoma of the urinary bladder. Cancer 66:543–548, 1990.

121. Hasui Y, Osada Y, Kitada S, Nishi S: Significance of invasion to the muscularis mucosa on the progression of superficial bladder cancer. Urology 43:782–786, 1994.

122. Angulo JC, Lopez JI, Grignon DJ, Sanchez-Chapado M: Muscularis mucosa differentiates two populations with different prognosis in stage T1 bladder cancer. Urology 45:47–53, 1995.

123. Cheng L, Weaver AL, Neumann RM, et al: Substaging of T1 bladder cancer based on depth of invasion. A new proposal. Cancer 86:1035–1043, 1999.

124. Platz CE, Cohen MB, Jones MP, et al: Is microstaging of early invasive cancer of the urinary bladder possible or useful? Mod Pathol 9:1035–1039, 1996.

125. Jimenez RE, Keane TE, Hardy HT, Amin MB: pT1 urothelial carcinoma of the bladder. Criteria for diagnosis, pitfalls, and clinical implications. Adv Anat Pathol 7:13–25, 2000.

126. Lamina propria microinvasion of bladder tumors, incidence

on stage allocation (pTa vs pT1). Recommended approach. Pathologists of the French Association of Urology Cancer Committee. World J Urol 11:161–164, 1993.

127. Esrig D, Freeman JA, Stein JP, Skinner DG: Early cystectomy for clinical stage T1 transitional cell carcinoma of the bladder. Semin Oncol 15:154–160, 1997.

128. Dixon JS, Gosling JA: Histology and fine structure of the muscularis mucosae of the human urinary bladder. J Anat 136:265–271, 1983.

129. Ro J, Ayala AG, el-Naggar AK: Muscularis mucosa of urinary bladder. Importance for staging and treatment. Am J Surg Pathol 11:668–673, 1987.

130. Keep JC, Piehl M, Miller A, Oyasu R: Invasive carcinomas of the urinary bladder. Evaluation of tunica muscularis mucosae involvement. Am J Clin Pathol 91:575–579, 1989.

131. Bochner BH, Nichols PW, Skinner DG: Overstaging of transitional cell carcinoma. Clinical significance of lamina propria fat within the urinary bladder. Urology 45:528–531, 1995.

132. Farrow GM, Utz DC: Observations on microinvasive transitional cell carcinoma of the urinary bladder. Clin Oncol 1:609–614, 1982.

133. Amin MB, Gomez JA, Young RH: Urothelial transitional cell carcinoma with endophytic growth patterns. A discussion of patterns of invasion and problems associated with assessment of invasion of 18 cases. Am J Surg Pathol 21:1057–1068, 1997.

134. Young RH, Zuckerberg LR: Microcystic transitional cell carcinomas of the urinary bladder. Report of 4 cases. Am J Clin Pathol 96:635–639, 1991.

135. Young RH, Eble JN: Unusual forms of carcinomas of the urinary bladder. Hum Pathol 22:948–965, 1991.

136. Drew PA, Furman J, Civantos F, Murphy WM: The nested variant of transitional cell carcinoma. An aggressive neoplasm with innocuous histology. Mod Pathol 9:989–994, 1996.

137. Eble JN, Young RH: Carcinoma of the urinary bladder. A review of its diverse morphology. Semin Diag Pathol 14:98–108, 1997.

138. Bell JT, Burney SW, Friedell GH: Blood vessel invasion in human bladder cancer. J Urol 105:675–678, 1971.

139. Heney NM, Proppe K, Prout Jr GR, et al: Invasive bladder cancer. Tumor configuration, lymphatic invasion and survival. J Urol 130:895–897, 1983.

140. Jewett HJ, King LR, Shelley WM: A study of 365 cases of infiltrating bladder cancer. Relation of certain pathological characteristics to prognosis after extirpation. J Urol 92:668–678, 1964.

141. McDonald JR, Thompson GJ: Carcinoma of the urinary bladder. A pathologic study with a special reference to invasiveness and vascular invasion. J Urol 60:435–445, 1948.

142. Larsen MP, Steinberg GD, Brendler CB, Epstein JI: Use of *Ulex europaeus* agglutinin I (UEAI) to distinguish vascular and "pseudovascular" invasion in transitional cell carcinoma of bladder with lamina propria invasion. Mod Pathol 3:83–88, 1990.

143. Ramani P, Birch BR, Harland SJ, Parkinson MC: Evaluation of endothelial markers in detecting blood and lymphatic channel invasion in pT1 transitional carcinoma of bladder. Histopathology 19:551–554, 1991.

144. Stein JP, Lieskovsky G, Ginsberg DA, et al: The T pouch. An orthotopic ileal neobladder incorporating a serosal lined ileal antireflux technique. J Urol 159:1836–1842, 1998.

145. Smith JA, Whitmore WF: Regional lymph node metastasis from bladder cancer. J Urol 126:591–593, 1981.

146. Whitmore WF: Bladder cancer. An overview. CA Cancer J Clin 38:213–223, 1988.

147. Laplante M, Brice M: The upper limits of hopeful application of radical cystectomy for vesical carcinoma. Does nodal metastasis always indicate incurability? J Urol 109:261–264, 1973.

148. Skinner DG: Management of invasive bladder cancer. A meticulous pelvic lymph node dissection can make a difference. J Urol 128:34–36, 1982.

149. Cote RJ, Chatterjee SJ: Molecular determinants of outcome in bladder cancer. Cancer J Sci Am 5:2–15, 1999.

150. Cordon-Cardo C: Mutation of cell cycle regulators. Biological and clinical implications for human neoplasia. Am J Pathol 147:545–560, 1995.

151. Hollstein M, Sidransky D, Vogelstein B, Harris CC: *p53* Mutations in human cancers. Science 253:49–53, 1991.

152. Lane DP: *p53*, Guardian of the genome. Nature 358:15–16, 1992.

153. Xiong Y, Hannon GJ, Zhang H, et al: *p21* Is a universal inhibitor of cyclin kinases. Nature 366:701–704, 1993.

154. Esrig D, Elmajian D, Groshen S, et al: Accumulation of nuclear *p53* and tumor progression in bladder cancer. N Engl J Med 331:1259–1264, 1994.

155. Sarkis AS, Dalbagni G, Cordon-Cardo C, et al: Nuclear overexpression of p53 protein in transitional cell bladder carcinoma. A marker for disease progression. J Natl Cancer Inst 85:53–59, 1993.

156. Lipponen PK: Overexpression of p53 nuclear oncoprotein in transitional cell bladder cancer and its prognostic value. Int J Cancer 85:53–59, 1993.

157. Cordon-Cardo C, Wartinger D, Petrylak D, et al: Altered expression of the retinoblastoma gene product. Prognostic indicator in bladder cancer. J Natl Cancer Inst 84:1251–1256, 1992.

158. Cote RJ, Dunn MD, Chatterjee SJ, et al: Elevated and absent *pRb* expression is associated with bladder cancer progression, and has cooperative effects with *p53*. Cancer Res 58:1090–1094, 1998.

159. Stein JP, Ginsberg DA, Grossfeld GD, et al: The effect of p21WAF1/CIP1 expression on tumor progression in bladder cancer. J Natl Cancer Inst 90:1072–1079, 1998.

160. Folkman J, Cole P, Zimmerman S: Tumor behavior in isolated perfused organs. In vitro growth and metastasis of biopsy material in rabbit thyroid and canine intestinal segment. Ann Surg 164:491–502, 1966.

161. Dickinson AJ, Fox SB, Persad RA, et al: Quantification of angiogenesis as an independent predictor of prognosis in invasive bladder carcinomas. Br J Urol 74:762–766, 1994.

162. Jaeger TM, Weidner N, Chew K, et al: Tumor angiogenesis correlates with lymph node metastases in invasive bladder cancer. J Urol 154:69–71, 1995.

163. Dameron KM, Volpert OV, Tainsky MA, Bouck N: Control of angiogenesis in fibroblasts by *p53* regulation of thrombospondin-1. Science 265:1582–1584, 1994.

164. Grossfeld GD, Ginsberg DA, Stein JP, et al: Thrombospondin-1 expression in bladder cancer. Association with p53 alterations, tumor angiogenesis, and tumor progression. J Natl Cancer Inst 89:219–227, 1997.

165. Crew JP: Vascular endothelial growth factor: An important angiogenic mediator in bladder cancer. Eur Urol 35:2–8, 1999.

166. O'Brien T, Cranston D, Fuggle S, et al: Different angiogenic pathways characterize superficial and invasive bladder cancer. Cancer Res 55:510–513, 1995.

167. Crew JP, O'Brien T, Bradburn M, et al: Vascular endothelial growth factor is a predictor of relapse and stage progression in superficial bladder cancer. Cancer Res 57:5281–5285, 1997.

168. Viekkola T, Karkkainen M, Claesson-Welsh L, Alitalo K: Regulation of angiogenesis via vascular endothelial growth factor receptors. Cancer Res 60:203–212, 2000.

169. Campbell SC, Volpert OV, Ivanovich M, Bouck NP: Molecular mediators of angiogenesis in bladder cancer. Cancer Res 58:1298–1304, 1998.

170. Lloyd KO: Philip Levine award lecture. Blood group antigens as markers for normal differentiation and malignant change in human tissues. Am J Clin Pathol 87:129–139, 1987.

171. Cordon-Cardo C, Lloyd KO, Finstad CL, et al: Immunoanatomic distribution of blood group antigens in the human urinary tract. Influence of secretor status. Lab Invest 55:444–454, 1986.

172. Sheinfeld J, Reuter VE, Melamed MR, et al: Enhanced bladder cancer detection with the Lewis X antigen as a marker of neoplastic transformation. J Urol 143:285–288, 1990.

173. Fradet Y, Cordon-Cardo C: Critical appraisal of tumor markers in bladder cancer. Semin Urol 11:145–153, 1993.

174. Ross JS, Cohen MB: Detecting recurrent bladder cancer. New

methods and biomarkers. Expert Rev Mol Diag 1:39–52, 2001.

175. Sarosdy MF, deVere White RW, Soloway MS, et al: Results of a multicenter trial using the BTA test to monitor for and diagnose recurrent bladder cancer. J Urol 154(2 pt 1):379–383, 1995.

176. Murphy WM, Rivera-Ramirez I, Medina CA, et al: The bladder tumor antigen (BTA) test compared to voided urine cytology in the detection of bladder neoplasms. J Urol 158:2102–2106, 1997.

177. Soloway MS, Briggman V, Carpinito GA, et al: Use of a new tumor marker, urinary NMP22, in the detection of occult or rapidly recurring transitional cell carcinoma of the urinary tract following surgical treatment. J Urol 156:363–367, 1996.

178. Sauter G, Gasser TC, Moch H, et al: DNA aberrations in urinary bladder cancer detected by flow cytometry and FISH. Urol Res 25(suppl 1):S37–S43, 1997.

179. Reeder JE, O'Connell MJ, Yang Z, et al: DNA cytometry and chromosome 9 aberrations by fluorescence in situ hybridization of irrigation specimens from bladder cancer patients. Urology 51(5A suppl):58–61, 1998.

180. Bush C, Price P, Norton J, et al: Proliferation in human bladder carcinoma measure by Ki-67 antiboby labeling. Its potential clinical importance. Br J Cancer 64:357–360, 1991.

181. Mao L, Schoenberg MP, Scicchitano M, et al: Molecular detection of primary bladder cancer by microsatellite analysis. Science 271:659–662, 1996.

182. Lance RS, Aldous WK, Blaser J, Thrasher JB: Telomerase activity in solid transitional cell carcinoma, bladder, washings, and voided urine. Urol Oncol 4:43–49, 1998.

183. Muller M, Krause H, Heicappell R, et al: Comparison of human telomerase RNA and telomerase activity in urine for diagnosis of bladder cancer. Clin Cancer Res 4:1949–1954, 1998.

184. Strohmeyer TG, Slamon DJ: Proto-oncogenes and tumor suppressor genes in human urological malignancies. J Urol 151:1479–1497, 1994.

185. Fradet Y: Markers of prognosis in superficial bladder cancer. Semin Urol 10:28–38, 1992.

186. Slamon DJ, Godolphin W, Jones LA, et al: Studies of the HER-2/neu proto-oncogene in human breast and ovarian cancer. Science 244:707–712, 1989.

187. Sato K, Moriyama M, Mori S, et al: An immunohistologic evaluation of c-erbB-2 gene product in patients with urinary bladder carcinoma. Cancer 70:2493–2498, 1992.

188. Mellon JK, Lunec J, Wright C, et al: c-erbB-2 in bladder cancer. Molecular biology, correlation with epidermal growth factor receptors and prognostic value. J Urol 155:321–326, 1996.

189. Neal DE, Marsh C, Bennett MK, et al: Epidermal-growth factor receptors in human bladder cancer. Comparison of invasive and surperficial tumours. Lancet 1:366–368, 1985.

190. Messing EM, Hanson P, Ulrich P, Erturk E: Epidermal growth factor—interactions with normal and malignant urothelium. In vivo and in situ studies. J Urol 138:1329–1335, 1987.

191. Stein JP, Grossfeld GD, Ginsberg DA, et al: Prognostic markers in bladder cancer. A contemporary review of the literature. J Urol 160:645–659, 1998.

192. Cohen MB, Griebling TL, Ahaghotu CA, et al: Cellular adhesion molecules in urologic malignancies. Am J Clin Pathol 107:56–63, 1997.

193. Lowe SW, Bodis S, McClatchey A, et al: p53 Status and the efficacy of cancer therapy in vivo. Science 266:807–810, 1994.

194. Lowe SW, Ruley HE, Jacks T, Housman DE: p53-Dependent apoptosis modulates the cytotoxicity of anticancer agents. Cell 74:957–967, 1993.

195. Bergh J, Norberg T, Sjogren S, et al: Complete sequencing of the p53 gene provides prognostic information in breast cancer patients, particularly in relation to adjuvant systemic therapy and radiotherapy. Nat Med 1:1029–1034, 1995.

196. Waldman T, Lengauer C, Kinzler KW, Vogelstein B: Uncoupling of S phase and mitosis induced by anticancer agents in cells lacking p21. Nature 381:713–716, 1996.

197. Fan S, Smith ML, Rivet II DJ, et al: Disruption of p53 func-

198. Hawkins DS, Derners W, Galloway DA: Inactivation of p53 enhances sensitivity to multiple chemotherapeutic agents. Cancer Res 56:892–898, 1996.

199. Wahl AF, Donaldson KL, Fairchild C, et al: Loss of normal p53 function confers sensitization to Taxol by increasing $G_2/M$ arrest and apoptosis. Nat Med 2:72–79, 1996.

200. Wang Q, Fan S, Eastman A, et al: UCN-01. A potent abrogator of $G_2$ checkpoint function in cancer cells with disrupted p53. J Natl Cancer Inst 88:956–965, 1996.

201. Cote RJ, Esrig D, Groshen S, et al: p53 and treatment of bladder cancer. Nature 385:123–125, 1997.

202. Deisseroth AB, DeVita VT: The cell cycle. Probing new molecular determinants of resistance and sensitivity to cytotoxic agents. Cancer J Sci Am 1:15–21, 1995.

203. Wang NP, Zee S, Zarbo RJ, et al: Coordinate expression of cytokeratins 7 and 20 defines unique subsets of carcinomas. Appl Immunohistochem Mol Morphol 3:99–107, 1995.

204. Baars JH, De Ruijter JL, Smedts F, et al: The applicability of a keratin 7 monoclonal antibody in routinely Papanicolaou-stained cytologic specimens for the differential diagnosis of carcinomas. Am J Clin Pathol 101:257–261, 1995.

205. Bassily NH, Vallorosi CJ, Akdas G, et al: Coordinate expression of cytokeratins 7 and 20 in prostate adenocarcinoma and bladder urothelial carcinoma. Am J Clin Pathol 113:383–388, 2000.

206. Chu P, Wu E, Weiss LM: Cytokeratin 7 and cytokeratin 20 expression in epithelial neoplasms. A survey of 435 cases. Mod Pathol 13:962–972, 2000.

207. Ordonez NG: Thrombomodulin expression in transitional cell carcinoma. Am J Clin Pathol 110:385–390, 1998.

208. Xu X, Sun TT, Prabodh K, et al: Uroplakin as a marker for typing metastatic transitional cell carcinoma on fine-needle aspiration specimens. Cancer Cytopathol 93:216–221, 2001.

209. Amin MB, Ro JY, El-Sharkawy T, et al: Micropapillary variant of transitional cell carcinoma of the urinary bladder. Am J Surg Pathol 18:1224–1232, 1994.

210. Smith JA, Herr HA, Middleton RG: Bladder carcinosarcoma. Histologic variation in metastatic lesions. J Urol 129:829–831, 1983.

211. Kusaba Y, Yushita Y, Suzu H, et al: Carcinosarcoma of the bladder. J Urol 131:118–119, 1984.

212. Young RH, Wick MR, Mills SE: Sarcomatoid carcinoma of the urinary bladder. A clinicopathologic analysis of 12 cases and review of the literature. Am J Clin Pathol 90:653–661, 1988.

213. Ro JY, Ayala AG, Wishnow KI: Sarcomatoid bladder carcinoma. Clinical, pathological, and immunohistochemical study of 44 cases. Surg Pathol 1:359–374, 1988.

214. Amin MB, Ro JY, Lee KM, et al: Lymphoepithelioma-like carcinoma of the urinary bladder. Am J Surg Pathol 18:466–473, 1994.

215. Gulley ML, Amin MB, Nicholls JM, et al: Epstein-Barr virus is detected in undifferentiated nasopharyngeal carcinoma but not in lymphoepithelioma-like carcinoma of the urinary bladder. Hum Pathol 26:1207–1214, 1995.

216. Holmang S, Borghede G, Johansson SL: Bladder carcinoma with lymphoepithelioma-like differentiation. A report of 9 cases. J Urol 159:779–782, 1998.

217. Blomjous CEM, Vos W, De Voogt HJ, et al: Small cell carcinoma of the urinary bladder. A clinicopathologic, morphometric, immunohistochemical, and ultrastructural study of 18 cases. Cancer 64:1347–1357, 1989.

218. Grignon DJ, Ro JY, Ayala AG, et al: Small cell carcinoma of the urinary bladder. A clinicopathologic analysis of 22 cases. Cancer 69:527–536, 1992.

219. Mills SE, Wolfe III JT, Weiss MA, et al: Small cell undifferentiated carcinoma of the urinary bladder. A light-microscopic, immunocytochemical, and ultrastructural study of 12 cases. Am J Surg Pathol 11:606–617, 1987.

220. Hailemariam S, Gaspert A, Komminoth P, et al: Primary, pure, large-cell neuroendocrine carcinoma of the urinary bladder. Mod Pathol 11:1016–1020, 1998.

221. Angulo JC, Lopez JI, Sanchez-Chapado ML: Small cell carci-

noma of the urinary bladder. A report of two cases with complete remission and a comprehensive literature review with emphasis on therapeutic decision. J Urol Pathol 5:9–28, 1996.

222. Tetu B, Ro JY, Ayala AG, et al: Small cell carcinoma of the prostate. Part I. A clinicopathologic study of 20 cases. Cancer 59:1803–1809, 1987.
223. Amin MB, Murphy WM, Reuter VE, et al: Controversies in the pathology of transitional cell carcinoma of the urinary bladder. Part I, Chapter 1. In: Reviews of Pathology, 1996, Vol. I. Editors: Rosen PP, Fechner RE. ASCP Press, Chicago, IL, pp 1–39.
224. Talbert WM, Young RH: Carcinoma of the urinary bladder with deceptively benign appearing foci. A report of three cases. Am J Surg Pathol 13:374–381, 1989.
225. Paz A, Rath-Wolfson L, Lask D, et al: The clinical and histological features of transitional cell carcinoma of the bladder with microcysts. Analysis of 12 cases. Br J Urol 79:722–725, 1997.
226. Murphy WM, Deana DG: The nested variant of transitional cell carcinoma. A neoplasm resembling proliferation of Brunn's nests. Mod Pathol 5:240–243, 1992.
227. Paulsen JC, Metawalli N, Wu B, Nachomovitz L: Transitional cell carcinoma of the urinary bladder with features of inverted papilloma. Mod Pathol 11:710–718, 1988.
228. Jacobo E, Loening S, Schmidt JD, Culp DA: Primary adenocarcinoma of the bladder. A retrospective study of 20 patients. J Urol 117:54–56, 1977.
229. Thomas DG, Ward AM, Williams JL: A study of 52 cases of adenocarcinoma of the bladder. Br J Urol 43:4–15, 1971.
230. Abenoza P, Manivel C, Fraley EE: Primary adenocarcinoma of urinary bladder. Clinicopathologic study of 16 cases. Urology 29:9–14, 1987.
231. Goyanna R, Emmett JL, McDonald JR: Extrophy of the bladder complicated by adenocarcinoma. J Urol 65:391–400, 1951.
232. Grignon DJ, Ro JY, Ayala AG, et al: Primary adenocarcinoma of the urinary bladder. A clinicopathologic analysis of 72 cases. Cancer 67:2165–2172, 1991.
233. Foschini MP, Baccarini P, Dal Monte PR, et al: Albumin gene expression in adenocarcinomas with hepatoid differentiation. Virchow Arch 433:537–541, 1998.
234. Burgues O, Ferrer J, Navarro S, et al: Hepatoid adenocarcinoma of the urinary bladder. An unusual neoplasm. Virchows Arch 435:71–75, 1999.
235. Ford TF, Watson GM, Cameron KM: Adenomatous metaplasia (nephrogenic adenoma) of urothelium. An analysis of 70 cases. Br J Urol 57:427–433, 1985.
236. Young RH, Scully RE: Nephrogenic adenoma. Am J Surg Pathol 10:268–275, 1986.
237. Saphir O: Signet-ring cell carcinoma of the bladder. Am J Surg Pathol 31:223–231, 1955.
238. Mostofi FK, Thomson RV, Dean Jr AL: Mucous adenocarcinoma of the urinary bladder. Cancer 8:741–758, 1955.
239. Grignon DJ, Ro JY, Ayala AG, et al: Primary signet-ring cell carcinoma of the urinary bladder. Am J Clin Pathol 95:13–20, 1991.
240. El-Bolkainy MN, Mokhtar NM, Ghoneim MA, Hussein MH: The impact of schistosomiasis on the pathology of bladder carcinoma. Cancer 48:2643–2648, 1981.
241. Sarma KP: Squamous cell carcinoma of the bladder. Int Surg 53:313–318, 1970.
242. Faysal MH, Freiha FS: Primary neoplasms in vesical diverticula. A report of 12 cases. Br J Urol 53:141–143, 1981.
243. Pearlman CK, Bobbitt RM: Carcinoma within a diverticulum of the bladder. J Urol 59:1127–1129, 1948.
244. Stuart WT: Carcinoma of the bladder associated with exstrophy. Report of a case and review of the literature. Va Med Mon 89:39–42, 1962.
245. Markl ID, Jones PA: Presence and location of TP53 mutation determines pattern of CDKNN2A/ARF pathway inactivation in bladder cancer. Cancer Res 58:5348–5353, 1999.
246. Del Mistro A, Koss LG, Braunstein J, et al: Condylomata acuminata of the urinary bladder. Natural history, viral typing, and DNA content. Am J Surg Pathol 12:205–215, 1988.
247. Newman DM, Brown JR, Jay AC, Pontius EE: Squamous cell carcinoma of the bladder. J Urol 100:470–473, 1968.

248. Richie JP, Waisman J, Skinner DG, Dretler SP: Squamous carcinoma of the bladder. Treatment by radical cystectomy. J Urol 115:670–672, 1976.
249. Jones WA, Gibbons RP, Correa Jr RJ, et al: Primary adenocarcinoma of the bladder. Urology 15:119–122, 1980.
250. Pallesen G: Neoplastic Paneth cells in adenocarcinoma of urinary bladder. A first case report. Cancer 47:1834–1837, 1981.
251. Wilson TG, Pritchett TR, Lieskovsky G, et al: Primary adenocarcinoma of bladder. Urology 38:223–226, 1991.
252. Sheldon CA, Clayman RV, Gonzalez R, et al: Malignant urachal lesions. J Urol 131:1–8, 1984.
253. Jacobs MA, Bavendam TG, Leach GE: Bladder leiomyoma. J Urol 34:56–57, 1989.
254. Mintz ER: Pedunculated neurofibroma of the bladder. J Urol 43:268–274, 1940.
255. Bolkier M, Ginesin Y, Lichtig C, Levin DR: Lymphangioma of bladder. J Urol 129:1049–1050, 1983.
256. Wyman HE, Chappell BS, Jones Jr WR: Ganglioneuroma of bladder. A report of a case. J Urol 63:526–532, 1950.
257. Mouradian J, Coleman JW, McGovern JH, Gray GF: Granular cell tumor (myoblastoma) of the bladder. J Urol 112:343–345, 1974.
258. Knoll LD, Segura JW, Scheithauer BW: Leiomyoma of the bladder. J Urol 136:906–908, 1986.
259. Bramwell SP, Pitts J, Goudie SE, Abel BJ: Giant leiomyoma of the bladder. Br J Urol 60:178–184, 1987.
260. Mills SE, Bova GS, Wick MR, Young RH: Leiomyosarcoma of the urinary bladder. A clinicopathologic and immunohistochemical study of 15 cases. Am J Surg Pathol 13:480–489, 1989.
261. Mackenzie AR, Whitmore Jr WF, Melamed MR: Myosarcomas of the bladder and prostate. Cancer 22:833–844, 1968.
262. Russo P, Brady MS, Conlon K, et al: Adult urological sarcoma. J Urol 147:1032–1036, 1992.
263. Maurer HM: The intergroup rhabdomyosarcoma study (NIH). Objectives and clinical staging classification. J Pediatr Surg 10:977–978, 1975.
264. Scholtmeijer RJ, Tromp CG, Hazebroeck FWJ: Embryonal rhabdomyosarcoma of the urogenital tract in childhood. Eur Urol 9:69–74, 1983.
265. Fellinger EJ, Garin-Chesa P, Su SL, et al: Biochemical and genetic characterization of the HBA71 Ewing's sarcoma cell surface antigen. Cancer Res 51:336–340, 1991.
266. Fellinger EJ, Garin-Chesa P, Triche TH, et al: Immunohistochemical analysis of Ewing's sarcoma cell surface antigen p30/32MIC2. Am J Surg Pathol 139:317–325, 1991.
267. Hendricksson C, Zetterlund CG, Boisen P, Pattersson S: Large rhabdomyosarcoma of the urinary bladder in an adult. Scand J Urol Nephrol 19:237–239, 1985.
268. Hays DM, Raney Jr RB, Lawrence Jr W, et al: Bladder and prostatic tumors in the Intergroup Rhabdomyosarcoma Study (IRS-I). Results of therapy. Cancer 50:1472–1482, 1982.
269. Bohne AW, Urwiller RD, Pantos TG: Leiomyosarcoma of the urinary bladder with review of the literature. Henry Ford Hosp Med Bull 10:445–448, 1962.
270. Reeves JFJ, Powell EB, Powell NB: Leiomyosarcoma of the bladder. Case report with autopsy. J Urol 97:486–489, 1967.
271. Gallagher L, Lind R, Oyasu R: Primary choriocarcinoma of the urinary bladder in association with undifferentiation carcinoma. Hum Pathol 11:793–795, 1984.
272. Jones EC, Young RH: Nonneoplastic and neoplastic spindle cell proliferations and mixed tumors of the urinary bladder. J Urol Pathol 2:105–134, 1994.
273. Jones EC, Clement PB, Young RH: Inflammatory pseudotumor of the urinary bladder. Am J Clin Pathol 17:264–274, 1994.
274. Ro JY, Ayala AG, Ordonez NG, et al: Pseudosarcomatous fibromyxoid tumor of the urinary bladder. Am J Clin Pathol 86:583–590, 1986.
275. Ro JY, el-Naggar AK, Amin MB, et al: Pseudosarcomatous fibromyxoid tumor of the urinary bladder and prostate. Immunohistochemical, ultrastructural, and DNA flow cytometric analyses of nine cases. Hum Pathol 24:1203–1210, 1993.
276. Nochomovitz LE, Orenstein JM: Inflammatory pseudotumor

of the urinary bladder—possible relationship to nodular fascitis. Am J Surg Pathol 9:366–373, 1985.

277. Wick MR, Brown BA, Young RH, Mills SE: Spindle-cell proliferations of the urinary tract. An immunohistochemical study. Am J Surg Pathol 12:379–389, 1988.

278. Proppe KH, Scully RE, Rosai J: Postoperative spindle cell nodules of genitourinary tract resembling sarcomas. A report of eight cases. Am J Surg Pathol 8:101–108, 1984.

279. Vekemans K, Vanneste A, Van Oyen P, et al: Postoperative spindle cell nodule of bladder. Urology 35:342–344, 1990.

280. Huang WL, Ro JY, Grignon DJ, et al: Postoperative spindle cell nodule of the prostate and bladder. J Urology 143:824–826, 1990.

281. Swartz DA, Johnson DE, Ayala AG, Watkins DL: Bladder leiomyosarcoma. A review of 10 cases with 5-year follow-up. J Urol 133:200–202, 1985.

282. Goodman AJ, Greany MG: Malignant fibrous histiocytoma of the bladder. Br J Urol 57:106–107, 1985.

283. Young RH, Rosenberg AE: Osteosarcoma of the urinary bladder. Report of a case and review of the literature. Cancer 59:174–178, 1987.

284. Stroup RM, Chang YC: Angiosarcoma of the bladder. A case report. J Urol 137:984–985, 1987.

285. Sutton R, Hopper IP, Munson KW: Haemangiopericytoma of the bladder. Br J Urol 63:548–554, 1989.

286. Ainsworth AM, Clark WH, Mastrangelo M, Conger KB: Primary malignant melanoma of the urinary bladder. Cancer 37:1928–1936, 1976.

287. Anichkov NM, Nikonov AA: Primary malignant melanomas of the urinary bladder. J Urol 128:813–815, 1982.

288. Van Ahlen H, Nicolas V, Lenz W, et al: Primary melanoma of urinary bladder. Urology 40:550–554, 1992.

289. Stein DS, Kendall AR: Malignant melanoma of the genitourinary tract. J Urol 132:859–868, 1984.

290. Freeman C, Berg JW, Cutler ST: Occurrence and prognosis of extranodal lymphomas. Cancer 29:252–260, 1972.

291. Chaitin BA, Manning JT, Ordonez NG: Hematologic neoplasms with initial manifestations in lower urinary tract. Urology 23:35–42, 1984.

292. Yang CH, Krzyzaniak K, Brown W, Kurtz SM: Primary carcinoid tumor of urinary bladder. Urology 26:594–597, 1985.

293. Colby TV: Carcinoid tumor of the bladder. Arch Pathol Lab Med 104:199–200, 1980.

294. Albores-Saavedra J, Maldonado ME, Ibarra J, Rodriguez HA: Pheochromocytoma of the urinary bladder. Cancer 23:1110–1118, 1969.

295. Kliewer KE, Wen DR, Cancilla PA, Cochran AJ: Paragangliomas. Assessment of prognosis by histologic, immunohistochemical, and ultrastructural techniques. Hum Pathol 20:29–39, 1989.

296. Hamond MEH, Henson DE: Urinary bladder, ureter, renal pelvis. In College of American Pathology: Cancer Protocol Manual, 2000. Available at http://www.cap.html.publications/cancerfactsheet.html.

297. Murphy WM: Recommendations for the reporting of urinary bladder specimens containing bladder neoplasm. With commentary. Pathol Case Rev 3:233–236, 1998.

298. Spevack L, Herschorn S, Srigley J: Inverted papilloma of the upper urinary tract. J Urol 153:1202–1204, 1995.

299. Uyama T, Nakamura S, Moriwaki S: Inverted papilloma of bladder. Two cases with questionable malignancy and squamous metaplasia. Urology 16:152–154, 1980.

300. Caro DJ, Tessler A: Inverted papilloma of the bladder. A distinct urological lesion. Cancer 42:708–713, 1978.

301. Goertchen R, Seidenschnur A, Stosiek P: Clinical pathology of inverted papillomas of the urinary bladder. A complex morphologic and catamnestic study (2) [German]. Pathologe 15:279–285, 1994.

302. Urakami S, Igawa M, Shirakawa H, et al: Biological characteristics of inverted papilloma of the urinary bladder. Br J Urol 77:55–60, 1996.

303. Wu TT, Wang JS, Huang JK, et al: Inverted papilloma of the urinary bladder. Chung Hua I Hsueh Tsa Chih 57:59–63, 1996.

304. de Knijff DW, Theunissen PH, Delaere KP: Inverted papil-

loma of the ureter with subsequent invasive bladder cancer. Acta Urol Belg 65:45–46, 1997.

305. Witjes JA, van Balken MR, van de Kaa CA: The prognostic value of a primary inverted papilloma of the urinary tract. J Urol 158:1500–1505, 1997.

306. Bissada NK, Cole AT, Fried FA: Extensive condylomas acuminata of the entire male urethra and the bladder. J Urol 112:201–203, 1974.

307. Isimbaldi G, Di Nuovo F, Sironi M, et al: Nephrogenic adenoma of the bladder. Morphological and immunophenotypic study with particular attention to differential diagnosis [Italian]. Pathologica 91:192–197, 1999.

308. Kilciler M, Tan O, Ozgok Y, et al: Nephrogenic adenoma of the bladder after intravesical bacillus Calmette-Guerin treatment. Urol Int 64:229–232, 2000.

309. Kajita Y, Mizutani Y, Okuno H, et al: Three cases of the nephrogenic adenoma of the bladder [Japanese]. Hinyokika Kiyo 44:669–670, 1998.

310. Ashida S, Yamamoto A, Oka N, et al: Nephrogenic adenoma of the bladder in a chronic hemodialysis patient. Int J Urol 6:208–210, 1999.

311. Greco A, Giammo A, Tizzani A: Nephrogenic adenoma arising from an urethral diverticulum in a female. Report of a case and review of the literature [Italian]. Minerva Urol Nefrol 51:39–43, 1999.

312. Peeker R, Aldenborg F, Fall M: Nephrogenic adenoma—a study with special reference to clinical presentation. Br J Urol 80:539–542, 1997.

313. Oliva E, Young RH: Clear cell adenocarcinoma of the urethra. A clinicopathologic analysis of 19 cases. Mod Pathol 9:513–520, 1996.

314. Gilcrease MZ, Delgado R, Vuitch F, Albores-Saavedra J: Clear cell adenocarcinoma and nephrogenic adenoma of the urethra and urinary bladder. A histopathologic and immunohistochemical comparison. Hum Pathol 29:1451–1456, 1998.

315. Assor D: A villous tumor of the bladder. J Urol 119:287–288, 1978.

316. Eble JN, Hull MT, Rowland RG, Hostetter M: Villous adenoma of the urachus with mucusuria. A light and electron microscopic study. J Urol 135:1240–1244, 1986.

317. Westney OL, Amundsen CL, McGuire EJ: Bladder endometriosis. Conservative management. J Urol 163:1814–1817, 2000.

318. Blaustein EBK, Kurmann RJ: Blaustein's Pathology of the Female Genital Tract. 4th ed. New York, Springer-Verlag, 1994.

319. Pinkert TC, Catlow CE, Strauss R: Endometriosis of the urinary bladder in a man with prostatic carcinoma. Cancer 43:1562–1567, 1979.

320. Nada W, Parker J, Wong F, et al: Laparoscopic excision of endocervicosis of the urinary bladder. J Am Assoc Gynecol Laparosc 71:135–137, 2000.

321. Clement PB, Young RH: Endocervicosis of the urinary bladder. A report of six cases of a benign mullerian lesion that may mimic adenocarcinoma. Am J Surg Pathol 16:533–542, 1992.

322. Young RH, Clement PB: Endocervicosis involving the uterine cervix. A report of four cases of a benign process that may be confused with deeply invasive endocervical adenocarcinoma. Int J Gynecol Pathol 19:322–328, 2000.

323. Parivar F, Bolton DM, Stoller M: Endocervicosis of the bladder. J Urol 153:1218–1219, 1995.

324. Tieng EB, Simon C, Sabanegh ES: Adult pseudosarcoma of the bladder. Urology 53:1228, 1999.

325. Jufe R, Molinolo AA, Fefer SA, Meiss RP: Plasma cell granuloma of the bladder: A case report. J Urol 131:1175–1176, 1984.

326. Noda S, Eto K: Histopathological studies on the cystic formation of the human urothelium. Kurume Med J 37:55–65, 1990.

327. Jarvi OH, Marin S: Intestinal mucosal heterotopia of an urethral caruncle. Acta Pathol Microbiol Immunol Scand 9:213–219, 1982.

328. Willett GD, Lack EE: Periurethral colonic-type polyp simulat-

ing urethral caruncle. A case report. J Reprod Med 35:1017–1018, 1990.

329. Wallin JE, Thompson SE, Zaidi A, Wong KH: Urethritis in women attending an STD clinic. Br J Vener Dis 57:50–54, 1981.

330. Elbadawi A, Malhoski WE, Frank IN: Mucinous urethral caruncle. Urology 12:587–590, 1978.

331. Godwin JT, Hanash K: Pathology of bilharzial bladder cancer. Prog Clin Biol Res 162:95–143, 1984.

332. Young RH: Pseudoneoplastic lesions of the urinary bladder and urethra. A selective review with emphasis on recent information. Semin Diag Pathol 14:133–146, 1997.

333. Bates AW, Dev S, Baithun SI: Malakoplakia and colorectal adenocarcinoma. Postgrad Med J 73:171–173, 1997.

334. Mitchell MA, Markovitz DM, Killen PD, Braun DK: Bilateral renal parenchymal malacoplakia presenting as fever of unknown origin. Case report and review. Clin Infect Dis 18:704–718, 1994.

335. Curran FT: Malakoplakia of the bladder. Br J Urol 59:559–563, 1987.

336. Long JP, Althausen AF: Malacoplakia. A 25-year experience with a review of the literature. J Urol 141:1328–1331, 1989.

337. Van der Voort HJ, Ten Velden JA, Wassenaar RP, Silberbusch J: Malacoplakia. Two case reports and a comparison of treatment modalities based on a literature review. Arch Intern Med 156:577–583, 1996.

338. Sugiyama T, Kaneko A, Saitoh Y, et al: A case of lupus cystitis—interstitial cystitis as a local manifestation of systemic lupus erythematosus in the bladder [Japanese]. Ryumachi 26:22–28, 1986.

339. Elbadawi A: Interstitial cystitis. A critique of current concepts with a new proposal for pathologic diagnosis and pathogenesis. Urology 49(5A suppl):14–40, 1997.

340. Theoharides TC, Pang X, Letourneau R, Sant GR: Interstitial cystitis. A neuroimmunoendocrine disorder. Ann N Y Acad Sci 840:619–634, 1998.

341. Sant GR, Theoharides TC, Letourneau R, Gelfand J: Interstitial cystitis and bladder mastocytosis in a woman with chronic urticaria. Scand J Urol Nephrol 31:497–500, 1997.

342. Smith BH, Dehner LP: Chronic ulcerating interstitial cystitis (Hunner's ulcer). A study of 28 cases. Arch Pathol Lab Med 93:76–81, 1972.

343. Maatman TJ, Novick AC, Montague DK, Levin HS: Radiation-induced cystitis following intracavitary irradiation for superficial bladder cancer. J Urol 130:338–339, 1983.

344. Suzuki K, Kurokawa K, Suzuki T, et al: Successful treatment of radiation cystitis with hyperbaric oxygen therapy. Resolution of bleeding event and changes of histopathological findings of the bladder mucosa. Int Urol Nephrol 30:267–271, 1998.

345. Pode D, Perlberg S, Steiner D: Busulfan-induced hemorrhagic cystitis. J Urol 130:347–348, 1983.

346. Jerkins GR, Noe HN, Hill D: Treatment of complications of cyclophosphamide cystitis. J Urol 139:923–925, 1988.

347. Algaba F: Papillo-polypoid cystitis. Focal cystitis with pseudoneoplastic aspect [Spanish]. Acta Urol Espan 15:260–264, 1991.

348. Buck E: Polypoid cystitis mimicking transitional cell carcinoma. J Urol 131:963, 1984.

349. Epstein JI (ed): Differential Diagnosis in Pathology: Urologic Disorders. New York, Igaku-Shoin Medical Medical Publishers, 1992.

350. Silverberg SG: Principles and Practice of Surgical Pathology and Cytopathology. Vol 3. 3rd ed. New York, Churchill Livingstone, 1997.

351. Crankson SJ, Ahmed S: Female bladder exstrophy. Int Urogynecol J Pelvic Floor Dysfunction 8:98–104, 1997.

352. Pieretti RV, Pieretti-Vanmarcke RV: Congenital bladder diverticula in children. J Pediatr Surg 34:468–173, 1999.

353. Baniel J, Vishna T: Primary transitional cell carcinoma in vesical diverticula. Urology 50:697–699, 1997.

354. Grigsby PW, Corn BW: Localized urethral tumors in women. Indications for conservative versus exenterative therapies. J Urol 147:1516–1520, 1992.

355. Foster RS, Garrett RA: Congenital posterior urethral polyps. J Urol 136:670–672, 1986.

356. Dalens B, Vanneuville G, Vincent L, Fabre JL: Congenital polyp of the posterior urethra and vesical calculus in a boy. J Urol 128:1034–1035, 1982.

357. Nellans RE, Stein JJ: Pedunculated polyp of posterior urethra. Urology 6:474–475, 1975.

358. Kesner KM: Extensive condylomata acuminata of male urethra. Management by ventral urethrotomy. Br J Urol 71:204–207, 1993.

# 32

# Surgical Pathology of the Prostate

David G. Bostwick

Despite its relatively small size, the prostate accounts for a substantial and disproportionate incidence of health problems in older men, including prostatitis, obstructive symptoms resulting from nodular hyperplasia, and cancer.

## ANATOMY AND HISTOLOGY

### Gross Anatomy

The prostate is composed of three zones: 1) peripheral zone, 2) central zone, and 3) transition zone.[1]

The peripheral zone contains about 70% of the volume of the prostate and is the most common site of prostatic intraepithelial neoplasia (PIN) and carcinoma. The central zone is a cone-shaped area that includes the entire base of the prostate and encompasses the ejaculatory ducts; it comprises about 25% of the volume of the prostate. The existence of the central zone has been questioned, and most authors now combine it with the peripheral zone (awkwardly referred to together as the *nontransition zone*). Digital rectal examination often includes a description of the left and right "lobes" based on palpation of the median furrow in the midline that divides the nontransition zone into left and right halves. The transition zone contains the smallest volume of the normal prostate, about 5%, but usually enlarges together with the anterior fibromuscular stroma to massive size as a result of benign prostatic hyperplasia and dwarfs the remainder of the prostate.

Running through the prostate is the prostatic urethra, which has a central 35° bend, creating proximal and distal segments of equal length. The verumontanum bulges from the posterior wall at the urethral bend and tapers distally to form the crista urethralis. Most prostatic ducts and the ejaculatory ducts empty into the urethra in this part of the mid and distal prostatic urethra, whereas the small periurethral glands have ducts throughout the length of the urethra. Just proximal to the verumontanum is a müllerian remnant, the utricle, a small 0.5-cm-long, epithelium-lined cul-de-sac. A circumferential sleeve of muscle surrounds the entire urethra. This muscular layer includes a proximal preprostatic smooth muscle sphincter that prevents retrograde ejaculation and a distal sphincter of striated and smooth muscle at the apex that is important in control of micturition.

The capsule of the prostate consists of an inner layer of smooth muscle and an outer covering of collagen, with marked variability in the relative amounts in different areas. At the apex, the acinar elements become sparse and the capsule becomes ill defined, composed of a mixture of fibrous connective tissue, smooth muscle, and striated muscle. Similarly, at the base, the smooth muscle of the prostate merges with the bladder neck musculature, and there is no distinct division at this site. As a result, the prostatic capsule is not a well-defined anatomic structure with constant features,[2] and it is not possible to determine the presence of extraprostatic extension of cancer at the apex and base.

The prostatic blood supply is furnished by one of the branches of the internal iliac artery. Veins drain directly into the prostatic plexus, and an extensive arborizing network is present in the capsule. The venous drainage empties into the internal iliac vein. Lymphatics from the prostate drain mainly into the internal iliac lymph nodes, with lesser drainage into the external iliac and sacral lymph nodes.

Prostatic nerves arise from paired neurovascular bundles that run along the posterolateral edge of the prostate from apex to base. Surgical sparing of these structures during radical prostatectomy may preserve sexual potency. Autonomic ganglia are clustered near the neurovascular bundles, sending out small nerve trunks that arborize over the surface of the prostate, penetrating through the capsule and branching to form an extensive network of nerve twigs within the prostate that are often in intimate contact with the walls of ducts and acini. Ganglion cells may be found occasionally within the substance of the prostate.[3]

The seminal vesicles are bounded by the prostate distally, the base of the bladder anteriorly, and

Denonvillier's fascia and the rectum posteriorly. Their anatomic distribution in this region is variable, and they occasionally are found within the capsule of the prostate gland. The seminal vesicles may be palpable on digital rectal examination and, when intimately associated with the prostate, may be mistaken for prostatic nodularity or induration. Of prostate biopsy specimens for nodularity, 20% contain fragments of seminal vesicle epithelium, a potential source of diagnostic confusion.

The seminal vesicle mucosa displays complex papillary folds and irregular convoluted lumina, and the lining cells are predominately secretory, with microvesicular lipid droplets and characteristic lipofuscin pigment granules (Fig. 32–1). The pigment is granular (1 to 2 $\mu$ diameter), abundant, golden brown, and refractile, increasing in amount with age; conversely, lipochrome pigment granules in prostatic epithelium are coarse-to-fine, generally smaller (0.25 to 4 $\mu$), scant or variable in amount, and poorly refractile or nonrefractile.[4] These cells express androgen receptors similar to the prostatic epithelium, but not prostate-specific antigen (PSA) or prostatic acid phosphatase (PAP).[4] The seminal vesicles begin to shrink in men in their 60s. The tall columnar cells lining the mucosa in young men are replaced slowly by flattened cuboidal cells. With advancing age, the stroma of the seminal vesicles becomes hyalinized and fibrotic. The flattening of the epithelium is accompanied by striking nuclear abnormalities, and highly atypical cells are present in about 75% of seminal vesicles in older men. When encountered in needle biopsy specimens, such pseudomalignant cytologic atypia may lead to a mistaken diagnosis of prostatic carcinoma. DNA content analysis reveals aneuploidy in 6.7% of seminal vesicles.[5]

Cowper's glands are small, paired bulbomembranous urethral glands that may be mistaken for prostatic carcinoma in biopsy specimens. These glands are composed of lobules of closely packed uniform acini lined by cytologically benign cells

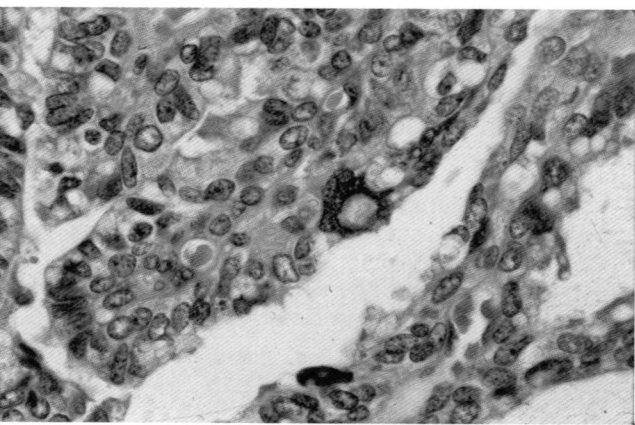

**FIGURE 32–1.** Seminal vesicle epithelium contains occasional bizarre giant cells and variable amounts of golden brown lipfuscin pigment.

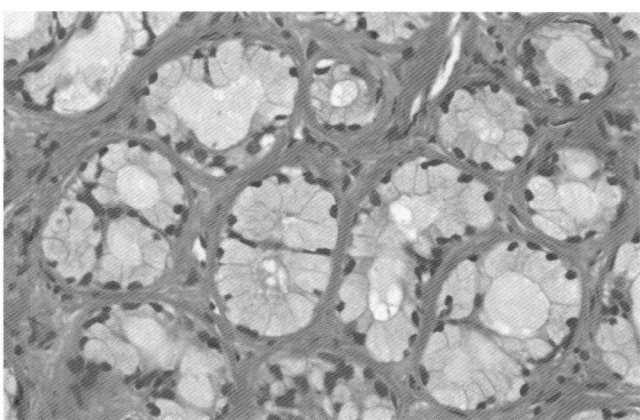

FIGURE 32–2. Cowper's gland. This biopsy specimen contained a small circumscribed lobulated aggregate of benign uniform acini with small dark basal nuclei.

with abundant apical mucinous cytoplasm. Nuclei are inconspicuous (Fig. 32–2). There is no PAP or PSA immunoreactivity,[6] although one study reported weak clumped PSA immunoreactivity.[7] Carcinoma of Cowper's glands is rare and is characterized by frank anaplasia of tumor cells.

## Normal Epithelium of the Prostate

The epithelium of the prostate is composed of three principal cell types: secretory cells, basal cells, and neuroendocrine cells (Fig. 32–3). The secretory luminal cells are cuboidal-to-columnar, with pale-to-clear cytoplasm, and produce PSA, PAP, acidic mucin, and other secretory products.

The basal cells possess the highest proliferative activity of the prostatic epithelium, albeit low, and are thought to contain a subset of stem cells that

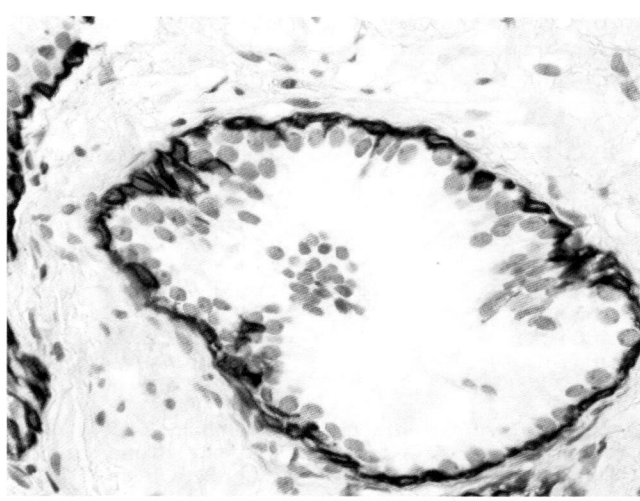

FIGURE 32–4. Intense cytoplasmic immunoreactivity in basal cells creates a continuous circumferential layer at the periphery of a benign prostatic acinus (antikeratin 34βE12 immunohistochemical stain).

repopulate the secretory cell layer. Basal cells retain the ability to undergo metaplasia, including squamous differentiation in the setting of infarction and myoepithelial differentiation in sclerosing adenosis. Basal cells are labeled selectively with antibodies to high-molecular-weight keratins, such as clone 34βE12 (Fig. 32–4), a property that is exploited immunohistochemically in separating benign acinar processes such as atrophy (which retains a basal cell layer) from adenocarcinoma (which lacks a basal cell layer)[8] (Table 32–1).

The neuroendocrine cells are the least common cell type of the prostatic epithelium and usually are not identified in routine H&E-stained sections except for rare cells with large eosinophilic granules[9–13] (Fig. 32–5). Although their function is unknown, neuroendocrine cells probably have an endocrine-paracrine regulatory role in growth and develop-

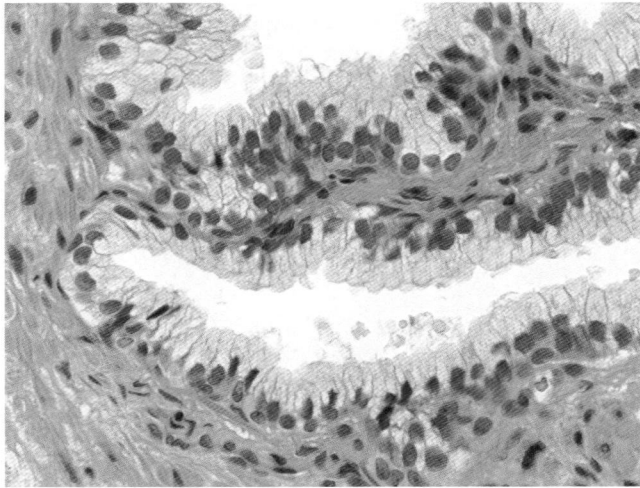

FIGURE 32–3. Benign prostatic epithelium. Although there is cell proliferation, spacing is uniform and nuclei are small without nucleolomegaly.

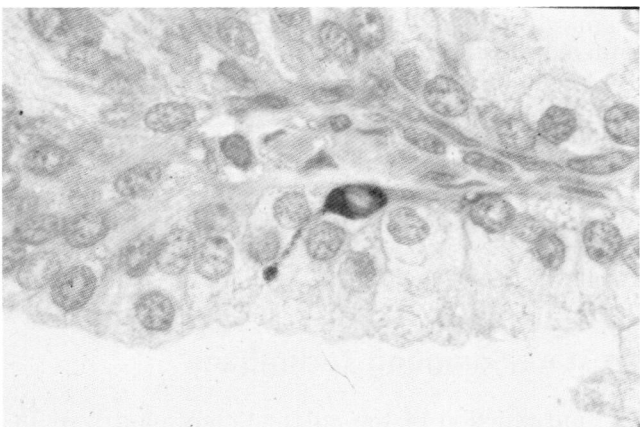

FIGURE 32–5. Neuroendocrine cell of the benign prostatic epithelium. Note the delicate slender cytoplasmic projections (antiserotonin immunohistochemical stain).

**TABLE 32–1.** Immunophenotype of Prostatic Basal Cells

| Biomarker | Function | Findings |
|---|---|---|
| PCNA* | Cell proliferation marker | 79% of labeled cells are basal cells |
| MIB-1 | Cell proliferation marker | 77% of labeled cells are basal cells |
| Ki-67 | Cell proliferation marker | 81% of labeled cells are basal cells |
| Androgen receptors | Nuclear receptors that are necessary for prostatic epithelial growth | Strong immunoreactivity; also present in cancer cells |
| Prostate-specific antigen | Enzyme that liquefies the seminal coagulum | Present in rare basal cells; mainly in secretory luminal cells |
| Keratin 8.12 | Keratins 13, 16 | Strong immunoreactivity |
| Keratin 4.62 | Keratin 19 | Moderate immunoreactivity |
| Keratin PKK1 | Keratins 7, 8, 17, 18 | Moderate immunoreactivity |
| Keratin 312C8-1 | Keratin 14 | Strong immunoreactivity |
| Keratin 34$\beta$E12 | Keratins 5, 10, 11 | Strong immunoreactivity; most commonly used for diagnostic purposes |
| Epidermal growth factor receptor | Membrane-bound 170-kd glycoprotein that mediates the activity of epidermal growth factor | Strong immunoreactivity; rare in cancer |
| CuZn superoxide dismutase | Enzyme that catalyzes superoxide anion radicals | Strong immunoreactivity |
| Type IV collagenase | Enzyme involved in extracellular matrix degradation | Strong immunoreactivity; decreased in cancer |
| Type VII collagen | Part of the hemidesmosomal complex | Strong immunoreactivity; lost in cancer |
| Integrins $\alpha$1, $\alpha$2, $\alpha$4, $\alpha$6, and v; $\beta$1 and $\beta$4 | Extracellular matrix adhesion molecules | Strong immunoreactivity; decreased in most with cancer, although $\alpha$6 and $\beta$1 are retained |
| Estrogen receptors | Hormone receptor | Moderate immunoreactivity |
| BCL2 | Oncoprotein that suppresses apoptosis | Strong immunoreactivity; also found in most cancers |
| c-erbB2 | Oncogene protein in the epidermal growth factor family | Strong immunoreactivity; also found in most cancers |
| Glutathione-S-transferase gene (GSTP1) | Enzyme that inactivates electrophilic carcinogens | Strong immunoreactivity; rare in cancer |
| C-CAM | Epithelial cell adhesion molecule | Strong immunoreactivity; absent in cancer |
| Transforming growth factor-$\beta$ | Growth factor that regulates cell proliferation and differentiation | Strong immunoreactivity; absent in cancer |
| Cathepsin B | Enzyme that degrades basement membranes; may be involved in tumor invasion and metastases | Present in many basal cells and rarely in luminal secretory cells; also found in cancer cells |
| Progesterone receptors | Hormone receptor | Moderate immunoreactivity |

* PCNA, proliferating cell nuclear antigen.

ment, similar to neuroendocrine cells in other organs, and contain multiple neuropeptides that can modulate cell growth and proliferation.[10-14] Serotonin and chromogranin are the best immunohistochemical markers of neuroendocrine cells in formalin-fixed sections of the prostate.

Melanin-like (Fontana-Masson–positive) and lipofuscin-like (Ziehl-Neelsen–positive, S-100 protein negative) pigment frequently is found in scattered foci in the normal and hyperplastic prostate[15] (Fig. 32–6). In blue nevus of the prostate, melanin pigment is contained within dendritic bipolar cells in the stroma,[16] whereas in prostatic melanosis, it is chiefly in the epithelium.

## Prostate Sampling Techniques

The introduction of the automatic spring-driven 18-gauge core biopsy gun began a new era in sampling of the prostate for histologic diagnosis. Inking the needle biopsy is useful for identifying the tissue cores in paraffin blocks, but this is performed infre-

quently. There is variation among laboratories in the number of serial sections obtained from prostate tissue blocks for routine examination[17-19]; I routinely obtain 6 sections on each of two slides, yielding a

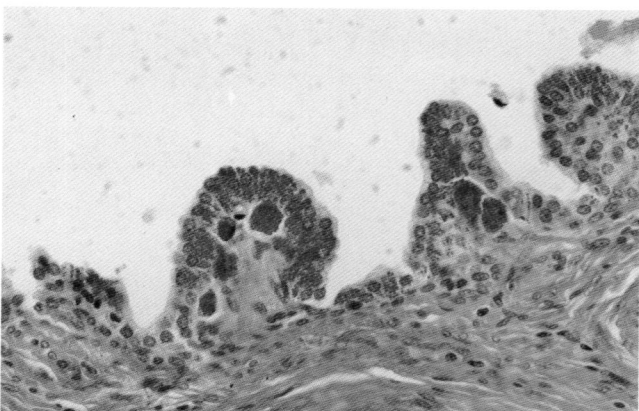

**FIGURE 32–6.** Melanin-like pigment in benign prostatic epithelium.

minimum of 12 sections. The first three sections and last three sections are placed on one slide and submitted for routine H&E staining; the intervening six sections are placed on a slide and saved for additional stains or special studies, such as immunohistochemistry for keratin 34βE12 or digital image analysis for DNA ploidy analysis. In my experience, recutting the block for additional levels is useful in about half of cases, with usually no more than four additional slides before the tissue specimen is exhausted. Most needle biopsy specimens consist only of tissue from the peripheral zone, seldom including the central or transition zones.

Transurethral resection of the prostate (TURP) specimens usually consist of tissue from the transition zone, urethra, periurethral area, bladder neck, and anterior fibromuscular stroma. The TURP specimen does not include tissue from the central or peripheral zone, and not all of the transition zone is removed. Well-differentiated adenocarcinoma found incidentally in TURP chips often has arisen in the transition zone. These tumors frequently are small and may be resected completely by TURP. Poorly differentiated adenocarcinoma in TURP chips usually represents part of a larger tumor that has invaded the transition zone from the peripheral zone. The Cancer Committee of the College of American Pathologists recommends a minimal submission of six cassettes for the first 30 g of tissue and one cassette for every 10 g thereafter.[20] Cautery artifact frequently is extensive in TURP specimens and often limits interpretation, particularly at the edges of the chips.

Fine-needle aspiration is popular for cytologic examination of the prostate in parts of Europe and around the world, but interest in this method in the United States has decreased because of the ease of acquisition and interpretation of the 18-gauge needle core biopsy. Both techniques have similar sensitivity in the diagnosis of prostate adenocarcinoma, and both are limited by small sample size; they are considered best as complementary techniques.[21, 22]

## INFLAMMATION

Patchy mild acute and chronic inflammation is present in most adult prostates and probably is a normal finding.[23] No difference exists in the extent of inflammation between African American and white men.[24] When the inflammation is severe, extensive, or clinically apparent, the term *prostatitis* is warranted. There is a wide spectrum of prostatitides, many of which are rare and poorly understood.[25]

Patients with prostatitis related to acquired immunodeficiency syndrome (AIDS) may be asymptomatic or present with acute prostatitis, chronic prostatitis, or abscess. Relapses are common despite prolonged antibiotic therapy. Infectious prostatitis occurs in 14% of AIDS patients and 3% of patients with AIDS-related complex or asymptomatic human immunodeficiency virus infection. Prostatitis in these patients may be due to a variety of pathogens, including *Escherichia coli, Klebsiella, Enterobacter, Serratia, Pseudomonas, Haemophilus parainfluenzae, Cryptococcus neoformans,* and *Mycobacterium tuberculosis.*[26]

## Acute Bacterial Prostatitis

Patients with acute bacterial prostatitis present with sudden onset of fever; chills; irritative voiding symptoms; and pain in the lower back, rectum, and perineum. The prostate is swollen, firm, tender, and warm. On microscopic examination, there are sheets of neutrophils surrounding prostatic glands, often with marked tissue destruction and cellular debris. The stroma is edematous and hemorrhagic, and microabscesses may be present. Diagnosis is based on culture of urine and expressed prostatic secretions; biopsy is contraindicated because of the potential for sepsis. Most cases of acute prostatitis are caused by bacteria responsible for other urinary tract infections, including *E. coli* (80% of infections), other *Enterobacteriaceae, Pseudomonas, Serratia, Klebsiella* (10% to 15%), and enterococci (5% to 10%). Abscess is a rare complication, usually occurring in immunocompromised patients, such as those with AIDS.

## Chronic Prostatitis

Chronic abacterial prostatitis is more common than bacterial prostatitis and rarely follows infection elsewhere in the urinary tract.[27] Patients often complain of painful ejaculation. Cultures of urine and expressed prostatic secretions are negative. The causative agent is unknown, but *Chlamydia, Ureaplasma,* and *Trichomonas* have been proposed. This form of prostatitis has a prolonged indolent course with relapses and remissions. Chronic bacterial prostatitis is a common cause of relapsing urinary tract infection and usually is caused by *E. coli*. Clinical diagnosis is difficult, often requiring multiple urine cultures obtained after prostatic massage. A prospective study of 368 biopsy specimens from 97 patients with chronic prostatitis and chronic pelvic pain revealed moderate or severe inflammation in only 5%, questioning current concepts of the pathophysiology of this disorder[28] (Fig. 32–7).

## Granulomatous Prostatitis

Granulomatous prostatitis is a group of morphologically distinct forms of chronic prostatitis, the pathogenesis of which often cannot be determined. It accounts for about 1% of benign inflammatory conditions of the prostate. Causes include infection, tissue disruption after biopsy, bacille Calmette-Guérin therapy, and others.[25] Most patients have a prior history of urinary tract infection. The prostate is hard, fixed, and nodular, and cancer usually is suspected clinically. Urinalysis often shows pyuria and hematuria. Granulomatous prostatitis probably

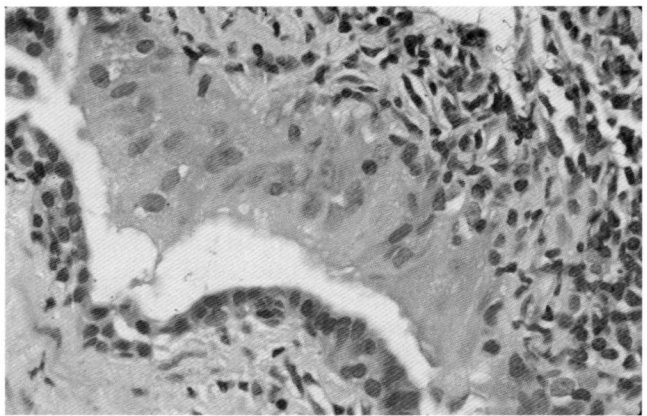

**FIGURE 32–7.** Inflammatory changes with epithelial metaplasia simulating high-grade PIN.

is caused by blockage of prostatic ducts and stasis of secretions, regardless of its etiology. The epithelium is destroyed, and cellular debris, bacterial toxins, and prostatic secretions escape into the stroma, including corpora amylacea, sperm, and semen, eliciting an intense localized inflammatory response (Fig. 32–8). This process is similar to intraprostatic sperm granuloma formation. Tissue eosinophilia may be prominent in prostates infested with parasites, systemic allergic or autoimmune disease, iatrogenic post-TURP prostatitis, or nonspecific granulomatous prostatitis. Fine-needle aspiration is a useful diagnostic test for granulomatous prostatitis, although other conditions share some cytologic findings.[29]

## IDIOPATHIC GRANULOMATOUS PROSTATITIS

Idiopathic (nonspecific) granulomatous prostatitis accounts for most cases of granulomatous prostatitis (69%). The granulomas usually are noncaseating and associated with parenchymal loss and marked fibrosis. Classification of eosinophilic and noneosinophilic types is probably of no clinical value. Ten percent of patients with idiopathic granulomatous prostatitis do not respond to conservative management, developing severe urethral obstruction that requires TURP. TURP is unsuccessful, however, in 50% of cases, with some patients requiring multiple procedures.

## INFECTIOUS GRANULOMATOUS PROSTATITIS

Infectious granulomatous prostatitis is an unusual form of granulomatous prostatitis and may be caused by bacteria, fungi, parasites, and viruses. *M. tuberculosis* infection of the prostate occurs only after pulmonary infection or miliary dissemination. Small 1- to 2-mm caseating granulomas coalesce within the prostatic parenchyma, forming yellow nodules and streaks. Brucellosis may mimic tuberculosis clinically and pathologically. Mycotic infections of the prostate are rare and invariably follow fungemia. Most deep mycoses induce necrotizing and non-necrotizing

granulomas and fibrosis; *Candida albicans* usually is associated only with acute inflammation. Granulomas caused by *Schistosoma haematobium* frequently are found in the prostate, bladder, and seminal vesicles in endemic areas such as Egypt. The organisms lodge in vesicular and pelvic venous plexus as the final habitat. The adult female schistosome migrates into the submucosa of the urinary bladder and prostatic stroma, where she lays eggs that induce granuloma formation and fibrosis. Herpes zoster infection may be associated with granulomatous prostatitis.

## POSTSURGICAL GRANULOMATOUS PROSTATITIS

Postsurgical granulomatous prostatitis can be identified years after TURP resulting from cauterization and surgical disruption of tissues. The granulomas characteristically are circumscribed and rimmed by palisading histiocytes with central fibrinoid necrosis. Multinucleated giant cells frequently are present. The striking histologic resemblance of postsurgical granulomatous prostatitis to rheumatoid nodule suggests a hypersensitivity reaction or cell-mediated immune response. Tissue eosinophilia is present in many cases. Treatment is unnecessary.

## BACILLE CALMETTE-GUÉRIN–INDUCED GRANULOMATOUS PROSTATITIS

Granulomatous prostatitis occurs in virtually all patients treated with intravesicular bacille Calmette-Guérin immunotherapy for superficial urothelial carcinoma of the bladder.[30] The granulomas characteristically are discrete, with or without necrosis, and often contain numerous acid-fast bacilli. No therapy is required.

## MALAKOPLAKIA

Malakoplakia is a granulomatous disease associated with defective intracellular lysosomal digestion of bacteria. It occasionally occurs in the prostate,[25] presenting as a diffuse indurated mass, clinically suggestive of prostatic carcinoma. *E. coli* commonly is isolated from urine cultures. On microscopic exami-

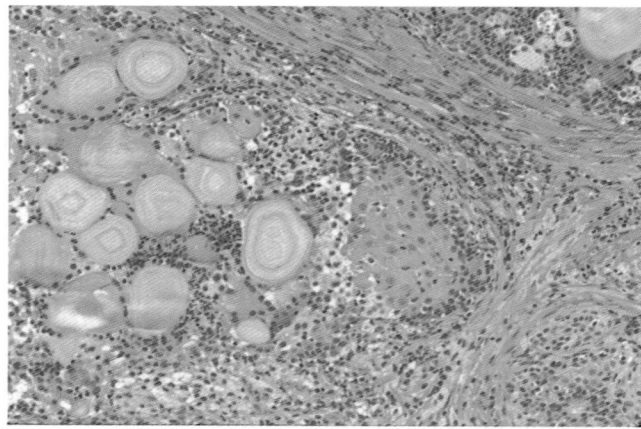

**FIGURE 32–8.** Granulomatous prostatitis with eosinophilic metasplasia of the epithelium *(left).*

nation, the prostate is effaced by sheets of macrophages admixed with lymphocytes and plasma cells. Intracellular and extracellular Michaelis-Gutmann bodies are identified, appearing as sharply demarcated spherical structures with concentric "owl's eyes" measuring 5 to 10 $\mu$ in diameter. Periodic acid–Schiff (PAS) stain is useful in identifying nonmineralized forms, and von Kossa stain is useful in identifying mineralized forms.

## XANTHOMA AND XANTHOGRANULOMATOUS PROSTATITIS

Xanthoma is a rare form of idiopathic granulomatous prostatitis that consists of a localized collection of cholesterol-laden histiocytes; it also may be seen in patients with hyperlipidemia.[31] Xanthoma occurs in older men and usually is an incidental finding in patients undergoing TURP or needle biopsy, although it may appear as a palpable nodule. Rare cases contain areas of typical granulomatous prostatitis, and the term *xanthogranulomatous prostatitis* is appropriate in such cases. Distinction from clear cell carcinoma (hypernephroid pattern) may be difficult, and immunohistochemical stains for PSA and PAP often assist with this diagnostic concern.[32]

## OTHER FORMS OF GRANULOMATOUS PROSTATITIS

Other rare causes of granulomatous prostatitis include sarcoidosis, rheumatoid nodule, polyarteritis nodosa, Wegener's granulomatosis, allergic (eosinophilic) prostatitis,[33] polytetrafluoroethylene (Teflon)-induced prostatitis,[34] silicone-induced prostatitis, and giant cell arteritis.

## Inflammation After Needle Biopsy

Contemporary transrectal 18-gauge needle biopsy of the prostate induces a predictable inflammatory response along a narrow track.[35] The biopsy track consists of a partially collapsed cavity, often filled with red blood cells, rimmed by mixed acute and chronic inflammation, including lymphocytes, macrophages, and occasional eosinophils (Fig. 32–9). There is a variable amount of hemosiderin pigment, granulation tissue, and fibrosis, usually limited to the edge of the cavity. Venous thrombosis and foreign body giant cell reaction are seen infrequently. Although tumor cells frequently are enmeshed within fibrous connective tissue, they are not seen within the cavity after 18-gauge biopsy.[35] Conversely, tumor occasionally is identified in the track after wider 14-gauge biopsy, particularly with perineal biopsy.[36]

Biopsy tracks in prostatectomies obtained 4 to 6 weeks after biopsy show fewer red blood cells and less acute inflammation than in those obtained earlier, but no other histologic differences are noted. There is no evidence of florid granulomatous prostatitis or fibrinoid necrosis, which often is seen after TURP. Biopsy specimens involving benign prostatic tissue and cancer are histologically similar.

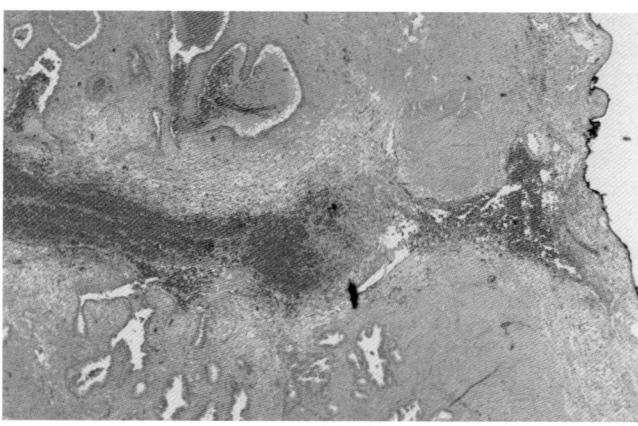

FIGURE 32–9. Line of hemorrhage denotes the needle track beneath the prostatic capsule on the right. This radical prostatectomy was obtained 2 weeks after sextant 18-gauge needle biopsies.

## METAPLASIA

### Squamous Metaplasia

Squamous metaplasia may result from a variety of insults to the prostate, including acute inflammation, infarction, radiation therapy, and androgen deprivation therapy. The changes may be focal or diffuse, appearing as intraductal syncytial aggregates of flattened cells with abundant eosinophilic cytoplasm or cohesive aggregates of glycogen-rich clear cells with shrunken hyperchromatic nuclei. Keratinization is unusual except at the edge of infarcts or areas of acute inflammation. Squamous metaplasia commonly involves the prostatic urethra in patients with indwelling catheters.

### Mucinous Metaplasia

Mucinous metaplasia refers to clusters of tall columnar cells or goblet cells that are observed infrequently in the prostatic acinar epithelium.[37] This finding is invariably microscopic and can be seen in the urothelium of large periurethral prostatic ducts, foci of urothelial metaplasia, atrophy, nodular hyperplasia, basal cell hyperplasia (BCH), and postatrophic hyperplasia (PAH). The cells contain acid mucin that stains with Mayer mucicarmine, alcian blue (pH 2.7), and PAS after diastase predigestion; luminal secretions with similar staining usually are present. There is no immunoreactivity for PSA and PAP.

### Neuroendocrine Cells with Eosinophilic Granules (Paneth Cell–Like Change)

Neuroendocrine cells with eosinophilic granules (NCEGs) are considered a distinct form of neuroendocrine differentiation in the prostatic epithelium and may represent a normal finding rather than metaplasia.[9] This finding is characterized by isolated cells or small groups of cells with prominent eosinophilic cytoplasmic granules, present on routine H&E-stained sections in 10% of serially sectioned radical prostatectomies. NCEG usually are present focally but occasionally are prominent and multifocal. NCEG invariably display intense cytoplasmic immunoreactivity for chromogranin, neuron-specific enolase, and serotonin. Many of these cells also express PSA and PAP. Lysozyme is negative. NCEG account for only a small percentage of cells with neuroendocrine differentiation in benign prostatic acini and adenocarcinoma. Most neuroendocrine cells have small granules that are not apparent on routinely stained sections.

## Urothelial Metaplasia

Urothelial metaplasia consists of urothelium within ducts, ductules, and acini beyond the normal urothelial-columnar junction, arising apparently as a result of metaplastic change. This junction is variable in location, creating difficulty in distinguishing metaplasia from normal urothelium in fragmented specimens, such as TURP and needle biopsy specimens. Consequently the diagnosis of metaplasia may be overused.

## Nephrogenic Metaplasia

Nephrogenic metaplasia most often occurs in adults in the urinary bladder, renal pelvis, ureter, and urethra; prostatic urethral involvement is rare, and extension into the prostatic parenchyma may create diagnostic confusion with adenocarcinoma. It usually follows instrumentation, urethral catheterization, infection, or calculi. Patients present with lower urinary tract symptoms, including hematuria, dysuria, obstruction, and urethral mass.[38, 39] Although the term *nephrogenic adenoma* is used commonly, it is a misnomer; this process is thought to be a reactive and metaplastic response to chronic inflammation or instrumentation and is not neoplastic.

Nephrogenic metaplasia appears as an exophytic papillary mass of cystic and solid tubules protruding from the urethral mucosa. The tubules may extend into the underlying prostate as a proliferation of small round-to-oval tubules, sometimes filled with colloid-like material. The lining consists of flattened or simple cuboidal cells, often with a distinctive hobnail appearance. Nuclei display finely granular uniform chromatin with inconspicuous nucleoli; occasional prominent nucleoli are observed. There frequently is chronic inflammation and edema of the stroma, but no desmoplasia is present. The tubules contain scant or moderate mucin that is positive with alcian blue and PAS stains. The basement membrane is accentuated with PAS stain. Epithelial membrane antigen is positive in the tubular epithelial cells, and high-molecular-weight keratin 34βE12 stains many of the basal cells. PSA, PAP, and carcinoembryonic antigen (CEA) are negative.[39]

## HYPERPLASIA

### Nodular Hyperplasia (Benign Prostatic Hyperplasia)

Enlargement of the prostate, also known as *nodular hyperplasia* or *BPH,* consists of overgrowth of the epithelium and fibromuscular tissue of the transition zone and periurethral area. Symptoms are caused by interference with muscular sphincteric function and by obstruction of urine flow through the prostatic urethra. These symptoms, referred to as *lower urinary tract symptoms,* include urgency, difficulty in starting urination, diminished stream size and force, increased frequency, incomplete bladder emptying, and nocturia.

Development of nodular hyperplasia includes three pathologic changes: 1) nodule formation, 2) diffuse enlargement of the transition zone and periurethral tissue, and 3) enlargement of nodules. In men younger than 70 years old, diffuse enlargement predominates; in men older than 70, epithelial proliferation and expansile growth of existing nodules predominates, probably as a result of androgenic and other hormonal stimulation. The proportion of epithelium to stroma increases as symptoms become more severe.[40]

On gross examination, BPH consists of variably sized nodules that are soft or firm, rubbery, and yellow-gray and bulge from the cut surface on transection. If there is prominent epithelial hyperplasia in addition to stromal hyperplasia, the abundant luminal spaces create soft and grossly spongy nodules that ooze a pale white, watery fluid. If the nodular hyperplasia is predominantly fibromuscular, there may be diffuse enlargement or numerous trabeculations without prominent nodularity. Degenerative changes include calcification and infarction. BPH usually involves the transition zone, but occasionally nodules arise from the periurethral tissue at the bladder neck. Protrusion of bladder neck nodules into the bladder lumen is referred to as *median lobe hyperplasia.*

On microscopic examination, BPH is composed of varying proportions of epithelium and stroma (fibrous connective tissue and smooth muscle). The most common are adenomyofibromatous nodules that contain all elements.

The diagnosis of BPH often is used in needle biopsy specimens when only normal benign peripheral zone prostatic tissue is present. The transition zone is sampled infrequently by needle biopsies unless the urologist specifically targets this area or there is massive nodular hyperplasia that compresses the peripheral zone. I require the presence of at least part of a nodule for the diagnosis of BPH in needle biopsy specimens, and this is unusual. Narrow 18-gauge biopsy specimens virtually never contain the entire nodule unless it is small and sampled fortuitously. Casual use of the term *nodular hyperplasia* for benign prostatic tissue may mislead the urologist into believing that a palpable nodule or hypoechoic focus of concern has been sampled and evaluated histologically.

Vascular insufficiency probably accounts for infarction of hyperplastic nodules, seen in 20% of resected cases. The center of the nodule undergoes hemorrhagic necrosis, often with reactive changes in the residual epithelium at the periphery, including squamous metaplasia and transitional cell metaplasia.

BPH is not a precursor of cancer, but there are many similarities.[41] Both display a parallel increase in prevalence with patient age according to autopsy studies, although cancer lags by 15 to 20 years. Both require androgens for growth and development, and both may respond to androgen deprivation treatment. Most cancers arise in patients with concomitant BPH, and cancer is found incidentally in a significant number (10%) of TURP specimens. BPH may be related to prostate cancer arising in the transition zone, perhaps in association with certain forms of hyperplasia.

## Atrophy and Postatrophic Hyperplasia

Atrophy is a near-constant microscopic finding in the prostate, consisting of small distorted glands with flattened epithelium, hyperchromatic nuclei, and stromal fibrosis. The prevalence and extent increase with advancing age, particularly after age 40.

Atrophy may be confused with adenocarcinoma because of prominent acinar architectural distortion, but it lacks significant nuclear and nucleolar enlargement. The nucleus-to-cytoplasmic ratio may be high as a result of scant cytoplasm, and nuclei are hyperchromatic.

Clusters of atrophic prostatic acini that display proliferative epithelial changes are referred to as *PAH*.[42] PAH is at the extreme end of the morphologic continuum of acinar atrophy that most closely mimics adenocarcinoma (Fig. 32–10). This continuum varies from mild acinar atrophy with a flattened layer of attenuated cells with scant cytoplasm to that of PAH, in which the lining cells are low cuboidal with moderate cytoplasm. There is no sharp division in this continuum between atrophy and PAH, challenging the utility of PAH as a distinct entity. The morphologic similarity of PAH and carcinoma creates the potential for misdiagnosis, however, sometimes resulting in unnecessary prostatectomy.[42, 43] I believe that PAH is a diagnostic category for atrophic acini that most closely mimic adenocarcinoma, recognizing that this is merely a descriptive term.

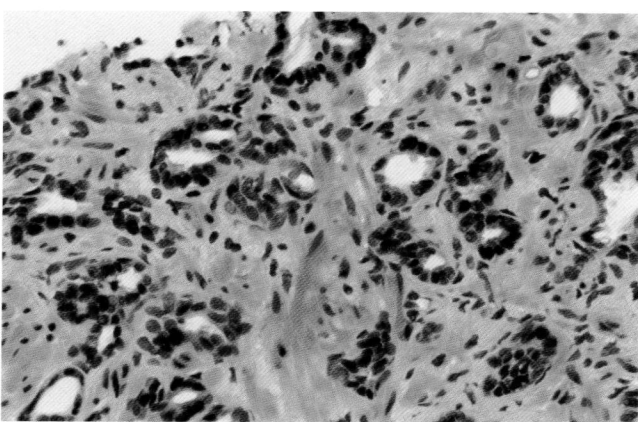

**FIGURE 32–10.** Atrophy and postatrophic hyperplasia of the prostate.

PAH consists of a microscopic lobular cluster of 5 to 15 small acini with distorted contours reminiscent of atrophy. One or more larger dilated acini usually are present within these round-to-oval clusters, and the small acini appear to bud off of the dilated acinus, imparting a lobular appearance to the lesion. The small acini are lined by a layer of cuboidal secretory cells with mildly enlarged nuclei with an increased nucleus-to-cytoplasmic ratio when compared with adjacent benign epithelial cells. The nuclei contain evenly distributed and finely granular chromatin, and nucleoli are usually small, although mildly enlarged basophilic nucleoli are present focally in 39% of cases.

PAH is distinguished from carcinoma by its characteristic lobular architecture, intact or fragmented basal cell layer, inconspicuous or mildly enlarged nucleoli, and adjacent acinar atrophy with stromal fibrosis or smooth muscle atrophy. Nucleolar changes are useful in separating PAH and carcinoma; mildly enlarged nucleoli may be present in PAH but only focally, and most cells have micronucleoli.

## Basal Cell Hyperplasia

There are three patterns of benign BCH: 1) typical BCH, 2) atypical BCH, and 3) basal cell adenoma.[44–46] BCH consists of a proliferation of basal cells two or more cells in thickness at the periphery of prostatic acini.[44–46] BCH sometimes appears as small nests of cells surrounded by compressed stroma, often associated with chronic inflammation. The nests may be solid or dilated cystically and occasionally are punctuated by irregular round luminal spaces, creating a cribriform pattern. BCH frequently involves only part of an acinus and sometimes protrudes into the lumen, retaining the overlying secretory cell layer; less commonly, there is symmetric duplication of the basal cell layer at the periphery of the acinus (Fig. 32–11). The basal

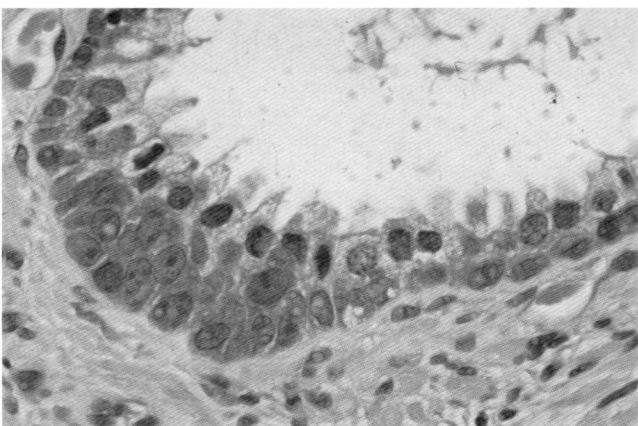

FIGURE 32–11. Eccentric pattern of basal cell hyperplasia.

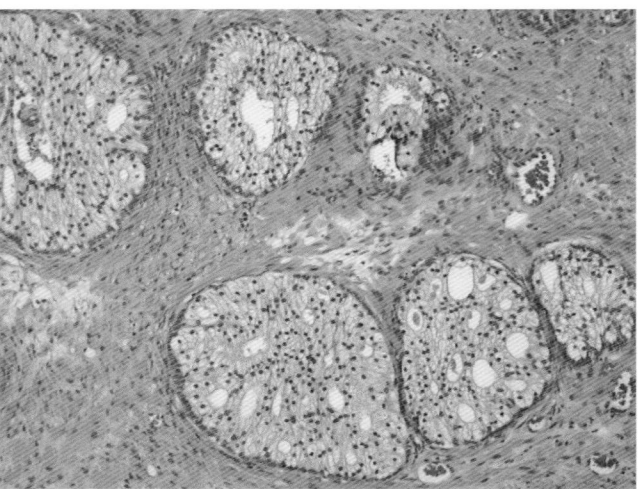

FIGURE 32–12. Cribriform hyperplasia.

cells are enlarged, ovoid or round, and plump (epithelioid), with large pale ovoid nuclei, finely reticular chromatin, and a moderate amount of cytoplasm. Nucleoli are usually inconspicuous (<1 $\mu$ in diameter) except in atypical BCH (see later). BCH also may appear as one or more large round, usually solitary circumscribed nodules of acini with BCH in the setting of nodular hyperplasia, referred to as *basal cell adenoma*.

Atypical BCH refers to BCH appearing as large prominent nucleoli. The nucleoli are round-to-oval and lightly eosinophilic. There is chronic inflammation in most cases, suggesting that nucleolomegaly is a reflection of reactive atypia. A morphologic spectrum of nucleolar size is observed in basal cell proliferations, and only those with more than 10% of cells exhibiting prominent nucleoli are considered atypical.[46] This lesion is significant because of the potential for misdiagnosis as adenocarcinoma.

BCH (typical and atypical forms) displays intense cytoplasmic immunoreactivity in virtually all of the cells with high-molecular-weight keratin 34$\beta$E12 and other basal cell–specific markers. Immunoreactivity for PSA, PAP, chromogranin, S-100 protein, and neuron-specific enolase is present in rare basal cells in most cases.

## Cribriform Hyperplasia

Clear cell change is common in BCH, often with a cribriform pattern; this is referred to by some as *cribriform hyperplasia* or *clear cell cribriform hyperplasia*. Cribriform hyperplasia, including clear cell cribriform hyperplasia, consists of a nodule of glands arranged in a distinctive cribriform pattern[47] (Fig. 32–12).

## Atypical Adenomatous Hyperplasia

Atypical adenomatous hyperplasia (AAH) is a localized proliferation of small acini within the prostate arising in intimate association with nodular hyper-

plasia[48–50] (Fig. 32–13). AAH varies in incidence from 19.6% (TURP specimens) to 24% (autopsy series in 20- to 40-year-old men).[51] Mean size of AAH is 0.03 cm$^3$, but mass-forming AAH measuring 21.1 cm$^3$ has been documented.[52]

AAH is distinguished from well-differentiated carcinoma by the presence of inconspicuous nucleoli, partially intact but fragmented basal cell layer, and infrequent crystalloids (Fig. 32–14). All measures of nucleolar size allow separation of AAH from adenocarcinoma, including mean nucleolar diameter, largest nucleolar diameter, and percentage of nucleoli greater than 1 $\mu$m in diameter. There apparently is widespread acceptance of Gleason's criterion of nucleolar diameter greater than 1 $\mu$m for separating well-differentiated cancer (Gleason primary grades 1 and 2) from other proliferative lesions, such as AAH.[53] Most Gleason pattern 1 cancers now are thought to represent foci of AAH.

AAH may be linked to a subset of prostate cancers that arise in the transition zone, but the evidence is circumstantial: increased incidence in association with carcinoma (15% in 100 prostates

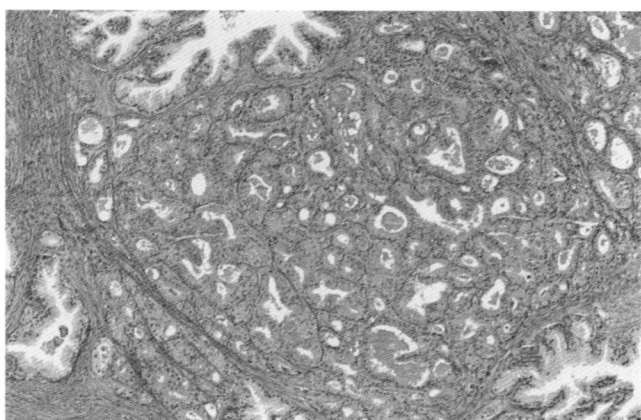

FIGURE 32–13. Atypical adenomatous hyperplasia. Note uniform round nuclei without prominent nucleoli.

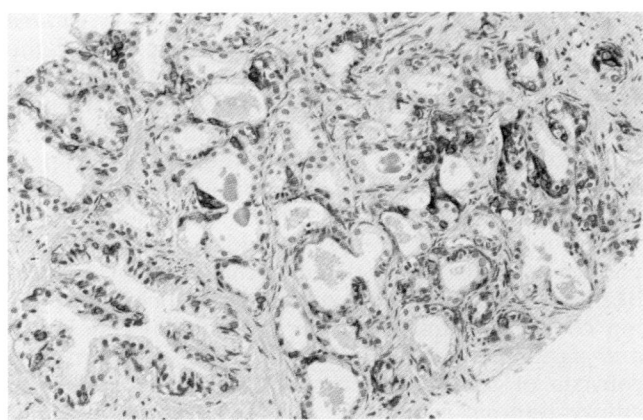

FIGURE 32–14. Keratin 34βE12 immunoreactivity in the fragmented basal cell layer of atypical adenomatous hyperplasia (anti-keratin 34βE12 immunohistochemical stain).

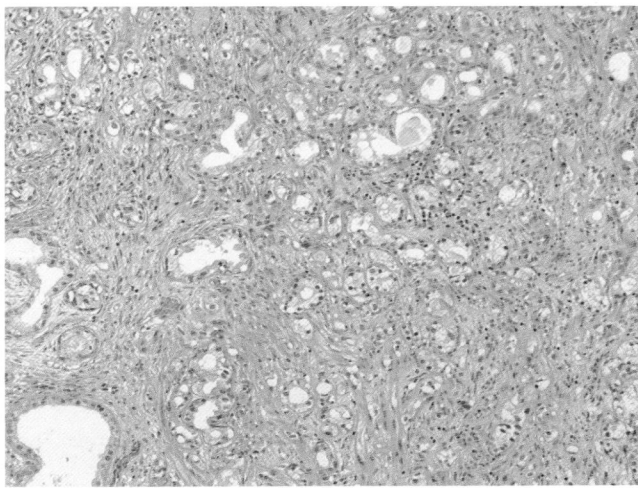

FIGURE 32–15. Sclerosing adenosis with benign acini set in a cellular stroma.

without carcinoma at autopsy and 31% in 100 prostates with cancer at autopsy), topographic relationship with small acinar carcinoma, age at peak incidence that proceeds that of carcinoma, increasing silver-staining nucleolar organizer region (AgNOR) count, increased nuclear area and diameter, a proliferative cell index that is similar to that of small acinar carcinoma but significantly higher than that of normal and hyperplastic prostatic epithelium, and rare cases with genetic instability.[54, 55] AAH has a higher proliferation rate than nodular hyperplasia, but the expression of BCL2, c-erbB-2, and c-erbB-3 is similar.[56]

## Sclerosing Adenosis

Sclerosing adenosis of the prostate, originally described as *adenomatoid* or *pseudoadenomatoid tumor,* consists of a benign, usually solitary circumscribed proliferation of small acini set in a dense spindle cell stroma.[57–59] It is present in about 2% of TURP specimens (Fig. 32–15).

The acini in sclerosing adenosis are predominantly well formed and small to medium size but may form minute cellular nests or clusters with abortive lumina. The cells lining the acini display a moderate amount of clear-to-eosinophilic cytoplasm, often with distinct cell margins (Fig. 32–16). The basal cell layer may be focally prominent and hyperplastic, particularly in acini thickly rimmed by cellular stroma. In some areas, the acini merge with the exuberant stroma of fibroblasts and loose ground substance. There is usually no significant cytologic atypia of the epithelial cells or stromal cells, but some cases may show moderate atypia.

The unique immunophenotype of sclerosing adenosis is a valuable diagnostic clue that distinguishes it from adenocarcinoma. The basal cells show immunoreactivity for S-100 protein and muscle-specific actin, in contrast to normal prostatic epithelium or carcinoma (Fig. 32–17); consequently, sclerosing adenosis is considered a form of metapla-

sia. The basal cell layer is intact or fragmented and discontinuous in sclerosing adenosis as shown with immunohistochemical stains for high-molecular-weight keratin 34βE12, compared with absence of staining in carcinoma. PSA and PAP are present within secretory luminal cells. Ultrastructural studies show myoepithelial differentiation in sclerosing adenosis, with collections of thin filaments and dense bodies.[59]

## Stromal Hyperplasia with Atypical Cells

Stromal hyperplasia with atypia consists of stromal nodules in the transition zone with increased cellularity and nuclear atypia.[60, 61] These may appear as solid stromal nodules (often erroneously referred to as *atypical leiomyoma*) or with atypical degenerative

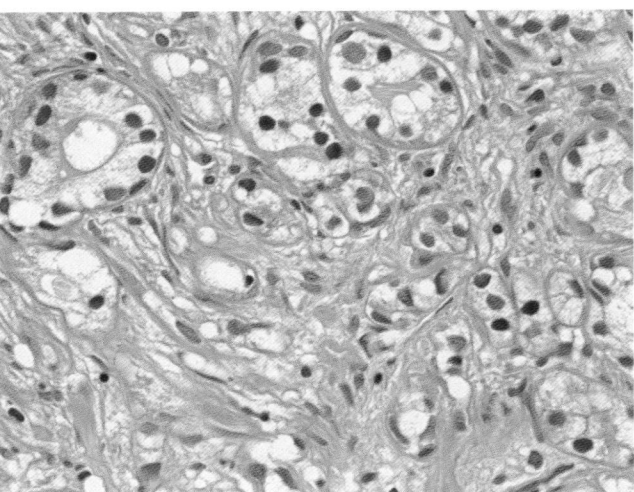

FIGURE 32–16. Sclerosing adenosis. Note prominent periacinar basement membrane thickening.

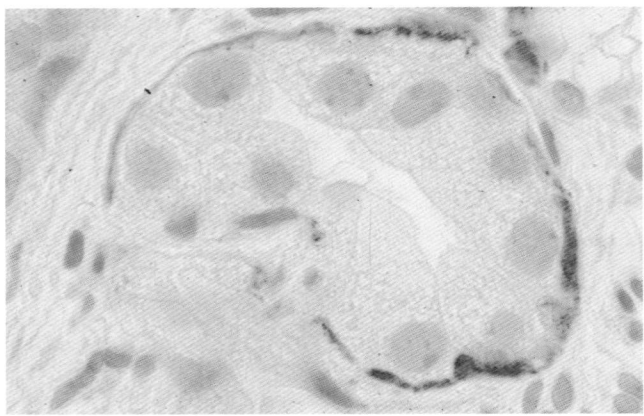

**FIGURE 32–17.** S-100 protein stain in sclerosing adenosis. There is prominent immunoreactivity in most of the basal cells.

smooth muscle cells interspersed with benign glands. Stromal nuclei are large, hyperchromatic, and rarely multinucleated or vacuolated, with inconspicuous nucleoli. There are no mitotic figures and no necrosis (Fig. 32–18).

## Verumontanum Mucosal Gland Hyperplasia

The epithelial lining of the verumontanum may become abundant and proliferative, but criteria for separating normal and hyperplastic mucosa are not well defined.[62] This is not usually a diagnostic problem.

## Hyperplasia of Mesonephric Remnants

Hyperplasia of mesonephric remnants is a proliferation of small tubules that is exceedingly rare in the prostate and periprostatic tissues, and the few re-

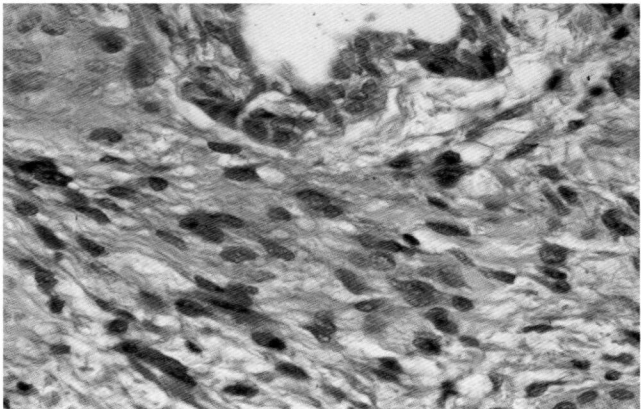

**FIGURE 32–18.** Stromal hyperplasia with atypical giant cells. Note prominent nuclear vacuolization.

ported cases lack cytologic atypia.[63–65] It shares many features with mesonephric hyperplasia of the female genital tract, including apparent infiltration of the stroma and neural spaces; lobular arrangement of small acini; or solid nests lined by a single cell layer of cuboidal or flat epithelium, prominent nucleoli, and eosinophilic intratubular material.

There are two histopathologic patterns, both with a lobular pattern and cuboidal cell lining. One pattern consists of small acini that contain colloid-like material reminiscent of thyroid follicles. The lining consists of a single layer of cuboidal cells without significant cytologic atypia. The second pattern consists of small acini or solid nests of cells with empty lumina, reminiscent of nephrogenic metaplasia. Acini may be atrophic or exhibit micropapillary projections lined by cuboidal cells. Prominent nucleoli are usually absent but are present in rare cases, compounding the diagnostic confusion. The diagnosis may be confirmed by cellular immunoreactivity for keratin 34βE12, although this is not a constant feature,[65] and lack of immunoreactivity for PSA and PAP.

## PROSTATIC CYSTS AND MISCELLANEOUS BENIGN PROCESSES

Cysts are unusual in the prostate. Giant multilocular prostatic cystadenoma is a large tumor composed of acini and cysts lined by prostatic-type epithelium set in a hypocellular fibrous stroma.[66–68] This rare tumor arises in men between ages 28 and 80 years as a large midline prostatic or extraprostatic mass causing urinary obstruction. The epithelial lining displays PSA immunoreactivity. Surgical excision is usually curative, although the tumor may recur if incompletely excised. Other benign cysts include seminal vesicle cyst, ejaculatory duct cyst,[69] and müllerian duct cyst.[70] Location often is useful, recognizing that seminal vesicle cyst is typically lateral, whereas müllerian duct cyst is midline. Phyllodes tumor is described later in the section on soft tissue tumors. Echinococcal cyst usually is associated with prominent inflammation, and organisms are often demonstrable.[71] Other benign processes include endometriosis,[72] benign adenofibroma of the ejaculatory duct,[73] and adenomatoid tumor of the ejaculatory duct.[74]

## PROSTATIC INTRAEPITHELIAL NEOPLASIA

High-grade PIN now is accepted as the most likely preinvasive stage of adenocarcinoma,[56, 75–79] more than a decade after its first formal description.[80, 81] PIN is characterized by cellular proliferations within preexisting ducts and acini with cytologic changes mimicking cancer, including nuclear and nucleolar

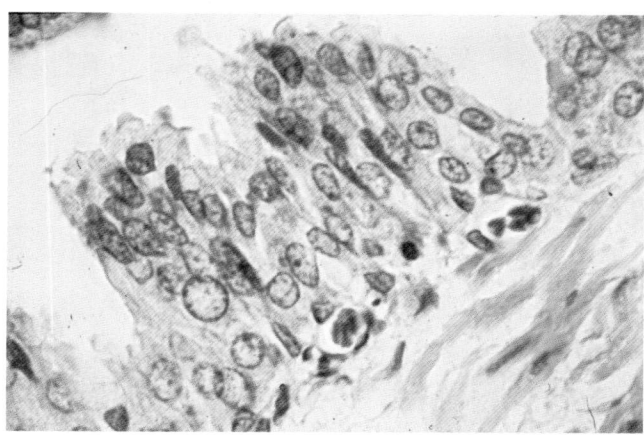

**FIGURE 32-19.** Low-grade PIN. There is marked variation in nuclear size and shape without nucleolomegaly. Compare with high-grade PIN in 30.

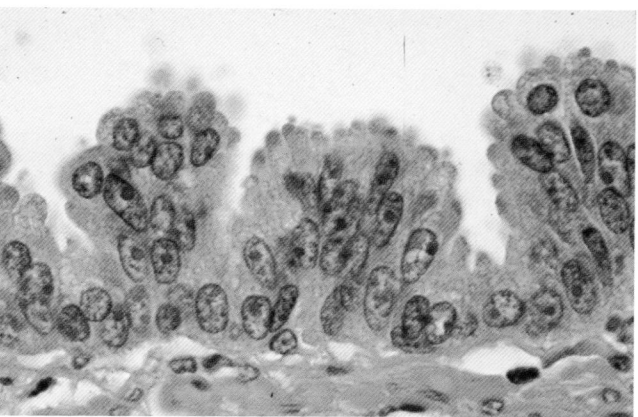

**FIGURE 32-21.** Tufting pattern of high-grade PIN. Small mounds of cells protrude into the lumen. This focus has a prominent basal cell layer at the periphery.

enlargement. It coexists with cancer in more than 85% of cases[82] but retains an intact or fragmented basal cell layer, in contrast to cancer, which lacks a basal cell layer.[81] The only method of detection is biopsy; PIN does not elevate total and free serum PSA concentration significantly and cannot be detected by ultrasonography.[83]

The incidence of PIN varies according to the population of men under study[75, 84-91] and increases with patient age.[92, 93] The lowest likelihood is in men participating in PSA screening and early detection studies, with an incidence of PIN in biopsy specimens ranging from 0.7% to 20%.[75, 84-91] Men have PIN in 4.4% to 25% of contemporary 18-gauge needle biopsy specimens obtained by urologists. Men undergoing TURP have the highest likelihood of PIN, varying from 2.8% to 33%.[90, 91] Select antikeratin antibodies, such as 34βE12 (high-molecular-weight keratin), may be used to stain tissue sections for the presence of basal cells, recognizing that PIN retains an intact or fragmented basal cell layer, whereas cancer does not.

## Diagnostic Criteria

PIN refers to the putative precancerous end of the continuum of cellular proliferations within the lining of prostatic ducts, ductules, and acini. *PIN* has been endorsed at multiple consensus meetings, and terms such as *dysplasia* and *intraductal carcinoma* are discouraged.[76]

There are two grades of PIN (low grade and high grade), although *PIN* usually is used to indicate high-grade PIN. The high level of interobserver variability with low-grade PIN limits its clinical utility, and many pathologists do not report this finding except in research studies, including my colleagues and me (Fig. 32-19). Interobserver agreement for high-grade PIN is good to excellent (Fig. 32-20).

There are four main patterns of high-grade PIN: 1) tufting, 2) micropapillary, 3) cribriform, and 4) flat[94] (Figs. 32-21 through 32-24). The tufting pattern is the most common, present in 97% of cases, although most cases have multiple patterns. There are no known clinically important differences be-

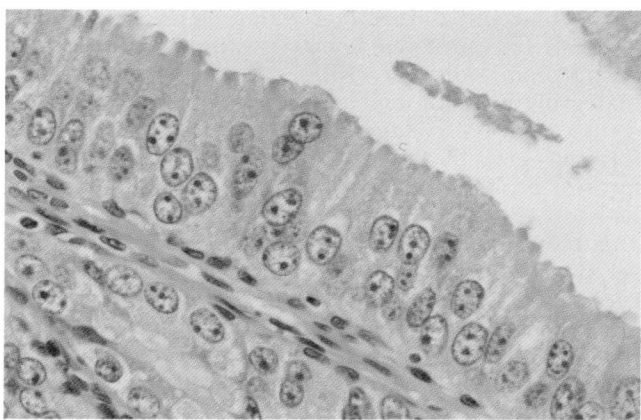

**FIGURE 32-20.** High-grade PIN. Nuclei are enlarged, with granular chromatin and nucleolomegaly.

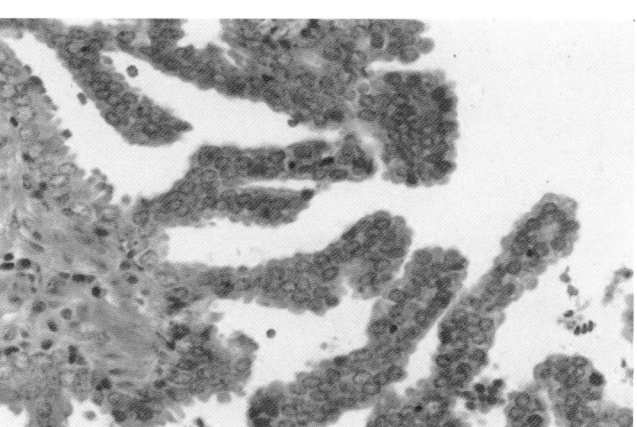

**FIGURE 32-22.** Micropapillary pattern of high-grade PIN. Elongated finger-like projections of epithelium protrude into the lumens.

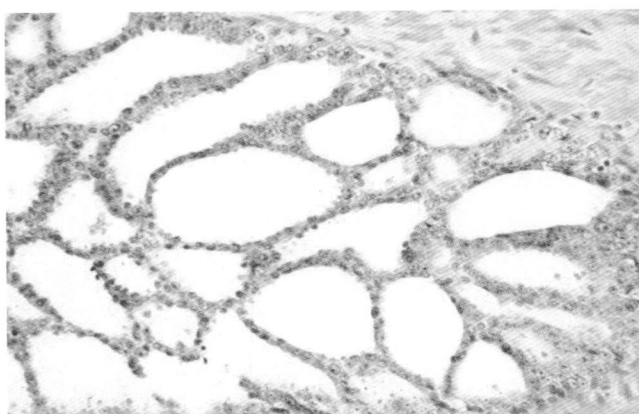

**FIGURE 32–23.** Cribriform pattern of high-grade PIN.

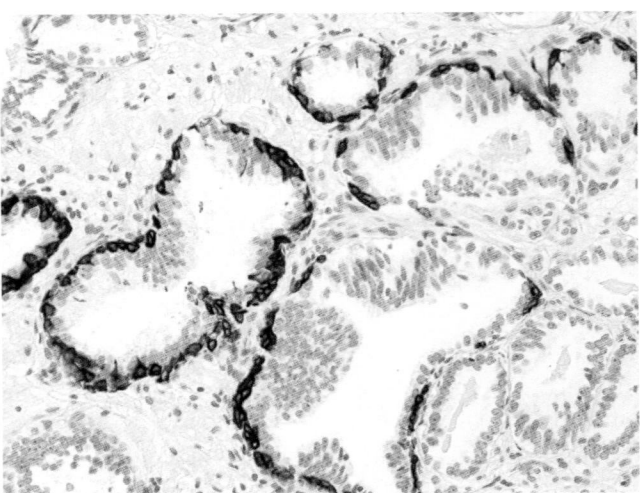

**FIGURE 32–25.** Keratin 34βE12 decorates the basal cells forming a discontinuous layer beneath the flat pattern of high-grade PIN (*left* and *top*); adenocarcinoma displays no immunoreactivity (*center, right,* and *bottom*) (anti-keratin 34βE12 immunohistochemical stain).

tween the architectural patterns of high-grade PIN, and their recognition seems to be of diagnostic utility only. Other unusual patterns of PIN include the signet ring cell pattern, small cell neuroendocrine pattern, mucinous pattern,[95] and microvacuolated (foamy gland) pattern.[96]

There is inversion of the normal orientation of epithelial proliferation with PIN; most proliferation normally occurs in the basal cell compartment, whereas in PIN, the greatest proliferation occurs on the luminal surface, similar to preinvasive lesions in the colon (tubular adenoma) and other sites.

PIN spreads through prostatic ducts in multiple different patterns, similar to prostatic carcinoma. In the first pattern, neoplastic cells replace the normal luminal secretory epithelium, with preservation of the basal cell layer and basement membrane. This pattern often has a cribriform or near-solid appearance. In the second pattern, there is direct invasion through the ductal or acinar wall, with disruption of the basal cell layer (Fig. 32–25). In the third pattern, neoplastic cells invaginate between the basal cell layer and columnar secretory cell layer ("pagetoid spread"), a rare finding.

Early stromal invasion, the earliest evidence of carcinoma, occurs at sites of acinar outpouching and basal cell disruption in acini with high-grade PIN. Such microinvasion is present in about 2% of high-power microscopic fields of PIN and is seen with equal frequency with all architectural patterns.[94]

PIN is associated with progressive abnormalities of phenotype and genotype that are intermediate between normal prostatic epithelium and cancer, indicating impairment of cell differentiation and regulatory control with advancing stages of prostatic carcinogenesis.[97] There is progressive loss of some markers of secretory differentiation, including PSA; PAP; secretory proteins; cytoskeletal proteins; and glycoproteins such as blood group antigens, neuroendocrine cells, p-cadherin, fibroblast growth factor-2, inhibin, prostate-specific transglutaminase, androgen receptor, insulin-like growth factor binding protein-3, telomerase, and p27KIP1. Other markers show progressive increase, including human glandular kallikrein 2 (hK2), *c-erbB-2* (*HER2-neu*) and *c-erbB-3* oncoproteins, *c-met* proto-oncogene, *BCL2* oncoprotein, mutator [RER(+)] phenotype, epidermal growth factor and epidermal growth factor receptor, type IV collagenase, Lewis Y antigen, transforming growth factor-α, apoptotic bodies, mitotic figures, proliferating cell nuclear antigen expression, Ki-67 expression, MIB-1 expression, tenascin-C, aneuploidy and genetic abnormalities,[98–100] microvessel density (MVD), Ep-Cam transmembrane glycoprotein, insulin-like growth factor binding protein rP1, and *p53* mutations. A model of prostatic carcinogenesis has been proposed based on the morphologic continuum of PIN and the multistep theory of carcinogenesis,[81] and animal models seem to confirm this model.[101, 102]

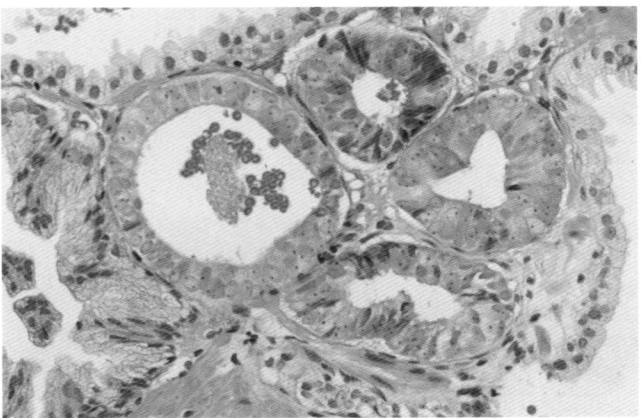

**FIGURE 32–24.** Flat pattern of high-grade PIN.

## Clinical Significance

PIN has a high predictive value as a marker for adenocarcinoma, and its identification warrants repeat biopsy for concurrent or subsequent invasive carcinoma.[103–111] The predictive value of high-grade PIN was evaluated in a retrospective case-control study of 100 patients with needle biopsy specimens with high-grade PIN and 112 biopsy specimens without PIN matched for clinical stage, patient age, and serum PSA.[105] Adenocarcinoma was identified in 36% of subsequent biopsy specimens from cases with PIN compared with 13% in the control group. The likelihood of finding cancer increased as the time interval from first biopsy specimen increased (32% incidence of cancer within 1 year compared with 38% incidence in follow-up biopsy specimens obtained after >1 year). High-grade PIN, patient age, and serum PSA concentration were jointly highly significant predictors of cancer, with PIN providing the highest risk ratio (14.9). These data underscore the strong association of PIN and adenocarcinoma and indicate that vigorous diagnostic follow-up is needed. High-grade PIN in TURP specimens also is an important predictive factor for prostate cancer.[90, 91]

## Effects of Therapy

There is a marked decrease in the prevalence and extent of high-grade PIN in cases after combination androgen deprivation therapy when compared with untreated cases.[112–114] Conversely, blockade of 5α-reductase with finasteride seems to have little or no effect on PIN, in contrast to other forms of androgen deprivation therapy.[115, 116] The prevalence and extent of PIN are decreased after radiation therapy.[117, 118]

## ADENOCARCINOMA

Prostate cancer is the most common cancer of men in the United States and is second only to lung cancer as a cause of cancer death. In 2002, 30,200 Americans will die of prostate cancer, and 189,000 new cases will be diagnosed.[119] For all men, the overall lifetime probability of developing clinical evidence of prostate cancer is greater than 1 in 6.[119a] Despite an 80% prevalence at autopsy by age 80 years, the clinical incidence is much lower, indicating that most men die with prostate carcinoma rather than from prostate carcinoma.

The incidence of prostate adenocarcinoma has risen dramatically, probably owing to early detection programs that employ digital rectal examination, serum PSA, and transrectal ultrasonography. As competing causes of mortality such as lung cancer and heart disease decline, men are living longer and increasing their risk of developing clinically apparent prostate cancer.

Prostate cancer has no specific presenting symptoms and usually is clinically silent, although it may cause lower urinary tract symptoms, mimicking nodular hyperplasia. Most cases today are found during screening or routine physical examination in men older than 40 years of age; digital rectal examination shows a nodular or diffusely enlarged prostate (clinical stage T2, T3, or T4), or serum PSA concentration is elevated, usually greater than 4 ng/mL (clinical stage T1c) (see later). Other clinical manifestations include incidental carcinoma in TURP specimens (clinical stage T1a carcinoma) and metastatic adenocarcinoma of unknown primary.

## Serum Prostate-Specific Antigen and Early Detection of Prostate Cancer

PSA is the most important, accurate, and clinically useful biochemical marker in the prostate.[120–122] It has contributed to an increase in the early detection rate of cancer and now is advocated for annual routine use in men older than age 40 who are at increased risk and in all men older than age 50. PSA is manufactured by the secretory epithelial cells and empties into the ductal system, where it catalyzes the liquefaction of the seminal coagulum after ejaculation. Serum levels are normally less than about 4.0 ng/mL but vary according to patient age, race, and other factors; any process that disrupts the normal architecture of the prostate allows diffusion of PSA into the stroma and microvasculature. Elevated serum PSA concentration is seen with prostatitis, with infarcts, with hyperplasia, and transiently after biopsy, but the most clinically important elevations are seen with prostate adenocarcinoma. Cancer produces less PSA per cell than benign epithelium, but the greater number and density of malignant cells and the stromal disruption associated with cancer account for the elevated serum PSA concentration.[123]

Serum PSA concentration is of proven value in detecting many cases of early prostate cancer. Cancer was present in 2.2% of a large series of healthy screened men with PSA concentration greater than 4.0 ng/mL.[121] The positive predictive value for PSA between 4.1 and 10.0 ng/mL was 22.4% to 26.5% and for PSA greater than 10.0 ng/mL was 50% to 67%.[120–122] A large multi-institutional study of 6630 men older than age 50 revealed PSA greater than 4.0 ng/mL in 15%; PSA was superior to digital rectal examination in detecting cancer (4.6% versus 3.2%), and the combination of these two tests was better (5.8%).[122] In addition to total serum PSA concentration, other derivatives of serum PSA have been described that may increase the predictive value for cancer by accounting for confounding variables, such as patient age, prostate volume, cancer volume, and amount: age-specific reference ranges, PSA den-

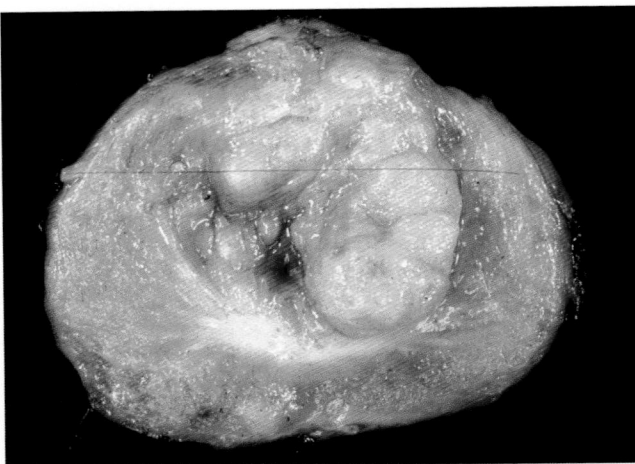

**FIGURE 32–26.** Prostate adenocarcinoma, gross appearance.

Atrophy
Postatrophic hyperplasia
Basal cell hyperplasia
Aypical adenomatous hyperplasia
Sclerosing adenosis
Nephrogenic metaplasia
Verumontanum mucosal gland hyperplasia
Hyperplasia of mesonephric remnants
High-grade prostatic intraepithelial neoplasia

sity, PSA velocity, PSA cancer density, PSA doubling time, free-to-total ratio, and complex PSA.

Serum PSA is an important tool in the management of prostate cancer. Elevation of PSA correlates with tumor recurrence and progression after surgery, radiation therapy, and androgen ablation therapy. Persistent elevation of PSA is associated with persistent carcinoma. PSA is a sensitive marker for tumor recurrence after treatment; it is useful for the early detection of metastases.

## Gross Pathology

Gross identification of prostate adenocarcinoma often is difficult in radical prostatectomy specimens, and definitive diagnosis requires microscopic examination. Adenocarcinoma tends to be multifocal, with a predilection for the peripheral zone. Grossly apparent tumor foci are at least 5 mm in greatest dimension and appear yellow-white with a firm consistency owing to stromal desmoplasia. Some tumors appear as yellow granular masses that stand in contrast with the normal spongy prostatic parenchyma (Fig. 32–26).

## Microscopic Features

Most prostate adenocarcinomas are composed of acini arranged in one or more patterns. The diagnosis relies on a combination of architectural and cytologic findings. The light microscopic features are usually sufficient for diagnosis, but rare cases may benefit from immunohistochemical studies (Table 32–2).

### ARCHITECTURE

Architectural features are assessed at low to medium power magnification and include variation in acinar spacing, size, and shape (Fig. 32–27). The arrangement of the acini is diagnostically useful and

is the basis of Gleason grade. Malignant acini usually have an irregular, haphazard arrangement, randomly scattered in the stroma in clusters or singly, usually with variation in spacing except in the lowest Gleason grades. The acini in suspicious foci are usually small or medium sized, with irregular contours that are in contrast to the smooth, round-to-elongate contours of benign and hyperplastic acini. Comparison with the adjacent benign prostatic acini is always of value.[124] Variation in acinar size is a particularly useful criterion, particularly when there are small irregular abortive acini with primitive lumina at the periphery of a focus of well-differentiated carcinoma.

### STROMA

The stroma in cancer frequently contains young collagen that appears lightly eosinophilic, although desmoplasia may be prominent. There sometimes is splitting or distortion of muscle fibers in the stroma, but this is an inconstant and unreliable feature by itself.

### CYTOLOGY

The cytologic features of adenocarcinoma include nuclear and nucleolar enlargement, and these are

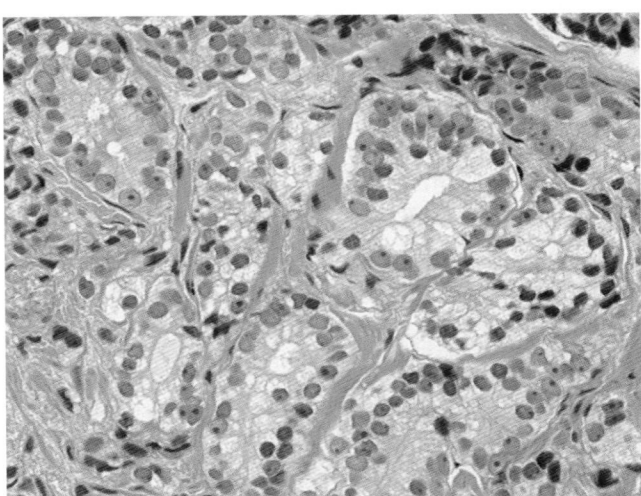

**FIGURE 32–27.** Gleason pattern 3 adenocarcinoma. There is greater variation in size, shape, and spacing of acini.

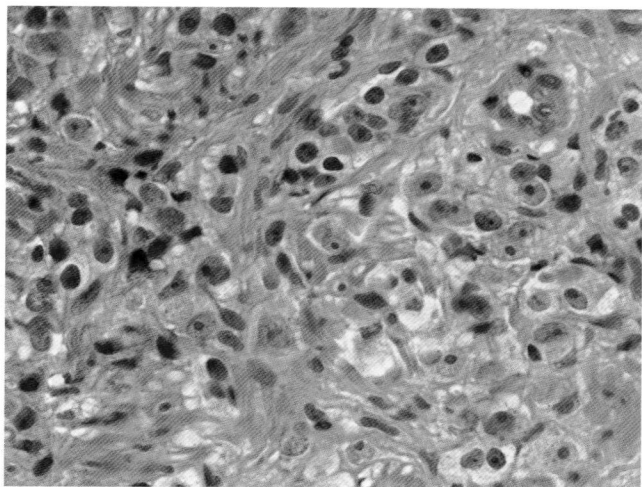

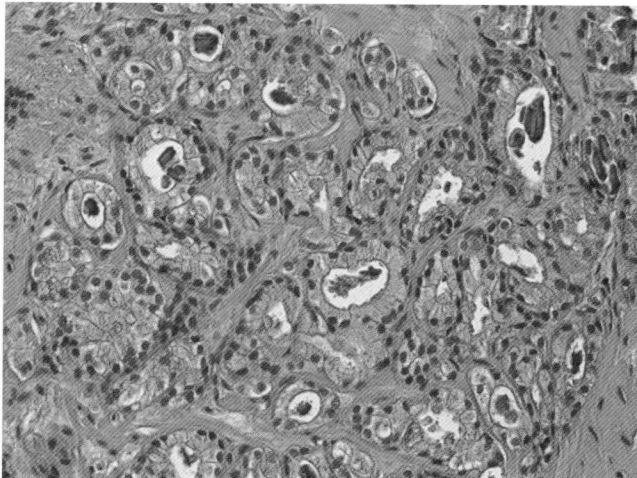

**FIGURE 32–28.** Gleason pattern 4 adenocarcinoma. The malignant acini are lined by cells with enlarged nuclei and prominent nucleioli.

**FIGURE 32–29.** Crystalloids in Gleason pattern 1 adenocarcinoma. We consider the presence of crystalloids to be a "soft" criterion for malignancy because they can be seen in AAH and other benign conditions.

present in most malignant cells (Fig. 32–28). Every cell has a nucleolus so that one searches for "prominent" nucleoli that are at least 1.25 to 1.50 $\mu$ in diameter or larger; however, I do not measure nucleoli routinely for diagnosis, so this determination is based on comparison with benign epithelial cells elsewhere in the specimen.[124] The identification of two or more nucleoli is virtually diagnostic of malignancy,[125] particularly when the nucleoli are located eccentrically in the nucleus; I find this criterion useful but employ it sparingly. Artifacts often obscure the nuclei and nucleoli, and overstaining of nuclei by hematoxylin creates one of the most common and difficult problems encountered in interpretation of suspicious foci. Differences in fixation and handling of biopsy specimens influence nuclear size and chromasia so that comparison with cells from the same specimen is important and serves as an internal control.

## LUMINAL MUCIN

Acidic sulfated and nonsulfated mucin often is seen in acini of adenocarcinoma, appearing as amorphous or delicate threadlike, faintly basophilic secretions in routine sections. This mucin stains with alcian blue and is shown best at pH 2.5, whereas the normal prostatic epithelium contains PAS-reactive neutral mucin. Acidic mucin is not specific for carcinoma.[126]

## CRYSTALLOIDS

Crystalloids are sharp needle-like eosinophilic structures that often are present in the lumina of well-differentiated and moderately differentiated carcinoma[127] (Fig. 32–29). They are not specific for carcinoma. They result from abnormal protein and mineral metabolism within benign and malignant

acini and probably are related to the hard eosinophilic proteinaceous secretions commonly found in the lumina of malignant acini. Ultrastructurally, crystalloids are composed of electron-dense material that lacks the periodicity of crystals, and x-ray microanalysis reveals abundant sulphur, calcium, and phosphorus and a small amount of sodium.[127] The presence of crystalloids in metastatic adenocarcinoma of unknown site of origin is strong presumptive evidence of prostatic origin, although it is an uncommon finding and is not conclusive.[128, 129]

## COLLAGENOUS MICRONODULES

Collagenous micronodules are a specific but infrequent and incidental finding in prostate adenocarcinoma, consisting of microscopic nodular masses of paucicellular eosinophilic fibrillar stroma that impinge on acinar lumina[130] (Fig. 32–30).

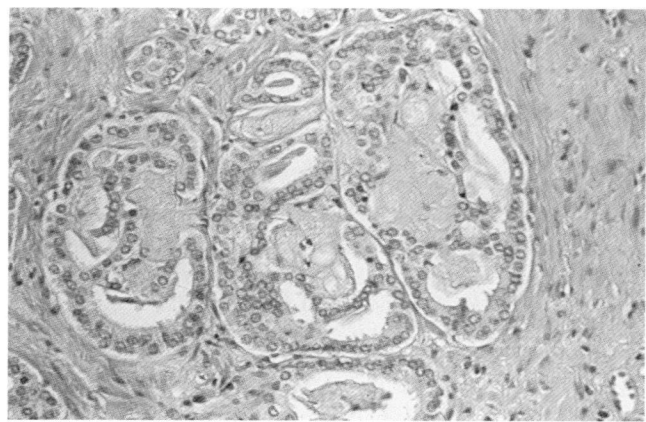

**FIGURE 32–30.** Collagenous micronodules in prostatic adenocarcinoma.

## PERINEURAL INVASION

Perineural invasion is common in adenocarcinoma and may be the only evidence of malignancy in biopsy specimens. This finding is strong presumptive evidence of malignancy but may occur rarely with benign acini.[131, 132] Complete circumferential growth, intraneural invasion, and ganglionic invasion are found only with cancer. This is probably not a useful predictive factor[133] (see later).

## VASCULAR AND LYMPHATIC INVASION

Microvascular invasion is a strong indicator of malignancy, and its presence correlates with histologic grade, although it sometimes is difficult to distinguish from fixation-associated retraction artifact of acini.[134]

## Immunohistochemistry

A few immunohistochemical studies are used commonly for diagnosis of prostate cancer. Studies of predictive factors are discussed elsewhere.

### BASAL CELL–SPECIFIC ANTIKERATIN 34βE12 (KERATIN 903, HIGH-MOLECULAR-WEIGHT KERATIN)

Basal cell–specific antikeratin 34βE12 stains virtually all of the normal basal cells of the prostate; there is no staining in the secretory and stromal cells. Basal cell layer disruption is present in 56% of cases of high-grade PIN, more commonly in glands adjacent to invasive carcinoma than in distant glands. The amount of disruption increases with increasing grades of PIN, with loss of more than one third of the basal cell layer in 52% of foci of high-grade PIN. Early carcinoma occurs at sites of acinar outpouching and basal cell layer disruption.[81] Prostate cancer cells do not react with this antibody, although it may stain other cancers. Basal cell layer disruption also occurs in inflamed acini, AAH, and PAH.[8, 42, 81]

In problem cases suspicious for adenocarcinoma, it may be useful to employ this immunohistochemical stain to evaluate the basal cell layer; however, this alone should not be the basis for a diagnosis of malignancy, particularly in small suspicious foci. This stain is of greatest utility in confirming the benignancy of a suspicious focus by showing an immunoreactive basal cell layer. It is also valuable after treatment for separating cancer and benign mimics of cancer (see later).

### PROSTATE-SPECIFIC ANTIGEN

Immunohistochemical staining for PSA is useful in identifying poorly differentiated prostate cancer in close proximity to the bladder and the rectum; it also can verify prostatic origin of metastatic carcinoma. The intensity of PSA immunoreactivity often varies from field to field within a tumor, and the correlation of staining intensity with tumor differentiation is inconsistent. PSA expression generally is greater in low-grade tumors than in high-grade tumors, but there is significant heterogeneity from cell to cell. Of poorly differentiated cancers, 1.6% are negative for PSA and PAP. The presence of PSA-immunoreactive tumor cells in poorly differentiated carcinoma suggests that these tumors retain subpopulations of cells with properties of normal secretory prostatic epithelial cells. Extraprostatic expression of PSA has been reported in many tissues and tumors, including periurethral gland adenocarcinoma in women, rectal carcinoid, and extramammary Paget's disease.

### PROSTATIC ACID PHOSPHATASE

PAP is a valuable immunohistochemical marker for identifying prostate cancer when used in combination with stains for PSA. There is more intense and uniform staining of tumor cells and the glandular epithelium of well-differentiated adenocarcinoma, whereas less intense and more variable staining was seen in moderately and poorly differentiated adenocarcinoma.

## Cancer Grade

Grade is one of the strongest predictors of biologic behavior in prostate cancer, including invasiveness and metastatic potential, but is not sufficiently reliable when used alone for predicting pathologic stage or outcome for individual patients. The Gleason score, recommended for routine use in all pretherapy specimens by the College of American Pathologists, is a scalar measurement that combines discrete primary and secondary groups (patterns or grades) into nine discrete groups (scores 2 to 10).[135] The primary grade is the most common or predominant grade; the secondary grade is the next most common but should comprise at least 5% of the tumor. It often is hard to apply this rule when the amount of cancer in the specimen is small; in such cases, there may be no secondary pattern, and the primary grade is doubled. Score should be reported on all cases as the histologic grade. Score and individual patterns should be reported, including the most frequent pattern followed by the worst pattern. (e.g., Gleason 7 [3 + 4]). In addition to individual specimen grading, global Gleason score should be given to encompass multiple biopsy specimens containing cancer. The relative percentage or proportion of high-grade cancer (Gleason primary pattern 4 and 5) also should be included, according to the World Health Organization.[135] Significant histologic changes in adenocarcinoma occur as a result of radiation and androgen deprivation therapy that make grading difficult and of questionable value. Interobserver and intraobserver variability have been reported with the Gleason grading system and other grading systems. Gleason[136] noted exact reproducibility of score in 50% of needle biopsy specimens, similar to the findings of others.

Gleason pattern 1 adenocarcinoma is uncommon and difficult to diagnose, particularly in biopsy specimens. It consists of a circumscribed mass of simple, monotonously replicated round acini that are uniform in size, shape, and spacing. Nuclear and nucleolar enlargement are moderate but allow separation from its closest mimic, AAH. Crystalloids are observed in more than half of cases.

Gleason pattern 2 is similar to pattern 1 except for the lack of circumscription of the focus, indicating the ability of the cancer to spread through the stroma. Slightly greater variation in acinar size and shape is observed, but the acinar contours are chiefly round and smoothly sculpted. Acinar packing is more variable than in pattern 1, and separation usually is less than one acinar diameter.

Gleason pattern 3 is the most common pattern of prostate adenocarcinoma and encompasses a wide and diverse group of lesions. The hallmark of pattern 3 adenocarcinoma is prominent variation in size, shape, and spacing of acini (Fig. 32–31). Despite this variation, the acini remain discrete and separate, in contrast to the fused acini of pattern 4 (see later). Acini are arranged haphazardly in the stroma, sometimes with prominent stromal fibrosis.

Gleason pattern 4 characteristically shows fusion of acini, with ragged infiltrating cords and nests at the edges (Fig. 32–32). In contrast to the simple entwined acinar tubules of pattern 3, this pattern consists of an anastomosing network of epithelium. Pattern 4 adenocarcinoma is considered poorly differentiated and is more malignant than pattern 3.

Gleason pattern 5 adenocarcinoma is characterized by fused sheets and masses of haphazardly arranged acini in the stroma, often displacing or overrunning adjacent tissues. In biopsy specimens, these cases raise the serious concern for anaplastic carcinoma or sarcoma. Cases with scattered acinar lumina indicative of glandular differentiation are included within this pattern. Comedocarcinoma is an

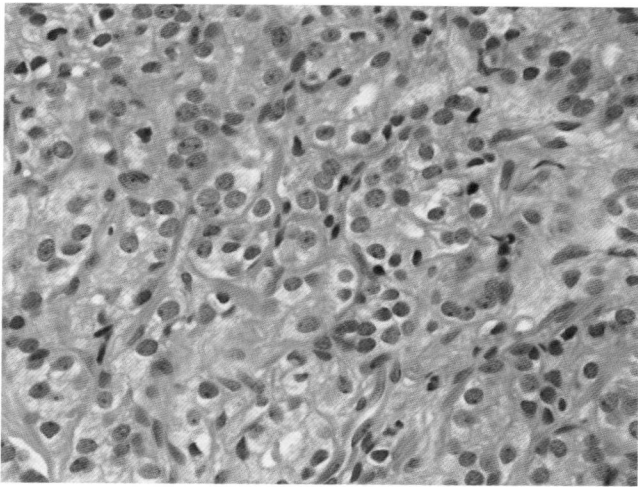

FIGURE 32–32. Gleason pattern 4 adenocarcinoma. There is prominent fusion and close packing of acini.

important subtype of this pattern, consisting of luminal necrosis within an otherwise cribriform pattern. Pattern 5 also includes rare histologic variants, such as signet ring cell carcinoma and small cell undifferentiated carcinoma.

Needle core biopsy underestimates tumor grade in 45% of cases and overestimates grade in 32%.[137–142] Exact correlation is present in about one third of biopsy specimens and about ± one Gleason unit in another one third. Grading errors are common in biopsy specimens with small amounts of tumor and low-grade tumor and probably are due to tissue sampling variation, tumor heterogeneity, and undergrading of needle biopsy specimens. Accuracy of biopsy is highest for the primary Gleason pattern, but the secondary pattern also provides useful predictive information, particularly when combined with the primary pattern to create the Gleason score. Gleason grading should be used for all needle biopsy specimens, even those with small amounts of tumor (Fig. 32–33).

On average, there are 2.7 (range, 1 to 5) different Gleason primary patterns (grades) in prostate cancer treated by radical prostatectomy.[143] More than 50% of cancers contain at least three different grades. The number of grades increases with greater cancer volume, the most common finding being high-grade cancer within the center of a larger, well-differentiated or moderately differentiated cancer occurring in approximately 53% of cases. Grade is an invariable component of most clinical nomograms in prostate cancer.

Reproducibility of this system has been reported to be a problem in some laboratories, as has been shown by Allsbrook and colleagues,[144] who reported on interobserver reproducibility of the Gleason grading system by 9 urologic pathologists and 41 general pathologists. In 35 of the 46 cases (about 70%), there was consensus among the urologic pathologists. Interobserver consensus among general pathologists

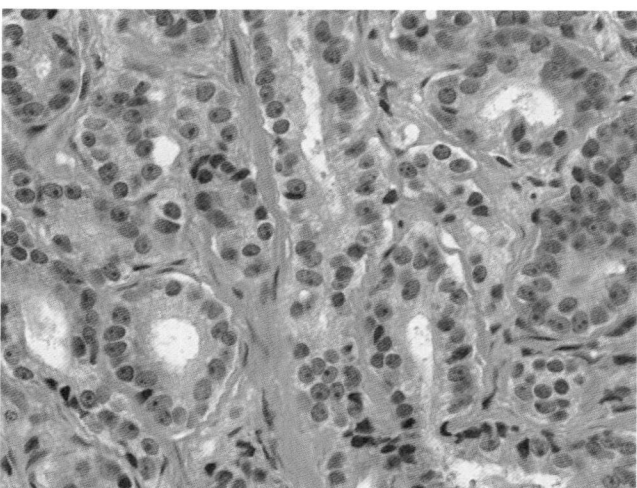

FIGURE 32–31. Gleason pattern 3 adenocarcinoma, large acinar type, consisting of an irregular aggregate of rigid angulated acini with variability of size, shape, and spacing. The epithelium may separate from the adjacent stroma, creating an artifactual space in some acini.

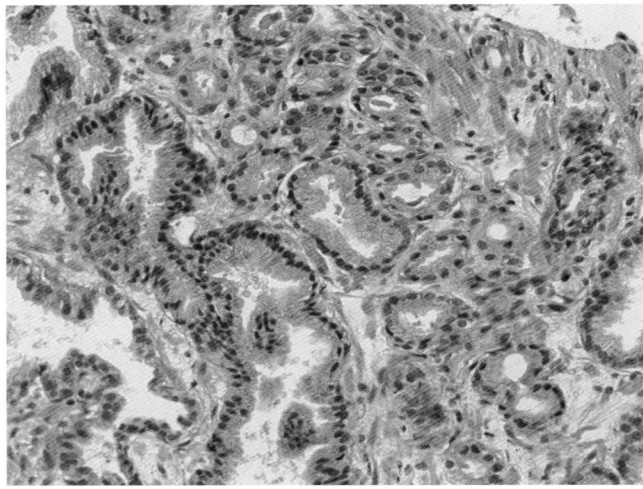

FIGURE 32–33. Minimum criteria for the diagnosis of cancer on needle biopsy. This tight cluster of small acini stands in contrast with the adjacent benign acini.

was overall at the low end of the moderate range ($\kappa$ = 0.435). There was consistent undergrading of Gleason's score 5 to 6 (47%), 7 (47%), and to lesser extent 8 (25%) among general pathologists.[145]

## Histologic Variants

The biologic behavior of histologic variants of adenocarcinoma may differ from typical acinar adenocarcinoma, and proper clinical management depends on accurate diagnosis and separation from tumors arising in other sites (Table 32–3).

### DUCTAL CARCINOMA (ADENOCARCINOMA WITH ENDOMETRIOID FEATURES, ENDOMETRIOID CARCINOMA)

Ductal carcinoma accounts for about 0.8% of prostate adenocarcinomas.[146] It typically arises as a poly-poid or papillary mass within the prostatic urethra and large periurethral prostatic ducts and may resemble histologically endometrial adenocarcinoma of the female uterus (Fig. 32–34). Most refer to this tumor as *adenocarcinoma with endometrioid features* or simply *ductal carcinoma*. The term *endometrial* should not be used in the prostate. My colleague and I reported that most cancers with papillary or cribriform pattern are located in the peripheral zone at a great distance from the urethra, indicating that the histologic findings are not specific.[146] Ductal carcinoma invariably displays intense cytoplasmic immunoreactivity for PAP and PSA. Focal CEA immunoreactivity is present occasionally. The prognosis of ductal carcinoma seems to be the same as typical acinar adenocarcinoma.

### MUCINOUS CARCINOMA (COLLOID CARCINOMA)

Pure mucinous carcinoma of the prostate is rare,[147, 148] although typical acinar adenocarcinoma often produces mucin focally, particularly after high-dose estrogen therapy. The clinical presentation of mucinous carcinoma is similar to typical acinar carcinoma, and there are no apparent differences in patient age, stage at presentation, cancer volume, serum PSA concentration, or pattern of metastases. This tumor may not respond well to endocrine therapy[149] or radiation therapy and is highly aggressive.[150, 151] Focal mucinous differentiation is observed in at least one third of cases of prostate carcinoma, but the accepted diagnosis of mucinous carcinoma arbitrarily requires that at least 25% of the tumor contains pools of extracellular mucin. Mucinous carcinoma consists of tumor cell nests and clusters floating in mucin, similar to mucinous carcinoma of the breast (Fig. 32–35). Three patterns of mucinous carcinoma have been described: 1) acinar carcinoma with luminal distention, 2) cribriform carcinoma with luminal distention, and 3) *colloid carcinoma* with cell nests embedded in mucinous lakes.[148] In some cases, the nuclei are low grade, with uniform finely granular chromatin and inconspicuous nucleoli, but

**TABLE 32–3.** Histologic Variants of Prostate Cancer

Adenocarcinoma with endometrioid features (ductal adenocarcinoma)
Mucinous carcinoma
Signet ring cell carcinoma
Adenocarcinoma with neuroendocrine differentiation
Neuroendocrine carcinoma
Squamous cell and adenosquamous cell carcinoma
Sarcomatoid carcinoma
Adenoid cystic carcinoma
Lymphoepithelioma-like carcinoma
Carcinoma with oncocytic features
Comedocarcinoma
Cribriform carcinoma
Pseudohyperplastic adenocarcinoma
Adenocarcinoma with microvacuolated cytoplasm (foamy cell carcinoma)
Adenocarcinoma with atrophic features
Adenocarcinoma with glomeruloid features

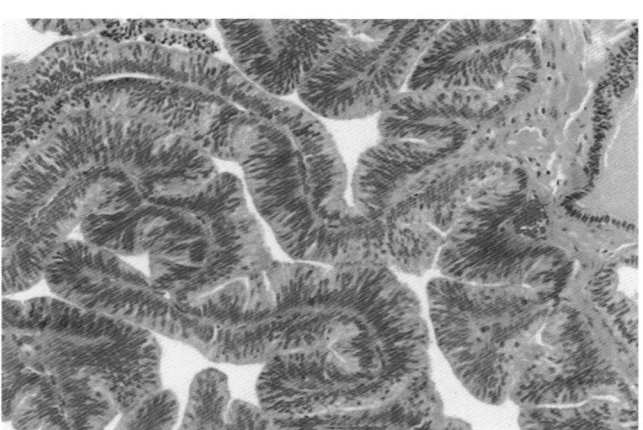

FIGURE 32–34. Ductal adenocarcinoma. This papillary proliferation filled the large periurethral prostatic ducts and protruded into the urethra.

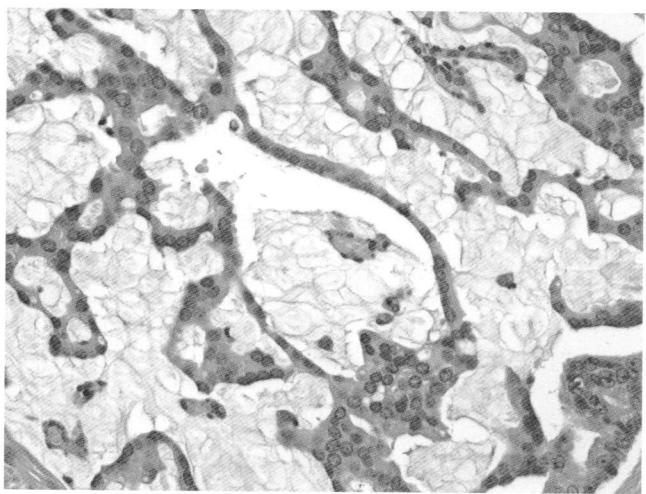

**FIGURE 32–35.** Mucinous (colloid) carcinoma, with pools of mucin punctuated by floating islands of cancer cells.

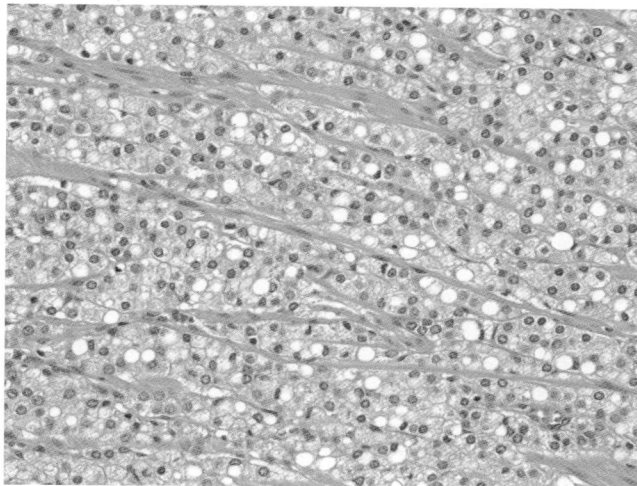

**FIGURE 32–36.** Signet ring cell carcinoma with pale blue mucinous luminal secretions.

their presence within mucin pools is diagnostic of malignancy. Mucinous carcinoma stains with PAS, alcian blue, and mucicarmine, similar to other prostatic mucin, but these stains are used rarely in practice. Most studies have found neutral mucin in benign acini and acidic mucin in malignant acini, although benign acini rarely produce small quantities of acidic mucin.[152] Some have suggested that acidic mucin is a useful supportive feature in the diagnosis of adenocarcinoma, present in about 60% of cases, but this has been refuted.[37]

## SIGNET RING CELL CARCINOMA

Signet ring cell carcinoma of the prostate is rare.[153–155] The clinical presentation is similar to typical acinar adenocarcinoma except that all are high stage. The prognosis is poor. The diagnosis of signet ring cell carcinoma arbitrarily requires that 25% or more of the tumor is composed of signet ring cells, although some authors require 50%. Most often, it is a minor component of Gleason pattern 5 carcinoma. Tumor cells show distinctive nuclear displacement by clear cytoplasm (Fig. 32–36). Signet ring cells are present in 2.5% of cases of acinar adenocarcinoma but rarely in sufficient numbers to be considered signet ring cell carcinoma.[154] Histochemical and immunohistochemical results with mucin, lipid, PSA, PAP, and CEA stains are variable, and the signet ring cell appearance may result from cytoplasmic lumina, mucin granules, and fat vacuoles.

## CARCINOMA WITH NEUROENDOCRINE DIFFERENTIATION (ADENOCARCINOMA WITH NEUROENDOCRINE CELLS, INCLUDING THOSE WITH LARGE EOSINOPHILIC GRANULES [PANETH CELL–LIKE CHANGE])

Virtually all prostate adenocarcinomas contain at least a few neuroendocrine cells, but special studies, such as histochemistry and immunohistochemistry,

usually are necessary to identify them.[10, 11, 13, 14, 110, 156] About 10% of adenocarcinomas contain cells with large eosinophilic granules (formerly referred to as *adenocarcinoma with Paneth cell–like change*), usually consisting of only rare foci of scattered cells and small clusters that may be overlooked.[9] The clinical features of adenocarcinoma with neuroendocrine differentiation are similar to typical acinar adenocarcinoma. Neuroendocrine differentiation in adenocarcinoma has no impact on prognosis so that there is no role for immunohistochemical stains for neuroendocrine markers in routine practice.

## NEUROENDOCRINE CARCINOMA (SMALL CELL CARCINOMA AND CARCINOID)

Most cases of neuroendocrine carcinoma have typical local signs and symptoms of prostate adenocarcinoma, although paraneoplastic syndromes are frequent in these patients, including Cushing's syndrome, malignant hypercalcemia, syndrome of inappropriate antidiuretic hormone (SIADH) secretion, and myasthenic (Eaton-Lambert) syndrome. Small cell carcinoma is aggressive and rapidly fatal.[157, 158] Neuroendocrine carcinoma of the prostate varies histopathologically from carcinoid-like pattern (low-grade neuroendocrine carcinoma) to small cell undifferentiated (oat cell) carcinoma (high-grade neuroendocrine carcinoma) (Fig. 32–37). These tumors are morphologically identical to their counterparts in the lung and other sites. Typical acinar adenocarcinoma is present, at least focally, in about half of cases, and transition patterns may be seen. In cases with solid Gleason 5 pattern suggestive of neuroendocrine carcinoma, immunohistochemical stains are recommended. A wide variety of secretory products may be detected within the malignant cells, including serotonin, calcitonin, adrenocorticotropic hormone, human chorionic gonadotropin, thyroid-stimulating hormone, bombesin, calcitonin gene–related peptide, and inhibin.[157] The same cells may express peptide hormones and PSA and PAP, but pure small cell

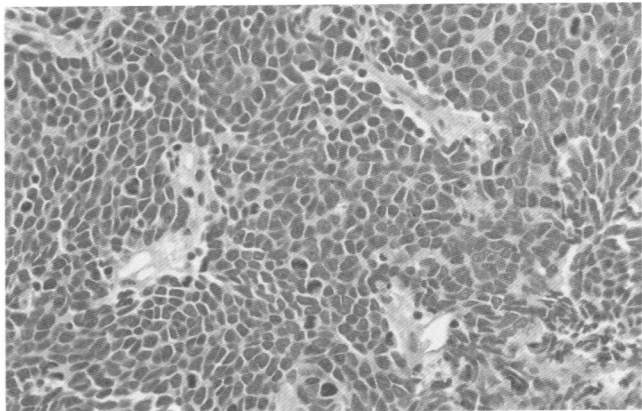

FIGURE 32–37. Small cell undifferentiated (oat cell) carcinoma of the prostate.

carcinoma usually does not display immunoreactivity for PSA. Serotonin, chromogranin, and synaptophysin are the most useful markers of neuroendocrine cells in formalin-fixed sections of prostate.[11, 13, 156] Ultrastructurally, small cell carcinoma and carcinoid tumor of the prostate contain a variable number of round regular membrane-bound neurosecretory granules. Well-defined cytoplasmic processes usually are present that contain neurosecretory granules.

## SQUAMOUS CELL AND ADENOSQUAMOUS CARCINOMA

Squamous cell carcinoma is rare in the prostate.[159–161] Adenosquamous carcinoma refers to the combination of squamous cell carcinoma and typical acinar carcinoma and is rare[162] (Fig. 32–38). Presenting signs and symptoms are similar to those of typical prostate adenocarcinoma, although there is often a history of hormonal therapy or radiation therapy.[161] Squamous cell carcinoma of the prostate also may

arise in patients with *Schistosoma haematobium*. Serum PSA and PAP concentrations usually are normal, even with metastases, and bone metastases typically are osteolytic rather than osteoblastic.[160] The prognosis is poor, with a mean survival of 14 months regardless of therapy. These tumors seem to be unresponsive to androgen deprivation therapy. Squamous cell carcinoma of the prostate is histopathologically similar to its counterpart in other organs, consisting of irregular nests and cords of malignant cells with keratinization and squamous differentiation, rarely with squamous pearls. Keratinizing squamous cell carcinoma of the prostate usually arises in the periurethral ducts and is rare; otherwise the site of origin of squamous cell carcinoma is unknown.[160] We require an absence of acinar differentiation for the diagnosis of squamous cell carcinoma and a lack of bladder involvement; mixed tumors are classified best simply as adenosquamous carcinoma. There may be PSA and PAP immunoreactivity in the acinar and squamous components of adenosquamous carcinoma.[162, 163]

## SARCOMATOID CARCINOMA (CARCINOSARCOMA, METAPLASTIC CARCINOMA)

*Sarcomatoid carcinoma* is considered by many to be synonymous with *carcinosarcoma*[164] (Fig. 32–39). Authors who separate these tumors define sarcomatoid carcinoma as an epithelial tumor showing spindle cell (mesenchymal) differentiation and carcinosarcoma as adenocarcinoma intimately admixed with heterologous malignant soft tissue elements. Regardless of terminology, these tumors are rare and aggressive. Patients tend to be older men who present with symptoms of urinary outlet obstruction, similar to typical adenocarcinoma. Serum PSA concentration may be normal at the time of diagnosis.[164] About half of patients have a prior history of typical acinar adenocarcinoma treated by radiation therapy or androgen deprivation therapy. Treatment is variable

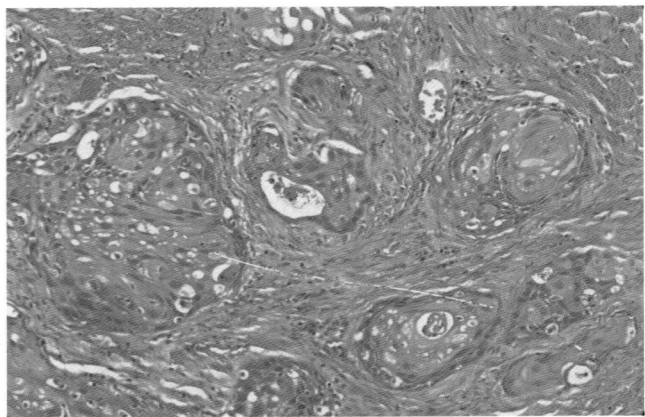

FIGURE 32–38. Adenosquamous cell carcinoma of the prostate. This tumor was identified many years after radiation therapy and androgen deprivation therapy for typical acinar adenocarcinoma. (Case courtesy of Dr. Manuel Doria, Chicago, IL.)

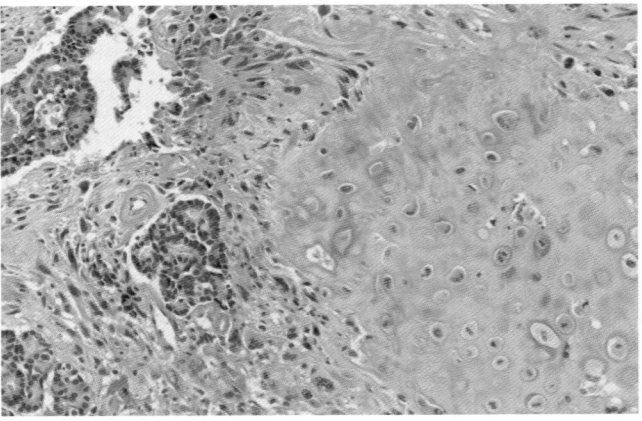

FIGURE 32–39. Sarcomatoid carcinoma (carcinosarcoma) of the prostate, consisting of an intimate admixture of adenocarcinoma and chondroblastic osteosarcoma.

and has no apparent influence on the poor prognosis. Pathologically the distinction between sarcomatoid carcinoma and carcinosarcoma often is difficult and of no apparent clinical significance. Metastases may consist of carcinoma or sarcoma or both, however, so that careful search of the primary tumor is useful to identify a component of carcinoma. Coexistent adenocarcinoma almost always is high grade. The most common soft tissue elements are osteosarcoma, with or without cartilaginous differentiation, and leiomyosarcoma.[164] The epithelial component displays cytoplasmic immunoreactivity for keratin, PSA, and PAP, similar to typical prostate adenocarcinoma. The soft tissue component usually displays immunoreactivity for vimentin, with variable staining for desmin, actin, and S-100 protein. Two cases arising after radiation therapy for typical acinar adenocarcinoma had increased expression of p53.[165]

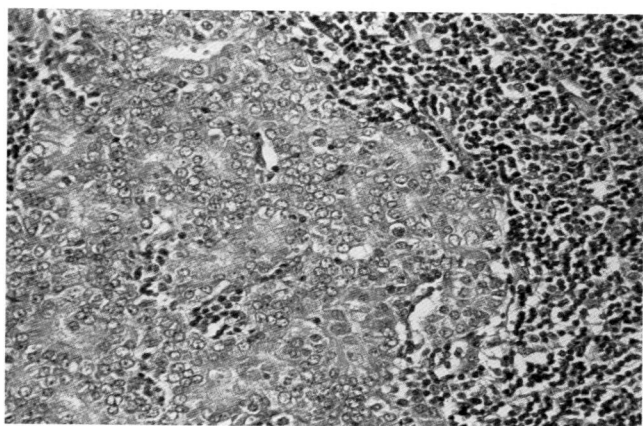

**FIGURE 32–40.** Lymphoepithelioma-like carcinoma of the prostate.

## ADENOID CYSTIC CARCINOMA/BASAL CELL CARCINOMA (BASAL CELL CARCINOMA, BASALOID CARCINOMA, ADENOID CYSTIC CARCINOMA, ADENOID CYSTIC-LIKE TUMOR, ADENOID BASAL CELL TUMOR)

Adenoid cystic carcinoma/basal cell carcinoma is rare, consisting of basal cell nests of varying size infiltrating the stroma. The malignant potential of adenoid cystic carcinoma/basal cell carcinoma is uncertain because of the small number of reported cases and limited follow-up, but some cases are malignant with extraprostatic extension and distant metastases. At present, adenoid basal cell tumor probably is considered best a tumor of low malignant potential.[166] There are two architectural patterns of adenoid cystic carcinoma/basal cell carcinoma: adenoid cystic and basaloid.[167] The adenoid cystic pattern consists of irregular clusters of crowded basal cells punctuated by round fenestrations, many of which contain mucinous material resembling salivary gland adenoid cystic carcinoma. The basaloid pattern consists of variably sized round basaloid cell nests with prominent peripheral palisading. These patterns frequently coexist, although pure forms have been described. Adenoid cystic carcinoma/basal cell carcinoma displays variable immunoreactivity with keratin 34βE12; there may be luminal cell staining or peripheral basal cell staining.[44, 46] Rare scattered cells show PSA and PAP immunoreactivity, but these may represent entrapped residual secretory luminal cells; other cells may show chromogranin staining. S-100 protein and neuron-specific enolase stains are negative.

## LYMPHOEPITHELIOMA-LIKE CARCINOMA

Carcinoma accompanied by a dense lymphocytic infiltrate is referred to as *lymphoepithelioma-like carcinoma* or *medullary carcinoma*.[168] This histologically distinctive tumor is identical to its counterpart in the head and neck region, although genitourinary cases are not associated with Epstein-Barr virus. The clinical significance of prostate lymphoepithelioma-like carcinoma is uncertain (Fig. 32–40).

## CARCINOMA WITH ONCOCYTIC FEATURES

Prostatic adenocarcinoma rarely has diffuse oncocytic change, consisting of tumor cells with abundant eosinophilic granular cytoplasm that reflects the presence of abundant mitochondria.[169, 170] Tumor cells display PSA immunoreactivity. The clinical behavior seems to be the same as typical acinar adenocarcinoma.

## COMEDOCARCINOMA

Comedocarcinoma is found invariably in association with other patterns of adenocarcinoma and probably does not warrant separation as a clinicopathologic entity. It is characterized by luminal necrosis within ducts expanded by malignant cells, similar to comedocarcinoma of the breast. This morphologic variant of adenocarcinoma is included in the Gleason grading system as poorly differentiated (grade 5) carcinoma based on the degree of acinar differentiation. There is a high frequency of aneuploidy in comedocarcinoma, suggesting aggressiveness. PSA and PAP are present in most tumor cells.

## CRIBRIFORM CARCINOMA

The cribriform pattern is found invariably in association with other patterns of adenocarcinoma and does not warrant separation as a clinicopathologic entity. This histologically distinct variant of Gleason grade 3 carcinoma is characterized by large intraductal epithelial cell masses punctuated by multiple small lumina. In contrast to cribriform PIN, cribriform carcinoma does not have a basal cell layer at the periphery of acini.[171, 172]

## PSEUDOHYPERPLASTIC CARCINOMA

At low magnification, pseudohyperplastic carcinoma, a low-grade carcinoma (Gleason primary pattern 2 or 3 cancer), may be mistaken for an exuberant hyperplastic nodule.[173] Pseudohyperplastic carcinoma is histologically distinctive but does not warrant separation as a clinicopathologic entity.

## ADENOCARCINOMA WITH MICROVACUOLATED CYTOPLASM (XANTHOMATOID CARCINOMA, FOAMY GLAND CARCINOMA)

Adenocarcinoma with microvacuolated cytoplasm is characterized by cells with abundant microvacuoles in the cytoplasm, displacing the nuclei basally. Diagnostic difficulty is encountered when this pattern predominates, owing to the small size and hyperchromasia of the nuclei that may be interpreted as benign. This is not a distinct clinicopathologic entity.

## ATROPHIC PATTERN OF ADENOCARCINOMA

Cancer acini with dilated lumina and flattened lining cells with modest-sized nucleoli are referred to as *atrophic* cancer.[173a, 174, 175] This is an unusual pattern that is mistaken easily for atrophy. Useful diagnostic features include the presence of adjacent typical acinar adenocarcinoma and identification of enlarged prominent nucleoli in at least some of the cells in the *atrophic* focus, but caution is warranted in rendering this difficult diagnosis based on needle biopsy specimens with only a small amount of cancer (Fig. 32–41).

## CARCINOMA WITH GLOMERULOID FEATURES

Prostate adenocarcinoma rarely contains focal or extensive glomeruloid pattern, characterized by round nests of cancer cells partially filling small cystic spaces, reminiscent of renal glomeruli.[176] This pattern is considered best Gleason primary pattern 3 cancer.

## Urothelial Carcinoma Involving the Prostate and Prostatic Urethra

Urothelial carcinoma of the prostate usually represents synchronous or metachronous spread from carcinoma in the bladder and urethra.[177] It involves

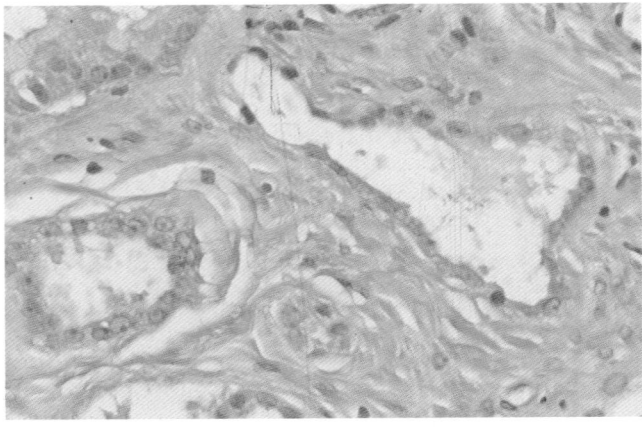

**FIGURE 32–41.** Atrophic pattern of adenocarcinoma.

the prostate and urethra in about 40% of radical cystoprostatectomy specimens for bladder carcinoma.[178] Patients usually present with symptoms of hematuria, urinary obstruction, or prostatitis. Serum PSA and PAP concentrations are not elevated. Diagnostic criteria are identical to those for urothelial cancer of the bladder and urethra. Carcinoma in situ (high-grade urothelial dysplasia or urothelial intraepithelial neoplasia) often is overlooked in specimens submitted for histologic examination.[179] It is usually multifocal, with bladder and urethral involvement; the prevalence varies from 4% to 32% in cystoprostatectomies for bladder cancer.

## Treatment Changes in Adenocarcinoma

Treatment changes in the benign and cancerous prostate create diagnostic challenges in pathologic interpretation, particularly in needle biopsy specimens and evaluation of possible extraprostatic metastases. It is crucial that the clinician provide the pertinent history of androgen deprivation or radiation therapy to assist the pathologist in rendering the correct diagnosis.

### ANDROGEN DEPRIVATION THERAPY

A variety of agents are used for androgen deprivation, and the histopathologic effects of most are similar[113, 114, 180–191] (Table 32–4). Hormonal treatment al-

**TABLE 32–4.** Androgen Deprivation Therapy: Histologic Features in the Prostate*

***Benign Epithelium***
Secretory cell layer
   Prominent acinar atrophy
   Decreased ratio of acini to stroma
   Enlargement and clearing of cytoplasm
   Prominent clear cell change
Basal cell layer
   Hyperplasia
   Prominent component of benign acini
   Squamous metaplasia
Stroma
   Edema in early stages; fibrosis in late stages
   Patchy condensation, resulting in focal hypercellularity
   Focal chronic inflammation (lymphohistiocytic)

***High-Grade Prostatic Intraepithelial Neoplasia***
Decrease in prevalence and extent
Nuclear shrinkage
Nuclear hyperchromasia
Nucleolar shrinkage
Other cytologic changes similar to benign secretory cell layer

***Prostatic Adenocarcinoma***
Loss of glandular architecture
Nuclear shrinkage
Nuclear hyperchromasia and pyknosis
Nucleolar shrinkage
Mucinous degeneration
Other cytologic changes similar to benign secretory cell layer

*There is some variability in these changes depending on the method of therapy.

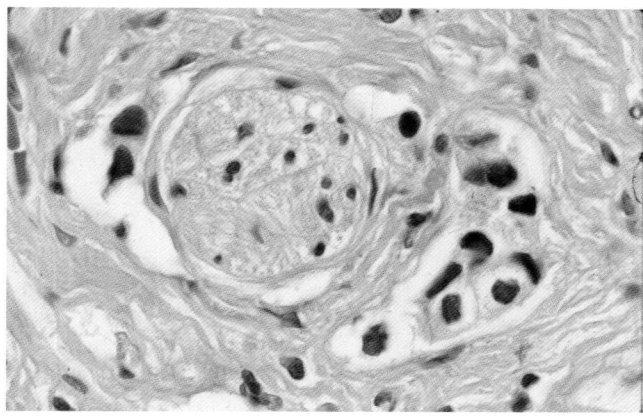

**FIGURE 32–42.** Perineural invasion by prostatic adenocarcinoma following androgen deprivation therapy.

ters the benign and cancerous prostatic epithelium, causing acinar atrophy, apoptosis (programmed cell death), cytoplasmic clearing, nuclear and nucleolar shrinkage, and chromatin condensation (Fig. 32–42). Squamous metaplasia and glycogenic acanthosis are common findings after orchiectomy and diethylstilbestrol therapy but are uncommon after contemporary forms of treatment. Cancer usually appears as sheets and ribbons of cells with clear cytoplasm and an infiltrative pattern reminiscent of lobular carcinoma of the breast. Tumor cell nuclei frequently are small and hyperchromatic, obscuring the nucleoli and creating a "nucleolus-poor" appearance in many areas.[191a]

Two international consensus conferences recommended that grading after hormonal therapy is of no practical value.[191, 192] The volume of prostate cancer is reduced by more than 40% after treatment, and there is a 20% to 25% decline in positive margins at radical prostatectomy.[190] Pathologic stage is similar in untreated and treated prostate adenocarcinoma, according to retrospective reports of radical prostatectomies, although there is a trend toward lower stage in treated cases. Occasional cases after therapy display the *vanishing cancer phenomenon,* in which no residual cancer was found in the radical prostatectomy specimen.[193]

PSA and PAP are retained in tumor cells after 3 months of therapy but decline with longer duration of therapy[194]; keratin 34$\beta$E12 remains negative, regardless of duration, indicating an absent basal cell layer.[194] No differences were found in expression of neuroendocrine differentiation markers, such as chromogranin, neuron-specific enolase, $\beta$-human chorionic gonadotropin, and serotonin after androgen deprivation therapy. Proliferating cell nuclear antigen immunoreactivity declines after androgen deprivation therapy, indicating that androgens regulate cyclically expressed proteins involved in cell proliferation. Quantitative comparative genomic hybridization studies of untreated and treated prostate cancer revealed similar level of genetic alterations, suggesting that untreated metastatic cancer contains

most of the chromosomal changes necessary for recurrence.[195]

### RADIATION THERAPY

Histologic changes of radiation injury in benign and hyperplastic epithelium include acinar atrophy and distortion, marked cytologic abnormalities of the epithelium, basal cell hyperplasia, stromal fibrosis, decreased ratio of acini to stroma, and vascular changes[118, 179, 196] (Table 32–5). PIN after radiation therapy retains characteristic features of untreated PIN, but the prevalence and extent decline.[118, 179] Histologic features that are helpful for the diagnosis of cancer after radiation therapy include infiltrative growth, perineural invasion, intraluminal crystalloids, blue mucin secretions, the absence of corpora amylacea, and the presence of concomitant high-grade PIN (Table 32–6; Fig. 32–43). For about 12 months after completion of external-beam irradiation, needle biopsy is of limited value because of ongoing tumor cell death. After this period, however, biopsy is a good method for assessing local tumor control, with a low level of sampling variation that is minimized by obtaining multiple specimens.[117, 118, 196–202] The changes after three-dimensional conformal therapy are similar to those after

**TABLE 32–5.** Histopathologic Findings in Benign Prostatic Tissue in Postirradiation Needle Biopsy Specimens at the Time of Prostate-Specific Antigen (Biochemical) Failure

| Histopathologic Findings | % Cases |
| --- | --- |
| Inflammation | 39 |
| Atrophy | 79 |
| Postatrophic hyperplasia | 18 |
| Acinar distortion | 54 |
| Decreased acinar-to-stromal ratio | 86 |
| Basal cell hyperplasia | 68 |
| Atypical basal cell hyperplasia | 57 |
| Hyperplastic (proliferative change) | 11 |
| Squamous metaplasia | 0 |
| Eosinophilic metaplasia | 21 |
| Stromal changes | |
|   Stromal fibrosis | 93 |
|   Stromal edema | 21 |
|   Stromal calcification | 21 |
|   Hemosiderin deposition | 0 |
|   Atypical fibroblasts | 25 |
|   Necrosis | 0 |
|   Granulation tissue formation | 0 |
| Myointimal proliferation | 11 |
| Cytologic changes | |
|   Nuclear pyknosis | 75 |
|   Nuclear enlargement | 86 |
|   Prominent nucleoli | 50 |
|   Bizarre nuclei | 54 |
|   Cytoplasmic vacuolization | 29 |
| Intraluminal contents | |
|   Crystalloids | 0 |
|   Mucin | 4 |
|   Eosinophilic granular secretions | 39 |
|   Corpora amylacea | 32 |

**TABLE 32–6.** Histopathologic Findings in Prostate Adenocarcinoma in Postirradiation Needle Biopsy Specimens at the Time of Prostate-Specific Antigen (Biochemical) Failure

| Histopathologic Findings | % Cases |
|---|---|
| **Gleason score** | |
| <7 | 17 |
| 7 | 48 |
| >7 | 35 |
| **Cancer involvement** | |
| ≤10% | 31 |
| 11–40% | 28 |
| 41–80% | 35 |
| 81–100% | 7 |
| **No. cancer foci** | |
| 1 | 36 |
| 2–4 | 50 |
| ≥5 | 14 |
| **Combined score of radiation effect\*** | |
| 0–2 (minimal) | 52 |
| 3–4 (moderate) | 38 |
| 5–6 (severe) | 10 |
| Infiltrative growth | 100 |
| Perineural invasion | 31 |
| Atrophic change | 10 |
| Nuclear pyknosis | 72 |
| Nuclear enlargement | 93 |
| Prominent nucleoli | 79 |
| **Cytoplasmic vacuolization** | |
| <10% | 45 |
| 10–50% | 45 |
| >50% | 10 |
| Inflammation | 0 |
| Stromal desmoplasia | 76 |
| Necrosis | 0 |
| **Intraluminal contents** | |
| Crystalloids | 3 |
| Mucin | 21 |
| Eosinophilic | 24 |
| Corpora amylacea | 0 |
| Concomitant high-grade PIN† | 7 |

\* Radiation effect was quantified using the scoring system described by Crook et al.[207]
† PIN, prostatic intraepithelial neoplasia.

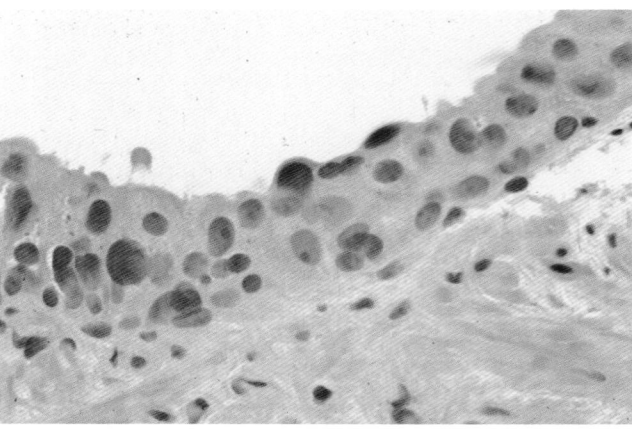

**FIGURE 32–43.** Radiation change of the prostatic epithelium mimicking high-grade PIN. There are marked nuclear abnormalities, including variation in size and shape and hyperchromasia.

ses, and death from prostate cancer than those with negative biopsy specimens. Postirradiation Gleason grade and DNA ploidy are independent prognostic factors in patients with prostate cancer who failed radiation therapy. Cancer grade usually shows little or no evidence of *dedifferentiation* after radiation therapy, however.[117, 118]

The severity and extent of radiation changes in the prostate may be of prognostic value in patients treated by external-beam therapy and brachytherapy[207, 208] and seem to vary according to radiation dose.[118, 209] No definitive method exists for assessment of tumor viability after irradiation.

## ULTRASOUND HYPERTHERMIA, MICROWAVE HYPERTHERMIA, LASER THERAPY, AND HOT WATER BALLOON THERMOTHERAPY

All forms of hyperthermia for nodular hyperplasia result in sharply circumscribed hemorrhagic coagulative necrosis that soon organizes with granulation tissue; the pattern and extent of injury are deter-

conventional external-beam therapy[118] (Fig. 32–44). The addition of androgen deprivation therapy has no appreciable histopathologic effect on the radiation-altered prostate.[118]

PSA, PAP and keratin 34βE12 expression in the prostatic epithelium are not altered by radiation therapy and often are of value in separating treated adenocarcinoma and its mimics. Prostate cancer after radiation therapy has increased *p53* nuclear accumulation and Ki-67 labeling index when compared with cancer without prior irradiation. Loss of *p21*^WAF1 function has been implicated in the failure of irradiation response.[203]

Persistent cancer in needle biopsy specimens after radiation therapy has a significant impact on patient management because positive needle biopsy specimens portend a worse prognosis.[118, 203, 203a, 204–206] Patients with positive biopsy specimens are more likely to have local recurrence, distant metasta-

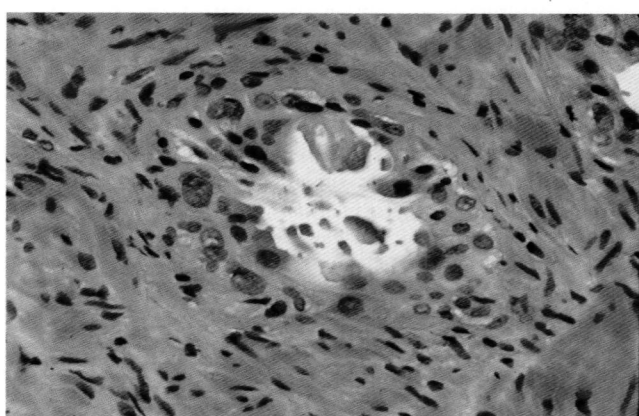

**FIGURE 32–44.** Radiation change of the prostatic epithelium, showing nuclear abnormalities involving the basal cell and secretory cell layers.

mined by the method of thermocoagulation employed, the duration of treatment, tissue perfusion factors, and the ratio of epithelium to stroma in the tissue being treated.[210, 211] Transurethral methods may be safer and more effective than transrectal methods because they seem to avoid injury to the rectal mucosa. When delivered transurethrally, laser thermocoagulation and microwave hyperthermia usually do not involve the peripheral zone or neighboring structures, presumably because of differences in tissue perfusion.[211, 212] Coagulation necrosis is greater in areas of predominantly epithelial nodular hyperplasia rather than predominantly stromal hyperplasia and the dense fibromuscular tissue of the bladder neck. Confluent coagulation necrosis occurs when multiple laser lesions are created in a single transverse plane.

## CRYOABLATION THERAPY (CRYOSURGERY)

Cryosurgical ablation refers to freezing of the prostate. Multiple cryoprobe needles filled with circulating liquid nitrogen transform the prostate into an iceball, resulting in substantial tissue destruction and death of benign and malignant cells. The flow of liquid nitrogen through the probes is adjusted to create the desired freezing pattern and extent of tissue destruction in the prostate; no liquid nitrogen comes in contact with the tissue.

Preliminary results with cryoablation for prostate cancer are encouraging, but the method still is considered experimental. After cryosurgery, the prostate shows typical features of repair, including marked stromal fibrosis and hyalinization, basal cell hyperplasia with ductal and acinar regeneration, squamous metaplasia, urothelial metaplasia, and stromal hemorrhage and hemosiderin deposition.[213–217] Coagulative necrosis is present between 6 and 30 weeks of therapy, but patchy chronic inflammation is more common. Focal granulomatous inflammation is associated with epithelial disruption resulting from corpora amylacea. Dystrophic calcification is infrequent and usually appears in areas with the greatest reparative response. Atypia and PIN are not seen in areas that otherwise show changes of postcryoablation therapy. Biopsy specimen after cryosurgery may reveal no evidence of recurrent or residual carcinoma, even in patients with elevated PSA. In some cases, the benign prostate and tumor appear unchanged, with no change in grade or definite evidence of tissue or immune response. As the postoperative interval increases, biopsy specimen is more likely to contain unaltered benign prostatic tissue.[217]

## Methods for Examination of Radical Prostatectomy Specimens

Accurate examination of radical prostatectomy specimens is crucial for predicting patient outcome and determining the need for adjuvant treatment. This issue has been addressed by the College of American Pathologists[20]; the Association of Directors of Anatomic and Surgical Pathology[218]; and a consensus conference sponsored by the American Cancer Society, World Health Organization, and Mayo Clinic.[219] Current guidelines for the evaluation of radical prostatectomy specimens emphasize information that should be included in the pathology report but leave the decision regarding partial or complete sampling to the pathologist[20] (Table 32–7).

Numerous methods for partial and complete sampling of prostatectomy specimens have been described, and the completeness of sampling affects the determination of pathologic stage.[20, 220–223] Haggman and colleagues[222] compared the results of partial sampling (sections of palpable tumor and two random sections of apex and base) with complete sampling and found a significant increase in positive surgical margins (12% versus 59%) and pathologic stage with complete sectioning. Others have shown that the presence and extent of extraprostatic extension in clinical stage T2 adenocarcinoma (and clinical staging error) were related directly to the number of tissue blocks submitted.[221] Donahue and Miller[223a] noted that 40% of patients had extraprostatic extension of cancer with standard study compared with 60% with whole-mount evaulation. Cohen and coworkers[224] found that partial sampling with alternate sections missed 15% of cases with extraprostatic extension that were identified by complete sampling. Partial sampling methods reportedly are equivalent to whole-mount sections for determining cancer volume,[221] but I question this finding.

All methods begin with weighing the specimen when fresh and measuring in three dimensions. For ultrasonographic measurements, radiologists often describe the shape of the prostate as a prolate ellipsoid (length × height × width × 0.532), but this is only a rough estimate that shows considerable variability. Separate measurements are made of the attached seminal vesicles.

Subsequent handling of the specimen can be performed when it is fresh or fixed. The fresh (or

**TABLE 32–7.** Examination of Radical Prostatectomy Specimens: Information to be Included in the Surgical Pathology Report

Histopathologic type of carcinoma
Histologic grade (Gleason score)
Location and size of cancer
Extraprostatic extension: extent and location
Seminal vesicle involvement
Surgical margin status
  Apex
  Base
  Neurovascular bundles
  Posterior prostate
  Anterior prostate
Lymph nodes
  Sites, number, and status
pTNM

fixed) prostate is inked by brief immersion in a small container of India ink or by painting the surface with different colors of ink to allow unequivocal identification of left and right sides. Subsequently the wet specimen is immersed briefly in acetone or Bouin's fixative and air dried or blotted dry. Some pathologists use different colors of ink for the anterior and posterior prostate, apex, and base to ensure proper orientation.

The apex and base are amputated at a thickness of about 3 mm, and these margins are submitted as 3- to 4-mm-thick conization slices in the vertical parasagittal plane[2]; alternatively, some pathologists prefer 1- to 2-mm-thick shave margins. For conization, the apex usually requires quadrant sectioning, and I routinely use abbreviations for the right anterior apex (RAX), left anterior apex (LAX), right posterior apex (RPX), and left posterior apex (LPX). Similarly the base is sampled, usually into left and right halves as left bladder base (LBB) and right bladder base (RBB). The remaining specimen is sectioned serially at 4 to 5 mm thickness by knife to create transverse sections perpendicular to the long axis of the prostate from its apex to the tip of the seminal vesicles. Partial and complete sampling differ by the amount of prostate tissue submitted after this point. According to a 1994 survey, 88% of pathologists preferred partial sampling, probably because of time and cost considerations.[225]

### GROSS IDENTIFICATION OF CANCER

Tumor foci apparent on gross examination usually are at least 5 mm in greatest dimension and appear yellow-white with a firm consistency owing to stromal desmoplasia. Some cancers appear as yellow granular masses that contrast sharply with the normal spongy prostatic parenchyma.

### PARTIAL (LIMITED) SAMPLING

Partial sampling results in histopathologic submission of a fraction of the prostate, usually less than 50%, including all grossly apparent cancer. Given the limitations of macroscopic identification of cancer, partial sampling protocols sometimes require submission of additional tissue to identify cancer (see "Vanishing Cancer Phenomenon").

### COMPLETE (TOTALLY EMBEDDED) SAMPLING

Complete sampling results in the entire prostate being submitted for histopathologic examination. Even this method is subject to sampling error, however, because generation of a single 5-$\mu$-thick section from each 4- to 5-mm tissue block still results in microscopic review of only 0.17% of all embedded tissue; theoretically, 15,600 slides would be required per case to review the entire specimen.[226] Two alternative methods exist for complete sampling: 1) routine sections and 2) whole-mount sections.

COMPLETE SAMPLING WITH ROUTINE SECTIONS. This method refers to submitting the entire prostate after cutting tissue samples sufficiently small to fit into routine cassettes, obviating the need for special handling required for whole-mount sections. Sections are obtained by slicing each transverse section into four quadrants; larger prostates often generate six or eight sections per transverse slice, whereas smaller prostates may generate only two sections per slice. This method of complete sampling yields a mean of 26 routine slides per case.[221] In rare cases with small prostates (<1 in 300 cases in my experience), intact transverse sections can fit into a cassette, allowing routine sections of whole mounts.

COMPLETE SAMPLING WITH WHOLE-MOUNT SECTIONS. This method refers to submitting the entire prostate as intact transverse serial slices without subdivision. This is the preferred method by some investigators but requires special handling of tissue samples that are larger than routine sections. This method may be optimal for teaching and research purposes but is used infrequently in routine practice.

## Predictive Factors in Prostate Cancer

Multifactorial analysis improves prediction of all outcome variables, including pathologic stage, cancer recurrence, and survival.[227] Factors recommended for routine reporting are listed in Table 32–8.[135]

### EXTRAPROSTATIC EXTENSION

The term *extraprostatic extension* (EPE) was accepted at an International Consensus Conference to replace other terms, including *capsular invasion, capsular penetration,* and *capsular perforation*.[219] Extension of cancer beyond the edge or capsule of the prostate is diagnostic of EPE. There are three criteria for EPE, depending on the site and composition of the extraprostatic tissue: 1) cancer in adipose tissue, 2) cancer in perineural spaces of the neurovascular bundles, and 3) cancer in anterior muscle. In patients treated by radical prostatectomy for clinically localized cancer, the frequency of EPE (stage pT3 cancer) was 23%,[228] 24%,[203] 41%,[229] 43%,[230] 45%,[1] or 52%. There is a strong association of tumor volume with extraprostatic extension and seminal vesicle invasion.[229] An autopsy study showed EPE in 2% of cancers less than 0.46 cc in volume, compared with 52% of larger cancers.[231] Patients with EPE have a worse prognosis than patients with organ-confined cancer.[203, 232] Cancer-specific survival 10 years after radical prostatectomy in patients with pT3 cancer was 54%,[233] 62%,[234] 70%,[235] or 80%[236]; at 15 years, survival was 69%.[236] Cancer-specific survival 10 years after definitive radiation therapy in patients with clinical stage T3 was 44%[237] or 59%[238]; at 15 years, survival was 36%,[237] 33%,[239] or 39%.[238] Many patients with EPE also have positive surgical margins,

**TABLE 32–8.** Classification of Prognostic Factors for Prostate Cancer: Recommendations from 1999 Consensus Conferences

### Category 1
Factors that have been proved to be prognostic or predictive based on evidence from multiple published trials and are recommended for routine reporting

| 1999 CAP* Conference | 1999 WHO† Conference |
| --- | --- |
| TNM stage | TNM stage |
| Histologic grade (Gleason) | Histologic grade (Gleason score and WHO nuclear grade) |
| Surgical margin status | Surgical margin status |
| Perioperative PSA‡ | Perioperative PSA |
| | Pathologic effects of treatment |
| | Location of cancer within prostate |

### Category 2
Factors that show promise as predictive factors based on evidence from multiple published studies but that require further evaluation before recommendation or are recommended despite incomplete data as diagnostic or prognostic markers

| 1999 CAP Conference | 1999 WHO Conference |
| --- | --- |
| DNA ploidy | DNA ploidy |
| Histologic type | Histologic type |
| Cancer volume in needle biopsy specimens (recommended) | Cancer volume in needle biopsy specimens (recommended) |
| Cancer volume in radical prostatectomy specimens (recommended) | Cancer volume in radical prostatectomy specimens (recommended) |

### Category 3
Factors that have some scientific evidence to support their adoption as diagnostic or prognostic agents but are not currently recommended; also, factors of uncertain significance

**1999 CAP Conference and 1999 WHO Conference**

Prostate-specific membrane antigen
Other serum tests (PSM, hK2, IGF)
Perineural invasion
Vascular/lymphatic invasion
Microvessel density (shows promise, but insufficient data)
Stromal factors, including transforming growth factor-$\beta$, integrins
Proliferation markers and apoptosis
Nuclear morphometry and karyometric analysis
Androgen receptors
Neuroendocrine markers
Genetic markers (show promise, but insufficient data)
All other factors that do not appear in categories 1 or 2

* CAP, College of American Pathologists.
† WHO, World Health Organization.
‡ PSA, prostate-specific antigen.

with a frequency of 41%,[203] 57%,[240] or 81%. The combination of EPE and positive margins predicts a worse prognosis than EPE alone.[203, 235, 241]

## LYMPH NODES

Staging pelvic lymph node biopsy often is performed before prostatectomy, and urologists may discontinue surgery if metastases are identified. Lymph node dissection is performed by an open or laparoscopic procedure. Radical perineal prostatectomy and lymph node dissection are performed as separate procedures because the surgical approaches are different, whereas radical retropubic prostatectomy and lymphadenectomy often are performed as a single procedure. The pathologist should evaluate the fibroadipose tissue obtained by lymphadenectomy carefully and submit all lymph nodes for pathologic examination. It may not be necessary to submit obvious adipose tissue, although it is my policy to do so. Sampling error by frozen section accounts for a false-negative rate of lymph node metastases of 2% to 3% in my experience (unpublished observations). The surgical pathology report should include the number and sites of all submitted lymph nodes and sites of involvement and the size of cancer foci. There is a low incidence of micrometastatic occult prostatic carcinoma in pelvic lymph nodes that cannot be detected by routine H&E staining.[242] Using immunohistochemical studies directed against cytokeratin, Moul and associates[242] found lymph node micrometastases in 3% of patients with clinically localized prostate adenocarcinoma, similar to the results of Gomella and colleagues.[243] The presence of extranodal extension is not associated with unfavorable survival, although nodal cancer volume was predictive of cancer-specific survival.[244]

## STAGE

The TNM (tumor, node, metastasis) system is the international standard for prostate adenocarcinoma staging[223, 245–247] (Table 32–9). The Commission on Cancer of the American College of Surgeons has required it for accreditation since 1995.[248] Such staging of early prostate adenocarcinoma separates patients into two groups: patients with palpable tumors and patients with nonpalpable tumors.[223, 245, 247] This reliance on palpability of the tumor as determined by digital rectal examination is unique among organ staging systems and is hampered by the low sensitivity, low specificity, and low positive predictive value of digital rectal examination. Refinements in staging led to the introduction of a stage of nonpalpable adenocarcinoma detected by elevated serum PSA concentration, referred to as *stage T1c*; however, this new stage was introduced without supportive clinical evidence, and studies show that it does not identify a distinct group of patients.[249, 250] The question remains whether patients who would benefit from early detection and intervention can be separated from those who would not benefit. PSA is responsible for a profound clinical stage migration in newly detected prostate cancer.[251]

## PATHOLOGY OF PROSTATE-SPECIFIC ANTIGEN–DETECTED ADENOCARCINOMA (CLINICAL STAGE T1c)

Before widespread clinical use of PSA, most organ-confined adenocarcinoma was discovered by digital rectal examination (clinical stage T2) or at the time of TURP (clinical stage T1). Routine use of serum PSA increased the detection rate and uncovered some adenocarcinomas that would not have been detected by digital rectal examination. There was a sevenfold increase in PSA-detected adenocarcinomas at the Mayo Clinic in the 3-year period from 1988 to 1991 (14 cases versus 118 cases).[252] There is no pathologic stage equivalent for clinical stage T1c, and such tumors invariably are upstaged at surgery, usually to pathologic stage T2 or T3. Oesterling and colleagues[252] found that clinical stage T1c adenocarcinoma and clinical stage T2a+b adenocarcinoma had similar maximal tumor diameters, frequencies of multifocality, tumor grades, DNA content results, pathologic stages, and tumor locations; they had different serum PSA values, tumor volumes, positive surgical margins, and prostate gland sizes, with the T1c tumors having higher values for each feature. These findings indicate that PSA detects adenocarcinoma that is clinically important and potentially curable. PSA-detected tumors that are visible on ultrasonography have similar pathologic features as those that are not visible.[253]

## SURGICAL MARGINS

Positive surgical margins are defined as cancer cells touching the inked surface of the prostate. Surgical

**TABLE 32–9.** Staging Prostate Adenocarcinoma

|  | American | TNM* |
|---|---|---|
| Nonpalpable cancer |  |  |
| ≤5% of TURP tissue†‡ | A1 | T1a |
| >5% of TURP tissue† | A2 | T1b |
| Cancer detected by biopsy (e.g., elevated prostate-specific antigen) | B0 | T1c |
| Palpable or visible cancer clinically confined within the capsule |  |  |
| ≤ Half of one lobe | B1 | T2a |
| > Half of one lobe, but not both lobes | B1 | T2b |
| Both lobes | B2 | T2c |
| Cancer with local extracapsular extension |  |  |
| Unilateral | C1 | T3a |
| Bilateral | C1 | T3b |
| Seminal vesicle invasion | C2 | T3c |
| Invasion of bladder neck, rectum, or external sphincter | C2 | T4a |
| Invasion of levator muscle or pelvic wall | C2 | T4b |
| Metastatic cancer |  |  |
| Single regional lymph node, ≤2 cm in greatest dimension | D1 | N1§ |
| Single regional lymph node, 2–5 cm, or multiple regional lymph nodes ≤5 cm | D1 | N2 |
| Single regional lymph node, >5 cm | D1 | N3 |
| Distant metastasis | D2 | M1 |
| Nonregional lymph node | D2 | M1a |
| Bone | D2 | M1b |
| Other sites | D2 | M1c |

* N0 or Nx M0 for T1–T4.
† Different definitions exist for substaging A1 and A2 cancers.
‡ TURP, transurethral resection of the prostate.
§ Nx, regional lymph nodes are not assessable; Mx, distant metastasis is not assessable.

margins are not included in pathologic staging.[203] Many studies have equated positive margins and extraprostatic extension erroneously, however, particularly in cases in which the surgeon has cut into the prostate and intraprostatic cancer.[219] The frequency of positive surgical margins has declined steadily, probably owing to refinements in surgical technique and earlier detection of cancer at smaller volume. Ohori and colleagues[230] found positive surgical margins in 24% of whole-mount radical prostatectomies obtained at their hospital before 1987, usually in the posterolateral region near the neurovascular bundles; by modifying surgery to approach the neurovasular bundles laterally and widely dissect the apex of the prostate, they observed a positive surgical margin rate of only 8% by 1993, despite similar volume, grade, and pathologic stage of cancer. Other reports noted a frequency of positive surgical margins of 29%,[203] 33%,[254] 46%,[255] and 57%,[256] with no difference in specimens from nerve-sparing and non–nerve-sparing operations.[255] Positive surgical margins are correlated strongly with cancer volume[229, 230, 235, 254, 257] and number of needle biopsy specimens containing cancer.[258, 259] Most positive surgical margins in prostates with cancer smaller than 4 cc are caused by surgical incision.[203, 257] Positive margins are located at the apex (48%), rectal and lateral surfaces (24%), bladder neck (16%), and superior pedicles (10%).[254] Surgical margin status is an important predictor of patient outcome after radical prostatectomy; it was the only predictor of cancer progression other than Gleason score[241, 249] or DNA ploidy[203] in patients without seminal vesicle invasion or lymph node metastases. The College of American Pathologists recommends that the presence, extent, and location of each margin reviewed should be reported specifically. There is no current agreement or recommendation, however, as to the specific method of quantifying the amount of cancer in these locations.

## LOCATION OF CANCER

The site of origin of cancer seems to be a significant prognostic factor. When it arises in the transition zone, it is apparently less aggressive than typical acinar adenocarcinoma arising in the peripheral zone. These adenocarcinomas are better differentiated than those in the peripheral zone, accounting for Gleason primary grade 1 and 2 tumors. The volume of low-grade tumors tends to be smaller than those arising in the peripheral zone, although frequent exceptions are seen. The confinement of transition zone adenocarcinoma to its anatomic site of origin may account in part for the favorable prognosis of clinical stage T1 tumors. The transition zone boundary may act as a relative barrier to tumor extension because malignant acini seem to fan out frequently along this boundary before invasion into the peripheral and central zones. The World Health Organization recommends that prostate biopsy specimens be submitted separately; the anatomic site of each prostate biopsy be labeled, at the discretion of the urologist; and pathologists report each specimen separately.[135] The anatomic site of carcinoma within each prostate biopsy specimen can be included in the pathology report and identified in the anatomic area specified by the urologist. The anatomic location of carcinoma within total prostatectomy specimens also should be specified in the pathology report whenever possible.

## CANCER VOLUME

Biopsy cancer volume depends on multiple factors, including prostate volume, cancer volume, cancer distribution, number of biopsy cores obtained, cohort of patients being evaluated, and technical competence of the investigator. The combined results from multiple studies indicate that the biopsy extent of tumor provides some predictive value for extent in radical prostatectomy specimens and probably should be reported, although its predictive value for an individual patient is limited.[249, 260–271] Reliance on this measure alone often may be misleading. There is a fair[265]-to-good[262] correlation between amount of cancer reported in biopsy specimens and amount of cancer subsequently found in radical prostatectomy specimens. This correlation is greatest for large cancers. High cancer burden on needle biopsy specimen is strongly suggestive of large-volume, high-stage cancer.[249, 260–263] Low tumor burden on needle biopsy specimen does not indicate low-volume, low-stage cancer. Cupp and associates[265] found that patients with less than 30% of needle cores replaced by cancer had a mean volume in the radical prostatectomy of 6.1 cc (range, 0.19 to 16.8 cc), indicating that the amount of tumor on transrectal needle biopsy specimen was not a good predictor of tumor volume. In another report, patients with less than 10% cancer in the biopsy specimen had a 30% risk of positive surgical margins, 27% risk of extraprostatic extension, and 22% risk of PSA biochemical progression; these risks were higher in patients with more than 10% cancer.[271] Patients with less than 3 mm cancer and Gleason score 6 or less on needle biopsy specimen had a 59% risk of cancer volume exceeding 0.5 cc.[261] Patients with less than 2 mm of cancer had 26% risk of extraprostatic cancer,[269] and patients with less than 3 mm had 52% risk.[268] The College of American Pathologists recommends that the volume of cancer in needle biopsy specimen should be reported as the percentage of tissue involved by cancer.

Measures of cancer volume are usually[272] but not always[249, 273] predictive of cancer recurrence after radical prostatectomy. The College of American Pathologists recommends that cancer volume be recorded in prostatectomy specimens, although there is no accepted universal approach.[20] Methods include computer-assisted morphometric determination,[262, 272, 273a] simple measurement of length × height × section thickness of the cancer (some measure the largest *index* focus, whereas others report the cumulative volumes),[274] greatest cancer dimension,[17, 275] grid method,[276] and visual estimate of the percentage of cancer.[277, 278] Measurements performed on fixed tissue sections may include a formalin shrinkage correction factor, which varies from about 1.25 to 1.5, representing tissue shrinkage of 18% to 33%; conversely, Schned and colleagues[279] showed that shrinkage correction is unnecessary. Cancer volume is a crucial element in definitions of clinically significant and insignificant prostate cancer.[274, 276]

## PERINEURAL INVASION

Perineural invasion is common in adenocarcinoma, present in 38% of biopsy specimens,[280] and may be the only evidence of malignancy in a needle core. Only half of patients with intraprostatic perineural invasion on biopsy specimen have extraprostatic extension. In univariate analysis, perineural invasion was predictive of extraprostatic extension, seminal vesicle invasion, and pathologic stage in patients treated by radical prostatectomy.[280, 281] In multivariate analysis, perineural invasion had no predictive value, however, after consideration of Gleason grade, serum PSA, and amount of cancer on biopsy specimen.[280] These findings indicate that there is no value in routinely reporting perineural invasion in biopsy specimens.

## VASCULAR AND LYMPHATIC INVASION

Microvascular invasion is a strong indicator of malignancy, and its presence correlates with histologic grade, although it sometimes is difficult to distinguish from fixation-associated retraction artifact of acini.[134, 282] Microvascular invasion also may be an important predictor of outcome and carries a fourfold greater risk of tumor progression and death.[282] Immunohistochemical stains directed against endothelial cells, such as factor VIII–related antigen, CD31, CD34, or *Ulex europaeus*, may increase the detection rate.[134] Microvascular invasion is present in 38% of radical prostatectomy specimens and is associated commonly with extraprostatic extension and lymph node metastases (62% and 67% of cases).[134, 282] It is not an independent predictor of progression, however, when stage and grade are included in the multivariate analysis.[282]

## MICROVESSEL DENSITY

MVD analysis offers promise for predicting pathologic stage and patient outcome in prostate cancer. Most prostatectomy studies found a positive correlation of MVD with pathologic stage.[283–285] In one study, the important difference in MVD between stage pT2 and pT3 were observed only for low-grade cancers, however, whereas the reverse was true in another study. MVD in cancer on biopsy specimen showed a positive correlation with matched prostatectomies and was an independent predictor of extraprostatic extension.[285, 286] The bulk of evidence favors the relationship of MVD and cancer stage, although variance exists between methods and patient cohorts. There generally is good agreement about prediction of cancer recurrence based on MVD.[287–290] In studies in which patients were treated by surgery or external-beam radiation therapy, MVD[287, 291, 292] and microvascular invasion[289] predicted biochemical (PSA) failure. MVD did not correlate with biochemical failure after controlling for stage (pT2 or pT3) and grade (Gleason grade ≥6) in patients treated by radical prostatectomy.[290]

## DNA PLOIDY

DNA ploidy analysis of prostate cancer provides important predictive information that supplements histopathologic examination. Patients with diploid tumors have a more favorable outcome than patients with aneuploid tumors. Among patients with lymph node metastases treated with radical prostatectomy and androgen deprivation therapy, patients with diploid tumors may survive 20 years or more, whereas patients with aneuploid tumors die within 5 years.[292a] The ploidy pattern of prostate cancer is often heterogeneous, however, creating potential problems with sampling error. A good correlation exists between DNA ploidy and histologic grade, and DNA ploidy adds clinically useful predictive information for some patients.[293–295] The incidence of aneuploidy in high-grade PIN varies from 32% to 68% and is lower than carcinoma, which shows aneuploidy in 55% to 62% of cases.[296] There is a high level of concordance of DNA content of PIN and cancer. About 70% of aneuploid cases of PIN are associated with aneuploid carcinoma; conversely, only 29% of cases of aneuploid cancer are associated with aneuploid PIN.[297] DNA ploidy pattern by flow cytometry correlates with cancer grade,[293] volume, and stage.[297a] Most low-stage tumors are diploid, and high-stage tumors are nondiploid, but numerous exceptions occur.[297b] The 5-year cancer-specific survival is about 95% for diploid tumors, 70% for tetraploid tumors, and 25% for aneuploid tumors.[298] Patients with diploid lymph node metastases treated by androgen deprivation therapy alone had longer progression-free survival and overall survival than patients with aneuploid metastases.[298a] Digital image analysis seems to have a high level of concordance (about 85%) with radical prostatectomy specimens evaluated by flow cytometry.[299]

## MORPHOMETRIC MARKERS

Morphometric markers provide useful predictive information in prostate cancer but still are considered research modalities.[135] Morphometric studies should employ objective, quantitative techniques that preferably are computer-assisted. There are no accepted standards for morphometric studies, and this is considered an important area for investigation. The most popular morphometric markers are nuclear size, nuclear shape, nuclear roundness, chromatin texture, size and number of nucleoli, and number of apoptotic bodies. Significant problems of reproducibility in nuclear roundness measurement have been described, and the results with different digitizing instruments are not comparable. Volume-weighted mean nuclear volume is independently predictive of cancer-specific survival in combination with Gleason score and clinical stage.[300] Four chromatin textural features discrimated androgen-responsive and unresponsive cancer in patients with metastases. Greater chromatin pattern heterogeneity correlated with shorter recurrence-free survival in patients treated by surgery.

## GENETIC INSTABILITY IN PROSTATE CANCER

Prostate carcinogenesis apparently involves multiple genetic changes, including loss of specific genomic sequences that may be associated with inactivation of tumor-suppressor genes and gain of some specific chromosome regions that may be associated with activation of oncogenes. The most common genetic alterations in PIN and carcinoma are gain of chromosome 7, particularly 7q31; loss of 8p and gain of 8q; and loss of 10q, 16q, and 18q.[301] Fluorescence in situ hybridization (FISH) studies showed that aneusomy of chromosome 7 is frequent in prostate cancer and associated with higher cancer grade, higher pathologic stage, and early patient death from prostate cancer.[302–305] Polymerase chain reaction analysis of microsatellite markers identified frequent imbalance of alleles mapped to 7q31 in prostate cancer.[306–311] Allelic imbalance of 7q31 was correlated strongly with cancer aggressiveness, progression, and cancer-specific death.[302] These findings suggest that genetic alterations of the 7q-arm play an important role in the development of prostate cancer.

The chromosome 8p-arm is one of the most frequently deleted regions in prostate cancer.[312–315] The rate of 8p22 loss ranged from 29% to 50% in PIN, 32% to 69% in primary cancer, and 65% to 100% in metastatic cancer.[313–315] Other frequently deleted 8p regions include 8p21 and 8p12.[312, 314] Emmert-Buck and associates[312] found loss of 8p12-21 in 63% of PIN foci and 91% of cancer foci using microdissected frozen tissue. My colleagues and I detected loss of 8p21-12 in 37% of PIN foci and 46% of cancer foci.[78] These findings suggest that more than one tumor-suppressor gene may be located on 8p, and inactivation of these tumor-suppressor genes may be important for the initiation of prostate cancer. In addition to loss of the 8p-arm, gain of the 8q-arm has been reported in prostate cancer.[195, 313, 316, 317] Bova and colleagues[315] found gain of 8q in 11% of primary cancers and 40% of lymph node metastases. Van Den Berg and coworkers[317a] found amplification of 8q DNA sequences in 75% of cancers metastatic to lymph nodes. Similarly, Visakorpi and associates[317] found gain of 8q far more frequently in locally recurrent cancer than in primary cancer. Cher and coworkers[318] also detected frequent gain of 8q in metastatic and androgen-independent prostate cancer. Using FISH, Qian and associates[319] observed that gain of chromosome 8 was the most frequent chromosomal anomaly in metastatic foci, and the frequency was much higher than in PIN and carcinoma. Jenkins and colleagues[316] identified c-myc gene amplification in 22% of metastatic foci, which was much more frequent than in primary cancer

(9%), suggesting that the 8q-arm may harbor a gene whose amplification and overexpression plays a key role in the progression and evolution of prostatic carcinoma. Gain of the chromosome 8 centromere or the 8q-arm occurs simultaneously with loss of portions of the 8p-arm in PIN and carcinoma.[195, 316, 317, 320] One simple genetic mechanism that could explain these prior observations is the presence of multiple copies of isochromosome 8q in cancer cells. Preliminary simultaneous FISH studies with probes specific for 8p, 8q, and the chromosome 8 centromere support this explanation. There is also a high frequency of allelic imbalance at 10p and 10q in prostate cancer.[321, 321a, 322] The most commonly deleted region on the 10q-arm includes bands 10q23-24, and allelic loss of this region may inactive the MXI-1 gene. The PTEN candidate gene in this region has been cloned.[323]

Chromosome 16 also had frequent allelic imbalance in prostate cancer. Allelic imbalance at 16q was present in about 30% of cases of clinically localized prostate cancer,[324] and there was a high frequency of allelic imbalance at 16q23-q24.[325, 326] The most commonly deleted region was located at 16q24.1-q24.2, and this deletion was associated significantly with cancer progression.[325, 327] The frequency of loss of 18q22.1 varied from 20% to 40%.[321] Other regions showing frequent allelic imbalance include 3p25-26, 5q12-23, 6q, 13q, 17p31.1, and 21q22.2-22.3.[327, 328] Loss of 10q, 16q, and 18q also has been reported in PIN.[78, 329]

### c-myc

Most studies suggest that c-myc plays a role in the regulation of prostate growth and carcinogenesis. There is substantial amplification with increasing grade of cancer, particularly in metastases,[316, 330] and myc expression correlates with growth of androgen-responsive prostate epithelium.[331]

## APOPTOSIS-SUPPRESSING ONCOPROTEIN BCL2

BCL2 is believed widely to be an apoptosis-suppressor gene. Overexpression of the protein in cancer cells may block or delay onset of apoptosis, selecting and maintaining long-living cells and arresting cells in the $G_0$ phase of the cell cycle.[332, 333] Expression of BCL2 normally is restricted to the basal cell layer of the normal and hyperplastic prostatic epithelium.[334, 334a] Overexpression of BCL2 is present is PIN, however.[334, 335] In cancer, the prevalence and expression pattern of BCL2 is controversial. One study found moderate heterogeneous BCL2 overexpression in localized cancer[334] that was correlated inversely with Gleason grade. Another report described a significant elevation of BCL2 in 45% of cases of primary cancer that was heterogeneous but did not correlate with grade. The area of cancer with high BCL2 expression was devoid of apoptotic cells. A study found that greater than 70% of prostate carcinomas were BCL2 negative, 18% had weak expression, and 11% exhibited strong expression.[336]

Expression of *BCL2* was correlated with high stage, metastases, and high grade. Androgen deprivation therapy decreased *BCL2* expression in cancer, suggesting that these cells develop resistance to apoptotic signals.[334, 337, 338]

### p53

Mutant *p53* expression is a late event in localized prostate cancer,[339–341] usually present in higher grade cancer[342–344] and elevated in untreated metastatic cancer,[345–347] hormone-refractory cancer,[340, 342, 347] and recurrent cancer.[345] Consequently, *p53* gene inactivation does not seem to be essential for the development of metastases and seems of limited prognostic value in patients with primary or metastatic cancer.[348]

### p21

The *WAF1/CIP1* gene encodes a *p21* cyclin-dependent kinase inhibitor that plays a role in the regulation of the cell cycle. On induction by *p53*, $p21^{WAF1/CIP1}$ binds to CDK2, resulting in down-regulation of CDK2 activity and $G_1$ growth arrest. Prostatic mutations in the *WAF1/CIP1* gene abrogate this apparent tumor-suppressor gene activity,[349] facilitating escape of $G_1/S$ checkpoint control with propagation into S-phase and maintenance of malignant potential. There is an increase in *WAF1/CIP1* polymorphisms in prostate cancer,[350] but no correlation exists between *WAF1/CIP1* expression and grade, stage, or cancer progression.[351]

### p27Kip1

The cyclin-dependent kinase inhibitor *p27Kip1* negatively regulates cell proliferation by mediating cell cycle arrest in $G_1$. *p27Kip1* expression decreases with higher Gleason score and seminal vesicle involvement by cancer.[352] *p27Kip1* expression is an independent predictor of treatment failure of node-negative cancer after radical prostatectomy.[352]

### OTHER FACTORS

A wide variety of other predictive factors have been evaluated in prostate cancer, but none are recommended at this time for routine use by the College of American Pathologists or the World Health Organization.

### COMBINING MULTIPLE PREDICTIVE FACTORS

The combination of predictive factors provides the greatest accuracy of predicting stage and outcome. The American Joint Committee on Cancer recommends use of neural network analysis to improve prostate cancer survival prediction.[353]

## Vanishing Cancer Phenomenon

In some radical prostatectomy specimens, there is minimal or no residual cancer within the specimen. This *vanishing cancer phenomenon* is increasing in incidence as more low-stage cancers are being treated by radical prostatectomy.[193] The inability to identify cancer in a prostate removed for needle biopsy–proven carcinoma does not indicate technical failure, although it is important to exclude the possibility of improper patient identification. DNA *fingerprinting* has been used as a research tool to compare the formalin-fixed paraffin-embedded biopsy specimen and prostatectomy tissues.[193] Substantial resources may be needed to identify minimal residual cancer, and exhaustive sectioning may fail. How many sections are reasonable to obtain in such cases? When can one stop sectioning if no cancer is found? I believe that it is appropriate for the pathologist to submit routine sections of the entire prostatectomy for histologic evaluation in such cases; however, after submission and examination of the entire prostate, further levels and block flipping probably are not necessary because any residual cancer at that point is likely to be extremely small and of no clinical significance.

## PROSTATIC SOFT TISSUE TUMORS

Interpretation of small prostatic biopsy specimens containing soft tissue proliferations often is difficult because of the potential for sampling error. Patient age and clinical history are essential in this setting. The serum PSA concentration usually is not significantly elevated.

## Benign Soft Tissue Tumors

### LEIOMYOMA AND FIBROMA

Leiomyoma and fibroma often are confused with nodular hyperplasia, and the distinction may be impossible in biopsy or TURP specimens. Leiomyoma is defined as a circumscribed solitary smooth muscle nodule greater than 1 cm in diameter.[61, 354, 355] It is histologically identical to leiomyoma occurring in the uterus and other sites. Fibroma is a similar nodule composed of collagen with few fibroblasts; fibroma may be indistinguishable from a pure stromal nodule of nodular hyperplasia. Some authors have questioned the existence of these tumors, preferring to consider them within the spectrum of nodular hyperplasia. Variants of leiomyoma include epithelioid leiomyoma,[356] cellular leiomyoma, atypical leiomyoma, and leiomyoblastoma.[354]

### POSTOPERATIVE SPINDLE CELL NODULE (POSTSURGICAL INFLAMMATORY MYOFIBROBLASTIC TUMOR)

Postoperative spindle cell nodule is a rare benign reparative process that occurs within months of surgery and consists of nodules of spindle cells arranged in fascicles with occasional or numerous mitotic figures (25 mitotic figures/10 high-power fields).[357] The cells have central elongate-to-ovoid nuclei, small prominent nucleoli, and abundant cytoplasm. Necrosis may be present but usually is not a prominent feature.

## INFLAMMATORY MYOFIBROBLASTIC TUMOR (INFLAMMATORY PSEUDOTUMOR, MYOFIBROBLASTOMA, LOW-GRADE INFLAMMATORY FIBROSARCOMA, SPINDLE CELL PROLIFERATION WITH NO PRIOR OPERATION, PSEUDOSARCOMA, NODULAR FASCIITIS, PSEUDOSARCOMATOUS FIBROMYXOID TUMOR)

Inflammatory myofibroblastic tumor is a rare benign pathologic entity of unknown origin that occurs in the bladder, prostate, urethra, and other sites without a history of prior surgery.[358] Patients range in age from 16 to 73 years (mean, 41 years), with a slight female predilection in the bladder. Mean tumor size is 3.6 cm, but tumors can measure 8 cm in diameter. The stroma is loose, edematous, and myxoid, with abundant small slitlike blood vessels resembling granulation tissue. Mitotic figures are infrequent (<3 mitotic figures/10 high-power fields); none are atypical. Ulceration and focal necrosis are present in most cases but are not prominent. There is strong vimentin immunoreactivity and rare immunoreactivity for smooth muscle actin, desmin, and keratin; S-100 protein and myoglobin are negative. Ultrastructural studies reveal myofibroblastic differentiation, including cytoplasmic microfilaments and dense bodies. Tumors usually are diploid, with a low S-phase fraction.

### OTHER BENIGN SOFT TISSUE TUMORS

Other benign tumors that arise in the prostate include hemangioma, lymphangioma, neurofibroma, neurilemoma, chrondroma, hemangiopericytoma, solitary fibrous tumor,[359, 360] and paraganglioma (pheochromocytoma).[361, 362]

## Malignant Soft Tissue Tumors

Sarcoma of the prostate accounts for less than 0.1% of prostatic neoplasms. One third occur in children, and most of these are rhabdomyosarcoma; leiomyosarcoma is most common in adults. Symptoms include prostatism and pelvic pain. Tumors may be 15 cm or more in diameter and usually are soft with focal necrosis.

### RHABDOMYOSARCOMA

Rhabdomyosarcoma has a peak incidence between birth and 6 years of age, but sporadic cases have been reported in men up to 80 years old. The prostate, bladder, and vagina account for 21% of cases in children, second only to head and neck origin. Serum PSA and PAP concentrations are normal. Three adults had hypercalcemia resulting from bone metastases.[363] The tumor usually is large and bulky, with a mean diameter of 9 cm. It usually involves

the prostate, bladder, and periurethral, perirectal, and perivesicular soft tissues. Urethral involvement may not be apparent cytoscopically. Symptoms include acute or chronic urethral obstruction, bladder displacement, and rectal compression. The prostate may be palpably normal, although large tumors often fill the pelvis and can be palpated suprapubically. Most are embryonal rhabdomyosarcoma, and the remainder are alveolar, botryoid, and spindle cell subtypes.[364] Tumor cells are arranged in sheets of immature round-to-spindle cells set in a myxoid stroma. Polypoid tumor fragments ("botryoid pattern") may fill the urethral lumen, covered by intact urothelium with condensed underlying tumor cells creating a distinctive cambium layer. Nuclei usually are pleomorphic and darkly staining. Scattered rhabdomyoblasts may be present, with eosinophilic cytoplasmic processes containing cross-striations (Fig. 32–45). Tumor cells display immunoreactivity for myoglobin, desmin, and vimentin but are negative for PSA and PAP. Ultrastructural study reveals two cell types, similar to rhabdomyosarcoma at other sites; large oval or elongate tumor cells contain segments of sarcomere with abundant glycogen, and smaller round cells contain abundant cytoplasmic organelles but lack myofibrils. All tumors appear to be aneuploid by flow cytometry.[365] Chemotherapy in combination with surgery and radiotherapy results in a 3-year survival rate of greater than 70%, according to the Intergroup Rhabdomyosarcoma Studies I and II[366]; long-term survival has been reported.

### LEIOMYOSARCOMA

Leiomyosarcoma presents as a large bulky mass that replaces the prostate and periprostatic tissues. It is the most common sarcoma in adults and accounts for 26% of all prostatic sarcomas. Patients range in age from 40 to 71 years (mean, 59 years), with sporadic reports in younger patients.[367] In a series of 23 cases from the Mayo Clinic, tumors ranged in size from 3.3 to 21 cm (mean, 9 cm). No tumors were grade 1, 7 were grade 2, 10 were grade 3, and 6 were grade 4.[367] The tumors were histologically similar to leiomyosarcoma at other sites. Prominent

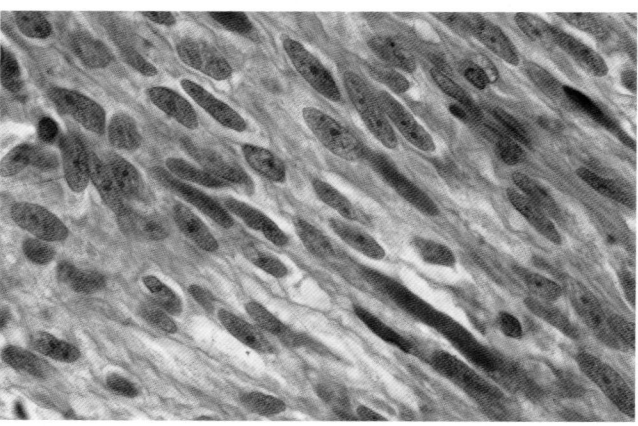

**FIGURE 32–45.** Rhabdomyosarcoma of the prostate.

sclerotic stroma was noted in two cases. Five tumors had epithelioid features, and one had a focal area reminiscent of neurilemoma. Necrosis may be extensive. Although the criteria for separating leiomyoma from low-grade leiomyosarcoma have not been defined precisely in the prostate, they probably are similar to those in other organs, including degree of cellularity, cytologic anaplasia, number of mitotic figures, amount of necrosis, vascular invasion, and size. Tumor cells usually display intense cytoplasmic immunoreactivity for smooth muscle–specific actin and vimentin and weak desmin immunoreactivity. Most are negative for cytokeratin (AE1/AE3) and S-100 protein, but exceptions have been described, particularly in tumors with epithelioid features in which keratin immunoreactivity may be seen.[367] Local recurrence and distant metastasis are frequent, and the prognosis is poor. Mean survival after diagnosis was less than 3 years in one series (range, 0.2 to 6.5 years), and most patients died from tumor.[367]

## PHYLLODES TUMOR (CYSTIC EPITHELIAL-STROMAL TUMOR, PHYLLODES TYPE OF ATYPICAL HYPERPLASIA, CYSTADENOLEIOMYOFIBROMA, CYSTOSARCOMA PHYLLODES)

Phyllodes tumor of the prostate is a rare lesion that should be considered a neoplasm rather than atypical hyperplasia because of the frequent early recurrences, infiltrative growth, and potential for extraprostatic spread in some cases.[367a] Dedifferentiation with multiple recurrences in some cases is further evidence of the potentially aggressive nature of this tumor.[367a] A benign clinical course has been emphasized in some reports, but the cumulative evidence in the literature indicates that some patients develop local recurrences and metastases.[367a] Patients with prostatic phyllodes tumor typically present with urinary obstruction, hematuria, and dysuria. There may be severe urinary obstruction, often occurring at a younger age than expected for typical prostatic hyperplasia. Most tumors range in size from 4 to 25 cm. At the time of TURP, the urologist may note an unusual spongy or cystic texture of the involved prostate. The diagnosis of phyllodes tumor usually is made on resected tissue, and it may be overlooked on needle biopsy specimen, in which it is difficult to appreciate the pattern of the tumor. Important diagnostic clues include diffuse infiltration, variably cellular stroma surrounding cysts, and compressed elongate channels that often have a leaflike configuration (Fig. 32–46). Prostatic phyllodes tumor exhibits a spectrum of histologic features, similar to its counterpart in the breast[367a] (Table 32–10). High-grade prostatic phyllodes tumor has a high stromal-to-epithelial ratio, prominent stromal cellularity and overgrowth, marked cytologic atypia, and increased mitotic activity. A sarcomatous component may arise within a low-grade tumor over time, invariably after multiple recurrences over many years.[367a] Immunohistochemical studies reveal intense cytoplasmic immunoreactivity in most stromal cells for vi-

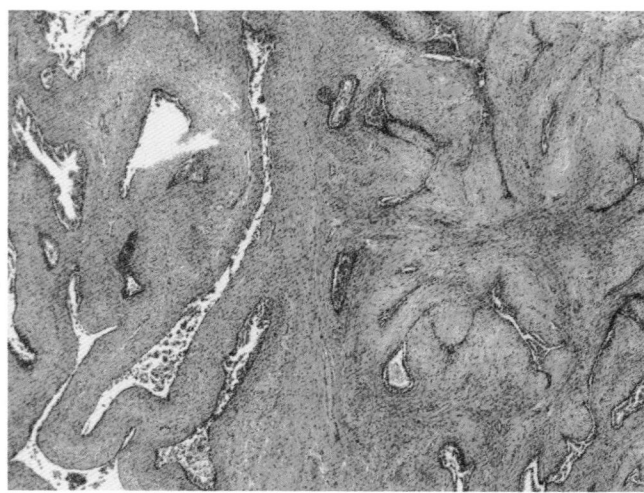

**FIGURE 32–46.** Low-grade phyllodes tumor of the prostate.

mentin and actin; in luminal epithelial cells for PSA, PAP, and keratin AE1/AE3; and in basal epithelial cells for high-molecular-weight keratin 34$\beta$E12; no staining was observed for desmin and S-100 protein.

### OTHER SARCOMAS

Other sarcomas reported in the prostate include fibrosarcoma, osteosarcoma, malignant fibrous histiocytoma, angiosarcoma, chondrosarcoma, neurofibrosarcoma, liposarcoma,[124] and synovial sarcoma.[368] Sarcoma of the prostate occasionally is unclassifiable, and I diagnose this as undifferentiated stromal sarcoma. Regardless of classification, the prognosis of most adult prostatic sarcomas is poor.

## OTHER RARE MALIGNANT TUMORS

### Malignant Lymphoma Involving the Prostate

Patients with malignant lymphoma involving the prostate usually are older men (mean age, 61 years), presenting with urinary obstructive symptoms.[369] Serum PSA concentration usually is not elevated. Secondary spread to the prostate by malignant lymphoma is much more frequent than primary lymphoma. The prevalence of primary prostatic lymphoma at autopsy is 0.2% of extranodal lymphomas. Prostatic lymphoma is diffuse or patchy within the stroma, with characteristic preservation of acini (Fig. 32–47). The infiltrate usually is extensive but may be irregular, often extending into the extraprostatic soft tissues. Tumor cell infiltration into the acinar epithelium is uncommon and rarely includes aggregates in the lumina. The most frequent lymphoma involving the prostate is diffuse non-Hodgkin's lymphoma, including small cleaved cell, large cell, and mixed cell types; Hodgkin's disease is rare,

**TABLE 32–10.** Phyllodes Tumor of the Prostate: Differential Diagnosis

| Characteristic Features | Phyllodes Tumor | Stromal Hyperplasia with Atypia (Leiomyoma-like Pattern)* | Stromal Hyperplasia with Atypia (Infiltrative Pattern)* | Leiomyosarcoma |
|---|---|---|---|---|
| *Clinical features* | | | | |
| Mean patient age (range) | | 68 y (57–80 y) | 69 y (59–80 y) | 61 y (41–78 y) |
| Presenting symptoms | Urinary obstructive symptoms, hematuria, or incidental finding | Urinary obstructive symptoms or incidental finding | Urinary obstructive symptoms or incidental finding | Urinary obstructive symptoms; perineal pain |
| Cystoscopic/macroscopic | | Stromal nodule | Stromal nodule | Mass measuring 3–21 cm in diameter (mean, 9 cm) |
| Serum PSA | Normal range | Normal range | Normal range | Normal range |
| *Architecture* | Biphasic pattern, including distorted cystically dilated or slitlike epithelial glands, often with leaflike projections, together with condensed stroma | Solid circumscribed expansile stromal nodule with abundant smooth muscle and atypical stromal cells | Ill-defined hyperplastic stromal nodule with atypical cells diffusely and uniformly infiltrating around typical hyperplasia acini; hypocellular loose myxoid matrix with large ectatic vessels | Large bulky nodular tumor composed of spindle cells |
| *Cytology* | Benign epithelium; variable number of bizarre stromal cells with vacuolated nuclei and multinucleation; mitotic figures and necrosis indicate higher grade | Bizarre giant stromal cells with vacuolated nuclei and frequent multinucleation; no mitotic figures or necrosis | Bizarre giant stromal cells with vacuolated nuclei and frequent multinucleation; no mitotic figures or necrosis | Spindle or epithelioid tumor cells with variable pleomorphism, mitotic figures, and frequent necrosis |
| *Immunohistochemistry* | | | | |
| Vimentin | Usually + + + | + | + + + | + + |
| Desmin | Usually −; rare + + + | + + + | Usually + | Usually −; rare + |
| Actin | + | + + + | + | Usually −; rare + |
| Estrogen receptors | − | − | − | NT† |
| Progesterone receptors | Usually −; rare + | Usually + + . | Usually + + + | NT |
| Androgen receptors | Usually −; rare + + | + + + | + + + | NT |
| Keratin AE1/AE3 | + + (epithelium) | − | − | Usually − (+ in 27% of cases) |
| Keratin 34βE12 | + + (epithelium) | − | − | NT |
| PSA | + + + | − | − | − |
| PAP | + + + | − | − | − |
| S-100 Protein | − | − | − | − |
| *Follow-up* | Frequent recurrences with late onset of stromal overgrowth | Benign; rare solitary recurrences | Benign; rare solitary recurrences | Malignant; mean of 22 mo to death (3–72 mo) |

† NT, not tested.
PAP, prostatic acid phosphatase; PSA, prostate-specific antigen.

with fewer than five documented cases. The prognosis of lymphoma involving the prostate usually is poor, regardless of patient age, stage of tumor, histologic classification, type of involvement (primary or secondary), or type of therapy.

## Leukemia Involving the Prostate

Chronic lymphocytic leukemia is the most common leukemia involving the prostate. The autopsy prevalence of prostatic involvement is about 20% of cases of leukemia. The clinical symptoms and histologic patterns in the prostate are similar to malignant lymphoma but are distinguished from lymphoma by the presence of blood involvement.

## Other Tumors

Other malignant tumors include multiple myeloma, germ cell tumor, Wilms' tumor, rhabdoid tumor, neuroblastoma, and metastases to the prostate.[124] Metastases are extremely rare, with involvement at autopsy in 0.5% to 2.2% of men dying of malignancies.

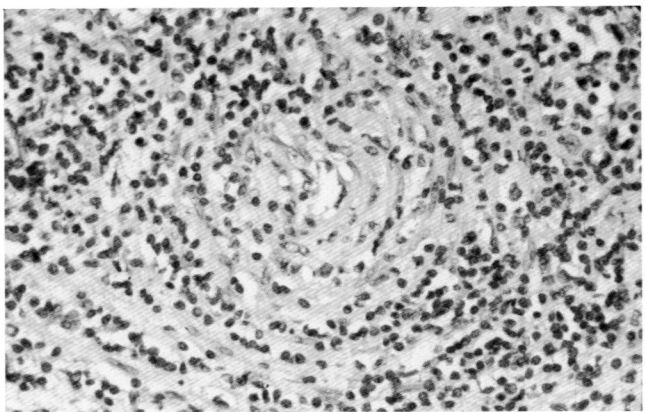

**FIGURE 32–47.** Malignant lymphoma, diffuse mixed small and large cell type, with prominent angiotropism.

## SEMINAL VESICLES

### Amyloidosis (Senile Seminal Vesicle Amyloidosis)

Localized amyloidosis of the seminal vesicles increases in frequency with patient age, present in 8% of men younger than 60 years and 34% of men older than 75 years.[370–373] It often extends bilaterally along the ejaculatory ducts, forming linear or massive nodular subepithelial deposits of amorphous eosinophilic fibrillar material.

### Seminal Vesiculitis

Seminal vesiculitis is an uncommon disorder that is associated with infection and inflammation of adjacent organs, including the prostate, bladder, ejaculatory ducts, vas deferens, and epididymis. Acute vesiculitis usually is caused by retrograde infection with or without indwelling catheter; ureteral or ejaculatory duct stenosis; or anatomic anomaly, calculi, or surgical trauma. Antibiotic therapy usually is effective. Chronic vesiculitis is associated with chronic prostatitis, and both respond poorly to antibiotic therapy. Schistosomiasis, usually secondary to *S. haematobium* infection of the bladder, involves the seminal vesicles more commonly than the prostate.

### Calcification

Calcification often follows seminal vesiculitis, particularly with tuberculosis. Calcification may be unilateral or bilateral and usually coexists with calcification of the vas deferens. The calcification is present in the muscular wall, often forming concentric rings; the mucosa is involved rarely. Osseous metaplasia also is observed rarely in the wall.

### Seminal Vesicle Cysts

Seminal vesicle cysts are rare and may be congenital or acquired. Congenital cyst is associated with ipsilateral renal agenesis in 80% of cases and commonly with ureteral ectopia, ureteral agenesis (Zinner's syndrome) and ipsilateral absence of the testis, or hemivertebrae. The cyst usually is unilateral and unilocular; lateral to the midline; and three times larger than the normal seminal vesicle, considerably smaller than müllerian duct cyst. Bilateral congenital cysts are rare and may be associated with absent vasa deferentia. Acquired cyst usually is associated with inflammation and obstruction of the ejaculatory ducts and seminal vesicles.

### Seminal Vesicle Adenocarcinoma

Primary neoplasms of the seminal vesicles are rare, including adenocarcinoma. Mean patient age is 62 years (range, 17 to 90 years), and presenting symptoms include urinary obstruction and hematospermia. The diagnosis of seminal vesicle adenocarcinoma requires the following: 1) tumor located primarily in the seminal vesicles; 2) no evidence of carcinoma in the prostate, bladder, or colon; 3) architectural features of adenocarcinoma, usually with papillary or sheetlike growth and mucinous differentiation; 4) in situ adenocarcinoma in the seminal vesicle epithelium; and 5) cytoplasmic immunoreactivity for CEA and absence of staining for PSA and PAP. Most cases are immunoreactive for CA 125 and cytokeratin 7.[374]

### Other Cancers Involving the Seminal Vesicles

Seminal vesicle involvement by prostate adenocarcinoma is common, observed in about 12% of radical prostatectomy specimens. There are three patterns of seminal vesicle invasion: 1) direct spread along the ejaculatory duct complex into the seminal vesicles, 2) prostatic capsular perforation followed by extension into the periprostatic soft tissues and spread into the seminal vesicles, and 3) isolated deposits of cancer in the seminal vesicles.[240, 375, 376] Bulky urothelial carcinoma of the bladder also may invade the seminal vesicles by direct extension or mucosal spread.[377] Mucosal involvement by in situ urothelial carcinoma is rare, present in only 1% of cases.

### Soft Tissue Tumors and Other Tumors

A variety of benign and malignant soft tissue tumors have been described in the seminal vesicles, including cystadenoma, phyllodes tumor, leiomyoma, fibroma, adenomyosis, mesonephric hamartoma, and sarcoma.[378]

## PROSTATIC URETHRA

### Inflammation

Men with urethritis may present with discharge or dysuria, but many have no symptoms. Causative agents include the entire spectrum of sexually transmitted diseases. Biopsy is uncommon. Polypoid urethritis is similar to polypoid cystitis, consisting of papillary broad-based exophytic masses of edematous granulation tissue invested with inflamed or ulcerated urothelium, often with metaplastic changes. It commonly occurs in association with indwelling catheter or calculi and usually resolves spontaneously after removal of the inciting agent. Malakoplakia usually affects the bladder, and urethral involvement is rare. It appears as an inflamed plaque or polypoid mucosal mass that mimics malignancy.

### Glandular and Squamous Metaplasia

Glandular and squamous metaplasia occur in the bladder and urethra as a result of chronic irritation from calculi, indwelling catheter, diverticuli, repeated instrumentation, and urinary tract infection. Glandular metaplasia may appear as colonic-type goblet cells or typical mucin-rich columnar cells. Nephrogenic metaplasia usually arises in the bladder, but occasional cases have been reported in the urethra, sometimes mimicking adenocarcinoma. Occasional cases occur in a urethral diverticulum. Urethritis cystica, urethritis glandularis, and Brunn's nests frequently coexist.

### Changes Associated with Urethral Stents

A report described the histologic changes associated with long-term external sphincter use. Findings included polypoid hyperplasia (11 cases), nonkeratinizing or keratinizing squamous metaplasia (2 and 7 cases), chronic inflammation (15 cases), foreign body giant cell reaction (2 cases), and microabscess formation (5 cases).[379]

### Urethral Polyps

Congenital urethral polyp (fibroepithelial polyp) arises in the prostatic urethra near the verumontanum (posterior urethral polyp) and is seen exclusively in boys, usually younger than 10 years old.

Patients present with hematuria, obstructive symptoms, and urethritis and cystitis. This polypoid mass of vascularized loose connective tissue and smooth muscle is covered by urothelium that often is eroded or ulcerated.

### Prostatic Urethral Polyp (Ectopic Prostatic Tissue, Benign Polyp with Prostatic-Type Epithelium)

Prostatic urethral polyp is one of the most common causes of hematuria in adolescents and young adults. It usually occurs in the prostatic urethra but rarely arises in the distal urethra and bladder. The polyp may be focal or extensive, consisting of delicate papillae with fibrovascular stalks and prostatic epithelial lining without cytologic atypia. The cells express PSA and PAP.

### Other Rare Urethral Neoplasms

The urethra is involved rarely with tumors that may involve the urinary bladder, including papilloma, inverted papilloma, leiomyoma, capillary hemangioma, paraganglioma, villous adenoma, condyloma acuminatum, urothelial carcinoma, squamous cell carcinoma, adenocarcinoma, malignant melanoma, and sarcoma.

## REFERENCES

1. McNeal JE, Bostwick DG: Anatomy of the prostate. Implications for disease. *In* Bostwick DG (ed): Pathology of the Prostate. New York, Churchill Livingstone, 1990, pp 1–14.
2. Ayala AG, Ro JY, Babaian R, et al: The prostatic capsule. Does it exist? Its importance in the staging and treatment of prostatic carcinoma. Am J Surg Pathol 13:21–30, 1989.
3. Sakamoto N, Hasegawa Y, Koga H, et al: Presence of ganglia within the prostatic capsule. Ganglion involvement in prostatic cancer. Prostate 40:167–171, 1999.
4. Shidham VB, Lindholm PF, Kajdacsy-Balla A, et al: Prostate-specific antigen expression and lipochrome pigment granules in the differential diagnosis of prostatic adenocarcinoma versus seminal vesicle-ejaculatory duct epithelium. Arch Pathol Lab Med 123:1093–1097, 1999.
5. Arber DA, Speights VO: Aneuploidy in benign seminal vesicle epithelium. An example of the paradox of ploidy studies. Mod Pathol 4:687–689, 1991.
6. Saboorian MH, Huffman H, Ashfaq R, et al: Distinguishing Cowper's glands from neoplastic and pseudoneoplastic lesions of prostate. Immunohistochemical and ultrastructural studies. Am J Surg Pathol 21:1069–1074, 1997.
7. Cina SJ, Silberman MA, Kahane H, Epstein JI: Diagnosis of Cowper's glands on prostate needle biopsy. Am J Surg Pathol 21:550–555, 1997.
8. Brawer MK, Peehl DM, Stamey TA, Bostwick DG: Keratin immunoreactivity in the benign and neoplastic human prostate. Cancer Res 45:3663–3667, 1985.
9. Adlakha H, Bostwick DG: Paneth cell-like change in prostatic adenocarcinoma represents neuroendocrine differentiation. Report of 30 cases. Hum Pathol 25:135–139, 1994.
10. Aprikian AG, Cordon-Cardo C, Fair WR, et al: Characterization of neuroendocrine differentiation in human benign pros-

tate and prostatic adenocarcinoma. Cancer 71:3952–3965, 1993.

11. Di Sant'Agnese PA: Neuroendocrine differentiation in carcinoma of the prostate. Diagnostic, prognostic, and therapeutic implications. Cancer 70:254–268, 1992.

12. Di Sant'Agnese PA, Cockett AT: The prostatic endocrine-paracrine (neuroendocrine) regulatory system and neuroendocrine differentiation in prostatic carcinoma. A review and future directions in basic research. J Urol 152:1927–1931, 1994.

13. Abrahamsson PA, Wadstrom LB, Alumets J, et al: Peptide-hormone- and serotonin-immunoreactive tumour cells in carcinoma of the prostate. Pathol Res Pract 182:298–307, 1987.

14. Bonkhoff H, Stein U, Remberger K: Multidirectional differentiation in the normal, hyperplastic and neoplastic human prostate. Simultaneous demonstration of cell specific epithelial markers. Hum Pathol 25:42–46, 1994.

14a. Di Sant'Agnese PA: Neuroendocrine cells of the prostate and neuroendocrine differentiation in prostatic carcinoma: a review of morphologic aspects. Urology 51(5A Suppl):121–124, 1998.

15. Brennick JB, O'Connell JX, Dickersin GR, et al: Lipofuscin pigmentation (so-called "melanosis") of the prostate. Am J Surg Pathol 18:446–454, 1994.

16. Ro JY, Grignon DJ, Ayala AG, et al: Blue nevus and melanosis of the prostate, electron-microscopic and immunohistochemical studies. Am J Clin Pathol 90:530–535, 1988.

17. Renshaw AA: Adequate tissue sampling of prostate core needle biopsies. Am J Clin Pathol 107:26–29, 1997.

18. Reyes AO, Humphrey PA: Diagnostic effect of complete histological sampling of prostate needle biopsy specimens. Am J Clin Pathol 109:416–422, 1998.

19. Brat DJ, Wills ML, Lecksell KL, Epstein JI: How often are diagnostic features missed with less extensive histologic sampling of prostate needle biopsy specimens? Am J Surg Pathol 23:257–262, 1999.

20. Henson DE, Hutter RVP, Farrow GM: Practice protocol for the examination of specimens removed from patients with carcinoma of the prostate gland. A publication of the Cancer Committee, College of American Pathologists. Arch Pathol Lab Med 118:779–783, 1994.

21. Al-Abadi H: Fine needle aspiration biopsy vs. ultrasound-guided transrectal random core biopsy of the prostate. Comparative investigations in 246 cases. Acta Cytol 41:981–986, 1997.

22. Maksem J: Fine needle aspiration of the prostate. In Foster C, Bostwick DG (eds): Pathology of the Prostate. Philadelphia, WB Saunders, 1999, pp 121–144.

23. Blumenfeld W, Tucci S, Narayan P: Incidental lymphocytic prostatitis. Selective involvement with nonmalignant glands. Am J Surg Pathol 16:975–981, 1992.

24. Zhang W, Sesterhenn IA, Connelly RR, et al: Inflammatory infiltrate (prostatitis) in whole mounted radical prostatectomy specimens from black and white patients is not an etiology for racial difference in prostate specific antigen. J Urol 163:131–136, 2000.

25. Lopez-Plaza I, Bostwick DG: Prostatitis. In Bostwick DG (ed): Pathology of the Prostate. New York, Churchill Livingstone, 1990, pp 15–30.

26. Selzman AA, Bennert KW, Kursh ED: Cryptococcal prostatitis causing urinary retention in an AIDS patient. A case report. J Urol Pathol 2:251–254, 1994.

27. Helpap B: Histological and immunohistochemical study of chronic prostatic inflammation with and without benign prostatic hyperplasia. J Urol Pathol 2:49–64, 1994.

28. True LD, Berger RE, Rothman I, et al: Prostate histopathology and the chronic prostatitis/chronic pelvic pain syndrome. A prospective biopsy study. J Urol 162:2014–2018, 1999.

29. Solano JG, Sanchez CS, Romero SM, Perez-Guillermo M: Diagnostic dilemmas in the interpretation of fine-needle aspirates of granulomatous prostatitis. Diagn Cytopathol 18:215–221, 1998.

30. Oates RD, Stilmant MM, Fredlund MC, et al: Granulomatous

prostatitis following bacillus Calmette-Guérin immunotherapy of bladder cancer. J Urol 140:751–754, 1988.

31. Sebo TJ, Bostwick DG, Farrow GM, et al: Prostatic xanthoma. A mimic of prostatic adenocarcinoma. Hum Pathol 25:386–389, 1994.

32. Presti B, Weidner N: Granulomatous prostatitis and poorly differentiated adenocarcinoma. Their distinction with the use of immunohistochemical methods. Am J Clin Pathol 95:330–334, 1991.

33. Stillwell TJ, Engen DE, Farrow GM: The clinical spectrum of granulomatous prostatitis. A report of 200 cases. J Urol 138:320–323, 1987.

34. Orozco RE, Peters RL: Teflon granuloma of the prostate mimicking adenocarcinoma. Report of two cases. J Urol Pathol 3:365–368, 1995.

35. Bostwick DG, Vonk J, Picado A: Pathologic changes in the prostate following contemporary 18-gauge needle biopsy. No apparent risk of local cancer seeding. J Urol Pathol 2:203–212, 1994.

36. Bastacky SS, Walsh PC, Epstein JI: Needle biopsy associated tumor tracking of adenocarcinoma of the prostate. J Urol 145:1003–1007, 1991.

37. Grignon DJ, O'Malley FP: Mucinous metaplasia in the prostate gland. Am J Surg Pathol 17:287–290, 1993.

38. Carcamo Valor PI, San Millan Arruti JP, Cozar Olmo JM, et al: Nephrogenic adenoma of the upper and lower urinary tract. Apropos of 22 cases. Arch Esp Urol 45:423–427, 1992.

39. Malpica A, Ro JY, Troncoso P, et al: Nephrogenic adenoma of the prostate gland. A clinicopathologic and immunohistochemical study of eight cases. Hum Pathol 25:390–395, 1994.

40. Shapiro E, Becich MJ, Hartanto V, et al: The relative proportion of stromal and epithelial hyperplasia is related to the development of symptomatic benign prostatic hyperplasia. J Urol 147:1293–1297, 1992.

41. Bostwick DG, Cooner WH, Denis L, et al: The association of benign prostatic hyperplasia and cancer of the prostate. Cancer 70:291–301, 1992.

42. Cheville JC, Bostwick DG: Post-atrophic hyperplasia of the prostate. A histologic mimick of prostatic adenocarcinoma. Am J Surg Pathol 19:1068–1076, 1995.

43. Amin MB, Tamboli P, Varma M, Srigley JR: Postatrophic hyperplasia of the prostate gland. A detailed analysis of its morphology in needle biopsy specimens. Am J Surg Pathol 23:925–931, 1999.

44. Grignon DJ, Ro JY, Ordonez NG, et al: Basal cell hyperplasia, adenoid basal cell tumor, and adenoid cystic carcinoma of the prostate gland. An immunohistochemical study. Hum Pathol 19:1425–1433, 1988.

45. Epstein JI, Armas OA: Atypical basal cell hyperplasia of the prostate. Am J Surg Pathol 16:1205–1214, 1992.

46. Devaraj LT, Bostwick DG: Atypical basal cell hyperplasia of the prostate. Immunophenotypic profile and proposed classification of basal cell proliferations. Am J Surg Pathol 17:645–659, 1993.

47. Frauenhoffer EE, Ro JY, El-Naggar AK, et al: Clear cell cribriform hyperplasia of the prostate. Immunohistochemical and flow cytometric study. Am J Clin Pathol 95:446–453, 1991.

48. Bostwick DG, Srigley J, Grignon D, et al: Atypical adenomatous hyperplasia of the prostate. Morphologic criteria for its distinction from well-differentiated carcinoma. Hum Pathol 24:819–832, 1993.

49. Bostwick DG, Algaba F, Amin MB, et al: Consensus statement on terminology. Recommendation to use atypical adenomatous hyperplasia in place of adenosis of the prostate. Am J Surg Pathol 18:1069–1070, 1994.

50. Bostwick DG, Qian J: Atypical adenomatous hyperplasia of the prostate. Relationship with carcinoma in 217 whole-mount radical prostatectomies. Am J Surg Pathol 19:506–518, 1995.

51. Brawn PN, Speights VO, Contin JU, et al: Atypical hyperplasia in prostates of 20 to 40 year old men. J Clin Pathol 42:383–386, 1989.

52. Humphrey PA, Zhu X, Crouch EC, et al: Mass-forming atypical adenomatous hyperplasia. J Urol Pathol 9:73–81, 1998.

53. Gleason DF: Atypical hyperplasia, benign hyperplasia, and well-differentiated adenocarcinoma of the prostate. Am J Surg Pathol 9:53–67, 1985.

54. Qian J, Bostwick DG, Jenkins RB: Chromosomal anomalies in atypical adenomatous hyperplasia and carcinoma of the prostate using fluorescence in situ hybridization. Urology 46:837–842, 1995.

55. Cheng L, Shan A, Cheville JC, et al: Atypical adenomatous hyperplasia of the prostate. A premalignant lesion? Cancer Res 58:389–391, 1998.

56. Haussler O, Epstein JI, Amin MB, et al: Cell proliferation, apoptosis, oncogene, and tumor suppressor gene status in adenosis with comparison to benign prostatic hyperplasia, prostatic intraepithelial neoplasia, and cancer. Hum Pathol 30:1077–1086, 1999.

57. Jones EC, Clement PB, Young RH: Sclerosing adenosis of the prostate gland. A clinicopathologic and immunohistochemical study of 11 cases. Am J Surg Pathol 15:1171–1180, 1991.

58. Collina G, Botticelli AR, Martinelli AM, et al: Sclerosing adenosis of the prostate. Report of three cases with electron microscopy and immunohistochemical study. Histopathology 20:505–510, 1992.

59. Grignon DJ, Ro JY, Srigley JR, et al: Sclerosing adenosis of the prostate gland. A lesion showing myoepithelial differentiation. Am J Surg Pathol 16:383–391, 1992.

60. Eble JN, Tejada E: Prostatic stromal hyperplasia with bizarre nuclei. Arch Pathol Lab Med 115:87–89, 1991.

61. Wang X, Bostwick DG: Prostate stromal hyperplasia with atypia. A study of 11 cases. J Urol Pathol 6:15–26, 1997.

62. Gagucas RJ, Brown RW, Wheeler TM: Verumontanum mucosal gland hyperplasia. Am J Surg Pathol 19:30–36, 1995.

63. Gikas PW, Del Buono EA, Epstein JI: Florid hyperplasia of mesonephric remnants involving prostate and periprostatic tissue. Possible confusion with adenocarcinoma. Am J Surg Pathol 16:454–459, 1992.

64. Pacelli A, Farrow GM, Bostwick DG: Mesonephric remnants of the prostate. Incidence and clinical significance. Mod Pathol 10:83A, 1997.

65. Jimenez RE, Raval MFT, Spanta R, et al: Mesonephric remnants hyperplasia. J Urol Pathol 9:83–92, 1998.

66. Maluf HM, King ME, DeLuca FR, et al: Giant multilocular prostatic cystadenoma. A distinctive lesion of the retroperitoneum in men. A report of two cases. Am J Surg Pathol 15:131–137, 1991.

67. Levy DA, Gogate PA, Hampel N: Giant multilocular prostatic cystadenoma. A rare clinical entity and review of the literature. J Urol 150:1920–1922, 1993.

68. Lim DJ, Hayden RT, Murad T, et al: Multilocular prostatic cystadenoma presenting as a large complex pelvic cystic mass. J Urol 149:856–859, 1993.

69. Mayersak JS: Urogenital sinus-ejaculatoy duct cyst. A case report with a proposed clinical classification and review of the literature. J Urol 142:1330–1332, 1989.

70. Hendry WF, Pryor JP: Müllerian duct (prostatic utricle) cyst. Diagnosis and treatment in subfertile males. Br J Urol 69:79–82, 1992.

71. DeKlotz RJ: Echinococcal cyst involving the prostate and seminal vesicles. A case report. J Urol 115:116–117, 1976.

72. Beckman EN, Pintado SO, Leonard GL, Sternberg WH: Endometriosis of the prostate. Am J Surg Pathol 9:374–379, 1985.

73. Mai KT, Walley VM: Adenofibroma of the ejaculatory duct. J Urol Pathol 2:301–305, 1994.

74. Fan K, Johnson DF: Adenomatoid tumor of ejaculatory duct. Urology 25:653–654, 1985.

75. Bostwick DG, Qian J, Frankel K: The incidence of high grade prostatic intraepithelial neoplasia in needle biopsies. J Urol 154:1791–1794, 1996.

76. Montironi R, Bostwick DG, Bonkhoff H, et al: Workgroup 1. Origins of prostate cancer. Cancer 78:362–365, 1996.

77. Cheng L, Shan A, Qian J, et al: Genetic heterogeneity in prostatic intraepithelial neoplasia and carcinoma. Mod Pathol 11:A78, 1998.

78. Bostwick DG, Shan A, Qian J, et al: Independent origin of multiple foci of prostatic intraepithelial neoplasia. Comparison with matched foci of prostate carcinoma. Cancer 83:1995–2002, 1998.

79. Bostwick DG: Prostatic intraepithelial neoplasia is a risk factor for prostate cancer. Semin Urol Oncol 17:187–198, 1999.

80. McNeal JE, Bostwick DG: Intraductal dysplasia. A premalignant lesion of the prostate. Hum Pathol 17:64–71, 1986.

81. Bostwick DG, Brawer MK: Prostatic intra-epithelial neoplasia and early invasion in prostate cancer. Cancer 59:788–794, 1987.

82. Qian J, Wollan P, Bostwick DG: The extent and multicentricity of high grade prostatic intraepithelial neoplasia in clinically localized prostatic adenocarcinoma. Hum Pathol 28:143–148, 1997.

83. Ramos CG, Carvahal GF, Mager DE, et al: The effect of high grade prostatic intraepithelial neoplasia on serum total and percentage of free prostate specific antigen levels. J Urol 162:1587–1590, 1999.

84. Feneley MR, Green JSA, Young MPA, et al: Prevalence of prostatic intraepithelial neoplasia (PIN) in biopsies from hospital practice and pilot screening. Clinical implications. Prostate Cancer and Prostatic Diseases 1:79–83, 1997.

85. Hoedemaeker RF, Kranse R, Rietbergen JB, et al: Evaluation of prostate needle biopsies in a population-based screening study. The impact of borderline lesions. Cancer 85:145–152, 1999.

86. Langer JE, Rovner ES, Coleman BG, et al: Strategy for repeat biopsy of patients with prostatic intraepithelial neoplasia detected by prostate needle biopsy. J Urol 155:228–231, 1996.

87. Wills ML, Hamper UM, Partin AW, et al: Incidence of high-grade prostatic intraepithelial neoplasia in sextant needle biopsy specimens. Urology 49:367–373, 1997.

88. Skjorten FJ, Berner A, Harvei S, et al: Prostatic intraepithelial neoplasia in surgical resections. Relationship to coexistent adenocarcinoma and atypical adenomatous hyperplasia of the prostate. Cancer 79:1172–1179, 1997.

89. Perachino M, Diciolo L, Barbetti V, et al: Results of rebiopsy for suspected prostate cancer in symptomatic men with elevated PSA levels. Eur Urol 32:155–159, 1997.

90. Pacelli A, Bostwick DG: The clinical significance of high-grade prostatic intraepithelial neoplasia in transurethral resection specimens. Urology 50:355–359, 1997.

91. Gaudin PB, Sesterhenn IA, Wojno KJ, et al: Incidence and clinical significance of high-grade prostatic intraepithelial neoplasia in TURP specimens. Urology 49:558–563, 1997.

92. Sakr WA, Haas GP, Cassin BJ, et al: The frequency of carcinoma and intraepithelial neoplasia of the prostate in young male patients. J Urol 150:379–385, 1993.

93. Billis A: Age and race distribution of high-grade prostatic intraepithelial neoplasia. An autopsy study in Brazil (South America). J Urol Pathol 5:1–7, 1996.

94. Bostwick DG, Amin MB, Dundore P, et al: Architectural patterns of high grade prostatic intraepithelial neoplasia. Hum Pathol 24:298–310, 1993.

95. Reyes AO, Swanson PE, Carbone JM, Humphrey PA: Unusual histologic types of high-grade prostatic intraepithelial neoplasia. Am J Surg Pathol 21:1215–1222, 1997.

96. Berman DM, Yang J, Epstein JI: Foamy gland high-grade prostatic intraepithelial neoplasia. Am J Surg Pathol 24:140–144, 2000.

97. Bostwick DG, Pacelli A, Lopez-Beltran A: Molecular biology of prostatic intraepithelial neoplasia. Prostate 29:117–134, 1996.

98. Weinberg DS, Weidner N: Concordance of DNA content between prostatic intraepithelial neoplasia and concomitant carcinoma. Evidence that prostatic intraepithelial neoplasia is a precursor of invasive prostatic carcinoma. Arch Pathol Lab Med 117:1132–1137, 1993.

99. Crissman JD, Sakr WA, Hussein ME, et al: DNA quantitation of intraepithelial neoplasia and invasive carcinoma of the prostate. Prostate 22:155–162, 1993.

100. Montironi R, Scarpelli M, Sisti S, et al: Quantitative analysis of prostatic intra-epithelial neoplasia on tissue sections. Anal Quant Cytol Histol 12:366–372, 1990.

101. Kasper S, Sheppard PC, Yan Y, et al: Development, progression, and androgen-dependence of prostate tumors in proba-

sin-large T antigen transgenic mice. A model for prostate cancer. Lab Invest 78:319–333, 1998.

102. Garabedian EM, Humphrey PA, Gordon JI: A transgenic mouse model of metastatic prostate cancer originating from neuroendocrine cells. Proc Natl Acad Sci U S A 95:15382–15387, 1998.
103. Aboseif S, Shinohara K, Weidner N, et al: The significance of prostatic intra-epithelial neoplasia. Br J Urol 76:355–359, 1995.
104. Krishnamurthi V, Klein EA, Levin HS: Probability of prostate cancer detection following diagnosis of prostatic intraepithelial neoplasia (PIN). J Urol 157(suppl):366, 1997.
105. Davidson D, Bostwick DG, Qian J, et al: Prostatic intraepithelial neoplasia is a risk factor for adenocarcinoma. Predictive accuracy in needle biopsies. J Urol 154:1295–1299, 1995.
106. Ellis WJ, Brawer MK: Repeat prostate needle biopsy. Who needs it? J Urol 153:1496–1498, 1995.
107. Weinstein MH, Epstein JI: Significance of high grade prostatic intraepithelial neoplasia on needle biopsy. Hum Pathol 24:624–629, 1993.
108. Keetch DW, Humphrey P, Stahl D, et al: Morphometric analysis and clinical follow-up of isolated prostatic intraepithelial neoplasia in needle biopsy of the prostate. J Urol 154:347–351, 1995.
109. Raviv G, Janssen TH, Zlotta AR, et al: Prostatic intraepithelial neoplasia. Influence of clinical and pathological data on the detection of prostate cancer. J Urol 156:1050–1055, 1996.
110. Berner A, Danielsen HE, Pettersen EO, et al: DNA distribution in the prostate. Normal gland, benign and premalignant lesions, and subsequent adenocarcinomas. Anal Quant Cytol Histol 15:247–252, 1993.
111. Shepherd D, Keetch DW, Humphrey PA, et al: Repeat biopsy strategy in men with isolated prostatic intraepithelial neoplasia on prostate needle biopsy. J Urol 156:460–463, 1996.
112. Balaji KC, Rabbani F, Tsai H, et al: Effect of neoadjuvant hormonal therapy on prostatic intraepithelial neoplasia and its prognostic significance. J Urol 162:753–757, 1999.
113. Ferguson J, Zincke H, Ellison E, et al: Decrease of prostatic intraepithelial neoplasia (PIN) following androgen deprivation therapy in patients with stage T3 carcinoma treated by radical prostatectomy. Urology 44:91–95, 1994.
114. Vaillancourt L, Tetu B, Fradet Y, et al: Effect of neoadjuvant endocrine therapy (combined androgen blockade) on normal prostate and prostate carcinoma. A randomized study. Am J Surg Pathol 20:86–93, 1996.
115. Yang XJ, Lecksell K, Short K, et al: Does long-term finasteride therapy affect the histologic features of benign prostatic tissue and prostate cancer on needle biopsy? Urology 53:696–700, 1999.
116. Slem CE, Cote RJ, Skinner EC, et al: The effect of finasteride on prostate gland peripheral zone histology and proliferation rates in men at high risk for prostate cancer. J Urol 157:228–232, 1997.
117. Cheng L, Cheville JC, Bostwick DG: Diagnosis of prostate cancer in needle biopsies after radiation therapy. Am J Surg Pathol 23:1173–1183, 1999.
118. Gaudin PB, Zelefsky MJ, Leibel SA, et al: Histopathologic effects of three-dimensional conformal external beam radiation therapy on benign and malignant prostate tissues. Am J Surg Pathol 23:1021–1031, 1999.
119. Greenlee RT, Murray T, Bolden S, Wingo PA: Cancer statistics, 2000. CA Cancer J Clin 50:7–33, 2000.
119a. American Cancer Society: Cancer facts and figures, 2002. Atlanta, American Cancer Society, Georgia p 4. www.cancer.org.
120. Brawer MK, Benson MC, Bostwick DG, et al: Prostate-specific antigen and other serum markers. Current concepts from the World Health Organization Second International Consultation on Prostate Cancer. Semin Urol Oncol 17:206–221, 1999.
121. Catalona WJ, Smith DS, Ratliff TL, et al: Measurement of prostate-specific antigen in serum as a screening test for prostate cancer. N Engl J Med 324:1156–1161, 1991.
122. Catalona WJ, Richie JP, Ahmann FR, et al: Comparison of digital rectal examination and serum prostate specific anti-gen in the early detection of prostate cancer. Results of a multicenter clinical trial of 6630 men. J Urol 151:1283–1290, 1994.
123. Blackwell KL, Bostwick DG, Zincke H, et al: Combining prostate specific antigen with cancer and gland volume to predict more reliably pathologic stage. The influence of prostate specific antigen cancer density. J Urol 151:1565–1570, 1994.
124. Bostwick DG, Dundore PA: Biopsy Pathology of the Prostate. London, Chapman & Hall Medical, 1997.
125. Helpap B: Observations on the number, size and location of nucleoli in hyperplastic and neoplastic prostatic disease. Histopathology 13:203–211, 1988.
126. Goldstein NS, Qian J, Bostwick DG: Mucin expression in atypical adenomatous hyperplasia of the prostate. Hum Pathol 26:887–891, 1995.
127. Del Rosario AD, Bui HX, Abdulla M, Ross JS: Sulfur-rich prostatic intraluminal crystalloids. A surgical pathologic and electron probe x-ray microanalytic study. Hum Pathol 24:1159–1167, 1993.
128. Molberg KH, Mikhail A, Vuitch F: Crystalloids in metastatic prostatic adenocarcinoma. Am J Clin Pathol 101:266–268, 1994.
129. Tressera F, Barastegui C: Intraluminal crystalloids in metastatic prostatic carcinoma. Am J Clin Pathol 103:665, 1995.
130. Bostwick DG, Wollan P, Adlakha K: Collagenous micronodules in prostate cancer. A specific but infrequent diagnostic finding. Arch Pathol Lab Med 119:444–447, 1995.
131. McIntire TL, Franzina DA: The presence of benign prostate glands in perineural spaces. J Urol 135:507–509, 1986.
132. Bastacky SI, Walsh PC, Epstein JI: Relationship between perineural tumor invasion on needle biopsy and radical prostatectomy capsular penetration in clinical stage B adenocarcinoma of the prostate. Am J Surg Pathol 17:336–341, 1993.
133. Egan AJM, Bostwick DG: Prediction of extraprostatic extension of prostate cancer based on needle biopsy findings. Perineural invasion lacks independent significance. Lab Invest 76:421, 1997.
134. Salamao DR, Graham SD, Bostwick DG: Microvascular invasion in prostate cancer correlates with pathologic stage. Arch Pathol Lab Med 119:1050–1054, 1995.
135. Bostwick DG, Foster CS: Predictive factors in prostate cancer. Current concepts from the 1999 College of American Pathologists Conference on Solid Tumor Prognostic Factors and the 1999 World Health Organization Second International Consultation on Prostate Cancer. Semin Urol Oncol 17:222–272, 1999.
136. Gleason DF: Histologic grading of prostate cancer. A perspective. Hum Pathol 23:273–279, 1992.
137. Bostwick DG: Gleason grading of prostatic needle biopsies. Correlation with grade in 316 matched prostatectomies. Am J Surg Pathol 18:796–803, 1994.
138. Kojima M, Troncoso P, Babaian RJ: Use of prostate-specific antigen and tumor volume in predicting needle biopsy grading error. Urology 45:807–812, 1995.
139. Thickman D, Speers WC, Philpott PJ, Shapiro H: Effect of the number of core biopsies of the prostate on predicting Gleason score of prostate cancer. J Urol 156:110–114, 1996.
140. Cookson MS, Fleshner NE, Soloway SM, Fair WR: Correlation between Gleason score of needle biopsy and radical prostatectomy specimen. Accuracy and clinical implications. J Urol 157:559–562, 1997.
141. Spires SE, Cibull ML, Wood DP, et al: Gleason histologic grading in prostatic carcinoma. Correlation of 18-gauge core biopsy with prostatectomy. Arch Pathol Lab Med 118:705–708, 1994.
142. Steinberg DM, Sauvageot J, Piantadosi S, Epstein JI: Correlation of prostate needle biopsy and radical prostatectomy Gleason grade in academic and community settings. Am J Surg Pathol 21:566–576, 1997.
143. Aihara M, Wheeler TM, Ohori M, Scardiono PT: Heterogeneity of prostate cancer in radical prostatectomy specimens. Urology 43:60–66, 1994.
144. Allsbrook WCJ, Lane RB, Lane CG, et al: Interobserver re-

producibility of Gleason's grading system. Urologic pathologists. Mod Pathol 11:75A, 1998.

145. Allsbrook WCJ, Mangold KA, Yang X, Epstein JI: The Gleason grading system. J Urol Pathol 10:141–157, 1999.

146. Bock BJ, Bostwick DG: Does prostatic ductal adenocarcinoma exist? Am J Surg Pathol 23:781–785, 1999.

147. Ro JY, Grignon DJ, Ayala AG, et al: Mucinous adenocarcinoma of the prostate. Histochemical and immunohistochemical studies. Hum Pathol 21:593–600, 1990.

148. McNeal JE, Alroy J, Villers A, et al: Mucinous differentiation in prostatic adenocarcinoma. Hum Pathol 22:979–988, 1991.

149. Efros MD, Fischer J, Mallouh C, et al: Unusual primary diagnostic malignancies. Urology 39:407, 1992.

150. Ishizu K, Yoshihiro S, Joko K, et al: [Mucinous adenocarcinoma of the prostate with good response to hormonal therapy. A case report]. Acta Urol Jpn 37:1057–1060, 1991.

151. Teichman JM, Shabaik A, Demby AM: Mucinous carcinoma of the prostate and hormonal sensitivity. J Urol 151:701–702, 1994.

152. Pinder SE, McMahon RFT: Mucins in prostatic carcinoma. Histopathology 16:43–46, 1990.

153. Alline KM, Cohen MB: Signet-ring cell carcinoma of the prostate. Arch Pathol Lab Med 116:99–102, 1992.

154. Guerin D, Hasan N, Keen CE: Signet ring cell differentiation in adenocarcinoma of the prostate. A study of five cases. Histopathology 22:367–371, 1993.

155. Torbenson M, Dhir R, Nangia A, et al: Prostatic carcinoma with signet ring cells. A clinicopathologic and immunohistochemical analysis of 12 cases, with review of the literature. Mod Pathol 11:552–559, 1998.

156. Bostwick DG, Dousa MK, Crawford BG, Wollan PC: Neuroendocrine differentiation in prostatic intraepithelial neoplasia and adenocarcinoma. Am J Surg Pathol 18:1240–1246, 1994.

157. Oesterling JE, Hauzear CG, Farrow GM: Small cell anaplastic carcinoma of the prostate. A clinical, pathological and immunohistological study of 27 patients. J Urol 147:804–809, 1992.

158. Abbas F, Civantos F, Benedetto P, Soloway MS: Small cell carcinoma of the bladder and prostate. Urology 46:617–630, 1995.

159. Little NA, Wiener JS, Walther PJ, et al: Squamous cell carcinoma of the prostate: 2 cases of a rare malignancy and review of the literature. J Urol 149:137–139, 1993.

160. Moskovitz N, Munichor M, Bolkier M, Livne PM: Squamous cell carcinoma of the prostate. Urol Int 51:181–183, 1993.

161. Miller VA, Reuter V, Scher HI: Primary squamous cell carcinoma of the prostate after radiation seed implantation for adenocarcinoma. Urology 46:111–113, 1995.

162. Gattuso P, Carson HJ, Candel A, Castelli MJ: Adenosquamous carcinoma of the prostate. Hum Pathol 26:123–126, 1995.

163. Devaney DM, Dorman A, Leader M: Adenosquamous carcinoma of the prostate. A case report. Hum Pathol 22:1046–1050, 1991.

164. Dundore PA, Nascimento AG, Cheville JC, et al: Carcinosarcoma of the prostate. Report of 22 cases. Cancer 76:1035–1042, 1995.

165. Delahunt B, Eble JN, Nacey JN, Grebe SK: Sarcomatoid carcinoma of the prostate. Progression from adenocarcinoma is associated with p53 over-expression. Anticancer Res 19:4279–4283, 1999.

166. Cohen RJ, Goldberg RD, Verhaart MJ, Cohen M: Adenoid cyst-like carcinoma of the prostate. Arch Pathol Lab Med 117:799–801, 1993.

167. Denholm SW, Webb JN, Howard GCW, Chisholm GD: Basaloid carcinoma of the prostate gland. Histogenesis and review of the literature. Histopathology 20:151–155, 1992.

168. Bostwick DG, Adlakha K: Lymphoepithelioma-like carcinoma of the prostate. J Urol Pathol 2:319–325, 1994.

169. Beer M, Occhionero F, Welsch U: Oncocytoma of the prostate. A case report with ultrastructural and immunohistochemical evaluation. Histopathology 17:370–372, 1990.

170. Pinto JA, Gonzalez JE, Granadillo MA: Primary carcinoma of the prostate with diffuse oncocytic changes. Histopathology 25:286–288, 1994.

171. Montironi R, Santinelli A, Galluzzi CM, Giannulis I: Prolifer-

ating cell nuclear antigen (PCNA) evaluation in the diagnostic quantitative pathology of cribriform adenocarcinoma of the prostate. In Vivo 7:343–346, 1993.

172. Amin MB, Schultz DS, Zarbo RJ: Analysis of cribriform morphology in prostate neoplasia using antibody to high molecular weight cytokeratins. Arch Pathol Lab Med 118:260–264, 1994.

173. Humphrey PA, Kaleem Z, Swanson PE, Vollmer RT: Pseudohyperplastic prostatic adenocarcinoma. Am J Surg Pathol 22:1239–1246, 1998.

173a. Egan AJ, Lopez-Beltran A, Bostwick DG: Prostatic adenocarcinoma with atrophic features: malignancy mimicking a benign process. Am J Surg Pathol 21:931–935, 1997.

174. Cina SJ, Epstein JI: Adenocarcinoma of the prostate with atrophic features. Am J Surg Pathol 21:289–295, 1997.

175. Kaleem Z, Swanson PE, Vollmer RT, Humphrey PA: Prostatic adenocarcinoma with atrophic features. A study of 202 consecutive completely embedded radical prostatectomy specimens. Am J Clin Pathol 109:695–703, 1998.

176. Pacelli A, Lopez-Beltran A, Egan AJ, Bostwick DG: Prostatic adenocarcinoma with glomeruloid features. Hum Pathol 29:543–546, 1998.

177. Cheville JC, Dundore PA, Bostwick DG, et al: Transitional cell carcinoma of the prostate. Clinicopathologic study of 50 cases. Cancer 82:703–707, 1998.

178. Frazier HA, Robertson JE, Dodge RK, Paulson DF: The value of pathologic factors in predicting cancer-specific survival among patients treated with radical cystectomy for transitional cell carcinoma of the bladder and prostate. Cancer 71:3993–4001, 1993.

179. Cheng L, Cheville JC, Pisansky TM, et al: Prevalence and distribution of prostatic intraepithelial neoplasia in salvage radical prostatectomy specimens after radiation therapy. Am J Surg Pathol 23:803–808, 1999.

180. Armas OA, Aprikian AG, Melemed J, et al: Clinical and pathological effects of neoadjuvant total androgen ablation therapy on clinically localized prostatic adenocarcinoma. Am J Surg Pathol 18:979–991, 1994.

181. Civantos F, Marcial MA, Banks ER, et al: Pathology of androgen deprivation therapy in prostate carcinoma. A comparative study of 173 patients. Cancer 75:1634–1641, 1995.

182. Ellison E, Chuang S-S, Zincke H, et al: Prostate adenocarcinoma after androgen deprivation therapy. A comparative study of morphology, morphometry, immunohistochemistry, and DNA ploidy. Pathol Case Rev 2:36–46, 1996.

183. Gaudin PB: Histopathologic effects of radiation and hormonal therapies on benign and malignant prostate tissues. J Urol Pathol 8:55–67, 1998.

184. Montironi R, Diamanti L: Morphologic changes in benign prostatic hyperplasia following chronic treatment with a 5-α-reductase inhibitor finasteride. Comparison with combination endocrine therapy. J Urol Pathol 4:123–135, 1996.

185. Montironi R, Bartels PH, Thompson D, et al: Androgen-deprived prostate adenocarcinoma. Evaluation of treatment-related changes vs no distinctive treatment effect with a Bayesian belief network. Eur Urol 30:307–315, 1996.

186. Murphy WM, Soloway MS, Barrows GH: Pathologic changes associated with androgen deprivation therapy for prostate cancer. Cancer 68:821–828, 1991.

187. Smith DM, Murphy WM: Histologic changes in prostate carcinomas treated with Leuprolide (luteinizing hormone-releasing hormone effect). Distinction from poor tumor differentiation. Cancer 73:1472–1477, 1994.

188. Tetu B, Srigley JR, Boivin JC, et al: Effect of combination endocrine therapy (LHRH agonist and flutamide) on normal prostate and prostatic adenocarcinoma. Am J Surg Pathol 15:111–120, 1991.

189. Reuter VE: Pathological changes in benign and malignant prostatic tissue following androgen deprivation therapy. Urology 49(suppl 3A):16–22, 1997.

190. Montironi R, Schulman CC: Pathological changes in prostate lesions after androgen manipulation. J Clin Pathol 51:5–12, 1998.

191. Grignon DJ, Bostwick DG, Civantos F, et al: Pathologic handling and reporting of prostate tissue specimens in patients

receiving neoadjuvant hormonal therapy. Report of the Pathology Committee. Mol Urol 3:193–198, 1999.

191a. Ellison E, Chuang SS, Zincke H, et al: Prostate adenocarcinoma after androgen deprivation therapy. A comparative study of morphology, morphometry, immunohistochemistry and DNA ploidy. Pathol Case Rev 1:74–83, 1996.

192. Algaba F, Epstein JI, Aldape HC, et al: Workgroup 5. Assessment of prostate carcinoma in core needle biopsy. Definition of minimal criteria for the diagnosis of cancer in biopsy material. Cancer 78:376–381, 1996.

193. Goldstein NS, Begin LR, Grody WW, et al: Minimal or no cancer in radical prostatectomy specimens. Report of 13 cases of the "vanishing cancer phenomenon." Am J Surg Pathol 19:1002–1009, 1995.

194. Patterson RF, Gleave ME, Jones EC, et al: Immunohistochemical analysis of radical prostatectomy specimens after 8 months of neoadjuvant hormonal therapy. Mol Urol 3:277–286, 1999.

195. Cher ML, Bova GS, Moore DH, et al: Genetic alterations in untreated metastases and androgen-independent prostate cancer deteted by comparative genomic hybridization and allelotyping. Cancer Res 56:3091–3102, 1996.

196. Bostwick DG, Egbert BM, Fajardo LF: Radiation injury of the normal and neoplastic prostate. Am J Surg Pathol 6:541–551, 1982.

197. Brawer MK, Nagle RB, Pitts W, et al: Keratin immunoreactivity as an aid to the diagnosis of persistent adenocarcinoma in irradiated human prostates. Cancer 63:454–460, 1989.

198. Grignon DJ, Sakr WA: Histologic effects of radiation therapy and total androgen blockade on prostate cancer. Cancer 75:1837–1841, 1995.

199. Helpap B, Koch V: Histological and immunohistochemical findings of prostatic carcinoma after external or interstitial radiotherapy. J Cancer Res Clin Oncol 117:608–614, 1991.

200. Siders DB, Lee F, Mayman DM: Diagnosis of prostate cancer altered by ionizing radiation with and without neoadjuvant antiandrogen hormonal ablation. *In* Foster CS, Bostwick DG (eds): Pathology of the Prostate. Philadelphia, WB Saunders, 1998, pp 315–326.

201. Siders DB, Lee F: Histologic changes of irradiated prostatic carcinoma diagnosed by transrectal ultrasound. Hum Pathol 23:344–351, 1992.

202. Wheeler JA, Zagars GK, Ayala AG: Dedifferentiation of locally recurrrent prostate cancer after radiation therapy. Evidence of tumor progression. Cancer 71:3783–3787, 1993.

203. Cheng L, Darson MF, Bergstralh EJ, et al: Correlation of margin status and extraprostatic extension with progression of prostate carcinoma. Cancer 86:1775–1782, 1999.

203a. Cheng L, Cheville JC, Bostwick DG: Diagnosis of prostate cancer in needle biopsies after radiation therapy. Am J Surg Pathol 23:1173–1183, 1999.

204. Kuban DA, Schellhammer PF: Prognostic significance of post-irradiation prostate biopsies. Oncology 7:29–38, 1993.

205. Letran JL, Brawer MK: Management of radiation failure for localized prostate cancer. Prostate Cancer and Prostatic Disease 1:119–127, 1998.

206. Prendergast NJ, Atkins MR, Schatte EC, et al: p53 immunohistochemical and genetic alterations are associated at high incidence with post-irradiation locally persistent prostate carcinoma. J Urol 155:1685–1692, 1996.

207. Crook JM, Bahadur YA, Robertson SJ, et al: Evaluation of radiation effect, tumor differentiation, and prostate specific antigen staining in sequential prostate biopsies after external beam radiotherapy for patients with prostate carcinoma. Cancer 79:81–89, 1997.

208. Goldstein NS, Martinez A, Vicini F, Stromberg J: The histology of radiation therapy effect on prostate adenocarcinoma as assessed by needle biopsy after brachytherapy boost. Correlation with biochemical failure. Am J Clin Pathol 110:765–775, 1998.

209. Sheaff MT, Baithun SI: Effects of radiation on the normal prostate gland. Histopathology 30:341–348, 1997.

210. Susani M, Maderbacher S, Kratzik C, Vingers L: Morphology of tissue destruction induced by focused ultrasound. Eur Urol 23(suppl 1):34–38, 1993.

211. Orihuela E, Motamedi M, Pow-Sang M, et al: Histopathological evaluation of laser thermocoagulation in the human prostate. Optimization of laser irradiation for benign prostatic hyperplasia. J Urol 153:1531–1536, 1995.

212. Bostwick DG, Larson T: Transurethral microwave thermal therapy. Pathologic findings in the canine prostate. Prostate 26:116–122, 1995.

213. Petersen DS, Milleman LA, Rose EF, et al: Biopsy and clinical course after cryosurgery for prostatic cancer. J Urol 120:308–311, 1978.

214. Shabaik A, Wilson S, Bidair M, et al: Pathologic changes in prostate biopsies following cryoablation therapy of prostate carcinoma. J Urol Pathol 3:183–194, 1995.

215. Borkowski P, Robinson MJ, Poppiti RJ Jr, Nash SC: Histologic findings in postcryosurgical prostatic biopsies. Mod Pathol 9:807–811, 1996.

216. Falconieri G, Lugnani F, Zanconati F, et al: Histopathology of the frozen prostate. The microscopic bases of prostatic carcinoma cryoablation. Pathol Res Pract 192:579–587, 1996.

217. Shuman BA, Cohen JK, Miller RJ Jr, et al: Histological presence of viable prostatic glands on routine biopsy following cryosurgical ablation of the prostate. J Urol 157:552–555, 1997.

218. Association of Directors of Anatomic and Surgical Pathology: Recommendations for the reporting of resected prostate carcinomas. Hum Pathol 27:321–323, 1996.

219. Sakr W, Wheeler T, Blute M, et al: Staging and reporting of prostate cancer. Sampling of the radical prostatectomy specimen. Cancer 78:366–368, 1996.

220. Hall GS, Kramer CE, Epstein JI: Evaluation of radical prostatectomy specimens. A comparative analysis of sampling methods. Am J Surg Pathol 16:315–324, 1992.

221. Schmid H-P, McNeal JE: An abbreviated standard procedure for accurate tumor volume estimation in prostate cancer. Am J Surg Pathol 16:184–191, 1992.

222. Haggman M, Norberg M, de la Torre M, et al: Characterization of localized prostatic cancer. Distribution, grading and pT-staging in radical prostatectomy specimens. Scand J Urol Nephrol 27:7–13, 1993.

223. Bostwick DG, Myers RP, Oesterling JE: Staging of prostate cancer. Semin Surg Oncol 10:60–73, 1994.

223a. Donohue RE, Miller GJ: Adenocarcinoma of the prostate: biopsy to whole mount Denver VA experience. Urol Clin North Am 18:449–452, 1991.

224. Cohen MB, Soloway MS, Murphy WM: Sampling of radical prostatectomy specimens. How much is adequate. Am J Clin Pathol 101:250–252, 1994.

225. True LD: Surgical pathology examination of the prostate gland. Practice survey by American Society of Clinical Pathologists. Am J Clin Pathol 10:572–579, 1994.

226. Humphrey PA: Complete histologic serial sectioning of a prostate gland with adenocarcinoma. Am J Surg Pathol 17:468–472, 1993.

227. Vollmer RT, Keetch DW, Humphrey PA: Predicting the pathology results of radical prostatectomy from preoperative information. A validation study. Cancer 83:1567–1580, 1998.

228. Theiss M, Wirth MP, Manseck A, Frohmuller HGW: Prognostic signfance of capsular invasion and capsular penetration in patients with clinically localized prostate cancer undergoing radical prostatectomy. Prostate 27:13–17, 1995.

229. Bostwick DG: Significance of tumor volume in prostate cancer. Urol Ann 8:1–22, 1994.

230. Ohori M, Wheeler TM, Kattan MW, et al: Prognostic significance of positive surgical margins in radical prostatectomy specimens. J Urol 154:1818–1824, 1995.

231. McNeal JE, Bostwick DG, Kindrachuk RA, et al: Patterns of progression in prostate cancer. Lancet 1:60–63, 1986.

232. Epstein JI, Partin AW, Suavageot J, Walsh PC: Prediction of progression following radical prostatectomy. A multivariate analysis of 721 men with long-term follow-up. Am J Surg Pathol 20:286–292, 1996.

233. Schellhammer P: Radical prostatectomy. Patterns of local failure and survival in 67 patients. Urology 31:191–197, 1988.

234. Stein A, deKernion JB, Dorey F, Smith RB: Adjuvant radio-therapy in patients post-radical prostatectomy with tumor extending through capsule or positive seminal vesicles. Urology 39:59–62, 1992.

235. Paulson DF, Moul JW, Walther PJ: Radical prostatectomy for clinical stage T1-2N0M0 prostatic adenocarcinoma. Long-term results. J Urol 144:1180–184, 1990.

236. Lerner SE, Blute ML, Zincke H: Primary surgery for clinical stage T3 adenocarcinoma of the prostate. *In* Vogelzang NJ, Scardino PT, Shipley WU, Coffey DS (eds): Comprehensive Textbook of Genitourinary Oncology. Baltimore, Williams & Wilkins, 1996, pp 803–811.

237. Scardino PT: Early detection of prostate cancer. Urol Clin North Am 16:635–655, 1989.

238. Scardino PT, Frankel JM, Wheeler TM, et al: The prognostic significance of post-irradiation biopsy results in patients with prostatic cancer. Urology 135:510–516, 1986.

239. Bagshaw MA, Cox RS, Ray GR: Status of radiation treatment of prostate cancer at Stanford University. Natl Cancer Inst Monogr 7:47–60, 1988.

240. Epstein JI, Carmichael M, Partin AW, Walsh PC: Is tumor volume an independent predictor of progression following radical prostatectomy? A multivariate analysis of 185 clinical stage B adenocarcinoma of the prostate with 5 years of fol-lowup. J Urol 149:1478–1485, 1993.

241. Epstein JI, Carmichael M, Walsh PC: Adenocarcinoma of the prostate invading the seminal vesicle. Definition and relation of tumor volume, grade, and margins of resection to progno-sis. J Urol 149:1040–1045, 1993.

242. Moul JW, Kahn DG, Lewis DJ, et al: Immunohistologic de-tection of prostate cancer pelvic lymph node micrometas-tases. Correlation to preoperative serum prostate-specific an-tigen. Urology 43:68–73, 1994.

243. Gomella LG, White JL, McCue PA, et al: Screening for occult nodal metastases in localized carcinoma of the prostate. J Urol 149:776–778, 1993.

244. Cheng L, Pisansky TM, Ramnani DM, et al: Extranodal ex-tension in lymph node-positive prostate cancer. Mod Pathol 13:113–118, 2000.

245. Schroder FH, Hermanek P, Denis L, et al: The TNM classifi-cation of prostate carcinoma. Prostate 4(suppl):129–138, 1992.

246. British Association of Urological Surgeons TNM Subcommit-tee, 1995: The TNM classification of prostate cancer. A dis-cussion of the 1992 classification. Br J Urol 76:279–285, 1995.

247. Montie JE: Staging of prostate cancer. Current TNM classifi-cation and future prospects for prognostic factors. Cancer 75:1814–1818, 1995.

248. Donaldson ES, Glenn JF: The 1995 staging requirement for approved cancer programs. Urology 47:455–456, 1996.

249. Epstein JI, Walsh PC, Carmichael M, Brendler CB: Pathologic and clinical findings to predict tumor extent of nonpalpable (stage T1c) prostate cancer. JAMA 271:368–374, 1994.

250. Scaletsky R, Koch MO, Eckstein CW, et al: Tumor volume and stage in carcinoma of the prostate detected by elevations in prostate specific antigen. J Urol 152:129–131, 1994.

251. Jhaveri FM, Klein EA, Kupelian PA, et al: Declining rates of extracapsular extension after radical prostatectomy. Evidence for continued stage migration. J Clin Oncol 17:3167–3172, 1999.

252. Oesterling JE, Suman VJ, Zincke H, Bostwick DG: PSA-de-tected (clinical stage T1c or B0) prostate cancer. Pathologi-cally significant tumors. Urol Clin North Am 20:687–693, 1993.

253. Ferguson JK, Bostwick DG, Suman V, et al: Prostate-specific antigen detected prostate cancer. Pathological characteristics of ultrasound visible versus ultrasound invisible tumors. Eur Urol 27:8–12, 1995.

254. Stamey TA, Villers AA, McNeal JE, et al: Positive surgical margins at radical prostatectomy. Importance of the apical dissection. J Urol 143:1166–1173, 1990.

255. Jones EC: Resection margin status in radical retropubic pros-tatectomy specimens. Relationship to type of operation, tu-mor size, tumor grade and local tumor extension. J Urol 144:89–93, 1990.

256. Catalona WJ, Dresner SM: Nerve-sparing radical prostatec-tomy. Extraprostatic tumor extension and preservation of erectile function. J Urol 134:1149–1151, 1985.

257. Voges G, McNeal JE, Redwine EA, et al: Morphologic analy-sis of surgical margins with positive findings in prostatec-tomy for adenocarcinoma of the prostate. Cancer 69:520–526, 1992.

258. Ackerman DA, Barry JM, Wicklund RA, et al: Analysis of risk factors associated with prostate cancer extension to the surgical margin and pelvic node metastasis at radical prosta-tectomy. J Urol 150:1845–1850, 1993.

259. Schmid HP, Ravery V, Billebaud T, et al: Early detection of prostate cancer in men with prostatism and intermediate prostate-specific antigen levels. Urology 47:699–703, 1996.

260. Hammerer P, Huland H, Sparanberg S: Digital rectal exami-nation, imaging, and systematic-sextant biopsy in identifying operable lymph node-negative prostatic carcinoma. Eur Urol 22:281–287, 1992.

261. Terris MK, McNeal JE, Stamey TA: Detection of clinically significant prostate cancer by transrectal ultrasound-guided systematic biopsies. J Urol Pathol 148:829–832, 1992.

262. Stamey TA, Freiha FS, McNeal JE, et al: Localized prostate cancer. Relationship of tumor volume to clinical significance for treatment of prostate cancer. Cancer 71:933–938, 1993.

263. Haggman M, Nybacka O, Nordin B, Busch C: Standardized in vitro mapping with multiple core biopsies of total prosta-tectomy specimens. Localization and prediction of tumor volume and grade. Br J Urol 74:617–625, 1994.

264. Irwin MB, Trapasso JG: Identification of insignificant pros-tate cancers. Analysis of preoperative parameters. Urology 44:862–868, 1994.

265. Cupp MR, Bostwick DG, Myers RP, Oesterling JE: The vol-ume of prostate cancer in the biopsy specimen cannot relia-bly predict the quantity of cancer in the radical prostatec-tomy specific antigen on an individual basis. J Urol 153:1543–1548, 1995.

266. Daneshgari F, Taylor GD, Miller GJ, Crawford ED: Com-puter simulation of the probability of detecting low volume carcinoma of the prostate with six random systematic core biopsies. Urology 5:609–612, 1995.

267. Humphrey PA, Baty J, Keetch D: Relationship between se-rum prostate specific antigen, needle biopsy findings, and histopathologic features of prostatic carcinoma in radical prostatectomy tissues. Cancer 75:1842–1849, 1995.

268. Weldon VE, Tavel FR, Neuwirth H, Cohen R: Failure of focal prostate cancer on biopsy to predict focal prostate cancer. The importance of prevalence. J Urol 154:1074–1077, 1995.

269. Bruce RG, Rankin WR, Cibull ML, et al: Single focus of adenocarcinoma in the prostate biopsy specimen is not pre-dictive of pathologic stage of disease. Urology 48:75–79, 1996.

270. Goto Y, Ohori M, Arakawa A, et al: Distinguishing clinically important from unimportant prostate cancers before treat-ment. Value of systematic biopsies. J Urol 156:1059–1063, 1996.

271. Ravery V, Schmid H-P, Toublanc M, Boccon-Gibod L: Is the percentage of cancer in biopsy cores predictive of extracap-sular diseae in T1-T2 prostate carcinoma? Cancer 78:1079–1084, 1996.

272. Noguchi M, Stamey TA, McNeal JE, Yemoto CEM: Assess-ment of morphometric measurements of prostate cancer vol-ume. Cancer 98:1056–1064, 2000.

273. Wheeler TM, Dillioglugil O, Kattan MW, et al: Clinical and pathological significance of the level and extent to capsular invasion in clinical stage T1-2 prostate cancer. Hum Pathol 29:856–862, 1998.

273a. Stamey TA, McNeal YE, Yemoto CM, et al: Biological deter-minants of cancer progression in men with prostate cancer. JAMA 281:1395–1400, 1999.

274. Babian RJ, Troncoso P, Steelhammer LC, et al: Tumor vol-ume and prostate specific antigen. Implications for early de-tection and defining a window of curability. J Urol 154:1808–1812, 1995.

275. Renshaw AA, Richie JP, Loughlin KR, et al: The greatest dimension of prostate carcinoma is a simple inexpensive pre-dictor of prostate specific antigen failure in radical prostatec-tomy specimens. Cancer 83:748–752, 1998.

276. Dugan JA, Bostwick DG, Myers RP, et al: The definition and preoperative prediction of clinically insignificant prostate cancer. JAMA 275:288–294, 1996.

277. Humphrey PA, Vollmer RT: Percentage carcinoma as a measure of prostatic tumor size in radical prostatectomy tissues. Mod Pathol 10:326–333, 1997.

278. Carvalhal GF, Humphrey PA, Thorson P, et al: Visual estimate of percentage of cancer is an independent predictor. Cancer 89:1308–1314, 2000.

279. Schned AR, Wheeler KJ, Hodorowski CA, et al: Tissue-shrinkage correction factor in the calculation of prostate cancer volume. Am J Surg Pathol 20:1501–1506, 1996.

280. Egan AJ, Bostwick DG: Prediction of extraprostatic extension of prostate cancer based on needle biopsy findings. Perineural invasion lacks significance on multivariate analysis. Am J Surg Pathol 21:1496–1500, 1997.

281. Hasson MO, Maksem J: The prostatic perineural space and its relation to tumor spread. An ultrastructural study. Am J Surg Pathol 4:143–148, 1980.

282. Bahnson RR, Dresner SM, Gooding W, Becich MJ: Incidence and prognostic significance of lymphatic and vascular invasion in radical prostatectomy specimens. Prostate 15:149–155, 1989.

283. Deering RE, Bigler SA, Brown M, Brawer MK: Microvascularity in benign prostatic hyperplasia. Prostate 26:111–115, 1995.

284. Wakui S, Furusato M, Itoh T, et al: Tumor angiogenesis in prostate carcinoma with and without bone marrow metastasis. A morphometric study. J Pathol 168:257–262, 1992.

285. Rogatsch H, Hittmair A, Reissigl A, et al: Microvessel density in core biopsies of prostatic adenocarcinoma. A stage predictor? J Pathol 182:205–210, 1997.

286. Bostwick DG, Wheeler TM, Blute M, et al: Optimized microvessel density analysis improves prediction of cancer stage from prostate needle biopsies. Urology 48:47–57, 1996.

287. Hall MC, Troncoso P, Pollack A, et al: Significance of tumor angiogenesis in clinically localized prostate carcinoma treated with external beam radiotherapy. Urology 44:869–875, 1994.

288. Vesalainen S, Lipponen PK, Talja MT, et al: Proliferating cell nuclear antigen and p53 expression as prognostic factors in T1-2MO prostatic adenocarcinoma. Int J Cancer 58:303–308, 1994.

289. McNeal JE, Yemoto CE: Significance of demonstrable vascular space invasion for the progression of prostatic adenocarcinoma. Am J Surg Pathol 20:1351–1360, 1996.

290. Gettman MT, Bergstralh EJ, Blute M, et al: Prediction of patient outcome in pathologic stage T2 adenocarcinoma of the prostate. Lack of significance for microvessel density analysis. Urology 51:79–85, 1998.

291. Weidner N, Carroll PR, Flax J, et al: Tumor angiogenesis correlates with metastasis ininvasive prostate carcinoma. Am J Pathol 143:401–409, 1993.

292. Fregene T, Khanuja P: Tumor-associated angiogenesis in prostate cancer. Anticancer Res 13:2377–2382, 1993.

292a. Zincke H, Bergstralh EJ, Larson-Keller JJ, et al: Stage D1 prostate cancer treated by radical prostatectomy and adjuvant hormonal treatment. Evidence for favorable survival in patients with DNA diploid tumors. Cancer 70:311–323, 1992.

293. Nativ O, Winkler HZ, Raz Y, et al: Stage C prostatic adenocarcinoma. Flow cytometric nuclear DNA ploidy analysis. Mayo Clin Proc 64:911–919, 1989.

294. Konchuba AM, Schellhammer PF, Kolm P, et al: Deoxyribonucleic acid cytometric analysis of prostate core biopsy specimens. Relationship to serum prostate specific antigen and prostatic acid phosphatase, clinical stage and histopathology. J Urol 150:115–119, 1993.

295. Shankey TV, Kallioniemi OP, Koslowski JM, et al: Consensus review of the clinical utility of DNA content cytometry in prostate cancer. Cytometry 14:497–500, 1993.

296. Amin MB, Schultz DS, Zarbo RJ: Computerized static DNA ploidy analysis of prostatic intraepithelial neoplasia. Arch Pathol Lab Med 117:794–798, 1993.

297. Barretton GB, Vogt T, Blasenbreu S: Comparison of DNA ploidy in prostatic intraepithelial neoplasia and invasive carcinoma of the prostate. An image cytometric study. Hum Pathol 25:506–513, 1994.

297a. Jones EC, McNeal J, Bruchovsky N, de Jong G: DNA content in prostatic adenocarcinoma. A flow cytometry study of the predictive value of aneuploidy for tumor volume, percentage Gleason grades 4 and 5, and lymph node metastases. Cancer 66:752–757, 1990.

297b. Tribukait B: DNA flow cytometry in carcinoma of the prostate for diagnosis, prognosis and study of tumor biology. Acta Oncol 30:187–192, 1991.

298. Deitch AD, deVere-White RW: Flow cytometry as a predictive modality in prostate cancer. Hum Pathol 23:352–359, 1992.

298a. Pollack A, Zagars GK: External beam radiotherapy dose response of prostate cancer. Int J Radiat Oncol Biol Phys 39: 1011–1018, 1997.

299. Takai K, Goellner JR, Katzmann JA, et al: Static image and flow DNA cytometry of prostatic adenocarcinoma. Studies of needle biopsy and radical prostatectomy specimens. J Urol Pathol 2:39–48, 1994.

300. Fujikawa K, Saski M, Arai Y, et al: Prognostic criteria in patients with prostate cancer. Gleason score versus volume-weighted mean nuclear volume. Clin Cancer Res 3:613–618, 1997.

301. Qian JQ, Jenkins RB, Bostwick DG: Determination of gene and chromosome dosage in prostatic intraepithelial neoplasia and carcinoma. Anal Quant Cytol Histol 20:373–380, 1998.

302. Takahashi S, Qian J, Brown JA, et al: Potential markers of prostate cancer aggressiveness detected by fluorescence in situ hybridization. Cancer 54:3574–3579, 1994.

303. Alcaraz A, Takahashi S, Brown JA, et al: Aneuploidy and aneusomy of chromosome 7 detected by fluorescence in situ hybridization are markers of poor prognosis in prostate cancer. Cancer Res 54:3998–4002, 1994.

304. Bandyk MG, Zhao L, Troncoso P, et al: A potential cytogenetic marker of human prostate cancer progression. Genes Chromosomes Cancer 9:19–27, 1994.

305. Takahashi S, Alcaraz A, Brown JA, et al: Aneusomies of chromosomes 8 and Y detected by fluorescence in situ hybridisation are prognostic markers for pathologic stage C $(pT_3N_0M_0)$ prostate carcinoma. Clin Cancer Res 2:137–145, 1996.

306. Zenklusen JC, Thomspon JC, Troncoso P, et al: Loss of heterozygosity in human primary prostate carcinoma. A possible tumor suppressor gene at 7q31.1. Cancer Res 54:6370–6373, 1994.

307. Latil A, Cussenot O, Fournier G, et al: Loss of heterozygosity at 7q31 is a frequent and early event in prostate cancer. Clin Cancer Res 1:385–389, 1995.

308. Takahashi S, Shan A, Ritland SR, et al: Frequent loss of heterozygosity at 7q31.1 in primary prostate cancer in association with tumor aggressiveness and progression. Cancer Res 55:4114–4119, 1995.

309. Collard JG, van de Poll M, Scheffer A, et al: Location of genes involved in invasion and metastasis on human chromosome 7. Cancer Res 47:6666–6670, 1987.

310. Zenklusen JC, Thompson JC, Klein-Szanto AJP, Conti CJ: Frequent loss of heterozygosity in human primary squamous cell and colon carcinomas at 7q331.1. Evidence for a broad range tumor suppressor gene. Cancer Res 55:1347–1350, 1995.

311. Jenkins RB, Qian JC, Lee HK, et al: A molecular cytogenetic analysis of 7q31 in prostate cancer. Cancer Res 58:759–766, 1998.

312. Emmert-Buck MR, Vocke CD, Pozzatti RO, et al: Allelic loss on chromosome 8p12–21 in microdissected intraepithelial neoplasia. Cancer Res 55:2959–2962, 1995.

313. MacGrogan D, Levy A, Bostwick D, et al: Loss of chromosome arm 8p loci in prostate cancer. Mapping by quantitative allelic imbalance. Gene Chromosomes Cancer 10:151–159, 1994.

314. Macoska JA, Trybus TM, Benson PD, et al: Evidence for three tumor suppressor gene loci on chromosome 8p in human prostate cancer. Cancer Res 55:5390–5395, 1995.

315. Bova GS, Fox WM, Epstein JI: Methods of radical prostatec-

tomy specimen processing. A novel technique for harvesting fresh prostate cancer tissue and review of processing techniques. Mod Pathol 6:201–207, 1993.

316. Jenkins RB, Qian J, Lieber MM, Bostwick DG: Detection of c-myc oncogene amplification and chromosomal anomalies in metastatic prostatic carcinoma by fluorescence in situ hybridization (FISH). Cancer Res 57:524–531, 1997.

317. Visakorpi T, Kallioniemi AH, Syvanen AC, et al: Genetic changes in primary and recurrent prostate cancer by comparative genomic hybridization. Cancer Res 55:342–347, 1995.

317a. Van Den Berg C, Guan XY, Von Hoff D, et al: DNA sequence amplification in human prostate cancer identified by chromosome microdissection: potential pronostic implications. Clin Cancer Res 1:11–18, 1995.

318. Cher ML, MacGrogan D, Bookstein R, et al: Comparative genomic hybridization, allelic imbalance and fluorescence in situ hybridization on chromosome 8 in prostate cancer. Genes Chromosomes Cancer 11:153–162, 1994.

319. Qian JQ, Bostwick DG, Takahashi S, et al: Chromosomal anomalies in prostatic intraepithelial neoplasia and carcinoma detected by fluorescence in situ hybridization. Cancer Res 55:5408–5414, 1995.

320. Joos S, Bergerheim US, Pan Y, et al: Mapping of chromosomal gains and losses in prostate cancer by comparative genomic hybridization. Genes Chromosomes Cancer 14:267–276, 1995.

321. Gray IC, Phillips SM, Lee SJ, et al: Loss of the chromosomal region 10q23-25 in prostate cancer. Cancer Res 55:4800–4803, 1995.

321a. Ittman M, Mansukhani A: Expression of fibroblast growth factors (FGFs) and FGF receptors in human prostate. J Urol 157:351–356, 1997.

322. Eagle LR, Yin X, Brothman AR, et al: Mutation of MXI1 gene in prostate cancer. Nat Genet 9:249–255, 1995.

323. Li J, Yen C, Liaw D, et al: PTEN, a putative protein tyrosine phosphatase gene mutated in human brain, breast and prostate cancer. Science 275:1943–1947, 1997.

324. Carter BS, Epstein JI, Isaacs WB: ras Gene mutations in human prostate cancer. Cancer Res 50:6830–6832, 1990.

325. Latil A, Cussenot O, Fournier G, et al: Loss of heterozygosity at chromosome 16q in prostate adenocarcinoma. Identification of three independent regions. Cancer Res 57:1058–1062, 1997.

326. Elo JP, Harkonen PO, Kyllonen AP, et al: Loss of heterozygosity at 16q24.1-q24.2 is significantly associated with metastatic and aggressive behavior of prostate cancer. Cancer Res 57:3356–3359, 1995.

327. Cunningham JM, Shan A, Wick MJ, et al: Allelic imbalance and microsatellite instability in prostatic adenocarcinoma. Cancer Res 56:4475–4482, 1996.

328. Bergheim USR, Kunimi K, Collins VP, Ekman P: Deletion of chromosome 8, 10 and 16 in human prostatic carcinoma. Genes Chromosomes Cancer 3:215–220, 1991.

329. Sakr WA, Macoska JA, Benson P, et al: Allelic loss in locally metastatic multisampled prostate cancer. Cancer Res 54:3273–3277, 1994.

330. Sato K, Qian J, Slezak JM, et al: Clinical significance of alterations of chromosome 8 in high-grade, advanced, nonmetastatic prostate carcinoma. J Natl Cancer Inst 91:1574–1580, 1999.

331. Kokonitis J, Takakura K, Hay N, Liao S: Increased androgen receptor activity and altered c-myc expression in prostate cancer cells after long-term androgen deprivation. Cancer Res 54:1566–1573, 1994.

332. Reed JC: Bcl-2 and the regulation of programmed cell death. J Cell Biol 124:1–6, 1994.

333. Reed JC: Prevention of apoptosis as a mechanism of drug resistance. Hematol Oncol Clin North Am 9:451–474, 1995.

334. Hockenbery D, Zutter M, Hickey W, et al: bcl-2 protein is topographically restricted to tissues characterized by apoptotic cell death. Proc Natl Acad Sci U S A 88:6961–6965, 1991.

334a. Foster CS, Ke Y: Stem cells in prostate epithelia. Int J Exp Pathol 78:311–329, 1997.

335. Tu H, Jacobs SC, Borkowski A, Kyprianou N: Incidence of apoptosis and cell proliferation in prostate cancer. Relationship with TGF-beta1 and bcl-2 expression. Int J Cancer 69:357–363, 1996.

336. Lipponen P, Vesalainen S: Expression of the apoptosis suppressing protein bcl-2 in prostatic adenocarcinoma is related to tumour malignancy. Prostate 32:9–16, 1997.

337. Colombel M, Symmans G, Gil S, et al: Detection of the apoptosis-suppressing oncoprotein bcl-2 in hormone-refractory human prostate cancer. Am J Pathol 143:390–400, 1993.

338. Colecchia M, Frigo B, Del Boca C, et al: Detection of apoptosis by the TUNEL technique in clinically localized prostatic cancer before and after combined endocrine therapy. J Clin Pathol 50:384–388, 1997.

339. Ittman M, Wieczorek R, Heller P, et al: Alterations in the p53 and MDC-2 genes are infrequent in clinically localized stage B prostate adenocarcinomas. Am J Pathol 145:287–293, 1994.

340. Hall MC, Navone NM, Troncoso P, et al: Frequency and characterization of p53 mutations in clinically localized prostate cancer. Urology 45:470–475, 1995.

341. Mottaz AE, Markwalder R, Fey MF, et al: Abnormal p53 expression is rare in clinically localized human prostate cancer. Comparison between immunohistochemical and molecular detection of p53 mutations. Prostate 31:209–215, 1997.

342. Navone NM, Troncoso P, Pisters LL, et al: p53 protein accumulation and gene mutation in the progression of human prostate carcinoma. J Natl Cancer Inst 85:1657–1669, 1993.

343. Kallakury BV, Figge J, Ross JS, et al: Association of p53 immunoreactivity with high Gleason tumor grade in prostate adenocarcinoma. Hum Pathol 25:92–97, 1994.

344. Fan K, Dao DD, Schultz M, Fink LM: Loss of heterozygosity and overexpression of p53 gene in human primary prostatic adenocarcinoma. Diagn Mol Pathol 3:265–270, 1994.

345. Moul JW, Bettencourt MC, Sesterhenn IA, et al: Protein expression of p53, bcl-2 and Ki-67 (MIB-1) as prognostic biomarkers in patients with surgically treated, clinically localized prostate cancer. Surgery 120:159–166, 1996.

346. Aprikian AG, Cordon-Cardo C, Fair WR, et al: Neuroendocrine differentiation in metastatic prostatic adenocarcinoma. J Urol 151:914–919, 1994.

347. Heidenberg HB, Sesterhenn IA, Gaddipati JP, et al: Alternation of tumor suppressor gene p53 in a high fraction of hormone refractory prostate cancer. J Urol 154:414–421, 1995.

348. Brooks JD, Bova GS, Ewing CM, et al: An uncertain role for p53 gene alterations in human prostate cancers. Cancer Res 56:3814–3822, 1996.

349. Gao X, Chen YQ, Wu N, et al: Somatic murations of the WAF1/CIP1 gene in primary prostate cancer. Oncogene 11:1395–1398, 1997.

350. Facher EA, Becich MJ, Deka A, Law JC: Association between human cancer and two polymorphisms occurring in the p21WAF1/CIP1 cyclin-dependent kinase inhibitor gene. Cancer 79:2424–2429, 1997.

351. Byrne RL, Horne CH, Robinson MC, et al: The expression of waf-1, p53 and bcl-2 in prostatic adenocarcinoma. Br J Urol 79:190–195, 1997.

352. Tsihlias J, Kapusta LR, DeBoer G, et al: Loss of cyclin-dependent kinase inhibitor p27Kip1 is a novel prognostic factor in localized human prostate adenocarcinoma. Cancer Res 58:542–548, 1998.

353. Burke HB, Goodman PH, Rosen DB, et al: Artificial neural networks improve the accuracy of cancer survival prediction. Cancer 79:857–862, 1997.

354. Persaud V, Douglas LL: Bizarre (atypical) leiomyoma of the prostate gland. West Indian Med J 31:217–220, 1982.

355. Yilmaz F, Sahin H, Hakverdi S, et al: Huge leiomyoma of the prostate. Scand J Urol Nephrol 32:223–224, 1998.

356. Schumacher S, Moll R, Muller SC, et al: Epithelioid leiomyoma of the prostate. Eur Urol 30:125–126, 1996.

357. Huang WL, Ro JY, Grignon DJ, et al: Postoperative spindle cell nodule of the prostate and bladder. J Urol 143:824–826, 1990.

358. Ro JY, el-Naggar AK, Amin MB, Ayala AG: Inflammatory

pseudotumor of the urinary bladder. Am J Surg Pathol 17:1193–1194, 1993.

359. Takeshima Y, Yoneda K, Sanda N, Inai K: Solitary fibrous tumor of the prostate. Pathol Int 47:713–717, 1997.

360. Westra WH, Grenko RT, Epstein J: Solitary fibrous tumor of the lower urogenital tract. A report of five cases involving the seminal vesicles, urinary bladder, and prostate. Hum Pathol 31:63–68, 2000.

361. Ostrowski ML, Wheeler TM: Paraganglia of the prostate. Location, frequency, and differentiation from prostatic adenocarcinoma. Am J Surg Pathol 18:412–420, 1994.

362. Boyle M, Gaffney EF, Thurston A: Paraganglioma of the prostatic urethra. A report of three cases and a review of the literature. Br J Urol 77:445–448, 1996.

363. Waring PM, Newland RC: Prostatic embryonal rhabdomyosarcoma in adults. A clinicopathologic review. Cancer 69:755–762, 1992.

364. Asmar L, Gehan EA, Newton WA, et al: Agreement among and within groups of pathologists in the classification of rhabdomyosarcoma and related childhood sarcomas. Report of an international study of four pathology classifications. Cancer 74:2579–2588, 1994.

365. Moroz K, Crespo P, de las Morenas A: Fine needle aspiration of prostatic rhabdomyosarcoma. A case report demonstrating the value of DNA ploidy. Acta Cytol 39:785–790, 1995.

366. Raney RB Jr, Gehan EA, Hays DM, et al: Primary chemotherapy with or without radiation therapy and/or surgery for children with localized sarcoma of the bladder, prostate, vagina, uterus, and cervix. A comparison of the results in Intergroup Rhabdomyosarcoma Studies I and II. Cancer 66:2072–2081, 1990.

367. Cheville JC, Dundore PA, Nascimento AG, et al: Leiomyosarcoma of the prostate. Report of 23 cases. Cancer 76:1422–1427, 1995.

367a. Bostwick DG, Qian J, Halling AC, et al: Phyllodes tumors of the prostate: long-term follow-up study of twenty cases. Submitted.

368. Fritsch M, Epstein JI, Perlman EJ, et al: Molecularly confirmed primary prostatic synovial sarcoma. Hum Pathol 31:246–250, 2000.

369. Bostwick DG, Iczkowski KA, Amin MB, et al: Malignant lymphoma involving the prostate. Report of 62 cases. Cancer 83:732–738, 1998.

370. Seidman JD, Shmookler BM, Connolly B, Lack EE: Localized amyloidosis of seminal vesicles. Report of three cases in surgically obtained material. Mod Pathol 2:671–675, 1989.

371. Cornwell GG III, Westermark GT, Pitkanen P, Westermark P: Seminal vesicle amyloid. The first example of exocrine cell origin of an amyloid fibril precursor. J Pathol 167:297–303, 1992.

372. Khan SM, Birch PJ, Bass PS, et al: Localized amyloidosis of the lower genitourinary tract. A clinicopathological and immunohistochemical study of nine cases. Histopathology 21:143–147, 1992.

373. Coyne JD, Kealy WF: Seminal vesicle amyloidosis. Morphological, histochemical and immunohistochemical observations. Histopathology 22:173–176, 1993.

374. Ormsby AH, Haskell R, Jones D, Goldblum JR: Primary seminal vesicle carcinoma. An immunohistochemical analysis of four cases. Mod Pathol 13:46–51, 2000.

375. Villers AA, McNeal JE, Redwine EA, et al: Pathogenesis and biological significance of seminal vesicle invasion in prostatic adenocarcinoma. J Urol 143:1183–1187, 1990.

376. Ohori M, Scardino PT, Lapin SL, et al: The mechanisms and prognostic significance of seminal vesicle involvement by prostate cancer. Am J Surg Pathol 17:1252–1261, 1993.

377. Ro JY, Ayala AG, el-Nagger A, Wishnow KI: Seminal vesicle involvement by in situ and invasive transition cell carcinoma of the bladder. Am J Surg Pathol 11:951–958, 1987.

378. Schned AR, Ledbetter JS, Selikowitz SM: Primary leiomyosarcoma of the seminal vesicle. Cancer 57:2202–2206, 1986.

379. Bailey DM, Foley SJ, McFarlane JP, et al: Histological changes associated with long-term urethral stents. Br J Urol 81:745–749, 1998.

# 33

# Penis and Scrotum

Mahul B. Amin    Pheroze Tamboli    Antonio L. Cubilla

## NEOPLASTIC LESIONS OF THE PENIS

### Benign Tumors

Hirsutoid papillomas (pearly penile plaques, papillomatosis of glans corona) are present in approximately 10% to 20% of normal males. On gross examination, they appear as multiple, 1- to 2-mm, pearly gray–white polypoid lesions characteristically arranged around the corona of the glans penis. Although they are termed papillomas, these lesions are not related to human papillomavirus (HPV) infection; rather, they are fibroepithelial polyps.[1]

Benign tumors such as hemangioma,[2] lymphangioma, leiomyoma, glomus tumor,[3] neurofibroma,[4] schwannoma,[5] and granular cell tumor[6] have been reported to involve the penis. Of these, the vascular lesions are the most common.

### Premalignant Lesions

Variable terminology has been used for premalignant lesions of the penis: low- and high-grade squamous intraepithelial lesion; mild, moderate, and severe dysplasia; penile intraepithelial neoplasia I, II, III; and dysplasia and carcinoma in situ.[7] We prefer the terms low- and high-grade squamous intraepithelial lesions. On the basis of histologic appearance, these may additionally be classified as squamous (usual), basaloid, and warty (condylomatous) (CD Fig. 33–1). Low-grade lesions often appear clinically as white patches or "leukoplakia." On microscopic examination, low-grade lesions show involvement of the lower to middle third of the squamous epithelium by atypical cells. High-grade lesions have atypical cells exhibiting a greater degree of atypia that involves two thirds or more of the epithelium. The atypical cells, by definition, are confined to the basement membrane and display loss of polarity, dyskeratosis, and enlarged pleomorphic hyperchromatic nuclei with irregular nuclear contours and nucleoli (CD Fig. 33–2). Normal and abnormal mitoses and koilocytotic atypia may also be present. Basaloid intraepithelial lesions show immature atypical basal cells, sometimes with prominent individual cell necrosis, and are usually associated with invasive basaloid carcinomas. Warty lesions generally have a characteristic papillary configuration but rarely may be flat. Hyperkeratosis, parakeratosis, and koilocytotic atypia are prominent.

Another area of controversy concerns the nomenclature of three lesions with similar histologic appearances but with different clinical presentations and biologic behaviors, that is, erythroplasia of Queyrat, Bowen's disease, and bowenoid papulosis. Clinical and pathologic features of the three entities are summarized in Table 33–1. Some experts believe that Bowen's disease and erythroplasia of Queyrat are different manifestations of the same disease, whereas others argue that they are distinct clinicopathologic entities. Some authors, including us, recommend use of the term *high-grade squamous intraepithelial lesion/squamous cell carcinoma in situ* because both lesions are essentially a form of carcinoma in situ.[8–10]

### ERYTHROPLASIA OF QUEYRAT

Tarnovsky originally described erythroplasia of Queyrat in 1891, but it was Queyrat[11] who coined the term *erythroplasia* in 1911. It usually occurs in the

**TABLE 33–1.** Distinguishing Features of Penile Preneoplastic Conditions

| Features | Erythroplasia of Queyrat | Bowen's Disease | Bowenoid Papulosis |
|---|---|---|---|
| Age | 4th and 5th decades | 5th and 6th decades | 3rd and 4th decades |
| Site | Glans, foreskin | Penile shaft | Penile shaft |
| Gross appearance | Erythematous plaque | Scaly plaque | Papules, usually multiple |
| Hyperkeratosis | − | + | + |
| Keratinocyte maturation | − | − | + |
| Involvement of sweat glands | − | − | + |
| Involvement of pilosebaceous units | − | + | − |
| Spontaneous regression | − | − | + |
| Progress to carcinoma | 10% | 5–10% | 0% |
| Associated second malignant neoplasm | +/− | + | − |

Modified from Ro JY, Amin MB, Ayala AG: Penis and scrotum. *In* Bostwick DG, Eble JN (eds): Urologic Surgical Pathology. Philadelphia, Mosby, 1997, pp 675–724.

fourth and fifth decade of life but has been reported among other age groups. Circumcision at an early age is thought to prevent its development. Invasive squamous cell carcinoma develops in approximately 10% of patients, and 2% develop distant metastases.[12] Gross examination shows an elevated, moist, velvety, erythematous plaque, usually on the glans penis or the prepuce.[12] The majority are solitary lesions; however, multiple lesions may also occur.[12] It has the same histologic features as squamous carcinoma in situ seen elsewhere; in addition, the underlying stroma may show a bandlike lymphocytic infiltrate. The clinical differential diagnosis of erythroplasia of Queyrat includes Zoon's balanitis, drug eruption, psoriasis, lichen planus, and other inflammatory processes; however, histologic distinction is straightforward.

## BOWEN'S DISEASE

Bowen's disease, first described by Bowen in 1912, designates squamous cell carcinoma in situ of both sun-exposed and nonexposed skin. This term is used for lesions that occur on the shaft and are not as grossly red as erythroplasia of Queyrat.[8, 9] Peak incidence is in the fifth and sixth decades, a decade earlier than erythroplasia of Queyrat.[9] Gross examination shows crusted, sharply demarcated, scaly white plaques; rarely, they may form papillomatous lesions. Histologic differences from erythroplasia of Queyrat, such as hyperkeratosis and involvement of pilosebaceous units, are a function of the differing anatomic locations.[8, 12] Approximately 5% to 10% of cases progress to invasive carcinoma. About one third of patients have been reported to develop cutaneous or extracutaneous malignant neoplasms; such a strong association with other cancers is not noted with erythroplasia of Queyrat.[12, 13]

## BOWENOID PAPULOSIS

Bowenoid papulosis is the term for multicentric squamous cell carcinoma in situ with an indolent clinical course, usually affecting young men.[14, 15] There is an association with HPV, most commonly types 16 and 18.[16] It is considered the male counter-

part of multifocal vulvovaginal dysplasia in young women. Multiple small (2 to 10 mm) soft papules are present, mainly on the penile shaft and occasionally on the glans or prepuce. The papules may coalesce to form plaques, resembling condyloma acuminata. On histologic examination, the typical changes of squamous cell carcinoma in situ are present, with the exception of greater maturation of keratinocytes in some cases (CD Fig. 33–3). The diagnosis of bowenoid papulosis should not be made on microscopic appearance alone; rather, the clinical presentation and gross appearance need to be taken into account because the natural history of this lesion differs significantly from that of Bowen's disease and erythroplasia of Queyrat. These lesions are treated conservatively by local excision, topical treatment, or laser treatment because they do not progress to invasive carcinoma if treated appropriately.[14] Spontaneous regression has been reported.[14]

## Malignant Tumors

### SQUAMOUS CELL CARCINOMA

Squamous cell carcinoma, the most common malignant tumor of the penis, exhibits a variety of morphologic patterns. Morphologic subtyping of these tumors does appear to have some prognostic significance, even though a small number of cases have been analyzed in each subset.[9, 17] Much of the work on histologic subtyping of penile squamous cell carcinoma has been done, by systematic and meticulous evaluation of penectomy specimens, at the Instituto Nacional del Cáncer in Paraguay. The pathologic parameters of importance for the pathologist to evaluate and the contents of the final report are listed in Tables 33–2 and 33–3, respectively.[9, 17–25]

#### *Epidemiology*

Squamous cell carcinoma of the penis is rare in the United States, Europe, and Japan. It is estimated that only 1100 new cases of squamous cell carcinoma of the penis and related male genital organs

**TABLE 33–2.** Evaluation of Penile Cancer

Tumor parameters
  Diagnosis
  Classification
  Presence or absence of invasion
  Depth of invasion
  Histologic grade
  Surgical margins of resection
Differential diagnosis
  Verruciform lesions
    Condyloma acuminatum and giant condyloma of Buschke-
      Löwenstein versus warty, verrucous, low-grade papillary
      carcinoma
  Hyperplastic lesions
    Squamous hyperplasia versus squamous carcinoma
Prognostic parameters

(excluding prostate and testis) will be diagnosed in the United States in the year 2000, with an estimated 300 patients dying of the disease.[26] These tumors are more common in Asia, Africa, and Latin America. In the United States, African Americans are more commonly affected, with a ratio of 2:1 compared with white men. It is less frequent in Jews and Moslems because males in both these religions undergo ritual circumcision at an early age.

Risk factors with the strongest association include poor hygiene and phimosis. Other risk factors include a history of genital warts, penile rash or trauma, late circumcision, smoking, and accumulation of smegma.[27, 28] HPV is also thought to play a role in the pathogenesis of this tumor; about a third of penile squamous cancers contain HPV DNA. HPV has also been detected in metastatic tumors. HPV type 16 is the most common, followed by type 18.[29, 30] Treatment with 8-methoxypsoralen and ultraviolet A phototherapy (PUVA) for psoriasis has also shown an increased risk for both penile and scrotal squamous cell carcinomas.[31]

### Clinical Features

Squamous cell carcinoma of the penis occurs in an older age group; the average age is 58 years.[32–35] The age distribution has ranged from children to men in their 90s, but it is rare in men younger than 40 years.[33] Patients usually present with a penile

**TABLE 33–3.** Contents of the Final Report: Penile Carcinoma

Histologic type
Pattern of growth
Histologic grade
Tumor size
Anatomic site of origin and extension
Depth of invasion (in millimeters and to include anatomic levels)
Vascular and perineural invasion
Surgical margins of resection
Associated lesions (e.g., carcinoma in situ, condyloma, squamous hyperplasia) and their extent

mass that may be exophytic or ulcerated. Other symptoms include pain, discharge, difficulty in micturition, bleeding, and inguinal lymphedenopathy due to metastases.[36]

### Classification of Penile Squamous Cell Carcinoma

Penile squamous cell carcinoma may be classified according to the site of origin, pattern of growth, and histologic appearance (Table 33–4). The aim of assessing these three parameters is to provide maximal prognostic information based on pathologic evaluation of the specimen.[9, 17]

SITE OF ORIGIN. The sites of origin and their relative frequencies are listed in Table 33–4.[32–35] Location of the tumor is important because it affects the prognosis; for example, tumors arising in the foreskin have the best prognosis, most likely owing to the superficial nature of the neoplasm. In some cases, particularly in larger tumors, it may be difficult to ascertain the site of origin because tumors arising in one site may spread to involve others.

PATTERN OF GROWTH. The patterns of growth observed in penile squamous cell carcinomas are superficial spreading, verruciform, vertical, mixed, and multicentric (see Table 33–4). These patterns are important because they correlate with prognosis.[37]

*Superficial spreading tumors* are flat; they grow widely and horizontally, predominantly with a prominent intraepithelial component and with superficial invasion[9, 17] (Fig. 33–1A). These tumors tend to grow slowly and may involve the glans, coronal sulcus, or foreskin; the majority involve

**TABLE 33–4.** Classification of Penile Squamous Cell Carcinoma

| Site | Frequency (%) |
|---|---|
| Glans | 48 |
| Foreskin | 21 |
| Coronal sulcus | 6 |
| Shaft | 2 |
| Multiple sites | 23 |
| **Pattern of Growth** | |
| Superficial spreading | 30–35 |
| Verruciform | 25 |
| Vertical | 20 |
| Mixed | 10–15 |
| Multicentric | 5 |
| **Histologic Subtype** | |
| Squamous cell carcinoma (usual type) | 70 |
| Verruciform | 20 |
| Papillary carcinoma NOS | 11 |
| Warty (condylomatous) carcinoma | 6 |
| Verrucous carcinoma | 3 |
| Basaloid squamous cell carcinoma | 8 |
| Sarcomatoid carcinoma | 2 |

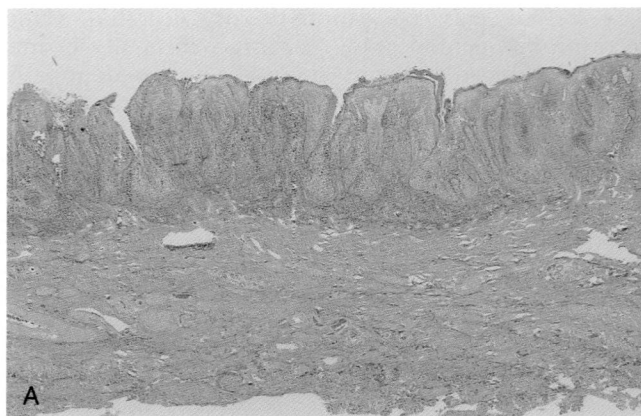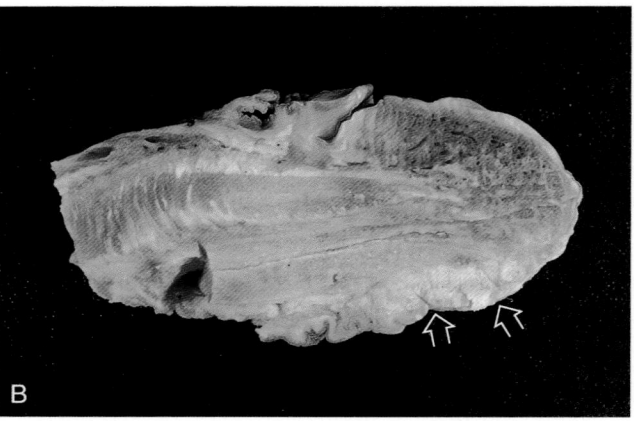

**FIGURE 33–1.** Squamous cell carcinoma of penis, superficial spreading type. *A.* The tumor chiefly involves the surface with a prominent intraepithelial component. *B.* Vertical cut section of penis shows a gray-white plaquelike tumor involving the glans penis *(arrows).*

more than one site. On gross examination, they involve most of the epithelial surface as an elevated, granular, or firm plaquelike mass, which may be ulcerated. The cut surface characteristically shows white or gray-white firm tumor growing in a band-like fashion (Fig. 33–1B). These tumors usually measure 2 to 3 cm in greatest dimension, with a vertical dimension of 1 to 10 mm. They tend to invade only the superficial layers of the penis (CD Fig. 33–4A); however, there may be progression to a vertical growth phase with deep invasion. On microscopic examination, most are well or moderately differentiated. Squamous cell carcinoma in situ is invariably present (CD Fig. 33–4B), as is squamous hyperplasia. These tumors rarely metastasize and have a relatively good prognosis. The main problem with this growth pattern is in achieving negative surgical margins, especially if partial penectomy is planned.

*Verruciform tumors* are low-grade tumors that exhibit an exophytic pattern of growth and most commonly involve the glans; the foreskin and coronal sulcus are rarely affected.[9, 17] Gross evaluation shows large, white to gray, exophytic masses with a papillary appearance and a well-defined base. On microscopic examination, three distinctive patterns are seen: verrucous, warty (condylomatous), and papillary not otherwise specified (NOS). Most tumors invade only into the lamina propria or into the corpus spongiosum.

Tumors with a *vertical growth* pattern invade vertically down, usually through the tunica albuginea deep into the corpus spongiosum or corpora cavernosa, surrounding the urethra or sometimes replacing it.[9, 17] They form large, fungating, often ulcerated masses. Hemorrhage and necrosis are common. Satellite tumor nodules may be present, often deep in the corpora cavernosa. These are often high-grade tumors, with a high rate of inguinal lymph node metastasis, and have the worst prognosis.

A *mixed pattern* of growth may have superficial spreading, verruciform, and vertical growth components in varying proportions. The gross appearance

varies according to the different patterns present: On microscopic examination, there may be a combination of low- and high-grade tumor.

Carcinoma is considered *multicentric* when there are two or more independent foci of carcinoma separated by benign tissue. These may be synchronous or metachronous and typically involve more than one anatomic compartment. Serial sectioning and meticulous examination of the entire penis helps in identification of these cases.[37] On gross appearance, they are superficial and typically involve several sites. On microscopic examination, the intervening mucosa is normal or may exhibit squamous hyperplasia.

HISTOLOGIC APPEARANCE. Penile carcimonas may be divided histologically into squamous cell carcinoma of usual type (70% of all squamous carcinoma), verruciform carcinomas (including papillary carcinoma NOS, warty carcinoma, and verrucous carcinoma), basaloid carcinoma, mixed carcinomas, and sarcomatoid carcinoma. The histologic types other than the usual type have a distinct morphologic appearance involving the majority of the tumor, arbitrarily defined as more than 80%. Squamous cell carcinoma (usual type) may occasionally exhibit small foci of the other patterns. Each of these histologic types is discussed individually in the following sections.

### Squamous Cell Carcinoma (Usual Type)

Squamous cell carcinoma (usual type) is histologically similar to that occurring in other organs. According to one report, 70% to 75% of these tumors are well differentiated, and 25% to 30% are moderately and poorly differentiated.[24] They are mostly nonpapillary, composed predominantly of nests or cords with variable amounts of keratinization (Fig. 33–2) (CD Fig. 33–5). High-grade tumors may be acantholytic, imparting a pseudoglandular appearance. These spaces are lined by flattened squamous cells and may be empty or contain kera-

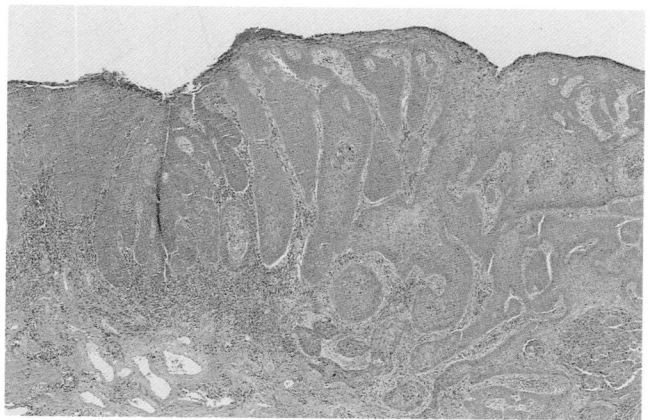

**FIGURE 33-2.** Squamous cell carcinoma of penis, usual type. Typical features of invasive, moderately differentiated squamous cell carcinoma are seen.

tin or inflammatory and necrotic debris. Small foci of spindle cells may also be seen in occasional poorly differentiated tumors. Stromal changes include mild to severe inflammatory infiltrate. The adjacent epithelium is frequently hyperplastic or dysplastic, or carcinoma in situ is present.

The differential diagnosis of squamous cell carcinoma (usual type) mainly includes pseudoepitheliomatous hyperplasia, extension of urothelial (transitional cell) carcinoma from the urethra, and metastasis of squamous cell carcinoma. Pseudoepitheliomatous hyperplasia lacks the irregular nests of cytologically atypical cells set in a desmoplastic stroma. The epithelium exhibits acanthosis with thin elongated rete ridges, which may appear "invasive" if cut tangentially. The associated dysplasia and carcinoma in situ are also lacking. Pseudoepitheliomatous hyperplasia may be seen adjacent to superfi-

cially invasive carcinoma; hence, the isolated presence of this feature should prompt one to consider whether the biopsy is representative of the main lesion. The distinction from poorly differentiated urothelial (transitional cell) carcinoma of the urethra with local extension to the glans is based on location of the tumor, absence of squamous intraepithelial changes, and presence of urothelial (transitional cell) carcinoma in situ. Adenosquamous carcinoma is a rare neoplasm of the penis that should be considered in the differential diagnosis of squamous cell carcinomas with acantholysis. In metastatic squamous cell carcinoma, neoplastic involvement is predominantly within the vascular sinusoids of the corpora cavernosa.

### Papillary Carcinoma, Not Otherwise Specified

Papillary carcinoma NOS is the most common carcinoma with a verruciform growth pattern, representing 11% of all squamous cancers. These tumors are mainly composed of papillae lined by malignant cells; they lack condylomatous features and have an irregular infiltrative border. They are low- to intermediate-grade tumors, with a 90% 5-year survival rate.[9, 17] They form large, cauliflower-like, firm, gray-white, granular masses most commonly on the glans and foreskin and rarely in the coronal sulcus. On cut section, they demonstrate a serrated surface, with a poorly delineated interface between tumor and the underlying stroma. Invasion into dartos and corpus spongiosum is common; invasion into corpora cavernosa or skin is rare.

On low-power microscopic examination, one sees a well-differentiated papillary tumor with acanthosis and hyperkeratosis (Fig. 33-3A). The papillae vary in length, and the central fibrovascular core may or may not reach the top of the papillae. The

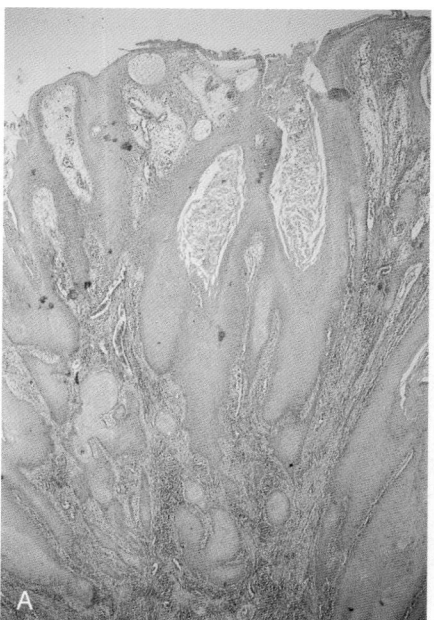
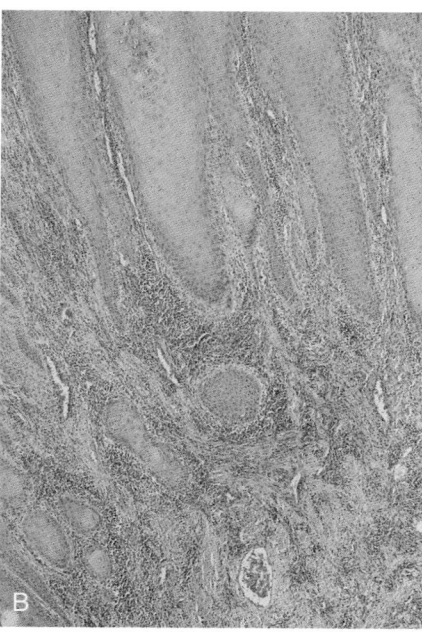

**FIGURE 33-3.** Squamous cell carcinoma of penis, papillary NOS type. *A.* Low-power view of a papillary tumor with hyperkeratosis and acanthosis. *B.* Intermediate-power view of base of tumor shows irregular nests of cells invading the underlying stroma.

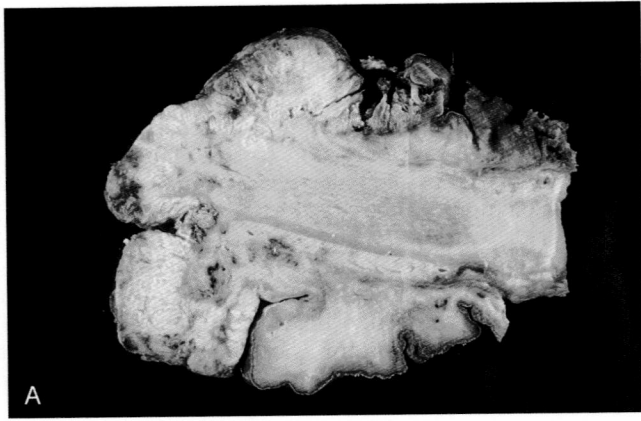
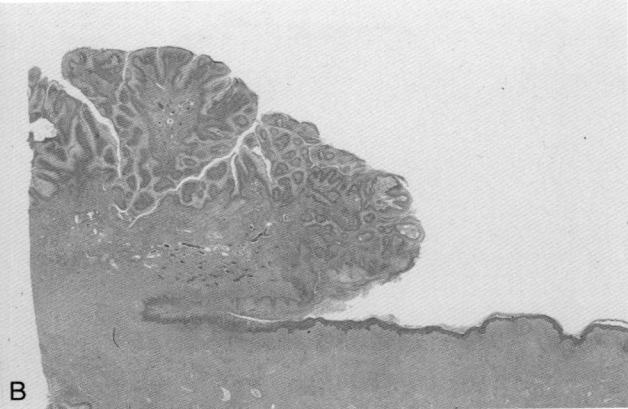

**FIGURE 33–4.** Squamous cell carcinoma of penis, warty type. *A.* A large tumor with an exophytic and endophytic growth pattern arises from the glans penis and invades the underlying tissue. *B.* Note the prominent exophytic and endophytic growth patterns.

base of the tumor is characteristically jagged, with irregular nests of cells invading the underlying stroma (Fig. 33–3*B*). Vascular and perineural invasion is rare. Microabscesses and acantholysis may also be present.

The differential diagnosis includes other squamous neoplasms with a verruciform growth pattern. Warty carcinomas show a greater degree of nuclear pleomorphism and have distinctive HPV-related changes. Verrucous carcinomas have minimal cytologic atypia or none, and they have a characteristic bulbous pushing border compared with the jagged and irregular one seen in most papillary carcinomas.

### Warty (Condylomatous) Carcinoma

Warty (condylomatous) carcinoma accounts for 6% of all squamous cancers and is similar to its vulvar counterpart; both are related to HPV infection. These tumors grow slowly; 10% of patients have metastases to inguinal lymph nodes at presentation. The 5-year survival rate is about 90%. The glans is involved most frequently, but the tumors

may be multicentric.[9, 17, 38] They form large (average, 4 cm) cauliflower-like, firm, gray-white masses, usually on the glans (Fig. 33–4*A*). On cut surface, exophytic and endophytic growth patterns are apparent (Fig. 33–4*B*). The tumor-host interface is well demarcated; a jagged or serrated appearance may be visible at the base (CD Fig. 33–6*A*). Invasion of the lamina propria and corpus spongiosum is common, whereas the corpora cavernosa are rarely invaded.

On microscopic examination, the characteristic feature is the presence of long papillae with a complex undulating appearance (Fig. 33–5*A*) (CD Fig. 33–6). The papillae are lined by cells with prominent koilocytotic nuclear atypia, a hallmark of this subtype, that is not seen in the other carcinomas with a verruciform growth pattern (Fig. 33–5*B*). Nuclei are large, wrinkled, and hyperchromatic. Binucleated and multinucleated cells are common. Numerous mitoses and foci of single-cell necrosis are present. The typical koilocytotic changes of HPV-related lesions are prominent and are a discriminating feature not seen in other squamous carcinomas

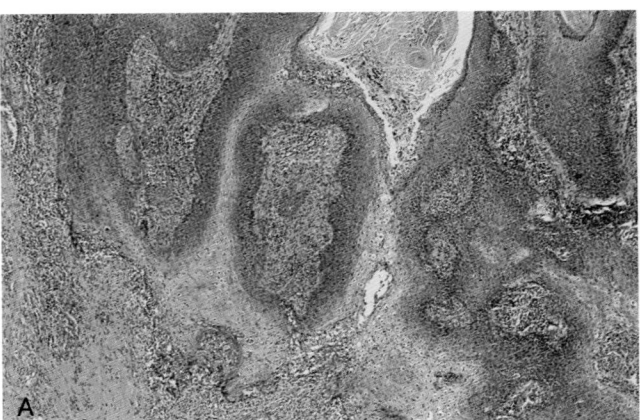
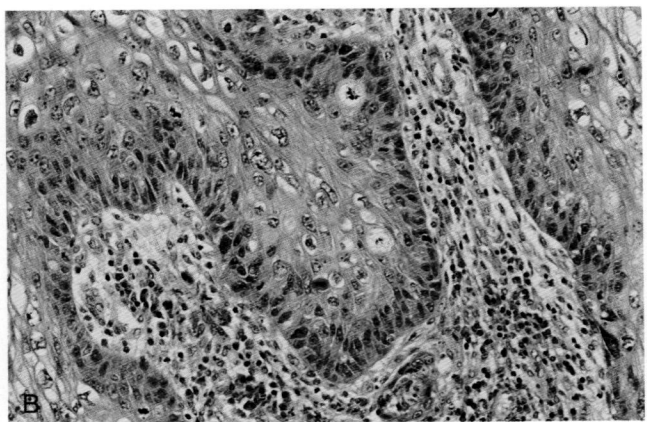

**FIGURE 33–5.** Squamous cell carcinoma of penis, warty type. *A.* Low-power view. *B.* High power view shows cells with prominent koilocytotic changes as well as nuclear anaplasia.

with a verruciform growth pattern. The majority of the tumors are low to intermediate grade. Prominent hyperkeratosis and atypical parakeratosis are usual. There is a striking similarity with benign condylomas, which are associated with about one third of the tumors.

Differential diagnosis includes the other carcinomas with a verruciform growth pattern, condyloma acuminatum, and giant condyloma of Buschke-Löwenstein. Papillary and verrucous carcinomas do not exhibit HPV-related changes. Condyloma acuminatum and giant condyloma of Buschke-Löwenstein are important in the differential diagnosis of warty carcinoma when there is limited or superficial sampling of the lesion. Giant condyloma of Buschke-Löwenstein may have similar HPV-induced cytologic features, but it has a lesser degree of nuclear atypia and, most importantly, does not show any stromal invasion. Condyloma acuminatum is identical to giant condyloma of Buschke-Löwenstein except for the difference in size.

### Verrucous Carcinoma

Verrucous carcinoma is a well-differentiated neoplasm that accounts for approximately 3% of all penile cancers. However, its true incidence is difficult to ascertain because condylomas and warty, papillary, and usual type squamous cell carcinomas have been diagnosed as verrucous carcinoma owing to a lack of consistent criteria for making this diagnosis.[9, 17, 39-42] Middle-aged patients are more commonly affected.[39-41] This carcinoma tends to grow slowly and does not metastasize if it is purely of verrucous type on histologic examination. Multiple recurrences may occur if the local excision is not adequate. Gross evaluation shows exophytic white to gray firm frequently ulcerated tumors (Fig. 33–6). Whereas the average size is 3 cm, larger and more destructive tumors may also be seen. They are usually unicentric, and the glans is the site most commonly involved.

On microscopic examination, it is a well-differentiated carcinoma with an exophytic and endo-

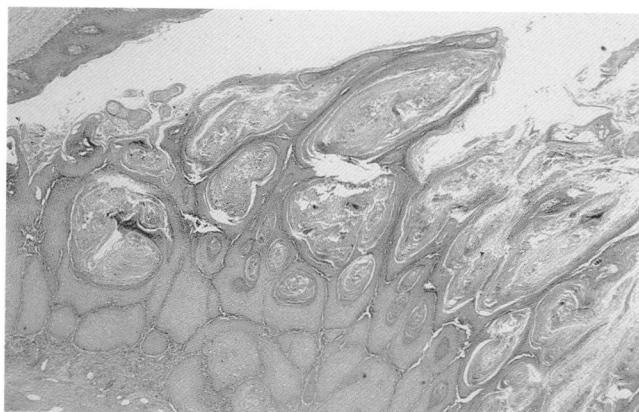

**FIGURE 33–7.** Squamous cell carcinoma of penis, verrucous type. Note the broad-based bulbous projections forming a regular pushing border. The surface shows acanthosis and papillomatosis.

phytic papillary growth pattern. A characteristic feature is the broad-based bulbous projections at the base of the tumor that deeply invaginate the lamina propria, forming a regular pushing border (Fig. 33–7). These projections constitute the invasive endophytic component; the irregular jagged nests characteristic of invasion in other forms of squamous cell carcinoma are absent in verrucous carcinoma. Prominent papillomatosis, hyperkeratosis, parakeratosis, and acanthosis are present. The papillae usually lack a central fibrovascular core. Vacuolated cells, distinct from the koilocytotic cells, may be seen on the surface. The cells have prominent intercellular bridges and exhibit no or minimal atypia, but rare mitoses may be seen at the base of the nests. A dense inflammatory infiltrate may be present at the tumor-stromal interface and may occasionally obscure it. A variable amount (usually focal) of squamous cell carcinoma (usual type) may be seen in tumors that are predominantly verrucous. The squamous cell carcinoma (usual type) component is manifest as invasive, irregular, jagged tongues of cytologically atypical cells. Tumors with mixed or hybrid verrucous and usual type patterns are more appropriately designated as mixed carcinomas.

The most important consideration in differential diagnosis is giant condyloma of Buschke-Löwenstein. By using strict morphologic criteria, these two lesions can easily be separated, even though some authors have included cases of giant condyloma of Buschke-Löwenstein as verrucous carcinoma.[41] Characteristic HPV-related changes seen in giant condyloma of Buschke-Löwenstein and warty carcinoma are lacking in verrucous carcinoma. Also, in verrucous carcinoma, papillae are shorter and lack a central fibrovascular core. Papillary carcinoma NOS exhibits more cytologic atypia and has an irregular invasive base.

### Basaloid Carcinoma

Basaloid carcinoma is an HPV-related carcinoma that is deeply invasive with a high frequency of

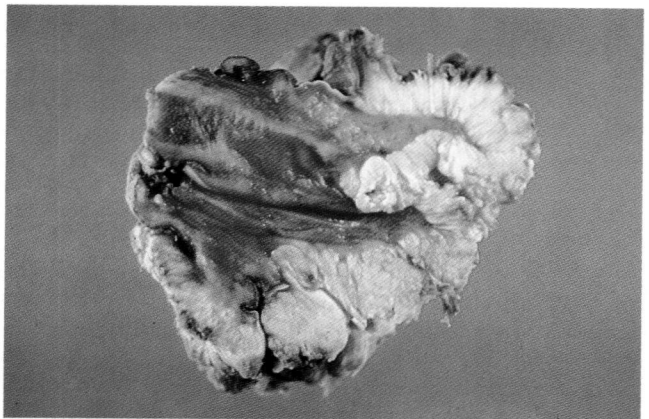

**FIGURE 33–6.** Squamous cell carcinoma of penis, verrucous type. An exophytic tumor is destroying the glans penis.

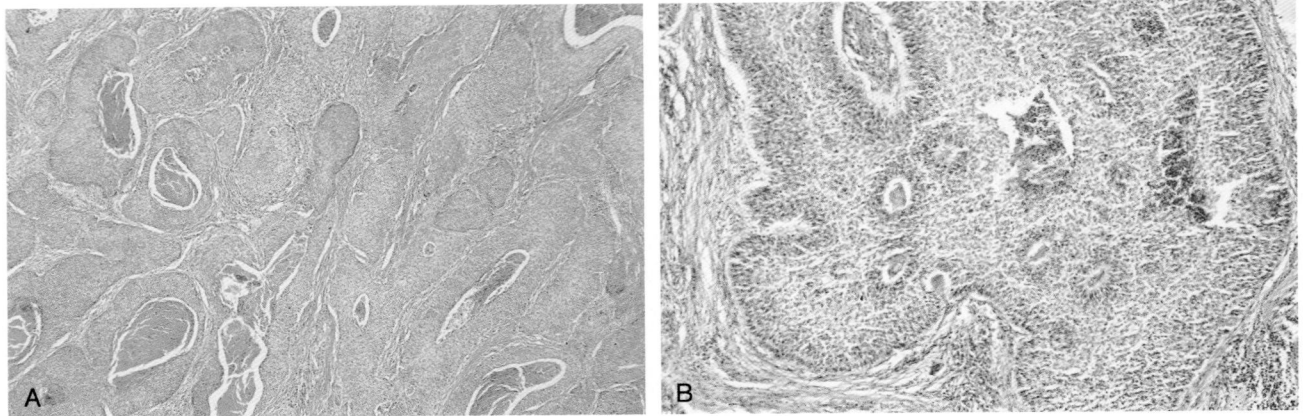

**FIGURE 33–8.** Squamous cell carcinoma of penis, basaloid type. *A.* Deeply invasive solid nest of malignant cells with basaloid features, with central comedonecrosis. *B.* High-power view of a nest of basaloid cells with central necrosis.

recurrence and lymph node metastasis. Patients range in age from 33 to 84 years (mean, 51 years).[43] These cancers have a poor prognosis; two thirds of patients present with metastases to inguinal lymph nodes.[43] They form large (average diameter, >4 cm) ulcerated, irregular, gray to red masses on the glans, commonly with focal necrosis. Secondary involvement of the coronal sulcus and foreskin is common; less frequently, there is infiltration of the skin of the shaft. On cut surface, the tumor has a rounded or slightly lobulated contour and is deeply invasive.

On microscopic examination, the tumor is characteristically composed of solid nests of small, poorly differentiated basaloid cells, with numerous foci of central comedonecrosis (Fig. 33–8). A vertical growth pattern is the most frequent, with extension into the deeper layers of the penis including the corpora cavernosa.[43] The cells are uniform, small, and sometimes spindled, with numerous mitoses. Cytoplasm is basophilic, and nucleoli are inconspicuous. The frequent individual cell necrosis may impart a "starry sky" appearance. Focal keratinization may be present, usually in the center of the nests. Perineural and vascular invasion is frequent.

Differential diagnosis includes urothelial (transitional cell) carcinoma and basal cell carcinoma. Urothelial (transitional cell) carcinomas exhibit a greater degree of nuclear pleomorphism and usually have an associated papillary component or urothelial (transitional cell) carcinoma in situ. Basal cell carcinoma typically involves the skin of the shaft, whereas basaloid carcinoma affects the glans. Nests of basal cell carcinoma are more regular, lack a high mitotic rate or single-cell necrosis, and show nuclear palisading.

### Sarcomatoid Carcinoma

Sarcomatoid carcinomas are predominantly composed of spindle cells and are aggressive tumors that frequently recur. They account for about 2% of penile carcinomas. Gross evaluation shows large (5 to 7 cm), bulky, gray-white or red fungating or polypoid masses, most commonly involving the glans.[44, 45] They characteristically show deep invasion into corpus spongiosum and corpora cavernosa. Small satellite tumor nodules are frequently seen in the corpora cavernosa or in the skin of the penis.

The characteristic microscopic finding is the biphasic histologic appearance, usually with the presence of a prominent malignant spindle cell component, arranged in fascicles and bundles resembling fibrosarcoma or leiomyosarcoma (CD Fig. 33–7). Sometimes the spindle cell component may resemble malignant fibrous histiocytoma with giant cells and pleomorphic epithelioid cells. Prominent necrosis and numerous mitoses are present. The squamous cell carcinoma component may be minimal or absent. In the absence of conventional squamous cell carcinoma, a prior history of carcinoma or presence of dysplasia or carcinoma in situ in the adjacent epithelium helps establish the diagnosis. Cytokeratin immunohistochemical stain can help confirm the diagnosis.

Differential diagnosis includes leiomyosarcoma and spindle cell melanoma. Leiomyosarcoma may be superficial or may arise deep in the corpora cavernosa; smooth muscle actin or muscle-specific actin immunohistochemical stains are confirmatory. Presence of lentiginous changes and melanosis in the adjoining mucosa and immunohistochemical stains for S-100 protein and HMB-45 are helpful in differentiation from melanoma.

### Mixed Carcinomas

Mixed carcinomas exhibit two or more different histologic patterns of squamous cell carcinoma. The most common form is a typical low-grade verrucous carcinoma with foci of moderate to high-grade squamous cell carcinoma (usual type). These tumors have also been referred to as hybrid carcinomas.[39, 40] These tumors show no significant differences in outcome, after similar treatment, compared with verrucous carcinoma.[39, 40] A mixed carcinoma composed of squamous cell carcinoma of usual type, basaloid carcinoma, or other types is also found occasionally.

### Patterns of Spread

Local spread starts with destruction of the prepuce and penile shaft, with the tunica albuginea acting as the first line of defense.[36] With progressive growth of the tumor, this barrier is compromised, and the tumor invades the corpus cavernosum. Fistula formation may lead to secondary involvement of the urethra.

Lymph node metastasis is the most common mode of distant spread of the tumor; the superficial inguinal lymph nodes are the first to be involved. Metastases to the contralateral nodes may occur because numerous anastomotic lymphatic channels crisscross the midline. At initial presentation, 58% of patients have palpable inguinal lymphadenopathy.[36] Lymph node metastases are found in 45% of patients with palpable inguinal lymphadenopathy and 20% of those with nonpalpable lymph nodes.[36] Secondary infection of the penile cancer is another cause of inguinal lymphadenopathy; for this reason, sentinel lymph node biopsy is commonly performed. However, controversy exists regarding the role of prophylactic bilateral inguinal lymphadenectomy.[18, 19, 21, 46–48]

In spite of the rich vascular channels found in the corpora cavernosa, hematogenous dissemination is rare. Visceral metastases at initial presentation are seen in less than 2% of patients. Metastases to the liver, lungs, and bone may be seen in untreated cases.[49]

### Prognostic Considerations

Prognostic factors and their importance are summarized in Table 33–5. Tumor stage and grade are the most important prognostic factors in determining lymph node metastases and overall survival.[20–25] The TNM system[50] and Jackson's staging system[51] are the most widely used staging systems. Depth of invasion determines the stage and hence the prognosis. Tumors invading Buck's fascia and corpora cavernosa have poorer prognosis because of their propensity to invade the rich supply of vascular channels.

Grading of penile carcinomas is based on the Broders classification, with division into well-differentiated, moderately differentiated, and poorly differentiated tumors. There is good correlation between histologic grade and stage; poorly differentiated tumors are usually high stage. Up to 80% of patients with well-differentiated tumors are long-term survivors. Histologic grade has also been correlated with lymph node metastases; in one series, lymph node metastases were observed in 24% of

**TABLE 33–5.** Prognosis: Penile Carcinoma

| Prognostic Factor | Good Prognosis | Intermediate Prognosis | Worse Prognosis |
|---|---|---|---|
| **Tumor Stage** | | | |
| Higher T stage | | | X |
| Lymph node metastasis | | | X |
| **Depth of Invasion** | | | |
| Into or beyond corpora cavernosa | | | X |
| **Tumor Grade** | | | |
| Well differentiated | X | | |
| Moderately differentiated | | X | |
| Poorly differentiated | | | X |
| **Vascular Invasion** | | | |
| Present | | | X |
| **Histologic Subtype** | | | |
| Papillary | | X | |
| Verrucous | X | | |
| Warty (condylomatous) | | X | |
| Basaloid | | | X |
| Sarcomatoid | | | X |
| **Location of Primary Tumor** | | | |
| Foreskin tumors | X | | |
| Glans | | X | |
| Coronal sulcus tumors | | | X |
| **Growth Pattern** | | | |
| Superficial spreading | X | | |
| Verruciform | X | | |
| Vertical | | | X |
| **Size** | | | |
| Larger size (non-verruciform) | | | X |

well-differentiated carcinomas compared with 46% of moderately differentiated and 82% of poorly differentiated carcinomas.[46] Another grading system in use is the one proposed by Maiche and colleagues[52] that is divided into four grades based on individual scores assigned to four features (i.e., degree of keratinization, mitotic activity, cellular atypia, and inflammatory infiltrate). This grading system has also shown a good correlation with stage.

Vascular invasion correlates well with lymph node metastases. Approximately 50% of tumors with vascular invasion metastasize to the lymph nodes, and vascular invasion can be demonstrated in two thirds of tumors that have metastasized.[9]

Location of the primary tumor is important, not only because of the different routes of tumor spread but because tumor grade varies; 50% of tumors of the shaft are poorly differentiated versus only 10% of those from the foreskin. Tumors arising in the coronal sulcus are more aggressive owing to their proclivity for invading the rich vascular network of the dartos muscle and Buck's fascia.

Growth pattern is important because tumors with a vertical growth pattern are uniformly aggressive and have a poorer prognosis. Verruciform and superficial spreading patterns have better prognosis.[9] Larger tumors are more aggressive, except for those with a verruciform growth pattern.[9]

The role of ancillary techniques, such as DNA flow cytometric analysis, proliferation markers, tumor suppressor genes, and oncogenes, remains under investigation. At present, all of these methods are used only for research purposes and do not have any clinical application.

## BASAL CELL CARCINOMA

Because the penile skin is generally not sun exposed, the incidence of basal cell carcinoma is low.[53, 54] Patients described with this tumor range in age from 37 to 79 years, and almost all are white.[53, 54] Whereas these tumors may arise anywhere on the penile skin, they involve the shaft in 56%, the glans in 30%, and the prepuce in 14%.[53, 54] Clinical presentation is usually as a small, irregular, ulcerated mass. On microscopic examination, features are similar to basal cell carcinoma seen elsewhere. The main differential diagnostic consideration is basaloid carcinoma. The clinical course is generally indolent, and these neoplasms are treated by local excision.

## PAGET'S DISEASE

Paget's disease rarely affects the penis and involves patients in their sixth and seventh decades of life. Its histologic features are similar to those of Paget's disease at other extramammary sites (CD Fig. 33–8), and it needs to be distinguished from squamous cell carcinoma in situ and malignant melanoma.[55, 56]

## MALIGNANT MELANOMA

Malignant melanoma of the penis is rare, with just over 100 cases having been reported.[57, 58] White men are affected most commonly, generally in their fifth and sixth decades. Interestingly, this group of patients is older than those affected by most cutaneous melanomas. The majority of melanomas are located on the glans, with occasional tumors occurring on the foreskin and shaft. Clinical presentation and histologic features are similar to those of malignant melanomas occurring in the skin and the mucosa. Differing histologic types, including nodular (CD Fig. 33–9), superficial spreading, and acral lentiginous, have been reported.[57] Prognosis depends on the depth of invasion and pathologic stage. Those invading to a depth of 0.75 mm or less have a more favorable prognosis, whereas those invading to 1.5 mm or more have a greater chance of metastasis. The main differential diagnosis includes lentiginous melanosis, which is characterized by multiple flat pigmented macules on the glans penis.[59] Malignant melanoma of soft parts has been reported rarely to involve the penis.[60]

## SARCOMAS OF THE PENIS

Sarcomas of the penis are uncommon tumors but are the second most common malignant neoplasm affecting the penis, representing less than 5% of all penile malignant neoplasms. Except for rhabdomyosarcoma, which is most commonly seen in children, the peak is in the fifth and sixth decades.[61] They are most commonly located on the penile shaft, except for Kaposi's sarcoma, which most commonly occurs on the glans. These tumors are histologically similar to their counterparts arising at other locations.

The most common sarcomas of the penis are of vascular origin, including Kaposi's sarcoma, epithelioid hemangioendothelioma, and angiosarcoma[62–64] (CD Fig. 33–10). Kaposi's sarcoma is usually associated with other systemic lesions and involves the skin of the shaft or glans. Of acquired immunodeficiency syndrome patients with Kaposi's sarcoma, about 20% have penile lesions.[62] Leiomyosarcomas may be superficial or deep. Superficial leiomyosarcomas form subcutaneous nodules. These are believed to arise from the smooth muscle of the glans penis or the dermis of the shaft. The deep type is less common, arising from the smooth muscle of corpora cavernosa. They tend to invade the urethra and metastasize early, leading to a poorer prognosis.[65] Embryonal rhabdomyosarcoma has been reported to occur in children, involving the penile shaft.[66] Rare cases of fibrosarcoma,[67] epithelioid sarcoma,[68] hemangiopericytoma, and malignant schwannoma have also been reported.

## METASTATIC TUMORS

Metastases to the penis are rare; the most common primary site is the prostate followed by the rectosigmoid colon (CD Figs. 33–11 and 33–12), urinary bladder, and kidney. Less common primary sites include the testes, ureters, lung, pancreas, nasopharynx, and bone.[69, 70] Most commonly, the metastases are located in the corpora cavernosa, filling the vascular sinusoids.[69] In rare instances, metastases to the penis may be the first sign of a neoplasm.[71] Metastases to the penis usually present with new-onset priapism, or they may present as an unusual penile lesion. Metastasis to the penis is usually a terminal event; most patients succumb to the disease.[69]

# NON-NEOPLASTIC LESIONS OF THE PENIS

## Infectious and Inflammatory Lesions

### SEXUALLY TRANSMITTED DISEASES

Sexually transmitted diseases affecting the penis include condyloma acuminatum, syphilis, granuloma inguinale, lymphogranuloma venereum, chancroid, molluscum contagiosum, and herpes simplex. Except for the first, the diagnosis of these infectious diseases is usually based on laboratory tests, but biopsy of these lesions is occasionally done because they may clinically mimic a neoplasm.

Condyloma acuminatum, which is caused by HPV, is the most common lesion of the penis to undergo biopsy because it forms a "tumor." Condylomas most commonly affect young adults, with a 5% incidence in the 20- to 40-year age group. The majority of these are sexually transmitted; a greater than average incidence is seen in men whose sexual partners have HPV-related lesions of the cervix.[72] Genital condylomas have also been reported in children, which should raise the suspicion of sexual abuse. HPV types 6 and 11 are most commonly associated with condylomas without dysplasia, whereas HPV types 16 and 18 are frequently associated with dysplastic condylomas.[73, 74] Autoinfection is common after the initial infection. Locations of penile condylomata acuminata, in decreasing order of frequency, are glans, foreskin, meatus, and shaft. Extension to the scrotal skin, perineum, urethra, and even urinary bladder may occur. In gross appearance, they are either flat or papillary cauliflower-like lesions. They are characterized microscopically by parakeratosis, hyperkeratosis, acanthosis, papillomatosis, and koilocytosis (Fig. 33–9). Because these may resemble seborrheic keratosis (CD Fig. 33–13), it is important to bear in mind that seborrheic keratosis does not affect non–hair-bearing skin of the glans penis. Bizarre cytologic atypia may be seen in treated cases, particularly those treated with podophyllin; these therapy-related changes need to be recognized to avoid making an erroneous diagnosis of dysplasia or carcinoma in situ.

Giant condyloma of Buschke-Löwenstein is a rare lesion that affects a slightly older population. The white to gray, firm cauliflower-like masses have an average diameter of 5 cm. The cut surface exhibits a well-circumscribed base, with a characteristic endophytic growth that in contrast to verrucous carcinoma may have elongated rete ridges, although broad bulbous extensions may be evident.[9, 75] It may

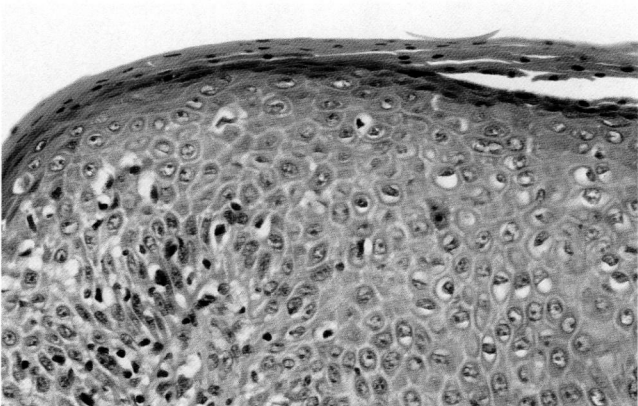

**FIGURE 33–9.** Condyloma acuminatum of penis. Flat condyloma (condyloma planum) exhibits hyperkeratosis, parakeratosis, acanthosis, and koilocytosis.

burrow deep into underlying tissue, causing erosion and ulceration of adjacent skin. Microscopic examination shows exuberant papillomatosis (Fig. 33–10A) and a conspicuous bulbous expansion at the base (Fig. 33–10B), in addition to all the features typically seen in condyloma acuminatum.[9, 75] The main differential diagnostic consideration is with verrucous and warty carcinoma; this distinction is discussed previously.

Syphilis of the penis is manifest in all its stages, (i.e., primary, secondary, and tertiary). The hard chancre is the classic lesion of primary syphilis but is seen uncommonly in this age. It forms a single, painless, round ulcer with well-defined margins and an indurated base, which is preceded by a small papule. A classic feature of syphilis is obliterative endarteritis with an accompanying dense plasma cell infiltrate; in primary syphilis, it is present at the base of the papule or ulcer. Condyloma latum is a gray maculopapule characteristic of secondary syphilis. In secondary syphilis, the endarteritis may be superficial or deep, and the associated plasma cell infiltrate often effaces the epidermal-dermal junction. Because plasma cell (Zoon's) balanitis may appear histologically similar, the diagnosis of syphilis may be confirmed by demonstrating the *Treponema pallidum* spirochete by use of a silver impregnation stain (e.g., Warthin-Starry, Steiner, or Dieterle).[76] Spirochetes are seen in the dermis, around and within the walls of dermal blood vessels, and between epidermal cells, especially in areas of neutrophilic exocytosis. Tertiary syphilis affecting the penis is manifest as the gumma, a mass composed of epithelioid histiocytes and multinucleated giant cells surrounding a zone of coagulative necrosis.[77]

Granuloma inguinale presents initially as a small, painless, nodular lesion that later forms an ulcer with abundant granulation tissue in the base.[78] Large destructive tumorlike nodules may be seen in untreated cases. Satellite lesions called pseudobuboes may be present. On microscopic examination, there is an extensive plasma cell infiltrate in the

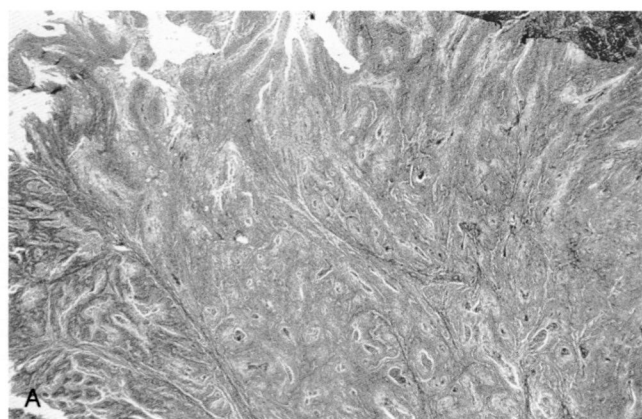
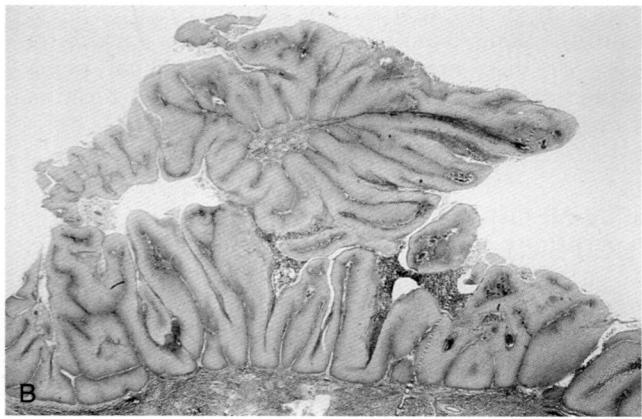

**FIGURE 33–10.** Giant condyloma of Buschke-Löwenstein. *A.* Exuberant papillary projections, with hyperkeratosis and parakeratosis at the tips of the papillae. *B.* Clinically, this lesion was larger than 5 cm; otherwise, the features are similar to those of condyloma acuminatum. (Courtesy of Abraham T. Philip, M.D., Boston, MA.)

granulation tissue with few lymphocytes and a diffuse infiltrate of neutrophils that may form microabscesses. Also present are mononuclear histiocytes with Donovan bodies; these are large, intracytoplasmic, encapsulated, bipolar bacilli that are best seen in smears and with a Giemsa stain. *Calymmatobacterium granulomatis* is the infectious agent, which stains with Warthin-Starry stain.[78]

Lymphogranuloma venereum is characterized by penile and inguinal lymph node infection. A transient painless nodule or ulcer may be seen on the penis. On microscopic examination, there is a flat base of granulation tissue with zonal marginal necrosis and a neutrophilic infiltrate. Non-necrotizing granulomas surrounded by plasma cells are present amid a lymphoplasmacytic infiltrate.[79] The adjacent skin shows pseudoepitheliomatous hyperplasia, which if pronounced may mimic a squamous malignant neoplasm. Inguinal lymph nodes initially show small neutrophilic microabscesses that eventually coalesce, forming the classic stellate lesions. Lymphoid hyperplasia and intense plasma cell infiltrate follow. Long-standing untreated cases have suppurative granulomas, followed by sinuses, fistulas, and eventually fibrosis. *Chlamydia trachomatis,* an obligate intracellular parasite, is the causative organism.[79]

Chancroid or soft chancre is caused by the gram-negative bacterium *Haemophilus ducreyi.*[80] It forms a painful ulcer with a soft base. A characteristic zonal pattern is seen microscopically; it consists of superficial necrosis, fibrin, and leukocytes, with underlying granulation tissue bordered by lymphocytes and plasma cells.[80]

Herpes simplex virus infection forms small vesicles that rupture to form painful ulcers. On microscopic examination, nuclei of infected epidermal cells show a typical ground-glass appearance with intranuclear eosinophilic inclusions, especially at the margins of the vesicles. The infected cells may also fuse to form multinucleated syncytial fragments. The histologic features are most often diagnostic, but immunohistochemical confirmation may be helpful in equivocal cases.

Molluscum contagiosum is caused by a poxvirus, which forms a 3 to 6-mm dome-shaped papule often with an area of central umbilication. Microscopic features are typical of those seen elsewhere[81] (CD Fig. 33–14).

## BALANITIS AND BALANOPOSTHITIS

Balanitis is inflammation of the glans. Balanoposthitis, inflammation of the glans and foreskin, usually affects uncircumcised men with poor hygiene, resulting from an inflammatory reaction due to accumulation of smegma; it may also occur secondary to bacterial and fungal infection, contact dermatitis, and other dermatologic conditions.[82] Both these conditions may result in phimosis.

## BALANITIS CIRCUMSCRIPTA PLASMACELLULARIS (PLASMA CELL BALANITIS, ZOON'S BALANITIS)

This inflammatory disorder almost exclusively affects uncircumcised men, usually elderly. It typically presents as a solitary, large, bright red moist patch on the glans or mucosa of the prepuce.[82, 83] It clinically resembles erythroplasia of Queyrat; hence, biopsy is almost always done. On microscopic examination, the distinction from carcinoma in situ is straightforward; this form of balanitis is characterized by a distinct bandlike infiltrate of plasma cells in the upper dermis. The dermis is edematous, with vertically oriented dilated capillaries, extravasated erythrocytes, and hemosiderin pigment. The epidermis is atrophic or may be partially ulcerated; the characteristic "lozenge keratinocytes" are diamond shaped and separated by intercellular edema[82, 83] (CD Fig. 33–15).

## BALANITIS XEROTICA OBLITERANS

Balanitis xerotica obliterans is an atrophic disorder of unknown etiology that is homologous to vulvar lichen sclerosus et atrophicus. It is usually localized to the glans and prepuce, especially around the meatus, and is characterized on gross evaluation by white papules or plaques. Microscopic features of the early lesion include epidermal atrophy, orthokeratotic hyperkeratosis, dermal edema, and interface dermatitis (CD Fig. 33–16). Later, the lesions show dense dermal fibrosis, inflammation in the upper dermis, and alternating areas of epithelial atrophy and hyperplasia. Complications include meatal stenosis, phimosis, and fissure formation. This condition has been associated with development of squamous carcinoma, but it has been argued that this association may be only coincidental.[82, 84]

## LIPOGRANULOMA (PARAFFINOMA)

Lipogranuloma of the penis is a foreign body inflammatory reaction that almost always results from the injection of paraffin, wax, silicone, or oil to enlarge the penis.[85] These patients present with localized areas of distortion or induration; the overlying skin appears normal. The diagnosis is easily established if the appropriate history is elicited, but lack of history may prompt a biopsy to rule out a neoplastic process. On microscopic examination, there is typical foreign body–type granulomatous inflammation, with variably sized lipid vacuoles set in dense fibrous tissue with a chronic inflammatory infiltrate (CD Fig. 33–17). Lipids can be demonstrated by oil red O stain.[85]

## VERRUCIFORM XANTHOMA

Verruciform xanthoma is a warty tumorlike lesion more commonly affecting the oral cavity that may rarely involve the penis. The clinical and microscopic appearances overlap considerably with those of condyloma acuminatum. On microscopic examination, the hallmark of the lesion is a xanthomatous infiltrate in the dermis, typically in between elongated rete ridges. Acanthosis, hyperkeratosis, and parakeratosis are also present.[86]

## FOURNIER'S GANGRENE/CORBUS' DISEASE

Fournier's gangrene is characterized by necrotizing fasciitis around the perineal region that may extend to involve adjacent skin of the anterior abdomen. Corbus' disease is the term sometimes used when there is massive involvement of the penis. This condition may be idiopathic, or it may be associated with various other debilitating diseases and human immunodeficiency virus infection.[87]

# Congenital and Acquired Malformations

## CONGENITAL MALFORMATIONS OF THE PENIS

Aphallia (penile agenesis) results from a failure of the genital tubercle to develop; it occurs in approximately 1 in 10,000,000 live births. The penile shaft is missing, whereas the scrotum is well developed, usually with descended testes. Most often, the urethra opens at the anal verge adjacent to a small skin tag; in the remainder, it opens into the rectum.[88]

Epispadias is the congenital absence of the dorsal wall of the urethra. The urethral opening is on the dorsum of the penis and is apparent as a groove or a cleft without any covering. This congenital malformation has an incidence of approximately 1 in 117,000 males.[89] The extent of the defect varies. Depending on the location, three types of epispadias are encountered: penopubic, penile, and glandular; penopubic is the most common type.[89]

In hypospadias, there is incomplete development of the anterior urethra, with the urethral opening being located anywhere on the ventral surface of the penis or on the perineum.[90] The incidence is approximately 1 per 300 live male births.

Miscellaneous congenital abnormalities include diphallus,[91] micropenis,[92] scrotal engulfment,[93] and concealed penis.[94]

## PENILE CYSTS

Epidermal inclusion cyst is the most common, varying from 0.1 to 1 cm in diameter, and is usually found on the penile shaft. Mucoid cysts arise from ectopic urethral mucosa and contain mucoid material. They are usually on the prepuce or glans and range in size from 0.2 to 2 cm; they tend to be unilocular and are lined by stratified columnar mucinous epithelium.[95] Median raphe cysts represent developmental defects in the embryogenesis of the genital tract and are most likely caused by incomplete closure of the genital fold. On histologic examination, these cysts are lined by pseudostratified columnar epithelium (CD Fig. 33–18). They may be unilocular or multilocular.[96]

## PEYRONIE'S DISEASE

Peyronie's disease (plastic induration of the penis, fibrous sclerosis of the penis, fibrous cavernitis) is characterized by the development of fibromatosis between the corpora cavernosa and the tunica albuginea, resulting in "penile bending" during erection.[97] This disease generally affects middle-aged or older men and is rare among those younger than 40 years. Diagnosis is usually made on clinical grounds; however, the presence of a "mass" may lead to a biopsy. It is microscopically similar to fibromatosis seen at other sites, although it tends to be less cellular and more sclerotic than most other types of superficial fibromatosis (CD Fig. 33–19). Rarely, calcification or ossification is seen. Approximately 10% of patients have other forms of fibromatoses, such as Dupuytren's contracture or palmar or plantar fibromatoses.[97]

## PHIMOSIS AND PARAPHIMOSIS

Phimosis is the inability to retract the foreskin behind the glans penis. It is normal in children younger than 5 years to not be able to retract the foreskin behind the glans. Phimosis may lead to urinary obstruction and ballooning of the foreskin. Histologic examination of the excised foreskin is usually nonspecific and variable; it may be normal or show edema, chronic or chronic active inflammation, vascular congestion, and fibrosis. Phimosis has also been associated with penile carcinoma; for this reason, foreskin resections from older patients should be examined thoroughly to rule out malignant and premalignant lesions.[98]

In paraphimosis, the foreskin is retracted behind the glans penis. This results in constriction of the glans, with concomitant vascular engorgement and edema that may eventually lead to such marked swelling of the glans that the foreskin can no longer be drawn forward, necessitating an emergency dorsal slit or circumcision.[98]

### CHORDEE

Chordee is a congenital or acquired condition that causes the penis to bend in a ventral, or dorsal, or lateral direction. Congenital chordee is most frequently associated with hypospadias; acquired chordee may follow trauma or be a result of Peyronie's disease.[99]

### MISCELLANEOUS LESIONS OF THE PENIS

Melanosis of the penis presents as flat pigmented macules with geographic, irregular borders located in the mucosa.[59] Its relationship with melanoma is unclear. Rare cases of Wegener's granulomatosis affecting the penis or distal urethra have been reported, some with destruction of the penis.[100] Tancho's nodules is another factitious condition resulting from implantation of glass beads in the glans penis.[101] Os penis, a rare acquired phenomenon produced by metaplasia, results in ossification of the penis; it is usually seen in the elderly and is associated with an underlying condition such as trauma, Peyronie's disease, diabetes, gout, venereal disease, or neoplasia.[102] Penile horn,[103] sarcoid of the glans,[104] and penile tuberculosis[105] have also been reported.

## NEOPLASTIC LESIONS OF THE SCROTUM

### Benign Tumors

The most common benign tumors of the scrotum are of mesenchymal origin, and these include cavernous and capillary hemangiomas,[106] angiokeratoma[107] (CD Fig. 33–20), lymphangioma,[108] and leiomyomas of the skin and dartos.[109] Rare cases of schwannoma,[110] neurofibroma,[4] juvenile xanthogranuloma,[111] lipoma, fibroma, fibrolipoma, myxoma and myxofibroma, and infantile fibromatosis of external genitalia[112] have also been reported. Benign cutaneous adnexal tumors of apocrine, eccrine, or hair follicle origin may also involve the scrotal skin.

### Locally Aggressive Tumors

Angiomyofibroblastomas, aggressive angiomyxomas,[113] and giant cell fibroblastoma[114] have been reported to occur in the scrotum. The histologic features of these tumors are similar to those found at other sites.

### Malignant Tumors

#### SQUAMOUS CELL CARCINOMA
##### General Considerations

The pathogenesis of squamous cell carcinoma of the scrotum is of great historical interest because it is the first malignant tumor to be directly linked to occupational exposure.[115] Currently, most cases reported in the United States are not associated with occupational exposure.[116] Sir Percivall Pott,[117] in 1775, reported its occurrence in chimney sweeps and speculated on the causal relationship of soot. Passey,[115] in 1922, finally proved that association. Risk factors include exposure to carcinogens in soot, tar, oils, and oil mist[118]; a dose-dependent exposure to PUVA therapy[31]; poor hygiene; HPV infection[119]; and the presence of multiple squamous cell carcinomas of the skin.[119]

##### Clinical Considerations

Squamous cell carcinoma is the most common malignant tumor of the scrotum. It has a low incidence in the United States.[119-121] The tumor mainly affects men in the sixth and seventh decades of life, with an age range of 46 to 87 years.[119, 121] It usually presents as a solitary lesion, in the form of a persistent slow-growing nodule, "wart," or pimple, which may ulcerate over time.[121] Multiple tumor nodules may be seen. Metachronous lesions have also been reported. Interestingly, the left side of the scrotum is more commonly involved in patients with a history of occupational exposure.[119] Metastases to ipsilateral inguinal lymph nodes are present at initial presentation in about 25% of patients, whereas about 50% have palpable lymphadenopathy.[120, 121]

##### Diagnostic Considerations

On gross evaluation, most tumors are ulcerated with raised rolled edges and an indurated base, which sometimes is necrotic. Rarely, tumors may invade into the testis or penis in patients with advanced disease.

Tumors exhibit the typical morphologic features of cutaneous squamous cell carcinomas. The majority of these are keratinizing and are well to moderately differentiated (CD Fig. 33–21). The adjacent epidermis usually exhibits hyperkeratosis, acanthosis, and dyskeratosis. Verrucous carcinoma may be seen rarely.[122] A spectrum of nuclear atypia including squamous cell carcinoma in situ may be seen in the adjacent epithelium. Bowenoid papulosis can involve the scrotum and is usually seen in cases that also affect the penis. HPV-related changes have also been reported.[119]

### Prognostic Considerations

The survival of patients correlates with the stage of the tumor, but the prognostic impact of histologic grade is unclear. Lowe's modification of Ray and Whitmore's staging system is the one that is most commonly used.[120, 121] Overall 5-year survival rates range from 22% to 52%.[120] Ray and Whitmore reported a 5-year survival rate of 70% for stage A disease and 44% for stage B disease.[120] However, patients with stage C and stage D disease had low rates of long-term survival.[120] In one study, older patients (>65 years) usually had nonlocalized cancers with a 17% 5-year survival, whereas younger patients usually had localized cancer with a 75% 5-year survival.[123]

## OTHER MALIGNANT TUMORS

Basal cell carcinoma of the scrotum is rare, and less than 30 cases have been reported, because the scrotal skin is not sun exposed.[124] Typical histologic features of basal cell carcinoma are seen; nodular, superficial, superficial multicentric, and fibroepithelioma of Pinkus types have been reported. In contrast to the nongenital forms, these tumors tend to be more aggressive. Of 24 reported cases, 13% (three cases) had lymph node or distant metastasis, and one patient died of disease.[124]

Paget's disease of the scrotum may be seen in patients with synchronous or metachronous visceral malignant neoplasms.[125] Microscopic features are identical to those seen elsewhere. Merkel cell carcinoma has also been reported.[126]

Malignant mesenchymal tumors are rare; leiomyosarcomas[109] and liposarcomas[127] are the most common. Other tumors that have been reported include malignant fibrous histiocytoma,[128] rhabdomyosarcoma, fibrosarcoma,[129] neurogenic sarcoma,[130] and Kaposi's sarcoma.[131] A number of cases reported as scrotal mesenchymal tumors actually arise in the paratesticular soft tissue and the spermatic cord and are not truly scrotal tumors in the strict anatomic sense.

Malignant melanomas, superficial spreading and nodular types, have been reported to rarely occur in the scrotal skin.[132]

Secondary tumors of the scrotal skin include metastases from carcinomas of the prostate, colon, stomach, and kidney.[133]

## NON-NEOPLASTIC LESIONS OF THE SCROTUM

### Infectious and Inflammatory Lesions

Condyloma acuminatum may involve the penoscrotal junction and the scrotum. The lesions may be pedunculated, papilloma-like, sessile, or flat (condyloma planum). The microscopic features are identical to those of condyloma lesions seen elsewhere.

Filariasis (elephantiasis) is relatively common in tropical and subtropical developing countries and the Pacific Islands while being extremely rare in the United States. The blockage of lymphatic drainage with resultant transudation of lymph, and secondary cellular proliferation in the connective tissue, may cause grotesque enlargement of the scrotum. On histologic examination, obliterative endolymphangitis (i.e., cellular proliferation of the walls of lymphatic vessels) is characteristic.[134]

Sexually transmitted diseases may also involve the scrotal skin, although they more commonly involve the penis.

Fournier's gangrene frequently involves the scrotum. The organisms implicated in its etiology include staphylococcal and streptococcal species, anaerobic bacteria, and other gram-negative bacteria.[87]

Lipogranuloma (paraffinoma), although more commonly seen to affect the penis, may also involve the scrotum.[85] The differential diagnosis includes sclerosing liposarcoma, metastatic signet ring cell carcinoma, and adenomatoid tumor. Marked variation in size of the vacuoles and the accompanying xanthogranulomatous inflammation and fibrosis are key features in differentiating lipogranuloma. The clinical history and immunohistochemical stains may help establish the diagnosis in difficult cases, especially with a small amount of tissue.

Verruciform xanthoma is rarely seen in the anogenital region and has histologic features identical to those found in the oral mucosa.[135]

Fat necrosis most commonly occurs in obese children and adolescents, usually after hypothermia. It presents as a swollen scrotum with firm and tender nodules, which are frequently bilateral.[136]

## Acquired and Congenital Malformations

Ectopic scrotum is a rare congenital malformation in which the hemiscrotum is in an anomalous position along the inguinal canal.[137] A suprainguinal location is more common than the infrainguinal or perineal locations. Accessory scrotum is defined as the presence of scrotal tissue in a location other than the normal. It is distinct from ectopic scrotum and occurs with normally developed scrotal sacs and testes. Another term that is sometimes used interchangeably albeit incorrectly is perineal lipoma with accessory scrotum.[138]

Fibrous hamartoma of infancy is a rare hamartomatous proliferation of myofibroblasts.[139] It typically occurs in the first year of life and most commonly involves the axilla or shoulder region of males. On microscopic examination, it is composed of varying amounts of adipose tissue, spindled myofibroblasts, and round mesenchymal cells arranged haphazardly.

Smooth muscle hamartoma of dartos is a rare hamartomatous lesion exhibiting a random proliferation of dermal smooth muscle bundles.[140]

## Metabolic and Degenerative Disorders

Epidermal inclusion cysts (keratinous cysts) are commonly seen in the scrotal skin as single or multiple nodules within or below the dermis.

Idiopathic scrotal calcinosis is an uncommon condition involving the scrotal skin, usually of children and young adults, that is characterized by the progressive development of multiple painless calcific nodules. These nodules vary in size from a few millimeters to large nodular bosselated masses. It is characterized histologically by granules and globules of dense calcification within the dermis, sometimes associated with a foreign body giant cell reaction[141] (CD Fig. 33–22). In most lesions, there is no lining epithelium; but in some, a flattened squamous lining, identical to that of epidermal inclusion cyst, may be present at least focally. A relationship between this entity and epidermal inclusion cyst has been demonstrated, suggesting that not all cases of scrotal calcinosis are idiopathic.[141]

## REFERENCES

1. Tannenbaum MH, Becker SW: Papillae of the corona of the glans penis. J Urol 93:391–395, 1965.
2. Senoh K, Miyazaki T, Kikuchi J, et al: Angiomatous lesions of the glans penis. Urology 17:194–196, 1981.
3. Macaluso JNJ, Sullivan JW, Tomberlin S: Glomus tumor of glans penis. Urology 25:409–410, 1985.
4. Ogawa A, Watanabe K: Genitourinary neurofibromatosis in a child presenting with an enlarged penis and scrotum. J Urol 135:755–757, 1986.
5. Mayersak JS, Viviano CJ, Babiarz JW: Schwannoma of the penis. J Urol 153:1931–1932, 1995.
6. Stone NN, Sun CC, Brutscher S, et al: Granular cell tumor of penis. J Urol 130:575, 1983.
7. Grossman B: Premalignant and early carcinomas of the penis and scrotum. Urol Clin North Am 19:221–226, 1992.
8. Kaye V, Zhang G, Dehner LP, et al: Carcinoma in situ of penis: is distinction between erythroplasia of Queyrat and Bowen's disease relevant? Urology 36: 479–482, 1990.
9. Young RH, Srigley JR, Amin MB, et al: The penis. *In* Tumors of the Prostate Gland, Seminal Vesicles, Male Urethra and Penis. Atlas of Tumor Pathology. Third Series, Fascicle 28. Washington, DC, Armed Forces Institute of Pathology, 2000, pp 403–487.
10. Ro JY, Amin MB, Ayala AG: Penis and scrotum. *In* Bostwick DG, Eble JN (eds): Urologic Surgical Pathology. Philadelphia, Mosby, 1997, pp 675–724.
11. Queyrat L: Erytroplasia du gland. Bull Soc Franc Derm Syph 22:378–382, 1911.
12. Graham JH, Helwig EB: Erythroplasia of Queyrat: a clinicopathologic and histochemical study. Cancer 32:1396–1414, 1973.
13. Callen JP, Headington JT: Bowen's and non-Bowen's squamous intraepithelial neoplasia of the skin: relationship to internal malignancy. Arch Dermatol 116:422–426, 1980.
14. Patterson JW, Kao GF, Graham JH, et al: Bowenoid papulosis: a clinicopathologic study with ultrastructural observations. Cancer 57:823–836, 1986.
15. Taylor DRJ, South DA: Bowenoid papulosis: a review. Cutis 27:92–98, 1981.
16. Ikenberg H, Gissmann K, Gross G, et al: Human papillomavirus type-16–related DNA in genital Bowen's disease and in bowenoid papulosis. Int J Cancer 32:563–565, 1983.
17. Cubilla AL, Barreto JE, Ayala G: The penis. *In* Sternberg SS (ed): Diagnostic Surgical Pathology. 2nd ed. New York, Raven Press, 1994, pp 1949–1974.
18. Fraley EE, Zhang G, Manivel C, et al: The role of ilioinguinal lymphadenectomy and significance of histological differentiation in the treatment of carcinoma of the penis. J Urol 142:1478–1482, 1989.
19. Ornellas AA, Seixas AL, de Moraes JR: Analysis of 200 lymphadenectomies in patients with penile carcinoma. J Urol 146:330–332, 1991.
20. Adeyoju AB, Thornhill J, Corr J, et al: Prognostic factors in squamous cell carcinoma of the penis and implications for management. Br J Urol 80:937–939, 1997.
21. McDougal WS: Carcinoma of the penis: improved survival by early regional lymphadenectomy based on the histologic grade and depth of invasion of the primary lesion. J Urol 154:1364–1366, 1995.
22. Pizzocaro G, Piva L, Bandieramonte G, et al: Up-to-date management of carcinoma of the penis. Eur Urol 32:5–15, 1997.
23. Sarin R, Norman AR, Steel GG, et al: Treatment results and prognostic factors in 101 men treated for squamous carcinoma of the penis. Int J Radiat Oncol Biol Phys 38:713–722, 1997.
24. Soria JC, Fizazi K, Piron D, et al: Squamous cell carcinoma of the penis: multivariate analysis of prognostic factors and natural history in a monocentric study with a conservative policy. Ann Oncol 8:1089–1098, 1997.
25. Theodorescu D, Russo P, Zhang S-F, et al: Outcomes of initial surveillance of invasive squamous cell carcinoma of the penis and negative nodes. J Urol 155:1626–1631, 1996.
26. Greenlee RT, Murray T, Bolden S, et al: Cancer statistics, 2000. CA Cancer J Clin 50:7–33, 2000.
27. Maden C, Sherman KJ, Beckman AM: History of circumcision, medical conditions and sexual activity and risk of penile cancer. J Natl Cancer Inst 85:19–24, 1993.
28. Brinton LA, Li JY, Rong SD, et al: Risk factors for penile cancer: results from a case-control study in China. Int J Cancer 47:504–509, 1991.
29. Sarkar FH, Miles BJ, Plieth DM, et al: Detection of human papillomavirus in squamous neoplasm of the penis. J Urol 147:389–392, 1992.
30. Wiener JS, Effert PJ, Humphrey PA, et al: Prevalence of human papillomavirus types 16 and 18 in squamous cell carcinoma of the penis: a retrospective analysis of primary and metastatic lesions by differential polymerase chain reaction. Int J Cancer 50:694–701, 1992.
31. Stern RS: Genital tumors among men with psoriasis exposed to psoralens and ultraviolet A radiation (PUVA) and ultraviolet B radiation. The Photochemotherapy Follow-up Study. N Engl J Med 322:1093–1097, 1990.
32. Fraley EE, Zhang G, Sazama R, et al: Cancer of the penis. Prognosis and treatment plans. Cancer 41:24–29, 1985.
33. Burgers JK, Badalament RA, Drago JR: Penile cancer: clinical presentation, diagnosis, and staging. Urol Clin North Am 19:247–256, 1992.
34. Jones WG, Fossa SD, Hamers H, et al: Penis cancer: a review by the joint radiotherapy committee of the European Organization for Research and Treatment of Cancer (EORTC) Genitourinary and Radiotherapy groups. J Surg Oncol 52:50–55, 1989.
35. Narayana AS, Olney LE, Loening SA, et al: Carcinoma of the penis. Analysis of 219 cases. Cancer 49:2185–2191, 1982.
36. Sufrin G, Huben R: Benign and malignant lesions of the penis. *In* Gillenwater JY, Grayhack JT, Howards SS, et al (eds): Adult and Pediatric Urology. Chicago, Year Book Medical, 1987, pp 1448–1483.
37. Cubilla AL, Barreto JE, Caballero C, et al: Pathologic features of epidermoid carcinomas of the penis. A prospective study of 66 cases. Am J Surg Pathol 17:753–763, 1993.
38. Cubilla AL, Velazquez E, Reuter V, et al: Warty (condylomatous) squamous cell carcinoma of the penis. Am J Surg Pathol 24:505–512, 2000.

39. Johnson DE, Lo RK, Srigley J, et al: Verrucous carcinoma of the penis. J Urol 133:216–218, 1985.

40. Masih AS, Stoler MH, Farrow GM, et al: Penile verrucous carcinoma: a clinicopathologic, human papillomavirus typing and flow cytometric analysis. Mod Pathol 5:48–55, 1992.

41. Kraus FT, Perez-Mesa C: Verrucous carcinoma: clinical and pathologic study of 105 cases involving oral cavity, larynx and genitalia. Cancer 19:26–38, 1966.

42. Robertson DI, Maung R, Duggan MA: Verrucous carcinoma of the genital tract: is it a distinct entity? Can J Surg 36:147–151, 1993.

43. Cubilla AL, Reuter VE, Gregoire L, et al: Basaloid squamous cell carcinoma of the penis: a distinctive human papilloma virus–related penile neoplasm: a report of 20 cases. Am J Surg Pathol 22:755–761, 1998.

44. Wood EW, Gardner WA, Brown FM: Spindle cell squamous carcinoma of the penis. J Urol 107:590–591, 1972.

45. Manglani KS, Manaligod JR, Ray B: Spindle cell carcinoma of the glans penis: a light and electron microscopic study. Cancer 46:2267–2272, 1980.

46. Horenblas S, van Tinteren H, Delemarre JFM, et al: Squamous cell carcinoma of the penis. III. Treatment of regional lymph nodes. J Urol 149:492–497, 1993.

47. Srinivas V, Joshi A, Agarwal B, et al: Penile cancer—the sentinel lymph node controversy. Urol Int 47:108–109, 1991.

48. Young MJ, Reda DJ, Waters WB: Penile carcinoma: a twenty-five year experience. Urology 38:529–532, 1991.

49. Johnson DE, Fuerst DE, Ayala AG: Cancer of the penis: experience with 153 cases. Urology 1:404–408, 1973.

50. Penis. AJCC Manual for Staging Cancer. 5th ed. Philadelphia, Lippincott-Raven, 1997, pp 215–217.

51. Jackson SM: The treatment of carcinoma of the penis. Br J Surg 53:33–35, 1966.

52. Maiche AG, Pyrhonen S, Karkinen M: Histological grading of squamous cell carcinoma of the penis: a new scoring system. Br J Urol 67:522–526, 1991.

53. Goldminz D, Scott G, Klaus S: Penile basal cell carcinoma. Report of a case and review of the literature. J Am Acad Dermatol 20:1094–1097, 1989.

54. McGregor DH, Tanimura A, Weigel JW: Basal cell carcinoma of penis. Urology 20:320–323, 1982.

55. Mitsudo S, Nakanishi I, Koss L: Paget's disease of the penis and adjacent skin. Its association with fatal sweat gland carcinoma. Arch Pathol Lab Med 105:518–520, 1981.

56. Helwig EB, Graham JH: Anogenital extramammary Paget's disease. A clinicopathological study. Cancer 16:387–403, 1963.

57. Johnson DE, Ayala AG: Primary melanoma of the penis. Urology 2:174–177, 1973.

58. Oldbring J, Mikulowski P: Malignant melanoma of the penis and male urethra. Report of nine cases and review of the literature. Cancer 59:581–587, 1987.

59. Barnhill RL, Albert LS, Shama SK, et al: Genital lentiginosis: a clinical and histopathologic study. J Am Acad Dermatol 22:453–460, 1990.

60. Saw D, Tse CH, Chan J, et al: Clear cell sarcoma of the penis. Hum Pathol 17:423–425, 1986.

61. Dehner LP, Smith BH: Soft tissue tumors of the penis. A clinicopathologic study of 46 cases. Cancer 25:1431–1447, 1970.

62. Lowe FC, Lattimer G, Metroka CE: Kaposi's sarcoma of the penis in patients with acquired immunodeficiency syndrome. J Urol 142:1475–1477, 1989.

63. Rasbridge SA, Parry JRW: Angiosarcoma of the penis. Br J Urol 63:440–441, 1989.

64. Weiss SW, Enzinger FM: Epithelioid hemangioendothelioma: a vascular tumor often mistaken for a carcinoma. Cancer 50:970–981, 1992.

65. Isa SS, Almaraz R, Magovern J: Leiomyosarcoma of the penis. Case report and review of the literature. Cancer 54:939–942, 1984.

66. Dalkin B, Zaontz MR: Rhabdomyosarcoma of the penis in children. J Urol 141:908–909, 1989.

67. Wilson LS, Lockhart JL, Bergman H, et al: Fibrosarcoma of the penis. Case report and review of the literature. J Urol 129:606–607, 1983.

68. Huang DJ, Stanisic TH, Hansen KK: Epithelioid sarcoma of the penis. J Urol 147:1370–1372, 1992.

69. Philip AT, Amin MB, Cubilla AL, et al: Secondary tumors of the penis: a study of 16 cases. Mod Pathol 12:104A, 1999.

70. Powell BL, Craig JB, Muss HB: Secondary malignancies of the penis and epididymis: a case report and review of the literature. J Clin Oncol 3:110–116, 1985.

71. Powell FC, Venencie PY, Winkelmann RK: Metastatic prostate carcinoma manifesting as penile nodules. Arch Dermatol 20:1604–1606, 1984.

72. Barrasso R, De Brux J, Croissant O, et al: High prevalence of papilloma virus–associated penile intraepithelial neoplasia in sexual partners of women with cervical intraepithelial neoplasia. N Engl J Med 317:916–923, 1987.

73. Nuovo GJ, Hochman HA, Eliezri HA, et al: Detection of human papillomavirus DNA in penile lesions histologically negative for condylomata. Analysis by in-situ hybridization and the polymerase chain reaction. Am J Surg Pathol 14:829–836, 1990.

74. O'Brien WM, Jenson AB, Lancaster WD, et al: Human papillomavirus typing of penile condyloma. J Urol 141:863–865, 1989.

75. Ananthakrishnan N, Ravindran R, Veliath AJ, et al: Lowenstein-Buschke tumor of penis: a carcinoma mimic. Br J Urol 53:460–465, 1981.

76. Jeerapaet P, Ackerman AB: Histologic patterns of secondary syphilis. Arch Dermatol 107:373–377, 1973.

77. Hay PE, Tam FW, Kitchen VS, et al: Gummatous lesions in men infected with human immunodeficiency virus and syphilis. Genitourin Med 66:374–379, 1990.

78. Davis CM: Granuloma inguinale: a clinical, histological and ultrastructural study. JAMA 211:632–636, 1970.

79. Smith MJ, Custer RP: The histopathology of lymphogranuloma venereum. J Urol 63:546–563, 1950.

80. McCarley ME, Cruz PD Jr, Sontheimer RD: Chancroid: clinical variants from an epidemic in Dallas County 1986–1987. J Am Acad Dermatol 19:330–337, 1988.

81. Oriel JD: Natural history of genital warts. Br J Vener Dis 47:1–13, 1971.

82. Vohra S, Badlani G: Balanitis and balanoposthitis. Urol Clin North Am 19:143–147, 1992.

83. Davis DA, Cohen PR: Balanitis circumscripta plasmacellularis. J Urol 153:424–426, 1995.

84. Ridley CM: Lichen sclerosus et atrophicus. Arch Dermatol 20:567–570, 1989.

85. Oertel YC, Johnson FB: Sclerosing lipogranuloma of male genitalia. Review of 23 cases. Arch Pathol 101:321–326, 1977.

86. Cuozzo DW, Vachher P, San P, et al: Verruciform xanthoma: a benign penile growth. J Urol 153:1625–1627, 1995.

87. Thambi Dorai CR, Kandasami P: Fournier's gangrene: its aetiology and management. Aust N Z J Surg 61:370–372, 1991.

88. Skoog SJ, Belman AB: Aphallia: its classification and management. J Urol 141:589–592, 1989.

89. Diamond DA, Ransley PG: Male epispadias. J Urol 154:2150–2155, 1995.

90. Duckett JW: Hypospadias. In Walsh PC, Retik AB, Vaughan ED Jr, et al (eds): Campbell's Urology. 7th ed. Philadelphia, WB Saunders, 1998, pp 2093–2116.

91. Hollowell JG, Witherington R, Ballagas AJ, et al: Embryologic considerations of diphallus and associated anomalies. J Urol 117:728–732, 1977.

92. Lee PA, Mazur T, Danish R, et al: Micropenis: I. Criteria, etiologies and classification. Johns Hopkins Med J 146:156–163, 1980.

93. Cohen-Addad N, Zarafu IW, Hanna MK: Complete penoscrotal transposition. Urology 26:149–152, 1985.

94. Marizels M, Zaontz M, Donovan J, et al: Surgical correction of the buried penis: description of a classification system and technique to correct the diagnosis. J Urol 136:268–271, 1986.

95. Cole LA, Helwig EB: Mucoid cysts of the penile skin. J Urol 115:397–400, 1976.

96. Golitz LE, Robin M: Median raphe canals of the penis. Cutis 27:170–172, 1981.

97. Enzinger FM, Weiss SW: Fibromatoses. In Enzinger FM,

Weiss SW (eds): Soft Tissue Tumors. 3rd ed. St. Louis, Mosby, 1995, pp 207–209.

98. Jordan GH, Schlossberg SM, Devine CJ: Surgery of the penis and urethra. In Walsh PC, Retik AB, Vaughan ED Jr, et al (eds): Campbell's Urology. 7th ed. Philadelphia, WB Saunders, 1998, pp 3330–3331.

99. Kaplan GW, Brock WA: The etiology of chordee. Urol Clin North Am 8:383–387, 1981.

100. Nielsen GP, Pilch BZ, Black-Schaffer WS, et al: Wegener's granulomatosis of the penis clinically simulating carcinoma. Report of a case. J Urol Pathol 4:265–272, 1996.

101. Gilmore WA, Weigand DA, Burgdorf WHC: Penile nodules in Southeast Asian men. Arch Dermatol 119:446–447, 1983.

102. Sarma DP, Weilbaecher TG: Human os penis. Urology 35:349–350, 1990.

103. Hassan AA, Orteza AM, Milam DF: Penile horn: review of the literature with 3 case reports. J Urol 97:315–317, 1967.

104. Vitenson JH, Wilson JM: Sarcoid of the glans penis. J Urol 108:284–286, 1972.

105. Walker D, Jordan WP: Tuberculous ulcer of the penis. J Urol 100:36–37, 1968.

106. Alter GJ, Trangove-Jones G, Horton CEJ: Hemangioma of penis and scrotum. Urology 42:205–208, 1993.

107. Imperial R, Helwig EB: Angiokeratoma of the scrotum (Fordyce type). J Urol 98:379–387, 1967.

108. Hagiwara K, Toyama K, Miyazato H, et al: A case of acquired lymphangioma due to a suspected old filariasis and review of literature. J Dermatol 21:358–362, 1994.

109. Newman PL, Fletcher CDM: Smooth muscle tumours of the external genitalia: clinicopathological analysis of a series. Histopathology 18:523–529, 1991.

110. Fernandez MJ, Martino A, Khan H, et al: Giant neurilemoma: unusual scrotal mass. Urology 30:74–76, 1987.

111. Goulding FJ, Traylor RA: Juvenile xanthogranuloma of the scrotum. J Urol 129:841–842, 1983.

112. Brock JWD, Jones C: Infantile fibromatosis of the external genitalia: diagnosis and management strategy. J Urol 149:357–358, 1993.

113. Tsang WY, Chan JK, Lee KC, et al: Aggressive angiomyxoma occurring in men. Am J Surg Pathol 16:1059–1065, 1992.

114. Dymock R, Allen PW, Gilbert EF: Giant cell fibroblastoma. A distinctive, recurrent tumor of childhood. Am J Surg Pathol 11:263–271, 1987.

115. Passey RD: Experimental soot cancer. Br Med J 2:1112, 1922.

116. Weinstein AL, Howe HL, Burnett WS: Sentinel health event surveillance: skin cancer of the scrotum in New York State. Am J Public Health 79:1513–1515, 1989.

117. Pott P: Cancer Scroti. In Hawes L, Clarke W, Collins R (eds): Chirurgical Observations Relative to the Cataract, the Polypus of the Nose, the Cancer of the Scrotum, the Different Kinds of Ruptures and the Mortification of Toes and Feet. London, Longerman, 1775, p 63.

118. Lee WR: Occupational aspects of scrotal cancer and epithelioma. Ann N Y Acad Sci 271:138–142, 1976.

119. Andrews PE, Farrow GM, Oesterling JE: Squamous cell carcinoma of the scrotum: long-term follow-up of 14 patients. J Urol 146:1299–1304, 1991.

120. Lowe FC: Squamous cell carcinoma of the scrotum. Urol Clin North Am 19:397–405, 1992.

121. Ray B, Whitmore WF: Experience with carcinoma of the scrotum. J Urol 117:741–745, 1977.

122. Lopez AE, Aliaga RM, Martinez MJ, et al: Scrotal verrucous carcinoma. Actas Urol Esp 19:169–173, 1995.

123. Roush GC, Kelly JA, Meigs JW, et al: Scrotal carcinoma in Connecticut metal workers. Am J Epidemiol 116:78–85, 1982.

124. Nahass GT, Blauvelt A, Leonardi CL, et al: Basal cell carcinoma of the scrotum: report of three cases and review of the literature. J Am Acad Dermatol 26:574–578, 1992.

125. Payne WG, Wells KE: Extramammary Paget's disease of the scrotum. Ann Plast Surg 33:669–671, 1994.

126. Best TJ, Metcalfe JB, Moore RB, et al: Merkel cell carcinoma of the scrotum. Ann Plast Surg 33:83–85, 1994.

127. Lissmer L, Kaneti J, Klain J, et al: Liposarcoma of the perineum and scrotum. Int Urol Nephrol 24:205–210, 1992.

128. Konety BR, Campanella SC, Hakam A, et al: Malignant fibrous histiocytoma of the scrotum. J Urol Pathol 5:51–55, 1996.

129. Lane D: Fibrosarcoma of the scrotum. Aust N Z J Surg 28:139, 1958.

130. Peters KM, Gonzalez JA: Malignant peripheral nerve sheath tumor of the scrotum: a case report. J Urol 155:649–650, 1996.

131. Vyas S, Manabe T, Herman JR, et al: Kaposi's sarcoma of scrotum. Urology 8:82–85, 1976.

132. Davis NS, Kim CA, Dever DP: Primary malignant melanoma of the scrotum: case report and literature review. J Urol 145:1056–1057, 1991.

133. Shetty MR, Khan F: Carcinoma of the rectum with scrotal metastases. Br J Urol 62:612, 1988.

134. Manson-Bahr PE, Apted FI: Filariasis. In Masson's Tropical Diseases. 18th ed. London, Baillière Tindall, 1983, pp 148–180.

135. Mohsin SK, Lee MW, Amin MB, et al: Cutaneous verruciform xanthoma: a report of five cases investigating the etiology and nature of xanthomatous cells. Am J Surg Pathol 22:479–487, 1998.

136. Hollander JB, Begun FP, Lee RD: Scrotal fat necrosis. J Urol 134:150–151, 1985.

137. Elder JS, Jeffs RD: Suprainguinal ectopic scrotum and associated anomalies. J Urol 127:336–338, 1982.

138. Sule JD, Skoog SJ, Tank ES: Perineal lipoma and the accessory labioscrotal fold: an etiological relationship. J Urol 151:475–477, 1994.

139. Popek EJ, Montgomery EA, Fourcroy JL: Fibrous hamartoma of infancy in the genital region: findings in 15 cases. J Urol 152:990–993, 1994.

140. Urbanek RW, Johnson WC: Smooth muscle hamartoma associated with Becker's nevus. Arch Dermatol 114:104–106, 1978.

141. Michl UH, Gross AJ, Loy V, et al: Idiopathic calcinosis of the scrotum—a specific entity of the scrotal skin. Scand J Urol Nephrol 28:213–217, 1994.

# Testis and Paratestis Including Spermatic Cord

Satish K. Tickoo   Pheroze Tamboli
Nancy E. Warner   Mahul B. Amin

Testicular cancer is relatively rare, accounting for less than 1% of malignant neoplasms affecting men.[1] Between 1990 and 1997, the annual incidence of testicular cancer in the United States was 2.9 per 100,000 among white men and approximately 0.8 per 100,000 among African American men.[2] The incidence varies according to geographic area; it is highest in Switzerland, Scandinavian countries, Germany, and New Zealand; intermediate in the United States; and lowest in Asia and Africa. In 2001, ap-

**TABLE 34–1.** Classification of Testicular and Paratesticular Tumors and Tumor-Like Lesions

***Germ cell tumors***
Precursor lesions
  Intratubular germ cell neoplasia, unclassified
  Intratubular germ cell neoplasia, specific types
Germ cell tumors of one histologic type
  Seminoma
    Variant: with syncytiotrophoblastic cells
  Spermatocytic seminoma
    Variants: with sarcomatous component; anaplastic type
  Embryonal carcinoma
  Yolk sac tumor (endodermal sinus tumor)
  Trophoblastic tumors
    Choriocarcinoma
    Placental site trophoblastic tumor
    Unclassified
  Teratoma
    Mature teratoma
      Variant: dermoid cyst
    Immature teratoma
    Teratoma with a secondary malignant component (specify)
    Monodermal teratoma
      Carcinoid
      Primitive neuroectodermal tumor
      Others
Germ cell tumors of more than one histologic type
  Mixed germ cell tumors (specify individual component and estimate its amount as percentage of the tumor)
  Polyembryoma
  Diffuse embryoma
Regressed ("burnt-out") germ cell tumors
  Scar only
  Scar with intratubular germ cell neoplasia
  Scar with minor residual germ cell tumor (teratoma, seminoma, or other)
***Sex cord–stromal tumors***
Sertoli–stromal cell tumors
  Sertoli cell tumor
    Variants: large cell calcifying; sclerosing
  Sertoli-Leydig cell tumor
  Leydig cell tumor
Granulosa–stromal cell tumors
  Granulosa cell tumor
    Types: adult; juvenile
Tumors in the fibroma-thecoma group
Mixed
Unclassified
Mixed germ cell–sex cord–stromal tumors
Gonadoblastoma
Unclassified
***Tumors of the rete testis***
Adenoma, adenofibroma, cystadenoma
Carcinoma
Miscellaneous (including unclassified tumors and tumors of uncertain cell type)
***Paratesticular tumors (including tumors of spermatic cord)***
Tumors of ovarian epithelial type
Adenomatoid tumor
Malignant mesothelioma
Desmoplastic small round cell tumor
Epididymal cystadenoma
Epididymal carcinoma
Melanotic neuroectodermal tumor (retinal anlage tumor)

Benign (or locally aggressive) soft tissue-type tumors
  Fibromatous tumors
  Vascular tumors
  Aggressive angiomyxoma
  Angiomyofibroblastoma
  Calcifying fibrous pseudotumor
  Others
Malignant soft tissue–type tumors
  Rhabdomyosarcoma
    Embryonal
      Variant: spindle cell
    Alveolar
    Others
  Liposarcoma
    Well-differentiated
    Pleomorphic/round cell
    Others
  Leiomyosarcoma
  Others
  Miscellaneous
***Hematopoietic tumors***
  Lymphoma
  Plasmacytoma
  Leukemia and granulocytic sarcoma
Secondary tumors
Tumor-like lesions
  Leydig cell hyperplasia
  Sertoli cell nodules
  Testicular tumor of the adrenogenital syndrome
  Seroid cell nodules with other disorders
  Adrenal cortical rests
  Torsion/infarct (of testis, of appendix testis, of appendix epididymis)
  Hematoma/hematocele
  Testicular appendages and Walthard nests
***Orchitis/epididymitis***
Infectious (bacterial, viral, granulomatous)
  Idiopathic granulomatous
  Granulomatous epididymitis
  Sarcoidosis
  Malakoplakia
***Rosai-Dorfman disease (sinus histiocytosis with massive lymphadenopathy)***
***Hydrocele-related changes***
***Inflammatory pseudotumor (proliferative funiculitis)***
***Fibrous pseudotumor***
***Meconium periorchitis***
***Mesothelial hyperplasia***
***Sclerosing lipogranuloma***
***Abnormalities related to sexual precocity***
***Idiopathic hypertrophy***
***Hyperplasia of the rete testis***
***Epidermoid cyst***
***Other cysts (parenchymal, rete, of tunics, epididymal)***
***Cystic dysplasia***
***Microlithiasis***
***Spermatocele***
***Sperm granuloma***
***Vasitis nodosa***
***Splenic-gonadal fusion***
***Others***

From Ulbright TM, Amin MB, Young RH: Tumors of the Testis, Adnexa, Spermatic Cord and Scrotum. Atlas of Tumor Pathology. Third Series, Fascicle 25. Washington, DC, Armed Forces Institute of Pathology, 1999.

proximately 7200 new cases were expected to be diagnosed in the United States.[2a] Most testicular tumors (>90%) are of germ cell origin, and most of these affect young men between the ages of 15 and 34 years.[3] A second peak in testicular cancers occurs in men between 80 and 90 years old, with metastasis being the most common tumor at that age. Since the 1970s, the availability of cisplatin-based chemotherapy has resulted in dramatic improvement in cure rates and survival among patients with testicular germ cell tumors.[4] More than 90% of men diagnosed with germ cell tumors are cured, and overall 5-year survival rates exceed 95%.[2] A wide range of non-neoplastic conditions also affect the testis, often presenting as space-occupying or mass lesions. Because radical orchiectomy is performed almost axiomatically for any testicular mass, non-neoplastic processes are encountered frequently in orchiectomy specimens.

## CLASSIFICATION

The list of testicular tumors and tumor-like conditions is exhaustive (Table 34–1). Table 34–2 lists the numerous classification systems that have been pro-

posed and used; the Third Series Armed Forces Institute of Pathology fascicle presents a modified and updated classification system that is clinically applicable (see under "treatment and prognosis," further on). Each classification system has been built on the previous system and is based primarily on the pioneering work of several early investigators, including Friedman and Moore,[5] Dixon and Moore,[6] Melicow,[7] and Mostofi and Price.[8] Another classification system proposed by the British Testicular Tumor Panel (BTTP) is used frequently in Europe and is based on the work of Collins and Pugh.[9] In the BTTP classification system, tumors are classified as seminoma or teratoma, with the latter divided into undifferentiated, intermediate, and trophoblastic. The Armed Forces Institute of Pathology classification is used widely in the United States and many other parts of the world and is preferred over the BTTP system for two reasons: 1) The BTTP system groups together different germ cell tumor subtypes that have potentially different biologic behavior (e.g., *malignant teratoma, intermediate*, includes teratoma and embryonal carcinoma, teratoma and yolk sac tumor, and teratoma with sarcomatous or carcinomatous components), and 2) the histologic categories in the BTTP system do not correlate with serum

**TABLE 34–2.** Comparison of Various Classification Schemes for Testicular Germ Cell Tumors

| AFIP (1999) | Mostofi (1980) | WHO (1977) | British Testicular Tumor Panel (Pugh, 1976) | Dixon & Moore (1952) |
|---|---|---|---|---|
| Seminoma | Seminoma | Seminoma | Seminoma | Group I seminoma |
| Spermatocytic seminoma | Spermatocytic seminoma | Spermatocytic seminoma | Spermatocytic seminoma | Not listed |
| Embryonal carcinoma | Embryonal carcinoma, adult type | Embryonal carcinoma | Malignant teratoma, undifferentiated | Group II embryonal carcinoma |
| Yolk sac tumor | Infantile embryonal carcinoma | Yolk sac tumor (endodermal sinus tumor) | Yolk sac tumor in children (orchioblastoma) | Not listed |
| Polyembryoma | Polyembryoma | Polyembryoma | Not listed | Not listed |
| Choriocarcinoma | Choriocarcinoma, pure | Choriocarcinoma, pure | Malignant teratoma, trophoblastic | Group V choriocarcinoma |
| Placental site trophoblastic tumor | | | | |
| Teratoma Mature Immature Monodermal | Teratoma Mature Immature | Teratoma Mature Immature | Teratoma, differentiated | Group III teratoma, pure ± seminoma |
| Teratoma with secondary malignant component (specify) | Teratoma with malignant areas other than S, EC, C* | Teratoma with malignant transformation | Malignant teratoma, intermediate | Group IV teratoma, with EC and/or C ± seminoma |
| Mixed germ cell tumor (specify components) | Embryonal carcinoma and teratoma (teratocarcinoma) | Embryonal carcinoma and teratoma (teratocarcinoma) | Malignant teratoma, intermediate | Group IV teratoma with EC and/or C ± seminoma |
| | Specify tumor type | Choriocarcinoma and other type | Malignant teratoma, trophoblastic | Group V choriocarcinoma with S and/or EC |
| | Specify tumor type | Other combinations | Combination tumors | Not listed |

* S, seminoma; EC, embryonal carcinoma; C, choriocarcinoma.
Adapted from Ro JY, Amin MB, Sahin AA, Ayala AG: Tumors and tumorous conditions of the male genital tract. Part B. Testicular neoplasms. *In* Fletcher CDM (ed): Diagnostic Histopathology of Tumors. 2nd ed. London, Churchill Livingstone, 2000, pp 733–838.

tumor markers that have become the cornerstone of management of testicular germ cell tumors in terms of monitoring of the disease and response to therapy.

## GERM CELL TUMORS

### General Considerations

The cause of germ cell tumors in most cases is unknown. Some of the known risk factors are discussed.

#### CRYPTORCHIDISM

Cryptorchidism is one of the best-established risk factors,[10] with approximately 3.5 to 5 times elevated risk of development of a testicular germ cell tumor compared with control populations,[11, 12] most commonly seminoma.[13] Testicular biopsies have been recommended in these high-risk patients to detect incipient neoplasia.[14] In a large series, only 1 of more than 1500 cryptorchid patients with testicular biopsy specimens that were negative for intratubular germ cell neoplasia developed testicular cancer over a follow-up period of 8 years,[14] in contrast to 50% of patients with intratubular germ cell neoplasia who developed invasive germ cell tumors over a 5-year period.[15]

#### FAMILIAL PREDISPOSITION

Familial basis and clustering among siblings have been reported in approximately 2% of first-degree male relatives of patients with testicular germ cell tumors.[16-18]

#### GERM CELL TUMOR IN CONTRALATERAL TESTIS

Patients with prior or current germ cell tumor are at a higher risk of having a concurrent or developing a metachronous tumor in the remaining testis. Approximately 1.9% to 5% of patients with germ cell tumor develop bilateral disease,[19-21] with an even greater risk if the second testis is cryptorchid or atrophic.[22, 23] Some urologists recommend a biopsy of the opposite testis at the time of initial orchiectomy.[24] In the United States, most urologists do not perform a contralateral biopsy because the finding of intratubular germ cell neoplasia in the opposite testis does not alter the overall management at that time and because regular follow-up would detect an invasive tumor at an early stage.

#### GONADAL DYSGENESIS AND ANDROGEN INSENSITIVITY SYNDROME

An approximately 30% risk of germ cell tumors is observed in men with gonadal dysgenesis who carry a Y chromosome.[25] Gonadoblastoma is the most frequent tumor type arising in this setting, and its presence predisposes to the development of invasive germ cell tumors, most commonly seminoma. Of patients with androgen insensitivity syndrome, 5% to 10% develop germ cell tumors. These tumors generally are diagnosed after the complete development of female secondary sexual characteristics.[26, 27]

#### INFERTILITY

The extent of increased risk of germ cell tumors in cases of male infertility is not clear. Because many cases are associated with cryptorchidism or gonadal dysgenesis, it is difficult to judge whether infertility itself is an independent risk factor. The frequency of intratubular germ cell neoplasia in subfertile men has been reported to be 0.4% to 1.1%.[22, 28]

### Histogenesis

The traditional model of histogenesis depicted germ cell tumors arising from the germ cell by two divergent pathways, one leading to terminally differentiated seminoma and the other to embryonal carcinoma, which subsequently could differentiate into all other nonseminomatous components. More recent evidence indicates, however, that seminoma is not terminally differentiated and may act as the precursor for many, if not all, nonseminomatous tumors. Evidence for such an alternative hypothesis includes 1) early carcinomatous differentiation in some cases of seminoma detected by ultrastructural evaluation,[29] 2) the finding of nonseminomatous elements at autopsy in patients dying of progressive tumors after treatment for pure testicular seminoma,[30, 31] 3) focal expression of immunohistochemical markers and blood-group antigens that are characteristic of embryonal carcinoma or yolk sac tumor in some cases of seminoma,[32, 33] and 4) presence of alpha-fetoprotein (AFP) mRNA detected by in situ hybridization in cases of typical seminoma with normal serum AFP levels.[34] Finally, it has been shown that most seminomas, but not embryonal carcinomas or yolk sac tumors, express c-kit protein (CD117).[35] However, seminomas with high clinical stage or atypical cytologic features often fail to express c-kit protein suggesting that such tumors may represent an early carcinomatous transition in seminoma.[36] Figure 34–1 shows the currently accepted tetrahedron histogenetic model of testicular germ cell neoplasia.

### Tumor Staging

Staging systems for testicular tumors are based predominantly on the initial work of Boden and Gibb.[37] Over the years, there have been multiple modifications by many of the major institutions treating testicular cancer. This situation has led to lack of standardized staging and different management protocols. The American Joint Committee on Cancer and the Union Internationale Contre le Cancer tumor-node-metastasis (TNM) system of classification

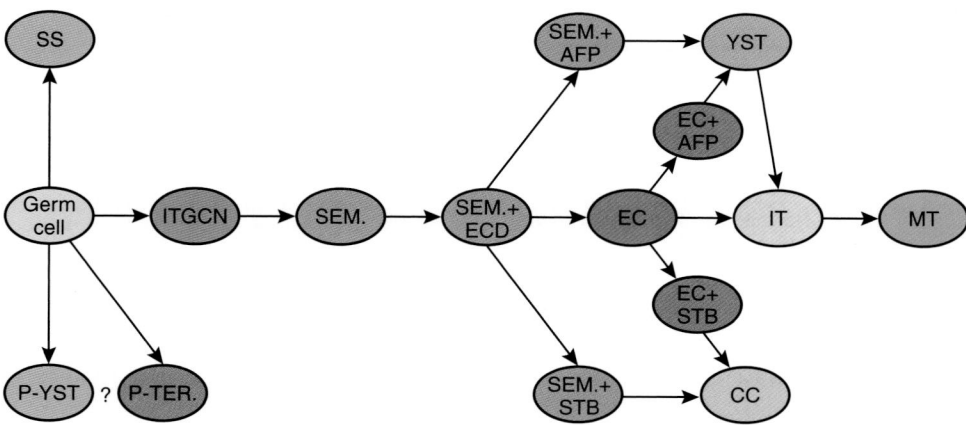

**FIGURE 34–1.** Modified model of histogenesis of testicular germ cell tumors. (SS-spermatocytic seminoma; P-YST-pediatric yolk sac tumor; P-TER.-pediatric teratoma; ITGCN-intratubular germ cell neoplasia; SEM.-seminoma; ECD-early carcinomatous differentiation; AFP-α-fetoprotein; STB-syncytiotrophoblasts; EC-embryonal carcinoma; IT-immature teratoma; MT-mature teratoma; YST-postpubertal yolk sac tumor; CC-choriocarcinoma). Adapted with permission from reference 65.

is an attempt to bring uniformity to the staging.[38] In the 1997 TNM classification, prognostically important factors, such as vascular invasion and tumor serum markers, were incorporated for the first time in the staging for any organ system (Table 34–3).

## Serum Tumor Markers

Serum tumor marker levels in germ cell tumors provide a simple, accurate, and reliable means for prognostication, evaluation of treatment adequacy, and monitoring relapses.[39, 40] The commonly used serum markers are AFP, β subunit of human chorionic gonadotropin (β-HCG), and lactate dehydrogenase isoenzyme 1. These markers are used in stratification of patients with clinical stage I disease for predicting occult metastasis and recurrent disease. In patients with metastatic disease, the levels of these markers provide prognostic information and indication of tumor burden.

AFP production is restricted to nonseminomatous germ cell tumors (Table 34–4), specifically yolk sac tumor. The presence of elevated serum AFP in seminomas may indicate a morphologically unrecognized nonseminomatous component in the testis, ev-

**TABLE 34–3.** AJCC and UICC Staging System for Testicular Cancer*

| TNM System (AJCC and UICC) | | Stage Grouping for AJCC and UICC System | |
|---|---|---|---|
| pTx | Unknown status of testis | Stage 0 | Tis, N0, M0, S0 |
| pT0 | No apparent primary (includes scars) | Stage IA | T1, N0, M0, S0 |
| pTis | Intratubular tumor, no invasion | Stage IB | T2–T4, N0, M0, S0 |
| pT1 | Testis and epididymis only; no vascular invasion | Stage IS | any T, N0, M0, S1–S3 |
| pT2 | Testis and epididymis with vascular invasion or through tunica albuginea to involve tunica vaginalis | Stage IIA | any T, N1, M0, S0–S1 |
| | | Stage IIB | any T, N2, M0, S0–S1 |
| pT3 | Spermatic cord | Stage IIC | any T, N3, M0, S0–S1 |
| pT4 | Scrotum | Stage IIIA | any T, any N, M1a, S0–S1 |
| | | Stage IIIB | any T, any N, M0–M1a, S2 |
| pNx | Unknown nodal status | Stage IIIC | any T, any N, M1a, S3 |
| pN0 | No regional node involvement | | any T, any N, M1b, any S |
| pN1 | Node mass or single nodes ≤2 cm; ≤5 nodes involved (no node >2 cm) | | |
| pN2 | Node mass >2 but <5 cm; or >5 nodes involved, none >5 cm; or extranodal tumor | | |
| pN3 | Node mass >5 cm | | |
| Mx | Unknown status of distant metastases | | |
| M0 | No distant metastases | | |
| M1a | Nonregional nodal or lung metastases | | |
| M1b | Distant metastasis other than nonregional nodal or lung | | |
| SX | No marker studies available | | |
| S0 | All marker levels normal | | |

| | LDH† | | β-HCG (mIU/mL) | | AFP (ng/mL) |
|---|---|---|---|---|---|
| S1 | <1.5 × N | and | <5000 | and | <1000 |
| S2 | 1.5–10 × N | or | 5000–50,000 | or | 1000–10,000 |
| S3 | >10 × N | or | >50,000 | or | >10,000 |

* AJCC, American Joint Committee on Cancer; UICC, Union Internationale Contre le Cancer.
† LDH, lactate dehydrogenase; N, normal value for assay.

**TABLE 34–4.** Serum Tumor Markers in Germ Cell Tumors

Typical seminoma
| | |
|---|---|
| LDH | Usually elevated, particularly in advanced disease |
| PLAP | Usually elevated |
| β-HCG | Normal to mildly elevated in some cases, owing to syncytiotrophoblasts |
| AFP | Normal; rarely minimal elevation |

Embryonal carcinoma
| | |
|---|---|
| LDH | Usually elevated, particularly in advanced disease |
| PLAP | Usually elevated |
| β-HCG | Normal to mildly elevated in some cases, owing to syncytiotrophoblasts |
| AFP | Normal; rarely minimal elevation |

Yolk sac tumor
| | |
|---|---|
| LDH | Usually elevated, particularly in advanced disease |
| PLAP | Usually elevated |
| β-HCG | Normal to mildly elevated in some cases, owing to syncytiotrophoblasts |
| AFP | Markedly elevated |

Choriocarcinoma
| | |
|---|---|
| LDH | Usually elevated, particularly in advanced disease |
| PLAP | Normal to mildly elevated |
| β-HCG | Markedly elevated |
| AFP | Normal |

Teratoma (pure)
| | |
|---|---|
| LDH | Normal to mildly elevated |
| PLAP | Usually elevated |
| β-HCG | Normal |
| AFP | Normal |

\* LDH, lactate dehydrogenase.

idence of early yolk sac tumor differentiation, or the presence of an occult metastasis, although some believe that low levels may be observed in pure seminomas.[41] Increased serum levels of β-HCG may be observed in choriocarcinomas or in any other germ cell tumor component that contains syncytiotrophoblastic giant cells, although the levels in the latter category are typically modest.

## Treatment and Prognosis

### INTRATUBULAR GERM CELL NEOPLASIA

Because progression to invasive tumor occurs in many cases, orchiectomy has been offered as a treatment option in patients with unilateral intratubular germ cell neoplasia, especially in patients with bilateral cryptorchidism, infertility, and ambiguous genitalia.[42] Low-dose radiation is an alternative mode of therapy, particularly for bilateral intratubular germ cell neoplasia.[42] Cisplatin-based chemotherapy may suppress intratubular germ cell neoplasia temporarily, but recurrence rates are high.[43] The prognosis for surgically treated cases, as expected, is excellent.

### SEMINOMA

After radical inguinal orchiectomy, most patients with stage I, IIA, and IIB disease are treated with radiation to retroperitoneal and ipsilateral pelvic lymph nodes. Cure rates exceeding 95% are expected (Table 34–5). Relapses occur in approximately 4% of patients with stage I disease and 10% with stage IIA or IIB disease.[44, 45] Subsequent chemotherapy after relapse cures more than 90% of these cases. Approximately 99% of cases with stages I, IIA, and IIB ultimately are cured.[3] Surveillance only may be another option for stage I seminoma,[46] although vascular invasion and large size (>6 cm) often are considered to be contraindications to this approach. With bulky retroperitoneal disease or supradiaphragmatic involvement, cisplatin-based chemotherapy is the preferred treatment. Disease-free survival rates exceeding 80% have been reported in such patients.[47]

### NONSEMINOMATOUS TUMORS

Nonseminomatous tumors include all germ cell tumors other than pure seminoma, either in pure form or in various combinations (with or without a classic seminoma component). Surveillance and nerve-sparing retroperitoneal lymph node dissection are the postorchiectomy options for stage I nonsemino-

**TABLE 34–5.** Commonly Used Management Strategies and Cure Rates for Testicular Germ Cell Tumors Postorchiectomy

| | Stage | | Treatment | Cure Rate (%) |
|---|---|---|---|---|
| Seminoma | I | | Radiation/surveillance | >95 |
| | II | Nonbulky | Radiation | >85 |
| | | Bulky\* | Chemotherapy | 80 |
| | III | | Chemotherapy | 80 |
| Nonseminomatous | I | Pathologically positive lymph nodes | RPLND†/surveillance Chemotherapy after RPLND | >95 |
| | II | Nonbulky | RPLND ± chemotherapy | 99 |
| | | Bulky | Chemotherapy, followed by RPLND | 80–90 |
| | III | | Chemotherapy, followed by RPLND | 70–80 |

\* >3 cm in diameter.
† RPLND, retroperitoneal lymph node dissection.

matous germ cell tumors. Approximately 20% of patients with clinical stage I disease (without angiolymphatic invasion or advanced local disease) are found to have lymph node involvement in the retroperitoneal lymph node dissection specimen.[3] If the lymph nodes are not involved by tumor, the patient is managed conservatively. If resected nodes are involved, management follows the principles for stage II disease. The strategy of surveillance is based on the premise that it is feasible to follow patients with nonseminomatous tumors by serum tumor markers, and if the patients relapse under observation, they can be treated effectively with chemotherapy. The presence of pure or extensive embryonal carcinoma and vascular invasion in the primary orchiectomy specimen usually are considered to be contraindications for surveillance alone.[48]

In stage II disease with a clinically small (<3 cm) retroperitoneal lymph node, retroperitoneal lymph node dissection is performed. On pathologic evaluation, if any positive node is found to be greater than 2 cm in size, or at least six lymph nodes are involved, or there is extranodal invasion, adjuvant chemotherapy generally is prescribed. Patients with stage IIC or III disease usually receive additional cisplatin-based chemotherapy. Patients with radiologic evidence of residual disease and normal serum markers after chemotherapy undergo surgical resection. About 45% of residual retroperitoneal masses exhibit necrosis or fibrosis alone on pathologic examination, and 40% have evidence of teratoma. A few masses still have viable nonteratomatous germ cell tumor, and these patients generally receive additional chemotherapy.[3]

## Genetics

Germ cell tumors nearly always are hyperdiploid and frequently are triploid or tetraploid.[49] Hyperdiploidy implies that chromosomal endoreduplication is an early event in germ cell transformation.[50] Germ cell tumors have at least one X and one Y chromosome, implying that transformation occurs in a germ cell before meiotic anaphase. Isochromosome of the short arm of chromosome 12, *i(12p)*, is a specific genetic marker of germ cell tumors, including intratubular germ cell neoplasia.[3, 50, 51] In the tumors not displaying i(12p), excess 12p genetic material has been found on marker chromosomes with aberrant banding, consisting of repetitive 12p segments.[3] Excess 12p genetic material is present in virtually all germ cell tumors and is believed to be one of the earliest genetic events in germ cell transformation. The i(12p) marker also is found in various malignant transformation components (somatic malignancies) in teratomas, establishing their clonal origin from the germ cells.[52] Widespread genetic losses also have been reported in testicular germ cell tumors. A homozygous deletion at band 12q22.2 commonly has been observed, suggesting the presence of a tumor-suppressor gene.[53]

**TABLE 34–6.** Diagnostic Utility of Immunohistochemistry in Common Testicular Neoplasms

| | GCT[1] | SCST[2] | Lymphoma | Metastatic Cancer |
|---|---|---|---|---|
| Pankeratin (AE1/AE3) | +/− | +/− | − | + |
| PLAP | + | − | − | − |
| EMA | −[7] | − | − | + |
| LCA | − | − | + | − |
| Inhibin/A103 | − | + | − | − |
| Vimetin | − | + | − | −/+ |

| | Seminoma | EC[3] | YST[4] | CC[5] |
|---|---|---|---|---|
| CAM 5.2 (CK8/18) | −/+[8] | +[9] | +[9] | + |
| CD30 | − | + | − | − |
| c-kit protein | +[9] | −[10] | − | − |
| AFP and A1-AT[6] | − | − | + | − |
| β-HCG | −[11] | −[11] | −[11] | +[12] |

[1] GCT, Germ cell tumors.
[2] SCST, Sex cord–stromal tumors.
[3] EC, Embryonal carcinoma.
[4] YST, Yolk sac tumor.
[5] CC, Choriocarcinoma.
[6] $\alpha_1$-antitrypsin.
[7] Syncytiotrophoblasts may be (+), rare EC also (+).
[8] If positive, usually focal and in a dotlike perinuclear pattern.
[9] Diffuse membranous.
[10] Rare cytoplasmic, when positive.
[11] Negative in tumor cells except syncytiotrophoblastic cells.
[12] Staining may be weak in cytotrophoblasts.

## Immunohistochemistry

The morphologic features in each subtype of germ cell tumor components are distinctive in most cases. Immunohistochemical evaluation may be required, however, 1) to differentiate germ cell tumors from non–germ cell tumors (e.g., sex cord–stromal tumors or metastases), 2) to confirm the germ cell nature of a tumor in metastatic sites, and 3) in the testis to distinguish between different germ cell tumor components. Table 34–6 provides an overview of the use of immunohistochemistry in the evaluation of testicular tumors.

## INTRATUBULAR GERM CELL NEOPLASIA

Intratubular germ cell neoplasia is the precursor lesion of all invasive germ cell tumors with the possible exceptions of spermatocytic seminoma, pediatric yolk sac tumor, and pediatric teratoma. It is characterized by the presence within seminiferous tubules of malignant germ cells that resemble seminoma cells. Because this form of intratubular germ cell neoplasia is found in all types of germ cell tumors, it also is referred to as *intratubular germ cell neoplasia, unclassified*. Intratubular germ cell neoplasia is found in almost all cases in which residual seminiferous tubules are identified around an invasive germ cell tumor. It also is present in 5% to 8% of cases of cryptorchidism,[54, 55] in 5% of patients with an invasive germ cell tumor in the contralateral testis,[56] and frequently in dysgenetic gonads. Although the lesion is conceptually akin to carcinoma in situ in other organs, the term *carcinoma in situ* is not preferred in the testis because intratubular germ cell neoplasia is not an epithelial lesion. Of patients with only intratubular germ cell neoplasia, 50% develop invasive germ cell tumors within 5 years,[57] and ultimately almost all develop invasive tumors.

Rarely, in cases with metastatic germ cell tumor, intratubular germ cell neoplasia may be found in the testis in association with a scar with or without calcification and without any recognizable invasive tumor. Such examples are believed to represent an invasive germ cell tumor in which the testicular primary has regressed ("burnt-out" germ cell tumors) (Fig. 34–2).[58] Frequently, intratubular germ cell neoplasia may involve the rete testis and rarely the epididymis in a pagetoid fashion (CD Figs. 34–1 through 34–3).

Microscopic examination shows the intratubular germ cell neoplasia cells lie adjacent to the basal portion of seminiferous tubules. The cells are large, with abundant clear cytoplasm and round, hyperchromatic, enlarged nuclei (Fig. 34–3). One or more prominent nucleoli are present. In formalin-fixed tissue, retraction artifact around these cells is frequent. Mitotic activity generally is not prominent. The

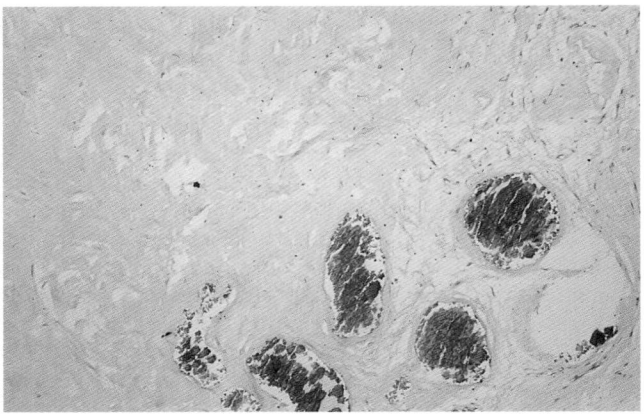

**FIGURE 34–2.** Burnt-out germ cell tumor. Testicular scar with calcification in a patient who had a metastatic germ cell tumor. Such lesions, particularly when associated with intratubular germ cell neoplasia but without any viable invasive germ cell tumor in the testis, are considered to represent a burnt-out germ cell tumor.

seminiferous tubules with intratubular germ cell neoplasia usually are abnormal, smaller than the surrounding uninvolved tubules, and often with a thickened basement membrane. These tubules usually lack any germ cells except in an early phase in which maturation may be preserved. Rarely, intratubular granulomatous reaction may be observed.

By convention, the term *intratubular germ cell neoplasia* is not used when the tumor cells fill the tubules. Terms such as *intratubular seminoma, intratubular spermatocytic seminoma*, and *intratubular embryonal carcinoma*, appropriate to the cell type present, are used. Occasionally, in cases of otherwise predominantly intratubular germ cell neoplasia, small foci of infiltrating seminoma-like cells are present beyond the confines of the tubular basement membranes. Such cases may be designated as *intratubular germ cell neoplasia, with early seminoma* or *intratubular*

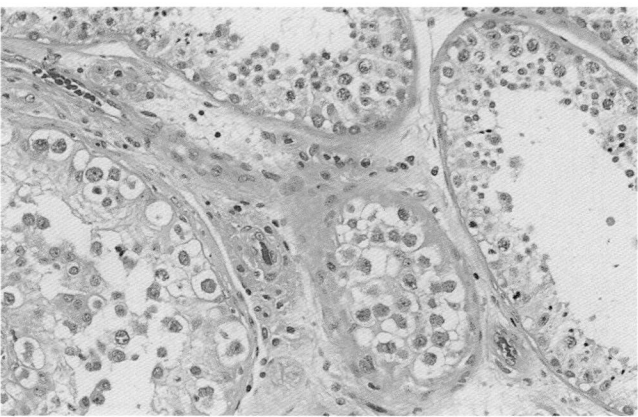

**FIGURE 34–3.** Intratubular germ cell neoplasia. The tubule on the lower left-hand side contains the neoplastic cells close to the tubular basement membrane, while the upper two tubules show normal spermatogenesis. The neoplastic cells have abundant clear cytoplasm and enlarged nuclei with prominent nucleoli.

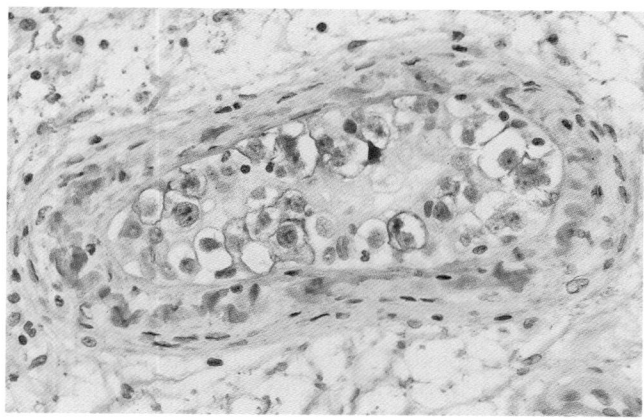

**FIGURE 34–4.** Intratubular germ cell neoplasia, placental alkaline phosphatase immunohistochemical stain. The neoplastic cells are highlighted by the membranous staining for PLAP.

*germ cell neoplasia, with extratubular extension* (CD Fig. 34–4).

Intratubular germ cell neoplasia cells, similar to seminoma, are rich in glycogen and are often positive for diastase-sensitive periodic acid–Schiff (PAS) reaction.[59] On immunohistochemistry, similar to seminoma, intratubular germ cell neoplasia exhibits membrane-associated positivity with placental-like alkaline phosphatase (PLAP) (Fig. 34–4) and c-kit protein.[35, 60]

## TYPICAL SEMINOMA (CLASSIC OR PURE SEMINOMA)

Pure seminoma is the most common testicular tumor, representing about 50% of all testicular germ cell tumors in more recent large series.[61, 62] These tumors occur at a mean age of 40.5 years, which is approximately a decade older than for nonseminomatous tumors.[62] Seminoma is extremely rare in children younger than age 10 years, uncommon in adolescents,[63] and uncommon in patients older than age 60 years.[64] Most patients present with self-identified testicular swelling, approximately 10% have acute groin pain, and fewer than 3% have symptoms secondary to metastatic disease, most commonly lumbar pain resulting from retroperitoneal involvement.[65] At the time of presentation, clinically about 75% of patients have disease limited to the testis, 20% have retroperitoneal involvement, and 5% have supradiaphragmatic or visceral metastases.[65]

Serum β-HCG levels are mildly elevated in 7% to 25% of patients with seminoma (owing to syncytiotrophoblastic cells), with the higher incidence being in patients with metastases.[66] Elevated serum β-HCG levels, although initially thought to be an adverse prognostic indicator,[67] now are believed to correlate more with metastatic status rather than prognosis.[68] AFP levels generally are not elevated in pure seminoma, and any elevations require thor-

ough sampling of the tumor for a nonseminomatous component.

## Gross Features

Seminomas average 3.5 to 5 cm in size, although tumors larger than 10 cm may be seen.[37] The testis is enlarged in most cases but rarely may appear normal or smaller in size. About 90% of seminomas are confined grossly to the testis. The cut surface reveals a well-circumscribed, lobulated cream or tan to light pink tumor that is soft and bulges above the surrounding parenchyma (Fig. 34–5 and CD Fig. 34–5) but may be firm and fibrous. Foci of necrosis may appear as granular yellow geographic areas and are common and conspicuous in larger tumors. Hemorrhagic necrosis is uncommon. Punctate foci of hemorrhage may indicate the presence of trophoblastic elements.

## Microscopic Features

Seminoma generally shows a diffuse sheetlike arrangement with lobularity created by thin fibrous septa (Fig. 34–6); less often, thick fibrous bands may subdivide the tumor into discrete nodules. Occasionally the tumor grows in cords or trabeculae, and rarely it may show a focal or predominant tubular growth pattern (tubular seminoma). A focal microcystic appearance with a collection of pink proteinaceous material may be seen focally as a result of edema. Most tumors obliterate the underlying parenchyma with no residual seminiferous tubules within the lesion; an interstitial growth pattern may be observed occasionally at the periphery (CD Fig. 34–6). Characteristically the fibrous septa contain varying amounts of mature lymphocytes, sometimes lymphoid aggregates with germinal center forma-

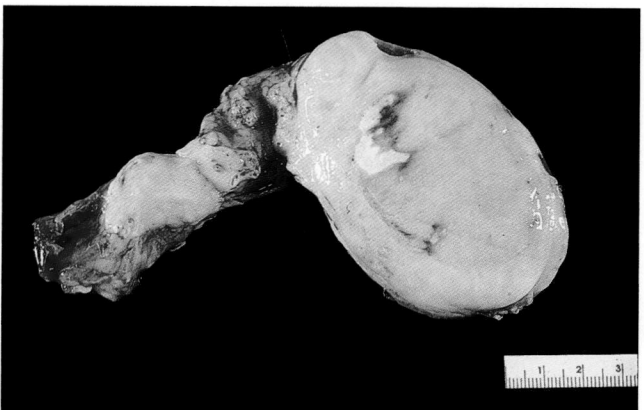

**FIGURE 34–5.** Seminoma (gross). The testicular parenchyma is almost completely replaced by the tumor with a homogeneous pale tan cut surface. Notice the irregular yellow area of necrosis in the center. Pure seminomas lack foci of hemorrhagic necrosis. A separate tumor nodule is seen in the spermatic cord.

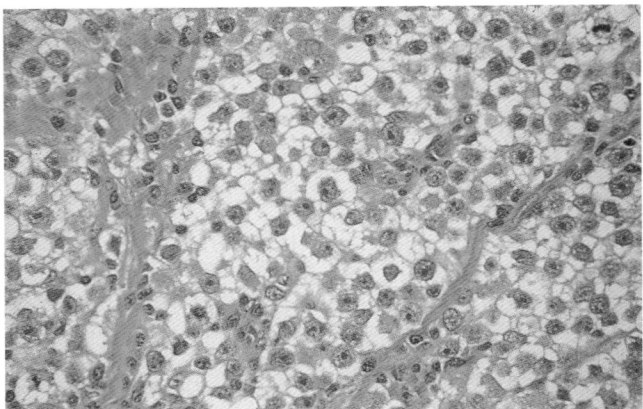

**FIGURE 34–6.** Seminoma. Note sheets of large relatively monotonous clear cells separated from one another by distinct cell membranes. The large central nucleus contains a prominent nucleolus. Thin fibrovascular septa containing lymphocytes divide the tumor cells into lobules.

tion, and rarely plasma cells and eosinophils. Less frequently, this infiltrate is between the tumor cells. Most of the mature lymphocytes are T lymphocytes, many with $\gamma/\delta$ phenotype.[69, 70] In 30% to 50% of cases, a granulomatous reaction may be present (Fig. 34–7), and rarely it may be so intense that it masks the underlying tumor.

Seminoma cells have a moderate amount of clear-to-pale eosinophilic cytoplasm, with distinct cell borders. The nuclei are central and large, with granular, evenly distributed chromatin and one or more prominent nucleoli. The nuclei may be round or have a flattened ("squared-off") appearance. In a well-fixed specimen, no nuclear overcrowding or syncytial growth is present (see Fig. 34–6). Mitotic activity usually is brisk. Currently, high mitotic activity is not believed to influence the prognosis, although in the past a high mitotic count ($\geq$3/high-

power field) was considered to be the criterion for the diagnosis of *anaplastic* seminoma.[71] Syncytiotrophoblasts are seen in a significant proportion of testicular seminomas, and these cells often are found around foci of hemorrhage. Lack of associated cytotrophoblasts distinguishes such cells from foci of choriocarcinoma.

## Immunohistochemical and Ultrastructural Features

Inadequately fixed or some well-fixed seminomas contain areas appearing more atypical than usual, immunostains may be necessary to rule out an embryonal carcinoma or yolk sac tumor component in such a tumor (see earlier under "immunohistochemistry") (Fig. 34–8). In brief, $\beta$-HCG and strong cytokeratin positivity is restricted to the syncytiotrophoblastic cells. Cytokeratins usually are negative in seminoma cells or sometimes show dotlike reactivity. Intense membranous cytokeratin positivity indicates early carcinomatous differentiation (Fig. 34–9 and CD Fig. 34–7). Ultrastructurally, seminoma cells appear primitive; are poor in organelles; contain abundant glycogen granules, and lack well-formed, epithelial-like cell junctions.

## Differential Diagnosis

When seminomas are not adequately fixed, artifactual morphologic alterations commonly create differential diagnostic problems. Seminomas are highly susceptible to significant cytologic alterations induced by improper or delayed fixation. The nuclei may become hyperchromatic, show nuclear membrane irregularities, and appear smudgy with loss of details. Because of the fragile nature of cytoplasm, cytoplasmic details and clarity are lost, and the cells

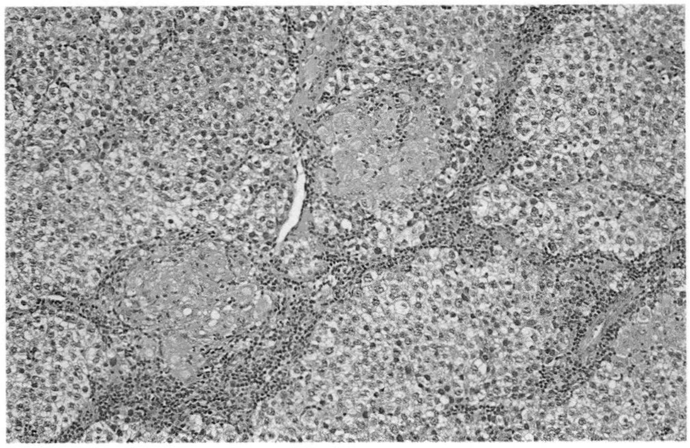

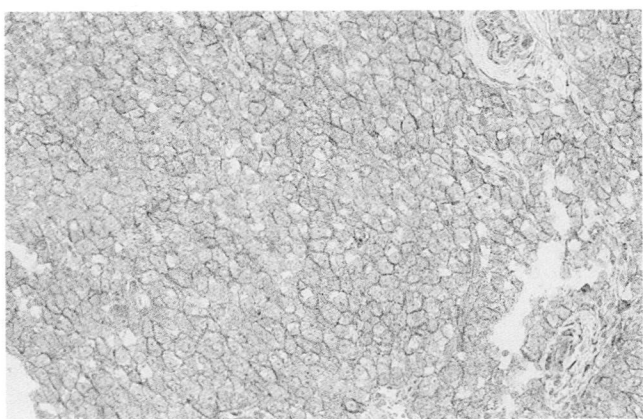

**FIGURE 34–7.** Seminoma. Besides the dense lymphocytic infiltrate there are two well-defined epithelioid granulomas in the fibrous septa. Granulomatous inflammation may be seen in approximately 50% of seminomas.

**FIGURE 34–8.** Seminoma, c-kit immunohistochemical stain. Membranous immunoreactivity with c-kit protein is a highly characteristic feature of both seminoma and intratubular germ cell neoplasia. Non-seminomatous germ cell tumors are either negative or rarely show focal cytoplasmic positivity.

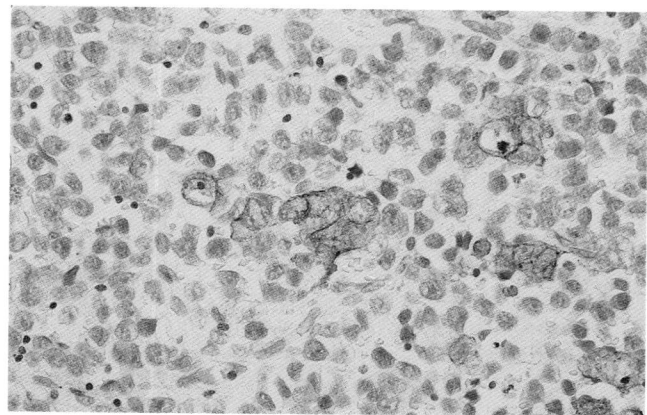

**FIGURE 34-9.** Seminoma with early carcinomatous differentiation, cytokeratin (Cam 5.2) immunohistochemical stain. Focal positivity in small clusters of cells for cytokeratin or CD30 (Ber-H2) indicates early carcinomatous differentiation.

appear overcrowded with eosinophilic cytoplasm. These nuclear and cytoplasmic alterations raise the question of *embryonal carcinoma*. In contrast to a typical seminoma, embryonal carcinoma has consistently a higher nuclear grade, irregular chromatin distribution, and syncytial arrangement of the cells. The cytoplasm often is amphophilic to basophilic, the cell borders are poorly defined, and glandular or papillary areas may be present. In problematic cases, use of immunostains is helpful (see Table 34–6).

Cases of otherwise typical seminoma with either focal or diffuse nuclear atypia and nuclear overlapping may show on immunohistologic evaluation small clusters with intense membrane-predominant cytokeratin or CD30 (Ber-H2) positivity (see Fig. 34–9 and CD Fig. 34–7). Such cases should be considered as seminomas with early transition to embryonal carcinoma and are designated as *seminomas with early carcinomatous differentiation*. The management of these tumors (whether as seminomas or as mixed germ cell tumors) is controversial and depends on the institution.

The solid pattern in *yolk sac tumors* also may mimic seminoma. This pattern usually is accompanied by other diagnostic patterns of yolk sac tumor, however, making the distinction usually easy. Yolk sac tumor cells generally have smaller nuclei with not prominent nucleoli and contain hyaline globules.[72] Edema and microcysts in a seminoma may raise the possibility of a reticular or microcystic pattern of yolk sac tumor. In seminoma, the cysts typically are irregular in outline and may contain edema fluid and free-floating cells. Yolk sac tumors are strongly cytokeratin positive and show immunoreactivity for AFP and $\alpha_1$-antitrypsin. Seminoma with syncytiotrophoblastic cells must be differentiated from *choriocarcinoma* and in our experience is sometimes a cause of miscategorization of germ cell tumors.

*Spermatocytic seminoma* may bear a superficial resemblance to typical seminoma, but on closer scru-

tiny the polymorphous cell population—its hallmark—is invariably evident. *Malignant lymphoma* may be confused with seminoma. Lymphomas of the testis usually are bilateral tumors, occur in older men, have an interstitial growth pattern, and lack intratubular germ cell neoplasia. Leukocyte common antigen and other lymphoid markers usually are positive, and PLAP is negative. Rarely, *metastatic tumors*, including renal cell carcinomas[73] and malignant melanomas, may create differential diagnostic problems. Frequent angiolymphatic invasion, interstitial growth pattern, and clinical history are important; immunostains are helpful (see Table 34–6).

Rarely, seminomas with conspicuous tubular architecture may resemble *Sertoli cell tumors* focally and superficially. The classic cytomorphology of seminoma cells is retained in tubular areas, however, and at least some areas have the typical sheet-like architecture. Because of a nested growth pattern, stromal fibrosis, and presence of lymphoid cells and intracytoplasmic glycogen, *clear cell sex cord–stromal tumor* may be mistaken for a seminoma and often is recognized as the correct diagnosis because of the lack of the expected response to radiation therapy for seminoma. The smaller, less pleomorphic nuclei and low mitotic count in the former and immunostains (see Table 34–6) help in this problematic differential diagnosis.[74] Finally, a florid and exuberant granulomatous response in a seminoma may obscure the neoplastic cells and lead to a misdiagnosis of *granulomatous orchitis*.

## SPERMATOCYTIC SEMINOMA

Although traditionally included among variants of seminoma, spermatocytic seminoma shows few features common to a typical seminoma. In contrast to seminoma, it tends to occur in older patients; does not occur as a primary tumor at any site other than the testis; does not have a histologically identical counterpart in the ovary; is not associated with intratubular germ cell neoplasia or other germ cell tumors, cryptorchidism, i(12p) positivity, or PLAP positivity; and metastasizes extremely rarely.[65] It was described as a distinct entity by Masson in 1946,[75] who considered it to mimic spermatogenesis, based on the polymorphous cell population and meiotic-like chromatin pattern in some cells. Although some authors were unable to identify the meiotic-specific structures and haploid DNA values in spermatocytic seminoma,[76] evidence suggests that in contrast to typical seminoma, cells in spermatocytic seminoma are capable of maturing to the stage of spermatogonia-spermatocyte.[77]

Spermatocytic seminoma is a rare entity (representing <1% of seminomas). The average age at presentation is 55 years. Bilateral tumors are present in approximately 9% of cases.[78] Rare cases of sarcomatous transformation have been reported; these may present with metastatic disease and are the cause of death in this tumor.[79] Otherwise the prognosis is excellent.

## Gross Features

The tumor usually is well circumscribed and multilobulated or multinodular. The cut surface typically is soft, with a gelatinous or mucoid consistency and areas of cystic change. Extension beyond the testis is rare; however, epididymal involvement has been described.[78]

## Microscopic Features

Cells are arranged in sheets, generally with scant fibrous stroma. Stroma may be prominent and when conspicuous is usually edematous. The intercellular edema imparts a pseudocystic or pseudoglandular appearance. Prominent intratubular growth is frequent at the periphery of the tumor; however, intratubular germ cell neoplasia is not present. Granulomatous reaction is exceedingly rare, and lymphocytic infiltration usually is absent or scant.

A three cell–type polymorphous neoplastic cell population (i.e., small, intermediate, and giant cells) is characteristic (Fig. 34–10 and CD Fig. 34–8).[65] The small, probably degenerate, cells (6 to 8 $\mu$m) resemble lymphocytes but have homogeneous and pyknotic nuclei with dense chromatin. The 15- to 20-$\mu$m intermediate cells are the most common cell type and have a round nucleus with finely granular chromatin and a moderate amount of cytoplasm. The large cells (50 to 100 $\mu$m), which often include multinucleated giant cells, are least common. Occasional intermediate and large cells have a filamentous or spireme chromatin similar to primary spermatocytes in meiotic prophase. Nucleoli may vary from inapparent to prominent. Intercellular borders are indistinct. The mitotic rate generally is brisk, and atypical mitoses may be present. In tumors with a sarcomatous component, the sarcoma frequently is undifferentiated, although cases with rhabdomyomatous differentiation have been described.[79, 80] An anaplastic variant that is morphologically unique with a preponderance of monomorphic cells bearing prominent nucleoli and resembling classic seminoma and embryonal carcinoma has been described; however, the prognosis is excellent, arguing against its representing a distinct entity.[81]

Spermatocytic seminomas generally do not stain for glycogen, and immunoreactivity for PLAP is absent,[82] although positivity in rare cells has been described.[83] Cytokeratin immunostains are negative, but dotlike cytoplasmic positivity with Cam 5.2 (similar to typical seminomas) may be present.[83]

## EMBRYONAL CARCINOMA

Embryonal carcinoma is a germ cell tumor composed of primitive anaplastic-appearing epithelial cells. Pure embryonal carcinoma is rare, constituting approximately 2% of all testicular germ cell tumors.[65] Approximately 40% of all testicular germ cell tumors have an embryonal carcinoma component,[65] however, and an embryonal carcinoma component is found in approximately 90% of mixed germ cell tumors.[61] In the older literature, the incidence of pure embryonal carcinoma was reported to be 20%[5, 8]; the apparent decline in frequency possibly reflects the recognition of other germ cell components, particularly yolk sac tumor elements that previously were diagnosed as embryonal carcinoma.

Pure embryonal carcinoma most commonly occurs in patients in their 20s and 30s, with an average age of 32 years.[61] It is extremely rare in prepubertal children.[84] Most patients (approximately 80%) present with testicular mass, with or without pain. About 10% present with symptoms resulting from metastases, and 10% present with hormonal symptoms, including gynecomastia. After clinical evaluation, only about 40% are found to have disease limited to the testis; in 40%, retroperitoneal lymph node involvement and in approximately 20% supradiaphragmatic or visceral involvement is discovered.[65] Approximately two thirds of the patients with a tumor composed predominantly of embryonal carcinoma have metastasis at diagnosis.[85]

Patients with pure embryonal carcinoma usually do not have elevated serum AFP levels. The reported frequent serum AFP elevations in patients with embryonal carcinoma in the past[86] were the result of the then unrecognized and now well-known frequent association of embryonal carcinoma with yolk sac elements. The reported immunoreactivity for AFP in an occasional pure embryonal carcinoma[87] perhaps is an indication of early transformation to yolk sac tumor.[65, 88]

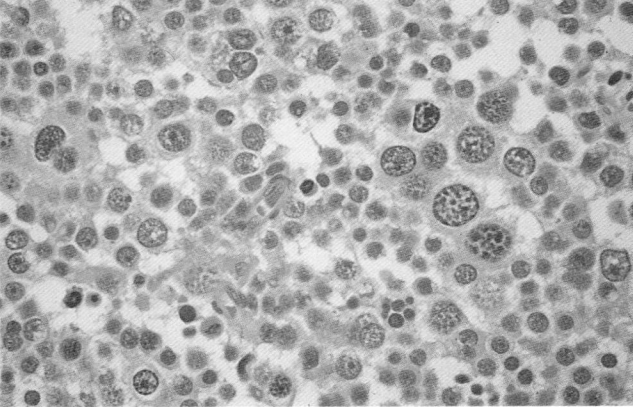

**FIGURE 34–10.** Spermatocytic seminoma. The tumor shows a proliferation of three cell types: large gigantic cells, a few small dark (pyknotic) cells, and a majority of intermediate cells. Note spireme-type chromatin in some of the larger cells.

## Gross Features

Pure embryonal carcinoma typically is a soft, pale gray-to-tan, granular tumor, rarely with firm areas and often with prominent foci of hemorrhage and necrosis (Fig. 34–11). The tumor outlines often are indistinct, and gross extension into testicular adnexa is present in approximately 25% of the tumors.[85]

## Microscopic Features

The primitive-looking cells of embryonal carcinoma are arranged in several architectural patterns, and often more than one pattern coexists[65] (Fig. 34–12 and CD Fig. 34–9). A *solid* pattern with the cells arranged in solid sheets and usually showing multiple foci of necrosis is most common and is present in almost all embryonal carcinomas. A *tubular* and *tubulopapillary* pattern is present in approximately three fourths of tumors. In this pattern, tumor cells form true glandular structures (Fig. 34–13) or display true papillary formations covering fibrovascular cores. Rarely a micropapillary pattern or papillae without cores but only piled-up epithelium may be observed. In the solid pattern, darkly staining, degenerate-looking cells with hyperchromatic, smudged nuclei often are present at the periphery of cell groups. These cells may be confused with syncytiotrophoblastic cells, raising the possibility of

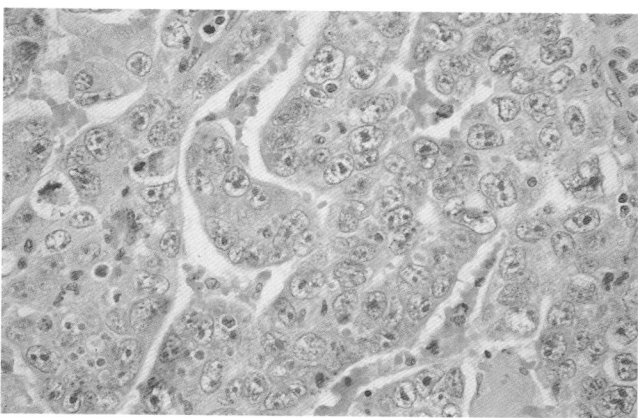

**FIGURE 34–12.** Embryonal carcinoma. Tumor cells are arranged in sheets and papillary formations. The cells lack distinct cell borders and have a syncytial appearance. Nuclei are large and overlapping, with irregular nuclear membranes and prominent nucleoli.

a choriocarcinoma.[65] Fibrous septations similar to those seen in seminoma are rare in embryonal carcinoma, as are lymphocytic infiltrate and granulomatous reaction.

The tumor cells in embryonal carcinoma contain abundant basophilic-to-amphophilic and, rarely, clear cytoplasm. Cytoplasmic borders characteristically are indistinct. The nuclei are large, with coarsely clumped chromatin and frequent nuclear membrane irregularities, with one or more prominent nucleoli. The nuclei often appear crowded and overlapped, resulting in a syncytial appearance. Mitotic figures, apoptotic bodies, and single cell necrosis are common (see Fig. 34–12 and CD Fig. 34–9).

Intratubular germ cell neoplasia is present in most cases with residual testicular parenchyma. Intratubular growth, particularly at the periphery of the tumor, is frequent. Often, embryonal carcinoma cells in these tubules show extensive necrosis that

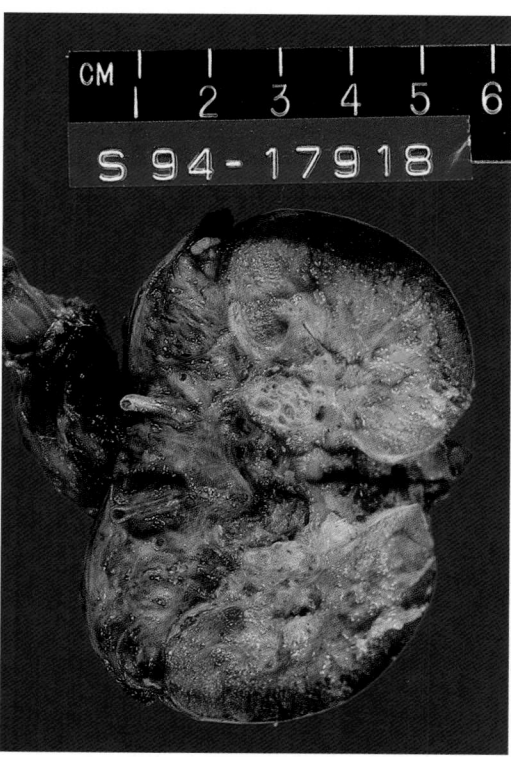

**FIGURE 34–11.** Embryonal carcinoma, gross. This bivalved testis shows a variegated mass with areas of hemorrhage and necrosis.

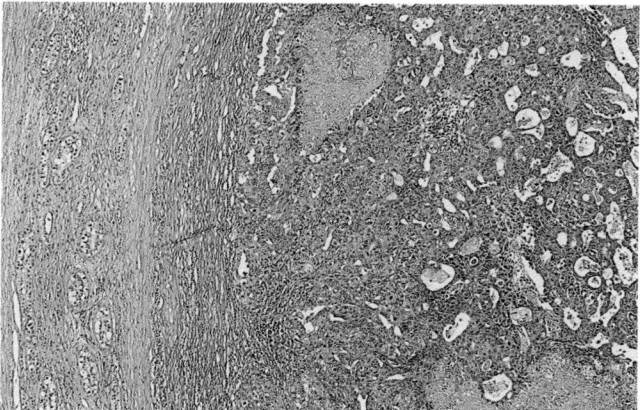

**FIGURE 34–13.** Embryonal carcinoma, tubular pattern. At low power, the darkly staining cells with hyperchromatic nuclei are characteristic of embryonal carcinoma. Note the extensive intratubular germ cell neoplasia in the adjacent testis.

frequently is associated with dystrophic calcification. The peritubular fibrosis helps distinguish intratubular growth from vascular invasion that frequently occurs in pure embryonal carcinoma and in mixed germ cell tumors with a predominant embryonal carcinoma component. Identification of vascular invasion is important because its presence excludes a patient from a "surveillance-only" approach and is associated with retroperitoneal lymph node metastasis in 50% of cases initially judged to have only clinical stage I disease.[89] Vascular invasion most often is easily recognizable at the periphery of the tumor, in the surrounding non-neoplastic testis, and frequently in the vascular channels running parallel to the tunica albuginea (CD Fig. 34–10). Vascular invasion needs to be distinguished from *pseudoinvasion* resulting from artifactual tumor implantation into vascular channels and from intratubular tumor, which sometimes can mimic true vascular invasion.[90]

Two controversial issues regarding embryonal carcinoma are the association of undifferentiated stroma and AFP immunoreactivity in pure embryonal carcinoma. An undifferentiated primitive-appearing spindle cell component may be seen in close association with the epithelial component of embryonal carcinoma. Although a minor component of such perithelial stroma is acceptable by most authorities as embryonal carcinoma,[65] many others believe this to be indicative of a teratomatous component. Presence of frequent foci of immature stroma requires careful evaluation for a teratomatous component. When the immature stromal foci are present only surrounding the epithelial component of embryonal carcinoma and do not form expansile nodules, such cases may be considered as pure "embryonal carcinoma with focal immature stromal component."[65, 91] Most AFP-positive foci in embryonal carcinomas probably represent admixed yolk sac tumor component, although rare cases of typical embryonal carcinoma do stain focally for AFP.[88]

## Immunohistochemical and Ultrastructural Features

Embryonal carcinomas usually show intense and diffuse immunoreactivity for PLAP, cytokeratins (AE1/AE3 and Cam 5.2), and CD30 (Ber-H2)[92] (Fig. 34–14 and CD Fig. 34–11). About 2% of cases react with epithelial membrane antigen (EMA).[93] Staining for c-kit protein generally is negative,[35] and β-HCG is demonstrable only in intermingled syncytiotrophoblastic cells (see Table 34–6).

On ultrastructural evaluation, embryonal carcinomas have features of poorly differentiated adenocarcinomas, with extracellular lumina even in solid patterns of the tumor. Stubby microvilli project into the luminal spaces, and tight junctional complexes with well-defined desmosomes are present between

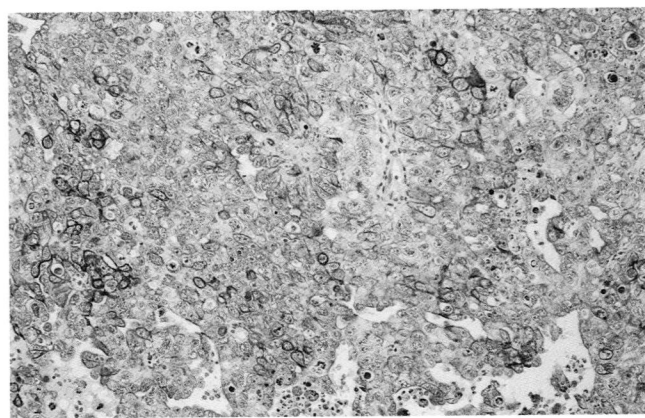

**FIGURE 34–14.** Embryonal carcinoma. Pancytokeratin immunohistochemical stain showing strong immunoreactivity.

cells around the lumina. The cytoplasm contains large numbers of ribosomes, rough endoplasmic reticulum, prominent Golgi apparatus, prominent mitochondria, glycogen granules, and scattered lipid droplets.[29]

## Differential Diagnosis

It is important to distinguish embryonal carcinoma from *seminoma* because of the markedly different therapeutic implications and biologic behavior (see earlier discussion). The solid and papillary patterns of embryonal carcinoma may be confused with similar patterns of *yolk sac tumor*. Yolk sac tumor typically shows myriad patterns within the same tumor, however. The cells in embryonal carcinoma have greater nuclear pleomorphism than yolk sac tumors. The presence of Schiller-Duval formations, hyaline globules, or basement membrane material favors yolk sac tumor. CD30 and AFP immunopanel is further discriminatory.

*Large cell lymphoma* (including Ki-1 lymphoma) sometimes may be confused with embryonal carcinoma; however, patients with lymphoma generally are older and usually have bilateral and extragonadal disease. Lymphomas have an interstitial growth pattern, lack intratubular germ cell neoplasia, and are negative for PLAP. Although Ki-1-positive lymphomas are positive for CD30 and rare cases may show focal expression of cytokeratin, diffuse and strong positivity for cytokeratins establishes the diagnosis of embryonal carcinoma over a large cell anaplastic lymphoma.[94]

One of the most difficult differential diagnoses is between embryonal carcinoma in an extratesticular site and *metastatic undifferentiated carcinoma*. In such situations, judicious use of mucin stains (positive in some metastatic carcinomas), immunohistochemistry (see Table 34–6), and clinical correlation are helpful.

# YOLK SAC TUMOR (ENDODERMAL SINUS TUMOR)

Yolk sac tumor is the most common testicular tumor of childhood, accounting for more than 80% of prepubertal germ cell tumors.[65, 95, 96] Mean age is 17 to 18 months, and with few exceptions, it almost always occurs as a pure neoplasm. In postpubertal patients, yolk sac tumor almost invariably is a component of a mixed germ cell tumor, and the reported frequency of yolk sac tumor among adult mixed germ cell tumors is 44%.[97] Yolk sac tumor remains the most commonly overlooked component of testicular germ cell tumors, however, because it is often focal and overlaps in its morphology with embryonal carcinoma.[65] The age range for adults with pure yolk sac tumor or a mixed germ cell tumor with yolk sac tumor component is 17 to 40 years, with rare cases occurring in the elderly.[65]

Yolk sac tumors in children show many other differences from those in adults. Compared with adult yolk sac tumors, childhood tumors are not associated with cryptorchidism, occur roughly equally in white and African American populations, are most often limited to the testis (84% to 94%),[95, 98] have a low incidence of retroperitoneal lymph node metastasis,[98] metastasize more commonly to the lung,[96, 98] are histologically pure, and usually lack intratubular germ cell neoplasia in the surrounding testis.[99] These differences suggest different histogenetic pathways for these morphologically similar tumors occurring in different age groups.

Children and adults most often present with a painless testicular mass. Most patients with childhood yolk sac tumor have stage I disease at presentation. There is some evidence that adults with a yolk sac tumor component in a mixed germ cell tumor have a higher frequency of stage I disease compared with those without such a component.[100] The presence of yolk sac tumor elements in metastatic testicular cancer has been associated with a poor prognosis.[101] These observations suggest that yolk sac tumor has lower metastatic potential and less chemosensitivity than embryonal carcinoma.[65, 102]

Of patients with a yolk sac tumor component in their tumors, 95% to 100% have elevated serum AFP.[103, 104] In most cases, the elevations are substantial (in the range of hundreds to thousands of nanograms per milliliter). Physiologic elevations in a relatively lower range may occur in normal young children,[65] and it is important not to overinterpret such elevations.

## Gross Features

Most pediatric yolk sac tumors are nonencapsulated gray-tan–to–yellow homogeneous tumors usually with a myxoid and variably cystic quality. Areas of hemorrhage and necrosis may be extensive in postpubertal cases, reflecting the association with other germ cell components.

## Microscopic Features

Yolk sac tumor shows marked heterogeneity in architecture and cytologic features on microscopic examination and typically exhibits a range of histologic patterns in a given case. Ulbright and coworkers[65] have modified Talerman's[105] originally described 9 histologic patterns of yolk sac tumor into the following 11 patterns:

1. The most common *reticular* or *microcystic* pattern (Fig. 34–15) is characterized by prominent cytoplasmic vacuoles creating a meshwork of sievelike spaces and an irregular labyrinthine arrangement of anastomosing cords of cells with loose spaces or microcysts. Occasionally the epithelial cords attenuate and disperse into surrounding stroma as single spindle cells. The stroma frequently is myxoid.
2. A *macrocystic* pattern (Fig. 34–16) results from coalescence of microcysts.
3. The *endodermal sinus* pattern (Fig. 34–17) is the most distinctive and is characterized by a papillary core of fibrous tissue containing a central small blood vessel, which is covered by a layer of cuboidal-to-columnar tumor cells. The entire structure is surrounded by a cystic space, which in turn is lined by flattened tumor cells. These glomeruloid structures are known as *Schiller-Duval bodies* (CD Fig. 34–12) and when cut tangentially may result in elongated fibrous tissue cores draped (festooned) by malignant epithelium.
4. In the *papillary* pattern, small irregular papillae, with or without fibrous cores, project into cystic spaces. Many detached papillae or cell clusters

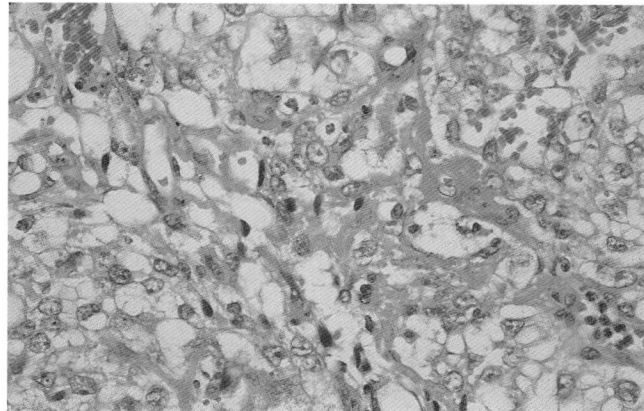

**FIGURE 34–15.** Yolk sac tumor, reticular microcystic and parietal pattern. The tumor cells have characteristic prominent cytoplasmic vacuoles creating a sievelike appearance and microcysts. Basement membrane material deposit characterizes the parietal pattern.

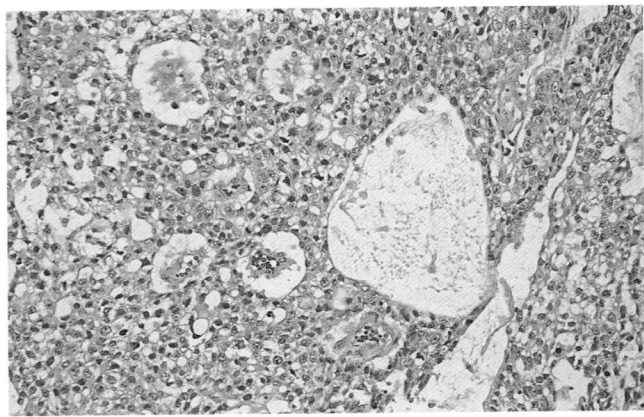

FIGURE 34–16. Yolk sac tumor, solid, microcystic and macrocystic pattern. Combination of multiple architectural patterns is frequently seen in yolk sac tumors.

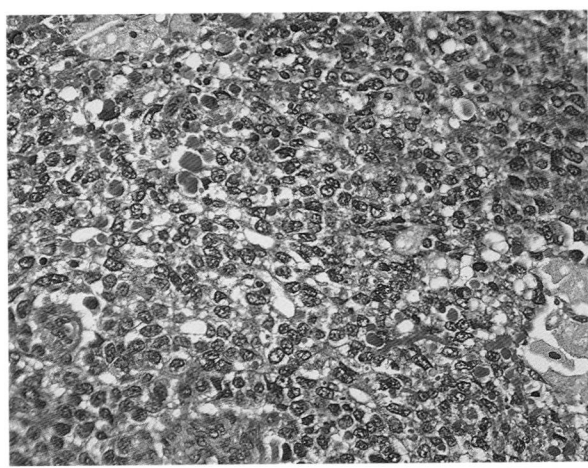

FIGURE 34–18. Yolk sac tumor, solid pattern. The sheetlike arrangement of cells may mimic a seminoma. Note the numerous intra and extracellular hyaline globules, a frequent occurrence in yolk sac tumors.

also are present in the cystic spaces that often are lined by cuboidal–to–low-columnar cells, occasionally with "hobnail" nuclear configuration.

5. The *solid* pattern (Fig. 34–18) consists of a sheet-like arrangement of polygonal cells, with eosinophilic-to-clear cytoplasm, well-defined cell borders, and relatively uniform nuclei. This pattern may be confused with seminoma (see under "differential diagnosis" of seminoma).

6. In the *glandular and alveolar* pattern, the glands and alveoli may be lined by flattened epithelium or columnar, pseudostratified epithelium with brush borders (enteric features) (CD Fig. 34–13). Rarely, basal cytoplasmic vacuoles, reminiscent of early secretory endometrium (endometrioid features), may be present.

7. The *myxoid* pattern is common and usually is associated with the reticular pattern, in which the epithelial cells of the latter acquire stellate

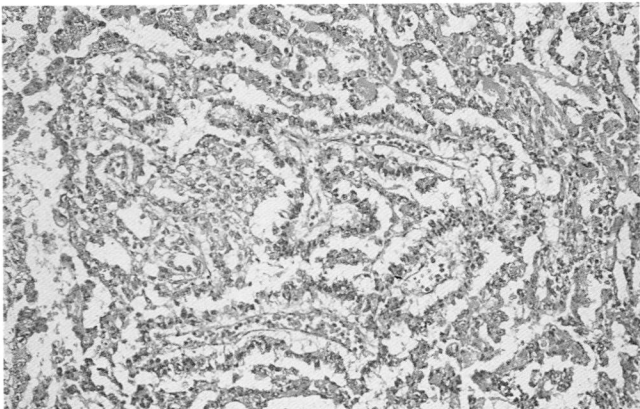

FIGURE 34–17. Yolk sac tumor, endodermal sinus (festoon-like) pattern. Central fibrovascular cores are surrounded by cuboidal to columnar tumor cells. When sectioned transversely these festoons may appear like glomeruloid structures (Schiller-Duval bodies).

and spindle profiles and gradually disperse into a myxoid, vacuolated stroma.

8. Rarely, yolk sac tumors have a cellular neoplastic *spindle cell* (sarcomatoid) component. The spindle cells retain cytokeratin positivity, supporting their derivation from the epithelial component of reticular yolk sac tumor.[106]

9. The *polyvesicular vitelline* pattern (CD Fig. 34–14) shows cysts often with an eccentric constriction, scattered in edematous to fibrous stroma. The cysts are lined by flattened-to-columnar epithelium, and the transition from the flattened to columnar epithelium usually occurs at the site of constriction.

10. The *hepatoid* pattern occurs in about 20% of yolk sac tumors[65, 72] and is evident as small clusters of cells with abundant eosinophilic cytoplasm and a large central nucleus with prominent nucleolus (hepatocyte-like). The cells may be arranged in nests, tubules, or trabeculae and may show bile canalicular formation. These areas are diffusely and strongly AFP positive and frequently show hyaline globules.

11. In the *parietal* pattern, a variable amount of eosinophilic basement membrane material is present in the extracellular space between tumor cells.[97] Patients with metastatic yolk sac tumor treated by chemotherapy may have recurrences with a pure parietal pattern.[65]

A characteristic, but inconsistent, feature of yolk sac tumor is the presence of hyaline eosinophilic globules; they may be seen only rarely in other testicular germ cell tumors.[97] The globules vary in size, ranging from 1 to more than 50 $\mu$m; tend to occur in clusters; and may be intracellular or extracellular in location (see Fig. 34–18). They are PAS positive and diastase resistant, and most often do not stain for AFP.

## Immunohistochemical and Ultrastructural Features

Yolk sac tumor stains for AFP, but the staining may be of a focal and patchy manner; the reported frequency ranges from 74% to 100% of the cases.[65, 93] $\alpha_1$-Antitrypsin is positive in about 50% of yolk sac tumors,[65] cytokeratin usually intensely marks almost all cases, and EMA and CD30 usually are negative.[107] Cytokeratin and vimentin are positive in spindle cell areas, and CD34, which is negative in seminoma and embryonal carcinoma, is positive in a few cases.[108]

Electron microscopic examination shows epithelial cells with tight junctional complexes and desmosomes and occasional extracellular lumina with apical microvilli. Irregularly shaped electron-dense basement membrane material frequently is seen in extracellular spaces and dilated cisterns of rough endoplasmic reticulum. Some cells show non-membrane-bound, densely osmophilic, homogeneous round cytoplasmic globules corresponding to the hyaline globules. Enteric glands have microvilli, associated rootlets, and a prominent glycocalyx.[65]

## Differential Diagnosis

Differentiation of the solid pattern of yolk sac tumor from pure *seminoma* is of great therapeutic and biologic importance and more crucial than its distinction from *embryonal carcinoma*. Differentiation of yolk sac tumor from seminoma and embryonal carcinoma has been discussed earlier.

Rare purely glandular yolk sac tumor may be confused with an *immature teratoma*. The enteric glands in yolk sac tumor often branch extensively, in contrast to the usually simple, oval-to-round glands that usually are surrounded by a smooth muscle layer in teratomas. A clinically major consideration is the distinction of *juvenile granulosa cell tumor* from a yolk sac tumor in infants. Both tumors show solid and cystic areas. The cells in juvenile granulosa cell tumors do not appear as primitive as in yolk sac tumor, however. The presence of other yolk sac tumor patterns is helpful. Juvenile granulosa cell tumor does not stain with AFP but stains with inhibin A.

## CHORIOCARCINOMA

Choriocarcinoma is a highly malignant tumor showing trophoblastic differentiation. Pure choriocarcinomas are rare, constituting less than 0.5% of testicular tumors.[8] Focal choriocarcinomatous elements are present, however, in approximately 16% of all mixed germ cell tumors.[61] In contrast to other testicular germ cell tumors, choriocarcinoma more commonly presents with metastases rather than with a testicular mass. Metastatic disease is found not only in the usual sites for other testicular tumors, but also frequently in areas of hematogenous spread without nodal involvement (i.e., lungs, liver, gastrointestinal tract, spleen, brain, and adrenals).[8, 65, 109, 110] About 10% of the cases present with gynecomastia as a result of the marked elevation of serum $\beta$-HCG levels.[65] Because of the structural similarities between $\beta$-HCG and thyroid-stimulating hormone, thyrotoxicosis also may occur in some.[65] Most patients with choriocarcinoma are in their teens or 20s. No cases have been reported in prepubertal boys.

## Gross Features

Typically the testis harboring a pure choriocarcinoma is of normal size or small and atrophic, reflecting the usually small size of the tumor. On cut section, the tumor is associated with extensive hemorrhage and necrosis, sometimes with ill-defined gray-tan–to–brown areas at the periphery. In mixed germ cell tumors, hemorrhagic and necrotic areas specifically need to be targeted to detect choriocarcinoma elements.

## Microscopic Features

The microscopic evaluation confirms the gross impression of extensively hemorrhagic and necrotic tissue, often with little viable tumor. The tumor characteristically is composed of an admixture of two distinct cell populations: 1) mononuclear cytotrophoblasts with clear-to-amphophilic cytoplasm and mild-to-moderate nuclear pleomorphism and 2) multinucleated syncytiotrophoblasts with smudged nuclear chromatin and abundant amphophilic cytoplasm, often with intracytoplasmic lumina occasionally containing red blood cells. In better differentiated areas, masses of cytotrophoblasts are capped by syncytiotrophoblasts (Fig. 34–19). In

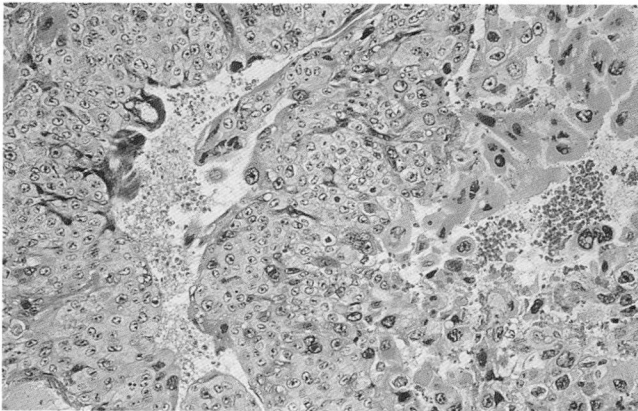

FIGURE 34–19. Choriocarcinoma. Two distinct cell populations are characteristic: the mononuclear cytotrophoblasts with clear to eosinophilic cytoplasm, capped by multinucleated syncytiotrophoblasts.

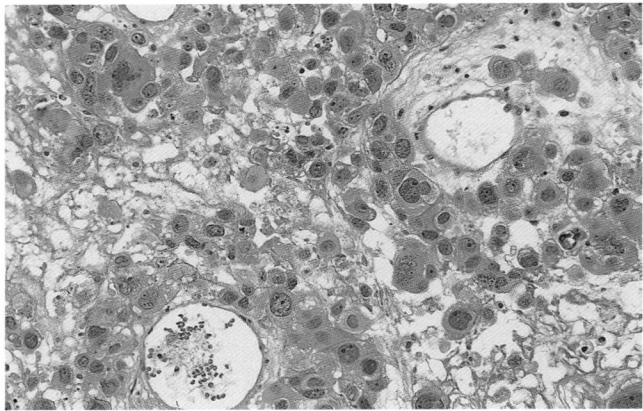

**FIGURE 34–20.** Placental site trophoblastic tumor. The tumor is composed of intermediate, predominantly mononuclear trophoblastic cells with abundant pink cytoplasm and hyperchromatic indented nuclei. (Courtesy of Thomas Ulbright, Indianapolis, IN.)

other instances, the intermingling is more random. In some cases, the cytotrophoblastic component predominates, and rarely syncytiotrophoblasts are so infrequent that a *monophasic* pattern is created (*monophasic choriocarcinoma*). Such a pattern is seen more commonly after chemotherapy. Syncytiotrophoblasts are mitotically inactive, whereas cytotrophoblasts generally show a high mitotic rate. Vascular invasion is a prominent and common feature in choriocarcinoma.

A rare form of trophoblastic tumor resembles placental-site trophoblastic tumor of the uterus[111] (Fig. 34–20) and has been reported in a 16-month-old boy. It consists of mostly mononucleate intermediate trophoblastic cells with a moderate amount of dense eosinophilic cytoplasm and hyperchromatic, smudged, and indented nuclei.

## Immunohistochemical and Ultrastructural Features

Stains for $\beta$-HCG are positive in all cases, more strongly in syncytiotrophoblasts and occasional large mononuclear forms that may represent transitional forms between syncytiotrophoblasts and cytotrophoblasts.[65, 112] $\beta$-HCG is weakly positive or negative in cytotrophoblasts (CD Fig. 34–15). Pregnancy-specific $\beta$1-glycoprotein and human placental lactogen also are positive in syncytiotrophoblasts and intermediate-sized trophoblasts but are negative in cytotrophoblasts.[65, 112]

On ultrastructural examination, syncytiotrophoblasts show prominent rough endoplasmic reticulum with dilated cisterns in a honeycomb pattern. Cytotrophoblasts contain only short profiles of tubular endoplasmic reticulum with numerous free ribosomes. Desmosome-like structures join adjacent cytotrophoblastic and syncytiotrophoblastic cells, and prominent interdigitating microvilli are present on the cell membranes of syncytiotrophoblasts.

## Differential Diagnosis

Choriocarcinoma with extensive hemorrhage and necrosis must be differentiated from testicular *hemorrhagic infarction* resulting from torsion or other causes. In contrast to choriocarcinoma, testicular infarction usually is painful, and the testis is swollen. The tubular outlines usually are identifiable, and intratubular germ cell neoplasia is not present. Differentiation from *other germ cell tumors* that contain syncytiotrophoblastic cells is important. The lack of a biphasic appearance and presence of hemorrhage and necrosis are helpful features.

## TERATOMA

Teratoma is a germ cell tumor that differentiates to form somatic tissue. Testicular teratoma in prepubertal patients differs from that in postpubertal patients in many ways. In young children, pure testicular teratoma is the second most common germ cell tumor (14% to 20% of cases). It is invariably benign even when histologically immature and is not associated with typical intratubular germ cell neoplasia, although rarely atypical germ cells that do not stain with PLAP and c-kit protein may be present. The mean age at diagnosis is 20 months, and occurrence in children older than 4 years is rare. In contrast, postpubertal testicular teratoma most commonly is a component of mixed germ cell tumor, being present in 50%[61, 65]; tumors with pure histology are rare. Pure teratomas in adults, even when mature (i.e., having a well-differentiated banal histology) have a malignant potential. Metastases from pure testicular teratomas may be teratomatous[65] (CD Fig. 34–16) or may have nonteratomatous components.[113–116] This phenomenon is explained by the hypothesis that a precursor element (probably embryonal carcinoma) present in the testicular primary metastasizes and differentiates to a teratoma at the metastatic sites.[65] A rare case of vascular invasion by mature teratoma is described,[117] and this is believed by some to represent intravascular maturation.[65] The incidence of metastasis in teratoma has been reported to range from 25% to 63%[6, 113]; the higher incidence has been attributed to referral bias. Serum tumor marker levels are not elevated in pure teratomas, although they may be elevated in some cases as a result of discordant morphology at a metastatic site.

## Gross Features

Pure teratomas usually are nodular with a variably cystic and solid cut surface. Cysts may contain keratinous or mucoid material or serous fluid. Gray-white translucent nodules of cartilage may be recognizable (Fig. 34–21). Hair is not seen[118] (see under "dermoid cyst"). Immature areas generally are soft and solid.

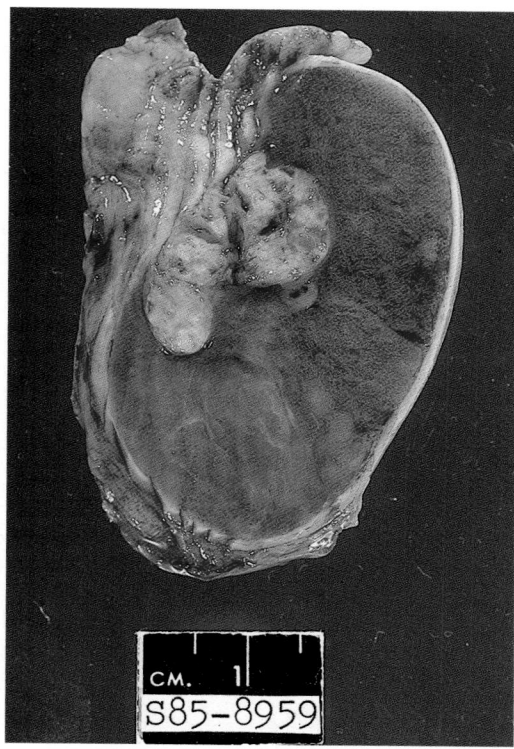

**FIGURE 34–21.** Teratoma (gross). This is a relatively small tumor showing cystic areas and glistening foci suggestive of cartilaginous tissue.

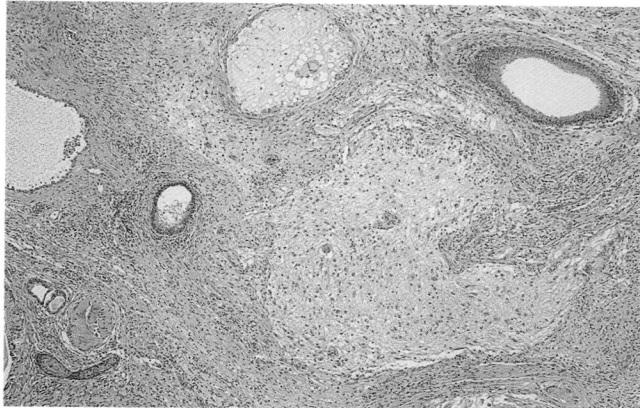

**FIGURE 34–22.** Mature teratoma. Glandular structures surrounded by smooth muscle and neuroglial tissue with the typical fibrillary background are seen.

## Microscopic Features

*Mature teratomas* contain elements resembling normal postnatal tissue, usually but not always from all three germ layers (Fig. 34–22 and CD Fig. 34–17). The ectodermal components usually consist of epidermis; endoderm is represented by enteric, respiratory, or other type of glandular mucosa and mucus glands; and the mesoderm is represented by muscle, cartilage, and bone. Foci of neural tissue, sometimes with ependymal differentiation, and cellular cartilage are common. The different components usually are organized to simulate the structure of normal organ systems (e.g., smooth muscle bundles surrounding enteric glands; smooth muscle, mucus glands, and cartilage surrounding respiratory mucosa) but may appear disorganized. Pigmented retinal-type epithelium, liver, salivary gland tissue, pancreatic tissue, and choroid plexus may occur infrequently.

*Immature teratomas* contain elements resembling embryonic tissue; these often accompany mature components. In testicular teratomas, presence of immaturity and the amount or grading of immature component is not of prognostic importance (in contrast to in ovarian teratomas). The immature elements are represented most commonly by nonspecific cellular, primitive-appearing spindle cells that may be arranged circumferentially around fetal-type

glands or may form sheets. Immature adipose tissue with myxoid background and prominent vascularity, neuroepithelium resembling embryonal nervous tissue and neural tubes (Fig. 34–23), immature hepatic cords, blastema with oval-to-spindle cells that may form primitive tubules (Wilms' tumor–like), and rarely embryonal rhabdomyoblastic foci are other forms of immaturity (see later for distinction from malignant transformation).

*Teratomas with secondary malignant component (malignant transformation)* are teratomas (usually immature) with various tumors of non–germ cell type. To designate *secondary malignant component* or *malignant transformation*, arbitrary criteria of "substantial (one half to whole field when viewed with a 4× objective)"[65] or as an "expansile nodule" size[52] are used. Sarcomas of different histologic types are the most common secondary tumors; rhabdomyosarcoma (Fig. 34–24 and CD Fig. 34–18) and primitive neuroectodermal tumor are the common types.[52] Epithe-

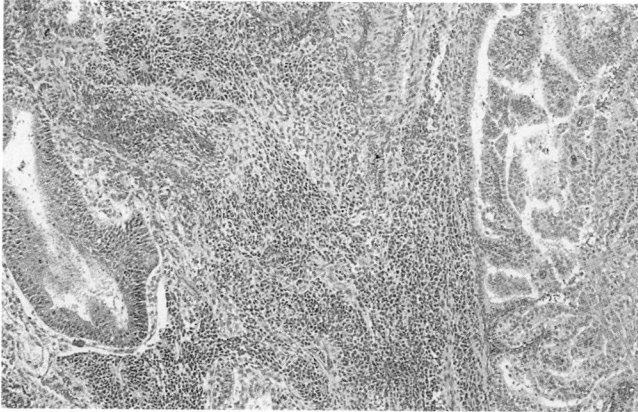

**FIGURE 34–23.** Immature teratoma component in a mixed germ cell tumor. The immature component is the form of small, blue, round cells (primitive neuroectodermal tumor-like cells). Note the pseudorosettes in the upper left hand corner.

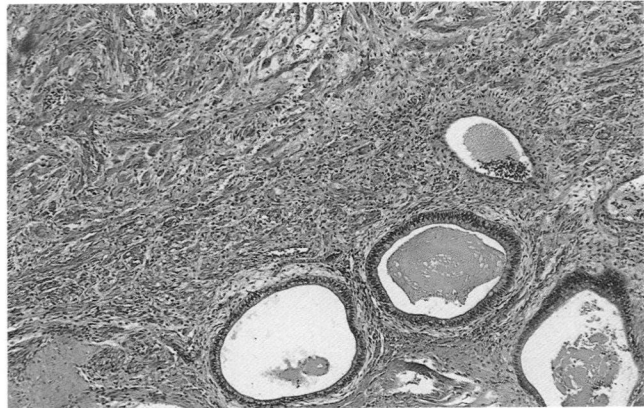

**FIGURE 34–24.** Teratoma with malignant transformation. Rhabdomyosarcoma is present adjacent to the glandular elements of mature teratoma.

lial somatic malignancies (e.g., adenocarcinoma and squamous cell carcinoma) also rarely may be present. The clinical significance of the malignant components is highly dependent on the site, whether primary or metastatic. The prognosis is worse when malignant transformation is present in the metastatic site.[119] Incomplete resection at the metastatic site is the most adverse prognostic factor.[52]

## Immunohistochemical Features

The immunoprofile of teratomatous elements is similar to that reported in the corresponding component it reproduces, although immunostains are rarely if ever required diagnostically. AFP may be focally positive in glandular elements and diffusely in hepatocellular areas. PLAP positivity has been reported in 4% to 27% of cases.[65]

## Differential Diagnosis

*Dermoid cyst,* the relationship of which with mature teratoma is controversial, consists of central keratinous material often containing hair, surrounded by a cyst wall composed of epidermis with skin appendages, including hair follicles and sebaceous glands.[118] The distinction from mature teratoma with predominant epidermal components is made by the absence of solid elements, any atypia or intratubular germ cell neoplasia, and the presence of hair.[65, 118] This separation is crucial because a metastasis from dermoid cyst has not been reported. *Epidermoid cyst* is not considered to be a teratoma, and histologic evaluation shows that it is composed of a cyst lined by keratinizing squamous epithelium. The nonlesional tissue should be sampled extensively because the presence of intratubular germ cell neoplasia goes against the diagnosis of an epidermoid cyst.

# MONODERMAL AND OTHER RARE TYPES OF TERATOMA

## Carcinoid Tumor

Primary carcinoid tumor of the testis is assumed to arise as a monodermal teratoma or to originate from argentaffin or enterochromaffin cells present in the gonad.[120] These extremely rare tumors occur either as pure neoplasms (approximately 75% of cases) or in association with testicular teratomas.[121–123]

Most carcinoid tumors are seen in patients older than the average age for other germ cell tumors (mean, 46 years; range, 10 to 83 years).[65, 121, 122] Patients present with unilateral testicular enlargement; only 12% of patients have symptoms related to the carcinoid syndrome.[65] Most carcinoid tumors have a benign clinical course, but all testicular carcinoids should be considered potentially malignant because approximately 8% have metastases.[122] Features that correlate with malignant behavior include large tumor size (>7 cm) and the presence of carcinoid syndrome. Smaller tumor size (<4 cm) and association with teratoma usually correlate with an indolent clinical course.[122]

### GROSS FEATURES

Pure carcinoid tumors are solid, well-circumscribed, pale yellow–to–brown tumors, ranging in size from 0.5 to 11 cm (mean, 3.5 cm).[122] The typical gross features of a teratoma are present when it is associated with a teratoma.

### MICROSCOPIC FEATURES

The tumor shows an insular, acinar, or trabecular pattern, with cells having uniformly round nuclei with finely dispersed chromatin (salt-and-pepper pattern). The cytoplasm is abundant and eosinophilic, often with distinct granularity. The tumor cells are positive on immunohistology for chromogranin, synaptophysin, neuron-specific enolase, and cytokeratin.

### DIFFERENTIAL DIAGNOSIS

The major differential diagnosis is with a *metastatic carcinoid tumor.* Association with teratomatous elements or absence of a primary lesion elsewhere indicates a primary testicular tumor. Bilaterality, multifocality, and angiolymphatic invasion favor a metastasis. Other differential diagnostic possibilities include a *Sertoli cell tumor;* however, attention to cytologic features and the use of appropriate immunohistochemical stains (inhibin or melan A/A103 positivity in sex cord–stromal tumors) should help in this differentiation.[124]

## Primitive Neuroectodermal Tumor

Most testicular primitive neuroectodermal tumors occur as a small component (representing immature teratoma) in mixed germ cell tumors.[65, 125] Sheets of small, poorly differentiated tumor cells, with foci showing primitive neural-type tubules lined by stratified epithelium, ependymal-type rosettes, or neuroblastic cells in an eosinophilic, fibrillary neuropil, are seen.[125] When present as a focal component in primary mixed germ cell tumors in the testis, primitive neuroectodermal tumor does not have an adverse prognosis.[126] The presence of primitive neuroectodermal tumor at metastatic sites and in patients previously treated with chemotherapy is associated with a high mortality, however.[126]

## MIXED GERM CELL TUMORS

Mixed germ cell tumor contains more than one germ cell tumor component in various combinations. It is the second most common testicular germ cell tumor, accounting for 40% to 45% of all primary germ cell tumors.[8, 127] The most common combinations are embryonal carcinoma and teratoma (26%); embryonal carcinoma and seminoma (16%); and embryonal carcinoma, yolk sac tumor, and teratoma (11%).[61] These tumors occur at a mean age of 30 years.[65] Prepubertal patients rarely have mixed germ cell tumors. Serum marker elevations are common and are a reflection of the components of the tumor (see Table 34–4).

### Gross Features

These tumors usually are variegated, reflecting a mixture of tumor types (Fig. 34–25). The different appearances within a tumor may have features suggestive of an individual tumor type (see "gross features" of each germ cell tumor).

### Microscopic Features

Individual components are identical to those in pure germ cell tumors (Fig. 34–26 and CD Fig. 34–19). Because the presence and amount of different components have prognostic implications (see "embryonal carcinoma" and "yolk sac tumor" earlier), it is important to list the components and their relative amounts in pathology reports (Table 34–7). Two distinctive patterns of mixed germ cell tumors are polyembryoma and diffuse embryoma. Although these patterns do not have any definite biologic significance other than those ascribable to individual components, because of their characteristic morphologic features, they are described separately.

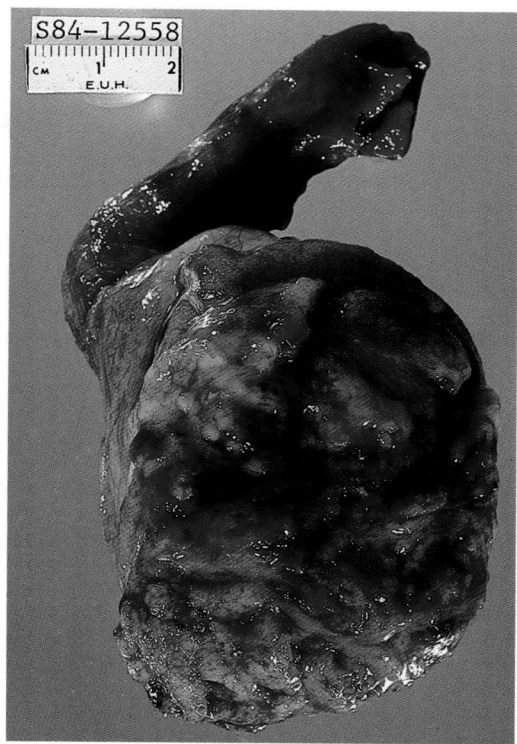

**FIGURE 34–25.** Mixed germ cell tumor (gross). Cut surface of the tumor shows variegated appearance with multiple foci of hemorrhage.

## POLYEMBRYOMA

In polyembryoma, embryonal carcinoma and yolk sac tumor components are arranged in a pattern resembling the presomitic embryo before day 18 of development.[128] Polyembryoma foci are always a part of a mixed germ cell tumor and most often are associated with teratoma. There are scattered embryoid bodies, with a central plate of one- to four-layer-thick, cuboidal-to-columnar cells (resembling

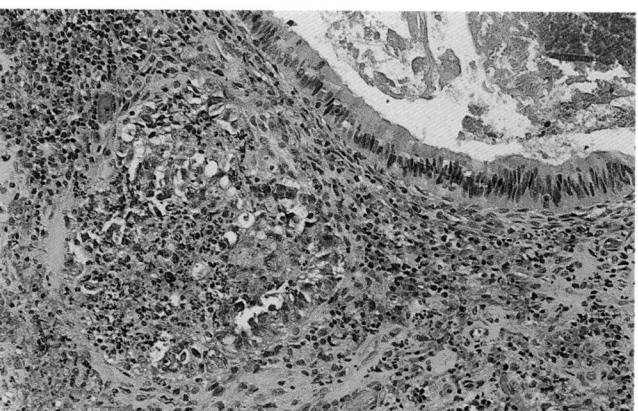

**FIGURE 34–26.** Mixed germ cell tumor, showing a combination of mature teratoma and embryonal carcinoma.

**TABLE 34–7.** Information to Be Recorded in a Surgical Pathology Report of a Testicular Germ Cell Tumor

---

***Primary Tumor***

Tumor size (cm)
Histologic type (pure or mixed; if mixed, list all components and their relative percentages)
Vascular invasion (present, absent, indeterminate)
Extent of tumor (confined to testis, through tunica albuginea involving tunica vaginalis, epididymis or spermatic cord involvement, scrotum [if resected])
Spermatic cord margin
Intratubular germ cell neoplasia*

***Metastatic Tumor†***

Number of lymph nodes examined
Number of lymph nodes positive
Size of largest metastasis (cm)
Extranodal extension (present, absent)
Histologic type (pure or mixed; if mixed, list all components and their relative percentages)

---

  \* Optional.
  † Information to be recorded when a viable tumor is present. Post-therapy resected nodes may contain fibrotic, necrotic, and xanthomatous areas. The presence or absence of a viable germ cell tumor must be recorded. Only lymph nodes with viable tumor are considered positive.

embryonal carcinoma); a "dorsal amnion–like cavity" lined by flat cells; and a "ventral yolk sac–like" vesicle composed of reticular and myxoid yolk sac tumor. The bodies generally are surrounded by a myxoid, embryonic-like mesenchyme.[65]

### DIFFUSE EMBRYOMA

In diffuse embryoma, an intimate mixture of orderly arranged embryonal carcinoma and yolk sac tumor occurs in roughly equal proportions. Yolk sac elements encircle foci of embryonal carcinoma as a parallel layer of flattened epithelium in a necklace or ribbon-like fashion.

## SEX CORD–STROMAL TUMORS

Sex cord–stromal tumors account for about 4% of all testicular neoplasms[65] but constitute almost 8% of the tumors in prepubertal boys.[129]

### Leydig Cell Tumor

Leydig cell tumor, the most common sex cord–stromal tumor of the testis, constitutes approximately 2% of all testicular neoplasms. These tumors may occur at any age, although a bimodal peak is observed; approximately 20% are detected in prepubertal boys, and about 25% are detected in men older than age 50 years. Only 3% occur bilaterally, and 15% extend beyond the testis at presentation.[130] Adults usually complain of testicular swelling, 30% have gynecomastia, and 20% have decreased li-

bido.[130] Children usually do not present with a mass lesion but with isosexual pseudoprecocity; the tumor often is detected after imaging studies.

The tumor is malignant in about 15% of cases. Other than the presence of metastasis, no single criterion predicts malignant behavior. Clinicopathologic features associated with an adverse outcome include older age (average age >60 years versus 40 years for all Leydig cell tumors), large size (6.9 cm mean size in malignant tumors versus 2.7 cm in benign tumors), infiltrative margins, angiolymphatic invasion, foci of necrosis, mitotic count of more than 3/10 high-power fields, and significant nuclear atypia.[130] The presence of at least four of these features strongly correlates with malignancy. Malignant Leydig cell tumors most often spread to regional lymph nodes, followed by lungs, liver, and bone.[131]

Testosterone and, uncommonly, androstenedione and dehydroepiandrosterone are secreted by Leydig cell tumors. Urinary 17-ketosteroids may be normal or high,[65] and estrogen levels may be elevated in some patients. Malignant tumors are rarely functional.

### GROSS FEATURES

The tumor is usually a sharply circumscribed solid mass, 3 to 5 cm in diameter, with a relatively typical yellow or yellow-tan–to–yellow-brown color (Fig. 34–27). Involvement of the entire testis or spread beyond the testis is rare; foci of hemorrhage or necrosis or both are seen in about 25% of tumors.

### MICROSCOPIC FEATURES

Diffuse and nodular growth patterns are most common; however, trabecular, tubular, or pseudofollicular patterns occasionally are present. Sheets and cords of cells are separated by fibrous bands of variable thickness that may have focal or conspicuous edematous or myxoid character. The tumor cells are large and polygonal with round nuclei and abundant eosinophilic cytoplasm (Fig. 34–28). Occasionally the cytoplasm is clear, vacuolated, or bubbly,

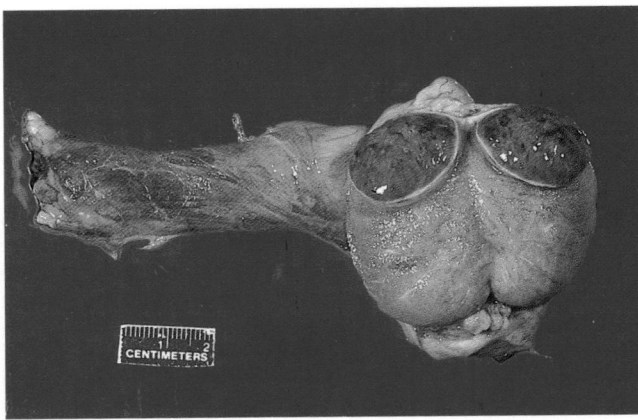

**FIGURE 34–27.** Leydig cell tumor (gross). A sharply circumscribed yellowish brown tumor.

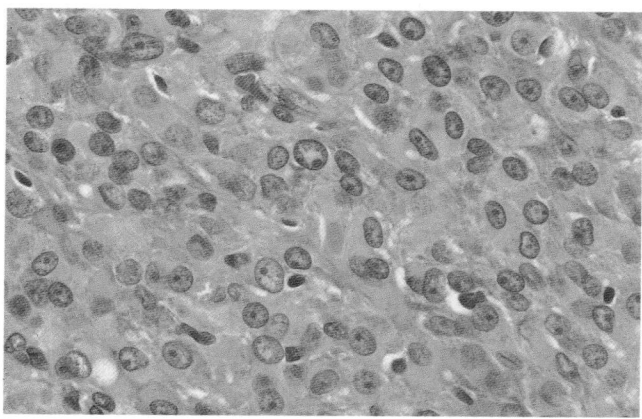

**FIGURE 34–28.** Leydig cell tumor. The tumor cells show a solid growth pattern, abundant pink granular cytoplasm, and minimally variable nuclei with prominent nucleoli. A crystalloid of Reinke is evident in the center.

owing to the presence of abundant lipid. Spindle cells with abundant pink cytoplasm may predominate in some cases. The nuclei typically have a single prominent nucleolus and rarely have nuclear grooves. Mitoses are rare but may be abundant when striking nuclear atypia is present. Reinke crystals—rod-shaped or oval-to-elongated pink cytoplasmic structures—considered pathognomonic, are seen in only one third of tumors. Lipofuscin is present in 10% to 15%.[130]

### IMMUNOHISTOCHEMICAL AND ULTRASTRUCTURAL FEATURES

Tumor cells are positive for inhibin (Fig. 34–29), melan A (A103), and vimentin; immunostaining for keratins and S-100 protein is negative or only focally positive.[132, 133] Ultrastructural features of steroid-producing cells are present and include the presence of abundant smooth endoplasmic reticulum, mitochondria with tubulocystic and lamellar cristae, and

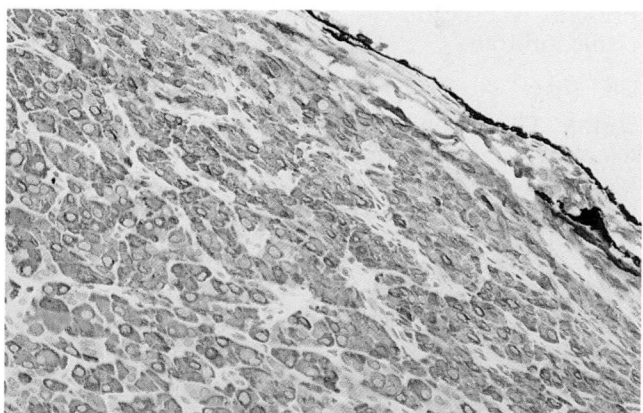

**FIGURE 34–29.** Leydig cell tumor. The tumor cells show diffuse and strong cytoplasmic positivity on immunohistochemical staining for inhibin.

abundant lipid droplets. In some cases, Reinke crystals showing a characteristic periodicity may be present.

### DIFFERENTIAL DIAGNOSIS

Leydig cell tumor may be confused with Leydig cell hyperplasia, large cell calcifying Sertoli cell tumor, testicular tumors of adrenogenital syndrome, malakoplakia, hepatoid yolk sac tumor, carcinoid tumor, lymphoma, and metastases to the testis. The absence of a discrete mass, an interstitial location of proliferating cells admixed with seminiferous tubules, and a background of testicular atrophy should suggest the diagnosis of *Leydig cell hyperplasia. Testicular tumors of adrenogenital syndrome* are bilateral, multifocal, and grossly dark brown. The cells show close resemblance to Leydig cell tumor; however, seminiferous tubules may be identified within the lesions, and Reinke crystals are absent. Multifocality and clinical history of adrenogenital syndrome are helpful in the diagnosis. *Large cell calcifying Sertoli cell tumors* usually are bilateral and multifocal and frequently show intratubular growth pattern at the periphery of the tumor. A tubular pattern, brisk acute inflammatory infiltrate, and prominent calcifications also are helpful in the diagnosis. Leydig cell tumor with myxoid stroma may be confused with *microcystic yolk sac tumor,* although an exclusively myxoid pattern is rare in yolk sac tumors. Overlap of Leydig cell tumor with *carcinoid tumor* may be superficially striking, but the distinctive architectural and nuclear characteristics of the latter and appropriate immunohistochemistry usually are diagnostic. Leydig cell tumors, particularly with scant cytoplasm and nuclear atypia, may be confused with *malignant lymphomas.* Lymphomas often are bilateral and have a characteristic interstitial pattern of growth. Bilaterality, multifocality, interstitial location, vascular invasion, prominent mitoses, clinical history, and immunostaining characteristics help in differentiation of Leydig cell tumor from *metastatic melanoma* and *carcinoma.*

## Sertoli Cell Tumor

Fewer than 1% of all testicular neoplasms are Sertoli cell tumors.[8, 134, 135] They occur at all ages, although it now is believed that bona fide cases of Sertoli cell tumors in children younger than 10 years old are quite rare.[65, 136, 137] Patients present with a scrotal mass that usually is unilateral.[8, 134, 137] Two variants, large cell calcifying Sertoli cell tumor and sclerosing Sertoli cell tumor, are described; only the former has unique clinical features to merit separate coverage from the usual form of Sertoli cell tumor. Evidence of hormonal production is rare in pure Sertoli cell tumors. Most Sertoli cell tumors are benign, but about 10% behave in a malignant fashion.[65] Large tumor size (>5 cm), presence of vascular invasion, mitotic rate of greater than 5/10 high-power fields, and solid and spindle cell architecture are reported to be associated more often with a malignant outcome.[138]

### GROSS FEATURES

Sertoli cell tumors are usually small (average size, 3.5 cm), well delineated, usually homogeneous, sometimes lobulated, yellow-tan or white tumors and usually are confined to the testis.[8, 137] With the exception of tumors in patients with Peutz-Jeghers syndrome or large cell calcifying Sertoli cell tumor, bilaterality is rare.

### MICROSCOPIC FEATURES

Tubular differentiation is the hallmark of most of the usual Sertoli cell tumors, and the extent usually parallels the degree of differentiation (Fig. 34–30). Some tumors may have a predominant solid growth pattern and only rare foci of tubular differentiation. The tubules vary in size and shape and may be round and hollow, solid, or elongated or may have a retiform pattern. Sclerosing Sertoli cell tumors have prominent stromal sclerosis throughout the tumor but otherwise have architectural patterns similar to the usual tumors[139] (CD Fig. 34–20). The tumor cells usually have moderate to occasionally abundant pale or eosinophilic cytoplasm. Most have bland cytologic features with a large vesicular nucleus and a prominent central nucleolus, but pleomorphism may be a feature in less differentiated tumors.[8, 138] Rarely, Sertoli cell tumors have a prominent malignant spindle cell component (sarcomatoid Sertoli cell tumor) that may show heterologous (e.g., osteosarcoma) differentiation.[140]

### IMMUNOHISTOCHEMICAL AND ULTRASTRUCTURAL FEATURES

Immunostains for cytokeratin and vimentin usually are positive in Sertoli cell tumors. S-100 protein, inhibin, and melan A (A103) staining is variable.[124, 132, 133] On ultrastructural evaluation, Sertoli cell tumors typically have a well-developed Golgi apparatus, variably prominent rough endoplasmic reticulum,

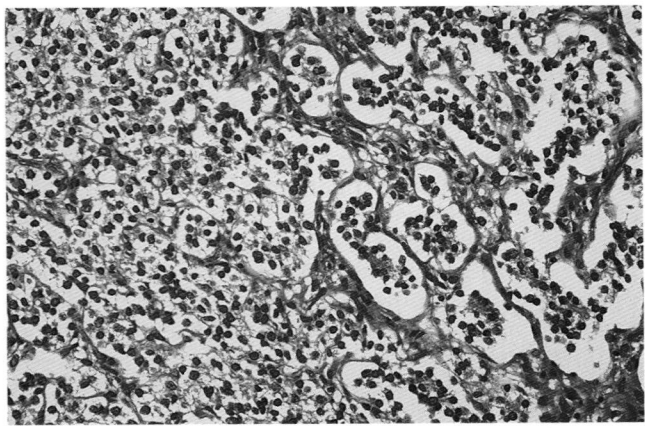

**FIGURE 34–30.** Sertoli cell tumor. Uniform cuboidal to columnar cells with clear cytoplasm are arranged in solid tubules and cords in this well-differentiated tumor.

lipid droplets, lateral desmosomes, and a peripheral investment of basement membrane. Rarely, *Charcot-Böttcher filaments* (parallel arrays of cytoplasmic filaments) are seen.

## Large Cell Calcifying Sertoli Cell Tumor

Large cell calcifying Sertoli cell tumor is a subtype of Sertoli cell tumor most commonly seen in the teens to early 20s (range, 2 to 51 years).[141–143] Patients frequently present with bilateral (40%) and multifocal (60%) disease.[142] Besides gynecomastia and sexual precocity, these tumors have unusual and interesting associations, including acromegaly, mucocutaneous pigmentation, sudden death, and Peutz-Jeghers syndrome.[142] A strong association with Carney's syndrome and its stigmata, including pituitary adenoma, cardiac myxoma, bilateral primary nodular adrenocortical hyperplasia, and lentigines, is known.[142, 144] Eight of 47 reported cases with large cell calcifying Sertoli cell tumor have been clinically malignant.[143] Malignant tumors usually occur in older patients and in patients without a syndrome (Peutz-Jeghers or Carney's). In contrast to benign tumors, these are unilateral and unifocal and show extratesticular spread, large size (>4 cm), vascular invasion, atypia, and necrosis.

Grossly, large cell calcifying Sertoli cell tumors are usually small (mean size, 2 cm), often multifocal, bilateral, and well-circumscribed tumors. Sectioning reveals firm, yellow-to-tan–to–white surface, often with fine-to-coarse granular calcific foci.

On microscopy, the tumor cells are large cuboidal-to-columnar with abundant eosinophilic cytoplasm and are arranged in diffuse sheets, nests, trabeculae, cords, tubules, or small groups separated by fibrous stroma. Foci of intratubular tumor with hyalinization of the basement membrane are present in about 50% of the tumors. A characteristic and frequent feature is the presence of conspicuous large basophilic, laminated calcific bodies (Fig. 34–31). Psammoma bodies and ossification also may be present. Many tumors show a prominent neutrophilic infiltrate.

### DIFFERENTIAL DIAGNOSIS

Sertoli cell tumors must be distinguished from *Sertoli cell nodules (Pick's adenoma)*, which are microscopic non-neoplastic congeners of immature tubules composed of Sertoli cells only that may be interspersed between Leydig cells and normal seminiferous tubules. A *typical seminoma* with clear cells and tubular pattern may mimic a Sertoli cell tumor; besides other cytoarchitectural features and intratubular germ cell neoplasia, PLAP, inhibin, and cytokeratin staining is helpful in making this distinction. *Juvenile granulosa cell tumors* may show superficial resemblance to Sertoli cell tumors. The former show prominent follicular differentiation that typically has irregular shape and size of the follicles, however,

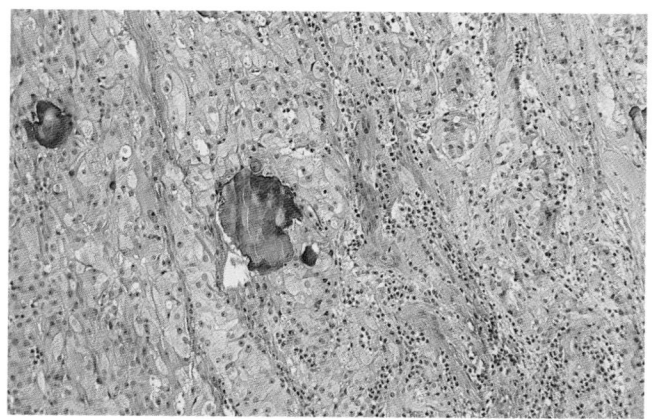

**FIGURE 34–31.** Large cell calcifying Sertoli cell tumor. The illustration shows nests and cords of large cells with eosinophilic granular cytoplasm and prominent calcifications. Notice the inflammatory infiltrate in the background, which is a frequent feature of this tumor.

compared with the generally more uniform tubules in Sertoli cell tumors. A diffuse architecture with eosinophilic or clear cytoplasm in some Sertoli cell tumors may resemble *Leydig cell tumor* (see "differential diagnosis" of Leydig cell tumor).

## Granulosa Cell Tumor

Similar to their ovarian counterparts, granulosa cell tumors have two distinct subtypes, adult and juvenile. The *adult-type granulosa cell tumor* is extremely rare, with fewer than 24 well-documented cases described in the literature.[65, 145] Patient age ranges from 20 to 53 years. Most patients present with a scrotal mass, some with a history of several years' duration. Twenty percent of cases are associated with gynecomastia. The tumors are lobulated, homogeneous, and yellow–to–yellow-gray and range in size from 1 to 13 cm. Microscopic examination reveals a microfollicular pattern with Call-Exner bodies or a solid pattern (CD Fig. 34–21). The nuclei are pale and oval-to-round with characteristic grooves.

The *juvenile form of granulosa cell tumor* is seen predominantly in infants and is the most common testicular tumor encountered in the first 6 months of life.[146, 147] Patients invariably present with a scrotal mass, and there is an association with undescended testis or gonadal dysgenesis.[147] The testis may measure 8 cm in diameter and is solid, cystic or solid and cystic in combination. The solid areas usually are yellow-orange, and the cysts are thin walled, containing viscid or gelatinous fluid. Microscopic examination shows variably prominent follicular and solid patterns. The follicles vary in size and may be quite large and typically contain basophilic or eosinophilic fluid that is mucicarmine and PAS positive. In solid areas, cells grow in sheets or nodules and in some cases are dispersed in a loose or myxoid stroma, simulating a reticular pattern of yolk sac

tumor (CD Fig. 34–22). The tumor cells are round-to-polyhedral with hyperchromatic nuclei and moderate-to-abundant eosinophilic cytoplasm. Mitoses usually are prominent.

Cytokeratins usually are negative or focally positive in granulosa cell tumors, and vimentin and inhibin usually are positive. All juvenile granulosa cell tumors are benign, whereas malignant outcome in adult granulosa cell tumors has been described.[145]

## Tumors of Fibroma-Thecoma Group

Tumors of fibroma-thecoma group are rare in testes and resemble their ovarian counterparts. Mean patient age is 30 years, and the outcome is uneventful.[65, 148]

## Mixed and Unclassified Sex Cord–Stromal Tumor

Some sex cord–stromal tumors contain histologic features of two or more of the above-described tumors and are considered mixed. Tumors similar to Sertoli-Leydig tumors of the ovary are rare in the testis. When the tumor lacks any specific differentiation but is deemed to be in the sex cord–stromal tumor category, the term *unclassified gonadal stromal tumor* is used. Unclassified sex cord–stromal tumors either have pure spindle cell morphology or are admixed with well-differentiated to poorly differentiated epithelial foci (CD Fig. 34–23). A clear cell variant, which almost invariably is confused with typical seminoma, has been described.[74] Because the clinical presentation and outcome are similar, mixed and unclassified tumors often are considered together. The tumors occur at all ages; however, a large proportion of tumors occurring in children are of the unclassified variety,[149] with 30% occurring in children younger than 1 year old.[137] Painless testicular enlargement is the most common presenting symptom, but gynecomastia is present in about 10% of patients.[65] The tumor behavior is mostly benign in prepubertal children, but about 25% of the cases in adults are malignant.[65]

On microscopy, the appearance of individual patterns in mixed tumors is similar to those in tumors with pure forms. In unclassified tumors, epithelial and stromal components are seen in varying proportions. The epithelial component consists of solid-to-hollow tubules or cords (resembling Sertoli cell elements), islands and masses of round-to-oval cells (resembling granulosa cells), or unclassifiable irregular interanastomosing trabeculae. The stromal component may range from densely cellular to fibrous. Mitoses usually are rare but may be prominent, particularly in the stromal component. Sarcomatoid patterns are frequent. The cells are variably positive for cytokeratin (even in stromal component), inhibin, S-100 protein, and desmin.

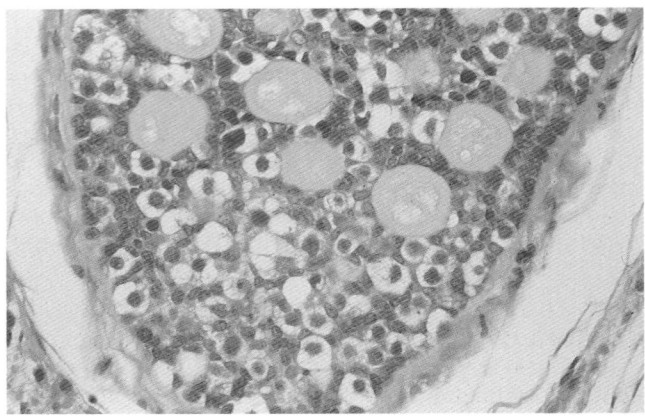

**FIGURE 34–32.** Gonadoblastoma. The tumor shows two cell types that are closely admixed: the smaller sex cord–stromal cells with eosinophilic hyaline material (Call-Exner-like bodies), and larger germ cells with abundant clear cytoplasm.

## MIXED GERM CELL–SEX CORD–STROMAL TUMORS

Mixed germ cell–sex cord–stromal tumors consist of neoplastic germ cells and sex cord–stromal components. There are two types of tumors in this category: gonadoblastoma and unclassified.

### Gonadoblastoma

Gonadoblastoma almost always is seen in dysgenetic gonads or undescended testis.[150, 151] About 80% of affected individuals are phenotypic females. Most patients are negative for sex chromatin, with karyotypes of 46,XY or mosaicism of 45,XO/46,XY.[152, 153] The gonads have features of mixed gonadal dysgenesis (unilateral streak gonad/streak testis and contralateral testis, or bilateral streak testes). About 40% are bilateral, and most patients are younger than age 20 years. The tumors may be considered to be in situ germ cell tumors because 50% develop invasive seminoma, and approximately 10% develop other germ cell tumor elements.[150]

The tumor is gray–to–yellow-brown when grossly appreciable; approximately 25% are microscopic.[150] Microscopic examination shows that the tumor is composed of germ cells resembling seminoma cells and immature Sertoli cell–like sex cord cells. The two components typically are admixed and are present within rounded-to-irregular nests that also often contain hyaline deposits of basement membrane material (Fig. 34–32). The sex cord (inhibin positive) cells often surround individual seminoma-like (PLAP positive) cells within the nests, similar to that in a primary ovarian follicle.[150, 154] Calcifications occur in 80% of cases, usually starting in the basement membrane–like material. The overgrowth of other germ cell tumors may lead to distortion and obliteration of foci of gonadoblastoma.

Coarse calcifications in an invasive germ cell tumor should raise the suspicion of origin from a gonadoblastoma.[150] The prognosis for patients with pure gonadoblastoma is excellent; when complicated by invasive germ cell tumor, prognosis depends on the characteristics of the invasive tumor.[155]

## Unclassified Mixed Germ Cell–Sex Cord–Stromal Tumor

Most examples of unclassified mixed germ cell–sex cord–stromal tumors possibly represent unclassified sex cord–stromal tumors with entrapped non-neoplastic germ cells or are examples of "collision" tumors.[156] True unclassified mixed germ cell–sex cord–stromal tumor is a rare entity[65, 157] (CD Fig. 34–24).

## HEMATOPOIETIC TUMORS

### Malignant Lymphoma

Malignant lymphoma accounts for approximately 5% of all testicular neoplasms and is the most common testicular neoplasm that is bilateral (6% to 38% of cases, usually metachronous) or that occurs in men older than age 60 years.[158, 159] Approximately two thirds of patients have localized disease, and others have associated lymphomas of lymph nodes, skin, central nervous system, Waldeyer's ring, or bones.[65] The actuarial 5-year disease-free survival is approximately 35% with a median of 13 months.[158] Localized tumors (stage I), unilateral tumors, and tumors with sclerosis have a more favorable outcome.

Gross examination shows partial or complete replacement of the testis by multiple confluent nodules or a single mass that is fleshy, with a cream, tan, or slightly pink homogeneous cut surface (Fig.

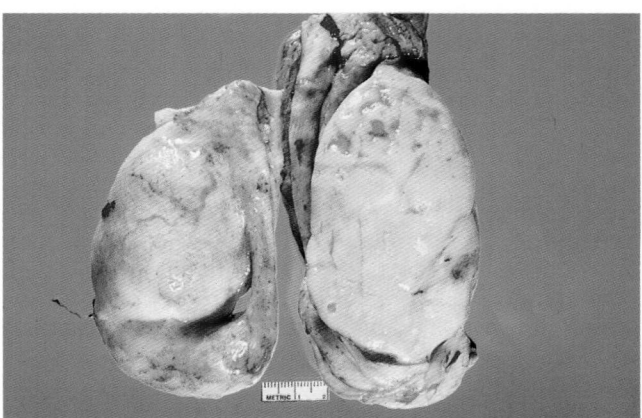

**FIGURE 34–33.** Malignant lymphoma (gross). Pale-tan fleshy tumor tissue completely replaces the testicular parenchyma and also involves the epididymis.

34–33). Gross epididymal and spermatic cord involvement is seen in 50% of cases.[158, 159] Histologic features include a tumor growth pattern that is typically interstitial with expansion of the intertubular spaces (Fig. 34–34). The seminiferous tubules usually are spared, but in many cases the tubules may be infiltrated by the tumor cells.[158]

Approximately 80% are diffuse large cell type, and 9% are small noncleaved cell type (using Working Formulation classification). Using the Kiel classification, 62% are centroblastic, 14% are immunoblastic, and 9% are Burkitt's type.[158] Most lymphomas that present in the testis are of B-cell phenotype. Cases of anaplastic (Ki-1) lymphoma, lymphoma of T cell or natural killer cell origin (similar to nasal type T cell/NK cell lymphoma), and rarely Hodgkin's disease have been reported.[65, 160, 161] T-cell lymphoma of lymphoblastic type is relatively common in children and young adults. Cytokeratin and PLAP are negative in lymphoma cells (useful in differentiation from seminoma and embryonal carcinoma), and leukocyte common antigen and other lymphoid markers are usually positive.

## Leukemic Infiltration

Sixty-five percent of patients with acute leukemias and 30% with chronic leukemia have involvement of the testis at autopsy.[162, 163] In current clinical practice, it is seen most commonly in biopsy specimens obtained to detect relapses after treatment in patients with acute lymphoblastic leukemia. The incidence of testicular infiltration by leukemia has increased as longer remissions from bone marrow and meningeal disease have been achieved.[164, 165] Testicular involvement is considered to be a harbinger of systemic relapse in such cases. Symptomatic testicular enlargement is seen in only 5% of cases. On microscopy, the pattern of leukemic infiltration is similar to that of lymphoma, predominantly intertubular, with rare tubular invasion and effacement.

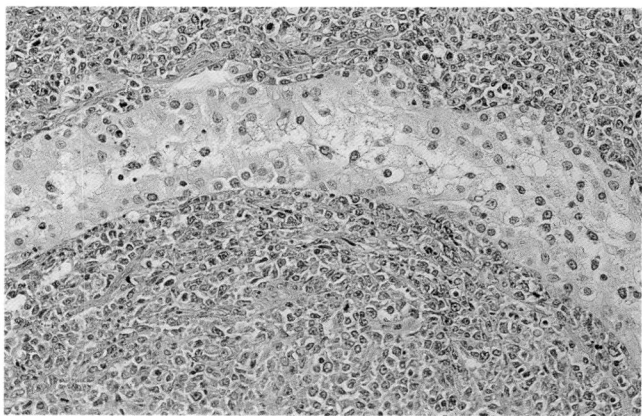

**FIGURE 34–34.** Malignant lymphoma. Large neoplastic lymphoid cells with the typical interstitial growth pattern, sparing the tubule in the middle.

## Multiple Myeloma and Plasmacytoma

The testis is involved in approximately 2% of cases of multiple myeloma, and it usually is identified only at autopsy.[166] In rare cases, testicular plasmacytoma may be an isolated finding, and in many of these it is the initial manifestation of a systemic disease.[167] The average age is about 55 years,[167] and bilaterality is seen in 20% to 30% of the cases. Gross appearance is similar to lymphoma except for less frequent involvement of the adnexa. The microscopic findings are similar to those at other sites, with interstitial involvement or effacement of the testicular parenchyma.

## METASTATIC TUMORS

Metastases to the testis, other than those from hematopoietic malignancies, are rare. In most cases (approximately 90%), patients are known to have a primary tumor.[168] Tumors from prostate (35%), lung (19%), skin (malignant melanoma) (9%), colon (9%), and kidney (7%) are the major sources of metastasis.[168] Age greater than 50 years, bilaterality, multifocality, interstitial growth, frequent vascular invasion, histology not conforming to germ cell or sex cord–stromal tumors, and clinical history all are helpful features to diagnose metastases.[65, 168, 169] In difficult cases, immunostaining (PLAP—usually negative in carcinomas; EMA—usually positive except in melanomas; and other appropriate markers) may prove helpful (see Table 34–6).

## TUMORS OF THE RETE TESTIS

### Benign Tumors

Benign tumorous lesions of rete testis rarely are described and include adenoma,[170] cystic dysplasia,[171] adenomatous hyperplasia,[172] adenofibroma,[173] and cystadenoma with sertoliform tubules.[174]

### Adenocarcinoma of the Rete Testis

Rete testis adenocarcinoma typically occurs in men older than age 30 years, who usually present with a painful scrotal mass and associated hydrocele.[65, 175, 176, 176a] The outcome usually is poor, with approximately 40% of patients dying within 1 year of the diagnosis.[176] The following criteria are required ideally to be met before a tumor is diagnosed as rete testis carcinoma: 1) absence of histologically similar extratesticular tumor, 2) tumor centered in testicular hilum, 3) morphology incompatible with any other type of testicular or paratesticular tumor, 4) presence of transition between unaffected rete testis and the tumor, and 5) a predominantly solid growth pattern.[175] The last two criteria are considered to be the least stringent for the diagnosis.[65] The tumors have a solid, tubular, papillary, or cribriform architecture, with columnar-to-cuboidal cells, nuclear stratification, and nuclei with moderate pleomorphism and frequent mitotic activity. The differential diagnoses include metastatic adenocarcinoma (particularly lung and prostate), paratesticular mesothelioma, and ovarian-type paratesticular epithelial tumors.

## TUMORS AND TUMOR-LIKE CONDITIONS OF PARATESTICULAR REGION (INCLUDING EPIDIDYMIS AND SPERMATIC CORD)

### Benign Conditions

#### ADRENAL RESTS

Ectopic adrenocortical tissue may occur in the spermatic cord, rete testis, epididymis, and tunica albuginea in about 4% of infants undergoing surgery for undescended testis or hernia.[177] Rarely, these rests may present as a mass lesion in adults.[178] The rests consist of small (usually <1 cm) yellow-orange nodules that appear on microscopic examination similar to normal adrenal cortex, predominantly zona fasciculata.

#### SPLENIC-GONADAL FUSION

Accessory splenic tissue may be seen adherent to the testis, epididymis, or spermatic cord or be present within tunica albuginea.[179] It may be connected to the abdominal spleen by a cord consisting of fibrous and splenic tissue (continuous type) or lack any connection (discontinuous type).[179] Enlargement may occur after splenectomy or in conditions that result in splenomegaly.

#### NODULAR AND DIFFUSE FIBROUS PROLIFERATION

A diffuse or localized, probably reactive, fibromatous proliferation can involve the tunics, epididymis, or spermatic cord. Numerous synonyms, including *nodular fibrous periorchitis, fibrous pseudotumor, reactive periorchitis*, and *fibrous mesothelioma*, have been used.[180, 181] The localized form consists of single or multiple nodules up to 9.5 cm in diameter, and in the diffuse form plaquelike diffuse thickening of the tunics is seen. The cut section is firm and white. Microscopic examination shows hyalinized collagen, with focal or massive calcification, in most cases. The histology in earlier lesions may be more cellular with granulation tissue–like fibrous proliferation and inflammation. Cellular lesions need to be differentiated from *sarcomas* and *infectious conditions*.

#### ADENOMATOID TUMOR

Adenomatoid tumor is the second most common paratesticular tumor after spermatic cord lipoma and is

of mesothelial origin. It may occur at any age, although it is quite rare in children.[65] Most patients present with a painless, firm, intrascrotal mass.[182] Adenomatoid tumor often involves the epididymis (usually the head) but may arise in testicular tunica or spermatic cord. Growth into testicular parenchyma is common, and despite infiltrative borders in some cases, the clinical course is benign.[65, 183, 184] The tumor almost always is solitary and unilateral. The gross tumor is a well-circumscribed, firm, tan-to-white nodule, typically smaller than 5 cm in diameter. On microscopic examination, a wide histologic spectrum, ranging from small to cystically dilated, round, oval, or slitlike tubules; signet ring–like cells; to cords and clusters of cells with intracytoplasmic vacuoles resembling epithelial units, vascular channels, or fat, may be seen (Fig. 34–35 and CD Fig. 34–25). The tubules are lined by flattened, cuboidal-to-columnar cells, with moderate-to-abundant eosinophilic or vacuolated cytoplasm. Usually a prominent fibrous-to-hyalinized stroma sometimes containing smooth muscle separates the tubules. Immunohistochemical and ultrastructural features are those of a mesothelium-derived tumor: positive for cytokeratins (CD Fig. 34–26), calretinin and thrombomodulin, and usually negative for carcinoembryonic antigen (CEA), Ber EP4, B72.3, and Leu M1, and the presence of long slender microvilli, intracellular canaliculi, desmosomes, and basal lamina on ultrastructural examination.[185]

The numerous differential diagnoses are a result of the protean histologic patterns seen in adenomatoid tumor. When tubular, *adenocarcinoma* and *mesothelioma* are in the differential diagnosis. Prominent vacuolation raises the possibilities of metastatic *signet ring cell carcinoma, liposarcoma*, or *histiocytoid hemangioma*. Primary intratesticular tumors, such as *yolk sac tumor* and *Sertoli cell tumor*, may be mimicked, at least superficially.

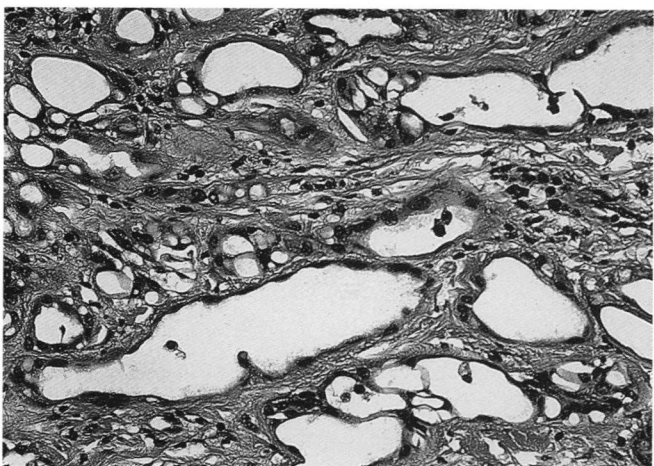

**FIGURE 34–35.** Adenomatoid tumor. Epithelial-like flat to cuboidal cells arranged in the form of tubules, irregular cysts, small cords and clusters, against the background of collagenous stroma.

## PAPILLARY CYSTADENOMA OF EPIDIDYMIS

Papillary cystadenoma of epididymis is a benign neoplasm accounting for almost one third of all primary epididymal tumors.[186-188] It is seen most often as an asymptomatic nodule in the head of the epididymis. There is a strong association with von Hippel–Lindau disease; two thirds of patients have von Hippel–Lindau disease, and more than one half of patients with von Hippel–Lindau disease develop (often bilaterally) papillary cystadenoma of epididymis.[186-188] The gross tumor is solid, cystic, or mixed solid and cystic and usually measures 1 to 2 cm in diameter. Cut surface is generally spongy with clear or green, yellow, or blood-tinged contents. Microscopy reveals a well-circumscribed mass composed of cells with clear (diastase-sensitive PAS positive) cytoplasm and variably sized tubules and cysts that may contain eosinophilic colloid-like contents. Intraluminal projections of papillae lined by single-layered or double-layered bland cuboidal-to-columnar cells are characteristic (Fig. 34–36).

## MESOTHELIAL CYSTS AND BENIGN CYSTIC MESOTHELIOMA

Thin-walled unilocular mesothelial cysts are found most commonly in the testicular tunics and less frequently in the epididymis and spermatic cord.[183, 189] These cysts are lined by flat-to-cuboidal mesothelial cells without cytologic atypia and are surrounded by hyalinized fibrous connective tissue. Multicystic structures with similar cytologic features have been designated *benign cystic mesotheliomas*.[189]

## AGGRESSIVE ANGIOMYXOMA

Lesions similar to those found in vulvovaginal regions of young women may occur in scrotum and spermatic cord. In contrast to the reported high recurrence rates in women (approximately 50%), aggressive angiomyxomas in men show a significantly lower recurrence rate (20%).[190, 191] On gross inspection, these are myxoid and gelatinous lesions that usually are unencapsulated, and even when grossly circumscribed, microscopic examination shows they are invariably infiltrative.

## ANGIOMYOFIBROBLASTOMA-LIKE TUMOR

Angiomyofibroblastoma-like tumors are well-circumscribed and morphologically and biologically similar to those occurring in the vulva of young to middle-aged women. These are described rarely in men in the scrotum and spermatic cord.[192]

## SCLEROSING LIPOGRANULOMA (PARAFFINOMA)

Sclerosing lipogranuloma is a distinctive granulomatous reaction that may occur in testicular and paratesticular locations. The features are similar to those described in Chapter 33.

## OTHER BENIGN TUMORS

Lipomas and lipomatous hypertrophy, which are difficult to distinguish from one another, constitute most paratesticular soft tissue masses.[193] Other benign tumors that may arise in the region include cutaneous myxoma, schwannoma, neurofibroma, giant cell tumor, hemangioma, and leiomyoma.[193]

# Malignant Tumors and Tumors of Uncertain Malignant Potential

## MESOTHELIAL TUMORS

### *Well-Differentiated Papillary Mesothelioma*

Well-differentiated papillary mesotheliomas are rare tumors of the tunica vaginalis of the testis[183, 194, 195] and are morphologically similar to well-differentiated papillary mesotheliomas of the peritoneum that generally occur in young women.[196] Most patients are in their 20s and 30s, presenting with unilateral or recurrent hydrocele.[194, 195] There is no firm association with asbestos exposure. Gross tumors are characterized by single or numerous nodules studding a hydrocele sac. Microscopic evaluation shows fibrous papillae covered by a single layer of flattened-to-cuboidal mesothelial cells that may show occasional basal vacuoles. The nuclear features are bland, and mitoses are absent or sparse.[194, 195] Psammoma bodies are seen occasionally.[194, 195] Well-differentiated papillary mesotheliomas are amenable to conservative surgical resection and have a favorable prognosis with no recurrences; however, the follow-up in most reported cases is not long.[195, 196] Because rare well-differentiated papillary mesotheliomas of the peritoneal cavity may evolve to diffuse malignant mesothelioma,[197] some experts consider all well-differentiated papillary mesotheliomas to be at least tumors of borderline malignancy.

### *Malignant Mesothelioma*

Malignant mesothelioma is the most common malignant neoplasm of the paratesticular region dis-

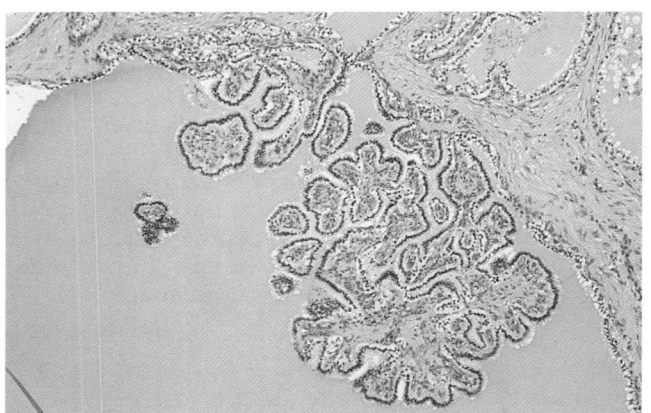

**FIGURE 34–36.** Papillary cystadenoma of epididymis. Papillary fronds are projecting into a cystic space containing eosinophilic colloid-like material. The bland-looking cells contain abundant clear cytoplasm.

playing an epithelial growth pattern.[183] The age at presentation ranges from 6 to 91 years (mean age, 53.5 years).[65, 198] Exposure to asbestos is the only known risk factor, with a confirmed positive history in 34% of cases.[183] Most patients present with clinical hydrocele. The gross tumor coats the tunica vaginalis in a diffuse or multinodular fashion, with or without invasion into surrounding structures. The microscopic features are similar to those seen at other sites. About 60% to 70% of cases are epithelial, and 30% to 40% are biphasic. Only one pure sarcomatous case has been reported.[199] Psammoma bodies may be present occasionally, as may be areas showing transition from normal to hyperplastic and neoplastic mesothelium. Mesotheliomas are positive for cytokeratins (AE1/AE3, Cam 5.2), WT-1, calretinin, cytokeratin 5/6, and thrombomodulin but negative for CEA, Leu M1, B72.3, Ber EP4, S-100, and E-cadherin.[183] This immunohistochemistry profile is of great value in the differential diagnosis from paratesticular *serous carcinoma* and *rete testis adenocarcinoma*. Distinction from *mesothelial hyperplasia* depends on the gross identification of a mass lesion, complex arborizing papillae with fibrovascular cores, invasive growth pattern, and cytologic atypia. The prognosis usually is guarded despite multimodal therapy; only 55% of patients survive beyond 2 years. Approximately 39% have local recurrences, and 56% to 65% develop metastases to retroperitoneum, lung, mediastinum, bone, or brain.[183]

## EPITHELIAL TUMORS

### Epididymal Carcinoma

Epididymal carcinoma is a rare tumor and has been reported only in adults (mean age, 47 years). The typical presentation is a scrotal mass, with or without hydrocele.[200] In contrast to epididymal papillary cystadenoma, no association with von Hippel–Lindau disease has been recorded. Epididymal carcinoma is an aggressive tumor, with about 50% of the patients ultimately dying of metastatic disease (e.g., retroperitoneal lymph nodes, lungs).[183, 188] On gross inspection, the epicenter of the mass must be in the epididymis with partial-to-complete destruction of epididymis and only limited, if any, involvement of the testis.[183] Microscopic features include invasive tubules, papillae, and sheets of cells with clear (diastase-sensitive PAS positive) to eosinophilic cytoplasm, with only mild-to-moderate atypia and rare mitotic figures.[183, 188]

### Ovarian-Type Epithelial Tumors

Ovarian-type epithelial tumors may occur in testicular tunics and rarely in the testis. They arise from either müllerian metaplasia of the mesothelium or paratesticular müllerian remnants (e.g., appendix testis); intratesticular tumors probably arise from embryonic mesothelial inclusions in the testis.[201, 202] Most cases have the features of papillary serous tumor of low malignant potential (serous borderline tumor) (Fig. 34–37 and CD Fig. 34–27), although

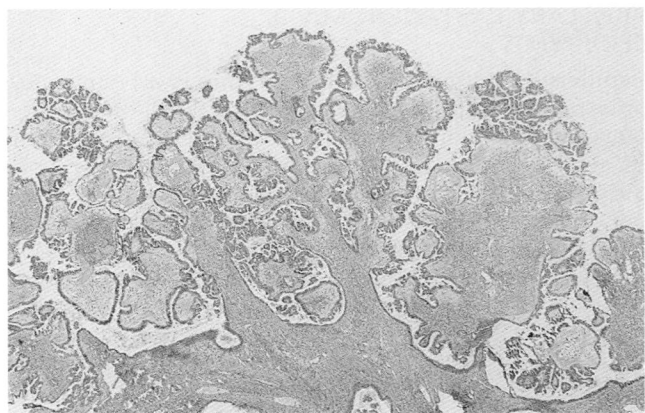

**FIGURE 34–37.** Papillary serous tumor of low malignant potential of tunica vaginalis, showing the typical morphologic features similar to those seen in the ovarian namesake.

serous carcinoma; benign, borderline, and malignant mucinous tumor; endometrioid carcinoma; Brenner's tumor; and clear cell carcinoma may occur rarely.[201] Morphologic evaluation shows they are identical to their namesakes in the ovary. The most difficult differential diagnostic consideration is between papillary serous tumor of low malignant potential and *malignant mesothelioma*. The differentiation is based on the greater degree of cellular budding and stratification, broader and branching papillae, and more prominent psammoma bodies in the former. Immunohistochemistry also is invaluable (see "malignant mesothelioma"). Although follow-up information is limited, patients with papillary serous tumor of low malignant potential seem to have an excellent prognosis, whereas patients with serous carcinoma, even if only focally invasive, have a guarded outcome.[203]

## MULTIPHENOTYPIC TUMORS

### Desmoplastic Small Round Cell Tumor

Desmoplastic small round cell tumor involves the paratesticular region as a primary tumor or in a secondary fashion.[202] They show the typical light microscopic features as seen in the abdominal tumors, with nests and islands of uniform small cells separated by a dense, variably cellular, fibrous or fibromyxoid stroma. Noted variations include tubules, pseudorosette formation, and cells containing abundant eosinophilic cytoplasm.[202] The cells have a characteristic polyimmunophenotypic profile (cytokeratin, desmin, and neuron-specific enolase positive). Although the behavior generally is aggressive, survival in patients with paratesticular tumors may be better than in patients with intra-abdominal tumors.[204]

### Melanotic Neuroectodermal Tumor of Infancy (Retinal Anlage Tumor, Melanotic Progonoma)

Melanotic neuroectodermal tumor of infancy most commonly involves the facial and skull bones of children within the first year of life; however, cases in paratesticular locations (mostly epididymal)

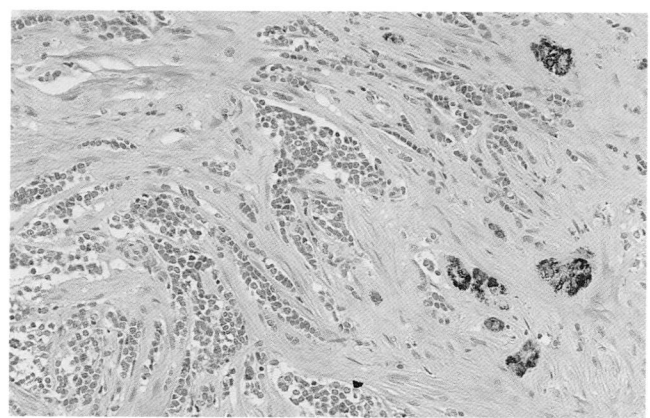

**FIGURE 34–38.** Melanotic neuroectodermal tumor. Nests of small, round, blue cells with hyperchromatic nuclei and scant cytoplasm, are associated with larger cells with abundant cytoplasm and melanin pigment.

are well documented.[202] Microscopic features include a characteristic dual population of cells; large melanin-containing, cuboidal-to-columnar epithelioid cells; and small neuroblastic cells (Fig. 34–38). On immunohistochemistry, the large cells stain for cytokeratins and HMB-45, and both cell types are neuron-specific enolase, synaptophysin, and Leu 7 positive. The clinical behavior usually is benign; however, tumors rarely may metastasize to inguinal and retroperitoneal lymph nodes.[205, 206]

## SARCOMAS

### Rhabdomyosarcoma

The paratesticular region is the most common site for rhabdomyosarcoma.[207] About 60% occur in the first 2 decades of life; mean age at presentation is 6.6 years. Any histologic subtype of rhabdomyosarcoma may occur in this location, although most cases are of embryonal subtype (about 90%), and within this subtype there is a predilection for spindle cell variant (leiomyomatous) histology[208]; approximately 6% are of alveolar subtype. The spermatic cord and paratesticular areas are involved predominantly or exclusively, and invasion into testicular parenchyma is rare.[209] Desmin, muscle-specific actin, myogenin, and myoD1 are positive and helpful in the differential diagnosis from other small round blue cell tumors and pleomorphic sarcomas. Prognosis depends largely on the extent (stage) of the disease at diagnosis. The 5-year event-free survival is approximately 80%, with the spindle cell variant having the best prognosis (>90%) with multimodal therapy.[210] The prognosis generally is much worse for stage III and IV disease.

### Leiomyosarcoma

Leiomyosarcoma represents about 30% of paratesticular sarcomas in adults.[207] Patient age ranges from 15 to 84 years (mean, 58 years). Origin in the spermatic cord is almost five times more frequent than in the epididymis. The histologic features are

identical to uterine tumors and may span a spectrum from extremely well-differentiated tumors that are distinguished from leiomyomas by virtue of mitotic activity and infiltrative growth only to markedly pleomorphic tumors that may require immunohistochemical staining to confirm a smooth muscle phenotype.[207] Although the criteria for separation from leiomyoma are not well defined, any mitotic activity, especially with nuclear atypia or necrosis, should be regarded as a sign of malignancy.[207] In young patients, an important differential diagnosis is with a *spindle cell rhabdomyosarcoma*.

### Liposarcoma

Liposarcoma probably is the most common sarcoma in the paratesticular location in adults.[207] Most cases are well differentiated (lipoma-like or sclerosing type), although myxoid and round cell, pleomorphic, and dedifferentiated subtypes may occur, albeit rarely. In some cases, the diagnosis is an unexpected finding at the time of examination of tissue surgically removed as "lipoma of the cord." The high frequency of local recurrence (79%) and the risk of dedifferentiation in well-differentiated tumors argues against the usage of the term *atypical lipoma* for paratesticular liposarcoma.[207] Occasionally an inguinal or paratesticular extension may be an initial manifestation in a retroperitoneal liposarcoma.

Other sarcomas reported from the paratesticular region include malignant fibrous histiocytoma (Fig. 34–39), fibrosarcoma, osteosarcoma, neurogenic sarcoma, angiosarcoma, Kaposi's sarcoma, malignant

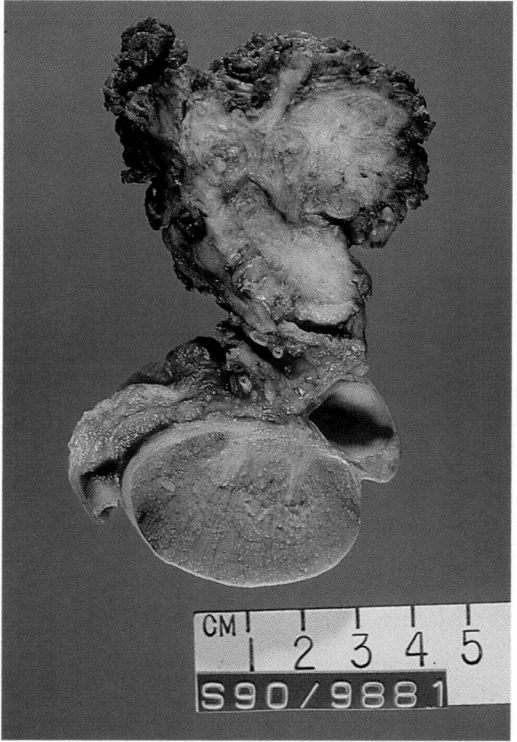

**FIGURE 34–39.** Malignant fibrous histiocytoma of the spermatic cord (gross).

solitary fibrous tumor, and rhabdoid tumor. Their pathologic features are similar to those in more common sites.

## INFECTIOUS AND INFLAMMATORY MIMICS OF TESTICULAR NEOPLASMS

### Orchitis

#### PYOGENIC ORCHITIS

In bacterial orchitis, the epididymis typically also is affected. The testis may show abscesses or may be fibrotic and adherent to the surrounding tissues, mimicking a neoplasm. *Escherichia coli* is the most common causative agent.

#### VIRAL ORCHITIS

About 25% of adults and fewer than 1% of children with *mumps* have testicular involvement and enlargement, raising the question of a neoplasm. The involvement is bilateral in about 20%, and the epididymis is affected in more than 80% of such cases.[65] On microscopic examination, it is characterized initially by edema and predominantly lymphocytic interstitial infiltrate. In later stages, intratubular inflammation and tubular destruction may be seen. Healing leads to patchy tubular hyalinization and interstitial fibrosis. *Coxsackie B virus* is the other relatively common cause for viral orchitis.

#### GRANULOMATOUS ORCHITIS

*Infectious granulomatous orchitis* may be due to tuberculosis, syphilis, leprosy, fungi, brucellosis, parasites, and rickettsia. Clinically, testicular involvement may resemble a neoplasm. *Idiopathic granulomatous orchitis* is the most common non-neoplastic lesion to mimic a neoplasm.[65] It is characterized grossly by a solid, nodular replacement of the normal testicular parenchyma, occasionally with focal necrosis. Microscopic examination shows the seminiferous tubules are filled with inflammatory cells composed predominantly of epithelioid histiocytes (Fig. 34–40), with variable plasma cells, neutrophils, and lymphocytes. Langhans's-type giant cells may be present, and sometimes eosinophils are prominent. The granulomatous response is at least in part secondary to the products of disintegrated sperm. A history of trauma to the region or urinary tract infection by gram-negative microorganisms frequently is available; ischemic and postobstructive causes also are proposed.

### Malakoplakia

Malakoplakia may involve the testis, either alone or in association with epididymis. It is usually unilateral.[211] Sectioning shows patchy, nodular or diffuse parenchymal replacement by usually yellow, and

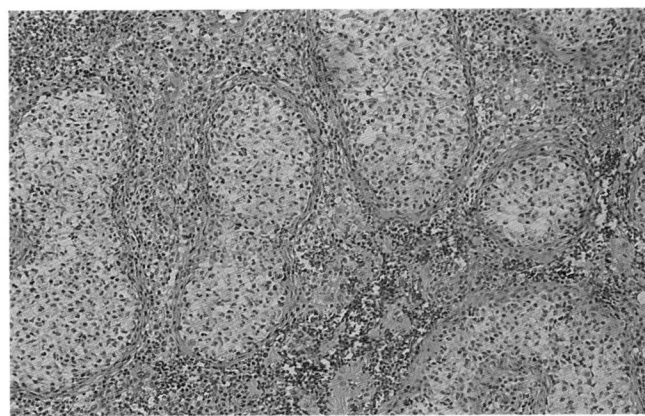

**FIGURE 34–40.** Idiopathic granulomatous orchitis. The seminiferous tubules are completely filled and expanded by granulomatous inflammation.

less commonly tan or brown, tissue. Microscopic examination shows the tubules and interstitium are replaced by abscesses and large histiocytes with granular eosinophilic cytoplasm (von Hansemann cells) occasionally containing targetoid, calcific, basophilic inclusions (Michaelis-Gutmann bodies), with a mixed inflammatory infiltrate. A prominent von Hansemann cell infiltrate may mimic a Leydig cell tumor. PAS, von Kossa and iron stains, and immunohistochemical histiocytic marker CD 68/KP1 help confirm the diagnosis. Two other proliferative histiocytic disorders that occasionally involve the testis are juvenile xanthogranuloma and Rosai-Dorfman disease.[212, 213]

## INFERTILITY-RELATED CHANGES

Infertility is a daunting problem that faces approximately 15% of couples. An abnormality in the male partner, so-called male factor infertility, accounts for about half of the cases (Table 34–8). Testicular biopsy as a means for investigating male infertility was introduced in 1940,[214] and for many years it was the gold standard for assessing spermatogenesis. The classification of impaired spermatogenesis into pretesticular, testicular, and post-testicular categories by Wong and colleagues[215–217] has been accepted widely, and it continues to be useful. Remarkable advances in reproductive technology occurred in the past decade, however, and new ways of managing male infertility have emerged. The most spectacular was the advent of in vitro fertilization by intracytoplasmic sperm injection (ICSI) directly into the ovum.[218] New techniques to assess spermatogenesis and to retrieve spermatozoa from the reproductive tract have been developed. Attention now is focused on azoospermia, which has two broad categories, obstructive (caused by a block in the excurrent ducts) and nonobstructive (caused by defective spermatogenesis). Therapeutic efforts are directed at correcting a block or obtaining sper-

**TABLE 34–8.** Principal Causes of Male Infertility

*Pretesticular*
Hypogonadotropism
  Prepubertal
  Postpubertal
Estrogen excess
  Endogenous
  Exogenous
Autoimmune

*Testicular*
Maturation arrest
Hypospermatogenesis
Absent germ cells (SCO*)
Genetic
  Klinefelter's
  Abnormal Y chromosome
Cryptorchidism
Iatrogenic
  Irradiation
  Chemotherapy
Mumps

*Post-Testicular*
Congenital (blocked ducts)
  Absence of vas
  Absence of seminal vesicle
Acquired
  Infection
  Vas ligation

\* SCO, Sertoli cell–only syndrome.

matozoa for ICSI. Needle aspiration has been eminently successful in obtaining viable spermatozoa and their precursors, and cytology has proved to be valuable in evaluating spermatogenesis.

Testicular biopsy continues to have a role in the management of infertility because it can assess the status of the germinal epithelium, the lamina propria, and the interstitium and confirm the diagnosis of obstructive azoospermia, with the possibility of surgical repair.[219] It is the surgical pathologist's responsibility to oversee processing of the testicular biopsy specimen and to recognize the abnormalities associated with infertility. These include hypospermatogenesis, maturation arrest, tubular hyalinization, mixed atrophy, Klinefelter's syndrome, cryptorchidism, Sertoli cell–only syndrome, and intratubular germ cell neoplasia, which has an increased incidence in the infertile man.

## Biopsy Specimen

The germinal epithelium is fragile and must be handled gently to avoid crush artifact. Ideally the pathologist should be present to receive the histopathologic specimen, ensuring prompt fixation in the correct fixative. It is best to place the specimen directly into fixative, preventing contact with a gauze sponge. The usual specimen is several millimeters in maximal diameter; a bit of tunica albuginea may be adherent. For light microscopy, a variety of fixatives has been recommended, including Bouin's, Stieve's,

and Zenker's.[220, 221] We prefer Bouin's solution. For routine sections, the specimen is embedded in paraffin and stained with H&E. Formalin should not be used as it causes irretrievable artifacts.

## Normal Testis

The ideal specimen contains two dozen or more cross-sections of tubules (Fig. 34–41). The normal seminiferous tubule is 180 $\mu$ or more in diameter. The normal germinal epithelium occupies about two thirds of the radius of the tubule; it is supported by a thin basal lamina. The germinal epithelium consists of differentiating gametes together with Sertoli cells. Spermatogenesis involves meiosis I and II, with differentiation of spermatocytes into spermatids and spermatozoa. In men, that process occurs in six stages, and each has its own particular association of seminiferous cells.[222] The cellular composition of the germinal epithelium along the length of a tubule varies according to these stages and is not uniform within a single cross-section of a particular tubule. In H&E section, the germ cells that can be recognized are the spermatogonia, primary spermatocytes, secondary spermatocytes, spermatids, and spermatozoa. If the testis is normal, all these types are found in the biopsy specimen.

The Sertoli cells are far outnumbered by the germ cells, and they appear sparse and inconspicuous in the normal germinal epithelium. They are diploid, nonmitotic cells. The nuclei are basal, with prominent nucleoli. Sertoli cells have an important function in spermatogenesis, surrounding the developing germ cells and forming compartments (known as *basal* and *adluminal*) in the germinal epithelium. These compartments contain the germ cells as they move from a basal position toward the lumen. Maturation of spermatids to spermatozoa occurs in the apical folds of the Sertoli cell cytoplasm. Sertoli cells are the sole target of follicle-stimulating hormone.

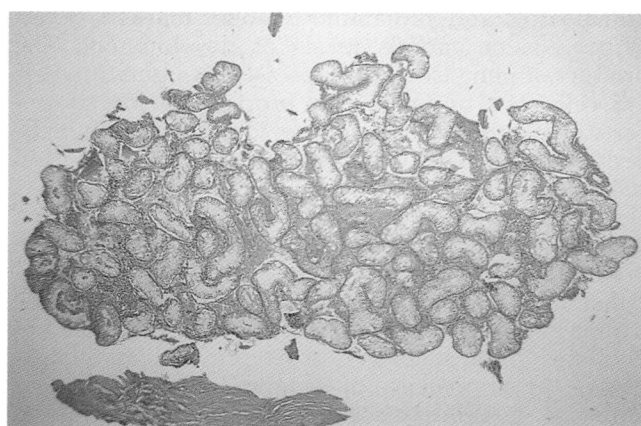

**FIGURE 34–41.** An adequate testicular biopsy, containing profiles of several dozen tubules. Note scrap of tunica albuginea in lower left. Sertoli cell–only syndrome. ×12.5 (Courtesy of Dr. Francis H. Straus.)

Under its influence, they secrete the androgen-binding protein required for spermatogenesis. Sertoli cells also secrete the glycoprotein inhibin B, an inhibitor of follicle-stimulating hormone secretion and a feedback regulator. Inhibin B is considered a useful marker of spermatogenesis. Sertoli cells also have a phagocytic function, and the cytoplasm may contain lipofuscin and lipid vacuoles. Oncocytic transformation has been observed in cryptorchid and retractile testes.[223, 224]

The interstitial cells of Leydig occur singly and in small clusters in the interstices between the tubules, together with small vessels and nerve twigs. Leydig cells also can be found in the tunica vaginalis and in the spermatic cord. Luteinizing hormone stimulates the Leydig cells to secrete testosterone, required for normal spermatogenesis. The hallmark of the functionally competent interstitial cell is the crystalloid of Reinke, although these are not found in every cell. Lipofuscin and lipid droplets also may be present. Proliferation of Leydig cells appropriately is termed hyperplasia when the proliferated cells fill and expand the interstitial space or form micronodules displacing the tubules.

The tubule is surrounded by a lamina propria consisting of a thin layer of collagen, reticulin, and smooth muscle in the form of peritubular contractile myoid cells.[225, 226] Spermatozoa in the testis are incapable of independent motility and must be propelled passively. Any process that damages the lamina propria has the potential for damaging the myoid cells, compromising the production and maturation of the spermatozoa. Varicocele and cryptorchidism have been cited as examples.[227] At puberty, the lamina propria acquires reticulin fibers, and the presence of reticulin differentiates tubular atrophy from hypoplasia.

Immunohistochemical markers promise to be a valuable adjunct in the identification of foci of spermatogenesis in a biopsy specimen. Male germ cells can be identified by immunohistochemical markers associated with genes *RBM* (RNA-binding motif),[228] *DAZ* (deleted in azoospermia), *CDY1* (chromodomain y1), and protamine-2. These markers detect germ cells at various levels of development. The product of gene *CK-18* is expressed in immature Sertoli cells, but normally this property is lost at puberty.[229] Sertoli cells also are identified with antibody to the *MIC2* gene product, which stains Sertoli cells but not germ cells.

Morphometry offers reproducible information that has proved useful in the evaluation and interpretation of testicular biopsy specimens.[225, 230] Parameters include tubular diameter, thickness of the lamina propria, and composition of the germinal epithelium.[231] The Johnsen[232] score provides an evaluation of the competence of the germinal epithelium in terms of its cellular constituents. The score ranges from 1 (no germ cells or Sertoli cells present) to 10 (complete spermatogenesis). After it was discovered that spermatocytes and round spermatids were capable of achieving pregnancy by ICSI, Yoshida and coworkers[233] proposed a modification known as the *seminiferous tubule score*, which recognizes and classifies the spermatocytes as primary or secondary and the spermatids as round and late forms. Identification and enumeration of mature spermatids are useful parameters in evaluating spermatogenesis. According to Silber,[221] the sperm count can be predicted by counting the total number of spermatids in at least 20 tubules and dividing the result by the number of tubules counted. From this information, the competence of the germinal epithelium can be established, avoiding an erroneous interpretation of adequate spermatogenesis, and an incorrect diagnosis of a block.

The intensive search for viable spermatozoa and spermatids has brought out the limitations of the biopsy method in analyzing infertility and azoospermia. Perhaps the most serious of these is the problem of sampling. It has become apparent that sections of a biopsy specimen from a patient with azoospermia may reveal tubules containing viable spermatozoa and spermatids side by side with tubules showing many of the most common histopathologic entities associated with infertility, including maturation arrest, Klinefelter's syndrome, irradiation damage, hyalinization resulting from mumps orchitis, cryptorchidism, and absence of germ cells (Sertoli cell–only syndrome). In this connection, sampling by means of needle aspiration has proved to be a useful method for assessing spermatogenesis,[234] mapping spermatogenesis,[235] and retrieving sperm for ICSI. Fine-needle aspiration does not permit, however, evaluation of tubules, tunica propria, or interstitial tissue.

It has become apparent that genetic abnormalities are an important cause of infertility.[236] The long arm of the Y chromosome is required for male fertility, and microdeletions in three different regions can cause severe spermatogenic defects, with a broad spectrum of associated histologic patterns ranging from Sertoli cell–only syndrome to maturation arrest and hypospermatogenesis. This is a rapidly expanding field, and continued explosive growth can be anticipated.

## Histopathology

### HYPOSPERMATOGENESIS (PROPORTIONAL HYPOPLASIA)

In hypospermatogenesis, all cell types of the germinal epithelium are present in the usual proportions, but the total number of cells of each type is reduced.[237] Consequently the thickness of the germinal epithelium is diminished (Fig. 34–42). In cases with minimal involvement, the tunica propria is unremarkable, and the Leydig cells are not affected. With advanced involvement, the tubular wall is thickened, the tubular lumina are reduced, and Leydig cells are increased.[238] A form of this disorder known as *hypospermatogenesis associated with primary spermatocyte sloughing* also has been described.[230] Pa-

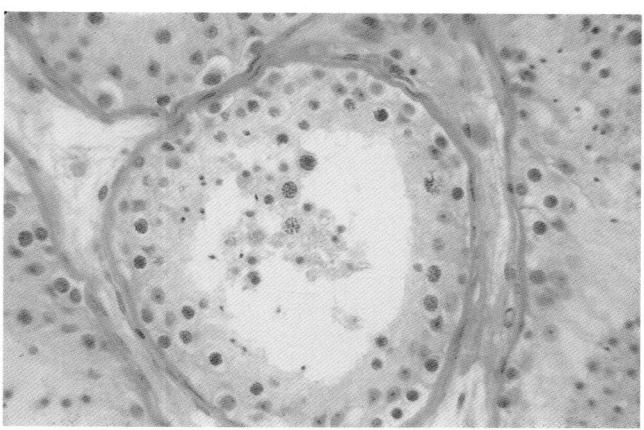

**FIGURE 34–42.** Hypospermatogenesis. All cell types are present, but number of cells and thickness of germinal epithelium are greatly reduced. ×250

tients with hypospermatogenesis have oligospermia. The cause has been ascribed to a primary defect in the stem cell population, which somehow is prevented from differentiation.[237] More recently, Sertoli cell failure has been implicated as the cause of the germ cell deficiency.[230] Other factors cited include hormonal dysfunction, androgen insensitivity, exposure to chemical or physical agents, and vascular malfunction.[230] In 5 of 25 patients in Soderstrom and Suominen's series,[237] the condition was found in only one testis.

## MATURATION ARREST

Maturation arrest is a block in maturation of germ cells at a particular stage; the precursor cells are normal or increased in number.[239] The arrest usually is at the level of the primary spermatocytes, although arrest at the level of spermatids or spermatogonia has been described. No abnormalities of Sertoli cells or tunica propria are apparent, and the Leydig cells appear unremarkable. The patient may have azoospermia or oligospermia. Patients with maturation arrest may benefit from testicular sperm extraction, which may yield occasional spermatids or spermatozoa that can be used successfully for ICSI.[221]

## TUBULAR HYALINIZATION

Tubular hyalinization is the end result of atrophy of germ cells and Sertoli cells, with sclerosis of the lamina propria and shrinkage of interstitium (Fig. 34–43). As the epithelium disappears, the tubular diameter decreases, and the wall becomes fibrotic and thickened. The end stage of the process is a shriveled, hyalinized tubular remnant that may have an ill-defined rim of nondescript cells at the periphery. The elastic fibers persist. Small clusters of Leydig cells may persist in the interstitium. These patients are azoospermic. A variety of causes are responsible,[230] including Klinefelter's syndrome, hypogonadotropic hypogonadism, viral orchitis result-

ing from mumps or coxsackie B virus, excess estrogen, radiation injury, and chemotherapy. The testis in the end stage is atrophic with hyalinized tubules. The involvement may be patchy, and a few normal tubules may persist.

## MIXED ATROPHY

Focal tubules containing only Sertoli cells may be encountered in a testis that otherwise has tubules with complete or incomplete spermatogenesis.[230, 240] This condition is known as *mixed atrophy*. As pointed out by Nistal and Paniagua,[230] many cases of mixed atrophy have been included under a variety of other diagnoses, including hypospermatogenesis, Sertoli cell–only syndrome with focal spermatogenesis, partial del Castillo's syndrome, cryptorchidism, retractile testes, chromosomal anomalies (Down's syndrome, Klinefelter's syndrome with mosaicism), partial androgen insensitivity, varicocele, and chemotherapy. Under these circumstances, diagnoses such as *Sertoli cell–only syndrome with focal spermatogenesis* have been rendered, leading to confusion, as described subsequently.

## KLINEFELTER'S SYNDROME

The classic patient with Klinefelter's syndrome is a phenotypic male with small testes, eunuchoid body habitus, gynecomastia, and azoospermia. It is a common condition, with an incidence cited as 1:600 live male births.[241] The usual cause is nondisjunction of the X chromosome in the mother and an extra X chromosome (47,XXY) in the offspring. Urinary gonadotropins are elevated, and plasma testosterone is low. At puberty, the testes fail to mature; instead, a distinctive form of tubular sclerosis occurs, characterized by hyalinization of tubules and failure of development of germinal epithelium (Fig. 34–44). Germ cells and Sertoli cells disappear gradually (Fig. 34–45). The tubules lose their lumina and become shrunken and sclerotic. The Leydig cells are hyperplastic, forming large clumps. This disorder is the result of chromosomal abnormality, and the usual karyotype is 47,XXY. Chromosomal variants of the

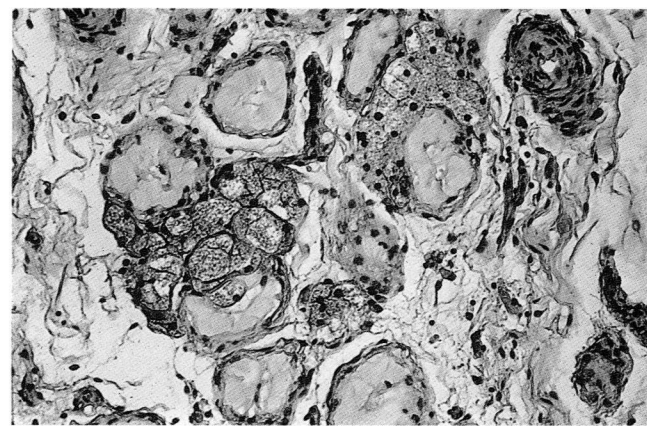

**FIGURE 34–43.** Tubular hyalinization following mumps orchitis. ×250

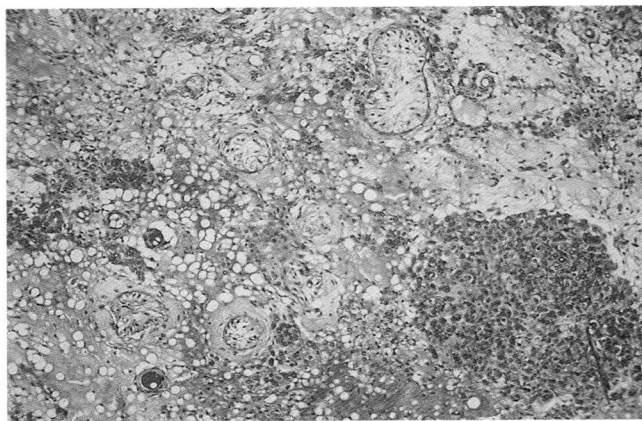

FIGURE 34–44. Klinefelter's syndrome with progressive tubular hyalinization and hyperplasia of Leydig cells. ×100

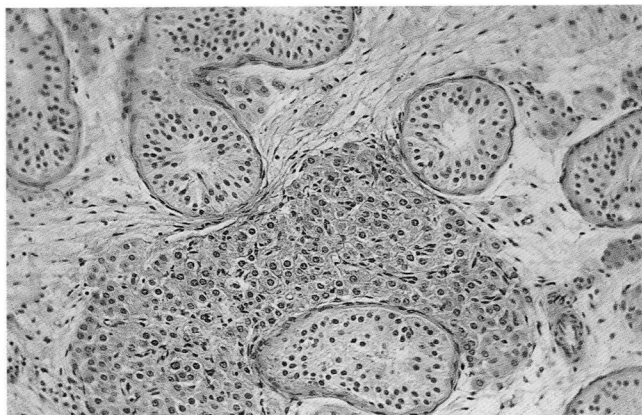

FIGURE 34–46. Cryptorchid testis. Small tubules deficient in germ cells and hyperplasia of Leydig cells. ×200

syndrome include mosaicism (47,XXY/46,XY). Although most patients are infertile, residual germ cells may be present, and these spermatogonia may be able to give rise to spermatozoa. Retrieval of such spermatozoa from the testis has been successful, and men with Klinefelter's syndrome have fathered children. The risk of chromosomal abnormality in the offspring is increased, however.[242] Investigation of the sex chromosome status of retrieved spermatozoa and counseling of prospective parents are advisable.[243]

## CRYPTORCHIDISM

The cryptorchid testis in the adult has small tubules lined by germinal epithelium that usually contains only spermatogonia and Sertoli cells.[244] The germ cells disappear gradually, and the tubules eventually undergo atrophy, with hyalinization and sclerosis. Leydig cells are abundant or frankly hyperplastic (Fig. 34–46). Elastic fibers in the tunica propria are sparse, and collagen is increased.[245] Eosinophilic granular change (accumulation of lysosomes) in the cytoplasm of the Sertoli cells has been re-

ported.[246, 247] Defective maturation has been suspected as the underlying abnormality of the germ cell in the cryptorchid testis and in the contralateral descended testis. Studies suggest that spermatogonia and primary spermatocytes fail to appear at the appropriate time in prepubertal life, resulting in a reduced total germ cell count.[248] Nonetheless, infertility is not absolute. Nistal and colleagues[249] showed that testicular biopsy specimens in some azoospermic men with cryptorchidism contain spermatogenic foci. The incidence of germ cell tumors is increased in the cryptorchid testis and in the contralateral descended testis.[230] The risk of cancer is 4 to 10 times higher in the cryptorchid testis. According to Dieckmann and Skakkebaek,[250] diagnosis is achieved best by surgical biopsy and immunostaining with PLAP.

## SERTOLI CELL–ONLY SYNDROME

In Sertoli cell–only syndrome, the tubules are lined only by Sertoli cells, and germ cells are entirely absent (Figs. 34–47 and 34–48). The diameter of the tubules is reduced. The Sertoli cells appear numer-

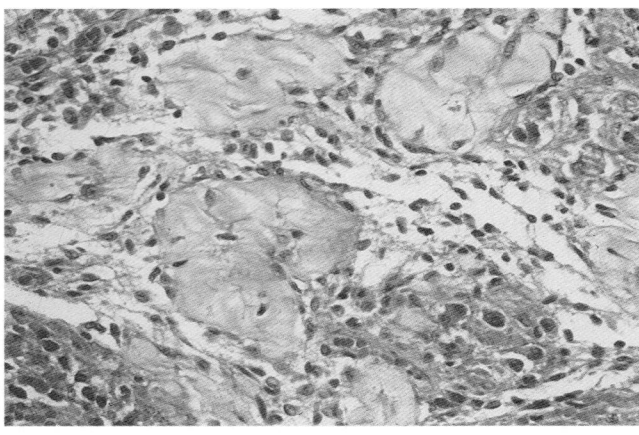

FIGURE 34–45. Klinefelter's syndrome. Sclerotic shrunken tubules and prominent Leydig cells. ×400

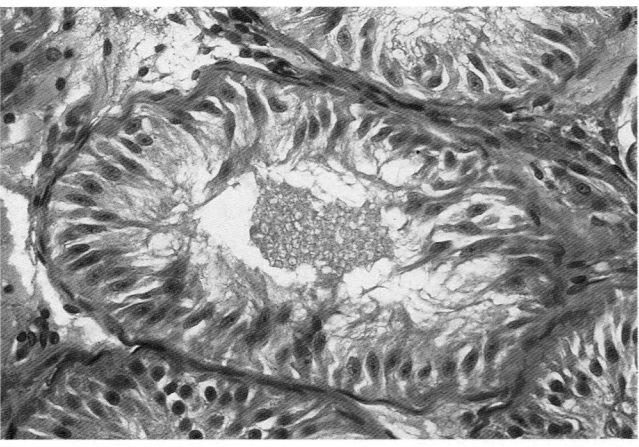

FIGURE 34–47. Sertoli cell–only syndrome. Tubule lined by Sertoli cells. No germ cells are evident. ×250

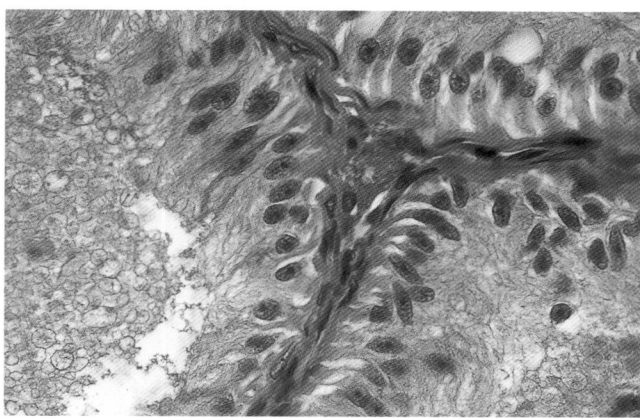

**FIGURE 34–48.** Sertoli cell–only syndrome. Sertoli cells have abundant cytoplasm and large nuclei, with prominent nucleoli. ×400

ous, with prominent nucleoli and abundant cytoplasm. Fat vacuoles may be present in the cytoplasm. The luminal border of the Sertoli cells may have an undulating margin that Sniffen and colleagues[251] described as resembling "windswept treetops." The lamina propria varies from normal to hyalinized. The Leydig cells appear unremarkable.

In the classic form of Sertoli cell–only syndrome, the loss of germ cells is total, permanent, and irreversible.[239, 252] The condition can be congenital or acquired, with multiple causes involved. Congenital factors include failure of germ cells to migrate to the gonad, cryptorchidism, Y chromosome abnormalities, and deficiency of follicle-stimulating hormone and luteinizing hormone. Factors in acquired loss of germ cells include radiation therapy, chemotherapy, exogenous estrogen, and gonadotropin-releasing hormone agonist. Some authors have recognized that Sertoli cell–only syndrome has at least two forms, designated *primary* and *secondary*. Nistal and Paniagua[230] have subclassified Sertoli cell–only syndrome into five forms, based on morphology and cause.

If one accepts the definition of Sertoli cell–only syndrome as the permanent, total, and irreversible loss of germ cells, conditions in which some tubules contain only Sertoli cells, while others contain germinal epithelium, do not qualify for the diagnosis. A variety of testicular disorders, most notably mixed atrophy, contain a mixture of tubules lined entirely by Sertoli cells, together with other tubules containing germinal epithelium exhibiting complete or incomplete spermatogenesis. Diagnosis of these conditions as Sertoli cell–only syndrome has led to confusion. The focal germ cell loss in such testes might be designated better by some other descriptive term, such as *Sertoli cell–only pattern*. Nomenclature is a matter of concern to the pathologist, whose goal is the correct diagnosis of the biopsy specimen and the correct identification of conditions offering the possibility of retrieval of a viable spermatozoon or spermatid. In this connection, immunohistochem-

istry and flow cytometry may be useful. The marker RBM is absent in Sertoli cell–only syndrome.[228] Flow cytometry of fine-needle aspiration material reveals only 2N populations of cells in Sertoli cell–only syndrome.[253]

## INTRATUBULAR GERM CELL NEOPLASIA

Intratubular germ cell neoplasia has been described in detail earlier in this chapter. It is important to be aware that male infertility is associated with an increased incidence of intratubular germ cell neoplasia. The association is so consistent that special attention should be given to the exclusion of intratubular germ cell neoplasia in all testicular biopsy specimens from infertile men. The diagnosis is made easily in an H&E section of the biopsy specimen, with confirmation by PLAP immunostain if necessary.

## REFERENCES

1. Brown LM, Pottern LM, Hoover RN, et al: Testicular cancer in the United States. Trends in incidence and mortality. Int J Epidemiol 15:164–170, 1986.
2. SEER Cancer Statistical Review, 1973–1997. Bethesda, MD, National Cancer Institute, 2001
2a. Greenlee RT, Hill-Harmon MB, Murray T, Thun M: Cancer statistics 2001. CA Cancer J Clin 51:15–36, 2001.
3. Bosl GJ, Motzer RJ: Testicular germ-cell cancer. N Engl J Med 337:242–253, 1997.
4. Feuer EJ, Frey CM, Brawley OW, et al: After a treatment breakthrough. A comparison of trial and population-based data for advanced testicular cancer. J Clin Oncol 12:368–377, 1994.
4a. Ro JY, Amin MB, Sahin AA, Ayala AG: Tumors and tumorous conditions of the male genital tract. Part B. Testicular neoplasms. *In* Fletcher CDM (ed): Diagnostic Histopathology of Tumors. 2nd ed. London, Churchill Livingstone, 2000, pp 733–838.
5. Friedman NB, Moore RA: Tumors of the testis. A report on 922 cases. Milit Surg 99:573–593, 1946.
6. Dixon FJ, Moore RA: Tumors of the Male Sex Organs. Atlas of Tumor Pathology. First Series, Fascicles 31b and 32. Washington, DC, Armed Forces Institute of Pathology, 1952.
7. Melicow MM: Classification of tumors of the testis. A clinical and pathological study based on 105 primary and 13 secondary cases in adults, and 3 primary and 4 secondary cases in children. J Urol 73:547–574, 1955.
8. Mostofi FK, Price EB Jr: Tumors of the Male Genital System. Atlas of Tumor Pathology. 2nd Series, Fascicle 8. Washington, DC, Armed Forces Institute of Pathology, 1973.
9. Collins DH, Pugh RCB: Classification and frequency of testicular tumors. Br J Urol 36(suppl):1–11, 1964.
10. United Kingdom Testicular Cancer Study Group: Aetiology of testicular cancer. Association with congenital abnormalities, age at puberty, infertility, and exercise. BMJ 308:1393–1399, 1994.
11. Giwercman A, Grindsted J, Hansen B, et al: Testicular cancer risk in boys with maldescended testis. A cohort study. J Urol 138:1214–1216, 1987.
12. Pottern LM, Brown LM, Hoover RN, et al: Testicular cancer risk among young men. Role of cryptorchidism and inguinal hernia. J Natl Cancer Inst 74:377–381, 1985.
13. Halme A, Kellokumpu-Lehtinen P, Lehtonen T, Teppo L: Morphology of testicular germ cell tumours in treated and untreated cryptorchidism. Br J Urol 64:78–83, 1989.
14. Giwercman A, Muller J, Skakkebaek NE: Carcinoma in situ of the undescended testis. Semin Urol 6:110–119, 1988.
15. Skakkebaek NE, Berthelsen JG, Giwercman A, Muller J: Carcinoma-in-situ of the testis. Possible origin from gonocytes

and precursor of all types of germ cell tumours except spermatocytoma. Int J Androl 10:19–28, 1987.

16. Patel SR, Kvols LK, Richardson RL: Familial testicular cancer. Report of six cases and review of the literature. Mayo Clin Proc 65:804–808, 1990.

17. Tollerud DJ, Blattner WA, Fraser MC, et al: Familial testicular cancer and urogenital developmental anomalies. Cancer 55:1849–1854, 1985.

18. Forman D, Oliver RT, Brett AR, et al: Familial testicular cancer. A report of the UK family register, estimation of risk and an HLA class 1 sib-pair analysis. Br J Cancer 65:255–262, 1992.

19. Osterlind A, Berthelsen JG, Abildgaard N, et al: Incidence of bilateral testicular germ cell cancer in Denmark, 1960–84. Preliminary findings. Int J Androl 10:203–208, 1987.

20. Scheiber K, Ackermann D, Studer UE: Bilateral testicular germ cell tumors. A report of 20 cases. J Urol 138:73–76, 1987.

21. Dieckmann KP, Boeckmann W, Brosig W, et al: Bilateral testicular germ cell tumors. Report of nine cases and review of the literature. Cancer 57:1254–1258, 1986.

22. Giwercman A, Berthelsen JG, Muller J, et al: Screening for carcinoma-in-situ of the testis. Int J Androl 10:173–180, 1987.

23. Ware SM, Heyman J, Al-Askari S, Morales P: Bilateral testicular germ cell malignancy. Urology 19:366–372, 1982.

24. Giwercman A, Skakkebaek NE: Carcinoma-in-situ (gonocytoma-in-situ) of the testis. In Burger H, de Krestser D (eds): The Testis. 2nd ed. New York, Raven Press, 1989, pp 475–491.

25. Rutgers JL, Scully RE: Pathology of the testis in intersex syndromes. Semin Diagn Pathol 4:275–291, 1987.

26. Manuel M, Katayama PK, Jones HW Jr: The age of occurrence of gonadal tumors in intersex patients with a Y chromosome. Am J Obstet Gynecol 124:293–300, 1976.

27. Rutgers JL, Scully RE: The androgen insensitivity syndrome (testicular feminization). A clinicopathologic study of 43 cases. Int J Gynecol Pathol 10:126–144, 1991.

28. Gondos B, Migliozzi JA: Intratubular germ cell neoplasia. Semin Diagn Pathol 4:292–303, 1987.

29. Srigley JR, Mackay B, Toth P, Ayala A: The ultrastructure and histogenesis of male germ neoplasia with emphasis on seminoma with early carcinomatous features. Ultrastruct Pathol 12:67–86, 1988.

30. Johnson DE, Appelt G, Samuels ML, Luna M: Metastases from testicular carcinoma. Study of 78 autopsied cases. Urology 8:234–239, 1976.

31. Bredael JJ, Vugrin D, Whitmore WF Jr: Autopsy findings in 154 patients with germ cell tumors of the testis. Cancer 50:548–551, 1982.

32. Czaja JT, Ulbright TM: Evidence for the transformation of seminoma to yolk sac tumor, with histogenetic considerations. Am J Clin Pathol 97:468–477, 1992.

33. Motzer RJ, Reuter VE, Cordon-Cardo C, Bosl GJ: Blood group-related antigens in human germ cell tumors. Cancer Res 48:5342–5347, 1988.

34. Yuasa T, Yoshiki T, Ogawa O, et al: Detection of alpha-fetoprotein mRNA in seminoma. J Androl 20:336–340, 1999.

35. Izquierdo MA, Van der Valk P, Van Ark-Otte J, et al: Differential expression of the c-kit proto-oncogene in germ cell tumours. J Pathol 177:253–258, 1995.

36. Tickoo SK, Hutchinson B, Bacik J, et al: Testicular seminoma: a clinicopathologic and immunohistochemical study of 105 cases with special reference to seminomas with atypical features. Int J Surg Pathol 10:23–32, 2002.

37. Boden G, Gibb R: Radiotherapy and testicular neoplasms. Cancer 2:1195–1197, 1951.

38. American Joint Committee on Cancer, Fleming ID, Cooper JS, Henson DE, et al (eds): AJCC Cancer Staging Manual. 5th ed. Philadelphia, Lippincott-Raven, 1997.

39. International Germ Cell Cancer Consensus Classification: A prognostic factor-based staging system for metastatic germ cell cancers. International Germ Cell Cancer Consensus Group. J Clin Oncol 15:594–603, 1997.

40. Bosl GJ: Germ cell tumor clinical trials in North America. Semin Surg Oncol 17:257–262, 1999.

41. Nazeer T, Ro JY, Amato RJ, et al: Histologically pure semi-

noma with elevated alpha-fetoprotein. A clinicopathologic study of ten cases. Oncol Rep 5:1425–1429, 1998.

42. Rorth M, Rajpert-De Meyts E, Andersson L, et al: Carcinoma in situ in the testis. Scand J Urol Nephrol 205(suppl):166–186, 2000.

43. Christensen TB, Daugaard G, Geertsen PF, von der Maase H: Effect of chemotherapy on carcinoma in situ of the testis. Ann Oncol 9:657–660, 1998.

44. Thomas GM, Rider WD, Dembo AJ, et al: Seminoma of the testis. Results of treatment and patterns of failure after radiation therapy. Int J Radiat Oncol Biol Phys 8:165–174, 1982.

45. Hamilton C, Horwich A, Easton D, Peckham MJ: Radiotherapy for stage I seminoma testis. Results of treatment and complications. Radiother Oncol 6:115–120, 1986.

46. Warde P, Gospodarowicz MK, Panzarella T, et al: Stage I testicular seminoma. Results of adjuvant irradiation and surveillance. J Clin Oncol 13:2255–2262, 1995.

47. Motzer RJ, Bosl GJ, Geller NL, et al: Advanced seminoma. The role of chemotherapy and adjunctive surgery. Ann Intern Med 108:513–518, 1988.

48. Hoskin P, Dilly S, Easton D, et al: Prognostic factors in stage I non-seminomatous germ-cell testicular tumors managed by orchiectomy and surveillance. Implications for adjuvant chemotherapy. J Clin Oncol 4:1031–1036, 1986.

49. Chaganti RS, Rodriguez E, Bosl GJ: Cytogenetics of male germ-cell tumors. Urol Clin North Am 20:55–66, 1993.

50. de Jong B, Oosterhuis JW, Castedo SM, et al: Pathogenesis of adult testicular germ cell tumors. A cytogenetic model. Cancer Genet Cytogenet 48:143–167, 1990.

51. Bosl GJ, Ilson DH, Rodriguez E, et al: Clinical relevance of the i(12p) marker chromosome in germ cell tumors. J Natl Cancer Inst 86:349–355, 1994.

52. Motzer RJ, Amsterdam A, Prieto V, et al: Teratoma with malignant transformation. Diverse malignant histologies arising in men with germ cell. J Urol 159:133–138, 1998.

53. Murty VV, Bosl GJ, Houldsworth J, et al: Allelic loss and somatic differentiation in human male germ cell tumors. Oncogene 9:2245–2251, 1994.

54. Pedersen KV, Boiesen P, Zetterlund CG: Experience of screening for carcinoma-in-situ of the testis among young men with surgically corrected maldescended testes. Int J Androl 10:181–185, 1987.

55. Giwercman A, Bruun E, Frimodt-Moller C, Skakkebaek NE: Prevalence of carcinoma in situ and other histopathological abnormalities in testes of men with a history of cryptorchidism. J Urol 142:998–1001, 1989.

56. von der Maase H, Rorth M, Walbom-Jorgensen S, et al: Carcinoma in situ of contralateral testis in patients with testicular germ cell cancer. Study of 27 cases in 500 patients. BMJ (Clin Res Ed) 293:1398–1401, 1986.

57. Skakkebaek NE, Berthelsen JG, Muller J: Carcinoma-in-situ of the undescended testis. Urol Clin North Am 9:377–385, 1982.

58. Bar W, Hedinger C: Comparison of histologic types of primary testicular germ cell tumors with their metastases. Consequences for the WHO and the British Nomenclatures? Virchows Arch A Pathol Anat Histol 370:41–54, 1976.

59. Coffin CM, Ewing S, Dehner LP: Frequency of intratubular germ cell neoplasia with invasive testicular germ cell tumors. Histologic immunocytochemical features. Arch Pathol Lab Med 109:555–559, 1985.

60. Burke AP, Mostofi FK: Placental alkaline phosphatase immunohistochemistry of intratubular malignant germ cells and associated testicular germ cell tumors. Hum Pathol 19:663–670, 1988.

61. Krag Jacobsen G, Barlebo H, Olsen J, et al: Testicular germ cell tumours in Denmark 1976–1980. Pathology of 1058 consecutive cases. Acta Radiol Oncol 23:239–247, 1984.

62. von Hochstetter AR, Hedinger CE: The differential diagnosis of testicular germ cell tumors in theory and practice. A critical analysis of two major systems of classification and review of 389 cases. Virchows Arch A Pathol Anat Histol 396:247–277, 1982.

63. Kay R: Prepubertal Testicular Tumor Registry. J Urol 150:671–674, 1993.

64. Thackray AC, Crane WA: Seminoma. *In* Pugh RC (ed): Pathology of the Testis. Oxford, Blackwell Scientific, 1976, pp 164–198.
65. Ulbright TM, Amin MB, Young RH: Tumors of the Testis, Adnexa, Spermatic Cord and Scrotum. Atlas of Tumor Pathology. Third Series, Fascicle 25. Washington, DC, Armed Forces Institute of Pathology, 1999.
66. Mann K, Siddle K: Evidence for free beta-subunit secretion in so-called human chorionic gonadotropin-positive seminoma. Cancer 62:2378–2382, 1988.
67. Fossa A, Fossa SD: Serum lactate dehydrogenase and human choriogonadotrophin in seminoma. Br J Urol 63:408–415, 1989.
68. Hori K, Uematsu K, Yasoshima H, et al: Testicular seminoma with human chorionic gonadotropin production. Pathol Int 47:592–599, 1997.
69. Wilkins BS, Williamson JM, O'Brien CJ: Morphological and immunohistological study of testicular lymphomas. Histopathology 15:147–156, 1989.
70. Zhao X, Wei YQ, Kariya Y, et al: Accumulation of gamma/delta T cells in human dysgerminoma and seminoma. Roles in autologous tumor killing and granuloma formation. Immunol Invest 24:607–618, 1995.
71. Mostofi FK: Testicular tumors. Epidemiologic, etiologic, and pathologic features. Cancer 32:1186–1201, 1973.
72. Ulbright TM, Roth LM, Brodhecker CA: Yolk sac differentiation in germ cell tumors. A morphologic study of 50 cases with emphasis on hepatic, enteric, and parietal yolk sac features. Am J Surg Pathol 10:151–164, 1986.
73. Ribalta T, Ro JY, Sahin AA, et al: Intrascrotally metastatic renal cell carcinoma. Report of two cases and review of the literature. J Urol Pathol 1:201–209, 1993.
74. Henley JD, Young RH, Ulbright TM: Clear cell sex cord-stromal tumors of the testis. A mimicker of seminoma (abstract). Mod Pathol 14:110A, 2001.
75. Masson P: Etude sur le seminome. Rev Can Biol 5:361–387, 1946.
76. Romanenko AM, Persidsky YV, Mostofi FK: Ultrastructure and histogenesis of spermatocytic seminoma. J Urol Pathol 1:387–395, 1993.
77. Stoop H, van Gurp R, de Krijger R, et al: Reactivity of germ cell maturation stage-specific markers in spermatocytic seminoma. Diagnostic and etiological implications. Lab Invest 81:919–928, 2001.
78. Burke AP, Mostofi FK: Spermatocytic seminoma. A clinicopathologic study of 79 cases. J Urol Pathol 1:21–32, 1993.
79. True LD, Otis CN, Delprado W, et al: Spermatocytic seminoma of testis with sarcomatous transformation. A report of five cases. Am J Surg Pathol 12:75–82, 1988.
80. Matoska J, Talerman A: Spermatocytic seminoma associated with rhabdomyosarcoma. Am J Clin Pathol 94:89–95, 1990.
81. Albores-Saavedra J, Huffman H, Alvarado-Cabrero I, Ayala AG: Anaplastic variant of spermatocytic seminoma. Hum Pathol 27:650–655, 1996.
82. Kraggerud SM, Berner A, Bryne M, et al: Spermatocytic seminoma as compared to classical seminoma. An immunohistochemical and DNA flow cytometric study. APMIS 107:297–302, 1999.
83. Cummings OW, Ulbright TM, Eble JN, Roth LM: Spermatocytic seminoma. An immunohistochemical study. Hum Pathol 25:54–59, 1994.
84. Hawkins EP, Finegold MJ, Hawkins HK, et al: Nongerminomatous malignant germ cell tumors in children. A review of 89 cases from the Pediatric Oncology Group, 1971–1984. Cancer 58:2579–2584, 1986.
85. Rodriguez PN, Hafez GR, Messing EM: Nonseminomatous germ cell tumor of the testicle. Does extensive staging of the primary tumor predict the likelihood of metastatic disease? J Urol 136:604–608, 1986.
86. Javadpour N: The role of biologic tumor markers in testicular cancer. Cancer 45(suppl):1755–1761, 1980.
87. Bosman FT, Giard RW, Nieuwenhuijen Kruseman AC, et al: Human chorionic gonadotrophin and alpha-fetoprotein in testicular germ cell tumours. A retrospective immunohistochemical study. Histopathology 4:673–684, 1980.
88. Wittekind C, Wichmann T, Von Kleist S: Immunohistological localization of AFP and HCG in uniformly classified testis tumors. Anticancer Res 3:327–330, 1983.
89. Hermans BP, Sweeney CJ, Foster RS, et al: Risk of systemic metastases in clinical stage I nonseminoma germ cell testis tumor managed by retroperitoneal lymph node dissection. J Urol 163:1721–1724, 2000.
90. Nazeer T, Ro JY, Kee KH, Ayala AG: Spermatic cord contamination in testicular cancer. Mod Pathol 9:762–766, 1996.
91. Shah VI, Amin MB, Linden MD, Zarbo RJ: Immunohistologic profile of spindle cell elements in non-seminomatous germ cell tumors (NSGCT). Histogenetic implications (abstract). Mod Pathol 11:96A, 1998.
92. Manivel JC, Jessurun J, Wick MR, Dehner LP: Placental alkaline phosphatase immunoreactivity in testicular germ-cell neoplasms. Am J Surg Pathol 11:21–29, 1987.
93. Niehans GA, Manivel JC, Copland GT, et al: Immuno-histochemistry of germ cell and trophoblastic neoplasms. Cancer 62:1113–1123, 1988.
94. Ferry JA, Ulbright TM, Young RH: Anaplastic large cell lymphoma presenting in the testis. J Urol Pathol 5:139–147, 1997.
95. Kaplan GW, Cromie WC, Kelalis PP, et al: Prepubertal yolk sac testicular tumors—report of the testicular tumor registry. J Urol 140:1109–1112, 1988.
96. Brosman SA: Testicular tumors in prepubertal children. Urology 13:581–588, 1979.
97. Talerman A: Endodermal sinus (yolk sac) tumor elements in testicular germ-cell tumors in adults. Comparison of prospective and retrospective studies. Cancer 46:1213–1217, 1980.
98. Grady RW, Ross JH, Kay R: Patterns of metastatic spread in prepubertal yolk sac tumor of the testis. J Urol 153:1259–1261, 1995.
99. Manivel JC, Simonton S, Wold LE, Dehner LP: Absence of intratubular germ cell neoplasia in testicular yolk sac tumors in children. A histochemical and immunohistochemical study. Arch Pathol Lab Med 112:641–645, 1988.
100. Freedman LS, Parkinson MC, Jones WG, et al: Histopathology in the prediction of relapse of patients with stage I testicular teratoma treated by orchidectomy alone. Lancet 2:294–298, 1987.
101. Logothetis CJ, Samuels ML, Trindade A, et al: The prognostic significance of endodermal sinus tumor histology among patients treated for stage III nonseminomatous germ cell tumors of the testes. Cancer 53:122–128, 1984.
102. Nseyo UO, Englander LS, Wajsman Z, et al: Histological patterns of treatment failures in testicular neoplasms. J Urol 133:219–220, 1985.
103. Talerman A, Haije WG, Baggerman L: Serum alphafetoprotein (AFP) in patients with germ cell tumors of the gonads and extragonadal sites. Correlation between endodermal sinus (yolk sac) tumor and raised serum AFP. Cancer 46:380–385, 1980.
104. Jacobsen GK: Alpha-fetoprotein (AFP) and human chorionic gonadotropin (HCG) in testicular germ cell tumours. A comparison of histologic and serologic occurrence of tumour markers. Acta Pathol Microbiol Immunol Scand (A) 91:183–190, 1983.
105. Talerman A: Germ cell tumors. *In* Talerman A, Roth LM (eds): Pathology of the Testis and Its Adnexa. New York, Churchill Livingstone, 1986, pp 29–65.
106. Michael H, Ulbright TM, Brodhecker CA: The pluripotential nature of the mesenchyme-like component of yolk sac tumor. Arch Pathol Lab Med 113:1115–1119, 1989.
107. Ferreiro JA: Ber-H2 expression in testicular germ cell tumors. Hum Pathol 25:522–524, 1994.
108. Shah VI, Amin MB, Linden MD, Zarbo RJ: Utility of a selective immunohistochemical (IHC) panel in the detection of components of mixed germ cell tumors (GCT) of testis (abstract). Mod Pathol 11:95A, 1998.
109. Barsky SH: Germ cell tumors of the testis. *In* Javadpour N, Barsky SH (eds): Surgical Pathology of Urologic Diseases. Baltimore, Williams & Wilkins, 1987, pp 224–246.
110. Bredael JJ, Vugrin D, Whitmore WF: Autopsy findings in 154

patients with germ cell tumors of the testis. Cancer 50:548–551, 1982.

111. Ulbright TM, Young RH, Scully RE: Trophoblastic tumors of the testis other than classic choriocarcinoma. "Monophasic" choriocarcinoma and placental site trophoblastic tumor. A report of two cases. Am J Surg Pathol 21:282–288, 1997.

112. Manivel JC, Niehans G, Wick MR, Dehner LP: Intermediate trophoblast in germ cell neoplasms. Am J Surg Pathol 11:693–701, 1987.

113. Leibovitch I, Foster RS, Ulbright TM, Donohue JP: Adult primary pure teratoma of the testis. The Indiana experience. Cancer 75:2244–2250, 1995.

114. Pugh RC, Cameron KM: Teratoma. *In* Pugh RC (ed): Pathology of the Testis. Oxford, Blackwell Scientific, 1976, pp 199–244.

115. Simmonds PD, Lee AH, Theaker JM, et al: Primary pure teratoma of the testis. J Urol 155:939–942, 1996.

116. Stevens MJ, Norman AR, Fisher C, et al: Prognosis of testicular teratoma differentiated. Br J Urol 73:701–706, 1994.

117. Mostofi FK, Sesterhenn IA: Pathology of germ cell tumors of testes. Prog Clin Biol Res 203:1–34, 1985.

118. Ulbright TM, Srigley JR: Dermoid cyst of the testis. A study of five postpubertal cases, including a pilomatrixoma-like variant, with evidence supporting its separate classification from mature testicular teratoma. Am J Surg Pathol 25:788–793, 2001.

119. Ahmed T, Bosl GJ, Hajdu SI: Teratoma with malignant transformation in germ cell tumors in men. Cancer 56:860–863, 1985.

120. Wurster K, Brodner O, Rossner JA, Grube D: A carcinoid occurring in the testis. Virchows Arch A Pathol Anat Histol 370:185–192, 1976.

121. Berdjis CC, Mostofi FK: Carcinoid tumors of the testis. J Urol 118:777–782, 1977.

122. Zavala-Pompa A, Ro JY, el-Naggar A, et al: Primary carcinoid tumor of testis. Immunohistochemical, ultrastructural, and DNA flow cytometric study of three cases with a review of the literature. Cancer 72:1726–1732, 1993.

123. Ordonez NG, Ayala AG: Primary malignant carcinoid of the testis. Arch Pathol Lab Med 106:539, 1982.

124. Iczkowski KA, Bostwick DG, Roche PC, Cheville JC: Inhibin A is a sensitive and specific marker for testicular sex cord-stromal tumors. Mod Pathol 11:774–779, 1998.

125. Nistal M, Paniagua R: Primary neuroectodermal tumour of the testis. Histopathology 9:1351–1359, 1985.

126. Michael H, Hull MT, Ulbright TM, et al: Primitive neuroectodermal tumors arising in testicular germ cell neoplasms. Am J Surg Pathol 21:896–904, 1997.

127. Pugh RCB, Thackray AC: Combined tumour. Br J Urol 36(suppl):45–51, 1964.

128. Evans RW: Developmental stages of embryo-like bodies in teratoma testis. J Clin Pathol 10:31–39, 1957.

129. Kaplan GW, Cromie WJ, Kelalis PP, et al: Gonadal stromal tumors. A report of the Prepubertal Testicular Tumor Registry. J Urol 136:300–302, 1986.

130. Kim I, Young RH, Scully RE: Leydig cell tumors of the testis. A clinicopathological analysis of 40 cases and review of the literature. Am J Surg Pathol 9:177–192, 1985.

131. Grem JL, Robins HI, Wilson KS, et al: Metastatic Leydig cell tumor of the testis. Report of three cases and review of the literature. Cancer 58:2116–2119, 1986.

132. Busam KJ, Iversen K, Coplan KA, et al: Immunoreactivity for A103, an antibody to melan-A (Mart-1), in adrenocortical and other steroid tumors. Am J Surg Pathol 22:57–63, 1998.

133. Amin MB, Young RH, Scully RE: Immunohistochemical profile of Sertoli and Leydig cell tumors of the testis (abstract). Mod Pathol 11:76A, 1998.

134. Collins DH, Symington T: Sertoli-cell tumor. Br J Urol 36:52–61, 1964.

135. Lawrence WD, Young RH, Scully RE: Sex cord stromal tumor. *In* Talerman A, Roth LM (eds): Pathology of the Testis and Its Adnexa. New York, Churchill Livingstone, 1986, pp 67–92.

136. Dubois RS, Hoffman WH, Krishnan TH, et al: Feminizing sex cord tumor with annular tubules in a boy with Peutz-Jeghers syndrome. J Pediatr 101:568–571, 1982.

137. Kaplan GW, Cromie WJ, Kelalis PP, et al: Gonadal stromal tumors. A report of the Prepubertal Testicular Tumor Registry. J Urol 136:300–302, 1986.

138. Young RH, Koelliker DD, Scully RE: Sertoli cell tumors of the testis, not otherwise specified. A clinicopathologic analysis of 60 cases. Am J Surg Pathol 22:709–721, 1998.

139. Zukerberg LR, Young RH, Scully RE: Sclerosing Sertoli cell tumor of the testis. A report of 10 cases. Am J Surg Pathol 15:829–834, 1991.

140. Gilcrease MZ, Delgado R, Albores-Saavedra J: Testicular Sertoli cell tumor with a heterologous sarcomatous component. Immunohistochemical assessment of Sertoli cell differentiation. Arch Pathol Lab Med 122:907–911, 1998.

141. Proppe KH, Scully RE: Large-cell calcifying Sertoli cell tumor of the testis. Am J Clin Pathol 74:607–619, 1980.

142. Tetu B, Ro JY, Ayala AG: Large cell calcifying Sertoli cell tumor of the testis. A clinicopathologic, immunohistochemical, and ultrastructural study of two cases. Am J Clin Pathol 96:717–722, 1991.

143. Kratzer SS, Ulbright TM, Talerman A, et al: Large cell calcifying Sertoli cell tumor of the testis. Contrasting features of six malignant and six benign tumors and a review of the literature. Am J Surg Pathol 21:1271–1280, 1997.

144. Carney JA, Gordon H, Carpenter PC, et al: The complex of myxomas, spotty pigmentation, and endocrine overactivity. Medicine (Baltimore) 64:270–283, 1985.

145. Jimenez-Quintero LP, Ro JY, Zavala-Pompa A, et al: Granulosa cell tumor of the adult testis. A clinicopathologic study of seven cases and a review of the literature. Hum Pathol 24:1120–1125, 1993.

146. Lawrence WD, Young RH, Scully RE: Juvenile granulosa cell tumor of the infantile testis. A report of 14 cases. Am J Surg Pathol 9:87–94, 1985.

147. Young RH, Lawrence WD, Scully RE: Juvenile granulosa cell tumor—another neoplasm associated with abnormal chromosomes and ambiguous genitalia. A report of three cases. Am J Surg Pathol 9:737–743, 1985.

148. Jones MA, Young RH, Scully RE: Benign fibromatous tumors of the testis and paratesticular region. A report of 9 cases with a proposed classification of fibromatous tumors and tumor-like lesions. Am J Surg Pathol 21:296–305, 1997.

149. Kay R: Prepubertal Testicular Tumor Registry. J Urol 150:671–674, 1993.

150. Scully RE: Gonadoblastoma. A review of 74 cases. Cancer 25:1340–1356, 1970.

151. Talerman A: The pathology of gonadal neoplasms composed of germ cells and sex cord stroma derivatives. Pathol Res Pract 170:24–38, 1980.

152. Rutgers JL: Advances in the pathology of intersex conditions. Hum Pathol 22:884–891, 1991.

153. Iezzoni JC, Von Kap-Herr C, Golden WL, Gaffey MJ: Gonadoblastomas in 45,X/46,XY mosaicism. Analysis of Y chromosome distribution by fluorescence in situ hybridization. Am J Clin Pathol 108:197–201, 1997.

154. Jorgensen N, Muller J, Jaubert F, et al: Heterogeneity of gonadoblastoma germ cells. Similarities with immature germ cells, spermatogonia and testicular carcinoma in situ cells. Histopathology 30:177–186, 1997.

155. Hart WR, Burkons DM: Germ cell neoplasms arising in gonadoblastomas. Cancer 43:669–678, 1979.

156. Ulbright TM, Srigley JR, Reuter VE, et al: Sex cord-stromal tumors of the testis with entrapped germ cells. A lesion mimicking unclassified mixed germ cell sex cord-stromal tumors. Am J Surg Pathol 24:535–542, 2000.

157. Talerman A: Tumors composed of germ cells and sex cord stromal derivatives. *In* Talerman A, Roth LM (eds): Pathology of the Testis and Its Adnexa. New York, Churchill Livingstone, 1987, pp 59–62.

158. Ferry JA, Harris NL, Young RH, et al: Malignant lymphoma of the testis, epididymis, and spermatic cord. A clinicopathologic study of 69 cases with immunophenotypic analysis. Am J Surg Pathol 18:376–390, 1994.

159. Sussman EB, Hajdu SI, Lieberman PH, Whitmore WF: Malignant lymphoma of the testis. A clinicopathologic study of 37 cases. J Urol 118:1004–1007, 1977.

160. Ferry JA, Ulbright TM, Young RH: Anaplastic large cell lymphoma presenting in the testis. J Urol Pathol 5:139–147, 1997.
161. Chan JK, Tsang WY, Lau WH, et al: Aggressive T/natural killer cell lymphoma presenting as testicular tumor. Cancer 77:1198–1205, 1996.
162. Givler RL: Testicular involvement in leukemia and lymphoma. Cancer 23:1290–1295, 1969.
163. Reid H, Marsden HB: Gonadal infiltration in children with leukaemia and lymphoma. J Clin Pathol 33:722–729, 1980.
164. Askin FB, Land VJ, Sullivan MP, et al: Occult testicular leukemia. Testicular biopsy at three years continuous complete remission of childhood leukemia. A Southwest Oncology Group Study. Cancer 47:470–475, 1981.
165. Nesbit ME, Robison LL, Ortega JA, et al: Testicular relapse in childhood acute lymphoblastic leukemia. Association with pretreatment patient characteristics and treatment. A report for Childrens Cancer Study Group. Cancer 45:2009–2016, 1980.
166. Young RH, Talerman A: Testicular tumors other than germ cell tumors. Semin Diagn Pathol 4:342–360, 1987.
167. Ferry JA, Young RH, Scully RE: Testicular and epididymal plasmacytoma. A report of 7 cases, including three that were the initial manifestation of plasma cell myeloma. Am J Surg Pathol 21:590–598, 1997.
168. Haupt HM, Mann RB, Trump DL, Abeloff MD: Metastatic carcinoma involving the testis. Clinical and pathologic distinction from primary testicular neoplasms. Cancer 54:709–714, 1984.
169. Tiltman AJ: Metastatic tumours in the testis. Histopathology 3:31–37, 1979.
170. Altaffer LF, Dufour DR, Castleberry GM, Steele SM: Coexisting rete testis adenoma and gonadoblastoma. J Urol 127:332–335, 1982.
171. Nistal M, Regadera J, Paniagua R: Cystic dysplasia of the testis. Light and electron microscopic study of three cases. Arch Pathol Lab Med 108:579–583, 1984.
172. Hartwick RW, Ro JY, Srigley JR, et al: Adenomatous hyperplasia of the rete testis. A clinicopathologic study of nine cases. Am J Surg Pathol 15:350–357, 1991.
173. Murao T, Tanahashi T: Adenofibroma of the rete testis. A case report with electron microscopy findings. Acta Pathol Jpn 38:105–112, 1988.
174. Jones MA, Young RH: Sertoliform rete cystadenoma. A report of two cases. J Urol Pathol 7:47–53, 1997.
175. Nochomovitz LE, Orenstein JM: Adenocarcinoma of the rete testis. Review and regrouping of reported cases and a consideration of miscellaneous entities. J Urogenit Pathol 1:11–40, 1991.
176. Nochomovitz LE, Orenstein JM: Adenocarcinoma of the rete testis. Consolidation and analysis of 31 reported cases with a review of the literature. J Urol Pathol 2:1–37, 1994.
176a. Sanchez-Chapado M, Angulo JC, Haas GP: Adenocarcinoma of the rete testis. Urology 46:468–475, 1995.
177. Mares AJ, Shkolnik A, Sacks M, Feuchtwanger MM: Aberrant (ectopic) adrenocortical tissue along the spermatic cord. J Pediatr Surg 15:289–292, 1980.
178. Czaplicki M, Bablok L, Kuzaka B, Janczewski Z: Heterotopic adrenal tissue. Int Urol Nephrol 17:177–181, 1985.
179. Gouw AS, Elema JD, Bink-Boelkens MT, et al: The spectrum of splenogonadal fusion. Case report and review of 84 reported cases. Eur J Pediatr 144:316–323, 1985.
180. Srigley JR, Hartwick RW: Tumors and cysts of the paratesticular region. Pathol Annu 25(pt 2):51–108, 1990.
181. Thompson JE, van der Walt JD: Nodular fibrous proliferation (fibrous pseudotumour) of the tunica vaginalis testis. A light, electron microscopic and immunocytochemical study of a case and review of the literature. Histopathology 10:741–748, 1986.
182. Walker AN, Mills SE: Surgical pathology of the tunica vaginalis testis and embryologically related mesothelium. Pathol Annu 23(pt 2):125–152, 1988.
183. Srigley JR, Hartwick RW: Tumors and cysts of the paratesticular region. Pathol Annu 25(pt 2):51–108, 1990.
184. Manson AL: Adenomatoid tumor of testicular tunica albuginea mimicking testicular carcinoma. J Urol 139:819–820, 1988.
185. Perez-Ordonez B, Srigley JR: Mesothelial lesions of the paratesticular region. Semin Diagn Pathol 17:294–306, 2000.
186. Price EB Jr: Papillary cystadenoma of the epididymis. A clinicopathologic analysis of 20 cases. Arch Pathol 91:456–470, 1971.
187. Kragel PJ, Pestaner J, Travis WD, et al: Papillary cystadenoma of the epididymis. A report of three cases with lectin histochemistry. Arch Pathol Lab Med 114:672–675, 1990.
188. Jones EC, Murray SK, Young RH: Cysts and epithelial proliferations of the testicular collecting system (including rete testis). Semin Diagn Pathol 17:270–293, 2000.
189. Weiss SW, Tavassoli FA: Multicystic mesothelioma. An analysis of pathologic findings and biologic behavior in 37 cases. Am J Surg Pathol 12:737–746, 1988.
190. Tsang WY, Chan JK, Lee KC, et al: Aggressive angiomyxoma. A report of four cases occurring in men. Am J Surg Pathol 16:1059–1065, 1992.
191. Iezzoni JC, Fechner RE, Wong LS, Rosai J: Aggressive angiomyxoma in males. A report of four cases. Am J Clin Pathol 104:391–396, 1995.
192. Laskin WB, Fetsch JF, Mostofi FK: Angiomyofibroblastoma-like tumor of the male genital tract. Analysis of 11 cases with comparison to female angiomyofibroblastoma and spindle cell lipoma. Am J Surg Pathol 22:6–16, 1998.
193. Folpe AL, Weiss SW: Paratesticular soft tissue neoplasms. Semin Diagn Pathol 17:307–318, 2000.
194. Mikuz G, Hopfel-Kreiner I: Papillary mesothelioma of the tunica vaginalis propria testis. Case report and ultrastructural study. Virchows Arch A Pathol Anat Histol 396:231–238, 1982.
195. Chetty R: Well differentiated (benign) papillary mesothelioma of the tunica vaginalis. J Clin Pathol 45:1029–1030, 1992.
196. Daya D, McCaughey WT: Well-differentiated papillary mesothelioma of the peritoneum. A clinicopathologic study of 22 cases. Cancer 65:292–296, 1990.
197. Burrig KF, Pfitzer P, Hort W: Well-differentiated papillary mesothelioma of the peritoneum. A borderline mesothelioma. Report of two cases and review of literature. Virchows Arch A Pathol Anat Histopathol 417:443–447, 1990.
198. Jones MA, Young RH, Scully RE: Malignant mesothelioma of the tunica vaginalis. A clinicopathologic analysis of 11 cases with review of the literature. Am J Surg Pathol 19:815–825, 1995.
199. Eimoto T, Inoue I: Malignant fibrous mesothelioma of the tunica vaginalis. A histologic and ultrastructural study. Cancer 39:2059–2066, 1977.
200. Jones MA, Young RH, Scully RE: Adenocarcinoma of the epididymis. A report of four cases and review of the literature. Am J Surg Pathol 21:1474–1480, 1997.
201. Young RH, Scully RE: Testicular and paratesticular tumors and tumor-like lesions of ovarian common epithelial and mullerian types. A report of four cases and review of the literature. Am J Clin Pathol 86:146–152, 1986.
202. Henley JD, Ferry J, Ulbright TM: Miscellaneous rare paratesticular tumors. Semin Diagn Pathol 17:319–339, 2000.
203. Jones MA, Young RH, Srigley JR, Scully RE: Paratesticular serous papillary carcinoma. A report of six cases. Am J Surg Pathol 19:1359–1365, 1995.
204. Roganovich J, Bisogno G, Cecchetto G, et al: Paratesticular desmoplastic small round cell tumor. Case report and review of the literature. J Surg Oncol 71:269–272, 1999.
205. De Chiara A, Van Tornout JM, Hachitanda Y, et al: Melanotic neuroectodermal tumor of infancy. A case report of paratesticular primary with lymph node involvement. Am J Pediatr Hematol Oncol 14:356–360, 1992.
206. Johnson RE, Scheithauer BW, Dahlin DC: Melanotic neuroectodermal tumor of infancy. A review of seven cases. Cancer 52:661–666, 1983.
207. Folpe AL, Weiss SW: Paratesticular soft tissue neoplasms. Semin Diagn Pathol 17:307–318, 2000.
208. Cavazzana AO, Schmidt D, Ninfo V, et al: Spindle cell rhabdomyosarcoma. A prognostically favorable variant of rhabdomyosarcoma. Am J Surg Pathol 16:229–235, 1992.

209. Kumar PV, Khezri AA: Pure testicular rhabdomyosarcoma. Br J Urol 59:282, 1987.

210. Ferrari A, Casanova M, Massimino M, et al: The management of paratesticular rhabdomyosarcoma. A single institutional experience with 44 consecutive children. J Urol 159: 1031–1034, 1998.

211. McClure J: Malakoplakia of the testis and its relationship to granulomatous orchitis. J Clin Pathol 33:670–678, 1980.

212. Townell NH, Gledhill A, Robinson T, Hopewell P: Juvenile xanthogranuloma of the testis. J Urol 133:1054–1055, 1985.

213. Foucar E, Rosai J, Dorfman R: Sinus histiocytosis with massive lymphadenopathy (Rosai-Dorfman disease). Review of the entity. Semin Diagn Pathol 7:19–73, 1990.

214. Charny CW: Testicular biopsy. Its value in male sterility. JAMA 115:1429–1432, 1940.

215. Wong T-W, Straus FH, Warner NE: Testicular biopsy in the study of male infertility. I. Testicular causes of infertility. Arch Pathol 95:151–159, 1973.

216. Wong T-W, Straus FH, Warner NE: Testicular biopsy in the study of male infertility. II. Posttesticular causes of infertility. Arch Pathol 95:160–164, 1973.

217. Wong T-W, Straus FH, Warner NE: Testicular biopsy in the study of male infertility. III. Pretesticular causes of infertility. Arch Pathol 98:1–8, 1974.

218. Palermo G, Joris H, Devroey P, Van Steirteghem A: Pregnancies after intracytoplasmic injection of single spermatozoon into an oocyte. Lancet 340:17–18, 1992.

219. Skakkebaek NE, Giwercman A, de Kretser D: Pathogenesis and management of male infertility. Lancet 343:1473–1479, 1994.

220. Damjanov I: Clinical evaluation of the infertile couple. *In* Damjanov I: Pathology of Infertility. St. Louis, Mosby, 1993, pp 7–23.

221. Silber SJ: Evaluation and treatment of male infertility. Clin Obstet Gynecol 43:854–888, 2000.

222. Heller CG, Clermont Y: Kinetics of the germinal epithelium in man. Recent Prog Horm Res 20:545–575, 1964.

223. Wong T-W, Straus FH, Foster LV: Cytoplasmic granular change of Sertoli cells in two cases of Sertoli-cell-only syndrome. Arch Pathol Lab Med 112:200–205, 1988.

224. Nistal M, Paniagua R, Diez-Pardo JA: Histologic classification of undescended testes. Hum Pathol 11:666–674, 1980.

225. Trainer TD: Testis and excretory duct system. *In* Sternberg SS (ed): Histology for Pathologists. 2nd ed. Philadelphia, Lippincott-Raven, 1997, pp 1019–1037.

226. Maekawa M, Kamimura K, Nagano T: Peritubular myoid cells in the testis. Their structure and function. Arch Histol Cytol 59:1–13, 1996.

227. Santamaria L, Martin R, Nistal M, Paniagua R: The peritubular myoid cells in the testes from men with varicocele. An ultrastructural immunohistochemical and quantitative study. Histopathology 21:423–433, 1992.

228. Maymon BB, Elliott DJ, Kleiman SE, et al: The contribution of RNA-binding motif (RBM) antibody to the histopathologic evaluation of testicular biopsies from infertile men. Hum Pathol 32:36–41, 2001.

229. Bar-Shira MB, Paz G, Elliott DJ, et al: Maturation phenotype of Sertoli cells in testicular biopsies of azoospermic men. Hum Reprod 15:1537–1542, 2000.

230. Nistal M, Paniagua R: Non-neoplastic diseases of the testis. *In* Bostwick DG, Eble JN (eds): Urological Surgical Pathology. St Louis, Mosby-Year Book, 1997, pp 458–465.

231. Makler A, Abramovici H: The correlation between sperm count and testicular biopsy using a new scoring system. Int J Fertil 23:300–304, 1978.

232. Johnsen SG: Testicular biopsy score count—a method of reg-

istration of spermatogenesis in human testes. Normal values and results in 335 hypogonadal males. Hormones 1:2–25, 1970.

233. Yoshida A, Miura K, Shirai M: Evaluation of seminiferous tubule scores obtained through testicular biopsy examinations of nonobstructive azoospermic men. Fertil Steril 68: 514–519, 1997.

234. Meng MV, Cha I, Ljung B-M, Turek PJ: Testicular fine-needle aspiration in infertile men. Correlation of cytologic pattern with biopsy histology. Am J Surg Pathol 25:71–79, 2001.

235. Turek PJ, Ljung B-M, Cha I, Conaghan J: Diagnostic findings from testis fine needle aspiration in mapping obstructed and nonobstructed azoospermic men. J Urol 163:1709–1716, 2000.

236. Krausz C, McElreavey K: Y chromosome and male infertility. Front Biosci 4:1–8, 1999.

237. Soderstrom KO, Suominen J: Human hypospermatogenesis. Histopathology and ultrastructure. Arch Pathol Lab Med 106:231–234, 1982.

238. Guarch R, Pesce C, Puras A, Lazaro L: A quantitative approach to the classification of hypospermatogenesis in testicular biopsies for infertility. Hum Pathol 23:1032–1037, 1992.

239. Soderstrom KO, Suominen J: Histopathology and ultrastructure of meiotic arrest in human spermatogenesis. Arch Pathol Lab Med 104:476–482, 1980.

240. Hatakeyama S, Takizama T, Kawara Y: Focal atrophy of the seminiferous tubule in the human testis. Acta Pathol Jpn 29: 901–905, 1979.

241. Chandrasoma PT, Taylor CR: Concise Pathology. 3rd ed. Stamford, CT, Appleton & Lange, 1998, p 231.

242. Hennebicq S, Pelletier R, Bergues U, Rousseaux S: Risk of trisomy 21 in the offspring of patients with Klinefelter's syndrome. Lancet 357:2104–2105, 2001.

243. Foresta C, Galeazzi C, Bettella A, et al: Analysis of meiosis in intratesticular germ cells from subjects affected by classic Klinefelter's syndrome. J Clin Endocrinol Metab 84:3807–3810, 1999.

244. Wong T-W, Straus FH, Jones TM, Warner NE: Pathological aspects of infertile testes. Urol Clin North Am 5:503–530, 1978.

245. Gotoh M, Miyake K, Mitsuya H: Elastic fibers in tunica propria of undescended and contralateral scrotal testes from cryptorchid patients. Urology 30:359–363, 1987.

246. Chan KW, Ma LT: Eosinophilic granular cells in a crytorchid testis. Arch Pathol Lab Med 111:877–879, 1987.

247. Nistal M, Garcia-Rodeja E, Paniagua R: Granular transformation of Sertoli cells in testicular disorders. Hum Pathol 22: 131–137, 1991.

248. Huff DS, Fenig DM, Canning DA, et al: Abnormal germ cell development in cryptochidism. Horm Res 55:11–17, 2001.

249. Nistal M, Riestra ML, Paniagua R: Correlation between testicular biopsies (prepubertal and post pubertal) and spermiogram in cryptorchid men. Hum Pathol 31:1022–1030, 2000.

250. Dieckmann KP, Skakkebaek NE: Carcinoma in situ of the testis. Review of biological and clinical features. Int J Cancer 83:815–822, 1999.

251. Sniffen RC, Howard RP, Simmons FA: The testis. III. Absence of germ cells; sclerosing tubular degeneration, "male climacteric". Arch Pathol 51:293–311, 1951.

252. Hinderer MG, Hedinger C: Sertoli-cell-only syndrome. Histology and pathogenesis [in German]. Schweiz Med Wochenschr 108:856–858, 1978.

253. Dey P, Mondal AK, Singh SK, Vohra H: Quantitation of spermatogenesis by DNA flow cytometry from fine-needle aspiration cytology material. Diagn Cytopathol 23:386–387, 2000.

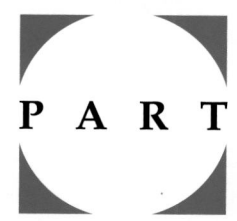

PART VII

# Female Reproductive System

# 35

# Vulva and Vagina

R. Tucker Burks    Juan C. Felix

## VULVA

### Anatomy

The vulva is composed of multiple anatomic structures, each with fairly distinctive characteristics. The mons pubis, consisting of hair-bearing skin and typically abundant subcutaneous adipose tissue, delineates the superior extent of the vulva overlying the symphysis pubis. Extending inferiorly and forming the lateral extent of the vulva are the labia majora, which are also composed of hair-bearing skin and subcutaneous tissue but are also richly innervated and vascularized. The papillary dermis is less well defined in the labia majora than it is in other skin regions and, theoretically, this may have some bearing on the biology of malignant disease progression, a point to be elaborated on later. The labial sulcus is an indentation that separates the labia majora from the labia minora, the latter being lined by keratinizing squamous epithelium without skin adnexal structures. The labia minora join superiorly at the clitoris, a highly vascularized, erectile structure overlaid by the prepuce and supported laterally by the frenulum.

In addition to typical skin adnexal constituents, Van der Putte effectively established mammary-like glands of the anogenital region as structures unique to the anogenital region and distinctive in their properties.[1] They are most numerous in the interlabial sulcus and share features in common with both eccrine and apocrine glands. They also express functionally active estrogen and progesterone receptors and, consequently, may simulate a variety of proliferative lesions and neoplasms that are otherwise native to the breast such as fibrocystic changes, ductal hyperplasia, intraductal papillomas, fibroadenomas, and adenocarcinomas. Because the glands contain myoepithelial cells, in addition to luminal epithelial cells, immunohistochemistry for actin positivity may prove useful in evaluating complex lesions. Given their unique characteristics, lesions arising from mammary-like glands should be distinguished from more classic lesions derived from skin adnexal structures (Fig. 35–1) (CD Figs. 35–1 to Fig. 35–3).

Other specialized glands of the vulva include vestibular glands, Bartholin's glands, and Skene's (paraurethral) glands. Bartholin's glands are located in the posterior third of the labia majora and discharge into the vestibule just external to the hymenal ring. The epithelial lining is location dependent. The acinar glands and proximal duct are lined by columnar to cuboidal mucinous epithelium. The middle to distal duct is lined by transitional epithelium. The distalmost portion of the duct then becomes replaced by squamous epithelium as the duct

FIGURE 35–1. Mammary-like glands. An intraductal papilloma-like structure is present within a cyst lined by thinned epithelial cells. Adjacent to the cyst are mammary duct and glandlike structures, some of which display apocrine-like features.

terminates into the vestibule (CD Figs. 35–4 to 35–8). The minor vestibular glands display similar features but lack the prominence and degree of organization characteristic of the Bartholin's glands and duct system and seldom have an identifiable duct.

Vulvar Intraepithelial Neoplasia and Superficially Invasive Squamous Cell Carcinoma

The term *vulvar intraepithelial neoplasia* (VIN) has been codified to describe varying degrees of squamous dysplasia of the vulva. The terminology was agreed on in 1985 by the International Society for the Study of Vulvar Disease[2] and has been adopted by the World Health Organization. It supplants other terms such as *bowenoid papulosis, erythroplasia of Queyrat, vulvar dysplasia,* and *carcinoma in situ* despite the protestations of some.[3] Trends have shown an increased incidence in VIN[4] accompanied by a decrease in the mean age of the patients affected.[4–11] These trends are somewhat contrary to those noted in vulvar squamous carcinoma, in which the incidence rate has not changed appreciably.[4] This discordance is likely due to the widespread adoption of ablative therapy for VIN before invasion occurs.

It is clear that the majority of high-grade VIN lesions arise in association with human papillomavirus infection, particularly HPV-16.[5, 6] Accordingly, discovery of VIN often precedes, follows, or is found concurrently with the disclosure of cervical intraepithelial neoplasia. However, unlike the case of cervical lesions, a significant number of VIN lesions arise from mechanisms that do not seem to require the oncogenic influence of HPV. Mutations of the p53 gene, by as of yet undetermined mechanisms, are postulated as causative.[7]

Other causative associations with VIN include herpes simplex virus type 2 (HSV-2), which has been proposed to work synergistically with HPV,[8] as well as cigarette smoking.[9, 10]

Clinically, the lesions have a variety of presentations. Some display a raised surface in the form of papules or plaques, whereas others may be macular. Pigmentation may be altered, with approximately 25% being pigmented and 50% being white. The remaining lesions may be gray, pink, or red (erythroplasia of Queyrat). The anal region is often involved, and detection may require anal colposcopy (CD Fig. 35–9).[11]

VIN 1 is a flat lesion that should be distinguished from exophytic condyloma (condyloma acuminata), the latter being associated almost exclusively with low-risk HPV types (6 and 11) and a negligible risk of progression to invasive carcinoma. Additionally, reactive cellular changes may mimic VIN 1. Accordingly, because of the subtlety of cytologic changes and overlapping features with reactive cellular changes that may mimic VIN 1,[12] its diagnosis usually requires the identification of koilocytic cells. Atypical basaloid keratinocytes and mitoses should be limited to the lower third of the epidermis, but cells displaying viropathic features usually extend toward the surface covered only by parakeratotic cells (Fig. 35–2) (CD Fig. 35–10). VIN 3 shows epithelial disorganization and full-thickness involvement of the epithelium by atypical basaloid cells, whereas VIN 2 shows features intermediate between VIN 1 and VIN 3 and is seldom observed in the absence of one or both of these bracketing lesions (see CD Fig. 35–10; CD Figs. 35–11 to 35–17). Microscopic distinction between VIN 2 or VIN 3 and squamous hyperplasia may at times be challenging. This is particularly the case when hyperplasia is accompanied by dense hyperkeratosis. In these instances, immunohistochemical studies with MIB-1 may be of assistance. High-grade VIN almost uni-

FIGURE 35–2. VIN 1. Numerous koilocytic cells are scattered throughout the acanthotic and parakeratotic epidermis. There is disarray of the keratinocytes and overlying parakeratosis. Mild chronic inflammatory cell infiltrate is present in the papillary dermis.

versally exhibits diffuse, transepithelial staining,[13] whereas squamous hyperplasia shows only mild to moderate basal positivity. Also of utility is in situ hybridization for HPV DNA, which is readily identifiable in VIN lesions of all grades but is not seen in hyperplasias.[14]

McLachlin and colleagues described "multinucleated atypia of the vulva," a lesion that may mimic VIN. It is observed most commonly in young women, is not related to HPV, and is distinct from VIN in its histopathologic appearance. The lesion is characterized by enlarged, multinucleate cells in the middle epithelial layer, lacking the superficial atypia seen in VIN. The nuclei of these cells have evenly dispersed chromatin and frequently contain nucleoli.[15] The actual incidence of VIN 1 and VIN 2 is not known because these lesions are not typically reported. Hereafter in this chapter, the term *VIN* will refer only to the more clinically relevant VIN 3.

Three histologic subtypes of VIN have been proposed.[6] Basaloid VIN is characterized by typically flat lesions composed of a fairly monomorphic group of small neoplastic cells that expand the epidermis, resulting in a rounded, bulging epidermal-dermal junction (Fig. 35–3) (see CD Figs. 35–14 and 35–15). Warty VIN is characterized by various degrees of exophytic architecture (Fig. 35–4) (see CD Figs. 35–16 and 35–17). The component cells typically display a marked degree of nuclear enlargement and pleomorphism, as well as multinucleation and increased numbers of atypical mitotic figures when compared with basaloid VIN. Differentiated (simplex) VIN[2, 16] is characterized by cellular atypia that is usually limited to the basal aspect of the epidermis, a feature that is distinctive from warty or basaloid VIN (Fig. 35–5). Lesions are typically flat and display tonguelike projections into the underlying dermis. The projections may be accompanied by squamous pearl formation. Although differentiated VIN may be seen in isolation, it is usually detected

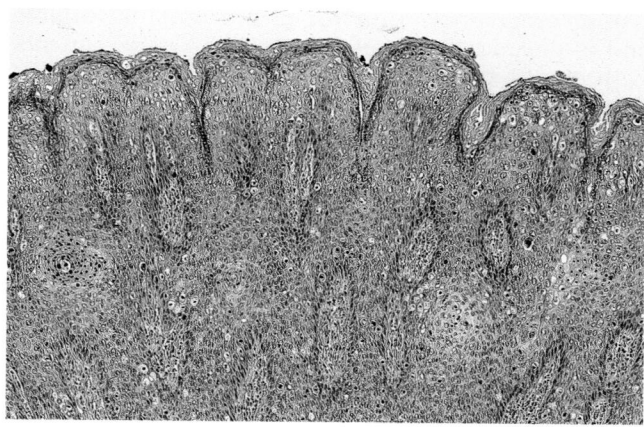

**FIGURE 35–4. Warty VIN 3.** A verruciform epidermal proliferation displays numerous apoptotic and dyskeratotic cells throughout the disorganized epidermis. Occasional mitotic figures are also present.

in association with invasive squamous carcinoma (CD Fig. 35–18).

Basaloid and warty VIN are not uncommonly found together and are most commonly seen in younger women, as compared with differentiated VIN. Additionally, HPV has been detected in the majority of cases of warty and basaloid VIN,[6] which distinguishes these lesions from differentiated VIN, in which HPV is seldom detected. HPV nucleic acids have been identified in VIN in patients over a broad age range, indicating that HPV may play a role in the development of vulvar squamous neoplasia at any point throughout life.[19] One intriguing finding has been the detection of HPV nucleic acids in some cases of lichen sclerosus–related VIN, thus linking two pathways of vulvar neoplasia.[19]

Because most VIN lesions are treated in some fashion, the risk of progression to invasive carcinoma is not well established.[20] It appears that the

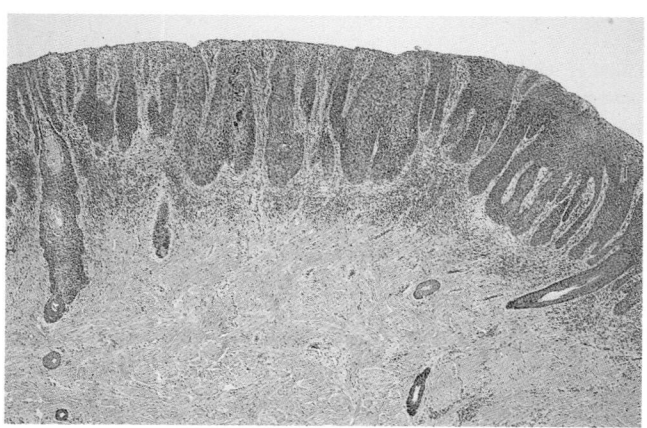

**FIGURE 35–3. Basaloid VIN 3.** A uniform basaloid population of atypical keratinocytes with a high nuclear-to-cytoplasmic ratio expands the rete pegs downward into the clinically inflamed papillary dermis.

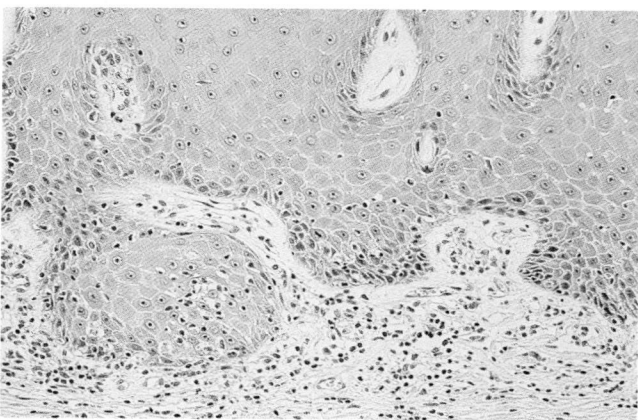

**FIGURE 35–5. Differentiated (Simplex) VIN 3.** Atypical keratinocytes characterized by enlarged nuclei with vesicular chromatin and prominent nucleoli are limited to the basal and parabasal portions of the otherwise organized epidermis. A clublike extension of the parabasal region protrudes into the chronically inflamed papillary dermis.

risk of progression to invasive carcinoma is variable and is dependent on several factors. Young patients with multifocal VIN 3 most frequently experience spontaneous regression, and progression to invasive squamous carcinoma has been reported in only a small subset (3% to 4%) of these cases.[21] It should be borne in mind that this low progression rate was observed in surgically treated women. Conversely, Jones and McClean suggested that older patients with multifocal VIN have a greater risk of progression to invasive disease.[22] Other factors associated with progression to invasive cancer include increasing age and basaloid lesions with low ploidy values.[19] Certain immunocompromised states have been shown to predispose to invasion.[23–25] Surprisingly, human immunodeficiency virus type 1 (HIV-1)–infected women do not appear to have an increased rate of progression to invasive disease, although this may be due to a lack of lengthy follow-up among these patients.[26, 27]

Surgical or ablative treatments are exercised in most cases and include Cavitron ultrasonic surgical aspiration, laser vaporization, surgical excision, and skinning vulvectomy (CD Figs. 35–19 and 35–20). Laser vaporization and Cavitron ultrasonic surgical aspiration are probably used less than in the past, because it has been shown by some that invasive disease may be underestimated, and invasion typically cannot be assessed with these techniques.[28, 29] Indeed, studies have shown foci of invasive disease in up to 20% of patients undergoing excision for biopsy-proven VIN.[30, 31] In addition, positive surgical margins determined in skinning vulvectomy specimens accurately predict disease recurrence, further underscoring the utility of this therapeutic choice.[32]

Progression to early invasion may be difficult to identify. This difficulty is compounded by the endophytic nature of VIN and its frequent involvement of skin appendages, both further complicated by poorly oriented excision specimens (CD Fig. 35–21). In this latter regard, multiple additional levels may be needed to avoid diagnostic misinterpretations. Evidence of early invasion includes loss of peripheral palisading of the basal cells; budding and small, detached nests of cells displaying maturation (characterized by increased eosinophilic cytoplasm); and an irregular infiltrative margin[33] (Fig. 35–6) (CD Figs. 35–22 to 35–25). Even after applying these criteria, assessment of invasion can be difficult, and investigators have attempted to find methods to assist in this assessment.

Expression of basement membrane zone proteins has been reported by some to be diminished to absent in foci of invasion.[34, 35] Although immunohistochemical stains for basement membrane zone proteins are promising, one must be cautious in asserting the presence of invasion on the basis of absent immunohistochemical staining alone. Johannson and colleagues proposed that matrix metalloproteinase (MMP) expression, specifically collagenase-3 (MMP-13), may be limited to invasive squamous carcinomas of the vulva and may not be present in

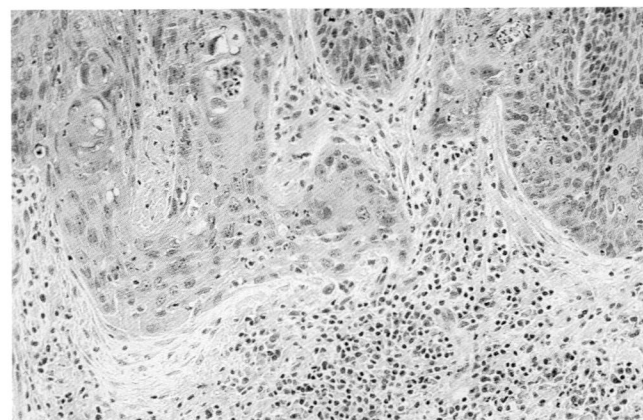

**FIGURE 35–6. VIN 3 with superficially invasive squamous carcinoma.** VIN 3 expands the rete pegs downward into the dermis. Centrally, an irregularity of the outline of the rete pegs is noted. Eosinophilia in this region is increased, which is indicative of cellular maturation and invasion.

in situ neoplasia.[36] Further study is needed, however, to determine the reliability of this diagnostic approach.

Despite these difficulties, it is critical to recognize invasion when it is present because it has been shown that lesions that invade to a depth greater than 1 mm may metastasize to regional lymph nodes.[37] This observation has led to defining stage IA invasive squamous cancer of the vulva (superficially invasive squamous cell carcinoma) as lesions with a maximal diameter of 2 cm and an invasive depth of 1 mm or less[38, 39] (Table 35–1). Although the prognostic significance of vascular space invasion in this setting is controversial, the presence of vascular space involvement by tumor should be reported because some investigators have found it to be associated with lymph node metastases.[37, 40, 41] It is further stipulated that superficially invasive squamous carcinoma does not include more than one

**TABLE 35–1.** FIGO (1995) Staging of Vulvar Carcinoma

| Stage | Findings |
| --- | --- |
| 0 | Carcinoma in situ; intraepithelial carcinoma |
| I | Tumor confined to vulva or perineum |
| | 2 cm or less in greatest dimension |
| | No nodal metastases |
| IA | Stromal invasion ≤1 mm |
| IB | Stromal invasion >1 mm |
| II | Tumor confined to vulva or perineum |
| | More than 2 cm in greatest dimension |
| | No nodal metastases |
| III | Tumor of any size with adjacent spread to urethra, vagina, or anus or with regional lymph node metastases |
| IVA | Tumor invades upper urethra, bladder mucosa, rectal mucosa, pelvic bone, or bilateral node metastases |
| IVB | Any distant metastasis, including pelvic lymph nodes |

vulvar site (e.g., right or left labia majora) in which these characteristics are displayed.[38]

Once invasion has been determined, it is critical to report an accurate measurement of invasive depth, particularly when the invasion is near the critical depth of 1 mm. It is fortunate that most minimally invasive vulvar lesions have intact overlying epithelium from which to measure. Precise measurement may be difficult, particularly in the context of markedly exophytic lesions. When adjacent benign epithelium is present, Wilkinson proposed obtaining a measurement of depth extending from the most superficial dermal peg of the normal epithelium to the invasive edge of the carcinoma.[42] An alternative approach that has been proposed measures the deepest invasive focus from the nearest in situ neoplastic disease in a manner analogous to that used in the cervix.[43] When the pathologist considers measuring the depth of invasion from an in situ component in an adnexal structure, there must be a high degree of confidence that the involved adnexa is the probable origin of the invasive focus. Without a strong degree of certainty regarding the origin of the invasive focus, the authors recommend measuring the invasion from the surface basal peg. When exophytic lesions are encountered, it may not be possible to provide an accurate and meaningful measurement of invasive depth. In such instances, a tumor thickness measurement may be helpful and is defined as the distance between the surface of the tumor, or granular cell layer in hyperkeratotic tumors, and the deepest point of invasion.[42] It should be made clear in the report that this is a measurement of thickness and not depth, as prognostic data are not available for this type of measurement.

## Squamous Cell Carcinoma of the Vulva

Squamous cell carcinoma of the vulva represents 85% to 95% of malignant vulvar neoplasms and 3% to 8% of gynecologic cancers overall.[44] Although the incidence of VIN has increased, that of squamous cell carcinoma has remained essentially unchanged.[4] Seventy-five percent of women with vulvar squamous cell carcinoma are older than 60 years of age,[45, 46] with a mean age of 66 years of age. In the United States, this translates to age-specific incidence rates that range from 1.5 to 20 patients per 100,000 women, the higher incidence representing women greater than 70 years of age.[47] The vast majority of vulvar squamous cell carcinomas, however, can be divided into two broad categories: older patients with non–HPV-related tumors and younger patients with HPV-related tumors.[7, 49]

The majority of squamous cell carcinomas are located in the labia (70%) and most typically involve the labia majora. The second most common site is the clitoris, representing 11% to 24% of cases.[50] Despite the fact that VIN is often multifocal, multifocal

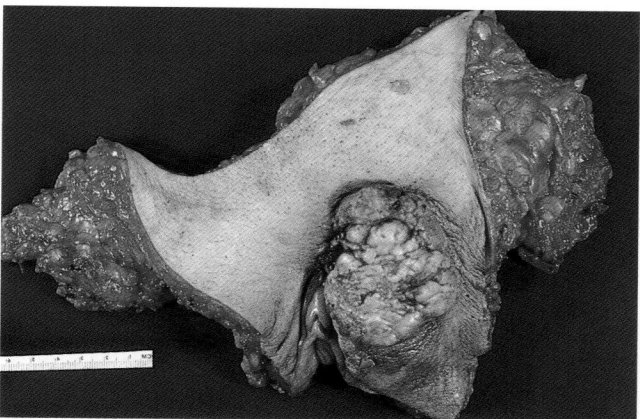

**FIGURE 35–7.** **Invasive vulvar carcinoma.** A radical vulvectomy specimen with invasive squamous cell carcinoma of the left labium majus. The lesion is bulky, irregular in shape and color, and characteristically deforms the normal labial architecture.

squamous carcinoma is rare; occasionally, "kissing" or "mirror image" tumors may arise.[50, 51] A subset of tumors may be associated with hypercalcemia,[52, 53] due in some instances to parathyroid hormone or parathyroid hormone–like substances secreted by the tumor cells.[53]

Grossly, squamous cell carcinoma may be plaquelike, exophytic and papillomatous or, more commonly, endophytic with central ulceration (Fig. 35–7). Microscopically, a variety of histologic patterns may be observed; however, as a rule, these lesions tend to be better differentiated than those found in the cervix. Infiltrative nests composed of polygonal cells with fairly abundant eosinophilic cytoplasm, round to oval nuclei with vesicular chromatin and prominent nucleoli, and focal to diffuse squamous pearl formation characterize the typical histologic pattern (Fig. 35–8) (CD Figs. 35–26 and 35–27). Intercellular bridges are usually readily observed. Squamous cell carcinomas of the vulva are

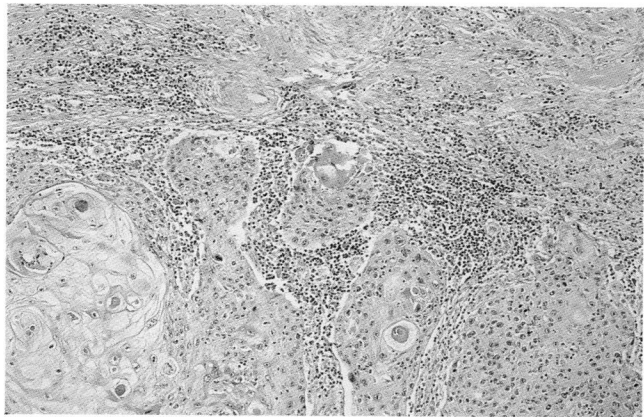

**FIGURE 35–8.** **Well-differentiated squamous carcinoma.** The carcinoma is characterized by an irregular infiltrative pattern of nests containing cells with abundant eosinophilic cytoplasm that also form keratin pearls. A chronic inflammatory cell stromal infiltrate is evident.

graded based on the degree of undifferentiated cells present, which are characterized as small cells with a high nuclear-to-cytoplasmic ratio that typically infiltrate the stroma as cords or in a finger-like fashion.[41] This scheme can be separated into three grades: Grade 1 exhibits no undifferentiated components, grade 2 has up to 50% of the tumor being composed of undifferentiated cells, and grade 3 has greater than 50% of the tumor composed of undifferentiated cells.[51]

Ambros and colleagues have drawn attention to a fibromyxoid stromal reaction that is seen in some examples of squamous cell carcinoma.[54] They found that this feature is associated with a significantly older age group, poorer survival rate, and more extensive lymph node metastases when compared with patients in whom this finding was absent. They later showed that this stromal response was associated with CD44 expression, a factor that serves as a receptor for hyaluronic acid, and suggested that its overexpression may result in altered hyaluronate metabolism with accelerated tumor cell migration and subsequent distal spread.[55] Tempfer and coworkers demonstrated that specific CD44v3 and CD44v6 variant isoform expressions, but not variants v5, v7, or v8, correlate with a worse prognosis.[56, 57]

Other, less commonly encountered, histologic patterns of squamous cell carcinoma include basaloid and warty variants, both of which are much more typically associated with HPV infection and a younger patient population (Table 35–2).[6, 48, 49, 58–60]

The basaloid and warty variants retain the microscopic characteristics observed in their respective in situ counterparts reviewed previously (see discussion of VIN) and display at least focal koilocytic nuclear atypia. Rounded infiltrative nests composed of mostly monomorphic cells with mild to moderate nuclear atypia mark infiltration of the basaloid type. Some squamous maturation may be observed, particularly in areas where the infiltrative pattern becomes more ragged, but squamous pearl formation is usually not seen. Warty carcinoma is distinguished from basaloid carcinoma by virtue of its exophytic papillary surface accompanied by usually marked cytologic atypia and more frequent atypical mitotic figures. Warty carcinoma tends to invade in irregular and pointed nests, usually eliciting a desmoplastic stromal response. These features help distinguish warty carcinoma from verrucous carcinoma, the latter lacking both significant cytologic atypia and an irregular infiltrative margin (CD Fig. 35–28).

Squamous cell carcinomas spread initially by contiguous growth and lymphatic invasion, and ultimately involve regional lymph nodes. Typically, nodal involvement is sequential with superficial inguinal nodes involved first followed by the femoral and pelvic nodes. On rare occasion, this orderly sequence is not upheld. With the exception of clitoral carcinomas in which bilateral nodal involvement is common, because of its unique lymphatic system, unilateral carcinoma usually metastasizes to ipsilateral lymph nodes.

It has become clear that p53 inactivation is a critical step in vulvar squamous tumorigenesis, either as a consequence of being targeted by HPV oncoproteins or undergoing a series of inactivating genetic events. These two pathways of p53 inactivation appear to be mutually exclusive processes, a logical dissociation because only one mechanism is required to inactivate this critical nuclear protein.[61–63] That there might not be any significant biologic differences between HPV-related and non–HPV-related carcinoma may be explained by the fact that allelotyping studies have shown that there are no appreciably different genetic losses between the two groups.[64]

Because clinically suspicious lymph nodes were found to correlate poorly with actual pathologic findings in the nodes, the International Federation of Gynecologists and Obstetricians adopted surgical pathologic staging that differs from clinical staging. This has led to better prognostic discrimination.[65] It should be noted, however, that even pathologic

**TABLE 35–2.** Comparison of Most Common Forms of Squamous Cell Carcinoma of the Vulva

| | Verrucous | Squamous | Basaloid, Warty |
|---|---|---|---|
| **Patient Profile** | *Elderly* | *Elderly* | *Younger* |
| Infiltrative pattern | Pushing, bulbous border | Infiltrative nests, cords, tentacles | Maturation of epithelial cells into infiltrative nests, cords, tentacles |
| HPV types | 6 and 11 | Most often negative | 16 and 18 |
| Associated VIN | None | Differentiated | Basaloid, Warty |
| Association with cigarette smoking | None | None | Positive |
| Miscellaneous | Must be distinguished from exophytic condyloma (condyloma acuminatum) and squamous carcinoma; rarely metastasizes | Typically well differentiated; metastasis to regional lymph nodes principal prognostic factor | Metastasizes to regional lymph nodes |
| Treatment | Excision only, radiation may cause malignant transformation | Excision or radiation | Excision or radiation |

HPV, human papillomavirus; VIN, vulvar intraepithelial neoplasia.

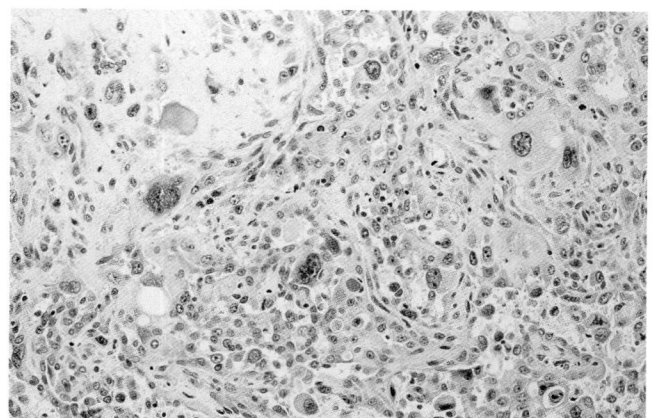

FIGURE 35–9. Giant cell squamous carcinoma. Scattered bizarre, pleomorphic, and multinucleate cells characterize this poorly differentiated squamous cell carcinoma.

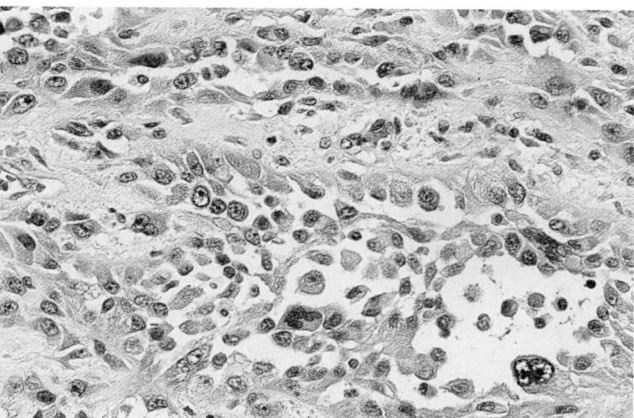

FIGURE 35–10. Acantholytic squamous cell carcinoma. Pseudoglandular spaces are lined by a single layer of cuboidal malignant epithelial cells of this poorly differentiated squamous carcinoma.

staging may suffer from false-negative lymph node evaluations; thus, it is recommended that all lymph node tissue, rather than "representative" portions of each node, be submitted by the pathologist.[66, 67]

The greatest tumor diameter and the presence or absence and distribution of lymph node involvement represent the only well-established independent prognostic factors in vulvar squamous cell carcinoma.[68] Five-year survival ranges from 90% to 100% in lymph node–negative cases compared with 30% to 70% in lymph node–positive cases. Five-year survival when pelvic lymph nodes are positive is estimated to be at approximately 25%. Hefler and associates reported that elevated levels of squamous cell carcinoma antigen were also an independent prognostic indicator; however, lymph node status was a variable not included in their multivariate analysis.[69]

## SARCOMATOID (SPINDLE CELL/GIANT CELL) CARCINOMA

Sarcomatoid carcinoma is a rare form of squamous cell carcinoma, characterized by the proliferation of malignant spindle[70–72] and giant cells[73] (Fig. 35–9) (CD Fig. 35–29). The malignant cells are immunoreactive for cytokeratin,[74] which helps distinguish this tumor from other mesenchymal spindle cell malignancies of the vulva, as well as from an amelanotic, spindle cell, malignant melanoma. Although only a few cases have been reported, this form of anaplastic carcinoma appears to be highly virulent and rapidly progressive.[70, 72, 75]

## ACANTHOLYTIC SQUAMOUS CELL CARCINOMA

Acantholytic squamous cell carcinoma is a rare variant, which is also referred to as *adenoid squamous carcinoma*.[76–78] It is characterized by the presence of pseudoglandular spaces lined by a single layer of flat to cuboidal cells. The spaces are thought to be artifacts of acantholysis, and occasionally dyskera-

totic cells may be found within (Fig. 35–10) (CD Figs. 35–30 and 35–31). These nonspecific features may be observed in well- or poorly differentiated tumors, and therefore their significance lies largely in the differential diagnoses invoked to include glandular malignancies involving the vulva.

## VERRUCOUS CARCINOMA

Verrucous carcinoma is a rare form of well-differentiated squamous cell carcinoma with distinctive biologic features. Generally, verrucous carcinoma affects older women, many in the eighth and ninth decades of life. Unlike squamous cell carcinomas of the usual variety, verrucous carcinoma infiltrates by a broad pushing margin and rarely metastasizes. Cytologic atypia should be mild and when present is limited to the base and parabasal regions of the tumor (Fig. 35–11) (CD Figs. 35–32 to 35–34). Mitoses are rare to absent. HPV is frequently detected in these tumors.[79] HPV-6 and HPV-11 have been dem-

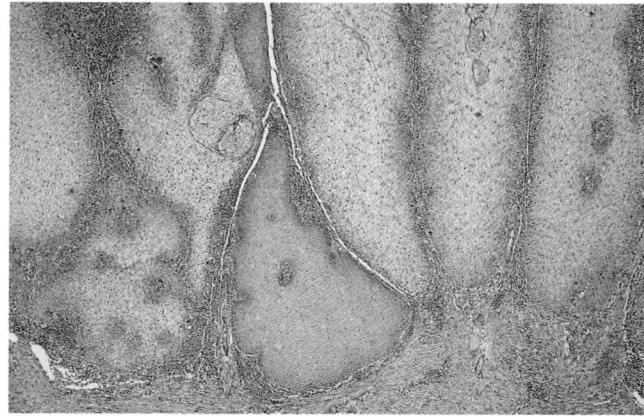

FIGURE 35–11. Verrucous carcinoma. The carcinoma is characterized by bulbous tumor projections that invade in a pushing fashion. The neoplastic epithelial cells lack significant anaplasia, and mitoses are rare. The leading edges of the tumor are bordered by a chronic inflammatory cell dermal infiltrate.

onstrated in the few available studies in which the HPV was typed.[80, 81] The presence of these "low-risk" viral types may explain, at least in part, their more indolent behavior.

Although some investigators have attempted to distinguish verrucous carcinoma from giant condyloma of Buschke,[82, 83] there seems to be little reason to do so.[84] Both characteristically contain a low-risk HPV genome,[80, 81, 85–87] display condylomatous features at least focally, and behave in a similar fashion.

The differential diagnosis includes condyloma acuminatum and warty carcinoma. Given the histologic similarity to condyloma acuminatum, superficial biopsy specimens lacking sampling of the pushing, infiltrative margin may lead to an erroneous diagnosis. Warty carcinoma displays greater cytologic atypia, more numerous and occasional atypical mitoses, and an infiltrative margin. Since nodal metastases are highly uncommon, wide local excision is the treatment of choice for verrucous carcinoma.

## Glandular Neoplasia

Benign and malignant glandular neoplasms of the vulva may arise from typical skin adnexal structures, mammary-like glands of the anogenital region, vestibular glands, and Bartholin's glands. Papillary hidradenoma, Bartholin's carcinoma, and Paget's disease are discussed in the following sections. Additional rare forms of glandular neoplasms are listed in Table 35–3.

### PAPILLARY HIDRADENOMA

Papillary hidradenoma (hidradenoma papilliferum) is a lesion that is predominantly limited to adult white women. Few women younger than 30 years of age have been reported with this tumor, and few, if any, black women are affected.[88] It presents as a well-circumscribed, unilateral, subcutaneous mass usually in the labium majus or, less commonly, the interlabial sulcus or labium minus. Central ulceration may be observed occasionally. Proposed to be derived from anogenital mammary-like glands,[89] the

**TABLE 35–3.** Miscellaneous Benign and Malignant Tumors of the Vulva

| Differentiation | Specific Type | References |
|---|---|---|
| Skeletal muscle | Rhabdomyoma | 281 |
| | Rhabdomyosarcoma | 282, 283 |
| Fibroblastic, fibrohistiocytic | Fibroma | 284 |
| | Benign fibrous histiocytoma | 285 |
| | Desmoid | 286, 287 |
| | Dermatofibrosarcoma protuberans | 288, 289 |
| | Malignant fibrous histiocytoma | 290 |
| Vascular | Hemangioma | 291 |
| | Pyogenic granuloma | 132 |
| | Angiokeratoma | 292, 293 |
| | Lymphangioma | 294 |
| | Lymphangiosarcoma | 295 |
| | Hemangiopericytoma | 296 |
| | Glomus tumor | 297, 298 |
| | Kaposi's sarcoma | 299 |
| | Epithelioid hemangioendothelioma | 300 |
| | Angiosarcoma | 301 |
| Neural | Schwannoma | 302, 303 |
| | Neurofibroma | 304, 305 |
| | Granular cell tumor | 306–309 |
| | Malignant schwannoma | 310, 311 |
| | Malignant granular cell tumor | 312 |
| Adipose tissue | Lipoma | 313 |
| | Liposarcoma | 314–316 |
| Uncertain histogenesis | Epithelioid sarcoma | 317–320 |
| | Alveolar soft part sarcoma | 321 |
| | Malignant rhabdoid tumor | 318, 319 |
| | Yolk sac (endodermal sinus) | 274, 275 |
| Skin adnexae | Syringoma | 254–256 |
| | Clear cell hidradenoma | 257 |
| | Trichoepithelioma | 258 |
| | Basal cell carcinoma | 259–263 |
| | Basosquamous (metatypical) carcinoma | 264 |
| | Adenosquamous carcinoma | 77, 91, 209, 265 |
| | Adenocarcinoma | 266–269 |
| | Sweat gland carcinoma | 268, 270, 271 |
| | Sebaceous carcinoma | 272, 273 |
| Lymphoid | Lymphoma | 276, 277 |
| Other | Metastatic tumors | 278–280 |

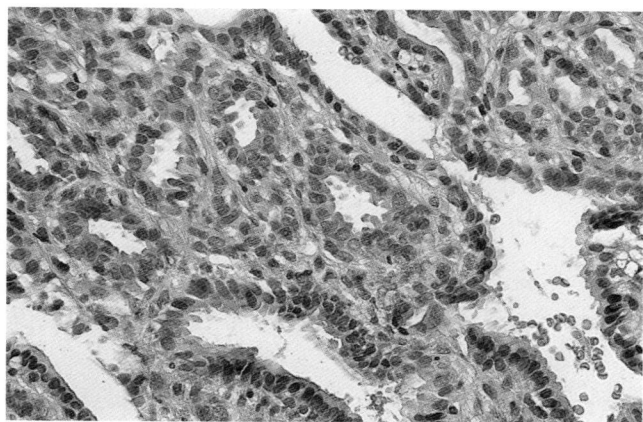

**FIGURE 35–12. Papillary hidradenoma.** High magnification of the papillary-glandular structures of the papillary hidradenoma. Focally, two cell layers can be identified; a subepithelial myoepithelial cell layer underlying cuboidal to columnar epithelial cells occasionally capped by apocrine snouts.

tumor bears features reminiscent of intraductal papillomas or nipple adenomas of the breast. Histological evaluation shows a proliferation of glandular elements, typically with a prominent papillary pattern. These papillae are typically lined by both an epithelial and a myoepithelial cell layer. The epithelial cells are cuboidal to columnar and may demonstrate apocrine features with luminal snouts (Fig. 35–12) (CD Figs. 35–35 to 35–37). Only rare cases of carcinoma arising in a papillary hidradenoma have been reported.[90, 91] Metastatic carcinoma may present clinically as a tumor presumed to be a papillary hidradenoma or Bartholin gland cyst and should be considered when a diagnosis of malignancy is being entertained.

## BARTHOLIN'S CARCINOMA

Bartholin's carcinoma represents 2% to 7% of vulvar malignancies[50] and most typically involves perimenopausal or postmenopausal women, although its occurrence in women as young as 14 years of age has been reported.[92] Clinically, they are often suspected to be Bartholin's cysts, their true nature being disclosed only after attempts to drain, marsupialize, or treat with antibiotics have failed. Indeed, in women older than 50 years of age, in whom an initial diagnosis of a Bartholin cyst is less common, excision of the gland is recommended.[93]

Because of the diverse histologic features of the Bartholin's gland, a variety of malignant neoplastic variants have been reported, with squamous cell carcinoma and adenocarcinoma being the most common types, each representing approximately 40% of cases. *Adenoid cystic carcinoma*, representing up to 15% of cases,[94–96] is the next most common type, with *transitional cell carcinoma, adenosquamous carcinoma*, and *anaplastic carcinoma* forming the remainder. Given the diversity of possible histopathologic features and the fact that these features are not unique to Bartholin's gland tumors, one must con-

sider the possibility that the tumor represents a metastasis from another site. Accordingly, it is recommended that strict criteria be applied when rendering a diagnosis of Bartholin's gland carcinoma:

1. The tumor should show a transition from benign to malignant epithelium.
2. The tumor must be centered in the area of the Bartholin gland and consist of epithelium consistent with Bartholin's gland origin.
3. There should be no evidence of a second primary with similar features elsewhere.[95]

In practice, however, the first criterion might not be met because tumors may replace the entire gland by the time of excision. Occasionally, one encounters cases in which VIN is present in contiguous vulvar epithelium and is observed descending into and perhaps replacing the glandular epithelium. These cases should be regarded as secondary involvement of the Bartholin gland. HPV-16 DNA has been detected in the majority of squamous cell carcinomas tested[97] and in some transitional cell carcinomas[98] of the Bartholin gland.

Given the deep location of Bartholin's carcinomas, they are often detected later and therefore present with advanced disease, including inguinofemoral nodal metastases in up to 50% of cases.[44] Accordingly, they are associated with a worse prognosis, as compared with most vulvar carcinomas, with an overall probability of a disease-free 5-year survival of 30%.[92, 95, 97] Adenoid cystic variants appear to follow a more indolent course that is characterized by local recurrences and rare examples of distant spread.[92, 99]

## PAGET'S DISEASE

Vulvar Paget's disease is a form of intraepithelial adenocarcinoma that is uncommonly associated with a synchronous or metachronous, invasive, local or regional tumor.[100] This varies from Paget's disease of the breast or perianal region, in which an infiltrative tumor is almost always present. The histogenesis of Paget's cells remains a source of debate but fundamentally must be considered to arise from a variety of potential sources, of which sweat glands and mammary-like glands are most suspect. Patients are most often postmenopausal and present with pruritus or, more rarely, bleeding. The lesions appear as red, well-demarcated, patches bearing a slight resemblance to eczema.

The Paget cells are distributed along the dermal-epidermal junction. They may be seen singly or in nests. Migration into the intermediate and superficial epidermis can also be seen. Foci of well-formed glands are occasionally encountered. A minor subtype of Paget's cells display signet ring features. Paget's cells usually contain abundant, clear cytoplasm. Most cells can be shown to contain mucin by special stains (mucicarmine, alcian blue with hyaluronidase pretreatment, and periodic acid–Schiff after diastase pretreatment). Nuclei are large and centrally located and display severe atypia with prominent nucleoli. Mitotic figures are seen occasionally (Fig. 35–13) (CD Fig. 35–38)

A multifocal nature of this disease has been suggested as the source of recurrent disease in the face of complete excision.[101] Recurrences are common, affecting residual skin and even grafts from other parts of the body. Preoperative intravenous administration of fluorescein and subsequent visualization via ultraviolet light has been recommended as an adjunct to aid the surgeon in delimiting the affected area.[102] Using immunohistochemistry to aid in the assessment of margins has been argued by some to be useful,[103] whereas others have failed to support this claim.[104] Paget's cells have been found to express immunoreactivity to low-molecular-weight cytokeratins, epithelial membrane antigen, and carcinoembryonic antigen (Fig. 35–14) (CD Fig. 35–39).

Expectedly, the prognosis is largely dependent on the origin of the Paget cells and the presence or absence of invasion. If derived from primary cells of the vulva and no invasion is present, an indolent course can be predicted, with an awareness of the risk of recurrences and the attendant necessity of reexcisions. When invasion occurs, it is almost always characterized by irregular nests or single Paget cells infiltrating the superficial dermis. Although desmoplasia is helpful when present, its absence is not exclusive of invasion. Care should be taken when making the diagnosis of invasion, as tangential sectioning can produce pseudoinvasive groups of Paget cells that may mimic invasion.[105] During the evolution of the disease, invasion may ultimately occur; this has been associated with a negative prognosis.[106] In general, however, invasion to less than 1 mm is associated with the same prognosis as noninvasive disease. There has been one report of a case of Paget's disease invasive to 1 mm associated with inguinofemoral lymph node metastases.[107]

A small but significant number of cases are associated with genital and extragenital malignancies,

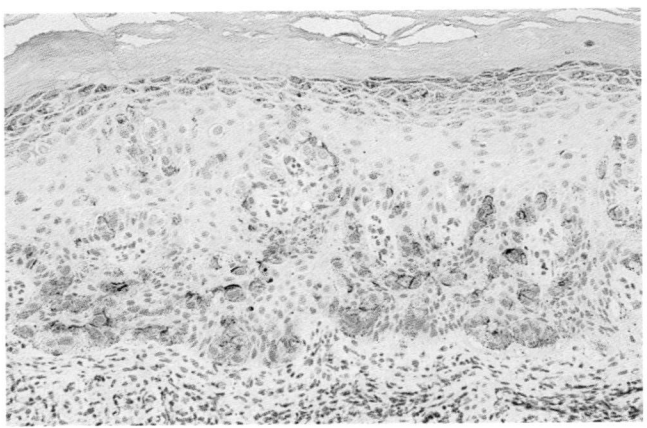

**FIGURE 35–14. Paget's disease.** Monoclonal carcinoembryonic antigen vividly decorates the Paget's cells.

including those of the breast,[108] urinary bladder, rectum (perianal involvement), Bartholin's gland, and other skin adnexal malignancies. Accordingly, other primary sites should be excluded in the process of managing affected patients. Goldblum and Hart have reported utility in using an immunophenotypic profile consisting of cytokeratins 7 and 20 (CK7 and CK20, respectively), and gross cystic disease fluid protein (GCDFP15) to assist in determining the origin of the Paget cells.[109, 110] Vulvar Paget's disease has a typical immunophenotypic profile of CK7+/ CK20−/GCDFP15+, whereas profiles of CK7−/ CK20+/ GCDFP15− or CK7+/CK20+/GCDFP15− suggest origin from another primary source such as the rectum or urinary bladder.[109, 110] In perianal Paget's disease, the presence of gastrointestinal-type glands and dirty luminal necrosis are additive features suggestive of a colorectal primary.[110] It should be noted that Toker cells and Merkel cells in the vulva are also immunoreactive for CK7 but can be distinguished from Paget cells by virtue of bland cytologic features.

In addition to other primary sources for Paget cells, malignant melanoma and other benign or malignant conditions should also be considered.[111] In addition to the aforementioned special stains and immunostains, immunoreactivity for carcinoembryonic antigen assists in confirming the diagnosis of Paget's disease, whereas HMB-45 and S-100 protein assist in the diagnosis of malignant melanoma (CD Figs. 35–40 and 35–41).

## Pigmented and Melanocytic Lesions

A variety of benign and malignant pigmented lesions may be observed in the vulva. They include dermatoses and pruritic lesions with pigment incontinence, VIN, ephelis, lentigo simplex, melanotic macules (melanosis), and melanocytic nevi.

Melanocytic nevi may be dermal, junctional, or compound and, significantly, are also well recognized for not uncommonly displaying atypical fea-

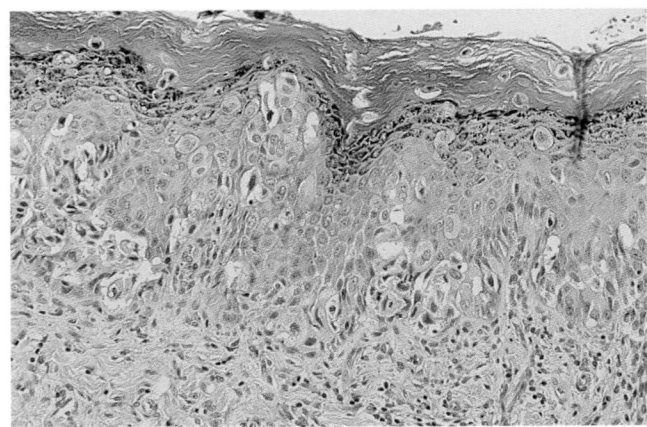

**FIGURE 35–13. Paget's disease.** Paget's cells are seen largely occupying the dermoepidermal junction. Occasional epidermotropism can be seen. The neoplastic cells are characterized by abundant clear cytoplasm and round to oval nuclei with vesicular chromatin and prominent nucleoli.

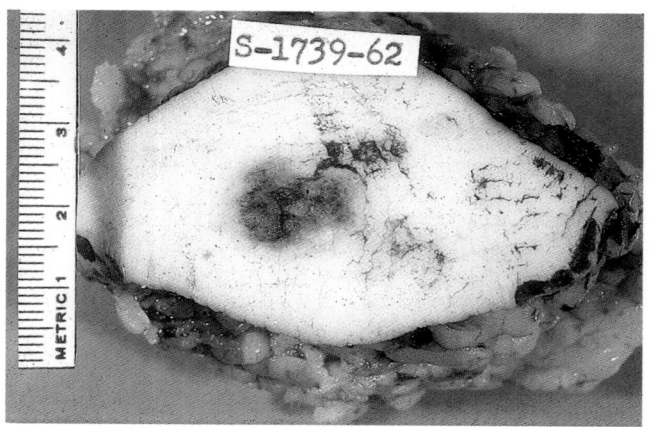

**FIGURE 35–15. Vulvar melanoma.** Hemivulvectomy specimen containing a central pigmented melanoma. The lesion is characteristic with irregular borders and central ulceration.

tures that may lead to the misdiagnosis of malignant melanoma. Particularly vexing cases were studied and described by Clark and colleagues,[112] who emphasized features that are useful in distinguishing *atypical melanocytic nevi of the genital type* from *dysplastic nevi* and *malignant melanoma.* The most significant distinguishing features are the clinical presentation and the presence of proliferative melanocytic activity that obscures the dermal-epidermal interface in atypical melanocytic nevi of the genital type.

Compared with melanomas found elsewhere on the body, vulvar *melanomas* are rare, composing approximately 2% of all melanomas, yet they represent between 2% and 10% of malignant vulvar tumors.[113, 114] The vast majority of the affected women are white and in their late reproductive to menopausal years. Cases of melanoma affecting prepubescent girls are exceedingly rare.[115] Approximately 10% have been estimated to arise from preexisting nevi. To compound this problem, genital nevi are often atypical and may represent a significant diagnostic challenge to the pathologist.[112]

Melanomas may be papular or macular, blue to black with irregular borders and, occasionally, central ulceration (Fig. 35–15). The clitoris, with its rich vascular supply, is a favored site for melanoma, but melanoma may arise at any vulvar site. Ragnarsson-Olding and colleagues observed that melanomas arising in mucosal (glabrous) areas of the vulva are more likely to be acral lentiginous than superficial spreading or nodular in pattern of growth, a finding opposite that observed in melanomas from other cutaneous sites.[116] For this reason, they posit that melanomas from these areas are more analogous to those that emerge from other glabrous skin sites such as those found on the palms, soles, and subungual areas. This assertion is further supported by their observation that although melanomas may be observed arising in association with nevi in hair-bearing vulvar sites, this is not observed in the vulvar mucosal sites.[116] Lentigo maligna and acral lentiginous patterns must be distinguished from Paget's disease (Table 35–4). One must be reminded that melanin pigment may be seen in Paget cells and that desmoplastic or amelanotic melanomas may lack both pigment and HMB-45 immunoreactivity (CD Figs. 35–42 to 35–46).

Prognosis is stage dependent and is generally poor. It is recommended that vulvar melanomas be staged surgically using the American Joint Committee on Cancer system, which incorporates both Breslow and Clark microstaging.[117] The Clark staging scheme may be applied only to melanomas of hair-bearing regions of the vulva because the papillary dermis is not well developed in mucosal regions of the vulva. In addition to staging, other characteristics have emerged as prognostically significant. Ragnarsson-Olding and colleagues suggest that macroscopic amelanosis and ulceration are useful predictors of a worse outcome.[118] Overall, the 5-year relative survival is 47%.[119]

## Soft Tissue Tumors

Soft tissue tumors of the vulva, particularly sarcomas, are extremely rare[120] and are summarized in Table 35–3. The most common form of soft tissue tumors, smooth muscle neoplasms, and aggressive angiomyxoma, a distinctive tumor that is unique to the female and male external genitalia, are discussed briefly.

**TABLE 35–4.** Comparison of Vulvar Malignant Melanoma and Paget's Disease

| General | Melanoma<br>*Typically Pigmented Lesions* | Paget's Disease<br>*Typically White Plaques* |
|---|---|---|
| Neoplastic cell distribution | Basal, intraepidermal, dermal | Basal, intraepidermal, dermal (when invasive) |
| Cytoplasmic melanin | +/− | +/− |
| Cytoplasmic mucin | − | + |
| HMB-45 | + | − |
| S-100 protein | + | − |
| CEA | − | + |
| Cytokeratin | − | + |

CEA, carcinoembryonic antigen.

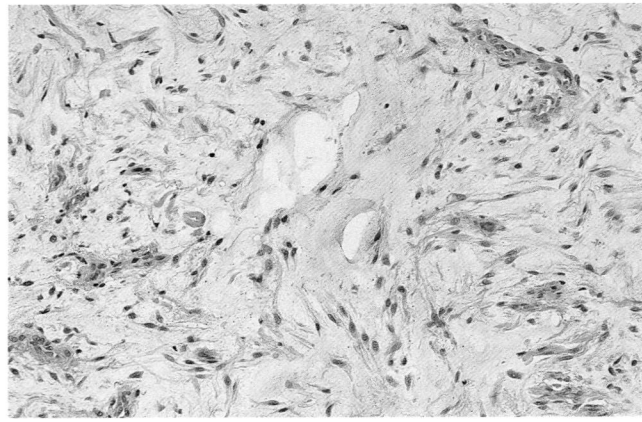

**FIGURE 35–16. Aggressive angiomyxoma.** The tumor is characterized by patches of myxoid tumor infiltrating the dermis and subcutaneous soft tissue. The tumor is comprised of small and medium-size vessels surrounded by a myxoid stroma that is populated by banal spindle to stellate stromal cells. Note the lack of perivascular hypercellularity which is a feature more typical of angiomyofibroblastoma.

### SMOOTH MUSCLE TUMORS

*Leiomyomas* are the most common mesenchymal neoplasms of the vulva. They have essentially the same characteristics as when observed elsewhere in the female genital tract. A propensity toward myxoid features, epithelioid features, and stromal hyalinization has been described.[121–123] Criteria to help distinguish between leiomyomas and leiomyosarcomas have been proposed. Mitotic activity greater than or equal to 5 to 10 mitoses per 10 high-power fields, as well as atypical mitotic figures, is of greatest importance. Extreme nuclear atypia is helpful, yet is present in only a few cases of malignancy. It should be noted, however, that although local recurrences are common among cases classified as leiomyosarcomas, distant metastases and death due to progressive disease have been reported only rarely.[123]

### AGGRESSIVE ANGIOMYXOMA

Aggressive angiomyxoma is a poorly circumscribed, locally aggressive, myofibroblastic tumor prone to inadequate resection and attendant morbidity. These lesions are composed of spindled to stellate stromal cells, thick-walled vessels of various caliber, and a myxoid extracellular matrix (Fig. 35–16) (CD Figs. 35–47 to 35–52). The differential diagnosis includes other neoplasms with myxoid features, chief among which is *angiomyofibroblastoma*. The neoplastic cells of aggressive angiomyxoma contain estrogen and progesterone receptors, suggesting a hormonal role in the development of the process.[124] Although desmin positivity was thought originally to distinguish angiomyofibroblastoma unequivocally from aggressive angiomyxoma, subsequent analysis has shown that weak desmin immunoreactivity may be observed in the stellate stromal cells in some examples of aggressive angiomyxoma.[125] The authors continue to use this stain because strong perivascular staining is still characteristic of angiomyofibroblastomas and is not seen in aggressive angiomyxomas.

## Infections of the Vulva

The vulva is a frequent site of infection, the most common form of which is viral (HPV and herpes simplex virus). Although other infectious causes may give rise to lesions evaluated by the surgical pathologist, the findings are often nonspecific or require additional tests to confirm the diagnosis. Both common and uncommon causative agents are summarized in Table 35–5.

### CONDYLOMA ACUMINATA

Condyloma acuminata are exophytic, verrucous lesions of the vulva that may arise singly, multiply, or as a coalescent, cauliflower-like mass resulting from infection with HPV (Fig. 35–17). Microscopically, the true acuminate lesion is characterized by finger-like papillae composed of a fibrovascular core and lined by squamous epithelial cells (CD Figs. 35–53 to 35–57). The squamous epithelium is acanthotic and invariably disorganized. Hyperkeratosis and focal parakeratosis frequently overlie the surface of the lesion. The nuclei of the squamous epithelial cells fail to attain maturation in the intermediate and superficial layers of the epithelium and are enlarged and frequently have an irregular contour. Unlike similar lesions in the cervix and vagina, lesions of the vulva frequently show no nuclear hyperchromasia of the involved cells. For this reason, classic koilocytic changes are sometimes not identified, a point of some significance when considering the differential diagnoses. Atypical mitotic figures are not a feature of these lesions. HPV-6 and HPV-11 are almost the exclusive viral types associated with typical examples of condyloma acuminatum.[126]

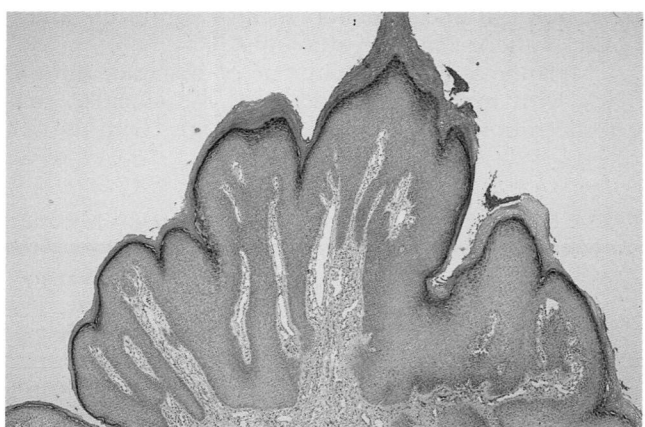

**FIGURE 35–17. Condyloma acuminatum.** Spire-shaped, exophytic papillary projections lined by hyperkeratotic and acanthotic epidermis. Koilocytic cells, characterized by enlarged hyperchromatic and wrinkled nuclei with associated cytoplasmic cavitation, are often difficult to appreciate.

**TABLE 35–5.** Vulvar Infections

| Etiologic Group | Disease | Agents | Clinical and Histologic Features | Miscellaneous | References |
|---|---|---|---|---|---|
| Viruses | Condyloma acuminatum | Human papillomavirus | Papillomatous lesions with koilocytes | Principal viral types 6, 11 (VIN types 16, 18) | 126 |
| | Herpes | Herpes simplex virus (HSV) | Vesicles with intranuclear "ground-glass" inclusions | Primarily HSV-2; occasionally HSV-1 | 350, 351, 367 |
| | Molluscum contagiosum | Poxvirus group | Umbilicated lesions containing "molluscum bodies" (intracytoplasmic inclusions) | Lesions may be extensive in immunosuppressed patients | 350, 364, 367 |
| | Shingles | Varicella zoster | Unilateral vesicles; infected cells multinucleated with intranuclear inclusions | Third dermatome | 360 |
| | | Cytomegalovirus | Intranuclear and intracytoplasmic inclusions | Immunosuppressed and infants predisposed | 351, 355 |
| Bacteria | Syphilis; condyloma latum | *Treponema pallidum* | Chancre (shallow ulcer) in primary infection; condyloma latum secondary manifestation with papules and plaques; perivascular lymphoplasmacytic endarteritis | Dark-field illumination for expressed fluid; immunofluorescence for scrapings; Warthin-Starry stain on tissue sections; serology | 350, 366 |
| | Chancroid | *Haemophilus ducreyi* | Ulcerative disease with nonspecific histologic features | Common in tropical and subtropical regions; uncommon in Europe and North America; gram-negative bacilli | 359, 366 |
| | Granuloma inguinale | *Calymmatobacterium granulomatis* | Inguinal lymphadenitis uncommon; papules and nodules with ulceration; granulation-like tissue with abundant histiocytes containing Donovan bodies | Tropical and subtropical regions; Giemsa and Warthin-Starry stains | 356 |
| | Lymphogranuloma venereum | *Chlamydia trachomatis* | Inguinal lymphadenitis typical, intracytoplasmic gram-negative bacteria; histologic features variable and nonspecific | Tropical and subtropical regions; serovars 1, 2, and 3; work-up directed toward excluding other causes | 363, 366 |
| | Tuberculosis | *Mycobacterium tuberculosis* | Typically in context of upper genital tract involvement; caseating granulomas bearing acid-fast bacilli | Atypical mycobacteria and sarcoidosis should be excluded, cultures taken | 358 |
| Protozoa | | *Trichomonas vaginalis* | Initiated in vagina with secondary involvement of vulva | Best detected in wet mount preparation due to motility, stains on routine pap | 245, 246 |
| Fungus | | *Candida* spp. | Pruritic, superficial infection | Seen on routine H&E but highlighted by PAS or silver stains | 243, 244 |
| Parasites | Pinworm | *Enterobius vermicularis* | Vulvovaginal pruritis | Cellulose tape–slide preparation used to demonstrate eggs | 357 |
| | Schistosomiasis | *Schistosoma mansoni* | Parasites in epidermis | Often refered to as swimmer's itch | 370 |

VIN; vulvar intraepithelial neoplasia; PAS; periodic acid–Schiff.

Accordingly, risk of progression to invasive squamous carcinoma is considered to be negligible.

The differential diagnosis includes fibroepithelial polyps, verruca vulgaris, squamous papillomas, seborrheic keratosis, and verrucous carcinoma. *Fibroepi-* *thelial polyps* are usually architecturally simple, lacking the complex exophytic features of condyloma acuminatum. They may, however, contain atypical and even bizarre stromal cells that raise concern over sarcomatous transformation.[127] *Squamous papillo-*

*mas* are distinguished from condyloma acuminatum by their lack of acanthosis, epithelial disorganization, and koilocytic changes. *Verruca vulgaris,* a lesion predominantly caused by HPV-2,[128] is uncommonly encountered in the vulva. It typically lacks the well-developed fibrovascular cores that extend to the tips of the exophytic projections seen in condyloma acuminatum (CD Figs. 35–58 and 35–59). The granular layer also tends to be better developed in verruca vulgaris with keratohyalin granules prominently displayed. In less typical examples of condyloma acuminatum, the features may mimic those of *seborrheic keratosis.* This is a point of some interest, as investigators have proposed that HPV may be present in seborrheic keratosis,[129] whereas others have disputed this claim.[130, 131] The authors are in agreement with Li and Ackerman, who indicate that careful application of diagnostic criteria permits one to distinguish between these two differential diagnoses.[131] Significantly, seborrheic keratosis should lack parakeratosis and be characterized by an expansion of basal cells rather than an expansion of the spinous keratinocyte layer, the latter being a feature of condyloma acuminatum (CD Figs. 35–60 to 35–64).

*Condyloma acuminata* should be differentiated from *verrucous carcinoma.* Architecturally, verrucous carcinomas are generally thicker lesions than condylomas, a characteristic that makes this lesion difficult to biopsy in an office setting and often results in an inadequate sample lacking the diagnostic basal portion. The base of this lesion is formed by broad, bulbous columns typically accompanied by a dermal chronic inflammatory cell infiltrate. In addition to these invasive characteristics, verrucous carcinoma can be distinguished from condyloma acuminatum by its lack of delicate fibrovascular cores extending to the tips of the squamous papillae (CD Fig. 35–65).[132]

## Noninfectious Inflammatory Lesions

A wide array of inflammatory processes that manifest as skin lesions may involve the vulva primarily or secondarily. These are addressed in Chapter 49. A limited number of lesions, however, bear special mention in this chapter. These are discussed in the following sections.

### PLASMA CELL VULVITIS (ZOON'S VULVITIS)

Plasma cell vulvitis is a rare condition of unknown cause characterized by a thinned epidermis, dilated vessels, extravasated red blood cells, hemosiderin deposition, and a dense dermal infiltrate predominantly consisting of plasma cells.[133, 134] An analogous lesion occurs on the penis (Zoon's balanitis, plasma cell balanitis). The diagnosis is one of exclusion from a differential diagnosis that includes syphilis and a variety of chronic dermatoses. Autoimmune disorders have been reported to be associated with the disease.[134, 135]

### VULVAR VESTIBULITIS

Vulvar vestibulitis is a poorly understood form of vulvodynia, leading to the symptoms of entry dyspareunia and intense, pinpoint pain in affected areas, resulting in significant psychologic and psychosexual dysfunction.[136, 137] Although most studies have emphasized the role of mild to moderate chronic inflammation involving the vestibular stroma and glands,[138, 139] some investigators have argued that inflammation may not play a specific role.[140] Others have suggested a pathologic role for increased innervation.[141, 142] Numerous studies have failed to establish HPV infection as a significant causative correlate.[143–147] Surgery in the form of local excision or laser ablation of the affected area appears to provide the best results.[148, 149] Alternatively, local instillation of α-interferon[149, 150] and behavioral intervention have also been used with some success.[151]

### VULVITIS GRANULOMATOSA

Vulvitis granulomatosa is a rare granulomatous inflammatory condition resembling cheilitis granulomatosa of Miescher.[152] The differential diagnosis includes other granulomatous inflammatory processes, including Crohn's disease and tuberculosis, and again is a diagnosis of exclusion.

### BEHÇET'S SYNDROME

Behçet's syndrome remains an enigmatic condition[153] characterized by the triad of oral, genital, and ocular lesions. The fact that the syndrome includes involvement of multiple systems is now appreciated. The underlying pathologic mechanism appears to be a vasculitis, which in the vulva manifests as painful ulcers. Microscopically, the findings are nonspecific but may include a necrotizing arteritis, chronic perivascular inflammation, and thrombosed arteries and veins. Treatment is directed toward the management of autoimmune disease, with varied success, and includes the administration of azathioprine and thalidomide.[153]

### FOX-FORDYCE DISEASE

Fox-Fordyce disease is a condition primarily affecting apocrine glands of the vulva, perianal region, and axillae of adolescent girls and persists until menopause, when some abatement of the disease may be observed. Rarely, prepubertal girls may be affected.[154] Improvement may also be observed during pregnancy or with the use of oral contraceptives. The lesions present as pruritic papules that correlate microscopically with keratinaceous plugs in hair follicles. These plugged follicles, in turn, disrupt the normal emission of sweat, the latter accumulating in dilated apocrine ducts and glands. The ducts and glands may rupture, eliciting a chronic inflammatory response. A variety of treatment methods have been used, ranging from electrocautery to antibiotic administration, with varying success. Given the apparent mechanism of disruption, keratolytic agents may hold the most promise for treatment.

## HIDRADENITIS SUPPURATIVA

Hidradenitis suppurativa is a potentially disfiguring inflammatory condition of the apocrine glands[155] or hair follicles,[156] or both, in the vulva and axillae. Initially, the apocrine glands are infiltrated by neutrophils, a process that eventually extends into the surrounding dermal tissues. A folliculitis has also been suggested as the initiating lesion but is less favored as a causative origin. The inflammation progresses to abscess formation, with tissue breakdown and ultimately sinus formation and scarring. A rare case of squamous carcinoma arising in association with hidradenitis suppurativa has been reported.[157] Surgical excision of the affected area appears to be the most effective form of therapy, with early intervention perhaps leading to better outcome.[158]

## BULLOUS DISEASES

A variety of bullous diseases may affect the vulva and typically require careful clinical correlation as well as immunofluorescent techniques to localize the precise site of disruption. These general conditions are discussed in greater detail in Chapter 49.

## Vulvar Cysts

Vulvar cysts can arise from a variety of epithelial structures with disparate embryologic derivation. Bartholin's cysts are described in the following sections. A summary of other epithelial cysts is provided in Table 35–6.

*Bartholin's cysts* present as firm, somewhat tender masses and, although they may occur at any age, they usually affect women in their reproductive years. Indeed, lesions presenting as Bartholin's cysts in postmenopausal women should be regarded with suspicion because Bartholin's carcinomas are more common in this age group. Bartholin's cysts result from blockage of the Bartholin duct. The cyst's epithelial lining reflects the cells of the acini and ducts of the Bartholin gland and thus may be mucinous, transitional, or squamous in type. In the context of long-standing inflammation, the cyst lining may be entirely denuded and replaced with inflammatory cells, histiocytes, and granulation tissue. Abscesses may develop, requiring marsupialization.

Epidermal inclusion cysts may occur in the vulva. They may be found in a wide anatomic distribution. Histologically they are indistinguishable from epidermal inclusion cysts elsewhere.

## Non-neoplastic Epithelial Disorders

Terminology relating to non-neoplastic epithelial disorders of the vulva was agreed to at the Ninth Congress of the International Society for the Study of Vulvar Disease in 1987.[159, 160] Significantly, the terminology replaces that of the vulvar dystrophies. Concurrent lesions should be reported separately.

### LICHEN SIMPLEX CHRONICUS AND SQUAMOUS HYPERPLASIA

Lichen simplex chronicus is a lesion that evolves in relation to itching and chronic irritation. The lesions are typically white but generally not well demarcated. Microscopically, the affected areas are characterized by acanthosis and hypergranulosis, with or without associated hyperkeratosis or parakeratosis, and a mild to moderate chronic inflammatory cell infiltrate in the papillary dermis with associated dermal sclerosis (CD Fig. 35–66). *Squamous hyperplasia* is also an acanthotic lesion but lacks a significant dermal inflammatory infiltrate and dermal sclerosis. Some have called into question the utility and appropriateness of the term *squamous hyperplasia*, suggesting that it lacks precision.[161, 162] Neither lesion displays keratinocyte atypia, and mitoses should be rare to absent and limited to the parabasal region (CD Fig. 35–67). The lesions may well represent spectrums of the same disease,[163] and indeed both are treated similarly by the application of topical corticosteroids and antipruritic agents.

Specific inflammatory dermatoses such as psoriasis and lichen planus should be excluded, an exercise that should not be understated,[162] as should infectious causes such as fungal infections. The latter are suggested by finding a neutrophilic infiltrate (exocytosis) in the epidermis. Special stains (Gomori-methenamine silver and periodic acid–Schiff) typically disclose the organisms in the keratinized surface of the epidermis. Vulvar intraepithelial neoplasia should also be excluded, the investigation of which may be enhanced by the use of DNA in situ hybridization techniques for the detection of HPV DNA.[14]

**TABLE 35–6.** Miscellaneous Vulvar Cysts

| Cyst | Cell Type | Derivation | Miscellaneous | References |
|---|---|---|---|---|
| Mesonephric (Gartner's) | Nonmucinous, columnar to cuboidal | Mesonephric (wolffian) duct remnant | Typically associated with smooth muscle cuff | 352, 354 |
| Mesothelial canal of Nuck | Flattened mesothelial cells | Persistent peritoneal diverticulum | Located near insertion of round ligament | 361, 362 |
| Mucous | Mucinous, columnar to cuboidal | Minor vestibular glands | Possible minor vestibular gland origin | 365, 368, 369 |
| Skene's | Transitional cells | Paraurethral glands | Often occurs in neonates | 353 |

Since the late 1990s, investigators have attempted to uncover a possible relationship between squamous hyperplasia and squamous carcinoma, since the former is often observed in the context of the latter. Assays to determine the clonality of squamous hyperplasia have been emphasized with contradictory results,[62, 164] hence a resolution to this question at present remains elusive.

## LICHEN SCLEROSUS

Lichen sclerosus is a chronic dermatitis of unknown cause, with a predilection for involvement of the vulva. Autoimmune, environmental, inflammatory, infectious, and metabolic associations have all been implicated as causative.[165, 166] The suffix "et atrophicus" may be confusing because the epidermis in lichen sclerosus may be either hyperplastic or atrophic, or both.[167, 168] Furthermore, studies have shown that lichen sclerosus may have a proliferative profile belying the histologic appearance of atrophy.[169–172]

The microscopic features are dependent on the stage of the lesion.[167, 168] Additional diagnostic criteria, particularly with respect to lesions early in development when atrophy is also absent, continue to emerge.[173] Carlson and colleagues have proposed as a minimal criterion the presence of a vacuolar interface reaction pattern, which is seen in conjunction with dermal sclerosis of any thickness, underneath which is a bandlike chronic inflammatory cell infiltrate.[174] The typical end-stage lesion is characterized by thinned epithelium, loss of skin adnexal structures, a band of densely sclerotic papillary dermis, and an attenuated to absent dermal chronic inflammatory cell infiltrate (Fig. 35–18) (CD Figs. 35–68 to 35–71).

There has been much debate as to the preneoplastic potential of lichen sclerosus resulting in the development of squamous cell carcinoma.[175, 177] This topic has been reviewed by Carlson and associates, who have concluded that patients with lichen sclerosus do have a small (4%) but real increased risk of developing squamous carcinoma. According to these investigators, the carcinomas arise from a pathway distinct from HPV-related carcinogenesis where p53 mutations are frequently observed. Although the mechanisms of such mutational events remain to be elucidated, the findings argue strongly for the condition having an independent neoplastic potential.[178]

Treatment for lichen sclerosus is variably effective but typically consists of potent topical corticosteroids such as clobetasol propionate and, to a lesser degree, topical sex steroids, the former being more effective than the latter.[179]

## Surgical Pathology Report

The surgical pathology report for vulvar specimens should include relevant diagnostic and prognostic information of both gross and microscopic features. Table 35–10 outlines a core of vital information that should be addressed in the report for neoplastic lesions. This information should form part of synoptic reports or be included routinely to enhance the clinical relevance of the surgical pathology report.

## VAGINA

### Embryology and Anatomy

To better understand vaginal anatomy and lesions found therein, one must appreciate its embryologic development. The müllerian system extends caudally to form the proximal third of the vagina, where it merges with the urogenital sinus, the latter forming the distal two thirds of the vagina. The mucinous müllerian epithelium of the proximal vagina is then replaced by the "advancing" squamous cells of the urogenital sinus,[180] a process perhaps facilitated by the stromal tissue of the vaginal wall.[181] Aberrations in the development of the vagina may give rise to an imperforate hymen, vaginal septa, vaginal agenesis, a solid noncanalized vagina, and stenosis. Persistent müllerian or mesonephric remnants may give rise to cysts lined by cuboidal to columnar mucinous and nonmucinous epithelium, respectively.

The vagina extends from the vestibule to the cervix and is lined by stratified, nonkeratinizing, squamous epithelium. The thickness and degree of cellular maturation of the epithelium is dependent on the hormonal milieu to which it is exposed (see "Inflammation"). Subjacent to the epithelium is the lamina propria, characterized by loose connective tissue containing spindle mesenchymal cells, nerves, vessels, and elastic fibers. The connective tissue becomes denser toward the muscularis propria and is composed of ill-defined muscular layers.

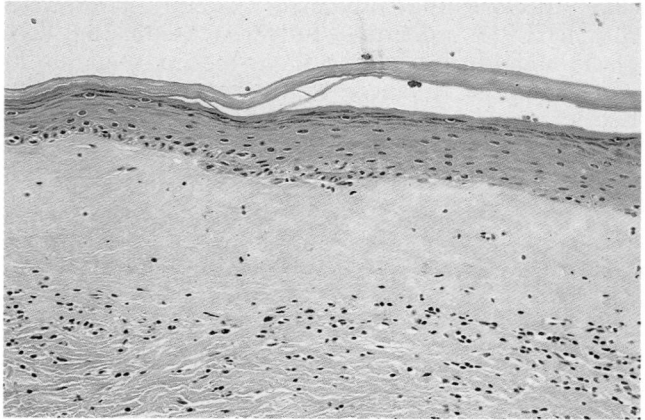

**FIGURE 35–18. Lichen sclerosus.** A small degree of orthokeratosis overlies a thinned epidermis, deep to which is a homogenized collagen band. Subjacent to the collagenous band is an infiltrate of chronic inflammatory cells.

## Vaginal Intraepithelial Neoplasia and Squamous Cell Carcinoma

Carcinoma of the vagina is encountered much less commonly than are carcinomas of the cervix or vulva. It is recommended that strict criteria be applied to appropriately designate a carcinoma as primary to the vagina. According to criteria promulgated by the International Federation of Gynecology and Obstetrics,[182] continuity with carcinomas of the cervix or vulva should lead to the carcinoma's being attributed to these latter sites. Even more restrictive are the criteria proposed by Murad and colleagues, who require additionally that spatially separate but synchronous tumors involving the vagina and cervix or vulva should be attributed to the latter sites.[183] With respect to squamous carcinomas of the lower genital tract, the authors find these latter criteria to be too restrictive because they fail to take into account the multifocality of HPV-related squamous neoplasia.[184] However, applying some or all of these criteria, it is not surprising then that primary vaginal squamous carcinomas represent only 1% of gynecologic malignancies[185, 186] but more than 90% of all vaginal malignancies.

When reviewed superficially, an association between HPV and the development of squamous cell carcinoma in the vagina does not appear to be as strong as that observed in the cervix. Thus far, only 21% to 64% of squamous carcinomas of the vagina have been shown to contain HPV DNA, most of which was HPV-16. However, it is likely that if a broader array of HPV types were studied, the HPV genome might well approach the 93% levels detected in cervical squamous cell carcinomas.[187] Lacking in the vaginal neoplasia model is the presence of immature squamous cell metaplasia, the favored "target" of HPV infection in the cervix, the exception being examples of vaginal adenosis (discussed in further detail later). Other causative factors, such as chronic irritation[188, 189] and ionizing radiation[190] (primarily from treatment of cervical cancer), have been demonstrated.

As in the vulva, condyloma acuminatum of the vagina is frequently observed in the context of other HPV-related lesions of the lower genital tract and rarely progresses to invasive carcinoma. The lesion is characterized by papillary projections lined by acanthotic squamous epithelium that may also display hyperkeratosis or parakeratosis, or both. A koilocytic viropathic effect is usually limited to the upper epithelial layers and is typically more easily recognized than condylomatous vulvar lesions (CD Figs. 35–72 to 35–74). The differential diagnosis includes *fibroepithelial polyp, squamous papilloma,* and *vaginal intraepithelial neoplasia (VAIN).* Condyloma acuminatum is distinguished from VAIN on the basis of the papillary architecture that is characteristic of the former but is not generally a feature of the latter. The cytologic atypia observed in rare examples of warty VAIN 3 distinguishes this lesion from condyloma acuminatum.

In situ neoplasia, analogous to that observed in the cervix, is also seen in the vagina, and is referred to as VAIN 1 to VAIN 3. Interestingly, the mean age of patients with VAIN 3 is approximately 53 years of age, which is 10 years older than the mean of patients diagnosed with CIN 3 at the same institution.[191] Discovery of the lesions is usually preceded by, or coincident with, cervical or vulvar squamous neoplasia.

As in the vulva, grading of the intraepithelial lesions is based on the degree to which atypical basaloid cells replace the epithelium. In VAIN 1, the atypical basaloid cells are limited to the basal third of the epithelium, but viropathic koilocytic atypia and scattered dyskeratotic cells may involve the remaining two thirds of the epithelial thickness. VAIN 3 is characterized by full-thickness involvement of atypical basaloid cells manifesting acanthosis, dyspolarity, anisonucleosis, coarse chromatin features, and usually brisk mitotic activity. Occasionally, atypical mitotic figures may be observed. VAIN 2 has features that are intermediate between VAIN 1 and VAIN 3 (CD Figs. 35–75 and 35–76).

HPV DNA has been detected in up to 100% of VAIN lesions assayed, with HPV-16 representing 75% of cases.[184] Most lesions are believed merely to persist or regress, with only a subset (5% to 9%) progressing to invasive disease despite close observation.[192–194] Proposed significant risk factors for persistence or progression derived through multivariate analysis include multifocal lesions and anogenital neoplastic syndrome, but not vaginal intraepithelial neoplasia grade, associated cervical neoplasia, or immunosuppression.[192]

## Squamous Cell Carcinoma

When invasion is present, advanced stage disease is often discovered. The lesions are usually located in the proximal third and posterior aspect of the vagina, that is, in the least accessible and readily observed location.[195] Corresponding to observations made between the mean ages of patients with VAIN 3 and CIN 3, patients with invasive squamous cell carcinoma of the vagina have a mean age of 64 years,[196] again approximately 10 years older[197] than that observed in cases of squamous cell carcinoma of the cervix. Patients may present with bleeding, dysuria, or pain[198] but are commonly asymptomatic. The tumors may be bulky and exophytic or ulcerated and infiltrative.

Early invasive disease is much less commonly identified than that found in the cervix and vulva, but it appears that invasive depths of less than 3 mm are associated with an excellent prognosis. Early infiltration is identified by applying the same criteria as those described for the vulva. Most squamous cell carcinomas are moderately differentiated, with ample evidence of squamous differentiation (CD Fig. 35–77).

Survival is dependent on the stage of the dis-

**TABLE 35-7.** Clinical Staging of Malignant Tumors of the Vagina

| AJC | FIGO | |
|---|---|---|
| Tx | | Primary tumor cannot be assessed |
| Tis | 0 | Carcinoma *in situ* (intraepithelial) |
| T1 | I | Confined to vaginal mucosa |
| T2 | II | Submucosal infiltration into parametrium, not extending to pelvic wall |
| | IIA* | Subvaginal infiltration, not into parametrium |
| | IIB* | Parametrial infiltration, not extending to pelvic wall |
| T3 | III | Tumor extending to pelvic wall |
| T4 | IV | Tumor extension to bladder or rectum or metastasis outside true pelvis |

AJC, American Joint Committee; FIGO, International Federation of Gynecology and Obstetrics. Proposed subdivision for stage II lesions.
(Perez CA, Arneson AN, Galakatos A, et al. Malignant tumors of the vagina. Cancer 31:36–44, 1973.)
From Perez CA, Gersell DJ, McGuire WP, Morris M: Vagina. *In* Hoskins WJ, Perez CA, Young RC (ed): Principles and Practice of Gynecologic Oncology. 2nd ed. Philadelphia; Lippincott-Raven, 1997, pp. 753–783.

ease, which is determined clinically (Table 35–7). Stage IV disease is associated with a dismal prognosis, whereas recent trends suggest advancements in effective care for lower stage disease. The preferred treatment for squamous cell carcinoma of the vagina is radiation therapy, although surgery and, even less commonly, chemotherapy are also used.[199]

Rare cases of verrucous carcinoma of the vagina have been reported.[200] They have the same histomorphologic features and biologic properties as those described in the vulva. Wide local excision is the treatment of choice. Other rare malignant tumors of the vagina are listed and referenced in Table 35–8.

## Benign Tumors of the Vagina

Benign tumors of the vagina are rare. Among them, condyloma acuminatum was discussed earlier. Fi-broepithelial polyps are polypoid projections of squamous cell–lined fibrous tissue. The squamous epithelium is well differentiated but seldom keratinized. The stroma is fibrous with evenly dispersed fibrocytes. Occasionally, focal stromal cells exhibit multinucleation and severe atypia. This finding does not alter the benign nature of this entity (CD Figs. 35–78 to 35–80). *Müllerian papillomas* consist of papillary nodules characterized by papillae and glands of cuboidal, flattened, or hobnail eosinophilic epithelium lacking atypical features.[201] A case describing the evolution of atypical cytologic features has been reported.[202] Focally, hyaline globules may be observed.[201] These tumors may be differentiated from yolk sac tumors and clear cell carcinomas by virtue of their innocuous cytologic features. *Mixed tumors* (spindle cell epitheliomas) consist of well-circumscribed, subepithelial neoplasms composed of a cellular to myxomatous benign spindle cell stroma in which occasional nests of benign squamous or glan-

**TABLE 35-8.** Rare Miscellaneous Benign and Malignant Tumors of the Vagina

| Differentiation | Specific Type | References |
|---|---|---|
| Epithelial | Villous adenoma | 323 |
| | Adenomatoid tumor | 324 |
| | Brenner tumor | 325 |
| | Carcinoid tumor | 326 |
| | Small cell carcinoma | 327, 328 |
| | Adenoid cystic carcinoma | 196 |
| | Adenoid basal cell carcinoma | 329 |
| | Adenocarcinoma arising in mesonephric duct remnants | 330 |
| Vascular | Hemangioma | 228 |
| | Glomus tumor | 331 |
| | Angiosarcoma | 332, 333 |
| | Epithelioid angiosarcoma | 332 |
| Neural, melanocytic | Neurofibroma | 334, 335 |
| | Paraganglioma | 336 |
| | Blue nevus | 337 |
| | Malignant schwannoma | 338 |
| Fibroblastic, Fibrohistiocytic | Fibrosarcoma | 339 |
| | Malignant fibrous histiocytoma | 340 |
| Other | Lymphoma | 341 |
| | Eosinophilic granuloma | 342 |
| | Malignant mixed mesodermal tumors | 215 |
| | Endometrial stromal sarcoma | 338 |
| | Alveolar soft part sarcoma | 343, 344 |
| | Yolk sac tumor (endodermal sinus tumor) | 214–216 |

**TABLE 35–9.** Clinicopathologic Features Distinguishing Embryonal Rhabdomyosarcoma from Fibroepithelial Polyp and Rhabdomyoma of the Vagina

| | Embryonal Rhabdomyosarcoma (Sarcoma Botryoides) | Fibroepithelial Polyp (Pseudosarcoma Botryoides) | Rhabdomyoma |
|---|---|---|---|
| Age at onset | Early childhood; adulthood rarely | Newborn to postmenopausal (mean 40 years) | Adulthood |
| Gross appearance | Multiple "grapelike" projections | Single or multiple edematous projections | Single polypoid or nodular mass |
| Cytologic features | Primitive rhabdomyoblasts with cambium layer, mitotic activity, and rare to occasional striated cells | Spindle, stellate, and occasional atypical and multinucleate stromal cells | Fetal or adult striated spindle cells without cytologic atypia |
| Behavior | Malignant | Benign | Benign |
| References | 282 | 345, 346 | 347–349 |

dular epithelium may be dispersed.[203] When the epithelial component consists of squamous nests, the features are reminiscent of Brenner's tumors of the ovary. Both müllerian papillomas and mixed tumors may recur but do not metastasize. Rare benign tumors of the vagina are listed in Table 35–9.

## Diethylstilbestrol-Related Malignancies

Before the era of in utero exposure to diethylstilbestrol (DES), clear cell carcinomas of the vagina and cervix were exceedingly rare, occurring almost exclusively in postmenopausal women. When young girls began presenting with clear cell carcinomas, an intensive effort disclosed the relationship between the malignancy and in utero DES exposure. Use of DES as an agent to reduce the risk of undesired abortions ceased thereafter, but it is estimated that as many as 3 million women were exposed in utero.[204]

DES is believed to exert its primary effect by interfering with the process of re-epithelialization of the lower müllerian system by the urogenital sinus. As a result, gross and microscopic anomalies occur, among them müllerian glandular epithelium, which is allowed to persist in the vagina in the form of adenosis (CD Fig. 35–81). In this context, it is the association of cells displaying tuboendometrioid differentiation rather than mucinous differentiation, whether atypical or not, that suggests that the former cell type gives rise to clear cell adenocarcinoma.[205] The molecular pathogenesis of this process remains enigmatic, however. It is clear that in utero DES exposure is critical but insufficient to establish malignancy, because the lifetime risk of developing cervicovaginal clear cell carcinoma is estimated to be only 1 in 1000 to 1 in 10,000.[206] However, concern for this population persists because the vagina of affected patients undergoes a process of squamous metaplasia identical to that observed in the cervix, thereby setting the stage for increased risk for developing HPV-related squamous or glandular neoplasia. To date, however, this concern has not been

realized, but the average age of exposed women is still young (38 years of age), necessitating continued, prudent follow-up.[204] One of the authors (RTB) has encountered a case of HPV 16–related adenocarcinoma in situ and VAIN 3 arising in vaginal adenosis (CD Fig. 35–82).

Vaginal clear cell carcinomas present as bulging submucosal masses in the middle or outer third of the vagina. They frequently have a yellow color that can often be appreciated through the vaginal epithelium. (Fig. 35–19) Microscopically, three patterns of clear cell carcinoma may be observed; papillary, tubulocystic, and solid. The hallmark hobnail cell is usually most evident in the papillary pattern. (Fig. 35–20) (CD Figs. 35–83 and 35–84) The tubulocystic pattern can be diagnostically challenging if care is not taken to closely observe the malignant nuclear characteristics; the differential diagnosis includes adenosis and atypical adenosis. A benign lesion sometimes observed in adenosis that should be distinguished from clear cell carcinoma is *microglandular hyperplasia*. Microglandular hyperplasia is characterized by microcystic architecture, glandular spaces di-

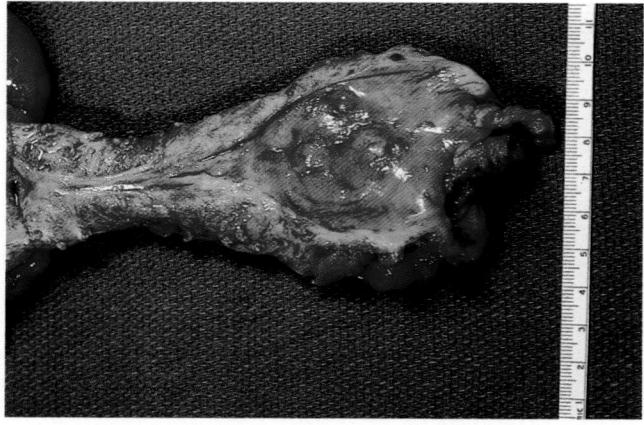

**FIGURE 35–19. Clear cell carcinoma of the vagina.** Radical hysterectomy and vaginectomy specimen containing a tumor seen bulging underneath the vaginal epithelium. The tumor is irregularly nodular, and its bright yellow color can be appreciated through the vaginal epithelium.

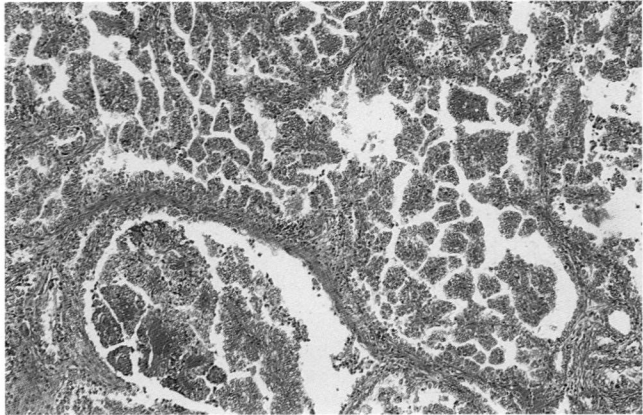

**FIGURE 35-20. Clear cell adenocarcinoma.** This pattern of clear cell adenocarcinoma is characterized by delicate papillary structures that are lined by cuboidal to columnar clear cells, as well as occasional hobnail cells. The cytoplasmic clearing, as seen in this example, may not be so evident in other examples in which the cytoplasm is eosinophilic.

vided by single cell layers as opposed to back-to-back glandular architecture, foci of squamous metaplasia, bland nuclear features, rare to absent mitotic figures, and a neutrophilic infiltrate (Fig. 35-21).

In addition to clear cell carcinoma, rare examples of vaginal adenocarcinoma with non–clear cell features have been described, including those with mucinous, endometrioid, and adenosquamous differentiation.[207–210] Clement and Benedet have also described a case of adenocarcinoma in situ of the vagina arising in adenosis,[211] perhaps the precursor lesion to these rare forms of infiltrative adenocarcinomas. As indicated in the case described previously, HPV may play a role in glandular as well as squamous neoplasia in a fashion analogous to that observed in the cervix.

## Yolk Sac Tumor (Endodermal Sinus Tumor)

A discussion of yolk sac tumor is included here because it bears some resemblance to clear cell carcinoma. As a group, germ cell tumors of the vagina are uncommon, with only a few cases of benign tumors being reported.[212, 213] Conversely, yolk sac tumors, although rare, have a curious predilection for this site and arise to the apparent virtual exclusion of other forms of malignant germ cell tumors.[214] The means by which germ cells reside in the vagina, thus giving rise to these tumors, is speculative.

Affected individuals are almost exclusively infants, and all are younger than 4 years of age at presentation.[214, 215] As in the ovary and testis, the tumors may display the same broad array of microscopic features (see Chapters 34 and 39). Immunohistochemistry greatly assists in distinguishing yolk sac tumors from clear cell adenocarcinomas; alpha-fetoprotein immunoreactivity in the absence of Leu-M1 staining assists in establishing the diagnosis of yolk sac tumor, whereas the opposite staining profile aids in establishing the diagnosis of clear cell adenocarcinoma.[216] Treatment consists of conservative surgery in combination with chemotherapy, with excellent prospects for long-term survival.[199]

## Malignant Melanoma

Malignant melanoma of the vagina, like other forms of mucosal melanomas, is rare, may be seen in all races, usually presents at an advanced stage, and is associated with a poor prognosis.[217, 218] Most affected women are older than 60 years of age. Vaginal melanomas are thought to arise from benign melanocytes, the latter having been found in 3% of benign postmortem vaginas studied.[219] When the benign melanocytes are aggregated in great enough num-

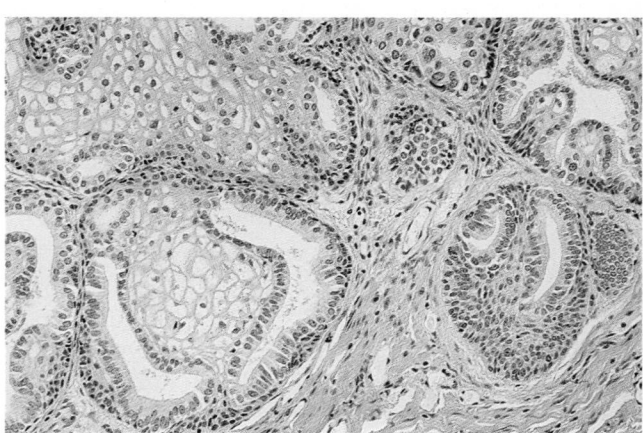

**FIGURE 35-21. Adenosis.** Not to be confused with clear cell carcinoma, adenosis is composed of simple glands with bland mucinous cells and frequent foci of squamous metaplasia.

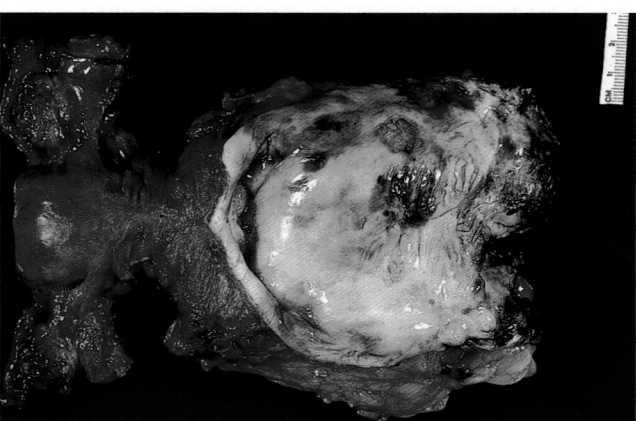

**FIGURE 35-22. Vaginal melanoma.** Radical hysterectomy and vaginectomy specimen for a vaginal melanoma. The vagina is opened posteriorly to reveal a deeply pigmented, irregular lesion in the anterior vaginal wall.

bers, to the extent that they present grossly as pigmented patches, the clinical term *melanosis* may be applied.[220] Vaginal melanosis is considered by many to be a premalignant lesion and may be treated aggressively by excision.[221, 222]

Grossly and microscopically, vaginal melanomas are similar to melanomas in other body sites (Fig. 35–22). Typically, they form nodular masses, which may or may not be pigmented, and are frequently ulcerated. When not ulcerated, the usual features of junctional activity and epidermotropism in the squamous epithelium are evident (Fig. 35–23). It is stated that when present, lateral junctional spread of the melanoma is a useful diagnostic clue.[223] On occasion, it may be necessary to apply immunohistochemistry to establish the correct diagnosis, for example, in amelanotic melanomas. Immunoreactivity for S-100 protein and HMB-45 aid in identifying melanomas, whereas carcinomas should not be immunoreactive for these markers but will show reactivity to cytokeratins (Fig. 35–24).

As in vulvar and skin melanomas, vaginal melanomas are microstaged. However, because the Clark's microstaging scheme[224] is by definition limited to skin lesions, that is, to the exclusion of mucosal lesions, Chung and colleagues[223] proposed microstaging according to millimeters of invasive depth (level I, tumor confined to the surface epithelium; level II, invasion of 1 mm or less; level III, 1 to 2 mm; and level IV, deeper than 2 mm). They found that nearly all melanomas in their study were level III or greater. It is not surprising, then, that the 5-year disease-free survival, regardless of extent of surgery, is less than 20%.[217, 218] The prognosis remains poor regardless of the therapy used, whether it be radical surgery, conservative surgery, or radiation.[199]

## Soft Tissue Tumors

Soft tissue tumors of the vagina are extremely rare, the most common type being leiomyoma.[225] These

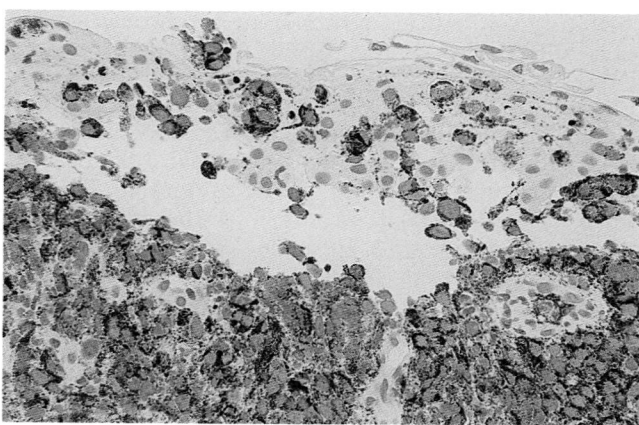

**FIGURE 35–24. Malignant melanoma.** HMB-45 immunostaining brilliantly decorates the malignant melanocytes of this vaginal melanoma.

tumors display the same histologic features as their counterparts in the myometrium. Features meriting the diagnosis of leiomyosarcoma include moderate to marked atypism and greater than or equal to 5 mitoses per 10 high-power fields.[226]

Among the remaining soft tissue tumors described in the vagina (see Table 35–9), embryonal rhabdomyosarcoma (sarcoma botryoides) is most significant and is described in further detail in the following section.

## Embryonal Rhabdomyosarcoma (Sarcoma Botryoides)

Embryonal rhabdomyosarcoma of the vagina is a rare malignancy of early childhood. More than 90% of affected girls are younger than 5 years of age. Rarely, adults may be affected. Patients present with rapid onset of grapelike masses arising focally or multifocally in the vagina.

Sectioning of the masses discloses edematous, myxoid cut surfaces with foci of hemorrhage. Microscopically, the tumors are composed of primitive, mitotically active, round to slightly spindled rhabdomyoblasts that tend to condense subjacent to intact epithelium and around vessels but are otherwise separated by a myxoid, extracellular matrix. Occasionally, one is able to identify differentiated rhabdomyoblasts characterized by cytoplasmic striations. The differential diagnosis includes two benign lesions, *fibroepithelial polyp* and *rhabdomyoma*, the features of which are compared in Table 35–9.

## Miscellaneous Tumorlike Lesions

*Prolapsed fallopian tubes* occur after vaginal or, less commonly, abdominal hysterectomies and present as painful, hyperemic, nodular masses at the vaginal cuff. Microscopically, they may display papillary ar-

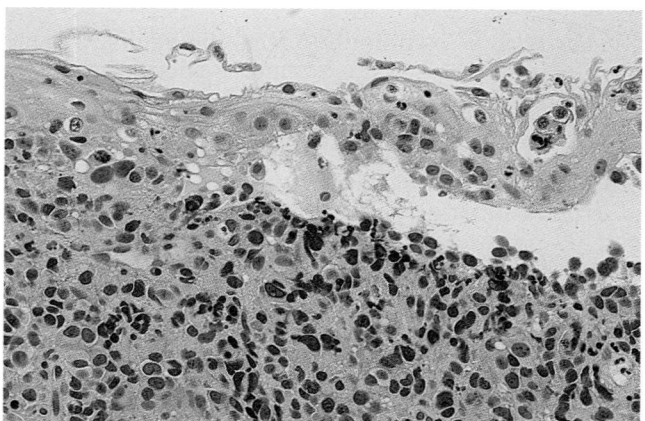

**FIGURE 35–23. Malignant melanoma.** This nodular variant of malignant melanoma displays a degree of epidermotropism as well as solid sheets of malignant melanocytes deep to the vaginal squamous epithelium.

chitecture or features reminiscent of chronic salpingitis with blunted and fused plicae and pseudoglands. Ciliated cells may be readily evident or difficult to find. Usually, there is also congestion and inflammation that may be accompanied with reactive nuclear atypia. The differential diagnosis includes endometriosis and adenocarcinoma. The absence of endometrial stroma and the presence of tubal architecture and epithelial constituents distinguish a prolapsed fallopian tube from endometriosis. The absence of cellular proliferation lacking stromal support, prominent mitotic activity with atypical mitoses, and moderate to severe nuclear atypia assist in excluding the diagnoses of serous or clear cell carcinoma.

On rare occasions, *postoperative spindle cell nodules* may arise in the vagina. Proppe and associates described four cases of vaginal lesions occurring up to 10 weeks after a surgical procedure.[229] The lesions

ranged up to 4 cm in greatest dimension and often had ulcerated surfaces. Microscopically, postoperative spindle cell nodules are characterized by a haphazard proliferation of spindle cells thrown into intersecting fascicles, focal to numerous mitoses, and a chronic inflammatory cell background infiltrate. Reflective of their infiltrative nature, several of the lesions reported by Proppe and associates were incompletely removed. None of the patients with vaginal lesions had additional treatment or recurrences after removal.[229]

## Inflammation

The hormonal milieu of the vagina significantly influences the histomorphologic features of the lining epithelial cells, which, in turn, affect the delicate ecology of its constituent microflora.[230]

The hypoestrogenic state of the newborn or postmenopausal woman is associated with an atrophic epithelium susceptible to erosion or infection, or both. In adolescent and mature women, adequate estrogen levels are associated with well-developed, glycogenated epithelium that is typically accompanied by an acid pH (approximately 4.5). The pH rises in postmenopausal women, a finding thought to be related to the estrogen hormone level status in these women.[231]

*Lactobacillus acidophilus* thrives in preference to other microorganisms at the optimal pH of 4.5. It is believed that *Lactobacillus acidophilus* inhibits the growth of other bacterial species, some of which are pathogenic, through its ability to generate $H_2O_2$. The $H_2O_2$ is thought to protect against colonization by catalase-negative anaerobic bacteria.[232, 233] Failure of this protective effect is best exemplified by *bacterial vaginosis*, in which overgrowth of noncommensal organisms produce symptoms.[234–240]

### Candida Albicans

*Candida albicans* commonly infects the vagina, resulting in intense pruritus; some patients may be asymptomatic. Predisposing factors include drug addiction, obesity, intake of birth control pills, pregnancy, antibiotic therapy, diabetes mellitus,[241] and orogenital sexual practices.[242, 243] The vaginal mucosa is usually intensely inflamed, and removable white patches with a "cottage cheese–like" appearance may be observed. *Candida albicans* is often readily diagnosed on routine Papanicolaou smears in which characteristic budding yeasts and pseudohyphae are seen. Microscopically, the organisms are usually limited to the surface of the vagina but may become invasive.[244] The cottage cheese–like patches consist of a mucous exudate with organisms and inflammatory cells. Other *Candida* species may infect the vagina, but they do so with considerably less frequency.

---

**TABLE 35–10.** Essential Components to Be Included in Surgical Pathology Report of Neoplastic Diseases of the Vulva and Vagina

**Vulva**

*Gross*
Description of surgical specimen
  Radical vulvectomy, hemivulvectomy, wide excision
Location of lesion
  Labial, forchette, clitoris
  Laterality, midline involved?
  Proximity to surgical margins
Lesion size
  Maximal diameter, gross thickness
Appearance of uninvolved skin
  Increased or decreased pigmentation
  Presence of atrophy
Presence of additional or satellite lesions

*Microscopic*
Cell type and grade
Depth of invasion and tumor thickness
Presence of vascular space involvement
Presence of precursor lesions (dysplasia)
Margin status

**Vagina**

*Gross*
Description of surgical specimen
  Vaginectomy, radical vaginectomy (+/− hysterectomy)
Location of lesion
  Proximal, middle, distal vagina
  Relationship to cervix, vulva, margins
Lesion size
  Maximal dimension
  Depth of invasion
  Proximity to surgical margins
Appearance of uninvolved mucosa
  Color and texture
  Presence, increased or decreased pigmentation

*Microscopic*
Cell type and grade
Depth of invasion
Presence of vascular space involvement
Presence of precursor lesion (dysplasia)
Margin status

## Trichomonas Vaginalis

Trichomonas vaginalis is a common causative agent for infective vaginitis. The organism accounts for almost all cases of protozoa-related vaginitis. At greatest risk are women with other venereal diseases.[245]

The organisms are usually detected either with wet mount preparations, permitting the visualization of the motile trichomonad, or with Papanicolaou smears in which the pear- or tear-shaped organisms resemble degenerate squamous epithelial cells. The polymerase chain reaction may also be used with great specificity and sensitivity to detect the organisms,[246] although the cost of such testing at this time is difficult to justify.

## Herpes Simplex Virus

HSV-2 is a common, sexually transmitted pathogen in the vagina. Rarely, HSV-1 may infect the vagina. HSV is significant in the lower genital tract for venereal transmission to sexual partners and for vertical transmission to newborns passing through the affected cervix and vaginal canal. Neonatal complications include severe infections of skin, eyes, mouth, and central nervous system; systemic dissemination; and death. Accordingly, patients approaching the time of parturition with clinical histories of genital HSV infection must be evaluated for active infection through careful examination, culture, and cervicovaginal Papanicolaou smears. If active infection is detected, cesarean section is highly advisable. There may be a role for polymerase chain reaction detection of HSV because many neonates are still infected when born to women who are asymptomatic but shedding HSV.[247]

When HSV is symptomatic, active infection is manifested by painful vesicular eruptions and ulceration. Microscopically, intraepidermal vesicle formation is preceded by balloon degeneration of the keratinocytes and acantholysis. The cells may fuse to form multinucleated cells. Mono- and multinucleated viral inclusions, seen best at the epithelial edge of the vesicle or ulcer, impart a basophilic or eosinophilic ground-glass appearance to enlarged and distorted nuclei. The underlying dermis displays an intense chronic active inflammatory cell infiltrate (CD Fig. 35–85).

## Emphysematous Vaginitis

Emphysematous vaginitis is an uncommon, poorly understood disease affecting women, most of whom are typically pregnant, in the second to fourth decades of life. Elicited by an unknown causative agent, cysts ranging up to 2 cm in greatest dimension form in the submucosa. The cysts may burst during sexual intercourse, resulting in a popping sound and the development of ulcers. Microscopically, histiocytes, multinucleated giant cells, and lymphocytes line the cysts; some cysts may also be lined with epithelial or endothelial cells.[215, 228] The lesions resolve within weeks to months postpartum without apparent permanent sequelae.[248]

## Desquamative Inflammatory Vaginitis

Desquamative inflammatory vaginitis is a rare disease of unknown cause. Some have related the disease to erosive lichen planus, but it is likely to be multifactorial in origin. It was originally defined as being limited to women with normal ovarian activity and estrogen levels to distinguish it from atrophic vaginitis[249]; however, others include women of all ages.[250, 251]

Microscopically, the disease is characterized by a thinned and hyperemic vaginal mucosa accompanied by edema and marked acute inflammation. Cervicovaginal smears disclose desquamated parabasal cells and neutrophils. The condition should be distinguished from postpartum vaginitis, which is due to estrogen deprivation.[252] Desquamative vaginitis is responsive to corticosteroids.[249, 251, 253] Data relating to responsiveness to estrogens and antibiotics are conflicting.[249, 250, 253]

## Fistulas

Fistulas connecting viscus organs, most commonly the urinary bladder and rectum, to the vagina may occur after surgery or irradiation or as a consequence of diverticular disease of the rectum, Crohn's disease, or neoplasia. The microscopic features are dependent on the cause of the fistula but, in general, are those of a tract lined by inflamed granulation tissue. Portions of the fistulous tract may be partially lined by epithelium native to the communicating organs. Of these, Crohn's-related fistulas deserve special mention, as they are least likely to respond to surgical repair. Diagnosis is made on exclusion of malignancy, on a history of radiation therapy, and on the basis of a predominance of deep chronic lymphocytic inflammation, which often includes granulomatous inflammation. Diagnosis is important in order to implement immunosuppressive therapy.

### REFERENCES

1. van der Putte SC: Mammary-like glands of the vulva and their disorders. Int J Gynecol Pathol 13:150–160, 1994.
2. Report of the ISSVD Terminology Committee. J Reprod Med 31:973–974, 1986.
3. Kiryu H, Ackerman AB: A critique of current classifications of vulvar diseases [see comments]. Am J Dermatopathol 12: 377–392, 1990.
4. Sturgeon SR, Brinton LA, Devesa SS, Kurman RJ: In situ and invasive vulvar cancer incidence trends (1973 to 1987). Am J Obstet Gynecol 166:1482–1485, 1992.
5. Bergeron C, Naghashfar Z, Canaan C, et al: Human papillomavirus type 16 in intraepithelial neoplasia (bowenoid papu-

losis) and coexistent invasive carcinoma of the vulva. Int J Gynecol Pathol 6:1–11, 1987.

6. Park JS, Jones RW, McLean MR, et al: Possible etiologic heterogeneity of vulvar intraepithelial neoplasia: A correlation of pathologic characteristics with human papillomavirus detection by in situ hybridization and polymerase chain reaction. Cancer 67:1599–1607, 1991.

7. Trimble CL, Hildesheim A, Brinton LA, et al: Heterogeneous etiology of squamous carcinoma of the vulva. Obstet Gynecol 87:59–64, 1996.

8. zur Hausen H: Human genital cancer: Synergism between two virus infections or synergism between a virus infection and initiating events? Lancet 2:1370–1372, 1982.

9. Ferenczy A: Intraepthelial neoplasia of the vulva. In Coppleson M (ed): Gynecologic Oncology. 3rd ed. Edinburgh, Churchill Livingstone, 1992, pp 443–463.

10. Wilkinson EJ, Cook JC, Friedrich EG, Massey JK: Vulvar intraepithelial neoplasia: Association with cigarette smoking. Colposc Gynecol Laser Surg 4:153–159, 1988.

11. Sonnex C, Scholefield JH, Kocjan G, et al: Anal human papillomavirus infection: A comparative study of cytology, colposcopy and DNA hybridisation as methods of detection. Genitourin Med 67:21–25, 1991.

12. Micheletti L, Barbero M, Preti M, et al: Vulvar intraepithelial neoplasia of low grade: A challenging diagnosis. Eur J Gynaecol Oncol 15:70–74, 1994.

13. Modesitt SC, Groben PA, Walton LA, et al: Expression of Ki-67 in vulvar carcinoma and vulvar intraepithelial neoplasia III: Correlation with clinical prognostic factors. Gynecol Oncol 76:51–55, 2000.

14. Felix JC, Wright TC: Analysis of lower genital tract lesions clinically suspicious for condylomata using in situ hybridization and the polymerase chain reaction for the detection of human papillomavirus. Arch Pathol Lab Med 118:39–43, 1994.

15. McLachlin CM, Mutter GL, Crum CP: Multinucleated atypia of the vulva: Report of a distinct entity not associated with human papillomavirus. Am J Surg Pathol 18:1233–1239, 1994.

16. Buscema J, Woodruff JD: Progressive histobiologic alterations in the development of vulvar cancer. Am J Obstet Gynecol 138:146–150, 1980.

17. Deleted.

18. Deleted.

19. Haefner HK, Tate JE, McLachlin CM, Crum CP: Vulvar intraepithelial neoplasia: Age, morphological phenotype, papillomavirus DNA, and coexisting invasive carcinoma. Hum Pathol 26:147–154, 1995.

20. Hording U, Junge J, Poulsen H, Lundvall F: Vulvar intraepithelial neoplasia III: A viral disease of undetermined progressive potential. Gynecol Oncol 56:276–279, 1995.

21. Fiorica JV, Cavanagh D, Marsden DE, et al: Carcinoma in situ of the vulva: 24 years' experience in southwest Florida. South Med J 81:589–593, 1988.

22. Jones RW, McLean MR: Carcinoma in situ of the vulva: A review of 31 treated and five untreated cases. Obstet Gynecol 68:499–503, 1986.

23. Caterson RJ, Furber J, Murray J, et al: Carcinoma of the vulva in two young renal allograft recipients. Transplant Proc 16:559–561, 1984.

24. Wilkinson EJ, Morgan LS, Friedrich EG Jr: Association of Fanconi's anemia and squamous-cell carcinoma of the lower female genital tract with condyloma acuminatum: A report of two cases. J Reprod Med 29:447–453, 1984.

25. Penn I: Cancers of the anogenital region in renal transplant recipients: Analysis of 65 cases. Cancer 58:611–616, 1986.

26. Spitzer M: Lower genital tract intraepithelial neoplasia in HIV-infected women: Guidelines for evaluation and management. Obstet Gynecol Surv 54:131–137, 1999.

27. Kuhn L, Sun XW, Wright TC Jr: Human immunodeficiency virus infection and female lower genital tract malignancy. Curr Opin Obstet Gynecol 11:35–39, 1999.

28. Wu AY, Sherman ME, Rosenshein NB, Erozan YS: Pathologic evaluation of gynecologic specimens obtained with the cavitron ultrasonic surgical aspirator (CUSA). Gynecol Oncol 44:28–32, 1992.

29. Ferenczy A, Wright JR, Richart RM: Comparison of $CO_2$ laser surgery and loop electrosurgical excision/fulguration procedure (LEEP) for the treatment of vulvar intraepithelial neoplasia (VIN). Int J Gynecol Cancer 4:22–28, 1994.

30. Chafe W, Richards A, Morgan L, Wilkinson E: Unrecognized invasive carcinoma in vulvar intraepithelial neoplasia (VIN). Gynecol Oncol 31:154–165, 1988.

31. Husseinzadeh N, Recinto C: Frequency of invasive cancer in surgically excised vulvar lesions with intraepithelial neoplasia (VIN 3). Gynecol Oncol 73:119–120, 1999.

32. Modesitt SC, Waters AB, Walton L, et al: Vulvar intraepithelial neoplasia III: Occult cancer and the impact of margin status on recurrence [see comments]. Obstet Gynecol 92:962–966, 1998.

33. Wilkinson EJ: Superficially invasive carcinoma of the vulva. In Wilkinson EJ (ed): Pathology of the Vulva And Vagina: Contemporary Issues in Surgical Pathology. New York, Churchill Livingstone, 1987, pp 103–117.

34. Ehrmann RL, Dwyer IM, Yavner D, Hancock WW: An immunoperoxidase study of laminin and type iv collagen distribution in carcinoma of the cervix and vulva. Obstet Gynecol 72:257–262, 1988.

35. Surico N, Priori L, Savoia P, et al: Distribution of integrins and extracellular matrix proteins in vulvar squamous cell carcinomas. Eur J Gynaecol Oncol 16:147–154, 1995.

36. Johansson N, Vaalamo M, Grenman S, et al: Collagenase-3 (MMP-13) is expressed by tumor cells in invasive vulvar squamous cell carcinomas. Am J Pathol 154:469–480, 1999.

37. Wilkinson EJ: Superficially invasive carcinoma of the vulva. Clin Obstet Gynecol 34:651–661, 1991.

38. Microinvasive Cancer of the Vulva: Report of the ISSVD Task Force. J Reprod Med 29:454–455, 1984.

39. Grant JM: Revised FIGO staging for early invasive carcinoma of the vulva and cervix [editorial; comment]. Br J Obstet Gynaecol 103:xxi–xxii, 1996.

40. Hoffman JS, Kumar NB, Morley GW: Microinvasive squamous carcinoma of the vulva: Search for a definition. Obstet Gynecol 61:615–618, 1983.

41. Sedlis A, Homesley H, Bundy BN, et al: Positive groin lymph nodes in superficial squamous cell vulvar cancer: A gynecologic oncology group study. Am J Obstet Gynecol 156:1159–1164, 1987.

42. Wilkinson EJ: Superficial invasive carcinoma of the vulva. Clin Obstet Gynecol 28:188–195, 1985.

43. Wells M, Jenkins M: Selected topics in the histopathology of the vulva. Curr Diagn Pathol 1:41–47, 1994.

44. Zaino RJ: Carcinoma of the vulva, urethra, and Bartholin's glands. In Wilkinson EJ (ed): Pathology of the Vulva and Vagina. New York, Churchill Livingstone, 1987, pp 119–153.

45. Green TH Jr: Carcinoma of the vulva: A Reassessment. Obstet Gynecol 52:462–469, 1978.

46. Benedet JL, Murphy KJ, Fairey RN, Boyes DA: Primary invasive carcinoma of the vagina. Obstet Gynecol 62:715–719, 1983.

47. Henson D, Tarone R: An epidemiologic study of cancer of the cervix, vagina, and vulva based on the Third National Cancer Survey in the United States. Am J Obstet Gynecol 129:525–532, 1977.

48. Crum CP, McLachlin CM, Tate JE, Mutter GL: Pathobiology of vulvar squamous neoplasia. Curr Opin Obstet Gynecol 9:63–69, 1997.

49. Kurman RJ, Toki T, Schiffman MH: Basaloid and warty carcinomas of the vulva: Distinctive types of squamous cell carcinoma frequently associated with human papillomaviruses [published erratum appears in Am J Surg Pathol 17:536, 1993. Am J Surg Pathol 17:133–145, 1993.

50. Ridley CM, Buckley CH, Fox H: Pathology of the vulva and associated structures. In Fox H (ed): Haines and Taylor Obstetrical and Gynaecological Pathology. 4th ed. New York, Churchill Livingstone, 1995, pp 51–133.

51. Wilkinson EJ: Premalignant and malignant tumors of the vulva. In Kurman RJ (ed): Blaustein's Pathology Of The Female Genital Tract, 4th ed. New York, Springer-Verlag, 1994, pp 87–129.

52. Niebyl JR, Genadry R, Friedrich EG Jr, et al: Vulvar carci-

noma with hypercalcemia. Obstet Gynecol 45:343–348, 1975.

53. Stewart AF, Romero R, Schwartz PE, et al: Hypercalcemia associated with gynecologic malignancies: Biochemical characterization. Cancer 49:2389–2394, 1982.

54. Ambros RA, Malfetano JH, Mihm MC Jr: Clinicopathologic features of vulvar squamous cell carcinomas exhibiting prominent fibromyxoid stromal response. Int J Gynecol Pathol 15:137–145, 1996.

55. Ambros RA, Kallakury BV, et al: Cytokine, cell adhesion receptor, and tumor suppressor gene expression in vulvar squamous carcinoma: Correlation with prominent fibromyxoid stromal response. Int J Gynecol Pathol 15:320–325, 1996.

56. Tempfer C, Sliutz G, Haeusler G, et al: CD44v3 and V6 variant isoform expression correlates with poor prognosis in early-stage vulvar cancer. Br J Cancer 78:1091–1094, 1998.

57. Tempfer C, Gitsch G, Haeusler G, et al: Prognostic value of immunohistochemically detected CD44 expression in patients with carcinoma of the vulva. Cancer 78:273–277, 1996.

58. Toki T, Kurman RJ, Park JS, et al: Probable nonpapillomavirus etiology of squamous cell carcinoma of the vulva in older women: A clinicopathologic study using in situ hybridization and polymerase chain reaction. Int J Gynecol Pathol 10:107–125, 1991.

59. Crum CP, Liskow A, Petras P, et al: Vulvar intraepithelial neoplasia (severe atypia and carcinoma in situ): A clinicopathologic analysis of 41 cases. Cancer 54:1429–1434, 1984.

60. Andersen WA, Franquemont DW, Williams J, et al: Vulvar squamous cell carcinoma and papillomaviruses: Two separate entities? Am J Obstet Gynecol 165:329–335, 1991.

61. Lee YY, Wilczynski SP, Chumakov A, et al: Carcinoma of the Vulva: HPV and p53 mutations. Oncogene 9:1655–1659, 1994.

62. Kim YT, Thomas NF, Kessis TD, et al: p53 mutations and clonality in vulvar carcinomas and squamous hyperplasias: Evidence suggesting that squamous hyperplasias do not serve as direct precursors of human papillomavirus-negative vulvar carcinomas. Hum Pathol 27:389–395, 1996.

63. Pilotti S, D'Amato L, Della Torre G, et al: Papillomavirus, p53 alteration, and primary carcinoma of the vulva. Diagn Mol Pathol 4:239–248, 1995.

64. Pinto AP, Lin MC, Mutter GL, et al: Allelic loss in human papillomavirus-positive and -negative vulvar squamous cell carcinomas. Am J Pathol 154:1009–1015, 1999.

65. Shanbour KA, Mannel RS, Morris PC, et al: Comparison of clinical versus surgical staging systems in vulvar cancer. Obstet Gynecol 80:927–930, 1992.

66. Wilkinson EJ, Hause LL, Hoffman RG, et al: Occult axillary lymph node metastases in invasive breast carcinoma: Characteristics of the primary tumor and significance of the Metastases. Pathol Annu 17(pt 2):67–91, 1982.

67. Wilkinson EJ, Hause L: Probability in lymph node sectioning. Cancer 33:1269–1274, 1974.

68. Homesley HD, Bundy BN, Sedlis A, et al: Assessment of current International Federation of Gynecology and Obstetrics staging of vulvar carcinoma relative to prognostic factors for survival (a Gynecologic Oncology Group Study). Am J Obstet Gynecol 164:997–1003, 1991.

69. Hefler L, Obermair A, Tempfer C, et al: Serum concentrations of squamous cell carcinoma antigen in patients with vulvar intraepithelial neoplasia and vulvar cancer. Int J Cancer 84:299–303, 1999.

70. Way S: Carcinoma of the vulva. Am J Obstet Gynecol 79:692–697, 1960.

71. Cockayne SE, Shah M, Slater DN, Harrington CI: Spindle and pseudoglandular squamous cell carcinoma arising in lichen sclerosus of the vulva. Br J Dermatol 138:695–697, 1998.

72. Copas P, Dyer M, Comas FV, Hall DJ: Spindle cell carcinoma of the vulva. Diagn Gynecol Obstet 4:235–241, 1982.

73. Wilkinson EJ, Croker BP, Friedrich EG Jr, Franzini DA: Two distinct pathologic types of giant cell tumor of the vulva: A report of two cases. J Reprod Med 33:519–522, 1988.

74. Santeusanio G, Schiaroli S, Anemona L, et al: Carcinoma of the vulva with sarcomatoid features: A case report with immunohistochemical study. Gynecol Oncol 40:160–163, 1991.

75. Steeper TA, Piscioli F, Rosai J: Squamous cell carcinoma with sarcoma-like stroma of the female genital tract: Clinicopathologic study of four cases. Cancer 52:890–898, 1983.

76. Lasser A, Cornog JL, Morris JM: Adenoid squamous cell carcinoma of the vulva. Cancer 33:224–227, 1974.

77. Underwood JW, Adcock LL, Okagaki T: Adenosquamous carcinoma of skin appendages (adenoid squamous cell carcinoma, pseudoglandular squamous cell carcinoma, adenocanthoma of sweat gland of lever) of the vulva: A clinical and ultrastructural study. Cancer 42:1851–1858, 1978.

78. Johnson WC, Helwig EB: Adenoid squamous cell carcinoma (adenoacanthoma): A clinicopathologic study of 155 patients. Cancer 19:1639–1650, 1966.

79. Rastkar G, Okagaki T, Twiggs LB, Clark BA: Early invasive and in situ warty carcinoma of the vulva: Clinical, histologic, and electron microscopic study with particular reference to viral association. Am J Obstet Gynecol 143:814–820, 1982.

80. Rando RF, Sedlacek TV, Hunt J, et al: Verrucous carcinoma of the vulva associated with an unusual type 6 human papillomavirus. Obstet Gynecol 67(3 suppl):70S–75S, 1986.

81. Crowther ME, Shepherd JH, Fisher C: Verrucous carcinoma of the vulva containing human papillomavirus-11: Case report. Br J Obstet Gynaecol 95:414–418, 1988.

82. Partridge EE, Murad T, Shingleton HM, et al: Verrucous lesions of the female genitalia. II. Verrucous carcinoma. Am J Obstet Gynecol 137:419–424, 1980.

83. Partridge EE, Murad T, Shingleton HM, et al: Verrucous lesions of the female genitalia. I. Giant condylomata. Am J Obstet Gynecol 137:412–418, 1980.

84. Gallousis S: Verrucous carcinoma: Report of three vulvar cases and review of the literature. Obstet Gynecol 40:502–507, 1972.

85. Rubben A, Traidl C, Baron JM, Grussendorf-Conen EI: Evaluation of non-radioactive temperature gradient sscp analysis and of temperature gradient gel electrophoresis for the detection of hpv 6-variants in condylomata acuminata and Buschke-Loewenstein tumours. Eur J Epidemiol 11:501–506, 1995.

86. Kato N, Ueno H, Tanaka H, Nishikawa T: Human papillomavirus type 6–associated Buschke-Lowenstein tumor (giant condyloma acuminatum). J Dermatol 20:773–778, 1993.

87. Rubben A, Beaudenon S, Favre M, et al: Rearrangements of the upstream regulatory region of human papillomavirus type 6 can be found in both Buschke-Lowenstein tumours and in condylomata acuminata. J Gen Virol 73(pt 12):3147–3153, 1992.

88. Woodworth H Jr, Dockerty MB, Wilson RB, Pratt JH: Papillary hidradenoma of the vulva: A clinicopathologic study of 69 cases. Am J Obstet Gynecol 110:501–508, 1971.

89. van der Putte SC: Anogenital "sweat" glands: Histology and pathology of a gland that may mimic mammary glands. Am J Dermatopathol 13:557–567, 1991.

90. Weilburg RD, Miller GV, Von Pohle KC: Paget's disease of the vulva associated with adenocarcinoma developing in a hidradenoma papilliferum. Am J Obstet Gynecol 98:294–295, 1967.

91. Bannatyne P, Elliott P, Russell P: Vulvar adenosquamous carcinoma arising in a hidradenoma papilliferum, with rapidly fatal outcome: Case report. Gynecol Oncol 35:395–398, 1989.

92. Leuchter RS, Hacker NF, Voet RL, et al: Primary carcinoma of the Bartholin gland: A report of 14 cases and review of the literature. Obstet Gynecol 60:361–368, 1982.

93. Burke TW, Eifel P, McGuire WP, Wilkinson EJ: Vulva. *In* Hoskins WJ, Perez CA, Young RC (eds): Principles and Practice of Gynecologic Oncology. 2nd ed. Philadelphia, Lippincott-Raven, 1997, pp 717–751.

94. Copeland LJ, Sneige N, Gershenson DM, et al: Bartholin gland carcinoma. Obstet Gynecol 67:794–801, 1986.

95. Chamlian DL Taylor HB: Primary carcinoma of Bartholin's gland: A report of 24 patients. Obstet Gynecol 39:489–494, 1972.

96. Wheelock JB, Goplerud DR, Dunn LJ, Oates JF: Primary carcinoma of the Bartholin gland: A report of ten cases. Obstet Gynecol 63:820–824, 1984.

97. Felix JC, Cote RJ, Kramer EE, et al: Carcinomas of Bartholin's gland: Histogenesis and the etiological role of human papillomavirus. Am J Pathol 142:925–933, 1993.

98. Scinicariello F, Rady P, Hannigan E, et al: Human papillomavirus type 16 found in primary transitional cell carcinoma of the Bartholin's gland and in a lymph node metastasis. Gynecol Oncol 47:263–266, 1992.

99. DePasquale SE, McGuinness TB, Mangan CE, et al: Adenoid cystic carcinoma of Bartholin's gland: A review of the literature and report of a patient. Gynecol Oncol 61:122–125, 1996.

100. Fanning J, Lambert HC, Hale TM, et al: Paget's disease of the vulva: Prevalence of associated vulvar adenocarcinoma, invasive Paget's disease, and recurrence after surgical excision. Am J Obstet Gynecol 180(1 pt 1):24–27, 1999.

101. Gunn RA, Gallager HS: Vulvar Paget's disease: A topographic study. Cancer 46:590–594, 1980.

102. Misas JE, Cold CJ, Hall FW: Vulvar Paget disease: Fluorescein-aided visualization of margins. Obstet Gynecol 77:156–159, 1991.

103. Bacchi CE, Goldfogel GA, Greer BE, Gown AM: Paget's disease and melanoma of the vulva: Use of a panel of monoclonal antibodies to identify cell type and to microscopically define adequacy of surgical margins. Gynecol Oncol 46:216–221, 1992.

104. Ganjei P, Giraldo KA, Lampe B, Nadji M: Vulvar Paget's disease: Is immunocytochemistry helpful in assessing the surgical margins? J Reprod Med 35:1002–1004, 1990.

105. Billings SD, Roth LM: Pseudoinvasive, nodular extramammary Paget's disease of the vulva. Arch Pathol Lab Med 122:471–474, 1998.

106. Crawford D, Nimmo M, Clement PB, et al: Prognostic factors in Paget's disease of the vulva: A study of 21 cases. Int J Gynecol Pathol 18:351–359, 1999.

107. Fine BA, Fowler LJ, Valente PT, Gaudet T: Minimally invasive Paget's disease of the vulva with extensive lymph node metastases. Gynecol Oncol 57:262–265, 1995.

108. Friedrich EG Jr, Wilkinson EJ, Steingraeber PH, Lewis JD: Paget's disease of the vulva and carcinoma of the breast. Obstet Gynecol 46:130–134, 1975.

109. Goldblum JR, Hart WR: Vulvar Paget's disease: A clinicopathologic and immunohistochemical study of 19 cases. Am J Surg Pathol 21:1178–1187, 1997.

110. Goldblum JR, Hart WR: Perianal Paget's disease: A histologic and immunohistochemical study of 11 cases with and without associated rectal adenocarcinoma. Am J Surg Pathol 22:170–179, 1998.

111. Kohler S, Rouse RV, Smoller BR: The differential diagnosis of pagetoid cells in the epidermis. Mod Pathol 11:79–92, 1998.

112. Clark WH Jr, Hood AF, Tucker MA, Jampel RM: Atypical melanocytic nevi of the genital type with a discussion of reciprocal parenchymal-stromal interactions in the biology of neoplasia. Hum Pathol 29(1 suppl 1):1–24, 1998.

113. Morrow CP, Rutledge FN: Melanoma of the vulva. Obstet Gynecol 39:745–752, 1972.

114. Chung AF, Woodruff JM, Lewis JL Jr: Malignant melanoma of the vulva: A report of 44 cases. Obstet Gynecol 45:638–646, 1975.

115. Egan CA, Bradley RR, Logsdon VK, et al: Vulvar melanoma in childhood. Arch Dermatol 133:345–348, 1997.

116. Ragnarsson-Olding BK, Kanter-Lewensohn LR, Lagerlof B, et al: Malignant melanoma of the vulva in a nationwide, 25-year study of 219 Swedish females: Clinical observations and histopathologic features. Cancer 86:1273–1284, 1999.

117. Trimble EL: Melanomas of the vulva and vagina. Oncology 10:1017–1023, 1996.

118. Ragnarsson-Olding BK, Nilsson BR, Kanter-Lewensohn LR, et al: Malignant melanoma of the vulva in a nationwide, 25-year study of 219 Swedish females: Predictors of survival. Cancer 86:1285–1293, 1999.

119. Ragnarsson-Olding B, Johansson H, Rutqvist LE, Ringborg U: Malignant melanoma of the vulva and vagina: Trends in incidence, age distribution, and long-term survival among 245 consecutive cases in Sweden 1960–1984. Cancer 71:1893–1897, 1993.

120. Curtin JP, Saigo P, Slucher B, Venkatraman ES, et al: Soft-tissue sarcoma of the vagina and vulva: A clinicopathologic study. Obstet Gynecol 86:269–272, 1995.

121. Tavassoli FA, Norris HJ: Smooth muscle tumors of the vulva. Obstet Gynecol 53:213–217, 1979.

122. Nielsen GP, Rosenberg AE, Koerner FC, et al: Smooth-muscle tumors of the vulva: A clinicopathological study of 25 cases and review of the literature. Am J Surg Pathol 20:779–793, 1996.

123. Newman PL, Fletcher CD: Smooth muscle tumours of the external genitalia: Clinicopathological analysis of a series [published erratum appears in Histopathology 19:198, 1991]. Histopathology 18:523–529, 1991.

124. Fetsch JF, Laskin WB, Lefkowitz M, et al: Aggressive angiomyxoma: A clinicopathologic study of 29 female patients. Cancer 78:79–90, 1996.

125. Granter SR, Nucci MR, Fletcher CD: Aggressive angiomyxoma: Reappraisal of its relationship to angiomyofibroblastoma in a series of 16 cases. Histopathology 30:3–10, 1997.

126. Brown DR, Bryan JT, Cramer H, Fife KH: Analysis of human papillomavirus types in exophytic condylomata acuminata by hybrid capture and southern blot techniques. J Clin Microbiol 31:2667–2673, 1993.

127. Nucci MR, Young RH, Fletcher CD: Cellular pseudosarcomatous fibroepithelial stromal polyps of the lower female genital tract: an underrecognized lesion often misdiagnosed as sarcoma. Am J Surg Pathol 24:231–240, 2000.

128. Jablonska S: Wart viruses: human papillomaviruses. Semin Dermatol 3:120–129, 1984.

129. Zhao YK, Lin YX, Luo RY, et al: Human papillomavirus (HPV) infection in seborrheic keratosis [see comments]. Am J Dermatopathol 11:209–212, 1989.

130. Zhu WY, Leonardi C, Kinsey W, Penneys NS: Irritated seborrheic keratoses and benign verrucous acanthomas do not contain papillomavirus DNA. J Cutan Pathol 18:449–452, 1991.

131. Li J, Ackerman AB: "Seborrheic keratoses" that contain human papillomavirus are condylomata acuminata. Am J Dermatopathol 16:398–405, 1994.

132. Kurman RJ, Norris HJ, Wilkinson E: Tumors of the vulva. In Rosai J, Sobin LH (eds): Tumors of the Cervix, Vagina, and Vulva. 3rd ed. Washington DC, Armed Forces Institute of Pathology, 1992, pp 179–255.

133. Souteyrand P, Wong E, MacDonald DM: Zoon's balanitis (balanitis circumscripta plasmacellularis). Br J Dermatol 105:195–199, 1981.

134. Scurry J, Dennerstein G, Brenan J, et al: Vulvitis circumscripta plasmacellularis: A clinicopathologic entity? J Reprod Med 38:14–18, 1993.

135. Salopek TG, Siminoski K: Vulvitis circumscripta plasmacellularis (Zoon's vulvitis) associated with autoimmune polyglandular endocrine failure. Br J Dermatol 135: 991–994, 1996.

136. White G, Jantos M. Sexual behavior changes with vulvar vestibulitis syndrome. J Reprod Med 1998; 43: 783–789.

137. Nunns D, Mandal D: Psychological and psychosexual aspects of vulvar vestibulitis. Genitourin Med 73:541–544, 1997.

138. Pyka RE, Wilkinson EJ, Friedrich EG Jr, Croker BP: The histopathology of vulvar vestibulitis syndrome. Int J Gynecol Pathol 7:249–257, 1988.

139. Chadha S, Gianotten WL, Drogendijk AC, et al: Histopathologic features of vulvar vestibulitis. Int J Gynecol Pathol 17: 7–11, 1998.

140. Lundqvist EN, Hofern PA, Olofsson JI, Sjoberg I: Is vulvar vestibulitis an inflammatory condition? A comparison of histological findings in affected and healthy women. Acta Derm Venereol 77:319–322, 1997.

141. Bohm-Starke N, Hilliges M, Falconer C, Rylander E: Increased intraepithelial innervation in women with vulvar vestibulitis syndrome. Gynecol Obstet Invest 46:256–260, 1998.

142. Westrom LV, Willen R: Vestibular nerve fiber proliferation in vulvar vestibulitis syndrome. Obstet Gynecol 91:572–576, 1998.

143. Wilkinson EJ, Guerrero E, Daniel R, et al: Vulvar vestibulitis

is rarely associated with human papillomavirus infection types 6, 11, 16, or 18. Int J Gynecol Pathol 12:344–349, 1993.

144. Prayson RA, Stoler MH, Hart WR: Vulvar vestibulitis: A histopathologic study of 36 cases, including human papillomavirus in situ hybridization analysis. Am J Surg Pathol 19:154–160, 1995.

145. Bergeron C, Moyal-Barracco M, Pelisse M, Lewin P. Vulvar vestibulitis: Lack of evidence for a human papillomavirus etiology. J Reprod Med 39:936–938, 1994.

146. Marks TA, Shroyer KR, Markham NE, et al: A clinical, histologic, and dna study of vulvodynia and its association with human papillomavirus. J Soc Gynecol Investig 2:57–63, 1995.

147. Origoni M, Rossi M, Ferrari D, et al: Human papillomavirus with co-existing vulvar vestibulitis syndrome and vestibular papillomatosis. Int J Gynaecol Obstet 64:259–263, 1999.

148. Bergeron S, Bouchard C, Fortier M, et al: The surgical treatment of vulvar vestibulitis syndrome: A follow-up study. J Sex Marital Ther 23:317–325, 1997.

149. Marinoff SC, Turner ML, Hirsch RP, Richard G: Intralesional alpha interferon: Cost-effective therapy for vulvar vestibulitis syndrome. J Reprod Med 38:19–24, 1993.

150. Bornstein J, Abramovici H: Combination of subtotal perineoplasty and interferon for the treatment of vulvar vestibulitis. Gynecol Obstet Invest 44:53–56, 1997.

151. Weijmar Schultz WC, Gianotten WL, van der Meijden WI, et al: Behavioral approach with or without surgical intervention to the vulvar vestibulitis syndrome: A prospective randomized and non-randomized study. J Psychosom Obstet Gynaecol 17:143–148, 1996.

152. Hackel H, Hartmann AA, Burg G: Vulvitis granulomatosa and anoperineitis granulomatosa. Dermatologica 182:128–131, 1991.

153. Yazici H, Yurdakul S, Hamuryudan V: Behçet's syndrome. Curr Opin Rheumatol 11:53–57, 1999.

154. Ranalletta M, Rositto A, Drut R: Fox-Fordyce disease in two prepubertal girls: Histopathologic demonstration of eccrine sweat gland involvement. Pediatr Dermatol 13:294–297, 1996.

155. Thomas R, Barnhill D, Bibro M, Hoskins W: Hidradenitis suppurativa: A case presentation and review of the literature. Obstet Gynecol 66:592–595, 1985.

156. Jemec GB, Hansen U: Histology of hidradenitis suppurativa. J Am Acad Dermatol 34:994–999, 1996.

157. Sparks MK, Kuhlman DS, Prieto A, Callen JP: Hypercalcemia in association with cutaneous squamous cell carcinoma: Occurrence as a late complication of hidradenitis suppurativa. Arch Dermatol 121:243–246, 1985.

158. Brown TJ, Rosen T, Orengo IF: Hidradenitis suppurativa. South Med J 91:1107–1114, 1998.

159. New nomenclature for vulvar disease. Report of the Committee on Terminology of the International Society for the Study of Vulvar Disease. J Reprod Med 35:483–484, 1990.

160. Lawrence WD: Non-neoplastic epithelial disorders of the vulva (vulvar dystrophies): Historical and current perspectives. Pathol Annu 28(pt 2):23-51, 1993.

161. O'Keefe RJ, Scurry JP, Dennerstein G, et al: Audit of 114 non-neoplastic vulvar biopsies. Br J Obstet Gynaecol 102:780–786 1995.

162. Ambros RA, Malfetano JH, Carlson JA, Mihm MC Jr: Non-neoplastic epithelial alterations of the vulva: Recognition assessment and comparisons of terminologies used among the various specialties. Mod Pathol 10:401–408, 1997.

163. Pincus SH, Stadecker MJ: Vulvar dystrophies and noninfectious inflammatory conditions. *In* Wilkinson EJ (ed): Contemporary Issues in Surgical Pathology: Pathology of the Vulva and Vagina. New York, Churchill Livingstone, 1987, pp 11–24.

164. Tate JE, Mutter GL, Boynton KA, Crum CP: Monoclonal origin of vulvar intraepithelial neoplasia and some vulvar hyperplasias. Am J Pathol 150:315–322, 1997.

165. Wakelin SH, Marren P: Lichen sclerosus in women. Clin Dermatol 15:155–169, 1997.

166. Powell JJ, Wojnarowska F: Lichen sclerosus. Lancet 1777–1783, 1999.

167. Ackerman AB, Ragaz A: Lichen sclerosus et atrophicus. The Lives of Lesions: Chronology in Dermatopathology. New York, Masson, 1984, pp 131–137.

168. Hewitt J: Histologic criteria for lichen sclerosus of the vulva. J Reprod Med 31:781–787, 1986.

169. Friedrich EG, Julian CG, Woodruff JD: Acridine-orange fluorescence in vulvar dysplasia. Am J Obstet Gynecol 90:128, 1964.

170. Woodruff JD, Borkowf HI, Holzman GB, et al: Metabolic activity in normal and abnormal vulvar epithelia. Am J Obstet Gynecol 91:809, 1965.

171. Newton JA, Camplejohn RS, McGibbon DH: A flow cytometric study of the significance of DNA aneuploidy in cutaneous lesions. Br J Dermatol 117:169–174, 1987.

172. Soini Y, Paakko P, Vahakangas K, et al: Expression of p53 and proliferating cell nuclear antigen in lichen sclerosus et atrophicus with different histological features. Int J Gynecol Pathol 13:199–204, 1994.

173. Fung MA, LeBoit PE: Light microscopic criteria for the diagnosis of early vulvar lichen sclerosus: A comparison with lichen planus. Am J Surg Pathol 22:473–478, 1998.

174. Carlson JA, Lamb P, Malfetano J, et al: Clinicopathologic comparison of vulvar and extragenital lichen sclerosus: Histologic variants, evolving lesions, and etiology of 141 cases. Mod Pathol 11:844–854, 1998.

175. Wallace HJ: Lichen sclerosus et atrophicus. Trans St Johns Hosp Dermatol Soc 57:9–30, 1971.

176. Hart WR, Norris HJ, Helwig EB: Relation of lichen sclerosus et atrophicus of the vulva to development of carcinoma. Obstet Gynecol 45:369–377, 1975.

177. Gomez Rueda N, Garcia A, Vighi S, et al: Epithelial alterations adjacent to invasive squamous carcinoma of the vulva. J Reprod Med 39:526–530, 1994.

178. Carlson JA, Ambros R, Malfetano J, et al: Vulvar lichen sclerosus and squamous cell carcinoma. A cohort, case control, and investigational study with historical perspective: Implications for chronic inflammation and sclerosis in the development of neoplasia. Hum Pathol, 29:932–948, 1998.

179. Bornstein J, Heifetz S, Kellner Y, et al: Clobetasol dipropionate 0.05% versus testosterone propionate 2% topical application for severe vulvar lichen sclerosus. Am J Obstet Gynecol 178(1 pt 1):80-84 1998.

180. Forsberg JG: Cervicovaginal epithelium: Its origin and development. Am J Obstet Gynecol 115:1025–1043, 1973.

181. Cunha GR: Epithelial-stromal interactions in development of the urogenital tract. Int Rev Cytol 47:137–194, 1976.

182. Kottmeier HL: Annual Report on the Results Of Treatment in Gynecological Cancer. Stockholm, Sweden, International Federation of Gynecology and Obstetrics, 1972.

183. Murad TM, Durant JR, Maddox WA, Dowling EA: The pathologic behavior of primary vaginal carcinoma and its relationship to cervical cancer. Cancer 35:787–794, 1975.

184. van Beurden M, ten Kate FW, Tjong A, et al: Human papillomavirus DNA in multicentric vulvar intraepithelial neoplasia. Int J Gynecol Pathol 17:12–16, 1998.

185. Daw E: Primary carcinoma of the vagina. J Obstet Gynaecol Br Commonw 78:853–856, 1971.

186. Herbst AL, Green TH Jr, Ulfelder H: Primary carcinoma of the vagina: An analysis of 68 cases. Am J Obstet Gynecol 106:210–218, 1970.

187. Bosch FX, Manos MM, Munoz N, et al: Prevalence of human papillomavirus in cervical cancer: A worldwide perspective. International Biological Study on Cervical Cancer (IBSCC) Study Group [see comments]. J Natl Cancer Inst 87:796–802, 1995.

188. Wade-Evans T: The aetiology and pathology of cancer of the vagina. Clin Obstet Gynaecol 3:229–241, 1976.

189. Haines M, Taylor CW: Gynaecological pathology. 2nd ed. Edinburgh, Churchill Livingstone, 1975.

190. Pride GL, Buchler DA: Carcinoma of vagina 10 or more years following pelvic irradiation therapy. Am J Obstet Gynecol 127:513–517, 1977.

191. Hummer WK, Mussey E, Decker DG, Dockerty MB: Carcinoma in situ of the vagina. Am J Obstet Gynecol 108:1109–1116, 1970.

192. Sillman FH, Fruchter RG, Chen YS, et al: Vaginal intraepithelial neoplasia: Risk factors for persistence, recurrence, and invasion and its management. Am J Obstet Gynecol 176:93–99,1997.

193. Cone R, Beckmann A, Aho M, et al: Subclinical manifestations of vulvar human papillomavirus infection. Int J Gynecol Pathol 10:26–35, 1991.
194. Aho M, Vesterinen E, Meyer B, et al: Natural history of vaginal intraepithelial neoplasia. Cancer 68:195–197, 1991.
195. Plentl AA, Friedman EA: Lymphatic system of the female genitalia: The morphologic basis of oncologic diagnosis and therapy. Philadelphia, WB Saunders, 1971.
196. Kurman RJ, Norris HJ, Wilkinson E: Tumors of the vagina. In Rosai J, Sobin LH (eds): Tumors of the Cervix, Vagina, and Vulva. 3rd ed. Washington DC, Armed Forces Institute of Pathology, 1992, pp 141–178.
197. Crum CP, Nuovo GJ: The cervix. In Sternberg SS (ed): Diagnostic Surgical Pathology. 2nd ed. New York, Raven Press, 1994, pp 2055–2090.
198. Johnston GA Jr, Klotz J, Boutselis JG: Primary invasive carcinoma of the vagina. Surg Gynecol Obstet 156:34–40, 1983.
199. Perez CA, Gersell DJ, McGuire WP, Morris M: Vagina. In Hoskins WJ, Perez CA, Young RC: Principles and Practice of Gynecologic Oncology. 2nd ed. Philadelphia, Lippincott-Raven, 1997, pp 753–783.
200. Crowther ME, Lowe DG, Shepherd JH: Verrucous carcinoma of the female genital tract: A review. Obstet Gynecol Surv 43:263–280, 1988.
201. Ulbright TM, Alexander RW, Kraus FT: Intramural papilloma of the vagina: Evidence of müllerian histogenesis. Cancer 48:2260–2266, 1981.
202. Dobbs SP, Shaw PA, Brown LJ, Ireland D: Borderline malignant change in recurrent müllerian papilloma of the vagina. J Clin Pathol 51:875–877, 1998.
203. Branton PA, Tavassoli FA: Spindle cell epithelioma, the so-called mixed tumor of the vagina: A clinicopathologic, immunohistochemical, and ultrastructural analysis of 28 cases. Am J Surg Pathol 17:509–515,1993.
204. Hatch EE, Palmer JR, Titus-Ernstoff L, et al: Cancer risk in women exposed to diethylstilbestrol in utero. JAMA 280:630–634, 1998.
205. Sedlis A, Robboy SJ: Diseases of the vagina. In Kurman RJ (ed): Blaustein's Pathology of the Female Genital Tract. 3rd ed. New York, Springer-Verlag, 1987, pp 97–140.
206. Giusti RM, Iwamoto K, Hatch EE: Diethylstilbestrol revisited: A review of the long-term health effects. Ann Intern Med 122:778–788, 1995.
207. Yaghsezian H, Palazzo JP, Finkel GC, et al: Primary vaginal adenocarcinoma of the intestinal type associated with adenosis. Gynecol Oncol 45:62–65, 1992.
208. DeMars LR, Van Le L, Huang I, Fowler WCL Primary non–clear-cell adenocarcinomas of the vagina in older DES-exposed women [see comments]. Gynecol Oncol 58:389–392, 1995.
209. Rhatigan RM, Mojadidi Q: Adenosquamous carcinomas of the vulva and vagina. Am J Clin Pathol 60:208–217, 1973.
210. Sulak P, Barnhill D, Heller P, et al: Nonsquamous cancer of the vagina. Gynecol Oncol 29:309–320, 1988.
211. Clement PB, Benedet JL: Adenocarcinoma in situ of the vagina: A case report. Cancer 43:2479–2485, 1979.
212. Kurman RJ, Prabha AC: Thyroid and parathyroid glands in the vaginal wall: Report of a case. Am J Clin Pathol 59:503–507, 1973.
213. Hirose R, Imai A, Kondo H, et al: Dermoid cyst of the paravaginal space. Arch Gynecol Obstet 249:39–41, 1991.
214. Schmidt WA: Pathology of the vagina. In Fox H (ed): Haines and Taylor Obstetrical and Gynaecological Pathology. 4th ed. New York, Churchill Livingstone, 1995, pp 135–223.
215. Zaino RJ, Robboy SJ, Bentley R, Kurman RJ: Diseases of the vagina. In Kurman RJ: Blaustein's Pathology of the Female Genital Tract. 4th ed. New York, Springer-Verlag, 1994, pp 131–183.
216. Zirker TA, Silva EG, Morris M, Ordonez NG: Immunohistochemical differentiation of clear-cell carcinoma of the female genital tract and endodermal sinus tumor with the use of alpha-fetoprotein and Leu-M1. Am J Clin Pathol 91:511–514, 1989.
217. Ragnarsson OB, Johansson H, Rutqvist LE, Ringborg U: Malignant melanoma of the vulva and vagina: Trends in incidence, age distribution, and long-term survival among 245 consecutive cases in Sweden 1960–1984. Cancer 71:1893–1897, 1993.
218. Weinstock MA: Malignant melanoma of the vulva and vagina in the United States: Patterns of incidence and population-based estimates of survival. Am J Obstet Gynecol 171:1225–1230, 1994.
219. Nigogosyan G, de la Pava S, Pickren JW: Melanoblasts in vaginal mucosa: Origin for primary malignant melanoma. Cancer 17:912–913, 1964.
220. Tsukada Y: Benign melanosis of the vagina and cervix. Am J Obstet Gynecol 124:211–212, 1976.
221. Lee RB, Buttoni L Jr, Dhru K, Tamimi H: Malignant melanoma of the vagina: A case report of progression from pre-existing melanosis. Gynecol Oncol 19:238–245, 1984.
222. Bottles K, Lacey CG, Goldberg J, et al: Merkel cell carcinoma of the vulva. Obstet Gynecol 63(3 suppl):61–65, 1984.
223. Chung AF, Casey MJ, Flannery JT, et al: Malignant melanoma of the vagina: Report of 19 cases. Obstet Gynecol 55:720–727, 1980.
224. Clark WH Jr, From L, Bernardino EA, Mihm MC: The histogenesis and biologic behavior of primary human malignant melanomas of the skin. Cancer Res 29:705–727, 1969.
225. Kaufman RH, Gardner HL: Tumors of the vulva and vagina: Benign mesodermal tumors. Clin Obstet Gynecol 8:953, 1965.
226. Tavassoli FA, Norris HJ: Smooth muscle tumors of the vagina. Obstet Gynecol 53:689–693, 1979.
227. Copeland LJ, Gershenson DM, Saul PB, et al: Sarcoma botryoides of the female genital tract. Obstet Gynecol 66:262–266, 1985.
228. Gompel C, Silverberg SG: The vagina. In Gompel C, Silverberg SG: Pathology in Gynecology and Obstetrics, 4th ed. Philadelphia, JB Lippincott, 1994, pp 46–71.
229. Proppe KH, Scully RE, Rosai J: Postoperative spindle cell nodules of genitourinary tract resembling sarcomas: A report of eight cases. Am J Surg Pathol 8:101–108, 1984.
230. Mardh PA: The vaginal ecosystem. Am J Obstet Gynecol 165:1163–1168, 1991.
231. Garcia-Closas M, Herrero R, Bratti C, et al: Epidemiologic determinants of vaginal pH. Am J Obstet Gynecol 180:1060–1066, 1999.
232. Skarin A, Sylwan J: Vaginal lactobacilli inhibiting growth of Gardnerella vaginalis, mobiluncus and other bacterial species cultured from vaginal content of women with bacterial vaginosis. Acta Pathol Microbiol Immunol Scand [B] 94:399–403, 1986.
233. Hillier SL, Krohn MA, Klebanoff SJ, Eschenbach DA: The relationship of hydrogen peroxide-producing lactobacilli to bacterial vaginosis and genital microflora in pregnant women. Obstet Gynecol 79:369–373, 1992.
234. Spiegel CA, Davick P, Totten PA, et al: Gardnerella vaginalis and anaerobic bacteria in the etiology of bacterial (nonspecific) vaginosis. Scand J Infect Dis Suppl 40:41–46, 1983.
235. Thomason JL, Schreckenberger PC, Spellacy WN, et al: Clinical and microbiological characterization of patients with non-specific vaginosis associated with motile, curved anaerobic rods. J Infect Dis 149:801–809, 1984.
236. Hammann R, Kronibus A, Lang N, Werner H: Quantitative studies on the vaginal flora of asymptomatic women and patients with vaginitis and vaginosis. Zentralbl Bakteriol Mikrobiol Hyg [A] 265:451–461, 1987.
237. Fredricsson B, Englund K, Weintraub L, et al: Bacterial vaginosis is not a simple ecological disorder. Gynecol Obstet Invest 28:156–160, 1989.
238. Levett PN: Bacterial vaginosis. West Indian Med J 38:126–132, 1989.
239. Hallen A, Pahlson C, Forsum U: Bacterial vaginosis in women attending STD clinic: Diagnostic criteria and prevalence of Mobiluncus spp. Genitourin Med 63:386–389, 1987.
240. Spiegel CA: Bacterial vaginosis. Clin Microbiol Rev 4:485–502, 1991.
241. Daus AD, Hafez ES: Candida albicans in women. Nurs Res 24:430–433, 1975.
242. Oates JK: Recurrent vaginitis and oral sex [letter]. Lancet 1:785, 1979.

243. White W, Spencer-Phillips PJ: Recurrent vaginitis and oral sex [letter]. Lancet 1:621, 1979.
244. Garcia-Tamayo J, Castillo G, Martinez AJ: Human genital candidiasis: Histochemistry, scanning and transmission electron microscopy. Acta Cytol 26:7–14, 1982.
245. Felman YM, Nikitas JA: Trichomoniasis, candidiasis, and *Corynebacterium vaginale* vaginitis. NY State J Med 79(10): 1563–1566, 1979.
246. Ryu JS, Chung HL, Min DY, et al: Diagnosis of trichomoniasis by polymerase chain reaction. Yonsei Med J 40:56–60, 1999.
247. Riley LE: Herpes simplex virus. Semin Perinatol 22:284–292, 1998.
248. Hoffman DB, Grundfest P: Vaginitis emphysematosa. Am J Obstet Gynecol 78:428–430, 1959.
249. Gardner HL: Desquamative inflammatory vaginitis: A newly defined entity. Am J Obstet Gynecol 102:1102–1105, 1968.
250. Sobel JD: Desquamative inflammatory vaginitis: A new subgroup of purulent vaginitis responsive to topical 2% clindamycin therapy. Am J Obstet Gynecol 171:1215–1220, 1994.
251. Oates JK, Rowen D: Desquamative inflammatory vaginitis: A review. Genitourin Med 66:275–279, 1990.
252. Wisniewski PM, Wilkinson EJ: Postpartum vaginal atrophy. Am J Obstet Gynecol 165(4 pt 2):1249–1254, 1991.
253. Edwards L, Friedrich EG Jr: Desquamative vaginitis: Lichen planus in disguise. Obstet Gynecol 71(6 pt 1):832–836, 1988.
254. Young AW Jr, Herman EW, Tovell HM: Syringoma of the vulva: Incidence, diagnosis, and cause of pruritus. Obstet Gynecol 55:515–518, 1980.
255. Isaacson D, Turner ML: Localized vulvar syringomas. J Am Acad Dermatol 1:352–356, 1979.
256. Tay YK, Tham SN, Teo R: Localized vulvar syringomas: An unusual cause of pruritus vulvae. Dermatology 192:62–63, 1996.
257. Lever WF, Castleman B: Clear cell myoepithelioma of the skin: Report of 10 cases. Am J Pathol 28:691–699, 1952.
258. Cho D, Woodruff JD: Trichoepithelioma of the vulva: A report of two cases. J Reprod Med 33:317–319, 1988.
259. Mizushima J, Ohara K: Basal cell carcinoma of the vulva with lymph node and skin metastasis: Report of a case and review of 20 Japanese cases. J Dermatol 22:36–42, 1995.
260. Cruz-Jimenez PR, Abell MR: Cutaneous basal cell carcinoma of vulva. Cancer 36:1860–1868, 1975.
261. Breen JL, Neubecker RD, Greenwald E, Gregori CA: Basal cell carcinoma of the vulva. Obstet Gynecol 46:122–129, 1975.
262. Nehal KS, Levine VJ, Ashinoff R: Basal cell carcinoma of the genitalia. Dermatol Surg 24:1361–1363, 1998.
263. Feakins RM, Lowe DG: Basal cell carcinoma of the vulva: A clinicopathologic study of 45 cases. Int J Gynecol Pathol 16: 319–324, 1997.
264. Schueller EF: Basal cell cancer of the vulva. Am J Obstet Gynecol 93:199, 1965.
265. Carson LF, Twiggs LB, Okagaki T, et al: Human papillomavirus DNA in adenosquamous carcinoma and squamous cell carcinoma of the vulva. Obstet Gynecol 72:63–67, 1988.
266. Cho D, Buscema J, Rosenshein NB, Woodruff JD: Primary breast cancer of the vulva. Obstet Gynecol 66(3 Suppl):79–81, 1985.
267. Di Bonito L, Patriarca S, Falconieri G: Aggressive "breast-like" adenocarcinoma of vulva. Pathol Res Pract 188:211–214, 1992.
268. van der Putte SC, van Gorp LH: Adenocarcinoma of the mammary-like glands of the vulva: A concept unifying sweat gland carcinoma of the vulva, carcinoma of supernumerary mammary glands and extramammary Paget's disease. J Cutan Pathol 21:157–163, 1994.
269. Kennedy JC, Majmudar B: Primary adenocarcinoma of the vulva, possibly cloacogenic: A report of two cases. J Reprod Med 38:113–116, 1993.
270. Wick MR, Goellner JR, Wolfe JT, Su WP: Vulvar sweat gland carcinomas. Arch Pathol Lab Med 109:43–47, 1985.
271. Rich PM, Okagaki T, Clark B, Prem KA: Adenocarcinoma of the sweat gland of the vulva: Light and electron microscopic study. Cancer 47:1352–1357, 1981.
272. Kawamoto M, Fukuda Y, Kamoi S, et al: Sebaceous carcinoma of the vulva. Pathol Int 45:767–773, 1995.
273. Jacobs DM, Sandles LG, LeBoit PE: Sebaceous carcinoma arising from Bowen's disease of the vulva. Arch Dermatol 122:1191–1193, 1986.
274. Ungerleider RS, Donaldson SS, Warnke RA, Wilbur JR: Endodermal sinus tumor: The Stanford experience and the first reported case arising in the vulva. Cancer 41:1627–1634, 1978.
275. Flanagan CW, Parker JR, Mannel RS, et al: Primary endodermal sinus tumor of the vulva: A case report and review of the literature. Gynecol Oncol 66:515–518, 1997.
276. Kaplan EJ, Chadburn A, Caputo TA: HIV-related primary non-Hodgkin's lymphoma of the vulva. Gynecol Oncol 61: 131–138, 1996.
277. Young RH, Harris NL, Scully RE: Lymphoma-like lesions of the lower female genital tract: A report of 16 cases. Int J Gynecol Pathol 4:289–299, 1985.
278. Dehner LP: Metastatic and secondary tumors of the vulva. Obstet Gynecol 42:47–57, 1973.
279. Menzin AW, De Risi D, Smilari TF, et al: Lobular breast carcinoma metastatic to the vulva: A case report and literature review. Gynecol Oncol 69:84–88, 1998.
280. Guidozzi F, Sonnendecker EW, Wright C: Ovarian cancer with metastatic deposits in the cervix, vagina, or vulva preceding primary cytoreductive surgery. Gynecol Oncol 49: 225–228, 1993.
281. di Sant'Agnese PA, Knowles DM: Extracardiac rhabdomyoma: A clinicopathologic study and review of the literature. Cancer 46:780–789, 1980.
282. Andrassy RJ, Hays DM, Raney RB, et al: Conservative surgical management of vaginal and vulvar pediatric rhabdomyosarcoma: A report from the Intergroup Rhabdomyosarcoma Study III. J Pediatr Surg 30:1034–1036, 1995.
283. Copeland LJ, Sneige N, Stringer CA, et al: Alveolar rhabdomyosarcoma of the female genitalia. Cancer 56:849–855, 1985.
284. LiVolsi VA, Brooks JJ: Soft tissue tumors of the vulva. In Wilkinson EJ (ed): Pathology of the Vulva and Vagina: Contemporary Issues in Surgical Pathology. New York, Churchill Livingstone, 1987, pp 209–238.
285. Wilkinson EJ: Benign diseases of the vulva. In Kurman RJ (ed): Blaustein's Pathology of the Female Genital Tract. 4th ed. New York, Springer-Verlag, 1994, pp 31–86.
286. Allen MV and Novotny, D. B. Desmoid Tumor of the Vulva Associated With Pregnancy. Arch Pathol Lab Med 1997,121(5):512–514.
287. Kfuri A, Rosenshein N, Dorfman H, Goldstein P: Desmoid tumor of the vulva. J Reprod Med 26:272–273, 1981.
288. Bock JE, Andreasson B, Thorn A, Holck S: Dermatofibrosarcoma protuberans of the vulva. Gynecol Oncol 20:129–135, 1985.
289. Leake JF, Buscema J, Cho KR, Currie JL: Dermatofibrosarcoma protuberans of the vulva. Gynecol Oncol 41:245–249, 1991.
290. Taylor RN, Bottles K, Miller TR, Braga CA: Malignant fibrous histiocytoma of the vulva. Obstet Gynecol 66(1):145–148, 1985.
291. Kaufman RH, Friedman K: Hemangioma of clitoris, confused with adrenogenital syndrome: Case report. Plast Reconstr Surg 62:452–454, 1978.
292. Blair C: Angiokeratoma of the vulva. Br J Dermatol 83:409–411, 1970.
293. Imperial R, Helwig EB: Angiokeratoma of the vulva. Obstet Gynecol 29:307–312, 1967.
294. Johnson TL, Kennedy AW, Segal GH: Lymphangioma circumscriptum of the vulva: A report of two cases. J Reprod Med 36:808–812, 1991.
295. Huey GR, Stehman FB, Roth LM, Ehrlich CE: Lymphangiosarcoma of the edematous thigh after radiation therapy for carcinoma of the vulva. Gynecol Oncol 20:394–401, 1985.
296. Zakut H, Lotan M, Lipnitzky M: Vulvar hemangiopericytoma: A case report and review of previous cases. Acta Obstet Gynecol Scand 64:619–621, 1985.

297. Katz VL, Askin FB, Bosch BD: glomus tumor of the vulva: A case report. Obstet Gynecol 67(3 suppl):43–45, 1986.

298. Kohorn EI, Merino MJ, Goldenhersh M: Vulvar pain and dyspareunia due to glomus tumor. Obstet Gynecol 67(3 suppl):41–42, 1986.

299. Macasaet MA, Duerr A, Thelmo W, et al: Kaposi sarcoma presenting as a vulvar mass. Obstet Gynecol 86(4 pt 2):695–697, 1995.

300. Strayer SA, Yum MN, Sutton GP: Epithelioid hemangioendothelioma of the clitoris: A case report with immunohistochemical and ultrastructural findings. Int J Gynecol Pathol 11:234–239, 1992.

301. Davos I, Abell MR: Soft tissue sarcomas of vulva. Gynecol Oncol 4:70–86, 1976.

302. Yamashita Y, Yamada T, Ueki K, et al: A case of vulvar schwannoma. J Obstet Gynaecol Res 22:31–34, 1996.

303. Woodruff JM, Marshall ML, Godwin TA, et al: Plexiform (multinodular) schwannoma: A tumor simulating the plexiform neurofibroma. Am J Surg Pathol 7:691–697, 1983.

304. Friedrich EG Jr, Wilkinson EJ: Vulvar surgery for neurofibromatosis. Obstet Gynecol 65:135–138, 1985.

305. Venter PF, Rohm GF, Slabber CF: Giant neurofibromas of the labia. Obstet Gynecol 57:128–130, 1981.

306. Wolber RA, Talerman A, Wilkinson EJ, Clement PB: Vulvar granular cell tumors with pseudocarcinomatous hyperplasia: A comparative analysis with well-differentiated squamous carcinoma. Int J Gynecol Pathol 10:59–66, 1991.

307. Degefu S, Dhurandhar HN, O'Quinn AG, Fuller PN: Granular cell tumor of the clitoris in pregnancy. Gynecol Oncol 19:246–251, 1984.

308. King DF, Bustillo M, Broen EN, Hirose FM: Granular-cell tumors of the vulva: A report of three cases. J Dermatol Surg Oncol 5:794–797, 1979.

309. Majmudar B, Castellano PZ, Wilson RW, Siegel RJ: Granular cell tumors of the vulva. J Reprod Med 35:1008–1014, 1990.

310. Lawrence WD, Shingleton HM: Malignant schwannoma of the vulva: A light and electron microscopic study. Gynecol Oncol 6:527–537, 1978.

311. Terada KY, Schmidt RW, Roberts JA: Malignant schwannoma of the vulva: A case report. J Reprod Med 33:969–972, 1988.

312. Robertson AJ, McIntosh W, Lamont P, Guthrie W: Malignant granular cell tumour (myoblastoma) of the vulva: report of a case and review of the literature. Histopathology 5:69–79, 1981.

313. Fukamizu H, Matsumoto K, Inoue K, Moriguchi T: Large vulvar lipoma. Arch Dermatol 118:447, 1982.

314. Brooks JJ, LiVolsi VA: Liposarcoma presenting on the vulva. Am J Obstet Gynecol 156:73–75, 1987.

315. Genton CY, Maroni ES: Vulval liposarcoma. Arch Gynecol 240:63–66, 1987.

316. Nucci MR, Fletcher CD: Liposarcoma (atypical lipomatous tumors) of the vulva: A clinicopathologic study of six cases. Int J Gynecol Pathol 17:17–23, 1998.

317. Hall DJ, Grimes MM, Goplerud DR: Epithelioid sarcoma of the vulva. Gynecol Oncol 9:237–246, 1980.

318. Perrone T, Swanson PE, Twiggs L, et al: Malignant rhabdoid tumor of the vulva: Is distinction from epithelioid sarcoma possible? A pathologic and immunohistochemical study [see comments]. Am J Surg Pathol 13:848–858, 1989.

319. Guillou L, Wadden C, Coindre JM, et al: "Proximal-type" epithelioid sarcoma: A distinctive aggressive neoplasm showing rhabdoid features. Clinicopathologic, Immunohistochemical, and Ultrastructural Study of a Series. Am J Surg Pathol 21:130–146, 1997.

320. Ulbright TM, Brokaw SA, Stehman FB, Roth LM: Epithelioid sarcoma of the vulva: Evidence suggesting a more aggressive behavior than extra-genital epithelioid sarcoma. Cancer 52:1462–1469, 1983.

321. Shen JT, D'ablaing G, Morrow CP: Alveolar soft part sarcoma of the vulva: Report of first case and review of literature. Gynecol Oncol 13:120–128, 1982.

322. Fletcher CD, Tsang WY, Fisher C, et al: Angiomyofibroblastoma of the vulva: A benign neoplasm distinct from aggressive angiomyxoma [see comments]. Am J Surg Pathol 16:373–382, 1992.

323. Fox H, Wells M, Harris M, et al: Enteric tumours of the lower female genital tract: A report of three cases. Histopathology 12:167–176, 1988.

324. Lorenz G: Adenomatoid tumor of the ovary and vagina [author's translation from German]. Zentralbl Gynakol 100:1412-1416, 1978.

325. Chen KT: Brenner tumor of the vagina. Diagn Gynecol Obstet 3:255–258, 1981.

326. Fukushima M, Twiggs LB, Okagaki T: Mixed intestinal adenocarcinoma-argentaffin carcinoma of the vagina. Gynecol Oncol 23:387–394, 1986.

327. Joseph RE, Enghardt MH, Doering DL, et al: Small cell neuroendocrine carcinoma of the vagina. Cancer 70(4):784–789, 1992.

328. Prasad CJ, Ray JA, Kessler S: Primary small cell carcinoma of the vagina arising in a background of atypical adenosis. Cancer 70:2484–2487, 1992.

329. Naves AE, Monti JA, Chichoni E: Basal cell–like carcinoma in the upper third of the vagina. Am J Obstet Gynecol 137:136–137, 1980.

330. Hinchey WW, Silva EG, Guarda LA, et al: Paravaginal wolffian duct (mesonephros) adenocarcinoma: A light and electron microscopic study. Am J Clin Pathol 80:539–544, 1983.

331. Spitzer M, Molho L, Seltzer VL, Lipper S: Vaginal glomus tumor: Case presentation and ultrastructural findings. Obstet Gynecol 66(suppl 3):86–88, 1985.

332. Prempree T, Tang CK, Hatef A, Forster S: Angiosarcoma of the vagina: A clinicopathologic report. A reappraisal of the radiation treatment of angiosarcomas of the female genital tract. Cancer 51:618–622, 1983.

333. Tohya T, Katabuchi H, Fukuma K, et al: Angiosarcoma of the vagina: A light and electronmicroscopy study. Acta Obstet Gynecol Scand 70:169–172, 1991.

334. Gold BM: Neurofibromatosis of the bladder and vagina. Am J Obstet Gynecol 113:1055–1056, 1972.

335. Dekel A, Avidan D, Bar Ziv J, et al: Neurofibroma of the vagina presenting with urinary retention: Review of the literature and report of a case. Obstet Gynecol Surv 43:325–327, 1988.

336. Pezeshkpour G: Solitary paraganglioma of the vagina: Report of a case. Am J Obstet Gynecol 139:219–221, 1981.

337. Tobon H, Murphy AI: Benign blue nevus of the vagina. Cancer 40:3174–3176, 1977.

338. Davos I, Abell MR: Sarcomas of the vagina. Obstet Gynecol 47:342–350, 1976.

339. Palmer JP, Biback SM: Primary cancer of the vagina. Am J Obstet Gynecol 67:377–397, 1954.

340. Webb MJ, Symmonds RE, Weiland LH: Malignant fibrous histiocytoma of the vagina. Am J Obstet Gynecol 119(2):190–192, 1974.

341. Harris NL, Scully RE: Malignant lymphoma and granulocytic sarcoma of the uterus and vagina: A clinicopathologic analysis of 27 cases. Cancer 53:2530–2545, 1984.

342. Issa PY, Salem PA, Brihi E, Azoury RS: Eosinophilic granuloma with involvement of the female genitalia. Am J Obstet Gynecol 137:608–612, 1980.

343. Chapman GW, Benda J, Williams T: Alveolar soft-part sarcoma of the vagina. Gynecol Oncol 18:125–129, 1984.

344. Kasai K, Yoshida Y, Okumura M: Alveolar soft part sarcoma in the vagina: Clinical features and morphology. Gynecol Oncol 9:227–236, 1980.

345. Miettinen M, Wahlstrom T, Vesterinen E, Saksela E: Vaginal polyps with pseudosarcomatous features: A clinicopathological study of seven cases. Cancer 51:1148–1151, 1983.

346. Ostor A, Fortune DW, Riley CB: Fibroepithelial polyps with atypical stromal cells (pseudosarcoma botryoides) of vulva and vagina: A report of 13 cases. Int J Gynecol Pathol 7:351–360, 1988.

347. Leone PG, Taylor HB: Ultrastructure of a benign polypoid rhabdomyoma of the vagina. Cancer 31:1414–1417, 1973.

348. Gad A, Eusebi V: Rhabdomyoma of the vagina. J Pathol 115:179–181, 1975.

349. Gold JH, Bossen EH: Benign vaginal rhabdomyoma: A light and electron microscopic study. Cancer 37:2283–2294, 1976.

350. Brown TJ, Yen-Moore A, Tyring SK: An overview of sexually

transmitted diseases. Part II [published erratum appears in J Am Acad Dermatol 2000 42(1 Pt 1):148]. J Am Acad Dermatol 41(5 Pt 1):661–677, 1999.

351. Brown TJ, Yen-Moore A, Tyring SK: An overview of sexually transmitted diseases. Part I. J Am Acad Dermatol 41:511–532, 1999.
352. Kang IK, Kim YJ, Choi KC: Ciliated cyst of the vulva. J Am Acad Dermatol 32:514–515, 1995.
353. Merlob P, Bahari C, Liban E, Reisner SH: Cysts of the female external genitalia in the newborn infant. Am J Obstet Gynecol 132:607–610, 1978.
354. Junaid TA, Thomas SM: Cysts of the vulva and vagina: A comparative study. Int J Gynaecol Obstet 19:239–243, 1981.
355. Friedmann W, Schafer A, Kretschmer R, Lobeck H: Disseminated cytomegalovirus infection of the female genital tract. Gynecol Obstet Invest 31:56–57, 1991.
356. Hart G: Donovanosis. Clin Infect Dis 25:24–30, 1997.
357. Sun T, Schwartz NS, Sewell C, et al: Enterobius egg granuloma of the vulva and peritoneum: Review of the literature. Am J Trop Med Hyg 45:249–253, 1991.
358. Agarwal J, Gupta JK: Female genital tuberculosis: A retrospective clinicopathologic study of 501 cases [published erratum appears in Indian J Pathol Microbiol 1994 37:238]. Indian J Pathol Microbiol 36:389–397, 1993.
359. Lagergard T: *Haemophilus ducreyi:* Pathogenesis and protective immunity. Trends Microbiol 3:87–92, 1995.
360. Brown D: Herpes zoster of the vulva. Clin Obstet Gynecol 15:1010–1014, 1972.
361. McElfatrick RA, Condon WB: Hydrocele of the canal of Nuck: A report of two adult cases. Rocky Mt Med J 72:112–113, 1975.
362. Anderson CC, Broadie TA, Mackey JE, Kopecky KK. Hydrocele of the canal of Nuck: Ultrasound appearance. Am Surg 61:959–961, 1995.
363. Burgoyne RA: Lymphogranuloma venereum. Prim Care 17(1):153–157, 1990.
364. Smith KJ, Yeager J, Skelton H: Molluscum contagiosum: Its clinical, histopathologic, and immunohistochemical spectrum. Int J Dermatol 38:664–672, 1999.
365. Newland JR, Fusaro RM: Mucinous cysts of the vulva. Nebr Med J 76:307–310, 1991.
366. Harms G, Matull R, Randrianasolo D, et al. Pattern of sexually transmitted diseases in a Malagasy population. Sex Transm Dis 21:315–320, 1994.
367. Elgart ML: Sexually transmitted diseases of the vulva. Dermatol Clin 10:387–403, 1992.
368. Woodruff JD, Friedrich EG Jr: The vestibule. Clin Obstet Gynecol 28:134–141, 1985.
369. Robboy SJ, Ross JS, Prat J, et al: Urogenital sinus origin of mucinous and ciliated cysts of the vulva. Obstet Gynecol 51:347–351, 1978.
370. McKee PH, Wright E, Hutt MS: Vulval schistosomiasis. Clin Exp Dermatol 8:189–194, 1983.

# 36

# Cervix

Juan C. Felix   Thomas C. Wright

The cervix marks the division between the lower and upper genital tract. This bulbous, predominantly fibrous organ is of great structural and functional importance to the uterus. The normal cervix is embryologically derived from the lower segment of the fused müllerian ducts. During the peripartum period and infancy, the cervix is entirely covered by mucinous glandular epithelium that is müllerian in origin. During childhood and adolescence, the cervix progressively acquires squamous epithelium, purportedly derived from the union of the müllerian duct with the urogenital sinus to eventually position the squamocolumnar junction near the ectocervical os. Structurally, the cervix functions as a diaphragm in the gravid uterus; it remains closed during the length of gestation only to physiologically dilate during labor to allow the passage of the fetus at maturity. Physiologically, the cervix acts as a selective barrier between the sterile endometrial cavity and the bacterial-laden vagina by preventing bacterial passage yet allowing optimal passage of spermatozoa into the upper genital for fertilization of an awaiting ovum during the periovulatory period.

As a consequence of its functional role in reproduction, the vast majority of the pathology of the cervix is a direct consequence of sexually transmitted diseases. Infections by different venereal pathogens are responsible for most of the inflammatory lesions of the cervix. Cumulative data regarding the role of human papillomavirus (HPV) infection in cervical carcinogenesis has now established this sexually transmitted agent as the cause of cervical neoplasia. Cervical cancer is now the most thoroughly studied model of virus-induced neoplasia in humans.

## THE ETIOLOGY OF CERVICAL CANCER AND ITS PRECURSOR LESIONS

Traditional risk factors influencing the acquisition of cervical cancer or its precursor lesions included early age of first sexual activity, multiple sexual partners, lower socioeconomic status, multiparity, cigarette smoking, oral contraceptive use and immunosupression.[1-3] These risk factors first pointed to the association between cervical cancer and its precursor lesions and a sexually transmitted agent. The concept that cervical cancer (and presumably its precursors) is a sexually transmitted disease is further substantiated by the epidemiologic characterization of the high-risk male. These studies document the relevance of the male partner's sexual history in determining a woman's risk for the development of cervical carcinoma and support the concept that a transmissible agent is responsible, in part, for the pathogenesis of cervical cancer.[4, 5]

Two large studies using the polymerase chain reaction (PCR) found that none of the standard sexual risk factors were independently associated with the development of invasive cervical cancer after controlling for the effect of HPV. These data suggest that sexual behavior risk factors are surrogates for HPV infection.[6, 7] In fact, overwhelming evidence exists defining a causal association between sexually acquired HPV infections and cervical cancer.[8, 9–11]

A variety of sexually transmitted pathogens including *Chlamydia trachomatis, Neisseria gonorrhea, Gardnerella vaginalis, Mycoplasma hominis, Trichomonas vaginalis,* and cytomegalovirus had been previously proposed as potential etiologic agents for cervical cancer. However, more recent studies, including a large case control study, of the prevalence of these pathogens in women with cervical cancer precursors have found that none are present more frequently in patients than in controls when analyzed independently of sexual activity. Therefore, the associations of infections by these particular pathogens with cervical cancer and its precursors seem to characterize the sexual history of the population at risk rather than playing an etiologic role themselves.[12–14]

Herpes simplex virus type 2 (HSV-2) previously received considerable attention in relation to the etiology of cervical intraepithelial neoplasia (CIN), with studies linking HSV-2 to CIN and cervical carcinoma biologically and epidemiologically.[15] Well-controlled, retrospective seroepidemiologic studies have shown that patients with cervical cancer and cervical cancer precursor lesions have a higher frequency of neutralizing antibodies against HSV-2 than do controls matched for race, age, and socioeconomic status.[16, 17] A recent case control study of 766 women with invasive cervical, and 1532 controls of women from Latin America found a possible interaction between HPV 16/18 and HSV-2 in the development of invasive cervical carcinoma. The presence of HSV-2 antibodies by themselves was associated with a relative risk of 1.6 for the development of invasive cervical cancer.[18] Although this relative risk was much less than that associated with the presence of HPV 16 or 18 DNA, it persisted independent of other risk factors. Most importantly, patients who had antibodies against HSV-2 and were also HPV 16/18 DNA positive had a two-fold greater risk for developing cervical cancer than patients who were only HPV 16/18 DNA positive, suggesting a possible interaction between the two viruses. Ultimately, as with other sexually transmitted diseases that may cause cervical cancer, research has challenged the belief that HSV-2 has a role in the direct causation of cervical cancer. In a prospective serologic study of Czechoslovakian women, with a follow-up of at least 4 years, no difference was found in the prevalence of HSV-2 antibody between patients with CIN and invasive carcinoma and matched controls. Furthermore, no differences were observed in the prevalence of HSV-2 antibody titers between patients having disease at entry and those developing disease during the study.[16]

## Human Papillomavirus

Papillomaviruses belong to the A genus of the Papovaviridae family. This family of viruses also includes SV40 virus and polyoma virus. Papillomaviruses are widely distributed and infect humans and animals (e.g., bovine, canine, rabbit, elk, and deer papillomaviruses have been identified). Although human and animal papillomaviruses share a similar genomic organization, they are species specific and do not cross-infect other species. Many types and subtypes of papillomaviruses may exist that infect a given species. Because the capsid proteins of papillomavirus are antigenically similar, papillomaviruses are not subdivided into serotypes based on structural antigenic features. Instead, they are subdivided into genotypes and subtypes that are based on the species that they infect and on their extent of DNA relatedness. A novel HPV is classified as a new type if the nucleotide sequence of the E6, E7, and L1 open reading frame (ORF) differs by more that 10% with the sequence of any previously described HPV type.[19] Although these different types are quite similar structurally, they demonstrate significant specificity with regard to the anatomic location of the epithelia that they infect and the type of lesions that they produce at the site of infection.

Twenty-three different types of HPV have been characterized that infect the female and male anogenital tract. These are HPV 6, 11, 16, 18, 30, 31, 33, 35, 39, 40, 42 to 45, 51 to 58 and 61. These 23 different HPV types are associated with a spectrum of anogenital diseases that range from condyloma acuminata to invasive squamous cell carcinoma. Based on their associations with either invasive cancer of the vulva, vagina or cervix, high-grade precursor lesions, or benign epithelial proliferations, the anogenital HPVs have been classified into three different oncogenic risk categories.[20] HPV types 6, 11, 16, and 53 are the most common types detected in women without cervical or vulvar disease.[21] HPV 6 is also the most common HPV type found in adult women or men with exophytic condylomas of the anogenital tract.[22] Exophytic condylomas that are not associated with HPV 6 are usually associated with HPV 11 but can be associated with HPV types 16 or 31. Exophytic, histologically low-grade lesions in adults are almost never associated with HPV 18 or with cutaneous HPV types such as 1 or 2. In children, however, 17% of exophytic condyloma acuminata are associated with HPV 2, which is a cutaneous type associated with common warts (verrucae vulgaris).[23] Small raised plaque-type warts on the penis are usually associated with HPV 6, 16, and 42.[24]

Using sensitive molecular methods such as PCR or hybrid capture II (HC II), HPV DNA can be identified in more than 80% of women with biopsy-confirmed CIN. Cervical lesions that are histologically low-grade, or CIN 1, are quite heterogeneous with regard to their associated HPV types and can be associated with almost any of the common anogenital HPV types.[25, 26] HPV 6 and 11 were the predominant types associated with CIN 1 in studies performed in the mid-1980s, but more recent studies have identified HPV 6 and 11 in only about 20% of cases of CIN 1. The most commonly detected HPVs in women with CIN 1 are novel or unrecognizable HPVs. HPV 16 and 18 combined have been detected in about 20% of cases of CIN 1. Infection with more than one type of HPV is common in women with CIN 1. In one study that analyzed lesional tissue using PCR, more than one type of HPV was detected in 22% of cases of CIN 1.[26] Using fluorescence in situ hybridization, it has been shown that infection of a single cell by two different HPV types can occur.[27]

High-grade dysplasia, or CIN 2 and CIN 3, is frequently associated with HPV 16. HPV 16 has been detected in 30% to 77% of women with CIN 2 and 3 in various studies.[25, 26] Approximately three fourths of high-grade lesions are associated with either HPV 16, 18, or members of the 30 s group (e.g., 31, 33, 35, 39). Unlike CIN 1, multiple types of HPV are uncommonly detected in women with CIN 2 or CIN 3.[26] The HPV types associated with CIN 2, CIN 3, and invasive cervical cancer are similar. HPV 16, 18, and 31 are the types most commonly identified in women with invasive cervical cancer from widely divergent geographic locations.[20] Other types that can be associated with invasive cervical cancer include HPV 45 and 56, other members of the 30s group, as well as HPV 51, 52, and 58.[20]

These associations between specific types of HPV and specific types of lesions have led to the classification of anogenital HPVs into three oncogenic risk groups.[20] The first group is termed low oncogenic risk viruses. Low oncogenic risk HPVs include types 6, 11, 42, 43, and 44, as well as most of the novel types of HPV. The low oncogenic risk viruses are commonly associated with condyloma acuminata and may sometimes be found in patients with CIN 1, but they are rarely associated with invasive cervical cancer. The second group of viruses is termed high oncogenic risk HPV types. These viruses are predominately HPV types 16, 18, and 31, which are the types commonly detected in women with CIN 2, CIN 3, and invasive cancer of the cervix, vulva, penis, and anus. HPV 45 and 56 are also frequently included in this group. The remaining types can be classified as being of intermediate oncogenic risk HPV types because they can be associated with CIN 2 and CIN 3 but are uncommonly detected in invasive anogenital cancers. Intermediate oncogenic risk types include HPV types 33, 35, 39, 51, and 52.

In vitro studies using tissue culture cells have provided an insight into the mechanism by which HPV *transforms* the cervical epithelium. The E6 and E7 ORFs represent the principal transforming genes of HPV.[28, 29] Expression of the E6 and E7 ORFs from high-oncogenic-risk HPVs such as 16 and 18 but not of low oncogenic risk HPVs such as 6 and 11 in established tissue culture cell lines causes the cells to become completely transformed.[30] A high efficiency of transformation of these already-immortalized tissue culture cell lines requires that both E6 and E7 be present. The two viral genes complement each other and are only weakly active when introduced alone. In addition to having in vitro transforming activity, both E6 and E7 are almost always actively transcribed in cervical cancers, suggesting that the over-regulated or unregulated expression of these genes is required for the maintenance of the transformed malignant phenotype.[31] This has been confirmed by studies demonstrating that inhibition of E6 and E7 expression by antisense mRNA leads to reversion to a nontransformed phenotype.[32] One way overexpression of the E6 and E7 ORFs might occur is through loss of E2 expression. The E2-encoded proteins regulate transcription of the early region, generally repressing E6 and E7 transcription.[33] In CIN 1 and in most cases of CIN 2 or CIN 3, HPV is episomal and the E2 ORF is intact.[34] However, in most cancers, the HPV DNA is integrated into cellular DNA.[35] Integration occurs in the E1/E2 region, leading to disruption and inactivation of these ORFs. Therefore, the control of E6 and E7 is lost, resulting in overexpression of E6 and E7 that is important for malignant transformation. These transforming genes appear to act by disrupting the normal control processes that regulate cellular growth. The E6 protein of HPV 16 binds to and causes the rapid degradation of the p53 protein, which is an important regulator of cellular growth and differentiation,[36–38] and the E7 protein appears to deregulate cell growth by binding to cyclin A, p107, and p105$^{RB}$ (retinoblastoma gene product). All of these factors are involved in regulating the progression of cells from the $G_1$ phase of the cell cycle into the S phase.[39, 40] This causes the loss of important cellular constraints to cell proliferation, thereby resulting in a loss of growth control.[41]

The above-mentioned model of cervical cancer pathogenesis based on E2 inactivation secondary to integration with resultant E6 and E7 overexpression is too simplistic and cannot fully explain the development of cervical cancer. For example, even though the vast majority of cervical cancers have HPV DNA integrated into the cellular DNA, in some invasive cancers, only episomal HPV DNA is detected.[34, 35] Likewise, fusion of HPV-associated transformed cervical epithelial cells with nontransformed cells results in the formation of nonmalignant hybrids despite the fact that there is continued overexpression of the E6 and E7 ORFs.[42] In vivo, there is, on average, a 10-year delay between an initial HPV infection and the development of cancer and only a small fraction of the patients exposed to high oncogenic risk HPVs will subsequently develop cancer. In vitro cultured human epithelial cells expressing the E6 and E7 ORFs are nonmalignant at early passages but become fully malignant at later passages.[43] This suggests that additional events or factors are probably important for the development of cervical cancer which may include induction of chromosomal instability with the development of aneuploidy, the site at which HPV integrates into the genome, and loss of cellular signals that regulate the expression of the E6 and E7 ORFs.[44]

## CERVICAL CANCER PRECURSOR LESIONS

Evidence strongly supports the premise that invasive cervical cancer is prefaced by an antecedent preinvasive phase. Epidemiologic data finds that these pre-invasive or precursor lesions (e.g., dyskaryosis, dysplasia, intraepithelial neoplasia, and squamous intraepithelial lesion) occur in women in their third to fifth decade of life. In contrast, the similar studies find that the peak age of invasive cervical cancer is in the fifth through seventh decade.[45-47] This lag has led investigators to postulate that the interval of progression from precursor lesions to invasive cancer is on the order of 10 to 15 years. The evidence is difficult to apply clinically in most instances, because the time from acquisition of the lesion is extremely difficult to assess for any given case. The progression of cervical cancer precursors to cervical cancer is also supported by histologic evidence of small foci of invasion emanating from otherwise usual cases of high-grade cervical cancer precursor lesions.

Whereas progression from high-grade precursor lesions to cervical cancer has been all but confirmed, progression of low-grade cervical cancer precursor lesions to high-grade cervical cancer precursors has now been almost completely dispelled.[48] Although many examples of concurrent low-grade and high-grade cervical cancer precursors have been documented, the association is believed to be coincidental. In situ hybridization frequently shows that different HPV types are found in concurrent lesions of different grades in the same cervix. This argues for separate infectious events rather than a progression from one lesion to the other. This molecular and morphologic data is supported by epidemiologic studies that find that most low-grade precursor lesions spontaneously regress, leaving only few lesions to persist and find only rare instances in which these lesions progress. Finally, it has been found that a high percentage of women who have high-risk HPV DNA but have no detectable lesions on their cervix will develop a high-grade cervical cancer precursor within 2 years.[12] These data validate the hypothesis that high-grade cervical cancer precursor lesions do not need to go through a lengthy low-grade phase but rather evolve rapidly into high-grade lesions.

### Terminology

Much controversy exists over the terminology used to refer to cervical cancer precursor lesions. The Bethesda System for the reporting of cervical cytology has created a uniform terminology that has been widely adopted in laboratories across the United States and is gaining acceptance worldwide.[49] This classification instituted a two-tiered system for evaluating cervical cancer precursors, substituting the previously used three- or four-tiered systems. Precursor lesions are divided into low-grade squamous intraepithelial lesions (LSIL) and high-grade squamous intraepithelial lesions (HSIL). The selection of a two-tiered classification over the previously used three-tiered classifications was made based largely on the desire to increase uniformity in reporting and a reduction in the interobserver variability found so pervasively in cytologic diagnoses. Subsequent molecular data showing that the high-grade lesions shared similar HPV types but differed from low-grade lesions provided some validation for this decision.[26] However ample clinical data continue to show that patients with moderate dysplasia (CIN 2) have different progression and regression rates than do patients with the severe dysplasia (CIN 3).[50-52] Caution has prevailed with regard to the Bethesda two-tiered system, and most laboratories include a three-tiered classification in addition to the Bethesda mandated two-tiered system.

Consensus does not exist when reporting cervical cancer precursor lesions that are identified in histologic sections. The two most common terms used to report cervical cancer precursor lesions in the United States are dysplasia and CIN, with CIN being significantly more prevalent. When initially proposed by Richart,[45, 53] the CIN classification was meant to describe lesions in a spectrum of progression from low-grade to high-grade lesions. Despite the current belief that progression does not occur from low-grade to high-grade lesions, the terminology offers the advantage of classifying lesions in a three-tiered scheme that is compatible with most clinical management algorithms. Finally, although initially criticized for erroneously designating these precursor lesions as neoplastic (intraepithelial *neoplasia*), recent data show that most cases of CIN III are clonal lesions and have aneuploid DNA, confirming their true neoplastic nature.[54-56] This is of particular relevance because in both prospective and retrospective studies, ploidy has been a good predictor of clinical behavior; the majority of cases of CIN that progress or persist have been aneuploid, whereas the majority of those that regress are diploid or polyploid.[57, 58]

Some authors have argued to create a two-tiered system (using the Bethesda System terminology) for both cytology and histopathology to facilitate the correlation between the two.[59] Strong arguments have been made in favor of such a classification. A two-tiered histologic diagnosis would reduce interobserver variability by the mere act of reducing the number of diagnostic options. In addition, the diagnosis could be directly correlated to the cytologic diagnosis without need for extrapolation. Desirable as these benefits might appear there are serious disadvantages to the two-tiered proposal. The benefit in the reduction of interobserver variability afforded by the two-tiered system serves mainly a cosmetic purpose. In this country, the critical decision to determine appropriate patient management is the differential between low grade (CIN 1) and high grade

(CIN 2). The problems caused by the interobserver variability between these two important diagnoses are not alleviated by the Bethesda proposed two-tiered category. In addition, when severe dysplasia was combined with carcinoma in situ into one category, CIN 3, studies had shown no difference in clinical characteristics or behavior between patients in the two groups. In contrast there are significant differences in the clinical characteristics and the clinical behavior of patients who have CIN 2 versus those who have CIN 3. Patients with CIN 2 are younger and have a significantly higher rate of regression than patients with CIN 3.[60] This distinct behavior has led to different therapeutic regimens for patients with these two diagnoses.

These authors continue to find a benefit in providing the clinician with the added information contained in a three-tiered system despite the risk of increasing interobserver variability. This is particularly important as medical therapy with immuno-modulators such as imiquimod (Aldara)[61, 62] have shown efficacy in the treatment of genital warts and are being proposed for the treatment of cervical cancer precursor lesions as an option to ablative therapy. These therapies are particularly attractive for patients who are at low risk of developing cervical cancer, such as patients with CIN 1 and some patients with CIN 2, but they are not as attractive for patients with significant risk for developing cervical cancer, such as patients with CIN 3 in whom a more cautious therapeutic option such as excision or ablation is proposed. In this chapter, we use the terminology suggested by the Bethesda System in describing cervical cytology and the CIN system for describing the histopathology of lesions.

## CYTOLOGY

The Pap smear continues to be the most widely used and most successful cancer-screening test in the world today. This simple test has reduced the incidence of cervical cancer in the United States by over 70% over the last 30 years.[63] Despite this great success, the sensitivity of the Pap smear has recently come into question. Two large meta-analyses of studies examining the performance of the conventional Pap smear have shown that the sensitivity of this test for the detection of all grades of cervical cancer precursor lesions is at best 50%.[64, 65] The realization of the fallibility of the conventional Pap smear and increasing concerns over the medicolegal liability of those performing it, have fueled technologic advances in the field. Two technologic modalities have emerged as practical and are approved by the Food and Drug Administration (FDA) for use in clinical practice. The first modality is that of computer-assisted screening devices. The second is that of liquid-based sample collection, followed by machine-made thin-layer slides.

Computer-assisted screening devices have been shown to reduce the incidence of false-negative re-sults in Pap tests.[66, 67] In addition, one instrument (the Autopap 300) is approved by the FDA for primary screening with the capability of rendering machine-only diagnoses of within normal limits for the 25% of the lowest-risk tests in a non-high risk screening population. Usage issues regarding the definition of the high-risk patient, unacceptability of many slides to be read by the device, combined with the increase in cost and low reimbursement rates by insurance carriers have delayed the widespread acceptance of this technology. Despite its slow penetrance of laboratories, computer-assisted screening devices offer tremendous promise for the future, particularly in times in which the number of human cytotechnologists are decreasing in numbers while demand for screeners is increasing.

Liquid-based, thin-layer cytology is founded on the immediate fixation of the cell sample into a fixative rather than on the application of the cell sample to a dry glass slide. This seminal change in the collection of the sample improves fixation and reduces drying artifacts over the conventional Pap smear and forms the basis of the improvement in the appearance of this test over the conventional test. Following fixation, the cell sample undergoes thorough mixing in order to create a homogeneous mixture of normal and abnormal components in the sample before giving rise to an aliquot of the sample that will be made into a slide. This mixing step has been shown to distribute abnormal cells effectively throughout the sample so that virtually all of the aliquots of the sample are diagnostically similar.[68] The success of this procedure not only increases diagnostic sensitivity but also allows for ancillary molecular testing from the residual cells in the collection vial for clinical testing. The procedure is completed by the placement of a thin layer of cell sample onto a glass slide. This process minimizes cell overlapping and obscuring of potentially diagnostic cells by blood, inflammatory cells, or other debris and significantly reduces the percentage of tests that are unsatisfactory or limited by factors that impede interpretation. A large body of data now exists showing a significant increase in the sensitivity of thin-layer cytology over conventional cytology for the diagnosis of cervical cancer precursor lesions.[69–73]

### Low-Grade Squamous Intraepithelial Lesions

LSILs are most prevalent in women in their early reproductive age (ages 16 to 26) or at the onset of sexual activity.[46, 74, 75, 76] They are uncommon in women in the remainder of their reproductive lives, only to become somewhat more common in mid to late menopause (age older than 58). The cytologic diagnosis of LSIL is made on the identification of abnormal squamous cells that have a cell size equivalent to a normal superficial or intermediate cell. Diagnostic abnormalities include enlargement of the

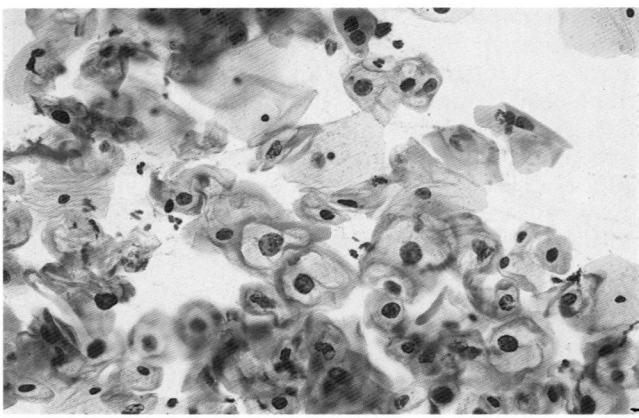

**FIGURE 36–1.** Low-grade squamous intraepithelial lesion. Numerous altered squamous cells are present that are the size of normal intermediate or superficial cells. The nuclei in these cells are enlarged, irregular, and hyperchromatic. In many instances, the cytoplasm shows margination concentrically around the nucleus to form a cleared out cavity with sharp internal borders.

nucleus, irregularity of the nuclear membrane, and irregular chromatin distribution. Additional features that aid in the diagnosis and are frequently seen include hyperchromasia, as well as cavitation of the cytoplasm immediately surrounding the nucleus to form a well-demarcated internal cytoplasmic border (Fig. 36–1). These cytoplasmic changes, commonly referred to as koilocytosis, should not be equated to a low-grade squamous epithelial lesion in the absence of the diagnostic nuclear features (CD Fig. 36–1). *Koilocytosis* is a descriptive term that implies infection by HPV. It should be made only in the presence of the diagnostic nuclear features and should not be used as a diagnosis.

### DIFFERENTIAL DIAGNOSIS OF LOW-GRADE SQUAMOUS INTRAEPITHELIAL LESIONS

The differential diagnosis of atypical cells resembling LSILs includes reactive and inflammatory squamous cells. Frequently, these changes are caused by infections with *Candida* or *Trichomonas* (CD Fig. 36–2). Squamous cells in these conditions often exhibit increased nuclear-to-cytoplasmic ratio, nuclear enlargement, increased chromatin content, and perinuclear halos that may mimic the true koilocytic cavity. The persistence of a smooth nuclear contour, evenly distributed chromatin, and the presence of small nucleoli are indicative of their benign nature. (CD Fig. 36–3). In perimenopausal and postmenopausal women, poorly maturing intermediate and parabasal squamous cells with perinuclear clearing may resemble LSILs (CD Fig. 36–4). Again in this instance, careful examination of the nuclear features will aid in the determination of these reactive or inflammatory lesions. In general, smooth nuclear membranes and evenly distributed chromatin will ascertain the benign nature of these mimics. When findings are inconclusive, the diagnosis of atypical

squamous cells of undetermined significance should be entertained (see later).

## High-Grade Squamous Intraepithelial Lesions

HSILs are most prevalent in women in their mid to late reproductive years (ages 26 to 48), although they may be seen at any age following the onset of sexual activity.[74, 77, 78] The cytological diagnosis of HSILs relies on the presence of abnormal squamous cells that are smaller than those seen in low-grade lesions. The average size of a high-grade squamous intraepithelial lesion is equivalent to that of a normal parabasal cell. Diagnostic abnormalities include nuclear enlargement, a marked increase in nuclear-to-cytoplasmic ratio, irregularity of the nuclear membrane, and irregular chromatin distribution. Commonly encountered features that aid the diagnosis also include marked hyperchromasia and abnormal nuclear shapes. (Fig. 36–2) (CD Fig. 36–5).

The differential diagnosis of HSIL can include reactive as well as inflammatory squamous cells commonly caused by infections with *Candida* or *Trichomonas* organisms. Notoriously, however, it will be inflamed or reactive immature squamous metaplasia that presents the greatest challenge to the cytopathologist. Unlike cells that are diagnostic of a HSIL, the cells seen with benign reactive immature squamous metaplastic epithelium almost always maintain a fine, evenly distributed chromatin and frequently contain prominent chromocenters or small nucleoli. In addition, although nuclear folds and nuclear grooves can be seen in metaplasia, true nuclear membrane irregularities are characteristic only of SILs and should not be tolerated as features of reactive cells (CD Fig. 36–6). Finally, the nuclear-to-cytoplasmic ratio in squamous metaplasia should

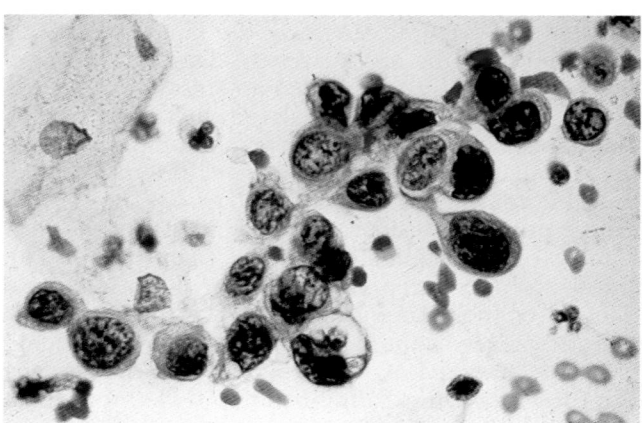

**FIGURE 36–2.** High-grade squamous intraepithelial lesion. Numerous altered squamous cells that are the size of normal parabasal cells are present. The nuclei in these cells are large, occupying most of the volume of the cell. In addition, the nuclei show hypercromasia, irregular nuclear clumping, and severe irregularities of the nuclear contour.

be significantly lower than 50%, whereas in HSILs, the nuclear-to-cytoplasmic ratio must approach 50% and is almost always greater. Inevitably, as in the differential diagnosis of LSIL, some difficult cases contain cells in which the cellular features are indeterminate between reactive squamous metaplasia and HSIL. It is these cases in which the authors most encourage the diagnosis of atypical squamous cells of undetermined significance because it is this group of atypical Pap smears that will yield the highest percentage of high grade lesions.[79, 80]

## Atypical Squamous Cells of Undetermined Significance

The diagnosis of atypical squamous cells of undetermined significance (ASCUS) is an undesirable but inevitable diagnosis that results from the morphologic variability of squamous cells in different physiologic and pathologic states. Although it is inevitable, the frequency with which the diagnosis of ASCUS is made should be minimized because its clinical management is fraught with controversy.[81] A general recommendation is that the frequency of an ASCUS diagnosis be kept under 5% of all Pap smears in a routine screening population or two and one half times the percent of all SILs diagnosed by the lab.[81, 82] The percentage of women with a cytologic diagnosis of ASCUS who harbor biopsy-proven dysplasia is generally accepted to be around 20%.[80, 83] Importantly, some series show that more cases of CIN 2 and CIN 3 are identified in patients with a cytologic diagnosis of ASCUS than are identified in patients with a cytologic diagnosis of HSIL.[84, 85] This fact underscores the importance of ASCUS and the significance of this diagnosis to the treating clinician. Although criteria exist to separate most cervical cancer precursor lesions from lesions that are reactive in nature, no single criteria or combination of criteria will effectively do so in all cases. Therefore, the category of ASCUS is reserved for lesions in which a clear distinction between reactive and neoplastic cells cannot be made. Paradoxically, the Bethesda System allows for the subclassification of ASCUS lesions into those in which a reactive process is favored and those in which a neoplastic origin is favored. The latter provision was instituted in an effort to aid in the clinical management of patients with this diagnosis. Although a few reports stratifying patients with a cytologic diagnosis of ASCUS who were at risk for having dysplasia using this system were extremely encouraging,[86, 87] the majority of reports thereafter failed to confirm a sufficiently high rate of distinction using this morphologic triage of patients to provide meaningful clinical application.[83, 84, 88, 89]

Results of two large clinical trials have shown that detection of high-oncogenic-risk HPV types using the HC II assay effectively separates patients with a cytologic diagnosis of ASCUS into a group with a high likelihood of having CIN 2 or CIN 3

and a group that is at no increased risk of harboring high-grade CIN. Patients with a diagnosis of ASCUS that are positive high-oncogenic-risk HPV have a significant risk of harboring high-grade CIN. In contrast, women with a diagnosis of ASCUS who are negative for high-oncogenic-risk HPV are at no increased risk of having a HSIL compared with women with a normal Pap smear result.[88, 90] The HPV test using the HC II test can be performed by collecting a sample of cells separately into a transport media or by using the residual cell sample from the liquid-based cytology sample. The option of using the residual cell sample offers the clinically desirable option of automatically testing the sample of patients with a cytologic diagnosis of ASCUS without the necessity of an additional patient visit or patient clinician interaction. If a patient is found to be HPV positive, she is referred to colposcopy for further diagnostic work-up. However, if the patient is negative for high-risk HPV, the risk of a HSIL is low enough to recommend screening at the routine interval. This triage strategy has been shown to reduce unnecessary colposcopic examinations in 45% to 60% of women with ASCUS, reducing the morbidity, anxiety, and cost associated with that procedure.[88, 90] Cost analyses of triage strategies have shown a cost savings in the management of patients using HPV testing rather than cytology-based or colposcopy-based strategies, which were used previously.[88] Results from the National Cancer Institute's sponsored ASCUS-Low Grade SIL Triage Study (ALTS) show a statistically significant improvement in the detection of CIN 2 and CIN 3 when patients were triaged to either immediate colposcopy or using HC II HPV detection when compared with patients followed with Pap smears.[90] These data have encouraged us to advocate the use of high-oncogenic-risk HPV testing in patients with a cytologic diagnosis of ASCUS to define the likelihood of dysplasia in the patient and the need for a colposcopic work-up. The criteria for the diagnosis of ASCUS are vaguely defined. Cells with an enlarged nucleus, purportedly to be two and one half to three times the size of a normal intermediate squamous cell nucleus, or cells that contain slight nuclear irregularities or hyperchromasia that are insufficient for a diagnosis of SIL are classified as ASCUS (Fig. 36–3) (CD Fig. 36–7).

## Cytology of Cervical Adenocarcinoma

Glandular lesions of the cervix are not as easily detected on cytologic examination as are squamous lesions.[91, 92] Speculation as to the reason for such decreased sensitivity of the Pap smear for adenocarcinoma of the cervix and its precursor lesions vary widely. It is possible that the cytologic features of early adenocarcinoma are so subtle that they are prey to not being recognized by the screening cytotechnologist or the diagnosing pathologist.[93] It is

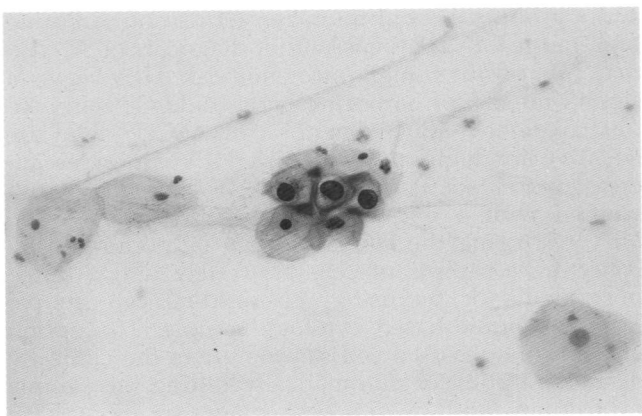

**FIGURE 36–3.** Atypical squamous cells of undetermined significance. The squamous cells shown exhibit an enlarged hyperchromatic nucleus. Despite the hyperchromasia, the nuclear membranes are smooth. The chromatin, although increased, is evenly dispersed throughout the nucleus.

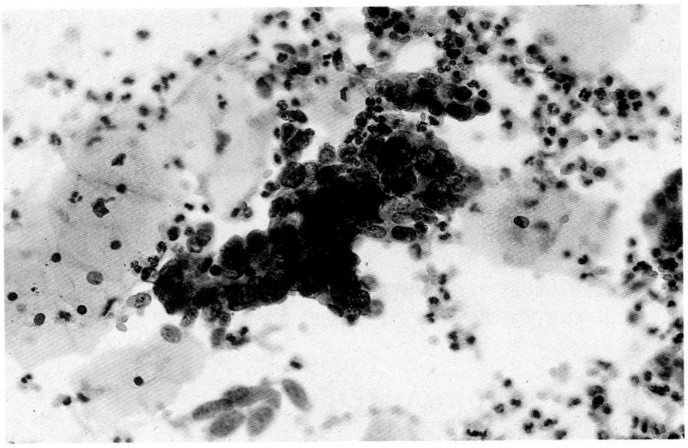

**FIGURE 36–4.** Cervical adenocarcinoma. A cluster of abnormal endocervical glandular cells is present centrally. The cells show marked crowding, as evidenced by nuclear overlapping and molding, as well as feathering. The nuclei are greatly enlarged and show irregular nuclear clumping and extreme hypercromasia.

also likely that the anatomic location of glandular lesions, preferentially found in the endocervical canal, makes them less likely to be adequately sampled.[93] The observed increase in the rate of diagnosis of adenocarcinoma in situ (AIS) has been explained to some extent by the advances in the design of Pap smear sampling devices that target the endocervical canal such as the cytobrush of the cervical broom device.

The cytologic characteristics that allow for a diagnosis of cervical adenocarcinoma include abundant glandular cellular material, marked crowding of endocervical glandular cells within clusters, architectural aberrations of glandular groups, and cytologic atypia.[93] The first of these criteria is helpful in that abundance of endocervical material on the slide draws attention to a possible abnormality [CD Figs. 36–8 and 36–9]. It has been our experience that virtually all cases of cervical adenocarcinoma contain at least several cellular groups of abnormal-appearing endocervical glandular cells. In most instances, the groups are larger than those expected with a normal endocervix. Examination of these cell groups at a higher magnification is essential for the recognition of the other more specific parameters. Marked cellular crowding is an essential component in the diagnosis of endocervical adenocarcinoma. Although normal endocervical cell clusters may appear crowded owing to gland folding or overlap (CD Fig. 36–10), true crowding as recognized by nuclear overlapping with occasional molding is seen only in adenocarcinoma or HSIL involving glands (CD Fig. 36–11). This crowding is the cytologic representation of the nuclear stratification seen in cervical adenocarcinoma. Stratification is also responsible for many of the architectural aberrations seen within cell clusters of glandular lesions on Pap smears such as crowded strips or glandular formations within endocervical cell clusters (CD Fig. 36–12). Feathering, a feature characterized by the irregular outlin-

ing of an endocervical gland cluster caused by nuclei protruding from edges of the cluster, is a result of the marked loss of cytoplasmic mucin and an increase in nuclear-to-cytoplasmic ratio also seen in adenocarcinoma (CD Fig. 36–13). If the architectural aberrations just mentioned are accompanied by nuclear enlargement, hyperchromasia, and coarsely granular clumping of the chromatin, then the findings are diagnostic of cervical adenocarcinoma (Fig. 36–4) (CD Fig. 36–14).

## Atypical Glandular Cells of Undetermined Significance

As with the squamous lesions of the cervix, some severe reactive changes as well as some high-grade squamous lesions present with features that that may mimic those of adenocarcinoma. When the features of such lesions are severe, the certainty of their histogenesis or their neoplastic nature can come into significant doubt. It is in these instances that the diagnosis of atypical glandular cells of undetermined significance (AGUS) should be entertained (Fig. 36–5). As in the case of atypical squamous cells of undetermined significance, the diagnosis of atypical glandular cells AGUS should be made only in instances when significant doubt exists as to the benign or neoplastic nature of cells in question. Cases of AGUS should represent significantly less than one half of 1% of all Pap smears diagnosed in a routine screening population.[94] As with ASCUS, the definition of AGUS is subjective and has a high degree of interobserver variability. Importantly, the percent of patients diagnosed with AGUS who have a significant biopsy-confirmed abnormality is nearly twice that as with a diagnosis of ASCUS. Also, patients with a diagnosis of AGUS harbor a much higher percentage of high-grade cervical cancer pre-

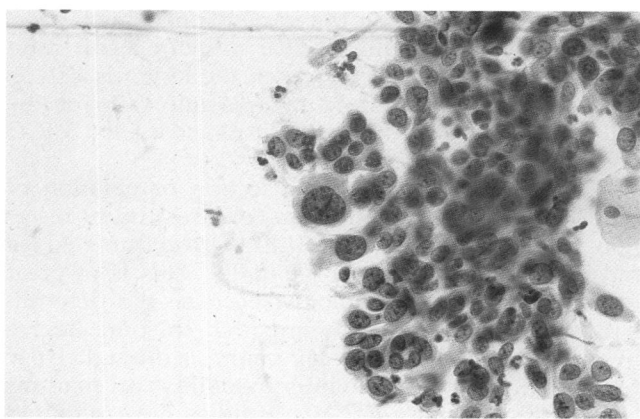

**FIGURE 36–5.** Atypical glandular cells of undetermined significance. The group of glandular cells shown exhibit moderate crowding, but no nuclear overlapping or molding is observed. The cells vary greatly in size, have lost their polarity, and show marked differences in nuclear size and shape. Despite the nuclear variability, the individual nuclei have evenly dispersed chromatin and smooth nuclear membranes.

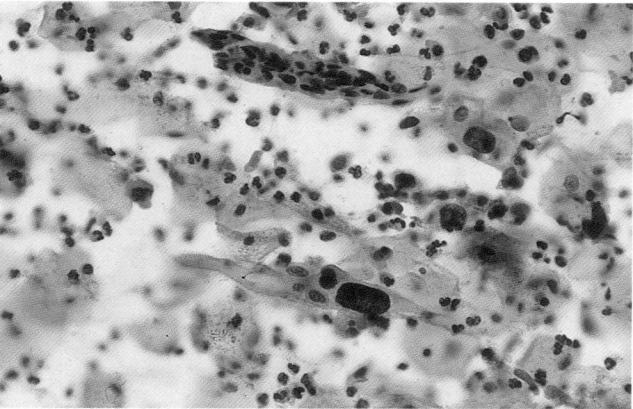

**FIGURE 36–6.** Invasive squamous carcinoma. Numerous markedly abnormal cells are present. The abnormal cells vary greatly in size and shape but are all characterized by extreme hyperchromasia and nuclear irregularities. The cytoplasm of some cells is keratinized and elongated (tadpole cells).

cursors and cervical cancer than do patients with a diagnosis of ASCUS.[95] The biopsy diagnosis of patients with a cytologic diagnosis of AGUS is varied and contains lesions that are squamous as well as glandular. Patients with a diagnosis of AGUS in whom a lesion is discovered more frequently have a high-grade squamous intraepithelial lesion rather than an adenocarcinoma.[96] Finally, in cases in which adenocarcinoma is diagnosed on biopsy, the most common location of the primary tumor is the cervix, followed by the endometrium, and finally, the ovary. Therefore, it is paramount that aberrations of glandular cell groups should be of great concern to the cytologist. Cytologic features most likely to elicit an appropriate diagnosis of AGUS include clusters or strips of endocervical cells displaying some degree of nuclear enlargement or hyperchromasia. When such changes are accompanied by some degree of crowding of cells but lack the architectural aberrations that are diagnostic of adenocarcinoma a diagnosis of AGUS should be strongly considered (CD Fig. 36–15).

## The Cytology of Cervical Cancer

The cytologic diagnosis of squamous cervical cancer can be made with a high degree of specificity, but its sensitivity has been questioned. Features that ensure the accurate diagnosis of cancer include numerous abnormal cells, a significant decrease in the normal cell population, and the presence of degenerated blood or necrotic debris (Fig. 36–6) (CD Fig. 36–16).[97] Caution should be observed in making a diagnosis of cancer in cases lacking most of these features, because HSIL can present with numerous abnormal cells, some of which can be large and have abnormal shapes that resemble those of cancer. Caution not to overcall these cases is clinically justi-

fied. The diagnostic management of patients with a cytologic diagnosis of HSIL is the same as that of patients with a cytologic diagnosis of cancer. Conversely, the erroneous diagnosis of cancer in a patient may result in unnecessarily aggressive workups in order to completely exclude such a serious presumptive diagnosis. The cytologic diagnosis of invasive adenocarcinoma has been shown to be more fraught with error than that of invasive squamous cancer. Studies have shown that the distinction between in situ and invasive adenocarcinoma has both a high false-positive rate as well as a high false-negative rate.[98]

## HISTOPATHOLOGY

CIN is characterized by abnormal cellular proliferation, maturation, and cytologic atypia. The cytologic abnormalities included hyperchromatic nuclei, abnormal chromatin distribution, nuclear pleomorphism, and increased nuclear-to-cytoplasmic ratio. Nuclear atypia is the hallmark of CIN. The nuclear borders are irregular, and the chromatin is coarse, granular (salt and pepper), or filamentous throughout the nuclear mass. Ultrastructurally, both the nuclear and cytoplasmic alterations of CIN are consistent with a progressive lack of normal differentiation.[99] There is a decrease in glycogen, tonofilaments, desmosomes, and specialized junctional units with decreasing histologic differentiation. These alterations are correlated with a progressive decrease in cellular adhesions, basal pseudopodia, and cell contact inhibition demonstrated by time-lapse cinematography in cells grown in vitro.[100, 101] The traditional grading of intraepithelial neoplasia is based on the proportion of the epithelium occupied by basaloid, undifferentiated cells, reflecting a progressive loss of epithelial maturation and

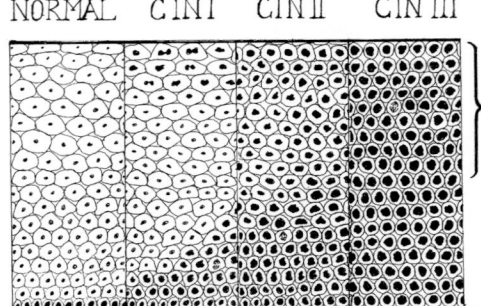

**FIGURE 36-7.** Cervical intraepithelial neoplasia grading scheme. This diagrammatic depiction of squamous epithelium shows both the classic grading scheme based on the content of parabasaloid cells as well as a newly proposed system based on cytology. In the classic scheme, dysplastic lesions containing atypical parabasaloid cells in the lower one third of the epithelium represents CIN I. Lesions that contain atypical parabasaloid cells in the lower two thirds of epithelium are considered CIN II and lesions with parabasaloid cells occupying greater than two thirds of the epithelium are diagnostic of CIN III. In the newly proposed scheme, cells in the upper half of the epithelium are evaluated for cell size and nuclear-to-cytoplasmic ratio. If the cells in the upper half of epithelium are the size of a superficial or intermediate cell with atypical nuclei then they are graded as CIN I. If the cells in the upper half of the epithelium are the size of parabasal cells with atypical nuclei, then they are either graded CIN II or CIN III. The distinction between CIN II and CIN III is made based on the nuclear-to-cytoplasmic ratio. If the nuclear-to-cytoplasmic ratio is 50% or less, the lesion is graded as CIN II. If this nuclear-to-cytoplasmic ratio is greater than 50%, then the lesion in graded as a CIN III.

decreasing glycogenization with increasing lesion severity.[47] Therefore, the epithelial alterations that comprise CIN were semiquantitatively classified into three categories: CIN grade 1—neoplastic, basaloid cells occupying the lower third of the epithelium; CIN grade 2—basaloid cells occupying the lower third to two thirds of the epithelium, and CIN grade 3—basaloid cells occupying two thirds to the full thickness of the epithelium (Fig. 36-7).

The classic grading system, albeit effective in many cases, is difficult to apply uniformly to all cervical biopsy specimens. Of particular concern are biopsy specimens in which the epithelium is tangentially cut or otherwise poorly oriented or where the epithelial layers are too few for the concept of "thirds" to be useful (Fig. 36-8). In these instances, these authors apply cytologic criteria to the cells in the superficial half of the epithelium to determine the grade of the lesion (see Fig. 36-7). In evaluating a biopsy specimen in this fashion, the pathologist abstracts the size of the cells composing the superficial half of the dysplastic area and evaluates their nuclear-to-cytoplasmic ratio. If the cells are the size of an intermediate or superficial cell and have nuclear to cytoplasmic ratios well under 50%, then the lesion is virtually always CIN 1. In contrast, if the cells in the upper half of the epithelium are the size of parabasal cells, then they will always represent a high-grade dysplasia, that is, CIN 2 or CIN 3. Further determination of grade among the high-grade

lesions can be made on the basis of their nuclear-to-cytoplasmic ratio. If the nuclear to cytoplasmic ratio is less than or equal to 50% then the lesion is CIN 2, whereas if the nuclear to cytoplasmic ratio of the cells is greater than 50%, the lesion is a CIN 3 (CD Figs. 36-17 to 36-23).

The therapy of CIN is resection or ablation of the lesion. In the United States, electrosurgical resection using loop electrodes (LEEP procedure) is the most common therapeutic modality. This is of great importance to the pathologist because the determination of margins may be impaired to some degree by the presence of thermal injury. Although early reports warned of the interpretability of margins with LEEP specimens,[102] later studies have reported that the interpretability of margins is comparable to that of cold-knife conization specimens.[103] These authors recognize that in rare instances thermal injury may preclude margin interpretation but find that in the vast majority of cases, the degree of thermal injury present has little detrimental effect on margin determination (CD Figs. 36-24 to 36-27)

## Cervical Intraepithelial Neoplasia Grade 1

CIN 1 is the cervical cancer precursor lesion with the highest rate of spontaneous regression and lowest rate of progression to cervical cancer. Nasiell and coworkers carried out one of the largest long-term studies of women with CIN in Sweden. In this study, 555 women with mild dysplasia were followed on average for 39 months.[104] Regression to normal occurred in 62% of the women with CIN 1, there was persistence in 22%, and in 16%, there was progression of mild dysplasia to severe dysplasia or carcinoma in situ. Several studies have substantiated these findings, confirming that greater than 60% of CIN 1 regress spontaneously and nearly all the rest

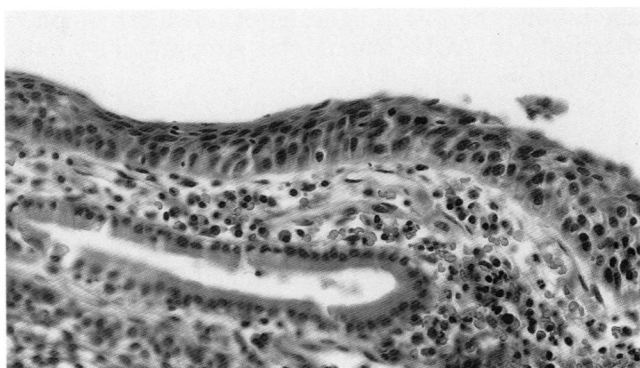

**FIGURE 36-8.** Cervical intraepithelial neoplasia. The epithelium in this lesion is thin, composed of four or fewer layers of squamous cells. Determining parabasaloid cells by thirds is extremely difficult. However, if the cells in the superficial half of the epithelium are evaluated for cell size and nuclear to cytoplasmic ratio, they show a cell size comparable to a parabasaloid cell with a nuclear cytoplasmic ratio of slightly less than 50%, making it a CIN II.

persist as CIN 1, whereas only rare lesions progress to carcinoma.[46, 105, 106]

It is now widely accepted that CIN 1 is the morphologic manifestation of productive HPV infections of the cervical squamous epithelium that can be caused by any of the anogenital types of HPV. These infections are almost always multifocal and cause distinct aberrations of the microarchitecture of the squamous epithelium. Normally, maturing squamous epithelium has a horizontal flow that resembles basket weave (Fig. 36–9). In contrast, HPV-induced lesions demonstrate an interruption in this smooth horizontal flow (Fig. 36–10). This change can be seen at a low magnification and should alert the pathologist as to the possible presence of a CIN 1. Confirmation of such a lesion depends on the diagnostic morphologic cellular changes. In productive HPV infection, large numbers of viral particles are produced and the infected squamous cells demonstrate the cytopathic effects of HPV.[107, 108] These cytopathic effects are now considered to be the most characteristic histologic features of CIN 1 and include significant nuclear enlargement, nuclear atypia, and perinuclear cytoplasmic cavitation of the cytoplasm with thickening of the cytoplasmic membrane. The diagnostic cells throughout most of the epithelium are large, comparable in cell volume to an intermediate or superficial cell. Nuclear atypia is characterized by enlargement, hyperchromasia, and irregularity of the nuclear membrane. Rarely, cells near the surface may have nuclei that are somewhat smaller and pyknotic. The combination of nuclear atypia and cytoplasmic cavitation has been termed koilocytosis or koilocytotic atypia (Fig. 36–11) (CD Fig. 36–28). Studies have shown that the E4 protein of HPV interacts with filaggrin, a cytokeratin-binding protein, and expression of the E4 protein in keratinocytes causes specific cytokeratin proteins to be lost from the cells and a collapse of the cytokeratin matrix.[109] This may lead to the cytoplasmic cavita-

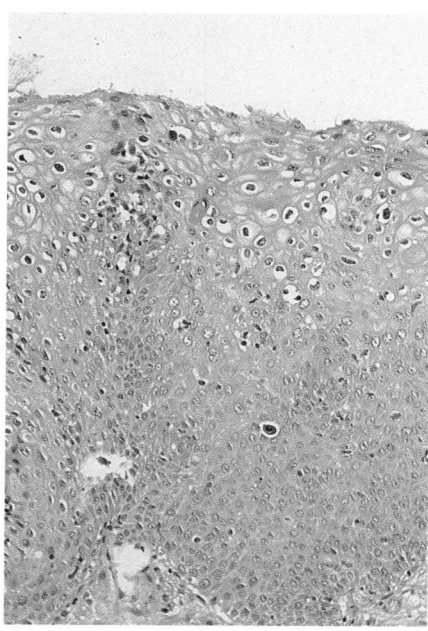

**FIGURE 36–10.** Cervical intraepithelial neoplasia grade 1. The squamous epithelium shown has a slight expansion of the basal row and lack of ordered maturation to superficial cells. The intermediate and superficial cells have also lost their polarity and there is an absence of horizontal flow. Near the surface the cells are the size of normal superficial cells. The nuclei in the superficial layers are larger, irregular, and hyperchromatic.

tion that is one of the features of koilocytosis. Mitotic spindle abnormalities that occur in productive HPV infections appear to interfere with the conduct of mitosis and cytokinesis. This leads to the polyploidy and binucleation that are usually present in productive HPV infections. Although the mechanism responsible for the interference by HPV of mitosis and cytokinesis is unknown, it has been shown that the capsid proteins of a closely related DNA tumor

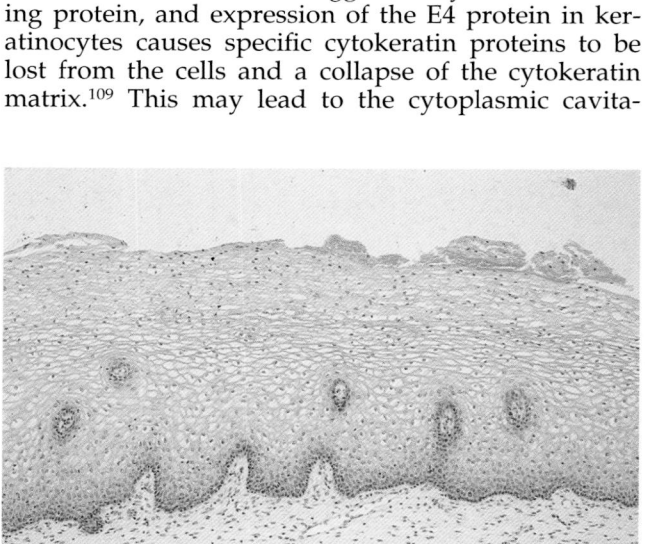

**FIGURE 36–9.** Normal squamous epithelium. The epithelium seen shows excellent polarity of the basal role with a rapid orderly maturation to superficial cells. The intermediate and superficial cells form a delicate, orderly mesh that gives the appearance of horizontal flow. The nuclei in the upper half of the epithelium are small and inconspicuous.

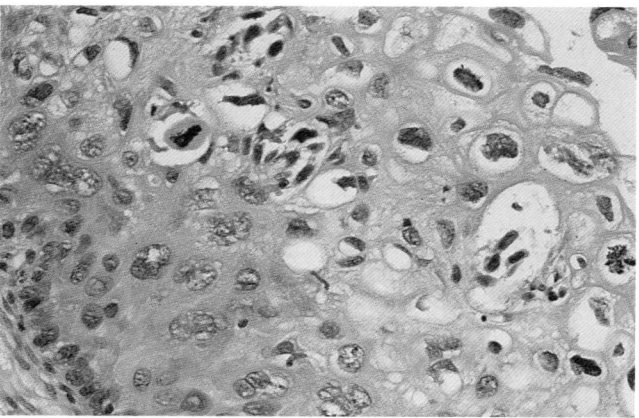

**FIGURE 36–11.** Koilocytes. The epithelium shown contains squamous cells with a markedly enlarged hyperchromatic nucleus with marked nuclear membrane irregularities. Prominent margination of the cytoplasm immediately surrounding the nucleus forming a sharp internal rim is present giving the appearance of a cavity surrounding the nucleus.

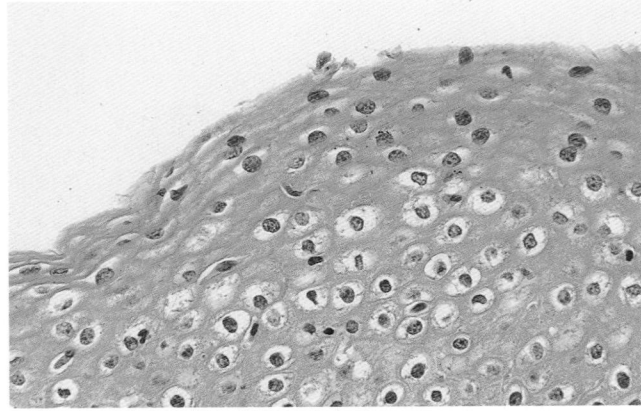

**FIGURE 36–12.** Benign reactive squamous epithelium. The squamous epithelium shown contains squamous cells with slightly enlarged nuclei that are surrounded by cytoplasmic clearing. In contrast to HPV induced changes, the nuclei are regular, contain smooth nuclear membranes, and have delicate evenly dispersed chromatin.

virus, polyoma, directly bind to the mitotic spindle of infected cells and may interfere with mitosis through this mechanism. Taken together, the histologic features of koilocytosis, nuclear atypia, architectural abnormalities, and multinucleation are pathognomonic of an HPV-infected epithelium at any site in the lower genital tract and are especially prominent in CIN 1 lesions.

## DIFFERENTIAL DIAGNOSIS

The most common problem in the differential diagnosis of CIN 1 is the overinterpretation of koilocytosis. This is due largely to the indiscriminate use of this term for squamous epithelium showing the slightest hint of cytoplasmic vacuolization in the absence of nuclear atypia. Normal metaplastic squamous epithelium with prominent glycogen vacuolization is often confused with CIN 1. In contrast to the focal distribution of koilocytes in CIN 1, the perinuclear clearing of normal squamous epithelium is not as sharply demarcated; the nuclei are not greatly enlarged or atypical (CD Fig. 36–29). Perinuclear clearing by itself may be associated with a variety of infectious microorganisms, notably *Trichomonas vaginalis*. In addition to the absence of severe nuclear atypia, normal stratification and maturation are maintained in such infections, whereas in HPV-associated lesions, there is some degree of cellular disorganization, particularly near the surface, and there is disturbance in the normal pattern of maturation. Nuclear changes associated with non-HPV induced lesions may be severe at times. Nuclear enlargement is particularly common with *Candida* infections, although they may be marked in other nonspecific inflammatory conditions. The distinction between these changes and those diagnostic of HPV-induced lesions is made based on the finer, more evenly distributed chromatin of the inflammatory le-

sions, as well as on the preservation of smooth nuclear contours (Fig. 36–12).

Studies from the United Kingdom measuring interobserver variability of histologic diagnosis of cervical lesions demonstrated that although agreement between pathologists was excellent for invasive lesions, and moderately good for CIN 2 and CIN 3, it was poor CIN 1.[109] The most significant discrepancies were in the ability of the pathologists to distinguish CIN 1 from reactive squamous proliferations. This suggests that the morphologic criteria routinely used to distinguish these two lesions have serious shortcomings. The importance of nuclear atypia in the distinction of CIN 1 from reactive lesions is confirmed by a number of studies. Correlation of HPV DNA with specific histologic findings has uniformly found that perinuclear halos in the absence of significant nuclear atypia are nonspecific features.[110, 111] Therefore, it appears clear that the identification of HPV-related changes and a diagnosis of CIN 1 should be made only when significant nuclear atypia accompanies perinuclear halos.

Because CIN I is a manifestation of productive HPV infection and reactive atypia is not, one approach that the pathologist can use as a quality control of their diagnosis of CIN 1 is to perform in situ hybridization (ISH) for HPV DNA on selected cervical biopsies (Fig. 36–13) (CD Figs. 36–30 and 36–31).[112, 113] Commercially available ISH kits have a sensitivity of approximately 50 copies of HPV DNA per cell and are sensitive enough to detect HPV DNA in approximately 80% of cervical lesions with the histologic features of CIN 1.[112, 114] Although HPV DNA can be detected in cervical swabs of cytologically normal women by PCR or Southern blot hybridization, HPV is not detected in normal or reactive epithelium by ISH.[112, 113] Therefore, these kits

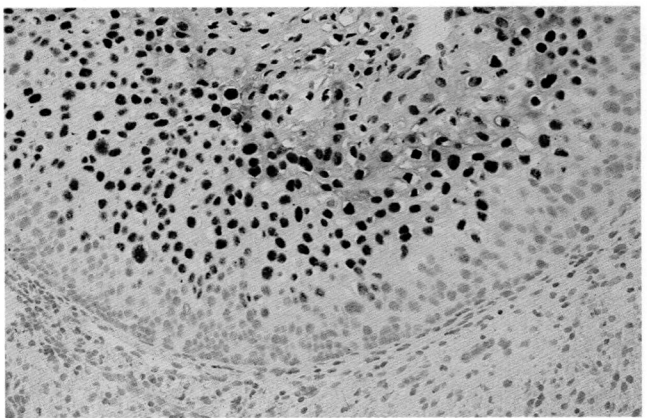

**FIGURE 36–13.** In situ hybridization for HPV. The image shown represents the results of in situ hybridization with biotinyllated HPV DNA probes. The squamous cells in the epithelium show positive reactivity to HPV probes as demonstrated by the red brown color of the nuclei (aminoethylcarbizole, AEC). Typical of HPV lesions, reactivity is seen in the intermediate and superficial layers of the squamous epithelium involved by HPV.

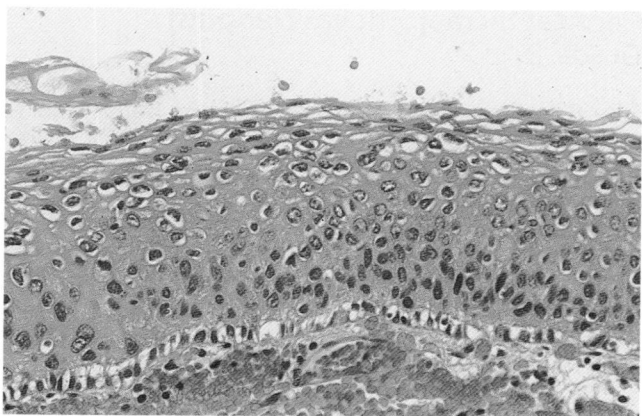

**FIGURE 36–14.** CIN II. The epithelium shows expansion of the parabasal layer with squamous cells containing atypical nuclei. The cells in the upper half of the epithelium lack appropriate maturation and are the size of parabasaloid cells. The nuclear to cytoplastic ratio is slightly less than 50%. The nuclei throughout the lesion show irregular nuclear outlines and irregular chromatin distribution.

can be used to distinguish CIN 1 from reactive processes that histologically mimic CIN 1. Because the ISH kits require a certain degree of technical expertise, pathologists should send specimens to be tested to reference laboratories if these tests are not performed routinely at their own institution. When ISH is used, it is important that the specimens be fixed in neutral buffered formalin or alcohol formalin and not be fixed in acidic fixatives such as Bouin's solution or Zenker's solution, which degrade the DNA and reduce sensitivity.[112, 115]

## Cervical Intraepithelial Neoplasia Grade 2

CIN 2 is associated with a more significant risk of progression to a higher grade lesion and to invasive carcinoma. Nasiell and coworkers prospectively followed 894 women with moderate dysplasia.[50] In this study, women with moderate dysplasia were followed without biopsy for an average of 51 months. Spontaneous regression occurred in 28% and progression to severe dysplasia or carcinoma in situ occurred in 50%, with the remainder of lesions persisting as CIN 2 throughout the study period. Other studies have shown an even greater rate of regression to normalcy of approximately 57% over a 2-year period.[60] These percentages are contrasted sharply with much lower regression rates of CIN 3 (see later).

Microscopically, CIN 2 is characterized by the presence of immature, parabasaloid cells involving the lower two thirds of the epithelium. In the vast majority of CIN 2 lesions, the nuclear-to-cytoplasmic ratio is increased yet remains below 50%. The cells frequently demonstrate significant variability in nuclear size and shape (anisonucleosis), loss of polarity, and variably increased numbers of mitotic figures (Fig. 36–14) (CD Fig. 36–32). Abnormal mitotic figures can be occasionally seen. When abnormal mitotic figures are clearly identified, the finding is of great use in distinguishing CIN 2 from the lower grade CIN 1 because they have been proposed as an excellent surrogate for the determination of aneuploidy.[112, 113, 116, 117]

### DIFFERENTIAL DIAGNOSIS

Immature squamous metaplasia, reparative squamous metaplasia, and atrophic squamous epithelium constitute the differential diagnosis of CIN 2. Immature squamous metaplasia can be distinguished from CIN 2 by its more orderly architecture, lack of anisonucleosis, and paucity of mitotic activity. In addition, immature squamous metaplasia is frequently associated with overlying glandular epithelium that is only rarely seen in CIN 2 (CD Fig. 36–33). Reactive squamous metaplasia is more problematic. Cases of severe reactive squamous metaplasia may exhibit significant irregularity in cell and nuclear size and a disorganized architecture (Fig. 36–15) (CD Figs. 36–34 and 36–35). In extreme cases, the distinction from CIN 2 may represent the most imposing challenge that the surgical pathologist may face. In these difficult cases, careful scrutiny of the nuclei provides the most useful information. Whereas the nuclei of CIN 2 is almost always hyperchromatic and contain irregularly distributed chromatin, reactive squamous metaplasia contains finer, more evenly distributed chromatin and frequently has small but prominent nucleoli, a feature almost always lacking in CIN 2. The presence of significant mitotic activity should greatly influence the decision in favor of CIN 2 because mitotic activity is extremely uncommon in squamous metaplasia.

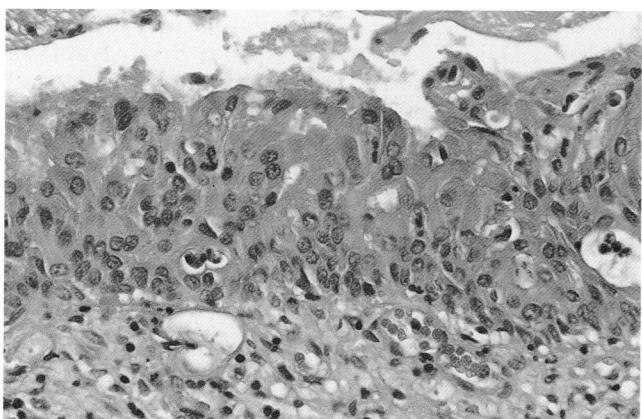

**FIGURE 36–15.** Immature squamous metaplasia. This epithelium shows squamous metaplastic cells exhibiting significant loss of polarity and lack of maturation. The nuclei are enlarged and slightly hyperchromatic but maintain smooth nuclear contour and even chromatin distribution. Careful scrutiny reveals the presence of endocervical glandular cells near the surface of the epithelium.

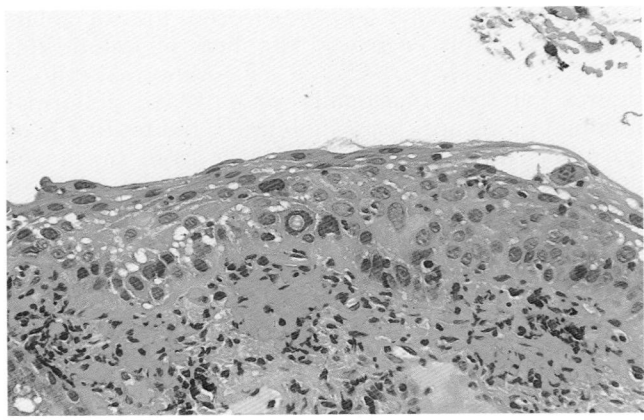

**FIGURE 36–16.** Reactive squamous metaplasia. The epithelium shown exhibits loss of polarity of the squamous metaplastic cells. The nuclei of the cells show moderate cell-to-cell variability as well as focal hyperchromasia. Careful examination reveals evenly dispersed chromatin in most cells, as well as absence of mitotic activity. Note the chronic inflammatory cells in both the submucosa and mucosa.

Some authors have suggested that the term atypical immature metaplasia be used to describe difficult lesions that are indeterminate between reactive squamous metaplasia and CIN 2.[118] We find that although there is merit in the associations found in these studies, the term atypical immature metaplasia has not gained wide acceptance and is extremely confusing to clinicians. For this reason, we discourage the use of atypical squamous metaplasia as a diagnostic term. In cases in which diagnostic ambiguity cannot be resolved, these authors recommend making a diagnosis of atypical squamous epithelium with a comment stating the unresolved differential diagnosis and a statement suggesting further follow-up. Finally, atrophic squamous epithelium can closely mimic CIN 2 owing to the small size of the cells throughout the height of the epithelium and its high nuclear-to-cytoplasmic ratio (Fig. 36–16) (CD Fig. 36–36). Distinction from dysplasia is made based on the uniformity in the size and shape of the nuclei in atrophy as in the absence of mitotic activity expected in these cases.

The difficulty in the differential diagnosis of CIN 2 and benign lesions again pose an area where continuous quality assurance measures may improve accuracy in diagnosis. As with CIN 1, virtually all cases of CIN 2 contain HPV. For this reason, the use of ISH with HPV probes can provide definitive proof of dysplasia in cases in which morphology alone is not diagnostic (CD Fig. 36–37). Hybridization with RNA or DNA probes directed to HPV are of greatest benefit when used to assess diagnostic accuracy retrospectively in groups of biopsies diagnosed as either CIN 2 or squamous metaplasia because most CIN 2 lesions will contain sufficient copies of HPV DNA to hybridize, whereas reactive or immature metaplasia and atrophic squamous epithelium will be uniformly negative.

## Cervical Intraepithelial Neoplasia Grade 3

CIN 3 is the cervical cancer precursor lesion that is most likely to progress to cervical cancer if it is left untreated. It is also the lesion least likely to regress.[51, 52, 119–121] In a prospective analysis, 71% of women with carcinoma in situ developed invasive carcinoma during a minimum follow-up period of 12 years.[120] In another study, CIN 3 progressed to invasive carcinoma in 29% of patients followed from 1 to 20 years, and the rate of progression increased directly with the length of follow-up, peaking at 34.6% in patients followed for 14 years.[52] Other long-term retrospective studies have demonstrated progression of carcinoma in situ to invasive cancer in 22% to 58% of cases.[52, 119]

The diagnosis of CIN 3 is established when atypical parabasaloid cells occupy greater than two thirds of the total epithelial thickness. The parabasaloid cells in CIN 3 have extremely high nuclear-to-cytoplasmic ratios almost always exceeding 50%. In addition, mitotic activity is generally high and mitotic figures should be expected in all but the smallest foci of CIN 3 (Fig. 36–17) (CD Fig. 36–38). Apoptosis is also frequently seen in CIN 3, has been suggested to be characteristic of this diagnosis,[122] and has been proposed to be a marker of progression to carcinoma.[123] The nuclei of CIN 3 share the properties of other CIN in that they contain irregularly distributed chromatin, hyperchromasia, and irregularities of the nuclear membrane. Although anisonucleosis is usually present, some CIN 3 lesions have extremely uniform-appearing nuclei. This is particularly the case in the basaloid-appearing CIN 3 lesions. Some investigators have subdivided CIN 3 into three cytologic subtypes: small cell anaplastic, large cell keratinizing, and large cell nonkeratinizing.[124] Again we believe that this distinction has little clinical significance and may cause confusion to

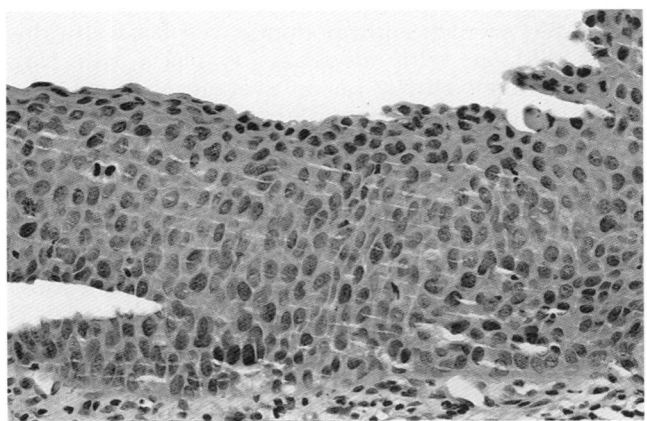

**FIGURE 36–17.** CIN III. The epithelium shown exhibits a complete lack of squamous maturation. The cells are small with a nuclear cytoplasmic ratio in excess of 50%. The nuclei are large and irregular, and contain dark irregularly distributed chromatin. Mitotic activity is abundant.

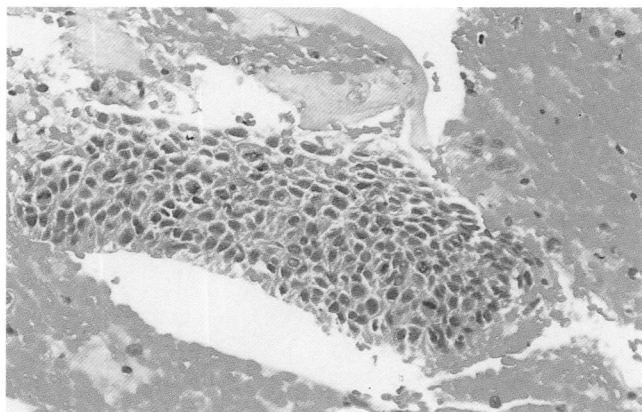

**FIGURE 36–18.** Endocervical curettage. This strip of atypical squamous cells in endocervical curettage contains small, parabasaloid cells with a high nuclear cytoplasmic ratio, hyperchromasia, and the presence of mitotic figures. The findings are diagnostic of high-grade dysplasia in endocervical curettage.

the clinician; so we discourage the use of this subclassification recommending that all cases be diagnosed solely as CIN 3.

The extremely high nuclear-to-cytoplasmic ratio seen in CIN 3 makes its identification extremely reliable when using cytologic criteria on biopsy specimens. This is of particular relevance, because many cases of CIN 3 occur in epithelial segments, with few layers making its division into thirds impossible. In these instances, identification of the parabasaloid cells with a nuclear-to-cytoplasmic ratio of greater than 50% in the upper half of the epithelium will ensure a diagnosis of CIN 3 (CD Fig. 36–39). Similarly, small strips of CIN III in endocervical curettage specimens can be distinguished from reactive mimics by this feature as well as by the presence of mitotic activity (Fig. 36–18) (CD Fig. 36–40).

### DIFFERENTIAL DIAGNOSIS

The differential diagnosis of CIN 3 is similar to that of CIN 2, and criteria for their distinction is similar. In the case of CIN 3, immature squamous metaplasia, particularly when occurring in a gland duct and cases of severe atrophy represent the most serious challenge to the surgical pathologist. In the case of immature squamous metaplasia involving glands, the absence of anisonucleosis, euchromasia, and even chromatin distribution are helpful features that distinguish them from CIN 3 (CD Fig. 36–41). Particularly helpful though is the high likelihood of encountering mitotic figures in CIN 3, which is contrasted to cases of squamous metaplasia in which mitotic figures are rare and limited to the basal areas. Transitional metaplasia of the cervix is a rarely encountered change that may also resemble CIN 3. The epithelium in this entity appears indistinguishable at times from normal urothelium. The small cell volume and moderate nuclear-to-cytoplasmic ratio give it a crowded appearance that may be confused

with high-grade dysplasia. Distinction between transitional metaplasia and CIN 3 is based on the regular nuclear membranes, even distribution of chromatin, nuclear grooves, and absence of mitotic activity seen in transitional metaplasia.[125] The immunophenotype of transitional metaplasia shares more similarities with urothelium than with squamous epithelium, expressing CK 13, CK 17, and CK 18 but not CK 20, a virtually identical pattern to normal urothelium.[126] Finally, profound atrophy alone or reactive changes in atrophic epithelium can be similarly distinguished from CIN 3 by the absence of mitotic activity and the more banal nuclear features generally seen in the atrophy (see CD Fig. 36–41). In difficult cases, the distinction between CIN 3 and atrophic epithelium can be greatly aided by the use of immunohistochemical markers directed at antigens of cell proliferation such as Ki-67 or MIB-1. Studies have shown that cervical epithelial cells in cases of atrophy display a low rate of proliferating cells and that these cells are limited to the basal rows. This is in contrast to cases of CIN 3, in which a high proportion of cervical cells stain positively for these markers throughout all epithelial layers.[127]

## Cervical Adenocarcinoma Precursors

It is now well accepted that, like squamous carcinoma, adenocarcinoma of the cervix has a precursor lesion: AIS. The mean age at diagnosis of women with AIS ranges from 39 to 46 years and is about 10 years lower than the mean age at which invasive adenocarcinoma of cervix is diagnosed.[128–130] The age relationship between AIS and invasive adenocarcinoma is similar to that of CIN 3 and invasive squamous cell carcinoma, and suggests that AIS is a precursor lesion.[131] However, unlike squamous lesions of the cervix in which high-grade precursors occur more frequently than invasive cancer, exactly the opposite relationship exists between AIS and invasive adenocarcinoma of the cervix. Invasive glandular lesions are more common than noninvasive glandular lesions. A number of reasons have been proposed for this apparent discrepancy including the fact that AIS is more difficult to detect both cytologically and colposcopically than is CIN and therefore might not be detected before the development of invasive adenocarcinoma. Additional support implicating AIS as a precursor of invasive adenocarcinoma comes from several anecdotal case reports and two small series of patients who had cytologic or histologic evidence of AIS several years before the detection of invasive adenocarcinoma.[132–134] In a cytologic study, Boddington and associates found that 6 of 13 women with invasive adenocarcinoma had previous Pap smears containing atypical endocervical cells 2 to 8 years before the diagnosis of cancer.[132] Similarly, Boon and colleagues found that 5 of 18 women with invasive adenocarcinoma had unrecognized AIS on cervical biopsies 3 to 7 years before detection of the invasive lesion.[133]

The proportion of AIS that occurs in association with CIN ranges from 24% to 75%.[130, 135–139] This suggests that the two types of lesions may share a common etiology. Using ISH, Tase and coworkers[140] examined eight cases of AIS for the presence of HPV DNA and found that five of the cases contained HPV and that, unlike CIN lesions analyzed with the same method, the majority of cases of AIS were associated with HPV 18 as opposed to HPV 16. Since this initial report, two other groups have analyzed AIS for the presence of HPV DNA and it appears clear that the majority of cases of AIS are associated with HPV DNA. Farnsworth and associates[141] detected HPV DNA in 89% of patients with AIS, and the ratio of HPV 18 to HPV 16 in positive cases was 2:1. In a series of eight cases, Griffin and colleagues[142] used PCR to detect HPV in 63% of patients with AIS, but HPV 18 was not detected. In contrast to AIS, an association between less severe atypical glandular lesions of the cervix and HPV has not been established. In the original study by Tase and associates,[131] only 2 of 36 cases of endocervical atypical hyperplasia contained HPV DNA.

AIS is characterized by the presence of architecturally normal endocervical glands that are lined by atypical columnar epithelial cells that cytologically resemble the cells of invasive adenocarcinoma but show no evidence of invasion (CD Figs. 36–42 and 36–43). These cells have markedly enlarged, elongated, hyperchromatic nuclei with granular chromatin. The amount of cytoplasm is greatly reduced, as is the intracellular mucin. The cells are crowded and pseudostratified or stratified, forming two or more rows, and can become cribriform within the glands. AIS may involve glands focally, multifocally, or diffusely. Typically some glands show an abrupt transition between normal epithelium and AIS (Fig. 36–19). Mitotic figures, including AMFs, are common. Architecturally, the glands of AIS can have numerous outpouchings and complex papillary infoldings, and may display a cribriform pattern focally (CD Fig. 36–44).

## Nondiagnostic Glandular Atypia

The terms endocervical glandular dysplasia, cervical intraepithelial glandular neoplasia, and atypical endocervical glandular hyperplasia have been proposed to describe lesions that are not diagnostic yet cause concern as to the possibility of AIS. Authors have gone as far as to suggest a causal association between these conditions and AIS despite the absence of studies more than coincidentally relating the two entities. Morphologic evidence suggests that AIS is not preceded by lesser degrees of glandular atypia. Commonly with AIS, the involved glands are observed to be only partially involved. In these cases, the transition from benign endocervical epithelium to AIS is abrupt, without evidence of incre-

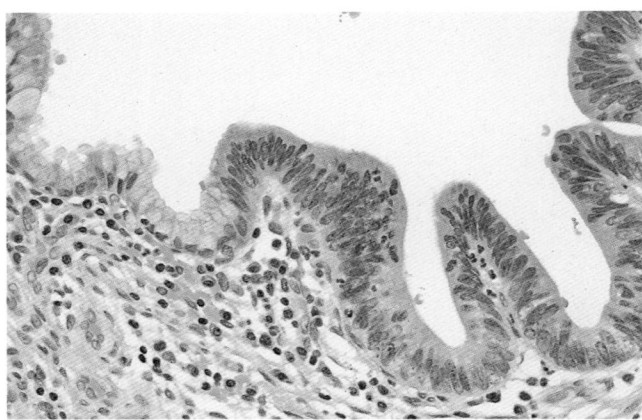

**FIGURE 36–19.** Adenocarcinoma in situ. An architectually normal endocervical gland is partially replaced by a stratified epithelium with enlarged, hyperchromatic, elongated nuclei. There is marked loss of polarity of the cells with respect to the basement membrane and mitotic activity is abundant. Note the abrupt transition between the neoplastic and normal glandular epithelium.

mental atypia (Fig. 36–19) (see CD Fig. 36–44). The fact that endocervical glandular dysplasia is virtually never associated with AIS in the same gland, but rather is found in separate, usually distant sites, is a strong argument against a causal association. Finally, there is no established clinical management for a diagnosis of these lesions other than further investigating the patient with additional biopsies. Because of the variability in the histologic criteria, coincidental relationship to AIS, absence of an association with HPV, and lack of clinical significance reported, these authors agree with Zaino's recommendation discouraging the use of the glandular dysplasia, glandular intraepithelial neoplasia, or atypical endocervical glandular hyperplasia as diagnostic terms.[143] In the rare instances that merit an ambiguous diagnosis, we prefer the descriptive term endocervical glandular atypia, followed by a comment stating the need for further follow-up rather than the use of the above-mentioned diagnostic terms.

As is the case with ASCUS, the existence of glandular atypia that is nondiagnostic is an inevitable reality. As in the case of ASCUS, the surgical pathologist should attempt to minimize the use of this nondiagnostic category, because the clinical management of lesions with this degree of atypia is widely variable. The histologic characteristics of cases of endocervical atypia include hyperchromasia of the nuclei and minimal pseudostratification. Endocervical glandular atypia virtually always lacks marked nuclear enlargement or coarse chromatin distribution. Architecturally, cribriform areas and papillary projections are rare to absent, and when they are present, they are almost always attributable to tangential sectioning of the gland or the presence of immature squamous metaplasia (CD Fig. 36–45). Mitotic figures and apoptotic bodies should be absent or extremely rare. Uncertainty as to whether a lesion represents AIS or not should be communicated to the treating clinician by the addition of a comment stating the ambiguity of the histology and the need for added biopsy material to exclude the possibility of AIS. Importantly, the occurrence of such a diagnosis should be rare and probably should not exceed 5% of the total number of AIS cases diagnosed in that particular population.

## DIFFERENTIAL DIAGNOSIS

The differential diagnosis of AIS includes invasive adenocarcinoma, reparative or reactive glandular changes secondary to inflammation, tubal metaplasia, radiation-induced atypia, viral infections, Arias-Stella reaction, microglandular hyperplasia, endocervical tunnel clusters, endometriosis, and mesonephric remnants. Distinction between AIS and microinvasive adenocarcinoma may be extremely difficult. Criteria differentiating in situ from invasive lesions have not proved to be consistently reproducible. Invasion should be suspected if the architecture of the abnormally lined glands is inconsistent with the architecture of non-neoplastic endocervix. These changes include exuberant glandular budding, an extensive cribriform pattern, foci in which the glands become confluent, small aberrantly shaped glands, and the formation of papillary projections from the endocervical surface (CD Figs. 36–46 and 36–47).[144] In addition, in AIS there should be no desmoplasia or stromal reaction around the involved glands. Unfortunately, few cases of early invasion demonstrate detectable evidence of desmoplasia, making it a very specific but poorly sensitive marker of invasion. Similarly, lesser degrees of stromal reaction should be considered with skepticism because these changes are not at all specific for invasion and can be seen in inflammatory conditions.

Endocervical glands develop a wide range of cytologic and architectural changes in response to inflammation. Despite its proposed origin from an inflammatory condition, severe reactive changes may occur in the virtual absence of active inflammation. Reactive or reparative changes are characterized by a predominantly single-cell lined epithelium with slight alteration in their polarity with respect to the basement membrane. The nuclei may become greatly enlarged and attain conspicuously prominent nucleoli, but have evenly distributed chromatin and lack significant hyperchromasia. Mitotic activity is rare, as is pseudostratification (CD Fig. 36–48). Care must be taken to distinguish between true pseudostratification and tangential sectioning through glands, which can appear as pseudostratification. Although intraglandular papillary projections should not occur in reactive or reparative processes, exaggerated endocervical papillary projections that project into the endocervical canal can occur. These stromal projections contain infiltrates of chronic inflammatory cells and are lined by a single layer of endocervical cells. This entity has been termed papillary endocervicitis (CD Figs. 36–49 and 36–50).[145]

Radiation-induced atypia is characterized by nuclear enlargement and pleomorphism, but the chromatin is characteristically smudged or shows distinct signs of degeneration. Atypia due to irradiation has much more cell-to-cell variation in size and shape than is typical of AIS or of atypias that are worrisome for AIS. The cytoplasm is frequently vacuolated or granular and may show amphophilia. Pseudostratification and mitotic figures are virtually always absent (CD Figs. 36–51 and 36–52). Tubal metaplasia is typically seen in areas of reactive or reparative endocervical glandular epithelium and may involve part of a gland, a whole gland, or many glands. In its most severely atypical forms, it resembles the cellular features of AIS. Careful scrutiny of the involved epithelium will reveal the typical tubal metaplastic epithelial types as well as the characteristic ciliation (CD Fig. 36–53). In addition, mitotic activity is extremely rare in tubal metaplasia and the presence of mitotic activity in such a focus should alert to the possibility of AIS as cases of ciliated adenocarcinomas of the cervix have been reported.[146] Intestinal metaplasia of the cervix is rare and is thought to occur as a result of a chronic inflammatory stimulus. Typically, intestinal-type cells, most commonly goblet cells, sporadically replace the normal endocervical-type glandular cells within the epithelium. The glands are lined by single cells, have minimal to no atypia, and lack significant mitotic activity (CD Figs. 36–54 and 36–55). Glands with the Arias-Stella reaction have a single layer of hyperchromatic, enlarged nuclei that frequently protrude into the gland lumen, that is, hobnail cells (CD Figs. 36–56 and 36–57). Typically, Arias-Stella reactions involve only a portion of a gland and mitotic activity is absent. Careful scrutiny of the surrounding stroma almost always reveals foci of stromal decidualization, a feature that greatly supports a diagnosis of Arias-Stella atypia.[147] Although microglandular hyperplasia can occasionally be confused with AIS owing to its glandular complexity and gland crowding, microglandular hyperplasia lacks significant nuclear atypia, lacks pseudostratification, and only rarely contains mitotic figures. Moreover, microglandular hyperplasia has a characteristic pattern of many small, closely packed, uniform glands that are unique to this entity (CD Figs. 36–58 and 36–59). Atypical forms of microglandular hyperplasia have been described that form solid masses of epithelium and have significant degrees of cytologic atypia.[145] These lesions almost always contain areas of typical microglandular hyperplasia that allow them to be identified as atypical forms of microglandular hyperplasia. Similarly, endometriosis of the cervix is usually readily recognizable and easily distinguished from AIS. Typical endometriosis of the cervix consists of endometrioid glands and is surrounded entirely or partially by endometrial stroma. The cells lining the glands are basally located endometrioid-type cells that can be pseudostratified with variable mitotic activity (CD Figs. 36–60 and 36–61). Mesonephric remnants can

**TABLE 36–1.** Modified World Health Organization Histologic Classification of Invasive Carcinomas of the Uterine Cervix

Squamous cell carcinoma
  Microinvasive squamous cell carcinoma
  Invasive squamous cell carcinoma
  Verrucous carcinoma
  Warty (condylomatous) carcinoma
  Papillary squamous cell (transitional) carcinoma
  Lymphoepithelioma-like carcinoma
Adenocarcinoma
  Mucinous adenocarcinoma
    Endocervical type
    Intestinal type
    Signet ring type
  Endometrioid adenocarcinoma
    Endometrioid adenocarcinoma with squamous metaplasia
  Clear cell adenocarcinoma
  Minimal deviation adenocarcinoma
    Endocervical type (adenoma malignum)
    Endometrioid type
  Well-differentiated villoglandular adenocarcinoma
  Serous adenocarcinoma
  Mesonephric carcinoma
Other epithelial tumors
  Adenosquamous carcinoma
  Glassy cell carcinoma
  Mucoepidermoid carcinoma
  Adenoid cystic carcinoma
  Adenoid basal carcinoma
  Carcinoid-like carcinoma
  Small cell carcinoma
  Undifferentiated carcinoma

be distinguished from AIS by their simpler architectural pattern with smaller rounder glands usually branching from a central duct. These remnants are typically located deep in the cervical stroma and are most often surrounded by smooth muscle cuffs. To complement these architectural features, mesonephric remnants are lined by cuboidal cells with bland, mitotically quiescent nuclei that allow them to be distinguished from AIS (CD Figs. 36–62 and 36–63). Mesonephric hyperplasia may be somewhat more troublesome, because in exaggerated cases, the lesions may be large and approach the endocervical surface. The architecture may show some disorganization, and the nuclei may become more prominent. Despite these features, mesonephric hyperplasia virtually never exhibits the degree of pseudostratification seen in AIS and mitotic activity is extremely rare (CD Figs. 36–64 and 36–65). Finally the so-called endocervical tunnel clusters are merely aggregates of cystically dilated endocervical glands lined by bland, attenuated endocervical glandular cells that should cause little concern as to their benign nature.

## INVASIVE CARCINOMA OF THE CERVIX

The World Health Organization (WHO) now recognizes three general categories of invasive carcinoma of the cervix. They are squamous cell carcinoma, adenocarcinoma, and other epithelial tumors (Table 36–1). The other epithelial tumor category now contains adenosquamous carcinoma, glassy cell carcinoma, adenoid basal cell carcinoma, and adenoid cystic carcinomas that previous classifications had classified as adenocarcinomas as well as carcinoid-like carcinoma and small cell carcinoma, which were previously classified as neuroendocrine carcinoma. The relative proportion of these different types of carcinoma varies from study to study, but in general, approximately 60% to 80% of invasive carcinomas of the cervix are classified as squamous cell carcinomas.[148–150]

Carcinoma of the cervix is a clinically staged tumor. The classification of the International Federation of Gynecologists and Obstetricians (FIGO) divides invasive tumors into four stages (Table 36–2).[151] Stage I includes all tumors confined to the cervix and is further divided into three categories; stage IA1, stage IA2, and stage IB. Stage II tumors extend beyond the cervix to the upper two thirds of the vagina (stage IIA) or into the parametrium but not to the pelvic sidewall (stage IIB). Stage III tu-

**TABLE 36–2.** FIGO Staging of Carcinoma of the Cervix Uteri

| Stage | |
|---|---|
| 0 | Carcinoma in situ, intraepithelial carcinoma |
| I | The carcinoma is strictly confined to the cervix or uterus |
| IA | Preclinical carcinomas of the cervix, that is those diagnosed microscopically |
| IA1 | Lesions detected microscopically that have less than 3 mm in depth and 7 mm in breadth |
| IA2 | Lesions detected microscopically with a depth of invasion between 3 mm and 5 mm and a horizontal spread of less than 7 mm |
| IB | Lesions of greater dimensions than stage IA2, whether seen clinically or not |
| II | The carcinoma extends beyond the cervix to the parametrium or upper vagina |
| IIA | Involvement of upper two thirds of the vagina with no obvious parametrial involvement |
| IIB | Involvement of the parametrium but no involvement of the pelvic sidewall |
| III | The carcinoma involves the lower third of the vagina or has extended to the pelvic wall. (All cases with hydronephrosis or nonfunctioning kidney are included unless they are known to be due to other causes) |
| IIIA | Involvement of the lower one third of the vaginal but no extension to the pelvic wall |
| IIIB | Extension to the pelvic wall, or hydronephrosis or nonfunctioning kidney |
| IV | The carcinoma has clinically extended beyond the true pelvis or has clinically involved the mucosa of the bladder or rectum |
| IVA | Spread of the growth to adjacent organs (rectal or bladder mucosa) |
| IVB | Spread to distant organs |

*Notes about the staging (selected):* Vascular space involvement does not affect the stage of squamous carcinoma but should be appended to the diagnosis, particularly for all stage I tumors, for purposes of prognosis determination and therapeutic decision-making.

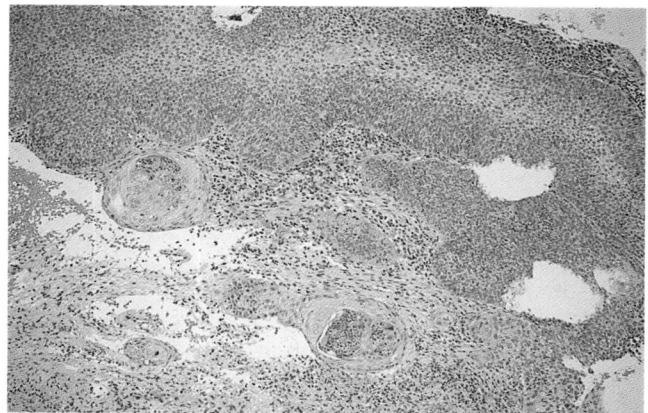

**FIGURE 36–20.** Microinvasive squamous carcinoma. This lesion shows CIN III with its characteristic parabasaloid appearance overlying nests of more eosinophilic squamous cells in an inflamed stroma.

mors include those that extend to the lower third of the vagina (stage IIIA) or involve the pelvic sidewall, cause hydronephrosis, or a nonfunctioning kidney (stage IIIB). Stage IV tumors extend beyond the true pelvis or have clinical involvement of the mucosa of the bladder or rectum.

## Microinvasive Cervical Carcinoma

The term microinvasive carcinoma of the cervix describes stage IA invasive carcinomas of the cervix that are discovered only upon microscopic examination. The 1995 FIGO staging for cervical cancer further defined stage IA cancers into stage IA1 and IA2 carcinomas. Stage IA1are defined as invasive carcinomas with measured invasion of stroma no greater than 3.0 mm in depth and no wider than 7.0 mm in breadth.[151] Stage IA2 tumors are those that invade deeper than 3 mm yet less than 5 mm and that are no greater than 7 mm in breadth.

## Microinvasive Squamous Carcinoma

Microinvasive squamous cell carcinomas of the cervix are generally found in women in their early 40s and are associated with large CIN 3 lesions that involve either the surface of the cervix or the endocervical crypts.[152] The prevalence of microinvasive squamous cell carcinoma of the cervix in the British Columbia cervical cancer registry is 4.8:100,000 women screened.[153] Most women with microinvasive squamous cell carcinoma have no symptoms and the lesion is detected during routine Pap smear screening. Microinvasion can easily be missed at the time of colposcopy for the evaluation of an abnormal Pap smear.[154] In one histopathologic analysis of shallow laser excisional conization specimens, microinvasive squamous cell carcinoma of the cervix was detected in 1% of patients thought to have only CIN 3 on

colposcopy.[155] Other studies of specimens obtained by loop electrosurgical excision have detected microinvasive squamous cell carcinoma of the cervix in 0.4% to 3.0% of patients being treated with loop excision for CIN.[156–159]

Microinvasive squamous cell carcinoma is characterized by the presence of malignant cells that penetrate through the basement membrane of the squamous epithelium into the cervical stroma. CIN 3 is almost invariably present. The cells in the microinvasive focus tend to paradoxically appear better differentiated than cells in the adjacent CIN 3. They have more abundant eosinophilic cytoplasm and their nuclei have more finely distributed chromatin and prominent nucleoli when compared with the associated CIN 3 (Figs. 36–20 and 36–21). Often, a conspicuous lymphoplasmocytic infiltrate surrounding the tips of the invasive epithelial prongs may be identified and there is frequently a surrounding desmoplastic response in the stroma (CD Figs. 36–66 and 36–67). The depth of invasion of the focus of microinvasion should be measured from the basement membrane of the immediately overlying epithelium to the deepest margin of the invading focus. Microinvasion frequently occurs at the tips of endocervical glands involved by CIN 3. When this is the case, the depth of invasion should be measured from the basement membrane of the gland from which the focus of invasion originates. In cases in which there is significant uncertainty as to the origin of the focus of microinvasion, the depth of invasion should be measured from the basement membrane of the overlying surface epithelium.

At the site of initial stromal invasion, disruption of the basement membrane has been identified using electron microscopy. Therefore, a number of studies have attempted to use immunohistochemistry and antibodies directed against basement membrane constituents such as laminin or type IV collagen as a

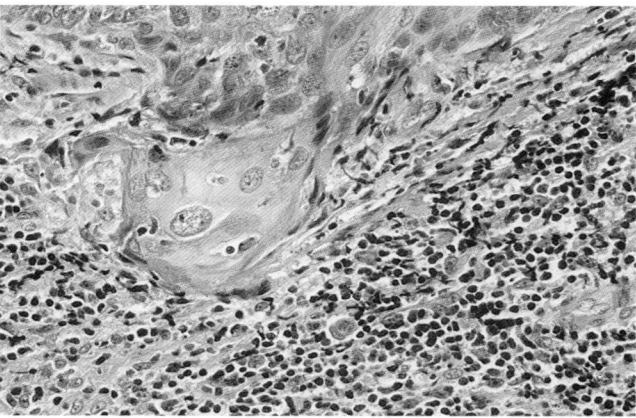

**FIGURE 36–21.** Microinvasive squamous carcinoma. High magnification of Figure 36–20 reveals the presence of malignant squamous cells with abundant eosinophilic cytoplasm and markedly enlarged nuclei breaching the basement membrane of squamous epithelium involved by CIN III.

**TABLE 36–3.** Pelvic Node Metastasis with Early Invasive Carcinoma According to Depth of Stromal Penetration

| Depth of Invasion (mm)* | Total Number of Patients | % of Patients with (+) Lymph Nodes |
|---|---|---|
| ≤3 | 382 | 0.5 |
| 3.1–5 | 399 | 5.3 |
| 5.1–10 | 329 | 15.8 |
| 10.1–15 | 179 | 23.5 |
| 15.1–20 | 121 | 38.0 |

* Depth of stromal invasion regardless of presence or absence of vascular invasion and confluency. Data from references 236–245.

way of enhancing the recognition of early stromal invasion in cervical lesions. In one of the first studies using this approach, Barsky and associates used antibodies against laminin and type IV collagen, and demonstrated that benign and in situ lesions from a number of sites including breast, pancreas, skin and prostate had a continuous basement membrane whereas microinvasive lesions at these sites had a loss of basement membrane staining.[160] However other investigators have found that small basement membrane disruptions (as defined by laminin and type IV collagen staining) frequently occur in both the normal cervical epithelium and in squamous intraepithelial lesions that lack microinvasion, especially in areas with severe stromal inflammatory infiltrates.[161, 162] In addition, foci of basement membrane staining frequently occur in areas of invasion and the amount of staining tends to increase as the degree of differentiation of the invading tumor increases.[163] In a recent test of the usefulness of type IV collagen immunoreactivity in assessing questionable early stromal invasion, Stewart and McNicol found the technique to be of limited diagnostic value.[164]

The reason for recognizing microinvasive squamous cell carcinoma of the cervix as a distinct clinical entity is that this lesion is associated with a low rate of recurrence and nodal metastases (Table 36–3).[165, 166] The data on risk factors for nodal metastases, recurrence, and death, although incomplete, suggest that lesions with 3 mm or less stromal penetration and without lymphovascular space involvement have virtually no potential for metastases or recurrence.[167] Takeshima and coworkers reported that lymph node metastases of IA1 cervical carcinoma occur in 1.2% of patients, whereas they occur in 6.8% of patients with IA2 carcinoma.[168] Buckley and colleagues reported similar findings with a rate of positive lymph nodes of 7.4% in patients with IA2 cervical cancers, a rate that more closely resembles that seen in stage IB carcinomas.[169] Therefore, patients with IA1 cervical carcinoma can be managed with less radical procedures than those required by more deeply invasive lesions.

The relationship between vascular space involvement and poor clinical outcome in women with early microinvasive squamous cell carcinoma is less well established than the relationship between depth of invasion and lymph node metastases. However vascular space involvement is reported to occur in 0% to 8% of early squamous cell carcinomas that invade less than 1 mm into the stroma and in 9% to 29% of tumors invading 1 to 3 mm into the stroma.[170–173] Several large series have correlated the presence of vascular space involvement with poor outcome in patients with microinvasive carcinoma.[170, 174] Therefore, it is the prevailing opinion in the United States that vascular space involvement should be assessed in women with microinvasive squamous cell carcinoma and that the presence of vascular space involvement prominently added to a comment in the pathology report. The diagnosis of vascular space involvement should be made on identifying malignant cells within an endothelial lined space (Fig. 36–22). Care should be taken not to mistake potential histologic mimics caused by stromal retraction from tumor nests, a phenomenon in which the spaces lack a true endothelial lining. Immunohistochemistry using antibodies specific for endothelial cells such as factor VIII, Ulex europaeus, or CD 41 may be of great aid in ensuring the true vascular nature of a space and is recommended in cases ambiguous by routine H&E examination.

## Microinvasive Adenocarcinoma of the Cervix

Microinvasive adenocarcinoma of the cervix is now a well-accepted entity. Initial reticence to accept the concept of microinvasion in adenocarcinomas of the cervix was derived from the extreme difficulty often involved in ascertaining this diagnosis. Unlike microinvasive squamous carcinomas in which the invasive nests protrude through well-defined basement membranes, it is uncommon to find cases of microinvasive adenocarcinoma in which the glandular

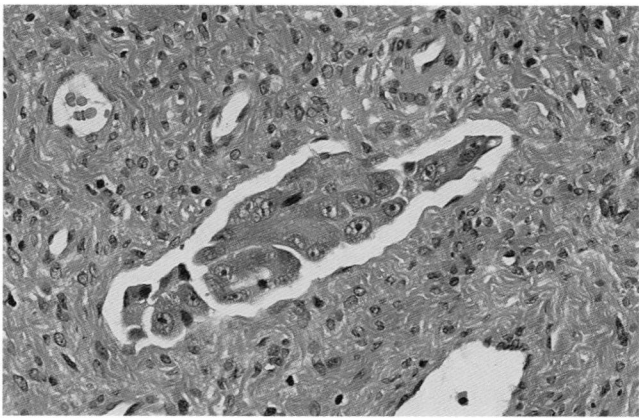

**FIGURE 36–22.** Vascular space involvement. Several vascular channels are present that are lined by characteristically flattened endothelial cells. The central space contains a cluster of malignant squamous cells.

cells disrupt any given gland basement membrane. In these cases, however, the appearance of the cells protruding through the glandular basement membrane resemble those seen in microinvasive squamous lesions showing paradoxical redifferentiation with more abundant eosinophilic cytoplasm and less hyperchromatic nuclei (Fig. 36–23) (CD Figs. 36–68 to 36–70). More commonly, the diagnostic features are more subjective, involving architectural derangements that are inconsistent with the architecture of non-neoplastic endocervical glands. The findings of areas of confluent glandular growth, complex intraglandular papillary formations, solid growth, or extensive cribriforming are all highly suggestive of microinvasion (see CD Figs. 36–46 and 36–47). Only occasionally is definitive evidence, mainly in the form of stromal desmoplasia, identified, ensuring the diagnosis (CD Figs. 36–71 to 36–74). As with microinvasive squamous carcinoma, the use of special studies to distinguish between AIS and microinvasive adenocarcinoma has proved of limited clinical value.[162] Significant clinical experience has been accrued over the last decade by several groups with interest in these tumors based on well-defined cases.

Several large studies now strongly suggest that the epidemiologic characteristics, behavior, and prognosis of microinvasive adenocarcinomas of the cervix are the same as those of microinvasive squamous carcinomas.[175–177] Kurian and al Nafussi[175] summarized their experience of 121 cases and concluded that AIS progresses to invasive adenocarcinoma with an estimated time to progression of 10 years. In their experience, microinvasive adenocarcinoma had an excellent prognosis when treated by simple hysterectomy. Ostor summarized a large experience with microinvasive adenocarcinomas. Defined as adenocarcinomas with less than 5 mm of invasion, he noted that only 2% of 219 cases with lymphadenectomies had lymph node metastases, a percentage comparable to their squamous counterparts. He also reported no recurrences in a selected group of 21 patients treated solely with cone biopsy.[178] Schorge and coworkers in the United States reported similar results for stage IA1 microinvasive adenocarcinomas.[177, 178] Finally, Nicklin and coworkers[179] failed to find metastases to adnexae and in particular, to the ovaries in 27 cases examined. Caution is to be observed, however, because two retrospective studies have shown a high incidence of residual AIS and invasive adenocarcinoma in patients undergoing hysterectomy following cone biopsies for AIS.[180, 181] A recent study by Goldstein and colleagues[182] found that found no residual disease in patients in which the cone biopsy margin demonstrated a free endocervical margin of 10 mm or greater. Despite these conflicting studies and although the experience worldwide is still limited, the current consensus is for optimism for the possibility of conservative therapy for women with microinvasive adenocarcinoma who are desirous of fertility. This latter possibility underscores the need for accurate evaluation and diagnosis of microinvasive adenocarcinoma, as well as the accurate determination and measurement of depth of invasion and status of the margin, with a statement indicating the distance of the nearest focus of disease from the endocervical margin. Owing to the difficulty in assessing the origin of the microinvasion in most cases, these authors recommend that microinvasion in cases of AIS be measured from the endocervical or cervical surface rather than attempting to determine an origin from a nearby gland.

## INVASIVE CERVICAL CANCER

Despite advances in detection and management, cervical cancer continues to be a significant health problem on a worldwide scale. Owing to widespread differences in the availability of screening programs and the prevalence of risk factors, there continue to be marked differences in the relative frequency of cervical cancer in developed and undeveloped countries. Cervical cancer is the most frequent type of cancer in women in the developing world whereas it is the 10th most frequent type in much of the developed world.[183] The average age of patients with invasive squamous cell carcinoma is 51.4 years, 15 to 23 years older than patients with CIN 3 and 8 years older than patients with microinvasive carcinoma.[183, 184] Cervical cancer occurs, however, at almost any age between 17 and 90 years. In recent years, there has been increasing recognition that cervical cancer can occur in women younger than 35 years of age. Women younger than 35 years of age account for approximately 24.5% of all patients with invasive cervical cancer at some institutions in the United States. In certain areas of the United Kingdom, increases in the incidence of invasive cervical cancer in women in this age group have been noted.[185] The increase in the United Kingdom is most likely related to multiple factors includ-

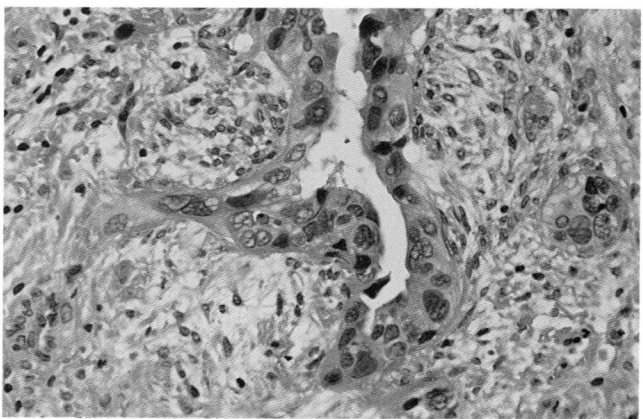

**FIGURE 36–23.** Microinvasive adenocarcinoma of the cervix. This rare case shows malignant glandular cells breaching the basement membrane of endocervical gland involved by in situ adenocarcinoma of the cervix. The cells rupturing the basement membrane are larger than those composing the in situ lesion and contain more abundant eosinophilic cytoplasm.

ing a failure to provide adequate cytologic screening programs for sexually active young women and to a change in the demographics of the population being screened.[186] The relative proportions and absolute incidences of squamous cell carcinomas and adenocarcinomas of the cervix have been changing in the United States and Western Europe over the last 40 years since the introduction of widespread cytologic screening programs. In the 1950s and 1960s, approximately 95% of all invasive cervical carcinomas were classified as squamous cell carcinomas and only 5% as adenocarcinomas.[187] However in series of invasive cervical cancers published since the early 1970s, squamous cell carcinomas have accounted for only 75% to 80% of the cases,[188–190] whereas the remainder, 20% to 25%, included various types of adenocarcinomas, adenosquamous carcinomas, and undifferentiated carcinomas.[191, 192] In the clinical series of Shingleton and coworkers,[193] the percentage of adenocarcinomas to total cervical cancers increased from 7% in the period from 1974 to 1978 to 19% in the period from 1979 to 1980. Similarly, in the clinical series of Hopkins and Morley, the percentage of adenocarcinomas to total cervical cancers increased from 19% in 1970 to 1973 to 27% in 1982 to 1985.[192] In the Finnish Cancer Registry, 88% of all cervical cancers were classified as squamous cell carcinoma and 6% as adenocarcinoma in 1953 to 1957, whereas 81% were classified as squamous cell carcinoma and 17% as adenocarcinoma in 1978 to 1982.[194] Similarly, many of the epidemiologic risk factors for the development of adenocarcinoma of the cervix are similar to those described for invasive squamous cell carcinomas.[148] Both are frequently associated with CIN,[195] and both are associated with a more than 5-year interval since the last Pap smear (relative risk of 2.7 and 3.6 for adenocarcinoma and squamous cell carcinomas respectively), multiple sexual partners (more than 10 partners has a relative risk of 10.9 and 2.9, respectively, for adenocarcinoma and squamous cell carcinoma), and a young age at first intercourse (intercourse under the age of 15 has a relative risk of 2.0 for both adenocarcinoma and squamous cell carcinoma).[148] In addition, HPV, particularly type 18, has been found in association with the majority of invasive adenocarcinomas.[196]

Although the use of oral contraceptives, particularly those with a large progestational component, for more than 10 years has been shown to be a risk factor for invasive cervical adenocarcinoma in some studies,[197, 198] these findings have not been confirmed by others. Most recent studies comparing the risk factors for invasive adenocarcinomas with those of squamous cell carcinomas have revealed no significant differences in oral contraceptive usage between the two groups of women.[199–201] Controlled prospective studies correlating the type of oral contraceptive or gestagen used, dosage, and duration of use with endocervical glandular changes are required before any relationship between oral contraceptives and progestins and endocervical adenocarcinoma can be substantiated. A genetic predisposition to invasive cervical adenocarcinoma has been documented in women with Peutz-Jeghers syndrome, in whom minimal deviation adenocarcinoma of the cervix occurs more frequently than in the general population.[202] It also appears that a generalized predisposition to the development of adenocarcinoma of the ovary and cervix can occur because dual primary cervical and ovarian adenocarcinomas develop in some women.[203]

## Invasive Squamous Carcinoma

### GROSS PATHOLOGY

Invasive squamous cell carcinomas of the cervix have a variety of macroscopic appearances. Tumors may be exophytic, creating large polypoid or papillary masses that frequently contain areas of hemorrhage and necrosis (Fig. 36–24) (CD Fig. 36–75). Squamous carcinomas may also be endophytic, revealing only an ulcer to the inspecting eye but expanding into the body of the cervix to occasionally give it a barrel-shape appearance (Fig. 36–25). The examining pathologist should make every effort to measure and report the three-dimensional size of the tumor grossly, while being aware that the extent of the grossly visible tumor may not reveal the true extent of the neoplasm. In instances in which the microscopic examination reveals a larger size of the tumor than that reported grossly, a microscopic measurement should be issued in the final microscopic diagnosis.

### MICROSCOPIC PATHOLOGY

The microscopic appearance of squamous carcinoma of the cervix is varied. Classically, squamous carcinomas are divided into keratinizing and nonkeratinizing types. Keratinizing carcinomas are defined as those tumors in which malignant cells produce extracellular keratin, most frequently in the form of keratin pearls (Fig. 36–26) (CD Figs. 36–76 and

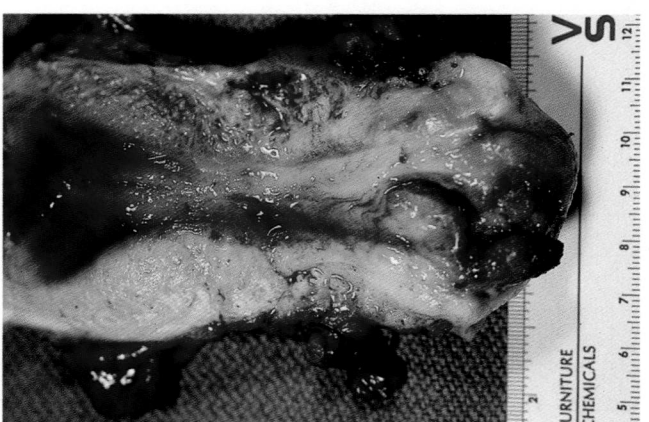

**FIGURE 36–24.** Invasive squamous carcinoma. This uterus has been bi-valved to reveal a hemorrhagic mass distorting the normal architecture of the ectocervix. The mass is nodular and contains areas of necrosis.

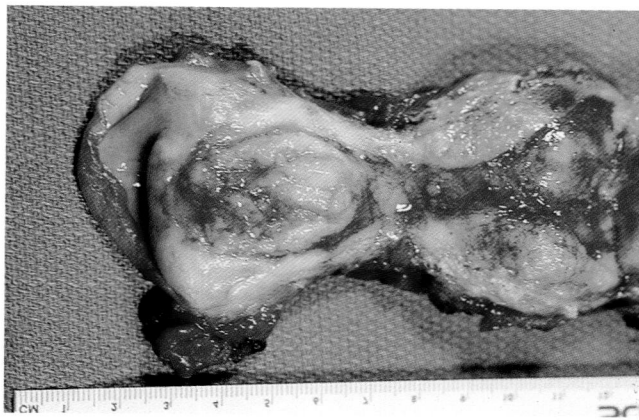

FIGURE 36–25. Invasive squamous cell carcinoma, predominantly endophytic. This uterus has been bi-valved to reveal a lesion occupying and expanding the endocervical canal of the uterus. Although minimal disruption to the ectocervical mucosa is present, the tumor dilates the endocervical area to form the characteristic barrel-shaped cervix.

36–77). The identification of a single keratin pearl is sufficient for classifying a tumor as keratinizing. Care should be taken not to mistake intracellular keratinization or degenerated dyskeratotic tumor cells as evidence of extracellular keratin. By exclusion, nonkeratinizing squamous cell carcinomas are those in which no evidence of extracellular keratin production can be identified (Fig. 36–27) (CD 36–78). In the experience of Wentz and Reagan,[203a] the best 5-year survival rate after radiation therapy was associated with large cell non-keratinizing carcinomas (68.3%), followed by the large cell keratinizing type (41.7%), whereas patients with small cell carcinomas had a 20% 5-year survival rate. Despite being divided into two general types, the microscopic appearance of squamous carcinomas is extremely varied. Most tumors contain nests or islands of malignant squamous cells that infiltrate deeply into

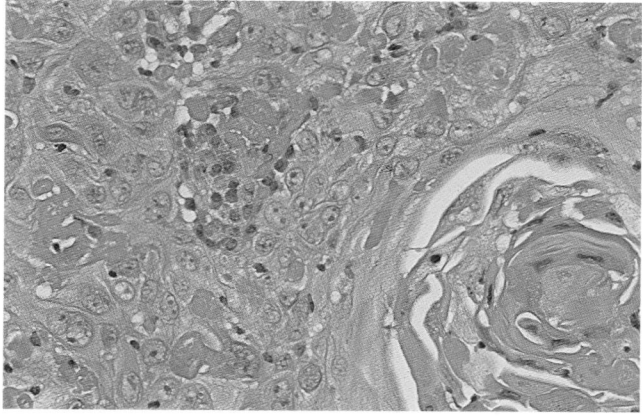

FIGURE 36–26. Keratinizing squamous carcinoma. Malignant cells are present that have abundant eosinophilic cytoplasm and contain abundant intracellular and extracellular keratin including a squamous pearl. The presence of extracellular keratin is required for the diagnosis of keratinizing squamous carcinoma.

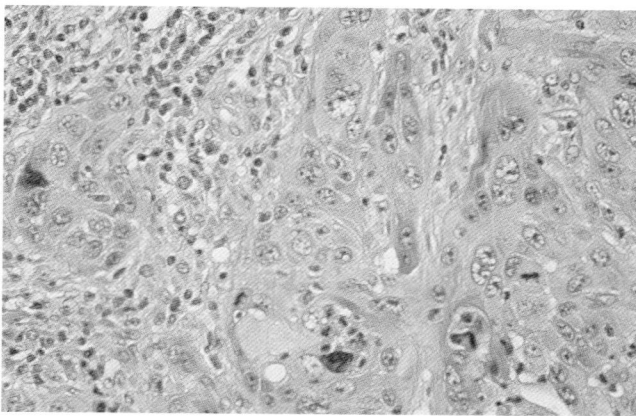

FIGURE 36–27. Nonkeratinizing squamous carcinoma. Nests of malignant squamous cells are present. Although cytoplasmic eosinophilia are seen, no extracellular keratin is present.

the fibrous stroma of the cervix. The nests of tumor are generally quite varied in size and shape, and frequently exhibit marked irregularities in their contour. Occasional nests may show central necrosis, giving a false appearance of glandular differentiation. Other features including confluent growth, pseudoreticular patterns, and single cell infiltration occur with frequency. Subtypes of squamous cell carcinoma have been described. These include warty carcinoma, verrucous carcinoma, basaloid carcinoma, transitional or papillary squamous carcinoma, clear cell squamous carcinoma and small cell carcinoma. With the exception of small cell carcinoma, evidence that these subtypes influence prognosis is controversial.

Prognostic variables other than stage and lymph node involvement have been proposed. The efficacy of grading systems to predict outcome for squamous cervical cancers has been questioned. Although some studies show predictive power,[204] others have failed to do so.[205] Clearly the use of grading systems using solely degrees of differentiation, as evidenced by the presence or absence of keratin, are of no clinical utility. This is particularly evident because many cases of heavily keratinized carcinomas exhibit marked nuclear atypia. Recent studies evaluating other parameters have shown that vascular space involvement by tumor, particularly when extensive, can predict lymph node involvement.[206] These authors believe that vascular space involvement, particularly if it is abundant, should be noted in the surgical pathology report. Relevant features to be included for completeness in the evaluation of cervical carcinoma can be seen in Table 36–4.

### SUBTYPES OF INVASIVE SQUAMOUS CARCINOMAS

Verrucous carcinomas of the cervix have been reported but are extremely rare. As in the vulva, they are characterized by their bland cytologic features that closely resemble condylomas and by the broad,

**TABLE 36–4.** Relevant Components of the Pathology Report of Cervical Neoplasms

***Gross Pathology:***
Size and shape of uterus and cervix
Description of ulcers or masses
Three-dimensional measurement of the tumor
Comment on the presence or absence of gross extra-cervical
   involvement

***Microscopic Pathology:***
Cell type:
Squamous carcinoma
   Keratinizing/non-keratinizing
Adenocarcinoma
   Mucinous/endometrioid/clear cell/serous
Others:
   Adenosquamous/small cell/glassy cell/adenoid cystic/adenoid
      basal/other rare tumors
Depth of invasion
   Report both absolute depth of invasion and percentage of
      total cervical wall involvement
Presence of vascular space involvement
Presence of paracervical tissue (parametrial) involvement

pushing borders of their interface with the stroma. Verrucous carcinoma is a slow-growing, locally invasive malignant tumor (CD Fig. 36–79). Because clinically it may be confused with cervical condyloma, it may become quite advanced and lead to death. Five of eight patients in one series of the cervix died of verrucous carcinoma or the cervix shortly after the diagnosis was made.[207] Warty carcinomas have a verrucous surface and contain numerous koilocytes in the superficial layers (CD Fig. 36–80). Distinction from verrucous carcinoma is made based on the irregular, infiltrative interface with the underlying cervical stroma. Warty carcinomas can be distinguished from condyloma acuminata of the cervix by the lack of fibrovascular cores in its papillary projections, its infiltrative interface with the stroma, and its high degree of cellular enlargement and nuclear atypia. Transitional carcinomas have a distinctive papillary surface. The papillae are slender and composed of central fibrovascular cores lined by transitional-like squamous cells that resemble grade 2 to 3 transitional cell carcinoma of the bladder (CD Fig. 36–81). Squamous differentiation can be seen at the base of transitional carcinomas, where their appearance is often indistinguishable from ordinary squamous carcinomas. Basaloid carcinomas are composed of nests of squamous cells with large basophilic nuclei and decreased amounts of cytoplasm. Characteristically, they exhibit pallisading of cells at the periphery of the nests and a high mitotic rate. They can be distinguished from small cell carcinomas by the more organized insular architecture, larger amount of cytoplasm, lower mitotic rate, fewer apoptotic bodies, and rarity of geographic necrosis (CD Figs. 36–82 and 36–83). Clear cell squamous carcinoma has an abundant, glycogen-laden cytoplasm and a large round nucleus with prominent nucleoli that closely resembles clear cell adeno-

carcinoma. Distinction from glandular clear cell carcinoma can be made by the identification of sharply demarcated, polygonal cell borders of the squamous neoplasm, as well as by the absence of the tubulocystic glandular patterns characteristic of clear cell adenocarcinomas (CD Figs. 36–84 and 36–85). Although data are lacking as to the relative behavior of clear cell squamous carcinoma, anecdotal reports and the combined experience of these authors seem to indicate that these tumors have a graver prognosis than do other types of squamous carcinomas.

## Invasive Adenocarcinoma of the Cervix

### GROSS PATHOLOGY

The gross appearance of invasive adenocarcinoma of the cervix is almost always indistinguishable from its squamous counterpart. Tumors may be exophytic or endophytic. They may be papillary or bulbous and invade in virtually identical pattern to squamous carcinomas. Occasionally, well-differentiated mucinous adenocarcinomas may present a soft, gelatinous appearance that may elicit suspicion as to its glandular nature (Fig. 36–28). As with squamous cancers, the inspecting pathologist must render a three-dimensional measurement of the gross lesion, followed by microscopic confirmation of the tumor size.

Gross differentiation of endocervical lesions from endometrial lesions is usually straightforward. Most cervical adenocarcinomas have their epicenter near the external os. In these instances, the origin of the tumor is clearly cervical (CD Figs. 36–86 and 36–87). There are instances, however, in which the tumor extends far into the endocervical canal to involve the internal os and part of the lower uterine segment (CD Fig. 36–88). In these cases, the distinction between a cervical versus an endometrial origin

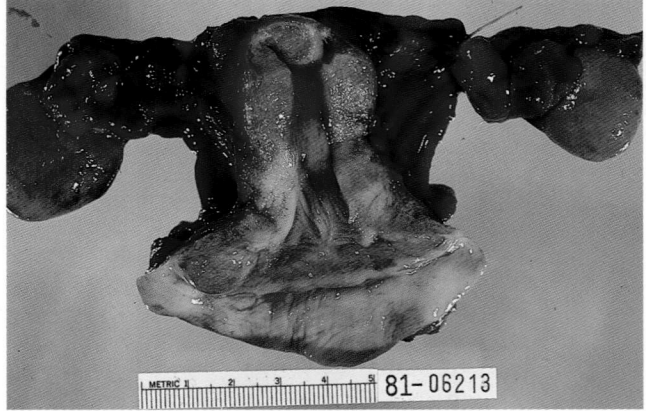

**FIGURE 36–28.** Invasive adenocarcinoma. This uterus has been opened anteriorly to reveal a mass distorting the normal contour of the cervix. The mass is polypoid and shows a gelatinous appearance. When seen, this appearance is characteristic of mucinous adenocarcinomas.

**TABLE 36–5.** Use of Histochemistry and Immunohistochemistry in Distinguishing Between Primary Endometrial and Cervical Adenocarcinomas

| | Percentage of Primary Tumors That Stain | |
|---|---|---|
| Stain or Antigen | *Endocervical* | *Endometrial* |
| Alcian blue[218] | 100% | 77% |
| CEA[198, 218] | 59%–80% (cytoplasmic) | 8%–50% (luminal) |
| Vimentin | 0% | 66% |
| IC5[198] | 90% (cytoplasmic) | 40% (luminal) |
| Mucus-antigens M1 and M3[218] | 56% | |
| 0 | | |

Data from references 246–249.

CEA, carcinoembryonic antigen; M1, M3 and IC5 are monoclonal antibodies derived against either endocervical adenocarcinoma cells or mucus-associated proteins.

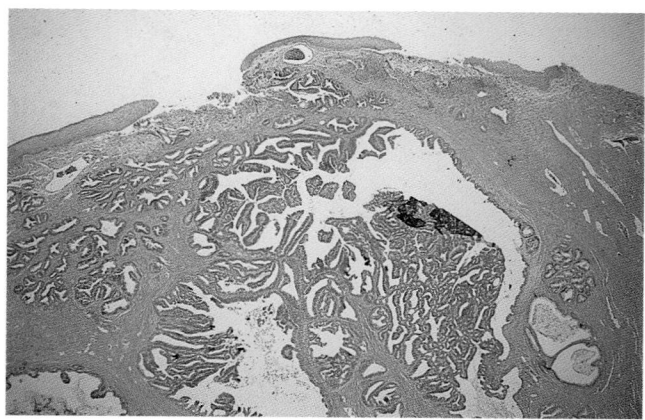

**FIGURE 36–29.** Invasive adenocarcinoma of the cervix. The normal stroma of the cervix is largely replaced by complex aggregates of abnormally shaped glandular structures. Papillary formations as well as confluent glandular aggregates are noted centrally.

of the tumor may be difficult. The differentiation in these cases can be greatly aided by a careful gross examination. If the epicenter of the tumor is external to the internal os, only to involve the lower uterine segment minimally, then the tumor is almost certainly cervical in origin. Conversely, if the majority of the tumor is in the lower uterine segment, only involving the cervix minimally, then an endometrial primary tumor should be strongly suspected. Microscopic confirmation of the gross inspection is essential in that typical histologic features of cervical cancer are extremely rare in endometrial cancers and may sway the diagnosis toward that direction in cases of ambiguous location of the lesion. Immunohistochemical studies have proved to be of variable use in the differential of these two tumors (Table 36–5). Finally, when the lesion is indeterminate in location, with the epicenter exactly at the internal os, then the diagnosis of carcinoma of the cervicouterine junction or carcinoma "corpus et colli" should be entertained (CD Fig. 36–89). This diagnosis carries the prognosis and metastatic spread patterns of both cervical carcinomas and endometrial carcinomas, and it should be treated surgically as cervical cancer.

## MICROSCOPIC PATHOLOGY

Adenocarcinomas of the cervix are an extremely heterogeneous group of tumors. Because these cell types and patterns are frequently admixed, the histologic classification of these tumors is based on the predominant cell type. The most common type of cervical adenocarcinoma is mucinous adenocarcinoma of the cervix.[199, 208, 209] Two types of mucinous carcinomas are seen commonly: the endocervical type and the intestinal type. Mucinous tumors are followed in frequency by endometrioid carcinomas. These two histologic types taken together account for 66% to 90% of all invasive cervical adenocarcinomas.[210]

Mucinous adenocarcinomas of the cervix, endocervical type, are typically composed of branching glands similar in architecture to normal endocervix of AIS. The glands are generally more compactly arranged than the in situ lesions, are more variable in size and shape, and usually penetrate deeply into the cervical stroma (Fig. 36–29) (CD Fig. 36–90). The diagnostic triad of adenocarcinoma consists of stratification, nuclear enlargement and atypia, and mitotic figures. The cells are columnar with variable but usually generous amounts of cytoplasmic mucin. The nuclei are large, often fusiform, and have coarse chromatin. Mitotic figures are almost always numerous and, characteristically of cervical adenocarcinomas, are found in the luminal border of the epithelium (jumping mitoses) (Fig. 36–30) (CD Fig. 36–91). The higher the grade of the tumor, the less

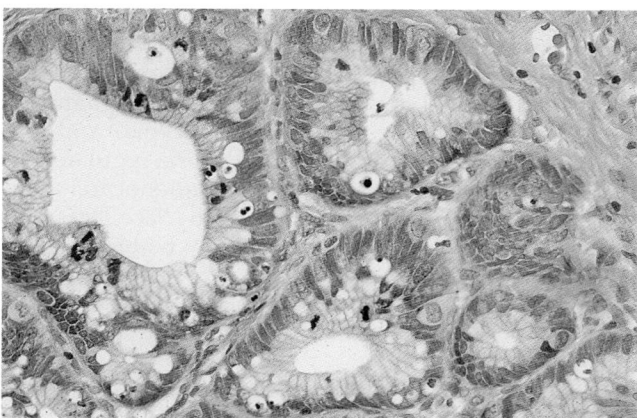

**FIGURE 36–30.** Cervical adenocarcinoma. The glands shown are lined by enlarged cells in a pseudostratified arrangement. The nuclei have lost their polarity with respect to the basement membrane, are enlarged, and hyperchromatic, and contain coarse chromatin. Mitotic figures and apoptotic bodies are abundant. Typically in adenocarcinoma of the cervix, mitotic figures are found near the apical border of the glandular epithelium.

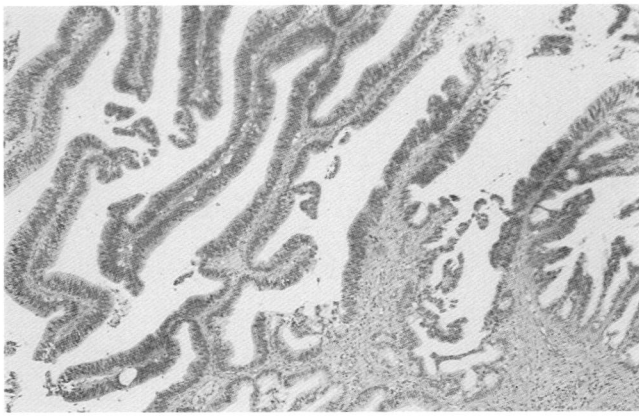

**FIGURE 36–31.** Villoglandular adenocarcinoma of the cervix. Slender papillary formations are characteristic of this tumor. The thin papillae are lined by stratified endocervical epithelium with hyperchromasia and mitotic activity. The degree of nuclear atypia is generally less than that found in other endocervical adenocarcinomas.

cytoplasmic mucin the cells contain and the more the tumor resembles an endometrioid adenocarcinoma. It is this latter characteristic that is undoubtedly the reason for the high degree of variability in the percentage of endometrioid tumors reported in various series. In mucinous carcinomas of the endocervical type, the cells are typically müllerian in appearance, that is, slender in shape with uniform amounts of mucin. In the intestinal types, the cells exhibit greater variation in size and shape and have clear evidence of intestinal differentiation in the way of goblet cells, Paneth cells, and argentaffin cells. The distinction is more of academic value, because little correlation has been found between cell types and behavior. The possible exception to this rule is the well-differentiated villoglandular adenocarcinoma of the cervix. This extremely well-differentiated variant characteristically presents as a predominantly exophytic tumor that is predominantly papillary. The papillae are slender and lined by very well-differentiated mucinous cells. Under high magnification, the cells are unequivocally malignant, as evidenced by stratification, nuclear atypia, and mitotic figures, but the nuclei are more regular and smaller than the usual mucinous adenocarcinoma (Fig. 36–31) (CD Figs. 36–92 and 36–93). This subset of carcinomas have a significantly better prognosis than adenocarcinomas of the usual type.[211] However, care should be observed that the entire tumor is of this bland histologic type because areas of very well-differentiated adenocarcinoma may be seen on the surface of higher grade neoplasms not deserving this diagnosis.

Endometrioid adenocarcinomas of the cervix are histologically identical to their counterparts in the endometrium. They are characterized by cylindrical glands that exhibit less branching than mucinous carcinomas. The glands are lined by stratified columnar epithelium with moderate to scant amounts of eosinophilic to amphophilic cytoplasm. Importantly, no intracytoplasmic mucin is present. The nuclei vary greatly in size and shape between tumors but are characteristically rounded with finer chromatin than the mucinous adenocarcinomas. Again as with intestinal variants, endometrioid tumors of the cervix behave clinically in the same fashion as mucinous adenocarcinomas of the usual type (CD Figs. 36–94 and 36–95).

## Variants of Invasive Cervical Adenocarcinomas

Several histologic variants are worthy of mention owing to their distinct or difficult appearance or their aggressive behavior. Minimal deviation adenocarcinoma is an extremely well-differentiated variant of mucinous adenocarcinoma of the endocervical type. These carcinomas can be recognized by their altered architecture and deeply penetrating glands. The glands of minimal deviation adenocarcinoma are enlarged and appear dilated, but rather than having a stretched lining, the lining is scalloped, with infoldings and areas of epithelial tufting (Fig. 36–32) (CD Figs. 36–96 and 36–97). The cells are single lined in most areas, but careful scrutiny of the tumor almost always reveals areas of stratification (Fig. 36–33). The cytology in most glands closely resembles normal or reactive endocervical cells, but again careful search almost always reveals nuclear enlargement, the presence of large nucleoli, and occasional mitotic figures (CD Fig. 36–98). Clear cell adenocarcinoma of the cervix is rare. It is indistinguishable from clear cell tumors of the endometrium or ovary. The cells typically contain abundant amounts of optically clear cytoplasm and large nuclei with prominent nucleoli. The architectural patterns include the tubulocystic as well as solid areas (CD Figs. 36–99 and 36–100). Although clear cell

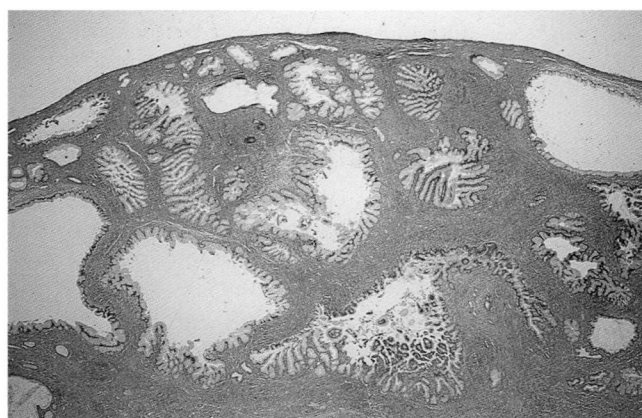

**FIGURE 36–32.** Minimal deviation adenocarcinoma. Enlarged irregularly shaped endocervical glands are noted penetrating deeply into the cervical stroma. The glands show internal papillary budding as well as scalloped external borders that characterize this lesion.

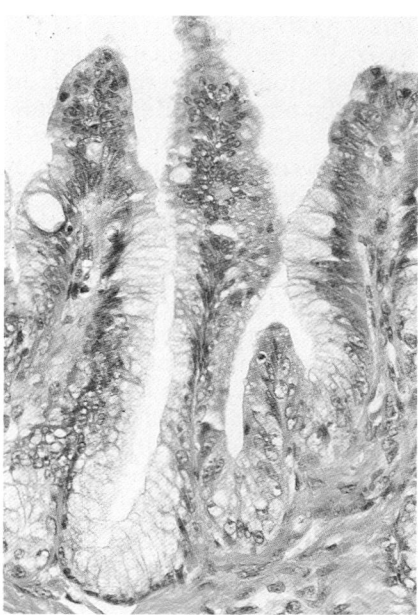

**FIGURE 36–33.** Minimal deviation adenocarcinoma. This detail enlargement of Figure 36–32 finds areas of minimally altered endocervical epithelium next to areas more easily diagnosed as adenocarcinoma.

adenocarcinoma of the cervix has been reported in young women with a history of in utero exposure to diethystilbestol (DES)[212, 213] these tumors can also develop in the absence of exposure to DES.[214, 215] Tumors that develop in the absence of DES exposure occur most commonly in postmenopausal women, whereas in patients who have been exposed to DES, the tumor generally develops in women who are young. Serous adenocarcinomas of the cervix are again extremely rare. They frequently occur in conjunction with endometrioid carcinomas. They are typical of serous carcinomas elsewhere. Generally, they are papillary tumors with broad fibrous papillae that are lined predominantly by a single layer of markedly atypical cells with variable amounts of eosinophilic cytoplasm. The nuclei classically exhibit marked loss of polarity, macronucleoli, and numerous, frequently abnormal mitotic figures (CD Figs. 36–101 and 36–102). In one report describing these tumors, none of the three tumors were deeply invasive, but two of the patients had pelvic node metastasis.[216] Mesonephric carcinomas of the cervix are extraordinarily rare neoplasms.[214] Their diagnosis should be made only when the tumor is predominantly located deep in the cervical stroma and the malignancy is accompanied by the presence of mesonephric hyperplasia (CD Figs. 36–103 and 36–104). Mesonephric carcinoma has a markedly disorganized architectural pattern with angulated glands that are lined by cuboidal to low columnar cells. Variable degrees of stratification may be present (CD Figs. 36–105 and 36–106). The cells contain scant apical cytoplasm that lacks cytoplasmic mucin. The nuclei are large, round, and contain finely gran-

ular chromatin. Occasionally, dense intraluminal eosinophilic secretions can be found. Their major differential diagnosis is mesonephric hyperplasia that can be distinguished by the organized lobular architecture around a central duct, as well as by the lack of cytologic atypia (see CD Figs. 36–64 and 36–65).[217]

## Other Epithelial Tumors of the Cervix

Tumors grouped into the category of other epithelial tumors often share histologic features with both squamous and glandular carcinomas. Tumors in this category generally have a poorer prognosis than squamous carcinomas or adenocarcinomas. Adenosquamous carcinoma of the cervix is a relatively common tumor, reported to represent 5% to 25% of all cervical carcinomas.[98, 199] They are defined as tumors that have evidence of malignant squamous and glandular differentiation (CD Fig. 36–107). These authors reserve the diagnosis of adenosquamous carcinomas for those tumors in which the two types of differentiation are intimately admixed. Tumors where separate areas of adenocarcinoma coexist with areas of squamous carcinomas we consider as separate, simultaneous primary or collision tumors (CD Fig. 36–108). Adenosquamous carcinomas have been reported to behave aggressively. These tumors have been shown to metastasize to pelvic lymph nodes twice as frequently as squamous cell carcinomas or adenocarcinomas.[193] Small cell carcinomas, which are also referred to as small cell neuroendocrine carcinomas of the cervix, are similar in morphology to small cell carcinomas of the lung. However, unlike small cell carcinomas of the lung, small cell carcinomas of the cervix are almost always found mixed with carcinomas of other epithelial cells types. Most commonly, small cell carcinoma is found adjacent or admixed with adenosquamous carcinoma, although they can be seen accompanying adenocarcinoma or squamous carcinoma. Pure small cell carcinomas of the cervix are rare. These tumors characteristically infiltrate in confluent growth patterns and often contain large areas of necrosis (CD Fig. 36–109). The cells are extremely small and contain small amounts of cytoplasm. The nuclei are often small but may be intermediate size, as with pulmonary tumors.[218] Regardless of cell size, the nuclei occupy a large percentage of the cell, often appear to overlap or even mold against the nuclei of adjacent cells, and have a finely stippled chromatin pattern (Fig. 36–34) (CD Fig. 36–110). Distinctively, small cell carcinomas have an extremely high rate of mitosis and very often an equally large number of apoptotic bodies. Immunohistochemical studies have shown that 40% to 60% of small cell carcinomas of the cervix express neuroendocrine markers (Fig. 36–35) (CD Fig. 36–111). Although neuron-specific enolase can be detected frequently, the frequent difficulties in the technical

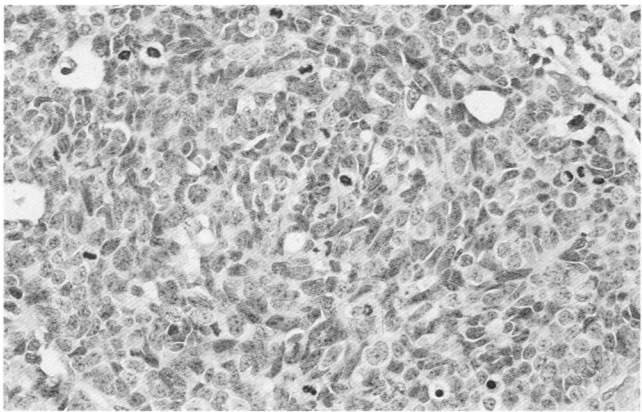

FIGURE 36–34. Small cell carcinoma of the cervix. Small malignant cells with abundant mitotic activity and numerous apoptotic bodies are present. Characteristically, the nuclei have finely glandular chromatin and nuclear molding.

interpretation of this stain as well as its purported lack of specificity make it an unreliable marker. However, synaptophysin is expressed in nearly as high a percentage of these tumors and is extremely specific and reliable. Finally although chromogranin is extremely specific, it is positive in only a small percentage of cervical small cell carcinomas. A diagnosis of small cell carcinomas confers the greatest effect in prognosis to the patient. Small cell carcinomas have been reported to have significantly higher recurrence rates and substantially higher mortality than other cervical carcinomas. Therefore, the diagnosis of small cell carcinomas of the cervix should be reserved exclusively for tumors believed to represent small cell neuroendocrine tumors and should not be used as a descriptive term for subtypes of squamous cell carcinomas not thought to be neuroendocrine in origin. Glassy cell carcinomas of the cervix are now recognized as high-grade variants of adenosquamous carcinomas that deserve special mention owing to their poor clinical behavior. They have been reported to have an extremely aggressive

clinical course, with a poor response to radiation and surgery.[219, 220] They are characterized by a predominantly solid growth pattern that is interrupted by a dense inflammatory infiltrate composed of plasma cells and eosinophils (CD Fig. 36–112). The cells are large and contain abundant homogeneously eosinophilic cytoplasm that gives them the characteristic glassy appearance. The nuclei are also characteristic in their uniformity; they are round, with marginated or finely dispersed chromatin and prominent macronucleoli (Fig. 36–36) (CD Fig. 36–113). Mucoepidermoid carcinoma is another tumor with both squamous and glandular differentiation. The distinction from adenosquamous carcinoma is based on the fact that mucoepidermoid carcinomas do not form well-defined glandular structures but rather have areas of tumor in which the cells contain intracytoplasmic mucin (CD Fig. 36–114).[221] The distinction is difficult at times and probably has little merit because they behave in a fashion similar to adenosquamous tumors. Adenoid cystic carcinoma of the cervix is histologically similar to its counterpart in the salivary glands. It exhibits a distinctive appearance granted to it by the nests of uniform but mitotically active basaloid cells that have a sievelike multicystic architecture. Within the cystic spaces, densely eosinophilic hyaline bodies are found in many of the lumens (CD Fig. 36–115). Like their salivary counterparts, the hyaline material is mucicarminophilic and periodic–acid Shiff positive and diastase resistant. Unlike salivary gland tumors, however, cervical adenoid cystic carcinomas contain few myoepithelial cells that would stain with antibodies to S-100 protein. Adenoid cystic carcinomas are rare tumors, accounting for fewer than 2% of cervical cancers, and behave aggressively. Lymphatic involvement is common, and the tumor behaves aggressively, with frequent local recurrences or metastatic spread.[222–224] Adenoid cystic carcinoma should be distinguished from adenoid basal carci-

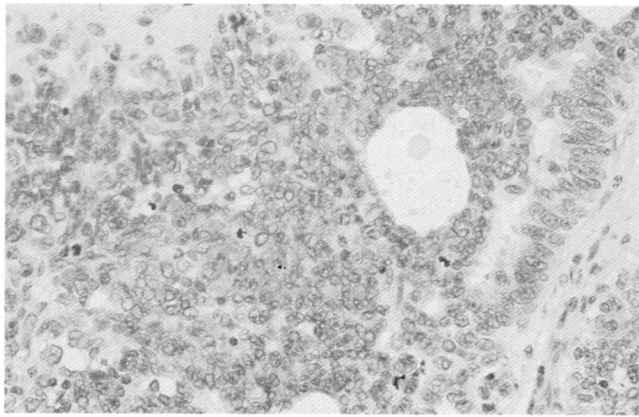

FIGURE 36–35. Small cell carcinoma of the cervix. Tumor cells show positive reactivity for synaptophysin.

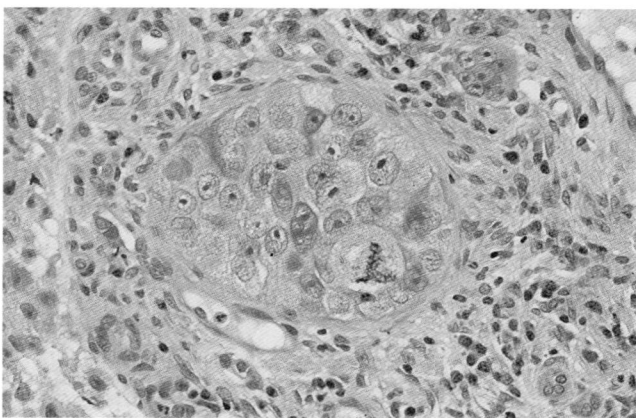

FIGURE 36–36. Glassy cell carcinoma. This tumor is characterized by malignant cells in a solid growth pattern that contain abundant, finely granular eosinophilic cytoplasm. The nuclei are round and contain prominent macronuclei. Mitotic activity including abnormal mitotic figures may be found.

noma. Adenoid basal carcinoma is formed by smaller nests of basaloid cells with fewer cystic spaces than those in adenoid cystic carcinoma. In addition adenoid basal carcinoma may have luminal necrotic debris but lacks the hyaline bodies of the adenoid cystic tumors. The cells are small, uniform, and tend to palisade at the periphery of the nests (CD Figs. 36–116 and 36–117). They also lack the mitotic rate characteristic of its more aggressive mimic. Adenoid basal carcinomas are rare tumors that occur more frequently in African-American women.[225] They are usually an incidental finding in cone biopsy specimens or uteri resected for the treatment of CIN lesions.

## Miscellaneous Tumors of the Cervix

Primary malignant melanoma is among the least common of the malignant tumors that arise in the cervix. Twenty-four patients have been reported.[226] The prognosis of primary malignant melanoma is poor, with only a 40% 5-year survival for patients with stage I disease and a 14% 5-year survival for patients with higher stage disease.[227] They are histologically identical to melanomas elsewhere. Primary choriocarcinoma in the cervix is rare and presumably results from a pre-existing cervical pregnancy or displaced intrauterine molar tissue. Nearly 50 such cases are recorded in the literature.[228] The gross and microscopic appearance, as well as the clinical course, is identical with those found in the uterine corpus. Both lymphomas and leukemias can involve the cervix. More often, these disorders are secondary

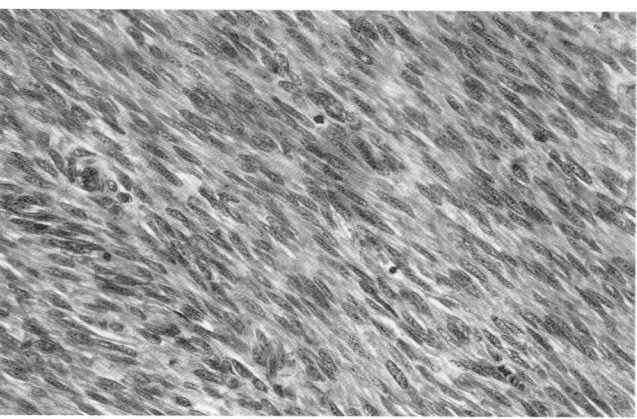

**FIGURE 36–38.** Leiomyosarcoma of the cervix. Typical malignant spindled cells with clearly identifiable smooth muscle features are identified. Note the abundant mitotic activity.

and are a manifestation of systemic disease. Leukemic infiltration of the cervix, especially of the granulocytic type, is a rather common occurrence at autopsy in women with leukemia. Secondary involvement of the cervix by lymphoma is reported in 6% of women dying with generalized disease.[229] Primary cervical lymphomas can occasionally arise in the cervix and usually present in premenopausal women as abnormal vaginal bleeding. Seventy percent of these tumors are of the diffuse large cell type and 20% are lower grade follicular lymphomas.[230] Malignant mesenchymal tumors that can arise in the cervix include leiomyosarcoma (Figs. 36–37 and 36–38), endometrial stromal sarcoma (Figs. 36–39 and

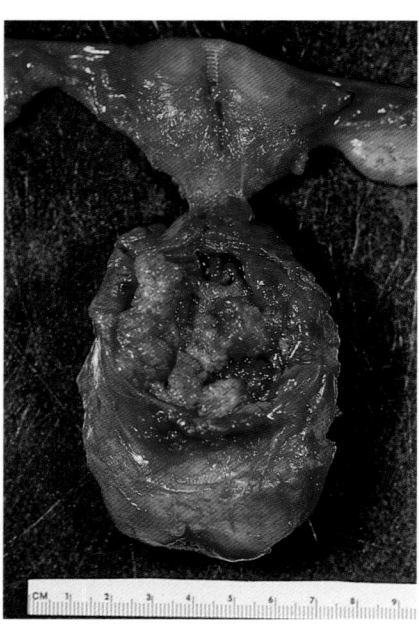

**FIGURE 36–37.** Leiomyosarcoma of the cervix. A friable, necrotic tumor mass greatly expands the cervix and erodes into the paracervical tissues.

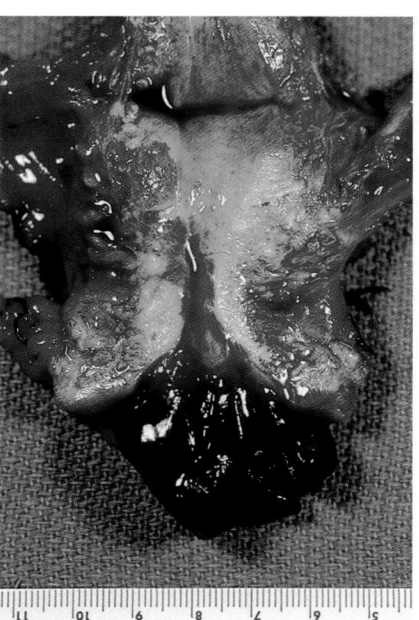

**FIGURE 36–39.** Endometrial stromal sarcoma of the cervix. This uterus has been bi-valved to reveal a hemorrhagic mass arising from and replacing the ectocervix. Note that the endometrial cavity is completely uninvolved.

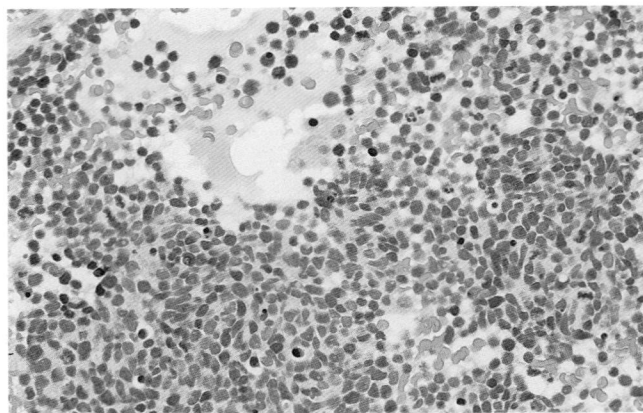

**FIGURE 36–40.** Endometrial stromal sarcoma of the cervix. Aggregates of small mesenchymal cells with endometrial stromal differentiation replace the normal cervical stroma.

36–40) embryonal rhabdomyosarcoma (botryoid type), alveolar soft part sarcoma, and osteosarcomas. Primary cervical sarcomas are very rare, and the most common form is the leiomyosarcoma, of which 20 cases have been reported. Primary cervical mixed epithelial and mesenchymal tumors include two reported cases of cervical adenosarcoma, rare cases of malignant mixed müllerian tumor, and a single reported case of Wilms' tumor. Primary cervical germ cell tumors have been described. These tumors include both the mature teratomas and yolk sac tumors.

## Metastatic Tumors Involving the Cervix

Direct extension from local pelvic tumor is the most common source of cervical involvement by secondary carcinoma, often originating in the endometrium, rectum, or bladder. Lymphatic or vascular metastases to the cervix are less frequent but may occur with ovarian carcinoma, endometrial adenocarcinoma, and uncommonly with transitional cell carcinoma of the bladder.[231] Another lesion that has a relatively high rate of cervical metastasis is choriocarcinoma. Sarcomas of the uterine corpus may also involve the cervix. Metastases to the cervix from distant primary foci are rare, the most common sites being the gastrointestinal tract (colon and stomach),[231, 232] the ovary,[231] and the breast.[233] Instances of metastatic carcinoma of the kidney, gallbladder, pancreas, lung, and thyroid,[231] as well as malignant melanoma have also been described.[232] On occasion, metastases may occur primarily as cervical involvement and pose a differential diagnostic problem. Unusual gross appearance or histologic patterns, for example, signet ring cell carcinoma or clear cell carcinoma, may provide a clue to the possibility of origin in a distant primary site.

## MISCELLANEOUS BENIGN CONDITIONS

Although innumerable benign conditions affect the cervix, most entities do not come to the attention of the surgical pathologist and are beyond the scope of this discussion. Rarely are infectious etiologies to cervicitis identified on cervical biopsy, even when using special stains. Therefore, inflammatory conditions of the cervix are grouped under the useful rubric of acute or chronic cervicitis, depending on the character of the inflammatory infiltrate. Two conditions are noteworthy: endocervical polyps and cervical leiomyomas. Endocervical polyps are common growths of the cervix. In a prospective study on women about to undergo hysterectomy, 2% of asymptomatic women were found to have endocervical polyps.[234] These benign growths are clinically associated with irregular and postcoital bleeding but more frequently are encountered incidentally at the time of speculum examination of the cervix. Endocervical polyps are polypoid fragments of endocervical tissue lined by the usual mucinous epithelial layer (CD Fig. 36–118). Microglandular hyperplasia is commonly seen involving areas of the polyp. Leiomyomas rarely involve the cervix. A recent study showed that although leiomyomas were present in 65% of uteri evaluated, only 0.6% of cervixes examined contained leiomyomas.[235] Because cervical leiomyomas are uncommon, they are often clinically mistaken for a malignancy and result in biopsies. Owing to their location in the cervical stroma (CD Fig. 36–119), occasional biopsies contain only small amounts of the leiomyomas, occasionally making them difficult to identify with certainty. Microscopically they are indistinguishable from uterine leiomyomas (CD Fig. 36–120).

## REFERENCES

1. Kjellberg L, Wang Z, Wiklund F, et al: Sexual behaviour and papillomavirus exposure in cervical intraepithelial neoplasia: A population-based case-control study. J Gen Virol 80(Pt 2): 391–398, 1999.
2. Kjellberg L, Hallmans G, Ahren AM, et al: Smoking, diet, pregnancy and oral contraceptive use as risk factors for cervical intra-epithelial neoplasia in relation to human papillomavirus infection. Br J Cancer 82:1332–1338, 2000.
3. Slattery ML, Robison LM, Schuman KL, et al: Cigarette smoking and exposure to passive smoke are risk factors for cervical cancer. JAMA 261:1593–1598, 1989.
4. Brinton LA: Epidemiology of Cervical Cancer—Overview. IARC Sci Publ 119:3–23, 1992.
5. Campion MJ, Singer A, Clarkson PK, McCance DJ: Increased risk of cervical neoplasia in consorts of men with penile condylomata acuminata. Lancet 1:943–946, 1985.
6. Bosch FX, Munoz N, de Sanjose S, et al: Risk factors for cervical cancer in Colombia and Spain. Int J Cancer 52:750–758, 1992.
7. Peng HQ, Liu SL, Mann V, et al: Human papillomavirus types 16 and 33, herpes simplex virus type 2 and other risk factors for cervical cancer in Sichuan Province, China. Int J Cancer 47:711–7166, 1991.
8. Walboomers JM, Jacobs MV, Manos MM, et al: Human pap-

illomavirus is a necessary cause of invasive cervical cancer worldwide [see comments]. J Pathol 189:12–19, 1999.

9. Bosch FX, Manos MM, Munoz N, et al: Prevalence of human papillomavirus in cervical cancer: A worldwide perspective. International Biological Study on Cervical Cancer (IBSCC) Study Group [see comments]. J Natl Cancer Inst 87:796–802, 1995.

10. Schiffman MH: Recent progress in defining the epidemiology of human papillomavirus infection and cervical neoplasia. J Natl Cancer Inst 84:394–398, 1992.

11. Schiffman MH, Bauer HM, Hoover RN, et al: Epidemiologic evidence showing that human papillomavirus infection causes most cervical intraepithelial neoplasia. J Natl Cancer Inst 85:958–964, 1993.

12. Koutsky LA, Galloway DA, Holmes KK: Epidemiology of genital human papillomavirus infection. Epidemiol Rev 10:122–163, 1988.

13. Vonka V, Kanka J, Roth Z: Herpes simplex type 2 virus and cervical neoplasia. Adv Cancer Res 48:149–191, 1987.

14. Cevenini R, Costa S, Rumpianesi F, et al: Cytological and histopathological abnormalities of the cervix in genital *Chlamydia trachomatis* infections. Br J Vener Dis 57:334–337, 1981.

15. Nahmias AJ, Naib ZM, Josey WE, et al: Prospective studies of the association of genital herpes simplex infection and cervical anaplasia. Cancer Res 33:1491–1497, 1973.

16. Vonka V, Kanka J, Hirsch I, et al: Prospective study on the relationship between cervical neoplasia and herpes simplex type-2 virus. II. Herpes simplex type-2 antibody presence in sera taken at enrollment. Int J Cancer 33:61–66, 1984.

17. Slattery ML, Overall JC, Abbott TM, et al: Sexual activity, contraception, genital infections, and cervical cancer: Support for a sexually transmitted disease hypothesis. Am J Epidemiol 130:248–258, 1989.

18. Hildesheim A, Mann V, Brinton LA, et al: Herpes simplex virus type 2: A possible interaction with human papillomavirus types 16/18 in the development of invasive cervical cancer. Int J Cancer 49:335–340, 1991.

19. de Villiers EM: Human pathogenic papillomavirus types: An update. Curr Top Microbiol Immunol 186:1–12, 1994.

20. Lorincz AT, Reid R, Jenson AB, et al: Human papillomavirus infection of the cervix: Relative risk associations of 15 common anogenital types. Obstet Gynecol 79:328–337, 1992.

21. Hildesheim A, Schiffman MH, Gravitt PE, et al: Persistence of type-specific human papillomavirus infection among cytologically normal women. J Infect Dis 169:235–240, 1994.

22. Felix JC, Wright TC: Analysis of lower genital tract lesions clinically suspicious for condylomata using in situ hybridization and the polymerase chain reaction for the detection of human papillomavirus. Arch Pathol Lab Med 118:39–43, 1994.

23. Obalek S, Misiewicz J, Jablonska S, et al. Childhood condyloma acuminatum: Association with genital and cutaneous human papillomaviruses. Pediatr Dermatol 10:101–106, 1993.

24. Barrasso R. HPV-related genital lesions in men. IARC Sci Publ 119:85–92, 1992.

25. Bergeron C, Barrasso R, Beaudenon S, et al: Human papillomaviruses associated with cervical intraepithelial neoplasia: Great diversity and distinct distribution in low- and high-grade lesions. Am J Surg Pathol 16:641–649, 1992.

26. Lungu O, Sun XW, Felix J, et al: Relationship of human papillomavirus type to grade of cervical intraepithelial neoplasia. JAMA 267:2493–2496, 1992.

27. Egawa K, Shibasaki Y, de Villiers EM: Double infection with human papillomavirus 1 and human papillomavirus 63 in single cells of a lesion displaying only an human papillomavirus 63–induced cytopathogenic effect. Lab Invest 69:583–588, 1993.

28. Kanda T, Furuno A, Yoshiike K: Human papillomavirus type 16 open reading frame E7 encodes a transforming gene for rat 3Y1 cells. J Virol 62:610–631, 1988.

29. Bedell MA, Jones KH, Laimins LA: The E6-E7 region of human papillomavirus type 18 is sufficient for transformation of NIH 3T3 and rat-1 cells. J Virol 61:3635–3640, 1987.

30. Yasumoto S, Burkhardt AL, Doniger J, DiPaolo JA: Human papillomavirus type 16 DNA-induced malignant transformation of NIH 3T3 cells. J Virol 57:572–577, 1986.

31. Schneider-Gadicke A, Schwarz E: Different human cervical carcinoma cell lines show similar transcription patterns of human papillomavirus type 18 early genes. EMBO J 5:2285–2292, 1986.

32. von Knebel, Doeberitz M, Bauknecht T, Bartsch D, zur Hausen H: Influence of chromosomal integration on glucocorticoid-regulated transcription of growth-stimulating papillomavirus genes E6 and E7 in cervical carcinoma cells. Proc Natl Acad Sci U S A 88:1411–1415, 1991.

33. Ward P, Parry GN, Yule R, et al: Human papillomavirus subtype 16a. Lancet 2:170, 1989.

34. Matsukura T, Koi S, and Sugase M: Both episomal and integrated forms of human papillomavirus type 16 are involved in invasive cervical cancers. Virology 172:63–72, 1989.

35. Fukushima M, Yamakawa Y, Shimano S, et al: The physical state of human papillomavirus 16 DNA in cervical carcinoma and cervical intraepithelial neoplasia. Cancer 66:2155–2161, 1990.

36. Finlay CA, Hinds PW, Levine AJ: The P53 proto-oncogene can act as a suppressor of transformation. Cell 57:1083–1093, 1989.

37. Eliyahu D, Michalovitz D, Eliyahu S, et al: Wild-type P53 can inhibit oncogene-mediated focus formation. Proc Natl Acad Sci U S A 86:8763–8767, 1989.

38. Scheffner M, Werness BA, Huibregtse JM, et al: The E6 oncoprotein encoded by human papillomavirus types 16 and 18 promotes the degradation of P53. Cell 63:1129–1136, 1990.

39. Dyson N, Howley PM, Munger K, Harlow E: The human papilloma virus-16 E7 oncoprotein is able to bind to the retinoblastoma gene product. Science 243:934–937, 1989.

40. Munger K, Phelps WC, Bubb V, et al: The E6 and E7 genes of the human papillomavirus type 16 together are necessary and sufficient for transformation of primary human keratinocytes. J Virol 63:4417–4421, 1989.

41. zur Hausen H: Human papillomaviruses in the pathogenesis of anogenital cancer. Virology 184:9–13, 1991.

42. Bosch FX, Schwarz E, Boukamp P, et al: Suppression in vivo of human papillomavirus type 18 E6-E7 gene expression in nontumorigenic hela x fibroblast hybrid cells. J Virol 64:4743–4754, 1990.

43. Hawley-Nelson P, Vousden KH, Hubbert NL, et al: HPV16 E6 and E7 proteins cooperate to immortalize human foreskin keratinocytes. EMBO J 8:3905–3910, 1989.

44. Woodworth CD, Bowden PE, Doniger J, et al: Characterization of normal human exocervical epithelial cells immortalized in vitro by papillomavirus types 16 and 18 DNA. Cancer Res 48:4620–4638, 1988.

45. Barron BA, Richart RM: A statistical model of the natural history of cervical carcinoma based on a prospective study of 557 cases. J Natl Cancer Inst 41:1343–1353, 1968.

46. Luthra UK, Prabhakar AK, Seth P, et al: Natural history of precancerous and early cancerous lesions of the uterine cervix. Acta Cytol 31:226–234, 1987.

47. Richart RM: Cervical intraepithelial neoplasia. Pathol Annu 8:301–328, 1973.

48. Kiviat NB, Critchlow CW, Kurman RJ: Reassessment of the morphological continuum of cervical intraepithelial lesions: Does it reflect different stages in the progression to cervical carcinoma? IARC Sci Publ 119:59–66, 1992.

49. The 1988 Bethesda System for Reporting Cervical/Vaginal Cytological Diagnoses. National Cancer Institute Workshop. JAMA 262:931–934, 1989.

50. Nasiell K, Nasiell M, Vaclavinkova V: Behavior of moderate cervical dysplasia during long-term follow-up. Obstet Gynecol 61:609–614, 1983.

51. Fidler HK, Boyes DA, Worth AJ: Cervical cancer detection in British Columbia. A progress report. J Obstet Gynaecol Br Commonw 75:392–404, 1968.

52. McIndoe WA, McLean MR, Jones RW, Mullins PR: The invasive potential of carcinoma in situ of the cervix. Obstet Gynecol 64:451–458, 1984.

53. Corfman PA, Richart RML: Cervical carcinogenesis; the application of experimentally derived concepts of carcinogene-

sis to an understanding of the development of cervical cancer in humans. Am J Obstet Gynecol 93:753–757, 1965.

54. Fu YS, Reagan JW, Richart RM: Definition of precursors. Gynecol Oncol 12(Pt 2):S220–S231, 1981.

55. Jakobsen A, Kristensen PB, Poulsen HK: Flow Cytometric Classification of biopsy specimens from cervical intraepithelial neoplasia. Cytometry 4:166–169, 1983.

56. Fu YS, Huang I, Beaudenon S, et al: Correlative study of human papillomavirus DNA, histopathology, and morphometry in cervical condyloma and intraepithelial neoplasia. Int J Gynecol Pathol 7:297–307, 1988.

57. Bibbo M, Dytch HE, Alenghat EL, et al: DNA ploidy profiles as prognostic indicators in CIN lesions. Am J Clin Pathol 92:261–265, 1989.

58. Fu YS, Braun L, Shah KV, et al: Histologic, nuclear DNA, and human papillomavirus studies of cervical condylomas. Cancer 52:1705–1711, 1983.

59. Richart RM: A modified terminology for cervical intraepithelial neoplasia. Obstet Gynecol 75:131–133, 1990.

60. Murthy NS, Sardana S, Narang N, et al: Biological behaviour of moderate dysplasia—a prospective study. Indian J Cancer 33:24–30, 1996.

61. Perry CM, Lamb HM: Topical imiquimod: A review of its use in genital warts. Drugs 58:375–390, 1999.

62. Syed TA, Ahmadpour OA, Ahmad SA, Ahmad SH: Management of female genital warts with an analog of imiquimod 2% in cream: A randomized, double-blind, placebo-controlled study. J Dermatol 25:429–433, 1998.

63. Pretorius R, Semrad N, Watring W, Fotheringham N: Presentation of cervical cancer. Gynecol Oncol 42:48–53, 1991.

64. Fahey MT, Irwig L, Macaskill P: Meta-analysis of Pap Test accuracy [see comments]. Am J Epidemiol 141:680–689, 1995.

65. Agency for Healthcare Policy and Research. Evidence Report/Technology Assessment No. 5, Evaluation of cervical cytology. 2-1-1999. Report No.: 99-E010.

66. Duggan MA: Papnet-assisted, primary screening of cervicovaginal smears. Eur J Gynaecol Oncol 21:35–42, 2000.

67. Wilbur DC, Prey, MU, Miller WM, et al: Detection of high grade squamous intraepithelial lesions and tumors using the autopap system: Results of a primary screening clinical trial. Cancer 87:354–358, 1999.

68. Hutchinson ML, Isenstein LM, Goodman A, et al: Homogeneous sampling accounts for the increased diagnostic accuracy using the Thinprep processor. Am J Clin Pathol 101:215–219, 1994.

69. Hutchinson ML, Zahniser DJ, Sherman ME, et al: Utility of liquid-based cytology for cervical carcinoma screening: Results of a population-based study conducted in a region of Costa Rica with a high incidence of cervical carcinoma [see comments]. Cancer 87:48–55, 1999.

70. Bolick DR, Hellman DJ: Laboratory implementation and efficacy assessment of the thinprep cervical cancer screening system. Acta Cytol 42:209–213, 1998.

71. Hatch KD: Multisite clinical outcome trial to evaluate performance of the Thinprep Pap Test. Obstet Gynecol 95(Suppl 1):S51, 2000.

72. Weintraub J, Morabia A: Efficacy of a liquid-based thin layer method for cervical cancer screening in a population with a low incidence of cervical cancer. Diagn Cytopathol 22:52–59, 2000.

73. Roberts JM, Gurley AM, Thurloe JK, et al: Evaluation of the ThinPrep Pap Test as an adjunct to the conventional pap smear. Med J Aust 167:466–469, 1997.

74. Carson HJ, DeMay RM: The mode ages of women with cervical dysplasia. Obstet Gynecol 82:430–434, 1993.

75. Meisels A: Cytologic diagnosis of human papillomavirus. Influence of age and pregnancy stage. Acta Cytol 36:480–482, 1992.

76. Burghardt E: Early histological diagnosis of cervical cancer. Major Probl Obstet Gynecol 6:391–401, 1973.

77. Fabiani G, Pittino M, D'Aietti V, et al: [Cervical dysplasias. Comparative study of the cytological picture, anatomo-pathologic and age stage]. Minerva Ginecol 39:629–632, 1987.

78. Cramer DW: The role of cervical cytology in the declining morbidity and mortality of cervical cancer. Cancer 34:2018–2027, 1974.

79. Geng L, Connolly DC, Isacson C, et al: Atypical immature metaplasia (AIM) of the cervix: Is it related to high-grade squamous intraepithelial lesion (HSIL)? Hum Pathol 30:345–351, 1999.

80. Sheils LA, Wilbur DC: Atypical squamous cells of undetermined significance. Stratification of the risk of association with, or progression to, squamous intraepithelial lesions based on morphologic subcategorization [see comments]. J Acta Cytol 41:1065–1072, 1997.

81. Solomon D, Frable WJ, Vooijs GP, et al: ASCUS and AGUS criteria. International Academy of Cytology Task Force Summary. Diagnostic cytology towards the 21st century: An international expert conference and tutorial. Acta Cytol 42:16–24, 1998.

82. Davey DD, Woodhouse S, Styer P, et al: Atypical epithelial cells and specimen adequacy: Current laboratory practices of participants in the College of American Pathologists Interlaboratory Comparison Program in cervicovaginal cytology. Arch Pathol Lab Med 124:203–211, 2000.

83. Kline MJ, Davey DD: Atypical squamous cells of undetermined significance qualified: A follow-up study. Diagn Cytopathol 14:380–384, 1996.

84. Kinney WK, Manos MM, Hurley LB, Ransley JE: Where's the high-grade cervical neoplasia? The importance of minimally abnormal Papanicolaou diagnoses. Obstet Gynecol 91:973–976, 1998.

85. Lonky NM, Sadeghi M, Tsadik GW, Petitti D: The clinical significance of the poor correlation of cervical dysplasia and cervical malignancy with referral cytologic results. Am J Obstet Gynecol 181:560–566, 1999.

86. Widra EA, Dookhan D, Jordan A, et al: Evaluation of the atypical cytologic smear. Validity of the 1991 Bethesda System. J Reprod Med 39:682–684, 1994.

87. Eltabbakh GH, Lipman JN, Mount SL, Morgan A: Significance of atypical squamous cells of undetermined significance on thinprep papanicolaou smears. Gynecol Oncol 79:44–49, 2000.

88. Manos MM, Kinney WK, Hurley LB, et al: Identifying women with cervical neoplasia: Using human papillomavirus DNA testing for equivocal Papanicolaou results [see comments]. JAMA 281:1605–1610, 1999.

89. Williams ML, Rimm DL, Pedigo MA, Frable WJ: Atypical squamous cells of undetermined significance: correlative histologic and follow-up studies from an academic medical center. Diagn Cytopathol 16:1–7, 1997.

90. Solomon D, Schiffman M, Tarone R: Comparison of three management strategies for patients with atypical squamous cells of undetermined significance: Baseline results from a randomized trial. J Natl Cancer Inst 93:293–299, 2001.

91. Ashfaq R, Gibbons D, Vela C, et al: ThinPrep Pap Test. Accuracy for glandular disease. Acta Cytol 43:81–85, 1999.

92. Raab SS: Can glandular lesions be diagnosed in pap smear cytology? Diagn Cytopathol 23:127–133, 2000.

93. Biscotti CV, Gero MA, Toddy SM, et al: Endocervical adenocarcinoma in situ: An analysis of cellular features. Diagn Cytopathol 17:326–332, 1997.

94. Soofer SB, Sidawy MK: Atypical glandular cells of undetermined significance: Clinically significant lesions and means of patient follow-up. Cancer 90:207–214, 2000.

95. Geier CS, Wilson M, Creasman W: Clinical evaluation of atypical glandular cells of undetermined significance. Am J Obstet Gynecol 184:64–69, 2001.

96. Duska LR, Flynn CF, Chen A, et al: Clinical evaluation of atypical glandular cells of undetermined significance on cervical cytology. Obstet Gynecol 91:278–282, 1998.

97. Reagan JW, Hamonic MJ, Wentz WB: Analytical study of the cells in cervical squamous cell cancer. Lab Invest 6:241–250, 1957.

98. Hayes MM, Matisic JP, Chen CJ, et al: Cytological aspects of uterine cervical adenocarcinoma, adenosquamous carcinoma and combined adenocarcinoma-squamous carcinoma: Appraisal of diagnostic criteria for in situ versus invasive lesions. Cytopathology 8:397–408, 1997.

99. Shingleton HM, Richart RM, Wiener J, Spiro D: Human cervical intraepithelial neoplasia: Fine structure of dysplasia and carcinoma in situ. Cancer Res 28:695–706, 1968.

100. Richart RM, Lerch V: Time-lapse cinematographic observations of normal human cervical epithelium, dysplasia, and carcinoma in situ. J Natl Cancer Inst 37:317–329, 1966.

101. Richart RM, Lerch V, Barron BA: A time-lapse cinematographic study in vitro of mitosis in normal human cervical epithelium, dysplasia, and carcinoma in situ. J Natl Cancer Inst 39:571–577, 1967.

102. Montz FJ, Holschneider CH, Thompson LD: Large-loop excision of the transformation zone: Effect on the pathologic interpretation of resection margins. Obstet Gynecol 81:976–982, 1993.

103. Felix JC, Muderspach LI, Duggan BD, Roman LD: The significance of positive margins in loop electrosurgical cone biopsies. Obstet Gynecol 84:996–1000, 1994.

104. Nasiell K, Roger V, Nasiell M: Behavior of mild cervical dysplasia during long-term follow-up. Obstet Gynecol 67:665–659, 1986.

105. Ho GY, Bierman R, Beardsley L, et al: Natural history of cervicovaginal papillomavirus infection in young women. N Engl J Med 338:423–428, 1998.

106. Lee SS, Collins RJ, Pun TC, Cheng DK, Ngan HY: Conservative treatment of low grade squamous intraepithelial lesions (LSIL) of the cervix. Int J Gynaecol Obstet 60:35–40, 1998.

107. Laverty CR, Russell P, Hills E, Booth N: The significance of noncondylomatous wart virus infection of the cervical transformation zone. A review with discussion of two illustrative cases. Acta Cytol 22:195–201, 1978.

108. Casas-Cordero M, Morin C, Roy M, et al: Origin of the koilocyte in condylomata of the human cervix: Ultrastructural study. Acta Cytol 25:383–392, 1981.

109. Doorbar J, Ely S, Sterling J, et al: Specific interaction between HPV-16 E1-E4 and cytokeratins results in collapse of the epithelial cell intermediate filament network. Nature 352:824–827, 1991.

110. Franquemont DW, Ward BE, Andersen WA, Crum CP: Prediction of 'high-risk' cervical papillomavirus infection by biopsy morphology. Am J Clin Pathol 92:577–582, 1989.

111. Ward P, Parry GN, Yule R, et al: Comparison between the polymerase chain reaction and slot blot hybridization for the detection of HPV sequences in cervical scrapes. Cytopathology 1:19–23, 1990.

112. Crum CP, Nuovo G, Friedman D, Silverstein SJ: A comparison of biotin and isotope-labeled ribonucleic acid probes for in situ detection of HPV-16 ribonucleic acid in genital precancers. Lab Invest 58:354–359, 1988.

113. Richart RM, Nuovo GJ: Human papillomavirus DNA in situ hybridization may be used for the quality control of genital tract biopsies. Obstet Gynecol 75:223–226, 1990.

114. Lorincz AT: Detection of human papillomavirus infection by nucleic acid hybridization. Obstet Gynecol Clin North Am 14:451–469, 1987.

115. Nuovo GJ, Silverstein SJ: Comparison of formalin, buffered formalin, and Bouin's fixation on the detection of human papillomavirus deoxyribonucleic acid from genital lesions. Lab Invest 59:720–724, 1988.

116. Winkler B, Crum CP, Fujii T, et al: Koilocytotic lesions of the cervix. The relationship of mitotic abnormalities to the presence of papillomavirus antigens and nuclear DNA content. Cancer 53:1081–1087, 1984.

117. Bergeron C, Ferenczy A, Shah KV, Naghashfar Z: Multicentric human papillomavirus infections of the female genital tract: Correlation of viral types with abnormal mitotic figures, colposcopic presentation, and location. Obstet Gynecol 69:736–742, 1987.

118. Crum CP, Egawa K, Fu YS, et al: Atypical immature metaplasia (AIM). A subset of human papilloma virus infection of the cervix. Cancer 51:2214–2219, 1983.

119. Koss LG, Stewart FW, Foote FW, et al: Some histological aspects of behavior of epidermoid carcinoma in situ and related lesions of the uterine cervix. Cancer 16:1160–1211, 2001.

120. Kottmeier HL: Evolution et traitment des epitheliomas. Rev Fran Gynecol d'Obstet 56:821–826, 1961.

121. Spriggs AI, Boddington MM: Progression and regression of cervical lesions. review of smears from women followed without initial biopsy or treatment. J Clin Pathol 33:517–522, 1980.

122. ter Harmsel B, Kuijpers J, Smedts F, et al: Progressing imbalance between proliferation and apoptosis with increasing severity of cervical intraepithelial neoplasia. Int J Gynecol Pathol 16:205–211, 1997.

123. Shoji Y, Saegusa M, Takano Y, et al: Correlation of apoptosis with tumour cell differentiation, progression, and HPV infection in cervical carcinoma. J Clin Pathol 49:134–138, 1996.

124. Reagan JW, Hamonic MJ: The cellular pathology in carcinoma in situ; a cytohistopathological correlation. Cancer 9:385–398, 1956.

125. Weir MM, Bell DA, Young RH: Transitional cell metaplasia of the uterine cervix and vagina: An underrecognized lesion that may be confused with high-grade dysplasia. A report of 59 cases [see comments]. Am J Surg Pathol 21:510–517, 1997.

126. Harnden P, Kennedy W, Andrew AC, Southgate J: Immunophenotype of transitional metaplasia of the uterine cervix. Int J Gynecol Pathol 18:125–129, 1999.

127. Bulten J, de Wilde PC, Schijf C, et al: Decreased expression of Ki-67 in atrophic cervical epithelium of post-menopausal women. J Pathol 190:545–553, 2000.

128. Bertrand M, Lickrish GM, Colgan TJ: The anatomic distribution of cervical adenocarcinoma in situ: Implications for treatment. Am J Obstet Gynecol 157:21–25, 1987.

129. Bousfield L, Pacey F, Young Q, et al: Expanded cytologic criteria for the diagnosis of adenocarcinoma in situ of the cervix and related lesions. Acta Cytol 24:283–296, 1980.

130. Luesley DM, Jordan JA, Woodman CB, et al: A retrospective review of adenocarcinoma-in-situ and glandular atypia of the uterine cervix. Br J Obstet Gynaecol 94:699–703, 1987.

131. Tase T, Okagaki T, Clark BA, et al: Human papillomavirus DNA in glandular dysplasia and microglandular hyperplasia: Presumed precursors of adenocarcinoma of the uterine cervix. Obstet Gynecol 73:1005–1008, 1989.

132. Boddington MM, Spriggs AI, Cowdell RH: Adenocarcinoma of the uterine cervix: Cytological evidence of a long preclinical evolution. Br J Obstet Gynaecol 83:900–903, 1976.

133. Boon ME, Baak JP, Kurver PJ, et al: Adenocarcinoma in situ of the cervix: An underdiagnosed lesion. Cancer 48:768–773, 1981.

134. Kashimura M, Shinohara M, Oikawa K, et al: An adenocarcinoma in situ of the uterine cervix that developed into invasive adenocarcinoma after 5 years. Gynecol Oncol 36:128–133, 1990.

135. Andersen ES, Arffmann E: Adenocarcinoma in situ of the uterine cervix: A clinico-pathologic study of 36 cases. Gynecol Oncol 35:1–7, 1989.

136. Christopherson WM, Nealon N, Gray LA: Noninvasive precursor lesions of adenocarcinoma and mixed adenosquamous carcinoma of the cervix uteri. Cancer 44:975–983, 1979.

137. Cullimore JE, Luesley DM, Rollason TP, et al: A prospective study of conization of the cervix in the management of cervical intraepithelial glandular neoplasia (CIGN)—a preliminary report. Br J Obstet Gynaecol 99:314–318, 1992.

138. Tobon H, Dave H: Adenocarcinoma in situ of the cervix. Clinicopathologic observations of 11 cases. Int J Gynecol Pathol 7:139–151, 1988.

139. Weisbrot IM, Stabinsky C, Davis AM: Adenocarcinoma in situ of the uterine cervix. Cancer 29:1179–1187, 1972.

140. Tase T, Okagaki T, Clark BA, et al: Human papillomavirus dna in adenocarcinoma in situ, microinvasive adenocarcinoma of the uterine cervix, and coexisting cervical squamous intraepithelial neoplasia. Int J Gynecol Pathol 8:8–17, 1989.

141. Farnsworth A, Laverty C, Stoler MH: Human papillomavirus messenger RNA expression in adenocarcinoma in situ of the uterine cervix. Int J Gynecol Pathol 8:321–330, 1989.

142. Griffin NR, Dockey D, Lewis FA, Wells M: Demonstration of low frequency of human papillomavirus DNA in cervical adenocarcinoma and adenocarcinoma in situ by the polymerase chain reaction and in situ hybridization. Int J Gynecol Pathol 10:36–43, 1991.

143. Zaino RJ: Glandular lesions of the uterine cervix. Mod Pathol 13:261–274, 2000.

144. Rollason TP, Cullimore J, Bradgate MG: A suggested columnar cell morphological equivalent of squamous carcinoma in situ with early stromal invasion. Int J Gynecol Pathol 8:230–236, 1989.
145. Young RH, Clement PB: Pseudoneoplastic glandular lesions of the uterine cervix. Semin Diagn Pathol 8:234–249, 1991.
146. Schlesinger C, Silverberg SG: Endocervical adenocarcinoma in situ of tubal type and its relation to atypical tubal metaplasia. Int J Gynecol Pathol 18:1–4, 1999.
147. Benoit JL, Kini SR: "Arias-Stella reaction"–like changes in endocervical glandular epithelium in cervical smears during pregnancy and postpartum states—a potential diagnostic pitfall. Diagn Cytopathol 14:349–355, 1996.
148. Brinton LA, Tashima KT, Lehman HF, et al: Epidemiology of cervical cancer by cell type. Cancer Res 47:1706–1711, 1987.
149. Clement PB, Scully RE: Carcinoma of the cervix: Histologic types. Semin Oncol 9:251–264, 1982.
150. Colgan TJ, Auger M, McLaughlin JR: Histopathologic classification of cervical carcinomas and recognition of mucin-secreting squamous carcinomas. Int J Gynecol Pathol 12:64–69, 1993.
151. Modifications in the staging for stage I vulvar and stage I cervical cancer. Report of the FIGO Committee on Gynecologic Oncology. International Federation of Gynecology and Obstetrics. Int J Gynaecol Obstet 50:215–216, 1995.
152. Tidbury P, Singer A, Jenkins D: CIN 3: The role of lesion size in invasion. Br J Obstet Gynaecol 99:583–586, 1992.
153. Benedet JL, Murphy KJ: Cervical cancer screening. Who needs a Pap test? How often? Postgrad Med 78:69–79, 1985.
154. Benedet JL, Anderson GH, Boyes DA: Colposcopic accuracy in the diagnosis of microinvasive and occult invasive carcinoma of the cervix. Obstet Gynecol 65:557–562, 1985.
155. McIndoe GA, Robson MS, Tidy JA, et al: Laser excision rather than vaporization: The treatment of choice for cervical intraepithelial neoplasia. Obstet Gynecol 74:165–168, 1989.
156. Bigrigg A, Haffenden DK, Sheehan AL, et al: Efficacy and safety of large-loop excision of the transformation zone. Lancet 343:32–34, 1994.
157. Bigrigg MA, Codling BW, Pearson P, et al: Colposcopic diagnosis and treatment of cervical dysplasia at a single clinic visit. Experience of low-voltage diathermy loop in 1000 patients. Lancet 336:229–231, 1990.
158. Hallam NF, West J, Harper C, et al: Large loop excision of the transformation zone (LLETZ) as an alternative to both local ablative and cone biopsy treatment: A series of 1000 patients. J Gynecol Surg 9:77–82, 1993.
159. Murdoch JB, Morgan PR, Lopes A, Monaghan JM: Histological incomplete excision of CIN after large loop excision of the transformation zone (LLETZ) merits careful follow up, not retreatment. Br J Obstet Gynaecol 99:990–993, 1992.
160. Barsky SH, Siegal GP, Jannotta F, Liotta LA: Loss of basement membrane components by invasive tumors but not by their benign counterparts. Lab Invest 49:140–147, 1983.
161. d'Ardenne AJ: Use of basement membrane markers in tumour diagnosis. J Clin Pathol 42:449–457, 1989.
162. Vogel HP, Mendelsohn G: Laminin immunostaining in hyperplastic, dysplastic, and neoplastic lesions of the endometrium and uterine cervix. Obstet Gynecol 69:794–799, 1987.
163. Ehrmann RL, Dwyer IM, Yavner D, Hancock WW: An immunoperoxidase study of laminin and type IV collagen distribution in carcinoma of the cervix and vulva. Obstet Gynecol 72:257–262, 1988.
164. Stewart CJ, McNicol AM: Distribution of type IV collagen immunoreactivity to assess questionable early stromal invasion. J Clin Pathol 45:9–15, 1992.
165. Copeland LJ, Silva EG, Gershenson DM, et al: Superficially invasive squamous cell carcinoma of the cervix. Gynecol Oncol 45:307–312, 1992.
166. Smiley LM, Burke TW, Silva EG, et al: Prognostic factors in stage 1B squamous cervical cancer patients with low risk for recurrence. Obstet Gynecol 77:271–275, 1991.
167. Sevin BU, Nadji M, Averette HE, et al: Microinvasive carcinoma of the cervix. Cancer 70:2121–2128, 1992.
168. Takeshima N, Yanoh K, Tabata T, et al: Assessment of the revised International Federation of Gynecology and Obstet-
169. Buckley SL, Tritz DM, Van Le L, et al: Lymph node metastases and prognosis in patients with stage IA2 cervical cancer. Gynecol Oncol 63:4–9, 1996.
170. Kolstad P: Follow-up study of 232 patients with stage Ia1 and 411 patients with stage Ia2 squamous cell carcinoma of the cervix (microinvasive carcinoma). Gynecol Oncol 33:265–272, 1989.
171. Leman MH, Benson WL, Kurman RJ, Park RC: Microinvasive carcinoma of the cervix. Obstet Gynecol 48:571–578, 1976.
172. Maiman MA, Fruchter RG, DiMaio TM, Boyce JG: Superficially invasive squamous cell carcinoma of the cervix. Obstet Gynecol 72(Pt 1):399–403, 1988.
173. Sedlis A, Sall S, Tsukada Y, et al: Microinvasive carcinoma of the uterine cervix: A clinical-pathologic study. Am J Obstet Gynecol 133:64–74, 1979.
174. Delgado G, Bundy BN, Fowler WC, et al: Prospective surgical pathological study of stage I squamous carcinoma of the cervix: A Gynecologic Oncology Group Study. Gynecol Oncol 35:314–320, 1989.
175. Kurian K, al Nafussi A: Relation of cervical glandular intraepithelial neoplasia to microinvasive and invasive adenocarcinoma of the uterine cervix: A study of 121 cases. J Clin Pathol 52:112–117, 1999.
176. Ostor A, Rome R, Quinn M: Microinvasive adenocarcinoma of the cervix: A clinicopathologic study of 77 women. Obstet Gynecol 89:88–93, 1997.
177. Schorge JO, Lee KR, Flynn CE, et al: Stage IA1 cervical adenocarcinoma: Definition and treatment. Obstet Gynecol 93:219–222, 1999.
178. Ostor AG: Early invasive adenocarcinoma of the uterine cervix. Int J Gynecol Pathol 19:29–38, 2000.
179. Nicklin JL, Perrin LC, Crandon AJ, Ward BG: Microinvasive adenocarcinoma of the cervix. Aust N Z J Obstet Gynaecol 39:411–413, 1999.
180. Muntz HG, Bell DA, Lage JM, et al: Adenocarcinoma in situ of the uterine cervix. Obstet Gynecol 80:935–939, 1992.
181. Wolf JK, Levenback C, Malpica A, et al:. Adenocarcinoma in situ of the cervix: Significance of cone biopsy margins. Obstet Gynecol 88:82–86, 1996.
182. Goldstein NS, Mani A: The status and distance of cone biopsy margins as a predictor of excision adequacy for endocervical adencarcinoma in situ. Am J Clin Pathol 109:727–732, 1998.
183. Parkin DM, Laara E, Muir CS: Estimates of the worldwide frequency of sixteen major cancers in 1980. Int J Cancer 41:184–197, 1988.
184. Cervical Cancer Screening Programs: Summary of the 1982 Canadian Task Force Report. Can Med Assoc J 127:581–589, 1982.
185. Cook GA, Draper GJ: Trends in cervical cancer and carcinoma in situ in Great Britain. Br J Cancer 50:367–375, 1984.
186. Silcocks PB, Moss SM: Rapidly progressive cervical cancer: Is it a real problem? Br J Obstet Gynaecol 95:1111–1116, 1988.
187. Mikuta JJ, Celebre JA: Adenocarcinoma of the cervix. Obstet Gynecol 33:753–756, 1969.
188. Devesa SS: Descriptive epidemiology of cancer of the uterine cervix. Obstet Gynecol 63:605–612, 1984.
189. Gallup DG, Abell MR: Invasive adenocarcinoma of the uterine cervix. Obstet Gynecol 49:596–603, 1977.
190. Horowitz IR, Jacobson LP, Zucker PK, et al: Epidemiology of adenocarcinoma of the cervix. Gynecol Oncol 31:25–31, 1988.
191. Davis JR, Moon LB: Increased incidence of adenocarcinoma of uterine cervix. Obstet Gynecol 45:79–83, 1975.
192. Hopkins MP, Schmidt RW, Roberts JA, Morley GW: Gland cell carcinoma (adenocarcinoma) of the cervix. Obstet Gynecol 72:789–795, 1988.
193. Shingleton HM, Gore H, Bradley DH, Soong SJ: Adenocarcinoma of the cervix. I. Clinical evaluation and pathologic features. Am J Obstet Gynecol 139:799–814, 1981.
194. Leminen A, Paavonen J, Forss M, et al: Adenocarcinoma of the uterine cervix. Cancer 65:53–59, 1990.
195. Maier RC, Norris HJ: Coexistence of cervical intraepithelial

neoplasia with primary adenocarcinoma of the endocervix. Obstet Gynecol 56:361–364, 1980.

196. Tenti P, Romagnoli S, Silini E, et al: Human papillomavirus types 16 and 18 infection in infiltrating adenocarcinoma of the cervix: PCR analysis of 138 cases and correlation with histologic type and grade. Am J Clin Pathol 106:52–56, 1996.

197. Jones MW, Silverberg SG: Cervical adenocarcinoma in young women: Possible relationship to microglandular hyperplasia and use of oral contraceptives. Obstet Gynecol 73:984–989, 1989.

198. Peters RK, Chao A, Mack TM, et al: Increased frequency of adenocarcinoma of the uterine cervix in young women in Los Angeles County. J Natl Cancer Inst 76:423–428, 1986.

199. Hurt WG, Silverberg SG, Frable WJ, et al: Adenocarcinoma of the cervix: Histopathologic and clinical features. Am J Obstet Gynecol 129:304–315, 1977.

200. Parazzini F, La Vecchia C, Negri E, et al: Risk factors for adenocarcinoma of the cervix: A case-control study. Br J Cancer 57:201–204, 1988.

201. Silcocks PB, Thornton-Jones H, Murphy M: Squamous and adenocarcinoma of the uterine cervix: A comparison using routine data. Br J Cancer 55:321–325, 1987.

202. Podczaski E, Kaminski PF, Pees RC, et al: Peutz-Jeghers syndrome with ovarian sex cord tumor with annular tubules and cervical adenoma malignum. Gynecol Oncol 42:74–78, 1991.

203. Young RH, Scully RE: Mucinous ovarian tumors associated with mucinous adenocarcinomas of the cervix. A clinicopathological analysis of 16 cases. Int J Gynecol Pathol 7:99–111, 1988.

203a. Wentz WB, Reagan JW: Clinical significance of postirradiation dysplasia of the uterine cervix. Am J Obstet Gynecol 106:812–817, 1970.

204. Chung CK, Stryker JA, Ward SP, et al: Histologic grade and prognosis of carcinoma of the cervix. Obstet Gynecol 57:636–642, 1981.

205. Larsson G, Alm P, Gullberg B, Grundsell H: Prognostic factors in early invasive carcinoma of the uterine cervix. A clinical, histopathologic, and statistical analysis of 343 cases. Am J Obstet Gynecol 146:145–153, 1983.

206. Roman L, Feli JC, Muderspach LI, et al: Influence of quantity of lymph-vascular space invasion on the risk of nodal metastases in women with early-stage squamous cancer of the cervix. Gynecol Oncol 68:220–225, 1998.

207. Lucas WE, Benirschke K, Lebherz TB: Verrucous carcinoma of the female genital tract. Am J Obstet Gynecol 119:435–440, 1974.

208. Kleine W, Rau K, Schwoeorer D, Pfleiderer A: Prognosis of the adenocarcinoma of the cervix uteri: A comparative study. Gynecol Oncol 35:145–149, 1989.

209. Saigo PE, Cain JM, Kim WS, et al: Prognostic factors in adenocarcinoma of the uterine cervix. Cancer 57:1584–1593, 1986.

210. Berek JS, Hacker NF, Fu YS, et al: Adenocarcinoma of the uterine cervix: Histologic variables associated with lymph node metastasis and survival. Obstet Gynecol 65:46–52, 1985.

211. Young RH, Scully RE: Villoglandular papillary adenocarcinoma of the uterine cervix. A clinicopathologic analysis of 13 cases. Cancer 63:1773–1779, 1989.

212. Herbst AL, Cole P, Norusis MJ, et al: Epidemiologic aspects and factors related to survival in 384 registry cases of clear cell adenocarcinoma of the vagina and cervix. Am J Obstet Gynecol 135:876–886, 1979.

213. Robboy SJ, Herbst AL, Scully RE: Clear-cell adenocarcinoma of the vagina and cervix in young females: Analysis of 37 tumors that persisted or recurred after primary therapy. Cancer 34:606–614, 1974.

214. Hart WR, Norris HJ: Mesonephric adenocarcinomas of the cervix. Cancer 29:106–113, 1972.

215. Kaminski PF, Maier RC: Clear cell adenocarcinoma of the cervix unrelated to diethylstilbestrol exposure. Obstet Gynecol 62:720–727, 1983.

216. Gilks CB, Clement PB: Papillary serous adenocarcinoma of the uterine cervix: A report of three cases. Mod Pathol 5:426–231, 1992.

217. Ferry JA, Scully RE: Mesonephric remnants, hyperplasia, and neoplasia in the uterine cervix. A study of 49 cases. Am J Surg Pathol 14:1100–1111, 1990.

218. Gilks CB, Young RH, Gersell DJ, Clement PB: Large cell neuroendocrine (corrected) carcinoma of the uterine cervix: A clinicopathologic study of 12 cases. Am J Surg Pathol 21:905–914, 1997.

219. Maier RC, Norris HJ: Glassy cell carcinoma of the cervix. Obstet Gynecol 60:219–224, 1982.

220. Seltzer V, Sall S, Castadot MJ, et al: Glassy cell cervical carcinoma. Gynecol Oncol 8:141–151, 1979.

221. Benda JA, Platz CE, Buchsbaum H, Lifshitz S: Mucin production in defining mixed carcinoma of the uterine cervix: A clinicopathologic study. Int J Gynecol Pathol 4:314–327, 1985.

222. Miles PA, Norris HJ: Adenoid cystic carcinoma of the cervix. An analysis of 12 cases. Obstet Gynecol 38:103–110, 1971.

223. Fowler WC, Miles PA, Surwit EA, et al: Adenoid cystic carcinoma of the cervix. report of 9 cases and a reappraisal. Obstet Gynecol 52:337–342, 1978.

224. King LA, Talledo OE, Gallup DG, et al: Adenoid cystic carcinoma of the cervix in women under age 40. Gynecol Oncol 32:26–30, 1989.

225. van Dinh T, and Woodruff JD: Adenoid cystic and adenoid basal carcinomas of the cervix. Obstet Gynecol 65:705–709, 1985.

226. Santoso JT, Kucera PR, Ray J: Primary malignant melanoma of the uterine cervix: Two case reports and a century's review. Obstet Gynecol Surv 45:733–740, 1990.

227. Jones HW, Droegemueller W, Makowski EL: A primary melanocarcinoma of the cervix. Am J Obstet Gynecol 111(7):959–963, 1971.

228. Tsukamoto N, Nakamura M, Kashimura M, Saito TL: Primary cervical choriocarcinoma. Gynecol Oncol 9:99–107, 1980.

229. Lathrop JC: Malignant pelvic lymphomas. Obstet Gynecol 30:137–145, 1967.

230. Muntz HG, Ferry JA, Flynn D, et al: Stage IE primary malignant lymphomas of the uterine cervix. Cancer 68:2023–2032, 1991.

231. Lemoine NR, Hall PA: Epithelial tumors metastatic to the uterine cervix. A study of 33 cases and review of the literature. Cancer 57:2002–2005, 1986.

232. Zhang YC, Zhang PF, Wei YH: Metastatic carcinoma of the cervix uteri from the gastrointestinal tract. Gynecol Oncol 15:287–290, 1983.

233. Way S: Carcinoma metastatic in the cervix. Gynecol Oncol 9:298–302, 1980.

234. Bajo J, Moreno-Calve FJ, Uguet-de-Resayre C, et al: Contribution of transvaginal sonography to the evaluation of benign cervical conditions. J Clin Ultrasound 27:61–64, 1999.

235. Tiltman AJ: Leiomyomas of the uterine cervix: A study of frequency. Int J Gynecol Pathol 17:231–234, 1998.

236. Copeland LJ, Silva EG, Gershenson DM, et al: Superficially invasive squamous cell carcinoma of the cervix. Gynecol Oncol 45:307–312, 1992.

237. Creasman WT, Fetter BF, Clarke-Pearson DL, et al: Management of stage IA carcinoma of the cervix. Am J Obstet Gynecol 153:164–172, 1985.

238. Delgado G, Bundy BN, Fowler WC Jr, et al: A prospective surgical pathological study of stage I squamous carcinoma of the cervix: A Gynecologic Oncology Group Study. Gynecol Oncol 35:314–320, 1989.

239. Hasumi K, Sakamoto A, Sugano H: Microinvasive carcinoma of the uterine cervix. Cancer 45:928–931, 1980.

240. Hopkins MP, Morley GW: Stage IB squamous cell cancer of the cervix: Clinicopathologic features related to survival. Am J Obstet Gynecol 164:1520–1527; discussion 1527–1529, 1991.

241. Leman MH Jr, Benson WL, Kurman RJ, Park RC: Microinvasive carcinoma of the cervix. Obstet Gynecol 48:571–578, 1976.

242. Maiman MA, Fruchter RG, DiMaio TM, Boyce JG: Superficially invasive squamous cell carcinoma of the cervix. Obstet Gynecol 72:399–403, 1988.

243. Sevin BU, Nadji M, Averette HE, et al: Microinvasive carcinoma of the cervix [review]. Cancer 70:2121–2128, 1992.

244. Simon NL, Gore H, Shingleton HM, et al: Study of superficially invasive carcinoma of the cervix. Obstet Gynecol 68: 19–24, 1986.

245. van Nagell JR Jr, Greenwell N, Powell DF, et al: Microinvasive carcinoma of the cervix. Am J Obstet Gynecol 145:981–991, 1983.

246. Kudo R, Sasano H, Koizumi M, et al: Immunohistochemical comparison of new monoclonal antibody IC5 and carcinoembryonic antigen in the differential diagnosis of adenocarcinoma of the uterine cervix. Int J Gynecol Pathol 9:325–336, 1990.

247. Maes G, Fleuren GJ, Bara J, Nap M: The distribution of mucins, carcinoembryonic antigen, and mucus-associated antigens in endocervical and endometrial adenocarcinomas. Int J Gynecol Pathol 7:112–122, 1988.

248. Tamimi HK, Gown AM, Kim-Deobald J, et al: The utility of immunocytochemistry in invasive adenocarcinoma of the cervix. Am J Obstet Gynecol 166:1655–1661; discussion 1661–1662, 1992.

249. Wahlstrom T, Lindgren J, Korhonen M, Seppala M: Distinction between endocervical and endometrial adenocarcinoma with immunoperoxidase staining of carcinoembryonic antigen in routine histological tissue specimens. Lancet 2:1159–1160, 1979.

# 37

# *Uterus*

Nilsa C. Ramirez   W. Dwayne Lawrence

## INTRODUCTION

### Embryology

In the female embryo with a normal genetic makeup (46XX), the primordial germ cells migrate from the yolk sac into the genital ridges close to the sixth gestational week[1]; the ovaries do not develop in the absence of the primordial germ cells.[1] The müllerian (or paramesonephric) ducts begin to form during the sixth gestational week.[1, 2] During the developmental stage, the lateral surface coelomic epithelium of the paired urogenital ridges invaginates in several areas; their coalescence results in the formation of the paired müllerian ducts.[1] As the female embryo develops, the caudad third of the ducts fuse by the end of the eighth gestational week, with the paired wolffian (mesonephric) ducts acting as guides during their caudad migration.[2] Around the ninth gestational week, the fused portion of the müllerian ducts can be identified as the uterine canal, a structure that eventually develops into the uterus, the cervix, and the upper one third of the vagina.[1, 3] The craniad portions of the müllerian ducts that fail to fuse develop into the fallopian tubes.[1] The uterine corpus further differentiates into the endometrium, the myometrium, and the serosa by the end of the 19th gestational week.[2] The recently developed endometrium consists of fibroblastic stroma associated with a single layer of surface columnar epithelium[4] until the 20th week of gestation, when the surface epithelium invaginates, resulting in the formation of glands.[3, 4] The uterus does not assume its adult form until the 24th gestational week.[2]

### Congenital Anomalies

Either isolated or combined with congenital anomalies of other systems, anomalies of the female reproductive system can result from numerical alterations or structural defects of the sex and somatic chromosomes. Commonly, these malformations are associated with defects in hormonal metabolic pathways that play crucial roles in their genesis. Many of these defective metabolic pathways are linked to the development of primary or secondary sexual characteristics or both. Maternal factors also may interfere with the normal development of the fetal reproductive organs. In utero exposure to androgenic or estrogenic hormones produced by benign or malignant maternal tumors, although rare, may result in such anomalies.[5] Use of exogenous hormones during pregnancy can be linked to developmental fetal anomalies involving different organ systems. An example of the latter was the use of diethylstilbestrol (DES), a synthetic nonsteroidal estrogen.[6] Female fetuses exposed to DES in utero were at a higher risk of developing structural anomalies of the reproductive tract and, later in life, neoplastic (vaginal clear cell carcinoma) and non-neoplastic (vaginal adenosis, cervical ectropion) conditions.[6]

Uterine congenital anomalies can be the result of abnormal fusion of the müllerian ducts, resulting in the persistence of fetal structures or in the failure of certain structures to develop. During embryogenesis, fusion of the müllerian ducts creates a temporary wall (septum) between the two lumina.[1] Normally, degeneration of the septum follows, with the consequent development of the endometrial cavity in continuity with the upper aspect of the vagina. Complete failure of the paired müllerian ducts to fuse results in the formation a double uterus (uterus didelphys) (CD Figs. 37–1 through 37–3) with a partially double vagina.[1] Partial fusion of the müllerian ducts engenders a single uterus with two cornual areas (uterus bicornis).[1] Persistence of a small fundal component of the septum, causing an indentation of the uterine wall in that area, results in a uterus arcuatus.[1] Muscular tissue occupies the lateral pelvic walls bilaterally when both müllerian ducts fail to develop.[1]

## Anatomy

The uterus, with the cervix, bilateral fallopian tubes, and ovaries lies in the pelvis. Each ovary is attached to the posterior surface of the broad ligament by a short peritoneal fold (mesovarium). The fallopian tubes are located in the upper free edge of each respective broad ligament. The broad ligaments are in continuity with the peritoneum covering most of the uterus except for an area in the lower anterior part.[6a] The body, or corpus, constitutes the major part of the uterus, and the portion above the level of the tubes is known as the *fundus*.[6a] The third and smallest part is the cervix, which projects into the upper vagina and meets the uterine body at a vertical angle. The uterus with the cervix lies at almost a right angle to the longitudinal axis of the vagina and is described as being anteverted in respect to the latter.[6a] The uterine surfaces are described as anterior (related to the urinary bladder) and posterior (related to the small intestine and the rectum). The right and left lateral uterine margins are attached to the broad ligaments.[6a] The cervix has intravaginal and supravaginal portions. The external cervical os opens into the upper vagina, and its lumen is continuous with the endocervical canal and the isthmus.[6a] The isthmus (or lower uterine segment) is a short segment between the endocervical canal and the uterine cavity.

## Endometrial Histology

The endometrial mucosa of the uterine corpus is divided into two main regions with distinct histologic characteristics: the basalis (stratum basale) (Fig. 37–1) and the functionalis (stratum spongiosum). The basalis corresponds to approximately the lower

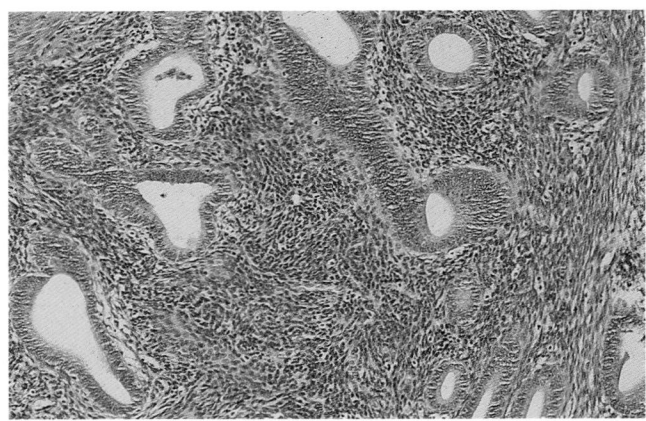

**Figure 37–1.** The endometrial basalis (stratum basalis). Note the spindle-shaped stromal cells and the glands lined by columnar pseudostratified cells.

one third of the endometrium; it meets the innermost aspect of the myometrium at the endomyometrial junction. The latter may be markedly irregular, as finger-like projections of the myometrium encounter sections of the basalis at different levels. The basalis retains essentially identical histologic features throughout the menstrual cycle because of a different sensitivity to hormonal stimulation than that of the functionalis. The glands of the basalis are straight and lined by columnar cells with pseudostratified, elongated nuclei; mitotic figures are rare. Mitotically inactive spindle-shaped cells characterize the stroma. The endometrial arteries in the basalis exhibit a subendothelial elastica similar to that present in myometrial arteries, a feature that contributes to their vasoconstrictive capabilities controlling bleeding during menstruation.[4] These arteries do not respond to progesterone and estrogen.[7] The small arteries of the functionalis lack a subendothelial elastica, however, and display morphologic changes throughout the menstrual cycle in response to the changing levels of progesterone and estrogen.[7] Because of its pivotal role in the regeneration of the functionalis after menstruation, the integrity of the basalis must be maintained.

The functionalis corresponds to approximately the upper two thirds of the full endometrial mucosal thickness. It is responsive to the cyclic hormonal influences that induce the sequential glandular and stromal changes associated with the menstrual cycle. During the proliferative phase of the menstrual cycle (ovarian follicular phase), the functionalis displays changes mainly associated with an estrogenic effect (Fig. 37–2). After ovulation, the secretory phase (ovarian luteal phase) is associated with rising levels of estrogen and progesterone; decline of the latter hormones is responsible eventually for the endometrial degeneration, necrosis, and eventual shedding associated with menstruation.

The mucosa of the isthmus (lower uterine segment) is usually out of synchrony with the function-

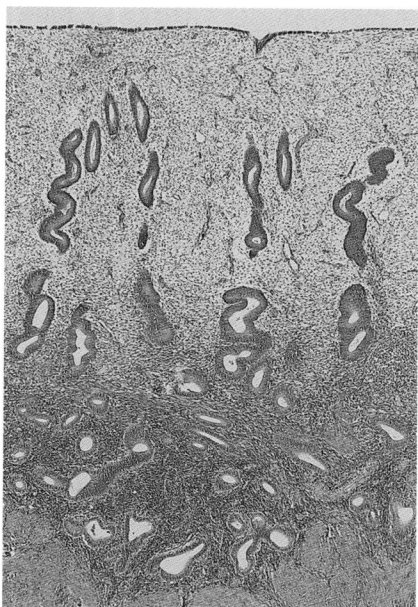

**Figure 37–2.** The endometrial mucosa. The stratum functionalis corresponds to approximately the upper two thirds of the mucosal thickness.

alis. Similar to the basalis, its glandular and stromal characteristics remain relatively constant throughout the menstrual cycle. The histologic features also are similar to those of the basalis; hybrid glands representing the transition from upper endocervical epithelium (mucinous) to endometrial epithelium also can be seen. Occasional isthmic glands show either pure tubal (ciliary) metaplasia or tuboendometrioid metaplasia of the epithelium. The mucosa of the basalis, the isthmus, and the endometrium of the peritubal ostia all contribute to the regeneration of the functionalis after menstruation.[4]

T lymphocytes and their subtypes and B lymphocytes normally can be seen in the endometrium. The presence of lymphoid follicles per se generally is not considered a pathologic finding because they can be seen permeating the stroma of normal endometrium usually in the basalis. Aggregates of B lymphocytes may be present in the basalis, but their presence in the functionalis[8, 9] seems to be unusual. Macrophages and T lymphocytes permeate the stroma[8, 9] throughout the menstrual cycle. Large granular lymphocytes, a subset of T lymphocytes, once were regarded to be "stromal granulocytes of undifferentiated endometrial cell origin"; they are more numerous in the late secretory phase of the menstrual cycle.[8, 9] Polymorphonuclear leukocytes occur in small numbers during the menstrual cycle but are more numerous during the late secretory–early menstrual part of the cycle and in association with more advanced glandular and stromal breakdown. Mast cells can permeate the endometrium; as the endometrium atrophies, the number of mast cells seems to decrease.[10]

## Endometrial Physiology

The endometrial histology of the newborn reflects the in utero influence of maternal circulating hormones, and these changes can persist for 1 month postpartum.[3] When the maternal hormonal effect subsides, the endometrium is characterized by an inactive pattern until the onset of puberty.

During the reproductive years, the nonpregnant endometrium is under the cyclic influence of estrogen and progesterone; their secretion, in turn, is regulated under normal circumstances by the interactions of the hypothalamus, the anterior pituitary gland, and the ovaries. This cyclic phenomenon is manifested as the menstrual cycle. In 1950, Noyes and colleagues[11] published their seminal observations describing an endometrial dating system, still widely used today, that was developed by determining time of ovulation using basal body temperature charting and comparing the derived clinical data with the histologic features of the corresponding endometrial biopsy specimens. In their system, the first day of menstruation defines the first day of the prototypical 28-day-long menstrual cycle, and ovulation occurs on day 14. The preovulatory phase (proliferative, or ovarian follicular, phase) can vary in length, accounting in large part for the difference in the length of the menstrual cycle observed among women. The proliferative phase endometrium lacks definitive, specific (day-to-day) histologic features, precluding precise dating. Certain histologic attributes, such as the degree of stromal edema, allow for the broad categorization of early, mid, and late proliferative events, however. The postovulatory phase (secretory, or ovarian luteal, phase) is relatively constant and is expected to last about 14 days. Although that assumption generally has been accepted, a study of 327 regularly cycling women revealed that only 26% of them had a 14-day-long luteal phase.[12] The histologic changes of the secretory phase are sufficiently predictable to allow the identification of key features roughly on a day-to-day basis. In the postmenopausal period, the failure of the hypothalamus-pituitary-ovarian complex to supply the necessary hormones to maintain the cycle (normally associated with the aging process) results in endometrial inactivity and eventual atrophy.

### HISTOLOGIC DATING: THE MENSTRUAL CYCLE

If we regard the first day of menstruation as the first day of the menstrual cycle, by day 5, the surface of the functionalis should be completely re-epithelialized.[4] During the menstrual cycle, the variations in the circulating levels of ovarian-derived estradiol and progesterone affect the intracellular concentrations of endometrial estrogen receptors and progesterone receptors. The synthesis of endometrial estrogen receptors and progesterone receptors is promoted by estradiol; progesterone inhibits the synthesis of endometrial estrogen receptors.[4] These

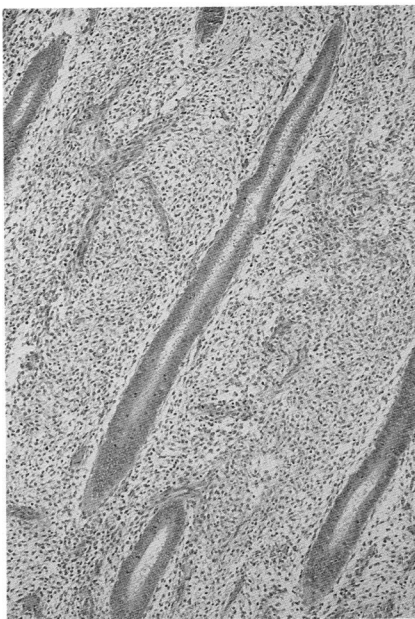

**Figure 37–3.** Proliferative phase endometrium. The glands are tubular, and there is mild stromal edema.

steroid receptors are located in the nuclei of endometrial epithelial and stromal cells. Because of its nature (ligand-specific receptor), the estrogen receptor may have a high affinity for sex steroid hormones; it can bind estrone and synthetic estrogens.[4] In the early proliferative phase (days 4 to 7), the endometrium is thin. The glands are short and tubular, lined by columnar cells with nuclear pseudostratification, increased nuclear-to-cytoplasmic ratio, coarse nuclear chromatin, and mitotic figures (Fig. 37–3). The edematous stroma contains spindled cells, with mitotic figures and noncoiled, thin-walled spiral arterioles. Ciliated cells begin to appear in the glandular epithelium at this time and are seen throughout the menstrual cycle, being more prominent during the proliferative phase, particularly near the uterine isthmus and in the surface epithelium.[13] The latter does not seem to respond strongly to progesterone, however, and retains basically the same histologic features during the menstrual cycle.[13]

In the midproliferative phase (days 8 to 10), the glands and the spiral arteries exhibit some degree of coiling. The columnar cells lining the glands still show nuclear pseudostratification, and the number of mitoses is increased. The spindled stroma is more edematous and mitotically active. During this phase, the plasma levels of estrogen peak, coinciding with increased endometrial mitotic activity and increased estrogen receptor concentrations.[4] The glands and the vessels seem to grow at a faster rate than those of the stroma.[4]

The late proliferative phase (days 11 to 14) is characterized by coiled, mitotically active glands that still exhibit nuclear pseudostratification. The stroma is not as edematous as in the early and midproliferative phases, however. The walls of the spiral arteries appear thicker. At the time of ovulation, the effect of the rising circulating levels of progesterone in the estrogen-primed endometrium is not immediately obvious. On days 14 and 15 of the cycle, postovulatory days 1 and 2, the endometrium resembles the late proliferative phase when examined by light microscopy. In the glandular epithelium, small and scattered, poorly formed subnuclear vacuoles appear on day 16 (postovulatory day 2) but occur in less than half of the glands. Some workers refer to the aforementioned histologic pattern as *interval* endometrium. To confirm ovulation by endometrial histology, more than half of the glands should show well-developed intracytoplasmic subnuclear glycogen vacuoles and palisading of their nuclei. At least half of the cells in a given gland should contain such subnuclear vacuoles. The glycogen vacuoles are the earliest histologic manifestation of ovulation and may be observed, using light microscopy, 36 hours after that event.[4]

On day 17 (postovulatory day 3), palisading of the nuclei, fewer mitotic figures, and prominent subnuclear vacuoles are seen in most glands, imparting a histologic picture reminiscent of "piano keys." The glycogen vacuoles migrate to a supranuclear location by day 18 (postovulatory day 4) (Fig. 37–4). Patchy early stromal edema can be seen between days 17 and 18 (postovulatory days 3 and 4); glandular mitotic figures, already uncommon at this time, typically are absent in secretory glands after day 19 (postovulatory day 5).

Between days 19 and 20 (postovulatory days 5 and 6), the supranuclear vacuolar contents (glycoproteins, mucopolysaccharides) are released into the glandular lumina by apocrine secretory activity.[4] The glands begin to show some tortuosity.

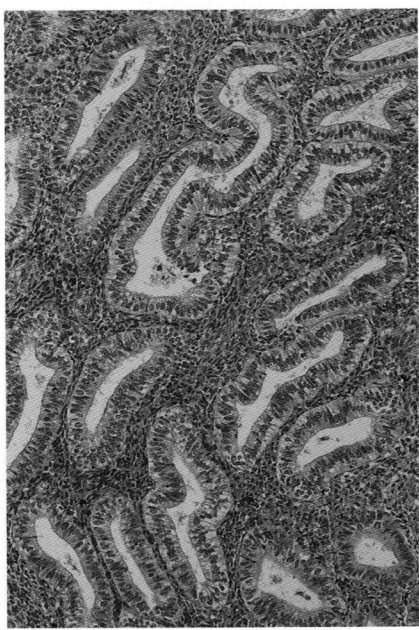

**Figure 37–4.** Secretory phase endometrium (days 17 to 18 of a 28-day cycle).

If fertilization occurs, implantation of the blastocyst typically coincides with day 21 (postovulatory day 7) during the maximal levels of glandular intraluminal secretions. On day 22 (postovulatory day 8), stromal edema reaches its peak. The glands are tortuous, have dilated lumina, have abundant secretions, and are lined by low columnar epithelium. On days 22 to 23 (postovulatory days 8 to 9), mitoses are seen in the perivascular stroma (Fig. 37–5). Predecidualization of the perivascular stroma, vascular endothelial proliferation (resulting in coiling of the spiral arterioles), and glandular intraluminal projections (*ferning*) are evident on day 23 (postovulatory day 9).

Prostaglandins $F_2$ and $E_2$ have been shown to mediate stromal edema and predecidualization and arteriolar coiling.[14] The level of cyclooxygenase, responsible for the synthesis of prostaglandins, increases around day 22 (postovulatory day 8) as a response to the elevated midluteal levels of circulating estradiol.[15]

By day 24 (postovulatory day 10), the glandular secretory *exhaustion* and the stromal predecidual reaction have become more prominent. "Islands" of predecidualized stroma often can be seen. Predecidualized stromal cells exhibit abundant eosinophilic cytoplasm, enlarged nuclei, and occasional multinucleation and are the precursors of the *true* decidual cells that develop if implantation of the blastocyst occurs. Predecidualized stromal cells have multiple properties, including phagocytosis.[4] The predecidualized cells are involved in extracellular collagenolysis and may contribute to the breakdown of the endometrial stroma during menstruation.[4]

On day 25 (postovulatory day 11), predecidualization of the subsurface endometrial stroma creates a bandlike pattern. The latter area is referred to as the *stratum compactum*, whereas the rest of the functionalis is referred to as the *stratum spongiosum* (Fig. 37–6). The glandular secretory exhaustion imparts to the luminal border a serrated, "saw-toothed" configuration.

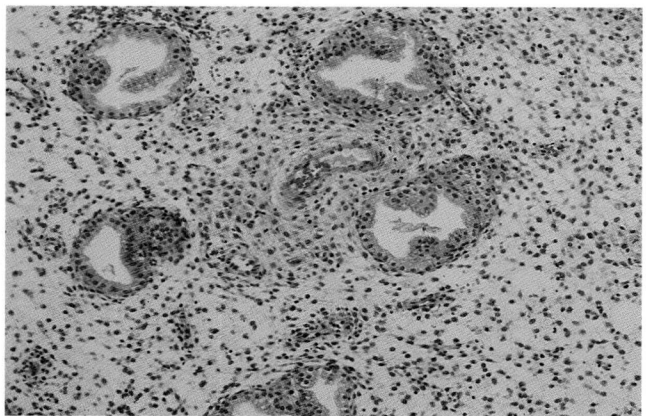

**Figure 37–5.** Secretory phase endometrium (days 22 to 23 of a 28-day cycle).

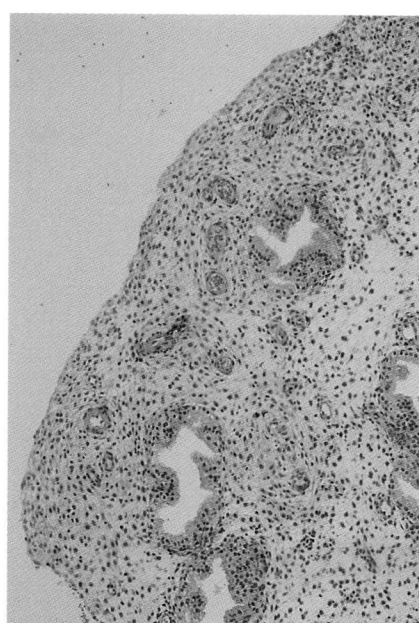

**Figure 37–6.** Secretory phase endometrium. The stratum compactum is noted in the subsurface endometrial stroma.

The upper two thirds of the functionalis undergoes predecidualization by days 26 and 27 (postovulatory days 12 and 13) (CD Fig. 37–4). Concurrently, the endometrial stroma is permeated by mononuclear cells with a kidney-shaped nucleus and granular eosinophilic cytoplasm that variously have been known as *metrial cells, metrial granulocytes, K cells,* or *stromal granulocytes.* The metrial granulocytes once were thought to be derived from undifferentiated stromal endometrial cells and to contain relaxin. More recent studies have shown, however, that these cells belong to the large granular T lymphocyte series; that they appear to be under hormonal control; and that if fertilization occurs, they may have a role in implantation and placentation.[9, 16, 17] The term *granular lymphocyte* seems to represent accurately the nature of these cells and is the term preferred by some workers (CD Fig. 37–5). Although the concentration of granular lymphocytes peaks on day 27 (postovulatory day 13), they can be seen, usually in smaller numbers, earlier in the cycle (CD Fig. 37–6).

Glandular cells from the functionalis and the basalis may engulf cellular debris of inflammatory cell origin on day 28 (postovulatory day 14) and days 1 and 2 of the cycle. The menstrual phase is estimated to last 3 to 5 days (average 4 days) (Fig. 37–7). Lysosomal autodigestion (the eventual result of the declining levels of estradiol and progesterone) mediates glandular, stromal, and vascular tissue degeneration.[4] The degenerating tissue consists of exhausted secretory glands mixed with predecidualized stroma, lymphocytes, and acute inflammatory cells. Prostaglandins are thought to contribute to the ischemic tissue necrosis and the vasomotor and expulsive mechanisms involved in menstruation.[4] Fibrinolytic

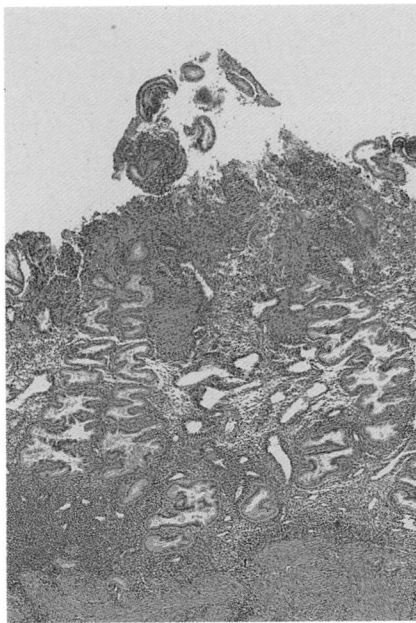

**Figure 37–7.** Menstrual endometrium.

activity in the menstrual fluid prevents clotting and facilitates the expulsion of the shedding endometrium.[4] Vasoconstriction of the endometrial arteries of the basalis and the radial and arcuate myometrial arteries helps control the extent of bleeding.[4] Shedding is more prominent in the first 2 days of the cycle (CD Fig. 37–7). Days 3 and 4 are characterized by proliferation of the residual glandular epithelium of the basalis in denuded areas, until the newly epithelialized areas merge with one another. Proliferation of endometrial stromal cells from the basalis also contributes to the replacement of the shedding endometrial stroma and to the re-epithelialization process. Additional assistance is provided by the isthmic mucosa and the mucosa of the peritubal ostia.[4] Re-epithelialization of the endometrial surface, attained by day 5 of the cycle, results in the cessation of bleeding.[4] The endometrial repair that occurs immediately after menstruation seems not to be influenced directly by circulating estrogen levels or by the number of endometrial estrogen receptors and progesterone receptors. At the time of menstruation, the levels of circulating estrogen and endometrial estrogen receptors and progesterone receptors are no different from their levels before menstruation.[4] The endometrial regeneration and the subsequent development of features seen in the proliferative phase characterize the beginning of a new menstrual cycle.

## ENDOMETRIUM

### Inflammatory Changes

Endometritis (inflammation of the endometrium) can be an acute or a chronic process and may involve the entire endometrium or only certain regions. Although it may be secondary to clinical procedures associated with cervical or endometrial instrumentation, often the cause of endometritis cannot be determined.

### ACUTE AND CHRONIC NONSPECIFIC ENDOMETRITIS

Acute endometritis can develop in the postpartum period after a vaginal delivery and most likely results from a polymicrobial bacterial ascending infection.[18] Risk factors for acute postpartum endometritis include delivery by cesarean section, manual removal of the placenta, chorioamnionitis, and premature rupture of membranes.[18] The most common bacteria include hemolytic *Streptococcus, Staphylococcus,* and *Clostridium welchii.*[19] In acute endometritis, the gross and microscopic findings are not specific for a particular infectious agent; a tissue culture may be necessary to identify the causative microorganism. The gross findings include endometrial congestion, petechiae, and areas of ulceration.[20] The histologic findings include a marked acute inflammatory cell infiltrate permeating the endometrium, with abscess formation accompanied by areas of necrosis, hemorrhage, and vascular thrombosis. Although necrosis, acute inflammation, hemorrhage, and vascular thromboses are histologic features of menstrual endometrium, from which acute endometritis should be distinguished, the acute inflammatory process is not that marked, and abscess formation is absent in the former.[19] Fragments of exhausted late secretory glands mixed with degenerating predecidualized stroma characterize menstrual endometrium. The endometrial glandular and stromal features associated with acute endometritis are not specific. Any pattern of endometrial histology (datable, pregnancy associated, hyperplastic, or malignant) can develop features of acute inflammation under the right circumstances. Occasionally, the inflammatory process can extend to the myometrium and result in an acute endomyometritis. Products of conception, including chorionic villi and fetal parts, also can undergo necrosis and become acutely inflamed; however, decidual necrosis, not associated with significant acute inflammation, can be seen in the postpartum period. Small areas of decidual necrosis with acute inflammation may be seen during pregnancy, and their presence is not considered a significant abnormal finding.[21] Occasionally, aggregates of polymorphonuclear leukocytes associated with cellular debris are noted in the lumina of otherwise unremarkable glands. This finding (when it is not associated with tissue permeation by acute inflammatory cells or with any other pathologic changes) is of no clinical significance; it most likely represents residual debris from a previous menstrual cycle.[37]

Chronic endometritis (CD Fig. 37–8) can develop after an acute infectious process and commonly is part of the spectrum of changes associated with pelvic inflammatory disease. In the latter setting, *Neisseria gonorrhoeae* and *Chlamydia trachomatis* are the most common causative agents cultured from the endometrium.[22-24] Despite careful clinical investigation, however, a causative agent often cannot be found. The histopathologic findings associated with chronic (nonspecific) endometritis include the presence of plasma cells usually accompanied by lymphocytes (either as a diffuse infiltrate or as lymphoid aggregates), reactive spindling of the endometrial stroma, and reactive glandular changes. Plasma cells represent evidence of antigenic stimulation, and they are required for the diagnosis of chronic endometritis. Polymorphonuclear leukocytes may contribute to the inflammatory spectrum of chronic endometritis, their presence varying from a focal mild infiltrate to a prominent and more diffuse process, even with microabscess formation. Additional microscopic findings include glandular and stromal dyssynchrony (precluding dating of the specimen), glandular and stromal breakdown, and endometrial epithelial metaplasias.[20, 21]

## SPECIFIC TYPES OF CHRONIC ENDOMETRITIS

### Infectious Endometritis

Acute (or chronic) endometritis caused by a particular infectious agent may exhibit histologic features that overlap with those described in the nonspecific endometritides. Nonetheless, there are occasional microscopic features that may implicate a particular microorganism in the genesis of a lesion. The presence of a granulomatous reaction in the endometrium (granulomatous endometritis) raises the question of infection by *Mycobacterium tuberculosis,* usually present as a manifestation of disseminated disease.[25] In tuberculous endometritis, the granulomas commonly are noncaseating, and conventional stains and methods (acid-fast, auramine-rhodamine) may fail to detect the presence of mycobacteria in tissue sections. Tissue culture may be the only sure method of identifying the infectious agent. Although uncommon in the United States, tuberculous endometritis is a complication of genital tuberculosis that can be associated with infertility, especially in regions of the world in which this condition is endemic.[25, 26] Granulomatous endometritis also may be seen in association with sarcoidosis.[27]

Other uncommon infectious causes of granulomatous endometritis include fungi (*Blastomyces dermatitidis,*[28] *Coccidioides immitis*[29]), parasites (*Schistosoma*[30]), and cytomegalovirus. Herpesvirus infection is associated with histologic evidence of viral cytopathic effect in the endometrial glands and stroma[31, 32]; it also has been described as occurring in the postpartum period.[32] In cases of cytomegalovirus, the viral cytopathic effect is noted in the glandular epithelium and in the vascular endothelium.[33] Human papillomavirus can infect the endometrium; the process is usually the result of secondary extension of the virus from the endocervix. The histologic features associated with the cytopathic effect of human papillomavirus in the endometrium, including the involvement of endometrial squamous metaplasia, consists of a spectrum of cellular changes similar to those identified in the cervix.[19]

Xanthogranulomatous endometritis (histiocytic endometritis)[34] and malacoplakia[35] have been reported in the endometrium. In rare instances, a florid reactive lymphoid inflammatory response associated with chronic endometritis may raise the question of a lymphoma. Reactive processes lack, however, the diffuse and extensive involvement of the uterus, a mass effect, and the monomorphic histopathologic and immunohistochemical features typical of a lymphoma. The presence of reactive germinal centers of various sizes and the common association with an acute inflammatory component should help in establishing the benign nature of this process.

### Noninfectious Endometritis

In certain cases, endometritis can result from diagnostic procedures. A foreign body–type granulomatous reaction may follow endometrial curettage, a transcervical endometrial laser ablation, a hysterosalpingogram, hysteroscopic diathermy ablation of the endometrium, or an examination whereby talc is introduced into the genital tract. The development of eosinophilic endomyometritis has been associated with a prior history of endometrial curettage.[36]

The type of response elicited in the endometrium by an intrauterine device (IUD) depends on several factors, one of the most important of which is its composition. IUDs can be manufactured from different components, and some models are able to release hormones into the surrounding endometrium. Also crucial is the length of time the device is in place. The associated endometritis can be acute or chronic, may involve the entire mucosa, or may be restricted to the area adjacent to the device. A granulomatous foreign body–type giant cell reaction also can be seen. IUD use has been linked strongly with the development of endometritis associated with *Actinomyces israelii,* a bacterial, rather than a fungal, organism. Microscopic findings in the latter condition include the presence of a chronic active inflammation (plasma cells, lymphocytes, and polymorphonuclear leukocytes) and aggregates of filamentous rods and tangled, delicate branching filamentous forms. The latter are the microscopic equivalent of the yellow flecks that have been observed grossly and designated as *sulfur granules.* Perforation of the uterine wall can be a complication related to the use of an IUD.

Because a granulomatous reaction in the endometrium may be associated with infectious and noninfectious conditions, clinicopathologic correlation always should be established when this reaction is encountered. Special stains for the aforementioned organisms may be helpful in ruling out infectious processes.

# Benign Noninflammatory Conditions of the Endometrium

## CHANGES ASSOCIATED WITH HORMONAL ALTERATIONS

### *Estrogen-Related Alterations*

Deviations from the usual fluctuations in sex steroid hormonal levels during the reproductive years and the perimenopausal and postmenopausal periods can result in abnormal patterns of uterine bleeding. *Dysfunctional uterine bleeding* (DUB) is a clinical term applied to cases in which either the length of the exposure to estrogen and progesterone or the levels of those hormones are anomalous. Uterine bleeding that results from organic conditions, such as a bleeding diathesis or uterine leiomyomas, should not be referred to as DUB.[19] Some clinicians use the term *abnormal uterine bleeding* to refer to the clinical symptoms of the latter group of patients.

Regardless of their cause, *anovulatory cycles* can be associated with the development of DUB. In the absence of progesterone exposure, the estrogen-primed endometrium fails to develop the secretory changes associated with the luteal phase of the menstrual cycle. Decreasing levels of estradiol production by the ovarian follicles eventually is responsible for the onset of uterine bleeding. The quantity of affected endometrial tissue can increase if the exposure to estradiol is sustained; bleeding and shedding occur when the endometrium outgrows its structural support.[37] Most workers believe that the duration of the exposure to estrogen (either endogenous or exogenous), regardless of the amount, determines the quantity and degree of tissue fragmentation.[37]

Microscopic evaluation of the endometrium in this clinical setting reveals proliferative phase glands and stroma, with areas of glandular and stromal disintegration, accompanied by tissue necrosis, intravascular fibrin thrombi, and thin-walled ectatic vessels[37]; this pattern of tissue fragmentation is known as *glandular and stromal breakdown* (CD Fig. 37–9). In such a background, the shedding stromal tissue may be encountered as spherical aggregates ("stromal blue balls"), sometimes ringed by circumferentially arranged glandular epithelial cells. This particular arrangement of fragmented and dehydrated stromal tissue may be seen in numerous conditions associated with endometrial shedding, including menstruation. Other features associated with breakdown of endometrial tissue (but not specific for any particular condition) include the presence of cellular debris permeating the stroma and located at the bases of the glands. The surface-type glandular epithelia often display a pattern associated with shedding known as *papillary syncytial change* (CD Fig. 37–10).[19, 37, 38] Also known as *papillary syncytial metaplasia* and *surface syncytial change*, most workers consider it to represent a degenerative/regenerative phenomenon, possibly the result of uneven tissue breakdown, and not a true metaplastic change. On histologic

evaluation, papillary syncytial change is characterized by aggregates of epithelial cells with copious eosinophilic cytoplasm that commonly assume a papillary configuration. Because the cellular borders appear blurred and ill-defined, the aggregate appears as a *syncytium.* The cytoplasm may be scantily vacuolated, and the nuclei show no significant atypia, although mitoses can be seen. Permeation of the cellular aggregates by acute inflammatory cells is a common finding in papillary syncytial change. The histologic features associated with glandular and stromal breakdown are not specific for any particular entity and may be encountered in numerous benign and malignant endometrial lesions that are undergoing shedding. Samples commonly may consist entirely of endometrial tissue with such an extensive degree of glandular and stromal breakdown that definitive histopathologic characterization of the endometrium may not be possible.

Another endometrial pattern associated with abnormal exposure to estrogen is known as *disordered proliferative endometrium* (DPE) (Fig. 37–8). Microscopic assessment of DPE reveals proliferative endometrium with focal, mildly dilated, and irregularly shaped glands; complex budding and branching are absent. The cytologic features of the epithelium lining the abnormal glands of DPE are virtually identical to those lining the proliferative glands of proliferative endometrium, in that significant epithelial atypia is absent. The stroma surrounding the glands is typically of proliferative type, being quite cellular and usually mitotically active. The focal nature of the changes should exclude the diagnosis of simple endometrial hyperplasia, which tends to be a more diffuse process. Some workers regard DPE, however, as part of the spectrum of changes associated with unopposed exposure to estrogen. In their view, DPE may represent an intermediate step between the changes identified in exuberant proliferative endometrium (lower end of the spectrum) and changes more characteristic of complex endometrial hyperplasia (upper end of the spectrum). Occasionally, fragments of endometrial basalis (the lower aspect of the endometrium abutting the myometrium) that

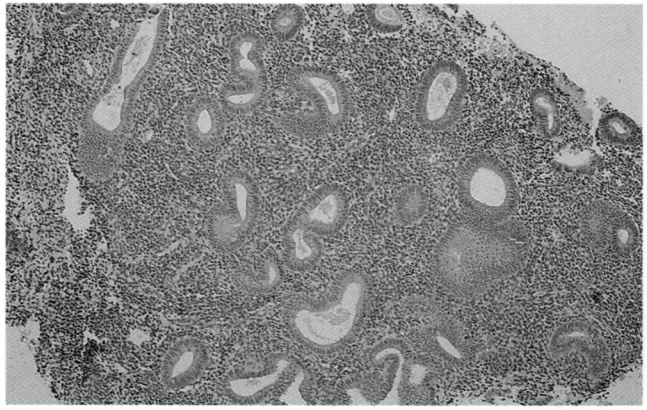

**Figure 37–8.** Disordered proliferative endometrium.

normally may show glands with mild architectural disarray, lined by proliferative-type epithelium, can be confused with DPE; however, the inactive and spindly appearance of the stroma, the thick-walled nature of the vessels, and interdigitating tongues of smooth muscle from the endomyometrial junction are helpful features in determining their origin from the basalis. The differential diagnosis of DPE also includes fragments from a disrupted hyperplastic-type endometrial polyp, especially if seen in a background of proliferative endometrium. In the absence of a polypoid configuration and surface epithelium on at least three sides, a single fragment from a hyperplastic endometrial polyp may be difficult to distinguish from DPE; however, the presence of thick-walled, "feeder-type" vessels, usually present in clusters within a more fibrous stroma, favors a disrupted hyperplastic polyp. The presence of multiple fragments from a hyperplastic polyp also imparts a more *diffuse* quality to the abnormal tissue present in the specimen, rather than *focality* more typical of DPE.

*Endometrial atrophy* results from minimal or absent stimulation of the endometrium by estrogen and can be manifested clinically as abnormal uterine bleeding. Such a histologic picture can be seen in association with the onset of menopause or secondary to therapeutic hormonal treatment. Studies have shown that atrophy is the most common finding in endometrial biopsy specimens obtained from patients with postmenopausal bleeding. In a study by Choo and colleagues,[39] endometrial atrophy accounted for 82% of all cases of postmenopausal bleeding. Microscopic evaluation of the usually scanty sample reveals free-lying strips of predominantly surface endometrial glandular epithelium mixed occasionally with fragmented inactive endometrial glands and stroma (Fig. 37–9). The lining of the glands is composed of mitotically inactive low cuboidal–to–low columnar epithelium. Although the atrophic glands may vary in size and still exhibit a tubular configuration, cystically dilated glands frequently are present in a focal or diffuse pattern, a condition termed *cystic atrophy*. The endometrium overlying a submucosal leiomyoma may undergo pressure-related atrophic changes, whereas the rest of the endometrium reveals a different histologic pattern, including datable glandular and stromal changes.

### Progesterone-Related Changes

The concept of a *luteal phase defect* (LPD) as developed by Jones[40] is typified by the inadequate secretory transformation of the endometrium as a result of insufficient progesterone secretion by the corpus luteum. The corpus luteum in a LPD, also known as *inadequate luteal phase*, may have developed abnormally or regressed prematurely, resulting in lower progesterone levels. LPD may occur sporadically in otherwise normally cycling women and become clinically evident as DUB; it is present in 3% to 5% of patients evaluated for infertility.[41] Classically, the clinical diagnosis of LPD is made using two consecutive endometrial biopsy specimens obtained during the luteal phase of each cycle. The day of the menstrual cycle in which each biopsy specimen is obtained is determined after establishing the time of ovulation by noting the luteinizing hormone surge and using the classic 28-day cycle as a reference. If the histologic changes in the endometrial biopsy specimens are out of phase by 2 or more days from the histologic changes expected for that particular day, the findings are considered to be consistent with a LPD (e.g., histologically typical day 21 endometrial changes in a biopsy specimen obtained on cyclic day 25). Because the endometrium may exhibit datable secretory features, correlation with the clinical data (expected versus actual histologic changes) is mandatory in this setting.[41]

A second category of histologic findings associated with LPD is characterized by dyssynchronous secretory endometrial changes. One pattern is typified by secretory endometrium with a difference of more than 2 days between the datable features exhibited by the glands and the datable features exhibited by the stroma (e.g., day 17 glands associated with day 23 stroma). The dyssynchrony in the glands may be focal, and the surrounding secretory glands may seem to be in synchrony with the stromal changes (CD Figs. 37–11 and 37–12). Cases occur in which there is dyssynchrony between the architectural and cytologic features of the glands. Other less invasive methods to assess LPD currently are under consideration and include serial measurements of serum progesterone levels during the luteal phase, assessment of endometrial thickness as determined by transvaginal ultrasonography, and measurements of proteins that may represent markers for luteal function or endometrial response, such as progestogen-associated endometrial protein.[42]

Another abnormality of the luteal phase can result from a persistent corpus luteum that fails to regress, providing continuous exposure of the endometrium to progesterone. The histologic pattern of

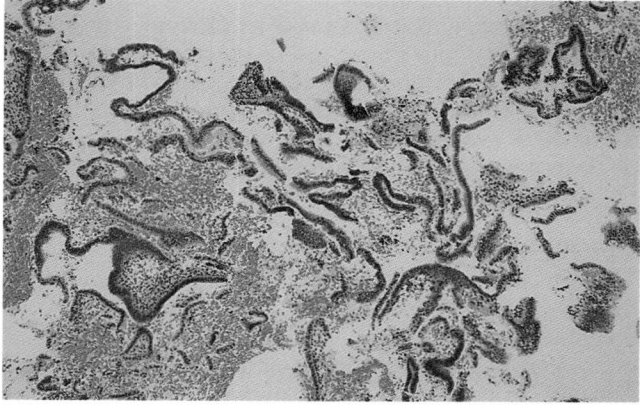

**Figure 37–9.** Endometrial biopsy from a patient with endometrial atrophy. The material obtained in these cases is usually very scant.

the endometrium manifested in this setting is known as *irregular shedding endometrium.*[37] The endometrium consists of endometrial fragments showing secretory and proliferative glands accompanied by evidence of breakdown and shedding. The secretory glands tend to be simple and irregular in shape, the glands may assume a star-shaped configuration as they involute,[37] and many of them exhibit signs of *secretory exhaustion.* The tubular proliferative glands appear inactive. The stroma varies in its appearance, showing densely packed, spindle-shaped cells associated mainly with the proliferative glands and alternating patchy edematous areas, possibly with an early predecidual reaction associated with the secretory glands. Evidence of glandular and stromal breakdown usually is present and may be extensive. To diagnose this entity, the biopsy material must be obtained at least 5 days after the start of bleeding.[37] It is important to correlate the histopathologic findings with the clinical findings in a particular patient before rendering this diagnosis. Other pathologic entities, including chronic endometritis and endometrial curettings associated with ectopic pregnancies, can exhibit histologic features similar to those of irregular shedding endometrium.

Occasionally, an endometrial biopsy specimen submitted with a clinical diagnosis of DUB is characterized by abnormally developed secretory glands with glandular and stromal breakdown (also known as *underdeveloped secretory endometrium* or *endometrial deficient secretory phase*).[37, 43] Although the secretory changes in these specimens are thought to be secondary to ovarian progesterone secretion, they are not developed as sufficiently as those of typical late secretory/early menstrual endometrium.[37, 43] The glandular and stromal components of abnormally developed secretory glands with glandular and stromal breakdown may exhibit architectural features more consistent with the early and mid secretory phase (mild glandular tortuosity and early stromal perivascular predecidual reaction), but the glandular lining may show secretory exhaustion or even hypersecretory features. Accompanying glandular and stromal breakdown commonly is noted as well as the presence of stellate-shaped secretory glands, a nonspecific architectural pattern representing involuting secretory glands. Although not entirely characteristic of a well-defined entity, the aforementioned abnormal secretory patterns are believed to represent the pathologic manifestations of DUB associated, at least to some degree, with abnormal levels of progesterone, possibly resulting from hormonal imbalances occurring during the luteal phase of the cycle.

## CHANGES ASSOCIATED WITH THE USE OF THERAPEUTIC DRUGS

When evaluating endometrial biopsy specimens or cytologic specimens, it is important to obtain the proper clinical information about the patient, particularly her age, menstrual history (last menstrual period), menopausal status, and any history of malig-nancy or systemic disease (especially diseases with an endocrinologic component). Information regarding the use of prescription drugs, especially those associated with endocrinologic manifestations, is crucial. Many of the drugs discussed in this section induce histopathologic patterns in the endometrium that are not pathognomonic for that particular drug. The proper clinical information must be submitted to permit clinicopathologic correlation at the time of interpretation of the biopsy specimen.

### Estrogen

Endometrial changes histologically similar to changes associated with abnormal endogenous estrogen metabolism are seen in cases of exogenous estrogen excess. Sustained unopposed exposure to estrogen, whether exogenous or endogenous in origin, may result in the development of one or all of the following: endometrial hyperplasia, low-grade endometrioid adenocarcinoma, and endometrial epithelial metaplasias.

### Combined Progesterone and Estrogen Therapy

The combined therapeutic use of estrogen and progesterone is exemplified by two major treatment modalities: oral contraceptives and postmenopausal hormone replacement therapy. The histopathologic appearance of the endometrium affected by oral contraceptives and hormone replacement therapy is influenced by the pattern of administration of the drug (sequential versus combined), the length of time the patient is exposed to the drug, the particular dose, the pretreatment status of the endometrium, and the time of the cycle in which the specimen is obtained.[19] In the combined modality of oral contraceptives, a pattern of inactive tubular glands with extensive predecidual stromal reaction may be seen after several months of treatment, even when earlier specimens in the same patient may have revealed a variety of histologic patterns. After the prolonged use of oral contraceptives, an atrophic pattern of endometrium may develop.[44] Although the methods of administration of oral contraceptives and hormone replacement therapy are similar, the hormonal concentrations used to prevent conception are different from those used to treat menopausal symptoms. A variety of histologic appearances ranging from datable secretory endometrium to hyperplasia and even atrophy have been identified in patients receiving hormone replacement therapy[19] (CD Fig. 37–13).

### Tamoxifen

Tamoxifen is a nonsteroidal antiestrogenic drug that is used widely as adjuvant chemotherapy in breast cancer patients. The antiestrogenic effect of tamoxifen is attributed to its ability to compete with estrogen for binding sites in tissues such as the breast; however, it also elicits a paradoxic estrogenic effect on the endometrium that seems to be related to the dose, the duration of the treatment, and the menopausal status of the patient.[45] The use of tamoxifen has been linked to an increased risk of developing adenomyosis, endometrial polyps, endometrial hyperplasia, endometrial carcinoma, and müllerian adenosarcoma.[45] Secretory-type glandular changes also may be observed superimposed on some of the previously described lesions.

### Clomiphene Citrate

Clomiphene is a nonsteroidal ovulatory stimulant with estrogenic and antiestrogenic activities but with no progestational capabilities. Clomiphene initiates a series of endocrinologic events that ultimately cause the development of multiple ovarian follicles. The influence of clomiphene on the endometrium may be difficult to assess; however, it is not unusual for the endometrial sample to reveal datable changes that correlate with the ones expected for that particular day of the cycle.[45] Conversely, there are reports of endometrial biopsy specimens from clomiphene-treated patients describing hypoestrogenic effects, glandular and stromal secretory phase alterations, and changes similar to those described with LPDs.[45–47]

### Danazol

Danazol is a derivative of testosterone that has been used in the treatment of endometriosis and endometrial hyperplasia. Although it can bind to three classes of intracellular steroid receptors (i.e., androgen, progesterone, and glucocorticoid receptors), its highest affinity is for binding the androgen receptor.[48] Danazol is known to suppress endometrial growth and to induce progestational changes in the endometrium[45, 49]; its prolonged use results in endometrial atrophy.[50]

### Gonadotropin-Releasing Hormone Agonists

Gonadotropin-releasing hormone agonists are commonly used to decrease the size of leiomyomas prior to surgery (myomectomy or hysterectomy) and also as part of stimulation protocols associated with in vitro fertilization.[50a] The compounds have been associated with various endometrial changes, including glandular-stromal dyssynchrony.[50a]

### Human Menopausal Gonadotropin and Human Chorionic Gonadotropin

Human menopausal gonadotropin and human chorionic gonadotropin are used concurrently as treatment for certain infertility conditions. There are no particular endometrial histologic patterns that characterize their use. Endometrial changes identified in this setting include normal secretory patterns, LPD-like patterns, and secretory changes more advanced than those expected for the clinically estimated day of the cycle.[51, 52]

### Progestins

When progestins are used alone, the endometrium exhibits histologic features similar to those identified with the use of oral contraceptives, including an atrophic pattern[45] (CD Fig. 37–14). With the use of the synthetic progestin levonorgestrel subcutaneous implant system (Norplant), the endometrial changes include atrophic glands accompanied by a predecidual stromal reaction.[53] An endometrial decidual-like reaction, not associated with the known use of exogenous or endogenous progestational agents, has been described in postmenopausal women[54]; termed *idiopathic postmenopausal decidual reaction,* its clinical significance is unknown.

### Mifepristone

Mifepristone is a synthetic steroid with potent antiglucocorticoid and antiprogestational properties[55, 56] that is used clinically for voluntary interruptions of pregnancy. The net effect of its action on the endometrium is to obstruct the effect of progesterone. The resulting histologic alterations depend on the time at which mifepristone was administered during the menstrual cycle.[55] When administered in a long-term, low-dose regimen, the endometrial changes include variations in the size and shape of the glands, variable epithelial linings (nonatypical), and mitotically active dense stroma; secretory changes also can be identified.[56]

## CHANGES ASSOCIATED WITH ENDOMETRIAL CURETTAGE, ENDOMETRIAL ABLATION, AND RADIATION

After an endometrial curettage, several histologic changes occur as a result of tissue removal. In addition to an organizing blood clot, the initial reactive and reparative process engenders an increase in the number of neutrophils permeating the tissue during the first 7 days after the procedure.[57] After some curettage procedures, an eosinophilic endomyometritis develops, characterized by numerous eosinophils and a resolving chronic inflammation that permeates the endometrium and the superficial aspect of the myometrium, mainly within the supportive connective tissue and around blood vessels.[36] The eosinophilic endomyometritis appears 18 hours after the procedure. Eosinophilic endomyometritis is considered to be reactive rather than allergic in nature[36]; at times, eosinophils may be a component of nonspecific endometrial inflammatory infiltrates.

Intrauterine synechiae (adhesions) can result from a traumatic curettage, which usually was performed for postabortal or postpartum bleeding. The exposure of the superficial myometrium after the removal of the basalis seems to trigger the formation of granulation tissue adhesions between the anterior and posterior uterine walls. Known as Asherman's syndrome, this condition may cause patients to seek medical consultation for amenorrhea, hypomenorrhea, or infertility. Hysteroscopy, hysterosalpingography, and sonography (in association with the patient's clinical history) help to establish the diagnosis. As might be expected, the amount of tissue obtained at the time of diagnostic endometrial curettage is small and consists mainly of smooth muscle bundles associated with fibrous connective tissue. Treatment modalities include resection of the adhesions using electrosurgery, prophylactic antibiotic treatment, and hormonal treatment to enhance endometrial growth. Intrauterine adhesions also may follow intrauterine infections or surgery but are unusual in these settings. Unusual complications associated with endometrial instrumentation include endometritis, pyomyoma, and uterine perforation.

When patients with DUB fail to respond to hormonal treatment modalities, endoscopic endometrial ablation using neodymium:yttrium aluminum garnet (Nd-YAG) laser photocoagulation can be performed as a safe, reliable, and less expensive alternative to a hysterectomy.[58, 59] During the first 3 months after the procedure, the endometrium exhibits necrosis and granulation tissue formation[60] accompanied by a foreign body–type granulomatous reaction.[61] Re-epithelialization of the endometrium may be completed by 3 months. Fibrosis of the endometrial stroma and areas of endometrial thinning, including some in which only low cuboidal surface epithelium overlies the myometrium, are evident later.[60, 61]

Radiation changes in the endometrium usually are secondary to modalities used in the treatment of uterine cancer, including tumors of the corpus and the cervix; the changes are nonspecific and affect benign and malignant tissues. The affected cells may increase in size and become pleomorphic. Cytoplasmic vacuolation is common. The nuclei become enlarged and hyperchromatic and may display various degrees of pleomorphism. Thrombosis of blood vessels is a relatively early finding followed subsequently by thickening of vessel walls. It is important to be aware of a history of radiation when evaluating a specimen, particularly because radiation changes superimposed on malignant neoplasms may affect the assessment of the histologic type of tumor and the degree of differentiation. Conversely, benign structures with radiation-induced histologic features may be misinterpreted as malignant if the pathologist is unaware of the history of prior radiation.

## NONEPITHELIAL METAPLASIAS AND RELATED CHANGES

Strictly defined, metaplasia is a process whereby one type of mature tissue is replaced by another type of mature tissue not indigenous to that organ or tissue. In the endometrium, nonepithelial metaplastic changes, consisting of smooth muscle, osseous (bone), cartilaginous, and adipocyte (adipose tissue) types, are uncommon. It is important to recognize these benign conditions and not to confuse them with malignant processes because osseous, cartilaginous, and adipocyte metaplasias can be mistaken for the heterologous components of a carcinosarcoma (malignant mixed müllerian tumor) of the uterus. Their benign histologic features are helpful, however, in elucidating their true nature. The presence of bone, cartilage, and glial tissue in the endome-

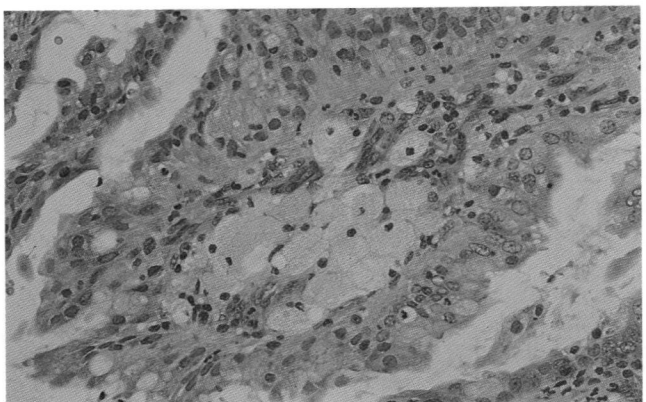

**Figure 37–10.** Endometrial stromal macrophages.

trium (or sometimes in the myometrium) can be the result of retained fetal tissue after a miscarriage or a voluntary interruption of pregnancy. Smooth muscle metaplasia of the endometrium can be confused with tissue from a smooth muscle or a stromal (benign or malignant) lesion.

The term *foam cells* or *foam cell change* applies to lipid-laden endometrial stromal cells[38]; however, their origin is controversial, and some workers favor a histiocytic origin for these cells[62] (Fig. 37–10). Although they usually are seen in association with well-differentiated endometrioid adenocarcinoma, they also may accompany endometrial hyperplasia, stromal sarcomas, benign endometrial polyps, and müllerian adenosarcomas. Because of the frequent association with endometrial malignancies, the presence of foam cells in endometrial curettage should be noted and followed by a thorough work-up of the sample.

## ENDOMETRIAL POLYPS

Endometrial polyps are benign lesions composed of endometrial glands and stroma that are believed by some workers to represent anomalous proliferations of the endometrial stratum basalis; their genesis has been linked to the effects of unopposed exposure to estrogen with the assumption that their estrogen and progesterone receptor status imitates that of the endometrial basalis. Mittal and coworkers[63] showed, however, by immunohistochemical methods, a reduction in the expression of estrogen and progesterone receptors in the endometrial stroma of functional and nonfunctional polyps as compared with those of normal endometrium. Their study also showed no significant difference in the expression of estrogen and progesterone receptors in the glands of endometrial polyps when compared with those of normal endometrium. Several workers have shown cytogenetic alterations that may support the neoplastic, rather than hyperplastic, nature of these lesions. The reported genetic alterations include inversion of 12p11.2q13,[64] rearrangement of 12q14-15,[65] and rearrangement of 6p21.[66] Considering the aforementioned findings and the variety of morphologic features exhibited by endometrial polyps, their evolution may involve more than one developmental pathway.

Endometrial polyps are more common in perimenopausal women, in whom they may present clinically as abnormal uterine bleeding, or they may be associated with infertility in women of reproductive age. Their true prevalence in the general population may be difficult to assess because endometrial polyps are believed to be asymptomatic in many instances. Studies have suggested that their presence may increase a woman's risk of subsequently developing endometrial adenocarcinoma.[67, 68] Although malignancies have been described to arise in the background of endometrial polyps, the incidence of this phenomenon is only approximately 0.5%.[68] The most common tumors seen in this setting include endometrioid, serous, and clear cell carcinomas and carcinosarcomas.

Endometrial polyps range in size from microscopic and barely visible with the naked eye to large lesions that may occupy the entire endometrial cavity. They can be sessile or pedunculated and even prolapse through the cervical os. Torsion of a polyp can be associated with tissue infarction and necrosis. Regarding their distribution within the endometrial cavity, endometrial polyps tend to be more common in the fundus and are multiple in approximately 20% of cases.[19]

The different types of endometrial polyps are categorized according to the microscopic features of the glandular and stromal components; they include hyperplastic, functional, atrophic, and mixed endocervical-endometrial polyps. Despite these distinctions, all polyps share certain histologic characteristics, as follows: a polypoid configuration with surface epithelium on at least three sides, a central (usually fibrotic) core that occasionally may contain smooth muscle bundles, and a vascular proliferation (mainly of thick-walled vessels). Endometrial polyps commonly exhibit histologic features that are out of synchrony with those of the surrounding endometrium.

The glands in most of the hyperplastic polyps display architectural and cytologic features similar to those of simple hyperplasia without atypia but are associated with a less cellular, fibrous stroma. Increased complexity of the glandular architectural patterns, various degrees of cytologic atypia, and superimposed epithelial metaplasias also can be seen. The differential diagnosis of hyperplastic polyps includes polypoid fragments from endometrial hyperplasia (simple and complex) and disordered proliferative endometrium. Endometrial hyperplasia may exhibit a polypoid configuration, and when tissue fragmentation is prominent, some areas may resemble hyperplastic polyps. Nonetheless, endometrial hyperplasia tends to be a diffuse process, and the specimens usually consist of abundant tissue displaying similar histologic features throughout. In disordered proliferative endometrium, the focus of architecturally altered glands, out of synchrony with

the rest of the endometrium, may resemble a hyperplastic polyp. In this situation, the evaluation of the tissue configuration and the stromal characteristics may be of help.

Also included in the differential diagnosis are uterine lesions that present with gross and microscopic features similar to those associated with endometrial polyps. These lesions include adenomyomas, adenofibromas, and adenosarcomas (see section on "Mixed Epithelial and Mesenchymal Lesions"). In the case of the adenomyomas, adenofibromas, and adenosarcomas, the histologic features of the stroma help to categorize the lesions, particularly adenosarcomas, in which the malignant nature of the stroma, with increased mitotic activity and periglandular hypercellularity, is more characteristic. Infrequently, the stroma of benign endometrial polyps may exhibit atypical cells that are similar to the multinucleated giant cells seen in vaginal and cervical benign fibroepithelial polyps with stromal atypia. The nuclei of these atypical cells are hyperchromatic and may be multilobated, and mitotic activity generally is absent. The stroma is not markedly cellular, and it lacks the distinctive periglandular "cuffing" arrangement described in typical müllerian adenosarcomas.

In functional polyps, the architectural and cytologic features of the glands are in synchrony with those in the remainder of the endometrium. The differential diagnosis includes polypoid fragments of functional endometrium. Secretory changes and stromal decidualization seem to be uncommon occurrences in endometrial polyps. Atrophic polyps (Fig. 37–11) show a glandular architecture that resembles endometrial cystic atrophy; the epithelium lining the glands is usually inactive or atrophic. Some workers regard these polyps as representing the inactive or atrophic phase of hyperplastic polyps (CD Fig. 37–15). The differential diagnosis of atrophic endometrial polyps includes fragments of endometrium with cystic atrophy and fragments of endometrial basalis. Tissue from the endometrial basalis is not unusual in endometrial curettings, and the presence of thick-walled vessels (actually from

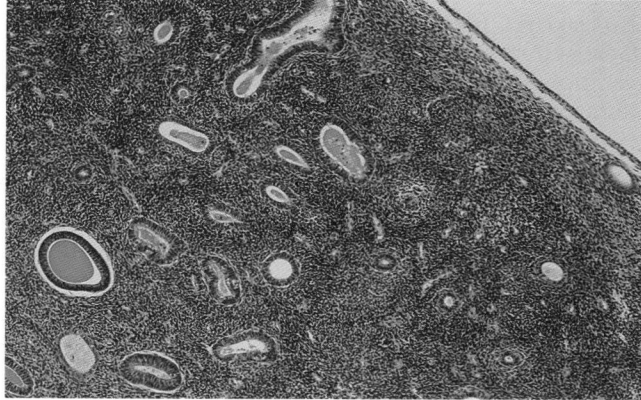

**Figure 37–11.** Endometrial mucosal polyp, atrophic type. The stroma is cellular and compact.

the endomyometrial junction) associated with fibrous stroma and inactive-appearing glands may raise the question of an atrophic polyp. The presence of interdigitating smooth muscle fibers (also from the endomyometrial junction) and the lack of surface epithelium on at least three sides should help indicate an origin from the basalis other than from a disrupted polyp. Mixed endometrial-endocervical polyps usually occur in the area of the upper endocervix and lower uterine segment mucosa and most likely originate from the latter. The benign glands may exhibit mild architectural disarray and cystic change. Endocervical mucinous epithelium may line some glands, whereas other glands are lined by a more endometrioid type of epithelium. It is common, however, to find hybrid glands, lined by a mixture of endocervical and endometrial epithelium, in these lesions.

An association between the long-term administration of tamoxifen, a nonsteroidal antiestrogenic drug used as adjuvant treatment in patients with breast cancer, and the subsequent development of endometrial polyps has been described in the literature.[69] Although tamoxifen has antiestrogenic action, it paradoxically has an estrogen effect on the endometrium. Tamoxifen-related endometrial polyps that develop in this setting are usually multiple, are often larger than those identified in patients not receiving the medication, and more frequently show areas of mucinous metaplasia.[70] Their microscopic features usually include hyperplastic glands, although foci of adenocarcinoma apparently arising within endometrial polyps are encountered more frequently in patients receiving tamoxifen.[70]

## Endometrial Hyperplasia

Current workers agree that most examples of endometrial hyperplasia are the result of prolonged exposure to unopposed estrogen, from either endogenous or exogenous sources, the latter often in the form of estrogen replacement therapy. Cases affecting younger women (<40 years old) often are accompanied by a history of chronic anovulation, hirsutism, obesity, and infertility; polycystic ovarian disease (Stein-Leventhal syndrome) is frequent in such patients. Women without the more overt manifestations of polycystic ovarian disease, but who are often obese, are thought to convert androstenedione to estrone in the peripheral adipose tissues. Older women, either perimenopausal or postmenopausal, who develop endometrial hyperplasia frequently do so in response to unopposed estrogen replacement therapy. Most cases, regardless of the age of the patient, come to diagnosis as a result of an investigative endometrial curettage; in such specimens, most of the problems of histopathologic interpretation discussed in this section are encountered.

There has been considerable controversy over the histopathologic classification and natural history of endometrial hyperplasias. Most investigators regard endometrial hyperplasia, using the simplest definition, to represent a heterogeneous group of abnormal proliferations of the endometrial glands and stroma, although in the more architecturally complex and cytologically atypical lesions, less emphasis is placed on the stroma. Despite the simplicity of the aforementioned definition, however, most workers probably would agree that there is considerable disparity and interobserver (and intraobserver) variation in the histopathologic interpretation of endometrial hyperplasias among different investigators (including established gynecologic pathologists), using essentially the same or comparable classifications.[71] All histopathologic classifications rely on artificial and arbitrary *breakpoints* in a probable continuum of nonuniformly progressive glandular architectural and cytologic atypicality. Although the degree of correlation among these arbitrarily contrived clinicopathologic categories of atypia and their subsequent biologic behavior is unknown, an accurate interpretation of the morphologic findings observed in a given specimen must be attempted until the utility of a particular classification is affirmed or disproved.

Until the latter is accomplished, our laboratories have conformed to the classification adopted by the International Society of Gynecological Pathologists, under the auspices of the World Health Organization (ISGP/WHO).[38] This classification has received worldwide approval to standardize the histopathologic diagnosis and clinical treatment of endometrial hyperplasia (Table 37–1).

In the diagnostic assessment of endometrial hyperplastic lesions, as in physiologic and other non-hyperplastic endometrial glandular changes, the two main histologic criteria to assess are the architectural and cytologic features. Hyperplastic endometrium is characterized by a proliferation of architecturally anomalous glands that may or may not be accompanied by significant atypical cellular changes; these changes may be focal or diffuse. Although the glandular alterations virtually always are accompanied by an increase in the stromal volume, the proportionally greater volume of the glandular component usually results in a significantly increased glandular-to-stromal ratio.

In the ISGP/WHO classification (see Table 37–1), the two major categories, endometrial hyperplasia and atypical endometrial hyperplasia, are distinguished by the presence or absence of cytologic

**TABLE 37–1.** Histologic Classification of (Tumors and) Related Lesions of the Uterine Corpus

1. Epithelial (tumors and) related lesions
  1.1. Endometrial hyperplasia
    1.1.1. Simple
    1.1.2. Complex (adenomatous)
  1.2. Atypical endometrial hyperplasia
    1.2.1. Simple
    1.2.2. Complex (adenomatous with atypia)

atypia within the glands; the major subcategories of each, simple and complex, are distinguished further by the degree of architectural disturbance within the glands. To assess cytologic atypia, the cytoplasmic and nuclear features must be evaluated; the former is important primarily because of the confusing endometrial epithelial changes (*metaplasias*[72]), whose superimposed cytoplasmic changes can cause a given hyperplastic lesion to appear more atypical, even approaching or mimicking adenocarcinoma. The worst offenders in this regard are the eosinophilic and ciliary metaplasias whose cytologic features may overlap. Nuclear features are the most reliable gauge of cytologic atypia, however. One always should attempt to compare the nuclei of a lesion in question with either normal or nonhyperplastic glands in the same specimen, if they are present, to provide for an "internal nuclear control." Some fixatives and processing procedures in individual laboratories may cause even physiologic nuclei to appear alarmingly atypical. To do so may prevent overdiagnosis of a given hyperplastic lesion.

A useful method to gauge the degree of architectural atypia in hyperplastic endometrial glands is to draw imaginary lines around their peripheral borders. By concentrating on the architectural features of the glands and attempting to ignore their cytologic features, their deviation from the normal architecture of physiologic endometrium can be evaluated. Architectural perturbations may be divided into simple and complex types. Both types are characterized by varying degrees of disturbances in glandular shape (degree of configurational irregularity) and by glandular proximity (degree of crowding).

The following histopathologic descriptions summarize the architectural and cytologic characteristics of each of the categories of the aforementioned ISGP/WHO classification system.

Simple glands of endometrial hyperplasia often are cystically dilated, with occasional noncomplex budding and mild-to-moderate glandular crowding (Fig. 37–12). Complex glands frequently are branched, with prominent papillary infoldings and marked glandular crowding. The cytologic changes encountered in association with simple and complex hyperplastic endometrial glands vary from changes that are similar to otherwise normal proliferative endometrium to severe atypia. The atypical epithelial changes in any particular gland are commonly focal. Glands of simple and complex hyperplasia are not expected to have significant atypical epithelial changes; rather, they often are lined by proliferative-type epithelium. It is common, however, to find in these nonatypical hyperplasias a degree of cellular stratification and mitotic activity that is greater than that ordinarily encountered in the lining of otherwise normal proliferative glands. Nonatypical endometrial hyperplasia also may exhibit focal or diffuse secretory changes, epithelial metaplasias, evidence of glandular and stromal breakdown, and chronic inflammation.

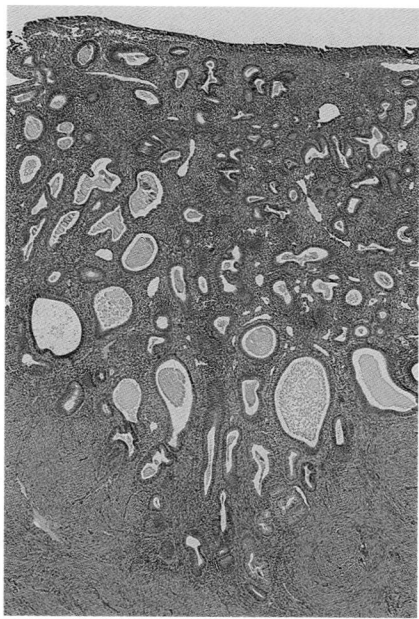

**Figure 37–12.** Endometrial hyperplasia, simple type.

Simple hyperplasia is characterized by glands with various degrees of cystic dilation that occasionally may exhibit noncomplex budding (CD Fig. 37–16). The lining epithelium consists of pseudostratified columnar cells with variable mitotic activity. The glandular crowding is mild to moderate. The term *cystic hyperplasia* used in older terminology is equivalent to the category of simple hyperplasia (CD Fig. 37–17).

Complex hyperplasia exhibits branched complex glands with papillary infoldings lined by stratified, mitotically active, "cigar-shaped" cells. The degree of stratification and the mitotic activity may vary. There may be marked crowding of the glands.

Atypical simple hyperplasia exhibits significant cytologic atypia. The glandular architecture is similar to that of simple hyperplasia, although the glands may be more irregular. The epithelial lining consists of atypical cells with round hyperchromatic nuclei and granular chromatin; nuclear pleomorphism and variability in size also can be present. Cellular stratification with loss of polarity is noted. There are variations in the degree of cellular atypia and mitotic activity.

Atypical complex hyperplasia architecturally resembles complex hyperplasia, but the glands may be more complex and crowded. The epithelial features are similar to those described in atypical simple hyperplasia.

The endometrial biopsy specimen in cases of endometrial hyperplasia usually consists of abundant tissue, all of which should be submitted for microscopic evaluation to ensure that the most atypical component of the lesion is identified. Patients with a histologic diagnosis of endometrial hyperplasia may be treated with progestational agents; in those cases, the endometrium may retain some degree of the glandular architectural abnormality, with the progestational effect being evident in the lining epithelium and the stroma. Cytologic atypia may persist, however, even after the hormonal treatment, and some areas of the hyperplastic endometrium may show virtually no response to treatment. It is important that a history of treated endometrial hyperplasia be submitted at the time of microscopic evaluation to evaluate the effect of the progestational agent properly. Examination of the original (nontreated) endometrial biopsy material and the subsequent biopsy specimens obtained throughout the course of treatment may aid in the interpretation of the changes induced by the medication and the assessment of its effectiveness.

Several studies have explored the epidemiologic implications of endometrial hyperplasia and its association with the subsequent development of endometrial adenocarcinoma. A study by Kurman and associates[73] identified the presence of epithelial atypia in cases of endometrial hyperplasia as the most important factor associated with the risk of subsequent development of endometrial adenocarcinoma. In their study, only 1.6% of the patients with simple hyperplasia and complex hyperplasia developed endometrial adenocarcinoma, compared with 22% of the patients with atypical simple hyperplasia and atypical complex hyperplasia. The type of endometrial adenocarcinoma usually seen in association with endometrial hyperplasia is the low-grade, low-stage endometrioid type.[73]

## Endometrial Epithelial Metaplasias and Related Changes

The term *epithelial metaplasia* applies to a process by which mature epithelium of one kind is transformed into mature epithelium of a different kind. The resultant metaplastic epithelium may not be of a type that is indigenous to the area in which the process occurs. The epithelial lining of the endometrial surface and glands may undergo focal or diffuse metaplastic changes as a response to environmental alterations.[72] Conditions associated with these changes include chronic endometritis, the use of an IUD, trauma, and a history of unopposed exposure to estrogen.[74] The nature of some of these epithelia may not be metaplastic as strictly defined here, however, but may represent reactive or reparative cytoplasmic or nuclear alterations of the native endometrial epithelium. Some workers favor the term *change* instead of *metaplasia* to describe them.[3] *Change* is believed to characterize them better because the former requires no commitment to a particular developmental mechanism, in contrast to the latter. According to the WHO,[38] endometrial epithelial metaplasias are classified as tumor-like lesions and are divided into nine types: 1) squamous metaplasia, 2) mucinous metaplasia, 3) ciliated cell (ciliary) metaplasia, 4) hobnail cell metaplasia, 5) clear cell change, 6) eosinophilic cell metaplasia, 7) surface syncytial change, 8) papillary change, and 9) Arias-Stella change.[38] Because metaplastic epithelium can occur in the background of endometrial hyperplasia and carcinoma, misinterpretation of their benign histologic features with those of neoplastic entities should be avoided. The metaplastic epithelium lacks any distinctive grossly identifiable features.

Metaplastic squamous epithelium[74] resembles the normal squamous mucosa seen in the cervix and the vagina (CD Fig. 37–18). It may exhibit immature and mature features, including keratinization and parakeratosis. The cells might assume different shapes, conforming to the architecture of the aggregate; large aggregates occasionally may undergo necrosis. When the squamous cells are arranged in nests of mainly spindle-shaped cells, the aggregate is referred to as a *morule*. The endometrium may be replaced by keratinizing squamous epithelium as a reaction to the presence of pus in the cavity (pyometra). The condition is known as *ichthyosis uteri*. Cases of endometrial hyperplasia and carcinoma (especially the endometrioid variety) may exhibit extensive squamous metaplasia.[74] Failure to recognize the latter may lead to the misinterpretation of those areas as solid aggregates of malignant cells. The differential diagnosis also includes the malignant squamous component associated with endometrioid endometrial carcinoma (formerly referred to as *adenosquamous carcinoma*) and the rare primary endometrial squamous cell carcinoma (especially in cases of ichthyosis uteri).

In *mucinous metaplasia*, the epithelium resembles the endocervical mucinous epithelium; rarely, gastrointestinal-type differentiation can be noted. This metaplasia is mainly focal, is unusual, and is seen mostly in association with endometrial hyperplasia and carcinoma.[74] Mucinous metaplasia should not be confused with mucinous endometrial adenocarcinoma.

The term *ciliated metaplasia* describes the replacement of the endometrial glandular lining by significant numbers of ciliated cells with round, nonatypical nuclei with a delicate chromatin pattern and eosinophilic cytoplasm. Ciliated cell metaplasia may be referred to as *tubal metaplasia*. The latter designation applies, however, only when the metaplastic process reveals the presence of the three types of cells (ciliated, secretory, and intercalary) indigenous to the mucosal lining of the fallopian tube. Ciliated cells can be seen normally as a component of the endometrium during the proliferative phase and on the surface endometrial epithelium.

The term *hobnail cell metaplasia* is applied to the process in which the metaplastic cells are "door knob–like" or "light bulb–like," with the bland nucleus located in the distal aspect. This change usually is seen in association with endometrial regeneration (e.g., after a curettage). Hobnail metaplasia may be seen in association with the Arias-Stella change and should not be confused with the malignant hobnail cells described in cases of clear cell and serous carcinomas.

Clear cell change (*clear cell metaplasia*) characterizes endometrial glands lined by benign cells with clear (glycogen-rich) cytoplasm. It usually is associated with pregnancy (intrauterine and ectopic). It should not be mistaken for clear cell carcinoma. In *eosinophilic cell metaplasia*, benign cells line the endometrial glands exhibiting bland nuclei and eosinophilic cytoplasm that occasionally may be granular. In the latter situation, the term *oncocytic metaplasia* may be used. The presence of eosinophilic cytoplasm is a feature that overlaps with other types of metaplasias, including the ciliated cell and squamous cell types.

The terms *surface papillary syncytial change, papillary syncytial change, papillary metaplasia, papillary change,* and *eosinophilic syncytial change* all have been used to describe the same entity.[3, 38, 72, 74] The WHO classification uses two terms (*surface syncytial change* and *papillary change*) and describes these changes as lesions that may coexist. We favor the more inclusive and descriptive term *papillary syncytial change.* The lesion usually is seen in the background of glandular and stromal breakdown and seems to represent a degenerative (or regenerative) process rather than a true metaplasia.[3] The cells have eosinophilic cytoplasm, nuclei that may exhibit degenerative or regenerative features (or both), and blurry cellular borders. The cells generally are arranged in aggregates (hence the term *syncytium*), may assume a papillary configuration, and commonly are permeated by acute inflammatory cells. The changes are not confined to the surface endometrium and can involve the endometrial glands. The differential diagnosis includes malignancies associated with a papillary configuration, such as serous papillary carcinoma.

The *Arias-Stella change* occurs when the endometrial cells assume a hobnail (door knob–like, light bulb–like) configuration, with enlarged, pleomorphic, and hyperchromatic nuclei, usually accompanied by clear (glycogen-rich) cytoplasm. Its presence is associated with elevated progesterone levels. Pregnancy (intrauterine and ectopic), gestational tropho-

blastic disease, and (rarely) exogenous progestational agents can induce the Arias-Stella reaction in the endometrium (CD Fig. 37–19). The differential diagnosis includes a clear cell carcinoma. The endocervical epithelium and the mucosa of the fallopian tube also can undergo this change.

## Endometrial Carcinoma

Most endometrial carcinomas are biologically indolent,[75] and their peak incidence is between the ages of 55 and 65, occurring only uncommonly before age 40 (Table 37–2). Table 37–3 provides an endometrial malignancy checklist for the pathologist to follow. Primary endometrial malignancies can be of epithelial, mesenchymal, or mixed epithelial-mesenchymal origin; however, 90% of all uterine malignancies are epithelial in nature. Most of them attempt to recapitulate the normal proliferative endometrium and are designated the *endometrioid* type. Some workers have suggested that two major types of endometrial carcinoma exist.[76, 77] Type I generally is observed in premenopausal and perimenopausal white women and is more likely to be associated with unopposed exposure to estrogen and a previous history of endometrial hyperplasia. The carcinoma is more likely to be minimally invasive or noninvasive, low grade, and of the endometrioid type. Type II carcinoma is more common in postmenopausal African American women and, in most cases, is not associated with a previous history of unopposed exposure to estrogen. Type II carcinomas are commonly high grade; deeply invasive; and of the serous, clear cell, or high-grade endometrioid with squamous differentiation (*adenosquamous*) types.

A strong association between endometrial carcinoma and unopposed exposure to estrogen has been established in numerous studies.[77] Persson and colleagues[78] showed that women receiving estrogenic hormone replacement therapy for more than 2 years experience a twofold to threefold increase in risk of developing endometrial carcinoma, whereas women

**TABLE 37–2.** Endometrial Carcinomas: Clinicopathologic Factors

| Histologic Type | Diagnosis | Prognosis |
|---|---|---|
| Endometrioid adenocarcinoma | FIGO grade I: at least 95% glands. Only ≤5% of the tumor should exhibit a solid component (excluding the solid squamous or morular component) <br> FIGO grade II: solid (nonsquamous, nonmorular) adenocarcinomatous component involves 6–50% of the tumor, with the rest consisting of malignant glands <br> FIGO grade III: glandular component constitutes <50% of the tumor | Good prognosis for well-differentiated lesions and histologically favorable types (mucinous, secretory). Prognostic factors include tumor size, histologic grade, depth of myometrial invasion, vascular space invasion, cervical involvement, lymph node metastasis, peritoneal cytology, and adnexal involvement |
| Serous adenocarcinoma | Resembles its ovarian counterpart. <br> Usually high nuclear grade, papillary and glandular patterns | Poor. Considered a high-grade tumor. Patients usually present with advanced disease |
| Clear cell adenocarcinoma | Resembles other clear cell carcinomas of müllerian origin. Various architectural patterns, including papillary, solid, and tubulocystic | Poor. Considered a high-grade tumor. Prognosis similar to that of serous adenocarcinoma |

**TABLE 37–3.** Endometrial Malignancy Checklist

Patient's name
Patient's identification number (social security number, hospital/clinic/office identification number)
Date of birth
Age
Date of procedure
Place procedure took place
Attending physician
Pertinent clinical information
    Previous surgical procedures (date, type of procedure, diagnosis—including any consultation reports)
    Menstrual history (last menstrual period, menopausal status)
    Gravida, para, abortus
    Medications (including exogenous hormonal treatment, length of treatment)
    Systemic conditions
    Clinical impression
Surgical pathology number
Intraoperative consultation result (frozen section diagnosis, gross diagnosis)
Type of surgical procedure
    Endometrial sample (biopsy, curettage, fractional curettage [endometrial/endocervical specimens])
    Hysterectomy (simple, radical)
    Hysterectomy with unilateral salpingectomy/salpingo-oophorectomy
    Hysterectomy with bilateral salpingectomy/salpingo-oophorectomy
    Other
        Biopsies (peritoneal, internal organs)
        Lymphadenectomy
        Pelvic/peritoneal washings
Total number of specimen containers
Types of specimens: uterus, uterus with unilateral/bilateral tubes, uterus with unilateral/bilateral ovaries, uterus with unilateral/
    bilateral tubes and ovaries
Special instructions by surgeon/clinician
Condition of specimen on receipt
    Fresh
    Fixative
    Unopened
    Opened
    Adequacy for evaluation
    Specific markings indicated by surgeon (stitches, ink)
Dimensions of specimen
    Weight
    Measurements
Tumor
    Gross evaluation
        Dimensions, color, consistency, configuration
        Anatomic location
            Anterior wall
            Posterior wall
            Isthmus
            Fundus
            Serosa
        Gross involvement of: myometrium, cervix, serosa, fallopian tubes, ovaries
        Additional pathologic findings (e.g., adenomyosis, leiomyomas, uterine rupture)
        Representative sections submitted
            Tumor, including deepest point of myometrial invasion, interface with uninvolved myometrium and endometrium, sections
                of upper endocervix/lower uterine segment endometrium
            Special studies: hormone receptors, electron microscopy, frozen tissue bank, flow cytometry, cytogenetics
        Photographs (if taken)
    Microscopic evaluation
        Histologic type of tumor:
            Endometrioid adenocarcinoma*
                Adenocarcinoma with squamous differentiation
                Secretory carcinoma
                Ciliated adenocarcinoma
                Villoglandular adenocarcinoma
            Mucinous adenocarcinoma
            Serous adenocarcinoma†
            Clear cell adenocarcinoma†
            Squamous cell carcinoma
            Undifferentiated carcinoma†
            Mixed epithelial carcinoma, including types
        Histologic grade (for endometrioid types only): I, II, or III*

**TABLE 37–3.** Continued

Extent of invasion
   Myometrial (maximum depth of invasion in mm; maximum thickness of myometrium in area of deepest invasion)
   Cervical: mucosal, stromal
   Serosa: distance of tumor from serosa
   Parametrial
   Lower uterine segment
Adnexal involvement: fallopian tubes, ovaries
Angiolymphatic invasion
Status of surgical margins of resection (cervical, parametrial)
   Distance from tumor to closest surgical margins of resection
Any additional pathologic findings (endometrial intraepithelial carcinoma; endometrial hyperplasia; cervical intraepithelial
   neoplasia; leiomyomas; adenomyosis)
Histologic findings in lymph nodes
   Diagnosis by specific clinical site (as submitted by clinician)
   Total number of lymph nodes (per clinical site) involved by metastatic neoplasm/total number of lymph nodes examined
   Presence of extracapsular invasion by tumor
   Any additional pathologic findings
Histologic findings in additional tissue samples submitted (including the presence of metastatic tumor, direct extension, or
   second primary; any additional pathologic findings)
Results of special studies (receptors, flow cytometry, cytogenetics)
Comment on any particular features of the tumor or pertinent clinicopathologic correlations

*Note:* Following the diagnosis of the resected specimens, the information should be used to provide proper staging using the TNM staging system (American Joint Committee on Cancer [AJCC])[426] and the FIGO staging system (International Federation of Gynecology and Obstetrics).[427] The AJCC staging and the FIGO staging should be included in the final report.
   * Cases of endometrioid adenocarcinoma of the uterine corpus should be grouped with regard to the degree of differentiation of the lesion.
   Grade I: Consists of at least 95% glands. Only ≤5% of the tumor should exhibit a solid component (excluding the solid squamous or morular component usually present in these tumors.
   Grade II: The solid (nonsquamous, nonmorular) adenocarcinomatous component involves 6–50% of the tumor, with the rest consisting of malignant glands.
   Grade III: The glandular component constitutes <50% of the tumor.
   Nuclear atypia of a higher grade than that expected for the architectural features of the lesion raises the FIGO grade I or II lesions by one additional grade.[38]
   † Because they are by definition high-grade tumors, serous clear cell and undifferentiated carcinomas do not have to be graded.[428]

receiving a combined type of hormone replacement therapy (estrogen and progesterone) experience no significant increase in their risk. Numerous conditions in which the common denominator is unopposed exposure to estrogen also have been linked to the subsequent development of endometrial carcinoma, including chronic anovulation (e.g., Stein-Leventhal syndrome)[77] and hormonally active ovarian tumors.[79] It is not surprising that constitutional factors associated with anomalous estrogen metabolism, such as obesity and infertility, also increase the risk of developing endometrial carcinoma. Hypertension and diabetes mellitus are other important risk factors.

Epidemiologic studies have suggested that the consumption of certain foods may increase the risk of developing endometrial carcinoma,[80] although there is no definitive evidence linking a particular diet with its subsequent development. Some studies have indicated a genetic predisposition for the development of endometrial carcinoma and breast carcinoma in relatives of patients with endometrial cancer.[81] Other studies suggest the existence of hereditary forms of endometrial carcinoma.[82]

## CLASSIFICATION OF ENDOMETRIAL CARCINOMA

The WHO/ISGP classification system of endometrial carcinoma uses the cell type of the tumor as the major discriminant.[38] In this system, the endometrioid variety is divided into a typical type with three different variants; six other separate types of epithelial malignancies also are described. Endometrioid adenocarcinoma accounts for approximately 80% of endometrial cancers.[83] Its gross findings are nonspecific (CD Figs. 37–20 and 37–21), varying from a diffuse thickening of the endometrial lining to a discrete, friable mass that may occupy the entire cavity (CD Fig. 37–22). The International Federation of Gynecology and Obstetrics (FIGO), in collaboration with the ISGP and WHO committees, developed a widely accepted histologic classification system based on a range of nuclear and architectural features.[38] Well-differentiated *endometrioid adenocarcinoma* (FIGO grade I) consists of at least 95% glands. Only 5% or less of the tumor should exhibit a solid component, excluding the solid squamous, or morular, component that commonly accompanies these lesions. The malignant glands are numerous and crowded, and although they may vary in size and complexity, they are commonly small. The cytologic features of well-differentiated endometrioid adenocarcinoma include nuclear atypia, although usually not marked, cellular stratification, and various degrees of mitotic activity. The cells display round nuclei, with coarse chromatin clumping and prominent nucleoli. It may be difficult to distinguish between an atypical endometrial hyperplasia and a well-differentiated endometrial adenocarcinoma. In these cases, the histologic evidence of stromal invasion by tumor may be the only factor favoring the diagnosis of malignancy. Overt stromal invasion may be manifested histologically by the presence of reactive fibrosis of the surrounding stroma or by the lack of intervening stroma between the glands (resulting in a "back-to-back" or *cribriform* glandular arrangement); the latter is a result of nondestructive *replacement* invasion of the stroma. Finally, if the nuclear atypia is sufficiently marked, the lesion may be classified as a FIGO II endometrioid adenocarcinoma even when the architectural background is that of a FIGO I lesion.

In *moderately differentiated endometrioid adenocarcinoma* (FIGO grade II), the solid adenocarcinomatous component involves 6% to 50% of the lesion and consists of malignant cells with varying degrees of mitotic activity (CD Fig. 37–23). The glandular component is more atypical than that observed in the FIGO I lesion, with increased architectural complexity and moderate cytologic atypia, cellular stratification, and mitotic activity that may include abnormal forms (Fig. 37–13). Notable (severe) nuclear atypia justifies raising a FIGO grade II to a grade III. *Poorly differentiated endometrioid adenocarcinoma* (FIGO III) is composed mainly of solid areas exhibiting markedly atypical malignant cells with a glandular component that constitutes less than 50% of the lesion. Endometrioid adenocarcinomas (mainly the well-differentiated ones) may display a papillary configuration and should not be confused with papillary serous carcinomas.

Despite its widespread use, the previously described FIGO/ISGP/WHO system has been criticized because of apparent difficulties in the reproducibility of the nuclear grading[71] and architectural system.[83] A Gynecologic Oncology Group (GOG) study comparing the prognostic value of nuclear versus architectural grading found, however, that the reproducibility of both parameters was similar, although the assessment of nuclear grade was a more laborious process.[84] In the GOG study, architectural grading was a better predictor of survival than nuclear grading and was similar to nuclear grading for predicting recurrence.[84]

Some workers have claimed that DNA ploidy seems to be a stronger prognostic factor than either nuclear or architectural grade and has the advantage of using a relatively objective and reproducible technique. In general, most studies evaluating DNA ploidy have shown that aneuploid endometrial carcinomas are notably more aggressive than diploid ones.[85] In a GOG study, Zaino and associates[86] found a significantly increased risk of disease-related death in patients with an aneuploid tumor type when compared with patients with a diploid tumor type. The same study identified a relationship between the ploidy status of the tumor and the depth of myometrial invasion; an absence of invasion was noted more frequently in diploid tumors.

Endometrial carcinomas exhibiting positivity for *estrogen and progesterone* receptors are known to have a better prognosis than tumors negative for these markers. The estrogen and progesterone receptor–positive tumors are more typically low-grade, low-stage endometrioid adenocarcinomas and are more likely to respond to hormonal therapy than receptor-negative tumors.[87, 88] Regarding tumor angiogenesis, a study by Wagatsuma and coworkers[89] showed that high microvessel count and tumor expression of the angiogenic factor c-met correlated with high surgical stage, high histologic grade, presence of lymph node metastases, and shorter patient survival in cases of endometrial carcinoma. Their study also identified tumor angiogenesis status as an independent prognostic indicator for endometrial carcinoma. Abnormal expression of p53 protein is more common in poorly differentiated endometrial carcinomas than in the well-differentiated types.[90–92]

The value of the FIGO/ISGP/WHO classification of endometrioid carcinoma becomes more evident when it is used in association with other parameters to determine the clinical staging of patients. For the purpose of surgical staging according to the FIGO system, it is necessary to assess the following parameters: tumor grade, depth of myometrial invasion (CD Fig. 37–24), lymphatic and blood vascular space invasion (CD Fig. 37–25), cervical involvement (CD Fig. 37–26), lymph node involvement, and adnexal involvement. When evaluating myometrial invasion, it is important to recognize the presence of coexistent adenomyosis because the latter may be involved by adenocarcinoma in 30% of cases.[93] Involvement of adenomyosis by endometrial carcinoma does not seem to affect the patient's prognosis[93, 94] (CD Fig. 37–27), even in the presence of outer third replacement of adenomyosis by tumor. The latter should not be misinterpreted as evidence of myometrial invasion, however, an error that may affect dramatically the staging of the tumor and the types of treatment options offered to the patient. Rarely, endometrial adenocarcinoma may arise from adenomyosis, without involving the mucosal lining of the endometrial cavity.[93, 95]

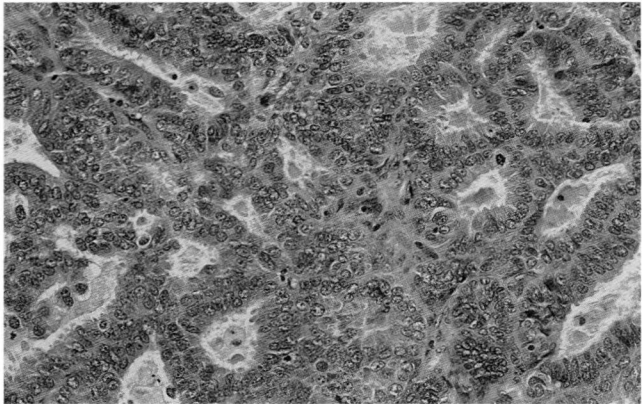

**Figure 37–13.** Section from an endometrioid adenocarcinoma, FIGO grade II. The malignant glands display high grade nuclei.

Endometrioid adenocarcinoma has several variants, but the ISGP/WHO classification recognizes only three: 1) adenocarcinoma with squamous differentiation variant, 2) secretory variant, and 3) ciliated cell variant.[38] Another variant is villoglandular adenocarcinoma, also referred as *papillary endometrioid carcinoma*.[96, 97] Endometrioid adenocarcinomas with squamous differentiation previously were designated as adenoacanthomas when the squamous component was *benign* and adenosquamous carcinomas when the squamous component also was *malignant*. The term *adenocarcinoma with squamous differentiation* currently is preferred when at least 10% of the tumor shows squamous differentiation (CD Fig. 37–28). The terminology was changed because the clinical behavior of *adenoacanthomas* and *adenosquamous carcinomas* seems to parallel the degree of differentiation of the glandular component and to be independent of the differentiation of the squamous component[98] (Fig. 37–14). The glandular component should be graded using the FIGO/ISGP/WHO classification and the squamous component noted as "with squamous differentiation." Nevertheless, the pathologist may choose to also include the optional terminology of "adenoacanthoma" or "adenosquamous carcinoma," depending on the interpretation of the degree of associated squamous atypia. The presence of peritoneal keratin granulomas has been noted in association with endometrioid carcinomas with squamous differentiation of the endometrium and ovary and with atypical polypoid adenomyomas.[100] Data on these patients suggest that the presence of keratin granulomas in the peritoneum is of no prognostic significance and should not be interpreted as evidence of metastatic (and viable) carcinoma.[100] The WHO classification has recommended that primary endometrial glassy cell carcinoma, a rare, aggressive lesion histologically similar to the primary endocervical variety of the same designation, be classified as a subtype of adenocarcinoma with squamous differentiation.[38, 101, 102]

The term *secretory variant of endometrioid adenocarcinoma* (secretory adenocarcinoma) is used when

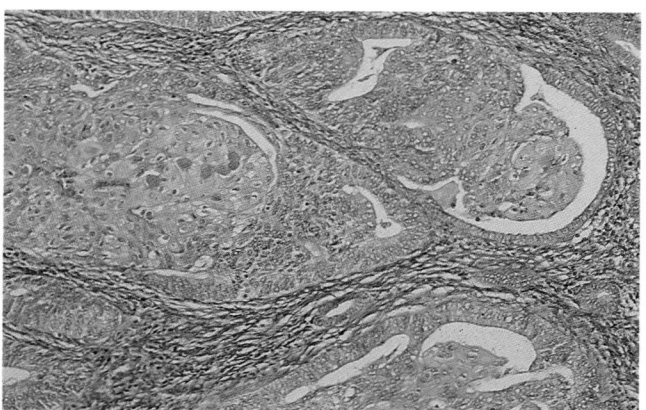

**Figure 37–14.** Endometrioid adenocarcinoma with squamous differentiation.

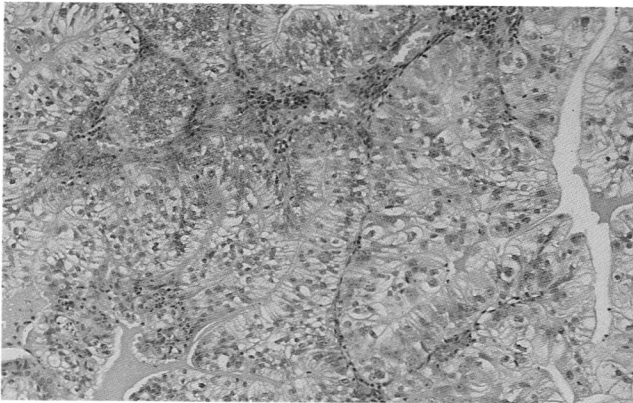

**Figure 37–15.** Endometrioid adenocarcinoma, secretory variant.

the endometrioid lesion exhibits superimposed secretory features similar to those present normally in the early secretory phase of the menstrual cycle[99, 103] (Fig. 37–15). The term *ciliated adenocarcinoma* may be applied to an endometrioid adenocarcinoma in which most of the cells have cilia (CD Fig. 37–29). The villoglandular adenocarcinoma probably is interpreted best to be a variant of well-differentiated endometrioid adenocarcinoma.[96, 97] Its architectural features consist of delicate papillary fronds with thin fibrovascular cores lined by cells with only mild-to-moderate cytologic atypia; marked cellular atypia, pleomorphism, and significant mitotic activity are not features of this lesion. It is important not to confuse this lesion with the more aggressive high-grade endometrial papillary serous carcinoma. A study[99] showed that endometrial endometrioid adenocarcinomas with mucinous, secretory, and ciliated cell differentiation and benign squamous cell differentiation in at least 10% of the tumor exhibited features similar to low-grade pure endometrioid adenocarcinoma and had a good prognosis. These features included expression of estrogen and progesterone receptors, low p53 immunoreactivity, and low cellular proliferation indices (Ki-67). In the same study, endometrial endometrioid adenocarcinoma with a high-grade malignant squamous component exhibited lack of expression of estrogen and progesterone receptors; many of the tumors expressed p53 immunoreactivity and had high cellular proliferation indices (Ki-67). These carcinomas had a prognosis similar to that of poorly differentiated endometrioid adenocarcinomas.[99]

A rare variant of endometrioid adenocarcinoma, referred to as *sertoliform endometrial adenocarcinoma*[104] (CD Fig. 37–30), exhibits microscopic areas that mimic ovarian Sertoli cell tumors in a manner analogous to the ovarian endometrioid carcinoma that resembles gonadal sex-cord stromal tumors. Two uterine stromal lesions that may be included in their differential diagnosis are so-called *uterine tumors resembling ovarian sex-cord tumors* and uterine stromal sarcomas with sex cord–like differentiation.[104]

Serous endometrial carcinoma accounts for ap-

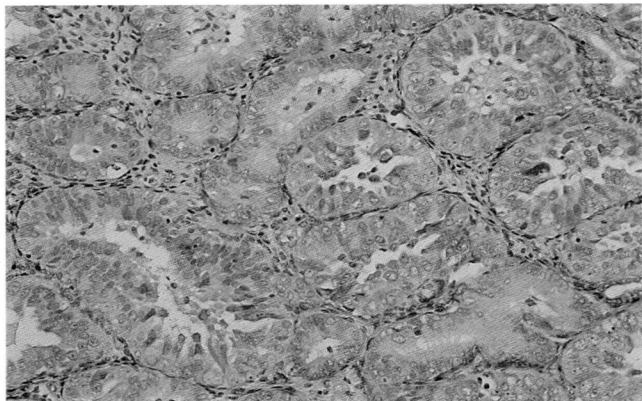

**Figure 37–16.** Endometrial serous carcinoma with a prominent glandular pattern. Note the well-formed glands but high-grade nuclear features.

proximately 5% to 10% of all endometrial carcinomas[105] and has a peak incidence in patients in their 50s and 60s. The clinical presentation is no different from that of other types of endometrial cancers. Although vaginal bleeding is typical, complaints of a serous or serosanguineous vaginal discharge are noted only occasionally. The gross findings also are nonspecific, but serous carcinomas tend to arise in small, atrophic uteri. Endometrial serous carcinomas histologically resemble their ovarian counterpart; they are characterized by papillary fronds of various degrees of complexity, with fibrovascular cores that also vary in size and shape. Occasionally, the malignant tumor can be found in solid sheets or in a predominantly glandular pattern, prompting the designation *serous carcinoma with predominant glandular pattern* (Fig. 37–16). The tumor cells almost always are markedly atypical, with large hyperchromatic nuclei and prominent eosinophilic macronucleoli. Various amounts of eosinophilic cytoplasm may accompany the largely pleomorphic cells, but sometimes they may assume a hobnail configuration. Mitoses are numerous, and abnormal forms are common. Psammoma bodies may be present; their presence in an abnormal (malignant) Papanicolaou smear sometimes may help elucidate the nature of the tumor. Areas of tumor necrosis may be extensive. The tumor has a tendency to invade the myometrium deeply and permeate the lymphatic and vascular channels extensively, with widespread dissemination being a relatively common finding at the time of diagnosis. Endometrial serous carcinomas frequently occur in a background of endometrial atrophy[77] and can arise in otherwise benign, and sometimes small, endometrial polyps. Uterine serous tumors have a poor prognosis and a low 5-year survival.[106–108]

Serum tumor markers may be helpful in following patients with serous carcinoma, considering that elevations of cancer antigen 125 (CA-125),[109] carcinoembryonic antigen (CEA),[110] and alpha fetoprotein[111] have been reported in association with serous carcinoma. Ploidy studies reveal that a high percentage

of serous carcinomas are aneuploid.[112, 113] High AgNOR counts and abnormal expression of p53 protein also have been reported.[114–116] The differential diagnosis of this lesion should include metastatic extrauterine serous papillary carcinoma and primary endometrial carcinomas with a papillary architecture, including variants of endometrioid adenocarcinomas, such as villoglandular adenocarcinomas, and papillary clear cell carcinomas. According to some studies, patients treated with tamoxifen for breast carcinoma who subsequently develop endometrial carcinoma are at risk for developing high-grade malignancies, including poorly differentiated endometrioid adenocarcinoma, serous carcinoma, clear cell carcinoma, malignant mixed müllerian tumors, leiomyosarcomas, and endometrial polyps more often associated with carcinoma.[117, 118] Some workers have suggested that a lesion known as *endometrial intraepithelial carcinoma* (endometrial carcinoma in situ[119, 120]) may represent a precursor of serous carcinomas. This microscopic lesion consists of large epithelial cells with pleomorphic nuclei and prominent eosinophilic macronucleoli, similar to the cellular changes seen in invasive serous tumors. It tends to involve the endometrial surface focally or to replace a few endometrial glands without disturbing their architecture (CD Fig. 37–31). It usually is seen in association with high-grade endometrial malignancies, most commonly serous carcinomas, arising in a background of either atrophic or weakly proliferative endometrium. Abnormal expression of p53 protein has been noted in endometrial intraepithelial carcinoma, a feature shared with overtly invasive uterine serous carcinomas.[121] Endometrial intraepithelial carcinoma has been reported in association with serous peritoneal carcinomatosis.[121] In these cases, the uterine in situ neoplasia was an incidental microscopic finding not associated with an invasive uterine neoplasm.

Clear cell endometrial carcinoma accounts for approximately 3% to 5% of all endometrial carcinomas[122–124] and displays histologic features similar to those of clear cell carcinomas arising in other parts of the female reproductive tract (Fig. 36–17). Their clinical presentation is similar to that of other pri-

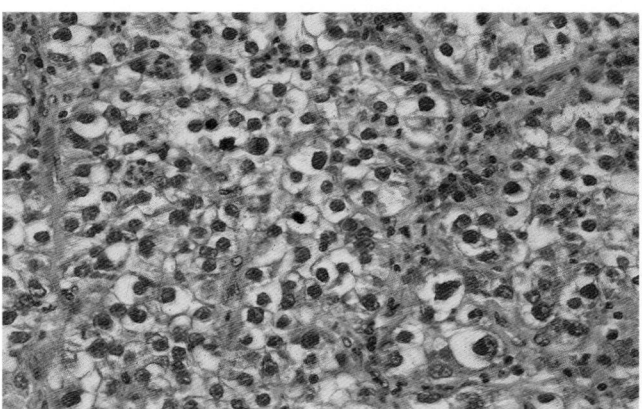

**Figure 37–17.** Endometrial clear cell carcinoma.

mary endometrial malignancies, and they tend to occur in postmenopausal women.[122, 123] Gross features are nonspecific. Most cells are large, with clear, glycogen-rich cytoplasm. A population of malignant cells with eosinophilic cytoplasm and cells with a hobnail configuration (similar to those described in serous tumors) may be present. The degree of nuclear atypia varies from moderate to severe; multinucleation and brisk mitotic activity associated with atypical mitotic figures are common findings. The malignant cells may be arranged in tubular, solid, cystic, or papillary patterns (CD Fig. 37–32) or in combinations of these patterns.[124] Psammoma bodies can be present in some tumors, usually in association with tumor areas showing a papillary configuration. Stromal hyalinization (secondary to deposition of basement membrane–like material) is a frequent and notable finding. Eosinophilic hyaline droplets are seen often,[123] but their presence is a nonspecific finding. Clear cell carcinomas have a poor prognosis, and neither the cytologic grade nor the type of architectural features seems to influence their prognosis.[124] Myometrial and vascular space invasion are common features.[110, 124] Similar to serous carcinomas, clear cell carcinomas can arise in the background of endometrial polyps and are estrogen independent.[125] A high percentage of clear cell carcinomas are aneuploid[113]; they frequently exhibit abnormal expression of p53 protein and a high (Ki-67) proliferative index.[90, 125] The differential diagnosis includes the secretory variant of endometrioid adenocarcinoma, hypersecretory endometrium (especially if associated with an Arias-Stella reaction), and serous carcinoma.

Mucinous endometrial carcinoma is a rare lesion.[126] Patients are usually postmenopausal and commonly present with a complaint of vaginal bleeding.[126] The tumor seems to behave similarly to low-grade endometrioid adenocarcinoma when matched for stage, grade, and depth of myometrial invasion[77]; it tends to be a well-differentiated lesion,[99, 126] with high estrogen and progesterone receptor expression and a good prognosis.[99] On histologic examination, these tumors resemble primary endocervical adenocarcinomas. Secondary endometrial involvement by a primary cervical malignancy should be ruled out before establishing the tumor as endometrial in origin. Minor foci of endocervical mucinous differentiation can be seen in 40% of endometrial endometrioid carcinomas.[127] Various workers have established the percentage of mucinous differentiation needed to define a tumor as a mucinous carcinoma to vary between 50%[127] and 70%.[126] The gross features of mucinous endometrioid carcinomas are nonspecific. Microscopically, the lesion exhibits a glandular architecture with various degrees of complexity and luminal aggregates of mucin; the latter, as in cases of endocervical adenocarcinoma, may be permeated by acute inflammatory cells. Cellular stratification and mitotic activity are not prominent features. The cells are columnar, with pale intracytoplasmic mucin and mild-to-mod-

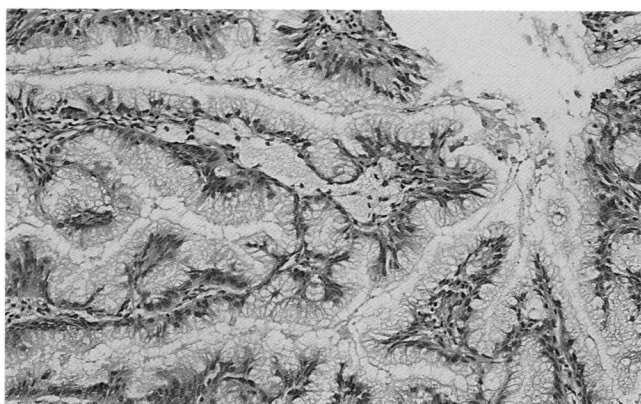

**Figure 37–18.** Endometrial mucinous adenocarcinoma, endocervical type.

erate nuclear atypia (Fig. 37–18). Intestinal mucinous differentiation also can occur[128] (CD Fig. 37–33). Positivity for mucicarmine and CEA is detected in most endometrial mucinous carcinomas, including the microglandular variant.[125, 129, 130] Vimentin positivity also may be expressed.[77] The most important differential diagnosis includes primary endocervical adenocarcinoma (CD Fig. 37–34); however, immunohistochemistry is generally not helpful in elucidating the origin of these tumors (endocervical versus endometrial) because they share many of these markers.

Regarding the presence of human papillomavirus DNA in mucinous endometrial carcinoma, a study by Anciaux and colleagues[131] showed the presence of human papillomavirus DNA in 61.5% of their cases of invasive cervical adenocarcinomas that did not contain areas of squamous differentiation. Human papillomavirus DNA also has been shown in endometrial adenocarcinomas, however.[132] Other lesions in the differential diagnosis include clear cell carcinoma, the secretory variant of endometrioid carcinoma, and otherwise typical endometrioid carcinomas with focal mucinous differentiation. A histologically bland variant of mucinous carcinomas may resemble closely microglandular hyperplasia of the endocervix. This pattern, referred to as *microglandular carcinoma of the endometrium*[129, 130] (CD Fig. 37–35), is characterized by microcystic spaces lined by mildly atypical cuboidal-to-columnar cells, alternating with solid tumor areas. Mitotic activity is infrequent, and the lesion usually is permeated by acute inflammatory cells. Endometrial mucinous adenocarcinomas also have been reported in association with tamoxifen-related endometrial neoplasia.[123, 134]

Occasionally, so-called surface epithelial changes[135] associated with endometrial adenocarcinomas, mainly of the endometrioid type, may be difficult to differentiate from endocervical microglandular hyperplasia, microglandular carcinoma, and endometrial epithelial (*metaplastic*) changes (CD Fig. 37–36). Surface epithelial changes may be focal or extensive, may exhibit a microglandular pattern or a papillary syncytial-like arrangement, and may be associated with metaplastic differentiation.[135] Cytologic atypicality in this lesion varies from mild to moderate and invariably is of a lesser degree than that of the underlying carcinoma. As recommended by the WHO classification, the rare *mucoepidermoid carcinoma* of the endometrium is classified as a variant of mucinous carcinoma.

Pure endometrial squamous cell carcinomas occur rarely. The patients usually are postmenopausal and present with vaginal bleeding.[136] The histologic features are otherwise similar to those of well-differentiated to poorly differentiated squamous malignancies involving other organs of the female reproductive tract (CD Fig. 37–37). When an endometrial squamous cell carcinoma is suspected, the presence of a concomitant malignant glandular component has to be ruled out. If the latter is present, the lesion most likely represents an endometrioid adenocarcinoma with malignant squamous differentiation (formerly known as *adenosquamous carcinoma*). The presence of a primary cervical squamous cell carcinoma extending into the endometrial cavity also should be excluded; nevertheless, there are reports of synchronous endocervical and endometrial squamous cell carcinomas.[137] The presence of human papillomavirus has been shown in a case of squamous cell carcinoma of the endometrium.[138] The WHO classification recommends that verrucous carcinoma of the endometrium[139] (an exceedingly rare lesion) be classified as a subtype of endometrial squamous cell carcinoma.[38] The prognosis of endometrial squamous cell carcinomas is poor.[136]

A mixed-type endometrial carcinoma is a lesion in which a second type of malignant component constitutes at least 10% of the tumor.[38] More than two components can be seen. Excluded from this designation are cases of adenocarcinoma with squamous differentiation. When reported, the different components of the mixed tumor should be mentioned, specifying which ones constitute the major and minor components.[38]

Carcinomas with histologic features similar to those of nasopharyngeal carcinomas have been described in numerous organs, including the cervix, vagina, and vulva. Vargas and Merino[140] described two cases of lymphoepithelioma-like endometrial carcinoma. The patients were postmenopausal and presented with a history of vaginal bleeding. An association with Epstein-Barr virus infection was not identified in either case, a finding shared by similar tumors occurring in the cervix, vulva, and vagina.

*Undifferentiated endometrial carcinomas* are lesions that fail to exhibit unequivocal glandular, squamous, or mesenchymal differentiation. The main histologic patterns recognized by the WHO classification include large cell, giant cell, spindle cell, and small cell. Unusual types of primary endometrial carcinomas include yolk sac tumor[141, 142] (CD Fig. 37–38), giant cell carcinoma[143] (CD Fig. 37–39), hepatoid adenocarcinoma,[144] choriocarcinoma,[145] and small cell neuroendocrine carcinoma.[146]

Tumors with histologic features of primary endometrial carcinomas can arise in the *lower uterine segment* (isthmus) and are classified as endometrial, rather than endocervical, in origin. Their incidence varies between 3% and 8% of all endometrial carcinomas.[147, 148] Grossly, they are bulky, involve the lower uterine segment, and may extend into the upper endocervix in a pattern reminiscent of an "hourglass." In two series,[147, 148] most of the tumors were high-grade endometrioid carcinomas with squamous differentiation, and all cases, independent of their histologic characteristics, showed myometrial invasion. The location of these tumors may influence the apparent poor outcome in these patients; however, most isthmic carcinomas seem to have other unfavorable prognostic indicators, such as an overall higher grade than typical primary carcinomas arising in the endometrium of the corpus, myometrial invasion, and the presence of vascular space invasion.[147, 148] Abnormal expression of p53 protein in isthmic carcinomas is associated with high-grade lesions in a manner similar to that of endometrial carcinomas of the uterine corpus.[148] The differential diagnosis includes extension of a primary endocervical lesion into the uterine isthmus.

The most common malignancies that metastasize to the endometrium are ovarian in origin. Nevertheless, in almost one fourth of the cases in which concomitant tumors are noted in the ovary and the endometrium, such a combination likely represents synchronous ovarian and endometrial carcinomas.[149] Both tumors are usually of the well-differentiated endometrioid type.[150, 151] Various studies of patients with synchronous endometrioid ovarian and endometrial tumors have suggested that genetic alterations, such as loss of heterozygosity and gene mutations, in only one tumor site represent patients with two separate synchronous primary tumors.[152, 153] Synchronous ovarian and endometrial primary tumors seem to have a better prognosis than would be expected if one were metastatic to the other.[150, 151] Outside of the female reproductive tract, carcinomas of the breast most commonly metastasize to the endometrium (CD Fig. 37–40), followed by gastric carcinoma and melanoma.[154] Occasionally, degenerative endometrial stromal changes may mimic metastatic carcinoma.[155] Degenerated epithelioid-type predecidual cells associated with glandular and stromal breakdown may be misinterpreted as representing metastatic breast carcinoma diffusely involving the endometrial stroma.[155]

Although unusual, endometrial adenocarcinoma can occur in association with an intrauterine pregnancy.[156–158] Almost 3% of women diagnosed with a malignancy of the reproductive tract have a coexistent pregnancy.[159] According to a study by Schammel and colleagues,[158] most endometrial malignancies are focal, well-differentiated endometrioid adenocarcinomas with absent or superficial myometrial invasion. They are likely to be discovered early in the gestation, often as an incidental finding associated with a miscarriage or a voluntary interruption of pregnancy. Cases diagnosed at the time of a live birth have been reported.[158] Rarely, the endometrial carcinomas associated with pregnancy may be of a higher grade and deeply invasive. Cases in which concomitant ovarian and endometrial carcinomas are present in association with an intrauterine pregnancy also have been reported.[160]

## Endometrial Stromal Lesions

Mesenchymal tumors of the uterus with histologic features reminiscent of endometrial stromal cells are classified as *endometrial stromal tumors*. The WHO recognizes three such lesions: 1) endometrial stromal nodule, 2) low-grade endometrial stromal sarcoma (LGESS) (formerly known as *endolymphatic stromal myosis*), and 3) high-grade endometrial stromal sarcoma (HGESS).[38] In a review of the literature, Oliva and associates[161] suggested that dividing endometrial stromal sarcomas into low-grade and high-grade lesions no longer is favored and that the term *endometrial stromal sarcoma* should be reserved only for LGESS. Oliva and associates[161] recommended retaining the use of the modifier *low grade*, however, to convey to clinicians the nature of the tumor. According to these authors, the rationale is the fact that mitotic counts no longer are used to differentiate between LGESS and HGESS. As previously postulated by Evans,[162] HGESS failed to show obvious endometrial stromal differentiation; many of these tumors may not be of endometrial stromal origin. The possibility that some HGESS represent monomorphic variants of malignant mixed müllerian tumors (carcinosarcomas) has been considered.[162] Some workers prefer the term *poorly differentiated endometrial sarcoma*, rather than *HGESS*, for these lesions.[161, 162]

The endometrial stromal nodule is an uncommon benign lesion. Symptoms include abnormal uterine bleeding that may be accompanied by pelvic pain. In a study by Tavassoli and Norris,[163] the patients ranged in age from the early 20s to the mid-70s. Most endometrial stromal nodules occur in the myometrium, and they are multiple in only approximately 5% of cases.[163, 164] Grossly, endometrial stromal nodules are soft and well circumscribed, with a yellow-to-tan coloration. Their cut surface is homogeneous and bulging; areas of cystic change, hemorrhage, and necrosis are unusual.[163, 164] According to several studies, the nodules range in size from 0.8 to 15 cm and have an average diameter of 4.0 to 5.7 cm.[163–167] Microscopic examination reveals cellular aggregates of oval to spindle-shaped cells with scant eosinophilic cytoplasm, similar to the stroma of proliferative phase endometrium.[163, 166] The tumor cells are associated with numerous small, thin-walled blood vessels; in many areas, the cells display a concentric arrangement around the vessels (CD Fig. 37–41). Vascular space invasion is absent. Hyalinized collagenous areas are noted; they may be arranged in plaques or in a perivascular fashion,

and they may undergo calcification.[163, 165–168] Stromal nodules lack infiltrative borders; the edges generally are smooth and seem to exert pressure on the surrounding myometrium or endometrium. Rarely, the edges may display focal finger-like projections with blunt contours that extend into the surrounding myometrium or endometrium, but this finding should not be interpreted as representing evidence of invasion.[163, 164] Mitotic activity is variable, and when present it usually amounts to fewer than 10 normal mitoses per 10 high-powered fields. Although stromal nodules with 15 normal mitoses per 10 high-powered fields have been described, the increased mitotic activity does not seem to be associated with a more aggressive behavior.[163, 164, 167]

Occasional findings include tumor cells arranged in epithelial-like cords and trabeculae (and glandlike structures) reminiscent of areas found in sex-cord stromal tumors of the ovary (CD Fig. 37–42) and foci of smooth muscle differentiation.[163–165] Lloreta and Pratt[169] were the first to report a stromal nodule associated with skeletal muscle differentiation. Other rare findings described within endometrial stromal nodules include the presence of benign endometrioid glands,[163] glands lined by clear cells,[166] and foci of mature and immature bone.[170] Clusters of histiocytes with foamy cytoplasm also have been noted.[167] Predecidual-type changes of the component stromal cells may be seen as a response to progestational stimulation.[171] Reticulin stains tend to highlight a pattern in which fibrils surround individual cells or clusters of a few tumor cells.[166, 170]

LGESS and HGESS (also known as poorly differentiated endometrial sarcomas) are more common in women in their 40s and early 50s.[162, 165, 166, 170] As a group, they represent less than 10% of all primary uterine sarcomas.[172] The gross appearance of an LGESS is variable. Rarely, a single well-circumscribed uterine nodule of LGESS may be mistaken for a leiomyoma, or an irregular polypoid mass may protrude into the endometrial cavity.[166] Another pattern is characterized by a diffuse involvement of the myometrium by tumor, in the absence of a discrete mass.[172] Ill-defined soft lesions with a yellow-to-tan coloration also can involve the myometrium, following a pattern that delineates the extensive involvement of vascular spaces by tumor (the reason for the older term *endolymphatic stromal myosis*[160, 166, 172] (CD Fig. 37–43). Cystic change, necrosis, and areas of intratumoral hemorrhage may be identified. Commonly, LGESS extensively invade the myometrium, extending to the serosa in approximately half of cases. Secondary involvement of the cervix by these tumors also has been described.[164] The LGESS exhibit histologic features that are identical to those of endometrial stromal nodules. The essential difference between the two lesions is the capacity of the LGESS to invade the surrounding myometrium, endometrium, and vascular spaces (CD Fig. 37–44), including the occasional extension of the tumor into extrauterine vessels. The differentiation between these two lesions at the microscopic level is based almost exclusively on the assessment of the tumor borders. In endometrial curettings, tissue disruption tends to hamper the evaluation of this parameter. In the latter cases, the WHO recommends that the diagnosis of *stromal tumor* be made, with a comment clarifying that the final diagnosis (benign versus malignant) is dependent on the submission of diagnostic material for that purpose (in most cases, a hysterectomy specimen).[38] In rare cases, the presence of rhabdoid-like cells in LGESS has been noted.[173]

HGESS (poorly differentiated endometrial sarcomas) frequently present as fungating, soft, tan-to-yellow masses protruding into the endometrial cavity[162] (CD Fig. 37–45). The involvement of the myometrium is usually extensive, and necrosis and hemorrhage commonly are noted.[162, 174] These tumors usually lack the more classic microscopic features associated with LGESS, mainly the vascular proliferation and the pattern of vascular and myometrial invasion; the poorly differentiated cells do not resemble endometrial stromal cells.[162] The tumor cells are elongated, with markedly pleomorphic nuclei and brisk mitotic activity (including abnormal forms) usually exceeding 10 mitoses per 10 high-powered fields[164, 174, 175] (CD Fig. 37–46). Multinucleated giant cells also may be seen.[162, 174, 175] The myometrial invasion is qualified as destructive.[162] Some of these tumors have shown areas suggestive of heterologous differentiation.[162] Despite the fact that most neoplasms classified as *HGESS* do not show a LGESS component,[162, 175] cases have been reported in which a coexisting pattern of LGESS is noted; these cases may represent dedifferentiation from a LGESS into a HGESS.[176–178] Oliva and coworkers[168] reported a series of endometrial stromal tumors with prominent myxoid and fibrous components; these tumors have to be differentiated from smooth muscle lesions with prominent fibrosis or myxoid change (myxoid leiomyoma, myxoid leiomyosarcoma), uterine myxomas (rare), and nerve sheath tumors, among others. Oliva and coworkers[168] also noted that focal myxoid and fibrous changes can be microscopic findings in benign and malignant endometrial stromal tumors.[168]

Regarding DNA content, stromal nodules appear to be diploid.[179, 180] Although most LGESS seem to be diploid, aneuploid cases have been reported.[177] HGESS usually exhibit chromosomal alterations.[177] Detection of estrogen and progesterone receptors in LGESS is a frequent finding; however, HGESS more often seem to lack estrogen and progesterone receptors.[177, 181, 182]

The immunohistochemical profile of endometrial stromal nodules and endometrial stromal sarcomas often is similar to that of smooth muscle tumors and myometrium, showing variable degrees of positive staining for vimentin, muscle-specific actin, $\alpha$ smooth muscle actin, desmin, and keratin.[167, 183–186] Epithelial membrane antigen is negative in endometrial stromal nodules and endometrial stromal sarcomas but can be variably positive in normal myometrium.[184] Other markers have been added in an attempt to differentiate smooth muscle lesions from endometrial stromal lesions. They include CD10 (a B-cell marker),[187, 188] h-caldesmon (a protein that regulates muscle contraction),[189, 190] and CD34 (a myeloid progenitor cell antigen).[191, 192] In one study,[188] immunopositive staining with CD10 was obtained in all six cases of endometrial stromal sarcoma examined. Of the smooth muscle tumors examined in that study, only one leiomyosarcoma exhibited immunopositive staining with CD10; all of the leiomyomas and the other 15 leiomyosarcomas in the study failed to show immunopositive staining with CD10. CD34 immunopositive staining has been described in gastrointestinal stromal tumors. In one study,[192] some uterine and extrauterine smooth muscle tumors also stained positive for CD34; however, when CD34 was tested in cases of endometrial stromal sarcoma, negative immunostaining was obtained.[191] In another study,[189] h-caldesmon showed immunopositive staining in all cases of uterine smooth muscle neoplasms (32 leiomyomas and 29 leiomyosarcomas) and 40 sections of uterine myometria evaluated. In the same study, negative immunostaining with h-caldesmon was obtained when the 24 endometrial stromal neoplasms (21 sarcomas, 3 nodules) and the 25 endometrial samples were evaluated.[189] Another study[190] demonstrated the utility of h-caldesmon in the distinction between smooth muscle lesions and endometrial stromal sarcomas.

Expression of p53 has been shown in LGESS and HGESS.[193] The differential diagnosis of an endometrial stromal nodule and LGESS includes adenomyosis with sparse glands,[194] cellular leiomyomas, intravascular adenomyosis,[161] intravenous leiomyomatosis, lymphoma, and metastatic neoplasms.

LGESS rarely may contain benign glands, usually of the endometrioid type (CD Fig. 37–47). Clement and Scully[195] have noted, however, that the presence of these glands may be misleading, especially if they are numerous or exhibit hyperplastic or malignant differentiation. Benign glands associated with a LGESS should be differentiated from an adenosarcoma, adenomyosis, endometriosis, or a LGESS arising in the background of the last two benign conditions. If the contained glands are malignant, the differential diagnosis includes an endometrial adenocarcinoma or a malignant mixed müllerian tumor.[195, 196] The differential diagnosis of a HGESS includes a leiomyosarcoma and a malignant mixed müllerian tumor (carcinosarcoma).

According to numerous studies, the surgical stage is the most significant prognostic factor regarding recurrence and survival in LGESS.[164] LGESS tend to grow slowly and commonly recur many years after the initial diagnosis.[162, 165, 166, 196] Pelvic or abdominal recurrences may occur in 50% of patients,[162, 164, 166, 171] and the recurrent tumor may exhibit histologic features different from those of the primary tumor (CD Fig. 37–48). Studies show that LGESS with significant levels of progesterone receptors respond more favorably to progesterone therapy[178, 181]; hormone receptor analysis should be performed routinely on tumor samples as part of the evaluation of these neoplasms. HGESS have a more aggressive clinical course. They tend to recur within 2 years of the initial treatment,[165, 166, 197] and hormonal therapy does not seem to be an effective treatment modality. In the case of endometrial stromal nodules, if the initial sampling cannot elucidate the status of the borders of the lesion, a hysterectomy and bilateral salpingo-oophorectomy is recommended. If that procedure is not an option, however, some workers recommend diagnostic imaging of the uterus.[164] If the lesion is morphologically benign, its resection may be attempted.[164]

The term *uterine tumor resembling ovarian sex-cord tumor* (UTROSCT) identifies a rare group of uterine neoplasms that, according to their WHO definition,[38] consist "predominantly or entirely" of sex cord–like structures associated with cells exhibiting endometrial stromal features (Fig. 37–19). It is not clear, however, from the previous definition what percentage of a tumor should exhibit sex cord–like areas to warrant that diagnosis. In the original study describing this entity, Clement and Scully[198] classified the tumors into group I (endometrial stromal tumors with focal areas resembling sex cord–like elements) and group II (tumors with a predominant or exclusive pattern of sex cord–like elements). The sex cord–like areas in UTROSCTs are reminiscent of those seen in ovarian granulosa cell and Sertoli cell tumors[198–200] and are characterized by the formation of cord–like structures, trabeculae, small nests, sertoliform tubules, and areas resembling Call-Exner bodies[198] (CD Fig. 37–49). The epithelioid cells show variable amounts of cytoplasm that may be eosinophilic, clear, or foamy.[198] Clusters of foam cells similar to those observed in the myometrium have been identified in these tumors.[199] A case of UTROSCT with osteoid metaplasia has been reported.[200] The fibrous stroma of the tumor varies in amount and degree of cellularity.[198] Smooth muscle is noted in association with the stroma in some tumors. Because similar histologic findings can be seen focally in other primary uterine lesions, it is believed that these neoplasms may originate from endometrial stromal cells, smooth muscle cells, or combinations of both.[198, 201, 202] The immunohistochemical profile of tumor areas resembling ovarian sex-cord elements includes positivity for vimentin, muscle-specific antigen, desmin, and keratin.[185, 186] They fail to stain with epithelial membrane antigen, however.[185, 186] Some studies have shown positive patterns of immunoreactivity for markers of ovarian sex cords (inhibin, CD99) and steroid cell (MART-1) differentiation in the sex cord areas of UTROSCTs; the latter finding is interpreted as strong evidence of true sex-cord differentiation in these tumors.[203–205] Positive immunoreactivity with inhibin (a hormone expressed by normal ovarian granulosa cells and ovarian sex-cord neoplasms) and CD99 (a marker for Ewing's sarcoma and primitive neuroectodermal tumors that also stains normal sex-cord elements) has been shown in UTROSCTs and in sex cord–like areas of uterine endometrial stromal tumors.[204, 205] Sex cord–like structures are known to occur as part of epithelioid smooth muscle tumors, so-called plexiform tumorlets, adenosarcomas, and leiomyomas. The stroma of these tumors has shown immunopositivity for smooth muscle antigens,[185, 186, 202] vimentin, desmin, cytokeratins, and (focally) epithelial membrane antigen.[206]

UTROSCTs often are accompanied by abnormal uterine bleeding and uterine enlargement in patients ranging in age from the reproductive years to the postmenopausal years.[198] These neoplasms usually are well circumscribed, soft, yellow, and range in diameter from 0.7 to 20 cm. They rarely show cystic change.[198] Although most UTROSCTs are benign, microscopic features associated with malignancy, such as infiltrative borders and vascular space invasion, can occur,[198, 207] and they can exhibit malignant biologic behavior.

## Mixed Epithelial and Mesenchymal Tumors

Uterine tumors composed of epithelial and mesenchymal elements are uncommon lesions, and their histogenesis is controversial. Currently, the various entities are classified best by characterization of the biphasic nature of their histologic features, as observed on hematoxylin and eosin–stained tissue sections.[38] The benign mixed tumors include adenofibroma, adenomyoma, and a variant of the latter, atypical polypoid adenomyoma.[38] Adenosarcoma and carcinofibroma are mixed tumors in which only one component is malignant; in carcinosarcoma (also known as *malignant mixed müllerian tumor, malignant mesodermal mixed tumor*), both components are malignant.[38] When the mesenchymal component of these lesions is of the homologous type, the differentiation is toward tissues indigenous to the uterus (smooth muscle, endometrial stroma, and fibroblasts). Differentiation of the mesenchymal component toward tissues not found normally in the uterus (cartilage,

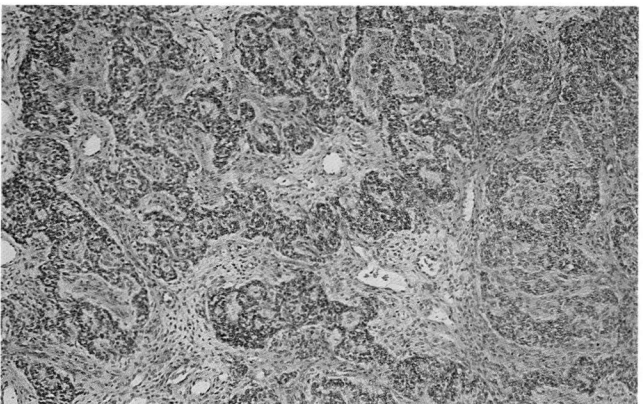

**Figure 37–19.** Uterine tumor resembling ovarian sex cord tumor.

skeletal muscle, bone, and adipose tissue) is referred to as *heterologous differentiation*. The homologous and heterologous components of these lesions can be benign or malignant. In general, these mixed tumors, both benign and malignant, tend to appear grossly as endometrial polypoid lesions and may prolapse through the endocervical canal. They usually are associated with complaints of irregular vaginal bleeding.

Adenofibromas can arise in the uterus[208, 209] and, less often, in the endocervix.[210] They seem to be more prevalent in the postmenopausal period.[209] In most cases, the adenofibroma is a polypoid sessile lesion that ranges in size from 2 to 20 cm; however, it may occupy the entire endometrial cavity.[172] The cut surface often exhibits numerous cystic spaces, imparting a spongelike appearance to the tissue.[172] The microscopic features include irregularly distributed glandular spaces and club-shaped papillary fronds lined by benign endometrioid epithelium that may be accompanied by other müllerian glandular epithelia (mucinous, tubal).[206] Squamous metaplasia is common, and secretory changes may occur.[38, 206] The lining epithelium can exhibit some degree of atypia; cases of adenocarcinoma arising in adenofibromas also have been described.[208, 211] In the latter cases, the rest of the endometrium should be examined carefully; in some cases, it may reveal hyperplasia or carcinoma.[208, 211] The cellular stroma usually is fibroblastic, lacks significant cellular atypia, and occasionally can be admixed with endometrial stromal cells or smooth muscle cells.[206] Skeletal muscle[212] and adipose tissue[213] differentiation of the benign stroma also has been described. The prominent periglandular hypercellular arrangement of the stromal cells (*periglandular cuffing*) characteristic of adenosarcoma is lacking in adenofibromas.[214] According to some workers, mitotic activity can occur in adenofibromas, and it usually does not exceed more than 3 mitoses per 10 high-power fields.[209] Other workers favor a mitotic count of 2 or more mitoses per 10 high-power fields as the minimal number acceptable for a diagnosis of adenosarcoma.[214, 215] Adenofibromas may recur if incompletely excised.[216] Although considered noninvasive tumors, reports of rare cases of myometrial, cervical, and vascular "invasion" by adenofibromas exist in the literature.[216, 217] The adenofibroma should be differentiated from other benign endometrial polyps and from an adenosarcoma.

The adenomyoma is a benign polypoid tumor arising in the endometrium and characterized by endometrial glands associated with a stromal component consisting mainly, or exclusively, of smooth muscle.[38] The glands are noncomplex and lack cytologic atypia. The stromal smooth muscle also lacks any significant cytologic atypia or mitotic activity. A central core of thick-walled vessels, similar to those seen in other endometrial polyps, also is a frequent feature. The variant designated as *atypical polypoid adenomyoma*[218] often arises in the area of the lower uterine segment, but it also may arise in the endo-

cervix.[219] The patients usually are premenopausal[219] (CD Fig. 37–50). Atypical polypoid adenomyomas infrequently are multiple and tend to average less than 2 cm in diameter.[219, 220] Grossly, they appear lobulated, well circumscribed, and rubbery tan or yellow-tan, and they may be pedunculated or sessile.[219] In addition to the distinctive vascular proliferation seen in endometrial polyps, glands with variable architectural complexity characterize this lesion.[219] The epithelium lining the glands is variably atypical and may be mitotically active; an infrequent association between these lesions and concomitant endometrial adenocarcinoma, and hyperplasia has been reported.[219, 221] The original report of atypical polypoid adenomyomas found that the glandular atypia in some of the cases was of sufficient severity to warrant the designation of so-called adenocarcinoma in situ. Endometrial adenocarcinoma also can arise from these lesions.[222, 223] Squamous metaplasia is a common occurrence (hence the name *atypical polypoid adenoacanthomyoma*), forming rounded, bland-appearing squamous morules or being less commonly associated with the formation of foreign body–type keratin granulomas; sometimes these metaplastic areas may undergo central necrosis[219] (CD Fig. 37–51). The stroma is composed of short interlacing smooth muscle bundles (Fig. 37–20) that may be mitotically active; when mitoses are present, there are usually less than 2 mitoses per 10 high-power fields.[219] These lesions can be confused easily with an invasive endometrioid adenocarcinoma, especially in disrupted specimens, because the atypical endometrioid glands are surrounded by smooth muscle, mimicking myometrial invasion. The lack of reactive changes around the atypical, but not frankly malignant, glands should help differentiate benign from malignant processes (CD Fig. 37–52). If the smooth muscle component accompanying the atypical glands is mitotically active, confusion with an adenosarcoma, or even a carcinosarcoma, can ensue.

Adenosarcomas typically arise from the endometrium and are encountered, less commonly, in the cervix.[214] They tend to occur in the postmenopausal

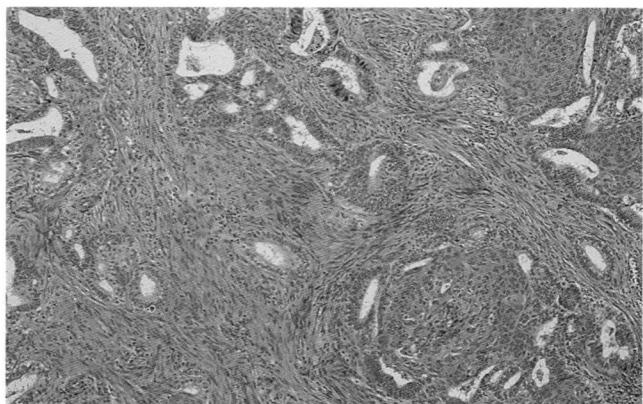

**Figure 37–20.** Atypical polypoid adenomyoma. This lesion may be confused with an area of myoinvasive adenocarcinoma.

period and frequently exist as a solitary endometrial polyp, although they can present as multiple polyps.[172] The cut surface is reminiscent of an adenofibroma, occasionally accompanied by areas of hemorrhage and necrosis.[172] Their development has been associated infrequently with a history of unopposed exposure to estrogen,[214] pelvic irradiation,[214] and the use of tamoxifen.[224-226] The epithelial component of adenosarcomas generally resembles the lining of proliferative phase endometrial glands, although other types of benign müllerian epithelium may be encountered.[206] Endometrioid glandular atypia, hyperplasia, and even adenocarcinoma have been reported in these lesions.[207, 214, 215] In the latter setting, it is common for hyperplasia and adenocarcinoma to be concomitant findings in other areas of the endometrium.[214, 227] The architectural configuration of the intraluminal papillary fronds and the associated glandular spaces resemble the pattern observed in müllerian adenofibromas. The glands vary from tubular to cleft-like to cystically dilated. The malignant stroma in most cases is similar to a stromal sarcoma, usually of the low-grade type, although fibrosarcoma or a combination of both also can occur[214] (Fig. 37–21). Smooth muscle differentiation of the stroma has been noted.[214] In one case report, the stromal component of a uterine adenosarcoma consisted of an angiosarcoma.[228] Varying degrees of nuclear atypia can exist in the sarcomatous component; hyalinized areas may occur. Although mitoses usually amount to 4 or more mitoses per 10 high-power fields,[209, 214, 229] some adenosarcomas may exhibit fewer mitotic figures, requiring extensive sampling to categorize the lesion properly.[209, 214] A count of 2 to 3 mitoses per 10 high-power fields in the proper glandular and stromal architectural and cytologic setting warrants the diagnosis of adenosarcoma.[172] A distinctive feature of adenosarcomas is the increased and often marked cellularity of the stroma in the areas encircling the atypical glands, a pattern described as *periglandular cuffing* (CD Figs. 37–53 and 37–54). Sex cord–like stromal elements, histologically similar to those observed in endometrial stromal tumors (see previous section), also have been encountered.[230-232] Myometrial invasion by tumor exhibiting epithelial and mesenchymal elements has been described in almost 20% of cases[214, 229, 233]; infrequently, the pattern of vascular space invasion may resemble the pattern associated with LGESS.[214] Heterologous mesenchymal elements, either benign or malignant, are present in about 20% of tumors.[209, 214, 229] In approximately 10% of adenosarcomas, there is an overgrowth of the stromal component, a variant that has been designated as *müllerian adenosarcoma with sarcomatous overgrowth* (CD Fig. 37–55), with the sarcomatous proliferation usually being of a higher grade than the primary component.[214, 229, 234] According to the WHO classification, the latter diagnosis should be applied only to an adenosarcoma in which continual fields of pure sarcoma constitute 20% or more of the total tumor area.[38] Either the sarcomatous component alone or a combination of the sarcomatous and epithelial components of adenosarcomas may recur in 25% to 40% of patients,[209, 214, 229] mainly in the area of the pelvis or the vagina; distant metastases are uncommon and observed in only 5% of cases.[172] Although adenosarcomas are considered to be tumors of relatively low malignant potential, poor prognostic factors associated with recurrence or metastases, or both, include myometrial invasion, sarcomatous overgrowth, extrauterine spread, and vascular space invasion.[209, 214, 229, 234] The differential diagnosis includes adenofibroma, pure homologous sarcoma (especially endometrial stromal type), and carcinosarcoma. Carcinofibroma is a rare tumor in which the malignant epithelial component is associated with a benign fibromatous stroma.[38, 235]

The most common malignant tumor of the uterus with a mesenchymal component is the carcinosarcoma or malignant mixed müllerian tumor;[38] however, it accounts for only about 1% to 2% of all uterine malignancies.[206] A strong association between a previous history of pelvic irradiation and the subsequent development of malignant mixed müllerian tumors has been reported in the literature.[236] Most patients are postmenopausal, are in their 50s, and present clinically with vaginal bleeding. Although almost all tumors originate in the endometrium, they rarely arise primarily in the endocervix. Malignant mixed müllerian tumors are usually polypoid, can be sessile or pedunculated, and tend to occupy the entire endometrial cavity (CD Fig. 37–56). The tumors often prolapse through the endocervical canal (CD Figs. 37–57 and 37–58), mimicking a primary cervical tumor, and in many cases, the extent of myometrial and endocervical involvement is evident grossly. Malignant mixed müllerian tumors are generally friable lesions with a variegated appearance; hemorrhage and necrosis are common findings. They have been reported to arise in association with endometrial polyps.[237, 238] Half of patients with malignant mixed müllerian tumors have clinical signs of extrauterine disease at the time

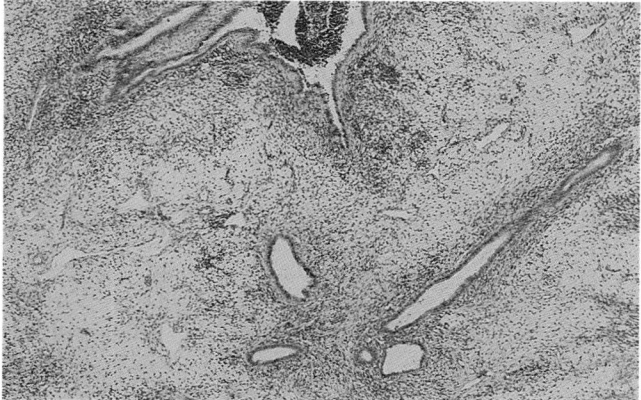

**Figure 37–21.** Müllerian adenosarcoma. The biphasic tumor reveals glands lined by benign müllerian epithelium. The malignant stroma shows increased periglandular cellularity (periglandular cuffing).

of diagnosis[239, 240] (CD Fig. 37–59). The biphasic nature of the lesion is evident microscopically, although either component may predominate in different areas of the tumor (CD Fig. 37–60). The epithelial component consists of a single type of carcinoma, usually an adenocarcinoma, or a combination of various types. The carcinomas are usually high grade, with endometrioid[241] and serous being the most common types; less common types include clear cell, mucinous, and squamous cell carcinomas.[206] The mesenchymal component of a malignant mixed müllerian tumor may be heterologous or homologous (Fig. 37–22). The most common malignant homologous components noted, either singly or in combination, include HGESS and fibrosarcoma,[206, 241] although tumors also may exhibit sarcomatous components resembling leiomyosarcoma, malignant fibrous histiocytoma, or undifferentiated sarcoma. Heterologous components may appear benign but more often are overtly malignant and may occur singly or in association with other heterologous mesenchymal derivatives. The most common heterologous cellular element seen in malignant mixed müllerian tumors is the rhabdomyoblast (rhabdomyosarcoma) (CD Fig. 37–61), followed by cartilage (chondrosarcoma), bone (osteosarcoma) (CD Fig. 37–62), and adipose tissue (liposarcoma).[206] Neuroendocrine differentiation also can occur in these tumors.[242] A relatively common histologic feature of malignant mixed müllerian tumors is the presence of hyaline droplets,[243] which may be single or multiple and measure 50 $\mu$ in diameter. These droplets can be found in either an intracellular or an extracellular location and typically are periodic acid–Schiff positive and diastase resistant aggregates of granular material that occur in both epithelial and mesenchymal cells.[243] They are not specific to malignant mixed müllerian tumors; similar hyaline droplets can be seen in other uterine malignancies (e.g., clear cell carcinomas).

The histogenesis of malignant mixed müllerian tumors is controversial. Some workers favor a common pluripotential stem cell origin capable of differentiating toward epithelial and mesenchymal elements.[244, 245] Others regard this tumor most likely to represent a metaplastic carcinoma, similar to the biphasic lesions that originate in other organs, such as the breast and the salivary glands.[241, 246] A third, but less popular, theory regards the malignant mixed müllerian tumor as an example of a collision tumor. Concurrent expression of cytokeratin, epithelial membrane antigen, vimentin, $\alpha_1$-antitrypsin, and $\alpha_1$-antichymotrypsin has been identified in the epithelial and mesenchymal components of malignant mixed müllerian tumors[172, 206]; however, it is common for the epithelial component to exhibit a strong and more uniform staining pattern with cytokeratin and epithelial membrane antigen and a patchy, less intense staining pattern with vimentin.[172, 206] Conversely, the stromal component usually reacts strongly and uniformly with vimentin and shows a patchy, usually weak staining pattern with cytokeratin and epithelial membrane antigen.[172, 206] Immunoreactivity to muscle markers (actin, myosin, myoglobin, and desmin) may be helpful in identifying the presence of muscle derivatives (including rhabdomyoblasts) in poorly differentiated areas. Heterologous differentiation (neuroendocrine, cartilage, bone) also can be highlighted using appropriate immunohistochemical markers.

Immunopositivity for proliferation markers and for p53 in the mesenchymal and the epithelial components of these tumors has been noted in several studies.[244–247] The presence of estrogen and progesterone receptors[248] and aneuploidy[245–247] has been shown.

Malignant mixed müllerian tumors are aggressive malignancies with a generally poor prognosis. The stage of the tumor at the time of diagnosis seems to be the most important prognostic factor associated with patient survival.[241, 245] Controversy still exists in the literature regarding the prognostic value of the degree of differentiation of the carcinomatous component[241]; however, the presence of heterologous elements and the differentiation of the sarcomatous component do not seem to influence patient survival.[241, 245] In the WHO classification, the terms *homologous* and *heterologous* are added to the diagnosis of malignant mixed müllerian tumor to qualify the lesion, although such subtyping is apparently of no clinical significance.[38] According to a large GOG study, most metastases from malignant mixed müllerian tumors consist of pure carcinoma, followed by mixed carcinoma and sarcoma, and, least commonly, pure sarcoma.[241] Despite the controversy regarding the nature of these tumors (metaplastic carcinoma versus true biphasic carcinosarcoma), uterine malignant mixed müllerian tumors seem to be clinically more aggressive than high-grade carcinomas.[249] The differential diagnosis of a malignant mixed müllerian tumor includes sarcomatoid carcinomas, carcinofibromas, adenosarcomas, pure homologous and heterologous sarcomas, and carcinomas with benign heterologous elements.

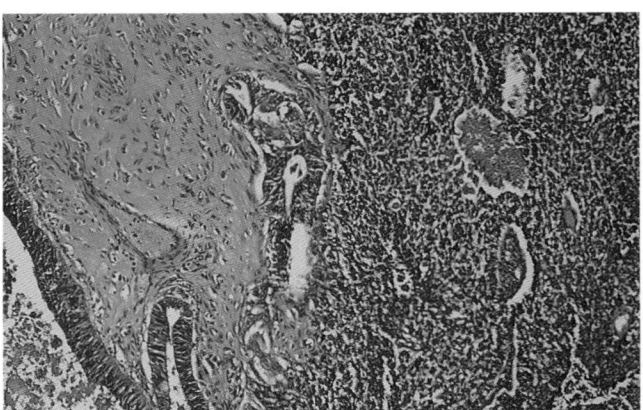

**Figure 37–22.** Carcinosarcoma.

## Miscellaneous Endometrial Lesions

### EXTRAMEDULLARY HEMATOPOIESIS

The presence of extramedullary hematopoiesis in the uterus is a rare finding. Immature blood precursors have been described in various organs normally not associated with the formation of blood elements, including the lungs, prostate, and skin, among others. Extramedullary hematopoiesis has been reported in the endometrium (CD Fig. 37–63) as an incidental finding in specimens obtained for a variety of clinical reasons in patients with concomitant hematologic disorders[250, 251] and in patients with no known hematologic conditions. We have observed several cases of endometrial extramedullary hematopoiesis, in addition to two cases exhibiting immature blood precursors in the cervix (one in a cervical polyp and the other in a cervix associated with an invasive uterine malignant mixed müllerian tumor with heterologous elements). In another of our cases, a mixed endometrial stromal and smooth muscle tumor exhibited multiple foci of extramedullary hematopoiesis. Immature blood precursors also have been described in leiomyomas.[252] We agree with the recommendations of various workers that the patient's attending physician should be alerted to this incidental finding and its potential association with the presence or subsequent development of hematologic disorders.

### PRIMITIVE NEUROECTODERMAL TUMOR

Although unusual, a primary primitive neuroectodermal tumor can develop in the endometrium of women of any age, although most cases occur in the postmenopausal period.[253–256] This lesion presents as a polypoid, soft gray endometrial mass typically with overt myometrial invasion. The histopathologic features include small cells ("blue cells") with round-to-elliptical hyperchromatic nuclei and a small amount of cytoplasm, areas of glial fibrillary differentiation, formation of true rosettes and pseudorosettes (Homer Wright rosettes appearing as perivascularly arranged cells), and occasionally the presence of ganglion cells. The typical immunohistochemical profile shows positivity with neuron specific enolase, glial fibrillary acidic protein, CD99, chromogranin, and S-100 protein. The clinical outcome seems to be related to the stage of the tumor.[255] A primary endometrial glioma also has been reported.[257]

### RARE TUMORS

Mature[258, 259] and immature[260, 261] primary endometrial teratomas are extremely rare lesions. Microscopically, they display identical features to those encountered in ovarian teratomas. The differential diagnosis includes the presence of residual embryonic remnants. Another rare tumor reported to occur in the uterus is Wilms' tumor.[262]

## MYOMETRIUM

### Mesenchymal Lesions

#### LEIOMYOMAS

The most common tumors of the uterus are leiomyomas, also popularly known as *fibroids*. These benign smooth muscle neoplasms frequently occur during the reproductive years and are unusual before the third decade.[176] During menopause, they frequently undergo atrophic changes.[3] Leiomyomas possess estrogen and progesterone receptors[263–267] and can respond with an increase in size when exposed to various hormonal treatment modalities. Clinically, rapidly growing leiomyomas have been described in association with pregnancy[268] and treatment with clomiphene citrate[269–271] and tamoxifen.[266, 272–274] Treatment with gonadotropin-releasing hormone agonists decreases their size.[265, 266, 275–277] Although several cytogenetic studies propose a monoclonal origin for uterine leiomyomas,[278–281] a study by Pandis and colleagues[278] suggested that some leiomyomas might be of multiclonal origin. Leiomyomas can cause a variety of clinical symptoms involving the female reproductive tract and the lower intestinal and lower urinary tracts. Their size, number, and location within the uterus may influence the magnitude of the symptoms, but they can be asymptomatic.

Leiomyomas typically are well-circumscribed, rubbery, white-tan nodules with a whorled, bulging cut surface. They range in size from microscopic to large tumors that distort the uterus or prolapse through the endocervical canal. If associated with pregnancy, they can cause miscarriages, placental abruption, and postpartum bleeding.[282] Leiomyomas can be single or multiple and may be located in the submucosal, intramyometrial (intramural), or subserosal aspects of the myometrial wall. Submucosal leiomyomas are capable of inducing pressure-related atrophy, hemorrhage, or ulceration of the overlying endometrium; they may present as sessile or pedunculated lesions protruding into the endometrial cavity. The subserosal leiomyomas may present as sessile or pedunculated lesions that protrude into the pelvic cavity, at times reaching sizes larger than the uterus itself (CD Fig. 37–64).

A leiomyoma is characterized microscopically by randomly arranged interlacing bundles of smooth muscle cells that, although grouped in a well-circumscribed manner, are out of synchrony with the architectural features of the surrounding myometrium. They usually appear slightly more cellular than the surrounding myometrium.[38] The spindle-shaped cells have variable amounts of eosinophilic cytoplasm and cigar-shaped nuclei with small nucleoli and are arranged in a background of fibrous connective tissue with scattered thick-walled blood vessels. Occasionally, leiomyomas exhibit areas with foci of hyalinization in a pattern reminiscent of the Verocay bodies observed in neurilemommas.[283]

In the myometrium, histiocytes are noted in the connective tissue interspersed between the smooth muscle bundles. In leiomyomas, histiocytes tend to permeate the lesion diffusely and seem to be more numerous than in the surrounding myometrium.[284] Mast cells seem to be more numerous in the smaller size leiomyomas and in leiomyomas with increased cellularity.[285] According to one study, the normal myometrium and cellular and bizarre leiomyomas contain more mast cells than otherwise common leiomyomas and leiomyosarcomas.[286] In the myometrium, mast cells seem uniformly distributed, whereas in common leiomyomas, they tend to display a more focal distribution.[286] Immunoreactivity with muscle-specific actin, desmin, $\alpha$ smooth muscle actin, and vimentin may be noted in the smooth muscle cells.[167, 287] Immunoreactivity with cytokeratin may be present in leiomyomas; the intensity and distribution of the staining seem to be related to the antibody used and the fixative in which the tissue is preserved.[287, 288] A protein that regulates muscle contraction, h-caldesmon has been shown to be immunopositive in uterine smooth muscle lesions (benign and malignant) and to be helpful in differentiating these lesions from endometrial stromal tumors.[189, 190] CD34 (a myeloid progenitor cell marker, a positive marker for gastrointestinal stromal tumors and other extrauterine smooth muscle tumors) also is immunopositive in uterine smooth muscle tumors.[191, 192] The presence of chromosomal imbalances has been shown in leiomyomas and leiomyosarcomas.[289] Leiomyomas and the myometrium synthesize many heparin-binding growth factors.[290] According to one study, when compared with the normal myometrium, leiomyomas exhibit decreased expression of heparin binding epidermal growth factor but increased expression of basic fibroblast growth factor.[290] Mitotic figures are rare in typical leiomyomas; however, during the secretory phase of the menstrual cycle, there seems to be some increase in mitotic activity.[291] Treatment with progestational agents and pregnancy can cause an increase in mitotic activity as well as cellular proliferation, nuclear atypia, edema, hemorrhage, and necrosis.[268] The most common degenerative change observed in leiomyomas is hyalinization,[172] but others may occur, including myxoid change, cystic change, edema or hydropic change, necrosis, hemorrhage, and calcifications. These degenerative changes may occur singly, but commonly, several of them are detected in a leiomyoma.

Depending on the patient's symptoms and desire to preserve her fertility, leiomyomas can be removed selectively by myomectomy, embolization of the uterine artery,[292] myolysis (coagulation) of the leiomyoma,[293] or hysterectomy. Leiomyomas may recur after a myomectomy.[294] Gonadotropin-releasing hormone agonists are used before a myomectomy to shrink leiomyomas; however, if the treatment is discontinued, the leiomyomas eventually may return to their original size.[295] Microscopic features seen within gonadotropin-releasing hormone–treated leiomyomas include thickening of vascular walls, degeneration, hyalinization, necrosis, areas of increased cellularity, irregular borders, and increased mitotic activity.[275, 296] In one study, mitotic activity in gonadotropin-releasing hormone agonist–treated leiomyomas was shown not to exceed 3 mitoses per 50 high-power fields.[296]

The histopathologic features of leiomyomas occasionally may deviate from the norm. Based on the predominant microscopic characteristics of a particular leiomyoma, several subtypes have been described.[38] The gross characteristics of these variants may be similar to those of otherwise common leiomyomas; they also may undergo degenerative changes. Cellular leiomyoma (Fig. 37–23) consists of markedly cellular bundles of spindle-shaped smooth muscle cells, associated with thick-walled vessels in a background of delicate fibrous connective tissue. According to the WHO, the degree of cellularity should be "significantly more" than that of the surrounding myometrium.[38] The margins are, in general, well circumscribed, although lesions with infiltrative borders have been described.[297] Cellular leiomyomas lack significant cytologic atypia, and mitotic activity in this lesion usually does not exceed 4 normal mitoses per 10 high-power fields.[297] Grossly, cellular leiomyomas may be yellow and have a softer consistency.[298] On microscopic evaluation, the differential diagnosis includes endometrial stromal nodule, LGESS, and leiomyosarcoma. Cellular leiomyomas lack the characteristic vascular pattern of the benign to low-grade endometrial stromal lesions (see previous section), although occasionally areas with small thin-walled vessels may be noted. Oliva and coworkers[167] identified a subset of cellular leiomyoma that they designated *highly cellular leiomyoma*, a leiomyoma whose cellularity is as marked as that of a low-grade endometrial stromal tumor. They described the presence of a fascicular pattern (usually in some portion of the tumor, often peripheral), large thick-walled muscular vessels, and artifactual cleft-like spaces as common features of highly cellular leiomyomas.[167] In contrast to cellular leiomyomas, leiomyosarcomas, even those with ab-

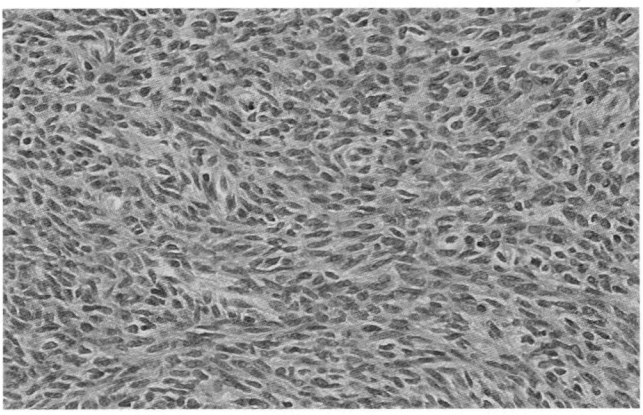

**Figure 37–23.** Cellular leiomyoma.

sent-to-minimal cytologic atypia, exhibit a mitotic count usually greater than 10 mitoses per 10 high-power fields.[299] Nevertheless, because of regional variations in histologic features, extensive sampling of cellular leiomyomas, certainly including the highly cellular leiomyoma, may be required to rule out endometrial stromal lesions and leiomyosarcomas.

The hemorrhagic cellular leiomyoma (also known as *apoplectic leiomyoma*) (CD Fig. 37–65) is a variant of leiomyoma seen during gestation, in the postpartum period, and in women taking oral contraceptives.[268, 300] Clinically, the most common complaint is abnormal uterine bleeding.[268] Grossly, the leiomyoma is well circumscribed, with irregularly distributed stellate areas of fresh hemorrhage and edema, occurring in one or more leiomyomas. Microscopic features include increased cellularity and variable mitotic activity, both changes largely confined to thin areas bordering the hemorrhagic foci, and occasional infarcts[268] (CD Fig. 37–66). Vascular abnormalities, including myxoid intimal change, can be seen in the vessels of the leiomyomas and in surrounding myometrial vessels.[268] Norris and associates[268] reported that 8 normal mitoses per 10 high-power fields may be identified in some cases. The tumors lack significant cellular atypia and infiltrative borders. The differential diagnosis is similar to that of cellular leiomyoma. Areas of "red degeneration" also can occur in otherwise typical leiomyomas during pregnancy. These are defined as grossly evident, well-delineated ischemic or hemorrhagic infarcts not associated with adjacent increased cellularity.[268]

Mitotically active leiomyomas (also known as *leiomyomas with increased mitotic index*) exhibit gross and histologic features comparable to those of otherwise common leiomyomas but usually are associated with more than 5 normal mitoses per 10 high-power fields.[268, 301–303] The maximal number of mitotic figures allowed by various workers for this entity has varied from 9 to 15 mitoses per 10 high-power fields[301–303]; a study by Bell and colleagues[299] defined tumors with a maximum of 20 mitoses per 10 high-power fields, no coagulative cell necrosis, and no significant cellular atypia as leiomyomas with increased mitotic index. Nevertheless, Bell and colleagues[299] noted that the clinical experience with that particular lesion, as defined by them, was limited. In a study by Prayson and Hart,[303] microscopic foci of vascular space invasion were noted in 15% of mitotically active leiomyomas.

Neoplasms with significant (moderate-to-severe) cellular atypia, associated with tumor cell necrosis and abnormal mitotic figures, do not qualify as mitotically active leiomyomas, even when the mitotic count is within the parameters described for this lesion. Mitotically active leiomyomas are more common in premenopausal women.[301–303] Numerous studies have suggested that the patient's hormonal status may be associated with the development of increased mitotic activity in these leiomyomas.[303–305]

Atypical leiomyomas are a controversial category and the diagnosis is eschewed by some observers. They tend to be more common in premenopausal women, are well circumscribed, and are characterized by moderate-to-severe cytologic atypia and 0 to 4 mitoses per 10 high-power fields. Tumor cell necrosis typically is absent in these lesions, although one study reported the presence of necrosis in some cases.[306] The cytologic atypia may be focal or diffuse; in some tumors, mitotic activity tends to occur adjacent to the atypical areas.[172] The atypical cells are variably pleomorphic, with hyperchromatic nuclei that occasionally may exhibit cytoplasmic pseudoinclusions[306, 307]; multinucleation is common. The sole presence of cytologic atypia does not represent evidence of malignancy in uterine smooth muscle tumors and may be associated with progestin therapy.[172] Based on their experience, Bell and colleagues[299] defined an atypical leiomyoma as a tumor with less than 20 mitoses per 10 high-power fields, *focal* moderate-to-severe cytologic atypia, and no evidence of coagulative tumor cell necrosis, but they admitted that the clinical experience and follow-up with this entity are limited. In the same study, Bell and colleagues[299] defined tumors with less than 10 mitotic figures per 10 high-power fields and exhibiting diffuse moderate-to-severe cytologic atypia and no coagulative cell necrosis as atypical leiomyomas with low risk of recurrence. Differentiating an atypical leiomyoma from a leiomyosarcoma may be difficult in some cases; extensive sampling of the tumor is always prudent.

In epithelioid leiomyomas, smooth muscle cells resemble epithelial cells (CD Figs. 37–67 and 37–68). Grossly, these tumors may be yellow and of a soft consistency.[3] In most cases, they are single[308] and average 7.0 cm in diameter.[172] Based on the more distinct histologic features of the epithelioid cells, leiomyomas can be classified into three subtypes: 1) plexiform leiomyoma, 2) leiomyoblastoma, and 3) clear cell leiomyoma.[38, 308] In plexiform leiomyoma, the cells are round to polygonal, with a small amount of eosinophilic cytoplasm and small round nuclei. They are arranged in cords and nests and generally are associated with varying degrees of stromal hyalinization. Microscopic plexiform leiomyomas, usually discovered as incidental findings, may be multiple and are referred to as *plexiform tumorlets*. The cells of leiomyoblastoma are round, with abundant granular eosinophilic cytoplasm and round nuclei that are larger than the nuclei observed in the other two subtypes.[3] Areas of stromal hyalinization may be present. Some workers are uncomfortable with the designation of these tumors as *leiomyoblastomas*, however, on the grounds that the term generally is used to describe a malignant neoplasm[297, 308–310] and may be confusing. Clear cell leiomyoma exhibits round-to-polygonal cells with copious amounts of clear cytoplasm and small round nuclei. Occasionally the cytoplasm displaces the nucleus to the side, resulting in a "signet ring–like" cellular configuration. Cytoplasmic glycogen can be detected in about half of cases, and lipid may be present in some tumors.[311] The clear cytoplasm has been ascribed to the presence of numerous dilated mitochondria by some[312] and to large aggregates of lysosomes by others.[310] Despite the previous classification, many epithelioid leiomyomas consist of a combination of the various cellular subtypes, including the presence of more typical spindle-shaped smooth muscle cells. The latter tumors are classified best as epithelioid leiomyomas. The differential diagnosis of epithelioid leiomyomas includes metastatic and primary endometrial carcinomas (in particular, clear cell carcinoma) involving the myometrium and endometrial stromal lesions.

The clinical behavior of epithelioid leiomyomas is difficult to forecast based solely on specific histologic criteria. According to a study by Kurman and Norris,[308] tumors that measure less than 5.0 cm in greatest dimension exhibit no more than 1 mitosis per 10 high-power fields, and lack significant cellular atypia and necrosis tend to behave in a benign fashion. Epithelioid smooth muscle tumors with more than 5 mitoses per 10 high-power fields probably are interpreted best as epithelioid leiomyosarcomas.[308] Tumors with histologic features between those of benign and malignant lesions perhaps should be regarded as epithelioid leiomyomas of uncertain malignant potential.[297] Plexiform leiomyomas[3] and plexiform tumorlets[313] seem to behave in a benign fashion.

Myxoid leiomyomas occur more commonly in women during the reproductive period[297] (CD Fig. 37–69). A myxoid leiomyoma is a well-circumscribed leiomyoma with significant myxoid change, also known as *myxoid degeneration*. Depending on the focal or diffuse nature of this change, the cut surface can be glistening with a mucoid consistency.[314] Microscopically, the latter areas consist of copious amounts of myxoid extracellular material that constitutes the background in which elongated smooth muscle cells are interspersed. The extracellular material is alcian blue positive, owing to an abundance of acid mucins[297] (CD Fig. 37–70). The smooth muscle cells lack atypical features and mitotic activity.[314] The presence of edema fluid in leiomyomas, also known as *hydropic change* or *degeneration*, is more common and sometimes may be difficult to differentiate from myxoid degeneration grossly and microscopically.[297] In those situations, special stains (alcian blue or colloidal iron) may be necessary to characterize the degenerative changes.[297] Myxoid leiomyoma should be differentiated from the myxoid variant of leiomyosarcoma.

A leiomyoma with a conspicuous vascular component may be classified as a vascular leiomyoma. The differential diagnosis includes uterine hemangiomas and arteriovenous malformations.[172] Hemangiomas of the uterus are uncommon; when present, they are most likely of the cavernous type.[172]

The term *lipoleiomyoma* is used to describe a leiomyoma with a mature adipose tissue component. These unusual lesions can be seen in association with otherwise common uterine leiomyomas, and they tend to occur in postmenopausal women.[315] Grossly, the cut surface may be tan and whorled, with focal, soft, light yellow areas. The uterine lesions have been reported to range in size from 1.2 to 11.0 cm. Microscopically, adipose tissue of variable amounts alternates with the spindle-shaped smooth muscle cells. If a significant vascular component is present, the term *angiolipoleiomyoma* is applied to the lesion. Although in most cases the smooth muscle component consists of spindle-shaped cells, Brooks and coworkers[316] described a bizarre epithelioid lipoleiomyoma of the uterus. The microscopic presence of adipose tissue also has been described in cases of disseminated peritoneal leiomyomatosis and in other types of leiomyomas.[172] The differential diagnosis of a lipoleiomyoma is a primary uterine lipoma (CD Fig. 37–71), an exceedingly rare lesion.[317]

Diffuse leiomyomatosis is an uncommon benign condition in which the myometrium is involved diffusely by numerous small leiomyomas. The distribution of the leiomyomas imparts a symmetric enlargement to the uterus and may cause a significant increase in weight.[281, 297] Many of these leiomyomas merge with each other and appear grossly as nodular protuberances of various sizes involving the myometrium rather than as well-circumscribed lesions. Microscopically, leiomyomas are composed of spindle-shaped smooth muscle cells that lack cellular atypia or mitotic activity. A case report suggested that, based on clonality analysis, this condition represents diffuse and uniform myometrial involvement by multiple leiomyomas.[281]

Disseminated peritoneal leiomyomatosis (also known as *leiomyomatosis peritonealis disseminata* or *diffuse peritoneal leiomyomatosis*) is an unusual benign condition. Disseminated peritoneal leiomyomatosis is characterized by the presence of multiple, histologically benign leiomyomas diffusely involving the surfaces of the omentum, the abdominopelvic organs, and the peritoneum,[316] clinically mimicking a disseminated malignant process. The patients are frequently women of reproductive age, although cases have been described in postmenopausal women, during the fetal period,[318] and in men.[319] This condition may be discovered as an incidental finding at the time of surgery (e.g., at cesarean section or during laparoscopic surgery). The patients usually are asymptomatic or complain of pelvic discomfort.[320, 321] Most cases have been associated with increased endogenous or exogenous steroid hormonal levels (e.g., during pregnancy, during use of oral contraceptives, and in association with steroid-secreting ovarian tumors).[317, 320, 321] The presence of estrogen and progesterone receptors has been shown in these lesions by various methods,[322, 323] and high levels of estrogen and progesterone receptor binding have been noted in them when compared with normal myometrium.[322]

The leiomyomas of disseminated peritoneal leiomyomatosis are rubbery, gray-tan, and well circumscribed, varying in size from 0.2 to 7.0 cm, although most tend to be within 1.0 to 2.0 cm in greatest dimension.[320, 321] Microscopically, they consist of interlacing bundles of spindle-shaped smooth muscle cells associated with connective tissue in a pattern reminiscent of benign uterine leiomyomas; a decidual reaction may be observed if the patient was recently pregnant.[320, 321] Mitotic activity and cytologic atypia are not significant. Microscopic foci of endometrial, endocervical, and adipose tissue have been reported[320, 321, 324, 325] as well as areas exhibiting sex cord–like patterns, similar to those sometimes observed in uterine leiomyomas.[326] Disseminated peritoneal leiomyomatosis rarely can be seen in association with endometriosis,[325] and a case of concomitant disseminated peritoneal leiomyomatosis, endometriosis, and multicystic mesothelioma has been reported.[327] At the ultrastructural level, leiomyomas of disseminated peritoneal leiomyomatosis may be composed exclusively of smooth muscle cells or may show a combination of smooth muscle cells, myofibroblasts, decidualized cells, and fibroblasts.[320, 321, 328] This condition most likely is the result of a metaplastic proliferation of the submesothelial undifferentiated connective tissue in response to variations in the hormonal milieu.[320, 321, 328, 329] A study pointed out that disseminated peritoneal leiomyomatosis displays cytogenetic features suggesting a monoclonal derivation of the individual lesions, and that their origin may be due to a mechanism similar to that of uterine leiomyomas.[318] In one study, 38% of all patients with disseminated peritoneal leiomyomatosis had a history of uterine leiomyomas.[320]

Treatment modalities vary from surgical resection of most lesions to subsequent hormonal therapy, depending on the extent of the disease and the specific needs of the patient. The leiomyomas may regress or become quiescent after the resolution of the hormonally altered state.[320, 321] The condition may recur, however, after similar alterations in the hormonal milieu, such as with a subsequent pregnancy.[321] The differential diagnosis includes metastatic leiomyosarcoma and benign metastasizing leiomyomas. Although distinctly rare, several cases of malignant transformation of disseminated peritoneal leiomyomatosis have been reported.[330–332] Lausen and associates[319] reported a case of malignant transformation occurring in a male patient.

The term benign metastasizing leiomyoma connotes a condition in which histologically benign uterine leiomyomas are believed to give rise to distant "metastases" that lack malignant histologic features. Although the metastases most commonly affect the lungs and the pelvic lymph nodes, other less common sites include the soft tissue of the lower limb,[333] bone,[334] and the heart.[335] Most such cases are diagnosed in retrospect, usually several years after a myomectomy or a hysterectomy for uterine leiomyomas. The patients may be asymptomatic, and undergo physical or radiologic evaluation as part of a routine checkup. In cases of pulmonary involve-

ment, the nodules may show up in chest radiographs obtained for reasons that vary from routine examinations to complaints of nonspecific dyspnea or coughing. At that time, single or multiple, typically bilateral, pulmonary smooth muscle nodules are noted, varying in size from 0.2 to 10.0 cm in greatest dimension.[336] Microscopically, the metastatic deposits consist of mature smooth muscle bundles that lack atypia or significant mitotic activity. Studies have shown estrogen and progesterone receptors in some specimens.[333, 336, 337] Treatment modalities include hysterectomy and bilateral salpingo-oophorectomy[338, 339] and hormonal therapy, including antiestrogenic and progestational agents.[336] The metastases are known to disappear or decrease in size during pregnancy[340] and menopause.[336] The cause of this condition is controversial, and various theories regarding its nature have been considered. One theory proposes distant metastases from a well-differentiated uterine leiomyosarcoma that either was missed initially or failed to show the conventional criteria established for the diagnosis of that type of malignancy.[336] Clonality analysis of various cases of benign metastasizing leiomyoma has determined a monoclonal origin for uterine and pulmonary tumors, favoring a metastatic process.[337, 341] In one study of 10 cases,[337] pulmonary lesions revealed low proliferation activity (Ki-67), frequent estrogen and progesterone receptor positivity, and p53 overexpression. A second theory favors metastases from intravenous leiomyomatosis. A third consideration is the multifocal origin of these lesions,[342] possibly in association with hormonal stimulation.

In intravascular leiomyomatosis, a histologically benign smooth muscle tumor, despite the absence of significant cellular atypia and mitotic activity, invades the uterine veins.[38, 343, 344] In one series, the average patient age was 46 years.[345] Most patients present with nonspecific clinical symptoms, including vaginal bleeding or a pelvic mass. The uterus may be grossly unremarkable. In some instances, the uterus appears enlarged, with numerous rubbery, gray-to-yellow nodules that may display well-to-poor circumscription; vascular space involvement may be evident grossly or may present only as a microscopic finding. Cylindrical-shaped tumor extensions into extrauterine pelvic veins can be noted in some cases. The vascular invasion may extend to involve the extrauterine pelvic veins, the inferior vena cava, and, in some instances, the right side of the heart.[346–348] Pulmonary metastases associated with this condition also have been reported.[345] An intravascular leiomyoma may originate from the smooth muscle of a venous wall[343] or may represent vascular space invasion from a leiomyoma.[343, 344] Microscopically, the tumor protrudes into the vascular space, and an endothelial lining usually is appreciated on its surface. The intravascular tumors display a variety of patterns, varying from a composition similar to common leiomyomas to a predominantly fibrous and hyalinized lesion; increased vascularity also may be a prominent feature.[172] Any variant of leiomyoma can occur as intravascular leiomyomatosis, and degenerative changes may be present.[349] The extent and the caliber of the uterine veins involved by the tumors are variable[345]; however, arteries are not affected. Leiomyomas occasionally may show nodular areas associated with surrounding retraction artifact mimicking an intravascular space suggestive of microscopic foci of intravascular leiomyomatosis.[350] In such cases, the use of immunohistochemical markers for detecting endothelial cells (Ulex europeus, factor VIII) may help elucidate the nature of this phenomenon.[350]

Small vascular space intrusions by the surrounding myometrium or by adenomyomatous elements (endometrial glands or stroma or both) occasionally are seen in hysterectomy specimens. The significance of such findings is unknown at this time; however, they should not be interpreted as evidence of intravascular leiomyomatosis. Also important is to differentiate intravascular leiomyomatosis from a leiomyosarcoma involving vascular spaces, especially if the histologic features of the intravascular leiomyoma are those of a bizarre or a mitotically active leiomyoma. Grossly evident vascular involvement of the uterine and extrauterine vessels by tumor can be seen in cases of endometrial stromal sarcoma, usually LGESS, and rarely in müllerian adenofibroma.[217] Intravascular leiomyomatosis usually follows a benign course, even when complete surgical excision may be difficult to attain or if lesions recur.[345, 349] Treatment modalities include hysterectomy with bilateral salpingo-oophorectomy, surgical removal of any visible lesions,[172, 345] and hormonal therapy.[343, 344, 347] Tamoxifen has been used in the treatment of this condition.[347]

A smooth muscle tumor of uncertain malignant potential is a leiomyoma that cannot be classified as either benign or malignant using the acceptable established criteria for those entities.[38] This tumor can be defined best against the background of the definitions of leiomyoma, leiomyosarcoma, and their variants. The use of this term should be accompanied by an explanation as to what features of the tumor seem to be unconventional. An example would be a markedly atypical tumor with increased cellularity but rare mitotic figures. Although Hendrickson and Kempson[351] described examples of leiomyomas of uncertain malignant potential, other workers defined some of the same lesions with similar criteria as benign. The controversial lesions that have been included within the uncertain malignant potential category encompass atypical leiomyomas, cellular leiomyomas, mitotically active leiomyomas, hemorrhagic cellular leiomyomas (apoplectic leiomyomas), tumors with any abnormal mitotic figures, and tumors with any degree of necrosis. Less controversial was the inclusion in the uncertain malignant potential category of tumors with infiltrating borders and 5 to 9 mitoses per 10 high-power fields and epithelioid and bizarre leiomyomas with 2 to 5 mitoses per 10 high-power fields. Smooth muscle tumors showing vascular invasion with 2 to 5 mitoses per 10

high-power fields and parasitic leiomyomas originating from the uterus with 5 to 9 mitoses per 10 high-power fields are neoplasms that have been classified as smooth muscle tumors of low malignant potential. Positive p53 immunoreactivity has been documented in cases designated as smooth muscle tumors of uncertain malignant potential.[352] Bell and associates[299] defined tumors with less than 10 mitoses per 10 high-power fields, absent or mild atypia, but with coagulative cell necrosis as smooth muscle tumors of low malignant potential. Nevertheless, these authors cautioned that the clinical follow-up experience with the last-mentioned lesions was limited and the differential diagnosis included a benign infarcted leiomyoma.[299]

Leiomyosarcomas are tumors composed of malignant smooth muscle cells. Clinically, they tend to occur in postmenopausal women and may be associated with nonspecific symptoms, including vaginal bleeding and pelvic discomfort. In the uterus, leiomyosarcomas constitute approximately one third of all primary sarcomas. It is postulated that leiomyosarcomas arise directly from the myometrium, although the issue regarding their origin from preexisting leiomyomas is controversial. Leiomyosarcomas of the uterus are generally solitary intramural lesions (CD Fig. 37–72); concomitant leiomyomas are observed in approximately 25% to 50% of cases,[353] and one may encounter patients in whom the history implies rapid growth.[354] Grossly, they present as a soft, tan hemorrhagic mass with ill-defined borders; according to one study,[355] leiomyosarcomas average 6.0 to 9.0 cm in diameter. They may involve the intramural aspect of the uterine wall or protrude into the endometrial cavity or, in some cases, may prolapse through the cervix. Microscopically, leiomyosarcomas can display varying degrees of differentiation, and geographic variation within the same tumor is not unusual. They frequently are cellular neoplasms composed of spindle-shaped cells with eosinophilic cytoplasm and hyperchromatic nuclei that may vary from elongated to markedly pleomorphic (Fig. 37–24). Multinucleation often is present

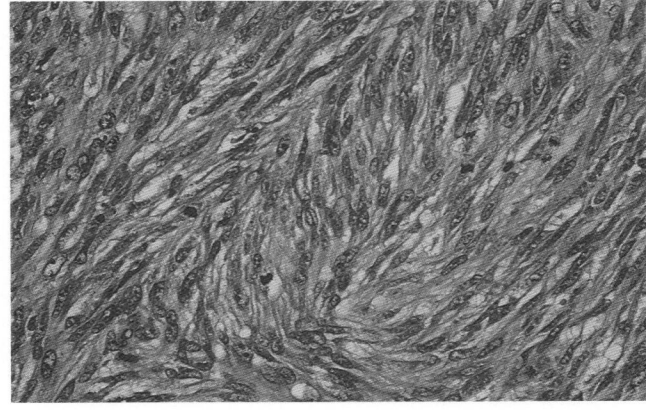

**Figure 37–24.** Leiomyosarcoma. Note the increased mitotic activity and nuclear atypia.

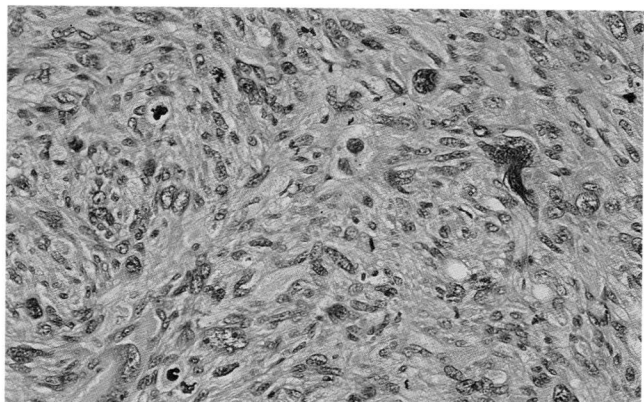

**Figure 37-25.** Leiomyosarcoma, high grade.

(Fig. 37-25), and cells resembling osteoclasts sometimes are noted.[356] Clear cell–type changes also have been described.[357] Nucleoli are prominent, and the chromatin is coarse and clumped. Mitotic activity tends to be brisk, and abnormal mitotic figures are frequent. In a study by Amada and colleagues,[358] the percentage of cells immunohistochemically positive for MIB-1 and other proliferation markers that reflect proliferative activity in tumor cells, was significantly higher in leiomyosarcomas than in bizarre and cellular leiomyomas. Frequent occurrence of loss of heterozygosity among tumor-suppressor genes has been reported in uterine leiomyosarcomas,[359] and other studies have shown p53 positivity to be more prevalent in leiomyosarcomas than in benign smooth muscle tumors.[352, 359] Most leiomyosarcomas are aneuploid.[289, 358, 360] Immunoreactivity with muscle-specific actins and desmin may be minimal or absent,[358] although immunopositivity for h-caldesmon has been shown in leiomyosarcomas.[189, 190] Positive immunostaining with cytokeratin and epithelial membrane antigen also can be observed.[361] Leiomyosarcomas display various degrees of necrosis, hemorrhage, and vascular space invasion. The margins with the surrounding myometrium are, in general, overtly infiltrative.

The main histopathologic criteria for the diagnosis of a leiomyosarcoma include the assessment of the degree of cellularity, mitotic activity, and cellular atypia.[306] The consensus among many workers is that evaluation of the previously described features in toto is necessary to define a tumor as a leiomyosarcoma. Other workers have advocated the number of mitotic figures as the single feature in uterine smooth muscle neoplasms indicative of a benign or malignant nature. Most would agree, however, that tumors with more than 5 mitoses per 10 high-power fields associated with significant cellular atypia, including pleomorphism, anaplasia, and multinucleation, should be diagnosed as leiomyosarcomas.[307] In their study, Bell and colleagues[299] defined tumors with more than 10 mitoses per 10 high-power fields, no coagulative cell necrosis, and diffuse moderate-to-severe cytologic atypia as leiomyosarcomas. They also defined tumors with any degree of mitotic activity, displaying diffuse moderate-to-severe cellular atypia and coagulative cell necrosis, as leiomyosarcomas.[299] These authors defined coagulative cell necrosis as the presence of individual necrotic ("ghost") cells in contact with viable tissue elements, including other malignant cells, supporting stroma, and blood vessels; in these ghost cells, the malignant nuclear features, including hyperchromasia and pleomorphism, are still distinguishable[299] (CD Figs. 37-73 and 37-74).

According to a study by Jones and Norris,[362] tumor features of uterine leiomyosarcomas that correlate with the subsequent development of metastases include tumor size, mitotic activity, cytologic atypia, necrosis, and cell type. These authors concluded that uterine leiomyosarcomas measuring less than 3 cm in greatest dimension tend not to metastasize.[362] Metastases may develop, however, 15 years after the initial diagnosis.[362] Myxoid and epithelioid leiomyosarcomas may behave in an aggressive manner but exhibit less mitotic activity and cytologic atypia than the more typical high-grade leiomyosarcomas. Postmenopausal women tend to have a worse prognosis than premenopausal women with uterine leiomyosarcomas.[3] Although rare, uterine leiomyosarcomas have been described in association with pregnancy[363-365]; in one reported case, the tumor was discovered at the time of cesarean section.[363]

To avoid misdiagnosing smooth muscle tumors, several important tenets should be followed. Any smooth muscle tumor that exhibits a different gross appearance in comparison to the surrounding leiomyomas or any other clinical or pathologic features that raise suspicion should result in a greater degree of tissue sampling (at least one block per 1 to 2 cm of the diameter of the tumor). The specimen should be fixed promptly in adequate amounts of fixative appropriate for the size of the specimen. Histologic sections should be thin and well stained. In counting mitoses, only unequivocal mitotic figures should be counted, taking care to exclude the numerous "mitoidic" figures that tempt the observer. Counting should be done in the areas of highest mitotic activity and performed at a magnification of 400×; at least four sets of 10 consecutive fields should be counted, and the highest set should be chosen to represent the mitotic index. Multiple sections should be taken from the tumor-myometrial interface so that any infiltrative borders of the smooth muscle tumor can be evaluated. The vessels within the tumor and those in the surrounding myometrium should be evaluated carefully for intravascular protrusions or invasion. The tumor should be examined carefully for tumor cell necrosis or coagulative tumor cell necrosis (as described by Bell and colleagues[299]). The degree of cytologic (nuclear) atypicality should be assessed; three degrees of atypia corresponding to mild, moderate, and severe may be assigned (some workers regard moderate and severe atypia as *significant nuclear atypicality*). The pathologist should be wary of making the diagnosis of leiomyosarcoma in a young (<30 years old) woman, a pregnant woman, or a woman taking oral contraceptives. Likewise, the pathologist should be wary of making the diagnosis of unequivocal benignancy in an older woman with any cellular or atypical smooth muscle tumor. At the time of frozen section, a conservative approach should be taken when the representative sections of a uterine smooth muscle tumor exhibit increased cellularity, cytologic atypia, necrosis, or mitotic activity. In the latter situation, the final diagnosis should be deferred to the permanent sections after extensive sampling, and the rationale for this decision should be discussed with the surgeon. Pertinent clinical information (e.g., history of rapid growth, medications, patient's age) should be obtained to establish the proper clinicopathologic correlation.

Some uterine leiomyosarcomas may include histologic features similar to those encountered in benign uterine leiomyomas. The uncommon myxoid variant of leiomyosarcoma grossly may appear well circumscribed, with a gelatinous cut surface, and ranges in diameter from 5 to 15 cm.[366, 367] Generally, the malignant cells are spindle shaped, lack significant cytologic atypia, and are observed in a myxoid (alcian blue and colloidal iron positive) background; mitotic activity frequently is low (<5 mitoses per 10 high-power fields)[367] (CD Fig. 37–75). Extensive sampling is needed, considering that in some tumors more cellular (nonmyxoid) areas can reveal atypical cytologic features and significant mitotic activity.[297] Myxoid leiomyosarcomas with high mitotic counts and significant cytologic atypia have been described.[368–370] Despite their well circumscribed gross appearance, myxoid leiomyosarcomas infiltrate the surrounding myometrium and blood vessels (Fig. 37–26). The latter feature seems to be more helpful in establishing the diagnosis of malignancy in tumors with bland cytologic features and few mitotic figures.[38] These tumors have been reported in patients 30 to 68 years old and may recur 6 months to 10 years after their diagnosis.[370] In epithelioid

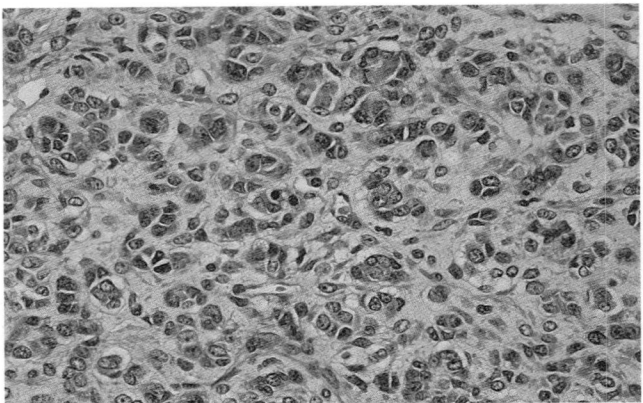

**Figure 37–27.** Epithelioid leiomyosarcoma.

leiomyosarcomas, the malignant cells exhibit epithelioid features similar to those described in the benign variant,[371] including the presence of clear cells,[357] and display fewer than average mitotic figures and moderate atypia[362] (Fig. 37–27; CD Figs. 37–76 and 37–77). Epithelioid leiomyosarcomas have been described in patients 20 years of age.[362] We encountered a primary leiomyosarcoma of the uterus in a 14-year-old girl; the microscopic features and immunohistochemical profile of the tumor were consistent with a mixed myxoid and epithelioid leiomyosarcoma (CD Fig. 37–78).

## Mixed Endometrial Stromal and Smooth Muscle Tumors

Uterine tumors exhibiting histologic features of endometrial stroma and smooth muscle are uncommon; they can be benign, malignant, or of uncertain malignant potential. The term *stromomyoma* has been used by some to refer to these lesions.[372–374] Their biphasic nature should be established on evaluation of the sections by light microscopy.[38] As might be expected, certain features in the immunohistochemical profile of an endometrial stromal tumor may overlap with those of a smooth muscle tumor; immunohistochemical studies may not be helpful when trying to qualify a lesion that seems to belong to this group of tumors by light microscopy. The assessment of their malignant potential should be established on evaluation of the malignant component with the highest grade.[38, 372, 375] The percentage of each component that should be present in a particular tumor to warrant this diagnosis has not been defined, although Tavassoli and Norris[372] suggested that lesions containing at least one third of each component should be present to classify the neoplasm as a mixed endometrial stromal and smooth muscle tumor. Oliva and coworkers[375] described a series of 15 cases of such tumors, in which the patients ranged in age from 29 to 68 years, and the clinical presentation did not differ from that of pure smooth muscle or endometrial stromal tumors.

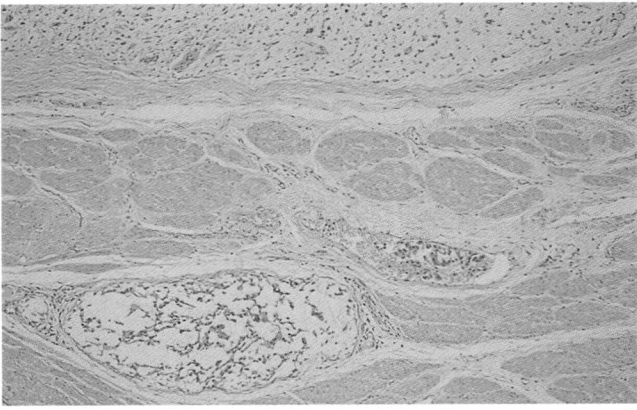

**Figure 37–26.** Myxoid leiomyosarcoma. The characteristic pattern of myometrial infiltration is appreciated.

The tumors ranged in diameter from 3.0 to 27.0 cm. Grossly, most of them were well circumscribed, and their cut surfaces frequently exhibited yellow-to-tan, soft areas associated with whorled firm areas.[375] Six of their cases had infiltrating borders more characteristic of LGESS. Microscopic features noted in most of their benign and malignant examples included the abrupt transition from one component to the other and the presence, in the smooth muscle component, of multiple, variably-sized nodules displaying central hyalinization and peripherally arranged, radiating thin collagen bundles ("starburst" pattern). The latter pattern, although a frequent feature of stromal tumors, is not characteristic of these tumors and can be seen in other neoplasms.[375] Sex cord–like areas also were identified in some mixed neoplasms. The differential diagnosis includes cellular leiomyomas, pure endometrial stromal tumors, and uterine tumors resembling ovarian sex-cord tumors.[375] Because of regional variations in cell types, mixed endometrial stromal and smooth muscle tumors may prove difficult to diagnose based on tissue samples obtained at the time of frozen section. Thorough sampling of a neoplasm of this nature is recommended to insure that all components are represented in the final diagnosis.

## Homologous and Heterologous Sarcomas

Pure mesenchymal tumors, other than smooth muscle lesions, representing the malignant counterpart of tissues indigenous to the uterus (homologous sarcomas) and tissues that normally do not occur in the uterus (heterologous sarcomas) (CD Fig. 37–79), are uncommon. Because they occur so rarely, significant data alluding to their clinical presentation, prognosis, and treatment are scarce. Many of the heterologous and homologous sarcomas described as occurring in the uterus can be present as a component of two relatively more common lesions: malignant mixed müllerian tumor and adenosarcoma. Therefore, it is necessary to rule out the presence of concomitant epithelial or additional mesenchymal components before making the exceedingly rare diagnosis of a pure uterine sarcoma. Pure sarcomas reported to occur in the uterus include angiosarcoma,[376, 377] rhabdomyosarcoma[378–380] (CD Fig. 37–80), liposarcoma,[381, 382] osteosarcoma,[383, 384] chondrosarcoma[385] (CD Fig. 37–81), malignant fibrous histiocytoma,[386] malignant rhabdoid tumor,[378] and alveolar soft part sarcoma.[388]

## Lymphomas

Primary lymphomas of the uterus are rare, and most of them arise in the cervix.[389, 390] Clinical symptoms are nonspecific and include pelvic discomfort and vaginal bleeding (Fig. 37–28). Grossly, lymphomas appear fleshy and are poorly circumscribed. Most

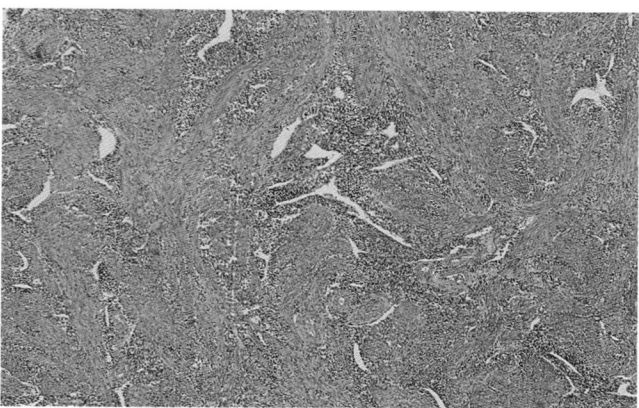
**Figure 37–28.** Primary uterine lymphoma involving the myometrium.

primary uterine lymphomas are of the diffuse large cell type with a B-cell phenotype[389, 390]; however, a diffuse large cell–type lymphoma with a peripheral T-cell phenotype has been described.[390] Other types of primary lymphomas are known to occur in the uterus and cervix, including Burkitt's lymphoma.[391] The differential diagnosis of a primary uterine lymphoma includes inflammatory pseudotumor of the uterus,[392] uterine leiomyomas with lymphoid infiltration,[393] lymphoma-like lesions of the endometrium,[394] and secondary involvement of the uterus by a disseminated lymphoma. Uterine leiomyomas with lymphoid infiltration are characterized by focal or diffuse aggregates of mostly lymphocytes mixed with plasma cells and rare eosinophils. Germinal centers may be observed as well as areas of sclerosis.[393] Grossly, such leiomyomas lack any distinctive features. The inflammatory pseudotumor of the uterus is an uncommon lesion that grossly may resemble a leiomyoma. Microscopically, it is characterized by myofibroblasts associated with a variably dense inflammatory cell infiltrate consisting of plasma cells, lymphocytes, and neutrophils.[392] Lymphoma-like lesions of the endometrium usually represent florid cases of chronic endometritis.[394] Multiple myeloma[395] and leukemias[396] may involve the uterus secondarily. Granulocytic sarcoma also has been described in the uterus and cervix.[391, 397]

## Adenomyosis

Adenomyosis is the result of invaginations of the uterine mucosa into the underlying myometrium. It consists of aggregates of benign endometrial glands and stroma within the myometrium that, on sectioning, appear dissociated from the endomyometrial junction. Because the endomyometrial junction may be irregular, the diagnosis of adenomyosis should be made when the foci are located at a distance of more than one half a low-power field from the deepest point of the endomyometrial junction.[38] Histologically, adenomyotic tissue usually resembles the mucosa of the basalis or proliferative endometrium and commonly is out of synchrony with the changes identified in the stratum functionalis (CD Fig. 37–82). The distribution of estrogen and progesterone receptors in adenomyotic tissue is similar to the findings noted in the basalis.[398] Nevertheless, secretory changes, features associated with exogenous hormones (e.g., oral contraceptives), endometrial hyperplasia, and carcinoma also can be identified. Careful analysis is necessary when carcinoma involves, and particularly replaces, adenomyosis to avoid confusion with foci of invasive cancer.[93, 94] Adenomyosis may be focal and superficial or extensive and deep; areas devoid of glands can be noted (CD Fig. 37–83). When the involvement is significant, the uterus can be diffusely enlarged, and the myometrium displays trabeculations and numerous small cystic spaces that can be filled with blood or small nodularities, some with areas of umbilication. The patient may experience nonspecific symptoms, including pelvic discomfort. Adenomyosis may be an isolated finding or can be seen in association with other uterine lesions, including leiomyomas.

## Myometrial Hypertrophy

In so-called myometrial hypertrophy, the uterus is evenly enlarged and shows an increase in weight and in the thickness of the myometrial wall.[172] No specific gross or microscopic features, such as seen in cases of adenomyosis, are noted. The weight of the uterus is affected by parity and menopausal status; according to one study, myometrial hypertrophy is present in the nulliparous uterus that weighs 130 g or more; the multiparous uterus with up to three pregnancies that weighs 210 g or more; and in the multiparous uterus with more than four pregnancies that weighs 250 g or more.[399]

## MISCELLANEOUS LESIONS

### Endometriosis, Endosalpingiosis, and Endocervicosis

Endometriosis is defined as the presence of endometrial glands or stroma or both in an ectopic location. Endometriotic foci undergo cyclic changes associated with the menstrual cycle, including bleeding. Uterine serosal involvement by endometriosis is common, at times extending into the underlying myometrium, and frequently is associated with fibrous adhesions. Uterine endometriosis regularly accompanies endometriosis of other pelvic organs, especially the ovaries, uterine ligaments, and peritoneum of the urinary bladder and rectosigmoid.[400] Grossly, endometriotic implants display a variety of appearances, including raised patchy areas; nodules and cysts; and areas of white, red-blue, or yellow-brown coloration. Foci of uterine endometriosis may undergo metaplastic epithelial changes, display epithe-

lial atypia, or undergo malignant transformation.[400] The clinical symptoms often are nonspecific and include vaginal bleeding and pelvic pain; infertility is noted in 30% of patients.[401]

Endosalpingiosis is defined as the presence of benign glands lined by tubal-type epithelium in the peritoneum, in subperitoneal areas, and within lymph nodes.[400] Endosalpingeal structures occasionally display architectural and cytologic atypia that raise the question of overt or borderline malignancy; they also can contain psammoma bodies. Endosalpingiosis is more prevalent in women of reproductive age, and although the condition is most likely of mesothelial origin, other theories regarding its cause have been proposed.[402] Usually a clinically silent incidental finding, endosalpingiosis commonly is detected in the serosa of the female reproductive organs. When clinically evident, minute white, yellow, or translucent fluid-filled cysts are noted.[400] Similar to endometriosis, it can involve the uterine serosa and the underlying myometrium (CD Figs. 37–84 and 37–85). These benign glandular structures should not be confused with metastatic carcinoma, particularly serous neoplasia, including primary peritoneal serous borderline tumor or carcinoma. Careful evaluation is necessary when the patient has a history of borderline serous ovarian or primary peritoneal neoplasia because in those cases, endosalpingiotic structures may be confused with implants of serous borderline tumor.[400, 403] In four cases of extensive cystic uterine endosalpingiosis resembling a neoplastic process described by Clement and Young,[404] two exhibited transmural involvement of the uterus by endosalpingiosis.

Benign peritoneal glands lined by endocervical mucinous epithelium, known as *endocervicosis*, are exceedingly rare, but they may involve the uterine serosa.[400] In such instances, caution should be exercised to rule out a metastatic well-differentiated, endocervical mucinous adenocarcinoma.

### Subinvolution of the Placental Bed Arteries

Subinvolution of the placental bed arteries may result in postpartum hemorrhage. This condition is characterized by the abrupt onset of bleeding 1 week to several months after delivery, with the peak incidence noted in the second postpartum week.[405] Normally the placental bed arteries undergo thrombosis, with organization of the clots and eventual shrinkage of the area.[406] The endometrium regenerates approximately 3 weeks after delivery.[407] The involuted placental bed arteries normally show regeneration of the vascular components, including the endothelium, and usually are not involved by extravillous (intermediate type) trophoblast.[405] In cases of subinvolution of the placental bed arteries, the uterus is soft, enlarged, and congested. Curettage material may not always contain tissue from the placental bed area; however, when present, the sub-involuted vessels appear dilated and distorted, with focal organizing nonocclusive thrombi. Hyaline material often replaces areas of the vascular walls, and regeneration of the components of the wall, including the endothelium, is absent.[405] In most cases, perivascular intramural and sometimes intravascular extravillous (intermediate type) trophoblast is associated with the subinvoluted vessels. Normal involuted vessels also may be identified in this area. Failure of the placental bed arteries to involute may be seen in older multiparous patients and may be a recurrent problem in subsequent pregnancies.[405]

## Adenomatoid Tumor

The adenomatoid tumor is a benign mesothelioma that can be seen in the serosal and subserosal and intramural aspects of the uterus, the round ligaments, and the fallopian tubes (CD Fig. 37–86). In the uterus, it is more common in the subserosa of the posterior myometrium.[408] Grossly, the adenomatoid tumor resembles a leiomyoma, or it may present as an ill-defined soft, white-tan mass. Although they frequently are single, multiple adenomatoid tumors may occur.[409] Grossly, cystic adenomatoid tumors of the uterine corpus have been encountered,[410] and Livingston and colleagues[411] described a diffuse uterine adenomatoid tumor with a serosal papillary cystic component. Adenomatoid tumors usually are incidental findings, occurring in 1.2% of uteri,[412] mainly in women of reproductive age. They average 0.5 to 3.5 cm in greatest dimension, although larger tumors with cystic gross features have been described.[410] It is possible for components of adenomatoid tumor to appear rarely in endometrial curettings.[413]

Microscopically, uterine adenomatoid tumors may exhibit three histologic patterns: 1) tubular (or "adenoid"), 2) plexiform, and 3) canalicular.[412] In the most common presentation, tubules lined by cuboidal or flattened cells with small round nuclei in a background of connective tissue appear to infiltrate the myometrium diffusely; however, these structures remain confined to a particular area and are not associated with infiltrative reactive features, such as desmoplasia. Cytoplasmic vacuoles or signet ring–like cellular features occasionally can be seen and may cause confusion with metastatic signet ring carcinoma.[408, 172] Mitotic activity is unusual. The cells exhibit immunoreactivity with antikeratin antibodies and fail to react when antibodies against CEA, epithelial membrane antigen, TAG-72, and CD-15 are used. In a study by Otis,[408] 9 of 11 uterine adenomatoid tumors exhibited focal weak immunopositivity for BER-EP4, an antibody against components of epithelial cells. The differential diagnosis includes a lymphangioma, a hemangioma, and the aforementioned metastatic carcinoma. In lymphangiomas and hemangiomas, the endothelial cells are immunopositive when antibodies against Ulex europeus and factor VIII are used; hemangiomas also exhibit blood within their vascular spaces.

## Metastatic Carcinoma

Metastatic carcinoma can involve the endometrium or the myometrium or both. As previously mentioned, the most common carcinoma that metastasizes to the uterus (other than those of genital tract origin) is of the breast, followed by carcinoma of the stomach and melanoma.[154, 414, 415] The myometrium may exhibit discrete, grossly evident metastatic lesions or diffuse microscopic foci of metastatic carcinoma; cystic degeneration of the metastatic lesions may be observed. In the endometrium, metastatic carcinoma tends to infiltrate the stroma around the glands, sparing the latter. Vaginal bleeding is reported regularly as the first clinical manifestation in these cases. Occasionally, benign endometrium undergoing glandular and stromal breakdown, such as menstrual endometrium or shedding endometrium associated with a defective corpus luteum, may be confused with carcinoma.[155] The presence of menstrual endometrium in uterine and parametrial blood vessels, a phenomenon rarely encountered in the face of otherwise ordinary menstruation, should not be confused with vascular space invasion by a malignancy.

## Arteritis

Although unusual, involvement of the uterus by a necrotizing arteritis displaying histologic features of polyarteritis nodosa may be the first manifestation of that systemic condition.[416–418] In these cases, uterine small and medium-sized arteries reveal segmental inflammatory changes ranging in chronology from acute to healed, all of which may coexist in the same vessel. In the acute stage, segmental fibrinoid necrosis may involve the full thickness of the wall in a circumferential fashion, associated with an inflammatory cell infiltrate consisting of polymorphonuclear leukocytes and mononuclear cells. In the healed stage, fibrosis results in thickening of the wall. So-called isolated necrotizing arteritis exhibits histologic features identical to those of polyarteritis nodosa but is self-limited and not associated with that systemic condition.[419] This rare entity has been described in various female genital organs, including the uterine corpus, the cervix, and the fallopian tubes and ovaries[419]; when present, the patient should be evaluated clinically to exclude systemic involvement by polyarteritis nodosa. Most patients are perimenopausal or postmenopausal; the clinical symptoms are nonspecific, and the prognosis is good.[419] In a study by Francke and associates,[419] immune complex deposits, including IgM, IgG, and C3, were identified in the vascular lesions of 7 of the 11 cases of isolated necrotizing arteritis of the female genital tract. Giant cell arteritis may involve the uterus, the cervix, the fallopian tubes, and the ovaries as a localized process or as part of systemic involvement in patients known to have the condition[420]; the uterus is involved frequently, either alone or in combination with the other reproductive organs. Such vascular lesions may be incidental findings in uteri removed for an unrelated reason.[420] In the myometrium, numerous blood vessels are permeated diffusely by a dense inflammatory cell infiltrate that almost obliterates the lumen. The infiltrate consists of lymphocytes, epithelioid histiocytes, multinucleated giant cells, eosinophils, and neutrophils. In these cases, it is important to evaluate the patients for any significant clinical history that may point to a systemic condition, including visual symptoms or the flulike symptoms associated with stiffness of the joints known as *polymyalgia rheumatica*. Marrogi and coworkers[420] reported that in 17 cases of giant cell arteritis of the female reproductive organs recorded in the literature, only about two thirds of them had clinical manifestations suggestive of a systemic vasculitis. These patients are usually postmenopausal and require only close follow-up when they fail to show any symptoms and their laboratory profiles, including erythrocyte sedimentation rate levels, are within the expected limits.

## Arteriovenous Malformations

Arteriovenous malformations of the uterus may involve the myometrium or the endometrium[421, 422] and are unusual. They may be congenital or acquired as the result of a previous curettage. The most common clinical presentation is vaginal bleeding. Microscopically, they can be localized or diffuse and consist of a combination of thick-walled and thin-walled vessels. Depending on their location, they may bleed into the myometrium or into the endometrial cavity.

## Myometrial Cysts

Occasionally, cysts may be identified in the myometrium. They have different causes and generally are benign. Adenomyotic glands may undergo cystic dilation and present grossly as a single cyst or as multiple scattered cystic structures involving the myometrial wall, many of them filled with bloody fluid. In an unusual case, submucosal adenomyosis underwent cystic change and presented as a polypoid mass that distorted the endometrial cavity and caused abnormal vaginal bleeding.[423] The spectrum of degenerative changes occurring in leiomyomas includes cystic change, in which one or several leiomyomas may undergo "cystification." In rare instances, myometrial cysts may arise from mesonephric or paramesonephric duct remnants. Surface mesothelial inclusion cysts can involve the outer myometrium and serosa. Brenner's tumor, believed to arise from metaplasia of entrapped peritoneal

mesothelium within the myometrium, has been reported.[424] In serosal and outer myometrial endometriosis, the endometrial glands also can undergo cystic change.

## Postoperative Spindle Cell Nodule

The postoperative spindle cell nodule is a reparative process that develops after a surgical incisional procedure. It has been described in numerous organs, including the endometrium.[425] Histologically, it is characterized by a population of closely packed spindle-shaped cells associated with capillaries and inflammatory cells, all of which impart a nodular fasciitis or "tissue culture"–like appearance. The interface with the surrounding tissues is irregular, and mitotic activity is common and quite brisk. Significant cytologic atypia is absent, however. In the original report of this lesion, postoperative spindle cell nodules were confused most often with a leiomyosarcoma. Care should be exercised to avoid its misdiagnosis as such or another type of sarcoma, particularly because the latter tend to be large, bulky tumors, and the postoperative spindle cell nodule more often is quite small in comparison.[425]

### REFERENCES

1. Sadler TW: Langman's Medical Embryology, 5th ed. Baltimore, Williams & Wilkins, 1985.
2. Robboy SJ, Bernhardt PF, Parmley T: Embryology of the female genital tract and abnormal sexual development. In Kurman RJ (ed): Blaustein's Pathology of the Female Genital Tract, 5th ed. New York, Springer-Verlag, 1995, pp 3–29.
3. Silverberg SJ, Kurman RJ: Atlas of Tumor Pathology. Tumors of the Uterine Corpus and Gestational Trophoblastic Disease. Third Series, Fascicle 3. Washington, DC, Armed Forces Institute of Pathology, 1992.
4. Ferenczy A: Anatomy and histology of the uterine corpus. In Kurman RJ (ed): Blaustein's Pathology of the Female Genital Tract, 5th ed. New York, Springer-Verlag, 1995, pp 327–366.
5. Scully RE: Ovarian tumors with functioning stroma. In Fox H (ed): Haines and Taylor Obstetrical and Gynaecological Pathology, 4th ed. New York, Churchill Livingstone, 1995, pp 983–996.
6. Herbst AL, Ulfelder H, Poskanzer DC: Adenocarcinoma of the vagina: Association of maternal stilbestrol therapy with tumor appearance in young women. 1971. Am J Obstet Gynecol 181:1574–1577, 1999.
6a. Hollinshead WH: Textbook of Anatomy, 3rd ed. Hagerstown, MD, Harper & Row, 1974.
7. Hendrickson MR, Kempson RL: Normal histology of the uterus and fallopian tube. In Sternberg SS: Histology for Pathologists, 2nd ed. Philadelphia, Lippincott-Raven, 1997, pp 879–929.
8. Marshall RJ, Jones DB: An immunohistochemical study of lymphoid tissue in human endometrium. Int J Gynecol Pathol 7:225–235, 1988.
9. Bulmer JN, Lunny DP, Hagin SV: Immunohistochemical characterization of stromal leucocytes in nonpregnant human endometrium. Am J Reprod Immunol Microbiol 17:83–90, 1988.
10. Crow J, Wilkins M, Howe S: Mast cells in the female genital tract. Int J Gynecol Pathol 10:230–237, 1991.
11. Noyes RW, Hertig AT, Rock J: Dating the endometrial biopsy (1950). Am J Obstet Gynecol 122:262–263, 1975.
12. Lenton EA, Landgren BM, Sexton L: Normal variation in the length of the luteal phase of the menstrual cycle. Identifica-

tion of the short luteal phase. Br J Obstet Gynaecol 91:685–689, 1984.

13. Masterton R, Armstrong EM, More IAR: The cyclical variation in the percentage of ciliated cells in the normal human endometrium. J Reprod Fertil 42:537–540, 1975.

14. Levitt MJ, Tobon H, Josimovich JB: Prostaglandin content of human endometrium. Fertil Steril 26:296–300, 1975.

15. Abel MH, Baird DT: The effect of 17 beta-estradiol and progesterone on prostaglandin production by human endometrium maintained in organ culture. Endocrinology 106:1599–1606, 1980.

16. Bulmer JN, Hollings D, Ritson A: Immunohistochemical evidence that endometrial stromal granulocytes are granulated lymphocytes. J Pathol 153:281–288, 1987.

17. King A, Wellings V, Gardner L: Immunohistochemical characterization of the unusual large granular lymphocytes in human endometrium throughout the menstrual cycle. Hum Immunol 24:195–205, 1989.

18. Casey BM, Cox SM: Chorioamnionitis and endometritis. Infect Dis Clin North Am 11:202–222, 1997.

19. Kurman RJ, Mazur MT: Benign diseases of the endometrium. In Kurman RJ (ed): Blaustein's Pathology of the Female Genital Tract, 5th ed. New York, Springer-Verlag, 1995, pp 367–409.

20. Silverberg SG, Gompel C: Pathology in Gynecology and Obstetrics, 4th ed. Philadelphia, JB Lippincott, 1994.

21. Mazur MT, Kurman RJ: Pregnancy, abortion, and ectopic pregnancy. In Mazur MT, Kurman RJ (eds): Diagnosis of Endometrial Biopsies and Curettings. A Practical Approach. New York, Springer-Verlag, 1995, pp 33–62.

22. Paavonen J, Aine R, Teisalak K, et al: Comparison of endometrial biopsy and peritoneal fluid cytology testing with laparoscopy in the diagnosis of acute pelvic inflammatory disease. Am J Obstet Gynecol 151:645–650, 1985.

23. Kiviat NB, Eschenbach DA, Paavonen JA, et al: Endometrial histopathology in patients with culture proved upper genital tract infection and laparoscopically diagnosed acute salpingitis. Am J Surg Pathol 14:167–175, 1990.

24. Hillier SL, Kiviat NB, Hawes SE: Role of bacterial vaginosis associated microorganisms in endometritis. Am J Obstet Gynecol 175:435–431, 1996.

25. Nogales-Ortiz F, Taranco I, Nogales FF Jr: The pathology of female genital tuberculosis. A 31 year study of 1436 cases. Obstet Gynecol 53:422–428, 1979.

26. Gini PC, Ikerionwu SE: Incidental tuberculous endometritis in premenstrual curettings from infertile women in eastern Nigeria. Int J Gynecol Obstet 31:141–144, 1990.

27. Ho KL: Sarcoidosis of the uterus. Hum Pathol 10:219–222, 1979.

28. Farber ER, Leahy MS, Meadows TR: Endometrial blastomycosis acquired by sexual contact. Obstet Gynecol 32:195–199, 1968.

29. Saw EC, Smale EI, Einstein H, et al: Female genital coccidioidomycosis. Obstet Gynecol 45:199–202, 1975.

30. Berry A: A cytopathological and histopathological study of bilharziasis of the female genital tract. J Pathol Bacteriol 91:325–338, 1966.

31. Duncan DA, Varner RE, Mazur MT: Uterine herpes virus infection with multifocal necrotizing endometritis. Hum Pathol 20:1021–1024, 1989.

32. Hollier LM, Scott LL, Murphree SS: Postpartum endometritis caused by herpes simplex virus. Obstet Gynecol 89(5 pt 2):836–838, 1997.

33. Mazur MT, Kurman RJ: Endometritis. In Mazur MT, Kurman RJ (eds): Diagnosis of Endometrial Biopsies and Curettings. A Practical Approach. New York, Springer-Verlag, 1995, pp 131–145.

34. Russack V, Lammers RJ: Xanthogranulomatous endometritis. Report of six cases and a proposed mechanism of development. Arch Pathol Lab Med 114:929–932, 1990.

35. Thomas W Jr, Sadeghieh B, Fresco R, et al: Malacoplakia of the endometrium, a probable cause of postmenopausal bleeding. Am J Clin Pathol 69:637–641, 1978.

36. Miko TL, Lampe LG, Thomazy VA: Eosinophilic endomyometritis associated with diagnostic curettage. Int J Gynecol Pathol 7:162–172, 1988.

37. Mazur MT, Kurman RJ: Dysfunctional uterine bleeding. In Mazur MT, Kurman RJ (eds): Diagnosis of Endometrial Biopsies and Curettings. A Practical Approach. New York, Springer-Verlag, 1995, pp 89–108.

38. Scully RE, Bonfiglio TA, Kurman RJ, et al: Histological Typing of Female Genital Tract Tumours. World Health Organization Histological Classification of Tumours, 2nd ed. New York, Springer-Verlag, 1994.

39. Choo YC, Mack C, Hsu C: Postmenopausal uterine bleeding from atrophic endometrium. Obstet Gynecol 66:225–228, 1985.

40. Jones GES: Some newer aspects of management of infertility. JAMA 141:1123–1129, 1949.

41. Leach RE, Ramirez NC: Endometrial biopsy. In Evans MI, Johnson MP, Moghissi KS (eds): Invasive Outpatient Procedures in Reproductive Medicine. Philadelphia, Lippincott-Raven, 1997, pp 171–184.

42. Eisenber E: Luteal phase defect. In Diamond MP, Osteen KG (eds): Endometrium and Endometriosis. Malden, MA, Blackwell Science, 1997, pp 84–90.

43. Noyes RW: The underdeveloped secretory endometrium. Am J Obstet Gynecol 77:929–945, 1959.

44. Charles D: Iatrogenic endometrial patterns. J Clin Pathol 17:205, 1964.

45. Mazur MT, Kurman RJ: Effects of hormones. In Mazur MT, Kurman RJ (eds): Diagnosis of Endometrial Biopsies and Curettings. A Practical Approach. New York, Springer-Verlag, 1995, pp 109–130.

46. Birkendfeld A, Navot D, Levij IS: Advanced secretory changes in the proliferative human endometrial epithelium following clomiphene citrate treatment. Fertil Steril 45:462–468, 1986.

47. Yeko TR, Bardawil WA, Nicosia SM: Histology of midluteal corpus luteum and endometrium from clomiphene citrate induced cycles. Fertil Steril 57:28–32, 1992.

48. Barbieri R: Danazol in the treatment of endometriosis. In Diamond MP, Osteen KG (eds): Endometrium and Endometriosis. Malden, MA, Blackwell Science, 1997, pp 96–201.

49. Fedele L, Marchiani M, Bianchi S: Endometrial patterns during danazol and buserelin therapy for endometriosis. Comparative structural and ultrastructural study. Obstet Gynecol 76:79–84, 1990.

50. Floyd WS: Danazol: Endocrine and endometrial effects. Int J Fertil 25:75–80, 1980.

50a. Tavaniotou A, Smitz J, Bourgain C, et al: Ovulation induction disrupts luteal phase defects. Ann NY Acad Sci 943:55–63, 2001.

51. Reshef E, Segars JH, Hill GA: Endometrial inadequacy after treatment with human menopausal gonadotropin. Fertil Steril 54:1012–1016, 1990.

52. Garcia JE, Acosta AA, Hsiu JG: Advanced endometrial maturation after ovulation induction with human menopausal gonadotropin/human chorionic gonadotropin for in vitro fertilization. Fertil Steril 41:31–35, 1984.

53. Croxatto HD, Diaz S, Pavez M: The endometrium during continuous use of Levonorgestrel. In Zatuchini GI, Goldsmith A, Sheldon JD, Sciarra JJ (eds): Long Acting Contraceptive Delivery Systems. Philadelphia, Harper & Row, 1984, p 290.

54. Clement PB, Scully RE: Idiopathic postmenopausal decidual reaction of the endometrium. Int J Gynecol Pathol 7:152–161, 1988.

55. Gemzell-Daniellson K, Svlander P, Swahn ML: Effects of a single post-ovulatory dose of RU486 on endometrial maturation in the implantation phase. Hum Reprod 9:2398–2404, 1994.

56. Murphy AA, Kettel LM, Morales AJ, et al: Endometrial effects of long term low dose administration of RU486. Fertil Steril 63:761–766, 1995.

57. Johanisson E, Fournier K, Roitton G: Regeneration of the human endometrium and presence of inflammatory cells following diagnostic curettage. Acta Obstet Gynecol Scand 60:451–457, 1981.

58. Golfarb HA: A review of 35 endometrial ablations using the Nd:YAG laser for recurrent menometrorrhagia. Obstet Gynecol 76:833–835, 1990.

59. Baggish MS, Sze EH: Endometrial ablation. A series of 568 patients treated over an 11 year period. Am J Obstet Gynecol 174:908–913, 1996.

60. Reid PC, Thurrell W, Smith JH: Nd:YAG laser endometrial ablation. Histological aspects of uterine healing. Int J Gynecol Pathol 11:174–179, 1992.

61. Ahosa AB, Boret F: Necrotising granulomas of the uterine corpus. J Clin Pathol 46:953–955, 1993.

62. Silver SA, Sherman ME: Morphologic and immunophenotypic characterization of foam cells in endometrial lesions. Int J Gynecol Pathol 17:140–145, 1998.

63. Mittal K, Schwartz L, Goswami S: Estrogen and progesterone receptor expression in endometrial polyps. Int J Gynecol Pathol 15:345–348, 1996.

64. Walter TA, Fan SX, Medchill MT: Inv (12p11.2q13) in an endometrial polyp. Cancer Genet Cytogenet 41:99–103, 1989.

65. Vanni R, Del Cin P, Marras S: Endometrial polyp. Another benign polyp characterized by 12q 13–15 changes. Cancer Genet Cytogenet 68:32–35, 1993.

66. Spelman F, Del Cin P, Van Roy N: Is t(6;20)(p21;q13) a characteristic chromosome change in endometrial polyps? Genes Chromosomes Cancer 31:318–319, 1991.

67. Armenia CC: Sequential relationship between endometrial polyps and carcinoma of the endometrium. Obstet Gynecol 30:524, 1967.

68. Salm R: The incidence and significance of early carcinomas in endometrial polyps. J Pathol 108:47, 1972.

69. Nuovo MA, Nuovo GJ, McCaffrey RM: Endometrial polyps in postmenopausal patients receiving Tamoxifen. Int J Gynecol Pathol 8:125–131, 1989.

70. Schlesinger C, Kamoi S, Ascher S: Endometrial polyps. A comparison study of patients receiving Tamoxifen with two control groups. Int J Gynecol Pathol 17:302–311, 1998.

71. Kendall BS, Ronnett BM, Isaacson CI, et al: Reproducibility of the diagnosis of endometrial hyperplasia, atypical hyperplasia, and well differentiated carcinoma. Am J Surg Pathol 22:1012–1019, 1998.

72. Hendrickson MR, Kempson RL: Endometrial epithelial metaplasias. Proliferations frequently misdiagnosed as adenocarcinoma. Report of 89 cases and proposed classification. Am J Surg Pathol 4:525–542, 1980.

73. Kurman RJ, Kaminski PF, Norris HJ: The behavior of endometrial hyperplasia. A long term study of "untreated hyperplasia" in 170 patients. Cancer 56:403–412, 1985.

74. Kurman RJ, Norris HJ: Endometrial hyperplasia and related cellular changes. *In* Kurman RJ (ed): Blaustein's Pathology of the Female Genital Tract, 5th ed. New York, Springer-Verlag, 1995, pp 411–438.

75. Visscher DW, Lawrence WD: Endometrial carcinoma. Current clinical and pathological concepts. Oper Tech Gynecol Surg 3:21–30, 1998.

76. Bokhman JV: Two pathogenetic types of endometrial carcinoma. Gynecol Oncol 15:10–17, 1983.

77. Kurman RJ, Zaino RJ, Norris HJ: Endometrial carcinoma. *In* Kurman RJ (ed): Blaustein's Pathology of the Female Genital Tract, 5th ed. New York, Springer-Verlag, 1995, pp 439–486.

78. Persson I, Adami HO, Bergkvist L: Risk of endometrial cancer after treatment with oestrogens alone or in conjunction with progestogens. Results of a prospective study. BMJ 298:147, 1989.

79. McDonald TW, Malkasian GD, Gaffey TA: Endometrial cancer associated with feminizing ovarian tumor and polycystic ovarian disease. Obstet Gynecol 49:654–658, 1977.

80. Gusberg SB: Current concepts in cancer. The changing nature of endometrial cancer. N Engl J Med 302:729, 1980.

81. Musubushi K, Nemoto H: Epidemiologic studies on uterine cancer at Cancer Institute Hospital, Tokyo, Japan. Cancer 30:268, 1972.

82. Sandles LG, Shulman LP, Elias S: Endometrial adenocarcinoma. Genetic analysis suggesting heritable site-specific uterine cancer. Gynecol Oncol 47:167–171, 1992.

83. Lax SF, Kurman RJ, Pizer ES, et al: A binary architectural grading system for uterine endometrial endometrioid carcinoma has superior reproducibility compared with FIGO grading and identified subsets of advanced-stage tumors with favorable and unfavorable prognosis. Am J Surg Pathol 24:1201–1208, 2000.

84. Zaino RJ, Silverberg SG, Norris HJ: The prognostic value of nuclear versus architectural grading in endometrial adenocarcinoma. A Gynecologic Oncology Group study. Int J Gynecol Pathol 13:29–36, 1994.

85. Nordstrom B, Strang P, Lindgren A: Carcinoma of the endometrium. Do the nuclear grade and DNA ploidy provide more prognostic information than do the FIGO and WHO classifications? Int J Gynecol Pathol 15:191–201, 1996.

86. Zaino RJ, Davis ATL, Ohlsson Wilhelm BM: DNA content is an independent prognostic indicator in endometrial adenocarcinoma. A GOG Study. Int J Gynecol Pathol 17:312–319, 1998.

87. Kadar N, Malfetano J, Homesley H: Steroid receptor concentrations in endometrial carcinoma. Effect on survival in surgically staged patients. Gynecol Oncol 50:281–286, 1993.

88. Nyholm HCJ, Nielsen AL, Lyndrup J: Estrogen and progesterone receptors in endometrial carcinoma. Comparison of immunohistochemical and biochemical analysis. Int J Gynecol Pathol 12:246–252, 1995.

89. Wagatsuma S, Konno R, Sato S: Tumor angiogenesis, hepatocyte growth factor, and c-Met expression in endometrial carcinoma. Cancer 82:520–530, 1998.

90. Geisler JP, Geisler HE, Wiemann MC, et al: p53 expression as a prognostic indicator of a 5-year survival in endometrial cancer. Gynecol Oncol 74:468–471, 1999.

91. Kohler M, Berchuk A, Davidoff A: Overexpression and mutation of p53 in endometrial carcinoma. Cancer Res 52:1622–1627, 1992.

92. Backe J, Gassel AM, Hauber K: p53 protein in endometrial cancer is related to proliferative activity and prognosis but not to expression of p21 protein. Int J Gynecol Pathol 16:361–368, 1997.

93. Jacques SM, Lawrence WD: Endometrial adenocarcinoma with variable level myometrial involvement limited to adenomyosis. A clinicopathologic study of 23 cases. Gynecol Oncol 37:401–407, 1990.

94. Mittal KB, Barwick KW: Endometrial adenocarcinoma involving adenomyosis without true myometrial invasion is characterized by frequent an preceding estrogen therapy, low histologic grades, and excellent prognosis. Gynecol Oncol 49:107–201, 1993.

95. Takai N, Akizuki S, Nasu K, et al: Endometrioid adenocarcinoma arising from adenomyosis. Gynecol Obstet Invest 48:141–144, 1999.

96. Zaino RJ, Kurman RJ, Brunetto VL, et al: Villoglandular adenocarcinoma of the endometrium. A clinicopathologic study of 61 cases. A Gynecologic Oncology Group study. Am J Surg Pathol 22:1379–1385, 1998.

97. Esteller M, Garcia A, Martinez-Palones JM, et al: Clinicopathologic features and genetic alterations in endometrioid carcinoma of the uterus with villoglandular differentiation. Am J Clin Pathol 111:336–342, 1999.

98. Zaino RJ, Kurman R, Herbold D, et al: The significance of squamous differentiation in endometrial carcinoma. Data from a Gynecologic Oncology Group. Cancer 68:2293, 1991.

99. Lax SF, Pizer ES, Ronnet BM, et al: Comparison of estrogen and progesterone receptor, Ki-67, and p53 immunoreactivity in uterine endometrioid carcinoma and endometrioid carcinoma with squamous, mucinous, secretory, and ciliated cell differentiation. Hum Pathol 299:924–931, 1998.

100. Kim KR, Scully RE: Peritoneal keratin granulomas with carcinomas of endometrium and ovary and atypical polypoid adenomyoma of endometrium. A clinicopathological analysis of 22 cases. Am J Surg Pathol 14:925–932, 1990.

101. Hachisuga T, Sugimori H, Kaku T, et al: Glassy cell carcinoma of the endometrium. Gynecol Oncol 36:134–138, 1990.

102. Christopherson WM, Alberhasky RC, Connelly P: Glassy cell carcinoma of the endometrium. Hum Pathol 13:418–421, 1982.

103. Tobon H, Watkins GJ: Secretory adenocarcinoma of the endometrium. Int J Gynecol Pathol 4:328–335, 1985.

104. Eichorn JH, Young RH, Clement PB: Sertoliform endometrial adenocarcinoma. A study of four cases. Int J Gynecol Pathol 15:119–126, 1996.

105. Hendrickson M, Ross J, Eifel P, et al: Uterine papillary serous carcinoma. A highly malignant form of endometrial adenocarcinoma. Am J Surg Pathol 6:93–108, 1982.

106. Carcangiu ML, Chambers JT: Early pathologic stage clear cell carcinoma and uterine papillary serous carcinoma of the endometrium. Comparison of clinicopathologic features and survival. Int J Gynecol Pathol 14:30–38, 1995.

107. Demopoulos RI, Genega E, Vamvakas E, et al: Papillary carcinoma of the endometrium. Morphometric predictors of survival. Int J Gynecol Pathol 25:110–115, 1995.

108. Cirisano FD, Robboy SJ, Dodge RK, et al: The outcome of stage I–II clinically and surgically staged papillary serous and clear cell endometrial cancers when compared with endometrioid carcinoma. Gynecol Oncol 77:55–65, 2000.

109. Abramovich D, Markman E, Kennedy A, et al: Serum CA-125 as a marker of disease activity in uterine papillary serous carcinoma. J Cancer Res Clin Oncol 125:697–698, 1999.

110. Fokuma K, Miyamura S, Thoya T, et al: Uterine papillary serous carcinoma with high levels of serum carcinoembryonic antigen. Response to combination chemotherapy. Cancer 59:403–405, 1987.

111. Kubo K, Lee GH, Yamauchi K, et al: Alpha fetoprotein producing papillary adenocarcinoma originating from a uterine body. A case report. Acta Pathol Jpn 41:399–403, 1991.

112. Sasano H, Comerford J, Wilkinson DS, et al: Serous papillary adenocarcinoma of the endometrium. Analysis of proto-oncogene amplification, flow cytometry, estrogen and progesterone receptors, and immunohistochemistry. Cancer 65:1545, 1990.

113. Konski AA, Domenico D, Irving D, et al: Clinicopathologic correlation of DNA flow cytometric content analysis (DFCA), surgical staging, and estrogen/progesterone receptor status in endometrial adenocarcinoma. Am J Clin Oncol 19:164–168, 1996.

114. Miller B, Umpierre S, Tornos C, et al: Histologic characterization of uterine papillary serous adenocarcinoma. Gynecol Oncol 56:425–429, 1995.

115. King SA, Adass AA, LiVolsi V, et al: Expression and mutation analysis of the p53 gene in uterine papillary serous carcinoma. Cancer 75:2700–2705, 1995.

116. Bancher Todesca D, Gitsch G, Williams KE, et al: p53 protein overexpression. A strong prognostic factor in uterine papillary serous carcinoma. Gynecol Oncol 71:59–63, 1998.

117. Magriples U, Naftolin F, Schuartz PE, et al: High grade endometrial carcinoma in Tamoxifen treated breast cancer patients. J Clin Oncol 11:485–490, 1993.

118. Silva EG, Tornos CS, Follen-Mitchell M: Malignant neoplasms of the uterine corpus treated for breast carcinoma. The effects of Tamoxifen. Int J Gynecol Pathol 13:248–258, 1994.

119. Ambros RA, Sherman ME, Zahn CM, et al: Endometrial intraepithelial carcinoma. A distinctive lesion specifically associated with tumors displaying serous differentiation. Hum Pathol 26:1260–1267, 1995.

120. Spiegel GW: Endometrial carcinoma in situ in postmenopausal women. Am J Surg Pathol 19:417–432, 1995.

121. Soslow RA, Pirog E, Isacson C: Endometrial intraepithelial carcinoma with associated peritoneal carcinomatosis. Am J Surg Pathol 24:726–732, 2000.

122. Webb GA, Lagios MD: Clear cell carcinoma of the endometrium. Am J Obstet Gynecol 156:1486–1491, 1987.

123. Christopherson WM, Alberhasky RC, Connelly PJ: Carcinoma of the endometrium. I. A clinicopathologic study of clear cell carcinoma and secretory carcinoma. Cancer 49:1511–1523, 1982.

124. Kanbour-Shakir A, Tobon H: Primary clear cell carcinoma of the endometrium. A clinicopathologic study of 20 cases. Int J Gynecol Pathol 10:67–78, 1991.

125. Lax SF, Pizer ES, Ronnett BM, et al: Clear cell carcinoma of the endometrium is characterized by a distinctive profile of p53, Ki-67, estrogen, and progesterone receptor expression. Hum Pathol 29:551–558, 1998.

126. Melhem MF, Tobon H: Mucinous adenocarcinoma of the endometrium. A clinico-pathological review of 18 cases. Int J Gynecol Pathol 6:347–355, 1987.

127. Ross JC, Eifel PJ, Cox RS, et al: Primary mucinous adenocarcinoma of the endometrium. A clinicopathological and histochemical study. Am J Surg Pathol 7:715, 1983.

128. Zheng W, Yang GC, Godwin TA, et al: Mucinous adenocarcinoma of the endometrium with intestinal differentiation. A case report. Hum Pathol 26:1385–1388, 1995.

129. Zaloudek C, Hayashi GM, Ryan IP, et al: Microglandular adenocarcinoma of the endometrium. A form of mucinous adenocarcinoma that may be confused with microglandular hyperplasia of the cervix. Int J Gynecol Pathol 16:52–59, 1997.

130. Fukunaga M: Mucinous endometrial adenocarcinoma simulating microglandular hyperplasia of the cervix. Pathol Int 50:541–545, 2000.

131. Anciaux D, Lawrence WD, Gregoire L: Glandular lesions of the uterine cervix. Prognostic implications of human papilloma virus status. Int J Gynecol Pathol 16:103–110, 1997.

132. O'Leary JJ, Landers R, Crowley M, et al: Human papilloma virus and mixed epithelial tumors of the endometrium. Hum Pathol 29:383–389, 1998.

133. Dallenbach-Hellweg G, Hahn U: Mucinous and clear cell adenocarcinomas of the endometrium in patients receiving antiestrogens (Tamoxifen) and gestagens. Int J Gynecol Pathol 14:7–15, 1995.

134. Dallenbach-Hellweg G, Schmidt D, Hellberg P, et al: The endometrium in breast cancer patients on Tamoxifen. Arch Gynecol Obstet 263:170–177, 2000.

135. Jacques SM, Qureshi F, Lawrence WD: Surface epithelial changes in endometrial adenocarcinoma. Diagnostic pitfalls in curettage specimens. Int J Gynecol Pathol 14:191–197, 1995.

136. Goodman A, Zukerberg LR, Rice LW, et al: Squamous cell carcinoma of the endometrium. A report of eight cases and review of the literature. Gynecol Oncol 61:54–60, 1996.

137. Teixeira M, de Magalhaes FT, Pardal de Oliveira F: Squamous cell carcinoma of the endometrium and cervix. Int J Gynecol Obstet 35:169–173, 1991.

138. Kataoka A, Nishida T, Sugiyama T, et al: Squamous cell carcinoma of the endometrium with human papilloma virus type 31 and without tumor suppressor gene p53 mutation. Gynecol Oncol 65:180–184, 1997.

139. Shidara Y, Karube A, Watanabe M, et al: A case report. Verrucous carcinoma of the endometrium—the difficulty of diagnosis and review of the literature. J Obstet Gynaecol Res 26:189–192, 2000.

140. Vargas MP, Merino MJ: Lymphoepithelioma-like carcinoma. An unusual variant of endometrial cancer. A report of two cases. Int J Gynecol Pathol 17:272–276, 1998.

141. Patsner B: Primary endodermal sinus tumor of the endometrium presenting as "recurrent" endometrial adenocarcinoma. Gynecol Oncol 80:93–95, 2000.

142. Spaqtz A, Bouron D, Pautier P, et al: Primary yolk sac tumor of the endometrium. A case report and review of the literature. Gynecol Oncol 70:285–288, 1998.

143. Jones MA, Young RH, Scully RE: Endometrial adenocarcinoma with a component of giant cell carcinoma. Int J Gynecol Pathol 10:260–270, 1991.

144. Hoshida V, Nagakawa T, Mano S, et al: Hepatoid adenocarcinoma of the endometrium associated with alpha feto protein production. Int J Gynecol Pathol 15:266–269, 1996.

145. Pesce C, Merino MJ, Chambers JT, et al: Endometrial carcinoma with trophoblastic differentiation. Cancer 68:1799–1802, 1991.

146. Van Hoeven KH, Hudock JA, Woodruff JM, et al: Small cell neuroendocrine carcinoma of the endometrium. Int J Gynecol Pathol 14:21–29, 1995.

147. Hachisuga T, Tsunehisa K, Enjoji M: Carcinoma of the lower uterine segment. Clinicopathologic analysis of 12 cases. Int J Gynecol Pathol 8:26–35, 1989.

148. Jacques SM, Qureshi F, Ramirez NC, et al: Tumors of the uterine isthmus. Clinicopathologic features and immunohistochemical characterization of p53 expression and hormone receptors. Int J Gynecol Pathol 16:18–44, 1997.

149. Tidy J, Mason WP: Endometrioid carcinoma of the ovary. A retrospective study. Br J Obstet Gynaecol 95:1165–1169, 1988.

150. Falkenberry SS, Steinhoff MM, Gordinier M, et al: Synchronous endometrioid tumors of the ovary and endometrium. A clinicopathologic study of 22 cases. J Reprod Med 41:713–718, 1996.
151. Sheu BC, Lin HH, Chen CK, et al: Synchronous primary carcinomas of the endometrium and ovary. Int J Gynecol Pathol 51:141–146, 1995.
152. Lin WM, Forgacs E, Warshal DP, et al: Loss of heterozygosity and mutational analysis in synchronous endometrial and ovarian carcinomas. Clin Cancer Res 4:2577–2583, 1999.
153. Shenson DL, Gallion HH, Powell DE, et al: Loss of heterozygosity and genomic instability in synchronous endometrioid tumors of the ovary and endometrium. Cancer 76:650–657, 1995.
154. Kumar NB, Hart WR: Metastasis to the uterine corpus from extragenital cancers. A clinicopathologic study of 63 cases. Cancer 50:2163, 1982.
155. Jacques SM, Qureshi F, Ramirez NC, et al: Unusual endometrial stromal changes mimicking metastatic carcinoma. Pathol Res Pract 192:33–36, 1996.
156. Ayhan A, Gunals S, Karaer C, et al: Endometrial adenocarcinoma in pregnancy. Gynecol Oncol 75:298–299, 1999.
157. Vaccarello L, Apte SM, Copeland LJ, et al: Endometrial carcinoma associated with pregnancy. A report of three cases and review of the literature. Gynecol Oncol 74:118–122, 1999.
158. Schammel DP, Mittal KR, Kaplan K, et al: Endometrial adenocarcinoma associated with intrauterine pregnancy. A report of five cases and a review of the literature. Int J Gynecol Pathol 14:327–335, 1998.
159. Zanotti KM, Belinson JL, Kennedy AW: Treatment of gynecologic cancers in pregnancy. Semin Oncol 27:686–698, 2000.
160. Foesterling DL, Blythe JC: Ovarian carcinoma, endometrial carcinoma, and pregnancy. Gynecol Oncol 72:425–426, 1999.
161. Oliva E, Clement PB, Young RH: Endometrial stromal tumors. An update on a group of tumors with a protean phenotype. Adv Anat Pathol 7:257–281, 2000.
162. Evans HL: Endometrial stromal sarcoma and poorly differentiated endometrial sarcoma. Cancer 50:2170, 1982.
163. Tavassoli FA, Norris HJ: Mesenchymal tumours of the uterus. VII. A clinicopathological study of 60 endometrial stromal nodules. Histopathology 5:1–10, 1981.
164. Chang LK, Crabtree GS, Lim-Tan SK, et al: Primary uterine endometrial stromal neoplasms. A clinicopathologic study of 117 cases. Am J Surg Pathol 14:415–438, 1990.
165. Fekete PS, Vellios F: The clinical and histologic spectrum of endometrial stromal neoplasms. A report of 41 cases. Int J Gynecol Pathol 3:198–212, 1984.
166. Norris HJ, Taylor HB: Mesenchymal tumors of the uterus. II. A clinical and pathologic study of 53 endometrial stromal tumors. Cancer 19:755–766, 1966.
167. Oliva E, Young RH, Clement PB, et al: Cellular benign mesenchymal tumors of the uterus. A comparative morphologic and immunohistochemical analysis of 33 highly cellular leiomyomas and six endometrial stromal nodules, two frequently confused tumors. Am J Surg Pathol 19:757–768, 1995.
168. Oliva E, Young RH, Clement PB, et al: Myxoid and fibrous endometrial stromal tumors of the uterus. A report of 10 cases. Int J Gynecol Pathol 18:310–319, 1999.
169. Lloreta J, Pratt J: Ultrastructure of an endometrial stromal nodule with skeletal muscle. Ultrastruct Pathol 17:405–410, 1993.
170. Jensen PA, Dockerty MB, Symmonds RE, et al: Endometrioid sarcoma ("stromal endometriosis"). Report of 15 cases including 5 with metastases. Am J Obstet Gynecol 95:79, 1966.
171. Baggish MS, Woodruff JD: Uterine stromatosis. Clinicopathologic features and hormone dependency. Obstet Gynecol 40:487, 1972.
172. Zaloudek C, Norris HJ: Mesenchymal tumors of the uterus. *In* Kurman RJ (ed): Blaustein's Pathology of the Female Genital Tract, 5th ed. New York, Springer-Verlag, 1995, pp 487–528.
173. McCluggage WG, Date A, Bharucha H, et al: Endometrial stromal sarcoma with sex cord like areas and focal rhabdoid differentiation. Histopathology 29:369–374, 1996.
174. Yoonessi M, Hart WR: Endometrial stromal sarcomas. Cancer 40:898, 1977.
175. Kempson RL, Hendrickson MR: Pure mesenchymal neoplasms of the uterine corpus. Selected problems. Semin Diagn Pathol 5:172, 1988.
176. Cheung AN, Ng WF, Chung LP, et al: Mixed low grade and high grade endometrial stromal sarcoma of uterus. Differences on immunohistochemistry and chromosome in situ hybridization. J Clin Pathol 49:604–607, 1996.
177. Cheung AN, Tin VP, Ngan HY, et al: Interphase cytogenetic study of endometrial stromal sarcoma by chromosome in situ hybridization. Mod Pathol 9:910–918, 1996.
178. Dunton CJ, Kelsten ML, Brooks SE, et al: Low grade stromal sarcoma. DNA flow cytometric analysis and estrogen progesterone receptor data. Gynecol Oncol 37:268–275, 1990.
179. August CZ, Bauer KD, Lurain J, et al: Neoplasms of endometrial stroma. Histopathologic and flow cytometric analysis with clinical correlation. Hum Pathol 20:232–237, 1989.
180. el-Naggar AK, Abdul-Karim FW, Silva EG, et al: Uterine stromal neoplasms. A clinicopathologic and DNA flow cytometric correlation. Hum Pathol 22:897–903, 1991.
181. Reich O, Regauer S, Urdl W, et al: Expression of estrogen and progesterone receptors in low grade endometrial stromal sarcomas. Br J Cancer 82:1030–1034, 2000.
182. Sabini G, Chumas JC, Mann WJ: Steroid hormone receptors in endometrial stromal sarcoma. A biochemical and immunohistochemical study. Am J Clin Pathol 97:381–386, 1992.
183. Binder SW, Nieberg RK, Cheng L, et al: Histologic and immunohistochemical analysis of nine endometrial stromal tumors. An unexpected high frequency of keratin protein positivity. Int J Gynecol Pathol 10:191–197, 1991.
184. Farhhod AI, Abrams J: Immunohistochemistry of endometrial stromal sarcoma. Hum Pathol 22:224–230, 1991.
185. Frankquemont DW, Frierson HF, Mills SE: An immunohistochemical study of normal endometrial stromal neoplasms. Am J Surg Pathol 15:861–870, 1991.
186. Lillemoe TJ, Perrone T, Norris HJ, et al: Myogenous phenotype of epithelial-like areas in endometrial stromal sarcomas. Arch Pathol Lab Med 115:215–219, 1991.
187. van Wering ER, van der Linden-Schrever BE, Szczepanski T, et al: Regenerative normal B-cell precursors during and after treatment of acute lymphoblastic leukemia. Implications for monitoring minimal residual disease. Br J Haematol 110:139–146, 2000.
188. Chu P, Arber DA: Paraffin-section detection of CD10 in 505 nonhematopoietic neoplasms. Frequent expression in renal cell carcinoma and ESS. Am J Clin Pathol 113:374–382, 2000.
189. Nucci MR, O'Connell JT, Huettner PC, et al: h-Caldesmon expression effectively distinguishes endometrial stromal tumors from uterine smooth muscle tumors. Am J Surg Pathol 25:455–463, 2001.
190. Rush DS, Tan J, Baergen RN, et al: h-Caldesmon, a novel smooth muscle specific antibody distinguishes between cellular leiomyoma and endometrial stromal sarcoma. Am J Surg Pathol 25:253–258, 2001.
191. Lindenmayer AE, Miettinen M: Immunophenotypic features of uterine stromal cells. CD34 expression in endocervical stroma. Virchows Arch 426:457–460, 1995.
192. Rizeq MN, van de Rijn M, Hendrickson MR, et al: A comparative immunohistochemical study of uterine smooth muscle neoplasms with emphasis on the epithelioid variant. Hum Pathol 25:671–677, 1994.
193. Blom R, Malstrom H, Guerrieri C: Endometrial stromal sarcoma of the uterus. A clinicopathologic, DNA flow cytometric, p53, and mdm-2 analysis of 17 cases. Int J Gynecol Cancer 9:98–104, 1999.
194. Goldblum JR, Clement PB, Hart WR: Adenomyosis with sparse glands. A potential mimic of low grade endometrial stromal sarcoma. Am J Clin Pathol 103:218–223, 1995.
195. Clement PB, Scully RE: Endometrial stromal sarcomas of the uterus with extensive endometrioid glandular differentiation. A report of three cases that caused problems in differential diagnosis. Int J Gynecol Pathol 11:163–173, 1992.
196. Berchuck SW, Nieberg RK, Cheng L, et al: Treatment of endometrial stromal tumors. Gynecol Oncol 36:60–65, 1990.

197. Larson B, Silfversward C, Nilsson B, et al: Endometrial stromal sarcoma of the uterus. A clinical and histopathological study. The Radiumhemmet series 1936–1981. Eur J Obstet Gynecol Reprod Biol 35:239–249, 1990.

198. Clement PB, Scully RE: Uterine tumors resembling ovarian sex cord tumors. A clinicopathologic analysis of fourteeen cases. Am J Clin Pathol 66:512–525, 1976.

199. Fekete PS, Vellios F, Patterson BD: Uterine tumor resembling an ovarian sex cord tumor. A report of an endometrial stromal tumor with foam cells and ultrastructural evidence of epithelial differentiation. Int J Gynecol Pathol 4:378–387, 1985.

200. Iwasaki I, Yu TJ, Takahashi A, et al: Uterine tumor resembling ovarian sex cord tumor with osteoid metaplasia. Acta Pathol Jpn 36:1391–1395, 1986.

201. Tang C, Toker C, Ances IG: Stromomyoma of the uterus. Cancer 43:308, 1979.

202. Devaney K, Tavassoli FA: Immunohistochemistry as a diagnostic aid in the interpretation of unusual mesenchymal tumors of the uterus. Arch Pathol Lab Med 4:225, 1991.

203. McCluggage WG: Value of inhibin staining in gynecological pathology. Int J Gynecol Pathol 20:79–85, 2001.

204. Krishnamurthy S, Jungbluth AA, Busam KJ, et al: Uterine tumors resembling ovarian sex cord tumors have an immunophenotype consistent with true sex cord differentiation. Am J Surg Pathol 22:1078–1082, 1998.

205. Baker RJ, Hildebrandt RH, Rouse RV, et al: Inhibin and CD99 (MIC2) expression in uterine stromal neoplasms with sex-cord-like-elements. Hum Pathol 30:671–679, 1999.

206. Clement PB, Scully RE: Tumors with mixed epithelial and mesenchymal elements. *In* Clement PB, Young RH (eds): Tumors and Tumorlike Lesions of the Corpus and Cervix. New York, Churchill Livingstone, 1993, pp 329–370.

207. Malfetano JH, Hussain M: A uterine tumor that resembles ovarian sex cord tumors. A low grade sarcoma. Obstet Gynecol 74:489, 1989.

208. Vellios F, Ng AB, Reagan JW: Papillary adenofibroma of the uterus. A benign mesodermal mixed tumor of müllerian origin. Am J Clin Pathol 60:543–551, 1973.

209. Zaloudek CJ, Norris HJ: Adenofibroma and adenosarcoma of the uterus. A clinicopathologic study of 35 cases. Cancer 48:354–366, 1981.

210. Agarwal PK, Husain N, Chandrawati C: Adenofibroma of uterus and endocervix. Histopathology 18:79–80, 1991.

211. Miller KN, McLure SP: Papillary adenofibroma of the uterus. Report of a case involved by adenocarcinoma and review of the literature. Am J Clin Pathol 97:806, 1992.

212. Sinkre P, Miller DS, Milchgrub S, et al: Adenomyofibroma of the endometrium with skeletal muscle differentiation. Int J Gynecol Pathol 19:280–283, 2000.

213. Horie Y, Ikawa S, Kadowaki K, et al: Lipoadenofibroma of the uterine corpus. Report of a new variant of adenofibroma (benign müllerian mixed tumor). Arch Pathol Lab Med 119:274–276, 1995.

214. Clement PB, Scully RE: Mullerian adenosarcoma of the uterus. A clinicopathological analysis of 100 cases with a review of the literature. Hum Pathol 21:363, 1990.

215. Czernobilsky B, Hohlweg-Majert P, Dallenbach-Hellweg G: Uterine adenosarcoma. A clinicopathologic study of 11 cases with a re-evaluation of histologic criteria. Arch Gynecol 233:281, 1983.

216. Ostor AG, Fortune DW: Benign and low grade variants of mixed mullerian tumours of the uterus. Histopathology 4:369, 1980.

217. Clement PB, Scully RE: Mullerian adenofibroma of the uterus with invasion of myometrium and pelvic veins. Int J Gynecol Pathol 9:363, 1990.

218. Mazur MT: Atypical polypoid adenomyomas of the endometrium. Am J Surg Pathol 5:473, 1981.

219. Young RH, Treger T, Scully RE: Atypical polypoid adenomyoma of the uterus. A report of 27 cases. Am J Clin Pathol 86:139, 1986.

220. Clement PB, Young RH: Atypical polypoid adenomyoma of the uterus associated with Turner's syndrome. A report of three cases, including a review of "estrogen associated" en-

dometrial neoplasms and neoplasms associated with Turner's syndrome. Int J Gynecol Pathol 6:104, 1987.

221. Mittal KR, Peng XC, Wallach RC, et al: Coexistent atypical polypoid adenomyoma and endometrial adenocarcinoma. Hum Pathol 26:574–576, 1995.

222. Longacre TA, Chung MH, Rouse RV, et al: Atypical polypoid adenomyofibromas (atypical polypoid adenomyomas) of the uterus. A clinicopathologic study of 55 cases. Am J Surg Pathol 20:11–20, 1996.

223. Sugiyama T, Ohta S, Nishida T, et al: Two cases of endometrial adenocarcinoma arising from atypical polypoid adenomyoma. Gynecol Oncol 71:141–144, 1998.

224. Arici DS, Aker H, Yildiz E, et al: Mullerian adenosarcoma of the uterus associated with Tamoxifen therapy. Arch Gynecol Obstet 262:105–107, 2000.

225. Kennedy MM, Baigire CF, Manek S: Tamoxifen and the endometrium. Review of 102 cases and comparison with HRT-related and non-HRT-related endometrial pathology. Int J Gynecol Pathol 18:130–137, 1999.

226. Clement PB, Oliva E, Young RH: Mullerian adenosarcoma of the uterine corpus associated with tamoxifen therapy. A report of six cases and a review of Tamoxifen associated endometrial lesions. Int J Gynecol Pathol 15:222–229, 1996.

227. Street B, Du T, Toit JP: Uterine adenosarcoma. Report of a case with two further primary malignant tumors. Gynecol Oncol 11:252, 1981.

228. Lack EE, Bitterman P, Sundeen JT: Mullerian adenosarcoma of the uterus with pure angiosarcoma. Case report. Hum Pathol 22:1289, 1991.

229. Kaku T, Silverberg SG, Major FJ, et al: Adenosarcoma of the uterus. A Gynecologic Oncology Group clinicopathologic study of 31 cases. Int J Gynecol Pathol 11:75–88, 1992.

230. Clement PB, Scully RE: Mullerian adenosarcoma of the uterus with sex cord like elements. A clinicopathological analysis of eight cases. Am J Clin Pathol 91:664, 1989.

231. Hirschfield L, Kahn LB, Chen S, et al: Mullerian adenosarcoma with ovarian sex cord-like differentiation. A light and electron microscopic study. Cancer 57:1197, 1986.

232. Raymundo Garcia C, Toro Rojas M, Morales Jiminez CM, et al: Uterine mullerian adenosarcoma with histiocytic (xanthomatous) mesenchymal component. Histopathology 6:363, 1991.

233. Ostor AG, Fortune DW: Benign and low grade variants of mixed mullerian tumour of the uterus. Histopathology 4:369–382, 1980.

234. Clement PB: Mullerian adenosarcomas of the uterus with sarcomatous overgrowth. A clinicopathological analysis of 10 cases. Am J Surg Pathol 13:28, 1989.

235. Imai H, Kitamura IH, Nananura T, et al: Mullerian carcinofibroma of the uterus. A case report. Acta Cytol 43:667–674, 1999.

236. Rodriguez J, Hart W: Endometrial cancers occurring 10 or more years after pelvic irradiation for carcinoma. Int J Gynecol Pathol 1:135–144, 1982.

237. Kahner S, Ferenczy A, Richart RM: Homologous mixed mullerian tumors (carcinosarcoma) confined to endometrial polyps. Am J Obstet Gynecol 121:278–279, 1975.

238. Barwick KW, LiVolsi VA: Heterologous mixed mullerian tumors confined to an endometrial polyp. Obstet Gynecol 53:512–514, 1979.

239. Macasaet MA, Waxman M, Fruchter RG, et al: Prognostic factors in malignant mesodermal (mullerian) mixed tumors of the uterus. Gynecol Oncol 20:32, 1985.

240. Lotocki R, Rosenshein NB: Mixed mullerian tumors of the uterus. Clinical and pathological correlations. Int J Gynaecol Obstet 20:237, 1982.

241. Silverberg SG, Major FJ, Blessing JA, et al: Carcinosarcoma (malignant mixed mesodermal tumor) of the uterus. A Gynecologic Oncology Group pathologic study of 203 cases. Int J Gynecol Pathol 9:1–9, 1990.

242. George E, Manivel JC, Dehner LP, et al: Malignant mixed mullerian tumors. An immunohistochemical study of 47 cases, with histogenetic considerations and clinical correlation. Hum Pathol l22:215, 1991.

243. Dictor M: Ovarian malignant mixed mesodermal tumor. The

occurrence of hyaline droplets containing alpha-1-antitrypsin. Hum Pathol 13:930, 1982.

244. Yanagibashi GI, Taki A, Udagawa TA, et al: Uterine carcinosarcoma is derived from a single stem cell. An in vitro study. Int J Cancer 72:821–827, 1997.

245. Iwasa Y, Haga H, Konishi I, et al: Prognostic factors in uterine carcinosarcoma. A clinicopathologic study of 25 patients. Cancer 82:512–519, 1998.

246. Abeln EC, Smit VT, Wessels JW, et al: Molecular genetic evidence for the conversion hypothesis of the origin of malignant mixed mullerian tumors. J Pathol 183:424–431, 1997.

247. Guerrieri BR, Stal O, Malstrom H, et al: Malignant mixed mullerian tumors of the uterus. A clinicopathologic, DNA flow cytometric, p53, and mdm-2 analysis of 44 cases. Gynecol Oncol 68:18–24, 1998.

248. Ansink AC, Cross PA, Scorer P, et al: The hormonal receptor status of uterine carcinosarcomas (mixed mullerian tumors). An immunohistochemical study. J Clin Pathol 50:328–331, 1997.

249. George E, Lillemoe TJ, Twiggs LB, et al: Malignant mixed mullerian tumor versus high grade endometrial carcinoma and aggressive variants of endometrial carcinoma. A comparative analysis of survival. Int J Gynecol Pathol 14:39–44, 1995.

250. Creagh TM, Bain BJ, Evans BJ, et al: Endometrial extramedullary hematopoiesis. J Pathol 176:99–104, 1995.

251. Sirgi KE, Swanson PE, Gersell DJ: Extramedullary hematopoiesis in the endometrium. Report of four cases and review of the literature. Am J Clin Pathol 101:643–646, 1994.

252. Schmid C, Beham A, Kratochvil P: Hematopoiesis in a degenerating uterine leiomyoma. Arch Gynecol Obstet 248:81–86, 1990.

253. Hendrickson MR, Scheithauer BW: Primitive neuroectodermal tumor of the endometrium. Report of two cases, one with electron microscopy observations. Int J Gynecol Pathol 5:249, 1986.

254. Rose PG, O'Toole RV, Keyhani-Rofagha S, et al: Malignant peripheral primitive neuroectodermal tumor of the uterus. J Surg Oncol 35:165, 1987.

255. Daya D, Lukka H, Clement PB: Primitive neuroectodermal tumors of the uterus. A report of four cases. Hum Pathol 23:1120, 1992.

256. Sinkre P, Albores-Saavedra J, Miller DS, et al: Endometrial endometrioid carcinomas associated with Ewing sarcoma/peripheral primitive neuroectodermal tumor. Int J Gynecol Pathol 19:127–132, 2000.

257. Young RH, Kleinman GM, Scully RE: Glioma of the uterus. Report of a case with comments on histogenesis. Am J Surg Pathol 5:695–699, 1981.

258. Takahashi O, Shibata S, Hazawa J, et al: Mature cystic teratoma of the uterine corpus. Acta Obstet Gynecol Scand 77:936–938, 1998.

259. Capello F, Barbato F, Tomasino RM: Mature teratoma of the uterine corpus with thyroid differentiation. Pathol Int 50:546–548, 2000.

260. Ansah-Boateng Y, Wells M, Poole DR: Coexistent immature teratoma of the uterus and endometrial adenocarcinoma complicated by gliomatosis peritonei. Gynecol Oncol 21:106–110, 1985.

261. Iwanawa S, Shimada A, Hasuo Y, et al: Immature teratoma of the uterine fundus. Kurume Med J 40:153–158, 1993.

262. Jiscoot P, Aertsens W, Degels MA, et al: Extrarenal Wilm's tumor of the uterus. Eur J Gynaecol Oncol 20:195–197, 1999.

263. Rein MS: Advances in uterine leiomyoma research. The progesterone hypothesis. Environ Health Perspect 108(suppl 5):791–793, 2000.

264. Hunter DS, Hodges LC, Vonier PM, et al: Estrogen receptor activation via activation function 2 predicts agonism of xenoestrogens in normal and neoplastic cells of the uterine myometrium. Cancer Res 59:3090–3099, 1999.

265. Englund K, Blank A, Gustavsson I, et al: Sex steroid receptors in human myometrium and fibroids. Changes during the menstrual cycle and gonadotropin-releasing hormone treatment. J Clin Endocrinol Metab 83:4092–4096, 1998.

266. Deligdisch L: Hormonal pathology of the endometrium. Mod Pathol 13:285–294, 2000.

267. Nisolle M, Gillerot S, Casanas-Roux F, et al: Immunohistochemical study of the proliferation index, oestrogen receptors and progesterone receptors A and B in leiomyomata and normal myometrium during the menstrual cycle and under gonadotrophin-releasing hormone agonist therapy. Hum Reprod 14:2844–2850, 1999.

268. Norris HJ, Hilliard GD, Irey NS: Hemorrhagic cellular leiomyomas ("apoplectic leiomyomas") of the uterus associated with pregnancy and oral contraceptives. Int J Gynecol Pathol 7:212–224, 1988.

269. Frankel T, Benjamin F: Rapid enlargement of a uterine fibroid after clomiphene therapy. J Obstet Gynaecol Br Commonw 80:764, 1973.

270. Felmingham JE, Corcoran R: Rapid enlargement of a uterine fibroid after clomiphene therapy (letter). Br J Obstet Gynaecol 82:431–432, 1975.

271. Lai FM, Wong FW, Allen PW: Diffuse uterine leiomyomatosis with hemorrhage. Arch Pathol Lab Med 115:834–837, 1991.

272. Schwartz LB, Rutkowski N, Horan C, et al: Use of transvaginal ultrasonography to monitor the effects of tamoxifen on uterine leiomyoma size and ovarian cyst formation. J Ultrasound Med 17:699–703, 1998.

273. Kang J, Baxi L, Heller D: Tamoxifen induced growth of leiomyomas. A case report. J Reprod Med 41:119–120, 1996.

274. Le Bouedec G, de Latour M, Dauplat J: Expansive uterine myoma during tamoxifen therapy. 11 cases. Presse Med 24:1694–1696, 1995.

275. Demopoulos RI, Jones KY, Mittal KR, et al: Histology of leiomyomata in patients treated with leuprolide acetate. Int J Gynecol Pathol 16:131–137, 1997.

276. Takeuchi H, Kobori H, Kikuchi I, et al: A prospective randomized study comparing endocrinological and clinical effects of two types of GnRH agonists in cases of uterine leiomyomas or endometriosis. J Obstet Gynaecol Res 26:325–331, 2000.

277. Scialli AR, Levi AJ: Intermittent leuprolide acetate for the nonsurgical management of women with leiomyomata uteri. Fertil Steril 74:540–546, 2000.

278. Pandis N, Heim S, Bardi G, et al: Chromosome analysis of 96 uterine leiomyomas. Cancer Genet Cytogenet 55:11–18, 1991.

279. Marshal RD, Fejzo ML, Friedman AJ, et al: Analysis of androgen receptor DNA reveals the independent clonal origins of uterine leiomyomata and the secondary nature of cytogenetic aberrations in the development of leiomyomata. Genes Chromosomes Cancer 11:1–6, 1994.

280. Hashimoto K, Azuma C, Kamiura T, et al: Clonal determination of uterine leiomyomas by analyzing differential inactivation of the X-chromosome-linked phosphoglycerokinase gene. Gynecol Obstet Invest 40:204–208, 1995.

281. Baschinsky DY, Isa A, Niemmen TH, et al: Diffuse leiomyomatosis of the uterus. A case report with clonality analysis. Hum Pathol 31:1429–1432, 2000.

282. Bajekal N, Li TC: Fibroids, infertility and pregnancy wastage. Hum Reprod Update 6:614–620, 2000.

283. Gisser SD, Young I: Neurilemmoma-like uterine myomas. An ultrastructural reaffirmation of their non-Schwannian nature. Am J Obstet Gynecol 129:389–392, 1977.

284. Adany R, Fodor F, Molnar P, et al: Increased density of histiocytes in uterine leiomyomas. Int J Gynecol Pathol 9:137–144, 1990.

285. Crow J, Wilkins M, Howe S, et al: Mast cells in the female genital tract. Int J Gynecol Pathol 10:230–237, 1991.

286. Orri A, Mori A, Zhai YL, et al: Mast cells in smooth muscle tumors of the uterus. Int J Gynecol Pathol 17:336–342, 1998.

287. Eyden BP, Hale RJ, Richmond I, et al: Cytoskeletal filaments in the smooth muscle cells of uterine leiomyoma and myometrium. An ultrastructural and immunohistochemical analysis. Virchows Arch A Pathol Anat Histopathol 420:51–58, 1992.

288. Brown DC, Theaker JM, Banks PM, et al: Cytokeratin expression in smooth muscle and smooth muscle tumors. Histopathology 11:477–486, 1987.

289. Levy B, Mukherjee T, Hirshhorn K: Molecular cytogenetic

analysis of uterine leiomyoma and leiomyosarcoma by comparative genomic hybridization. Cancer Genet Cytogenet 121: 1–8, 2000.

290. Mangrulkar RS, Ono M, Ishikawa M, et al: Isolation and characterization of heparin-binding growth factors in human leiomyomas and normal myometrium. Biol Reprod 53:636–646, 1995.

291. Andersen J: Factors in fibroid growth. Baillieres Clin Obstet Gynaecol 12:225–243, 1998.

292. Vanshisht A, Studd JW, Carey AH, et al: Fibroid embolisation. A technique not without significant complications. Br J Obstet Gynaecol 107:1166–1170, 2000.

293. Golfarb HA: Myoma coagulation (myolysis). Obstet Gynecol Clin North Am 27:421–430, 2000.

294. Fauconnier A, Chapron C, Babaki-Fard K, et al: Recurrence of leiomyomata after myomectomy. Hum Reprod Update 6: 595–602, 2000.

295. Letterie GS, Coddington CC, Winkel CA, et al: Efficacy of a gonadotropin releasing hormone agonist in the treatment of uterine leiomyomata. Long term follow up. Fertil Steril 51: 951–956, 1989.

296. August C, Kepic T, Meier L, et al: Histologic findings in uterine leiomyomata of women treated with gonadotropin-releasing hormone agonist. Am J Clin Pathol 97:448, 1992.

297. Clement PB: Pure mesenchymal tumors. In Clement PB, Young RH (eds): Tumors and Tumorlike Lesions of the Corpus and Cervix. New York, Churchill Livingstone, 1993, pp 265–328.

298. Hendrickson MR, Kempson RL: The uterine corpus. In Sternberg SS (ed): Diagnostic Surgical Pathology. New York, Raven Press, 1994, pp 2091–2194.

299. Bell WS, Kempson RL, Hendrickson MR: Problematic uterine smooth muscle neoplasms. Am J Surg Pathol 18:535–558, 1994.

300. Myles JL, Hart WR: Apoplectic leiomyomas of the uterus. A clinicopathologic study of five distinctive hemorrhagic leiomyomas associated with oral contraceptive usage. Am J Surg Pathol 9:798–805, 1985.

301. Perrone T, Dehner LP: Prognostically favorable "mitotically active" smooth muscle tumors of the uterus. A clinicopathologic study of ten cases. Am J Surg Pathol 12:1–8, 1988.

302. O'Connor DM, Norris HJ: Mitotically active leiomyomas of the uterus. Hum Pathol 21:223–227, 1990.

303. Prayson RA, Hart WR: Mitotically active leiomyomas of the uterus. Am J Clin Pathol 97:14–20, 1992.

304. Kawaguchi K, Fujii S, Konoshi I, et al: Mitotic activity in uterine leiomyomas during the menstrual cycle. Am J Obstet Gynecol 160:637–641, 1989.

305. Tiltman AJ: The effect of progestins on the mitotic activity of uterine fibromyomas. Int J Gynecol Pathol 4:89–96, 1985.

306. Burns B, Curry RH, Bell MEA: Morphologic features of prognostic significance in uterine smooth muscle tumors. A review of eighty-four cases. Am J Obstet Gynecol 135:109, 1979.

307. Kempson RL, Hendrickson MR: Pure mesenchymal neoplasms of the uterine corpus. Selected problems. Semin Diagn Pathol 5:172–198, 1988.

308. Kurman RJ, Norris HJ: Mesenchymal tumors of the uterus. VI. Epithelioid smooth muscle tumors including leiomyoblastoma and clear cell leiomyoma. Cancer 37:1853–1865, 1976.

309. Evans HL: Smooth muscle neoplasms of the uterus other than ordinary leiomyoma. A study of 46 cases, with emphasis on diagnostic criteria and prognostic factors. Cancer 62: 2239, 1988.

310. Mazur MT, Priest JT: Clear cell leiomyoma (leiomyoblastoma) of the uterus. Ultrastructural observations. Ultrastruct Pathol 10:249, 1986.

311. Rywlin AM, Recher L, Benson J: Clear cell leiomyoma of the uterus. Report of 2 cases of a previously undescribed entity. Cancer 17:100, 1964.

312. Hyde KE, Geisinger KR, Jones TL: The clear cell variant of uterine epithelioid leiomyoma. An immunohistochemical and ultrastructural study. Arch Pathol Lab Med 113:551, 1989.

313. Kaminski PF, Tavassoli FA: Plexiform tumorlet. A clinical and pathologic study of 15 cases with ultrastructural observations. Int J Gynecol Pathol 3:124–134, 1984.

314. Mazur MT, Kraus FT: Histogenesis of morphologic variations in tumors of the uterine wall. Am J Surg Pathol 4:59, 1980.

315. Shintaku M: Lipoleiomyomatous tumors of the uterus. A heterogeneous group? Histopathologic study of five cases. Pathol Int 46:498–502, 1996.

316. Brooks JJ, Well GB, Yeh IT, et al: Bizarre epithelioid lipoleiomyoma of the uterus. Int J Gynecol Pathol 11:144–149, 1992.

317. Willson JR, Peale AR: Multiple peritoneal leiomyomas associated with a granulosa cell tumor of the ovary. Am J Obstet Gynecol 64:204, 1952.

318. Quade BJ, McLachlin CM, Soto-Wright V, et al: Disseminated peritoneal leiomyomatosis. Clonality analysis by X chromosome inactivation and cytogenetics of a clinically benign smooth muscle proliferation. Am J Pathol 150:2153–2166, 1997.

319. Lausen I, Jensen OJ, Andersen E, et al: Disseminated peritoneal leiomyomatosis with malignant change, in a male. Virchows Arch A Pathol Anat Histopathol 417:173–175, 1990.

320. Minassian SS, Frangipane W, Polin JI, et al: Leiomyomatosis peritonealis disseminata. A case report and literature review. J Reprod Med 31:997–1000, 1986.

321. Tavassoli FA, Norris HJ: Peritoneal leiomyomatosis (leiomyomatosis peritonealis disseminata). A clinicopathologic study of 20 cases with ultrastructural observations. Int J Gynecol Pathol 1:59–74, 1982.

322. Sutherland JA, Wilson EA, Edger DE, et al: Ultrastructure and steroid binding studies in leiomyomatosis peritonealis disseminata. Am J Obstet Gynecol 136:992, 1980.

323. Fujii S, Nakashima N, Okamura H, et al: Progesterone induced smooth muscle like cells in subperitoneal nodules produced by estrogen. Am J Obstet Gynecol 139:164, 1981.

324. Kaplan CK, Bernishke K, Johnson KC: Leiomyomatosis peritonealis disseminata with endometrium. Obstet Gynecol 55: 119, 1980.

325. Kuo T, London S, Dinh T: Endometriosis occurring in leiomyomatosis peritonealis disseminata. An ultrastructural study and histogenetic consideration. Am J Surg Pathol 4: 197–204, 1980.

326. Ma KF, Chow LT: Sex cord like pattern leiomyomatosis peritonealis disseminata. A hitherto undescribed feature. Histopathology 21:389–391, 1992.

327. Zotatis G, Nayar R, Hicks DG: Leiomyomatosis peritonealis disseminata, endometriosis, and multicystic mesothelioma. An unusual association. Int J Gynecol Pathol 17:178–182, 1998.

328. Nogales FF, Matilla A Carrascal E: Leiomyomatosis peritonealis disseminata. An ultrastructural study. Am J Clin Pathol 69:452, 1978.

329. Goldberg MF, Hurt WG, Frable WJ: Leiomyomatosis peritonealis disseminata. Report of a case and review of the literature. Obstet Gynecol 49:46, 1977.

330. Raspagliesi F, Quattrone P, Grosso G, et al: Malignant degeneration in leiomyomatosis peritonealis disseminata. Gynecol Oncol 61:272–277, 1996.

331. Fulcher AS, Szucs RA: Leiomyomatosis peritonealis disseminata complicated by sarcomatous transformation and ovarian torsion. Presentation of two cases and review of the literature. Abdom Imaging 23:L640–644, 1998.

332. Morizaki A, Hayashi H, Ishikawa M: Leiomyomatosis peritonealis disseminata with malignant transformation. Int J Gynaecol Obstet 66:43–45, 1999.

333. Horiuchi K, Yabe H, Mukai M, et al: Multiple smooth muscle tumors arising in deep soft tissue of lower limbs with uterine leiomyomas. Am J Surg Pathol 22:897–901, 1998.

334. Gatti J, Morvan G, Henin D, et al: Leiomyomatosis metastasizing to the spine. Am J Bone Joint Surg 65:1163–1165, 1983.

335. Takemura G, Takatsu Y, Kaitani H, et al: Metastasizing uterine leiomyoma. A case with cardiac and pulmonary metastasis. Pathol Res Pract 192:622–629, 1996.

336. Jautzke G, Muller-Ruchholtz E, Thalmann U: Immunohistochemical detection of estrogen and progesterone receptors in multiple and well differentiated leiomyomatous lung tumors

in women with uterine leiomyomas (so-called benign metastasizing leiomyomas). A report of 5 cases. Pathol Res Pract 192:215–223, 1996.

337. Kayser K, Zink S, Schneider T, et al: Benign metastasizing leiomyoma of the uterus. Documentation of clinical, immunohistochemical and lectin-histochemical data of ten cases. Virchows Arch 437:284–292, 2000.
338. Abell MR, Little ER: Benign metastasizing uterine leiomyoma. Multiple lymph nodal metastases. Cancer 36:2206–2213, 1975.
339. Banner AS, Carrington CB, Emory WB, et al: Efficacy of oophorectomy in lymphangioleiomyomatosis and benign metastasizing leiomyoma. N Engl J Med 305:204–209, 1981.
340. Horstmann JP, Pietra GG, Harman JA, et al: Spontaneous regression of pulmonary leiomyomas during pregnancy. Cancer 39:314–321, 1977.
341. Tietze L, Gunther K, Horbe A, et al: Benign metastasizing leiomyoma. A cytogenetically balanced but clonal disease. Hum Pathol 31:126–128, 2000.
342. Cho KR, Woodruff JD, Epstein JI: Leiomyoma of the uterus with multiple extrauterine smooth muscle tumors. A case report suggesting multifocal origin. Hum Pathol 20:8083, 1989.
343. Norris HJ, Parmley T: Mesenchymal tumors of the uterus. V. Intravenous leiomyomatosis. A clinical and pathological study of 14 cases. Cancer 36:2164, 1975.
344. Nogales FF, Navarro N, de Victoria JMM, et al: Uterine intravascular leiomyomatosis. An update and report of seven cases. Int J Gynecol Pathol 6:331, 1987.
345. Mulvany NJ, Slavin JL, Ostor AG, et al: Intravenous leiomyomatosis of the uterus. A clinicopathologic study of 22 cases. Int J Gynecol Pathol 13:1–9, 1994.
346. Ling FT, David TE, Merchant N, et al: Intracardiac extension of intravenous leiomyomatosis in a pregnant woman. A case report and review of the literature. Can J Cardiol 16:73–79, 2000.
347. Lo KW, Lau TK: Intracardiac leiomyomatosis. Case report and literature review. Arch Gynecol Obstet 264:209–210, 2001.
348. Andrade LA, Torresan RZ, Sales JF, et al: Intravenous leiomyomatosis of the uterus. A report of three cases. Pathol Oncol Res 4:44–47, 1998.
349. Clement PB, Young RH, Scully RE: Intravenous leiomyomatosis of the uterus. A clinicopathological analysis of 16 cases with unusual histologic features. Am J Surg Pathol 12:932–945, 1988.
350. Clement PB, Young RH, Scully RE: Diffuse, perinodular, and other patterns of hydropic degeneration within and adjacent to uterine leiomyomas. Problems in the differential diagnosis. Am J Surg Pathol 16:26–32, 1992.
351. Hendrickson MR, Kempson RL: Pure mesenchymal neoplasms of the uterine corpus. In Fox H (ed): Haines and Taylor Obstetrical and Gynaecological Pathology, 4th ed. New York, Churchill Livingstone, 1995, pp 519–586.
352. Jeffers MD, Farquharson MA, Richmond JA, et al: p53 immunoreactivity and mutation of the p53 gene in smooth muscle tumors of the uterine corpus. J Pathol 177:65–70, 1995.
353. Taylor HB, Norris HJ: Mesenchymal tumors of the uterus. IV. Diagnosis and prognosis of leiomyosarcomas. Arch Pathol 82:40–44, 1966.
354. Vardi JR, Tovell HMM: Leiomyosarcoma of the uterus. Clinicopathologic study. Obstet Gynecol 56:428–434, 1980.
355. Barter JF, Smith EB, Szpak CA, et al: Leiomyosarcoma of the uterus. Clinicopathologic study of 21 cases. Gynecol Oncol 21:220–227, 1985.
356. Watanabe K, Hiraki H, Ohishi M, et al: Uterine leiomyosarcoma with osteoclast-like giant cells. Histopathological and cytological observations. Pathol Int 46:656–660, 1996.
357. Silva AG, Tornos C, Ordonez NG, et al: Uterine leiomyosarcoma with clear cell areas. Int J Gynecol Pathol 14:174–178, 1995.
358. Amada S, Nakano H, Tsuneyoshi M: Leiomyosarcoma versus bizarre and cellular leiomyoma of the uterus. A comparative study based on the MIB-1 and proliferating cell nuclear

antigen indices, p53 expression, DNA flow cytometry, and muscle specific actins. Int J Gynecol Pathol 14:134–142, 1995.
359. Zhai YL, Nikaido T, Orii A, et al: Frequent occurrence of loss of heterozygosity among tumor suppressor genes in uterine leiomyosarcoma. Gynecol Oncol 75:453–459, 1999.
360. Nordal RR, Kristensen GB, Kaern J, et al: The prognostic significance of stage, tumor size, cellular atypia, and DNA ploidy in uterine leiomyosarcoma. Acta Oncol 34:797–802, 1995.
361. Miettinen M: Immunoreactivity for cytokeratin and epithelial membrane antigen in leiomyosarcoma. Arch Pathol Lab Med 112:637, 1988.
362. Jones MW, Norris HJ: Clinicopathologic study of 28 uterine leiomyosarcomas with metastasis. Int J Gynecol Pathol 14:243–249, 1995.
363. Younis JS, Okon E, Anteby SO: Uterine leiomyosarcoma in pregnancy. Arch Gynecol Obstet 247:155–160, 1990.
364. Lau TK, Wong WS: Uterine leiomyosarcoma associated with pregnancy. Report of two cases. Gynecol Oncol 53:245–247, 1994.
365. Bekkers RL, Massuger LF, Berg PP, et al: Uterine malignant leiomyoblastoma (epithelioid leiomyosarcoma) during pregnancy. Gynecol Oncol 72:433–436, 1999.
366. King ME, Dickerson GR, Scully RE: Myxoid leiomyosarcoma of the uterus. A report of six cases. Am J Surg Pathol 6:589–598, 1982.
367. Peacock G, Archer S: Myxoid leiomyosarcoma of the uterus. Case report and review of the literature. Am J Obstet Gynecol 160:1515–1519, 1989.
368. Pounder DJ, Prema VI: Uterine leiomyosarcoma with myxoid stroma. Arch Pathol Lab Med 109:762–764, 1985.
369. Kunzel KE, Mills NZ, Muderspaach LI, et al: Case report. Myxoid leiomyosarcoma of the uterus. Gynecol Oncol 48:277–280, 1993.
370. Schneider D, Halperin R, Segal M, et al: Myxoid leiomyosarcoma of the uterus with unusual malignant histologic pattern—a case report. Gynecol Oncol 59:156–158, 1995.
371. Prayson RA, Goldblum JR, Hart WR: Epithelioid smooth-muscle tumors of the uterus. A clinicopathologic study of 18 patients. Am J Surg Pathol 21:383–391, 1997.
372. Tavassoli FA, Norris HJ: Mesenchymal tumours of the uterus. VII. A clinicopathological study of 60 endometrial stromal nodules. Histopathology 5:1–10, 1981.
373. Roth LM, Senteny GE: Stromomyoma of the uterus. Ultrastruct Pathol 9:137–143, 1985.
374. Erhan Y, Baygum M, Ozdemir N: The coexistence of stromomyoma and uterine tumor resembling ovarian sex cord tumors. Report of a case and immunohistochemical study. Acta Obstet Gynecol Scand 71:390–393, 1992.
375. Oliva E, Clement PB, Young RH, et al: Mixed endometrial stromal and smooth muscle tumors of the uterus. Am J Surg Pathol 22:997–1005, 1998.
376. Mendez LE, Joy S, Angoli R, et al: Primary uterine angiosarcoma. Gynecol Oncol 75:272–276, 1999.
377. Schammel DP, Tavassoli FA: Uterine angiosarcomas. A morphologic and immunohistochemical study of four cases. Am J Surg Pathol 22:246–250, 1998.
378. Scheidt P, Moerman PH, Vergote I: Rhabdomyosarcoma of the corpus of the uterus. A case report. Eur J Gynaecol Oncol 21:371–373, 2000.
379. Okada DH, Rowland JB, Petrovic LM: Uterine pleomorphic rhabdomyosarcoma in a patient receiving Tamoxifen therapy. Gynecol Oncol 75:509–513, 1999.
380. Takano M, Kikuchi Y, Aida S, et al: Embryonal rhabdomyosarcoma of the uterine corpus in a 76 year old patient. Gynecol Oncol 75:490–494, 1999.
381. Schmidt C, Doroszewski AW: Liposarcoma of the uterus—a case report. Geburtshilfe Frauenheilkd 56:262–264, 1996.
382. Scneebauer J, Brinninger G, Halabi M, et al: Liposarcoma of the uterus. Gynakol Geburtshilfliche Rundsch 36:90–91, 1996.
383. Emoto M, Iwasaki H, Kawarabayashi T, et al: Primary osteosarcoma of the uterus. Report of a case with immunohistochemical analysis. Gynecol Oncol 54:385–388, 1994.
384. DeYoung B, Bitterman P, Lack EE: Primary osteosarcoma of the uterus. Report of a case with immunohistochemical study. Mod Pathol 5:212–215, 1992.

385. Kofinas AD, Suarez J, Calame RJ, et al: Chondrosarcoma of the uterus. Gynecol Oncol 19:231–237, 1984.

386. Karseladze AI, Zakharova TI, Navarro S, et al: Malignant fibrous histiocytoma of the uterus. Eur J Gynaecol Oncol 21:588–590, 2000.

387. Cho KR, Rosenchein NB, Epstein JI: Malignant rhabdoid tumor of the uterus. Int J Gynecol Pathol 8:381–387, 1989.

388. Nielsen GP, Oliva E, Young RH: Alveolar soft part sarcoma of the female genital tract. A report of nine cases and review of the literature. Int J Gynecol Pathol 14:283–292, 1995.

389. Vang R, Medeiros LJ, Ha CS, et al: Non-Hodgkin's lymphomas involving the uterus. A clinicopathological analysis of 26 cases. Mod Pathol 13:219–228, 2000.

390. Masunaga A, Abe M, Tsujii E, et al: Primary uterine T-cell lymphoma. Int J Gynecol Pathol 17:376–379, 1998.

391. Harris NL, Scully RE: Malignant lymphoma and granulocytic sarcoma of the uterus and vagina: A clinicopathologic analysis of 27 cases. Cancer 53:2530–2545, 1984.

392. Gilks BC, Taylor GP, Clement PB: Inflammatory pseudotumor of the uterus. Int J Gynecol Pathol 6:275–286, 1987.

393. Ferry JA, Harris NL, Scully RE: Uterine leiomyomas with lymphoid infiltration simulating lymphoma. A report of seven cases. Int J Gynecol Pathol 8:263–270, 1989.

394. Young RH, Harris NL, Scully RE: Lymphoma like lesions of the lower female genital tract. A report of 16 cases. Int J Gynecol Pathol 4:289–299,1985.

395. Smith NL, Baird DB, Strausbauch PH: Endometrial involvement by multiple myeloma. Int J Gynecol Pathol 16:173–175, 1997.

396. Barcos M, Lane W, Gomez GA: An autopsy study of 1206 acute and chronic leukemias (1958 to 1982). Cancer 60:827, 1987.

397. Oliva E, Ferry JA, Young RH, et al: Granulocytic sarcoma of the female genital tract. A clinicopathologic study of 11 cases. Am J Surg Pathol 21:1156–1165, 1997.

398. Tamaya T, Motoyama T, Ohono Y, et al: Steroid receptor levels and histology of endometriosis and adenomyosis. Fertil Steril 31:396–400, 1979.

399. Langlois PL: The size of the normal uterus. J Reprod Med 4:220–228, 1970.

400. Clement PB: Diseases of the peritoneum (including endometriosis). *In* Kurman RJ (ed): Blaustein's Pathology of the Female Genital Tract, 5th ed. New York, Springer-Verlag, 1995, pp 647–704.

401. Cramer DW: Epidemiology of endometriosis in adolescents. *In* Wilson EA (ed): Endometriosis. New York, Alan Liss, 1987, p 5.

402. Zinsser KR, Wheeler JE: Endosalpingiosis in the omentum. A study of autopsy and surgical material. Am J Surg Pathol 6:109–117, 1982.

403. Bell DA, Scully RE: Serous borderline tumors of the peritoneum. Am J Surg Pathol 14:230–239, 1990.

404. Clement PB, Young RH: Florid cystic endosalpingiosis with tumor like manifestations. A report of four cases including the first reported cases of transmural endosalpingiosis of the uterus. Am J Surg Pathol 23:166–175, 1999.

405. Andrew AC, Bulmer JN, Wells M, et al: Subinvolution of the uteroplacental arteries in the human placental bed. Histopathology 15:395–405, 1989.

406. Ober WB, Grady HG: Subinvolution of the placental site. Bull N Y Acad Med 37:713–730, 1961.

407. Paalman RJ, McElin TW: Noninvolution of the placental site. Am J Obstet Gynecol 78:898–907, 1959.

408. Otis CN: Uterine adenomatoid tumors. Immunohistochemical characteristics with emphasis on Ber-EP4 immunoreactivity and distinction from adenocarcinoma. Int J Gynecol Pathol 15:146–151, 1996.

409. Srigley JR, Colgan TJ: Multifocal and diffuse adenomatoid tumor involving uterus and fallopian tube. Ultrastruct Pathol 12:351–355, 1988.

410. Palacios J, Suarez Manrique A, Ruiz Villaespesa A, et al: Cystic adenomatoid tumor of the uterus. Int J Gynecol Pathol 10:296–301, 1991.

411. Livingston EG, Guis MS, Pearl ML, et al: Diffuse adenomatoid tumor of the uterus with a serosal papillary cystic component. Int J Gynecol Pathol 11:288–292, 1992.

412. Tiltman AJ: Adenomatoid tumors of the uterus. Histopathology 4:437–443, 1980.

413. Carlier MT, Dardick I, Lagace AF, et al: Adenomatoid tumor of the uterus. Presentation in uterine curettings. Int J Gynecol Pathol 5:69–74, 1986.

414. Kumar A, Schneider V: Metastases to the uterus from extrapelvic primary tumors. Int J Gynecol Pathol 2:134, 1983.

415. Gupta D, Balsara G: Extrauterine malignancies. Role of Pap smears in diagnosis and management. Acta Cytol 43:806–813, 1999.

416. Pilch H, Schaffer U, Gunzel S, et al: Asymptomatic necrotizing arteritis of the female genital tract. Eur J Obstet Gynecol Reprod Biol 91:191–196, 2000.

417. Lombard CM, Moore MH, Seifer DB: Diagnosis of systemic polyarteritis nodosa following total abdominal hysterectomy and bilateral salpingo-oophorectomy. A case report. Int J Gynecol Pathol 5:63–68, 1986.

418. Ganesa R, Ferriman SR, Mejer L, et al: Vasculitis of the female genital tract with clinicopathologic correlation. A study of 46 cases with follow-up. Int J Gynecol Pathol 19:258–265, 2000.

419. Francke ML, Mihaescu A, Chaubert P: Isolated necrotizing arteritis of the female genital tract. A clinipathologic and immunohistochemical study of 11 cases. Int J Gynecol Pathol 17:193–200, 1998.

420. Marrogi AJ, Gersell DJ, Kraus FT: Localized asymptomatic giant cell arteritis of the female genital tract. Int J Gynecol Pathol 10:51–58, 1991.

421. Hickey M, Frasier IS: Clinical implications of disturbances of uterine vascular morphology and function. Baillieres Best Pract Res Clin Obstet Gynaecol 14:937–951, 2000.

422. Wiebe ER, Switzer P: Arteriovenous malformations of the uterus associated with medical abortion. Int J Gynaecol Obstet 71:155–158, 2000.

423. Dobashi Y, Fiedler PN, Carcangiu ML: Polypoid cystic adenomyosis of the uterus. Report of a case. Int J Gynecol Pathol 11:240–243, 1992.

424. Arhelger RB, Bocian JJ: Brenner tumor of the uterus. Cancer 38:1741–1743, 1976.

425. Clement PB: Postoperative spindle cell nodule of the endometrium. Arch Pathol Lab Med 112:566–568, 1988.

426. Fleming ID, Cooper JS, Henson DE, et al (eds): AJCC Manual for Staging of Cancer, 5th ed. Philadelphia, Lippincott-Raven, 1997.

427. Peterson F: Annual Report of the Results of Treatment in Gynecological Cancer. Stockholm, International Federation of Gynecology and Obstetrics, 1991.

428. Silverberg SG: Protocol for the examination of specimens from patients with carcinomas of the endometrium: A basis for checklists. Cancer Committee, College of American Pathologists. Arch Pathol Lab Med 123:28–32, 1999.

# Fallopian Tubes and Broad Ligament

Nilsa C. Ramirez   W. Dwayne Lawrence

## FALLOPIAN TUBES

The fallopian tubes act as conduits that provide the appropriate environment for the bidirectional transportation of the ovum and the spermatozoa. After fertilization occurs, the fallopian tubes subsequently transport the developing blastocyst into the endometrial cavity where, normally, implantation may take place. Anatomic or chemical alterations in the milieu necessary for these processes can result in infertility or in an ectopic pregnancy. Clinically significant tubal lesions usually are associated with inflammatory processes or ectopic gestations. Nevertheless, primary benign and malignant tumors can involve the fallopian tubes.

## Embryology

In the female embryo, fusion of the müllerian (paramesonephric) ducts is accomplished around the ninth gestational week.[1] The fused caudad third of the müllerian ducts (known as the *genital canal* or *uterovaginal canal*) develops into the uterus, cervix, and upper one third of the vagina. The nonfused cephalad two thirds of the müllerian ducts become the fallopian tubes.[1]

### CONGENITAL ANOMALIES

Isolated congenital anomalies of the fallopian tube are uncommon. However, they can be seen in association with other uterine defects, resulting from the abnormal development or fusion of the paired müllerian ducts. Conditions associated with fusion include in utero exposure to diethylstilbestrol, a syn-

thetic nonsteroidal estrogen,[2] and chromosomal alterations associated with abnormal gonadal development. Reports exist in the literature of congenital unilateral duplication of the fallopian tube,[3] unilateral absence of a fallopian tube and the ipsilateral ovary,[4] absence of the proximal segment of the fallopian tube,[5] and bilateral absence of the muscular layer of the ampullary tubal region.[6] Accessory fallopian tubes[7] also have been described.

### EMBRYOLOGIC RESTS

Embryologic rests occasionally can be found in the fallopian tubes, mainly as incidental findings in tubal ligation and hysterectomy specimens. Hilar cells have been described in the tubal mucosa and near the fimbriated end.[8] Mesonephric duct remnants commonly are encountered and may present clinically as cysts (CD Fig. 38–1). They consist of a variable number of microscopic tubules surrounded by smooth muscle bundles and lined by a single layer of cuboidal to low-columnar ciliated and nonciliated epithelium (Fig. 38–1). Paramesonephric müllerian duct remnants also occur; they too can undergo cystic dilatation. Smooth muscle bundles encircle these tubular structures, and their epithelial lining resembles that of the fallopian tube, occasionally displaying plica-like structures. *Hydatid of Morgagni* is the name given to a paramesonephric duct cyst located in the fimbriated end of the tube. These lesions can be pedunculated, can be multiple, can undergo torsion, and in some cases may be associated with infertility. Adrenal rests may be present in the wall of the fallopian tube (Fig. 38–2). A case of ectopic pancreatic tissue has been reported in the fallopian tube.[9]

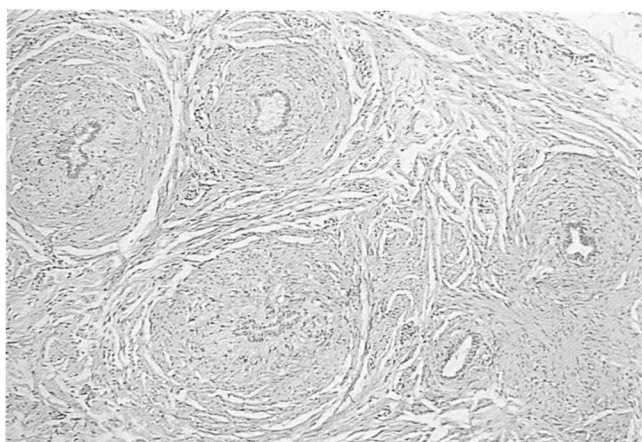

**FIGURE 38–1.** Mesonephric duct remnants.

## Anatomy

The major portion of each fallopian tube lies in the free upper border of each broad ligament and is surrounded mainly by peritoneum.[9a] When the fallopian tube is fully developed, its extrauterine aspect may measure 8.0 to 15.0 cm in length.[10] The fallopian tube is divided into four morphologically different segments. The intramural (or interstitial) segment corresponds to the proximal portion of the tube that lies within the myometrium. In this area, the tube opens into the endometrial cavity through its uterine ostium; this segment ranges from 1.0 to 3.5 cm in length and from 0.2 to 0.4 cm in luminal diameter. The next segment is the isthmus, varying in length from 2.0 to 3.0 cm, with a luminal diameter that may vary from less than 0.1 cm to 0.2 cm. Following the isthmus is the longest segment of the tube, the ampulla. The ampulla varies in length from 5.0 to 8.0 cm and has a luminal diameter of 0.1 to 0.2 cm. The more distal segment is the funnel-shaped infundibulum, where the finger-like fimbriae originate and where the tube opens into the peritoneal cavity through its ostium (the abdominal ostium). In this segment, the length of the tube and its diameter average 1.0 cm.[10] The fimbriae are extensions of the infundibular wall lined by tubal epithelium that is continuous with the peritoneum of the outer surface of the tube. One of the fimbriae (fimbria ovarica) is larger than the others and is attached to the ovary, holding it in close proximity to the abdominal ostium.[10]

## Histology and Physiology

The full thickness of the fallopian tube wall consists of three regions: 1) the serosa, 2) the muscularis, and 3) the mucosa. The serosa consists of an outer mesothelial cell layer overlying a thin layer of vascularized connective tissue. The middle region corresponds to the muscularis, where smooth muscle

bundles associated with interstitial connective tissue are arranged into two layers—a thicker inner circular one and a thinner outer longitudinal one. An additional third layer of smooth muscle bundles (the inner longitudinal layer) can be seen involving the area from the intramural portion of the tube into the ampulla.[10] The muscularis is thicker at the isthmus. The mucosa rests on the muscularis; throughout the length of the tube, it varies in thickness. Such alterations in the mucosal configuration form the foldings known as *plicae;* the latter vary in architecture and in number, from relatively few blunt plicae at the isthmus to numerous slender, long, and complex plicae at the ampulla. The mucosa consists of a vascularized loose connective tissue lamina propria overlaid by epithelium. This epithelium is simple, nonstratified, and composed of three types of columnar cells. The most numerous ones are the secretory cells, accounting for approximately 55% to 65% of the cell population.[10] They have an oval nucleus with dense chromatin, small nucleoli, and eosinophilic cytoplasm. Secretory cells are associated with the formation of tubal luminal fluid, a mixture of multiple substances[11] including immunoglobulins,[12] amylase, and electrolytes. The ciliated cells represent almost 20% to 30% of the population.[10] Although the synchronized movement of the cilia has an important role in transporting the ovum toward the uterine cavity, other factors (e.g., tubal motility) play an important role in this process. Ciliated cells have eosinophilic cytoplasm, oval to round nuclei with granular chromatin, and a small nucleolus.[10] The third type of columnar cell is the intercalary or peg cell, believed to represent a type of secretory cell. Receptors for immunoglobulin A and secretory component are expressed by the epithelial cells.[12] Small numbers of lymphocytes permeate the connective tissue of the lamina propria, most of them of the T cell suppressor/cytotoxic subgroup.[13] Scattered plasma cells are seen normally, but they increase in number in the presence of infection.[12] During preg-

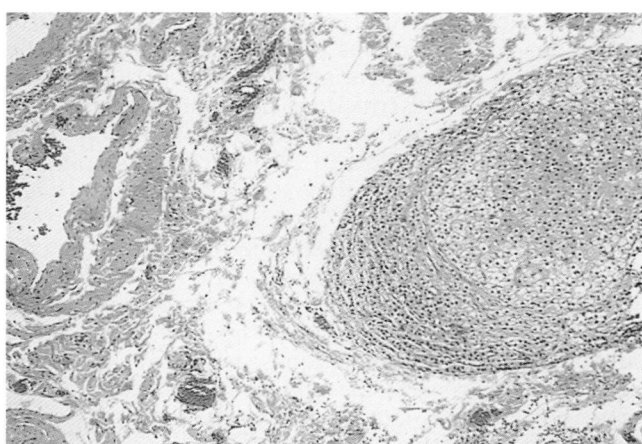

**FIGURE 38–2.** Adrenal rest present in the wall of fallopian tube. Notice clear cells with abundant cytoplasm.

nancy (intrauterine and ectopic), the lamina propria may undergo a decidual reaction. Cyclic variations in the circulating levels of estrogen and progesterone associated with the menstrual cycle influence the tubal epithelium. Estrogen receptors are present in the epithelium of the fallopian tube,[14] and an increase in the levels of circulating estrogen is associated with the formation of cilia and with an increase in the function of the secretory epithelium.[15, 16] An increase in the levels of serum progesterone leads to the loss of cilia in the tubal epithelium.[17] Ciliated cells can be seen in the fetal tubal mucosa.[18]

## Inflammatory Changes

Bacterial infections are the most common cause of acute and chronic (resolving) salpingitis. As a likely consequence of these inflammatory processes, irreversible damage to the fallopian tube may result in infertility or in an increased risk of developing an ectopic tubal pregnancy.[19]

Inflammatory processes that involve the fallopian tubes are mainly the result of ascending infection. Salpingitis of infectious origin is an important sign of pelvic inflammatory disease, a condition associated with sexually transmitted diseases. Acute pelvic inflammatory disease is polymicrobial in most cases,[20] with aerobic and anaerobic bacteria participating in the process. Organisms such as *Chlamydia trachomatis* and *Neisseria gonorrhoeae* may be accompanied by bacteria that usually can be found colonizing the lower female genital tract, including *Escherichia coli, Bacteroides, Peptostreptococcus,* and *Pseudomonas aeruginosa.*[21, 22]

On gross inspection, the acutely inflamed tube is distended with a thickened edematous wall; there is acute inflammation and vascular congestion, and the lumen commonly is filled with purulent exudate. The serosa may be involved by a fibrinous or fibrinopurulent exudate. On microscopic examination, acute inflammatory cells permeate the full thickness of the tubal wall associated with varying degrees of edema. Tissue necrosis also can be seen (Fig. 38–3). Mucosal ulceration and inflammation result in plical adhesions. Complications of this process include the formation of a tubo-ovarian abscess and pyosalpinx. The previously described microscopic findings are nonspecific and can be seen in association with polymicrobial infections. In cases of acute salpingitis associated with *N. gonorrhoeae,* the luminal purulent exudate may be copious.

The manner by which the different bacteria spread varies among organisms. In the case of *N. gonorrhoeae,* the bacteria spread by a mechanism that involves direct interaction with the epithelium of the tubal mucosa.[23] Menstruation seems to facilitate the spread of *N. gonorrhoeae* and *C. trachomatis*[24]; however, the spread of other microorganisms does not seem to be influenced by menstruation. The clinical onset of symptoms associated with tubal infection by *N. gonorrhoeae* is sudden, with fever occurring

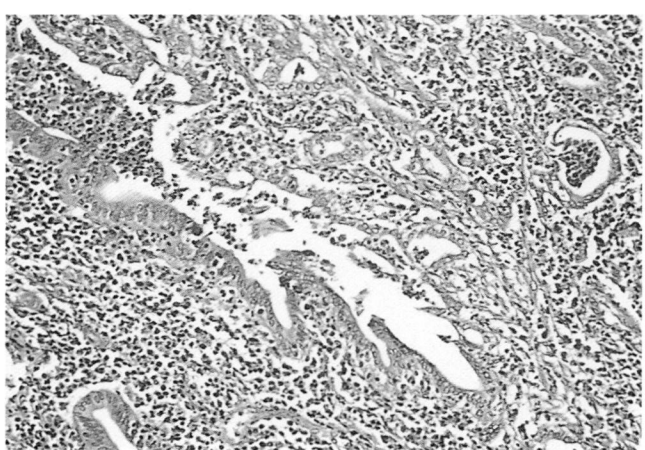

**FIGURE 38–3.** Acute gonococcal salpingitis. Notice extensive neutrophilic exudate infiltrating the tubal epithelium, with microabscess formation.

during or after the menstrual period. In the case of tubal infection by *C. trachomatis*, the onset of symptoms is not as abrupt and may occur at any time during the menstrual cycle.

An acute (or mixed acute and chronic) inflammatory infiltrate of variable intensity has been observed permeating the tubal mucosa a few days postpartum.[25] In these cases, tissue cultures are negative. Similar histologic changes can be seen in association with menstruation and have been termed *physiologic salpingitis.*[26]

### CHRONIC SALPINGITIS

Chronic salpingitis may be the end result of unresolved, most typically recurrent, episodes of acute salpingitis (CD Fig. 38–2). Microscopic findings in these cases include blunting and fibrosis of the plicae, with permeation by a variably intense chronic inflammatory cell infiltrate consisting of lymphocytes, plasma cells, and occasionally histiocytes (CD Fig. 38–4). Squamous metaplasia of the tubal epithelium may occur. Fusion of the tubal plicae after resolution of the acute inflammatory process may result in the formation of follicle-like spaces of various sizes, a histologic pattern of chronic salpingitis known as *follicular salpingitis* (salpingitis follicularis) (Fig. 38–4). The gross distortion of the fallopian tube may be minimal or marked, depending on the degree of fibrosis, the presence of luminal occlusion, and the extent of the formation of fibrous serosal adhesions. *Hydrosalpinx* may develop after purulent salpingitis, when resorption of the pus is followed by the formation of a transudate. In these cases, there is tubal dilatation, and the fimbriated end is obliterated; fibrous serosal adhesions are common. The tubal wall is thin and associated with attenuated mucosal plicae and variable flattening of the epithelial lining. In the thin areas of the wall, the muscular layer may have undergone atrophy, with replacement of the muscle by fibrous tissue.[27]

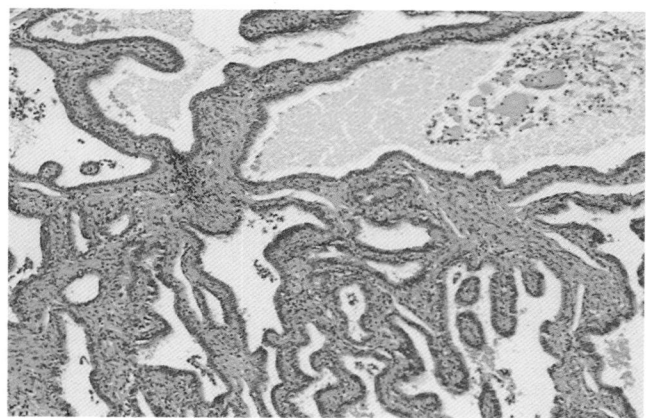

**FIGURE 38–4.** Section from the wall of a fallopian tube exhibiting plical blunting and fusion, resulting in chronic "follicular" salpingitis (salpingitis follicularis).

*Tubo-ovarian adhesions* and the formation of a *tubo-ovarian abscess* are complications associated with acute salpingitis. Enlarged fallopian tubes (resulting from pyosalpinx, hydrosalpinx, or a tubo-ovarian abscess) may undergo torsion, resulting in further complications, including necrosis and rupture. Occasionally, *psammoma bodies* can be seen in cases of chronic salpingitis; however, their presence is a nonspecific finding. These structures also can be seen in otherwise normal fallopian tubes or in association with primary tubal serous carcinoma. In cases of chronic salpingitis, the tubal epithelium may develop reactive atypia that may be severe enough (as in cases of tubal involvement by tuberculosis or by Crohn's disease) to simulate a malignancy.[28, 29] Mucosal involvement by *Liesegang's rings* (eosinophilic, acellular, ringlike structures) was reported in a case of chronic salpingitis.[30]

## GRANULOMATOUS SALPINGITIS

Granulomatous salpingitis may be noninfectious or associated with infectious agents known to trigger that type of inflammatory response. The most common causative microorganism is *Mycobacterium tuberculosis*.[31] Bilateral involvement of the fallopian tubes generally occurs in the setting of disseminated tuberculosis, the result of hematogenous spread of the mycobacteria. Concurrent endometrial involvement is noted in approximately 80% of cases. Sterility is a complication of this condition. The gross tubal changes may simulate chronic salpingitis of various causes; however, it is not unusual for the abdominal ostia to remain patent in these cases.[32] Serosal tubercules sometimes can be identified grossly. Microscopic evaluation reveals caseating and noncaseating granulomas, mainly mucosal (although transmural involvement by the granulomas can be seen), and a chronic inflammatory cell infiltrate (Fig. 38–5). In the endometrium, caseating granulomas are rare. As a result of the cyclic shedding associated with the menstrual cycle, the granu-

lomas slough off before the caseation necrosis develops or may not form at all. There is evidence of chronic salpingitis, such as plical fusion, fibrosis, and reactive epithelial atypia that may be marked,[33] and areas of calcification. The incidence of tuberculous salpingitis parallels that of tuberculosis.[31] The presence of acid-fast bacilli must be ruled out, however, in patients with either unilateral or bilateral granulomatous salpingitis that lack the classic caseation necrosis accompanied by Langhans'-type giant cells.[31] In immunosuppressed women in whom the condition is clinically suspected, special procedures (acid-fast, auramine-rhodamine) are necessary because these patients may be unable to mount a granulomatous response, and the histologic changes may appear to be mild and nonspecific.

Actinomycosis of the fallopian tubes is an uncommon complication of intrauterine contraceptive device placement or its prolonged use[34] associated with a granulomatous response. "Sulfur granules" may be seen on gross or microscopic examination in the purulent luminal exudate. The condition is bilateral in almost half of the cases. The development of fistulous tracts between organs (including the skin), adhesions, and tubo-ovarian abscesses can accompany this infectious process and may mimic a malignancy. Other infectious agents that can cause granulomatous salpingitis include parasites such as *Schistosoma mansoni*,[35] *Schistosoma haematobium*,[35] *Enterobius vermicularis*,[36] *Cysticercus*,[37] and *Echinococcus granulosus*[38] and fungi such as *Blastomyces*[39] and *Coccidioides*.[40]

Systemic conditions associated with granulomatous salpingitis include Crohn's disease[41] and sarcoidosis.[42] Amyloidosis of the fallopian tube[43] also has been described. After tubal diathermy[44] (for tubal ligation), palisading granulomas with central areas of necrosis can develop.

Foreign bodies can reach the tube as the result of surgical procedures or the use of contrast media

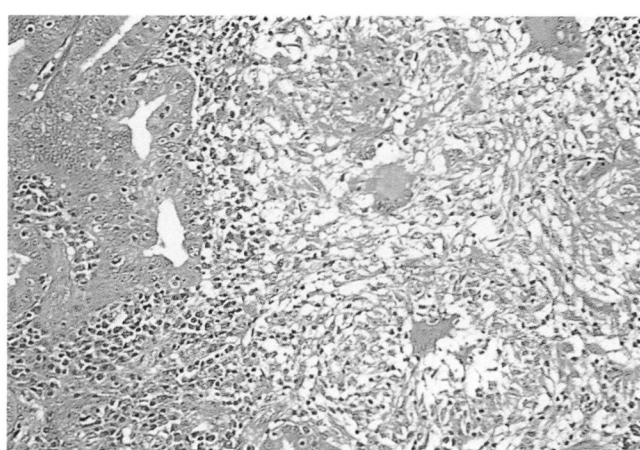

**FIGURE 38–5.** Granulomatous salpingitis in a patient with tuberculosis. Note noncaseating granuloma with multinucleated giant cells.

in radiologic studies. These foreign substances include starch and lipid material used in hysterosalpingograms. It is important to correlate the presence of such substances with the patient's clinical history to avoid confusion with infectious processes or malignancies. Polyvinylpyrrolidone, a component of certain blood substitutes, is a mucicarmine-positive foreign substance. After ingestion by histiocytes, deposition of this substance has been described in numerous organs *(mucicarminophilic histiocytosis),* including the fallopian tube.[45] In these cases, a clinical history of prior treatment with a blood substitute containing polyvinylpyrrolidone is crucial because the differential diagnosis includes tubal involvement by a signet ring cell carcinoma.[45]

Xanthogranulomatous inflammation[46] and malacoplakia[47] also have been described in the fallopian tube. In both conditions, histologic features similar to those identified in other organs involved by these processes are noted.

## SALPINGITIS ISTHMICA NODOSA AND TUBAL DIVERTICULA

Salpingitis isthmica nodosa (SIN) is characterized on gross examination by single or multiple nodular areas of variable sizes, mainly in the isthmic portion of the fallopian tube. The nodularities may extend into the adjacent uterine cornu or involve the ampulla. They are associated with a smooth overlying serosa, and their cut surfaces may reveal numerous minute cavities or umbilicated areas involving the tubal wall. SIN is seen in women between the ages of 25 and 60[48] and frequently is bilateral. Its cause is unknown, but several theories have been proposed. One theory favors SIN to be the outcome of a reparative response to previous infectious processes. Although tubal infections usually involve the ampulla, this area is affected by SIN only in approximately one third of the cases.[49] Another more likely theory proposes that SIN is the result of an acquired defect in the tubal wall associated with the development of mucosal invaginations (diverticula) that manifest grossly as nodularities. On microscopic evaluation, the nodular areas correspond to points of mucosal invaginations into the surrounding muscular layer, creating diverticula, in a fashion similar to that of adenomyosis. The muscle surrounding the diverticula appears thickened and concentrically arranged; there is no peridiverticular scarring. Because of tissue sectioning, the diverticular mucosa appears detached from the luminal aspect of the tube; it may display similar histologic features as those of the luminal mucosa, metaplastic changes, or endometriosis. A significant chronic inflammatory infiltrate is uncommon. These diverticula may be single or multiple and can be arranged in a circumferential or focal fashion (CD Fig. 38–4). They may involve the tubal wall at different levels, from the inner aspect to the full thickness (Fig. 38–6). SIN can be seen in association with infertility and ectopic pregnancy.[19, 50]

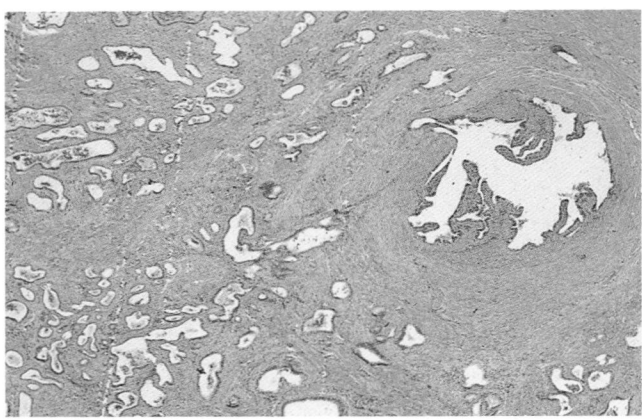

**FIGURE 38–6.** Cross-section from a fallopian tube exhibiting multiple mucosal diverticula, arranged in a circumferential fashion and involving the full thickness of the wall.

## Ectopic Pregnancy

In the United States, ectopic pregnancy is the leading cause of maternal death in the first trimester of pregnancy and the second overall cause of maternal death.[51] An ectopic pregnancy is the result of implantation of the maturing blastocyst at a site other than the mucosa of the endometrial cavity. Tubal alterations resulting from inflammation, congenital anomalies, or previous surgery may be associated with the development of tubal or extratubal pregnancies. Although ectopic pregnancies have been described in numerous organs, including the uterine cornu, ovaries,[52] abdominal cavity,[53] liver,[54] and spleen,[55] in more than 95% of cases they occur in the fallopian tubes (CD Fig. 38–5), where they appear to be more common on the right side.[19] Simultaneous bilateral tubal ectopic pregnancies have been reported.[19, 56] Coexisting intrauterine and tubal pregnancies *(heterotopic pregnancies)* are estimated to occur in 1 out of every 10,000 to 30,000 pregnancies.[57] An increase in their incidence has been noted in association with ovulation induction and the use of techniques of assisted reproduction (e.g., embryo transfer and in vitro fertilization), especially if tubal disease is present.[58]

A relationship between a prior history of pelvic inflammatory disease and the subsequent development of ectopic pregnancies has been shown by many workers.[19] Tubal damage is a consequence of the reactive and reparative processes that result from previous acute and chronic inflammatory episodes, mainly caused by bacterial infections. Other predisposing factors include a history of prior abdominal or pelvic surgery (including tubal ligations and reanastomosis), hormonal anomalies in the periovulatory and early luteal phase of the menstrual cycle, congenital uterine and tubal anomalies, and a history of acute salpingitis. Some predisposing factors, such as previous voluntary interruption of pregnancy and endometriosis, are controversial, with some studies favoring them and others failing to show a significant relationship with the subsequent development of ectopic pregnancies.[19] The role of the intrauterine contraceptive device as a predisposing factor has been debated. More recent studies have failed to show a significant association between the use of intrauterine devices and the subsequent development of ectopic pregnancies.[19]

Tubal pregnancies usually occur in women in their late 20s, although the reported ages of patients have ranged from 14 to 46.[19] Clinical presentation includes lower abdominal pain that might be localized to the right or left lower quadrant or associated with abnormal uterine bleeding. Signs and symptoms of an acute abdomen are common, and acute appendicitis is frequently in the differential diagnosis. Patients may be in hypovolemic shock secondary to a ruptured ectopic pregnancy at the time of presentation. Assessment of the serum levels of human chorionic gonadotropin, ultrasonographic pelvic studies, and pertinent clinical information help establish the diagnosis.

In 90% of cases of ectopic pregnancy, some degree of tubal pathology seems to be the common factor linking the numerous conditions predisposing to its development.[19, 59] It is not unusual to identify various pathologic conditions in the same surgical specimen. Chronic salpingitis is the most common condition identified in this setting,[19] and follicular salpingitis can be detected in 20% of those cases. Hydrosalpinx was identified on histologic evaluation in approximately 32% of the cases of chronic salpingitis in a retrospective study of 571 tubal pregnancies performed at our former institution. Most of the cases of hydrosalpinx (58%) also were associated with the presence of hematosalpinx (luminal blood). The number of tubal pregnancies reported to arise in the background of SIN is variable (most likely the result of data collection methods and specimen sampling), with studies reporting values that fluctuate from rare to 43% of all cases.[19] In our study, 18% of the cases of uterine cornual (interstitial) ectopic pregnancies were associated with mucosal diverticula but lacked the gross nodularities usually noted in SIN. The latter may reflect a propensity for mucosal diverticula to develop in the intramural (cornual) portion of the fallopian tube.

The gross findings in a case of tubal pregnancy are influenced by the pathologic changes present in the tube before implantation (CD Fig. 38–6). The tubal ampulla hosts 75% to 80% of pregnancies,[60] a third of which are estimated to rupture.[61] Ten percent to 15% of pregnancies occur in the isthmus,[60] and approximately 5% occur in the fimbriae.[60] Commonly the salpingectomy specimen is dilated in the ampullary region, and the cut surface reveals luminal blood mixed with placental tissue. The bloody contents may impart a hemorrhagic discoloration to the wall in that area (Fig. 38–7). Embryonal tissue may be identified on gross or microscopic examination in many cases. Tubes with hydrosalpinx may resemble a cyst and be preoperatively confused with an ovarian cyst.

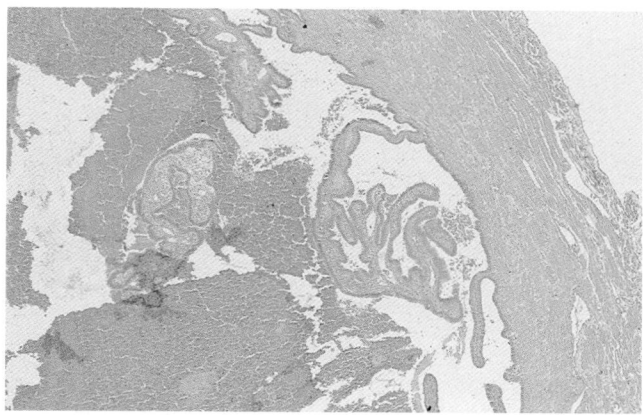

**FIGURE 38–7.** Chronic salpingitis with hydrosalpinx and hematosalpinx, findings often associated with cases of tubal ectopic pregnancy.

Implantation and placentation seem to follow a course similar to the one observed in the uterus.[62] By light microscopy, extravillous (intermediate type) trophoblast invades the tubal wall in a manner similar to that identified in intrauterine pregnancies. A study by Egarter and Husslein[63] indicated, however, that tubal pregnancies seem to develop at a slower rate than intrauterine pregnancies and that they display variations in their growth rate, as opposed to the similar growth rate noted among intrauterine pregnancies. In another study, ectopic chorionic villi were found to display architectural anomalies and a decrease in ramification and new villi formation.[64] Also, a delay in ectopic villous development was noted after the fourth week of gestation when compared with normal intrauterine villi.[64] Tubal trophoblast does not differentiate into chorion frondosum and chorion laeve.[62] The site of implantation (mucosal, intramural, or transmural) may determine the extent of the tissue involved by the ectopic pregnancy and the subsequent rupture of the tubal wall. The latter seems to be influenced by various factors, including the increased luminal pressure generated by the developing products of conception. Tubal rupture occurs close to the 8th week of gestation; however, cornual (interstitial) pregnancies rupture around the 12th week of gestation (CD Fig. 38–7). In some cases, granulation tissue formation already is noted at the rupture site, and marked reactive serosal changes are common in this setting. Decidual reactions can be seen in the mucosal and connective tissue areas, including those associated with SIN and tubal diverticula, and, when present, in foci of endometriosis (CD Figs. 38–8 and 38–9). Products of conception have to be shown on histologic examination to establish the diagnosis of ectopic pregnancy. Immature chorionic villi may fill the lumen, but sometimes only rare trophoblastic cells are present within the luminal blood, requiring extensive sampling to find them. In cases of tubal abortion, it may be necessary to submit numerous tissue

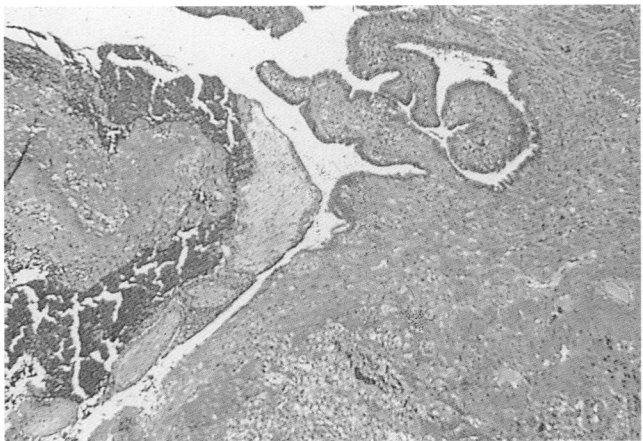

**FIGURE 38–8.** Implantation of an ectopic pregnancy in the wall of a fallopian tube.

sections. In the absence of luminal products of conception, tissue from the placental implantation site still may remain in the wall. It is not unusual to see chorionic villi in direct contact with the muscularis, a finding similar on histologic examination to the type of implantation observed in cases of placenta accreta (Fig. 38–8).

The endometrium associated with cases of ectopic pregnancy can display several histologic patterns. The clinician should be notified immediately of the absence of products of conception (chorionic villi, trophoblast, placental implantation site tissue, or fetal parts) in endometrial curettings from pregnant patients. Gestation-associated endometrial patterns (hypersecretory endometrium with or without an Arias-Stella reaction or a decidual cast) are common in cases of ectopic pregnancy. Other "nongestational" patterns (e.g., datable endometrium, acute and chronic endometritis, or "irregular shedding-like" patterns) also may be encountered (CD Fig. 38–10). We retrospectively examined 240 endometrial curettage specimens obtained at the time of admission from patients eventually diagnosed with an ectopic pregnancy.[19] Most cases (66%) revealed gestation-associated histologic patterns. We also noted the presence (in 3% of all cases) of fragments of hyalinized extravillous (intermediate) trophoblast, consistent on histologic examination with fragments from a placental site nodule. The latter represents hyalinized placental implantation site tissue retained from a previous (remote) intrauterine pregnancy. These fragments display positive diffuse immunostaining for placental alkaline phosphatase,[65, 66] cytokeratin, and epithelial membrane antigen.[65] Focal positive immunostaining is obtained with human placental lactogen[65, 66] and human chorionic gonadotropin[65] in some cases. It is important to recognize the true nature of these residua and to avoid their misinterpretation as a marker of current intrauterine implantation, especially in the background of the aforementioned gestation-associated patterns. Pla-

cental site nodules also have been described in ectopic locations, including the fallopian tube and the broad ligament;[67, 68] these lesions are the result of remote ectopic pregnancies and usually are described as incidental microscopic findings in specimens obtained for other medical reasons.

The treatment in cases of tubal ectopic pregnancies is determined based on the clinical findings at the time of evaluation (rupture, tubal abortion, viability of the tube) with consideration of the patient's desire to conceive in the future. Laparoscopically assisted surgical procedures usually are performed. A total salpingectomy might be done in cases of ruptured or severely distorted tubal pregnancies. A linear salpingostomy can be an option for the retrieval of the products of conception in an intact fallopian tube. Conservative laparoscopic surgical procedures may be complicated, however, by persistent viable trophoblast in 3% to 20% of cases, ultimately requiring more surgery or a pharmacologic approach.[69] Methotrexate (an inhibitor of DNA and RNA synthesis commonly used in the treatment of gestational trophoblastic disease) has been used in cases of unruptured tubal pregnancies. Methotrexate also is used in cases in which surgery is contraindicated and for postoperative persistent trophoblast. The failure rate associated with this treatment is 5% to 11%, and these patients ultimately undergo a surgical procedure to remove the products of conception. In one study,[69] 12 surgical specimens from failed methotrexate-treated tubal pregnancies were compared with tubal pregnancies from maternal age–matched and gestational age–matched controls. Of the methotrexate-treated cases, 67% revealed significant trophoblastic atypia (irregular enlarged nuclei, smudged chromatin, and prominent nucleoli) compared with 25% of the control cases. There were no significant statistical differences regarding the degree of villous necrosis, villous morphology, trophoblastic vacuolization, or embryonic development between the two groups. The presence of atypical trophoblast in failed methotrexate-treated tubal pregnancies might be confused with early gestational trophoblastic disease. It is important for the surgical pathologist to obtain a proper clinical history in these cases to avoid misdiagnosis.

The term *chronic ectopic pregnancy* is used to define remote, involuted ectopic pregnancies. Many of these cases are clinically silent incidental findings removed at the time of surgery for an unrelated ailment; others are clinically evident, but their true nature is not clear until histopathologic evaluation is performed. Detectable levels of β-subunit human chorionic gonadotropin are absent. It is not unusual for patients to deny a past history of tubal ectopic pregnancies. Microscopic evaluation reveals necrotic ("ghost") villi, associated with areas of calcification and, occasionally, viable-appearing extravillous (intermediate) trophoblast.[70]

When patients with a history of tubal pregnancies are treated conservatively, the risk of a subsequent ectopic pregnancy in the same fallopian tube does not seem to be increased significantly.[19, 71] The pathologic features present in the tube (or tubes) seem to determine a patient's risk of developing a recurrent ectopic pregnancy.[71] Ectopic pregnancies also may display chromosomal anomalies and evidence of overt gestational trophoblastic disease (partial moles, complete moles, and choriocarcinoma). Choriocarcinoma can develop in association with any type of pregnancy, and 2.5% of all gestational engendered choriocarcinomas follow an ectopic pregnancy.[72] Tubal abortions are common; products of conception expelled from the tube in this setting may be responsible for the development of extratubal gestations.

## Infertility

Because the main function of the fallopian tubes is to provide an adequate environment for fertilization to occur and to transport the developing zygote, alterations in their function can impair fertility significantly. Tubal-associated infertility accounts for more than 50% of the causes of female infertility.[73] Among the most common causes are anatomic deformities that interfere with motility or cause partial or complete obstruction of the lumen in different regions of the tubes; such causes include acute and chronic inflammatory processes, SIN, endometriosis, prior tubal ligation and reanastomosis, peritubal and periadnexal adhesions, and history of tubal pregnancy. After sterilization procedures, the fallopian tubes tend to display histologic changes that include chronic inflammatory infiltrates with pseudopolyp formation, plical attenuation, and proximal luminal dilatation.[74] These changes seem to be associated with the length of time from the completion of the sterilization procedure and may affect the success rate of subsequent reanastomotic surgery.[74] Other causes of tubal infertility include congenital anomalies. Patients with Kartagener's syndrome (immotile cilia syndrome) are not infertile but have impaired fertility.[75] The presence of accessory fallopian tubes, accessory ostia, and hydatids of Morgagni (especially when multiple) may interfere with fertility.

## Endometriosis and Endosalpingiosis

Endometriosis commonly involves the peritoneum of the fallopian tubes, where it may become evident as raised patchy areas, nodules, or cysts that may be pigmented or nonpigmented and associated with adhesion formation. Classically defined as the presence of endometrial-type glands and stroma in an extrauterine location, endometriosis also can involve any area of the full thickness of the tubal wall. Endometriotic foci in the muscularis induce the concentric proliferation of the smooth muscle around them. When such changes are clinically significant, gross nodularities reminiscent of those associated

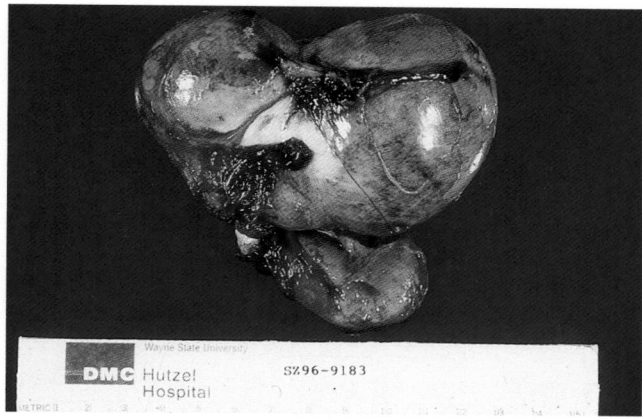

**FIGURE 38–9.** Dilated ovarian endometrioma adherent to the tubal serosa. Endometriosis was also noted in the tubal wall.

with SIN may develop. Mucosal endometriosis may result in luminal occlusion and contribute to infertility. Endometriotic foci may undergo a decidual reaction, hypersecretory glandular changes, and the Arias-Stella reaction as a response to intrauterine and ectopic pregnancies. Chronic nonspecific salpingitis can be seen in association with ovarian endometriosis in one third of cases[76] (Fig. 38–9). In pseudoxanthomatous salpingitis (pigmentosis tubae, pseudoxanthomatous salpingiosis), lipofuscin-laden macrophages (pseudoxanthomatous cells) infiltrate the tubal mucosa, a condition that can be associated with pelvic endometriosis.[77] So-called necrotic pseudoxanthomatous nodules are lesions characterized by central necrosis surrounded by palisading pseudoxanthomatous cells or fibrous tissue that may or may not be associated with endometrial-type tissue[78]; they can develop in tubal endometriosis and should be distinguished from granulomatous lesions of infectious origin or those associated with tubal diathermy.[44] The uterine mucosa normally may extend into the interstitial portion of the fallopian tube and sometimes may involve the isthmic portion. This finding should not be interpreted as mucosal endometriosis. Endometriosis also can develop after a tubal ligation, usually in the area of the proximal stump.[79]

In endosalpingiosis, glandular structures lined by serous, or tubal-type, epithelium are noted in the peritoneal and subperitoneal areas of the fallopian tubes. The process is benign and may represent mesothelium or mesothelial inclusion cysts with metaplastic tubal epithelial changes.

## Benign Lesions

Serosal *mesothelial inclusion cysts* are usually small (1 to 2 mm) clear or light tan cysts present on the serosal and subserosal aspects of the tubes. They usually are incidental findings of no clinical significance. When the mesothelial epithelium of the inclu-

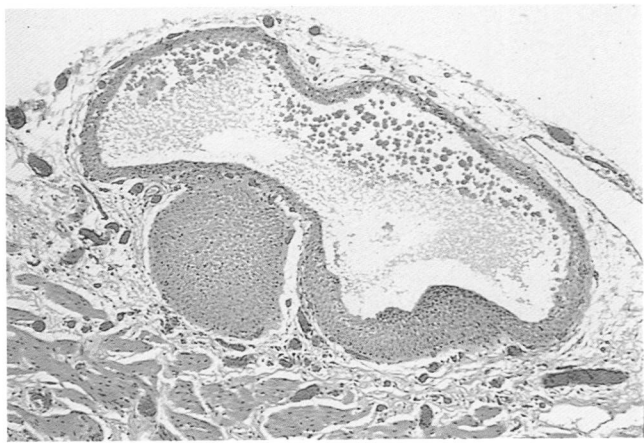

**FIGURE 38–10.** Mesothelial inclusion cyst (Walthard's cell rests) with transitional metaplasia of lining epithelium.

sions undergoes transitional-type metaplasia, the resulting structures are referred to as *Walthard's cell rests* (Fig. 38–10). These gross structures are yellow-tan and may undergo cystic change (CD Fig. 38–11). *Cystadenomas* of serous, endometrioid, and mucinous types rarely can arise primarily in the fallopian tubes.[80, 81]

The *adenomatoid tumor,* a benign mesothelioma that involves the serosa and subserosal areas of the fallopian tubes and round ligaments, is the most common benign tumor of the fallopian tube. It also can comprise the full thickness of the tubal wall. The gross tumor is a yellow-to-white nodule that usually does not exceed 2 cm in its greatest dimension, but it also can present as an incidental finding. On microscopic examination, they are identical to adenomatoid tumors of other sites, including the uterus. Adenomatoid tumors display small tubular and slitlike spaces lined by cuboidal or flattened cells with small round nuclei (Fig. 38–11). They are

associated with connective tissue that may be hyalinized; intraluminal and intracellular alcian blue–positive (hyaluronidase digestible) material may be noted. Although the lesions may be large enough to occlude the lumen, they are usually confined to a particular area and are not associated with infiltrative reactive features, such as desmoplasia. Cytoplasmic vacuoles or signet ring–like cellular features can be seen occasionally; however, mitoses are unusual. The cells exhibit an immunohistochemical profile similar to those of adenomatoid tumors elsewhere.[82] The adenomatoid tumor should be differentiated from metastatic involvement of the fallopian tube by an adenocarcinoma.

The *metaplastic papillary tumor* of the fallopian tube is a rare lesion usually detected as a microscopic incidental finding at the time of pregnancy, or postpartum.[83, 84] The polypoid tumor arises from the mucosa and projects into the tubal lumen. It is characterized by papillary projections with fine connective tissue cores lined by a single or double layer of large columnar cells with abundant eosinophilic cytoplasm and large vesicular nuclei with small nucleoli (Fig. 38–12 and CD Fig. 38–12). Formation of small cystic structures may be noted. Mitotic figures are rare. Mucicarmine-positive cytoplasmic vacuoles are present. Malignant features, such as invasion and significant cytologic atypia, are absent. Ultrastructural analysis of one of these lesions suggests a metaplastic origin.[84] The reported cases have followed a benign clinical course, but the differential diagnosis includes a primary tubal adenocarcinoma. The tubal epithelium may undergo other *metaplastic* changes as well. Squamous metaplasia can be seen in association with chronic salpingitis, and mucinous and transitional (urothelial)[85] metaplasias of the tubal mucosa may be isolated findings. Tubal endocervical-type mucinous metaplasia can be seen in association with mucinous cervical and ovarian tumors, especially in women with Peutz-Jeghers syndrome.[81] *Epithelial papillomas* may arise in the tubal

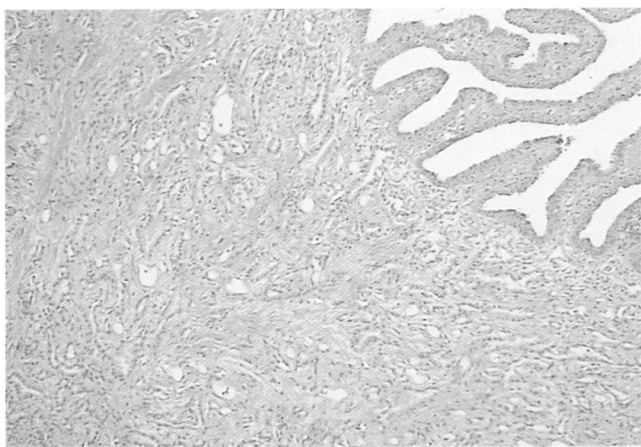

**FIGURE 38–11.** Adenomatoid tumor of fallopian tube comprised of small, uniform glandular structures lined by a single layer of cuboidal cells occupying the myosalpinx.

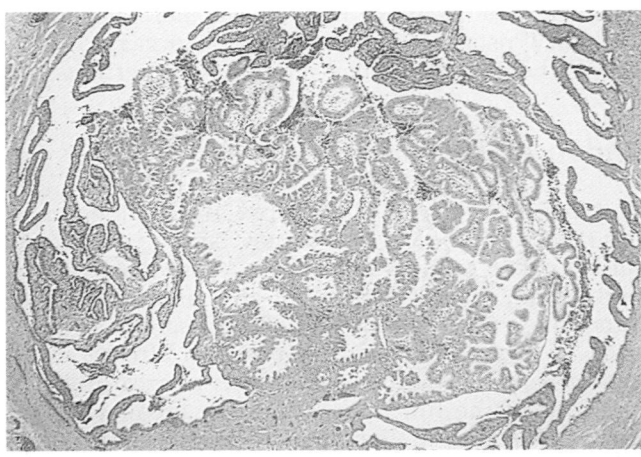

**FIGURE 38–12.** Metaplastic papillary tumor showing admixture of conventional tubal epithelium and metaplastic columnar epithelium with prominent oncocytic cytoplasm.

mucosa but are exceedingly rare.[86] They are usually microscopic lesions characterized by a central connective tissue core that arborizes into thin papillary projections lined by nonciliated columnar or oncocytic epithelium.

*Leiomyomas* can develop in the fallopian tube, where they are considered to arise from the muscularis or from the walls of the blood vessels. They are not as common as their uterine counterparts but display similar histologic features. Although rare, *adenomyomas*,[87] *cystadenofibromas*,[76] and *adenofibromas*[76] have been noted in the fallopian tubes. Tubal hemangiomas,[88, 89] lipomas,[90] angiomyolipomas,[91] and angiofibroblastomas[92] also have been described.

*Teratomas* of the fallopian tube are rare tumors. They have been described in the serosal, intramural, and luminal aspects of the tube.[93–96] They commonly are cystic and range in size from 1.0 to 12.0 cm in greatest dimension. On histologic evaluation, tubal teratomas resemble their ovarian counterpart and most likely are the product of the anomalous development of migrating ova. Malignant tubal teratomas also have been described.[97–100] A mixed malignant germ cell tumor of the fallopian tube composed of immature teratoma and yolk sac tumor has been reported.[101]

*Isolated necrotizing arteritis* that displays histologic features identical to those of polyarteritis nodosa can involve the fallopian tube. Although this arteritis is self-limited and to date has not been associated with the systemic condition,[102, 103] patients still should be evaluated appropriately to exclude systemic involvement by polyarteritis nodosa.[104] *Giant cell arteritis* may involve the uterus, the cervix, the fallopian tubes, and the ovaries as a localized process or as part of systemic involvement in patients known to have the condition.[105]

*Hyperplasia* of the tubal epithelium can occur in association with acute and chronic salpingitis,[28] unopposed exposure to endogenous or exogenous estrogen,[106] use of tamoxifen,[107] and carcinomas of the female reproductive tract (particularly ovarian serous tumors of borderline malignancy or of low malignant potential).[108, 109] Hyperplasia also can be an incidental finding in fallopian tubes, not associated with any of the previously described conditions.[110] The prevalence of these changes varies from study to study; for example, hyperplastic epithelial changes in tubal ligation specimens have varied from 19%[111] to 66%.[110] The spectrum of the cytologic and architectural atypia displayed by the hyperplastic epithelium ranges from mild to marked. Some authors have categorized cases of markedly atypical hyperplastic epithelium as serous carcinoma in situ.[112] In a study by Yanai-Inbar and Silverberg,[110] mild atypical hyperplasia (which they named *mild mucosal epithelial proliferation*) was noted more often in tubal ligation specimens. Moderate-to-marked atypical hyperplasia (moderate-to-marked mucosal epithelial proliferation) more often accompanied a variety of non-neoplastic and neoplastic lesions of the female genital tract and seemed to be a more

widespread lesion. Yanai-Inbar and Silverberg[110] recommended use of the term *hyperplasia* only to refer to cases displaying moderate-to-marked atypical tubal epithelial hyperplasia. In general, the hyperplastic epithelium is characterized by varying degrees of nuclear pleomorphism and hyperchromatism, epithelial tufting, papillarity, and stratification. Mitotic activity is variable. In most cases, the changes are bilateral.[110] Clear cell hyperplasia of the tubal epithelium was described in association with an ectopic pregnancy.[113]

## Malignant Lesions

Primary malignant neoplasms of the fallopian tube are rare. The most common type is invasive serous papillary carcinoma; serous carcinoma in situ and serous tumors of borderline malignancy also may occur. The *in situ stage of serous carcinoma* is an unusual finding, most often encountered in association with an invasive tubal serous papillary carcinoma. The malignant cells resemble those of the invasive component of the tumor, exhibiting large hyperchromatic and pleomorphic nuclei, prominent (usually multiple) nucleoli, and scant cytoplasm, but are limited to the mucosa by an intact basement membrane. There is cellular stratification, with formation of small papillary projections, and mitotic activity is brisk. The degree of cellular and architectural changes and the mitotic activity present in serous carcinoma in situ is greater than that seen with marked atypical hyperplasia of the tubal epithelium.

Tubal *serous papillary carcinoma* is an aggressive, invasive tumor, but it is estimated to represent only 0.5% of all gynecologic cancers.[114] Such patients usually are postmenopausal and older than age 50.[114] Bilaterality is present in 30% of cases.[115] Clinical signs and symptoms are nonspecific and include pelvic pain, a pelvic mass, and vaginal bleeding; a clear or serosanguineous vaginal discharge has been known to occur with these tumors.[116] The tube is markedly dilated, and on sectioning, the lumen may be filled completely with friable, gray-tan hemorrhagic tumor (Fig. 38–13; CD Fig. 38–13). The tumor may extend into the uterus or involve the adjacent ovary. In these cases, it might be difficult to establish the unequivocal (tubal, endometrial, or ovarian) origin of the tumor. In many instances, however, histologic evaluation reveals a clear-cut transition between benign and malignant tubal epithelium, a finding, when accompanied by more extensive tumor in the tube than in the ovary, that can help establish the tubal origin. In the absence of the latter features, however, the ovary should be favored as the primary site because primary ovarian serous papillary carcinomas are more common than their tubal counterpart. In cases of endometrial involvement, the pattern of uterine tumor invasion and the amount of tumor also can help elucidate the origin of the lesion.

Histologic features of serous carcinomas include

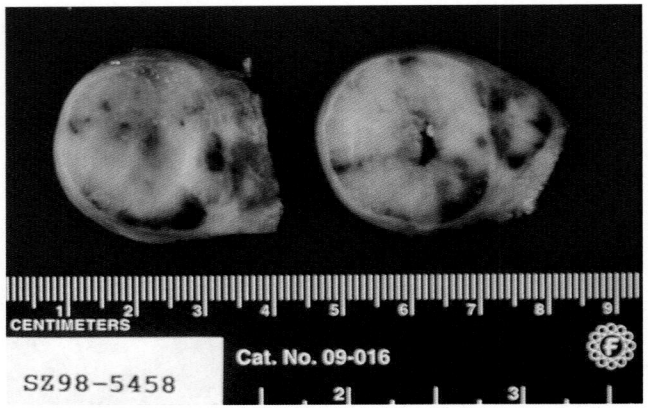

CENTIMETERS

Cat. No. 09-016

SZ98-5458

**FIGURE 38–13.** Section from the wall of a fallopian tube involved by a primary serous adenocarcinoma. Note the almost total occlusion of the lumen due to the carcinoma in this area.

a papillary architecture, with fibrous connective tissue cores lined by malignant cells displaying stratification and tufting, although in many areas the lining may consist of a single layer of cells (Table 38–1). Glandular and solid patterns are frequent. Gross and microscopic evidence of necrosis is common. High-grade cellular features are usual findings, including nuclear pleomorphism, hyperchromasia, and multinucleation, and there is brisk mitotic activity, with numerous abnormal mitotic figures. Psammoma bodies are not uncommon. Transmural invasion may be associated with malignant adhesions between adjacent pelvic structures.

Most primary serous tubal carcinomas are aneuploid,[117] and overexpression of the tumor-suppressor gene *p53* has been reported in more than 50% of

cases.[117, 118] In a study by Heselmeyer and colleagues,[117] recurrent nonrandom patterns of chromosomal aberrations were detected in 11 cases of tubal serous papillary carcinoma, using the comparative genomic hybridization technique. The most common aberration was a gain of chromosome arm 3q,[117] a finding that was present in all of the serous tumors, all of which also displayed positive *p53* immunoreactivity. The authors tested a case of primary endometrioid tubal carcinoma that showed only 6 aberrations compared with the average 20.9 identified in the serous tumors. The endometrioid carcinoma was the only case in their study that failed to show a gain of the long arm of chromosome 3 or to display immunopositivity for *p53*. All 12 cases were negative for human papillomavirus genomes.

Other less common types of primary epithelial malignancies have been described in the fallopian tubes and include squamous cell,[119] adenosquamous,[120] mucinous,[81] glassy cell,[121] endometrioid,[122] clear cell,[123] and transitional[124] types. Mucinous and endometrioid tumors of borderline malignancy can arise as primary tubal lesions.[80] A synchronous mucinous adenocarcinoma of the endocervix and fallopian tubes has been described.[125] Rarely, endometrioid carcinomas of the tube may display features resembling an adnexal tumor of probable wolffian origin.[126]

In general, fallopian tube malignancies have a poor prognosis (Table 38–2). In one study of 19 patients with primary carcinoma of the fallopian tube,[114] 63% of patients were International Federation of Gynecology and Obstetrics (FIGO) stage III and IV at the time of diagnosis; the 5-year survival rate for this group of patients was 0. A staging system for fallopian tube tumors developed by

**TABLE 38–1.** Fallopian Tube Malignancy Checklist*

Patient's name
Patient's identification number (social security number, hospital/clinic/office identification number)
Date of birth
Age
Date of procedure
Place procedure took place
Attending physician
Pertinent clinical information
  Previous surgical procedures (date, type of procedure, diagnosis—including any consultation reports)
  Menstrual history (last menstrual period, menopausal status)
  Gravida, para, abortus
  Medications (including exogenous hormonal treatment, length of treatment)
  Systemic conditions
  Clinical impression
Surgical pathology number
Intraoperative consultation result (frozen section diagnosis, gross diagnosis)
Type of surgical procedure:
  Biopsy (specify site)
  Tubal resection (unilateral, bilateral), including fimbriated end
  Hysterectomy with unilateral salpingectomy/salpingo-oophorectomy
  Hysterectomy with bilateral salpingectomy/salpingo-oophorectomy
  Other
    Biopsies (peritoneal, internal organs)
    Lymphadenectomy
    Pelvic/peritoneal washings

**TABLE 38–1.** Fallopian Tube Malignancy Checklist* *Continued*

Total number of specimen containers
Type of specimen: fallopian tube, uterus with unilateral/bilateral tube, uterus with unilateral/bilateral tube, and ovary
Special instructions by surgeon/clinician
Condition of specimen on receipt
  Fresh
  Fixative
  Unopened
  Opened
  Adequacy for evaluation
  Specific markings indicated by surgeon (stitches, ink)
Dimensions of specimen
  Weight
  Measurements
Tumor
  Gross evaluation
    Bilateral, unilateral
    Dimensions, color, consistency, configuration
    Anatomic location
      Interstitial (cornual) area
      Isthmus
      Ampulla
      Fimbriated end
      Serosa
      Intraluminal
      Tubo-ovarian area
    Gross involvement of ovaries†
    Additional pathologic findings (e.g., cysts, separate ovarian tumor)
    Representative sections submitted:
      Tumor, including areas involving serosa, interface with uninvolved tubal tissue, areas of perforation, areas of tubo-ovarian involvement, serosal/tubo-ovarian adhesions, any separate tumor nodules, uninvolved ovary, surgical margins of resection (if applicable), tumor involving any other organs submitted (e.g., uterus, omentum)
      Special studies: hormonal receptors, electron microscopy, frozen tissue bank, flow cytometry, cytogenetic
    Photographs (if taken)
  Microscopic evaluation
    Histologic type of tumor
      Carcinoma in situ
      Serous adenocarcinoma
      Endometrioid adenocarcinoma
      Mucinous adenocarcinoma
      Clear cell adenocarcinoma
      Squamous cell carcinoma
      Transitional cell carcinoma
      Undifferentiated carcinoma
    Extent of invasion
      Carcinoma in situ
      Invasive carcinoma confined to the lumen
      Invasive carcinoma confined to the fimbriated end
      Invasion of the mucosa, muscularis, or serosa
    Perforation of the wall
    Involvement of the ovary
    Angiolymphatic invasion
    Status of surgical margins of resection (if applicable)
    Any additional pathologic findings (in the tube or any other organ submitted)
    Histologic findings in lymph nodes
      Diagnosis by specific clinical site (as submitted by clinician)
      Total number of lymph nodes (per clinical site) involved by metastatic neoplasm/total number of lymph nodes examined
      Presence of extracapsular invasion by tumor
      Any additional pathologic findings
    Histologic findings in additional tissue samples submitted (including the presence of metastatic tumor, direct extension, or second primary; any additional pathologic findings)
    Results of special studies (receptors, flow cytometry, cytogenetics)
    Comment on any particular features of the tumor or pertinent clinicopathologic correlation

*Note: After the diagnosis of the resected specimens, the information should be used to provide proper staging using the TNM staging system (American Joint Committee on Cancer) and the FIGO staging system (International Federation of Gynecology and Obstetrics)[158]. The pAJCC staging and the FIGO staging should be included in the final report.[31, 127, 151, 159]
†It may be difficult to distinguish whether a tumor that involves the fallopian tube and the ipsilateral ovary is an ovarian or a tubal primary.

**TABLE 38-2.** Prognosis

| Neoplasm | Diagnosis | Prognosis |
|---|---|---|
| Serous carcinoma | High-grade carcinoma with nuclear pleomorphism, hyperchromasia, brisk mitotic activity, and necrosis. Architectural patterns include papillary, glandular, and solid. Transition from benign to malignant tubal epithelium can help establish unequivocal tubal origin | Poor. Most patients are at an advanced stage at the time of diagnosis |

FIGO is used widely, although even well-established and acceptable staging systems may not be useful in predicting the natural history of tubal carcinomas. According to one study,[80] cancers arising in the fimbriated end of the tube may have a worse prognosis than cancers arising from the tubal wall, most likely as a result of their relationship with the peritoneal cavity. These authors criticized the ability of the current FIGO staging system to stage tubal malignancies adequately.[80, 127] Despite the proximity of such tumors to the peritoneal cavity, their fimbrial origin hampers access to the tubal wall, precluding the establishment of tubal wall invasion required for FIGO stage I. For that purpose, the authors recommended a new category for such neoplasms: stage I(F).[80]

Treatment modalities for primary tubal malignancies include hysterectomy with bilateral salpingo-oophorectomy, associated when necessary with chemotherapy or radiation therapy or both. The CA-125 marker is a membrane glycoprotein present in the epithelium of benign, malignant, and ectopic endometrium, endocervix, fallopian tubes, peritoneum, pleura, pericardium, and müllerian ducts.[128] Serum levels of CA-125 are elevated in cases of tubal carcinoma and can aid in the evaluation of recurrence or progression of the disease. Elevations of this serum marker should be interpreted with some caution, however, because they also can be noted in association with numerous benign and malignant gynecologic and nongynecologic conditions.[128]

Unusual primary malignancies of the fallopian tubes include malignant mixed müllerian (mesodermal) tumors (carcinosarcomas)[129] and pure sarcomas.[130-133] In malignant mixed müllerian tumors, epithelial and mesenchymal elements are malignant. They can display homologous or heterologous elements. The term *homologous* is used when the mesenchymal tumor components are malignant counterparts of tissues indigenous to the tubes, such as leiomyosarcoma. *Heterologous* is used when the malignant components are counterparts of tissues not normally present in the tubal wall, such as chondrosarcoma or rhabdomyosarcoma. Leiomyosarcoma is the most common pure primary sarcoma to arise in the fallopian tubes.[132, 133] A case of primary tubal pure embryonal rhabdomyosarcoma has been reported.[131] Secondary involvement of the fallopian tubes by metastatic carcinoma is a more common phenomenon than involvement by a primary malig-nancy. The most common metastatic malignancies are of ovarian origin.

## Torsion and Prolapse

Torsion of the adnexal structures is infrequent and can be due to a variety of causes. Often asymptomatic, adnexal torsion might present clinically as chronic lower abdominal pain or as an acute abdomen.[134] Although enlargement of an ovary or a tube is often a predisposing factor, the entire adnexa and a normal ovary or fallopian tube can undergo torsion.[135] Accessory fallopian tubes or paratubal structures also may undergo torsion.[136] Torsion is seen more often in women of reproductive age, but postmenopausal women and children may experience it.[134] Torsion of normal ovaries or fallopian tubes or both has been reported in children and seems to show a predilection for the right side.[137-139] Cases in which absent uterine adnexal structures are not associated with urinary tract defects often are considered likely to represent asymptomatic torsion with subsequent resorption of the adnexal tissue.[4, 140, 141] A case of antenatal torsion of the fallopian tube and ovary also has been described.[142]

The torsed structures undergo gross and microscopic changes that most likely reflect the manner and the acute or chronic nature of the time frame in which the event took place. Intermittent pain can reflect episodes of torsion followed by untwisting of the tissue over time. Edema and hemorrhage result from vascular events, such as occlusion and thrombosis. Eventually, tissue necrosis (gangrene) develops; granulation tissue formation may follow. The previously described gross and microscopic changes tend to involve the normal structures and any pathologic entity, such as ectopic pregnancy or carcinoma, that is associated with the development of the torsion.

## Paratubal Lesions

Paramesonephric and mesonephric duct remnants as well as mesothelial inclusion cysts (including Walthard's cell rests) may undergo cystic dilatation and clinically present as paratubal lesions. The so-called adnexal tumor of probable wolffian origin (see later) usually arises in the broad ligament[143, 144] but also may originate in association with the fallopian tube.

## BROAD LIGAMENT

As a consequence of the midline fusion of the paramesonephric ducts, bilateral transverse folds of pelvic peritoneum are created and are known as the *broad ligaments of the uterus*.[9a] They extend from the lateral aspect of the uterus to the pelvic wall. Numerous structures are located within the connective tissue of these double layers of peritoneum known as the *parametrium*. They include the following: fallopian tubes (upper free edge), round ligaments of the uterus, ovarian ligaments, and uterine, tubal, and ovarian vessels.[9a] The ovaries are located on the posterior aspect of the broad ligaments. The broad ligament can be divided into three parts: 1) mesovarium, 2) mesosalpinx, and 3) mesometrium.[9a] The mesovarium is the peritoneal fold between the anterior border of the ovary and the posterior surface of the broad ligament. The mesosalpinx encompasses the area between the mesovarium and the fallopian tube. Most of the broad ligament corresponds to the area below the mesovarium, the mesometrium.[9a] Microscopic examination shows that the peritoneum consists of a single layer of cuboidal mesothelial cells associated with underlying connective tissue that is continuous with the peritoneum covering other pelvic structures and the pelvic walls.

Paramesonephric (müllerian) and mesonephric (wolffian) duct remnants can be found within the parametrial soft tissue. Adrenal rests consisting of adrenal cortical–type tissue can be identified in the broad ligaments as small soft yellow nodules or as incidental microscopic findings. Functional adrenal cortical adenomas may arise from these remnants.[145]

### Endometriosis and Endosalpingiosis

Endometriosis of the ligamentous structures associated with the uterus (broad ligaments, round ligaments) is a common finding.[146] The lesions can be pigmented and nodular or cystic; they may be complicated by adhesion formation. The histologic features of the endometriotic foci are similar to those encountered in other areas of the body. The smooth muscle of the ligamentous tissue can surround the endometriotic foci in a concentric arrangement, similar to the phenomenon in the fallopian tube or the peritoneum, resulting in grossly visible nodularities. Endometriotic foci can undergo histologic changes associated with the hormonal fluctuations of the menstrual cycle and pregnancy, although they frequently are out of synchrony. Displacement of the ureters[147] has been reported in association with endometriosis of the broad ligament. Endosalpingiosis and mesothelial inclusion cysts also may occur in the broad ligament.

### Mesonephric Duct Remnants

Remnants of the paramesonephric and mesonephric ducts are common in the broad ligament, and their histologic features are similar to those encountered in the fallopian tube. They may undergo cystic dilatation and metaplastic changes. A case of an endometrial stromal sarcoma involving the broad ligament and arising in endometriosis of a paramesonephric duct cyst has been reported.[148]

### Cysts

Benign, malignant, and infectious lesions of the broad ligament have the potential to undergo cystic dilatation as a result of degeneration, increased production of luminal fluid content, or bleeding. Such cysts, independent of their nature, may undergo torsion and rupture, with possible catastrophic complications. A rare case of a broad ligament cyst presenting clinically as a groin hernia has been reported.[149] Cysts of the broad ligament may masquerade as primary lesions of the ovary, fallopian tubes, or uterus on evaluation by radiologic or ultrasonographic means, potentially resulting in inappropriate preoperative assessment and selection of the wrong surgical procedure.

### Leiomyomas

Primary leiomyomas of the broad ligament are uncommon; however, they are the most common solid tumor occurring in the area. Although histologic evaluation shows they exhibit features similar to those of their uterine counterpart, the possibility that they may represent uterine lesions (most likely subserosal) that parasitize the ligamentous tissue and eventually detach from their origin cannot be excluded completely. In cases of uterine intravenous leiomyomatosis, the gross involvement of the periuterine vessels may simulate lesions of the broad ligament. A case mimicking Meigs' syndrome has been reported in association with a broad ligament leiomyoma.[150]

### Neoplastic Lesions

Primary benign and malignant neoplasms of the broad ligament are rare; however, virtually every entity described in association with the ovary and fallopian tube has been described in the broad ligament. Overall, müllerian-type tumors seem to be the most common epithelial neoplasms in this area, with serous cystadenoma being the most common lesion.[151] Serous tumors of borderline malignancy (low malignant potential) also occur with some frequency. Regarding primary müllerian-type carcinomas, the most common types appear to be endometrioid and clear cell types followed by serous adenocarcinomas. Endometriosis has been described in association with several tumors arising in the broad ligament.[152]

The female adnexal tumor of probable wolffian origin (FATPWO) is a rare neoplasm that arises primarily in the broad ligament, in the retroperitoneal area, in the ovary, or as a pedunculated lesion attached to the fallopian tube. Because most arise in the broad ligament, where mesonephric duct remnants are common, a wolffian origin for these tumors has been favored.[143, 144] Patients range in age from 15 to 81. The tumor usually presents as a unilateral, predominantly solid mass, with a tan or yellow cut surface averaging 12 cm in size. Hemorrhage and necrosis are unusual; calcifications can be present. Microscopic examination shows FATPWOs may be solid or cystic or display a combination of both patterns (Fig. 38–14 and CD Fig. 38–14). The tumor cells usually are epithelioid, with relatively bland, round nuclei, although spindled cells also can be identified. The cells may be arranged in tubules with eosinophilic secretions or in solid sheets. Mitotic activity may be found but usually is not marked. The stroma is fibrous and of variable amount. The immunohistochemical profile of the tumor favors a wolffian origin, according to some workers.[153] In one study of 25 FATPWOs,[153] all of the tumors exhibited positivity for pan–cytokeratin (AE1/3,CK1) and vimentin; focal staining with cytokeratin 7 was noted in 88% of the cases. Epithelial membrane antigen positivity was present in 12% of cases; keratin 903 positivity in 17% of cases; estrogen receptor positivity in 28% of cases; progesterone receptor positivity in 24% of cases; inhibin positivity in 68% of cases; and calretinin positivity in 91% of cases. The differential diagnosis mainly includes Sertoli–stromal cell tumors and metastatic carcinomas. FATPWOs with malignant behavior have been described, but most of these tumors follow a benign clinical course.[143, 144, 153] Although aggressive behavior has been associated with malignant histologic features, tumors with bland histologic features have been noted to behave in an aggressive fashion.

Leiomyosarcoma is the most common primary sarcoma of the broad ligament.[154] Rare sarcomas, including Ewing's sarcoma,[155] alveolar rhabdomyosarcoma,[156] and alveolar soft part sarcoma,[157] have been described as primary tumors of the broad ligament. Metastatic lesions from virtually anywhere in the body, especially the urogenital tract, may involve the broad ligament secondarily and present as the initial symptom of metastatic disease.

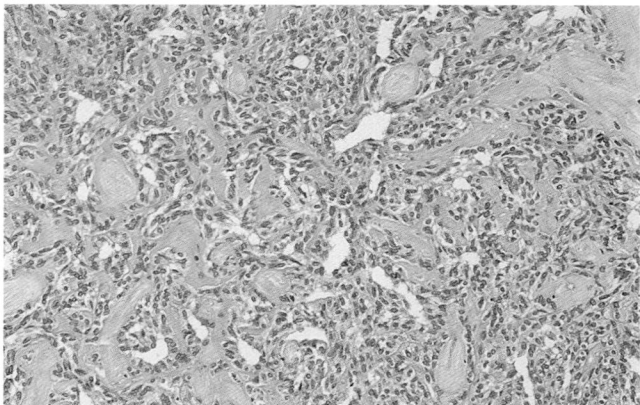

**FIGURE 38–14.** Microscopic section from a female adnexal tumor of probable wolffian origin (FATPWO) arising in the broad ligament.

# REFERENCES

1. Sadler TW: Langman's Medical Embryology. 5th ed. Baltimore, Williams & Wilkins, 1985.
2. DeCherney AH, Cholst I, Naftolin F: Structure and function of the fallopian tubes following exposure to diethylstilbestrol (DES) during gestation. Fertil Steril 36:741–745, 1981.
3. Daw E: Duplication of the uterine tube. Obstet Gynecol 42:137–138, 1973.
4. Georgy FM, Viechnicki MB: Absence of an ovary and uterine tube. Obstet Gynecol 44:441–442, 1974.
5. Silverman HV, Greenberg EI: Absence of segment of the proximal portion of a fallopian tube. Obstet Gynecol 62:905–915, 1983.
6. Tulusan AH: Complete absence of the muscular layer of the ampullary part of the fallopian tubes. Arch Gynecol 234:279–281, 1984.
7. Beyth V, Kopolovic J: Accessory tubes. A possible contributing factor in infertility. Fertil Steril 38:382–383, 1982.
8. Lewis JD: Hilus cell hyperplasia of ovaries and tubes. Obstet Gynecol 24:728–731, 1964.
9. Mason TE, Quagliariello JR: Ectopic pancreas in the fallopian tube. Obstet Gynecol 48:705–735, 1976.
9a. Hollinshead WH: Textbook of Anatomy. 3rd ed. Hagerstown, MD, Harper & Row, 1974.
10. Woodruff JD, Pauerstein CJ: The Fallopian Tube. Structure, Function, Pathology and Management. Baltimore, Williams & Wilkins, 1969.
11. Mastroianni Jr L, Comis J: Capacitation, ovum maturation, fertilization and preimplantation development in the oviduct. Gynecol Invest 6:226–233, 1975.
12. Kutteh WH, Hatch KD, Blackwell RE, et al: Secretory immune system of the female reproductive tract. I. Immunoglobulin and secretory component-containing cells. Obstet Gynecol 71:56–60, 1988.
13. Morris H, Emms H, Visser T, et al: Lymphoid tissue of the normal fallopian tube—a form of mucosal associated lymphoid tissue (MALT)? Int J Gynecol Pathol 5:11–22, 1986.
14. Jansen RPS: Endocrine response in the fallopian tube. Endocr Rev 5:525–551, 1984.
15. Flickinger GL, Meulcher EK, Mikhail G: Estradiol receptor in the human fallopian tube. Fertil Steril 25:900–903, 1974.
16. Gaddum-Rose P, Rumery RE, Blandau RT, et al: Studies on the mucosa of postmenopausal oviducts. Surface appearance, ciliary activity, and the effect of estrogen treatment. Fertil Steril 26:951–969, 1975.
17. Donnez J, Casanas-Roux F, Caprasse J, et al: Cyclic changes in ciliation, cell height, and mitotic activity in human tubal epithelium during reproductive life. Fertil Steril 43:554–559, 1985.
18. Patek E, Nilsson L: Scanning electron microscopic observations on the ciliogenesis of the infundibulum of the human fetal and adult fallopian tube epithelium. Fertil Steril 24:819–831, 1973.
19. Ramirez NC, Lawrence WD, Ginsberg KA: Ectopic pregnancy. A 5-year recent study and literature review of the last 50 years. J Reprod Med 41:733–740, 1996.
20. Eschenbach DA: New concepts of obstetric and gynecologic infection. Arch Intern Med 142:2039–2044, 1982.

21. Chow AW, Malkasian KL, Marshall JR, et al: The bacteriology of acute pelvic inflammatory disease. Am J Obstet Gynecol 122:876–879, 1975.
22. Sweet RL: Anaerobic infections of the female genital tract. Am J Obstet Gynecol 122:891–901, 1975.
23. Ward ME, Watt PJ, Robertson JN: The human fallopian tube. A laboratory model for gonococcal infection. J Infect Dis 129:650–659, 1974.
24. Sweet RL, Blankfort-Doyle M, Robbie MO, et al: The occurrence of chlamydial and gonococcal salpingitis during the menstrual cycle. JAMA 255:2062–2064, 1986.
25. Rubu A, Czernobilsky B: Tubal ligation. A bacteriologic, histologic and clinical study. Obstet Gynecol 36:199–203, 1970.
26. Nassberg S, McKay DG, Hertig AT: Physiologic salpingitis. Am J Obstet Gynecol 67:130, 1954.
27. David A, Garcia CR, Czernobilsky B: Human hydrosalpinx. Histologic study and chemical composition of the fluid. Am J Obstet Gynecol 105:400–411, 1969.
28. Cheung ANY, Young RH, Scully RE: Pseudocarcinomatous hyperplasia of the fallopian tube associated with salpingitis. Report of 14 cases. Am J Surg Pathol 18:1125–1130, 1994.
29. Brooks JJ, Wheeler JE: Granulomatous salpingitis secondary to Crohn's disease. Obstet Gynecol 49(1 suppl):31–33, 1977.
30. Clement PB, Young RH, Scully RE: Liesegang rings in the female genital tract. A report of three cases. Int J Gynecol Pathol 8:271–276, 1989.
31. Wheeler JE: Diseases of the fallopian tube. In Kurman RJ (ed): Blaustein's Pathology of the Female Genital Tract. 5th ed. New York, Springer-Verlag, 2002, pp 617–648.
32. Schaefer G: Tuberculosis of the female genital tract. Clin Obstet Gynecol 13:965–998, 1970.
33. Pauerstein CJ, Woodruff JD: Cellular patterns in proliferative and anaplastic disease of the fallopian tube. Am J Obstet Gynecol 96:486–492, 1966.
34. Dische FE, Burt JM, Davison NJH: Tubo-ovarian actinomycosis associated with intra-uterine contraceptive devices. J Obstet Gynaecol Br Commonw 81:724–729, 1974.
35. Gelfand M, Ross MD, Blair DM: Distribution and extent of schistosomiasis in female pelvic organs with special reference to the genital tract, as determined at autopsy. Am J Trop Med Hyg 20:846–849, 1971.
36. Symmers WSC: Pathology of oxyuriasis. Arch Pathol 50:475–516, 1950.
37. Abraham JL, Spore WW, Benirschke K: Cysticercosis of the fallopian tube. Histology and microanalysis. Hum Pathol 13:665–670, 1982.
38. Georgakopoulos PA, Gogas CG, Sariyannis HG: Hydatid disease of the female genitalia. Obstet Gynecol 55:555–559, 1980.
39. Murray JJ, Clark CA, Lands RH: Reactivation blastomycosis presenting as a tuboovarian abscess. Obstet Gynecol 64:828–830, 1984.
40. Bylund DJ, Nanfro JJ, Marsh WL: Coccidioidomycosis of the female genital tract. Arch Pathol Lab Med 110:232–235, 1986.
41. Wlodarski FM, Trainer TD: Granulomatous oophoritis and salpingitis associated with Crohn's disease of the appendix. Am J Obstet Gynecol 122:527–528, 1975.
42. Kay S: Sarcoidosis of the fallopian tubes. J Obstet Gynaecol Br Emp 63:871, 1956.
43. Copeland W, Hawley PC, Teteris NJ: Gynecologic amyloidosis. Am J Obstet Gynecol 1153:555–556, 1985.
44. Roberts JT, Roberts GT, Maudsley RF: Indolent granulomatous necrosis in patients with previous tubal diathermy. Am J Obstet Gynecol 129:112–113, 1977.
45. Kuo T-T, Hsueh S: Mucicarminophilic histiocytosis. A polyvinyl pyrrolidone (PVP) storage disease simulating signet-ring cell carcinoma. Am J Surg Pathol 8:419–428, 1984.
46. Ladefoged C, Lorentzen M: Xanthogranulomatous inflammation of the female genital tract. Histopathology 13:541–551, 1988.
47. Aikat BK, Radhakrishnan VV, Rao MS: Malacoplakia—a report of two cases with review of the literature. Indian J Pathol Bacteriol 16:64–70, 1973.
48. Benjamin CL, Beaver DC: Pathogenesis of salpingitis isthmica nodosa. Am J Clin Pathol 21:212–222, 1951.
49. Majmudar B, Henderson PH, Semple E: Salpingitis isthmica nodosa. A risk factor for tubal pregnancy. Obstet Gynecol 62:73–78, 1986.
50. Saracoglu FO, Mungan T, Tanzer F: Salpingitis isthmica nodosa in infertility and ectopic pregnancy. Gynecol Obstet Invest 34:202–205, 1992.
51. Trends in ectopic pregnancies. United States, 1970–1985. Stat Bull Metrop Insur Co 68:24–30, 1987.
52. Raziel A, Golan A, Pansky M, et al: Ovarian pregnancy. A report of 20 cases in one institution. Am J Obstet Gynecol 163:1182–1185, 1990.
53. Martin JR, Sessums JK, Martin RW, et al: Abdominal pregnancy. Current concepts of management. Obstet Gynecol 71:549–557, 1988.
54. Barbosa JA, de Freitas LA, Mota MA: Primary pregnancy of the liver. A case report. Pathol Res Pract 187:329–331, 1991.
55. Yackel DB, Pantom ONM, Martin DJ, et al: Splenic pregnancy—case report. Obstet Gynecol 71 (3 pt 2):471–473, 1988.
56. Adair CD, Benrubi GI, Sanchez-Ramos L, et al: Bilateral tubal ectopic pregnancies after bilateral partial salpingectomy. A case report. J Reprod Med 39:131–133, 1994.
57. Winer AE, Bergman WD, Fields C: Combined intra- and extrauterine pregnancy Am J Obstet Gynecol 74:170–178, 1957.
58. Dimitry ES, Subak-Sharpe R, Mills M: Nine cases of heterotopic pregnancies in 4 years of in vitro fertilization. Fertil Steril 53:107–110, 1990.
59. Dubuisson JB, Aubriot FX, Cardone V, et al: Tubal causes of ectopic pregnancy. Fertil Steril 46:970–972, 1986.
60. Breen JL: A 21 yr survey of 654 ectopic pregnancies. Am J Obstet Gynecol 106:1004–1019, 1969.
61. Hu CY, Cheng FK: Tubal pregnancy. Pathologic analysis of 300 cases. Chin Med J 76:517–528, 1958.
62. Randall S, Buckley HC, Fox H: Placentation of the fallopian tube. Int J Gynecol Pathol 6:132–139, 1987.
63. Egarter C, Husslein P: Proliferative activity of ectopic trophoblastic tissue. Hum Reprod 10:2441–2444, 1995.
64. Demir R, Demir N, Ustenel I: The fine structure of normal and ectopic (tubal) human placental villi as revealed by scanning and transmission electron microscope. Zentralbl Pathol 140:427–442, 1995.
65. Huettner PC, Gersell DJ: Placental site nodule. A clinicopathologic study of 38 cases. Int J Gynecol Pathol 13:191–198, 1994.
66. Shih IM, Seidman JD, Kurman RJ: Placental site nodule and characterization of distinctive types of intermediate trophoblast. Hum Pathol 30:687–694, 1999.
67. Kouvidou C, Karaylanni M, Liapi-Avgeri G, et al: Old ectopic pregnancy remnants with morphological features of placental site nodule occurring in fallopian tube and broad ligament. Pathol Res Pract 196:329–332, 2000.
68. Campello TR, Fittipaldi H, O'Valle F, et al: Extrauterine (tubal) placental site nodule. Histopathology 32:562–565, 1998.
69. Doss BJ, Ramirez NC, Lawrence WD: Failed methotrexate-treated ectopic pregnancies. Clinicopathologic correlations. Int J Surg Pathol 5:83–94, 1997.
70. Jacques SM, Qureshi F, Ramirez NC: Retained trophoblastic tissue in fallopian tubes. A consequence of unsuspected ectopic pregnancies. Int J Gynecol Pathol 16:219–224, 1997.
71. Stock RJ: Histopathology of the fallopian tubes with recurrent tubal pregnancy. Obstet Gynecol 75:9–14, 1990.
72. Lurain JR, Brewer JI, Torok EE: Gestational trophoblastic disease. Treatment results at the Brewer Trophoblastic Disease Center. Obstet Gynecol 60:354–360, 1982.
73. Miller JH, Weinberg RK, Canino NL, et al: The pattern of infertility diagnoses in women of advanced reproductive age. Am J Obstet Gynecol 181:952–957, 1999.
74. Stock RJ: Histopathologic changes in fallopian tubes subsequent to sterilization procedures. Int J Gynecol Pathol 2:13–27, 1983.
75. Halbert SA, Patton DL, Zartskie PW, et al: Function and structure of cilia in the fallopian tube of an infertile woman with Kartagener's syndrome. Hum Reprod 12:55–58, 1997.
76. Czernobilsky B, Silverstein A: Salpingitis in ovarian endometriosis. Fertil Steril 30:45–49, 1978.

77. Seidman JD, Oberer S, Bitterman P: Pathogenesis of pseudoxanthomatous salpingitis. Mod Pathol 6:53–55, 1993.

78. Clement PB, Young RH, Scully RE: Necrotic pseudoxanthomatous nodules of ovary and peritoneum in endometriosis. Am J Surg Pathol 12:390–397, 1988.

79. Stock RJ: Post salpingectomy endometriosis. A reassessment. Obstet Gynecol 60:560–570, 1982.

80. Alvarado-Cabrero I, Navani SS, Young RH, et al: Tumors of the fimbriated end of the fallopian tube. A clinicopathologic analysis of 20 cases, including nine carcinomas. Int J Gynecol Pathol 16:189–196, 1997.

81. Seidman JD: Mucinous lesions of the fallopian tube. A report of seven cases. Am J Surg Pathol 18:1205–1212, 1994.

82. Mainguene C, Hugol D, Hofman P, et al: Adenomatoid tumors of the uterus. Study of 5 cases with immunohistochemical and ultrastructural confirmation of the mesothelial origin. Arch Anat Cytol Pathol 44:174–179, 1996.

83. Bartnik J, Powell WS, Mouber-Katz S, et al: Metaplastic papillary tumor of the fallopian tube. Case report, immunohistochemical features and review of the literature. Arch Pathol Lab Med 113:545–547, 1989.

84. Keeney G, Thrasher TV: Metaplastic papillary tumor of the fallopian tube. A case report with ultrastructure. Int J Gynecol Pathol 7:86–92, 1988.

85. Egan MAJ, Russell P: Transitional (urothelial) cell metaplasia of the fallopian tube mucosa. Morphological assessment of three cases. Int J Gynecol Pathol 15:72–76, 1996.

86. Gisser SD: Obstructing fallopian tube papilloma. Int J Gynecol Pathol 5:179–182, 1986.

87. Gilks CB, Clement PB, Hart WR, et al: Uterine adenomyomas excluding atypical polypoid adenomyomas and adenomyomas of endocervical type. A clinicopathologic study of 30 cases of underemphasized lesion that may cause diagnostic problems with brief consideration of adenomyomas of other female genital tract sites. Int J Gynecol Pathol 19:195–205, 2000.

88. Ebrahimi T, Okagaki T: Hemangioma of the fallopian tube. Am J Obstet Gynecol 115:864–865, 1973.

89. Joglekar VM: Hemangioma of the fallopian tube. Br J Obstet Gynaecol 86:823–825, 1979.

90. Carinelli I, Senzani F, Bruni M, et al: Lipomatous tumors of uterus, fallopian tube, and ovary. Clin Exp Obstet Gynecol 7:215–218, 1980.

91. Katz DA, Thom D, Bogard P, et al: Angiomyolipoma of the fallopian tube. Am J Obstet Gynecol 148:341–343, 1984.

92. Kobayashi T, Suzuki K, Arai T, et al: Angiomyofibroblastoma arising from the fallopian tube. Obstet Gynecol 94(5 pt 2):833–834, 1999.

93. Mazzarella P, Okagaki T, Richard RM: Teratoma of the uterine tube. A case report and review of the literature. Obstet Gynecol 39:381–388, 1972.

94. Alenghat E, Sassone M, Talerman A: Mature, solid teratoma of the fallopian tube. J Reprod Med 27:484–486, 1982.

95. Hoda SA, Huvos AG: Struma salpingitis associated with struma ovarii. Am J Surg Pathol 17:1187–1189, 1993.

96. Yoshioka T, Tanaka T: Mature solid teratoma of the fallopian tube. Case report. Eur J Obstet Gynaecol Reprod Biol 89:205–206, 2000.

97. Baginski L, Yazigi R, Sandstand J: Immature (malignant) teratoma of the fallopian tube. Am J Obstet Gynecol 160:671–672, 1989.

98. Nasu K, Matsui N, Kawano Y, et al: Adenocarcinoma arising from a mature cystic teratoma of the ovary. A case report of successful treatment with cisplatin-based chemotherapy. Gynecol Obstet Invest 41:143–146, 1996.

99. Astall EC, Brewster JA, Lonsdale R: Malignant carcinoid tumour arising in a mature teratoma of the fallopian tube. Histopathology 36:282–283, 2000.

100. Doss BJ, Jacques SM, Qureshi F, et al: Immature teratomas of the genital tract in older women. Gynecol Oncol 73:433–438, 1999.

101. Li S, Zimmerman RL, LiVolsi VA: Mixed malignant germ cell tumor of the fallopian tube. Int J Gynecol Pathol 18:183–185, 1999.

102. Francke ML, Mihaescu A, Chaubert P: Isolated necrotizing arteritis of the female genital tract. A clinicopathologic and immunohistochemical study of 11 cases. Int J Gynecol Pathol 17:193–200, 1998.

103. Pilch H, Schaffer U, Gunzel S, et al: Asymptomatic necrotizing arteritis of the female genital tract. Eur J Obstet Gynaecol Reprod Biol 91:191–196, 2000.

104. Lombard CM, Moore MH, Seifer DB: Diagnosis of systemic polyarteritis nodosa following total abdominal hysterectomy and bilateral salpingo-oophorectomy. A case report. Int J Gynecol Pathol 5:63–68, 1986.

105. Ganesa R, Ferriman SR, Mejer L, et al: Vasculitis of the female genital tract with clinicopathologic correlation. A study of 46 cases with follow-up. Int J Gynecol Pathol 19:258–265, 2000.

106. Stern J, Buscema J, Parmley T, et al: Atypical epithelial proliferations in the fallopian tube. Am J Obstet Gynecol 140:309–312, 1981.

107. Pickel H, Reich O, Tammussino K: Bilateral atypical hyperplasia of the fallopian tube associated with tamoxifen. A report of two cases. Int J Gynecol Pathol 17:284–285, 1998.

108. Robey SS, Silva EG: Epithelial hyperplasia of the fallopian tube. Its association with serous borderline tumors of the ovary. Int J Gynecol Pathol 8:214–220, 1989.

109. Yanai-Inbar I, Siriaunkgul S, Silverberg SG: Mucosal epithelial proliferations of the fallopian tube. A particular association with ovarian serous tumor of low malignant potential? Int J Gynecol Pathol 14:107–113, 1995.

110. Yanai-Inbar I, Silverberg SG: Mucosal epithelial proliferations of the fallopian tube. Prevalence, clinical associations, and optimal strategy for histopathologic assessment. Int J Gynecol Pathol 19:139–144, 2000.

111. Dallenbach-Hellweg G, Nichoff B: Epithelium of the tubes in correlation with histological findings in endometrium and ovary. Virchows Arch A Pathol Anat Histopathol 354:66–79, 1971.

112. Bannatyne P, Russell P: Early adenocarcinoma of the fallopian tubes. A case for multifocal tumorigenesis. Diagn Gynecol Obstet 3:49–60, 1981.

113. Tziortziotis DV, Bouros AC, Ziogas VS, et al: Clear cell hyperplasia of the fallopian tube epithelium associated with ectopic pregnancy. Report of a case. Int J Gynaecol Obstet 17:79–80, 1997.

114. Schneider C, Wight E, Perucchini D, et al: Primary carcinoma of the fallopian tube. A report of 19 cases with literature review. Eur J Gynaecol Oncol 21:578–582, 2000.

115. Schiller HM, Silverberg SG: Staging and prognosis in primary carcinoma of the fallopian tube. Cancer 28:389–395, 1971.

116. Rabinovich A: Primary carcinoma of the fallopian tube. Study of 11 cases. Eur J Obstet Gynaecol Reprod Biol 91:169–175, 2000.

117. Heselmeyer K, Hellstrom AC, Blegen H, et al: Primary carcinoma of the fallopian tube. Comparative genomic hybridization reveals high genetic instability and a specific, recurrent pattern of chromosomal aberrations. Int J Gynecol Pathol 17:245–254, 1998.

118. Hellstrom AC, Blegen H, Malec M, et al: Recurrent fallopian tube carcinoma. p53 mutation and clinical course. Int J Gynecol Pathol 19:145–151, 2000.

119. Cheung AN, So KF, Ngan HY, et al: Primary squamous cell carcinoma of the fallopian tube. Int J Gynecol Pathol 13:92–95, 1994.

120. Moore DH, Woosley JT, Reddick RL, et al: Adenosquamous carcinoma of the fallopian tube. A clinicopathologic case report with verification of the diagnosis by immunohistochemical and ultrastructural studies. Am J Obstet Gynecol 157(4 pt 1):903–905, 1987.

121. Herbold DR, Axelrod JH, Bobowski SJ, et al: Glassy cell carcinoma of the fallopian tube. A case report. Int J Gynecol Pathol 7:384–390, 1988.

122. Navani SS, Alvarado-Cabrero I, Young RH, et al: Endometrioid carcinoma of the fallopian tube. A clinicopathologic analysis of 26 cases. Gynecol Oncol 63:371–378, 1996.

123. Voet RL, Lifshitz S: Primary clear cell adenocarcinoma of the fallopian tube. Light microscopic and ultrastructural findings. Int J Gynecol Pathol 1:292–298, 1982.

124. Koshiyama M, Konishi I, Yoshide M, et al: Transitional cell carcinoma of the fallopian tube. A light and electron microscopy study. Int J Gynecol Pathol 13:175–180, 1994.

125. Jackson-York G, Ramzy I: Synchronous papillary mucinous adenocarcinoma of the endocervix and fallopian tubes. Int J Gynecol Pathol 11:63–67, 1992.

126. Daya D, Young RH, Scully RE: Endometrioid carcinoma of the fallopian tube resembling an adnexal tumor of probable wolffian origin. A report of six cases. Int J Gynecol Pathol 11:122–130, 1992.

127. Alvarado-Cabrero I, Young RH, Vamvakas EC, et al: Carcinoma of the fallopian tube. A clinicopathological study of 105 cases with observations on staging and prognostic factors. Gynecol Oncol 72:367–379, 1999.

128. Molina R, Filella X, Jo J, et al: CA-125 in biological fluids. Int J Biol Mark 13:224–230, 1998.

129. Hom LC, Werschik C, Bilek K, et al: Diagnosis and clinical management in malignant mullerian tumors of the fallopian tube. A report of four cases and review of recent literature. Arch Gynecol Obstet 258:47–53, 1996.

130. Kohler U, Horn LC, Marzotko E, et al: Primary dedifferentiated leiomyosarcoma of the fallopian tube. Zentralbl Gynakol 119:237–240, 1997.

131. Buchwalter CL, Jenison EL, Fromm M, et al: Pure embryonal rhabdomyosarcoma of the fallopian tube. Gynecol Oncol 67:95–101, 1997.

132. Ebert A, Goetzbe B, Herbst H, et al: Primary leiomyosarcoma of the fallopian tube. Ann Oncol 6:618–619, 1995.

133. Jacoby AF, Fuller AF, Thor AD, et al: Primary leiomyosarcoma of the fallopian tube. Gynecol Oncol 51:404–407, 1993.

134. Lomano JM, Trelford JD, Ullery JC: Torsion of the uterine adnexa causing an acute abdomen. Obstet Gynecol 35:221–225, 1969.

135. Moravec WD, Angerman NS, Reale FR, et al: Torsion of the uterine adnexa. A clinicopathologic correlation. Int J Gynaecol Obstet 18:7–14, 1980.

136. Barlow B, Fajolu O, Leblanc W: Hydatid torsion. Am J Dis Child 132:1216–1217, 1978.

137. Ward MJA, Frazier TG: Torsion of normal uterine adnexa in childhood. Case report. Pediatrics 61:573–574, 1978.

138. Evans JP: Torsion of the normal uterine adnexa in premenarchal girls. J Pediatr Surg 13:195–196, 1978.

139. Farrell TP, Boal DK, Teele RL, et al: Acute torsion of normal uterine adnexa in children. Sonographic demonstration. Am J Radiol 139:1223–1225, 1982.

140. Nissen ED, Kent DR, Nissen SE, et al: Unilateral tubo-ovarian autoamputation. J Reprod Med 19:151, 1977.

141. Sebastian JA, Baker RL, Cordray D: Asymptomatic infarction and separation of ovary and distal uterine tube. Obstet Gynecol 41:531, 1973.

142. Dresler S: Antenatal torsion of a normal ovary and fallopian tube. Am J Dis Child 131:236, 1972.

143. Kariminejad MH, Scully RE: Female adnexal tumor of probable wolffian origin. A distinctive pathologic entity. Cancer 31:671–677, 1973.

144. Daya D: Malignant female adnexal tumor of probable wolffian origin with review of the literature. Arch Pathol Lab Med 118:310–312, 1994.

145. Adashi EY, Rosenshein NB, Parmley TH, et al: Histogenesis of the broad ligament adrenal rest. Int J Gynaecol Obstet 18:102–104, 1980.

146. Jenkins S, Olive DL, Haney AF: Endometriosis. Pathogenetic implications of the anatomic distribution. Obstet Gynecol 67:335–338, 1986.

147. Nackley AC, Yeko TR: Ureteral displacement associated with pelvic peritoneal defects and endometriosis. J Am Assoc Gynecol Laparosc 7:131–133, 2000.

148. Persaud V, Anderson MF: Endometrial stromal sarcoma of the broad ligament arising in an area of endometriosis in a paramesonephric cyst. Case report. Br J Obstet Gynaecol 84:149–152, 1977.

149. Pridjian G, Pridjian AK: Paraovarian cyst presenting as a groin hernia. A case report. J Reprod Med 37:100–102, 1992.

150. Bown RS, Marley JL, Cassoni AM: Pseudo-Meigs' syndrome due to broad ligament leiomyoma. A mimic of metastatic ovarian carcinoma. Clin Oncol 10:192–201, 1998.

151. Scully RE, Young RH, Clement PB: Tumors of the Ovary, Maldeveloped Gonads, Fallopian Tube, and Broad Ligament. Atlas of Tumor Pathology. Fascicle 23. Washington, DC, Armed Forces Institute of Pathology, 1996.

152. Aslani M, Scully RE: Primary carcinoma of the broad ligament. Report of four cases and review of the literature. Cancer 64:1540–1545, 1989.

153. Devouassoux-Shisheboran M, Silver SA, Tavassoli FA: Wolffian adnexal tumor, so-called female adnexal tumor of probable Wolffian origin (FATWO). Immunohistochemical evidence in support of a Wolffian origin. Hum Pathol 30:856–863, 1999.

154. Pekin T, Eren F, Pekin O: Leiomyosarcoma of the broad ligament. Case report and literature review. Eur J Gynaecol Oncol 21:318–319, 2000.

155. Longway SR, Lind HM, Haghighi P: Extraskeletal Ewing's sarcoma arising in the broad ligament. Arch Pathol Lab Med 110:1058–1061, 1986.

156. Copeland LJ, Sneige N, Striger CA, et al: Alveolar rhabdomyosarcoma of the female genitalia. Cancer 56:849–855, 1985.

157. Nielsen GP, Oliva E, Young RH, et al: Alveolar soft-part sarcoma of the female genital tract. A report of nine cases and review of the literature. Int J Gynecol Pathol 14:283–292, 1995.

158. Peterson F: Annual Report of the Results of Treatment in Gynecological Cancer. Stockholm, International Federation of Gynecology and Obstetrics, 1991.

159. Scully RE, Henson DE, Nielsen ML, et al: Protocol for the examination of specimens from patients with carcinoma of the fallopian tube. A basis for checklists. Arch Pathol Lab Med 123:33–38, 1999.

# 39

# Ovaries

Debra Budwit Novotny

**NEOPLASTIC LESIONS**
Classification
General Considerations
Surface Epithelial Tumors
Sex Cord–Stromal Tumors
Germ Cell Tumors
Mixed Germ Cell and Sex Cord–Stromal Tumors
Miscellaneous Tumors
Metastatic Tumors

**NON-NEOPLASTIC LESIONS**
Congenital Abnormalities
Inflammatory Diseases
Cysts
Pregnancy-Associated Lesions
Stromal Hyperplasia and Hyperthecosis
Massive Ovarian Edema and Fibromatosis
Other Surface and Stromal Proliferations
Stromal Metaplasias
Infertility

## NEOPLASTIC LESIONS

### Classification

The classification of ovarian tumors used in this chapter is that formulated and accepted by the World Health Organization and the International Society of Gynecological Pathologists with minor modifications[1] (Table 39–1). This scheme is largely based on morphology with consideration of embryology and presumed histogenesis, that is, surface epithelium, sex cord–stroma, germ cells, or other cells of origin.

### General Considerations

Pathogenesis, staging, grading, prognostic features, and therapy are discussed as warranted for the respective broad categories of ovarian tumors.

#### PROCESSING OF SPECIMENS

Specimens submitted for evaluation of an ovarian mass are processed to provide the necessary pathology information for appropriate staging, histologic typing, and grading.[2] The ovarian or adnexal mass is weighed and measured in three dimensions. If it is present, the fallopian tube is identified. The external surface of the mass is evaluated for areas of rupture; tumor excrescences are marked with ink. The mass should be serially sectioned at 1- to 2-cm intervals; ideally, one section per 1 to 2 cm of greatest tumor diameter is submitted for histologic examination. These sections should principally sample solid and thickened areas and the bases of papillary excrescences of tumor to evaluate for stromal invasion. Sections should also be submitted from any surface growths and to demonstrate the relationship of the fallopian tube to the tumor.

Staging procedures for an ovarian tumor may also include several other specimens. The contralateral ovary and tube are also processed as described. Involvement of the uterus should be documented; when it is present, it is usually noted on serosal surfaces. The omentum is measured; one to three sections are submitted from areas of grossly evident tumor, or at least three sections are submitted from the firmest palpable regions. Abdominal and pelvic peritoneal biopsy specimens are submitted separately according to site and are processed in toto. Additional slide levels are obtained from these small biopsy specimens as warranted, particularly for primary staging procedures. Lymph node dissections are also submitted separately and are processed as such with all lymph nodes evaluated from each region. Ascites and peritoneal washings obtained during surgery are also submitted for evaluation of the presence of malignant cells.

#### CONTENTS OF FINAL REPORT

In general, surgical pathology reports of ovarian tumors should include the surgical procedures performed and specimens submitted. Descriptors of the primary ovarian neoplasm include histologic type, grade, size or greatest tumor dimension, integrity of the capsule, and presence or absence of surface growths. Involvement of other submitted specimens should be indicated. Tumor implants are character-

**TABLE 39–1.** Histologic Classification of Ovarian Tumors*

Surface epithelial tumors
  Serous tumors
    Benign (cystadenoma, papillary cystadenoma, adenofibroma, cystadenofibroma)
    Low malignant potential (borderline, atypically proliferating)
    Malignant (adenocarcinoma, cystadenocarcinoma)
  Mucinous tumors, endocervical-like and intestinal types
    Benign (cystadenoma, adenofibroma, cystadenofibroma)
    Low malignant potential (borderline, atypically proliferating)
    Malignant (adenocarcinoma, cystadenocarcinoma)
  Endometrioid tumors
    Benign (adenoma, cystadenoma, adenofibroma, cystadenofibroma)
    Low malignant potential (borderline, atypically proliferating)
    Malignant
      Adenocarcinoma
      Adenocarcinoma with squamous differentiation
    Carcinosarcoma (malignant mixed mesodermal or müllerian tumor)
      Homologous
      Heterologous
    Adenosarcoma
    Endometrioid stromal sarcoma
  Clear cell tumors
    Benign
    Low malignant potential (borderline, atypically proliferating)
    Adenocarcinoma
  Transitional cell tumors
    Benign Brenner tumor
    Brenner tumor of low malignant potential (borderline, proliferating)
    Malignant Brenner tumor
    Transitional cell carcinoma (non-Brenner type)
  Squamous cell tumors
  Mixed epithelial tumors
  Undifferentiated carcinoma
  Other

Sex cord-stromal tumors
  Granulosa cell tumors
    Adult type
    Juvenile type
  Thecoma-fibroma group
    Thecoma
    Luteinized thecoma
    Fibroma
    Fibrosarcoma
    Sclerosing stromal tumor
    Stromal tumor with minor sex cord elements
    Unclassified

  Sertoli-Leydig cell tumors (androblastomas)
    Sertoli cell tumor
    Sertoli-Leydig cell tumor
      Well differentiated
      Intermediate differentiation
      Poorly differentiated (sarcomatoid)
      With heterologous elements
      Retiform
      Mixed
  Gynandroblastoma
  Sex cord tumor with annular tubules
  Steroid cell tumors (lipid cell tumors)
    Stromal luteoma
    Hilus cell tumor (Leydig cell tumor)
    Steroid cell tumor, not otherwise specified
  Unclassified

Germ cell tumors
  Dysgerminoma
  Endodermal sinus tumor (yolk sac tumor)
    Usual
    Polyvesicular vitelline
    Hepatoid
    Glandular
  Embryonal carcinoma
  Polyembryoma
  Choriocarcinoma
  Teratomas
    Immature
    Mature
      Monodermal or specialized
        Struma ovarii
        Dermoid
        Carcinoid
        Strumal carcinoid
        Mucinous carcinoid (adenocarcinoid)
        Neuroectodermal tumor
        Sebaceous tumor
        Other
      With malignant transformation
  Mixed germ cell tumors

Mixed germ cell and sex cord–stromal tumors
  Gonadoblastoma
  Unclassified

Miscellaneous tumors
  Small cell carcinoma, hypercalcemic and pulmonary types
  Tumors of rete ovarii
  Tumors of probable wolffian origin
  Soft tissue tumors
  Malignant lymphoma and leukemia

Metastatic tumors

* Classification as formulated by the World Health Organization and the International Society of Gynecological Pathologists with modifications.

ized as invasive or noninvasive, a distinction of particular importance for epithelial tumors of low malignant potential (LMP). Lymph node dissections are reported as the number of positive nodes found for the total number of nodes examined from each of the respective locations.

Checklists have been proposed as guidelines for the reporting of surgical pathology tumor specimens with the goal of ensuring inclusion of necessary pathology information for appropriate staging, treatment, and prognosis and to assist with standardization of reports within and between institutions.[3, 4] A sample checklist for surgical pathology reports of ovarian tumors is shown in Table 39–2.

## Surface Epithelial Tumors

This group of tumors is the most numerous and accounts for approximately two thirds of all ovarian neoplasms.[5] These tumors are considered to be derived from ovarian surface or germinal epithelium that develops embryologically from coelomic lining epithelium. Most tumors may develop from surface

## TABLE 39–2. Contents of the Final Report: Ovarian Cancer

Case No.:                              Operative procedure:

Diagnosis (include histologic type with percentage of each type if mixed, histologic grade, tumor size, presence of surface involvement, sites of extension, and metastases):

WHO* histologic type (include percentage of subtypes if mixed):

Histologic grade:

FIGO or GOG grade for epithelial tumors:
  Grade 1 or well differentiated
  Grade 2 or moderately differentiated
  Grade 3 or poorly differentiated

Proposed universal grade for epithelial tumors:
  Architectural pattern (>50% predominant growth pattern):
    Glandular = 1
    Papillary = 2
    Solid = 3
  Nuclear pleomorphism:
    Slight = 1
    Moderate = 2
    Marked = 3
  Mitotic count:
    <10/10 HPF = 1
    10–24/10 HPF = 2
    ≥25/10 HPF = 3
  Overall grade (sum of above scores):
    Grade 1 or well-differentiated = 3–5 points
    Grade 2 or moderately differentiated = 6–7 points
    Grade 3 or poorly differentiated = 8–9 points

Immature teratomas:
  Low-power (×40) fields of immature elements (neuroepithelium) per slide:
    Grade 1 = <1
    Grade 2 = 1–<3
    Grade 3 = >3

Right ovary:
  Size (3 dimensions):          ×        ×        cm
  Weight:       g
  Capsule:      intact      ruptured (spontaneously, surgically)
  Surface tumor:    present    absent
  Lymphovascular space invasion:    present    absent

Left ovary:
  Size (3 dimensions):          ×        ×        cm
  Weight:       g
  Capsule:      intact      ruptured (spontaneously, surgically)
  Surface tumor:    present    absent
  Lymphovascular space invasion:    present    absent

Tumor involvement of other sites:
  Right fallopian tube:      positive      negative
  Left fallopian tube:      positive      negative
  Uterine serosa:      positive      negative
  Omentum:      positive      negative
  Other organs (specify):      positive      negative

  Peritoneal biopsy specimens:
  Right pelvic sidewall:      positive      negative
  Left pelvic sidewall:      positive      negative
  Right paracolic gutter:      positive      negative
  Left paracolic gutter:      positive      negative
  Bladder peritoneum:      positive      negative
  Cul-de-sac:      positive      negative
  Diaphragm:      positive      negative
  Other sites (specify):      positive      negative

  Lymph nodes (indicate number of nodes positive for metastases of total number of nodes examined from each site, and extranodal extension if present):
  Right obturator:            Left obturator:
  Right external iliac:       Left external iliac:
  Right internal iliac:       Left internal iliac:
  Right common iliac:       Left common iliac:
  Right pelvic, NOS:        Left pelvic, NOS:
  Para-aortic:
  Other (specify):

  Ancillary studies (when indicated):
  Immunohistochemical diagnostic studies:
  Estrogen and progesterone receptors:
  DNA ploidy:
  Molecular markers:

---

*WHO, World Health Organization; FIGO, International Federation of Gynecology and Obstetrics; GOG, Gynecologic Oncology Group; HPF, high-power field; NOS, not otherwise specified.

inclusion cysts that increase with age, presumably as the consequence of repeated ovulations. This surface germinal epithelium may exhibit various paths of müllerian differentiation in tumors and metaplastic conditions, resembling the fallopian tube (serous), endometrial (endometrioid), or endocervical (mucinous) epithelium, among others. More than one epithelial cell type may be present in any tumor, but two or more components should compose at least 10% of the neoplasm for it to be classified as a mixed epithelial tumor.

Most surface epithelial tumors are benign, and the carcinomas represent the majority of malignant ovarian cancers. Within each of the histologic subtypes of epithelial tumors, some exhibit morphologic and clinical features intermediate between those of benign and frankly malignant tumors. These neoplasms have been described as LMP tumors, borderline tumors, and atypically proliferating tumors.[6-16] These tumors lack the significant destructive stromal invasion in the primary ovarian masses that is characteristically seen in overtly malignant tumors and have substantially better prognoses than carcinomas do. Nonetheless, they may present at high stage with peritoneal implants, may recur, and occasionally may be associated with synchronous or metachronous invasive implants possibly attributable to malignant transformation or de novo peritoneal neoplasia.[17] Lymph node involvement has been reported to occur in approximately one fifth of cases.[18] In view of this and the familiarity of clinical colleagues with established terminology, these neoplasms are referred to as low malignant potential, or LMP, tumors in this chapter.

Patients with ovarian carcinoma may present with abdominal distention secondary to large tumor masses or malignant ascites. Presenting symptoms may also be attributable to mass effects on nearby organs, such as the bladder and rectum. Abnormal bleeding through the vagina may result from direct involvement by invasive disease.

The International Federation of Gynecology and Obstetrics staging scheme for ovarian carcinomas is listed in Table 39–3. Different grading systems have been used for the various histologic subtypes of ovarian carcinoma. The Pathology Committee of the Gynecologic Oncology Group (GOG) uses a system for grading ovarian carcinomas that incorporates both architectural and cytologic features.[19] GOG grading criteria are discussed later for the respective histologic types of carcinoma. Shimizu, Silverberg, and colleagues[20, 21] have proposed a universal grading system for ovarian carcinoma that can be applied regardless of histologic tumor type, similar to the Nottingham system of Elston and Ellis for the grading of breast cancer. The proposed universal grading system combines architectural, nuclear, and mitotic features for the assignment of an overall grade as presented in Table 39–4. In their series of 461 patients, the overall tumor grade significantly correlated with survival in both early and advanced stages of disease for all histologic types except clear cell adenocarcinoma and retained its prognostic significance in multivariate analysis.[21]

The mainstay of therapy for surface epithelial tumors is surgery. Conservative surgical resection is curative for benign tumors. LMP tumors and recurrences may also be surgically managed for those

**TABLE 39–3.** International Federation of Gynecology and Obstetrics (FIGO) Staging for Ovarian Carcinoma

| | |
|---|---|
| Stage I | Growth limited to the ovaries. |
| IA | Growth limited to one ovary; no ascites present containing malignant cells; no tumor on the external surface; capsule intact. |
| IB | Growth limited to both ovaries; no ascites present containing malignant cells; no tumor on the external surfaces; capsules intact. |
| IC* | Stage IA or IB tumor, but with tumor on the surface of one or both ovaries; or with capsule(s) ruptured; or with ascites present containing malignant cells or with positive peritoneal washings. |
| Stage II | Growth involving one or both ovaries with pelvic extension. |
| IIA | Extension and/or metastases to the uterus and/or tubes. |
| IIB | Extension to other pelvic tissues. |
| IIC* | Stage IIA or IIB tumor, but with tumor on the surface of one or both ovaries; or with capsule(s) ruptured; or with ascites present containing malignant cells or with positive peritoneal washings. |
| Stage III | Tumor involving one or both ovaries with peritoneal implants outside the pelvis and/or positive retroperitoneal or inguinal lymph nodes. Superficial liver metastasis equals stage III. Tumor is limited to the true pelvis but with histologically proven malignant extension to small bowel or omentum. |
| IIIA | Tumor grossly limited to the true pelvis with negative nodes but with histologically confirmed microscopic seeding of abdominal peritoneal surfaces. |
| IIIB | Tumor of one or both ovaries with histologically confirmed implants of abdominal peritoneal surfaces, none exceeding 2 cm in diameter; nodes are negative. |
| IIIC | Abdominal implants greater than 2 cm in diameter and/or positive retroperitoneal or inguinal nodes. |
| Stage IV | Growth involving one or both ovaries, with distant metastases. If pleural effusion is present, there must be positive cytologic findings to allot a case to stage IV. Parenchymal liver metastasis equals stage IV. |

*Notes on staging: To evaluate the impact on prognosis of the different criteria for allotting cases to stage IC or IIC, it would be of value to know if rupture of the capsule was spontaneous or caused by the surgeon and if the source of malignant cells detected was peritoneal washings or ascites.

From SGO Handbook: Staging of Gynecologic Malignancies. 2nd ed. Chicago, Society of Gynecologic Oncologists, 1997, pp 32–33.

**TABLE 39–4.** Proposed Universal Grading System for Ovarian Carcinomas

Architectural pattern (>50% predominant growth pattern)
 Glandular = 1
 Papillary = 2
 Solid = 3

Nuclear pleomorphism

| | |
|---|---|
| Slight = 1 | Relatively uniform vesicular nuclei (variation in diameter no greater than 2:1), low nuclear-to-cytoplasmic ratio, no chromatin clumping or prominent nucleoli |
| Moderate = 2 | Intermediate variation in nuclear size (between 2:1 and 4:1) and shape, nucleoli recognizable but small, some chromatin clumping, no bizarre cells |
| Marked = 3 | Marked variation in nuclear size (greater than 4:1) and shape, high nuclear-to-cytoplasmic ratio, prominent chromatin clumping, thick nuclear membranes, large eosinophilic nucleoli, possibly bizarre cells present |

Mitotic count (HPF = high-power field equivalent to Nikon Optiphot ×10 wide field ocular and ×40 objective, with field diameter of 0.663 mm and field area of 0.345 mm²)
 Slight = 1 (<10 mitoses/10 HPF)
 Moderate = 2 (10–24 mitoses/10 HPF)
 Marked = 3 (≥25 mitoses/10 HPF)

Overall grade (sum of above scores)
 Grade 1 or well differentiated = 3–5 points
 Grade 2 or moderately differentiated = 6–7 points
 Grade 3 or poorly differentiated = 8–9 points

patients with noninvasive disease. For frankly invasive tumors, adjuvant chemotherapy or radiation therapy is warranted and may be followed by additional laparotomies to assess for residual disease and need for further therapy.

## SEROUS TUMORS

### Clinical Features

These tumors represent one fourth to one half of all ovarian neoplasms. Approximately 60% are benign and are most common in women between the ages of 30 and 40 years. Nearly 15% are LMP tumors occurring in women between the ages of 30 and 60 years. The remaining 25% are carcinomas and usually occur in women 40 to 70 years old.

### Macroscopic Findings

Benign serous tumors are usually cystic (cystadenomas) and are characteristically unilocular (Fig. 39–1) or paucilocular; the thin-walled cysts contain thin watery fluid, although the fluid may be thick and gelatinous. External surfaces and the cyst wall linings are usually smooth, but papillary excrescences may be present (papillary cystadenomas). The tumors may have solid, firm, whitish tan areas and robust polypoid growths when a pronounced fibroblastic stromal component is present (adenofibromas [CD Fig. 39–1], cystadenofibromas [CD Fig. 39–2]). Benign serous tumors can be large and may be bilateral in up to 20% of cases.

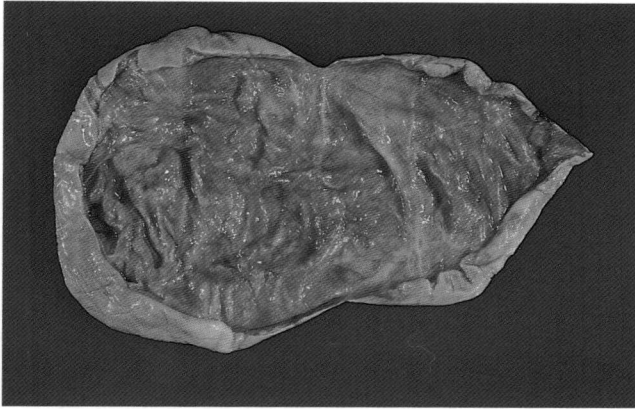

**FIGURE 39–1.** Serous cystadenoma. This unilocular thin-walled cyst has a smooth external surface and cyst wall lining. The cysts are usually filled with thin, watery fluid.

Serous LMP tumors (Fig. 39–2) have some similarities to benign neoplasms but are usually somewhat more architecturally complex and contain more extensive, exuberant, and finer papillary excrescences. They are bilateral in approximately one third of patients.

Serous adenocarcinomas (Fig. 39–3) are usually large, variably multiloculated cystic or solid masses with frequent foci of hemorrhage and necrosis. Polypoid growths are complex and friable. Bilateral tumors are present in approximately two thirds of cases.

### Microscopic Findings

The cyst walls (Fig. 39–4) and papillary fronds (CD Fig. 39–3) of benign serous tumors are lined by a single layer of nonstratified to pseudostratified columnar, eosinophilic, predominantly ciliated cells resembling fallopian tube epithelium. This epithelium may become greatly attenuated and nondescript as a result of pressure by cyst contents. The papillae of cystadenofibromas are relatively simple with readily

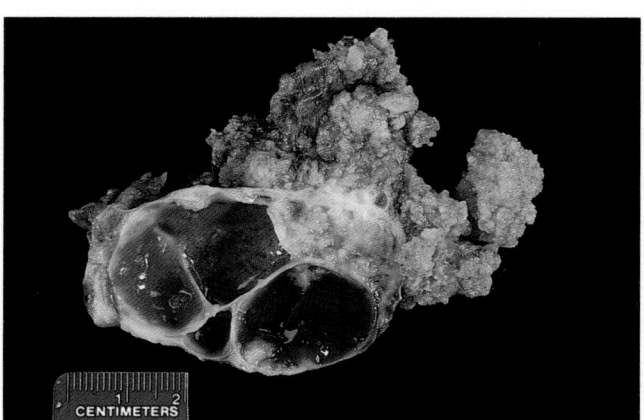

**FIGURE 39–2.** Serous tumor of low malignant potential. This paucilocular cystic mass has numerous exuberant papillary excrescences covering a large part of the external surface and along some of the cyst wall linings.

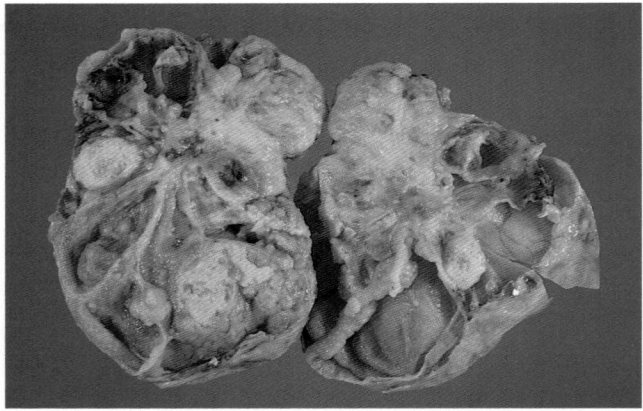

**FIGURE 39–3.** Serous adenocarcinoma. The tumor is composed of admixed cystic and solid components with areas of polypoid soft excrescences.

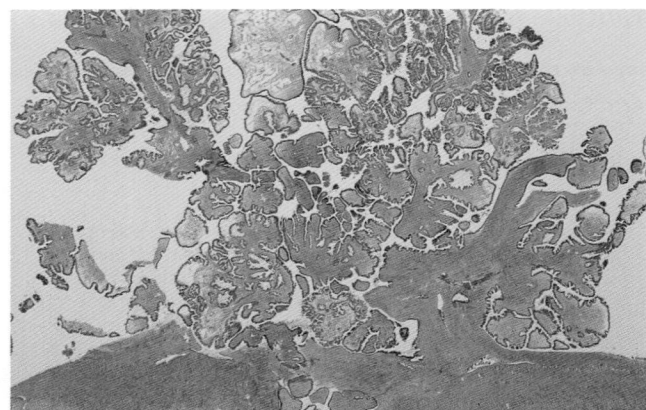

**FIGURE 39–5.** Serous tumor of low malignant potential. The papillae consist of complex, arborizing branches with fibrovascular cores that may be hyalinized. Note the lack of invasion of the underlying cyst wall. (Original magnification ×20.)

identifiable fibrous or edematous stromal cores (CD Figs. 39–4 and 39–5). At most, focal cellular stratification and mild cytologic atypia may be present.

The papillae of serous LMP tumors (Fig. 39–5) exhibit complex branching patterns lined by stratified epithelium often several cell layers in thickness. This architectural complexity may be manifest as apparent detached cellular clusters "free floating" within cyst lumina on essentially two-dimensional histologic sections (CD Fig. 39–6). Cells are predominantly columnar and often ciliated. Varying degrees of cytologic atypia and mitotic figures are present (Fig. 39–6). Psammoma bodies, calcific laminated concretions, are frequently present.

The absence of significant destructive stromal invasion is the sine qua non that distinguishes serous LMP tumors from well-differentiated adenocarcinomas.[7, 22] LMP tumors may exhibit complex, extensive glandular stromal invaginations simulating invasion, but these invaginations are smooth in contour and orderly and lack a stromal response. In contrast, de-

structive stromal invasion is manifest by infiltrating, irregularly shaped glands, cell clusters, or single cells with an associated desmoplastic stromal response. Caution must be exercised in not overinterpreting desmoplastic autoimplants within the ovarian tumor as evidence of stromal invasion.[23] These autoimplants resemble noninvasive desmoplastic implants described later. Rarely, foci of microinvasion, defined as measuring less than 3 mm in maximal extent, and lymphatic involvement may be identified in otherwise typical serous LMP tumors.[24, 25] These microinvasive foci (CD Figs. 39–7 and 39–8) are characterized by single cells or small clusters of cells, often with abundant eosinophilic cytoplasm and surrounded by cleftlike spaces, within the stroma of the tumor. A stromal response is usually absent. The prognosis of these tumors seems to be similar to that of typical serous LMP tumors; however, the significance of microinvasion warrants further study.

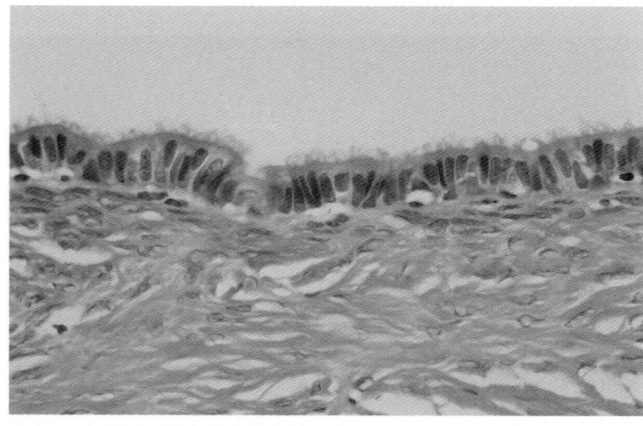

**FIGURE 39–4.** Serous cystadenoma. The cyst wall is lined by a single layer of columnar, eosinophilic, predominantly ciliated cells resembling fallopian tube epithelium. (Original magnification ×600.)

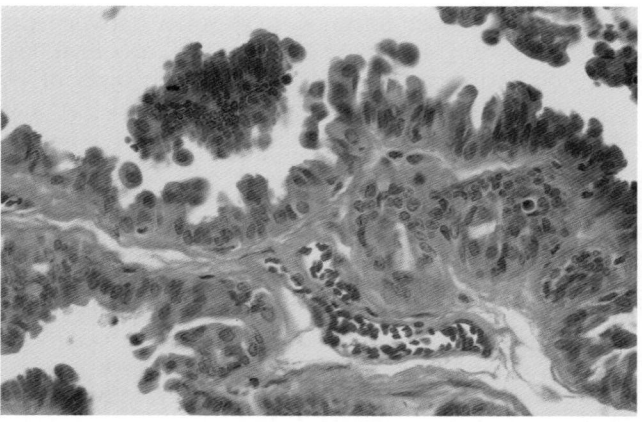

**FIGURE 39–6.** Serous tumor of low malignant potential. The papillae are lined by variably stratified, eosinophilic columnar cells with scattered cilia. There is mild to focally moderate cytologic atypia, and mitotic figures are discernible. (Original magnification ×400.)

The majority of serous LMP tumors are confined to the ovaries (stage I), but one quarter to one half may be associated with peritoneal implants involving the pelvis (stage II) and upper abdomen (stage III), and rare patients may present with stage IV disease. These implants may be invasive or noninvasive; the noninvasive implants are further subclassified as epithelial or desmoplastic.[22, 26–29] Noninvasive implants maintain smooth, circumscribed interfaces with underlying normal tissues when they involve peritoneal surfaces (CD Fig. 39–9) or are within the septa of omental fat lobules. Noninvasive epithelial implants are composed of papillary proliferations of columnar or cuboid serous cells resembling those of the primary ovarian tumor. They may be present on peritoneal surfaces or within smoothly contoured subperitoneal invaginations lined by mesothelium (CD Fig. 39–10). Noninvasive desmoplastic implants are composed of small papillary fronds, glands, cell clusters, or single cells embedded in a dense fibrous stroma, often associated with psammoma bodies, inflammatory cells, fibrin, and hemorrhage (CD Fig. 39–11). Although the desmoplastic stromal response is pronounced in these implants, there is no destructive invasion of the surrounding tissues. Conversely, invasive implants exhibit irregular infiltration of underlying normal tissues by irregularly shaped glands with marked cytologic atypia resembling low-grade serous carcinoma. The classification of an ovarian neoplasm as a serous LMP tumor is made solely on the basis of the histologic features of the primary neoplasm regardless of the nature of the implants. The recognition of invasive implants is of prognostic importance in that these patients have a disease course similar to that of patients with frank invasion identified in the primary ovarian tumors. In some reported series, more than 80% of patients with ovarian serous LMP tumors associated with invasive implants died of their disease.[22, 26, 28] True implants of serous tumor should be distinguished from benign glandular serous inclusions, also called benign müllerian inclusions or endosalpingiosis, to avoid inappropriate upstaging of patients.[18, 30–32] Endosalpingiosis is characterized by subperitoneal or intranodal (CD Fig. 39–12) glands lined by a simple layer of columnar, predominantly ciliated cells without cytologic atypia (CD Fig. 39–13), and it does not exhibit the complex papillary architecture with apparent detached cell clusters observed in tumor implants. Of additional note, some patients may present with peritoneal foci of serous neoplasia resembling implants of LMP tumor with little or no involvement of the ovaries, so-called serous borderline or LMP tumors of the peritoneum.[33, 34]

A group of serous tumors has been described and designated micropapillary serous carcinoma of the ovary.[35, 36] These are low-grade carcinomas that are frequently associated with serous LMP tumors, from which they may arise. These tumors exhibit a filigree morphologic pattern of complex micropapillae with minimal fibrovascular support arising directly from large, thick central cores or cyst walls

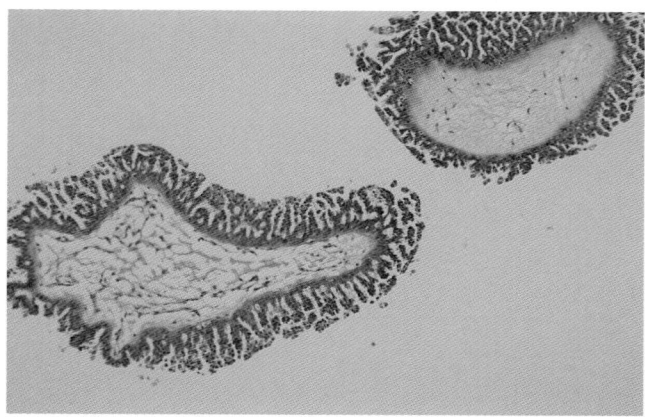

FIGURE 39–7. Serous tumor with micropapillary pattern. (Original magnification ×100.)

(Fig. 39–7). The constituent cells are round to cuboid with high nuclear-to-cytoplasmic ratios and only infrequent cilia. In the first series of 26 cases,[35] nine tumors contained areas of stromal invasion. In the other study,[36] all 7 of 11 patients who developed recurrent invasive carcinoma or died of disease had associated invasive implants at initial presentation. Whether a micropapillary pattern in an ovarian serous tumor in the absence of invasion in either the primary tumor or associated implants portends a more aggressive course remains to be elucidated, and such lesions are better classified as LMP tumors rather than frank carcinomas.

Serous adenocarcinomas must have unequivocal evidence of destructive stromal invasion greater than 3 mm in extent. Histologic features depend on the degree of differentiation[37, 38] (Figs. 39–8 and 39–9). Complex, branching papillae are delicate and irregular and are lined by variably stratified, eosinophilic, cuboid to low columnar cells often forming micropapillae, yielding a slitlike appearance to glandular luminal spaces. Less well differentiated areas

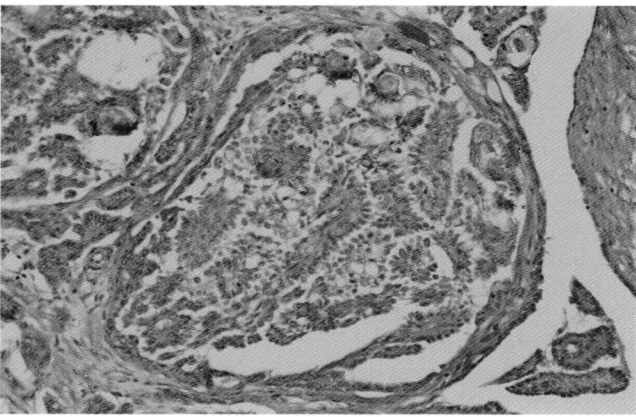

FIGURE 39–8. Serous adenocarcinoma, well differentiated. The tumor consists of well-formed, delicate branching papillae lined by cuboid to low columnar cells. Several psammoma bodies are present. (Original magnification ×200.)

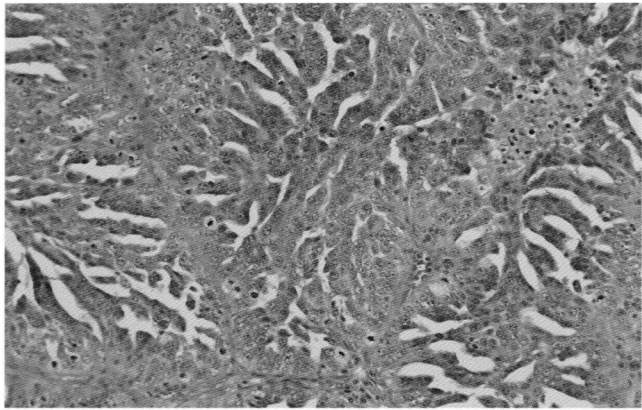

**FIGURE 39–9.** Serous adenocarcinoma, poorly differentiated. These tumors consist predominantly of solid masses of high-grade, pleomorphic cells, although areas with retained characteristic slitlike luminal spaces as seen here assist with recognition. (Original magnification ×200.)

are composed of irregularly shaped infiltrating glands, solid nests, or single cells with an associated dense desmoplastic stroma. Psammoma bodies may be present in one third to one half of cases and are more frequent in better differentiated tumors. Grading criteria used by the GOG are as follows:

Grade 1 or well-differentiated tumors have well-formed papillae and glands with less than 5% solid growth. Nuclei exhibit mild dispolarity, stratification, anisonucleosis, and hyperchromasia.

Grade 2 or moderately differentiated carcinomas have more architecturally complex papillae and glands. Areas of solid growth are more than 5% but less than 50% of the tumor, and there is greater nuclear atypia.

Grade 3 or poorly differentiated tumors consist predominantly of solid tumor growth and exhibit pronounced nuclear pleomorphism.

A rare form of low-grade serous carcinoma called serous psammocarcinoma of the ovary and peritoneum has been described.[39] This tumor shows invasion of underlying stroma, psammoma bodies in at least 75% of the papillae, no significant solid epithelial component more than 15 cells in diameter, and only mild to moderate nuclear atypia. It has a good prognosis more closely approximating that of serous LMP tumors.

As with LMP tumors, invasive serous neoplasia of the peritoneum with minimal ovarian involvement has been described, so-called serous surface papillary carcinoma or extraovarian primary peritoneal serous papillary carcinoma.[40–44] It remains unclear whether the prognosis for these tumors is different from that for patients with ovarian serous cancer of similar grade and stage. Pending further elucidation of the behavior of these lesions, the GOG has designated cases of extraovarian primary peritoneal serous papillary carcinoma when there is

no focus of ovarian stromal invasion greater than 5 mm by 5 mm in greatest extent. Of pathogenetic interest, multiple tumor masses in patients with disseminated primary ovarian serous carcinoma are monoclonal in molecular studies, suggesting unifocal origin,[45] whereas tumor masses in serous carcinoma of probable primary peritoneal origin with secondary ovarian involvement exhibit different genetic patterns, supporting multifocal independent origins.[46]

### Differential Diagnosis

The differential diagnosis of serous carcinomas includes other ovarian epithelial tumors that may have a papillary architecture, such as endometrioid and clear cell carcinomas. The papillary fronds present in some endometrioid carcinomas have a more villous character, are usually longer and more regular than those present in serous tumors, and are typically lined by columnar cells with smooth communal luminal borders. The presence of squamous differentiation is usually associated with endometrioid tumors, but such areas have also been reported in serous carcinomas.[47] Poorly differentiated serous tumors may contain areas with retained characteristic slitlike luminal spaces, whereas a more microglandular pattern with smooth communal luminal borders may be observed in endometrioid carcinomas, although this distinction can be difficult and mixed epithelial carcinomas do occur. In clear cell carcinomas, the papillae frequently have a ramifying anastomosing network of hyalinized stromal cores and are lined by clear and hobnail cells, although hobnail cells may be present in serous carcinomas. The frequent presence of other typical architectural growth patterns in clear cell carcinomas is also useful. Although luminal and apical mucin may be present in serous tumors, significant intracytoplasmic mucin as seen in mucinous neoplasms is absent.

The rare retiform variant of Sertoli-Leydig cell tumor contains papillae and irregular slitlike glandular spaces and thus may be difficult to distinguish from serous carcinoma. These tumors, however, arise in women younger than 20 years, which is rare for serous carcinoma, and often contain other areas more typical of Sertoli-Leydig cell tumor.[48] Although the constellation of clinical, gross, and microscopic findings permits distinction of most cases of malignant mesothelioma from serous carcinoma, immunohistochemistry may be useful for difficult cases.[49, 50] Mesotheliomas exhibit strong cytoplasmic and perinuclear staining for high-molecular-weight cytokeratin and a peripheral membranous staining pattern for epithelial membrane antigen (EMA); they are usually negative for Leu-M1, B72.3, carcinoembryonic antigen (CEA), CA-125, S-100 protein, and placental alkaline phosphatase. The majority of serous carcinomas are immunoreactive with these antibodies, although only a small percentage may be positive for carcinoembryonic antigen.

Metastatic carcinoma to the ovary must be distinguished from primary serous carcinoma, particularly primary serous carcinoma of the endometrium with secondary involvement of the ovaries. In the setting of known uterine serous carcinoma, extensive involvement of ovarian lymphovascular channels and foci of ovarian surface tumor favor metastatic disease to the ovaries, although synchronous neoplasia may have developed in some cases.

## MUCINOUS TUMORS

### Clinical Features

These tumors make up one tenth to one fourth of ovarian neoplasms.[51, 52] Approximately 80% or more are benign cystadenomas and occur in women between the ages of 20 and 50 years. The remaining 20% of mucinous tumors are nearly equally distributed between LMP tumors and carcinomas and arise in women between 30 and 60 years of age. About 5% of patients with mucinous ovarian tumors may present with pseudomyxoma peritonei with viscous pools of mucin filling and distending the peritoneal cavities. Studies support a primary appendiceal origin for the mucinous tumor in the majority of these cases; however, whether the ovarian and appendiceal tumors represent related or independent primary neoplasms in some cases remains controversial.[53-56] Molecular studies have demonstrated genetic differences between the tumors in some cases, supporting separate primaries at least in these relatively few instances.[57] Some patients with mucinous ovarian tumors may have a concomitant mucinous cervical adenocarcinoma, and an increased incidence has been reported in patients with Peutz-Jeghers syndrome.[58-60]

### Macroscopic Findings

Mucinous tumors may attain massive proportions, measuring up to 50 cm in greatest diameter and weighing 5 kg or more (Fig. 39–10). Cystadenomas have smooth external surfaces and unlike their serous counterparts tend to be multiloculated. The cysts have smooth linings and are usually filled with

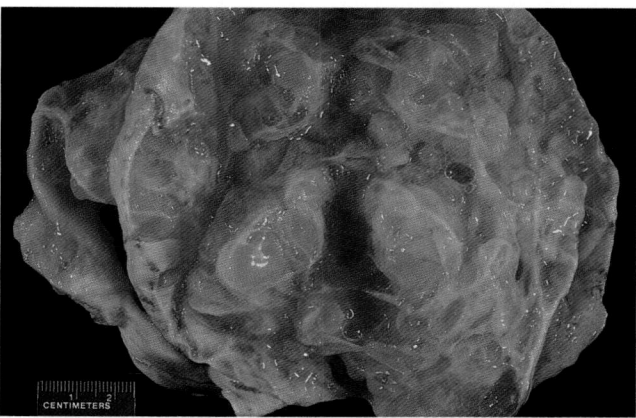

**FIGURE 39–10.** Mucinous tumor. As a group, these tumors are typically large and multiloculated with thick, gelatinous cyst contents. Histologic sampling of the cysts with thicker linings and walls revealed a mucinous tumor of low malignant potential.

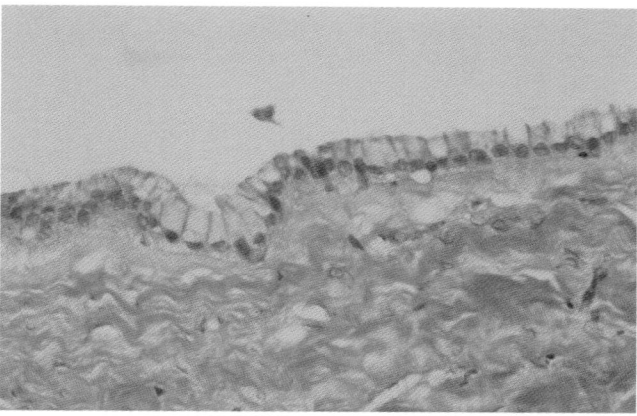

**FIGURE 39–11.** Mucinous cystadenoma. The cyst wall is lined by a single layer of uniform, columnar cells resembling endocervical epithelium. (Original magnification ×400.)

thick viscous secretions, although some may contain thinner, more watery fluid resembling serous tumors. Cystadenomas are bilateral in up to 5% of cases. LMP tumors and invasive carcinomas more often contain thicker papillary cyst linings and solid areas. Hemorrhage and necrosis more commonly occur in the malignant lesions but can be present in benign and LMP tumors. Bilateral neoplasms are present in approximately 10% of patients with LMP tumors and in about 20% of mucinous adenocarcinoma cases.

### Microscopic Findings

Benign cystadenomas are lined by a single layer of simple mucinous epithelium usually resembling that of the endocervix, composed of tall, columnar cells with basally oriented nuclei and abundant intracytoplasmic mucin (Fig. 39–11). Intestinal-type epithelium with scattered goblet cells may infrequently be present. Uncommonly, these tumors may contain a pronounced stromal component and are designated mucinous adenofibromas or cystadenofibromas.[61]

Approximately 85% of mucinous LMP tumors are of the intestinal type[62] (Fig. 39–12). These tumors are composed of cysts and glands and may have pronounced secondary cyst formations and glandular stromal invaginations. Finely branching filiform papillae may be present. The lining epithelium exhibits cellular stratification up to two or three layers, mild to moderate nuclear atypia, and frequent mitotic figures. Goblet cells are typically present, and argyrophil and Paneth cells may also be seen. These intestinal mucinous LMP tumors may be difficult to distinguish from well-differentiated adenocarcinomas (Fig. 39–13) because stromal invasion may not be demonstrable in the setting of complex glandular growths and the absence of a desmoplastic response. For cases lacking frank stromal invasion, Hart and Norris[62] with subsequent modifications by Hart[6] have proposed the following criteria for the diagnosis of mucinous intraglandular car-

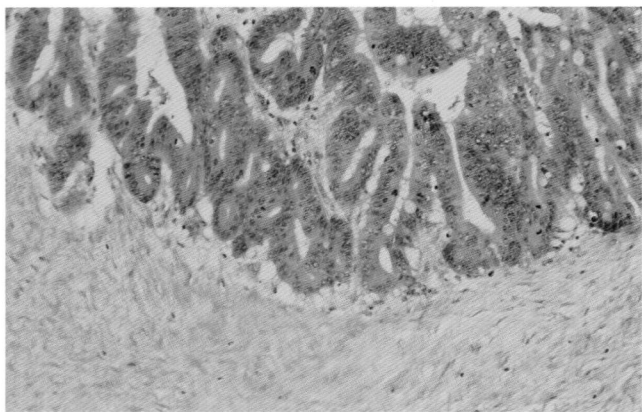

**FIGURE 39–12.** Mucinous tumor of low malignant potential, intestinal type. The lining epithelium exhibits small, filiform papillae, stratification up to three cell layers, mild to moderate cytologic atypia, scattered goblet cells, and mitotic figures. (Original magnification ×200.)

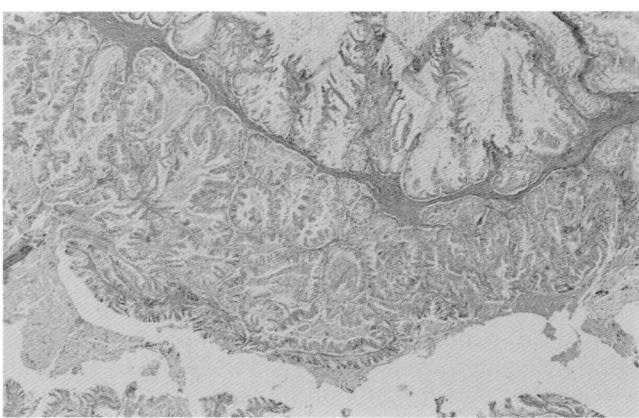

**FIGURE 39–14.** Mucinous intraglandular carcinoma. Complex papillary (top) and cribriform glandular (bottom) growth patterns are evident. (Original magnification ×40.)

cinoma: 1) stratification of atypical epithelial cells to four or more cell layers in thickness, 2) complex cribriform glandular or papillary growth patterns without stromal cores (Fig. 39–14), and 3) markedly atypical cytologic features (Fig. 39–15). These and subsequent studies[51] have confirmed the prognostic utility of these criteria, although other studies have not.[52, 63] In a later study by Hoerl and Hart[64] of primary ovarian mucinous adenocarcinomas with long-term follow-up, all 30 patients with stage I intraglandular carcinoma or tumors with stromal microinvasion not exceeding 1 mm had an excellent prognosis without evidence of tumor after mean follow-up intervals of 5 to 6 years.

Endocervical-like or müllerian neoplasms make up approximately 15% of mucinous LMP tumors.[65, 66] These neoplasms are composed predominantly of endocervical-type epithelium and may also have so-called indifferent eosinophilic cells that are polygonal and contain abundant cytoplasm. There are no morphologic areas of intestinal differentiation. They

contain complex papillae that resemble those of serous LMP tumors (CD Fig. 39–14). Luminal and stromal acute inflammatory infiltrates are characteristically present. Associated endometriosis has been noted in about 20% of cases. Other differences from intestinal mucinous LMP tumors include a high incidence of bilaterality in almost half of the cases, discrete peritoneal implants or lymph node involvement in one fifth of patients, but yet an excellent prognosis; marked stratification of the eosinophilic cells may be present (CD Fig. 39–15). Thus, the criteria of Hart and Norris for distinguishing intestinal LMP mucinous tumors from low-grade carcinomas are not useful for endocervical-like LMP neoplasms.

Guidelines for grading of mucinous adenocarcinomas used by the GOG are as follows:

Grade 1 or well-differentiated carcinomas may show either epithelial stratification of four or more cell layers with moderate to marked cytologic atypia or stromal invasion with an associated desmoplastic stromal response. Solid growth is less than 5%. The presence

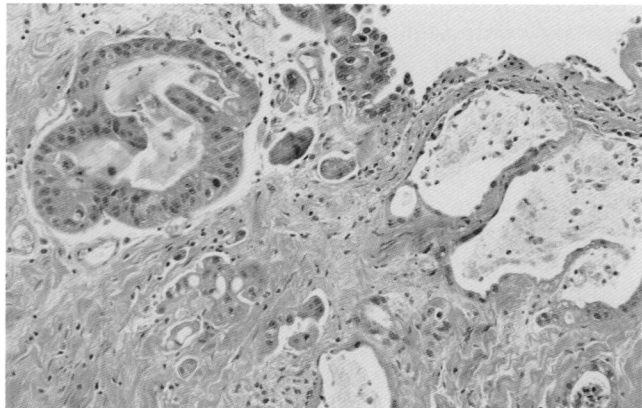

**FIGURE 39–13.** Mucinous adenocarcinoma with stromal invasion. Irregular glands, small nests, and single cells infiltrate the stroma. (Original magnification ×200.)

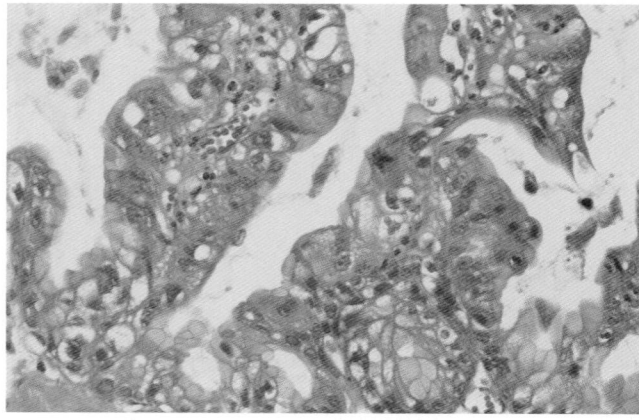

**FIGURE 39–15.** Mucinous intraglandular carcinoma. Note the pronounced cytologic atypia. (Original magnification ×400.)

or absence of stromal invasion should be clearly stated.

Grade 2 or moderately differentiated carcinomas have more complex and smaller glands, greater stratification, and areas of solid growth more than 5% but less than 50% of the tumor.

Grade 3 or poorly differentiated carcinomas have large sheets of solid tumor growth without glands or stroma composing more than 50% of the tumor. Cytologic atypia is marked, and multinucleated tumor cells are frequent.

Ovarian mucinous tumors may rarely contain solid mural nodules that are sarcoma-like and may be reactive in nature with an excellent prognosis,[67, 68] high-grade sarcoma,[69] or anaplastic carcinoma.[70]

### Differential Diagnosis

Mucinous adenocarcinoma may be difficult to distinguish from endometrioid adenocarcinoma, Sertoli-Leydig cell tumor with heterologous elements, and metastatic mucinous carcinomas from various sites. Although endometrioid carcinomas may contain abundant mucin, it is typically extracellular and apical in distribution with less than 10% of cells containing intracellular mucin. The presence of squamous differentiation also strongly supports a diagnosis of endometrioid carcinoma. Sertoli-Leydig cell tumors frequently contain heterologous elements, particularly gastrointestinal-type mucinous epithelium.[71] When the mucinous component is pronounced, it may resemble benign or LMP mucinous tumors more than carcinoma. The presence of typical Sertoli-Leydig cell elements helps to distinguish this tumor.

Metastatic mucinous carcinomas may be particularly difficult to distinguish from primary ovarian mucinous tumors. Primary sites of origin include the gastrointestinal tract,[72–74] appendix,[75, 76] cervix,[60] pancreas,[77] and biliary system.[78] Features favoring metastatic disease to the ovaries include a concomitant extraovarian neoplasm, bilateral ovarian involvement, tumor implants on external ovarian surfaces, multinodular involvement of ovarian parenchyma, and extensive lymphovascular space invasion.[79] Additional microscopic features typically associated with primary colon cancers include a garland or cribriform growth pattern, segmental destruction of glands, intraluminal "dirty" necrosis, absence of squamous metaplasia, and nuclear grade disproportionately high relative to the degree of gland formation.[73, 74] In more problematic cases, immunohistochemistry with use of differential cytokeratins 7 and 20[80, 81] and HAM-56[82, 83] may be useful. Most primary ovarian mucinous adenocarcinomas are immunoreactive for both cytokeratins, whereas colonic adenocarcinomas have a predominant cytokeratin 7 negative, cytokeratin 20 positive immunophenotype. Nonmucinous primary endometrioid and serous adenocarcinomas of the ovary are cytokeratin 7 positive, cytokeratin 20 negative. Strong membranous immunostaining for HAM-56 has been observed in up to three quarters of primary ovarian mucinous tumors and in 90% or more of other epithelial ovarian primaries, whereas most colon carcinomas are negative or exhibit focal weak cytoplasmic immunostaining when positive.

Pseudomyxoma peritonei of usual appendiceal origin with secondary ovarian involvement is characterized by abundant pools of extracellular mucin with extensive dissection through the ovarian stroma, so-called pseudomyxoma ovarii (CD Figs. 39–16 and 39–17). A stromal response to the dissecting mucin is usually absent. Glands and free-floating groups of mucinous epithelium with goblet cells are usually found (CD Figs. 39–18 and 39–19). In contrast, primary mucinous LMP tumors and carcinomas may be associated with focal disruption of glands and cysts with stromal extravasation of mucin in one quarter to one third of cases, often with associated stromal xanthogranulomatous and foreign body giant cell responses. Ovaries involved by pseudomyxoma peritonei of appendiceal origin are also negative for HAM-56 and cytokeratin 7, as discussed before.

## ENDOMETRIOID TUMORS

### Clinical Features

The majority of endometrioid tumors are carcinomas[84–87] and compose approximately one fifth of malignant ovarian tumors. They arise in women 40 years of age and older. Bilateral carcinomas are present in approximately 40% of patients. There is associated endometriosis in 10% to 20% of cases.[88–90] Other than adenofibromas, benign endometrioid tumors are rare,[91–93] and LMP tumors are uncommon; their criteria for diagnosis remain controversial, and their clinical significance remains unclear.[92, 94–96]

### Macroscopic Findings

Endometrioid adenocarcinomas may be cystic or solid, and they are more frequently solid than their serous or mucinous counterparts (Fig. 39–16). Cyst contents are often hemorrhagic. Friable solid or papillary growths may be present within cysts. Solid adenofibromatous components are often present and may predominate.

### Microscopic Findings

Endometrioid tumors are composed of tubulovillous glands similar to those of uterine corpus endometrial benign, hyperplastic, and malignant proliferations. Benign adenofibromas or cystadenofibromas consist of simple glands lined by bland columnar cells embedded in a fibroblastic stroma. Squamous differentiation may be present. Various criteria have been used to classify endometrioid LMP tumors. Rare tumors exhibit papillary villoglandular, well-differentiated fronds protruding into a cyst without invasion of the cyst wall. Most described cases are adenofibromatous and consist of

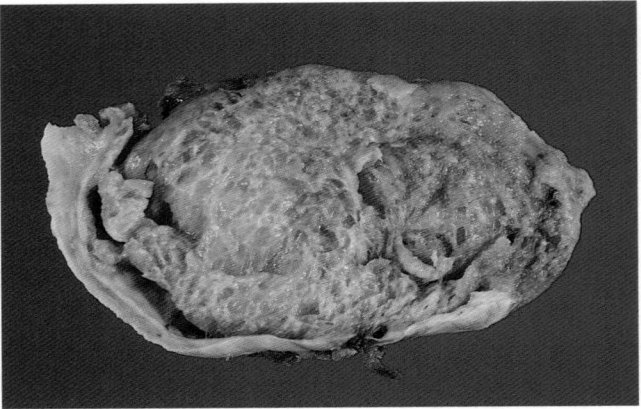

**FIGURE 39–16.** Endometrioid adenocarcinoma with a predominantly solid cut surface.

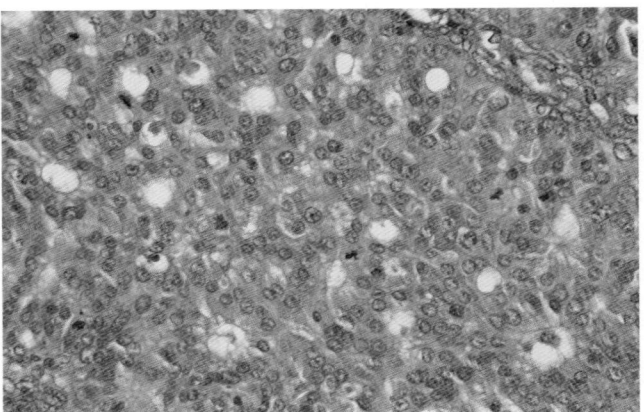

**FIGURE 39–18.** Endometrioid adenocarcinoma, poorly differentiated. Tumors composed of a predominant solid growth pattern may retain areas having a microglandular appearance as demonstrated here. Compare with Figure 39–9 of serous adenocarcinoma with slitlike luminal spaces. (Original magnification ×200.)

atypically proliferating, closely packed glands or epithelial nests with a cribriform pattern within a fibromatous stroma. The glands may have the appearance of low-grade adenocarcinoma, but destructive stromal invasion is absent. Squamous differentiation may also be present in these tumors. Bell and Scully[94] required the epithelial component to be no more than low grade in which glands are usually lined by pseudostratified or stratified cells with atypical nuclei containing irregularly clumped chromatin and at least focally conspicuous nucleoli. Snyder and colleagues[95] proposed quantitative criteria, classifying endometrioid LMP tumors as those containing areas of atypical epithelial proliferation measuring greater than 5 mm in dimension in the absence of stromal invasion. They also placed tumors with greater degrees of epithelial atypia in this category, including those with malignant cytologic features, when stromal invasion is absent. Nonetheless, the prognosis of these tumors in all series is excellent, inasmuch as they are amenable to surgical management without adjuvant therapy.

Endometrioid adenocarcinomas are composed of tubular glands or villous papillae lined by pseudostratified or stratified columnar eosinophilic cells with smooth communal luminal borders (Fig. 39–17). Nuclear atypia usually parallels the degree of gland formation. Poorly differentiated tumors may retain a microglandular appearance in areas (Fig. 39–18). Squamous differentiation may be seen in 25% to 50% of cases (Fig. 39–19). Abundant mucin secretion may be present and is typically luminal and apical in distribution. Intracellular mucin is present in only a minority of cells. Basal vacuolization similar to that seen in early secretory phase endometrium may be present. Cases with abundant, eosinophilic, so-called oxyphilic epithelium have been reported.[97]

Guidelines for grading of endometrioid adenocarcinomas used by the GOG are as follows:

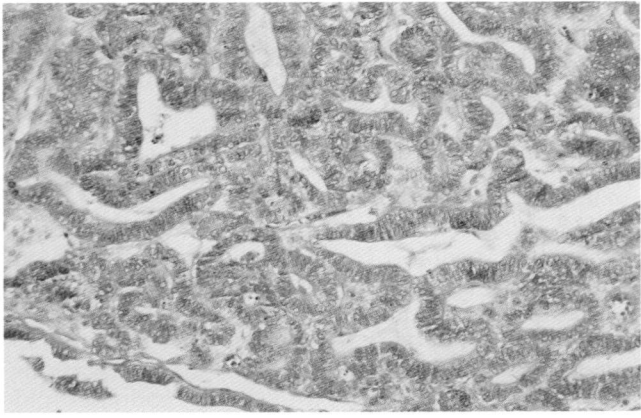

**FIGURE 39–17.** Endometrioid adenocarcinoma, well differentiated. The tumor is composed of confluent or crowded irregularly shaped glands lined by columnar cells with smooth communal borders. (Original magnification ×200.)

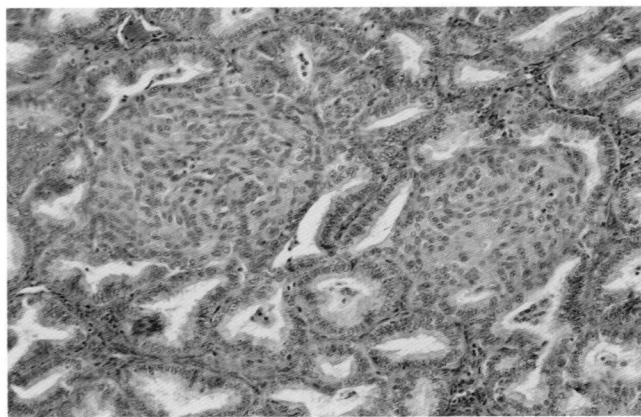

**FIGURE 39–19.** Endometrioid adenocarcinoma with squamous differentiation. The tumor consists of well-formed glands with associated squamous morular aggregates. (Original magnification ×200.)

Grade 1 or well-differentiated tumors resemble the typical villoglandular carcinoma of the uterine corpus. The glands are well formed. Less than 5% of the tumor is solid.

Grade 2 or moderately differentiated carcinomas have more complex glands with increased stratification. Solid tumor nests compose more than 5% but less than 50% of the tumor.

Grade 3 or poorly differentiated tumors have poorly formed glands, nests, and large sheets of cells with more than 50% solid growth.

Squamous differentiation may be present in all three grades, and these areas are excluded from the assessment of percentage of solid growth.

### Differential Diagnosis

The differential diagnosis of endometrioid adenocarcinomas includes serous and mucinous carcinomas as previously discussed. Poorly differentiated tumors lacking definitive evidence of endometrioid differentiation are best classified as serous or undifferentiated in the absence of distinguishing features. The presence of adenofibromatous components and squamous differentiation favor a diagnosis of endometrioid adenocarcinoma. Metastatic gastrointestinal adenocarcinomas more often mimic endometrioid adenocarcinomas than their mucinous counterparts do. Useful gross, microscopic, and immunohistochemical distinguishing features are discussed earlier in the section on mucinous adenocarcinomas.

Endometrioid adenocarcinomas may also be difficult to distinguish from sex cord–stromal tumors, particularly Sertoli-Leydig cell tumors, when they contain small tubular glands, solid tubules, discrete trabeculae, islands, and thin cords of cells.[98, 99] Endometrioid adenocarcinomas may also contain luteinized stromal cells resembling Leydig cells. Small glands with eosinophilic secretions in endometrioid carcinomas may mimic Call-Exner bodies, but they lack the characteristic pale nuclei with longitudinal linear grooves of granulosa cell tumors. Features supporting a diagnosis of endometrioid carcinoma include the presence of areas with more usual appearing larger glands, foci of squamous differentiation, intraluminal mucin, and adenofibromatous components. Immunohistochemistry may be useful in problematic cases. Unlike most sex cord–stromal tumors, endometrioid carcinomas exhibit positive immunostaining for EMA, OM-1, and B72.3[100] and are negative for inhibin.[101]

Endometrioid adenocarcinomas may coexist in the ovary and uterine corpus and in most cases probably represent synchronous neoplasms.[102, 103] Ovarian metastases are likely in the setting of deep myometrial invasion with lymphovascular space invasion, luminal involvement of a fallopian tube, bilateral ovarian involvement, and tumor involving ovarian surfaces or lymphatics. Metastasis to the endometrium from an ovarian primary is uncommon. In some cases, synchronous tumors of the endometrium and ovary may be distinguished as distinct primaries or related neoplasms by molecular genetic studies.[104]

Rare tumors that may resemble endometrioid carcinoma include the endometrioid-like yolk sac tumor[105] and the ovarian tumor of probable wolffian origin.[106]

### Other Endometrioid Tumors

Uncommon neoplasms included in the category of ovarian endometrioid tumors are carcinosarcoma, adenosarcoma, and endometrioid stromal sarcoma. Carcinosarcomas (malignant mixed mesodermal or müllerian tumors)[107–111] occur in postmenopausal women. In gross appearance, they are usually solid with hemorrhage and necrosis. At microscopic examination, they contain malignant epithelial and mesenchymal components. The mesenchymal component may be homologous or heterologous, including cartilage, skeletal muscle, bone, and fat. The epithelial component usually consists of endometrioid or serous adenocarcinoma, although other histologic types may be present. Adenosarcomas[112, 113] consist of benign proliferating endometrial glands within a malignant cellular stroma that characteristically exhibits periglandular condensation or cuffing. Endometrioid stromal sarcomas[114, 115] are often solid or solid and cystic with soft, tannish yellow cut surfaces. They microscopically resemble stromal sarcomas of the uterine corpus and are composed of uniform, small, round to oval cells and a regularly distributed network of small arterioles. Ovarian metastases from a uterine primary stromal sarcoma should be excluded.[116]

## CLEAR CELL TUMORS

### Clinical Features

Clear cell benign and LMP tumors are rare.[91, 117, 118] The majority are carcinomas[119–126] and make up approximately 5% or more of ovarian cancers. They occur most frequently in women 40 to 70 years of age and may be bilateral in 10% to 20% of cases. Associated endometriosis is present in up to one quarter of cases.

### Macroscopic Findings

Benign and LMP clear cell tumors are adenofibromatous and as such are solid or solid with small cystic spaces. Adenocarcinomas are mixed solid and cystic masses that may be large. Tumor masses may arise in the walls of endometriotic cysts (CD Fig. 39–20). They are whitish yellow to tan and may have associated hemorrhage and necrosis (Fig. 39–20).

### Microscopic Findings

Benign clear cell adenofibromas are composed of glands lined by flattened to cuboid clear cells embedded in variable amounts of fibrous stroma. The glands of LMP tumors are lined by slightly strati-

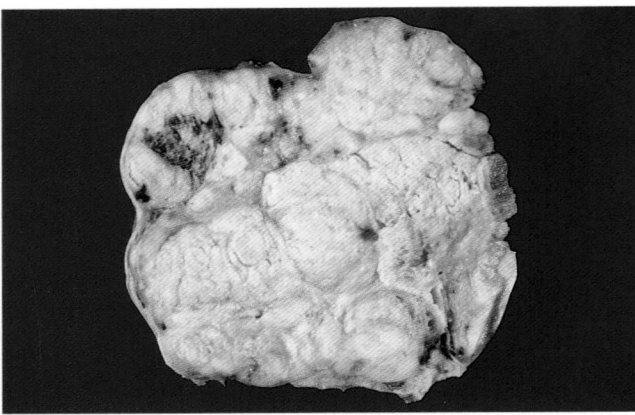

**FIGURE 39–20.** Clear cell adenocarcinoma. The tumor is predominantly solid with focal areas of hemorrhage and necrosis.

fied, more atypical cells, and destructive stromal invasion is absent.

Clear cell adenocarcinomas exhibit a variety of growth patterns, including solid, tubulocystic, and papillary (CD Figs. 39–21 to 39–23). Most tumors contain a mixture of these patterns. Papillary areas characteristically contain ramifying networks of hyalinized stromal cores (CD Fig. 39–24). The cells are large and contain voluminous amounts of clear or occasionally eosinophilic cytoplasm that is typically glycogen rich and may contain fat (Fig. 39–21). Luminal and apical mucin may also be present. Up to one quarter of cases may contain hyaline globules. Nuclei are typically pleomorphic, being enlarged and hyperchromatic with irregular contours. They are usually eccentric and may appear to be extruding from the cells, yielding a so-called hobnail appearance (CD Fig. 39–25). Clear cell adenocarcinomas are considered high-grade neoplasms.

### Differential Diagnosis

The differential diagnosis of clear cell adenocarcinomas includes papillary serous and endometrioid

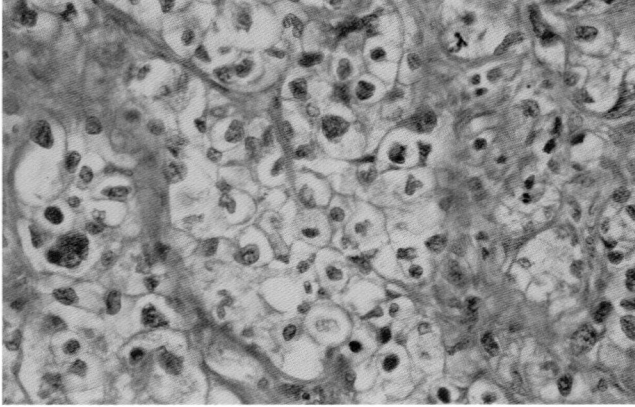

**FIGURE 39–21.** Clear cell adenocarcinoma. The cells contain abundant clear cytoplasm and pleomorphic nuclei. (Original magnification ×400.)

adenocarcinomas, as previously discussed. Clear cell adenocarcinomas are more often confused with endodermal sinus (yolk sac) tumors.[127] Clinicopathologically, clear cell adenocarcinomas occur principally in older women, whereas endodermal sinus tumors, like most primitive germ cell tumors, arise in patients younger than 30 years. Both neoplasms may contain solid or tubular areas composed of clear cells and periodic acid–Schiff–positive, diastase-resistant hyaline globules. Differences in papillae provide useful diagnostic clues. The papillae of clear cell adenocarcinomas are often complex and have hyalinized stromal cores, whereas those of endodermal sinus tumors tend to be single and simple with a looser stroma containing a central vessel (Schiller-Duval bodies). Although immunostaining for α-fetoprotein (AFP) has traditionally been considered to support a diagnosis of endodermal sinus tumor, it has been demonstrated in many ovarian tumors of diverse origin including clear cell adenocarcinomas. Zirker and colleagues[128] found a panel using both Leu-M1 and AFP to be useful for this differentiation. In their study, approximately 95% of clear cell adenocarcinomas were immunoreactive for Leu-M1 compared with about 30% of endodermal sinus tumors. Positive immunostaining for AFP was present in approximately 86% and 18% of endodermal sinus tumors and clear cell carcinomas, respectively. All tumors that showed immunostaining only for Leu-M1 were clear cell carcinomas, and similarly all tumors that were positive only for AFP were endodermal sinus tumors. Positive or negative immunostaining for both markers was not diagnostically useful.

Clear cell adenocarcinomas may also be confused with juvenile granulosa cell tumors, which may contain follicles lined by hobnail cells resembling the tubulocystic pattern of clear cell carcinoma. The uncommon oxyphilic variant of clear cell carcinoma[129] may be difficult to distinguish from both hepatoid yolk sac tumor[130] and hepatoid carcinoma.[131] The diagnosis of these cases may be facilitated by clinicopathologic features and the presence of more typical tumor foci in clear cell adenocarcinomas with admixed growth patterns.

Although metastatic renal cell carcinoma to the ovary is rare, it may be difficult to distinguish from primary clear cell adenocarcinoma.[132] The pronounced sinusoidal vascular network in renal cell carcinomas is absent in clear cell adenocarcinomas. Renal cell carcinomas also lack hobnail cells and intraluminal mucin secretion, features that may be found in clear cell adenocarcinomas.

## BRENNER AND OTHER TRANSITIONAL CELL TUMORS

The classification[133] of these tumors has changed largely because of the recognition of transitional cell carcinomas unassociated with a Brenner component with distinctive clinicopathologic features. This category includes benign Brenner tumor, LMP Brenner tumor, malignant Brenner tumor, and transitional cell carcinoma.

### Clinical Features

Benign Brenner tumors[134-136] constitute approximately 2% of all ovarian neoplasms. They occur in women between 40 and 70 years of age and are unilateral in about 95% of cases. Some patients may present with manifestations of hyperestrogenism resulting from a functioning stromal component.[137] LMP and malignant Brenner tumors[138-142] are uncommon and arise in women who are usually older than those with benign tumors.

Transitional cell carcinomas[142-144] make up only about 1% of ovarian carcinomas and principally occur in postmenopausal women. These tumors have been reported to behave more aggressively than malignant Brenner tumors of similar stage,[142] yet they are much more responsive to chemotherapy and are associated with improved survival of patients compared with most other ovarian carcinomas of similar stage and grade.[133, 143, 144]

### Macroscopic Features

Benign Brenner tumors are usually small but may measure up to 10 cm in diameter. They are circumscribed, solid, firm masses with gray-white to tannish yellow whorled cut surfaces frequently containing minuscule to conspicuous cystic spaces (Fig. 39–22). Gritty calcifications may be evident on sectioning. On occasion, mucinous cyst formation may be prominent in so-called metaplastic Brenner tumors[140] (CD Fig. 39–26). LMP tumors are usually cystic with papillomatous masses protruding into cystic spaces. Malignant Brenner tumors and transitional cell carcinomas may be solid or solid and cystic masses.

### Microscopic Features

Benign Brenner tumors consist of small, round to oval, solid and cystic nests of epithelial cells resembling transitional epithelium, surrounded by abundant fibrous stroma with frequent foci of calcification (Fig. 39–23). The cystic spaces contain eosinophilic secretions or mucin. The epithelial cells are

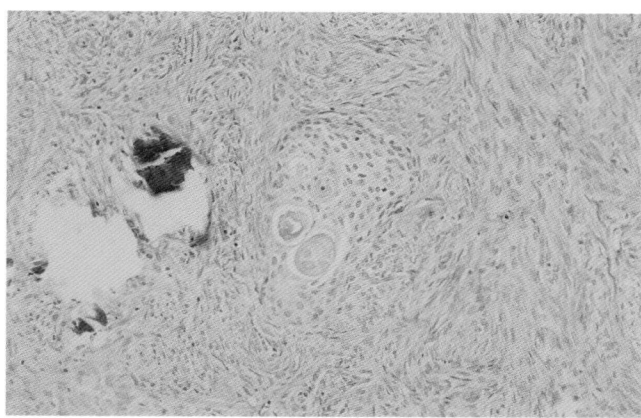

**FIGURE 39–23.** Brenner tumor. The central nest of bland transitional cells contains a few cysts filled with eosinophilic secretions. The surrounding stroma is focally calcified. (Original magnification ×200.)

oval or polygonal, containing pale cytoplasm and uniform nuclei with longitudinal linear grooves. The epithelial cells may appear squamoid or clear with glycogenation. Metaplastic Brenner tumors or mixed mucinous and Brenner tumors contain grossly apparent cysts lined by bland mucinous epithelium, with benign Brenner components in or adjacent to cyst walls (CD Fig. 39–26).

Proliferating and LMP tumors are composed of cysts containing protruding papillae lined by stratified transitional cells. Roth and colleagues[140, 141] considered proliferating Brenner tumors to be those composed of epithelium resembling grade 1 papillary noninvasive transitional cell carcinoma, whereas LMP tumors have higher grade 3 epithelium. Stromal invasion is absent, and a typical Brenner tumor component must be present. The GOG uses similar criteria for LMP tumors. The prognosis for both proliferating and LMP Brenner tumors is excellent.

Malignant Brenner tumors must have stromal invasion with a desmoplastic response, and areas of benign, metaplastic, or proliferating Brenner tumor must be identified. Well-differentiated tumors have low-grade atypia, whereas poorly differentiated tumors resemble high-grade transitional cell carcinoma.

Primary transitional cell carcinomas by definition lack components of benign, metaplastic, or proliferating Brenner tumors. The predominant malignant component closely resembles transitional carcinoma of the urinary tract (Figs. 39–24 and 39–25), although foci of squamous or adenocarcinomatous differentiation may be present in up to half of cases. Tumor grade is assigned in accordance with World Health Organization and Armed Forces Institute of Pathology criteria for transitional cell carcinoma of the urinary bladder.

### Differential Diagnosis

Diagnostic difficulties are most frequent with transitional cell carcinomas and are due largely to

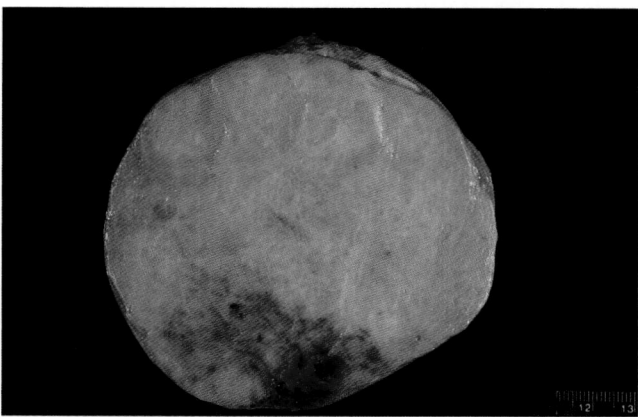

**FIGURE 39–22.** Brenner tumor. The tumor is circumscribed and solid and has a tan-yellow cut surface with a few scattered, small cysts.

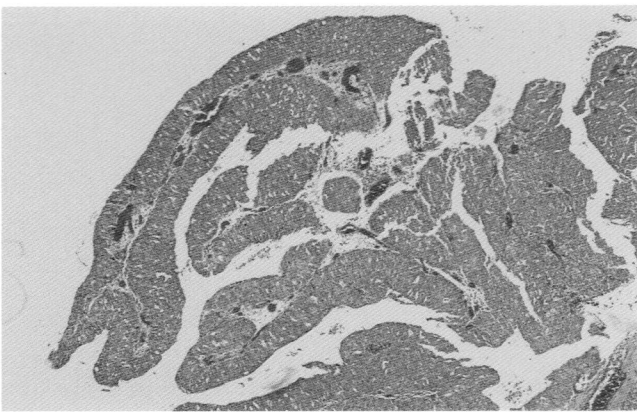

**FIGURE 39–24.** Transitional cell carcinoma. Papillae lined by stratified epithelium project into the cystic space. Note the absence of large areas of tumor necrosis. (Original magnification ×40.)

recognizing such neoplasms arising in organs outside of the urinary tract. Consequently, these neoplasms may be misclassified as poorly differentiated serous, endometrioid, or undifferentiated carcinomas. The most helpful histopathologic feature is the presence of undulating papillary folds lined by stratified epithelium exhibiting transitional-type cytologic features and projecting into cystic spaces in an invasive cystic and solid carcinoma. The cystic spaces into which the papillae project typically do not contain large areas of tumor necrosis, a finding usually present in undifferentiated and other poorly differentiated carcinomas, although this distinction may be difficult. Rare metastatic transitional cell carcinomas[145] may also mimic primary ovarian neoplasms. Deep invasion of the urinary tract tumor and other general features of metastatic tumor to the ovaries, as previously discussed, may favor a diagnosis of metastatic transitional cell carcinoma. Immunohistochemistry with cytokeratin 20 may be of diagnostic utility. Soslow and coworkers[146] observed positive cytokeratin 20 immunostaining in most urinary tract

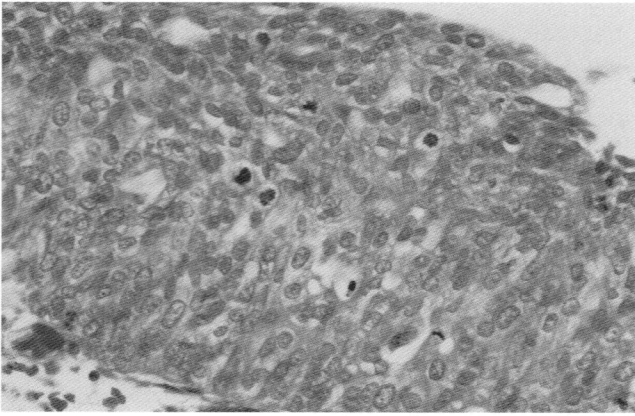

**FIGURE 39–25.** Transitional cell carcinoma. Stratified epithelium consists of moderately atypical transitional cells with several mitotic figures. (Original magnification ×400.)

transitional cell carcinomas, but not in those of female genital tract origin.

## MIXED EPITHELIAL TUMORS

A tumor is classified as mixed epithelial if there are two or more components each making up at least 10% of the tumor. The components should be specified. Serous tumors with abundant extracellular mucin have been erroneously designated mixed seromucinous tumors. Tumors should be classified as having a mucinous component only when significant intracellular mucin can be demonstrated.

Mixed epithelial tumors may be benign, of low malignant potential, or carcinomas. Mixed epithelial-papillary cystadenoma of borderline (LMP) malignancy is a specifically recognized subtype.[147] These tumors arise in younger patients with an average age of 35 years, may be bilateral in approximately one quarter of cases, and are associated with endometriosis in one half of patients. These tumors are composed histologically of complex branching papillae similar to those of serous LMP tumors but are lined by admixtures of endocervical-like mucinous, serous, and endometrioid cells. Acute inflammatory infiltrates are typically present in the lumina, stroma, and epithelium. They behave like other müllerian-type LMP tumors.

## UNDIFFERENTIATED CARCINOMA

Undifferentiated carcinomas[148] have clinical features similar to those of poorly differentiated serous carcinomas. They are bilateral in approximately half of cases. Gross evaluation shows that they are predominantly solid and frequently contain areas of necrosis, hemorrhage, and cystic degeneration. Microscopic examination shows that these tumors are composed of confluent masses, irregular nests, and single epithelial cells surrounded by a desmoplastic stroma. The cells may be highly pleomorphic, and tumor giant cells are often present. This diagnosis is made in the absence of more clearly defined differentiated areas in a well-sampled tumor.

## OTHER EPITHELIAL TUMORS

Other epithelial tumors that may arise in the ovary are rare. Reported cases include primary squamous cell carcinoma,[149] adenoid cystic and basaloid carcinomas,[150] and non–small cell neuroendocrine carcinomas.[151] Small cell carcinomas and other tumors of uncertain histogenesis are discussed in later sections.

## IMMUNOHISTOCHEMISTRY OF SURFACE EPITHELIAL TUMORS

Common immunohistochemical reactions observed in ovarian neoplasms are summarized in Table 39–5. Ovarian surface epithelial tumors are immunoreactive for epithelial markers such as pancytokeratins, EMA, CD15 (Leu-M1), and B72.3.[152, 153] High-molecular-weight cytokeratins can detect areas of early squamous differentiation in endometrioid tumors, which may be useful in the distinction from serous tumors.[154, 155] CA 125 is frequently positive in ovar-

**TABLE 39–5.** Expected or Common Immunohistochemical Reactions in Ovarian Neoplasms

| Histologic Type of Neoplasm | Positive Immunoreactivities* |
| --- | --- |
| Surface epithelial tumors | Pancytokeratins, EMA, CD15 (Leu-M1), B72.3, CA-125 |
| Serous | S-100 protein, vimentin |
| Mucinous | CEA |
| Endometrioid | High-molecular-weight cytokeratin (areas of squamous differentiation) |
| Clear cell | Vimentin |
| Brenner–transitional cell | CEA |
| Sex cord–stromal tumors | Vimentin, inhibin, smooth muscle actin, estrogen, progesterone, testosterone |
| Germ cell tumors | hPLAP, AFP, $\beta$-hCG, cytokeratin, CD30 (Ki-1) |

*EMA, Epithelial membrane antigen; CEA, carcinoembryonic antigen; hPLAP, human placental alkaline phosphatase; AFP, $\alpha$-fetoprotein; hCG, human chorionic gonadotropin.

ian carcinomas, particularly in serous tumors, but much less so in mucinous tumors, which may be immunoreactive in less than 20% of cases.[156, 157] S-100 protein immunoreactivity among epithelial tumors is similar to that of CA-125; many serous and some endometrioid and clear cell tumors are S-100 positive, whereas mucinous tumors are typically negative.[158] A reverse distribution is observed for carcinoembryonic antigen, which is positive in most cases of mucinous carcinoma, frequently present in transitional cell and some endometrioid neoplasms, but usually negative in serous tumors.[159, 160] Estrogen and progesterone receptors are frequently expressed in ovarian epithelial neoplasms. Additional potentially useful distinguishing markers are discussed in the differential diagnosis section for the respective neoplasms.

## MOLECULAR BIOLOGY AND OTHER STUDIES OF SURFACE EPITHELIAL TUMORS

Since the late 1980s, the literature has been replete with reports on the molecular biology of ovarian cancer, principally surface epithelial tumors. Most of these investigations have sought to elucidate mechanisms of ovarian cancer development and progression or identify potential molecular prognostic markers, as discussed later. As the molecular basis of ovarian cancer becomes further understood, potential clinical applications include genetic screening and early diagnosis of high-risk patients and novel biologic and gene therapies.[161–163]

Initial karyotypic and cytogenetic studies of ovarian carcinoma in general have revealed complex chromosome alterations that frequently involve chromosomes 1, 3, 11, and 17; multiple abnormalities usually occur in any one tumor.[161, 164] Chromosome alterations become more complex and atypical as the stage and grade of tumor increase. Consistently observed allelic deletions or loss of heterozygosity is considered presumptive evidence that these loci may contain tumor suppressor genes. DNA allelic deletions and loss of heterozygosity have been reported in ovarian carcinomas, with many occurring at known tumor suppressor and other genetic loci, such as chromosome 3[165–167]; chromosome 6, including the c-myc and estrogen receptor loci[165, 166, 168, 169]; chromosome 11, including the c-Ha-ras-1, WT1, and WT2 loci[165, 166, 168, 170–173]; chromosome 13, including the BRCA2 gene[174, 175]; chromosome 17, including p53, BRCA1, and other tumor suppressors and HER2-neu loci[168, 176–178]; and chromosome 18 near the DCC locus.[179] Loss of the X chromosome has also been frequently observed.[180] Loss of heterozygosity tends to increase with higher tumor stage and grade. Many studies have also demonstrated similar findings of loss of heterozygosity between primary and metastatic lesions, suggesting that loss of heterozygosity preceded metastasis.[161]

In further investigations, alterations in specific genes have been identified in hereditary and sporadic ovarian carcinomas; these include proto-oncogenes, tumor suppressor genes, and DNA mismatch repair genes. Proto-oncogenes encode proteins that promote cell growth, and mutations in these genes enhance cellular proliferation. Conversely, tumor suppressor genes encode proteins that inhibit cell growth; hence, alteration of these genes also augments cellular proliferation. Deficiencies in DNA mismatch repair genes are thought to cause replication errors that may result in altered expression of growth regulatory genes.[161, 162]

Hereditary ovarian and breast-ovarian cancer syndromes make up approximately 10% or more of ovarian cancer cases. Investigators have identified a specific gene on chromosome 17q, designated BRCA1, that may account for the majority of familial cases of breast cancer as well as hereditary early-onset breast and ovarian cancer.[181–184] An additional second gene has been discovered on chromosome 13q, designated BRCA2, which is also associated with an increased risk of familial breast and ovarian cancer.[185, 186] BRCA1[187] and BRCA2 are thought to be tumor suppressor genes. CMM86 is another putative tumor suppressor gene located on chromosome 17 near BRCA1 and is linked with familial breast-ovarian cancer.[188] The Lynch syndrome II includes patients with hereditary ovarian, breast, endometrial, and nonpolyposis colon cancer and may be associated with genes located on chromosomes 2 and 3.[189, 190] Genetic analysis of patients with familial site-specific ovarian cancer has provided preliminary evidence of rare autosomal dominant genes in some families.[191]

The majority of ovarian cancers are sporadic and are thought to arise as a result of acquired alterations in proto-oncogenes, tumor suppressor genes, and other genes that regulate DNA repair and cellular growth.[161, 162, 192] Abnormalities of the HER2-neu proto-oncogene are frequently observed in ovarian carcinomas. *HER2-neu* is also located on chromosome 17 and encodes a transmembrane glycoprotein of the tyrosine kinase class, c-*erb*-b2, which is related to but distinct from the epidermal growth factor receptor gene c-*erb*-b1. Amplification or overexpression of *HER2-neu* has been reported in one quarter to one third of ovarian carcinomas; it has been associated with well-differentiated lesions, endometrioid carcinomas, high-stage tumors, and poor survival.[193–197] The c-*myc* proto-oncogene is also frequently altered in sporadic ovarian cancers. It is located on chromosome 6 and encodes a DNA-binding protein associated with the regulation of cellular proliferation. Amplification of c-*myc* has been described in approximately one third of advanced stage ovarian carcinomas.[198, 199] Other proto-oncogenes less commonly altered in ovarian cancers include *ras* genes, usually the K-*ras* oncogene (guanosine triphosphate–binding protein gene),[200–202] c-*fms* (colony-stimulating factor receptor gene),[203, 204] and *AKT2* (serine-threonine protein kinase).[205] Of note, although it is infrequent in most ovarian invasive carcinomas, some investigators have reported K-*ras* mutation in up to half of epithelial LMP tumors,[202, 206] suggesting that the majority of these neoplasms may result from distinct neoplastic processes rather than representing earlier stages in the progression of an ovarian carcinoma sequence.

The *p53* tumor suppressor gene is located on chromosome 17p and is a frequent genetic alteration in ovarian and many other solid neoplasms. It encodes a DNA-binding protein that interferes with transcriptional regulators, thus inhibiting cellular proliferation. The wild-type p53 protein is rapidly degraded and as such is not detected in normal cells. Mutations with allelic losses result in the production of nonfunctional p53 proteins that are more resistant to degradation and accumulate in the cell, thus permitting their detection by immunohistochemical methods. Overexpression of mutant p53 as manifested by nuclear immunoreactivity may be seen in up to half of invasive ovarian carcinomas, but it has been detected in less than 5% of LMP tumors.[207–209] Its overexpression in ovarian carcinomas has been associated with aggressive tumor behavior and diminished survival of patients.[210–212] In addition to *BRCA1* and *BRCA2* discussed before, other putative tumor suppressor genes implicated in ovarian carcinogenesis include *OVCA1* and *OVCA2,* which are also located on the short arm of chromosome 17.[213]

The clinical utility of flow cytometric analysis of DNA content (ploidy) and proliferation (S phase fraction) has been extensively studied in ovarian epithelial tumors.[214–224] Many studies have reported associations of DNA aneuploidy and high S phase fraction with advanced tumor stage and histologic grade. There is no well-defined relationship between DNA content and histologic subtype, although most serous carcinomas are DNA aneuploid. Most LMP tumors are DNA diploid. Results are conflicting concerning the prognostic significance of aneuploidy in

LMP tumors and potential risk for relapse or progression. Endometrioid and mucinous adenocarcinomas tend to have low S phase fractions compared with other histologic subtypes. Although there are conflicting results in the literature concerning the relationship between DNA ploidy and clinical outcome measures, many studies have found DNA ploidy to be of independent prognostic significance by multivariate analysis; DNA diploidy is associated with higher chemotherapy response rates, longer disease-free intervals, and increased survival. Some studies have found that S phase fraction may also be an independent prognostic indicator; low S phase fractions are associated with favorable outcomes.

The primary role of cytology for ovarian neoplasms is in the evaluation of ascites and peritoneal washings for the presence of malignant cells,[225] the results of which are incorporated into the International Federation of Gynecology and Obstetrics staging system (see Table 39–3). Patients with positive results of fluid cytology generally have a worse prognosis than do those with negative results; however, this difference has not been shown to be independent of stage. Interpretation of these fluids may be hampered by the presence of reactive mesothelial cells, endosalpingiosis, and other benign processes.[226] Although still controversial, cytologic evaluation of ovarian cystic lesions by fine-needle aspiration is becoming a more commonly used diagnostic tool, particularly in certain clinical settings.[227–230] Aspiration of ovarian masses is usually performed under ultrasound guidance or during laparoscopy. Some consider its general use contraindicated because of the risk of potentially spilling malignant cells into the peritoneal cavity and reported less than optimal accuracy rates, usually because of high false-negative results in the setting of malignancy. Nonetheless, evaluation of ovarian cystic lesions by experienced pathologists may be useful in clinical situations in which retention of ovarian function is desired (e.g., young women with functional cysts, evaluation of cysts associated with assisted reproductive technologies). Although aspiration of solid or partially solid ovarian masses is generally contraindicated, it may be the diagnostic procedure of choice when the patient is not a surgical candidate or has inoperable disease and in the setting of confirming suspected recurrent disease.

## PROGNOSIS OF SURFACE EPITHELIAL TUMORS

Relevant pathologic prognostic features of ovarian neoplasms are summarized in Table 39–6.

The overall prognosis of ovarian carcinoma remains relatively poor; 5-year survival rates range from 30% to 40% in most series. This is attributable in large part to the paucity of early symptoms with presentation at advanced stage for many patients. Stage is generally considered to be the most important prognostic factor for ovarian carcinoma. The 5-year survival rates are approximately 85% for stage

**TABLE 39–6. Prognostic Features: Ovarian Neoplasms**

**Surface Epithelial Tumors**
Low malignant potential versus frankly invasive carcinoma
Histologic grade
Histologic type
DNA ploidy
S phase fraction
*HER2-neu* amplification/c-erb-b2 overexpression
*p53* overexpression

**Sex Cord–Stromal Tumors**
Granulosa cell tumors
   Tumor size
   Degree of cytologic atypia
   Mitotic rate

Sertoli-Leydig cell tumors
   Histologic grade
   Heterologous elements
   Retiform variant

Steroid cell tumor, not otherwise specified
   Tumor size
   Presence of hemorrhage or necrosis
   Nuclear atypia
   Mitotic rate

**Germ Cell Tumors**
Histologic type and amount of malignant components

Immature teratomas
   Tumor size
   Histologic grade

I, 60% for stage II, 25% for stage III, and 10% for stage IV cancers.[231, 232]

The distinction of LMP tumors from frankly invasive carcinomas is of significant prognostic importance, including those cases with extraovarian disease.[13, 233, 234] The 5-year survival rate for serous LMP tumors is nearly 99% for stage I, and it remains high at greater than 90% when all stages are considered. Survival at 5 years for mucinous LMP tumors is approximately 90% to 95% for stage I and 80% to 90% overall for all stages.

Tumor grade and, to a lesser extent, histologic subtype are also associated with prognosis in at least univariate analyses.[235–237] The proposed universal grading system[20, 21] for ovarian carcinomas discussed before retains its significance in multivariate analysis in the initial studies of its application. Tumor grade is closely correlated with survival. Patients with low-stage, high-grade carcinomas do significantly worse than those with better differentiated low-stage tumors. Overall, patients with endometrioid and mucinous adenocarcinomas tend to do better than those with serous carcinomas, and poor outcomes are observed with clear cell and undifferentiated carcinomas. When corrected for stage, however, the common carcinoma subtypes (serous, mucinous, endometrioid, and clear cell) do not have significantly different outcomes.[123, 126, 238] Although tumor grade correlates better with survival than histologic type does, the histologic type is a better predictor of response to chemotherapy and type of chemotherapy.[239]

The prognostic significance or potential value of DNA ploidy, S phase fraction, overexpression of *HER2-neu* (c-*erb*-b2) oncogene, and *p53* tumor suppressor gene is discussed earlier. Other clinical factors associated with prognosis include volume of residual disease after tumor debulking, presence and volume of ascites, age of the patient,[240] spontaneous preoperative rupture of tumor capsule,[241] and level of serum CA 125.[242]

## Sex Cord–Stromal Tumors

This group of tumors accounts for approximately 5% to 10% of all ovarian neoplasms and for the majority of hormonally functioning ovarian tumors.[243, 244] They contain varying mixtures of sex cord and gonadal stromal elements that exhibit differentiation resembling ovarian cells (e.g., granulosa cells), testicular cells (e.g., Sertoli and Leydig cells), and intermediate or indifferent cells.

### GRANULOSA CELL TUMORS

#### Clinical Features

Approximately 1% to 2% of all ovarian tumors are granulosa cell tumors. Most arise in postmenopausal women, but they may occur in children and young women.[245–251] Three quarters of cases are estrogenic, and the others are nonfunctioning or rarely androgenic.[252] Patients who do not have signs or symptoms of hyperestrogenism or virilization may present with abdominal swelling or pain due to tumor rupture. Two types have been described, adult granulosa cell tumors and juvenile granulosa cell tumors. The juvenile granulosa cell tumors most often occur in children and women younger than 20 years; in children, they are usually associated with isosexual pseudoprecocity. Both types are usually unilateral and low stage, and they may be treated in many cases with conservative surgery. These are low-grade malignant neoplasms with good prognoses; low-stage tumors have 10-year survival rates of greater than 90% in some series.[245, 246, 253–255] Late recurrences even as long as 20 years may develop, necessitating long-term follow-up.

#### Macroscopic Findings

These tumors vary considerably in size, ranging from microscopic to large tumors with an average diameter in the 10- to 15-cm range. They are usually encapsulated with a smooth external surface. Cut surfaces are typically solid and soft, tan to yellow; they may have hemorrhagic or necrotic areas, particularly in large neoplasms (Fig. 39–26). They may also be extensively cystic, resembling cystadenomas, often in the androgenic tumors.[252]

#### Microscopic Findings

Microscopic features of granulosa cell tumors are highly variable, even within the same neoplasm.

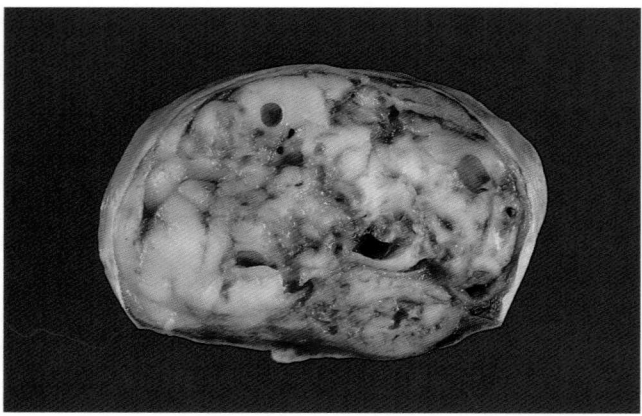

**FIGURE 39–26.** Adult granulosa cell tumor. The mass is encapsulated and has a lobulated, soft, yellow-tan cut surface with cystic degeneration and focal hemorrhage.

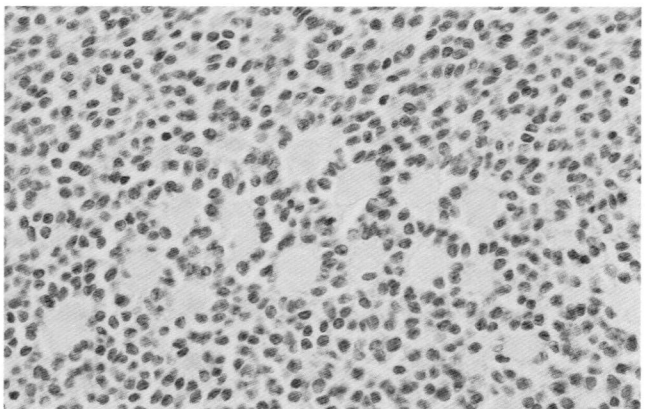

**FIGURE 39–27.** Adult granulosa cell tumor, microfollicular pattern with Call-Exner bodies. The tumor cells are small and uniform with scant cytoplasm. Nuclei contain scattered linear longitudinal grooves. (Original magnification ×400.)

Architectural growth patterns include microfollicular (CD Fig. 39–27), macrofollicular (CD Fig. 39–28), insular (CD Fig. 39–29), trabecular (CD Fig. 39–30), tubular, moiré silk (watered silk), and diffuse (sarcomatoid) (CD Fig. 39–31). The microfollicular pattern is the most readily recognized and consists of small cystic cavities often containing eosinophilic secretions lined by well-differentiated granulosa cells. These microfollicular structures are reminiscent of ovarian follicles and are called Call-Exner bodies (Fig. 39–27). Macrofollicular areas consist of larger cysts. Insular patterns are composed of islands of cells, and trabecular areas consist of anastomosing bands of tumor. The watered-silk pattern exhibits geographic or parallel arrays of intertwining or undulating thin cords of cells. Diffuse areas are characterized by sheets of oval or spindled cells, yielding a so-called sarcomatoid appearance to the tumor.

Adult granulosa cell tumors may exhibit any or all of these patterns. The cells in these tumors are typically uniform, round or oval to angular, with scant cytoplasm, although abundant eosinophilic cytoplasm may occasionally be present. The nuclei characteristically contain longitudinal grooves or folds, imparting a so-called coffee-bean appearance (see Fig. 39–27). Chromatin is bland and nucleoli are inconspicuous. Mitotic figures are usually infrequent. Pleomorphic bizarre nuclei representing probable degenerative changes may uncommonly be seen.[256] In contrast, juvenile granulosa cell tumors usually consist of diffuse or macrofollicular growth patterns, with mucin-positive intrafollicular secretions. Unlike in the adult forms, cells often contain abundant eosinophilic cytoplasm, nuclei are somewhat rounder and rarely grooved, nucleoli may be conspicuous, and mitotic figures are frequent and may be atypical[250, 251] (Fig. 39–28).

### Differential Diagnosis

Granulosa cell tumors, particularly the adult form, may be distinguished from cellular thecomas and fibromas with reticulin stains. Reticulin is abundant around individual cells in these tumors, whereas granulosa cell tumors contain scant reticulin surrounding groups or nests of cells. Poorly differentiated, predominantly solid surface epithelial tumors, particularly endometrioid and clear cell adenocarcinomas, may be difficult to distinguish from granulosa cell tumors. These carcinomas typically have more pleomorphic nuclei and frequent mitotic figures. Other clinicopathologic features and immunohistochemistry may be useful in problematic cases, as previously discussed. Unlike carcinomas, granulosa cell tumors may exhibit dotlike paranuclear staining rather than diffuse immunoreactivity for cytokeratin,[257] are negative for EMA,[258] and are usually positive for inhibin.[101, 259, 260] Granulosa cell tumors are also immunoreactive for vimentin, smooth muscle actin,[261] and MIC2,[262] and in about half of the cases for S-100 protein.[258] The differential diagnosis of granulosa cell tumors, particularly the juvenile type, also includes malignant germ cell tu-

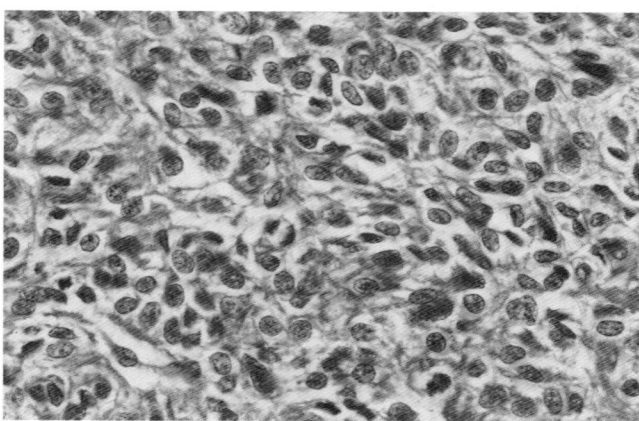

**FIGURE 39–28.** Juvenile granulosa cell tumor. Compared with the adult form, the cells are larger and contain more abundant eosinophilic to vacuolated cytoplasm. The nuclei are oval to round with scattered nucleoli, and nuclear grooves are inconspicuous. (Original magnification ×600.)

mors, carcinoid tumor, and small cell carcinoma of the hypercalcemic type, as discussed in later sections on these neoplasms.

### Prognosis

As indicated before, adult granulosa cell tumor is a low-grade malignant neoplasm with a favorable prognosis at and beyond 10 years,[245, 246, 253–255] with a propensity for late recurrences. The overall prognosis is predominantly related to tumor stage. Patients with stage I tumors have an excellent prognosis, with a 10-year survival rate approaching or greater than 90%, but this rate falls to approximately 30% to 50% for high-stage tumors. Other factors associated with prognosis include tumor rupture, tumor size greater than 5 cm in diameter, and degree of cytologic atypia. Mitotic rates as few as three mitoses or more per 10 high-power fields have also been correlated with prognosis[245, 246, 255]; however, the significance of high mitotic activity diminishes when it is corrected for stage. Cellular atypia and high mitotic rates have also been associated with earlier recurrences within 10 years of diagnosis.[263] The prognostic influence of histologic pattern is unclear. Initial reports suggested that those tumors with a follicular or trabecular pattern have increased survival rates compared with those with a more diffuse or sarcomatoid pattern; however, the prognostic significance of histologic pattern alone has not been confirmed in subsequent investigations.[245–247, 253, 254]

Juvenile granulosa cell tumors also have a highly favorable prognosis, with stage being the most important factor.[249–251] In contrast to the adult type, most recurrences develop within 3 years of diagnosis, yet higher survival rates have been reported. Mitotic rate and cytologic atypia also correlate with prognosis for all stages, but not within the subset of stage I tumors.[250]

## THECOMA-FIBROMA TUMORS

### Thecoma

CLINICAL FEATURES. Typical thecomas occur in postmenopausal women in more than 80% of cases. Many tumors are associated with estrogenic manifestations, although some may be androgenic.[264, 265] They are usually unilateral but may be bilateral in less than 3% of cases. These are benign neoplasms, although rare malignant tumors have been reported.[266]

MACROSCOPIC FINDINGS. Thecomas range in size from very small to large tumors with smooth external surfaces. Cut surfaces are typically solid and firm, and they characteristically have yellow areas indicative of lipid-containing cells interspersed with gray-white, more fibrotic areas (Fig. 39–29). Cystic degeneration is occasionally present.

MICROSCOPIC FINDINGS. Thecomas are composed of fascicles and aggregates of spindled to rounded cells with centrally placed, blunt-ended nuclei and moderate amounts of ill-defined cytoplasm that may be extensively vacuolated (Fig. 39–30).

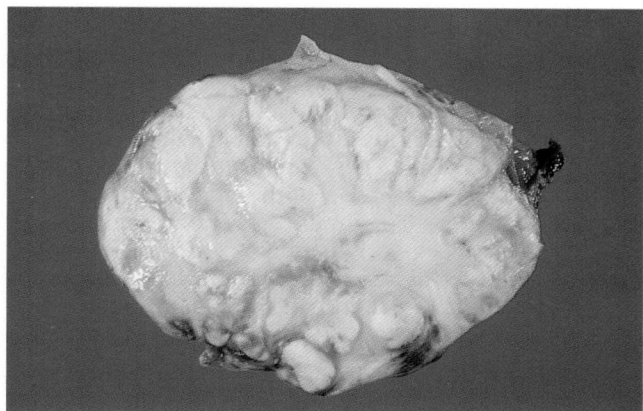

**FIGURE 39–29.** Thecoma with admixed lobulated yellow and firm white areas.

Nuclei are round to oval without significant atypia. Mitotic figures are infrequent. Sheets and nests of theca cells are often separated by collagenous bands of fibrotic stroma. Hyaline plaques are frequently present and may be conspicuous (see Fig. 39–30). Focal calcification is occasionally observed.

DIFFERENTIAL DIAGNOSIS. Thecomas may occasionally be confused with solid granulosa cell tumors, for which reticulin stains are useful, as previously discussed.

### Luteinized Thecoma

Luteinized thecomas contain large clusters or single cells with abundant eosinophilic granular or vacuolated luteinized cytoplasm.[267, 268] They usually occur in younger patients than typical thecomas do. In some cases, they have been associated with sclerosing peritonitis of abdominal and pelvic cavities.[269, 270] In this clinical setting, the tumors may be bilateral and hypercellular with high mitotic activity resembling fibrosarcomas (CD Figs. 39–32 and 39–33).

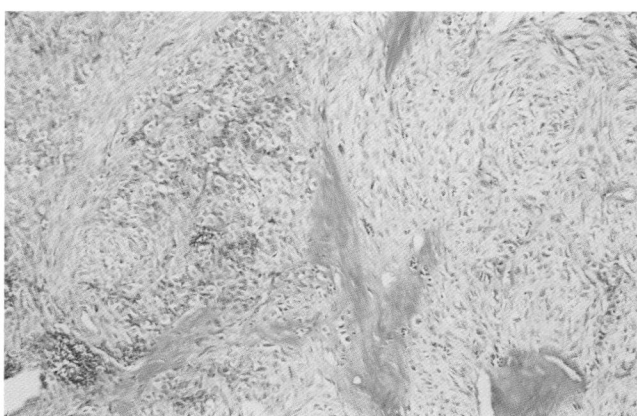

**FIGURE 39–30.** Thecoma. Cells are spindle shaped to rounded and contain abundant pale cytoplasm. Note the hyalinized fibrous plaques. (Original magnification ×100.)

### Fibroma

CLINICAL FEATURES. Fibromas are relatively common, composing approximately 5% of all ovarian tumors. They typically occur in patients older than 40 years,[271] although they may arise in younger patients with basal cell nevus syndrome.[272] Large tumors may be associated with ascites and pleural effusion (Meigs' syndrome),[273, 274] although these findings may occur in patients with other solid ovarian tumors and tumorlike conditions. Fibromas are usually unilateral and are benign tumors cured by surgical resection.

MACROSCOPIC FINDINGS. Fibromas are typically solid and firm with uniformly lobulated, predominantly gray-white cut surfaces. Myxoid changes with focal cystic degeneration may be seen. Focal yellow areas and calcification may be present, resembling thecomas or Brenner tumors grossly. Cellular fibromas may be softer with areas of hemorrhage or necrosis.[275]

MICROSCOPIC FINDINGS. Fibromas are composed of interlacing fascicles and storiform patterns of spindled fibroblast-like cells with abundant collagen production (Fig. 39–31). Hyalinized areas, focal calcifications, and edema may be present. Cytologic atypia is absent or minimal, and mitotic figures are inconspicuous. Cellularity may vary even within the same tumor. Neoplasms with high cellularity are referred to as cellular fibromas if the mitotic rate is not more than three mitoses per 10 high-power fields; more mitotically active tumors are considered fibrosarcomas.[275] Fibromas and thecomas rarely contain sex cord elements composing less than 5% of the tumor and are designated stromal tumors with minor sex cord elements.[276] Their behavior more closely approximates that of usual fibromas or thecomas.

DIFFERENTIAL DIAGNOSIS. Fibromas are most often confused with thecomas. Fat-containing cells may be present in fibromas and as such are not useful in this distinction. A spectrum may exist between both of these tumors of ovarian stromal origin; in such cases, these tumors may be designated fibrothecoma or thecoma-fibroma. As noted before, fibrosarcomas may be differentiated from cellular fibromas by increased mitotic activity and cytologic atypia. Rare smooth muscle and neural tumors of the ovary may be distinguished from fibromas by standard histologic criteria and immunohistochemical profiles.

### Fibrosarcoma

Fibrosarcomas are rare primary ovarian neoplasms and resemble fibrosarcomas of other sites. They exhibit high cellularity, cytologic atypia, and more than three mitoses per 10 high-power fields.[275]

### Sclerosing Stromal Tumor

CLINICAL FEATURES. Sclerosing stromal tumors are distinctive neoplasms that predominantly occur in women younger than 30 years.[277, 278] They are occasionally estrogenic and only rarely androgenic. These are unilateral benign tumors.

MACROSCOPIC FINDINGS. These are typically well-circumscribed, predominantly solid neoplasms with frequent edematous or cystic areas. Cut surfaces are gray-white with yellow flecks. They vary in size, with an average diameter of approximately 10 cm.

MICROSCOPIC FINDINGS. These tumors are characterized microscopically by lobules or pseudolobules separated by collagenous or edematous stromal bands (Fig. 39–32). The lobules are typically highly vascular and consist of a dual cell population; spindled cells produce collagen, and round or oval cells contain eosinophilic or vacuolated, lipid-laden cytoplasm. Mitotic figures are inconspicuous. The tumor cells have been reported to show immunohistochemical and electron microscopic evidence of smooth muscle differentiation.[279, 280]

DIFFERENTIAL DIAGNOSIS. The characteristic highly vascular pseudolobules and paucity of hya-

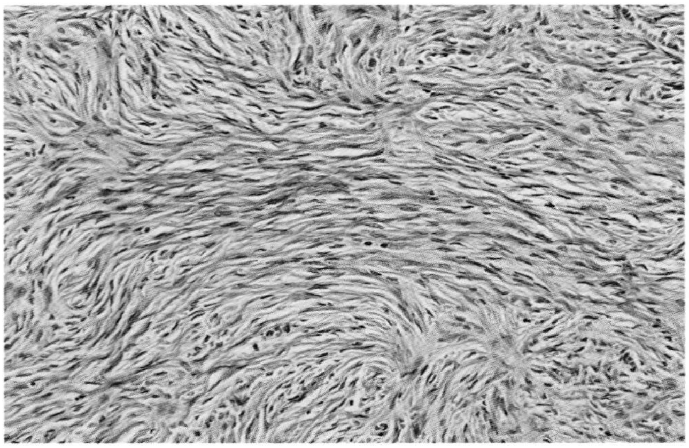

FIGURE 39–31. Fibroma composed of bundles of spindled cells with elongated, sharp-ended nuclei and abundant collagen. (Original magnification ×200.)

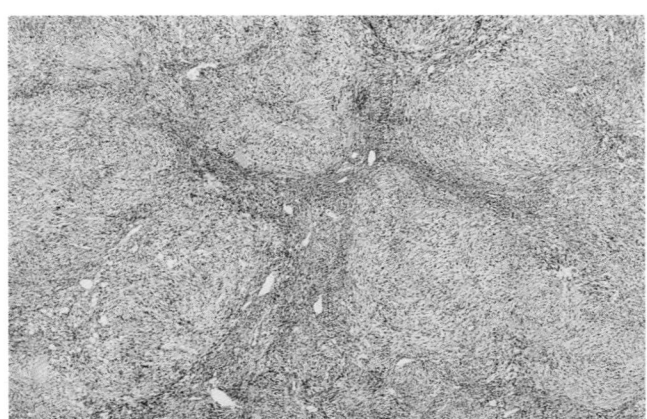

FIGURE 39–32. Sclerosing stromal tumor. Low-power magnification demonstrates typical pseudolobulated appearance. (Original magnification ×20.)

line plaques in sclerosing stromal tumors help distinguish these neoplasms from relatively more uniform fibromas and thecomas. The lipid-laden vacuolated cells of sclerosing stromal tumors may resemble signet ring cell tumors of metastatic mucinous adenocarcinomas, which may be differentiated by appropriate stains.

## SERTOLI AND SERTOLI-LEYDIG CELL TUMORS

These tumors have also been called arrhenoblastomas and androblastomas. They include tumors composed of only Sertoli cells[281, 282] and those composed of admixtures of Sertoli and Leydig cells. Tumors composed purely of Leydig cells are included among steroid cell tumors as discussed in a later section.

### Clinical Features

These tumors are uncommon, constituting far less than 1% of all ovarian neoplasms, and occur predominantly in patients between 20 and 40 years of age.[283–285] Approximately 40% of patients present with features of excess androgen secretion. Occasional tumors produce estrogen, and the remaining are nonfunctioning. The majority of tumors are unilateral; they are bilateral in only 2% of cases. These are typically benign neoplasms, although 10% to 15% of tumors are clinically malignant and have been poorly differentiated or of intermediate differentiation with retiform areas, or have contained heterologous mesenchymal elements.

### Macroscopic Findings

Sertoli-Leydig cell tumors vary greatly in size, with an average diameter of approximately 10 cm. They are lobulated, firm, predominantly solid masses with smooth external surfaces and tan to yellow cut surfaces. Retiform variants and those with heterologous elements may have prominent cysts. Hemorrhage and necrosis are uncommon except in poorly differentiated tumors.

### Microscopic Findings

Sertoli only tumors are composed of hollow and solid tubules lined by cuboid to columnar mature Sertoli cells with pale cytoplasm and bland nuclei. The fibrotic stroma contains only rare or no Leydig cells.

Sertoli-Leydig cell tumors vary widely in their microscopic appearances and have been divided into six general categories: well-differentiated, intermediate-differentiated, poorly differentiated, with heterologous elements, retiform, and mixed.[48, 71, 284–289] Well-differentiated or grade 1 tumors have hollow or solid tubules (Fig. 39–33) composed of bland-appearing Sertoli cells interspersed with variable numbers of Leydig cells that occasionally contain Reinke crystalloids. Grade 2 tumors of intermediate differentiation exhibit a wide variety of growth patterns. Typically, they consist of immature Sertoli cells arranged in lobulated sheets, aggregates, or

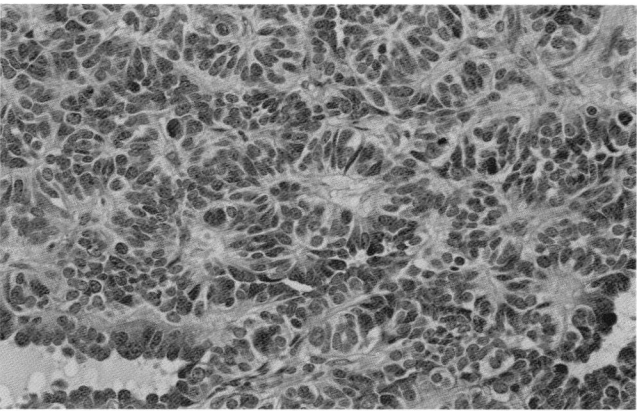

**FIGURE 39–33.** Sertoli-Leydig cell tumor with hollow and solid tubules. (Original magnification ×400.)

cords (CD Fig. 39–34) resembling embryonic testicular sex cords. The stroma usually contains clusters of recognizable Leydig cells (Fig. 39–34) but may be composed of indifferent spindled cells with discernible mitoses. Variably sized cysts containing eosinophilic material may be present (CD Fig. 39–35). Grade 3 poorly differentiated (CD Fig. 39–36) or sarcomatoid tumors are predominantly composed of diffusely infiltrating spindled cells with nuclear atypia and high mitotic activity, resembling fibrosarcoma or poorly differentiated carcinoma. These lesions may be identified as Sertoli-Leydig cell tumors by the additional presence of tubules or cords of Sertoli cells and aggregates of Leydig cells with more diagnostic patterns of these tumors.

Tumors of intermediate or poor differentiation may contain heterologous elements in approximately 20% of cases. The most common element consists of cysts lined by gastrointestinal mucinous epithelium often containing goblet and neuroendocrine cells (CD Figs. 39–37 and 39–38). This mucinous epithelium is benign appearing in most cases but may be of low malignant potential or low-grade adenocarci-

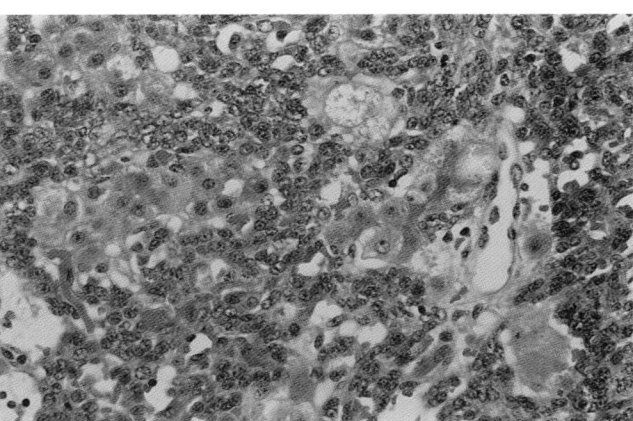

**FIGURE 39–34.** Sertoli-Leydig cell tumor of intermediate differentiation. Aggregates of immature, small Sertoli cells are admixed with clusters of Leydig cells containing abundant eosinophilic granular cytoplasm. (Original magnification ×400.)

noma. Cartilage, bone, skeletal muscle, smooth muscle, and fat may also be present. Tumors with a retiform pattern resemble the rete tubules of the testis and ovary. These areas are composed of elongated branching tubules with irregular slitlike spaces that may contain blunt papillae with hyalinized or edematous cores (CD Fig. 39–39). The spaces are lined by low cuboid cells with round, usually uniform nuclei and scant cytoplasm. Mixed tumors with combinations of these patterns also occur. Like granulosa cell tumors, Sertoli-Leydig cell tumors may contain cells with bizarre and multiple nuclei presenting probable degenerative changes,[256] and those that arise in pregnant patients may be extensively edematous.[290]

### Differential Diagnosis

The differential diagnosis of Sertoli-Leydig cell tumors is long and complex. Most difficulties occur with poorly differentiated and retiform tumors and those with heterologous elements. They may be difficult to distinguish from endometrioid adenocarcinomas, tumors that usually occur in older patients without symptoms of excess androgen or estrogen production. Useful histologic and immunohistochemical differentiating criteria were previously discussed for endometrioid tumors.[98, 99]

Retiform tumors with papillae may be confused with serous LMP tumors, low-grade adenocarcinomas, and papillary areas of endodermal sinus (yolk sac) tumors. To further complicate matters, all of these tumors may be associated with elevated serum AFP levels.[291, 292] Extensive tumor sampling, with particular attention to areas between the retiform areas, should reveal other diagnostic features of Sertoli-Leydig cell tumors.

When tumors are composed predominantly of heterologous elements, they may be confused with cystic teratomas but only rarely contain neuroectodermal tissues that are common in these tumors. Squamous and respiratory epithelium and skin adnexal structures have not been reported in Sertoli-Leydig cell tumors. They may also simulate cystic mucinous tumors or metastatic adenocarcinoma when abundant gastrointestinal glands are present; however, more diagnostic areas of Sertoli-Leydig cell differentiation are found between and around these glands with adequate sampling. The differential diagnosis also includes sarcoma and carcinosarcoma when mesenchymal heterologous elements are extensive. Immunohistochemistry may be useful in problematic cases. Sertoli cell components are immunoreactive for keratin and often for inhibin but are negative for EMA, CA 19-9, CA 125, carcinoembryonic antigen, S-100 protein, and placental alkaline phosphatase.[101, 293] Some tumors may also be positive for AFP.[291]

### Prognosis

The prognosis of Sertoli cell and Sertoli-Leydig cell tumors as a group is generally favorable. For most young women, a unilateral salpingo-oophorec-tomy is adequate therapy in the absence of adverse prognostic features. Prognosis correlates closely with stage, rupture, and degree of differentiation or subtype.[281, 284–286] In a large series of 207 cases reported by Young and Scully,[285] all of the well-differentiated tumors were benign; however, 11% of those with intermediate differentiation, 59% of the poorly differentiated tumors, and 19% of cases with heterologous elements behaved in a malignant fashion. The presence of a retiform pattern may also be associated with aggressive behavior in approximately 25% of cases.[48] Recurrences of malignant Sertoli-Leydig cell tumors usually appear early, within 1 year of initial therapy in about two thirds of patients.[285]

## GYNANDROBLASTOMA

Gynandroblastoma is an extremely rare neoplasm that consists of admixtures of Sertoli-Leydig cell and granulosa-theca cell tumor elements. This tumor tends to be overdiagnosed because minor components of each tumor may be present in the other. This diagnosis should be reserved for those tumors that consist of at least 10% of the lesser component. Some patients may present with androgenic or estrogenic manifestations.[294–297]

## SEX CORD TUMOR WITH ANNULAR TUBULES

Sex cord tumor with annular tubules is a distinctive neoplasm that is associated with Peutz-Jeghers syndrome (familial gastrointestinal polyposis, mucocutaneous melanin pigmentation) in approximately one third of cases.[298–301] Tumors tend to be bilateral, small, multifocal, and focally calcified in those patients with this syndrome; those without the syndrome tend to have unilateral, larger, rarely calcified tumors that may behave in a malignant fashion in approximately 20% of cases. About half of all cases are associated with relative hyperestrogenism.

Microscopic examination shows that these tumors contain characteristic, sharply circumscribed aggregates of simple and complex ring-shaped tubules resembling testicular structures (CD Fig. 39–40). The tubules are composed of columnar cells with pale, lipid-containing cytoplasm, and the nuclei are arranged in an antipodal fashion (Fig. 39–35) (CD Fig. 39–41). The spaces of the tubules contain densely eosinophilic, hyalinized basement membrane–like material. Other areas of the tumor resemble granulosa cell tumors. Its other clinicopathologic features warrant its designation as a distinctive neoplasm.

## STEROID CELL TUMORS

Steroid (lipid) cell tumors are defined as those composed of large cells that simulate luteinized stromal cells, Leydig cells, or adrenal cortical cells. Many but not all of these tumors contain intracellular lipid; hence, steroid cell tumor is the term preferred to lipid cell tumor. The three categories of these tumors are stromal luteoma,[302] hilus (Leydig) cell tumor,[303, 304] and steroid cell tumor not otherwise specified.[305, 306]

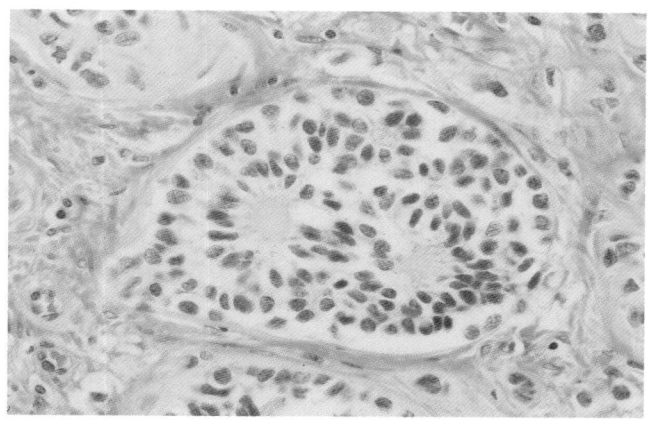

**FIGURE 39–35.** Sex cord tumor with annular tubules. The tubules contain dense eosinophilic material. Note the antipodal arrangement of nuclei in the cells. (Original magnification ×400.)

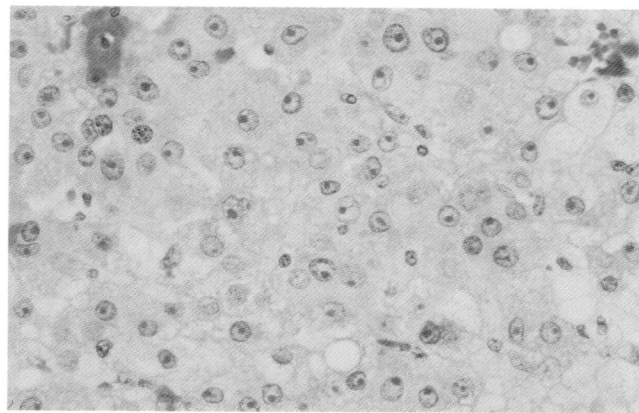

**FIGURE 39–36.** Hilus cell tumor. (Original magnification ×400.)

### Stromal Luteoma

CLINICAL FEATURES. These tumors constitute approximately 20% of steroid cell tumors. They occur predominantly in postmenopausal women with associated estrogenic manifestations in more than half of cases; approximately 10% may be androgenic. They are unilateral benign neoplasms.

MACROSCOPIC FINDINGS. Stromal luteomas arise from and are confined to the ovarian stroma. They are well-circumscribed small neoplasms measuring less than 3 cm in greatest dimension with tan-yellow to brown cut surfaces.

MICROSCOPIC FINDINGS. These tumors consist of sheets and cords of luteinized cells with abundant eosinophilic cytoplasm that frequently contains lipochrome pigment. Nuclei are bland, and mitotic figures are inconspicuous. They frequently coexist with areas of stromal hyperplasia in the same or contralateral ovary. Degenerative changes consisting of irregular round or slitlike spaces may be present.

### Hilus (Leydig) Cell Tumor

CLINICAL FEATURES. These tumors make up approximately 15% of steroid cell tumors and arise principally in postmenopausal women. Most of these neoplasms are androgenic, and the remainder are usually nonfunctioning; estrogenic tumors are relatively uncommon. They are typically unilateral, benign neoplasms.

MACROSCOPIC FINDINGS. Most of these tumors arise from the ovarian hilum; few originate in the stroma. They are well-circumscribed tumors that vary greatly in size, although most measure less than 5 cm in diameter. Cut surfaces are yellow-orange to brown and may have hemorrhagic foci.

MICROSCOPIC FINDINGS. These tumors consist of large, uniform, rounded or polygonal cells with central nuclei containing conspicuous single or multiple nucleoli (Fig. 39–36). Cytoplasm is abundant,

eosinophilic, and finely granular to foamy; it may contain lipochrome pigment. Reinke crystalloids are demonstrable in approximately half of hilar cases and must be present in those of nonhilar origin. Mitoses are not discernible. Degenerative changes similar to those seen in stromal luteomas may be present.

### Steroid Cell Tumor, Not Otherwise Specified

CLINICAL FEATURES. These are the most common steroid cell tumors, composing approximately 60% of this category. They may occur in patients of any age. Most are androgenic, and the remainder are estrogenic or nonfunctioning. Few tumors have been associated with Cushing's syndrome.[307] They are usually unilateral; however, one quarter or more may have a malignant course with extraovarian spread.

MACROSCOPIC FINDINGS. Steroid cell tumors not otherwise specified are well-circumscribed neoplasms that vary greatly in size. Cut surfaces are predominantly solid and yellow-orange to red-brown; they may contain areas of hemorrhage, necrosis, and cystic degeneration (Fig. 39–37).

MICROSCOPIC FINDINGS. These tumors are composed of nests or diffuse aggregates of cells separated by a highly vascular stroma. The cells are large and round or polygonal, and they contain abundant eosinophilic to pale vacuolated cytoplasm in which lipochrome pigment may be observed (Fig. 39–38). Reinke crystalloids are absent. Nuclei are centrally located, with conspicuous nucleoli.

PROGNOSIS. Morphologic features associated with malignant behavior include tumors greater than 7 cm in diameter, necrosis, hemorrhage, pronounced nuclear atypia, and two mitoses or more per 10 high-power fields.[306]

### Differential Diagnosis of Steroid Cell Tumors

The differential diagnosis of tumors in this category includes other tumors in which extensive lu-

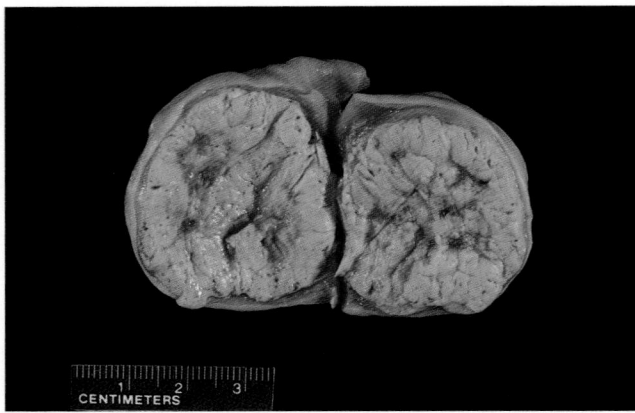

**FIGURE 39–37.** Steroid cell tumor, not otherwise specified. The tumor mass is circumscribed and has a lobulated yellow cut surface. This tumor arose in a 17-year-old woman with markedly elevated serum testosterone levels.

teinization may be present, such as granulosa cell tumor, thecoma, lipid-rich Sertoli cell tumor, and sclerosing stromal tumor. Other eosinophilic and clear cell tumors may also be considered, including oxyphilic endometrioid carcinoma; hepatoid carcinoma; hepatoid endodermal sinus tumor; ovarian clear cell carcinoma; and metastatic carcinomas of renal, adrenal, or hepatic origin. In contrast to steroid cell tumors, pregnancy-associated proliferations such as luteomas and hyperreactio luteinalis are often bilateral and multiple as discussed in a subsequent section. Steroid cell tumors are immunoreactive for vimentin in three quarters of cases, for cytokeratins in one third to one half, and for actin in one quarter to one third.[308]

## UNCLASSIFIED SEX CORD–STROMAL TUMORS

Approximately 10% of sex cord–stromal tumors do not demonstrate unequivocal patterns of ovarian or

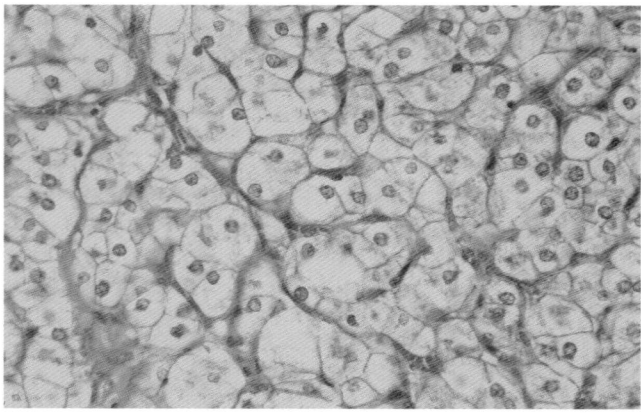

**FIGURE 39–38.** Steroid cell tumor, not otherwise specified. The cells contain abundant pale cytoplasm. (Original magnification ×400.)

testicular differentiation and as such are considered unclassified. Classification may be particularly difficult in those tumors that occur in pregnant patients, when the morphologic appearance may be confounded by extensive edema and luteinization.[290]

## IMMUNOHISTOCHEMISTRY OF SEX CORD–STROMAL TUMORS

Various steroid hormones, their precursors, and related biosynthesis enzymes may be immunohistochemically demonstrated in this group of neoplasms and generally reflect the morphologic appearance and hormonal activity of the tumor in most cases.[309–311] Immunoreactivity for the α-subunit of inhibin has been demonstrated as a marker of sex cord–stromal differentiation and may be useful in the diagnostic distinction of problematic cases as previously discussed.[101, 259, 260] Other immunohistochemical profiles of differential diagnostic utility are discussed earlier for selected specific sex cord–stromal tumors.

## MOLECULAR BIOLOGY OF SEX CORD–STROMAL TUMORS

Few genetic studies have been conducted in nonepithelial ovarian tumors. Trisomy 12 is frequently observed in sex cord–stromal tumors, including adult and juvenile granulosa cell tumors and those in the thecoma-fibroma group,[312–315] although this cytogenetic abnormality has also been reported as a common finding in serous LMP tumors.[314] DNA ploidy analysis studies have shown that the majority of adult granulosa cell tumors are diploid or near-diploid, whereas up to nearly half of juvenile granulosa cell tumors are aneuploid.[316–320] The independent prognostic value of DNA ploidy or proliferation in these tumors has not been convincingly demonstrated.

# Germ Cell Tumors

Germ cell tumors constitute approximately 20% to 30% of all ovarian neoplasms. They are thought to be derived from primitive totipotential germ cells and may appear undifferentiated (dysgerminoma) or as high-grade anaplastic carcinoma (embryonal carcinoma), or they may exhibit some degree of differentiation resembling extraembryonic yolk sac (endodermal sinus tumor), trophoblast (choriocarcinoma), or combinations of the three embryonic germ layers (teratoma). Most germ cell tumors occur in children and adolescents and account for two thirds to three quarters of all ovarian tumors in these age groups.[321] About 95% of germ cell tumors are benign mature cystic teratomas curative by surgical resection. The remainder are malignant tumors warranting adjuvant radiation, chemotherapy, or both. Advances in chemotherapeutic regimens for malignant germ cell tumors have yielded overall 5-year survival rates of greater than 95%.[322, 323]

# DYSGERMINOMA

## Clinical Features

Dysgerminomas account for approximately 1% of all ovarian neoplasms and about half of malignant germ cell tumors. More than 80% occur in patients younger than 30 years; they are somewhat more common in the right ovary than in the left, and they are bilateral in 10% to 15% of cases.[324, 325] Approximately 5% of cases are associated with abnormal gonadal development and may arise from an underlying gonadoblastoma. These are typically hormonally nonfunctioning tumors; most patients present with symptoms of an abdominopelvic mass.

## Macroscopic Findings

Dysgerminomas are typically well-circumscribed, large tumors with smooth or cerebriform external surfaces. Cut surfaces are solid, lobulated, and soft; they may be tan, gray, yellow, pink, or red (Fig. 39–39). Areas of hemorrhage, necrosis, or cystic degeneration may be present, which should be extensively sampled to evaluate for other germ cell components.

## Microscopic Findings

These tumors are composed of well-defined nests or bands of tumor cells separated by fibrous septa (Fig. 39–40) infiltrated by numerous mature lymphocytes with occasional lymphoid follicles and non-necrotizing granulomas. The tumor cells are large, uniform, and rounded, and they contain abundant pale to finely granular eosinophilic glycogen-rich cytoplasm with distinct cell borders. Nuclei are typically large, centrally located, and vesicular with coarse chromatin; they contain prominent single or multiple nucleoli (Fig. 39–41). Mitotic figures are frequent. Rare dysgerminomas may appear anaplastic with highly pleomorphic nuclei and mitotic rates in excess of 30 mitotic figures per 10 high-power fields.[326] Like testicular seminomas, ovarian dysgerminomas may contain foci of differentiation toward other germ cell elements.[327–329] About 3% of dysger-

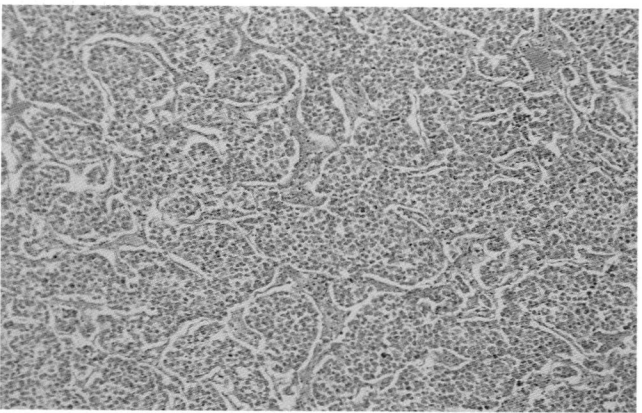

**FIGURE 39–40.** Dysgerminoma. The tumor cells are arranged in nests separated by fibrous septa. (Original magnification ×100.)

minomas contain scattered human chorionic gonadotropin (hCG)–positive syncytiotrophoblastic giant cells adjacent to blood vessels with associated elevated serum hCG levels, but they lack the concomitant presence of cytotrophoblast to warrant a diagnosis of mixed germ cell tumor with choriocarcinoma.[327] The presence of abortive yolk sac elements may be associated with elevated serum AFP levels.[328] The presence of these and other admixed germ cell components significantly affects prognosis as discussed later. Focal calcification in a dysgerminoma should prompt a search for an underlying gonadoblastoma.

## Differential Diagnosis

The differential diagnosis of dysgerminoma includes other malignant neoplasms with diffuse growth patterns, such as endodermal sinus tumor, embryonal carcinoma, clear cell carcinoma, and other poorly differentiated primary or metastatic carcinomas. Characteristic clinical presentations, the presence of more diagnostic areas, and immunohistochemical profiles are useful in distinguishing these

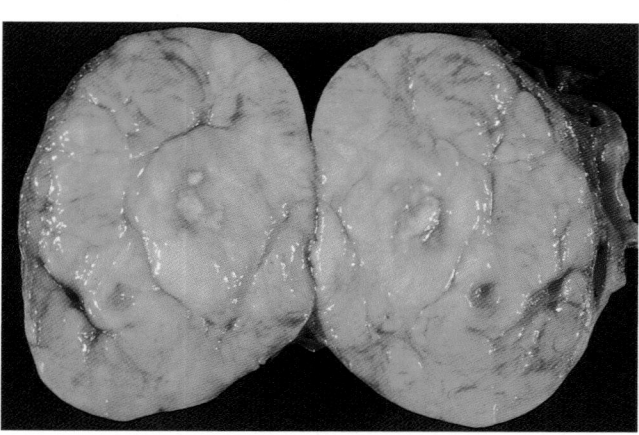

**FIGURE 39–39.** Dysgerminoma. The tumor has a lobulated, soft, yellow-tan cut surface with focal necrosis.

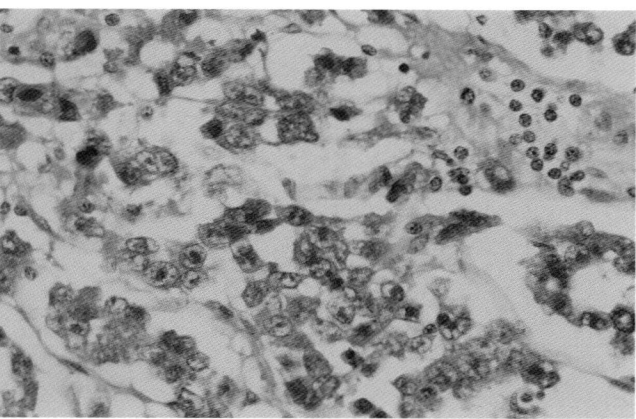

**FIGURE 39–41.** Dysgerminoma. Nuclei are large and vesicular and contain prominent nucleoli. Note the lymphocytes within the stroma at upper right. (Original magnification ×400.)

tumors. These tumors may also resemble large cell lymphomas involving the ovary, but the absence of glycogen in lymphomas and distinctive immunophenotypes help separate these neoplasms.

### Prognosis

The majority of dysgerminomas are unilateral, and 5-year survival rates for low-stage pure tumors are nearly 100%. Like testicular seminomas, these tumors are exquisitely radiosensitive; however, because of advances in chemotherapeutic regimens, adjuvant multidrug chemotherapy after surgical resection is preferred.[322] The 5-year survival rates of higher stage tumors are greater than 80%.

## ENDODERMAL SINUS TUMOR (YOLK SAC TUMOR)

### Clinical Features

Endodermal sinus tumor is a malignant germ cell tumor that exhibits differentiation toward extraembryonic endoderm and mesoderm, recapitulating embryonic yolk sac development.[330] These tumors are most common in children and adolescents, occurring only rarely in patients older than 40 years.[331–337] The typical presentation is that of a large abdominopelvic mass frequently associated with the sudden onset of pain, and serum AFP levels are almost invariably elevated. Rare patients may present with virilization.[338] Virtually all ovarian endodermal sinus tumors are unilateral, although they are aggressive neoplasms; one third to nearly one half of patients present with extraovarian disease involving the peritoneum or retroperitoneal lymph nodes.

### Macroscopic Findings

Endodermal sinus tumors are typically large encapsulated tumors with an average diameter of approximately 15 cm. Cut surfaces are usually solid or solid and cystic, soft, and tan-yellow to gray, with frequent areas of hemorrhage and necrosis (Fig. 39–

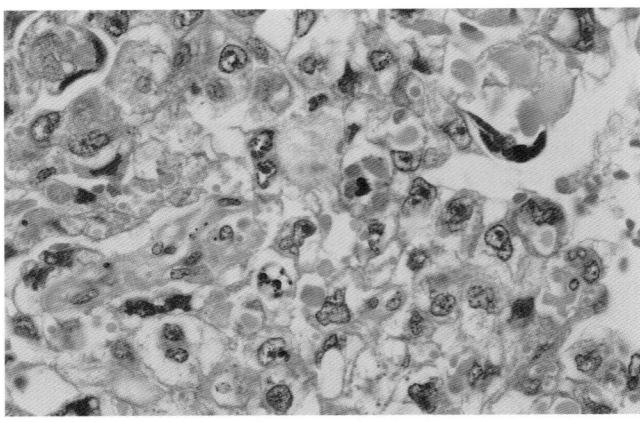

**FIGURE 39–43.** Endodermal sinus (yolk sac) tumor. The tumor cells are large with abundant clear to granular cytoplasm and contain markedly pleomorphic nuclei. Note the densely eosinophilic hyaline globules. (Original magnification ×600.)

42). The polyvesicular-vitelline variant may have a microcystic gross appearance.

### Microscopic Findings

Endodermal sinus tumors consist of tumor cells with moderately abundant clear to finely granular cytoplasm containing glycogen and occasionally lipid. Nuclei are large, pleomorphic with irregular borders, and hyperchromatic and contain prominent nucleoli (Fig. 39–43). Mitotic figures are numerous and may be atypical. Extracellular or intracellular hyaline globules are frequently present and are usually immunoreactive for $\alpha_1$-antitrypsin or AFP.

Endodermal sinus tumors exhibit a myriad of architectural growth patterns. Most tumors contain one or more areas with a reticular or papillary pattern. The most common pattern is reticular (Fig. 39–44) or microcystic composed of interconnecting spaces lined by flattened to cuboid tumor cells. The endodermal sinus or papillary pattern (CD Fig. 39–42) consists of characteristic Schiller-Duval bodies

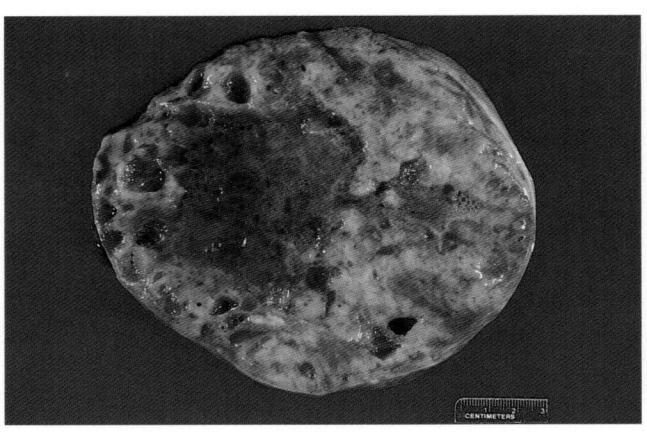

**FIGURE 39–42.** Endodermal sinus (yolk sac) tumor. This large tumor has a variegated solid and cystic cut surface with hemorrhage and focal necrosis.

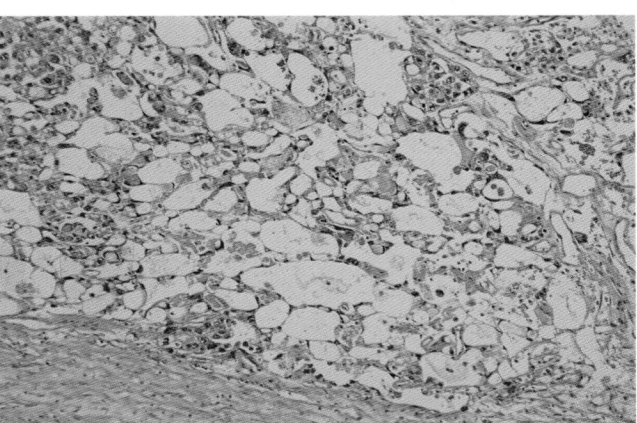

**FIGURE 39–44.** Endodermal sinus (yolk sac) tumor, reticular pattern. (Original magnification ×100.)

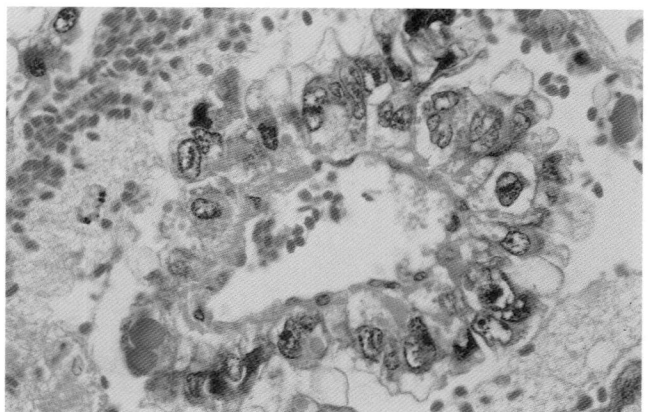

**FIGURE 39–45.** Endodermal sinus (yolk sac) tumor with Schiller-Duval body. (Original magnification ×600.)

(CD Fig. 39–43), which are thought to recapitulate embryonic structures in the rat placenta. Schiller-Duval bodies (Fig. 39–45) consist of rounded to elongated papillae with fibrovascular cores containing a single central vessel and are covered by a single layer of columnar or cuboid tumor cells. The parietal pattern is characterized by extracellular basement membrane–like material analogous to Reichert membrane of parietal yolk sac origin.[336] The polyvesicular-vitelline pattern is composed of small cysts or vesicles with eccentric constrictions lined by flattened to cuboid cells, separated by a densely compact spindled cell stroma.[339] Hepatoid areas simulate hepatocellular carcinoma and are composed of nests of large polyhedral cells with abundant eosinophilic cytoplasm.[127] Predominantly glandular areas may exhibit intestinal differentiation[340] or resemble endometrioid adenocarcinomas[105] (CD Fig. 39–44). Less common patterns include solid (CD Fig. 39–45), myxomatous, and adenofibromatous areas. Primitive mesenchyme-like components may be prominent in some endodermal sinus tumors, especially after chemotherapy.[341] Rarely, these tumors may contain cells that resemble lipoblasts, syncytiotrophoblastic giant cells, luteinized stromal cells, granulomatous inflammation, or foci of extramedullary hematopoiesis.[332, 336, 341]

### Differential Diagnosis

Endodermal sinus tumors are most often confused with clear cell carcinoma, as previously discussed. Endometrioid-like endodermal sinus tumor[105] may resemble endometrioid carcinoma, and those with a hepatoid pattern should be distinguished from hepatoid carcinoma.[131] The differential diagnosis also includes other malignant germ cell tumors (particularly embryonal carcinoma), juvenile granulosa cell tumor, Sertoli-Leydig cell tumors, and steroid (lipid) cell tumors. The clinical presentation of endodermal sinus tumor in young patients with markedly elevated serum AFP levels, combined with extensive tumor sampling to reveal characteristic microscopic patterns, permits the proper diagnosis of these neoplasms in most cases.

### Prognosis

Although endodermal sinus tumors are highly aggressive malignant neoplasms, the advent of multiagent combination chemotherapy has resulted in long-term survival rates in at least 80% of stage I patients and in more than 50% of patients with advanced stage disease.[335] Clinical stage is the most important prognostic factor.[337] A study also found that stage I endodermal sinus tumors with three or four histologic subtype patterns had a better prognosis than did those with only one or two patterns.[342]

## EMBRYONAL CARCINOMA

Embryonal carcinoma is an extremely rare neoplasm in the ovary compared with its testicular counterpart. It usually presents as a mixed component of other germ cell tumors, most often endodermal sinus tumor, with which it shares some features.[334] Sufficient clinicopathologic differences exist between the two neoplasms to warrant their separate designations.[343, 344]

These tumors occur in children and adolescents with a median age of 14 years. Patients usually present with an abdominopelvic mass associated with pain. More than half of patients present with precocious puberty. Other presentations include abnormal bleeding through the vagina, amenorrhea, and hirsutism. Serum levels of hCG or AFP, or both, are frequently elevated.

At gross evaluation, the tumors are often large, ranging from 10 to 25 cm, and have smooth external surfaces. Cut surfaces are solid, soft, and tan-gray to yellow, with frequent areas of hemorrhage and necrosis. Microscopic examination shows that they are composed of solid masses, nests, and occasional papillae or abortive glands of large anaplastic cells (CD Fig. 39–46). Cytoplasm is pale and eosinophilic or amphophilic; it may contain large vacuoles. Nuclei are large and vesicular or hyperchromatic, and they contain single or multiple prominent nucleoli. Mitoses are frequent and may be atypical. Multinucleated syncytiotrophoblast-like tumor giant cells are frequently present. Necrosis is a common feature (CD Fig. 39–47). As with other malignant germ cell tumors, prognosis has improved with multiagent chemotherapeutic regimens.

## POLYEMBRYOMA

Polyembryoma is an exceedingly rare, highly malignant neoplasm consisting of embryoid bodies resembling early human embryos.[345, 346] It is usually a unilateral solid neoplasm with cut surfaces revealing areas of hemorrhage and necrosis. Well-formed embryoid bodies are composed of an embryonic disk lined by endoderm-like epithelium on one side and by ectoderm-type cells on the other. Amniotic and yolk sac cavities are situated on opposite sides of the embryonic disk. Most of these tumors are combined with other germ cell tumor components and may be associated with elevated serum levels of hCG or AFP.[347]

## CHORIOCARCINOMA

Primary pure choriocarcinoma of the ovary is rare.[348–351] It is more frequently present as a component of mixed germ cell tumors or as metastatic disease of corpus origin. The majority of pure primary ovarian tumors occur in children and women younger than 20 years. Serum hCG level is invariably elevated with frequent hormonal manifestations.

At gross evaluation, these tumors are usually solid soft masses with abundant hemorrhage. The microscopic diagnosis of choriocarcinoma requires the presence of both cytotrophoblast and syncytiotrophoblast cells (CD Fig. 39–48), the latter of which are strongly positive for hCG. The dual trophoblast populations are intimately admixed and frequently associated with hemorrhagic areas. Choriocarcinoma should be distinguished from other malignant germ cell tumors (dysgerminoma, embryonal carcinoma, endodermal sinus tumor) that may contain foci of syncytiotrophoblast cells but lack cytotrophoblasts. Rare, poorly differentiated carcinomas, which occur in older women, may also contain areas of choriocarcinomatous differentiation and produce hCG.[352, 353]

## TERATOMA

Teratomas are composed of mixtures of tissues derived from the three embryonic germ layers. They are divided into mature and immature forms. Mature teratomas are composed entirely of mature-appearing tissues and are considered benign neoplasms curable by surgical resection. Any degree of immaturity warrants a diagnosis of immature teratoma; thus, thorough histologic sampling is necessary for these tumors. Most tumors consist of tissues from at least two germ layers, but ectodermal, mesodermal, and endodermal derivatives can usually be demonstrated in any one tumor with adequate sampling. Occasional tumors may consist predominantly or exclusively of one tissue type and are designated monodermal teratomas. Teratomas are considered to be of parthenogenetic origin, arising from a single germ cell after the first meiotic division.[354]

### *Immature Teratoma*

CLINICAL FEATURES. Immature teratomas account for approximately 20% of malignant germ cell tumors. They occur most commonly in patients younger than 20 years who typically present with an abdominopelvic mass frequently associated with pain.[355] These are usually unilateral neoplasms, although one third of patients may present with extraovarian spread as peritoneal implants and occasional lymphatic or hematogenous dissemination.

MACROSCOPIC FINDINGS. These neoplasms are typically large with smooth external surfaces. Cut surfaces are predominantly solid and gray-tan or pink, with focal areas of hemorrhage and necrosis

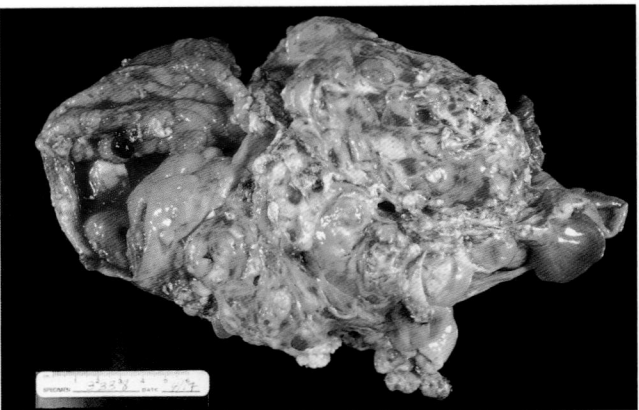

**FIGURE 39–46.** Immature teratoma with a variegated solid and cystic cut surface.

(Fig. 39–46). Small cysts or large cystic areas may also be present. Approximately one quarter may contain grossly apparent dermoid cysts, and about 10% of patients may have a dermoid cyst or other benign neoplasm in the contralateral ovary.[356]

MICROSCOPIC FINDINGS. Immature teratomas are composed of mature and variable amounts of immature tissues. The most common immature component is neuroectodermal and usually consists of tubules (Fig. 39–47), rosettes, or solid masses (CD Fig. 39–49) of primitive neuroepithelial cells. Mesodermal components as manifest by immature cartilage, skeletal muscle, or other tissues are also common. Occasional tumors are composed predominantly of endodermal derivatives.[357]

The clinical behavior of immature teratomas is related to the amount of immature elements, which are graded on a scale of 1 to 3.[355, 358] Grade 1 tumors have abundant mature tissues but also exhibit some immaturity that may involve any element. Immature neural tissue or neuroepithelium is rare and is limited to less than an aggregate area of one low-power microscopic field (×40; ×4 objective and ×10 ocu-

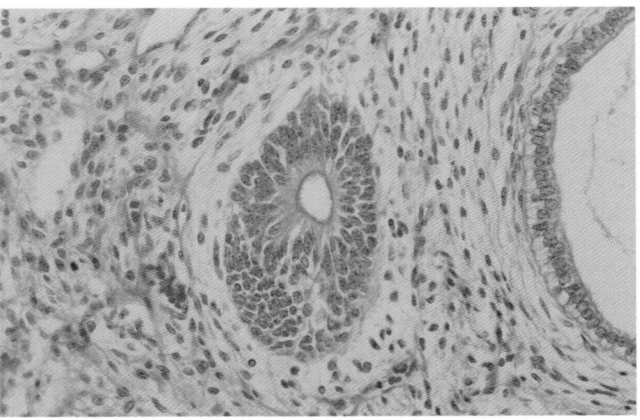

**FIGURE 39–47.** Immature teratoma with tubule of immature neuroepithelium. (Original magnification ×400.)

lar) in any slide. Mitotic activity is low. Grade 2 tumors have a greater degree of immature tissue or neuroepithelium than grade 1 neoplasms, but the aggregate area of immature tissue does not exceed three low-power fields in any one slide of tumor. Mitotic activity is moderate. Grade 3 tumors contain abundant immature tissues or neuroepithelium in more than three low-power fields per tumor slide. Mitotic activity is high.

Consideration should be given to the degree of immaturity of all tissue components in grading teratomas, although immature neuroepithelium is the most common and reproducible immature element. A two-tiered grading schema (low grade versus high grade) for immature teratomas has been proposed to enhance reproducibility, with grade 2 and grade 3 tumors combined into the high-grade category.[358] When present, metastatic foci are often mature, often as glial tissue, although they may consist of other mature elements and behave in a benign fashion; as such, they are graded separately from the primary neoplasm.[359-361]

DIFFERENTIAL DIAGNOSIS. As indicated, immature teratomas must be distinguished from benign mature teratomas, which may be achieved by extensive histologic sampling, particularly when the mature teratomas are predominantly solid neoplasms. The differential diagnosis also includes heterologous carcinosarcomas (mixed müllerian or mesodermal tumors), which occur in postmenopausal patients and lack neuroepithelial tissues, and monodermal neuroectodermal tumors discussed in a later section.

PROGNOSIS. Survival has been associated with stage and tumor size but more closely with histologic grade as described before.[355] In the past, survival was poor for high-grade neoplasms and for those tumors with immature implants. With the advent of multiagent chemotherapy after surgical resection, long-term remission and increased survival rates have been achieved in 90% or more of patients.[362-364]

### Mature Teratoma

CLINICAL FEATURES. Mature teratomas are the most common germ cell tumors; approximately 95% of tumors in this category and about 30% of all ovarian tumors are mature teratomas. They most commonly arise in children and young adults but affect a wide age range and may occur in postmenopausal women. The usual presentation is that of an abdominopelvic mass that may be associated with pain due to rupture or torsion, and leakage of cyst contents may elicit a foreign body giant cell reaction to keratin or other components.[365] These benign neoplasms are curative by conservative surgical resection, although malignant transformation may occur in approximately 2% of cases as discussed later. They are bilateral in approximately 10% of cases.

MACROSCOPIC FINDINGS. The majority of mature teratomas are cystic and are commonly referred to as dermoid cysts, although predominantly solid

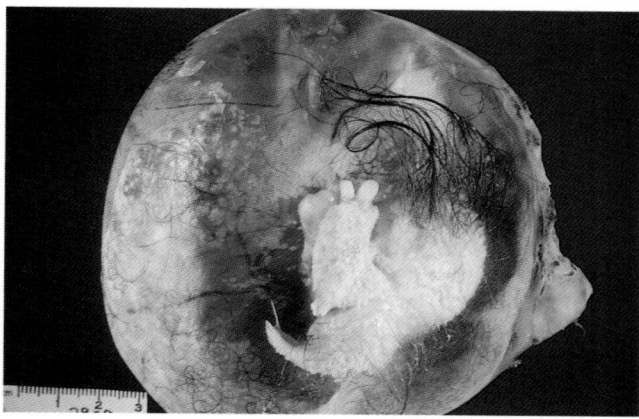

FIGURE 39–48. Mature cystic teratoma. The tumor is predominantly cystic. Note Rokitansky protuberance at the right from which brunette hair and teeth are emanating.

tumors do occur.[366] They vary in size from microscopic to large globular masses with smooth external surfaces. The cystic cavities are frequently filled with grumous keratinous and sebaceous material and hair. One or more solid masses known as Rokitansky protuberances or nodules may protrude from the cyst walls and frequently contain grossly recognizable hair, teeth, and bone (Fig. 39–48). These nodules contain the greatest variety of tissue types and should be sampled for histologic examination. Any other solid areas and those with hemorrhage or necrosis should also be sampled to exclude immature elements or malignant transformation.

MICROSCOPIC FINDINGS. These tumors are composed of mature tissues usually from all three embryonic germ layers.[367] Ectodermal derivatives predominate and consist of keratinized squamous epithelium containing hair and other skin adnexal structures (Fig. 39–49), mature glial tissue, or other organized neural structures. Common mesodermal tissues include cartilage (CD Fig. 39–50), bone, mus-

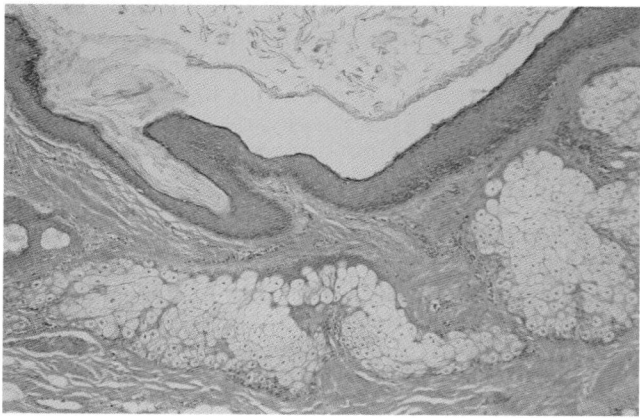

FIGURE 39–49. Mature cystic teratoma. Keratin-filled cyst is lined by stratified squamous epithelium with skin adnexal structures. (Original magnification ×100.)

cle, and fat; endodermal derivatives composed of gastrointestinal (CD Fig. 39–51) and respiratory epithelium are frequently encountered. Other organoid tissues may also be present. Mitoses are absent or infrequent.

Approximately 2% of otherwise mature cystic teratomas may exhibit malignant transformation in one of the tissue components, a complication that usually occurs in those tumors detected in older patients.[368–373] The most common cancer encountered is squamous cell carcinoma, followed by carcinoid and adenocarcinoma. Other rare malignant neoplasms have also been described. These malignant neoplasms may be confined to the teratoma or may penetrate the capsule and invade locally with a relatively poor prognosis.

### Monodermal Teratomas

Although thyroid tissue may be encountered in approximately one fifth of mature cystic teratomas, the designation of struma ovarii is reserved for those tumors that are composed predominantly or exclusively of this tissue component.[374–378] It is the most common monodermal teratoma, but overall, it is a rare neoplasm representing less than 1% of ovarian solid tumors. It occurs in a wide age range, with a peak incidence in women 40 to 50 years old. Most patients are asymptomatic, whereas others present with signs and symptoms of an abdominopelvic mass. Approximately one third of patients may present with ascites, and hyperthyroidism is occasionally attributable to functioning ovarian thyroid tumor tissue or concomitant primary thyroid disorders.[375] More than 90% of tumors are unilateral. Approximately 40% of cases are associated with extraovarian spread, and malignant change is known to occur.[376–378] The incidence of malignant change is difficult to determine because of the inconsistent criteria used among authors. Nonetheless, cases of struma ovarii with histologically malignant thyroid tissue are rarely clinically malignant, and extraovarian spread may be a late event with a prolonged clinical course.[378] In gross appearance, these are predominantly solid or solid and cystic neoplasms that vary greatly in size. Occasional neoplasms may be largely cystic, confounding the diagnosis.[379] Cut surfaces resemble thyroid tissue, appearing firm or gelatinous, frequently nodular, and tan to red-brown (CD Fig. 39–52). Hemorrhagic areas may be present. Microscopic examination shows that they are composed of thyroid tissue (CD Fig. 39–53) and may exhibit a wide spectrum of thyroid histopathologic features, including normal thyroid, non-neoplastic goiter, nonspecific lymphocytic and Hashimoto's thyroiditis, adenoma, and follicular and papillary carcinomas. Some tumors may have predominant solid or trabecular growth patterns resembling other ovarian tumors.[380] The presence of other characteristic features, such as colloid-containing calcium oxalate crystals, and positive immunoreactivity for thyroglobulin may help distinguish struma ovarii in problematic cases.

Pure epidermoid cysts are uncommon[381, 382] and in many cases may not be true monodermal neoplasms, as suggested by the frequent presence of nests of transitional epithelium in the cyst walls. They lack the skin adnexal structures and other tissues seen in mature cystic teratomas.

Pure primary ovarian carcinoid tumors[383–385] occur predominantly in postmenopausal women. Patients present with an abdominopelvic mass, and approximately one third with insular tumors, usually those with large neoplasms, will have carcinoid syndrome. Other presentations include profound constipation[386] and hormonal manifestations due to functioning stroma. These are unilateral neoplasms, although in approximately 15% of cases the contralateral ovary may contain a mature cystic teratoma, mucinous neoplasm, or Brenner tumor. At gross evaluation, pure carcinoid tumors are solid tumors with smooth external surfaces and tan to yellow homogeneous cut surfaces (CD Fig. 39–54). At microscopic examination (CD Fig. 39–55), insular carcinoid tumors[383] resemble those arising from the midgut (appendix, jejunum, ileum) and consist of discrete islands and nests of small uniform cells with round nuclei containing coarse chromatin, inconspicuous to small nucleoli, and rare mitotic figures. Small acini lined by columnar cells with more abundant cytoplasm are often present. Trabecular tumors[384, 385] resemble foregut (stomach) and hindgut (rectum) carcinoids and consist of ribbons of cuboid to columnar cells separated by fibrous stroma. Uncommon carcinoid tumors may exhibit pleomorphic architectural and cytologic features.[387] Primary carcinoid tumors may be difficult to distinguish from metastatic carcinoid.[388] Features favoring metastatic disease include detection of a probable primary lesion in the gastrointestinal tract or other site, bilateral ovarian involvement, multinodular ovarian growth, extraovarian metastases, and persistent carcinoid syndrome after removal of the ovarian tumor. A variety of neuroendocrine markers, including chromogranin, serotonin, pancreatic polypeptide, glucagon, enkephalin, somatostatin, and other less common peptides, have been immunohistochemically demonstrated in pure and mixed ovarian carcinoid tumors.[389]

Strumal carcinoids are tumors composed of admixtures of carcinoid and thyroid tissue.[390–393] The majority are benign and only rarely behave in a malignant fashion. Approximately 10% are bilateral. The carcinoid component consists of trabecular, insular, or mixed patterns. The strumal component may resemble normal or adenomatous thyroid tissue. These tumors are immunoreactive for thyroglobulin and neuroendocrine markers.

Mucinous carcinoids (adenocarcinoids) of the ovary are rare and resemble the tumors that are more frequently encountered in the appendix.[394, 395] They consist of small glands and acini lined by cuboid cells or cuboid cells with pale cytoplasm, goblet cells, and argyrophil or argentaffin cells. Occasional tumors contain foci of poorly differentiated

**TABLE 39–7.** Immunohistochemistry of Germ Cell Tumors*

| Tumor | PLAP | CK | EMA | AFP | hCG | CD30 | A1AT | CEA |
|---|---|---|---|---|---|---|---|---|
| Dysgerminoma-seminoma | +++ | ± | − | − | − | − | − | − |
| Endodermal sinus (yolk sac) tumor | ++ | ++++ | − | +++ | − | − | ++ | ± |
| Choriocarcinoma | ++ | ++++ | ++ | − | ++++ | − | + | + |
| Embryonal carcinoma | +++ | ++++ | − | + | + | +++ | ± | − |

*PLAP, Placental alkaline phosphatase; CK, cytokeratins; EMA, epithelial membrane antigen; AFP, $\alpha$-fetoprotein; hCG, human chorionic gonadotropin; A1AT, $\alpha_1$-antitrypsin; CEA, carcinoembryonic antigen.

adenocarcinoma with signet ring cells resembling metastatic Krukenberg tumor. Mucinous carcinoids are more likely to be associated with a malignant course than are other types of ovarian carcinoid tumors.

Ovarian neuroectodermal tumors are uncommon and resemble central nervous system neoplasms.[396, 397] They include tumors resembling differentiated ependymoma, primitive neuroectodermal tumor, medulloblastoma, medulloepithelioma, neuroblastoma, and anaplastic glioblastoma multiforme. They affect a wide age range but occur predominantly in women younger than 40 years. They are typically large, variably cystic, and solid friable neoplasms. Extraovarian spread is common with the primitive and anaplastic types. Differentiated ependymomas have a favorable prognosis, whereas the other types have an aggressive behavior. The differential diagnosis of neuroectodermal tumors includes surface epithelial and small cell carcinomas, sex cord–stromal tumors, and immature teratomas. Clinical features, thorough tumor sampling to exclude other more diagnostic areas, and immunohistochemical panels to include glial fibrillary acidic protein are useful in problematic cases.

Ovarian sebaceous tumors arising in dermoid cysts are rare.[398] The reported cases have all been unilateral. They histologically resemble sebaceous neoplasms of the skin ranging from adenoma to carcinoma. Most of these patients have had a favorable outcome, with only one known recurrence.

## MIXED GERM CELL TUMORS

Approximately 10% of germ cell tumors contain mixtures of malignant histologic types.[399, 400] The most common combination consists of dysgerminoma and endodermal sinus tumor, although many other mixtures may occur.[401] The therapy and prognosis for patients with mixed germ cell tumors may depend on both the amount and the histologic type of the neoplastic elements, warranting extensive sampling of these tumors. The relative composition of the various histologic types should be included in the surgical pathology report.

## IMMUNOHISTOCHEMISTRY OF GERM CELL TUMORS

Useful expected immunohistochemistry reaction patterns of germ cell tumors that may occur in pure or mixed forms are summarized in Table 39–7.[402–405] Expression of placental alkaline phosphatase in the absence of EMA immunoreactivity appears to be a pattern characteristic of germ cell tumors. The distinction of dysgerminomas from other germ cell tumors is of particular therapeutic and prognostic importance. Unlike other germ cell tumors, dysgerminomas are usually negative for cytokeratin, although approximately 10% of these tumors may be cytokeratin positive. Dysgerminomas are also usually negative for AFP, hCG, and CD30 in the majority of tumor cells, which assists in the distinction from other subtypes. Endodermal sinus tumors and choriocarcinomas are most often positive for AFP and hCG, respectively. Endodermal sinus tumors are also often immunoreactive for $\alpha_1$-antitrypsin, particularly in the hyaline globules. CD30 (Ki-1, Ber-H2) has been reported to be a relatively specific marker for testicular embryonal carcinomas,[403–405] a finding that may be extrapolated to those that arise in the ovary. Lack of immunoreactivity for EMA, leukocyte common antigen (CD45), and S-100 protein assists in the distinction of germ cell tumors from carcinomas, lymphomas, and melanoma, respectively.

## MOLECULAR BIOLOGY OF GERM CELL TUMORS

Relatively few such studies have been reported for ovarian germ cell tumors. Dysgerminoma shares the same chromosome marker as seminoma, an isochromosome i(12p), and may also exhibit apparent nonrandom gains of chromosomes 7 and 12.[406] DNA cytometry analyses have shown that these tumors are aneuploid to near-tetraploid,[406, 407] and variation in DNA index does not correlate with clinical outcome measures.[407] Most ovarian immature teratomas have normal 46,XX karyotypes, and the presence of karyotypic abnormalities correlates with tumor grade and possibly prognosis.[408]

# Mixed Germ Cell and Sex Cord–Stromal Tumors

## GONADOBLASTOMA

Gonadoblastomas, rare neoplasms composed of germ cell and sex cord–stromal derivatives, usually occur in children and adolescents with underlying abnormal gonadal development.[409] Most patients have pure or mixed gonadal dysgenesis, and a Y chromosome is present in more than 90% of patients. Nearly 40% are bilateral. They are usually small tumors and may be apparent only at microscopic examination, although large tumors may also occur. At gross evaluation, they are solid, gray-white to yellow-brown tumors with various degrees of calcification. The macroscopic appearance may vary if concomitant malignant germ cell elements are present. Microscopic examination shows intimate admixtures of nests of mitotically active primitive germ cells and sex cord–stromal derivatives resembling immature Sertoli and granulosa cells. Leydig cells or luteinized stromal cells are frequently present. Globular aggregates or bands of hyaline basement membrane–like material and calcification are usually found and may be extensive (CD Figs. 39–56 to 39–58). Approximately half or more of cases may give rise to a malignant germ cell tumor, most frequently dysgerminoma, although other histologic types may be encountered.[410, 411] Pure gonadoblastomas are benign, whereas those that harbor a malignant germ cell tumor have a prognosis associated with the respective components.

## UNCLASSIFIED MIXED GERM CELL AND SEX CORD–STROMAL TUMOR

This category includes mixed germ cell and sex cord–stromal tumors with clinicopathologic features that differ from gonadoblastoma.[412, 413] These tumors arise in genotypically normal children younger than 10 years. The tumors are unilateral and usually achieve large dimensions. They consist microscopically of admixtures of germ cell and sex cord–stromal derivatives arranged in diffuse masses, long ramifying cords and trabeculae, or tubules, but they usually lack the hyaline basement membrane–like material and calcification frequently observed in gonadoblastoma. These tumors are usually benign, although malignant germ cell components may occasionally be present.

## Miscellaneous Tumors

The ovarian tumors discussed here include those of uncertain histogenesis, tumors not specific to the ovary, and other miscellaneous neoplasms.

### SMALL CELL CARCINOMA OF THE HYPERCALCEMIC TYPE

#### Clinical Features

Primary ovarian small cell carcinomas of the hypercalcemic type are highly aggressive malignant neoplasms that occur in women younger than 40 years.[414–418] Although most reports suggest that this tumor is a poorly differentiated carcinoma, the histogenesis remains unclear. Approximately two thirds of patients present with hypercalcemia that is probably due to the secretion of a parathyroid hormone–related protein. The neoplasms are usually unilat-

eral, although one third of patients present with extraovarian disease. Approximately one third of patients with stage IA disease may achieve long-term survival; however, the prognosis for more advanced stages is extremely poor.

#### Macroscopic Findings

These neoplasms are usually large, with an average diameter of 15 cm. Cut surfaces are solid to lobulated, soft, and gray-white to tan. Areas of hemorrhage and necrosis are frequent.

#### Microscopic Findings

These tumors are composed of diffuse sheets of small cells admixed with variable numbers of characteristic follicle-like spaces containing eosinophilic fluid. Small nests, cords, and single tumor cells may also be present. The tumor cells are typically small with scant cytoplasm; small round nuclei contain coarse chromatin and discernible single small nucleoli and are highly mitotically active. Approximately half or more of cases may also contain larger cells with abundant eosinophilic cytoplasm and large nuclei with prominent nucleoli. These cells may predominate in some tumors, and the cytoplasm may contain globular hyaline inclusions imparting a rhabdoid appearance to the cells. In approximately 10% to 15% of cases, the cystic spaces are lined by mucinous epithelial cells.

Immunohistochemical staining reveals that tumor cells are usually immunoreactive for cytokeratins, most frequently low-molecular-weight cytokeratin, and may also be positive for EMA, vimentin, neuron-specific enolase, chromogranin A, parathyroid hormone–related protein, and occasionally parathyroid hormone. They are negative for S-100 protein, B72.3, and desmin.[415, 418] Ultrastructural study shows that the cells have specialized cell junctions with occasional desmosomes and abundant dilated rough endoplasmic reticulum; dense-core granules of neurosecretory-secretory type are generally absent.[417] These tumors are DNA diploid, a feature of differential diagnostic utility, as discussed next.[419]

#### Differential Diagnosis

This tumor should be distinguished from primary ovarian small cell carcinoma of the pulmonary type, which resembles small cell neuroendocrine carcinoma of the lung and other organs.[420, 421] These tumors usually arise in perimenopausal or postmenopausal women, are bilateral in approximately half of cases, and are not associated with hypercalcemia. They differ microscopically from the small cell carcinomas of hypercalcemic type by the absence or paucity of follicle-like spaces, evenly dispersed chromatin, and inconspicuous nucleoli. They may coexist with endometrioid carcinoma or other epithelial tumors. Immunohistochemical profiles may overlap between the two types, although vimentin is absent in pulmonary-type carcinomas. Also in contrast to hypercalcemic-type carcinomas, they may be DNA aneuploid. Metastatic small cell carcinoma should be distinguished from both types, for which clinical findings usually suffice.

Small cell carcinoma of the hypercalcemic type is commonly misinterpreted as a granulosa cell tumor, particularly the juvenile type. Small cell carcinomas lack the characteristic nuclear grooves of adult granulosa cell tumors and are more mitotically active. The follicles of juvenile granulosa cell tumors contain mucin, whereas the spaces of small cell carcinoma of the hypercalcemic type do not, although the cells of small cell carcinoma of the hypercalcemic type may occasionally contain intracytoplasmic mucin that is absent in granulosa cell tumors. The cells of juvenile granulosa cell tumors have moderate to abundant eosinophilic cytoplasm and larger nuclei than those of small cell carcinoma. Hypercalcemic small cell carcinomas that contain foci of larger cells usually have other areas composed of more typical small cells with scant cytoplasm. Juvenile granulosa cell tumors also contain fibrothecomatous areas that are absent in small cell carcinomas.

Other primary and metastatic small cell tumors may be considered in the differential diagnosis, including lymphoma, melanoma, sarcoma, primitive neuroectodermal tumor, tumor of probable wolffian origin, and intra-abdominal desmoplastic small round cell tumor.

## TUMORS OF RETE OVARII

Neoplasms of rete ovarii are uncommon and usually occur in postmenopausal women.[422] Most lesions are cystadenomas that arise in the hilum, vary in size up to more than 20 cm, and are usually unilocular thin-walled cysts filled with thin clear or straw-colored fluid. The cyst walls are composed of fibrovascular tissue and smooth muscle bundles. The cyst linings typically form thin crevices lined by low columnar to cuboid or flattened cells that are only rarely ciliated. These microscopic features permit distinction from serous cystadenomas. Rete adenomas are usually incidental microscopic findings and are composed of closely packed small tubules and occasional cysts containing small papillae. A rare carcinoma has been reported.

## TUMORS OF PROBABLE WOLFFIAN ORIGIN

These rare ovarian tumors[106, 423] are similar to those that more commonly occur in the broad ligament and fallopian tube, so-called female adnexal tumors of probable wolffian origin.[424, 425] They are solid or partially cystic, firm, gray-white to tan-yellow tumors. They consist microscopically of closely packed solid or hollow tubules that are delineated by periodic acid–Schiff stains of surrounding basement membranes. Diffuse, sievelike, or adenomatoid-appearing areas may also be present; these patterns are useful diagnostic features in distinguishing these tumors from Sertoli cell tumors. The tumor cells are small and oval to spindled; they contain bland nuclei and scant eosinophilic cytoplasm. They usually behave in a benign fashion.

## SOFT TISSUE TUMORS

Benign and malignant soft tissue tumors may arise in the ovary. Primary ovarian sarcomas are rare, representing approximately 3% of all ovarian neoplasms.[426] They usually arise in older women, although they may also occur in children and adolescents. Sarcomas may be due to overgrowth of this component from more complex neoplasms, such as malignant mixed müllerian tumors, teratomas, and other germinal neoplasms, although many are directly derived from ovarian stromal elements. They resemble their counterparts in other sites.

The most common soft tissue tumors are benign fibromas, which were discussed previously. Primary fibrosarcomas are rare and are separated from cellular fibromas primarily on the basis of mitotic activity of four mitoses or more per 10 high-power fields, as well as by their often large size and aggressive clinical course.[275, 427–429]

Leiomyomas are uncommon and constitute approximately 1% of benign ovarian tumors.[430–433] They resemble their counterparts in other sites and may be mitotically active. Primary leiomyosarcomas are rare and exhibit cytologic atypia and necrosis in addition to increased mitotic activity[434, 435] (CD Figs. 39–59 and 39–60).

Ovarian myxomas occur in premenopausal women as unilateral, asymptomatic masses.[436, 437] They have characteristic histologic features of myoma with frequent areas of cystic degeneration. This tumor should be distinguished from low-grade myxoid sarcoma and other myxoid lesions, such as edematous fibroma and massive ovarian edema.

Ovarian hemangiomas are usually incidental neoplasms that tend to be unilateral, small, hilar in location, and cavernous in type.[438] They may be associated with hemangiomas in other body locations. They should be distinguished from normal vascular hilar tissue and vascular lipid cell tumors.

Other rare benign and malignant mesenchymal tumors have been described in the ovary primarily as case reports. Other sarcomas include rhabdomyosarcoma,[439–441] chondrosarcoma,[442] osteosarcoma,[443–446] angiosarcoma,[447] and malignant schwannoma.[448]

## MALIGNANT LYMPHOMA AND LEUKEMIA

Ovarian involvement by disseminated disease may be found in approximately one quarter of patients with malignant lymphoma and in up to one half of patients with leukemia. With the exception of Burkitt's lymphoma that frequently involves the ovaries, less than 1% of patients with malignant lymphoma present with ovarian involvement, and rare primary ovarian lymphomas have been reported.[449–454] Ovarian involvement by lymphoma may be unilateral or bilateral with nearly equal frequency; bilateral disease is usually an indication of systemic disease.

The ovaries appear grossly as smooth or nodular solid masses with homogeneous, fleshy, gray-white to yellow-tan cut surfaces (CD Fig. 39–61). Areas of necrosis or cystic degeneration may be present, particularly in large masses. The tumors microscopically resemble those in nodal sites (CD Fig. 39–62); however, tumor cells in the ovary may grow in nests and cords with varying degrees of stromal sclerosis. The majority of cases involving the ovary have B cell immunophenotypes. The differential diagnosis of ovarian involvement by hematolymphoid lesions includes dysgerminoma, granulosa cell tumor, primary and metastatic small cell carcinomas and undifferentiated carcinomas, other metastatic carcinomas (particularly those of breast origin), and melanoma. Problematic cases may be distinguished by immunohistochemical panels that include leukocyte common antigen (CD45), B and T cell–associated markers, placental alkaline phosphatase, inhibin, cytokeratins, synaptophysin, chromogranin, S-100 protein, and HMB-45.

## OTHER MISCELLANEOUS TUMORS

Other rare tumors that may arise in or involve the ovary include hepatoid carcinoma resembling hepatocellular carcinoma,[131, 455] adenomatoid tumor,[456] mesothelioma,[457, 458] and intra-abdominal desmoplastic small round cell tumor[459–461] (CD Figs. 39–63 and 39–64). The last entity occurs in young patients and consists of nests of small cells in a desmoplastic stroma; the tumor cells are typically immunoreactive for cytokeratin and desmin.

## Metastatic Tumors

The ovary is a common site of metastatic disease.[462, 463] Approximately 5% to 10% of malignant ovarian tumors represent metastases. Recognizing metastatic tumors to the ovary can be a conundrum for the gynecologist and pathologist, because the metastases often mimic primary ovarian tumors clinically, grossly, and histologically. Metastatic ovarian tumors can present before, concomitantly with, or after the discovery of the primary neoplasm. Failure to recognize metastasis to the ovary can lead to unnecessary surgery, inappropriate radiation or chemotherapy, and delay in the identification of the primary tumor.

Features that should alert the gynecologist and pathologist to the possibility of ovarian metastases include a prior or concomitant extraovarian neoplasm, bilateral ovarian disease because metastases may involve both ovaries in two thirds to three quarters of cases, tumor implants on external ovarian surfaces, multinodular involvement of ovarian parenchyma, extensive lymphovascular space invasion, and a pattern of extraovarian disease that is not characteristic of ovarian cancer (e.g., hepatic or pulmonary parenchymal disease in the absence of peritoneal spread).[79] In adults, the most common sources of ovarian metastases are the gastrointestinal tract (particularly the colon, stomach, and appendix), breast, uterine corpus, and cervix, among others, as discussed in the following. In children younger than 15 years, the most common primary sites are neuroblastoma, rhabdomyosarcoma, Ew-

ing's sarcoma, malignant rhabdoid tumor of the kidney, and carcinoid.[463]

## GASTROINTESTINAL TRACT PRIMARY TUMORS

The ovary is a frequent site of metastasis from colon cancer, being involved in up to 10% of patients. Most patients present with signs and symptoms attributable to the intestinal primary tumor; however, up to one fifth of patients present with an ovarian mass or masses.[464] Although most ovarian metastases from the large intestine resemble typical moderately differentiated colon carcinoma (Fig. 39–50), some tumors may mimic primary ovarian mucinous and endometrioid carcinomas. Useful distinguishing morphologic features[73, 74] and immunohistochemical profiles[80–83] were previously discussed in the differential diagnosis sections for the respective ovarian carcinomas. Other metastatic tumors that may resemble primary mucinous ovarian neoplasms include those originating from the appendix,[53–56, 75, 76] pancreas,[77] biliary tract,[78] and cervix.[60] Of interest, metastatic ovarian cancer may be associated with stromal luteinization with endocrine manifestations, a finding more commonly seen with colonic and gastric carcinomas than with other primary tumors.[465]

Krukenberg tumor is an eponym used to describe ovarian carcinomas that are usually metastatic, often bilateral, and composed of abundant mucin-containing signet ring cells with associated marked stromal proliferation.[72, 466–468] Rare primary ovarian Krukenberg tumors have been reported.[469] Most of these metastatic tumors arise in the stomach; other less common primary sites include the colon, breast, pancreas, gallbladder, urinary bladder, and cervix. Patients tend to be relatively young; the majority of tumors occur in women between the ages of 40 and 50 years, although many are younger than 40 years. Gross evaluation shows that the tumors are solid, with smooth external surfaces and

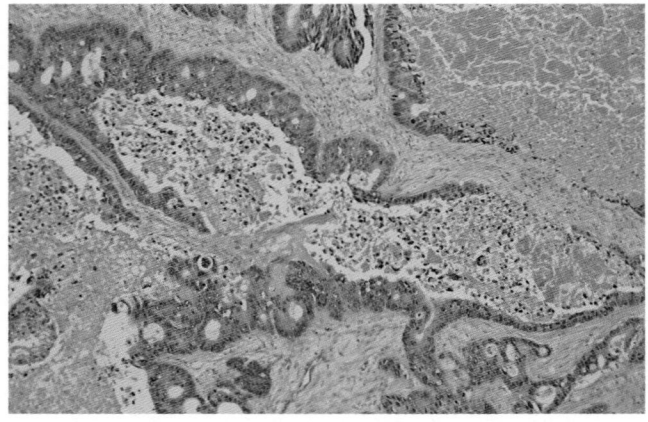

**FIGURE 39–50.** Ovary with metastatic colon carcinoma. Note the segmental gland destruction, garland or cribriform growth pattern, and "dirty" intraluminal necrosis. (Original magnification ×100.)

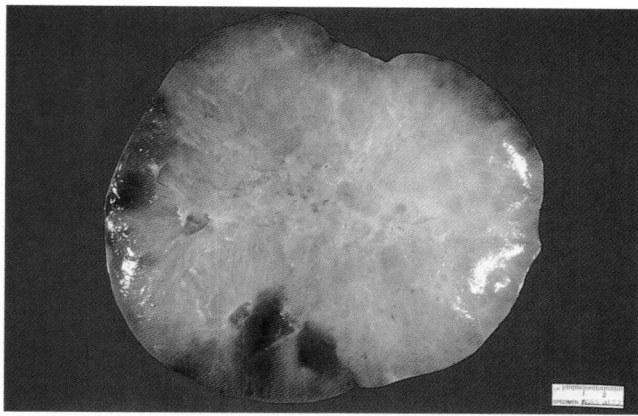

**FIGURE 39–51.** Ovary with metastatic signet ring cell carcinoma (Krukenberg tumor). The ovary is greatly enlarged by solid tumor with a glistening mucoid cut surface.

smooth to lobulated, firm to fleshy cut surfaces with a mucoid appearance (Fig. 39–51). At microscopic examination, the signet ring cells may infiltrate singly or in nests and are surrounded by a densely cellular or edematous stroma that may be luteinized (Fig. 39–52). Occasional Krukenberg tumors may have a tubular growth pattern resembling Sertoli-Leydig cell tumor.[470] The differential diagnosis also includes fibroma-thecomas, sclerosing stromal tumor, steroid cell tumor, clear cell carcinomas containing signet ring cells, and primary and metastatic mucinous carcinoids.

Metastatic carcinoids were discussed earlier in the section on specialized monodermal teratomas. In contrast to primary ovarian carcinoid, metastatic tumors tend to be bilateral with associated extraovarian disease. Carcinoids represent about 2% of ovarian metastases. The most common primary site is the ileum, although other gastrointestinal tract sites and the lung may be origins. Approximately half of patients present with carcinoid syndrome. In addi-

tion to primary carcinoid, the differential diagnosis includes granulosa cell tumor, Sertoli-Leydig cell tumors, Brenner tumor, and various adenocarcinomas.[79, 388] The diagnosis is facilitated by characteristic histologic features and immunohistochemical panels that include neuroendocrine markers.

## BREAST PRIMARY TUMORS

Ovarian involvement by metastatic breast cancer is common, occurring in one quarter to one third of patients during their disease course.[471, 472] Metastatic tumors are bilateral in most cases. The ovaries may be enlarged, but in many cases they may be grossly normal with metastatic disease detected only by microscopic examination. Unlike some of the tumors discussed before, metastatic breast cancer uncommonly presents as presumed primary ovarian neoplasia.[79] Lobular carcinomas (Fig. 39–53) are more likely to metastasize to the ovaries than is ductal carcinoma, but metastatic ductal carcinomas occur more commonly owing to their higher frequency.[473] A diffuse pattern of infiltration by small cords, nests, or acini of cells is usually present. Clinical history, morphologic findings, and immunohistochemical panels that include gross cystic disease fluid protein-15 (BRST-2)[474] may assist in the identification of these tumors.

## OTHER GYNECOLOGIC PRIMARY TUMORS

Ovarian metastases from endometrial primary carcinomas have been reported to occur in one third to nearly one half of cases.[475, 476] Endometrioid carcinomas involving both the corpus and the ovaries are likely to represent synchronous independent tumors in the majority of cases,[79, 102, 103] but metastatic ovarian endometrioid carcinomas of corpus origin do occur, and metastases to the corpus of primary ovarian endometrioid carcinomas are rare.[103] As previously mentioned, ovarian metastases from an endometrial primary are favored in the setting of deep myometrial invasion with lymphatic space in-

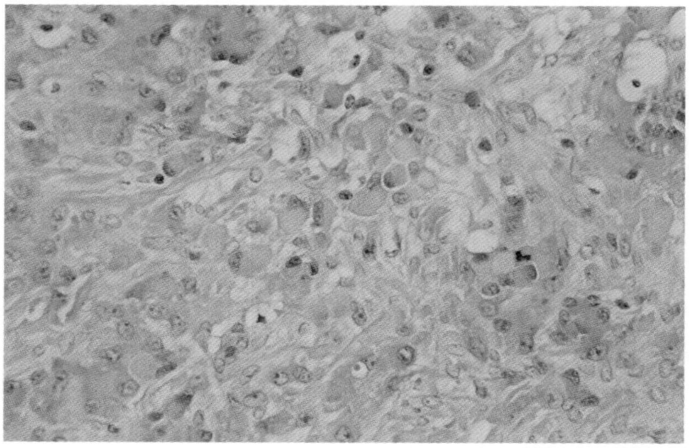

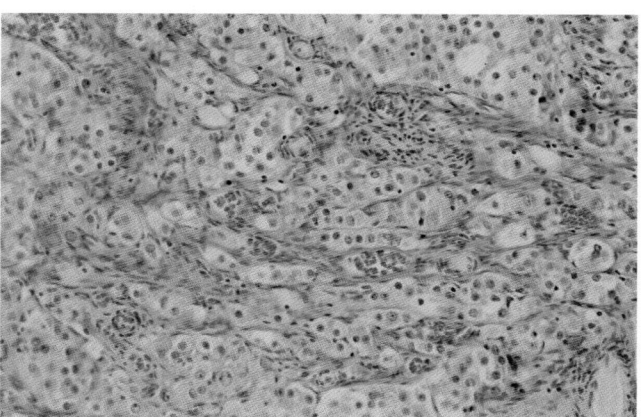

**FIGURE 39–52.** Krukenberg tumor composed of diffusely infiltrating signet ring cells. The primary tumor was in the stomach. (Original magnification ×400.)

**FIGURE 39–53.** Ovary with metastatic breast cancer, pleomorphic lobular type. Linear strands of single cells or "Indian file" pattern of infiltration is present in areas. (Original magnification ×200.)

volvement, luminal involvement of the fallopian tubes, bilateral ovarian disease, small size of ovarian tumor, and presence of tumor on ovarian surfaces or within lymphatics. Molecular genetic studies may also be useful in the distinction between synchronous and independent endometrioid tumors of the ovaries and corpus.[104]

Endometrial stromal sarcomas and uterine leiomyosarcomas may also metastasize to the ovaries, the former more than the latter.[116] Metastatic endometrial stromal sarcomas may be confused with granulosa cell tumors, Sertoli-Leydig cell tumors, or thecoma-fibroma. Ovarian mucinous adenocarcinomas may be associated with similar tumors of the cervix.[58-60] In such cases, it may be difficult to distinguish whether these represent synchronous independent or related neoplasms. It is uncommon for cervical tumors other than adenocarcinomas to metastasize to the ovaries.[477] The ovary may also be involved by primary fallopian tube carcinoma, usually by direct extension.[462]

### OTHER PRIMARY TUMORS

Renal cell carcinomas may metastasize to the ovary and be confused with primary clear cell carcinoma.[132] The characteristic sinusoidal vascular and organoid growth patterns of renal cell carcinoma in the absence of other features of clear cell adenocarcinoma aid in this distinction. Transitional cell carcinomas of urinary tract origin must also be distinguished from primary ovarian tumors.[145, 146] Pulmonary carcinomas may involve the ovaries but are rarely symptomatic.[478] Metastases from malignant melanoma[479, 480] and various sarcomas[116] may also involve the ovary. Other primary tumors that may metastasize to the ovary are rare and are largely the subject of case reports.

## NON-NEOPLASTIC LESIONS

### Congenital Abnormalities

Congenital lesions of the ovary are rare. Absent ovaries with residual streak gonads are usually encountered in patients with abnormal karyotypes and gonadal dysgenesis syndromes.[481] Streak gonads consist of thin, fibrous bands of ovarian stromal and hilar tissue and lack oocytes. Congenital absence of an ovary may rarely be an incidental finding in an otherwise normal woman.[482] Accessory or supernumerary[483] and ectopic[484] ovaries may also be encountered. Ectopic adrenal cortical rests (CD Fig. 39-65) may be found in periadnexal tissue and rarely within the ovary.[485] Splenic-gonadal fusion[486] and uterus-like masses[487] have also been described.

### Inflammatory Diseases

#### INFECTIOUS DISEASES

Inflammation of the ovaries is most commonly due to bacterial infection from ascending pelvic inflammatory disease[488] with involvement of the adjacent fallopian tubes, resulting in bilateral tubo-ovarian abscesses. The infections are typically polymicrobial, with a preponderance of anaerobic organisms or aerobic streptococci and enterococci.[489] Pelvic inflammatory disease attributable to *Actinomyces* infection is usually associated with intrauterine contraceptive devices, although most infections that occur in users of intrauterine contraceptive devices are caused by other organisms.[490, 491] Sequelae of tubo-ovarian infections range from nearly complete resolution with scattered adhesions to extensive fibrous organization forming tubo-ovarian complexes of solid and cystic masses (CD Fig. 39-66). Rarely, recurrent chronic infection may result in xanthogranulomatous oophoritis forming a solid pseudotumor composed of foamy histiocytes, multinucleated giant cells, and other chronic inflammatory cells.[492] Malacoplakia may rarely involve the ovary as a consequence of bacterial infection.[493] At histologic examination, there are diffuse aggregates of histiocytes with foamy to eosinophilic granular cytoplasm containing characteristic Michaelis-Gutmann bodies consisting of small, basophilic phagolysosomes filled with incompletely digested bacteria. These are mineralized bodies that contain calcium and iron. Ovarian abscesses in the absence of tubal infection are uncommon and occur as a result of lymphatic or hematogenous dissemination from another site or by direct extension from inflammatory processes involving other nongynecologic pelvic organs.[494, 495]

Ovarian tuberculosis is usually a result of extension from adjacent involved fallopian tubes.[496] Ovarian parenchymal disease is present in up to 10% of cases involving the female genital tract. Characteristic necrotizing granulomas are usually confined to the cortex. The diagnosis should be confirmed by demonstration of acid-fast bacilli to exclude other organisms and other granulomatous processes.

Cytomegalovirus oophoritis is a rare, incidental finding in immunocompromised patients as part of a more generalized infection.[497, 498] At histologic examination, there are areas of coagulative necrosis with associated inflammation. Cytomegalovirus inclusions may be detected in surrounding endothelial and stromal cells (CD Fig. 39-67).

Except in endemic regions, other bacterial, fungal, viral, and parasitic infections are exceedingly rare in the ovary.

#### NONINFECTIOUS INFLAMMATORY DISORDERS

Noninfectious granulomas involving the ovaries have a variety of causes. Starch granules from surgical gloves may elicit a foreign body–type granulomatous response, which can be recognized by the characteristic Maltese cross particles revealed by polarized light.[499] Prior surgical or ablative procedures may result in noninfectious ovarian granulomas without starch granules, presumably representing reaction to traumatic tissue destruction.[500, 501] A foreign body–type granulomatous response may also be elicited by talc,[502] keratin derived from mature cystic teratomas and corpus or ovarian endometrioid carcinomas with squamous differentiation,[503] and bowel contents from colo-ovarian fistulas.[504] Ovarian granulomas may also be encountered in sarcoidosis[505] and Crohn's disease.[506, 507]

Autoimmune oophoritis is often associated with premature ovarian failure and thus is one cause of infertility.[508–512] Patients frequently have other associated disorders thought to be autoimmune in nature. Circulating antibodies to granulosa and theca cells and other steroid-producing cells have been detected in most of these patients. The ovaries are usually normal in size but may be enlarged and cystic. At microscopic examination, there is a chronic inflammatory infiltrate composed predominantly of lymphocytes and plasma cells concentrated within and around developing follicles. Eosinophils, histiocytes, and granulomas may also be present.

## Cysts

### SURFACE EPITHELIAL INCLUSION CYSTS

Surface epithelial inclusion cysts (also called germinal inclusion cysts, müllerian inclusion cysts, or ovarian endosalpingiosis) are thought to arise from cortical invaginations of surface epithelium after successive ovulations.[513, 514] As such, they are most numerous in postmenopausal women, although inclusions may be found in patients of any age. Most measure up to 1 cm in diameter. They are lined by a single layer of epithelium usually composed of columnar, often ciliated cells resembling tubal epithelium or by cuboid to flattened nondescript cells. The cysts with attenuated or absent linings may be designated simple cysts. Endometrioid- or endocervical-type epithelium may also be seen. Associated psammoma bodies may be present. They are generally of no clinical significance; however, there is evidence to support that such inclusion cysts are the origin of surface epithelial neoplasms.[515, 516]

### FOLLICULAR CYSTS

In general, normally developing follicles may attain sizes up to 1 cm in diameter. Cystic follicles measure between 1 and 2.5 cm in diameter, and cysts of greater size are designated follicular cysts. They are common and occur at any age from fetal life to rarely in postmenopausal women.[517–521] Follicular cysts are usually asymptomatic, but patients may present with adnexal masses or with symptoms of hyperestrogenism. In gross appearance, the cysts are single or multiple, unilocular, thin walled with smooth linings and are filled with serous to serosanguineous fluid; they usually do not exceed 10 cm in diameter. Microscopic examination shows that the cyst walls are lined by an internal layer of granulosa cells and an external layer of thecal cells, either of which may be luteinized.

### CORPUS LUTEUM CYSTS

The majority of corpus luteum cysts occur after ovulation in women of reproductive age. They are usually single, unilocular, between 2.5 and 5 cm in diameter, with yellow to yellow-orange serpiginous walls and smooth internal surfaces. They are filled with serosanguineous fluid to thick clotted blood. At microscopic examination, the cysts are lined by thick layers of large, luteinized granulosa cells. Corpus luteum cysts associated with pregnancy often contain extracellular and intracellular hyaline globules and focal calcification. A potential complication of corpus luteum cysts as well as of follicular cysts is rupture with resultant hemoperitoneum.[522]

### POLYCYSTIC OVARIAN DISEASE (STEIN-LEVENTHAL SYNDROME)

The pathogenesis of polycystic ovarian disease is complex and remains to be fully elucidated.[523–526] There is evidence to suggest abnormal regulation of enzymes involved in ovarian androgen biosynthesis, possibly influenced by insulin, growth factors, and luteinizing hormone.[526] Polycystic ovarian disease is characterized by abnormal gonadotropin secretion with relatively low follicle-stimulating hormone and high luteinizing hormone serum levels or ratios, hyperandrogenism, hyperestrogenism due to increased peripheral conversion of androgens to estrogens, chronic anovulation with oligomenorrhea or secondary amenorrhea, and sclerocystic ovaries. Polycystic ovarian disease is estimated to affect nearly 4% to 7% of women,[527] who often present at 20 to 30 years of age with hirsutism and infertility. Patients may have a disordered proliferative or hyperplastic endometrium, and infrequently well-differentiated endometrial adenocarcinoma may occur.[528, 529] The ovaries are usually somewhat enlarged but may be normal in size. Cut sections reveal subcortical cysts generally less than 1 cm in diameter beneath a frequently thickened and fibrotic surface layer (Fig. 39–54). The underlying stroma is tan to yellow with usually ab-

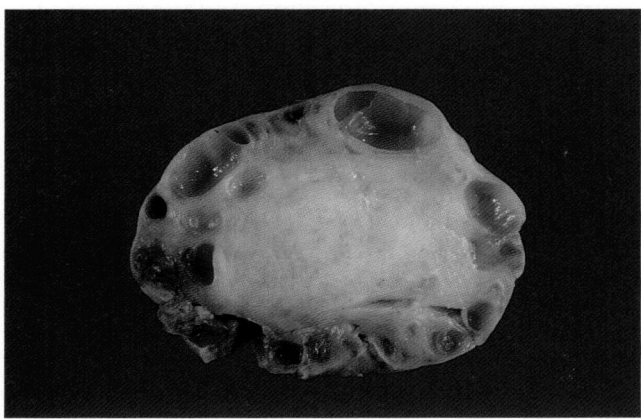

**FIGURE 39–54.** Polycystic ovarian disease. The cut surface demonstrates numerous subcortical cystic follicles and tan to yellow underlying stroma. Note the absence of corpus luteum and corpus albicans.

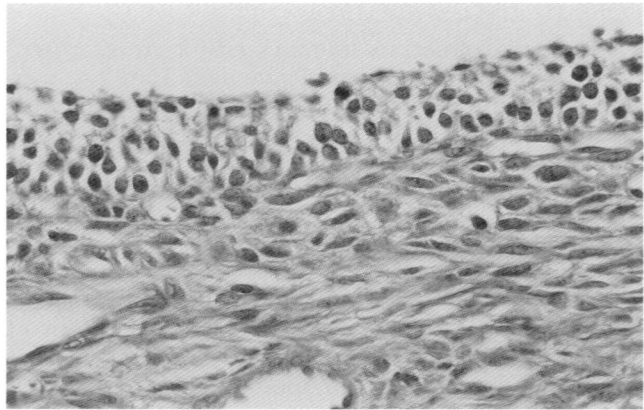

**FIGURE 39–55.** Polycystic ovarian disease. The subcortical cysts are lined by an inner layer of granulosa cells *(top)* and outer layers of theca cells. (Original magnification ×400.)

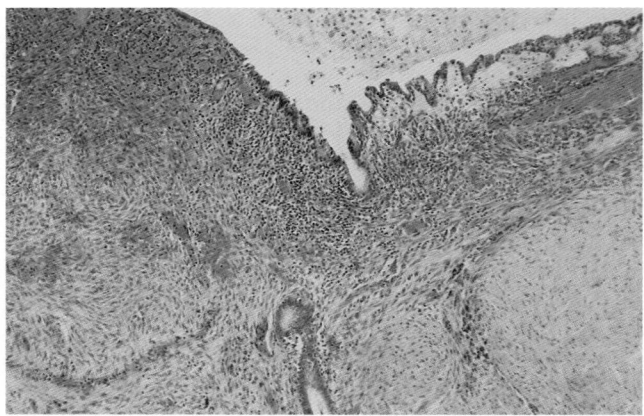

**FIGURE 39–57.** Endometriosis. The wall of this cyst contains all three components diagnostic of endometriosis: endometrial glands, endometrial stroma, and hemosiderin-laden macrophages. (Original magnification ×100.)

sent corpus luteum and corpus albicans. Microscopic examination shows numerous subcortical follicles lined by an inner layer of granulosa cells and outer layer of luteinized theca cells (Fig. 39–55), and the surrounding and underlying stroma is often hyperplastic and may be luteinized.[530, 531]

## ENDOMETRIOSIS

Endometriosis consists of endometrial glands or stroma in ectopic locations outside of the uterine corpus.[532, 533] The ovary is the most commonly involved site and is often associated with infertility. Endometriotic foci vary in size and frequently have varying amounts of remote and recent hemorrhage because of their retained responsiveness to menstrual cycle hormone changes. Endometriotic cysts or endometriomas are most commonly encountered in the ovaries and are typically filled with thick, brown hemorrhagic contents resulting in so-called chocolate cysts (Fig. 39–56).

Histologic findings diagnostic of endometriosis

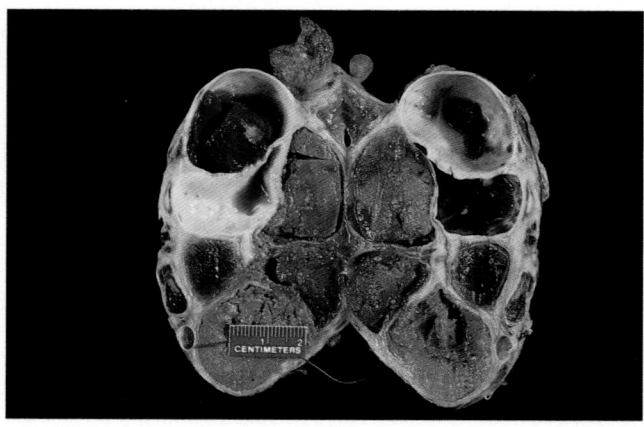

**FIGURE 39–56.** Endometriosis. The ovary has been extensively replaced by thick-walled cysts filled with tenacious, red to brown hemorrhagic cyst contents.

should include at least two of three criteria: endometrial lining epithelium or glands, endometrial stroma, and hemosiderin-laden macrophages (Fig. 39–57). It is often difficult to microscopically identify diagnostic glands or stroma in lesions that are large or of long duration. Cyst linings may become attenuated and obscured by hemosiderin-laden macrophages and organizing fibrous tissue, findings that are consistent with but not diagnostic of endometriosis. The endometrial cells of cyst linings may exhibit pronounced reactive atypia.[534, 535] Any polypoid excrescences or solid areas arising from cyst walls should be evaluated histologically for hyperplastic and neoplastic lesions, usually endometrioid adenocarcinoma, that may arise in the setting of endometriosis.[534, 536, 537]

## PAROVARIAN CYSTS

Parovarian and paratubal cysts (CD Fig. 39–68) in the hilar region are common and are derived from mesonephric (wolffian) and paramesonephric (müllerian) remnants or from peritoneal mesothelial inclusions.[538, 539] Mesonephric cysts are lined by cuboidal, predominantly nonciliated epithelium and may have more prominent muscular walls. Paramesonephric cysts are lined by columnar ciliated and nonciliated cells; the most common is the hydatid cyst of Morgagni located at the fimbriated end of the fallopian tube. Most cysts greater than 3 cm in diameter are of mesothelial origin.

## Pregnancy-Associated Lesions

Lesions of the ovary associated with pregnancy may present as masses that mimic ovarian neoplasms.[540] These include large solitary luteinized follicle cyst, hyperreactio luteinalis, pregnancy luteoma, and granulosa cell proliferations, among others.

## LARGE SOLITARY LUTEINIZED FOLLICLE CYST OF PREGNANCY AND THE PUERPERIUM

Large solitary luteinized follicle cyst of pregnancy and the puerperium is a rare lesion. It presents as a unilateral, large, solitary follicular cyst that is thought to develop as a consequence of hCG hyperstimulation.[541] Unlike other follicular cysts, these cysts may attain massive sizes with a reported median diameter of 25 cm. They are lined by single to multiple layers of luteinized cells with pronounced anisopoikilocytosis. The nuclei typically exhibit focal marked pleomorphism and hyperchromasia, which may represent degenerative changes (CD Fig. 39–69). None of the reported cases has been associated with endocrine abnormalities.

### HYPERREACTIO LUTEINALIS

Hyperreactio luteinalis (theca-lutein cysts) is characterized by multiple luteinized follicular cysts involving both ovaries.[542, 543] These lesions are usually associated with disorders with high serum levels of hCG, such as choriocarcinoma, hydatidiform molar gestations, and multiple gestations. The ovarian masses usually regress post partum but may persist for several months. The ovaries may be greatly enlarged by multiple, variably sized cysts filled with serous or bloody fluid (Fig. 39–58). Histologic examination reveals large follicular cysts lined by luteinized granulosa and theca cells, usually with associated pronounced stromal luteinization and edema (Fig. 39–59).

### PREGNANCY LUTEOMA

Pregnancy luteomas result from solid, nodular, hyperplastic proliferations of luteinized theca or stromal cells.[544, 545] Most reported lesions have occurred in multiparous women as incidental findings at the time of cesarean section or tubal ligation, although they may attain large tumorlike sizes.[540] There may be associated hirsutism or virilization in about one fourth of patients. At gross evaluation,

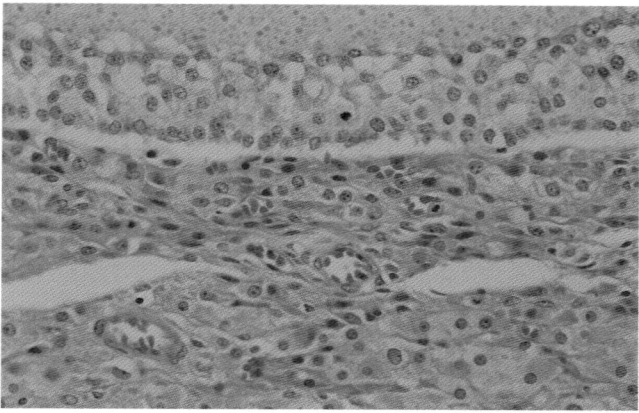

**FIGURE 39–59.** Hyperreactio luteinalis. A large follicle cyst is lined by luteinized inner granulosa cells *(top)* and theca cells *(middle)*, surrounded by luteinized stromal cells *(bottom)*. (Original magnification ×400.)

they are composed of multiple circumscribed, nodular masses of soft, yellow-orange to brown tissue with frequent hemorrhagic foci (Fig. 39–60). At microscopic examination, the nodules are composed of uniform large luteinized cells with abundant eosinophilic granular cytoplasm (Fig. 39–61). The nuclei may exhibit focal pleomorphism, and mitotic figures may be frequent with occasional atypical forms. These are benign ovarian lesions that regress to normal size within weeks after delivery.

### GRANULOSA CELL PROLIFERATIONS

Focal proliferations of granulosa cells resembling small tumors may occasionally be incidental findings, usually in the ovaries from pregnant women.[546] They have microscopic architectural and cytologic features that resemble adult granulosa cell tumors. Relatively small size and multifocality in a pregnant patient suggest that these are likely to represent non-neoplastic proliferations in this clinical setting.

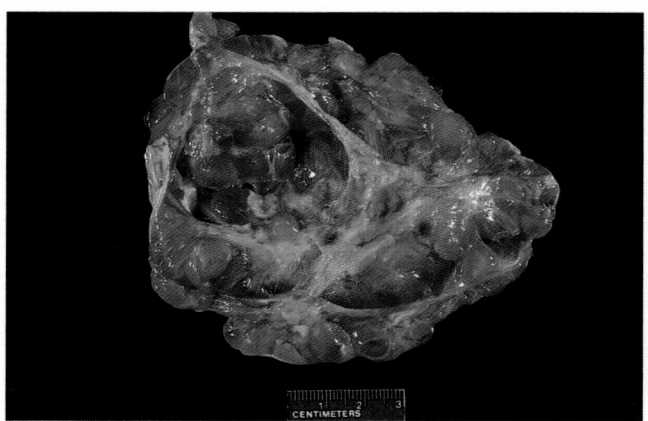

**FIGURE 39–58.** Hyperreactio luteinalis. The ovary is enlarged and replaced by numerous variably sized, thin-walled cysts.

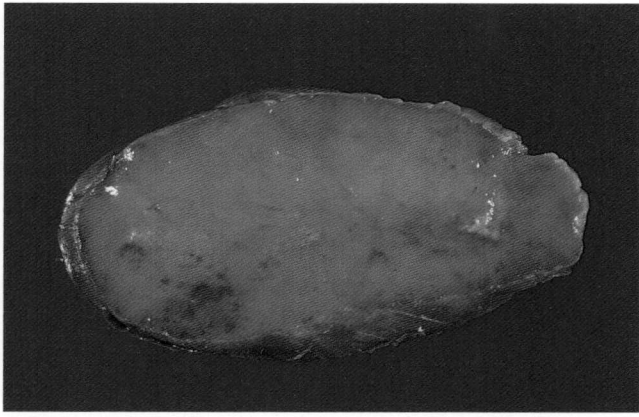

**FIGURE 39–60.** Pregnancy luteoma. The cut surface demonstrates solid nodular masses of red to tan-brown tissue.

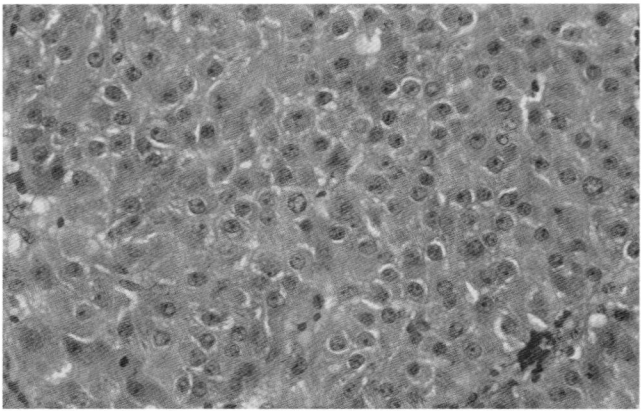

**FIGURE 39–61.** Pregnancy luteoma composed of large luteinized cells with abundant eosinophilic cytoplasm. (Original magnification ×400.)

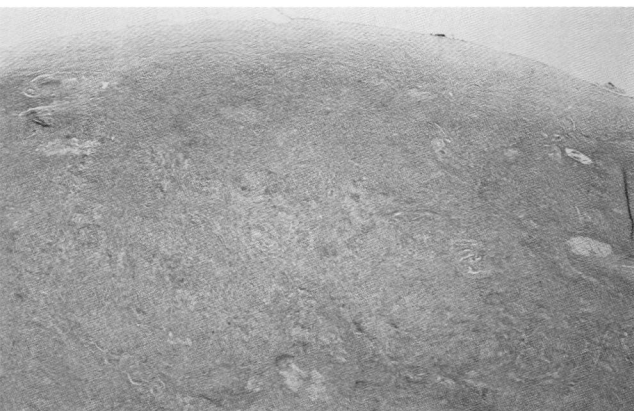

**FIGURE 39–63.** Stromal hyperplasia. There is diffuse proliferation of basophilic stromal cells surrounding residual atretic follicles and other normal structures. (Original magnification ×20.)

## ECTOPIC PREGNANCY

Ovarian ectopic pregnancy is rare.[547] More than 95% of ectopic pregnancies occur in the fallopian tube. A diagnosis of ovarian ectopic pregnancy requires the exclusion of tubal involvement and the demonstration of trophoblast within ovarian cortical tissue. Fetal parts are not usually found.

## Stromal Hyperplasia and Hyperthecosis

Ovarian cortical stromal proliferation is common in women older than 40 years. When this process is of moderate to marked degree, a designation of stromal hyperplasia is warranted. Stromal hyperthecosis refers to the condition of clusters of luteinized cells scattered throughout the hyperplastic stroma. Significant stromal hyperplasia or hyperthecosis[548] is characterized by bilaterally enlarged ovaries with homogeneous yellow-white to tan surfaces (Fig. 39–62). Microscopic examination reveals diffuse or nod-

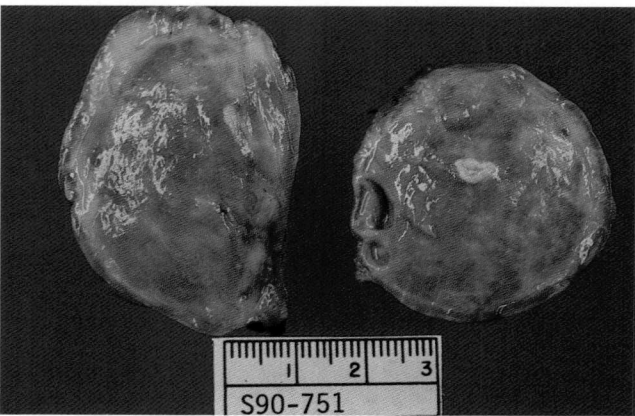

**FIGURE 39–62.** Stromal hyperplasia. Both ovaries are enlarged and have relatively homogeneous tan-brown cut surfaces.

ular proliferations of stromal cells surrounding residual follicle structures and encroaching on the medulla (Fig. 39–63). Luteinized cells of hyperthecosis contain abundant granular eosinophilic to vacuolated cytoplasm and produce androgens, as evidenced by immunohistochemical studies.[549] Stromal hyperthecosis may be associated with androgenic or estrogenic manifestations; estrogenic manifestations presumably result from peripheral conversion of ovarian androgens.

## Massive Ovarian Edema and Fibromatosis

Massive ovarian edema and fibromatosis are probably related entities that share clinical and pathologic features.[550, 551] Both may cause tumorlike enlargement of the ovaries and occur in women younger than 40 years who present with abdominal pain, menstrual abnormalities, or androgenic manifestations. Massive ovarian edema results from excessive accumulation of ovarian stromal edema, possibly as a result of impaired lymphatic and venous drainage from torsion of the mesovarium. Most cases are unilateral and usually involve the right ovary. The ovary is greatly enlarged, with soft, spongy cut surfaces that exude watery fluid. At histologic examination, there is pronounced, diffuse stromal edema surrounding follicles and other normal structures, with relative sparing of the superficial cortex. Vascular and lymphatic dilatation is usually present. Nearly half of the cases may have clusters of luteinized stromal cells, which may account for associated endocrine manifestations in some cases.

The differential diagnosis includes ovarian primary and metastatic tumors, which may be edematous or myxomatous. Ovarian fibromatosis is also usually unilateral and is characterized by proliferating stromal cells with varying amounts of collagen surrounding follicles and other normal structures.

Occasional cases may also contain luteinized cells. Fibromatosis may precede the development of massive ovarian edema.[551] In contrast to ovarian fibromatosis, fibromas are discrete mass lesions that are usually nonfunctioning and occur in older women.

## Other Surface and Stromal Proliferations

Reactive mesothelial hyperplasia of the peritoneum is a common reaction to injury of various causes and may be encountered on the ovarian surface and within periovarian adhesions. In most circumstances, mesothelial hyperplasia is not usually associated with nodular proliferations, atypia, or necrosis, and macrophages are often admixed with the mesothelial cells. Florid mesothelial proliferations may also be found in association with ovarian tumors and may mimic neoplastic foci by forming nests, cords, and glandlike arrangements of atypical mesothelial cells.[552]

Cortical stromal nodules are common incidental findings usually encountered in the ovaries from postmenopausal women. They are composed of nodular surface proliferations of ovarian stromal tissue with variable amounts of hyalinization covered by a single layer of surface epithelium. They should be distinguished from serous surface papillomas and adenofibromas.

Hilus cell hyperplasia is a common finding in the ovaries of postmenopausal women, presumably as a result of elevated gonadotropins.[553] Microscopic examination shows nodular or diffuse proliferations of hilus cells that may be atypical, and occasional mitotic figures may be present. This process should be distinguished from the discrete mass lesion of a hilus cell tumor.

## Stromal Metaplasias

A variety of benign stromal metaplasias have been described in the ovary. Foci of stromal decidual reaction may be found, usually in the ovaries of pregnant women,[554, 555] although occasional decidualized stromal areas may also be encountered in the ovaries of nonpregnant premenopausal and postmenopausal women of unknown etiology. Ectopic decidua may be misinterpreted as carcinoma. Other benign ovarian stromal metaplasias include those composed of smooth muscle,[261] adipose tissue,[556] and rarely heterotopic bone.[557]

## Infertility

A variety of disorders involving the ovary may result in reproductive failure,[558] including abnormal gonadal development, pelvic inflammatory disease, autoimmune oophoritis, polycystic ovarian disease, and endometriosis, as previously discussed. Other causes of premature ovarian failure include true menopause and hypergonadotropic resistant ovaries.[559–561] In true premature menopause, the ovaries are characteristically small with depleted oocytes and follicles. Hypergonadotropic resistant ovaries contain oocytes and primordial follicles but few fully developed follicles; proposed causes of this disorder include deficiencies or defects of and antibodies to follicle-stimulating hormone and luteinizing hormone receptors. Ovarian biopsy specimens may be obtained in the evaluation of infertile women.[562, 563] Serial sections of such biopsy specimens should be evaluated for the presence and quantity of follicles, follicle maturation, evidence of ovulation as manifested by corpora lutea and albicantia, and nature of the stroma.

## REFERENCES

1. Scully RE, Young RH, Clement PB: Tumors of the Ovary, Maldeveloped Gonads, Fallopian Tube, and Broad Ligament. Atlas of Tumor Pathology. Third Series, Fascicle 23. Washington, DC, Armed Forces Institute of Pathology, 1998.
2. Ovary and fallopian tube. *In* Hruban RH, Westra WH, Phelps TH, Isacson C: Surgical Pathology Dissection. An Illustrated Guide. New York, Springer-Verlag, 1996, pp 130–135.
3. Rosai J: Standardized reporting of surgical pathology diagnoses for the major tumor types. A proposal. Am J Clin Pathol 100:240–255, 1993.
4. Robboy SJ, Bentley RC, Krigman H, et al: Synoptic reports in gynecologic pathology. Int J Gynecol Pathol 13:161–174, 1994.
5. Koonings PP, Campbell K, Mishell DR Jr, et al: Relative frequency of primary ovarian neoplasms: a 10-year review. Obstet Gynecol 74:921–926, 1989.
6. Hart WR: Ovarian epithelial tumors of borderline malignancy (carcinomas of low malignant potential). Hum Pathol 8:541–549, 1977.
7. Katzenstein A-LA, Mazur MT, Morgan TE, et al: Proliferative serous tumors of the ovary. Histologic features and prognosis. Am J Surg Pathol 2:339–355, 1978.
8. Russell P: The pathological assessment of ovarian neoplasms. III: The malignant "epithelial" tumors. Pathology 11:493–532, 1979.
9. Scully RE: Common epithelial tumors of borderline malignancy (carcinomas of low malignant potential). Bull Cancer (Paris) 69:228–238, 1982.
10. Colgan TJ, Norris HJ: Ovarian epithelial tumors of low malignant potential. A review. Int J Gynecol Pathol 1:367–382, 1983.
11. Barnhill D, Heller P, Brzozowski P, et al: Epithelial ovarian carcinoma of low malignant potential. Obstet Gynecol 65:53–59, 1985.
12. Ulbright TM, Roth LM: Common epithelial tumors of the ovary. Proliferating and of low malignant potential. Semin Diagn Pathol 2:2–15, 1985.
13. Bostwick DG, Tazelaar HD, Ballon SC, et al: Ovarian epithelial tumors of borderline malignancy. A clinical and pathologic study of 109 cases. Cancer 58:2052–2065, 1986.
14. Kliman L, Rome RM, Fortune DW: Low malignant potential tumors of the ovary: a study of 76 cases. Obstet Gynecol 68:338–344, 1986.
15. Rice LW, Berkowitz RS, Mark SD, et al: Epithelial ovarian tumors of borderline malignancy. Gynecol Oncol 39:195–198, 1990.
16. Russell P: Surface epithelial-stromal tumors of the ovary. *In* Kurman RJ (ed): Blaustein's Pathology of the Female Genital Tract. 4th ed. New York, Springer-Verlag, 1994, pp 705–782.
17. Silva EG, Tornos C, Zhuang Z, et al: Tumor recurrence in stage I ovarian serous neoplasms of low malignant potential. Int J Gynecol Pathol 17:1–6, 1998.

18. Leake JF, Rader JS, Woodruff JD, et al: Retroperitoneal lymphatic involvement with epithelial ovarian tumors of low malignant potential. Gynecol Oncol 42:124–130, 1991.
19. Benda JA, Zaino R: GOG Pathology Manual. Buffalo, NY, Gynecologic Oncology Group, 1994.
20. Shimizu Y, Kamoi S, Amada S, et al: Toward the development of a universal grading system for ovarian epithelial carcinoma. I. Prognostic significance of histopathologic features—problems involved in the architectural grading system. Gynecol Oncol 70:2–12, 1998.
21. Shimizu Y, Kamoi S, Amada S, et al: Toward the development of a universal grading system for ovarian epithelial carcinoma. Testing of a proposed system in a series of 461 patients with uniform treatment and follow-up. Cancer 82:893–901, 1998.
22. DeNictolis M, Montironi R, Tommasoni S, et al: Serous borderline tumors of the ovary. A clinicopathologic, immunohistochemical, and quantitative study of 44 cases. Cancer 70:152–160, 1992.
23. Bell DA, Young RH, Scully RE: Ovarian desmoplastic implants (autoimplantation) involving serous borderline tumors: a mimic of serous carcinoma (abstract). Mod Pathol 8:85A, 1995.
24. Tavassoli FA: Serous tumor of low malignant potential with early stromal invasion (serous LMP and microinvasion). Mod Pathol 1:407–414, 1988.
25. Bell DA, Scully RE: Ovarian serous borderline tumors with stromal microinvasion: a report of 21 cases. Hum Pathol 21:396–403, 1990.
26. McCaughey WTE, Kirk ME, Lester W, et al: Peritoneal epithelial lesions associated with proliferative serous tumours of the ovary. Histopathology 8:195–208, 1984.
27. Michael H, Roth LM: Invasive and noninvasive implants in ovarian serous tumors of low malignant potential. Cancer 57:1240–1247, 1986.
28. Bell DA, Weinstock MA, Scully RE: Peritoneal implants of ovarian serous borderline tumors: histologic features and prognosis. Cancer 62:2212–2222, 1988.
29. Gershenson DM, Silva EG: Serous ovarian tumors of low malignant potential with peritoneal implants. Cancer 65:578–585, 1990.
30. Ehrmann RL, Federschneider JM, Knapp RC: Distinguishing lymph node metastases from benign glandular inclusions in low-grade ovarian carcinoma. Am J Obstet Gynecol 136:737–746, 1980.
31. Zinsser KR, Wheeler JE: Endosalpingiosis in the omentum. A study of autopsy and surgical material. Am J Surg Pathol 6:109–117, 1982.
32. Bell DA, Scully RE: Clinicopathologic features of lymph node (LN) involvement with ovarian serous borderline tumors (OBST) (abstract). Mod Pathol 5:61A, 1992.
33. Bell DA, Scully RE: Serous borderline tumors of the peritoneum. Am J Surg Pathol 14:230–239, 1990.
34. Biscotti CV, Hart WR: Peritoneal serous micropapillomatosis of low malignant potential (serous borderline tumors of the peritoneum). A clinicopathologic study of 17 cases. Am J Surg Pathol 16:467–475, 1992.
35. Burks RT, Sherman ME, Kurman RJ: Micropapillary serous carcinoma of the ovary. A distinctive low-grade carcinoma related to serous borderline tumors. Am J Surg Pathol 20:1319–1330, 1996.
36. Seidman JD, Kurman RJ: Subclassification of serous borderline tumors of the ovary into benign and malignant types. A clinicopathologic study of 65 advanced stage cases. Am J Surg Pathol 20:1331–1345, 1996.
37. Kent SW, McKay DG: Primary cancer of the ovary. An analysis of 349 cases. Am J Obstet Gynecol 80:430–438, 1960.
38. Aure JC, Høeg K, Kolstad P: Clinical and histologic studies of ovarian carcinoma. Long-term follow-up of 990 cases. Obstet Gynecol 37:1–9, 1971.
39. Gilks CB, Bell DA, Scully RE: Serous psammocarcinoma of the ovary and peritoneum. Int J Gynecol Pathol 9:110–121, 1990.
40. Gooneratne S, Sassone M, Blaustein A, et al: Serous surface papillary carcinoma of the ovary. A clinicopathologic study of 16 cases. Int J Gynecol Pathol 1:258–269, 1982.
41. White PF, Merino MJ, Barwick KW: Serous surface papillary carcinoma of the ovary: a clinical, pathologic, ultrastructural, and immunohistochemical study of 11 cases. Pathol Annu 20:403–418, 1985.
42. Dalrymple JC, Bannatyne P, Russell P, et al: Extra-ovarian peritoneal serous papillary carcinoma. A clinicopathologic study of 31 cases. Cancer 64:110–115, 1989.
43. Truong LD, Maccato ML, Awalt H, et al: Serous surface carcinoma of the peritoneum: a clinicopathologic study of 22 cases. Hum Pathol 21:99–110, 1990.
44. Mulhollan TJ, Silva EG, Tornos C, et al: Ovarian involvement by serous surface papillary carcinoma. Int J Gynecol Pathol 13:120–126, 1994.
45. Tsao SW, Mok CH, Knapp RC, et al: Molecular genetic evidence of a uniform origin for human serous ovarian carcinomas. Gynecol Oncol 48:5–10, 1993.
46. Muto MC, Welch WR, Mok SCH, et al: Evidence for a multifocal origin of papillary serous carcinoma of the peritoneum. Cancer Res 55:490–492, 1995.
47. Ulbright TM, Roth LM, Sutton GP: Papillary serous carcinoma of the ovary with squamous differentiation. Int J Gynecol Pathol 9:86–94, 1990.
48. Young RH, Scully RE: Ovarian Sertoli-Leydig cell tumors with a retiform pattern: a problem in histopathologic diagnosis. A report of 25 cases. Am J Surg Pathol 7:755–771, 1983.
49. Bollinger DJ, Wick MR, Dehner LP, et al: Peritoneal malignant mesothelioma versus serous papillary adenocarcinoma. A histochemical and immunohistochemical comparison. Am J Surg Pathol 13:659–670, 1989.
50. Khoury N, Raju U, Crissman JD, et al: A comparative immunohistochemical study of peritoneal and ovarian serous tumors, and mesotheliomas. Hum Pathol 21:811–819, 1990.
51. Chaitin BA, Gershenson DM, Evans HL: Mucinous tumors of the ovary. A clinicopathologic study of 70 cases. Cancer 55:1958–1962, 1985.
52. Watkin W, Silva EG, Gershenson DM: Mucinous carcinoma of the ovary. Pathologic prognostic factors. Cancer 69:208–212, 1992.
53. Young RH, Gilks CB, Scully RE: Mucinous tumors of the appendix associated with mucinous tumors of the ovary and pseudomyxoma peritonei. A clinicopathological analysis of 22 cases supporting an origin in the appendix. Am J Surg Pathol 15:415–429, 1991.
54. Kahn MA, Demopoulos RI: Mucinous ovarian tumors with pseudomyxoma peritonei. A clinicopathologic study. Int J Gynecol Pathol 11:15–23, 1992.
55. Seidman JD, Elsayed AM, Sobin LH, et al: Association of mucinous tumors of the ovary and appendix. A clinicopathologic study of 25 cases. Am J Surg Pathol 17:22–34, 1993.
56. Prayson RA, Hart WR, Petras RE: Pseudomyxoma peritonei. A clinicopathologic study of 19 cases with emphasis on site of origin and nature of associated ovarian tumors. Am J Surg Pathol 18:591–603, 1994.
57. Chuaqui RF, Zhuang Z, Emmert-Buck MR, et al: Genetic analysis of synchronous mucinous tumors of the ovary and appendix. Hum Pathol 27:165–171, 1996.
58. LiVolsi VA, Merino MJ, Schwartz PE: Coexistent endocervical adenocarcinoma and mucinous adenocarcinoma of ovary: a clinicopathologic study of four cases. Int J Gynecol Pathol 1:391–402, 1983.
59. Kaminski PF, Norris HJ: Coexistence of ovarian neoplasms and endocervical adenocarcinoma. Obstet Gynecol 64:553–556, 1984.
60. Young RH, Scully RE: Mucinous ovarian tumors associated with mucinous adenocarcinomas of the cervix. A clinicopathological analysis of 16 cases. Int J Gynecol Pathol 7:99–111, 1988.
61. Bell DA: Mucinous adenofibromas of the ovary. A report of 10 cases. Am J Surg Pathol 15:227–232, 1991.
62. Hart WR, Norris HJ: Borderline and malignant mucinous tumors of the ovary. Histologic criteria and clinical behavior. Cancer 31:1031–1045, 1973.
63. DeNictolis M, Montironi R, Tommasoni S, et al: Benign, borderline, and well-differentiated malignant intestinal mucinous tumors of the ovary: a clinicopathologic, histochemical,

immunohistochemical, and nuclear quantitative study of 57 cases. Int J Gynecol Pathol 13:10–21, 1994.

64. Hoerl HD, Hart WR: Primary ovarian mucinous cystadeno-carcinomas. A clinicopathologic study of 49 cases with long-term follow-up. Am J Surg Pathol 22:1449–1462, 1998.

65. Rutgers JL, Scully RE: Ovarian müllerian mucinous papillary cystadenomas of borderline malignancy: a clinicopathological analysis of 30 cases. Cancer 61:340–348, 1988.

66. Siriaunkgul S, Robbins KM, McGowan L, et al: Ovarian mucinous tumors of low malignant potential. A clinicopathologic study of 54 tumors of intestinal and müllerian type. Int J Gynecol Oncol 14:198–208, 1995.

67. Prat J, Scully RE: Ovarian mucinous tumors with sarcoma-like mural nodules. A report of seven cases. Cancer 44:1333–1344, 1979.

68. Baergen RN, Rutgers JL: Mural nodules in common epithelial tumors of the ovary. Int J Gynecol Pathol 13:62–72, 1994.

69. Prat J, Scully RE: Sarcomas in ovarian mucinous tumors. A report of two cases. Cancer 44:1327–1331, 1979.

70. Prat J, Young RH, Scully RE: Ovarian mucinous tumors with foci of anaplastic carcinoma. Cancer 50:300–304, 1982.

71. Young RH, Prat J, Scully RE: Ovarian Sertoli-Leydig cell tumors with heterologous elements. I. Gastrointestinal epithelium and carcinoid: a clinicopathologic analysis of thirty-six cases. Cancer 50:2448–2456, 1982.

72. Holtz F, Hart WR: Krukenberg tumors of the ovary. A clinicopathological analysis of 27 cases. Cancer 50:2438–2447, 1982.

73. Lash RH, Hart WR: Intestinal adenocarcinomas metastatic to the ovaries. A clinicopathological evaluation of 22 cases. Am J Surg Pathol 11:114–121, 1987.

74. Daya D, Nazerali L, Frank GL: Metastatic ovarian carcinoma of large intestinal origin simulating primary ovarian carcinoma. A clinicopathologic study of 25 cases. Am J Clin Pathol 97:751–758, 1992.

75. Merino MJ, Edmonds P, LiVolsi V: Appendiceal carcinoma metastatic to the ovaries and mimicking primary ovarian tumors. Int J Gynecol Pathol 4:110–120, 1985.

76. Ronnett BM, Kurman RJ, Shmookler BM, et al: The morphologic spectrum of ovarian metastases of appendiceal adenocarcinomas. A clinicopathologic and immunohistochemical analysis of tumors often misinterpreted as primary ovarian tumors or metastatic tumors from other gastrointestinal sites. Am J Surg Pathol 21:1144–1155, 1997.

77. Young RH, Hart WR: Metastases from carcinomas of the pancreas simulating primary mucinous tumors of the ovary: a report of seven cases. Am J Surg Pathol 13:748–756, 1989.

78. Young RH, Scully RE: Ovarian metastases from carcinoma of the gallbladder and extrahepatic bile ducts simulating primary tumors of the ovary: a report of six cases. Int J Gynecol Pathol 9:60–72, 1990.

79. Young RH, Scully RE: Metastatic tumors of the ovary: a problem-oriented approach and review of the recent literature. Semin Diagn Pathol 8:250–276, 1991.

80. Wauters C, Smedts F, Gerrits L, et al: Keratins 7 and 20 as diagnostic markers of carcinomas metastatic to the ovary. Hum Pathol 26:852–855, 1995.

81. Loy TS, Calaluce RD, Keeney GL: Cytokeratin immunostaining in differentiating primary ovarian carcinoma from metastatic colonic adenocarcinoma. Mod Pathol 11:1040–1044, 1996.

82. Fowler LJ, Maygarden SJ, Novotny DB: Human alveolar macrophage-56 and carcinoembryonic antigen monoclonal antibodies in the differential diagnosis between primary ovarian and metastatic gastrointestinal carcinomas. Hum Pathol 25:666–670, 1994.

83. Younes M, Katikaneni PR, Lechago LV, et al: HAM56 antibody: a tool in the differential diagnosis between colorectal and gynecologic malignancy. Mod Pathol 7:396–400, 1994.

84. Long ME, Taylor HC Jr: Endometrioid carcinoma of the ovary. Am J Obstet Gynecol 90:936–950, 1964.

85. Czernobilsky B, Silverman BB, Mikuta JJ: Endometrioid carcinoma of the ovary. A clinicopathologic study of 75 cases. Cancer 26:1141–1152, 1970.

86. Kurman RJ, Craig JM: Endometrioid and clear cell carcinoma of the ovary. Cancer 29:1653–1664, 1972.

87. Kline RC, Wharton JT, Atkinson EN, et al: Endometrioid carcinoma of the ovary. Retrospective review of 145 cases. Gynecol Oncol 39:337–346, 1990.

88. Corner GW Jr, Hu YC, Hertig AT: Ovarian carcinoma arising in endometriosis. Am J Obstet Gynecol 59:760–774, 1950.

89. Mostoufizadeh M, Scully RE: Malignant tumors arising in endometriosis. Clin Obstet Gynecol 23:951–963, 1980.

90. Depriest PD, Banks ER, Powell DE, et al: Endometrioid carcinoma of the ovary and endometriosis: the association in post-menopausal women. Gynecol Oncol 47:71–75, 1992.

91. Kao GF, Norris HJ: Unusual cystadenofibromas: endometrioid, mucinous, and clear cell types. Obstet Gynecol 54:729–736, 1979.

92. Roth LM, Czernobilsky B, Langley FA: Ovarian endometrioid adenofibromatous and cystadenofibromatous tumors: benign, proliferating, and malignant. Cancer 48:1838–1845, 1981.

93. Hughesdon PE: Benign endometrioid tumours of the ovary and the müllerian concept of ovarian epithelial tumours. Histopathology 8:977–990, 1984.

94. Bell DA, Scully RE: Atypical and borderline endometrioid adenofibromas of the ovary. Am J Surg Pathol 9:205–214, 1985.

95. Snyder RR, Norris HJ, Tavassoli F: Endometrioid proliferative and low malignant potential tumors of the ovary. A clinicopathologic study of 46 cases. Am J Surg Pathol 12:661–671, 1988.

96. Norris HJ: Proliferative endometrioid tumors and endometrioid tumors of low malignant potential of the ovary. Int J Gynecol Pathol 12:134–140, 1993.

97. Pitman MB, Young RH, Clement PB, et al: Endometrioid carcinoma of the ovary and endometrium, oxyphilic cell type. A report of nine cases. Int J Gynecol Pathol 13:290–301, 1994.

98. Roth LM, Liban E, Czernobilsky B: Ovarian endometrioid tumors mimicking Sertoli and Sertoli-Leydig cell tumors. Sertoli-form variant of endometrioid carcinoma. Cancer 50:1322–1331, 1982.

99. Young RH, Prat J, Scully RE: Ovarian endometrioid carcinomas resembling sex-cord stromal tumors. A clinicopathologic analysis of 13 cases. Am J Surg Pathol 6:513–522, 1982.

100. Aguirre P, Thor AD, Scully RE: Ovarian endometrioid carcinomas resembling sex cord–stromal tumors. An immunohistochemical study. Int J Gynecol Pathol 8:364–373, 1989.

101. Pelkey TJ, Frierson HF Jr, Mills SE, et al: The diagnostic utility of inhibin staining in ovarian neoplasms. Int J Gynecol Pathol 17:97–105, 1998.

102. Zaino RJ, Unger ER, Whitney C: Synchronous carcinomas of the uterine corpus and ovary. Gynecol Oncol 19:329–335, 1984.

103. Ulbright TM, Roth LM: Metastatic and independent cancers of the endometrium and ovary: a clinicopathologic study of 34 cases. Hum Pathol 16:28–34, 1985.

104. Shenson DL, Gallion HH, Powell DE, et al: Loss of heterozygosity and genomic instability in synchronous endometrioid tumors of the ovary and endometrium. Cancer 76:650–657, 1995.

105. Clement PB, Young RH, Scully RE: Endometrioid-like yolk sac tumor of the ovary. A clinicopathological analysis of eight cases. Am J Surg Pathol 11:767–778, 1987.

106. Young RH, Scully RE: Ovarian tumors of probable wolffian origin: a report of 11 cases. Am J Surg Pathol 7:125–135, 1983.

107. Dehner LP, Norris HJ, Taylor HB: Carcinosarcomas and mixed mesodermal tumors of the ovary. Cancer 27:207–216, 1971.

108. Barwick KW, LiVolsi VA: Malignant mixed mesodermal tumors of the ovary. A clinicopathologic assessment of 12 cases. Am J Surg Pathol 4:37–42, 1980.

109. Morrow CP, d'Ablaing G, Brady LW, et al: A clinical and pathologic study of 30 cases of malignant mixed müllerian epithelial and mesenchymal ovarian tumors: a Gynecologic Oncology Group study. Gynecol Oncol 18:278–292, 1984.

110. Dictor M: Malignant mixed mesodermal tumor of the ovary: a report of 22 cases. Obstet Gynecol 65:720–724, 1985.

111. Terada KY, Johnson TL, Hopkins M, et al: Clinicopathologic features of the ovarian mixed mesodermal tumors and carcinosarcomas. Gynecol Oncol 32:228–232, 1989.

112. Clement PB, Scully RE: Extrauterine mesodermal (müllerian) adenosarcoma. Am J Clin Pathol 69:276–283, 1978.

113. Kao GF, Norris HJ: Benign and low grade variants of mixed mesodermal tumor (adenosarcoma) of the ovary and adnexal region. Cancer 42:1314–1324, 1978.

114. Silverberg SG, Fernandez FN: Endolymphatic stromal sarcomas of the ovary. A report of three cases and literature review. Gynecol Oncol 12:129–138, 1981.

115. Young RH, Prat J, Scully RE: Endometrioid stromal sarcomas of the ovary. A clinicopathologic analysis of 23 cases. Cancer 53:1143–1155, 1984.

116. Young RH, Scully RE: Sarcomas metastatic to the ovary: a report of 21 cases. Int J Gynecol Pathol 9:231–252, 1990.

117. Roth LM, Langley FA, Fox H, et al: Ovarian clear cell adenofibromatous tumors. Benign, of low malignant potential, and associated with invasive clear cell carcinoma. Cancer 53:1156–1163, 1984.

118. Bell DA, Scully RE: Benign and borderline clear cell adenofibromas of the ovary. Cancer 56:2922–2931, 1985.

119. Scully RE, Barlow JF: "Mesonephroma" of ovary. Tumor of müllerian nature related to the endometrioid carcinoma. Cancer 20:1405–1417, 1967.

120. Czernobilsky B, Silverman BB, Enterline HT: Clear cell carcinoma of the ovary. A clinicopathologic analysis of pure and mixed forms and comparison with endometrioid carcinoma. Cancer 25:762–772, 1970.

121. Shevchuk MM, Winkler-Monsanto B, Fenoglio CM, et al: Clear cell carcinoma of the ovary: a clinicopathologic study with review of the literature. Cancer 47:1344–1351, 1981.

122. Brescia RJ, Dubin N, Demopoulous RI: Endometrioid and clear cell carcinoma of the ovary. Factors affecting survival. Int J Gynecol Pathol 8:132–138, 1989.

123. Crozier MA, Copeland LJ, Silva EG, et al: Clear cell carcinoma of the ovary: a study of 59 cases. Gynecol Oncol 35:199–203, 1989.

124. Kennedy AW, Biscotti CV, Hart WR, et al: Ovarian clear cell adenocarcinoma. Gynecol Oncol 32:342–349, 1989.

125. Montag AG, Jenison EL, Griffiths CT, et al: Ovarian clear cell carcinoma. A clinicopathologic analysis of 44 cases. Int J Gynecol Pathol 8:85–96, 1989.

126. Kennedy AW, Biscotti CV, Hart WR, et al: Histologic correlates of progression-free interval and survival in ovarian clear cell adenocarcinoma. Gynecol Oncol 50:334–338, 1993.

127. Klemi PJ, Meurmann L, Gronroos M, et al: Clear cell (mesonephroid) tumor of the ovary with characteristics resembling endodermal sinus tumor. Int J Gynecol Pathol 1:95–100, 1982.

128. Zirker TA, Silva EG, Morris M, et al: Immunohistochemical differentiation of clear-cell carcinoma of the female genital tract and endodermal sinus tumor with the use of alpha-fetoprotein and Leu-M1. Am J Clin Pathol 91:511–514, 1989.

129. Young RH, Scully RE: Oxyphilic clear cell carcinoma of the ovary: a report of nine cases. Am J Surg Pathol 11:661–667, 1987.

130. Prat J, Bahn AK, Dickersin GR, et al: Hepatoid yolk sac tumor of the ovary (endodermal sinus tumor with hepatoid differentiation). A light microscopic, ultrastructural and immunohistochemical study of seven cases. Cancer 50:2355–2368, 1982.

131. Ishikura H, Scully RE: Hepatoid carcinoma of the ovary: a report of five cases of newly described tumor. Cancer 60:2775–2784, 1987.

132. Young RH, Hart WR: Renal cell carcinoma metastatic to the ovary: a report of three cases emphasizing possible confusion with ovarian clear cell adenocarcinoma. Int J Gynecol Pathol 11:96–104, 1992.

133. Roth LM, Gersell DJ, Ulbright TM: Ovarian Brenner tumors and transitional cell carcinoma. Recent developments. Int J Gynecol Pathol 12:128–133, 1993.

134. Jorgensen EO, Dockerty MB, Wilson RB, et al: Clinicopathologic study of 53 cases of Brenner's tumors of the ovary. Am J Obstet Gynecol 108:122–127, 1970.

135. Erlich CE, Roth LM: The Brenner tumor. A clinicopathologic study of 57 cases. Cancer 27:332–342, 1971.

136. Silverberg SG: Brenner tumor of the ovary. A clinicopathologic study of 60 tumors in 54 women. Cancer 28:588–596, 1971.

137. Ming SC, Goldman H: Hormonal activity of Brenner tumors in postmenopausal women. Am J Obstet Gynecol 83:666–673, 1962.

138. Roth LM, Sternberg WH: Proliferating Brenner tumors. Cancer 27:687–693, 1971.

139. Miles PA, Norris HJ: Proliferative and malignant Brenner tumors of the ovary. Cancer 30:174–186, 1972.

140. Roth LM, Dallenbach-Hellweg G, Czernobilsky B: Ovarian Brenner tumors. I. Metaplastic, proliferating, and of low malignant potential. Cancer 56:582–591, 1985.

141. Roth LM, Czernobilsky B: Ovarian Brenner tumours. II. Malignant. Cancer 56:592–601, 1985.

142. Austin RM, Norris HJ: Malignant Brenner tumor and transitional cell carcinoma of the ovary. A comparison. Int J Gynecol Pathol 6:29–39, 1987.

143. Robey SS, Silva EG, Gershenson DM, et al: Transitional cell carcinoma in high-grade high-stage ovarian carcinoma. An indicator of favorable response to chemotherapy. Cancer 63:839–847, 1989.

144. Silva EG, Robey-Cafferty SS, Smith TL, et al: Ovarian carcinomas with transitional cell carcinoma pattern. Am J Clin Pathol 93:457–470, 1990.

145. Young RH, Scully RE: Urothelial and ovarian carcinomas of identical cell types. Problems in interpretation. A report of three cases and review of the literature. Int J Gynecol Pathol 7:197–211, 1988.

146. Soslow RA, Rouse RV, Hendrickson MR, et al: Transitional cell neoplasms of the ovary and urinary bladder: a comparative immunohistochemical analysis. Int J Gynecol Pathol 15:257–265, 1996.

147. Rutgers JL, Scully RE: Ovarian mixed-epithelial papillary cystadenomas of borderline malignancy. A clinicopathological analysis. Cancer 61:546–554, 1988.

148. Silva EG, Tornos C, Bailey MA, et al: Undifferentiated carcinoma of the ovary. Arch Pathol Lab Med 115:377–381, 1991.

149. Pins MR, Young RH, Daly WJ, et al: Primary squamous cell carcinoma of the ovary. Report of 37 cases. Am J Surg Pathol 20:823–833, 1996.

150. Eichhorn JH, Scully RE: "Adenoid cystic" and basaloid carcinoma of the ovary. Evidence for a surface epithelial lineage. A report of 12 cases. Mod Pathol 8:731–740, 1995.

151. Eichhorn JH, Lawrence WD, Young RH, et al: Ovarian neuroendocrine carcinomas of non–small-cell type associated with surface epithelial adenocarcinomas. A study of five cases and review of the literature. Int J Gynecol Pathol 15:303–314, 1996.

152. Puts JJG, Moesker O, Aldeweireldt J, et al: Application of antibodies to intermediate filament proteins in simple and complex tumors of the female genital tract. Int J Gynecol Pathol 6:257–274, 1987.

153. Thor A, Ohuchi N, Szpak CA, et al: Distribution of oncofetal antigen tumor-associated glycoprotein-72 defined by monoclonal antibody B72.3. Cancer Res 46:3118–3124, 1986.

154. Moll R, Pitz S, Levy R, et al: Complexity of expression of intermediate filament proteins, including glial filament protein, in endometrial and ovarian adenocarcinomas. Hum Pathol 22:989–1001, 1991.

155. Viale G, Gambacorta M, Dell'Orto P, et al: Coexpression of cytokeratins and vimentin in common epithelial tumours of the ovary: an immunohistochemical study of eighty-three cases. Virchows Arch A Pathol Anat Histopathol 413:91–101, 1988.

156. Koelma IA, Nap M, Rodenburg GJ, et al: The value of tumour marker CA 125 in surgical pathology. Histopathology 11:287–294, 1987.

157. Neunteufel W, Breitenecker GL: Tissue expression of CA 125 in benign and malignant lesions of ovary and fallopian tube: a comparison with CA 19-9 and CEA. Gynecol Oncol 32:297–302, 1989.

158. Lin M, Hanai J, Wada A, et al: S-100 protein in ovarian tumors. A comparative immunohistochemical study of 135 cases. Acta Pathol Jpn 41:233–239, 1991.

159. Charpin C, Bhan AK, Zurawski VR, et al: Carcinoembryonic antigen (CEA) and carbohydrate determinant 19-9 (CA 19-9) localization in 121 primary and metastatic ovarian tumors. An immunohistochemical study with the use of monoclonal antibodies. Int J Gynecol Pathol 1:231–245, 1982.

160. Khalifa MA, Sesterhenn IA: Tumor markers of epithelial ovarian neoplasms. Int J Gynecol Pathol 9:217–230, 1990.

161. Baker VV: Molecular biology and genetics of epithelial ovarian cancer. Obstet Gynecol Clin North Am 21:25–40, 1994.

162. Gallion HH, Pieretti M, DePriest PD, et al: The molecular basis of ovarian cancer. Cancer 76:1992–1997, 1995.

163. Depasquale SE, Giordano A, Donnenfeld AE: The genetics of ovarian cancer: molecular biology and clinical application. Obstet Gynecol Surv 53:248–256, 1998.

164. Gallion HH, Powell DE, Smith LW, et al: Chromosome abnormalities in human epithelial ovarian malignancies. Gynecol Oncol 38:473–477, 1990.

165. Ehlen T, Dubeau L: Loss of heterozygosity on chromosomal segments 3p, 6q, and 11p in human ovarian carcinomas. Oncogene 5:219–223, 1990.

166. Zheng, Robinson WR, Ehlen T, et al: Distinction of low grade from high grade human ovarian carcinomas on the basis of losses of heterozygosity on chromosomes 3, 6, and 11 and *HER-2/neu* gene amplification. Cancer Res 51:4045–4051, 1991.

167. Jones MH, Nakamura Y: Deletion mapping of chromosome 3p in female genital tract malignancies using microsatellite polymorphisms. Oncogene 7:1631–1634, 1992.

168. Lee JH, Kavanaugh JJ, Wildrick DM, et al: Frequent loss of heterozygosity on chromosomes 6q, 11 and 17 in human ovarian carcinomas. Cancer Res 50:2724–2728, 1990.

169. Foulkes WD, Fagoussis J, Stamp GW, et al: Frequent loss of heterozygosity on chromosome 6 in human ovarian carcinoma. Br J Cancer 67:551–559, 1993.

170. Lee JH, Kavanaugh JJ, Wharton JT, et al: Allele loss at the c-Ha-*ras*-1 locus in human ovarian cancer. Cancer Res 49:1220–1222, 1989.

171. Viel A, Giannini F, Tumiotto L, et al: Chromosomal localisation of two putative 11p oncosuppressor genes involved in human ovarian tumours. Br J Cancer 66:1030–1036, 1992.

172. Foulkes WD, Campbell IG, Stamp GW, et al: Loss of heterozygosity and amplification on chromosome 11q in human ovarian cancer. Br J Cancer 67:268–273, 1993.

173. Kiechle-Schwarz, M, Bauknecht T, Weinker T, et al: Loss of constitutional heterozygosity on chromosome 11p in human ovarian cancer. Positive correlation with grade of differentiation. Cancer 72:2423–2432, 1993.

174. Yang-Feng TL, Han H, Chen KC, et al: Allelic loss in ovarian cancer. Int J Cancer 54:546–551, 1993.

175. Kim TM, Benedict WF, Xu HJ, et al: Loss of heterozygosity on chromosome 13 is common only in the biologically more aggressive subtypes of ovarian epithelial tumors and is associated with normal retinoblastoma gene expression. Cancer Res 54:605–609, 1994.

176. Eccles DM, Russell SE, Haites NE, et al: Early loss of heterozygosity on 17q in ovarian cancer. The Abe Ovarian Cancer Genetics Group. Oncogene 7:2069–2072, 1992.

177. Jacobs IJ, Smith SA, Wiseman RW, et al: A deletion unit on chromosome 17q in epithelial ovarian tumors distal to the familial breast/ovarian cancer locus. Cancer Res 53:1218–1221, 1993.

178. Schildkraut JM, Collins NK, Dent GA, et al: Loss of heterozygosity on chromosome 17q11–21 in cancers of women who have both breast and ovarian cancer. Am J Obstet Gynecol 172:908–913, 1995.

179. Chenevix-Trench G, Leary J, Kerr J, et al: Frequent loss of heterozygosity on chromosome 18 in ovarian adenocarcinoma which does not always include the *DCC* locus. Oncogene 7:1059–1065, 1992.

180. Thompson FH, Emerson J, Alberts D, et al: Clonal chromosomal abnormalities in 54 cases of ovarian carcinoma. Cancer Genet Cytogenet 73:33–45, 1994.

181. Miki Y, Swensen J, Shattuck-Eidens D, et al: A strong candidate for the breast and ovarian cancer susceptibility gene *BRCA1*. Science 226:66–71, 1994.

182. Futreal P, Liu Q, Shattuck-Eidens D, et al: *BRCA1* mutations in primary breast and ovarian cancer carcinomas. Science 266:120–122, 1994.

183. Castilla LH, Couch FJ, Erdos MR, et al: Mutation in the *BRCA1* gene in families with early onset breast and ovarian cancer. Nat Genet 8:387–391, 1994.

184. Narod SA, Ford D, Devilee P, et al: An evaluation of genetic heterogeneity in 145 breast cancer families. Am J Hum Genet 56:254–264, 1995.

185. Wooster R, Neuhausen SL, Mangion J, et al: Localization of a breast cancer susceptibility gene, *BRCA2*, to chromosome 13q12–13. Science 265:2088–2090, 1994.

186. Wooster R, Bignell G, Lancaster J, et al: Identification of the breast cancer susceptibility gene *BRCA2*. Nature 378:789–792, 1995.

187. Holt JT, Thompson ME, Szabo C, et al: Growth retardation and tumour inhibition by *BRCA1*. Nat Genet 12:298–302, 1996.

188. Narod SA, Feuntuen J, Lynch HT, et al: Familial breast-ovarian cancer locus on chromosome 17q12–q23. Lancet 338:82–83, 1991.

189. Aaltonen LA, Peltomaki P, Leach FS, et al: Clues to the pathogenesis of familial colon cancer. Science 260:812–816, 1993.

190. Claus EB, Schwartz PE: Familial ovarian cancer: update and clinical applications. Cancer 76:1998–2003, 1995.

191. Houlston RS, Collins A, Slack J, et al: Genetic epidemiology of ovarian cancer: segregation analysis. Ann Hum Genet 55:291–299, 1991.

192. Berchuck A, Kohler MF, Boente MP, et al: Growth regulation and transformation of ovarian epithelium. Cancer 71:545–551, 1993.

193. Slamon DJ, Godolphin W, Jones LA, et al: Studies of the *Her-2/neu* proto-oncogene in human breast and ovarian cancer. Science 244:707–712, 1989.

194. Berchuck A, Kamel A, Whitaker R, et al: Overexpression of *Her-2/neu* is associated with poor survival in advanced epithelial ovarian cancer. Cancer Res 50:4087–4091, 1990.

195. Huettner PC, Carney WP, Naber SP, et al: *Neu* oncogene expression in ovarian tumors: a quantitative study. Mod Pathol 5:250–256, 1992.

196. Seidman JD, Frisman DM, Norris HJ: Expression of the *HER-2/neu* proto-oncogene in serous ovarian neoplasms. Cancer 70:2875–2860, 1992.

197. Meden H, Marx D, Rath W, et al: Overexpression of the oncogene c-*erb*B2 in primary ovarian cancer. Evaluation of the prognostic value in a Cox proportional hazards multiple regression. Int J Gynecol Pathol 13:45–53, 1994.

198. Baker VV, Borst MP, Dixon D, et al: C-*myc* amplification in ovarian cancer. Gynecol Oncol 38:340–342, 1990.

199. Sasano H, Garrett CT: Oncogenes in gynecologic tumors. Curr Top Pathol 85:357–372, 1992.

200. Ennomoto T, Inoue M, Perantoni AO, et al: K-*ras* activation in neoplasms of the human female reproductive tract. Cancer Res 50:6139–6145, 1990.

201. Yang-Feng TL, Li SB, Leung WY, et al: Trisomy 12 and K-*ras*-2 amplification in human ovarian tumors. Int J Cancer 48:678–681, 1991.

202. Teneriello MG, Ebina M, Linnoila R, et al: *p53* and Ki-*ras* gene mutations in epithelial ovarian neoplasms. Cancer Res 53:3103–3108, 1993.

203. Kacinski BM, Carter D, Mittal K, et al: Ovarian adenocarcinomas express *fms*-complementary transcripts and fms antigen, often with coexpression of CSF-1. Am J Pathol 137:135–147, 1990.

204. Baiocchi G, Kavanaugh JJ, Talpaz M, et al: Expression of macrophage colony stimulating factor and its receptor in gynecologic malignancies. Cancer 67:990–996, 1991.

205. Bellacosa A, DeFeo D, Godwin AK, et al: Molecular alterations of the *Akts* oncogene in ovarian and breast carcinomas. Int J Cancer 64:280–285, 1995.

206. Mok SCH, Bell DA, Knapp RC, et al: Mutations of Ki-*ras*

proto-oncogene in human ovarian epithelial tumors of borderline malignancy. Cancer Res 53:1489–1492, 1993.

207. Marks JR, Davidoff AM, Kerns B, et al: Overexpression and mutations of *p53* in epithelial ovarian cancer. Cancer Res 51: 2979–2984, 1991.

208. Frank TS, Bartos RE, Haefner HK, et al: Loss of heterozygosity and overexpression of the *p53* gene in ovarian carcinoma. Mod Pathol 7:3–8, 1994.

209. Berchuck A, Kohler MF, Hopkins MP, et al: Overexpression of the *p53* tumor suppressor gene is not a feature of benign and early-stage borderline ovarian epithelial tumors. Gynecol Oncol 52:232–236, 1994.

210. Bosari S, Viale G, Radaelli U, et al: p53 accumulation in ovarian carcinomas and its prognostic implications. Hum Pathol 24:1175–1179, 1993.

211. Hartmann LC, Podratz KC, Keeney GL, et al: Prognostic significance of p53 immunostaining in epithelial ovarian cancer. J Clin Oncol 12:64–69, 1994.

212. Levesque MA, Katsaros D, Yu H, et al: Mutant p53 protein overexpression is associated with poor outcome in patients with well or moderately differentiated ovarian carcinoma. Cancer 75:1327–1338, 1995.

213. Schultz DC, Vanderveer L, Berman DB, et al: Identification of two candidate tumor suppressor genes on chromosome 17p13.3. Cancer Res 56:1997–2002, 1996.

214. Friedlander ML, Hedley DW, Swanson C, et al: Prediction of long-term survival by flow cytometric analysis of cellular DNA content in patients with advanced ovarian cancer. J Clin Oncol 6:282–290, 1988.

215. Rodenburg CJ, Cornelisse CJ, Heintz PAM, et al: Tumor ploidy as a major prognostic factor in advanced ovarian cancer. Cancer 59:317–323, 1987.

216. Kallioniemi OP, Punnonen R, Mattila J, et al: Prognostic significance of DNA index, multiploidy and S-phase fraction in ovarian cancer. Cancer 61:334–339, 1988.

217. Volm M, Kleine W, Pfleiderer A: Flow-cytometric prognostic factors for the survival of patients with ovarian carcinoma. A 5-year follow-up study. Gynecol Oncol 35:84–89, 1989.

218. Barnabei VM, Miller DS, Bauer KD, et al: Flow cytometric evaluation of epithelial ovarian cancer. Am J Obstet Gynecol 162:1584–1590, 1990.

219. Brescia RJ, Barakat RA, Beller U, et al: The prognostic significance of nuclear DNA content in malignant epithelial tumors of the ovary. Cancer 65:141–147, 1990.

220. Bell DA: Flow cytometry of ovarian neoplasms. Curr Top Pathol 85:337–356, 1992.

221. Lage JM, Weinberg DS, Huettner PC, et al: Flow cytometric analysis of nuclear DNA content in ovarian tumors. Association of ploidy with tumor type, histologic grade and clinical stage. Cancer 69:2668–2675, 1992.

222. Seidman JD, Norris HJ, Griffin JL, et al: DNA flow cytometric analysis of serous ovarian tumors of low malignant potential. Cancer 71:3947–3951, 1993.

223. Gajewski WH, Fuller AF Jr, Pastel-Ley C, et al: Prognostic significance of DNA content in epithelial ovarian cancer. Gynecol Oncol 53:5–12, 1994.

224. Rice LW, Mark SD, Berkowitz RS, et al: Clinicopathologic variables, operative characteristics, and DNA ploidy in predicting outcome in ovarian epithelial carcinoma. Obstet Gynecol 86:379–385, 1995.

225. Yoshimura S, Scully RE, Taft PD, et al: Peritoneal fluid cytology in patients with ovarian cancer. Gynecol Oncol 17:161–167, 1984.

226. Sneige N, Fanning CV: Peritoneal washing cytology in women: diagnostic pitfalls and clues for correct diagnosis. Diagn Cytopathol 8:632–642, 1992.

227. Moran O, Menczer J, Ben-Baruch G, et al: Cytologic examination of ovarian cyst fluid for the distinction between benign and malignant tumors. Obstet Gynecol 82:444–446, 1993.

228. Trimbos JB, Hacker NF: The case against aspirating ovarian cysts. Cancer 72:828–831, 1993.

229. Ganjei P, Dickinson B, Harrison TA, et al: Aspiration cytology of neoplastic and non-neoplastic ovarian cysts: is it accurate? Int J Gynecol Pathol 15:94–101, 1996.

230. Mulvany NJ: Aspiration cytology of ovarian cysts and cystic neoplasms. A study of 235 aspirates. Acta Cytol 40:911–920, 1996.

231. Haapasalo H, Collan Y, Atkin NB: Major prognostic factors in ovarian carcinomas. Int J Gynecol Cancer 1:155–162, 1991.

232. Nguyen HN, Averette HE, Hoskins W, et al: National survey of ovarian carcinoma IV. Critical assessment of current International Federation of Gynecology and Obstetrics staging system. Cancer 72:3007–3011, 1993.

233. Baak JP, Chan KK, Stolk JG, et al: Prognostic factors in borderline and invasive ovarian tumours of the common epithelial type. Pathol Res Pract 182:755–774, 1987.

234. Kurman RJ, Trimble CL: The behavior of serous tumors of low malignant potential. Are they ever malignant? Int J Gynecol Pathol 12:120–127, 1993.

235. Sorbe B, Frankendal BO, Veress B: Importance of histologic grading in the prognosis of epithelial ovarian carcinoma. Obstet Gynecol 59:576–582, 1982.

236. Malkasian GD, Melton LJ, O'Brien PC, et al: Prognostic significance of histologic classification and grading of epithelial malignancies of the ovary. Am J Obstet Gynecol 149:274–284, 1984.

237. Swenerton KD, Hislop TG, Spinelli J, et al: Ovarian carcinoma. A multivariate analysis of prognostic factors. Obstet Gynecol 65:264–270, 1985.

238. Czernobilsky B: Endometrioid neoplasia of the ovary. A reappraisal. Int J Gynecol Pathol 1:203–210, 1982.

239. Shimizu Y, Kamoi S, Amada S, et al: The grader and the typer should be friends: a study of comparative value of histopathologic grading and typing of ovarian epithelial carcinoma. Mod Pathol 11:115A, 1998.

240. Thigpen T, Brady MF, Omura GA, et al: Age as a prognostic factor in ovarian carcinoma. The Gynecologic Oncology Group experience. Cancer 71:606–614, 1993.

241. Sjovall K, Nilsson B, Einhorn N: Different types of rupture of the tumor capsule and the impact on survival in early ovarian carcinoma. Int J Gynecol Cancer 4:333–336, 1994.

242. Sevelda P, Schemper M, Spona J: CA 125 as an independent prognostic factor for survival in patients with epithelial ovarian cancer. Am J Obstet Gynecol 161:1213–1216, 1989.

243. Young RH, Scully RE: Ovarian sex cord–stromal tumors. Recent advances and current status. Clin Obstet Gynecol 11: 93–134, 1984.

244. Tavassoli FA: Ovarian tumors with functioning manifestations. Endocr Pathol 5:137–148, 1994.

245. Fox H, Agrawal K, Langley FA: A clinicopathologic study of 92 cases of granulosa cell tumor of the ovary with special reference to the factors influencing prognosis. Cancer 35:231–241, 1975.

246. Stenwig JT, Hazekamp JT, Beecham JB: Granulosa cell tumors of the ovary. A clinicopathological study of 118 cases with long term follow-up. Gynecol Oncol 7:136–152, 1979.

247. Evans AT, Gaffey TA, Malkasian GD Jr, et al: Clinicopathologic review of 118 granulosa and 82 theca cell tumors. Obstet Gynecol 55:231–238, 1980.

248. Lack EE, Perez-Atayde AR, Murthy ASK, et al: Granulosa theca cell tumors in premenarchal girls. A clinical and pathologic study of ten cases. Cancer 48:1846–1854, 1981.

249. Zaloudek C, Norris HJ: Granulosa tumors of the ovary in children. A clinical and pathologic study of 32 cases. Am J Surg Pathol 6:503–512, 1982.

250. Young RH, Dickersin GR, Scully RE: Juvenile granulosa cell tumor of the ovary. A clinicopathologic analysis of 125 cases. Am J Surg Pathol 8:575–596, 1984.

251. Biscotti CV, Hart WR: Juvenile granulosa cell tumors of the ovary. Arch Pathol Lab Med 113:40–46, 1989.

252. Nakashima N, Young RH, Scully RE: Androgenic granulosa cell tumors of the ovary. A clinicopathologic analysis of 17 cases and review of the literature. Arch Pathol Lab Med 108: 786–791, 1984.

253. Norris HJ, Taylor HB: Prognosis of granulosa-theca tumors of the ovary. Cancer 21:255–263, 1968.

254. Bjørkholm E, Silfersward C: Prognostic factors in granulosa cell tumors. Gynecol Oncol 11:261–274, 1981.

255. Malmstrom H, Hogberg T, Risberg B, et al: Granulosa cell

tumors of the ovary: prognostic factors and outcome. Gynecol Oncol 52:50–55, 1994.

256. Young RH, Scully RE: Ovarian sex cord–stromal tumors with bizarre nuclei. A clinicopathologic analysis of seventeen cases. Int J Gynecol Pathol 1:325–335, 1983.

257. Otis CN, Powell JL, Barbuto D, et al: Intermediate filament proteins in adult granulosa cell tumors. An immunohistochemical study of 25 cases. Am J Surg Pathol 16:962–968, 1992.

258. Costa MJ, Derose PB, Roth LM, et al: Immunohistochemical phenotype of ovarian granulosa cell tumors: absence of epithelial membrane antigen has diagnostic value. Hum Pathol 25:60–66, 1994.

259. Zheng W, Sung J, Hanna I, et al: α and β subunits of inhibin/activin as sex cord–stromal differentiation markers. Int J Gynecol Pathol 16:263–271, 1997.

260. Kommoss F, Oliva E, Bhan AK, et al: Inhibin expression in ovarian tumors and tumor-like lesions: an immunohistochemical study. Mod Pathol 11:656–664, 1998.

261. Santini D, Ceccarelli C, Leone O, et al: Smooth muscle differentiation in normal human ovaries, ovarian stromal hyperplasia and ovarian granulosa-stromal cell tumors. Mod Pathol 8:25–30, 1995.

262. Loo KT, Leung AKF, Chan JKC: Immunohistochemical staining of ovarian granulosa cell tumours with MIC2 antibody. Histopathology 27:388–390, 1995.

263. Miller BE, Barron BA, Wan JY, et al: Prognostic factors in adult granulosa cell tumor of the ovary. Cancer 79:1951–1955, 1997.

264. Sternberg WH, Gaskill CJ: Theca-cell tumors. With a report of twelve new cases and observations on the possible etiologic role of ovarian stromal hyperplasia. Am J Obstet Gynecol 59:575–587, 1950.

265. Bjørkholm E, Silfersward C: Theca-cell tumors. Clinical features and prognosis. Acta Radiol Oncol Radiat Phys Biol 19:241–244, 1980.

266. Waxman M, Vuletin JC, Urcuyo R, et al: Ovarian low grade stromal sarcoma with thecomatous features. A critical reappraisal of the so-called "malignant thecoma." Cancer 44:2206–2217, 1979.

267. Zhang J, Young RH, Arseneau J, et al: Ovarian stromal tumors containing lutein or Leydig cells (luteinized thecomas and stromal Leydig cell tumors)—a clinicopathological analysis of fifty cases. Int J Gynecol Pathol 1:270–285, 1982.

268. Roth LM, Sternberg WH: Partly luteinized theca cell tumor of the ovary. Cancer 51:1697–1704, 1983.

269. Clement PB, Young RH, Hanna W, et al: Sclerosing peritonitis associated with luteinized thecomas of the ovary. A clinicopathological analysis of six cases. Am J Surg Pathol 18:1–13, 1994.

270. Werness BA: Luteinized thecoma with sclerosing peritonitis. Arch Pathol Lab Med 120:303–306, 1996.

271. Dockerty MB, Masson JC: Ovarian fibromas: a clinical and pathologic study of two hundred and eighty-three cases. Am J Obstet Gynecol 47:741–752, 1944.

272. Gorlin RJ: Nevoid basal cell carcinoma syndrome. Medicine (Baltimore) 66:98–113, 1987.

273. Meigs JV: Fibroma of the ovary with ascites and hydrothorax—Meig's syndrome. Am J Obstet Gynecol 67:962–987, 1954.

274. Samanth KK, Black WC: Benign ovarian stromal tumors associated with free peritoneal fluid. Am J Obstet Gynecol 107:538–545, 1970.

275. Prat J, Scully RE: Cellular fibromas and fibrosarcomas of the ovary: a comparative clinicopathologic analysis of seventeen cases. Cancer 47:2663–2670, 1981.

276. Young RH, Scully RE: Ovarian stromal tumors with minor sex cord elements: a report of seven cases. Int J Gynecol Pathol 2:227–234, 1983.

277. Chalvardjian A, Scully RE: Sclerosing stromal tumors of the ovary. Cancer 31:664–670, 1973.

278. Gee DC, Russell P: Sclerosing stromal tumours of the ovary. Histopathology 3:367–376, 1979.

279. Saitoh A, Tsutsumi Y, Osamura RY, et al: Sclerosing stromal tumor of the ovary. Immunohistochemical and electron-microscopic demonstration of smooth-muscle differentiation. Arch Pathol Lab Med 113:372–376, 1989.

280. Shaw JA, Dabbs DJ, Geisinger KR: Sclerosing stromal tumor of the ovary. An ultrastructural and immunohistochemical analysis with histogenetic considerations. Ultrastruct Pathol 16:363–377, 1992.

281. Tavassoli FA, Norris H: Sertoli tumors of the ovary. A clinicopathologic study of 28 cases with ultrastructural observations. Cancer 46:2281–2297, 1980.

282. Young RH, Scully RE: Ovarian Sertoli cell tumors. A report of ten cases. Int J Gynecol Pathol 2:349–363, 1984.

283. Roth LM, Anderson MC, Govan ADT, et al: Sertoli-Leydig cell tumors. A clinicopathologic study of 34 cases. Cancer 48:187–197, 1981.

284. Zaloudek C, Norris HJ: Sertoli-Leydig tumors of the ovary. A clinicopathologic study of 64 intermediate and poorly differentiated neoplasms. Am J Surg Pathol 8:405–418, 1984.

285. Young RH, Scully RE: Ovarian Sertoli-Leydig cell tumors: a clinicopathological analysis of 207 cases. Am J Surg Pathol 9:543–569, 1985.

286. Young RH, Scully RE: Well-differentiated ovarian Sertoli-Leydig cell tumors: a clinicopathological analysis of 23 cases. Int J Gynecol Pathol 3:277–290, 1984.

287. Prat J, Young RH, Scully RE: Ovarian Sertoli-Leydig cell tumors with heterologous elements. II. Cartilage and skeletal muscle: a clinicopathological analysis of twelve cases. Cancer 50:2465–2475, 1982.

288. Roth LM, Slayton RE, Brady LW, et al: Retiform differentiation in ovarian Sertoli-Leydig cell tumors. A clinicopathologic study of six cases from a Gynecologic Oncology Group study. Cancer 55:1093–1098, 1985.

289. Talerman A: Ovarian Sertoli-Leydig cell tumor (androblastoma) with retiform pattern. A clinicopathologic study. Cancer 60:3056–3064, 1987.

290. Young RH, Dudley AG, Scully RE: Granulosa cell, Sertoli-Leydig cell and unclassified sex cord–stromal tumors associated with pregnancy. A clinicopathological analysis of thirty-six cases. Gynecol Oncol 18:181–205, 1984.

291. Gagnon S, Tetu B, Silva EG, et al: Frequency of α-fetoprotein production by Sertoli-Leydig cell tumors of the ovary: an immunohistochemical study of eight cases. Mod Pathol 2:63–67, 1989.

292. Higuchi Y, Kouno T, Teshima H, et al: Serous papillary cystadenocarcinoma associated with alpha-fetoprotein production. Arch Pathol Lab Med 108:710–712, 1984.

293. Costa MJ, Morris RJ, Wilson R, et al: Utility of immunohistochemistry in distinguishing ovarian Sertoli–stromal cell tumors from carcinosarcomas. Hum Pathol 23:787–797, 1992.

294. Neubecker RD, Breen JL: Gynandroblastoma. A report of five cases, with discussion of the histogenesis and classification of ovarian tumors. Am J Clin Pathol 38:60–69, 1962.

295. Novak ER: Gynandroblastoma of the ovary. Review of 8 cases from the Ovarian Tumor Registry. Obstet Gynecol 30:709–715, 1967.

296. Anderson MC, Rees DA: Gynandroblastoma of the ovary. Br J Obstet Gynaecol 82:68–73, 1975.

297. Chalvardjian A, Derzko C: Gynandroblastoma. Its ultrastructure. Cancer 50:710–721, 1982.

298. Scully RE: Sex cord tumor with annular tubules. A distinctive ovarian tumor of the Peutz-Jeghers syndrome. Cancer 25:1107–1121, 1970.

299. Hart WR, Kumar N, Crissman JD: Ovarian neoplasms resembling sex cord tumors with annular tubules. Cancer 45:2352–2363, 1980.

300. Anderson MC, Govan ADT, Langley FA, et al: Ovarian sex cord tumours with annular tubules. Histopathology 4:137–145, 1980.

301. Young RH, Welch WR, Dickersin GR, et al: Ovarian sex cord tumor with annular tubules: review of 74 cases including 27 with Peutz-Jeghers syndrome and four with adenoma malignum of the cervix. Cancer 50:1384–1402, 1982.

302. Hayes MC, Scully RE: Stromal luteoma of the ovary: a clinicopathological analysis of 25 cases. Int J Gynecol Pathol 6:313–321, 1987.

303. Roth LM, Sternberg WH: Ovarian stromal tumors containing

Leydig cells. II. Pure Leydig cell tumors, nonhilar type. Cancer 32:952–960, 1973.

304. Paraskevas M, Scully RE: Hilus cell tumor of the ovary. A clinicopathological analysis of 12 Reinke crystal-positive and nine crystal-negative cases. Int J Gynecol Pathol 8:299–310, 1989.

305. Taylor HB, Norris HJ: Lipid cell tumors of the ovary. Cancer 20:1953–1962, 1967.

306. Hayes MC, Scully RE: Ovarian steroid cell tumors, not otherwise specified (lipid cell tumors): a clinicopathological analysis of 63 cases. Am J Surg Pathol 11:835–845, 1987.

307. Young RH, Scully RE: Ovarian steroid cell tumors associated with Cushing's syndrome: a report of three cases. Int J Gynecol Pathol 6:40–48, 1987.

308. Seidman JD, Abbondanzo SL, Bratthauer GL: Lipid cell (steroid cell) tumor of the ovary: immunophenotype with analysis of potential pitfall due to endogenous biotin-like activity. Int J Gynecol Pathol 14:331–338, 1995.

309. Kurman RJ, Ganjei P, Nadji M: Contributions of immunocytochemistry to the diagnosis and study of ovarian neoplasms. Int J Gynecol Pathol 3:3–26, 1984.

310. Costa MJ, Morris R, Sasano H: Sex steroid biosynthesis enzymes in ovarian sex-cord stromal tumors. Int J Gynecol Pathol 13:109–119, 1994.

311. Sasano H: Functional pathology of human ovarian steroidogenesis. Normal cycling ovary and steroid-producing neoplasms. Endocr Pathol 5:81–89, 1994.

312. Fletcher JA, Gibas Z, Donovan K, et al: Ovarian granulosa-stromal cell tumors are characterized by trisomy 12. Am J Pathol 138:515–520, 1991.

313. Schofield DE, Fletcher JA: Trisomy 12 in pediatric granulosa-stromal cell tumors. Demonstration by a modified method of fluorescence in situ hybridization on paraffin-embedded material. Am J Pathol 141:1265–1269, 1992.

314. Persons DL, Hartmann LC, Herath JF, et al: Fluorescence in situ hybridization analysis of trisomy 12 in ovarian tumors. Am J Clin Pathol 102:775–779, 1994.

315. Halperin D, Visscher DW, Wallis T, et al: Evaluation of chromosome 12 copy number in ovarian granulosa cell tumors using interphase cytogenetics. Int J Gynecol Pathol 14:319–323, 1995.

316. Chadha S, Cornelisse CJ, Schaberg A: Flow cytometric DNA ploidy analysis of ovarian granulosa cell tumors. Gynecol Oncol 36:240–245, 1990.

317. Suh KS, Silverberg SG, Rhame JG, et al: Granulosa cell tumor of the ovary. Histopathologic and flow cytometric analysis with clinical correlation. Arch Pathol Lab Med 114:496–501, 1990.

318. Swanson SA, Norris HG, Kelsten ML, et al: DNA content of juvenile granulosa tumors determined by flow cytometry. Int J Gynecol Pathol 9:101–109, 1990.

319. Jacoby AF, Young RH, Colvin RB, et al: DNA content in juvenile granulosa cell tumors of the ovary. A study of early- and advanced-stage disease. Gynecol Oncol 46:97–103, 1992.

320. Evans MP, Webb MJ, Gaffey TA, et al: DNA ploidy of ovarian granulosa cell tumors. Lack of correlation between DNA index or proliferative index and outcome in 40 patients. Cancer 75:2295–2298, 1995.

321. Lack EE, Young RH, Scully RE: Pathology of ovarian neoplasms in childhood and adolescence. Pathol Annu 27:281–356, 1992.

322. Gershenson DM: Update on malignant ovarian germ cell tumors. Cancer 71:1581–1590, 1993.

323. Pfleiderer A: Therapy of ovarian malignant germ cell tumors and granulosa tumors. Int J Gynecol Pathol 12:162–165, 1993.

324. LaPolla JP, Benda J, Vigliotti AP, et al: Dysgerminoma of the ovary. Obstet Gynecol 69:859–867, 1987.

325. Bjorkholm E, Lundell M, Gyftodimos A, et al: Dysgerminoma: the Radiumhemmet series 1927–1984. Cancer 65:38–44, 1990.

326. Gillespie JJ, Arnold LK: Anaplastic dysgerminoma. Cancer 42:1886–1889, 1978.

327. Zaloudek CJ, Tavassoli FA, Norris HJ: Dysgerminoma with syncytiotrophoblastic giant cells. A histologically and clinically distinctive subtype of dysgerminoma. Am J Surg Pathol 5:361–367, 1981.

328. Parkash V, Carcangiu ML: Transformation of ovarian dysgerminoma to yolk sac tumor. Evidence for a histogenetic continuum. Mod Pathol 8:881–887, 1995.

329. Lifshitz-Mercer B, Walt H, Kushnir I, et al: Differentiation potential of ovarian dysgerminoma. An immunohistochemical study of 15 cases. Hum Pathol 26:62–66, 1995.

330. Nogales FF: Embryologic clues to human yolk sac tumors. A review. Int J Gynecol Pathol 12:101–107, 1993.

331. Huntington RW, Bullock WK: Yolk sac tumors of the ovary. Cancer 25:1357–1367, 1970.

332. Kurman RJ, Norris HJ: Endodermal sinus tumor of the ovary. A clinical and pathologic analysis of 71 cases. Cancer 38:2404–2419, 1976.

333. Gonzalez-Crussi F, Roth LM: The human yolk sac and yolk sac carcinoma. Hum Pathol 7:675–691, 1976.

334. Langley FA, Govan ADT, Anderson MC, et al: Yolk sac and allied tumours of the ovary. Histopathology 5:389–401, 1981.

335. Gershenson DM, Del Junco G, Herson J, et al: Endodermal sinus tumor of the ovary: the M.D. Anderson experience. Obstet Gynecol 61:194–202, 1983.

336. Ulbright TM, Roth LM, Brodhecker CA: Yolk sac differentiation in germ cell tumors. A morphologic study of 50 cases with emphasis on hepatic, enteric, and parietal yolk sac features. Am J Surg Pathol 10:151–164, 1986.

337. Kawai M, Kano T, Furuhashi Y, et al: Prognostic factors in yolk sac tumors of the ovary. A clinicopathologic analysis of 29 cases. Cancer 67:184–192, 1991.

338. Stewart KR, Casey MJ, Condos B: Endodermal sinus tumor of the ovary with virilization. Light and electron microscopic study. Am J Surg Pathol 5:385–391, 1981.

339. Nogales FF Jr, Matilla A, Nogales-Ortiz F, et al: Yolk sac tumors with pure and mixed polyvesicular vitelline patterns. Hum Pathol 9:553–566, 1978.

340. Cohen MB, Friend DS, Molnar JJ, et al: Gonadal endodermal sinus (yolk sac) tumor with pure intestinal differentiation: a new histologic type. Pathol Res Pract 182:609–616, 1987.

341. Michael H, Ulbright TM, Brodhecker CA: The pluripotential nature of the mesenchyme-like component of yolk sac tumor. Arch Pathol Lab Med 113:1115–1119, 1989.

342. Sasaki H, Furusato M, Teshima S, et al: Prognostic significance of histopathological subtypes in stage I pure yolk sac tumour of the ovary. Br J Cancer 69:529–536, 1994.

343. Neubecker RD, Breen JL: Embryonal carcinoma of the ovary. Cancer 15:546–556, 1962.

344. Kurman RJ, Norris HJ: Embryonal carcinoma of the ovary. A clinicopathologic entity distinct from endodermal sinus tumor resembling embryonal carcinoma of the adult testis. Cancer 38:2420–2433, 1976.

345. Nakashima N, Murakami S, Fukatsu T, et al: Characteristics of "embryoid body" in human gonadal germ cell tumors. Hum Pathol 19:1144–1154, 1988.

346. King ME, Hubbell MJ, Talerman A: Mixed germ cell tumor of the ovary with a prominent polyembryoma component. Int J Gynecol Pathol 10:88–95, 1991.

347. Takeda A, Ishizuka T, Goto T, et al: Polyembryoma of ovary producing alpha-fetoprotein and HCG: immunoperoxidase and electron microscopic study. Cancer 14:1878–1889, 1982.

348. Gerbie MV, Brewer JI, Tamini H: Primary choriocarcinoma of the ovary. Obstet Gynecol 46:720–723, 1975.

349. Jacobs AJ, Newland JR, Green RK: Pure choriocarcinoma of the ovary. Obstet Gynecol Surv 37:603–609, 1982.

350. Axe SR, Lein VR, Woodruff JD: Choriocarcinoma of the ovary. Obstet Gynecol 66:111–114, 1985.

351. Vance RP, Geisinger KR: Pure nongestational choriocarcinoma of the ovary. Report of a case. Cancer 56:2321–2325, 1985.

352. Civantos F, Rywlin A: Carcinomas with trophoblastic differentiation and secretion of chorionic gonadotrophins. Cancer 29:789–798, 1972.

353. Oliva E, Andrada E, Pezzica E, et al: Ovarian carcinomas with choriocarcinomatous differentiation. Cancer 72:2441–2446, 1993.

354. Linder D, McCaw BK, Hecht F: Parthenogenic origin of benign ovarian teratomas. N Engl J Med 292:63–66, 1975.

355. Norris HJ, Zirkin HJ, Benson WL: Immature (malignant) teratoma of the ovary. A clinical and pathologic study of 58 cases. Cancer 37:2359–2372, 1976.

356. Yanai-Inbar I, Scully RE: Relation of ovarian dermoid cysts and immature teratomas: an analysis of 350 cases of immature teratoma and 10 cases of dermoid cyst with microscopic foci of immature tissue. Int J Gynecol Pathol 6:203–212, 1987.

357. Nogales FF, Ruiz Avila I, Concha A, et al: Immature endodermal teratoma of the ovary. Embryologic correlations and immunhistochemistry. Hum Pathol 24:364–370, 1993.

358. O'Connor DM, Norris HJ: The influence of grade on the outcome of stage I ovarian immature (malignant) teratomas and the reproducibility of grading. Int J Gynecol Pathol 13:283–289, 1994.

359. Robboy SJ, Scully RE: Ovarian teratoma with glial implants on the peritoneum. Hum Pathol 1:643–653, 1970.

360. Nogales FF Jr, Favara BE, Major FJ, et al: Immature teratoma of the ovary with a neural component ("solid" teratoma). A clinicopathologic study of 20 cases. Hum Pathol 7:625–642, 1976.

361. Nielsen SNJ, Scheithauer BW, Gaffey TA: Gliomatosis peritonei. Cancer 56:2499–2503, 1985.

362. Gershenson DM, Del Junco G, Silva EG, et al: Immature teratoma of the ovary. Obstet Gynecol 68:624–629, 1986.

363. Koulous JP, Hoffman JS, Steinhoff MM: Immature teratoma of the ovary. Gynecol Oncol 34:46–49, 1989.

364. Kawai M, Kano T, Furuhashi Y, et al: Immature teratoma of the ovary. Gynecol Oncol 40:133–137, 1991.

365. Pantoja E, Noy MA, Axtmayer RW, et al: Ovarian dermoids and their complications. Comprehensive historical review. Obstet Gynecol Surv 30:1–20, 1975.

366. Thurlbeck WM, Scully RE: Solid teratoma of the ovary. A clinicopathological analysis of 9 cases. Cancer 13:804–811, 1960.

367. Blackwell, WJ, Dockerty MB, Masson JC, et al: Dermoid cysts of the ovary. Clinical and pathologic significance. Am J Obstet Gynecol 51:151–172, 1946.

368. Peterson WF: Malignant degeneration of benign cystic teratomas of the ovary. A collective review of the literature. Obstet Gynecol Surv 12:793–830, 1957.

369. Kelley RR, Scully RE: Cancer developing in dermoid cysts of the ovary. A report of 8 cases including a carcinoid and a leiomyosarcoma. Cancer 14:989–1000, 1961.

370. Climie ARW, Heath LP: Malignant degeneration of benign cystic teratomas of the ovary. Review of the literature and report of a chondrosarcoma and carcinoid tumor. Cancer 22:824–832, 1968.

371. Krumerman MS, Chung A: Squamous carcinoma arising in benign cystic teratoma of the ovary. A report of four cases and review of the literature. Cancer 39:1237–1242, 1977.

372. Genadry R, Parmley R, Woodruff JD: Secondary malignancies in benign cystic teratomas. Gynecol Oncol 8:246–251, 1979.

373. Hirakawa T, Tsuneyoshi M, Enjoji M: Squamous cell carcinoma arising in mature cystic teratoma of the ovary. Clinicopathologic and topographic analysis. Am J Surg Pathol 13:397–405, 1989.

374. Woodruff JD, Rauh JT, Markley RI: Ovarian struma. Obstet Gynecol 27:194–201, 1966.

375. Kempers RD, Dockerty MB, Hoffman DL, et al: Struma ovarii—ascitic, hyperthyroid and asymptomatic syndromes. Ann Intern Med 72:883–893, 1970.

376. Hasleton PS, Kelehan P, Whittaker JS, et al: Benign and malignant struma ovarii. Arch Pathol Lab Med 102:180–184, 1978.

377. Pardo-Mindan FJ, Vazquez JJ: Malignant struma ovarii. Light and electron microscopic study. Cancer 51:337–343, 1983.

378. Devaney K, Snyder R, Norris HJ, et al: Proliferative and histologically malignant struma ovarii: a clinicopathologic study of 54 cases. Int J Gynecol Pathol 12:333–343, 1993.

379. Szyfelbein WM, Young RH, Scully RE: Cystic struma ovarii. A frequently unrecognized tumor. A report of 20 cases. Am J Surg Pathol 18:785–788, 1994.

380. Szyfelbein WM, Young RE, Scully RE: Struma ovarii simulating ovarian tumors of other types. A report of 30 cases. Am J Surg Pathol 19:21–29, 1995.

381. Nogales FF, Silverberg SG: Epidermoid cysts of the ovary: a report of five cases with histogenetic considerations and ultrastructural findings. Am J Obstet Gynecol 124:523–528, 1976.

382. Young RH, Prat J, Scully RE: Epidermoid cyst of the ovary. A report of three cases with comments on histogenesis. Am J Clin Pathol 73:272–276, 1980.

383. Robboy SJ, Norris HJ, Scully RE: Insular carcinoid primary in the ovary. A clinicopathologic analysis of 48 cases. Cancer 36:404–418, 1975.

384. Robboy SJ, Scully RE, Norris HJ: Primary trabecular carcinoid of the ovary. Obstet Gynecol 49:202–207, 1977.

385. Talerman A, Evans MI: Primary trabecular carcinoid tumor of the ovary. Cancer 50:1403–1407, 1982.

386. Motoyama T, Katayama Y, Watanabe H, et al: Functioning ovarian carcinoids induced severe constipation. Cancer 70:513–518, 1992.

387. Czernobilsky B, Segal M, Dgani R: Primary ovarian carcinoid with marked heterogeneity of microscopic features. Cancer 54:585–589, 1984.

388. Robboy SJ, Scully RE, Norris HJ: Carcinoid metastatic to ovary. A clinicopathologic analysis of 35 cases. Cancer 33:798–811, 1974.

389. Sporrong B, Falkmer S, Robboy SJ, et al: Neurohormonal peptides in ovarian carcinoids: an immunohistochemical study of 81 primary carcinoids and of intraovarian metastases from six mid-gut carcinoids. Cancer 49:68–74, 1982.

390. Greco MA, LiVolsi VA, Pertschuk LP, et al: Strumal carcinoid of the ovary. Cancer 43:1380–1388, 1979.

391. Robboy SJ, Scully RE: Strumal carcinoid of the ovary: an analysis of 50 cases of a distinctive tumor composed of thyroid tissue and carcinoid. Cancer 46:2019–2034, 1980.

392. Snyder RR, Tavassoli FA: Ovarian strumal carcinoid: immunohistochemical, ultrastructural, and clinicopathologic observations. Int J Gynecol Pathol 5:187–201, 1986.

393. Stagno PA, Petras RE, Hart WR: Strumal carcinoids of the ovary. An immunohistologic and ultrastructural study. Arch Pathol Lab Med 111:440–446, 1987.

394. Alenghat E, Okagaki T, Talerman A: Primary mucinous carcinoid tumor of the ovary. Cancer 58:777–783, 1986.

395. Wolpert HR, Fuller AF, Bell DA: Primary mucinous carcinoid tumor of the ovary. A case report. Int J Gynecol Pathol 8:156–162, 1989.

396. Aguirre P, Scully RE: Malignant neuroectodermal tumor of the ovary, a distinctive form of monodermal teratoma. Report of five cases. Am J Surg Pathol 6:283–292, 1982.

397. Kleinman GM, Young RH, Scully RE: Primary ovarian neuroectodermal tumors. A report of 25 cases. Am J Surg Pathol 17:764–778, 1993.

398. Chumas JC, Scully RE: Sebaceous tumors arising in ovarian dermoid cysts. Int J Gynecol Pathol 10:356–363, 1991.

399. Kurman RJ, Norris HJ: Malignant mixed germ cell tumors of the ovary. A clinical and pathologic analysis of 30 cases. Obstet Gynecol 48:579–589, 1976.

400. Gershenson DM, Del Junco G, Copeland LJ, et al: Mixed germ cell tumors of the ovary. Obstet Gynecol 64:200–206, 1984.

401. Young RH: New and unusual aspects of ovarian germ cell tumors. Am J Surg Pathol 17:1210–1224, 1993.

402. Niehans GA, Manivel JC, Copland GT, et al: Immunohistochemistry of germ cell and trophoblastic neoplasms. Cancer 62:1113–1123, 1988.

403. Pallesen G, Hamilton-Dutoit SJ: Ki-1(CD30) antigen is regularly expressed by tumor cells of embryonal carcinoma. Am J Pathol 133:446–450, 1988.

404. Ferreiro JA: Ber-H2 expression in testicular germ cell tumors. Hum Pathol 25:522–524, 1994.

405. Suster S, Moran CA, Dominguez-Malagnon H, et al: Germ cell tumors of the mediastinum and testis: a comparative immunohistochemical study of 120 cases. Hum Pathol 29:737–742, 1998.

406. Gibas Z, Talerman A: Analysis of chromosome aneuploidy

in ovarian dysgerminoma by flow cytometry and fluorescence in situ hybridization. Diagn Mol Pathol 2:50–56, 1993.

407. Oud PS, Soeters RP, Pahlplatz MMM: DNA cytometry of pure dysgerminomas of the ovary. Int J Gynecol Pathol 7: 258–267, 1988.

408. Ihara T, Ohama K, Satoh H, et al: Histologic grade and karyotype of immature teratoma of the ovary. Cancer 54: 2988–2994, 1984.

409. Scully RE: Gonadoblastoma. A review of 74 cases. Cancer 25: 1340–1356, 1970.

410. Govan ADT, Woodcock AS, Gowing NFC, et al: A clinico-pathological study of gonadoblastoma. Br J Obstet Gynecol 84:222–228, 1977.

411. Hart WE, Burkons DM: Germ cell neoplasms arising in go-nadoblastomas. Cancer 43:669–678, 1979.

412. Talerman A: A distinctive gonadal neoplasm related to go-nadoblastoma. Cancer 30:1219–1224, 1972.

413. Lacson AG, Gillis DA, Shawwa A: Malignant mixed germ cell–sex cord–stromal tumors of the ovary associated with isosexual precocious puberty. Cancer 61:2122–2133, 1988.

414. Dickersin GR, Kline IW, Scully RE: Small cell carcinoma of the ovary with hypercalcemia. A report of eleven cases. Cancer 49:188–197, 1982.

415. Aguirre P, Thor AD, Scully RE: Ovarian small cell carci-noma: histogenetic considerations based on immunohisto-chemical and other findings. Am J Clin Pathol 92:140–149, 1989.

416. Scully RE: Small cell carcinoma of hypercalcemic type. Int J Gynecol Pathol 12:148–152, 1993.

417. Dickersin GR, Scully RE: An update on the electron micros-copy of small cell carcinoma of the ovary with hypercal-cemia. Ultrastruct Pathol 17:411–422, 1993.

418. Young RH, Oliva E, Scully RE: Small cell carcinoma of the ovary, hypercalcemic type. A clinicopathological analysis of 150 cases. Am J Surg Pathol 18:1102–1116, 1994.

419. Eichhorn JH, Bell DA, Young RH, et al: DNA content and proliferative activity in ovarian small cell carcinomas of the hypercalcemic type. Implications for diagnosis, prognosis, and histogenesis. Am J Clin Pathol 98:579–586, 1992.

420. Eichhorn JH, Young RH, Scully RE: Primary ovarian small cell carcinoma of the pulmonary type. A clinicopathologic, immunohistologic, and flow cytometric analysis of 11 cases. Am J Surg Pathol 16:926–938, 1992.

421. Eichorn JH, Young RH, Scully RE: Nonpulmonary small cell carcinomas of extragenital origin metastatic to the ovary. Cancer 71:177–186, 1993.

422. Rutgers JL, Scully RE: Cysts (cystadenomas) and tumors of the rete ovarii. Int J Gynecol Pathol 7:330–342, 1988.

423. Hughesdon PE: Ovarian tumours of wolffian or allied na-ture: their place in ovarian oncology. J Clin Pathol 35:526–535, 1982.

424. Kariminejad MH, Scully RE: Female adnexal tumor of proba-ble wolffian origin. A distinctive pathological entity. Cancer 31:671–677, 1973.

425. Rahilly MA, Williams ARW, Krausz T, et al: Female adnexal tumour of probable wolffian origin. A clinicopathological and immunohistochemical study of three cases. Histopathol-ogy 26:69–74, 1995.

426. Shakfeh SM, Woodruff JD: Primary ovarian sarcomas. Report of 46 cases and review of the literature. Obstet Gynecol Surg 42:331–349, 1987.

427. Kraemer BB, Silva EG, Sniege N: Fibrosarcoma of ovary. A new component in the nevoid basal-cell carcinoma syn-drome. Am J Surg Pathol 8:231–236, 1984.

428. Miles PA, Kiley KC, Mena H: Giant fibrosarcoma of the ovary. Int J Gynecol Pathol 4:83–87, 1985.

429. Anderson B, Turner DA, Benda J: Ovarian sarcoma. Gynecol Oncol 26:183–192, 1987.

430. Fallahzadeh H, Dockerty MB, Lee RA: Leiomyoma of the ovary: report of five cases and review of the literature. Am J Obstet Gynecol 113:394–398, 1972.

431. Matamala MF, Nogales FF, Aneiros J, et al: Leiomyomas of the ovary. Int J Gynecol Pathol 7:190–196, 1988.

432. Kandalaft PL, Esteban JM: Bilateral massive ovarian leiomy-omata in a young woman. A case report with review of the literature. Mod Pathol 5:586–589, 1992.

433. Prayson RA, Hart WR: Primary smooth-muscle tumors of the ovary. A clinicopathologic study of four leiomyomas and two mitotically active leiomyomas. Arch Pathol Lab Med 116:1068–1071, 1992.

434. Friedman HD, Mazur MT: Primary ovarian leiomyosarcoma. An immunohistochemical and ultrastructural study. Arch Pathol Lab Med 115:941–945, 1991.

435. Nogales FF, Ayala A, Ruiz-Avila I, et al: Myxoid leiomyosar-coma of the ovary: analysis of three cases. Hum Pathol 22: 1268–1273, 1991.

436. Eichhorn JH, Scully RE: Ovarian myxoma: clinicopathologic and immunocytologic analysis of five cases and a review of the literature. Int J Gynecol Pathol 10:156–169, 1991.

437. Costa MJ, Thomas W, Majmudar B, et al: Ovarian myxoma: ultrastructural and immunohistochemical findings. Ultra-struct Pathol 16:429–438, 1992.

438. Alvarez M, Cerezo L: Ovarian cavernous hemangioma. Arch Pathol Lab Med 110:77–78, 1986.

439. Guerard MJ, Arguelles MA, Ferenczy A: Rhabdomyosarcoma of the ovary: ultrastructural study of a case and review of the literature. Gynecol Oncol 15:325–339, 1983.

440. Chen YF, Leung CS, Ma L: Primary embryonal rhabdomyo-sarcoma of the ovary in a 4-year-old girl. Histopathology 15: 303–311, 1989.

441. Tsujimura T, Kawano K: Rhabdomyosarcoma coexistent with ovarian mucinous cystadenocarcinoma: a case report. Int J Gynecol Pathol 11:58–62, 1992.

442. Talerman A, Auerbach WM, Van Meurs AJ: Primary chon-drosarcoma of the ovary. Histopathology 5:319–324, 1981.

443. Hirakawa T, Tsuneyoshi M, Enjoji M, et al: Ovarian sarcoma with histologic features of telangiectatic osteosarcoma of bone. Am J Surg Pathol 12:567–572, 1988.

444. Hines JF, Compton DM, Stacy CC, et al: Pure primary osteo-sarcoma of the ovary presenting as an extensively calcified adnexal mass: a case report and review of the literature. Gynecol Oncol 39:259–263, 1990.

445. Ngwalle KE, Hirakawa T, Tsuneyoshi M, et al: Osteosarcoma arising in a benign dermoid cyst of the ovary. Gynecol On-col 37:143–147, 1990.

446. Sakata H, Hirahara T, Ryu A, et al: Primary osteosarcoma of the ovary. A case report. Acta Pathol Jpn 41:311–317, 1991.

447. Ongkasuwan C, Taylor JE, Tang C-K, et al: Angiosarcomas of the uterus and ovary: clinicopathologic report. Cancer 49: 1469–1475, 1982.

448. Stone GC, Bell DA, Fuller A, et al: Malignant schwannoma of the ovary. Report of a case. Cancer 58:1575–1582, 1986.

449. Chorlton I, Norris HJ, King FM: Malignant reticuloendothe-lial disease involving the ovary as a primary manifestation. A series of 19 lymphomas and 1 granulocytic sarcoma. Can-cer 34:397–407, 1974.

450. Rotmensch J, Woodruff JD: Lymphoma of the ovary. Report of twenty new cases and update of previous series. Am J Obstet Gynecol 143:870–875, 1982.

451. Osborne BM, Robboy SJ: Lymphomas or leukemia presenting as ovarian tumors. An analysis of 42 cases. Cancer 52:1933–1943, 1983.

452. Linden MD, Tubbs RR, Fishleder AJ, et al: Immunotypic and genotypic characterization of non-Hodgkin's lymphomas of the ovary. Am J Clin Pathol 89:156–162, 1988.

453. Ferry JA, Young RH: Malignant lymphoma, pseudolym-phoma, and hematopoietic disorders of the female genital tract. Pathol Annu 26(pt 1):227–263, 1991.

454. Monterroso V, Jaffe ES, Merino MJ, et al: Malignant lympho-mas involving the ovary: a clinicopathologic analysis of 39 cases. Am J Surg Pathol 17:154–170, 1993.

455. Young RH, Gersell DJ, Clement PB, et al: Hepatocellular carcinoma metastatic to the ovary: a report of three cases discovered during life with discussion of the differential di-agnosis of hepatoid tumors of the ovary. Hum Pathol 23: 574–580, 1992.

456. Young RH, Silva EG, Scully RE: Ovarian and juxtaovarian adenomatoid tumors: a report of six cases. Int J Gynecol Pathol 10:364–371, 1991.

457. Addis BJ, Fox H: Papillary mesothelioma of ovary. Histopa-thology 7:287–298, 1983.

458. Daya D, McCaughey WTE: Pathology of the peritoneum. A review of selected topics. Semin Diagn Pathol 8:277–289, 1991.

459. Gerald WL, Miller HK, Battifora H, et al: Intra-abdominal desmoplastic small round-cell tumor: report of 19 cases of a distinctive type of polyphenotypic malignancy affecting young individuals. Am J Surg Pathol 15:499–513, 1991.

460. Young RH, Eichhorn JH, Dickersin GR, et al: Ovarian involvement by the intra-abdominal desmoplastic small round cell tumor with divergent differentiation. A report of three cases. Hum Pathol 23:454–464, 1992.

461. Zaloudek C, Miller TR, Stern JL: Desmoplastic small cell tumor of the ovary. A unique polyphenotypic tumor with an unfavorable prognosis. Int J Gynecol Pathol 14:260–265, 1995.

462. Mazur MT, Hsueh S, Gersell DJ: Metastases to the female genital tract. Analysis of 325 cases. Cancer 53:1978–1984, 1984.

463. Young RH, Kozakewich HPW, Scully RE: Metastatic ovarian tumors in children: a report of 14 cases and review of the literature. Int J Gynecol Pathol 12:8–19, 1993.

464. Harcourt KF, Dennis DL: Laparotomy for "ovarian tumors" in unsuspected carcinoma of the colon. Cancer 21:1244–1246, 1968.

465. Scully RE, Richardson GS: Luteinization of the stroma of metastatic cancer involving the ovary and its endocrine significance. Cancer 14:827–840, 1961.

466. Woodruff JD, Novak ER: The Krukenberg tumor. Study of 48 cases from the Ovarian Tumor Registry. Obstet Gynecol 15:351–360, 1960.

467. Hale RW: Krukenberg tumor of the ovaries. A review of 81 records. Obstet Gynecol 32:221–225, 1968.

468. Wong PC, Ferenczy A, Fan L-D, et al: Krukenberg tumors of the ovary. Ultrastructural, histochemical, and immunohistochemical studies of 15 cases. Cancer 57:751–760, 1986.

469. Joshi VV: Primary Krukenberg tumor of ovary. Review of literature and case report. Cancer 22:1199–1207, 1968.

470. Bullon A Jr, Arseneau J, Prat J, et al: Tubular Krukenberg tumor. A problem in histopathologic diagnosis. Am J Surg Pathol 5:225–232, 1981.

471. Gagnon Y, Tetu B: Ovarian metastases of breast carcinoma. A clinicopathologic study of 59 cases. Cancer 64:892–898, 1989.

472. Young RH, Carey RW, Robboy SJ: Breast carcinoma masquerading as a primary ovarian neoplasm. Cancer 48:210–212, 1981.

473. Harris M, Howell A, Chrissohou M, et al: A comparison of the metastatic pattern of infiltrating lobular carcinoma and infiltrating duct carcinoma of the breast. Br J Cancer 50:23–30, 1984.

474. Monteagudo C, Merino MJ, LaPorte N, et al: Value of gross cystic disease fluid protein-15 in distinguishing metastatic breast carcinomas among poorly differentiated neoplasms involving the ovary. Hum Pathol 22:368–373, 1991.

475. Bunker ML: The terminal findings in endometrial carcinoma. Am J Obstet Gynecol 77:530–538, 1959.

476. Beck RP, Latour JPA: Necropsy reports on 36 cases of endometrial carcinoma. Am J Obstet Gynecol 77:530–538, 1963.

477. Young RH, Gersell DJ, Roth LM, et al: Ovarian metastases from cervical carcinomas other than pure adenocarcinomas. A report of twelve cases. Cancer 71:407–418, 1993.

478. Young RH, Scully RE: Ovarian metastases from cancer of the lung: problems in interpretation—a report of seven cases. Gynecol Oncol 21:337–350, 1985.

479. Fitzgibbons PL, Martin SE, Simmons TJ: Malignant melanoma metastatic to the ovary. Am J Surg Pathol 11:959–964, 1987.

480. Young RH, Scully RE: Malignant melanoma metastatic to the ovary: a clinicopathologic analysis of 20 cases. Am J Surg Pathol 15:849–860, 1991.

481. Robboy SJ, Bernhardt PF, Parmley T: Embryology of the female genital tract and disorders of abnormal sexual development. *In* Kurman RJ (ed): Blaustein's Pathology of the Female Genital Tract. 4th ed. New York, Springer-Verlag, 1994, pp 3–29.

482. Dare FO, Makinde OO, Makinde ON, et al: Congenital absence of an ovary in a Nigerian woman. Int J Gynecol Obstet 29:377–378, 1989.

483. Cruikshank SH, Van Drie DM: Supernumerary ovaries: update and review. Obstet Gynecol 60:126–129, 1982.

484. Lachman MF, Berman MM: The ectopic ovary: a case report and review of the literature. Arch Pathol Lab Med 115:233–235, 1991.

485. Symonds DA, Driscoll SG: An adrenal cortical rest within the fetal ovary: report of a case. Am J Clin Pathol 60:562–564, 1973.

486. Meneses MF, Ostrowski ML: Female splenic-gonadal fusion. Hum Pathol 20:486–488, 1989.

487. Rahilly MA, Al-Nafussi A: Uterus-like mass of the ovary associated with endometrioid carcinoma. Histopathology 18:549–551, 1991.

488. McCormack WM: Pelvic inflammatory disease. N Engl J Med 330:115–119, 1994.

489. Landers DV, Sweet RL: Current trends in the diagnosis and treatment of tuboovarian abscess. Am J Obstet Gynecol 151:1098–1110, 1985.

490. Bhagavan BS, Gupta PK: Genital actinomycosis and intrauterine contraceptive devices. Hum Pathol 9:567–578, 1978.

491. Schmidt WA: IUDs, inflammation, and infection: assessment after two decades of IUD use. Hum Pathol 13:878–881, 1982.

492. Pace EH, Voet RL, Melancon JT: Xanthogranulomatous oophoritis: an inflammatory pseudotumor of the ovary. Int J Gynecol Pathol 3:398–402, 1984.

493. Klempner LB, Giglio PG, Niebles A: Malacoplakia of the ovary. Obstet Gynecol 69:537–540, 1987.

494. Willson JB, Black JR III: Ovarian abscess. Am J Obstet Gynecol 90:34–43, 1964.

495. Wetchler SJ, Dunn LJ: Ovarian abscess. Report of a case and review of the literature. Obstet Gynecol Surv 40:476–485, 1985.

496. Nogales-Ortiz F, Taracon I, Nogales FF: The pathology of female genital tract tuberculosis. Obstet Gynecol 53:422–428, 1979.

497. Subietas A, Deppisch LM, Astarloa J: Cytomegalovirus oophoritis: ovarian cortical necrosis. Hum Pathol 8:285–292, 1977.

498. Williams DJ, Connor P, Ironside JW: Pre-menopausal cytomegalovirus oophoritis. Histopathology 16:405–407, 1990.

499. Nissin F, Ashkenazy M, Borenstein R, et al: Tuberculoid cornstarch granulomas with caseous necrosis. A diagnostic challenge. Arch Pathol Lab Med 105:86–88, 1981.

500. Herbold DR, Frable WJ, Kraus FT: Isolated noninfectious granuloma of the ovary. Int J Gynecol Pathol 2:380–391, 1984.

501. Kernohan NM, Best PV, Jandial V, et al: Palisading granuloma of the ovary. Histopathology 19:279–280, 1991.

502. Mostofa SAM, Bargeron CB, Flower RW, et al: Foreign body granulomas in normal ovaries. Obstet Gynecol 66:701–702, 1985.

503. Kim KR, Scully RE: Peritoneal keratin granulomas with carcinomas of endometrium and ovary and atypical polypoid adenomyoma of endometrium. A clinicopathological analysis of 22 cases. Am J Surg Pathol 14:925–932, 1990.

504. Gilks CB, Clement PB: Colo-ovarian fistula. A report of two cases. Obstet Gynecol 69:533–537, 1987.

505. Chalvardjian A: Sarcoidosis of the female genital tract. Am J Obstet Gynecol 132:78–80, 1978.

506. Wlodarski FM, Trainer TD: Granulomatous oophoritis and salpingitis associated with Crohn's disease of the appendix. Am J Obstet Gynecol 122:527–528, 1975.

507. Brady K, Yavner DL, Glantz C, et al: Crohn's disease presenting as a tubo-ovarian abscess. A case report. J Reprod Med 33:928–930, 1988.

508. Gloor E, Hurlimann J: Autoimmune oophoritis. Am J Clin Pathol 81:105–109, 1984.

509. Apler MM, Garner PR: Premature ovarian failure: its relationship to autoimmune disease. Obstet Gynecol 66:27–30, 1985.

510. Damewood MD, Zacur HA, Hoffmann GJ, et al: Circulating antiovarian antibodies in premature ovarian failure. Obstet Gynecol 68:850–854, 1986.

511. Sedmak DD, Hart WR, Tubbs RR: Autoimmune oophoritis: a histopathologic study of involved ovaries with immunologic characterization of the mononuclear cell infiltrate. Int J Gynecol Pathol 6:73–81, 1987.

512. Bannatyne P, Russell P, Shearman RP: Autoimmune oophoritis: a clinicopathologic assessment of 12 cases. Int J Gynecol Pathol 9:191–207, 1990.

513. Mulligan RM: A survey of epithelial inclusions in the ovarian cortex of 470 patients. J Surg Oncol 8:61–66, 1976.

514. Blaustein A, Kantius M, Kaganowicz A, et al: Inclusions in ovaries of females aged day 1–30 years. Int J Gynecol Pathol 1:145–153, 1982.

515. Scully RE: Ovary. In Henson DE, Albores-Saavedra J (eds): The Pathology of Incipient Neoplasia. Philadelphia, WB Saunders, 1986, pp 279–293.

516. Mittal KR, Zeleniuch-Jacquotte A, Cooper JL, et al: Contralateral ovary in unilateral ovarian carcinoma: a search for preneoplastic lesions. Int J Gynecol Pathol 12:59–63, 1993.

517. Meizner I, Levy A, Katz M, et al: Fetal ovarian cysts: prenatal ultrasonographic detection and postnatal evaluation and treatment. Am J Obstet Gynecol 164:874–878, 1991.

518. Towne BH, Mahour GH, Woolley MM, et al: Ovarian cysts and tumors in infancy and childhood. J Pediatr Surg 10:311–320, 1975.

519. Kosloske AM, Goldthorn JF, Kaufman E, et al: Treatment of precocious pseudopuberty associated with follicular cysts of the ovary. Am J Dis Child 138:147–149, 1984.

520. Piver MS, Williams LJ, Marcuse PM: Influence of luteal cysts on menstrual function. Obstet Gynecol 35:740–751, 1970.

521. Strickler RC, Kelly RW, Askin FB: Postmenopausal ovarian follicle cyst: an unusual case of estrogen excess. Int J Gynecol Pathol 3:318–322, 1984.

522. Hallatt JG, Steele CH Jr, Snyder M: Ruptured corpus luteum with hemoperitoneum: a study of 173 surgical cases. Am J Obstet Gynecol 149:5–9, 1984.

523. McKenna TJ: Pathogenesis and treatment of polycystic ovarian syndrome. N Engl J Med 318:558–562, 1988.

524. Insler V, Lunenfeld B: Pathophysiology of polycystic ovarian disease. New insights. Hum Reprod 6:1025–1029, 1991.

525. Frank S: Polycystic ovarian syndrome. N Engl J Med 333:853–861, 1995.

526. Homburg R: Polycystic ovary syndrome—from gynaecological curiosity to multisystem endocrinopathy. Hum Reprod 11:29–39, 1996.

527. Futterweit W: Polycystic Ovarian Disease. Clinical Perspectives in Obstetrics and Gynecology. New York, Springer-Verlag, 1985.

528. Fechner RE, Kaufman RH: Endometrial adenocarcinoma in Stein-Leventhal syndrome. Cancer 34:444–452, 1974.

529. Smyczek-Gargya B, Geppert M: Endometrial cancer associated with polycystic ovaries in young women. Pathol Res Pract 188:946–948, 1992.

530. Green JA, Goldzieher JW: The polycystic ovary. IV. Light and electron microscope studies. Am J Obstet Gynecol 91:173–181, 1965.

531. Hughesdon PE: Morphology and morphogenesis of the Stein-Leventhal ovary and of so-called "hyperthecosis." Obstet Gynecol Surv 37:59–77, 1982.

532. Clement PB: Pathology of endometriosis. Pathol Annu 25:245–295, 1990.

533. Olive DL, Schwartz LB: Endometriosis. N Engl J Med 328:1759–1769, 1993.

534. Czernobilsky B, Morris WJ: A histologic study of ovarian endometriosis with emphasis on hyperplastic and atypical changes. Obstet Gynecol 53:318–323, 1979.

535. Ballouk F, Ross JS, Wolf BC: Ovarian endometriotic cysts. An analysis of cytologic atypia and DNA ploidy patterns. Am J Clin Pathol 102:415–419, 1994.

536. Mostoufizadeh M, Scully RE: Malignant tumors arising in endometriosis. Clin Obstet Gynecol 23:951–963, 1980.

537. La Grenade A, Silverberg SG: Ovarian tumors associated with atypical endometriosis. Hum Pathol 19:1080–1084, 1988.

538. Genadry R, Parmley T, Woodruff JD: The origin and clinical behavior of the parovarian tumor. Am J Obstet Gynecol 129:873–880, 1977.

539. Samaha M, Woodruff JD: Paratubal cysts: frequency, histogenesis, and associated clinical features. Obstet Gynecol 65:691–693, 1985.

540. Clement PB: Tumor-like lesions of the ovary associated with pregnancy. Int J Gynecol Pathol 12:108–115, 1993.

541. Clement PB, Scully RE: Large solitary luteinized follicle cyst of pregnancy and puerperium. A clinicopathologic analysis of eight cases. Am J Surg Pathol 4:431–438, 1980.

542. Caspi E, Schreyer P, Bukovsky J: Ovarian lutein cysts in pregnancy. Obstet Gynecol 42:388–398, 1973.

543. Wajda KJ, Lucas JG, Marsh WL Jr: Hyperreactio luteinalis. Benign disorder masquerading as an ovarian neoplasm. Arch Pathol Lab Med 113:921–925, 1989.

544. Sternberg WH, Barclay DL: Luteoma of pregnancy. Am J Obstet Gynecol 95:165–181, 1966.

545. Norris HJ, Taylor HB: Nodular theca-lutein hyperplasia of pregnancy (so-called "pregnancy luteoma"). A clinical and pathologic study of 15 cases. Am J Clin Pathol 47:557–566, 1967.

546. Clement PB, Young RH, Scully RE: Ovarian granulosa cell proliferations of pregnancy. A report of nine cases. Hum Pathol 19:657–662, 1988.

547. Grimes HG, Nosal RA, Gallagher JC: Ovarian pregnancy: a series of 24 cases. Obstet Gynecol 61:174–180, 1983.

548. Stearns HC, Sneeden VD, Fearl JD: A clinical and pathologic review of ovarian stromal hyperplasia and its possible relationship to common diseases of the female reproductive system. Am J Obstet Gynecol 119:375–381, 1974.

549. Sasano H, Fukunaga M, Rojas M, et al: Hyperthecosis of the ovary. Clinicopathologic study of 19 cases with immunohistochemical analysis of steroidogenic enzymes. Int J Gynecol Pathol 8:311–320, 1989.

550. Roth LM, Deaton RL, Sternberg WH: Massive ovarian edema. A clinicopathologic study of five cases including ultrastructural observations and review of the literature. Am J Surg Pathol 3:11–21, 1979.

551. Young RH, Scully RE: Fibromatosis and massive edema of the ovary, possibly related entities: a report of 14 cases of fibromatosis and 11 cases of massive edema. Int J Gynecol Pathol 3:153–178, 1984.

552. Clement PB, Young RH: Florid mesothelial hyperplasia associated with ovarian tumors: a potential source of error in tumor diagnosis and staging. Int J Gynecol Pathol 12:51–58, 1993.

553. Sternberg WH: The morphology, androgenic function, hyperplasia, and tumours of the human ovarian hilus cells. Am J Pathol 25:493–521, 1949.

554. Rewell RE: Extra-uterine decidua. J Pathol 105:219–222, 1972.

555. Bersch W, Alexy E, Heuser HP, et al: Ectopic decidua formation in the ovary (so-called deciduoma). Virchows Arch A Pathol Anat Histopathol 360:173–177, 1973.

556. Honore LH, O'Hara KE: Subcapsular adipocytic infiltration of the human ovary: a clinicopathological study of eight cases. Eur J Obstet Gynaecol Reprod Biol 10:13–20, 1980.

557. Shipton EA, Meares SD: Heterotopic bone formation in the ovary. Aust N Z J Obstet Gynaecol 5:100–102, 1965.

558. Young RH, Scully RE: Ovarian pathology of infertility. In Kraus FT, Damjanov I, Kaufman N (eds): Pathology of Reproductive Failure. Monographs in Pathology No. 33. Baltimore, Williams & Wilkins, 1991, pp 104–139.

559. Koninck PR, Brosens IA: The "gonadotropin-resistant ovary" syndrome as a cause of secondary amenorrhea and infertility. Fertil Steril 28:926–931, 1977.

560. Russell P, Bannatyne P, Sherman RP, et al: Premature hypergonadotropic ovarian failure: Clinicopathological study of 19 cases. Int J Gynecol Pathol 1:185–201, 1982.

561. Aiman J, Smentek C: Premature ovarian failure. Obstet Gynecol 66:9–14, 1985.

562. Steele SJ, Beilby JOW, Papadaki L: Visualization and biopsy of the ovary in the investigation of amenorrhea. Obstet Gynecol 36:899–902, 1970.

563. Stevenson CS: The ovaries in infertile women. A clinical and pathologic study of 81 women having ovarian surgery at laparotomy. Fertil Steril 21:411–425, 1970.

# 40

# *Gestational Pathology*

Cynthia G. Kaplan

Examination of gestational material is a common and important function of surgical pathology in any hospital in which obstetric deliveries and care of women and newborns occur. These specimens range from scant endometrial tissue obtained by curettage in spontaneous abortion to well-developed placentas and include samples for the evaluation of trophoblastic disease and the miniautopsies of midtrimester losses. Unfortunately, gestational specimens are often somewhat neglected in a busy surgical pathology laboratory. Frozen sections are infrequent, and there is often little rush for results. This does not imply, however, that the evaluation of pregnancy-related specimens should be less thorough. Many pregnancies are highly valued because infertility and late childbearing are common. A wealth of information can be gleaned from gestational tissue, usually far beyond what is typically reported. There are often clinical implications.[1-7] Gross evaluation and proper choice of material for histologic examination are particularly important in gestational pathology. Many important diagnoses are made entirely by gross examination, and a few well-chosen histologic sections are all that is necessary for microscopic evaluation.

## SPECIMEN HANDLING

### Placenta

Traditionally, not every placenta has been routinely examined in surgical pathology; whether the placenta is submitted is at the discretion of the obstetrician. With the recognition of the wealth of information that can be gleaned relating to perinatal disease and medicolegal complications, many more placentas are being seen in the pathology laboratory (Table 40–1). It is neither necessary nor practical to perform a microscopic examination on every placenta.

**TABLE 40–1.** Common Placental Changes in Clinical Situations

*Prematurity*
Ascending infection
Villus ischemic change
Retroplacental hemorrhage
Circumvallation
Marginal hemorrhage
Shape abnormalities
Hydrops
Decidual vascular disease
Chronic villitis of unknown etiology

*Growth Retardation*
Villus ischemic change or infarcts
Maternal vascular disease
Chronic villitis of unknown etiology
Hematogenous infection
Dysmaturity
Single umbilical artery
Velamentous cord insertion

*Stillbirth*
Villus ischemic change or infarcts
Retroplacental hemorrhage
Cord occlusion, hemorrhage
Hematogenous infection
Ascending infection, severe
Massive intervillous fibrin, maternal floor infarction
Fetal vascular thrombosis
Chronic villitis of unknown etiology
Hydrops
Dysmaturity

*Bleeding*
Retroplacental hemorrhage
Marginal hemorrhage
Circumvallation
Ascending infection
Retromembranous hemorrhage
Marginal previa
Ruptured velamentous vessel

Every institution needs to establish a clear protocol and set of indications for placental triage (Fig. 40–1). The College of American Pathologists' guideline[8] provides information that can be modified according to institutional needs (Table 40–2). Nearly all potential legal cases will be included if similar guidelines are followed. Education of the pathology and obstetric staff is necessary in the implementation of such a plan.

Gross examination of the placenta is extremely important because it is a guide for histologic sectioning and a clue to microscopic lesions.[9, 10] The examination includes evaluation of the cord, membranes, fetal surface, maternal surface, and villus parenchyma. Histologic sampling includes these regions and several regions of the most grossly normal villus tissue. This examination should be carefully documented and include certain features (Table 40–3). Gross aspects of the placenta are available only from the report. Photography of unusual or extensive lesions is useful. Methods of placental examination have varied widely among pathologists.[11]

## Spontaneous Abortion

Spontaneous pregnancy loss is common. At least one in seven recognized pregnancies is affected, which makes "products of conception" one of the most frequent specimens in pathology laboratories.[12–14] These specimens are also variable, ranging from blood clot with scant fragments of tissue to intact sacs, placentas, and fetuses. More complete and well-preserved specimens obviously lend themselves to more detailed evaluation. Such specimens are examined to determine whether there is evidence of intrauterine pregnancy, to identify the cause of recurrent loss, to identify specific syndromes, and to predict malignant potential. Much parental guilt may be relieved because the parents can usually be reassured that a particular event in their lives did not cause the loss of the pregnancy.

Ideally, the specimen is received fresh so that material for special procedures can be obtained, if desired. The fresh state also makes it simpler to choose appropriate material for histologic sampling and to separate the loose, often abundant blood clot from tissue. Finding an embryo, gestational sac fragments, villi, or implantation site is generally considered diagnostic of intrauterine pregnancy and should be documented.[3, 15] Histologic sectioning of large amounts of loose soft clot is rarely rewarding

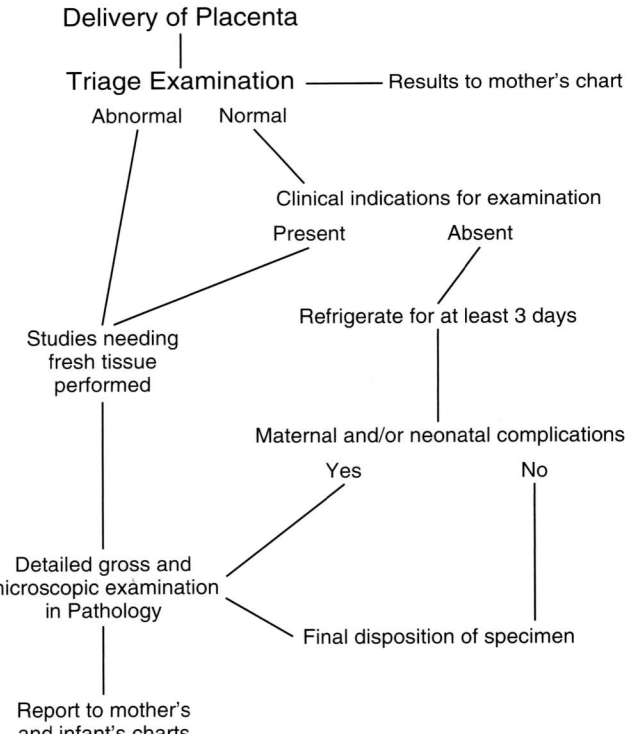

**FIGURE 40–1.** Placental triage scheme. (Adapted from Langston C, Kaplan C, Macpherson T, et al: Practice guideline for the examination of the placenta: developed by the Placental Pathology Practice Guideline Development Task Force of the College of American Pathologists. Arch Pathol Lab Med 121:449–476, 1997.)

**TABLE 40–2.** Indications for Examination of the Placenta

| Maternal Indications | |
|---|---|
| *Recommended* | *Other* |
| Systemic disorders with clinical concerns for the mother or infant | Premature delivery from 35–37 wk gestation |
| Premature delivery <35 wk | Severe, unexplained polyhydramnios |
| Peripartum fever or infection | History of substance abuse |
| Unexplained third trimester or excessive bleeding | Gestational age >41 wk |
| Clinical concern for infection during the pregnancy | Severe maternal trauma |
| Severe oligohydramnios | Prolonged (>24 h) rupture of membranes |
| Unexplained or recurrent pregnancy complications | |
| Invasive procedures with suspected placental injury | |
| Abruption | |
| Nonelective pregnancy termination | |
| Thick or viscid meconium | |

| Fetal and Neonatal Indications | |
|---|---|
| *Recommended* | *Other* |
| Admission or transfer to other than a level 1 nursery | Birth weight >95th percentile |
| Stillborn or perinatal death | Asymmetric growth |
| Hydrops fetalis | Multiple gestation without other indications |
| Compromised clinical condition (cord pH <7, Apgar score <7 at 5 min, ventilatory assistance >10 min, hematocrit <35%) | Vanishing twin beyond first trimester |
| Birth weight <10th percentile | |
| Seizures | |
| Infection or sepsis | |
| Major congenital anomalies, dysmorphic phenotype, or abnormal karyotype | |
| Discordant twin growth (>20% weight difference) | |
| Multiple gestation with same-sex infants, fused placentas | |

| Placental Indications | |
|---|---|
| *Recommended* | *Other* |
| Physical abnormality (e.g., mass, vascular thrombosis, abnormal color, retro-placental hematoma, malodor, extensive infarction) | Abnormalities of placental shape |
| Small or large placental size for gestational age | Long cord (>100 cm) |
| Umbilical cord lesions (e.g., thrombosis, torsion, true knot, single artery) | Marginal or velamentous cord insertion |
| Total umbilical cord length <32 cm at term | |

Adapted from Langston C, Kaplan C, Macpherson T, et al: Practice guideline for the examination of the placenta: developed by the Placental Pathology Practice Guideline Development Task Force of the College of American Pathologists. Arch Pathol Lab Med 121:449–476, 1997.

in finding evidence of intrauterine gestation; however, granular degenerating blood clot often contains villi or an implantation site. Intact gestational sacs are not uncommon, particularly in spontaneously passed material. They may be encased in firmer blood clot or within a decidual cast (Fig. 40–2). In general, nonfetal tissue is more abundant than fetal tissue. Villus tissue is finely papillary and often held together by a smooth, shiny membrane constituting the remnants of the gestational sac. Both intrauterine and ectopic pregnancies often contain sheets of decidua and endometrial tissue. These tend to be smooth on one side and slightly undulating on the other but never with the sheen of fetal membranes (CD Fig. 40–1). Such tissues rarely contain an implantation site. Examining the specimen under the dissecting microscope or by suspension in saline may help identify villus tissue (CD Fig. 40–2).

Even in these times of cost containment, histologic examination has been found to be a necessary part of evaluation of the products of conception because errors in gross evaluation are made even by careful, experienced observers.[16] Specimens containing only the implantation site cannot be identified by gross examination. The number of histologic cassettes required varies with the specimen. If an obvious sac, embryo, or part of an embryo is present, documentation of pregnancy requires only one block. More information about the potential cause is obtained if decidual tissue is submitted to help look for extraembryonic causes of pregnancy loss. Evaluation of the embryo is useful[17–20]; however, it is often disrupted or disintegrated, leaving only the placental tissues. Maceration and procedural disruption of fetuses in later demise diminish their utility as well.

**TABLE 40–3. Contents of the Final Report: Placenta**

**Gross**

The following placental aspects should be observed as part of the examination. Items in *italics* should always be included in the gross report. Others are included if present and/or abnormal.

*Umbilical cord: length, diameter,* twist, *insertion,* velamentous vessels (intactness)
Site of membrane rupture
*Type of membrane insertion*
Subchorionic fibrin
*Coloration and other membrane or surface abnormalities*
*Trimmed weight (without cord, membranes, soft clot)*
*Dimensions of disk*
Abnormalities of shape including succenturiate lobes
*Intactness of maternal surface*
*Color and consistency of villus tissue*
Retroplacental and retromembranous hemorrhage
Presence of infarcts, thromboses, abnormal fibrin deposition
Calcification

**Microscopic**

The placenta should be evaluated in a systematic manner including observation of the following. Microscopic description, if performed, includes maturation, inflammation, and other significant deviations from normal.

Umbilical cord: vessel number and remnants, inflammation, thrombosis, muscle necrosis, pigmented macrophages, Wharton jelly
Membranes: inflammation, pigments, amniotic changes
Fetal surface: vessels and membranes as above
Decidua (membranes and base of placenta): inflammation, vessel changes, necrosis, thrombosis
Villus tissue: maturation, inflammation
Intervillous processes

**Diagnoses**

The only placentas diagnosed as "no pathologic diagnosis" are those at term without other findings. Preterm gestationally appropriate development is noted. Other significant findings are noted. It is often helpful to separate diagnoses into the following:

Placenta
Fetal membranes
Umbilical cord

## Special Procedures

Cytogenetic abnormalities occur in about 50% of early spontaneous abortions, and submission of material for karyotyping is occasionally indicated.[13] With macerated fetuses and embryos, it is the placental villus tissue that most readily grows in tissue culture. It is usually representative of the fetus or embryo. If the specimen is maintained fresh and refrigerated, villus tissue cultures can be established even a week after the specimen was passed. If cytogenetic analysis is desired, a piece of the sac or other villi should be sent in an attempt to eliminate maternal tissue. For specimens with grossly hydropic villi (CD Fig. 40–3), flow cytometry for DNA ploidy is most easily performed on fresh specimens.[21] Fluorescent in situ hybridization offers an alternative means of cytogenetic evaluation, particularly when one suspects certain lesions. Tissue may also be saved frozen for potential DNA analysis, particularly in unusual or undefined cases. New immunologic and in situ hybridization techniques that can be used on fixed tissue are particularly helpful with unexpected findings.[19, 22–25] Cultures, electron microscopy, and other procedures may be important in selected cases.

## BASIC PLACENTAL AND VILLOUS DEVELOPMENT

The villus tissue undergoes remarkable change during the course of gestation, and all pathologic processes need to be evaluated in that context and with experience in normal development.[5, 26–28] Early key features are villus vascularization and percentage of nucleated red blood cells. Villus size, trophoblastic pattern, and vascular distribution are more useful later in gestation.

The principal component of the placenta is the

## Trophoblastic Disease

Specimens from suspected trophoblastic disease most commonly come from the evacuation of an ultrasonically diagnosed mole. These are evaluated similarly to typical spontaneous abortion specimens, with ample sectioning and cytogenetic analysis or flow cytometry.[21] One should carefully look for an embryo or fetus and cord or membranes; these usually preclude the diagnosis of complete hydatidiform mole.[22] The nonvillus tissue will show the implantation site abnormalities. Occasional specimens are re-evacuations with a prior diagnosis. These should be amply sectioned to look for villus tissue and occasionally myometrial changes.

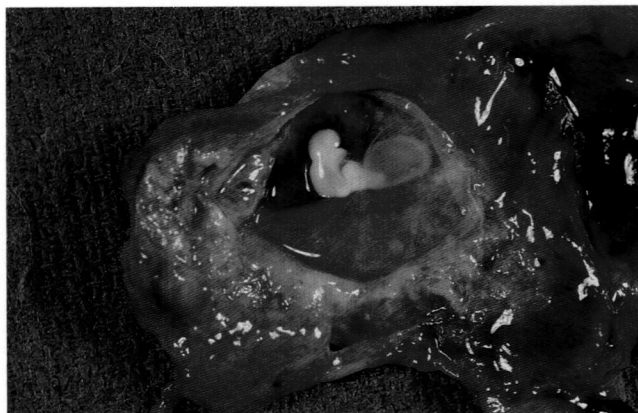

**FIGURE 40–2.** Intact gestational sac found within a mass of hemorrhage in a spontaneous abortion. The sac has been opened to reveal the macerated embryo and yolk sac inside.

**TABLE 40–4.** Characteristics of Trophoblastic Cells

| Cell Type | Predominant Site | Role | Histologic Characteristics | Hormone Production* | Keratin Staining |
|---|---|---|---|---|---|
| Cytotrophoblast | Villous (central) | Generation of cells for syncytium | Uninucleated Clear cytoplasm | None | + |
| Syncytiotrophoblast | Villous (peripheral) | Maternal-fetal exchange, hormone production | Multinucleated Irregular shape Dense cytoplasm Small, dark nuclei | HCG | + |
| Intermediate trophoblast | Extravillous | Invasion of implantation site, maternal vessels | Uninucleated or multinucleated Polygonal Amphophilic cytoplasm Enmeshed in fibrin | HPL Some HCG | + |

* HCG, Human chorionic gonadotropin; HPL, human placental lactogen.

trophoblast (Table 40–4). This is the earliest cell to differentiate in the morula at 4 to 5 days after fertilization. Implantation occurs at 5 to 6 days, and the blastocyst becomes totally surrounded by endometrium (interstitial). Endometrial stroma throughout the uterus undergoes decidual changes. Decidua between the blastocyst and myometrium is decidua basalis, that covering the surface defect is decidua capsularis, and that lining the rest of the uterus is decidua parietalis (vera) (CD Fig. 40–4).

The fetal-maternal circulation is initiated at about 9 days with formation of lacunae in the syncytiotrophoblast. Intermediate trophoblast invades maternal vessels, destroying muscle and elastica—physiologic change (CD Fig. 40–5). In the second trimester, there is a second wave of trophoblastic invasion into the myometrial segments of vessels. Placental villus tissue is not normally present in the myometrium. A layer of decidual tissue separates the anchoring villi from muscle. Lacunae in the syncytium link with eroded maternal vessels by days 12 to 13. Primary villi are cores of cytotrophoblast covered by syncytium (14 days). Avascular extraembryonic mesenchyme from the embryonic body stalk invades, forming secondary villi (15 days). Capillaries form within the villi, coalesce, and connect to the fetus by the vessels differentiating from the inner chorion and the embryonic body stalk. The establishment of the capillary network forms tertiary villi by the third developmental week. The umbilical cord forms in the region of the body stalk where the embryo is attached to the chorion. This area contains the allantois, evolving umbilical vessels, omphalomesenteric duct, and vitelline vessels. The expanding amnion surrounds these, covering the umbilical cord. Most of the embryonic structures and the right umbilical vein eventually disappear, leaving two arteries and one vein.

Red blood cells are first derived from the yolk sac. These are all nucleated (CD Fig. 40–6). As the liver and other mesenchymal tissues in the embryo begin to take over erythropoiesis in the fifth week (seventh menstrual week), non-nucleated red blood cells appear. One can estimate gestational age by the percentage of nucleated red blood cells until 12 menstrual weeks (Table 40–5). At this time, essentially all red blood cells are non-nucleated.[29]

As the placenta grows, the villi branch. Primary stem villi divide, forming secondary and tertiary stem villi, all of which contain collagen and muscularized vessels. Each primary stem forms a fetal lobule, supplied by a branch of a fetal surface vessel. There is no fetal cross-circulation between villus districts. In situ, most villi float free in the intervillous space supplied by blood injected from maternal spiral arterioles into the center of the lobules. The villi at the base of the placenta, anchoring villi, retain large cords of cytotrophoblast capped by syncytiotrophoblast. The peripheral syncytiotrophoblast degenerates and is replaced by fibrin (Nitabuch layer). Implantation generally occurs in the upper part of the uterus and protrudes into the endometrial cavity as the conceptus grows. The entire gestational sac is initially covered by chorionic villi; however, as it enlarges, the surface thins, forming the placental membranes composed of decidua capsularis, atrophied chorion, and amnion. The definitive placenta

**TABLE 40–5.** Correlation of Gestational Age and Percentage of Nucleated Red Blood Cells

| Gestational Age (d) | Estimated Percentage of Nucleated Red Blood Cells |
|---|---|
| 48 | 97 |
| 53 | 75 |
| 59 | 58 |
| 63 | 42 |
| 69 | 28 |
| 71 | 18 |
| 76 | 10 |
| 78 | 4 |
| 81 | 1 |

Adapted from Salafia CM, Weigl CA, Foye GJ: Correlation of placental erythrocyte morphology and gestational age. Pediatr Pathol 8: 495–502, 1988.

is left at the base. Eventually there is apposition of the membranes to the decidua vera of the opposite uterine wall, but no true fusion.

The general gross morphologic features of the placenta are established by the end of the first trimester. Further change is predominantly growth and histologic maturation of villi. Villus maturation entails several features. Villus size and stromal content diminish, with an increased percentage of the area occupied by blood vessels. Syncytiotrophoblast nuclei become aggregated into "knots" and their cytoplasm thins in areas, forming vasculosyncytial membranes (CD Figs. 40–7 and 40–8). The initially prominent cytotrophoblastic layer becomes difficult to see with light microscopy by term but is still detectable with electron microscopy.

## LESIONS OF THE UMBILICAL CORD (EXCLUDING INFECTION AND MECONIUM)

### Vessels and Remnants

The umbilical cord normally contains three blood vessels—two arteries and the persisting left umbilical vein. Absence of one umbilical artery occurs in about 1% of deliveries (CD Fig. 40–9). In 95% of placentas, the two arteries fuse or connect in the last few centimeters above the fetal surface,[30] and the absence of one artery should be confirmed at several points. About 20% of infants missing one artery have other major congenital anomalies, involving any organ system. Abnormalities are generally apparent in the neonatal period, except for an increase in inguinal hernias. "Nonmalformed infants" with absence of one umbilical artery may be slightly small and have increased perinatal mortality.[29] Cord accidents have been frequent in this group.[31]

Remnants of the allantois are common in the cord, particularly near the fetal end. These are usually located between the arteries and show a transitional-type epithelium (CD Fig. 40–10). Omphalomesenteric remnants may be ductal (gastrointestinal epithelium) or vascular. Vascular remnants can be single or multiple and have no muscular wall (CD Figs. 40–11 and 40–12).

### Length, Twist, and Thrombosis

An obvious feature of the umbilical cord is its length. Cord length increases throughout gestation, but growth slows in the third trimester.[2, 5] Both abnormally long and short cords have significant clinical correlates. Fetal activity apparently increases cord length, and long cords (>70 cm) are associated with knots and fetal entanglements. It is not clear whether entanglements occur because the cord is long or whether length increases owing to traction

when entanglement occurs. Long cords may be associated with later hyperactivity.[2] Most knots and entanglements are not associated with problems, but they do occasionally cause fetal distress and death. The presence of differential congestion or thrombosis suggests that an obstruction was functionally significant (Fig. 40–3). The vein is more readily compressed, leading to congestion on the placental side. One should be cautious in attributing death to a cord problem and rule out other causes.

Short cords occur in disorders with poor fetal movement (oligohydramnios, arthrogryposis). They have been associated with subsequent poor neurologic development, which could be due to in utero problems that compromise fetal mobility. A minimal cord length of 32 cm is thought to be necessary for normal vaginal delivery. Undue traction potentially causes fetal distress, cord tearing, and possibly abruption.[30] Despite the importance of an accurate cord length, the pathologist is at a disadvantage in this because the amount of cord left on the infant or taken for analysis of cord gases is often unknown. Measuring the umbilical cord length is ideally done in the delivery room.[8, 10]

The umbilical cord usually twists counterclockwise (CD Fig. 40–13). The number of helixes is variable, averaging 11. These are well developed by 11 weeks of gestation. The etiology of this is unclear. Adverse perinatal outcome with cords that lack twisting or that have abnormal twisting is not established. Some cords show excessive twisting, and this is at times apparently the cause of fetal death, as may be torsion at the fetal end.[30]

Hemolytic discoloration of the cord in a liveborn infant suggests vascular thrombosis (CD Fig. 40–14). An occlusive thrombus in one artery can occur without fetal problems because the usual arterial anastomoses allow perfusion of the whole placenta. Thrombosis of a cord vessel causes necrosis of the

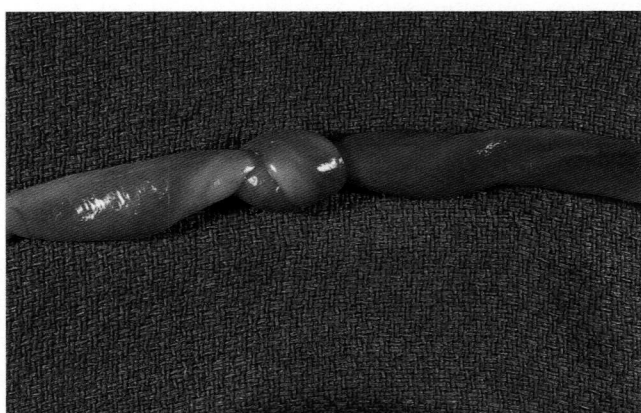

**FIGURE 40–3.** Tight true knot in an umbilical cord associated with fetal demise. Note the congestion on one side of the knot. This indicates that the knot was physiologically significant. Early thrombosis was present on histologic section.

wall because flow is its only nutrient source. Most hemorrhages in the cord are artifacts of trauma during delivery of the placenta and cord clamping. True vascular ruptures occurring before the infant is delivered usually result in fetal death.

## Insertion

Location of the cord insertion into the placenta disk is due to the plane of implantation and differential placental growth. The cord may insert into central villus tissue, at the margin of the disk, or into the membranes (velamentous) (CD Fig. 40–15). Velamentous and marginal insertions are considered abnormal, and infants with such cord insertions are slightly smaller on average. Velamentous vessels, unsupported by Wharton jelly, are at risk for compression and tearing, particularly those over the cervical os (vasa praevia). Rupture of a velamentous vessel before fetal delivery leads to rapid, often catastrophic, fetal blood loss. Velamentous vessels also occur with succenturiate lobes and occasionally at the edge of an otherwise normal placenta. In "furcate" cord insertions, the vessels divide and lose their protective Wharton jelly before reaching the placental surface (CD Fig. 40–16). The cord is sometimes partially encased by a fold of amnion at its placental end, an amniotic web. This may tightly bind the cord to the placental surface, limiting the mobility of the cord (CD Fig. 40–17).

## ABNORMALITIES OF THE FETAL MEMBRANES (NONINFECTIOUS)

### Extrachorial Placentation

The peripheral membranes normally insert at the peripheral margin of the placenta, which is usually the peripheral limit of the vascular plate. In extrachorial placentation, villus tissue extends peripherally beyond the vascular plate. These placentas tend to be thick. Circummarginate placentas show a small ridge of fibrin where the membranes contact the placental surface (CD Fig. 40–18). Circumvallation is similar; however, there is a redundant, doubled-back membrane fold at the site of membrane insertion (CD Fig. 40–19). Hemorrhage often occurs in this marginal area. Either process may involve all or part of the circumference, and the width of the extension varies from 1 cm to occasionally more than 8 cm. In general, there are no pathologic sequelae to circummargination. Prematurity and chronic bleeding are associated with circumvallation. The origin of extrachorial placentation is unclear. Possibilities include abnormally deep implantation, secondary growth lines, and loss of amniotic fluid pressure.[5, 32]

### Amnion Nodosum and Squamous Metaplasia

Yellow nodules of compressed squames and hair on the membranes are amnion nodosum[32] (CD Figs. 40–20 and 40–21). Although amnion nodosum is variable, it is often better developed late in pregnancy when more fetal cells have been shed. Earlier in pregnancy, it appears as fibrinous deposits. Amnion nodosum is associated with severe, long-standing oligohydramnios, a setting in which pulmonary hypoplasia commonly develops. Squamous metaplasia is a normal variant frequently seen near the cord insertion. The amnion undergoes metaplasia, developing a granular layer and keratinized cells (CD Fig. 40–22). The white nodules cannot be readily removed with scraping, in contrast to amnion nodosum. Neither of these processes should be confused with the remnant of the yolk sac, a 4-mm calcified yellow nodule between the amnion and chorion usually seen at the placental periphery (see CD Fig. 40–18).

### Amniotic Rupture, Bands, and Adhesions

On occasion, the amnion ruptures before delivery. The resulting amniotic bands can entrap and disrupt fetal tissues, leading to anomalies including amputations, abdominal wall and neural tube defects, and clefts (CD Fig. 40–23). The surface of the placenta is dull where the amnion has been lost and may be discolored by old hemorrhage. The actual bands are composed of amnion, often necrotic. Histologic examination shows absent amnion with squames embedded in the chorion. This change is critical because separation of the amnion is a common artifact of delivery. Similar chorionic changes are noted in true extra-amniotic pregnancies in which the fetus is outside the amniotic cavity.

### Abnormal Coloration Including Meconium

Color and translucency of the membranes vary, depending on pigmentation, edema, cellular content, and amount of attached decidua. Ascending infection, the most common cause of opacified membranes, is discussed under "Infection." Red-brown thickenings and yellow areas with iron-laden macrophages mark old hemorrhage behind the membranes (CD Fig. 40–24). This usually results from confined bleeding in small areas of decidual necrosis. Long dead embryos and fetuses may appear as yellow plaques in the membranes. Green coloration of the placental surface is often interpreted to be meconium staining; however, severe infection and old hemorrhage may also produce a greenish appearance, particularly in preterm fetuses.

Meconium passage by the fetus is a common cause of discolored membranes, particularly in the last half of the third trimester.[33] Gross findings range from fresh mucoid material on the fetal surface to deep staining of the underlying chorion (CD Figs. 40–25 and 40–26). At times, there is only a slight opacity. At microscopic examination, fresh meconium contains hair, squames, pigment, and mucin-positive material (CD Fig. 40–27). Meconium is taken up by macrophages in the amnion and chorion of the fetal surface and peripheral membranes and in the umbilical cord (Fig. 40–4) (CD Fig. 40–28). These cells have a brown, sometimes vacuolated appearance but may be difficult to see, especially in the cord. The pigment is iron negative. Bile stains have also been suggested to demonstrate them.[1] In the peripheral membranes, pigment is eventually seen in the decidua. In vitro studies suggest that meconium is rapidly found in macrophages of the amnion (1 hour) and chorion (3 hours).[34] Meconium exposure may cause the amnion to rapidly become necrotic or appear pseudostratified. The exact time course in vivo is unknown, but it is clear that meconium reaches macrophages in hours, not days. Whether the macrophages ever disappear from the surface chorion or cord is unknown. The amount of amniotic fluid and meconium passed may affect what is observed. Experience suggests that membrane edema is seen in 3 hours, and the appearance of large numbers of pigmented macrophages in the chorion requires 6 to 12 hours.[1]

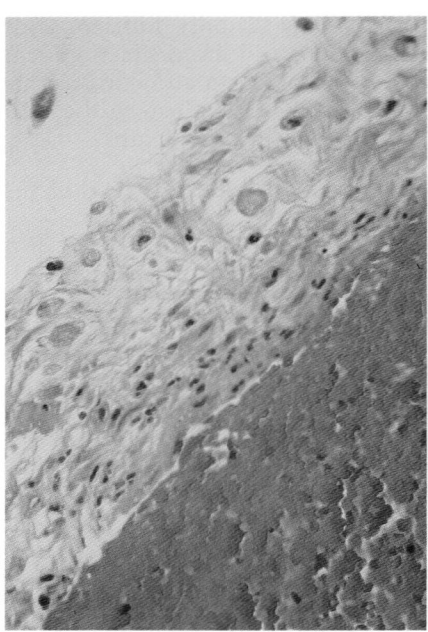

**FIGURE 40–5.** Section of umbilical cord showing an umbilical artery with necrosis of muscle cells. Cells are rounded and eosinophilic with pyknotic nuclei. Meconium macrophages are present, and there is minimal acute inflammation.

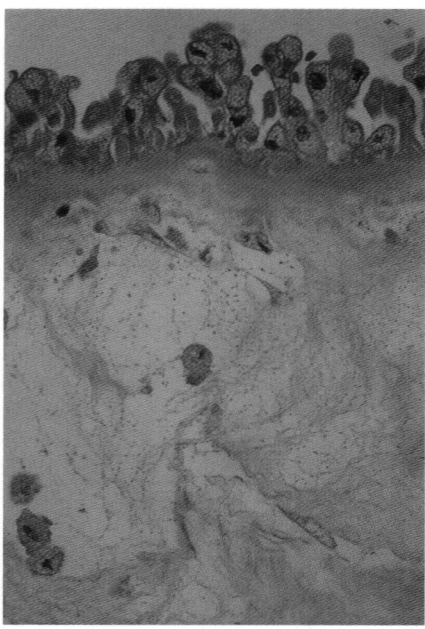

**FIGURE 40–4.** Fetal surface with meconium staining reveals vacuolated, heaped up amnion and pigment-filled macrophages in the edematous connective tissue. These changes indicate that the meconium has been present several hours.

Meconium passage by the fetus has often been taken as a sign of fetal "stress." Although some infants in distress do pass meconium, grossly discolored amniotic fluid is noted by the obstetrician in at least 10% of term deliveries, and careful examination reveals that a few meconium macrophages are common in term placentas. The majority of such infants have not had prior significant hypoxic episodes. As the fetus matures, meconium is passed in response to many stimuli. However, the presence of significant amounts of meconium in the amniotic fluid creates its own problems. The infant may aspirate this material before or during birth. Meconium in the amniotic fluid causes vasoconstriction of umbilical cord vessels[35] and may be toxic to the vascular muscle cells of the cord.[36] Necrosis of the peripheral muscle cells of the arterial wall is occasionally seen after a day or more of meconium exposure (Fig. 40–5). Necrosis generally means that there has been a severe hypoxic insult to the infant.

The relationship among meconium, amniotic sac infection, and inflammation is not entirely clear. They are often seen together.[37] Meconium-stained amniotic fluid may be more susceptible to infection. Inflammation in the cord is occasionally seen with meconium-stained fluid in the absence of other signs of infection.[38] However, not all green fluid represents meconium; infection and at times old hemorrhage may give this appearance, particularly in preterm infants.

# ABNORMALITIES OF THE PLACENTAL DISK

## Shape and Site

At term, the typical placenta is round to ovoid, 18 to 20 cm in diameter by 1.5 to 2.5 cm thick. Unusual placental shapes or implantation sites may reflect uterine cavity abnormalities, such as septate uteri, scars, and leiomyomas. Lateral uterine sulcal implantations may lead to bilobate placentas—two equal lobes with the cord velamentously inserted between them (CD Fig. 40–29). Failure of some of the peripheral villi to atrophy leads to succenturiate lobes (CD Fig. 40–30), and some placentas appear to be composed of many small, connected lobes. These variations in shape, often with considerable marginal infarction and fibrin deposition, are generally not of pathologic significance, aside from the issues of velamentous vessels, placenta previa, and placenta accreta. Rarely, one sees a diffuse, thin placenta with few free membranes—placenta membranaceae. This may derive from a shallow implantation with persistence of most of the peripheral villi.[5]

## Weight

Weighing the placenta is fraught with methodologic problems, and some have discounted its value.[6] Fresh refrigerated placentas lose a small amount of weight with storage, and formalin fixation slightly increases the weight.[5] The amount of blood and the presence of cord, membranes, and clot also have effects. The value of placental weight information lies largely at the extremes, considering gestational age and the infant's weight. A relatively heavy or light placenta often indicates a microscopic abnormality. Although tables of normal placental weights by gestational age exist,[2] the fetal-to-placental ratio is often more useful. At 20 weeks, the placenta is one third to one fourth of the infant's weight; it falls to approximately one seventh at term.[39]

## Subchorionic and Intervillous Fibrin

As pregnancy progresses, fibrin and thrombotic material under the fetal surface increase. Subchorionic fibrin deposition has been associated with fetal activity and eventual outcome.[2] *Breus mole* describes massive nodular subchorionic hematomas seen in both live births and spontaneous abortion[4–6] (CD Fig. 40–31). Some previllous fibrin deposition is seen in virtually all mature placentas. There are conditions associated with excessive fibrin deposition.[5, 40] Massive intervillous fibrin deposition exists when fibrin surrounds more than half the villus tissue (CD Figs. 40–32 and 40–33). Excessive fibrin deposition at the maternal floor around basal villi is

maternal floor infarction. These two processes often overlap in gross and microscopic appearance. Both are associated with stillbirth, growth retardation, and preterm delivery. They may recur in subsequent pregnancies. The etiology is unknown but may relate to abnormal clotting. Cysts lined by X cells, a form of trophoblast, are often found on the surface and in septa of term placentas (CD Fig. 40–34). Some are identified only by microscopy, but they may reach many centimeters and may be filled with old or recent hemorrhage. Cysts occur in areas of abundant fibrin deposition, whether it is normal or abnormal.

## Infarcts

True infarcts, villus regions that have lost their maternal blood supply, are common in placentas. Infarcts are firmer than adjacent tissue and appear granular owing to the remaining villus ghosts. Over time, they progress from red to yellow and white[5, 9, 40, 41] (Fig. 40–6) (CD Figs. 40–35 and 40–36). Cavitation and hemorrhage may occur. Infarction is common at the placental margin, and a small (1 to 2 cm) lesion is generally insignificant. Central infarcts suggest maternal vascular problems. The earliest infarcts show only villus vascular congestion and collapse, with diminution of the intervillous space. Over time, nuclear staining of trophoblast and finally of the entire villus is lost (CD Fig. 40–37). Fibrin is laid down in the intervillous space, but true organization never occurs. A slight infiltrate of neutrophils may be present at the edge of infarcts. Old infarcts and regions of previllous fibrin are at times difficult to differentiate.

## Retroplacental and Other Hemorrhage

Hemorrhages on the maternal surface arise from areas of premature placental separation.[5] The blood is

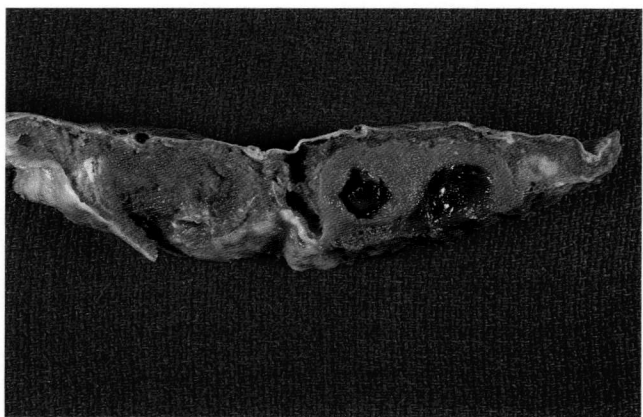

**FIGURE 40–6.** Cross-section of placenta showing several infarcts of varying ages and compression of the villus tissue by fresh hemorrhage. The mother had severe preeclampsia and a growth-retarded infant.

largely maternal, but some fetal blood may be present. It is preferable to use descriptive terminology rather than abruptio placentae, a clinical expression. Finding retroplacental hemorrhage may correspond to clinical abruption; however, many such lesions are clinically unsuspected.

Retroplacental hemorrhages occur both centrally and at the placental margin, overlying regions of villus tissue (CD Fig. 40–38). Marginal hemorrhage is peripheral aggregation of blood extending onto the membranes, not villi. The gross appearance of retroplacental hemorrhage depends on the duration and degree of blood trapping. When blood is confined behind the placenta, the clot compresses the villus tissue. If the pregnancy continues, the area develops infarction because the blood supply has been lost. The blood eventually breaks down, becoming brown to yellow. If the blood has egress through the vagina or into the amniotic fluid, the villus tissue may not be compressed, although infarction of the devascularized villi will eventually occur. Recent, sometimes massive clinical abruptions may show little or no gross or histologic change, appearing much like a normally separated placenta. Large amounts of blood clot are often received with such specimens. Aside from changes of early infarction, intravillous hemorrhage and intervillous fibrin deposition at the base are early clues (CD Fig. 40–39). Necrotic decidua may lead to a plane of placental separation.[41] Hypertensive disorders, smoking, and possibly cocaine use are associated with marginal and retroplacental hemorrhages. Ascending infection is also associated with placental separation,[42] through either decidual necrosis or chronic bleeding. Maternal trauma is a well-established cause of premature placental separation, and abuse is now recognized as a common cause.[43] Trauma does not have to be directly abdominal to initiate separation, which begins at the time of the event, although symptoms may be delayed.

## Intervillous Thrombi

Intervillous thrombi occur in the intervillous space, both in central villus tissue and at the base, and differ from subchorionic thrombosis, infarct, and retroplacental hemorrhage. The earliest thrombi are red clots that progress to laminated thrombi and old, glistening white lesions (CD Fig. 40–40). They are seen more frequently in conditions with large, friable placentas. They may be caused by coagulation at areas of villus damage.[40]

## Chorangiomas and Other Nontrophoblastic Tumors

Chorangiomas are similar to other hemangiomas and are better designated hamartomas. These lesions are most common under the chorionic surface[6, 44] (CD Fig. 40–41). They have a variety of gross appearances. Chorangiomas may be red, tan, or white; fleshy or hemorrhagic; and discrete or blending imperceptibly with the surrounding tissue (CD Fig. 40–42). They are often confused with other gross lesions, including infarcts and thrombi. The histologic pattern is variable as to size and perfusion of vessels and the presence of necrosis. The surface trophoblast of chorangiomas often appears hyperplastic (CD Fig. 40–43). They are often found at microscopic examination. The smallest lesions look like extremely large villi with diffusely increased capillaries, somewhat overlapping with chorangiosis. Large lesions may lead to heart failure and nonimmune hydrops. Platelet trapping also occurs. On occasion, the infants have other hemangiomas.

Other tumors of the placenta are uncommon.[7] Metastases from maternal tumors are rare, with breast carcinoma and melanoma the most common. Leukemias may be seen in the intervillous space. Fetal tumors, such as neuroblastomas and melanocytic lesions, are found on occasion.[45]

## MICROSCOPIC VILLUS ABNORMALITIES

Microscopic evaluation of villus tissue is a difficult part of placental examination.[46] Assessing whether villus structure and form are appropriate for a given gestational age takes experience gained from looking at many normal and abnormal placentas. Awareness of the clinical history, particularly gestational age, is critical in making these assessments. The placenta responds to many insults by subtle variations[5, 40] in villus maturation. Microscopic villus abnormalities are often suggested by the gross examination of the placenta. Villus color usually correlates with histologic maturation, darkening as gestation progresses. Pale villus areas are often atrophic or agglutinated villi. A generally soft consistency can indicate chorangiosis, edema, or hypoplastic villi. Hydropic placentas are usually pale, coarse, and friable.[9]

Table 40–6 outlines the histologic findings in the disorders of villus maturation and form. Ischemic villus change is due to reduced maternal blood flow to the placenta (Fig. 40–7). It is an extremely common finding in histologically examined placentas and is seen in many cases of otherwise unexplained preterm labor, premature rupture of membranes, and growth retardation. There is usually no history of maternal vascular disease.[2, 41, 47] Ischemic change in early or recurrent losses should raise the consideration of anticardiolipin syndromes.[5] There are many causes of hydrops in the fetus, both immune and nonimmune (Fig. 40–8). Some placentas have specific features of the disease of origin.[5] Dysmature placentas are associated with congenital anomalies and are usually seen in infants with trisomy 18 (CD Fig. 40–44). Villitis and intervillositis of unknown etiology are associated with unexplained fetal

**TABLE 40–6.** Guide to Normal and Abnormal Villus Morphology

***Normal Maturation***
Villi: primary (trophoblastic), secondary (+mesenchyme), tertiary (+vessels)
Villus maturation
  Decreasing size
  Decreasing stroma
  Increasing vascularity with vasculosyncytial membranes
  Increasing trophoblastic "knots" with less apparent cyto-
    trophoblast
Placental circulation
  Injection of blood into central villus areas
  Under surface, base—ischemic
  Margins—ischemic
  Some variation in pattern is expected normally, depending
    on location
Use *low power* to assess pattern
  Regular distribution of villus sizes, stems to terminal villi
  Tangential cuts lead to some small villi at all gestations
  Distribution of intermediate and terminal villi in normal and
    abnormal maturation

***Ischemic Change (Common Placental Finding; Decreased Maternal Perfusion of Placenta)***
Correlate morphology with gestational age
Small size with increased exaggerated knotting
Poor branching leads to two villus populations, large stems
  and small terminal villi
Empty maternal intervillous space
Frequent in premature infants but usually not suggested by
  gross or clinical findings

***Hydrops and Edema***
Large villi
Diminished knotting with increased visible cytotrophoblasts
Often increased nucleated red blood cells
Edema with vacuolated macrophages (Hofbauer cells)
Immature-type intermediate villi show vacuolated stroma that
  suggests edema, but is not

***Miscellaneous Villus Changes***
Hypoplasia—sparse but not ischemic
Chorangiosis
  Increased villus size
  Increased numbers of blood vessels in the central parts of
    the villi
  Diffuse or focal
Dysmaturity
  Irregular pattern with mixtures of maturation patterns
  Congenital anomalies
  Diabetes mellitus
Villus atrophy—lack of fetal perfusion
  Fibrosed villi with viable surface trophoblasts
  Early change is degenerating blood vessels with red blood
    cell fragmentation
Chronic villitis, nonspecific
  Foci in normal villus background (specific infections have
    generalized change)
  Lymphocytes, histiocytes, neutrophils; plasma cells rare
  Agglutinated villi

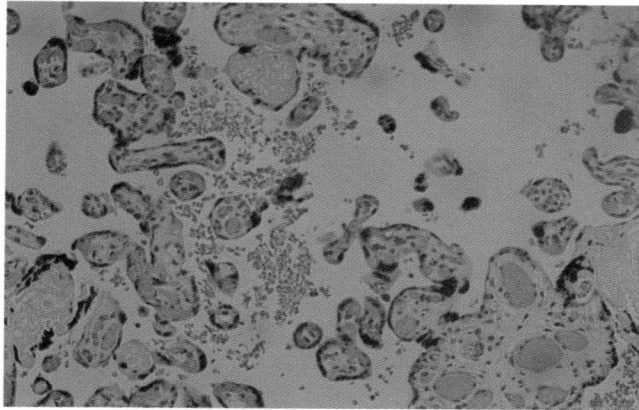

**FIGURE 40–7.** Ischemic villus tissue at 32 weeks showing extremely small villi with dark, smudgy syncytiotrophoblast. The field appears sparse with two populations—highly branched terminal villi and large stems.

lumens in each villus."[51] This definition is difficult to apply, and a gestalt approach is frequently used. Infants whose placentas have extensive chorangiosis demonstrate increased perinatal morbidity, mortality, and anomalies. The change appears in the placentas of infants born at high altitude and appears to be related to tissue hypoxia.[52]

The villus tissue undergoes specific alterations after intrauterine demise. Atrophy is associated with cessation of the fetal circulation.[53] These atrophic changes consist of contraction of the fetal blood vessels generally. Larger vessels subdivide into multiple lumina, appearing to have ingrowth of fibroblasts (CD Fig. 40–48). Shrinkage of capillaries in peripheral villi may be less obvious (CD Fig. 40–49). Cellular debris in and around blood vessels is seen within hours. By 1 to 2 weeks, the villus stroma is avascular and fibrotic (Fig. 40–10). Trophoblast covering such villi remains relatively intact because it is nourished by the maternal blood supply. This change is distinct from infarction, in which villi be-

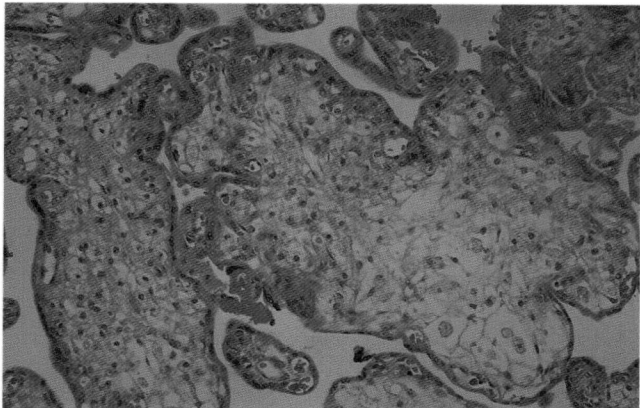

**FIGURE 40–8.** Term placenta with hydrops shows edematous large villi with prominent immature-appearing trophoblastic covering.

growth retardation and occasionally intrauterine death[48-50] (CD Figs. 40–45 and 40–46). The process may be recurrent, often with increasing severity. The etiology is unclear, although immunologic and possibly infectious factors are involved. Chorangiosis (Fig. 40–9) (CD Fig. 40–47) has been formally defined as "at least 10 different fields in 10 different placental areas with 10 villi that have 10 capillary

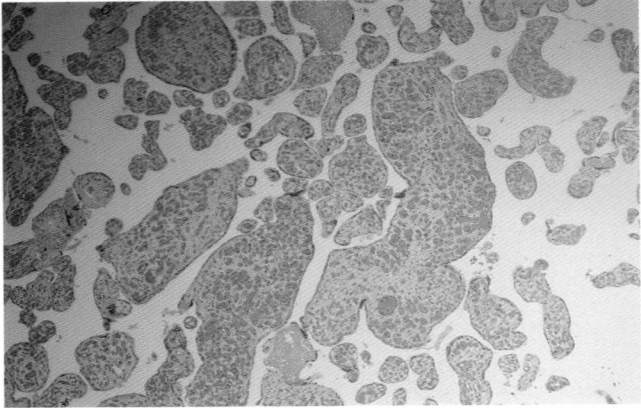

**FIGURE 40–9.** Severe chorangiosis with enlarged villi showing large numbers of capillary cross-sections.

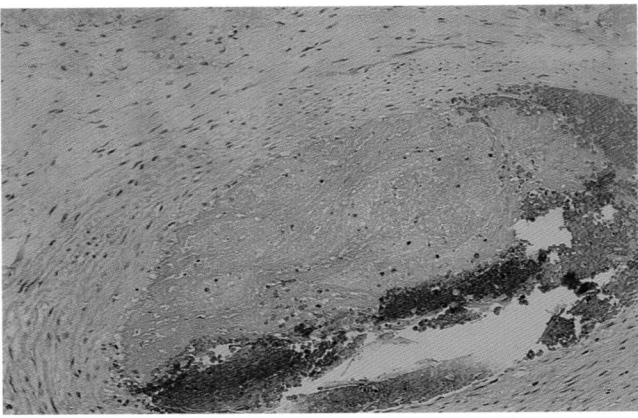

**FIGURE 40–11.** Fetal surface vessel with recent thrombosis.

come pale-staining ghosts with early loss of trophoblastic staining. Fibroblasts in atrophic villi are viable for weeks, and tissue culture can be established. Areas of villus atrophy can be seen in liveborn infants and imply interference with fetal blood flow to these villi (CD Fig. 40–50). Large vessels feeding such areas may show thrombosis and obliteration of the lumen with red blood cell fragmentation. Thromboses of fetal blood vessels are frequently recognized in situations without fetal demise. Thrombi are seen in several forms—fibrin-platelet aggregates, dense fibrin on the vessel wall, well-developed occlusive thrombi, and fibrotic lesions that may calcify (Fig. 40–11) (CD Fig. 40–51). Maternal diabetes has long been recognized to predispose to fetal thrombosis. Other fetal and maternal thrombotic disorders are increasingly recognized as causes of gestational and perinatal morbidity and mortality.[54–56] Vascular occlusion and distal atrophy are not infrequently seen when one examines placentas from infants with problems in labor or the neonatal period.[57, 58] Infants

with these placental changes have shown other vascular lesions, including porencephalic cysts and gut atresias. These changes indicate preexisting abnormal fetal perfusion of the placenta.

It is difficult at term to identify circulating nucleated red blood cells in villus vessels, and finding them easily is distinctly abnormal. Recognized causes for increased nucleated red blood cells include anemia, congenital infection, and maternal diabetes. Chronic intrauterine hypoxia is also associated with increased circulating nucleated red blood cells from increased production of erythropoietin.[1, 5, 58]

## INFECTION

The most common route of infection is ascending—from the vagina through the cervix to the amniotic cavity, leading to inflammation of the placental membranes—chorioamnionitis. Amniotic sac infections occasionally follow invasive procedures (e.g., amniocentesis) or come from the fallopian tube or directly from the endometrium. Infection of the fetus also occurs hematogenously. Organisms (bacteria, viruses, parasites) in the maternal blood stream may reach the fetus through the villi. Villitis is the usual pathologic change in this setting.[48, 59]

### Ascending Infection

Ascending infection is extremely common; minimal degrees of infection are frequent in term placentas.[60] It often occurs with intact membranes, although membrane rupture facilitates infection. Bacteria, *Candida*, and herpes simplex virus are the usual agents. Acute inflammation in the membranes is not associated with any process other than ascending infection (e.g., meconium, hypertension), and its presence indicates that some organism has contaminated the amniotic cavity.[5] Although typical hospital cultures may be negative, organisms are recovered in the

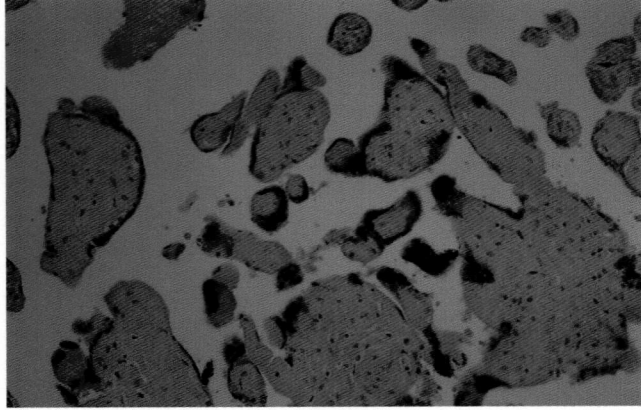

**FIGURE 40–10.** Villus tissue showing the changes associated with cessation of the fetal circulation. The vessels are obliterated, but the trophoblast is viable from the maternal circulation.

majority of cases with sensitive specific culture techniques. *Mycoplasma, Ureaplasma,* anaerobes, and certain aerobes are found frequently and are relatively nonpathogenic for the fetus.[48, 61] Organisms may enter the lungs from fetal aspiration of amniotic fluid. Infants with early sepsis usually have ascending infections in their placentas, but the majority (95%) of infants with placental changes of ascending infection do not have sepsis. There is some but not complete correlation with severity of the process.[62] Unfortunately, the inflammatory process itself creates problems. It may directly weaken the membranes. Bacteria and inflammatory cells release phospholipids. This leads to prostaglandin production that initiates uterine contractions and cervical dilatation.[48] As gestational age at delivery decreases, the incidence of chorioamnionitis increases. Ascending infection accounts for at least 40% of preterm delivery through premature rupture of membranes and preterm labor.[63] Unfortunately, treatment of intrauterine infection with antibiotics has not been particularly successful in delaying delivery.[64]

Inflammation in large fetal blood vessels may cause abnormal intrauterine heart patterns through changes in umbilical vascular reactivity with potential hypoxia.[65, 66] A continuing area of research relates to systemic effects of cytokines released by the inflammatory process. Neurologic problems and cerebral palsy are more common in infants with chorioamnionitis, particularly preterm infants.[67]

In severe amniotic sac infections, the fetal surface is green and opaque (Fig. 40–12) (CD Fig. 40–52) with an indistinct vascular pattern. Mild processes are difficult to identify by gross examination.[9] Some placentas smell foul. At microscopic examination, inflammation of the fetal surface is often seen first, progressing from aggregation of maternal neutrophils in the intervillous space under the chorion to invasion of the chorion and amnion (Fig. 40–13) (CD Figs. 40–53 and 40–54). The maternal response is often accompanied by a fetal response of neutrophils migrating toward the amnion from surface

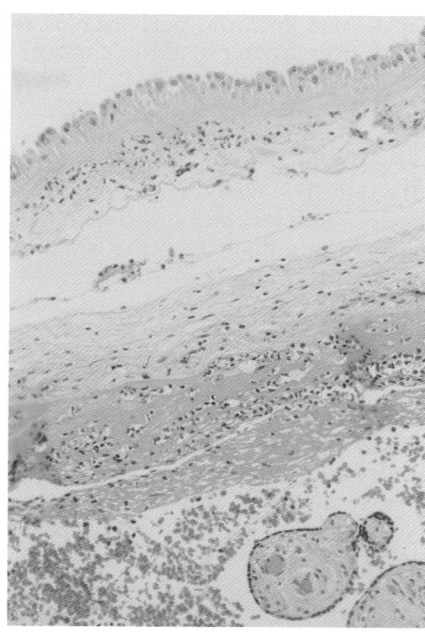

**FIGURE 40–13.** Mild chorioamnionitis is shown in the fetal surface. Cells have migrated from the maternal intervillous space under the plate to aggregate in the subchorionic fibrin and extend into the chorion and amnion.

vessels.[59] Similar changes occur in the cord, usually first from the vein (Fig. 40–14). Cells eventually move from all three vessels into Wharton jelly—funisitis. In the membranes, neutrophils infiltrate the chorion and amnion (CD Fig. 40–55). The point of rupture, often the center of the roll, usually has the most severe reaction, frequently with necrosis.[5, 48, 59] The degree of inflammation can differ widely in areas of the surface, peripheral membranes, and cord. Various observers use different criteria for the minimal level of inflammation diagnosed as ascending infection.[48, 59, 60] The lowest suggested criterion has been an aggregation of five neutrophils under the subchorionic fibrin of the plate.[60] The membranes

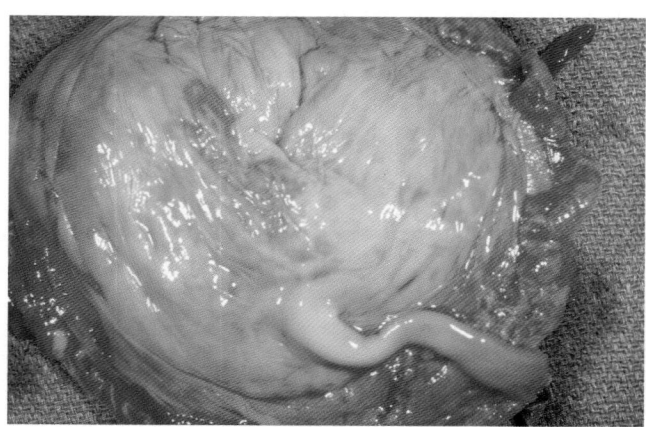

**FIGURE 40–12.** Immature placenta with severe chorioamnionitis. The surface is opaque and slightly yellow-green from infiltration by neutrophils.

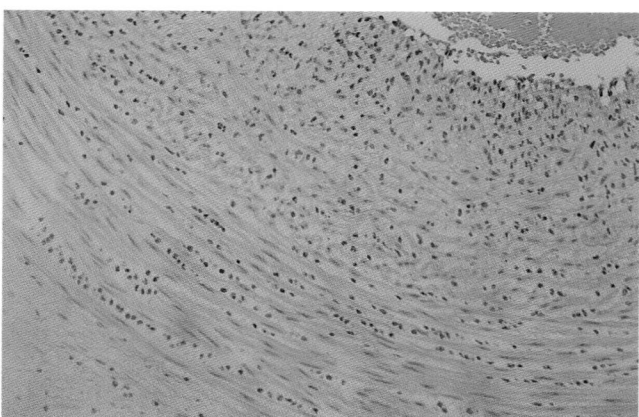

**FIGURE 40–14.** Umbilical vasculitis showing fetal neutrophils migrating from the lumen into the wall. This change is usually seen first in the vein.

first show a diffuse decidual perivascular reaction or a bandlike infiltrate at the decidua-chorion interface. Even a few neutrophils infiltrating a vessel wall in the cord is significant. The severity of the inflammation should be evident from the diagnosis rendered in the report. Some have used chorioamnionitis grades I, II, and III.[2] These correspond to my preferred terms of subchorionic intervillositis, chorionitis, and chorioamnionitis.[59] Features such as necrosis or bacteria should also be noted. Necrosis and neutrophil breakdown indicate processes of longer duration. The exact time course for ascending infection is unknown; it is difficult to identify the true time of amniotic sac contamination. Chorioamnionitis often precedes rupture of membranes or onset of labor. Naeye's work suggested that it may take several days to evolve a circumferential reaction.[2] Clinical signs frequently do not correlate with placental findings. Many asymptomatic mothers have well-developed pathologic changes. The specific infecting agent may alter the pattern of inflammation. Fusobacteria lead to severe necrotizing inflammation with organisms visible on routine and bacterial stains.[48] *Candida* infection produces distinctive nodular yellow fungal microabscesses on the cord surface[5, 9, 59] (CD Figs. 40–56 to 40–58). Group B streptococcal infections usually show associated chorioamnionitis, although some fulminant infections show a paucity of inflammation with abundant organisms.[48] Herpes is extremely uncommon today with newer obstetric protocols; cases show a chronic chorioamnionitis with plasma cells.

Necrotizing funisitis is a mixed or chronic inflammatory process surrounding the vessels of the cord. Necrosis and calcification are common (CD Fig. 40–59). At gross evaluation, these cords are nonpliable and show a "barber pole" configuration. This nonspecific finding apparently results from a long-standing antenatal infection, usually ascending, by an organism of low virulence. The infants are usually premature but do not have sepsis.[30, 68]

## Hematogenous Infection

Intrauterine hematogenous infections include the classic TORCH infections of toxoplasmosis, rubella, and cytomegalovirus as well as a wide variety of others including syphilis, varicella, and tuberculosis. Chronic villus inflammation is the typical lesion.[5, 48, 59, 69] Villitis may reflect the initial placental invasion during maternal septicemia or systemic fetal dissemination. The origin of the inflammatory cells is likely to be both fetal and maternal. Hematogenous infections usually show varied pathologic changes with a mix of lesions in different stages. The most active ones are proliferative with a variety of inflammatory cells including lymphocytes, histiocytes, and sometimes neutrophils and plasma cells. The cells fill and distort the villi. Vasculitis and vascular obliteration are often prominent because many viruses infect endothelial cells. Frank necrosis, particularly of tropho-

blast, can occur. Resolution of the inflammatory process leaves scarred, atrophic villi. Abnormalities of villus maturation are also associated with hematogenous infections, particularly those starting early in gestation. Hydrops may be present. Not all clinically diagnosed fetal infections show specific placental changes.

Villus changes also vary somewhat with the specific agent and are well described.[5, 48, 59, 69] The pathologic process of rubella is known from studies during previous epidemics and is similar to that of villitis of unknown etiology. Cytomegalovirus infection often has distinctive morphologic changes with plasmacytic villitis, typical cytomegalovirus intranuclear and intracytoplasmic inclusions, and fibrotic villi with hemosiderin (Fig. 40–15) (CD Fig. 40–60). Varicella has a more granulomatous picture. Infection with human parvovirus B19, the agent of fifth disease or erythema infectiosum, can be diagnosed from the placenta. Second trimester infections will most likely cause problems for the fetus; this is when erythropoietic cells are most rapidly dividing and are susceptible to the virus. The placenta shows hydrops similar to that seen in isoimmunization. There are numerous circulating erythroblasts, some of which contain intranuclear eosinophilic inclusions with central clearing and chromatic condensation at the periphery (CD Fig. 40–61). Unlike in other congenital infections, no inflammatory reaction occurs in the placenta.

In toxoplasmosis, the placenta is often heavy with enlarged and somewhat fibrotic villi. An inflammatory infiltrate is less prominent than in rubella or cytomegalovirus infection. *Toxoplasma* cysts are more often found in the membranes than in villus lesions. Syphilis is not uncommon today. Classically, the placenta is heavy and edematous with villus fibrosis, plasmacytic villitis, and obliterative endarteritis. Chorioamnionitis and chronic funisitis are also common in syphilis. Organisms may be found with silver stain in the placenta and cord in

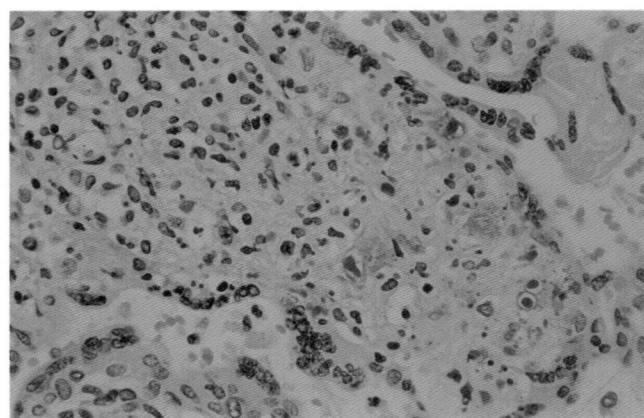

**FIGURE 40–15.** Chronic villitis associated with cytomegalovirus infection. There are lymphocytes, histiocytes, cellular debris, and intranuclear and intracytoplasmic inclusions. Inclusions are typically found in the more active areas of inflammation.

severe cases. There is a wide range of involvement in documented maternal infection, and the placenta often appears normal with early maternal treatment. *Listeria monocytogenes* probably also infects by the hematogenous route, but the pattern is different. The characteristic lesion is a necrotizing abscess with infarction; neutrophils are the predominant cell type. Lesions are soft and yellow-white, ranging from a few millimeters to several centimeters. They are seen on the maternal surface and scattered through the villus tissue. There is also usually severe chorioamnionitis with green amniotic fluid. Organisms are typically found in the amnion or the cord. In placentas, 99% of the villitis observed cannot be attributed to a specific organism and falls into the category of villitis of unknown etiology.

The pathologic process of human immunodeficiency virus infection is currently being explored, and our knowledge will continue to evolve as new treatment regimens are evaluated. Virus has been identified in cells of the placenta at times. A variety of pathologic lesions have been described, without a clearly specific pattern emerging. Many placentas appear to be normal, however.[70]

## DECIDUAL LESIONS

Familiarity with the normal vascular alterations of pregnancy is important for recognizing decidual vascular disease.[5, 41] Such lesions are usually present only focally, even in clinically severe cases, and appropriate placental sampling is necessary.[71, 72] Atherosis is the classic lesion of preeclampsia. It consists of fibrinoid change in vessel walls with finely vacuolated "lipid"-filled intimal cells (CD Fig. 40–62). Thrombosis is common. This vessel change is also seen in anticardiolipin syndrome. Lack of physiologic change is also considered a feature of preeclampsia. It can be seen only in regions where vessels should have been invaded by trophoblast (decidua basalis and capsularis). In chronic hypertension, uterine vessel changes are similar to those seen elsewhere; intimal hyperplasia is the most prominent feature (CD Fig. 40–63). Acute decidual inflammation is common with ascending infection. In otherwise unremarkable placentas, a slight decidual infiltrate of lymphocytes is not uncommon. More substantial chronic inflammation in the decidua is often associated with basal chronic villitis. Decidual necrosis in the absence of inflammation is also common, with unclear implications.

## MULTIPLE GESTATION

A substantial portion of perinatal morbidity and mortality arises from multiple gestations, and nearly all placentas from twins and higher multiple births should be examined histologically.[5, 68, 73, 74] Twin placentas demonstrate the whole range of disorders seen in singletons as well as their own special path-

ologic processes. The following discussion alludes to twins, but the same principles apply to examining the placentas of higher multiple births.

The critical first step in examining the placenta of a multiple birth is determination of chorionicity.[5, 9, 73] Dichorionic means that two placentas have formed; monochorionic indicates a shared placenta. Any gestation arising from two fertilized eggs is dichorionic, because each conceptus has its own placenta. The placentas may be totally separate; however, limitations of uterine space frequently lead to a single disk. Monozygotic (identical) twins, in whom the fertilized egg splits early in development, can have several types of placenta. Dichorionic placentas result from splits before 3 days of development because all the cells of the conception are essentially undifferentiated. As cells become developmentally committed, these portions can no longer divide. The chorion differentiates first, and two separate embryos and amnions develop within a single chorion. Such a diamniotic monochorionic placenta is diagnostic of monozygotic twins. Later splits are infrequent, resulting in monoamniotic and conjoined twins. Two thirds of monozygotic twins are monochorionic; the rest are dichorionic. Testing for genetic traits is required to differentiate monozygotic dichorionic twins from dizygotic like-sexed twins. Of naturally occurring twins in the United States, about 80% of monochorionic like-sexed pairs are dizygotic on the basis of relative incidences of monozygotic and dizygotic twins.

Completely separate placentas, always dichorionic, are examined as singleton placentas. In fused placentas, gross determination of chorionicity is simple. Dichorionic dividing membranes are thicker and more opaque than monochorionic ones, with a ridge where they meet the placental surface (Fig. 40–16) (CD Fig. 40–64). If one tries to completely remove dichorionic dividing membranes by separating the layers, the placental surface is disrupted. In contrast, monochorionic membranes show no ridge and are easily separated, leaving a continuous chorionic

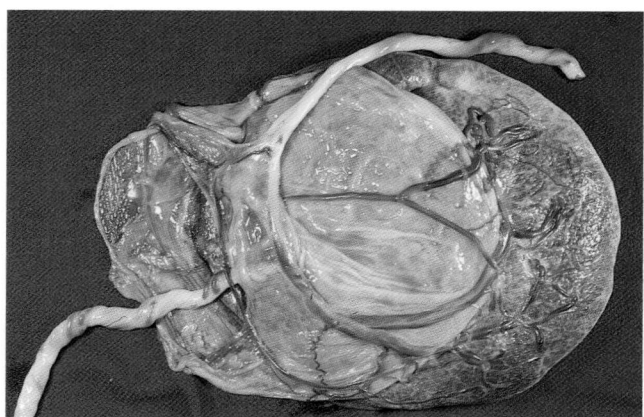

**FIGURE 40–16.** Diamniotic dichorionic twin placenta with velamentous insertion of one cord into the thick dividing membranes.

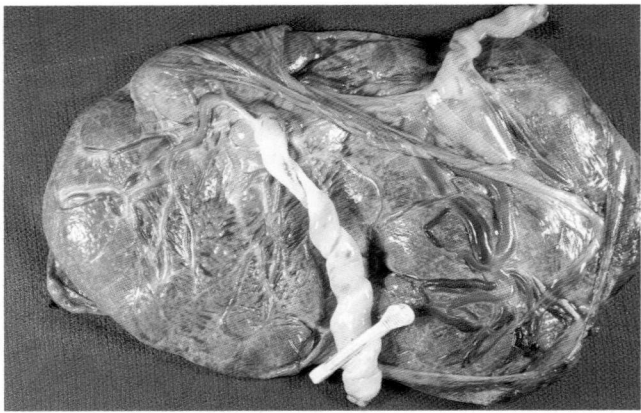

**FIGURE 40–17.** Diamniotic monochorionic placenta showing the single chorionic plate with the delicate dividing membranes in a roll on the surface. Vascular anastomoses are present.

plate (Fig. 40–17) (CD Figs. 40–64 and 40–65). One should histologically confirm chorionicity. T sections (T-shaped sections) include a point where the dividing membranes abut the placental surface, or a roll of the dividing membranes may be made (CD Figs. 40–66 and 40–67). The dividing membranes have three or four layers in dichorionic twins—amnion from each side and two layers of chorion that often fuse. Dividing membranes of diamniotic monochorionic placentas show only two amnions. The presence of any chorionic tissue in the dividing membranes indicates dichorionic placentation.

Monochorionic placentas virtually always show one or more vascular anastomoses, artery to artery, artery to vein, and vein to vein. Arteries always pass over veins on the placental surface. By tracing large superficial vessels, one can often see the vascular connections between the sides. Vessels can also be injected. A deep anastomosis is likely when one sees a vessel dipping into the villus tissue without a returning mate next to a similar configuration from the other side. Vascular anastomoses lead to the specific problems of monochorionic twins, and it is important to document them. Unbalanced cross-circulation may cause transfusion syndrome. In the classic chronic form, the donor is growth retarded with oligohydramnios and the recipient is larger and plethoric with polyhydramnios. The donor's placenta is pale from anemia, whereas the recipient's is deep red and congested. There may be subtle differences in villus configuration between the twins. Premature delivery is common in severe chronic transfusion syndrome. Acute transfusion syndromes also occur if one fetus bleeds through anastomoses into the placenta of the other, as when pressure drops after one is delivered. Intertwin anastomoses are often complicated, and it is likely that flow between them varies during pregnancy. In symptomatic cases of transfusion syndrome, laser obliteration of anastomoses and repetitive amniocentesis have been used with some success.[75] If one twin dies, chronic transfusion will cease, although the survivor has a sub-

stantial risk of vascular disruptive anomalies (e.g., gut atresia, porencephalic cysts).[76] This may relate to circulatory change similar to that seen in acute transfusions. Damage apparently occurs near the time of death.

Abnormalities of cord insertion and single umbilical arteries are more common in all twins. Velamentous insertion can occur in the dividing membranes of dichorionic twins and is prone to problems. There may also be considerable differences in the relative placental size between infants, particularly in higher multiple births. When a dead fetus in a multiple gestation is retained many months, a compressed fetus papyraceus forms (CD Fig. 40–68). Chorionicity of the dividing membranes can often be determined, and radiographs help determine gestational age. Such compressed fetuses may result from transfusion syndrome, anomalies, cord problems, and, frequently today, reductions of higher multiple births.

## ABORTION SPECIMENS

### Examination and Histology

There are many causes of spontaneous abortions, some more frequent at certain points in gestation. The often used dividing point of 20 weeks bears no relationship to pathologic entities, because the causes of spontaneous loss in the first half of pregnancy are similar to the causes of obstetric complications in the last half. Induced terminations done for fetal abnormality require efforts to document disorders. Obtaining a history is imperative. Unfortunately, the commonly used dilatation and evacuation method of termination fragments the specimen so that recognition of certain anomalies may be impossible.

In spontaneous abortions, the viability of the gestation at time of the loss is a key feature. This information can be obtained from both the embryo or fetus and the placenta. Extraembryonic causes of early pregnancy loss (e.g., abnormal hormonal function of the corpus luteum, abnormal uterine form, abnormal endometrial function) tend to produce nonmacerated specimens with well-developed embryos; intrinsic embryonic causes are associated with intrauterine death and long retention, classically of 3 to 4 weeks before spontaneous passage.[13, 77] The natural time course is often altered today by rapid ultrasound recognition of nonviability and immediate evacuation of the pregnancy. Changes of intrauterine demise are often less striking (CD Fig. 40–69). If an embryo or fetus is present, it should be evaluated.[17–19] Fixation before detailed examination is often useful. In small intact specimens, crown-rump length is the most useful measurement. In larger fragmented fetuses, hand and foot lengths are measured. Maceration is assessed grossly by the color and texture of the embryo or fetus. Macerated specimens are tan to gray-brown, opaque, and soft. Nonmacerated embryos tend to be normally developed relative to gestational age; macerated ones range from markedly growth disorganized to relatively normal in appearance. One should look for malformations. Often the limbs are the most useful and intact (CD Fig. 40–70). With care, many viscera in a fetus can be identified. In macerated fetuses, sectioning of lung and kidney may be most useful. Placental tissue should always be submitted.

In early losses, it is common to not identify an embryo. This may be due to disruption or degeneration, even in an intact sac. The embryo's prior existence can be postulated from the placental tissue. Villus stroma is derived from the extraembryonic mesenchyme, which in turn comes from the primary embryonic tissue[26]; thus, villus stroma indicates that embryonic tissue was once present but has now disintegrated. The remnant of the secondary yolk sac is frequently still identifiable without the embryo. It is important to understand the expected placental changes with intrauterine demise.[14, 77, 78] In general, one sees hydropic villi or villi with stromal fibrosis and vascular obliteration. The difference between the two villus patterns reflects villous development at the time of death. Before the establishment of the extraembryonic circulation, the villi become hydropic; the fibrous pattern results from problems after villus vascularization. Hydropic change is due to inability of fluid to drain from villi. Such villi are characterized by loose, sometimes cystic stroma with rudimentary or absent blood vessels. Trophoblast is largely attenuated, with loss of the inner cytotrophoblast (CD Fig. 40–71). Hydropic morphology is most commonly associated with an empty sac and embryonic death occurring before 6 to 7 menstrual weeks.[14, 78] The fibrotic pattern shows smaller villi that may have two layers of trophoblast. Blood vessels are present, usually collapsed or undergoing obliteration, and may contain intact and fragmented red blood cells (CD Figs. 40–72 and 40–73). This pattern occurs when the embryo dies after 7 to 8 menstrual weeks. Table 40–7 is a scheme for developmental dating. In using this guideline, it must be considered that the capsular villi never become vascularized and always eventually become hydropic. To accurately assess the developmental age at embryonic death, one needs to look for the most advanced region. In incomplete specimens, one may get falsely early gestational ages because the tissue present may not represent the status of the more central villus tissue.[3]

## Cytogenetic Considerations

Cytogenetic abnormalities occur in about 50% of early spontaneous abortions, predominantly trisomy (27%), polyploidy (10%), and monosomy X (9%). Trisomy 16 accounts for about one third of trisomies.[13, 79] In those spontaneous abortions that are empty sacs, growth-disordered embryos, or embryos with focal defects, the frequency of abnormal karyo-

**TABLE 40–7.** Morphologic Markers Useful in Dating First Trimester Spontaneous Abortions

| Developmental/Menstrual Age (wk) | Morphologic Feature |
|---|---|
| 12 d/3.5 | Syncytiotrophoblastic lacunar network |
| 2/4 | Primary villi of cytotrophoblast and syncytiotrophoblast Secondary yolk sac |
| 3/5 (early) | Secondary villi with mesenchymal cores |
| 3/5 (late) | Tertiary villi with vasculature |
| 3–4/5–6 | Yolk sac hematopoiesis established |
| 4.5/6.5 | Yolk sac nucleated erythrocytes in placental capillaries |
| 6–7/8–9 | Non-nucleated erythrocytes from liver begin to replace nucleated erythrocytes |
| 9/11 | Yolk sac present as remnant |
| 10/12 | Essentially all non-nucleated red blood cells circulate |
| 10/12 | Apposition of amnion and chorion |

Adapted from Kaplan CG: Embryonic pathology of the placenta. In Lewis SH, Perrin E (eds): Pathology of the Placenta. 2nd ed. Philadelphia, Churchill Livingstone, 1999, pp 89–106.

type rises to 60% to 80%.[18] Thus, if one finds an abnormal embryo or placental morphologic features associated with embryonic death, one can predict the likely presence of a chromosome abnormality without actual karyotype. The occurrence of abnormal karyotypes in future pregnancies is either random or, for trisomies, related to maternal age.[80] Thus, there is little clinical value to be gained from chromosome analysis of an isolated spontaneous abortion, although such information may be important to a family and their understanding of the loss. New techniques may eventually simplify the analysis of karyotype in spontaneous abortion. In situ studies in interphase nuclei for just three chromosomes—16, X, and Y—will identify many trisomies, triploidy, and monosomy X.[19] A few chromosomally abnormal pregnancies continue into the second and third trimesters. At this time, the typical phenotypes in the fetus may be recognized. Macerated fetuses, even those not obviously malformed, have a high frequency of chromosome abnormalities.

It has long been debated whether one can determine a precise cytogenetic abnormality in a spontaneous abortion by placental morphologic features.[81–86] Most reports agree that except for triploidy, one cannot predict a specific abnormal karyotype from the placenta, and many of the spontaneous abortions that are found to be triploid do not show the distinctive histologic features. The villus changes commonly seen in aneuploidy relate to early time and long duration of intrauterine loss. The ability to predict a normal karyotype from morphologic features would also be useful because such patients may have subsequent reproductive problems. The presence of fetal anucleated erythrocytes or an umbilical cord, less villus hydrops, infarcts, and chronic inflammation have been associated with normal karyotype.[85, 86] These features probably relate to more advanced development in many karyotypically normal spontaneous abortions.

## Other Causes of Early Spontaneous Abortion

The rate of twinning in spontaneous abortions has been found to be three times that in live births. Spontaneously aborted twin embryos are virtually all monozygotic, and nearly all show abnormal development.[87] Marked variation in the appearance of the villi may sometimes be explained by multiple gestations with varying time of death. The role of infection in loss in the first trimester is less well documented than its role in early delivery beginning in the second trimester. Infection probably causes less than 5% of losses in the first trimester.[88] Organisms such as *Ureaplasma* have been cultured more frequently from patients with spontaneous abortion,[89] but no specific histologic pattern has been identified. Acute and chronic inflammatory patterns are common in spontaneous abortion and were seen in patients with both positive and negative cultures. On occasion, specimens show clear evidence of infection with viruses (e.g., cytomegalovirus) (CD Fig. 40–74) or bacteria such as *Listeria.*

Proper functioning of the maternal hormones and the trophoblast is necessary for the continuation of a pregnancy. Trophoblast helps maintain the endocrine milieu, initiates implantation, and invades uterine vessels. Reduced trophoblastic penetration into decidua and spiral arteries has been found in the majority of spontaneously expelled abortuses[85, 90] (Fig. 40–18). Trophoblastic columns are thin, and physiologic vascular changes may be absent. This possibly relates to maternal hypertensive disorders or genetic abnormalities in the embryo.

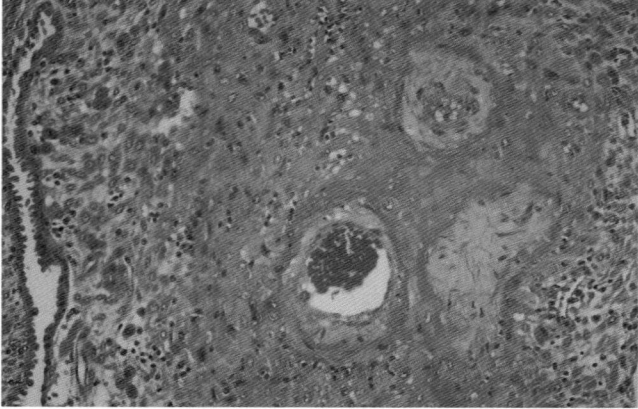

**FIGURE 40–18.** Implantation site tissue in a spontaneous abortion reveals numerous trophoblastic cells and the decidua. The maternal decidual vessels are abnormal, however; they appear inadequately transformed and show intimal proliferation.

Placental pathologic features associated with maternal anticardiolipin antibodies are well recognized and include vascular changes in the decidual blood vessels and ischemic villus changes.[5] This disorder more often causes problems after the first trimester, although some early gestational loss is recognized. Heritable thrombotic disorders appear to also play a role in fetal loss.[54–56] Although clinical data suggest that there may be other immunologic abnormalities associated with spontaneous abortion, few histopathologic features have been described except for immunologic marking of cells in the decidua.[5]

Three or more consecutive spontaneous abortions characterize habitual abortion. A variety of factors are associated, including anatomic, structural, genetic, hormonal, autoimmune, and infectious. Precise dating of the loss by use of the developmental scheme is particularly helpful in assessing the etiology of recurrent loss.

## Minimal Diagnostic Criteria for Intrauterine Pregnancy

It is now recognized that chorionic villi are not necessary for a diagnosis of intrauterine pregnancy.[15] A uterine site of implantation is equally definitive. This change includes trophoblastic cells and typical alterations of blood vessels and stroma by trophoblast. Typically, one sees dense perivascular fibrin deposition containing largely uninucleated and occasionally multinucleated intermediate trophoblastic cells. Vessels are invaded by trophoblast, often with intraluminal cells. Such areas stand out at low power from the bland decidual tissue and loose fibrin of blood clot. If it is unclear whether certain cells are trophoblastic, a keratin stain can be used (CD Fig. 40–75). This will stain trophoblastic cells (and endometrial glandular cells, if present, as an internal control) but not decidual cells. One should be wary of isolated multinucleated giant cells admixed with blood because macrophages are frequently present from cervical material. It is also possible that isolated trophoblastic cells (or possibly even a villus) could have derived from an ectopic pregnancy, particularly a cornual one.

Pathologists have often felt compelled to exhaustively search a specimen to document intrauterine pregnancy, submitting and leveling blood clot and obvious decidual tissue in an attempt to find an implantation site or villi. This usually proves futile if the original selection of material was inappropriate. It is also often clinically unnecessary with today's sensitive diagnostic modalities.

## GESTATIONAL TROPHOBLASTIC DISEASE

Gestational trophoblastic disease is an abnormal proliferation of trophoblastic tissue, reflecting its in-

**TABLE 40–8.** World Health Organization Histopathologic Classification of Gestational Trophoblastic Disease

Hydatidiform mole
    Partial hydatidiform mole
    Complete hydatidiform mole
Invasive mole
Choriocarcinoma
Placental site trophoblastic tumor
Miscellaneous trophoblastic lesion
    Exaggerated placental site
    Placental site nodules and plaques
Unclassified lesions

Adapted from Silverberg SG, Kurman RJ: Tumors of the Uterine Corpus and Gestational Trophoblastic Disease. Atlas of Tumor Pathology. Third Series, Fascicle 3. Washington, DC, Armed Forces Institute of Pathology, 1992.

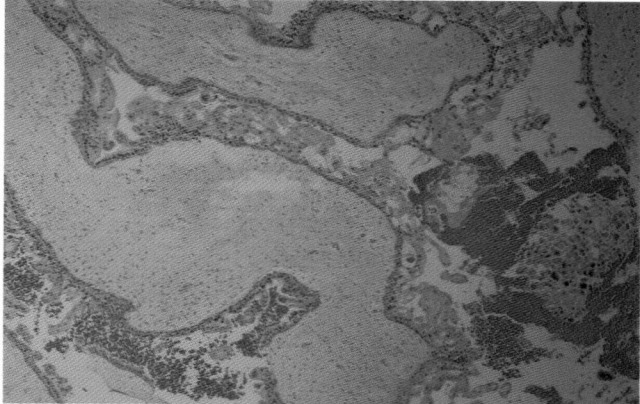

**FIGURE 40–19.** Complete hydatidiform mole with abundant trophoblastic proliferation on the surface and edematous stroma.

herent capacity for invasiveness. Some lesions contain villus structures, others do not. Historically, gestational trophoblastic disease was classified into three well-defined types—hydatidiform mole, invasive mole, and choriocarcinoma. The current World Health Organization classification of trophoblastic disease is presented in Table 40–8.[91, 92] There are additional categories, some of which overlap with spontaneous abortion and implantation site reactions. The surgical pathology of gestational trophoblastic disease has also undergone remarkable changes. The advent of sensitive tests for human chorionic gonadotropin (HCG) and of effective chemotherapy for obliteration of trophoblastic disease has somewhat lessened the critical nature of pathologic diagnosis in these disorders. Serial serum values are easily followed in questionable cases. Ultrasonography with early diagnosis and evacuation has also led to more specimens that do not fit with the classically described entities.

## Hydatidiform Mole

Hydatidiform moles are now divided into complete and partial forms.[22, 23] The classic complete hydatidiform mole is readily recognized. It is composed of free translucent vesicles ("bunches of grapes") without recognizable placenta or fetus (CD Fig. 40–76). All villi are dilated to varying degrees, ranging from a few millimeters to several centimeters. The villi are histologically largely avascular, and larger ones show central cisternae. No blood is present in the occasional vessel. Proliferation of cytotrophoblast and syncytiotrophoblast is present on the surface of the villi, showing a haphazard, often circumferential arrangement (Fig. 40–19) (CD Fig. 40–77). The typical polar cap of syncytiotrophoblast overlying cytotrophoblastic that is noted on young avascular villi of early pregnancy is not present. Free aggregates of trophoblastic cells are common. The placental site reaction tends to be exaggerated with numerous giant cells in the myometrium (CD Fig. 40–78). Early

complete moles may be difficult to recognize, showing few of the classically described morphologic features.[93] They are characterized by richly cellular vasculogenic stroma with focal necrobiotic cells. Vessels may be present but are empty of blood. Edema is present early in the stroma, gradually collecting into the more characteristic cisterns. Even in early moles, the trophoblast is hyperplastic, with both layers involved.

A syndrome of partial hydatidiform mole has been distinguished from complete mole.[23, 94] Here there is organization of the villus tissue into a placenta, and a fetus or embryo is often found (CD Fig. 40–79). The villi display a variable pattern. Some are edematous with cisterns (molar), whereas others are small and sometimes fibrotic (Fig. 40–20) (CD Fig. 40–80). Capillaries are frequently present and may contain blood. Surface trophoblast, predominantly syncytiotrophoblast, is somewhat hyperplastic, often with a vacuolated appearance to the cytoplasm (CD Fig. 40–81). The outlines of the villi tend to be irregular and maplike, leading to the frequent

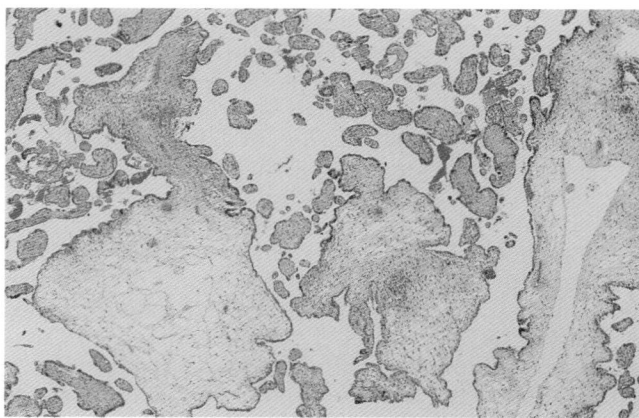

**FIGURE 40–20.** Partial hydatidiform mole with two populations of villi with tortuous outlines, trophoblastic inclusions, and edema in the larger ones. This mole was associated with a karyotype of 69,XXY.

finding of stromal trophoblastic inclusions on section.

Cytogenetic studies reveal that partial moles are usually triploid (69,XXX, XXY, and XYY) from double fertilization by two sperm. The typical true hydatidiform mole is diploid or tetraploid and consists wholly of chromosomes of paternal origin (androgenetic). Thus, both types of moles have a predominance of paternal genes, which is implicated in causing the hydropic change. Flow cytometry of molar pregnancies can also determine the ploidy of an individual case; however, only those triploids with paternal origin of the extra chromosome set are molar.[22, 23]

Treatment of all moles is by uterine evacuation. The concentration of the $\beta$ subunit of HCG is rarely above 100,000 mIU in a partial mole. HCG levels are followed, looking for a plateau or rise that indicates persistent disease requiring chemotherapy. The incidence of such disease is 10% to 20% after a complete mole but 5% or less after a partial mole. Choriocarcinoma is extremely rare after a partial mole. The majority of patients with complete and partial moles later have normal pregnancies.

## Invasive Mole

Invasive mole is probably the most common form of persistent trophoblastic disease, but it is rarely diagnosed by histologic examination. Persistent HCG elevations indicate its presence, and most cases are adequately treated by chemotherapy. Invasive moles are occasionally seen as pathologic specimens when complications necessitate hysterectomy (CD Fig. 40–82). In such cases, histologic examination shows villi, typical of a classic mole, extending into the uterine wall. The diagnosis cannot usually be made on evacuated material.

## Choriocarcinoma

Choriocarcinoma is a true malignant neoplasm of trophoblastic cells.[91, 92, 95] Approximately 50% follow molar pregnancies. The remainder occur after spontaneous abortions and ectopic or intrauterine pregnancies. In gross appearance, choriocarcinoma is an extremely hemorrhagic lesion in both primary and metastatic sites. Microscopic examination shows a haphazard mixture of cytotrophoblast and syncytiotrophoblast (CD Figs. 40–83 and 40–84). The syncytiotrophoblast may be extensively vacuolated. In general, anaplasia is not striking but may be present. No molar villi are seen, and their presence precludes the diagnosis. Patients with choriocarcinoma usually present with bleeding after a molar or other pregnancy. Treatment with multiagent chemotherapy is usually curative, and later normal pregnancy is possible. Choriocarcinoma follows some term pregnancies, and several reports have found foci of choriocarcinoma in term placentas more frequently than was previously thought[96, 97] (CD Fig. 40–85).

## Placental Site Trophoblastic Tumor

Placental site trophoblastic tumor is an uncommon lesion composed of confluent uninucleated and multinucleated intermediate trophoblastic cells that invade myometrium and blood vessels, mimicking a normal implantation site with abundant fibrin.[92, 98] The cells have abundant clear to eosinophilic cytoplasm (CD Figs. 40–86 and 40–87). Placental site trophoblastic tumors secrete predominantly human placental lactogen and a small amount of HCG. This tumor tends to present with irregular bleeding and a uterine mass, and it may perforate the uterus. Differentiation from normal and exaggerated placental sites may be difficult; however, placental site trophoblastic tumors usually follow term pregnancies, not early ones. About 10% to 15% of cases behave in a malignant fashion. Treatment is surgical because there is a poor response to chemotherapy.

## Placental Site Lesions

As described previously, the placental site is largely composed of intermediate trophoblastic cells. These cells are involved in several benign placental site processes.[92, 98] The exaggerated placental site reaction (syncytial endometritis) is usually seen shortly after a pregnancy (CD Fig. 40–88). It contains multinucleated and uninucleated intermediate cells. Although there may be large masses of cells, the underlying architecture is retained. Placental site nodules and plaques are much less cellular and show hyalinized material surrounding the intermediate cells (CD Figs. 40–89 and 40–90). These are remnants of former gestations and may be found years later.

## OTHER PREGNANCY-RELATED LESIONS

### Retained Products of Conception

Placental tissue remaining in the uterus after delivery or spontaneous abortion leads to incomplete uterine contraction and continued bleeding. Evacuation of such material is usually therapeutic. One often finds hyalinized, infarcted placental tissue along with the placental site, usually with some degree of subinvolution.

### Subinvolution of the Placental Site

The placental site normally involutes in the weeks after delivery with obliteration of the blood vessel lumina through contraction and thrombosis[5] (Fig. 40–21). Postpartum bleeding may be related to fail-

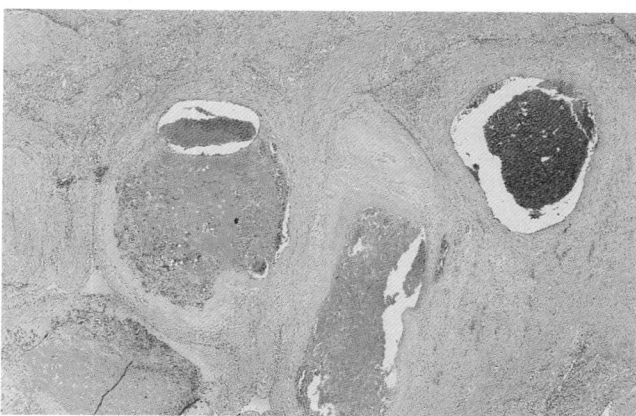

FIGURE 40–21. Subinvolution of the placental site. The placental site vessels are not fully involuted and show open, only partially thrombosed lumina. This curettage specimen was associated with continued hemorrhage 2 weeks after delivery.

ure of this physiologic process to occur, with open vessel lumina with incompletely formed thrombi. Bleeding may be delayed and occur days or even weeks later. This diagnosis is made only in the absence of retained placental tissue.

## Placenta Accreta

If invasion of the placental tissue fails to stop before the myometrium is reached, an abnormally adherent placenta results. Placenta accreta goes to the myometrium, placenta increta invades the myometrium, and placenta percreta perforates the myometrium.[5, 7] The absence of decidua between the base of the placenta and the myometrium is necessary for the diagnosis of placenta accreta. The large cells noted at the base of such placentas are usually trophoblastic, not decidual. It is unusual to make a diagnosis of these processes on a delivered placenta or material obtained by curettage, but it is much easier in hysterectomy specimens (CD Figs. 40–91 and 40–92). The occurrence of placenta accreta seems to be increasing, possibly owing to the increased numbers of cesarean deliveries.

## MEDICOLEGAL ASPECTS

Lawyers are increasingly turning to the placenta for information in medicolegal cases related to poor pregnancy outcomes for the mother and infant.[58, 99] Cases involving meconium staining, infection, prematurity, or bleeding and cases resulting in hysterectomy or fetal or maternal death are common. The legal nature of a case may not be apparent at the time of specimen examination; thus, it is important in all gestational specimens to institute "universal precautions," which includes good documentation of gross aspects and appropriate sectioning.

## REFERENCES

1. Altshuler G: Role of the placenta in perinatal pathology (revisited). Pediatr Pathol Lab Med 16:207–233, 1996.
2. Naeye RL: Disorders of the Placenta, Fetus, and Neonate: Diagnosis and Clinical Significance. St. Louis, CV Mosby, 1992.
3. Kaplan CG: Embryonic pathology of the placenta. *In* Lewis SH, Perrin E (eds): Pathology of the Placenta. 2nd ed. Philadelphia, Churchill Livingstone, 1999, pp 89–106.
4. Lewis SH, Benirschke K: Overview of placental pathology and justification for examination of the placenta. *In* Lewis SH, Perrin E (eds): Pathology of the Placenta. 2nd ed. Philadelphia, Churchill Livingstone, 1999, pp 1–47.
5. Benirschke K, Kaufmann P: Pathology of the Human Placenta. 3rd ed. New York, Springer-Verlag, 1995.
6. Fox H: Pathology of the Placenta. Philadelphia, WB Saunders, 1997.
7. Rushton DH: Pathology of the placenta. *In* Wigglesworth JS, Singer DB (eds): Textbook of Fetal and Perinatal Pathology. 2nd ed. Malden, MA, Blackwell Science, 1998, pp 145–199.
8. Langston C, Kaplan C, Macpherson T, et al: Practice guideline for the examination of the placenta: developed by the Placental Pathology Practice Guideline Development Task Force of the College of American Pathologists. Arch Pathol Lab Med 121:449–476, 1997.
9. Kaplan C: Color Atlas of Gross Placental Pathology. New York, Igaku-Shoin, 1994.
10. Kaplan C: Postpartum examination of the placenta. Clin Obstet Gynecol 39:535–548, 1996.
11. Gersell DJ: ASCP survey on placental examination. J Clin Pathol 109:127–143, 1998.
12. Ellish NJ, Saboda K, O'Connor J, et al: A prospective study of early pregnancy loss. Hum Reprod 11:406–412, 1996.
13. Warburton D, Fraser CF: Spontaneous abortion risks in man: data from reproductive histories collected in a medical genetics center. Am J Hum Genet 16:1–25, 1964.
14. Rushton DI: The classification and mechanism of spontaneous abortion. Perspect Pediatr Pathol 8:269–287, 1984.
15. O'Connor DM, Kurman RJ: Intermediate trophoblast in uterine curetting in the diagnosis of ectopic pregnancy. Obstet Gynecol 72:665–670, 1988.
16. Heatley MK, Clark J: The value of histopathologic examination of conceptual products. Br J Obstet Gynaecol 102:256–258, 1995.
17. Poland BJ, Miller JR, Harris M, Livingston J: Spontaneous abortion: a study of 1961 women and their conceptuses. Acta Obstet Gynecol Scand Suppl 102:1–32, 1981.
18. Kalousek DK, Pantzar T, Tsai M, Paradice B: Early spontaneous abortion: morphologic and karyotypic findings in 3,912 cases. Birth Defects Orig Artic Ser 29:53–61, 1993.
19. Kalousek DK: Pathology of abortion: the embryo and the previable fetus. *In* Gilbert-Barness E (ed): Potter's Pathology of the Fetus and Infant. St. Louis, CV Mosby, 1997, pp 106–127.
20. Laurini RN: Abortion from a morphological viewpoint. *In* Huisjes HJ, Lind T (eds): Early Pregnancy Failure. New York, Churchill Livingstone, 1990, pp 79–113.
21. Lage JM, Wolf NG: Gestational trophoblastic disease: new approaches to diagnosis. Clin Lab Med 15:631–664, 1995.
22. Gschwendtner A, Neher A, Kreczy A, et al: DNA ploidy determination of early molar pregnancies by image analysis: comparison to histologic classification. Arch Pathol Lab Med 122:1000–1004, 1998.
23. Szulman AE: Trophoblastic diseases: complete and partial hydatidiform moles. *In* Lewis SH, Perrin E (eds): Pathology of the Placenta. 2nd ed. Philadelphia, Churchill Livingstone, 1999, pp 259–281.
24. Paradinas FJ, Fisher RA, Browne P, Newlands ES: Diploid hydatidiform moles with fetal red blood cells in molar villi: pathology, incidence, and prognosis. J Pathol 181:183–188, 1997.
25. Kalousek DK, Robinson W, Harrington B, et al: Molecular biology of the placenta with focus on special placental studies of infants with intrauterine growth retardation. *In* Lewis SH,

Perrin E (eds): Pathology of the Placenta. 2nd ed. Philadelphia, Churchill Livingstone, 1999, pp 343–365.

26. Popek EJ: Normal anatomy and histology of the placenta. *In* Lewis SH, Perrin E (eds): Pathology of the Placenta. 2nd ed. Philadelphia, Churchill Livingstone, 1999, pp 49–88.

27. Moore KL, Persaud TVN: The Developing Human. 6th ed. Philadelphia, WB Saunders, 1998.

28. Benirschke K: Anatomical relationship between fetus and mother. Ann N Y Acad Sci 731:9–20, 1994.

29. Salafia CM, Weigl CA, Foye GJ: Correlation of placental erythrocyte morphology and gestational age. Pediatr Pathol 8: 495–502, 1988.

30. Heifetz SA: Pathology of the umbilical cord. *In* Lewis SH, Perrin E (eds): Pathology of the Placenta. 2nd ed. Philadelphia, Churchill Livingstone, 1999, pp 107–135.

31. Kaplan C, August D, Mizrachi H: Single umbilical artery and cord accidents. Mod Pathol 3:87a, 1990.

32. Lewis SH, Gilbert-Barness E: Placental membranes. *In* Lewis SH, Perrin E (eds): Pathology of the Placenta. 2nd ed. Philadelphia, Churchill Livingstone, 1999, pp 137–159.

33. Beebe LAA, Altshuler G: The epidemiology of placental features: associations with gestational age and neonatal outcome. Obstet Gynecol 87:771–778, 1996.

34. Miller PW, Coen RW, Benirschke K: Dating the time interval from meconium passage to birth. Obstet Gynecol 66:459–462, 1985.

35. Altshuler G, Orizawa M, Molnar-Nadasdy G: Meconium-induced umbilical cord vascular necrosis and ulceration: a potential link between the placenta and poor pregnancy outcome. Obstet Gynecol 79:760–766, 1992.

36. Altshuler G, Hyde S: Meconium induced vasoconstriction: a potential cause of cerebral and other fetal hypoperfusion and of poor pregnancy outcome. J Child Neurol 4:137–142, 1989.

37. Piper JM, Newton ER, Berkus MD, et al: Meconium: a marker for peripartum infection. Obstet Gynecol 91:741–745, 1998.

38. Burgess AM, Hutchins GM: Inflammation of the lungs, umbilical cord and placenta associated with meconium passage in utero: review of 123 autopsied cases. Pathol Res Pract 192: 1121–1128, 1996.

39. Molteni RA, Stys SJ, Battaglia FC: Relationship of fetal and placental weight in human beings: fetal/placental weight ratios at various gestational ages and birth weight distributions. J Reprod Med 21:327–334, 1978.

40. Redline RW: Disorders of the placental parenchyma. *In* Lewis SH, Perrin E (eds): Pathology of the Placenta. 2nd ed. Philadelphia, Churchill Livingstone, 1999, pp 160–184.

41. Salafia CM, Pijnenborg R: Disorders of the decidua and maternal vasculature. *In* Lewis SH, Perrin E (eds): Pathology of the Placenta. 2nd ed. Philadelphia, Churchill Livingstone, 1999, pp 185–212.

42. Darby MJ, Caritis SN, Shen-Schwartz S: Placental abruption in the preterm gestation: an association with chorioamnionitis. Obstet Gynecol 74:88–92, 1989.

43. Pearlman MD, Tintinatti JE, Lorenz RP: Blunt trauma during pregnancy. N Engl J Med 323:1608–1613, 1990.

44. Shanklin DR: Chorangiomas and other tumors. *In* Lewis SH, Perrin E (eds): Pathology of the Placenta. 2nd ed. Philadelphia, Churchill Livingstone, 1999, pp 295–315.

45. Ball RA, Genest D, Sander M, et al: Congenital melanocytic nevi with placental infiltration by melanocytes: a benign condition that mimics metastatic melanoma. Arch Dermatol 134: 711–714, 1998.

46. Khong TY, Staples A, Bendon RW, et al: Observer reliability in assessing placental maturity by histology. J Clin Pathol 48: 420–423, 1995.

47. Arias F, Rodriquez L, Rayne SC, et al: Maternal placental vasculopathy and infection: two distinct subgroups among patients with preterm labor and preterm ruptured membranes. Am J Obstet Gynecol 168:585–591, 1993.

48. Hyde SR, Altshuler GA: Infectious disorders of the placenta. *In* Lewis SH, Perrin E (eds): Pathology of the Placenta. 2nd ed. Philadelphia, Churchill Livingstone, 1999, pp 317–342.

49. Jacques SM, Qureshi F: Chronic intervillositis of the placenta. Arch Pathol Lab Med 117:1032–1035, 1993.

50. Gersell DJ: Chronic villitis, chronic chorioamnionitis, and maternal floor infarction. Semin Diagn Pathol 10:251–266, 1993.

51. Altshuler G: Chorangiosis: an important placental sign of neonatal morbidity and mortality. Arch Pathol Lab Med 108:71–74, 1984.

52. Reshetnikova OS, Burton GJ, Milovanov AP, et al: Increased incidence of placental chorioangioma in high-altitude pregnancies: hypobaric hypoxia as a possible etiologic factor. Am J Obstet Gynecol 174:557–561, 1996.

53. Genest DR: Estimating the time of death in stillborn fetuses: II. Histologic evaluation of the placenta. Obstet Gynecol 80: 585–592, 1992.

54. Preston FE, Rosendaal FR, Walker ID, et al: Increased fetal loss in women with heritable thrombophilia. Lancet 348:913–966, 1996.

55. Brenner B, Blumenfeld Z: Thrombophilia and fetal loss. Blood Res 11:72–79, 1997.

56. Arias F, Romero R, Joist H, et al: Thrombophilia: a mechanism of disease in women with adverse pregnancy outcome and thrombotic lesions in the placenta. J Matern Fetal Med 7: 277–286, 1998.

57. Kraus FT: Cerebral palsy and thrombi in placental vessels of the fetus: insights from litigation. Hum Pathol 28:246–248, 1997.

58. Kaplan C: Forensic aspects of the placenta. Perspect Pediatr Pathol 19:20–42, 1995.

59. Blanc WA: Pathology of the placenta, membranes and umbilical cord in bacterial, fungal and viral infections. *In* Naeye RL, Kissane JM, Kaufman N (eds): Perinatal Disease. Baltimore, Williams & Wilkins, 1981, pp 67–132.

60. Salafia CM, Weigl C, Silberman L: The prevalence and distribution of acute placental inflammation in uncomplicated term pregnancies. Obstet Gynecol 73:383–389, 1989.

61. Romero R, Salafia CM, Athanassiadis, AP, et al: The relationship between acute inflammatory lesions of the preterm placental and amniotic fluid microbiology. Am J Obstet Gynecol 166:1382–1388, 1992.

62. van Hoeven KH, Anyaegbunam A, Hochster H, et al: Clinical significance of increasing histologic severity of acute inflammation in the fetal membranes and umbilical cord. Pediatr Pathol Lab Med 16:731–744, 1996.

63. Belady PH, Farkouh LJ, Gibbs RS: Intraamniotic infection and premature rupture of the membranes. Clin Perinatol 24:43–57, 1997.

64. Gibbs RS, Eschembach DA: Use of antibiotics to prevent preterm birth. Am J Obstet Gynecol 177:375–380, 1997.

65. Hyde S, Smotherman J, Moore JL, et al: A model of bacterially induced umbilical vein spasm, relevant to fetal hypoperfusion. Obstet Gynecol 73:966–970, 1989.

66. Salafia CM, Mangam HE, Weigl CA, et al: Abnormal fetal heart rate patterns and placental inflammation. Am J Obstet Gynecol 160:140–147, 1989.

67. Grether JK, Nelson KB: Maternal infection and cerebral palsy in infants of normal birth weight. JAMA 278:207–211, 1997.

68. Jacques SM, Qureshi F: Necrotizing funisitis: a study of 45 cases. Hum Pathol 23:1278–1283, 1992.

69. Kaplan C: Viral infections and the placenta. Semin Diagn Pathol 10:232–250, 1993.

70. Anderson VM: The placental barrier to maternal HIV infection. Obstet Gynecol Clin North Am 24:797–820, 1997.

71. Khong TY, Chambers HM: Alternative method of sampling placentas for the assessment of uteroplacental vasculature. J Clin Pathol 45:925–927, 1992.

72. Meekins JW, Pijnenborg R, Hanssens M, et al: A study of placental bed spiral arteries and trophoblast invasion in normal and severe pre-eclamptic pregnancies. Br J Obstet Gynaecol 101:669–674, 1994.

73. Baldwin VJ: Pathology of Multiple Pregnancy. New York, Springer-Verlag, 1994.

74. Baldwin VJ: Placental pathology and multiple gestation. *In* Lewis SH, Perrin E (eds): Pathology of the Placenta. 2nd ed. Philadelphia, Churchill Livingstone, 1999, pp 213–257.

75. Dennis LG, Winkler CL: Twin-to-twin transfusion syndrome: aggressive therapeutic amniocentesis. Am J Obstet Gynecol 177:342–349, 1997.

76. Benirschke K: Intrauterine death of a twin: mechanisms, implications for surviving twin and placental pathology. Semin Diagn Pathol 10:222–231, 1993.
77. Szulman AE: Examination of the early conceptus. Arch Pathol Lab Med 115:696–700, 1991.
78. Szulman AE: Embryonic death: pathology and forensic implications. Perspect Pediatr Pathol 19:43–58, 1995.
79. Boue J, Boue A, Lazar P: Retrospective and prospective epidemiologic studies of 1500 karyotypes from spontaneous human abortions. Teratology 12:11–26, 1975.
80. Warburton D, Kline J, Stein Z, et al: Does the karyotype of a spontaneous abortion predict the karyotype of a subsequent abortus? Evidence from 271 women with two karyotyped spontaneous abortions. Am J Hum Genet 41:465–483, 1987.
81. Philippe E, Boue J: Le placenta dans les aberrations chromosomiques léthales. Ann Anat Pathol 14:249–266, 1969.
82. Honore LH, Dill FJ, Poland BJ: Placental morphology in spontaneous human abortuses with normal and abnormal karyotypes. Teratology 14:151–166, 1976.
83. Van Lijnschoten G, Arends JW, Thunnissen FBJM, Geraedts JPM: A morphometric approach to the relation of karyotype, gestational age and histologic features in early spontaneous abortions. Placenta 15:189–200, 1994.
84. Novak R, Agamanolis D, Dasu S, et al: Histologic analysis of placental tissue in first trimester abortions. Pediatr Pathol 8:477–482, 1988.
85. Salafia C, Maier D, Vogel C, et al: Placental and decidual histology in spontaneous abortions: detailed description and correlations with chromosome number. Obstet Gynecol 82:295–303, 1993.
86. Genest DR, Roberts D, Boyd T, Bieber F: Fetoplacental histology as a predictor of karyotype: a controlled study of spontaneous first trimester abortions. Hum Pathol 26:201–209, 1995.
87. Livingston JE, Poland BJ: A study of spontaneously aborted twins. Teratology 21:139–148, 1980.
88. Simpson JL, Gray RH, Queenan JT, et al: Further evidence that infection is an infrequent cause of first trimester spontaneous abortion. Hum Reprod 11:2058–2060, 1996.
89. Joste NE, Kundsin RB, Genest DR: Histology and *Ureaplasma urealyticum* culture in 63 cases of first trimester abortion. Am J Clin Pathol 102:729–732, 1994.
90. Hustin J, Jauniaux E, Schaaps JP: Histologic study of the materno-embryonic interface in spontaneous abortion. Placenta 11:477–486, 1990.
91. Silverberg SG, Kurman RJ: Tumors of the Uterine Corpus and Gestational Trophoblastic Disease. Atlas of Tumor Pathology. Third Series, Fascicle 3. Washington, DC, Armed Forces Institute of Pathology, 1992.
92. Heller D: Gestational trophoblastic disease. *In* Lewis SH, Perrin E (eds): Pathology of the Placenta. 2nd ed. Philadelphia, Churchill Livingstone, 1999, pp 283–294.
93. Keep D, Zaragoza MV, Hassold T, et al: Very early complete hydatidiform mole. Hum Pathol 27:708–713, 1996.
94. McFadden DE, Pantzar JT: Placental pathology of triploidy. Hum Pathol 27:1018–1020, 1996.
95. Baergen RN: Gestational choriocarcinoma. Gen Diagn Pathol 143:127–141, 1997.
96. Fukunaga M, Nomura K, Ushigome S: Choriocarcinoma in situ at first trimester: report of two cases indicating an origin of trophoblast of a stem villus. Virchows Arch 429:185–188, 1996.
97. Flam F: Choriocarcinoma in the term placenta: a difficult diagnosis. Eur J Gynaecol Oncol 17:510–511, 1996.
98. Baergen RN: Trophoblastic lesions of the placental site. Gen Diagn Pathol 143:143–158, 1997.
99. Naeye RL: The placenta: medicolegal considerations. *In* Lewis SH, Perrin E (eds): Pathology of the Placenta. 2nd ed. Philadelphia, Churchill Livingstone, 1999, pp 387–399.

# 41

# *Lymph Nodes*

Karen L. Chang    Daniel A. Arber    Lawrence M. Weiss

Enlarged peripheral lymph nodes are among the tissues most frequently examined by biopsy in both children and adults. Enlarged lymph nodes are often readily accessible and may yield diagnoses of disorders from which they are distant, thereby obviating the necessity for biopsy at less amenable sites. Lymph node biopsy specimens may yield evidence of benign reactive lymphadenopathies, infectious processes, metabolic disorders, and metastatic tumors, or these nodes may be the sites of primary lymph node neoplasms, namely, malignant lymphomas.

Despite many technical advances in pathology, specifically in the areas of lymph node diseases, complete clinical information is absolutely essential to arrive at an accurate diagnosis. This point cannot be emphasized enough, for a pertinent history often guides the pathologist to a proper and narrow set of differential diagnoses. Relevant history is particularly important when the amount of tissue submit-

ted for microscopic examination is small, such as in fine-needle aspiration biopsy or radiographically guided needle biopsies.

## SPECIMEN TYPES

### Excisional Lymph Node Biopsy

An excised lymph node biopsy specimen should be received fresh (not in fixative), intact, and preferably sterile. Placing the specimen on a dry towel or sponge introduces morphologic artifacts. If a long time between removal in the operating room and receipt in the surgical pathology laboratory is anticipated, the node should be placed in sterile saline, with the caveat that this may introduce undesirable histologic artifacts into any subsequent frozen section studies.

One should first harvest tissue for sterile studies, which may include microbiologic cultures and cytogenetic studies, if clinically indicated.[1] For cases expected to be diagnostically difficult, the pathologist should prepare touch imprints and smear preparations, the results of which may help guide how to process the remainder of the tissue. Cytologic features are demonstrated in touch and rapidly fixed scrape preparations as well as or even better than in paraffin sections. As an alternative, one may wish to prepare a rapid frozen section, which can help determine adequacy of the tissue, establish a tentative diagnosis, and determine which special studies may be particularly useful to obtain. Only a small piece of tissue should be frozen, and if necessary, this piece may be kept frozen for possible future frozen section immunohistochemical studies or molecular studies. Fresh tissue for potential future studies (flow cytometry and molecular studies) should also be taken at this time. If a metastatic tumor is a possibility, a small piece could also be appropriately fixed for electron microscopy, which has diagnostic utility for some sarcomas.

Frozen section diagnosis of hematolymphoid disorders can be reliable, as long as one recognizes the technique's limitations, the primary one being the lack of cytologic detail. Distinctions that can be made in high-quality frozen sections include benign versus malignant, hematolymphoid versus nonhematolymphoid, Hodgkin's versus non-Hodgkin's lymphoma, and low-grade versus high-grade non-Hodgkin's lymphoma. One should provide as much of a diagnosis that is necessary for immediate clinical decisions, and of course, one should avoid making distinctions that are not needed rapidly. In addition, one should defer making the diagnosis when significant doubt exists.

### Needle Core Biopsies

Advances in radiographic techniques often allow procurement of tissue with minimal morbidity. Many patients undergo ultrasonography-guided needle core biopsy or percutaneous needle biopsy for their primary tissue diagnosis of lymphoma.[2] The cores are often few in number and small in size. Therefore, rapid cytologic and frozen section assessments are not recommended. For these tissues, the choice of ancillary techniques may be severely limited because of the tissue requirements for cytogenetics, molecular studies, or flow cytometric studies. Paraffin section immunohistochemistry may be the only feasible adjunct technique.

### Fine-Needle Aspiration Biopsy

Fine-needle aspiration biopsy is often used for the evaluation of lymphadenopathy.[3] This technique may help answer numerous clinical questions, including whether a suspected enlarged lymph node is indeed lymphoid tissue or whether there is metastatic tumor. Fine-needle aspiration can also be used to obtain material for special studies, including culture, immunophenotyping studies, and molecular studies.[4] The cytologic preparations can also lead to diagnoses of reactive hyperplasia, infectious lymphadenitis, transformation of lymphoma, and residual or recurrent lymphoma.[5, 6] Diagnosis and staging of Hodgkin's disease and non-Hodgkin's lymphomas can also be accomplished with use of fine-needle aspiration biopsy. The efficacy of the technique varies with the clinical setting. Fine-needle aspiration biopsy is probably best used in cases in which reactive hyperplasia is suspected and is probably least effective in cases in which the initial diagnosis of a non-Hodgkin's lymphoma is the primary clinical consideration.

## TISSUE FIXATIVES

Prompt and proper tissue fixation is more important than choice of fixative in the preparation of optimal histologic sections. The sections should be thinly cut and not underfixed (underfixation may hinder morphologic interpretation) or overfixed (overfixation may hinder immunohistochemical studies). If formalin is used as the primary fixative, it should be freshly prepared and at the proper pH. Some pathologists use a second fixative, usually a metal-based fixative such as B5, for fixation of lymph nodes to better evaluate nuclear features. H&E-stained sections are usually adequate for morphologic interpretation, but some pathologists supplement this with reticulin–van Gieson (to evaluate the architecture), Giemsa (to better visualize the nuclear features), and methyl green–pyronin stains (to get a rough estimate of the RNA content of the cytoplasm).

## SPECIAL STUDIES

### Paraffin Section Immunohistochemistry

Paraffin section immunohistochemical studies are an important adjunct technique to standard morphologic examination, particularly for diagnostically difficult cases. The particular antibodies used for any one case depend on the differential diagnosis suggested by the morphologic features.

Many of the important leukocyte antigens easily detectable in paraffin sections are listed in Table 41–1. Some suggested panels are given in Table 41–2. Immunohistochemical stains may provide an indication of cell lineage and may help identify the immunologic compartments of the lymph node. In some cases, the immunohistochemical stains can provide an assessment of malignancy, with use of specific

**TABLE 41–1.** Commonly Used Major Leukocyte Antigens Detectable in Paraffin Sections*

| Antibody | Predominant Hematolymphoid Cell Expression |
|---|---|
| ALK | Anaplastic large cell lymphomas that express t(2;5) |
| Bcl-1 | Mantle cell lymphoma |
| Bcl-2 | Non–germinal center B cells, most T cells, most follicular lymphomas, many low-grade and some higher grade B cell lymphomas |
| DBA.44 | Hairy cells, B cells |
| Elastase | Granulocytic tumors, leukemia |
| Epithelial membrane antigen | Plasma cells and plasma cell neoplasms, many cases of nodular L&H lymphocyte predominance, anaplastic large cell lymphoma, and T cell–rich B cell lymphoma |
| EBV latent membrane protein | Some EBV-infected cells, including EBV⁺ Hodgkin cells, post-transplantation lymphoproliferative disorders, and EBV-associated infectious mononucleosis |
| Fascin | Dendritic cells, Reed-Sternberg cells |
| Granzyme B | Natural killer cells and cytotoxic T cells |
| Hemoglobin A | Nucleated erythroid cells (benign and neoplastic) |
| HLA-DR | B cells, interdigitating cells, Langerhans cells, immature granulocytes and erythroid cells |
| Immunoglobulin light and heavy chains | Plasma cells, plasma cell and plasmacytoid neoplasms, some follicular and marginal zone lymphomas |
| Ki-67 (MIB-1) | Proliferating cells |
| Lysozyme | Histiocytes-monocytes and myeloid cells (benign and neoplastic) |
| Myeloperoxidase | Myeloid cells (benign and neoplastic) |
| Perforin | Cytotoxic T cells and natural killer cells |
| TdT | Thymic lymphoid cells, lymphoblastic neoplasms, and some myeloid neoplasms |
| TIA-1 | Cytotoxic T cells and natural killer cells |
| CD1a | Thymocytes, some T lymphoblastic lymphomas, and Langerhans cells |
| CD2 | T cells and T cell lymphomas |
| CD3 | T cells and many T cell lymphomas |
| CD4 | Histiocytes and histiocytic neoplasms, T helper cells, and many T cell lymphomas |
| CD5 | T cells and many T cell lymphomas, B small lymphocytic lymphoma/chronic lymphocytic leukemia, mantle cell lymphoma |
| CD7 | T cells, some T cell neoplasms, some myeloid leukemias |
| CD8 | T cytotoxic-suppressor cells, some T cell lymphomas |
| CD10 (CALLA) | Precursor B cells and B lymphoblastic neoplasms, many follicular lymphomas |
| CD15 | Myeloid cells, Hodgkin's disease, rare non-Hodgkin's lymphomas |
| CD16 | Natural killer cells and neoplasms; some myeloid cells |
| CD20 | B cells and B cell lymphomas, nodular L&H lymphocyte predominance |
| CD21 | Follicular dendritic cells and neoplasms; mantle and marginal zone B cells |
| CD23 | Mantle zone B cells and most B small lymphocytic lymphoma/chronic lymphocytic leukemia |
| CD30 | Activated lymphoid cells, Hodgkin's disease, anaplastic large cell lymphoma |
| CD34 | Progenitor cells, some myeloid and lymphoblastic neoplasms |
| CD35 | Follicular dendritic cells and neoplasms |
| CD43 | T cells, myeloid cells, mast cells, T cell lymphomas, some B cell lymphomas, myeloid leukemia, mast cell neoplasms |
| CD45/CD45RB | All hematolymphoid cells, nodular L&H lymphocyte predominance; relatively low expression in anaplastic large cell lymphoma and lymphoblastic neoplasms; not on Reed-Sternberg cells |
| CD45RA | B cells and subset of T cells, B cell lymphomas, nodular L&H lymphocyte predominance |
| CD45RO | Most T cells, histiocytes, myeloid cells, T cell lymphomas |
| CD56 | Natural killer cells and subset of T cell lymphomas |
| CD57 | Subset of T cells and natural killer cells, subset of T cell lymphomas |
| CD61 | Megakaryocytes (including dysplastic and neoplastic forms) |
| CD68 | Histiocytes, myeloid cells, mast cells and neoplasms, some non-Hodgkin's lymphomas |
| CD79a | Immature and mature B cells and lymphomas, plasma cells and plasma cell neoplasms |
| CD99 | Lymphoblastic lymphoma-leukemia |
| CD117 | Immature myeloid cells |
| CD138 | Plasma cells, plasma cell lesions |

*These antibodies are also reactive in frozen sections.

antibodies (e.g., Bcl-2 expression in neoplastic follicles) or groups of antibodies (e.g., aberrant CD20 and CD43 coexpression in low-grade B cell lymphomas or immunoglobulin light chain restriction).[7-22] One may also use these stains to highlight the presence of a particular cell population (e.g., immunoblasts or Reed-Sternberg cells) or particular nodal structure (e.g., follicles) or to measure cell proliferation of different cell populations.[23-26] An even wider range of antibodies can be used in cell suspension studies or acetone-fixed frozen sections[27, 28] (Table 41–3).

## Flow Cytometry

Flow cytometric studies are particularly useful for quantifying immunoglobulin light chain ratios and

**TABLE 41–2.** Suggested Panels for the Diagnosis of Lymphoma

Is the tumor a hematolymphoid or nonhematolymphoid neoplasm?
 Keratin, S-100, CD45/CD45RB (initial panel)
 (CD30, CD20, and CD43) (second line)
Is this a non-Hodgkin's lymphoma or Hodgkin's disease?
 CD15, CD20, CD30, CD43, CD45/45RB, (EBV latent membrane protein)
Is this classical Hodgkin's or nodular L&H lymphocyte predominant Hodgkin's disease?
 CD15, CD20, CD30, CD43, CD45/45RB, CD57, EBV latent membrane protein, (epithelial membrane antigen), (fascin)
Is this reactive follicular hyperplasia or follicular lymphoma?
 Bcl-2, CD10, CD20, CD43, (immunoglobulin light chains)
Is this follicular lymphoma or another lymphoma?
 Bcl-2, CD5, CD10, CD20, CD23, CD43, (CD21)
Is this extranodal diffuse B cell lymphoma or lymphoid hyperplasia?
 Bcl-2, CD20, CD43, (immunoglobulin light chains, if plasmacytoid)
Is this small lymphocytic lymphoma or another lymphoma?
 Bcl-2, CD5, CD20, CD23, CD43
Is this marginal zone B cell lymphoma or marginal zone B cell hyperplasia?
 Bcl-2, CD20, CD43
Is this mantle cell lymphoma or another lymphoma?
 Bcl-1, Bcl-2, CD5, CD10, CD20, CD23, CD43
Is this a benign or malignant plasmacytoid proliferation?
 Immunoglobulin light chains, CD20, CD43, CD138, (CD79a)
Is this plasmacytoma or a plasmacytoid lymphoma?
 CD20, CD43, CD45/45RB, immunoglobulin light chains, immunoglobulin heavy chains
Is this B cell lymphoma or peripheral T cell lymphoma?
 CD3, CD20, CD43, CD30 (initial panel)
 (CD2, CD45RO, CD45RA, CD79a as second panel)
 (CD4, CD5, CD7, CD8 if needed)
Is this peripheral T cell lymphoma or hyperplasia?
 CD2, CD3, CD4, CD5, CD7, CD8
Is this lymphoblastic lymphoma or another lymphoma?
 CD1, CD3, CD43, CD79a, CD99, TdT
Is this lymphoblastic lymphoma or thymoma?
 CD1, CD43, CD79a, CD99, keratin, TdT
Is this lymphoblastic lymphoma or blastic variant of mantle cell lymphoma?
 Bcl-1, CD1, CD3, CD5, CD20, CD43, CD79a, CD99, TdT
Is this lymphoblastic leukemia or myeloid leukemia?
 CD3, CD10, CD20, CD43, myeloperoxidase, CD79a, TdT
Is this acute promyelocytic leukemia or another acute nonlymphocytic leukemia?
 CD7, CD43, CD79a, HLA-DR, myeloperoxidase

**TABLE 41–3.** Selected Useful Major Leukocyte Antigens Detectable Only in Suspensions or Frozen Sections*

| Antibody | Predominant Hematolymphoid Expression |
|---|---|
| CD11c | Histiocytes and histiocytic neoplasms, M4 and M5 myeloid leukemia, hairy cell leukemia, marginal zone lymphoma |
| CD19 | B cells, precursor B cells, and their neoplasms |
| CD22 | B cells and B cell lymphomas |
| CD25 (TAC) | Activated lymphoid cells, adult T cell lymphoma-leukemia, hairy cell leukemia, most anaplastic large cell lymphomas, most Hodgkin's disease, subsets of other B and T cell lymphomas |
| CD38 | Plasma cells and plasma cell neoplasms, B and T precursor cells and lymphoblastic neoplasms |

*The antibodies from Table 42–1 are also reactive in frozen sections.

## Frozen Section Immunohistochemistry

Frozen section immunohistochemical studies have the advantage of allowing correlation of staining with architecture. However, morphologic features are less than optimally preserved, making it difficult to assign accurate staining profiles to rare cell populations such as Reed-Sternberg cells, particularly when there is staining of adjacent cells. Historically, the increased number of monoclonal antibodies reacting in cell suspension or frozen sections allowed a pathologist to apply additional criteria for malignancy.[27] These criteria included the aberrant absence of immunoglobulin (common in diffuse large cell B cell lymphoma) or other B lineage antigens (uncommon in B cell lymphoma) and the aberrant absence of T lineage antigens in peripheral T cell lymphoma. In addition, these studies were useful in the subclassification of lymphomas. For example, the low-grade B cell lymphomas were more easily subclassified by their differential expression of CD5, CD10, and CD23.[33, 34] However, innovations in paraffin section immunohistochemistry and monoclonal antibody technology have essentially obviated the need for frozen section immunohistochemistry because many antibodies formerly useful only in frozen sections are now available in paraffin tissues.[35-40] Paraffin section immunohistochemistry has two main advantages over other immunologic methods: the tissue does not require special handling, and cytologic and architectural features are well preserved, allowing concurrent interpretation.[41, 42]

Despite the many technical and interpretive advantages of paraffin section immunohistochemistry, frozen section immunohistochemistry still has great clinical utility because some antibodies still work optimally on unfixed or acetone-fixed cells. Thus, frozen sections may offer additional help for diagnosis and subclassification should paraffin section his-

for performing double-labeling studies.[29] Flow cytometric studies can also be used to determine cell proliferation and DNA content, which show correlation with lymphoma grade as well as with specific prognosis.[30-32] Flow cytometry, which is also applicable to fluid specimens such as those obtained by aspiration biopsy, has the advantage of greater sensitivity than immunocytochemical studies on cell smears.[4] Disadvantages of flow cytometry include difficulty in obtaining adequate numbers of cells in fibrotic tissues (particularly in extranodal sites), inability to visualize the individual cells that stain (although one can "gate" on certain populations by differential cell size), and inability to relate the results to specific architectural compartments.

tology and immunohistochemistry be insufficient to establish a definitive diagnosis.

## Molecular Studies

Molecular studies may be extremely useful in the diagnosis and classification of lymphoid neoplasms, particularly for cases in which immunohistochemistry is inconclusive. The detection of clonal immunoglobulin light and heavy chain gene and T cell receptor gene rearrangements offers strong proof of malignancy, with the caveat that the identification of a monoclonal population is not completely synonymous with malignancy.[43–48] Southern blot hybridization has a sensitivity of approximately 1% to 5% for detection of antigen receptor gene rearrangements. However, the test has practical limitations, including the requirement for frozen tissue and a completion time of approximately 2 weeks. Sufficient DNA may be obtained by fine-needle aspiration biopsy.[49]

Polymerase chain reaction (PCR) is the preferred technique for detecting clonality because of its higher sensitivity, faster test time, and ability to use paraffin tissue. In cases with detectable gene rearrangements, the sensitivity of PCR for the detection of lymphoma cells may be high, but there is also a potential for false-positive results because of contamination during the analysis. Both Southern blot hybridization and PCR can be used to accurately assign stage for patients with known lymphoma and to identify recurrent or residual disease; PCR has a higher potential sensitivity.[43]

## Cytogenetic Studies

Cytogenetic studies may be extremely useful in the diagnosis and classification of lymphoid proliferations in selected cases. Certain lymphomas are associated with characteristic cytogenetic abnormalities, usually translocations[50] (see later section on "Non-Hodgkin's Lymphoma").

Cytogenetic abnormalities may be detected by classic metaphase analysis after brief cell culture, by fluorescent in situ hybridization (FISH) on cells in interphase, by Southern blotting, or by PCR. Classic cytogenetics requires fresh, sterile tissue but does not require foreknowledge of any particular abnormality. Classic cytogenetics may reveal a characteristic translocation, but the actual breakpoint may occur in widely varying locations in the genome at the molecular level. Thus, Southern blot hybridization and PCR analysis may give false-negative results, depending on the specific translocation. Both Southern blot hybridization and PCR analysis require foreknowledge of the specific translocation. For Southern blot hybridization, a specific probe that hybridizes to the area of the genome just adjacent to the translocation must be available; for PCR analysis, the sequence of DNA flanking both sides of the translocation must be known. FISH can be per-

formed on paraffin sections, but one can examine the section for only one specific translocation at a time.[51] Thus, the number of detectable abnormalities is much lower than for classic cytogenetics. Whereas chromosome translocations are specific for neoplasia when they are detected by classic cytogenetics, FISH, and Southern blotting, this may not be the case when the translocation is detected by the highly sensitive PCR. For example, the t(14;18) has been detected by highly sensitive PCR methods in tissues with reactive follicular hyperplasia from patients without a history of lymphoma.[52]

## NONHEMATOPOIETIC LESIONS IN LYMPH NODES

The following nonhematopoietic lesions may be found in lymph nodes:

*Metastatic Tumors*

Carcinoma
Malignant melanoma
Germ cell tumor
Sarcoma
Unknown primary site
Childhood tumors

*Congenital Rests and Inclusions*

Epithelial: salivary gland, müllerian, breast, thyroid
Mesothelial
Nevomelanocytic: ordinary nevus, blue nevus

*Primary Mesenchymal Lesions*

Lipomatosis
Vascular: vascular transformation of sinuses, nodular spindle cell vascular transformation, bacillary angiomatosis, Kaposi's sarcoma, intranodal hemangioma and variants, lymphangioma, hemangioendothelioma and variants, angiosarcoma
Myofibroblastic: inflammatory pseudotumor, mycobacterial pseudotumor, mediastinal spindle cell pseudotumor, palisaded myofibroblastoma
Smooth muscle: intranodal leiomyoma, angiomyomatous hamartoma and variants, leiomyomatosis, lymphangiomyomatosis, angiomyolipoma, smooth muscle proliferation of the nodal hilum
Protein deposition: amyloid, para-amyloid, proteinaceous lymphadenopathy

## Metastatic Tumors

The most common nonhematopoietic lesions involving lymph nodes are metastatic tumors, including carcinoma, melanoma, germ cell tumors, and less frequently certain types of sarcoma. The presence of lymph node metastases typically signifies an adverse prognosis; thus, removal of local lymph nodes, often followed by formal lymph node dissection, is common practice in most standard surgical cancer resections. In any lymph node dissection, all lymph nodes should be grossly identified and submitted for microscopic examination. The number of involved lymph nodes and the total number of examined lymph nodes should be documented. Lymph nodes involved by metastatic tumor usually show total or subtotal replacement and may show tumor in adjacent perinodal lymphatics and soft tissues. The subcapsular sinuses are usually the locus of early tumor involvement. In general, the prognosis is inversely proportional to the number of involved nodes. The presence of extracapsular soft tissue extension may indicate a need for subsequent radiation therapy.[53] Investigators have shown that the detection of involved lymph nodes is enhanced with the use of adjunct immunohistochemistry to detect occult foci of tumor, but whether their detection affects prognosis has not yet been convincingly demonstrated.[54]

Sentinel lymph node dissection is a minimally invasive surgical technique that is now routine for staging of breast cancer in patients without palpable lymphadenopathy.[55] It is based on the hypothesis that the histologic character of the first draining lymph node accurately predicts the histologic character of the rest of the axillary lymph nodes. The sensitivity of this technique relies on careful histologic and immunohistochemical examination of the sentinel lymph node.[56, 57] For cases that have no lymph node tumor detected at frozen section, it is recommended that the pathologist examine one section each with H&E and cytokeratin stains from at least two levels, 40 $\mu$m apart, of the paraffin block. These levels should be prepared for each half of a bisected sentinel lymph node, for a total of eight sections. These parameters provide optimal histologic sensitivity at permanent section, with minimal labor and financial burden to the laboratory.[58]

In addition, sentinel lymph nodes are used in the diagnosis of micrometastatic melanoma. In one large study of melanoma patients, sentinel lymph node status was the most significant prognostic factor for recurrence in patients with clinically negative nodes.[59]

A patient without a prior history of malignant disease will often have an enlarged lymph node that contains an undifferentiated malignant neoplasm with no clear differentiating features. Even if some differentiating features are present, the differential diagnosis can be broad. For example, signet ring cells can be found in carcinomas, lymphomas, and malignant melanomas. Although electron microscopy may be helpful in selected cases, the majority of cases can be resolved with the use of histochemical stains, such as mucin, and immunohistochemical studies performed in paraffin-embedded tissues.

Leukocyte common antigen (CD45) identifies more than 90% of malignant lymphomas.[60] CD30 (a marker of Hodgkin's disease, anaplastic large cell lymphoma, and some other lymphomas), the B lineage marker CD20, and the T cell–myeloid marker CD43 identify the majority of CD45$^-$ hematolymphoid tumors.[23, 61, 62] Keratin stains almost all cases of carcinoma, whereas S-100 protein is a sensitive (but not completely specific) marker for malignant melanoma. Use of a panel of immunohistochemical stains, rather than any single antibody, is important for an accurate diagnosis because many tumors have overlapping reactivities and one needs to cross-validate staining reactions. For example, melanomas as well as many breast carcinomas stain for S-100 protein. A strongly keratin-positive, S-100 protein–positive tumor is most likely breast carcinoma and not malignant melanoma. However, a keratin-negative, S-100 protein–positive tumor that also stains for the melanoma markers Melan A and HMB-45 should be diagnosed as malignant melanoma and not breast carcinoma. Placental alkaline phosphatase is a relatively sensitive (but not completely specific) marker for germ cell tumors.

The pathologist may occasionally encounter cases of metastatic carcinoma of unknown primary site. The best clue to the possible primary site is the anatomic location of the involved lymph node. Location in the neck should raise consideration of a primary carcinoma within the upper aerodigestive tract. Location in the axilla in a woman should raise strong consideration of breast carcinoma. Involvement of the supraclavicular region should raise consideration of an abdominal primary. Paraffin section immunohistochemistry can be helpful in determining the possible primary site. The chosen panel depends on the clinical situation (Table 41–4). Vimentin is positive in endometrial, ovarian, renal cell, and thyroid neoplasms. If a primary breast carcinoma is suspected, S-100 protein, estrogen receptor, and gross cystic disease fluid protein 15 may be useful. If a thyroid primary is suspected, a thyroglobulin (positive in papillary and follicular carcinoma) or calcitonin (positive in medullary carcinoma) may help. Prostate-specific antigen and prostatic acid phosphatase confirm a prostate origin. Keratin antibodies with specific reactivities may also be of diagnostic use. The expression of keratin subsets in tumors mimics the coordinate keratin subset expression in normal tissues and thus can be extremely useful in determining the primary site of origin.[63] Furthermore, the cytokeratin profile of a primary tumor appears to be preserved in any metastasis or recurrence. Keratin 7 and keratin 20 are the most frequently used keratin subset pairs for determining the primary site of origin for an undifferentiated carcinoma (Table 41–5). The pattern of keratin positivity may give a clue about the neoplasm. Most epithelial neoplasms show strong diffuse cytoplasmic reactivity, but small cell neuroendocrine neoplasms may show a dotlike cytoplasmic positivity.

**TABLE 41–4.** Suggested Panels for Unknown Primary Malignant Neoplasms

Hematolymphoid vs. nonhematolymphoid
  Keratin S-100, CD45/CD45RB (brief)
  (CD30, CD20, and CD43 as second line)
Carcinoma, unknown primary
  Keratin 7, keratin 20, canalicular CEA, (GFAP), (PSA/PAcP), (GCDFP-15), (CAM 5.2/AE1)
Is this breast carcinoma?
  ER/PR, GCDFP-15, Bcl-2, S-100, (keratin 7, keratin 20)
Metastatic breast carcinoma vs. metastatic lung carcinoma
  ER, TTF-1, GCDFP-15, Bcl-2, (S-100) (in general, not CEA, vimentin, keratin 7, keratin 20)
Metastatic breast carcinoma vs. nonmucinous ovarian carcinoma
  GCDFP-15 (in general, not ER, S-100, CEA, vimentin, keratin 7, keratin 20)
Small cell carcinoma of lung vs. Merkel cell carcinoma
  Keratin 8/18, keratin 20, TTF-1
Carcinoid of gastrointestinal tract vs. carcinoid of lung
  Keratin 7, keratin 8/18, keratin 19, TTF-1
Neuroendocrine carcinoma
  Chromogranin, synaptophysin, neuron-specific enolase, (keratin 7, keratin 20)
Mesothelioma vs. carcinoma
  CEA, CD15, Ber-EP4, B72.3, calretinin, thrombomodulin, TTF-1
Is this melanoma?
  S-100, vimentin, HMB-45, Melan A
Spindled cutaneous neoplasm
  Vimentin, keratin, S-100, (smooth muscle actin, collagen IV, factor XIII)
Sarcoma, unknown type
  Vimentin, keratin, desmin, actin, smooth muscle actin, collagen IV, (CD31), (CD34), (CD/17), (vWF), (Ulex)
In this small round blue cell tumor of childhood?
  CD99, CD45/RB, vimentin, neurofilament, chromogranin, synaptophysin, desmin, actin, TdT
Germ cell tumor
  Placental alkaline phosphatase, keratin (hCG, AFP, EMA, CD30)
Neural vs. meningioma
  GFAP, S-100, EMA, (CD57), (neurofilament)

AFP, α-Fetoprotein; CEA, carcinoembryonic antigen; EMA, epithelial membrane antigen; ER, estrogen receptor; GCDFP-15, gross cystic disease fluid protein 15; GFAP, glial fibrillary acidic protein; hCG, human chorionic gonadotropin; PAcP, prostatic acid phosphatase; PR, progesterone receptor; PSA, prostate-specific antigen; TTF-1, thyroid transcription factor 1; vWF, von Willebrand factor.

Metastatic papillary carcinoma of the thyroid may appear bland. In a patient with no known thyroid lesion, one needs to differentiate this from the rare entity of ectopic thyroid tissue in lymph nodes, which lacks papillae, psammoma bodies, and nuclear atypia.[64] Lymph node metastases of Spitz nevus, cellular blue nevus, or malignant melanoma are usually confined to the subcapsular sinuses in these circumstances, thus distinguishing them from benign neval rests.[65]

Benign entities that may be confused with metastatic carcinoma include hyperplastic endothelial cells of postcapillary venules, nodal megakaryocytes resembling anaplastic nuclear changes, and histiocytic granulomas. In these cases, immunohistochemical studies are extremely useful.[66]

## Congenital Rests and Inclusions

### EPITHELIAL-TYPE INCLUSIONS

Salivary gland inclusions, müllerian inclusions, breast epithelial inclusions, thyroid inclusions, and rare epithelial tumors constitute primary epithelial lesions present in lymph nodes. In general, the key to distinguishing these from malignant neoplasms is the lack of cytologic atypia.

Salivary gland tissue, including ducts and acini, may be present in adjacent lymph nodes as well as in lower cervical lymph nodes. Pathologic dilatation of these ducts may lead to benign lymphoepithelial cysts in human immunodeficiency virus (HIV)–infected patients. In addition, these benign salivary gland inclusions may give rise to tumors, such as benign Warthin tumor. Other benign salivary gland tumors as well as malignant salivary gland tumors may rarely arise in adjacent lymph nodes.

Benign inclusions of müllerian epithelium are found in 5% to 40% of intra-abdominal lymph nodes of women.[67] Such inclusions have also been rarely described in the intra-abdominal lymph nodes of men. One sees bland, often ciliated columnar cells in the lymph node capsule or cortex (Fig. 41–1). They may also be called endosalpingiosis, but when endometrial stroma is also seen, a diagnosis of endometriosis should be rendered.[68] Rarely, the stromal component predominates or may be the only component present. The most common example of this is the extensive decidualization that occurs during pregnancy in so-called deciduosis of lymph nodes.[69] The pathogenesis of these lesions is still unclear. A

**TABLE 41–5.** Differential Cytokeratin 7 and Cytokeratin 20 Expression of Selected Carcinomas*

| Cytokeratin 7 Positive Cytokeratin 20 Positive | Cytokeratin 7 Positive Cytokeratin 20 Negative | Cytokeratin 7 Negative Cytokeratin 20 Positive | Cytokeratin 7 Negative Cytokeratin 20 Negative |
|---|---|---|---|
| Ovarian mucinous carcinoma | Breast carcinoma | Colorectal adenocarcinoma | Hepatocellular carcinoma |
| Pancreatic adenocarcinoma | Endometrial carcinoma | | Prostatic adenocarcinoma |
| Transitional cell carcinoma | Epithelial mesothelioma | | Renal cell carcinoma |
| | Lung adenocarcinoma | | Small cell neuroendocrine carcinoma |
| | Ovarian serous adenocarcinoma | | Squamous cell carcinoma |
| | Thymoma | | |

*This general guide to cytokeratin expression should not be considered absolute because a subset of each malignant neoplasm may not show the most common differential keratin expression.

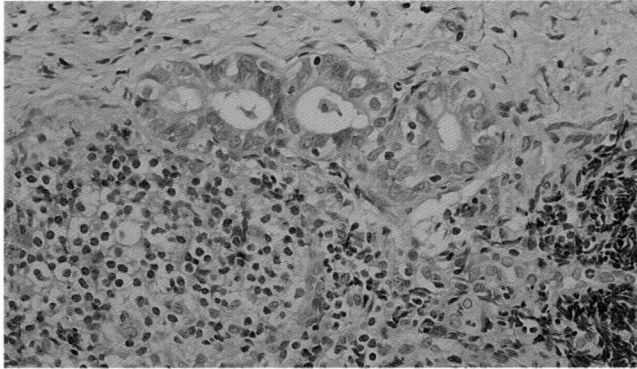

FIGURE 41–1. Müllerian inclusion. The lymph node capsule contains a common type of benign inclusion, which has bland nuclear features and cilia.

metaplastic phenomenon is favored, but congenital, implantation, and metastatic origins are also possible.

Benign inclusions of breast tissue may be encountered rarely in axillary nodes.[70] They are usually found in the intracapsular or subcapsular region of the lymph node. Rare primary carcinomas have been reported arising within these inclusions.

The occurrence of ectopic thyroid tissue in cervical lymph nodes is a point of controversy because distinguishing bland-appearing metastases of papillary carcinoma of the thyroid from benign ectopic thyroid tissue may be difficult. For the diagnosis of ectopic thyroid tissue in lymph nodes to be made confidently over metastatic carcinoma, the inclusions should consist entirely of bland thyroid follicles of relatively small size without any papillae, psammoma bodies, or nuclear atypia.[64] In cases in which the thyroid gland is also removed, complete serial sections of the gland have failed to identify tumor, thus confirming that ectopic thyroid tissue in the lymph node does truly occur. Intranodal squamous epithelial cells, which originate from metaplastic calyceal urothelium, may also be mistaken for metastatic carcinoma in patients undergoing nephrectomy for Wilms' tumor or other renal malignant neoplasms.[66]

### MESOTHELIAL INCLUSIONS

Benign mesothelial inclusions in lymph nodes are exceedingly rare but have been reported in mediastinal, pelvic, and abdominal lymph nodes.[66, 71–74] Lymphatic dissemination is probably the route by which the mesothelial cells reach the lymphatic nodes. These cells may be mistaken for metastatic carcinoma, mesothelioma, or melanoma. Immunohistochemical studies are useful for evaluating these inclusions.

### BENIGN NEVUS CELL RESTS

Benign nevus cell rests have been most often reported in axillary lymph nodes, but they have also been reported in inguinal and cervical lymph nodes.[75] They have been identified in 0.3% to 6% of axillary lymph nodes by light microscopic examination and in a slightly higher percentage of cases when adjunct S-100 protein immunohistochemical staining is performed. The bland epithelioid nevus cells, which may include blue neval cells, usually occur as nests and cords within the lymph node capsule, with occasional extension into the perinodal adipose tissues[76] (Fig. 41–2). Rarely, cutaneous nevi may be found near the area of drainage.[77] Although a "benign" metastatic origin cannot be excluded, the location of neval nests within the lymph node capsule and not the subcapsular sinuses strongly favors the theory that they represent an arrest of migration toward their final destination. This phenomenon should be distinguished from metastasis of Spitz nevus, cellular blue nevus, and malignant melanoma to lymph nodes because the metastatic cells are found in the subcapsular sinuses in those circumstances.[65]

## Primary Mesenchymal Lesions

### LIPOMATOSIS

The most common mesenchymal lesion found in lymph nodes is lipomatosis, which is often an incidental finding in lymph node dissections but may rarely manifest as lymphadenopathy. In this entity, the lymph node parenchyma is almost totally replaced by adipose tissue, with only a thin rim of residual lymphoid tissue and capsule remaining.

### VASCULAR

#### Vascular Transformation of Lymph Node Sinuses

The differential diagnosis of primary vascular lesions of lymph nodes includes vascular transformation of lymph node sinuses, an unusual vasoproliferative lesion that is most often found in intraabdominal lymph nodes removed in lymphoma staging procedures and in axillary lymph nodes removed after radical mastectomy.[78–80] The etiology of vascular transformation of lymph node sinuses is

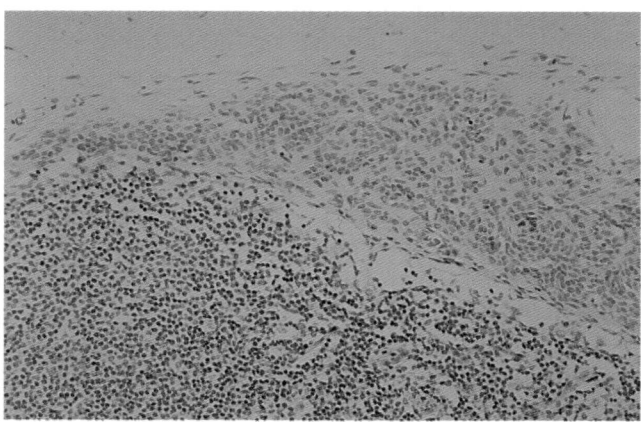

FIGURE 41–2. Nevus cell inclusion. The lymph node capsule contains a nest of nevus cells, which have a slightly organoid configuration.

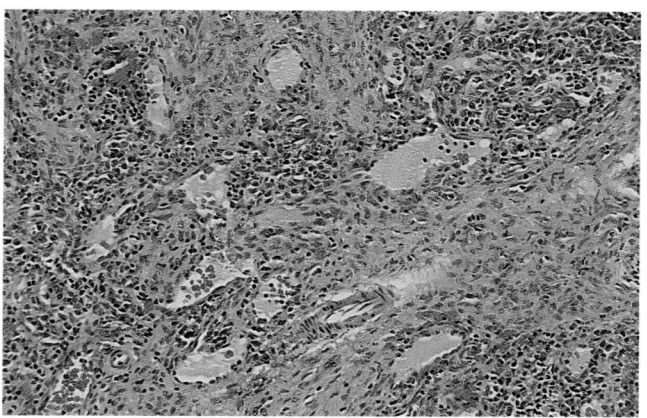

**FIGURE 41–3.** Vascular transformation of sinuses. A proliferation of dilated blood vessels is seen in the lymph node sinuses. Bland endothelial cells line the vessels.

not known but may be related to extranodal venous obstruction, with shunting of blood through anastomoses between blood vessels and lymphatic sinuses.[80] The vascular proliferation is usually confined to subcapsular sinuses but may also involve intermediate and medullary sinuses (Fig. 41–3). The lesion consists of endothelium-lined blood-filled spaces associated with varying degrees of fibrosis. The vessels may form anastomosing narrow clefts or plexiform channels. Hilar veins of the affected nodes may be thrombosed. Vascular transformation of sinuses must be distinguished from Kaposi's sarcoma.[78] In contrast to Kaposi's sarcoma, vascular transformation of sinuses is limited to the sinuses, often contains fibrosis and well-developed vascular channels, lacks well-formed spindle cell fascicles, and does not involve the lymph node capsule.

### Nodular Spindle Cell Vascular Transformation of Lymph Nodes

Nodular spindle cell vascular transformation of lymph nodes is a variant of vascular transformation of lymph node sinuses.[81] Because of its nodular configuration, spindle cell composition, cellularity, and occasional high mitotic activity, this lesion can be confused with Kaposi's sarcoma. Its propensity to occur in sites draining carcinomas also leads to its confusion with metastatic sarcomatoid carcinomas. Nodular spindle cell vascular transformation of lymph nodes is usually seen in retroperitoneal lymph nodes excised in association with radical nephrectomies for renal cell carcinoma, but it can also be present in association with other malignant tumors. On occasion, it is seen in superficial lymph nodes in patients with no history of malignant neoplasm.

### Nodal Bacillary Angiomatosis

Another primary vascular lesion of lymph nodes is nodal bacillary angiomatosis.[82] This reactive vascular proliferation occurs almost exclusively in individuals with the acquired immunodeficiency syndrome (AIDS). It is characterized by proliferation of small blood vessels and endothelial cells in skin, visceral organs, and occasionally lymph nodes, which may be the sole site of involvement. The *Bartonella* species has also been found to be the causative agent of bacillary angiomatosis.[83–85] Involved lymph nodes show coalescing nodules of proliferating vessels lined by plump endothelial cells with reactive nuclear changes. Neutrophils are usually scattered around the vessels. There is often abundant amorphous interstitial material that represents numerous short bacilli, demonstrable by Warthin-Starry or Giemsa stains. There is no association with the Kaposi's sarcoma–associated human herpesvirus 8 (HHV-8).[86]

### Kaposi's Sarcoma

Kaposi's sarcoma is the most common primary vascular tumor to involve lymph nodes. It most often occurs as a complication of HIV infection, primarily in homosexual men, and is also seen in children and young adults in Africa.[87] In addition, nodal Kaposi's sarcoma is a rare complication of classic Kaposi's sarcoma occurring in Mediterranean populations. Rare reports of its lymphadenopathic form have also been described as a complication of organ transplantation.[88, 89] The histologic appearance of Kaposi's sarcoma in lymph nodes resembles that in skin and other organs. The normal lymph node architecture may be completely effaced or may show subtle sinusoidal or subcapsular infiltration, with variable extension to the capsule or into the paracortical areas (Fig. 41–4). On occasion, the lymph node shows Castleman's disease–like changes. In addition, Kaposi's sarcoma may be associated with multicentric Castleman's disease.[90] All forms of Kaposi's sarcoma have been shown to be associated with HHV-8 (also known as Kaposi's sarcoma–associated herpesvirus).[91–95] The differential diagnosis of Kaposi's sarcoma includes vascular transformation of sinuses, nodular spindle cell vascular transformation of lymph nodes (both discussed previously), and mycobacterial pseudotumor (discussed later).

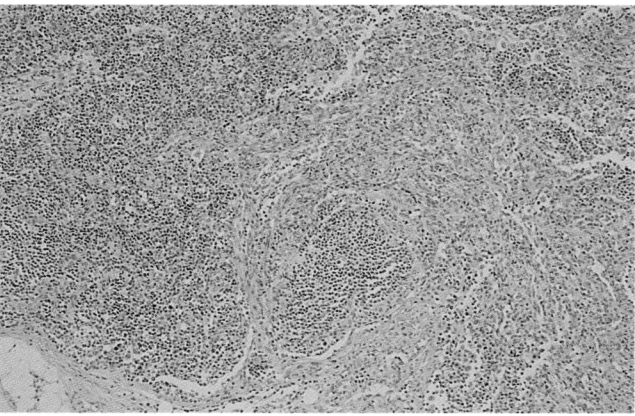

**FIGURE 41–4.** Kaposi's sarcoma. A bland spindled cell proliferation surrounds primary follicles.

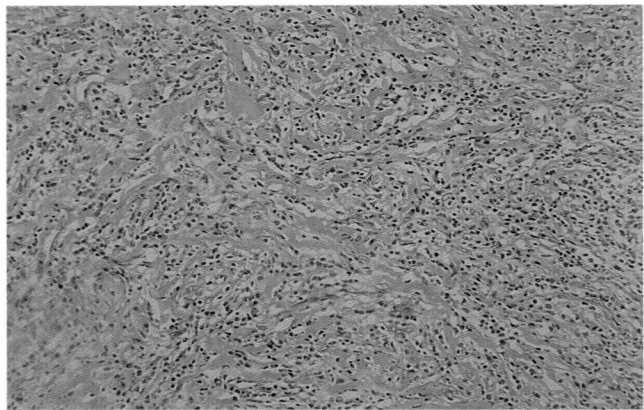

**FIGURE 41–5.** Inflammatory pseudotumor. The nodal parenchyma contains areas of fibrosis admixed with numerous reactive lymphocytes and scattered histiocytes.

### Other Vascular Tumors

Other vascular tumors that can primarily involve the lymph node are extremely rare and include intranodal hemangioma, epithelioid hemangioma, and lymphangioma.[96] Epithelioid hemangioma, also known as angiolymphoid hyperplasia with eosinophils, comprises well-formed epithelioid endothelium-lined vascular channels with admixed small lymphocytes and eosinophils. Other vascular tumors are hemangioendothelioma (including polymorphous and the spindle and epithelioid varieties) and angiosarcoma.[90, 96, 97]

## MYOFIBROBLASTIC AND SMOOTH MUSCLE PROLIFERATIONS

### Inflammatory Pseudotumor

Inflammatory pseudotumor is a rare but distinctive lesion that probably represents a reactive proliferation of mesenchymal cells.[98–101] It usually affects young adults; clinical presentation may include lymphadenopathy and systemic symptoms such as fever. Affected lymph nodes are moderately enlarged and show a proliferation of blood vessels, spindled cells (comprising fibroblasts and some myofibroblasts), and histiocytes, with variable numbers of acute and chronic inflammatory cells (Fig. 41–5). Typically, one also sees an inflammatory reaction in larger blood vessels. The process preferentially affects the lymph node capsule and hilum. The lesion is benign but rarely may recur. It probably represents the end stage of a variety of inflammatory lesions that may affect the lymph node. PCR studies show no heavy chain or T cell receptor chain gene rearrangements.[99, 102] A histologically similar lesion is mycobacterial spindle cell pseudotumor, which contains numerous acid-fast bacilli in the proliferating histiocytes, unlike inflammatory pseudotumor, which is negative for acid-fast bacilli.[103]

### Mycobacterial Pseudotumor

Mycobacterial pseudotumor, an exuberant spindle cell lesion induced in lymph nodes by mycobacteria, has been reported exclusively in patients infected with HIV.[103–106] It presents with lymph node enlargement and is characterized histologically by a proliferation of spindled cells, closely mimicking intranodal Kaposi's sarcoma (Fig. 41–6). However, its spindle cells have a loose storiform pattern, unlike the compact fascicles of spindled cells in Kaposi's sarcoma. Although Kaposi's sarcoma does not usually have concomitant mycobacterial infection, rare cases of Kaposi's sarcoma with acid-fast bacilli have been reported. The spindled cells of mycobacterial pseudotumor usually stain for S-100 protein and CD68, unlike those of Kaposi's sarcoma.

### Mediastinal Spindle Cell Pseudotumors

Rare cases of reactive mediastinal spindle cell pseudotumors associated with anthracosis and anthracosilicosis have been reported.[107] The histologic appearance includes a prominent storiform pattern of intertwining spindle cells, sometimes with extracapsular or perineural involvement. Nodular hyaline scars and polarizable material are also seen. Despite the presence of extracapsular or perineural spindled proliferations, the reported lesions have followed a benign clinical course.

### Palisaded Myofibroblastoma

Palisaded myofibroblastoma (hemorrhagic spindle cell tumor with amianthoid fibers) is a rare benign primary lymph node tumor of myofibroblastic or smooth muscle origin.[108, 109] It is a well-demarcated lesion, almost always seen in inguinal lymph nodes; other sites may rarely be affected. One sees fascicular proliferation of bland spindled cells with focal nuclear palisading and stellate configurations of distinctive amianthoid fibers, an unusual type of collagen that may calcify. Hemorrhagic areas are also present. Collagen type IV uniformly stains all of the amianthoid fibers, whereas type II collagen and actin staining are limited to the peripheral portion of the amianthoid fiber collections. The tumor cells do not stain for desmin. Metaplastic bone formation has been described.[110–113]

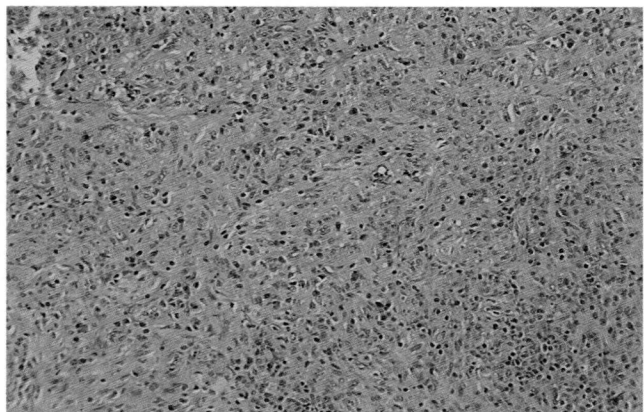

**FIGURE 41–6.** Mycobacterial pseudotumor. This lymph node shows a loose storiform collection of inflammatory cells, including plasma cells, and small blood vessels.

*Other Smooth Muscle Proliferations*

Intranodal leiomyoma, angiomyomatous hamartoma, leiomyomatosis, lymphangiomyomatosis, angiomyolipoma, and smooth muscle proliferation in the nodal hilum are among the wide variety of rare smooth muscle tumors, proliferations, and malformations that may primarily involve the lymph node.[114] Some of the lesions, such as angiomyolipoma, lymphangiomyomatosis, and vascular leiomyomatosis (so-called primary nodal leiomyomatosis), may represent manifestations of tuberous sclerosis and are HMB-45 positive.[115] Smooth muscle proliferation of the nodal hilum is primarily found in inguinal lymph nodes and consists of an irregular proliferation of smooth muscle cells, accompanied by fibrosis. It is usually limited to the hilum.[116] A similar lesion, which may involve the entire lymph node, is angiomatous hamartoma, an irregular smooth muscle proliferation associated with blood vessels.[96] Leiomyomatosis usually occurs in the intra-abdominal lymph nodes of women and may represent a "benign" metastasis of otherwise benign uterine leiomyoma, a manifestation of leiomyomatosis peritonealis disseminata, or a metaplastic phenomenon related to endometriosis.[117]

## PROTEIN DEPOSITION

### Amyloid

Amyloid deposition is often seen in lymph nodes of patients with systemic amyloidosis.[118] Amyloid deposition may also be seen in the lymph nodes of patients with plasmacytoma, lymphoplasmacytic lymphoma, and Castleman's disease.[119] Amyloid lymphadenopathy in the absence of systemic amyloidosis or lymphoproliferative disorder is unusual. Despite the varied clinical presentations, the morphologic appearance of amyloid in the lymph nodes is consistent. The amorphous eosinophilic amyloid material is usually found in the walls of the vessels and may also be found partially involving or completely obliterating follicles, or it may be present diffusely throughout the parenchyma (Fig. 41–7).

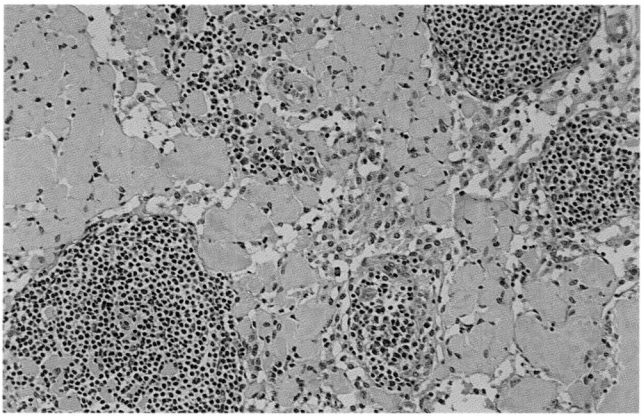

**FIGURE 41–7.** Amyloidosis. Globules of acellular amorphous material surround dormant follicles. This showed apple-green birefringence with Congo red stain.

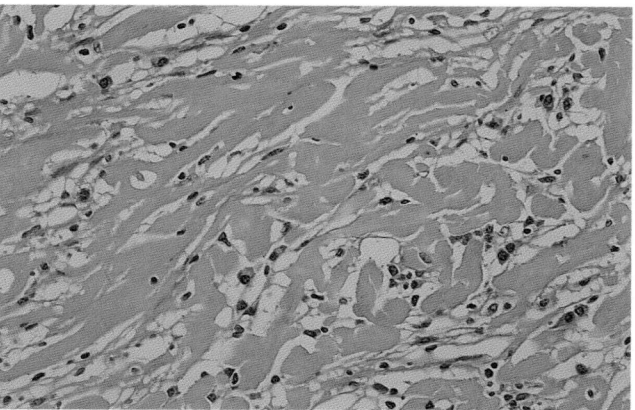

**FIGURE 41–8.** Proteinaceous lymphadenopathy. This lymph node also contains abundant acellular material, but unlike amyloid, the material does not show Congo red staining or restricted light chain staining.

Similar to amyloid in other parts of the body, one should see a characteristic apple-green birefringence with Congo red histochemical staining.

### Para-amyloid

Para-amyloid refers to a sclerosis commonly seen in lymph nodes from the inguinal and pelvic region. By light microscopy, it appears similar to amyloid. However, para-amyloid is periodic acid–Schiff (PAS) positive and Congo red negative. It is an inflammatory or abnormal immune reaction product seen in lymph nodes from patients with angioimmunoblastic lymphadenopathy or Hodgkin's disease, or it may be due to iatrogenic causes.

### Proteinaceous Lymphadenopathy

Proteinaceous lymphadenopathy is a rare disease of unknown etiology.[120, 121] It has also been called angiocentric sclerosing lymphadenopathy. It is thought to be an unusual variant of plasma cell dyscrasia. Patients present with generalized lymphadenopathy and polyclonal hypergammaglobulinemia. The normal nodal architecture is obliterated by deposition of a nonamyloid material, which usually lines vessel walls and appears to be composed of bundles of fine reticulin fibers, which show an "onion skin" effect around the vessels (Fig. 41–8). Lymphocytes are rarely seen. Unlike light chain deposition disease or multiple myeloma, proteinaceous lymphadenopathy is paucicellular and shows generalized angiosclerosis. Also, no monotypic light chain population and no Congo red staining are seen in proteinaceous lymphadenopathy.

## REACTIVE LYMPHADENOPATHIES

Lymph nodes process antigens and present altered antigens to B or T lymphocytes.[122] The altered antigens may stimulate proliferation of B or T cells, sinus histiocytes, or specialized accessory cells in one or more of the lymph node compartments, leading to expansion of these compartments and subsequent nodal enlargement or lymphadenopathy. The diversity of lymph node proliferations is due to the range of the population's age and immunologic makeup, an individual's past experience with the offending antigen, and the duration of the proliferation.

Fine-needle aspiration biopsy is an effective method for evaluating reactive lymphadenopathy, both by excluding malignancy and by suggesting a specific etiology to a reactive condition. Material may also be obtained for microbiologic and flow cytometric studies. A definitive diagnosis of reactive lymphadenopathy should be made only with adequate clinical history and the opportunity for adequate clinical follow-up. After a diagnosis of reactive lymphadenopathy, a patient may have persistent or increasing lymphadenopathy. In this setting, one should repeat the aspiration biopsy or perform a surgical biopsy.

Reactive lymph node proliferations are generally divided into two categories, lymphadenitis and lymphoid hyperplasia. Lymphadenitis, which may be acute or chronic, indicates that an infectious agent is probably present. The typical etiologic agents are pyogenic bacteria, particularly streptococci and staphylococci. Acute lymphadenitis is most commonly caused by local septic infections that spread to lymph nodes. The surgical pathologist rarely encounters acute lymphadenitis, because the primary site of infection (tonsils, skin, oral cavity) is usually known and biopsy of draining lymph nodes is not performed. Chronic lymphadenitis is a general term that encompasses numerous disorders instigated by a variety of infectious agents. Granulomatous disorders and lymph node enlargement caused by viruses, rickettsiae, and various mycoses and other agents are forms of chronic lymphadenitis but are usually designated by the name of the etiologic agent if it is known (e.g., tuberculous lymphadenitis, toxoplasmic lymphadenitis).

In contrast to lymphadenitis, lymphoid hyperplasia indicates a response to antigenic stimulation without evidence of infectious involvement. Lymphoid hyperplasias can be divided into three groups on the basis of the normal lymph nodal compartments. These include 1) follicular hyperplasia (preferential stimulation of B cell component), 2) reactive paracortical hyperplasia (preferential stimulation of the paracortex, the site where most of the T cells are located), and 3) reactive histiocytic hyperplasia (preferential expansion of the mononuclear phagocyte system, including phagocytic histiocytes). Combinations of these patterns are frequently seen because it is unusual for one part of the lymph node to be stimulated without another part being affected. In some diseases, necrosis is the predominant histologic pattern.

The major reactive lymphadenopathies, according to their predominant pattern, are as follows. Granulomatous disorders are considered separately.

### Follicular

Nonspecific reactive follicular hyperplasia
Rheumatoid arthritis
Sjögren's syndrome
Kimura's disease
Toxoplasmosis
Syphilis
Castleman's disease
HIV-associated lymphadenopathy
Progressive transformation of germinal centers

### Paracortical

Nonspecific reactive paracortical hyperplasia
Viral: Epstein-Barr, cytomegalovirus, herpesvirus
Drug-induced and postvaccinial
Dermatopathic lymphadenitis

### Sinus

Sinus histiocytosis
Monocytoid B cell hyperplasia
Hemophagocytic syndrome
Sinus histiocytosis with massive lymphadenopathy
Whipple's disease
Exogenous lipids

### Extensive necrosis

Complete necrosis-infarction
Kikuchi's histiocytic necrotizing lymphadenitis
Systemic lupus erythematosus
Kawasaki's disease

### Granulomatous

Noninfectious
Infectious: nonsuppurative, suppurative, cat-scratch disease, lymphogranuloma venereum, *Yersinia* lymphadenitis

## Follicular Hyperplasia

### NONSPECIFIC REACTIVE FOLLICULAR HYPERPLASIA

Follicular hyperplasia is the most common type of reactive lymphoid proliferation. It is especially common in children and adolescents but is found in all age groups.[123] The etiology of reactive follicular hyperplasia is often unknown. However, some diseases that show reactive follicular hyperplasia have additional distinctive morphologic features that may prompt confirmatory laboratory tests. Nonspecific reactive hyperplasia involving younger patients often resolves spontaneously without further consequences for the patient. However, older individuals with nonspecific reactive hyperplasia often have involvement of multiple lymph nodes; the hyperplasia has been associated with concurrence or subsequent development of malignant lymphoma in a significant subset of cases.

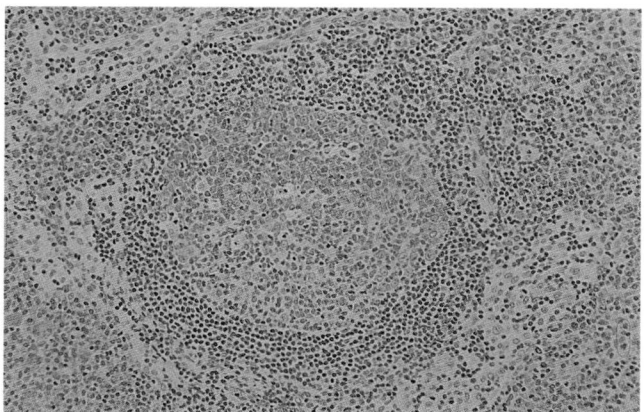

**FIGURE 41–9.** Reactive germinal center. This reactive follicle exhibits polarization, that is, a dark zone at the top with gradation to a light zone at the bottom. The tingible body macrophages impart a starry sky appearance.

Follicular hyperplasia represents stimulation of the B cell compartment of the lymph node. The unstimulated follicle is known as a primary follicle, which consists primarily of small B lineage lymphocytes enmeshed in a tight network of dendritic reticulum cells. When stimulated, the follicle becomes known as a secondary follicle. Follicular hyperplasia refers to an increase in the number and size of follicles, which show variation in shape. Fusion of adjacent germinal centers may result in large, bizarre geographic structures. The hyperplastic follicles consist of expanded germinal centers with thin or attenuated mantle zones (Fig. 41–9). The hyperplastic germinal centers usually contain mixtures of small and large cleaved and noncleaved (B lineage) cells, scattered polyclonal plasma cells, and admixed small T lymphocytes, but they may consist almost exclusively of large transformed cells. Hyperplastic germinal centers have numerous mitotic figures and a "starry sky" appearance, which is also indicative of a high proliferative rate. The dendritic meshwork becomes enlarged, as highlighted by appropriate immunohistochemical studies (CD21 or CD35). Polarity of the germinal centers, which is a feature of benign follicles, is seen in most follicles. At one pole (the "dark zone") of the follicle is a predominance of large transformed germinal center cells that have a high mitotic rate, interspersed with tingible body macrophages. The other pole (the "light zone") contains primarily small cleaved cells and dendritic reticulum cells.[124] Few, if any, tingible body macrophages are present among these cells. The germinal centers and mantle zones are distinct from one another, except in some cases of florid follicular hyperplasia, such as in lymph nodes of HIV-infected individuals.[125] In those cases, small lymphocytes infiltrate and disrupt germinal centers, a phenomenon known as follicle lysis. The mantle zone may be attenuated or totally absent. Fine-needle aspiration smears of reactive follicular hyperplasia show a polymorphous population of lymphoid cells with scattered tingible body macrophages.

Distinguishing follicular hyperplasia from follicular lymphoma may be extremely difficult. Some useful (but not entirely foolproof) criteria are listed in Table 41–6.[126] No single criterion can be used to distinguish between follicular hyperplasia and follicular lymphoma in an individual case. However, the pathologist's consideration of all the listed morphologic features will help lead to the correct diagnosis. Suboptimal sections may compound the difficulties encountered in the differential diagnosis. Clinical information, such as the rarity of follicular lymphomas in patients younger than 40 years, may offer a clue.

The most reliable morphologic criteria for distinguishing follicular hyperplasia from follicular lymphoma are the distribution and density of follicles per unit area and the observation of polarity.[127, 128] These factors are readily determined by scanning the slide under low magnification. Neoplastic follicles also tend to be closely apposed, with a "back-to-back" appearance. Neoplastic follicles tend to have more uniform size and shape than benign follicles. The interfollicular areas of lymphoma may have neoplastic cells. In addition, the interfollicular areas of lymphoma are smaller and have plasma cells more frequently than the corresponding areas of follicular hyperplasia. Polarity is absent in neoplastic follicles. The absence of tingible body macrophages, a lower mitotic rate, and attenuation or complete absence of mantle zones favor a neoplastic diagnosis. An exception is follicular large cell lymphoma, which may have a high mitotic rate and a starry sky appearance, thereby resembling hyperplastic germinal centers. Diffuse lymphomatous areas are usually also present and mantle zones are absent, helping to

**TABLE 41–6.** Follicular Hyperplasia Versus Lymphoma

| Reactive Follicular Hyperplasia | Follicular Lymphoma |
| --- | --- |
| Follicles limited to subcortical region | Follicles distributed evenly throughout nodal parenchyma |
| Follicles do not extend beyond capsule | Follicles extend beyond capsule |
| Low density of follicles | High density of follicles |
| Follicles of uneven size and shape | Follicles of similar size and shape |
| Mixture of cell types in germinal center | Monomorphic or polymorphic population |
| Tingible body macrophages present | Tingible body macrophages rarely seen |
| Low to high mitotic rate | Low to moderate mitotic rate |
| Mantle zone distinct | Mantle zone indistinct or absent |
| Cell polarization often seen | Cell polarization absent |
| Large interfollicular areas | Compressed interfollicular areas |
| No diffuse effacement seen | Contains areas of diffuse effacement |

distinguish this least common subtype of follicular lymphoma from follicular hyperplasia. For cases in which the morphologic criteria do not establish a definitive diagnosis, immunohistochemistry and molecular studies may be useful.[39, 47, 129]

Immunohistochemical staining for Bcl-2 protein is often helpful in distinguishing between follicular hyperplasia and follicular lymphoma. In contrast to Bcl-2⁻ reactive follicular hyperplasia (Fig. 41–10), staining for Bcl-2 is positive in more than 90% of cases of follicular lymphoma (Fig. 41–11), with the exception of the large cell subtype, in which Bcl-2 is expressed in approximately three quarters of cases.[39, 130, 131] CD10 immunohistochemical staining and flow cytometric intensity are also much stronger in follicular lymphoma than in most follicular hyperplasias.[132, 133] In addition, about 85% to 90% of follicular lymphomas have the structural cytogenetic t(14;18), which is absent in follicular hyperplasia.[130] If fresh or frozen tissue is unavailable to study clonality, additional lymph node biopsy may be required. A staging bone marrow biopsy may show involvement by lymphoma and may help confirm a lymph node impression of lymphoma.

The differential diagnosis of follicular hyperplasia also includes mantle cell lymphoma, especially with a mantle zone pattern, and rarely small lymphocytic lymphoma/chronic lymphocytic leukemia with proliferation centers. In mantle cell lymphoma, the follicular structures may show two patterns. First, there may be expanded mantles of small lymphoid cells, some of which have irregular nuclear contours (mantle zone derived); these expanded mantles surround benign germinal centers. Second, one may see a diffuse proliferation of mantle zone cells around small "naked" germinal centers.[134] The expanded mantle zones and naked germinal centers are not usually seen in follicular hyperplasia. Paraffin section immunohistochemistry usually shows aberrant expression of CD43 and CD5 with CD20 in mantle cell lymphoma.[23, 135] In small lymphocytic lymphoma/chronic lymphocytic leukemia, the pro-

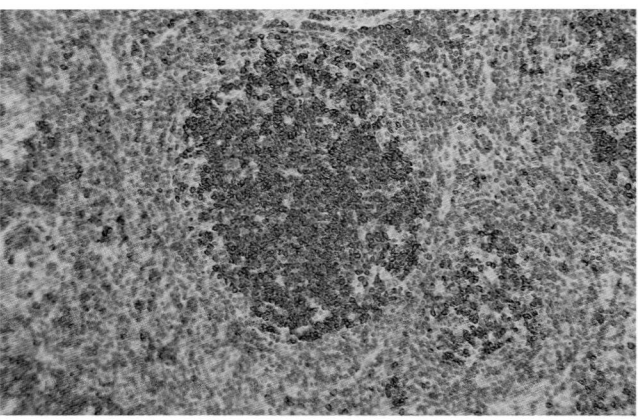

**FIGURE 41–11.** Follicular lymphoma, Bcl-2 stain. The majority of cells in this follicle show the characteristic cytoplasmic staining for Bcl-2. The slightly irregular nuclear outlines are highlighted.

liferation centers contain small and large transformed monoclonal B cells but do not contain cleaved cells and tingible body macrophages, which are present in reactive follicles.[128] Also, the proliferation centers have no mantle zones, which are usually present in follicular hyperplasia. This entity also shows abnormal coexpression of CD20 with CD5 and CD43 by paraffin immunohistochemistry. In addition, CD23 staining is usually also seen.

If low-magnification examination of the lymph node shows slightly expanded interfollicular areas, high-power examination may reveal the polymorphous infiltrate of interfollicular Hodgkin's disease, which may be masked by prominent follicular hyperplasia.[136] Paraffin immunohistochemical staining with CD15 and CD30 may highlight Reed-Sternberg cells.

## RHEUMATOID LYMPHADENOPATHY AND SJÖGREN'S LYMPHADENOPATHY

In rheumatoid arthritis and Sjögren's syndrome, lymphadenopathy is common and may be generalized.[137] There may be waxing and waning in the size of the lymph nodes. These chronically ill patients, particularly those with Sjögren's syndrome, have an increased risk of developing B cell lymphoma.[138] A lymph node biopsy may be performed because the nodes can reach a considerable size and the possibility of lymphoma cannot be excluded clinically.

The lymph nodes of patients with rheumatoid arthritis and Sjögren's syndrome show follicular hyperplasia and interfollicular plasmacytosis. Follicular hyperplasia is generalized throughout the entire node.[139, 140] Prominent germinal centers, some of which are polarized, contain tingible body macrophages and numerous mitoses. Mantle zones may be attenuated. The sinuses may be compressed by the enlarged germinal centers, and they usually contain some polymorphonuclear leukocytes. Interfollicular plasmacytosis is prominent. The plasma cells are polyclonal. Immunoblasts and vascular proliferation in the interfollicular areas are usually not prominent.

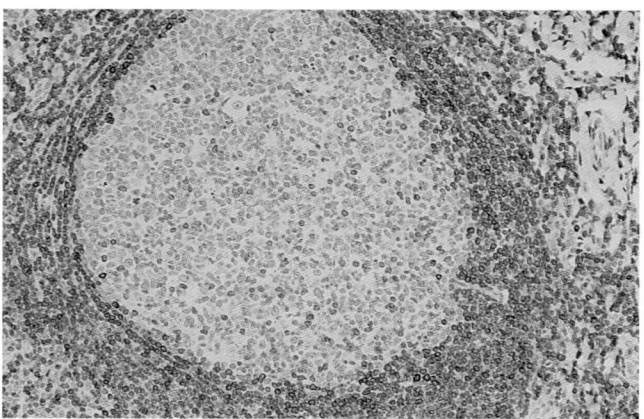

**FIGURE 41–10.** Reactive germinal center, Bcl-2 stain. This shows staining of the normal T lymphocytes in the mantle zone and only scattered admixed T cells in the germinal center.

Lymph Nodes

1491

The histologic changes in rheumatoid arthritis and Sjögren's syndrome are identical, with one exception. The lymph nodes of patients with Sjögren's syndrome may have a sinusoidal or paracortical monocytoid B cell proliferation that can cause distortion of the nodal architecture.[141] Sometimes, one cannot distinguish on morphologic grounds alone between benign (polyclonal) monocytoid B cell proliferations and malignant (monoclonal) low-grade monocytoid B cell lymphomas that are associated with Sjögren's syndrome. Immunophenotypic or genotypic studies may be helpful in these cases.

The differential diagnosis also includes secondary syphilis and the plasma cell variant of Castleman's disease. In addition to follicular hyperplasia and interfollicular plasmacytosis, lymph nodes of patients with secondary syphilis also have thickened capsules and fibrous trabeculae. The last two features are absent in lymph nodes of patients with rheumatoid arthritis or Sjögren's syndrome.[79, 142] On histologic examination, the plasma cell variant of Castleman's disease may be indistinguishable from the changes associated with rheumatoid arthritis or Sjögren's syndrome.[143] Clinical history and laboratory tests will enable the pathologist to differentiate among the disorders.[137]

## KIMURA'S LYMPHADENOPATHY

Kimura's disease is a rare chronic inflammatory disorder with a benign clinical course. It is endemic throughout Asia and is uncommon in the United States.[144, 145] Its etiology is unknown. The disease is seen predominantly in young to middle-aged men, who present with deep-seated masses involving the subcutaneous tissue of the head and neck region; the submandibular or parotid glands and regional lymph nodes may also be involved. In unusual cases, solitary lymph node enlargement may be the initial presentation.[144] The patients also have peripheral blood eosinophilia and elevated levels of serum immunoglobulin E.

The individual histologic features are not pathognomonic for the disease, but the total histologic picture should alert the pathologist to consider this disorder in the differential diagnosis. Lymph nodes from these patients show moderate to florid follicular hyperplasia with a paracortical and sinusoidal infiltrate of eosinophils, plasma cells, and mast cells. The germinal centers are highly vascularized and may contain polykaryocytes of the Warthin-Finkeldey type, proteinaceous material, and eosinophilic abscesses. Partial necrosis of germinal centers may also be seen. The paracortex may also contain Warthin-Finkeldey–type cells and eosinophilic abscesses. In addition, the paracortex contains a proliferation of postcapillary venules. The sinuses and paracortex often show partial or nearly total obliteration by dense sclerosis. Immunophenotyping studies show immunoglobulin E in the germinal centers and on the surface of nondegranulated mast cells in the paracortex.[144, 145]

The sclerosis and eosinophilia of Kimura's disease may lead to confusion with Hodgkin's disease. However, the presence of Reed-Sternberg cells and the loss of normal architecture in Hodgkin's disease (except in the interfollicular type) are not seen in Kimura's disease. Massive eosinophilia in lymph nodes may also be seen in allergic or drug reactions.[142] Marked eosinophilia and eosinophilic abscesses are also seen in parasitic infestation of lymph nodes. The florid follicular hyperplasia and Warthin-Finkeldey giant cells of Kimura's disease help distinguish it from the other disorders, including Langerhans cell histiocytosis, which preferentially involves the sinuses. Finally, the morphologic features of Kimura's disease are often mistaken for angiolymphoid hyperplasia with eosinophilia (epithelioid hemangioma); however, this entity contains histiocytoid or epithelioid endothelial cells, which are not found in Kimura's disease.

## TOXOPLASMIC LYMPHADENITIS

Toxoplasma gondii has a worldwide distribution and is present in approximately 50% of adults in the United States. Acute acquired toxoplasmosis has a varied clinical presentation ranging from no symptoms to influenza-like symptoms to an infectious mononucleosis–like picture (including atypical lymphocytes in the peripheral blood). The typical presentation is isolated posterior cervical lymphadenopathy. Less commonly, multiple nodes may become enlarged.

Toxoplasmic lymphadenitis has a characteristic triad of histologic findings, including 1) marked follicular hyperplasia, 2) interfollicular epithelioid histiocytes present singly or in small clusters, and 3) sinuses that are filled with or partially distended by monocytoid B cells and plasma cells[146] (Fig. 41–12). An important caveat is that not all three criteria are present in all cases. The follicles contain mostly large, transformed lymphoid cells, numerous tingible body macrophages, and numerous mitotic figures. The histiocytes may abut and encroach on the

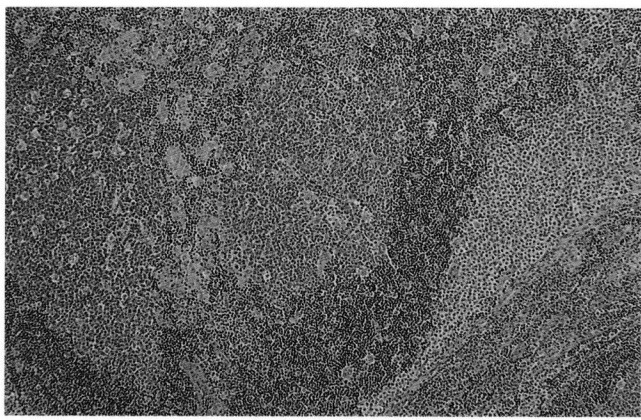

FIGURE 41–12. Toxoplasmic lymphadenitis. Note the characteristic triad of reactive follicular hyperplasia, clusters of epithelioid histiocytes, and a proliferation of reactive monocytoid B cells.

germinal centers, resulting in ragged edges. The histiocytes do not form granulomas. Multinucleated giant cells and necrosis are not present. Scattered neutrophils are usually seen among the monocytoid B cells. Parasitic cysts have only rarely been reported in lymph nodes. Fine-needle aspiration may also show a polymorphous population of cells and, rarely, histiocytes with intracellular organisms resembling *T. gondii*.[147] The triad of histologic or cytologic findings is consistent with a diagnosis of toxoplasmic lymphadenitis, but the definitive diagnosis requires confirmation by serologic studies.

The differential diagnosis of toxoplasmic lymphadenitis includes two conditions seen in HIV-associated lymphadenopathy: florid reactive follicular hyperplasia and sinusoidal-parafollicular monocytoid B cell proliferation.[125, 148] Epithelioid histiocyte clusters are not usually seen in HIV-associated lymphadenopathy, whereas follicular lysis and hemorrhage, which are features of HIV-associated lymphadenopathy, are not seen in toxoplasmosis. The degree of follicular hyperplasia is much greater in HIV-associated lymphadenopathy. Interfollicular Hodgkin's disease must also be distinguished from toxoplasmic lymphadenitis. Coexistence of the two disorders has been reported but is unusual.[149] Both diseases may show prominent follicular hyperplasia and single or small clusters of epithelioid histiocytes. However, eosinophils are not usually seen in toxoplasmic lymphadenitis but are often present in Hodgkin's disease, so their presence should alert the pathologist to the possibility of interfollicular Hodgkin's disease. Monocytoid B cell proliferations, a characteristic feature of toxoplasmic lymphadenitis, have not been described in interfollicular Hodgkin's disease. Immunohistochemical studies are also useful; CD15 and CD30 highlight the Reed-Sternberg cells of interfollicular Hodgkin's disease. The histologic features of toxoplasmosis have also been described in patients with leishmaniasis.[150]

## SYPHILITIC LYMPHADENITIS

Surgical pathologists rarely encounter lymph nodes for primary or secondary syphilis.[142] However, the pathologist should be aware of the characteristic but not specific histologic findings in syphilitic or luetic lymphadenitis, the incidence of which is on the rise. In most of the reported cases, biopsy of the inguinal lymph nodes was performed, although lymphadenopathy is often generalized in secondary syphilis. Luetic lymphadenitis is characterized histologically by follicular hyperplasia and interfollicular plasmacytosis resembling that seen in rheumatoid arthritis.[79, 142] It differs from rheumatoid arthritis in that the capsule and trabeculae are thickened and infiltrated by plasma cells. Perivenular plasmacytosis and clusters of epithelioid histiocytes and epithelioid granulomas with multinucleated giant cells may be present. Endarteritis, phlebitis, and occasionally abscesses are noted. The histologic impression of syphilitic lymphadenitis is confirmed by demonstration of the causative spirochetes by the Warthin-Starry silver stain or by immunohistochemistry. Serologic tests are also available. In lymph nodes, the spirochetes are often found within and around the walls of postcapillary venules and sometimes within germinal centers.[142]

## CASTLEMAN'S DISEASE

Castleman's disease has also been termed angiofollicular lymph node hyperplasia or giant lymph node hyperplasia.[143, 151–153] The original report of this entity described solitary lesions that were confined to the mediastinum, which is still the most frequent site of involvement. The disease has also been reported in other anatomic sites, including the abdominal and retroperitoneal cavities (the second most common site), the pulmonary parenchyma, the axillary and cervical regions, the skeletal muscle, and rarely the kidney.[143] The disease is most commonly localized but rarely may be multicentric or systemic.[152–155]

### Localized Castleman's Disease

Localized Castleman's disease has two main histologic patterns, the hyaline vascular type and the plasma cell type.[143] Rarely, one may see a mixture of both types.[156] The two major forms of the disease vary not only in their histologic appearance but also in their clinical presentation. Another type, known as stromal-rich Castleman's disease, has also been reported.[157]

**HYALINE VASCULAR TYPE.** More than 90% of cases of Castleman's disease have the hyaline vascular histologic appearance.[143] The disease has no sex predilection. Patients range in age from 8 to 69 years, with a median age at diagnosis of 33 years. Patients are generally asymptomatic unless the tumor mass abuts or partially obstructs a vital structure, such as a bronchus. The lesions generally occur as a single mass and have been reported to range in size from 1.5 to 16 cm. In unusual instances, it may be associated with non-Hodgkin's lymphoma.

The hyaline vascular type of Castleman's disease has two prominent microscopic features (Fig. 41–13). First, variably sized mantle zones, often arranged in concentric rings referred to as onion skin layers, surround regressively transformed, involuted, or atrophic germinal centers. The germinal centers are depleted of lymphocytes and consist predominantly of dendritic reticulum cells and some endothelial cells. In some cases, the palisading, small mantle zone lymphocytes nearly completely obscure the atrophic germinal centers. When this histologic feature predominates, the term *lymphoid variant of the hyaline vascular type* is used.[143] One may also find more than one small germinal center within a single follicle. Second, one sees prominent interfollicular vascularity and no sinuses. The increased vascularity accounts for the reported profuse bleeding during surgery. The vessels are often hyalinized and can be seen entering the germinal center from the interfollicular zone. The histologic picture is that of a "lolli-

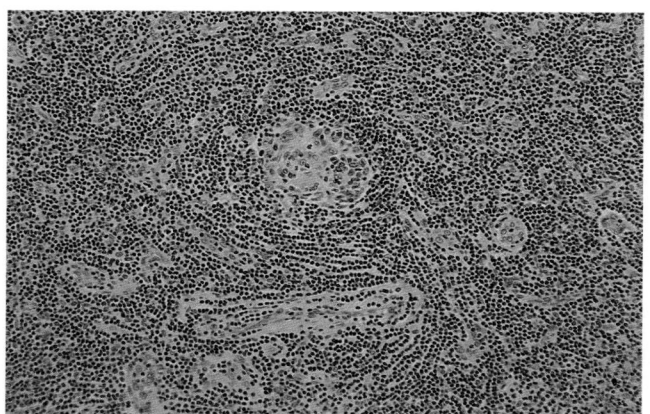

FIGURE 41–13. Castleman's disease, hyaline vascular type. A hyaline vascular follicle is shown. The mantle zone lymphocytes lie in a concentric ring (so-called onion skin pattern) around the reactive germinal center. There is a proliferation of small blood vessels.

pop," with abnormal germinal centers that superficially resemble Hassall corpuscles and a penetrating hyalinized vessel entering at right angles to the follicle.[143] The interfollicular areas contain small lymphocytes, occasional eosinophils, some plasma cells, and a few immunoblasts. Clusters of T lineage plasmacytoid cells are often found.[158] Large, dense fibrotic masses may be seen around larger vessels, usually in interfollicular areas. Rare cases are associated with follicular dendritic cell tumors.[159]

The differential diagnosis of the hyaline vascular type of Castleman's disease includes the Castleman's disease–like lesions seen in HIV-infected patients with persistent generalized lymphadenopathy.[153, 160] In both diseases, small germinal centers may be present, but in Castleman's disease, the interfollicular vascularity is greater and the cellular polymorphism and interfollicular plasmacytosis are less pronounced. Also, the mantle zones are prominent in Castleman's disease, whereas they tend to be small or even absent in HIV-related adenopathy. Another entity in the differential diagnosis of Castleman's disease is an unusual regressive germinal center described in the lymph nodes of organ transplant recipients.[161] The follicles in these immunocompromised patients are composed predominantly of follicular dendritic cells with rare to absent lymphocytes and no tingible body macrophages. Unlike hyaline vascular Castleman's disease, the regressive germinal centers lack a broad lymphocyte mantle with an onion skin appearance.

Immunohistochemical stains in paraffin sections can aid in the diagnosis of Castleman's disease. The CD21/CD35 cluster of antibodies, which stain follicular dendritic cells, highlight the distinctive follicular dendritic meshwork of Castleman's disease. In this disease, the follicular dendritic network loses its cohesion and is loosely arranged but not totally disrupted.[39] Fascin immunohistochemical staining also reveals abnormal syncytial networks of follicular

dendritic cells.[162] This is in contrast to follicular lymphoma, which has decreased or absent fascin staining in the follicles, and it is also in contrast to follicular hyperplasia, which has normal or increased numbers of fascin-positive follicular dendritic cells.

PLASMA CELL TYPE. Approximately 10% of Castleman's disease cases are of the plasma cell type. Patients with this type of Castleman's disease range in age from 8 to 62 years (median age is 22 years).[163] No sex predilection has been noted.[156] There are significant differences between the two types of Castleman's disease. In contrast to patients with the hyaline vascular type, those with the plasma cell type frequently have a variety of unexplainable symptoms and abnormal laboratory test results. These include anemia (often microcytic), polyclonal hypergammaglobulinemia, thrombocytosis, and a number of other abnormalities, which somewhat mysteriously all return to normal after excision of the solitary lesion.[143, 153] The plasma cell variant often consists of a group of enlarged nodes rather than the single, rounded mass characteristic of the hyaline vascular type. The plasma cell variant most often occurs in an abdominal location, particularly the small bowel mesentery, but the anterior mediastinum may be alternatively involved.

Histologic examination shows the nodal architecture to be partially preserved; sinuses are usually absent. Follicular hyperplasia is prominent, and occasional atrophic germinal centers may be present. Mantle zones are usually intact and are always surrounded by sheets of plasma cells (Fig. 41–14). The plasma cells are polyclonal in most cases, although monoclonal plasma cells have occasionally been reported.[164] The vascular proliferation characteristic of the hyaline vascular variant is inconspicuous or absent.

In the differential diagnosis of the plasma cell variant of Castleman's disease are follicular hyperplasias with prominent interfollicular plasmacytosis, including those associated with rheumatoid ar-

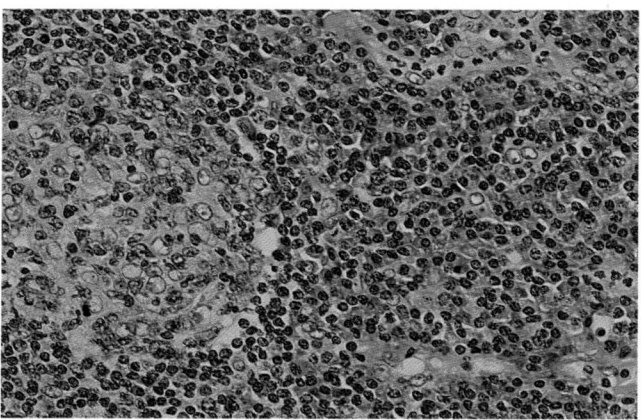

FIGURE 41–14. Castleman's disease, plasma cell type. An atrophic follicle is surrounded by numerous plasma cells, all of which are polyclonal.

thritis and other autoimmune disorders, and syphilis.[152, 153, 165] There is a greater degree of obliteration of sinuses in Castleman's disease than in other disorders. The thick, fibrosed capsule and trabeculae seen in syphilis are lacking in the plasma cell variant of Castleman's disease. The diagnosis of the plasma cell variant of Castleman's disease should not be conclusively made until other disorders are excluded through clinical findings and laboratory tests.[153]

TRANSITIONAL TYPE. The transitional or mixed variant of Castleman's disease is uncommon. Patients are usually asymptomatic and have a localized lesion.[156] On histologic examination, the lesion resembles the hyaline vascular type except for rare foci of plasma cells and possibly some hyperplastic germinal centers. Marked interfollicular plasmacytosis with hyaline vascular germinal centers is even less common.

STROMAL-RICH TYPE. The interfollicular areas of Castleman's disease may rarely contain an overgrowth of stromal elements, such as myoid cells, follicular dendritic cells, and dendritic histiocytes, with or without an increase in blood vessels. On histologic examination, the interfollicular zones are enlarged, occupying more than 75% of the size of the mass, and composed of abundant stromal elements. Correct identification of these various stromal proliferations is clinically important because of differences in their biologic behavior.[157] Sinuses are usually obliterated but may be seen at the periphery of the lesion.

### Systemic (Multicentric) Castleman's Disease

Systemic (multicentric) Castleman's disease is perhaps better termed systemic lymphoproliferative disorder with morphologic features of Castleman's disease.[152] Frizzera defined this disorder by a combination of four clinicopathologic criteria: 1) the characteristic histologic features of the plasma cell type of the disease; 2) a predominantly lymphadenopathic disease involving multiple lymph node sites, mostly peripheral nodes; 3) the various manifestations of multisystem involvement; and 4) an idiopathic nature.[153]

Patients with multicentric Castleman's disease are older (median age is 57 years) than those with the localized disease, the majority are male, peripheral lymph nodes are always involved, and the development of malignant neoplasms is common. The clinical course of this disorder varies. It may behave like a chronic disease with a persistent or relapsing pattern, or it may behave like an unremitting aggressive lymphoproliferative disorder that may be fatal.[155, 166] The disorder may be associated with Kaposi's sarcoma or with polyneuropathy, organomegaly, endocrinopathy, M protein, and skin changes (POEMS or Crow-Fukase syndrome).[167, 168] Lymph nodes with similar histologic changes have also been reported in patients with AIDS.[169] Unlike unicentric Castleman's disease, the systemic form is not amenable to surgical treatment alone and usually requires multimodality therapy, including chemotherapy.[166, 170] Other organs frequently involved by the systemic disorder include bone marrow, liver, kidney, skin, and central and peripheral nervous system.

The histologic changes of multicentric Castleman's disease resemble those of the plasma cell variant of the localized lesion, except follicles with hyaline vascular–type germinal centers may be present. In contrast to the plasma cell variant of the localized disease, there is greater architectural preservation of the node, and dilated sinuses are often filled with deeply stained lymph fluid. The germinal centers vary from regressively transformed to hyperplastic. The interfollicular areas show plasmacytosis, but the plasma cells may be admixed with immunoblasts, and some areas may show vascular proliferation. The plasma cells in most cases are polyclonal, although cases with monoclonal plasma cells have also been reported.[152, 164]

Molecular studies may show a small clonal population of T or B cells but most often show germline configuration of the lymphocyte antigen receptor genes.[171] Evidence of the Kaposi's sarcoma–associated herpesvirus (HHV-8) has been identified in many cases, particularly in those associated with HIV infection but also in approximately 40% of HIV-negative patients with systemic Castleman's disease.[95, 172–175]

Before the rare diagnosis of multicentric Castleman's disease is made, other disorders that cause similar histologic changes must be excluded.[153] The differential diagnoses include autoimmune disorders, HIV-related lymphadenopathy, nodal or disseminated Kaposi's sarcoma, and reactive clinical processes secondary to other malignant neoplasms.[152–154, 167] Clinical history and laboratory findings are essential in the differential diagnosis.

## HIV-RELATED LYMPHADENOPATHY

The systemic presence of enlarged lymph nodes is a frequent finding in HIV-infected patients and is known as persistent generalized lymphadenopathy.[176] Persistent generalized lymphadenopathy is defined as 1) lymph node enlargement of at least 3 months' duration, 2) absence of any illness or drug use known to cause lymph node enlargement, and 3) histologic evidence of follicular hyperplasia in the node examined by biopsy.[177] Biopsy of enlarged lymph nodes in patients with HIV infection should be done to determine whether the adenopathy is due to lymphoid hyperplasia, infection, lymphoma, or Kaposi's sarcoma. Associated hepatosplenomegaly may be present. HIV-related lymphadenopathy is often associated with a heterogeneous Epstein-Barr virus (EBV) population.[178–180]

Lymph nodes show a variety of histologic patterns that correspond to the temporal progression of the disease. The histologic appearance seems to correlate with the immune status and the prognosis of

HIV-positive patients.[125, 148, 181–183] "Explosive" reactive follicular hyperplasia and a combination of reactive follicular hyperplasia with follicular involution are the most common patterns seen in lymph nodes examined by biopsy.[125, 182, 184] Follicular involution alone is seen in clinically more advanced disease. Lymphocyte depletion is usually seen in the disease's final stages, usually identified post mortem. Patients with lymph nodes showing follicular involution and lymphocyte depletion tend to develop some of the stigmata of AIDS, whereas those whose lymph nodes demonstrate follicular hyperplasia appear to have a less symptomatic course.[125, 181, 182]

Explosive reactive follicular hyperplasia consists of variably sized follicles, some of which are extremely large. The follicles are evenly distributed throughout the cortex and medulla and sometimes extend into the capsule.[182–184] The large germinal centers are composed predominantly of transformed large noncleaved and small noncleaved follicle center cells. They have a high mitotic rate and a prominent starry sky appearance. The mantle zones are attenuated or entirely absent, and the naked germinal centers are surrounded by cells of the interfollicular areas, which are also depleted. Coalescence of adjacent follicles may result in the formation of giant-sized germinal centers, which may have bizarre outlines referred to as geographic follicles.[182, 184] A characteristic but not specific finding is the invagination of small mantle zone lymphocytes into the germinal centers, which is termed follicle lysis. Follicle lysis manifests as irregular clusters of germinal center cells among sheets of small mantle zone lymphocytes. The absence of mantle zones and the irregular clusters of large germinal center cells may impart the appearance of large cell lymphoma.[183] Extravasation of red blood cells from germinal center vessels is also encountered.[182] Multinucleated giant cells, some of the Warthin-Finkeldey type, may be seen in follicles or paracortical areas.[148] The paracortical areas have a decreased CD4:CD8 ratio, similar to that seen in the peripheral blood in these patients. Another characteristic but nonspecific finding is the distention of sinuses filled with polyclonal monocytoid B cells, usually accompanied by scattered neutrophils.[148, 182–185] The monocytoid B cell proliferation may also be seen in paracortical areas, sometimes partially encircling germinal centers.[185] The interfollicular areas contain a polymorphous inflammatory cell infiltrate of lymphocytes, plasma cells, eosinophils, immunoblasts, and histiocytes as well as a vascular proliferation with prominent endothelial cells.[182, 184] Focal dermatopathic changes, often without demonstrable melanin, may be identified. The constellation of histologic changes is not specific but should alert the pathologist to the possibility that the patient may have HIV infection.

Biopsy specimens that are obtained later in the disease course may contain changes of follicular involution, with or without explosive follicular hyperplasia.[125, 182, 183] Follicular involution is characterized by small germinal centers, which are also referred to as regressively transformed or "burned-out" germinal centers.[148, 169, 181, 184] The germinal centers consist primarily of concentrically arranged dendritic reticulum cells and a few residual lymphocytes, mimicking the small compact follicles seen in the hyaline vascular type of Castleman's disease. As in Castleman's disease, hyalinized vessels may enter the small germinal centers at right angles, giving rise to the characteristic "lollipop" appearance.[181] Mantle zones may be absent or greatly disrupted. The interfollicular areas are prominent and expanded. Lymphocytes are decreased in number. Morphologic features of the plasma cell variant of Castleman's disease may also be seen in follicular involution, including focal or diffuse plasmacytosis, increased numbers of histiocytes and immunoblasts in interfollicular areas, and vascular proliferation with prominent endothelial cells.[125, 148, 181] Sinus histiocytosis may be present or absent. Fibrosis of the capsule with obliteration of the subcapsular sinus is common. Medullary fibrosis may also be present.[181]

The lymph nodes in mixed follicular hyperplasia and follicular involution are usually enlarged and show histologic features of both follicular hyperplasia and involution.[125, 183] The percentage of involuted follicles is usually less than 50%. The interfollicular areas, which contain a mixture of lymphocytes, plasma cells, immunoblasts, and histiocytes, are larger than those in nodes with florid follicular hyperplasia.[183] Monocytoid B cells in sinuses and paracortex are usually also present.

Biopsy of lymph nodes characteristic of lymphocyte depletion is not usually done because they are small, but they are often obtained at autopsy. There is nodal and capsular fibrosis. Follicles and germinal centers are not seen, and there is severe lymphocyte depletion.[125, 184] The remaining medulla and sinuses may contain plasma cells and histiocytes, the latter often with phagocytosed blood cells, predominantly erythrocytes. The presence of many histiocytes may appear granulomatous. In these cases, an acid-fast stain often shows numerous *Mycobacterium avium-intracellulare* organisms.

Fascin immunohistochemical staining is strongly positive within the interdigitating dendritic cells of the hyperplastic follicles. There may be focal disruption of the fascin-positive dendritic framework. Cases that progress to partial follicular involution have loss of follicular dendritic staining for fascin.[186]

The differential diagnosis of HIV-associated lymphadenopathy includes the hyaline vascular and multicentric types of Castleman's disease, as previously discussed. In addition, lymph nodes of HIV-associated lymphadenopathy may have concurrent infections or concurrent malignant neoplasms. In particular, Kaposi's sarcoma may be a focal finding in the lymph node capsule, especially in lymph nodes with Castleman's disease–like hyaline vascular follicles or lymphocyte depletion. Areas of non-Hodgkin's lymphoma may also be present.

## PROGRESSIVE TRANSFORMATION OF GERMINAL CENTERS

Progressive transformation of germinal centers is an uncommon nonspecific reactive process that is usually associated with follicular hyperplasia in the same lymph node. Its close resemblance to nodular lymphocyte predominant Hodgkin's disease is a frequent cause of cancer overdiagnosis. In fact, an etiologic relationship between progressively transformed germinal centers and nodular lymphocyte predominant Hodgkin's disease has been proposed.[187-191] Progressive transformation may occur before, concurrently with, or after the onset of nodular lymphocyte predominant Hodgkin's disease. Both disorders have a tendency to recur, and subsequent biopsy examination may show either one or the other process.

Progressively transformed germinal centers are often interspersed among benign hyperplastic follicles. The transformed germinal centers are large (three to four times the size of a hyperplastic follicle) and oval (Fig. 41–15). Because of their large size, progressively transformed germinal centers are best identified under low-magnification microscopic examination. The fully developed transformed germinal center consists predominantly of small non-neoplastic lymphocytes with remnants of scattered, residual germinal center cells and dendritic cells.[187, 189, 190] Various stages of transformation may be seen. The earlier lesions consist of germinal centers fragmented by the infiltrating small lymphocytes, and as the name implies, the germinal center cells are progressively replaced until only a few remain.

Progressive transformation of germinal centers and nodular lymphocyte predominant Hodgkin's disease have a similar appearance under low magnification, and both consist predominantly of small B lymphocytes.[187-190, 192] Nodular lymphocyte predominant Hodgkin's disease more commonly has epithelioid histiocytes within or surrounding the nodules, but occasional cases of transformed germinal centers may also have epithelioid histiocytes in the periphery of the nodules. Residual large germinal center cells within the transformed germinal center may closely resemble the popcornlike lymphocytic and histiocytic (L&H) cells of nodular lymphocyte predominant Hodgkin's disease. Both of these cell types stain for CD20 and not for CD15.[187] There is no difference with respect to staining for CD30 or CD21. One distinguishing feature is that the nodules of nodular lymphocyte predominant Hodgkin's disease generally replace the entire lymph node or at least displace any residual reactive follicles to the periphery, unlike progressive transformation, which does not have a mass effect. In addition, progressively transformed nodules have well-circumscribed, confluent sheets of CD20+ small lymphocytes, whereas the nodules of lymphocyte predominance have an irregular, "broken-up" CD20 staining pattern.[193] The most useful clue that the large cells are L&H cells is the presence of T cells (CD4+, CD57+) forming a wreathlike configuration around the L&H cells. T cells do not show the same ring formation around residual large germinal center cells.[194] Also, L&H cells stain with anti–epithelial membrane antigen, whereas residual germinal center cells do not.

Occasional cases of follicular small cleaved cell lymphoma (particularly the floral variant) and mantle cell lymphoma may be mistaken for progressive transformation of germinal centers. The neoplastic follicles of both lymphomas are never as large as the nodules of transformed germinal centers. Both lymphomas are monoclonal B cell processes. The follicular hyperplasia that is associated with progressive transformation of germinal centers is usually not seen in either lymphoma. Follicular small cleaved cell lymphoma is composed of irregular small cleaved cells, and mantle cell lymphoma is composed of cells with slightly irregular nuclear contours. This is in contrast to the round, regular small lymphocytes of progressively transformed follicle centers.

## Reactive Paracortical Hyperplasia

The paracortex is the primary venue of small T lymphocytes. It also contains postcapillary venules, which bring circulating T cells to the paracortex, and a network of interdigitating reticulum cells, which are not easily seen without immunohistochemical stains. The monotonous paracortical or interfollicular region of an unstimulated lymph node appears less prominent than the circumscribed follicles of polymorphous cellular germinal centers. When stimulated, the paracortical region expands to include an increased number of small and large B and T cells, immunoblasts, plasma cells, eosinophils, and histiocytes. The cellular composition varies according to

**FIGURE 41–15.** Progressive transformation of germinal centers. The progressively transformed germinal center is expanded and ill-defined, in contrast to the adjacent reactive follicle.

the nature of the stimulus and its duration. The presence of immunoblasts among the small paracortical T cells lends a mottled appearance to the expanded area, which is usually accompanied by a proliferation of postcapillary venules lined by prominent endothelial cells. The large transformed cells may be of T or B cell type, the latter having migrated from hyperplastic follicles that may have been present at an earlier stage of the process. Germinal centers and sinuses are usually preserved but displaced by the expanded paracortex. Fine-needle aspiration biopsy of reactive paracortical hyperplasia shows a polymorphous population of cells. Benign paracortical hyperplasia is almost always accompanied by some degree of reactive follicular hyperplasia and reactive sinus hyperplasia. A specific etiology can be identified only in a minority of cases, but some disorders have additional characteristic or even diagnostic features.

## VIRAL AND POSTVACCINIAL LYMPHADENITIS

Viral lymphadenitis is a common cause of reactive paracortical hyperplasia. Marked variation in the microscopic appearance of viral lymphadenitis is a consequence of the different times of biopsy during the course of the disease.[195] The most characteristic finding of viral lymphadenitis is paracortical expansion by a proliferation of immunoblasts, admixed with small, predominantly T lineage lymphocytes, plasma cells, plasmacytoid cells, and a brisk proliferation of postcapillary venules with prominent, hyperplastic endothelial cells. The immunoblasts show variation in size and degree of cytoplasmic basophilia and may even be mildly atypical. The overall nodal architecture is usually intact but may be severely distorted. If the lymph node is fragmented, partial architectural preservation may be difficult to discern. In the early stages of the disease, one sees florid reactive follicular hyperplasia, which diminishes inversely as disease progresses with markedly rising numbers of mitotically active immunoblasts (Fig. 41–16). Foci of necrosis may also be seen, either within the germinal centers or in the paracortical regions. The sinuses are usually dilated and filled by monocytoid B cells or a mixture of monocytoid B cells, immunoblasts, and histiocytes. Hemophagocytosis may be identified. In advanced cases, the paracortical cells may spill over into the sinuses, resulting in dilatation of the sinuses. In some cases, the sinuses may be compressed by the paracortical dilatation. Also in advanced cases, the paracortical cells may obliterate the follicles, leading to diffuse effacement of the nodal architecture.

The differential diagnosis of viral lymphadenitis includes Hodgkin's disease and non-Hodgkin's lymphoma.[196-198] The paracortical immunoblasts may be binucleated and appear identical to Reed-Sternberg cells, thus suggesting the possibility of Hodgkin's disease. The additional presence of occasional eosin-

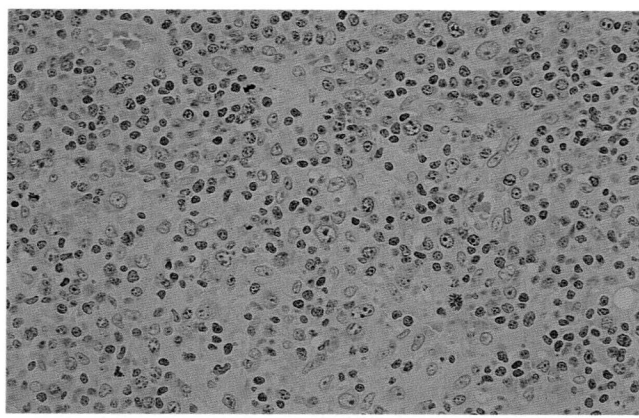

**FIGURE 41–16.** Infectious mononucleosis. There is a mixture of lymphocytes, monocytoid B cells, immunoblasts, and histiocytes, none of which shows cytologic atypia. In clinically advanced disease, sheets of immunoblasts may be mistaken for large cell lymphoma.

ophils may also support that diagnosis. Although binucleated immunoblasts and Reed-Sternberg cells may be morphologically indistinguishable, the surrounding cellular milieu may help distinguish between the two diseases. The telltale mottled appearance of the paracortex is characteristic of viral disorders but is not seen in Hodgkin's disease. Immunohistochemical staining of the binucleated cells may be of additional help. True Reed-Sternberg cells in Hodgkin's disease stain for CD15 and CD30. The Reed-Sternberg cell mimickers of viral lymphadenitis are CD15⁻, but they are often CD30⁺.[196, 199-201] Both are EBV positive, but a spectrum of cell types are EBV positive in infectious mononucleosis, and only the Reed-Sternberg cells and Reed-Sternberg variants are EBV positive in Hodgkin's disease.

In some cases, the immunoblasts form clusters or sheets, thus suggesting the diagnosis of large cell immunoblastic lymphoma.[198] Distinguishing viral lymphadenitis from this malignant disease can be particularly problematic when the biopsy sample of the lymph node is fragmented. Low-magnification examination shows portions of the node with benign reactive change in viral lymphadenitis, whereas large cell lymphomas more typically efface the entire lymph node. Large cell lymphomas may partially involve a lymph node on occasion, but the presence of a mottled paracortex with a polymorphous infiltrate in areas not involved by lymphoma would be unusual. Immunohistochemical stains for CD20 highlight large confluent sheets of large cells in lymphoma, whereas a mixture of B lineage and T lineage cells is seen in viral lymphadenitis. Demonstration of clonality may help to establish a diagnosis of malignancy, although oligoclonal proliferation of T cells has been demonstrated in some cases of viral lymphadenitis.

### Infectious Mononucleosis

Infectious mononucleosis is the prototypic reactive paracortical hyperplasia. Clinical and serologic findings as well as the presence of atypical lymphocytes in the peripheral blood usually lead to the diagnosis. Thus, the surgical pathologist is confronted with a tissue specimen of infectious mononucleosis only in rare patients whose disease is clinically aberrant or whose adenopathy is persistent. Because of the rareness of infectious mononucleosis cases among surgical pathologists, the disease in its late stages may easily be confused with malignant neoplasms.[196, 197, 199, 200] Immunohistochemical study of EBV latent membrane protein and EBV in situ hybridization studies generally have positive results and are therefore not useful in distinguishing between infectious mononucleosis and Hodgkin's disease, except as noted before.[202, 203] Anaplastic large cell lymphoma is also in the differential diagnosis of infectious mononucleosis. Both lesions have large immunoblasts that show immunohistochemical staining for CD30 and CD43. However, in contrast to the reactive lesion, the malignant cells of anaplastic large cell lymphoma are positive for anaplastic lymphoma kinase (ALK) protein and CD3 (majority of cases) and are present predominantly as large clusters in the sinuses or as a diffuse proliferation. The malignant cells do not usually stain for CD20, which is positive in the large immunoblasts of infectious mononucleosis.

### Cytomegalovirus Infection

Cytomegalovirus (CMV) infections in immunocompromised and nonimmunosuppressed individuals may resemble changes seen in infectious mononucleosis. In addition, CMV infections may show pronounced follicular hyperplasia with a monocytoid B cell proliferation, with no paracortical expansion.[195] The morphologic features are similar to those of other viral lymphadenitides. Characteristic cellular CMV inclusions together with serologic, immunohistochemical, and in situ hybridization techniques establish a specific diagnosis of CMV infection.[204, 205] The differential diagnosis of cytomegaloblastic lymphadenitis includes Hodgkin's disease because the eosinophilic nuclear inclusions of CMV may mimic the eosinophilic nucleoli of Reed-Sternberg cells. Both entities stain for CD15. However, in situ hybridization or paraffin immunohistochemistry studies for CMV DNA or antigen, respectively, should distinguish between the two entities.[206]

### Herpesvirus Infection

Herpes simplex or herpes zoster infections may cause regional lymphadenopathy.[207, 208] However, biopsy of these nodes is rarely done because such infections are usually easily diagnosed clinically by the presence of a characteristic vesicular skin lesion. The histologic changes are similar to those described in other viral disorders. There is a prominent paracortical polymorphous infiltrate in which immunoblasts may predominate. Reed-Sternberg–like cells may also be present. Characteristic viral inclusions may be found at the edge of necrotic areas. The diagnosis can be confirmed by immunohistochemical stains and in situ hybridization.

### Postvaccinial Lymphadenitis

Clinical history is also important in establishing the etiology of viral lymphadenitis. Postvaccinial lymphadenitis, an entity more commonly seen in the past when vaccination against smallpox was routinely required for international travel, shows morphologic changes identical to infectious mononucleosis. Most patients present with painful enlargement of the left cervical lymph nodes, which drain the site of vaccination.[195] A similar histologic picture may be seen in regional lymph nodes after intramuscular or subcutaneous inoculation of attenuated measles virus vaccine or tetanus toxoid.[209] The characteristic Warthin-Finkeldey giant cells of measles may also be seen.

## DRUG-INDUCED HYPERSENSITIVITY REACTIONS

Phenytoin (Dilantin) is the most common drug to be associated with lymphadenopathy, but other drugs including the anticonvulsant carbamazepine may also cause enlargement of lymph nodes in susceptible individuals.[210–214] Cervical lymphadenopathy is common, and patients may also have axillary and inguinal lymphadenopathy. The onset of lymphadenopathy is generally 2 to 3 weeks after phenytoin is started, but the time of onset may be greatly extended. Lymphadenopathy usually subsides within 2 weeks of stopping the medication but may recur on reintroduction of the drug. In addition to lymphadenopathy, patients may also have fever, rash, gingival hyperplasia, hepatosplenomegaly, or sometimes joint pains. Some patients, especially those taking phenytoin, may be asymptomatic. Subsequent development of Hodgkin's and non-Hodgkin's lymphomas has been described in patients receiving long-term phenytoin therapy.[137]

Marked paracortical expansion is due to a diffuse polymorphous proliferation of lymphocytes, immunoblasts, plasma cells, eosinophils, and histiocytes. If biopsy of the lymph node is performed in the early stages of enlargement, one may see follicular hyperplasia in addition to paracortical expansion, but biopsy specimens in the later stages of the disease show attrition or collapse of follicles that is due to expansion of the paracortex. The morphologic changes are nonspecific and are similar to those seen in postvaccinial lymphadenopathy or infectious mononucleosis. One may also see a proliferation of high endothelial vessels; this, in combination with many immunoblasts, may call to mind immunoblastic-angioimmunoblastic lymphadenopathy, except reactive germinal centers are often still present. Such proliferations may be interpreted as representing abnormal immune reactions. When sheets of immunoblasts are present, the proliferation may resemble large cell lymphoma.[79] Binucleate immunoblasts may be indistinguishable from Reed-Sternberg cells, thus mimicking Hodgkin's disease. Low-magnification examination shows partial preservation of the normal nodal architecture, which is more commonly seen in benign proliferations than in lymphomas.

## DERMATOPATHIC LYMPHADENITIS

Dermatopathic lymphadenitis is a reactive condition that may be seen in lymph nodes draining areas near skin lesions. The skin disorders may be benign (such as psoriasis) or malignant (such as mycosis fungoides).[215, 216] Histologic findings identical to those in patients with skin lesions have also been reported in individuals without apparent skin disorders. Dermatopathic changes in patients with mycosis fungoides are an ominous prognostic sign whether or not the node is involved by the neoplastic T cells.

Gross evaluation shows the lymph node to be slightly enlarged; a streaky dark pigment may be seen. On histologic examination, the overall nodal architecture is preserved. The hallmark morphologic feature of dermatopathic lymphadenitis is the expanded paracortex, which contains numerous interdigitating cells, Langerhans cells, histiocytes, and eosinophils, resulting in a characteristic "mottled" appearance at low magnification. Large transformed lymphoid cells (immunoblasts) and plasma cells may also be present in the paracortex. A minority of histiocytes show phagocytosis of melanin, cholesterol, or hemosiderin.[217] Small lymphoid cells, some of which may have irregular nuclear contours, are also present. Interdigitating dendritic cells and Langerhans cells are usually prominent and can be recognized by their distinctive nuclei, which have complex and delicately folded membranes, and their characteristic immunohistochemical staining for S-100 protein, HLA-DR, and CD1.[39, 218] The follicles, which may be atrophic or hyperplastic, are often displaced to the outer cortex by the paracortical expansion. The cytologic features are also discernible by fine-needle aspiration.[219, 220]

Because the small lymphocytes of dermatopathic lymphadenitis may have irregular nuclear contours, they cannot always be reliably distinguished from early nodal involvement by mycosis fungoides. Early involvement by this cutaneous T cell lymphoma can be ascertained morphologically with confidence only when at least partial effacement of the lymph node is present.[216] The evaluation of lymph nodes in patients with known or suspected mycosis fungoides is found in the discussion of mycosis fungoides later in this chapter. The differential diagnosis of dermatopathic changes also includes Langerhans cell histiocytosis, Hodgkin's disease, and monocytic leukemia. The Langerhans cells of Langerhans cell histiocytosis are usually present in the sinuses, with spillover into the paracortex. This is unlike dermatopathic lymphadenitis, in which the Langerhans cells are predominantly in the paracortex. The paracortical location and bland histiocyte morphology of dermatopathic lymphadenitis are easily distinguished from Hodgkin's disease or monocytic leukemia. Immunohistochemical studies may be needed for cases in which the histologic preparation is poor.

## Sinus Hyperplasia

### NONSPECIFIC SINUS HISTIOCYTOSIS

Sinus histiocytosis is a common nonspecific finding in lymph node biopsy specimens.[128] It may be accompanied by follicular or interfollicular hyperplasia. It may be seen in lymph nodes draining sites of inflammation or tumors, especially breast and gastrointestinal carcinomas.[221] It is also frequently seen in lymph nodes from the abdomen and in those draining the extremities. There are frequent reports of sinus histiocytosis, with or without granulomatous changes, in lymph nodes draining sites of prostheses.[222–224]

On histologic examination, the sinuses are dilated and filled with histiocytes, which are large cells with ample cytoplasm and bland-appearing nuclei. Red cell phagocytosis and hemosiderin deposition may be seen in the cytoplasm after transfusions or in cases of hemolytic anemia, and lymph nodes from the mediastinum usually contain sinus histiocytes with anthracotic pigment.[225] Strongly birefringent particles resembling polyethylene may also be seen after joint replacement surgery.[226] A rare variant of sinus histiocytosis contains signet ring–like histiocytes, which show no nuclear atypia, thus distinguishing the entity from metastatic signet ring cell carcinoma.[227, 228] The clear cytoplasmic vacuoles do not stain for mucin but may contain lipid.

### MONOCYTOID B CELL HYPERPLASIA

Clusters of reactive monocytoid B cells can be identified in approximately 10% of lymph nodes associated with reactive lesions, including toxoplasmosis, HIV-associated lymphadenopathy, suppurative granulomatous lymphadenitis, and viral lymphadenitis.[185, 229–231] The cells are moderate in size, usually with small nuclei that have slightly irregular nuclear contours and bland chromatin (Fig. 41–17). The cytoplasm is abundant and clear to pale. There are usually admixed neutrophils and plasma cells, and occasionally there are immunoblasts. CD20 immunohistochemical staining highlights the distinct cell borders with adjacent cells, in contrast to poorly processed lymphoid cells that have perinuclear clearing because of retraction of the cytoplasm, in which the CD20 staining appears perinuclear rather than around the circumference of the cytoplasm.

The differential diagnosis of monocytoid B cell hyperplasia includes marginal zone B cell lymphoma, which was originally called monocytoid B cell lymphoma in its earlier descriptions. Unlike the lymphoma, monocytoid B cell hyperplasia involves only a small portion of the lymph node, shows no

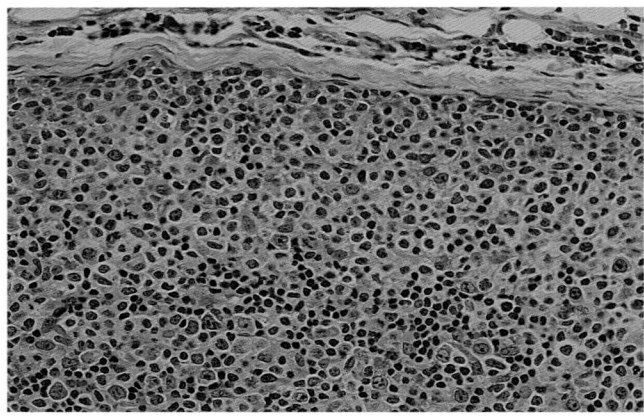

**FIGURE 41–17.** Monocytoid B cell hyperplasia. The sinuses are filled with medium-sized cells with small bland nuclei and abundant clear cytoplasm. There are occasional activated large cells.

involvement of the paracortex, has less nuclear atypia and a lower mitotic rate, and is usually not associated with another lymphoma type. In addition, reactive monocytoid B cells do not stain for Bcl-2 protein, which is positive in a high percentage of monocytoid B cell lymphomas.[131] Furthermore, monocytoid B cells have polytypic light chain expression by immunohistochemistry, whereas marginal zone lymphoma cells show light chain restriction.

## HEMOPHAGOCYTIC SYNDROMES

Infection-associated hemophagocytic syndrome is a benign, potentially reversible but often fatal disorder that occurs primarily in immunocompromised patients.[232–234] Older terms for this entity include histiocytic medullary reticulosis and virus-associated hemophagocytic syndrome. The syndrome has been described in transplant recipients and in patients with acute lymphoblastic leukemia and T cell lymphomas as well as in individuals with congenital immunodeficiency.[235–237] The clinical findings include high fever, constitutional symptoms, anemia, lymphadenopathy, hepatosplenomegaly, abnormal liver function test results, and coagulopathy. Many cases are associated with EBV.[238]

Lymph nodes from these patients show dilated sinuses filled with bland-appearing histiocytes that contain phagocytosed red blood cells. The histiocyte cytoplasm may also contain neutrophils, lymphocytes, and platelets, all of which are typically not as prominent as the red cells (Fig. 41–18). The normal nodal architecture is usually intact, but the lymph node may also show vascular proliferation and a generalized depletion of lymphocytes. In some cases, the entire nodal architecture may be completely effaced.

The differential diagnosis of infection-associated hemophagocytic syndrome includes familial hemophagocytic lymphohistiocytosis, which can be distinguished on clinical grounds.[128, 239, 240] Most patients with familial hemophagocytic lymphohistiocytosis

are younger than 1 year and have impaired cellular and humoral immunity.[241] These patients often have involvement of the lymph nodes and bone marrow. Spleen, liver, and central nervous system are also affected. Some investigators hypothesize that familial hemophagocytic lymphohistiocytosis and infection-associated hemophagocytic syndrome represent the same disease, with familial hemophagocytic lymphohistiocytosis affecting individuals with familial immunodeficiencies.

The differential diagnosis of infection-associated hemophagocytic syndrome also includes malignant histiocytosis and malignant lymphomas associated with benign hemophagocytosis, metastatic carcinoma, and metastatic melanoma.[235, 242] Most previously reported cases of malignant histiocytosis were probably examples of infection-associated hemophagocytic syndrome. Cases of malignant histiocytosis in which the cells had malignant cytologic features were most likely examples of anaplastic large cell lymphomas, which often have a sinusoidal localization in lymph nodes.[243–245] In these lymphomas, erythrophagocytosis is not prominent, but when it is present, it is almost exclusively in benign histiocytes and not in the cytologically malignant cells. Furthermore, the sinusoidal cells of anaplastic large cell lymphoma show immunohistochemical staining for CD30, unlike the benign phagocytosing histiocytes of infection-associated hemophagocytic syndrome. Carcinoma and malignant melanoma preferentially metastasize to the lymph node sinuses; when this is prominent, it may be confused with hemophagocytic syndrome. Cytokeratin immunohistochemistry highlights metastatic carcinoma cells, with the caveat that normal lymph node dendritic cells show a spiderlike keratin staining pattern that is unlike the exclusively membrane, pericellular staining of carcinoma cells. S-100 protein shows a similar dendritic pattern of staining in the normal lymph node, but it shows nuclear staining in the malignant cells of metastatic melanoma.

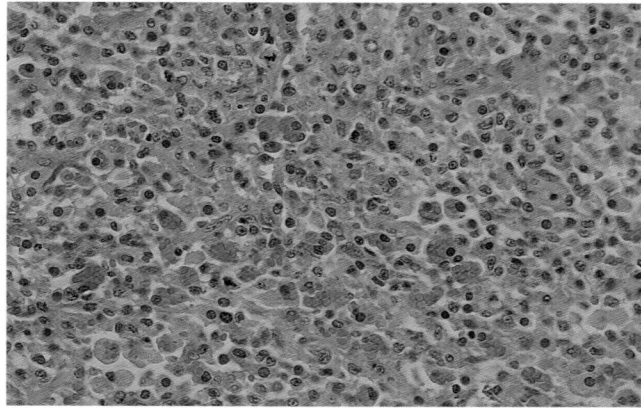

**FIGURE 41–18.** Infection-associated hemophagocytic syndrome. The sinuses contain numerous histiocytes showing erythrophagocytosis.

Far less likely, monocytoid B cell proliferations and hairy cell leukemia in lymph nodes may mimic infection-associated hemophagocytic syndrome.[231, 235, 246] However, monocytoid B cell lymphomas, reactive monocytoid B cell proliferations, and hairy cell leukemia are not associated with hemophagocytosis and resemble the syndrome only in their sinusoidal and parafollicular pattern of nodal involvement.

## SINUS HISTIOCYTOSIS WITH MASSIVE LYMPHADENOPATHY

Sinus histiocytosis with massive lymphadenopathy, also known as Rosai-Dorfman disease, is a rare idiopathic disorder.[247–249] Males are slightly more often affected than are females. The disease is seen in all age groups, but most cases occur in the first 2 decades of life. Massive bilateral cervical adenopathy is the most common presentation; other sites of involvement include inguinal, axillary, and mediastinal nodes. Approximately 40% of patients have extranodal involvement. The eponym Rosai-Dorfman disease has been used for this form of sinus histiocytosis. Hepatosplenomegaly is not common. Abnormal laboratory findings include polyclonal hypergammaglobulinemia, elevated erythrocyte sedimentation rate, and anemia. The etiology of the disorder is unknown, but recent findings suggest that it is a disorder of altered immunity.

On gross evaluation, the lymph node is markedly enlarged and usually multinodular.[249] Microscopic examination shows a markedly thickened capsule with pericapsular fibrosis. The sinuses are markedly dilated (Fig. 41–19) by highly characteristic histiocytic cells, which have a vesicular nucleus with a central, small, distinct nucleolus (Fig. 41–20). The cytoplasm is abundant and contains numerous intact lymphocytes (emperipolesis). Less frequently, the histiocytes engulf plasma cells, neutrophils, and even red cells. Some histiocytes may contain atypical hyperchromatic nuclei with a prominent nucleolus. The cytologic features of the histiocytes may be recognized by fine-needle aspiration.[250, 251] Also charac-

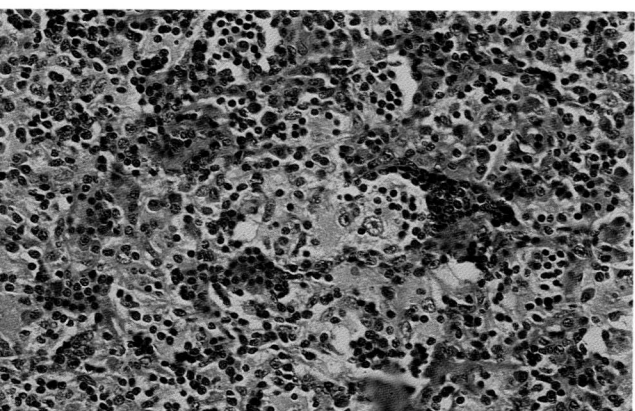

**FIGURE 41–20.** Sinus histiocytosis with massive lymphadenopathy, high power. The distinctive histiocytes have a vesicular nucleus, one or several prominent nucleoli, and abundant cytoplasm exhibiting lymphophagocytosis. There are numerous admixed plasma cells.

teristic of this entity is a heavy plasma cell infiltrate in the medullary cords. In many cases, only remnants of intersinusoidal lymphoid tissue remain. Follicles are not prominent. The sinusoidal histiocytes stain for S-100 protein and CD68, similar to the cells of Langerhans cell histiocytosis but unlike the histiocytes of reactive sinus histiocytosis.[248, 252] However, CD1 and R4/23 (a monoclonal antibody with high specificity for follicular dendritic cells) are not positive in sinus histiocytosis with massive lymphadenopathy, helping to distinguish it from Langerhans cell histiocytosis.[253–255] Another difference from Langerhans cell histiocytosis is the lack of Birbeck granules in sinus histiocytosis with massive lymphadenopathy. Molecular studies show a germline configuration for both the immunoglobulin heavy chain gene and the T cell receptor β-chain gene.[248]

## WHIPPLE'S DISEASE

Whipple's disease is a bacterial infection of the small intestine caused by *Tropheryma whippelii*.[256, 257] The patients are usually middle-aged men, who may be asymptomatic or who may present with variable symptoms, including weight loss, diarrhea, and arthralgias.[258] Symptomatic patients often have steatorrhea, hypoalbuminemia, and low serum carotene levels. Abdominal lymph nodes are frequently involved, and peripheral lymphadenopathy may be seen in about 50% of patients. Lymph node biopsy specimens show dilated sinuses filled with pale-staining, finely vacuolated, PAS-positive histiocytes. Non-necrotizing granulomas and interspersed extracellular lipid vacuoles are also common findings. The strong and characteristic intracellular diastase-resistant PAS positivity is due to the causative sickle-form bacilli.[258, 259]

The differential diagnosis of Whipple's disease includes infection by *M. avium-intracellulare*, which also has PAS-positive histiocytes. However, an acid-

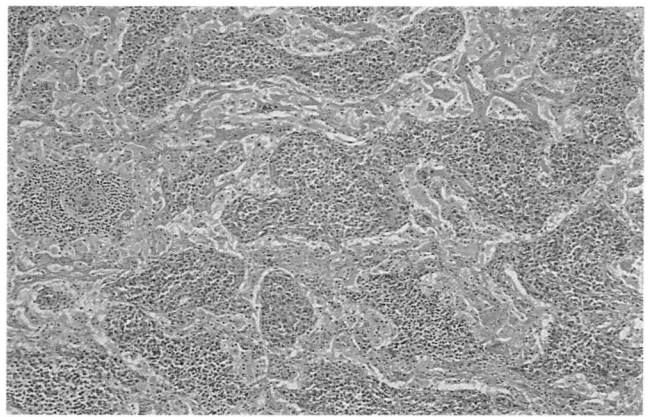

**FIGURE 41–19.** Sinus histiocytosis with massive lymphadenopathy, low power. The sinusoidal pattern is highly characteristic.

fast stain distinguishes between these two infections because of the abundant acid-fast bacilli in the mycobacterial infection and lack of staining for acid-fast bacilli in Whipple's disease. Another entity in the differential diagnosis is lymphadenopathy due to deposition of exogenous lipids, which can be distinguished by clinical history.

## LYMPHADENOPATHY DUE TO DEPOSITION OF EXOGENOUS LIPIDS

Lymphangiography, a radiologic technique once used routinely for the staging of Hodgkin's disease, is now used uncommonly. Thus, nodes showing the changes caused by injection of the radiopaque lipid-based contrast media are rarely seen on biopsy examination. The most prominent histologic finding is sinuses containing large vacuoles, which result from dissolution of the injected medium during tissue processing[260] (Fig. 41–21). Histiocytes and multinucleated foreign body–type giant cells surround the vacuoles and may be scattered throughout the lymph node parenchyma. Eosinophils may be seen within the sinuses and in medullary cords.

The differential diagnosis includes normal lymph nodes of the porta hepatis and celiac axis, which may show lipophagic vacuolization of sinus histiocytes and multinucleated giant cells. However, the vacuoles are much smaller than those associated with lymphangiography, and the lymph nodes often also contain lipid granulomas. Lymph node sinuses in cases of pneumatosis intestinalis contain large gas vacuoles surrounded by a granulomatous reaction.[128] Other entities that may mimic lymphangiography effect include fungal infections, tuberculous lymphadenitis, and sarcoidosis. Grocott-Gomori methenamine silver stain and stains for acid-fast bacilli aid in the diagnosis of the first two conditions, respectively. Sarcoidosis generally contains well-defined granulomas without any vacuoles.

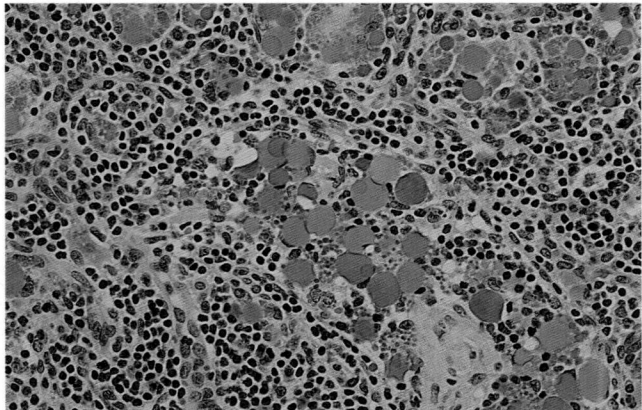

**FIGURE 41–21.** Sinus histiocytes with foreign material. Numerous histiocytes engulf radiographic contrast material. The variation in size, shape, and quantity of this polarizable matter is a clue to its nature.

## Benign Lymphadenopathy with Prominent Necrosis

Focal areas of necrosis are common in many of the benign lymphadenopathies or lymphadenitides. However, extensive necrosis is a primary or characteristic finding in some clinical settings, including in some patients with AIDS, lymphoma, Kikuchi's histiocytic necrotizing lymphadenitis, systemic lupus erythematosus, and Kawasaki's disease.

### COMPLETE LYMPH NODE NECROSIS

Complete lymph node necrosis may manifest as liquefactive necrosis or coagulative necrosis. Liquefactive necrosis consists of karyorrhectic debris, neutrophil fragments, and possibly abscess formation. This is usually more frequently encountered during postmortem examinations, but in surgical specimens, particularly those from immunocompromised patients, it may be due to fungal infection (such as histoplasmosis) or a wide variety of bacteria.

Coagulative necrosis is due to vascular compromise, and the most common cause in lymph nodes is malignant lymphoma, usually non-Hodgkin's lymphoma of large cell type.[261] The affected lymph node may have a partially viable outer rim, but most of the node shows ghosts of lymphoid cells and few inflammatory cells. One may see venous thrombosis or granulation tissue in the pericapsular adipose tissue. Immunohistochemical stains identify the cell lineage; the cellular membrane antigens remain immunologically viable despite the histologic appearance of cell death.

### HISTIOCYTIC NECROTIZING LYMPHADENITIS

Histiocytic necrotizing lymphadenitis, also known as histiocytic necrotizing lymphadenitis without granulocytic infiltration, Kikuchi-Fujimoto disease, and Kikuchi's disease, is a benign, self-limited, well-defined clinicopathologic disorder first described in the 1970s.[262–266] Although it was first recognized in Japan, numerous cases have now been reported in other parts of the world.[264, 267–270]

The patients are generally healthy young women. The age of patients at presentation covers a spectrum from adolescence to the elderly, with a median age at diagnosis of 30 years. The male-to-female ratio is approximately 1:4.[271] No trend in occupation, lifestyle, or underlying disease has been implicated. Lymphadenopathy of several months' duration is the only symptom in most patients. Isolated cervical lymphadenopathy is common, but less often, other lymph nodes may be primarily affected; rarely, two or more lymph node sites are involved. Reported symptoms may also include a mild fever associated with upper respiratory symptoms, weight loss, nausea, vomiting, myalgia, arthralgia, chills, night sweats, and rarely a malar rash.[272] The peripheral blood of these patients usually shows no abnormalities, although neutropenia, lymphocytosis, and circulating atypical lymphocytes have been reported.[128] Serologic studies usually show no evidence of an infectious etiology, although one group has reported three cases in which serologic studies suggested infection with *Yersinia enterocolitica*.[262, 264] The disorder may be a forme fruste of systemic lupus erythematosus because a small number of patients later develop lupus and the lesions are histologically similar.[264]

Lymph nodes appear grossly normal, perhaps with a slight increase in size. On microscopic examination, the nodal architecture is only partially effaced, and the uninvolved lymphoid tissue is usually normal, with dormant nonhyperplastic follicles. Discrete foci of necrosis are scattered throughout the paracortex and less often in the cortex. These necrotic foci usually consist of large deposits of an eosinophilic substance (probably representing fibrin) and marked karyorrhectic debris (Fig. 41–22). In rare cases, the foci may contain little eosinophilic amorphous material.[262-265, 268] Also present within the well-circumscribed necrotic areas are viable cells consisting of histiocytes that exhibit phagocytosis and occasionally contain foamy cytoplasm, reactive immunoblasts (some binucleated), and plasmacytoid monocytes. The absence of intact neutrophils, plasma cells, and eosinophils in areas of extensive necrosis is a useful diagnostic feature. Immediately adjacent to the foci of necrosis, one generally sees a proliferation of reactive immunoblasts. The sinuses may be focally distended by monocytoid B lymphocytes, but this is not a usual finding.[264] The lymph node capsule may be thickened adjacent to the necrotic foci. Plasma cells are usually sparse or absent. The remainder of the lymph node usually contains immunoblasts scattered among small paracortical lymphocytes, imparting a mottled appearance not unlike that seen in viral infections. Follicles are usually not prominent.

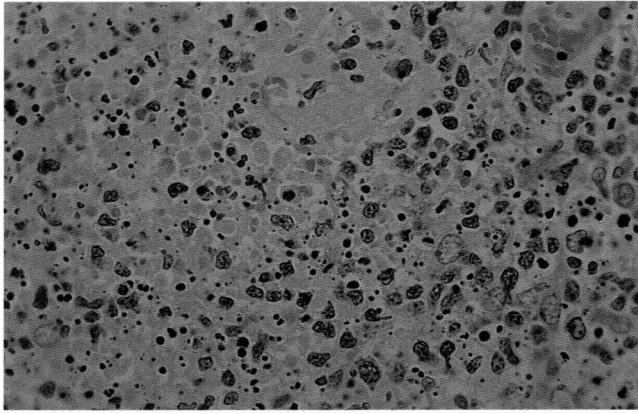

**FIGURE 41–22.** Kikuchi's histiocytic necrotizing lymphadenitis. There is abundant necrosis with karyorrhectic debris and histiocytes with twisted nuclei. Note the absence of polymorphonuclear neutrophils.

Immunohistochemical studies show a predominance of T cells and macrophages within involved areas of the lymph node.[267, 269, 270] In lesions detected and sampled early, helper-inducer T cells may predominate, whereas the majority of biopsy specimens taken late after presentation appear to contain cytotoxic-suppressor T cells.[273] There is some evidence that the karyorrhectic debris may be derived from T lineage–associated plasmacytoid cells.[269]

Distinguishing histiocytic necrotizing lymphadenitis from non-Hodgkin's lymphoma is important because of great differences in treatment and prognosis. Each has a characteristic clinical history that differs from the other. The abundant karyorrhectic debris and sheets of macrophages seen in histiocytic necrotizing lymphadenitis may impart a superficial appearance of a high-grade lymphoma. However, one must keep in mind that the only lymphomas to have a large amount of karyorrhexis are Burkitt's-type and large cell immunoblastic lymphoma. The monotonous and malignant cells of these lymphomas are not seen in lymph nodes with histiocytic necrotizing lymphadenitis. In nodal non-Hodgkin's lymphoma, the infarcted areas are generally rimmed by granulation tissue and may contain the ghosts of the malignant cells.[261, 274] Compared with non-Hodgkin's lymphoma, histiocytic necrotizing lymphadenitis shows more heterogeneity of the large cells, has a more patchy appearance, and contains many more plasmacytoid monocytes. In the development of the typical necrotic lesion, one stage is termed the proliferative phase and is characterized by foci of a mixture of immunoblasts, histiocytes, and plasmacytoid monocytes. It is in this stage that the differential diagnosis from lymphoma may be particularly difficult to make.

The differential diagnosis of histiocytic necrotizing lymphadenitis also includes Hodgkin's disease. The necrosis associated with Hodgkin's disease usually contains neutrophils. The background polymorphous inflammatory infiltrate of Hodgkin's disease is highly characteristic. Many Reed-Sternberg cells may surround the necrotic foci in Hodgkin's disease, and these can be immunophenotypically distinguished from the atypical large (often binucleate) cells seen in Kikuchi's disease by CD15 staining in the Reed-Sternberg cells only.

Histiocytic necrotizing lymphadenitis may also be confused with lymph nodes that have manifestations of infectious agents, such as *Y. enterocolitica*, the agent of lymphogranuloma venereum, or the cat-scratch disease organism, because they are associated with stellate areas of necrosis (stellate microabscesses). In these entities, the presence of neutrophils in and around the necrotic foci allows easy separation from histiocytic necrotizing lymphadenitis.

Lymph node biopsy specimens from patients with Kawasaki's disease also contain neutrophils in association with the areas of necrosis. In addition, fibrin thrombi in small vessels are usually a promi-

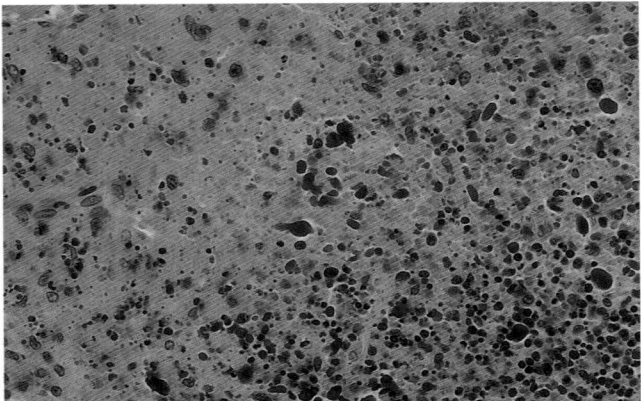

**FIGURE 41–23.** Lupus lymphadenopathy. This lymph node shows coagulative necrosis with karyorrhectic debris adjacent to a reactive area with plasma cells.

nent feature of Kawasaki's disease lymph nodes but not of lymph nodes with histiocytic necrotizing lymphadenitis.[275]

Lymph nodes involved by histiocytic necrotizing lymphadenitis and lymph nodes involved by systemic lupus erythematosus have similar morphologic features, particularly the presence of discrete necrotic foci and eosinophilic deposits. Histologic features that favor systemic lupus erythematosus are the presence of basophilic necrotic material, which is often deposited in vessel walls and sometimes forms hematoxyphilic bodies, and the presence of more than occasional plasma cells.[262] However, distinguishing between histiocytic necrotizing lymphadenitis and systemic lupus erythematosus may be impossible on a purely morphologic basis, so clinical investigation should be undertaken. Some investigators hypothesize that histiocytic necrotizing lymphadenitis represents a self-limited autoimmune condition resembling systemic lupus erythematosus.[262]

The etiology of histiocytic necrotizing lymphadenitis is unknown. Search for an infectious etiology has not yielded any conclusive evidence. However, human herpesvirus 6 was reported to be isolated from 5 of 12 patients with the typical clinicopathologic picture of histiocytic necrotizing lymphadenitis.[276] In addition, the presence of DNA sequences of Kaposi's sarcoma–associated herpesvirus (KSHV/HHV-8) has been reported in 6 of 26 patients with histiocytic necrotizing lymphadenitis. None of the patients was positive for HIV or was otherwise immunocompromised.[277]

The prognosis for most patients with histiocytic necrotizing lymphadenitis is excellent.[264] Spontaneous resolution of the disease usually occurs within 1 to 4 months. One patient has been described with development of recurrent lymphadenopathy in which repeated biopsy also showed histiocytic necrotizing lymphadenitis. At least two patients subsequently had development of systemic lupus erythematosus, and thus it seems prudent for all patients to remain under clinical surveillance.[262]

## SYSTEMIC LUPUS ERYTHEMATOSUS

Thirty percent to 60% of patients with systemic lupus erythematosus have lymphadenopathy, especially of cervical nodes. Patients with autoimmune disorders have an increased risk for development of lymphoma, and thus biopsy of enlarged lymph nodes in these patients is often done. The lymph nodes are usually no larger than 3 cm. Fragmentation of the lymph node during removal is common because the node may be extensively necrotic. On histologic examination, normal nodal architecture is effaced, with extensive necrosis (sometimes coagulative type).[128, 137, 278] Some cases may instead show discrete foci of necrosis with karyorrhectic debris and absence of neutrophils, similar to Kikuchi's disease, but with plasmacytosis.[264, 278] These cases may have residual follicles, showing reactive hyperplasia with plasmacytosis. Other common histologic features of lupus include necrotic or thrombosed blood vessels and the presence of hematoxylin bodies, which are amorphous hematoxyphilic PAS-positive (and Feulgen-positive) structures of altered DNA, 5 to 12 mm in diameter[128] (Fig. 41–23). Clinical history and serologic studies are necessary to confirm the histologic diagnosis of lupus erythematosus.

## MUCOCUTANEOUS LYMPH NODE SYNDROME (KAWASAKI'S DISEASE)

Kawasaki's disease, also known as mucocutaneous lymph node syndrome, is an acute, multisystem vasculitic disorder seen in young children.[128, 137, 275, 279, 280] It is characterized clinically by prolonged fever, erythematous rash, lesions of the conjunctiva and oral mucosa, cervical adenopathy, and coronary arteritis. One percent to 3% of children die of coronary arteritis during the acute phase of the disease. A smaller percentage may die several years after apparent recovery. Lymph nodes in these patients show extensive geographic necrosis with prominent fibrinoid thrombosis of small blood vessels outside the necrotizing foci (Fig. 41–24). T lineage lymphocytes and histiocytes infiltrate the blood vessel walls.[281] The

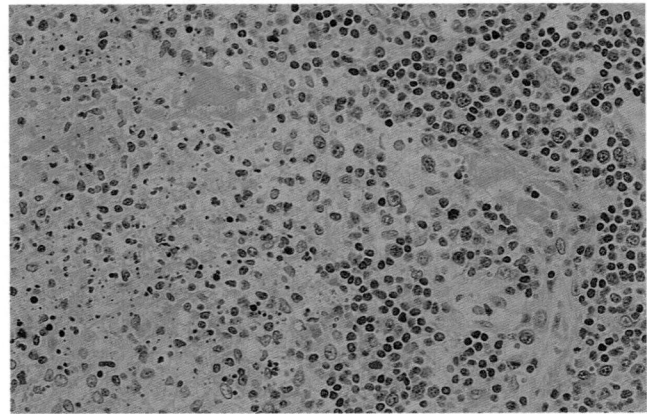

**FIGURE 41–24.** Kawasaki's disease. The small blood vessels contain numerous fibrin thrombi, adjacent to an area of necrosis.

necrosis may be indistinguishable from that seen in lymph nodes of patients with systemic lupus erythematosus, which can be excluded from the differential diagnosis on clinical grounds. The presence of neutrophils and the geographic rather than discrete foci of necrosis also separate Kawasaki's syndrome from Kikuchi's disease, another necrotizing lymphadenitis. The etiology of Kawasaki's syndrome is unknown, but its clinical and epidemiologic features are most consistent with an infectious cause.[282] There have been rare reports of lymphoid malignant neoplasms after the diagnosis of Kawasaki's disease.[283]

## Granulomatous Disorders

### NONINFECTIOUS GRANULOMATOUS LYMPHADENOPATHY

There are numerous causes of noninfectious granulomatous lymphadenopathy, including sarcoidosis.[284] Non-necrotizing granulomas may also be found in mesenteric lymph nodes of patients with Crohn's disease and in nodes draining sites of carcinomas.[284, 285] They are also found in lymph nodes of patients with berylliosis.[284, 285] These granulomas may also be a prominent feature of some non-Hodgkin's lymphomas.[286] These granulomas have also been described in Hodgkin's disease; because of their number, they may mask Reed-Sternberg cells present in the small amount of intervening lymphoid tissue.[287] In addition, granulomas are common in uninvolved lymph nodes of Hodgkin's disease patients.

### Sarcoidosis

Sarcoidosis is a multisystemic granulomatous disease in which the etiology and pathogenic mechanisms are not known.[284] In contrast, the clinical presentation, course of the disease, and laboratory and histologic features are well recognized.[284] Sarcoidosis is characterized histologically by discrete, non-necrotizing epithelioid granulomas (Fig. 41–25). One may

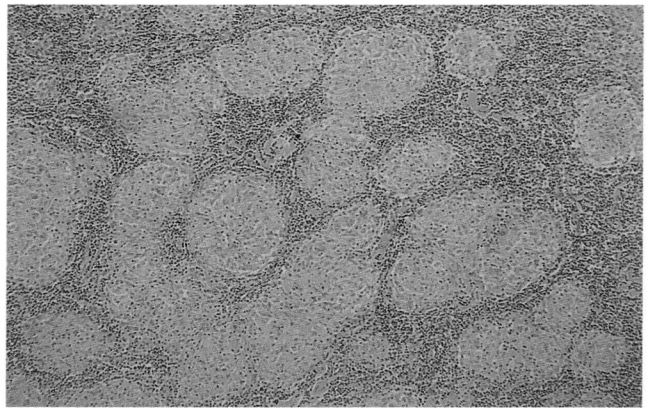

FIGURE 41–25. Sarcoidosis. Multiple epithelioid granulomas are evenly distributed throughout the lymph node parenchyma. Their presence is not specific for sarcoidosis.

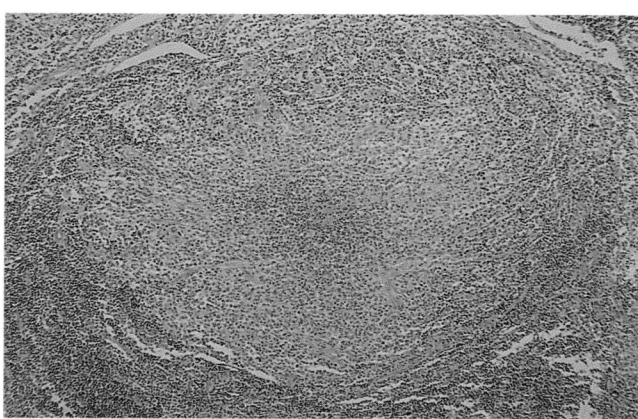

FIGURE 41–26. Necrotizing granuloma. The central area of this granuloma is necrotic and is surrounded by reactive histiocytes.

occasionally see small foci of central fibrinoid necrosis. The granulomas may be surrounded by sclerosis, and older granulomas may become progressively hyalinized. Langerhans giant cells may or may not be present. Asteroid bodies, Schaumann bodies, and crystals of calcium oxalate are rarely seen within giant cells and are not specific for sarcoidosis. One may see Hamazaki-Wesenberg bodies, which are small, needlelike, PAS-positive, acid-fast structures found in the cytoplasm of giant cells.[137]

Sarcoidlike granulomas are not specific, and thus the diagnosis of sarcoidosis is one of exclusion. Staining for acid-fast bacilli and fungi should always be carried out to exclude an infectious etiology of any granulomatous lymphadenitis. The granulomas in tuberculosis usually but not always have areas of necrosis surrounded by epithelioid histiocytes and Langhans giant cells; fungal infections show similar necrosis of granulomas or sometimes suppurative granulomas and, rarely, non-necrotizing epithelioid granulomas. Immunohistochemical stains may be needed to exclude Hodgkin's disease or non-Hodgkin's lymphoma.

### INFECTIOUS GRANULOMATOUS LYMPHADENITIS

Necrotizing or caseating granulomas (Fig. 41–26) are seen in mycobacterial or fungal infections; suppurative granulomas are characteristic of disorders such as cat-scratch disease,[137, 288, 289] lymphogranuloma venereum,[137, 290] tularemia,[128, 137] *Yersinia* infection,[128, 137, 291] and certain fungal infections.[128] Special stains for acid-fast organisms and fungi or silver stains and microbiologic culture of lymph node biopsy specimens may be useful for establishing a specific etiologic diagnosis.

### Tuberculosis

*Mycobacterium tuberculosis* reemerged late in the 20th century as an important and viable pathogen in developed countries, years after it was thought to be under control. There has been a dramatic increase in the number of cases, particularly in urban settings, owing in part to complacency as well as to the growing number of drug-resistant strains. Lymph node involvement, usually of the cervical neck, accompanies lung involvement. Tuberculous lymphadenopathy accounts for 40% of nonrespiratory infections. Tuberculous lymphadenopathy and sarcoidosis are histologically identical, with the exception of more frequent caseating granulomas in tuberculous lymphadenopathy. Tuberculous mycobacteria can be identified by acid-fast stains in the areas of necrosis or by PCR studies.

### Atypical Mycobacterial Infections

Atypical mycobacterial infections are a more common cause of isolated granulomatous lymphadenitis than is tuberculosis. Compared with tuberculosis, there may be fewer granulomatous changes and a greater degree of acute inflammation with abscess formation.[292] Lymph nodes from immunocompromised patients may have a foamy histiocytic infiltration in the paracortex and possibly involving the entire lymph node. An acid-fast stain shows copious amounts of acid-fast bacilli in the histiocytes. In some cases, the fibroblasts may be spindled and increased in number, mimicking inflammatory pseudotumor, which contains no acid-fast organisms.[98, 103] Cases with spindled fibroblasts and abundant acid-fast organisms may represent mycobacterial pseudotumor, which is discussed in an earlier section.

### Lepromatous Lymphadenitis

Depending on the lepromatous patient's immunity status, one may see different morphologic features.[293, 294] In patients with intact cellular immunity, the lymph nodes show reactive paracortical hyperplasia but are not involved by leprosy. In patients with borderline leprosy, the paracortex contains numerous noncaseating granulomas. Fite stains may or may not identify any acid-fast organisms. In patients with defective cellular immunity, one sees numerous foamy macrophages in the paracortex. These macrophages contain numerous organisms and may form clumps, but true granulomas are not formed. In this lepromatous form, one may also see reactive follicular hyperplasia with abundant plasma cells.

### Fungal Infections

Systemic fungal infections may involve lymph nodes. However, the most common fungal cause of solitary lymphadenitis is histoplasmosis.[295, 296] Lymph nodes usually show a granulomatous reaction. One may instead see acute inflammation with abscess formation. Microbiologic cultures are the best method of organism identification. However, PAS or Grocott-Gomori methenamine silver stains may highlight the organisms in tissue sections.

### Pneumocystis carinii

Rare cases of granulomatous lymphadenitis caused by this protozoal organism have been reported in patients with AIDS.[297]

### Cat-Scratch Disease and Lymphogranuloma Venereum

Cat-scratch disease is a self-limited disorder characterized by development of regional lymphadenopathy, usually but not always occurring after a cat scratch or flea bite distal to the affected lymph node. Lymph nodes in the axilla, groin, and neck are the most commonly affected sites. Most cases of cat-scratch disease resolve spontaneously within several months, but some patients have severe complications including encephalitis, neuroretinitis, and follicular conjunctivitis. The accepted etiologic agent of cat-scratch disease is *Bartonella henselae* (formerly *Rochalimaea henselae*), which is a fastidious gram-negative bacterium that shares etiologic responsibility with *Bartonella quintana* for bacillary angiomatosis and culture-negative endocarditis.[298]

Early on, the lymph nodes of patients with cat-scratch disease show florid follicular hyperplasia and distended sinuses and paracortexes filled with monocytoid B cells. There may be small foci of necrosis and small clusters of neutrophils surrounded by histiocytes. The early lesions usually start near the subcapsular sinuses. The small developing abscesses may also involve germinal centers, which contributes to the pronounced degree of follicular hyperplasia. The causative organisms are most likely to be detected in the early stages, especially within walls of capillaries, histiocytes, and areas of necrosis. As the disease progresses, one also sees granulomas within or adjacent to the monocytoid B cell proliferation. The granulomas consist of a central area of suppurative necrosis surrounded by palisading histiocytes and fibroblasts. The suppurative granulomas may extend into the medullary region. In the full-blown disease state, one sees discrete stellate microabscesses rimmed by epithelioid histiocytes. Plasma cells and immunoblasts fill the sinuses and paracortex and also surround the microabscesses. The lymph node capsule is often fibrotic. In the later stages of the disease, the neutrophils gradually disappear, necrotic areas are no longer suppurative, and the organisms are not detectable. The lymph node may frequently contain all stages of development of the suppurative granulomas.

The organisms of cat-scratch disease are positive with a Warthin-Starry silver impregnation stain, which helps to distinguish it from other histologically similar lesions caused by other microorganisms (particularly lymphogranuloma venereum).[288, 299] Detection with antibodies to *B. henselae* and amplification of *B. henselae* DNA in affected tissue are the two mainstays in the laboratory diagnosis of cat-scratch disease and are useful for evaluating the clinical course of the disease and the efficacy of antibiotic therapy.[83, 300–302]

The differential diagnosis of cat-scratch disease includes the morphologically identical lymphogranuloma venereum, which is a sexually transmitted disease caused by *Chlamydia* and is diagnosed most frequently in inguinal lymph nodes.[290] One may see

and in lower socioeconomic groups of developed nations, there is an increase in childhood cases (particularly in boys) and a decrease of incidence in the young adult group.[328, 329] The Hodgkin's disease incidence pattern parallels the degree of economic development.[330-332] The incidence of Hodgkin's disease is low in all age groups studied in several Asian countries.[329, 333]

In the United States, Hodgkin's disease shows a slight male predominance (male-to-female ratio of 1.3:1), with the exception of the nodular sclerosis subtype, which is more common in young women.[326] Children and young adults more often have the nodular sclerosis and lymphocytic predominant subtypes. The older age group tends to more often have the mixed cellularity and lymphocytic depletion subtypes.[325, 334-336] In developing countries, mixed cellularity and lymphocytic depletion subtypes predominate in both childhood and adult groups. There is probably an increase in incidence of the mixed cellularity subtype in patients with AIDS, especially in the group with a history of intravenous drug use.[337-339]

Genetic susceptibility and familial aggregation seem to have an etiologic role in the development of Hodgkin's disease.[340-344] There appears to be an increased risk of Hodgkin's disease to first-degree relatives of Hodgkin's disease patients, particularly in siblings of young adult patients. This risk is magnified even more in same-sex siblings.[344-346] An increased risk of Hodgkin's disease in monozygotic twins of Hodgkin's disease cases has also been reported.[347] There are also reports of associations between HLA type and risk of Hodgkin's disease, independent of EBV status.[341, 343, 348]

Epidemiologic data show that Hodgkin's disease in young patients shares some characteristics with the disease epidemiology of certain viral infections such as poliomyelitis and infectious mononucleosis, suggesting the involvement of a viral agent.[349, 350] Retroviruses, human herpesvirus 6, and EBV have been suggested as putative etiologic agents.[337, 338, 351-357] Only EBV has emerged as a strong etiologic factor, with abundant serologic, immunophenotypic, and molecular data to support the epidemiologic hypothesis.[350, 358-369] Approximately 40% to 50% of Hodgkin's disease cases has been associated with EBV in the neoplastic cells, but an etiologic role has not yet been clearly established.[367, 370] The type of Hodgkin's disease most frequently associated with EBV is the mixed cellularity type, whereas the lymphocyte predominant type is usually negative.

The most common clinical presentation is a young adult with an asymptomatic, slowly growing mass, most often in the cervical neck, high neck, or axilla.[371-373] The inguinal and femoral lymph nodes and mediastinum are less common sites of presentation. Approximately 25% of patients have constitutional symptoms (so-called B symptoms), including unexplained fevers (including intermittent fevers known as Pel-Ebstein fevers), recurrent drenching night sweats during the previous month, and unex-plained weight loss (>10% of body weight) during the previous 6 months. Pruritus or pain after alcohol ingestion may also occur. Laboratory studies can usually document a deficiency in cellular immunity.

## Disease Staging

Hodgkin's disease spreads in a highly predictable manner. From the initial involvement of one lymph node, the disease spreads through lymphatic channels to adjacent lymphoid tissues before disseminating to distant organs and nonadjacent sites. The pattern of disease at presentation appears to be associated with the histologic subtype.[373]

The staging of Hodgkin's disease follows the Cotswolds staging classification, which includes minor modifications of the Ann Arbor classification and is outlined in Table 41–7.[371, 374-376] Clinical staging includes history, physical examination, plain chest radiography, and computed tomography and magnetic resonance imaging of chest and abdomen. Routine pathologic staging procedures include bilateral bone marrow biopsies. Staging laparotomy for gross examination of the spleen and liver is no longer routinely performed in many institutions owing to long-term increased risk of acute leukemia

**TABLE 41–7.** The Cotswolds Modification of the Ann Arbor Staging Classification

| Stage | Description |
|---|---|
| I | Involvement of a single lymph node region (I) or of a single extralymphatic organ or site (I$_E$) |
| II | Involvement of two or more lymph node regions on the same side of the diaphragm (II) [right and left hilum: one area each, independent of mediastinum; number of anatomic nodal areas to be indicated by a subscript (II$_4$)] or localized involvement of an extralymphatic organ or site and of one or more lymph node regions on the same side of the diaphragm (II$_E$) |
| III | Involvement of lymph node regions on both sides of the diaphragm (III), or localized involvement of an extralymphatic organ or site (III$_E$) or spleen (III$_S$) or both (III$_{SE}$) III$_1$ = with or without splenic hilar, celiac, or portal nodes III$_2$ = with para-aortic iliac, or mesenteric nodes |
| IV | Diffuse or disseminated involvement of one or more extralymphatic organs or tissues, with or without associated lymph node involvement |

Use suffixes to denote the absence (A) or presence (B) of fever >38°C or night sweats in the last month, and/or unexplained loss of >10% body weight in the 6 months preceding admission.

| | |
|---|---|
| E | Extranodal involvement by contiguity, encompassable in the nodal radiation field |
| X | Bulky disease, >⅓ widening of mediastinum at T5-6 level, or >10 cm maximum dimension of nodal mass |
| CR(u) | Unconfirmed/uncertain complete remission (residual imaging abnormality) |

**TABLE 41–8.** Hodgkin's Disease Classifications

| Jackson and Parker | Lukes | Rye | WHO Classification |
|---|---|---|---|
| Paragranuloma | L&H nodular<br>L&H diffuse | Lymphocyte predominance | Nodular lymphocyte predominant Hodgkin's lymphoma |
| Granuloma | Nodular sclerosis | Nodular sclerosis | Classical Hodgkin's lymphoma<br>  Nodular sclerosis (grades 1 and 2)<br>  Lymphocyte-rich |
|  | Mixed | Mixed cellularity | Mixed cellularity |
| Sarcoma | Diffuse fibrosis<br>Reticular | Lymphocyte depletion | Lymphocyte depletion |

and infections,[376–380] but it may still be performed when detection of disease might alter therapy.[381] Selected subgroups of patients who generally do not need splenectomy are female patients in clinical stage IA, female patients younger than 26 years in clinical stage IIA with limited nodal disease, and male patients in clinical stage IA with the lymphocyte predominant subtype of Hodgkin's disease.

## Disease Classification and Histology

In 1966, Lukes and Butler[321] proposed a pathologic classification of Hodgkin's disease that still forms the basis of current classification schemas. Emerging biologic, clinical, and pathologic findings imposed necessary modifications, including updates proposed by participants of a 1966 conference held in Rye, New York; the International Lymphoma Study Group and its 1994 Revised European-American Lymphoma (REAL) classification; and the 2001 World Health Organization (WHO) Lymphoma Classification (Table 41–8). The original classification recognized six categories of Hodgkin's disease: nodular L&H, diffuse L&H, nodular sclerosis, mixed cellularity, diffuse fibrosis, and reticular.[321] The Rye modification combined the categories of nodular and diffuse L&H into a new category of lymphocyte predominant; diffuse fibrosis and reticular were combined into lymphocyte depletion.[321] Subsequent to the original classification, the L&H forms of Hodgkin's disease were shown to have different clinicopathologic and biologic behavior compared with the other subtypes of Hodgkin's disease.[382–384] Thus, in the WHO classification, nodular lymphocyte predominant Hodgkin's disease is separated from the other forms of Hodgkin's disease, which are lumped into a category of classical Hodgkin lymphoma. The other forms of lymphocyte predominance are now termed lymphocyte-rich (nodular or diffuse) within the category of classical Hodgkin's lymphoma. In addition, the subtype of nodular sclerosis is subdivided into two grades. Furthermore, the newest classification proposes the term *Hodgkin lymphoma* to replace Hodgkin's disease. This recognizes the entity as a true neoplasm and also follows current lexicographic fashion to dismiss the possessive in all med-

ical eponyms. In this chapter, we retain the term *Hodgkin's disease.*

## NODULAR LYMPHOCYTE PREDOMINANT (L&H) TYPE (WITH OR WITHOUT DIFFUSE AREAS)

In contrast to the Reed-Sternberg cells of classical Hodgkin's disease, the L&H cells of nodular lymphocyte predominant are clonally derived from germinal center B cells that have retained their immunoglobulin coding capacity in most cases.[177, 382, 385] At low-power magnification, one sees numerous large neoplastic nodules that closely resemble those of progressively transformed germinal centers (Fig. 41–28). Part of the lymph node may also contain hyperplastic germinal centers, but the neoplastic and reactive follicles are rarely interspersed. The neoplastic follicles are generally closely apposed, but their outlines may be obscure. A diffuse architecture may be focally present. The capsule is usually intact. Fibrosis is uncommon. The nodules contain numerous small lymphocytes and histiocytes as well as a distinctive cell termed the L&H cell, which has a large lobulated nucleus with a high nuclear-to-cytoplasmic ratio (Fig. 41–29). The L&H cell has also been called an "elephant foot" cell or "popcorn"

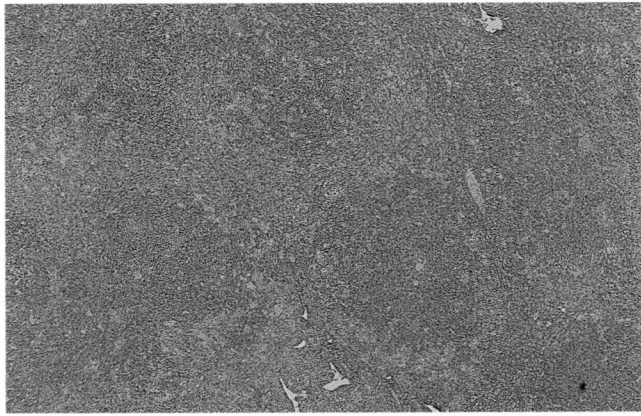

**FIGURE 41–28.** L&H lymphocyte predominant Hodgkin's disease, low power. Large confluent tumor nodules are present. There are no intervening reactive germinal centers.

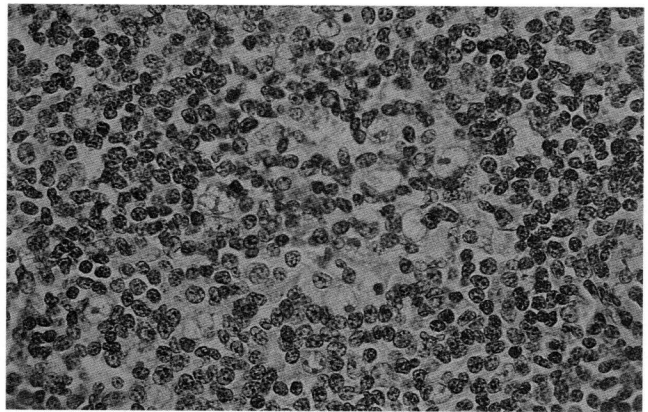

**FIGURE 41-29.** L&H lymphocyte predominant Hodgkin's disease, high power. Several L&H cells are seen, including polylobulated ones. The background small lymphocytes are B lineage.

cell. Its nuclear chromatin is fine, and nucleoli are inconspicuous. L&H cells may be prominent and even form aggregates. The histiocytes are epithelioid type and found preferentially in the outer rim of the nodular infiltrates, usually as small clusters. Well-formed granulomas have been described in rare cases. Eosinophils, plasma cells, and neutrophils are rare in lymphocyte predominant subtype, in contrast to classical Hodgkin's disease.

Whether a purely diffuse form of lymphocyte predominance exists has been debated because at least a minimal degree of nodularity is identified when the whole lymph node is examined. Thus, it would be prudent to avoid the diagnosis of diffuse lymphocyte predominance on small biopsy specimens or without immunophenotyping. If no nodular areas are seen, one must exclude the diagnoses of T cell–rich large B cell lymphoma and lymphocyte-rich classical Hodgkin's disease. Diffuse large B cell lymphoma should be diagnosed only when the large atypical cells occupy the majority of the lymph node parenchyma and, in particular, form sheets outside the nodules.

## CLASSICAL HODGKIN'S DISEASE

The diagnosis of classical Hodgkin's disease is made by identification of Reed-Sternberg cells and variants (Hodgkin cells) in a characteristic cellular milieu (Fig. 41–30). Thus, attention to the atypical cells as well as to the background non-neoplastic cells is necessary for the appropriate histologic diagnosis of Hodgkin's disease. The Reed-Sternberg cell is a large cell with a polyploid nucleus or multiple nuclei. Each lobe or nucleus contains a single large inclusion-like eosinophilic nucleolus, with a diameter up to 10 $\mu$m. The paranucleolar chromatin is clear, and the nuclear membrane is thick. Colorful terms such as "owl's eye" and "pennies on a platter" have been applied to the various appearances of Reed-Sternberg cells. Mononuclear variants are similar to the classic Reed-Sternberg cells but have a single nucleus and a large eosinophilic nucleolus. In all types

of classical Hodgkin's disease, one can see apoptotic Hodgkin cells ("mummified" cells), which have degenerated nuclei and shrunken, highly eosinophilic cytoplasm. Hodgkin cells generally comprise less than 1% of the cellularity in any involved tissue. For many years, the presence of at least one classic Reed-Sternberg cell was considered essential for a definitive diagnosis of Hodgkin's disease. This was not a practical requirement, particularly when the tissue sample was less than optimally fixed. In addition, the amount of tissue submitted for diagnosis has been decreasing as invasive procedures become more sophisticated, placing an additional burden on the pathologist to identify a rare cell. Fortunately, morphologic identification of a Reed-Sternberg cell is no longer considered de rigueur because adjunct immunohistochemistry studies may yield a characteristic phenotype to support a definitive diagnosis of Hodgkin's disease.

Hodgkin's disease has a polymorphous cellular background. Small, round lymphocytes predominate, but one also sees histiocytes, eosinophils, plasma cells, neutrophils, fibroblasts, and immunoblasts. No cellular atypia is seen. A spectrum of lymphoid size and atypia should raise consideration of diagnoses other than Hodgkin's disease. The histiocytes may be epithelioid type. Well-formed granulomas may be found.[386] Rarely, foamy histiocytes may predominate. Eosinophils may vary from few to numerous, even forming eosinophilic abscesses. Plasma cells are usually scattered throughout the lymph node parenchyma, and their presence in large clusters or sheets should raise doubt about the diagnosis of Hodgkin's disease. Neutrophils are usually minimal in number; they are most often found in patients with B symptoms. Fibroblasts are also few but occasionally may be so numerous as to simulate fibrous histiocytoma.

### Nodular Sclerosis Type

Nodular sclerosis is the most frequently diagnosed subtype of Hodgkin's disease, composing about 60% to 70% of cases in Western populations.

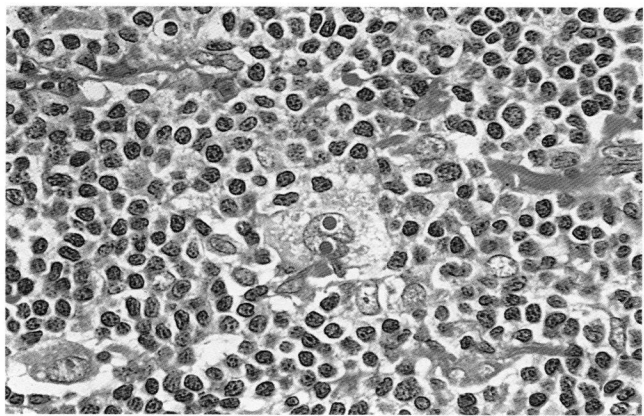

**FIGURE 41-30.** Reed-Sternberg cell. The characteristic owl's eye nucleoli are seen in a minority of Hodgkin cells.

In addition to the general features described for classical Hodgkin's disease, the nodular sclerosis subtype also contains fibrous bands and lacunar cells.[321] The sclerotic bands usually extend from a thickened capsule to separate the lymphoid parenchyma into nodules (Fig. 41–31). The bands are composed of dense collagen with interspersed small lymphocytes. The amount of sclerosis may be extremely scant. Cases in which no fibrous bands are detected may represent the cellular phase of nodular sclerosis, "follicular" Hodgkin's disease, or the follicular variant of lymphocyte-rich classical Hodgkin's disease.[387, 388] The nodules are usually composed of lacunar cells, which are mononuclear Reed-Sternberg cells that have abundant amphophilic cytoplasm (at least in metal-based fixatives) that is retracted to the nucleus in formalin-fixed sections (Fig. 41–32). The lacunar cells vary from few to numerous.[389] Eosinophils are generally abundant.

The WHO Lymphoma Classification Project adopted subclassification of nodular sclerosis into two grades on the basis of prognostic data from the British National Lymphoma Investigation group.[390–394] Cases are classified as grade 2 if they meet two of the following three criteria: 1) more than 25% of the cellular nodules show reticular or pleomorphic lymphocyte depletion, 2) more than 80% of the cellular nodules show fibrohistiocytic lymphocyte depletion, and 3) more than 25% of the cellular nodules contain numerous bizarre and highly anaplastic-appearing Hodgkin cells without lymphocyte depletion.[391] Cases of nodular sclerosis not meeting two of these criteria are classified as grade 1.

### Mixed Cellularity Type

Mixed cellularity Hodgkin's disease accounts for approximately 30% of Hodgkin's disease cases in the Western countries and up to 60% of Hodgkin's disease cases in developing countries.[330] The capsule is usually intact, without extension of the lymphoid

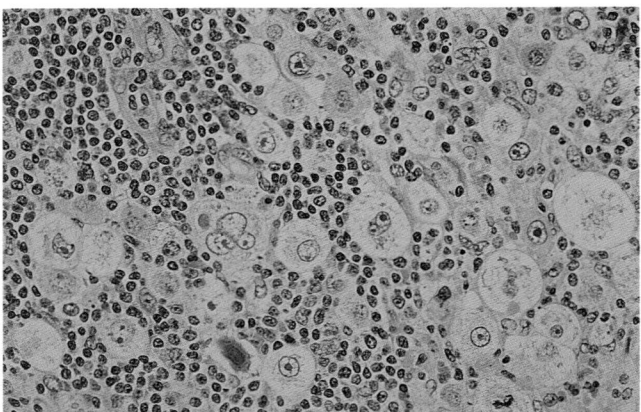

**FIGURE 41–32.** Hodgkin's disease, nodular sclerosing type. Numerous lacunar cells are seen.

proliferation into the surrounding soft tissues. One may see a vague nodularity, but even a small amount of fibrous bands warrants categorization as nodular sclerosis. Reed-Sternberg cells and variants are abundant, but lacunar cells are rare (Fig. 41–33). The background cells are similar to those of nodular sclerosis.

### Lymphocyte Depletion Type

Lymphocyte depletion Hodgkin's disease accounts for less than 5% of cases of Hodgkin's disease, particularly in developed countries. This term encompasses the diffuse fibrosis and reticular categories of the original Lukes-Collins classification. In the diffuse fibrosis type, one sees abundant reticulin collagen fibrosis surrounding individual Hodgkin cells and not surrounding nodules of cells as is seen in nodular sclerosis subtype (Fig. 41–34). The background stroma also contains few lymphocytes. In the reticular subtype, one sees large clusters or sheets of Hodgkin cells, mimicking large cell non-

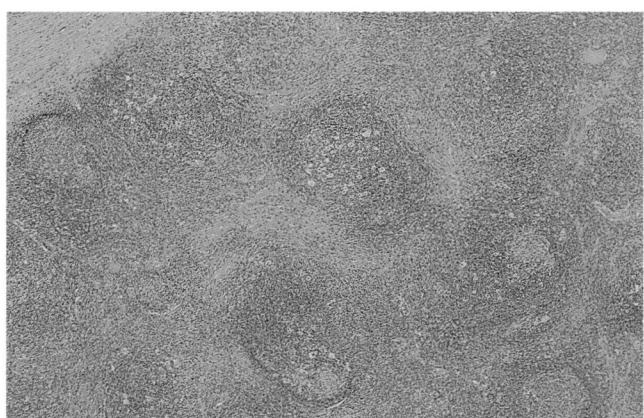

**FIGURE 41–31.** Hodgkin's disease, nodular sclerosing type. Broad fibrous bands separate the tumor nodules. The upper left and lower right corners contain a reactive germinal center.

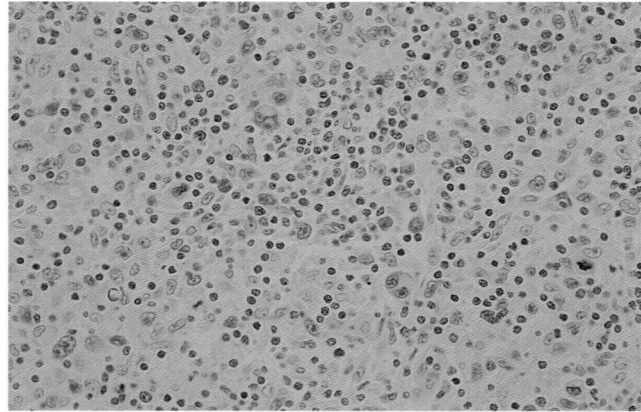

**FIGURE 41–33.** Hodgkin's disease, mixed cellularity type. Several mononuclear Hodgkin cells and rare classic Reed-Sternberg cells are present. The polymorphous background cells include mature lymphocytes, histiocytes, and plasma cells.

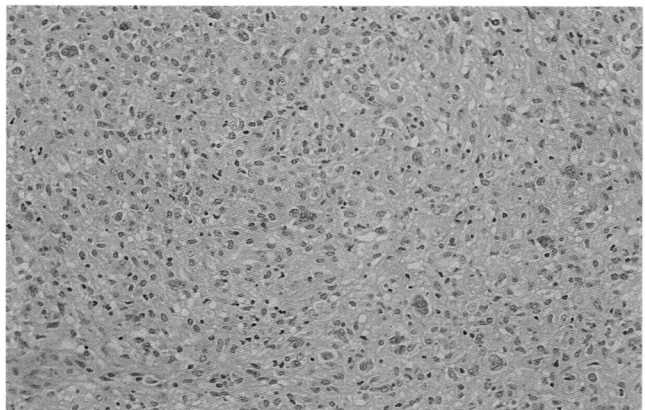

FIGURE 41–34. Hodgkin's disease, lymphocyte depletion type. Several neoplastic cells are present in a background of histiocytes and fibrosis. Few small lymphoid cells are seen.

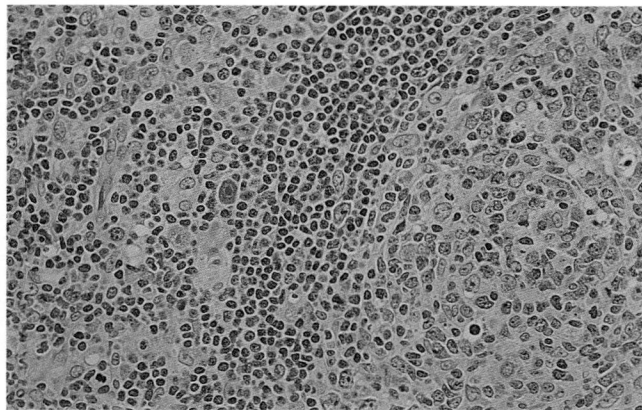

FIGURE 41–36. Hodgkin's disease, interfollicular. A Reed-Sternberg variant is present in a polymorphous background adjacent to the mantle of a reactive germinal center.

Hodgkin's lymphoma or syncytial variant of nodular sclerosis. The reticular variant has the typical classical Hodgkin's immunophenotype, which distinguishes it from non-Hodgkin's lymphoma, and does not have any fibrous bands, which distinguishes it from the syncytial variant of nodular sclerosis.

### Lymphocyte-Rich Types (Nodular and Diffuse)

The morphologic and immunophenotypic features of lymphocyte-rich Hodgkin's disease are similar to those of other types of classical Hodgkin's disease, with two important differences. First, lymphocytes are more abundant in the lymphocyte-rich type than in the other types (Fig. 41–35). Second, the background small lymphocytes of lymphocyte-rich classical Hodgkin's disease are generally B lineage and not T lineage, as is seen in the other categories of classical Hodgkin's disease.

### Other Subtypes of Classical Hodgkin's Disease

Interfollicular Hodgkin's disease contains numerous reactive germinal centers with Hodgkin cells in the interfollicular areas[389] (Fig. 41–36). Rather than a specific subtype, this most likely represents focal nodal involvement. The importance of this variant is distinguishing it from reactive follicular hyperplasia.

The syncytial variant of nodular sclerosis Hodgkin's disease contains sheets of Reed-Sternberg cells, often so numerous that the typical cellular background of Hodgkin's disease is diminished or obscured[389] (Fig. 41–37). Because of the large number of malignant cells, one may suspect non-Hodgkin's lymphoma, malignant melanoma, or carcinoma. Immunohistochemical stains may be needed to definitively establish a diagnosis of classical Hodgkin's disease. The syncytial variant falls into the grade 2

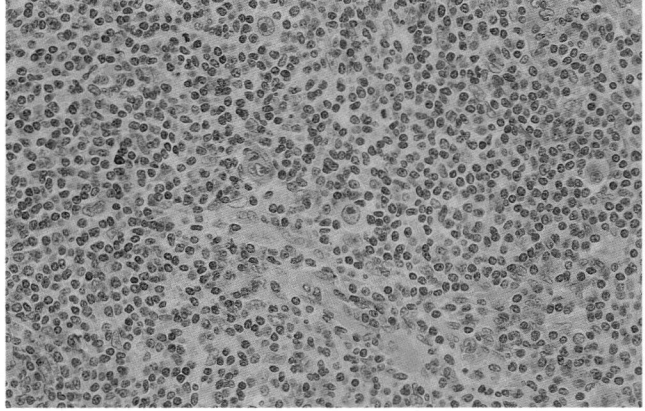

FIGURE 41–35. Classic lymphocyte predominance Hodgkin's disease. Reed-Sternberg variants are present amid numerous small lymphocytes.

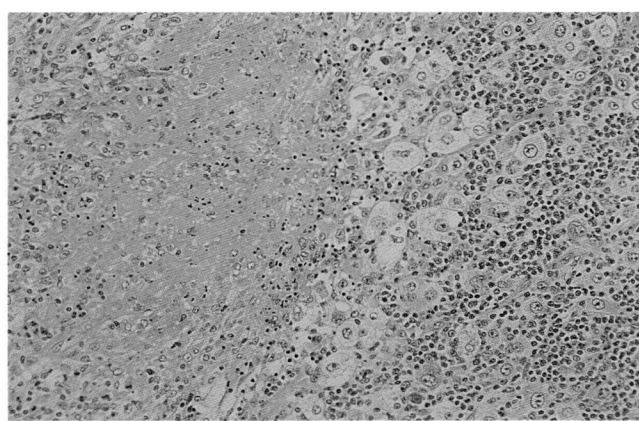

FIGURE 41–37. Hodgkin's disease, nodular sclerosing type, syncytial type. Large clusters of lacunar cells are present, adjacent to an area of necrosis.

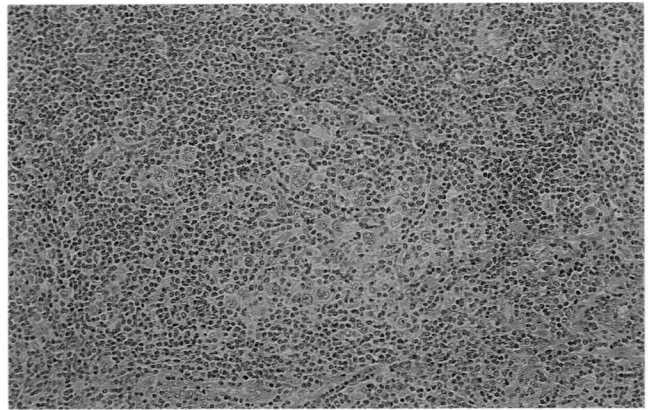

**FIGURE 41–38.** Hodgkin's disease, follicular. Reed-Sternberg cells and Hodgkin variants are found within the follicle.

nodular sclerosis category of the WHO classification and thus may be associated with a poorer prognosis.

A fibroblastic variant of Hodgkin's disease has been described in which numerous fibroblasts are present in the lymph node parenchyma, but no collagen deposition is seen.[395] These cases most likely correspond to the fibrohistiocytic areas of grade 2 nodular sclerosis classical Hodgkin's disease in the WHO classification.

Rarely, Hodgkin's disease may have a follicular pattern.[388] As the name implies, one sees numerous follicles without any fibrous bands, thus distinguishing it from nodular sclerosis Hodgkin's disease (Fig. 41–38). The Reed-Sternberg cells are confined to the follicles, which are predominantly composed of small B lineage lymphocytes. The Hodgkin cells have the immunophenotype of classical Hodgkin's disease, with the additional expression of B cell antigens. These cases most likely correspond to the nodular variant of lymphocyte-rich classical Hodgkin's disease.

### PATHOLOGY OF POST-TREATMENT AND RELAPSED CLASSICAL HODGKIN'S DISEASE AND HODGKIN'S DISEASE AT AUTOPSY

Lymph nodes successfully treated for classical Hodgkin's disease show dense collagenous fibrosis, a sparse lymphocytic infiltrate, and possibly foamy macrophages and fibroblasts. No Hodgkin cells are present. The lymph node may contain large acellular or hypocellular scars, which may cause a clinically apparent mass.

Recurrences of classical Hodgkin's disease in untreated sites usually retain the original histologic features.[396, 397] The numbers of eosinophils, histiocytes, and Hodgkin cells may increase in the specimens of relapsed disease. Disease relapse in previously treated areas may have significantly different histologic features, including greater numbers and greater atypia of the Hodgkin cells.[396, 398] However, the histologic features have no bearing on the subse-

quent disease course and response to therapy. In general, the patient's disease at autopsy is similar to that of post-treatment or recurrent Hodgkin's disease, showing effects reflective of treatment.[399]

## Pathology Evaluation of Hodgkin's Disease in Lymph Nodes

At the time of surgery, touch or scrape preparations may be more useful than actual frozen sections for the recognition of Hodgkin cells. Fine-needle aspiration biopsy may be a means of diagnosing and staging Hodgkin's disease; in one study, the accuracy for diagnosis of Hodgkin's disease was above 90%.[400] On low magnification, the aspirate smears usually show a dispersed population of lymphoid cells in which scattered large cells are evident. At high magnification, these cells have bilobed or polylobulated nuclei with prominent nucleoli and moderately abundant cytoplasm. Immunohistochemical studies of the cell block may be helpful for confirmation. Fine-needle aspiration studies are of less use in subclassifying Hodgkin's disease, although one study reported an accuracy of 58%.[400] Fine-needle aspiration may be of great use in the diagnosis of recurrent Hodgkin's disease because Hodgkin cells are sometimes more easily identified in this setting.

### ANCILLARY STUDIES FOR THE DIAGNOSIS OF HODGKIN'S DISEASE

The most useful ancillary study for the diagnosis of Hodgkin's disease is paraffin section immunohistochemistry. Electron microscopy, frozen section immunohistochemistry, flow cytometry, and molecular studies have limited utility for the diagnosis of Hodgkin's disease. Electron micrographs show nonspecific features; the Reed-Sternberg cells appear as transformed lymphocytes without any viral or other pathognomonic inclusions. Frozen sections usually yield suboptimal histologic features; coupled with the rarity of the Reed-Sternberg cells, these results may be difficult to interpret. Flow cytometric studies rely on assessment of a homogeneous population of thousands of cells. Because of the infrequency of Reed-Sternberg cells, attempts to demonstrate an abnormal phenotype are generally unsuccessful. In fact, by demonstrating the reactive, non-neoplastic nature of the abundant background lymphocytes, the results of flow cytometry may mislead a pathologist into making a benign lymph node diagnosis.

The most important use of molecular studies in Hodgkin's disease is to exclude a non-Hodgkin's lymphoma, many of which have characteristic gene rearrangements.[401] Most cases of typical classical Hodgkin's disease show no gene rearrangements. However, cases with a large number of Hodgkin cells may show rearrangements of the immunoglobulin heavy chain gene.[402–404] One group identified the t(2;5), a translocation typically found in T cell–null cell anaplastic large cell lymphoma, but other studies have not confirmed this finding.[405–407] Highly

**TABLE 41–9.** Immunophenotype and Genetic Features of Malignant Lymphoma Cells in Paraffin Sections

| | CD45 (%) | CD15 (%) | CD30 (%) | CD20 (%) | CD3 (%) | CD4 (%) | EMA (%) | EBV (%) |
|---|---|---|---|---|---|---|---|---|
| Classical Hodgkin's disease | 10 | 90 | 90 | 24 | 5 | 5 | 0 | 40–50 |
| Nodular lymphocyte pre-dominance | 90 | 10 | <5 | 92 | 0 | 0 | 40 | <1 |
| B cell lymphoma | >95 | <5 | 5 | 94 | <1 | 0 | <10 | Var* |
| T cell lymphoma | 90 | 20 | 40 | 0 | >99 | >90 | 0 | Var† |

CD, Cluster designation; EMA, epithelial membrane antigen; EBV, Epstein-Barr virus.

*Five percent to 20% Western Burkitt, 95% African Burkitt, 60% to 90% AIDS-associated lymphoma, 95% post-transplantation lymphomas, 5% sporadic B cell lymphomas.

†More than 95% extranodal T-NK cell lymphoma; 10% sporadic T cell lymphomas.

sensitive PCR studies have identified small monoclonal immunoglobulin gene rearrangements, particularly in cases expressing B lineage antigens such as CD20.[408] EBV-encoded small nuclear RNA (EBER) in situ hybridization is a reliable test to identify the EBV in a large subset of cases.[364, 409] Cytogenetic studies are often not useful in the routine diagnosis of Hodgkin's disease because of the scarcity of Hodgkin cells and their slow growth in cell culture. Successful studies usually show complex hyperdiploid karyotypes without consistent structural abnormalities.[410]

Paraffin section immunohistochemical studies are superior to frozen section immunohistochemical studies for the diagnosis of Hodgkin's disease because of optimal morphologic preservation.[411] The characteristic phenotype of Reed-Sternberg cells of classical Hodgkin's disease is given in Table 41–9.[23, 26, 60, 62, 411–420] The Reed-Sternberg cells are usually positive for CD15 and CD30 and negative for CD45/45RB. Among lineage-specific markers, CD20 stains a subset of Reed-Sternberg cells in approximately 25% of cases of classical Hodgkin's disease. CD3 is almost always negative in Reed-Sternberg cells. Using only these five markers (CD15, CD30, CD45/45RB, CD20, CD3), one can resolve the majority (>90%) of cases of classical Hodgkin's disease (Fig. 41–39). Other markers that usually stain

Reed-Sternberg cells in paraffin sections include fascin, CD40, CD70, and restin. EBV latent membrane protein usually stains the EBV-positive cases of classical Hodgkin's disease, particularly mixed cellularity Hodgkin's disease.[370] Despite their relatively low mitotic activity, the Reed-Sternberg cells and Hodgkin cells are Ki-67 positive.[39, 421] Reed-Sternberg cells are usually negative for CD43 and CDw75 (LN-1). However, as Table 41–9 indicates, exceptions are seen with all stains, and thus there is great case-to-case variation. The phenotype is often preserved in any recurrences but may show variation.[422, 423] The background lymphocytes are predominantly T cells, usually of helper subtype, and show ringing around the Reed-Sternberg cells. In frozen sections, Reed-Sternberg cells are also positive for HLA-DR, CD25, CD71, and CD138.[411, 424]

The typical phenotype of L&H cells of nodular lymphocyte predominant Hodgkin's disease is also given in Table 41–9.[385] In contrast to the Reed-Sternberg cells of classical Hodgkin's disease, L&H cells usually stain for CD20 and CD45/45RB and not for CD15 or CD30 (Fig. 41–40). L&H cells also stain for epithelial membrane antigen and CD79a, both of which are negative in Reed-Sternberg cells. The L&H cells are usually present in a background of disrupted nodules of small B lymphocytes, often containing large numbers of CD57+ lymphocytes.

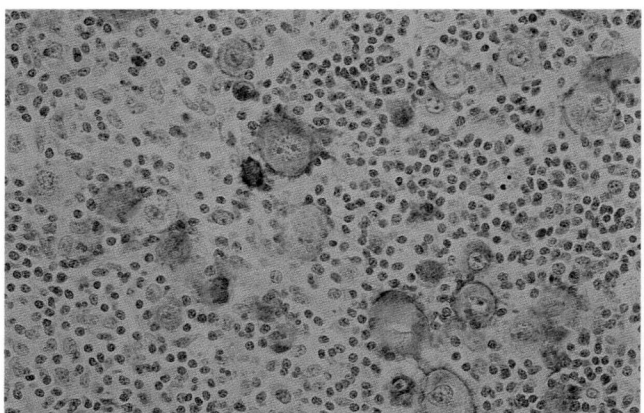

**FIGURE 41–39.** Hodgkin's disease, CD15 stain. Membranous and paranuclear staining of Hodgkin cells is seen.

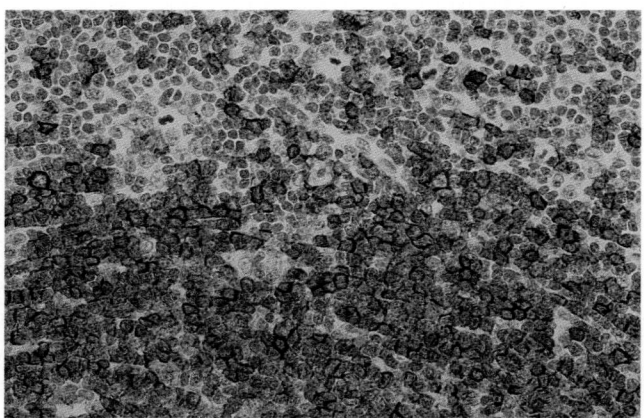

**FIGURE 41–40.** L&H lymphocyte predominant Hodgkin's disease, CD20 stain. CD20 rims the cytoplasm of the L&H cells and also stains the background small lymphocytes.

This is in contrast to the T lineage background lymphocytes in nodules of nodular sclerosis Hodgkin's disease. A characteristic feature of nodular L&H is the presence of a wreathlike configuration of the CD57+ small lymphocytes around L&H cells. In contrast to Reed-Sternberg cells, fascin, CD74, and CD138 do not stain L&H cells.[424] EBV latent membrane protein is negative in virtually all cases of nodular lymphocyte predominance.

## DIFFERENTIAL DIAGNOSIS OF HODGKIN'S DISEASE

A wide variety of reactive and neoplastic conditions may be confused with Hodgkin's disease. Carcinoma (Fig. 41–41), malignant melanoma, germ cell tumor, sarcoma, reactive lymphoid hyperplasia, and non-Hodgkin's lymphoma may be mistaken for classical Hodgkin's disease or nodular lymphocyte predominant Hodgkin's disease.

Reactive immunoblastic proliferations may be confused with classical Hodgkin's disease. In reactive immunoblastic lymph node proliferations, one sees numerous immunoblasts with large nuclei and prominent nucleoli in the paracortex. There are also numerous plasma cells and lymphoplasmacytoid cells. Binucleated immunoblasts, resembling Reed-Sternberg cells, may be present. The immunoblasts tend to be evenly scattered in reactive immunoblastic proliferations, unlike the clustering of Reed-Sternberg cells seen in Hodgkin's disease. The typical background of classical Hodgkin's disease includes only scattered plasma cells and no lymphoplasmacytoid cells. Immunohistochemical studies of reactive immunoblastic proliferations show staining of many of the immunoblasts for CD45/45RB and not for CD15, with a mixture of CD20+, CD3+, and CD30+ cells. In contrast, Reed-Sternberg cells stain for CD15 and CD30 and not for CD45/45RB. As discussed before, CD20 stains a subset of Reed-Sternberg cells

in approximately 25% of cases of classical Hodgkin's disease.

Another reactive lesion that may be confused with classical Hodgkin's disease is necrotizing granulomatous lymphadenitis. In necrotizing granulomatous lymphadenitis, the necrotic areas are lined by histiocytes that have bland cytologic features and that stain with CD68 but not with CD15 or CD30. A moderate number of cases of classical Hodgkin's disease also contain necrotic foci. However, in these cases, Hodgkin cells in addition to histiocytes surround the necrosis.

Progressive transformation of germinal centers may be confused with nodular lymphocyte predominance. Both have enlarged and disrupted nodular configurations. Progressive transformation usually has widely spaced round nodules, with intervening reactive germinal centers. In contrast, nodular lymphocyte predominant cells have closely apposed nodules with only rare (if any) hyperplastic follicles. If hyperplastic follicles are present, they are pushed to the periphery of the neoplastic lymph node. The pattern of CD20 immunohistochemical staining differs between the two entities. In progressive transformation, CD20 highlights well-circumscribed nodules of small confluent B cells. In contrast, nodular lymphocyte predominant cells have an irregular distribution of CD20 positivity ("moth-eaten") with additional CD20 staining of large L&H cells. In addition, the distribution of T cells differs between the two entities. CD3 shows only scattered positivity in the nodules of progressive transformation but highlights numerous irregular aggregates and clumps of small lymphocytes in lymphocyte predominant Hodgkin's disease.

Cases of nodular sclerosis Hodgkin's disease (syncytial variant or type 2) may be confused with metastatic carcinoma, melanoma, germ cell tumor, or sarcoma. Clues to the correct diagnosis of Hodgkin's disease are the presence of eosinophils, localization of neoplastic cells next to necrotic areas, and subtotal lymph node involvement. Immunohistochemical stains are often confirmatory; the majority of carcinomas stain for keratin, melanomas for S-100 protein and Melan A, and germ cell tumors for placental alkaline phosphatase. One caveat is that CD30, which is positive in more than 95% of Reed-Sternberg cells in classical Hodgkin's disease, also stains the majority of embryonal carcinomas. Thus, keratin immunohistochemical stain may also be necessary to differentiate between Hodgkin's disease (keratin negative) and embryonal carcinoma (keratin positive).

Cases of classical Hodgkin's disease (nodular sclerosis and lymphocyte depletion) with exuberant fibroblastic proliferations may be confused with sarcoma. The spindled cells of sarcomas usually show marked nuclear atypia, unlike the bland spindled cells of Hodgkin's disease. Again, immunohistochemical studies may help by highlighting rare Reed-Sternberg cells. Sarcomas do not show any staining with CD30. CD15 stains only benign leukocytes that are admixed with malignant sarcoma cells.

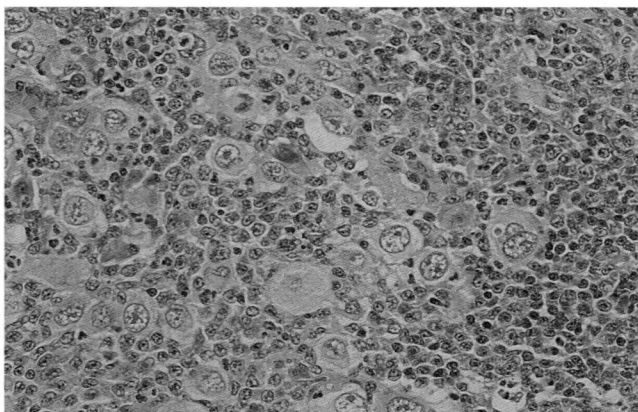

**FIGURE 41–41.** Nasopharyngeal carcinoma. The individual tumor cells and the background small lymphoid cells mimic Hodgkin's disease. However, the nucleolar membranes are less distinct than those of Reed-Sternberg cells. In addition, the cytoplasm of the carcinoma cells is more abundant and eosinophilic than that of Hodgkin cells.

Distinguishing Hodgkin's disease from non-Hodgkin's lymphoma may be extremely difficult. Myriad non-Hodgkin's lymphomas may be confused with both classical Hodgkin's disease and nodular lymphocyte predominant Hodgkin's disease. Small lymphocytic lymphoma may be mistaken for lymphocyte-rich classical Hodgkin's disease. Lymph nodes involved by small lymphocytic lymphoma show small lymphocytes with occasional admixed larger cells (paraimmunoblasts), often forming pseudofollicular centers, which are pale-staining areas at low magnification. Eosinophils and plasma cells are generally not present. Similarly, lymphocyte-rich classical Hodgkin's disease contains numerous small lymphocytes, but the background also contains Reed-Sternberg cells and eosinophils and lacks the admixed paraimmunoblasts. Immunohistochemical studies of small lymphocytic lymphoma show the small lymphoid cells to stain for CD20, CD43 (aberrantly coexpressed on the CD20+ cells), CD5, and CD23. The small lymphoid cells of lymphocyte-rich classical Hodgkin's disease stain predominantly for CD20 but do not show coexpression of CD43 or CD5. In addition, immunohistochemical stains for CD30 and CD15 help highlight the Reed-Sternberg cells of Hodgkin's disease. Rare cases of small lymphocytic lymphoma may have Reed-Sternberg–like cells.[425]

Peripheral T cell lymphomas (particularly polymorphous types) show histologic features similar to those of classical Hodgkin's disease (particularly mixed cellularity type). Both entities result in diffuse effacement of the nodal architecture and are composed of a mixed cellular proliferation with eosinophils, histiocytes (including epithelioid histiocytes), and plasma cells. The most striking difference is the range of size and cytologic atypia in the lymphoid cells of peripheral T cell lymphoma, compared with the benign homogeneous background of Hodgkin's disease. In peripheral T cell lymphoma, the lymphoid cells range from small to large, and all the cells have irregular nuclear outlines and an abnormal chromatin pattern. In addition, the mitotic rate in peripheral T cell lymphoma is generally higher than that seen in Hodgkin's disease. Paraffin immunohistochemical studies can be useful because the large atypical cells of peripheral T cell lymphoma are CD45/45RB+, in contrast to Reed-Sternberg cells and Hodgkin variants, which are CD45/45RB−. CD3 positivity of the small lymphoid cells is seen in both disorders. Thus, one must exercise great care to observe the cytoplasmic CD3 staining pattern in a range of morphologically atypical cells for peripheral T cell lymphoma, which differs from the staining of a homogeneously small and mature lymphoid population for Hodgkin's disease. This differential diagnosis may be aided by frozen section immunohistochemistry or flow cytometric studies, which may show aberrant loss of mature T cell antigens. If the morphologic and immunologic features are not conclusive, molecular studies may be necessary to distinguish between the entities. The observation of a sizable rearrangement of the $\beta$ or $\gamma$ T cell receptor gene strongly favors a diagnosis of peripheral T cell lymphoma.

T cell–rich/histiocyte-rich B cell lymphoma is another non-Hodgkin's lymphoma that may be confused with both classical Hodgkin's disease (particularly mixed cellularity and lymphocyte rich) and lymphocyte predominant Hodgkin's disease. T cell–rich/histiocyte-rich B cell lymphoma contains numerous small mature T cells and numerous histiocytes. The neoplastic component (large atypical mononuclear B lineage cells) represents a fraction of the cells and is dispersed throughout the reactive background, in a distribution similar to that of the malignant cells of classical Hodgkin's disease. The malignant cells of lymphocyte predominance tend to stay clustered in the nodules but may be more dispersed in the diffuse variant. The large neoplastic cells of T cell–rich/histiocyte-rich B cell lymphoma may have binucleated or multinucleated cells resembling either Reed-Sternberg cells or L&H cells. Immunohistochemical stains help distinguish among these entities.[426] CD20 is virtually always positive in the malignant cells of T cell–rich/histiocyte-rich B cell lymphoma. As discussed previously, CD20 also stains a subset of cells in approximately 25% of cases of classical Hodgkin's disease. Usually, the number of CD20+ cells is less than in T cell–rich/histiocyte-rich B cell lymphoma, but the distribution of CD20+ cells in the background is similar among the three entities. The presence of CD15 and CD30 staining and the lack of CD45 staining establish the diagnosis of classical Hodgkin's disease; these three stains have opposite reactivities in the non-Hodgkin's lymphomas. Differentiation of T cell–rich B cell lymphoma from lymphocyte predominant Hodgkin's disease (nodular with or without diffuse) may be extremely difficult, even with the aid of immunohistochemical stains. There are rare cases of concurrence of the two neoplasms.[427] The most useful immunohistochemical stains in this differential are CD20 and CD57. Although CD20 stains the neoplastic elements of both entities, the pattern of staining differs in that CD20 also stains the majority of the small lymphoid cells in the nodules of nodular lymphocyte predominant Hodgkin's disease, in contrast to only scattered cells in T cell–rich/histiocyte-rich B cell lymphoma. In addition, CD57 stains many more background cells in nodular lymphocyte predominant than in T cell–rich/histiocyte-rich B cell lymphoma.

Cases of the syncytial variant of nodular sclerosis Hodgkin's disease may be mistaken for large B cell lymphoma. Both may show a significant amount of sclerosis, particularly in the mediastinum, which is the most frequent site of occurrence for the syncytial variant of nodular sclerosis. The demonstration of CD45 positivity and CD15 negativity strongly favors large B cell lymphoma over Hodgkin's disease, with the caveat that CD20 is positive in 10% to 20% of cases of Hodgkin's disease. Rarely, one may encounter composite lymphoma, which is composed of

Hodgkin's disease and B cell lymphoma, or a discordant lymphoma, which is the simultaneous occurrence of non-Hodgkin's lymphoma and Hodgkin's disease at different sites.[428] Furthermore, non-Hodgkin's lymphomas may arise in patients successfully treated for Hodgkin's disease, and conversely, Hodgkin's disease may occur in patients with a history of non-Hodgkin's lymphomas.[429, 430]

Follicular lymphoma and nodular lymphocyte predominance may also be confused. However, size of nodules (smaller in follicular lymphoma) and the presence of extracapsular extension (often in follicular lymphoma, never in nodular lymphocyte predominance) offer clues to distinguishing between the entities. The cellular composition of the nodules is also different; follicular lymphoma shows marked atypia in the majority of cells, and nodular lymphocyte predominant nodules contain rare large atypical (L&H) cells amid a background of normal-appearing small lymphoid cells. Immunohistochemical and molecular studies may be helpful in the minority of cases that cannot be resolved by light microscopy. The atypical lymphoid cells of follicular lymphoma stain for Bcl-2, which is negative in L&H cells. CD20 highlights nearly every cell in the follicles of follicular lymphoma, with some spillover into the interfollicular areas. In nodular lymphocyte predominant sections, CD20 stains the large L&H cells and shows a moth-eaten appearance of positivity to the background lymphoid cells. Immunoglobulin heavy chain gene rearrangements or t(14;18) translocations are found in approximately 85% of follicular lymphomas and never in nodular lymphocyte predominant Hodgkin's disease.[431, 432]

Anaplastic large cell lymphoma is also in the differential diagnosis of classical Hodgkin's disease. Both neoplasms contain numerous large, highly atypical cells with prominent nucleoli and show CD30 staining in the malignant cells. The entity of Hodgkin's-related anaplastic large cell lymphoma, described in the late 1980s and early 1990s, has since been shown to be a highly aggressive form of Hodgkin's disease, probably nodular sclerosis, grade 2.[177, 433, 434] Clinical features may be useful in distinguishing between anaplastic large cell lymphoma and Hodgkin's disease. Anaplastic large cell lymphoma frequently involves the skin, an unusual site for Hodgkin's disease, and is more common in children. Preferential localization to sinuses favors anaplastic large cell lymphoma over Hodgkin's disease, because Hodgkin's disease usually involves sinuses only when there is extensive paracortical involvement. The presence of abundant neutrophils and plasma cells also favors anaplastic large cell lymphoma over Hodgkin's disease, which usually has more numerous eosinophils. Immunohistochemical stains are essential for distinguishing between the two entities. Both stain for CD30. CD45 is negative in Hodgkin cells and may be negative in up to one third of cases of anaplastic large cell lymphoma.[60] The expression of epithelial membrane antigen or T lineage–associated antigens such as CD43 favors anaplastic large cell lymphoma, and the expression of CD15 favors Hodgkin's disease. In addition, ALK1, the protein overexpressed with the t(2;5), is positive in a large number of cases of anaplastic large cell lymphoma and is never positive in Hodgkin's disease.[435, 436] Molecular studies may be helpful because the t(2;5) strongly favors anaplastic large cell lymphoma; however, ALK1 positivity correlates well with t(2;5).[437-439]

## NON-HODGKIN'S LYMPHOMA

Non-Hodgkin's lymphoma is a term for the general category of all lymphoid neoplasms other than Hodgkin's disease. Thus, it is unique among pathologic taxonomy by being defined not by what it *is* but by what it is *not*. There are approximately 40,000 new cases each year of non-Hodgkin's lymphoma, approximately five times more than of Hodgkin's disease. The rate has been increasing by 3% to 4% per year.[324, 440] A rise in the number of HIV-associated cases accounts for part of the increase.[441] Environmental exposures, such as to hair dyes, herbicides, and organic chemicals, may also contribute to the increase.[442-444] A subset of cases is associated with human T-lymphotropic virus (HTLV) 1, and other subsets of cases are associated with EBV.[370, 445] Non-Hodgkin's lymphomas occur in both children and adults, with an overall male-to-female ratio of 1.3:1. Although more common in adults, non-Hodgkin's lymphoma accounts for a relatively high percentage of cancer in childhood.

Non-Hodgkin's lymphoma usually presents as painless, localized, or generalized enlargement of lymph nodes, with or without hepatosplenomegaly. However, masses may present initially in the tonsil, mediastinum, or abdomen. Localized or generalized lesions may involve any or all organs or organ systems. Constitutional B symptoms may occur, but not as frequently as in Hodgkin's disease. The signs and symptoms of non-Hodgkin's lymphoma may occur acutely or may have been present for a long time, occasionally years. Progression of disease is generally not as orderly and predictable as in Hodgkin's disease, but the Ann Arbor system is still used for the staging of non-Hodgkin's lymphoma.[446, 447]

Non-Hodgkin's lymphoma applies to a wide variety of neoplasms of different cell lineages frozen at different stages of ontologic development. Eighty percent to 90% of cases of non-Hodgkin's lymphoma are B lineage neoplasms. Most of these B cell non-Hodgkin's lymphomas are related to cells of the germinal center, but less frequently, they are related to cells of the B cell mantle or marginal zone or B cell populations native to extranodal tissues.[448] Most of the remainder of cases represent T lineage neoplasms, including neoplasms of immature (thymic) as well as mature T cell phenotype (post-thymic or peripheral). A small minority of cases are of natural killer (NK) cell lineage, indeterminate lineage (also known as null cell type), and true histiocytic lineage.

**TABLE 41–10.** Common Chromosome Translocations Found in Non-Hodgkin's Lymphomas

| Translocation | Lymphoma | Involved Genes |
|---|---|---|
| t(2;5)(p23;q35) | Anaplastic large cell lymphoma | *ALK* and *NPM* |
| t(9;14)(p13;q32) | Lymphoplasmacytoid lymphoma | *PAX5* and *IGH* |
| t(11;14)(q13;q32) | Mantle cell lymphoma | *PRAD1/CCND1/BCL1* and *IgH* |
| t(11;18)(q21;q21) | Low-grade B cell lymphoma of MALT type | *API2* and *MLT* |
| t(14;18)(q32;q21) | Follicular lymphoma; some diffuse large cell lymphomas | *IGH* and *BCL2* |
| i(7)(q10); +8 | Hepatosplenic $\gamma\delta$ T cell lymphoma | |
| t(2;8)(p12;q24) | Burkitt's lymphoma | *Ig$\kappa$* and c-*myc* |
| t(8;14)(q24;q32) | Burkitt's lymphoma | c-*myc* and *IGH* |
| t(8;22)(q24;q11) | Burkitt's lymphoma | c-*myc* and *Ig$\lambda$* |
| t(3;v)(q27;v) | Diffuse large B cell lymphoma | *BCL6/LAZ3* and variable |

See text and Chapter 43 for chromosome studies in small lymphocytic lymphoma.

In general, non-Hodgkin's lymphomas are monoclonal proliferations.[44] Thus, B cell lymphomas expressing immunoglobulin usually show only one of the light chains, so-called light chain restriction. Monoclonal immunoglobulin gene rearrangements are usually detectable. For T cell lymphomas, there is no immunologic marker of monoclonality that is analogous to light chain analysis in B cell lymphomas. However, most (if not all) T cell lymphomas have T cell receptor gene rearrangements. Aberrant clonal rearrangements of the $\beta$-chain T cell receptor gene may be detectable in a minority of cases of B cell lymphomas, particularly the immature lymphoblastic neoplasms. Similarly, aberrant monoclonal immunoglobulin heavy chain gene rearrangements may be detectable in a minority of T cell lymphomas, again particularly in the immature lymphoblastic neoplasms. Many types of non-Hodgkin's lymphomas are associated with characteristic cytogenetic abnormalities, usually balanced translocations (Table 41–10). A cellular oncogene is typically translocated adjacent to one of the antigen receptor genes.

## Classification

Various classifications of non-Hodgkin's lymphoma have been used in the past several decades. As new laboratory methods have emerged, the classification schemas have become increasingly more sophisticated. The earliest classification was based on morphology, which still forms the basis of all classification schemes.[449] The Working Formulation classification of 1982 (Table 41–11) was devised as a system of "translation" between six different classifications but became a classification scheme in its own right.[450] It included 10 major categories of lymphoma, organized into three histologic grades: low grade, with a median survival of 6.0 years; intermediate grade, with a median survival of 3.5 years; and high grade, with a median survival of 1.4 years. The Working Formulation has been widely used throughout the United States and Canada for more than 15 years, and many oncologists and patholo-

gists still prefer that system. The updated Kiel classification of 1988 (Table 41–12) combined cytologic and immunologic data into a classification that recognized several cytologic types of B and T cell lymphoma.[451] The updated Kiel classification has been widely used throughout Europe. The newest and most widely accepted classification is the WHO classification of hematologic malignant neoplasms (Table 41–13), based on the 1994 REAL classification (Table 41–14), which itself is based on the Working Formulation and Kiel classifications.[177, 452]

Complicating the difficulties in classification is the fact that a minority of lymphomas may have different histologic appearances in different anatomic sites. These lymphomas are called discordant

**TABLE 41–11.** Working Formulation of Non-Hodgkin's Lymphomas for Clinical Use

***Low Grade***
Small lymphocytic
    Consistent with chronic lymphocytic leukemia; plasmacytoid
Follicular predominantly small cleaved cell
    Diffuse areas, sclerosis
Follicular mixed small cleaved and large cell
    Diffuse areas, sclerosis

***Intermediate Grade***
Follicular predominantly large cell
    Diffuse areas, sclerosis
Diffuse mixed, small and large cell
    Sclerosis
Diffuse mixed, small and large cell
    Sclerosis, epithelioid cell component
Diffuse large cell
    Cleaved cell, noncleaved cell, sclerosis

***High Grade***
Large cell, immunoblastic
    Plasmacytoid, clear cell, polymorphous, epithelioid cell component
Lymphoblastic
    Convoluted, nonconvoluted
Small noncleaved cell
    Burkitt's, follicular areas

***Miscellaneous***
Composite, mycosis fungoides, histiocytic, extramedullary
Plasmacytoma, unclassifiable, other

**TABLE 41–12.** Updated Kiel Classification of Non-Hodgkin's Lymphomas

| B Cell | T Cell |
|---|---|
| Low grade | Low grade |
| Lymphocytic | Lymphocytic |
| Chronic lymphocytic and prolymphocytic leukemia | Chronic lymphocytic leukemia |
| | Prolymphocytic leukemia |
| Hairy cell leukemia | |
| Lymphoplasmacytic/cytoid | Lymphoepithelioid |
| Plasmacytic | Angioimmunoblastic |
| Centroblastic/centrocytic | Pleomorphic, small cell |
| High grade | High grade |
| Centroblastic | Pleomorphic, medium and large cell |
| Immunoblastic | Immunoblastic |
| Large cell anaplastic | Large cell anaplastic |
| Burkitt's lymphoma | Lymphoblastic |
| Rare types | Rare types |

lymphomas. Rarely, lymphomas may have two or more distinctly different histologic appearances at the same site (including coexisting non-Hodgkin's lymphoma and Hodgkin's disease); such lymphomas are called composite lymphomas.[427, 428, 453, 454] In addition, a low-grade lymphoma may transform over

**TABLE 41–13.** WHO Classification of Lymphomas

Precursor B cell neoplasm
  Precursor B lymphoblastic lymphoma-leukemia
Mature (peripheral) B cell lymphomas
  B cell small lymphocytic lymphoma
  Lymphoplasmacytic lymphoma
  Splenic marginal zone lymphoma (± villous lymphocytes)
  Plasma cell myeloma/plasmacytoma
  Extranodal marginal zone B cell lymphoma of MALT type
  Nodal marginal zone B cell lymphoma (± monocytoid B cells)
  Follicular lymphoma
  Mantle cell lymphoma
  Diffuse large B cell lymphoma
Precursor T cell neoplasm
  Precursor T lymphoblastic lymphoma-leukemia
Mature (peripheral) T cell lymphomas
  Adult T cell lymphoma-leukemia (HTLV1+)
  Extranodal NK-T cell lymphoma, nasal type
  Enteropathy-type T cell lymphoma
  Hepatosplenic γδ T cell lymphoma
  Subcutaneous panniculitis–like T cell lymphoma
  Mycosis fungoides/Sézary's syndrome
  Anaplastic large cell lymphoma, T-null cell, primary cutaneous type
  Peripheral T cell lymphoma, not otherwise characterized
  Angioimmunoblastic T cell lymphoma
  Anaplastic large cell lymphoma, T-null cell, primary systemic type
Hodgkin's lymphoma (Hodgkin's disease)
  Nodular lymphocyte predominant Hodgkin's lymphoma
  Classical Hodgkin's lymphoma
    Nodular sclerosis Hodgkin's lymphoma (grades 1 and 2)
    Lymphocyte-rich classical Hodgkin's lymphoma
    Mixed cellularity Hodgkin's lymphoma
    Lymphocyte depletion Hodgkin's lymphoma

**TABLE 41–14.** List of Lymphoid Neoplasms Recognized by the International Lymphoma Study Group

**B Cell Neoplasms**
I. Precursor B cell neoplasm: Precursor B lymphoblastic leukemia-lymphoma
II. Peripheral B cell neoplasms
  1. B cell chronic lymphocytic leukemia/prolymphocytic leukemia/small lymphocytic lymphoma
  2. Lymphoplasmacytoid lymphoma/immunocytoma
  3. Mantle cell lymphoma
  4. Follicle center lymphoma, follicular
     Provisional cytologic grades: I (small cell), II (mixed small and large cell), III (large cell)
     Provisional subtype: diffuse, predominantly small cell type
  5. Marginal zone B cell lymphoma
     Extranodal (MALT-type ± monocytoid B cells)
     Provisional subtype: Nodal (± monocytoid B cells)
  6. Provisional entity: Splenic marginal zone lymphoma (± villous lymphocytes)
  7. Hairy cell leukemia
  8. Plasmacytoma/plasma cell myeloma
  9. Diffuse large B cell lymphoma
     Subtype: Primary mediastinal (thymic) B cell lymphoma
  10. Burkitt's lymphoma
  11. Provisional entity: High-grade B cell lymphoma, Burkitt-like

**T Cell and Putative NK Cell Neoplasms**
I. Precursor T cell neoplasm: Precursor T lymphoblastic lymphoma-leukemia
II. Peripheral T cell and NK cell neoplasms
  1. T cell chronic lymphocytic leukemia/prolymphocytic leukemia
  2. Large granular lymphocyte leukemia (LGL)
     T cell type
     NK cell type
  3. Mycosis fungoides/Sézary's syndrome
  4. Peripheral T cell lymphoma, unspecified
     Provisional cytologic categories: medium-sized cell, mixed medium and large cell, large cell, lymphoepithelioid cell
     Provisional subtype: Hepatosplenic γδ T cell lymphoma
     Provisional subtype: Subcutaneous panniculitic T cell lymphoma
  5. Angioimmunoblastic T cell lymphoma (AILD)
  6. Angiocentric lymphoma
  7. Intestinal T cell lymphoma (± enteropathy associated)
  8. Adult T cell lymphoma-leukemia (ATL/L)
  9. Anaplastic large cell lymphoma (ALCL), CD30+, T and null cell types
  10. Provisional entity: Anaplastic large cell lymphoma, Hodgkin's-like

**Hodgkin's disease**
I. Lymphocyte predominance
II. Nodular sclerosis
III. Mixed cellularity
IV. Lymphocyte depletion
V. Provisional entity: Lymphocyte-rich classical Hodgkin's disease

time to a higher grade lymphoma. Finally, some lymphomas have overlap with leukemic counterparts; it is likely that both represent the same biologic entity with different clinical manifestations.

Fine-needle aspiration biopsy may be used for the primary diagnosis of non-Hodgkin's lymphoma, but the technique has limitations for diagnosis as well as for classification.[455-457] Fine-needle aspiration biopsy is more easily applied to the staging of non-Hodgkin's lymphoma, allowing easy, widespread sampling of different sites. It may also be used to diagnose recurrent or residual disease or to identify large cell transformation in a patient with a history of low-grade lymphoma. For most non-Hodgkin's lymphomas, fine-needle aspiration yields a monotonous lymphoid cell population. The monotony applies primarily to the chromatin pattern, which shows remarkable cell-to-cell uniformity. The nuclear size is also uniform, albeit slightly less than the chromatin pattern. Some lymphomas are composed of a heterogeneous mixture of neoplastic cells (e.g., peripheral T cell lymphoma); these may be difficult to recognize by fine-needle aspiration unless highly bizarre or pleomorphic cells are identified. Supplemental immunophenotypic and molecular studies are of great utility for establishing a primary diagnosis of non-Hodgkin's lymphoma but may not aid in precise classification.[455] The distinction between low-grade and high-grade lymphomas can usually be made. In some series, approximately 90% of non-Hodgkin's lymphomas have been correctly diagnosed, with the correct assignment of grade in virtually all cases.[456, 457]

Prognostic factors in non-Hodgkin's lymphoma include histologic grade and stage and clinical factors such as age, sex, Karnofsky performance index, number of nodal and extranodal sites of disease, size of tumor, and $\beta_2$-microglobulin and lactate dehydrogenase levels.[458-465] In addition, a variety of immunobiologic factors may be of importance in determining prognosis, including proliferative rate, cytotoxic T cell response, loss of molecules of immune recognition, loss of cell adhesion antigens, gain of drug resistance molecules, acquisition of aneuploidy, gain of specific oncogenes, and loss of specific tumor suppressor genes.[13, 464, 466]

## Follicular Lymphoma

Follicular lymphomas are neoplasms of B cell derivation with a component of follicular architecture. In the United States, follicular lymphoma accounts for approximately 40% of cases of non-Hodgkin's lymphoma.[440, 441] The mean age at occurrence is 55 years; only rare cases are reported in childhood and few cases before the age of 40 years.[467] An approximately equal number of cases occur in males and females. Patients usually present with one or several enlarged lymph nodes, often of long duration. The majority of patients also present with bone marrow, liver, or spleen involvement. Peripheral blood involvement also occurs frequently, either at presentation or during the course of disease.

Follicular lymphoma usually behaves in an indolent fashion; it occasionally regresses spontaneously, progression is slow, and numerous relapses occur over time, seemingly independent of treatment.[468, 469] Thus, most cases of follicular lymphoma

are not treated aggressively. An exception to this is the large cell variant, which is often treated with standard anthracycline-based chemotherapy with curative intent.[464] Approximately 40% to 50% of cases of follicular lymphoma transform to a diffuse large cell lymphoma. When this occurs, survival is usually less than 1 year, although some patients undergo remissions with aggressive chemotherapy.

By definition, all cases of follicular lymphoma have true follicular architecture, at least focally within the tumor.[470] The follicles are usually evenly dispersed throughout the entire lymph node parenchyma, often with extension into the perinodal adipose tissue (Fig. 41–42). Sometimes there are also areas of diffuse effacement of architecture (most often seen in the large cell type). The presence of diffuse areas may adversely affect prognosis, particularly in the mixed and large cell variants.[464, 471] On occasion, the follicular areas may be only focally appreciated, with the remainder of the lymph node showing diffuse architectural effacement. Rarely, follicular lymphoma may focally involve a lymph node with otherwise normal architecture; in this case, adjacent lymph nodes may show a greater degree of lymphomatous involvement.

The follicles are classically round and relatively homogeneously sized. On occasion, the follicle shapes are highly irregular. Mantles are usually absent; if present, they consist of a thin rim of mantle cells. Most cases of follicular lymphoma have compressed interfollicular regions, with resultant back-to-back arrangement of the follicles. Sometimes the follicles coalesce. However, in some cases, the interfollicular areas may be normal and the follicles clearly distinct. In rare cases, the marginal zones (the areas just outside of the mantle zone) may be expanded by a proliferation of monocytoid cells forming a pale collar around the neoplastic follicles; in these cases, the proliferating monocytoid cells are part of the lymphomatous process.[472, 473]

The cytologic features are equally important to the architectural features for establishing a morphologic diagnosis of follicular lymphoma. The cells in

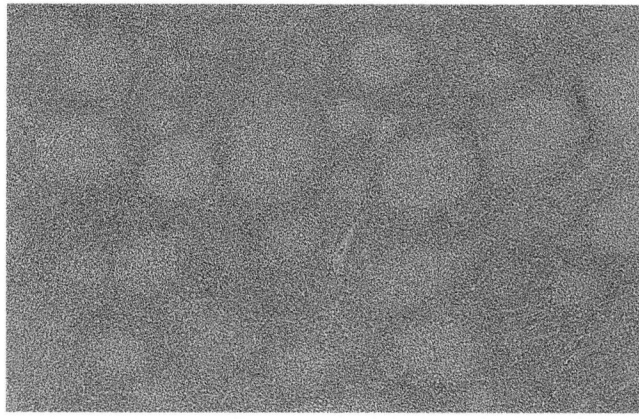

**FIGURE 41–42.** Follicular lymphoma. The follicles are closely packed, lack polarity, and are relatively uniform in size.

the follicles are varying mixtures of small cleaved cells, large cleaved cells, and large noncleaved cells. All of these cells have an origin from the follicular center.[474-476] Small cleaved cells are slightly larger than mature lymphocytes and have nuclei that are elongated and contorted, with highly irregular nuclear outlines, coarse chromatin, and inconspicuous nucleoli (Fig. 41–43). These cells are also called centrocytes. Older terms for small cleaved cells include germinocytes, poorly differentiated lymphocytes, and small cleaved follicular center cells (Fig. 41–44). Large cleaved cells have similar features, but the nuclear size is approximately two to three times that of small cleaved cells. Large noncleaved cells are slightly larger and have rounded nuclear outlines, a vesicular chromatin pattern, and one to several moderately sized nucleoli, often apposed to the nuclear membrane. A moderate amount of amphophilic or slightly basophilic cytoplasm is typically present. The large cells are also called centroblasts and have in the past been referred to as germinoblasts, histocytes, large follicular center cells, and large lymphoid cells. All of these cells also have an origin from the follicular center.

The WHO classification divides follicular lymphoma into three grades.[450, 452] Grade 1 and grade 2 correspond to low-grade follicular small cleaved type and low-grade follicular mixed small cleaved and large cell type, respectively, of the Working Formulation. Grade 3 corresponds to intermediate-grade follicular large cell type of the Working Formulation. The following criteria have been proposed for assigning grade: 1 to 5 centroblasts (large cells) per high-power field, grade 1; 6 to 15 centroblasts per high-power field, grade 2; more than 15 centroblasts per high-power field, grade 3.[452, 477] In actual practice, the distinction of these grades of lymphoma may be arbitrary, at least partially owing to poor reproducibility even among experienced hema-

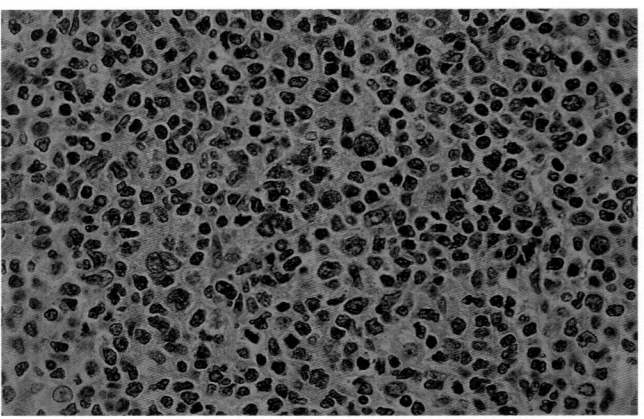

**FIGURE 41–44.** Follicular lymphoma, mixed small cleaved cell and large cell type (centroblastic). A mixture of highly atypical cells is present.

topathologists and the variation in area covered by a high-power field with different microscopes. Approximately two thirds of cases of follicular lymphoma are grade 1, about 25% of cases are diagnosed as grade 2, and about 10% are classified as grade 3. A low-power appearance of a pale follicle may be a clue to grade 3. Tingible body macrophages and a brisk mitotic rate may also be seen in grade 3 follicular lymphoma.

Areas of diffuse lymphomatous effacement are often present in follicular lymphoma and may have an impact on prognosis. The diffuse areas should be classified separately, as discussed later (see "Diffuse Large B Cell Lymphoma"). The following criteria are suggested in the WHO classification scheme: if less than 25% of the lymphoma has diffuse areas, the lymphoma should be considered follicular; if less than 25% of the lymphoma has follicular areas, it should be considered predominantly diffuse; and if the follicular area accounts for 25% to 75% of the lymphoma, it should be considered follicular and diffuse.[452]

There have been reports of rare cytologic and architectural variants of follicular lymphoma. These include the so-called signet ring cell variant of follicular lymphoma, which is characterized by the presence of clear or eosinophilic cytoplasmic inclusions[478] (Fig. 41–45). In addition, follicular lymphoma may rarely have small round nuclei (termed follicular small lymphocytic lymphoma),[479] cerebriform nuclei reminiscent of the cells of mycosis fungoides,[480] multilobated nuclei,[481] plasmacytoid nuclear and cytoplasmic features,[482] immunoblastic features,[483] and blastic nuclei resembling the nuclei of lymphoblastic leukemia.[484] In addition, a floral variant of follicular lymphoma is characterized by prominent mantle zones that invaginate irregularly into the follicle centers, resulting in a flowerlike appearance.[485, 486] Finally, rare cases of follicular lymphoma may contain a prominent (>5%) proliferation of extrafollicular monocytoid B cells, which appear to have adverse prognostic impact.[473]

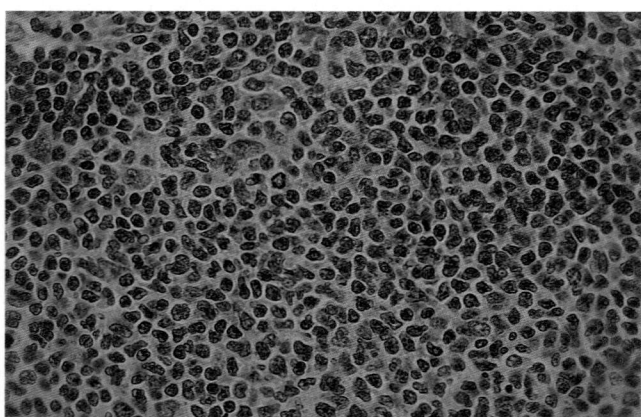

**FIGURE 41–43.** Follicular lymphoma, predominantly small cleaved cell (centrocytic) type. The majority of cells have irregular nuclear outlines and condensed chromatin, but occasional cells with more open chromatin are also present. No tingible body macrophages are seen. This cellular composition is not seen in reactive follicular hyperplasia.

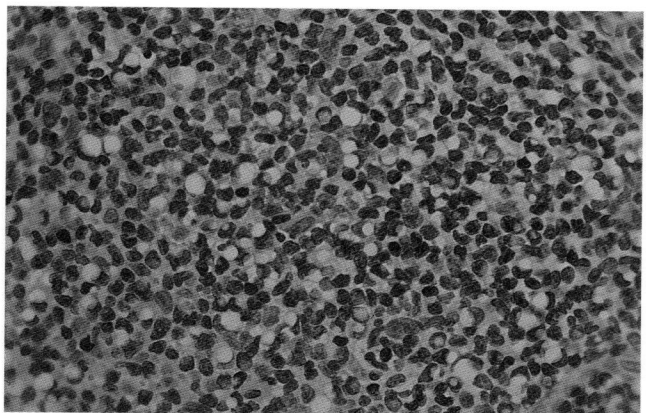

**FIGURE 41–45.** Follicular lymphoma, signet ring cell type. The tumor cells contain large cytoplasmic vacuoles, mimicking gastric adenocarcinoma.

Fine-needle aspiration smears of follicular lymphoma show vague nodular aggregates at low magnification. High magnification may show hyperchromatic nuclei with wrinkled or indented nuclear outlines (small cleaved cells) or rounded or cleaved vesicular nuclei with irregularly thick and thin nuclear membranes (large cells). Cytologic identification of the mixed cell type may be difficult, but immunophenotyping and molecular studies may help to establish a diagnosis of follicular lymphoma.

Immunohistochemical studies demonstrate that all follicular lymphomas are of B lineage, expressing multiple B lineage antigens in both paraffin and frozen sections, including CD20 and CD79a.[39, 412, 474, 487, 488] The CD20 stains all the cells in the follicles and a high percentage of cells in the interfollicular areas. Approximately 90% of follicular lymphomas express monotypic immunoglobulins by flow cytometry or frozen section immunohistochemistry, usually immunoglobulin M or immunoglobulin G.[489] Ten percent of cases, predominantly the large cell subtype, are immunoglobulin negative by the same methods. Monotypic immunoglobulin may also be detected in paraffin sections in a significant proportion of cases (Fig. 41–46), but this procedure is somewhat less sensitive than frozen section studies. In contrast to Bcl-2⁻ reactive follicular hyperplasia, the Bcl-2 oncoprotein is expressed by the neoplastic cells in approximately 90% of cases (see Fig. 41–11); again, the exception is the large cell subtype, in which Bcl-2 is seen in approximately 75% of cases.[130, 131, 490] The neoplastic cells express CD10 in about 60% of cases and are almost always negative for CD23 and CD5.[133, 491] Aberrant coexpression CD43 is rare.[23, 135] T lineage antibodies do not stain the neoplastic cells but demonstrate a significant population of T cells within the neoplastic follicles. A subset of these cells express the NK cell–associated marker CD57. Stains such as CD21 and CD35 demonstrate a rich network of follicular dendritic cells, similar to that seen in non-neoplastic follicles. In addition, Bcl-6 expression is common in follicular lymphomas.[492, 493]

Almost all cases of follicular lymphomas have a detectable immunoglobulin heavy chain rearrangement by Southern blot analysis; approximately 35% to 50% of the cases have the same rearrangements detectable by PCR analysis.[388, 494, 495] In addition, evidence of the t(14;18) can be found by a variety of techniques in about 90% of cases.[488, 496–499] At the molecular level, the t(14;18) involves translocation of the BCL2 gene on chromosome 18 into the immunoglobulin heavy chain gene on chromosome 14, leading to Bcl-2 deregulation and overexpression.[497, 500] Most translocations involve the major breakpoint region, but 5% to 10% of cases involve a minor cluster region that requires detection by a different set of PCR primers and Southern blot probes. Evidence of the t(14;18) can also be detected by sensitive molecular techniques in a high proportion of peripheral blood and bone marrow specimens from patients with follicular lymphoma, consistent with the disseminated nature of the disease.[501] The t(14;18) has also been detected by PCR analysis in normal peripheral blood and in reactive lymph nodes, suggesting that this translocation can occur in small numbers of cells without the development of malignant lymphoma.[502–504] The presence of other cytogenetic abnormalities, such as abnormalities involving chromosome regions 1p21–22 and 6q23–26 and the short arm of chromosome 17, may be associated with adverse prognosis.[505] Mutations of the tumor suppressor gene TP53 have been identified in a subset of cases of large cell transformation.[506, 507] Deletions involving chromosome 9p21 at p15 and p16 have been associated with histologic progression in follicular lymphoma.[508]

Follicular lymphoma may be confused with mantle cell lymphoma or marginal cell lymphoma. Mantle cell lymphoma has a nodular subtype in which the germinal centers as well as the mantle zone regions are replaced by a homogeneous population of neoplastic mantle cells. The cells are small with slightly irregular nuclear contours. One sees few admixed large cleaved and noncleaved cells. Im-

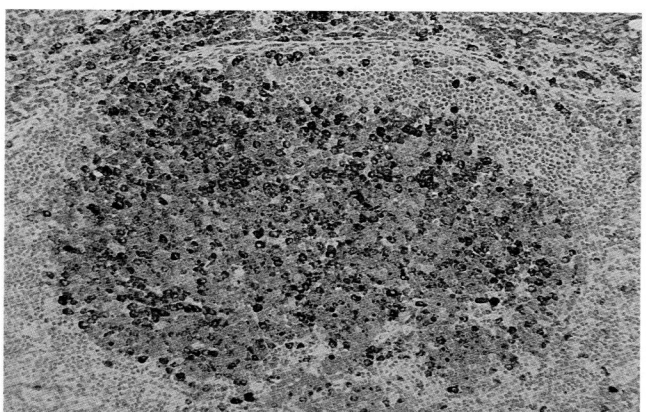

**FIGURE 41–46.** Follicular lymphoma, κ stain. Strong cytoplasmic positivity is seen in the tumor cells. The λ stain was negative.

munohistochemical studies are helpful for distinguishing between follicular lymphoma and mantle cell lymphoma. The cells of mantle cell lymphoma show aberrant coexpression of CD5 or CD43, both of which are rare findings in follicular lymphoma. In addition, molecular studies show t(14;18) in a high percentage of follicular lymphoma cases and t(11;14) in many cases of mantle cell lymphoma. In marginal zone lymphomas, neoplastic cells may colonize reactive germinal centers, mimicking follicular lymphoma. Low-power magnification scanning may show otherwise typical areas of marginal zone lymphoma, and high-power magnification will help identify a moderate to abundant amount of pale cytoplasm and the lack of cleaved nuclei. Bcl-2 immunohistochemistry may not be that useful for distinguishing between the two entities; both lymphomas are Bcl-2+, and follicles colonized by marginal cell lymphoma are also Bcl-2+. However, aberrant CD43 coexpression is identified in approximately 30% of cases of marginal zone lymphoma and in almost no cases of follicular lymphoma.[135] Molecular studies for the t(14;18) may also be helpful because marginal zone lymphomas do not have that translocation. Also in the differential diagnosis of follicular lymphoma is reactive follicular hyperplasia (see Table 41–6) and nodular L&H lymphocyte predominant Hodgkin's disease, as discussed in the sections on those entities.

The floral variant of follicular lymphoma mimics progressive transformation of germinal centers. However, in contrast to progressive transformation of germinal centers, the floral variant of follicular lymphoma shows involvement of all nodules without the presence of any reactive germinal centers, contains a homogeneous proliferation of large transformed lymphocytes with a markedly decreased or absent population of phagocytic histiocytes, and shows extension of abnormal cells into the perinodal adipose tissue. In addition, Bcl-2 and monotypic immunoglobulin light chain immunohistochemical staining, immunoglobulin gene rearrangements, and t(14;18) are not seen in progressive transformation of germinal centers.[485, 486]

## Small Lymphocytic Lymphoma

In the Working Formulation, the low-grade category of small lymphocytic lymphoma included several clinicopathologic entities characterized by a diffuse proliferation of relatively small lymphoid cells, including small lymphocytic lymphoma/chronic lymphocytic leukemia, marginal zone B cell lymphoma (particularly the extranodal variants), lymphoplasmacytic lymphoma/immunocytoma, and some cases of mantle cell lymphoma. As these entities became more clearly delineated, the single Working Formulation category did not adequately encompass the increasingly broader spectrum of behavior, immunophenotype, and prognosis. On the basis of the REAL classification proposal, the WHO classification now recognizes these as separate categories of B cell lymphoma.[177, 452] In this section, we have adopted the more limited WHO classification definition of small lymphocytic lymphoma as the nodal equivalent of classical B cell chronic lymphocytic leukemia. The two diseases are considered different stages of the same disease, and the distinction between the two is arbitrary. One group has recommended the designation *chronic lymphocytic leukemia* if patients have more than 5000/mm$^3$ circulating lymphocytes and more than 30% lymphocytes in the marrow, but this is not universally applied.[509]

Small lymphocytic lymphoma is seen almost exclusively in adults older than 40 years, with a median age of approximately 60 years.[510–513] Most patients present with generalized lymphadenopathy. Many of these patients have or develop peripheral blood involvement during their disease course. Pathologic stage IV disease is seen in approximately 80% of patients at presentation, usually because of bone marrow involvement but also with frequent liver and spleen involvement. The clinical course is indolent; spontaneous regression occurs in 15% of untreated patients, progression is slow, and numerous relapses occur over time seemingly independent of treatment.[468] Ten percent to 20% of patients undergo histologic transformation to large cell lymphoma (Richter's syndrome).[468, 514] As previously discussed, rare cases may transform to a lymphoma with a Hodgkin's-like histologic appearance or even true Hodgkin's disease.[425, 515]

The diagnosis of small lymphocytic lymphoma is often made at low-magnification microscopy by appreciating nearly diffuse nodal effacement, perinodal adipose tissue infiltration, and pale proliferation centers (also known as pseudofollicles).[488, 516, 517] The mitotic rate is generally low, but higher numbers may be found in the proliferation centers. At high magnification, the predominant cell type is a small lymphoid cell with condensed chromatin (Fig. 41–47). The cells are usually round but may exhibit

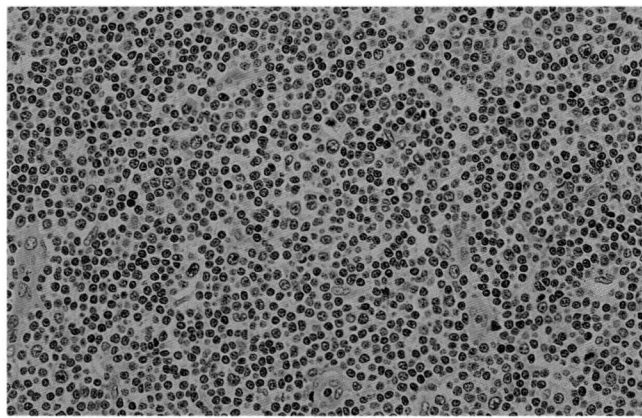

**FIGURE 41–47.** Small lymphocytic lymphoma. The majority of cells are small with round nuclear contours and mature chromatin, but there are also larger cells with prominent nucleoli evenly distributed throughout the nodal parenchyma.

a mild degree of nuclear irregularity. Nucleoli are generally small but may be moderately sized in some cases. Cytoplasm is generally scant. In some cases, the small lymphoid cells have plasmacytoid features. In addition to the small cells, one also always sees a population of larger cells. These cells may be medium sized, termed prolymphocytes or paraimmunoblasts (Fig. 41–48), or the cells may be large, termed immunoblasts. Both larger cell types have round nuclei with a vesicular chromatin pattern and medium to large nucleoli. The aggregation of these large cells gives rise to the proliferation centers appreciated at low magnification. Other cell types, including eosinophils, neutrophils, and histiocytes, are not found in any appreciable number. The proliferation centers are particularly identified in cases associated with peripheral blood lymphocytosis.[517] Rarely, paraimmunoblasts may predominate; this is then termed the paraimmunoblastic variant of small lymphocytic lymphoma.[518] These cases have a worse prognosis than other cases of small lymphocytic lymphoma do, but it is still better than for cases of de novo diffuse large cell lymphoma. However, when immunoblasts predominate and form sheets, this indicates transformation to a higher grade lymphoma, and the prognosis becomes significantly worse. Fine-needle aspiration biopsy smears of small lymphocytic lymphoma show a preponderance of small lymphoid cells with round, regular nuclear membranes and clumped chromatin, with occasional admixed cells of similar size with an open chromatin pattern and a prominent nucleolus, representing prolymphocytes.

Small lymphocytic lymphomas are B lineage neoplasms. They express the B cell markers CD20 and CD79a in paraffin sections, but the reactivity for CD20 is usually weak.[39, 61, 412, 487] Immunoglobulin expression with light chain restriction is seen in virtually all cases by flow cytometry, but the level of immunoglobulin expression is typically low.[513, 519, 520]

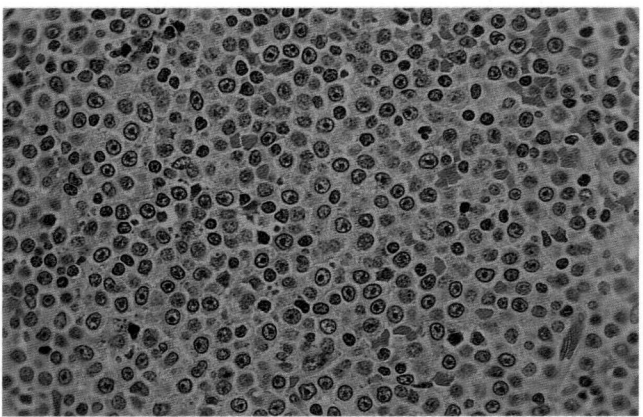

**FIGURE 41–48.** Small lymphocytic lymphoma, paraimmunoblasts. Cases of small lymphocytic lymophoma always have admixed paraimmunoblasts, whether in clusters or as individual cells. The paraimmunoblasts have slightly more open chromatin and small nucleoli. The nuclei are still round and regular.

Both $\mu$ and $\delta$ heavy chains are characteristically present. Results of immunoglobulin studies in paraffin sections are usually negative unless the cells exhibit some plasmacytoid features, but the cells usually have faint immunoglobulin expression in frozen sections. Aberrant expression of the paraffin T/myeloid marker CD43 is found in about 80% of cases. Aberrant expression of CD5 is found in about 90% of cases by flow cytometry, frozen section immunohistochemistry, and paraffin immunohistochemistry.* In contrast to mantle cell lymphoma, CD23 is usually positive, and in contrast to follicular lymphoma, CD10 is usually negative.[33, 133, 491, 517, 524] CD22 antigen is weakly expressed on chronic lymphocytic leukemia/small lymphocytic lymphoma (>90%).[525] The most common cytogenetic abnormalities in small lymphocytic lymphoma are probably deletions of chromosome bands 13q14 and 11q.[513, 526] Translocations involving 17p have also been described and may be associated with poor response to chemotherapy and poor clinical outcome.[527] Trisomy of chromosome 12 is found in about one third of cases and is more commonly associated with cases with atypical features or undergoing transformation to a higher grade process.[513, 528] Monoclonal rearrangement of the immunoglobulin heavy and light chain genes is seen in virtually all cases.

The differential diagnosis of small lymphocytic lymphoma includes reactive lymphoid proliferations, follicular lymphoma, and other small cell B lineage lymphomas. By morphology, small lymphocytic lymphoma can usually be distinguished from reactive lymphoid proliferations; small lymphocytic lymphoma has a somewhat monotonous cellular population, with lack of normal architectural compartmentalization. Paraffin section immunohistochemical studies of small lymphocytic lymphoma show a diffuse B cell infiltrate, most often with aberrant CD43 and CD5 coexpression; in frozen section immunohistochemistry studies, light chain restriction is usually seen. These are in contrast to a well-compartmentalized pattern in reactive infiltrates. Flow cytometric studies also show a monotypic population in small lymphocytic lymphoma as well as characteristic dim CD20 and surface immunoglobulin positivity, reactivity of CD5 and CD23, and lack of FMC7 expression.[519] Prominent proliferation centers may be mistaken for the neoplastic follicles of follicular lymphoma. However, the proliferation centers are always more poorly defined than neoplastic follicles and lack small cleaved cells. Immunohistochemistry may show scattered follicular dendritic cells, but the network is never as well developed as in follicular lymphoma. CD10 staining is usually positive in follicular lymphoma and is usually negative in small lymphocytic lymphoma, which may be difficult to distinguish from other diffuse small cell B lineage lymphomas. The presence of proliferation

*References 20, 23, 27, 135, 491, 521–523.

centers or CD23 positivity favors small lymphocytic lymphoma over the other neoplasms. The presence of scattered larger cells also distinguishes small lymphocytic lymphoma from mantle cell lymphoma, which has a monotonous small cell population, whereas the identification of a t(11;14) favors mantle cell lymphoma. In addition, flow cytometry of mantle cell lymphoma shows FMC7 positivity, bright CD20 and surface immunoglobulin positivity, and no expression of CD23.[519] The cells of marginal zone B cell lymphoma generally have more abundant cytoplasm than the cells of small lymphocytic lymphoma do and commonly have extranodal sites of involvement. In addition, marginal zone B cell lymphomas have aberrant CD43 expression in only about 30% of cases and usually do not coexpress CD5. Although small lymphocytic lymphoma may show mild plasmacytoid features, marked plasmacytic differentiation with Dutcher bodies and Russell bodies is more commonly seen in lymphoplasmacytic lymphoma.[513] Clinically, patients with lymphoplasmacytic lymphoma often have large M protein spikes or even symptoms of Waldenström's macroglobulinemia. A recently described rare signet ring cell variant of small lymphocytic lymphoma may be confused with metastatic carcinoma, but immunohistochemical study helps to differentiate the lymphoma from the carcinoma.[529] The diffuse nature as well as the CD5 and CD43 coexpression also distinguishes this rare variant from the signet ring cell variant of follicular lymphoma.

## Marginal Zone B Cell Lymphoma

The normal marginal zone is the area circumferentially adjacent to the mantle zone and distal to the germinal center of a reactive (secondary) follicle. The marginal zone is most easily visualized in the spleen and is not easy to appreciate in normal lymph nodes outside of the abdominal region. Normal marginal zone B cells may differentiate into either monocytoid B cells or plasma cells. Marginal zone B cell lymphoma, also known as marginal zone lymphoma, is theoretically the neoplastic counterpart to those normal marginal zone B cells. It is a low-grade lymphoma and in the proposed WHO classification of lymphoid neoplasms encompasses three entities: nodal marginal zone B cell lymphoma (with or without monocytoid B cells), splenic marginal zone B cell lymphoma (with or without villous lymphocytes), and extranodal marginal zone B cell lymphoma of mucosa-associated lymphoid tissue (MALT) type.[246, 452, 530-535] The last term, which applies to marginal zone lymphomas occurring in extranodal sites other than the spleen, may be misleading, because this lymphoma may occur in extranodal sites that are not usually thought of as mucosa associated.[530, 531, 536, 537] A common term in the United States for extranodal marginal zone B cell lymphoma of MALT-type is MALToma. The splenic marginal zone lymphoma is more thor-

oughly discussed in the chapter on splenic diseases.[177] Some authors suggest that nodal marginal zone lymphomas be divided into nodal marginal zone lymphoma of splenic type and nodal marginal zone lymphoma of MALT type.[532] In the Working Formulation, all variants of marginal zone B cell lymphoma were probably classified as low grade, small lymphocytic, with or without plasmacytoid differentiation.[450]

Nodal marginal zone B cell lymphoma is most often a disease of the elderly, with a median age of about 60 years; the male-to-female ratio is about 1:2.[488, 512, 538, 539] Patients usually present with isolated or generalized lymphadenopathy. Bone marrow involvement occurs in approximately 40% of cases, splenomegaly in 20%, hepatomegaly in 15%, and involvement of the peripheral blood in 5%. Bone marrow or peripheral blood involvement adversely affects prognosis.[540] Nodal marginal zone B cell lymphoma has a high rate of early relapse, and overall survival is similar to or slightly worse than that of follicular lymphoma. Transformation to large cell lymphoma occurs in approximately 10% of patients and is another poor prognostic sign.[539] MALTomas typically occur in patients with a long history of autoimmune disease or antigenic stimulation, such as Sjögren's syndrome, Hashimoto's thyroiditis, or *Helicobacter* gastritis.[530, 541-543] Many different extranodal organs may be affected, particularly the gastrointestinal tract, salivary glands, and conjunctiva.* Even organs without true mucosa, such as thyroid, soft tissue, and skin, may be affected. Patients with MALToma tend to have recurrence in other extranodal sites. If lymph nodes are involved, they tend to be regional nodes draining an area affected by MALToma.

At low magnification, involved lymph nodes may have partially or completely effaced architecture.[545] Partial involvement preferentially affects the marginal zones. Lymph nodes may be involved by another lymphoma, usually follicular type.[473, 539] At high magnification, the typical neoplastic cells have small to medium-sized nuclei with round to slightly irregular nuclear outlines, condensed chromatin, and indistinct nucleoli (Fig. 41-49). The marginal zone cells are also termed monocytoid B cells. A highly characteristic feature is the presence of moderately abundant clear to pale cytoplasm. The cell membranes are often distinct and highlighted when two cells with clear or pale cytoplasm abut one another. Immunoblasts are often scattered among the neoplastic B cells. Lymphoid cells with plasmacytoid features (including Dutcher bodies) and mature plasma cells may also be present, either admixed with the other cells or segregated, often next to the capsule or trabeculae. In some cases, one may see scattered neutrophils, similar to what one may see in reactive monocytoid proliferations. Nodal marginal zone lymphoma may have a more prominent

---

*References 530, 531, 537, 541, 542, 544.

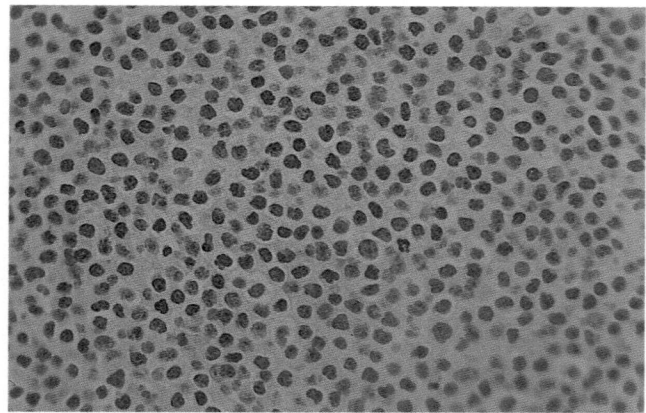

**FIGURE 41–49.** Marginal zone B cell lymphoma. Medium-sized cells with small nuclei and abundant clear cytoplasm are present. The nuclei have bland chromatin and slightly irregular nuclear contours.

monocytoid B cell population than that seen in a MALT lymphoma.

The diagnosis of marginal zone lymphoma should be made only when the lymphoma is composed almost exclusively of small cells, regardless of anatomic site. The presence of large cells in any appreciable quantity should result in the diagnosis of diffuse large B cell lymphoma, even in a MALT-related site; "high-grade MALT lymphoma" should not be used. The specific cutoff for the proportion of large cells requiring a diffuse large B cell lymphoma diagnosis is not specified in the WHO classification, but more than 5% large cells has been suggested. For lymphomas composed of both small cells and large cells, *diffuse large B cell lymphoma (with or without areas of marginal zone/MALT-type lymphoma)* is the suggested terminology. For cases of MALT lymphoma in which large lymphoid cells do not form clusters or sheets, an alternative term is *MALT lymphoma with increased large cells.* The clinical behavior of such cases is not yet known.

By definition, these lymphomas are B lineage, and almost all cases express surface immunoglobulin.[39, 412] About half of cases also express cytoplasmic immunoglobulin, which is detectable in paraffin sections, particularly in those cases with plasmacytoid differentiation.[39, 546] About one third of cases show aberrant CD43 coexpression.[135] CD5, CD10, and CD23 are usually negative.[491, 532] Monoclonal immunoglobulin heavy and light chain gene rearrangements are usually detectable, but *BCL1* and *BCL2* genes are germline.[546] Trisomy 3 has been detected in a majority of both nodal and extranodal cases, and numerical abnormalities of chromosomes 12 and 18 have also been found.[547–549] Detection of the t(11;18)(q21;q21) has been found in a high number of MALTomas and has been associated with decreased likelihood of transformation to a high-grade tumor.[550, 551] The t(11;18) has not been detected in cases of splenic marginal zone lymphoma and has only rarely been detected in cases of nodal marginal

zone lymphoma, suggesting that the entities are biologically different.[552–555]

Marginal zone B cell lymphoma must be distinguished from other low-grade to intermediate-grade B cell lymphomas. Unlike small lymphocytic lymphoma, marginal zone B cell lymphoma does not have proliferation centers and has cells with more abundant pale cytoplasm. Coexpression of CD5 is usually seen in small lymphocytic lymphoma but is present in only 10% of cases of marginal zone B cell lymphoma.[39, 491, 523] Marginal zone B cell lymphoma may be difficult to distinguish from lymphoplasmacytic lymphoma because both may show marked plasmacytoid differentiation, including Dutcher bodies. The presence of cells with more abundant pale cytoplasm excludes lymphoplasmacytic lymphoma. Mantle cell lymphoma contains a more homogeneous population of cells and lacks large transformed cells, and the cells have a greater degree of nuclear irregularities. Again, coexpression of CD5 is usually seen, unlike in marginal zone B cell lymphoma.[523] Marginal zone B cell lymphoma may be difficult to distinguish from some cases of follicular lymphoma because the cells of marginal zone B cell lymphoma may colonize reactive germinal centers (Fig. 41–50). Attention should be given to the cytologic features of cells, both within and outside the germinal centers. Truly small cleaved cells are absent within the germinal centers, whereas typical marginal zone B cells are found both within and outside the germinal centers. However, true follicular lymphoma may also have marginal zone B cell areas.[473, 539] Marginal zone B cell lymphoma may be difficult to distinguish histologically from lymph node involvement by hairy cell leukemia. However, the clinical circumstances are different; lymph node involvement by hairy cell leukemia rarely occurs without marked splenomegaly and obvious changes in the blood or bone marrow. Immunohistochemical studies may help demonstrate positivity for tartrate-resistant acid phosphatase activity and DBA.44 in

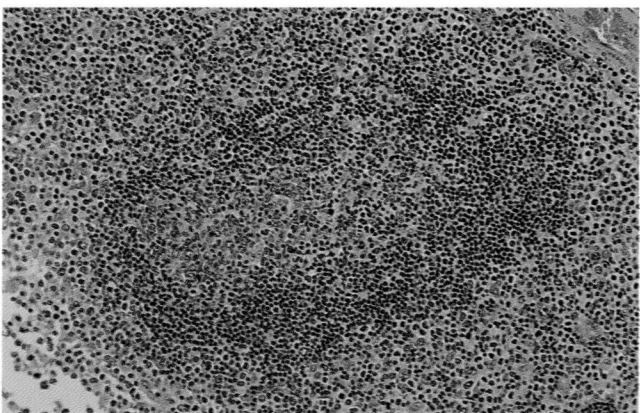

**FIGURE 41–50.** Marginal zone B cell lymphoma with follicular colonization. Most of the lymphoma cells form an arc around the reactive follicle, but some of the small lymphoma cells are also present in the mantle and germinal center.

hairy cell leukemia; these are usually negative in marginal zone lymphomas.[556] Furthermore, hairy cell leukemia shows positivity for CD25 and CD103 by flow cytometry, distinguishing it from other CD5⁻ B lineage lymphoproliferative disorders.[519, 557]

## Lymphoplasmacytic Lymphoma

Lymphoplasmacytic lymphoma is a low-grade lymphoma of small lymphocytes, plasma cells, and transitional forms between the two. This must be distinguished from other lymphoma subtypes that show differentiation to plasma cells, including mantle cell lymphoma, follicular lymphoma, and MALT/marginal zone lymphoma. Lymphoplasmacytic lymphoma corresponds to low-grade small lymphocytic with plasmacytoid differentiation in the Working Formulation and lymphoplasmacytic immunocytoma in the updated Kiel classification.[177, 450, 451, 512] It comprises approximately 2% to 3% of non-Hodgkin's lymphomas in the United States. Most patients are elderly. Some patients present with symptoms of Waldenström's macroglobulinemia, with high amounts of a monoclonal serum paraprotein of immunoglobulin M type, often with symptoms of hyperviscosity; others present with symptoms resembling small lymphocytic lymphoma, with generalized lymphadenopathy with or without splenomegaly.[510] The clinical course is generally indolent, but transformation to large cell lymphoma (usually an immunoblastic lymphoma with plasmacytoid features) may occur in 5% to 10% of cases and indicates a poor prognosis.[513]

Lymphoplasmacytic lymphoma is a diagnosis of exclusion because most other diffuse B cell lymphomas may show plasmacytic differentiation. On histologic examination, the lymphomatous node is diffusely effaced. Germinal centers may occasionally be seen, but proliferation centers are not present. The cell composition includes a mixture of small lymphocytes, plasmacytoid lymphocytes, and plasma cells. Scattered plasmacytoid immunoblasts may also be found (Fig. 41–51). Occasional cases may contain numerous plasmacytoid immunoblasts (polymorphous immunocytoma); these cases may be classified as diffuse mixed small and large cell with plasmacytoid differentiation in the Working Formulation because they may be more aggressive. Dutcher bodies are frequently present and easily identified, and Russell bodies may also be present. Scattered epithelioid histiocytes may be present, occasionally in such large numbers as to obscure the lymphoma or to simulate a T cell lymphoma.[558] Mast cells may also be numerous. Rare cases may contain abundant numbers of histiocytes with crystals of monotypic immunoglobulin.[559]

Immunophenotypic studies show consistent presence of monotypic cytoplasmic and surface immunoglobulin of M type, usually easily demonstrated in paraffin sections. This is in contrast to myeloma, in which the heavy chain is usually im-

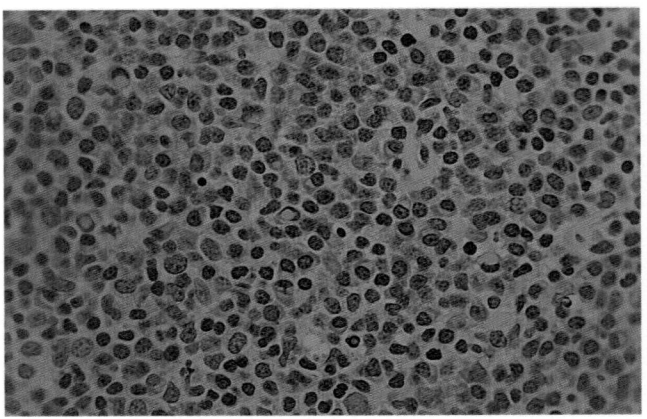

**FIGURE 41–51.** Lymphoplasmacytic lymphoma. There is a range of lymphoplasmacytic differentiation. Note the numerous Dutcher bodies in this field.

munoglobulin G or immunoglobulin A. Lymphoplasmacytic lymphomas usually express B lineage markers and often show aberrant coexpression of CD43 in paraffin sections.[23, 33, 135, 560] The neoplastic cells usually do not stain for or express CD5, CD10, or CD23, but rare exceptions may occur. Monoclonal gene rearrangement of the immunoglobulin heavy and light chain genes is detected in virtually all cases. A subset of cases may have a t(9;14) or a del(7q).[561–564] Eighty percent of the t(9;14) abnormalities can be detected by FISH study.[563]

Lymphoplasmacytic lymphoma may be confused with reactive lymphoplasmacytic proliferations, other diffuse B lineage lymphomas with plasma cells, Hodgkin's disease, and T cell lymphoma. The presence of more than rare numbers of Dutcher bodies favors lymphoplasmacytic lymphoma over a reactive lymphoplasmacytic proliferation. Paraffin immunohistochemical staining for cytoplasmic immunoglobulins shows polytypic staining in reactive proliferations and a monotypic population in lymphoplasmacytic lymphoma. All other diffuse B lineage lymphomas may have lymphoplasmacytic differentiation; thus, for the diagnosis of lymphoplasmacytic lymphoma to be made, the neoplasm must lack evidence of other types of lymphomas. The presence of proliferation centers indicates a diagnosis of small lymphocytic lymphoma rather than lymphoplasmacytic lymphoma, despite lymphoplasmacytic features. The presence of areas of neoplastic monocytoid B cells indicates a diagnosis of marginal zone B cell lymphoma. The presence of a homogeneous population of lymphoplasmacytoid cells with irregular nuclei is rare in mantle cell lymphoma; thus, that diagnosis must be supported by immunophenotypic studies demonstrating Bcl-1 positivity and molecular studies showing t(11;14). Even rare cases of follicular lymphoma may have lymphoplasmacytic features with numerous Dutcher bodies. The presence of follicles of neoplastic cells and the characteristic cleaved nuclei help to distinguish this from lymphoplasmacytic lymphoma. Hodgkin's disease and peripheral T cell lymphoma may have scattered plasma cells and epithelioid histiocytes, thus simulating lymphoplasmacytic lymphoma. However, the plasma cells are polyclonal, and both neoplasms feature neoplastic elements (Reed-Sternberg cells in Hodgkin's disease and a spectrum of atypical lymphoid cells in peripheral T cell lymphoma) not seen in lymphoplasmacytic lymphoma.

## Mantle Cell Lymphoma

Mantle cell lymphoma is composed of neoplastic cells showing differentiation toward normal mantle B cells.[565-569] The current terminology is relatively new, but the entity has been recognized for many years. It was known as diffuse predominantly small cleaved cell lymphoma in the Working Formulation, centrocytic lymphoma in the updated Kiel classification, and intermediately differentiated lymphocytic lymphoma in the modified Rappaport classification.[451, 565] Most hematopathologists and hematologists consider it to be an intermediate-grade lymphoma because of its relatively poor overall survival. However, its clinical features are more similar to the low-grade lymphomas in that there is no plateau in survival (patients are incurable) and relapses occur independently of time.[514, 568-571]

Mantle cell lymphoma comprises between 6% and 12% of lymphomas in the United States.[450, 514, 568] It occurs most commonly in elderly adults and is rare in children. The male-to-female ratio is about 2:1. Patients frequently present in stage IV, with generalized lymphadenopathy. Commonly involved sites include spleen, Waldeyer ring, bone marrow, and peripheral blood. It may also present as multiple polypoid masses in the intestine, known as lymphomatous polyposis.[572-575] Progression or transformation to large cell lymphoma is rare, but transformation to a "blastic" variant is not uncommon and portends a poor prognosis.[33, 570]

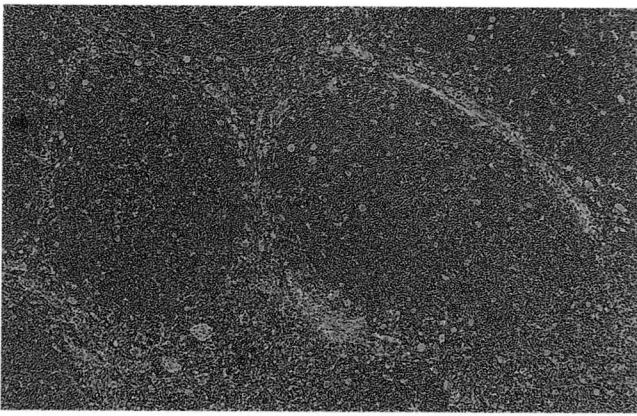

**FIGURE 41–53.** Mantle cell lymphoma, nodular pattern. Large crowded nodules of uniform lymphoid cells are present. No mantle zone or germinal center is visible.

Three different architectural patterns may be seen.[567, 568, 576] The most common is a diffusely effaced architecture. Another pattern is the mantle zone pattern in which the neoplastic infiltrate replaces the mantle zone of reactive follicles, leaving naked germinal centers surrounded by thickened cuffs of neoplastic cells (Fig. 41–52). The last and least common pattern is a nodular pattern, in which the neoplastic cells replace the mantle and spill over to "colonize" the germinal centers (Fig. 41–53). One may also see a mixture of these patterns.[577] The predominant cell type in mantle cell lymphoma, regardless of architectural pattern, is a small to medium-sized lymphoid cell with condensed chromatin, inconspicuous nucleoli, and highly irregular nuclear outlines (Fig. 41–54). In some cases, particularly those with suboptimal fixation, the indented nuclear contours may not be easily appreciated. A cytoplasmic stain, such as Bcl-2 antibody, may help to highlight the nuclear abnormalities. The neoplastic popu-

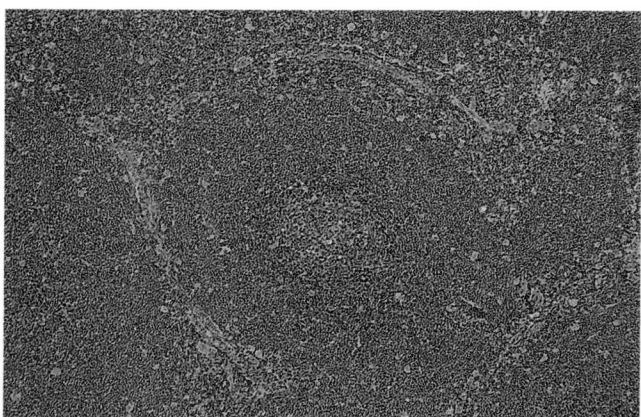

**FIGURE 41–52.** Mantle cell lymphoma, mantle zone pattern. A mantle zone architecture is present, with expanded mantle zones, surrounding a small reactive germinal center. The mantle zone is circumferentially uniform, unlike the mantle of reactive follicular hyperplasia, which has a crescent configuration.

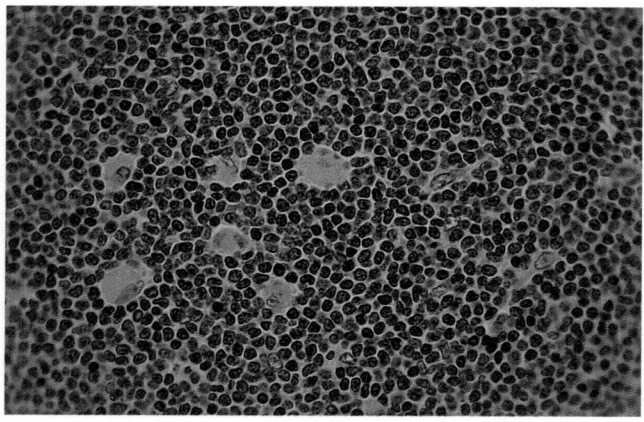

**FIGURE 41–54.** Mantle cell lymphoma, high power. A monotonous population of small lymphoid cells with irregular nuclear contours is seen. There are rare single histiocytes. The spectrum of cell size seen in small lymphocytic lymphoma is not present.

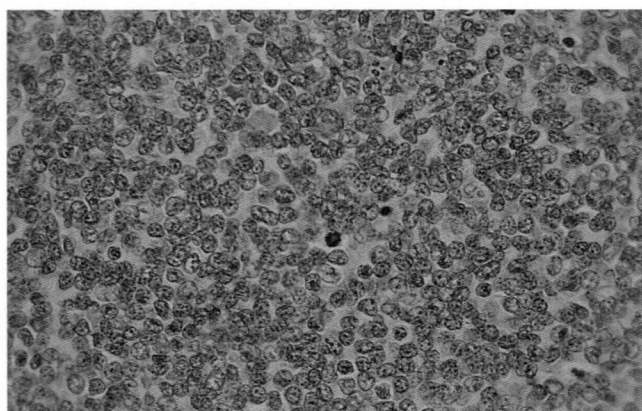

**FIGURE 41–55.** Mantle cell lymphoma, blastic variant, high power. The lymphoid cells have irregular nuclear outlines and fine chromatin. The mitotic rate is high. The cells were TdT negative.

lation is highly homogeneous and monotonous in almost all cases. One may rarely identify scattered large cells, usually in small clusters; these cells may represent residual germinal center cells from follicles that have been nearly completely replaced by neoplastic cells. In addition, scattered epithelioid histiocytes may be present and are helpful in suggesting the diagnosis of mantle cell lymphoma. Fine-needle aspiration biopsy smears of mantle cell lymphoma show small lymphoid cells with round and irregular nuclear contours. The chromatin pattern is usually less lumped or coarse than that seen in small lymphocytic or small cleaved cell lymphoma.[578, 579] The WHO classification system does not recommend subclassification or grading of mantle cell lymphoma; rather, different cytologic types and patterns should be mentioned in any diagnostic report.[452]

Three variants of mantle cell lymphoma have been described. The blastic (or lymphoblastoid) variant is the most common. The majority of blastic mantle lymphoma cells have fine chromatin, simulating lymphoblastic lymphoma[570, 580] (Fig. 41–55). The mitotic rate is high, and the prognosis is worse than in usual-type mantle cell lymphoma. The centroblastic variant has larger than usual neoplastic cells and more dispersed chromatin than is ordinarily seen.[451] The pleomorphic (or anaplastic) variant has neoplastic cells that are focally larger and more hyperchromatic than usual; the malignant cells also have prominent nuclear clefts.[451, 581, 582]

Mantle cell lymphoma, a B lineage lymphoma, expresses the B cell markers CD20 and CD79a in paraffin sections.[412, 487, 488] It also expresses monotypic surface immunoglobulin, which is most easily demonstrated by flow cytometry or frozen section immunohistochemistry. Interestingly, there is a slight predilection for λ as opposed to κ light chain restriction.[520] Aberrant coexpression of the paraffin section marker CD43 is seen in about 94% of cases, and aberrant coexpression of CD5 is seen in about

80% of cases.[23, 135, 523] CD10 and CD23 are usually negative but may occasionally be positive.[520] By flow cytometry, FMC7 is expressed with strong fluorescence intensity in 75% of cases of mantle cell lymphoma.[519, 520] A relatively specific feature for mantle cell lymphoma is reactivity with antibodies to cyclin D1[569, 583, 584] (Fig. 41–56). Cyclin D1 antibodies that have 75% sensitivity in paraffin sections are commercially available.[583, 584]

Monoclonal rearrangements of the immunoglobulin heavy and light chain genes are present in virtually all cases. Approximately 60% of cases are associated with t(11;14)(q13;q32), involving juxtaposition of the BCL1 locus of chromosome 11 with an immunoglobulin heavy chain gene enhancer sequence of chromosome 14.[585–590] The translocation results in deregulation and overexpression of the PRAD1/CCND1 gene. Classic cytogenetics, FISH, and Southern blotting can detect this translocation, and the majority of the translocations can be detected by PCR.[591] Overexpression of this gene can be detected in virtually all cases of mantle cell lymphoma by Northern blot analysis.[592] The degree of karyotypic complexity has a strong impact on prognosis. Deletions of 13q14, 11q, and 17p and total or partial +12 are also frequently seen in cases of mantle cell lymphoma; the last is putatively associated with a shorter survival.[590, 593–595] BCL6 mutations are virtually absent in mantle cell lymphoma, in contrast to higher frequency of BCL6 mutations in follicular lymphoma, lymphoplasmacytic lymphoma, MALToma, and diffuse large B cell lymphoma.[493]

The differential diagnosis of mantle cell lymphoma with a diffuse pattern includes other diffuse low-grade to intermediate-grade B cell lymphomas.[568] Small lymphocytic lymphoma and mantle cell lymphoma may easily be confused. Both lymphoma types have a spectrum of nuclear shapes ranging from round and regular to somewhat irregular nuclear outlines. However, small lymphocytic lymphoma usually has proliferation centers and is composed of a mixture of cell types, whereas mantle

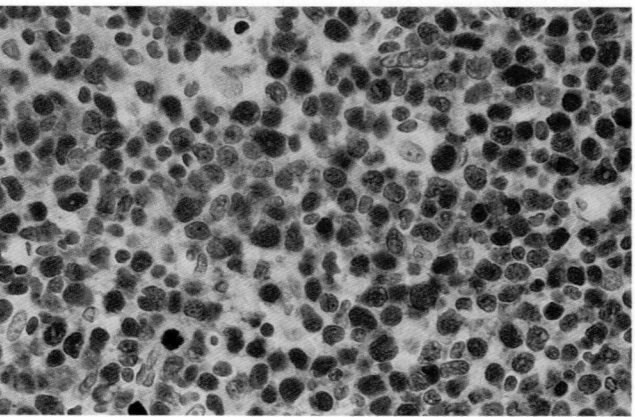

**FIGURE 41–56.** Mantle cell lymphoma, cyclin D1/Bcl-1 immunohistochemical stain. The nuclei of the tumor cells show strong staining. This pattern is restricted to mantle cell lymphoma.

cell lymphoma never has proliferation centers and is composed of a homogeneous population of small cells. Large cells with vesicular chromatin are not part of the neoplastic proliferation of mantle cell lymphoma. Both lymphomas are B lineage with aberrant CD43 and CD5 coexpression, but evidence of cyclin D1 overexpression or the t(11;14) would greatly favor mantle cell lymphoma. In addition, small lymphocytic lymphoma is usually CD23⁺ and FMC7⁻; mantle cell lymphoma has the opposite profile of CD23⁻ and FMC7⁺.[487, 519] The homogeneous population of cells in mantle cell lymphoma is also unlike the mixture of cells generally present in lymphoplasmacytoid lymphoma and marginal zone B cell lymphoma. In addition, CD5 or CD43 coexpression or evidence of cyclin D1 protein overexpression or the t(11;14) strongly favors mantle cell lymphoma.[487, 567–569]

When mantle cell lymphoma has a mantle zone or nodular pattern, the differential diagnosis includes follicular lymphoma. The mantle zone pattern of mantle cell lymphoma shows the architectural and cytologic characteristics of reactive germinal centers. In the nodular pattern of mantle cell lymphoma, the nodules are generally somewhat larger than the follicles of follicular lymphoma because they encompass both the region of the germinal center and the mantle zone. In addition, the follicles of follicular lymphoma virtually always include at least some large cells, whereas the cells of mantle cell lymphoma are usually more homogeneous, without large cells. Again, immunophenotypic studies may be useful for distinguishing these entities because follicular lymphoma is generally Bcl-2⁺ and CD43⁻.[131, 135]

The blastic variant of mantle cell lymphoma may easily be confused with lymphoblastic lymphoma. The presence of areas of typical mantle cell lymphoma within the same specimen or a history of mantle cell lymphoma favors blastic mantle cell lymphoma. In addition, the cells of mantle cell lymphoma are terminal deoxynucleotidyl transferase (TdT) negative, whereas TdT is almost always positive in lymphoblastic malignant neoplasms. Furthermore, the cytogenetic finding of t(11;14) or cyclin D1 expression favors a diagnosis of blastic mantle cell lymphoma.[50] Leukemic phase of blastic mantle cell lymphoma may be difficult to distinguish from other B lineage leukemias with blasts.[596, 597] This differential diagnosis is discussed in greater detail in Chapter 43.

## Diffuse Large B Cell Lymphoma

Diffuse large B cell lymphomas are aggressive lymphomas that have a diffuse architecture and a significant component of large lymphoid cells. This WHO terminology encompasses several entities of the Working Formulation, including intermediate-grade diffuse mixed small and large, intermediate-grade diffuse large cell, and high-grade large cell immuno-

blastic lymphomas.[450, 598] The centroblastic and B immunoblastic lymphomas of the updated Kiel classification also fall into this WHO classification term.[451]

Diffuse large B cell lymphomas comprise approximately one third of all non-Hodgkin's lymphomas and occur in all age groups, with a median age at presentation of 55 years.[450] The male-to-female ratio is about 1.2:1. Most cases are primary (de novo) lymphomas; approximately two thirds of these present with a single enlarged lymph node, one third at a single extranodal site.[599] A minority of patients have a history of a previous low-grade B cell lymphoma. The most commonly associated antecedent lymphoma is follicular lymphoma, but cases of small lymphocytic lymphoma, marginal zone B cell lymphoma, and lymphoplasmacytoid lymphoma also have a propensity for transformation to large cell lymphoma. Some patients have a history of immunodeficiency—congenital, iatrogenic (including after transplantation), or HIV associated; these are discussed further in the section "Immunodeficiency-related Lymphoproliferations." The International Prognostic Index for aggressive lymphomas was designed for large cell lymphoma and stratifies patients into several prognostic groups.[463] These lymphomas are generally treated with multidrug chemotherapy, with response rates above 80% and survival rates of about 60%.[600, 601] Relapses generally occur early, with a plateau in survival seen after a few years. A study suggests that previously unrecognized molecular heterogeneity in large cell lymphomas contributes to the marked differences in response to therapy and survival.[602] Using DNA microarray technology, the investigators identified two molecularly different gene expression patterns in diffuse large B cell lymphoma, indicative of different stages of B cell differentiation. Those with a so-called germinal center B cell–like ("resting") pattern had a better overall survival than did those with an "activated" B cell–like pattern. This gene expression profiling may provide important therapeutic and prognostic information in the future.

Large cell lymphoma arising in the mediastinum may have distinct clinicopathologic features; it occurs in younger adults with a male-to-female ratio of about 1:1.5.[603–610] Locally aggressive behavior may be a problem, but these neoplasms are responsive to aggressive therapies and have overall survivals similar to those of other large cell lymphomas.[611, 612]

By definition, diffuse large B cell lymphomas have a diffuse architecture. However, follicular areas may be focally present in a minority of cases as part of a residual follicular lymphoma that has undergone transformation. Similarly, areas of other low-grade lymphomas may be seen, presumably also preceding the development of large cell lymphoma in such cases. The diffuse large cell lymphoma may involve only part of the lymph node, for instance, only the sinuses (sinusoidal large cell lymphoma) or only the paracortical areas. Approximately half of cases have some type of sclerosis, including broad bands surrounding large areas of tumor, a fine scle-

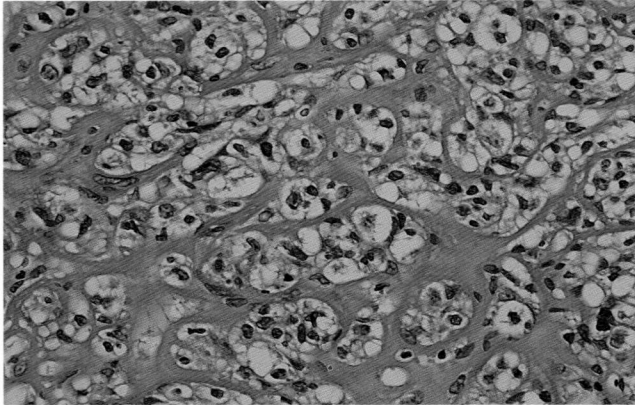

**FIGURE 41–57.** Sclerosing large cell lymphoma. There is hyaline sclerosis, which surrounds individual tumor cells and clusters of tumor cells.

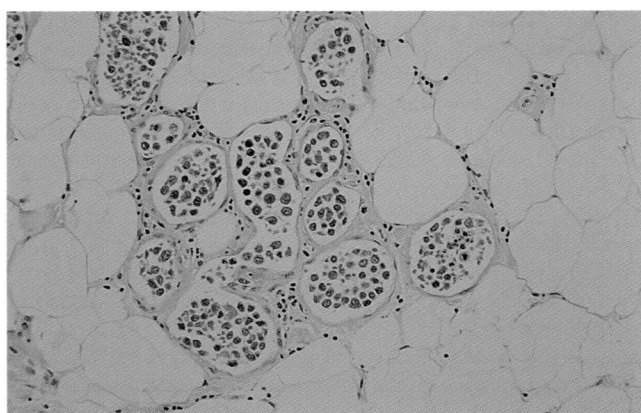

**FIGURE 41–59.** Diffuse large cell B cell lymphoma, intravascular pattern. The lymphoma cells are confined to the small vessels, which are packed with tumor cells.

rosis enveloping single cells (Fig. 41–57), and a compartmentalizing fibrosis enclosing clusters of cells (Fig. 41–58); the last is particularly common in mediastinal large cell lymphoma.[604] A rare variant of large cell lymphoma is intravascular or angiotropic lymphoma, which has an exclusively or predominantly intravascular component and is most often found in soft tissue or extranodal sites[613–615] (Fig. 41–59).

As the name indicates, these lymphomas have a significant component of large cells, although the exact percentage of cells required to distinguish this from diffuse lymphomas of small cells is not specified in the WHO classification. A figure frequently cited for diffuse large B cell lymphoma is more than 25%. There are several types of large cells, including large cleaved and noncleaved cells (also known as centroblasts and already described in the section on follicular lymphoma), multilobated large cells, and immunoblasts (Fig. 41–60). Multilobated cells have more than three lobes and usually have a chromatin

pattern intermediate between large cleaved and noncleaved cells. Immunoblasts have round to oval vesicular nuclei with one (sometimes more) prominent central nucleolus. Cytoplasm is generally abundant and plasmacytoid or pale to clear. The large cells of mediastinal large cell lymphoma are often distinctive, with nuclei resembling large cleaved or noncleaved cells or multilobated cells and abundant clear to pale-staining cytoplasm.[616] Each of these cell types, or combinations thereof, accounted for a different category of large cell lymphoma in older classifications, but they have been put into the general category of diffuse large B cell lymphoma in the WHO classification because there were no clear differences in survival among the categories.[450, 452, 598] Diffuse large B cell lymphomas always contain other types of cells, including small reactive T cells, atypical small B cells (not usually present, but part of the neoplastic process when they are present), histiocytes, eosinophils, plasma cells, and rarely neutrophils. Fine-needle aspiration smears of diffuse large

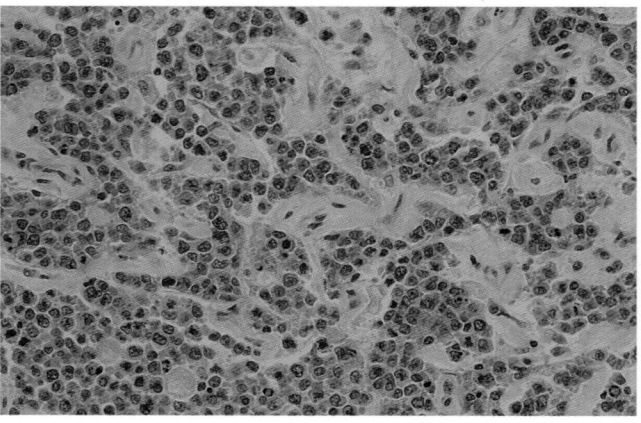

**FIGURE 41–58.** Diffuse large cell B cell lymphoma, primary in the mediastinum. A compartmentalizing fibrosis is present, as is typical of large cell lymphomas primary in this site.

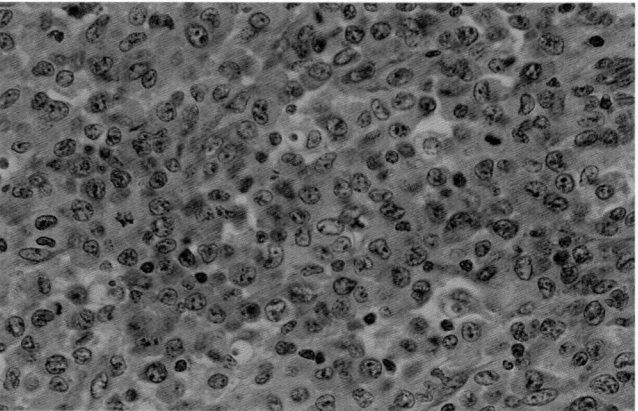

**FIGURE 41–60.** Diffuse large cell B cell lymphoma. A mixture of large cleaved (centroblastic/centrocytic) and large noncleaved (centroblastic monomorphous) cells is present. The cytoplasm may be scant or plasmacytoid, as in this example.

B cell lymphoma may show a dispersed population of cells with rounded or cleaved vesicular nuclei with irregularly thick and thin nuclear membranes, with one to multiple small nucleoli. The immunoblastic-type large lymphoma cells have a single, more prominent nucleolus and may have more abundant cytoplasm. Rarely, large cell lymphomas may form a rosettelike structure or have myxoid or fibrillary stroma.[617, 618] In addition, neoplastic large B cells may be signet ring type (with either clear or eosinophilic inclusions), may have microvillus-like cytoplasmic projections, or extremely rarely may be spindled.[604, 619, 620]

Numerous histologic variants have been described. The WHO classification recognizes six different morphologic variants (Table 41–15). The centroblastic variant is the same as the diffuse large cell variant or mixed small cleaved and large cell variant of the Working Formulation and is identical to the centroblastic lymphoma of the updated Kiel classification. The immunoblastic variant is the same as the high-grade large cell immunoblastic variant of the Working Formulation. T cell–rich B cell lymphoma has scattered large B lineage lymphoma cells amid a large reactive component of small T cells[621–623] (Fig. 41–61). In histiocyte-rich B cell lymphoma, histiocytes predominate as the reactive component.[624] Lymphomatoid granulomatosis type is an EBV-positive B cell proliferation associated with an exuberant T cell reaction that presents in extranodal sites, most commonly the lung.[625–629] Other frequent sites of involvement include kidney, skin, central nervous system, and liver. The patterns of necrosis in lymphomatoid granulomatosis and T-NK cell lymphoma appear similar. Lymphomatoid granulomatosis is discussed in Chapter 15 and is briefly covered with T-NK cell lymphomas (see later section, "Extranodal T Cell Lymphomas"). Anaplastic large B cell lymphoma is considered a variant of diffuse large B cell lymphoma that has highly anaplastic morphology.[433, 630] The category of anaplastic large cell lymphoma originally embraced B lineage neoplasms, but the B lineage cases were removed from the category of anaplastic large cell lymphoma in the WHO classification. This was because of differences in clin-

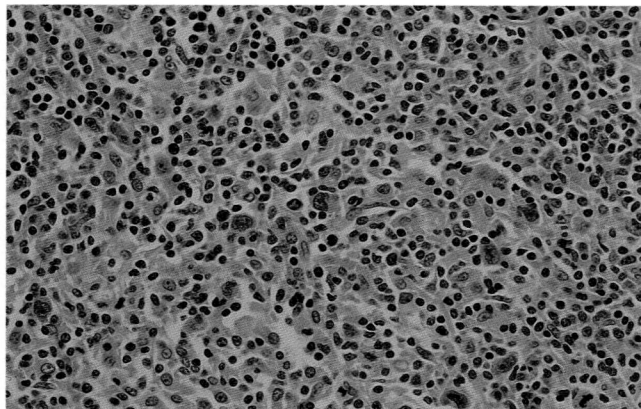

**FIGURE 41–61.** T cell–rich B cell lymphoma. Large neoplastic cells represent a minority of the cell population.

ical presentation and behavior and in cytotoxic cell marker expression compared with anaplastic large cell lymphoma of T cell or null cell lineage. In addition, the anaplastic large B cell lymphoma cases lack the t(2;5) translocation and ALK protein immunoreactivity that are characteristic of anaplastic large cell lymphoma of T cell or null cell lineage (discussed later). The plasmablastic variant of diffuse large B cell lymphoma is associated with HIV infection and is discussed further in the section on immunodeficiency-related lymphoproliferative disorders.[631–634]

By definition, these lymphomas are B lineage neoplasms, with staining for CD20 and CD79a.[39, 412] CD20 stains are particularly helpful in highlighting the minority B cell component in T cell–rich/histiocyte-rich B cell lymphoma. Almost all large cell lymphomas are positive for CD45, with the exception being some cases of plasmacytoid immunoblastic lymphoma.[60] About two thirds express surface immunoglobulin detectable in frozen sections or by flow cytometry,[10, 519] and a subset express cytoplasmic immunoglobulin detectable in paraffin sections, particularly cases of plasmacytoid immunoblastic lymphoma. Aberrant coexpression of CD43 or CD5 is found in about 20% and 5% of cases, respectively.[23, 523 135] Virtually all cases have detectable immunoglobulin heavy or light chain gene rearrangement.[635] About 30% of cases have evidence of a t(14;18), particularly those cases with a history of follicular lymphoma.[497] BCL1 gene rearrangements are generally not found. Rearrangement involving BCL6 (LAZ3), an oncogene on chromosome 3q27, is found in about 40% of cases, particularly cases presenting in extranodal sites.[493, 636, 637] The presence of a BCL6 rearrangement has been correlated with better overall survival as well as survival without disease progression. Primary mediastinal large B cell lymphomas commonly overexpress the MAL gene, whereas other diffuse large B cell lymphomas do not, providing further evidence that this is a distinct clinicopathologic entity.[637a] The prognostic significance of a t(14;18) in large cell lymphomas is still not clear, but its identification should suggest a

**TABLE 41–15.** Morphologic Variants and Subtypes of Diffuse Large B Cell Lymphoma in WHO Classification

*Morphologic Variants*
Centroblastic
Immunoblastic
T cell/histiocyte-rich
Lymphomatoid granulomatosis type
Anaplastic large B cell
Plasmablastic

*Subtypes*
Mediastinal (thymic) large B cell lymphoma
Primary effusion lymphoma
Intravascular large B cell lymphoma

search for history or coexistence of follicular lymphoma. A subset of cases have been reported to have evidence of c-*myc* rearrangements and probably represent misclassified cases of Burkitt-like lymphoma. There may also be a prognostic role for Ki-67 in these lymphomas.[466, 638, 639]

The differential diagnosis of the large cell lymphomas includes reactive lymphoid proliferations, other non-Hodgkin's lymphomas, nonhematopoietic neoplasms, classical Hodgkin's disease, and L&H lymphocyte predominance Hodgkin's disease. The last three were discussed earlier in their respective sections. The differential diagnosis with true histiocytic tumor and extramedullary myeloid tumor is discussed later. Features that differentiate large B cell lymphoma from small noncleaved cell lymphoma (Burkitt-like lymphoma) and peripheral T cell lymphoma are also discussed later in this chapter. Reactive immunoblastic proliferations and histiocytic necrotizing lymphadenitis (Kikuchi's disease) are the reactive conditions most easily confused with diffuse large cell lymphoma. Clinical history is extremely helpful for these differential diagnoses; a tonsillar lesion in an adolescent with viral symptoms suggests infectious mononucleosis, and an enlarged cervical lymph node in an otherwise asymptomatic young female patient raises the possibility of Kikuchi's disease. Compared with diffuse large B cell lymphoma, reactive lymphoid proliferations usually have greater architectural preservation (at least focally within the lymph node) and a greater degree of cellular polymorphism. In reactive proliferations, immunohistochemical studies usually demonstrate a predominance of T cells and a modest number of B cells. B lineage large cell lymphomas generally have a monomorphous appearance, with sheets of B lineage cells seen on immunohistochemical studies. A prominent exception is T cell–rich/histocyte-rich B cell lymphoma, which lacks a spectrum of B cell atypia and is composed of a mixture of small T cells (or histiocytes) and large B cells, without medium or small B cells.

Other non-Hodgkin's lymphomas that may be confused with the large cell lymphomas are the paraimmunoblastic variant of small lymphocytic lymphoma and the centroblastic variant of mantle cell lymphoma. The paraimmunoblastic variant of small lymphocytic lymphoma is usually preceded by small lymphocytic lymphoma/chronic lymphocytic leukemia, and thus clinical history may be extremely useful. In morphologic appearance, the cells of the paraimmunoblastic variant of small lymphocytic lymphoma are smaller and have less prominent nucleoli and less abundant cytoplasm than the cells of large B cell lymphoma. In the centroblastic variant of mantle cell lymphoma, the cells are also smaller than the cells of diffuse large B cell lymphoma. However, the distinction may be difficult to make by morphologic appearance alone, and additional studies may be required. Immunohistochemical studies generally demonstrate CD5 positivity, and

molecular studies often demonstrate evidence of a t(11;14) or cyclin D1 expression in the centroblastic variant of mantle cell lymphoma.

## Burkitt's Lymphoma and Burkitt Cell Leukemia

In the WHO categorization scheme, the category of Burkitt's lymphoma encompasses the high-grade, small noncleaved cell lymphoma (Burkitt's and non-Burkitt's subtypes) of the Working Formulation and Burkitt's lymphoma of the updated Kiel classification.[450, 451] The neoplastic cells of Burkitt's lymphoma are biologically equivalent to the French-American-British L3 cells of acute lymphoblastic leukemia.

The WHO classification lists three clinical and genetic subtypes of Burkitt's lymphoma: endemic, sporadic, and immunodeficiency associated.[452] The immunodeficiency-associated Burkitt's lymphomas frequently involve bone marrow and lymph nodes and are discussed further in the section on immunodeficiency-related lymphoproliferations. The endemic form, which occurs in equatorial Africa, affects young children (particularly boys), who present with jaw tumors or other extranodal masses.[640] Sporadic Burkitt's lymphoma occurs in children and young adults, most commonly with involvement of the lower abdomen or Waldeyer ring.[641–644] In most series, the Burkitt's and non-Burkitt's subtypes of small noncleaved cell lymphoma in the Working Formulation did not have marked clinical differences or survival differences, and thus they were combined into a single category in the WHO classification.[645, 646] Burkitt's lymphoma is an extremely aggressive lymphoma treated primarily by multidrug chemotherapy, although there may be a role for bone marrow transplantation.[645, 647] Survival rates are now in the range of 80%; relapses, if they occur, usually arise in the first year.

Burkitt's lymphoma usually shows diffuse architectural effacement; rare cases show focal germinal center involvement.[648] The characteristic low-power appearance is a starry sky pattern imparted by a high mitotic rate, numerous apoptotic cells, and evenly dispersed tingible body macrophages (Fig. 41–62). Viewing at high magnification shows a homogeneous population of medium-sized cells with round nuclei, vesicular chromatin, several moderately sized nucleoli, and a moderate amount of basophilic cytoplasm that tends to square off as it abuts adjacent cells ("jigsaw puzzle" configuration) (Fig. 41–63). Two morphologic variants of Burkitt's lymphoma are recognized in the WHO classification: Burkitt-like tumors and tumors with plasmacytoid differentiation.[452] The tumors with plasmacytoid differentiation are associated with the AIDS population. The Burkitt-like tumors have more cell size heterogeneity and slightly fewer but more prominent nucleoli than those of typical Burkitt's lymphoma. The Burkitt-like tumors were formerly

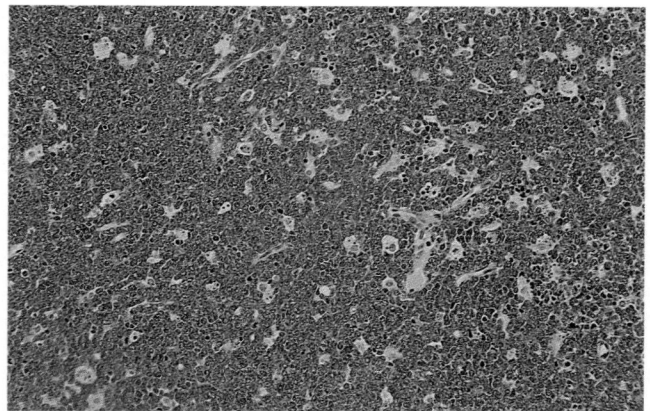

**FIGURE 41–62.** Burkitt-type lymphoma, low power. A starry sky pattern is present.

classified as small, noncleaved, non-Burkitt's lymphomas in the Working Formulation. Fine-needle aspiration smears of Burkitt's lymphoma usually show a homogeneous population of medium-sized cells with round nuclei, coarsely reticulated chromatin, and several nucleoli. The cytoplasm is basophilic and relatively abundant and usually contains small vacuoles on air-dried smears. Again, the variant formerly known as non-Burkitt's type contains similarly sized rounded nuclei with slightly finer chromatin and some cells with only one small but prominent nucleolus.

All cases of Burkitt's lymphoma are B lineage neoplasms and almost always express monotypic immunoglobulins.[16, 39] CD20, CD79a, and CD10 are positive in virtually all cases.[412] Aberrant CD43 coexpression may be identified in a majority of cases.[23] CD5 and CD23 are usually negative, but rare CD5+ Burkitt lymphoma cases have been reported.[39, 649] Immunoglobulin heavy and light chain gene rearrangements can be detected in virtually all cases. The Ki-67 fraction should be above 99% for all

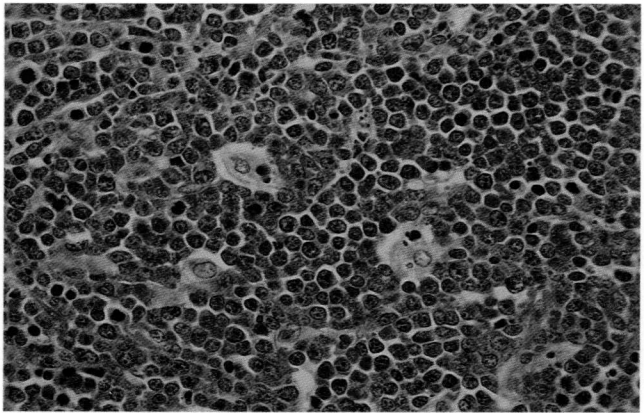

**FIGURE 41–63.** Burkitt-type lymphoma, high power. The tumor cells are homogeneous in size and chromatin pattern.

cases of Burkitt's lymphoma or Burkitt-like lymphoma.[638, 639] In contrast to lymphoblastic lymphoma, TdT is negative.

Burkitt's lymphoma cases have a translocation involving the c-*myc* gene on chromosome 8. The t(8;14) involving the immunoglobulin heavy chain gene is found in 85% of cases.[650, 651] A t(2;8) involving the κ gene is found in 10% of cases. The t(8;22) involving the λ gene is found in 5% of cases.[652, 653] In fact, the chromosome 8 translocation or c-*myc* rearrangement is considered the "gold standard" for the diagnosis of Burkitt's lymphoma. The actual site of translocation differs between endemic and sporadic Burkitt's lymphoma.[654–657] Variations in the translocations make them poor targets for detection by routine PCR techniques, although newer PCR techniques are being developed.[658] In addition, Southern blot analysis for c-*myc* has sensitivity in only 80% to 85% of cases owing to the heterogeneity of the breakpoints. FISH studies may be performed on paraffin-embedded tissues.[659] EBV is associated with nearly all cases of endemic Burkitt's lymphoma and only 20% to 25% of sporadic Burkitt's lymphoma occurring in Europe and North America.[370] The percentage of EBV-positive cases of sporadic Burkitt's lymphoma rises to approximately 50% to 80% in South America and parts of the Middle East.

The differential diagnosis of Burkitt's lymphoma includes lymphoblastic lymphoma and diffuse large B cell lymphoma, particularly those formerly classified as large cell immunoblastic lymphoma in the Working Formulation. Compared with diffuse large B cell lymphoma, Burkitt's lymphoma generally has more cellular homogeneity, has less host cells other than histiocytes, and more consistently has a starry sky appearance. Cell size has not proved to be a reliable and reproducible criterion in the discrimination between Burkitt's lymphoma and diffuse large B cell lymphomas. In questionable cases, Ki-67 immunohistochemical staining may help; the highest percentages of Ki-67 stain in Burkitt's lymphoma.[638]

## Mature T Cell Lymphoma

Mature T cell lymphomas, also known as peripheral T cell lymphomas or post-thymic T cell lymphomas, are a general category of non-Hodgkin's lymphomas that have morphologic and immunohistochemical features consistent with mature T cells. The term encompasses subsets of intermediate-grade to high-grade lymphomas in the Working Formulation, including diffuse predominantly small cleaved, mixed small cleaved and large cell, and large cell lymphoma and large cell immunoblastic lymphoma.[450] In the updated Kiel classification, peripheral T cell lymphoma encompasses at least eight categories of T cell lymphoma.[451] The classification of T cell lymphomas in the older systems had many imperfections. In contrast to B cell lymphomas, cytologic grade did not appear to correlate with progno-

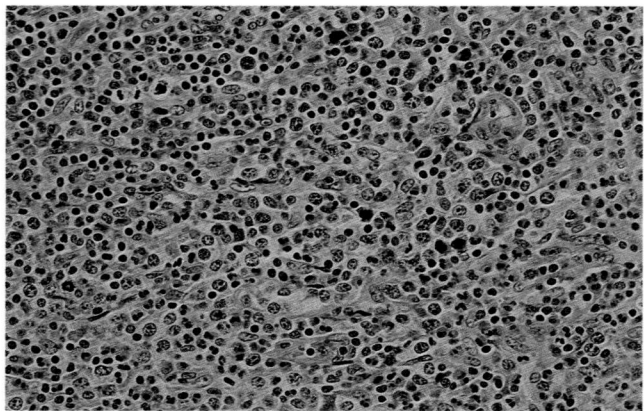

**FIGURE 41–64.** Peripheral T cell lymphoma. A spectrum of lymphoid atypia is present in a mixed inflammatory background.

sis.[660–662] In many studies, stage of disease emerged as a more important factor than cytologic subtype. In addition, cytologic features alone did not distinguish among different disease entities. In fact, clinical presentation was found to be important in the classification of T cell malignant neoplasms. Thus, the REAL and WHO classifications divided the mature T cell lymphomas into several clinicopathologic entities as well as a general category of peripheral T cell lymphoma, not otherwise characterized.[177, 452] The first part of this discussion covers peripheral T cell lymphoma, not otherwise characterized. The second part of this section discusses several clinicopathologic entities of mature T cell lymphomas. Anaplastic large cell lymphoma, which is probably the single most common subtype of T cell lymphoma, is discussed separately. The leukemic or systemic groups of T cell malignant neoplasms are discussed in Chapter 43.

## PERIPHERAL T CELL LYMPHOMA, NOT OTHERWISE CHARACTERIZED

Peripheral T cell lymphomas account for only approximately 10% of cases of diffuse non-Hodgkin's lymphoma. They occur at all ages but particularly in the elderly; the median age is 60 years.[660, 663–665] The male-to-female ratio is approximately 1.5 : 1. Patients usually present with generalized lymphadenopathy and may have a history of autoimmune disease. Constitutional symptoms are common, and patients are often anemic. Approximately two thirds of patients have stage III or stage IV disease, often with involvement of extranodal organs such as skin, spleen, and liver. The clinical course is variable, ranging from an indolent course to rapid demise. Peripheral T cell lymphoma is usually treated similarly to B lineage large cell lymphoma with aggressive multidrug chemotherapy.[666] Patients with peripheral T cell lymphoma have a worse prognosis than do equivalent patients with B cell lymphoma, particularly if treatment is suboptimal.[667]

Peripheral T cell lymphomas show focal or diffuse architectural effacement. Focal involvement (T zone pattern) shows changes in the paracortical areas, with sparing of the follicles. As the follicles become obliterated, the involvement becomes more diffuse. Vascularity is often prominent, with numerous high endothelial venules. The neoplastic population comprises a spectrum of cellular atypia, with a range of nuclear size and nuclear shapes (Fig. 41–64). In general, the small cells have highly irregular nuclei with condensed chromatin; the large cells may have round or irregular nuclei, condensed or vesicular chromatin, and prominent nucleoli. Cytoplasm is often pale or clear and may be scant or abundant. Characteristically, one can identify an exuberant host infiltrate, which is composed of small round lymphocytes, epithelioid and nonepithelioid histiocytes, eosinophils, neutrophils, and plasma cells. Rarely, one may see hemophagocytosis in benign histiocytes, either within the neoplasm or at distant sites. Also rarely, Reed-Sternberg–like cells and Touton-like tumor giant cells have been reported in cases of T cell lymphoma.[668–670] A particular type of peripheral T cell lymphoma known as lymphoepithelioid T cell lymphoma (Lennert's lymphoma) is placed in the category of "peripheral T cell lymphoma, not otherwise specified" in the WHO classification. It has the distinctive histologic feature of the presence of numerous epithelioid histiocytes throughout the lymph node, as single cells or small clusters, but not forming discrete granulomas[671] (Fig. 41–65). The neoplastic component may be masked by the epithelioid histiocytes unless the tissue is carefully examined for cytologically malignant cells.

By definition, these lymphomas express one or more definitive T cell antigens in the absence of B antigen expression. The T cell antigen receptor lacks mutually exclusive subunits that are analogous to immunoglobulin light chains; thus, there is no surrogate test for T cell clonality based on antibody studies. In theory, one could use a panel of T cell antigen receptor variable region antibodies to recognize dominant specific T cell antigen receptor usage, with

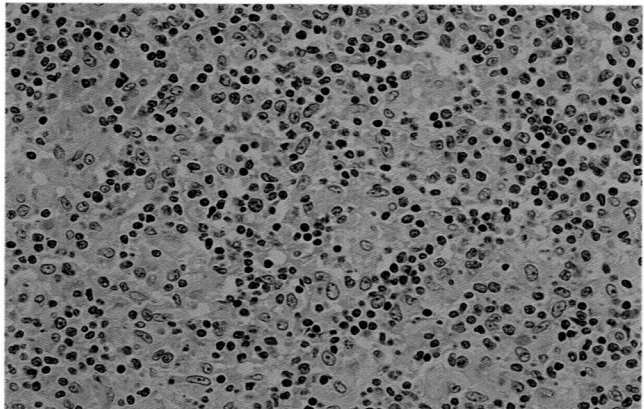

**FIGURE 41–65.** Lymphoepithelioid T cell (Lennert's) lymphoma. Sheets of epithelioid histiocytes may mask the tumor cell population.

any dominance highly suggestive of a clonal population. However, the limited availability and sensitivity of variable region antibodies precludes their use in practice. Currently, at best, one can use a relatively small panel of pan–T cell antigens to aid the diagnosis of T cell lymphoma. In paraffin and frozen sections, the majority of mature, reactive T cells express the pan–T cell markers CD2, CD3 (Fig. 41–66), CD5, and βF1, and more than 50% express CD7.[39, 672] In contrast, peripheral T cell lymphoma cells frequently show pan–T antigen loss, defined as staining of less than 50% of total T cells. In one large study, nearly 75% of peripheral T cell lymphomas exhibited loss of one or more pan–T antigens, including CD7 (56%), CD5 (46%), F1 (23%), CD3 (19%), and CD2 (18%).[22, 673–675] A helper (CD4+ CD8−) phenotype is usually seen, but a suppressor-cytotoxic (CD4− CD8+) phenotype may also be present. The identification of a mature T cell population that is also CD4− CD8− (seen in about one sixth of cases) or CD4+ CD8+ (seen rarely) also constitutes evidence for a diagnosis of T cell lymphoma. CD4− CD8− or CD4+ CD8+ phenotypes are also a relatively common phenomenon in T lymphoblastic neoplasms. CD95, an antibody implicated in aggressive behavior in malignant neoplasms, is frequently expressed in NK and T cell lymphomas but rarely in B cell lymphomas.[676] By immunohistochemistry, approximately 90% of peripheral T cell lymphomas express CD45 and nearly all express CD43.[23, 60] The B-associated antigen CD20 is almost always negative.[412] A subset of T cell lymphomas expresses CD56, the neural cell adhesion molecule; these cases have a predilection for involvement of unusual extranodal sites and are discussed further in the section on extranodal T cell lymphomas.[677, 678]

Southern blot analysis of the T cell receptor β-chains detects more than 90% of T cell malignant neoplasms but usually does not detect gene rearrangement in malignant neoplasms of γδ T cells or NK cells.[679] PCR-based assays for T cell clonality are usually directed against T cell receptor γ-chain or β-chain and can be performed on paraffin-embedded tissue.

Fine-needle aspiration biopsy diagnosis of peripheral T cell lymphoma may be extremely difficult because a mixed population is usually seen.[680] The identification of highly bizarre or anaplastic cells favors a diagnosis of malignancy. Immunohistochemical or molecular studies are extremely helpful in confirming a diagnosis of lymphoma and are essential for the recognition of T cell lineage.

The differential diagnosis of peripheral T cell lymphoma includes reactive paracortical proliferations, B cell lymphoma, and Hodgkin's disease. The last differential is discussed in the section on Hodgkin's disease. Distinguishing paracortical hyperplasia from peripheral T cell lymphoma may be extremely difficult by morphology and often requires immunohistochemical studies to demonstrate an aberrant T cell immunophenotype or molecular studies to demonstrate a monoclonal T cell population. On histologic examination, paracortical hyperplasia appears mottled at low magnification because of the mixture of discrete cell types, including small lymphocytes, immunoblasts, histiocytes, and granulocytes. Peripheral T cell lymphoma shows a continuous spectrum of cellular atypia, from small to large lymphoid cells. Peripheral T cell lymphoma is more likely to show complete architectural effacement, but an exclusive paracortical (T zone) distribution may occur. However, the intervening follicles are usually atrophic in lymphoma, whereas they are usually highly hyperplastic in a reactive proliferation. The differential diagnosis of Lennert's lymphoma includes lymphoplasmacytic lymphoma, which may occasionally have extensive infiltrates of epithelioid histiocytes. The B cell phenotype of lymphoplasmacytic lymphoma can easily be determined by flow cytometry or immunohistochemistry. The absence of well-formed granulomas or necrosis makes lymphoepithelioid T cell lymphoma easy to distinguish from granulomatous lymphadenitis.

Although the morphologic features of peripheral T cell lymphoma appear to be distinctive, the histologic differentiation between B and T cell lymphomas is extremely difficult in practice.[681] Features that favor a peripheral T cell lymphoma are a diffuse proliferation of atypical lymphoid cells, the presence of a spectrum of lymphoid atypia, the presence of more than occasional eosinophils, and a paracortical distribution. However, immunohistochemical or molecular studies are necessary to confirm any histologic suspicions. The presence of CD3+ or CD2+ atypical cells is a good indication of a T cell lymphoma, but staining for CD45RO or CD43 alone should not be used as definitive evidence of a T cell lymphoma because both are reactive in some B cell lymphomas and myeloid leukemias.[23, 135] However, positivity for CD45RO or CD43 in the absence of staining for the reliable B lineage markers CD20 and CD79a or the myeloid marker myeloperoxidase is strong presumptive evidence of T cell lymphoma.

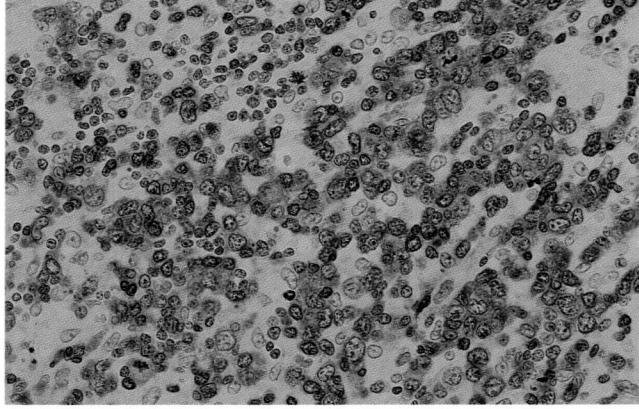

**FIGURE 41–66.** Peripheral T cell lymphoma, CD3 stain. The atypical lymphoid cells are labeled with this T lineage marker. The CD20 stain was negative.

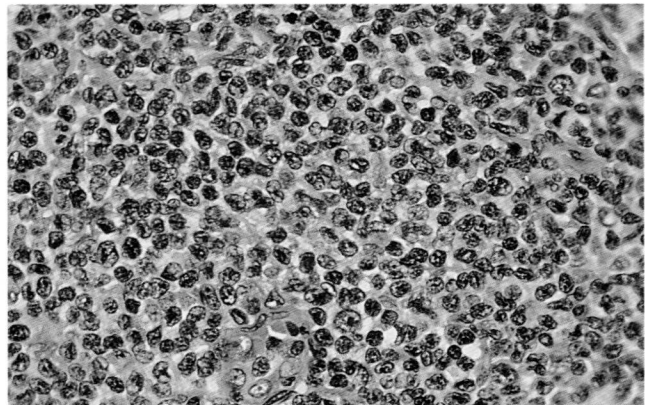

FIGURE 41–67. Mycosis fungoides. Sheets of tumor cells are present in this lymph node of a patient with skin lesions.

## SUBTYPES OF PERIPHERAL T CELL LYMPHOMA

### Adult T Cell Lymphoma-Leukemia

Adult T cell lymphoma-leukemia is a specific clinicopathologic variant first described in southwestern Japan but also described in other, mostly equatorial, areas.[682, 683] It is caused by HTLV-1.[684] Patients usually present with generalized lymphadenopathy and hypercalcemia. Less commonly, lymphomatous, chronic, and smoldering forms may occur.[685] The peripheral blood has characteristic malignant lymphoid cells, with highly convoluted nuclear outlines. Involved lymph nodes show histologic features similar to those described for peripheral T cell lymphoma; marked nuclear pleomorphism is often seen.[445] The tumor cells are characteristically positive for CD25 by flow cytometry or frozen section immunohistochemistry. Molecular studies show clonal integration of HTLV-1 in the tumor cells as well as T cell receptor gene rearrangements.

### Mycosis Fungoides

Mycosis fungoides is a peripheral T cell lymphoma that primarily involves the skin or, rarely, another epithelial site.[114] It is composed of small cerebriform lymphoid cells that have a CD4+ helper T cell phenotype.[686] Patients with mycosis fungoides often have lymph node enlargement that is due to dermatopathic lymphadenitis, but the neoplastic cells may also involve the lymph node.[687] Lymph node involvement begins as subtle infiltrates of atypical cells in the paracortex, admixed with the dendritic cells and macrophages of the dermatopathic areas. The histologic diagnosis of mycosis fungoides can generally be made only when large aggregates of cerebriform cells are found in the paracortex or when architectural effacement is present (Fig. 41–67). The presence of clonal T cell receptor gene rearrangements may more reliably make the distinction between mycosis fungoides and dermatopathic lymphadenitis. Transformation to large cell lymphoma may occur and confers a poor prognosis.[688] The term *Sézary's syndrome* is used when the mycosis fungoides cells are present in the peripheral blood. Patients with Sézary's syndrome often have lymphadenopathy.

### Angioimmunoblastic T Cell Lymphoma

Angioimmunoblastic T cell lymphoma is also known as AILD-like T cell lymphoma. It is a peripheral T cell lymphoma with clinical and histologic features similar to those of AILD.[689, 690] Some pathologists consider all cases of AILD to represent angioimmunoblastic T cell lymphoma ab initio, whereas others view AILD as a possible polyclonal or preneoplastic T cell disorder. Lymphoma should be suspected when there are clusters and small sheets of atypical lymphoid cells, particularly around vessels (Fig. 41–68). A firm diagnosis of angioimmunoblastic T cell lymphoma can be made when there are large sheets of atypical lymphoid cells, immunohistochemical evidence of an aberrant T cell immunophenotype, or molecular evidence of a sizable (more than 1% to 5%) monoclonal T cell population.[311] As in AILD, germinal centers are usually absent. However, there are rare cases with angioimmunoblastic proliferation, hyperplastic germinal centers with ill-defined borders, and frequent interfollicular tingible body macrophages.[691]

### Extranodal T Cell Lymphomas

Excluding mycosis fungoides, nearly one third of T cell lymphomas arise as primary tumors in extranodal sites, and these lymphomas are biologically different from their nodal counterparts.[692, 693] As such, the WHO classification of lymphoid neoplasms includes extranodal T cell lymphomas: extranodal T-NK cell lymphoma (nasal and nasal type), enteropathy-type T cell lymphoma, subcutaneous panniculitis–like T cell lymphoma, and hepatosplenic $\gamma\delta$ T cell lymphoma, all of which are discussed later. Also included in the WHO classifica-

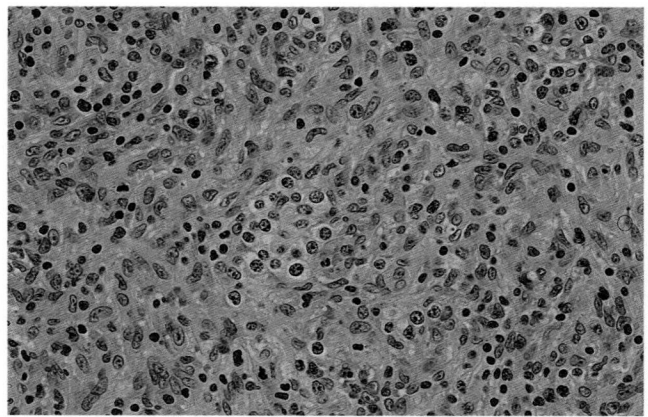

FIGURE 41–68. Angioimmunoblastic lymphadenopathy–like peripheral T cell lymphoma. The overall features resemble angioimmunoblastic lymphadenopathy, but there are clusters of atypical cells with clear cytoplasm.

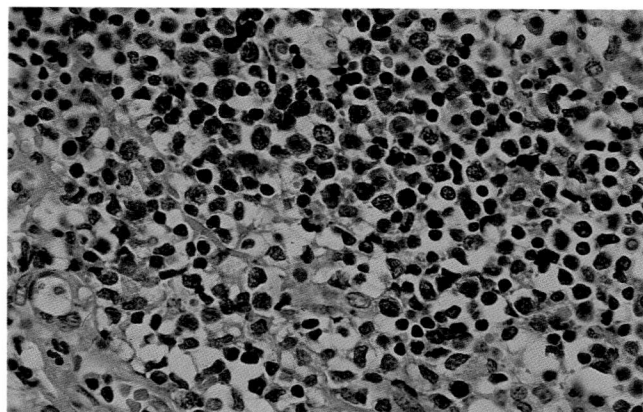

**FIGURE 41-69.** Nasal T-NK cell lymphoma. Clusters of lymphoma cells are admixed with apoptotic cells.

tion is primary cutaneous anaplastic large cell lymphoma, which is discussed in conjunction with its nodal counterpart in the following section. For these extranodal lymphomas, cytologic features usually are not specific, and there are no normal morphologic or immunologic counterparts to help define the neoplastic nature of these T cell processes. Most extranodal T cell lymphomas, particularly extranodal T-NK cell lymphoma, enteropathy-type T cell lymphoma, and subcutaneous panniculitis-like T cell lymphoma, appear to be derived from cytotoxic T cells, which express perforin, T cell intracellular antigen 1 (TIA-1), and granzyme B by paraffin immunohistochemistry.[694-697] Mature T cell neoplasms involving primarily the blood and bone marrow are discussed in Chapter 43.

The term *extranodal T-NK cell lymphoma (nasal and nasal type)* refers to a group of rare and highly aggressive hematolymphoid malignant neoplasms that frequently present in extranodal sites, including the nasal area and the upper aerodigestive system, and non-nasal areas, such as the skin and the gastrointestinal tract.[628, 698-702] On the basis of clinicopathologic features, the neoplasm may be classified into nasal T-NK lymphoma, nasal-type (occurring in other extranodal sites, such as skin, subcutis, and gastrointestinal tract) NK cell lymphoma, or NK cell lymphoma-leukemia. It has also been called angiocentric T cell lymphoma. A subset of cases previously reported as lymphomatoid granulomatosis may also represent nasal T-NK lymphoma. This lymphoma is more common in Asian populations and occurs sporadically in the United States. There is a strong association with EBV.[370, 698-700, 703-705] The cytologic features range from small or medium-sized cells to large transformed cells. Histologic progression often occurs with time.[706] The characteristic histologic feature is an angiocentric and angiodestructive infiltrate of atypical cells in the wall of blood vessels, nearly always with extensive necrosis of the surrounding tissues (Fig. 41-69). Nasal T-NK cell lymphoma has a characteristic immunophenotype,

CD2+ CD56+ (Fig. 41-70), but is usually negative for surface CD3. Cytoplasmic CD3 can be detected in paraffin sections. Except for CD56, it generally lacks markers of NK cell lineage.[707] Clonal T cell receptor gene rearrangement is not found.[708] The differential diagnosis includes blastic or monomorphic NK cell lymphoma-leukemia, CD56+ peripheral T cell lymphoma, and enteropathy-associated T cell lymphoma.[693]

Enteropathy-type T cell lymphoma, also known as intestinal T cell lymphoma, is a rare type of lymphoma derived from the intestinal intraepithelial T lymphocytes.[709] Affected patients often have a history of celiac sprue. Patients often present with an acute abdomen, and ulcers are often found in the jejunum. The base of the ulcer contains an infiltrate of atypical lymphoid cells, and atypical cells are often found in the adjacent nonulcerated mucosa. An aberrant T cell phenotype is usually present, along with expression of human mucosal lymphocyte antigen (HML-1), a marker of normal mucosa-associated T lymphocytes.[710]

Subcutaneous panniculitis-like T cell lymphoma was originally described as an uncommon form of cutaneous lymphoma occurring primarily within the interstitium of fat lobules in the subcutis and mimicking lobular panniculitis.[711-713] Patients usually have multiple subcutaneous tumors or plaques involving the extremities or trunk. Constitutional symptoms are commonly present, most likely caused by systemic hemophagocytic syndrome, which is also often present. Systemic dissemination of lymphoma does not usually occur. The neoplastic cells are usually small with slightly irregular nuclear contours and may cause widening of the intralobular septa (Fig. 41-71). Large cell transformation is infrequent. There is often an admixture of histiocytes, which sometimes form noncaseating granulomas. Karyorrhectic debris is often seen. As mentioned before, hemophagocytosis by benign histiocytes may be seen. Fat necrosis with foamy macrophages is a constant finding. The tumors show a characteristic staining pattern of CD8+ suppressor T cells rimming

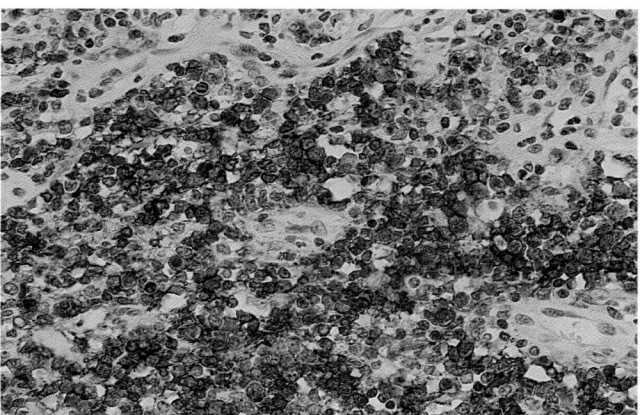

**FIGURE 41-70.** Nasal T-NK cell lymphoma, CD56 stain. The tumor cells show membranous staining of CD56.

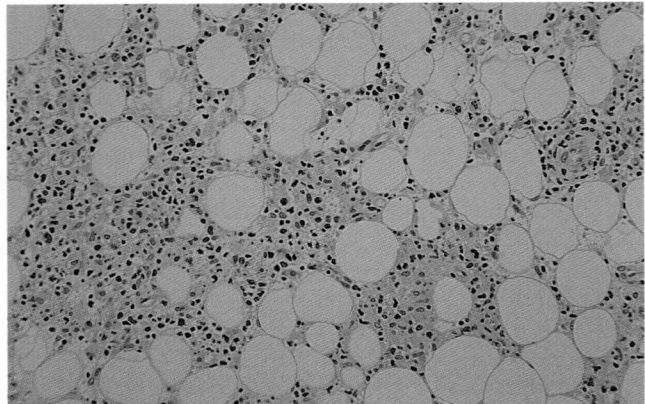

FIGURE 41–71. Subcutaneous panniculitic T cell lymphoma. Unlike in fat necrosis, which contains numerous histiocytes, the cells here have a spectrum of cytologic atypia.

the non-neoplastic adipocytes. The cells stain immunohistochemically with markers of cytotoxic granules, including TIA-1 and perforin.[712] Clonal T cell gene rearrangements are frequently found. EBV has not been identified in cases of subcutaneous panniculitis–like T cell lymphoma. The differential diagnosis includes another CD8+ primary cutaneous lymphoma, epidermotropic cytotoxic T cell lymphoma, which has a tendency for metastases and affects the epidermis with variable degrees of spongiosis, intraepidermal blistering, and necrosis.[714]

Hepatosplenic γδ T cell lymphoma is a rare but distinct clinicopathologic entity that most commonly affects young men.[693, 715–718] Unlike the extranodal T-NK cell lymphomas, this tumor is a more systemic disease and is thought to be derived from functionally immature cytotoxic cells. Patients usually present with massive splenomegaly, and most patients have hepatomegaly, cytopenias, and constitutional B symptoms. The clinical course is aggressive, and prognosis is extremely poor. Consistent cytogenetic abnormalities of i(7)(q10) and trisomy 8 have been reported. The neoplastic cells are T lineage and in frozen sections stain for antibodies to the T cell receptor δ-chain and have T cell receptor γ-chain rearrangements. The tumor cells are EBV negative. Hepatosplenic γδ T cell lymphoma can be distinguished from the cytologically similar large granular lymphocytosis by its different clinical setting. Hepatosplenic γδ T cell lymphoma can also be distinguished from aggressive NK cell leukemia-lymphoma, which is usually EBV positive and does not show T cell receptor gene rearrangements.

## Anaplastic Large Cell Lymphoma

Anaplastic large cell lymphoma was first described in 1985 as a neoplasm of highly pleomorphic lymphoid cells in a predominantly sinusoidal pattern.[242, 630, 719, 720] Virtually all tumors were subsequently found to express CD30 antigen, and a high percent-

age were found to have a cytogenetic t(2;5) abnormality. It was recognized as an entity in the B cell and T cell categories in the updated Kiel classification.[451] In the Working Formulation, these cases were usually classified as high-grade, immunoblastic, polymorphous lymphoma, but there was no truly equivalent category.[450] Cases of anaplastic large cell lymphoma of B lineage were shown to differ from morphologically similar cases of T and null cell lineage in many aspects, including their clinical and molecular features, clinical behavior, and expression of cytotoxic cell markers.[433, 630] In fact, the B lineage anaplastic large cell lymphomas had many features more similar to diffuse large B cell lymphoma. Thus, in the REAL and WHO classification schemas, any lymphomas with morphologic features of anaplastic large cell lymphoma but of B lineage phenotype were included within the category of diffuse large B cell lymphoma. Like the REAL classification, the WHO classification recognizes only T and null cell types of anaplastic large cell lymphoma.[177, 452] In addition, two subtypes of anaplastic large cell lymphoma are recognized in the WHO classification, the primary systemic type and the primary cutaneous type. For most cases, the two types can easily be distinguished on the basis of clinical features. However, some forms of systemic anaplastic large cell lymphoma may present initially in the skin, with the other sites of disease appearing only subsequently.

Anaplastic large cell lymphoma constitutes approximately 2% to 3% of all non-Hodgkin's lymphomas.[630, 721, 722] The primary systemic cases commonly involve lymph nodes, with or without involvement of a variety of extranodal sites, including the gastrointestinal tract and soft tissue.[723] This presentation has a bimodal age distribution, with one peak in children and the second in older adults.[724] These cases have aggressive clinical behavior but show good response to multidrug chemotherapy and no tendency toward spontaneous regression. In the second type of presentation, which occurs primarily in adults, there are solitary or multiple skin papules and nodules without extracutaneous involvement, similar to lymphomatoid papulosis. There is most likely a clinical, histologic, and biologic continuum between primary cutaneous anaplastic large cell lymphoma and lymphomatoid papulosis.[630, 725–727] This form of the disease is indolent and has a highly favorable prognosis, not requiring systemic therapy. Spontaneous regression with subsequent relapse is a characteristic feature of some cases. Systemic dissemination may eventually occur, heralding a more aggressive course. In the third type of presentation, in patients with a history of another type of lymphoma, including mycosis fungoides, mature T cell lymphoma, follicular lymphoma, and Hodgkin's disease, there is transformation to anaplastic large cell lymphoma; the prognosis in these cases is unfavorable.[728, 729]

Involved lymph nodes may show partial or complete effacement of the normal nodal architec-

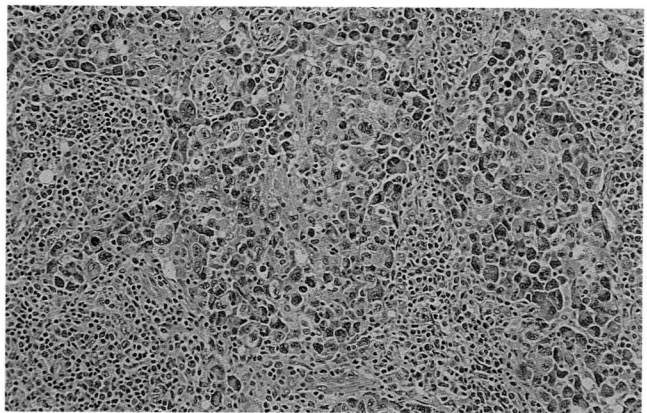

**FIGURE 41–72.** Anaplastic large cell lymphoma. The tumor cells have a characteristic sinusoidal pattern of infiltration.

ture. There is characteristically preferential infiltration of the sinuses, commonly with extension to the paracortical regions (Fig. 41–72). Often, one sees fibrosis of the lymph node capsule, with focal extension of fibrosis into the parenchyma. The mitotic rate is high, and a starry sky pattern may be present. Different cytologic variants have been described.[720, 730, 731] The most common cytologic subtype is the pleomorphic or classic type, which has numerous highly anaplastic cells, often with multilobated nuclei or multinucleated giant tumor cells. The tumor cells have been described as doughnut-like and wreathlike. Nucleoli are large but not as large as in Reed-Sternberg cells. In the monomorphic subtype, the tumor cells are homogeneous with large round to oval nuclei and fairly abundant basophilic cytoplasm without a paranuclear hof. Multinucleation is not seen. Both subtypes usually have a mixed population of host reactive cells, including small lymphocytes, histiocytes, plasma cells, eosinophils, and neutrophils. In some cases, morphologic features intermediate between the pleomorphic and monomorphic types may be identified. The small cell variant is composed of atypical small cells with marked nuclear irregularity, dense chromatin, and scanty cytoplasm.[732] There may be a minority of large cells interspersed singly or in clusters or forming a perivenular cuff. The large cells have distinct small nucleoli and a moderate amount of clear to weakly basophilic cytoplasm. The number of large cells varies from field to field and may be increased in subsequent biopsy specimens.[733] Rare leukemic cases of the small cell variant have been reported.[734] The lymphohistiocytic variant is the least common morphologic variant and has an extremely unusual appearance. Involved lymph nodes contain numerous reactive cells, including ovoid histiocytes with eccentrically placed round nuclei and abundant eosinophilic cytoplasm. In addition, there are isolated tumor cells that are medium sized to large with coarse or vesicular chromatin, small but distinct nucleoli, and basophilic cytoplasm. The malignant cells do not appear frankly atypical and are often ob-

scured by an abundance of reactive cells.[735] Other rare variants include a giant cell variant, a neutrophil-rich variant, and a sarcomatoid variant.[736] The REAL classification included a category of Hodgkin's-like variant of anaplastic large cell lymphoma, which most likely included cases of an anaplastic variant of nodular sclerosing Hodgkin's disease as well as cases of anaplastic large cell lymphoma, pleomorphic type with Reed-Sternberg–like cells.[737]

About one half to two thirds of cases of systemic anaplastic large cell lymphomas possess a t(2;5) involving the *ALK* gene on chromosome 2p23 and the *NPM* gene on chromosome 5q35.[438, 439, 720, 738–743] The incidence of this translocation in anaplastic large cell lymphoma is higher in children than in adults and in systemic cases compared with cutaneous or extranodal cases. It was almost never identified in the B lineage cases formerly classified as anaplastic large cell lymphoma of B cell lineage. Antibodies to the ALK protein, including p80 and ALK1, are available for detection by paraffin section immunohistochemistry.[435–437, 439, 744, 745] The antibody shows strong nuclear and cytoplasmic staining in the majority of the cases of the pleomorphic subtype and in a lower percentage of the cases of other subtypes of anaplastic large cell lymphoma, somewhat proportionally to the number of large tumor cells in the neoplasm (Fig. 41–73). The small anaplastic cells of the small cell variant are usually characterized by nucleus-restricted ALK expression.[745] In addition, the antibody stains some cases with variants of the t(2;5).[746, 747] Patients with anaplastic large cell lymphomas that express ALK have been found to have improved 5-year survivals over patients whose tumors are ALK negative.[437]

The other immunohistochemical hallmark of anaplastic large cell lymphoma is the expression of CD30 in all or nearly all of the neoplastic cells[62, 242, 719] (Fig. 41–74). Only two thirds of cases show staining for CD45; this is the lowest rate of CD45 positivity of any of the major subtypes of non-Hodgkin's lymphoma.[60] Therefore, a CD30 stain should be obtained in any CD45/45RB⁻ large cell neoplasm for

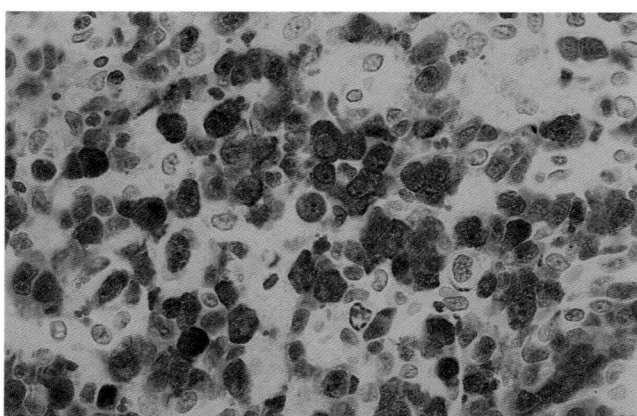

**FIGURE 41–73.** Anaplastic large cell lymphoma, ALK stain. Nearly all of the tumor nuclei show intense staining.

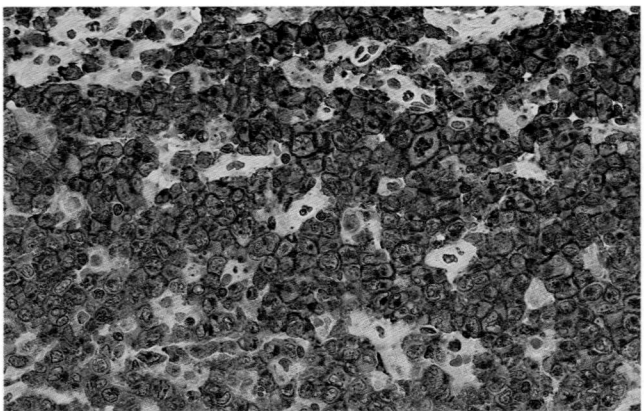

**FIGURE 41–74.** Anaplastic large cell lymphoma, CD30 stain. The tumor nuclei usually show strong and diffuse membranous staining as well as focal paranuclear staining.

which lymphoma is a diagnostic possibility. Most cases are of T lineage, expressing CD43, CD3, and CD45RO and showing aberrant T cell phenotypes in frozen section studies.[23, 135, 242, 719] Approximately one third of cases are of null cell lineage, although CD43 is still usually positive. In addition, HLA-DR, CD25, CD71 (the transferrin receptor), and TIA-1 are often positive.[695, 748] As mentioned previously, B lineage cases are no longer considered within the definition of anaplastic large cell lymphoma. Epithelial membrane antigen is usually positive in systemic cases and negative in cutaneous cases and may be used as a surrogate for ALK.[749] The cutaneous lymphocyte antigen HECA-452 is usually positive in the cutaneous cases.[726] Occasional cases may be CD15+, and rare cases may be keratin positive.[750, 751] Bcl-6 protein expression can be identified in approximately 40% of T-null anaplastic large cell lymphomas, which appears to be the only T cell neoplasm to express this protein.[752]

Anaplastic large cell lymphoma may be difficult to distinguish from a wide variety of neoplasms, including metastatic carcinoma and malignant melanomas (both of which are discussed in the section on metastatic neoplasms), classical Hodgkin's disease (discussed in the section on Hodgkin's disease), other large cell lymphomas, and malignant histiocytosis. The anaplastic histologic appearance and diffuse CD30 positivity are usually sufficient to differentiate anaplastic large cell lymphoma from most non-Hodgkin's lymphomas, which usually show no staining or only focal staining for CD30. Only rare cases of non-Hodgkin's lymphoma other than anaplastic large cell lymphoma exhibit diffuse CD30 positivity, including mediastinal large B cell lymphoma.[753] In addition, the specificity of t(2;5) for anaplastic large cell lymphoma is high. Virtually all cases having both CD30 and t(2;5) are anaplastic large cell lymphoma of T or null cell lineage.[747, 754] The specificity of the paraffin section p80 and ALK1 antibodies is similar to or slightly less than that of the molecular studies.[437]

Many of the cases originally diagnosed as malignant histiocytosis have been found to be anaplastic large cell lymphoma when studied by use of modern techniques.[245] Immunohistochemical positivity for CD30 and ALK antibodies and molecular studies for t(2;5) help establish the diagnosis of anaplastic large cell lymphoma over malignant histiocytosis. Rare cases of inflammatory pseudotumors have been reported to have chromosome rearrangement involving 2p23 and to stain for ALK protein by immunohistochemistry.[755]

## Lymphoblastic Lymphoma

Lymphoblastic neoplasms are composed of cells frozen at the level of immature lymphoid cells, either T lineage thymocytes or immature B lineage bone marrow lymphoid cells. They are considered high-grade lymphomas in the Working Formulation.[450] The updated Kiel classification separates lymphoblastic neoplasms into B and T cell types.[451] The WHO classification lists them as precursor B cell and precursor T cell lymphoblastic leukemia-lymphomas.[177, 452] The cells of lymphoblastic lymphoma are equivalent to the neoplastic cells of acute lymphoblastic leukemia. The lymphoblastic lymphomas and the lymphoblastic leukemias are considered different clinical presentations of the same biologic disease. When more than 10% blasts are found in the peripheral blood or more than 25% of the bone marrow contains lymphoblasts, many clinicians prefer the designation acute lymphoblastic leukemia, but the cutoff between the lymphoblastic lymphoma and lymphoblastic leukemia is arbitrary.[756–759]

Lymphoblastic lymphoma has a median age of incidence of 17 years and a male-to-female ratio of 2 : 1.[450, 756, 757, 760, 761] It accounts for approximately one third of non-Hodgkin's lymphomas in childhood, but it occurs in all age groups. Approximately 50% of the patients present with a symptomatic mediastinal mass, often associated with pleural or pericardial effusions, or supradiaphragmatic lymphadenopathy. Most of the lymphoblastic lymphomas presenting in the mediastinum have a T cell phenotype, with only rare reports of B lineage mediastinal lymphoblastic lymphoma. The precursor B cell lymphoblastic lymphomas have a tendency to involve skin.[762] Lymphoblastic leukemia has a tendency to have an immature B cell phenotype. Lymphoblastic lymphoma has an aggressive clinical course and often involves peripheral blood, bone marrow, central nervous system, and gonads. The tumor responds well to multidrug chemotherapeutic regimens similar to or identical with those given for acute lymphoblastic leukemia. Adverse prognostic factors include high stage, involvement of the central nervous system, and high serum lactate dehydrogenase level.[756]

Lymph nodes involved by lymphoblastic lymphoma show diffuse effacement of the normal nodal architecture, capsular destruction, and extensive infiltration of the adjacent soft tissues. The neoplasm is a monotonous infiltrate of small to medium-sized cells with a fine chromatin pattern, inconspicuous nucleoli, and a small amount of cytoplasm (Fig. 41–75). The nuclear contours may be highly irregular (convoluted variant) or round to oval (nonconvoluted variant). Approximately 10% of cases have cells that may be slightly larger than usual, with larger nuclei with one or two small nucleoli.[763] There is a high mitotic rate, and a starry sky pattern may be focally present. There are usually few host cells. Occasional cases may have scattered plasma cells or eosinophils. Fine-needle aspiration smears of lymphoblastic lymphoma show a monomorphous population of medium-sized lymphoid cells with a fine chromatin pattern and inconspicuous nucleoli. The cytologic appearance is identical to acute lymphoblastic leukemia in bone marrow aspirate smears or peripheral blood smears.

TdT can be identified in virtually all lymphoblastic lymphomas by frozen or paraffin section immunohistochemistry, immunocytochemistry, or flow cytometry[764, 765] (Fig. 41–76). Approximately 80% of cases are positive for CD45. This rate of CD45 positivity is lower than that seen in all cases of non-Hodgkin's lymphomas except anaplastic large cell lymphoma.[39, 60] Approximately 85% of lymphoblastic lymphomas are T lineage neoplasms, which almost always express CD43, CD2, CD7, and cytoplasmic or surface CD3.[8, 23, 675, 766] Nearly half of cases are CD45RO+.[60] The B cell marker CD79a may be positive in a subset of cases.[39, 767] These tumors have a range of T cell antigen expression that is consistent with the different stages of thymocyte maturation.[768] Approximately 20% of the T lineage cases may also show strong expression of the NK cell markers CD16 and CD57, which in one study occurred more often in female patients and had a more aggressive clinical course.[769, 770] Approximately 15% of lymphoblastic lymphomas are B lineage neoplasms.[8, 766] These tumors have phenotypes that mimic the normal stages of B cell development. Nearly all B lineage cases express CD19 (frozen section immunohis-

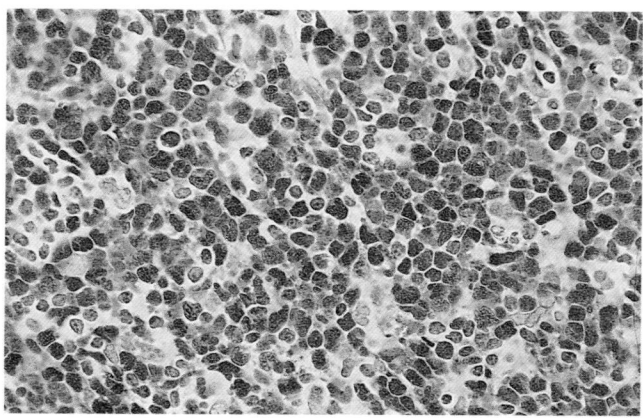

**FIGURE 41–76.** Lymphoblastic lymphoma, TdT immunohistochemical stain. The tumor cells show strong nuclear reactivity with cell-to-cell variation.

tochemistry or flow cytometry) or CD79a (paraffin immunohistochemistry), but because they are immature, only 40% to 50% of cases express CD20.[412, 771–773] CD10 (also known as common acute lymphoblastic leukemia antigen [CALLA]) is expressed in approximately 90% of precursor B cell lymphoblastic lymphoma-leukemia by flow cytometry, with nearly equal sensitivity by paraffin immunohistochemistry.[133, 766] CD10 is also expressed in approximately one fourth of precursor T acute lymphoblastic leukemia (27%). CD99, the MIC2 antigen, is positive in the majority of acute lymphoblastic leukemias, with precursor B lineage more commonly positive than T lineage acute lymphoblastic leukemia.[774] CD34 is also frequently positive by flow cytometry and immunohistochemistry.[774] Cytoplasmic immunoglobulin may be positive (often designated pre-B) or negative (often designated pre-pre-B). Cases reported in 1990 as surface immunoglobulin–positive lymphoblastic lymphoma, in retrospect, probably represent the earliest recognized cases of blastic mantle cell lymphoma, an entity that was subsequently described.[570, 580, 775] However, rare cases of lymphoblastic lymphoma are both TdT positive and express monotypic light chains.[776]

Monoclonal T cell receptor β-chain gene rearrangements can be detected in approximately 90% of cases of T lineage lymphoblastic lymphomas. In addition, approximately 25% of T lineage cases may have immunoglobulin heavy chain gene rearrangements.[777, 778] Monoclonal immunoglobulin heavy chain gene rearrangements can be detected in virtually all B lineage lymphoblastic lymphomas, but light chain gene rearrangements are detectable in only approximately 40% of such cases. T cell receptor β-chain gene rearrangements may be detected in approximately 25% of cases of B lineage lymphoblastic lymphoma.[777, 778] An unusual syndrome of T lymphoblastic lymphoma, marrow myeloid hyperplasia, and peripheral eosinophilia has been described in association with t(8;13).[779–781] Other molec-

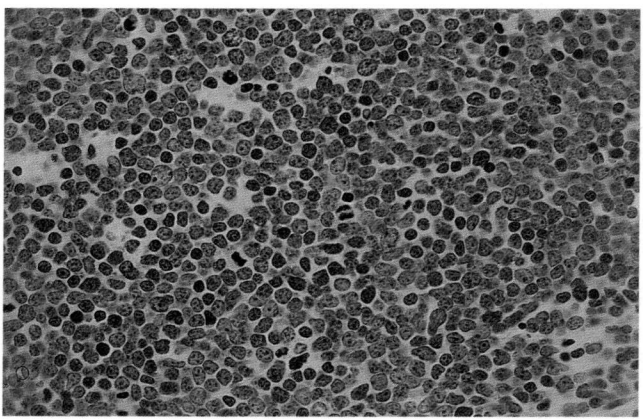

**FIGURE 41–75.** Lymphoblastic lymphoma. A diffuse, monotonous proliferation of medium-sized cells with fine chromatin and indistinct nucleoli is present. Note the high mitotic rate.

ular findings in lymphoblastic neoplasms are discussed in Chapter 43.[782]

Lymphoblastic lymphoma may be mistaken for many other tumors, including other types of non-Hodgkin's lymphoma, extramedullary myeloid tumor, thymoma, and small cell undifferentiated carcinoma. Lymphoblastic lymphoma may be confused morphologically with Burkitt-type or Burkitt-like lymphoma. The cells of lymphoblastic lymphoma have a finer chromatin pattern than those of Burkitt-type or Burkitt-like lymphoma, which has more distinct nucleoli and a greater amount of cytoplasm that may square off with adjacent cells. The blastic variant of mantle cell lymphoma may be morphologically identical to lymphoblastic lymphoma. Areas of more typical mantle cell lymphoma (if present) and a past history of mantle cell lymphoma (if known) are helpful, but immunohistochemical studies may be necessary. TdT is probably the most useful marker in the differential diagnosis of lymphoblastic lymphoma versus other non-Hodgkin's lymphomas, because it is positive in virtually all cases of lymphoblastic lymphoma and negative in all other types of non-Hodgkin's lymphoma.[764] In addition to TdT, lineage determination may be useful because most cases of lymphoblastic lymphoma are of T lineage.

Extramedullary myeloid tumor may have morphologic features similar to those of lymphoblastic lymphoma, including single-file pattern of infiltration in fibrous tissue and a fine chromatin pattern. The presence of eosinophils or cells with more than scant cytoplasm favors the diagnosis of extramedullary myeloid tumor. Myeloperoxidase is a relatively sensitive marker for extramedullary myeloid tumor, but rare cases may be negative. One must keep in mind that approximately 10% of cases of extramedullary myeloid tumor are TdT positive. Bone marrow examination should be recommended in any ambiguous cases. The proliferating thymocytes of thymoma are morphologically and immunohistochemically similar to the cells of lymphoblastic lymphoma.[783] However, thymomas have a population of epithelial cells, which are scattered larger cells with vesicular chromatin. Keratin immunohistochemical staining helps to highlight the network of epithelial cells throughout a thymoma, with the caveat that occasional residual thymic epithelial cells can be seen in mediastinal masses of lymphoblastic lymphoma. Adjunct immunohistochemical stains are recommended over flow cytometric study, which may yield highly confusing data by detecting an immature T cell phenotype in thymoma, without detection of an epithelial population. Small cell undifferentiated carcinoma and Merkel cell carcinoma may be mistaken for lymphoblastic lymphoma, particularly when the technical preparations are less than optimal. Keratin immunohistochemical staining helps to establish the diagnosis of carcinoma. Finally, other small round blue cell tumors of childhood, such as neuroblastoma, Ewing's sarcoma, peripheral neural ectodermal tumor, and rhabdo-

myosarcoma, may be confused histologically with lymphoblastic lymphoma. Appropriate immunohistochemical stains, as discussed in Chapter 46, are usually needed.

## Immunodeficiency-Related Lymphoproliferations

Patients with congenital, acquired, or iatrogenically induced immunodeficiencies have an increased incidence of lymphoproliferative disorders over the general population.[784, 785] The incidence and specific types of lymphoproliferative disorders vary with the specific type of immunodeficiency. However, they frequently occur or originate in extranodal sites, are B cell lineage, and have rapid clinical progression. Many of the lymphoproliferations are EBV-associated non-Hodgkin's lymphomas and have diffuse aggressive histologic features.

Patients with primary or congenital immunodeficiencies may develop reactive hyperplasias, atypical lymphoid hyperplasias, or malignant lymphomas. Lymphoproliferative disorders most commonly arise in patients with X-linked lymphoproliferative syndrome, ataxia-telangiectasia, common variable immunodeficiency, Wiskott-Aldrich syndrome, and severe combined immunodeficiency.[786–788] An intermediate-grade to high-grade diffuse non-Hodgkin's lymphoma (usually extranodal) may develop in approximately 65% of patients with X-linked lymphoproliferative syndrome, 15% of patients with Wiskott-Aldrich syndrome, and 5% of patients with common variable immunodeficiency syndrome. Patients with common variable immunodeficiency more often have lymphadenopathy that reveals chronic granulomatous inflammation, reactive hyperplasia, or atypical lymphoid hyperplasia.[789] Approximately 10% of patients with ataxia-telangiectasia and 3% of patients with severe combined immunodeficiency develop non-Hodgkin's lymphoma or Hodgkin's disease. The non-Hodgkin's lymphomas in ataxia-telangiectasia reflect the lymphomas occurring in the normal population, whereas those in severe combined immunodeficiency are usually intermediate-grade to high-grade lymphomas that arise in multiple extranodal sites. The cases of Hodgkin's disease are usually of mixed cellularity or lymphocyte depletion subtypes.

Lymphoproliferative disorders may also arise in patients with HIV infection. Benign lymphadenopathies associated with HIV infection were discussed earlier in the chapter. Approximately 3% of HIV-infected patients develop non-Hodgkin's lymphoma, accounting for approximately 10% of cases of non-Hodgkin's lymphoma currently diagnosed in the United States.[441] These lymphomas are usually B lineage and may be systemic (nodal or extranodal) or primarily involve the central nervous system or the body cavity. The body cavity–based lymphomas are termed primary effusion lymphomas[790, 791] (Fig. 41–77). The primary effusion lymphomas contain the Kaposi's sarcoma–associated herpesvirus (HHV-8). The most common morphologic types of lymphoma arising in the setting of HIV infection are Burkitt-type and Burkitt-like lymphomas and diffuse large B cell lymphoma[632, 792] (Fig. 41–78). The Burkitt-type and Burkitt-like lymphomas are usually node based and occur in patients at an early stage of HIV infection, whereas the diffuse large B cell lymphomas tend to involve extranodal sites in patients who already have a diagnosis of AIDS. The molecular lesions also differ between the small noncleaved cell and large cell immunoblastic cases.[793] HIV-infected patients occasionally develop other types of malignant lymphoma, including Hodgkin's disease and T cell lymphomas.[339] Plasmablastic lymphoma is a rare AIDS-related non-Hodgkin's lymphoma that is generally limited to the oral cavity and jaw at the time of diagnosis, although extension to distant sites frequently occurs at a later stage.[631–634] The morphologic features are similar to those of diffuse large B cell lymphomas, but these tumors have an unusual immunohistochemical profile (Fig. 41–79). The cells are negative for CD45/45RB and CD20, but they are positive for the plasma cell–reactive antibody VS38c and usually positive for CD79a antibody. There is moderate association with EBV. Most cases have cytoplasmic immunoglobulin and a monoclonal immunoglobulin heavy chain gene rearrangement.

Patients with iatrogenic causes of immunosuppression are also susceptible to the development of lymphoproliferative disorders. The most common clinical setting is after organ transplantation, but patients treated for a collagen-vascular disease may also occasionally develop lymphoproliferations. Patients who are receiving immunosuppression after organ transplantation are at greatly increased risk for the development of post-transplantation lymphoproliferative disorders, with the specific risk dependent on age, the type of organ transplant, and the drug regimen used. According to the WHO classifi-

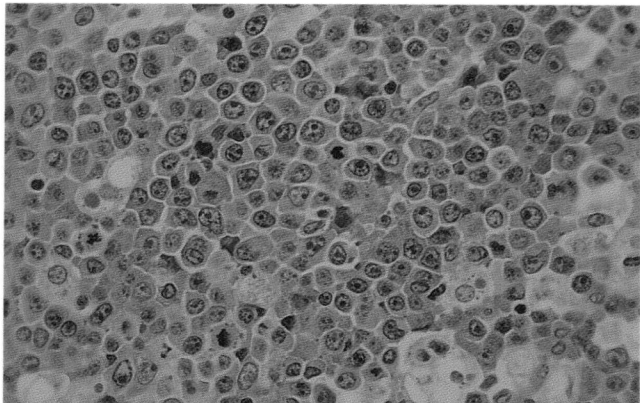

**FIGURE 41–78.** Diffuse large cell lymphoma, patient with HIV infection. The tumor nuclei have vesicular chromatin and prominent nucleoli. The cytoplasm has a plasmacytoid appearance.

cation, these lesions are categorized into several types. The early lesions include reactive plasmacytic hyperplasia and infectious mononucleosis–like lesions.[794] In plasmacytic hyperplasia, there is expansion of the paracortical areas predominantly by plasmacytoid lymphocytes and plasma cells; plasmacytoid immunoblasts are usually difficult to find. Cytologic atypia is minimal. Follicles may be hyperplastic, show regression, or be absent.[794] The lesions are usually polyclonal, and one generally sees regression of the lesion with reduction in immunosuppression. Another category of post-transplantation lymphoproliferative disorders includes polymorphic lesions, in which there is disruption of the normal nodal architecture. One sees the entire range of B lymphocyte forms, including small lymphocytes, plasma cells, small lymphoplasmacytoid forms, plasmacytoid immunoblasts, and small and large cleaved and noncleaved lymphoid cells. There may be some necrosis. Cytologic atypia may also be seen. The clinical course is variable, with partial to

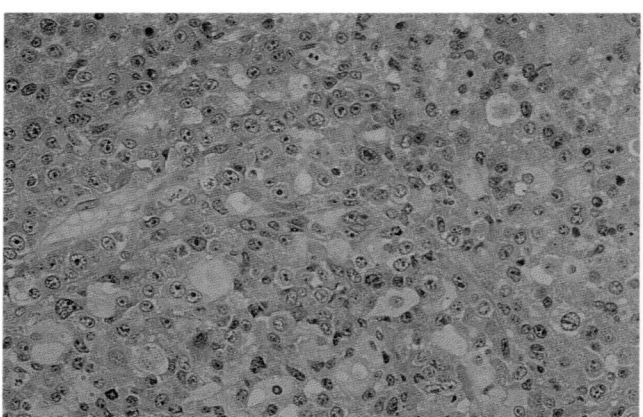

**FIGURE 41–77.** Body cavity–based lymphoma. This shows pleomorphic tumor cells with few admixed small lymphocytes. Immunohistochemical studies may be needed to distinguish this from carcinoma or mesothelioma.

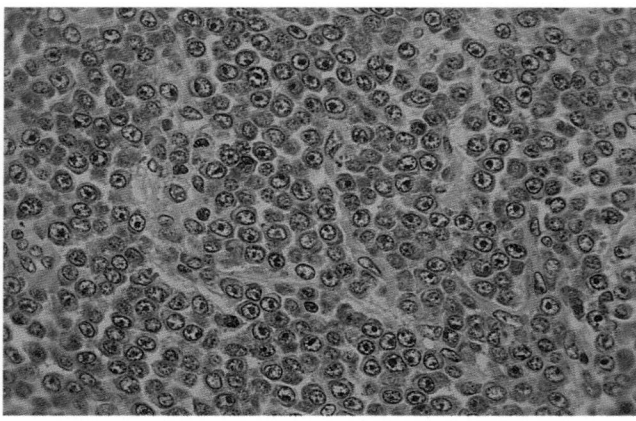

**FIGURE 41–79.** Plasmablastic lymphoma. Similar to the cells in Figure 41–78, the tumor cells have vesicular nuclear chromatin, prominent nucleoli, and abundant plasmacytoid cytoplasm. The tumor cells did not stain for CD20 or CD79a.

complete regression after immunosuppression reduction or progression despite therapy. Disease progression appears to correlate with *BCL6* gene mutation.[795] Monomorphic lesions, which are generally subtyped by the specific histologic type of lymphoma, constitute another category of post-transplantation lymphoproliferative disorders. These lesions have marked disturbance of underlying architecture and significant cytologic atypia. Most of the malignant neoplasms are diffuse large B cell lymphomas (encompassing the diffuse large cell lymphomas and large cell immunoblastic categories of the Working Formulation), with the remainder multiple myeloma.[794] Rare cases of Burkitt-type or Burkitt-like lymphomas have been reported in transplant recipients.[785] Molecular studies demonstrate that almost all the polymorphic B cell lesions and all of the monomorphic lesions harbor monoclonal B cell populations and are almost all EBV associated.[794, 796] The monomorphic lymphomas have additional genetic mutations that apparently confer a more neoplastic phenotype. T cell lymphomas arising after organ transplantation are rare and tend to occur much later after transplantation than their B cell counterparts do. The T cell lesions include lymphoblastic lymphoma, peripheral T cell lymphoma, and anaplastic large cell lymphoma. The final category of post-transplantation lymphoproliferative disorders is "other types, rare," which includes Hodgkin's disease–like lesions and plasmacytoma-like lesions.[452]

Patients with collagen-vascular disease who are treated with methotrexate are also at increased risk for development of malignant lymphomas, including both non-Hodgkin's lymphoma and Hodgkin's disease.[797–799] These lymphomas are usually EBV negative and are classified according to their specific histologic subtype. Nontransplantation iatrogenically induced lymphoproliferative disorders have also been described in association with patients receiving other immunomodulatory therapy, including cyclosporine, corticosteroids, and azathioprine.[785] Some of these lymphomas have undergone regression on withdrawal of the drug.

## OTHER NEOPLASMS

### Langerhans Cell Histiocytosis (Histiocytosis X)

Langerhans cell histiocytosis encompasses a group of closely related clinicopathologic disorders with a common proliferating element, the Langerhans cell.[800–804] It is also known as histiocytosis X and Langerhans cell granulomatosis. There are many different classification schemes, but generally there are three main and sometimes overlapping clinical syndromes. Unifocal disease (solitary eosinophilic granuloma) accounts for approximately two thirds of cases. Multifocal unisystem disease (Hand-Schüller-Christian syndrome) and multifocal multisystem disease (Letterer-Siwe syndrome) are the other two common syndromes.[801, 805] Lymph nodes may be the site of involvement in any of the three clinical presentations. In addition, Langerhans cell histiocytosis may be diagnosed in lymph nodes draining the site of disease or, rarely, adjacent to a focus of malignant lymphoma.[806–808]

Regardless of the clinical presentation, the morphologic features of involved lymph nodes are consistent. Affected lymph nodes are generally slightly enlarged. The lymph node architecture is almost always intact. Focal involvement of the sinuses is usually seen. The paracortex may exhibit dermatopathic changes. In advanced cases, one may see partial or complete nodal effacement by numerous sinusoidal Langerhans cells, resulting in marked sinus distention. The proliferation of Langerhans cells may extend into the perinodal tissues.

Langerhans cell histiocytosis lesions have a wide spectrum of histologic changes, but a constant feature is a sinusoidal proliferation of Langerhans cells in the appropriate cellular background[809] (Fig. 41–80). Langerhans cells have a single large nucleus with a characteristic folded or grooved nucleus ("coffee-bean" appearance) with small inconspicuous nucleoli. The nuclear chromatin is usually bland. Slight cytologic atypia may be seen. The cells are approximately 12 to 15 $\mu$m in diameter, with a moderate amount of eosinophilic cytoplasm. Mitotic activity varies from lesion to lesion but is generally low. The background cells include mononuclear and multinucleated histiocytes, abundant eosinophils, neutrophils, and small lymphocytes. Plasma cells are rare or absent. Small clusters of eosinophils may be associated with necrosis, forming so-called eosinophilic microabscesses. Rare cases may contain Langerhans cells with unequivocally malignant cytologic features; these have been called malignant histiocytosis X or malignant Langerhans cell histiocytosis.[810]

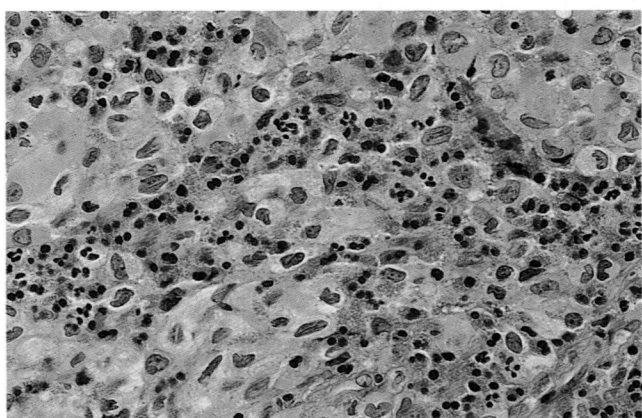

**FIGURE 41–80.** Langerhans cell histiocytosis. A mixture of Langerhans cells, histiocytes, and eosinophils is present. The Langerhans cell nuclei show characteristic grooves and folding.

The ultrastructural, enzyme histochemical, and immunohistochemical features of Langerhans cells of Langerhans cell histiocytosis are virtually identical to those of normal Langerhans cells. By immunohistochemistry, Langerhans cells virtually always express CD1 and S-100 protein, and a portion of the neoplastic cells express CD68 and anti–placental alkaline phosphatase.[811-813] In addition, peanut agglutinin lectin, vimentin, CDw75, and LN-3 also stain Langerhans cells. CD1 staining has the greatest diagnostic utility, because CD1 expression is limited to reactive and neoplastic Langerhans cells, immature thymocytes, and T lineage lymphoblastic neoplasms. Other histiocytic and dendritic cells lack CD1 expression.[814] The Langerhans cells do not stain with CD30 or CD15. In addition, CD45/45RB is generally negative in paraffin sections but positive in frozen sections.[811, 815] Langerhans cells contain the characteristic Birbeck granules by electron microscopy. These granules are racket-shaped organelles approximately 200 to 400 nm long and 33 nm wide, with an osmiophilic core and a double outer sheath.[816]

Langerhans cell histiocytosis has been shown to be a monoclonal proliferation, as evidenced by its pattern of X chromosome inactivation in the X-linked human androgen receptor gene.[817] Molecular hybridization studies show a germline configuration for the immunoglobulin heavy chain gene as well as the $\beta$-, $\gamma$-, and $\delta$-chains of the T cell receptor genes.[817, 818] DNA ploidy studies of paraffin-embedded tissues of localized or disseminated Langerhans cell histiocytosis show a normal diploid population in most cases.[819, 820]

Lymph node involvement by Langerhans cell histiocytosis should be distinguished from other diseases that involve the sinuses, including metastatic adenocarcinoma, metastatic malignant melanoma, sinusoidal malignant lymphoma, sinus histiocytosis with massive lymphadenopathy, and reactive sinus hyperplasia. Identification of the characteristic Langerhans cell cleaved nucleus as well as the characteristic cellular milieu helps to establish the diagnosis of Langerhans cell histiocytosis. The cells of sinus histiocytosis with massive lymphadenopathy have rounded nuclei with vesicular chromatin and prominent nucleoli and abundant cytoplasm, which differs from the folded, grooved nuclei of Langerhans cell histiocytosis. Also in contrast to Langerhans cell histiocytosis, sinus histiocytosis with massive lymphadenopathy lymph nodes shows phagocytosis and increased numbers of plasma cells and lacks eosinophils. The malignant cytology of cells of the metastatic malignant neoplasms and sinusoidal malignant lymphoma contrasts with the bland cytology of Langerhans cell histiocytosis. Dermatopathic lymphadenitis contains large numbers of Langerhans cells in the paracortex and not in the sinuses, as is the case in Langerhans cell histiocytosis. In dermatopathic lymphadenopathy, numerous melanin-containing histiocytes and interdigitating reticulum cells are admixed with the proliferating cells.[809]

## Dendritic Cell Neoplasms

Dendritic cell neoplasms other than those derived from Langerhans cells include follicular dendritic cell tumors, interdigitating dendritic cell tumors, and indeterminate tumors.[821-826] Follicular dendritic cell tumors have a tendency to recur, either locally or at multiple sites, although the prognosis has generally been good. Interdigitating cell tumors are more aggressive; approximately half of patients die of their disease. Indeterminate tumors have generally responded to chemotherapy, and it is not known whether these tumors have different clinical behavior from Langerhans cell histiocytosis.

### FOLLICULAR DENDRITIC TUMORS

Follicular dendritic tumors are rare neoplasms arising from follicular dendritic cells in lymphoid tissue. They occur primarily in young or middle-aged adults, with a median age of 43 years and a male-to-female ratio of 1 : 1.[159] Half of patients present with isolated cervical lymphadenopathy, but axillary and supraclavicular lymph nodes may be involved. Extranodal presentations are seen in approximately 30% of cases. Tonsil, oral cavity, gastrointestinal tract, intra-abdominal soft tissue, and breast are favored extranodal sites of involvement. Approximately 10% to 20% of cases are associated with Castleman's disease, mostly with the hyaline vascular type but also rarely with the plasma cell variant.[826-828] Recurrences are common, and metastases occur in approximately one fourth of patients.[829] A wide range of tumor sizes has been reported, with a median size of approximately 5 cm. The retroperitoneum harbors the largest tumors, with dimensions up to 20 cm. The tumors are usually well-circumscribed, solid, pink or tan-gray masses. The smaller lesions, which occur primarily in the lymph nodes or tonsils, have no hemorrhage or necrosis. The larger lesions, which occur primarily in the mediastinum or in the abdomen but have also been reported in the cervical neck and axilla, have grossly visible areas of hemorrhage and necrosis. On microscopic examination, the tumors are composed of storiform or whorled bundles of spindled cells with ovoid to spindled bland nuclei (Fig. 41–81). Rarely, the tumor has a denser, more fibroblastic appearance (Fig. 41–82). The nuclear membrane is thin, the chromatin is usually vesicular or granular, and the nucleolus is distinct but small. Cytoplasm is eosinophilic and somewhat fibrillar. The tumor cells have indistinct borders. Rare cases have nuclear pseudoinclusions or multinucleated giant cells. A characteristic feature of these tumors is the admixture of small lymphocytes between the tumor cells and in perivascular spaces. Mitotic activity has a considerable range; approximately two thirds of cases have between 0 and 9 mitotic figures per 10 high-power fields, and one third of cases have 10 or more mitotic figures per 10 high-power fields. High-grade

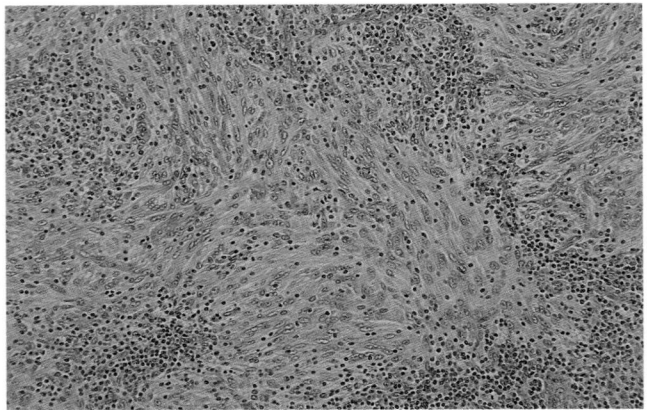

**FIGURE 41–81.** Follicular dendritic cell tumor. Fascicles of spindled cells are seen. The spindled cell nuclei are bland. Note the admixed clusters of small lymphocytes.

morphologic features, including nuclear pleomorphism, high mitotic activity, abnormal mitoses, and necrosis, are more often seen in deep-seated lesions. Specimens from recurrences or metastases may show increased cytologic atypia, nuclear pleomorphism, and mitotic activity compared with the original tumor.[821, 828] Rare cases show histologic changes after chemotherapy or radiotherapy, including squamous metaplasia of the tumor cells, increased nuclear atypia, and sheets of foamy histiocytes.[829] By electron microscopy, the tumor cells contain characteristic thin cytoplasmic processes that are connected to one another by numerous desmosomes.

The neoplastic cells have an immunohistochemical profile similar to normal follicular dendritic cells, with consistent staining for vimentin, CD21 (C3b complement receptor), CD35 (C3d complement receptor), and R4/23 (a nonclustered follicular dendritic cell–specific marker).[159] In addition, the cells usually stain for epithelial membrane antigen, which usually does not stain normal follicular dendritic cells. The cells also show weak S-100 protein staining; absent to weak CD45/45RB staining; and variable expression of CD68, muscle-specific actin, and desmoplakin. The tumor cells do not stain for CD20, CD1a, desmin, HMB-45, or the high-molecular-weight keratins. The tumors are usually EBV negative.[159]

The differential diagnosis of follicular dendritic cell tumors includes interdigitating dendritic cell tumors (discussed later), thymoma, spindle cell carcinoma, malignant melanoma, and sarcoma. CD21 and CD35 immunohistochemical staining has high specificity for follicular dendritic cell tumors. In addition, keratin positivity is seen in thymomas, in spindle cell carcinomas, and in a moderate number of epithelioid leiomyosarcomas but not in follicular dendritic cell tumors. S-100 protein positivity is seen in malignant melanomas and follicular dendritic cell tumors. However, additional stains for HMB-45 and Melan A (both positive in melanoma and both negative in follicular dendritic cell tumors) help to estab-

lish the correct diagnosis. There is no association with HHV-8.[830] Rare tumors that may be related to follicular dendritic cell tumors have been reported in the liver and spleen. These tumors have an immunohistochemical profile of dendritic follicular cells and, interestingly, are often EBV positive.[831] These cases may represent a subset of inflammatory pseudotumors. Some pathologists use the presence of well-formed fascicles, concentric whorls, cellular atypia, and decreased numbers of plasma cells to make the diagnosis of follicular dendritic cell tumors over inflammatory pseudotumors.[831]

## INTERDIGITATING DENDRITIC CELL TUMORS

Interdigitating dendritic cell tumors (also known as interdigitating dendritic cell sarcomas) are extremely uncommon neoplasms of dendritic cell origin.[823, 825] These tumors have been described in adults as well as in teenagers and have an aggressive clinical course. The clinical presentations in the few reported cases have varied from solitary lymph node enlargement to systemic disease including hepatosplenomegaly.

The tumors have a range of morphologic features, appearing similar to follicular dendritic cell tumors or even large cell lymphomas. The spindled cells are often found in the paracortex. Electron microscopic studies show interdigitating cell processes without well-formed desmosomes, unlike follicular dendritic cell tumors, and no Birbeck granules, unlike Langerhans cell histiocytosis. Immunohistochemical studies are needed to establish the diagnosis of interdigitating dendritic cell tumors and are necessary to differentiate them from follicular dendritic cell tumors. Interdigitating dendritic tumors usually stain for vimentin and CD68 and not for B or T lineage antigens, similar to follicular dendritic cell tumors. However, in contrast to follicular dendritic cell tumors, the reported interdigitating dendritic cell tumors are often positive for CD45 and S-

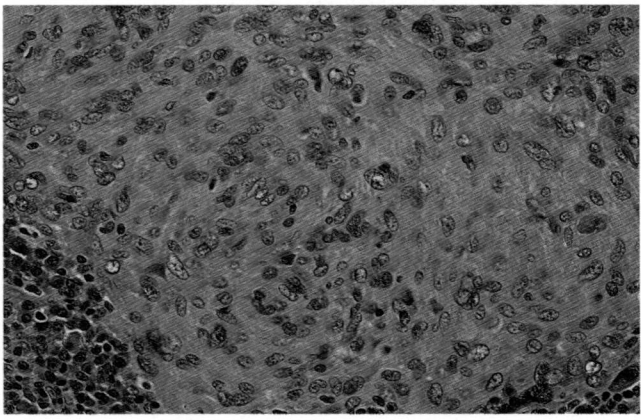

**FIGURE 41–82.** Follicular dendritic cell tumor. This spindled cell proliferation is less organized and more fibrotic than in the tumor illustrated in Figure 41–81. It also had collections of small lymphocytes.

100 protein and never stain for the follicular dendritic markers CD21 and CD35. Some reports of interdigitating tumors include CD1[+] tumors; however, we consider those to be indeterminate tumors, as discussed next.

## INDETERMINATE CELL NEOPLASMS

Indeterminate cell neoplasms (also known as indeterminate cell histiocytosis) are rare lesions that show differentiation toward indeterminate cells, a normal cell with morphologic and immunologic similarities to normal Langerhans cells, but lack Birbeck granules.[824, 832, 833] The tumors have been described primarily in adults. The patients usually present with single or multiple cutaneous lesions; rare patients present with lymphadenopathy. Some of the cases have been associated with low-grade B cell lymphomas.[824]

At low-power microscopy, the lesion is dermal based, occasionally with epidermal extension. The cells are large, with highly irregularly shaped nuclei and abundant cytoplasm. Multinucleated and foam cells may be present. By electron microscopy, the cells have numerous dendritic processes that interdigitate with those from adjacent cells but importantly do not contain Birbeck granules. By immunohistochemistry, the tumor cells stain for vimentin, CD45, CD1, S-100 protein, fascin, and macrophage-associated antigens. The diagnosis of indeterminate cell tumors can be made only with immunohistochemical and ultrastructural data.

## True Histiocytic Lymphoma and Malignant Histiocytosis

True histiocytic lymphoma and malignant histiocytosis describe a rare neoplasm in which the malignant cells show lineage consistent with histiocytes.[834, 835] Historically, the diagnosis of malignant histiocytosis was made when the morphologic and cytochemical features of the tumor cells were considered those of histiocytes. In retrospect, neither the appearance nor the cytochemical studies were unique to the neoplasm. With use of more modern ancillary techniques that have high specificity, the majority of cases of malignant histiocytosis reported in the past have since been shown to be lymphoid in nature.[244, 245, 836-838] We prefer to use the term *true histiocytic lymphoma* for this category of neoplasms because the term *malignant histiocytosis* has been used inconsistently in the past.[839]

True histiocytic lymphoma accounts for less than 0.5% of all hematolymphoid neoplasms and occurs most commonly in adults.[840] Patients generally present with fever, fatigue, and weakness and may have weight loss, lymphadenopathy, skin lesions, or splenomegaly. Laboratory test results are usually unremarkable. Lymph nodes are commonly involved, but extranodal sites of involvement have been reported.[839, 841] Rarely, true histiocytic lympho-

mas have been reported in association with or after a non-Hodgkin's lymphoma.[842, 843]

The normal lymph node architecture may be partially or completely effaced by a proliferation of cytologically malignant cells that resemble histiocytes.[839] The neoplastic cells vary in size and have a large, eccentrically placed, oval nucleus with a prominent irregular nucleolus and abundant eosinophilic cytoplasm (Fig. 41-83). Bizarre multinucleated tumor cells, multiple nucleoli, vacuolated cytoplasm, and hemophagocytosing tumor cells may also be seen. Spindle cell sarcoma-like areas and a prominent foam cell component have also been described in some cases. Mitotic activity is high. The tumor cells have no unique morphologic characteristics, and thus immunophenotypic and molecular studies are absolutely essential for diagnosis.

To make the diagnosis of true histiocytic lymphoma, one must establish strong immunologic evidence of histiocytic lineage, with complete absence of specific T and B lineage markers.[834, 835, 839] In addition, the tumor must have molecular evidence of a germline configuration for the T cell receptor and immunoglobulin genes.[27, 243, 244] By paraffin section immunohistochemistry, the tumor cells of true histiocytic lymphoma should express CD68, lysozyme, and $\alpha_1$-antitrypsin; they should not stain with CD30, CD1a, any B lineage or T lineage-specific antibodies, any of the antikeratin antibodies, or HMB-45.[834, 840, 844] S-100 protein staining has been reported in a minority of cases.[839] In addition, rare cases have been reported to be CD56[+].[702] Frozen section immunohistochemical studies and flow cytometric studies should show reactivity of the malignant cells with CD45 and multiple histiocytic markers but with none of the T or B lineage markers.[834]

True histiocytic lymphoma may be confused with anaplastic large cell lymphoma, B cell sinusoidal large cell lymphoma, anaplastic carcinomas showing hemophagocytosis, malignant lymphomas associated with benign erythrophagocytosis, follicu-

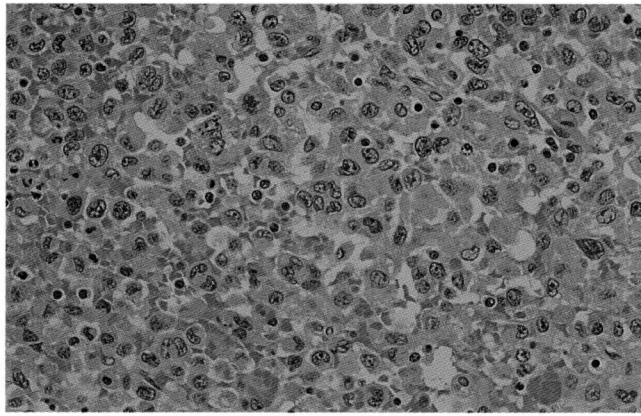

**FIGURE 41-83.** True histiocytic tumor. The cells have pleomorphic nuclei and abundant cytoplasm. Hemophagocytosis is seen. The diagnosis of a true histiocytic lymphoma was made after a large panel of immunohistochemical and molecular studies.

lar dendritic cell neoplasms, hepatosplenic T cell lymphoma, infection-associated hemophagocytic syndrome, storage diseases such as Gaucher's disease and Niemann-Pick disease, and familial hemophagocytic lymphohistiocytosis. In fact, the early reports of malignant histiocytosis have since been reclassified as anaplastic large cell lymphoma, B or T cell lymphomas, or infection-associated hemophagocytic syndrome. The strict morphologic, phenotypic, and molecular criteria of true histiocytic lymphoma along with clinical presentation help separate true histiocytic lymphoma from the other entities in the differential diagnosis.[839, 844–846]

Other entities historically associated with so-called malignant histiocytosis include histiocytic medullary reticulosis and regressing atypical histiocytosis. In addition, cases of malignant histiocytosis have been reported in association with mediastinal germ cell tumors, including malignant teratoma with or without yolk sac differentiation.[847] The histiocytic nature of these cases has generally not been rigorously tested; thus, it is not certain whether these cases represent true histiocytic lymphomas. Cases of histiocytic medullary reticulosis, first described in 1939, were also noted to have great clinical and morphologic overlap with cases of malignant histiocytosis.[234, 235] Cases of histiocytic medullary reticulosis have also been restudied with use of newly available diagnostic techniques and have been found to represent a heterogeneous category of entities, including Hodgkin's disease, non-Hodgkin's lymphomas (T cell lymphoma with or without hemophagocytosis, anaplastic large cell lymphoma, Lennert's lymphoma), and hyperimmune reactions. Cases of regressing atypical histiocytosis are now considered to fall in the category of lymphomatoid papulosis/anaplastic large cell lymphoma, cutaneous type, and not a true histiocytic lymphoma.[311]

## Extramedullary Myeloid Tumors

Myeloid leukemias involving extramedullary sites are known as extramedullary myeloid tumors, granulocytic sarcomas, or chloromas.[848, 849] There are several modes of clinical presentation.[850–852] Patients with known acute myeloid leukemia may develop lymph node involvement. Myeloid leukemia in the lymph node may be the first sign of blastic transformation in a patient with known chronic myelogenous leukemia, other myeloproliferative disorder, or myelodysplastic syndrome. Finally, nodal involvement by myeloid leukemia may occur in a patient with no known history of leukemia.

The cells of extramedullary myeloid tumor may involve the sinusoidal, interfollicular, or perinodal spaces of a lymph node or may diffusely efface the normal nodal architecture. Eosinophilic myelocytes are often admixed with the malignant cells, which have intermediately sized round or lobated nuclei, fine delicate or vesicular chromatin, and small to prominent nucleoli (Fig. 41–84). The cytoplasm is usually minimal in amount. However, occasional cases may have cells that have a moderate amount of cytoplasm and intracytoplasmic granules. The tumor usually has a high mitotic rate, and interspersed tingible body macrophages may lend a starry sky appearance. Touch imprints or frozen sections, if available, can be examined cytochemically for myeloperoxidase or Sudan black B.[848] In tissues, the Leder stain (chloroacetate esterase reaction) is positive in approximately 75% of cases, but the number of positive blasts can be low. Immunohistochemistry is extremely useful, with CD68, antimyeloperoxidase, CD117 (c-kit), CD43, CD15, and antilysozyme each positive in a high percentage of cases.[39, 849, 853] Flow cytometric expression of CD34, CD33, CD13, and CD117 is also seen. Approximately 15% of cases of acute myelogenous leukemia are also TdT positive.

The diagnosis of extramedullary myeloid tumor may be difficult to make in a patient with chronic myelomonocytic leukemia.[854] Older terms for such tumors are plasmacytoid T cell lymphoma and plasmacytoid monocytic lymphoma.[855] On histologic examination, the neoplasms may lack cytologic evidence of granulocyte maturation, such as cytoplasmic granulation or eosinophilic myelocytes, and the Leder stains for chloroacetate esterase are usually negative. Immunohistochemical studies, which yield results similar to those described before, may be necessary to establish the correct diagnosis.

When one sees an immature proliferation of cells in a lymph node from a patient with known myeloid leukemia, myeloproliferative disorder, or myelodysplastic syndrome, the diagnosis of extramedullary myeloid tumor may easily be made. However, when such malignant changes occur in a lymph node as the initial presentation of a myeloid malignant neoplasm, the diagnosis may be difficult to make. The differential diagnosis of extramedullary myeloid tumor includes non-Hodgkin's lym-

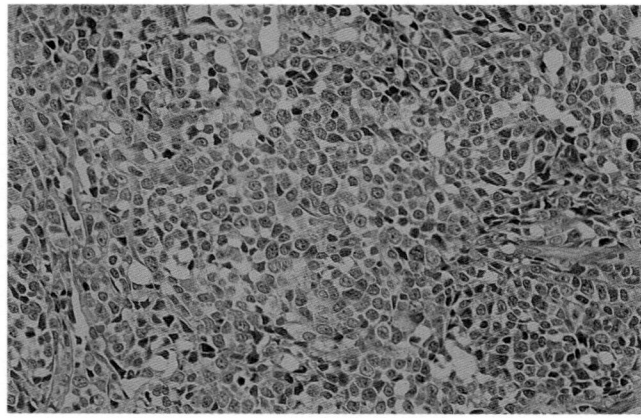

**FIGURE 41–84.** Extramedullary myeloid tumor. A monomorphous population of large cells with fine chromatin replaces the nodal parenchyma. Occasional myelocytes offer a subtle clue to the correct diagnosis.

phoma, especially lymphoblastic, Burkitt's, or large cell subtypes. The larger size and more prominent nucleoli of myeloid cells compared with lymphoblasts and the finer chromatin pattern compared with cells of large cell lymphoma help distinguish between these entities. Identifying eosinophilic metamyelocytes or cytoplasmic granules also favors a myeloid process. Cytochemical and immunohistochemical studies are extremely useful in the differential diagnosis.

## Miscellaneous Neoplasms

Hairy cell leukemia may involve the lymph nodes, but rarely without concomitant involvement of the bone marrow and spleen.[557] The outer cortex of the lymph node is preferentially involved (Fig. 41–85), and the morphologic appearance and immunologic profile are the same as those of hairy cell leukemia involving other sites.[556] Regional lymph nodes near a site of solitary plasmacytoma may be involved by plasmacytoma.[856]

Primary plasmacytoma of lymph node is extremely rare.[857, 858] Rare cases of plasmacytoma of lymph node are associated with amyloidosis.[859] The patients with primary plasmacytoma appear to have a more favorable outcome compared with patients with other extramedullary plasmacytomas and only rare progression to multiple myeloma.

Lymph nodes may rarely be involved in cases of systemic mastocytosis.[860] The mast cell infiltrate is found predominantly in the medullary cords and perivascular areas and is composed of bland cells with small oval or indented nuclei, fine chromatin, and a moderate amount of pale cytoplasm (Fig. 41–86). Eosinophils and sclerosis typically accompany the mast cell clusters. By immunohistochemistry, mast cells stain for CD43, CD68, CD117 (c-kit), and tryptase but not for CD20, which differentiates them from monocytoid B cells and cells of hairy cell leukemia.[861, 862] In addition, they do not stain for CD3.

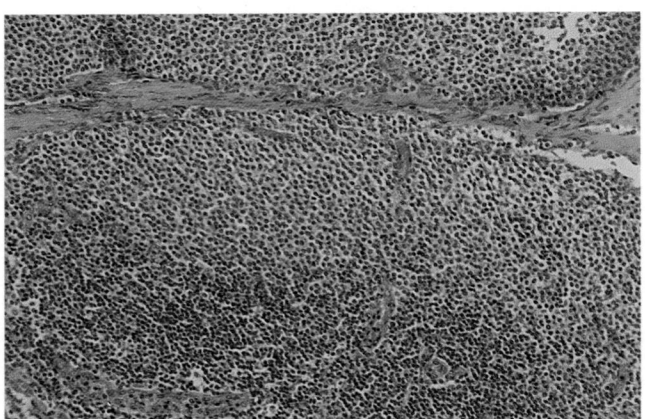

**FIGURE 41–85.** Hairy cell leukemia. The lymph node sinuses are distended by a monotonous infiltrate of small round cells with ample cytoplasm.

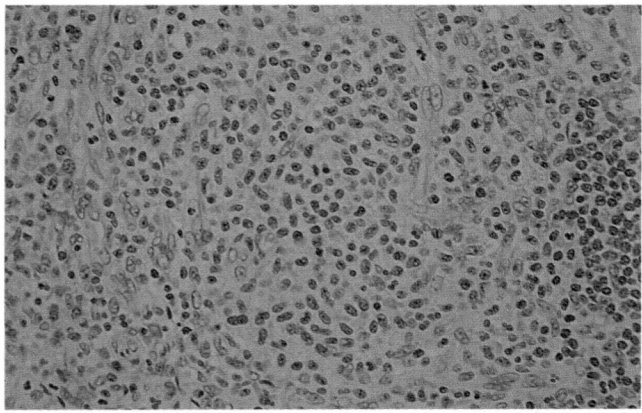

**FIGURE 41–86.** Mast cell disease. The lymph node parenchyma contains a proliferation of medium-sized cells with round to oval nuclei and abundant cytoplasm. Only the occasional nuclear irregularity may help differentiate this from hairy cell leukemia involving the lymph node and monocytoid B cell proliferations. Immunohistochemical studies are usually needed.

Giemsa, chloroacetate esterase, and toluidine blue stains are used to identify mast cell granules.

## REFERENCES

1. Rouse RV, Warnke RA: Special application of tissue section immunologic staining in the characterization of monoclonal antibodies and in the study of normal and neoplastic tissues. In Weir DM, Herzenberg LA, Blackwell CC (eds): Handbook of Experimental Immunology. 4th ed. Edinburgh, Blackwell, 1986, pp 116.1–116.10.
2. Zinzani PL, Colecchia A, Festi D, et al: Ultrasound-guided core-needle biopsy is effective in the initial diagnosis of lymphoma patients. Haematologica 83:989–992, 1998.
3. Pitts WC, Weiss LM: The role of fine needle aspiration biopsy in diagnosis and management of hematopoietic neoplasms. In Knowles DM (ed): Neoplastic Hematopathology. Baltimore, Williams & Wilkins, 1992, pp 385–405.
4. Henrique RM, Sousa ME, Godinho MI, et al: Immunophenotyping by flow cytometry of fine needle aspirates in the diagnosis of lymphoproliferative disorders: a retrospective study. J Clin Lab Anal 13:224–228, 1999.
5. Sneige N, Dekmezian R, El Naggar A, et al: Cytomorphologic, immunocytochemical and nucleic acid flow cytometric study of 50 lymph nodes by fine needle aspiration. Comparison with results obtained by subsequent excisional biopsy. Cancer 67:1003–1007, 1991.
6. Das DK: Value and limitations of fine-needle aspiration cytology in diagnosis and classification of lymphomas: a review. Diagn Cytopathol 21:240–249, 1999.
7. Chan LC, Pegram SM, Greaves MF: Contribution of immunophenotype to the classification and differential diagnosis of acute leukaemia. Lancet 1:475–479, 1985.
8. Cossman J, Chused TM, Fisher RI, et al: Diversity of immunological phenotypes of lymphoblastic lymphoma. Cancer Res 43:4486–4490, 1983.
9. Davey FR, Gatter KC, Ralfkiaer E, et al: Immunophenotyping of non-Hodgkin's lymphomas using a panel of antibodies on paraffin-embedded tissues [published erratum appears in Am J Pathol 130:9, 1988]. Am J Pathol 129:54–63, 1987.
10. Doggett RS, Wood GS, Horning S, et al: The immunologic characterization of 95 nodal and extranodal diffuse large cell lymphomas in 89 patients. Am J Pathol 115:245–252, 1984.
11. Dorfman RF, Gatter KC, Pulford KAF, et al: An evaluation of the utility of anti-granulocyte and anti-leukocyte monoclonal antibodies in the diagnosis of Hodgkin's disease. Am J Pathol 123:508–519, 1986.

12. Warnke RA, Gatter KC, Falini B, et al: Diagnosis of human lymphoma with monoclonal anti-leukocyte antibodies. N Engl J Med 309:1275–1281, 1983.
13. Grogan TM: Immunobiologic correlates of prognosis in lymphoma. Semin Oncol 5:58–74, 1993.
14. Clark JR, Williams ME, Swerdlow SH: Detection of B- and T-cells in paraffin-embedded tissue sections. Diagnostic utility of commercially obtained 4KB5 and UCHL-1. Am J Clin Pathol 93:58–69, 1990.
15. Strickler JG, Weiss LM, Copenhaver CM: Monoclonal antibodies reactive in routinely processed tissue sections of malignant lymphoma, with emphasis on T-cell lymphomas. Hum Pathol 18:808–814, 1987.
16. Garcia CF, Weiss LM, Warnke RA: Small noncleaved cell lymphoma: an immunophenotypic study of 18 cases and comparison with large cell lymphoma. Hum Pathol 17:454–461, 1986.
17. Gelb AB, Rouse RV, Dorfman RF, et al: Detection of immunophenotypic abnormalities in paraffin-embedded B-lineage non-Hodgkin's lymphomas. Am J Clin Pathol 102:825–834, 1994.
18. Kurec AS, Cruz VE, Barrett D, et al: Immunophenotyping of acute leukemias using paraffin-embedded tissue sections. Am J Clin Pathol 93:502–509, 1990.
19. Norton AJ, Issacson PG: Lymphoma phenotyping in formalin-fixed and paraffin wax–embedded tissues. I. Range of antibodies and staining patterns. Histopathology 14:437–446, 1989.
20. Said JW, Stoll PN, Shintaku P, et al: Leu-22: a preferential marker for T-lymphocytes in paraffin sections. Staining profile in T- and B-cell lymphomas, Hodgkin's disease, other lymphoproliferative disorders, myeloproliferative diseases, and various neoplastic processes. Am J Clin Pathol 91:542–549, 1989.
21. Poppema S, Hollema H, Visser L, et al: Monoclonal antibodies (MT1, MT2, MB1, MB2, MB3) reactive with leukocyte subsets in paraffin-embedded tissue sections. Am J Pathol 127:418–429, 1987.
22. Weiss LM, Crabtree GS, Rouse RV, et al: Morphologic and immunologic characterization of 50 peripheral T-cell lymphomas. Am J Pathol 118:316–324, 1985.
23. Arber DA, Weiss LM: CD43: a review. Appl Immunohistochem 1:88–96, 1993.
24. Schmid C, Sargent C, Isaacson PG: L and H cells of nodular lymphocyte predominant Hodgkin's disease show immunoglobulin light-chain restriction. Am J Pathol 139:1281–1289, 1991.
25. Warnke RA: The distinction of Hodgkin's disease from B cell lymphoma. Semin Diagn Pathol 9:284–290, 1992.
26. Said JW: The immunohistochemistry of Hodgkin's disease. Semin Diagn Pathol 9:265–271, 1992.
27. Picker LJ, Weiss LM, Medeiros LJ, et al: Immunophenotypic criteria for the diagnosis of non-Hodgkin's lymphoma. Am J Pathol 128:181–201, 1987.
28. Stein H, Lennert K, Feller AC, et al: Immunohistological analysis of human lymphoma: correlation of histological and immunological categories. Adv Cancer Res 42:67–147, 1984.
29. Borowitz MJ, Bray R, Gascoyne R, et al: U.S.-Canadian Consensus recommendations on the immunophenotypic analysis of hematologic neoplasia by flow cytometry: data analysis and interpretation. Cytometry 30:236–244, 1997.
30. Braylan RC, Benson NA, Nourse VA: Cellular DNA of human neoplastic B-cells measured by flow cytometry. Cancer Res 44:5010–5016, 1984.
31. Costa A, Mazzini G, Delbino G, et al: DNA content and kinetic characteristics of non-Hodgkin's lymphoma: determined by flow cytometry and autoradiography. Cytometry 2:185–188, 1981.
32. Shackney SE, Skramstad KS, Cunningham RE, et al: Dual parameter flow cytometry studies in human lymphomas. J Clin Invest 66:1281–1294, 1980.
33. Zukerberg LR, Medeiros LJ, Ferry JA, et al: Diffuse low-grade B-cell lymphomas: four clinically distinct subtypes defined by a combination of morphologic and immunophenotypic features. Am J Clin Pathol 100:373–385, 1993.
34. Chan JKC, Banks PM, Cleary ML, et al: A proposal for classification of lymphoid neoplasms (by the International Lymphoma Study Group). Histopathology 25:517–526, 1994.
35. Taylor CR, Shi SH, Cote RJ: Antigen retrieval for immunohistochemistry. Status and need for greater standardization. Appl Immunohistochem 4:144–166, 1996.
36. Shi SR, Cote RJ, Taylor CR: Antigen retrieval immunohistochemistry: past, present and future. J Histochem Cytochem 45:327–343, 1997.
37. Cattoretti G, Pileri S, Parravicini C, et al: Antigen unmasking on formalin-fixed, paraffin embedded tissue sections. J Pathol 171:83–98, 1993.
38. Cuevas EC, Bateman AC, Wilkins BS, et al: Microwave antigen retrieval in immunocytochemistry: a study of 80 antibodies. J Clin Pathol 47:448–452, 1994.
39. Chu PG, Chang KL, Arber DA, et al: Practical applications of immunohistochemistry for hematolymphoid disorders: an updated review. Ann Diagn Pathol 3:104–133, 1999.
40. Pileri SA, Roncador G, Ceccarelli C, et al: Antigen retrieval techniques in immunohistochemistry: comparison of different methods. J Pathol 183:116–123, 1997.
41. Spier CM, Grogan TM, Lippman SM, et al: The aberrancy of immunophenotype and immunoglobulin status as indicators of prognosis in B cell diffuse large cell lymphoma. Am J Pathol 133:118–126, 1988.
42. Mason DY, Biberfeld P: Technical aspects of lymphoma immunohistology. J Histochem Cytochem 28:731–745, 1980.
43. Weiss LM, Spagnolo DV: Assessment of clonality in lymphoid proliferations. Am J Pathol 142:1579–1582, 1993.
44. Sklar J, Weiss LM: Application of antigen receptor gene rearrangements to the diagnosis and characterization of lymphoid neoplasms. Annu Rev Med 39:315–334, 1988.
45. Cossman J, Aehnbauer B, Garrett C, et al: Gene rearrangements in the diagnosis of lymphoma/leukemia: guidelines for use based on a multiinstitutional study. Am J Clin Pathol 95:347–354, 1991.
46. Cossman J, Uppenkamp M, Sundeen J, et al: Molecular genetics and the diagnosis of lymphoma. Arch Pathol Lab Med 134:117–127, 1988.
47. Davis RE, Warnke RA, Dorfman RF, et al: Utility of molecular genetic analysis for the diagnosis of neoplasia in morphologically and immunophenotypically equivocal hematolymphoid lesions. Cancer 67:2890–2899, 1991.
48. Stevenson GT, Cragg MS: Molecular markers of B-cell lymphoma. Semin Cancer Biol 9:139–147, 1999.
49. Hu E, Horning S, Flynn S, et al: Diagnosis of B cell lymphoma by analysis of immunoglobulin gene rearrangements in biopsy specimens obtained by fine needle aspiration. J Clin Oncol 4:278–283, 1986.
50. Schlegelberger B, Zwingers T, Harder L, et al: Clinicopathogenetic significance of chromosomal abnormalities in patients with blastic peripheral B-cell lymphoma. Blood 94:3114–3120, 1999.
51. Anastasi J: Interphase cytogenetic analysis in the diagnosis and study of neoplastic disorders. Am J Clin Pathol 95(suppl):S22–S28, 1991.
52. Aster JC, Kobayashi Y, Shiota M, et al: Detection of the t(14;18) at similar frequencies in hyperplastic lymphoid tissues from American and Japanese patients. Am J Pathol 141:291–299, 1992.
53. Fisher ER, Gregorio RM, Redmond C, et al: Pathologic findings from the National Surgical Adjuvant Breast Project (Protocol No. 4). III. The significance of extranodal extension of axillary metastasis. Am J Clin Pathol 65:439–444, 1976.
54. Wells CA, Heryet A, Brochier J, et al: The immunocytochemical detection of axillary micrometastases in breast cancer. Br J Cancer 50:193–197, 1984.
55. Rubio IT, Korourian S, Cowan C, et al: Sentinel lymph node biopsy for staging breast cancer. Am J Surg 176:532–537, 1998.
56. Turner RR, Ollila DW, Krasne DL, et al: Histopathologic validation of the sentinel lymph node hypothesis for breast carcinoma. Ann Surg 226:271–276, 1997.
57. Giuliano AE, Dale PS, Turner RR, et al: Improved axillary staging of breast cancer with sentinel lymphadenectomy. Ann Surg 222:394–399, 1995.

58. Turner RR, Ollila DW, Stern S, et al: Optimal histopathologic examination of the sentinel lymph node for breast carcinoma staging. Am J Surg Pathol 23:263–267, 1999.

59. Gershenwald JE, Thompson W, Mansfield PF, et al: Multi-institutional melanoma lymphatic mapping experience: the prognostic value of sentinel lymph node status in 612 stage I or II melanoma patients. J Clin Oncol 17:976–983, 1999.

60. Weiss LM, Arber DA, Chang KL: CD45: a review. Appl Immunohistochem 1:166–181, 1993.

61. Cartun RW, Coles FB, Pastuszak WT: Utilization of monoclonal antibody L26 in the identification and confirmation of B-cell lymphomas. A sensitive and specific marker applicable to formalin- and B5-fixed, paraffin-embedded tissues. Am J Pathol 129:415–421, 1987.

62. Chang KL, Arber DA, Weiss LM: CD30: a review. Appl Immunohistochem 1:244–255, 1993.

63. Wang NP, Zee S, Zarbo RJ, et al: Coordinate expression of cytokeratins 7 and 20 defines unique subsets of carcinomas. Appl Immunohistochem 3:99–107, 1995.

64. Rosai J, Carcangiu ML, DeLellis RA: Tumors of the Thyroid Gland. Atlas of Tumor Pathology. Third Series, Fascicle 5. Washington, DC, Armed Forces Institute of Pathology, 1992.

65. Rodriguez HA, Ackerman LV: Cellular blue nevus: clinicopathologic study of forty-five cases. Cancer 21:393–405, 1968.

66. Weeks DA, Beckwith JB, Mierau GW: Benign nodal lesions mimicking metastasis from pediatric renal neoplasms: a report of the National Wilms' Tumor Study Pathology Center. Hum Pathol 21:1239–1244, 1990.

67. Karp LA, Czernobilsky B: Glandular inclusions in pelvic and abdominal paraaortic lymph nodes, a study of autopsy and surgical material in males and females. Am J Clin Pathol 52: 212–218, 1969.

68. Clement PB: Pathology of endometriosis. Pathol Annu 1:245–295, 1990.

69. Mills SE: Decidual and squamous metaplasia in abdomino-pelvic lymph nodes. Int J Gynecol Pathol 2:209–215, 1983.

70. Holdsworth PJ, Hopkinson JM, Leveson SH: Benign axillary epithelial lymph node inclusions—a histological pitfall. Histopathology 13:226–228, 1988.

71. Rutty GN, Lauder I: Mesothelial cell inclusions within mediastinal lymph nodes. Histopathology 25:483–487, 1994.

72. Cohn DE, Folpe AL, Gown AM, et al: Mesothelial pelvic lymph node inclusions mimicking metastatic thyroid carcinoma. Gynecol Oncol 68:210–213, 1998.

73. Suarez VD, Izquierdo Garcia FM: Embolization of mesothelial cells in lymphatics: the route to mesothelial inclusions in lymph nodes? Histopathology 33:570–575, 1998.

74. Parkash V, Vidwans M, Carter D: Benign mesothelial cells in mediastinal lymph nodes. Am J Surg Pathol 23:1264–1269, 1999.

75. Bautista NC, Cohen S, Anders KH: Benign melanocytic nevus cells in axillary lymph nodes. A prospective incidence and immunohistochemical study with literature review. Am J Clin Pathol 102:102–108, 1994.

76. Epstein JL, Erlandson RA, Rosen PP: Nodal blue nevi: a study of three cases. Am J Surg Pathol 8:907–915, 1984.

77. McCarthy SW, Palmer AA, Bale PM, et al: Nevus cells in lymph nodes. Pathology 6:351–358, 1971.

78. Chan JKC, Warnke RA, Dorfman RF: Vascular transformation of sinuses in lymph nodes: a study of its morphologic spectrum and distinction from Kaposi's sarcoma. Am J Surg Pathol 15:732–743, 1991.

79. Dorfman RF, Warnke RA: Lymphadenopathy simulating the malignant lymphomas. Hum Pathol 5:519–550, 1974.

80. Haferkamp O, Rosenau W, Lennert K: Vascular transformation of lymph node sinuses due to venous obstruction. Arch Pathol 92:81–83, 1971.

81. Cook PD, Czerniak B, Chan JKC, et al: Nodular spindle cell vascular transformation of lymph nodes: a benign process occurring predominantly in retroperitoneal lymph nodes draining carcinomas that can simulate Kaposi's sarcoma or metastatic tumor. Am J Surg Pathol 19:1010–1020, 1995.

82. Chan JKC, Lewin KJ, Lombard CD, et al: The histopathology of bacillary angiomatosis of lymph nodes. Am J Surg Pathol 14:430–437, 1991.

83. Zangwill KM, Hamilton DH, Perkins BA, et al: Cat scratch disease in Connecticut: epidemiology, risk factors, and evaluation of a new diagnostic test. N Engl J Med 329:8–13, 1993.

84. Koehler JE, Quinn FD, Berger GT, et al: Isolation of *Rochalimaea* species from cutaneous and osseous lesions of bacillary angiomatosis. N Engl J Med 327:1625–1631, 1992.

85. Koehler JE, Sanchez MA, Garrido CS, et al: Molecular epidemiology of *Bartonella* infections in patients with bacillary angiomatosis-peliosis. N Engl J Med 337:1876–1883, 1997.

86. Relman DA, Fredricks DN, Yoder KE, et al: Absence of Kaposi's sarcoma–associated herpesvirus DNA in bacillary angiomatosis-peliosis lesions. J Infect Dis 180:1386–1389, 1999.

87. Finkbeiner WE, Egbert BM, Groundwater JR, et al: Kaposi's sarcoma in young homosexual men, a histopathologic study with particular reference to lymph node involvement. Arch Pathol Lab Med 106:261–264, 1982.

88. Yokois NU, Perlman ER, Colombani P, et al: Kaposi's sarcoma presenting as a protracted multisystem illness in an adolescent liver transplant recipient. Liver Transplant Surg 3: 541–544, 1997.

89. Wang AY, Li PK, To KF, et al: Coexistence of Kaposi's sarcoma and tuberculosis in a renal transplant recipient. Transplantation 66:115–118, 1998.

90. Chen KTK: Multicentric Castleman's disease and Kaposi's sarcoma. Am J Surg Pathol 8:287–293, 1984.

91. Chang Y, Cesarman E, Pessin MS, et al: Identification of herpesvirus-like DNA sequences in AIDS-associated Kaposi's sarcoma. Science 266:1865–1869, 1994.

92. Chang Y, Moore PS: Kaposi's sarcoma (KS)–associated herpesvirus and its role in KS. Infect Agents Dis 5:215–222, 1996.

93. Moore PS, Kingsley LA, Holmberg SD, et al: Kaposi's sarcoma–associated herpesvirus infection prior to onset of Kaposi's sarcoma. AIDS 10:175–180, 1996.

94. Kennedy MM, Cooper K, Howells DD, et al: Identification of HHV8 in early Kaposi's sarcoma: implications of Kaposi's sarcoma pathogenesis. Mol Pathol 51:14–20, 1998.

95. Dupin N, Fisher C, Kellam P, et al: Distribution of human herpesvirus-8 latently infected cells in Kaposi's sarcoma, multicentric Castleman's disease, and primary effusion lymphoma. Proc Natl Acad Sci U S A 96:4546–4551, 1999.

96. Chan JK, Frizzera G, Fletcher CD, et al: Primary vascular tumors of lymph nodes other than Kaposi's sarcoma: analysis of 39 cases and delineation of two new entities. Am J Surg Pathol 16:335–350, 1992.

97. Cho NH, Yang WI, Lee WJ: Spindle and epithelioid haemangioendothelioma of the inguinal lymph nodes. Histopathology 30:595–598, 1997.

98. Perrone T, De Wolf-Peeters C, Frizzera G: Inflammatory pseudotumor of lymph nodes. A distinctive pattern of nodal reaction. Am J Surg Pathol 12:351–361, 1988.

99. Davis RE, Warnke RA, Dorfman RF: Inflammatory pseudotumor of lymph nodes. Additional observations and evidence for an inflammatory etiology. Am J Surg Pathol 15: 744–756, 1991.

100. Moran CA, Suster S, Abbondanzo SL: Inflammatory pseudotumor of lymph nodes: a study of 25 cases with emphasis on morphological heterogeneity. Hum Pathol 28:332–338, 1997.

101. Coffin CM, Humphrey PA, Dehner LP: Extrapulmonary inflammatory myofibroblastic tumor: a clinical and pathological survey. Semin Diagn Pathol 15:85–101, 1998.

102. Menke DM, Griesser H, Araujo I, et al: Inflammatory pseudotumors of lymph node origin show macrophage-derived spindle cells and lymphocyte-derived cytokine transcripts without evidence of T-cell receptor gene rearrangements. Implications for pathogenesis and classification as an idiopathic retroperitoneal fibrosis-like sclerosing immune reaction. Am J Clin Pathol 105:430–439, 1996.

103. Chen KTK: Mycobacterial spindle cell pseudotumor of lymph nodes. Am J Surg Pathol 16:276–281, 1992.

104. Suster S, Moran CA, Blanco M: Mycobacterial spindle-cell pseudotumor of the spleen. Am J Clin Pathol 101:539–542, 1994.

105. Wolf DA, Wu CD, Medeiros LJ: Mycobacterial pseudotumors of lymph node. A report of two cases diagnosed at the time

of intraoperative consultation using touch imprint preparation. Arch Pathol Lab Med 119:811–814, 1995.

106. Logani S, Lucas DR, Cheng JD, et al: Spindle cell tumors associated with mycobacteria in lymph nodes of HIV-positive patients: "Kaposi sarcoma with mycobacteria" and "mycobacterial pseudotumor." Am J Surg Pathol 23:656–661, 1999.

107. Argani P, Ghossein R, Rosai J: Anthracotic and anthrasilicotic spindle cell pseudotumors of mediastinal lymph nodes: report of five cases of a reactive lesion that simulates malignancy. Hum Pathol 29:851–855, 1998.

108. Suster S, Rosai J: Intranodal hemorrhagic spindle cell tumor with "amianthoid" fibers. Report of six cases of a distinctive mesenchymal neoplasm of the inguinal region that simulates Kaposi's sarcoma. Am J Surg Pathol 13:347–357, 1989.

109. Weiss SW, Gnepp DR, Bratthauer GL: Palisaded myofibroblastoma. A benign mesenchymal tumor of lymph node. Am J Surg Pathol 13:341–346, 1989.

110. Creager AJ, Garwacki CP: Recurrent intranodal palisaded myofibroblastoma with metaplastic bone formation. Arch Pathol Lab Med 123:433–436, 1999.

111. Hisaoka M, Hashiomoto H, Daimaru Y: Intranodal palisaded myofibroblastoma with so-called amianthoid fibers: a report of two cases with a review of the literature. Pathol Int 48:307–312, 1998.

112. Eyden BP, Harris M, Greywoode GI, et al: Intranodal myofibroblastoma: report of a case. Ultrastruct Pathol 20:79–88, 1996.

113. Rossi A, Bulgarini A, Rondanelli E, et al: Intranodal palisaded myofibroblastoma: report of three new cases. Tumori 81:464–468, 1995.

114. Warnke RA, Weiss LM, Chan JKC, et al: Tumors of the Lymph Nodes and Spleen. Atlas of Tumor Pathology. Third Series, Fascicle 14. Washington, DC, Armed Forces Institute of Pathology, 1995.

115. Chan JK, Tsang WY, Pau MY, et al: Lymphangiomyomatosis and angiomyolipoma: closely related entities characterized by hamartomatous proliferation of HMB-45–positive smooth muscle. Histopathology 22:445–455, 1993.

116. Channer JL, Davies JD: Smooth muscle proliferation in the hilum of superficial lymph nodes. Virchow Arch A Pathol Anat Histopathol 406:261–270, 1985.

117. Abell MR, Littler ER: Benign metastasizing uterine leiomyoma: multiple lymph node metastasis. Cancer 36:2206–2213, 1975.

118. MacKenzie DH: Amyloidosis presenting as lymphadenopathy. Br Med J 2:1449–1450, 1963.

119. Ordi J, Grau JM, Junque A, et al: Secondary (AA) amyloidosis associated with Castleman's disease. Report of two cases and review of the literature. Am J Clin Pathol 100:393–397, 1993.

120. Michaeli J, Niesvizky R, Siegel D, et al: Proteinaceous (angiocentric sclerosing) lymphadenopathy: a polyclonal stemic, nonamyloid deposition disorder. Blood 86:1159–1162, 1995.

121. Osborne BM, Butler JJ, MacKay B: Proteinaceous lymphadenopathy with hypergammaglobulinaemia. Am J Surg Pathol 3:137–145, 1979.

122. Hall JG: The functional anatomy of lymph nodes. In Stansfeld AG (ed): Lymph Node Biopsy Interpretation. Edinburgh, Churchill Livingstone, 1985, pp 1–25.

123. Segal GH, Perkins SL, Kjeldsberg CR: Benign lymphadenopathies in children and adolescents. Semin Diagn Pathol 12:288–302, 1995.

124. Liu Y-J, Johnson GD, Gordon J, et al: Germinal center in T-cell–dependent antibody responses. Immunol Today 13:17–21, 1992.

125. Chadburn A, Metroka C, Mouradian J: Progressive lymph node histology and its prognostic value in patients with acquired immunodeficiency syndrome and AIDS-related complex. Hum Pathol 20:579–587, 1989.

126. Rappaport H, Winter WJ, Hicks EB: Follicular lymphoma: a re-evaluation of its position in the scheme of malignant lymphoma, based on a survey of 253 cases. Cancer 9:792–821, 1956.

127. Nathwani BN, Winberg CD, Diamond LW, et al: Morpho-

logic criteria for the differentiation of follicular lymphoma from florid reactive follicular hyperplasia: a study of 80 cases. Cancer 48:1794–1806, 1981.

128. Symmers W: The lymphoreticular system. In Henry K, Symmers W St C (eds): Systemic Pathology. Edinburgh, Churchill Livingstone, 1992.

129. Stein H: The immunologic and immunochemical basis for the Kiel classification. In Lennert K (ed): Malignant Lymphomas Other Than Hodgkin's Disease. Berlin, Springer-Verlag, 1978.

130. Ngan B, Chen-Levy Z, Weiss LM, et al: Expression in non-Hodgkin's lymphoma of the bcl-2 protein associated with the t(14;18) chromosomal translocation. N Engl J Med 318:1638–1644, 1988.

131. Lai R, Arber DA, Chang KL, et al: Frequency of bcl-2 expression in non-Hodgkin's lymphoma. A study of 798 cases with comparison of marginal zone lymphoma and monocytoid B cell hyperplasia. Mod Pathol 11:864–869, 1998.

132. Almasri NM, Iturraspe JA, Braylan RC: CD10 expression in follicular lymphoma and large cell lymphoma is different from that of reactive lymph node follicles. Arch Pathol Lab Med 122:539–544, 1998.

133. Arber DA, Weiss LM: CD10: a review. Appl Immunohistochem 5:125–140, 1997.

134. Weisenburger DD: Mantle-zone lymphoma. An immunohistologic study. Cancer 53:1073–1080, 1984.

135. Lai R, Weiss LM, Chang KL, et al: Frequency of CD43 expression in non-Hodgkin's lymphoma. A survey of 742 cases and further characterization of rare CD43+ follicular lymphomas. Am J Clin Pathol 111:488–494, 1999.

136. Doggett RS, Colby TV, Dorfman RF: Interfollicular Hodgkin's disease. Am J Med 78:22–28, 1983.

137. Schnitzer B: Reactive lymphoid hyperplasia. In Jaffe ES (ed): Surgical Pathology of the Lymph Nodes and Related Organs. Philadelphia, WB Saunders, 1985, pp 22–56.

138. Symmons DP: Neoplasms of the immune system in rheumatoid arthritis. Am J Med 78:22–28, 1985.

139. Nosanchuk JS, Schnitzer B: Follicular hyperplasia in lymph nodes from patients with rheumatoid arthritis. Cancer 24:343–354, 1969.

140. Kondratowicz GM, Symmons DP, Bacon PA, et al: Rheumatoid lymphadenopathy: a morphological and immunohistochemical study. J Clin Pathol 43:106–113, 1990.

141. McCurley TJ, Collins D, Ball E, et al: Nodal and extranodal lymphoproliferative disorders in Sjögren's syndrome: a clinical and immunopathologic study. Hum Pathol 21:482–492, 1990.

142. Hartsock RJ, Halling LW, King FM: Luetic lymphadenitis: a clinical and histologic study of 20 cases. Am J Clin Pathol 53:304–314, 1970.

143. Keller AR, Hochholzer L, Castleman B: Hyaline-vascular and plasma-cell types of giant lymph node hyperplasia of mediastinum and other locations. Cancer 29:670–683, 1972.

144. Hui PK, Chan JKC, Ng CS, et al: Lymphadenopathy in Kimura's disease. Am J Surg Pathol 13:177–186, 1989.

145. Kuo TT, Shih LY, Chan HL: Kimura's disease. Involvement of regional lymph nodes and distinction from angiolymphoid hyperplasia with eosinophilia. Am J Surg Pathol 12:843–854, 1988.

146. Stansfeld AG: The histologic diagnosis of toxoplasmic lymphadenitis. J Clin Pathol 14:565–573, 1961.

147. Gupta RK: Fine needle aspiration cytodiagnosis of toxoplasmic lymphadenitis. Acta Cytol 41:1031–1034, 1997.

148. Brynes RK, Chan WC, Spira TJ, et al: Value of lymph node biopsy in unexplained lymphadenopathy in homosexual men. JAMA 250:1313–1317, 1983.

149. McCabe RE, Brooks RG, Dorfman RF, et al: Clinical spectrum in 107 cases of toxoplasmic lymphadenopathy. Rev Infect Dis 9:754–774, 1987.

150. Daneshbod K: Localized lymphadenitis due to leishmania simulating toxoplasmosis. Value of electron microscopy for differentiation. Am J Clin Pathol 69:462–467, 1978.

151. Castleman B, Iverson I, Menendez VP: Localized mediastinal lymph node hyperplasia resembling thymoma. Cancer 9:822–830, 1956.

152. Frizzera G, Peterson BA, Bayrd ED, et al: A systemic lymphoproliferative disorder with morphologic features of Castleman's disease: clinical findings and clinicopathologic correlations in 15 patients. J Clin Oncol 3:1202–1216, 1985.

153. Frizzera G: Castleman's disease and related disorders. Semin Diagn Pathol 5:346–364, 1988.

154. Frizzera G: Castleman's disease: more questions than answers. Hum Pathol 16:202–205, 1985.

155. Weisenburger DD, Nathwani BN, Winberg CD, et al: Multicentric angiofollicular lymph node hyperplasia: a clinicopathologic study of 16 cases. Hum Pathol 16:162–172, 1985.

156. Flendrig JA: Benign giant lymphoma: clinicopathologic correlation study. In Clark RL, Curnley R (eds): The Year Book of Cancer. Chicago, Year Book Medical, 1970, pp 296–299.

157. Lin O, Frizzera G: Angiomyoid and follicular dendritic cell proliferative lesions in Castleman's disease of hyaline-vascular type: a study of 10 cases. Am J Surg Pathol 21:1295–1306, 1997.

158. Harris NL, Bhan AK: "Plasmacytoid T cells" in Castleman's disease: immunohistologic phenotype. Am J Surg Pathol 11:109–113, 1987.

159. Perez-Ordonez B, Rosai J: Follicular dendritic cell tumor: review of the entity. Semin Diagn Pathol 15:144–154, 1998.

160. Oksenhendler E, Duarte M, Soulier J, et al: Multicentric Castleman's disease in HIV infection: a clinical and pathological study of 20 patients. AIDS 10:61–67, 1996.

161. Yamakawa M, Ikeda I, Masuda A, et al: An unusual regressive germinal center, the "FDC-only lymphoid follicle," in lymph nodes of organ transplant recipients. Am J Surg Pathol 23:536–545, 1999.

162. Said JW, Pinkus JL, Shintaku IP, et al: Alterations in fascin-expressing germinal center dendritic cells in neoplastic follicles of B-cell lymphomas. Mod Pathol 11:1–5, 1998.

163. Smir BN, Greiner TC, Weisenburger DD: Multicentric angiofollicular lymph node hyperplasia in children: a clinicopathologic study of eight patients. Mod Pathol 9:1135–1142, 1996.

164. Radaszkiewicz T, Hansmann ML, Lennert K: Monoclonality and polyclonality of plasma cells in Castleman's disease of the plasma cell variant. Histopathology 14:11–24, 1989.

165. Frizzera G, Massarelli G, Banks PM, et al: A systemic lymphoproliferative disorder with morphologic features of Castleman's disease: pathological findings in 15 patients. Am J Surg Pathol 7:211–231, 1983.

166. Herrada J, Cabanillas F, Rice L, et al: The clinical behavior of localized and multicentric Castleman disease. Ann Intern Med 128:657–662, 1998.

167. Dickson D, Ben-Ezra JM, Reed F, et al: Multicentric giant lymph-node hyperplasia, Kaposi's sarcoma, and lymphoma. Arch Pathol Lab Med 109:1013–1018, 1985.

168. Bitter MA, Komaiko W, Franklin WA: Giant lymph node hyperplasia with osteoblastic bone lesions and the POEMS (Takatsuki's) syndrome. Cancer 56:188–194, 1985.

169. Centers for Disease Control: Persistent, generalized lymphadenopathy among homosexual males. MMWR 31:249–251, 1982.

170. Bowne WB, Lewis JJ, Filippa DA, et al: The management of unicentric and multicentric Castleman's disease: a report of 16 cases and a review of the literature. Cancer 85:706–717, 1999.

171. Hanson CA, Frizzera G, Patton DF, et al: Clonal rearrangement for immunoglobulin and T-cell receptor genes in systemic Castleman's disease: association with Epstein-Barr virus. Am J Pathol 131:84–91, 1988.

172. Soulier J, Grollet L, Oksenhendler E, et al: Kaposi's sarcoma–associated herpesvirus-like DNA sequences in multicentric Castleman's disease. Blood 86:1276–1280, 1995.

173. Cesarman E, Knowles DM: The role of Kaposi sarcoma–associated herpesvirus (KSHV/HHV-8) in lymphoproliferative diseases. Semin Cancer Biol 3:165–174, 1999.

174. Chadburn A, Cesarman E, Nador RG, et al: Kaposi's sarcoma–associated herpesvirus sequences in benign lymphoid proliferations not associated with human immunodeficiency virus. Cancer 80:788–797, 1997.

175. Teruya-Feldstein J, Zauber P, Setsuda JE, et al: Expression of human herpesvirus-8 oncogene and cytokine homologues in an HIV-seronegative patient with multicentric Castleman's disease and primary effusion lymphoma. Lab Invest 78:1637–1642, 1998.

176. Said JW: Human immunodeficiency virus–related lymphoid proliferations. Semin Diagn Pathol 14:48–53, 1997.

177. Harris NL, Jaffe ES, Stein H, et al: A revised European-American classification of lymphoid neoplasms. A proposal from the International Lymphoma Study Group. Blood 84:1361–1392, 1994.

178. Ometto L, Menen C, Masiero S, et al: Molecular profile of Epstein-Barr virus in human immunodeficiency virus type 1–related lymphadenopathies and lymphomas. Blood 90:313–322, 1997.

179. Shibata D, Weiss LM, Hernandez AM, et al: Epstein-Barr virus–associated non-Hodgkin's lymphoma in patients infected with the human immunodeficiency virus. Blood 81:2102–2109, 1993.

180. Brousset P, Schlaifer D, Roda D, et al: Characterization of Epstein-Barr virus–infected cells in benign lymphadenopathy of patients seropositive for human immunodeficiency virus. Hum Pathol 27:263–268, 1996.

181. Ioachim HL, Cronin W, Roy M, et al: Persistent lymphadenopathies in people at high risk for HIV infection. Clinicopathologic correlations and long-term follow-up in 79 cases. Am J Clin Pathol 93:208–218, 1990.

182. Knowles DN, Chadburn A: Lymphadenopathy and the lymphoid neoplasms associated with the acquired immune deficiency syndrome (AIDS). In Knowles DM (ed): Neoplastic Hematopathology. Baltimore, Williams & Wilkins, 1992, pp 773–835.

183. Pileri S, Rivano MT, Raise E, et al: The value of lymph node biopsy in patients with acquired immunodeficiency syndrome (AIDS) and the AIDS-related complex (ARC): a morphological and immunohistochemical study of 90 cases. Histopathology 10:1107–1129, 1986.

184. Ewing EP, Chandler FW, Spira TJ, et al: Primary lymph node pathology in AIDS and AIDS-related lymphadenopathy. Arch Pathol Lab Med 109:977–981, 1985.

185. Sohn CC, Sheibani K, Winberg CD, et al: Monocytoid B lymphocytes: their relation to the patterns of the acquired immunodeficiency syndrome (AIDS) and AIDS-related lymphadenopathy. Hum Pathol 16:979–985, 1985.

186. Said JW, Pinkus JL, Yamashita J, et al: The role of follicular and interdigitating dendritic cells in HIV-related lymphoid hyperplasia: localization of fascin. Mod Pathol 10:421–427, 1997.

187. Burns BF, Colby TV, Dorfman RF: Differential diagnostic features of nodular L&H Hodgkin's disease, including progressive transformation of germinal centers. Am J Surg Pathol 8:253–261, 1984.

188. Hansmann ML, Fellbaum C, Hui PK, et al: Progressive transformation of germinal centers with and without association to Hodgkin's disease. Am J Clin Pathol 93:219–226, 1990.

189. Osborne BM, Butler JJ: Clinical implications of progressive transformation of germinal centers. Am J Surg Pathol 8:725–733, 1984.

190. Poppema S, Kaiserling E, Lennert K: Hodgkin's disease with lymphocyte predominance, nodular type (nodular paragranuloma) and progressively transformed germinal centers—a cytohistological study. Histopathology 3:295–308, 1979.

191. Ferry JA, Zukerberg LR, Harris NL: Florid progressive transformation of germinal centers. A syndrome affecting young men, without early progression to nodular lymphocyte predominance Hodgkin's disease. Am J Surg Pathol 16:252–258, 1992.

192. Osborne BM, Butler JJ, Gresik MV: Progressive transformation of germinal centers: comparison of 23 pediatric patients to the adult population. Mod Pathol 5:135–140, 1992.

193. Nguyen PL, Ferry JA, Harris NL: Progressive transformation of germinal centers and nodular lymphocyte predominance Hodgkin's disease: a comparative immunohistochemical study. Am J Surg Pathol 23:27–33, 1999.

194. Poppema S, Visser L, Leij LD: Reactivity of presumed anti-natural killer cell antibody Leu 7 with intrafollicular T-lymphocytes. Clin Exp Immunol 54:834–837, 1983.

195. Hartsock RJ: Postvaccinial lymphadenitis: hyperplasia of lymphoid tissue that simulates malignant lymphomas. Cancer 21:632–649, 1968.

196. Childs CC, Parham DM, Berard CW: Infectious mononucleosis: the spectrum of morphologic changes simulating lymphoma in lymph nodes and tonsils. Am J Clin Pathol 53:304–314, 1987.

197. Tindle BH, Parker JW, Lukes RJ: "Reed-Sternberg cells" in infectious mononucleosis. Am J Clin Pathol 58:607–617, 1972.

198. Otteman LA, Greipp PR, Ruiz-Arguelles GJ, et al: Infectious mononucleosis mimicking a B cell immunoblastic lymphoma associated with an abnormality in regulatory T cells. Am J Med 78:885–890, 1985.

199. Abbondanzo SL, Sato N, Straus SE, et al: Acute infectious mononucleosis. CD30 (Ki-1) antigen expression and histologic correlations. Am J Clin Pathol 93:698–702, 1990.

200. Fellbaum C, Hansmann ML, Parwaresch MR, et al: Monoclonal antibodies on Hodgkin's and Reed-Sternberg cells of Hodgkin's disease. An immunocytochemical study on lymph node cytospins using monoclonal antibodies. Histopathology 11:1229–1242, 1988.

201. Reynolds DJ, Banks PM, Gulley ML: New characterization of infectious mononucleosis and a phenotypic comparison with Hodgkin's disease. Am J Pathol 146:379–388, 1995.

202. Spector SA, Hsia K, Denaro F, et al: Use of molecular probes to detect human cytomegalovirus and human immunodeficiency virus. Clin Chem 35:1581–1587, 1999.

203. Malik UR, Oleksowicz L, Dutcher JP, et al: Atypical clonal T-cell proliferation in infectious mononucleosis. Med Oncol 13:207–213, 1996.

204. Strickler JG, Fedeli F, Horwitz CA, et al: Infectious mononucleosis in lymphoid tissue. Histopathology, in situ hybridization, and differential diagnosis. Arch Pathol Lab Med 117:269–278, 1993.

205. Shin SS, Berry GJ, Weiss LM: Infectious mononucleosis. Diagnosis by in situ hybridization in two cases with atypical features. Am J Surg Pathol 15:625–631, 1991.

206. Rushin JM, Riordan GP, Heaton RB, et al: Cytomegalovirus-infected cells express Leu-M1 antigen: a possible source of diagnostic error. Am J Pathol 136:989–995, 1990.

207. Tamaru J, Atsuo M, Horie H, et al: Herpes simplex lymphadenitis. Report of two cases with review of the literature. Am J Surg Pathol 14:571–577, 1990.

208. Gaffey MJ, Ben-Ezra J, Weiss LM: Herpes simplex lymphadenitis. Am J Clin Pathol 95:709–714, 1991.

209. Dorfman RF, Herweg J: Live, attenuated measles virus vaccine: Inguinal lymphadenopathy complicating administration. JAMA 198:320–321, 1966.

210. Gams RA, Neal JA, Conrad FG: Hydantoin-induced pseudolymphoma. Ann Intern Med 69:557–568, 1968.

211. Saltzstein SL, Ackerman LV: Lymphadenopathy induced by anticonvulsant drugs clinically and pathologically mimicking malignant lymphomas. Cancer 12:164–182, 1959.

212. Shuttleworth D, Graham-Brown RA, Williams AJ, et al: Pseudo-lymphoma associated with carbamazepine. Clin Exp Dermatol 9:421–423, 1984.

213. Abbondanzo SL, Irye NS, Frizzera G: Dilantin-associated lymphadenopathy: spectrum of histopathologic patterns. Am J Surg Pathol 19:675–686, 1995.

214. Segal GH, Cough JD, Tubbs RR: Autoimmune and iatrogenic causes of lymphadenopathy. Semin Oncol 20:611–626, 1993.

215. Gould E, Porto R, Albores-Saavedra J, et al: Dermatopathic lymphadenitis. The spectrum and significance of its morphologic features. Arch Pathol Lab Med 112:1145–1150, 1988.

216. Burke JS, Colby TV: Dermatopathic lymphadenopathy. Comparison of cases associated and unassociated with mycosis fungoides. Am J Surg Pathol 5:343–352, 1981.

217. Rausch E, Kaiserling E, Goos M: Langerhans cells and interdigitating reticulum cells in the thymus-dependent region in human dermatopathic lymphadenitis. Virchows Arch B Cell Pathol 25:327–343, 1977.

218. Weiss LM, Beckstead JH, Warnke RA, et al: Leu 6 expressing lymph node cells are dendritic cells and closely related to interdigitating cells. Hum Pathol 17:179–184, 1986.

219. Sudilovsky D, Cha I: Fine needle aspiration cytology of dermatopathic lymphadenitis. Acta Cytol 42:1341–1346, 1998.

220. Iyer VK, Kapila K, Verma K: Fine needle aspiration cytology of dermatopathic lymphadenitis. Acta Cytol 42:1347–1351, 1998.

221. Black MM, Speer F: Sinus histiocytosis of lymph node in cancer. Surg Gynecol Obstet 106:163–175, 1958.

222. Albores-Saavedra J, Vuitch F, Delgado R, et al: Sinus histiocytosis of pelvic lymph nodes after hip replacement. A histiocytic proliferation induced by cobalt-chromium and titanium. Am J Surg Pathol 18:83–90, 1994.

223. Vaamonde R, Cabrera JM, Vaamonde-Martin RJ, et al: Silicone granulomatous lymphadenopathy and siliconomas of the breast. Histol Histopathol 12:1003–1011, 1997.

224. Truong LD, Cartwright J, Goodman D, et al: Silicone lymphadenopathy associated with augmentation mammoplasty: morphologic features of nine cases. Am J Surg Pathol 12:484–491, 1988.

225. Listinsky CM: Common reactive erythrophagocytosis in axillary lymph nodes. Hum Pathol 89:189–192, 1988.

226. Shear KG, Bloebaum RD, Avent JM, et al: Analysis of lymph nodes for polyethylene particles in patients who have had a primary joint replacement. J Bone Joint Surg Am 78:497–504, 1996.

227. Gould E, Perez J, Albores-Saavedra J, et al: Signet ring cell sinus histiocytosis: a previously unrecognized histologic condition mimicking metastatic adenocarcinoma in lymph nodes. Am J Clin Pathol 92:509–512, 1989.

228. Frost AR, Shek YH, Lack EE: "Signet ring" sinus histiocytosis mimicking metastic adenocarcinoma: report of two cases with immunohistochemical and ultrastructural study. Mod Pathol 5:497–500, 1992.

229. Dorfman RF, Remington JS: Value of lymph node biopsy in the diagnosis of toxoplasmosis. N Engl J Med 289:878–881, 1973.

230. Plank L, Hansmann ML, Fischer R: The cytological spectrum of the monocytoid B-cell reaction: recognition of its large cell type. Histopathology 23:425–431, 1993.

231. Sheibani K, Fritz RM, Winberg CD, et al: "Monocytoid" cells in reactive follicular hyperplasia with and without multifocal histiocytic reactions: an immunohistochemical study of 21 cases including suspected cases of toxoplasmosis lymphadenitis. Am J Clin Pathol 81:453–458, 1984.

232. Risdall RJ, Brunning RD, Hernandez JJ: Bacteria-associated hemophagic syndrome. Cancer 54:2968–2972, 1984.

233. Risdall RJ, McKenna RW, Nesbitt ME, et al: Virus associated hemophagocytic syndrome. A benign histiocytic proliferation distinct from malignant histiocytosis. Cancer 44:993–1002, 1979.

234. Scott RB, Robb-Smith AHT: Histiocytic medullary reticulosis. Lancet 2:194–198, 1939.

235. Falini B, Pileri S, DeSolas I, et al: Peripheral T-cell lymphoma associated with hemophagocytic syndrome. Blood 75:434–444, 1990.

236. Jaffe ES, Costa J, Fauci AS, et al: Malignant lymphoma and erythrophagocytosis simulating malignant histiocytosis. Am J Med 75:741–749, 1983.

237. Karcher D, Head DR, Mullins JD: Malignant histiocytosis occurring in patients with acute lymphoblastic leukemia. Cancer 41:1967–1973, 1978.

238. Wong KF, Chan JK, Lo ES, et al: A study of the possible etiologic association of Epstein-Barr virus with reactive hemophagocytic syndrome in Hong Kong Chinese. Hum Pathol 27:1239–1242, 1996.

239. Ost A, Nilsson-Ardnor S, Henter JI: Autopsy findings in 27 children with haemophagocytic lymphohistiocytosis. Histopathology 32:310–316, 1998.

240. Arico M, Janka G, Fischer A, et al: Hemophagocytic lymphohistiocytosis. Report of 122 children from the International Registry. Leukemia 10:197–203, 1998.

241. Ladisch S, Holiman B, Poplack DG, et al: Immunodeficiency in familial erythrophagocytic lymphohistiocytosis. Lancet 1:581–583, 1978.

242. Stein H, Mason DY, Gerdes J, et al: The expression of the Hodgkin's disease associated antigen Ki-1 in reactive and

neoplastic tissue: evidence that Reed-Sternberg cells and histiocytic malignancies are derived from activated lymphoid cells. Blood 66:848–858, 1985.

243. Weiss LM, Picker LJ, Copenhaver CM, et al: Large-cell hematolymphoid neoplasms of uncertain lineage. Hum Pathol 19:967–973, 1988.

244. Weiss LM, Trela MJ, Cleary M, et al: Frequent immunoglobulin and T cell receptor gene rearrangement in "histiocytic" neoplasms. Am J Pathol 121:369–373, 1985.

245. Wilson MS, Weiss LM, Gatter KC, et al: Malignant histiocytosis: a reassessment of cases previously reported in 1975 based upon paraffin section immunophenotyping studies. Cancer 66:530–536, 1990.

246. Sheibani K, Burke JS, Swartz WG, et al: Monocytoid B cell lymphoma. Clinicopathologic study of 21 cases of a unique type of low grade lymphoma. Cancer 62:1531–1538, 1988.

247. Rosai J, Dorfman RF: Sinus histiocytosis with massive lymphadenopathy: a pseudolymphomatous benign disorder. Analysis of 34 cases. Cancer 30:1174–1188, 1972.

248. Foucar E, Rosai J, Dorfman RF: Sinus histiocytosis with massive lymphadenopathy (Rosai-Dorfman disease). Review of the entity. Semin Diagn Pathol 7:19–73, 1990.

249. Rosai J, Dorfman RF: Sinus histiocytosis with massive lymphadenopathy: a newly recognized benign clinicopathologic entity. Arch Pathol 87:63–70, 1969.

250. Stastny KF, Wilderson ML, Hamati HF, et al: Cytologic features of sinus histiocytosis with massive lymphadenopathy. A report of three cases. Acta Cytol 41:871–876, 1997.

251. Deshpande V, Verma K: Fine needle aspiration cytology of Rosai-Dorfman disease. Cytopathology 9:329–335, 1998.

252. Eisen RN, Buckley PJ, Rosai J: Immunophenotypic characterization of sinus histiocytosis with massive lymphadenopathy (Rosai-Dorfman disease). Semin Diagn Pathol 7:74–82, 1990.

253. Naiem M, Gerdes J, Abdulaziz A, et al: Production of a monoclonal antibody reactive with human dendritic cells and its use in the immunohistological analysis of lymphoid tissue. J Clin Pathol 36:167–175, 1983.

254. Parwaresch MR, Radzun HJ, Hansmann M-L, et al: Monoclonal antibody Ki-M4 specifically recognizes human dendritic cells (follicular dendritic cells) and their possible precursors in blood. Blood 62:585–590, 1983.

255. Bonetti F, Chilosi M, Menestrina F, et al: Immunohistological analysis of Rosai-Dorfman histiocytosis. A disease of S-100$^+$ CD1$^-$ histiocytes. Virchows Arch A Pathol Anat Histopathol 411:129–135, 1987.

256. Dobbins WO, Ruffin JM: A light and electron microscope study of bacterial invasion in Whipple's disease. Am J Pathol 51:225–242, 1967.

257. Relman DA, Schmidt TM, McDermott RP, et al: Identification of the uncultured bacillus of Whipple's disease. N Engl J Med 327:293–301, 1992.

258. Fleming JL, Wiesner RH, Shorter RG: Whipple's disease: clinical, biochemical, and histopathologic features and assessment of treatment in 29 patients. Mayo Clin Proc 63:539–551, 1988.

259. Sieracki JC, Fine G: Whipple's disease—observations on systemic involvement: II. Gross and histologic observations. Arch Pathol 67:81–93, 1959.

260. Ravel R: Histopathology of lymph nodes after lymphangiography. Am J Clin Pathol 46:335–340, 1966.

261. Cleary KR, Osborne BM, Butler JJ: Lymph node infarction foreshadowing malignant lymphoma. Am J Surg Pathol 6:435–442, 1982.

262. Dorfman RF, Berry GJ: Kikuchi's histiocytic necrotizing lymphadenitis: an analysis of 108 cases with emphasis on differential diagnosis. Semin Diagn Pathol 5:329–345, 1988.

263. Chamulak GA, Brynes RK, Nathwani BN: Kikuchi-Fujimoto disease mimicking malignant lymphoma. Am J Surg Pathol 14:514–523, 1990.

264. Fujimoto Y, Kozima Y, Yamaguchi K: Cervical subacute necrotizing lymphadenitis. A new clinicopathologic entity. Naika 20:920–927, 1972.

265. Kikuchi M: Lymphadenitis showing focal reticulum cell hyperplasia with nuclear debris and phagocytes: a clinico-pathological study [in Japanese]. Nippon Ketsueki Gakkai Zasshi 35:379–380, 1972.

266. Kuo T: Kikuchi's disease (histiocytic necrotizing lymphadenitis). A clinicopathologic study of 79 cases with an analysis of histologic subtypes, immunohistology, and DNA ploidy. Am J Surg Pathol 19:798–809, 1995.

267. Turner RR, Martin J, Dorfman RF: Necrotizing lymphadenitis: a study of 30 cases. Am J Surg Pathol 7:115–123, 1983.

268. Pileri S, Kikuchi M, Helbron D, et al: Histiocytic necrotizing lymphadenitis without granulocytic infiltration. Virchows Arch A Pathol Anat Histol 395:257–271, 1982.

269. Feller AC, Lennert K, Stein H, et al: Immunohistology and aetiology of histiocytic necrotizing lymphadenitis: report of three instructive cases. Histopathology 7:825–829, 1983.

270. Unger PD, Rappaport KM, Strauchen JA: Necrotizing lymphadenitis (Kikuchi's disease): report of four cases of an unusual pseudolymphomatous lesion and immunologic marker studies. Arch Pathol Lab Med 111:1031–1034, 1987.

271. Dorfman RF: Histiocytic necrotizing lymphadenitis of Kikuchi and Fujimoto. Arch Pathol Lab Med 111:1026–1029, 1987.

272. Aqel N, Henry K, Woodrow D: Skin involvement in Kikuchi's disease: an immunocytochemical and immunofluorescence study. Virchows Arch 430:349–352, 1997.

273. Sumiyoshi Y, Kikuchi M, Takeshita M, et al: Immunohistologic studies of Kikuchi's disease. Hum Pathol 24:1114–1119, 1993.

274. Menasce LP, Banerjee SS, Edmondson D, et al: Histiocytic necrotizing lymphadenitis (Kikuchi-Fujimoto disease): continuing diagnostic difficulties. Histopathology 33:248–254, 1998.

275. Giesker DW, Pastuszak WT, Forouhar FA, et al: Lymph node biopsy for early diagnosis in Kawasaki disease. Am J Surg Pathol 6:493–501, 1982.

276. Kurata T, Iwasaki T, Sata T, et al: Viral pathology of human herpesvirus 6 infection. In Proceedings of the International Conference on Immunobiology and Prophylaxis of Human Herpesvirus Infections. New York, Plenum, 1990, pp 39–41.

277. Huh J, Kang GH, Gong G, et al: Kaposi's sarcoma–associated herpesvirus in Kikuchi's disease. Hum Pathol 29:1091–1096, 1998.

278. Medeiros LJ, Kaynor B, Harris NL: Lupus lymphadenitis: report of a case with immunohistologic studies on frozen sections. Hum Pathol 20:295–299, 1989.

279. Kawasaki T: Acute febrile mucocutaneous syndrome with lymphoid involvement with specific desquamation of fingers and toes in children. Jpn J Allergy 16:178–222, 1967.

280. Yamagihara R, Todd JK: Acute febrile mucocutaneous lymph node syndrome. Am J Dis Child 134:603–614, 1980.

281. Jason J, Gregg L, Han A, et al: Immunoregulatory changes in Kawasaki disease. Clin Immunol Immunopathol 84:296–306, 1997.

282. Rowley AH, Eckerley CA, Jack HM, et al: IgA plasma cells in vascular tissue of patients with Kawasaki syndrome. J Immunol 159:5946–5955, 1997.

283. Murray JC, Bomgaars LR, Carcamo B, et al: Lymphoid malignancies following Kawasaki disease. Am J Hematol 50:299–300, 1995.

284. Bascom R, Johns CJ: The natural history and management of sarcoidosis. Adv Intern Med 31:213–241, 1986.

285. Cook MG: The size and histological appearances of mesenteric lymph nodes in Crohn's disease. Gut 13:970–972, 1972.

286. Hollingsworth HC, Longo DL, Jaffe ES: Small noncleaved cell lymphoma associated with florid epithelioid granulomatous response: a clinicopathologic study of seven patients. Am J Surg Pathol 17:51–59, 1993.

287. Braylan RC, Long JC, Jaffe ES, et al: Malignant lymphoma obscured by concomitant extensive epithelioid granulomas: report of three cases with similar clinicopathologic features. Cancer 39:1146–1155, 1977.

288. Wear DJ, Margileth AM, Hadfield TL, et al: Cat-scratch disease: a bacterial infection. Science 221:1403–1404, 1983.

289. Stastny JF, Wakely RE, Frable WJ: Cytologic features of necrotizing granulomatous inflammation consistent with cat-scratch disease. Diagn Cytopathol 15:108–115, 1996.

290. Walzer PD, Armstrong D: Lymphogranuloma venereum presenting as supraclavicular and inguinal lymphadenopathy. Sex Transm Dis 4:12–14, 1977.

291. Schapers RFM, Reif R, Lennert K, et al: Mesenteric lymphad-

enitis due to *Yersinia enterocolitica.* Virchows Arch A Pathol Anat Histol 390:127–138, 1981.

292. Reid JD, Wolinsky E: Histopathology of lymphadenitis caused by atypical mycobacteria. Am Rev Respir Dis 99:8–12, 1969.

293. Ridley DS, Jopling WH: Classification of leprosy according to immunity: a five-group system. Int J Lepr Other Mycobact Dis 34:255–273, 1966.

294. Binford CH: Pathology—the doorway to the understanding of leprosy. Am J Clin Pathol 51:681–698, 1969.

295. Goodwin RA, Shapiro JL, Thurman GH, et al: Disseminated histoplasmosis: clinical and pathologic correlations. Medicine (Baltimore) 59:1–33, 1980.

296. Bonner JR, Alexander WJ, Dismukes WE, et al: Disseminated histoplasmosis in patients with the acquired immune deficiency syndrome. Arch Intern Med 144:2178–2181, 1984.

297. Barnett RN, Hull JG, Vortel V: *Pneumocystis carinii* in lymph nodes and spleen. Arch Pathol Lab Med 88:175–180, 1969.

298. Maurin M, Birtles R, Raoult D: Current knowledge of *Bartonella* species. Eur J Clin Microbiol 16:487–506, 1997.

299. Catchpole RM, Variakojis D, Vardiman JW, et al: Cat-scratch disease. Identification of bacteria in seven cases of lymphadenitis. Am J Surg Pathol 10:276–281, 1986.

300. Not T, Canciani M, Buratti E, et al: Serologic response to *Bartonella henselae* in patients with cat scratch disese and in sick and healthy children. Acta Paediatr 88:284–289, 1999.

301. Sander A, Posselt M, Bohm N, et al: Detection of *Bartonella henselae* DNA by two different PCR assays and determination of the genotypes of strains involved in histologically defined cat scratch disease. J Clin Microbiol 37:993–997, 1999.

302. Litwin CM, Martins TB, Hill HR: Immunologic response to *Bartonella henselae* as determined by enzyme immunoassay and Western blot analysis. Am J Clin Pathol 108:202–209, 1997.

303. Hadfield TL, Lamy Y, Wear DJ: Demonstration of *Chlamydia trachomatis* in inguinal lymphadenitis of lymphogranuloma venereum: a light microscopy, electron microscopy and polymerase chain reaction study. Mod Pathol 8:927–929, 1995.

304. Frizzera G, Moran EM, Rappaport H: Angioimmunoblastic lymphadenopathy: diagnosis and clinical course. Am J Med 59:803–818, 1975.

305. Lukes RJ, Tindle BH: Immunoblastic lymphadenopathy: a hyperimmune entity resembling Hodgkin's disease. N Engl J Med 292:1–8, 1975.

306. Frizzera G, Kaneko Y, Sakurai M: Angioimmunoblastic lymphadenopathy and related disorders: a retrospective look in search of definitions. Leukemia 3:1–5, 1989.

307. Pirker R, Schwarzmeier JD, Radaszkiewicz T, et al: B-immunoblastic lymphoma arising in angioimmunoblastic lymphadenopathy. Acta Haematol 75:105–109, 1986.

308. Abruzzo LV, Schmidt K, Weiss LM, et al: B cell lymphoma evolving from AILD: a case with oligoclonal gene rearrangements associated with Epstein-Barr virus. Blood 82:241–246, 1993.

309. Watanabe S, Sato Y, Shimoyama M, et al: Immunoblastic lymphadenopathy, angioimmunoblastic lymphadenopathy, and IBL-like T-cell lymphoma. A spectrum of T-cell neoplasia. Cancer 58:2224–2232, 1986.

310. Watanabe S, Shimosato Y, Shimoyama M, et al: Adult T cell lymphoma with hypergammaglobulinemia. Cancer 46:2472–2483, 1980.

311. Weiss LM, Strickler JG, Dorfman RF, et al: Clonal T-cell populations in angioimmunoblastic lymphadenopathy and angioimmunoblastic lymphadenopathy–like lymphoma. Am J Pathol 122:392–397, 1986.

312. Steinberg AD, Seldin MF, Jaffe ES, et al: NIH Conference. Angioimmunoblastic lymphadenopathy with dysproteinemia. Ann Intern Med 108:575–584, 1988.

313. Hodgkin T: On some morbid appearances of the absorbent glands and spleen. Med Chir Trans 17:68–114, 1832.

314. Wilks S: Cases of enlargement of the lymphatic glands and spleen (or Hodgkin's disease), with remarks. Guys Hosp Rep 11:56–67, 1865.

315. Kaplan HS: Hodgkin's disease: unfolding concepts concerning its nature, management and prognosis. Cancer 45:2439–2474, 1980.

316. Kaplan HS: Hodgkin's disease: biology, treatment, prognosis. Blood 57:813–822, 1981.

317. Ohshima K, Ishiguro M, Ohgami A, et al: Genetic analysis of sorted Hodgkin and Reed-Sternberg cells using comparative genomic hybridization. Int J Cancer 82:250–255, 1999.

318. Stein H, Hummel M: Cellular origin and clonality of classic Hodgkin's lymphoma: immunophenotypic and molecular studies. Semin Hematol 36:233–241, 1999.

319. Deng F, Lu G, Li G, et al: Hodgkin's disease: immunoglobulin heavy and light chain gene rearrangements revealed in single Hodgkin/Reed-Sternberg cells. Mol Pathol 52:37–41, 1999.

320. Cossman J, Annunziata CM, Barash S, et al: Reed-Sternberg cell genome expression supports a B-cell lineage. Blood 94:411–416, 1999.

321. Lukes RJ, Butler JJ: The pathology and nomenclature of Hodgkin's disease. Cancer Res 26:1063–1081, 1966.

322. Lukes RJ: Criteria for involvement of lymph node, bone marrow, spleen, and liver in Hodgkin's disease. Cancer Res 31:1755–1767, 1971.

323. Ries LAG, Kosary CL, Hankey BF, et al: SEER Cancer Statistics Review: 1973–1994. Bethesda, MD, US Department of Health and Human Services, National Institutes of Health, National Cancer Institute, 1997. NIH publication 97–2789.

324. Boring CC, Squires TS, Tong T: Cancer statistics. Ca Cancer J Clin 43:7–26, 1993.

325. Chen YZ, Zheng T, Chou MC, et al: The increase of Hodgkin's disease incidence among young adults. Experience in Connecticut. Cancer 79:2209–2218, 1997.

326. MacMahon B: Epidemiology of Hodgkin's disease. Cancer Res 26:1189–1200, 1966.

327. MacMahon B: Epidemiological evidence on the nature of Hodgkin's disease. Cancer 10:1045–1054, 1957.

328. Vianna NJ, Thind IS, Louria DB, et al: Epidemiologic and histologic patterns of Hodgkin's disease in blacks. Cancer 40:3133–3139, 1977.

329. Correa P, O'Conor GT: Geographic pathology of lymphoreticular tumors: summary of survey from the geographic pathology committee of the International Union Against Cancer. J Natl Cancer Inst 50:1609–1617, 1973.

330. Correa P, O'Conor GT: Epidemiologic patterns of Hodgkin's disease. Int J Cancer 8:192–201, 1971.

331. Hartge P, Devesa SS, Fraumeni JF: Hodgkin's disease and non-Hodgkin's lymphomas. Cancer Surv 19/20:423–453, 1994.

332. Glaser SL: Hodgkin's disease in black populations: a review of the epidemiologic literature. Semin Oncol 17:643–659, 1990.

333. Horn JW, Devesa SS, Burhansstipanov L: Cancer incidence, mortality and survival among racial and ethnic minority groups in the United States. *In* Schottenfeld D, Fraumeni JF (eds): Cancer Epidemiology and Prevention. New York, Oxford Press, 1996, p 192.

334. Chakravarti A, Halloran SL, Bale SJ, et al: Etiological heterogeneity in Hodgkin's disease: HLA linked and unlinked determinants of susceptibility independent of histological concordance. Genet Epidemiol 3:407–415, 1986.

335. Gutensohn NM, Shapiro DS: Social class risk factors among children with Hodgkin's disease. Int J Cancer 30:433–435, 1982.

336. Cozen W, Katz J, Mack T: Risk patterns of Hodgkin's disease in Los Angeles vary by cell type. Cancer Epidemiol Biomarkers Prev 1:261–268, 1992.

337. Roithman S, Tourani J-M, Andrieu J-M: Hodgkin's disease in HIV-infected intravenous drug abusers. N Engl J Med 323:275–276, 1990.

338. Garnier G, Taillan B, Michiels JF: HIV-associated Hodgkin disease. Ann Intern Med 115:233–233, 1991.

339. Schoeppel SL, Hoppe RT, Dorfman RF, et al: Hodgkin's disease in homosexual men with generalized lymphadenopathy associated with individuals at risk for the acquired immune deficiency syndrome. Ann Intern Med 102:68–70, 1985.

340. Robertson SJ, Lowman JT, Grufferman S, et al: Familial Hodgkin's disease. A clinical and laboratory investigation. Cancer 59:1314–1319, 1987.

341. Bowers TK, Moldow CF, Bloomfield CD, et al: Familial Hodgkin's disease and the major histocompatibility complex. Vox Sang 33:273–277, 1977.

342. Donhuijsen-Ant R, Abken H, Bornkamm G, et al: Fatal Hodgkin and non-Hodgkin lymphoma associated with persistent Epstein-Barr virus in four brothers. Ann Intern Med 109:946–952, 1988.

343. Marshall WH, Barnard JM, Buehler SK, et al: HLA in familial Hodgkin's disease: results and new hypothesis. Int J Cancer 19:450–455, 1977.

344. Grufferman S, Cole P, Smith PG, et al: Hodgkin's disease in siblings. N Engl J Med 296:248–250, 1977.

345. Razis DV, Diamond HD, Craver LF: Familial Hodgkin's disease: its significance and implications. Ann Intern Med 51:933–971, 1959.

346. Grufferman S, Barton JW, Eby NL: Increased sex concordance of sibling pairs with Behçet's disease, Hodgkin's disease, multiple sclerosis and sarcoidosis. Am J Epidemiol 126:365–369, 1987.

347. Mack TM, Cozen W, Shibata DK, et al: Concordance in identical twins suggests genetic susceptibility to young adult Hodgkin's disease. N Engl J Med 332:413–418, 1994.

348. Sasazuki T, McDevitt HO, Grumet FC: The association between genes in the major histocompatibility complex and disease susceptibility. Annu Rev Med 28:425–452, 1977.

349. Gutensohn N, Cole P: Childhood social environment and Hodgkin's disease. N Engl J Med 304:135–140, 1981.

350. Gutensohn N, Cole P: Epidemiology of Hodgkin's disease in the young. Int J Cancer 19:595–604, 1977.

351. Chezzi C, Dettori G, Manzari V, et al: Simultaneous detection of reverse transcriptase and high weight RNA in tissue of patients with Hodgkin's disease and patients with leukemia. Proc Natl Acad Sci USA 73:4649–4652, 1976.

352. Tesch H, Jucker M, Kronke M, et al: Analysis of HTLV-1 in Hodgkin's disease. Leuk Lymphoma 4:371–374, 1991.

353. Komaroff AL: Human herpesvirus-6 and human disease. Am J Clin Pathol 93:836–837, 1990.

354. Krueger GRF, Ablashi DV, Salahuddin SZ, et al: Diagnosis and differential diagnosis of progressive lymphoproliferation and malignant lymphoma in persistent active herpesvirus infection. J Virol Methods 21:255–264, 1988.

355. Torelli G, Marasca R, Luppi M, et al: Human herpesvirus-6 in human lymphomas: identification of specific sequences in Hodgkin's lymphomas by polymerase chain reaction. Blood 77:2251–2258, 1991.

356. Josephs SF, Buchbinder A, Streicher HZ, et al: Detection of human B-lymphotropic virus (human herpesvirus 6) sequences in B cell lymphoma tissues of three patients. Leukemia 2:132–135, 1988.

357. Jarrett R, Onions D: Viruses and Hodgkin's disease. Leukemia 6:14–17, 1992.

358. Munoz N, Davidson RJL, Witthoff B, et al: Viruses and Hodgkin's disease. Int J Cancer 22:10–13, 1978.

359. Rosdahl N, Larsen S, Clemmesen J: Hodgkin's disease in patients with previous infectious mononucleosis: 30 years' experience. Br Med J 2:253–256, 1974.

360. Mueller N, Evans A, Harris NA, et al: Hodgkin's disease and Epstein-Barr virus: altered antibody pattern before diagnosis. N Engl J Med 320:689–695, 1989.

361. Weiss LM, Strickler JG, Warnke RA, et al: Epstein-Barr viral DNA in tissues of Hodgkin's disease. Am J Pathol 129:86–91, 1987.

362. Weiss LM, Mohaved LA, Warnke RA, et al: Detection of Epstein-Barr viral genomes in Reed-Sternberg cells of Hodgkin's disease. N Engl J Med 320:502–506, 1989.

363. Anagnostopoulos I, Herbst H, Niedobitek G, et al: Demonstration of monoclonal EBV genomes in Hodgkin's disease and Ki-1–positive anaplastic large cell lymphoma by combined Southern blot and in situ hybridization. Blood 74:810–816, 1989.

364. Wu TC, Mann RB, Charache P, et al: Detection of EBV gene expression in Reed-Sternberg cells of Hodgkin's disease. Int J Cancer 46:801–804, 1990.

365. Brousset P, Chittal S, Schlaifer D, et al: Detection of Epstein-Barr virus messenger RNA in Reed-Sternberg cells of Hodgkin's disease by in situ hybridization with biotinylated probes on specially processed modified acetone methyl benzoate xylene (ModAMeX) sections. Blood 77:1781–1786, 1991.

366. Herbst H, Steinbrecher E, Niedobitek G, et al: Distribution and phenotype of Epstein-Barr virus–harboring cells in Hodgkin's disease. Blood 80:484–491, 1992.

367. Weiss LM, Chen Y-Y, Liu X-F, et al: Epstein-Barr virus and Hodgkin's disease: a correlative in situ hybridization and polymerase chain reaction study. Am J Pathol 139:1259–1265, 1991.

368. Pallesen G, Hamilton DS, Rowe M, et al: Expression of Epstein-Barr virus latent gene products in tumour cells of Hodgkin's disease [see comments]. Lancet 337:320–322, 1991.

369. Armstrong AA, Gallagher A, Krajewski AS, et al: The expression of the EBV latent membrane protein (LMP-1) is independent of CD23 and bcl-2 in Reed-Sternberg cells in Hodgkin's disease. Histopathology 21:72–73, 1992.

370. Weiss LM, Chang KL: The association of the Epstein-Barr virus with hematolymphoid neoplasia. Adv Anat Pathol 3:1–15, 1996.

371. Kaplan H: Hodgkin's Disease. Cambridge, MA, Harvard University Press, 1980.

372. Rosenberg SA, Kaplan HS: Evidence for an orderly progression in the spread of Hodgkin's disease. Cancer Res 26:1225–1231, 1966.

373. Mauch PM, Kalish LA: Patterns of presentation of Hodgkin's disease. Implications for etiology and pathogenesis. Cancer 71:2062–2071, 1993.

374. Lister TA, Crowther D, Sutcliffe SB, et al: Report of a committee convened to discuss the evaluation of staging of patients with Hodgkin's disease: Cotswolds meeting. J Clin Oncol 7:1630–1636, 1989.

375. Lister TA, Crowther D: Staging for Hodgkin's disease. Semin Oncol 17:696–703, 1990.

376. Urba WJ, Longo DL: Hodgkin's disease. N Engl J Med 326:678–687, 1992.

377. Leibenhaut MH, Hoppe RT, Efron B, et al: Prognostic indicators of laparotomy findings in clinical stage I–II supradiaphragmatic Hodgkin's disease. J Clin Oncol 7:81–91, 1989.

378. Mauch P, Larson D, Osteen R: Prognostic factors for positive surgical staging in patients with Hodgkin's disease. J Clin Oncol 8:257–265, 1990.

379. Mauch P, Somers R: Controversies in the use of diagnostic staging laparotomy and splenectomy in the management of Hodgkin's disease. Ann Oncol 3:41–43, 1992.

380. Moormeier JA, Williams SF, Golomb HM: The staging of Hodgkin's disease. Hematol Oncol Clin North Am 3:237–251, 1989.

381. Ng AK, Weeks JC, Mauch PM, et al: Laparotomy versus no laparotomy in the management of early-stage, favorable-prognosis Hodgkin's disease: a decision analysis. J Clin Oncol 17:241–252, 1999.

382. Mason DY, Banks PM, Chan J, et al: Nodular lymphocyte predominance Hodgkin's disease. A distinct clinicopathological entity. Am J Surg Pathol 18:526–530, 1994.

383. Diehl V, Sextro M, Fanklin J, et al: Clinical presentation, course, and prognostic factors in lymphocyte-predominant Hodgkin's disease and lymphocyte-rich classical Hodgkin's disease: report from the European Task Force on Lymphoma Project on Lymphocyte-Predominant Hodgkin's Disease. J Clin Oncol 17:776–783, 1999.

384. Orlandi E, Lazzarino M, Brusamolino E, et al: Nodular lymphocyte predominance Hodgkin's disease: long-term observation reveals a continuous pattern of recurrence. Leuk Lymphoma 26:359–368, 1997.

385. Chan WC: Cellular origin of nodular lymphocyte-predominant Hodgkin's lymphoma: immunophenotypic and molecular studies. Semin Hematol 36:242–252, 1999.

386. Sacks EL, Donaldson SS, Gordon J, et al: Epithelioid granulomas associated with Hodgkin's disease: clinical correlations in 55 previously untreated patients. Cancer 41:562–567, 1978.

387. Lukes RJ: Relationship of histologic features to clinical stages in Hodgkin's disease. Am J Roentgenol 90:944–955, 1963.

388. Ashton-Key M, Thorpe PA, Allen JP, et al: Follicular Hodgkin's disease. Am J Surg Pathol 19:1294–1299, 1995.

389. Strickler JG, Michie SA, Warnke RA, et al: The "syncytial variant" of nodular sclerosing Hodgkin's disease. Am J Surg Pathol 10:470–477, 1986.

390. Ferry JA, Linggood RM, Convery KM, et al: Hodgkin's disease, nodular sclerosis type: implications of histologic subclassification. Cancer 71:457–463, 1993.

391. MacLennan KA, Bennett MH, Tu A, et al: Relationship of histopathologic features to survival and relapse in nodular sclerosing Hodgkin's disease: a study of 1,659 patients. Cancer 64:1686–1693, 1989.

392. Georgii A, Fischer R, Hubner K, et al: Classification of Hodgkin's disease biopsies by a panel of four histopathologists. Report of 1,140 patients from the German National Trial. Leuk Lymphoma 9:365–370, 1993.

393. Wijlhuizen TJ, Vrints LW, Jairam R, et al: Grades of nodular sclerosis (NSI-NSII) in Hodgkin's disease: are they of independent prognostic value? Cancer 63:1150–1153, 1989.

394. Baur AS, Meuge-Marow C, Michel G, et al: Prognostic value of follicular dendritic cells in nodular sclerosing Hodgkin's disease. Histopathology 32:512–520, 1998.

395. Colby TV, Hoppe RT, Warnke RA: Hodgkin's disease: a clinicopathologic study of 659 cases. Cancer 49:1848–1858, 1982.

396. Colby TV, Warnke RA: The histology of the initial relapse of Hodgkin's disease. Cancer 45:289–292, 1980.

397. Strum SB, Rappaport H: Consistency of histologic subtypes in Hodgkin's disease in simultaneous and sequential biopsy specimens. Natl Cancer Inst Monogr 36:253–260, 1973.

398. Dolginow D, Colby TV: Recurrent Hodgkin's disease in treated sites. Cancer 48:1124–1126, 1981.

399. Colby TV, Hoppe RT, Warnke RA: Hodgkin's disease at autopsy: 1972–1977. Cancer 47:1852–1862, 1981.

400. Das DK, Gupta SK, Datta BM, et al: Fine needle aspiration cytodiagnosis of Hodgkin's disease and its subtypes. I. Scope and limitations. Acta Cytol 34:329–336, 1989.

401. Weiss LM, Chang KL: Molecular biologic studies of Hodgkin's disease. Semin Diagn Pathol 9:272–278, 1992.

402. Weiss LM, Strickler JG, Hu E, et al: Immunoglobulin gene rearrangements in Hodgkin's disease. Hum Pathol 17:1009–1014, 1986.

403. Schmid C, Pan L, Diss T, et al: Expression of B-cell antigens by Hodgkin's and Reed-Sternberg cells. Am J Pathol 139:701–707, 1991.

404. Kuzu I, Delsol G, Jones M, et al: Expression of the Ig-associated heterodimer (mb-1 and B29) in Hodgkin's disease. Histopathology 22:141–144, 1993.

405. Orscheschek K, Mere H, Hell J, et al: Large-cell anaplastic lymphoma–specific translocation (t[2;5][p23;q35]) in Hodgkin's disease—indication of a common pathogenesis? Lancet 345:87–90, 1995.

406. Weiss LM, Lopategui JR, Sun L-H, et al: Absence of the t(2;5) in Hodgkin's disease. Blood 85:2845–2847, 1995.

407. Ladanyi M, Cavalchire G, Morris SW, et al: Reverse transcriptase polymerase chain reaction for the Ki-1 anaplastic large cell lymphoma–associated t(2;5) translocation in Hodgkin's disease. Am J Pathol 145:1296–1300, 1994.

408. Tamaru J, Hummel M, Zemlin M, et al: Hodgkin's disease with a B-cell phenotype often shows a VDJ rearrangement and somatic mutations in the $V_H$ genes. Blood 84:708–715, 1994.

409. Chang KL, Chen Y-Y, Shibata D, et al: In situ hybridization methodology for the detection of EBV EBER-1 RNA in paraffin-embedded tissues, as applied to normal and neoplastic tissues. Diagn Mol Pathol 1:246–255, 1992.

410. Cabanillas F: A review and interpretation of cytogenetic abnormalities identified in Hodgkin's disease. Hematol Oncol 6:271–274, 1988.

411. Chittal SM, Caveriviere P, Schwarting R, et al: Monoclonal antibodies in the diagnosis of Hodgkin's disease: the search for a rational panel. Am J Surg Pathol 12:9–21, 1988.

412. Chang KL, Arber DA, Weiss LM: CD20: a review. Appl Immunohistochem 4:1–15, 1996.

413. Arber DA, Weiss LM: CD15: a review. Appl Immunohistochem 1:17–30, 1993.

414. Enblad G, Sundstrom C, Glimerlius B: Immunohistochemical characteristics of Hodgkin and Reed-Sternberg cells in relation to age and clinical outcome. Histopathology 22:535–541, 1993.

415. Hall PA, d'Ardenne AJ, Stansfeld AG: Paraffin section immunohistochemistry. II. Hodgkin's disease and large cell anaplastic (Ki1) lymphoma. Histopathology 13:161–169, 1988.

416. Agnarsson BA, Kadin ME: The immunophenotype of Reed-Sternberg cells. A study of 50 cases of Hodgkin's disease using fixed frozen tissues. Cancer 63:2083–2087, 1989.

417. Medeiros LJ, Weiss LM, Warnke RA, et al: Utility of combining antigranulocyte with antileukocyte antibodies in differentiating Hodgkin's disease from non-Hodgkin's lymphoma. Cancer 62:2475–2481, 1988.

418. Pinkus GS, Thomas P, Said JW: Leu-M1—a marker for Reed-Sternberg cells in Hodgkin's disease. An immunoperoxidase study of paraffin-embedded tissues. Am J Pathol 119:244–252, 1985.

419. Ree HJ, Neiman RS, Martin AW, et al: Paraffin section markers for Reed-Sternberg cells. A comparative study of peanut agglutinin, Leu-M1, LN-2, and Ber H2. Cancer 63:2030–2036, 1989.

420. Sheibani K, Battifora H, Burke JS, et al: Leu-M1 antigen in human neoplasms. An immunohistologic study of 400 cases. Am J Surg Pathol 10:227–236, 1986.

421. Arber DA, Windisch LB, Griffin SH: Paraffin-section evaluation of proliferative activity in Hodgkin's disease. Lack of correlation with CD15, CD30, or Epstein-Barr virus latent membrane protein expression. Appl Immunohistochem 3:245–249, 1995.

422. Chu W-S, Abbondanzo SL, Frizzera G: Inconsistency of the immunophenotype of Reed-Sternberg cells in simultaneous and consecutive specimens from the same patients. A paraffin section evaluation in 56 patients. Am J Pathol 141:11–17, 1992.

423. Vasef MA, Alsabeh R, Medeiros LJ, et al: Immunophenotype of Reed-Sternberg and Hodgkin's cells in sequential biopsy specimens of Hodgkin's disease. A HIER-based study. Am J Clin Pathol 108:54–59, 1997.

424. Carbone A, Gloghini A, Gattei V, et al: Reed-Sternberg cells of classical Hodgkin's disease react with plasma cell–specific monoclonal antibody B-B4 and express human syndecan-1. Blood 89:3787–3794, 1997.

425. Momose H, Jaffe ES, Shin SS, et al: Chronic lymphocytic leukemia/small lymphocytic lymphoma with Reed-Sternberg–like cells and possible transformation to Hodgkin's disease. Mediation by Epstein-Barr virus. Am J Surg Pathol 16:859–867, 1992.

426. McBride JA, Rodriguez J, Luthra R, et al: T-cell–rich B large-cell lymphoma simulating lymphocyte-rich Hodgkin's disease. Am J Surg Pathol 20:193–201, 1996.

427. Delabie J, Greiner TC, Chan WC, et al: Concurrent lymphocyte predominance Hodgkin's disease and T-cell lymphoma. A report of three cases. Am J Surg Pathol 20:355–362, 1996.

428. Gonzalez CL, Medeiros LJ, Jaffe ES: Composite lymphoma. A clinicopathologic analysis of nine patients with Hodgkin's disease and B-cell non-Hodgkin's lymphoma. Am J Clin Pathol 96:81–89, 1991.

429. Zarate-Osorno A, Medeiros LJ, Longo DL, et al: Non-Hodgkin's lymphomas arising in patients successfully treated for Hodgkin's disease. A clinical, histologic, and immunophenotypic study of 14 cases. Am J Surg Pathol 16:885–895, 1992.

430. Zarate-Osorno A, Medeiros LJ, Kingma DW, et al: Hodgkin's disease following non-Hodgkin's lymphoma. A clinicopathologic and immunophenotypic study of nine cases. Am J Surg Pathol 17:123–132, 1993.

431. Lorenzen J, Hansmann ML, Pezzella F, et al: Expression of the bcl-2 oncogene product and chromosomal translocation t(14;18) in Hodgkin's disease. Hum Pathol 23:1205–1209, 1992.

432. Said JW, Sassoon AF, Shintaku IP, et al: Absence of bcl-2 major breakpoint region and $J_H$ gene rearrangement in lymphocyte predominance Hodgkin's disease: results of Southern blot analysis and polymerase chain reaction. Am J Pathol 138:261–264, 1991.

433. Benharroch D, Meguerian-Bedoyan Z, Lamant L, et al: ALK-positive lymphoma: a single disease with a broad spectrum of morphology. Blood 91:2076–2084, 1998.

434. Rosso R, Paulli M, Magrini U, et al: Anaplastic large cell lymphoma, CD30/Ki-1 positive, expressing the CD15/Leu-M1 antigen. Immunohistochemical and morphological relationships to Hodgkin's disease. Virchow's Arch A Pathol Anat Histopathol 416:229–235, 1990.

435. Pittaluga S, Wlodarska I, Pulford K, et al: The monoclonal antibody ALK1 identifies a distinct morphological subtype of anaplastic large cell lymphoma associated with 2p23/ALK rearrangements. Am J Pathol 151:343–351, 1997.

436. Pulford K, Lamant L, Morris SW, et al: Detection of anaplastic lymphoma kinase (ALK) and nucleolar protein nucleophosmin (NPM)–ALK proteins in normal and neoplastic cells with the monoclonal antibody ALK1. Blood 89:1394–1404, 1997.

437. Cataldo KA, Jalal SM, Law ME, et al: Detection of t(2;5) in anaplastic large cell lymphoma: comparison of immunohistochemical studies, FISH, and RT-PCR in paraffin-embedded tissue. Am J Surg Pathol 23:1386–1392, 1999.

438. Kadin ME, Morris SW: The t(2;5) in human lymphomas. Leuk Lymphoma 29:249–256, 1998.

439. Lamant L, Meggetto F, Al Saati T, et al: High incidence of the t(2;5)(p23;q35) translocation in anaplastic large cell lymphoma and its lack of detection in Hodgkin's disease. Comparison of cytogenetic analysis, reverse transcriptase–polymerase chain reaction, and P-80 immunostaining. Blood 87:284–291, 1996.

440. Devesa SS, Fears T: Non-Hodgkin's lymphoma time trends: United States and International Data. Cancer Res 52(suppl):5432–5440, 1992.

441. Gail MH, Pluda JM, Rabkin CS, et al: Projections of the incidence of non-Hodgkin's lymphoma related to acquired immunodeficiency syndrome. J Natl Cancer Inst 83:695–701, 1991.

442. Scherr PA, Hutchison GB, Neiman RS: Non-Hodgkin's lymphoma and occupational exposure. Cancer Res 52(suppl):5503–5509, 1992.

443. Hoar SK, Blair A, Holmes FF, et al: Agricultural herbicide and risk of lymphoma and soft tissue sarcoma. JAMA 256:1141–1147, 1986.

444. Cantor KP, Blair A, Everett G, et al: Hair dye use and risk of leukemia and lymphoma. Am J Public Health 78:570–571, 1988.

445. Jaffe ES, Blattner WA, Blayney DW, et al: The pathologic spectrum of adult T-cell leukemia/lymphoma in the United States. Human T-cell leukemia/lymphoma virus–associated lymphoid malignancies. Am J Surg Pathol 8:263–275, 1984.

446. Rosenberg SA: Validity of the Ann Arbor Staging Classification for the non-Hodgkin's lymphomas. Cancer Treat Rep 61:1023–1027, 1977.

447. Vlachaki MT, Ha CS, Hagemeister FB, et al: Long-term outcome of treatment for Ann Arbor stage 1 Hodgkin's disease: patterns of failure, late toxicity and second malignancies. Int J Radiat Oncol Biol Phys 39:609–616, 1997.

448. Lukes RJ, Collins RD: Immunologic characterization of human malignant lymphomas. Cancer 34:1488–1503, 1974.

449. Rappaport H: Tumors of the Hematopoietic System. Atlas of Tumor Pathology. First Series, Fascicle 8. Washington, DC, Armed Forces Institute of Pathology, 1966.

450. Non-Hodgkin's lymphoma pathologic classification project. National Cancer Institute sponsored study of classifications of non-Hodgkin's lymphomas: summary and description of a Working Formulation for clinical usage. Cancer 49:2112–2135, 1982.

451. Stansfeld AG, Diebold J, Kapanci Y, et al: Updated Kiel classification for lymphomas (letter). Lancet 1:292–293, 1988.

452. Jaffe ES, Harris NL, Stein H, Vardiman JW (eds): World Health Organization Classification of Tumours. Pathology and Genetics of Tumours of Haematopoietic and Lymphoid Tumors. Lyon, IARC Press, 2001.

453. Kim H, Hendrickson MR, Dorfman RF: Composite lymphoma. Cancer 40:959–976, 1977.

454. Fend F, Quintanilla-Martinez L, Kumar S, et al: Composite low grade B-cell lymphomas with two immunophenotypically distinct cell populations are true biclonal lymphomas. A molecular analysis using laser capture microdissection. Am J Surg Pathol 154:1857–1866, 1999.

455. Young NA, Al-Saleem T, Ehya H, et al: Utilization of fine-needle aspiration cytology and flow cytometry in the diagnosis and subclassification of primary and recurrent lymphoma. Cancer 25:252–261, 1998.

456. Russell J, Skinner J, Orell S, et al: Fine needle aspiration cytology in the management of lymphoma. Aust N Z J Med 13:365–368, 1983.

457. Stewart CJ, Duncan JA, Farquharson M, et al: Fine needle aspiration cytology diagnosis of malignant lymphoma and reactive lymphoid hyperplasia. J Clin Pathol 51:197–203, 1998.

458. Velasquez WS, Jagannath S, Tucker SL, et al: Risk classification as the basis for clinical staging of diffuse large-cell lymphoma derived from 10-year survival data. Blood 74:551–557, 1989.

459. Shipp MA, Yeap BY, Harrington DP, et al: The m-BACOD combination chemotherapy regimen in large-cell lymphoma: analysis of the completed trial and comparison with the M-BACOD regimen. J Clin Oncol 8:84–93, 1990.

460. Hoskins PJ, Ng V, Spinelli JJ, et al: Prognostic variables in patients with diffuse large-cell lymphoma treated with MACOP-B. J Clin Oncol 9:220–226, 1991.

461. Dixon DO, Neilan B, Jones SE, et al: Effect of age on therapeutic outcome in advanced diffuse histiocytic lymphoma: the Southwest Oncology Group experience. J Clin Oncol 4:295–305, 1986.

462. Coiffier B, Gisselbrecht C, Vose JM, et al: Prognostic factors in aggressive malignant lymphomas: description and validation of a prognostic index that could identify patients requiring a more intensive therapy. J Clin Oncol 9:211–219, 1991.

463. The International Non-Hodgkin's Lymphoma Prognostic Factors Project. A predictive model for aggressive non-Hodgkin's lymphoma. N Engl J Med 329:987–994, 1993.

464. Bartlett NL, Rizeq M, Dorfman RF, et al: Follicular large-cell lymphoma: intermediate or low grade? J Clin Oncol 12:1349–1357, 1994.

465. Mok TS, Steinberg J, Chan AT, et al: Application of the international prognostic index in a study of Chinese patients with non-Hodgkin's lymphoma and a high incidence of primary extranodal lymphoma. Cancer 82:2439–2448, 1998.

466. Grogan TM, Lippman SM, Spier CM, et al: Independent prognostic significance of a nuclear proliferation antigen in diffuse large cell lymphomas as determined by the monoclonal antibody Ki-67. Blood 71:1157–1160, 1988.

467. Pinto A, Hutchison RE, Grant LH, et al: Follicular lymphomas in pediatric patients. Mod Pathol 3:308–313, 1990.

468. Horning SJ, Rosenberg SA: The natural history of initially untreated low grade non-Hodgkin's lymphomas. N Engl J Med 311:1471–1475, 1984.

469. Rosenberg SA: The low-grade non-Hodgkin's lymphomas: challenges and opportunities. J Clin Oncol 3:299–310, 1985.

470. Isaacson P: Malignant lymphomas with a follicular growth pattern. Histopathology 28:487–495, 1996.

471. Hu E, Weiss LM, Hoppe RT, et al: Follicular and diffuse mixed small cleaved and large cell lymphoma—a clinicopathologic study. J Clin Oncol 3:1183–1187, 1985.

472. Slovak ML, Weiss LM, Nathwani BN, et al: Cytogenetic studies of composite lymphomas: monocytoid B-cell lymphoma and other non-Hodgkin's lymphomas. Hum Pathol 24:1086–1094, 1993.

473. Nathwani BN, Anderson JR, Armitage JO, et al: Clinical significance of follicular lymphoma with monocytoid B cells. Hum Pathol 30:263–268, 1999.

474. Garcia CF, Warnke RA, Weiss LM: Follicular large cell lymphoma. An immunophenotype study. Am J Pathol 123:425–431, 1986.

475. Jaffe E, Shevach E, Frank M, et al: Nodular lymphoma: evidence for origin from follicular B lymphocytes. N Engl J Med 290:813–819, 1974.

476. Leech JH, Glick AD, Waldron JA, et al: Malignant lympho-

mas of follicular center cell origin in man. I. Immunologic studies. J Natl Cancer Inst 54:11–21, 1975.

477. Mann RB, Berard CW: Criteria for the cytologic subclassification of follicular lymphomas: a proposed alternative method. Hematol Oncol 1:187–192, 1982.

478. Kim H, Dorfman RF, Rappaport H: Signet-ring lymphoma: a rare morphologic and functional expression of nodular (follicular) lymphoma. Am J Surg Pathol 2:119–132, 1978.

479. Chang KL, Arber DA, Shibata D, et al: Follicular small lymphocytic lymphoma: a rare but distinct clinicopathologic entity. Am J Surg Pathol 18:999–1009, 1994.

480. Nathwani BN, Sheibani K, Winberg CD, et al: Neoplastic B cells with cerebriform nuclei in follicular lymphomas. Hum Pathol 16:173–180, 1985.

481. van der Putte SC, Schuurman HJ, Rademakers LH, et al: Malignant lymphoma of follicular center cell with marked nuclear lobation. Virchows Arch B Cell Pathol 46:93–107, 1984.

482. Vago JF, Hurtubise PE, Redden-Borowski MN, et al: Follicular center-cell lymphoma with plasmacytic differentiation, monoclonal paraprotein, and peripheral blood involvement. Recapitulation of normal B-cell development. Am J Surg Pathol 9:764–770, 1985.

483. Chan JK, Hui PK, Ng CS: Follicular immunoblastic lymphoma: neoplastic counterpart of the intrafollicular immunoblast? Pathology 22:103–105, 1990.

484. Come SE, Jaffe ES, Andersen JC, et al: Non-Hodgkin's lymphomas in leukemic phase: clinicopathologic correlations. Am J Med 69:667–674, 1980.

485. Goates JJ, Kamel OW, LeBrun DP, et al: Floral variant of follicular lymphoma. Immunological and molecular studies support a neoplastic process. Am J Surg Pathol 18:37–47, 1994.

486. Osborne BM, Butler JJ: Follicular lymphoma mimicking progressive transformation of germinal centers. Am J Clin Pathol 88:264–269, 1987.

487. Kurtin PJ, Hobday KS, Ziesmer S, et al: Demonstration of distinct antigenic profiles of small B-cell lymphomas by paraffin section immunohistochemistry. Am J Clin Pathol 112:319–329, 1999.

488. Swerdlow SH: Small B-cell lymphomas of the lymph nodes and spleen: practical insights to diagnosis and pathogenesis. Mod Pathol 12:125–140, 1999.

489. Warnke R, Levy R: The immunopathology of follicular lymphomas: a model of B-lymphocyte homing. N Engl J Med 298:481–486, 1978.

490. Pezzella F, Tse AG, Cordell JL, et al: Expression of the bcl-2 oncogene protein is not specific for the 14;18 chromosomal translocation. Am J Pathol 137:225–232, 1990.

491. de Leon ED, Alkan S, Huang JC, et al: Usefulness of an immunohistochemical panel in paraffin-embedded tissues for the differentiation of B-cell non-Hodgkin's lymphomas of small lymphocytes. Mod Pathol 11:1046–1051, 1998.

492. Raible MD, Hsi ED, Alkan S: Bcl-6 protein expression by follicle center lymphomas. A marker for differentiating follicle center lymphomas from other low-grade lymphoproliferative disorders. Am J Clin Pathol 112:101–107, 1999.

493. Capello D, Vitolo D, Pasqualucci L, et al: Distribution and pattern of *BCL-6* mutations throughout the spectrum of B-cell neoplasia. Blood 95:651–659, 2000.

494. Abdel-Reheim FA, Edwards E, Arber DA: Utility of a rapid polymerase chain reaction panel for the detection of molecular changes in B-cell lymphoma. Arch Pathol Lab Med 120:357–363, 1996.

495. Segal GH, Jorgensen T, Scott M, et al: Optimal primer selection for clonality assessment by polymerase chain reaction analysis: II. Follicular lymphomas. Hum Pathol 25:1276–1282, 1994.

496. Yunis JJ, Oken MM, Kaplan ME, et al: Distinctive chromosomal abnormalities in histologic subtypes of non-Hodgkin's lymphoma. N Engl J Med 307:1231–1236, 1982.

497. Weiss LM, Warnke RA, Sklar J, et al: Molecular analysis of the t(14;18) chromosomal translocation in malignant lymphomas. N Engl J Med 317:1185–1189, 1987.

498. Yunis JJ, Mayer MG, Amesen MA: bcl-2 and other genomic alterations in the prognosis of large-cell lymphoma. N Engl J Med 320:1047–1054, 1989.

499. Horsman DE, Gascoyne RD, Coupland RW, et al: Comparison of cytogenetic analysis, Southern analysis, and polymerase chain reaction for the detection of t(14;18) in follicular lymphoma. Am J Clin Pathol 103:472–478, 1995.

500. Tsujimoto T, Cossman J, Jaffe E, et al: Involvement of the bcl-2 gene in human follicular lymphoma. Science 288:1440–1443, 1985.

501. Berinstein NL, Reis MD, Ngan BY, et al: Detection of occult lymphoma in peripheral blood and bone marrow of patients with untreated early-stage and advanced-stage follicular lymphoma. J Clin Oncol 11:1344–1352, 1993.

502. Limpens J, de Jong D, van Krieken JHJM: Bcl-2/J$_H$ rearrangements in benign lymphoid tissues with follicular hyperplasia. Oncogene 6:2271–2276, 1991.

503. Ohshima K, Masahiro K, Kobari S, et al: Amplified bcl-2/JH rearrangements in reactive lymphadenopathy. Virchows Arch B Cell Pathol 85:2528–2536, 1993.

504. Limpens J, Stad R, Vos C, et al: Lymphoma-associated translocation t(14;18) in blood B cells of normal individuals. Blood 85:2528–2536, 1995.

505. Tilly H, Rossi A, Stamatoullas A, et al: Prognostic value of chromosomal abnormalities in follicular lymphoma. Blood 84:1043–1049, 1994.

506. LoCoco F, Gaidano G, Louie DC, et al: p53 mutations are associated with histologic transformation of follicular lymphoma. Blood 92:2289–2295, 1994.

507. Sander CA, Yano T, Clark HM, et al: p53 mutation is associated with progression in follicular lymphoma. Blood 82:1994–2004, 1993.

508. Elenitoba-Johhson KS, Gascoyne RD, Lim MS, et al: Homozygous deletions at chromosome 9p21 involving p16 and p15 are associated with histologic progression in follicle center lymphoma. Blood 91:4677–4685, 1998.

509. Cheson BD, Bennett JM, Rai KR, et al: Guidelines for clinical protocols for chronic lymphocytic leukemia: recommendations of the National Cancer Institute–sponsored working group. Am J Hematol 29:152–163, 1988.

510. Pangalis GA, Boussiotis VA, Kittas C: Malignant disorders of small lymphocytes. Small lymphocytic lymphoma, lymphoplasmacytic lymphoma, and chronic lymphocytic leukemia: their clinical and laboratory relationship. Am J Clin Pathol 99:402–408, 1993.

511. Morrison WH, Hoppe RT, Weiss LM, et al: Small lymphocytic lymphoma. J Clin Oncol 7:598–606, 1989.

512. Coiffier B, Thieblemont C, Felman P, et al: Indolent nonfollicular lymphomas: characteristics, treatment, and outcome. Semin Hematol 36:198–208, 1999.

513. Pangalis GA, Angelopoulou MK, Vassilakopoulos TP, et al: B-chronic lymphocytic leukemia, small lymphocytic lymphoma, and lymphoplasmacytic lymphoma, including Waldenström's macroglobulinemia: a clinical, morphologic, and biologic spectrum of similar disorders. Semin Hematol 36:104–114, 1999.

514. Berger F, Felman P, Sonet A, et al: Nonfollicular small B-cell lymphomas: a heterogeneous group of patients with distinct clinical features and outcome. Blood 83:2829–2835, 1994.

515. Brecher M, Banks PM: Hodgkin's disease variant of Richter's syndrome. Report of eight cases. Am J Clin Pathol 93:333–339, 1990.

516. Ben-Ezra J, Burke JS, Swartz WG, et al: Small lymphocytic lymphoma: a clinicopathologic analysis of 268 cases. Blood 73:579–587, 1989.

517. Dick FR, Maca RD: The lymph node in chronic lymphocytic leukemia. Cancer 41:283–292, 1978.

518. Pugh WC, Manning JT, Butler JJ: Paraimmunoblastic variant of small lymphocytic lymphoma/leukemia. Am J Surg Pathol 12:907–917, 1988.

519. Di Giuseppe JA, Borowitz MJ: Clinical utility of flow cytometry in the chronic lymphoid leukemias. Semin Oncol 25:6–10, 1998.

520. Tworek JA, Singleton TP, Schnitzer B, et al: Flow cytometric and immunohistochemical analysis of small lymphocytic lymphoma, mantle cell lymphoma, and plasmacytoid small lymphocytic lymphoma. Am J Clin Pathol 110:582–589, 1998.

521. Ngan BY, Picker LJ, Medeiros LJ, et al: Immunophenotypic diagnosis of non-Hodgkin's lymphoma in paraffin sections. Co-expression of L60 (Leu-22) and L26 antigens correlates with malignant histologic findings. Am J Clin Pathol 91:579–583, 1989.

522. Contos MJ, Kornstein MJ, Innes DJ, et al: The utility of CD20 and CD43 in subclassification of low-grade B-cell lymphoma on paraffin sections. Mod Pathol 5:631–633, 1992.

523. Arber DA, Weiss LM: CD5: a review. Appl Immunohisto-chem 3:1–22, 1995.

524. Dorfman DM, Pinkus GS: Distinction between small lympho-cytic and mantle cell lymphoma by immunoreactivity for CD23. Mod Pathol 7:326–331, 1994.

525. Mason DY, Stein H, Gerdes J, et al: Value of monoclonal anti-CD22 (p135) antibodies for the detection of normal and neoplastic B lymphoid cells. Blood 69:836–840, 1987.

526. Dohner H, Stilgenbauer S, James MR, et al: 11q deletions identify a new subset of B-cell chronic lymphocytic leukemia characterized by extensive nodal involvement and inferior prognosis. Blood 89:2516–2522, 1997.

527. Callet-Bauchu E, Salles G, Gazzo S, et al: Translocations in-volving the short arm of chromosome 17 in chronic B-lym-phoid disorders: frequent occurrence of dicentric rearrange-ments and possible association with adverse outcome. Leukemia 13:460–468, 1999.

528. Knuutila S, Elonen E, Teerenhovi L, et al: Trisomy 12 in B cells of patients with B-cell chronic lymphocytic leukemia. N Engl J Med 314:865–869, 1986.

529. Ramnani D, Lindberg G, Gokaslan ST, et al: Signet-ring cell variant of small lymphocytic lymphoma with a prominent sinusoidal pattern. Ann Diagn Pathol 3:220–226, 1999.

530. Isaacson PG: Lymphomas of mucosa-associated lymphoid tissue (MALT). Histopathology 16:617–619, 1990.

531. Isaacson PG, Wright DH: Malignant lymphoma of mucosa associated lymphoid tissue. A distinctive B cell lymphoma. Cancer 52:1410–1416, 1983.

532. Campo E, Miquel R, Krenacs L, et al: Primary nodal mar-ginal zone lymphomas of splenic and MALT type. Am J Surg Pathol 23:59–68, 1999.

533. Mollejo M, Lloret E, Marguez J, et al: Lymph node involve-ment by splenic marginal zone lymphoma: morphological and immunohistochemical features. Am J Surg Pathol 21:772–780, 1997.

534. Nathwani BN, Drachenberg MR, Hernandez AM, et al: Nodal monocytoid B-cell lymphoma (nodal marginal-zone B-cell lymphoma). Semin Hematol 36:128–138, 1999.

535. Banks PM, Isaacson PG: MALT lymphomas in 1997. Where do we stand? Am J Clin Pathol 111:S75–S83, 1999.

536. Isaacson P, Spencer J: Malignant lymphoma of mucosa-asso-ciated lymphoid tissue. Histopathology 11:445–462, 1987.

537. Burke JS: Are there site-specific differences among the MALT lymphomas—morphologic, clinical? Am J Clin Pathol 111:S133–S143, 1999.

538. Shin SS, Sheibani K: Monocytoid B-cell lymphoma. Am J Clin Pathol 99:421–425, 1993.

539. Ngan BY, Warnke R, Wilson M, et al: Monocytoid B-cell lymphoma: a study of 36 cases. Hum Pathol 22:409–421, 1991.

540. Traweek ST, Sheibani K: Monocytoid B-cell lymphoma. The biologic and clinical implications of peripheral blood in-volvement. Am J Clin Pathol 97:591–598, 1992.

541. Shin SS, Sheibani K, Fishleder A, et al: Monocytoid B-cell lymphoma in patients with Sjögren's syndrome: a clinico-pathologic study of 13 patients. Hum Pathol 22:422–430, 1991.

542. Parsonnet J, Hansen S, Rodriguez L, et al: *Helicobacter pylori* infection and gastric lymphoma [see comments]. N Engl J Med 330:1267–1271, 1994.

543. Royer B, Cazals-Hatem D, Sibilia J, et al: Lymphomas in patients with Sjögren's syndrome are marginal zone B-cell neoplasms, arise in diverse extranodal and nodal sites, and are not associated with viruses. Blood 90:766–775, 1997.

544. Pelstring RJ, Essell JH, Kurtin PJ, et al: Diversity of organ site involvement among malignant lymphomas of mucosa-associated tissues. Am J Clin Pathol 96:738–745, 1991.

545. Nathwani BN, Mohrmann RL, Brynes RK, et al: Monocytoid B-cell lymphomas: an assessment of diagnostic criteria and a perspective on histogenesis. Hum Pathol 23:1061–1071, 1992.

546. Chan JKC: Antibiotic-responsive gastric lymphoma? Adv Anat Pathol 1:33–37, 1994.

547. Brynes RK, Almaguer PD, Leathery KE, et al: Numerical cytogenetic abnormalities of chromosomes 3, 7, and 12 in marginal zone B-cell lymphoma. Mod Pathol 10:995–1000, 1996.

548. Wotherspoon AC, Finn TM, Isaacson PG: Trisomy 3 in low-grade primary B-cell lymphomas of mucosa-associated lym-phoid tissue (MALT). Blood 85:2000–2004, 1995.

549. Dierlamm J, Rosenberg C, Stul M, et al: Characteristic pat-tern of chromosomal gains and losses in marginal zone B cell lymphoma detected by comparative genomic hybridiza-tion. Leukemia 11:747–758, 1997.

550. Auer IA, Gascoyne RD, Connors JM, et al: t(11;18)(q21;q21) is the most common translocation in MALT lymphoma. Ann Oncol 8:979–985, 1997.

551. Ott G, Katzenberger T, Greiner A, et al: The t(11;18)(q21;q21) chromosome tranlocation is a frequent and specific aberra-tion in low-grade but not high-grade malignant non-Hodg-kin's lymphomas of the mucosa-associated lymphoid tissue (MALT)–type. Cancer Res 57:3944–3948, 1997.

552. Rosenwald A, Ott G, Stilgenbauer S, et al: Exclusive detec-tion of the t(11;18)(q21;q21) in extranodal marginal zone B cell lymphomas (MZBL) of MALT type in contrast to other MZBL and extranodal large B cell lymphomas. Am J Surg Pathol 155:1817–1821, 1999.

553. Bertoni F, Cotter FE, Zucca E: Molecular genetics of extrano-dal marginal zone (MALT-type) B-cell lymphoma. Leuk Lymphoma 35:57–68, 1999.

554. Dierlamm J, Baens M, Wlodarska I, et al: The apoptosis inhibitor gene *AP12* and a novel 18q gene, *MLT*, are recur-rently rearranged in the t(11;18)(q21;q21) associated with mucosa-associated lymphoid tissue lymphomas. Blood 93:3601–3609, 1999.

555. Stoffel A, Rao PH, Louie DC, et al: Chromosome 18 break-point in t(11;18)(q21;q21) translocation associated with MALT lymphoma is proximal to *BCL2* and distal to *DCC*. Genes Chromosomes Cancer 24:156–159, 1999.

556. Hoyer JD, Li CY, Yam LT, et al: Immunohistochemical dem-onstration of acid phosphatase isoenzyme 5 (tartrate-resis-tant) in paraffin sections of hairy cell leukemia and other hematologic disorders. Am J Clin Pathol 108:308–315, 1997.

557. Chang KL, Stroup R, Weiss LM: Hairy cell leukemia. Cur-rent status. Am J Clin Pathol 97:719–738, 1992.

558. Patsouris E, Noël H, Lennert K: Lymphoplasmacytic/lym-phoplasmacytoid immunocytoma with a high content of epi-thelioid cells: histologic and immunohistochemical findings. Am J Surg Pathol 14:660–670, 1990.

559. Harada M, Shimada M, Fukayama M, et al: Crystal-storing histiocytosis associated with lymphoplasmacytic lymphoma mimicking Weber-Christian disease: immunohistochemical, ultrastructural, and gene-rearrangement studies. Histopathol-ogy 33:459–464, 1998.

560. Strickler JG, Audeh MW, Copenhaver CM, et al: Immuno-phenotypic differences between plasmacytoma/multiple my-eloma and immunoblastic lymphoma. Cancer 61:1782–1786, 1988.

561. Offit K, Parsa NZ, Filippa D, et al: t(9;14)(p13;q32) denotes a subset of low-grade non-Hodgkin's lymphoma with plasma-cytoid differentiation. Blood 80:2594–2599, 1992.

562. Offit K, Louie DC, Parsa NZ, et al: del(7)(32) is associated with a subset of small lymphocytic lymphoma with plasma-cytoid features. Blood 86:2365–2370, 1995.

563. Iida S, Rao PH, Ueda R, et al: Chromosomal rearrangement of the PAX-5 locus in lymphoplasmacytic lymphoma with t(9;14)(p13;q32). Leuk Lymphoma 34:25–33, 1999.

564. Hernandez JM, Mecucci C, Michaux L, et al: del(7q) in chronic B-cell lymphoid malignancies. Cancer Genet Cytoge-net 93:147–151, 1997.

565. Weisenburger DD, Kim H, Rappaport H: Malignant lym-phoma, intermediate lymphocytic type: a clinicopathologic study of 42 cases. Cancer 48:1415–1425, 1981.

566. Banks PM, Chan J, Cleary ML, et al: Mantle cell lymphoma. A proposal for unification of morphologic, immunologic, and molecular data. Am J Surg Pathol 16:637–640, 1992.

567. Weisenburger DD, Armitage JO: Mantle cell lymphoma—an entity comes of age. Blood 87:4483–4494, 1996.

568. Kurtin PJ: Mantle cell lymphoma. Adv Anat Pathol 5:376–398, 1998.

569. Campo E, Raffeld M, Jaffe ES: Mantle-cell lymphoma. Semin Hematol 36:115–127, 1999.

570. Lardelli P, Bookman MA, Sundeen J, et al: Lymphocytic lymphoma of intermediate differentiation. Morphologic and immunophenotypic spectrum and clinical correlations. Am J Surg Pathol 14:752–763, 1990.

571. Fisher RI, Dahlberg S, Nathwani BN, et al: A clinical analysis of two indolent lymphoma entities: mantle cell lymphoma and marginal zone lymphoma (including the mucosa-associated lymphoid tissue and monocytoid B-cell categories): a Southwest Oncology Group study. Blood 85:1075–1082, 1995.

572. O'Briain DS, Kennedy MJ, Daly PA, et al: Multiple lymphomatous polyposis of the gastrointestinal tract: a clinicopathologically distinctive form of non-Hodgkin's lymphoma of centrocytic type. Am J Surg Pathol 13:691–699, 1989.

573. Moynihan MJ, Bast MA, Chan WC, et al: Lymphomatous polyposis. A neoplasm of either follicular mantle or germinal center cell origin. Am J Surg Pathol 20:442–452, 1996.

574. Breslin NP, Urbanski SJ, Shaffer EA: Mucosa-associated lymphoid tissue (MALT) lymphoma manifesting as multiple lymphomatosis polyposis of the gastrointestinal tract. Am J Gastroenterol 94:2540–2545, 1999.

575. Hashimoto Y, Nakamura N, Kuze T, et al: Multiple lymphomatous polyposis of the gastrointestinal tract is a heterogenous group that includes mantle cell lymphoma and follicular lymphoma: analysis of somatic mutation of immunoglobulin heavy chain gene variable region. Hum Pathol 30:581–587, 1999.

576. Argatoff LH, Connors JM, Klasa RJ, et al: Mantle cell lymphoma: a clinicopathologic study of 80 cases. Blood 89:2067–2078, 1997.

577. Weisenburger DD, Kim H, Rappaport H: Mantle zone lymphoma. A follicular variant of intermediate lymphocytic lymphoma. Cancer 49:1429–1438, 1982.

578. Koo CH, Rappaport H, Sheibani K, et al: Imprint cytology of non-Hodgkin's lymphomas. Based on a study of 212 immunologically characterized cases. Hum Pathol 20(suppl):1–137, 1989.

579. Rassidakis GZ, Tani E, Svedmyr E, et al: Diagnosis and subclassification of follicle center and mantle cell lymphomas on fine-needle aspirates: a cytologic and immunocytochemical approach based on the Revised European-American Lymphoma (REAL) classification. Cancer 87:216–223, 1999.

580. Laszlo T, Matolcsy A: Blastic transformation of mantle cell lymphoma: genetic evidence for a clonal link between the two stages of the tumour. Histopathology 35:355–359, 1999.

581. Ott MM, Ott G, Kuse R, et al: The anaplastic variant of centrocytic lymphoma is marked by frequent rearrangements of the Bcl-1 gene and high proliferation indices. Histopathology 24:329–334, 1994.

582. Lennert K, Feller AC: Histopathology of Non-Hodgkin's Lymphomas (based on the updated Kiel Classification). 2nd ed. Berlin, Springer-Verlag, 1992.

583. Zukerberg LR, Yang W-I, Arnold A, et al: Cyclin D1 expression in non-Hodgkin's lymphomas. Detection by immunohistochemistry. Am J Clin Pathol 103:756–760, 1995.

584. Chan JK, Miller KD, Munson P, et al: Immunostaining for cyclin D1 and the diagnosis of mantle cell lymphoma: is there a reliable method? Histopathology 34:266–270, 1999.

585. Raffeld M, Jaffe ES: bcl-1, t(11;14), and mantle cell–derived lymphomas. Blood 78:259–263, 1991.

586. Leroux D, LeMarc'hadour F, Gressin R, et al: Non-Hodgkin's lymphomas with t(11;14)(q13;q32): a subset of mantle zone/intermediate lymphocytic lymphoma? Br J Haematol 77:346–353, 1991.

587. Williams ME, Swerdlow SH, Rosenberg CL, et al: Chromosome 11 translocation breakpoints at the PRAD1/cyclin D1 gene locus in centrocytic lymphoma. Leukemia 7:241–245, 1993.

588. Rimokh R, Berger F, Delsol G, et al: Rearrangement and overexpression of the BCL-1/PRAD-1 gene in intermediate lymphocytic lymphomas and in t(11q13)-bearing leukemias. Blood 81:3063–3067, 1993.

589. Rimokh R, Berger F, Delsol G, et al: Detection of the chromosomal translocation t(11;14) by polymerase chain reaction in mantle cell lymphomas. Blood 83:1871–1875, 1994.

590. Matutes E, Carrara P, Coignet L, et al: Cytogenetic profile of lymphoma of follicle mantle lineage: correlation with clinicobiologic features. Blood 93:1372–1380, 1999.

591. Matutes E, Carrara P, Coignet L, et al: FISH analysis for BCL-1 rearrangements and trisomy 12 helps the diagnosis of atypical B cell leukaemias. Leukemia 13:1721–1726, 1999.

592. Rosenberg CL, Wong E, Petty E, et al: Overexpression of PRAD1, a candidate BCL1 breakpoint region oncogene, in centrocytic lymphomas. Proc Natl Acad Sci U S A 88:9638–9642, 1991.

593. Stilgenbauer S, Winkler D, Ott G, et al: Molecular characterization of 11q deletions points to a pathogenic role of the ATM gene in mantle cell lymphoma. Blood 94:3262–3264, 1999.

594. Wlodarska I, Pittaluga S, Hagemeijer A, et al: Secondary chromosome changes in mantle cell lymphoma. Haematologica 84:594–599, 1999.

595. Espinet B, Sole F, Woessner S, et al: Translocation (11;14)(q13;q32) and preferential involvement of chromosomes 1, 2, 9, 13, and 17 in mantle cell lymphoma. Cancer Genet Cytogenet 111:92–98, 1999.

596. Wong KF, Chan JK, So JC, et al: Mantle cell lymphoma in leukemic phase: characterization of its broad cytologic spectrum with emphasis on the importance of distinction from other chronic lymphoproliferative disorders. Cancer 86:850–857, 1999.

597. Singleton TP, Anderson MM, Ross CW, et al: Leukemic phase of mantle cell lymphoma, blastoid variant. Am J Clin Pathol 111:495–500, 1999.

598. Kwak LW, Wilson M, Weiss LM, et al: Clinical significance of morphologic subdivision in diffuse large cell lymphoma. Cancer 68:1988–1993, 1991.

599. Mann RB: Are there site-specific differences among extranodal aggressive B-cell neoplasms? Am J Clin Pathol 111:S144–S150, 1999.

600. Armitage JO: Treatment of non-Hodgkin's lymphoma. N Engl J Med 328:1023–1030, 1993.

601. Urba WJ, Duffey PL, Longo DL: Treatment of patients with aggressive lymphomas: an overview. J Natl Cancer Inst Monogr 10:29–37, 1990.

602. Alizadeh AA, Eisen MB, Davis RE, et al: Distinct types of diffuse large B-cell lymphoma identified by gene expression profiling. Nature 403:503–511, 2000.

603. Addis BJ, Isaacson PG: Large cell lymphoma of the mediastinum: a B-cell tumour of probable thymic origin. Histopathology 10:379–390, 1986.

604. Perrone T, Frizzera G, Rosai J: Mediastinal diffuse large-cell lymphoma with sclerosis: a clinicopathologic study of 60 cases. Am J Surg Pathol 10:176–191, 1986.

605. Yousem SA, Weiss LM, Warnke RA: Primary mediastinal non-Hodgkin's lymphomas: a morphologic and immunologic study of 19 cases. Am J Clin Pathol 83:676–680, 1985.

606. Davis RE, Dorfman RF, Warnke RA: Primary large cell lymphoma of the thymus: a diffuse B-cell neoplasm presenting as primary mediastinal lymphoma. Hum Pathol 21:1262–1268, 1990.

607. Lamarre L, Jacobson JO, Aisenberg AC, et al: Primary large cell lymphoma of the mediastinum. Am J Surg Pathol 13:730–739, 1989.

608. Abou-Elella AA, Weisenburger DD, Vose JM, et al: Primary mediastinal large B-cell lymphoma: a clinicopathologic study of 43 patients from the Nebraska Lymphoma Study Group. J Clin Oncol 17:784–790, 1999.

609. Paulli M, Strater J, Gianelli U, et al: Mediastinal B-cell lymphoma: a study of its histomorphologic spectrum based on 109 cases. Hum Pathol 30:178–187, 1999.

610. Suster S, Moran CA: Pleomorphic large cell lymphomas of the mediastinum. Am J Surg Pathol 20:224–232, 1996.

784. Elenitoba-Johnson KS, Jaffe ES: Lymphoproliferative disorders associated with congenital immunodeficiencies. Semin Diagn Pathol 14:35–47, 1997.

785. Knowles DM: Immunodeficiency-associated lymphoproliferative disorders. Mod Pathol 12:200–217, 1999.

786. Filipovich AH, Mathus A, Kamat D, et al: Primary immunodeficiencies: genetic risk factors for lymphoma. Cancer Res 52(suppl):5465S–5467S, 1992.

787. Maia DM, Garwacki CP: X-linked lymphoproliferative disease: pathology and diagnosis. Pediatr Dev Pathol 2:72–77, 1999.

788. Kroft SH, Finn WG, Singleton TP, et al: Follicular large cell lymphoma with immunoblastic features in a child with Wiskott-Aldrich syndrome: an unusual immunodeficiency-related neoplasm not associated with Epstein-Barr virus. Am J Clin Pathol 110:95–99, 1998.

789. Sander CA, Medeiros LM, Weiss LM, et al: Lymphoproliferative lesions in patients with common variable immunodeficiency syndrome. Am J Surg Pathol 16:1170–1182, 1992.

790. Ansari MQ, Dawson DB, Nador R, et al: Primary body cavity–based AIDS-related lymphomas. Am J Clin Pathol 105:221–229, 1996.

791. Cesarman E, Nador RG, Aozasa K, et al: Kaposi's sarcoma–associated herpesvirus in non-AIDS related lymphomas occurring in body cavities. Blood 88:645–656, 1996.

792. Davi F, Delecluse HJ, Guiet P, et al: Burkitt-like lymphomas in AIDS patients: characterization within a series of 103 human immunodeficiency virus–associated non-Hodgkin's lymphomas. J Clin Oncol 16:3788–3795, 1998.

793. Ballerini P, Gaidano G, Gong JZ, et al: Multiple genetic lesions in AIDS-related non-Hodgkin lymphoma. Blood 81:166–176, 1993.

794. Knowles DN, Cesarman E, Chadburn A, et al: Correlative morphologic and molecular genetic analysis demonstrates three distinct categories of posttransplantation lymphoproliferative disorders. Blood 85:552–565, 1995.

795. Cesarman E, Chadburn A, Liu YF, et al: bcl-6 gene mutations in posttransplantation lymphoproliferative disorders predict response to therapy and clinical outcome. Blood 92:2294–2302, 1998.

796. Chadburn A: Molecular pathology of the post-transplantation lymphoproliferative disorders. Semin Diagn Pathol 14:15–26, 1997.

797. Kamel OW, van de Rijn M, LeBrun DP, et al: Lymphoproliferative lesions in patients with rheumatoid arthritis and dermatomyositis: frequency of Epstein-Barr virus and other features associated with immunosuppression. Hum Pathol 25:638–643, 1994.

798. Kamel OW, van de Rijn M, Colby TV, et al: Hodgkin's disease in patients receiving long-term, low-dose methotrexate therapy. Am J Surg Pathol 20:1279–1287, 1996.

799. Kamel OW: Iatrogenic lymphoproliferative disorders in nontransplantation settings. Semin Diagn Pathol 14:27–34, 1997.

800. Becroft DMO, Dix MR, Gillman JC, et al: Benign sinus histiocytosis with massive lymphadenopathy: transient immunological defects in a child with mediastinal involvement. J Clin Pathol 26:463–469, 1973.

801. Lieberman PH, Jones CR, Steinman RM, et al: Langerhans cell (eosinophilic) granulomatosis: a clinicopathologic study encompassing 50 years. Am J Surg Pathol 20:519–552, 1996.

802. The French Langerhans' Cell Histiocytosis Group: A multicentre retrospective survey of Langerhans' cell histiocytosis: 348 cases observed between 1983 and 1993. Arch Dis Child 75:17–24, 1996.

803. Huang F, Arceci R: The histiocytoses of infancy. Semin Perinatol 23:317–331, 1999.

804. Howarth DM, Gilchrist GS, Mullan BP, et al: Langerhans cell histiocytosis: diagnosis, natural history, management, and outcome. Cancer 85:2278–2290, 1999.

805. Lichtenstein L: Histiocytosis X: integration of eosinophilic granuloma of bone, Letterer-Siwe disease and Schüller-Christian disease as related manifestations of a single nosologic entity. Arch Pathol 56:84–102, 1953.

806. Motoi M, Helbron D, Kaiserling E, et al: Eosinophilic granuloma of lymph nodes: a variant of histiocytosis X. Histopathology 4:585–606, 1980.

807. Burns BF, Colby TV, Dorfman RF: Langerhans' cell granulomatosis (histiocytosis X) associated with malignant lymphomas. Am J Surg Pathol 7:529–533, 1983.

808. Egeler RA, Neglia JP, Puccetti DM, et al: Association of Langerhans cell histiocytosis with malignant neoplasms. Cancer 71:865–873, 1993.

809. Favara BE, Steele A: Langerhans cell histiocytosis of lymph nodes: a morphological assessment of 43 biopsies. Pediatr Pathol Lab Med 17:769–787, 1997.

810. Ben-Ezra J, Bailey A, Azumi N, et al: Malignant histiocytosis X. A distinct clinicopathologic entity. Cancer 68:1050–1060, 1991.

811. Azumi N, Sheibani K, Swartz WG, et al: Antigenic phenotype of Langerhans cell histiocytosis. An immunohistochemical study demonstrating the value of LN-2, LN-3 and vimentin. Hum Pathol 19:1376–1382, 1988.

812. Hage C, Willman CL, Favara BE, et al: Langerhans' cell histiocytosis (histiocytosis X): immunophenotype and growth fraction. Hum Pathol 24:840–845, 1993.

813. Ruco LP, Pulford KAF, Mason D: Expression of macrophage-associated antigens in tissues involved by Langerhans' cell histiocytosis (histiocytosis X). Am J Clin Pathol 92:273–279, 1989.

814. Krenacs L, Tiszlavicz L, Krenacs T, et al: Immunohistochemical detection of CD1a antigen in formalin-fixed and paraffin-embedded tissue sections with monoclonal antibody O10. J Pathol 171:99–104, 1993.

815. Beckstead JH, Wood GS, Turner RR: Histiocytosis X cells and Langerhans' cells: enzyme histochemical and immunologic similarities. Hum Pathol 15:826–833, 1984.

816. Mierau GW, Favara BE, Brenman JM: Electron microscopy in histiocytosis X. Ultrastruct Pathol 3:137–142, 1982.

817. Willman CL, Busque L, Griffith BB, et al: Langerhans'-cell histiocytosis (histiocytosis X)—a clonal proliferative disease. N Engl J Med 331:154–160, 1994.

818. Yu RC, Chu AC: Lack of T-cell receptor gene rearrangements in cells involved in Langerhans cell histiocytosis. Cancer 75:1162–1166, 1995.

819. Rabkin MS, Wittwer CT, Kjeldsberg CR, et al: Flow-cytometric DNA content of histiocytosis X (Langerhans cell histiocytosis). Am J Pathol 131:183–189, 1988.

820. Ornvold K, Carstensen H, Larsen JK, et al: Flow cytometric DNA analysis of lesions from 18 children with Langerhans cell histiocytosis (histiocytosis X). Am J Pathol 136:1301–1307, 1990.

821. Monda L, Warnke R, Rosai J: A primary lymph node malignancy with features suggestive of dendritic reticulum cell differentiation. Am J Surg Pathol 122:562–572, 1986.

822. Weiss LM, Berry GJ, Dorfman RF, et al: Spindle cell neoplasms of lymph nodes of probable reticulum cell lineage. True reticulum cell sarcoma? Am J Surg Pathol 14:405–414, 1990.

823. Nakamura S, Hara K, Suchi T, et al: Interdigitating cell sarcoma. A morphologic, immunohistologic, and enzyme-histochemical study. Cancer 61:562–568, 1988.

824. Vasef MA, Zaatari GS, Chan WC, et al: Dendritic cell tumors associated with low-grade B-cell malignancies. Report of three cases. Am J Clin Pathol 104:696–701, 1995.

825. Fonseca R, Yamakawa M, Nakamura S: Follicular dendritic cell sarcoma and interdigitating reticulum cell sarcoma: a review. Am J Hematol 59:161–167, 1998.

826. Andriko JW, Kaldjian EP, Tsokos M, et al: Reticulum cell neoplasms of lymph nodes: a clinicopathologic study of 11 cases with recognition of a new subtype derived from fibroblastic reticular cells. Am J Surg Pathol 22:1048–1058, 1998.

827. Chan JKC, Tsang WYW, Ng CS: Follicular dendritic cell tumor and vascular neoplasm complicating hyaline-vascular Castleman's disease. Am J Surg Pathol 18:517–525, 1994.

828. Perez-Ordonez B, Erlandson RA, Rosai J: Follicular dendritic cell tumor. Report of 13 additional cases of a distinctive entity. Am J Surg Pathol 20:944–955, 1996.

829. Chan JKC, Fletcher CDM, Nayler S, et al: Follicular dendritic cell sarcoma. Clinicopathologic analysis of 17 cases suggest-

ing a malignant potential higher than currently recognized. Cancer 79:294–313, 1997.

830. Nayler SJ, Taylor L, Cooper K: HHV-8 is not associated with follicular dendritic cell tumours. Mol Pathol 51:168–170, 1998.

831. Arber DA, Weiss LM, Chang KL: Detection of Epstein-Barr virus in inflammatory pseudotumor. Semin Diagn Pathol 15:155–160, 1998.

832. Berti E, Gianotti R, Alessi E: Unusual cutaneous histiocytosis expressing an intermediate immunophenotype between Langerhans' cells and dermal macrophages. Arch Dermatol 124:1250–1253, 1988.

833. Kolde G, Brocker E-B: Multiple skin tumors of indeterminate cells in an adult. J Am Acad Dermatol 15:591–597, 1986.

834. Hanson CA, Jaszcz W, Kersey JH, et al: True histiocytic lymphoma: histopathologic, immunophenotypic and genotypic analysis. Br J Haematol 73:187–198, 1989.

835. Kamel OW, Gocke CD, Kell DL, et al: True histiocytic lymphoma: a study of 12 cases based on current definition. Leuk Lymphoma 18:81–86, 1995.

836. Ornvold K, Carstensen H, Junge J, et al: Tumours classified as "malignant histiocytosis" in children are T-cell neoplasms. APMIS 100:558–566, 1992.

837. Salter DM, Krajewski AS, Dewar AE: Immunophenotype analysis of malignant histiocytosis of the intestine. J Clin Pathol 39:8–15, 1986.

838. Isaacson P, Wright DH, Jones DB: Malignant lymphoma of true histiocytic (monocyte-macrophage) origin. Cancer 51:80–91, 1983.

839. Copie-Bergman C, Wotherspoon AC, Norton AJ, et al: True histiocytic lymphoma. A morphologic, immunohistochemical and molecular genetic study of 13 cases. Am J Surg Pathol 22:1386–1392, 1998.

840. Ralfkiaer E, Delsol G, O'Connor NTJ, et al: Malignant lymphomas of true histiocytic origin. A clinical, histological, immunophenotypic and genotypic study. J Pathol 160:9–17, 1990.

841. Arai E, Su WPD, Roche PC, et al: Cutaneous histiocytic malignancy. Immunohistochemical re-examination of cases previously diagnosed as cutaneous "histiocytic lymphoma" and "malignant histiocytosis." J Cutan Pathol 20:115–120, 1993.

842. Alvaro T, Bosch R, Salvado MT, et al: True histiocytic lymphoma of the stomach associated with low-grade B-cell mucosa-associated lymphoid tissue (MALT)–type lymphoma. Am J Surg Pathol 20:1406–1411, 1996.

843. Martin-Rodilla C, Fernandez-Acenero J, Pena-Mayor L, et al: True histiocytic lymphoma as a second neoplasm in a follicular centroblastic-centrocytic lymphoma. Pathol Res Pract 193:319–322, 1997.

844. Bucksy P, Favara B, Feller AC: Malignant histiocytosis and large cell anaplastic (Ki-1) lymphoma in childhood: guidelines for differential diagnosis—report of the Histiocyte Society. Med Pediatr Oncol 22:200–203, 1994.

845. Chang C-S, Wang C-H, Su I-J, et al: Hematophagic histiocytosis: a clinicopathologic analysis of 23 cases with special reference to the association with peripheral T-cell lymphoma. J Formos Med Assoc 93:421–428, 1994.

846. Okada Y, Nakanishi I, Nomura H, et al: Angiotropic B-cell lymphoma with hemophagocytic syndrome. Pathol Res Pract 190:718–727, 1994.

847. DeMent SH: Association between mediastinal germ cell tumors and hematologic malignancies: an update. Hum Pathol 21:699–703, 1990.

848. Neiman RS, Barcos M, Berard C, et al: Granulocytic sarcoma: a clinicopathologic study of 61 biopsied cases. Cancer 48:1426–1437, 1981.

849. Traweek ST, Arber DA, Rappaport H, et al: Extramedullary myeloid cell tumors. An immunohistochemical and morphologic study of 28 cases. Am J Surg Pathol 17:1011–1019, 1993.

850. Meis JM, Butler JJ, Osborne BM, et al: Granulocytic sarcoma in nonleukemic patients. Cancer 58:2697–2709, 1986.

851. Muller S, Sangster G, Crocker J, et al: An immunohistochemical and clinicopathological study of granulocytic sarcoma (chloroma). Hematol Oncol 4:101–112, 1986.

852. Hancock JC, Prchal JT, Bennett JM, et al: Trilineage extramedullary myeloid cell tumor in myelodysplastic syndrome. Arch Pathol Lab Med 121:520–523, 1997.

853. Roth MJ, Medeiros LJ, Elenitoba-Johnson K, et al: Extramedullary myeloid cell tumors. An immunohistochemical study of 29 cases using routinely fixed and processed paraffin-embedded tissue sections. Arch Pathol Lab Med 119:790–798, 1995.

854. Elenitoba-Johnson K, Hodges GF, King TC, et al: Extramedullary myeloid cell tumors arising in the setting of chronic myelomonocytic leukemia. A report of two cases. Arch Pathol Lab Med 120:62–67, 1996.

855. Baddoura FK, Hanson C, Chan WC: Plasmacytoid monocytic proliferation associated with myeloproliferative disorders. Cancer 69:1457–1467, 1992.

856. Addis BJ, Isaacson P, Billings JA: Plasmacytosis of lymph nodes. Cancer 46:340–346, 1980.

857. Lin BT, Weiss LM: Primary plasmacytoma of lymph nodes. Hum Pathol 28:1083–1090, 1997.

858. Hussong JW, Perkins SL, Schnitzer B, et al: Extramedullary plasmacytoma. A form of marginal zone cell lymphoma? Am J Clin Pathol 111:111–116, 1999.

859. Kahn H, Strauchen JA, Gilbert HS, et al: Immunoglobulin-related amyloidosis presenting as recurrent isolated lymph node involvement. Arch Pathol Lab Med 115:948–950, 1991.

860. Travis WD, Li CY: Pathology of the lymph node and spleen in systemic mast cell disease. Mod Pathol 1:4–14, 1988.

861. Li WV, Kapadia SB, Sonmez-Alpan E, et al: Immunohistochemical characterization of mast cell disease in paraffin sections using tryptase, CD68, myeloperoxidase, lysozyme, and CD20 antibodies. Mod Pathol 9:982–988, 1996.

862. Yang F, Tran T-A, Carlson JA, et al: Paraffin section immunophenotype of cutaneous and extracutaneous mast cell disease: comparison to other hematopoietic neoplasms. Am J Surg Pathol 24:703–709, 2000.

# Spleen

Daniel A. Arber

The spleen offers certain diagnostic challenges to the surgical pathologist and hematopathologist. Although it may be enlarged in a variety of conditions, a definite primary cause for its enlargement may not be evident by histologic examination alone. In addition, certain tumorous proliferations unique to the spleen have been recognized. Despite this, many tumors and proliferations of the spleen are similar if not identical to those of other organs. This chapter focuses on the features of common splenic lesions as well as on the proliferations unique to the spleen.

Splenectomy specimens are the most common spleen specimens studied by most pathologists. The spleen may be removed therapeutically, incidentally, or diagnostically. Therapeutic splenectomy is often performed in patients with splenomegaly related to a systemic disease or in patients with traumatic rupture of the organ. When the surgical pathologist is provided with the appropriate clinical indication for the splenectomy, these cases generally give little difficulty. However, incidental tumorous proliferations may be found in such specimens, or unexpected dis-

eases involving the spleen may be identified. Similar proliferations may be found in the incidentally removed spleen during surgery for other diseases. The diagnostic splenectomy is performed in a search for a primary tumor diagnosis or to identify a metastatic lesion. With the now common use of advanced imaging techniques to stage malignant neoplasms, smaller splenic tumors are identified and removed to exclude the possibility of metastasis. Many of these are incidental, nonmalignant proliferations.

Although splenectomy remains common, needle biopsy and even fine-needle aspiration of the spleen are becoming more common. These procedures are most often performed in patients with a radiologically discrete lesion that is anatomically accessible to biopsy, thus reducing the risk of hemorrhage from the procedure. Needle biopsies and aspirations of the spleen have limitations similar to those in other organs, but these procedures may identify metastatic disease and even lymphomatous proliferations and therefore reduce the need for splenectomy in some patients. Partial splenectomy specimens or fragmented spleens from laparoscopic procedures are occasionally encountered, and these types of specimens will probably increase in the coming years.

## THE NORMAL SPLEEN

There is variation in the size of the normal adult spleen that is directly related to the patient's height and body weight. The weight of the spleen is greatest in young adults; it decreases from approximately the age of 25 years until the middle of the fourth decade, and then it remains stable until approximately the age of 60 years, after which it gradually decreases with age.[1] A series of medical-legal autopsy cases found a mean normal spleen weight of 156 g with a 95% confidence interval range of 53 to 361 g.[2] Normal spleen weights of more than 400 g are unusual, with the exception of large individuals.

A smooth fibrous capsule covers the spleen and is surfaced by a single layer of mesothelial cells. The histology of the splenic parenchyma is fairly complex and has been described in detail elsewhere,[3-6] but it can be divided into two general compartments of the red and white pulp (Fig. 42–1). The red pulp, the larger of these two compartments, is composed of the splenic sinuses, cords, and small vessels. A single layer of plump cells, which are often termed *littoral cells*, lines the sinuses. These cells are thought to have features of both endothelium and histiocytes. The sinuses are surrounded by the cords of Billroth, which form the reticular structure of the red pulp. Both the sinuses and cords contain red blood cells and only a sparse number of lymphocytes and plasma cells. Histiocytes within the cords remove the damaged or aging red blood cells.

The white pulp is the primary lymphocyte component of the spleen. It contains the lymphoid nodules, or malpighian corpuscles, and the periarterial

lymphatic sheaths. The lymphoid nodules are composed mostly of B lymphocytes, whereas the periarterial lymphocytes are of T lineage. Distinct zones of the white pulp nodules are not present in the normal adult spleen but are seen in the white pulp of children and antigenically stimulated adults. In these settings, three white pulp zones are apparent. A small lymphocyte mantle zone surrounds a central germinal center containing small, medium, and large lymphocytes, with or without histiocytes. This pattern is similar in appearance and cellular makeup to a reactive germinal center of lymph nodes. The reactive white pulp of the spleen, however, differs from the reactive lymph node by the presence of a third zone, outside of the mantle zone, termed the *splenic marginal zone*. The marginal zone is composed of a band of small to medium-sized lymphocytes with moderately abundant pale cytoplasm. T cells are admixed with the B cell nodules, particularly in the germinal centers and at the periphery of the marginal zone. In some adult patients, acellular eosinophilic material and small clusters of histiocytes may be present within the central white pulp. The periarterial lymphatic sheath cells are usually small T lymphocytes and do not demonstrate the zonal distribution of the B cell nodules.

## SPECIMEN HANDLING

Because of its tendency to autolyze rapidly, the spleen should be received fresh and be weighed and sampled immediately. The fresh spleen can easily be sliced into 1-cm sections. If it is removed as part of a staging procedure, however, even thinner sections may be desirable. Although many splenic proliferations form large nodular lesions, many do not. For this reason, the splenic parenchyma should be carefully examined, and any suggestion of accentuation of the white pulp should be sampled. Even with distinct lesions, the remainder of the cut surface should be examined carefully and sampled. Some proliferations diffusely involve the spleen, however, and the parenchyma exhibits a homogeneous, often bloody cut surface. In these cases, random sections are usually sufficient for evaluation. Either B5 or formalin fixation of thin sections (2 mm or less) is acceptable for histologic examination; however, the use of formalin requires adequate fixation (overnight fixation if the specimen is received late in the day) before tissue processing.

If certain tumors are suspected, particularly hematopoietic tumors, fresh tissue should be harvested for ancillary studies. These might include fresh tissue for flow cytometric immunophenotyping and frozen tissue for immunohistochemical or molecular genetic studies. Touch or scrape preparations are also often useful. These should be performed on the fresh specimen. The cut surface of the spleen should be washed and dabbed dry with a towel to remove excess blood before the touch and scrape preparations are made.

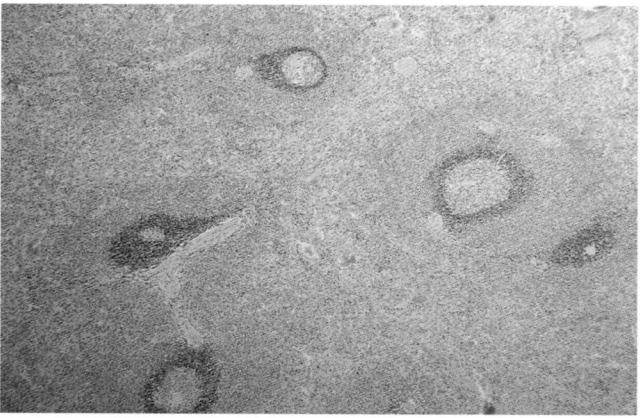

**FIGURE 42–1.** The normal spleen in a child and the reactive spleen in an adult demonstrate evenly spaced white pulp that contains a central germinal center, a surrounding mantle zone of small dark-staining lymphocytes, and an outer pale-staining marginal zone. These three white pulp zones are not distinct in the nonstimulated adult spleen. The intervening red pulp contains the splenic cords and sinuses with few lymphoid cells, except for small aggregates of lymphocytes surrounding small vessels.

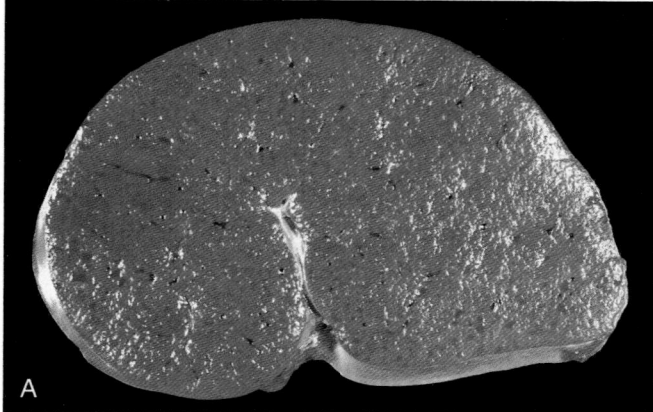
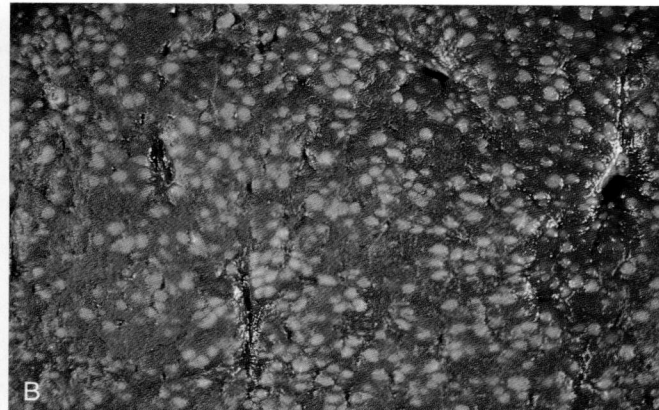
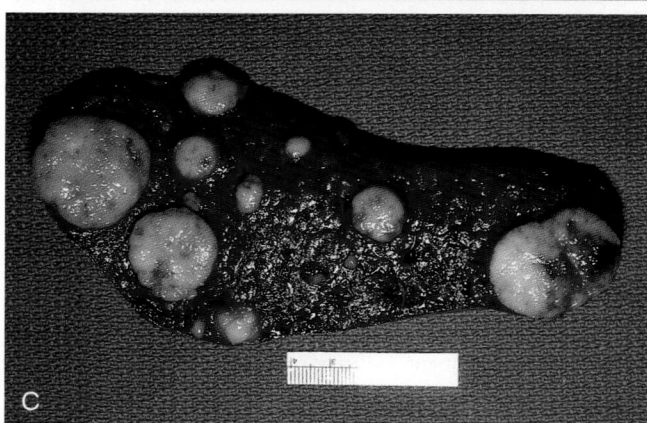

**FIGURE 42-2.** Three main gross patterns of splenic disease are identifiable on the splenic cut surface. *A.* The diffuse pattern shows splenic enlargement with a homogeneous cut surface, as seen in this 5000-g spleen from a patient with chronic myelogenous leukemia. *B.* The miliary pattern demonstrates multiple small tan-white nodules that are present throughout the spleen, as seen in this specimen from a patient with chronic lymphocytic leukemia. *C.* The nodular pattern represents distinct tumor nodules, either single or multiple, as seen in this patient with splenic involvement by large B cell lymphoma. Mixtures of these patterns may also be present.

## GROSS AND MICROSCOPIC PATTERNS OF DISEASE

Gross and microscopic patterns of splenic involvement have historically been used to develop a differential diagnosis for splenic neoplasms,[7-12] and key features of the spleen examination and report are listed in Table 42-1. Gross evaluation shows three main patterns of disease: diffuse, miliary, and nodular (Fig. 42-2). Diffuse refers to a diffuse expansion of the spleen with a homogeneous cut surface. This pattern often correlates with diffuse red pulp disease with decreased or lost white pulp and is often seen with metabolic disease, red blood cell disor-

TABLE 42-1. **Contents of the Final Report: Spleen**

***Gross Examination***
Weight
External examination of capsule
Cut surface pattern (1-cm or thinner sections throughout)
  Nodular
  Diffuse
  Miliary
  Mixed
Gross lesion sampling as indicated
Touch or scrape preparation slides, and save fresh or frozen tissue as indicated by gross examination and clinical information

***Microscopic Examination***
Low-magnification pattern of disease
  Nodular
  Primarily red pulp involvement (with or without residual white pulp)
  Expanded white pulp
High magnification features of nodular disease

Cyst or inflammatory proliferation?
Vascular proliferation?
Lymphoid proliferation?
Metastatic disease?
High magnification features of red pulp disease
  Entrapped abnormal red blood cells of a red blood cell disorder?
  Hemophagocytosis or abnormal (Gaucher or Niemann-Pick) histiocytes?
  Blast cells, hairy cells, or atypical T cell population of a hematopoietic neoplasm?
  Extramedullary hematopoiesis with atypical megakaryocyte clusters of a chronic myeloproliferative disorder?
  Increase in B cells associated with expansion of the white pulp (suggestive of low-grade B cell lymphona)?
High magnification features of expanded white pulp
  Three distinct zones of reactive follicles?
  Biphasic pattern of splenic marginal zone lymphoma?
  Central white pulp evidence of other lymphoma (with or without a prominent marginal zone)?

**TABLE 42-2.** Gross and Microscopic Patterns of Splenic Involvement

| Diffuse or Predominantly Red Pulp Disease | Miliary or Predominantly White Pulp Disease | Predominantly Nodular Disease |
|---|---|---|
| Hemophagocytic syndromes | Reactive hyperplasia | Cysts |
| Infectious mononucleosis* | Infectious mononucleosis* | Abscess |
| Malaria | Granulomatous inflammation* | Granulomatous inflammation (especially tuberculosis and tertiary syphilis)* |
| Metabolic diseases (especially Gaucher's and Niemann-Pick diseases) | Human immunodeficiency virus infection | Localized reactive lymphoid hyperplasia |
| Red blood cell disorders (including hereditary spherocytosis) | Bacillary splenitis | Inflammatory pseudotumor |
| Peliosis | Idiopathic thrombocytopenic purpura | Hamartoma |
| Hemangiomatosis | Chronic lymphocytic leukemia/small lymphocytic lymphoma | Hemangioma |
| Lymphangiomatosis | Prolymphocytic leukemia | Littoral cell angioma |
| Mast cell disease† | Follicular center cell lymphoma, grades 1 and 2 | Epithelioid hemangioendothelioma |
| Acute leukemias | Mantle cell lymphoma | Angiosarcoma |
| Hairy cell leukemia | Splenic marginal zone lymphoma | Metastatic tumors |
| Chronic myeloproliferative disorders | Lymphoplasmacytic lymphoma* | Large B cell lymphoma |
| Chronic myelomonocytic leukemia | Early involvement by large B cell lymphoma | Hodgkin's disease |
| Lymphoblastic lymphoma | | Follicular center cell lymphoma, grade 3 |
| Hepatosplenic $\gamma \delta$ T cell lymphoma | | Some peripheral T cell lymphomas |
| Large granular lymphocytosis | | |
| Lymphoplasmacytic lymphoma* | | |
| Some peripheral T cell lymphomas | | |
| Rare large B cell lymphomas | | |

* More than one pattern may occur with these diseases.
† Mast cell disease may also demonstrate a multifocal gross "scarring" pattern that does not fit into the other categories.

ders, leukemic infiltrations other than chronic lymphocytic leukemia, and some T cell neoplasms. The miliary pattern is one of punctate round to irregular white areas evenly distributed across the splenic cut surface. These areas generally correlate with white pulp expansions, including florid white pulp hyperplasia, infectious diseases, chronic lymphocytic leukemia, and low-grade B cell lymphomas. Early splenic involvement by large B cell lymphoma may also give this pattern. The nodular pattern represents single to multiple gross tumor nodules that are usually not encapsulated. These most often correlate with cysts, vascular tumors, large cell lymphoma, Hodgkin's disease, and metastatic carcinoma, but gross nodules may also be seen in some reactive conditions. Mixtures of these patterns also occur, especially a mixed nodular and miliary pattern in low-grade lymphomas with nodular areas of large cell transformation. Rarely, vague nodules may be superimposed on an otherwise diffuse pattern. These may represent aggregates of blast cells, megakaryocytes, or sea-blue histiocytes in patients with extensive red pulp involvement by a chronic myeloproliferative disorder or an unusually dense accumulation of hairy cells in a patient with hairy cell leukemia.[13, 14] Subcapsular, wedge-shaped areas of infarction that are massively enlarged in an otherwise diffuse pattern are also frequently present in the spleen.

Microscopic pattern schemes are similar to the gross miliary and diffuse patterns and have employed categories of white pulp versus red pulp lesions. Most malignant lymphomas of B lineage and chronic lymphocytic leukemia are in the predominantly white pulp distribution group; T cell lymphomas and most other leukemias are generally assigned to the predominantly red pulp disease group. Even microscopic patterns of involvement may be misleading, such as large B cell lymphomas with a predominantly red pulp pattern, so these types of schemes must be used only as guidelines and not as absolutes. Table 42-2 lists the most common patterns of splenic involvement by various diseases.

## CONGENITAL AND ACQUIRED DISORDERS

### Ectopic Splenic Tissue

Up to 19% of humans have accessory spleens,[15, 16] which enlarge after splenectomy. The gross and histologic features of the accessory spleen are similar to those of the normal spleen with both red and white pulp components. After trauma to the spleen, autotransplantation of splenic tissue (splenosis) may occur, forming multiple dark red nodules within the splenic mesentery.[17-19] The nodules of splenosis are similar to accessory spleens but are usually multiple and frequently are composed of only red pulp. Because of the similarities between splenosis and accessory spleen, the distinction between them often depends on the clinical history and intraoperative findings. Rare cases of intrahepatic splenic tissue have also been reported, apparently enlarging with functional red and white pulp after splenectomy.[20]

Splenic-gonadal fusion (CD Fig. 42–1) occurs in males with attachment of the spleen or an accessory spleen to the left testicle in two different manners.[21] Continuous splenic-gonadal fusion indicates a cord-like attachment between the spleen and gonad, with fibrous and splenic tissue identified within the cord. *Discontinuous fusion* is the term for a direct attachment of an accessory spleen to the gonad. Subsets of patients with splenic-gonadal fusion also have congenital defects of the extremities and mandible.

## Cysts

Cysts of the spleen are found in less than 1% of splenectomy specimens[21a] and may be congenital or acquired. They are often asymptomatic, but large cysts may present as an abdominal mass with pain. Splenic cysts are most frequently detected in men in the third decade of life. Although they vary in size, the average reported size is 10 cm.[22]

Splenic cysts may be classified as primary or secondary, which have also been termed *true or false cysts,* respectively.[22] Both cyst types are usually unilocular, but small primary cysts may be multilocular (Fig. 42–3) (CD Fig. 42–2). Primary cysts have a firm, roughened, and trabecular gross appearance to the lining that is similar to normal endocardium. The cyst wall is composed of thick fibrous tissue with an epithelial lining. This lining is usually mesothelial or squamous, but lining cells may be present only focally. The squamous lining of some primary cysts probably represents a metaplastic change, and subdividing these cases by type of epithelial lining does not appear warranted.[23] Because the lining epithelium may be only focally present, multiple sections of the cyst wall may be needed to identify lining cells and to classify the cyst properly. Primary cysts may be parasitic or nonparasitic. Primary parasitic (echinococcal) cysts are relatively uncommon in Western countries, but parasite scolices are usually identifiable. Nonparasitic cysts probably arise from congenital inclusions and include small subcapsular lesions that have previously been interpreted as solitary lymphangiomas of the spleen.[24, 25]

Secondary splenic cysts are more common than primary ones, representing approximately 80% of all splenic cysts. They are usually associated with abdominal trauma and are probably acquired. The grossly smooth lining of the secondary cyst differs from the characteristic trabecular gross appearance of the primary cyst. No epithelial lining is identifiable in secondary cysts, and the wall is composed of thick fibrous tissue that may contain calcification and hemosiderin.

## INFECTIOUS DISEASES

### Hemophagocytic Syndromes

The hemophagocytic syndromes may be primary or secondary. Primary hemophagocytic lymphohistiocytosis is either familial or sporadic and is an autosomal recessive, usually fatal disorder of early infancy.[26–30] Specific diagnostic criteria are defined for this disorder; these are the presence of fever of undetermined etiology for at least 1 week, splenomegaly, cytopenias, hypofibrinogenemia or hypertriglyceridemia, and tissue evidence of hemophagocytosis.[31] The most common sites of hemophagocytosis are bone marrow, spleen, and lymph node, but not all may be involved. Secondary hemophagocytic syndromes are usually related to an infection or malignant neoplasm, but they may also be associated with other disorders (immune deficiencies, Chédiak-Higashi disease, Langerhans cell histiocytosis, rheumatoid arthritis, necrotizing lymphadenitis) and even lipid-rich parenteral hyperalimentation.[26] Infection-related hemophagocytic syndromes were originally described in association with viruses,[32] including cytomegalovirus, Epstein-Barr virus, and other herpesviruses, but hemophagocytic syndromes also occur with other types of infections, including bacterial.[33] Primary hemophagocytic lymphohistiocytosis is also commonly elicited by a viral infection, which makes the clinical distinction between the primary and secondary forms difficult.

Despite the cause, the hemophagocytic syndromes have similar morphologic features (Fig. 42–4). In a series of children with hemophagocytic lymphohistiocytosis, the spleen was the most commonly affected organ with involvement in 71% of patients.[27] The spleen is usually massively enlarged for the patient's age. Mononuclear histiocytes expand the red pulp, and the white pulp lymphocytes are reduced in number or may be absent. Erythrophagocytosis may be evident in the red pulp on histologic sections, but this feature is not always obvious on H&E-stained sections alone. Hemophagocytosis is usually more easily identified on imprint slides. On

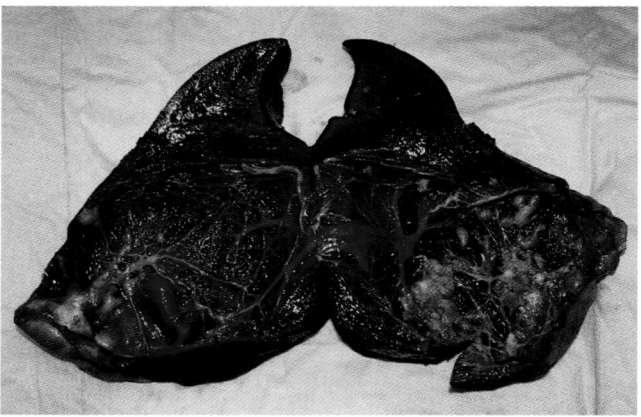

**FIGURE 42–3.** Primary cyst of the spleen. The lining of the collapsed cyst has a trabecular pattern.

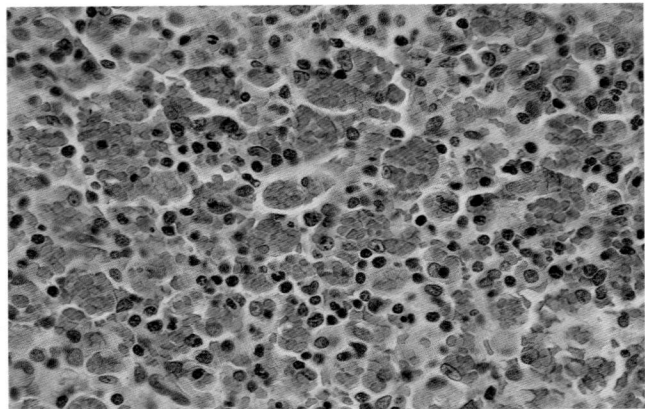

**FIGURE 42–4.** Hemophagocytic syndrome showing marked erythrophagocytosis.

imprints, phagocytosed red blood cells and platelets are most commonly seen, but intracellular lymphocytes and granulocytes may also be identified. Distinguishing primary from secondary disease is generally not possible by morphologic examination alone, with the exception of cases of malignant neoplasia–associated hemophagocytosis. T cell lymphomas, including hepatosplenic γδ T cell lymphoma, are the most common malignant neoplasms associated with hemophagocytosis. Atypical lymphoid cells may be evident adjacent to or admixed with the non-neoplastic phagocytosing histiocytes. Immunohistochemical studies may identify an atypical T cell population (CD3+) within the areas of hemophagocytosis, and patients with hemophagocytosis should be examined carefully to exclude an underlying malignant neoplasm.

## Abscesses

Splenic abscesses are uncommon and are usually associated with sepsis or endocarditis, contiguous spread, infection after abdominal trauma with possible splenic rupture, and functional asplenia of sickle cell disease.[34–38] Streptococci, staphylococci, *Escherichia coli,* and salmonellae are the most common organisms associated with splenic abscesses, and infections are polymicrobial in more than half of cases. Numerous other bacteria and fungi may be associated with abscess formation, however, and appropriate cultures should be obtained in all cases. The abscesses may be single or multiple. Single lesions are most easily recognized before splenectomy; they usually have a thick fibrous capsule and are surrounded by normal splenic parenchyma with white pulp hyperplasia. A fibrous capsule may not be present around smaller abscesses in patients with multiple lesions. Abscesses, particularly in patients with sickle cell anemia, are usually treated with splenectomy.

## Epstein-Barr Virus and Infectious Mononucleosis

The features of Epstein-Barr virus–associated hemophagocytic syndrome are not specific for this virus (see earlier). Infectious mononucleosis, usually due to Epstein-Barr virus infection, is associated with splenomegaly in virtually all cases, although it may be clinically apparent in only half of cases. The spleen is diffusely enlarged without discrete masses. The white pulp may be expanded or depleted but shows a spectrum of cellular changes that may suggest splenic involvement by malignant lymphoma.[39–43] The lymphoid infiltrate involves the white pulp and some of the red pulp. It includes a spectrum of small, medium, and large atypical lymphoid cells, many with plasmacytoid features, as well as cells that may have morphologic features suggestive of Reed-Sternberg cells and their mononuclear variants (Fig. 42–5). Individual cell necrosis, larger areas of necrosis, and epithelioid granulomas are also common in infectious mononucleosis. Many of the lymphoid cells have a T suppressor immunophenotype and may express CD30. The expression of CD30, an activation antigen also expressed by the neoplastic cells of Hodgkin's disease and anaplastic large cell lymphoma, may lead to overinterpretation of these specimens as neoplastic. The spectrum of plasmacytoid cells, the presence of individual cell necrosis, and the lack of tumor nodules, however, are features of infectious mononucleosis that are not seen in Hodgkin's disease and are rare in large cell lymphomas. In some cases, in situ hybridization using probes directed against Epstein-Barr virus EBER-1 RNA may help confirm the diagnosis. Although the Reed-Sternberg cells of some cases of Hodgkin's disease may be Epstein-Barr virus positive, the background lymphoid cells in Hodgkin's disease are usually negative in contrast to the marked positivity of many different cell types in infectious mononucleosis.[43, 44]

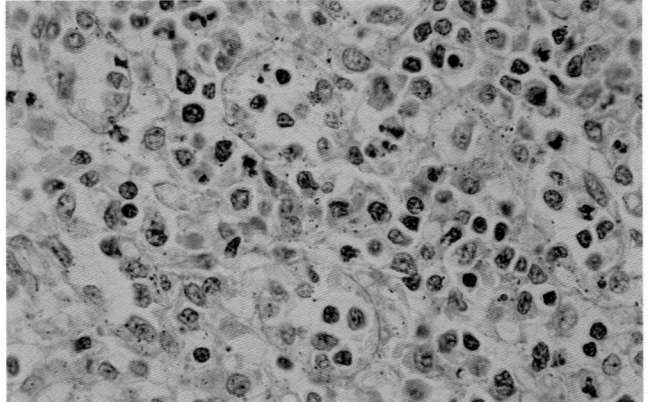

**FIGURE 42–5.** Epstein-Barr virus–associated infectious mononucleosis showing a spectrum of plasmacytoid lymphocytes and individual cell necrosis in the red pulp.

Numerous reports indicate an increased frequency of splenic rupture in patients with infectious mononucleosis. This disorder and malaria are the most frequent causes of infection-related splenic rupture.[39, 45] Rare cases of spontaneous splenic rupture in infectious mononucleosis have been described, but most are associated with at least minor abdominal trauma. Infiltration of the splenic capsule and trabeculae by the polymorphous plasmacytoid cell proliferation is commonly seen in the ruptured splenectomy specimen.[39, 40]

## Granulomatous Diseases

Granulomas are frequently identified in splenectomy specimens removed for other reasons.[46, 47] As in other organs, necrotizing granulomas (CD Fig. 42–3) involving the spleen may occur with mycobacterial infections, histoplasmosis, and infectious mononucleosis, and noncaseating granulomas may be seen in sarcoidosis, brucellosis, and syphilis. Miliary tuberculosis may cause a gross splenic cut surface pattern similar to that seen in reactive white pulp hyperplasia, but the small nodules of tuberculosis are usually yellow in contrast to the gray-white gross appearance of small reactive white pulp lymph follicles. It is now uncommon to find the large tumor nodules caused by late-stage infectious diseases, such as tuberculosis and tertiary syphilis.

Granulomas are also common in the spleen without an associated infectious disease. They are common in and around the white pulp in association with splenic involvement by almost any type of non-Hodgkin's lymphoma and in Hodgkin's disease. Splenic granulomas are frequent in patients with Hodgkin's disease,[48, 49] even when the spleen is not involved; therefore, granulomas alone should not be misinterpreted as representing splenic involvement by Hodgkin's disease. Granulomas of the spleen are also reported to be increased in association with chronic uremia and selective immunoglobulin A deficiency.[46]

Splenic lipogranulomas not associated with disease are found at autopsy in half of patients in North America, are usually seen only in adulthood, and are presumably related to dietary intake.[50, 51] These granulomas are composed of clusters of vacuolated histiocytes surrounded by lymphocytes and plasma cells. Granulomas are also seen after lymphangiograms and contain epithelioid, foreign body–type histiocytes.

## Other Infections: Malaria and Human Immunodeficiency Virus Infection

Although not commonly seen by the surgical pathologist, parasitic diseases such as malaria, leishmaniasis, and schistosomiasis may result in massive splenomegaly. Worldwide, malaria is one of the most common causes of splenomegaly, particularly in the chronic stage. The spleen is massively enlarged and the malarial pigment imparts a dark brown-black color to the cut surface. Scarring or evidence of rupture may be evident grossly. Microscopic examination reveals heavy pigment deposition, and aggregates of red blood cells containing the parasites occlude vessels in the acute form of the disease.

A variety of opportunistic infections and neoplasms may involve the spleen of patients with the acquired immunodeficiency syndrome (AIDS), but these are not lesions that are generally specific to the spleen. Gross lesions, including white pulp accentuation, granulomas, and infarcts, may be evident in half of cases. The microscopic features of the AIDS spleen are variable and may include white pulp depletion; histiocyte, plasma cell, or immunoblastic proliferations of the white pulp, red pulp, or both; and nonspecific cord congestion of the red pulp.[52] The white pulp changes in AIDS are similar to those of lymph nodes. In the early stages of the disease, the white pulp demonstrates expanded germinal centers and marginal zones, resulting in splenomegaly.[53] Cellular depletion of the white pulp and the periarterial lymphoid sheaths occurs in the later stages of the disease.[53] The late-stage AIDS spleen may have features that are indistinguishable from those of patients with severe combined immunodeficiency or Wiskott-Aldrich syndrome[54] or of patients who have received chemotherapy.

Spleens from patients with AIDS may also have an increase in perivascular and nodular amyloid-like material. Small accumulations of eosinophilic, fibrinous material are seen in the white pulp follicles of many spleens, and this finding is nonspecific. However, in AIDS, larger nodular aggregates of relatively acellular, fibrillar-appearing amorphous material may be confused with amyloid. This material does not demonstrate the characteristic apple-green birefringence of amyloid with the Congo red stain and does not show features of amyloid by electron microscopy.[55] These hyalinized nodules of the spleen probably represent areas of regression of previous AIDS-associated follicle hyperplasia. Another feature of late human immunodeficiency virus infection is increased numbers of S-100 protein–positive macrophages in the red pulp. The most frequent opportunistic infections to directly involve the AIDS spleen are due to *Mycobacterium avium-intracellulare* and cytomegalovirus, and the most frequent AIDS-associated neoplasms seen in the spleen are malignant lymphomas and Kaposi's sarcoma.[52]

Human immunodeficiency virus–positive patients who are also infected with *Bartonella henselae* may have splenic involvement by bacillary angiomatosis, which has been termed *bacillary peliosis* or *bacillary splenitis*.[56–59] The spleen is moderately enlarged and demonstrates a miliary gross pattern of involve-

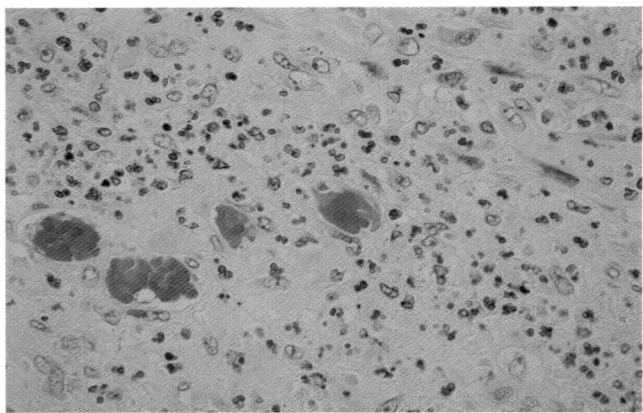

**FIGURE 42–6.** Bacillary angiomatosis. Aggregates of neutrophils are admixed with a proliferation of plump, bland vascular cells.

ment on the cut surface, with coalescing, bulging, fleshy nodules up to 2 cm in diameter. A lobular proliferation of branching vessels with plump lining cells and admixed neutrophils, lymphocytes, and histiocytes is present (Fig. 42–6), similar to the cutaneous lesions of this infection. In addition, areas of blood-filled, dilated vascular spaces are present as well as suppurative nodules surrounded by histiocytes. Numerous bacilli may be identified on Warthin-Starry stain, especially in the areas of vascular proliferation and dilatation. Rare cases of bacillary angiomatosis, including splenic involvement, have been reported without associated immunosuppression.[60]

## Splenic Rupture

Splenic rupture is frequently associated with other diseases but is usually accompanied by some degree of trauma. Rupture is most commonly associated with severe trauma, infectious mononucleosis (see earlier), malaria, peliosis, amyloidosis, and malignant neoplasms.[61–66] Malignant neoplasms reported with rupture include acute and chronic leukemias, multiple myeloma, malignant lymphomas, angiosarcoma, and metastatic malignant melanoma and carcinoma of varying types. Even when trauma is considered the sole cause of splenic rupture, the spleen demonstrates changes different from those in nonruptured control spleens.[63–67] The ruptured spleen is generally heavier than control spleens and has an increased lymphoid component. The white pulp is expanded with germinal center formation commonly present in adult patients, compared with the inactive white pulp of the usual adult spleen. Numbers of CD4+ parafollicular T cells are increased in ruptured spleens compared with control spleens. These findings suggest that some type of unrecognized immunologic stimulation in these patients may predispose them to traumatic rupture of the spleen.

## METABOLIC DISEASES

Many different congenital enzymatic abnormalities may result in the accumulation of metabolic products in histiocytes, causing the so-called storage diseases.[68] When these abnormalities involve the spleen, splenomegaly results from the massive accumulation of histiocytes in the red pulp. The spleen has a homogeneous, pale cut surface. Gaucher's, Niemann-Pick, Tay-Sachs, Fabry's, Wolman's, von Gierke's, and Tangier diseases and Hunter's, Hurler's, and Hermansky-Pudlak syndromes may involve the spleen. Most of these occur in infancy or childhood, although an adult type (type 1) of Gaucher's disease is relatively common. The precise diagnosis of any of these disorders requires detection of the specific enzymatic or molecular genetic defect,[69] and a detailed description of the morphologic and biochemical abnormalities of each disease is beyond the scope of this chapter. The interested reader is referred to other texts that deal with this subject in great detail.[68]

In general, Gaucher's and Niemann-Pick diseases are the most common to involve the spleen (Fig. 42–7). The histiocytes of Gaucher's disease are most easily evaluated on touch imprints and have a characteristic, fine "tissue paper" character to their cytoplasm, in contrast to the multivacuolated cytoplasm of the Niemann-Pick histiocyte. Ceroid (sea-blue) histiocytes, with dirty brown, granular cytoplasm on tissue sections and blue-green cytoplasm on Wright-Giemsa–stained imprints, and less distinctive histiocytes are seen with other storage diseases and are generally nonspecific. Ceroid histiocytes may also be seen in association with chronic myeloproliferative disorders, red blood cell disorders, and autoimmune diseases.[70] The Gaucher and ceroid histiocytes contain diastase-resistant, periodic acid–Schiff—positive material. The Gaucher cell cytoplasm is autofluorescent and may stain for lipid and iron. The ceroid histiocyte is characteristically positive with acid-fast stains and iron stains, and unfixed tissue stains with oil red O. The Niemann-Pick histiocytes are faintly periodic acid–Schiff positive and are positive for oil red O or other fat stains.

## RED BLOOD CELL DISORDERS

A variety of red blood cell disorders result in splenomegaly.[71] The mechanism of splenomegaly of each of these is similar. Abnormal hemoglobin production or abnormalities of red blood cell surface spectrin or related proteins cause the cell to lose its normal pliability, which is necessary for the cells to pass through the cords of Billroth into the splenic sinuses. This disruption of the normal circulation of red blood cells results in expansion of the splenic red pulp cords with fairly open sinuses. Splenomegaly due to this mechanism occurs in hereditary spherocytosis and elliptocytosis, in hemoglobinopa-

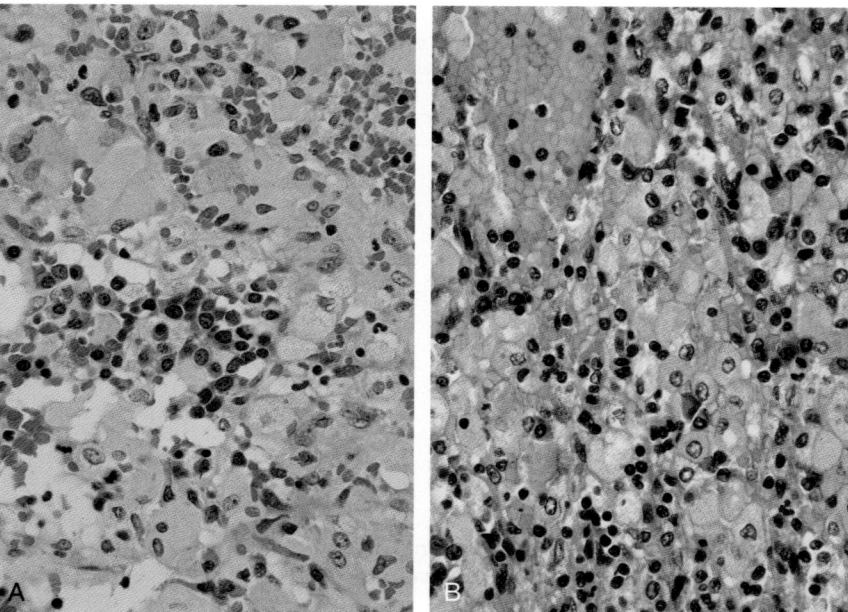

**FIGURE 42-7.** Red pulp involvement by (*A*) Gaucher's disease with histiocytes with abundant fine cytoplasms and (*B*) Niemann-Pick disease with multivacuolated histiocytes.

thies, in autoimmune hemolytic anemia, and with parasitic infection of red blood cells.

Hereditary spherocytosis is one of the most common of these disorders to result in splenectomy. This is usually an autosomal dominant disorder that results in diffuse expansion of the red pulp with engorged cords and open sinuses. A similar pattern is seen with all of the red blood cell disorders, although the degree of splenomegaly may vary and splenectomy is not usually performed for the hemoglobinopathies. Sickle cell anemia will also result in splenomegaly, often massive, in infants and young children before the spleen infarcts and eventually involutes. In late childhood and adulthood, the spleen has become nonfunctional and is small and fibrotic. Gamna-Gandy bodies (CD Fig. 42-4), areas of old infarction that show fibrosis with calcification and hemosiderin deposition, are numerous in the nonfunctional spleen of patients with sickle cell anemia.

## AUTOIMMUNE DISORDERS

As in hereditary spherocytosis, the diagnosis of idiopathic thrombocytopenic purpura (ITP) is usually well established before splenectomy. Hypersplenism due to other causes, including vascular proliferations and lymphoproliferative disorders, may also result in thrombocytopenia and may be mistaken for ITP. Therefore, morphologic evaluation of all splenectomy specimens for suspected ITP is essential.

The cut surface of the ITP spleen is usually unremarkable except for a possible accentuation of the white pulp. At microscopic examination, the white pulp is usually hyperplastic with germinal center formation and distinct mantle and marginal zones.

Such changes are not usually seen in normal adult spleens but are common with ITP as well as with other autoimmune disorders, including Felty's syndrome, or after antigenic stimulation.[72] In ITP, the red pulp demonstrates an increased number of foamy macrophages that may contain recognizable, engulfed platelets.[73] Small collections of lymphocytes and plasma cells are also commonly present in the red pulp.

The morphologic findings in the spleen may be more subdued if corticosteroid therapy was given before splenectomy.[74] In these cases, the reactive white pulp changes and red pulp lymphoplasmacytoid aggregates are usually absent, but platelet-containing foamy macrophages are still evident.

## VASCULAR AND LYMPHATIC PROLIFERATIONS

Vascular lesions are the most common primary proliferations of the spleen and occur in a variety of forms. Some are diffuse proliferations, whereas others may form single or multiple tumors. Diffuse proliferations are less common and include peliosis, hemangiomatosis, and lymphangiomatosis. The immunophenotypic features of some of these proliferations are summarized in Table 42-3.

### Peliosis

Peliosis of the spleen is a rare, generally diffuse proliferation of small vascular spaces that is usually an incidental finding in adults.[75, 76] It is most commonly associated with prior use of anabolic steroids,

**TABLE 42–3.** Immunophenotype of the Lining Cells of Splenic Vascular Tumors

| Diagnosis | CD31, vWF, Ulex* | CD34 | CD68 | CD21 | CD8 |
|---|---|---|---|---|---|
| Littoral cell angioma | + | − | + | + | − |
| Hemangioma | + | + | ∓ | − | − |
| Hamartoma | + | ± | − | − | + |
| Angiosarcoma | + | ± | ∓ | − | ∓ |

*vWF, von Willebrand factor (factor VIII–related antigen); Ulex, *Ulex europaeus.*

but it may also be seen in association with malignant neoplasms, tuberculosis, and aplastic anemia. It is frequently present with hepatic peliosis but may be an isolated finding. The spleen is usually not enlarged. The gross cut surface may demonstrate small (less than 1 mm), dilated vascular spaces or may be unremarkable.

At microscopic examination, numerous round to oval blood-filled cavities are lined by a single layer of flattened cells (Fig. 42–8). Prominent fibrosis of the surrounding splenic cords is not evident. The vascular proliferation of peliosis may be confused with dilated sinuses related to splenic congestion. In contrast to passive congestion of the spleen, which primarily involves the central red pulp, peliosis involves both the central red pulp and areas immediately around the white pulp, including the marginal zone. Some cases have a distinct perifollicular pattern of involvement.[77] In contrast to the usual peliosis, bacillary peliosis, as described before, demonstrates accompanying vascular and suppurative lesions.

## Hemangiomas

Splenic hemangiomas are usually asymptomatic, incidental findings but may cause splenomegaly with associated abdominal discomfort or hypersplenism.[22, 78, 79] Hemangiomas are most commonly localized, causing single or multiple discrete nodules, but they may also form diffuse proliferations (hemangiomatosis). The gross splenic cut surface contains cystic, blood-filled spaces of varying sizes. Splenic hemangiomas are histologically identical to hemangiomas of other sites. A cavernous component is almost always present, and a single, flattened layer of bland endothelium lines the vascular spaces. Focal papillary areas may be present in regions of organizing thrombus, but the lining cells remain bland without nuclear enlargement or mitotic activity. Fibrosis is commonly present between the vascular spaces, and rare cases may demonstrate calcification.

Diffuse hemangiomatosis[80, 81] is much less common than localized vascular tumors but may occur at any age and be associated with systemic hemangiomatosis. The spleen is usually massively enlarged and may have a distorted, irregular external surface because of parenchymal scarring. The entire splenic cut surface is involved by the vascular proliferation (CD Fig. 42–5).

Massive splenomegaly, cavernous vascular spaces, and fibrosis are features that help differentiate hemangiomatosis from peliosis. The immunohistochemical detection of vascular antigens, such as CD31, CD34, von Willebrand factor, and *Ulex europaeus,* confirms the vascular nature of hemangiomas but is not usually necessary.

## Lymphangiomas

Lymphangiomas of the spleen, also considered to be common tumors, are reported to occur in localized or diffuse forms.[22, 78, 82] Both are described as having features of lymphangiomas of other sites with a proliferation of cystic, thin-walled lymphatic spaces lined by a single layer of flattened to plump cells. The cystic spaces are filled with mostly acellular, eosinophilic proteinaceous material with occasional lymphocytes, red blood cells, and histiocytes.

The localized lesions are the most common and are usually incidental findings representing a single cyst or a cluster of several small cysts in a capsular location (CD Fig. 42–6). The subcapsular location and the lack of prominent blood-filled spaces help in excluding a hemangioma. Most of these localized lesions probably do not represent true lymphangiomas, however. Immunohistochemical studies have demonstrated that most localized subcapsular lesions with features of lymphangiomas are actually small, incidental mesothelial cysts with keratin-positive lining cells.[25] However, because of the lack of clinical significance to the differentiation of mesothelial cyst from lymphangioma in most cases, it is probably unnecessary to routinely perform immunohistochemical studies on all of these fairly commonly identified, incidental proliferations.

Diffuse or multiple lymphangiomas of the spleen (lymphangiomatosis), however, are rare true

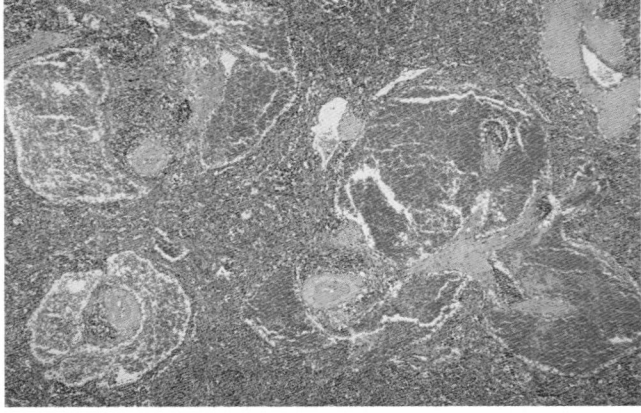

**FIGURE 42–8.** Peliosis of the spleen with dilated, blood-filled spaces separated by normal-appearing red pulp.

lymphatic tumors that frequently involve other organs but may be localized to the spleen.[82-86] Lymphangiomatosis is most commonly identified in children or young adults but may occur at any age. The spleen is usually massively enlarged. The cut surface has a spongy multicystic appearance with cysts up to 3 cm in diameter containing pink-brown thick fluid (CD Fig. 42–7). The thin-walled cystic spaces are lined by bland, flattened cells; pink-staining fluid in the spaces may contain varying numbers of red blood cells. The lining cells are positive for von Willebrand factor and negative for keratin.

## Littoral Cell Angioma

Unlike most splenic vascular tumors, littoral cell angioma is unique to the spleen. Littoral cell angioma is a fairly recently described tumor that differs in morphologic features and by immunophenotype from traditional hemangiomas; it is presumably derived from the normal splenic littoral cell.[79, 87] The tumor may occur at any age and frequently causes mild to moderate splenic enlargement, although the lesion is often an incidental finding. It usually forms multiple nodules that are grossly distinct and vary

from 0.2 to 9.0 cm. At gross evaluation, as with hemangiomas, dark, spongy hemorrhagic spaces are present (Fig. 42–9) (CD Fig. 42–8).

The microscopic features differ from those of the usual hemangioma, however. The vascular spaces are lined by plump to tall cells with enlarged nuclei and small nucleoli. Despite the nuclear enlargement, nuclear pleomorphism and mitotic figures are not present. The lining cells also form tufts or micropapillary structures, and lining cells and histiocytes are present within the lumina. These sloughed cells may demonstrate evidence of hemophagocytosis with intracellular pigment. The lining cells of littoral cell angioma have a unique immunophenotype that is useful in differentiating this tumor from other splenic proliferations. The cells express the vascular-associated antigen CD31 and are immunoreactive for von Willebrand factor and with *Ulex europaeus*. They lack expression of CD34 on the actual lining cells and do not express CD8, an antigen normally expressed by sinus lining cells. The cells demonstrate a unique pattern of expression of the histiocyte-associated antigen CD68 and the complement receptor CD21, both of which can be detected in paraffin sections.[79] This immunophenotype appears to be unique to littoral cell angioma.

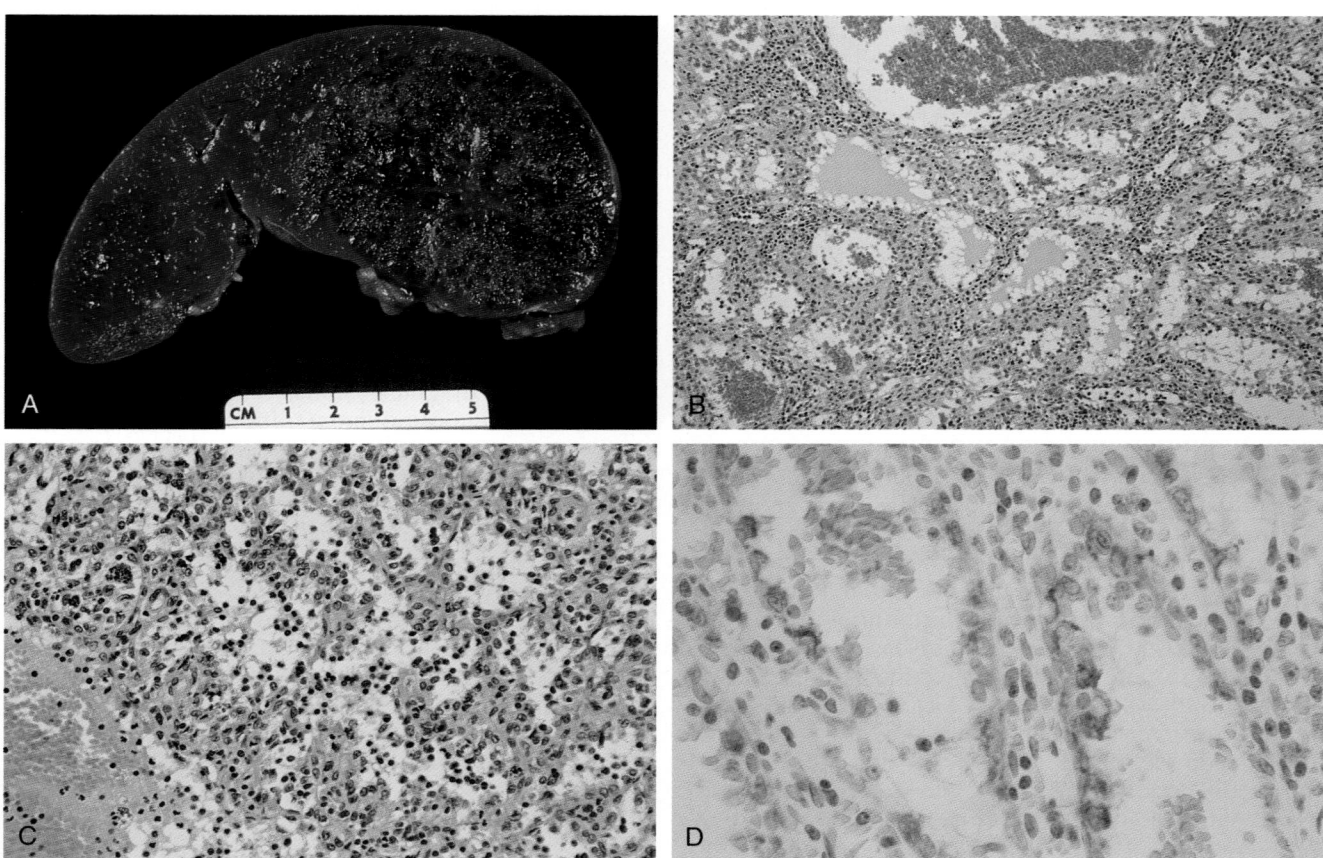

**FIGURE 42–9.** *A.* Littoral cell angioma of the spleen characteristically forms a hemorrhagic mass in the spleen. The microscopic pattern varies from cystic *(B)* to micropapillary *(C)* with enlarged lining cells that slough into the luminal spaces. The lining cells are usually positive for CD21 *(D)* as well as for CD31 and CD68.

The primary tumors in the differential diagnosis with littoral cell angioma are hemangioma and angiosarcoma. The nuclear enlargement with papillary structures helps distinguish littoral cell angioma from hemangioma; the lack of true nuclear pleomorphism, mitotic figures, and necrosis help exclude angiosarcoma. A subgroup of hemangiomas and angiosarcomas may express CD68, and this marker should not be used alone to make a diagnosis of littoral cell angioma. Hemangiomas and angiosarcomas are generally CD21-negative.

## Kaposi's Sarcoma, Epithelioid Hemangioendothelioma, and Angiosarcoma

Kaposi's sarcoma involving the spleen is most commonly associated with human immunodeficiency virus infection. The proliferation may diffusely replace the splenic parenchyma or may form isolated purple nodules that are usually less than 1 cm.[53] The spindled cell proliferation is similar to that in other sites, with irregular tumor nodules that invade the red pulp.

Epithelioid hemangioendothelioma is considered a borderline or low-grade angiosarcoma and has only rarely been reported in spleens of children and adults.[88-90] As with angiosarcoma, the patients usually present with anemia and may have evidence of hypersplenism or hyposplenism. The spleen is moderately to markedly enlarged and contains large, usually circumscribed, white or variegated white and red tumor nodules. At microscopic examination, the tumor in sharply demarcated from the surrounding splenic tissue and is composed of lobules of epithelioid cells with admixed small vessels surrounded by fibrous bands. Intracellular lumina may be evident within the pale, eosinophilic cytoplasm of some of the epithelioid cells. These cells have indistinct cytoplasmic borders and enlarged nuclei with nucleoli. Mitotic figures are present, but there is usually less than 1 mitosis per 10 high-power fields. Necrosis is not present in most cases. Immunohistochemical studies for vascular markers such as von Willebrand factor, CD31, and CD34 identify small slitlike vascular spaces and intracellular lumina and help in excluding other epithelioid and spindled cell tumors. In contrast to usual high-grade angiosarcomas, these tumors are often incidental findings; several reported cases have been localized to the spleen without recurrence after splenectomy.

High-grade angiosarcoma of the spleen most commonly occurs in adults; it is associated with prominent splenomegaly, cytopenias, and abdominal pain and is often accompanied by splenic rupture.[79, 91, 92] Because the disease is frequently disseminated at the time of diagnosis, it may be difficult to determine whether a lesion represents a primary splenic tumor or metastasis. The spleen usually weighs more than 500 g, and the cut surface shows

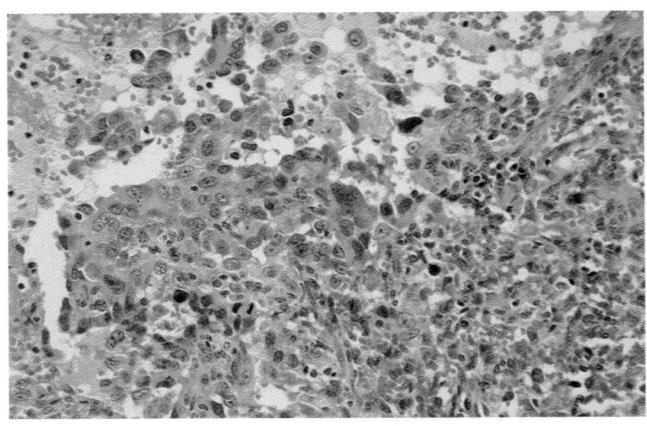

**FIGURE 42-10.** High-grade angiosarcoma of the spleen with cytologic atypia and necrosis.

a diffuse, variable appearance with both tumor nodules and hemorrhagic cysts. The tumor may have a varied microscopic appearance, but cytologic atypia and areas of necrosis are consistently present, and frequent mitoses are easily identified in most cases (Fig. 42-10). The most common pattern is one of irregular anastomosing blood-filled channels lined by plump endothelial cells with cytologic atypia. Areas with tufting or papillary proliferations of the endothelial cells may be present, and the low-power appearance of the proliferation may be poorly delineated from the surrounding non-neoplastic red pulp. Rarely, a predominantly cavernous pattern may mimic a hemangioma, but the lining cells demonstrate obvious cytologic evidence of malignancy. Some tumors are more difficult to identify as angiosarcoma because of a predominantly solid and sarcomatous pattern that resembles other high-grade sarcomas. Careful examination of multiple sections of the tumor may reveal areas of obvious vascular proliferation with blood-filled spaces lined by tumor cells, but for diagnosis, some cases may require immunohistochemical demonstration of vascular antigen expression, such as CD31, CD34, von Willebrand factor, or *Ulex europaeus*. Rare cases of splenic angiosarcoma with cytochemical or immunohistochemical evidence of sinus lining cell differentiation have been reported,[93-96] suggesting a malignant counterpart to splenic littoral cell angioma. Whether cases of this type differ from the usual type of high-grade angiosarcoma of the spleen is not clear. In general, high-grade angiosarcomas of the spleen have a poor prognosis; most patients die within 1 year of diagnosis.

## HAMARTOMA

Splenic hamartomas, also known as splenomas or spleen-in-spleen syndrome, may occur at any age.[97-100] They are rare proliferations that are usually incidental findings, although rare cases have been associated with abdominal pain, cytopenias, and

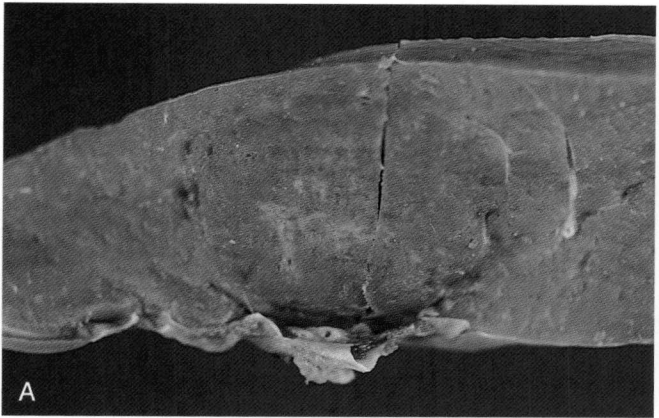 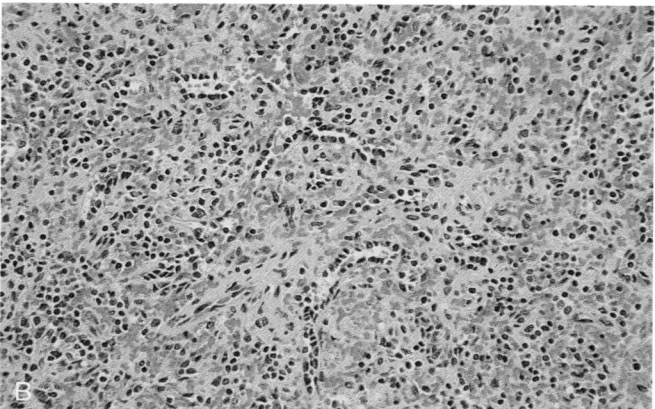

FIGURE 42–11. *A.* Hamartoma of the spleen with the characteristic bulging cut gross surface. *B.* The hamartoma microscopically resembles normal red pulp with increased fibrosis.

even splenic rupture. Up to 30% of patients with hamartomas have hematologic evidence of hypersplenism. Splenic hamartomas may be single or multiple and form bulging, nonencapsulated masses on the cut surface of the spleen (Fig. 42–11) (CD Fig. 42–9). In general, they have a gross appearance similar to the normal splenic cut surface or may be slightly lighter in color. Larger lesions may contain areas of scarring.

In contrast to the obvious, bulging gross lesion of a hamartoma, the microscopic proliferation is usually difficult to delineate. Splenic hamartomas are reduplications of red pulp and therefore merge almost indistinguishably with the surrounding normal red pulp tissue. The lining cells of splenic hamartomas are plump, similar to the surrounding red pulp, but more fibrosis is usually present in the underlying splenic cords in hamartomas in comparison to normal red pulp. True white pulp is not present within a hamartoma, but poorly defined aggregates of lymphocytes may be seen.

The lining cells of a splenic hamartoma are immunophenotypically similar to normal sinus lining cells and are CD8+.[79, 101] This feature may be useful in differentiating a hamartoma from a hemangioma, which would not express this antigen. The lack of cavernous spaces in the lesion and the lack of defined tumor borders are other features that are helpful in excluding hemangioma. The presence of scarring and cordal fibrosis in hamartomas may rarely cause confusion with inflammatory pseudotumor of the spleen, but the identification of sinus lining cells throughout the lesion helps exclude inflammatory pseudotumor.

## INFLAMMATORY PSEUDOTUMOR AND LOCALIZED REACTIVE LYMPHOID HYPERPLASIA

Localized reactive lymphoid hyperplasia[102] is an uncommon incidental finding in spleens that are usu-

ally not enlarged. A well-defined but uncircumscribed white or gray-white nodule of 1.0 cm or less is present grossly, or a small lesion may be evident only microscopically. The spleen, in general, shows evidence of white pulp hyperplasia with a distinct nodule of reactive lymphoid tissue with germinal center formation and associated fibrosis (CD Fig. 42–10). In patients with known Hodgkin's disease, these nodules should be thoroughly sectioned to exclude malignancy.

Inflammatory pseudotumor, also known as inflammatory myofibroblastic tumor, may occur at virtually any site and at any age.[103, 104] Tumors of the spleen and liver, however, may differ from inflammatory pseudotumors of other sites.[105, 106] The lesions may be asymptomatic incidental findings, or the patients may present with abdominal pain with or without a mass.[107, 108] Patients may also have clinical symptoms of fever, weight loss, and malaise, and they may have anemia, leukocytosis, thrombocytosis, polyclonal hypergammaglobulinemia, or elevations of the erythrocyte sedimentation rate. Findings of infectious disease evaluations for prolonged symptoms are often negative. The lesions are usually single, up to 12 cm, and form well-circumscribed but unencapsulated tumors. The gross tumors differ from hamartomas by having a firm tan-white surface, often with areas of hemorrhage or necrosis that clearly differ from the surrounding, uninvolved splenic parenchyma. The microscopic lesions contain prominent fibrosis that may be sclerotic or may contain plump fibroblasts. Varying numbers of lymphocytes and plasma cells, sometimes with germinal center formation, are present and often include immunoblasts. Infiltrates or aggregates of neutrophils, eosinophils, and foamy histiocytes are also frequently present. Small vessels are often scattered throughout the proliferation of inflammatory cells.

Immunohistochemical and molecular genetic studies suggest that inflammatory pseudotumors of the liver and spleen differ from those of other sites. These studies have found that up to two thirds of splenic tumors demonstrate evidence of Epstein-Barr virus in the numerous plump spindle cells (Fig. 42–12) that is not present in the surrounding, uninvolved splenic tissue and is not usually found in inflammatory pseudotumor of lymph node.[105, 109] Various studies have demonstrated an increased number of follicular dendritic cells in some hepatic and splenic cases of inflammatory pseudotumor, and many of these cells harbor monoclonal DNA of the Epstein-Barr virus.[105, 106, 110] Cases of this type may be further designated as inflammatory pseudotumor, follicular dendritic cell type.[104] Although 15% to 20% of inflammatory pseudotumors, in general, are known to recur, they are not reported to metastasize. Therefore, the significance of clonality in these lesions is unclear.

Inflammatory pseudotumors must be differentiated from Hodgkin's disease, which may have a similar cellular background. Reed-Sternberg cells or cells with the characteristic immunophenotype of Hodgkin's cells (CD45⁻, CD30⁺, and CD15⁺) are not present in inflammatory pseudotumor, but scattered CD30⁺ immunoblasts may be present. The high number of follicular dendritic cells in some lesions may suggest follicular dendritic cell sarcoma, but the characteristic storiform pattern with nuclear atypia and frequent mitosis of follicular dendritic cell tumor is not present in inflammatory pseudotumor. Inflammatory fibrosarcoma,[111] which is considered by some authors to be within the spectrum of inflammatory myofibroblastic tumors, may also mimic inflammatory pseudotumor, and care must be take to exclude an underlying malignant spindle cell proliferation. Inflammatory fibrosarcoma is reportedly Epstein-Barr virus negative,[112] most commonly occurs in children or young adults, and forms multinodular or infiltrative gross tumors. The spindle cell proliferation is more cellular and organized with cytologic atypia, which are not prominent features of inflammatory pseudotumor. Infectious diseases, most notably mycobacterial infections in patients with AIDS, may also cause inflammatory lesions of the spleen that are histologically similar to inflammatory pseudotumor with spindled cells, histiocytes, and other inflammatory cells.[113]

## MAST CELL DISEASE

Mast cell disease includes localized and systemic forms. Systemic mast cell disease or mastocytosis is further subdivided into benign and malignant forms. The malignant forms usually do not include cutaneous involvement and are more often associated with other hematologic malignant neoplasms.[114, 115]

Splenomegaly is present in more than 70% of patients with systemic mastocytosis. The enlarged spleen of mast cell disease has a thickened capsule. The cut surface may have a diffuse pattern of apparent red pulp expansion with white pulp atrophy or may show gross areas of thickened trabeculae or scarring. Two microscopic patterns occur, and the white pulp may be normal or atrophic with either. One is a diffuse, predominantly red pulp infiltrate of mast cells that are fairly uniform in size with abundant granular to clear cytoplasm. The second and most common pattern is one of stellate fibrosis scattered throughout all splenic compartments, including the fibrous trabeculae and periarteriolar sheaths, and in and around follicles. The mast cells form clusters of monotonous cells, and the characteristic basophilic cytoplasmic mast cell granules may be washed out in appearance or absent. Spindled fibrous areas may predominate and often mask the mast cell infiltrate. Eosinophils and plasma cells are often admixed with the mast cells. The low-magnification pattern of multiple stellate areas of scarring or fibrosis in a spleen should be a clue to investigate further for possible mast cell disease (Fig. 42–13) (CD Fig. 42–11).

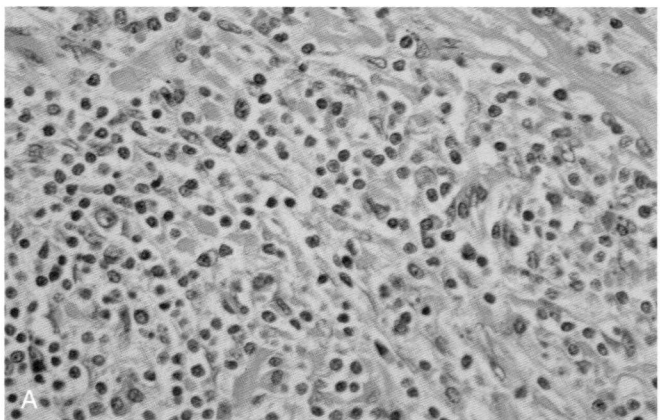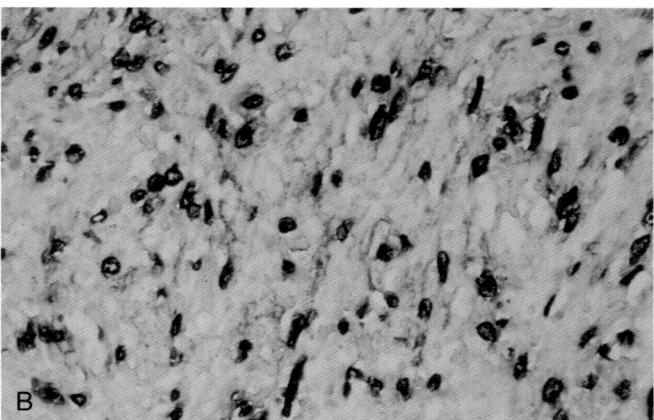

**FIGURE 42–12.** Inflammatory pseudotumor of spleen. *A.* A mixture of lymphoid cells and fibroblasts is present. *B.* Double-labeling immunohistochemistry and in situ hybridization studies demonstrate that most of the spindled cell nuclei are positive for the Epstein-Barr virus (black) and also immunoreact as dendritic cells (brown).

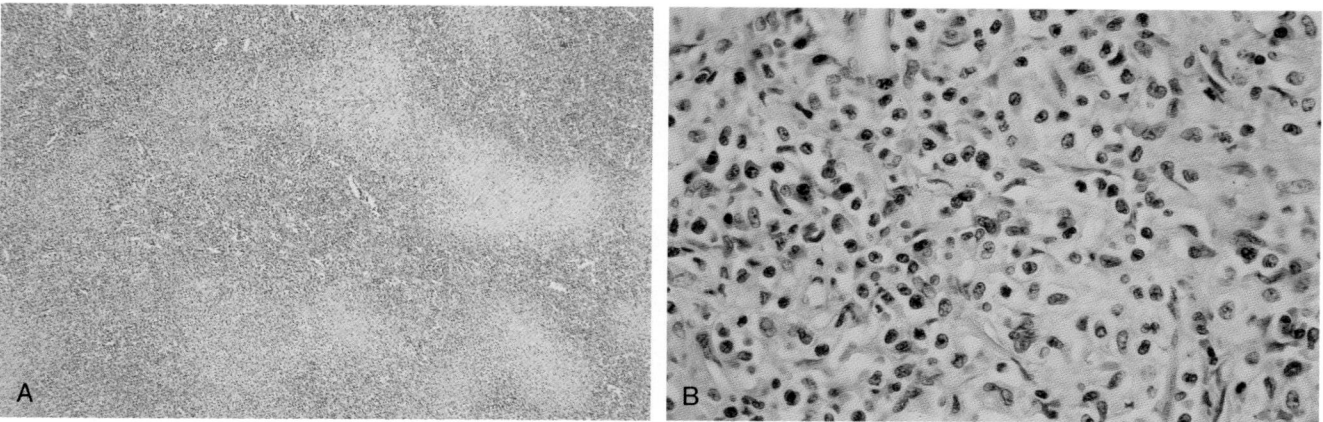

**FIGURE 42–13.** Mast cell disease in the spleen usually forms multiple pale-staining, stellate areas of fibrosis (A) throughout the spleen. B. These areas contain collections of cells with clear to slightly granular cytoplasm with associated eosinophils.

Immunohistochemical studies are helpful in paraffin sections to confirm the presence of increased mast cells within areas of fibrosis. Mast cells express CD45, CD68, and CD43 but do not express more specific T cell markers, B cell markers, or myeloperoxidase. CD117 (c-kit) and tryptase are more specific for mast cells and are useful as second-line markers when a diagnosis of mast cell disease is suspected.[116–118a] Cytochemical methods that characteristically identify non-neoplastic mast cells, such as those using chloracetate esterase and toluidine blue, are often pH dependent when used to detect neoplastic mast cells.[119]

The spleen should be carefully examined for other neoplastic proliferations once a diagnosis of mast cell disease is made. Chronic myeloproliferative disorders, acute myeloid leukemias, and myelodysplastic syndromes are the neoplasms most often associated with mast cell disease, but solid tumors and non-Hodgkin's lymphomas have also been associated with this disease.[114, 120]

## HEMATOPOIETIC PROLIFERATIONS

### Primary Lymphoproliferative Disorders

Any type of malignant lymphoma may involve the spleen and may present as a primary splenic lymphoma; however, most lymphomas represent disseminated disease and are not localized to the spleen.[7, 10, 121, 122] Virtually any type of lymphoma may present as a primary splenic lymphoproliferative disorder (CD Fig. 42–12). Although only representing a fraction of splenic lymphomas, splenic marginal zone lymphoma and hepatosplenic γδ T cell lymphoma are unique to the spleen (or spleen and liver in the latter case). Both typically present with massive splenomegaly without lymphadenopathy.

### SPLENIC MARGINAL ZONE LYMPHOMA

Splenic marginal zone lymphoma is a low-grade B cell lymphoma that is unique to the spleen but that often secondarily involves the splenic hilar lymph nodes.[106, 122–126] It is thought to be distinct from the other so-called marginal zone cell lymphomas (monocytoid B cell lymphoma and lymphomas of mucosa-associated lymphoid tissues).[127] It was originally described as a splenic lymphoma with clinical and peripheral blood findings mimicking hairy cell leukemia.[128]

The disease characteristically affects elderly adults and causes massive splenomegaly. An abnormal peripheral blood lymphocytosis is present in a subgroup of patients. The spleen usually weighs more than 1000 g and has a miliary cut surface with minute, irregular foci of white pulp accentuation (Fig. 42–14).

Splenic marginal zone lymphoma has a characteristic biphasic histologic pattern of white pulp lymphoid infiltrate. A monotonous population of small lymphoid cells in the central white pulp may overrun and replace a central germinal center or may surround non-neoplastic central white pulp cells. An outer white pulp zone of neoplastic cells simulates the normal splenic marginal zone with a rim of medium-sized cells with slightly open chromatin and moderately abundant clear cytoplasm. Nuclear pleomorphism is not evident in either component. Plasmacytoid differentiation is usually not a prominent feature. Smaller aggregates of lymphoma cells are scattered throughout the red pulp, forming small nodules. The central white pulp small lymphocyte component of splenic marginal zone lymphoma is easily overlooked, but it also represents a clonal B cell proliferation and is a helpful clue in the diagnosis. The neoplastic cells of splenic marginal zone lymphoma are CD20+ B cells that express bcl-2 protein, although at lower levels than in most of the other low-grade B cell lymphomas.[129] The cells do not aberrantly coexpress CD5 or CD43, usual find-

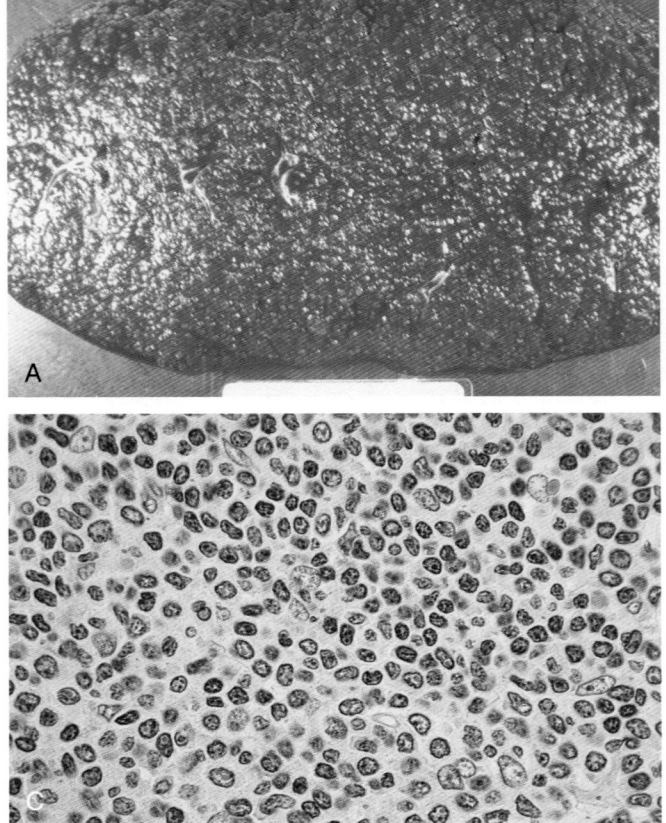

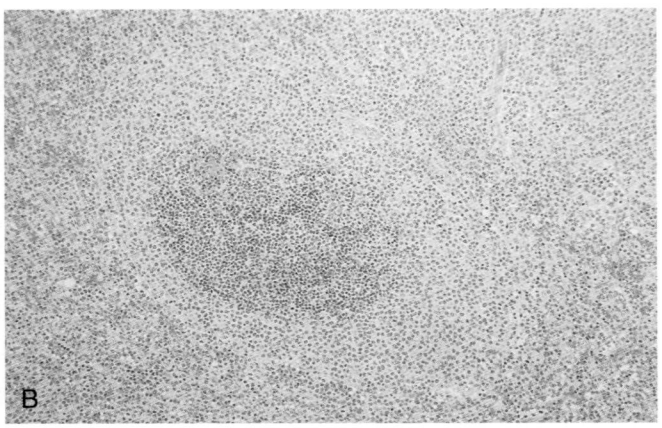

**FIGURE 42–14.** *A.* A massively enlarged spleen with a miliary gross pattern of involvement by splenic marginal zone lymphoma. *B.* The proliferation shows the characteristic biphasic pattern of splenic white pulp involvement by splenic marginal zone lymphoma. The central white pulp contains small, dark-staining lymphocytes; the outer "marginal" zone contains cells with more abundant cytoplasm. *C.* Higher magnification shows the small lymphoid component on the right and the cells with more abundant cytoplasm on the left. Both components are part of the clonal neoplasm.

ings in chronic lymphocytic leukemia or mantle cell lymphoma, and are usually cyclin D1 negative.

Examination of the peripheral blood of patients with splenic lymphoma is useful because many patients with splenic marginal zone lymphoma have the peripheral blood changes of the clinical syndrome termed *splenic lymphoma with villous lymphocytes*[130–132] (Fig. 42–15). The patients have a moder-

ate lymphocytosis composed of medium-sized cells with moderately abundant cytoplasm. Most patients with splenic lymphoma with villous lymphocytes have splenic marginal zone lymphoma,[133] although a subgroup may have peripheral blood involvement by other B cell lymphomas. Flow cytometric immunophenotyping of the peripheral blood is useful in excluding cases of chronic lymphocytic leukemia

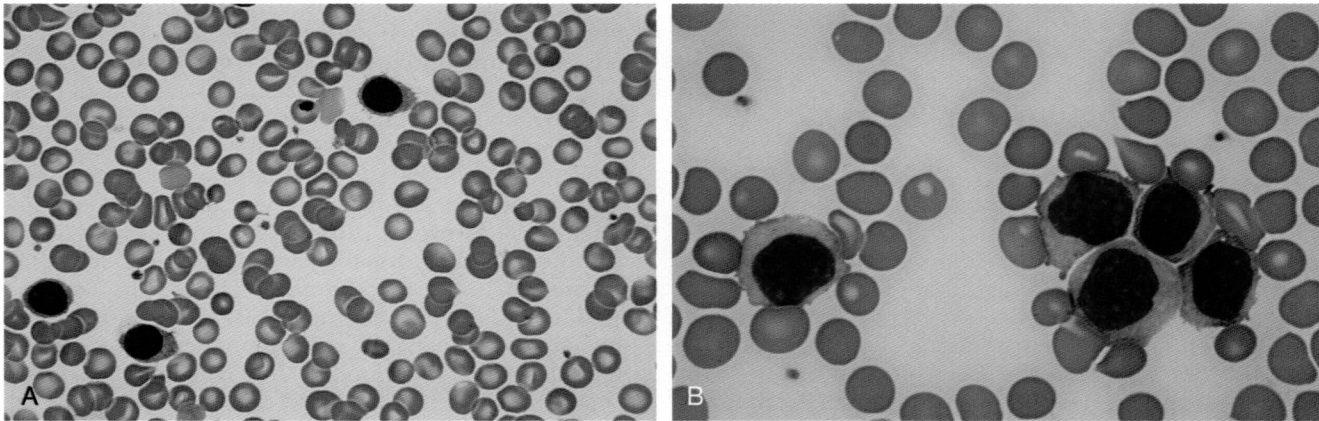

**FIGURE 42–15.** *A.* Splenic lymphoma with circulating villous lymphocytes. Although most patients with splenomegaly and these cells in the peripheral blood have splenic marginal zone lymphoma, other lymphoma types may have similar peripheral blood features. *B.* These atypical lymphoid cells in the peripheral blood do not have a villous appearance, but they also represent peripheral blood involvement by splenic marginal zone cell lymphoma.

and mantle cell lymphoma (both CD5$^+$) or follicular center cell lymphoma (often CD10$^+$). The peripheral blood immunophenotype coupled with the spleen morphology is often sufficient to make a diagnosis without additional studies. An expanded marginal zone is commonly seen in reactive conditions and may also accompany splenic involvement by other lymphomas (see later). This finding alone, therefore, is not sufficient for a diagnosis of splenic marginal zone lymphoma.

## HEPATOSPLENIC γδ T CELL LYMPHOMA

Hepatosplenic γδ T cell lymphoma is a primary splenic lymphoma that also usually involves the liver and bone marrow at the time of presentation.[106, 134–138] It was originally described as erythrophagocytic Tγ lymphoma[139] and is usually a neoplastic proliferation of γδ T cells. Overall, γδ T cells are much less common than αβ T cells in healthy adults, but they are normally relatively increased in the spleen and are preferentially located in the red pulp.[140]

Hepatosplenic γδ T cell lymphoma most commonly occurs in young adults with a marked male predominance. Rare cases have also been reported after solid organ transplantation.[141, 142] The patients present with fever, weight loss, and jaundice in addition to hepatosplenomegaly. Pancytopenia from hypersplenism is common, and some patients will have circulating lymphoma cells in the peripheral blood.

The spleen usually weighs more than 1000 g and has a homogeneous cut surface. The red pulp is expanded by a diffuse proliferation of cells with reduced to absent white pulp elements. The lymphoma cells expand the splenic sinuses and are medium in size with moderately abundant agranular cytoplasm (Fig. 42–16) (CD Fig. 42–13). The cells have slightly irregular nuclear contours with open nuclear chromatin. Some cases exhibit evidence of hemophagocytosis and may have been interpreted as malignant histiocytosis in the past. The neoplastic

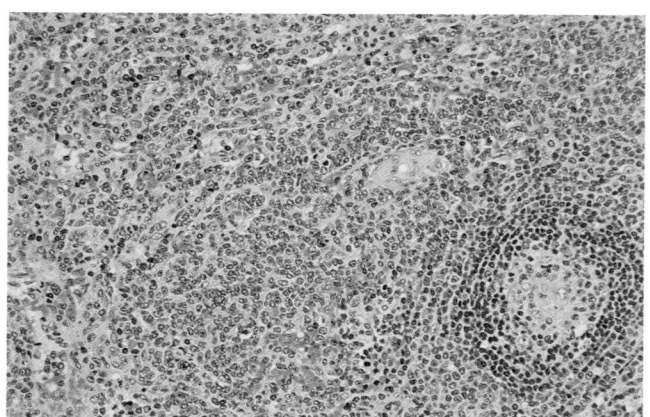

**FIGURE 42–16.** Hepatosplenic γδ T cell lymphoma. The lymphoma primarily involves the splenic red pulp; the white pulp, on the lower right, is somewhat atrophic.

cells express the T cell–associated antigens CD2, CD3, CD5, CD7, CD43, and CD45RO and are immunoreactive with antibodies directed against T cell receptor γ-chain and δ-chain. The cells are usually CD4$^-$ and CD8$^-$ as well as βF1$^-$, an antibody directed against the T cell receptor β-chain. The cells usually show immunoreactivity with natural killer (NK) cell–associated markers, such as CD16, CD56, and T cell intracellular antigen 1 (TIA-1), and are negative for B lineage–associated markers as well as for granzyme B and perforin. The tumors always demonstrate T cell receptor γ-chain rearrangements, but detection of T cell receptor β-chain rearrangements is variable. Several reports have identified the combined cytogenetic abnormality of isochromosome 7q and trisomy 8 in hepatosplenic γδ T cell lymphoma.[143–145] In general, this is an aggressive disease with a poor response to chemotherapy and with short survival.

## Other Lymphoproliferative Disorders Secondarily Involving the Spleen

Any lymphoproliferative disorder that involves lymph node or bone marrow may also involve the spleen.[122] A more detailed description of each is given in the chapters 41 and 43, but key features that relate to splenic involvement are discussed here. Features in the differential diagnosis with splenic marginal zone lymphoma and hepatosplenic γδ T cell lymphoma are given in Tables 42–4 and 42–5.

Hairy cell leukemia usually occurs in elderly adults with pancytopenia and splenomegaly. Patients have peripheral blood, bone marrow, and splenic involvement at diagnosis, usually without lymphadenopathy. The clinical and peripheral blood findings of patients with hairy cell leukemia overlap with those of splenic marginal zone lymphoma. In contrast to most low-grade lymphomas in the spleen, including splenic marginal zone lymphoma, hairy cell leukemia primarily involves the splenic red pulp with decreased or absent white pulp elements (Fig. 42–17). This low-power feature is usually sufficient to exclude most other B lineage chronic lymphoproliferative disorders. Dilated, blood-filled spaces may be present in the red pulp in hairy cell leukemia. The red blood cell "lakes" can be confused with cavernous hemangiomas. The patterns of infiltration of hairy cell leukemia, a B cell proliferation, and hepatosplenic γδ T cell lymphoma are similar, but immunophenotyping of the tumor cells quickly resolves this differential diagnosis. Immunophenotyping studies of the spleen, peripheral blood, or bone marrow in hairy cell leukemia demonstrate a monoclonal B lineage neoplasm without expression of CD5, CD10, or CD43. The cells express CD11c, CD25, and CD103 and are immunoreactive with the paraffin section DBA44 and TRAP antibodies. Weak expression of cyclin D1, a nuclear antigen

**TABLE 42–4.** Common Immunophenotypic Findings in Splenic Marginal Zone Lymphoma and Other Lymphoproliferative Disorders in the Differential Diagnosis

| Diagnosis | CD19/CD20 | CD5 | CD10 | CD23 | CD43 | CD103 | Cyclin D1 | DBA44 |
|---|---|---|---|---|---|---|---|---|
| SMZL | + | – | – | – | – | ∓ | – | ± |
| HCL | + | – | – | – | – | + | ± | + |
| CLL/SL | +† | + | – | + | + | – | – | – |
| B-PLL | + | ± | – | ± | ± | – | – | ∓ |
| LPL | ± | – | – | – | ± | – | ∓ | ∓ |
| MCL | + | + | – | – | + | – | + | – |
| FCCL | + | – | + | – | – | – | – | – |

\* SMZL, Splenic marginal zone lymphoma; HCL, hairy cell leukemia; CLL/SL, chronic lymphocytic leukemia/small lymphocytic lymphoma; B-PLL, B cell prolymphocytic leukemia; LPL, lymphoplasmacytic lymphoma; MCL, mantle cell lymphoma; FCCL, follicular center cell lymphoma.

† CD20 expression is characteristically dim.

commonly expressed by mantle cell lymphoma, has also been reported.[146, 147] The cytochemical detection of tartrate-resistant acid phosphatase is also a fairly specific finding in hairy cell leukemia.

Chronic lymphocytic leukemia/small lymphocytic lymphoma and mantle cell lymphoma are CD5+, monoclonal B cell tumors that frequently involve the spleen and cause enlargement of the white pulp (Fig. 42–18) (CD Fig. 42–14) to such a degree that white pulp aggregates may fuse to form microscopic dumbbell shapes. Increased numbers of neoplastic B cells in the red pulp are also evident, and this finding helps in excluding a reactive condition. The morphologic features of both diseases are similar to those in lymph node, but large aggregates of epithelioid histiocytes may be present with mantle cell lymphoma and may obscure the diagnosis in some cases. Prolymphocytoid transformation of chronic lymphocytic leukemia and prolymphocytic leukemia may show increased numbers of the medium-sized prolymphocytes with more open nuclear chromatin than small lymphocytes located at the periphery of the expanded white pulp. This pattern may cause confusion with splenic marginal zone lymphoma.

Lymphoplasmacytic lymphoma may massively enlarge the spleen and cause the clinical syndrome of Waldenström's macroglobulinemia. Although lymphoplasmacytic lymphoma may have a white pulp pattern of involvement similar to that of the other low-grade B cell lymphomas, it may also demonstrate a diffuse red pulp pattern of involvement (CD Fig. 42–15). This pattern may simulate hairy cell leukemia, but plasmacytoid features, including nuclear inclusions (Dutcher bodies), are not usually found in hairy cell leukemia.

Follicular lymphoma in the spleen is usually a predominantly white pulp disease. Early involvement may simulate non-neoplastic germinal centers and may be easily overlooked. Immunohistochemical demonstration of bcl-2 protein expression in the follicular lymphoma cells is helpful, because non-neoplastic germinal center B cells are bcl-2 negative. Follicular lymphoma in the spleen may also show evidence of marginal zone differentiation. Marginal zone differentiation or marginal zone hyperplasia may accompany almost any type of malignant lymphoma in the spleen but is apparently most common with follicular center cell lymphomas[148–150] (Fig. 42–19). The expanded marginal zone, which may be

**TABLE 42–5.** Common Features of Hepatosplenic γδ T Cell Lymphoma and Other T and Natural Killer Cell Proliferations in the Differential Diagnosis

| Feature | Hepatosplenic γδ T Cell Lymphoma | T Cell LGL* | NK Cell LGL | Angiocentric NK and T Cell Lymphoma | Aggressive NK Cell Leukemia and Lymphoma |
|---|---|---|---|---|---|
| Cytoplasmic granules | – | ∓ | + | + | + |
| CD2 | + | + | + | + | + |
| mono CD3 | + | + | – | – | – |
| poly CD3 | + | + | + | + | + |
| CD56 | + | ∓ | + | + | + |
| CD57 | – | ± | ∓ | – | – |
| βF1 | – | + | – | – | – |
| TCRδ1 | + | – | – | – | – |
| TCR GR | + | + | – | – | + |
| EBV RNA | – | – | – | + | + |

\* LGL, Large granular lymphocytosis; mono CD3, monoclonal CD3/Leu-4; poly CD3, polyclonal CD3ε; TCR, T cell receptor; GR, gene rearrangement; EBV, Epstein-Barr virus; NK, natural killer.

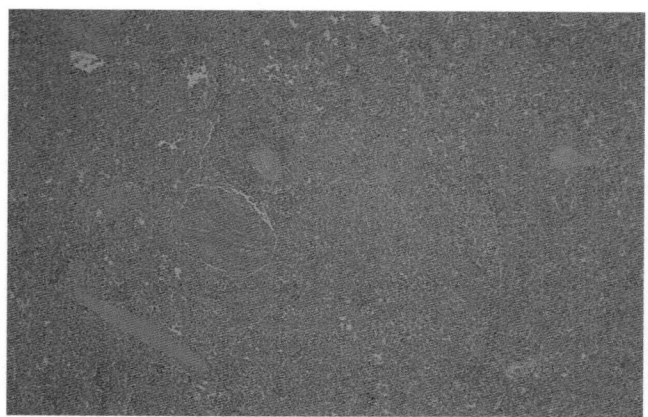

**FIGURE 42–17.** Hairy cell leukemia diffusely involves the splenic red pulp with loss of the white pulp. Dilated, blood-filled sinuses, also termed *red blood cell lakes,* are commonly present.

clonal, may lead to an incorrect diagnosis of splenic marginal zone lymphoma in these cases. Careful examination of the central white pulp for changes more characteristic of follicular center cell lymphoma is imperative. Although the areas of marginal zone differentiation in cases of splenic follicular lymphoma may be clonal, the clone is apparently derived from the follicular center cell lymphoma and is probably best termed *follicular center cell lymphoma with marginal zone differentiation* rather than composite lymphoma. Follicular center cell lymphomas with predominantly large cells often form nodular tumor masses in addition to the predominantly white pulp lymphoma pattern in the surrounding spleen.

Most diffuse large B cell lymphomas and some large cell types of peripheral T cell lymphoma form large tumor nodules with histologic changes similar to those of lymph nodes (CD Fig. 42–16). Rare cases of diffuse large B cell lymphoma have a red pulp distribution that mimics splenic involvement by leu-

kemia or hepatosplenic $\gamma\delta$ T cell lymphoma. The immunohistochemical detection of CD20 on the tumor cells easily confirms the diagnosis. Some authors have suggested that cases of red pulp large B cell lymphoma are a variant of angiotropic B cell lymphoma[151] (Fig. 42–20). Some peripheral T cell lymphomas predominantly involve the red pulp and may simulate hepatosplenic $\gamma\delta$ T cell lymphoma. These lymphomas are usually disseminated, in contrast to $\gamma\delta$ T cell lymphoma, and are lymphomas of $\alpha\beta$ T cells, features helpful in the differential diagnosis. Because of the great variation in and overlap of patterns of splenic involvement by B and T cell lymphomas, it is not possible to accurately predict the lineage of a lymphoid proliferation by its pattern alone. Immunophenotyping studies of either the primary site of involvement or the splenic infiltrate are necessary to assign lineage.

Splenic involvement by large granular lymphocytic leukemia, angiocentric NK and T cell lymphoma, and aggressive NK cell leukemia and lymphoma may cause confusion with hepatosplenic $\gamma\delta$ T cell lymphoma. Large granular lymphocytosis of T or NK type usually occurs in an older age group without the massive splenomegaly of hepatosplenic $\gamma\delta$ T cell lymphoma. Touch preparations of the spleen and review of the peripheral blood smear are helpful in identifying the granular lymphocytes of large granular lymphocytosis that are not seen in hepatosplenic $\gamma\delta$ T cell lymphoma. Although large granular lymphocytosis primarily involves the red pulp (CD Fig. 42–17), it spares the white pulp, which is usually atrophic or absent in spleens involved by hepatosplenic $\gamma\delta$ T cell lymphoma.[152, 153] Angiocentric NK and T cell lymphoma and aggressive NK cell leukemia and lymphoma are usually positive for the Epstein-Barr virus by in situ hybridization, and this virus is not usually identifiable in hepatosplenic $\gamma\delta$ T cell lymphoma. Also, NK cell malignant neoplasms do not express surface CD3 and are negative on study with monoclonal antibodies directed against this antigen. Both NK and T cells are positive for cytoplasmic CD3, detected by the polyclonal antibody usually used in paraffin sections.

Multiple myeloma may involve the spleen but is usually an incidental finding. Small aggregates of plasma cells are present in the red pulp and may mimic changes of autoimmune disorders. The plasma cells in multiple myeloma, however, may demonstrate cytologic atypia and are monotypic by immunohistochemistry. Although the plasma cells of multiple myeloma usually do not greatly involve the spleen, amyloidosis may extensively involve this organ.[154] Extensive splenic involvement by amyloid is associated with peripheral blood changes of hyposplenism, including the presence of Howell-Jolly bodies. In these cases, the splenic cords and white pulp areas show extensive Congo red–positive amyloid deposits.

Splenomegaly is common in multicentric Castleman's disease (angiofollicular lymph node hyperpla-

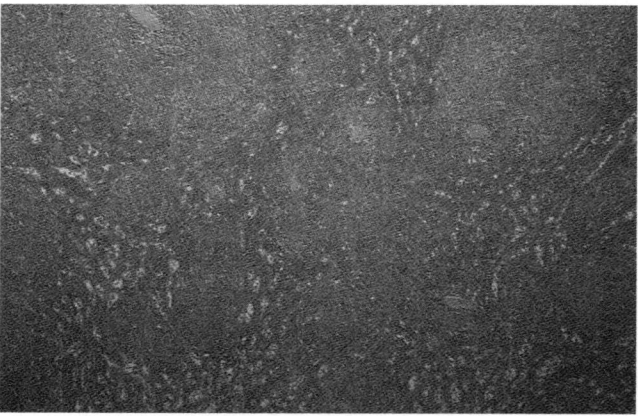

**FIGURE 42–18.** Small lymphocytic lymphoma/chronic lymphocytic leukemia involving the spleen causes monotonous expansions of the splenic white pulp by small lymphocytes with admixed prolymphocytes.

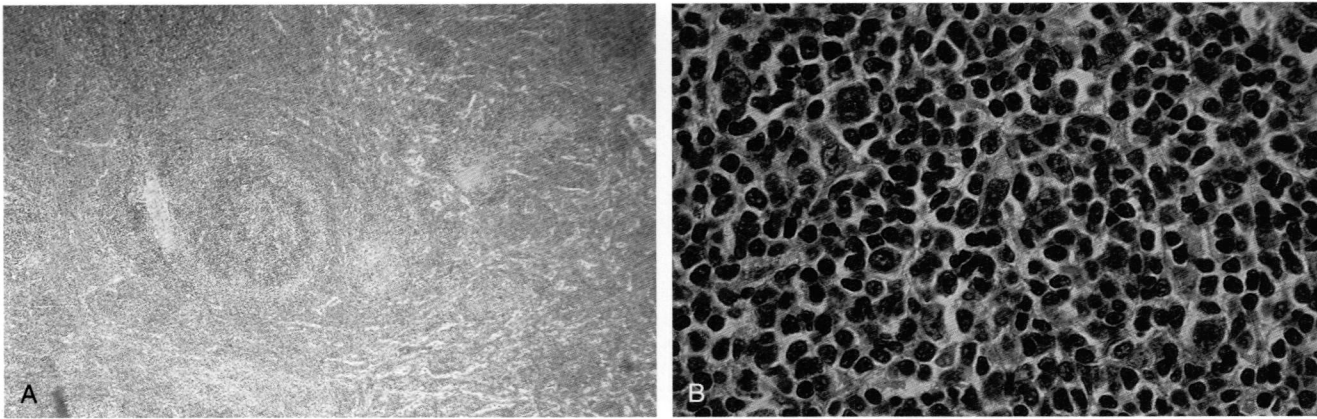

**FIGURE 42–19.** Follicular lymphoma involving the spleen. *A.* A prominent marginal zone is present on low power. *B.* High magnification of the central white pulp shows a mixture of small cleaved cells and large cells that are characteristic of follicular lymphoma.

sia) and may represent involvement by either the hyaline vascular or plasma cell type of the disease.[155, 156] Both types may result in normal to moderately enlarged spleens with an expansion of the white pulp. The hyaline vascular type shows white pulp changes that are similar to those of lymph nodes, with germinal center atrophy, intervening vessels, and concentric layering of mantle cells around the central white pulp. The plasma cell type of Castleman's disease may include reactive germinal centers and contains numerous plasma cells that may expand the marginal zone. Either type may demonstrate fibrosis of the white pulp, of the marginal zone, or around the periarteriolar lymphoid sheath with accompanying hemosiderin deposition.

Hodgkin's disease also forms tumor nodules in the spleen that are grossly similar to those of large cell lymphoma.[8] In early splenic involvement by Hodgkin's disease, only minute accentuations of the splenic white pulp may be evident grossly. The identification of mononuclear Hodgkin's cells with the characteristic immunophenotype of classic Hodgkin's disease (CD45⁻, CD15⁺, CD30⁺) is sufficient for a diagnosis of involvement. Foci of granulomas, however, may be seen in the spleen of patients with Hodgkin's disease without evidence of Reed-Sternberg cells or their mononuclear variants, and this finding alone should not be used as evidence of splenic involvement by the disease. Lymphocyte predominance Hodgkin's disease rarely involves the spleen but forms nodular aggregates of disease.[157]

## Histiocytic Tumors

Most histiocytic and dendritic proliferations are rare and uncommonly involve the spleen. Most cases previously diagnosed as malignant histiocytosis probably represent T cell lymphomas,[158, 159] but rare cases of true histiocytic lymphoma are described.[160] These tumors lack immunologic and molecular genetic evidence of B or T cell lineage and usually involve other sites before involving the spleen. Similar to large cell lymphoma, the histiocytic lymphomas are composed of large cells with pleomorphic nuclei, chromatin clearing, and prominent nucleoli.

Langerhans cell histiocytosis (histiocytosis X) is a disseminated disease of childhood that involves the spleen in a diffuse, red pulp pattern. In adults, it may rarely form a discrete, incidental tumor nodule in the spleen[161] and is frequently associated with Hodgkin's disease, non-Hodgkin's lymphoma, acute myeloid leukemia, or carcinomas.[162–164] All presentations of the disease show the characteristic aggregates of cells with folded nuclei and nuclear grooves as well as admixed eosinophils (CD Fig. 42–18). The histiocytic cells demonstrate Birbeck granules by electron microscopy and CD1 expression by immunohistochemistry.

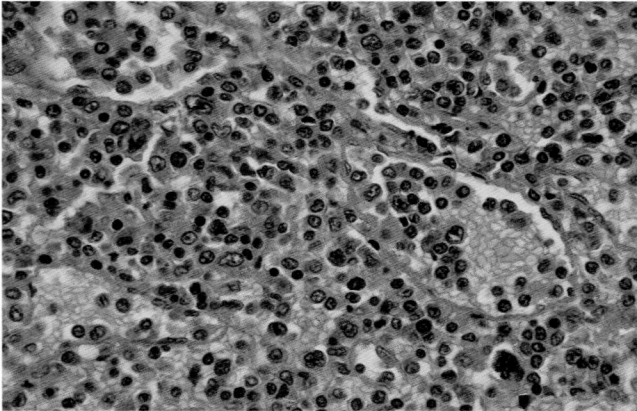

**FIGURE 42–20.** Splenic red pulp involvement by large B cell lymphoma with no white pulp nodules. The pattern of involvement may cause confusion with leukemic infiltrates or T cell lymphomas. The large cells showed immunoreactivity for CD20, confirming their B lineage.

## Chronic Myeloproliferative Disorders

The chronic myeloproliferative disorders frequently cause splenomegaly with a diffuse red pulp pattern of involvement. There is great morphologic overlap between the diseases (Fig. 42–21), and any of them may cause splenomegaly secondary to an increase in blast cells.

Myelofibrosis with myeloid metaplasia, also termed *agnogenic myeloid metaplasia* or *primary osteomyelofibrosis*, is almost always associated with splenomegaly that is usually massive.[14, 165] The spleen usually weighs 1000 g or more. It has a thickened capsule with areas of capsular fibrosis, and gross areas of infarction are often present. The cut surface is usually homogeneous and red to brown. Some cases may demonstrate grossly nodular lesions. At microscopic examination, the white pulp is reduced and widely separated by the markedly expanded red pulp. The red pulp contains extensive extramedullary hematopoiesis that most commonly shows a granulocyte predominance but may show an erythroid predominance. The granulocytes expand the red pulp cords; the erythroid clusters expand the sinuses. Clusters of small, dysplastic, and immature megakaryocytes are present in either the cords or sinuses and are a prominent feature of this disorder. In some patients, large aggregates of megakaryocytes are present and correspond to the gross nodular lesions. Red pulp fibrosis, secondary to congestion, is frequently present in massively enlarged spleens. Some cases may demonstrate evidence of red pulp plasmacytosis. Splenectomy in patients with myelofibrosis is reportedly associated with an increased risk of blast crisis.[166]

Chronic myelogenous leukemia and the spent phase of polycythemia (rubra) vera have morphologic overlap with myelofibrosis, and the splenic features alone are not sufficient for precise classification of the type of myeloproliferative disorder. In chronic myelogenous leukemia, the red pulp is expanded and shows a predominance of maturing myeloid cells. Other evidence of extramedullary hematopoiesis is less pronounced. Blast cells within the red pulp may be increased, and a rapidly enlarging spleen is a feature of accelerated phase or blast crisis of chronic myelogenous leukemia. Immunohistochemical studies for CD34 are often useful in these cases, and in any chronic myeloproliferative disorder with suspected blast crisis, to confirm the presence of increased numbers of blast cells in the red pulp. In the spent phase of polycythemia vera, the spleen may show changes identical to those of myelofibrosis with myeloid metaplasia.[167]

In essential thrombocythemia and the erythrocytotic or early phase of polycythemia vera, splenomegaly is less pronounced and is not related to extramedullary hematopoiesis. In essential thrombocythemia, the spleen may even be small and atrophic. When it is enlarged, the red pulp is expanded by platelet-filled macrophages.[168] In the erythrocytotic phase of polycythemia vera, the red pulp is expanded because of massive congestion of the cords and sinuses, and only minimal extramedullary hematopoiesis is evident.[167]

Some cases of chronic myelomonocytic leukemia have features more suggestive of a myeloproliferative disorder than of a myelodysplastic syndrome. In these cases, splenomegaly is present. The splenic infiltrate involves the red pulp with decreased or absent white pulp. Monocytoid cells predominate, expanding the cord with less involvement of the sinuses. Similar to splenic involvement by chronic myelogenous leukemia, extramedullary hematopoiesis is present but is less prominent than that seen in myelofibrosis with myeloid metaplasia. Dilated, blood-filled spaces similar to peliosis or the red blood cell lakes of hairy cell leukemia are also often present and may cause a vaguely nodular gross ap-

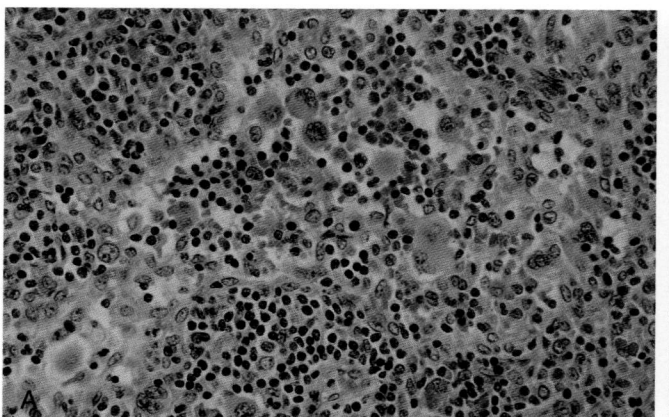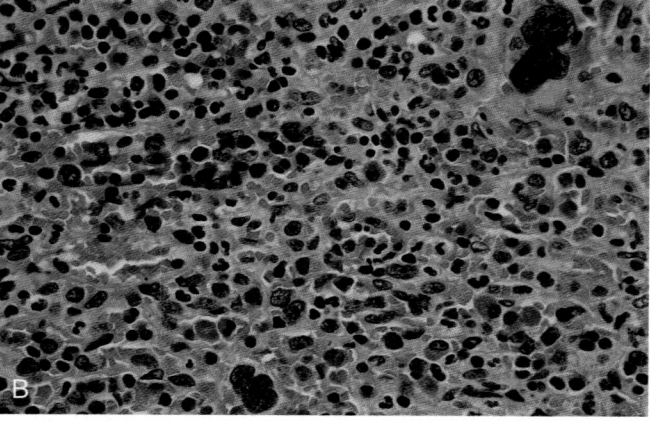

**FIGURE 42–21.** Splenomegaly secondary to chronic myeloproliferative disorders is often due to extramedullary hematopoiesis in the red pulp. Although there is great overlap of the morphologic features of these diseases, the megakaryocytes of chronic myelogenous leukemia *(A)* tend to cluster and are small. This is in contrast to the megakaryocytes of myelofibrosis with myeloid metaplasia and polycythemia vera *(B)*, which display more nuclear atypia and may contain more cytoplasm.

pearance.[169] Other types of myelodysplasia may cause splenomegaly with red pulp expansion with extramedullary hematopoiesis. The red blood cell precursors may show obvious evidence of dysplasia with irregular nuclear contours or nuclear lobations. Some patients may also demonstrate aggregates of plasma cells in the red pulp.[170]

Because of the great overlap of morphologic features between the various myeloproliferative disorders in the spleen, the precise classification of the disorders should be based on a variety of parameters that include cytogenetic studies and peripheral blood and bone marrow findings. Those features are described in Chapter 44.

## Acute Leukemias

Acute leukemias are rarely primary splenic neoplasms, but the spleen may be the first organ examined that shows blast cell transformation of a preexisting myeloproliferative or myelodysplastic syndrome. Acute myeloid and lymphoblastic leukemias expand the splenic red pulp, involving both the cords and sinuses (CD Fig. 42–19). They may be overlooked in poorly fixed sections because the neoplastic cells may mimic monocytes or lymphocytes in the red pulp. Touch preparations, including air-dried smears for cytochemistry, and fresh tissue submitted for flow cytometry are helpful for the proper classification of leukemic infiltrates. However, immunohistochemical studies on paraffin sections usually provide sufficient information to determine whether the leukemic infiltrate is of immature B (CD79a[+] and terminal deoxynucleotidyl transferase positive), immature T (CD2[+], CD3[+], and terminal deoxynucleotidyl transferase positive), or myeloid (myeloperoxidase) lineage. CD34 expression, when it is present, provides further evidence of an immature cell infiltrate. Blast cells of any type are CD43[+]. CD43 antibodies are frequently used as an initial screen for T cells, but a variety of cell types may express this antigen. The detection of a large population of CD43[+] abnormal cells in the spleen should raise suspicion for an acute leukemic infiltrate.

Patients receiving granulocyte colony-stimulating factor may demonstrate a proliferation of immature myeloid cells in the red pulp that may be morphologically indistinguishable from splenic involvement by acute myeloid leukemia and chronic myelogenous leukemia.[171] These spleens, however, are usually normal or only slightly enlarged, in contrast to most cases of chronic myelogenous leukemia.

Lymphoblastic lymphoma and acute lymphoblastic leukemia have identical features of splenic involvement, usually with extensive red pulp infiltration by a population of immature lymphoid cells. Some cases may show less extensive red pulp disease with predominantly subendothelial and adventitial periarterial trabecular involvement.[172] A high mitotic rate is often present, and its detection may help in raising the suspicion of a lymphoblastic process. Detection of nuclear terminal deoxynucleotidyl transferase, with associated CD79a or CD3 expression, in the cellular infiltrate is diagnostic of lymphoblastic leukemia and lymphoma.

## SARCOMAS

Other than angiosarcomas, primary splenic sarcomas are extremely rare. Malignant fibrous histiocytoma, fibrosarcoma, leiomyosarcoma, and rhabdosarcoma have been reported as primary splenic tumors.[22, 173, 174] The tumors usually form large, poorly circumscribed nodular gross lesions and often contain areas of necrosis. The diagnostic criteria for these tumors are similar to those of soft tissue sarcomas. The rare Epstein-Barr virus–positive smooth muscle tumors that occur in some patients with acquired immunodeficiency or after solid organ transplantation may also involve the spleen, but they also affect other organs.[175]

## CARCINOMAS AND METASTATIC TUMORS

Case reports of primary splenic carcinomas include a squamous cell carcinoma arising in a cyst,[176] a mucinous cystadenocarcinoma that presumably arose from ectopic pancreas or from an invagination of peritoneal surface epithelium,[177] and a carcinosarcoma possibly representing a malignant mixed müllerian tumor arising from peritoneal mesothelium.[178] Splenic involvement by carcinoma is much more often due to either metastasis or direct extension of tumor into the spleen, but either form of splenic involvement is relatively uncommon.[179]

One third of metastatic tumors microscopically involve the spleen without gross lesions and may infiltrate venous sinusoids or trabecular vessels or form microscopic nodules of the red or white pulp.[179–181] Grossly visible metastases usually form tumor nodules, often with necrosis. Some cases may show complete replacement of the splenic parenchyma. Virtually any tumor will metastasize, but lung and breast carcinomas were the most common to involve the spleen in one autopsy study.[179] Although metastatic splenic lesions are usually accompanied by metastases to other sites, solitary spleen metastases may be treated with splenectomy.[182]

## REFERENCES

1. DeLand FH: Normal spleen size. Radiology 97:589–592, 1970.
2. Sprogoe-Jakobsen S, Sprogoe-Jakobsen U: The weight of the normal spleen. Forensic Sci Int 88:215–223, 1997.
3. van Krieken JHJM, te Velde J: Spleen. In Sternberg SS (eds): Histology for Pathologists. 2nd ed. Philadelphia, Lippincott-Raven, 1997, pp 675–685.
4. Bishop MA, Lansing LS: The spleen: a correlative overview of normal and pathologic anatomy. Hum Pathol 13:334–342, 1982.

5. Weiss L: The structure of the normal spleen. Semin Hematol 2:205–228, 1965.
6. Rappaport H: The pathologic anatomy of the splenic red pulp. In Lennert K, Harms D (eds): The Spleen. Berlin, Springer-Verlag, 1970, pp 24–41.
7. Davey FP, Skarin AT, Moloney WC: Pathology of splenic lymphoma. Am J Clin Pathol 59:95–103, 1973.
8. Burke JS: Surgical pathology of the spleen: an approach to the differential diagnosis of splenic lymphomas and leukemias. Part I. Diseases of the white pulp. Am J Surg Pathol 5:551–563, 1981.
9. Burke JS: Surgical pathology of the spleen: an approach to the differential diagnosis of splenic lymphomas and leukemias. Part II. Diseases of the red pulp. Am J Surg Pathol 5:681–694, 1981.
10. Kraemer BB, Osborne BM, Butler JJ: Primary splenic presentation of malignant lymphoma and related disorders. A study of 49 cases. Cancer 54:1606–1619, 1984.
11. Audouin J, Diebold J, Schvartz H, et al: Malignant lymphoplasmacytic lymphoma with prominent splenomegaly (primary lymphoma of the spleen). J Pathol 155:17–33, 1988.
12. van Krieken JHJM, Feller AC, te Velde J: The distribution of non-Hodgkin's lymphoma in the lymphoid compartments of the human spleen. Am J Surg Pathol 13:757–765, 1989.
13. Hogan SF, Osborne BM, Butler JJ: Unexpected splenic nodules in leukemic patients. Hum Pathol 20:62–68, 1989.
14. Falk S, Mix D, Stutte H-J: The spleen in osteomyelofibrosis. A morphologic and immunohistochemical study of 30 cases. Virchows Arch A Pathol Anat Histopathol 416:437–442, 1990.
15. Eraklis AJ, Filler RM: Splenectomy in childhood: a review of 1413 cases. J Pediatr Surg 7:382–388, 1972.
16. Wadham BM, Adams PB, Johnson MA: Incidence and location of accessory spleens. N Engl J Med 304:1111, 1981.
17. Fleming CR, Dickson ER, Harrison EG Jr: Splenosis: autotransplantation of splenic tissue. Am J Med 61:414–419, 1976.
18. Pearson HA, Johnston D, Smith KA, et al: The born-again spleen: return of splenic function after splenectomy for trauma. N Engl J Med 298:1389–1392, 1978.
19. Carr NJ, Turk EP: The histological features of splenosis. Histopathology 21:549–553, 1992.
20. Davidson LA, Reid IN: Intrahepatic splenic tissue. J Clin Pathol 50:532–533, 1997.
21. Putschar WGJ, Manion WC: Splenic-gonadal fusion. Am J Pathol 32:15–33, 1956.
21a. McClure RD, Altemeier WA: Cysts of the spleen. Ann Surg 116:98–102, 1942.
22. Garvin DF, King FM: Cysts and nonlymphomatous tumors of the spleen. Pathol Annu 16:61–80, 1981.
23. Bürrig K-F: Epithelial (true) splenic cysts. Pathogenesis of the mesothelial and so-called epidermoid cyst of the spleen. Am J Surg Pathol 12:275–281, 1988.
24. Fowler RH: Nonparasitic benign cystic tumors of the spleen. Int Abstr Surg 96:209–227, 1953.
25. Arber DA, Strickler JG, Weiss LM: Splenic mesothelial cysts mimicking lymphangiomas. Am J Surg Pathol 21:334–338, 1997.
26. Favara BE, Feller AC: Contemporary classification of histiocytic disorders. Med Pediatr Oncol 29:157–166, 1997.
27. Öst Å, Nilsson-Ardnor S, Henter J-I: Autopsy findings in 27 children with haemophagocytic lymphohistiocytosis. Histopathology 32:310–316, 1998.
28. Soffer D, Elimelech O, Rosen N, et al: Familial hemophagocytic lymphohistiocytosis in Israel. II. Pathologic findings. Cancer 54:2423–2431, 1984.
29. Loy TS, Diaz-Arias AA, Perry MC: Familial erythrophagocytic lymphohistiocytosis. Semin Oncol 18:34–39, 1991.
30. Arico M, Janka G, Fischer A, et al: Hemophagocytic lymphohistiocytosis. Report of 122 children from the International Registry. Leukemia 10:197–203, 1996.
31. Henter J-I, Elinder G, Öst Å, et al: Diagnostic guidelines for hemophagocytic lymphohistiocytosis. Semin Oncol 18:29–33, 1991.
32. Risdall RJ, McKenna RW, Nesbit ME, et al: Virus-associated hemophagocytic syndrome. A benign histiocytic proliferation distinct from malignant histiocytosis. Cancer 44:993–1002, 1979.
33. Risdall RJ, Brunning RD, Hernandez JI, et al: Bacteria-associated hemophagocytic syndrome. Cancer 54:2968–2972, 1984.
34. Paris S, Weiss SM, Ayers WH Jr, et al: Splenic abscess. Am Surg 60:358–361, 1994.
35. Chun CH, Raff MJ, Contreras L, et al: Splenic abscess. Medicine (Baltimore) 59:50–65, 1980.
36. Chulay JD, Lankerani MR: Splenic abscess. Report of 10 cases and review of the literature. Am J Med 61:513–522, 1976.
37. Al-Salem AH, Qaisaruddin S, Jam'a AA, et al: Splenic abscess and sickle cell disease. Am J Hematol 58:100–104, 1998.
38. Brook I, Frazier EH: Microbiology of liver and spleen abscesses. J Med Microbiol 47:1075–1080, 1998.
39. Smith EB, Custer RP: Rupture of the spleen in infectious mononucleosis. A clinicopathologic report of seven cases. Blood 1:317–333, 1946.
40. Sakulsky SB, Wallace RB, Silverstein MN, et al: Ruptured spleen in infectious mononucleosis. Arch Surg 94:349–352, 1967.
41. Farley DR, Zietlow SP, Bannon MP, et al: Spontaneous rupture of the spleen due to infectious mononucleosis. Mayo Clin Proc 67:846–853, 1992.
42. Asgari MM, Begos DG: Spontaneous splenic rupture in infectious mononucleosis: a review. Yale J Biol Med 70:175–182, 1997.
43. Strickler JG, Fedeli F, Horwitz CA, et al: Infectious mononucleosis in lymphoid tissue. Histopathology, in situ hybridization, and differential diagnosis. Arch Pathol Lab Med 117:269–278, 1993.
44. Reynolds DJ, Banks PM, Gulley ML: New characterization of infectious mononucleosis and a phenotypic comparison with Hodgkin's disease. Am J Pathol 146:379–388, 1995.
45. Aldrete JS: Spontaneous rupture of the spleen in patients with infectious mononucleosis. Mayo Clin Proc 67:910–912, 1992.
46. Neiman RS: Incidence and importance of splenic sarcoid-like granulomas. Arch Pathol Lab Med 101:518–521, 1977.
47. Kuo T, Rosai J: Granulomatous inflammation in splenectomy specimens. Clinicopathologic study of 20 cases. Arch Pathol 98:261–268, 1974.
48. Kadin ME, Donaldson SS, Dorfman RF: Isolated granulomas in Hodgkin's disease. N Engl J Med 283:859–861, 1970.
49. O'Connell MJ, Schimpff SC, Kirschner RH, et al: Epithelioid granulomas in Hodgkin's disease. A favorable prognostic sign? JAMA 233:886–889, 1975.
50. Cruickshank B: Follicular (mineral oil) lipidosis: I. Epidemiologic studies of involvement of the spleen. Hum Pathol 15:724–730, 1984.
51. Cruickshank B, Thomas MJ: Mineral oil (follicular) lipidosis: II. Histologic studies of spleen, liver, lymph nodes, and bone marrow. Hum Pathol 15:731–737, 1984.
52. Klatt EC, Meyer PR: Pathology of the spleen in acquired immunodeficiency syndrome. Arch Pathol Lab Med 111:1050–1053, 1987.
53. Falk S, Müller H, Stutte H-J: The spleen in acquired immunodeficiency syndrome (AIDS). Pathol Res Pract 183:425–433, 1988.
54. Vermi W, Blanzuoli L, Kraus MD, et al: The spleen in the Wiskott-Aldrich sydrome. Histopathologic abnormalities of the white pulp correlate with the clinical phenotype of the disease. Am J Surg Pathol 23:182–191, 1999.
55. Markowitz GS, Factor SM, Borczuk AC: Splenic para-amyloid material: a possible vasculopathy of the acquired immunodeficiency syndrome. Hum Pathol 29:371–376, 1998.
56. Slater LN, Welch DF, Min K-W: Rochalimaea henselae causes bacillary angiomatosis and peliosis hepatis. Arch Intern Med 152:602–606, 1992.
57. Perkocha LA, Geaghan SM, Yen TSB, et al: Clinical and pathological features of bacillary peliosis hepatis in association with human immunodeficiency virus infection. N Engl J Med 323:1581–1586, 1990.
58. Koehler JE, Sanchez MA, Garrido CS, et al: Molecular epidemiology of Bartonella infections in patients with bacillary angiomatosis-peliosis. N Engl J Med 337:1876–1883, 1997.

59. Tsang WYW, Chan JKC: Bacillary angiomatosis. A "new" disease with a broadening clinicopathologic spectrum. Histol Histopathol 7:143–152, 1992.

60. Tappero JW, Koehler JE, Berger TG, et al: Bacillary angiomatosis and bacillary splenitis in immunocompetent adults. Ann Intern Med 118:363–365, 1993.

61. Karakousis CP, Elias EG: Spontaneous (pathologic) rupture of spleen in malignancies. Surgery 76:674–677, 1974.

62. Bauer TW, Haskins GE, Armitage JO: Splenic rupture in patients with hematologic malignancies. Cancer 48:2729–2733, 1981.

63. Barnard H, Dreef EJ, van Krieken JHJM: The ruptured spleen. A histological, morphometrical and immunohistochemical study. Histol Histopathol 5:299–304, 1990.

64. Gupta PB, Harvey L: Spontaneous rupture of the spleen secondary to metastatic carcinoma. Br J Surg 80:613, 1993.

65. Gupta R, Singh G, Bose SM, et al: Spontaneous rupture of the amyloid spleen. A report of two cases. J Clin Gastroenterol 26:161, 1998.

66. Üstün C, Sungur C, Akbas O, et al: Spontaneous splenic rupture as the initial presentation of plasma cell leukemia: a case report. Am J Hematol 57:266–267, 1998.

67. Farhi DC, Ashfaq R: Splenic pathology after traumatic injury. Am J Clin Pathol 105:474–478, 1996.

68. Scriver CR, Beaudet AL, Sly WS, Valle D (eds): The Metabolic and Molecular Bases of Inherited Disease. 7th ed. New York, McGraw-Hill, 1995.

69. NIH Technology Assessment Panel on Gaucher Disease: Gaucher disease. Current issues in diagnosis and treatment. JAMA 275:548–553, 1996.

70. Wolf BC, Neiman RS: Disorders of the Spleen. Philadelphia, WB Saunders, 1989.

71. Blaustein AU, Diggs LW: Pathology of the spleen. In Blaustein A (ed): The Spleen. New York, McGraw-Hill, 1963, pp 45–178.

72. Laszlo J, Jones R, Silberman HR, et al: Splenectomy for Felty's syndrome. Clinicopathological study of 27 patients. Arch Intern Med 138:597–602, 1978.

73. Firkin BG, Wright R, Miller S, et al: Splenic macrophages in thrombocytopenia. Blood 33:240–245, 1969.

74. Hassan NMR, Neiman RS: The pathology of the spleen in steroid-treated immune thrombocytopenic purpura. Am J Clin Pathol 84:433–438, 1985.

75. Taxy JB: Peliosis: a morphologic curiosity becomes an iatrogenic problem. Hum Pathol 9:331–340, 1978.

76. Tada T, Wakabayashi T, Kishimoto H: Peliosis of the spleen. Am J Clin Pathol 79:708–713, 1983.

77. Gugger M, Gebbers J-O: Peliosis of the spleen: an immune-complex disease? Histopathology 33:387–389, 1998.

78. Morgenstern L, Rosenberg J, Geller SA: Tumors of the spleen. World J Surg 9:468–476, 1985.

79. Arber DA, Strickler JG, Chen Y-Y, et al: Splenic vascular tumors: a histologic, immunophenotypic, and virologic study. Am J Surg Pathol 21:827–835, 1997.

80. Shiran A, Naschitz JE, Yeshurun D, et al: Diffuse hemangiomatosis of the spleen: splenic hemangiomatosis presenting with giant splenomegaly, anemia, and thrombocytopenia. Am J Gastroenterol 85:1515–1517, 1990.

81. Ruck P, Horny H-P, Xiao J-C, et al: Diffuse sinusoidal hemangiomatosis of the spleen. A case report with enzyme-histochemical, immunohistochemical, and electron-microscopic findings. Pathol Res Pract 190:708–714, 1994.

82. Morgenstern L, Bello JM, Fisher BL, et al: The clinical spectrum of lymphangiomas and lymphangiomatosis of the spleen. Am Surg 58:599–604, 1992.

83. Marymont JV, Knight PJ: Splenic lymphangiomatosis: a rare cause of splenomegaly. J Pediatr Surg 22:461–462, 1987.

84. Avigad S, Jaffe R, Frand M, et al: Lymphangiomatosis with splenic involvement. JAMA 236:2315–2317, 1976.

85. Chan KW, Saw D: Distinctive, multiple lymphangiomas of spleen. J Pathol 131:75–81, 1980.

86. O'Sullivan DA, Torres VE, de Groen PC, et al: Hepatic lymphangiomatosis mimicking polycystic liver disease. Mayo Clin Proc 73:1188–1192, 1998.

87. Falk S, Stutte HJ, Frizzera G: Littoral cell angioma. A novel splenic vascular lesion demonstrating histiocytic differentiation. Am J Surg Pathol 15:1023–1033, 1991.

88. Suster S: Epithelioid and spindle-cell hemangioendothelioma of the spleen. Report of a distinctive splenic vascular neoplasm of childhood. Am J Surg Pathol 16:785–792, 1992.

89. Kaw YT, Duwaji MS, Kinsley RE, et al: Hemangioendothelioma of the spleen. Arch Pathol Lab Med 116:1079–1082, 1992.

90. Budke HL, Breitfeld PP, Neiman RS: Functional hyposplenism due to a primary epithelioid hemangioendothelioma of the spleen. Arch Pathol Lab Med 119:755–757, 1995.

91. Falk S, Krishnan J, Meis JM: Primary angiosarcoma of the spleen. A clinicopathologic study of 40 cases. Am J Surg Pathol 17:959–970, 1993.

92. Sordillo EM, Sordillo PP, Hajdu SI: Primary hemangiosarcoma of the spleen: report of four cases. Med Pediatr Oncol 9:319–324, 1981.

93. Takato H, Iwamoto H, Ikezu M, et al: Splenic hemangiosarcoma with sinus endothelial differentiation. Acta Pathol Jpn 43:702–708, 1993.

94. Rosso R, Paulli M, Gianelli U, et al: Littoral cell angiosarcoma of the spleen—case report with immunohistochemical and ultrastructural analysis. Am J Surg Pathol 19:1203–1208, 1995.

95. Rosso R, Gianelli U, Chan JKC: Further evidence supporting the sinus lining cell nature of splenic littoral cell angiosarcoma (letter). Am J Surg Pathol 20:1531, 1996.

96. Meybehm M, Fischer HP: Littoralzellangiosarkom der Milz. Morphologische, immunohistochemische Befunde und Überlegungen zur Histogenese eines seltenen Milztumors. Pathologe 18:401–405, 1997.

97. Silverman ML, LiVolsi VA: Splenic hamartoma. Am J Clin Pathol 70:224–229, 1978.

98. Morgenstern L, McCafferty L, Rosenberg J, et al: Hamartomas of the spleen. Arch Surg 119:1291–1293, 1984.

99. Falk S, Stutte HJ: Hamartomas of the spleen: a study of 20 biopsy cases. Histopathology 14:603–612, 1989.

100. Steinberg JJ, Suhrland M, Valensi Q: The spleen in the spleen syndrome: the association of splenoma with hematopoietic and neoplastic disease—compendium of cases since 1864. J Surg Oncol 47:193–202, 1991.

101. Zukerberg LR, Kaynor BL, Silverman ML, et al: Splenic hamartoma and capillary hemangioma are distinct entities. Immunohistochemical analysis of CD8 expression by endothelial cells. Hum Pathol 22:1258–1261, 1991.

102. Burke JS, Osborne BM: Localized reactive lymphoid hyperplasia of the spleen simulating malignant lymphoma. A report of seven cases. Am J Surg Pathol 7:373–380, 1983.

103. Coffin CM, Watterson J, Priest JR, et al: Extrapulmonary inflammatory myofibroblastic tumor (inflammatory pseudotumor). A clinicopathologic and immunohistochemical study of 84 cases. Am J Surg Pathol 19:859–872, 1995.

104. Chan JKC: Inflammatory pseudotumor: a family of lesions of diverse nature and etiologies. Adv Anat Pathol 3:156–171, 1996.

105. Arber DA, Kamel OW, van de Rijn M, et al: Frequent presence of the Epstein-Barr virus in inflammatory pseudotumor. Hum Pathol 26:1093–1098, 1995.

106. Delsol G, Diebold J, Isaacson PG, et al: Pathology of the spleen: report of the workshop of the VIIIth meeting of the European Association for Haematopathology, Paris 1996. Histopathology 32:172–179, 1998.

107. Cotelingam JD, Jaffe ES: Inflammatory pseudotumor of the spleen. Am J Surg Pathol 8:375–380, 1984.

108. Thomas RM, Jaffe ES, Zarate-Osorno A, et al: Inflammatory pseudotumor of the spleen. A clinicopathologic and immunophenotypic study of eight cases. Arch Pathol Lab Med 117:921–926, 1993.

109. Arber DA, Weiss LM, Chang KL: Detection of Epstein-Barr virus in inflammatory pseudotumor. Semin Diagn Pathol 15:155–160, 1998.

110. Selves J, Meggetto F, Brousset P, et al: Inflammatory pseudotumor of the liver. Evidence for follicular dendritic reticulum cell proliferation associated with clonal Epstein-Barr virus. Am J Surg Pathol 20:747–753, 1996.

111. Meis JM, Enzinger FM: Inflammatory fibrosarcoma of the mesentery and retroperitoneum. A tumor closely simulating inflammatory pseudotumor. Am J Surg Pathol 15:1146–1156, 1991.

112. Meis-Kindblom JM, Kjellström C, Kindblom L-G: Inflammatory fibrosarcoma: update, reappraisal and perspective on its place in the spectrum of inflammatory myofibroblastic tumors. Semin Diagn Pathol 15:133–143, 1998.

113. Suster S, Moran CA, Blanco M: Mycobacterial spindle-cell pseudotumor of the spleen. Am J Clin Pathol 101:539–542, 1994.

114. Horny H-P, Ruck MT, Kaiserling E: Spleen findings in generalized mastocytosis. A clinicopathologic study. Cancer 70:459–468, 1992.

115. Travis WD, Li C-Y: Pathology of lymph node and spleen in systemic mast cell disease. Mod Pathol 1:4–14, 1988.

116. Arber DA, Tamayo R, Weiss LM: Paraffin section detection of the c-kit gene product (CD117) in human tissues: value in the diagnosis of mast cell disorders. Hum Pathol 28:498–504, 1998.

117. Hughes DM, Kurtin PJ, Hanson CA, et al: Identification of normal and neoplastic mast cells by immunohistochemical demonstration of tryptase in paraffin sections. J Surg Pathol 1:87–96, 1995.

118. Horny H-P, Sillaber C, Menke D, et al: Diagnostic value of immunostaining for tryptase in patients with mastocytosis. Am J Surg Pathol 22:1132–1140, 1998.

118a. Yang F, Tran T-A, Carlson JA, et al: Paraffin section immunophenotype of cutaneous and extracutaneous mast cell disease: comparison to other hematopoietic neoplasms. Am J Surg Pathol 24:703–709, 2000.

119. Klatt EC, Lukes RJ, Meyer PR: Benign and malignant mast cell proliferations. Diagnosis and separation using a pH-dependent toluidine blue stain in tissue section. Cancer 51:1119–1124, 1983.

120. Travis WD, Li C-Y, Bergstralh EJ: Solid and hematologic malignancies in 60 patients with systemic mast cell disease. Arch Pathol Lab Med 113:365–368, 1989.

121. Falk S, Stutte HJ: Primary malignant lymphomas of the spleen. A morphologic and immunohistochemical analysis of 17 cases. Cancer 66:2612–2619, 1990.

122. Arber DA, Rappaport H, Weiss LM: Non-Hodgkin's lymphoproliferative disorders involving the spleen. Mod Pathol 10:18–32, 1997.

123. Schmid C, Kirkham N, Diss T, et al: Splenic marginal zone cell lymphoma. Am J Surg Pathol 16:455–466, 1992.

124. Pawade J, Wilkins BS, Wright DH: Low-grade B-cell lymphomas of the splenic marginal zone: a clinicopathologic and immunohistochemical study of 14 cases. Histopathology 27:129–137, 1995.

125. Mollejo M, Menárguez J, Lloret E, et al: Splenic marginal zone lymphoma: a distinctive type of low-grade B-cell lymphoma—a clinicopathological study of 13 cases. Am J Surg Pathol 19:1146–1157, 1995.

126. Hammer RD, Glick AD, Greer JP, et al: Splenic marginal zone lymphoma. A distinct B-cell neoplasm. Am J Surg Pathol 20:613–626, 1996.

127. Sol Mateo M, Mollejo M, Villuendas R, et al: Analysis of the frequency of microsatellite instability and p53 gene mutation in splenic marginal zone and MALT lymphomas. J Clin Pathol Mol Pathol 51:262–267, 1998.

128. Neiman RS, Sullivan AL, Jaffe R: Malignant lymphoma simulating leukemic reticuloendotheliosis. A clinicopathologic study of ten cases. Cancer 43:329–342, 1979.

129. Lai R, Arber DA, Chang KL, et al: Frequency of bcl-2 expression in non-Hodgkin's lymphoma: a study of 778 cases with comparison of marginal zone lymphoma and monocytoid B-cell hyperplasia. Mod Pathol 11:864–869, 1998.

130. Melo JV, Robinson SF, Gregory C, et al: Splenic B cell lymphoma with "villous" lymphocytes in the peripheral blood: a disorder distinct from hairy cell leukemia. Leukemia 1:294–299, 1987.

131. Mulligan SP, Matutes E, Dearden C, et al: Splenic lymphoma with villous lymphocytes: natural history and response to therapy in 50 cases. Br J Haematol 78:206–209, 1991.

132. Troussard X, Valensi F, Duchayne E, et al: Splenic lymphoma with villous lymphocytes: clinical presentation, biology and prognostic factors in a series of 100 patients. Br J Haematol 93:731–736, 1996.

133. Isaacson PG, Matutes E, Burke M, et al: The histopathology of splenic lymphoma with villous lymphocytes. Blood 84:3828–3834, 1994.

134. Gaulard P, Zafrani ES, Mavier P, et al: Peripheral T-cell lymphoma presenting as predominant liver disease: a report of three cases. Hepatology 6:864–868, 1986.

135. Gaulard P, Bourquelot P, Kanavaros P, et al: Expression of the α/β and γ/δ T-cell receptors in 57 cases of peripheral T-cell lymphomas. Identification of a subset of γ/δ T-cell lymphomas. Am J Pathol 137:617–628, 1990.

136. Cooke CB, Krenacs L, Stetler-Stevenson M, et al: Hepatosplenic T-cell lymphoma: a distinct clinicopathologic entity of cytotoxic γδ T-cell origin. Blood 88:4265–4274, 1996.

137. Salhany KE, Feldman M, Kahn MJ, et al: Hepatosplenic γδ T-cell lymphoma: ultrastructural, immunophenotypic, and functional evidence for cytotoxic T lymphocyte differentiation. Hum Pathol 28:674–685, 1997.

138. Chang KL, Arber DA: Hepatosplenic γδ T-cell lymphoma—not just alphabet soup. Adv Anat Pathol 5:21–29, 1998.

139. Kadin ME, Kamoun M, Lamberg J: Erythrophagocytic Tγ lymphoma. A clinicopathologic entity resembling malignant histiocytosis. N Engl J Med 304:648–653, 1981.

140. Bordessoule D, Gaulard P, Mason DY: Preferential localisation of human lymphocytes bearing γδ T cell receptors to the red pulp of the spleen. J Clin Pathol 43:461–464, 1990.

141. Ross CW, Schnitzer B, Sheldon S, et al: Gamma/delta T-cell prosttransplantation lymphoproliferative disorder primarily in the spleen. Am J Clin Pathol 102:310–315, 1994.

142. Kraus MD, Crawford DF, Kaleem Z, et al: T γ/δ hepatosplenic lymphoma in a heart transplant patient after an Epstein-Barr virus positive lymphoproliferative disorder. A case report. Cancer 82:983–992, 1998.

143. Wang C-C, Tien H-F, Lin M-T, et al: Consistent presence of isochromosome 7q in hepatosplenic T γ/δ lymphoma: a new cytogenetic-clinicopathologic entity. Genes Chromosomes Cancer 12:161–164, 1995.

144. Yao M, Tien H-F, Lin M-T, et al: Clinical and hematological characteristics of hepatosplenic T γ/δ lymphoma with isochromosome for long arm of chromosome 7. Leuk Lymphoma 22:495–500, 1996.

145. Jonveaux P, Daniel MT, Martel V, et al: Isochromosome 7q and trisomy 8 are consistent primary, non-random chromosomal abnormalities associated with hepatosplenic T γ/δ lymphoma. Leukemia 10:1453–1455, 1996.

146. Bosch F, Jares P, Campo E, et al: PRAD-1/cyclin D1 gene overexpression in chronic lymphoproliferative disorders: a highly specific marker of mantle cell lymphoma. Blood 84:2726–2732, 1994.

147. de Boer CJ, van Krieken JHJM, Kluin-Nelemans HC, et al: Cyclin D1 messenger RNA overexpression as a marker of mantle cell lymphoma. Oncogene 10:1833–1840, 1995.

148. Moskow JM, Weiss LM, Rappport H, Arber DA: Marginal zone pattern in malignant lymphomas involving the spleen. Mod Pathol 7:116A, 1994.

149. Alkan S, Ross CW, Hanson CA, et al: Follicular lymphoma with involvement of the splenic marginal zone: a pitfall in the differential diagnosis of splenic marginal zone cell lymphoma. Hum Pathol 27:503–506, 1996.

150. Piris MA, Mollejo M, Campo E, et al: A marginal zone pattern may be found in different varieties of non-Hodgkin's lymphoma: the morphology and immunohistology of splenic involvement by B-cell lymphomas simulating splenic marginal zone lymphoma. Histopathology 33:230–239, 1998.

151. Köbrich U, Falk S, Karhoff M, et al: Primary large cell lymphoma of the splenic sinuses: a variant of angiotropic B-cell lymphoma (neoplastic angioendotheliomatosis)? Hum Pathol 23:1184–1187, 1992.

152. Loughran TP Jr, Starkebaum G, Clark E, et al: Evaluation of splenectomy in large granular lymphocytic leukaemia. Br J Haematol 67:135–140, 1987.

153. Griffiths DFR, Jasani B, Standen GR: Pathology of the spleen

in large granular lymphocytic leukaemia. J Clin Pathol 42: 885, 1989.

154. Boyko WJ, Pratt R, Wass H: Functional hyposplenism, a diagnostic clue in amyloidosis. Report of six cases. Am J Clin Pathol 77:745–748, 1982.

155. Frizzera G, Massarelli G, Banks PM, et al: A systemic lymphoproliferative disorder with morphologic features of Castleman's disease. Pathological findings in 15 patients. Am J Surg Pathol 7:211–231, 1983.

156. Weisenburger DD: Multicentric angiofollicular lymph node hyperplasia. Pathology of the spleen. Am J Surg Pathol 12: 176–181, 1988.

157. Chang KL, Kamel OW, Arber DA, et al: Pathologic features of nodular lymphocyte predominance Hodgkin's disease in extranodal sites. Am J Surg Pathol 19:1313–1324, 1995.

158. Wilson MS, Weiss LM, Gatter KC, et al: Malignant histiocytosis. A reassessment of cases previously reported in 1975 based on paraffin section immunophenotyping studies. Cancer 66:530–536, 1990.

159. Ornvold K, Carstensen H, Junge J, et al: Tumours classified as "malignant histiocytosis" in children are T-cell neoplasms. APMIS 100:558–566, 1992.

160. Ralfkiaer E, Delsol G, O'Conner NTJ, et al: Malignant lymphomas of true histiocytic origin. A clinical, histological, immunophenotypic and genotypic study. J Pathol 160:9–17, 1990.

161. Lam KY, Chan ACL, Wat MS: Langerhans cell histiocytosis forming an asymptomatic solitary nodule in the spleen. J Clin Pathol 49:262–264, 1996.

162. Burns BF, Colby TV, Dorfman RF: Langerhans' cell granulomatosis (histiocytosis X) associated with malignant lymphomas. Am J Surg Pathol 7:529–533, 1983.

163. Neumann MP, Frizzera G: The coexistence of Langerhans' cell granulomatosis and malignant lymphoma may take different forms: report of seven cases with a review of the literature. Hum Pathol 17:1060–1065, 1986.

164. Egeler RM, Neglia JP, Puccetti DM, et al: Association of Langerhans' cell histiocytosis with malignant neoplasms. Cancer 71:865–873, 1993.

165. Thiele J, Klein H, Falk S, et al: Splenic megakaryocytopoiesis in primary (idiopathic) osteomyelofibrosis. An immunohistological and morphometric study with comparison of corresponding bone marrow features. Acta Haematol 87:176–180, 1992.

166. Barosi G, Ambrosetti A, Centra A, et al: Splenectomy and risk of blast transformation in myelofibrosis with myeloid metaplasia. Blood 91:3630–3636, 1998.

167. Wolf BC, Banks PM, Mann RB, et al: Splenic hematopoiesis in polycythemia vera. A morphologic and immunohistochemical study. Am J Clin Pathol 89:69–75, 1988.

168. Rappaport H: Tumors of the Hematopoietic System. Atlas of Tumor Pathology. Second Series, Fascicle 8. Washington, DC, Armed Forces Institute of Pathology, 1966.

169. Diebold J, Audouin J: Peliosis of the spleen. Report of a case associated with chronic myelomonocytic leukemia, presenting with spontaneous splenic rupture. Am J Surg Pathol 7: 197–204, 1983.

170. Kraus MD, Bartlett NL, Fleming MD, et al: Splenic pathology in myelodysplasia. A report of 13 cases with clinical correlation. Am J Surg Pathol 22:1255–1266, 1998.

171. Vasef MA, Neiman RS, Meletiou SD, et al: Marked granulocytic proliferation induced by granulocyte colony-stimulating factor in the spleen simulating a myeloid leukemic infiltrate. Mod Pathol 11:1138–1141, 1998.

172. Kostich ND, Rappaport H: Diagnostic significance of the histologic changes in the liver and spleen in leukemia and malignant lymphoma. Cancer 18:1214–1232, 1965.

173. Wick MR, Smith SL, Scheithauer BW, et al: Primary nonlymphoreticular malignant neoplasms of the spleen. Am J Surg Pathol 6:229–242, 1982.

174. Feakins RM, Norton AJ: Rhabdomyosarcoma of the spleen. Histopathology 29:577–579, 1996.

175. Le Bail B, Morel D, Mérel P, et al: Cystic smooth-muscle tumor of the liver and spleen associated with Epstein-Barr virus after renal transplantation. Am J Surg Pathol 20:1418–1425, 1996.

176. Elit L, Aylward B: Splenic cyst carcinoma presenting in pregnancy. Am J Hematol 32:57–60, 1989.

177. Morinaga S, Ohyama R, Koizumi J: Low-grade mucinous cystadenocarcinoma in the spleen. Am J Surg Pathol 16:903–908, 1992.

178. Westra WH, Anderson BO, Klimstra DS: Carcinosarcoma of the spleen. An extragenital malignant mixed müllerian tumor? Am J Surg Pathol 18:309–315, 1994.

179. Marymont JH, Gross S: Patterns of metastatic cancer in the spleen. Am J Clin Pathol 40:58–66, 1963.

180. Cummings OW, Mazur MT: Breast carcinoma diffusely metastatic to the spleen. A report of two cases presenting as idiopathic thrombocytopenic purpura. Am J Clin Pathol 97: 484–489, 1992.

181. Fakan F, Michal M: Nodular transformation of splenic red pulp due to carcinomatous infiltration. A diagnostic pitfall. Histopathology 25:175–178, 1994.

182. Klein B, Stein M, Kuten A, et al: Splenomegaly and solitary spleen metastasis in solid tumors. Cancer 60:100–102, 1987.

# Bone Marrow

Daniel A. Arber

The bone marrow biopsy specimen differs from biopsy material from most other organs because a proper evaluation of the bone marrow requires the incorporation of a variety of specimen types to arrive at an accurate and complete diagnosis. Bone marrow studies should be evaluated in conjunction with clinical data, review of peripheral blood smears, and complete blood count data as well as with bone marrow aspirate smears or imprints. Many cases also benefit from cytochemical evaluation, immunophenotyping, and molecular genetic and cytogenetic studies, and the results of all of these should be considered in making a final diagnosis. This chapter emphasizes this multifactorial approach to bone marrow evaluation and attempts to highlight the specimen types that require the use of ancillary techniques for accurate diagnosis. Complete clinical information is essential for the proper triage of material for microbiology cultures, flow cytometry, cytogenetics, and molecular genetic studies because these methods usually require fresh tissue.

## SPECIMEN HANDLING

Most bone marrow specimens are sternal aspirates or iliac crest aspirates with or without biopsy. Details of the procedure and of specimen preparation are well described elsewhere.[1-4] Aspirate smears are usually made at the bedside but may also be made in the laboratory after the procedure. Bone marrow aspirate material may be immediately placed into "purple top" tubes containing ethylenediamine-tetraacetic acid (EDTA) for the preparation of smears at a later time. This method limits the clotting of the

aspirate specimen and allows material to be submitted for ancillary studies or even particle sections. Whether the smears are made at the bedside or from EDTA tubes, the aspirate should be grossly evaluated for the presence of bone marrow particles. Such particles should be removed and placed on a slide for the actual smear preparation. The absence of particles on a smear limits its diagnostic usefulness in many cases, and such smears often show changes of peripheral blood. Many pediatric patients, however, will not demonstrate gross particles in the aspirate material despite numerous bone marrow elements in the specimen.

Similar to the preparation of peripheral blood smears,[5] only a small amount of bone marrow material needs to be gently smeared across the slide. Different methods may be employed, such as the use of coverslips to gently smear the particles. An alternative method is to place a small drop of particulate marrow toward the labeled end of a slide.[2] The outer portion of the drop, away from the label, is then touched with the edge of a second slide, and the marrow is gently "pulled" across the original slide with the edge of the second slide. Large drops of marrow on a slide result in thick and bloody smears that are difficult to interpret. Smears made with too much pressure distort or destroy the marrow cells. Multiple air-dried smears should be prepared, although the actual number depends on the number of marrow particles in the specimen and the clinical indication for the procedure. At least three extra smears for cytochemical studies should be made for patients suspected of having acute leukemia. Although touch preparations or imprints are suggested for all specimens with a bone marrow biopsy, they are essential in cases with a "dry tap" in which the aspirated material has the appearance of peripheral blood.[6]

Representative aspirate smears and imprints are stained with a Romanovsky stain. The actual stain type varies among laboratories and includes Giemsa, Wright-Giemsa, and May-Grünwald-Giemsa stains. The author prefers the Wright-Giemsa stain. Rapid review of these smears helps in determining the need for ancillary studies, such as cytochemistry, immunophenotyping, cytogenetic analysis, and molecular genetic study.

Clot biopsy sections are often made from coagulated aspirate material. This material contains predominantly blood as well as small marrow particles that can be embedded and processed for sections stained with H&E or periodic acid–Schiff. Despite the absence of clotting of EDTA-anticoagulated aspirate specimens, the bone marrow particles that are left after smears are made can be filtered and embedded for histologic evaluation.[7] This method provides a more concentrated collection of marrow particles but may not yield any material in some pediatric patients.

Trephine core biopsy is not performed for all patients, but these specimens are essential in the evaluation of patients suspected of having disease that may only focally involve the bone marrow, such as malignant lymphoma, and are preferred in all patients. Bilateral bone marrow biopsies are recommended for patients undergoing bone marrow staging.[8] Imprint slides from the biopsy specimens may be made either at the bedside or in the laboratory. To make them in the laboratory, the bone marrow core is submitted fresh, on saline-dampened gauze, with the imprints made immediately to allow adequate fixation of the biopsy specimen. Otherwise, the imprints are made at the bedside, and the biopsy specimen is submitted in fixative. Many laboratories prefer mercuric chloride–based fixatives for bone marrow specimens, but distribution of this substance to hospital wards and offices is often not advisable. Submission of the bone marrow biopsy material in formalin, followed by fixation in mercuric chloride in the laboratory, provides results similar to those obtained with primary mercuric chloride fixation. After fixation, the core biopsy specimen is decalcified and processed for H&E-stained or periodic acid–Schiff–stained sections.

## THE NORMAL BONE MARROW AND AN APPROACH TO BONE MARROW EVALUATION

It is often easiest to evaluate a bone marrow specimen by comparing the specimen to what would be expected in the normal bone marrow.[9, 10] The initial evaluation on low magnification of the biopsy specimen is of the marrow cellularity. Estimates of cellularity on aspirate material are described[11] but may

be unreliable in variably cellular marrows.[12] The normal cellularity varies with age, and evaluation of cellularity must always be made in the context of the patient's age.[13] The marrow is approximately 80% cellular in children through age 10 years; it then slowly declines in cellularity until age 30 years, when it remains about 50% cellular. The marrow cellularity declines again in elderly patients to about 30% at 70 years. Because of the variation in cellularity by age, the report should clearly indicate whether the stated cellularity in a given specimen is normocellular, hypocellular, or hypercellular.

Estimates of cellularity may be inappropriately lowered by several factors. Subcortical bone marrow is normally hypocellular, and these areas should be ignored in the cellularity estimate. Superficial core biopsies may contain only these subcortical areas, and such biopsy specimens should be considered inadequate for cellularity evaluation. Technical artifacts may also cause a false lowering of marrow cellularity. Tears made in the section during processing and cutting as well as artifactual displacement of marrow from bony trabeculae should not be considered in the estimate.

After the marrow cellularity has been evaluated, the cellular elements must be considered. The three main bone marrow cell lines, maturing granulocytes, erythroid precursors, and megakaryocytes, should be evaluated first. Maturing granulocytes are the most common cell type in the normal marrow with a 2:1 or 3:1 granulocyte-to-erythroid ratio; the higher ratio is more common in women.[10] All stages of granulocyte and erythroid maturation are normally present, with blast cells usually less than 3%. The various stages of maturation are best evaluated on the aspirate smear material, but the location of immature cell clusters is best evaluated on the core biopsy specimen. Immature clusters of myeloid and erythroid cells normally occur adjacent to bony trabeculae. Megakaryocytes are easily identifiable on smear and biopsy material in the normal marrow and should consist of predominantly mature forms with hypersegmented nuclei.

Lymphocytes normally represent 10% to 15% of cells on aspirate smears, but lymphoid precursors and mature lymphocytes may be normally increased in children and the elderly, respectively. The lymphoid precursors, or hematogones,[14] are not obvious in the biopsy material of children, despite being evident on aspirate smears. Lymphoid aggregates, however, are common in biopsy material of elderly patients and are nonparatrabecular in location. These cells are predominantly T lymphocytes. Cells that are present at a lower frequency in the bone marrow include monocytes, plasma cells, mast cells, eosinophils, basophils, and osteoblasts. These cells normally represent less than 5% of marrow cells on smears.[10]

Cells and proliferations that do not normally occur in the marrow, including histiocyte accumulations or granulomas, fibrosis, serous atrophy, and neoplastic cells, should be systematically assessed in

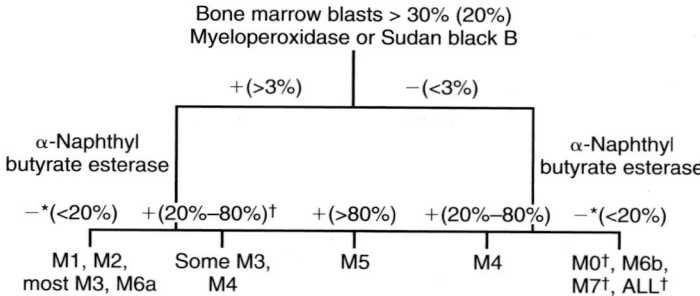

**FIGURE 43–1.** Algorithm of the cytochemical evaluation of acute leukemia. A pecentage of bone marrow blasts of 20% may be used, as proposed in new classifications.

*Staining of less than 20% of cells or punctate perinuclear staining of any percentage of cells is considered a negative result for α-naphthyl butyrate esterase.

†These cases require immunophenotyping for diagnosis.

all specimens. The bony trabeculae should also be evaluated for evidence of osteopenia, osteoblastic proliferations, and changes of Paget's disease. Iron stores of the normal marrow are predominantly in histiocytes within marrow particles, but red blood cell iron incorporation is normally seen on oil immersion in scattered cells that usually demonstrate one or two siderotic granules adjacent to the nucleus.

## NEOPLASTIC AND PROLIFERATIVE PROCESSES

### Ancillary Techniques Useful in Bone Marrow Evaluation

Ancillary techniques are essential for the proper diagnosis of many bone marrow neoplasms. Because therapy is now often specific for the exact lineage of the neoplastic cells and prognosis is often directly related to genetic changes of the neoplasm, these tests are vital for the proper evaluation of patients. Despite the advances in immunophenotyping and cancer genetics, morphologic evaluation remains the initial step in the bone marrow study, and morphologic changes can reliably suggest further studies to identify clinically significant immunophenotypic and genetic findings in some cases. These morphologic features are discussed with the specific diseases, as are the specific findings of the various ancillary tests. The general utility and applications of ancillary testing, however, are discussed here.

#### CYTOCHEMISTRY

Despite the widespread use of immunophenotyping in the diagnosis of hematopoietic neoplasms, cytochemical studies are still of diagnostic importance.[15] This is particularly true of the acute leukemias; however, a large menu of cytochemical tests is probably not necessary for most leukemias. Figure 43–1 provides a practical algorithm of diagnostic cytochemical tests for acute leukemia. However, many leukemia types require the use of cytochemistry in conjunction with immunophenotyping studies for precise classification. Myeloperoxidase or Sudan black B staining, by cytochemistry, remains the hallmark of a diagnosis of acute myeloid leukemia (AML) in most cases. Some cases, such as minimally

differentiated AML and monoblastic leukemias, are myeloperoxidase negative. The use of nonspecific esterase cytochemistry, such as α-naphthyl butyrate esterase, is still the primary means of identifying monocytic differentiation for classification purposes. Cytochemistry is of limited value in the diagnosis of acute lymphoblastic leukemia (ALL). Whereas negative results of peroxidase cytochemical studies are expected in ALL, they do not sufficiently exclude a myeloid leukemia and should not be used as the sole evidence of lymphoid lineage. Periodic acid–Schiff staining, frequently showing "chunky" positivity in lymphoblast cytoplasm, is also not sufficiently specific to be used diagnostically.

The Prussian blue stain for iron is a histochemical stain that is commonly employed on bone marrow specimens.[16] Although it may be used for clot or biopsy material, it is most reliable and useful for bone marrow aspirate smears as long as sufficient particles are present on the smear.[17] Iron staining is useful in identifying reticuloendothelial iron stores in the evaluation of a patient for iron deficiency or overload, but it also helps in the evaluation of red blood cell iron incorporation. Iron stores are often graded from 0 to 6+,[18] as summarized in Table 43–1, and such grading correlates well with other chemical measures of iron. The identification of an increase in iron within erythroid precursors, particularly in the form of ringed sideroblasts, helps in the

**TABLE 43–1.** Histologic Grading of Iron Storage in Bone Marrow Aspirate Material

| Grade | Characteristic |
| --- | --- |
| 0 or negative | No iron identified under oil immersion |
| 1+ | Small iron-positive particles visible only under oil immersion |
| 2+ | Small, sparsely distributed iron particles usually visible under low magnification |
| 3+ | Numerous small particles present in histiocytes throughout the marrow particles |
| 4+ | Larger particles throughout the marrow with tendency to aggregate into clumps |
| 5+ | Dense, large clumps of iron throughout the marrow |
| 6+ | Large deposits of iron, both intracellular and extracellular, that obscure cellular detail in the marrow particles |

Adapted from Reference 18.

diagnosis of myelodysplasia and AML with associated dysplasia. The other cytochemical test that is commonly used on bone marrow specimens is the detection of tartrate-resistant acid phosphatase in hairy cell leukemia,[19] although this cytochemical study should be used in conjunction with immunophenotypic studies.

## IMMUNOPHENOTYPING

Immunophenotyping studies are essential for the proper diagnosis of lymphoblastic malignant neoplasms and help in the classification of mature lymphoid neoplasms and some myeloid neoplasms. In addition, these studies can provide a characteristic immunologic "fingerprint" of an acute leukemia that may be useful in the subsequent evaluation of residual disease.

### Flow Cytometry and Immunocytochemistry

Some antibodies that are useful in the immunophenotypic evaluation of blastic proliferations by flow cytometry and immunocytochemistry are listed in Table 43–2. The best markers for lymphomas are discussed in Chapter 41. Several consensus reports and reviews regarding the use of flow cytometric immunophenotyping in hematologic malignant neoplasms[20–26] offer guidelines to the use of this methodology on peripheral blood and bone marrow specimens.

Both flow cytometry and immunocytochemistry primarily detect surface antigens, although some cytoplasmic antigens may also be detected. Flow cytometry has the advantage of allowing the evaluation of several thousand cells in a rapid manner, and it has the ability to assess the expression of multiple antigens on a single cell. Also, the use of CD45 versus side scatter gating strategies allows only cells with specific characteristics (such as blast cells or lymphoid cells) to be evaluated, and this method greatly increases the ability to detect residual disease in a specimen.[27] Although the same antibodies that are available for flow cytometry can be used for immunocytochemistry, the number of slides available for the latter technique limits the number of antibodies that can be studied on a given sample. Advantages of immunocytochemistry are that it allows the direct visualization of the marker on the tumor cell and does not require the instrumentation needed for flow cytometry.

### Immunohistochemistry

Immunohistochemistry on paraffin sections of the clot or core biopsy material is ideal for the assessment of focal lesions that may not be available as aspirate material submitted for flow cytometry, owing to sampling differences or dry taps. This includes focal marrow involvement by malignant lymphoma. This method is also useful for the characterization of tumors that are not routinely assessed by flow cytometry, such as metastatic carci-

**TABLE 43–2.** Selected Useful Flow Cytometry and Immunocytochemistry Markers in Acute Leukemia

| |
|---|
| General |
|   CD45 |
| Myeloid |
|   CD11c |
|   CD13 |
|   CD15 |
|   CD33 |
|   CD65 |
|   CD117 |
|   Cytoplasmic myeloperoxidase |
| Myelomonocytic |
|   CD14 |
|   CD36 |
| Megakaryocyte |
|   CD41 |
|   CD61 |
| Immature B lineage |
|   CD10 |
|   CD19 |
|   CD22 |
|   TdT |
| Mature B lineage |
|   CD19 |
|   CD20 |
|   $\kappa$ and $\lambda$ light chains |
| T lineage |
|   CD2 |
|   CD5 |
|   CD7 |
|   CD4/CD8 |
|   TdT |
|   Cytoplasmic CD3 |
| Others |
|   CD34 |
|   CD56 |
|   HLA-DR |

nomas and small round cell tumors of childhood.

Because of limitations in the detection of some antigens by paraffin section immunohistochemistry, flow cytometric immunophenotyping is preferred for the evaluation of lymphoproliferative disorders and acute leukemias. When such material is not available, immunohistochemistry may still provide diagnostic information.[28–30] Useful antibodies for the evaluation of lymphomatous proliferations are discussed in more detail in Chapter 41. Paraffin section antibodies useful for the evaluation of acute leukemia proliferations are given in Table 43–3.

As with all immunophenotyping studies, pertinent positive and negative findings should be obtained with a panel of antibodies because the detection of a single antigen is usually never sufficiently lineage specific. For example, whereas terminal deoxynucleotidyl transferase (TdT) is usually detectable in lymphoblastic malignant neoplasms, it is also present in a subgroup of myeloid leukemias. Initial immunophenotyping panels that are useful in the evaluation of acute leukemias are listed in Table 43–4.

**TABLE 43–3.** Selected Useful Paraffin Section Antibodies in Acute Leukemia

Immature B cell
CD10
CD79a
TdT
T cell
CD2
CD3
CD5
TdT
Myeloid
Myeloperoxidase
Lysozyme
Others
CD34
HLA-DR

## MOLECULAR GENETIC AND CYTOGENETIC ANALYSIS

Molecular genetic and cytogenetic studies on bone marrow specimens offer valuable information in certain clinical situations, and the prognostic significance of karyotypic changes in acute leukemia are now well established. In general, routine karyotype analysis is the preferred first-line test in newly diagnosed leukemias and when myelodysplasia is suspected, because a multitude of acquired genetic abnormalities may be detected by this method. When cryptic or masked translocations are suspected, when a precise genetic breakpoint with prognostic implications needs to be confirmed, or when residual disease testing is needed, molecular genetic tests are useful. This testing also helps in identifying gene rearrangement in lymphomas that are not readily identifiable by karyotype analysis and in detecting some lymphoma translocations that may not be consistently found by karyotype analysis. Details about the specific molecular genetic abnormalities associated with bone marrow diseases are discussed with those diseases.

**TABLE 43–4.** Suggested Initial Immunophenotyping Panels for Acute Leukemia Depending on the Type of Material Available

| Lineage | Fresh Tissue Flow Cytometry and Immunocytochemistry | Paraffin Section Immunohistochemistry |
|---|---|---|
| Myeloid | CD13 CD33 | Myeloperoxidase |
| Lymphoid | CD2 CD5 CD7 CD10 CD19 Tdt | CD3 CD10 CD79a TdT |
| Others | CD34 HLA-DR | CD34 |

**TABLE 43–5.** Some of the Common Cytogenetic and Molecular Genetic Abnormalities in Acute Myeloid Leukemia and Myelodysplasia

| Translocation | Involved Genes | Most Common Disease Type |
|---|---|---|
| inv(3)/t(3;3)(q21;q26) | RPN1/EVI1 | Myelodysplasia |
| t(3;21)(q26;q22) | EVI1, EAP, or MDS1/AML1 | Myelodysplasia |
| t(3;5)(q25;q34) | NPM/MLF1 | Myelodysplasia, M2, M6 |
| t(8;21)(q22;q22) | AML1/ETO | M2 |
| t(6;9)(p23;q34) | DEK/CAN | M1, M2, M4 |
| t(7;11)(p15;p15) | NUP98/HOXA9 | M2, M4 |
| t(15;17)(q22;q21) | PML/RARα | M3 |
| t(11;17)(q23;q21) | PLZF/RARα | M3 |
| t(11;17)(q13;q21) | NuMA/RARα | M3 |
| t(5;17)(q31;q21) | NPM/RARα | M3 |
| inv(16)/t(16;16)(p13;q22) | CBFβ/MYH11 | M4Eo |
| t(9;11)(p22;q23) | AF9/MLL | M5 |
| Other 11q23 abnormalities | MLL | M4, M5 |
| t(1;22)(p13;q31) | ?/PDGFβ | M7 |

A large number of cytogenetic abnormalities occur with acute leukemias; some of them are summarized in Tables 43–5 and 43–6. The most common groups of abnormalities are those that disrupt transcription factors, tyrosine kinase translocations, retinoic acid translocations, and 11q23 abnormalities.[31, 32]

Translocations that involve genes that encode transcription factor proteins are some of the most common in acute leukemia. Of these, the core binding factor, a transcription factor involved in normal hematopoiesis, is one of the best described.[33] The core binding factor is formed by an aggregate of different proteins that include the AML1 protein, en-

**TABLE 43–6.** Some of the Common Cytogenetic and Molecular Genetic Abnormalities in Acute Lymphoblastic Leukemia

| Type of Leukemia | Translocation | Involved Genes |
|---|---|---|
| Precursor B cell ALL (L1, L2) | t(9;22)(q34;q11) t(12;21)(p13;q22) t(1;19)(q23;p13) t(17;19)(q22;p13) t(4;11)(q21;q23) Other 11q23 abnormalities | BCR/ABL TEL/AML1 E2A/PBX E2A/HLF AF4/MLL MLL |
| B cell ALL (L3) | t(8;14)(q24;q32) t(2;8)(p12;q24) t(8;22)(q24;q11) | IGH/MYC IGκ/MYC IGλ/MYC |
| T cell ALL (L1, L2) | 1q32 abnormalities t(8;14)(q24;q11) t(11;14)(p15;q11) t(11;14)(p13;q11) t(10;14)(q24;q11) del 9(p21) t(1;7)(p34;q34) | TAL1 TCRα/MYC TCRδ/RBTN1 TCRδ/RBTN2 TCRδ/HOX11 p16 and p15 TCRβ/LCK |

coded by the *AML1* gene on chromosome band 21(q22), and the core binding factor $\beta$-subunit protein, which is encoded on chromosome band 16(q22). Disruption of either one of these chromosome regions, as seen in t(8;21), t(3;21), t(12;21), inv(16), and t(16;16), results in the development of acute leukemia. These abnormalities may cause loss of the normal transactivation domain on the AML protein or cause disruption of the normal configuration of the core binding factor. Either mechanism blocks the usual interactions that trigger normal hematopoiesis. The leukemia types of each abnormality vary. The AML1/ETO fusion product of t(8; 21)(q22;q22) usually results in a de novo AML with maturation (M2); AML1/EVI-1, AML1/EAP, and AML1/MDS1 fusion products of t(3;21)(q26;q22) usually result in myelodysplasia-associated processes; the TEL/AML1 fusion product of t(12; 21)(p13;q22) is usually seen in pediatric ALL; and the CBF/MYH11 fusion product of inv(16)(p13q22) or t(16;16)(p13;q22) is usually seen with de novo acute myelomonocytic leukemia with abnormal eosinophils (M4Eo). Despite the great variability in the morphologic and immunophenotypic features of these leukemias, they all have a similar molecular genetic mechanism that is at least in part related to the development of the leukemic process.

Translocations resulting in the development of a tyrosine kinase fusion protein are a second group of abnormalities in leukemias. These include the BCR/ABL proteins of t(9;22)(q32;q11) in chronic myelogenous leukemia (CML) and some cases of AML, the TEL/PDGFR$\beta$ protein of t(5;12)(q33;p13) in some cases of chronic myelomonocytic leukemia (CMML), and the TEL/ABL fusion protein of t(9;12)(q32;p13) of some acute and chronic leukemias. These tyrosine kinase proteins interact with other proteins to activate the *RAS* signaling pathway, which may result in abnormal myeloid proliferation.

The t(15;17)(q22;q11.2) is the most common retinoic acid translocation and is present in the majority of acute promyelocytic leukemias. This translocation results in a PML/RARA fusion protein. Other less common translocations also occur in acute promyelocytic leukemia and involve the *RARA* gene. Fusion proteins involving RARA negatively inhibit the poorly understood normal functions of the *RARA* gene, apparently resulting in the development of acute leukemia. This mechanism of leukemia transformation is unique to the acute promyelocytic leukemias. All-*trans*-retinoic acid overrides the negative inhibitory effect of the leukemic fusion protein, making it a unique therapeutic agent for this disease.

Translocations involving chromosome band 11q23 are common, and at least 30 different translocation partners may occur with this chromosome region in acute leukemia. Most translocations involve the *MLL* gene that is also known as *ALL1* and *HRX*.[34] The *MLL* gene is believed to function as a homeotic transcription regulator, but how translocations involving this gene cause leukemia is not well understood. The type of leukemia differs with the different *MLL* translocations. The t(4;11)(q21;q23) results in an AF4/MLL fusion protein. This translocation is usually associated with precursor B cell ALL, often with aberrant CD15 expression, and is extremely common in infants. The t(9;11)(p22;q23) results in a AF9/MLL fusion protein and is more commonly associated with AMLs in adults with monocytic features. Translocations involving the *MLL* gene also occur in therapy-related AMLs and are common after chemotherapy with topoisomerase II inhibitors. These leukemias also usually demonstrate monocytic features.

The lymphoid malignant neoplasms also demonstrate evidence of immunoglobulin or T cell receptor gene rearrangements that may be useful markers of clonality. Such tests are usually not necessary to make a diagnosis of malignancy in cases of acute leukemia, and because lineage infidelity is common in ALLs, these tests may not be useful in defining cell lineage. A unique gene rearrangement in an ALL may be sequenced, however, and patient-specific polymerase chain reaction (PCR) primers and probes, which have been shown to be useful for the monitoring of residual disease, may be devel-

**TABLE 43–7.** French-American-British (FAB) Cooperative Group Classification of Myelodysplastic Syndromes

| Syndrome | Peripheral Blood Monocytosis of >1 × 10⁹/mm³ | Peripheral Blood Blasts | | Bone Marrow Blasts | Ringed Sideroblasts > 15% of Erythroid Cells |
|---|---|---|---|---|---|
| Refractory anemia | − | <1% | *and* | <5% | − |
| Refractory anemia with ringed sideroblasts | − | <1% | *and* | <5% | + |
| Refractory anemia with excess blasts | − | >1% but <5% | *or* | ≥5% but ≤20% | +/− |
| Refractory anemia with excess blasts in transformation | − | ≥5% | *or* | >20% but <30% (or Auer rod +)† | +/− |
| Chronic myelomonocytic leukemia | + | <5% | *and* | ≥20% | +/− |
| Chronic myelomonocytic leukemia in transformation* | + | ≥5% | *or* | >20% but <30% | +/− |

* Not included in the original FAB classification, but generally accepted as a category.
† The presence of Auer rods with any blast cell count is considered evidence of refractory anemia with excess blasts in transformation.

oped. These methods are not available in most medical centers for routine use. The mature lymphoid malignant neoplasms also demonstrate gene rearrangements, and many are associated with unique cytogenetic translocations. These are discussed in more detail with each disease and in Chapter 41.

Cytogenetic studies are essential to identify the abnormality associated with a given leukemia, although t(12;21) and some *MLL* translocations may be missed by routine karyotype analysis. PCR methods are useful for confirming a precise translocation site and are potentially useful in following up patients for residual disease. Some translocations, including t(8;21) and possibly inv(16), may persist in low numbers after treatment. Detection of these abnormalities by routine PCR methods does not necessarily predict relapse. For this reason, quantitative PCR methods may be of more value in the future for the detection of residual disease after therapy.[35]

## Myelodysplastic Syndromes and Acute Leukemia

Pathologists traditionally use the classification systems for acute leukemia and myelodysplastic syndromes developed by the French-American-British (FAB) cooperative group[36-40]; these systems are summarized in Tables 43–7 and 43–8. However, these schemes do not include some of the clinically significant genetic findings of these diseases that have been described in recent years, and many of the categories of disease are not considered to be of clinical relevance with modern therapeutic approaches. The World Health Organization (WHO) recently published an updated classification system for all hematopoietic tumors, including acute and chronic leukemias and myelodysplastic syndromes.[41] The WHO categories that relate to most bone marrow disease is given in Table 43–9.[42]

**TABLE 43–8.** French-American-British (FAB) Cooperative Group Classification of Acute Leukemia

*Acute Myeloid Leukemia*

| | |
|---|---|
| M0 | Minimally differentiated acute myeloid leukemia |
| M1 | Myeloblastic leukemia without maturation |
| M2 | Myeloblastic leukemia with maturation |
| M3 | Promyelocytic leukemia |
| M3v | Microgranular variant |
| M4 | Myelomonocytic leukemia |
| M4Eo | Myelomonocytic leukemia with eosinophils |
| M5a | Monoblastic leukemia (poorly differentiated) |
| M5b | Monocytic leukemia (differentiated) |
| M6 | Erythroleukemia |
| M7 | Megakaryoblastic leukemia |

*Acute Lymphoblastic Leukemia*

L1
L2
L3 (Burkitt's)

**TABLE 43–9.** World Health Organization Classification of Primary Bone Marrow Disorders

Chronic myeloproliferative diseases
  Chronic myelogenous leukemia
  Chronic neutrophilic leukemia
  Chronic eosinophilic leukemia/hypereosinophilic syndrome
  Chronic idiopathic myelofibrosis
  Polycythemia vera
  Essential thrombocythemia
  Myeloproliferative disease, unclassified

Myelodysplastic/myeloproliferative diseases
  Chronic myelomonocytic leukemia
  Atypical chronic myeloid leukemia
  Juvenile myelomonocytic leukemia
  Myelodysplastic/myeloproliferative diseases, unclassifiable

Myelodysplastic syndromes
  Refractory anemia
  Refractory anemia with ringed sideroblasts
  Refractory cytopenia with multilineage dysplasia
  Refractory anemia with excess blasts
  Myelodysplastic syndrome associated with isolated del(5q) chromosome abnormality
  Myelodysplastic syndrome, unclassified

Acute myeloid leukemia (AML)
  Acute myeloid leukemias with recurrent cytogenetic abnormalities
    AML with t(8;21)(q22;q22) (*AML1/ETO*)
    Acute promyelocytic leukemia; (AML with t(15;17)(q22;q12) and variants, *PML/RARα*)
    AML with inv(16)(p13q22) or t(16;16)(p13;q22), (*CBFβ/MYH11*)
    AML with 11q23 (*MLL*) abnormalities

  Acute myeloid leukemia with multilineage dysplasia
    With prior myelodysplastic syndrome
    Without prior myelodysplastic syndrome

  Acute myeloid leukemia and myelodysplastic syndrome, therapy related
    Alkylating agent related
    Topoisomerase II–inhibitor related

  Acute myeloid leukemia not otherwise categorized
    AML, minimally differentiated
    AML, without maturation
    AML, with maturation
    Acute monoblastic and myelomonocytic leukemia
    Acute monocytic leukemia
    Acute erythroid leukemia
    Acute megakaryocytic leukemia
    Acute basophilic leukemia
    Acute panmyelosis with myelofibrosis

Acute leukemia of ambiguous lineage

Acute lymphoblastic leukemias (part of the lymphoid neoplasms classification)
  Precursor B lymphoblastic leukemia-lymphoma
  Precursor T lymphoblastic lymphoma-leukemia
  Burkitt's lymphoma–Burkitt cell leukemia

**TABLE 43–10.** Proposed Classification of Myelodysplasia

| Type of Anemia | Peripheral Blood Blasts | | Bone Marrow Blasts | Prominent Multilineage Dysplasia | Ringed Sideroblasts >15% of Erythroid Cells |
|---|---|---|---|---|---|
| Refractory anemia | <1% | *and* | <5% | − | − |
| Refractory anemia with ringed sideroblasts | <1% | *and* | <5% | − | + |
| Refractory anemia with multi-lineage dysplasia | <1% | *and* | <5% | + | +/− |
| Refractory anemia with excess blasts, type 1 | >1% but <5% | *or* | ≥5% but ≤10% | + | +/− |
| Refractory anemia with excess blasts, type 2 | >1% but <5% | *or* | ≥10% but ≤20% (or Auer rod +)† | + | +/− |
| Refractory anemia with excess blasts in transformation | ≥5% | | NA‡ | + | +/− |

* This includes the subtype of 5q− syndrome as described in the text.
† The presence of Auer rods with any blast cell count is considered evidence of refractory anemia with excess blasts type 2.
‡ Cases with a bone marrow blast cell count of greater than 20% are considered acute leukemia in this system.
Treatment-related myelodysplasia might fulfill criteria for any of the categories, but it is considered a separate category on the basis of the poor prognosis of patients with a history of previous therapy. Chronic myelomonocytic leukemia is *not* classified as a pure myelodysplastic syndrome in this system.

The classification, especially for AMLs, is complicated and controversial. Tables 43–10 and 43–11 summarize what the author believes to be a clinically useful pathologic classification system for these disorders that incorporates some proposals made in the development of the WHO classification. This system allows the addition of cytogenetic and molecular genetic results that may provide clinically important information. It is noteworthy that the WHO group has proposed changing the percentage of blast cells required for a diagnosis of AML to 20% or greater. This change reflects findings of similar outcomes for patients with myelodysplasia with high blast cell counts and patients with AML treated in a similar fashion.[43] Therefore, the proposed classification system of Tables 43–10 and 43–11 also uses a 20% blast cell cutoff for acute leukemia, and this change affects the categories of myelodysplasia in the proposed system. Details of the proposed classification system, its FAB counterparts, and other entities described in the literature are addressed later.

## MYELODYSPLASIA

Myelodysplasia, previously termed *preleukemia,* is a clonal neoplastic proliferation of the bone marrow that may be primary or may follow toxic exposures or therapy.[37, 44] Primary myelodysplasia is relatively common in elderly patients, is associated with persistent cytopenia, and frequently progresses to bone marrow failure, with resulting infections, or to AML. As a rule, the degree of trilineage dysplasia and percentage of blast cells correlate with the aggressiveness of the disease.

**TABLE 43–11.** Proposed Pathologic Classification of Acute Leukemia

| Type of Leukemia | Subtypes* | FAB Equivalents |
|---|---|---|
| Acute myeloid leukemia de novo types | Acute myeloid leukemia, not otherwise specified (NOS) | M0, M1, M2 |
| | Acute myeloid leukemia with maturation and changes suggestive of t(8;21) | M2 |
| | Acute promyelocytic leukemia | M3 |
| | Acute myeloid leukemia with monocytic features, NOS | M4, M5a, M5b |
| | Acute myeloid leukemia with abnormal eosinophils suggestive of inv(16) or t(16;16) | M4Eo |
| | Acute megakaryoblastic leukemia | M7 |
| Myelodysplasia-associated types | Treatment-related acute myeloid leukemia | RAEB-T, M0–M2, M4–M7 |
| | Acute myeloid leukemia arising from myelodysplasia | RAEB-T, M0–M2, M4–M7 |
| | Acute myeloid leukemia with associated myelodysplasia (including acute erythroleukemia subtypes) | RAEB-T, M0–M2, M4–M7 |
| Acute lymphoblastic leukemia-lymphoma | Precursor B cell acute lymphoblastic leukemia/lymphoma | L1, L2 |
| | T cell acute lymphoblastic leukemia/lymphoma | L1, L2 |
| | Burkitt's leukemia/lymphoma | L3 |
| Biphenotypic acute leukemia | Mixed myeloid/precursor B cell type | — |
| | Mixed myeloid/T cell type | — |

* All pathologic subtypes should be combined with results of cytogenetic studies that define clinically significant information.

Evaluation of the peripheral blood smear is just as important as evaluation of the bone marrow in patients with suspected myelodysplasia, and features of dysplasia are identified in the peripheral blood of most patients with this disease[45] (CD Fig. 43–1). These patients have significant cytopenias, which almost always includes anemia and an elevation of the red blood cell distribution width. The anemia is often macrocytic. The red cells frequently demonstrate a dimorphic appearance with macrocytes and hypochromic teardrop-shaped cells. The white blood cell count is often low, with or without circulating blast cells. The neutrophils often demonstrate abnormalities of nuclear lobation and abnormal cytoplasmic granulation. The nuclei are often mature, with the chromatin of a segmented neutrophil, but fail to demonstrate normal segmentation. Abnormal bilobed neutrophil nuclei with mature and clumped nuclear chromatin and only a thin band of nucleoplasm connecting the lobes are termed *pseudo–Pelger–Huët cells*. Neutrophils may also show loss of normal cytoplasmic granulation with zonal, hypogranular areas with a "washed out" appearance, and some may have abnormal cytoplasmic vacuoles. Platelets are often decreased; many show loss of normal platelet granules.

Similar dysplastic changes are evident in the bone marrow (Fig. 43–2). The marrow is usually hypercellular but may be normocellular or even hypocellular. The erythroid series is usually hyperplastic and left-shifted with abnormally large, megaloblastoid erythroid cells with smudged or thick ropy nuclear chromatin and dark basophilic cytoplasm with or without cytoplasmic vacuoles. Nuclear-cytoplasmic asynchrony is also common, as are bilobated or multilobated erythroid precursors and cells with irregular nuclear contours. Siderotic granules may be evident even on Romanovsky-stained smears, and Howell-Jolly–like nuclear fragments may be present in the cytoplasm. The granulocyte

series may show changes similar to those described in the blood. In addition, myeloblasts are often increased to 3% or more. Some blasts may have cytoplasmic granules in a more uneven distribution than promyelocytes, and these cells should be counted as blasts rather than promyelocytes when they are the prominent immature cell type. Megakaryocyte dysplasia is also common in the marrow. The most specific findings are nuclear hyperchromasia and hypolobation, but hyperlobated megakaryocyte nuclei with detached nuclear segments may also be identified.

Another morphologic feature that has been associated with myelodysplasia is the detection of aggregates of immature cells away from the bony trabeculae.[46] Normal foci of regeneration, in non–bone marrow transplant patients, are located adjacent to bone. Such aggregates of immature cells away from bony trabeculae are termed ALIPs, for *a*bnormal *l*ocalized *i*mmature *p*recursors. Detection of such aggregates is associated with a significantly poor prognosis.[47] Bone marrow fibrosis is not usually found in association with myelodysplasia, but rare cases occur and may be confused with myeloproliferative disorders.[47–50] Fibrosis in myelodysplasia is associated with a worse prognosis.

### Refractory Anemia and Refractory Anemia with Ringed Sideroblasts

Refractory anemia and refractory anemia with ringed sideroblasts cause persistent anemia that may be macrocytic, but it may be morphologically subtle. The characteristic features of dysplasia mentioned before may not be obvious in the blood or bone marrow. These patients have erythroid hyperplasia and often demonstrate mild dyserythropoiesis without other evidence of dysplasia. Blast cells are often not increased and are less than 5% in the bone marrow and 1% or less in the peripheral blood, by definition.[37] Iron staining of an aspirate smear may re-

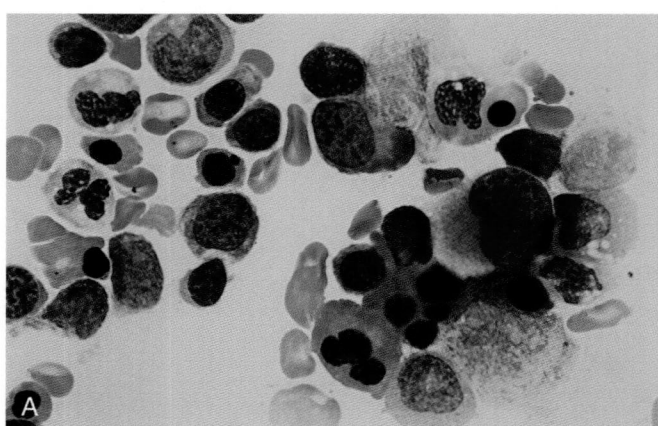
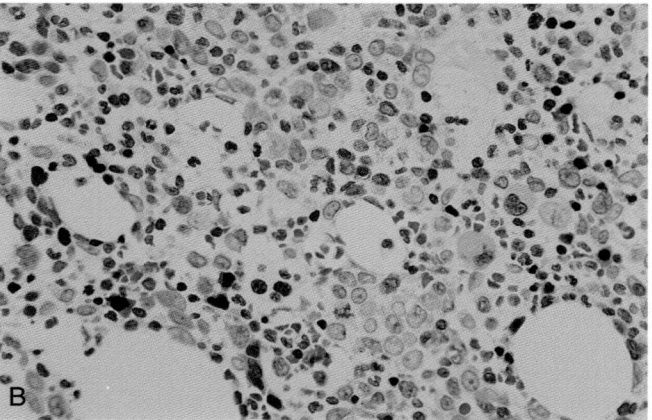

**FIGURE 43–2.** Myelodysplasia. *A.* The bone marrow aspirate material demonstrates dyserythropoiesis with abnormal nucleation of red blood cell precursors. A small megakaryocyte with a hypolobated nucleus is also present. *B.* The bone marrow biopsy specimen may contain aggregates of immature-appearing cells that are not adjacent to bone trabeculae, often referred to as abnormal localized immature precursors (ALIPs).

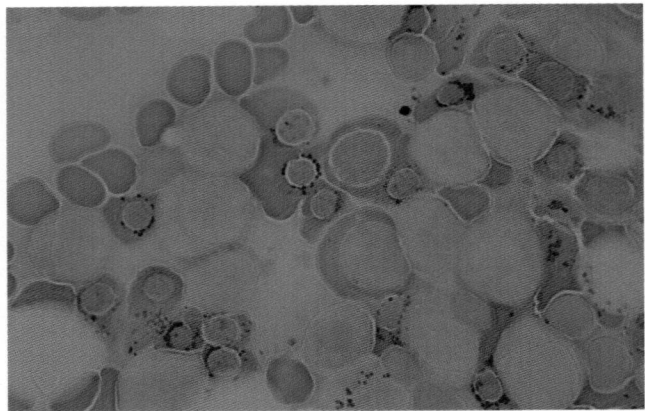

**FIGURE 43–3.** An iron stain of a bone marrow aspirate smear showing numerous ringed sideroblasts in a case of refractory anemia with ringed sideroblasts.

veal an increase in red blood cell iron incorporation, and more than 15% of erythroid precursors are ringed sideroblasts (ringing around at least one third of the nucleus) in cases of refractory anemia with ringed sideroblasts (Fig. 43–3).

In the absence of ringed sideroblasts, a descriptive diagnosis with a request for cytogenetic studies may be indicated before a definite diagnosis of myelodysplasia can be made. The detection of characteristic clonal cytogenetic abnormalities, such as 5q or 20q deletions, monosomy 7, and trisomy 8, or of complex cytogenetic abnormalities is diagnostic of refractory anemia in this setting.[51–53] In the absence of a clonal cytogenetic abnormality, the persistence of anemia with the exclusion of other causes may be sufficient for an eventual clinical diagnosis of refractory anemia. Refractory anemia and refractory anemia with ringed sideroblasts are the most indolent of the myelodysplastic syndromes.

SIDEROBLASTIC ANEMIAS. Not all anemias with increases in ringed sideroblasts (sideroblastic anemias) are clonal myelodysplastic syndromes. Hereditary, congenital, and acquired sideroblastic anemias may occur, and a fairly complex classification system of these disorders has been proposed.[54] Ringed sideroblasts are usually due to a mitochondrial disorder or a defect in normal heme synthesis. Acquired causes of ringed sideroblasts include myelodysplastic syndromes, but these cells also result from direct toxic exposure to chloramphenicol, isoniazid, lead, copper, ethanol, and cycloserine.[55–57] Toxins inhibit mitochondrial protein synthesis or δ-aminolevulinate synthesis of the heme pathway.

Of the hereditary sideroblastic anemias, X-linked sideroblastic anemia is one of the best studied. This disease primarily affects males and causes a microcytic hypochromic anemia with ringed sideroblasts that may be confused with a hemoglobinopathy. Many of these patients carry a point mutation in the δ-aminolevulinate synthase 2 gene *(ALAS2)* on chromosome band region X(p11). Distinguishing these disorders from true myelodysplasias may be difficult, but they should be suspected in children or young adult patients because refractory anemia with ringed sideroblasts is extremely unusual in those age groups.

Patients with anemia and ringed sideroblasts but no evidence of granulocyte or megakaryocyte dysplasia often have no cytogenetic abnormalities on routine karyotype analysis and are less likely to progress to a myelodysplasia with increased numbers of blasts or to acute leukemia.[58] Cases with prominent multilineage dysplasia or an increase in blast cell numbers are best classified as one of the other subtypes of myelodysplasia described in the following.

THE 5Q− SYNDROME. One morphologically and clinically distinct subtype of refractory anemia is the 5q− syndrome.[59–61] This syndrome most frequently occurs in elderly women who present with a macrocytic anemia and normal platelet counts. The bone marrow of these patients has less than 5% blast cells and usually no obvious dysplastic changes of the granulocyte series. Mild dyserythropoiesis is common, but the marked erythroid hyperplasia of other myelodysplasias is infrequent. The most striking feature of these patients is the presence of increased numbers of abnormal megakaryocytes (Fig. 43–4). More than 50% of megakaryocytes of these patients have monolobated or bilobated nuclei. These morphologic findings, when they are seen in conjunction with a deletion of chromosome band 5 (q13;q33) as the sole cytogenetic abnormality, are associated with a good prognosis with a low risk of transformation to acute leukemia. Patients with an increase in blast cell numbers or with karyotype abnormalities in addition to 5q− do not share this good prognosis and should not be considered to have the 5q− syndrome. Ringed sideroblasts are also uncommon in this syndrome, and their presence usually correlates with additional karyotype abnormalities.

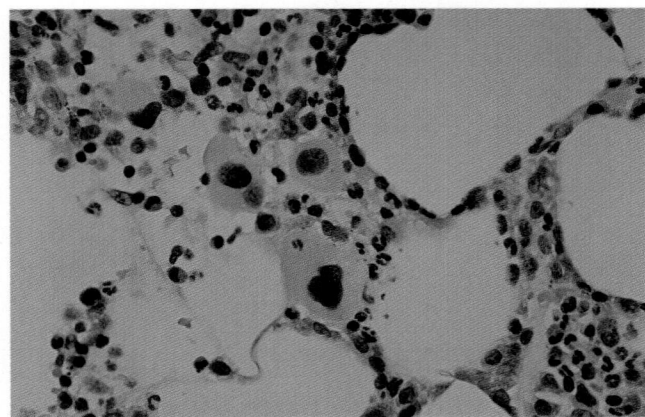

**FIGURE 43–4.** The 5q− syndrome. Clusters of small, hypolobated megakaryocytes are present on the biopsy specimen.

### Refractory Anemia with Multilineage Dysplasia

Refractory anemia with multilineage dysplasia[62, 63] with or without ringed sideroblasts was previously included in the categories of refractory anemia and refractory anemia with ringed sideroblasts or called unclassified. The presence of prominent multilineage dysplasia (two or more cell lines), even without an increase in blast cell numbers, is associated with a more aggressive behavior than is refractory anemia or refractory anemia with ringed sideroblasts and with more severe cytopenias. The median survival (24 months in one study) is intermediate between that of refractory anemia and refractory anemia with excess blasts.[62] Therefore, separation of these cases into a distinct subtype of myelodysplasia appears warranted.

### Refractory Anemia with Excess Blasts

Refractory anemia with excess blasts is also associated with anemia and trilineage dysplasia, but in addition it demonstrates an increase in myeloblasts (CD Fig. 43–2). Blast cells represent 5% or more (but less than 20%) of bone marrow nucleated cells or more than 1% (but less than 5%) of peripheral blood white cells. Although abnormalities of red blood cell incorporation of iron, including the presence of ringed sideroblasts, are frequently present, this finding does not affect the classification of myelodysplastic syndromes with increased numbers of blast cells. The proposed classification further subdivides refractory anemia with excess blasts into type 1 and type 2: type 1 includes patients with less than 10% blasts, and type 2 includes patients with 10% or more blasts but less than 20% blasts. Patients with less than 10% blasts but with Auer rods present are also considered to have type 2 refractory anemia with excess blasts (see later).

### Refractory Anemia with Excess Blasts in Transformation

Refractory anemia with excess blasts in transformation to acute leukemia is defined in the FAB classification as the presence of 20% or more blasts (but less than 30%) in the bone marrow or the presence of 5% or more blasts in the peripheral blood. Because the proposed classification considers cases with 20% or more peripheral blood or bone marrow blasts to represent AML, its definition of refractory anemia with excess blasts in transformation is restricted to the presence of 5% or more blasts in the peripheral blood. The presence of Auer rods in blast cells of either the peripheral blood or the bone marrow is also considered evidence of refractory anemia with excess blasts in transformation in the FAB classification and of type 2 refractory anemia with excess blasts in the proposed classification, even if the overall number of blast cells is not increased. This criterion is somewhat controversial, because some studies have found no correlation between the presence of Auer rods and aggressive behavior of myelodysplasia.[64] Because of the possible differences in the behavior of cases diagnosed as refractory anemia with excess blasts in transformation solely on the basis of the presence of Auer rods, the author recommends that the criteria for the diagnosis be clearly stated in the report. The category of refractory anemia with excess blasts in transformation is not included in the WHO classification.

### Myelodysplastic Syndromes with 17p Abnormalities

Myelodysplastic syndromes with 17p abnormalities are reported to have distinct morphologic features, but they have variable numbers of blast cells and may fit into any of the previously described categories of myelodysplastic syndrome.[65] They are associated with *TP53* mutations, which are otherwise uncommon in myelodysplastic syndromes.[66] The abnormalities may occur with unbalanced translocations, deletions, or monosomy 17. Myelodysplasias with these abnormalities have frequent pseudo–Pelger-Huët cells, abnormal monolobated neutrophils, and neutrophils with vacuolated cytoplasm. Although these features are common in patients with 17p abnormalities, they may also be seen with other cytogenetic abnormalities, and cytogenetic studies are still needed in these cases.

### Hypocellular Myelodysplastic Syndrome

Some authors have considered hypocellular myelodysplastic syndrome to be a distinct entity.[67, 68] Definition of a myelodysplastic syndrome with a cellularity of less than 30% as hypocellular myelodysplasia is somewhat arbitrary and may not represent a truly hypocellular marrow in elderly patients. For this reason, some have advocated the use of age-specific cutoffs for this diagnosis.[67] Other than the low cellularity of the bone marrow of these patients, the morphologic features allow classification into the preceding categories. Because differences in the blast cell counts and other features of the specific disease categories are seen in hypocellular myelodysplasia, the author recommends use of the preceding categories with a comment that the marrow is hypocellular rather than making a nonspecific diagnosis of hypocellular myelodysplasia.

### Therapy-Related Myelodysplastic Syndromes

Therapy-related myelodysplastic syndromes may be categorized as in the preceding, but they are usually more rapidly progressive diseases and can be considered a distinct type of myelodysplastic syndrome.[69–73] This type of myelodysplasia as well as therapy-related AML may be further subdivided by the previously administered therapeutic agent. Myelodysplastic syndrome and AML that follow treatment with topoisomerase II inhibitors are most often associated with balanced translocations involving chromosome bands 11(q23) and 21(q22),[74] although other more typical de novo leukemia translocations may occur in these patients. The interval between treatment and disease is relatively short; myelodysplastic syndrome and AML occur in 2 to 3 years. Many patients treated with topoisomerase II inhibitors progress directly to AML without the obvious dysplastic changes seen in AML and myelodysplastic syndrome that follow alkylating agent therapy. Myelodysplastic syndrome and AML that follow treatment with alkylating agents have a longer latent period of 7 years or more and are associated with chromosome 5 or chromosome 7 deletion or unbalanced 11(q23) and 21(q22) rearrangements. Therapy-related myelodysplasia with 17p deletions, with morphologic features as described before and *p53* mutations, has also been reported after alkylating agent therapy for lymphoma and hydroxyurea treatment of essential thrombocythemia.[75, 76]

### Cytogenetic Analysis

Cytogenetic analysis is one of the most important ancillary studies to be performed in the evaluation of myelodysplastic syndromes.[77] In cases of morphologically subtle refractory anemia, the detection of a characteristic clonal karyotype abnormality, such as monosomy 7, 5q deletions, and trisomy 8, clearly establishes the diagnosis. The type of cytogenetic abnormality also has prognostic significance. Several prognostic scoring systems for myelodysplasia have been proposed, some of which include cytogenetic studies.[78-80] The International Prognostic Scoring System for myelodysplasia[80] is now widely used. Rather than the disease categories described, this system uses a combination of the peripheral blood findings, blast cell count, and cytogenetic findings to place patients into prognostic categories. This system is summarized in Table 43–12.

Cytogenetic studies are therefore essential in the proper characterization of myelodysplastic syndromes. Because gains and losses of chromosomes are common features of myelodysplastic syndromes, these abnormalities are difficult to detect with most molecular studies, and traditional karyotyping remains the standard for initial assessment. Fluorescent in situ hybridization (FISH) studies, however, are ideal for following up these patients once the abnormality is identified. Because the blast cells in virtually all cases of myelodysplasia are myeloblasts, immunophenotyping studies are of limited utility in characterizing the cells but may be of value in quantitation of blast cells. The detection of increased numbers of CD34+ blast cells by flow cytometry or immunohistochemistry[47, 81, 82] may complement the morphologic evaluation of these cases. In contrast to cytogenetic studies, immunophenotyping studies are rarely essential in the diagnosis or classification of myelodysplasias.

## ACUTE MYELOID LEUKEMIA WITH OR WITHOUT ASSOCIATED MYELODYSPLASIA

AML is defined, by use of FAB criteria,[38] as a proliferation of myeloblasts that represent 30% or more of nucleated marrow cells or 30% or more of nonerythroid precursor cells if erythroid precursors represent 50% or more of marrow nucleated cells (FAB M6). The proposed classification and the WHO classification of AML lower the number of blast cells required for diagnosis of acute leukemia to 20%. This change would result in an AML diagnosis in cases previously considered in the FAB classification to be refractory anemia with excess blasts in transformation. During a transition period to the use of any classification system that changes the blast cell count to 20% for acute leukemia, cases with 20% to 30% blast cells should be clearly designated by criteria of both the traditional FAB classification and the new system to avoid confusion.

The FAB classification of AML is useful in defining some distinct disease types, such as acute promyelocytic leukemia. However, this system does not incorporate the presence of associated dysplastic changes that are commonly seen in adult AML patients and includes disease categories of questionable clinical significance. Many de novo AMLs are associated with well-defined cytogenetic translocations that have prognostic significance. AML of adults increases in frequency with age and may have abnormalities similar to the de novo AMLs of childhood or, more commonly, have complex cytogenetic abnormalities that are more suggestive of myelodysplasia. The latter cases also frequently have associated dysplastic changes in the non–blast cell populations or a history suggestive or diagnostic of preexisting myelodysplasia. AML, therefore, may be divided into two broad categories (see Table 43–11): de novo AMLs, which can be subdivided into different types; and AML of the elderly, with or without associated dysplastic changes. A variety of types of AML are described here, in contrast to the more

**TABLE 43–12.** International Prognostic Scoring System for Myelodysplasia*

| Variable/score | 0 | 0.5 | 1.0 | 1.5 | 2.0 |
|---|---|---|---|---|---|
| Bone marrow blasts (%) | <5 | 5–10 | ** | 11–20 | 21–30 |
| Karyotype | Normal, del(5q), or del(20q) | All other abnormalities | Complex (≥3 abnormalities) or chromosome 7 abnormalities | ** | ** |
| Cytopenias | 0 or 1 | 2 or 3 | ** | ** | ** |

* Risk groups for survival or acute myeloid leukemia evolution are low (score 0), intermediate-1 (score 0.5–1.0), intermediate-2 (score 1.5–2.0), and high (score ≥2.5).

limited categories of the proposed classification in Table 43–11. Although the proposed classification offers a way to classify the different pathologic types of AML, it is still useful to understand the morphologic variants that have been described and to understand the lack of specificity of some of those variants. The primary criticisms of the FAB classification of AML have focused on its inability to incorporate cytogenetic changes or to separate cases with dysplastic features from those without, and other groups and individuals have tried to incorporate those features into AML classifications.[83–85]

Of the ancillary studies in AML, detection of cytogenetic abnormalities that define prognostically significant disease groups is probably the most important.[86–89] Cytochemical evaluation should be a routine part of the diagnostic work-up of the AMLs, with the addition of immunophenotyping studies to identify cases of minimally differentiated AML. Although immunophenotyping is not essential for the diagnosis of AML in many cases, it is beneficial in identifying certain disease groups, which are described later, and in identifying aberrant blast cell immunophenotypes that can be used to monitor follow-up specimens for minimal residual disease. The use of molecular genetic studies, particularly PCR-based tests, in the follow-up of these patients is of somewhat limited value. As previously mentioned, some AML-associated translocations will continue to be PCR positive even after remission is achieved, and these findings are not predictors of relapse. In contrast, the detection of t(15;17) after therapy in acute promyelocytic leukemia is usually predictive of relapse. Other molecular methods that are less sensitive, such as FISH analysis, are currently more suitable for the evaluation of residual disease for many of these disease groups. The development of quantitative PCR methods to evaluate the number of cells with a particular abnormality over time will make PCR analysis more useful in the future.

### Minimally Differentiated AML

Minimally differentiated AML is termed *M0* in the FAB classification.[40, 90–92] The blasts do not demonstrate Auer rods or cytoplasmic granules and lack evidence of myeloid or monocytic differentiation by cytochemical analysis (Fig. 43–5). Therefore, they are negative for myeloperoxidase, Sudan black B, and nonspecific esterase by cytochemistry. Detection of myeloperoxidase expression by immunophenotypic studies is acceptable for this diagnosis. These cases are frequently TdT positive, and this finding coupled with the negative cytochemistry results may lead to an incorrect diagnosis of ALL if adequate immunophenotyping studies are not performed. Detection of myeloid-associated antigens, such as CD13, CD33, CD65, and CD117, in the absence of lymphoid-specific markers, such as CD3, CD19, CD20, and CD79a, is critical for making the correct diagnosis of a myeloid lineage leukemia. Other less restrictive criteria for the diagnosis of AML M0 have been reported that allow nonspecific esterase posi-

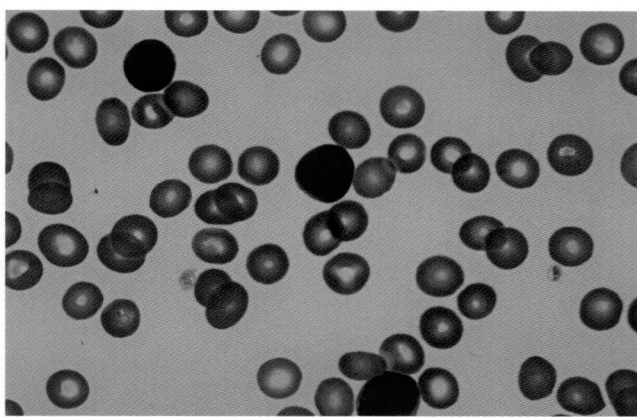

**FIGURE 43–5.** Minimally differentiated AML (M0). The peripheral blood shows blasts with scant cytoplasm. Immunophenotyping studies are needed to confirm the myeloid lineage of the cells.

tivity and expression of one or more lymphoid antigens. Such cases often have complex cytogenetic abnormalities or karyotypes suggestive of associated myelodysplastic syndromes and often demonstrate morphologic evidence of myelodysplasia. The author prefers to diagnose such cases as AML unclassified or as AML with associated myelodysplastic changes (see later).

### AML Without or with Maturation

AMLs without or with maturation are termed *M1 and M2 leukemias*, respectively, in the FAB system (CD Fig. 43–3). M2 leukemias are distinguished by the presence of maturation to the promyelocyte level of differentiation in at least 10% of cells. The blast cells are otherwise similar in the two groups, with the exception of the t(8;21) AMLs discussed later, and include cells with indented nuclei and large nucleoli. The blast cell cytoplasm may contain varying numbers of cytoplasmic granules, and Auer rods may be seen in either leukemia type. Blast cells are usually defined as having 20 or fewer cytoplasmic granules. Some blasts, however, may have more granules and should be considered blast cells if they retain the immature nuclear features of other more typical blasts, rather than the more mature nucleus of a normal promyelocyte. These cells also do not demonstrate the characteristic perinuclear clearing of granules, or hof, of normal promyelocytes. By definition, 3% or more of the blast cells are positive for myeloperoxidase and less than 20% of cells are positive for nonspecific esterase by cytochemistry.

### AML with t(8;21)

Differentiating M1 from M2 leukemias is of little significance in most cases, except for the identification of leukemias that may have the cytogenetic abnormality t(8;21)(q22;q22).[86–88] This translocation involves the *ETO* gene of chromosome 8 and the *AML1* gene of chromosome 21 that encodes a component of the core binding factor involved in normal hematopoiesis.[93] These leukemias have a generally

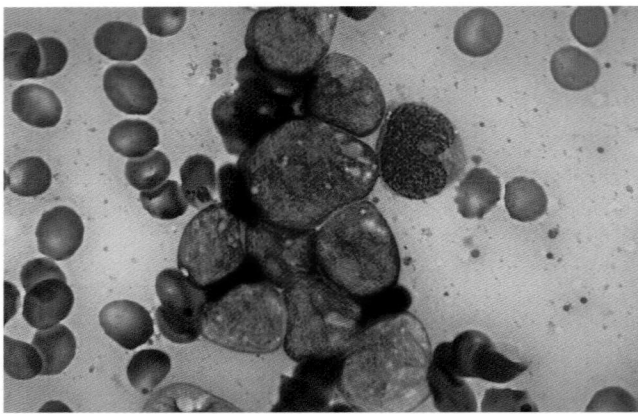

**FIGURE 44–6.** AML (M2) with t(8;21). The blasts have numerous cytoplasmic granules including large, chunky, salmon-colored granules that are characteristic of leukemias with this cytogenetic abnormality.

better prognosis than do other AMLs and demonstrate a characteristic M2 morphology[94] (Fig. 43–6) (CD Fig. 43–4). The blast cells have large salmon-colored granules, which may be mistaken for promyelocytes. These cells should be counted as blast cells, and the identification of these unique cells is sufficient to suggest this cytogenetic translocation (although it must be confirmed).

These cases also have characteristic immunophenotypic features. Approximately two thirds of t(8;21) AMLs aberrantly express the B lineage–associated antigen CD19 on the blast cells that are also characteristically CD34+.[95–97] The combination of salmon-colored granules in an M2 leukemia with CD19 and CD34 expression is fairly specific for this cytogenetic translocation, but CD19 expression alone in an AML is not sufficient for this diagnosis.[98] Up to half of t(8;21) leukemias also express the CD56 antigen, a marker more commonly seen on natural killer (NK) cell lymphocytes.[99] CD56 expression in t(8;21) leukemia is reported to be associated with a shortened time of remission and decreased survival.

Rare t(8;21) AMLs are negative for the commonly used myeloid-associated antigens CD13 and CD33 but are positive for myeloperoxidase by cytochemistry.[97]

The AML1/ETO fusion protein is easily detected by reverse transcriptase–PCR (RT-PCR),[100] but patients may remain RT-PCR positive even while they are in remission. Therefore, a positive RT-PCR test result does not necessarily indicate an increased risk of relapse, and this finding limits the use of routine RT-PCR testing for residual disease in these patients.[101]

### AML with Maturation and Increased Basophils

AML with maturation and increased basophils has been described as a specific type of AML (M2-baso) associated with abnormalities of the short arm of chromosome 12 or t(6;9)(p23;q34). Basophils may also be associated with t(9;22)-positive AMLs, including myeloid blast crisis of CMLs. Basophils in t(6;9) AML may be seen with other FAB types of AML as well, including M1 and M4 (CD Fig. 43–5).[102] In addition to basophilia, t(6;9)-positive AMLs are associated with relative erythroid hyperplasia and dysplastic bone marrow changes.

Although the presence of an increase in basophils in an AML may suggest any one of these cytogenetic abnormalities, no morphologic subtype of disease is specific for any one of these cytogenetic abnormalities, and a diagnosis of M2-baso is not of significance without appropriate cytogenetic studies. Therefore, the author considers the presence of basophils in an AML a clue of possible abnormalities to be further investigated, but not a marker of a specific AML type.

### Acute Promyelocytic Leukemia

Acute promyelocytic leukemia, or FAB M3, is another example of morphologic features that correlate with karyotypic and prognostic features[103] (Fig. 43–7). These patients have a high occurrence of dis-

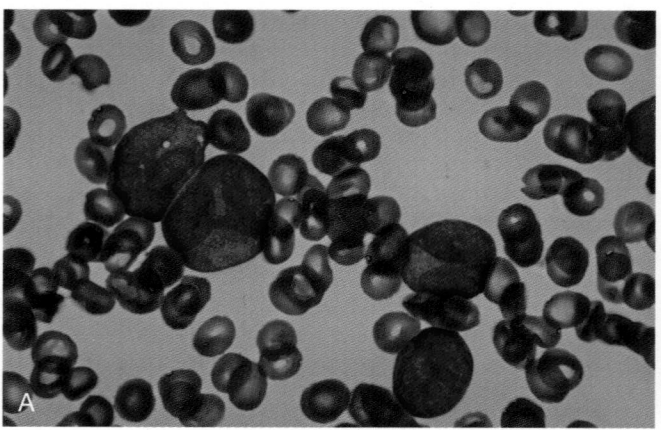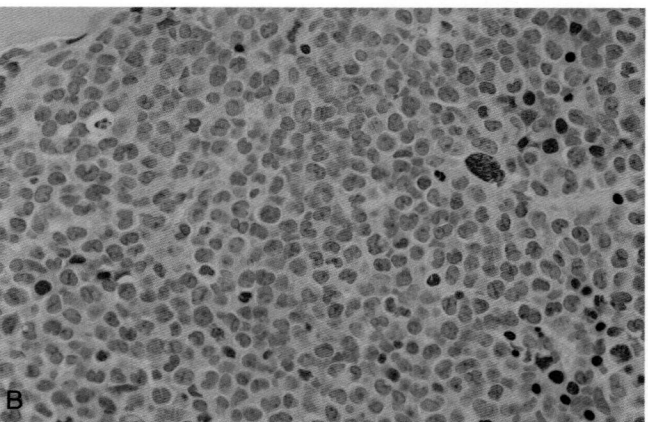

**FIGURE 44–7.** Acute promyelocytic leukemia (M3). *A.* The aspirate smear material contains numerous cells with folded, "monocytoid" nuclei and fine cytoplasmic granules. *B.* The biopsy specimen shows sheets of cells with abundant pink cytoplasm.

seminated intravascular coagulopathy and generally respond favorably to therapeutic regimens that include all-*trans*-retinoic acid.[104] In acute promyelocytic leukemia, abnormal promyelocytes predominate and are counted as blast cells. Different morphologic variants have been described.[105, 106] In the most common type, the cells demonstrate abundant cytoplasmic granules, and cells with numerous Auer rods, termed faggot cells, may be identified. Some cases, however, do not demonstrate obvious cytoplasmic granules, may have basophilic cytoplasm, and have folded immature nuclei that may be mistaken for monocytes. These are referred to as the microgranular variant of acute promyelocytic leukemia, or M3v. Both types are strongly myeloperoxidase positive in virtually all cells by cytochemistry, but a subpopulation of cells may also be positive for nonspecific esterase, which might suggest an incorrect diagnosis of acute myelomonocytic leukemia. Immunophenotyping studies confirm the myeloid lineage of the cells and usually demonstrate the blast cells to be negative for HLA-DR, an antigen that is usually expressed in the other types of AML.[98, 107] The blasts may also aberrantly express the T cell–associated antigen CD2, usually without CD7 expression. Apart from the morphologic features of typical acute promyelocytic leukemia, no one feature is sufficient for the diagnosis. A combination of findings of strong myeloperoxidase positivity with loss of HLA-DR, however, can help in identifying cases of the microgranular variant.

The majority of cases of acute promyelocytic leukemia, including the microgranular variant, have the cytogenetic abnormality t(15;17)(q22;p21), which fuses the retinoic acid receptor-α *(RARα)* gene of chromosome 17 to the promyelocytic leukemia gene *(PML)* of chromosome 15. Cytogenetic detection of t(15;17) by routine karyotyping or molecular methods is essential to further define the disease, because variant translocations may occur in cases of acute promyelocytic leukemia. The best described variant translocations involve the *RARα* gene on chromosome 17 with the *PLZF* gene at 11q23, the *NuMA* gene at 11q13, and the *NPM* gene at 5q35. Although most of these variant translocations are responsive to all-*trans*-retinoic acid, translocations involving the *PLZF* gene and abnormalities that do not involve the *RARα* gene are not responsive and require different treatment.[108, 109] Monitoring of t(15;17) can be easily performed by RT-PCR analysis,[110] and the presence of this abnormality by RT-PCR after treatment correlates with an increased risk of relapse.[111, 112]

### Acute Myelomonocytic and Acute Monoblastic Leukemias

Acute myelomonocytic and acute monoblastic leukemias (M4 and M5) have cytochemical evidence of monocytic origin by cytochemistry using nonspecific esterase stains. These include α-naphthyl butyrate esterase and α-naphthyl acetate esterase. The acetate esterase reaction is inhibited by sodium fluoride in monocytic cells. The designation M4 in the

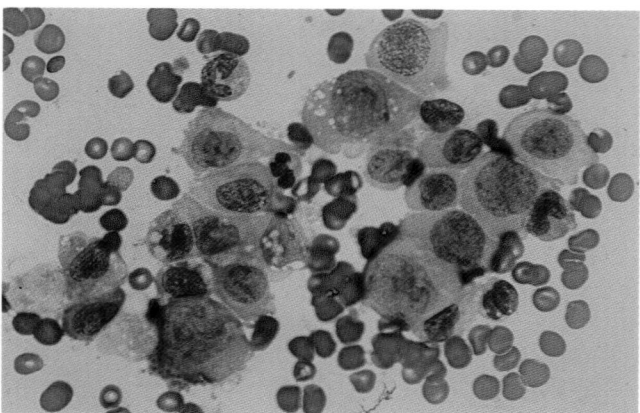

**FIGURE 43–8.** Acute monoblastic leukemia (M5b). The blasts have round to slightly indented nuclei with abundant vacuolated cytoplasm. More prominent nuclear folds are present in some cases.

FAB classification is given when 20% to 80% of blast cells are positive for nonspecific esterase; M5 is diagnosed when more than 80% of blast cells are positive (Fig. 43–8) (CD Fig. 43–6). A subpopulation of cells are also myeloperoxidase positive, especially in M4, but some monoblastic leukemias are entirely negative for myeloperoxidase and Sudan black B. Monoblastic leukemias may be further subdivided into those without maturation with immature cells with abundant cytoplasm and round immature nuclei (M5a) and those with monocytic maturation with folded nuclei (M5b). Immature monocytic cells, including promonocytes that demonstrate immature nuclear chromatin with nucleoli but have nuclear folds with or without cytoplasmic vacuoles of mature monocytes, are counted as blast cells in these types of leukemias. More pronounced maturation may be evident in the peripheral blood of patients with acute monocytic leukemias, making subtyping of these leukemias on blood specimens unreliable. The peripheral blood finding may suggest CMML, and chronic monocytic proliferations in the blood should not be diagnosed without excluding an acute leukemia by bone marrow examination.

Some patients with acute monoblastic leukemia present with extramedullary myeloid tumors, and gingival infiltrates by monoblasts are classically associated with this type of AML.[113, 114] Despite these clinical presentations, there is great overlap between these leukemias and other AMLs, with a few exceptions.

AML WITH ABNORMAL EOSINOPHILS. Acute myelomonocytic leukemia with abnormal eosinophils (M4Eo) demonstrates an increase in eosinophils that have abnormal, large basophilic granules[115] (Fig. 43–9) (CD Fig. 43–7). These eosinophils are weakly positive for chloracetate esterase, in contrast to normal eosinophils in other leukemias, but this cytochemical study is usually not necessary for the diagnosis. The significance of the finding of abnormal eosinophils is that it is associated with the

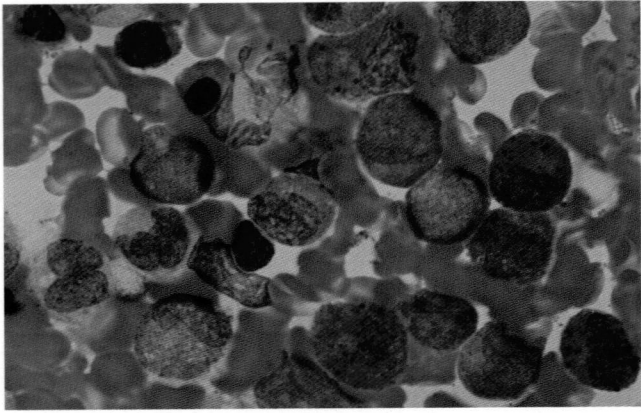

FIGURE 43–9. Acute myelomonocytic leukemia with abnormal eosinophils and inversion of chromosome 16 (M4Eo). Numerous eosinophils are present, and some contain abnormal, basophilic granules that are characteristic of this disorder.

presence of inv(16)(p13q22) or other abnormalities that involve this region of chromosome 16, including t(16;16)(p13;q22).[115–117] These abnormalities result in fusion of the core binding factor β-subunit gene (CBFβ) to the smooth muscle myosin heavy chain gene (SMMHC or MYH11), both on chromosome 16. Disruptions of the core binding factor, an important element of normal hematopoiesis, are also caused by the AML1/ETO fusion of t(8;21) leukemias, and both leukemia types have an improved prognosis compared with other AMLs. Some AMLs have abnormal eosinophils but do not fulfill the FAB cytochemical criteria for M4. Despite this, the cases have similar clinical outcomes and the same cytogenetic abnormalities. These cases are sometimes referred to as M2Eo and are covered in the proposed classification as a more general category of AML with abnormal eosinophils suggestive of inv(16) or t(16;16).

AML WITH 11Q23 ABNORMALITIES. Some acute monoblastic leukemias are associated with various cytogenetic translocations or cryptic abnormalities involving the MLL gene of chromosome band 11q23.[118, 119] The t(9;11)(p22;q23), involving the AF9 gene on chromosome 9, is most commonly associated with a monoblastic morphology, but various 11q23 abnormalities may be associated with other types of AML and ALL. Abnormalities involving the MLL gene generally confer a poor prognosis, but patients with t(9;11) appear to do better than those with other MLL translocations.[120] Administration of topoisomerase II inhibitors may also induce MLL breakpoints[121] and result in therapy-related AMLs with abnormalities of 11q23 and monoblastic features. Rearrangements of the MLL gene may not be evident by routine karyotype analysis in all cases. Various FISH, multiplex PCR, and Southern blot methods are performed in a few laboratories but are less available than testing for other translocations. PCR methods will miss some translocations and may detect evidence of an MLL abnormality in healthy patients when sensitive methods are em-

ployed.[122] Therefore, the use of PCR analysis for the monitoring of residual disease in patients with these leukemias is still controversial.[123]

### Acute Erythroid Leukemia

Acute erythroid leukemia is designated M6 in the FAB classification and has many features in common with the myelodysplastic syndromes (Fig. 43–10). Two types of erythroid leukemia occur.[38, 124, 125] The first form is the one described by the FAB. These leukemias have 50% or more bone marrow erythroid precursors. Myeloblasts represent 30% or more of the nonerythroid cell elements of the marrow. These blasts are otherwise similar to the myeloblasts of the other AMLs. This type of AML is also referred to as M6a.

The second type of M6 has been termed pure erythroid leukemia, erythremic myelosis, Di Guglielmo's disease, or M6b. This is a proliferation of immature cells with erythroid features,[125] and some of these cases were probably classified as myelodysplasias in the past. The immature cells have basophilic cytoplasm, similar to the erythroid pronormoblast, and often have cytoplasmic vacuoles. Although dysplastic erythroid changes are common in both types of erythroid leukemia, they are most striking in M6b. The immature cells are negative for myeloperoxidase and Sudan black B as well as for most myeloid-associated markers, such as CD13. The cells are usually positive for α-naphthyl acetate esterase and acid phosphatase, and the cytoplasmic vacuoles are positive for periodic acid–Schiff. Increases in red blood cell iron incorporation and ringed sideroblasts may be identified by iron stains. The cells may immunoreact for CD33, glycophorin A, or hemoglobin A. The diagnoses of M6a and M6b, however, are made primarily by morphologic features. Complex cytogenetic abnormalities, including those common to myelodysplastic syndromes, are common in acute erythroleukemia.[126]

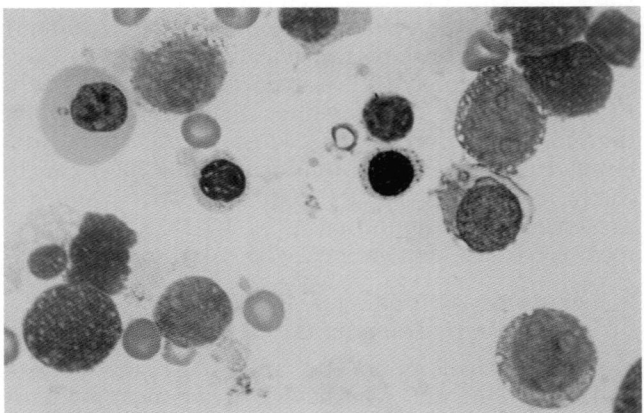

FIGURE 43–10. Acute erythroid leukemia (M6). The bone marrow contains a spectrum of abnormal cells that include dysplastic erythroid precursors with nuclear cytoplasmic asynchrony, red blood cell precursors with siderotic granules, and immature cells with vacuolated, basophilic cytoplasm.

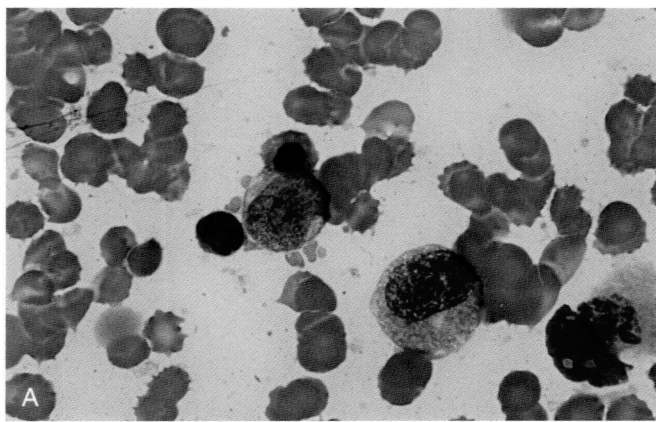 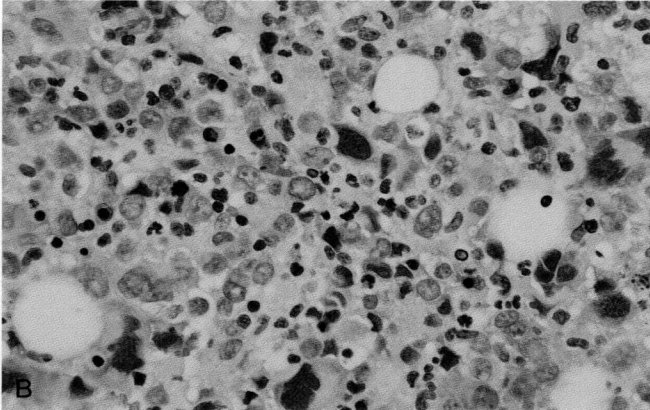

**FIGURE 43–11.** Acute megakaryoblastic leukemia (M7). *A.* The aspirate smears are often acellular but may contain blast cells with friable cytoplasm similar to a mature megakaryocyte. This feature is not sufficiently specific for the diagnosis, and a megakaryocytic immunophenotype should be demonstrated. *B.* The biopsy material is usually fibrotic with immature cells and abnormal megakaryocytes.

### Acute Megakaryoblastic Leukemia

Acute megakaryoblastic leukemia (FAB M7) is a leukemia of immature cells with megakaryocyte features that occurs in young children (1 to 3 years of age) or in adults[39, 127, 128] (Fig. 43–11). Maturing megakaryocytes are often easy to identify admixed with the immature cell population. The immature cells may be so poorly differentiated to suggest an ALL. The blasts have fairly uniform, fine nuclear chromatin with varying amounts of basophilic cytoplasm. The cytoplasm often forms blebs or pseudopods, but this feature alone is not sufficient for a diagnosis of M7.

Similar to M6 leukemia, this leukemia is often associated with myelodysplastic changes and also commonly has associated bone marrow fibrosis resulting in a dry tap. When blast cells are available for evaluation, they are negative for myeloperoxidase and Sudan black B but may be positive for acid phosphatase and α-naphthyl acetate esterase (sodium fluoride sensitive). Immunophenotyping studies are positive for CD13 and CD33 in some cases. Detection of platelet/megakaryocyte–associated antigens, such as CD41, CD42, and CD61, or the detection of platelet peroxidase by electron microscopy[129] is essential for the diagnosis. In the author's experience, detection of at least two megakaryocytic markers is needed to make a diagnosis of M7, because many other types of AML may express one of these markers.[98] Because of the common presence of fibrosis in this type of leukemia, immunohistochemical markers may be necessary for the diagnosis. CD61, von Willebrand factor, and *Ulex europaeus* are commonly positive in the immature cells by this method. There may be morphologic, immunophenotypic, and molecular genetic overlap between M6 and M7 in some cases, suggesting that these diseases are closely related.[130, 131] Associated dysplastic changes are seen with M7, particularly in adults, and cytogenetic overlap with myelodysplasias, including chromosome 7 deletions and trisomy

8, are common.[132] Cytogenetic abnormalities of pediatric M7 include trisomy 21 (see later) and t(1; 22)(p13;q13), possibly involving the N-*ras* gene on chromosome 1 and the *PDGFβ* gene on chromosome 22.[133–135]

### Therapy-Related AML and AML with Associated Myelodysplastic Changes

Except for M6 and M7 leukemias, therapy-related AML and AML with associated myelodysplastic changes are probably best categorized outside of the FAB system. Therapy-related AML is associated with the same cytogenetic abnormalities that follow treatment with alkylating agents and topoisomerase II inhibitors in the therapy-related myelodysplastic syndromes described earlier. Although not treatment related, AMLs arising from myelodysplasia or with associated myelodysplastic changes are similar diseases and are the major types of AML in elderly patients. Although many patients have a recognized myelodysplasia before development of AML, some elderly patients present, seemingly *de novo*, as AML with associated dysplastic changes of the nonblastic marrow elements.[136] These cases tend to have complex cytogenetic abnormalities with deletions and trisomies, similar to the myelodysplastic syndromes, and a poor prognosis. It is not clear whether there is any clinical significance for further subdividing these cases into the traditional FAB subtypes of AML, and the proposed classification does not automatically subtype these leukemias.

TRANSIENT MYELOPROLIFERATIVE DISORDER OF DOWN'S. Myeloproliferative disorders associated with Down's syndrome include proliferations that occur in neonates that have the overall features of myelodysplastic syndromes or AMLs, particularly acute megakaryoblastic leukemia.[137–139] Some of these proliferations will spontaneously regress, and it is not possible to predict, by morphologic features, which cases are transient. Even with regression in the neonatal period, some Down's syndrome pa-

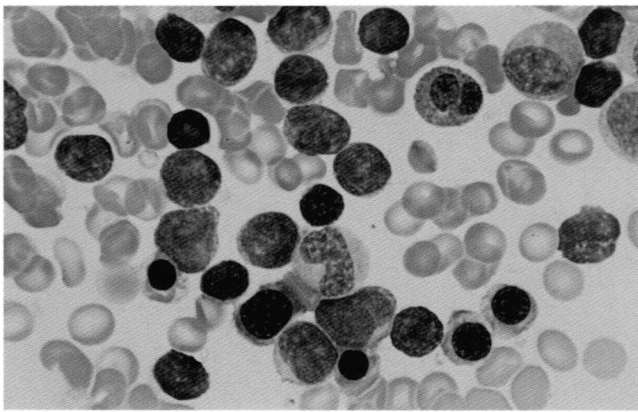

**FIGURE 43–12.** ALL (L1). The blast cells are uniform in size with scant cytoplasm. This case represents a T cell ALL, but the morphologic features do not help in predicting the immunophenotype.

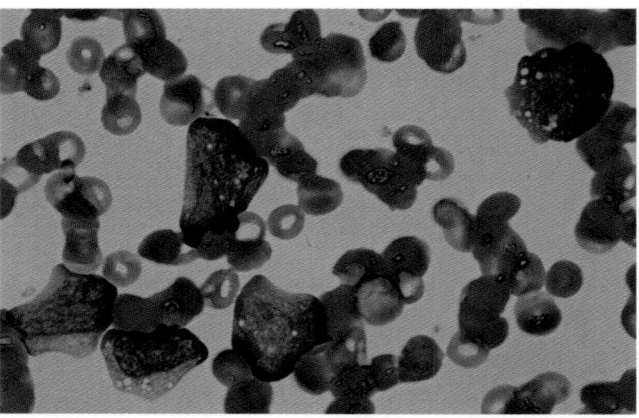

**FIGURE 43–14.** Burkitt's leukemia-lymphoma (L3). The blasts have multiple nucleoli, basophilic cytoplasm, and abundant cytoplasmic vacuoles. The cells demonstrated a mature B cell immunophenotype with surface immunoglobulin expression and no TdT expression. Cytoplasmic vacuoles are not required for this diagnosis.

tients will develop acute megakaryoblastic leukemia between ages 1 and 4 years.

## ACUTE LYMPHOBLASTIC LEUKEMIA

ALL is the most common malignant neoplasm in children, with relatively high cure rates, but it also affects adults with a more dismal prognosis.[140] ALL is divided into three morphologic groups (L1, L2, L3) in the FAB classification, without consideration of the immunophenotype of the blast cell population (Figs. 43–12 to 43–14).

L2 morphology may be associated with a worse prognosis, at least in children, but this may be related to other immunophenotypic and cytogenetic factors and is not necessarily an independent prognostic factor.[141, 142] Blasts with abundant cytoplasm, irregular nuclear membranes, and prominent nucleoli should represent 25% or more of total blast cells

before a diagnosis of L2 is made.[143] Because of similarities to minimally differentiated AML (M0), it is critical to perform immunophenotyping studies on all cases suggestive of ALL before such a diagnosis is made. The proposed classification system separates the lymphoblastic leukemias by immunophenotype, and it recognizes the great overlap between these diseases and the malignant lymphomas.

### Precursor B Cell ALL

Precursor B cell ALL is a proliferation of immature B cells and represents the majority of all ALLs. The blasts have fine nuclear chromatin, small indistinct nucleoli, and scant, slightly basophilic cytoplasm. The blast cells are often homogeneous in size and shape, but some cases may show marked variation in nuclear size and have abundant cytoplasm (L2 morphology). Subclassification into immunologic subtypes usually defines cases as pro–B cell if they are CD10⁻, common–B cell if they are CD10⁺ but negative for cytoplasmic μ-chains, and pre–B cell if they are positive for both cytoplasmic μ-chains and CD10.[144] When cytogenetic findings are taken into account, these immunophenotypic subtypes add little additional information. For this reason, the author prefers the general term of *precursor B cell ALL*, which covers all subtypes. Morphologic features do not help in the prediction of certain cytogenetic abnormalities, and cytogenetic studies are essential to identify prognostically significant disease groups.[145, 146]

### Precursor T Cell ALL

Precursor T cell ALL represents 15% to 20% of all ALL cases and is immunophenotypically identical to most cases of lymphoblastic lymphoma.[147, 148] Patients frequently present with a mediastinal mass consisting of T lymphoblasts. In most cases, the blast cells are morphologically indistinguishable from precursor B cell tumors. Subclassification of T cell ALL

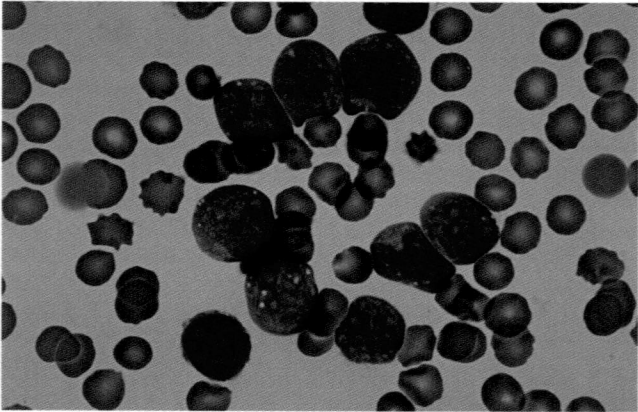

**FIGURE 43–13.** ALL (L2). The blast cells are variable in size with multiple nucleoli and moderately abundant cytoplasm. Some contain vacuoles, but the number of vacuoles is not sufficient for a diagnosis of L3. This leukemia was of a precursor B cell type in an infant with t(4;11). These cells lacked expression of CD10 and were positive for CD15. This immunophenotype and cytogenetic abnormality are common in infant leukemias.

by immunophenotype is also described,[144] but it is not necessary. Rare cases of T cell ALL have basophilic cytoplasm and cytoplasmic vacuoles that may erroneously suggest L3 leukemia if immunophenotyping to assign lineage is not performed.

### Burkitt's Leukemia-Lymphoma

Burkitt's leukemia-lymphoma, also known as mature B cell ALL, includes most cases of FAB L3 ALL, although some precursor lymphoid neoplasms may demonstrate the characteristic cytoplasmic vacuoles of L3 leukemia. Burkitt's leukemia is a mature B cell proliferation that demonstrates large leukemic cells with clumped nuclear chromatin and multiple nucleoli. The cells have moderately abundant basophilic cytoplasm with or without cytoplasmic vacuoles. The vacuoles contain lipid that is positive for oil red O, but these vacuoles are not required for a diagnosis of Burkitt's leukemia (CD Figs. 43–8 and 43–9). Because of similarities in morphologic features, immunophenotype, and karyotype between these leukemias and Burkitt's lymphoma,[149] they are combined as different presentations of a single disease. This designation, however, applies only to cases with a mature B cell immunophenotype.

### Immunophenotyping

Immunophenotyping studies are essential in the work-up of ALLs. Immunophenotyping excludes minimally differentiated AML (M0), which has similar morphologic features, and allows the proper classification of the ALL into the three immunologic types of precursor B cell, T cell, and Burkitt's leukemia.[150, 151] Precursor B cell ALLs are almost always positive for CD19, CD22, CD79a, and TdT and are usually positive for CD45 and CD10. The cells are CD20[-] in more than half of cases, and surface immunoglobulin expression is generally not detectable. Loss of expression or weak expression of CD45 is associated with an improved prognosis.[152, 153] Loss of expression of CD10 is generally an indicator of poor prognosis in precursor B cell ALL,[154, 155] is seen commonly in ALL of infants, and is often associated with 11q23 abnormalities in infants. Rare cases of precursor B cell ALL express both TdT and surface immunoglobulin light chains.[156] These cases should not be confused with Burkitt's leukemias, which are negative for TdT. Precursor T cell ALL does not always express surface CD3, but cytoplasmic CD3 is usually detectable, and other T cell antigens, such as CD2, CD5, and CD7, are usually expressed, as is TdT (CD Fig. 43–10). Double expression of CD4 and CD8 may be present. CD10 expression is present in some cases of T cell ALL and is associated with a good prognosis.[150] Burkitt's leukemia is a mature, monoclonal B cell proliferation that expresses surface immunoglobulin light and heavy chains as well as CD20 and often CD10, but not TdT.

A high percentage of precursor B and T cell ALLs express at least one myeloid-associated antigen, and some express both CD13 and CD33.[151, 157] Although such aberrant antigen expression is useful in following up the patient for residual disease, it should not be taken as an indication of biphenotypic acute leukemia (see later). When myeloid antigens are expressed in ALL, they are usually present only on a subset of the blast cells. Virtually all of the blast cells express antigens more typical of ALL, and the detection of a subset of cells with myeloid antigen expression does not appear to have clinical significance.[157]

### Cytogenetic and Molecular Genetic Studies

Cytogenetic and molecular genetic studies identify prognostically significant disease groups in ALL.[145, 146] The Philadelphia chromosome is present in approximately 20% of adult cases and in less than 5% of pediatric ALL cases and confers a worse prognosis. This translocation, t(9;22)(q34;q11), produces a BCR/ABL fusion transcript. A p190 protein product is more commonly formed in ALL, in contrast to the p210 product seen in most patients with Philadelphia chromosome–positive CML. Philadelphia chromosome–positive ALL often demonstrates aberrant expression of myeloid-associated antigens.[151, 158]

Translocations involving chromosome band 11q23 are of prognostic significance that differs with the different translocations, but the most common 11q23 translocation in ALL, t(4;11)(q21;q23), confers a poor prognosis. Most of these translocations involve the *MLL* gene, and these cases have a higher frequency of loss of CD10 and aberrant expression of myeloid antigens than other ALLs do.[159] Some cytogenetic abnormalities that have prognostic significance are not detectable by standard karyotyping. Some 11q23 abnormalities involve deletions that cannot be readily visualized, and t(12;21) is not usually detectable by karyotyping. The t(12;21)(p13;q22) is the most common cytogenetic abnormality in childhood ALL, present in at least 20% of cases, and identifies a group of patients with an improved prognosis.[160] Molecular genetic studies, such as Southern blot analysis, FISH, and PCR, are necessary for identifying these abnormalities. However, as mentioned earlier, some abnormalities of the *MLL* gene are detectable in a small number of cells in some healthy patients, and the use of PCR alone for the detection of *MLL* rearrangements remains controversial.[122, 123]

In children, DNA ploidy analysis also provides information related to prognosis.[161, 162] Hyperdiploid ALLs (>50 chromosomes or DNA index ≥1.16) have improved survival over other ploidy groups. Immunoglobulin and T cell receptor gene rearrangements may both occur in a single leukemia and do not necessarily correlate well with the immunophenotype.[163] The identification of these rearrangements, however, allows the identification of patient-specific clones that can be monitored for residual disease by PCR analysis.[164] The development of patient-specific PCR primers is a labor-intensive process and is not routinely available in most laboratories.

## BIPHENOTYPIC ACUTE LEUKEMIA

The definition of biphenotypic or mixed lineage acute leukemia is controversial. Some hematopathologists require two morphologically distinct populations of blast cells, one expressing myeloid antigens and the other lymphoid antigens. In the author's experience, such cases are extremely rare. More commonly, two morphologic populations are present—one expressing a purely myeloid or lymphoid immunophenotype and the second demonstrating a mixed immunophenotype. The number of antigens expressed to constitute a mixed immunophenotype is also controversial; some require only expression of any two myeloid-associated and two lymphoid-associated antigens, no matter how nonspecific.

The European Group for the Immunologic Classification of Leukemias has proposed a scoring system for biphenotypic leukemias that weighs the antigen expression according to its specificity.[144] The author's modification of this scoring system is presented in Table 43–13. More than two points must be present for two different lineages before a case is designated biphenotypic. The use of such a system limits the number of cases that are called biphenotypic and increases the number of cases of ALL with myeloid antigen expression and AML with lymphoid antigen expression. This system should also be used in conjunction with cytogenetic analysis, however. For example, biphenotypic acute leukemias with t(9;22) may not differ from Philadelphia chromosome–positive ALLs.[158]

## Chronic Myeloproliferative Disorders

The chronic myeloproliferative disorders are clonal stem cell proliferations that demonstrate bone marrow hypercellularity with varying degrees of mar-

**TABLE 43–13.** Modified Scoring System for Biphenotypic Acute Leukemia*

| Points | B Lineage | T Lineage | Myeloid Lineage |
|---|---|---|---|
| 2 | CD79a<br>cIgM<br>cCD22 | c/sCD3<br>Anti-TCRα/β<br>Anti-TCRγ/δ | Myeloperoxidase cytochemistry |
| 1 | CD19<br>CD10<br>CD20 | CD2<br>CD5<br>CD8<br>CD10 | CD13<br>CD33<br>CD65<br>Anti-MPO<br>CD117 |
| 0.5 | TdT<br>CD24 | TdT<br>CD7<br>CD1a | CD11c<br>CD14<br>CD15 |

*More than 2 points each for the myeloid and one of the lymphoid lineages is required for a diagnosis of biphenotypic acute leukemia; c, cytoplasmic; s, surface.
Modified from Bene MC, Castoldi G, Knapp W, et al: Proposal for the immunologic classification of acute leukemias. Leukemia 9:1783–1786, 1995.

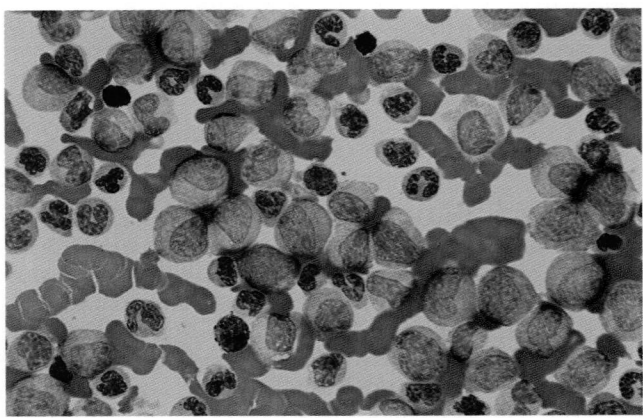

**FIGURE 43–15.** CML. The peripheral blood white blood cell count is markedly elevated with increased numbers of granulocytes, including many myelocytes.

row fibrosis. They show great morphologic overlap but generally differ by which cell line is most proliferative. Although detailed descriptions of the morphologic features of the various chronic myeloproliferative disorders are useful in suggesting a specific disease,[165] precise classification requires correlation of morphologic features with clinical, hematologic, and cytogenetic findings. A definite diagnosis cannot usually be made by morphologic examination alone.

## CHRONIC MYELOGENOUS LEUKEMIA

CML[166, 167] is the most common of the chronic myeloproliferative disorders and can occur at any age, although it is uncommon in children. It is defined by the presence of the Philadelphia chromosome or molecular genetic evidence of the BCR/ABL fusion product. In contrast to the t(9;22) of acute leukemias, which usually demonstrate the p190 BCR/ABL fusion protein, CML almost always demonstrates the p210 fusion protein of this translocation.[168] CML is primarily a proliferation of granulocytic cells, although multiple cell lines demonstrate the Philadelphia chromosome. The peripheral blood findings are those of an elevated white blood cell count with granulocytes at all stages of maturation (Fig. 43–15). Segmented neutrophils may show abnormal nuclear segmentation. Myelocytes and metamyelocytes are present in high numbers in the peripheral blood, and basophils are also increased in most cases. Abnormal basophils with washed-out granules may be identified. Platelets are usually elevated. The bone marrow is markedly hypercellular with a cellularity approaching 100% in most untreated cases (Fig. 43–16A). The myeloid-to-erythroid ratio of the bone marrow is markedly elevated, often greater than 10:1. Megakaryocytes are increased in number; clusters of small megakaryocytes with hypolobated nuclei are usually present. Some degree of reticulin fibrosis is usually demonstrated in these cases, and marked increases in reticulin and collagen marrow fibrosis are associated with a decreased survival.[169] Pseudo-Gaucher histiocytes are common in CML, re-

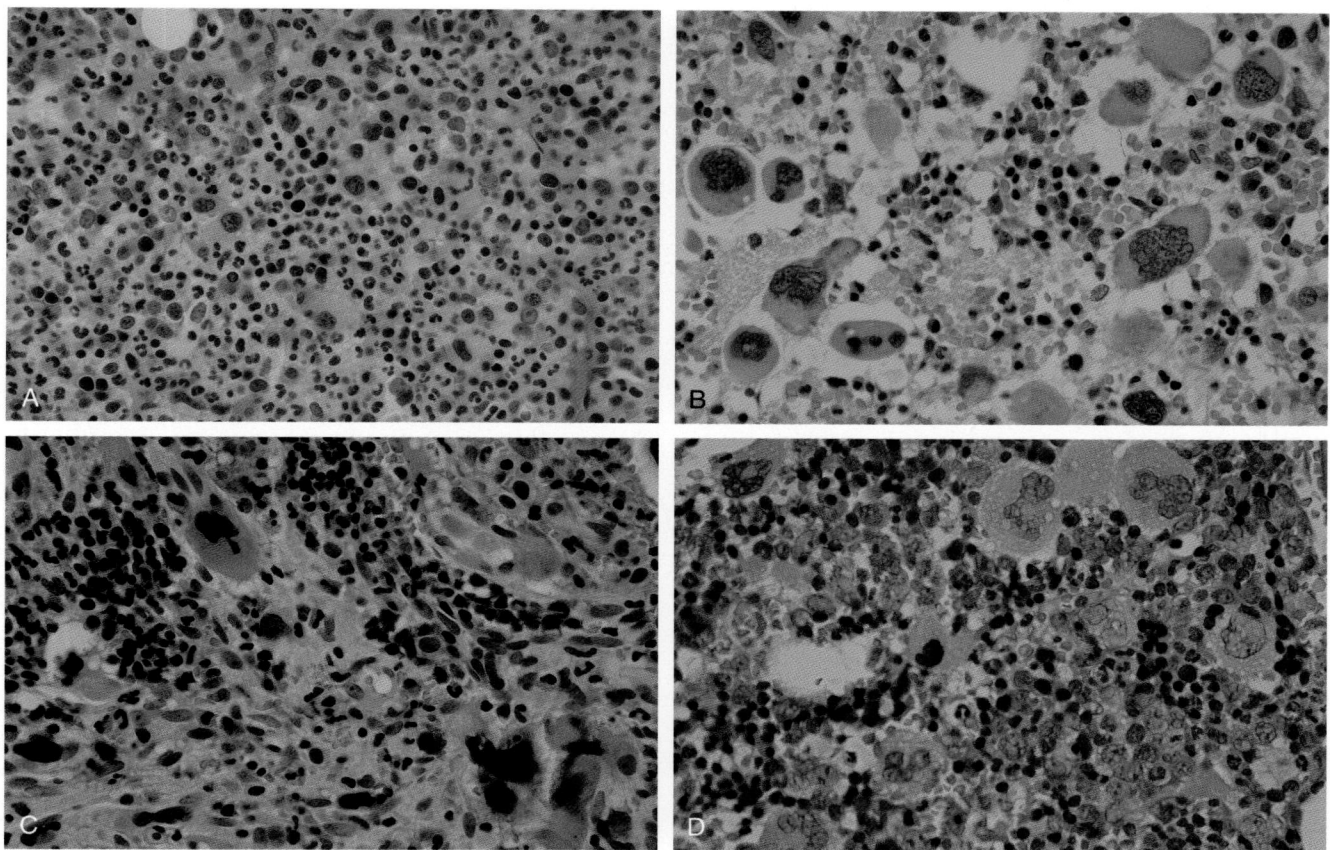

**FIGURE 43-16.** Bone marrow biopsy specimens of the various chronic myeloproliferative disorders in chronic phase. *A.* CML is markedly hypercellular with a high myeloid-to-erythroid ratio and clusters of small megakaryocytes. *B.* The megakaryocytes of essential thrombocythemia are larger with more abundant cytoplasm. *C.* The marrow of myelofibrosis with myeloid metaplasia is often more fibrotic with atypical megakaryocytes that commonly have hyperchromatic nuclei. Trabecular bone is often thickened in this disorder as well. *D.* The proliferative phase of polycythemia vera may look similar to essential thrombocythemia with large megakaryocytes, but an increased number of erythroid precursors are evident. The spent phase of polycythemia vera is usually indistinguishable from the marrow of myelofibrosis with myeloid metaplasia.

portedly present in 37% to 70% of cases.[170] These histiocytes have abundant fibrillar birefringent cytoplasm, and their presence has been associated with an improved survival.[169] Leukemoid reactions in patients with infectious or other reactive conditions may demonstrate features similar to CML. These reactive proliferations, however, do not usually show the basophilia, degree of marrow cellularity, or megakaryocyte clustering characteristic of CML. However, cytogenetic and molecular genetic studies are indicated if the differential diagnosis includes CML.

CML usually presents in a chronic phase, which is essentially defined by the lack of features of accelerated or blastic phase. The chronic phase of CML in many patients will eventually transform to a more aggressive phase of disease. Any one of a variety of parameters defines the accelerated phase of CML, but the criteria for the aggressive phase of CML are inconsistent in the literature.[171, 172] Most criteria for a diagnosis of accelerated phase require the presence of either 10% or 15% or more blasts in

the peripheral blood or bone marrow or the presence of 20% or more blast cells plus promyelocytes in the blood or marrow. Other criteria for the accelerated phase include the development of myelofibrosis; acquisition of additional chromosome abnormalities (clonal evolution); elevations of basophil and eosinophil numbers to 20% or more of blood cells; and any of the following that do not respond to conventional therapies: persistence of anemia or thrombocytopenia, marked white blood cell count elevations, platelet count of 1,000,000/mm³ or more, or increasing splenomegaly. The blastic phase, or blast crisis, of CML is usually defined by the presence of 30% or more blast cells plus promyelocytes in the peripheral blood or bone marrow (CD Fig. 43–11). The development of extramedullary myeloid tumors (granulocytic sarcomas, chloromas) is also usually sufficient for the blastic phase, but some criteria consider the presence of these tumors evidence of the accelerated phase.

Detection of the t(9;22)(q34;q11) by karyotype analysis, FISH, or RT-PCR is essential for the diagnosis of CML. Detection of this abnormality confirms the clonal or neoplastic nature of the proliferation, excludes a leukemoid reaction that may mimic CML, and helps exclude other chronic myeloproliferative disorders. Immunophenotyping studies are of little value in the chronic phase of CML but are helpful in defining the blast cell population of accelerated and blastic phases of this disease.[173, 174] The majority of blast crisis cases express myeloid-associated antigens without lymphoid markers and are easily classified as myeloid blast crisis by immunophenotyping studies, but some myeloid blast crisis cases may be myeloperoxidase negative by cytochemistry. Although most blast transformations of CML are proliferations of myeloblasts, approximately one-third of cases are lymphoid blast crises. Most cases of lymphoid blast crisis are of precursor B cell lineage, but rare cases of T cell blast crisis occur. Lymphoid blast crisis is reported to have a better prognosis than myeloid blast crisis, and lymphoid blast crisis has traditionally been defined as a blast cell proliferation that is positive for TdT. More detailed immunophenotyping of these cases usually demonstrates expression of other precursor B cell markers, such as CD19 and CD10, but expression of myeloid-associated antigens, such as CD13 and CD33, is also common. Cases with a lymphoid immunophenotype, regardless of the expression of myeloid antigens, have an improved survival[174] and are probably best classified as having lymphoid blast crisis.

Bone marrow specimens of CML patients treated with interferon-$\alpha$[175] may be morphologically normal with normocellularity and a normal myeloid-to-erythroid ratio. Although cytogenetic remission may also occur with this therapy, the normal morphology does not necessarily indicate a complete cytogenetic response, and karyotype analysis is still indicated.

Neutrophilic CML,[176] also known as chronic neutrophilic leukemia, appears to be a less aggressive variant of CML. This disease is associated with a proliferation of more mature granulocytes, usually at the segmented neutrophil stage of development. These patients have less severe clinical symptoms and are slower to progress to a blastic stage. At least some of these patients also have evidence of the Philadelphia chromosome, but the BCR/ABL fusion protein, at 230 kd, is larger than that usually seen in CML.

Philadelphia chromosome–negative CML is a rare occurrence, and such a diagnosis should be made with caution. Cryptic *BCR/ABL* translocations may occur that cannot be identified by routine karyotype analysis. When this is suspected, molecular genetic studies are indicated, such as FISH or RT-PCR analysis. When results of these studies are negative, other diagnostic considerations must be considered. Re-review of cytogenetic and molecular genetic Philadelphia chromosome–negative CML cases has resulted in most being reclassified as CMML or atypical CML (described later).[177]

**TABLE 43–14.** Criteria for Essential Thrombocythemia

Platelet count > 600,000/mm³
No cause of reactive thrombocytosis
Hematocrit < 40% or normal red cell mass (<36 mL/kg in males and <32 mL/kg in females)
Normal red blood cell mean corpuscular volume, serum ferritin, or marrow iron stain
Collagen fibrosis absent or less than one third of biopsy area without both splenomegaly and leukoerythroblastic reaction
No cytogenetic or morphologic evidence of myelodysplasia
No Philadelphia chromosome or *BCR/ABL* gene rearrangement

## ESSENTIAL THROMBOCYTHEMIA

Essential thrombocythemia is a bone marrow proliferation that primarily demonstrates an elevation in peripheral blood platelet number. The platelet count is usually above 1,000,000/mm³, and it must be above 600,000/mm³ with use of the Polycythemia Vera Study Group criteria for essential thrombocythemia[178] (Table 43–14). Modified criteria for this disease have also been proposed, some of which allow platelet counts between 400,000 and 600,000/mm³.[179, 180] Essential thrombocythemia probably represents two different diseases, one clonal and one reactive, even with use of the listed criteria.[181] Without the ability to perform clonality assays, however, it is not possible to differentiate between the two groups. Patients with the nonclonal form of the disease may include those with abnormalities of the thrombopoietin gene and appear to be at a decreased risk for development of thrombosis.[181, 182] Both types show similar peripheral blood and bone marrow features. The thrombocytosis may be accompanied by abnormal, large platelets. Leukocytosis, when present, is usually mild without the prominent leftward shift or associated increase in basophils seen in CML. The marrow is usually slightly to moderately hypercellular with increased numbers of megakaryocytes occurring in clusters (Fig. 43–16B). The megakaryocytes tend to be large with abundant cytoplasm and multilobated nuclei,[183] and they are larger than those seen in reactive conditions and CML. The myeloid-to-erythroid ratio is nearly normal, and marrow fibrosis is minimal. Thrombotic and hemorrhagic complications are the most frequent with this disease,[184] and transformation to acute leukemia occurs in 5% or less of patients.[75, 185] With time, marked marrow fibrosis may occur, producing a "spent" phase similar to that seen in polycythemia vera, but this is also a relatively uncommon event.

The value of ancillary studies in essential thrombocythemia is similar to that for CML. The detection of clonal cytogenetic abnormalities is useful in determining that the morphologic changes represent a neoplastic rather than a reactive process, but most cases do not demonstrate cytogenetic abnormalities. Although rare Philadelphia chromosome–positive essential thrombocythemia cases are described in the literature, they appear to have a higher frequency of blast transformation than do other types of essential thrombocythemia, and most authors consider such cases to be unusual variants of CML. Red blood cell mass studies may be necessary to exclude cases of polycythemia vera with associated thrombocytosis that might mimic essential thrombocytosis. Reactive causes of megakaryocyte hyperplasia and thrombocytosis (discussed later) must be excluded.

## MYELOFIBROSIS WITH MYELOID METAPLASIA

Myelofibrosis with myeloid metaplasia, also known as agnogenic myeloid metaplasia and idiopathic myelofibrosis, occurs with a slight male predominance in elderly patients and usually presents with leukoerythroblastic peripheral blood, massive splenomegaly, and marrow fibrosis.[186-188] The peripheral blood changes include the presence of large teardrop-shaped red blood cells; a granulocyte left-shift, often including rare myeloblasts; and giant platelets that are larger than a red blood cell (Fig. 43–17). Basophilia may be present, and bare megakaryocyte nuclei are often seen in the blood and bone marrow. Although spleen enlargement occurs with many chronic myeloproliferative disorders, the splenomegaly of myelofibrosis with myeloid metaplasia is much more than usually seen in the other diseases, and it may cause severe discomfort and wasting syndromes. The bone marrow may be hypercellular, particularly early in the disease when marrow fibrosis is less prominent. The myeloid-to-erythroid ratio is slightly increased, and megakaryocyte numbers are increased (Fig. 43–16C). Most patients show marked marrow fibrosis, which may include collagen fibrosis. Clusters of atypical megakaryocytes remain prominent in association with the fibrosis, and megakaryocyte clusters may be evident in the sinusoid. Sclerosis of bone trabeculae also occurs in many patients. Lymphoid aggregates, of predominantly T cells, occur commonly in association with myelofibrosis with myeloid metaplasia.

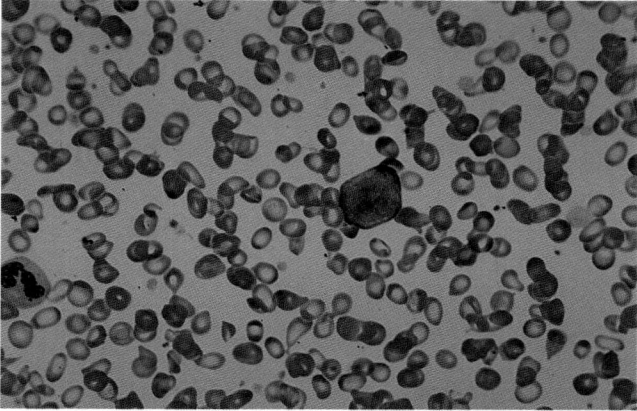

**FIGURE 43–17.** The peripheral blood changes of myelofibrosis with myeloid metaplasia characteristically show a triad of marked red blood cell poikilocytosis with abundant teardrop-shaped cells, a granulocyte leftward shift with rare blast cells, and abnormal giant platelets.

**TABLE 43–15.** Italian Criteria for Myelofibrosis with Myeloid Metaplasia

***Required Criteria***
Diffuse bone marrow fibrosis
Absence of the Philadelphia chromosome or BCR/ABL in peripheral blood

***Optional Criteria\****
Splenomegaly of any grade
Anisopoikilocytosis with teardrop-shaped red blood cells
Presence of circulating immature myeloid cells
Presence of circulating nucleated red blood cells
Presence of clusters of megakaryocytes and abnormal megakaryocytes in bone marrow sections
Myeloid metaplasia

\* Three optional criteria are needed if one is splenomegaly, and four are required if splenomegaly is not present.
Adapted from Barosi G, Ambrosetti A, Finelli C, et al: The Italian Consensus Conference on Diagnostic Criteria for Myelofibrosis with Myeloid Metaplasia. Br J Haematol 104:730–737, 1999.

The diagnostic criteria proposed by an Italian consensus conference are listed in Table 43–15. They require the presence of diffuse marrow fibrosis and the absence of the Philadelphia chromosome, plus any other two optional criteria when splenomegaly is present or four optional criteria when splenomegaly is absent.[189] The most frequent causes of death in these patients are marrow failure (22%), including anemia, infections, and hemorrhage; transformation to AML (15%); and portal hypertension related to massive splenomegaly (11%).[190]

Ancillary studies help exclude the Philadelphia chromosome of CML; approximately 35% of patients demonstrate a cytogenetic abnormality, with deletions of chromosome arms 20q and 13q most common.[190, 191] Other ancillary studies are of limited utility, with the exception of immunophenotyping of the blast cells of the cases that undergo blast transformation. The spent phase of polycythemia vera may have identical morphologic features.

## POLYCYTHEMIA VERA

Polycythemia vera is a clonal proliferation, usually occurring in elderly patients with a male predominance, that presents as an expansion of the red blood cell mass.[192, 193] Because of the morphologic overlap between this disease and other myeloproliferative and reactive conditions, detailed criteria are described for this disorder[193-195] (Table 43–16). The spleen is usually enlarged and erythropoietin levels are usually decreased in this disease.[196] Two morphologic phases of disease occur.[197]

The proliferative or erythrocytotic phase may show elevations of red blood cells, white blood cells, mostly left-shifted granulocytes, and platelets. The peripheral blood basophil count may be slightly elevated, but not as much as is usually seen in CML. Platelet counts may exceed 600,000/mm$^3$, which may cause confusion with essential thrombocythemia. Some patients may have associated iron deficiency with microcytic red blood cells. The bone marrow is usually moderately hypercellular with all

**TABLE 43–16.** Criteria for the Diagnosis of Polycythemia Vera*

*Major*
Red blood cell mass of >36 mL/kg in males or >32 mL/kg in females
Arterial oxygen saturation of >92%
Splenomegaly on palpation

*Minor*
Thrombocytosis/platelet count of >400,000/mm³
White blood cell count of >12,000/mm³ with no fever or infection
Raised neutrophil alkaline phosphatase level of >100
Raised unsaturated vitamin $B_{12}$–binding capacity of >2200 pg/mL

* After secondary causes of polycythemia are excluded, the diagnosis requires all three major or two major and two minor criteria.

cell lines involved (Fig. 43–16D). In contrast to some other chronic myeloproliferative disorders, however, the erythroid series is relatively normal or increased. Clusters of atypical megakaryocytes are common, similar to those seen in essential thrombocythemia. Marrow fibrosis may be minimal in this stage of the disease.

The spent phase of polycythemia vera is associated with marked marrow fibrosis; peripheral blood and bone marrow changes are similar or identical to those seen in myelofibrosis with myeloid metaplasia with leukoerythroblastic peripheral blood changes, splenomegaly, and marrow fibrosis. Differentiation between these two diseases may not be possible without a history of the earlier phase of polycythemia vera.

Because of the overlap in features between essential thrombocythemia and polycythemia vera, some cases may be resolved only by red blood cell mass studies. Red blood cell mass may be decreased in polycythemia vera patients who also have iron deficiency, and the studies may have to be repeated after iron therapy if polycythemia vera is suspected. Reactive or secondary polycythemia must also be excluded and may be related to smoking, lung and renal disease, erythropoietin-producing tumors, congenital conditions causing erythropoietin overproduction, and exogenous administration of erythropoietin. The atypical megakaryocytic hyperplasia of polycythemia vera is not seen in these conditions. Approximately 10% of polycythemia vera patients will transform to AML within 15 years, and up to half will develop acute leukemia during 20 years.[193]

Again, the absence of a Philadelphia chromosome is essential for the diagnosis. Other karyotype abnormalities may be detected in up to half of cases; chromosome 20q deletions are the most common.[198, 199] These abnormalities are not specific for polycythemia vera, however.[200] Various point mutations occur in association with polycythemias, particularly in the congenital or familial forms.[201]

### OTHER CHRONIC MYELOPROLIFERATIVE DISORDERS

Other chronic myeloproliferative disorders have been described and include chronic neutrophilic leukemia, chronic eosinophilic leukemia, and unclassifiable cases. All cases should be studied for the Philadelphia chromosome to exclude unusual presentations of CML, and, as mentioned before, variant BCR/ABL fusion proteins are detected in some cases of chronic neutrophilic leukemia, suggesting that these are variants of CML. Many Philadelphia chromosome–negative cases will fall into the category of atypical CML (described later).

Chronic eosinophilic leukemia and idiopathic hypereosinophilic syndrome[202] are defined as an unexplained peripheral blood proliferation of more than 1500/mm³ of eosinophils for 6 months or more with bone marrow eosinophilia, associated hypercellularity, and associated tissue damage. Tissue damage is usually cardiac, presumably related to release of eosinophil granule contents. Other causes of eosinophilia, including parasite infections, allergies, and elevations of eosinophil numbers associated with other malignant neoplasms, including CML, must be excluded. Once it is determined that the proliferation is related to a chronic myeloproliferative disorder, idiopathic hypereosinophilic syndrome is probably not an appropriate term, and even cases without clonal cytogenetic abnormalities have demonstrated clonality by analysis of X chromosome inactivation patterns.[203] A variety of clonal cytogenetic abnormalities are reported in chronic eosinophilic leukemia, but t(5;12)(q33;p13) and other abnormalities involving chromosome band 5q33 are most commonly associated with this disorder. Myeloproliferative syndromes with translocations involving 8p11 may also be associated with eosinophilia.[204] These disorders are frequently associated with non-Hodgkin's lymphomas, including T lymphoblastic lymphoma, and appear to transform to acute leukemia more commonly than chronic eosinophilic leukemia does. The fibroblast growth factor receptor 1 gene (*FGFR1*) of chromosome band 8q11 most commonly fuses with the *ZNF198* gene of 13q12 for a t(8;13)(q11;q12), but other 8q11 translocations may occur.[205]

Other patients may present with bone marrow hypercellularity suggestive of a chronic myeloproliferative disorder that does not fit well into any of the other categories after correlation with cytogenetic and other laboratory studies. Rare cases of unclassified myeloproliferative disorder are associated with mast cell disease, and this possibility should be excluded. Other cases may be best classified as CMML or atypical CML,[177] as described later.

### Mixed Myeloproliferative and Myelodysplastic Syndromes

Some proliferations have features of both myeloproliferative and myelodysplastic syndromes.[206, 207] They present with cytopenias and dysplastic changes of any cell line, similar to the myelodysplastic syndromes, and elevated white blood cell counts, hypercellular marrows with fibrosis, and organomegaly, features more commonly associated with

**TABLE 43–17.** Helpful Features in the Differential Diagnosis of Chronic Phase of CML, Atypical CML, and CMML in Adults

| Feature | CML | Atypical CML | CMML |
|---|---|---|---|
| Philadelphia chromosome/*BCR/ABL* | + | – | – |
| Peripheral blood white cell count | +++ | ++ | + |
| Peripheral blood basophils | ≥2% | <2% | <2% |
| Peripheral blood monocytes | <3% | 3%–10% | Usually >10% |
| Peripheral blood promyelocytes, myelocytes, and metamyelocytes | >20% | 10%–20% | ≤10% |
| Peripheral blood blasts | <2% | >2% | <2% |
| Granulocyte dysplasia | – | ++ | + |
| Bone marrow erythroid hyperplasia | – | – | + |

myeloproliferative disorders. The presence of fibrosis alone in a case that is otherwise typical of myelodysplasia is not sufficient to use this category. The three best defined mixed myeloproliferative and myelodysplastic syndromes are atypical CML, CMML, and juvenile myelomonocytic leukemia (JMML). Features that help in differentiating the chronic phase of CML from atypical CML and CMML in adults are listed in Table 43–17.

## ATYPICAL CHRONIC MYELOGENOUS LEUKEMIA

Atypical CML[208, 209] is a Philadelphia chromosome–negative and *BCR/ABL*-negative proliferative disorder that affects elderly patients with an apparent male predominance. Patients have some features of usual CML with splenomegaly, an elevated white blood cell count of predominantly granulocytic cells, anemia, and normal or decreased platelet counts. However, atypical CML patients are usually older, and some may have an initial presentation more typical of myelodysplasia with a low white blood cell count with evolution into atypical CML.[210] The white blood cells are shifted to the left with immature granulocytes, including blast cells, promyelocytes, and myelocytes, representing 10% to 20% of cells. Monocytes are usually less than 10% of peripheral blood cells. The bone marrow is hypercellular, with an elevated myeloid-to-erythroid ratio, and marrow fibrosis may be prominent. In contrast to usual CML, basophilia is not prominent, usually less than 2% of peripheral blood white cells; the myeloid-to-erythroid ratio is usually less than 10:1, and there is no evidence of the Philadelphia chromosome by either routine karyotype or molecular studies for the BCR/ABL fusion product. Although some abnormalities of granulocyte nuclear lobation may be seen in CML, atypical CML usually has more typical dysplastic changes that may involve all cell lines (trilineage dysplasia). Granulocytes may show typical pseudo–Pelger-Huët changes and cytoplasmic hypogranularity. Dyserythropoiesis and megakaryocyte dysplasia are common, and megakaryocytes may be reduced in number with associated thrombocytopenia. Atypical CML appears to be a more aggressive disease than usual CML, and progression occurs within 2 years.[210, 211] Patients may develop acute leukemia or may have bone marrow failure secondary to marked fibrosis.

Cytogenetic and molecular genetic studies are essential in the diagnosis of atypical CML to exclude t(9;22) or the BCR/ABL fusion product of usual-type CML. There is no known defining cytogenetic abnormality for atypical CML, but del(20)(q11) and trisomy 8 have been reported.[206, 211] Other ancillary studies, particularly immunophenotyping studies, do not usually help unless blast cell numbers are elevated.

## CHRONIC MYELOMONOCYTIC LEUKEMIA

CMML was originally defined as a myelodysplastic syndrome in the FAB classification, but it has features similar to those of atypical CML and is best classified as a mixed myeloproliferative-myelodysplastic syndrome. Patients often have both dysplastic changes and elevated white blood cell counts with splenomegaly. The disease may be divided into myelodysplastic and myeloproliferative subtypes on the basis of a white blood cell count of 13,000/mm$^3$ or higher for the myeloproliferative type and less than that number for the myelodysplastic type.[208] Although the patients with the higher white blood cell counts have a higher incidence of splenomegaly, both types may demonstrate prominent dysplastic changes, and the use of a white blood cell cutoff to separate the subtypes is somewhat arbitrary.[212]

The diagnosis requires a monocyte count of at least 1000/mm$^3$ in the peripheral blood. The monocytes may be abnormal in appearance with bizarre nuclei and even cytoplasmic granules. Promonocytes, with more immature nuclear chromatin, may be present in the blood, but monoblasts are usually not present or represent less than 2% of peripheral blood cells. The peripheral blood may demonstrate cytopenias and dysplastic changes more typical of the myelodysplastic syndromes, or dysplastic changes may be minimal. Although an elevated peripheral blood monocyte count is necessary for the diagnosis of CMML, such a diagnosis should never be made without examination of the bone marrow. Some AMLs with monocytic blasts may show peripheral blood changes similar to those of CMML because of maturation of the blast cell population in the peripheral blood. The bone marrow of CMML is usually hypercellular and may demonstrate monocytic or granulocytic hyperplasia (Fig. 43–18) (CD Fig. 43–12). When granulocytic hyperplasia is prominent, it may be difficult to distinguish the abnormal

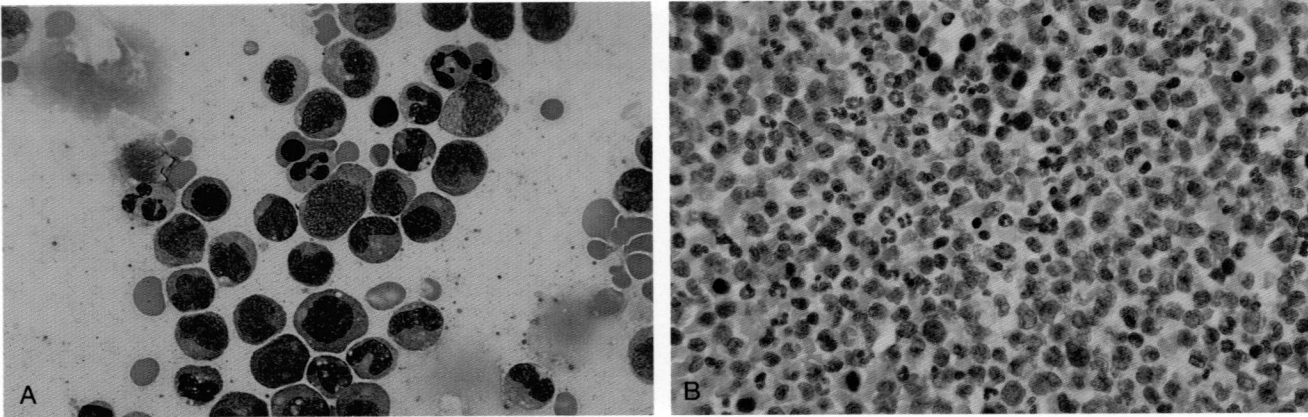

**FIGURE 43–18.** CMML. *A.* Numerous monocytes, including some with the appearance of myelocytes, are present in the bone marrow aspirate. *B.* The biopsy specimen is hypercellular with abundant monocytes present.

monocyte population from myelocytes. Erythroid precursors and megakaryocytes may demonstrate prominent dysplastic changes, but these cell types are often normal in appearance. Ringed sideroblasts are present in increased numbers in some cases. Blast cell and promonocyte counts may be elevated to 20%, and an elevation in blast cell numbers is associated with a poorer prognosis.[213, 214] When bone marrow blast and promonocyte counts are more than 20%, cases have been considered CMML in transformation. Such cases are now diagnosed as AMLs in the proposed classification of acute leukemias and the WHO. The designation CMML in transformation is probably still appropriate for cases with more than 5% peripheral blood blasts but less than 20% bone marrow blasts.

Ancillary studies help in the differential diagnosis of CMML. Cytochemistry for nonspecific esterase on the peripheral blood and bone marrow confirms the presence of an increase in monocytes and can help differentiate abnormal monocytes of CMML from myelocytes in CML and atypical CML. Cytogenetic and molecular genetic studies, particularly the absence of the Philadelphia chromosome and *BCR/ABL*, help in excluding CML. A subset of cases will have the t(5;12)(q33;p13) involving the *PDGFRβ* and *TEL* genes.[215–217] The resulting tyrosine kinase fusion protein activates the *RAS* signal transduction pathway. Mutations of *RAS* are detected in approximately one third of CMML cases. Although detection of *RAS* mutations is not generally useful for diagnosis, abnormalities involving the *RAS* pathway are thought to be the mechanism for this and other chronic myeloproliferative disorders, including CML. Mutations of *RAS* are not usually seen in CML, but the BCR/ABL fusion protein is also a tyrosine kinase protein that activates the *RAS* pathway.

The differential diagnosis between atypical CML and CMML may be difficult but is critical because of the worse prognosis of patients with atypical CML compared with CMML. CMML may be distin-

guished from atypical CML by peripheral blood features,[208] but some overlap with atypical CML may occur (see Table 43–17). Monocyte counts are slightly elevated in atypical CML but do not usually exceed 10%, whereas monocyte counts in CMML are usually above 10%. The degree of granulocyte dysplasia in CMML is also not as pronounced as is usually seen in atypical CML. Atypical CML demonstrates an increase in immature granulocytic cells, including blast cells, promyelocytes, and myelocytes, of up to 20% in the peripheral blood; these cell types are almost always below 10% in the blood of patients with CMML.

## PEDIATRIC MYELODYSPLASIA AND JUVENILE MYELOMONOCYTIC LEUKEMIA

Children may develop any of the myelodysplastic syndromes described for adults,[218–221] although refractory anemia with ringed sideroblasts is uncommon. These cases must be differentiated from known forms of AML with low blast counts that include many of the AMLs with t(8;21) or inv(16).[222] These types of AML do not usually have associated dysplasia and should be considered acute leukemias and not myelodysplasias. JMML and infantile monosomy 7 syndrome have also been described as pediatric myelodysplastic syndromes but demonstrate features of both myelodysplasia and myeloproliferative syndromes. Some favor use of FAB criteria and terminology for these disorders,[223] which would place them under the diagnosis of CMML. Because they appear to be clinically distinct from adult CMML, however, the author favors use of different terminology for these cases.

JMML, also known as juvenile CML, is rare, but it is the most common myeloproliferative-myelodysplastic syndrome of children.[224] Children with JMML are more often boys and develop the disease by age 4 years in most cases. The children usually have elevations of fetal hemoglobin and detectable I antigen. Skin lesions often precede the diagnosis, and these children present with an elevated white blood cell count, of granulocytes and monocytes, that may be identical to that in CMML of adults. Thrombocytopenia is also often present, and organomegaly is common. Dysplastic changes and marrow hypercellularity are also common, similar to adult CMML. Overlap with adult atypical CML also occurs, and the criteria for atypical CML and CMML are probably not appropriate in children.[225] Proposed criteria for the diagnosis of JMML require clinical findings of hepatosplenomegaly, lymphadenopathy, pallor, fever, and rash.[221] Proposed laboratory criteria are the absence of the Philadelphia chromosome, monocytosis of greater than $1000/mm^3$, and less than 20% bone marrow blast cells. In contrast to adult CMML, JMML has an aggressive clinical course. Infantile monosomy 7 syndrome[226] is clinically similar to JMML and probably represents a subgroup of JMML patients.[227]

Cytogenetic abnormalities other than monosomy 7, which may occur with any of the myelodysplastic syndromes, are not specific for JMML. Similar to adult CMML, *RAS* mutations occur in approximately 20% of cases of JMML.[228] There is also an association between JMML and neurofibromatosis type 1,[220] and mutations of the *NF1* gene may occur in up to 15% of patients without evidence of the disease.[228] Abnormalities of the *NF1* gene result in deregulation of the normal *RAS* signaling pathways.

## OTHER MYELOPROLIFERATIVE-MYELODYSPLASTIC SYNDROMES

Some cases demonstrate features of both myelodysplasia and myeloproliferative syndromes and do not fit well into any of the previously mentioned categories. Many of these cases have typical features of myelodysplasia as well as an atypical finding more suggestive of a myeloproliferative disorder, such as marked marrow fibrosis and hypercellularity or organomegaly. Such cases may be termed mixed myeloproliferative-myelodysplastic syndromes, not further classifiable, with a comment describing the atypical findings. One such syndrome has features of refractory anemia with ringed sideroblasts and thrombocythemia.[206] These cases have no sex predilection or specific cytogenetic abnormality and must be differentiated from the 5q− syndrome myelodysplasias. A mixed myeloproliferative-myelodysplastic disorder associated with isochromosome 17q has been described; it occurs with a male predominance in adults and is associated with severe hyposegmentation of neutrophil nuclei, monocytosis, and a high rate of transformation to AML.[229]

## Plasma Cell Disorders

### MULTIPLE MYELOMA

Multiple myeloma is a clonal proliferation of plasma cells that usually express monoclonal immunoglobulin G or immunoglobulin A or monotypic κ or λ immunoglobulin light chains without an associated heavy chain.[230, 231] The disease usually affects older adults; reports in children or young adults are extremely uncommon.[232] The disease occurs in men slightly more commonly than in women and in blacks more frequently than in whites. There are different diagnostic clinical criteria for multiple myeloma.[233, 234] Most rely on the detection of a serum monoclonal paraprotein level of 3 g/dL or more or a light chain immunoglobulin level of 1 g/24 h in the urine, the radiologic detection of bone lesions, and the presence of an increase in bone marrow plasma cells. Patients frequently have anemia and may have hypercalcemia. Although the monoclonal protein results in an elevated total serum protein level, normal immunoglobulin levels are low. The detection of more than 30% monotypic plasma cells in the marrow is usually sufficient for the diagnosis, but 10% to 30% marrow plasma cells is often enough for a clinical diagnosis if other parameters, such as anemia, renal insufficiency, or hypercalcemia, are present.

The peripheral blood of patients with multiple myeloma characteristically shows a normocytic anemia. Thrombocytopenia and leukopenia are usually not present. Rouleaux formation of the red blood cells is common and is often associated with a blue background on the smears (CD Fig. 43–13). Both of these findings are related to the raised serum monoclonal protein level. Circulating plasma cells are seen in some patients but, when present, are usually only a small number of white blood cells. The bone marrow is either normocellular or hypercellular with varying numbers of plasma cells[235] (Fig. 43–19). Plasma cell counts are most reliably performed with aspirate material or imprints. The plasma cells vary in their morphologic appearance, ranging from small well-differentiated cells that are similar to normal plasma cells to poorly differentiated or plasmablastic forms with large central nucleoli or immature nuclear chromatin that might cause confusion with lymphoma cells or myeloblasts. Binucleated and trinucleated plasma cells are commonly identified in multiple myeloma. Cytoplasmic inclusions, including vacuoles, granules, and crystals, may occur in the plasma cells (CD Fig. 43–14). Various morphologic grades of neoplastic plasma cells are described[236, 237] that center on the number of "plasmablasts" present. Plasmablasts are defined as having fine reticular nuclear chromatin with little or no chromatin clumping.[238] The nucleus is enlarged and may have a large nucleolus with a high nuclear-to-cytoplasmic ratio and minimal or no cytoplasmic hof. Some authors have used a cutoff of less than 10% plasmablasts for well-differentiated disease and 50% or more plasmablasts for poorly differentiated disease.[237] The presence of only 2% or more plasmablasts, however, correlates with a poor prognosis.[238, 239] Other marrow elements are usually normal in appearance but may be reduced in number in patients with extensively involved marrow. Osteosclerosis is rarely seen in multiple myeloma[240]; some cases are associated with the POEMS syndrome

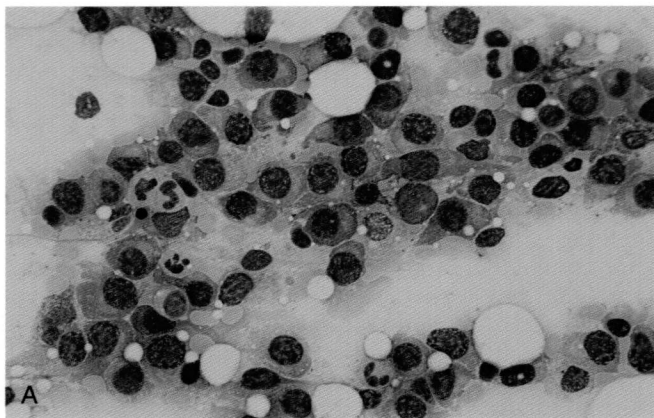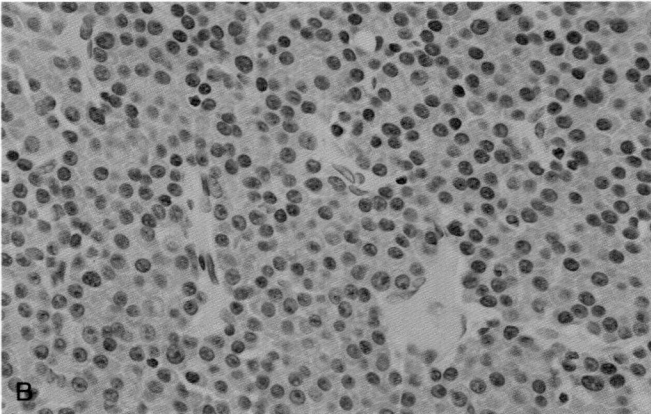

**FIGURE 43-19.** Sheets of plasma cells are present in the bone marrow aspirate *(A)* and the biopsy material *(B)* in a case of multiple myeloma.

of polyneuropathy, organomegaly, endocrinopathy, monoclonal gammopathy, and skin lesions.[241]

Multiple myeloma may be further subdivided into indolent and smoldering types.[234] Indolent multiple myeloma is defined by greater than 30% plasma cells with no clinical symptoms or associated disease features, lower paraprotein levels, and no or only limited bone lesions. Smoldering myeloma has similar features, with between 10% and 30% plasma cells. Therefore, the plasma cell count is an essential element of the bone marrow report. The bone marrow cellularity and plasma cell count should be given for all specimens, and when possible, a direct comparison between specimens and the previous marrow is recommended to properly evaluate response to therapy.

Solitary plasmacytoma differs from multiple myeloma by being a solitary soft tissue or bone lesion with no systemic symptoms of multiple myeloma and less than 10% plasma cells in the bone marrow. *Plasma cell leukemia* is the term used when 20% or more of peripheral blood white cells are plasma cells. This usually occurs with aggressive disease and is associated with short survival. These patients usually have anemia, thrombocytopenia, lymphadenopathy, and organomegaly. However, the detection of lower numbers of monotypic peripheral blood plasma cells is common in multiple myeloma, and levels as low as 4% are associated with shortened survival.[242]

In the setting of more than 30% plasma cells in a patient with a known monoclonal gammopathy, immunophenotyping studies may not be necessary. Protein electrophoresis studies are recommended for all patients with suspected multiple myeloma,[243, 244] and the results of these studies coupled with an increase in bone marrow plasma cells are often sufficient for diagnosis. However, when the differential diagnosis is with a reactive plasmacytosis, immunophenotyping studies may be extremely helpful. The detection of a monoclonal plasma cell population is often difficult by routine flow cytometry because plasma cells do not usually express surface immuno-

globulin light chains. Detection of cytoplasmic light chains is possible by flow cytometry, but this technique is more difficult to perform than routine surface studies. These studies are often coupled with detection of CD38, an activation marker present on most plasma cells as well as on T cells and other cell types, or CD138 (anti–syndecan 1), an antigen more specific for plasma cells.[242, 245] Paraffin section immunohistochemistry[246] to detect immunoglobulin light chains is often more helpful than flow cytometry for the determination of clonality as well as for the detection of residual clonal disease. Although plasma cells represent the end-stage maturation of B cells, they frequently will not immunoreact for CD20, and the use of CD20 antibodies to evaluate plasma cell populations is unreliable. Although CD79a detects a higher percentage of plasma cells than CD20 does, many cases are also negative for this antigen. Other paraffin section markers that may be useful in multiple myeloma include CD138, which marks neoplastic and non-neoplastic plasma cells, and CD56, which is usually not expressed by non-neoplastic plasma cells.[247] DNA labeling indices or proliferative rates are also used in some centers to evaluate the aggressiveness of multiple myeloma cases.[248]

Immunoglobulin heavy chain gene rearrangements are present in multiple myeloma, but they are often more difficult to detect by PCR analysis than in other lymphoid malignant neoplasms because the plasma cells undergo somatic hypermutation of the immunoglobulin heavy chain gene.[248] When PCR-detectable gene rearrangements are present, this test may be useful in monitoring patients after bone marrow transplantation. Approximately 40% of multiple myeloma cases demonstrate cytogenetic abnormalities.[249, 250] A variety of cytogenetic translocations may be detected in multiple myeloma and often involve the immunoglobulin heavy chain region of chromosome 14.[251] Up to 30% of multiple myeloma cases demonstrate t(11;14)(q13;q32), which involves the *BCL1/CCND1* gene on chromosome 11 that is also translocated in mantle cell lymphoma, although the breakpoint sites within the *CCND1* gene differ in multiple myeloma and mantle cell lymphoma.[252] The t(4;14)(p16;q32) is present in approximately 25% of myelomas and involves the *MMSET* gene (multiple myeloma SET domain) of chromosome 4.[253] Partial or complete deletions of chromosome 13 and abnormalities of chromosome 1 are the other most common cytogenetic findings in multiple myeloma. The chromosome 13 and 11q13 abnormalities are associated with a worse prognosis.[249] The role of human herpesvirus 8 infection of bone marrow dendritic cells in multiple myeloma[254] remains controversial, and tests for this virus in multiple myeloma are not currently indicated for the diagnosis or follow-up of this disease.

## MONOCLONAL GAMMOPATHY OF UNDETERMINED SIGNIFICANCE

Monoclonal gammopathy of undetermined significance is a relatively indolent disease that occurs in the absence of evidence of multiple myeloma, other chronic lymphoproliferative disorders, or amyloidosis.[255] Like multiple myeloma, it is more common in elderly and male patients and is the most common cause of a monoclonal serum protein.

By definition, patients with monoclonal gammopathy of undetermined significance have a serum paraprotein level of less than 3 g/dL and less than 10% bone marrow plasma cells; they do not have anemia, renal failure, hypercalcemia, or other clinical parameters of multiple myeloma. These patients do not require treatment, but 20% to 25% will eventually progress to myeloma, Waldenström's macroglobulinemia, amyloidosis, or another chronic lymphoproliferative disorder.[255, 256] The only pathologic finding is an increase of plasma cells of less than 10% in the bone marrow, but a recognizable plasma cell increase may not be present. The plasma cells are usually normal in appearance, and polyclonal plasma cells are usually admixed with the monoclonal cells.[257] This mixture of polyclonal and monoclonal cells may make interpretation of immunohistochemical studies difficult, and such studies are not usually indicated.

## WALDENSTRÖM'S MACROGLOBULINEMIA

Waldenström's macroglobulinemia, or primary macroglobulinemia, is a clinical syndrome of an immunoglobulin M monoclonal gammopathy that is associated with splenomegaly or hepatomegaly in 40% of cases.[258–260] These patients are usually elderly and there is a slight male predominance, but in contrast to multiple myeloma, Waldenström's macroglobulinemia is extremely unusual in African-American men. The patients have an increased risk of hemorrhage as well as a high frequency of hyperviscosity syndrome and cryoglobulinemia. This syndrome is characteristically associated with bone marrow and organ involvement by a malignant lymphoma with plasmacytoid features, particularly lymphoplasmacytic lymphoma (Fig. 43–20) (CD Fig. 43–15). As with

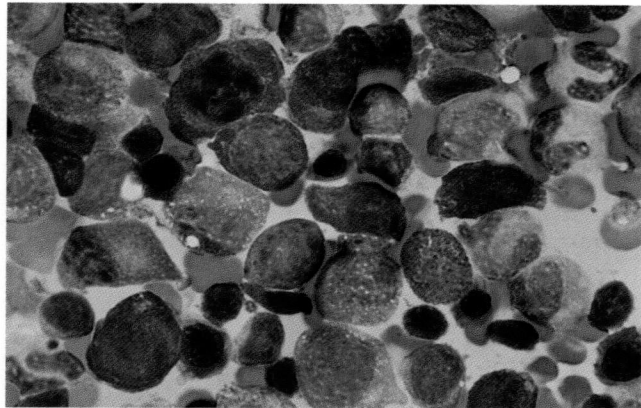

**FIGURE 43–20.** The bone marrow aspirate smear contains an increase in lymphocytes as well as obvious plasma cells in a case of lymphoplasmacytic lymphoma that presented as Waldenström's macroglobulinemia.

multiple myeloma, the monoclonal protein level is 3 g/dL or more.

A normocytic anemia is the most common peripheral blood finding in Waldenström's macroglobulinemia, and rouleaux formation with the characteristic blue background associated with increased paraprotein is also frequently identified. Peripheral blood involvement by the associated lymphoproliferative disorder is frequently present and may have the appearance of an increase in small lymphocytes, similar to chronic lymphocytic leukemia (CLL), or it may show an increase in lymphoplasmacytic cells. Virtually any type of malignant lymphoma may involve the bone marrow in Waldenström's macroglobulinemia, although lymphoplasmacytic lymphoma is the most common type. The pattern may be nodular, interstitial, diffuse, or a mixture of more than one pattern. The lymphocytes are generally small on smears; some show eccentric, basophilic cytoplasm, similar to the cytoplasm of plasma cells, while often retaining the nuclear features of mature lymphocytes (plasmacytoid lymphocytes). Some cases, however, demonstrate a frank plasma cell component. Intranuclear inclusions in some of the lymphoid cells (Dutcher bodies) are usually present, and mast cells are usually increased in number.

Because any type of malignant lymphoma may be associated with Waldenström's macroglobulinemia, the bone marrow in these cases should be diagnosed as involved by the specific type of lymphoma. A comment should acknowledge that the findings are consistent with the clinical setting of Waldenström's macroglobulinemia.

Paraffin section immunohistochemistry often helps in identifying a monotypic plasma cell population for Waldenström's macroglobulinemia and allows for the exclusion of a reactive lymphoplasmacytic population in the bone marrow. The detection of immunoglobulin M heavy chains helps in excluding multiple myeloma, which usually expresses only immunoglobulin A, immunoglobulin G, or light chain and is not positive for immunoglobulin M. Flow cytometric immunophenotyping may also be useful in identifying a monoclonal B cell population and in the subclassification of the precise lymphoproliferative disorders. The lymphoplasmacytic lymphoma that is most commonly associated with Waldenström's macroglobulinemia is usually CD5-; it differs further from CLL by its bright CD20 and immunoglobulin light chain expression and expression of FMC7. These studies are useful on both peripheral blood and bone marrow specimens. Even if morphologic evidence of peripheral blood involvement is not apparent, flow cytometric studies may still detect a small monotypic B cell population. Gene rearrangement studies may help, because all of the malignant lymphomas associated with Waldenström's macroglobulinemia are B cell malignant neoplasms. Up to half of lymphoplasmacytic lymphomas are associated with the t(9;14)(p13;q32) involving the immunoglobulin heavy chain gene of chromosome 14 and the *PAX5* gene of chromosome 9.[261] Most laboratories, however, do not currently offer PCR testing for this translocation.

### HEAVY CHAIN DISEASES

The heavy chain diseases are rare monoclonal proliferations expressing immunoglobulin A, immunoglobulin M, or immunoglobulin G without an associated light chain. $\alpha$-Heavy chain disease primarily involves the gastrointestinal tract in young people with an extensive lymphoplasmacytic or plasmacytic infiltrate and rarely involve the bone marrow.[262] $\mu$-Heavy chain disease usually has features identical to those of CLL, although vacuolated plasma cells have been described as a characteristic finding in the bone marrow.[263] $\gamma$-Heavy chain disease may be associated with any type of malignant lymphoma and often produce a syndrome similar to Waldenström's macroglobulinemia with associated bone marrow involvement.[264]

### AMYLOIDOSIS

Amyloidosis represents a heterogeneous group of disorders that can be divided into those derived from light chain (usually $\lambda$) fibrils (AL) and those caused by deposition of amyloid protein A (AA). $\beta_2$-Microglobulin- and transthyretin-derived (formerly known as prealbumin) amyloid may also occur.[265-267] AL amyloidosis is often termed *primary*; AA amyloidosis is generally a secondary disease. Amyloidosis can be clinically divided into systemic and nonsystemic types. The systemic type is further divided into those cases associated with plasma cell dyscrasias; reactive amyloidosis related to infections, autoimmune disorders, and malignant neoplasms; familial amyloidosis; dialysis-associated amyloidosis; and senile systemic amyloidosis. All types show the characteristic deposition of homogeneous, acellular eosinophilic material that demonstrates apple-green birefringence when it is polarized with Congo red stain.

Most cases of primary amyloidosis are considered plasma cell dyscrasias with an associated monoclonal gammopathy, although many do not demonstrate evidence of multiple myeloma or Waldenström's macroglobulinemia. Patients frequently have nephrotic syndrome, congestive heart failure, orthostatic hypotension, or peripheral neuropathy.[268] The bone marrow biopsy appears to be more reliable than the aspirate smear in identifying amyloid deposits,[269] but amyloid may be identifiable in the marrow in only one third of patients with known systemic disease.[270] Amyloid deposition in the marrow may be in the form of sheets of the material, or deposits may be evident only in the walls of thickened blood vessels. Plasma cells are often increased in the bone marrow but may appear polyclonal in up to one third of cases despite the presence of a monoclonal serum protein.[270] The bone marrow biopsy is often performed specifically to confirm or exclude amyloid deposits, which can be easily resolved with the Congo red stain.

## Lymphoid Proliferations

### LYMPHOCYTIC LEUKEMIAS OF B LINEAGE

#### *Chronic Lymphocytic Leukemia*

CLL is a monoclonal B cell proliferation of predominantly small lymphocytes involving the peripheral blood that is morphologically and immunophenotypically identical to small lymphocytic lymphoma[271, 272] (Fig. 43–21). CLL occurs more commonly in older adults, with a male predominance, and patients usually have generalized lymphadenopathy. The white blood cell count is normal or elevated with an absolute lymphocytosis. The diagnostic criteria for CLL are variable but generally require a lymphocyte count of at least 5000/mm³ or more with at least 30% bone marrow small lymphocytes.[273] Bone marrow examination is not required for this diagnosis, however. Demonstration of the characteristic immunophenotype of CLL is critical. When this immunophenotype is present in conjunc-

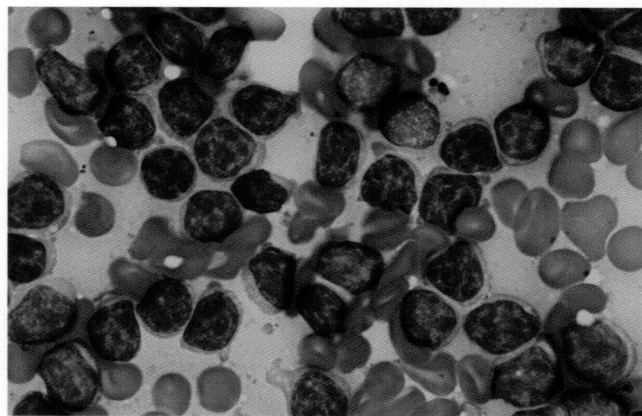

**FIGURE 43–21.** CLL in the bone marrow showing a proliferation of small to medium-sized lymphocytes with clumped nuclear chromatin and scant cytoplasm.

tion with bone marrow involvement, a diagnosis of CLL can be made with peripheral blood lymphocyte counts of less than 5000/mm³.

The peripheral blood shows predominantly small lymphocytes with scant, basophilic cytoplasm and mature, clumped nuclear chromatin, but scattered large lymphoid cells and prolymphocytes with nucleoli may be present. Anemia and thrombocytopenia are usually not present but are associated with a shortened survival when they occur, and these parameters are included in the Rai and Binet staging systems.[273, 274] The bone marrow is almost always involved in CLL, and although the absolute number of small lymphocytes identified on an aspirate smear has significance, the bone marrow biopsy pattern of infiltration is also important[275] (Fig. 43–22). This pattern of infiltration may be nodular, interstitial, diffuse, or mixed. The pattern of infiltration has prognostic significance; the nodular pattern is associated with the best prognosis, and the diffuse pattern is associated with a worse prognosis.[276, 277] As in the blood, the bone marrow lymphocytes are predominantly small, but large cells are commonly present in small numbers. A heterogeneous pattern of small lymphocytes with admixed larger cells is a characteristic feature of CLL on histologic sections. Aggregates of large cells or prolymphocytes with prominent nucleoli in the bone marrow may reflect transformation to a higher grade lymphoprolifera-

tive disorder, but transformation of CLL is usually determined by peripheral blood changes.

Morphologic variants of CLL can occur and include cases with cleaved cells, plasmacytoid cells, large cells, and increased prolymphocyte numbers (CD Figs. 43–16 and 43–17). The presence of large cells or prolymphocytes of between 10% and 55% of peripheral blood at presentation has been termed mixed cell type of CLL or mixed CLL–prolymphocytic leukemia.[278] Although such designations may identify patients with slightly more aggressive disease, they are not made by all hematopathologists and are not part of the National Cancer Institute–sponsored working group guidelines for CLL.[273] Cases with cleaved small lymphocytes or plasmacytoid cells that have the characteristic immunophenotype of CLL should be classified as CLL and are believed to behave like CLL cases with typical morphologic features. CLL may undergo prolymphocytoid transformation or Richter's transformation, and such transformation is often associated with a poor prognosis. In prolymphocytoid transformation, a patient with preexisting CLL develops more than 55% peripheral blood prolymphocytoid cells, which have more abundant cytoplasm than usual CLL lymphocytes and have prominent nucleoli[273, 278] (Fig. 43–23). A paraimmunoblastic variant has been described in which the prolymphocytoid cells have a single prominent nucleolus giving an appearance similar to

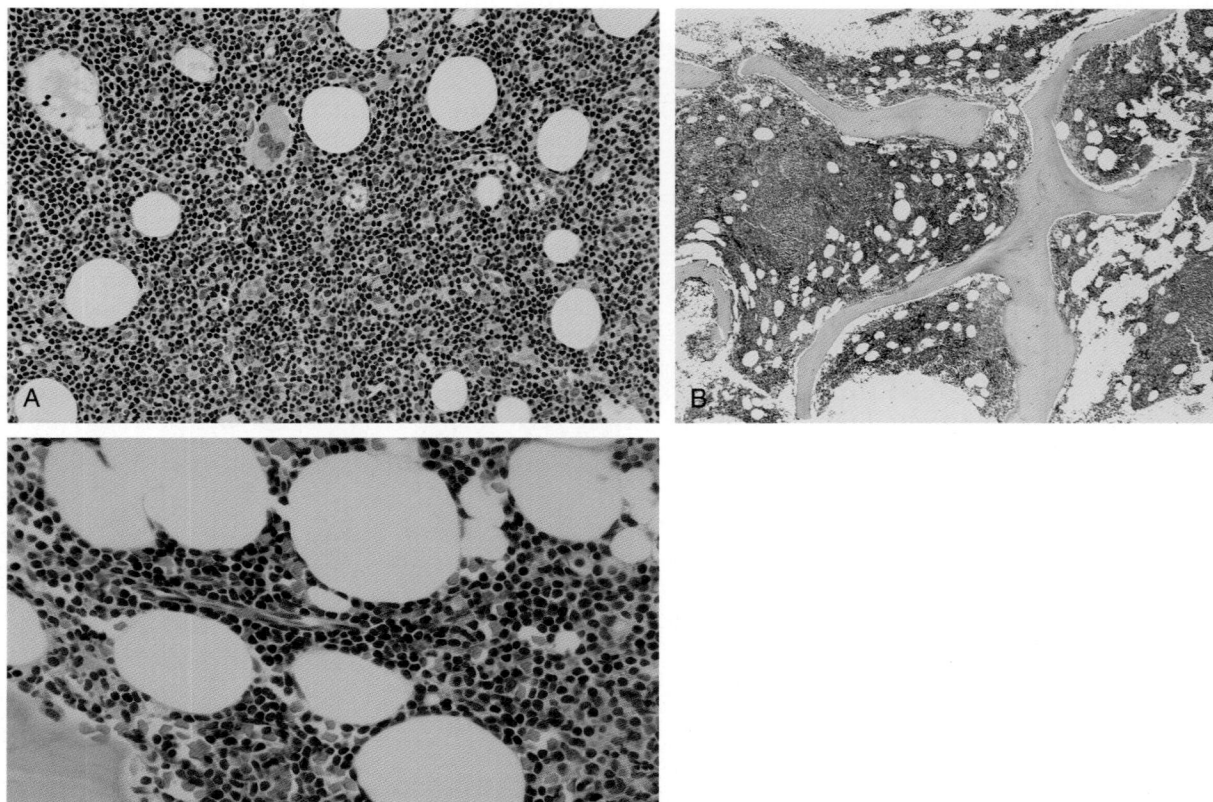

**FIGURE 43–22.** The major patterns of bone marrow infiltration by CLL are diffuse *(A)*, nodular *(B)*, and interstitial *(C)*.

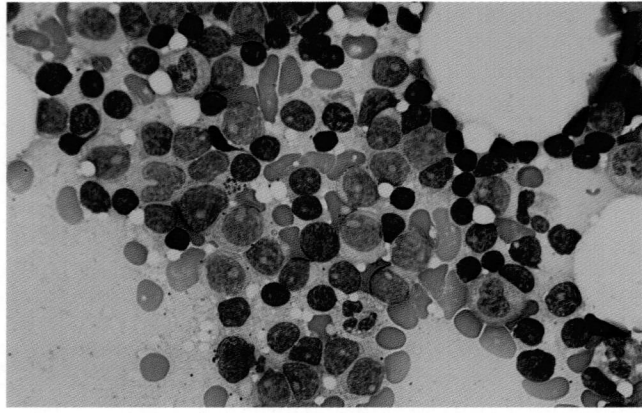

FIGURE 43–23. CLL with increased prolymphocytes. Note the increased numbers of bone marrow cells with moderately abundant cytoplasm and nucleoli. The presence of more than 55% of such cells in the peripheral blood is characteristic of prolymphocytoid transformation.

immunoblast nuclei on histologic sections.[279] Richter's transformation refers to the development of any higher grade lymphoma in a patient with CLL, but it usually represents development of a large B cell lymphoma with or without immunoblastic features. Transformation of CLL is generally associated with aggressive clinical behavior and short survival.[280–282]

Autoimmune disorders frequently occur in patients with CLL and should not be overlooked. These include autoimmune hemolytic anemia, idiopathic thrombocytopenic purpura, red cell aplasia, and neutropenia.[283, 284] A careful search for erythroid precursors should be made on all CLL bone marrow specimens, because red cell aplasia may be easily overlooked.

Immunophenotyping studies are now considered essential for the initial diagnosis of all chronic lymphoproliferative disorders that involve the blood. The term *CLL* is now reserved for cases of B lineage neoplasms that have a characteristic immunophenotype.[285–287] CLL demonstrates monoclonal immunoglobulin light and heavy chains, but this expression, as well as the expression of CD20, is characteristically weak. These cells also express B lineage–associated markers CD19 and CD79a, and they express CD23 and the T cell–associated markers CD5 and CD43. They are almost always negative for FMC7. Weak light chain and CD20 expression and aberrant expression of CD5 are critical in the diagnosis of CLL. Cases with morphologic features of CLL but strong light chain expression or no expression of CD5 may be termed *atypical CLL*. CD5⁻ CLL is rare, however, and peripheral blood involvement by other lymphoma types, such as marginal zone and follicular lymphomas, should be excluded. Atypical CLL cases behave in a manner different from that of the usual-type CLL, often more aggressively, and they are more often associated with splenomegaly.[288, 289] CD38 expression is also associated with more aggressive disease.[290] Bright light

chain expression and loss of CD5 commonly occur with prolymphocytoid transformation of CLL.

Gene rearrangement studies identify an immunoglobulin heavy chain rearrangement in virtually all cases of CLL. Lack of mutation of immunoglobulin heavy chain variable region genes has been shown to be associated with more aggressive disease and atypical morphologic features.[290, 291] In order of frequency, deletions of chromosome band 13q14, 11q23 deletions, trisomy 12, 6q21 deletions, and deletions or mutations of the *TP53* gene on 17p are the most common cytogenetic abnormalities in CLL.[292–296] Trisomy 12 is commonly seen in cases with atypical features (such as mixed CLL–prolymphocytic leukemia morphology), bright surface immunoglobulin expression, or transformation to a higher grade process.

### B Cell Prolymphocytic Leukemia

B cell prolymphocytic leukemia (B-PLL) occurs in older patients with no history of CLL and demonstrates a male predominance. Patients usually have splenomegaly without peripheral lymphadenopathy and have a markedly elevated white blood cell count.[297] The peripheral blood shows at least 55% prolymphocytes, but this disease differs from prolymphocytoid transformation of CLL by the lack of preexisting CLL.[278] Anemia and thrombocytopenia are commonly present. The bone marrow is usually extensively involved in an interstitial, diffuse, or mixed pattern by small and medium-sized lymphocytes with prominent nucleoli[298] (Fig. 43–24). The nodular bone marrow pattern that is often seen in CLL is uncommon in B-PLL. The medium-sized cells tend to have clearing of nuclear chromatin, and mitotic figures are frequent. Admixed larger cells are also common. The peripheral blood and bone marrow cells are monotypic B cells with bright immunoglobulin light chain expression and variable CD5 expression. They are usually positive for FMC7. Immunoglobulin heavy chain gene rearrangements are usually detectable, and cytogenetic abnormalities similar to those in CLL may be identified, including abnormalities of chromosome 12.[299] Mutations of

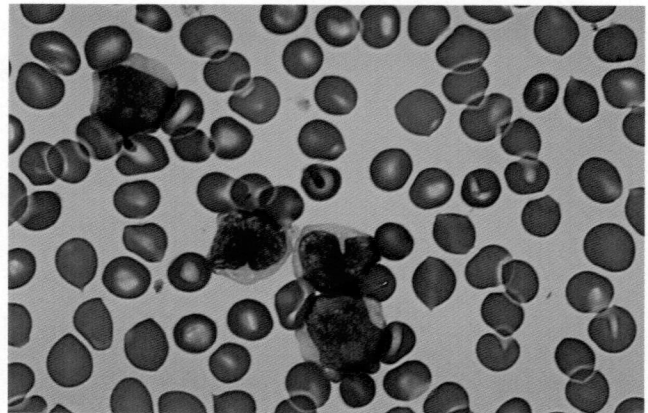

FIGURE 43–24. B-PLL shows cells with abundant cytoplasm and a prominent central nucleolus.

*TP53* are reported to be much higher in B-PLL than in other B cell malignant neoplasms.[300]

The differential diagnosis of B-PLL includes T cell prolymphocytic leukemia (T-PLL), mixed CLL–prolymphocytic leukemia, prolymphocytoid transformation of CLL, blood and bone marrow involvement by large cell lymphoma and mantle cell lymphoma, and even acute leukemia. The clinical history helps exclude transformation of CLL or large cell lymphoma in most cases, and the prolymphocyte count distinguishes mixed CLL–prolymphocytic leukemia (≤55% peripheral blood prolymphocytes) from B-PLL (>55% peripheral blood prolymphocytes). Mantle cell lymphoma involving the peripheral blood and bone marrow may be difficult to distinguish from prolymphocytic leukemia, but it usually does not demonstrate the characteristic single, central nucleolus of prolymphocytic leukemia. Cytogenetic or molecular genetic studies for t(11;14) of mantle cell lymphoma or immunophenotypic studies for cyclin D1/bcl-1 help in identifying cases of mantle cell lymphoma, and these studies are discussed in more detail later. Immunophenotyping studies easily distinguish B-PLL from a T cell malignant neoplasm or an acute leukemia.

## Hairy Cell Leukemia

Hairy cell leukemia is a rare monoclonal B cell disorder that usually affects elderly men in the sixth decade of life.[301, 302] The common clinical presentation of these patients is pancytopenia and splenomegaly without associated lymphadenopathy. The anemia is usually normocytic and normochromic. Monocytopenia is almost always present. Abnormal lymphocytes are usually few in the peripheral blood but have cytoplasmic projections or "hairs" (Fig. 43–25). This feature is nonspecific, and villous cytoplasmic projections of lymphocytes may be artifactual and may be seen with other lymphoproliferative disorders.

The abnormal cell population has slightly basophilic cytoplasm, and the cell nucleus is round, slightly indented, or reniform. The nuclear chromatin is smooth without the characteristic chromatin clumping seen in CLL or normal small lymphocytes. Nucleoli are indistinct or absent in the hairy cells. Platelets are usually decreased in number. The bone marrow is virtually always involved in hairy cell leukemia, but the pattern of involvement is interstitial and may be subtle on H&E sections. The bone marrow also demonstrates fine reticulin fibrosis,

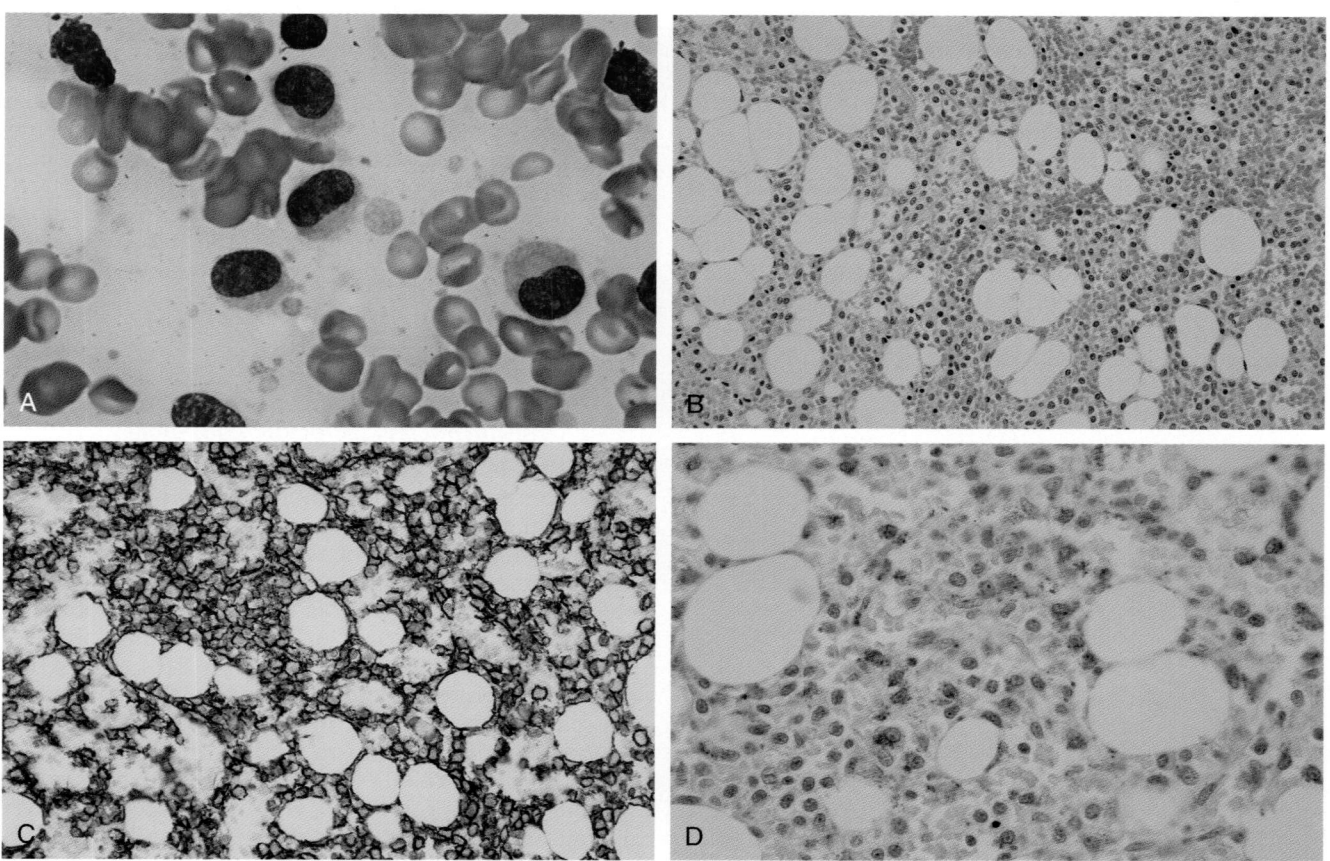

**FIGURE 43–25.** Hairy cell leukemia. *A.* The bone marrow aspirate is often paucicellular but may contain cells with reniform nuclei and moderately abundant cytoplasm that is often friable, giving a "hairy" appearance. *B.* The bone marrow biopsy specimen shows an interstitial infiltrate of small cells with clear cytoplasm. The cells stain for CD20 *(C)* and tartrate-resistant acid phosphatase *(D)* by immunohistochemistry.

making aspiration difficult in many cases. Because of the limited material available by aspiration in many cases, the bone marrow biopsy is often necessary for the diagnosis.[303] The marrow may be normocellular or hypercellular, but normal hematopoietic elements are commonly reduced in number. Small lymphocytes, similar to those seen in the blood, are identified on aspirate smears or touch imprints. The bone marrow biopsy specimen shows an interstitial infiltration by small cells with moderately abundant clear to slightly eosinophilic cytoplasm without nucleoli. The cells with oval or reniform nuclei and abundant cytoplasm often have a "fried-egg" appearance. When the cells are admixed with other bone marrow cells, they may be mistaken for erythroid precursors.

Hairy cell leukemia variant is a chronic lymphoproliferative disorder that has features of hairy cell leukemia and B-PLL.[304] The white blood cell count is usually elevated, as in B-PLL. The lymphoid cells have cytoplasmic projections, as in hairy cell leukemia, but also demonstrate a prominent central nucleolus, as in B-PLL (Fig. 43–26).

Immunophenotyping studies performed on peripheral blood or bone marrow in hairy cell leukemia demonstrate a monoclonal B cell population, without expression of CD5 or CD10. The cells are usually positive for CD11c, CD25, and CD103 and demonstrate bright surface immunoglobulin heavy and light chains and bright CD20.[305-307] By cytochemical methods, the cells are positive for tartrate-resistant acid phosphatase[19] (CD Fig. 43–18). Because of the high frequency of dry taps in patients with hairy cell leukemia, immunohistochemical studies on bone marrow biopsy material may be necessary.[308] The interstitial small lymphocyte infiltrate immunoreacts for CD20, confirming the B lineage of the cells. DBA.44 is also positive on the hairy cells; it is negative on the cells of CLL.[309] Hairy cells do not aberrantly coexpress CD43, but they may be weakly positive for cyclin D1.[310] A paraffin section antibody directed against tartrate-resistant

acid phosphatase has become available (see Fig. 43–25D).[311] Cytogenetic studies do not usually help because of limited growth of the specimens. Although no specific abnormality has been described for hairy cell leukemia, clonal abnormalities involving chromosome 5, including trisomy 5, are reported in 40% of cases.[312] Immunoglobulin heavy chain gene rearrangements are consistently detected in hairy cell leukemia.

The differential diagnosis of hairy cell leukemia in the blood includes splenic marginal zone cell lymphoma and splenic lymphoma with villous lymphocytes, hairy cell leukemia variant, and other chronic lymphoproliferative disorders including CLL. Immunophenotyping easily excludes CLL and mantle cell lymphoma by the lack of CD5 expression in hairy cell leukemia. There is overlap between the immunophenotype of splenic lymphoma with villous lymphocytes and hairy cell leukemia, although splenic lymphoma with villous lymphocytes is more frequently CD103⁻ and is usually negative for tartrate-resistant acid phosphatase. The pattern of bone marrow infiltration differs between hairy cell leukemia and most lymphomas. In general, lymphomas form sinusoidal aggregates, nodules, or sheets in the bone marrow, in contrast to the interstitial pattern of bone marrow involvement by hairy cell leukemia. CD25 expression is reportedly less common in hairy cell leukemia variant than in the usual-type hairy cell leukemia,[313] but the morphologic feature of a prominent nucleolus in hairy cell leukemia variant is the primary means of differentiating these two diseases. There is also morphologic and immunophenotypic overlap between hairy cell leukemia variant and splenic lymphoma with villous lymphocytes, and distinguishing the two on peripheral blood alone is not always possible (CD Fig. 43–19).

## T CELL LEUKEMIAS

### T Cell Prolymphocytic Leukemia and T Cell Chronic Lymphocytic Leukemia

T-PLL is a clonal T cell proliferation that occurs most commonly in the elderly, with a slight male predominance.[278, 314, 315] The disease also occurs frequently in younger patients with ataxia telangiectasia.[316] Patients have a markedly elevated white blood cell count as well as organomegaly and lymphadenopathy. Nodular or maculopapular skin lesions are also common. The peripheral blood white blood cell count is usually above 100,000/mm³ with a predominance of medium-sized cells with abundant basophilic cytoplasm and a single prominent nucleolus (Fig. 43–27). These cells are virtually identical to B cell prolymphocytes. The prolymphocyte nucleus may be round or slightly convoluted. Normocytic anemia and thrombocytopenia are common. The bone marrow may not be involved to the degree that would be expected by the marked elevation in peripheral blood prolymphocytes. The pattern of involvement may be interstitial, diffuse, or

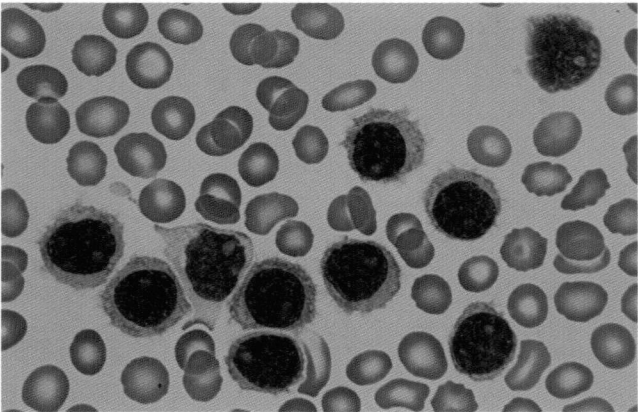

**FIGURE 43–26.** The peripheral blood cells of hairy cell leukemia variant have the friable cytoplasm typical of hairy cell leukemia and the prominent nucleolus of prolymphocytic leukemia.

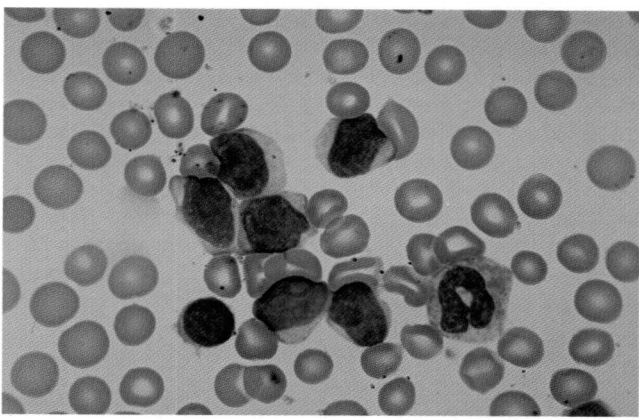

**FIGURE 43–27.** T-PLL in the peripheral blood is indistinguishable from B-PLL with abundant cytoplasm and a prominent central nucleolus.

mixed, and reticulin fibrosis is frequently present[298] (Fig. 43–28). In general, T-PLL is an aggressive disease with short survival. However, a subpopulation of patients with T-PLL, including many with ataxia telangiectasia, have an initially indolent disease course that eventually transforms to the more typical aggressive disease.[317]

Immunophenotyping is necessary to distinguish T-PLL from B-PLL, and it is often helpful in excluding acute leukemia. T cell–associated antigens CD2, CD3, CD5, and CD7 are expressed by T-PLL, and surface CD3 is present. Most cases are CD4+, but a subset of cases express CD8 or both CD4 and CD8. The absence of both CD20 and immunoglobulin light chain expression excludes B-PLL. The lack of TdT and CD1 expression as well as the presence of surface CD3 excludes most cases of T cell ALL. T cell receptor gene rearrangements are uniformly detectable in T-PLL. Cytogenetic abnormalities in T-PLL include inv(14)(q11;q32) and t(14;14)(q11;q32) involving the *TCL1* gene in the region of the T cell receptor α and δ chains, i(8q), and trisomy 8.[317, 318] Abnormalities of chromosome region 11q22-23, in-

volving the *ATM* tumor suppressor gene that is consistently mutated in ataxia telangiectasia, are present in some patients with T-PLL even in the absence of ataxia telangiectasia.[319]

### T-CLL and Small Cell Variant of T-PLL

Many cases that were originally termed T cell CLL are now included in the category of large granular lymphocytosis. Some T cell chronic lymphoproliferative disorders have cells with morphologic features similar to B cell CLL without the prominent nucleolus typical of usual-type prolymphocytic leukemia.[320, 321] Some consider these to represent cases of true T cell CLL; others term them small cell variants of T-PLL (CD Fig. 43–20). Although the median age and white blood cell count are lower in these patients than in those with the usual-type T-PLL, the immunophenotypic and cytogenetic features are similar to those in T-PLL and there is a similarly aggressive clinical course.

### Large Granular Lymphocytosis

Elevations of the number of peripheral blood large granular lymphocytes may be reactive, such as after viral infections, or they may be clonal neoplasms of T cells or NK cells. Patients with prolonged elevations of large granular lymphocytes with associated neutropenia frequently have the clonal disease of large granular lymphocytic (LGL) leukemia.[322–326] These patients are usually elderly, may have associated infections or a previously diagnosed autoimmune disorder, and may have mild to moderate splenomegaly, but they rarely have lymphadenopathy.

The peripheral blood white blood cell count is normal to slightly elevated, and neutrophil counts are usually decreased. Large granular lymphocytes predominate, usually above 2000/mm³, for 6 months or more. The cells have clear to pale-staining cytoplasm with multiple azurophilic cytoplasmic granules (Fig. 43–29); they are medium to large with mature round to indented nuclei without prominent nucleoli. Anemia and thrombocytopenia are present

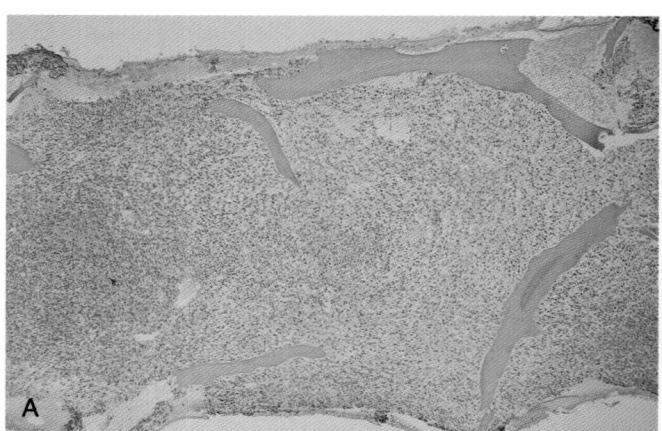
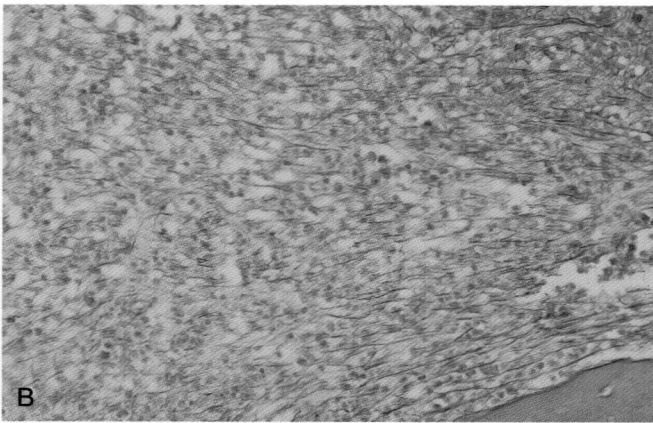

**FIGURE 43–28.** The bone marrow biopsy specimen of T-PLL shows a diffuse infiltration of lymphoid cells *(A)* and an increase in reticulin fibrosis *(B)*.

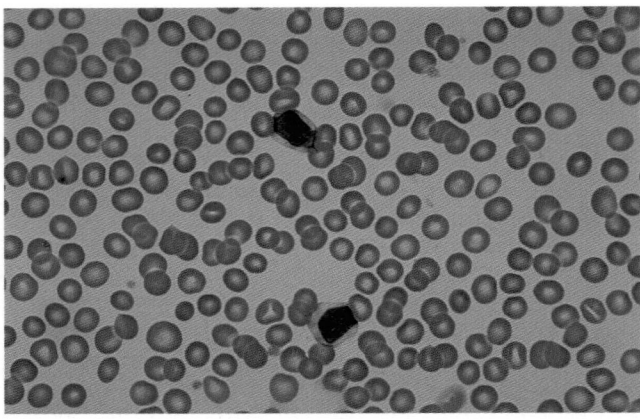

**FIGURE 43–29.** The lymphocytes of large granular lymphocytosis have abundant cytoplasm with a variable number of cytoplasmic granules.

in some patients. Rouleaux formation may be present, related to a polyclonal hypergammaglobulinemia that occurs in some of these patients. The bone marrow is usually slightly hypercellular with a mild interstitial infiltration of large granular lymphocytes or small nonparatrabecular aggregates that may be difficult to identify on H&E sections[327] (CD Fig. 43–21). Other hematopoietic elements are normal or may be slightly decreased in number.

LGL leukemia is further subdivided into T cell and NK cell types. The T cell proliferations express CD2, surface and cytoplasmic CD3, and CD8, but they may also express NK-associated markers such as CD16, CD56, and CD57. The T cell type of LGL leukemia is the most common, accounting for approximately 85% of cases. These cases have T cell receptor gene rearrangements, a finding that helps in excluding a reactive T cell large granular lymphocyte proliferation.[328] The NK cell type of LGL leukemia is negative for surface CD3 but may express CD8 and is usually positive for CD16 and CD56. These cases do not demonstrate T cell receptor gene rearrangements and require prolonged evidence of the proliferation for a diagnosis of leukemia. NK cell proliferations that are associated with a leukocytosis of more than 11,000/mm³ are more likely to be associated with persistent disease.[329] T cell LGL leukemia is usually an indolent disease with an increase in infections secondary to the associated neutropenia, but T cell LGL leukemia with CD56 expression may behave more aggressively.[330] NK cell LGL leukemia is less common than T cell LGL leukemia, but some reports indicate a more aggressive clinical course. Because reactive large granular lymphocyte proliferations are indistinguishable from LGL leukemia, gene rearrangement studies are essential in the T cell proliferations, and evidence of prolonged elevations in NK cell proliferations are necessary before a definite diagnosis can be made. Rare blastic NK cell leukemias have cells that resemble myeloblasts and demonstrate an aggressive clinical course.[331] These cases are uncommon but should be distinguished

from both the mature LGL leukemias and the AMLs with CD56 expression.

As mentioned, the CD3⁺ T cell LGL leukemia cases demonstrate T cell receptor gene rearrangements that involve both of the commonly tested β- and γ-chains. In contrast to some of the other T cell and NK cell–T cell lymphoproliferative disorders, LGL leukemias are negative for the Epstein-Barr virus and the human T cell lymphotropic virus type I (HTLV-I). Cytogenetic abnormalities are not usually detected in LGL leukemia.

### Adult T Cell Leukemia-Lymphoma

Adult T cell leukemia-lymphoma (ATLL) is a clonal T cell proliferation that is associated with HTLV-I infection.[278, 332] This infection is more common in southwest Japan, west Africa, the Caribbean, and the southeastern United States. It is rare in other locations. Most patients are adults with lymphadenopathy, with or without organomegaly. Skin lesions and hypercalcemia are also common. Approximately one third of patients present without lymphadenopathy but have 10% or more abnormal cells in the blood and are considered leukemic. The remaining patients present with lymphoma or a mixture of leukemia and lymphoma.

The peripheral blood shows a marked elevation in the white blood cell count because of leukemic cells. The abnormal lymphocytes are medium in size and have a characteristic hyperlobated, "flowerlike" nucleus or a multilobated "knobby" nucleus with moderate to scant, slightly basophilic cytoplasm. Hyperlobated nuclei may be rare or absent in some cases; small, uniform CLL-like cells are seen more commonly in the chronic or smoldering form of the disease.[333] Mild anemia and thrombocytopenia are seen in some cases. The bone marrow is frequently normocellular, with minimal and focal interstitial or diffuse involvement seen in approximately half of the cases.[332, 334] This bone marrow involvement is usually nonparatrabecular and may be subtle despite the extensive peripheral blood involvement seen in many of these patients. Patients with hypercalcemia commonly show prominent osteoclastic activity and bone resorption.

Acute, chronic, and smoldering types of ATLL are described.[278, 335] In the acute form, many atypical lymphocytes with abnormal nuclear lobations are present in the blood. In the chronic form, the lymphoid population is more uniform, with only rare nuclear folds or bilobated forms present. Smoldering ATLL has 3% or less abnormal peripheral blood cells with changes similar to those seen in the chronic form of the disease. The acute form is an aggressive disease; the chronic and smoldering forms of ATLL are more indolent diseases that may progress to an acute disease.

The leukemic cells of ATLL express CD2, surface CD3, and CD5; are usually CD4⁺ and CD25⁺; and frequently do not express CD7 or CD8. They also lack TdT expression, excluding a T cell ALL. The CD25 expression differs from many of the other chronic T cell proliferations. The lack of CD7 in ATLL is considered useful in the differential diagnosis of T-PLL, which is usually CD7+.[336] The detection of HTLV-I and T cell receptor gene rearrangements helps in establishing the diagnosis of ATLL. Cytogenetic abnormalities, including multiple trisomies, loss of sex chromosomes, translocations involving 14q, and deletions of 6q, have been reported in ATLL.[337]

### Sézary Syndrome and Other T Cell Proliferations

Other T cell lymphomas may involve the blood and bone marrow, producing a leukemic peripheral blood picture. They are usually easily recognized and diagnosed if the appropriate clinical information of previous lymphoma or clinical evidence of mycosis fungoides is relayed to the pathologist. Sézary syndrome is a leukemic manifestation of mycosis fungoides that occurs most commonly in middle-aged men.[338] The patients have the characteristic generalized erythroderma of mycosis fungoides and may have lymphadenopathy, organomegaly, and other dermatologic problems.

The peripheral blood shows an elevated white blood cell count because of circulating Sézary cells. These cells may be subdivided into large and small cell types.[339, 340] The large cell type should be present for diagnosis, because small Sézary cells may be identified in patients with non-neoplastic dermatosis. The Sézary cell has scant to moderately abundant pale or slightly basophilic cytoplasm that may contain vacuoles. The nucleus is enlarged with an irregular "cerebriform" appearance with multiple nuclear indentations. The nuclear chromatin may be focally dense or hyperchromatic, and nucleoli are not prominent (Fig. 43–30). The small cell variant has dense chromatin and less conspicuous nuclear indentations. The bone marrow is usually normocellular with subtle focal nodular or interstitial involvement by small irregular lymphocytes, or it may be uninvolved.[341, 342] Large transformed cells may be

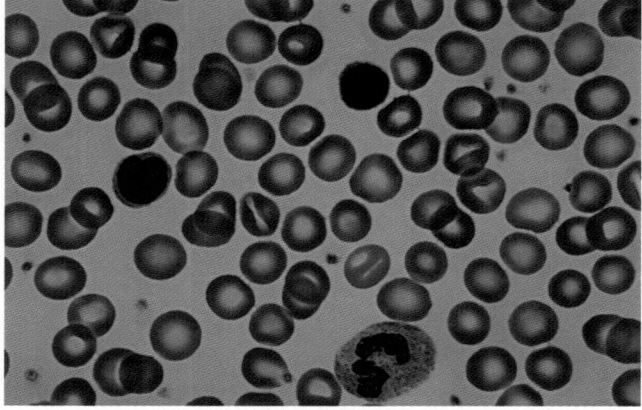

**FIGURE 43–30.** In Sézary syndrome, the peripheral blood cells have dense nuclear chromatin, and many have irregular, cerebriform nuclei.

admixed with the small irregular cells. Aggregates of cytologically normal lymphocytes should not be overinterpreted as definite evidence of bone marrow involvement. Bone marrow eosinophilia may be present even in the absence of bone marrow involvement by lymphoma.

Immunophenotyping demonstrates a mature T cell immunophenotype with surface CD3 expression, and the Sézary cells are usually CD4+ and CD8-. Although the Sézary cells and the cells of ATLL are CD4+ T cells with irregular nuclear contours, they differ by the lack of flowerlike nuclei, hypercalcemia, evidence of HTLV-I, and CD25 expression in most cases of Sézary syndrome. T cell receptor gene rearrangements are present in Sézary syndrome and may be useful in excluding reactive T cell proliferations. Gene rearrangement studies, however, must be correlated with other pathologic and clinical findings because T cell receptor gene rearrangements may be detected in the peripheral blood of some patients with benign inflammatory skin lesions.[343] Clonal cytogenetic abnormalities are present in the peripheral blood of more than half of patients with Sézary syndrome, but there is a wide variation in the specific types of abnormalities.[344]

The term *Sézary cell leukemia* has been used to describe clonal peripheral blood T cell disorders with convoluted cell nuclei similar to those seen in Sézary syndrome.[345, 346] In contrast to Sézary syndrome, these patients do not have erythema or other evidence of skin involvement at presentation. Immunophenotyping and cytogenetic analysis of these cases suggest that they represent morphologic variants of T-PLL.

## LYMPHOMAS

Any type of B or T lineage malignant lymphoma may involve the peripheral blood and bone marrow.[347, 348] Details of the different lymphoma types are described in Chapter 41, and not all lymphoma types are covered in this chapter. A primary diagnosis of malignant lymphoma can be made on bone marrow material by criteria similar to those used for lymph nodes. Immunophenotyping studies are often useful in confirming the presence of lymphoma and in subclassifying the process.[287, 349] The evaluation of the bone marrow in patients with a known diagnosis of malignant lymphoma is critical in the staging of the disease. When the bone marrow is involved by lymphoma, specific information that should be mentioned in the report includes the type of lymphoma, pattern of involvement, and percentage of involvement in terms of percentage of all nucleated marrow cells.[350] Discordance between bone marrow and lymph node lymphoma type is common; lower grade lymphoma is commonly identified in the bone marrow of patients with higher grade lymphoma elsewhere.[351, 352] Because the detection of low-grade lymphoma in the bone marrow of a patient with a history of intermediate- or high-grade lymphoma confers a worse prognosis,[353] a small lymphocyte proliferation in the bone marrow should not be au-

**TABLE 43–18.** Immunophenotypic Findings of Peripheral Blood Bone Marrow B Cell Lymphoid Proliferations*

| Feature | CCL | PLL | MCL | FCCL | HCL | MZL/SLVL |
|---|---|---|---|---|---|---|
| CD19 | + | + | + | + | + | + |
| CD20 | Weak +/− | + | + | + | + | + |
| Light chains | Weak +/− | + | + | + | + | + |
| CD5 | + | −/+ | + | − | − | − |
| CD10 | − | − | −/+ | + | − | − |
| CD23 | + | −/+ | − | +/− | − | − |
| CD43 | + | −/+ | + | − | − | −† |
| CD103 | − | − | − | − | + | −/+ |
| Cyclin D1/Bcl-1 | − | − | + | − | Weak +/− | − |
| DBA44 | − | −/+ | − | − | + | + |
| FMC7 | − | + | + | −/+ | + | + |

CLL, Chronic lymphocytic leukemia; PLL, B cell prolymphocytic leukemia; MCL, mantle cell lymphoma; FCCL, follicular center cell lymphoma; HCL, hairy cell leukemia; MZL/SLVL, marginal zone lymphoma/splenic lymphoma with circulating villous lymphocytes; +, positive; +/−, usually positive; −/+, usually negative; −, negative.
*Approximately 40% of nonsplenic marginal zone cell lymphomas are CD43+.

tomatically assumed to be evidence of lack of involvement in a patient with an intermediate- or high-grade lymphoma elsewhere, and a designation of atypical or indeterminate lymphoid aggregate may be necessary in some cases (see later).

Immunohistochemistry, flow cytometric immunophenotyping, and gene rearrangement studies are useful in the primary diagnosis of peripheral blood and bone marrow involvement by lymphoma.[354] Table 43–18 summarizes some of the most useful features of various lymphomas and other B cell lymphoproliferative disorders in the blood and marrow. Flow cytometry is of less value in the evaluation of residual disease in the bone marrow, and findings are often negative when the morphologic or immunohistochemical evaluation identifies evidence of residual disease.[355] Gene rearrangement studies help in the evaluation of residual disease, but the routine use of consensus primers usually limits the PCR methods for immunoglobulin heavy chain and T cell receptor chains to a detection level of one rearranged cell in 100 to 1000 cells. Because of this, tumor-specific primers made from the patient's original lymphoma specimen may be developed to increase the level of detection to one cell in 10,000 or 100,000, but this method is not currently offered in most institutions.[356] PCR testing for specific translocations, such as t(14;18) of follicular lymphoma or t(11;14) of mantle cell lymphoma, detects much lower amounts of residual disease without the expense of tumor-specific primers.

### Follicular Center Cell Lymphomas

Follicular center cell lymphomas may show significant involvement of the peripheral blood that may mimic another chronic lymphoproliferative disorder. Cells with cleaved nuclei are usually identifiable, but subclassification of lymphoproliferative disorders by peripheral blood morphology is often difficult (CD Fig. 43–22). Follicular lymphomas usually involve the bone marrow in a paratrabecular pattern (Fig. 43–31), although a diffuse pattern of involvement that includes paratrabecular disease may be present with extensive bone marrow involvement.[347, 348] An increase in reticulin fibrosis in association with the lymphoid aggregates is common, and this fibrosis often limits the ability to aspirate lymphoma cells for smears or immunophenotyping studies. Small collections of lymphoid cells immediately adjacent to bone trabeculae without intervening marrow or adipose tissue should be considered evidence of bone marrow involvement in a patient with known follicular center cell lymphoma and should be considered highly suggestive of lymphoma in patients without known lymphoma. These aggregates contain a mixture of small cells with irregular nuclei and a variable number of large lymphoid cells. Predominantly small cleaved cell lymphoma (grade I of the WHO Classification of Lymphoid Neoplasms) is the most common type of follicular lymphoma seen in the bone marrow, but the other types occur.

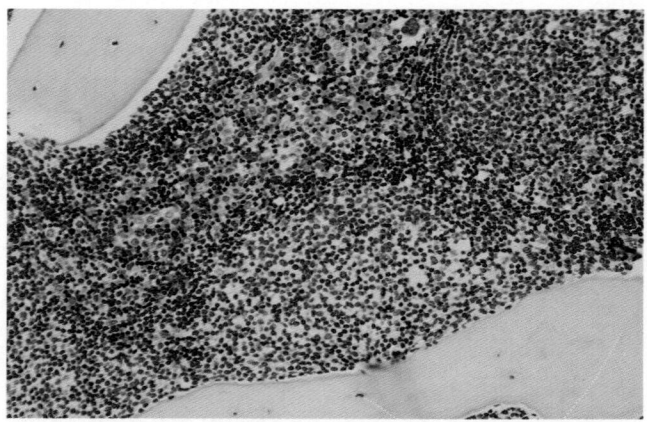

**FIGURE 43–31.** Follicular lymphoma preferentially involves the bone marrow in a paratrabecular pattern. Any lymphoid aggregate of the bone marrow in this location should be considered highly suggestive of lymphoma, and this pattern in a patient with a history of follicular lymphoma is diagnostic of bone marrow involvement by the disease.

Immunophenotyping of peripheral blood or bone marrow suspected of being involved by follicular lymphoma can be extremely helpful.[287] The lymphoid cells are monoclonal B cells that often express CD10 but do not express CD5. The lack of CD5 expression excludes most cases of CLL or mantle cell lymphoma involving blood, and the detection of CD10 on the cell population is usually sufficient to strongly suggest a follicular center cell lymphoma. Absence of CD10 does not exclude follicular center cell lymphoma, however. Immunophenotyping of bone marrow specimens to look for focal or residual involvement by known follicular lymphoma is less helpful. The bone marrow biopsy morphology is frequently positive even when flow cytometric immunophenotyping does not detect a clonal B cell population. In patients with known follicular lymphoma and characteristic paratrabecular lymphoid aggregates in the bone marrow, paraffin section immunophenotyping is not necessary for a diagnosis of bone marrow involvement and may actually cause unnecessary confusion when only small aggregates are present. Follicular lymphomas characteristically have large numbers of associated, non-neoplastic T cells, and a small paratrabecular lymphoid aggregate may show a mixture of T and B cells by immunohistochemistry that might incorrectly suggest a reactive aggregate. In patients without a history of lymphoma and large aggregates in the bone marrow, paraffin section immunohistochemistry may help. The B cells should not aberrantly coexpress CD5 or CD43 and are frequently positive for CD10 and bcl-2 protein.

Molecular genetic or cytogenetic studies may help confirm a diagnosis of follicular center cell lymphoma involving the blood or bone marrow. The immunoglobulin heavy chain gene rearrangement of a significant number of follicular lymphomas cannot be detected by the PCR method. Most follicular lymphomas demonstrate t(14;18)(q32;q21) involving the immunoglobulin heavy chain gene on chromosome 14 and the *BCL2* gene on chromosome 18.[357] The major breakpoint region or minor cluster region of this translocation can be detected by PCR analysis in most cases.[358, 359]

### Mantle Cell Lymphoma

Mantle cell lymphoma frequently involves the peripheral blood and bone marrow[360–362] (CD Fig. 43–23). In the blood, there may be an increase in small to medium-sized lymphocytes, which vary from cells with round nuclei with small nuclear chromocenters to cells with irregular and cleaved nuclei. A separate population of prolymphocytes is not seen, but the leukemic cell population may mimic *de novo* prolymphocytic leukemia. A similar cell population is seen on bone marrow aspirate smears, with other hematopoietic elements relatively reduced. The biopsy specimen may be normocellular or hypercellular with nodular, interstitial, paratrabecular, diffuse, and mixed patterns of involvement. In the author's experience, a mixed nodular and paratrabecular pattern is common in this disease. The lymphoid cells are homogeneous in size with generally scant cytoplasm and small nuclear chromocenters. Epithelioid histiocytes are commonly admixed with the lymphoma cells, but admixed large lymphoid cells are not a feature of mantle cell lymphoma. Rare cases of mantle cell lymphoma involving the bone marrow have lymphoma cells surrounding a reactive germinal center, similar to the mantle zone pattern seen in the lymph nodes. The blastic type of mantle cell lymphoma has cells with fine nuclear chromatin that may be mistaken for lymphoblastic leukemia-lymphoma when there is a diffuse pattern of marrow involvement. The immunophenotypic findings are useful in excluding a lymphoblastic process.

Immunophenotyping of the blood and marrow shows a monoclonal B cell population with bright light chain and CD20 expression, in contrast to CLL, and the cells characteristically express CD5, CD43, and FMC7 without expression of CD23. In contrast to lymphoblastic malignant neoplasms, blastic mantle cell lymphoma is negative for TdT. The cells express the bcl-2 protein and often demonstrate nuclear expression of cyclin D1/bcl-1. The detection of CD5, FMC7, and cyclin D1 on a monoclonal B cell population is specific for this disease. Although cyclin D1 staining is technically difficult and cannot be demonstrated in all cases, detailed staining methods are now described, and such staining is probably indicated before performance of molecular genetic studies for t(11;14).[363] If the diagnosis of mantle cell lymphoma is already established, not all of these studies may be necessary. Demonstration of a predominance of B cells with aberrant coexpression of CD43 in a questionable lymphoid infiltrate is usually sufficient for the confirmation of bone marrow involvement by previously diagnosed disease.

Immunoglobulin heavy chain gene rearrangements are usually easily detectable in mantle cell lymphoma by PCR analysis. The t(11;14)(q13;q32), involving the immunoglobulin heavy chain gene on chromosome 14 and the *BCL1/CCND1/PRAD1* gene on chromosome 11, is present in most cases of mantle cell lymphoma.[364] However, the PCR test most commonly used for this translocation detects only the major translocation cluster of t(11;14) and is positive in only 40% to 50% of cases.[365]

### Other Non-Hodgkin's Lymphomas

Bone marrow involvement by small lymphocytic lymphoma and lymphoblastic lymphoma is similar to that described for CLL and ALL, respectively. Morphologic and immunophenotypic features similar to those used in lymph nodes and other sites may be used in the diagnosis of bone marrow involvement by other lymphoma types, including large cell lymphoma (see Chapter 41). Some patients without a history of lymphoma demonstrate bone marrow involvement by small lymphoid cells that are predominantly of B lineage but do not have diagnostic immunophenotypic features of CLL–

small lymphocytic lymphoma, mantle cell lymphoma, or follicular lymphoma. Such cases are best categorized as bone marrow involvement by unclassified B cell lymphoma. Further work-up of these patients often reveals evidence of lymphoma at other sites that is more suitable for classification, often of marginal zone type.

### Hodgkin's Disease

Although eosinophilia is common in Hodgkin's disease, peripheral blood involvement by neoplastic cells is not. The bone marrow is most frequently involved in patients with a known diagnosis of Hodgkin's disease, but a primary diagnosis of the disease can be made on a bone marrow specimen. Any type of Hodgkin's disease may involve the marrow, although involvement by the lymphocyte predominance type is uncommon.[366] Bone marrow eosinophilia, lymphohistiocytic aggregates, and granulomas may occur in patients with Hodgkin's disease, and their presence does not definitely indicate bone marrow involvement by the disease.[367] Identification of Reed-Sternberg cells or their mononuclear variants, usually in association with marrow fibrosis, is required for the diagnosis (Fig. 43–32). These cells are large, may be multinucleated, and have large eosinophilic nucleoli. Diagnostic cells are usually not easily identified on bone marrow aspirate smears but may be present on imprints. Specimens showing large, atypical lymphohistiocytic aggregates without obvious Hodgkin's cells should have multiple H&E-stained levels cut through to exclude the presence of disease.

Immunohistochemical studies on the biopsy material help in confirming the presence of mononuclear Reed-Sternberg cell variants. These cells should be CD45⁻ and CD15⁺ and CD30⁺.[285] This immunophenotype is typical of classic Hodgkin's disease, including nodular sclerosis, mixed cellularity, and lymphocyte-depleted types. CD15 expression by normal hematopoietic cells must not be overinterpreted as a positive result, and expression in neoplastic cells of the marrow may be perinuclear and weak.

The background small lymphocytes are CD3⁺ T cells. CD20 expression by large neoplastic cells may be seen in any type of Hodgkin's disease, but strong, uniform staining for CD20 with CD45 expression and no CD15 or CD30 expression is the characteristic immunophenotype of nodular lymphocyte predominance Hodgkin's disease. In the bone marrow, however, it is usually not possible to distinguish nodular lymphocyte predominance Hodgkin's disease from bone marrow involvement by T cell–rich large B cell lymphoma. Subclassification of the types of classic Hodgkin's disease is also not usually possible on bone marrow material alone.

Ancillary studies other than immunohistochemistry are of limited value in Hodgkin's disease. Although Hodgkin's cells have a characteristic immunophenotype, it is usually not detectable by flow cytometry. *In situ* hybridization for the Epstein-Barr virus is positive in Hodgkin's cells in approximately 40% of cases.[368] Immunohistochemical detection of the Epstein-Barr virus latent membrane protein, however, is a reliable means of detecting Epstein-Barr virus–positive cells in Hodgkin's disease without the use of *in situ* hybridization. Microdissected Hodgkin's cells may demonstrate evidence of immunoglobulin heavy chain gene rearrangements,[369] but these studies are generally negative on whole bone marrow specimens. Therefore, unless a non-Hodgkin's lymphoma is in the differential diagnosis, flow cytometric immunophenotyping and gene rearrangement studies do not help in the evaluation of a bone marrow specimen for Hodgkin's disease.

### THE NON-NEOPLASTIC LYMPHOID AGGREGATE

The identification of lymphoid aggregates in the bone marrow often causes diagnostic problems, particularly in patients with a history of malignant lymphoma. Because discordance in morphology may occur between the original lymphoma and the bone marrow disease, these aggregates cannot be ignored simply because they are morphologically different from the original disease. Non-neoplastic lymphoid

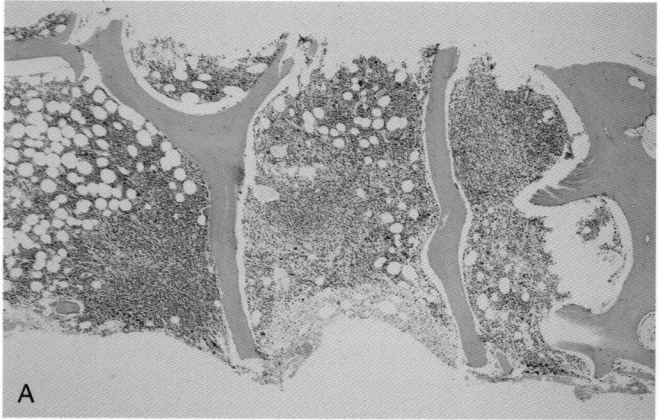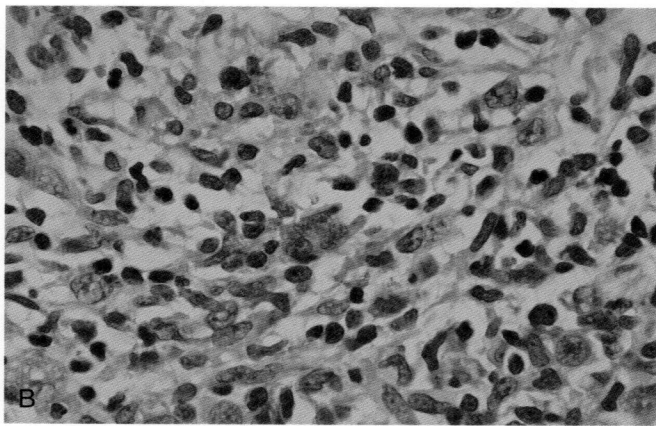

**FIGURE 43–32.** Hodgkin's disease involves the bone marrow with patchy areas of associated fibrosis (A). The fibrous areas must contain classic Reed-Sternberg cells or their mononuclear variants (B).

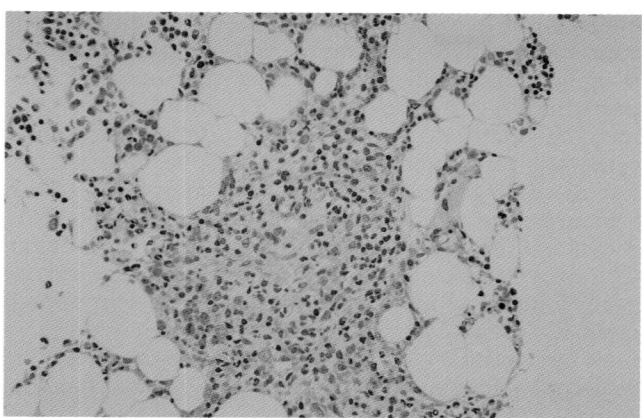

**FIGURE 43–33.** A non-neoplastic lymphoid aggregate in a bone marrow clot section. These aggregates are more common on clot section, are nonparatrabecular when they are present on biopsy section, are usually well circumscribed, and often contain admixed histiocytes.

aggregates are common in elderly patients and are more common on clot biopsy material because more marrow is usually present for evaluation in the clot than in the trephine biopsy material.[370–372] These non-neoplastic aggregates are usually small and uniformly round without irregular infiltration into the surrounding marrow (Fig. 43–33). They are often associated with small capillaries that may be identified within the aggregate. The lymphoid cells are usually small, but a few admixed large cells and histiocytes may be present. The majority of lymphocytes in a non-neoplastic or reactive lymphoid aggregate are T cells that immunoreact with CD3, CD43, and bcl-2 but not CD20. Germinal center formation with predominantly B cells may also occur and is usually a clue to a reactive or autoimmune process.[372–374] Rare cases of mantle cell lymphoma involving the bone marrow, however, have associated reactive-appearing germinal centers surrounded by a neoplastic mantle zone.

The neoplastic lymphoid aggregate is often monotonous and irregular in appearance and may show irregular infiltration into the surrounding marrow. Aggregates of small lymphocytic lymphoma and follicular lymphoma, however, often show a heterogeneous mixture of small cells with admixed larger cells. As mentioned before, a paratrabecular aggregate without identifiable marrow or fat between the aggregate and the bone in a patient with a history of follicular lymphoma should be considered evidence of bone marrow involvement by lymphoma. In other situations, immunohistochemical or molecular genetic studies may be useful. The neoplastic aggregates of B cell lymphoma characteristically demonstrate a marked increase in CD20+ B cells.[7, 375] Aberrant coexpression of CD5 or CD43 in this B cell population is usually sufficient for a diagnosis of involvement by lymphoma. Coexpression requires an increase in B cells, and virtually every lymphoid cell should immunoreact for CD5 or CD43. Although an increased number of bcl-2+ lym-

phoid cells is present in most neoplastic aggregates compared with non-neoplastic aggregates, non-neoplastic T lymphocytes and mantle B lymphocytes are bcl-2+. Therefore, bcl-2 staining should not be used alone to distinguish neoplastic from reactive proliferations.[376] The molecular detection of a gene rearrangement or a translocation known to be associated with a type of lymphoma may also be useful in characterizing an atypical lymphoid aggregate,[354] but these studies should be correlated with the morphologic and immunophenotypic findings.

In some cases, the nature of the aggregates cannot be defined with certainty, and this should be clearly stated in the report. In these instances, the author uses the term *atypical lymphoid aggregates of undetermined (or unknown) significance*. An international workshop to standardize response criteria for non-Hodgkin's lymphoma proposed a category of "indeterminate" for involvement by lymphoma for cases in which lymphoid aggregates are increased in number or size without cytologic or architectural atypia.[350]

## Granulomatous and Histiocytic Disorders

### GRANULOMAS OF BONE MARROW

Although aggregates of histiocytes may be present on aspirate smears, granulomas are best identified with bone marrow trephine and clot biopsy material.[377–379] Granulomas in the bone marrow should be approached in a fashion similar to those in other sites. There are generally two types of granulomas considered in the marrow. The lipogranuloma is a collection of histiocytes surrounding adipose tissue and is usually not associated with disease. Epithelioid granulomas without associated adipose tissue may have admixed lymphocytes, plasma cells, neutrophils, or eosinophils and may have associated necrosis. Mycobacteria and fungal organisms should be excluded by special stains in all cases with epithelioid granulomas, and fresh bone marrow aspirate material should be submitted for culture in all patients being evaluated for infectious diseases. Patients with immunodeficiency syndromes may have abundant atypical mycobacteria even when well-formed granulomas are not present. In such cases, special stains for organisms are indicated when any increase in histiocytes is noted. Although fungi and mycobacteria are the most common infectious causes of bone marrow granulomas, brucellosis, leprosy, and viral infections may also cause bone marrow granulomas. Occasional infectious granulomas, particularly in Q fever, contain a central clear space surrounded by fibrin that may be mistaken for an incidental lipogranuloma.[380] Similar "fibrin ring granulomas" have also been described with cytomegalovirus infection.[381]

Noninfectious granulomas, including those of sarcoidosis, drug reactions, and collagen-vascular disease and those associated with neoplasms, cannot be reliably distinguished from infectious granulomas, and appropriate histochemical stains for organisms are indicated in these patients. Bone marrow granulomas are common in patients with Hodgkin's disease and non-Hodgkin's lymphomas and may be present in the absence of bone marrow involvement by the neoplasm.[382] Although noninfectious granulomas are common in these diseases, these patients are also at risk for the development of infectious diseases and may have infectious granulomas as well as hematologic malignant disease. In Hodgkin's disease, multiple step sections through the biopsy specimen should be examined before a diagnosis of granulomas without involvement by Hodgkin's disease is made, because only rare Hodgkin's cells may be present in the specimen.

### HEMOPHAGOCYTIC SYNDROMES

Hemophagocytosis may be related to primary or secondary syndromes and is discussed in more detail in Chapter 42. Primary hemophagocytic lymphohistiocytosis is a rare, fatal childhood disorder that may be familial or sporadic.[383] It is usually elicited by a viral infection. Bone marrow involvement may be evident in only 40% of cases that have extensive disease elsewhere.[384] Secondary hemophagocytosis may be related to infection or neoplasia.[385–387] All types frequently involve multiple organs, including the bone marrow, and have similar morphologic features (Fig. 43–34).

Hemophagocytosis consists most prominently of erythrophagocytosis that may be best visualized on aspirate smears or imprint slides. The histiocytes have characteristically bland nuclear features without mitoses or atypia. Hemophagocytosis may be associated with T cell malignant neoplasms, and many of these cases in the past were interpreted as malignant histiocytosis. The neoplastic T cells are usually distinct from the reactive-appearing histiocytes that are engulfing other hematopoietic cells, which may include phagocytosis of neoplastic cells. In some cases, the bone marrow may demonstrate evidence of hemophagocytosis without definite marrow involvement by the T cell neoplasm that is prominent in another site. Other marrow elements, particularly granulocytes and erythroid precursors, may be relatively decreased in number. Lymphoid cells, including immunoblasts, may be increased in the marrow in association with hemophagocytosis. The presence of immunoblasts does not necessarily indicate the presence of an associated lymphoma. Cytologic atypia of the lymphoid cells should be easily identified in lymphoma-associated hemophagocytosis. Gene rearrangement studies may help in making a primary diagnosis of lymphoma on a bone marrow specimen that has extensive hemophagocytosis.

### STORAGE DISEASES

Various storage diseases may involve the bone marrow, but these diseases are generally rare and should be diagnosed and classified by identification of the enzymatic defect characteristic of each disease.[388] Gaucher's and Niemann-Pick disease are the most common storage diseases encountered in the bone marrow, and both may cause the accumulation of patchy or diffuse aggregates of large histiocytes with abundant cytoplasm and small nuclei.[389] On smears, Gaucher's cells have slightly basophilic cytoplasm that is often compared with crumpled tissue paper, in contrast to the finely vacuolated cytoplasm of the characteristic cells of Niemann-Pick disease (CD Fig. 43–24). Small histiocytes with more basophilic cytoplasm and vacuoles are often termed *sea-blue histiocytes* and are also seen in Niemann-Pick disease. None of these cell types is specific for a given disease, and sea-blue histiocytes may also be seen in association with lipid disorders, infectious diseases, red blood cell disorders, and myeloproliferative disorders. Therefore, the accumulation of histiocytes of these types may suggest a storage disease, but the actual diagnosis should be based on biochemical or molecular genetic testing specific for these diseases.

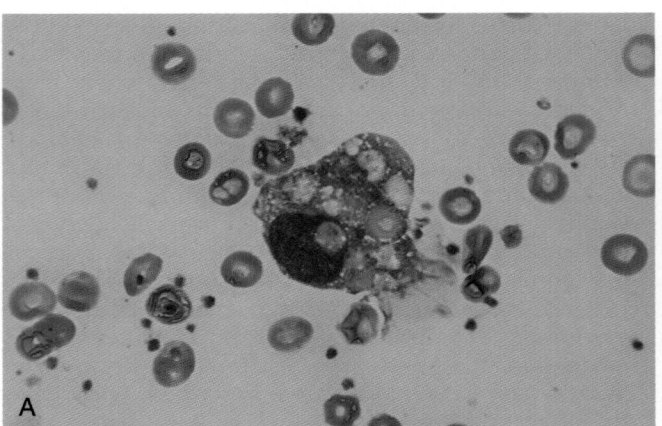 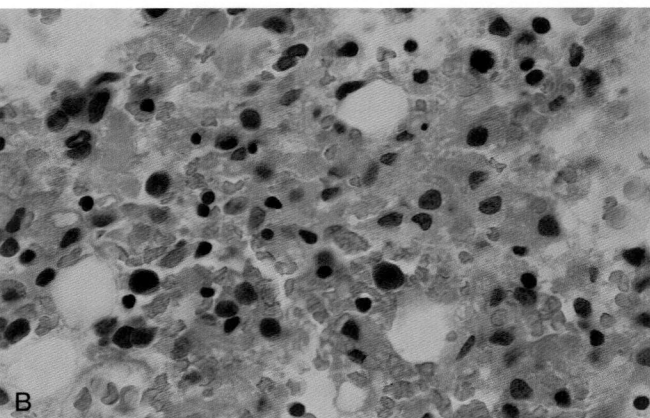

**FIGURE 43–34.** Hemophagocytic syndrome. *A.* Large histiocytes engulfing red blood cells are identified on touch preparations or aspirate smears. *B.* Sheets of histiocytes may be present on the bone marrow biopsy specimen.

## NONLEUKEMIC HISTIOCYTIC DISORDERS

Histiocytic disorders, other than acute and chronic leukemias, are rare in the bone marrow. Langerhans cell histiocytosis, sinus histiocytosis with massive lymphadenopathy, and true histiocytic lymphoma generally present in other organs and only rarely and focally involve the marrow. These disorders are covered in more detail in Chapter 41.

So-called malignant histiocytosis or true histiocytic lymphoma involving the marrow is controversial. Most cases seem to represent extramedullary presentations of acute monoblastic leukemia without obvious peripheral blood involvement, similar to other extramedullary myeloid tumors, and may have minimal or no evidence of bone marrow involvement.[390, 391] Cases of hemophagocytic syndrome (with or without associated malignant disease), anaplastic large cell lymphoma, and other malignant lymphomas with bone marrow involvement have previously been interpreted as malignant histiocytosis.[392, 393] Because of the historic heterogeneity of diseases covered by this term as well as the current lack of specific features that distinguish malignant histiocytosis of the bone marrow from monoblastic leukemia, the author does not use this term in the diagnosis of primary bone marrow proliferations.

## Mast Cell Disease

Generalized mast cell disease, or mastocytosis, may be subdivided into systemic mast cell disease, which is usually associated with skin lesions and a good prognosis, and malignant mast cell disease, which does not characteristically involve the skin, is often associated with other hematologic malignant neoplasms, and has a generally poor prognosis.[394] Either type may involve the bone marrow.[395, 396]

On aspirate smear material, mast cells are usually admixed with hematopoietic cells within the marrow particle, and an increase in the cells may be overlooked (CD Fig. 43–25). Other abnormalities of marrow cells, however, may be best identified on the smears. The most common histologic pattern of bone marrow involvement is one of patchy paratrabecular or perivascular stellate aggregates of fibrosis with admixed mast cells, lymphocytes, and eosinophils (Fig. 43–35). The mast cells are easily overlooked in these aggregates and may have a spindled appearance similar to that of fibroblasts or histiocytes, or they may represent small round cells with slightly granular, basophilic cytoplasm that may be mistaken for lymphocytes or plasma cells. When relatively normal surrounding marrow elements and cellularity accompany this pattern of infiltration, it is most commonly associated with systemic mast cell disease. However, this perivascular and paratrabecular pattern of mast cells may also be associated with surrounding marrow changes of AML, myelodysplasia, or a chronic myeloproliferative disorder (often unclassifiable), features more common in malignant mast cell disease.[397–399] Sheets of atypical mast cells

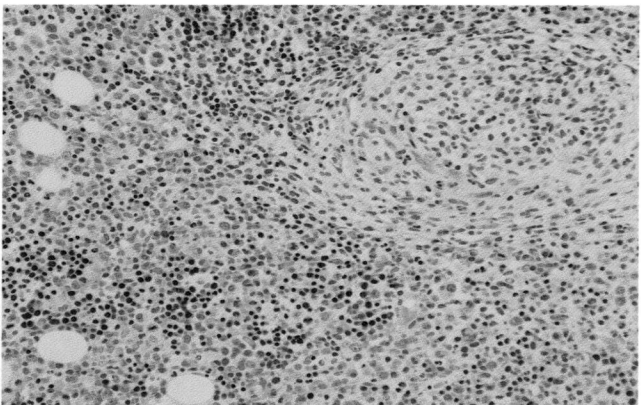

**FIGURE 43–35.** Mast cell disease in a patient with myelodysplasia. A focus of marrow fibrosis contains mast cells admixed with eosinophils. The surrounding bone marrow is hypercellular, and myelodysplastic changes were evident on the bone marrow aspirate smears.

may rarely be evident on bone marrow sections. This pattern is more commonly associated with peripheral blood involvement by mast cells (mast cell leukemia) and is another feature of malignant mast cell disease. Osteosclerosis may be seen with any pattern of marrow involvement.

On tissue sections, mast cells are usually positive for Giemsa, toluidine blue, and chloracetate esterase, but some of these cytochemical reactions are pH dependent in neoplastic mast cells.[400] Immunohistochemical studies show the mast cells to be positive for CD43, CD68, CD117 (c-kit), and tryptase; tryptase is the most specific marker for these cells.[401–403a]

Except for cases of mast cell leukemia, the peripheral blood changes of mast cell disease are not specific.[399] In systemic mast cell disease, the peripheral blood is often normal, whereas cytopenias are common in malignant mast cell disease. Because many cases of mast cell disease are associated with other hematologic malignant neoplasms, the peripheral blood often demonstrates evidence of those diseases rather than of the mast cell disease.

## Metastatic Tumors

Metastatic tumors in the bone marrow may be identified in staging procedures or may be unexpected findings in a patient undergoing an evaluation for abnormal blood counts.[404] A bone marrow biopsy may be a relatively easy way to identify and classify a pediatric tumor without resection of the primary mass. The most common nonhematologic malignant neoplasms to involve the bone marrow are prostate carcinoma, breast carcinoma, lung carcinoma, neuroblastoma, Ewing's sarcoma/peripheral neuroectodermal tumor, rhabdomyosarcoma, and malignant melanoma.[405, 406] Tumor is often not easily identifiable on aspirate smears, but when present, it is more

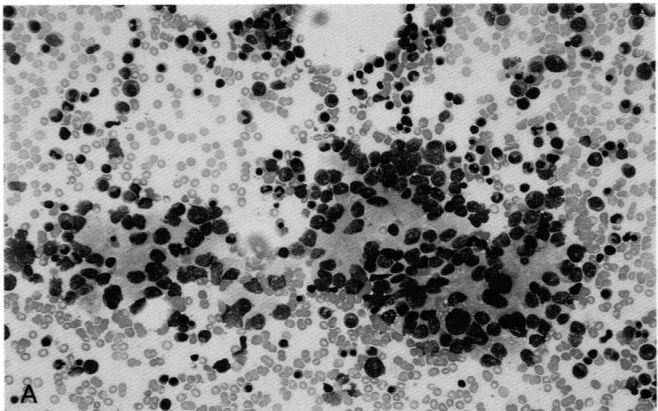
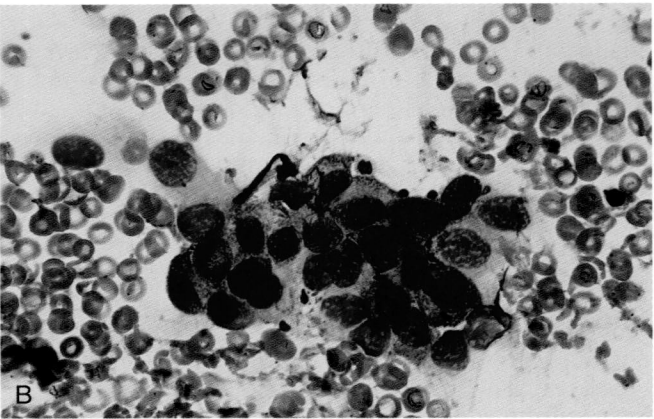

**FIGURE 43–36.** *A.* Neuroblastoma on a bone marrow aspirate showing rosette formation. *B.* Clumps of metastatic lobular breast carcinoma are identified at the feathered edge of a bone marrow aspirate smear.

often seen on the feathered edges of the smears as small clumps of cells (Fig. 43–36). When the primary tumor type is unknown, immunohistochemical studies may be useful to identify the tumor type. In adults, the majority of metastatic tumors are carcinomas or malignant melanoma, although sarcomas may rarely involve the marrow. Immunohistochemical study for keratin and S-100 protein is useful as an initial screen to identify keratin-positive carcinoma and keratin-negative, S-100 protein–positive malignant melanoma. When clinically indicated, additional immunohistochemical studies may be useful to identify estrogen receptor–positive breast or gynecologic carcinomas, prostate-specific antigen–positive prostate tumors, and chromogranin-positive small cell carcinomas.

Pediatric sarcomas in the bone marrow display an immunohistochemical staining profile similar to that seen in other sites, and primary diagnosis can be made on a bone marrow biopsy specimen in many cases. The small blue round cell tumors may be confused with acute leukemic infiltrates of the marrow. An initial immunohistochemical panel that includes vimentin, keratin, desmin, CD99, myeloperoxidase, and TdT often helps in the evaluation of these tumors. Although CD99 is characteristic of Ewing's sarcoma/peripheral neuroectodermal tumor, ALL is also positive for this marker. TdT staining helps in this differential diagnosis and is positive in ALL but negative in Ewing's sarcoma/peripheral neuroectodermal tumor. Details of the morphologic, immunohistochemical, and molecular genetic features of these tumors are described in Chapters 7 and 46.

The routine use of immunohistochemical studies is usually not necessary in the evaluation or staging of post-therapy marrow of patients with these diseases. Metastatic tumor cells are usually large, occur in aggregates, and have associated fibrosis with or without necrosis in the marrow. When foci of fibrosis are present without obvious tumor, selected immunohistochemical studies may be useful to further

exclude tumor cells within the fibrous stroma. Lobular carcinoma of the breast, however, often infiltrates the bone marrow as individual small cells without associated fibrosis and may be easily overlooked on H&E-stained sections alone[407] (CD Fig. 43–26). Because the detection of these individual cells within the marrow appears to have prognostic significance, the author routinely stains bone marrow biopsy and clot sections from patients with lobular carcinoma for keratin. The identification of keratin-positive cells by immunohistochemistry allows the re-review of the suspicious area on the routine section and usually identification of individual tumor cells on those sections.

Peripheral blood involvement by metastatic tumor, termed *carcinocythemia,* is extremely uncommon and usually represents a late event with short survival.[408] Other abnormalities of the blood in patients with metastatic carcinoma are generally nonspecific and include anemia, leukoerythroblastosis, leukocytosis, and microangiopathic hemolytic anemia.

## APPROACH TO THE NON-NEOPLASTIC BONE MARROW

### The Aplasias

A decrease in bone marrow cellularity for a patient's age may be related to a variety of causes. Artifactual hypocellularity due to sampling of only subcortical marrow should not be misinterpreted, and an accurate estimate of marrow cellularity cannot be made on small biopsy specimens that contain only the subcortical marrow space. True hypocellularity may be due to a decrease in all marrow cell lines or decreases in only selected cell lines.

#### APLASTIC ANEMIA

Aplastic anemia may be acquired or congenital and represents a decrease in granulocytic, erythroid, and megakaryocytic cells.[409, 410] Criteria for aplastic anemia include 1) a bone marrow of less than 25% cellularity or less than 50% cellularity with less than 30% hematopoiesis and 2) two of the following three peripheral blood findings: a neutrophil count of less than 500/mm$^3$, a platelet count of less than 20,000/mm$^3$, or anemia with a corrected reticulocyte count of less than 1%.

The peripheral blood demonstrates pancytopenia without obvious abnormalities of the circulating cells.[411] Aspirate smears usually show small particles containing histiocytes, mast cells, lymphocytes, and plasma cells with no or rare normal hematopoietic cells. The biopsy specimens in these patients are variably hypocellular. Some have only rare hematopoietic cells, representing less than 5% of the marrow cellularity; others have large areas of markedly hypocellular marrow admixed with more normocellular areas. Interstitial small lymphocytes and plasma cells, as well as well-formed lymphoid aggregates, are common. Aplastic marrow may be seen after toxic exposures or viral infections, including parvovirus infection, and either may result in only a transient aplasia. This is the case in patients who have received chemotherapy or radiation therapy. The post-therapy biopsy often demonstrates transient marrow aplasia that is usually associated with marrow edema and eosinophilic proteinaceous fluid accumulation in the marrow.

Other diseases may mimic aplastic anemia. Hypocellular acute leukemias and hypocellular myelodysplastic syndromes have a similar appearance and may result in inaspirable material for evaluation,[412, 413] and a subset of patients with apparent aplastic anemia will progress to myelodysplasia or acute leukemia.[414] The identification of an increase in CD34$^+$ immature cells in the marrow (>5%) is helpful in the identification of these diseases. Cytogenetic studies are also useful in the differential diagnosis of marrow aplasia versus myelodysplasia to identify cytogenetic abnormalities commonly associated with myelodysplastic syndromes. Patients with Fanconi's anemia may develop marrow aplasia and may also progress to myelodysplasia and acute leukemia.[415] Hairy cell leukemia may mimic aplastic anemia, but the identification of increased numbers of interstitial B lymphocytes in the marrow of hairy cell leukemia excludes aplastic anemia.

## PAROXYSMAL NOCTURNAL HEMOGLOBINURIA

Paroxysmal nocturnal hemoglobinuria may cause a pancytopenia and marrow aplasia similar to aplastic anemia or may result in an erythroid hyperplasia.[416] Paroxysmal nocturnal hemoglobinuria is characterized by recurrent episodes of hematuria that are secondary to intravascular hemolysis. It is a stem cell disorder that is often related to somatic mutation of the X-linked *PIG-A* gene.[417] This mutation results in a deficiency of the glycosylphosphatidylinositol-anchoring proteins of decay-accelerating factor (*DAF* or CD55) and the membrane inhibitor of reactive lysis (*MIRL* or CD59) on red blood cells, granulocytes, monocytes, and platelets. Loss of these proteins results in the increased sensitivity of the red blood cells to the lytic action of complement. The antigen loss may be detected by flow cytometric evaluation.[418]

Paroxysmal nocturnal hemoglobinuria is characterized by the presence of chronic hemolytic anemia, and positive sucrose hemolysis and Ham test results are useful in confirming this diagnosis. The defects of paroxysmal nocturnal hemoglobinuria may also be present in patients with acute leukemias and myelodysplasia, suggesting an association of paroxysmal nocturnal hemoglobinuria with these diseases.[419]

## SEROUS FAT ATROPHY

Serous degeneration, also known as serous fat atrophy, is associated with a hypocellular marrow and represents mucinous or gelatinous degeneration of the fatty marrow elements[420, 421] (Fig. 43–37). On aspirate material, pink to blue staining may be seen surrounding fat cells. On the biopsy material, the fat cells are decreased in size and are surrounded by amorphous pink material. Such degeneration in the marrow represents a systemic change in the total body adipose tissue. Serous fat atrophy is seen with a variety of diseases that are associated with malnutrition and emaciation, including anorexia nervosa, chronic renal disease, malignant neoplasms, acquired immunodeficiency syndrome, and tuberculosis.

## RED CELL APLASIAS

Aplasia of a single cell line in the bone marrow is less common than the trilineage aplasias. Pure red cell aplasia may be congenital or acquired. Diamond-Blackfan anemia is an autosomal recessive disorder that is often associated with other abnormalities, and the anemia becomes apparent shortly after birth with persistent elevations of hemoglobin F, i antigen, and red blood cell macrocytosis.[422]

Other red cell aplasias are secondary to drug or toxin exposure and infections, or they may occur in

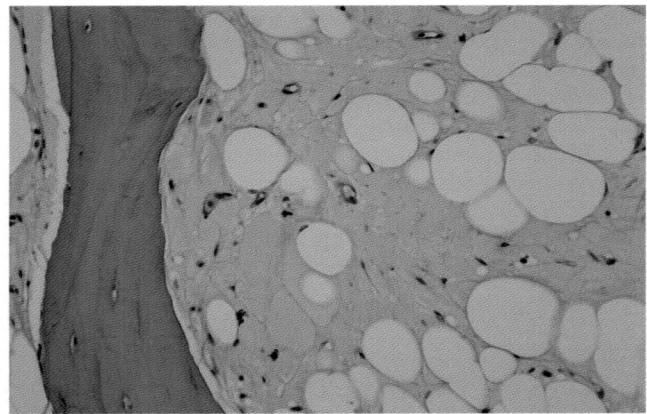

**FIGURE 43–37.** Serous fat atrophy in a bone marrow biopsy specimen.

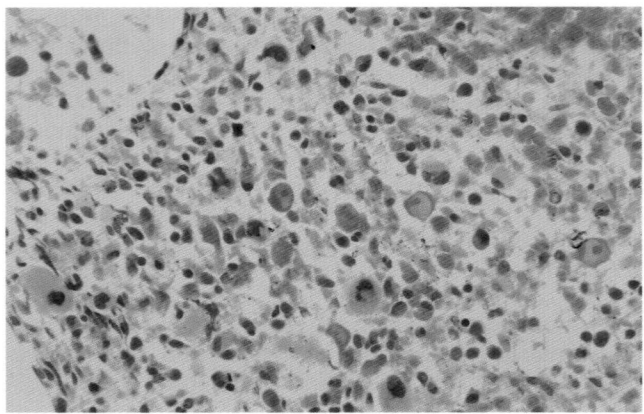

FIGURE 43–38. Bone marrow biopsy specimen from a child with parvovirus infection. The erythroid precursors are enlarged with nuclear clearing.

association with thymoma or CLL.[423] Parvovirus infection causes erythema infectiosum (fifth disease) in children and infects red blood cell precursors, which may result in a red cell aplasia.[424, 425] The virus causes the few residual erythroblasts to enlarge, and one may see large intranuclear inclusions (Fig. 43–38).

All causes of red cell aplasia produce similar morphologic features, with the exception of the characteristic nuclear inclusions of parvovirus infection. All demonstrate a marked decrease in red blood cell precursors with only rare scattered erythroblasts present. A transient red cell aplasia (transient erythroblastopenia of childhood) has been described in young children that is not yet known to be associated with any viral or toxic insult.[426, 427]

### GRANULOCYTE APLASIA

Granulocyte aplasia may be congenital or acquired.[428, 429] Congenital causes include Shwachman-Diamond syndrome, Kostmann's syndrome, and cyclic neutropenia. Acquired granulocytopenia may be secondary to drugs, infections, hypersplenism, and autoimmune disease. Acquired granulocytopenias are secondary to peripheral destruction or redistribution of granulocytes, and bone marrow examination of these patients may not demonstrate a decrease in granulocytic cells.[430] Although parvovirus infection is usually associated with red cell aplasia, it may also cause chronic neutropenia.[431] The congenital causes of granulocyte aplasia result in a decrease in bone marrow granulocytes that are usually normal in appearance; however, maturation arrest at the promyelocyte and myelocyte stage is seen in Kostmann's syndrome.[429]

### MEGAKARYOCYTE APLASIA

Megakaryocyte aplasia is uncommon, and most cases of megakaryocyte-poor thrombocytopenia probably represent an unusual form of myelodysplasia primarily involving that cell lineage.[432, 433] In newborns, megakaryocyte hypoplasia is associated with the TAR (thrombocytopenia with absent radius) syndrome.[434]

## The Hyperplasias

Non-neoplastic hyperplasias of one or more bone marrow cell lines are often related to changes outside of the marrow and must be correlated with peripheral blood findings, other appropriate laboratory data, and clinical information. Patients recovering from toxic insults, including chemotherapy and radiation therapy, demonstrate trilineage bone marrow hyperplasia. In a similar fashion, destruction of a particular cell line outside of the marrow, as in some autoimmune diseases, results in hyperplasia of the corresponding cell line in the marrow. Because the bone marrow changes may represent a reaction to events elsewhere in the body, the bone marrow specimen alone is often not diagnostic of the patient's underlying disease process.

### ERYTHROID HYPERPLASIA

Erythroid hyperplasias represent a response to peripheral red blood cell loss or destruction or are related to the ineffective production of normal red blood cells, as in hemoglobinopathies. The causes of erythroid hyperplasia are best addressed in combination with peripheral blood features of the red blood cells.[435, 436] In general, ancillary laboratory testing is needed to precisely characterize the cause of the erythroid hyperplasia. Dyserythropoiesis, particularly mild irregularities of the nuclear contours of erythroid precursors, is common in cases of florid erythroid hyperplasia and should not be overinterpreted as evidence of myelodysplasia.

#### Erythroid Hyperplasia Associated with Normocytic Anemia

Hemorrhage, hemolytic anemia, intrinsic bone marrow disease (including aplastic anemia and malignant neoplasms), and anemia of chronic disease are the most common causes of erythroid hyperplasia associated with normocytic anemia in patients with no history of a toxic insult, chemotherapy, or hemoglobinopathy. After hemorrhage or with hemolytic anemia, the peripheral blood demonstrates an increase in polychromatophilic red blood cells because of reticulocytosis. Hemolytic anemias may demonstrate microspherocytes and fragmented red blood cells in the peripheral blood. The bone marrow changes of the various causes of normocytic anemia with erythroid hyperplasia are similar, with an increase in red blood cell precursors. This increase is usually accompanied by a left-shift in erythroid precursors with increased numbers of pronormoblasts. Such a left-shift should not be interpreted as megaloblastic change, which represents an enlargement of both myeloid and erythroid precursors. Iron staining of a bone marrow aspirate smear and laboratory iron studies are appropriate in normocytic anemias of unknown cause, because the early stages of iron deficiency may present as a normocytic anemia with erythroid hyperplasia. Combined anemias, such as vitamin $B_{12}$ or folate deficiency coupled with iron deficiency or thalassemia, may also present with normocytic red blood cell indices.

### Erythroid Hyperplasia Associated with Macrocytic Anemia

Erythroid hyperplasia associated with macrocytic anemia may be related to megaloblastic anemia or to other causes. Megaloblastic anemias are due to deficiencies of vitamin $B_{12}$ or folate and demonstrate peripheral blood changes that include macrocytic anemia and hypersegmentation of neutrophils.[437, 438] Bone marrow examination is not usually performed for this diagnosis. The bone marrow aspirate characteristically shows a left-shift of erythroid cells with enlarged pronormoblasts and normoblasts with fine nuclear chromatin that may be mistaken for myeloblasts. The erythroid series in the marrow also demonstrates multinucleation and nuclear-cytoplasmic asynchrony. The maturing granulocyte series is also abnormal in megaloblastic anemia with enlarged or "giant" metamyelocytes and band neutrophils present. Megakaryocytes may show hypersegmentation of nuclei. These features should be correlated with vitamin $B_{12}$ and folate levels and may be confused with changes of myelodysplasia or acute leukemia. Cases of severe hemolytic anemia or hemorrhage result in a macrocytic anemia with a high reticulocyte count and marked left-shift of erythroid precursors of the marrow.

Congenital dyserythropoietic anemia results in an erythroid hyperplasia, and types I and III are associated with a macrocytic anemia (type II may be normocytic)[439] (CD Fig. 43–27). Congenital dyserythropoietic anemia is associated with abnormal bone marrow erythroid cells with intranuclear bridging and varying degrees of multinucleated erythroid cells. The most bizarre multinucleated cells are present in type III, more than one third binucleated cells in type II, and intranuclear chromatin bridges and less than one third binucleated cells in type I. Type II is also termed HEMPAS (hereditary erythroblastic multinuclearity with a positive acidified serum test result), which differs from paroxysmal nocturnal hemoglobinuria by a negative response to the sucrose hemolysis test.

Other disorders may result in erythroid hyperplasia with macrocytic anemia.[438, 440] These include alcohol ingestion, liver disease, cytotoxic drugs, hypothyroidism, pulmonary disease, aplastic anemia, and myelodysplasia. Anemias related to these disorders may not have an associated marrow hyperplasia.

### Erythroid Hyperplasia Associated with Microcytic Anemia

Iron deficiency is the most common cause of erythroid hyperplasia associated with microcytic anemia.[441, 442] Although early iron deficiency may result in a normocytic anemia, untreated patients develop a microcytic anemia with hypochromic red blood cells and prominent anisopoikilocytosis with elliptic or elongated red blood cells. Thrombocytosis is also often present. Iron staining of bone marrow aspirate material and serum iron or ferritin studies are usually diagnostic of iron deficiency. Lead toxicity may also result in a similar peripheral blood and bone marrow pattern and may be accompanied by iron deficiency.[443] Coarse basophilic stippling of peripheral blood red cells and bone marrow erythroid cells is seen in lead toxicity and not in the usual case of iron deficiency. Thalassemias and hemoglobin E disease and trait also result in a microcytic anemia; however, the total red blood cell count of the peripheral blood is often normal in thalassemia in comparison to the decrease in red blood cells of iron deficiency.[441] Some anemias of chronic disease and hereditary sideroblastic anemias also result in a microcytic anemia. Despite the cause, all demonstrate an erythroid hyperplasia in the marrow and cannot be reliably distinguished without iron studies and other appropriate laboratory tests.

OTHER CAUSES OF ERYTHROID HYPERPLASIA. Polycythemia vera and myelodysplasia are two neoplastic conditions that may be confused with non-neoplastic causes of erythroid hyperplasia. Non-neoplastic causes of erythroid hyperplasia must be excluded for a diagnosis of polycythemia vera, and diagnostic criteria are well established for that disorder. Mild dyserythropoietic changes in a patient with erythroid hyperplasia should not be used as the sole criterion for a diagnosis of myelodysplasia, and the identification of dysplastic changes of other cell lines with exclusion of vitamin $B_{12}$ or folate deficiency is recommended before a diagnosis of myelodysplasia is made. In patients with persistent anemia and only mild dysplastic changes confined to the erythroid series, the detection of a cytogenetic abnormality characteristic of myelodysplasia may be the only means of making a definite diagnosis of myelodysplasia.

## WHITE BLOOD CELL HYPERPLASIAS

### Neutrophilia

Peripheral blood neutrophilia is usually not associated with bone marrow granulocytic hyperplasia and usually results from demargination of neutrophils or a shift of neutrophils to the blood from other organs. Bone marrow granulocytic hyperplasia is usually a response to an infection, allergic reaction (usually with eosinophilia), toxic event, or drug reaction or occurs in association with neoplasia. The ratio of granulocytes to erythroid precursors may increase with a left-shift of myeloid cells. With infectious disease, the peripheral blood neutrophils often demonstrate toxic granulation and Döhle bodies. In neoplastic conditions, granulocytic hyperplasia of the marrow may not be associated with marrow involvement by the neoplasm.[444] Although organisms, including parasites, may rarely be identifiable in the bone marrow smears or biopsy material, the cause of the granulocytic hyperplasia is usually not apparent.

The primary differential diagnosis of non-neoplastic granulocytic hyperplasia is with CML or another chronic myeloproliferative disorder. The lack of basophilia or clusters of atypical megakaryocytes often help in excluding CML, but cytogenetic studies for t(9;22) are recommended when the etiology of the hyperplasia is not clear on clinical grounds.

### Monocytosis

A reactive monocytosis is a nonspecific finding that may be seen with infections, sarcoidosis, collagen-vascular diseases, hematologic disorders, and malignant neoplasms.[445, 446] The hematologic disorders include hemolytic anemia, and reactive monocytes may be increased in the peripheral blood or bone marrow in patients with Hodgkin's disease, non-Hodgkin's lymphoma, and carcinomas. Neoplastic monocytes in the peripheral blood with acute myelomonocytic leukemia and CMML may have features similar to reactive monocytes, and bone marrow examination is necessary to confirm and classify the leukemic process in those patients.

### Eosinophilia

The most common cause of peripheral blood or bone marrow eosinophilia worldwide is parasitic infection, although drugs and allergic reactions are the most common causes in developed countries.[447] Other causes of eosinophilia are asthma, inflammatory bowel disease, vasculitides, and malignant neoplasms. Reactive eosinophilia may be prominent in patients with colon carcinoma, Hodgkin's disease, T cell lymphomas, and chronic myeloproliferative disorders. Abnormal eosinophils are present in AMLs associated with chromosome 16 abnormalities.[115, 117]

### Basophilia and Mast Cell Hyperplasia

Non-neoplastic peripheral blood and bone marrow basophilia is usually mild and is commonly overshadowed by a more noticeable eosinophilia. It is most commonly associated with allergic or inflammatory conditions, including asthma, allergic rhinitis, nasal polyposis, and atopic dermatitis.[448] Significant increases in basophils, often abnormal, are seen in the peripheral blood and bone marrow of patients with CML and acute leukemias that are associated with t(9;22) and t(6;9).

Elevations of non-neoplastic bone marrow mast cell counts are common in association with chronic lymphoproliferative disorders in the marrow. These mast cells are evenly dispersed throughout the marrow particles and do not form the aggregates and foci of fibrosis that are seen with bone marrow involvement by mast cell disease.

### Lymphocytosis

Reactive lymphocytosis is most commonly related to viral infections, particularly infectious mononucleosis and viral hepatitis, and it may also

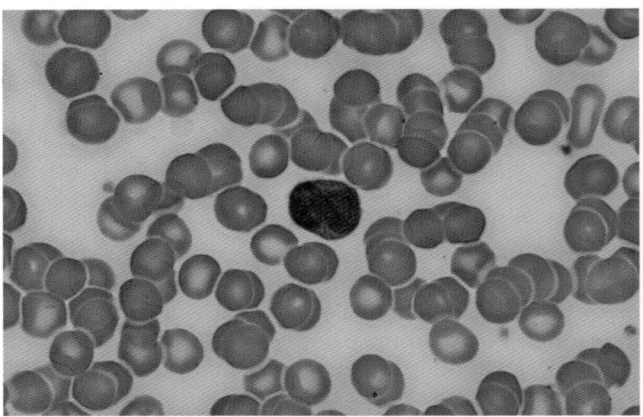

**FIGURE 43–39.** A binucleated peripheral blood lymphocyte in a woman with polyclonal B cell lymphocytosis.

be seen with bacterial infections. The reactive cells are usually CD8+ T cells and are large with abundant cytoplasm. In children, a reactive lymphocytosis with cleaved and irregular T lymphocyte nuclei may be seen with *Bordetella pertussis* infection.[449] Transient T cell lymphocytosis may also occur with trauma, acute cardiac disease, and epinephrine administration.[450, 451]

B cell lymphocytosis is less common than T cell lymphocytosis. Persistent polyclonal B lymphocytosis occurs most frequently in young and middle-aged female patients and is associated with smoking, elevated serum immunoglobulin M, and presence of the HLA-DR7 antigen.[452, 453] The patients have a persistent lymphocytosis, usually between 4000 and 14,000/mm$^3$, with binucleated peripheral blood lymphocytes. Lymphocytosis in the bone marrow may include bilobed lymphocytes (Fig. 43–39), and nodular lymphoid aggregates may be present. The polyclonal B cells are positive for CD19/CD20/CD22, do not usually express CD5, and are FMC7 positive. The chromosome abnormality i(3q) is reported in a majority of patients, but the clinical course is benign. Immunoglobulin heavy chain gene rearrangements are not detected in these cases. Rare cases of CD5+ reactive B lymphocytosis have also been described.[454]

## MEGAKARYOCYTIC HYPERPLASIAS

Non-neoplastic megakaryocytic hyperplasias are associated with either thrombocytopenia or thrombocytosis. Thrombocytopenia-associated megakaryocytic hyperplasia is usually caused by an autoimmune disorder, particularly idiopathic (or immune) thrombocytopenic purpura. The bone marrow in these cases shows an increased number of normal-appearing megakaryocytes; however, small, more immature megakaryocytes may also be present.

Non-neoplastic megakaryocytic hyperplasia associated with thrombocytosis may occur with chronic infections, in the recovery phase of acute infections, with collagen-vascular disease, with hemolytic anemias, with iron deficiency anemia, and in association with malignant neoplasms. A rebound thrombocytosis may occur after recovery from thrombocytopenia and after splenectomy. Reactive thrombocytosis must be differentiated from the chronic myeloproliferative disorders, particularly essential thrombocythemia. Reactive thrombocytosis rarely demonstrates a platelet count as high as 1,000,000/mm³, and the atypical megakaryocytes of the chronic myeloproliferative disorders are usually not present in reactive conditions. Even when the platelet count exceeds 1,000,000/mm³ in reactive conditions, the number of bone marrow megakaryocytes is less than that usually seen in chronic myeloproliferative disorders with high platelet counts.[455]

## HYPERPLASIAS RELATED TO GROWTH FACTORS

Bone marrow hyperplasia related to growth factor administration is most often related to erythropoietin, granulocyte colony-stimulating factor (G-CSF), and granulocyte-macrophage colony-stimulating factor (GM-CSF).[456] Administration of growth factor should always be documented in the clinical information for bone marrow specimens. The erythroid hyperplasia caused by erythropoietin does not usually cause diagnostic dilemmas. However, some difficulty may be encountered when changes related to G-CSF or GM-CSF are not recognized. These factors usually result in peripheral blood neutrophilia, but leukoerythroblastosis, monocytosis, or eosinophilia may occur. Toxic granulation of neutrophils with Döhle bodies may mimic an infectious leukocytosis. The bone marrow may demonstrate a granulocyte hyperplasia with a left-shift that may range from a hypocellular marrow with aggregates of left-shifted immature cells, mimicking a hypocellular acute leukemia, to a hypercellular marrow with granulocytic hyperplasia, mimicking a chronic myeloproliferative disorder or maturation arrest (Fig. 43–40).

Although granulocyte maturation occurs over time after growth factor administration, a single marrow specimen may demonstrate a predominance of immature myeloid cells, usually at the promyelocyte and myelocyte stages of differentiation. These findings may suggest a diagnosis of *de novo* acute promyelocytic leukemia or of relapsed AML. The promyelocytes in these specimens are usually large with a prominent perinuclear hof, do not contain Auer rods, and are not associated with increased numbers of myeloblasts. A predominance of such cells in a specimen should raise the suspicion of G-CSF or GM-CSF therapy. Even when a history of growth factor therapy is known in a patient with a history of AML, the differential diagnosis between relapse and growth factor effect may be difficult. In such cases, immunophenotyping studies to identify an aberrant phenotype characteristic of the patient's original leukemia may help, as may cytogenetic studies to identify a leukemic clone. Alternatively, an aspirate specimen may be obtained several days after the growth factor is stopped to see whether the immature cell population has disappeared (loss of growth factor effect) or increased (relapsed leukemia effect). Patients receiving megakaryocytic growth factors are less likely to undergo bone marrow biopsy after therapy, but these agents result in a proliferation of megakaryocyte precursors.[457]

## Other Non-Neoplastic Marrow Changes

### FIBROSIS

Fibrosis of the bone marrow may occur in association with a variety of neoplastic and non-neoplastic conditions, but it is a nonclonal proliferation of fibroblasts.[458] Fibrosis is usually of the reticulin type, as detected by silver stains, in the early stages, but it may progress to a collagen fibrosis that is detectable by trichrome stains. Reticulin fibrosis of the bone marrow is normally absent or minimal but increases

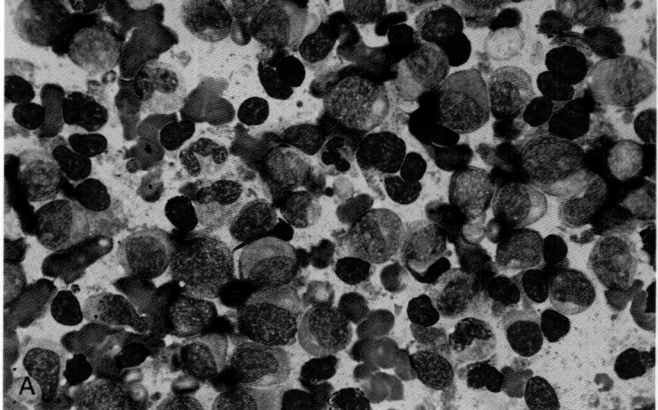 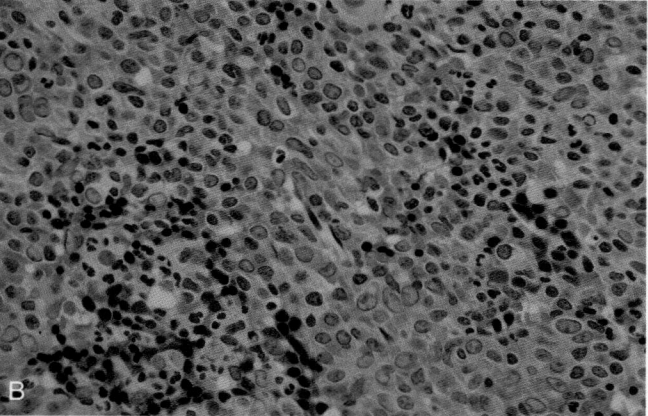

**FIGURE 43–40.** Growth factor administration may cause a marked granulocyte predominance and left-shift on the bone marrow aspirate smear *(A)* and biopsy specimen *(B)* that may be mistaken for residual acute leukemia or a chronic myeloproliferative disorder if growth factor administration is not suspected.

**TABLE 43–19.** Conditions Associated with Bone Marrow Fibrosis

---

Fibrosis associated with malignant neoplasms*
  Myelofibrosis with myeloid metaplasia
  Other chronic myeloproliferative disorders
  Acute megakaryoblastic leukemia
  Other acute myeloid leukemias
  Acute lymphoblastic leukemia
  Hairy cell leukemia
  Mast cell disease
  Malignant lymphoma, particularly of follicular center
    cell origin
  Hodgkin's disease
  Carcinoma

Fibrosis associated with non-neoplastic conditions
  Renal osteodystrophy
  Primary hyperparathyroidism
  Hypoparathyroidism
  Vitamin D deficiency

---

  * Fibrosis may be present even in the absence of marrow involvement by the neoplasm.

slightly with age.[459] Extensive marrow fibrosis typically causes an erythroblastosis of the peripheral blood that is characterized by a left-shift of granulocytes, enlarged platelets, teardrop-shaped red blood cells, and nucleated red blood cells. Diffuse fibrosis usually results in the inability to aspirate marrow particles. Bone marrow fibrosis is common in chronic myeloproliferative disorders, and extensive fibrosis with peripheral blood erythroblastosis is typical of myelofibrosis with myeloid metaplasia. Many other neoplasms involving the marrow, including some acute leukemias, malignant lymphomas, and metastatic tumors, result in focal or diffuse marrow fibrosis (Table 43–19).

Marrow fibrosis may also be associated with non-neoplastic conditions, especially inflammatory or reparative changes and metabolic disorders. Renal osteodystrophy and primary hyperparathyroidism cause extensive marrow fibrosis with a relative decrease in normal marrow elements (Fig. 43–41). Extensive bone remodeling with abundant osteo-

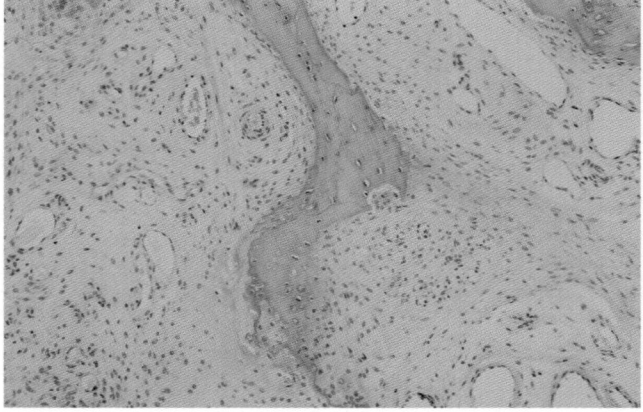

**FIGURE 43–41.** Prominent osteoblast proliferation and bone marrow fibrosis in a patient with primary hyperparathyroidism.

blasts is also common, and multinucleated giant cells may be present. Because bone marrow fibrosis is a reactive proliferation of fibroblasts triggered by growth factor production of neoplastic cells or hormonal changes related to metabolic disease, treatment of the underlying disease process usually resolves the fibrosis.

### NECROSIS

Bone marrow necrosis is an expected finding after chemotherapy for hematopoietic tumors, and early post-therapy bone marrow specimens may be acellular with only fibrinous, eosinophilic necrotic material present. With time, regenerative changes are admixed with the fibrinous necrosis. Other forms of bone marrow necrosis that are not treatment related are uncommon,[460, 461] but they are generally assumed to be associated with infarction or related to infectious diseases, such as necrotizing granulomas of tuberculosis. Zonal areas of tumor necrosis with ghosts of tumor cell nuclei may be seen in bone marrow of patients with sickle cell crisis; with hematopoietic malignant neoplasms, such as acute leukemia or malignant lymphoma; or adjacent to areas of viable metastatic tumor, even before chemotherapy. On smears, necrotic cells are smudged without clear cell borders and are difficult to further classify. With extensive bone marrow necrosis, patients may have bone pain and fever.

### ABNORMALITIES OF BONE TRABECULAE

The bone trabeculae should be evaluated in all bone marrow biopsy specimens, even when other abnormalities are apparent in the specimen.[462] Thinning of the trabeculae, usually due to osteoporosis, is the most common abnormality identified. Thickened trabeculae may be seen in association with metabolic disorders or neoplasia. The thickened bone of Paget's disease is associated with an increase in both osteoclasts and osteoblasts. The increase in osteoblasts with associated bone resorption and scalloping is seen more commonly in Paget's disease than in myelofibrosis with myeloid metaplasia, another relatively common cause of thickened bone trabeculae, and marrow fibrosis of myelofibrosis is usually not a prominent feature of Paget's disease. Osteosclerotic lesions may also be seen with mast cell disease, multiple myeloma (as part of the POEMS syndrome), metastatic carcinoma, renal failure, and osteopetrosis and at fracture sites, including sites of previous marrow biopsy.

## THE BONE MARROW REPORT

Table 43–20 lists the suggested elements to include in the bone marrow report. Many elements of the report, as well as which tests are performed, are determined by the initial morphologic findings and clinical situation; therefore, the clinical indication for the bone marrow examination should be included. Available complete blood cell count data should also

**TABLE 43–20. Contents of the Final Report: Bone Marrow**

Clinical information
Peripheral blood examination
  Complete blood count data
  Red blood cell changes
    Red blood cell number and size
    Hypochromasia, if present
    Description of anisocytosis and poikilocytosis and description or granules of inclusions, if present
    Presence of increased polychromasia, if present
  White blood cell changes
    White blood cell number
    Description of cell types with relative hyperplasias, cytopenias, or left-shift
    Description of dysplastic or toxic changes
    Presence or absence of blast cells, atypical or neoplastic lymphoid cells, or other abnormal cell populations
  Platelet changes
    Platelet number
    Platelet morphology, including granulation and size
Bone marrow aspirate smear or imprint
  Red blood cell precursors
    Relative percentage
    Normal maturation versus left-shift
    Dyplastic changes
  Granulocyte precursors
    Relative percentage
    Normal maturation versus left-shift
    Dysplastic changes
    Percentage of blasts and description of blasts if elevated
  Megakaryocytes
    Relative number
    Description of morphology, including size and nuclear features
  Description of other cell types including elevations of lymphocytes, plasma cells, monocytes, mast cells, eosinophils, and basophils
  Differential cell count, if indicated
Bone marrow trephine or clot biopsy
  Marrow cellularity, including percentage and comparison to normal cellularity for age

Proportions of myeloid to erythroid cells
Relative number of megakaryocytes
Features of bone trabeculae
Degree of fibrosis, if present
Abnormal cellular infiltrates, including granulomas, lymphoid cell infiltrates, plasma cells, and metastatic tumor
  Percentage of marrow involvement
  Location and pattern (particularly neoplastic lymphoid infiltrates)
  Cell type (lymphoma cell type or differentiation of plasma cell infiltrate)
Cytochemistry results, if indicated
  Iron stain results for reticuloendothelial stores and red blood cell incorporation, including presence and percentage of ringed sideroblasts
  Cytochemical studies for acute leukemia or hairy cell leukemia, including stains performed and results
Immunophenotyping results, if indicated
  Method used (e.g., flow cytometry, immunocytochemistry, immunohistochemistry)
  Antibodies and antigens studied
  Cell population studied (e.g., blast cells, lymphoid cells, plasma cells)
  Specimen type studied (peripheral blood, bone marrow aspirate, bone marrow biopsy)
  Results for each antibody and antigen and interpretation of total findings
Molecular genetic and cytogenetic studies, if indicated
  Method used (e.g., karyotype analysis, polymerase chain reaction, Southern blot, fluorescence in situ hybridization)
  Test performed (e.g., *BCR/ABL,* immunoglobulin heavy chain gene rearrangements)
  Interpretation of results
Diagnosis
  Tissue examined
  Diagnostic interpretation, incorporating all results
  Classification system used clearly indicated in the diagnosis

be included as well as review of the peripheral blood smear.

The bone marrow aspirate and biopsy examinations describe the three main cell lines of the marrow and, as appropriate, other abnormal cellular elements. In the case of infiltrative lesions in the marrow, the cell type and percentage of involvement are included. Results of all ancillary studies are ideally included in the final report and correlated with the final diagnosis. This may require amending the report when studies are sent out to other laboratories or adding results that are not available at the time of the initial report, such as molecular genetic or cytogenetic results. This approach allows a single report that clearly interprets all available data and addresses all findings, including seemingly contradictory data that may be easily explained when all of the information is considered together.

## REFERENCES

1. Foucar K: Bone marrow examination techniques. *In* Bone Marrow Pathology. Chicago, ASCP Press, 1995, pp 25–36.
2. Brynes RK, McKenna RW, Sundberg RD: Bone marrow aspiration and trephine biopsy. An approach to a thorough study. Am J Clin Pathol 70:753–759, 1978.
3. Hyun BH, Gulati GL, Ashton JK: Bone marrow examination: techniques and interpretation. Hematol Oncol Clin North Am 2:513–523, 1988.
4. Brunning, RD, McKenna, RW: Appendix: bone marrow specimen processing. *In* Tumors of the Bone Marrow. Atlas of Tumor Pathology. Third Series, Fascicle 9. Washington, DC, Armed Forces Institute of Pathology, 1994, pp 475–489.
5. Perkins SL: Examination of the blood and bone marrow. *In* Lee GR, Foerster J, Lukens J, et al (eds): Wintrobe's Clinical Hematology. 10th ed. Baltimore, Williams & Wilkins, 1999, pp 9–35.
6. James LP, Stass SA, Schumacher HR: Value of imprint preparations of bone marrow biopsies in hematologic diagnosis. Cancer 46:173–177, 1980.
7. Arber DA, Johnson RM, Rainer PA, et al: The bone marrow agar section: a morphologic and immunohistochemical evaluation. Mod Pathol 6:592–598, 1993.
8. Wang J, Weiss LM, Chang KL, et al: Diagnostic utility of bilateral bone marrow examination—significance of morphologic and ancillary technique study in malignancy. Cancer 94:1522–1531, 2002.
9. Brown DC, Gatter KC: The bone marrow trephine biopsy: a review of normal histology. Histopathology 22:411–422, 1993.
10. Bain BJ: The bone marrow aspirate of healthy subjects. Br J Haematol 94:206–209, 1996.
11. Fong TP, Okafor LA, Schmitz TH, et al: An evaluation of

cellularity in various types of bone marrow specimens. Am J Clin Pathol 72:812–816, 1979.

12. Gruppo RA, Lampkin BC, Granger S: Bone marrow cellularity determination: comparison of the biopsy, aspirate, and buffy coat. Blood 49:29–31, 1977.

13. Hartsock RJ, Smith EB, Petty CS: Normal variations with aging of the amount of hematopoietic tissue in bone marrow from the anterior iliac crest. A study made from 177 cases of sudden death examined by necropsy. Am J Clin Pathol 43:326–331, 1965.

14. Longacre TA, Foucar K, Crago S, et al: Hematogones: a multiparameter analysis of bone marrow precursor cells. Blood 73:544–552, 1989.

15. Scott CS, Den Ottolander GJ, Swirsky D, et al: Recommended procedures for the classification of acute leukaemias. Leuk Lymphoma 11:37–49, 1993.

16. Sundberg RD, Broman H: The application of the Prussian blue stain to previously stained films of blood and bone marrow. Blood 10:160–166, 1955.

17. Fong TP, Okafor LA, Thomas W Jr, et al: Stainable iron in aspirated and needle-biopsy specimens of marrow: a source of error. Am J Hematol 2:47–51, 1977.

18. Gale E, Torrance J, Bothwell T: The quantitative estimation of total iron stores in human bone marrow. J Clin Invest 42:1076–1082, 1963.

19. Yam LT, Li CY, Lam KW: Tartrate-resistant acid phosphatase isoenzyme in the reticulum cells of leukemic reticuloendotheliosis. N Engl J Med 284:357–360, 1971.

20. Rothe G, Schmitz G: Consensus protocol for the flow cytometric immunophenotyping of hematopoietic malignancies. Leukemia 10:877–895, 1996.

21. Stelzer GT, Marti G, Hurley A, et al: U.S.-Canadian consensus recommendations on the immunophenotypic analysis of hematologic neoplasia by flow cytometry: standardization and validation of laboratory procedures. Cytometry 30:214–230, 1997.

22. Stewart CC, Behm FG, Carey JL, et al: U.S.-Canadian consensus recommendations on the immunophenotypic analysis of hematologic neoplasia by flow cytometry: selection of antibody combinations. Cytometry 30:231–235, 1997.

23. Borowitz MJ, Bray R, Gascoyne R, et al: U.S.-Canadian consensus recommendations on the immunophenotypic analysis of hematologic neoplasia by flow cytometry: data analysis and interpretation. Cytometry 30:236–244, 1997.

24. Braylan RC, Atwater SK, Diamond L, et al: U.S.-Canadian consensus recommendations on the immunophenotyic analysis of hematologic neoplasia by flow cytometry: data reporting. Cytometry 30:245–248, 1997.

25. Davis BH, Foucar K, Szczarkowski W, et al: U.S.-Canadian consensus recommendations on the immunophenotypic analysis of hematologic neoplasia by flow cytometry: medical indications. Cytometry 30:249–263, 1997.

26. Jennings CD, Foon KA: Recent advances in flow cytometry: application to the diagnosis of hematologic malignancy. Blood 90:2863–2892, 1997.

27. Borowitz MJ, Guenther KL, Shults KE, et al: Immunophenotyping of acute leukemia by flow cytometric analysis. Use of CD45 and right-angle light scatter to gate on leukemic blasts in three-color analysis. Am J Clin Pathol 100:534–540, 1993.

28. Arber DA, Jenkins KA: Paraffin section immunophenotyping of acute leukemias in bone marrow specimens. Am J Clin Pathol 106:462–468, 1996.

29. Loyson SAJ, Rademakers LHPM, Joling P, et al: Immunohistochemical analysis of decalcified paraffin-embedded human bone marrow biopsies with emphasis on MHC class I and CD34 expression. Histopathology 31:412–419, 1997.

30. Pileri SA, Ascani S, Milani M, et al: Acute leukaemia immunophenotyping in bone-marrow routine sections. Br J Haematol 105:394–401, 1999.

31. Strout MP, Caligiuri MA: Developments in cytogenetics and oncogenes in acute leukemia. Curr Opin Oncol 9:8–17, 1997.

32. Sawyers CL: Molecular genetics of acute leukaemia. Lancet 349:196–200, 1997.

33. Downing JR: The AML1-ETO chimaeric transcription factor in acute myeloid leukaemia: biology and clinical significance. Br J Haematol 106:296–308, 1999.

34. DiMartino JF, Cleary ML: MLL rearrangements in haematological malignancies: lessons from clincal and biological studies. Br J Haematol 106:614–624, 1999.

35. Liu Yin JA, Tobal K: Detection of minimal residual disease in acute myeloid leukaemia: methodologies, clinical and biological significance. Br J Haematol 106:578–590, 1999.

36. Bennett JM, Catovsky D, Daniel MT, et al: Proposals for the classification of the acute leukaemias. French-American-British (FAB) co-operative group. Br J Haematol 33:451–458, 1976.

37. Bennett JM, Catovsky D, Daniel MT, et al: Proposals for the classification of the myelodysplastic syndromes. Br J Haematol 51:189–199, 1982.

38. Bennett JM, Catovsky D, Daniel MT, et al: Proposed revised criteria for the classification of acute myeloid leukemia. A report of the French-American-British Cooperative Group. Ann Intern Med 103:626–629, 1985.

39. Bennett JM, Catovsky D, Daniel M-T, et al: Criteria for the diagnosis of acute leukemia of megakaryocytic lineage (M7). A report of the French-American-British Cooperative Group. Ann Intern Med 103:460–462, 1985.

40. Bennett JM, Catovsky D, Daniel M-T, et al: Proposal for the recognition of minimally differentiated acute myeloid leukaemia (AML-M0). Br J Haematol 78:325–329, 1991.

41. Vardiman JW, Head D: Society for Hematopathology: the myelodysplastic syndromes (MDS) and related disorders. Mod Pathol 12:101–106, 1999.

42. Jaffe ES, Harris NL, Stein H, Vardiman JW (eds): World Health Organization Classification of Tumours. Pathology and Genetics of Tumours of Haematopoietic and Lymphoid Tissues. Lyon, IARC Press, 2001.

43. Estey E, Thall P, Beran M, et al: Effect of diagnosis (refractory anemia with excess blasts, refractory anemia with excess blasts in transformation, or acute myeloid leukemia [AML]) on outcome of AML-type chemotherapy. Blood 90:2969–2977, 1997.

44. Heaney ML, Golde DW: Myelodysplasia. N Engl J Med 340:1649–1660, 1999.

45. Hast R, Nilsson I, Widell S, et al: Diagnostic significance of dysplastic features of peripheral blood polymorphs in myelodysplastic syndromes. Leuk Res 13:173–178, 1989.

46. De Wolf–Peeters C, Stessens R, Desmet V, et al: The histological characterization of ALIP in the myelodysplastic syndromes. Pathol Res Pract 181:402–407, 1986.

47. Orazi A, Cattoretti G, Solligo D, et al: Therapy-related myelodysplastic syndromes: FAB classification, bone marrow histology, and immunohistology in the prognostic assessment. Leukemia 7:838–847, 1993.

48. Pagliuca A, Layton DM, Manoharan A, et al: Myelofibrosis in primary myelodysplastic syndromes: a clinico-morphological study of 10 cases. Br J Haematol 71:499–504, 1989.

49. Lambertenghi-Deliliers G, Orazi A, Luksch R, et al: Myelodysplastic syndrome with increased marrow fibrosis: a distinct clinico-pathological entity. Br J Haematol 78:161–166, 1991.

50. Ohyashiki K, Sasao I, Ohyashiki JH, et al: Cytogenetic and clinical findings of myelodysplastic syndromes with a poor prognosis. Cancer 70:94–99, 1992.

51. Fenaux P, Morel P, Lai J-L: Cytogenetics of myelodysplastic syndromes. Semin Hematol 33:127–138, 1996.

52. Verhoef GEG, Boogaerts MA: Cytogenetics and its prognostic value in myelodysplastic syndromes. Acta Haematol 95:95–101, 1996.

53. Mecucci C: Molecular features of primary MDS with cytogenetics changes. Leuk Res 22:293–302, 1998.

54. Koc S, Harris JW: Sideroblastic anemias: variations on imprecision in diagnostic criteria, proposal for an extended classification of sideroblastic anemias. Am J Hematol 57:1–6, 1998.

55. Bridges KR: Sideroblastic anemia: a mitochondrial disorder. J Pediatr Hematol Oncol 19:274–278, 1997.

56. May A, Fitzsimons EJ: Sideroblastic anaemia. Baillieres Clin Haematol 7:851–878, 1994.

57. Fitzsimons EJ, May A: The molecular basis of the sideroblastic anemias. Curr Opin Hematol 3:167–172, 1996.

58. Garand R, Gardais J, Bizet M, et al: Heterogeneity of acquired idiopathic sideroblastic anaemia (AISA). Leuk Res 16:463–468, 1992.
59. Van den Berghe H, Cassiman J-J, David G, et al: Distinct haematological disorder with deletion of long arm of no. 5 chromosome. Nature 251:437–438, 1974.
60. Boultwood J, Lewis SWJS: The 5q− syndrome. Blood 84:3253–3260, 1994.
61. Lewis S, Oscier D, Boultwood J, et al: Hematological features of patients with myelodysplastic syndromes associated with a chromosome 5q deletion. Am J Hematol 49:194–200, 1995.
62. Rosati S, Mick R, Xu F, et al: Refractory cytopenia with multilineage dysplasia: further characterization of an 'unclassifiable' myelodysplastic syndrome. Leukemia 10:20–26, 1996.
63. Matsuda A, Jinnai I, Yagaski F, et al: Refractory anemia with severe dysplasia: clinical significance of morphological features in refractory anemia. Leukemia 12:482–485, 1998.
64. Seymour JF, Estey EH: The prognostic significance of Auer rods in myelodysplasia. Br J Haematol 85:67–76, 1993.
65. Lai J-L, Preudhomme C, Zandecki M, et al: Myelodysplastic syndromes and acute myeloid leukemia with 17p deletion. An entity characterized by specific dysgranulopoiesis and a high incidence of p53 mutations. Leukemia 9:370–381, 1995.
66. Sugimoto K, Hirano N, Toyoshima H, et al: Mutations of the p53 gene in myelodysplastic syndrome (MDS) and MDS-derived leukemia. Blood 81:3022–3026, 1993.
67. Tuzuner N, Cox C, Rowe JM, et al: Hypocellular myelodysplastic syndromes (MDS): new proposals. Br J Haematol 91:612–617, 1995.
68. Goyal R, Qawi H, Ali I, et al: Biologic characteristics of patients with hypocellular myelodysplastic syndromes. Leuk Res 23:357–364, 1999.
69. Pui C-H, Behm FG, Raimondi SC, et al: Secondary acute myeloid leukemia in children treated for acute lymphoid leukemia. N Engl J Med 321:136–142, 1989.
70. Neugut AI, Robinson E, Nieves J, et al: Poor survival of treatment-related acute nonlymphocytic leukemia. JAMA 264:1006–1008, 1990.
71. Pedersen-Bjergaard J, Daugaard G, Hansen SW, et al: Increased risk of myelodysplasia and leukaemia after etoposide, cisplatin, and bleomycin for germ-cell tumours. Lancet 338:359–363, 1991.
72. Miller JS, Arthur DC, Litz CE, et al: Myelodysplastic syndrome after autologous bone marrow transplantation: An additional late complication of curative cancer therapy. Blood 83:3780–3786, 1994.
73. Darrington DL, Vose JM, Anderson JR, et al: Incidence and characterization of secondary myelodysplastic syndrome and acute myelogenous leukemia following high-dose chemoradiotherapy and autologous stem-cell transplantation for lymphoid malignancies. J Clin Oncol 12:2527–2534, 1994.
74. Pui C-H, Ribeiro RC, Hancock ML, et al: Acute myeloid leukemia in children treated with epipodophyllotoxins for acute lymphoblastic leukemia. N Engl J Med 325:1682–1687, 1991.
75. Sterkers Y, Preudhomme C, Lai J-L, et al: Acute myeloid leukemia and myelodysplastic syndromes following essential thrombocythemia treated with hydroxyurea: high proportion of cases with 17p deletion. Blood 91:616–622, 1998.
76. Merlat A, Lai J-L, Sterkers Y, et al: Therapy-related myelodysplastic syndrome and acute myeloid leukemia with 17p deletion. A report on 25 cases. Leukemia 13:250–257, 1999.
77. Pfeilstöcker M, Reisner R, Nösslinger T, et al: Cross-validation of prognostic scores in myelodysplastic syndromes on 386 patients from a single institution confirms importance of cytogenetics. Br J Haematol 106:455–463, 1999.
78. Aul C, Gattermann N, Heyll A, et al: Primary myelodysplastic syndromes: analysis of prognostic factors in 235 patients and proposals for an improved scoring system. Leukemia 6:52–59, 1992.
79. Morel P, Hebbar M, Lai J-L, et al: Cytogenetic analysis has strong independent prognostic value in de novo myelodysplastic syndromes and can be incorporated in a new scoring system: a report on 408 cases. Leukemia 7:1315–1323, 1993.
80. Greenberg P, Cox C, LeBeau M, et al: International scoring system for evaluating prognosis in myelodysplastic syndromes. Blood 89:2079–2088, 1997.
81. Oertel J, Kleiner S, Huhn D: Immunotyping of blasts in refractory anaemia with excess of blasts. Br J Haematol 84:305–309, 1993.
82. Oriani A, Annaloro C, Soligo D, et al: Bone marrow histology and CD34 immunostaining in the prognostic evaluation of primary myelodysplastic syndromes. Br J Haematol 92:360–364, 1996.
83. Second MIC Cooperative Study Group: Morphologic, immunologic, and cytogenetic (MIC) working classification of the acute myeloid leukemias. Report of the Workshop held in Leuven, Belgium, September 15–17, 1986. Cancer Genet Cytogenet 30:1–15, 1988.
84. Barnard DR, Kalousek DK, Wiersma SR, et al: Morphologic, immunologic, and cytogenetic classification of acute myeloid leukemia and myelodysplastic syndrome in childhood: a report from the Childrens Cancer Group. Leukemia 10:5–12, 1996.
85. Head DR: Revised classification of acute myeloid leukemia. Leukemia 10:1826–1831, 1996.
86. Fenaux P, Preudhomme C, Lai JL, et al: Cytogenetics and their prognostic value in de novo acute myeloid leukaemia: report on 283 cases. Br J Haematol 73:61–67, 1989.
87. Dastugue N, Payen C, Lafage-Pochitaloff M, et al: Prognostic significance of karyotype in de novo adult acute myeloid leukemia. Leukemia 9:1491–1498, 1995.
88. Bloomfield CD, Lawrence D, Byrd JC, et al: Frequency of prolonged remission duration after high-dose cytarabine intensification in acute myeloid leukemia varies by cytogenetic subtype. Cancer Res 58:4173–4179, 1998.
89. Grimwade D, Walker H, Oliver F, et al: The importance of diagnostic cytogenetics on outcome in AML: analysis of 1,612 patients entered into the MRC AML 10 trial. Blood 92:2322–2333, 1998.
90. Venditti A, Del Poeta G, Buccisano F, et al: Minimally differentiated acute myeloid leukemia (AML-M0): comparison of 25 cases with other French-American-British subtypes. Blood 89:621–629, 1997.
91. Villamor N, Zarco M-A, Rozman M, et al: Acute myeloblastic leukemia with minimal myeloid differentiation: phenotypical and ultrastructural characteristics. Leukemia 12:1071–1075, 1998.
92. Cohen PL, Hoyer JD, Kurtin PJ, et al: Acute myeloid leukemia with minimal differentiation. A multiparameter study. Am J Clin Pathol 109:32–38, 1998.
93. Nisson PE, Watkins PC, Sacchi N: Transcriptionally active chimeric gene derived from the fusion of the *AML1* gene and a novel gene on chromosme 8 in t(8;21) leukemic cells. Cancer Genet Cytogenet 63:81–88, 1992.
94. Nakamura H, Kuriyama K, Sadamori N, et al: Morphological subtyping of acute myeloid leukemia with maturation (AML-M2): homogeneous pink-colored cytoplasm of mature neutrophils is most characteristic of AML-M2 with t(8;21). Leukemia 11:651–655, 1997.
95. Kita K, Nakase K, Miwa H, et al: Phenotypical characteristics of acute myelocytic leukemia associated with the t(8;21)(q22;q22) chromosomal abnormality: frequent expression of immature B-cell antigen CD19 together with stem cell antigen CD34. Blood 80:470–477, 1992.
96. Hurwitz CA, Raimondi SC, Head D, et al: Distinctive immunophenotypic features of t(8;21)(q22;q22) acute myeloblastic leukemia in children. Blood 80:3182–3188, 1992.
97. Arber DA, Glackin C, Lowe G, et al: Presence of t(8;21)(q22;q22) in myeloperoxidase-positive, myeloid surface antigen–negative acute myeloid leukemia. Am J Clin Pathol 107:68–73, 1997.
98. Khalidi HS, Medeiros LJ, Chang KL, et al: The immunophenotype of adult acute myeloid leukemia: high frequency of lymphoid antigen expression and comparison of immunophenotype, French-American-British classification, and karyotypic abnormalities. Am J Clin Pathol 109:211–220, 1998.
99. Baer MR, Stewart CC, Lawrence D, et al: Expression of the neural cell adhesion molecule CD56 is associated with short

remission duration and survival in acute myeloid leukemia with t(8;21)(q22;q22). Blood 90:1644–1648, 1997.

100. Downing JR, Head DR, Curcio-Brint AM, et al: An *AML/ETO* fusion transcript is consistently detected by RNA-based polymerase chain reaction in acute myelogenous leukemia containing the (8;21)(q22;q22) translocation. Blood 81:2860–2865, 1993.

101. Jurlander J, Caligiuri MA, Ruutu T, et al: Persistence of the *AML1/ETO* fusion transcript in patients treated with allogeneic bone marrow transplantation for t(8;21) leukemia. Blood 88:2183–2191, 1996.

102. Alsabeh R, Brynes RK, Slovak ML, et al: Acute myeloid leukemia with t(6;9) (p23;q34). Association with myelodysplasia, basophilia, and initial CD34 negative immunophenotype. Am J Clin Pathol 107:430–437, 1997.

103. Lo Coco F, Nervi C, Avvisati G, et al: Acute promyelocytic leukemia: a curable disease. Leukemia 12:1866–1880, 1998.

104. Tallman MS, Andersen JW, Schiffer CA, et al: All-*trans*-retinoic acid in acute promyelocytic leukemia. N Engl J Med 337:1021–1028, 1997.

105. McKenna RW, Parkin J, Bloomfield CD, et al: Acute promyelocytic leukaemia: a study of 39 cases with identification of a hyperbasophilic microgranular variant. Br J Haematol 50:201–214, 1982.

106. Neame PB, Soamboonsrup P, Leber B, et al: Morphology of acute promyelocytic leukemia with cytogenetic or molecular evidence for the diagnosis: characterization of additional microgranular variants. Am J Hematol 6:131–142, 1997.

107. Guglielmi C, Martelli MP, Diverio D, et al: Immunophenotype of adult and childhood acute promyelocytic leukaemia: correlation with morphology, type of PML gene breakpoint and clinical outcome. A cooperative Italian study on 196 cases. Br J Haematol 102:1035–1041, 1998.

108. Melnick A, Licht JD: Deconstructing a disease: RARα, its fusion partners, and their roles in the pathogenesis of acute promyelocytic leukemia. Blood 93:3167–3215, 1999.

109. Grimwade D: The pathogenesis of acute promyelocytic leukaemia: evaluation of the role of molecular diagnosis and monitoring in the management of the disease. Br J Haematol 106:591–613, 1999.

110. Miller Jr WH, Kakizuka A, Frankel SR, et al: Reverse transcription polymerase chain reaction for the rearranged retinoic acid receptor α clarifies diagnosis and detects minimal residual disease in acute promyelocytic leukemia. Proc Natl Acad Sci USA 89:2694–2698, 1992.

111. Miller WH, Levine K, DeBlasio A, et al: Detection of minimal residual disease in acute promyelocytic leukemia by a reverse transcription polymerase chain reaction assay for the PML/RAR-alpha fusion mRNA. Blood 82:1689–1694, 1993.

112. Lo Coco F, Diverio D, Falini B, et al: Genetic diagnosis and molecular monitoring in the management of acute promyelocytic leukemia. Blood 94:12–22, 1999.

113. Tobelem G, Jacquillat C, Chastang C, et al: Acute monoblastic leukemia: a clinical and biologic study of 74 cases. Blood 55:71–76, 1980.

114. Scott CS, Stark AN, Limbert HJ, et al: Diagnostic and prognostic factors in acute monocytic leukaemia: an analysis of 51 cases. Br J Haematol 69:247–252, 1988.

115. LeBeau MM, Larson RA, Bitter MA, et al: Association of an inversion of chromosome 16 and abnormal marrow eosinophils in acute myelomonocytic leukemia. N Engl J Med 309:630–636, 1983.

116. Larson RA, Williams SF, LeBeau MM, et al: Acute myelomonocytic leukemia with abnormal eosinophils and inv(16) or t(16;16) has a favorable prognosis. Blood 68:1242–1249, 1986.

117. Liu PP, Hajra A, Wijmenga C, et al: Molecular pathogenesis of the chromosome 16 inversion in the M4Eo subtype of acute myeloid leukemia. Blood 85:2289–2302, 1995.

118. Baer MR, Stewart CC, Lawrence D, et al: Acute myeloid leukemia with 11q23 translocations: myelomonocytic immunophenotype by multiparameter flow cytometry. Leukemia 12:317–325, 1998.

119. Satake N, Maseki N, Nishiyama M, et al: Chromosome abnormalities and *MLL* rearrangements in acute myeloid leukemia of infants. Leukemia 13:1013–1017, 1999.

120. Mrozek K, Heinonen K, Lawrence D, et al: Adult patients with de novo acute myeloid leukemia and t(9;11)(p22;q23) have a superior outcome to patients with other translocations involving band 11q23: a Cancer and Leukemia Group B study. Blood 90:4532–4538, 1997.

121. Aplan PD, Chervinsky DS, Stanulla M, et al: Site-specific DNA cleavage within the MLL breakpoint cluster region induced by topoisomerase II inhibitors. Blood 87:2649–2658, 1996.

122. Schnittger S, Wörmann B, Hiddemann W, et al: Partial tandem duplications of the MLL gene are detectable in peripheral blood and bone marrow of nearly all healthy donors. Blood 92:1728–1734, 1998.

123. Hunger SP, Cleary ML: What significance should we attribute to the detection of MLL fusion transcripts? Blood 93:709–711, 1998.

124. Davey FR, Abraham N Jr, Brunetto VL, et al: Morphologic characteristics of erythroleukemia (acute myeloid leukemia; FAB-M6): a CALGB study. Am J Hematol 49:29–38, 1995.

125. Garand R, Duchayne E, Blanchard D, et al: Minimally differentiated erythroleukaemia (AML M6 'variant'): a rare subset of AML distinct from AML M6. Br J Haematol 90:868–875, 1995.

126. Olopade OI, Thangavelu M, Larson RA, et al: Clinical, morphologic, and cytogenetic characteristics of 26 patients with acute erythroblastic leukemia. Blood 80:2873–2882, 1992.

127. Ribeiro RC, Oliveira MSP, Dairclough D, et al: Acute megakaryoblastic leukemia in children and adolescents: a retrospective analysis of 24 cases. Leuk Lymphoma 10:299–306, 1993.

128. Gassmann W, Löffler H: Acute megakaryoblastic leukemia. Leuk Lymphoma 18(suppl 1):69–73, 1995.

129. Breton-Gorius J, Reyes F, Duhamel G, et al: Megakaryoblastic acute leukemia: identification by the ultrastructural demonstration of platelet peroxidase. Blood 51:45–60, 1978.

130. Helleberg C, Knudsen K, Hansen PB, et al: CD34⁺ megakaryoblastic leukaemic cells are CD38⁻, but CD61⁺ and glycophorin A⁺: improved criteria for diagnosis of AML-M7? Leukemia 11:830–834, 1997.

131. Linari S, Vannucchi AM, Ciolli S, et al: Coexpression of erythroid and megakaryocytic genes in acute erythroblastic (FAB M6) and megakaryoblastic (FAB M7) leukaemias. Br J Haematol 102:1335–1337, 1998.

132. Cuneo A, Mecucci C, Kerim S, et al: Multipotent stem cell involvement in megakaryoblastic leukemia: cytologic and cytogenetic evidence in 15 patients. Blood 74:1781–1790, 1989.

133. Lion T, Haas OA, Harbott J, et al: The translocation t(1;22)(p13;q13) is a nonrandom marker specifically associated with acute megakaryocytic leukemia in young children. Blood 79:3325–3330, 1992.

134. Chan WC, Carroll A, Alvarado CS, et al: Acute megakaryoblastic leukemia in infants with t(1;22)(p13;q13) abnormality. Am J Clin Pathol 98:214–221, 1992.

135. Lu G, Altman AJ, Benn PA: Review of the cytogenetic changes in acute megakaryoblastic leukemia: one disease or several? Cancer Genet Cytogenet 67:81–89, 1993.

136. Gahn B, Haase D, Unterhalt M, et al: De novo AML with dysplastic hematopoiesis: cytogenetic and prognostic significance. Leukemia 10:946–951, 1996.

137. Yumura-Yagi K, Hara J, Kurahashi H, et al: Mixed phenotype of blasts in acute megakaryocytic leukaemia and transient abnormal myelopoiesis in Down's syndrome. Br J Haematol 81:520–525, 1992.

138. Kurahashi H, Hara J, Yumura-Yagi K, et al: Transient abnormal myelopoiesis in Down's syndrome. Leuk Lymphoma 8:465–475, 1992.

139. Zipursky A, Brown EJ, Christensen A, et al: Transient myeloproliferative disorder (transient leukemia) and hematologic manifestations of Down syndrome. Clin Lab Med 19:157–167, 1999.

140. Cortes JE, Kantarjian HM: Acute lymphoblastic leukemia. A comprehensive review with emphasis on biology and therapy. Cancer 76:2393–2417, 1995.

141. Rubin CM, LeBeau MM, Mick R, et al: Impact of chromo-

somal translocations on prognosis in childhood acute lymphoblastic leukemia. J Clin Oncol 9:2183–2192, 1991.

142. Lilleyman JS, Hann IM, Stevens RF, et al: Cytomorphology of childhood lymphoblastic leukaemia: a prospective study of 2000 patients. Br J Haematol 81:52–57, 1992.

143. Bennett JM, Catovsky D, Daniel MT, et al: The morphologic classification of acute lymphoblastic leukaemia: concordance among observers and clinical correlations. Br J Haematol 47:553–561, 1981.

144. Bene MC, Castoldi G, Knapp W, et al: Proposal for the immunologic classification of acute leukemias. Leukemia 9:1783–1786, 1995.

145. Chessells JM, Swansbury GJ, Reeves B, et al: Cytogenetics and prognosis in childhood lymphoblastic leukaemia: results of MRC UKALL X. Br J Haematol 99:93–100, 1997.

146. Wetzler M, Dodge RK, Mrózek K, et al: Prospective karyotype analysis in adult acute lymphoblastic leukemia: the Cancer and Leukemia Group B experience. Blood 93:3983–3993, 1999.

147. Gassmann W, Löffler H, Thiel E, et al: Morphological and cytochemical findings in 150 cases of T-lineage acute lymphoblastic leukaemia in adults. Br J Haematol 97:372–382, 1997.

148. Uckun FM, Sensel MG, Sun L, et al: Biology and treatment of childhood T-lineage acute lymphoblastic leukaemia. Blood 91:735–746, 1998.

149. Dayton VD, Arthur DC, Gajl-Peczalska KJ, et al: L3 acute lymphoblastic leukemia. Comparison with small noncleaved cell lymphoma involving the bone marrow. Am J Clin Pathol 101:130–139, 1994.

150. Boucheix C, David B, Sebban C, et al: Immunophenotype of adult acute lymphoblastic leukemia, clinical parameters, and outcome: an analysis of a prospective trial including 562 tested patients (LALA87). Blood 84:1603–1612, 1994.

151. Khalidi HS, Chang KL, Medeiros LJ, et al: Acute lymphoblastic leukemia. Survey of immunophenotype, French-American-British classification, frequency of myeloid antigen expression, and karyotypic abnormalities in 210 pediatric and adult cases. Am J Clin Pathol 111:467–476, 1999.

152. Behm FG, Raimondi SC, Schell MJ, et al: Lack of CD45 antigen on blast cells in childhood acute lymphoblastic leukemia is associated with chromosomal hyperdiploidy and other favorable prognostic features. Blood 79:1011–1016, 1992.

153. Borowitz MJ, Shuster J, Carroll AJ, et al: Prognostic significance of fluorescence intensity of surface marker expression in childhood B-precursor acute lymphoblastic leukemia. A Pediatric Oncology Group study. Blood 89:3960–3966, 1997.

154. Vannier JP, Bene MC, Faure GC, et al: Investigation of the CD10 (cALLA) negative acute lymphoblastic leukaemia: further description of a group with a poor prognosis. Br J Haematol 72:156–160, 1989.

155. Basso G, Putti MC, Cantù-Rajnoldi A, et al: The immunophenotype in infant acute lymphoblastic leukaemia: correlation with clinical outcome. An Italian multicentre study (AIEOP). Br J Haematol 81:184–191, 1992.

156. Vasef MA, Brynes RK, Murata-Collins JL, et al: Surface immunoglobulin light chain–positive acute lymphoblastic leukemia of FAB L1 or L2 type. A report of 6 cases in adults. Am J Clin Pathol 110:144–149, 1998.

157. Czuczman MS, Dodge RK, Stewart CC, et al: Value of immunophenotype in intensively treated adult acute lymphoblastic leukemia: Cancer and Leukemia Group B study 8364. Blood 93:3931–3939, 1999.

158. Schenk TM, Keyhani A, Bottcher S, et al: Multilineage involvement of Philadelphia chromosome positive acute lymphoblastic leukemia. Leukemia 12:666–674, 1998.

159. Pui C-H, Behm FG, Downing JR, et al: 11q23/MLL rearrangement confers a poor prognosis in infants with acute lymphoblastic leukemia. J Clin Oncol 12:909–915, 1994.

160. Rubnitz JE, Behm FG, Pui C-H, et al: Genetic studies of childhood acute lymphoblastic leukemia with emphasis on p16, MLL, and ETV6 gene abnormalities: results of St. Jude Total Therapy Study XII. Leukemia 11:1201–1206, 1997.

161. Trueworthy R, Shuster J, Crist W, et al: Ploidy of lympho-blasts is the strongest predictor of treatment outcome in B-progenitor cell acute lymphoblastic leukemia of childhood: a Pediatric Oncology Group study. J Clin Oncol 10:606–613, 1992.

162. Ito C, Kumagai M, Manabe A, et al: Hyperdiploid acute lymphoblastic leukemia with 51 to 65 chromosomes: a distinct biological entity with a marked propensity to undergo apoptosis. Blood 93:315–320, 1999.

163. Pelicci P-G, Knowles DM II, Dalla Favera R: Lymphoid tumors displaying rearrangements of both immunoglobulin and T cell receptor genes. J Exp Med 162:1015–1024, 1985.

164. Cavé H, van der Werff ten Bosch J, Suciu S, et al: Clinical significance of minimal residual disease in childhood acute lymphoblastic leukemia. N Engl J Med 339:591–598, 1998.

165. Georgii A, Vykoupil K-F, Buhr T, et al: Chronic myeloproliferative disorders in bone marrow biopsies. Pathol Res Pract 186:3–27, 1990.

166. Sawyers CL: Chronic myeloid leukemia. N Engl J Med 340:1330–1340, 1999.

167. Faderl S, Talpaz M, Estrov Z, et al: The biology of chronic myeloid leukemia. N Engl J Med 341:164–172, 1999.

168. Melo JV: The molecular biology of chronic myeloid leukaemia. Leukemia 10(suppl 2):S4–S9, 1996.

169. Thiele J, Kvasnicka HM, Titius BR, et al: Histological features of prognostic significance in CML—an immunohistochemical and morphometric study (multivariate regression analysis) on trephine biopsies of the bone marrow. Ann Hematol 66:291–302, 1993.

170. Büsche G, Majewski H, Schlué J, et al: Frequency of pseudo-Gaucher cells in diagnostic bone marrow biopsies from patients with Ph-positive chronic myeloid leukaemia. Virchows Arch 430:139–148, 1997.

171. Arlin ZA, Silver RT, Bennett JM: Blastic phase of chronic myeloid leukemia (blCML): a proposal for standardization of diagnostic and response criteria. Leukemia 4:755–757, 1990.

172. Ross DW, Brunning RD, Kantarjian HM, et al: A proposed staging system for chronic myeloid leukemia. Cancer 71:3788–3791, 1993.

173. Khalidi HS, Brynes RK, Medeiros LJ, et al: The immunophenotype of blast transformation of chronic myelogenous leukemia: a high frequency of mixed lineage phenotype in "lymphoid" blasts and a comparison of morphologic, immunophenotypic, and molecular findings. Mod Pathol 11:1211–1221, 1998.

174. Cervantes F, Villamor N, Esteve J, et al: 'Lymphoid' blast crisis of chronic myeloid leukaemia is associated with distinct clinicohaematological features. Br J Haematol 100:123–128, 1998.

175. Facchetti F, Tironi A, Marocolo D, et al: Histopathological changes in bone marrow biopsies from patients with chronic myeloid leukaemia after treatment with recombinant alpha-interferon. Histopathology 31:3–11, 1997.

176. Pane F, Frigeri F, Sindona M, et al: Neutrophilic-chronic myeloid leukemia: a distinct disease with a specific molecular marker (BCR/ABL with C3/A2 junction). Blood 88:2410–2414, 1996.

177. Wiedemann LM, Karhi KK, Shivji MKK, et al: The correlation of breakpoint cluster region rearrangement and p210 phl/abl expression with morphological analysis of Ph-negative chronic myeloid leukemia and other myeloproliferative diseases. Blood 71:349–355, 1988.

178. Murphy S, Peterson P, Iland H, et al: Experience of the Polycythemia Vera Study Group with essential thrombocythemia: a final report on diagnostic criteria, survival, and leukemic transition by treatment. Semin Hematol 34:29–39, 1997.

179. Kutti J, Wadenvik H: Diagnostic and differential criteria of essential thrombocythemia and reactive thrombocytosis. Leuk Lymphoma 22(suppl 1):41–45, 1996.

180. Michiels JJ, Juvonen E: Proposal for revised diagnostic criteria of essential thrombocythemia and polycythemia vera by the Thrombocythemia Vera Study Group. Semin Thromb Hemost 23:339–347, 1997.

181. Harrison CN, Gale RE, Machin SJ, et al: A large proportion of patients with a diagnosis of essential thrombocythemia do

not have a clonal disorder and may be at lower risk of thrombotic complications. Blood 93:417–424, 1999.

182. Nimer SD: Essential thrombocythemia: another "heterogenous disease" better understood? Blood 93:415–416, 1999.

183. Thiele J, Schneider G, Hoeppner B, et al: Histomorphometry of bone marrow biopsies in chronic myeloproliferative disorders with associated thrombocytosis—features of significance for the diagnosis of primary (essential) thrombocythaemia. Virchows Arch A Pathol Anat 413:407–417, 1988.

184. Besses C, Cervantes F, Pereira A, et al: Major vascular complications in essential thrombocythemia: a study of the predictive factors in a series of 148 patients. Leukemia 13:150–154, 1999.

185. Mesa RA, Silverstein MN, Jacobsen SJ, et al: Population-based incidence and survival figures in essential thrombocythemia and agnogeneic myeloid metaplasia: an Olmsted county study, 1976–1995. Am J Hematol 61:10–15, 1999.

186. Hasselbalch H: Idiopathic myelofibrosis: a clinical study of 80 patients. Am J Hematol 34:291–300, 1990.

187. Thiele J, Kvasnicka H-M, Werden C, et al: Idiopathic primary osteo-myelofibrosis: a clinico-pathological study on 208 patients with special emphasis on evolution, differentiation from essential thrombocythemia and variable of prognostic impact. Leuk Lymphoma 22:303–317, 1996.

188. Manoharan A: Idiopathic myelofibrosis: a clinical review. Int J Hematol 68:355–362, 1998.

189. Barosi G, Ambrosetti A, Finelli C, et al: The Italian Consensus Conference on Diagnostic Criteria for Myelofibrosis with Myeloid Metaplasia. Br J Haematol 104:730–737, 1999.

190. Dupriez B, Morel P, Demory JL, et al: Prognostic factors in agnogenic myeloid metaplasia: a report of 195 cases with a new scoring system. Blood 88:1013–1018, 1996.

191. Reilly JT, Snowden JA, Spearing RL, et al: Cytogenetic abnormalities and their prognostic significance in idiopathic myelofibrosis: a study of 106 cases. Br J Haematol 98:96–102, 1997.

192. Gruppo Italiano Studio Policitemia: Polycythemia vera: the natural history of 1213 patients followed for 20 years. Ann Intern Med 123:656–664, 1995.

193. Murphy S: Diagnostic criteria and prognosis in polycythemia vera and essential thrombocythemia. Semin Hematol 36(suppl 2):9–13, 1999.

194. Berlin NI: Diagnosis and classification of the polycythemias. Semin Hematol 12:339–351, 1975.

195. Pearson TC, Messinezy M: The diagnostic criteria for polycythaemia rubra vera. Leuk Lymphoma 22:87–93, 1996.

196. Messinezy M, Pearson TC: Diagnosis of polycythaemia. J Clin Pathol 51:1–4, 1998.

197. Ellis JT, Peterson P, Geller SA, et al: Studies of the bone marrow in polycythemia vera and the evolution of myelofibrosis and second hematologic malignancies. Semin Hematol 23:144–155, 1986.

198. Diez-Martin JL, Graham DL, Pettit RM, et al: Chromosomes studies in 104 patients with polycythemia vera. Mayo Clin Proc 66:287–299, 1991.

199. Asimakopoulos FA, Gilbert JGR, Aldred MA, et al: Interstitial deletion constitutes the major mechanism for loss of heterozygosity on chromosome 20q in polycythemia vera. Blood 88:2690–2698, 1996.

200. Asimakopoulos FA, Green AR: Deletions of chromosome 20q and the pathogenesis of myeloproliferative disorders. Br J Haematol 95:219–226, 1996.

201. Prchal JF, Prchal JT: Molecular basis for polycythemia. Curr Opin Hematol 6:100–109, 1999.

202. Bain BJ: Eosinophilic leukemias and the idiopathic hypereosinophilic syndrome. Br J Haematol 95:2–9, 1996.

203. Chang H-W, Leong K-H, Koh D-R, et al: Clonality of isolated eosinophils in the hypereosinophilic syndrome. Blood 93:1651–1657, 1999.

204. Macdonald D, Aguiar RCT, Mason PJ, et al: A new myeloproliferative disorder associated with chromosmal translocations involving 8p11: a review. Leukemia 9:1628–1630, 1995.

205. Reiter A, Sohal J, Kulkarni S, et al: Consistent fusion of ZNF198 to the fibroblast growth factor receptor-1 in the (t8;13)(p11;q12) myeloproliferative syndrome. Blood 92:1735–1742, 1998.

206. Neuwirtová R, Mociková K, Musiolová J, et al: Mixed myelodysplastic and myeloproliferative syndromes. Leuk Res 20:717–726, 1996.

207. Oscier D: Atypical chronic myeloid leukemias. Pathol Biol (Paris) 45:587–593, 1997.

208. Bennett JM, Catovsky D, Daniel M-T, et al: The chronic myeloid leukaemias: guidelines for distinguishing chronic granulocytic, atypical chronic myeloid, and chronic myelomonocytic leukaemia. Proposals by the French-American-British cooperative leukaemia group. Br J Haematol 87:746–754, 1994.

209. Dobrovic A, Morley AA, Seshadri R, et al: Molecular diagnosis of Philadelphia negative CML using the polymerase chain reaction and DNA analysis: clinical features and course of M-bcr negative and M-bcr positive. Leukemia 5:187–190, 1991.

210. Oscier DG: Atypical chronic myeloid leukaemia, a distinct clinical entity related to the myelodysplastic syndrome? Br J Haematol 92:582–586, 1996.

211. Martiat P, Michaux J-L, Rodhain J: Philadelphia-negative (Ph⁻) chronic myeloid leukemia (CML): comparison with Ph⁺ CML and chronic myelomonocytic leukemia. Blood 78:205–211, 1991.

212. Germing U, Gattermann N, Minning H, et al: Problems in the classification of CMML—dysplastic versus proliferative type. Leuk Res 22:871–878, 1998.

213. Fenaux P, Beuscart R, Lai J-L, et al: Prognostic factors in adult chronic myelomonocytic leukemia: an analysis of 107 cases. J Clin Oncol 6:1417–1424, 1988.

214. Storniolo AM, Moloney WC, Rosenthal DS, et al: Chronic myelomonocytic leukemia. Leukemia 4:766–770, 1990.

215. Golub TR, Barker GF, Lovett M, et al: Fusion of PDGF receptor to a novel ets-like gene, tel, in chronic myelomonocytic leukemia with t(5;12) chromosomal translocation. Cell 77:307–316, 1994.

216. Sawyers CL, Denny CT: Chronic myelomonocytic leukemia: tel-a-kinase what ets all about. Cell 77:171–173, 1994.

217. Gilliland DG: Molecular genetics of human leukemia. Leukemia 12:S7–S12, 1998.

218. Passmore SJ, Hann IM, Stiller CA, et al: Pediatric myelodysplasia: a study of 68 children and a new prognostic scoring system. Blood 85:1742–1750, 1995.

219. Groupe Français de Cytogénétique Hématologique: Forty-four cases of childhood myelodysplasia with cytogenetics, documented by the Groupe Français de Cytogénétique Hématologique. Leukemia 11:1478–1485, 1997.

220. Luna-Fineman S, Shannon K, Atwater SK, et al: Myelodysplastic and myeloproliferative disorders of childhood: a study of 167 patients. Blood 93:459–466, 1999.

221. Emanuel PD: Myelodysplasia and myeloproliferative disorders in childhood: an update. Br J Haematol 105:852–863, 1999.

222. Chan GCF, Wang WC, Raimondi SC, et al: Myelodysplastic syndrome in children: differentiation from acute myeloid leukemia with a low blast count. Leukemia 11:206–211, 1997.

223. Niemeyer CM, Aricó M, Basso G, et al: Chronic myelomonocytic leukemia in childhood: a retrospective analysis of 110 cases. Blood 89:3534–3543, 1997.

224. Aricò M, Biondi A, Pui C-H: Juvenile myelomonocytic leukemia. Blood 90:479–488, 1997.

225. Hasle H: Atypical chronic myeloid leukaemia and chronic myelomonocytic leukaemia in children. Br J Haematol 89:428–429, 1995.

226. Luna-Fineman S, Shannon KM, Lange BJ: Childhood monosomy 7: epidemiology, biology, and mechanistic implications. Blood 85:1985–1999, 1995.

227. Hasle H, Arico M, Basso G, et al: Myelodysplastic syndrome, juvenile myelomonocytic leukemia, and acute myeloid leukemia associated with complete or partial monosomy 7. Leukemia 13:376–385, 1999.

228. Side L, Emanuel PD, Taylor B, et al: Mutations of the NF1 gene in children with juvenile myelomonocytic leukemia without clinical evidence of neurofibromatosis, type 1. Blood 92:267–272, 1998.

229. McClure RF, DeWald GW, Hoyer JD, et al: Isolated isochro-

mosome 17q: a distinct type of mixed myeloproliferative disorder/myelodysplastic syndrome with an aggressive clinical course. Br J Haematol 106:445–454, 1999.

230. Bataille R, Harousseau J-L: Multiple myeloma. N Engl J Med 336:1657–1664, 1997.

231. Varterasian ML: Advances in the biology and treatment of multiple myeloma. Curr Opin Oncol 11:3–8, 1999.

232. Bergsagel D: The incidence and epidemiology of plasma cell neoplasms. Stem Cells 13:1–9, 1995.

233. Durie BGM: Staging and kinetics of multiple myeloma. Semin Oncol 13:300–309, 1986.

234. Greipp PR: Advances in the diagnosis and management of myeloma. Semin Hematol 29:24–45, 1992.

235. Bartl R, Frisch B: Clinical significance of bone marrow biopsy and plasma cell morphology in MM and MGUS. Pathol Biol (Paris) 47:158–168, 1999.

236. Bartl R, Frisch B, Fateh-Moghadam A, et al: Histologic classification and staging of multiple myeloma: a retrospective and prospective study of 674 cases. Am J Clin Pathol 87:342–355, 1987.

237. Sukpanichnant S, Cousar JB, Leelasiri A, et al: Diagnostic criteria and histologic grading in multiple myeloma: histologic and immunohistologic analysis of 176 cases with clinical correlation. Hum Pathol 25:308–318, 1994.

238. Rajkumar SV, Fonseca R, Lacy MQ, et al: Plasmablastic morphology is an independent predictor of poor survival after autologous stem-cell transplantation for multiple myeloma. J Clin Oncol 17:1551–1557, 1999.

239. Greipp PR, Leong T, Bennett JM, et al: Plasmablastic morphology—an independent prognostic factor with clinical and laboratory correlates: Eastern Cooperative Oncology Group (ECOG) myeloma trial E9486 report by the ECOG Myeloma Laboratory Group. Blood 91:2501–2507, 1998.

240. Lacy MQ, Gertz MA, Hanson CA, et al: Multiple myeloma associated with diffuse osteosclerotic bone lesions: a clinical entity distinct from osteosclerotic myeloma (POEMS syndrome). Am J Hematol 56:288–293, 1997.

241. Miralles D, O'Fallon JR, Talley NJ: Plasma-cell dyscrasia with polyneuropathy. The spectrum of POEMS syndrome. N Engl J Med 327:1919–1923, 1992.

242. Witzig TE, Gertz MA, Lust JA, et al: Peripheral blood monoclonal plasma cells as a predictor of survival in patients with multiple myeloma. Blood 88:1780–1787, 1996.

243. Kyle RA: Sequence of testing for monoclonal gammopathies. Serum and urine assays. Arch Pathol Lab Med 123:114–118, 1999.

244. Alexanian R, Weber D, Liu F: Differential diagnosis of monoclonal gammopathies. Arch Pathol Lab Med 123:108–113, 1999.

245. Wijdenes J, Vooijs WC, Clement C, et al: A plasmocyte selective monoclonal antibody (B-B4) recognizes syndecan-1. Br J Haematol 94:318–323, 1996.

246. Petruch UR, Horny H-P, Kaiserling E: Frequent expression of haemopoietic and non-haemopoietic antigens by neoplastic plasma cells: an immunohistochemical study using formalin-fixed, paraffin-embedded tissue. Histopathology 20:35–40, 1992.

247. Rawstron A, Barrans S, Blythe D, et al: Distribution of myeloma plasma cells in peripheral blood and bone marrow correlates with CD56 expression. Br J Haematol 104:138–143, 1999.

248. Davies FE, Jack AS, Morgan GJ: The use of biological variables to predict outcome in multiple myeloma. Br J Haematol 99:719–725, 1997.

249. Tricot G, Barlogie B, Jagannath S, et al: Poor prognosis in multiple myeloma is associated only with partial or complete deletions of chromosome 13 or abnormalities involving 11q and not with other karyotype abnormalities. Blood 86:4250–4256, 1995.

250. Seong C, Delasalle K, Hayes K, et al: Prognostic value of cytogenetics in multiple myeloma. Br J Haematol 101:189–194, 1998.

251. Nishida K, Tamura A, Nakazawa N, et al: The Ig heavy chain gene is frequently involved in chromosomal translocations in multiple myeloma and plasma cell leukemia as detected by in situ hybridization. Blood 90:526–534, 1997.

252. Ronchetti D, Finelli P, Richelda R, et al: Molecular analysis of 11q13 breakpoints in multiple myeloma. Blood 93:1330–1337, 1999.

253. Chesi M, Nardini E, Lim RSC, et al: The t(4;14) translocation in myeloma dysregulates both FGFR3 and a novel gene, MMSET, resulting in IgH/MMSET hybrid transcripts. Blood 92:3025–3034, 1998.

254. Said JW, Rettig MR, Heppner K, et al: Localizaion of Kaposi's sarcoma–associated herpesvirus in bone marrow biopsy samples from patients with multiple myeloma. Blood 90:4278–4282, 1997.

255. Kyle RA: Monoclonal gammopathy of undetermined significance. Curr Top Microbiol Immunol 210:375–383, 1996.

256. Blade J, Lopez-Guillermo A, Rozman C, et al: Malignant transformation and life expectancy in monoclonal gammopathy of undetermined significance. Br J Haematol 81:391–394, 1992.

257. Ocqueteau M, Orfao A, Almeida J, et al: Immunophenotypic characterization of plasma cells from monoclonal gammopathy of undetermined significance patients: implications for the differential diagnosis between MGUS and multiple myeloma. Am J Pathol 152:1655–1665, 1998.

258. Dimopoulos MA, Alexanian R: Waldenström's macroglobulinemia. Blood 83:1452–1459, 1994.

259. Andriko J-AW, Aguilera NSI, Chu WS, et al: Waldenström's macroglobulinemia: a clinicopathologic study of 22 cases. Cancer 80:1926–1935, 1997.

260. Pangalis GA, Angelopoulou MK, Vassilakopoulos TP, et al: B-chronic lymphocytic leukemia, small lymphocytic lymphoma, and lymphoplasmacytic lymphoma, including Waldenström's macroglobulinemia: a clinical, morphologic, and biologic spectrum of similar disorders. Semin Hematol 36:104–114, 1999.

261. Iida S, Rao PH, Nallasivam P, et al: The t(9;14)(p13;q32) chromosomal translocation associated with lymphoplasmacytoid lymphoma involves the PAX-5 gene. Blood 88:4110–4117, 1996.

262. Fine KD, Stone MJ: Heavy chain disease, Mediterranean lymphoma, and immunoproliferative small intestinal disease. Am J Gastroenterol 94:1139–1152, 1999.

263. Franklin EC: μ-Chain disease. Arch Intern Med 135:71–72, 1975.

264. Fermand J-P, Brouet J-C, Danan F, et al: Gamma heavy chain "disease": heterogeneity of the clinicopathologic features. Report of 16 cases and review of the literature. Medicine (Baltimore) 68:321–335, 1989.

265. Kisilevsky R: Amyloid and amyloidoses: differences, common themes, and practical considerations. Mod Pathol 4:514–518, 1991.

266. Husby G: Nomenclature and classification of amyloid and amyloidoses. J Intern Med 232:511–512, 1992.

267. Gillmore JD, Hawkins PN, Pepys MB: Amyloidosis: a review of recent diagnostic and therapeutic developments. Br J Haematol 99:245–256, 1997.

268. Kyle RA: Primary systemic amyloidosis. J Intern Med 232:523–524, 1992.

269. Krause JR: Value of bone marrow biopsy in the diagnosis of amyloidosis. South Med J 70:1072–1079, 1977.

270. Wu SSH, Brady K, Anderson JJ, et al: The predictive value of bone marrow morphologic characteristics and immunostaining in primary (AL) amyloidosis. Am J Clin Pathol 96:95–99, 1991.

271. Oscier D: Chronic lymphocytic leukaemia. Br J Haematol 105:1–3, 1999.

272. Caligaris-Cappio F, Hamblin TJ: B-cell chronic lymphocytic leukemia: a bird of a different feather. J Clin Oncol 17:399–408, 1999.

273. Cheson BD, Bennett JM, Grever M, et al: National Cancer Institute–sponsored working group guidelines for chronic lymphocytic leukemia: revised guidelines for diagnosis and treatment. Blood 87:4990–4997, 1996.

274. Hallek M, Kuhn-Hallek I, Emmerich B: Prognostic factors in chronic lymphocytic leukemia. Leukemia 11:S4–S13, 1997.

275. Montserrat E, Villamor N, Reverter J-C, et al: Bone marrow assessment in B-cell chronic lymphocytic leukaemia: aspirate

or biopsy? A comparative study in 258 patients. Br J Haematol 93:111–116, 1996.

276. Pangalis GA, Roussou PA, Kittas C, et al: Patterns of bone marrow involvement in chronic lymphocytic leukemia and small lymphocytic (well-differentiated) non-Hodgkin's lymphoma. Its clinical significance in relation to their differential diagnosis and prognosis. Cancer 54:702–708, 1984.

277. Rozman C, Montserrat E, Rodríguez-Fernández JM, et al: Bone marrow histologic pattern—the best single prognostic parameter in chronic lymphocytic leukemia: a multivariate survival analysis of 329 cases. Blood 64:642–648, 1984.

278. Bennett JM, Catovsky D, Daniel M-T, et al: Proposals for the classification of chronic (mature) B and T lymphoid leukaemias. J Clin Pathol 42:567–584, 1989.

279. Pugh WC, Manning JT, Butler JJ: Paraimmunoblastic variant of small lymphocytic lymphoma/leukemia. Am J Surg Pathol 12:907–917, 1988.

280. Enno A, Catovsky D, O'Brien M, et al: 'Prolymphocytoid' transformation of chronic lymphocytic leukaemia. Br J Haematol 41:9–18, 1979.

281. Kjeldsberg CR, Marty J: Prolymphocytic transformation of chronic lymphocytic leukemia. Cancer 48:2447–2457, 1981.

282. Harousseau JL, Flandrin G, Tricot G, et al: Malignant lymphoma supervening in chronic lymphocytic leukemia and related disorders. Richter's syndrome: a study of 25 cases. Cancer 48:1302–1308, 1981.

283. Diehl LF, Ketchum LH: Autoimmune disease and chronic lymphocytic leukemia: autoimmune hemolytic anemia, pure red cell aplasia, and autoimmune thrombocytopenia. Semin Oncol 25:80–97, 1998.

284. Prisch O, Maloum K, Doghiero G: Basic biology of autoimmune phenomena in chronic lymphocytic leukemia. Semin Oncol 25:34–41, 1998.

285. Harris NL, Jaffe ES, Stein H, et al: A revised European-American classification of lymphoid neoplasms: a proposal from the International Lymphoma Study Group. Blood 84:1361–1392, 1994.

286. Matutes E, Owusu-Ankomah K, Morilla R, et al: The immunological profile of B-cell disorders and proposal of a scoring sytem for diagnosis of CLL. Leukemia 8:1640–1645, 1994.

287. DiGiuseppe JA, Borowitz MJ: Clinical utility of flow cytometry in the chronic lymphoid leukemias. Semin Oncol 25:6–10, 1998.

288. Geisler CH, Larsen JK, Hansen NE, et al: Prognostic importance of flow cytometric immunophenotyping of 540 consecutive patients with B-cell chronic lymphocytic leukemia. Blood 78:1795–1802, 1991.

289. Criel A, Michaux L, De Wolf–Peeters C: The concept of typical and atypical chronic lymphocytic leukaemia. Leuk Lymphoma 33:33–45, 1999.

290. Damle RN, Wasil T, Fais F, et al: Ig V gene mutation status and CD38 expression as novel prognostic indicators in chronic lymphocytic leukemia. Blood 94:1840–1847, 1999.

291. Hamblin TJ, Davis Z, Gardiner A, et al: Unmutated Ig $V_H$ genes are associated with a more aggressive form of chronic lymphocytic leukemia. Blood 94:1848–1854, 1999.

292. Bigoni R, Roberti MG, Bardi A, et al: Chromosome aberrations in atypical chronic lymphocytic leukemia: a cytogenetic and interphase cytogenetic study. Leukemia 11:1933–1940, 1997.

293. Döhner H, Stilgenbauer S, Benner A, et al: Genomic aberrations and survival in chronic lymphocytic leukemia. N Engl J Med 343:1910–1916, 2000.

294. Criel A, Verhoef G, Vlietinck R, et al: Further characterization of morphologically defined typical and atypical CLL: a clinical, immunophenotypic, cytogenetic and prognostic study on 390 cases. Br J Haematol 97:383–391, 1997.

295. Geisler CH, Philip P, Christensen BE, et al: In B-cell chronic lymphocytic leukaemia chromosome 17 abnormalities and not trisomy 12 are the single most important cytogenetic abnormalities for the prognosis: a cytogenetic and immunophenotypic study of 480 unselected newly diagnosed patients. Leuk Res 21:1011–1023, 1997.

296. Döhner H, Stilgenbauer S, Bentz M, et al: Chromosome aberrations in B-cell chronic lymphocytic leukemia: reassessment based on molecular cytogenetic analysis. J Mol Med 77:266–281, 1999.

297. Galton DAG, Goldman JM, Wiltshaw E, et al: Prolymphocytic leukaemia. Br J Haematol 27:7–23, 1974.

298. Nieto LH, Lampert IA, Catovsky D: Bone marrow histological patterns in B-cell and T-cell prolymphocytic leukemia. Hematol Pathol 3:79–84, 1989.

299. Brito-Babapulle V, Pittman S, Melo JV, et al: Cytogenetic studies on prolymphocytic leukemia. 1. B-cell prolymphocytic leukemia. Hematol Pathol 1:27–33, 1987.

300. Lens D, De Schouwer PJJC, Hamoudi RA, et al: p53 abnormalities in B-cell prolymphocytic leukemia. Blood 89:2015–2023, 1997.

301. Chang KL, Stroup R, Weiss LM: Hairy cell leukemia. Current status. Am J Clin Pathol 97:719–738, 1992.

302. Pettitt AR, Zuzel M, Cawley JC: Hairy cell leukaemia: biology and management. Br J Haematol 106:2–8, 1999.

303. Burke JS: The value of the bone-marrow biopsy in the diagnosis of hairy cell leukemia. Am J Clin Pathol 70:876–884, 1978.

304. Catovsky D, O'Brien M, Melo JV, et al: Hairy cell leukemia (HCL) variant: an intermediate disease between HCL and B prolymphocytic leukemia. Semin Oncol 11:362–369, 1984.

305. Robbins BA, Ellison DJ, Spinosa JC, et al: Diagnostic application of two-color flow cytometry in 161 cases of hairy cell leukemia. Blood 82:1277–1287, 1993.

306. Juliusson G, Lenkei R, Liliemark J: Flow cytometry of blood and bone marrow cells from patients with hairy cell leukemia: phenotype of hairy cells and lymphocyte subsets after treatment with 2-chlorodeoxyadenosine. Blood 83:3672–3681, 1994.

307. Matutes E, Morilla R, Owusu-Ankomah K, et al: The immunophenotype of hairy cell leukemia (HCL). Proposal for a scoring system to distinguish HCL from B-cell disorders with hairy or villous lymphocytes. Leuk Lymphoma 14:57–61, 1994.

308. Kreft A, Büsche G, Bernhared J, et al: Immunophenotype of hairy-cell leukaemia after cold polymerization of methyl-methacrylate embeddings from 50 diagnostic bone marrow biopsies. Histopathology 30:145–151, 1997.

309. Salomon-Nguyen F, Valensi F, Troussard X, et al: The value of the monoclonal antibody, DBA44, in the diagnosis of B-lymphoid disorders. Leuk Res 20:909–913, 1996.

310. Bosch F, Campo E, Jares P, et al: Increased expression of the PRAD-1/CCND1 gene in hairy cell leukaemia. Br J Haematol 91:1025–1030, 1995.

311. Hoyer JD, Li C-Y, Yam LT, et al: Immunohistochemical demonstration of acid phosphatase isoenzyme 5 (tartrate-resistant) in paraffin sections of hairy cell leukemia and other hematologic disorders. Am J Clin Pathol 108:308–315, 1997.

312. Haglund U, Juliusson G, Stellan B, et al: Hairy cell leukemia is characterized by clonal chromosome abnormalities clustered to specific regions. Blood 83:2637–2645, 1994.

313. de Totero D, Tazzari PL, Lauria F, et al: Phenotypic analysis of hairy cell leukemia: "variant" cases express the interleukin-2 receptor $\beta$ chain, but not the $\alpha$ chain (CD25). Blood 82:528–535, 1993.

314. Matutes E, Brito-Babapulle V, Swansbury J, et al: Clinical and laboratory features of 78 cases of T-prolymphocytic leukemia. Blood 78:3269–3274, 1991.

315. Bartlett NL, Longo DL: T–small lymphocyte disorders. Semin Hematol 36:164–170, 1999.

316. Taylor AMR, Metcalfe JA, Thick J, et al: Leukemia and lymphoma in ataxia telangiectasia. Blood 87:423–438, 1996.

317. Garand R, Goasguen J, Brizard A, et al: Indolent course as a relatively frequent presentation of T-prolymphocytic leukaemia. Groupe Français d'Hématologie Cellulaire. Br J Haematol 103:488–494, 1998.

318. Brito-Babapulle V, Pomfret M, Matutes E, et al: Cytogenetic studies on prolymphocytic leukemia. II. T cell prolymphocytic leukemia. Blood 70:926–931, 1987.

319. Stoppa-Lyonnet D, Soulier J, Garand R, et al: Inactivation of the ATM gene in T-cell prolymphocytic leukemias. Blood 91:3920–3926, 1998.

320. Hoyer JD, Ross CW, Li C-Y, et al: True T-cell chronic lymphocytic leukemia: a morphologic and immunophenotypic study of 25 cases. Blood 86:1163–1169, 1995.

321. Matutes E, Catovsky D: Similarities between T-cell chronic lymphocytic leukemia and the small-cell variant of T-prolymphocytic leukemia. Blood 87:3520–3521, 1996.

322. Pandolfi F, Loughran TP Jr, Starkebaum G, et al: Clinical course and prognosis of the lymphoproliferative disease of granular lymphocytes. A multicenter study. Cancer 65:341–348, 1990.

323. Loughran TP Jr: Clonal disease of large granular lymphocytes. Blood 82:1–14, 1993.

324. Scott CS, Richards SJ, Sivakumaran M, et al: Transient and persistent expansions of large granular lymphocytes (LGL) and NK-associated (NKa) cells: the Yorkshire Leukaemia Group study. Br J Haematol 83:504–515, 1993.

325. Oshimi K, Yamada O, Kaneki T, et al: Laboratory findings and clinical courses of 33 patients with granular lymphocyte-proliferative disorders. Leukemia 7:782–788, 1993.

326. Zambello R, Semenzato G: Large granular lymphocytosis. Haematologica 83:936–942, 1998.

327. Agnarsson BA, Loughran TP Jr, Starkebaum G, et al: The pathology of large granular lymphocyte leukemia. Hum Pathol 20:644–651, 1989.

328. Loughran TP Jr, Starkebaum G, Aprile JA: Rearrangement and expression of T-cell receptor genes in large granular lymphocyte leukemia. Blood 71:822–824, 1988.

329. Sivakumaran M, Richards SJ: The clinical relevance of fluctuations in absolute lymphocyte counts during follow-up of large granular lymphocyte proliferations. Blood 88:1899–1900, 1996.

330. Gentile TC, Uner AG, Hutchison RE, et al: CD3+, CD56+ aggressive variant of large granular lymphocyte leukemia. Blood 84:2315–2321, 1994.

331. DiGiuseppe JA, Louie DC, Williams JE, et al: Blastic natural killer cell leukemia/lymphoma: a clinicopathologic study. Am J Surg Pathol 21:1223–1230, 1997.

332. Jaffe ES, Cossman J, Blattner WA, et al: The pathologic spectrum of adult T-cell leukemia/lymphoma in the United States. Am J Surg Pathol 8:263–275, 1984.

333. Tsukasaki K, Imaizumi Y, Tawara M, et al: Diversity of leukaemic cell morphology in ATL correlates with prognostic factors, aberrant immunophenotype and defective HTLV-1 genotype. Br J Haematol 105:369–375, 1999.

334. Kikuchi M, Takeshita M, Ohshima K, et al: Pathology of adult T-cell leukemia/lymphoma and HTLV-1 associated organopathies. Gann Monogr Cancer Res 39:69–80, 1992.

335. Yamaguchi K, Nishimura H, Kohrogi H, et al: A proposal for smoldering adult T-cell leukemia: a clinicopathologic study of five cases. Blood 62:758–766, 1983.

336. Ginaldi L, Matutes E, Farahat N, et al: Differential expression of CD3 and CD7 in T-cell malignancies: a quantitative study by flow cytometry. Br J Haematol 93:921–927, 1996.

337. Kamada N, Sakurai M, Miyamoto K, et al: Chromosome abnormalities in adult T-cell leukemia/lymphoma: a karyotype review committee report. Cancer Res 52:1481–1493, 1992.

338. Diamandidou E, Cohen PR, Kurzock R: Mycosis fungoides and Sézary syndrome. Blood 88:2385–2409, 1996.

339. Vonderheid EC, Sobel EL, Nowell PC, et al: Diagnostic and prognostic significance of Sézary cells in peripheral blood smears from patients with cutaneous T cell lymphoma. Blood 66:358–366, 1985.

340. Schechter GP, Sausville EA, Fischmann AB, et al: Evaluation of circulating malignant cells provides prognostic information in cutaneous T cell lymphoma. Blood 69:841–849, 1987.

341. Salhany KE, Greer JP, Cousar JB, et al: Marrow involvement in cutaneous T-cell lymphoma. A clinicopathologic study of 60 cases. Am J Clin Pathol 92:747–754, 1989.

342. Graham SJ, Sharpe RW, Steinberg SM, et al: Prognostic implications of a bone marrow histopathologic classification system in mycosis fungoides and the Sézary syndrome. Cancer 72:726–734, 1993.

343. Weinberg JM, Jaworsky C, Benoit BM, et al: The clonal nature of circulating Sézary cells. Blood 86:4257–4262, 1995.

344. Thangavelu M, Finn WG, Yelavarthi KK, et al: Recurring structural chromosome abnormalities in peripheral blood lymphocytes of patients with mycosis fungoides/Sézary syndrome. Blood 89:3371–3377, 1997.

345. Pawson R, Matutes E, Brito-Babapulle V, et al: Sézary cell leukaemia: a distinct T cell disorder or a variant form of T prolymphocytic leukaemia? Leukemia 11:1009–1013, 1997.

346. Brito-Babapulle V, Maljaie SH, Matutes E, et al: Relationship of T leukaemias with cerebriform nuclei to T-prolymphocytic leukaemia: a cytogenetic analysis with in situ hybridization. Br J Haematol 96:724–732, 1997.

347. McKenna RW, Hernandez JA: Bone marrow in malignant lymphoma. Hematol Oncol Clin North Am 2:617–635, 1988.

348. Lambertenghi-Deliliers G, Annaloro C, Soligo D, et al: Incidence and histologic features of bone marrow involvement in malignant lymphomas. Ann Hematol 65:61–65, 1992.

349. Fineberg S, Marsh E, Alsonso F, et al: Immunophenotypic evaluation of the bone marrow in non-Hodgkin's lymphoma. Hum Pathol 24:636–642, 1993.

350. Cheson BD, Horning SJ, Coiffier B, et al: Report of an international workshop to standardize response criteria for non-Hodgkin's lymphomas. J Clin Oncol 17:1244–1253, 1999.

351. Robertson LE, Redman JR, Butler JJ, et al: Discordant bone marrow involvement in diffuse large-cell lymphoma: a distinct clinical-pathologic entity associated with a continuous risk of relapse. J Clin Oncol 9:236–242, 1991.

352. Crisan DC, Mattson JC: Discordant morphologic features in bone marrow involvement by malignant lymphomas: use of gene rearrangement patterns for diagnosis. Am J Hematol 49:299–309, 1995.

353. Colan MG, Bast M, Armitage JO, et al: Bone marrow involvement by non-Hodgkin's lymphoma: the clinical significance of morphologic discordance between lymph node and bone marrow. J Clin Oncol 8:1163–1172, 1990.

354. Crotty PL, Smith BR, Tallini G: Morphologic, immunophenotypic, and molecular evaluation of bone marrow involvement in non-Hodgkin's lymphoma. Diagn Mol Pathol 7:90–95, 1998.

355. Naughton MJ, Hess JL, Zutter MM, et al: Bone marrow staging in patients with non-Hodgkin's lymphoma. Is flow cytometry a useful test? Cancer 82:1154–1159, 1998.

356. van Belzen N, Hupkes PE, Doekharan D, et al: Detection of minimal disease using rearranged immunoglobulin heavy chain genes from intermediate- and high-grade malignant B cell non-Hodgkin's lymphoma. Leukemia 11:1742–1752, 1997.

357. Weiss LM, Warnke RA, Scklar J, et al: Molecular analysis of the t(14;18) chromosomal translocation in malignant lymphomas. N Engl J Med 317:1185–1189, 1987.

358. Abdel-Reheim FA, Edwards E, Arber DA: Utility of a rapid polymerase chain reaction panel for the detection of molecular changes in B-cell lymphoma. Arch Pathol Lab Med 120:357–363, 1996.

359. Segal GH, Jorgensen T, Scott M, et al: Optimal primer selection for clonality assessment by polymerase chain reaction analysis: II. Follicular lymphomas. Hum Pathol 25:1276–1282, 1994.

360. Wasman J, Rosenthal NS, Farhi DC: Mantle cell lymphoma. Morphologic findings in bone marrow involvement. Am J Clin Pathol 106:196–200, 1996.

361. Cohen PL, Kurtin PJ, Donovan KA, et al: Bone marrow and peripheral blood involvement in mantle cell lymphoma. Br J Haematol 101:302–310, 1998.

362. Wong K-F, Chan JKC, So JCC, et al: Mantle cell lymphoma in leukemic phase. Characterization of its broad cytologic spectrum with emphasis on the importance of distinction from other chronic lymphoproliferative disorders. Cancer 86:850–857, 1999.

363. Chan JKC, Miller KD, Munson P, et al: Immunostaining for cyclin D1 and the diagnosis of mantle cell lymphoma: is there a reliable method? Histopathology 34:266–270, 1999.

364. Rosenberg CL, Wong E, Petty EM, et al: *PRAD1*, a candidate *BCL1* oncogene: mapping and expression in centrocytic lymphoma. Proc Natl Acad Sci USA 88:9638–9642, 1991.

365. Rimokh R, Berger F, Delsol G, et al: Detection of the chro-

mosomal translocation t(11;14) by polymerase chain reaction in mantle cell lymphomas. Blood 83:1871–1875, 1994.

366. Chang KL, Kamel OW, Arber DA, et al: Pathologic features of nodular lymphocyte predominance Hodgkin's disease in extranodal sites. Am J Surg Pathol 19:1313–1324, 1995.

367. Kadin ME, Donaldson SS, Dorfman RF: Isolated granulomas in Hodgkin's disease. N Engl J Med 283:859–861, 1970.

368. Weiss LM, Chen Y-Y, Liu X-F, et al: Epstein-Barr virus and Hodgkin's disease. A correlative in situ hybridization and polymerase chain reaction study. Am J Pathol 139:1259–1265, 1991.

369. Hummel M, Ziemann K, Lammert H, et al: Hodgkin's disease with monoclonal and polyclonal populations of Reed-Sternberg cells. N Engl J Med 333:901–906, 1995.

370. Rywlin AM, Ortega RS, Dominguez CJ: Lymphoid nodules of bone marrow: normal and abnormal. Blood 43:389–400, 1974.

371. Liu PI, Takanari H, Yatani R, et al: Comparative studies of bone marrow from the United States and Japan. Ann Clin Lab Sci 19:345–351, 1989.

372. Thiele J, Zirbes TK, Kvasnicka HM, et al: Focal lymphoid aggregates (nodules) in bone marrow biopsies: differentiation between benign hyperplasia and malignant lymphoma—a practical guideline. J Clin Pathol 52:294–300, 1999.

373. Farhi DC: Germinal centers in the bone marrow. Hematol Pathol 3:133–136, 1989.

374. Rosenthal NS, Farhi DC: Bone marrow findings in connective tissue disease. Am J Clin Pathol 92:650–654, 1989.

375. Bluth RF, Casey TT, McCurley TL: Differentiation of reactive from neoplastic small-cell lymphoid aggregates in paraffin-embedded marrow particle preparations using L-26 (CD20) and UCHL-1 (CD45RO) monoclonal antibodies. Am J Clin Pathol 99:150–156, 1993.

376. Ben-Ezra JM, King BE, Harris AC, et al: Staining for Bcl-2 protein helps to distinguish benign from malignant lymphoid aggregates in bone marrow biopsies. Mod Pathol 7:560–564, 1994.

377. Bodem CR, Hamory BH, Taylor HM, et al: Granulomatous bone marrow disese. A review of the literature and clinicopathologic analysis of 58 cases. Medicine (Baltimore) 62:372–383, 1983.

378. Bhargava V, Farhi DC: Bone marrow granulomas: clinicopathologic findings in 72 cases and review of the literature. Hematol Pathol 21:44–50, 1988.

379. Vilalta-Castel E, Valdes-Sanchez MD, Teno-Esteban C, et al: Significance of granulomas in bone marrow: a study of 40 cases. Eur J Haematol 41:12–16, 1988.

380. Srigley JR, Geddie WR, Vellend H, et al: Q-fever. The liver and bone marrow pathology. Am J Surg Pathol 9:752–758, 1985.

381. Young JR, Goulian M: Bone marrow fibrin ring granulomas and cytomegalovirus infection. Am J Clin Pathol 99:65–68, 1993.

382. Yu HC, Rywlin AM: Granulomatous lesions of the bone marrow in non-Hodgkin's lymphoma. Hum Pathol 13:905–910, 1982.

383. Arico M, Janka G, Fischer A, et al: Hemophagocytic lymphohistiocytosis. Report of 122 children from the International Registry. Leukemia 10:197–203, 1996.

384. Öst Å, Nilsson-Ardnor S, Henter J-I: Autopsy findings in 27 children with haemophagocytic lymphohistiocytosis. Histopathology 32:310–316, 1998.

385. McKenna RW, Risdall RJ, Brunning RD: Virus associated hemophagocytic syndrome. Hum Pathol 12:395–398, 1981.

386. Risdall RJ, Brunning RD, Hernandez JI, et al: Bacteria-associated hemophagocytic syndrome. Cancer 54:2968–2972, 1984.

387. Takeshita M, Kikuchi M, Ohshima K, et al: Bone marrow findings in malignant histiocytosis and/or malignant lymphoma with concurrent hemophagocytic syndrome. Leuk Lymphoma 12:79–89, 1993.

388. Scriver CR, Beaudet AL, Sly WS, Valle D: The Metabolic and Molecular Bases of Inherited Disease. 7th ed. New York, McGraw-Hill, 1995.

389. Volk BW, Adachi M, Schneck L: The pathology of sphingolipidoses. Semin Hematol 9:317–348, 1972.

390. Favara BE, Feller AC: Contemporary classification of histiocytic disorders. Med Pediatr Oncol 29:157–166, 1997.

391. Elghetany MT: True histiocytic lymphoma: is it an entity? Leukemia 11:762–764, 1997.

392. Wilson MS, Weiss LM, Gatter KC, et al: Malignant histiocytosis. A reassessment of cases previously reported in 1975 based on paraffin section immunophenotyping studies. Cancer 66:530–536, 1990.

393. Ornvold K, Carstensen H, Junge J, et al: Tumours classified as "malignant histiocytosis" in children are T-cell neoplasms. APMIS 100:558–566, 1992.

394. Bain BJ: Systemic mastocytosis and other mast cell neoplasms. Br J Haematol 106:9–17, 1999.

395. Horny H-P, Parwaresch MR, Lennert K: Bone marrow findings in systemic mastocytosis. Hum Pathol 16:808–814, 1985.

396. Lawrence JB, Friedman BS, Travis WD, et al: Hematologic manifestations of systemic mast cell disease: a prospective study of laboratory and morphologic features and their relation to prognosis. Am J Med 91:612–624, 1991.

397. Prokocimer M, Polliack A: Increased bone marrow mast cells in preleukemic syndromes, acute leukemia, and lymphoproliferative disorders. Am J Clin Pathol 75:34–38, 1981.

398. Travis WD, Li C-Y, Bergstralh EJ: Solid and hematologic malignancies in 60 patients with systemic mast cell disease. Arch Pathol Lab Med 113:365–368, 1989.

399. Horny H-P, Ruck M, Wehrmann M, et al: Blood findings in generalized mastocytosis: evidence of frequent simultaneous occurrence of myeloproliferative disorders. Br J Haematol 76:186–193, 1990.

400. Klatt EC, Lukes RJ, Meyer PR: Benign and malignant mast cell proliferations. Diagnosis and separation using a pH-dependent toluidine blue stain in tissue section. Cancer 51:1119–1124, 1983.

401. Arber DA, Tamayo R, Weiss LM: Paraffin section detection of the c-*kit* gene product (CD117) in human tissues: value in the diagnosis of mast cell disorders. Hum Pathol 28:498–504, 1998.

402. Escribano L, Orfao A, Díaz-Agustin B, et al: Indolent systemic mast cell disease in adults: immunophenotypic characterization of bone marrow mast cells and its diagnostic implications. Blood 91:2731–2736, 1998.

403. Horny H-P, Sillaber C, Menke D, et al: Diagnostic value of immunostaining for tryptase in patients with mastocytosis. Am J Surg Pathol 22:1132–1140, 1998.

403a. Yang F, Tran T-A, Carlson JA, et al: Paraffin section immunophenotype of cutaneous and extracutaneous mast cell disease. Comparison to other hematopoietic neoplasms. Am J Surg Pathol 24:703–709, 2000.

404. Wong KF, Chan JKC, Ma SK: Solid tumour with initial presentation in the bone marrow—a clinicopathologic study of 25 adult cases. Hematol Oncol 11:35–42, 1993.

405. Anner RM, Drewinki B: Frequency and significance of bone marrow involvement by metastatic solid tumors. Cancer 39:1337–1344, 1977.

406. Papac RJ: Bone marrow metastases. A review. Cancer 74:2403–2413, 1994.

407. Lyda MH, Tetef M, Carter NH, et al: Keratin immunohistochemistry detects clinically significant metastases in bone marrow biopsy specimens in women with lobular breast carcinoma. Am J Surg Pathol 24:1593–1599, 2000.

408. Gallivan MVE, Lokich JJ: Carcinocythemia (carcinoma cell leukemia). Report of two cases with English literature review. Cancer 53:1100–1102, 1984.

409. Guinan EC: Clinical aspects of aplastic anemia. Hematol Oncol Clin North Am 11:1025–1044, 1997.

410. Young NS: Acquired aplastic anemia. JAMA 282:271–278, 1999.

411. Camitta BM, Thomas ED, Nathan DG, et al: A prospective study of androgens and bone marrow trasplantation for treatment of severe aplastic anemia. Blood 53:504–514, 1979.

412. Nagai K, Kohno T, Chen Y-X, et al: Diagnostic criteria for hypocellular acute leukemia: a clinical entity distinct from overt acute leukemia and myelodysplastic syndrome. Leuk Res 20:563–574, 1996.

413. Orazi A, Albitar M, Heerema NA, et al: Hypoplastic myelo-

dysplastic syndromes can be distinguished from acquired aplastic anemia by CD34 and PCNA immunostaining of bone marrow biopsy specimens. Am J Clin Pathol 107:268–274, 1997.

414. Tooze JA, Marsh JCW, Gordon-Smith EC: Clonal evolution of aplastic anaemia to myelodysplasia/acute myeloid leukaemia and paroxysmal nocturnal haemoglobinuria. Leuk Lymphoma 33:231–241, 1999.
415. Alter BP: Fanconi's anemia and malignancies. Am J Hematol 53:99–110, 1996.
416. Parker CJ: Molecular basis of paroxysmal nocturnal hemoglobinuria. Stem Cells 14:396–411, 1996.
417. Takeda J, Miyata T, Kawagoe K, et al: Deficiency of the GPI anchor caused by a somatic mutation of the *PIG-A* gene in paroxysmal nocturnal hemoglobinuria. Cell 73:703–711, 1993.
418. Iwamoto N, Kawaguchi T, Nagakura S, et al: Markedly high population of affected reticulocytes negative for decay-accelerating factor and CD59 in paroxysmal nocturnal hemoglobinuria. Blood 85:2228–2232, 1995.
419. Iwanaga M, Furukawa K, Amenomori T, et al: Paroxysmal nocturnal haemoglobinuria clones in patients with myelodysplastic syndromes. Br J Haematol 102:465–474, 1998.
420. Seaman JP, Kjeldsberg CR, Linker A: Gelatinous transformation of the bone marrow. Hum Pathol 9:685–692, 1978.
421. Mehta K, Gascon P, Robboy S: The gelatinous bone marrow (serous atrophy) in patients with acquired immunodeficiency syndrome. Evidence of excess sulfated glycosaminoglycan. Arch Pathol Lab Med 116:504–508, 1992.
422. Krijanovski OI, Sieff CA: Diamond-Blackfan anemia. Hematol Oncol Clin North Am 11:1061–1077, 1997.
423. Erslev AJ, Soltan A: Pure red-cell aplasia: a review. Blood Rev 10:20–28, 1996.
424. Krause JR, Penchansky L, Knisely AS: Morphological diagnosis of parvovirus B19 infection. A cytopathic effect easily recognized in air-dried, formalin-fixed bone marrow smears stained with hematoxylin-eosin or Wright-Giemsa. Arch Pathol Lab Med 116:178–180, 1992.
425. Brown KE, Young NS: Parvovirus B19 in human disease. Annu Rev Med 48:59–67, 1997.
426. Cherrick T, Karayalcin G, Lanzkowsky P: Transient erythroblastopenia of childhood. Prospective study of fifty patients. Am J Pediatr Hematol Oncol 16:320–324, 1994.
427. Farhi DC, Leubbers EL, Rosenthal NS: Bone marrow biopsy findings in childhood anemia. Prevalence of transient erythroblastopenia of childhood. Arch Pathol Lab Med 122:638–641, 1998.
428. Young NS: Agranulocytosis. JAMA 271:935–938, 1994.
429. Welte K, Boxer LA: Severe chronic neutropenia: pathophysiology and therapy. Semin Hematol 34:267–278, 1997.
430. Jonsson OG, Buchanan GR: Chronic neutropenia during childhood: a 13-year experience in a single institution. Am J Dis Child 145:232–235, 1991.
431. McClain K, Estrov E, Chen H, et al: Chronic neutropenia of childhood: frequent association with parvovirus infection and correlations with bone marrow culture studies. Br J Haematol 85:57–62, 1993.
432. Pearson HA, McIntosh S: Neonatal thrombocytopenia. Clin Haematol 7:111–122, 1995.
433. Stoll DB, Blum S, Pasquale D, et al: Thrombocytopenia with decreased megakaryocytes. Evaluation and prognosis. Ann Intern Med 94:170–175, 1981.
434. Hall JG, Levin J, Kuhn JP, et al: Thrombocytopenia with absent radius (TAR). Medicine (Baltimore) 48:411–439, 1969.
435. Walters MC, Abelson HT: Interpretation of the complete blood count. Pediatr Clin North Am 43:599–622, 1996.
436. Peterson P, Cornacchia MF: Anemia: pathophysiology, clinical features, and laboratory evaluation. Lab Med 30:463–467, 1999.
437. Toh B-H, van Driel IR, Gleeson PA: Pernicious anemia. N Engl J Med 337:1441–1448, 1997.
438. Green R: Macrocytic and marrow failure anemias. Lab Med 30:595–599, 1999.
439. Wickramasinghe SN: Dyserythropoiesis and congenital dyserythropoietic anaemias. Br J Haematol 98:785–797, 1997.
440. Hoffbrand V, Provan D: ABC of clinical haematology. Macrocytic anaemias. Br Med J 314:430–433, 1997.
441. Meredith JL, Rosenthal NS: Differential diagnosis of microcytic anemias. Lab Med 30:538–542, 1999.
442. Provan D: Mechanisms and management of iron deficiency anaemia. Br J Haematol 105:16–26, 1999.
443. Griggs RC: Lead poisoning: hematologic aspects. Prog Hematol 4:117–137, 1964.
444. Kitamura H, Kodama F, Odagiri S, et al: Granulocytosis associated with malignant neoplasms: a clinicopathologic study and demonstration of colony-stimulating activity in tumor extracts. Hum Pathol 20:878–885, 1989.
445. Maldonado JE, Hanlon DG: Monocytosis: a current appraisal. Mayo Clin Proc 40:248–259, 1965.
446. Johnston RB Jr: Monocytes and macrophages. N Engl J Med 318:747–752, 1988.
447. Rothenberg ME: Eosinophilia. N Engl J Med 338:1592–1600, 1998.
448. Denburg JA: Basophil and mast cell lineages in vitro and in vivo. Blood 79:846–860, 1992.
449. Kubic VL, Kubic PT, Brunning RD: The morphologic and immunophenotypic assessment of the lymphocytosis accompanying *Bordetella pertussis* infection. Am J Clin Pathol 95:809–815, 1991.
450. Thommasen HV, Boyko WJ, Montaner JSG, et al: Absolute lymphocytosis associated with nonsurgical trauma. Am J Clin Pathol 86:480–483, 1986.
451. Teggatz JR, Parkin J, Peterson L: Transient atypical lymphocytosis in patients with emergency medical conditions. Arch Pathol Lab Med 111:712–714, 1987.
452. Agrawal S, Matutes E, Voke J, et al: Persistent polyclonal B-cell lymphocytosis. Leuk Res 18:791–795, 1994.
453. Mossafa H, Malaure H, Maynadie M, et al: Persistent polyclonal B lymphocytosis with binucleated lymphocytes: a study of 25 cases. Br J Haematol 104:486–493, 1999.
454. Lush CJ, Vora AJ, Campbell AC, et al: Polyclonal CD5+ B-lymphocytosis resembling chronic lymphocytic leukaemia. Br J Haematol 79:119–120, 1991.
455. Buss DH, O'Connor ML, Woodruff RD, et al: Bone marrow and peripheral blood findings in patients with extreme thrombocytosis. A report of 63 cases. Arch Pathol Lab Med 115:475–480, 1991.
456. Schmitz LL, McClure JS, Litz CE, et al: Morphologic and quantitative changes in blood and marrow cells following growth factor therapy. Am J Clin Pathol 101:67–75, 1994.
457. Hofmann WK, Ottmann OG, Hoelzer D: Megakaryocytic growth factors: Is there a new approach for management of thrombocytopenia in patients with malignancies? Leukemia 13:14–18, 1999.
458. McCarthey DM: Fibrosis of the bone marrow: content and causes. Br J Haematol 59:1–7, 1985.
459. Beckman EN, Brown AW Jr: Normal reticulin level in iliac bone marrow. Arch Pathol Lab Med 114:1241–1243, 1990.
460. Brown CH III: Bone marrow necrosis. A study of seventy cases. Johns Hopkins Med J 131:189–203, 1972.
461. Conrad ME, Carpenter JT: Bone marrow necrosis. Am J Hematol 7:181–189, 1979.
462. Gruber HE, Stauffer ME, Thompson ER, et al: Diagnosis of bone disease by core biopsies. Semin Hematol 18:258–278, 1981.

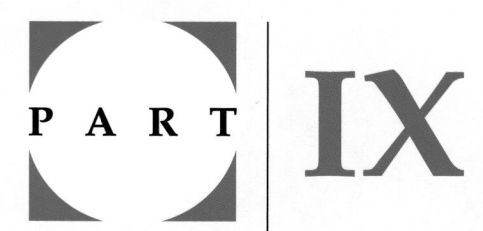

# PART IX

# Endocrine System

# 44

# *Thyroid and Parathyroid*

John K. C. Chan

# A. The Thyroid Gland

## NEOPLASTIC LESIONS

### Classification

The primary tumors of the thyroid gland, grouped according to the line of differentiation, include the following.[1]

### *Tumors of Thyroid Follicular Epithelium*

Follicular adenoma, including Hürthle cell adenoma

Follicular carcinoma, including Hürthle cell carcinoma

Papillary carcinoma

**TABLE 44–1. Immunohistochemical Staining Profile of the Various Thyroid Neoplasms**

| Tumor Type | Cytokeratin | Pan-neuroendocrine Markers (such as synaptophysin, chromogranin) | Thyroglobulin | Calcitonin | Thyroid Transcription Factor 1 | Other Markers |
|---|---|---|---|---|---|---|
| Papillary carcinoma; follicular adenoma-carcinoma; poorly differentiated thyroid carcinoma; columnar cell carcinoma | Positive | Negative | Positive | Negative | Positive | — |
| Medullary carcinoma | Positive | Positive | Negative | Positive | Positive | Carcinoembryonic antigen (CEA)+; S-100+ sustentacular cells may be present in hereditary form |
| Mixed follicular-parafollicular carcinoma | Positive | Positive | Positive | Positive | Positive | — |
| Anaplastic carcinoma | Variable (positive in ~50% of cases) | Negative | Negative | Negative | Usually negative | — |
| Angiosarcoma | Variable (usually negative, but sometimes positive) | Negative | Negative | Negative | Negative | Positive for endothelial markers, such as CD31, CD34, factor VIII |
| Malignant lymphoma | Negative | Negative | Negative | Negative | Negative | Leukocyte common antigen+ and other lymphoid markers+ |
| Carcinoma showing thymus-like element (CASTLE) | Positive | Negative | Negative | Negative | Negative | CD5+ |
| Intrathyroid parathyroid tumor | Positive | Positive | Negative | Negative | Negative | Parathyroid hormone+ |
| Paraganglioma | Negative | Positive | Negative | Negative | Negative | S-100+ sustentacular cells; CEA− |

Poorly differentiated thyroid carcinoma, including insular carcinoma

Anaplastic carcinoma, squamous cell carcinoma, and carcinosarcoma

Rare tumor types: columnar cell carcinoma, mucoepidermoid carcinoma, sclerosing mucoepidermoid carcinoma with eosinophilia, mucinous carcinoma

### Tumors Showing C Cell or Simultaneous Follicular and C Cell Differentiation

Medullary carcinoma

Collision tumor: follicular and medullary carcinomas or papillary and medullary carcinomas

Mixed follicular-parafollicular carcinoma (differentiated thyroid carcinoma, intermediate type)

### Ectopic Tumors

Ectopic thymoma

Spindle epithelial tumor with thymus-like element (SETTLE)

Carcinoma showing thymus-like element (CASTLE)

Intrathyroid parathyroid adenoma and carcinoma

### Tumors of Hematolymphoid Cells

Malignant lymphoma
Plasmacytoma
Langerhans cell histiocytosis

### Mesenchymal and Other Tumors

Benign and malignant mesenchymal tumors, such as solitary fibrous tumor, smooth muscle tumor, peripheral nerve sheath tumor, angiosarcoma

Paraganglioma
Teratoma

The most common primary thyroid cancer is papillary carcinoma, which accounts for 60% to 80% of all cases, followed by follicular carcinoma, which accounts for 10% to 20% of cases. Most thyroid tumors can be readily diagnosed on morphologic assessment alone. Nonetheless, in some circumstances, especially with medullary carcinoma or unusual-looking tumors, immunohistochemical studies are required for a definitive classification. The immunohistochemical profiles of the more common thyroid tumors are shown in Table 44–1.[2–5]

## General Considerations

### PATHOGENESIS

Some risk factors for development of thyroid cancer have been identified; radiation exposure is the best documented factor.[6] External radiation was once popularly used to treat patients with a variety of benign disorders of the head and neck region, such as acne, tinea capitis, cervical tuberculous lymphadenitis, and thymic enlargement; such patients have an increased chance of developing thyroid cancer. Cancer patients treated with radiation have been shown to have an excess of thyroid cancer compared with control subjects. Survivors of the Hiroshima atomic bomb have a high risk for development of thyroid cancer; persons who were younger than 10 years when they were exposed have an excess relative risk of 9.46. The Chernobyl nuclear accident in 1986 provides further evidence of the importance of radiation in thyroid carcinogenesis; in some exposed areas, the incidence of thyroid cancer in children increased from 0.5 per million per year to 96.4 per million per year. The clinicopathologic features of the Chernobyl accident–associated thyroid cancers are listed in Table 44–2.

Iodine deficiency and endemic goiter are associated with an increased risk of thyroid carcinoma and angiosarcoma. It has been postulated that the tumors may result from prolonged stimulation of the thyroid tissues by thyroid-stimulating hormone.[7]

Hashimoto's thyroiditis and lymphocytic thyroiditis are associated with an increased risk for malignant lymphoma. In addition, sclerosing mucoepidermoid carcinoma with eosinophilia almost always arises in a setting of fibrosing Hashimoto's thyroiditis. Hashimoto's thyroiditis may slightly increase the risk for development of papillary carcinoma.[8]

**TABLE 44–2.** Features of Chernobyl Nuclear Accident–Associated Thyroid Cancer

It is caused by exposure to radioactive iodine fallout; the accident occurred on April 26, 1986.

Most cases are papillary carcinomas (~95%). The papillary carcinomas often show a follicular, solid, or mixed follicular-papillary-solid pattern, contrasting with the typical papillary pattern seen in sporadic papillary carcinomas in children.

The incidence of thyroid cancer in areas around Chernobyl has increased 6- to 500-fold compared with previous years, depending on the distance from the accident site. The greatest number of cases occur in areas where the thyroid radiation dose is ≥0.5 gy.

The tumors show greater aggressiveness at presentation, such as extrathyroidal extension, venous invasion, and lymph node metastasis. Thus, treatment often entails total thyroidectomy and lymph node dissection.

Lymphocytic thyroiditis and antithyroperoxidase antibody are more common than in sporadic cases.

Age at diagnosis is usually ≤14 years, which is younger than for the sporadic thyroid cancers in children not related to a nuclear accident.

The time interval between the nuclear accident and the diagnosis of thyroid cancer is ~6–7 years.

Subjects younger than 5 years or in utero at the time of the nuclear accident account for the majority of cases.

Papillary carcinomas occurring in this setting show a much higher frequency of *RET/PTC* (especially *RET/PTC3*) gene rearrangement compared with sporadic cases.

Thyroid cancer can occur as a component of some heritable syndromes.[8, 9] Medullary carcinoma is a key component of multiple endocrine neoplasia type 2 (MEN 2) or familial medullary thyroid carcinoma. Thyroid adenoma or carcinoma sometimes occurs as a component of MEN type 1 (MEN 1). Some patients with familial adenomatous polyposis develop thyroid cancer, most commonly papillary carcinoma of the cribriform-morular variant (so-called familial adenomatous polyposis–associated thyroid carcinoma). Thyroid tumors also constitute a component of Cowden's disease and may include follicular adenoma, follicular carcinoma, and papillary carcinoma. There are also less well defined familial nonmedullary thyroid cancer syndromes.

## GRADING AND STAGING

The TNM staging is the most widely used staging system for thyroid cancer (Table 44–3). There are no universally accepted grading systems for thyroid cancers, although the histologic grade may be implied from the histologic type (e.g., low grade for

**TABLE 44–3.** Staging of Thyroid Tumors

**TNM Staging**

**Primary Tumor (T)**
All categories may be subdivided: (a) solitary; (b) multifocal—the largest is measured for classification

| | |
|---|---|
| TX | Primary tumor cannot be assessed |
| T0 | No evidence of primary tumor |
| T1 | Tumors ≤1 cm, limited to the thyroid |
| T2 | Tumor 1–4 cm, limited to the thyroid |
| T3 | Tumor >4 cm, limited to the thyroid |
| T4 | Tumor of any size extending beyond thyroid capsule |

**Lymp Node (N)**

| | |
|---|---|
| NX | Regional lymph nodes cannot be assessed |
| N0 | No regional lymph node metastasis |
| N1 | Regional lymph node metastasis |
| N1a | Metastasis in ipsilateral cervical lymph nodes |
| N1b | Metastasis in bilateral, midline or contralateral cervical, or upper mediastinal lymph nodes |

**Distant Metastasis (M)**

| | |
|---|---|
| MX | Presence of distant metastasis cannot be assessed |
| M0 | No distant metastasis |
| M1 | Distant metastasis |

**Stage Grouping**

**Papillary or Follicular Carcinoma**

| Stage | <45 y | ≥45 y |
|---|---|---|
| I | Any T, any N, M0 | T1, N0, M0 |
| II | Any T, any N, M1 | T2, N0, M0<br>T3, N0, M0 |
| III | — | T4, N0, M0<br>Any T, N1, M0 |
| IV | — | Any T, any N, M1 |

**Medullary Carcinoma**

| Stage | TNM status |
|---|---|
| I | T1, N0, M0 |
| II | T2, N0, M0<br>T3, N0, M0<br>T4, N0, M0 |
| III | Any T, N1, M0 |
| IV | Any T, any N, M1 |

**Anaplastic Carcinoma**
All cases are stage IV (i.e., any T, any N, any M)

papillary and follicular carcinomas, and high grade for anaplastic carcinoma).

## PROGNOSTIC FEATURES

The different types of thyroid cancers have a number of significant prognostic factors in common.

- Age younger than 40 years is a highly favorable prognostic factor.[10]
- Small tumor size (especially <1 cm) is a favorable prognostic factor.
- Tumor stage (intrathyroid tumor versus presence of extrathyroidal extension; presence or absence of metastasis) is a highly significant prognostic factor.[10–12]

According to the Surveillance, Epidemiology, and End Results study,[10] the 10-year relative survival rates of the major thyroid carcinomas are as follows: papillary carcinoma, 0.98; follicular carcinoma, 0.92; medullary carcinoma, 0.80; and anaplastic carcinoma, 0.13. Papillary carcinoma and follicular carcinoma are sometimes lumped together in one category of "differentiated thyroid carcinoma" in clinical studies, but this is not advisable because they show different clinical and biologic features.

## THERAPY

The mainstay of therapy for thyroid tumors is surgical excision, and the extent of surgery depends on the tumor type. For thyroid carcinomas that can take up iodine (such as follicular carcinoma, papillary carcinoma, and poorly differentiated thyroid carcinoma), radioactive iodine is sometimes administered after total thyroidectomy so that residual microscopic tumor can be eradicated. Thyroxine is also commonly given postoperatively to suppress thyroid-stimulating hormone activity in the hope of reducing tumor recurrence. External radiation therapy and chemotherapy are often reserved for uncontrollable disease or highly aggressive tumors.

## TISSUE PROCUREMENT

### Fine-Needle Aspiration

In recent years, fine-needle aspiration cytology has become the first-line screening or diagnostic procedure for patients presenting with a thyroid mass.[13, 14] The technique is popular because the procedure is simple and relatively nontraumatic, with good acceptance by patients. In experienced hands, the false-positive rate (~0%) and false-negative rate (7% to 10%) are low.[15] The diagnostic categories and their rationale are listed in Table 44–4. By use of the cytologic diagnosis for triage, patients with a diagnosis of tumor or who are suspected of having tumor can be selected for early operation. Those shown on cytologic assessment to have non-neoplastic lesions (such as cyst or colloid nodule) can be followed up; repeated fine-needle aspiration may be required during follow-up to rule out a missed neoplasm.[15, 16]

### Core Needle Biopsy

Core or large needle biopsy is performed in some centers either as the sole procedure or as a complementary procedure to fine-needle aspiration for the initial investigation of thyroid nodules.[17–22] The procedure is more traumatic than fine-needle aspiration, but the yield is generally higher, permitting more accurate diagnosis to be made in some cases.

**TABLE 44–4.** Diagnostic Categories from Fine-Needle Aspiration Cytology of the Thyroid

| Cytologic Diagnosis | Rationale |
| --- | --- |
| Inadequate for diagnosis | With the exception of cyst (which can be hypocellular, with only macrophages being identified), the minimal criterion for adequacy of a specimen is the presence of 5–6 groups of thyroid follicular epithelium with >10 cells per group. |
| Benign, e.g., nodular goiter, cyst, Hashimoto's thyroiditis | Nodular goiter can usually be recognized by features such as abundant thick colloid, low cellularity, large follicles, and honeycombed arrangement of nuclei in the epithelial fragments. |
| Follicular lesion | It can be difficult to make a distinction between cellular adenomatoid nodule and follicular neoplasm. In such situations, the descriptive term *follicular lesion* is applicable. |
| Follicular neoplasm | It is not possible to make a distinction between follicular carcinoma and follicular adenoma on the basis of fine-needle aspiration cytology because diagnosis of follicular carcinoma requires demonstration of vascular or capsular invasion. |
| Suspicious of malignancy | A diagnosis of "suspicious of malignancy" is justified if there are cytologic features suggestive of but not diagnostic of malignancy. |
| Malignant neoplasm, e.g., papillary carcinoma, medullary carcinoma, anaplastic carcinoma, lymphoma | Papillary carcinoma, medullary carcinoma, anaplastic carcinoma, and malignant lymphoma can often be diagnosed on the basis of fine-needle aspiration samples because they exhibit distinctive cytologic and sometimes architectural features. Immunohistochemical studies on the aspirate smears or cell blocks prepared from the aspirated materials are particularly helpful in supporting a diagnosis of medullary carcinoma or lymphoma. Definitive treatment can proceed on the basis of the cytologic diagnosis. A diagnosis of follicular carcinoma cannot be made from fine-needle aspiration cytology. |

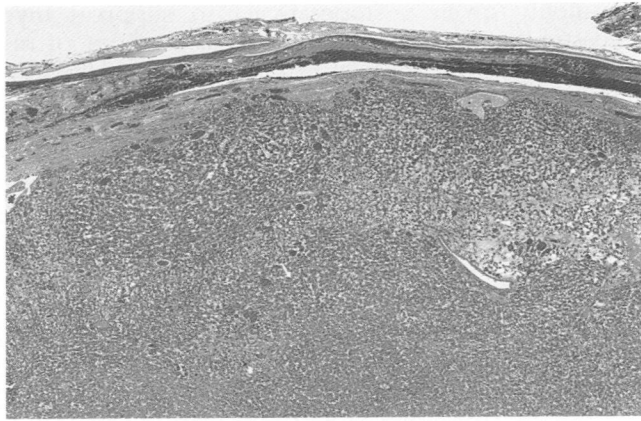

**FIGURE 44–1.** Follicular adenoma. The tumor is enveloped by a thin fibrous capsule. There is no capsular or vascular invasion.

### Surgical Excision

Surgical excision is the standard treatment of thyroid tumors, providing ample tissue for histologic examination and special studies. It is most important to sample the specimen adequately so that an accurate diagnosis can be reached and all prognostic information can be provided. Sampling is most critical for encapsulated follicular neoplasm because a diagnosis of follicular carcinoma can be missed owing to the focal nature of the invasive foci. Some authors recommend a minimum of 10 blocks.[23] Others recommend at least five blocks initially, with five or more additional blocks being taken if the tumor is found to be cellular on initial histologic examination.[24] Most blocks should be taken from the peripheral portions of the tumor, including the interface with the normal thyroid, rather than from the central portion. For optimal assessment of the capsule in all histologic sections, after bisection of the nodule through the equator, radial cuts are made to produce wedge-shaped pieces, like cutting slices of an orange.[25]

### Intraoperative Frozen Section

Diagnosis of thyroid tumors is usually not difficult on frozen sections; the greatest difficulty lies in the distinction between follicular adenoma and follicular carcinoma because the invasive component is often focal and thus not seen in random frozen sections. Touch preparations form an important adjunct at intraoperative assessment and are particularly helpful for recognizing the characteristic nuclear features of papillary carcinoma and medullary carcinoma.

The role of intraoperative frozen section has much diminished in recent years because of the widespread use of fine-needle aspiration cytology for preoperative screening or diagnosis. It is currently used mostly when fine-needle aspiration findings are suggestive of malignancy or are inconclusive. Intraoperative frozen section is of limited use and cost-effectiveness for follicular neoplasms because of the high deferral rate ("follicular neoplasm; defer diagnosis to permanent sections").[26–29] After frozen section is performed, the remaining tissue should be fixed and further sampled for histologic examination.

## Follicular Adenoma

### CLINICAL CONSIDERATIONS

#### Presentation

Follicular adenoma occurs most commonly in adult women aged 20 to 50 years, although no age or sex is exempt. Most patients present with a painless thyroid nodule ("cold" nodule on iodine scan). Rare tumors show increased iodine uptake ("hot" nodules) and may be associated with hyperthyroidism. Follicular adenomas are benign and are adequately treated by lobectomy.

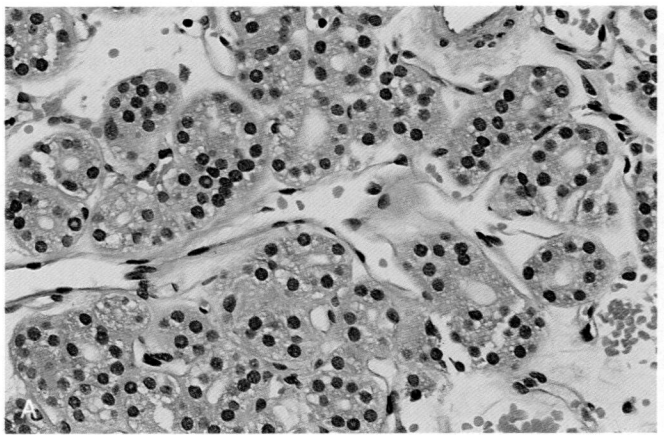
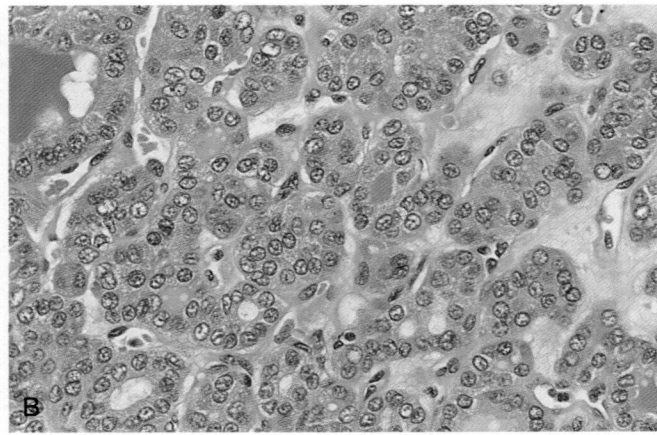

**FIGURE 44–2.** Follicular adenoma. *A.* This tumor is composed of small follicles lined by cells with uniform dark nuclei. *B.* This tumor shows a trabecular to microfollicular growth pattern and comprises cells with mildly atypical nuclei.

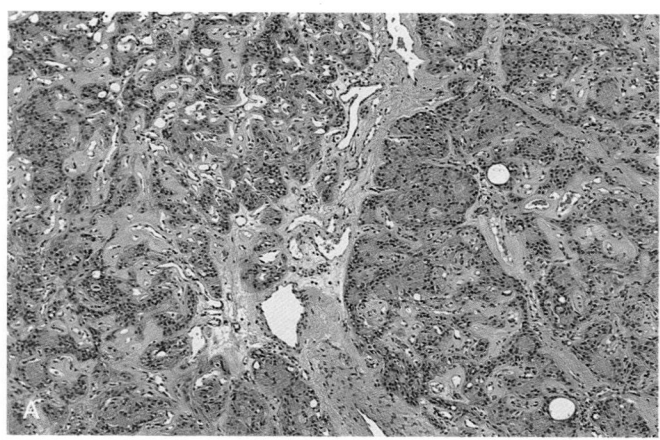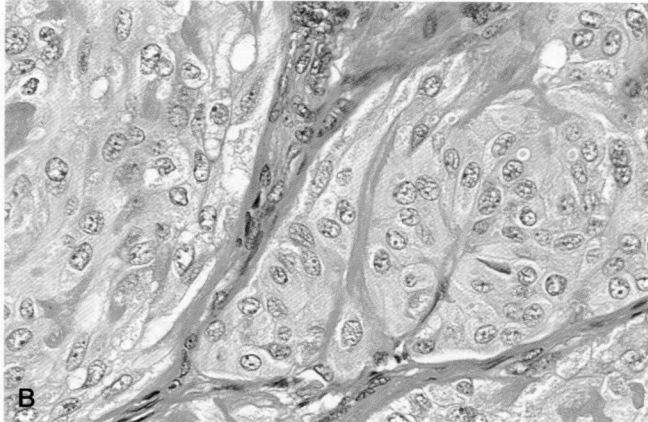

**FIGURE 44–3.** Hyalinizing trabecular adenoma. *A.* The tumor typically forms wavy trabeculae interspersed with lumpy hyaline material. There are interspersed small cystic spaces representing abortive follicle formation. *B.* The tumor cells possess pale oval nuclei that are sometimes grooved, mimicking the cytologic features of papillary carcinoma. Perinucleolar haloes are present. Some tumor cells contain distinctive cytoplasmic "yellow bodies" that stain dull pink and are surrounded by a halo.

### Macroscopic Findings

Follicular adenomas are almost invariably solitary. They are round or oval and are enveloped in a fibrous capsule, which is often thin. The cut surface shows homogeneous tan-brown fleshy tumor, sometimes with a glistening quality. Secondary changes such as hemorrhage and cystic degeneration may be present. Hürthle cell adenomas are typically mahogany brown.

## DIAGNOSTIC CONSIDERATIONS

### Microscopic Findings

Follicular adenoma is typically enclosed in a fibrous capsule of variable thickness, often with compression of the surrounding thyroid tissue (Fig. 44–1). It can show a wide spectrum of architectural features, but a follicular pattern is most common.

The lining cells often have uniform, dark, round nuclei, although occasional enlarged hyperchromatic nuclei can be interspersed (Fig. 44–2).

The many histologic variants of follicular adenoma are listed in Table 44–5 (Figs. 44–3 to 44–10). By definition, capsular or vascular invasion must be absent; if invasion is found, the tumor has to be diagnosed as follicular carcinoma.[23, 30–56] The nature of hyalinizing trabecular adenoma has been most controversial. The hyalinizing trabecular pattern is not specific for follicular adenoma; it can be observed in papillary carcinoma and follicular carcinoma as well as focally in various thyroid lesions, such as colloid nodule and thyroiditis.[57–59] Some investigators consider hyalinizing trabecular adenoma to represent a peculiar variant of papillary carcinoma because of merging with typical papillary carcinoma in some cases, similarities in cytologic

## TABLE 44–5. Variants of Follicular Adenoma

| Variant* | Defining Morphologic Features | Entity for Which the Variant May be Mistaken |
|---|---|---|
| Macrofollicular | Most follicles in the neoplasm are large. | Nodular goiter |
| Microfollicular | Most follicles in the neoplasm are small. | Poorly differentiated (insular) carcinoma |
| Trabecular (embryonal) | The tumor cells form straight trabeculae separated by a delicate vasculature. | Poorly differentiated (insular) carcinoma Medullary carcinoma |
| Hyalinizing trabecular | The tumor forms wavy trabeculae with interspersed microcystic spaces representing abortive follicle formation. The elongated tumor cells are aligned perpendicularly in the trabeculae. The nuclei are often grooved and show pseudoinclusions. Unique cytoplasmic yellow bodies are present. Lumpy hyaline material is interspersed throughout the tumor. Calcified colloid may be present. | Papillary carcinoma Paraganglioma Medullary carcinoma |

*Table continued on following page*

**TABLE 44–5.** Variants of Follicular Adenoma (*Continued*)

| Variant* | Defining Morphologic Features | Entity for Which the Variant May be Mistaken |
|---|---|---|
| Hürthle cell | Follicular neoplasm; most tumor cells have abundant oxyphilic cytoplasm because of accumulation of mitochondria.<br>Nucleoli are often distinct. Some nuclei can be grooved.<br>The tumor often shows a microfollicular or trabecular pattern of growth. | Medullary carcinoma, oxyphilic variant<br>Papillary carcinoma, oxyphilic variant |
| Clear cell | Follicular neoplasm; the tumor cells possess clear cytoplasm because of ballooning of mitochondria, accumulation of lipid or glycogen, or deposition of intracellular thyroglobulin.<br>The clear cytoplasm often retains a finely reticulated or granular quality, instead of being water-clear. | Other primary thyroid neoplasms with clear cell change<br>Metastatic renal cell carcinoma<br>Intrathyroid parathyroid neoplasm |
| Signet ring cell | The tumor cells exhibit discrete cytoplasmic vacuoles that displace the nuclei to one side.<br>The cytoplasmic vacuoles are thyroglobulin immunoreactive and often show the staining properties of mucosubstances. They correspond ultrastructurally to intracellular lumina lined by microvilli.<br>Signet ring cell changes can be focal or diffuse, and this pattern may merge into microcystic spaces filled with extracellular mucin. | Metastatic adenocarcinoma |
| Mucinous | The tumor shows abundant extracellular basophilic mucinous material, often accompanied by a microcystic or reticular growth pattern in the follicular epithelium.<br>Some tumor cells may exhibit signet ring appearance. | Metastatic adenocarcinoma |
| Follicular adenoma with papillary hyperplasia (papillary variant of follicular adenoma) | The tumor is encapsulated and partially cystic. It is composed of papillae and follicles lined by cells with uniform, round, and hyperchromatic nuclei regularly aligned at the base. | Papillary carcinoma |
| Hot adenoma (toxic adenoma) | Follicular adenoma producing symptoms of hyperthyroidism.<br>On histologic examination, the follicles often show papillary infoldings, similar to the follicles seen in Graves' disease. | — |
| Adenolipoma | Follicular adenoma accompanied by a stroma containing adipose cells | — |
| Follicular adenoma with bizarre nuclei | An otherwise typical follicular adenoma with interspersed huge monstrous cells | Follicular carcinoma<br>Anaplastic carcinoma |
| Atypical adenoma | Follicular neoplasm shows generalized nuclear atypia, giant cells, or unusual histologic patterns (such as spindle cell fascicles) but lacks vascular and capsular invasion after thorough sampling. It pursues a benign course. | Follicular carcinoma<br>Medullary carcinoma<br>Anaplastic carcinoma |

* All tumors have to be assessed for vascular or capsular invasion, which, if present, is indicative of a diagnosis of follicular carcinoma.

features, and similarities in immunohistochemical profile (such as expression of high-molecular-weight cytokeratin and basement membrane deposition) [49, 56, 59, 60] (see Fig. 44–3). Nonetheless, a study showed the cytokeratin profile of hyalinizing trabecular adenoma (high-molecular-weight cytokeratin and cytokeratin 19 are often negative or only focally positive) to be different from that of papillary carcinoma, and thus it does not support a histogenetic link between the two tumors.[61] Recent molecular

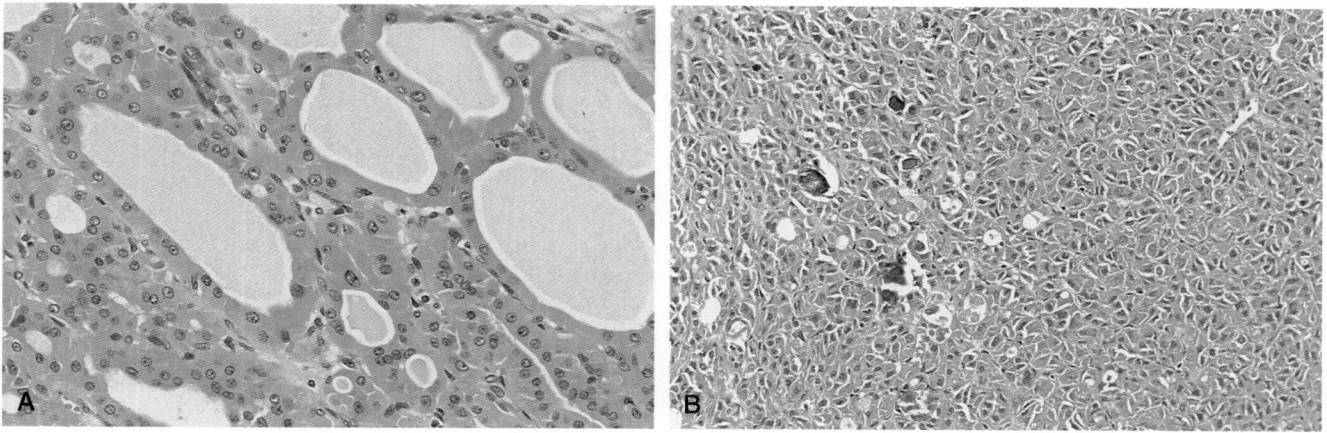

FIGURE 44–4. Hürthle cell adenoma. *A.* This tumor shows a follicular growth pattern. The cells possess abundant eosinophilic granular cytoplasm. Nucleoli are often but not invariably distinct in Hürthle cells. *B.* This tumor shows a solid to trabecular growth pattern. The calcified colloid (*left field*) can potentially be mistaken for psammoma bodies. In contrast to psammoma bodies, they occur within follicular lumina rather than in the stroma.

studies demonstrated a high frequency of *RET/PTC* translocation, suggesting a histogenetic relationship of hyalinizing trabecular adenoma with papillary carcinoma.[61a–61c]

### Immunohistochemistry

Follicular adenomas are immunoreactive for cytokeratin and thyroglobulin but not for calcitonin and pan-neuroendocrine markers. Hyalinizing trabecular adenoma is peculiar in that it often shows an unusual cell membrane pattern of staining for Ki-67.

### Molecular Biology

Mutations in the *ras* gene are found in some follicular adenomas, at a frequency lower than in follicular carcinomas.[62, 63] Hemizygous deletion of the Cowden disease gene, *PTEN*, is found in 26% of follicular adenomas.[64] Activating mutations of the genes coding for the thyrotropin receptor and α-subunit of the stimulatory G protein have been detected in some follicular adenomas, especially the hyperfunctioning ones.[62, 65–70]

### Differential Diagnosis

COLLOID (ADENOMATOID) NODULE. It can be difficult to distinguish between follicular adenoma and adenomatoid nodule (hypercellular colloid nodule); the distinction is sometimes arbitrary. In general, adenomatoid nodules are multiple, lack a well-defined fibrous capsule, and are composed of follicles morphologically similar to those in the surrounding thyroid tissue.

PAPILLARY CARCINOMA. Pale or clear nuclei are not uncommonly encountered in follicular ade-

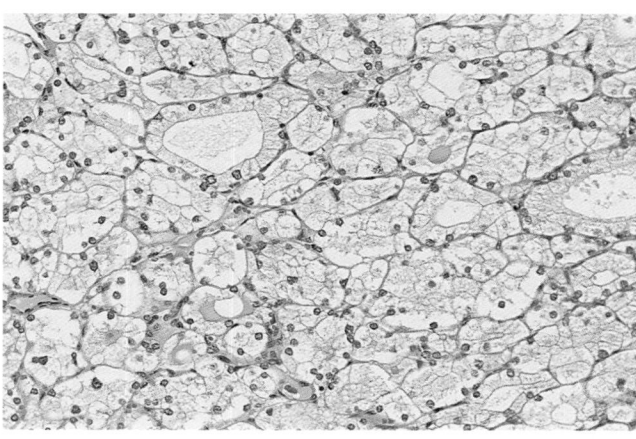

FIGURE 44–5. Follicular adenoma, clear cell variant. The clear cytoplasm is not water-clear but retains a finely reticulated quality.

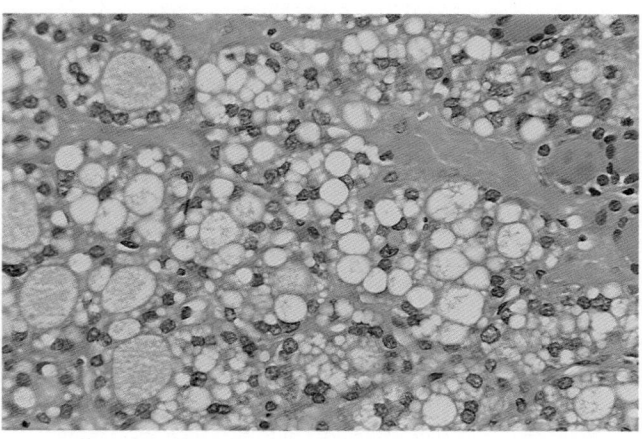

FIGURE 44–6. Follicular adenoma, signet ring cell variant.

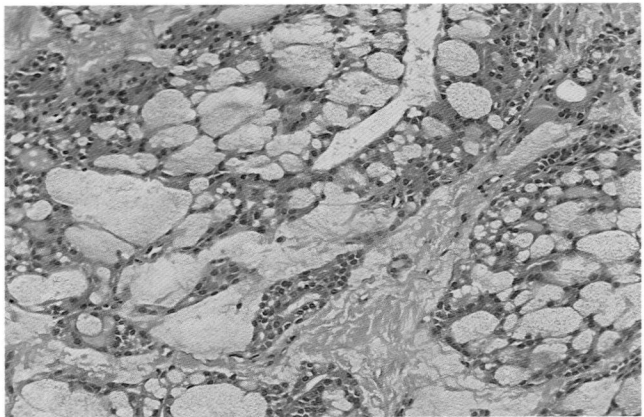

**FIGURE 44–7.** Follicular adenoma, mucinous variant. Intercellular pools of mucin are evident.

nomas, most probably owing to delayed fixation because they are often most prevalent in the central portions of the tumor (Fig. 44–11). Other cytologic features of papillary carcinoma, such as nuclear crowding and nuclear grooving, are lacking, however.

INTRATHYROID PARATHYROID TUMOR. Parathyroid adenoma can sometimes arise within the thyroid gland and thus can be mistaken for microfollicular adenoma, clear cell follicular adenoma, or Hürthle cell adenoma. The presence of clear cells is a most useful clue that the tumor in question might be of parathyroid origin. The diagnosis can be confirmed by the clinical information (hypercalcemia) and positive immunostaining for parathyroid hormone.

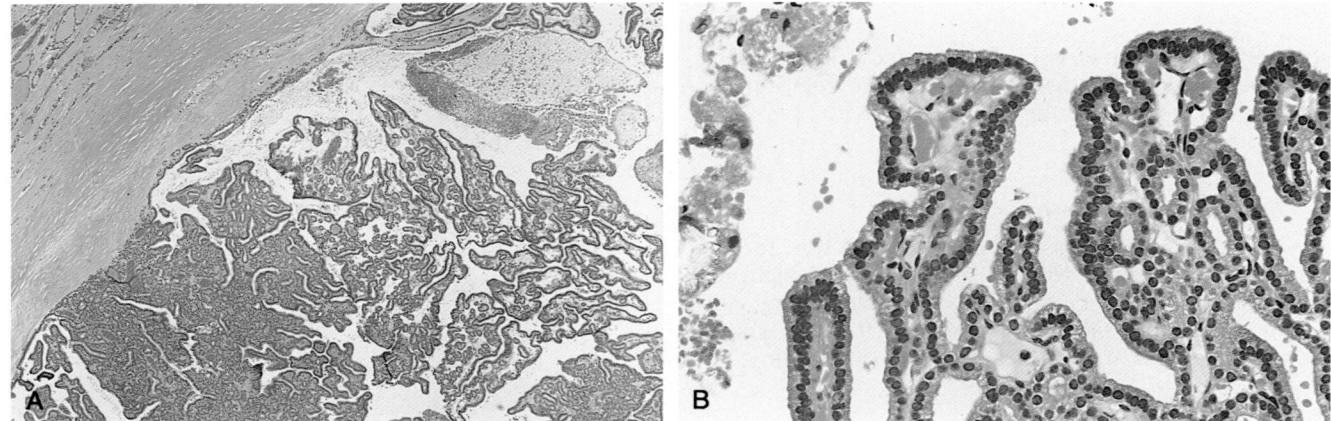

**FIGURE 44–8.** Follicular adenoma with papillary hyperplasia, so-called papillary adenoma. *A.* The tumor is surrounded by a well-defined fibrous capsule. Arborizing papillae are present. *B.* In contrast to papillary carcinoma, the tumor cells have regularly aligned, basal, dark-staining nuclei.

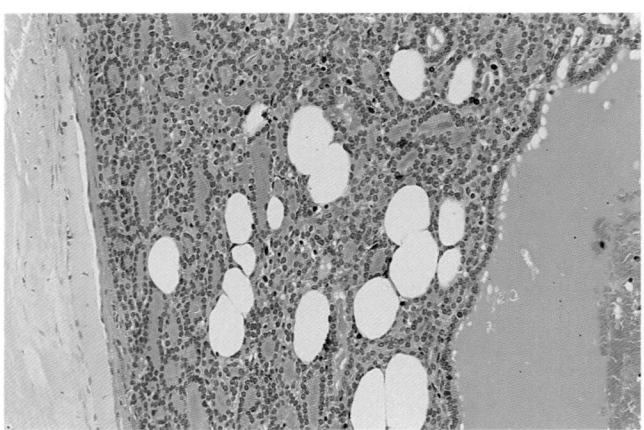

**FIGURE 44–9.** Follicular adenoma, adenolipoma variant.

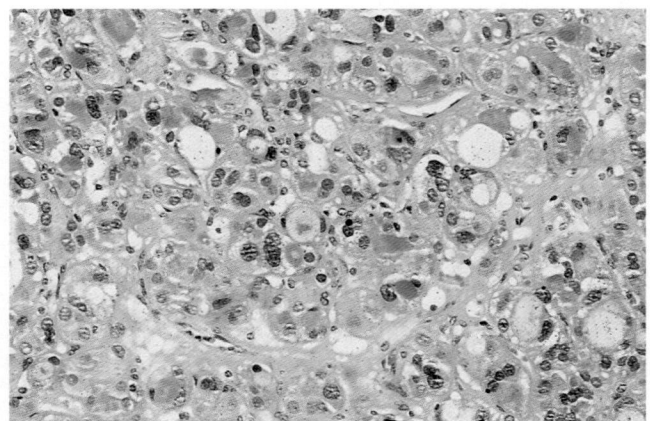

**FIGURE 44–10.** Atypical follicular adenoma. Many tumor cells have enlarged hyperchromatic nuclei.

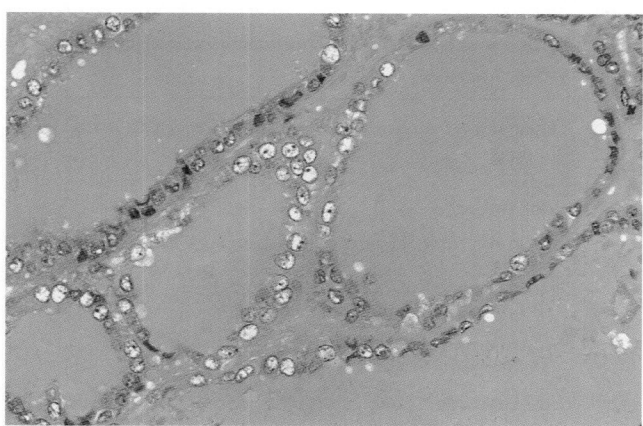

**FIGURE 44–11.** Follicular adenoma showing nuclear clearing. Although the nuclei show clearing, they are not crowded and do not exhibit grooves. This is a common finding confined to the central portion of follicular adenoma, where fixation is delayed.

## Follicular Carcinoma

### CLINICAL CONSIDERATIONS

#### Presentation

Follicular carcinoma is a malignant thyroid neoplasm showing follicular cell differentiation but lacking the diagnostic features of papillary carcinoma.[1] It generally occurs in patients with a mean age higher than that of those with follicular adenoma. It usually manifests as a solitary thyroid mass or, less commonly, as metastatic tumor, in particular in bone.[71–74] The main mode of spread is hematogenous (predilection sites are bone and lung) rather than lymphatic.[75] The differences in clinicopathologic and biologic features between follicular carcinoma and papillary carcinoma are listed in Table 44–6.

#### Macroscopic Findings and Major Subtypes of Follicular Carcinoma

Follicular carcinoma is categorized into minimally invasive and widely invasive types, which show different clinical outcome (Table 44–7). The minimally invasive type is more common.[1, 24, 44, 76–80]

Minimally invasive carcinomas are macroscopically indistinguishable from follicular adenoma, although the capsule tends to be thicker. Vascular or capsular invasion is identified only on histologic assessment (Fig. 44–12). The prognosis is excellent, and thus treatment can be conservative.[24, 72, 73, 81–88]

The less common widely invasive follicular carcinoma shows obvious invasion of the adjacent thyroid parenchyma (Fig. 44–13). The tumor can extend into the perithyroid tissues, and plugging of blood vessels by tumor may also be evident.[1, 44] There is a significant risk of distant metastasis, and the prognosis is much worse than for minimally invasive follicular carcinoma.[44, 89] Of note, many cases reported in the literature as "widely invasive follicular carcinomas" are now reclassifiable as poorly differentiated thyroid carcinomas.

**TABLE 44–6.** Comparison Between Papillary and Follicular Carcinoma

| | Papillary Carcinoma | Follicular Carcinoma |
|---|---|---|
| Frequency | >70% of thyroid cancers | <20% of thyroid cancers |
| Age | Wide age range (mean, 43 y) | Minimally invasive type: mean, 48 y<br>Widely invasive type: mean, 55 y |
| Presentation | Slow-growth thyroid mass; cervical lymphadenopathy; incidental finding | Slow-growing thyroid mass; fast-growing thyroid mass (less common); distant metastasis (such as bone) |
| Multifocal disease | Common | Uncommon |
| Clinical behavior | Tumor is locally invasive; typically spreads by lymphatic route to lymph nodes (~40%).<br>Distant metastasis (such as to lungs) is rare.<br>The tumor is indolent; the cancer-related mortality is only 6.5%—often confined to older patients with extensive extrathyroid disease or distant metastasis. | Tumor spreads predominantly by bloodstream; bone is the predilection site.<br>Lymph node metastasis is uncommon.<br>The cumulative mortality rates of the minimally invasive and widely invasive types are 3% and 32%, respectively. |
| Basis of diagnosis | Diagnosis is mostly based on the nuclear characteristics (crowded, ground-glass, grooved nuclei with pseudoinclusions), and demonstration of invasion is not required for the diagnosis. Therefore, this tumor is diagnosable by fine-needle aspiration cytology. | A follicular neoplasm demonstrating vascular or capsular invasion, and nuclear features of papillary carcinoma must be lacking. Therefore, distinction from follicular adenoma cannot be made on fine-needle aspiration cytology; only a diagnostic label of "follicular neoplasm" can be given. |
| Genetic basis | Overexpression of *RET* proto-oncogene due to fusion with *PTC1*, *PTC2*, or *PTC3* gene, or overexpression of *NTRK1* gene due to fusion with other genes such as *TPM3* | Somatic mutation of *ras* oncogene in ~50% of cases, most commonly involving codon 61 CAA → CGA (Gln → Arg). t(2;3)(q13;p25) resulting in *PAX8-PPARγ1* fusion is found in >50% of cases. |

**TABLE 44–7.** Categories of Follicular Carcinoma

|  | **Minimally Invasive** | **Widely Invasive** |
| --- | --- | --- |
| Definition | Totally encapsulated tumor with no gross invasion; vascular or capsular invasion is identified on histologic examination. | Tumor shows obvious invasion of adjacent thyroid tissue. |
| Age | Younger (mean, ~48 y) | Older (mean, ~56 y) |
| Metastases | Regional lymph node or distant metastasis is rare and occurs late if it does. | Regional lymph node metastasis occurs in 13%–24% of cases. Distant metastasis (such as to lung, bone, brain, liver) is common (29%–60%). |
| Outcome | Excellent prognosis. The long-term mortality is only 3%–5%. | Long-term mortality is 30%–50%. |
| Treatment | Curable by lobectomy or subtotal thyroidectomy, with or without suppressive dose of thyroxine. For high-risk patients, such as old patients and those with large tumors, total thyroidectomy and radioactive iodine therapy may have to be considered. | Total thyroidectomy, radioactive iodine, and suppressive dose of thyroxine |

## DIAGNOSTIC CONSIDERATIONS

### Microscopic Findings

Follicular carcinomas are often surrounded by a thick, dense fibrous capsule, although some widely invasive follicular carcinomas may not have a fibrous capsule (see Figs. 44–12 and 44–13). The tumors comprise cuboid cells forming closely packed follicles, trabeculae, or solid sheets. The follicles are mostly small, but large follicles can also be present. The tumor cells often have uniform, dark-staining or pale-staining, round nuclei, but significant nuclear atypia can be observed in some cases (Fig. 44–14). The cytoplasm is eosinophilic, oxyphilic, or clear. Mitotic figures range from being scanty to easily found. Secondary changes such as hemorrhage, hemosiderin deposition, sclerosis, edema, necrosis, and cystic change are not uncommon. The tumors may show variant histologic features like those listed for follicular adenomas[31, 34, 90–93] (see Table 44–5).

The only feature that distinguishes a follicular carcinoma from a follicular adenoma is the presence of vascular or capsular invasion.[1] Strict criteria must be applied in the assessment of invasion.[94–98] The histologic features that should heighten the suspicion for follicular carcinoma are listed in Table 44–8, but they are by themselves insufficient for a diagnosis of malignancy.

To qualify for vascular invasion, the following two criteria must be satisfied[24]:

- Involved blood vessels have to be located within or outside the fibrous capsule.
- The intravascular polypoid tumor plug has to be covered by endothelium; if it is not endothelialized, it must be associated with thrombus formation (Fig. 44–15; see also Fig. 44–12).

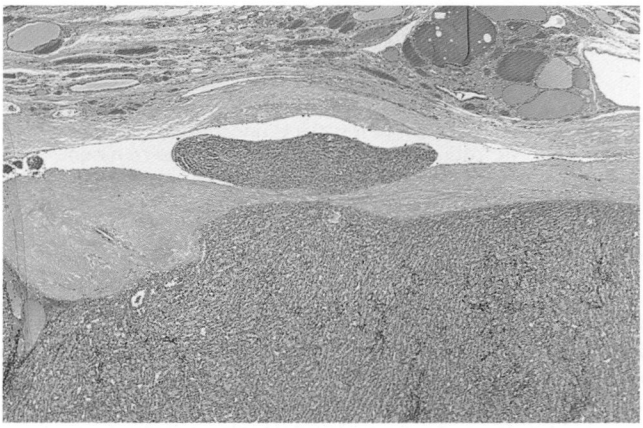

**FIGURE 44–12.** Follicular carcinoma, minimally invasive type. The tumor is typically surrounded by a thick fibrous capsule. Vascular invasion is present (*upper field*).

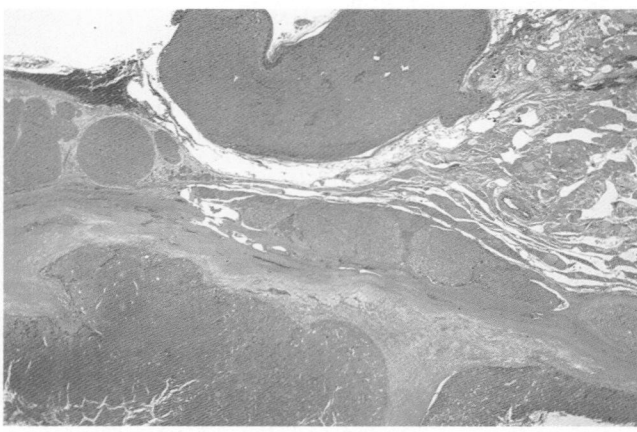

**FIGURE 44–13.** Follicular carcinoma, widely invasive type. There is frank invasion of the thyroid tissue in the form of multiple cellular tumor nodules. The upper field shows vascular invasion.

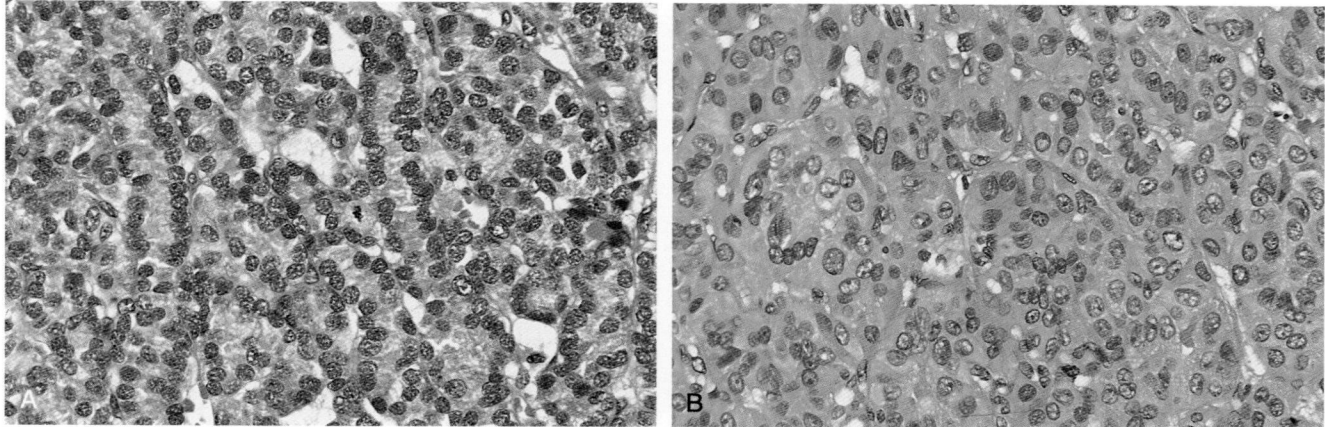

**FIGURE 44–14.** Follicular carcinoma. *A.* This tumor shows a trabecular growth pattern and comprises cells with fairly uniform, dark, round nuclei. *B.* This tumor exhibits generalized nuclear atypia. This is a feature that should alert one to the possibility of carcinoma for a follicular neoplasm.

An invasive bud frequently pushes into the fibrous capsule and then into a capsular blood vessel lumen (Fig. 44–16). Mere bulging of follicles against the thin-walled capsular vessels is not sufficient for a designation of vascular invasion (Fig. 44–17). Retraction spaces around tumor islands should not be mistaken for vascular invasion, and they can be recognized by the lack of endothelial lining. The presence of ragged clusters of nonendothelialized tumor within blood vessels does not count for vascular invasion. This is believed to result from artifactual

dislodgment of tumor during sectioning of the specimen.[24] Intravascular endothelial hyperplasia occurring in capsular blood vessels should also not be mistaken for vascular invasion; the intravascular polypoid plug is formed by plump spindly endothelial cells and pericytes instead of follicular epithelial cells[99] (Fig. 44–18).

To qualify for capsular invasion, there must be complete transgression of the fibrous capsule by tumor. That is, the tumor bud must have extended beyond an imaginary line drawn through the exter-

---

**TABLE 44–8.** Key Points and Caveats in Diagnosis of Follicular Adenoma and Carcinoma

There is a tendency to overdiagnose follicular carcinoma. To qualify for follicular carcinoma, the following criteria must be satisfied:
- Follicular neoplasm lacking nuclear features of papillary carcinoma
- Capsular or vascular invasion, which must be unequivocal

Histologic features in a follicular neoplasm warranting more careful sampling to look for invasion (these features are not diagnostic of carcinoma per se):
- Thick fibrous capsule
- High cellularity, i.e., tumors that are predominantly solid, trabecular, or microfollicular
- Diffuse nuclear atypia (as opposed to presence of occasional bizarre cells)
- Readily identifiable mitotic figures
- Perpendicularly aligned neoplastic follicles or mushroom-shaped tumor bud in fibrous capsule
- Hürthle cell neoplasm (~35% of all Hürthle cell neoplasms are malignant, a percentage higher than that of non–Hürthle cell neoplasms)

Do not mistake capsular rupture associated with prior fine-needle aspiration as true capsular invasion. Capsular rupture can be recognized by the following features:
- Tumor buds within fibrous capsule (at most one or two sites) are tiny and lack a "mushroom" contour.
- Tumor buds are associated with blood, chronic inflammatory cells, and hemosiderin deposit.
- Tumor cells often have a degenerated appearance.
- Hemorrhagic track (with or without reparative features) is often identifiable in the vicinity.

If prominent delicate fibrovascular septa are present, consider the alterantive possibilities:
- Medullary carcinoma
- Intrathyroid parathyroid neoplasm
- Paraganglioma

If a Hürthle cell neoplasm appears unusual, it may represent oxyphilic variant of the following tumors:
- Medullary carcinoma
- Intrathyroid parathyroid neoplasm
- Papillary carcinoma

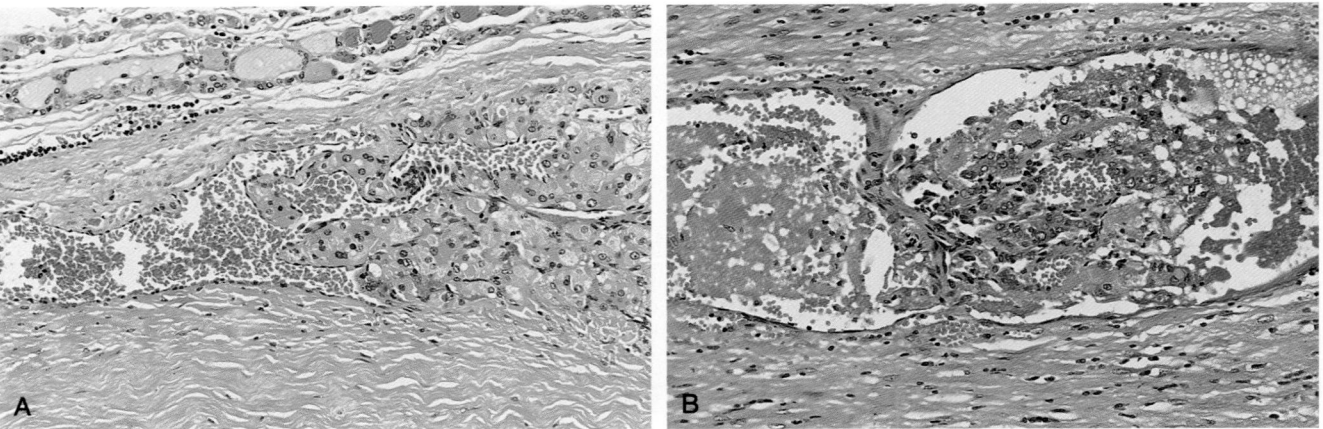

**FIGURE 44–15.** Follicular carcinoma showing vascular invasion. *A.* A tumor plug projects into a capsular blood vessel, and it is clothed by endothelium. *B.* The intravascular tumor plug has a jagged outline and is not clothed by endothelium. However, this satisfies the criterion for vascular invasion because there is associated fibrin thrombus (*left field*).

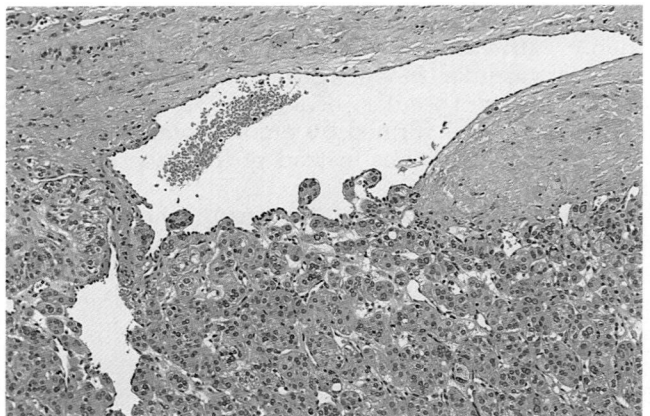

**FIGURE 44–16.** Follicular carcinoma. The tumor (*lower field*) extends into the fibrous capsule and then projects into a vascular lumen in the capsule.

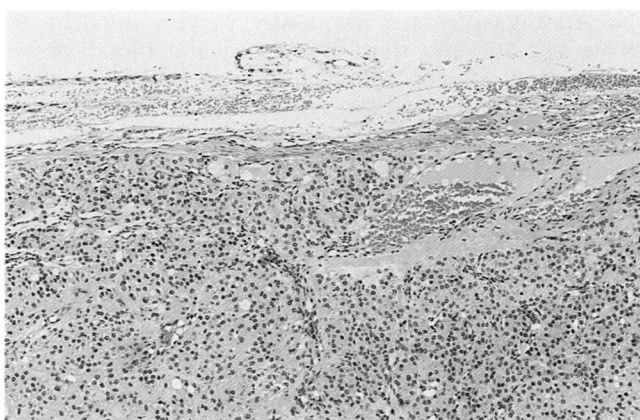

**FIGURE 44–17.** Follicular adenoma. Bulging of tumor against blood vessels within the tumor proper does not constitute vascular invasion.

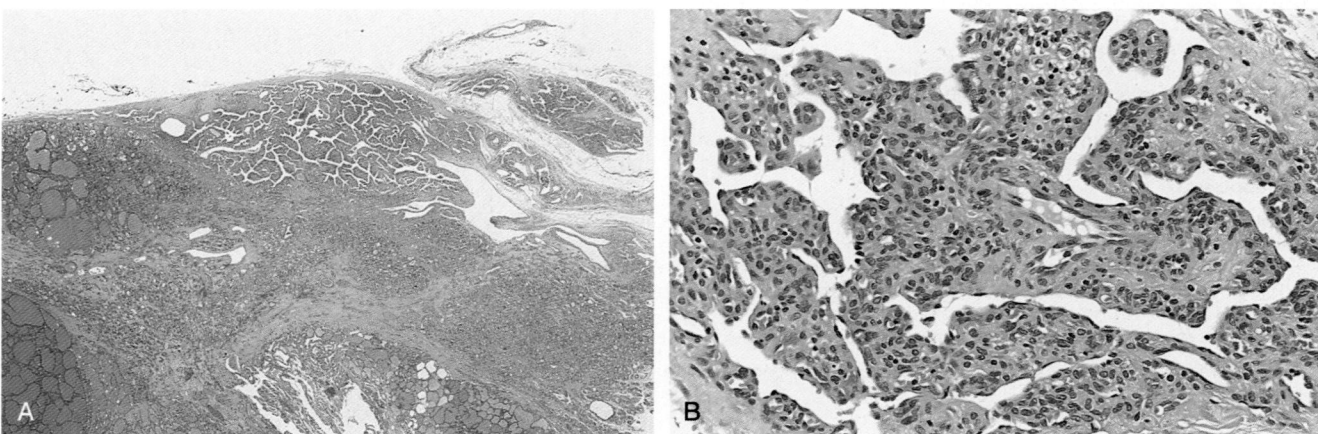

**FIGURE 44–18.** Follicular adenoma with intravascular endothelial hyperplasia in the capsule, mimicking vascular invasion. *A.* Cellular proliferation is seen in the capsular blood vessel (*upper field*). *B.* Closer examination reveals that the intravascular proliferation consists of small blood vessels and not tumor cells.

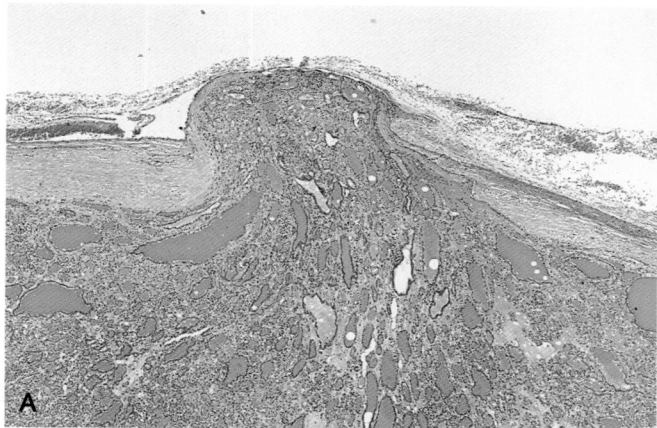
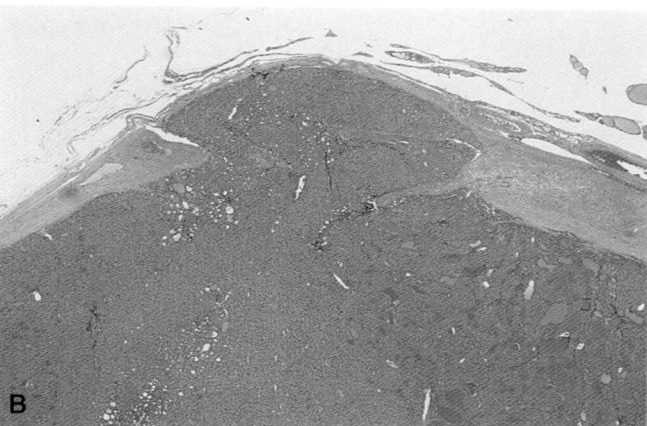

FIGURE 44–19. Follicular carcinoma showing capsular invasion. *A.* In this case, there is total penetration of the fibrous capsule. The invasive bud does not have a fibrous cap. *B.* In this case, the invasive bud has penetrated the fibrous capsule, reaching beyond an imaginary line drawn along the external contour of the capsule. This invasive bud is clothed by a newly formed, thin fibrous cap.

nal contour of the capsule (Fig. 44–19). The invasive bud may be "naked" (without a fibrous capsule) or clothed by a thinner, newly formed fibrous capsule[24, 71, 78, 100] (Fig. 44–19). A tumor bud that shows incomplete penetration of the capsule despite examination of multiple levels of the tissue block can be disregarded. Follicles entrapped in the capsule by a sclerotic process are often aligned parallel to the fibers of the capsule (Fig. 44–20), whereas follicles oriented perpendicular to the fibers or forming a mushroom-shaped bud are more indicative of an active invasive process, mandating examination of multiple levels and multiple blocks for more definite evidence of capsular invasion (Fig. 44–21). Fine-needle aspiration can result in capsular rupture, mimicking capsular invasion; see Table 44–8 for features supportive of this interpretation[101] (Fig. 44–22).

### Hürthle Cell Carcinoma

Hürthle cell carcinoma is a variant of follicular carcinoma characterized by mitochondria-rich cells,[75] although some investigators consider it to be a distinct entity.[45] There is new evidence that the pattern of chromosome allelic alteration in Hürthle cell carcinomas differs from that of conventional follicular carcinomas.[102]

On gross evaluation, the tumor is bright brown. A size of 4 cm or larger is strongly correlated with malignancy.[103] On histologic examination, the tumor shows a trabecular, microfollicular, diffuse, or rarely papillary growth pattern. The tumor cells possess abundant brightly eosinophilic granular cytoplasm, which can exhibit partial to complete clearing as a result of ballooning of the mitochondria (Fig.

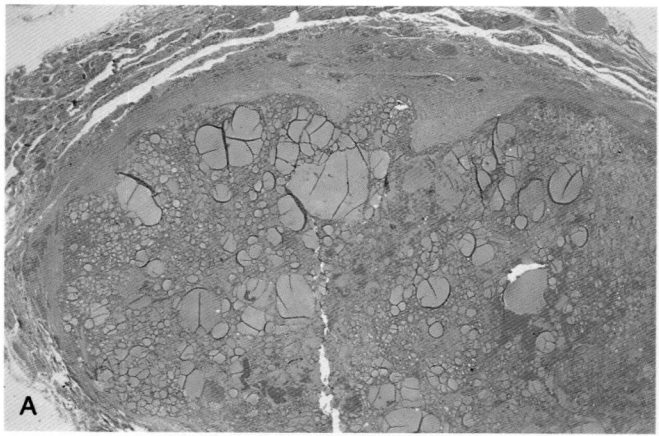
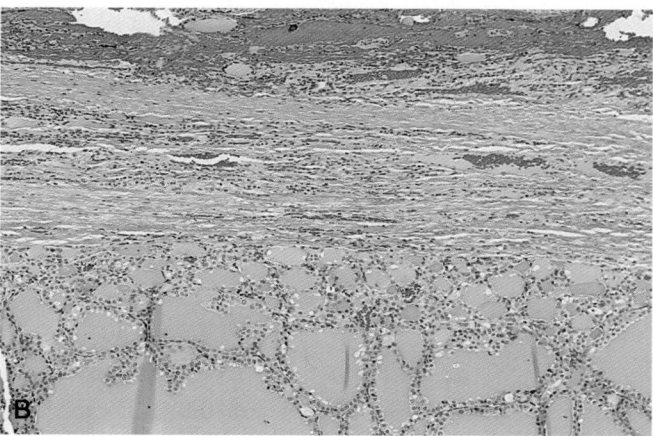

FIGURE 44–20. Follicular adenoma. *A.* Bosselations of the tumor on the inner aspect of the fibrous capsule should not be interpreted as capsular invasion. *B.* In the fibrous capsule, there are atrophic follicles aligned in the direction of the fibrous capsule. This phenomenon results from passive entrapment of follicles in the fibrotic process and does not indicate capsular invasion.

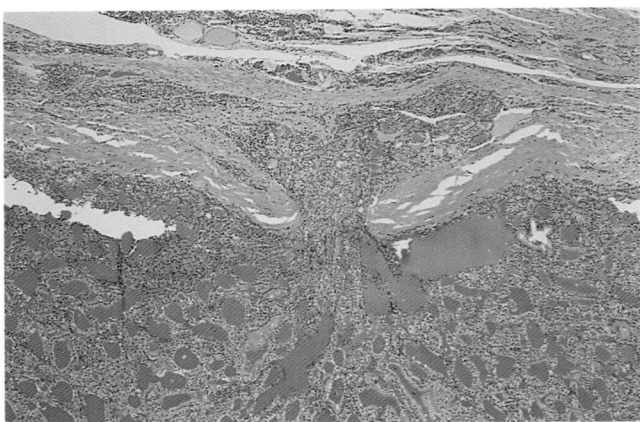

**FIGURE 44–21.** Follicular carcinoma. Not uncommonly, an invasive bud takes the shape of a mushroom, indicating an active invasive process. This field, however, is insufficient to qualify for full capsule penetration because the bud has not extended beyond the external contour of the fibrous capsule. Nonetheless, this finding should prompt careful examination of deeper levels and multiple blocks for more definite evidence of capsular or vascular invasion.

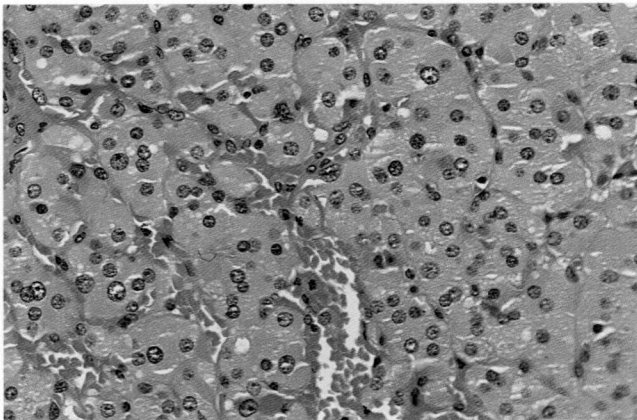

**FIGURE 44–22.** Follicular adenoma with fine-needle aspiration–associated capsular rupture. The bud in the fibrous capsule is small and accompanied by hemorrhage and chronic inflammatory cells.

44–23). The nuclei are round or sometimes grooved. The chromatin is granular to coarse, and nucleoli are often prominent. Some degree of nuclear pleomorphism is common. The colloid can undergo calcification and thus may be mistaken for psammoma bodies. Hürthle cell neoplasms are particularly prone to infarction after fine-needle aspiration.[101, 104–106]

Some previous studies have proposed aggressive treatment for all Hürthle cell neoplasms, irrespective of whether invasion could be demonstrated histologically, on the basis of the belief that all were potentially malignant.[107–110] However, many later studies have challenged this misconception and shown that the behavior of Hürthle cell neoplasms can be accurately predicted by histologic features (i.e., whether there is vascular or capsular invasion, as in follicular neoplasms).* Only those showing invasion are diagnosed as carcinoma (see Fig. 44–15A). Such tumors can recur locally, metastasize to regional lymph nodes, or show distant metastasis (especially to bone and lungs).[71, 98, 100, 119, 120] When a Hürthle cell neoplasm shows some but inconclusive evidence of invasion, the term *Hürthle cell tumor of uncertain malignant potential* is sometimes applied. Clinical follow-up shows a benign evolution in all cases. It may therefore be more appropriate to simply label such cases "Hürthle cell adenoma."[100, 121]

The overall mortality rate of Hürthle cell carcinomas is 30% to 70%.[71, 98, 100] Compared with conventional follicular carcinomas, Hürthle cell carcinomas take up radioactive iodine less satisfactorily;

they show a higher frequency of extrathyroidal extension, local recurrence, and metastasis to lymph nodes, and the survival rate is lower.[75, 96, 100, 122, 123] However, with stratification by the extent of invasion, the differences are obliterated.[75] It has been suggested that the presence of a solid or trabecular pattern in more than 75% of the tumor area identifies a poorly differentiated subgroup with worse prognosis—30% died of disease or were alive with recurrent disease, compared with a 2.5% mortality rate for the non–poorly differentiated subgroup.[124]

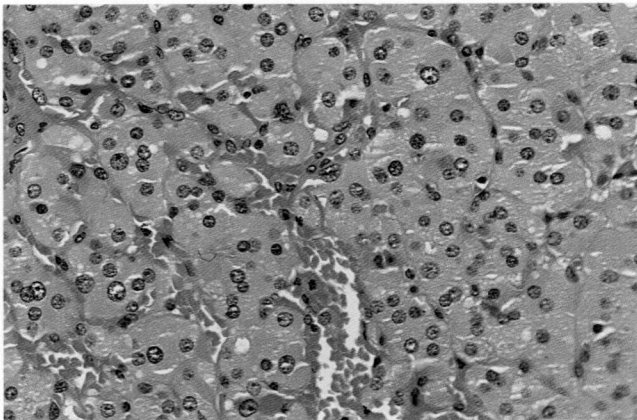

**FIGURE 44–23.** Hürthle cell carcinoma. The tumor comprises trabeculae of tumor cells with abundant eosinophilic granular cytoplasm. There is mild nuclear pleomorphism.

---

*References 71, 94, 95, 98, 100, 107, 111–119.

### Immunohistochemistry

Follicular carcinoma is immunoreactive for cytokeratin and thyroglobulin but not for pan-neuroendocrine markers.[125] Immunohistochemical studies are rarely required for diagnosis of this tumor with the exception of two scenarios:

- Unusual-looking thyroid neoplasm—thyroglobulin immunoreactivity confirms the presence of thyroid follicular cell differentiation and is helpful for distinction from medullary carcinoma.
- Metastatic neoplasm suspected to represent metastatic follicular carcinoma—thyroglobulin immunoreactivity confirms the thyroid origin of the carcinoma.

### Molecular Biology and Special Studies

Clonal chromosome abnormalities, such as nondisjunctional chromosome loss and deletions in 3p25 → pter, are common in follicular carcinomas.[126–129] Comparative genomic hybridization studies reveal frequent DNA copy number changes; loss of chromosome 22 is associated with the widely invasive type and old age at presentation.[130] Molecular studies show frequent loss of heterozygosity on chromosomes 3p (86%), 17p (72%), and 10q (57%); 17p change is correlated with mortality.[131, 132]

A high frequency of activating point mutations in the family of *ras* genes is found in follicular carcinomas, although similar mutations can also be found in some follicular adenomas.[62, 63] N-*ras* mutation is found in 50% of follicular carcinomas, most commonly involving codon 61 with CAA → CGA (Gln → Arg); this mutation is observed in approximately 25% of anaplastic carcinomas but not in papillary carcinomas.[133] H-*ras* codon 12 mutation is found in 33% of follicular carcinomas.[134] Alteration in the *TP53* gene is uncommon, but its presence is associated with an increased risk of metastasis.[135] Recently, t(2;3)(q13; p25), which results in fusion of *PAX8* gene with peroxisome proliferator–activated receptor gamma 1 (*PPARγ1*) gene, has been shown to be a characteristic genetic aberration of follicular carcinoma. The fusion transcript is detected in 5 of 8 follicular carcinomas, but not in 20 follicular adenomas, 10 papillary carcinomas, and 10 cases of multinodular hyperplasia.[135a]

### Differential Diagnosis

FOLLICULAR ADENOMA. The current "gold standard" for distinguishing between follicular carcinoma and follicular adenoma is identification of vascular or capsular invasion in follicular carcinoma (see "Microscopic Findings"). Although some antibodies, such as Leu-7, thyroid peroxidase (monoclonal antibody 47), HBME-1, tissue polypeptide antigen, dipeptidyl aminopeptidase IV (CD26), and topoisomerase II, have been reported to stain follicular carcinomas and follicular adenomas with different frequencies,[136–142] the discriminatory power is not high enough for routine diagnostic application. Various tumor markers, such as carcinoembryonic antigen, oncogene products (Ras p21, c-Myc), cyclin D1, cyclin-dependent kinase inhibitor (p27), proliferation marker (Ki-67), epidermal growth factor, P-glycoprotein, high-mobility group I HMGI(Y) protein, and telomerase activity, have not been shown to be sufficiently discriminatory either.[121, 125, 143–149] DNA ploidy analysis also fails to distinguish follicular carcinoma from follicular adenoma.[150–154]

HASHIMOTO'S THYROIDITIS AND DYSHORMONOGENESIS. In Hashimoto's thyroiditis or dyshormonogenetic goiter, multiple cellular hyperplastic nodules can be present, raising a concern for follicular carcinoma. However, vascular invasion is not found, and the different cellular nodules often exhibit different cellularities and follicle size.

MEDULLARY CARCINOMA. Some variants of medullary carcinoma can mimic follicular or Hürthle cell carcinoma. The presence of prominent delicate fibrovascular septa should always raise the possibility of medullary carcinoma. If there is any uncertainty about the diagnosis, immunohistochemical studies should be performed.

PAPILLARY CARCINOMA. Some follicular carcinomas may show nuclear clearing, mimicking papillary carcinomas. However, this phenomenon is often confined to the central portion of the tumor, where there is delayed fixation. Hürthle cell carcinomas can show nuclear grooving, but this is often a focal phenomenon and other cytologic features of papillary carcinoma are lacking.

## PROGNOSTIC CONSIDERATIONS

The most important prognostic factors for follicular carcinoma are age, degree of invasiveness, and presence or absence of distant metastasis.

AGE. The prognosis is excellent for patients younger than 30 to 40 years.*

MINIMALLY INVASIVE VERSUS WIDELY INVASIVE TYPE. The prognosis of the widely invasive follicular carcinoma is much worse than that of the minimally invasive type (see Table 44–7). Tumor invasion of the soft tissues of the neck is associated with a particularly unfavorable prognosis.[44, 82, 96, 111, 123]

METASTASIS. Distant metastasis at presentation is a highly unfavorable prognostic factor.†

SEX. Some studies have shown the male sex to be associated with a worse outcome.[82, 100, 156]

HISTOLOGIC TYPE OR PATTERN. As a group, Hürthle cell carcinomas have a worse prognosis than that of conventional follicular carcinomas.[71, 75, 100, 123] Presence of a solid or trabecular pattern in more than 75% of the tumor area is associated with a worse prognosis.[124]

---

*References 44, 71, 78, 82, 100, 111, 123, 155, 156.

†References 44, 71, 81, 100, 111, 123, 156–158.

TUMOR SIZE. Some studies have reported a large tumor (>4 cm) to be associated with a worse prognosis.[78, 100, 123, 155, 156]

VASCULAR INVASION. Follicular carcinomas showing capsular invasion alone in the absence of vascular invasion have a negligible risk of metastasis.[81, 121, 156, 159]

E-CADHERIN EXPRESSION. Lack of E-cadherin expression is reported to be an unfavorable prognostic factor.[160]

DNA ANEUPLOIDY. Whereas some studies suggest that aneuploid follicular carcinomas are more aggressive, other studies have not been able to confirm this observation.[150, 151, 161]

P53 ABERRATION. Presence of p53 aberration may confer an increased chance of metastasis.[124, 135]

## Papillary Carcinoma

### CLINICAL CONSIDERATIONS

#### Presentation

Papillary carcinoma can occur in patients of any age, including children. The mean age is 43 years, and there is a female predilection[162-165] (see Table 44–6). The patients usually present with a thyroid mass or cervical lymph node metastasis. Small papillary carcinoma can also be discovered incidentally in thyroid glands excised for various reasons (latent papillary carcinoma).[166, 167]

#### Macroscopic Findings

The macroscopic appearances of papillary carcinoma are highly variable, mirroring the myriad histologic patterns that this tumor can assume. The classic examples exhibit firm to hard white-tan tumors with invasive borders. The tumor often has a granular quality on the cut surface due to the presence of papillae. The presence of psammoma bodies can impart a gritty sensation on cutting of the tumor. Tumors with a predominantly follicular architecture are often tan-brown and fleshy, similar to follicular neoplasms. Some tumors can be encapsulated. Cystic change can occur.

### DIAGNOSTIC CONSIDERATIONS

#### Microscopic Findings

Papillary carcinoma is defined as a malignant epithelial tumor showing evidence of follicular cell differentiation, typically with papillary and follicular structures as well as characteristic nuclear changes.[1, 168, 169] The diagnosis is based on the nuclear characteristics, which include large size, pallor, ground-glass appearance, irregular outline, deep grooves, and pseudoinclusions[169-172] (Fig. 44–24).

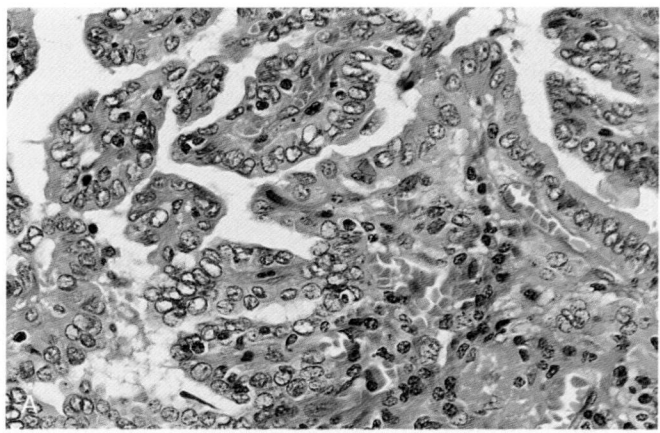
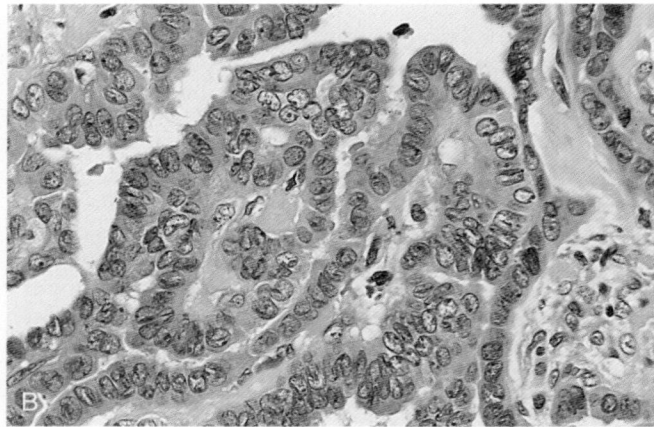
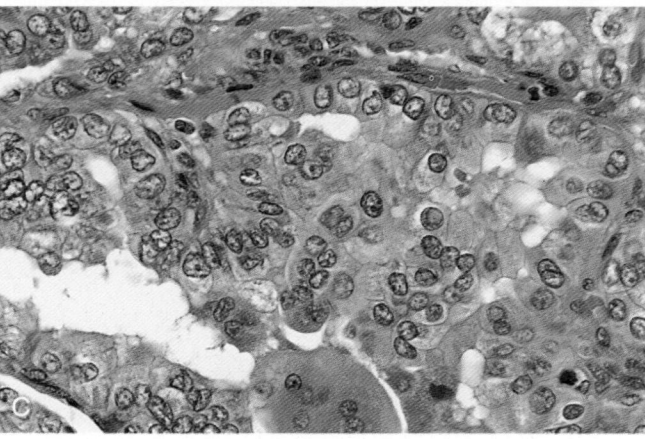

**FIGURE 44–24.** Papillary carcinoma showing the spectrum of cytologic features. *A.* The papillae are covered by cells with pale nuclei, some of which are optically clear (*left field*). The nuclei also exhibit crowding. *B.* The nuclei are comparatively chromatin rich, although still pale. They are ovoid, with grooving and distinct nucleoli. Note the lack of polarity. *C.* The nuclei are pale, and some nuclear pseudoinclusions are seen. Portion of a multinucleated histiocyte is seen in the lumen (*lower field*).

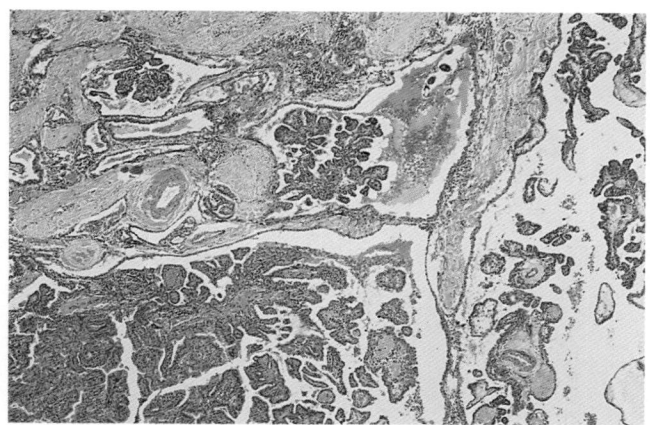

**FIGURE 44–25.** Papillary carcinoma. A typical example showing infiltrative growth, prominent branching papillae, and sclerotic stroma.

Papillary carcinomas are usually infiltrative, but some may be circumscribed or even encapsulated (Fig. 44–25).

The papillae are usually arborizing, with delicate fibrovascular cores (Fig. 44–26A; see also Fig. 44–25). However, the papillae can be broad, with the cores being formed by fibrocellular, edematous, or hyalinized tissue, which may contain foamy macrophages, adipose cells, or small neoplastic follicles.[38, 173, 174] Micropapillae comprising cellular tufts are sometimes formed. Follicles are frequently present. They vary in size and contour but are commonly elongated or irregularly shaped and contain dark-staining colloid. Some follicles can be large and markedly distended with colloid. Intrafollicular hemorrhage is common. There is often an intricate blending of the follicles and papillae, resulting in a complex tubulopapillary pattern (Fig. 44–26B). Less common patterns are microglandular, cribriform, anastomosing tubular, trabecular, and solid.[171, 175] Multinucleated histiocytes with deeply eosinophilic cytoplasm can be found in the luminal space of some follicles and papillae in approximately 50% of cases and can aid in the diagnosis of papillary carcinoma because they are extremely rare in other thyroid lesions or tumors[176] (see Fig. 44–24C).

There is commonly an abundant sclerotic stroma,[177, 178] and desmoplastic stroma is often confined to the invasive fronts[170] (Fig. 44–27; see also Fig. 44–25). The stroma commonly shows patchy infiltration of lymphocytes, plasma cells, and macrophages. Psammoma bodies are found in the stalks of the papillae, in the fibrous stroma, or among the tumor cells in about 50% of cases; they are virtually pathognomonic of papillary thyroid carcinoma[170, 179, 180] (see Fig. 44–26A).

The nuclei of papillary carcinoma are characteristically large, crowded, ovoid, ground-glass ("Orphan Annie" eye), and grooved and contain small distinct nucleoli[171, 181] (see Fig. 44–24). Nuclear pseudoinclusions may be identified in a small proportion of tumor cells[181–184] (see Fig. 44–24C). Mitotic figures are usually sparse. In some papillary carcinomas, the typical nuclear features may not be well developed, and thus the diagnosis of papillary carcinoma would have to depend on the architectural features and on the identification of foci showing more typical nuclear features (Fig. 44–28).

The neoplastic cells are cuboid, polygonal, columnar, flattened, dome shaped, or hobnailed. The cytoplasm is lightly eosinophilic to amphophilic, but it can be oxyphilic or clear.[31, 34, 185–187] Cytoplasmic mucin can be demonstrated by histochemical stains in a proportion of cases.[188, 189] Focal squamous differentiation is common, and such foci usually do not exhibit the characteristic nuclear features of papillary carcinoma (Fig. 44–29).

Many variants of papillary carcinoma have been recognized, but only some are of prognostic signifi-

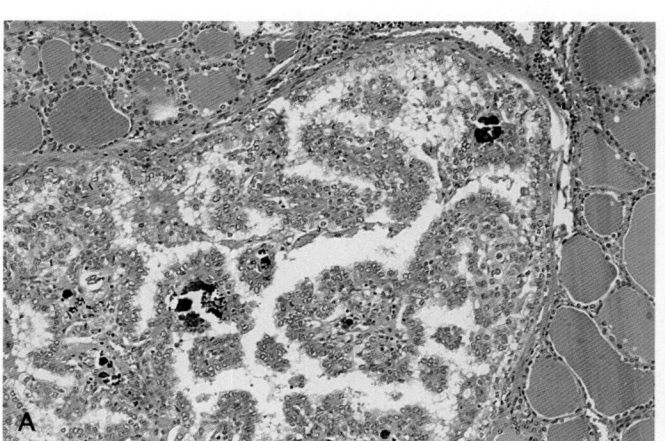
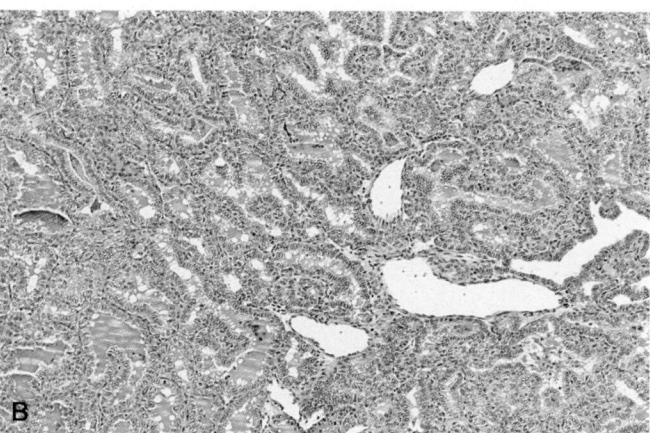

**FIGURE 44–26.** Papillary carcinoma. *A.* Arborizing papillae are evident. Psammoma bodies are seen in the cores of some papillae. *B.* Complex tubulopapillary architecture is a common growth pattern.

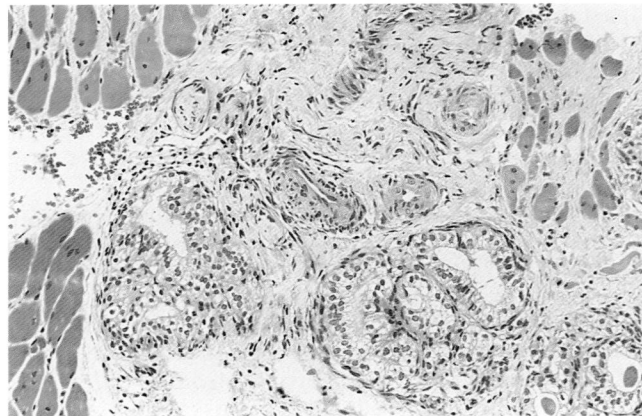

**FIGURE 44–27.** Papillary carcinoma with extrathyroidal extension. The tumor extends into the skeletal muscle of the anterior neck and is accompanied by a desmoplastic stroma.

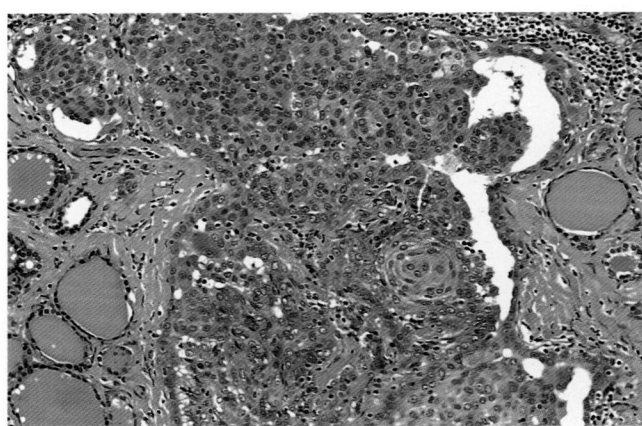

**FIGURE 44–29.** Papillary carcinoma showing focal squamous metaplasia.

cance.* They are listed in Table 44–9 (Figs. 44–30 to 44–42).

### Latent Papillary Carcinoma

Latent papillary carcinomas are cancers incidentally found in thyroidectomy specimens or at autopsy. In autopsy series, they are found in approximately 5% to 10% of cases, but the frequency ranges from as high as 36% in Finland to as low as 1.2% in Switzerland.[171, 248–257] Latent papillary carcinomas usually appear after puberty, and the prevalence does not show a significant increase with age thereafter.[250, 258–260] A small proportion of cases can show regional lymph node metastasis, but the deposits are often microscopic and probably remain dormant

*References 45, 72, 76, 164, 165, 170, 171, 180, 185, 190–247.

even without excision.[261] The lack of female predominance in latent papillary carcinomas and the dissociation between the prevalence rates of latent and clinical thyroid carcinomas suggest that most latent papillary carcinomas remain dormant and do not grow to become clinically apparent tumors.[180, 250, 254, 262] Because latent papillary carcinomas are innocuous, no additional therapy is required.

Latent papillary carcinomas are almost always tiny and commonly show a predominantly follicular architecture. Most cases exhibit an invasive stellate contour and sclerosis; others comprise a circumscribed or encapsulated collection of neoplastic follicles without intratumoral sclerosis[245, 263] (Figs. 44–43 and 44–44).

### Immunohistochemistry

The immunohistochemical profile of papillary carcinoma is listed in Table 44–1. The staining for

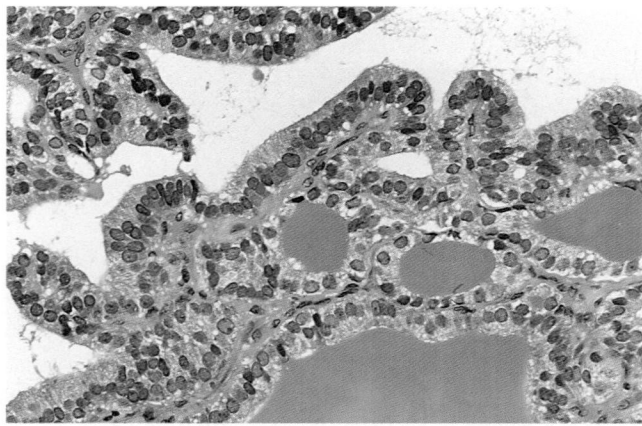

**FIGURE 44–28.** Papillary carcinoma. In this tumor, the nuclear features of papillary carcinoma are poorly developed. A diagnosis of papillary carcinoma is made because the tumor exhibits a papillary architecture and frank invasion into the soft tissues of the neck.

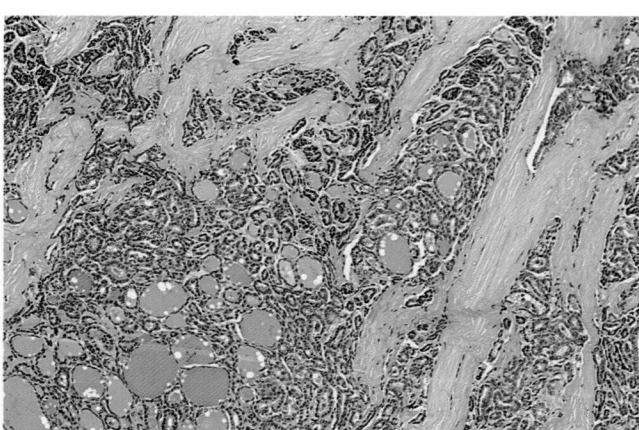

**FIGURE 44–30.** Papillary carcinoma, follicular variant. This tumor is composed exclusively of follicles. It is infiltrative and accompanied by a sclerotic stroma, and thus recognition of the malignant nature of the neoplasm is easy.

**TABLE 44-9.** Variants of Papillary Carcinoma

| Variant* | Defining Morphologic Features | Entity for Which the Variant May Be Mistaken | Clinical Significance |
|---|---|---|---|
| Follicular variant | Composed exclusively or almost exclusively of follicles<br>The follicles are often elongated and irregularly shaped, with abortive papillae.<br>The colloid is often dark staining. | Follicular adenoma<br>Follicular carcinoma | No prognostic implications |
| Encapsulated variant | Tumor with a distinct fibrous capsule<br>Capsular or vascular invasion may or may not be present. | Follicular adenoma<br>Follicular carcinoma | Highly favorable prognosis: no tumor relapse after nodulectomy or lobectomy |
| Cystic variant | Prominent cyst formation<br>There may or may not be neoplastic papillae projecting into the cystic space. | Cystic degeneration of colloid nodule | No prognostic implications |
| Encapsulated follicular variant | Encapsulated tumor composed exclusively or almost exclusively of follicles | Follicular adenoma<br>Follicular carcinoma | Highly favorable prognosis: no tumor relapse after treatment |
| Diffuse sclerosing variant | Diffuse extensive involvement of one or both lobes without forming a gross tumor nodule<br>Thyroid parenchyma shows sclerosis and lymphoid infiltration. Tumor islands are often small and dispersed, with many lying within lymphatic spaces.<br>Tumor commonly shows squamous metaplasia and prominent psammoma body formation. | Thyroiditis, especially because of the diffuse nature of the process and frequent presence of circulating antithyroid antibodies | Some studies have reported this variant to be more aggressive, with frequent lymph node and sometimes distant metastases, but outcome is still favorable because of the young age of patients (favorable prognostic factor).<br>Some studies have not shown this variant to exhibit a high metastatic rate. |
| Diffuse follicular variant | Diffuse involvement of the entire thyroid without formation of discrete tumor nodules, and composed entirely of follicles<br>No fibrosis | Colloid goiter | More aggressive, with frequent lymph node and distant metastases, but outcome is still favorable because of the young age of patients (favorable prognostic factor) and good response to radioactive iodine therapy. |
| Macrofollicular variant | Presence of many large follicles, mimicking colloid nodule | Nodular goiter | No prognostic implications |
| Tall cell variant | >50% of tumor cells with a height of more than twice the breadth<br>Tumor cells often possess oxyphilic cytoplasm. | Columnar cell carcinoma | As a group, tall cell variant is more aggressive than conventional papillary carcinoma, with larger tumors, more frequent extrathyroidal extension, higher recurrence rate, and higher mortality (reported 9%–25%).<br>For intrathyroidal tumors occurring in young patients, however, the prognosis appears to be similar to that of conventional papillary carcinoma. |
| Oxyphil cell variant | >50% of tumor cells with abundant oxyphilic cytoplasm | Hürthle cell adenoma or carcinoma | No prognostic implications |
| Solid variant | >50% of tumor showing a solid growth pattern<br>The sheets and nests of tumor are often traversed by delicate fibrovascular septa. | Poorly differentiated (insular) carcinoma | No prognostic implications |

*Table continued on following page*

**TABLE 44–9.** Variants of Papillary Carcinoma *Continued*

| Variant* | Defining Morphologic Features | Entity for Which the Variant May Be Mistaken | Clinical Significance |
|---|---|---|---|
| Trabecular variant | >5% of tumor showing a trabecular growth pattern | Follicular adenoma or carcinoma, trabecular (embryonal) type | Some studies have shown this variant to have a less favorable outcome. |
| Cribriform-morular variant | An intricate admixture of cribriform structures, closely packed small follicles, papillae, and squamoid islands (morulas)<br>Colloid is usually scanty or absent.<br>Some tumor cells in the morula contain nuclei with a lightly eosinophilic homogeneous appearance caused by biotin accumulation.<br>The tumor cell nuclei are often more hyperchromatic and pseudostratified compared with classic papillary carcinoma. | Columnar cell carcinoma<br>Tall cell variant of papillary carcinoma | Familial adenomatous polyposis should be excluded because the papillary carcinomas associated with the syndrome commonly exhibit histologic features of this variant.<br>By itself, the variant has no prognostic implications. |
| Variant with nodular fasciitis–like stroma | Presence of abundant nodular fasciitis–like or fibromatosis-like reactive stroma<br>The papillary carcinoma component can be masked by the stromal component or shows peculiar architectural features reminiscent of fibrocystic disease or phyllodes tumor of the breast. | Nodular fasciitis<br>Fibromatosis<br>Benign mesenchymal neoplasm | No prognostic implications |
| Warthin tumor–like variant | Presence of broad papillae covered by oxyphilic neoplastic cells, with the cores being packed with lymphoid cells, reminiscent of Warthin tumor of salivary gland | Hashimoto's thyroiditis | No prognostic implications |
| Papillary microcarcinoma | Small tumor, <1 cm | Multifocal fibrosing thyroiditis<br>Hyperplastic adenomatoid nodule | Highly favorable prognosis<br>Virtually all patients remain well on long-term follow-up.<br>The rare patients who have an unfavorable outcome are those with lymphadenopathy >3 cm and a nonencapsulated type of primary lesion. |
| Dedifferentiated papillary carcinoma | Papillary carcinoma accompanied by an anaplastic carcinoma or poorly differentiated thyroid carcinoma, indicating transformation to a higher-grade neoplasm | — | High mortality rate |

* All variants show the typical nuclear characteristics of papillary carcinoma, at least in some areas of the tumor.

thyroglobulin is patchy, and it is often absent in areas of squamous differentiation. The main application of immunohistochemical staining is in confirmation of the thyroid origin of metastatic carcinoma, such as cystic metastasis of papillary thyroid carcinoma in a cervical lymph node. Although staining for high-molecular-weight cytokeratin or cytokeratin 19 has been suggested to be of value in supporting a diagnosis of papillary carcinoma versus benign thyroid lesions in difficult cases,[264–267] the results are not consistent enough for routine application.

### Cytogenetics and Molecular Biology

The key molecular change in papillary carcinoma involves activation of the proto-oncogene *RET* or *NTRK1* by intrachromosome inversion or chromosome translocation.[268–270] Constitutive activation of RET (a receptor tyrosine kinase) occurs through fu-

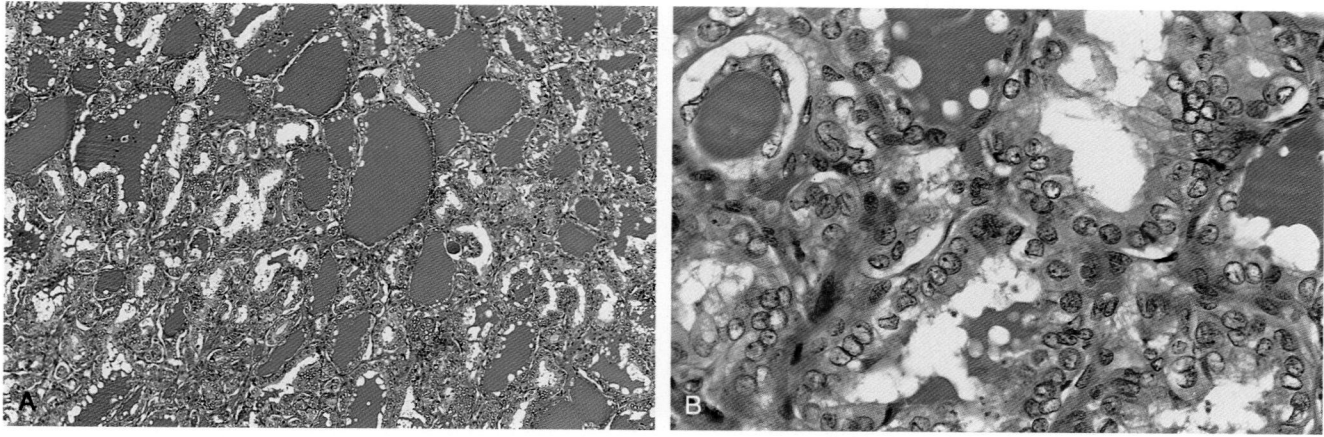

**FIGURE 44–31.** Papillary carcinoma, encapsulated follicular variant. *A.* The encapsulated tumor is composed exclusively of follicles, rendering distinction from follicular adenoma or follicular carcinoma difficult. The clues to diagnosis are dark-staining colloid, elongated follicles, and presence of abortive papillae. *B.* The follicles are lined by cells with crowded, pale, and grooved nuclei, compatible with papillary carcinoma.

sion of the *RET* gene with a gene commonly expressed in thyroid epithelial cells, such as *PTC1* through inv(10)(q11.2q21), *PTC2* through t(10;17) (q11.2;q23), and *PTC3* through cytogenetically undetectable paracentric inversion within 10q11.2.[271–277]

The *RET/PTC* translocation occurs in approximately 30% to 40% of papillary carcinomas, but the frequency is higher in children and young patients, Chernobyl accident–associated tumors, and patients who received external radiation during child-

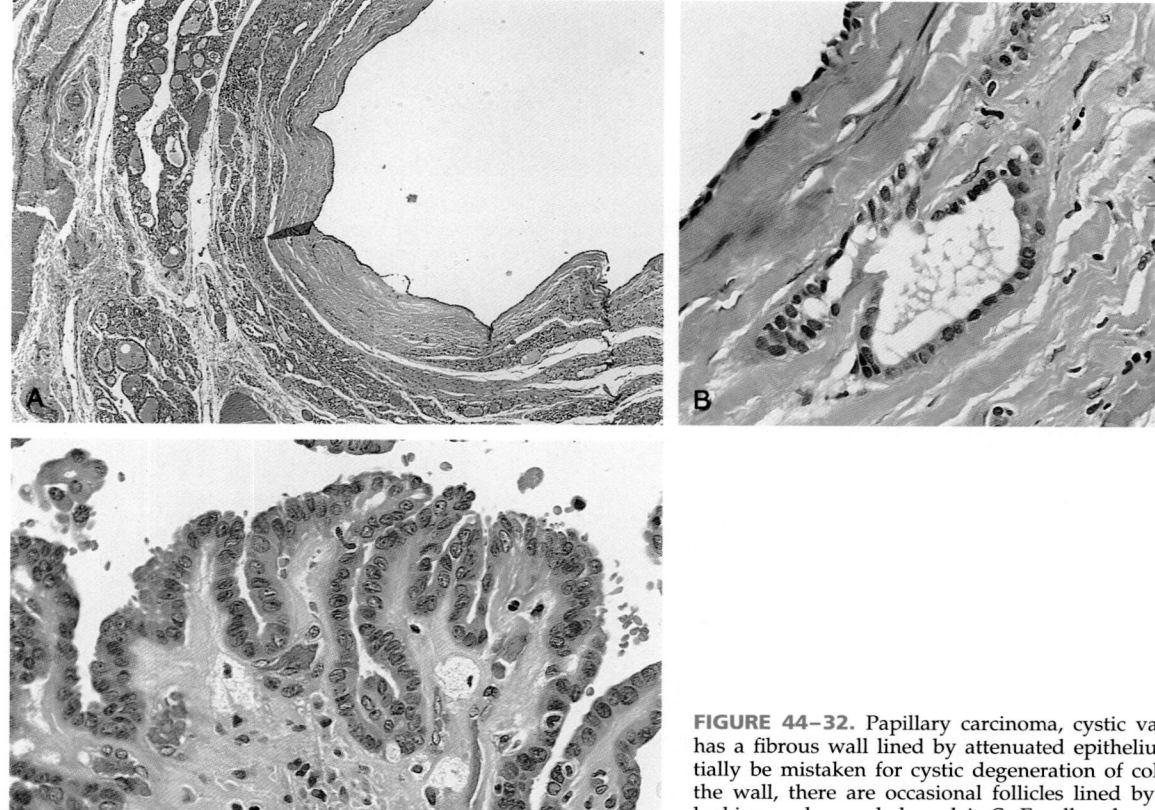

**FIGURE 44–32.** Papillary carcinoma, cystic variant. *A.* The cyst has a fibrous wall lined by attenuated epithelium and can potentially be mistaken for cystic degeneration of colloid nodule. *B.* In the wall, there are occasional follicles lined by cells with active-looking and crowded nuclei. *C.* Focally, short papillae lined by cells exhibiting features of papillary carcinoma are identified, permitting the correct diagnosis to be made.

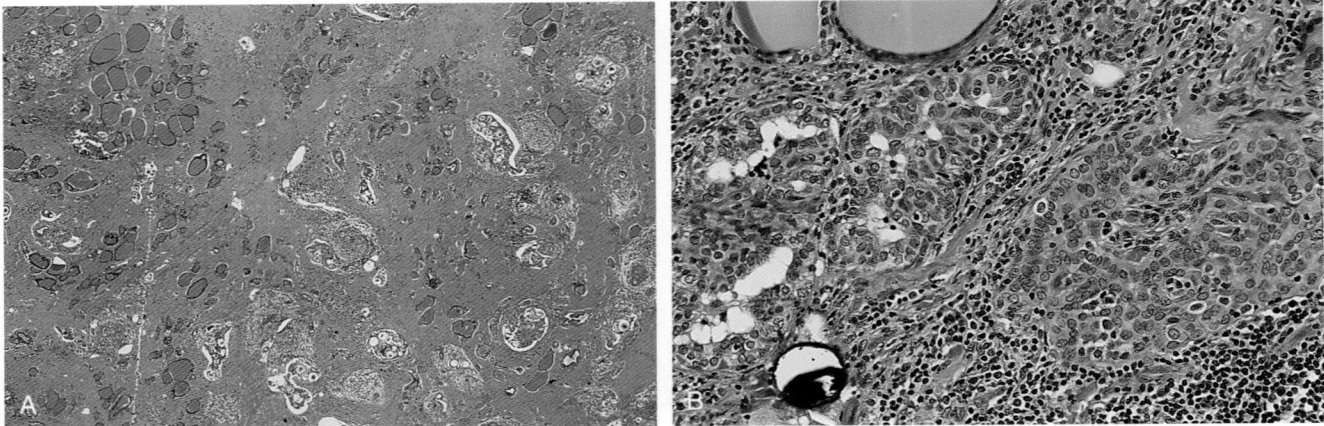

**FIGURE 44–33.** Papillary carcinoma, diffuse sclerosing variant. *A.* The thyroid gland shows sclerosis and chronic inflammation, mimicking thyroiditis. However, linear scratches on the slide suggest the presence of calcified psammoma bodies. *B.* Hiding within the gland are islands of papillary carcinoma. A psammoma body is seen in the left lower field.

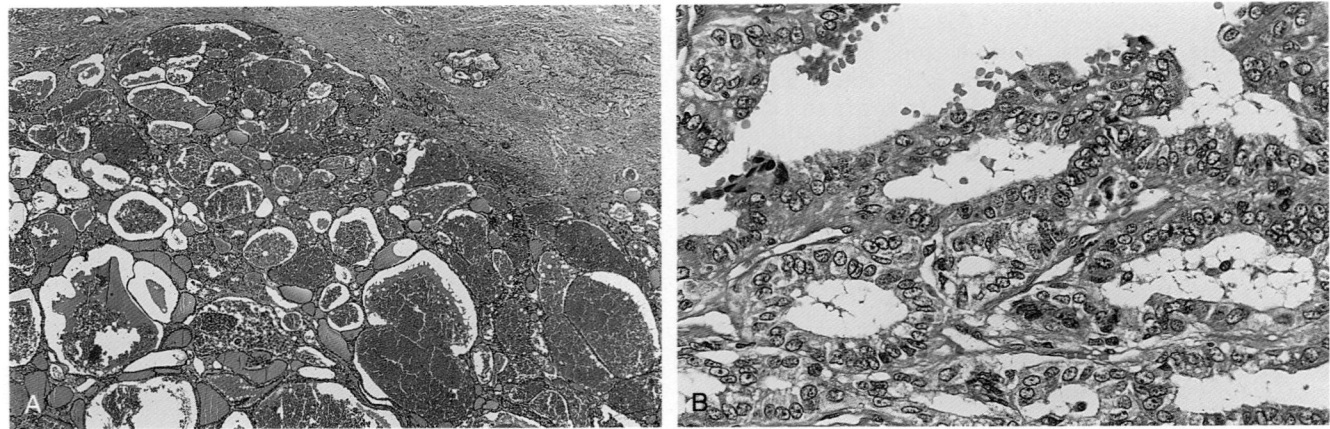

**FIGURE 44–34.** Papillary carcinoma, diffuse follicular variant. *A.* The neoplasm shows extensive involvement of the thyroid without discrete nodule formation or sclerosis and thus can be mistaken for a diffuse goiter, especially because some follicles are large. *B.* Careful examination of the smaller follicles reveals cytologic features of papillary carcinoma.

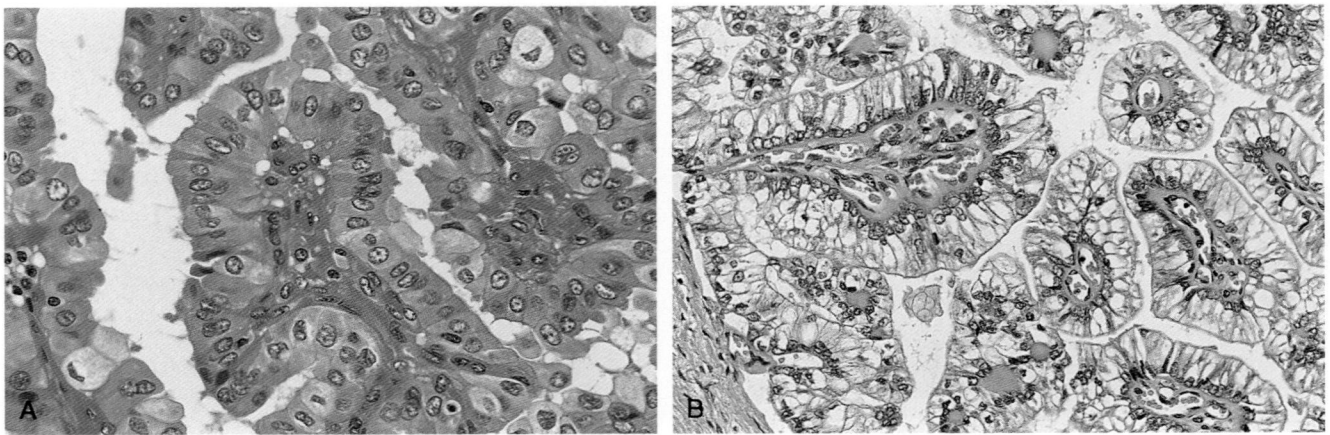

**FIGURE 44–35.** Papillary carcinoma, tall cell variant. *A.* The neoplastic cells are tall columnar and exhibit oncocytic cytoplasmic features. The nuclear features are no different from those of conventional papillary carcinoma. *B.* In this unusual example, the cells show cytoplasmic clearing.

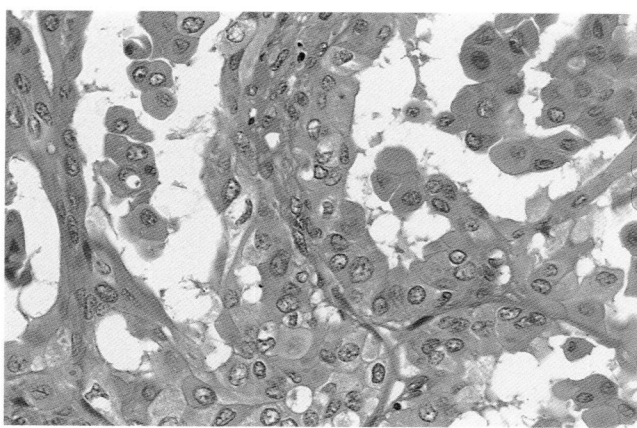

**FIGURE 44–36.** Papillary carcinoma, oncocytic variant. The cuboid and polygonal tumor cells possess abundant eosinophilic granular cytoplasm.

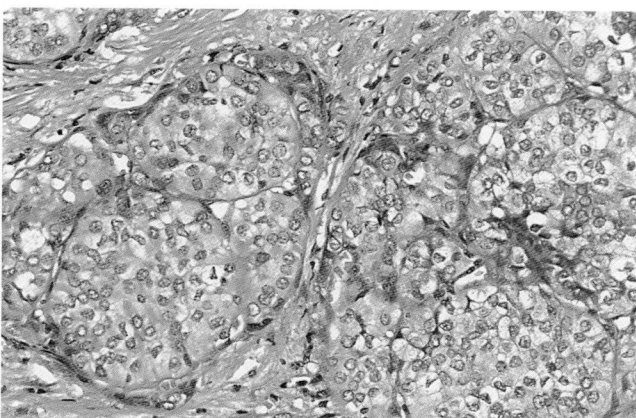

**FIGURE 44–37.** Papillary carcinoma, solid variant. Solid islands of tumor are often traversed by delicate capillaries. The characteristic nuclear features of papillary carcinoma are present.

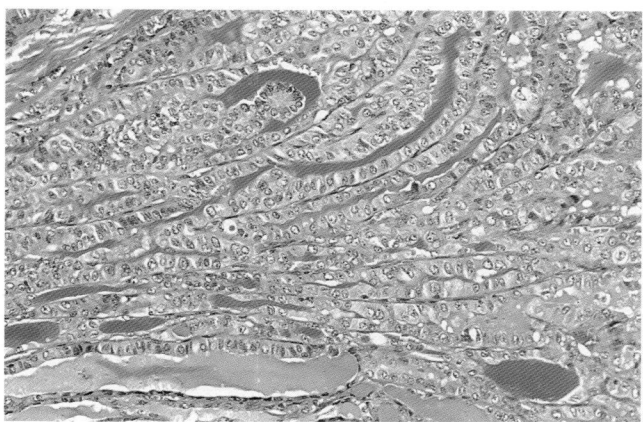

**FIGURE 44–38.** Papillary carcinoma, trabecular variant.

hood.[62, 278–296] Activation of the *NTRK1* gene product (a receptor for nerve growth factor) occurs through fusion with widely expressed "housekeeping" genes, such as *TPM3* (tropomyosin gene), *TPR*, and *TAG*.[268, 280, 281, 285, 297–299]

### Differential Diagnosis

The main criteria and problems in diagnosis of papillary carcinoma are listed in Table 44–10.[300] Some immunohistochemical markers, such as expression of high-molecular-weight cytokeratin (34$\beta$E12, cytokeratin 1), cytokeratin 19, vimentin, mesothelium-associated antibody HBME-1, Leu-7 (CD57), CD15 (Leu-M1), or CD44, and loss of expression of thyroid peroxidase or retinoblastoma protein have been reported to be of value in distin-

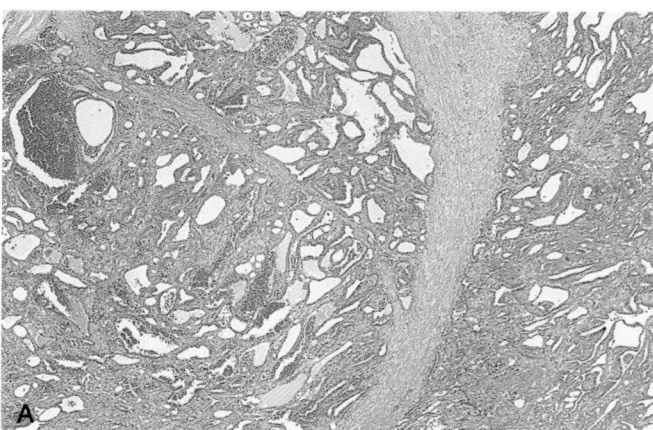

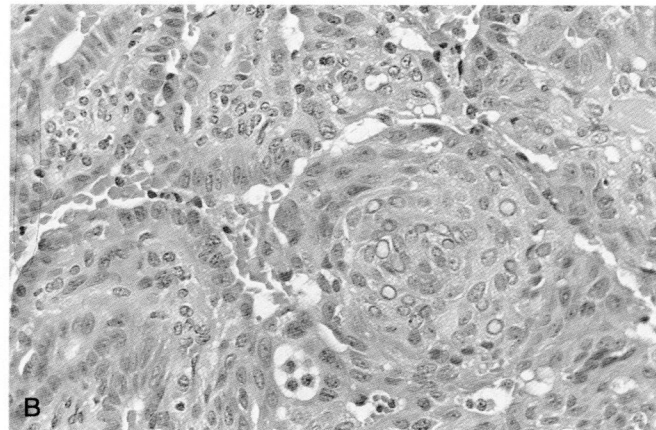

**FIGURE 44–39.** Papillary carcinoma, cribriform-morular variant. *A.* There is an intricate blend of cribriform structures, empty follicles, and solid foci. *B.* Papillae merge into a morular structure. Highly characteristic homogeneous, lightly eosinophilic biotin inclusions are seen in the nuclei of the morula. The tumor cells are often more chromatin rich than in a usual case of papillary carcinoma.

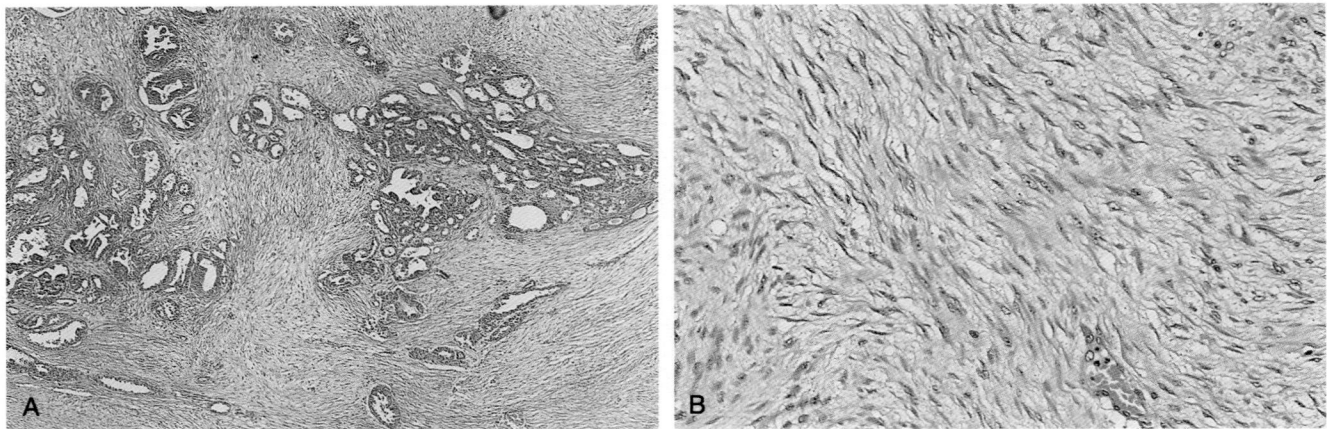

**FIGURE 44–40.** Papillary carcinoma, variant with nodular fasciitis–like stroma. *A.* The interaction of the abundant fibrocellular stroma with the papillary carcinoma results in a peculiar pattern mimicking sclerosing adenosis of the breast. *B.* The stroma comprises loose fascicles of active-looking myofibroblasts, mimicking nodular fasciitis or fibromatosis.

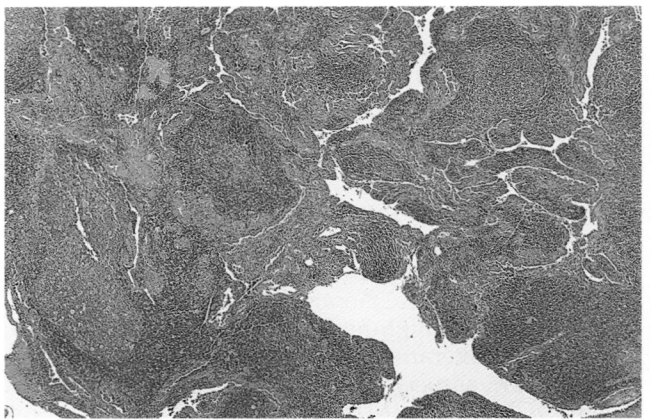

**FIGURE 44–41.** Papillary carcinoma, Warthin tumor–like variant. The resemblance to Warthin tumor of the salivary gland is striking. The neoplastic cells show oncocytic change.

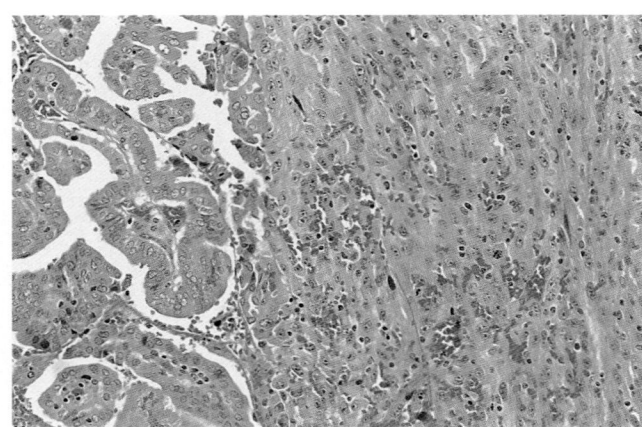

**FIGURE 44–42.** Papillary carcinoma, dedifferentiated variant. Papillary carcinoma component is shown on the left; the anaplastic carcinoma comprising pleomorphic spindly cells is shown on the right.

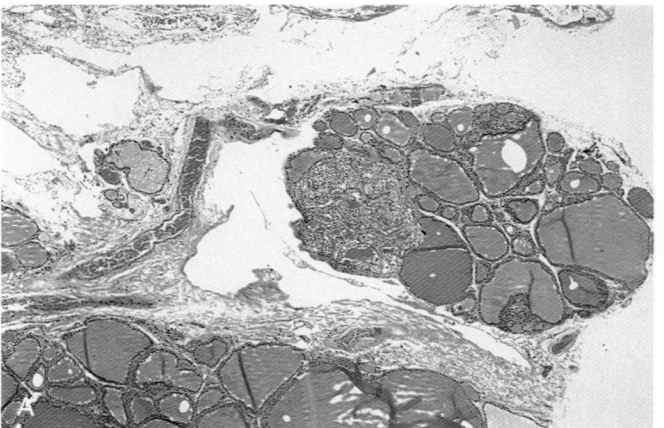

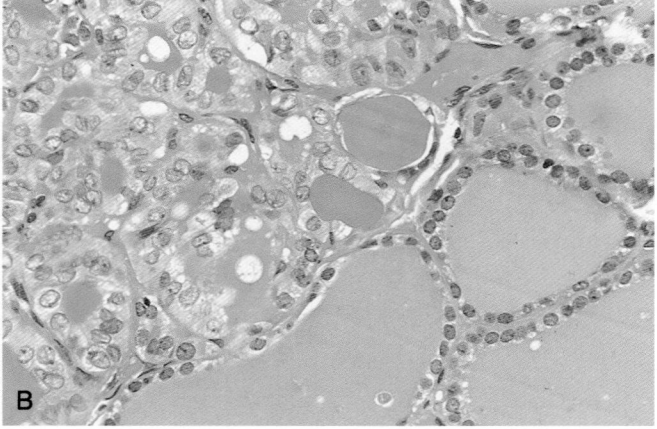

**FIGURE 44–43.** Latent papillary carcinoma as an incidental finding. *A.* Near the central field, there is a collection of small follicles representing latent papillary carcinoma. It is not accompanied by a sclerotic stroma. *B.* The follicles are lined by cells with large pale nuclei lacking polarity (*left field*), characteristic of papillary carcinoma. Note the abrupt difference in nuclear features compared with the adjoining normal follicles (*right field*).

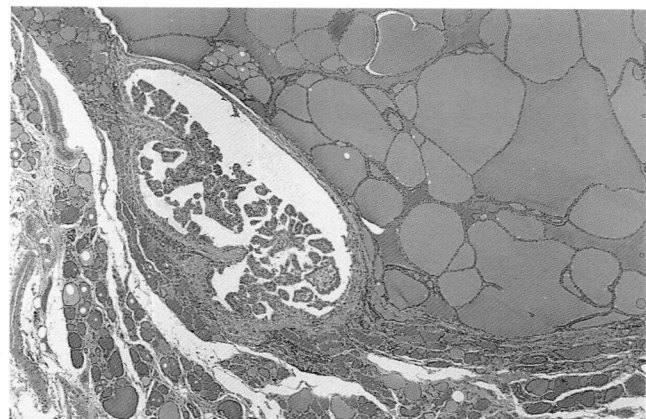

**FIGURE 44–44.** Latent papillary carcinoma as an incidental finding. This microcarcinoma shows a papillary architecture.

guishing papillary carcinoma from benign thyroid lesions and other thyroid tumors, but so far none of these makers is reliable enough to aid in routine diagnosis of papillary carcinoma.[138, 139, 265, 266, 301–314] Future studies are required to determine whether overexpression of *RET* by in situ hybridization or immunohistochemistry can aid in the diagnosis of papillary carcinoma. Currently, morphologic assessment remains the gold standard in rendering a diagnosis of papillary carcinoma.

COLLOID NODULE. In contrast to papillary carcinoma, the papillae found in colloid or adenoma-toid nodules are often broad, with small follicles in the loose core. The cells are usually columnar, with dark round nuclei regularly aligned at the base of the cells. In some colloid or adenomatoid nodules, there can be collections of follicles with pale or clear nuclei, raising a concern for papillary carcinoma. However, a diagnosis of papillary carcinoma (follicular variant) should not be made unless there are totally convincing nuclear features (see Figs. 44–24 and 44–31 and Table 44–10). The neoplastic follicles of papillary carcinoma should show an abrupt change from the surrounding benign follicles, often accompanied by enlargement of the nuclei (see Fig. 44–43). In contrast, the atypical follicles of adenomatoid nodule typically show gradual transition with the surrounding benign follicles.

FOLLICULAR ADENOMA WITH PAPILLARY HYPERPLASIA. Distinguishing features from papillary carcinoma are the same as those for colloid nodule.

FOLLICULAR ADENOMA. Some follicular adenomas may have some pale or clear nuclei, raising the possibility of follicular variant of papillary carcinoma. The nuclear clearing is often artifactual because of delayed fixation, with "blowing up" of the nuclei (see Fig. 44–11). Convincing nuclear features must be present in rendering a diagnosis of papillary carcinoma in an encapsulated follicular neoplasm because there is no harm in missing an encapsulated papillary carcinoma, which has an excellent prognosis (see Table 44–9).

**TABLE 44–10.** Key Points and Caveats in Diagnosis of Papillary Carcinoma

Diagnostic criteria for papillary carcinoma are based on a constellation of features, no single one of which is pathognomonic. For a noninvasive tumor, the diagnostic label "papillary carcinoma" should be applied only when the typical cytologic features are well developed.

Basic criteria
  • Cytologic features: ovoid nuclei that are crowded, without polarization, clear or pale, and grooved, with or without pseudoinclusions
  • Demonstration of vascular or capsular invasion is not required

Strong supporting feature, if present
  • Psammoma bodies

Other supporting histologic features
  • Papillae (including abortive papillae)
  • Follicles that are elongated or irregularly shaped
  • Dark-staining colloid
  • Multinucleated histiocytes in lumina of follicles or papillae

Deceptively "benign" patterns warranting serious consideration of the possibility of papillary carcinoma:
  • "Colloid nodule" with delicate papillary budding in some follicles, or psammoma bodies, or many clear nuclei (papillary carcinoma, macrofollicular variant)
  • Hashimoto's or lymphocytic thyroiditis–like picture, but with many "knife marks" on the histologic section due to presence of psammoma bodies (diffuse sclerosing variant of papillary carcinoma)
  • "Follicular adenoma" with many elongated follicles and dark-staining colloid or abortive papillae (papillary carcinoma, encapsulated follicular variant)
  • "Degenerate cyst," but with occasional small papillary tufts projecting into the lumen or some follicles in the fibrous wall lined by cells with high nuclear-to-cytoplasmic ratio (cystic variant of papillary carcinoma)
  • Spindle cell proliferation resembling nodular fasciitis or fibromatosis (papillary carcinoma variant with exuberant nodular fasciitis–like stroma)

COLUMNAR CELL CARCINOMA. See later.

MEDULLARY CARCINOMA WITH PSEUDOPAPILLARY PATTERN. See later.

## PROGNOSTIC CONSIDERATIONS

Papillary carcinoma is an indolent neoplasm. According to a long-term follow-up study from the Mayo Clinic, the cancer-related mortality is only 6.5%.[164] The tumor is locally invasive and has a propensity to metastasize to regional lymph nodes, but distant metastasis is uncommon and often late (~10%).[73, 192, 193, 315, 316]

The most significant prognostic factors are age, stage, and tumor size. To aid in prediction of outcome and selection of therapy, a number of parameters (such as age, metastasis, extent of primary cancer, and tumor size) are taken into consideration to divide patients into low-risk and high-risk groups.[317-320] The low-risk group has an excellent prognosis, and conservative therapy can be considered. The high-risk group has a worse outcome, and thus more aggressive therapy is required.

AGE. Young age is an important favorable prognostic factor. Few patients younger than 40 years die of papillary carcinoma.[164, 165, 241, 321-329]

SEX. The male sex is often associated with a worse prognosis.[226, 323, 325, 326, 329-332]

TUMOR SIZE. Risk of death from papillary carcinoma increases with the size of the primary tumor.[164] Microcarcinomas (<1 to 1.5 cm) have an excellent prognosis, whereas tumors larger than 4 cm fare worse.[78, 164, 241, 325, 333]

TUMOR STAGE. Extrathyroidal extension worsens the prognosis, which is even worse when there is invasion of the esophagus or trachea.[164, 325, 327, 334, 335] Presence of distant metastasis is a highly unfavorable prognostic feature.[157] Papillary carcinoma is unique among carcinomas in that most studies have not found lymph node metastasis to be of prognostic significance.*

TUMOR ENCAPSULATION. Encapsulated papillary carcinomas have an excellent prognosis. There is no recurrence after excision of the tumor.[72, 192, 196]

HISTOLOGIC VARIANTS. The prognostic significance of the variants is listed in Table 44–9.[340]

COMPLETENESS OF EXCISION. Incomplete tumor excision increases the probability of recurrence.[319, 341]

HISTOLOGIC FEATURES. The histologic features shown in some studies to be associated with a worse prognosis are marked cellular atypia (multilayered cells with marked variation in cellular and nuclear size and shape, uneven distribution of chromatin) and trabecular growth pattern[237, 331, 332, 342] (Fig. 44–45). High tumor grade (grade 2), as defined by the presence of marked nuclear atypia, tumor

---

*References 77, 164, 321, 324, 325, 328, 329, 336–339.

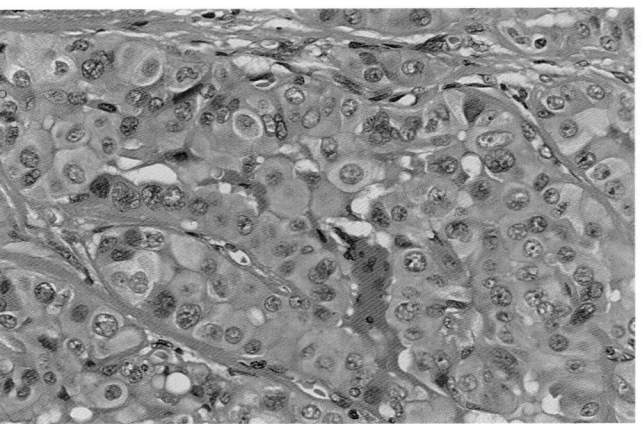

FIGURE 44–45. Papillary carcinoma with marked cellular atypia (grade 2). Some studies have shown this feature to be associated with a worse prognosis.

necrosis, or vascular invasion, has been reported to be associated with a worse prognosis.[339, 343]

STROMAL REACTION. Chronic thyroiditis in the background thyroid tissue and stromal bone formation have been reported to be favorable prognostic factors.[178, 329]

VASCULAR INVASION. Invasion of sizable blood vessels is an unfavorable prognostic factor.[77, 192]

IMMUNOHISTOCHEMICAL FEATURES. High density of S-100 protein–positive histiocytes is a favorable prognostic factor.[344] The features associated with a worse prognosis are Leu-M1 positivity, epithelial membrane antigen positivity, p53 protein immunoreactivity, lack of E-cadherin expression, and low-level expression of retinoblastoma protein.[160, 303, 345-348]

TUMOR ANGIOGENESIS. Whereas some studies have suggested that a high microvessel count (intratumoral microvessel count as highlighted by immunostaining for vascular markers) correlates with a worse prognosis, other studies cannot confirm this finding.[349-351]

DNA PLOIDY. Multiploidy or aneuploidy is an unfavorable prognostic factor.[178, 352]

N-RAS MUTATION. N-ras mutation at codon 61, which is uncommon, is associated with a more aggressive behavior.[353]

## Poorly Differentiated Thyroid Carcinoma

### CLINICAL CONSIDERATIONS

#### Presentation

Poorly differentiated thyroid carcinoma shows histologic and biologic features intermediate between differentiated thyroid carcinomas and anaplastic carcinomas.[342, 354-357] It retains sufficient differentiation to form small follicular structures and to produce thyroglobulin, but it lacks the usual morphologic characteristics of papillary and follicular carcinoma.[358] The morphologic spectrum of poorly differentiated thyroid carcinoma is broad, and insular carcinoma is the best characterized form.[354] An alternative designation of "primordial cell carcinoma" has also been proposed in view of the cytoarchitectural resemblance to the fetal thyroid.[355]

Poorly differentiated carcinomas can arise de novo or transform from differentiated thyroid carcinomas, either after repeated recurrences or with the two components being discovered simultaneously at diagnosis.[238, 359] They can further transform to anaplastic carcinoma.

The tumor predominantly affects middle-aged and elderly adults, with a mean age of 54 years.[89, 354, 355, 358] Women are more commonly affected than are men (male-to-female ratio = 1:2). Most patients present with an enlarging thyroid mass, and there may be a preceding history of long-standing goiter. Rare patients present with bone metastasis. The disease is often locally advanced at presentation, with extrathyroidal extension in more than 50% of cases.[89] Lymph node and distant metastases are already present at presentation in approximately 40% and approximately 30% of cases, respectively.[89, 354, 358]

### Macroscopic Findings

The tumor is partially encapsulated or frankly invasive. It is often large, with a mean size of 4.7 cm.[358] The cut surface is solid, firm, and fleshy, often punctuated by areas of necrosis and hemorrhage.

## DIAGNOSTIC CONSIDERATIONS

### Microscopic Findings

Insular carcinoma typically grows in the form of large solid nests (insulae) decorated with variable numbers of small abortive follicles (Fig. 44–46). It is common to observe retraction artifacts around the tumor islands. The frequent presence of coagulative necrosis results in a characteristic "peritheliomatous" appearance. The tumor can also form diffuse sheets, trabeculae, festoons, and papillae (Fig. 44–47). Vascular invasion is common.[354, 360] Some cases may show transition with typical papillary carcinoma or follicular carcinoma. The tumor cells are relatively small, with uniform round, hyperchromatic nuclei, indistinct nucleoli, and scanty cytoplasm[355] (Fig. 44–48). Some mitotic figures can often be identified.

There is a morphologic range of poorly differentiated thyroid carcinomas that do not fit the histologic description of insular carcinoma. They are composed of large cells growing in a trabecular, cribriform, solid, or focally follicular pattern[355] (Fig. 44–48*B*).

### Immunohistochemistry

Poorly differentiated thyroid carcinoma is immunoreactive for cytokeratin, thyroglobulin, and thyroid transcription factor 1. The positive staining for thyroglobulin may be confined to the abortive follicles and isolated cells in the form of paranuclear globules.[354, 355, 361] There is reduced expression of the cyclin-dependent kinase inhibitor p27 and a higher Ki-67 index compared with differentiated thyroid carcinomas.[357, 362] Positive staining for Bcl-2 is common (84%), contrasting with the infrequent positive staining in anaplastic carcinomas (14%).[363]

### Molecular Biology

Approximately half of the cases of poorly differentiated thyroid carcinomas show immunoreactivity for p53 protein, whereas this feature is uncommon in well-differentiated thyroid carcinomas but common in anaplastic carcinomas. Thus, it appears that *TP53* gene mutation may play a role in the genesis of some cases.[363, 364] The finding of point mutations in the *ras* oncogene in a proportion of cases suggests

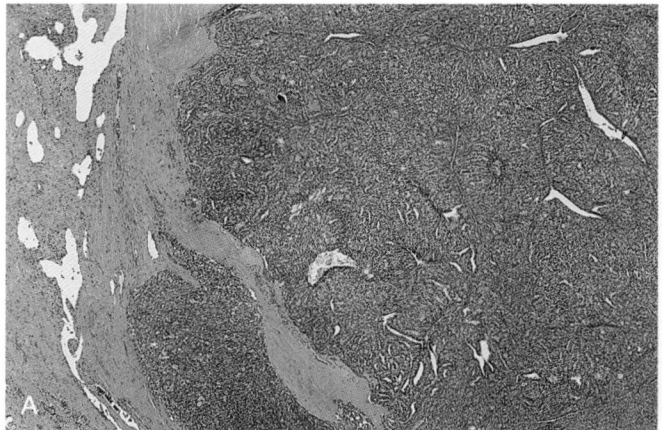
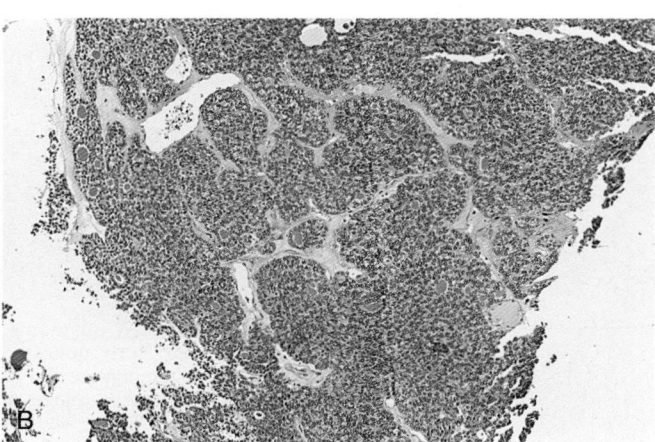

**FIGURE 44–46.** Insular carcinoma. *A.* The tumor is infiltrative and highly cellular. *B.* The tumor frequently forms islands punctuated by small follicles.

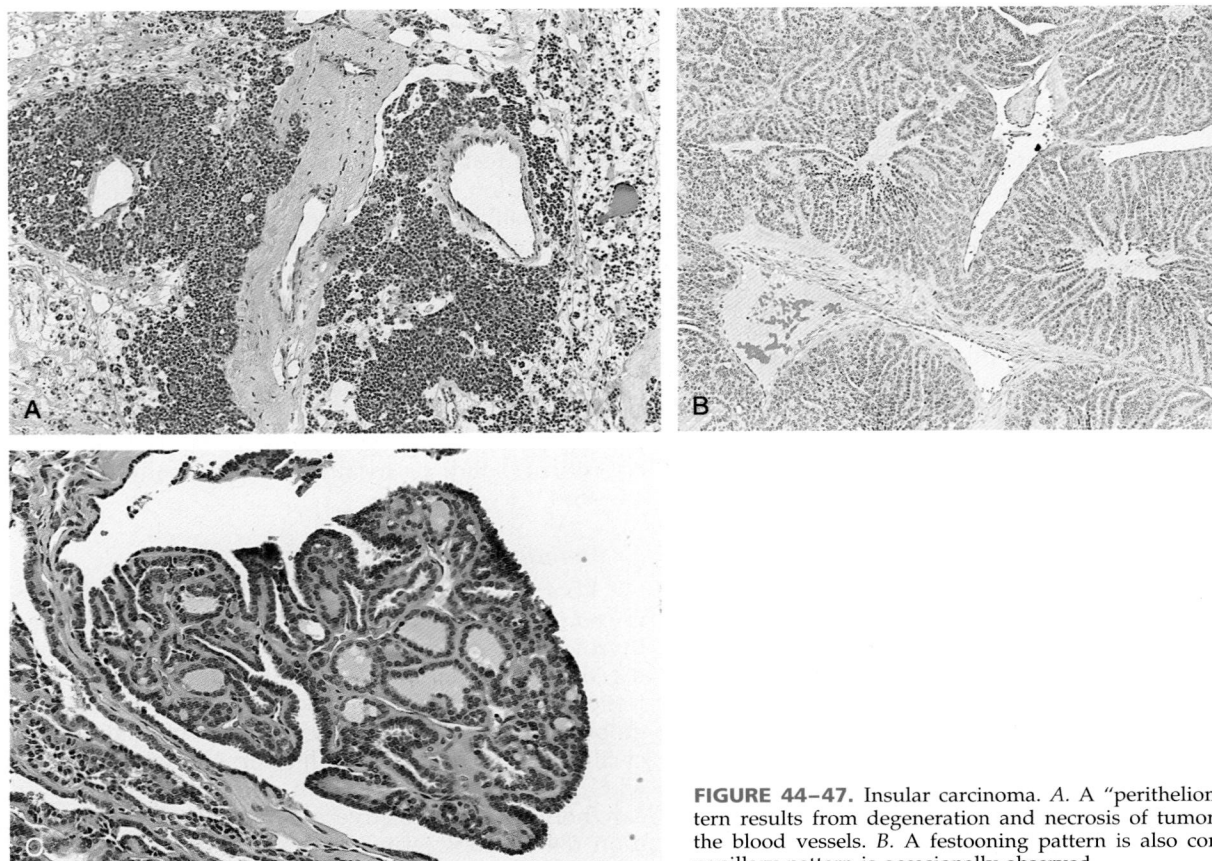

**FIGURE 44–47.** Insular carcinoma. *A.* A "peritheliomatous" pattern results from degeneration and necrosis of tumor away from the blood vessels. *B.* A festooning pattern is also common. *C.* A papillary pattern is occasionally observed.

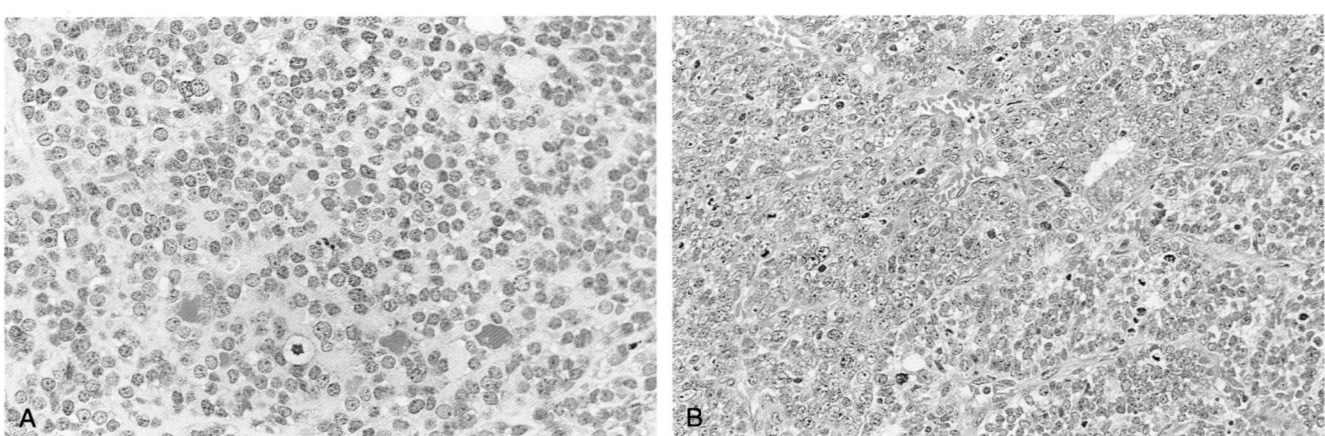

**FIGURE 44–48.** Poorly differentiated carcinoma. *A.* In insular carcinoma, the tumor cells are typically small and monotonous, with fairly uniform dark-staining nuclei. Some mitotic figures can often be identified. Note the focal differentiation into small follicles. *B.* In this poorly differentiated thyroid carcinoma, the right lower field shows cytologic features characteristic of insular carcinoma. In the left upper field, the cells are slightly larger and more pleomorphic, with brisk mitotic activity. This component is still a form of poorly differentiated rather than anaplastic carcinoma because there is organoid arrangement of the tumor cells and immunoreactivity for thyroglobulin.

a relationship with follicular carcinoma in such cases.[89, 365]

### Differential Diagnosis

MEDULLARY CARCINOMA. Insular carcinoma may mimic medullary carcinoma as a result of the growth pattern and amyloid-like sclerosis. The distinction can be readily made by immunostaining for thyroglobulin and calcitonin (see Table 44–1).

ANAPLASTIC THYROID CARCINOMA. Poorly differentiated carcinoma lacks the prominent nuclear pleomorphism and frequent mitoses of anaplastic carcinoma and furthermore shows abortive follicles and thyroglobulin immunoreactivity.

SOLID VARIANT OF PAPILLARY CARCINOMA. See Table 44–9.

## PROGNOSTIC CONSIDERATIONS

Recurrence or metastasis develops in approximately 60% of cases after treatment.[89, 354, 355] In contrast to the rapidly fatal course of anaplastic carcinoma, poorly differentiated carcinoma causes death after several years (mean survival, 3.9 years). The long-term survival rate is around 40%.[89, 354–356, 366] Death is often attributable to metastasis rather than to uncontrollable local disease. The treatment usually consists of total thyroidectomy, radioactive iodine, and suppressive thyroxine.[354] Radiotherapy and chemotherapy may also be considered in view of the unfavorable prognosis. Poor prognostic factors include advanced age, large tumor size, extrathyroidal extension, lymph node metastasis, and presence of an anaplastic carcinoma component.[356]

Whether the presence of a minor component of poorly differentiated carcinoma worsens the prognosis of an otherwise typical differentiated thyroid carcinoma remains controversial.[360, 367–369] The outcome will probably be worsened if the poorly differentiated carcinoma component is found in the invasive portions of the tumor but not if the component is confined to an encapsulated tumor.

# Anaplastic (Undifferentiated) Carcinoma

## CLINICAL CONSIDERATIONS

### Presentation

Anaplastic carcinoma is predominantly a disease of older adults with a mean age of 67 years; there is a slight female predominance.[238, 370–372] The patients present with a rapidly enlarging thyroid mass or metastatic tumor in cervical lymph nodes or distant sites. The mass lesion is frequently accompanied by hoarseness, dysphagia, and dyspnea. Some patients have a history of long-standing goiter or well-differentiated thyroid carcinoma.[238, 359, 370, 373, 374] Squamous cell carcinoma and carcinosarcoma can be considered variants of anaplastic carcinoma.

### Macroscopic Findings

Anaplastic thyroid carcinoma typically shows infiltration of the perithyroid soft tissues and adjacent structures, such as the larynx and pharynx. The tumor is fleshy, with areas of necrosis and hemorrhage.

## DIAGNOSTIC CONSIDERATIONS

### Microscopic Findings

Anaplastic thyroid carcinoma is characterized by highly pleomorphic tumor cells that lack any organoid growth pattern[238, 374] (Fig. 44–49). The tumor grows in diffuse sheets, irregular islands, cords, and fascicles. The tumor cells are large and are polygonal, ovoid, or spindly; some foci can show squamous differentiation[229] (Fig. 44–50). A pseudoangiomatoid pattern resembling angiosarcoma can be seen in some cases (Fig. 44–51). Mitotic figures are frequent, and coagulative tumor necrosis is often extensive (see Fig. 44–49). There is a tendency for the tumor cells to permeate and replace the walls of blood vessels, obliterating their lumina[238] (Fig. 44–52). There are commonly some admixed inflammatory cells, particularly neutrophils.

A component of papillary carcinoma, follicular carcinoma, or poorly differentiated thyroid carcinoma can be found in approximately 50% of cases, suggesting that the anaplastic carcinoma arises through a process of "dedifferentiation"[238, 354, 366, 373–377] (Fig. 44–53).

The morphologic variants of anaplastic carcinoma are listed in Table 44–11 (Figs. 44–54 and 44–55).[300, 373, 378–391] True "small cell" anaplastic carcinomas are extremely rare; most cases diagnosed as such in the past represent malignant lymphoma, medullary carcinoma, or poorly differentiated thyroid carcinoma.[238, 373, 374, 392–396]

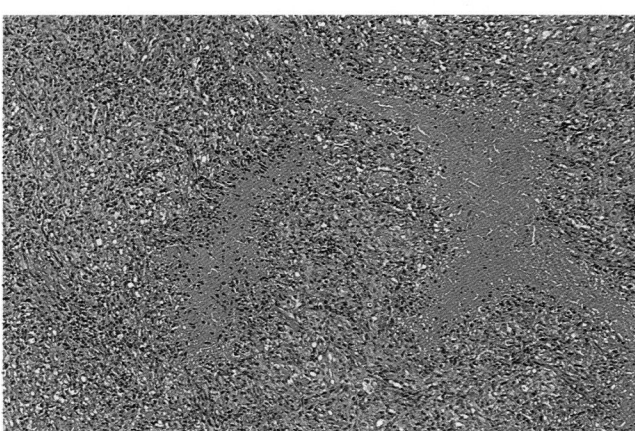

**FIGURE 44–49.** Anaplastic carcinoma. The tumor is solid growing, lacking organoid features. Coagulative necrosis is a common finding.

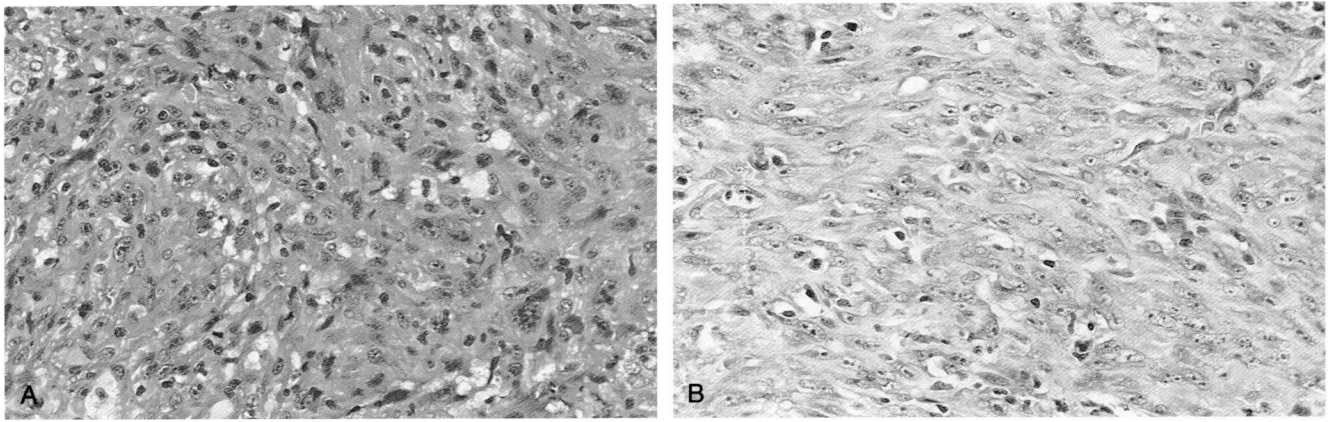

FIGURE 44–50. Anaplastic carcinoma. *A.* This tumor is composed of ovoid and plump spindly cells with significant nuclear pleomorphism. Many tumor cells possess multiple large nucleoli. *B.* This tumor is composed of spindly cells with distinct nucleoli.

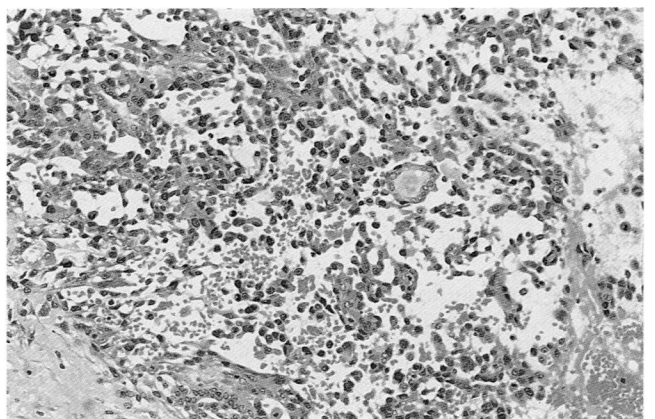

FIGURE 44–51. Anaplastic carcinoma. This tumor shows cellular dehiscence and interstitial hemorrhage, mimicking angiosarcoma.

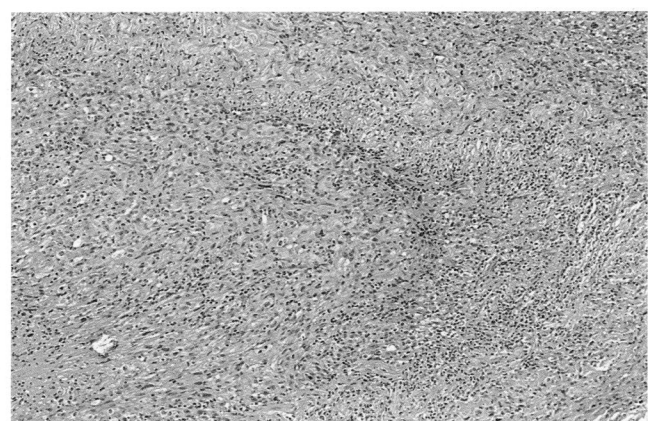

FIGURE 44–52. Anaplastic carcinoma. A highly characteristic feature is obliteration of the wall and lumen of large blood vessels by tumor cells.

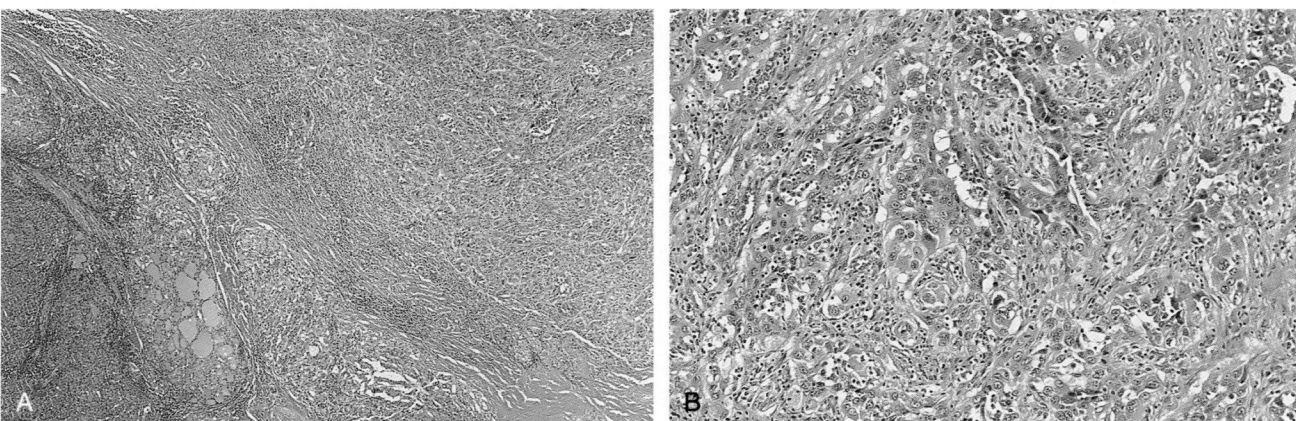

FIGURE 44–53. Anaplastic carcinoma. *A.* A component of Hürthle cell neoplasm (*left field*) is found in this anaplastic carcinoma. *B.* At the interface between the two components, there are highly atypical Hürthle cells that merge into the anaplastic carcinoma, suggesting transformation of Hürthle cell neoplasm into anaplastic carcinoma.

**TABLE 44–11.** Variants of Anaplastic Thyroid Carcinoma

| Variant* | Defining Morphologic Features | Entity for Which the Variant May be Mistaken |
|---|---|---|
| Angiomatoid variant | Presence of irregular cleftlike tumor cell–lined spaces mimicking vascular spaces | Angiosarcoma |
| Osteoclastic variant | Reactive osteoclastic giant cells are interspersed in an otherwise typical anaplastic carcinoma | Giant cell tumor of larynx (thyroid cartilage) |
| Paucicellular variant | Low-cellularity tumor with large areas of sclerosis and infarction. A sprinkling of lymphocytes is often present. Focally, spindly tumor cells with mild to moderate nuclear atypia can be identified. These spindle cells also obliterate the wall and lumina of blood vessels. | Riedel's thyroiditis |
| Lymphoepithelioma-like variant | Irregular infiltrative islands and sheets of syncytial-appearing pleomorphic tumor cells, heavily intermingled with lymphocytes and plasma cells | CASTLE |
| Squamous cell carcinoma | Identical to squamous cell carcinoma occurring in other sites | CASTLE |
| Adenosquamous carcinoma | Squamous cell carcinoma with areas of mucin production | — |
| Carcinosarcoma | Anaplastic carcinoma accompanied by a sarcomatous component with muscle, fat, cartilage, or bone differentiation | — |

\* None of these variants has clinical or prognostic significance.

### Immunohistochemistry

In anaplastic carcinoma, epithelial markers cannot be consistently demonstrated, except in areas of squamous differentiation. Cytokeratin is positive in only approximately half of the cases, whereas epithelial membrane antigen is positive in only 33% to 55%.[238, 370, 372, 397, 398] Vimentin is positive in 50% to 100% but has no diagnostic value.[372, 397]

Thyroglobulin and thyroid transcription factor 1 are negative in the anaplastic carcinoma component, but immunostaining for these markers can sometimes highlight the preexisting differentiated thyroid carcinoma component if it is present.[2, 3, 370, 393, 399] Calcitonin is negative.[238, 370] Focal immunoreactivity

for factor VIII–related antigen has been reported, possibly indicating focal divergent endothelial differentiation.[398]

### Molecular Biology

Aberrations in the p53 pathways have been implicated in the transformation of differentiated thyroid carcinoma to anaplastic carcinoma.[364, 377, 400–404] The anaplastic carcinoma component commonly shows strong immunoreactivity for p53 protein, whereas the differentiated thyroid carcinoma component is negative. The β-catenin gene commonly shows somatic mutations in anaplastic carcinoma and may thus play a key role in the development of this tumor type.[405]

### Differential Diagnosis

The main pitfalls in diagnosis of anaplastic carcinoma are listed in Table 44–12.

SARCOMA. Anaplastic carcinomas composed predominantly of spindly cells are difficult to distinguish from sarcomas. However, because primary sarcomas of the thyroid are rare, they should be diagnosed only when there is strong proof of a definite line of differentiation, such as smooth muscle or nerve sheath differentiation.[238]

LARGE CELL LYMPHOMA. Large cell lymphoma can be distinguished from anaplastic carcinoma by the poor cellular cohesion, presence of plasmacytoid or amphophilic cytoplasm, infiltration of thyroid follicular epithelium, stuffing of follicular lumina by tumor cells, and immunohistochemical expression of leukocyte markers.

METASTATIC CARCINOMA. Clinical correlation is required to distinguish anaplastic carcinoma from

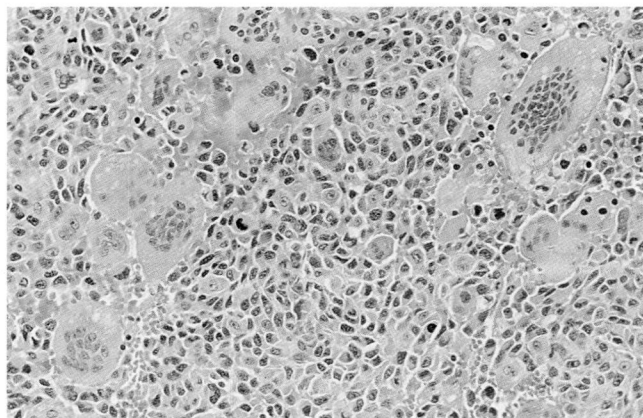

FIGURE 44–54. Anaplastic carcinoma, osteoclastic variant. Non-neoplastic osteoclast giant cells are dispersed among the highly pleomorphic ovoid tumor cells.

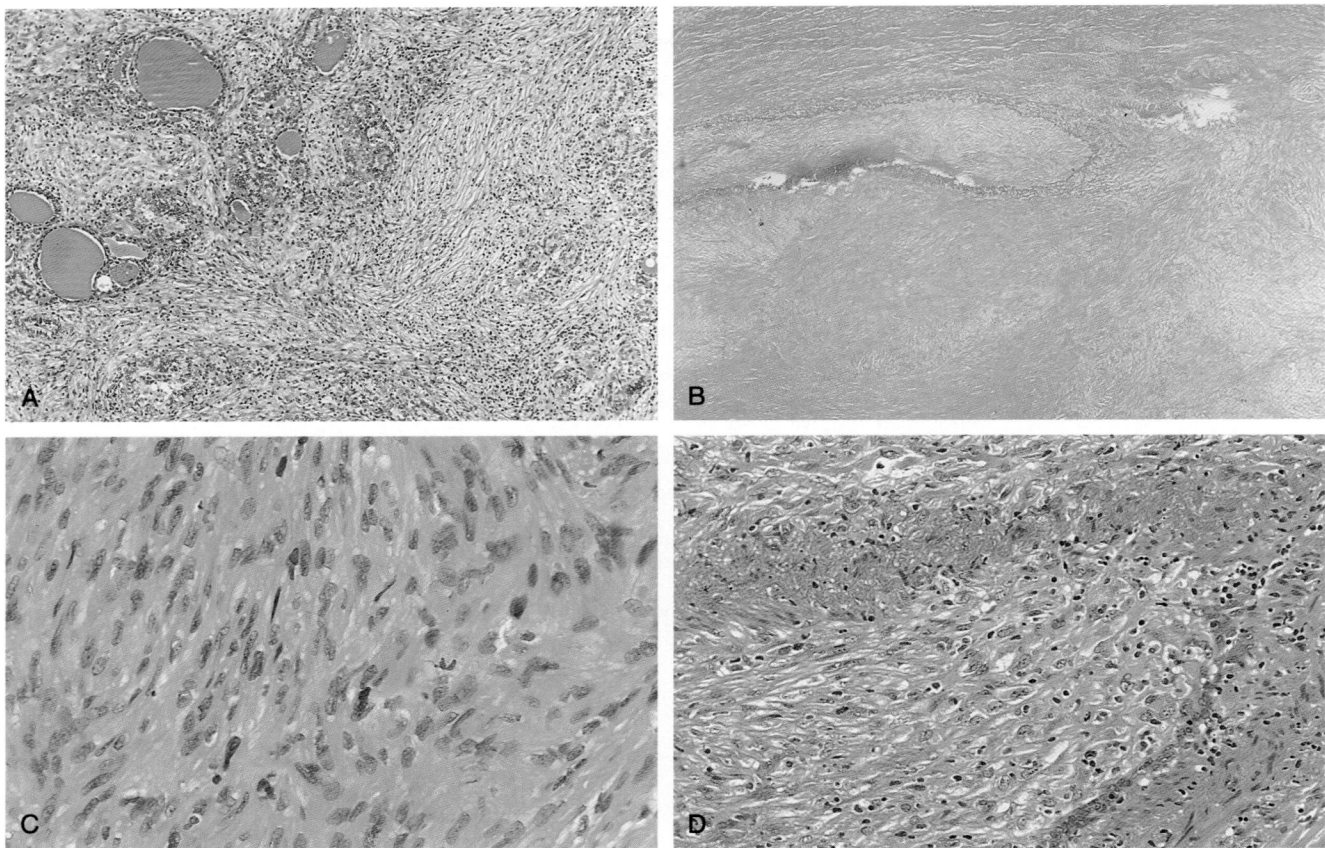

**FIGURE 44–55.** Anaplastic carcinoma, paucicellular variant. *A.* The tumor infiltrates and replaces the thyroid parenchyma. The extremely low cellularity, fibrosis, and sprinkling of chronic inflammatory cells impart an impression of thyroiditis. *B.* In areas, there is dense fibrous tissue with ghost shadows of blood vessels, indicating prior infarction of the tissue. *C.* Careful scrutiny of the less hypocellular areas reveals myofibroblast-like spindly cells that are in fact tumor cells. Mild nuclear atypia is evident. *D.* Identification of blood vessels showing obliteration by atypical spindly cells provides the best clue to the diagnosis of anaplastic carcinoma.

metastatic carcinoma, although metastatic carcinoma should be suspected if the bulk of the tumor lies within lymphovascular spaces. The presence of a component of differentiated thyroid carcinoma strongly favors the diagnosis of anaplastic carcinoma.

PARATHYROID CARCINOMA. Parathyroid carcinoma presenting as a thyroid mass is not uncommonly misdiagnosed as anaplastic thyroid carcinoma. The distinction is important because parathyroid carcinoma is a much more indolent neoplasm. Histologic clues to the correct diagnosis are presence of clear cells, mixture of cell types, paucity of mitotic figures, and prominent delicate vasculature.

RIEDEL'S THYROIDITIS. The paucicellular variant of anaplastic carcinoma can be mistaken for Riedel's thyroiditis, which has a favorable prognosis. Features favoring the diagnosis of a paucicellular variant of anaplastic carcinoma are presence of infarction, cytologic atypia (albeit focal and often subtle), vascular occlusion by spindle cells, discrete interface

with the adjacent tissue, and cytokeratin immunoreactivity.

ANGIOSARCOMA. See later.

SOLID VARIANT OF PAPILLARY CARCINOMA. The solid variant of papillary carcinoma can be distinguished from anaplastic carcinoma by the typical nuclear features, lack of bizarre cells, and paucity of mitotic figures.

POORLY DIFFERENTIATED THYROID CARCINOMA. Poorly differentiated thyroid carcinoma usually shows definite cellular organization into islands with microfollicles, relatively small cells, fairly uniform nuclei, lack of bizarre cells, and thyroglobulin immunoreactivity.

THYMIC AND RELATED TUMORS. See later.

## PROGNOSTIC CONSIDERATIONS

Anaplastic carcinoma is inoperable in about half of the cases because of extensive local disease. Regional lymph node and distant metastases (mostly lungs, sometimes bones) are common. The cause of death

**TABLE 44–12.** Main Pitfalls in Diagnosis of Anaplastic Thyroid Carcinoma

| Main Diagnostic Pitfall | Entities That May Cause the Diagnostic Confusion |
| --- | --- |
| Benign lesions mimicking anaplastic thyroid carcinoma | Reparative cellular atypia in benign tumor attributable to infarction or fine-needle aspiration injury<br>Florid granulation tissue formation resulting from organization of infarcted tumor<br>Inflammatory pseudotumor |
| Low-grade malignant tumors mimicking anaplastic thyroid carcinoma | Papillar carcinoma, solid variant<br>Mucoepidermoid carcinoma<br>Sclerosing mucoepidermoid carcinoma with eosinophilia<br>Thymic and branchial pouch–related tumors (ectopic thymoma, SETTLE, CASTLE)<br>Parathyroid carcinoma<br>Malignant lymphoma |
| Anaplastic thyroid carcinoma variant potentially misdiagnosed as benign or low-grade malignant lesions | Paucicellular variant, which may be mistaken for Riedel's thyroiditis<br>Lymphoepithelioma-like carcinoma variant, which may be mistaken for CASTLE or malignant lymphoma |

is usually upper airway obstruction from extensive local disease or a combination of the effects of local and metastatic disease.[406] The median survival is only 3 to 4 months, and the 5-year survival rate is 5% to 10%.[366, 377, 407–409] The rare patients who can achieve a cure usually have relatively small (<5 cm) tumors confined to the thyroid gland and have been treated with aggressive local intervention.[374, 406, 407, 410–412] Unfavorable prognostic factors for anaplastic carcinoma include large tumor size (>6 cm), extension of tumor beyond the neck, old age at diagnosis, male gender, and dyspnea as a presenting symptom.[406]

## Columnar Cell Carcinoma

### CLINICAL AND PROGNOSTIC CONSIDERATIONS

Although columnar cell carcinoma was originally reported as an aggressive neoplasm,[413] studies have shown that aggressive behavior is observed only in the frankly invasive tumors. For invasive tumors, there is slight male predilection and the mean age is 55.6 years.[413–422] There is a high frequency of regional lymph node and distant metastases. The mortality rate, which is at least 75%, is high. In contrast, for encapsulated tumors, there is marked female predominance and patients are younger (mean, 42.7 years).[414, 422–425] Most patients remain well on follow-up.

There are divergent views on the nature of columnar cell carcinoma: a distinct tumor type versus a variant of thyroid carcinoma. In fact, occasional cases show merging with tall cell papillary carcinoma.[419, 421, 422, 426, 427] There is also some morphologic overlap with the cribriform-morular variant of papillary carcinoma and familial adenomatous polyposis–associated thyroid carcinoma.

### DIAGNOSTIC CONSIDERATIONS

#### Microscopic Findings

Columnar cell carcinoma shows heterogeneous growth patterns, including papillary, complex glandular, cribriform, and solid. The cells are tall columnar and characteristically show marked nuclear pseudostratification and hyperchromasia, reminiscent of colorectal adenocarcinoma or endometrioid adenocarcinoma (Fig. 44–56). Subnuclear vacuoles and diffuse cytoplasmic clearing can sometimes oc-

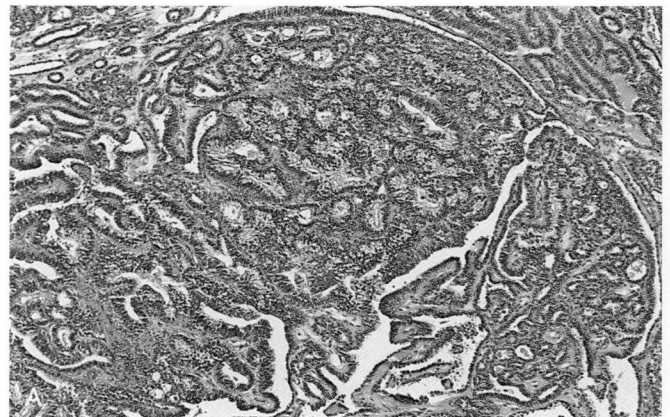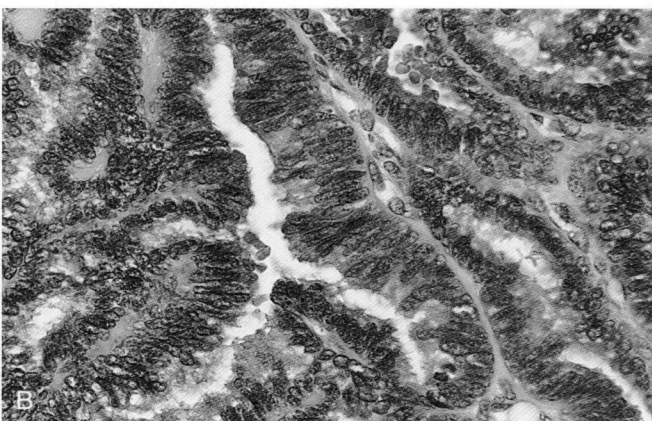

**FIGURE 44–56.** Columnar cell carcinoma. *A.* Complex tubulopapillary structures characterize the growth pattern of this tumor. *B.* The lining cells are markedly pseudostratified cells and possess chromatin-rich nuclei.

cur. Short fascicles of spindle cells can also be present. The follicular epithelial nature of the tumor is evidenced by thyroglobulin immunoreactivity.

### Differential Diagnosis

Columnar cell carcinoma can be distinguished from tall cell papillary carcinoma by the features of taller cells, striking nuclear pseudostratification, nuclear hyperchromasia, and lack of oxyphilic change.

## Mucoepidermoid Carcinoma

### CLINICAL AND PROGNOSTIC CONSIDERATIONS

This is a rare tumor showing female predominance. The mean age is 37.9 years.[428–441a] The patients present with a thyroid mass. Lymph node metastasis is common (60%), but distant metastasis is rare (13%). This is a low-grade malignant neoplasm; most patients remain well after treatment.

The nature of mucoepidermoid carcinoma is controversial: origin from ultimobranchial body,[442] origin from thyroglossal duct,[436] or merely a metaplastic variant of papillary carcinoma. In some cases, a component of conventional papillary carcinoma can be identified.[434, 435, 437–441a]

### DIAGNOSTIC CONSIDERATIONS

The tumor comprises tumor cell islands that infiltrate a sclerotic stroma. The tumor cells are squamoid to squamous, and there are interspersed mucin-secreting cells (Fig. 44–57A). In areas, a cribriform pattern with elongated lumina containing colloidlike material can be found. The nuclei are hyperchromatic or pale; nuclear pleomorphism is mild to moderate (Fig. 44–57B). Comedo-type necrosis or psammoma bodies can sometimes be found. The tumor usually does not show immunoreactivity for thyroglobulin while the papillary carcinoma compo-

nent, if present, is immunoreactive for thyroglobulin.[428–432, 435, 438, 441a]

## Sclerosing Mucoepidermoid Carcinoma with Eosinophilia

### CLINICAL AND PROGNOSTIC CONSIDERATIONS

Sclerosing mucoepidermoid carcinoma with eosinophilia is a low-grade malignant neoplasm that usually arises in a background of fibrosing Hashimoto's thyroiditis.[443] It affects adults with a mean age of 55 years, and there is a marked female predominance.[436, 441a, 443–447] Regional or distant metastases are uncommon, and the outcome is generally favorable.[436, 441a, 443–446]

### DIAGNOSTIC CONSIDERATIONS

#### Microscopic Findings and Immunohistochemistry

Sclerosing mucoepidermoid carcinoma with eosinophilia is typically infiltrative, and there may be extrathyroidal extension. Anastomosing cords and nests of tumor cells are associated with a sclerotic stroma infiltrated by eosinophils. The tumor cells are polygonal, with mild to moderate nuclear pleomorphism and distinct nucleoli. There can sometimes be foci of squamous differentiation and small pools of mucin (Fig. 44–58). Tumor cell dehiscence may produce a pseudoangiomatous appearance. The tumor cells are immunoreactive for cytokeratin but not for thyroglobulin and calcitonin.

### Differential Diagnosis

The most important reasons to recognize sclerosing mucoepidermoid carcinoma with eosinophilia are not to mistake it for the vastly more aggressive anaplastic or squamous carcinomas of the thyroid on the one hand and not to misdiagnose it as be-

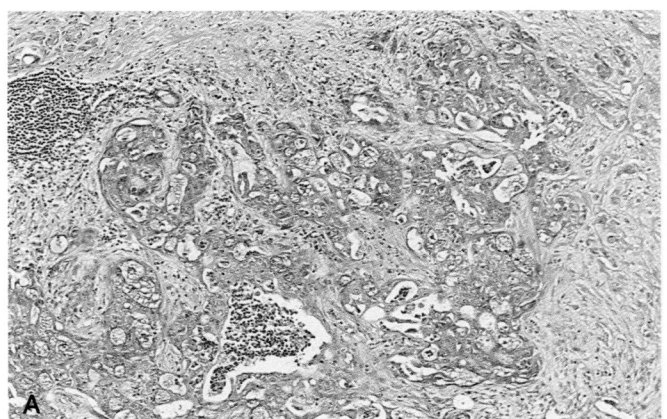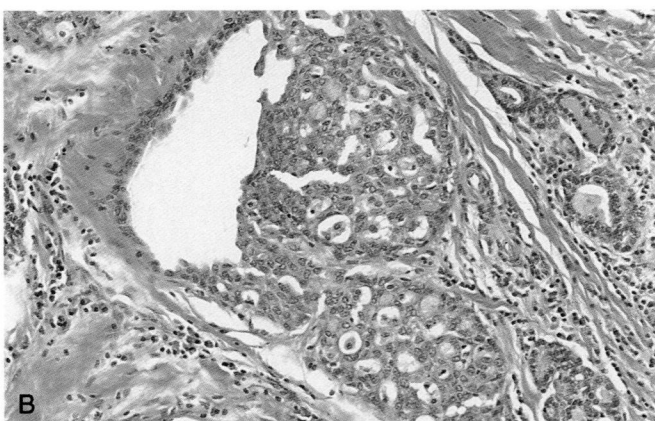

**FIGURE 44–57.** Mucoepidermoid carcinoma. *A.* Irregular islands of tumor infiltrate a desmoplastic stroma. Multiple mucin-containing cystic spaces are interspersed within the tumor islands. *B.* The tumor cells often have bland-looking and pale-staining nuclei.

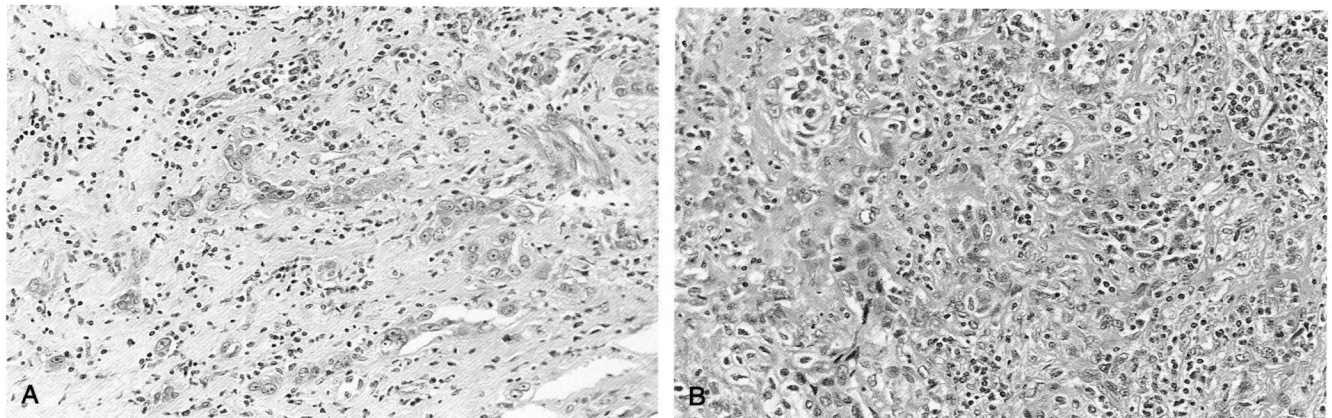

**FIGURE 44–58.** Sclerosing mucoepidermoid carcinoma with eosinophilia. *A.* Cords of polygonal tumor cells with distinct nucleoli infiltrate a sclerotic stroma richly infiltrated by eosinophils and lymphocytes. *B.* Irregular islands of squamoid cells are intermingled with eosinophils and lymphocytes. The mucinous component is usually difficult to appreciate without recourse to mucin stain.

nign squamous metaplasia on the other. In contrast to anaplastic or squamous cell carcinoma, the growth pattern is more diffuse with formation of cords or large islands; nuclear atypia is generally not striking, and the inflammatory component is usually eosinophilic rather than neutrophilic.

## Mucinous Carcinoma

Primary mucinous carcinoma of the thyroid is extremely rare; only four cases have been reported in the literature.[448–451] It is histologically identical to colloid carcinoma of other sites, except that thyroglobulin is usually positive.

## Medullary Thyroid Carcinoma

### CLINICAL CONSIDERATIONS

#### Presentation

Medullary thyroid carcinoma is a malignant neoplasm exhibiting parafollicular C cell differentiation.[452] The patients are mostly adults with slight female predominance.[453–464] Most patients present with a thyroid mass or cervical lymphadenopathy.[465] Some patients may have diarrhea or, more rarely, Cushing's syndrome.[454, 466] The stage distribution at presentation is as follows: stage I, 21%; stage II, 21%; stage III, 47%; and stage IV, 12%.[467] In some centers, routine screening of the calcitonin level in patients with nodular thyroid disease allows early diagnosis of unsuspected sporadic medullary thyroid carcinoma.[468–470]

Approximately 20% to 30% of medullary carcinomas are heritable (autosomal dominant with high penetrance).[453, 455] The tumor often appears at an earlier age, multicentrically and bilaterally, and on a background of C cell hyperplasia[454–461, 471–473] (Table 44–13). Germline mutation in the *RET* gene is the underlying molecular event.[462–464] Thyroidectomy is usually performed for the mutant *RET* gene carriers identified through screening of family members, and the medullary carcinomas diagnosed in such circumstances are often small and at an early stage.

#### Macroscopic Findings

Medullary carcinoma has a predilection for the middle third of the lateral lobe, where normal C cells are most prevalent.[460] It is infiltrative, circumscribed, or encapsulated[474, 475] (Fig. 44–59). It is firm and grayish white, tan, or reddish brown. Hemorrhage and necrosis can be seen in larger tumors.[476]

### DIAGNOSTIC CONSIDERATIONS

#### Microscopic Findings

Medullary carcinoma typically grows in the form of sheets, packets, or irregular islands tra-

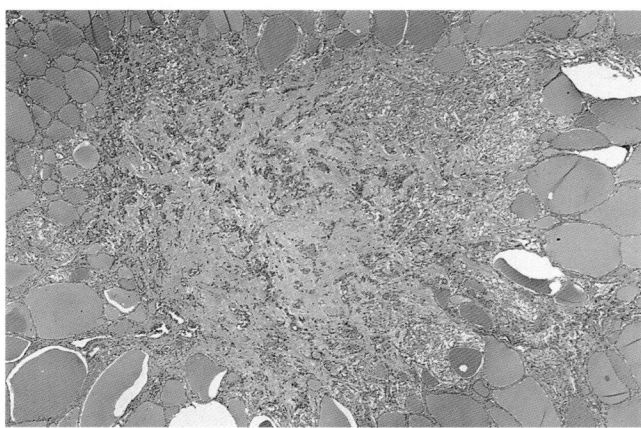

**FIGURE 44–59.** Medullary carcinoma. This tumor exhibits invasive borders, but other cases can have circumscribed borders.

**TABLE 44–13.** Sporadic and Hereditary Forms of Medullary Thyroid Carcinoma (MTC)

| | Sporadic MTC | Familial MTC | MEN 2A | MEN 2B |
|---|---|---|---|---|
| | | | **Hereditary MTC** | |
| Mean age at diagnosis | 44–50 y | 29–43 y | 21–38 y | 12–23 y |
| Sex ratio | Male-female 1:1.4 | ←——————————— Male-Female 1:1.1 ———————————→ | | |
| Other components of the syndrome | Nil | Nil | Pheochromocytoma Parathyroid hyperplasia | Pheochromocytoma Mucosal neuromas Marfanoid appearance |
| Germline mutation in *RET* proto-oncogene | Nil | Mutation involving exon 10, 11, 13, or 14 | Mutation involving exon 10 or 11 | Mutation involving exon 16 (codon 918), with ATG → ACG (methionine → threonine) |
| Bilaterality and C cell hyperplasia in the background | Uncommon | ←——————————— Frequent ———————————→ | | |
| Metastases at diagnosis | Lymph node: 40%–50% Distant: 12% | Lymph node: 10%–20% Distant: 0% | Lymph node: 14% Distant: 0%–3% | Lymph node: 38% Distant: 20% |
| Tumor-related mortality | ~30% | ~0% (most indolent among the various types) | 0%–17% | 50% (most aggressive) |

MEN, multiple endocrine neoplasia.

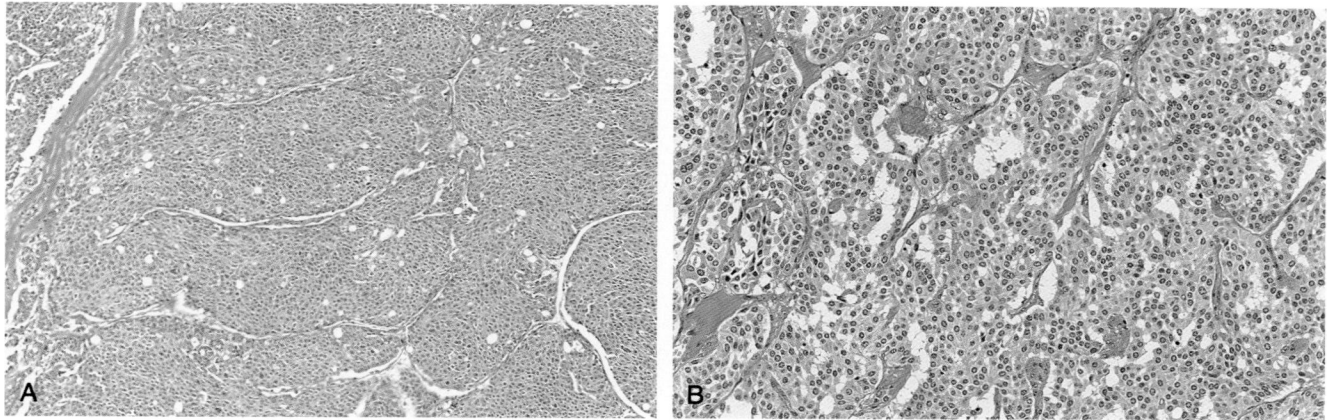

**FIGURE 44–60.** Medullary carcinoma. *A* and *B.* Medullary carcinoma typically grows in the form of sheets and islands traversed by delicate fibrovascular septa.

versed by delicate fibrovascular septa[477, 478] (Fig. 44–60). On occasion, a trabecular, pseudopapillary, whorled, rosette, tubular, microglandular, or cribriform pattern can be observed.[455, 475] Cellular dehiscence and interstitial edema are common (Fig. 44–61*A*). The tumor cells are polygonal or spindly. Their round or oval nuclei exhibit finely stippled chromatin and indistinct nucleoli. The nuclei often appear uniform, with occasional interspersed larger hyperchromatic nuclei (Fig. 44–61*B*). The cytoplasm is finely granular. Cytoplasmic mucin is demonstrable in some tumor cells in up to 50% of cases[189, 479] (Fig. 44–62).

Amyloid, in the form of globules or massive deposits, is found in 80% to 85% of cases[476] (Fig. 44–63). It may show calcification or foreign body giant cell reaction. In microcarcinomas, amyloid is less common, being found in 27% of cases[480] (Fig. 44–64).

Many histologic variants of medullary carcinoma have been recognized, but most are of no prognostic importance (Fig. 44–65; Table 44–14). It is usually not too difficult to render a correct diagnosis for such variants because a component of conventional medullary carcinoma can often be identified on careful search.[476, 478, 481–497]

### Immunohistochemistry

A diagnosis of medullary carcinoma should always be confirmed by immunohistochemistry. Almost all cases are immunoreactive for calcitonin, and a low percentage of positive cells is correlated with a more aggressive behavior[493, 498–501] (Fig. 44–66*A*). If the staining is equivocal or difficult to interpret, immunostaining with a pan-neuroendocrine marker such as chromogranin can readily confirm the diagnosis (Fig. 44–66*B*). Carcinoembryonic antigen is positive in 88% to 100% of cases; this is a highly useful diagnostic marker for poorly differentiated or small cell medullary carcinoma, when calcitonin may be negative.[476, 478, 489, 493, 501, 502]

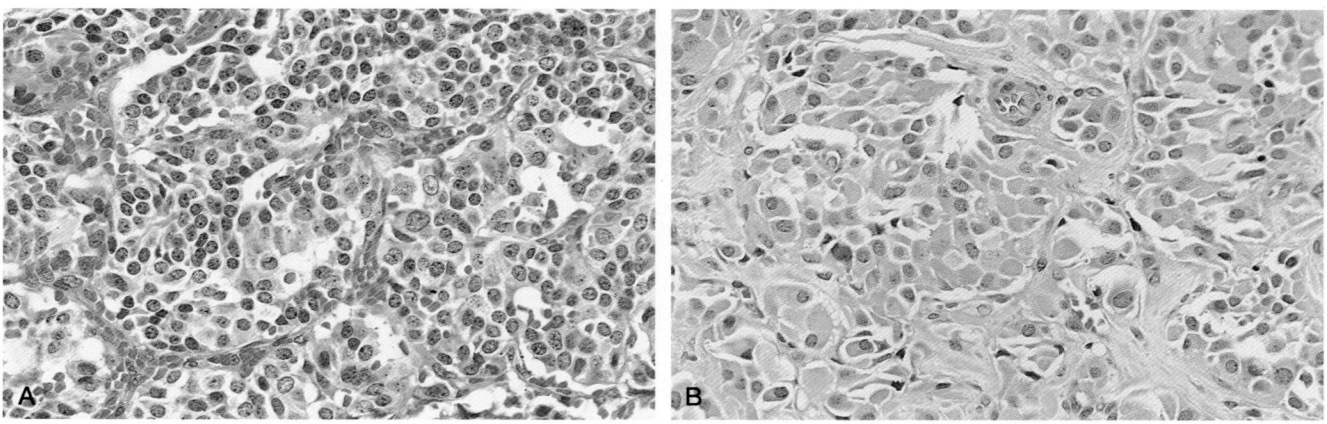

**FIGURE 44–61.** Medullary carcinoma. *A.* The tumor cells are polygonal and exhibit finely granular chromatin and finely granular cytoplasm. Note the characteristic delicate fibrovascular septa. *B.* Cellular dehiscence is a common feature within the tumor islands.

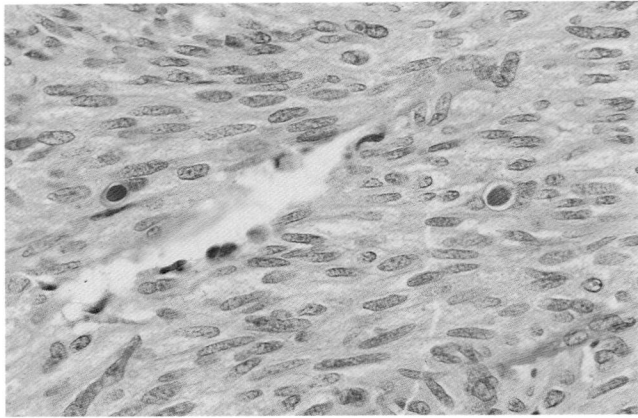

**FIGURE 44–62.** Medullary carcinoma. Staining with periodic acid–Schiff shows presence of mucin vacuoles in some tumor cells.

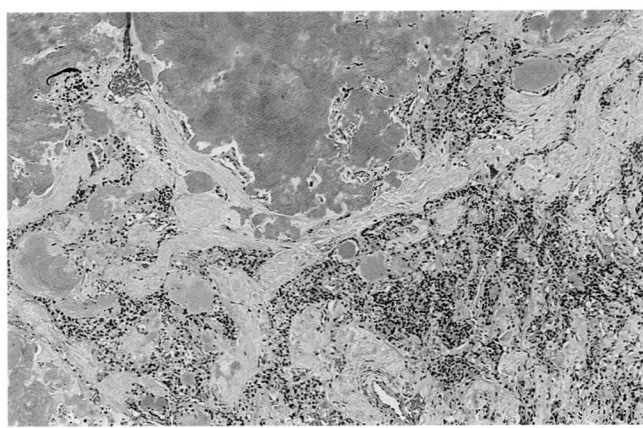

**FIGURE 44–63.** Medullary carcinoma. Abundant amyloid deposits (*upper field*) are evident in this tumor.

**TABLE 44–14.** Variants of Medullary Thyroid Carcinoma

| Variant* | Defining Morphologic Features | Entities for Which the Variant May Be Mistaken |
|---|---|---|
| Glandular-follicular | Presence of glandular or follicular structures which may contain eosinophilic secretion in the lumina<br>The cytoplasm toward the luminal aspect is often more deeply eosinophilic due to polarization of neurosecretory granules. | Follicular adenoma or carcinoma<br>Poorly differentiated (insular) thyroid carcinoma |
| Papillary | Presence of pseudopapillae due to cellular dehiscence, and only rarely are there true papillary formations | Papillary carcinoma |
| Oxyphilic | Tumor cells with abundant eosinophilic granular cytoplasm due to accumulation of mitochondria | Hürthle cell neoplasm |
| Clear cell | Presence of tumor cells with water-clear cytoplasm | Other clear cell tumors |
| Spindle cell | Presence of spindly tumor cells arranged in fascicles or whorls | Mesenchymal tumors |
| Pigmented | Presence of brown melanin pigment in some tumor cells | — |
| Squamous | Presence of squamous differentiation | Squamous cell carcinoma |
| Small cell | Tumor composed predominantly of small cells, often with nuclear molding, resembling small cell carcinoma of lung | Malignant lymphoma |
| Giant cell (anaplastic) | Presence of large cells with bizarre and pleomorphic nuclei, but mitotic figures are rare | Anaplastic carcinoma |
| Neuroblastoma-like | Presence of fibrillary matrix or rosettes, resembling neuroblastoma | Malignant lymphoma<br>Metastatic neuroblastoma<br>Peripheral primitive neuroectodermal tumor |
| Carcinoid-like | Histologic features resembling intestinal carcinoid, with tumor islands, trabeculae, or glands separated by fibrohyaline stroma | Metastatic carcinoid<br>Paraganglioma<br>Follicular neoplasm |
| Hyalinizing trabecular adenoma–like | Wavy trabeculae of tumor cells, which merge into abundant extracellular hyaline material, mimicking hyalinizing trabecular adenoma | Hyalinizing trabecular adenoma<br>Paraganglioma |
| Paraganglioma-like | Tumor forming packets delineated by a delicate vasculature | Paraganglioma |

* The listed variants have no clinical or prognostic significance, except the small cell type, which is more aggressive. The prognostic implication of the giant cell variant is still unsettled.

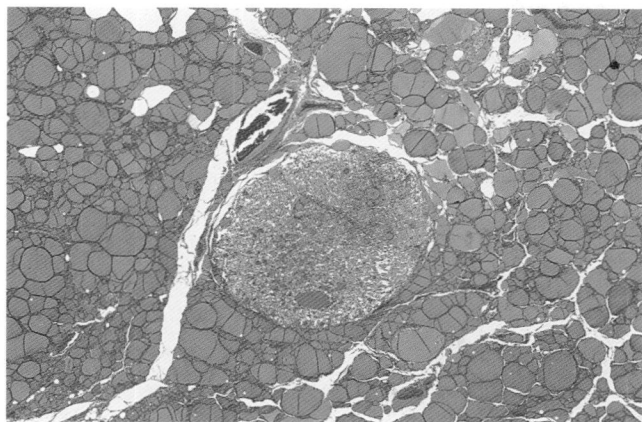

**FIGURE 44–64.** Medullary carcinoma as an incidental finding. As is characteristic of microcarcinoma, amyloid is often absent or scanty.

S-100 protein–positive sustentacular cells are usually absent, except in the setting of multiple endocrine neoplasia or familial medullary carcinoma, when 62.5% of cases can show a population of sustentacular cells.[503]

The hereditary form of medullary carcinoma typically arises in a background of C cell hyperplasia, which has been classified into a diffuse type and a nodular type. However, there are no universally accepted criteria for the diffuse type of C cell hyperplasia, and a similar degree of C cell proliferation can be seen in normal subjects, around various types of thyroid tumors, and in thyroiditis[504–509] (Fig. 44–67). The nodular type of C cell hyperplasia is defined as "complete obliteration of follicular space by C cells with production of solid intrafollicular aggregates," but distinction from a minute medullary carcinoma or intrathyroid spread of medullary carcinoma can be difficult[507, 510] (Fig. 44–68).

### Molecular Biology

The *RET* proto-oncogene on chromosome 10q11 plays a key role in the genesis of medullary carcinoma. The *RET* gene, which comprises 21 exons, encodes a receptor tyrosine kinase with a cysteine-rich extramembrane domain, a transmembrane domain, and an intracellular tyrosine kinase component. Germline mutations of *RET* are found in patients with MEN 2 or familial medullary thyroid carcinoma. The mutations result in constitutive activation of the receptor owing to dimerization or alteration in the tyrosine kinase substrate specificity.[274, 511, 512] In MEN 2A, the mutations involve the cysteine-rich region of the extracellular domain, resulting in substitution of cysteine by another amino acid, the most common being TGC → CGC (Cys → Arg) at codon 634.[513, 514] The sites of mutation are more varied in familial medullary thyroid carcinoma.[274] MEN 2B is always caused by the same mutation in codon 918 of exon 16: ATG → ACG

(Met → Thr).[513–515] Molecular study is currently the most reliable way to diagnose the hereditary form of medullary thyroid carcinoma—germline mutation in *RET* can be conveniently demonstrated on DNA extracted from peripheral blood leukocytes or paraffin-embedded nontumor tissues. After exons 10, 11, and 16 are amplified by the polymerase chain reaction, mutation screening can be performed by the single-stranded conformation polymorphism or heteroduplex technique; the site of mutation can be confirmed by DNA sequencing or restriction endonuclease cleavage. If the patient is confirmed to show germline mutation in *RET*, all family members should be screened to detect carriers of the *RET* mutation, who should be counseled, offered thyroidectomy, and closely followed up.[516–518]

In sporadic medullary carcinomas, somatic mutations in *RET* are found in 26% to 69% of cases, most commonly involving codon 918 of exon 16 (ATG → ACG).[514, 519–522]

### Differential Diagnosis

POORLY DIFFERENTIATED (INSULAR) THYROID CARCINOMA. See earlier.

HYALINIZING TRABECULAR ADENOMA. Hyalinizing trabecular adenoma can mimic medullary carcinoma architecturally, but long wavy trabeculae are most uncommon in medullary carcinoma, and the nuclear features (nuclear grooves, nuclear pseudoinclusions, perinucleolar haloes) are also different.

PARAGANGLIOMA. There is significant morphologic overlap between paraganglioma and medullary carcinoma, such as packeting pattern, rich vascularity, and granular cytoplasm. Paraganglioma differs in being negative for cytokeratin, calcitonin, and carcinoembryonic antigen.

METASTATIC NEUROENDOCRINE CARCINOMA. Metastatic neuroendocrine carcinoma (carcinoid and atypical carcinoid) from the bronchus or intra-abdominal sites can present initially as thyroid tumor and is often misdiagnosed as medullary carcinoma.[523] The neuroendocrine carcinoma forms nests, ribbons, islands, rosettes, and sheets traversed by delicate fibrovascular stroma. Clues to the diagnosis are predominantly interstitial growth, multiple tumor foci, absence of C cell hyperplasia, presence of peculiar protrusions into thyroid follicles in the form of subepithelial cell balls, and lack of amyloid. The tumor cells lack immunoreactivity for calcitonin and carcinoembryonic antigen.

HÜRTHLE CELL NEOPLASM. Medullary carcinoma with oncocytic change is not uncommonly misdiagnosed as Hürthle cell neoplasm. The most helpful clue is the presence of the delicate fibrovascular septa; identification of areas of conventional medullary carcinoma is also helpful.

ANAPLASTIC CARCINOMA. Bizarre and highly atypical cells may occur in an otherwise typical medullary carcinoma; this tumor can be distin-

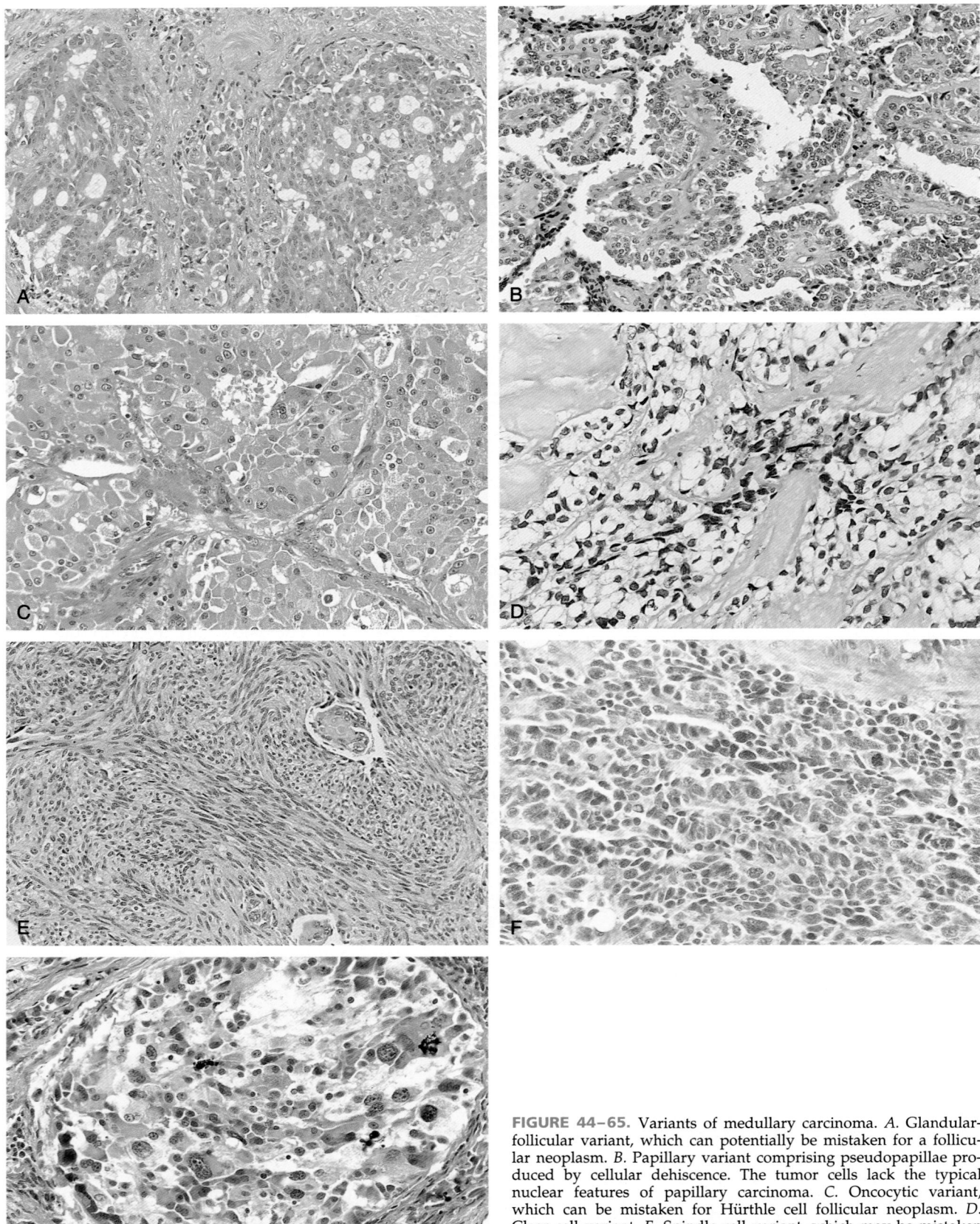

**FIGURE 44–65.** Variants of medullary carcinoma. *A.* Glandular-follicular variant, which can potentially be mistaken for a follicular neoplasm. *B.* Papillary variant comprising pseudopapillae produced by cellular dehiscence. The tumor cells lack the typical nuclear features of papillary carcinoma. *C.* Oncocytic variant, which can be mistaken for Hürthle cell follicular neoplasm. *D.* Clear cell variant. *E.* Spindle cell variant, which may be mistaken for a mesenchymal neoplasm. *F.* Small cell variant. *G.* Giant cell variant.

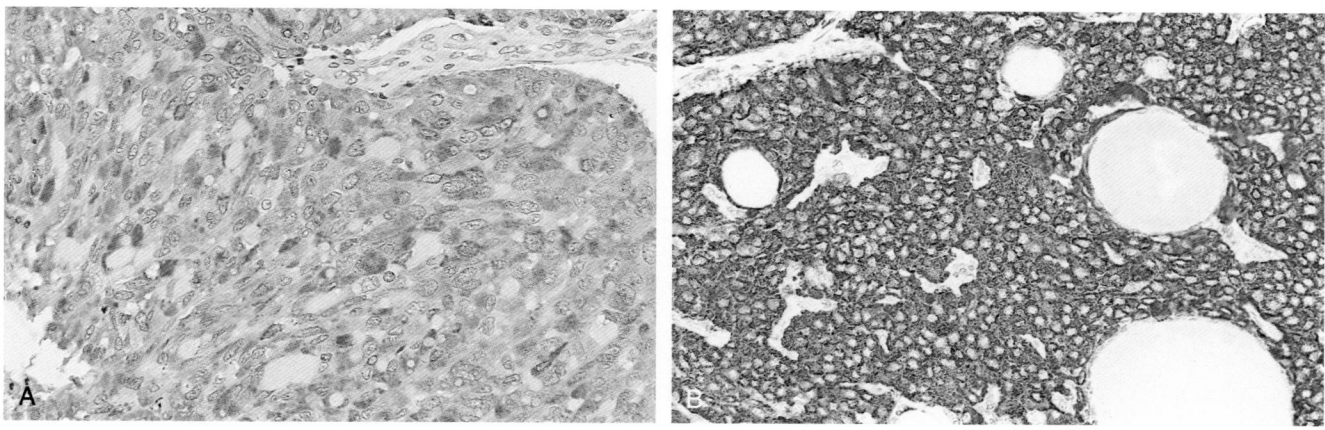

**FIGURE 44-66.** Medullary carcinoma, immunohistochemical staining. *A.* All tumor cells show positive staining for calcitonin. *B.* Strong positive granular staining for chromogranin is observed.

guished from anaplastic carcinoma by the presence of many bland-looking cells among the bizarre cells and the paucity of mitotic figures.

PARATHYROID NEOPLASM. See later.

## PROGNOSTIC CONSIDERATIONS

The tumor tends to spread by lymphatics to lymph nodes of the neck (one third to two thirds) and upper mediastinum.[454, 465, 524] Local recurrence develops in about one third of cases after treatment.[465] Late in the course, the tumor may metastasize to other sites, such as lungs, liver, adrenal, and bone, although distant metastasis is already present in 8% of patients at presentation.[524] Patients may still survive for many years despite the presence of distant metastases. The 5-year, 10-year, and 15-year survival rates are 65% to 87%, 51% to 78%, and 65%, respectively,[453, 465, 525-527] indicating that this tumor is indo-

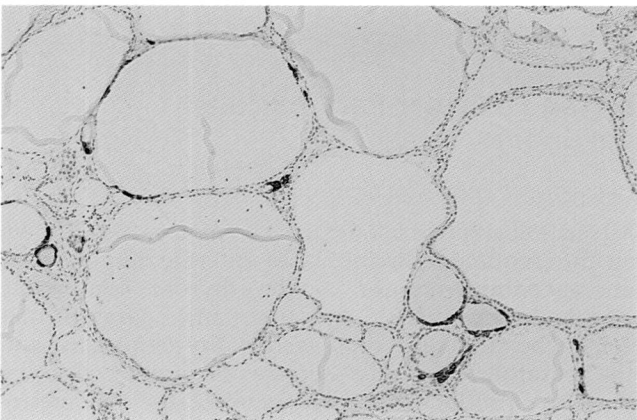

**FIGURE 44-67.** C cell hyperplasia, diffuse type, found adjacent to a follicular adenoma. This form of C cell hyperplasia cannot be appreciated in conventional histologic sections. Immunostaining for calcitonin shows increased isolated C cells (stained brown). These cells lie within the basal lamina of the follicles.

lent and not rapidly lethal. However, there is still an excess mortality 10 years after a diagnosis of medullary carcinoma.[527] Because medullary carcinoma is not radiosensitive, adequate surgical clearance (total thyroidectomy) is the mainstay of primary treatment.[528, 529]

Tumor stage is the single most important prognostic factor on multivariate analysis.[453, 473, 524-527]

STAGE OF DISEASE. Extrathyroidal extension is associated with a high risk of recurrence, disease progression, and worsened survival.[526, 529, 530] Presence of lymph node metastasis at diagnosis greatly worsens the prognosis, with 10-year survival dropping from 86% to 95% (node negative) to 46% to 55% (node positive).* Distant metastasis is associated with a poor survival.[529]

AGE. Older patients (>50 to 60 years) have a worse outcome.†

SEX. Some studies have shown the female sex to be associated with a better prognosis,[493, 526] but this factor loses prognostic significance on multivariate analysis according to some series.[524, 525]

MEDULLARY CARCINOMA OF MEN 2. MEN 2A-associated medullary carcinoma has a better prognosis than the sporadic variety does; MEN 2B-associated medullary carcinoma is associated with a worse prognosis.[455, 471, 527, 531] Nonetheless, this factor is apparently not significant after multivariate analysis according to one study.[453]

TUMOR SIZE. Small tumors less than 1 cm have an excellent prognosis.[461, 468, 474, 527, 532] Unfavorable outcome in microcarcinomas is virtually confined to patients who are symptomatic (such as palpable microcarcinoma, diarrhea, or metastatic disease at presentation).[532]

---

*References 455, 465, 493, 524, 526, 528, 530.

†References 453, 455, 465, 473, 493, 524, 526, 528.

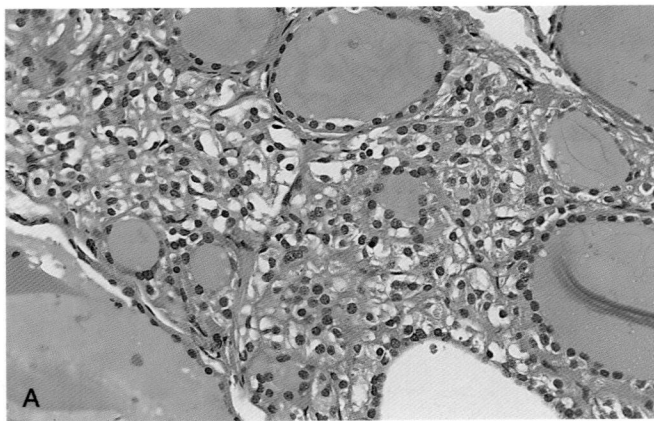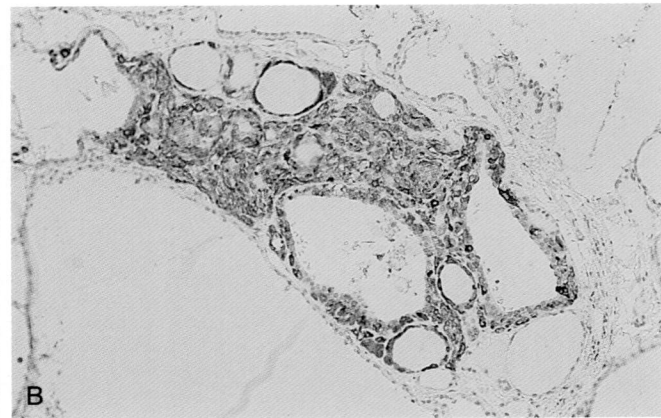

**FIGURE 44–68.** C cell hyperplasia, nodular type, associated with MEN 2A. *A.* Small nodular clusters of cells are found among the follicles, sometimes obliterating their lumina. *B.* A corresponding field stained for calcitonin clearly delineates the hyperplastic C cells.

BIOCHEMICAL CURE. Achievement of biochemical cure predicts good survival (98% at 10 years versus 70% for those not achieving biochemical cure).[525, 530]

HISTOLOGIC FEATURES. Features associated with a worse prognosis include high mitotic count (more than 1 mitotic figure per 25 high-power fields), coagulative necrosis, absence of amyloid, and small cell variant[474, 475, 486, 526, 527, 533] (Fig. 44–69).

IMMUNOHISTOCHEMICAL FEATURES. Calcitonin-poor medullary carcinomas fare worse than calcitonin-rich tumors.[534–536] The calcitonin content of the tumor may decrease at relapse. Strong expression of CD15/Leu-M1 is correlated with a higher risk of local recurrence and tumor mortality.[537, 538] Low expression of chromogranin B or Bcl-2 is associated with a more aggressive course.[539, 540]

N-MYC EXPRESSION. Increased expression of N-*myc* has been reported to be an unfavorable prognostic factor.[541]

TUMOR ANGIOGENESIS. A high microvessel count is associated with a poorer prognosis.[542]

DNA PLOIDY. Aneuploid tumors behave more aggressively than diploid ones do.[493, 527, 543, 544]

## Collision Tumor

Collision tumors are neoplasms comprising two components: medullary carcinoma and a carcinoma of follicular cell derivation (follicular carcinoma or papillary carcinoma).[545–552] The two components can be intermingled, contiguous, or separate. Most probably represent coincidental occurrence of two neoplasms in proximity.

## Mixed Follicular-Parafollicular Carcinoma

### CLINICAL CONSIDERATIONS

Mixed follicular-parafollicular carcinoma, also known as differentiated carcinoma of intermediate type, is an uncommon tumor of the thyroid comprising closely intermingled follicular and parafollicular cells. The follicular cells secrete thyroglobulin, and the parafollicular cells secrete calcitonin or other hormone products such as somatostatin and neurotensin; on occasion, both hormone products can be produced by the same cell.[553–556] The patients have a median age of 48 years. They present with a thyroid nodule, and lymph node involvement is common (~75%). The mean size of the tumor is 3.7 cm.[556]

**FIGURE 44–69.** Medullary carcinoma showing "aggressive" histologic features, such as diffuse cellular atypia, coagulative necrosis, and mitotic figures.

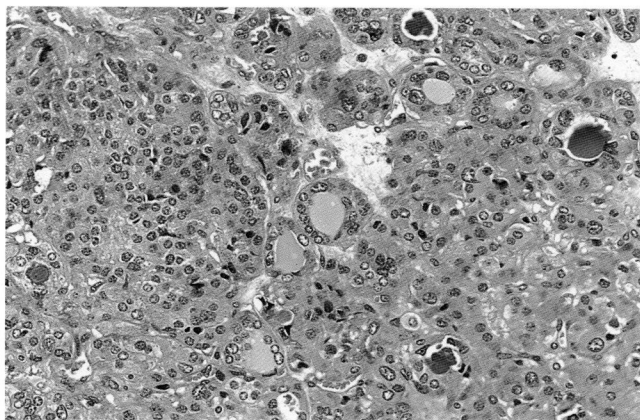

**FIGURE 44–70.** Mixed follicular-parafollicular carcinoma. It shows a solid growth interspersed with follicles.

## DIAGNOSTIC CONSIDERATIONS

### Microscopic Findings

Mixed follicular-parafollicular carcinomas are often completely or partially encapsulated. They show solid, nested, or cribriform growth with intermingled follicles[553, 557–559] (Fig. 44–70). It is important not to mistake entrapped thyroid follicles in a conventional medullary carcinoma for a mixed follicular-parafollicular carcinoma. Cytologic comparison of the cells lining the follicles with those of the surrounding follicles is most helpful. The most definitive evidence of follicular differentiation is identification of follicles in metastatic deposits. Amyloid is occasionally present. On ultrastructural examination, neurosecretory granules, follicular cells, cells with intermediate features, and indifferent cells are identified.[553]

### Immunohistochemistry

Thyroglobulin immunoreactivity is characteristically seen in the follicular and cribriform areas and sometimes in the solid component; calcitonin immunoreactivity is most conspicuous in the solid areas[553, 555] (Fig. 44–71). Rare cells with dual hormone production can be identified in some cases.

### Differential Diagnosis

This tumor histologically mimics the less well differentiated examples of follicular carcinoma or insular carcinoma. Immunohistochemical confirmation is therefore essential for diagnosis. However, the possibilities of entrapped benign follicles and diffusion of thyroglobulin from surrounding thyroid tissue have to be excluded.

### Molecular Biology

Although it has been thought that mixed follicular-parafollicular carcinoma results from an uncommitted stem cell capable of differentiating toward both follicular cells and C cells, molecular studies have failed to confirm such a hypothesis.[556] Studies of gene mutation, allelic loss, and clonal composition on microdissected tumor tissue show that the follicular and parafollicular components belong to different clones.[560] Furthermore, the follicular component is often oligoclonal or polyclonal.

## PROGNOSTIC CONSIDERATIONS

Mixed follicular-parafollicular carcinomas spread by both the lymphatic and hematogenous routes and are more aggressive than differentiated thyroid carcinomas. In the series of 18 patients reported by Ljungberg,[553] 6 developed metastasis, and 4 died of the tumor 1 month to 15 years after surgery. According to the review of Papotti and colleagues,[556] 56% of patients (N = 25) were alive with disease or dead of disease up to 10 years after diagnosis. The results contrast with those of otherwise typical med-

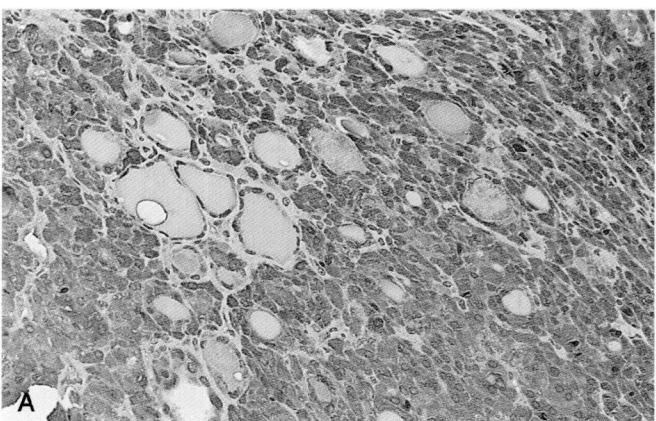
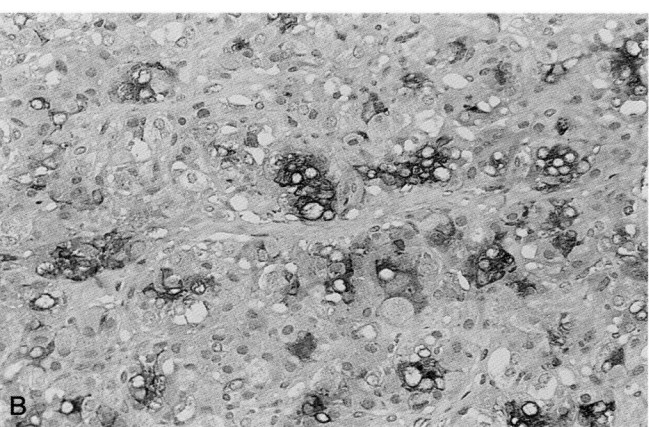

**FIGURE 44–71.** Mixed follicular-parafollicular carcinoma, immunohistochemical staining. *A.* The solid component shows immunoreactivity for calcitonin. *B.* Thyroglobulin immunoreactivity is confined to the follicles.

**TABLE 44–15.** Clinicopathologic Features of Thymic and Related Branchial Pouch Tumors in the Thyroid

| | Ectopic Thymoma | Spindle Epithelial Tumor with Thymus-like Element (SETTLE) | Carcinoma Showing Thymus-like Element (CASTLE) |
|---|---|---|---|
| Age | Middle age | Children and young adults, with a mean age of 18 y | Middle and old age, with a mean age of 49 y |
| Sex | F > M | M > F | M ≤ F |
| Presentation | Thyroid mass | Thyroid mass | Thyroid mass, with or without cervical node enlargement |
| Pathology | Encapsulated tumor with jigsaw puzzle–type lobulation<br>Composed of a variable admixture of pale-staining plump epithelial cells and small lymphocytes | The tumor is demarcated into incomplete lobules by sclerotic stroma. It is highly cellular, with compact interlacing to reticulated fascicles of spindle cells merging imperceptibly into epithelial structures that can be in the form of cords, tubules, or papillae. The spindle cells possess elongated bland-looking nuclei with fine chromatin; mitosis is infrequent.<br>In some cases, discrete glandular structures lined by mucinous or respiratory-type epithelium are found.<br>Lymphocytes are sparse or absent. | The tumor usually involves the lower pole of the thyroid and invades in pushing fronts. Variably sized, often smooth-contoured lobules of tumor cells are demarcated by desmoplastic fibrous stroma.<br>The tumor cells have indistinct cell borders, vesicular nuclei, and prominent nucleoli or show a squamous or squamoid appearance.<br>The tumor cells and fibrous septa show scanty to heavy infiltration by lymphocytes and plasma cells. |
| Immunohistochemistry | Epithelial component is cytokeratin positive<br>Lymphoid component comprises mostly immature T cells (TdT+). | Both glandular and spindle cell components are cytokeratin positive<br>CD5 negative | Cytokeratin and CD5 positive |
| Clinical behavior | Benign in all reported cases | Behavior is unpredictable, but a significant proportion of patients develop delayed distant metastasis (~70% with long-term follow-up), especially to the lungs.<br>Even in the presence of metastasis, this indolent tumor can pursue a protracted course for many years before killing the patient. | Extrathyroidal extension is common. Regional lymph node metastasis occurs in about half of the cases.<br>The tumor is indolent; most patients enjoy long survivals after surgery or radiation therapy, although occasional cases can pursue a more aggressive course. |

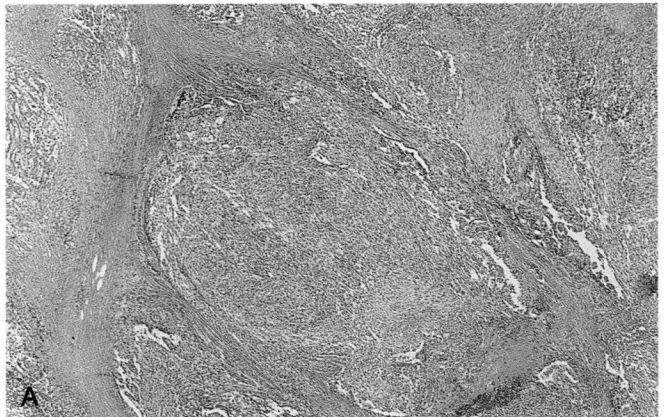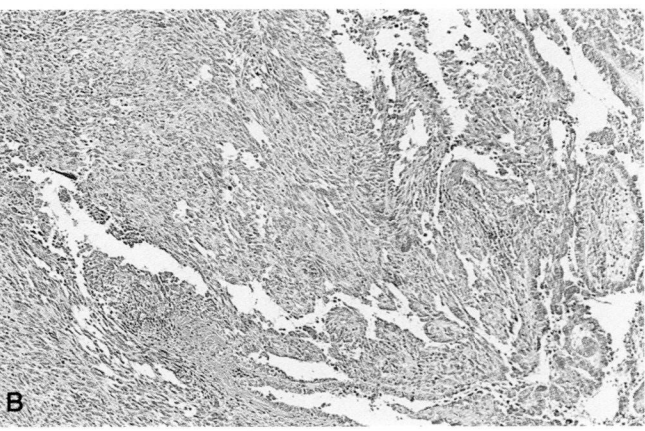

**FIGURE 44–72.** Spindle epithelial tumor with thymus-like element. *A.* The tumor forms lobules demarcated by sclerotic septa, reminiscent of the architectural features of thymoma. *B.* Compact and reticulated fascicles of spindly cells merge imperceptibly into tubulopapillary epithelial structures (*right field*). This tumor type shows cytoarchitectural resemblance to synovial sarcoma.

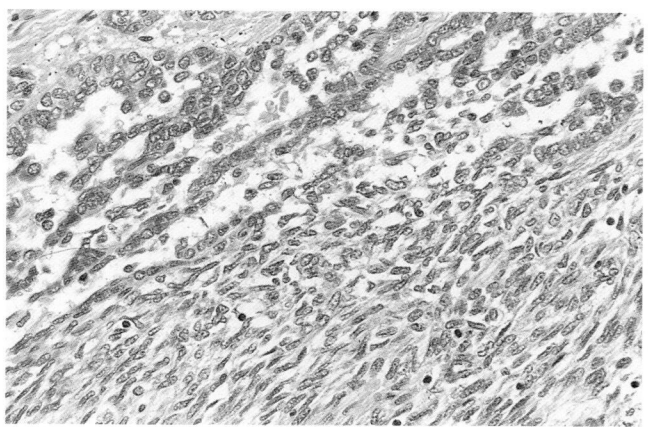

**FIGURE 44–73.** Spindle epithelial tumor with thymus-like element. The spindly cells have fairly uniform nuclei and scanty cytoplasm. The glandular structures (*left upper field*) exhibit bland-looking, pale-staining nuclei.

ullary carcinoma shown on immunohistochemical staining to be thyroglobulin positive, which has a prognosis similar to or better than that of conventional medullary carcinoma.[561]

## Thymic and Related Branchial Pouch Tumors of the Thyroid

### CLINICAL CONSIDERATIONS

The occasional presence of sequestered thymic tissue or branchial pouch remnants in the thyroid gland may explain the occurrence of ectopic thymic tumors in the thyroid. These rare tumors include ectopic thymoma, spindle epithelial tumor with thymus-like element (SETTLE), and carcinoma showing thymus-like element (CASTLE); their clinicopathologic features are summarized in Table 44–15 (Figs. 44–72 to 44–74).[562–581]

### DIAGNOSTIC CONSIDERATIONS

Ectopic thymoma is histologically identical to the mediastinal counterpart. For CASTLE, the morphologic features and expression of CD5 (a lymphocyte-associated marker commonly expressed in thymic carcinomas but not in nonthymic carcinomas) strongly suggest that this is an intrathyroid thymic carcinoma.[582–584] The histogenesis of SETTLE currently remains elusive.[581]

The most important reason for recognizing this group of neoplasms is that they are benign to low-grade malignant and should not be mistaken for lymphoma or the vastly more aggressive anaplastic carcinoma. Follicular dendritic cell tumor can also potentially be misdiagnosed as CASTLE.[585]

## Intrathyroid Parathyroid Tumor

Because the parathyroid glands are close to or are embedded in the thyroid gland, parathyroid adenoma or carcinoma can occur as primary thyroid tumor.[586, 587] These tumors are not uncommonly misdiagnosed as follicular adenoma, follicular carcinoma, or anaplastic carcinoma (Fig. 44–75A). A parathyroid origin should be suspected when there are clear cells, prominent delicate vasculature, and regimentation of nuclei along the vascular septa. The diagnosis can be confirmed by immunostaining for parathyroid hormone (Fig. 44–75B).

## Malignant Lymphoma

### CLINICAL CONSIDERATIONS

#### Presentation

Primary lymphoma of the thyroid accounts for approximately 5% of all thyroid cancers.[588] It affects mostly adults, and there is a female predominance (male-to-female ratio = 1:2.5).[589–599] Hashimoto's

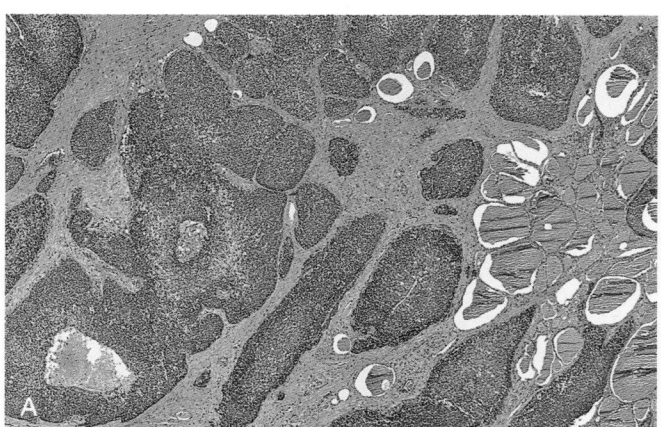
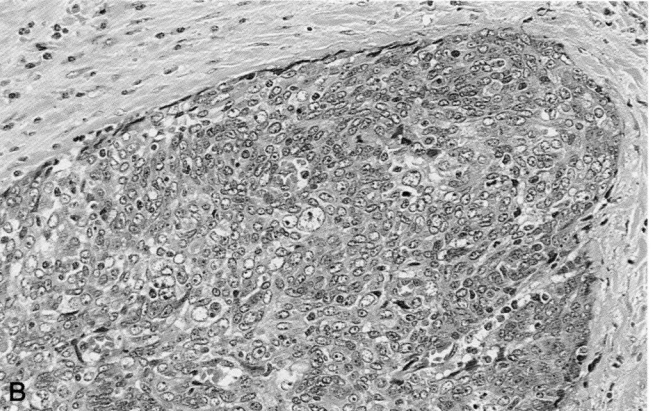

**FIGURE 44–74.** Carcinoma showing thymus-like element. *A.* The tumor invades the thyroid predominantly in the form of smooth-contoured cell islands, different from the extensive permeative growth of anaplastic carcinoma. *B.* The tumor island comprises squamoid cells with moderate nuclear atypia. The cytoarchitectural features are identical to those of squamous cell carcinoma of the thymus.

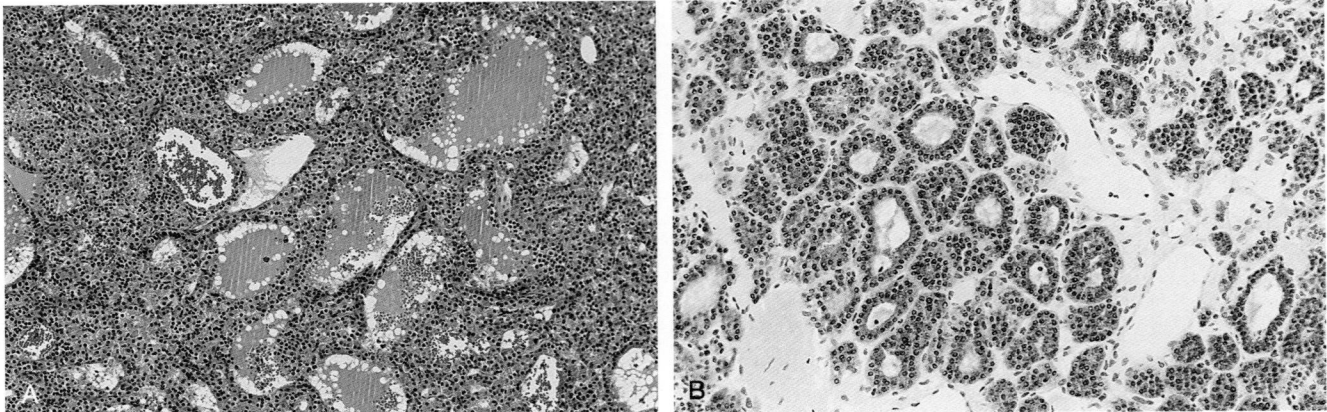

**FIGURE 44–75.** Intrathyroid parathyroid adenoma. *A.* The presence of follicle structures creates a strong mimicry of follicular neoplasm. *B.* The diagnosis can be readily confirmed by positive immunoreactivity for parathyroid hormone.

thyroiditis and lymphocytic thyroiditis are recognized predisposing factors.[589, 593, 598]

Some patients present with a rapidly enlarging thyroid mass, which may be accompanied by dysphagia or hoarseness, simulating the presentation of anaplastic carcinoma. Others present with gradual enlargement of the thyroid gland or a slow-growing thyroid nodule. The tumor can be confined to the thyroid or show extrathyroidal extension. Regional lymph nodes are sometimes involved.

### Macroscopic Findings

The lymphoma forms a noncircumscribed rubbery to soft mass in one or both lobes of the thyroid. The cut surfaces are slightly bulging, fleshy, light tan, and often homogeneous, with or without necrosis and hemorrhage. The size ranges from less than 1 cm to 19.5 cm.[592, 600]

## DIAGNOSTIC CONSIDERATIONS

### Histologic Types

Hodgkin's lymphoma of the thyroid is extremely rare.[601] Among non-Hodgkin's lymphomas, diffuse large B cell lymphoma and extranodal marginal zone B cell lymphoma of mucosa-associated lymphoid tissue (MALT) type constitute almost all cases.[589, 596, 599, 602] Exceptional examples of follicular lymphoma, intravascular lymphomatosis, and T cell lymphomas have been reported.[599, 603–607]

### Extranodal Marginal Zone B Cell Lymphoma of MALT Type

The histologic features of extranodal marginal zone B cell lymphoma involving the thyroid are similar to those of this lymphoma type occurring elsewhere. Within the diffuse lymphomatous infiltrate, some reactive lymphoid follicles are often interspersed (Fig. 44–76A). The lymphoma cells are small to medium sized, resembling small lymphocytes, centrocytes, or monocytoid B cells; the cellular composition is often mixed. Plasma cells, often in

groups, are commonly found among the lymphoma cells. Invasion of the thyroid follicles by lymphoma cells results in formation of lymphoepithelial lesions and plugging of the follicular lumina by lymphoma cells[589, 599, 608] (Fig. 44–77; see also Fig. 44–76B). Colonization of the reactive lymphoid follicles can result in a pattern reminiscent of follicular lymphoma (see Fig. 44–76C).[599, 608, 609] Immunohistochemical staining shows expression of B markers; CD5, CD10, CD23, and cyclin D1 are negative.[599, 607] Monotypic immunoglobulin can be demonstrated in the plasma cells in approximately 30% of cases.[608, 610]

### Diffuse Large B Cell Lymphoma with or Without a Component of Extranodal Marginal Zone B Cell Lymphoma

Diffuse large B cell lymphoma accounts for more than 60% of all thyroid lymphomas. In some cases, there is a component of extranodal marginal zone B cell lymphoma, suggesting transformation from it.[590, 591, 593, 599, 611, 612] The lymphomatous growth effaces the architecture of the thyroid tissue (Fig. 44–78A). The lymphoma cells are large, with round vesicular nuclei, distinct nucleoli, and a moderate amount of amphophilic cytoplasm that may sometimes be plasmacytoid (Fig. 44–78B). Mitotic figures and apoptotic bodies are common. Invasion of the thyroid epithelium to produce lymphoepithelial lesions is common, whereas plugging of follicular lumina by lymphoma cells is much less frequent.[590, 592, 599, 613] Vascular invasion can sometimes be identified[590, 592] (Fig. 44–78C). Immunohistochemical analysis shows positive staining for leukocyte common antigen and B markers.

### Differential Diagnosis

HASHIMOTO'S THYROIDITIS. When Hashimoto's thyroiditis shows a florid chronic inflammatory cell infiltrate, it can be difficult to tell whether there is superimposed extranodal marginal zone B cell lym-

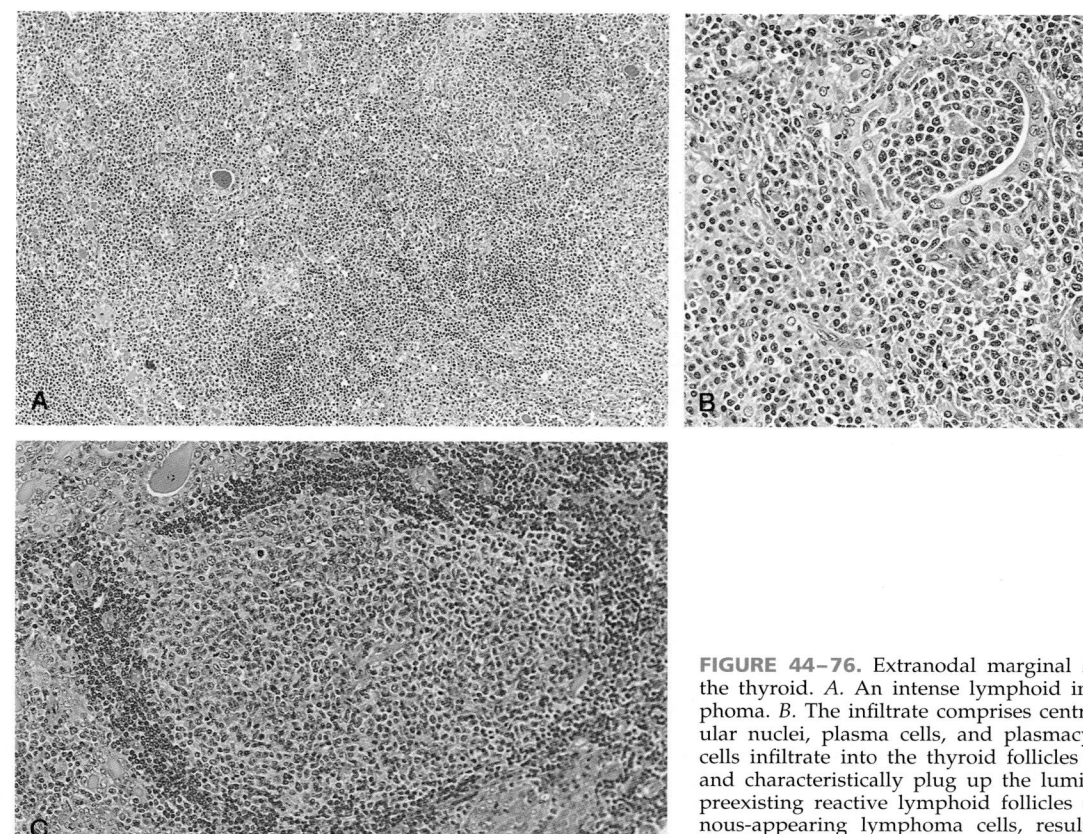

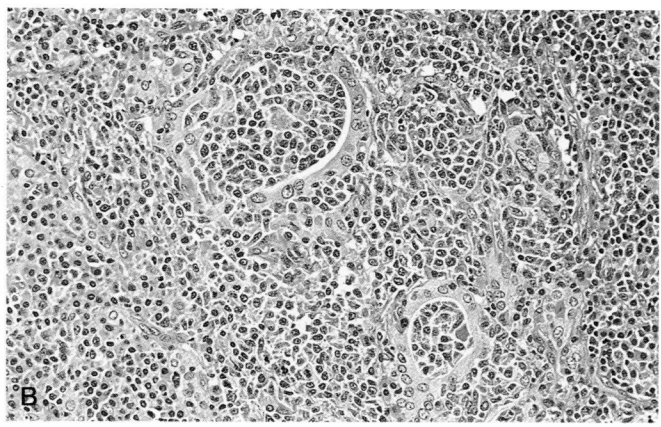

FIGURE 44–76. Extranodal marginal zone B cell lymphoma of the thyroid. *A.* An intense lymphoid infiltrate characterizes lymphoma. *B.* The infiltrate comprises centrocyte-like cells with irregular nuclei, plasma cells, and plasmacytoid cells. The lymphoid cells infiltrate into the thyroid follicles (lymphoepithelial lesions) and characteristically plug up the lumina of the follicles. *C.* The preexisting reactive lymphoid follicles are colonized by monotonous-appearing lymphoma cells, resulting in a resemblance to follicular lymphoma.

phoma.[608] A dense lymphoid infiltrate, broad bands of centrocyte-like cells or clear cells, and prominent lymphoepithelial lesions are histologic features strongly favoring a diagnosis of lymphoma, which can be further supported by immunohistochemical studies to demonstrate sheets of B cells, aberrant coexpression of CD43, or light chain restriction.[300]

ANAPLASTIC CARCINOMA. Features favoring a diagnosis of lymphoma are lack of cellular cohesion, plasmacytoid cytoplasm, presence of lymphoepithelial lesions, and plugging of follicular lumina by tumor cells. The diagnosis can be readily confirmed by immunohistochemical studies (see Table 44–1).

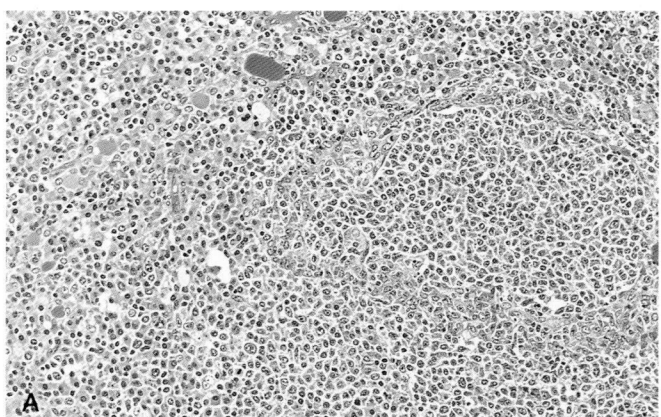

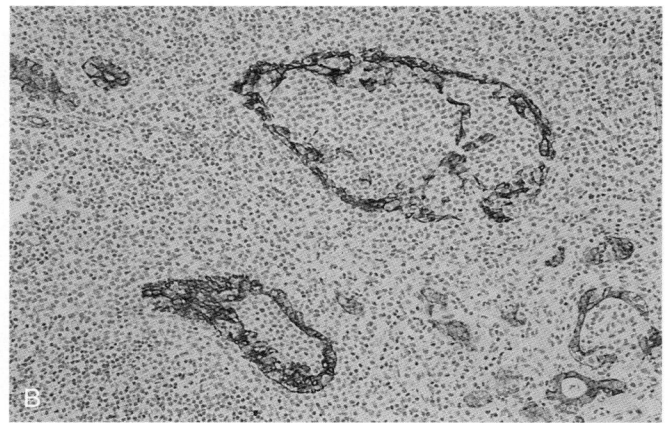

FIGURE 44–77. Extranodal marginal zone B cell lymphoma of the thyroid. *A.* The lymphoma cells show prominent infiltration and expansion of the thyroid follicles to produce lymphoepithelial lesions (*right field*). *B.* Cytokeratin immunostaining of a corresponding field clearly shows follicular destruction and expansion by the neoplastic infiltrate.

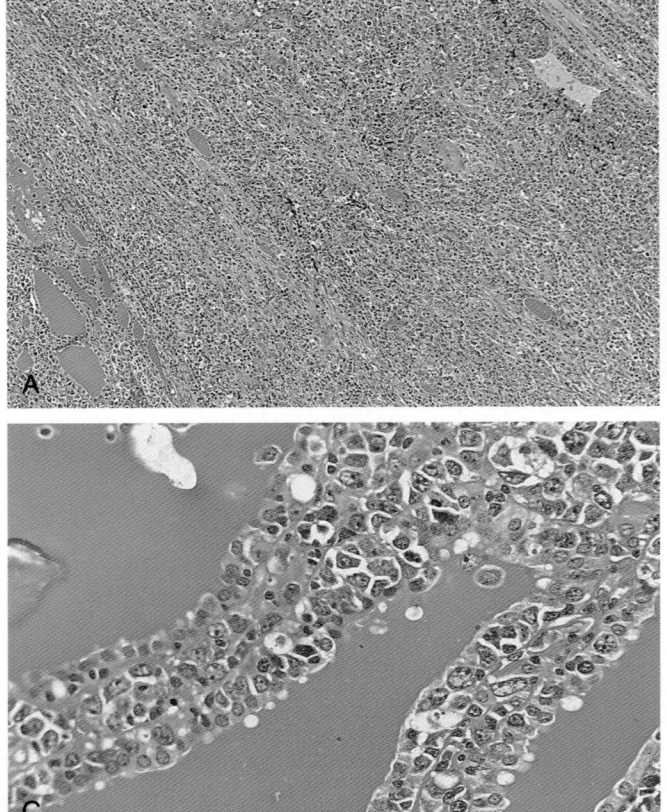

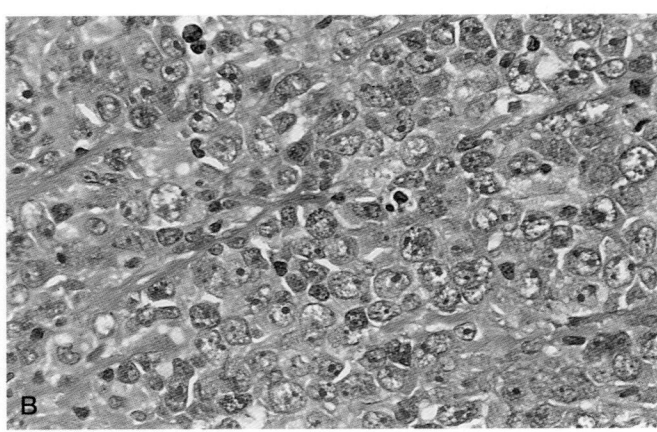

**FIGURE 44–78.** Diffuse large B cell lymphoma of the thyroid. *A.* The neoplasm is permeative and destructive. Residual follicles are evident in the left lower field. *B.* The noncohesive neoplastic cells are large and possess round or irregular nuclei, distinct nucleoli, and amphophilic cytoplasm. *C.* The neoplastic cells commonly infiltrate the epithelial lining of the follicles, but they rarely aggregate within the central colloid material.

## PROGNOSTIC CONSIDERATIONS

The 5-year survival rate for thyroid lymphoma is 50% to 79%.* The most important prognostic factors are tumor stage and histologic type.

TUMOR STAGE. Stage $II_E$ or higher is associated with a much worse prognosis than is stage $I_E$ disease; almost all mortalities are confined to the stage $II_E$ and higher group.[591, 592, 599] Most studies have also shown extrathyroidal extension to worsen the prognosis, with a 5-year survival of 40% compared with 85% for intrathyroidal tumor.[590–593, 596, 599]

HISTOLOGIC TYPE. Although some studies have not found the histologic type to correlate with prognosis,[589, 591, 593, 594, 616] other studies have shown the prognosis of extranodal marginal zone B cell lymphoma of MALT type to be much superior to that of diffuse large B cell lymphoma.[590, 599, 612, 617] According to the series from the Armed Forces Institute of Pathology, none of 30 patients with pure extranodal marginal zone B cell lymphoma died of lymphoma, whereas 20 (26%) of 77 patients with a diffuse large B cell lymphoma component died of the disease.[599] There is no difference in outcome for diffuse large B cell lymphoma with or without an identifiable com-

ponent of extranodal marginal zone B cell lymphoma, similar to the findings in other mucosal sites such as the stomach, although conflicting results are reported by Skacel and coworkers.[599, 618]

AGE. Advanced age (older than 60 to 65 years) has been shown in some studies to be associated with a worse prognosis.[590, 591]

TUMOR SIZE. A large tumor (>10 cm) is reported to be associated with a worse prognosis according to some but not all studies.[590, 596, 599]

VASCULAR INVASION. Vascular invasion is associated with a worse prognosis.[592, 599]

HISTOLOGIC FEATURES. High mitotic count and high apoptotic count are associated with a worse prognosis.[599] Tumor necrosis is associated with a worse prognosis according to one study but not another.[592, 599]

## Plasmacytoma of the Thyroid

Plasmacytoma of the thyroid is uncommon, and the prognosis is excellent[592, 619] (Table 44–16). The neoplastic infiltrate comprises a monotonous population of mature-looking, immature-looking, pleomorphic, or plasmablastic plasma cells. It has been suggested that thyroid plasmacytoma may represent an ex-

---

*References 589–591, 593, 600, 610, 611, 614, 615.

**TABLE 44–16.** Comparison Between Plasmacytoma and Malignant Lymphoma of Thyroid

| | Plasmacytoma | Malignant Lymphoma |
|---|---|---|
| Sex | Slight male predominance (male-female 1.4 : 1) | Female predominance (male-female 1 : 2.5) |
| Age (mean) | 58 y | 62 y |
| Presentation | Usually slowly growing thyroid mass | Rapidly or slowly growing thyroid mass |
| 5-year survival | More favorable: 85% | Less favorable: overall ~60%, but much more favorable for extranodal marginal zone B cell lymphoma of MALT type |

treme (mature) form of extranodal marginal zone B cell lymphoma with prominent plasmacytic differentiation.[600, 620] The major differential diagnoses are inflammatory pseudotumor (plasma cell granuloma)[621, 622] and malignant lymphoma.

## Langerhans Cell Histiocytosis (Histiocytosis X)

### CLINICAL AND PROGNOSTIC CONSIDERATIONS

The thyroid gland can be involved by Langerhans cell histiocytosis as the sole lesion or as part of disseminated disease. The patients show a wide age range (median, 37 years), and there is no sex predilection.[623–628] The disease presents either as an incidental finding in the thyroid removed for other reasons or at autopsy or as a large thyroid. The prognosis is excellent for disease limited to the thyroid but poor for patients with disseminated disease.

### DIAGNOSTIC CONSIDERATIONS

The thyroid is infiltrated by Langerhans cells in a patchy or extensive pattern, and there can be extrathyroidal extension. The Langerhans cells possess grooved or highly contorted nuclei, thin nuclear membrane, delicate chromatin, and moderate amount of eosinophilic cytoplasm. They can infiltrate and destroy the thyroid follicular epithelium. There are variable numbers of admixed eosinophils, sometimes with formation of eosinophil abscesses. The diagnosis should be confirmed by positive immunostaining for S-100 protein and CD1a.

## Angiosarcoma

### CLINICAL AND PROGNOSTIC CONSIDERATIONS

#### Presentation

Angiosarcoma of the thyroid, also known as malignant hemangioendothelioma, is rare. It affects mostly old patients with a slight male predominance.[629] The patients usually present with rapid onset of a neck mass, which may cause difficulties in breathing and swallowing. They may have a history of long-standing goiter. Some patients may present with distant metastasis.

Angiosarcoma of the thyroid is extremely aggressive, and metastatic spread is common, such as to the lung, pleura, lymph node, adrenal, gastrointestinal tract, and bone.[629] The median survival is only 3.5 months, and the rare survivors all have small tumors lacking extrathyroidal extension.[630]

#### Macroscopic Findings

The tumor is usually solitary and infiltrative, with a fleshy gray-tan appearance punctuated by areas of necrosis and hemorrhage. There can be a central cavity filled with coagulated or fluid blood.[629]

### DIAGNOSTIC CONSIDERATIONS

#### Microscopic Findings

Angiosarcomas of the thyroid are often poorly differentiated. The tumors grow in solid sheets and irregular anastomosing channels that contain blood. The tumor cells often exhibit significant nuclear pleomorphism; some of them have cytoplasmic vacuolation. Some cases can show epithelioid morphologic features, with polygonal tumor cells and abundant eosinophilic hyaline cytoplasm[630–632] (Fig. 44–79).

#### Immunohistochemistry

A diagnosis of angiosarcoma has to be substantiated by positive immunohistochemical staining for

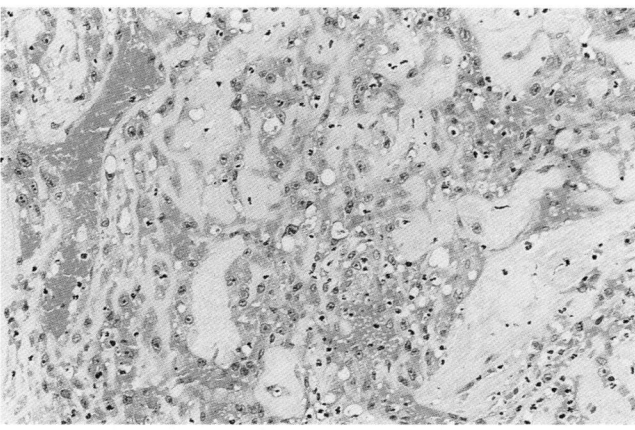

**FIGURE 44–79.** Epithelioid angiosarcoma. Cords and islands of polygonal cells with voluminous hyaline cytoplasm show cytoplasmic vacuoles and occasional irregular narrow vascular channels.

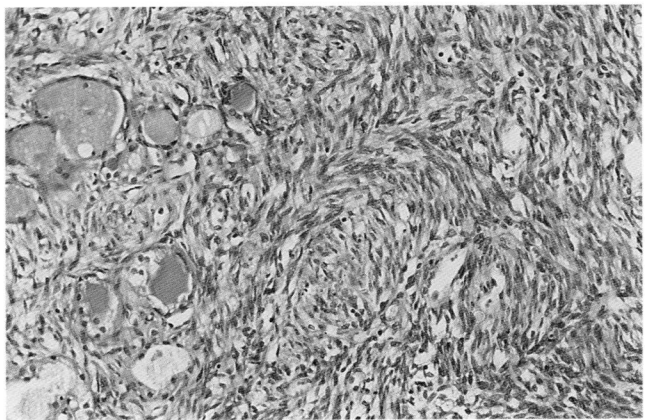

**FIGURE 44–80.** Solitary fibrous tumor. Nondescript spindly cells with scanty cytoplasm and in close interaction with delicate collagen fibrils characterize solitary fibrous tumor. Some entrapped follicles are seen in the peripheral portion of the tumor.

endothelial markers, such as factor VIII–related antigen, CD31, and CD34.[397, 398] Some cases can exhibit immunoreactivity for cytokeratin.[631]

### Differential Diagnosis

Because anaplastic carcinoma can exhibit angiosarcoma-like morphologic features focally (angiomatoid carcinoma), distinction between anaplastic carcinoma and pure angiosarcoma can be difficult.[633–635] The distinction is not too important from a clinical point of view, however, because both are highly aggressive neoplasms with similar survival figures.

Fine-needle aspiration changes such as reactive vascular proliferation or pseudoangiosarcomatous change in the damaged thyroid follicular epithelium can mimic angiosarcoma.

Sclerosing mucoepidermoid carcinoma with eosinophilia can exhibit a pseudoangiomatous pattern, focally mimicking angiosarcoma.

## Solitary Fibrous Tumor

Solitary fibrous tumor can rarely occur as a primary thyroid tumor.[636–639] All patients have remained well after surgical excision.

The histologic features are identical to those of the pleural counterpart. The tumor is well circumscribed, although some thyroid follicles can be entrapped in the periphery. It shows alternating hypercellular and hypocellular areas, with haphazardly distributed bland-looking spindly or stellate cells intimately intermingled with delicate to thick collagen fibers (Fig. 44–80). A pericytomatous vascular pattern is common. The tumor cells are immunoreactive for CD34 but are negative for cytokeratin and S-100 protein.

## Other Mesenchymal Tumors

Smooth muscle tumors of the thyroid gland are rare, and most are malignant.[640] Leiomyomas are encapsulated and confined to the thyroid gland, with no cellular atypia, necrosis, or mitotic activity. Leiomyosarcomas often affect older patients and are often larger. On histologic examination, they exhibit cellular pleomorphism, mitotic activity, necrosis, hemorrhage, invasive growth, and extrathyroidal extension. The diagnosis has to be confirmed by immunohistochemical or ultrastructural studies, especially for distinction from anaplastic carcinoma. These tumors are aggressive; most patients die within 2 years. Metastases to the lungs and other sites develop early in the course of disease.[640–645]

Rare mesenchymal tumors reported to occur in the thyroid include hemangioma, lymphangioma, peripheral nerve sheath tumors, fibrosarcoma, liposarcoma, chondrosarcoma, osteosarcoma, and follicular dendritic cell sarcoma.[624, 646–654]

## Paraganglioma

### CLINICAL CONSIDERATIONS

Rarely, paragangliomas can occur within the thyroid gland, probably from the inferior laryngeal paraganglia. There is a female predominance, and most patients are aged between 40 and 60 years.[262, 655] The patients present with a neck mass. The tumors are circumscribed or can extend into the adjacent larynx or trachea. All patients have remained well after surgical excision.

### DIAGNOSTIC CONSIDERATIONS

The tumors usually have a size of approximately 2 cm.[262, 656] Alveolar packets of ovoid cells with finely granular cytoplasm are surrounded by an inconspicuous layer of sustentacular cells (Fig. 44–81; see Table 44–1). The stroma is typically richly vascular-

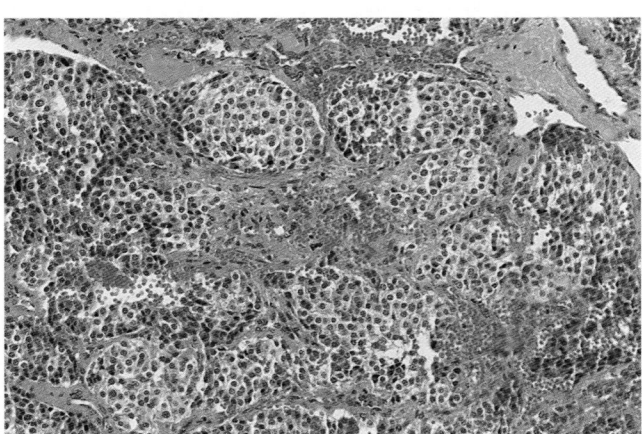

**FIGURE 44–81.** Paraganglioma. Oval islands of tumor are separated by a richly vascularized stroma. This tumor can potentially be mistaken for medullary carcinoma.

ized. Tumors with enlarged, hyperchromatic, or bizarre nuclei can potentially be misdiagnosed as a malignant neoplasm. Other major differential diagnoses are medullary carcinoma and hyalinizing trabecular adenoma.

## Teratoma

### CLINICAL AND PROGNOSTIC CONSIDERATIONS

There are two distinct age peaks for the occurrence of thyroid teratomas. The first and higher peak is in the newborn period to the age of 2 years; the second smaller peak is in older children and adults, mostly between the ages of 20 and 50 years.[600, 657–662] These tumors are more common in females than in males. Most patients present with a large thyroid or neck mass, which may be accompanied by respiratory difficulties.

Thyroid teratomas occurring before the age of 2 years usually pursue a benign course after surgical excision, although some patients may die of respiratory obstruction. Thyroid teratomas occurring in adults are more likely to be malignant, with local recurrence, cervical lymph node metastasis, and pulmonary metastasis. Nonetheless, long-term survival is possible with aggressive treatment including chemotherapy and surgery.[600, 663, 664]

### DIAGNOSTIC CONSIDERATIONS

The teratomas are most often immature, although some may be of the mature type. Tissues from the various germ layers are present, and neuroectodermal tissue may be prominent. The presence of neural tissue provides a strong point against the differential diagnosis of anaplastic carcinoma.

Tumors occurring in neonates and infants are often immature (grade 1 or 2), but they are sometimes mature. Those occurring in adults most often show grade 3 immaturity ("malignant").[600]

## Metastatic Malignant Neoplasms in Thyroid

Because the thyroid gland is rich in blood vessels and lymphatics, it is not infrequently involved by metastatic cancer in patients with carcinomatosis, most commonly due to pulmonary carcinoma (usually adenocarcinoma), breast carcinoma, malignant melanoma, and renal cell carcinoma.[665–669] The metastatic deposits are often small and asymptomatic and are associated with obvious widespread metastatic tumor elsewhere.[665]

Renal cell carcinoma can metastasize to the thyroid gland as the initial manifestation of the tumor or as the first evidence of relapse many years after resection of the renal primary.[31, 665] It can potentially be misdiagnosed as primary clear cell tumor of the

---

**TABLE 44–17. Contents of the Final Report: Thyroid Excision Specimens**

Specimen type/operation procedure

Diagnosis
  Histologic type, and variant if applicable
  Histologic grade, if relevant

Other tumor features
  Tumor location (right lobe, left lobe, isthmus)
  Tumor size
  Solitary or multicentric
  Encapsulated or nonencapsulated
  Capsular invasion (absent, present, extensive)
  Vascular invasion (absent, present, extensive)
  Extrathyroidal extension (structures invaded, if applicable)
  Mitotic activity

Surgical margins: free, close to surgical margin (specify distance), or margin involved (specify site)

Non-neoplastic thyroid: normal, nodular goiter, lymphocytic thyroiditis, Hashimoto's thyroiditis, atrophy, fibrosis

Lymph nodes
  Number of lymph nodes found, and their location (level)
  Number of involved lymph nodes
  Size of largest metastatic deposit
  Presence or absence of extracapsular extension

---

thyroid, but it can be recognized by the presence of multiple tumor nodules, distinct cell membranes, water-clear cytoplasm, sinusoidal vascular pattern, fresh hemorrhage in the glandular lumina, and negative immunostaining for thyroglobulin.[31]

## Contents of the Final Surgical Pathology Report

In the surgical pathology report of thyroid excision specimens for tumors, it is important to include all information relevant for staging and prognostication in addition to the diagnosis[15, 45, 46] (Table 44–17).

## NON-NEOPLASTIC LESIONS

### Incidental and Insignificant Findings in the Thyroid Gland

Skeletal muscle fibers may be intermingled with the thyroid follicles in the region beneath the thyroid capsule. Adipose cells and hyaline cartilage rest are occasionally found incidentally in the thyroid gland.[670] Ectopic parathyroid tissue, ectopic thymic tissue, and ectopic salivary gland tissue can also sometimes be found within the thyroid.

Rarely, there can be columnar ciliated epithelium replacing part of the follicular epithelium.[670] The thyroid follicular epithelium can also undergo squamous metaplasia or oncocytic metaplasia.[671]

Crystals are commonly found in the colloid of the thyroid follicles. They are most commonly seen in nodular goiters, but they can be seen in various non-neoplastic and neoplastic lesions of the thyroid. The crystals vary in geometric shapes and are most often composed of calcium oxalate.[672–674]

Solid cell nests, common incidental findings in the thyroid, are often detected at low-magnification scanning as a blue-staining cellular focus.[671, 675–679] They appear as a small collection of solid epithelial islands resembling transitional epithelium (Fig. 44–82). Some islands can show cystic change and contain mucinous substance. The epithelial cells possess oval grooved nuclei. The solid cell nests are believed to be remnants of ultimobranchial bodies, and many scattered C cells are associated with these nests.[508, 677]

Palpation granuloma (palpation thyroiditis) is a common incidental finding of no consequence and is believed to result from the mechanical trauma of palpation.[680] One or two thyroid follicles appear to have ruptured and are replaced by histiocytes and multinucleated histiocytes. They are not associated with fibrous scarring.

## Cysts

The most common cyst of the thyroid gland is degenerate cyst resulting from cystic degeneration of nodular goiter. Cystic degeneration can also occur in various thyroid tumors, such as follicular adenoma. The cystic variant of papillary carcinoma is characterized by the presence of a prominent cystic component lined by neoplastic cells.

Thyroglossal duct cyst represents cystic dilatation of the persistent thyroglossal duct. The patient usually presents in the first 3 decades of life with a swelling in the midline of the neck that typically moves upward with swallowing. The cyst is usually situated below the hyoid bone but above the thyroid isthmus. When it is complicated by infection, there can be tenderness and pain. Histologic examination shows the cyst to be lined by respiratory or stratified squamous epithelium. The wall consists of fibrous tissue, which may be infiltrated by chronic inflammatory cells. Mucous glands can be present in the wall. Some thyroid follicles are often but not invariably identified in the vicinity. Rarely, carcinomas can develop in a thyroglossal duct cyst. Papillary carcinoma is the most common histologic type, but squamous cell carcinoma can also rarely occur in this setting.[681–683]

Multiple branchial cleft–like cysts are rarely found in association with Hashimoto's thyroiditis. The cysts are lined by squamous or respiratory epithelium and are surrounded by a band of dense lymphoid infiltrate.[684] Postulated pathogenetic mechanisms include metaplastic and cystic change of the thyroid follicles in the setting of thyroiditis and origin from developmental rests.[684, 685]

## Thyroid Tissue in the Lateral Neck

### LATERAL ABERRANT THYROID

Thyroid tissue occurring in the lateral neck separate from the thyroid gland has often been referred to as lateral aberrant thyroid. This can occur in several circumstances[46]: 1) sequestered nodule in nodular goiter; the nodule may still be connected by a narrow strand of tissue to the main gland; 2) regrowth of thyroid tissue that has been implanted in the soft tissues of the neck from prior surgery; and 3) sequestered thyroid tissue involved by Hashimoto's thyroiditis or Graves' disease. It is most important, however, to rule out the possibility of metastatic thyroid carcinoma (most commonly papillary carcinoma) in cervical lymph nodes.

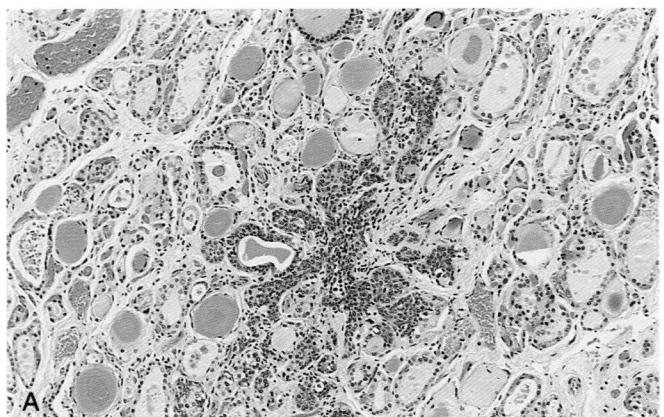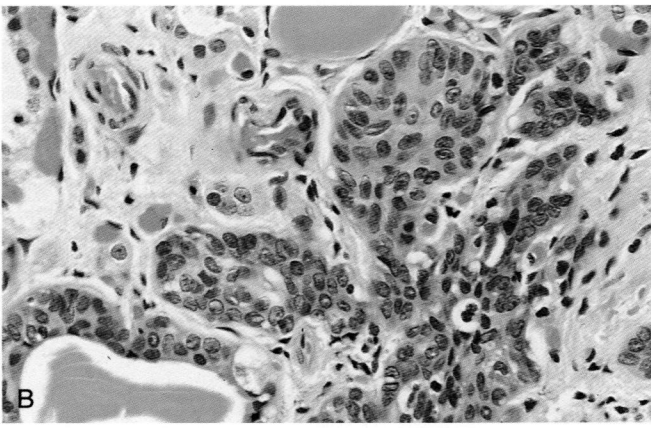

**FIGURE 44–82.** Solid cell nest of the thyroid. *A.* Small, blue-staining islands of epithelium are disposed in a stellate configuration among the thyroid follicles. Occasional epithelial islands show cyst formation with secretion. *B.* The epithelial cells resemble transitional epithelium, and nuclear grooves are common.

## THYROID INCLUSIONS IN CERVICAL LYMPH NODE

Benign thyroid follicles can rarely occur in cervical lymph nodes. Nonetheless, this belief is not universally accepted; some investigators consider all thyroid tissues within lymph nodes to represent metastasis from clinically undetected thyroid carcinoma.[686] Because the distinction between benign thyroid inclusions and metastasis from an occult thyroid carcinoma can be extremely difficult owing to the almost normal histologic appearances of some thyroid carcinomas, strict criteria must be used in the diagnosis of benign thyroid inclusions[46, 687, 688]:

- They consist of only a small conglomerate of thyroid follicles.
- They are limited to the periphery of one or two lymph nodes.
- Nuclear features of papillary carcinoma are lacking, that is, nuclei are not enlarged, with fine chromatin and inconspicuous nucleoli.
- Psammoma bodies are absent.
- There is lack of a desmoplastic reaction.

## METASTATIC THYROID CARCINOMA IN CERVICAL LYMPH NODE

Papillary carcinoma commonly metastasizes to lymph nodes, whereas follicular carcinoma rarely does. Cervical lymph node metastasis is sometimes the first clinical manifestation of an occult papillary thyroid carcinoma—the thyroid primary is almost always located on the ipsilateral side. The node can be cystic or show sudden enlargement because of hemorrhage. On histologic examination, a diagnosis of metastatic papillary thyroid carcinoma can be obvious because of presence of recognizable lymph node tissue and papillary carcinoma. However, in some cases, the cyst wall is formed by dense fibrous tissue with scanty lymphoid tissue underneath and lined by attenuated nondescript cells, and thus it may be mistaken for a branchial cyst (Fig. 44–83). Careful search may be required to uncover small papillae projecting into the lumen or some elongated follicles in the wall, with the cells exhibiting the typical nuclear features of papillary carcinoma (Fig. 44–83B, C). A diagnosis can be readily confirmed by positive immunostaining for thyroglobulin.

## MIMICKER OF METASTATIC THYROID CARCINOMA IN CERVICAL LYMPH NODE

A sequestered thyroid nodule involved by florid Hashimoto's thyroiditis can potentially be mistaken for metastatic thyroid carcinoma in lymph node because the lymphoplasmacytic infiltrate with germinal center formation imparts a lymph node–like appearance and the thyroid follicles can exhibit nuclear atypia or pallor. However, subcapsular sinuses, a hallmark of lymph node, are lacking.

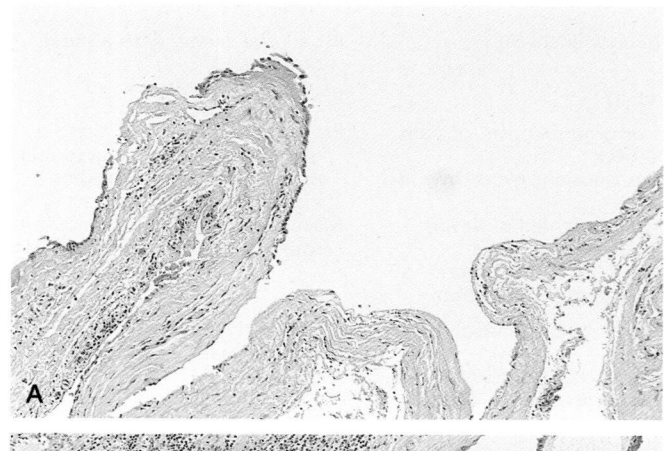
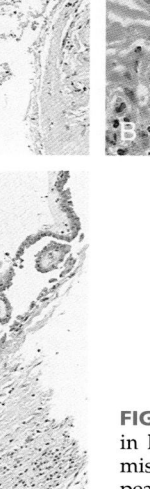
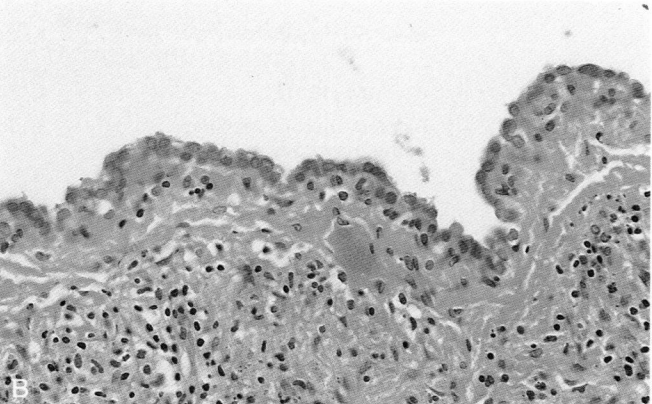

**FIGURE 44–83.** Cystic metastasis of papillary thyroid carcinoma in lymph node. *A.* This cyst excised from the lateral neck can be mistaken for a developmental cyst because of its innocuous appearance. The wall is formed by fibrous tissue with only focal lining by attenuated epithelium. *B.* In areas, more plump and slightly pseudostratified epithelial cells are seen lining the cyst. *C.* On careful search, a small focus with papillary structures is found, clinching the diagnosis of metastatic papillary carcinoma.

# Thyroiditis

## ACUTE THYROIDITIS

Acute thyroiditis is rare. It is caused by bacterial infection, such as *Staphylococcus, Streptococcus pyogenes,* and *Haemophilus influenzae.* The patients are often immunosuppressed, or there is a regional infective focus, such as piriform sinus fistula. They present with painful swelling of the thyroid and fever. Histologic examination shows polymorph infiltration associated with destruction of the thyroid follicles.

## INFECTIOUS GRANULOMATOUS THYROIDITIS

Granulomatous inflammation can be produced in the thyroid by some infective processes, such as tu-

berculosis, actinomycosis, and fungal infection. The patients are often immunocompromised. Granulomas with or without caseation are found in the thyroid, although they can be poorly formed in immunocompromised hosts. The main differential diagnoses are sarcoidosis and de Quervain's thyroiditis.

## DE QUERVAIN'S THYROIDITIS (SUBACUTE GRANULOMATOUS THYROIDITIS)

de Quervain's thyroiditis is thought to be caused by viral infection, although no specific virus has been incriminated. The main features are summarized in Table 44–18.[689, 690] In contrast to the randomly distributed granulomas in infectious granulomatous thyroiditis, the granulomas in de Quervain's thyroiditis are centered around residual colloid (Fig. 44–84).

**TABLE 44–18.** Major Types of Thyroiditis

| | Hashimotos' Thyroiditis | de Quervain's Thyroiditis | Riedel's Thyroiditis |
|---|---|---|---|
| Nature of disease process | Autoimmune thyroiditis, with autoantibodies against thyroglobulin, thyroid peroxidase, thyrotropin receptor, and iodine transporter, as well as cell-mediated immunity against thyroid tissue components | A subacute thyroiditis<br>Possibly related to viral infection or postviral inflammatory process | An inflammatory fibrosclerosing lesion<br>A small proportion of patients subsequently develop inflammatory fibrosclerosis of other sites, e.g., retroperitoneal fibrosis, mediastinal fibrosis, orbital pseudotumor, sclerosing cholangitis |
| Age | Most commonly 45–65 y | Most commonly 30–50 y | Broad age range, with a mean of 48 y |
| Sex | F >> M (15:1) | F > M (4:1) | F > M (5:1) |
| Presentation | Painless thyroid swelling<br>Some may have evidence of hypothyroidism, whereas some may have transient hyperthyroidism | Sudden or gradual onset of pain in the neck<br>May have transient hyperthyroidism<br>Can be accompanied by fever and systemic symptoms<br>May have a history of preceding upper respiratory infection | Recent enlargement of thyroid gland, which may be accompanied by pressure symptoms, e.g, dyspnea, dysphagia<br>Most patients are euthyroid, but some can be hypothyroid |
| Pattern of involvement of the thyroid gland | Diffuse, with involvement of both lobes<br>No extrathyroidal extension | Unilateral or bilateral involvement<br>Usually a patchy process (1 cm to several centimeters in diameter), but there is no extrathyroidal extension | Focal involvement of thyroid, associated with extrathyroidal extension |
| Antithyroid antibodies in serum | Always | Usually negative | Approximatelly two thirds of patients |
| Major histologic features | Lymphoplasmacytic infiltration<br>Follicular infiltration and destruction by lymphocytes<br>Widespread oncocytic change in thyroid epithelium | Disrupted follicles<br>Histiocytes and multinucleated giant cells around pools of residual colloid<br>Lymphocytic infiltration<br>Patchy fibrosis | Invasive process, and may entrap skeletal muscle fibers<br>Focal replacement of thyroid parenchyma by hypocellular fibrous tissue<br>Patchy chronic inflammation with or without lymphoid follicle formation<br>Phlebitis |
| Clinical outcome | Gradual loss of thyroid function, i.e., hypothyroidism | May have transient hyperthyroidism<br>Disease usually resolves in a few months | Disease appears to be self-limited<br>Prognosis after subtotal removal of the fibrotic mass is excellent |

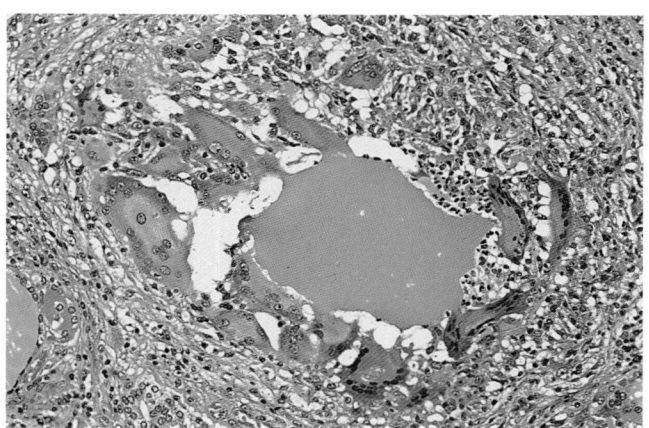

**FIGURE 44–84.** de Quervain's thyroiditis. The thyroid shows infiltration by chronic inflammatory cells and mild fibrosis. The most characteristic feature is the presence of foreign body–type giant cells engulfing colloid material, indicating that there has been destruction of follicles.

## HASHIMOTO'S THYROIDITIS

### Clinical Considerations

Hashimoto's thyroiditis, also known as struma lymphomatosa, is the prototype of autoimmune thyroiditis. The salient clinical features are summarized in Table 44–18.[689–691] There is an increased risk for development of malignant lymphoma and papillary carcinoma.

The thyroid is usually symmetrically enlarged, with a firm or rubbery consistency. The cut surface is tan or tan-brown, with a homogeneous or vaguely lobulated appearance.

### Diagnostic Considerations

On histologic examination, there is heavy infiltration of the interstitium and some thyroid follicles by lymphocytes and plasma cells. Reactive lymphoid follicles are often present. There is loss of thyroid follicles, and the remaining ones are often small. The thyroid follicular epithelium shows extensive oncocytic (Hürthle cell) change and can have enlarged or pale nuclei (Fig. 44–85). Those examples with heavy lymphoplasmacytic infiltration can be difficult to distinguish from extranodal marginal zone B cell lymphoma or plasmacytoma arising in Hashimoto's thyroiditis; see the relevant sections for distinguishing features.

Nodular Hashimoto's thyroiditis refers to the presence of superimposed nodules comprising closely packed small follicles or trabeculae, most of which are lined by Hürthle cells (Fig. 44–86). The multiplicity of nodules and the frequent presence of isolated pleomorphic nuclei can potentially lead to an erroneous diagnosis of Hürthle cell carcinoma. Vascular invasion is absent, however.

The fibrosing variant accounts for 12.5% of all cases of Hashimoto's thyroiditis. It is defined by the presence of broad bands of dense hyaline fibrous tissue occupying more than one third of the thyroid gland, separating islands of thyroid parenchyma exhibiting typical histologic features of Hashimoto's thyroiditis (oxyphilic change, follicular cell damage, and lymphoid infiltration)[692] (Fig. 44–87). Squamous metaplasia in the thyroid follicles is common. Clinically, the thyroid gland feels firm or hard, and pressure symptoms can be present. The antithyroid antibody titers are often high. Clinical evidence of hypothyroidism is present in approximately 50% of cases.

## LYMPHOCYTIC THYROIDITIS AND PAINLESS THYROIDITIS

The term *lymphocytic thyroiditis* is often applied when there is diffuse or multifocal lymphoplasmacytic infiltration in the absence of oncocytic change in the thyroid follicular epithelium. There is no significant atrophy of the thyroid follicles. However, during the active phase, there can be follicular destruction and hyperplastic change in the follicles.

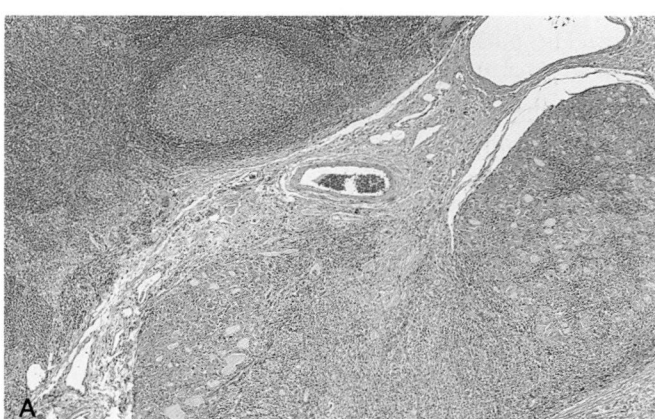

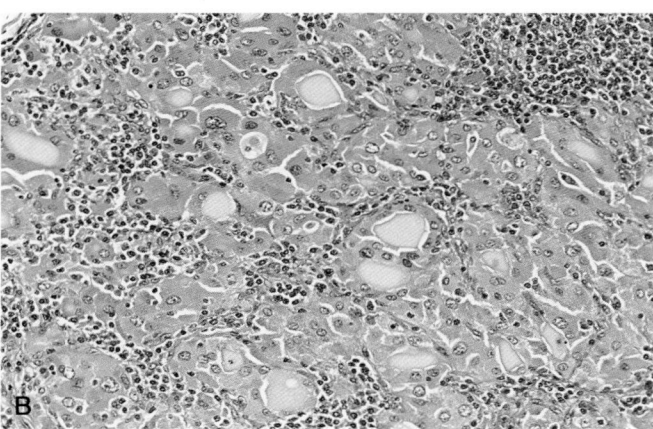

**FIGURE 44–85.** Hashimoto's thyroiditis. *A.* There is frequently an accentuated lobulated architecture. Lymphoid infiltration with lymphoid follicle formation is evident. The pink appearance in areas not infiltrated by lymphoid cells results from oncocytic change in the follicular epithelium. *B.* The follicles are typically small and lined by oncocytic (Hürthle) cells. There are many intermingled lymphocytes and plasma cells.

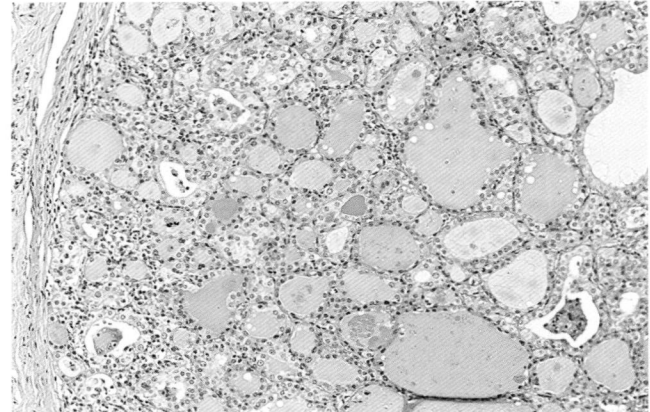

**FIGURE 44–86.** Nodular Hashimoto's thyroiditis. In the background Hashimoto's thyroiditis, variably sized nodules composed of follicles lined by Hürthle cells are present. These nodules contain few lymphoplasmacytic cells.

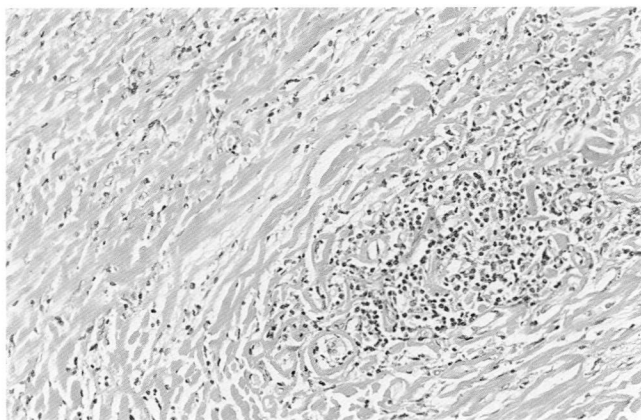

**FIGURE 44–88.** Riedel's thyroiditis. The fibroproliferative process replaces the thyroid parenchyma and extends into the surrounding tissue. In addition to a sprinkling of chronic inflammatory cells, small aggregates of lymphocytes are present.

The disease is believed to have an autoimmune basis.

The clinical counterpart is variously known as painless thyroiditis, silent thyroiditis, juvenile thyroiditis, or postpartum thyroiditis, depending on the clinical scenario.[693–698] In most patients, there is transient hyperthyroidism followed by hypothyroidism and spontaneous evolution. Some patients present with thyroid swelling. The entire clinical course usually lasts less than 1 year. Only rarely do the patients eventually become hypothyroid.

### RIEDEL'S THYROIDITIS

The main features of Riedel's thyroiditis are summarized in Table 44–18 (Fig. 44–88).[689, 699–701] The clinical impression is usually that of thyroid cancer because of the presence of a stony hard thyroid mass. Riedel's thyroiditis is rare; for unknown reasons, its incidence has decreased dramatically during the

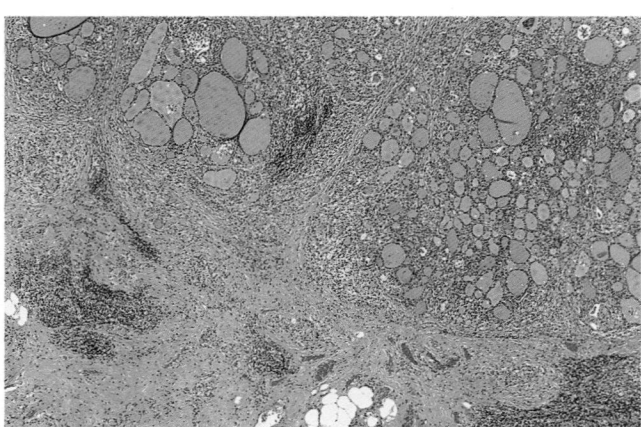

**FIGURE 44–87.** Fibrosing Hashimoto's thyroiditis. Broad fibrous bands traverse the thyroid gland involved by Hashimoto's thyroiditis. In contrast to Riedel's thyroiditis, the process does not extend beyond the thyroid capsule.

past few decades.[701] Although steroid treatment may sometimes be effective, surgical excision is usually required to relieve the pressure symptoms and to exclude malignancy.

The most important differential diagnosis is paucicellular variant of anaplastic carcinoma because of marked differences in outcome (see "Anaplastic Carcinoma").[381] Riedel's thyroiditis can also be distinguished from fibrosing Hashimoto's thyroiditis by the features of extrathyroidal extension of the fibroproliferative process, presence of phlebitis, and relatively normal surviving thyroid tissue.[700]

### FOCAL LYMPHOCYTIC THYROIDITIS (NONSPECIFIC LYMPHOCYTIC THYROIDITIS)

Focal lymphoid infiltration in the thyroid gland is a fairly common incidental finding in thyroidectomy specimens and at autopsy.[702–705] This is also a common finding in the vicinity of various thyroid tumors, especially papillary carcinoma. The lymphoid cells tend to be localized to the interlobular areas, with little evidence of destruction of thyroid follicles. The pathogenesis is unknown, but the lesion is probably of no consequence.

### MULTIFOCAL FIBROSING THYROIDITIS

Multifocal fibrosing thyroiditis is a peculiar form of thyroiditis characterized by many microscopic foci of stellate cellular fibrosis with some entrapped thyroid follicles, mimicking the low-magnification architecture of papillary microcarcinoma.[45] The pathogenesis is not known.

## Graves' Disease

### CLINICAL CONSIDERATIONS

Graves' disease is the most common cause of hyperthyroidism. It is an organ-specific autoimmune disease produced by thyroid-stimulating antibodies—

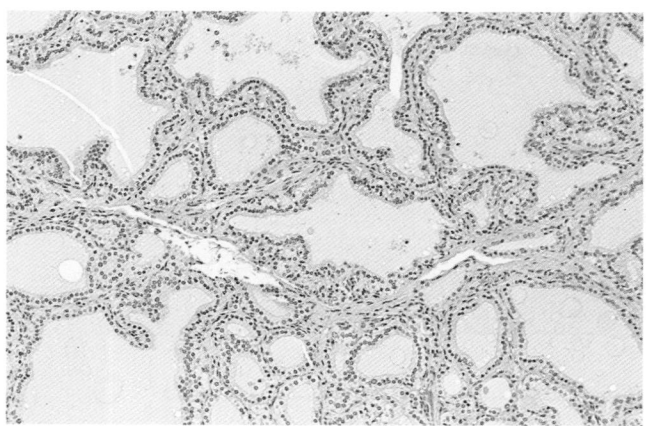

**FIGURE 44–89.** Graves' disease. The follicles are mostly medium sized and lined by columnar cells that form papillary infoldings.

thyrotropin receptor antibody, which stimulates hormone production, and thyroid growth–stimulating immunoglobulin, which promotes parenchymal hyperplasia.

Graves' disease mostly affects adults in their 20s and 30s with a marked female predominance. The patients present with hyperthyroidism, diffuse swelling of the thyroid gland, and exophthalmos.

## DIAGNOSTIC CONSIDERATIONS

Thyroid gland involved by Graves' disease is typically diffusely and symmetrically enlarged, with a meaty quality on the cut surface. An accentuated lobular architecture is evident histologically. The follicles are mostly medium sized. The lining columnar cells form papillary projections into the luminal spaces, with some lumina appearing star shaped (Fig. 44–89). The nuclei often show some variation in size, and some can appear pale. Colloid is scanty, pale, and scalloped. There is a patchy light lymphoid infiltrate in the interstitium.

The typical histologic features are now rarely seen in surgical pathology practice because the patients have been treated with drugs to control the hyperthyroidism before the operation. With such treatment, the follicles show greater variation in size, and some follicles may appear involuted. The follicular epithelium becomes less tall, and colloid can often be seen. Nonetheless, the hyperplastic appearance with papillary infoldings is often still evident in focal areas.

## Nodular Goiter

### CLINICAL CONSIDERATIONS

#### Presentation

Nodular goiter is the most common thyroid lesion encountered in surgical pathology practice. It is characterized by nodule formation in the thyroid, with hyperplastic as well as involuted areas.

The endemic form (endemic goiter) is due to iodine deficiency in the diet or water and hence a low production of thyroid hormones, leading to compensatory increase in thyroid-stimulating hormone, which stimulates the thyroid follicles to undergo hyperplasia (parenchymatous goiter). Subsequently, some follicles undergo involution with massive accumulation of colloid (diffuse colloid goiter), and nodule formation supervenes. The sporadic form of nodular goiter is of unknown pathogenesis.

The patients usually present with an enlarged multinodular thyroid gland, which may be accompanied by compression symptoms. Extension into the mediastinum can occur, producing additional symptoms related to the mediastinal location. There can be pain and sudden enlargement of the thyroid gland due to hemorrhage. Some patients present with a solitary thyroid mass, but additional nodules are often evident on ultrasound examination. Most patients are euthyroid, but rare patients may have hyperthyroidism (toxic nodular goiter).

#### Macroscopic Findings

The thyroid gland is enlarged, sometimes to an enormous size. The external contour is often distorted. There are multiple nodules, which often lack fibrous capsules (Fig. 44–90A). The nodules exhibit variable appearances ranging from colloid-rich with brown color and glistening quality to solid, tan, and fleshy. Secondary changes such as fibrosis, hemorrhage, cystic degeneration, and calcification are common. In some cases, there is an apparently solitary nodule surrounded by a thin capsule, making distinction from follicular neoplasm difficult (Fig. 44–90B). Careful examination of the background thyroid often reveals multiple vague nodules with a colloid-rich quality.

### DIAGNOSTIC CONSIDERATIONS

#### Microscopic Findings

In most cases, multiple, variably sized nodules are evident. The different nodules often exhibit different degrees of cellularity and variations in follicle size (Fig. 44–91).

The typical nodule comprises large follicles lined by regular low cuboidal epithelium and distended with colloid (colloid nodule) (Fig. 44–92). There are frequently some broad papillae projecting into the large follicles, so-called Sanderson polsters (Fig. 44–93). In contrast to papillary carcinoma, the papillae have broad edematous cores and are lined by columnar cells with dark round nuclei regularly aligned at the base of the cells. Smaller "daughter" follicles are present in the cores of these papillae. Hemosiderin-laden macrophages are commonly found within the follicular lumina or in the interstitium, providing evidence of prior hemorrhage. Patchy fibrosis and calcification are common (Fig. 44–94A). Some areas may undergo infarction, with only "ghost" follicles being identifiable. There can be

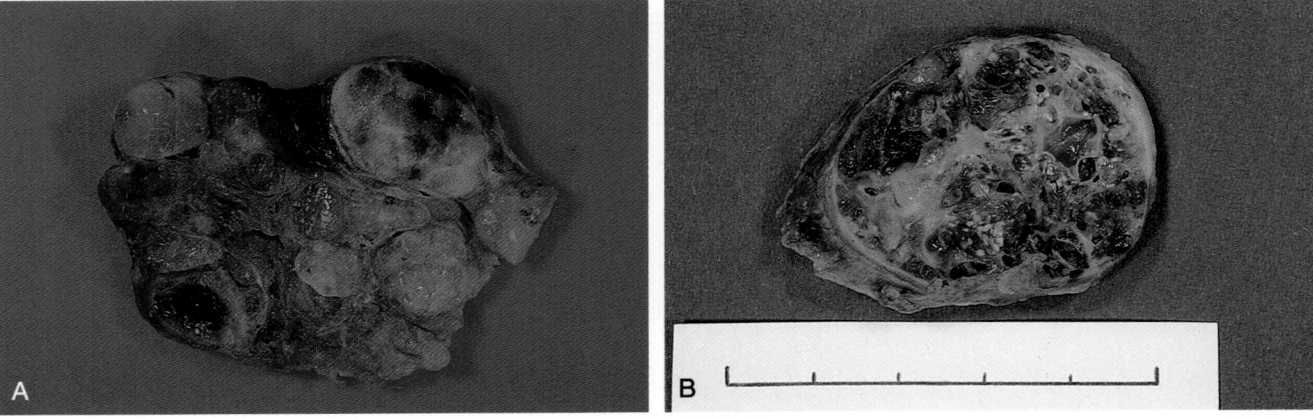

**FIGURE 44–90.** Nodular goiter. *A.* In this case, multiple nodules with a glistening colloid (gelatinous) quality are evident. *B.* In this case, the nodule is apparently solitary and enveloped by a thin capsule. It has a variegated appearance with colloidlike areas, small cysts, hemorrhagic areas, fibrosis, and calcification.

interspersed cysts comprising a fibrous wall with or without lining by attenuated epithelium (Fig. 44–94*B*). The lining epithelium and entrapped follicles in the fibrous wall may show reactive atypia or squamous metaplasia. In some cysts, collections of residual large follicles project into the cyst lumen.

Some nodules can be highly cellular, being composed of small follicles and trabeculae (Fig. 44–95; see also Fig. 44–92*C*). The nuclei of the thyroid epithelial cells appear uniform or atypical. Oncocytic, clear cell, and signet ring change can occur. There can also be areas resembling hyalinizing trabecular adenoma.[57] These cellular nodules (adenomatoid nodules) can be difficult to distinguish from follicular neoplasm or even insular carcinoma. When the follicles exhibit large pale nuclei, the additional differential diagnosis of papillary carcinoma may be raised; these follicles show gradual transition with the normal or benign follicles, and they lack the sharp demarcation from the non-neoplastic follicles as seen in papillary carcinoma.

### Differential Diagnosis

**FOLLICULAR ADENOMA.** The distinction between nodular goiter presenting as a solitary nodule and follicular adenoma can be difficult and sometimes arbitrary. The distinction is not critical, however, as long as there is no capsular or vascular invasion. In general, an adenoma is solitary, is completely enveloped by a fibrous capsule, is expansile and produces a compression effect on the surrounding tissues, and shows cytoarchitectural features dissimilar from the surrounding parenchyma.

**FOLLICULAR CARCINOMA.** See earlier.

**PAPILLARY CARCINOMA.** See earlier

**INSULAR CARCINOMA.** See earlier.

**DYSHORMONOGENESIS.** For young patients not living in areas of endemic goiter and presenting with large multinodular goiter, the possibility of dyshormonogenesis should be entertained.

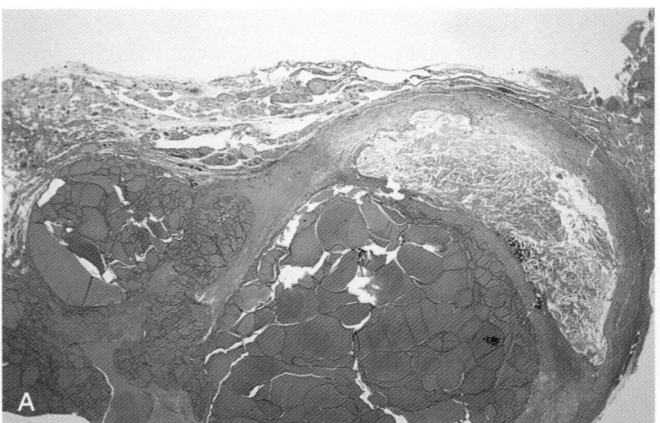
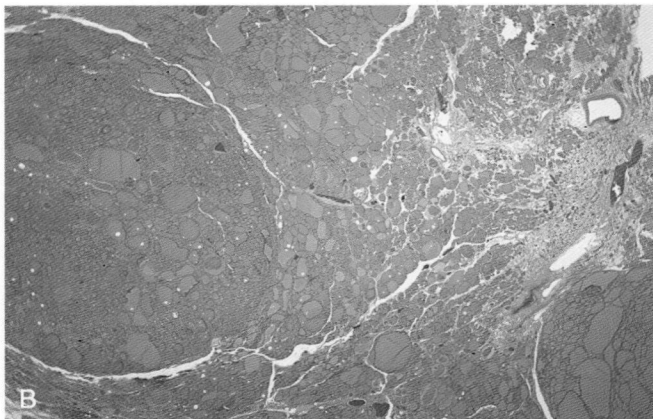

**FIGURE 44–91.** Nodular goiter. Multiple nodules with variable cellularities and follicle sizes are seen. *A.* In this case, most follicles are large. *B.* In this case, there are large as well as small follicles.

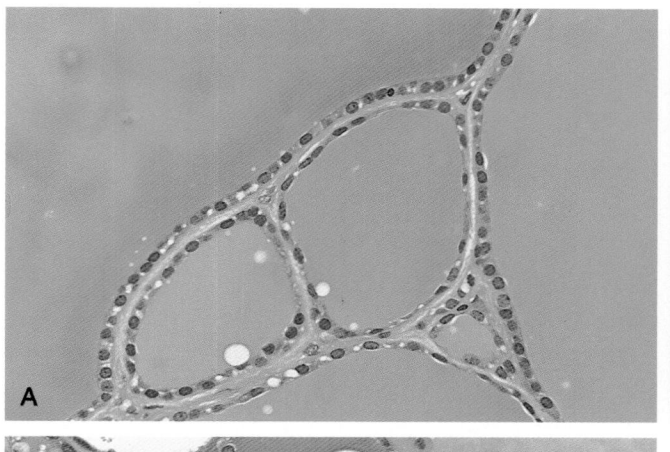
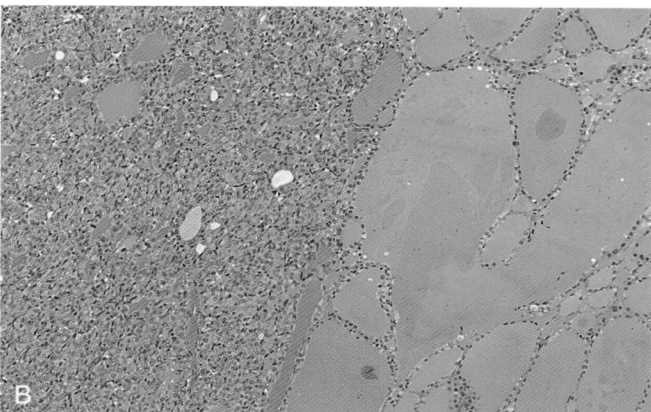
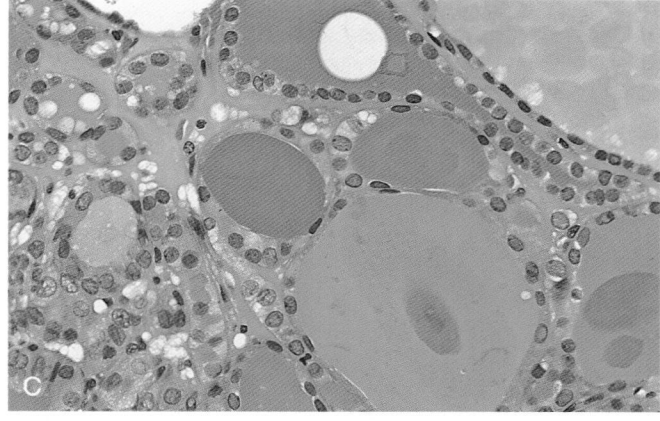

**FIGURE 44–92.** Nodular goiter. *A.* The large follicles are distended with colloid and are lined by uniform cells with small dark nuclei. *B.* Small and closely packed follicles (*left field*) can be found in some nodules. *C.* Although the cells lining the smaller follicles may have pale nuclei (*left field*), raising the possibility of papillary carcinoma, they show gradual transition with the benign follicles in the right field instead of forming a distinct neoplastic population.

## Dyshormonogenetic Goiter

### CLINICAL CONSIDERATIONS

Dyshormonogenesis is a form of familial goiter caused by genetic enzyme defects in thyroid hormone synthesis.[297] The patients usually present with congenital hypothyroidism or early-onset goiter. However, some patients may not present until middle age.[706] The enlarged multinodular thyroid can weigh up to 600 g. There can be a slightly increased risk for thyroid carcinoma.[706]

### DIAGNOSTIC CONSIDERATIONS

#### Microscopic Findings

The most salient feature of dyshormonogenetic goiter is the presence of highly cellular nodules ex-

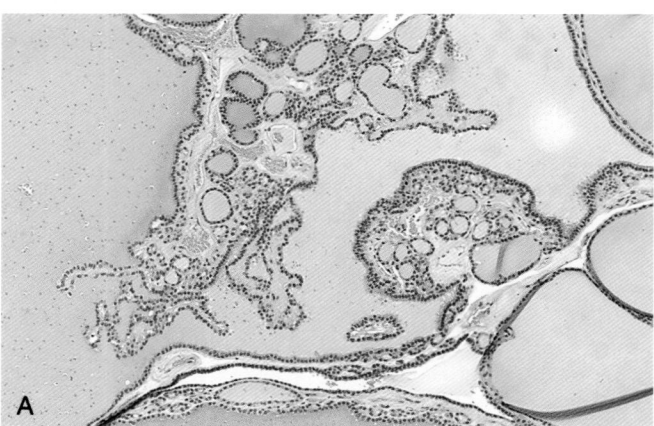
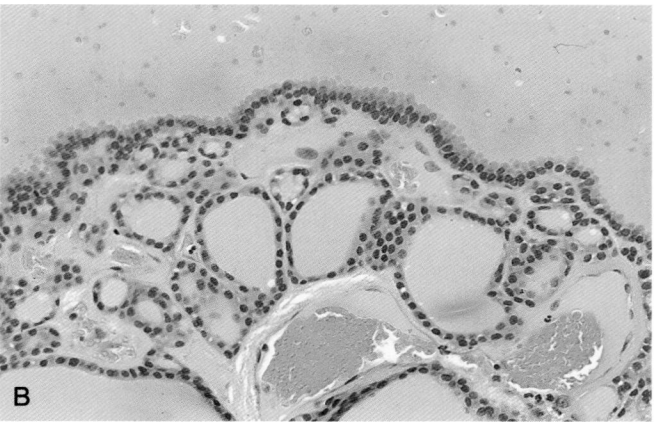

**FIGURE 44–93.** Nodular goiter. *A.* Sanderson polsters and papillary structures project into a large colloid-filled follicle. *B.* Sanderson polster is a broad protuberance with daughter follicles in the core. The lining cells have uniform and regularly aligned nuclei.

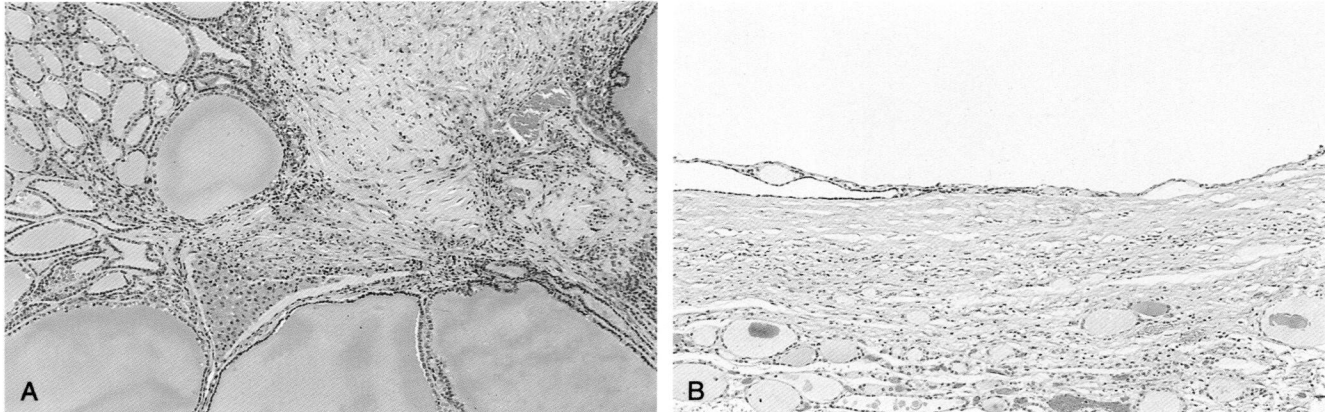

**FIGURE 44–94.** Nodular goiter. *A.* Nodular goiter showing patchy fibrosis, with infiltration of histiocytes and chronic inflammatory cells. *B.* Cystic degeneration in nodular goiter. The cyst has a fibrous wall lined by attenuated epithelium.

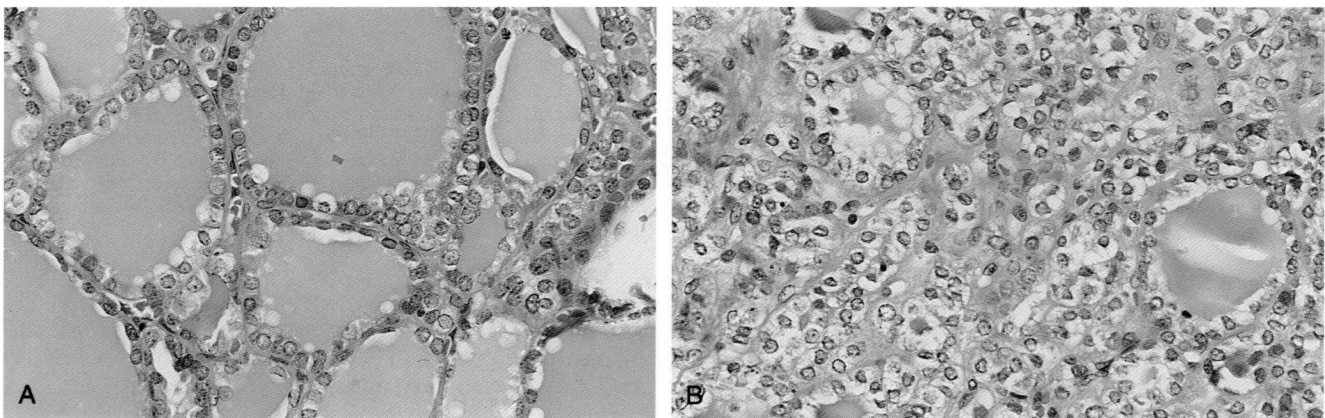

**FIGURE 44–95.** Nodular goiter with cellular nodules (adenomatoid nodules). *A.* The follicles are small, and distinction from follicular neoplasm can be difficult. *B.* A solid appearance can also be produced.

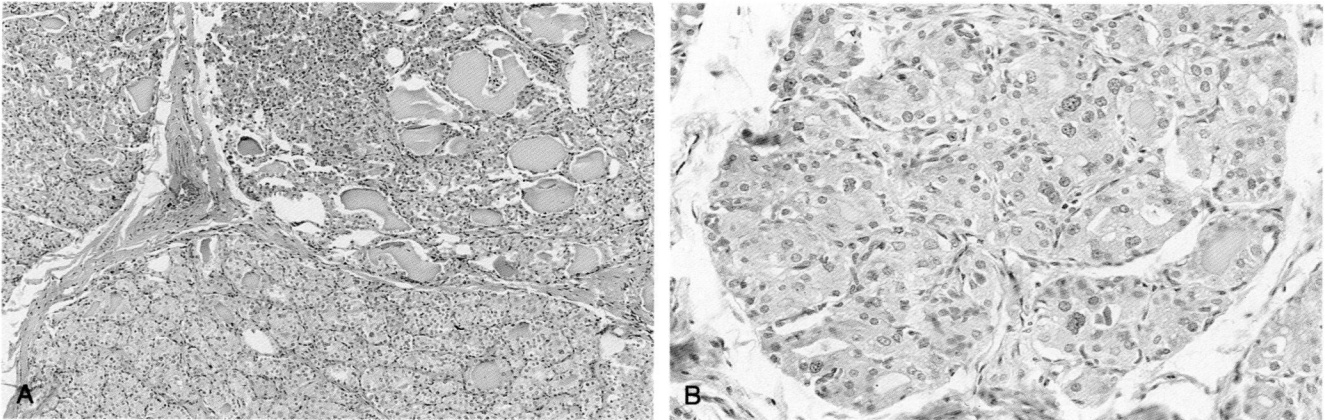

**FIGURE 44–96.** Dyshormonogenesis. *A.* A multinodular pattern is evident. *B.* The follicles are often small with no or scanty colloid. There are interspersed cells with large hyperchromatic nuclei.

hibiting a variety of architectural features (Fig. 44–96*A*). The nodules can show a microfollicular, trabecular, solid, papillary, insular, or mixed growth pattern. Follicles, when present, are small and frequently devoid of colloid. There are commonly interspersed cells with large hyperchromatic nuclei or vesicular nuclei. Cells with hyperchromatic pleomorphic nuclei are most commonly found in the internodular tissue in association with streaming of follicles (Fig. 44–96*B*). There is often prominent fibrosis between the nodules. Because of the presence of multiple highly cellular nodules, cellular atypia, and pseudoinfiltrative pattern created by the fibrosis, dyshormonogenetic goiter can be mistaken for follicular carcinoma.[706]

### Differential Diagnosis

FOLLICULAR CARCINOMA. In contrast to follicular carcinoma, the different nodules exhibit different degrees of cellularity and architectural features, and genuine vascular invasion is lacking.[707]

NODULAR GOITER. In contrast to nodular goiter, there is scanty colloid, less degenerative change, presence of prominent nuclear atypia, and absence of normal internodular tissue.[706]

THYROID TREATED WITH RADIOACTIVE IODINE. The thyroid glands in patients treated with radioactive iodine can be indistinguishable from dyshormonogenetic goiter histologically. The clinical history is essential for making the distinction.

## Fine-Needle Aspiration–Associated Changes in the Thyroid Gland

Fine-needle aspiration of the thyroid gland can lead to a variety of histologic changes, some mundane and some potentially causing diagnostic problems.[101, 106]

### TISSUE INJURY

In the track of the needle pass, a linear hemorrhagic track or an irregularly shaped hematoma is formed (Fig. 44–97*A*). The thyroid follicles in the vicinity can undergo partial disruption or necrosis.

### REPARATIVE CHANGE

Organization of the hematoma and damaged tissue leads to granulation tissue formation, chronic inflammatory cell infiltration, hemosiderin deposition, and subsequently fibrous scarring.

### TISSUE INJURY OR REPAIR-ASSOCIATED REACTIVE CHANGES THAT MAY LEAD TO A MISDIAGNOSIS OF MALIGNANCY

The stromal reparative reaction to the trauma of fine-needle aspiration can be exuberant. Active-looking plump spindly myofibroblasts are admixed with thin-walled blood vessels, histiocytes, and hemosiderin (Fig. 44–97*B*). The lesion can be mistaken for Kaposi's sarcoma or other sarcomas; the term *post–fine-needle aspiration spindle cell nodule* has also been applied to this lesion.[708]

Tumor infarction complicating fine-needle aspiration can be accompanied by exuberant fibrogranulation tissue that begins in the peripheral zone and gradually extends inward. This reparative process can potentially be mistaken for anaplastic carcinoma, attributable to the poorly defined contour of the lesion and reactive atypia of the spindly cells (Fig. 44–98).

Organization of the fine-needle aspiration–associated hematoma can result in an exuberant, Masson tumor–like reaction, which can potentially be mistaken for angiosarcoma.[709]

The follicles around the areas of tissue injury or infarction can exhibit reactive atypia, such as nuclear enlargement and prominent nucleoli, and can potentially be mistaken for high-grade carcinoma. These reactive follicles can show anastomosis and intrafol-

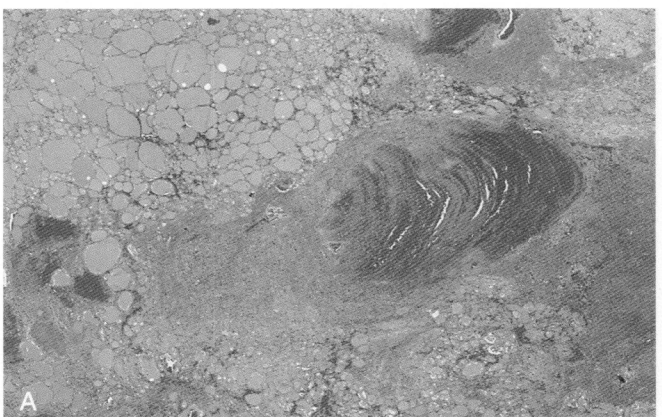
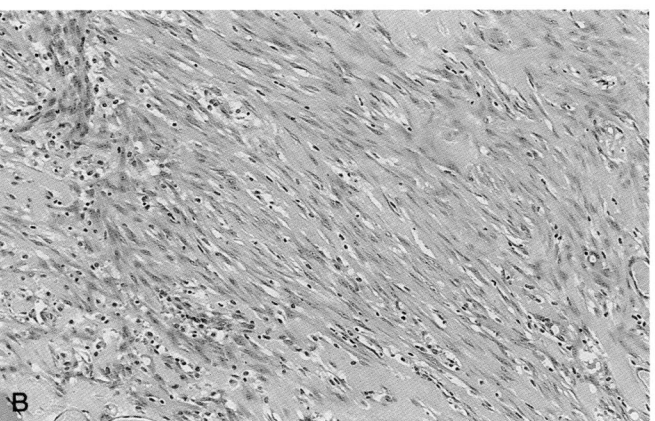

**FIGURE 44–97.** Fine-needle aspiration–associated changes in the thyroid. *A.* A linear hemorrhagic needle track is evident. *B.* Exuberant fibroblastic-myofibroblastic reaction in an area of tissue injury, so-called post–fine-needle aspiration spindle cell nodule.

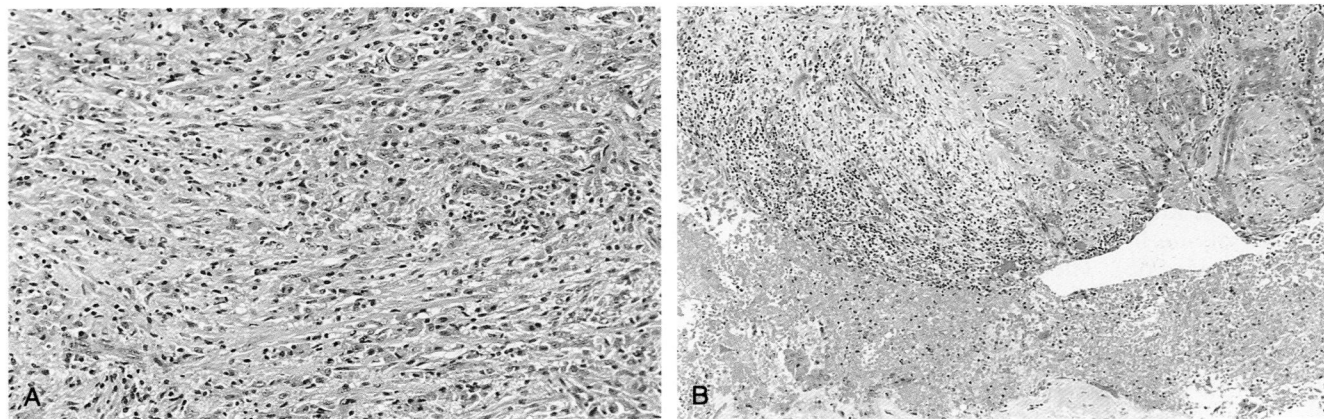

**FIGURE 44–98.** Fine-needle aspiration–associated infarction of papillary carcinoma. *A.* In most areas of the resection specimen, there is prominent myofibroblastic proliferation associated with histiocytes and deposits of hematoidin and hemosiderin. This represents organization of the infarct. *B.* Residual papillary carcinoma is identified focally (*right upper field*). Note the adjacent reparative reaction and infarcted tumor (*lower field*).

licular hemorrhage, resulting in an angiosarcoma-like appearance[106, 709, 710] (Fig. 44–99).

### TUMOR IMPLANTATION IN NEEDLE TRACK

At the site of needle puncture of the fibrous capsule of a thyroid neoplasm, some tumor islands can herniate into the capsule. This phenomenon (capsular rupture) can potentially lead to an erroneous interpretation of capsular invasion (see Fig. 44–22 and Table 44–8).

### TUMOR INFARCTION

Among the various types of thyroid tumors, Hürthle cell tumor is particularly prone to undergo infarction after fine-needle aspiration, probably because of the high energy requirements of the mitochondria-rich tumor cells[104] (Fig. 44–100). Papillary carcinoma also occasionally undergoes infarction after fine-nee-

dle aspiration (see Fig. 44–98). It can be difficult to arrive at a definitive diagnosis in the excision specimen if the tumor shows complete infarction.

## Amyloid Goiter

The thyroid gland is a common site for deposition of amyloid in systemic amyloidosis, but this usually does not result in enlargement of the thyroid or clinical symptoms. However, on occasion, amyloid deposits are so extensive that the patients present with a nontender, rapidly enlarging neck mass, which may be associated with dysphagia, dyspnea, and hoarseness. There is usually no clinical or biochemical evidence of thyroid dysfunction.[711, 712]

On histologic examination, amyloid is deposited between and around the follicles, accompanied by

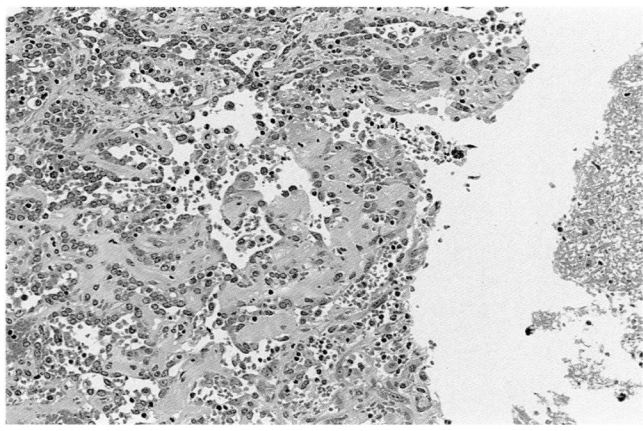

**FIGURE 44–99.** Fine-needle aspiration–associated reactive cellular atypia. Around the hemorrhagic needle track, the follicles anastomose to produce branching clefts, which in association with the extravasated blood mimic angiosarcoma.

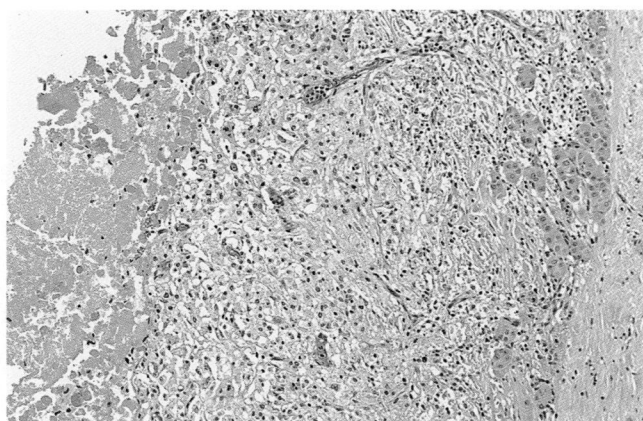

**FIGURE 44–100.** Fine-needle aspiration–associated infarction of Hürthle cell adenoma. Virtually the entire tumor has undergone infarction. Necrotic ghost cells are seen in the left field, and only a thin rim of viable tumor is seen in the right field. The intervening zone shows histiocytic infiltration and reparative changes.

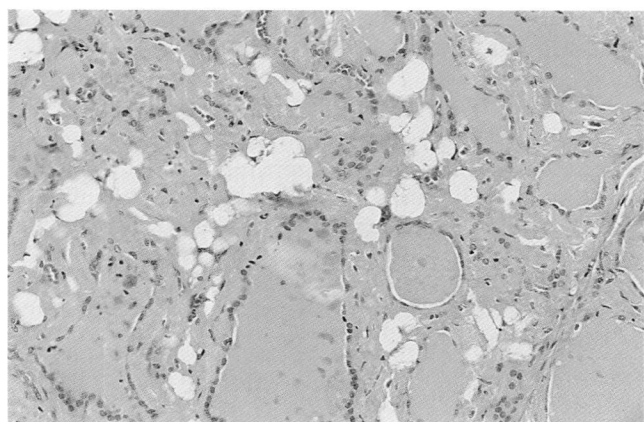

**FIGURE 44–101.** Amyloid goiter. There is interstitial deposition of eosinophilic-staining amyloid. Commonly, there are interspersed adipose cells. The follicles are atrophic and lined by attenuated epithelium.

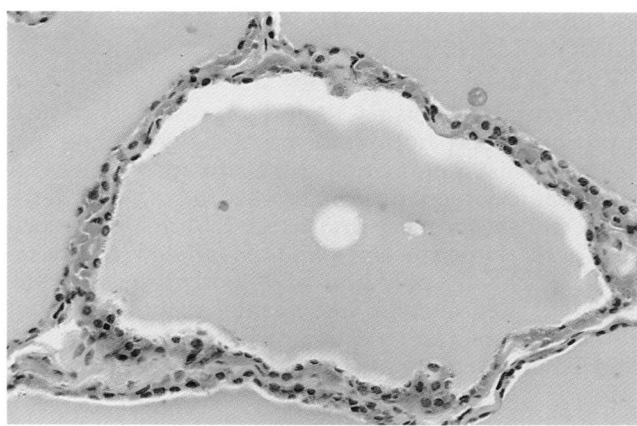

**FIGURE 44–102.** Black thyroid associated with minocycline intake. The follicular epithelial cells contain bright brown granules in the cytoplasm.

atrophy of the follicles (Fig. 44–101). Amyloid is also deposited in the blood vessel walls. Adipose cells are commonly interspersed within the amyloid. The amyloid can be of AA or AL type.

## Black Thyroid

Black thyroid is an uncommon but dramatic condition caused by administration of minocycline, a form of tetracycline. There are no clinical symptoms. On gross evaluation, the thyroid is black. On histologic examination, the follicular cells contain fine, dark brown granules, and ultrastructural analysis shows the pigment to be located in lysosomes (Fig.

44–102). The pigment is currently believed to result from oxidative interaction between thyroid peroxidase and the drug; it resembles neuromelanin in histochemical properties.[713–720] Of interest, when a tumor arises in a black thyroid, the tumor is often nonpigmented.[721–723]

## Uncommon Lesions of the Thyroid Gland

Exceptional examples of Rosai-Dorfman disease, malacoplakia, extramedullary hematopoiesis, and inflammatory pseudotumor (plasma cell granuloma) have been reported in the thyroid.[621, 724–730]

# B. The Parathyroid Gland

## NEOPLASTIC LESIONS

### Classification

Few tumor types are known to affect the parathyroid gland, and they include the following:

Parathyroid adenoma
  Typical
  Variants
    Lipoadenoma
    Papillary variant
    Water-clear variant
    Follicular variant
    Oxyphil variant
Parathyroid carcinoma (functional or nonfunctional)

Parathyroid neoplasm of uncertain malignant potential

### General Considerations

#### PATHOGENESIS

Parathyroid adenomas and carcinomas usually occur sporadically, but they can sometimes occur as a component of multiple endocrine neoplasia (MEN 1 and MEN 2) or familial idiopathic hyperparathyroidism.[731–733] Radiation to the head and neck region has also been implicated as a possible etiologic factor of parathyroid adenoma.[734, 735] Parathyroid carcinoma can occasionally supervene on parathyroid adenoma or parathyroid hyperplasia.[736]

## HYPERPARATHYROIDISM AS THE MAIN CLINICAL MANIFESTATION OF PARATHYROID NEOPLASMS

Parathyroid neoplasms typically present with features of hyperparathyroidism, although some patients are asymptomatic. There are three forms of hyperparathyroidism: primary, secondary, and tertiary. Only the primary and tertiary forms are associated with hypercalcemia and its related complications, such as polyuria and polydipsia, muscle weakness, renal stone, and mental disturbance, but all three forms can be associated with hyperparathyroid bone disease manifesting as bone pain or fracture.[733, 737–748]

### Primary Hyperparathyroidism

Primary hyperparathyroidism is defined as overproduction of parathyroid hormone as a result of intrinsic abnormality of the parathyroid glands. In more than 85% of cases, the underlying pathologic process is a parathyroid neoplasm. The remaining cases result from primary parathyroid hyperplasia, which can be sporadic or syndromatic (Table 44–19).

### Secondary Hyperparathyroidism

Secondary hyperparathyroidism is defined as compensatory hyperplasia of parathyroid glands with overproduction of parathyroid hormone due to hypocalcemia. As a result, the serum calcium concentration is often normalized. Nonetheless, the parathyroid hormone can stimulate bone resorption, resulting in parathyroid bone disease. Underlying disorders include chronic renal failure (the most common), malabsorption, vitamin D deficiency, and renal tubular acidosis.

### Tertiary Hyperparathyroidism

Tertiary hyperparathyroidism is defined as autonomous parathyroid hyperfunction supervening on secondary hyperparathyroidism. As a result, the serum calcium concentration is elevated. The autonomous parathyroid hyperfunction is most often caused by nodular hyperplasia; it is only uncommonly due to superimposed parathyroid adenoma or carcinoma.

## Parathyroid Adenoma

### CLINICAL CONSIDERATIONS

#### Presentation

Parathyroid adenoma is the most common cause of primary hyperparathyroidism (>85%).[749, 750] It occurs in patients with a mean age of 56 to 62 years. Women are more commonly affected than are men. Approximately 50% of patients are asymptomatic, being incidentally found to have hypercalcemia on routine blood chemistry.[750, 751] Others present with renal stone (30%) or parathyroid bone disease (20%), but simultaneous renal and skeletal disease is extremely rare.[750–755] Surgical excision of the single involved parathyroid gland is curative.[749, 756]

Although parathyroid adenoma typically involves a single gland, occasionally two of the four glands are simultaneously involved (double adenoma) on both sides or on the same side of the

---

**TABLE 44–19.** Syndromes Associated with Hyperparathyroidism

| | MEN 1 | MEN 2A | Familial Isolated Hyperparathyroidism |
|---|---|---|---|
| Endocrine organ disease | Parathyroid hyperplasia or neoplasm<br>Thyroid nodule or follicular adenoma<br>Adrenal nodule or adenoma<br>Islet cell tumor<br>Pituitary adenoma<br>Thymic carcinoid<br>Bronchial carcinoid | Parathyroid hyperplasia or neoplasm<br>Thyroid medullary carcinoma<br>Pheochromocytoma | Parathyroid hyperplasia or neoplasm |
| Other clinical features | Facial angiofibromas<br>Collagenomas<br>Multiple lipomas | Lichen amyloidosis (some cases) | Some kindreds also have jaw tumors (hyperparathyroidism–jaw tumor syndrome) |
| Natural history of hyperparathyroidism | Hyperparathyroidism is commonly the first presentation.<br>Serum calcium level tends to be lower than that of parathyroid adenoma, but incidence of renal or bone involvement is similar. | Hyperparathyroidism occurs in 20%–30% of cases and is usually mild and asymptomatic. | Hyperparathyroidism is often diagnosed at an early age.<br>Incidence of renal stone is high.<br>Recurrent or persistent hyperparathyroidism is common. |
| Genetic basis | Germline mutation in *MEN1* locus on chromosome 11q13 | Germline gain-of-function mutation in *RET* proto-oncogene on chromosome 10q11 | Genetic locus linked to 1q21–32 (*HPT-JT* or *HRPT2* gene) |

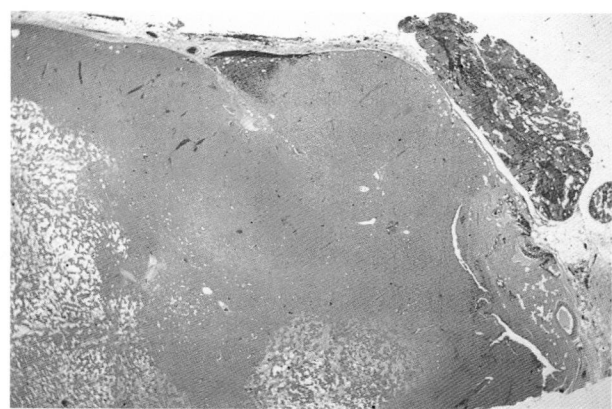

**FIGURE 44–103.** Parathyroid adenoma. The well-circumscribed tumor exhibits a solid growth pattern punctuated by edematous areas (*left field*). Residual normal parathyroid tissue is seen in the right upper field.

neck.[751, 757–760] These patients are often symptomatic and have a significantly higher parathyroid hormone level and tumor weight than with solitary adenoma. Because distinction from asymmetric primary hyperplasia of the parathyroid glands can be difficult, strict criteria must be applied for its diagnosis[757, 758]:

- Two enlarged parathyroid glands are confirmed histologically to be hypercellular.
- The remaining parathyroid glands are confirmed intraoperatively to be normal (preferably confirmed histologically by biopsy).
- No clinical evidence or family history of multiple endocrine neoplasia or familial hyperparathyroidism is found.
- Permanent cure of hypercalcemia is achieved by excision of the two enlarged glands alone.

Parathyroid adenomas can sometimes cause problems in their localization because of occurrence in ectopic locations, such as the mediastinum, thyroid, or esophagus.[761–766] When they occur within the thyroid gland, they can potentially be mistaken for thyroid follicular adenoma or medullary carcinoma.[761, 767]

### *Macroscopic Findings*

Parathyroid adenomas usually weigh less than 1 g, with size ranging from less than 1 cm to several centimeters.[768] The degree of hypercalcemia is generally correlated with the weight of the tumor.[768] Parathyroid adenoma forms a solitary circumscribed nodule, which is usually soft and orange-brown or reddish yellow to mahogany brown. Hemorrhage or cystic degeneration can sometimes be seen. The unaffected parathyroid glands are normal in size or small.

## DIAGNOSTIC CONSIDERATIONS

### *Microscopic Findings*

Parathyroid adenomas are typically well circumscribed and solitary, although exceptionally they may be multinodular (Fig. 44–103). Vague lobulation may be present.[769, 770] A thin rim of compressed parathyroid tissue can be present at the periphery. In contrast to the normal parathyroid gland, interspersed adipose cells are absent or scanty.

The tumor cells form solid sheets, cords, acini, follicles, and microcysts traversed by a delicate capillary or sinusoidal network (Fig. 44–104). They are polygonal, and the cytoplasm can be clear, eosinophilic, or oxyphilic. The nuclei are usually dark, round, and uniform, but there can be interspersed nuclei that are large, hyperchromatic, or even bizarre[768] (Fig. 44–105). The nuclei also show a tendency to be polarized toward the vascular aspect of the cells (Fig. 44–106). Mitotic figures are rare or absent. Vague nodular foci are sometimes seen within the tumor.[771]

Fibrosis, hemorrhage, infarction, or cystic change can occur, but there should not be coagulative tumor necrosis; if it is present, coagulative tumor ne-

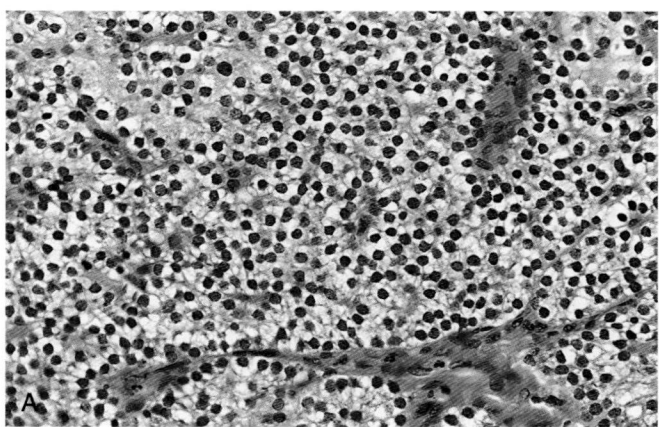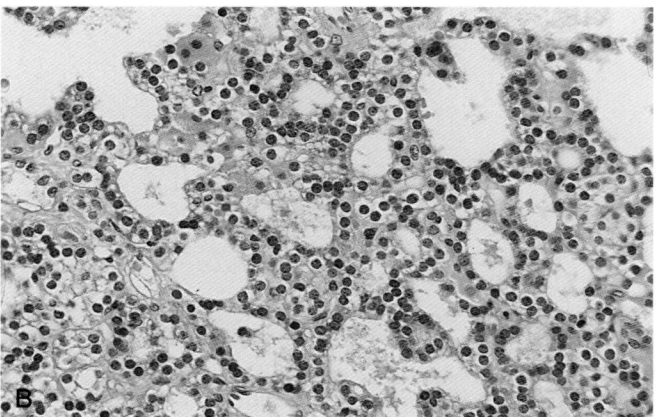

**FIGURE 44–104.** Parathyroid adenoma. *A.* Clear cells grow in a diffuse pattern and are characteristically traversed by delicate blood vessels. *B.* The tumor shows a complex acinar growth pattern.

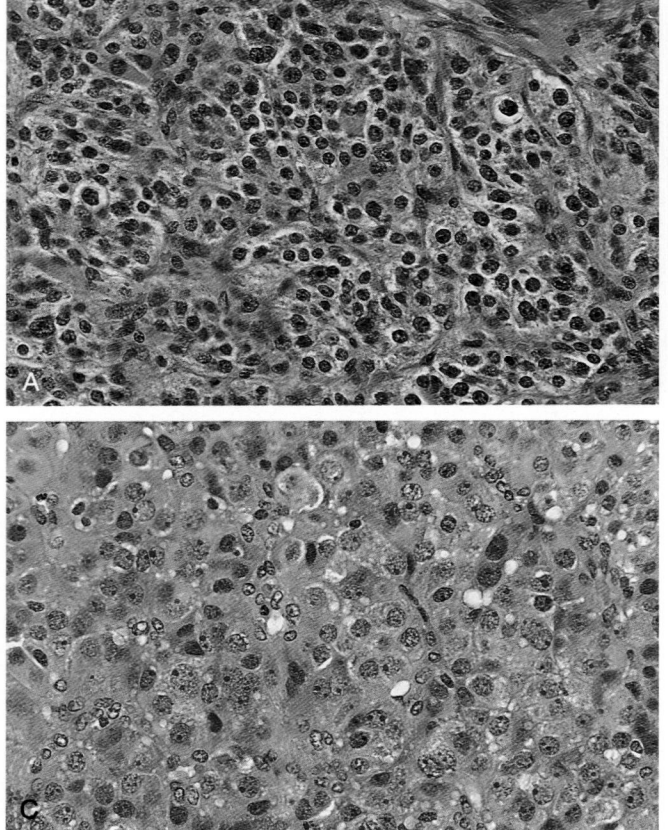

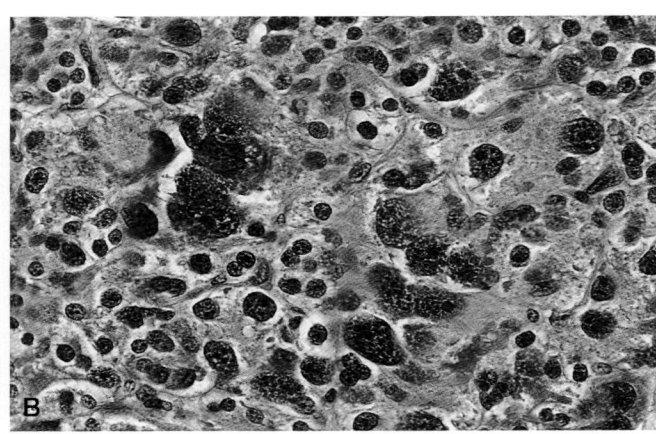

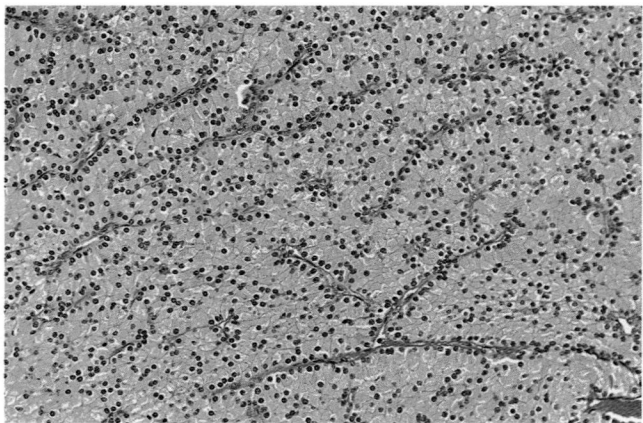

FIGURE 44–105. Parathyroid adenoma. *A.* The tumor cells possess clear or eosinophilic cytoplasm. The nuclei appear uniform and dark staining. *B.* In focal areas, there are cells with large hyperchromatic nuclei. Presence of these large nuclei is not indicative of malignancy. *C.* In this example, most nuclei are mildly atypical.

crosis strongly suggests parathyroid carcinoma. Rare cases show a lymphoid infiltrate in the peripheral portion in the form of lymphoid follicles or in the parenchyma in the form of isolated cells.[772, 773]

FIGURE 44–106. Parathyroid adenoma. A characteristic feature commonly seen in the normal parathyroid gland, parathyroid adenoma, and parathyroid carcinoma is palisading of nuclei along the vascular pole of the cells.

Rarely, intrafollicular or interstitial amyloid can be found[767, 774, 775] (Fig. 44–107). The morphologic variants are listed in Table 44–20 (Figs. 44–107 to 44–109).[775–788]

### Immunohistochemistry

The tumor cells of parathyroid adenoma are immunoreactive for cytokeratin, pan-neuroendocrine markers (such as synaptophysin, chromogranin, and neurofilament), and parathyroid hormone.[789–791] The Ki-67 proliferative index is low (0.5% to 5.1%, with a mean of 2% to 3%), but the nodular foci may show a higher index.[771, 792–794]

Immunohistochemical staining for parathyroid hormone is rarely required for diagnostic purposes, except when there are difficulties in distinction from a thyroid follicular adenoma or when the tumor occurs in an ectopic location.

### Molecular Biology and Genetics

Molecular evidence of monoclonality can be demonstrated in most parathyroid adenomas by use of X-linked restriction fragment length polymorphism studies.[795–797] Furthermore, some cases exhibit tumor-specific DNA alterations in the parathyroid hormone gene.[795]

**TABLE 44–20.** Morphologic Variants of Parathyroid Adenoma

| Variant | Major Pathologic Findings | Potential Diagnostic Pitfall |
|---|---|---|
| Lipoadenoma ("parathyroid hamartoma") | Often large size; chief and oxyphil cells are intermingled with many mature adipose cells, which occupy 20%–90% of the tissue area; loose fibromyxoid stroma can be present in some cases | Without information on the gross appearance (circumscribed and large), it can be mistaken histologically for normal parathyroid |
| Papillary | Prominent papillary pattern | May be mistaken for papillary thyroid carcinoma |
| Water-clear cell | Composed of tumor cells with clear cytoplasm and distinct cell membranes | — |
| Follicular | Prominent follicular-acinar pattern | May be mistaken for follicular thyroid neoplasm |
| Oxyphilic | Composed entirely of oxyphilic cells with abundant eosinophilic granular cytoplasm | May be mistaken for Hürthle cell neoplasms of thyroid |

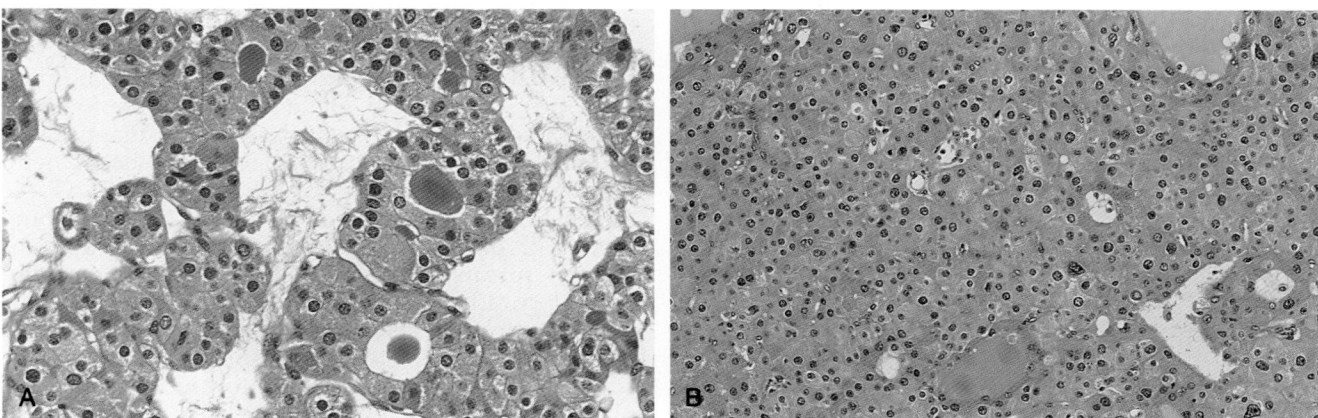

FIGURE 44–107. Parathyroid adenoma, oxyphilic type. *A.* The tumor cells form trabeculae and acini. Amyloid is found in the lumina of the acini. *B.* This example shows a diffuse growth pattern. In contrast to Hürthle (oxyphilic) cells of the thyroid, the cell membranes are typically distinct.

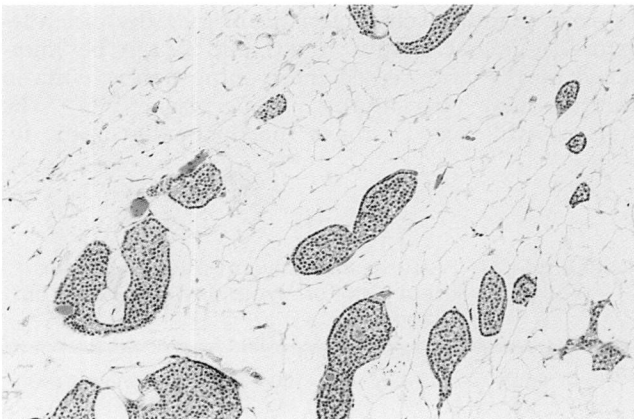

FIGURE 44–108. Parathyroid lipoadenoma. Islands of parathyroid parenchymal cells are interspersed among abundant adipose cells. The circumscribed border of the large tumor is seen in the left upper field.

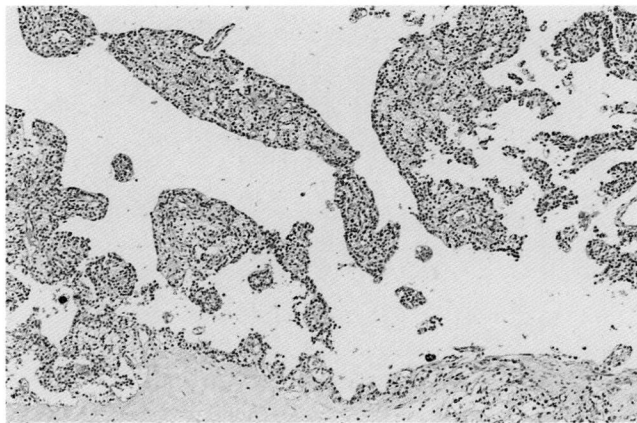

FIGURE 44–109. Parathyroid adenoma, papillary variant. The papillary processes are not genuine papillae but represent pseudopapillae formed by dehiscence of the tumor tissue.

On cytogenetic analysis, rare cases of parathyroid adenoma show pericentric inversion of chromosome 11, which results in translocation of the cyclin D1 (PRAD1) gene with the parathyroid hormone gene, causing overexpression of cyclin D1 and hence increased cellular proliferation.[795, 796, 798–801] Immunohistochemical expression of cyclin D1 occurs at a higher frequency (~25% of cases), suggesting deregulation of cyclin D1 by mechanisms other than pericentric chromosome inversion in such cases.[798, 802] The MEN 1–associated MEN1 gene shows somatic mutation in 10% to 23% of sporadic parathyroid adenomas.[803, 804] Chromosome abnormalities identified by comparative genomic hybridization include loss of 11p, 11q, 1p, and 1q and gain of 16p and 19p.[805]

### Differential Diagnosis

PRIMARY OR SECONDARY PARATHYROID HYPERPLASIA. In parathyroid hyperplasia, all the parathyroid glands should be enlarged, although they are unevenly enlarged in some cases. Not uncommonly, the individual enlarged glands have a multinodular appearance.

PARATHYROID CARCINOMA. See subsequent section.

THYROID FOLLICULAR ADENOMA. When the parathyroid tumor is inside the thyroid gland and shows a microfollicular pattern, it can be mistaken for a follicular adenoma. Parathyroid adenoma is immunoreactive for parathyroid hormone, whereas thyroid follicular adenoma is immunoreactive for thyroglobulin.

OXYPHIL CELL NODULE. Oxyphil cell nodules are a common incidental finding in the parathyroid gland, especially in an older subject. They are small and commonly multifocal (Fig. 44–110).

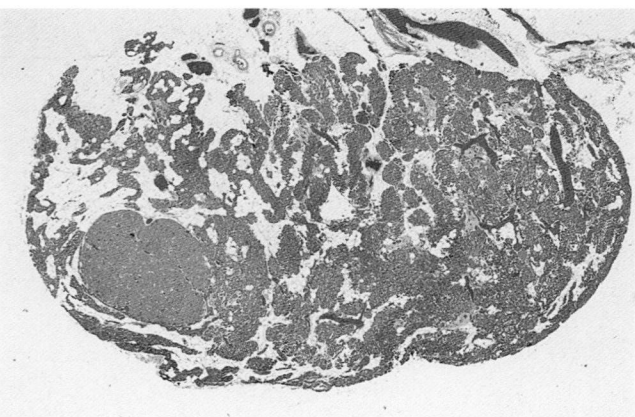

**FIGURE 44–110.** Oxyphil cell nodule. Small nodule composed entirely of oxyphilic cells is a common incidental finding in the parathyroid gland.

### Intraoperative Frozen Section Diagnosis of Parathyroid Adenoma

Intraoperative frozen section evaluation of patients presenting with hyperparathyroidism aims to achieve the following[806, 807]:

• Confirm that the tissue removed for examination indeed represents parathyroid tissue, not lymph node, thyroid, or ectopic thymus.
• Determine whether the abnormal parathyroid tissue represents parathyroid adenoma (removal of the diseased gland alone is sufficient), parathyroid hyperplasia (removal of 3.5 glands is required), or parathyroid carcinoma (en bloc radical excision is required).[749, 756]

The gland should be measured, weighed, and examined histologically. It is usually easy to confirm that the excised tissue is parathyroid gland on histologic examination, except that a small biopsy specimen of lymph node may occasionally be misinterpreted as parathyroid tissue because of artifactual spaces created by freezing that mimic adipose cells.[808] A parathyroid gland with few or no interspersed adipose cells is supportive of a diagnosis of "hypercellular parathyroid gland, consistent with parathyroid adenoma or hyperplasia" (Table 44–21). Some investigators consider lipid staining (Sudan II or IV, oil red O) on frozen sections or imprint smears to be helpful in identifying an abnormal parathyroid gland[797, 809–812] because the normal parathyroid cells contain abundant intracytoplasmic lipid droplets, whereas the hyperplastic or adenomatous cells are often devoid of intracytoplasmic lipid. An exception is the oxyphil cell, which always contains no or scanty intracytoplasmic lipid droplets.[770] Adenomatous or hyperplastic glands may occasionally contain intracytoplasmic lipid, albeit weakly and focally.[813–816]

After it is confirmed that the parathyroid gland is hypercellular, the next step is to determine whether it represents an adenoma or hyperplastic process. Although a compressed rim of normal parathyroid gland is characteristic of parathyroid adenoma, it is not always found and it can be mimicked by the compressed intervening parenchyma in multinodular parathyroid hyperplasia.[817, 818] The most reliable way to make the distinction is by de-

**TABLE 44–21.** Features Indicative of a Hypercellular (Neoplastic or Hyperplastic) Parathyroid Gland

Weight: single gland weighing >100 mg (normal weight, ~30 mg)
Adipose cells in gland: few or absent (on average, ~17% of a normal parathyroid gland is composed of adipose cells)
Intracytoplasmic lipid droplets as demonstrated by lipid stain: absent or scanty

termining the status of the other parathyroid glands. If they are all normal in size or small, a diagnosis of adenoma is favored. If all are enlarged, a diagnosis of parathyroid hyperplasia is favored. Simple inspection is not reliable because some hyperplastic processes affect the glands unequally; it is preferable to take an incisional biopsy specimen of one or more glands for histologic confirmation to ascertain whether they are normal-suppressed or hyperplastic.[819]

Intraoperative assay of the parathyroid hormone level is an alternative way for guiding the extent of surgery, taking advantage of the fact that the hormone has a short half-life.[807, 820–822] If preoperative imaging studies can identify an enlarged parathyroid gland, a more limited unilateral procedure can be performed in place of bilateral neck exploration. Approximately 15 minutes after removal of the enlarged gland, a serum sample is taken for parathyroid hormone assay. A significant drop in the hormone level (>50%) suggests successful removal of the hypersecreting tissue, and thus cure is reasonably ensured. The other parathyroid glands have to be explored for hyperplasia if the parathyroid hormone level remains elevated after removal of one enlarged gland.

## Parathyroid Carcinoma

### CLINICAL CONSIDERATIONS

#### Presentation

Parathyroid carcinomas are rare, constituting only about 2% of all parathyroid neoplasms. Compared with parathyroid adenoma, the patients with parathyroid carcinoma have a lower mean age (45 to 54 years), there is no sex predilection, and virtually all patients are symptomatic because of the high serum calcium level (3.5 to 4 mmol/L). Only rare tu-

**TABLE 44–22.** Clues for Recognizing Parathyroid Carcinoma Versus Parathyroid Adenoma

| Clinical Clues* | Clues at Operation |
| --- | --- |
| High serum calcium level (>3.5 mmol/L or 14 mg/dL) | Firm consistency |
| Simultaneous parathyroid bone disease and renal stone (found in ~40%) | Thick capsule |
| Palpable neck mass (found in ~40%) | Adherence and invasion to adjacent organs, e.g., thyroid, muscle, nerve, esophagus |
| Vocal cord paralysis | |
| Presence of metastasis | |

* The clinical clues actually reflect a large tumor or a tumor with invasive properties.

mors are nonfunctional.* The clues for recognizing the malignant nature of a parathyroid neoplasm are listed in Table 44–22.

#### Macroscopic Findings

The carcinomas are usually hard because of the presence of fibrous trabeculae. The size ranges from 1 cm to several centimeters.[752] They are often much larger than parathyroid adenomas, with an average weight of 12 g (versus less than 1 g for parathyroid adenoma).[768] They can be circumscribed or invasive. Necrosis and calcification can be present.[834]

### DIAGNOSTIC CONSIDERATIONS

#### Microscopic Findings

The tumor shows frank invasive features or is surrounded by a thick fibrous capsule[736] (Fig. 44–111). It comprises polygonal cells forming solid sheets, trabeculae, acini, and packets.[755] In some

---

*References 731, 736, 752–754, 767, 823–833.

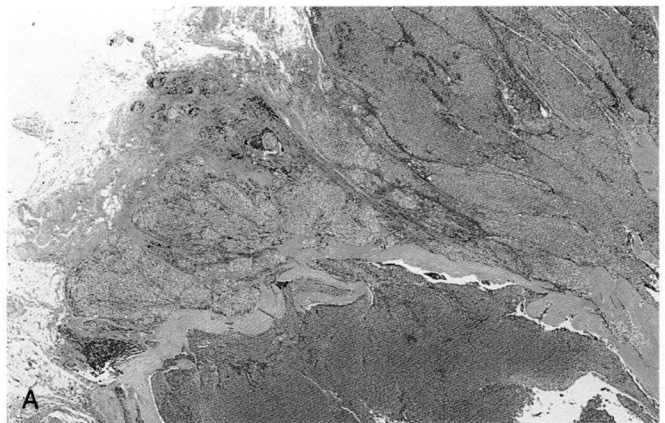 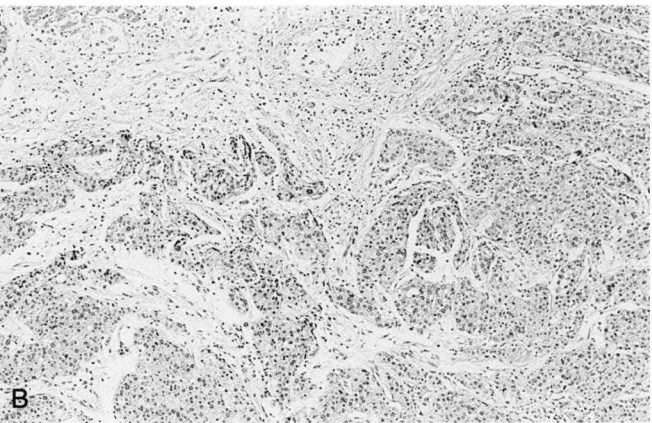

**FIGURE 44–111.** Parathyroid carcinoma. *A.* The tumor shows frank infiltration into the surrounding fibrofatty tissue. *B.* In this example, the tumor grows in the form of irregular infiltrative islands. The stroma is desmoplastic.

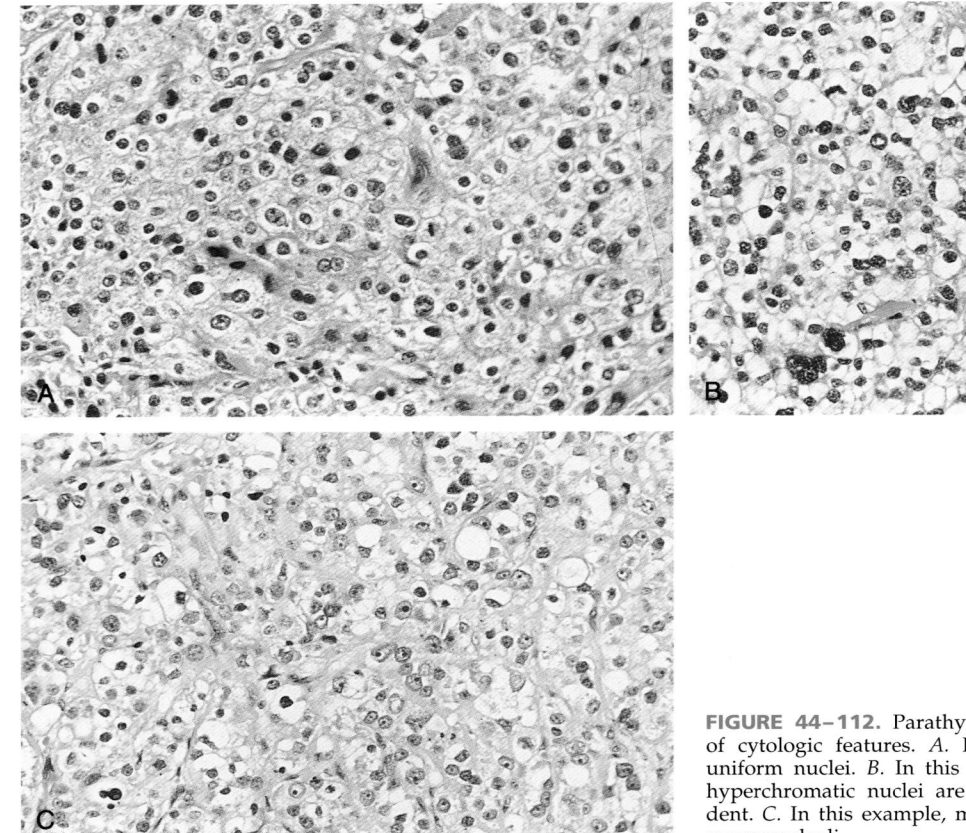

**FIGURE 44–112.** Parathyroid carcinoma showing the spectrum of cytologic features. *A.* In this example, the cells have fairly uniform nuclei. *B.* In this example, interspersed cells with large hyperchromatic nuclei are present. Mitotic figures are also evident. *C.* In this example, many tumor cells are atypical and have macronucleoli.

cases, the nuclei are uniform and bland-looking, with or without interspersed large hyperchromatic or bizarre nuclei[731] (Fig. 44–112). In other cases, the nuclei are overtly pleomorphic (Fig. 44–112C). Nucleoli are sometimes prominent.[835] The cytoplasm is clear, lightly eosinophilic, or oxyphilic.[834, 836, 837] On occasion, monotonous small cells with high nuclear-to-cytoplasmic ratio can dominate (Fig. 44–113). Coagulative necrosis can be present.[835]

The features for diagnosing parathyroid carcinoma are outlined in Table 44–23.[838] Stringent criteria must be used in the assessment of capsular or vascular invasion, similar to those applied for follicular neoplasms of the thyroid. Broad fibrous septa

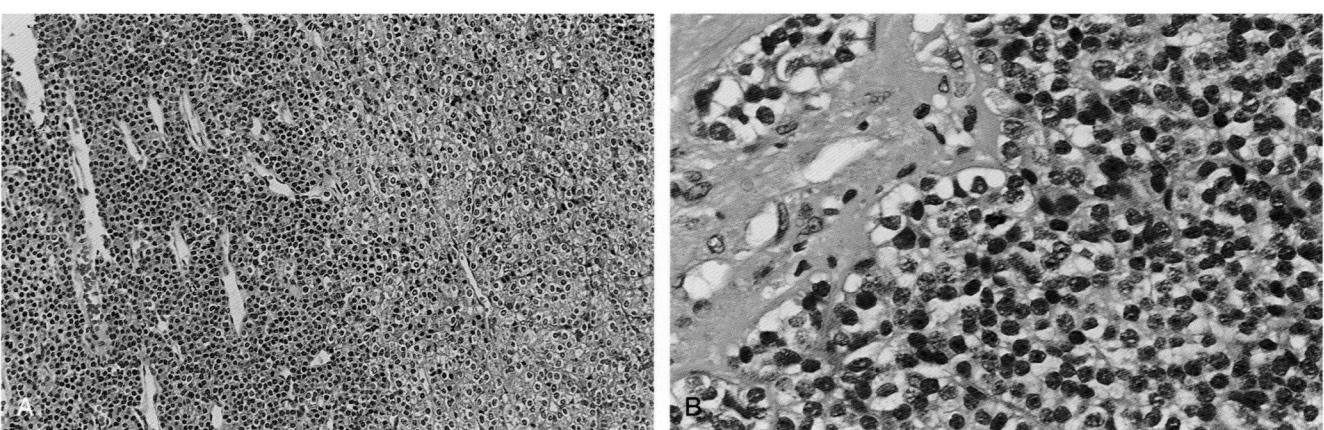

**FIGURE 44–113.** Parathyroid carcinoma. *A.* Monotonous small cells are seen in the left field of this tumor. *B.* Higher magnification shows small cells with high nuclear-to-cytoplasmic ratio. A mitotic figure is seen near the central field.

**TABLE 44–23.** Histologic Criteria for Diagnosis of Parathyroid Carcinoma in a Parathyroid Neoplasm

| Absolute Criteria of Malignancy | Features Associated with Malignancy |
| --- | --- |
| Presence of any one of the following criteria is sufficient for a diagnosis of malignancy:<br>　—Invasion into surrounding tissues<br>　　• Thyroid<br>　　• Esophagus<br>　　• Nerves<br>　　• Soft tissues<br>　—Regional or distant metastasis | When the absolute criteria are lacking, at least 2 and preferably 3 or more of the following features have to be present to establish a diagnosis of malignancy:<br>　—Vascular invasion<br>　—Capsular invasion<br>　—Broad fibrous bands splitting the parenchyma and delineating expansile nodules<br>　—Coagulative tumor necrosis<br>　—Mitotic count >5 per 10 high-power fields<br>　—Sheetlike monotonous small cells with high nuclear-to-cytoplasmic ratio<br>　—Generalized cellular atypia<br>　—Frequent macronucleoli |

Ancillary studies that may help in supporting a diagnosis of parathyroid carcinoma over adenoma:
Immunostaining for Ki-67: high Ki-67 index (mean Ki-67 index for carcinoma is 6.1%–8.4%; that for adenoma is 2.0%–3.3%)
Immunostaining for retinoblastoma protein (lack of nuclear staining in tumor cells, provided that appropriate internal positive control is found) or molecular analysis of retinoblastoma gene in tumor (allelic loss)
Immunostaining for p27: low percentage of positive cells (mean labeling index 13.9% for carcinoma versus 56.8% for adenoma)

In some cases, there are some features associated with malignancy, but they are insufficient for a definite diagnosis of carcinoma to be made. A designation "parathyroid neoplasm of uncertain malignant potential" may be appropriate in such circumstances.

traversing the tumor must be accompanied by expansile nodules before they are considered significant to distinguish them from the focal scarring due to previous hemorrhage or surgery[752] (Fig. 44–114). Although mitotic figures have been emphasized as being the single most important criterion of malignancy,[752] they are now recognized as being significant only when they are present in considerable numbers[736, 838–840] (see Fig. 44–112B). Conversely, some carcinomas may show no or few mitotic figures.[752, 835, 838]

### Immunohistochemistry

The tumor cells of parathyroid carcinoma are immunoreactive for cytokeratin, pan-neuroendocrine

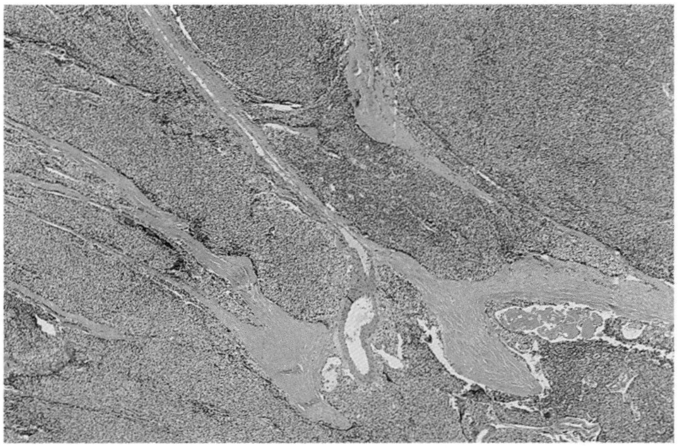

**FIGURE 44–114.** Parathyroid carcinoma. The tumor is traversed by dense fibrous bands associated with expansile nodules of tumor tissue.

markers, and parathyroid hormone. Immunostaining for parathyroid hormone is most helpful for confirming a diagnosis of nonfunctioning or ectopic parathyroid carcinoma.

### Molecular Biology

In most parathyroid carcinomas, allelic loss of the retinoblastoma *(RB)* tumor suppressor gene is found.[800, 838, 841] On immunohistochemical staining, lack of immunoreactivity for the RB protein occurs in 20% to 88% of cases.[792, 841, 842] Cyclin D1 overexpression is also common (91% of cases).[798, 802] There is commonly reduced expression of the cyclin-dependent kinase inhibitor protein p27 (mean labeling index of 14% versus 57% for parathyroid adenoma).[794]

### Differential Diagnosis

The main problem in diagnosis of parathyroid carcinoma is to recognize its malignant nature. The difficulty lies in the fact that some apparently bland-looking tumors may declare themselves to be malignant by subsequent recurrence or metastasis.[836, 843] In some cases, the malignant nature of the tumor is obvious by virtue of the frankly invasive growth, significant cellular pleomorphism, and frequent mitoses. However, in other cases, it is essential to consider a number of features to render a diagnosis of malignancy (see Table 44–23).

Immunostaining for the proliferation marker Ki-67 can sometimes be helpful because the index is higher in parathyroid carcinoma than in adenoma.[792–794] Nonetheless, it cannot be used as the sole criterion because there is overlap in the counts between adenomas and carcinomas.[844] Whereas a high Ki-67 index (>5%) suggests a diagnosis of carcinoma, a low index does not exclude this possibility. The role of flow cytometric analysis of DNA in the diagnosis of parathyroid carcinoma remains controversial.[845-848] A study employing a static DNA fluorometric method has reported a high nuclear DNA content and aneuploidy to favor a diagnosis of parathyroid carcinoma over parathyroid adenoma.[849]

When there are some but inconclusive features associated with malignancy, the designation "parathyroid neoplasm of uncertain malignant potential" or "atypical parathyroid adenoma" can be applied.[850] Follow-up with regular monitoring of the serum calcium level will be helpful for such patients. Firm data on the outcome of these cases are lacking.

## PROGNOSTIC CONSIDERATIONS

### General Behavior

Parathyroid carcinoma generally pursues an indolent clinical course. It can invade contiguous structures, particularly the thyroid.[754, 830, 851] Surgery is the mainstay of treatment. Local recurrence develops in approximately one third of patients, usually within 3 years[833]; this occurrence may be reduced by postoperative radiotherapy.[826] About one third of patients develop metastasis, usually relatively late in the course; the favored sites are regional lymph nodes of the neck and mediastinum, lungs, liver, and bones. The relapse usually manifests as recurrent hypercalcemia, and symptomatic control or even occasionally cure can still be achieved by further operations.* The 5-year and 10-year survival rates are 60% and 40%, respectively. Death is usually caused by metabolic complications of hypercalcemia rather than by organ replacement by tumor.[752-754, 834, 853]

### Prognostic Factors

Data on prognostic factors of parathyroid carcinoma are limited. Adequate en bloc excision (removal of the tumor, adjacent thyroid lobe, paratracheal soft tissues and lymph nodes, and ipsilateral thymus) on recognition of the malignant nature of the tumor at the initial operation offers the best chance of cure.[824, 827, 833, 852] Nonfunctioning parathyroid carcinomas appear to behave more aggressively than functioning ones.[823] The triad of macronucleoli, more than 5 mitoses per 50 high-power fields, and necrosis is correlated with a more aggressive outcome. High nuclear DNA content is correlated with a less favorable survival.[835]

## Contents of the Final Surgical Pathology Report

The checklist of contents of the final report of parathyroid carcinoma excision specimens is listed in Table 44–24.

---

*References 753, 754, 823, 828, 830, 843, 852.

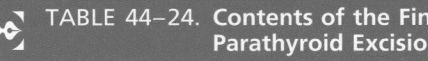

**TABLE 44–24. Contents of the Final Report: Parathyroid Excision Specimens**

Specimen type/operation procedure

Diagnosis
  Histologic diagnosis

Other tumor features
  Tumor location
  Tumor size
  Encapsulated or nonencapsulated
  Capsular invasion (absent, present, extensive)
  Vascular invasion (absent, present, extensive)
  Tissues or structures invaded by the carcinoma
  Mitotic count
  Immunohistochemical expression of RB, cyclin D1, p27 (optional)

Surgical margins: free, close to surgical margin, or margin involved (specify site)

Non-neoplastic parathyroid: normal, diffuse hyperplasia, nodular hyperplasia

Lymph nodes
  Number of lymph nodes found, and their location (level)
  Number of involved lymph nodes
  Size of largest metastatic deposit
  Presence or absence of extracapsular extension

## NON-NEOPLASTIC LESIONS

## Primary Parathyroid Chief Cell Hyperplasia

### CLINICAL CONSIDERATIONS

Primary parathyroid chief cell hyperplasia is a de novo hyperplastic process involving all the parathyroid glands, producing the clinical features of primary hyperparathyroidism.[737, 756, 769, 854] Approximately 80% of cases are sporadic; the other cases occur as a component of MEN 1, MEN 2, familial isolated hyperparathyroidism, or hyperparathyroidism–jaw tumor syndrome. The condition is more common in females than in males. Treatment consists of subtotal parathyroidectomy (removal of 3.5 glands); the remaining gland is sometimes autoimplanted in the forearm.

### DIAGNOSTIC CONSIDERATIONS

Although all parathyroid glands are involved, they may be unevenly enlarged, with some glands apparently having a "normal size"—and hence leading to a misdiagnosis of parathyroid neoplasm. The combined weight of the parathyroid glands ranges from less than 1 g to 10 g.

In primary chief cell hyperplasia, the parathyroid glands are hypercellular, with marked reduction in interposed adipose cells. The proliferated parathyroid cells include predominantly chief cells, but water-clear cells and oxyphil cells are often present. The parathyroid cells show a solid, trabecular, follicular, or cordlike growth. In areas, it is common to see the characteristic palisading of the nuclei along the vascular septa. The pathologic process is initially diffuse, but with time, nodules will supervene on the background of diffuse hyperplasia. The various nodules often show different cellular compositions and different patterns of cellular organization.

## Primary Water-Clear Cell Hyperplasia

### CLINICAL CONSIDERATIONS

Water-clear cell hyperplasia is a rare form of primary parathyroid hyperplasia. It shows no familial incidence or association with multiple endocrine neoplasia. Of interest, for unknown reasons, this entity has virtually disappeared in the past few decades.[737, 738, 855, 856]

The condition occurs mostly in older adults, but any age can be affected. It is slightly more common in males than in females. The patients present with features of primary hyperparathyroidism. In general, the hypercalcemia is more severe than in chief cell hyperplasia.

### DIAGNOSTIC CONSIDERATIONS

In water-clear cell hyperplasia, the parathyroid glands are usually markedly enlarged; the combined weight of the gland is frequently above 10 g. The upper glands are often larger than the lower ones. On histologic examination, the hyperplastic parathyroid cells are large and possess water-clear cytoplasm. They form solid sheets and acini.

## Secondary Parathyroid Hyperplasia

### CLINICAL CONSIDERATIONS

Secondary parathyroid hyperplasia is a hyperplastic condition of the parathyroid glands in response to hypocalcemia or hyperphosphatemia. The most common cause is chronic renal failure. The patients present with features of secondary hyperparathyroidism (mostly with parathyroid bone disease) or tertiary hyperparathyroidism (mostly with complications of hypercalcemia). Treatment consists of subtotal parathyroidectomy.

### DIAGNOSTIC CONSIDERATIONS

There is uniform or uneven enlargement of all parathyroid glands, indistinguishable from that seen in primary parathyroid hyperplasia. A multinodular pattern is seen in the majority of cases. The proliferation involves chief cells, clear cells, and oxyphil cells, which are arranged in sheets, trabeculae, or acini (Fig. 44–115). There can be fibrous bands

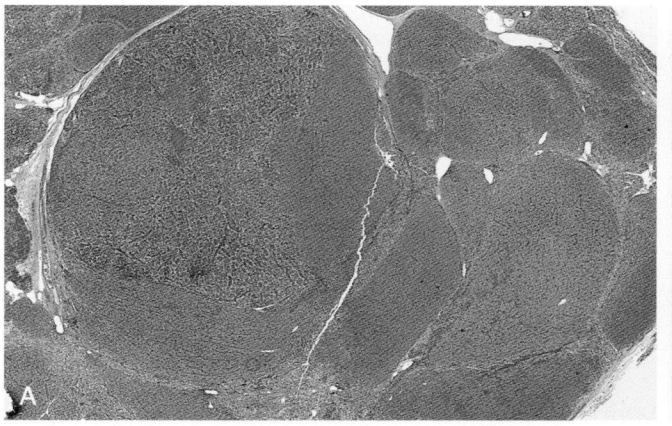

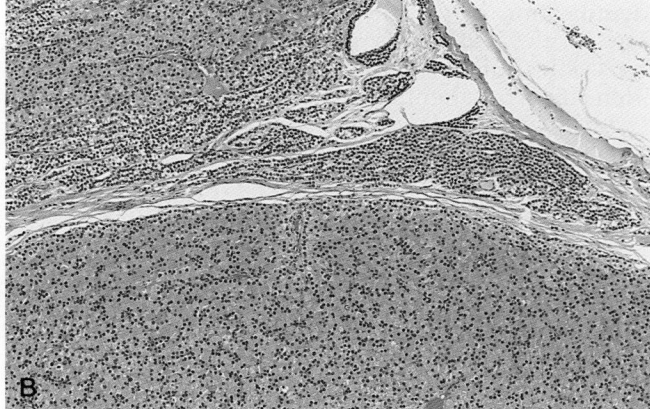

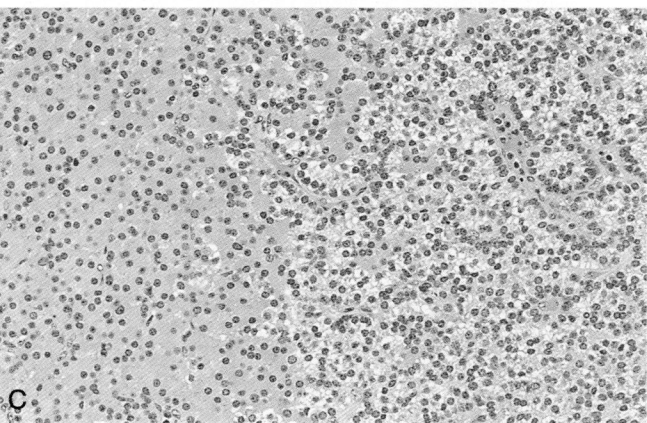

**FIGURE 44–115.** Secondary parathyroid hyperplasia in chronic renal failure. *A.* The enlarged parathyroid gland is converted into multiple hyperplastic nodules. *B.* The nodules show different cell compositions. This field may give a false impression of an adenoma surrounded by compressed residual parathyroid tissue. *C.* The nodules often show a mixture of cell types.

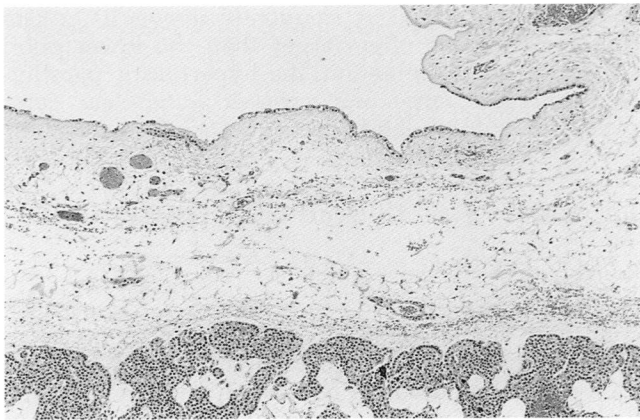

**FIGURE 44–116.** Parathyroid cyst. The cyst is lined by a single layer of parathyroid cells. Normal parathyroid tissue is identified in the wall (*lower field*).

around the nodules, hemosiderin deposition, and cystic change. Calcification can be present.

## Parathyroid Cyst

Parathyroid cyst manifests clinically as a mass lesion or hypercalcemia, but it can also be an incidental finding. Its size can range from a few millimeters to 10 cm. The wall is thin and translucent.[857] A diagnosis can be made by fine-needle aspiration, either by identification of parathyroid cells or by demonstration of elevated levels of parathyroid hormone in the cystic fluid.[858] On histologic examination, it is often lined by attenuated parathyroid cells and surrounded by islands of normal, hyperplastic, or adenomatous parathyroid tissue (Fig. 44–116). That is, some cases represent cystic change of a parathyroid adenoma and are thus associated with hypercalcemia.

## Periparathyroid Salivary Heterotopia–Cyst Unit

An uncommon lesion occurring in a periparathyroid location is the salivary heterotopia–cyst unit.[859] It is usually small, measuring 1 to 6 mm, comprising small lobules of salivary acini and cysts. The cysts are lined by flattened, ciliated, or columnar cells, without parathyroid cell lining. The salivary heterotopia–cyst unit has been postulated to be of third and fourth-fifth branchial pouch derivation.

## Amyloidosis

The parathyroid glands can be involved in systemic amyloidosis. The glands are enlarged and histologically show deposition of amyloid in blood vessel walls and the interstitium.[860] When there is abundant amyloid deposition, parenchymal cells may be lost, leading to the development of mild hypocalcemia.

## REFERENCES

1. Hedinger C, Williams ED, Sobin LH: Histological Typing of Thyroid Tumors. WHO International Histological Classification of Tumors. 2nd ed. Berlin, Springer-Verlag, 1988.
2. Ordonez NG: Thyroid transcription factor-1 is a marker of lung and thyroid carcinomas. Adv Anat Pathol 7:123–127, 2000.
3. Katoh R, Kawaoi A, Miyagi E, et al: Thyroid transcription factor-1 in normal, hyperplastic, and neoplastic follicular thyroid cells examined by immunohistochemistry and nonradioactive in situ hybridization. Mod Pathol 13:570–576, 2000.
4. Chan JKC: Tumors of the thyroid and parathyroid glands. In Fletcher CDM (ed): Diagnostic Histopathology of Tumors. 2nd ed. Edinburgh, Churchill Livingstone, 2000, pp 959–1056.
5. Katoh R, Miyagi E, Nakamura N, et al: Expression of thyroid transcription factor-1 (TTF-1) in human C cells and medullary thyroid carcinomas. Hum Pathol 31:386–393, 2000.
6. Figge J, Jennings T, Gerasimov G: Radiation and thyroid cancer. In Wartofsky L (ed): Thyroid Cancer, A Comprehensive Guide to Clinical Management. Totowa, NJ, Humana Press, 2000, pp 85–116.
7. Figge J: Epidemiology of thyroid cancer. In Wartofsky L (ed): Thyroid Cancer, A Comprehensive Guide to Clinical Management. Totowa, NJ, Humana Press, 2000, pp 77–81.
8. Williams ED: The aetiology of thyroid tumours. Clin Endocrinol Metab 8:193–207, 1979.
9. Feilotter H, Mulligan L: Endocrine cancers. In Foulkes WD, Hodgson SV (eds): Inherited susceptibility to cancer: clinical, predictive and ethical perspectives. Cambridge, UK, Cambridge University Press, 1998, pp 326–354.
10. Gilliland FD, Hunt WC, Morris DM, Key CR: Prognostic factors for thyroid carcinoma. A population-based study of 15,698 cases from the Surveillance, Epidemiology and End Results (SEER) program 1973–1991. Cancer 79:564–573, 1997.
11. Brierley JD, Panzarella T, Tsang RW, et al: A comparison of different staging systems predictability of patient outcome. Thyroid carcinoma as an example. Cancer 79:2414–2423, 1997.
12. Gemsenjager E, Heitz PU, Martina B: Selective treatment of differentiated thyroid carcinoma. World J Surg 21:546–551, discussion 551–552, 1997.
13. Oertel YC, Oertel JE: Diagnosis of malignant epithelial thyroid lesions: fine needle aspiration and histopathologic correlation. Ann Diagn Pathol 2:377–400, 1998.
14. Oertel YC: Fine-needle aspiration and the diagnosis of thyroid cancer. Endocrinol Metab Clin North Am 25:69–91, 1996.
15. Silver CE, Owen RP: Year 2000 update: what the head and neck surgeon expects of the pathologist. Pathol Case Rev 5:183–188, 2000.
16. Chang HY, Lin JD, Chen JF, et al: Correlation of fine needle aspiration cytology and frozen section biopsies in the diagnosis of thyroid nodules. J Clin Pathol 50:1005–1009, 1997.
17. Quinn SF, Nelson HA, Demlow TA: Thyroid biopsies: fine-needle aspiration biopsy versus spring-activated core biopsy needle in 102 patients. J Vasc Interv Radiol 5:619–623, 1994.
18. Munn JS, Castelli M, Prinz RA, Walloch JL: Needle biopsy of nodular thyroid disease. Am Surg 54:438–443, 1988.
19. Lo Gerfo P: The value of coarse needle biopsy in evaluating thyroid nodules. Thyroidology 6:1–4, 1994.
20. Wang C, Guyton SP, Vickery AL Jr: A further note on the large needle biopsy of the thyroid gland. Surg Gynecol Obstet 156:508–510, 1983.
21. Miller JM: Evaluation of thyroid nodules. Accent on needle biopsy. Med Clin North Am 69:1063–1077, 1985.
22. Broughan TA, Esselstyn CB Jr: Large-needle thyroid biopsy: still necessary. Surgery 100:1138–1141, 1986.

23. Lang W, Georgii A, Stauch G, Kienzle E: The differentiation of atypical adenomas and encapsulated follicular carcinomas in the thyroid gland. Virchows Arch Pathol Anat 385:125–141, 1980.

24. Franssila KO, Ackerman LV, Brown CL: Follicular carcinoma. Semin Diagn Pathol 2:101–122, 1985.

25. Yamashina M: Follicular neoplasms of the thyroid. Total circumferential evaluation of the fibrous capsule. Am J Surg Pathol 16:392–400, 1992.

26. McHenry CR, Raeburn C, Strickland T, Marty JJ: The utility of routine frozen section examination for intraoperative diagnosis of thyroid cancer. Am J Surg 172:658–661, 1996.

27. Gibb GK, Pasieka JL: Assessing the need for frozen sections: still a valuable tool in thyroid surgery. Surgery 118:1005–1009, discussion 1009–1010, 1995.

28. Sabel MS, Staren ED, Gianakakis LM, et al: Use of fine-needle aspiration biopsy and frozen section in the management of the solitary thyroid nodule. Surgery 122:1021–1026, discussion 1026–1027, 1997.

29. Mulcahy MM, Cohen JI, Anderson PE, et al: Relative accuracy of fine-needle aspiration and frozen section in the diagnosis of well-differentiated thyroid cancer. Laryngoscope 108:494–496, 1998.

30. Deligdisch L, Subhani Z, Gordon RE: Primary mucinous carcinoma of the thyroid gland: report of a case and ultrastructural study. Cancer 45:2564–2567, 1980.

31. Carcangiu ML, Sibley RK, Rosai J: Clear cell change in primary thyroid tumors. A study of 38 cases. Am J Surg Pathol 9:705–722, 1985.

32. Schroder S, Husselmann H, Bocker W: Lipid-rich cell adenoma of the thyroid gland. Report of a peculiar thyroid tumour. Virchows Arch A Pathol Anat Histopathol 404:105–108, 1984.

33. Toth K, Peter I, Kremmer T, Sugar J: Lipid-rich cell thyroid adenoma: histopathology with comparative lipid analysis. Virchows Arch A Pathol Anat Histopathol 417:273–276, 1990.

34. Schroder S, Bocker W: Clear-cell carcinomas of thyroid gland: a clinicopathological study of 13 cases. Histopathology 10:75–89, 1986.

35. Vuitch F, Leavitt A: Papillary variant of follicular adenoma of thyroid (abstract). Mod Pathol 3:104A, 1990.

36. Hjorth L, Thomsen LB, Nielsen VT: Adenolipoma of the thyroid gland. Histopathology 10:91–96, 1986.

37. Laforga JB, Vierna J: Adenoma of thyroid gland containing fat (thyrolipoma). Report of a case. J Laryngol Otol 110:1088–1089, 1996.

38. Gnepp DR, Ogorzalek JM, Heffess CS: Fat-containing lesions of the thyroid gland. Am J Surg Pathol 13:605–612, 1989.

39. Gherardi G: Signet ring cell 'mucinous' thyroid adenoma: a follicle cell tumour with abnormal accumulation of thyroglobulin and a peculiar histochemical profile. Histopathology 11:317–326, 1987.

40. Mendelsohn G: Signet-cell–simulating microfollicular adenoma of the thyroid. Am J Surg Pathol 8:705–708, 1984.

41. Rigaud C, Peltier F, Bogomoletz WV: Mucin producing microfollicular adenoma of the thyroid. J Clin Pathol 38:277–280, 1985.

42. Alsop JE, Yerbury PJ, O'Donnell PJ, Heyderman E: Signet-ring cell microfollicular adenoma arising in a nodular ectopic thyroid. A case report. J Oral Pathol 15:518–519, 1986.

43. Hazard JB, Kenyon R: Atypical adenoma of the thyroid. Arch Pathol 58:554–563, 1954.

44. Lang W, Choritz H, Hundeshagen H: Risk factors in follicular thyroid carcinomas. A retrospective follow-up study covering a 14-year period with emphasis on morphological findings. Am J Surg Pathol 10:246–255, 1986.

45. Rosai J, Carcangiu ML, DeLellis RA: Tumors of the Thyroid Gland. Atlas of Tumor Pathology. Third Series, Fascicle 5. Washington, DC, Armed Forces Institute of Pathology, 1992.

46. Rosai J: Ackerman's Surgical Pathology. 8th ed. St. Louis, CV Mosby, 1996.

47. Hirokawa M, Carney JA: Cell membrane and cytoplasmic staining for MIB-1 in hyalinizing trabecular adenoma of the thyroid gland. Am J Surg Pathol 24:575–578, 2000.

48. Hirokawa M, Shimizu M, Manabe T, et al: Hyalinizing trabecular adenoma of the thyroid: its unusual cytoplasmic immunopositivity for MIB1. Pathol Int 45:399–401, 1995.

49. Papotti M, Riella P, Montemurro F, et al: Immunophenotypic heterogeneity of hyalinizing trabecular tumours of the thyroid. Histopathology 31:525–533, 1997.

50. Rothenberg HJ, Goellner JR, Carney JA: Hyalinizing trabecular adenoma of the thyroid gland: recognition and characterization of its cytoplasmic yellow body. Am J Surg Pathol 23:118–125, 1999.

51. Carney JA, Ryan J, Goellner JR: Hyalinizing trabecular adenoma of the thyroid gland. Am J Surg Pathol 11:583–591, 1987.

52. Sambade C, Sarabando F, Nesland JM, Sobrinho-Simoes M: Hyalinizing trabecular adenoma of the thyroid (case of the Ullensvang course). Hyalinizing spindle cell tumor of the thyroid with dual differentiation (variant of the so-called hyalinizing trabecular adenoma). Ultrastruct Pathol 13:275–280, 1989.

53. Katoh R, Jasani B, Williams ED: Hyalinizing trabecular adenoma of the thyroid. A report of three cases with immunohistochemical and ultrastructural studies. Histopathology 15:211–224, 1989.

54. Bronner MP, LiVolsi VA, Jennings TA: PLAT: paraganglioma-like adenoma of the thyroid. Surg Pathol 1:383–389, 1988.

55. Schmid KW, Mesewinkel F, Bocker W: Hyalinizing trabecular adenoma of the thyroid—morphology and differential diagnosis. Acta Med Austriaca 23:65–68, 1996.

56. Chetty R, Beydoun R, LiVolsi VA: Paraganglioma-like (hyalinizing trabecular) adenoma of the thyroid revisited. Pathology 26:429–431, 1994.

57. Chan JKC, Tse CCH, Chiu HS: Hyalinizing trabecular adenoma–like lesion in multinodular goiter. Histopathology 16:611–614, 1990.

58. Li M, Rosai J, Carcangiu ML: Hyalinizing trabecular adenoma of the thyroid: a distinct tumor type or a pattern of growth? Evaluation of 28 cases (abstract). Mod Pathol 8:54A, 1995.

59. Fonseca E, Nesland JM, Sobrinho-Simoes M: Expression of stratified epithelial-type cytokeratins in hyalinizing trabecular adenomas supports their relationship with papillary carcinomas of the thyroid. Histopathology 31:330–335, 1997.

60. Li M, Carcangiu ML, Rosai J: Abnormal intracellular and extracellular distribution of basement membrane material in papillary carcinoma and hyalinizing trabecular tumors of the thyroid: implication for deregulation of secretory pathways. Hum Pathol 28:1366–1372, 1997.

61. Hirokawa M, Carney JA, Ohtsuki Y: Hyalinizing trabecular adenoma and papillary carcinoma of the thyroid gland express different cytokeratin patterns. Am J Surg Pathol 24:877–881, 2000.

61a. Papotti M, Volante M, Giuliano A, et al: *RET/PTC* activation in hyalinizing trabecular tumors of the thyroid. Am J Surg Pathol 24:1615–1621, 2000.

61b. Cheung CC, Boerner SL, MacMillan CM, et al: Hyalinizing trabecular tumor of the thyroid: a variant of papillary carcinoma proved by molecular genetics. Am J Surg Pathol 24:1622–1626, 2000.

61c. LiVolsi VA: Hyalinizing trabecular adenoma of the thyroid: adenoma, carcinoma or neoplasm of uncertain malignant potential? Am J Surg Pathol 24:1683–1684, 2000.

62. Schlumberger MJ: Papillary and follicular thyroid carcinoma (review). N Engl J Med 338:297–306, 1998.

63. Wright PA, Lemoine NR, Mayall ES, et al: Papillary and follicular thyroid carcinomas show a different pattern of ras oncogene mutation. Br J Cancer 60:576–577, 1989.

64. Dahia PL, Marsh DJ, Zheng Z, et al: Somatic deletions and mutations in the Cowden disease gene, PTEN, in sporadic thyroid tumors. Cancer Res 57:4710–4713, 1997.

65. Porcellini A, Ciullo I, Pannain S, et al: Somatic mutations in the VI transmembrane segment of the thyrotropin receptor constitutively activate cAMP signalling in thyroid hyperfunctioning adenomas. Oncogene 11:1089–1093, 1995.

66. Porcellini A, Ciullo I, Laviola L, et al: Novel mutations of

thyrotropin receptor gene in thyroid hyperfunctioning adenomas. Rapid identification by fine needle aspiration biopsy. J Clin Endocrinol Metab 79:657–661, 1994.

67. Krohn K, Fuhrer D, Holzapfel HP, Paschke R: Clonal origin of toxic thyroid nodules with constitutively activating thyrotropin receptor mutations. J Clin Endocrinol Metab 83:130–134, 1998.

68. Pinducciu C, Borgonovo G, Arezzo A, et al: Toxic thyroid adenoma: absence of DNA mutations of the TSH receptor and G$_s$ alpha. Eur J Endocrinol 138:37–40, 1998.

69. Tonacchera M, Chiovato L, Pinchera A, et al: Hyperfunctioning thyroid nodules in toxic multinodular goiter share activating thyrotropin receptor mutations with solitary toxic adenoma. J Clin Endocrinol Metab 83:492–498, 1998.

70. Esapa C, Foster S, Johnson S, et al: G protein and thyrotropin receptor mutations in thyroid neoplasia. J Clin Endocrinol Metab 82:493–496, 1997.

71. Crile G Jr, Pontius KI, Hawk WA: Factors influencing the survival of patients with follicular carcinoma of the thyroid gland. Surg Gynecol Obstet 160:409–413, 1985.

72. Schroder S, Bocker W, Dralle H, et al: The encapsulated papillary carcinoma of the thyroid. A morphologic subtype of the papillary thyroid carcinoma. Cancer 54:90–93, 1984.

73. Shaha AR, Shah JP, Loree TR: Differentiated thyroid cancer presenting initially with distant metastasis. Am J Surg 174:474–476, 1997.

74. Lo CY, Lorentz TG, Wan KY: Follicular carcinoma of the thyroid gland in Hong Kong Chinese. Br J Surg 82:1095–1097, 1995.

75. Evans HL, Vassilopoulou-Sellin R: Follicular and Hürthle cell carcinomas of the thyroid: a comparative study. Am J Surg Pathol 22:1512–1520, 1998.

76. Woolner LB: Thyroid carcinoma: pathologic classification with data on prognosis. Semin Nucl Med 1:481–502, 1971.

77. Franssila KO: Prognosis in thyroid carcinoma. Cancer 36:1138–1146, 1975.

78. Schroder S, Pfannschmidt N, Dralle H, et al: The encapsulated follicular carcinoma of the thyroid. A clinicopathologic study of 35 cases. Virchows Arch A Pathol Anat Histopathol 402:259–273, 1984.

79. Lang W, Georgii A: Minimal invasive cancer in the thyroid. Clin Oncol 1:527–537, 1982.

80. Crile G Jr, Hawk WA: Carcinomas of the thyroid. Cleve Clin Q 38:97–104, 1971.

81. van Heerden JA, Hay ID, Goellner JR, et al: Follicular thyroid carcinoma with capsular invasion alone: a nonthreatening malignancy. Surgery 112:1130–1136, discussion 1136–1138, 1992.

82. Rossi RL, Nieroda C, Cady B, Wool MS: Malignancies of the thyroid gland. The Lahey Clinic experience. Surg Clin North Am 65:211–230, 1985.

83. Brooks JR, Starnes HF, Brooks DC, et al: Surgical therapy for thyroid carcinoma: a review of 1249 solitary thyroid nodules. Surgery 104:940–946, 1988.

84. Van Nguyen K, Dilawari RA: Predictive value of AMES scoring system in selection of extent of surgery in well differentiated carcinoma of thyroid. Am Surg 61:151–155, 1995.

85. Shah JP, Loree TR, Dharker D, Strong EW: Lobectomy versus total thyroidectomy for differentiated carcinoma of the thyroid: a matched-pair analysis. Am J Surg 166:331–335, 1993.

86. Wax MK, Briant TD: Completion thyroidectomy in the management of well-differentiated thyroid carcinoma. Otolaryngol Head Neck Surg 107:63–68, 1992.

87. Loh KC: Familial nonmedullary thyroid carcinoma: a meta-review of case series. Thyroid 7:107–113, 1997.

88. Lerch H, Schober O, Kuwert T, Saur HB: Survival of differentiated thyroid carcinoma studied in 500 patients. J Clin Oncol 15:2067–2075, 1997.

89. Pilotti S, Collini P, Mariani L, et al: Insular carcinoma: a distinct de novo entity among follicular carcinomas of the thyroid gland. Am J Surg Pathol 21:1466–1473, 1997.

90. Molberg K, Albores-Saavedra J: Hyalinizing trabecular carcinoma of the thyroid gland. Hum Pathol 25:192–197, 1994.

91. Gonzalez-Campora R, Fuentes-Vaamonde E, Hevia-Vazquez A, et al: Hyalinizing trabecular carcinoma of the thyroid gland: report of two cases of follicular cell thyroid carcinoma with hyalinizing trabecular pattern. Ultrastruct Pathol 22:39–46, 1998.

92. McCluggage WG, Sloan JM: Hyalinizing trabecular carcinoma of thyroid gland. Histopathology 28:357–362, 1996.

93. Ishimaru Y, Fukuda S, Kurano R, et al: Follicular thyroid carcinoma with clear cell change showing unusual ultrastructural features. Am J Surg Pathol 12:240–246, 1988.

94. LiVolsi VA: Current concepts in follicular tumors of the thyroid. Monogr Pathol 35:118–137, 1993.

95. Gosain AK, Clark OH: Hürthle cell neoplasms. Malignant potential. Arch Surg 119:515–519, 1984.

96. Watson RG, Brennan MD, Goellner JR, et al: Invasive Hürthle cell carcinoma of the thyroid: natural history and management. Mayo Clin Proc 59:851–855, 1984.

97. Evans HL: Follicular neoplasms of the thyroid. A study of 44 cases followed for a minimum of 10 years, with emphasis on differential diagnosis. Cancer 54:535–540, 1984.

98. Bronner MP, LiVolsi VA: Oxyphilic (Askanazy/Hürthle cell) tumors of the thyroid: microscopic features predict biologic behavior. Surg Pathol 1:137–150, 1988.

99. Baloch ZW, LiVolsi VA: Intravascular Kaposi's-like spindle cell proliferation of the capsular vessels of follicular-derived thyroid carcinomas. Mod Pathol 11:995–998, 1998.

100. Carcangiu ML, Bianchi S, Savino D, et al: Follicular Hürthle cell tumors of the thyroid gland. Cancer 68:1944–1953, 1991.

101. Chan JK, Tang SK, Tsang WY, et al: Histologic changes induced by fine-needle aspiration. Adv Anat Pathol 3:71–90, 1996.

102. Segev DL, Saji M, Phillips GS, et al: Polymerase chain reaction–based microsatellite polymorphism analysis of follicular and Hürthle cell neoplasms of the thyroid. J Clin Endocrinol Metab 83:2036–2042, 1998.

103. Chen H, Nicol TL, Zeiger MA, et al: Hürthle cell neoplasms of the thyroid: are there factors predictive of malignancy? Ann Surg 227:542–546, 1998.

104. Kini SR, Miller JM: Infarction of thyroid neoplasms following aspiration biopsy (abstract). Acta Cytol 30:591, 1986.

105. Jones JD, Pittman DL, Sandes LR: Necrosis of thyroid nodules after fine needle aspiration. Acta Cytol 29:29–31, 1985.

106. LiVolsi VA, Merino MJ: Worrisome histologic alterations following fine-needle aspiration of the thyroid (WHAFFT). Pathol Annu 29:99–120, 1994.

107. Flint A, Lloyd RV: Hürthle-cell neoplasms of the thyroid gland. Pathol Annu 25:37–52, 1990.

108. Thompson NW, Dunn EL, Batsakis JG, Nishiyama RH: Hürthle cell lesions of the thyroid gland. Surg Gynecol Obstet 139:555–560, 1974.

109. Gundry SR, Burney RE, Thompson NW, Lloyd R: Total thyroidectomy for Hürthle cell neoplasm of the thyroid. Arch Surg 118:529–532, 1983.

110. Miller RH, Estrada R, Sneed WF, Mace ML: Hürthle cell tumors of the thyroid gland. Laryngoscope 93:884–888, 1983.

111. Jorda M, Gonzalez-Campora R, Mora J, et al: Prognostic factors in follicular carcinoma of the thyroid. Arch Pathol Lab Med 117:631–635, 1993.

112. Rosen IB, Luk S, Katz I: Hürthle cell tumor behavior: dilemma and resolution. Surgery 98:777–783, 1985.

113. Heppe H, Armin A, Calandra DB, et al: Hürthle cell tumors of the thyroid gland. Surgery 98:1162–1165, 1985.

114. Arganini M, Behar R, Wu TC, et al: Hürthle cell tumors: a twenty-five-year experience. Surgery 100:1108–1115, 1986.

115. Caplan RH, Abellera RM, Kisken WA: Hürthle cell tumors of the thyroid gland. A clinicopathologic review and long-term follow-up. JAMA 251:3114–3117, 1984.

116. Gonzalez-Campora R, Herrero-Zapatero A, Lerma E, et al: Hürthle cell and mitochondrion-rich cell tumors. A clinicopathologic study. Cancer 57:1154–1163, 1986.

117. Saull SC, Kimmelman CP: Hürthle cell tumors of the thyroid gland. Otolaryngol Head Neck Surg 93:58–62, 1985.

118. Bondeson L, Bondeson AG, Ljungberg O, Tibblin S: Oxyphil tumors of the thyroid: follow-up of 42 surgical cases. Ann Surg 194:677–680, 1981.

119. Wasvary H, Czako P, Poulik J, Lucas R: Unilateral lobectomy

for Hürthle cell adenoma. Am Surg 64:729–732, discussion 732–733, 1998.

120. Grant CS, Barr D, Goellner JR, Hay ID: Benign Hürthle cell tumors of the thyroid: a diagnosis to be trusted? World J Surg 12:488–495, 1988.

121. Erickson LA, Jin L, Goellner JR, et al: Pathologic features, proliferative activity, and cyclin D1 expression in Hürthle cell neoplasms of the thyroid. Mod Pathol 13:186–192, 2000.

122. Tollefsen HR, Shah JP, Huvos AG: Hürthle cell carcinoma of the thyroid. Am J Surg 130:390–394, 1975.

123. Shaha AR, Loree TR, Shah JP: Prognostic factors and risk group analysis in follicular carcinoma of the thyroid. Surgery 118:1131–1136, discussion 1136–1138, 1995.

124. Papotti M, Torchio B, Grassi L, et al: Poorly differentiated oxyphilic (Hürthle cell) carcinomas of the thyroid. Am J Surg Pathol 20:686–694, 1996.

125. Davila RM, Bedrossian CW, Silverberg AB: Immunocytochemistry of the thyroid in surgical and cytologic specimens. Arch Pathol Lab Med 112:51–56, 1988.

126. Roque L, Clode A, Belge G, et al: Follicular thyroid carcinoma: chromosome analysis of 19 cases. Genes Chromosomes Cancer 21:250–255, 1998.

127. Pierotti MA, Bongarzone I, Borello MG, et al: Cytogenetics and molecular genetics of carcinomas arising from thyroid epithelial follicular cells. Genes Chromosomes Cancer 16:1–14, 1996.

128. Tung WS, Shevlin DW, Kaleem Z, et al: Allelotype of follicular thyroid carcinomas reveals genetic instability consistent with frequent nondisjunctional chromosomal loss. Genes Chromosomes Cancer 19:43–51, 1997.

129. Roque L, Castedo S, Clode A, Soares J: Deletion of 3p25 → pter in a primary follicular thyroid carcinoma and its metastasis. Genes Chromosomes Cancer 8:199–203, 1993.

130. Hemmer S, Wasenius VM, Knuutila S, et al: DNA copy number changes in thyroid carcinoma. Am J Pathol 154:1539–1547, 1999.

131. Grebe SK, McIver B, Hay ID, et al: Frequent loss of heterozygosity on chromosomes 3p and 17p without VHL or p53 mutations suggests involvement of unidentified tumor suppressor genes in follicular thyroid carcinoma. J Clin Endocrinol Metab 82:3684–3691, 1997.

132. Zedenius J, Wallin G, Svensson A, et al: Deletions of the long arm of chromosome 10 in progression of follicular thyroid tumors. Hum Genet 97:299–303, 1996.

133. Oyama T, Suzuki T, Hara F, et al: N-ras mutation of thyroid tumor with special reference to the follicular type. Pathol Int 45:45–50, 1995.

134. Bouras M, Parvaz P, Berger N, et al: Ha-ras oncogene (codon 12) mutation in thyroid carcinogenesis: analysis of 60 benign and malignant thyroid tumors. Ann Biol Clin 53:549–555, 1995.

135. Sapi Z, Lukacs G, Sztan M, et al: Contribution of p53 gene alterations to development of metastatic forms of follicular thyroid carcinoma. Diagn Mol Pathol 4:256–260, 1995.

135a. Kroll TG, Sarraf P, Pecciarini L, et al: *PAX8-PPAR* gamma 1 fusion oncogene in human thyroid carcinoma. Science 289:1357–1360, 2000.

136. Ghali VS, Jimenez EJ, Garcia RL: Distribution of Leu-7 antigen (HNK-1) in thyroid tumors: its usefulness as a diagnostic marker for follicular and papillary carcinomas. Hum Pathol 23:21–25, 1992.

137. De Micco C, Ruf J, Chrestian MA, et al: Immunohistochemical study of thyroid peroxidase in normal, hyperplastic, and neoplastic human thyroid tissues. Cancer 67:3036–3041, 1991.

138. Sack MJ, Astengo-Osuna C, Lin BT, et al: HBME-1 immunostaining in thyroid fine-needle aspirations: a useful marker in the diagnosis of carcinoma. Mod Pathol 10:668–674, 1997.

139. Miettinen M, Karkkainen P: Differential reactivity of HBME-1 and CD15 antibodies in benign and malignant thyroid tumours. Preferential reactivity with malignant tumours. Virchows Arch 429:213–219, 1996.

140. Tuccari G, Barresi G: Tissue polypeptide antigen in thyroid tumours of follicular cell origin: an immunohistochemical reevaluation for diagnostic purposes. Histopathology 16:377–381, 1990.

141. Kotani T, Asada Y, Aratake Y, et al: Diagnostic usefulness of dipeptidyl aminopeptidase IV monoclonal antibody in paraffin-embedded thyroid follicular tumours. J Pathol 168:41–45, 1992.

142. Aratake Y, Kotani T, Tamura K, et al: Dipeptidyl aminopeptidase IV staining of cytologic preparations to distinguish benign from malignant thyroid diseases. Am J Clin Pathol 96:306–310, 1991.

143. Johnson TL, Lloyd RV, Thor A: Expression of *ras* oncogene p21 antigen in normal and proliferative thyroid tissues. Am J Pathol 127:60–65, 1987.

144. Johnson TL, Lloyd RV, Burney RE, Thompson NW: Hürthle cell thyroid tumors. An immunohistochemical study. Cancer 59:107–112, 1987.

145. Mizukami Y, Nonomura A, Hashimoto T, et al: Immunohistochemical demonstration of epidermal growth factor and c-myc oncogene product in normal, benign and malignant thyroid tissues. Histopathology 18:11–18, 1991.

146. Erickson LA, Jin L, Wollan PC, et al: Expression of p27kip1 and Ki-67 in benign and malignant thyroid tumors. Mod Pathol 11:169–174, 1998.

147. Loy TS, Gelven PL, Mullins D, Diaz-Arias AA: Immunostaining for P-glycoprotein in the diagnosis of thyroid carcinomas [see comments]. Mod Pathol 5:200–202, 1992.

148. Chiappetta G, Tallini G, De Biasio MC, et al: Detection of high mobility group I HMGI(Y) protein in the diagnosis of thyroid tumors: HMGI(Y) expression represents a potential diagnostic indicator of carcinoma. Cancer Res 58:4193–4198, 1998.

149. Umbricht CB, Saji M, Westra WH, et al: Telomerase activity: a marker to distinguish follicular thyroid adenoma from carcinoma. Cancer Res 57:2144–2147, 1997.

150. Backdahl M, Wallin G, Akensten U, et al: Nuclear DNA measurements in follicular thyroid adenomas. Eur J Surg Oncol 15:125–129, 1989.

151. Hruban RH, Huvos AG, Traganos F, et al: Follicular neoplasms of the thyroid in men older than 50 years of age. A DNA flow cytometric study. Am J Clin Pathol 94:527–532, 1990.

152. Schurmann G, Mattfeldt T, Feichter G, et al: Stereology, flow cytometry, and immunohistochemistry of follicular neoplasms of the thyroid gland. Hum Pathol 22:179–184, 1991.

153. Oyama T, Vickery AL Jr, Preffer FI, Colvin RB: A comparative study of flow cytometry and histopathologic findings in thyroid follicular carcinomas and adenomas. Hum Pathol 25:271–275, 1994.

154. Joensuu H, Klemi P, Eerola E: DNA aneuploidy in follicular adenomas of the thyroid gland. Am J Pathol 124:373–376, 1986.

155. Schmidt RJ, Wang CA: Encapsulated follicular carcinoma of the thyroid: diagnosis, treatment and results. Surgery 100:1068–1076, 1986.

156. Segal K, Arad A, Lubin E, et al: Follicular carcinoma of the thyroid. Head Neck 16:533–538, 1994.

157. Zohar Y, Strauss M: Occult distant metastases of well-differentiated thyroid carcinoma. Head Neck 16:438–442, 1994.

158. Marcocci C, Pacini F, Eliseri R, et al: Clinical and biologic behavior of bone metastasis from differentiated thyroid carcinoma. Surgery 106:960–966, 1989.

159. Goldstein NS, Czako P, Neill JS: Metastatic minimally invasive (encapsulated) follicular and Hürthle cell thyroid carcinoma: a study of 34 patients. Mod Pathol 13:123–130, 2000.

160. von Wasielewski R, Rhein A, Werner M, et al: Immunohistochemical detection of E-cadherin in differentiated thyroid carcinomas correlates with clinical outcome. Cancer Res 57:2501–2507, 1997.

161. Joensuu H, Klemi P, Eerola E, Tuominen J: Influence of cellular DNA content on survival in differentiated thyroid cancer. Cancer 58:2462–2467, 1986.

162. Beaugie JM, Brown CL, Doniach I, Richardson JE: Primary malignant tumours of the thyroid: the relationship between histological classification and clinical behaviour. Br J Surg 63:173–181, 1976.

163. Hirabayashi RN, Lindsay S: Carcinoma of the thyroid gland: a statistical study of 390 patients. J Clin Endocrinol Metab 21:1596–1610, 1961.

164. McConahey WM, Hay ID, Woolner LB, et al: Papillary thyroid cancer treated at the Mayo Clinic, 1946 through 1970: initial manifestations, pathologic findings, therapy, and outcome. Mayo Clin Proc 61:978–996, 1986.

165. Meissner WA, Adler A: Papillary carcinoma of the thyroid, a study of the pattern in 226 patients. Arch Pathol 66:518–525, 1958.

166. Verge J, Guixa J, Alejo M, et al: Cervical cystic lymph node metastasis as first manifestation of occult papillary thyroid carcinoma: report of seven cases. Head Neck 21:370–374, 1999.

167. al-Talib RK, Wilkins BS, Theaker JM: Cystic metastasis of papillary carcinoma of the thyroid—an unusual presentation. Histopathology 20:176–178, 1992.

168. Hedinger C, Sobin L: Histological Typing of Thyroid Tumors. Geneva, World Health Organization, 1974.

169. Hedinger C, Williams ED, Sobin LH: The WHO histological classification of thyroid tumors: a commentary on the second edition. Cancer 63:908–911, 1989.

170. Carcangiu ML, Zampi G, Rosai J: Papillary thyroid carcinoma: a study of its many morphologic expressions and clinical correlates. Pathol Annu 20:1–44, 1985.

171. Chan JK: Papillary carcinoma of thyroid: classical and variants. Histol Histopathol 5:241–257, 1990.

172. Rosai J, Carcangiu ML: Pitfalls in the diagnosis of thyroid neoplasms. Pathol Res Pract 182:169–179, 1987.

173. Bruno J, Ciancia EM, Pingitore R: Thyroid papillary adenocarcinoma; lipomatous-type. Virchows Arch A Pathol Anat Histopathol 414:371–373, 1989.

174. Vestfrid MA: Papillary carcinoma of the thyroid gland with lipomatous stroma: report of a peculiar histological type of thyroid tumour. Histopathology 10:97–100, 1986.

175. Chan JK, Loo KT: Cribriform variant of papillary thyroid carcinoma. Arch Pathol Lab Med 114:622–624, 1990.

176. Guiter GE, DeLellis RA: Multinucleate giant cells in papillary thyroid carcinoma. A morphologic and immunohistochemical study. Am J Clin Pathol 106:765–768, 1996.

177. Isarangkul W: Dense fibrosis. Another diagnostic criterion for papillary thyroid carcinoma. Arch Pathol Lab Med 117:645–646, 1993.

178. Yamashita H, Noguchi S, Murakami N, et al: DNA ploidy and stromal bone formation as prognostic indicators of thyroid papillary carcinoma in aged patients: a retrospective study. Acta Pathol Jpn 43:22–27, 1993.

179. Johannessen JV, Sobrinho-Simoes M: The origin and significance of thyroid psammoma bodies. Lab Invest 43:287–296, 1980.

180. Vickery AL, Carcangiu ML, Johannessen JV: Papillary carcinoma. Semin Diagn Pathol 2:90–100, 1985.

181. Chan JK, Saw D: The grooved nucleus. A useful diagnostic criterion of papillary carcinoma of the thyroid. Am J Surg Pathol 10:672–679, 1986.

182. Glant MD, Berger EK, Davey DD: Intranuclear cytoplasmic inclusions in aspirates of follicular neoplasms of the thyroid. A report of two cases. Acta Cytol 28:576–580, 1984.

183. Oyama T: A histopathological, immunohistochemical and ultrastructural study of intranuclear cytoplasmic inclusions in thyroid papillary carcinoma. Virchows Arch A Pathol Anat Histopathol 414:91–104, 1989.

184. Scopa CD, Melachrinou M, Saradopoulou C, Merino MJ: The significance of the grooved nucleus in thyroid lesions. Mod Pathol 6:691–694, 1993.

185. Hazard JB: Nomenclature of thyroid tumors. In Young S, Inman DR (eds): Thyroid Neoplasia. London, Academic Press, 1968, pp 3–37.

186. Dickersin GR, Vickery AL Jr, Smith SB: Papillary carcinoma of the thyroid, oxyphil cell type, "clear cell" variant: a light- and electron-microscopic study. Am J Surg Pathol 4:501–509, 1980.

187. Variakojis D, Getz ML, Paloyan E, Straus FH: Papillary clear cell carcinoma of the thyroid gland. Hum Pathol 6:384–390, 1975.

188. Chan JK, Tse CC: Mucin production in metastatic papillary carcinoma of the thyroid. Hum Pathol 19:195–200, 1988.

189. Mlynek ML, Richter HJ, Leder LD: Mucin in carcinomas of the thyroid. Cancer 56:2647–2650, 1985.

190. Chen KT, Rosai J: Follicular variant of thyroid papillary carcinoma: a clinicopathologic study of six cases. Am J Surg Pathol 1:123–130, 1977.

191. Rosai J, Zampi G, Carcangiu ML: Papillary carcinoma of the thyroid. A discussion of its several morphologic expressions, with particular emphasis on the follicular variant. Am J Surg Pathol 7:809–817, 1983.

192. Carcangiu ML, Zampi G, Pupi A, et al: Papillary carcinoma of the thyroid. A clinicopathologic study of 241 cases treated at the University of Florence, Italy. Cancer 55:805–828, 1985.

193. Franssila KO: Is the differentiation between papillary and follicular thyroid carcinoma valid? Cancer 32:853–864, 1973.

194. Moreno A, Rodriguez JM, Sola J, et al: Encapsulated papillary neoplasm of the thyroid: retrospective clinicopathological study with long term follow up. Eur J Surg 162:177–180, 1996.

195. Vickery AL Jr: Thyroid papillary carcinoma. Pathological and philosophical controversies. Am J Surg Pathol 7:797–807, 1983.

196. Evans HL: Encapsulated papillary neoplasms of the thyroid. A study of 14 cases followed for a minimum of 10 years. Am J Surg Pathol 11:592–597, 1987.

197. Chan JK, Carcangiu ML, Rosai J: Papillary carcinoma of thyroid with exuberant nodular fasciitis–like stroma. Report of three cases. Am J Clin Pathol 95:309–314, 1991.

198. Michal M, Chlumska A, Fakan F: Papillary carcinoma of thyroid with exuberant nodular fasciitis–like stroma. Histopathology 21:577–579, 1992.

199. Mizukami Y, Nonomura A, Matsubara F, et al: Papillary carcinoma of the thyroid gland with fibromatosis-like stroma. Histopathology 20:355–357, 1992.

200. Terayama K, Toda S, Yonemitsu N, et al: Papillary carcinoma of the thyroid with exuberant nodular fasciitis–like stroma. Virchows Arch 431:291–295, 1997.

201. Acosta J, Rodriguez JM, Sola J, et al: Nodular fasciitis–type papillary thyroid carcinoma. Presentation of a new case. Eur J Surg Oncol 24:80–81, 1998.

202. Mizukami Y, Kurumaya H, Kitagawa T, et al: Papillary carcinoma of the thyroid gland with fibromatosis-like stroma: a case report and review of the literature. Mod Pathol 8:366–370, 1995.

203. Chan JK, Tsui MS, Tse CH: Diffuse sclerosing variant of papillary carcinoma of the thyroid: a histological and immunohistochemical study of three cases. Histopathology 11:191–201, 1987.

204. Hayashi Y, Sasao T, Takeichi N, et al: Diffuse sclerosing variant of papillary carcinoma of the thyroid. A histopathological study of four cases. Acta Pathol Jpn 40:193–198, 1990.

205. Fujimoto Y, Obara T, Ito Y, et al: Diffuse sclerosing variant of papillary carcinoma of the thyroid. Clinical importance, surgical treatment, and follow-up study. Cancer 66:2306–2312, 1990.

206. Albareda M, Puig-Domingo M, Wengrowicz S, et al: Clinical forms of presentation and evolution of diffuse sclerosing variant of papillary carcinoma and insular variant of follicular carcinoma of the thyroid. Thyroid 8:385–391, 1998.

207. Carcangiu ML, Bianchi S: Diffuse sclerosing variant of papillary thyroid carcinoma. Clinicopathologic study of 15 cases [see comments]. Am J Surg Pathol 13:1041–1049, 1989.

208. Carcangiu ML, Bianchi S, Rosai J: Diffuse sclerosing papillary carcinoma: report of 8 cases of a distinctive variant of thyroid malignancy (abstract). Lab Invest 56:10A, 1987.

209. Soares J, Limbert E, Sobrinho-Simoes M: Diffuse sclerosing variant of papillary thyroid carcinoma. A clinicopathologic study of 10 cases. Pathol Res Pract 185:200–206, 1989.

210. Schroder S, Bay V, Dumke K, et al: Diffuse sclerosing variant of papillary thyroid carcinoma. S-100 protein immunocytochemistry and prognosis. Virchows Arch A Pathol Anat Histopathol 416:367–371, 1990.

211. Gomez-Morales M, Aneiros J, Alvaro T, Navarro N: Langer-

hans' cells and prognosis of thyroid carcinoma (letter). Am J Clin Pathol 91:628–629, 1989.

212. Gomez-Morales M, Alvaro T, Munoz M, et al: Diffuse sclerosing papillary carcinoma of the thyroid gland: immunohistochemical analysis of the local host immune response. Histopathology 18:427–433, 1991.

213. Sobrinho-Simoes M, Soares J, Carneiro F: Diffuse follicular variant of papillary carcinoma of the thyroid: report of eight cases of a distinct aggressive type of thyroid tumor. Surg Pathol 3:189–203, 1990.

214. Mizukami Y, Nonomura A, Michigishi T, et al: Diffuse follicular variant of papillary carcinoma of the thyroid. Histopathology 27:575–577, 1995.

215. Hawk WA, Hazard JB: The many appearances of papillary carcinoma of the thyroid. Cleve Clin Q 43:207–215, 1976.

216. Johnson TL, Lloyd RV, Thompson NW, et al: Prognostic implications of the tall cell variant of papillary thyroid carcinoma. Am J Surg Pathol 12:22–27, 1988.

217. Ostrowski ML, Merino MJ: Tall cell variant of papillary thyroid carcinoma: a reassessment and immunohistochemical study with comparison to the usual type of papillary carcinoma of the thyroid. Am J Surg Pathol 20:964–974, 1996.

218. Ruter A, Dreifus J, Jones M, et al: Overexpression of p53 in tall cell variants of papillary thyroid carcinoma. Surgery 120:1046–1050, 1996.

219. Apel RL, Asa SL, LiVolsi VA: Papillary Hürthle cell carcinoma with lymphocytic stroma. "Warthin-like tumor" of the thyroid [see comments]. Am J Surg Pathol 19:810–814, 1995.

220. Vera-Sempere FJ, Prieto M, Camanas A: Warthin-like tumor of the thyroid: a papillary carcinoma with mitochondrion-rich cells and abundant lymphoid stroma. A case report. Pathol Res Pract 194:341–347, 1998.

221. Ozaki O, Ito K, Mimura T, et al: Papillary carcinoma of the thyroid. Tall-cell variant with extensive lymphocyte infiltration. Am J Surg Pathol 20:695–698, 1996.

221a. Baloch ZW, LiVolsi VA: Warthin-like papillary carcinoma of the thyroid. Arch Pathol Lab Med 124:1192–1195, 2000.

222. Nakamura T, Moriyama S, Nariya S, et al: Macrofollicular variant of papillary thyroid carcinoma. Pathol Int 48:467–470, 1998.

223. Albores-Saavedra J, Gould E, Vardaman C, Vuitch F: The macrofollicular variant of papillary thyroid carcinoma: a study of 17 cases. Hum Pathol 22:1195–1205, 1991.

224. Albores-Saavedra J, Housini I, Vuitch F, Snyder WH 3rd: Macrofollicular variant of papillary thyroid carcinoma with minor insular component. Cancer 80:1110–1116, 1997.

225. Sobrinho-Simoes MA, Nesland JM, Holm R, et al: Hürthle cell and mitochondrion-rich papillary carcinomas of the thyroid gland: an ultrastructural and immunocytochemical study. Ultrastruct Pathol 8:131–142, 1985.

226. Tscholl-Ducommun J, Hedinger CE: Papillary thyroid carcinomas. Morphology and prognosis. Virchows Arch Pathol Anat 396:19–39, 1982.

227. Beckner ME, Heffess CS, Oertel JE: Oxyphilic papillary thyroid carcinomas. Am J Clin Pathol 103:280–287, 1995.

228. Berho M, Suster S: The oncocytic variant of papillary carcinoma of the thyroid: a clinicopathologic study of 15 cases. Hum Pathol 28:47–53, 1997.

229. Katoh R, Sakamoto A, Kasai N, Yagawa K: Squamous differentiation in thyroid carcinoma. With special reference to histogenesis of squamous cell carcinoma of the thyroid. Acta Pathol Jpn 39:306–312, 1989.

230. Cameselle-Teijeiro J, Chan JK: Cribriform-morular variant of papillary carcinoma: a distinctive variant representing the sporadic counterpart of familial adenomatous polyposis–associated thyroid carcinoma? Mod Pathol 12:400–411, 1999.

231. Yamashita T, Hosoda Y, Kameyama K, et al: Peculiar nuclear clearing composed of microfilaments in papillary carcinoma of the thyroid. Cancer 70:2923–2928, 1992.

232. Harach HR, Williams GT, Williams ED: Familial adenomatous polyposis associated thyroid carcinoma: a distinct type of follicular cell neoplasm. Histopathology 25:549–561, 1994.

233. Cetta F, Toti P, Petracci M, et al: Thyroid carcinoma associated with familial adenomatous polyposis. Histopathology 31:231–236, 1997.

234. Perrier ND, van Heerden JA, Goellner JR, et al: Thyroid cancer in patients with familial adenomatous polyposis. World J Surg 22:738–742, discussion 743, 1998.

235. Soravia C, Sugg SL, Berk T, et al: Familial adenomatous polyposis–associated thyroid cancer: a clinical, pathological, and molecular genetics study. Am J Pathol 154:127–135, 1999.

236. Cetta F, Pelizzo MR, Curia MC, Barbarisi A: Genetics and clinicopathological findings in thyroid carcinomas associated with familial adenomatous polyposis. Am J Pathol 155:7–9, 1999.

237. Mizukami Y, Noguchi M, Michigishi T, et al: Papillary thyroid carcinoma in Kanazawa, Japan: prognostic significance of histological subtypes. Histopathology 20:243–250, 1992.

238. Carcangiu ML, Steeper T, Zampi G, Rosai J: Anaplastic thyroid carcinoma. A study of 70 cases. Am J Clin Pathol 83:135–158, 1985.

239. Kawahara E, Ooi A, Oda Y, et al: Papillary carcinoma of the thyroid gland with anaplastic transformation in the metastatic foci. An immunohistochemical study. Acta Pathol Jpn 36:921–927, 1986.

240. D'Antonio A, De Chiara A, Santoro M, et al: Warthin-like tumour of the thyroid gland: RET/PTC expression indicates it is a variant of papillary carcinoma. Histopathology 36:493–498, 2000.

241. Ito J, Noguchi S, Murakami N, Noguchi A: Factors affecting the prognosis of patients with carcinoma of the thyroid. Surg Gynecol Obstet 150:539–544, 1980.

242. Chen KT: Minute (less than 1 mm) occult papillary thyroid carcinoma with metastasis (letter). Am J Clin Pathol 91:746, 1989.

243. Kasai N, Sakamoto A: New subgrouping of small thyroid carcinomas. Cancer 60:1767–1770, 1987.

244. Laskin WB, James LP: Occult papillary carcinoma of the thyroid with pulmonary metastases. Hum Pathol 14:83–85, 1983.

245. Sampson RJ, Key CR, Buncher CR, Iijima S: Smallest forms of papillary carcinoma of the thyroid. A study of 141 microcarcinomas less than 0.1 cm in greatest dimension. Arch Pathol 91:334–339, 1971.

246. Strate SM, Lee EL, Childers JH: Occult papillary carcinoma of the thyroid with distant metastases. Cancer 54:1093–1100, 1984.

247. Sugitani I, Yanagisawa A, Shimizu A, et al: Clinicopathologic and immunohistochemical studies of papillary thyroid microcarcinoma presenting with cervical lymphadenopathy. World J Surg 22:731–737, 1998.

248. Fukunaga FH, Yatani R: Geographic pathology of occult thyroid carcinomas. Cancer 36:1095–1099, 1975.

249. Harach HR, Franssila KO, Wasenius VM: Occult papillary carcinoma of the thyroid. A "normal" finding in Finland. A systematic autopsy study. Cancer 56:531–538, 1985.

250. Sampson RJ: Prevalence and significance of occult thyroid cancer. In DeGroot LJ, Frohman LA, Kaplan DL (eds): Radiation-Associated Thyroid Carcinoma. New York, Grune & Stratton, 1977, pp 137–153.

251. Arellano L, Ibarra A: Occult carcinoma of the thyroid gland. Pathol Res Pract 179:88–91, 1984.

252. Bondeson L, Ljungberg O: Occult thyroid carcinoma at autopsy in Malmo, Sweden. Cancer 47:319–323, 1981.

253. Fukunaga FH, Lockett LJ: Thyroid carcinoma in the Japanese in Hawaii. Arch Pathol 92:6–13, 1971.

254. Lang W, Borrusch H, Bauer L: Occult carcinomas of the thyroid. Evaluation of 1,020 sequential autopsies. Am J Clin Pathol 90:72–76, 1988.

255. Ludwig G, Nishiyama RH: The prevalence of occult papillary thyroid carcinoma in 100 consecutive autopsies in an American population. Lab Invest 34:320–321, 1976.

256. Ottino A, Pianzola HM, Castelletto RH: Occult papillary thyroid carcinoma at autopsy in La Plata, Argentina. Cancer 64:547–551, 1989.

257. Sobrinho-Simoes MA, Sambade MC, Goncalves V: Latent thyroid carcinoma at autopsy: a study from Oporto, Portugal. Cancer 43:1702–1706, 1979.

258. Mills SE, Allen MS Jr: Congenital occult papillary carcinoma of the thyroid gland. Hum Pathol 17:1179–1181, 1986.

259. Komorowski RA, Hanson GA: Occult thyroid pathology in the young adult: an autopsy study of 138 patients without clinical thyroid disease. Hum Pathol 19:689–696, 1988.

260. Franssila KO, Harach HR: Occult papillary carcinoma of the thyroid in children and young adults. A systemic autopsy study in Finland. Cancer 58:715–719, 1986.

261. Rassel H, Thompson LD, Heffess CS: A rationale for conservative management of microscopic papillary carcinoma of the thyroid gland: a clinicopathologic correlation of 90 cases. Eur Arch Otorhinolaryngol 255:462–267, 1998.

262. LaGuette J, Matias-Guiu X, Rosai J: Thyroid paraganglioma: a clinicopathologic and immunohistochemical study of three cases. Am J Surg Pathol 21:748–753, 1997.

263. Schroder S, Pfannschmidt N, Bocker W, et al: Histopathologic types and clinical behaviour of occult papillary carcinoma of the thyroid. Pathol Res Pract 179:81–87, 1984.

264. Fonseca E, Nesland JM, Hoie J, Sobrinho-Simoes M: Pattern of expression of intermediate cytokeratin filaments in the thyroid gland: an immunohistochemical study of simple and stratified epithelial-type cytokeratins. Virchows Arch 430:239–245, 1997.

265. Raphael SJ, McKeown-Eyssen G, Asa SL: High-molecular-weight cytokeratin and cytokeratin-19 in the diagnosis of thyroid tumors. Mod Pathol 7:295–300, 1994.

266. Raphael SJ, Apel RL, Asa SL: Brief report: detection of high-molecular-weight cytokeratins in neoplastic and non-neoplastic thyroid tumors using microwave antigen retrieval. Mod Pathol 8:870–872, 1995.

267. Schelfhout LJ, Van Muijen GN, Fleuren GJ: Expression of keratin 19 distinguishes papillary thyroid carcinoma from follicular carcinomas and follicular thyroid adenoma. Am J Clin Pathol 92:654–658, 1989.

268. Pierotti MA, Vigneri P, Bongarzone I: Rearrangements of RET and NTRK1 tyrosine kinase receptors in papillary thyroid carcinomas. Recent Results Cancer Res 154:237–247, 1998.

269. Smanik PA, Furminger TL, Mazzaferri EL, Jhiang SM: Breakpoint characterization of the ret/PTC oncogene in human papillary thyroid carcinoma. Hum Mol Genet 4:2313–2318, 1995.

270. Santoro M, Carlomagno F, Hay ID, et al: Ret oncogene activation in human thyroid neoplasms is restricted to the papillary cancer subtype. J Clin Invest 89:1517–1522, 1992.

271. Sozzi G, Bongarzone I, Miozzo M, et al: A t(10;17) translocation creates the RET/PTC2 chimeric transforming sequence in papillary thyroid carcinoma. Genes Chromosomes Cancer 9:244–250, 1994.

272. Minoletti F, Butti MG, Coronelli S, et al: The two genes generating RET/PTC3 are localized in chromosomal band 10q11.2. Genes Chromosomes Cancer 11:51–57, 1994.

273. Fugazzola L, Pierotti MA, Vigano E, et al: Molecular and biochemical analysis of RET/PTC4, a novel oncogenic rearrangement between RET and ELE1 genes, in a post-Chernobyl papillary thyroid cancer. Oncogene 13:1093–1097, 1996.

274. Ponder BAJ: Multiple endocrine neoplasia type 2. In Vogelstein B, Kinzler KW (eds): The Genetic Basis of Human Cancer. New York, McGraw-Hill, 1998, pp 475–487.

275. Klugbauer S, Demidchik EP, Lengfelder E, Rabes HM: Molecular analysis of new subtypes of ELE/RET rearrangements, their reciprocal transcripts and breakpoints in papillary thyroid carcinomas of children after Chernobyl. Oncogene 16:671–675, 1998.

276. Klugbauer S, Demidchik EP, Lengfelder E, Rabes HM: Detection of a novel type of RET rearrangement (PTC5) in thyroid carcinomas after Chernobyl and analysis of the involved RET-fused gene RFG5. Cancer Res 58:198–203, 1998.

277. Bongarzone I, Butti MG, Fugazzola L, et al: Comparison of the breakpoint regions of ELE1 and RET genes involved in the generation of RET/PTC3 oncogene in sporadic and in radiation-associated papillary thyroid carcinomas. Genomics 42:252–259, 1997.

278. Williams GH, Rooney S, Thomas GA, et al: RET activation in adult and childhood papillary thyroid carcinoma using a reverse transcriptase-n-polymerase chain reaction approach on archival-nested material. Br J Cancer 74:585–589, 1996.

279. Lam AK, Montone KT, Nolan KA, Livolsi VA: Ret oncogene activation in papillary thyroid carcinoma: prevalence and implication on the histological parameters. Hum Pathol 29:565–568, 1998.

280. Delvincourt C, Patey M, Flament JB, et al: Ret and trk proto-oncogene activation in thyroid papillary carcinomas in French patients from the Champagne-Ardenne region. Clin Biochem 29:267–271, 1996.

281. Kitamura Y, Minobe K, Nakata T, et al: Ret/PTC3 is the most frequent form of gene rearrangement in papillary thyroid carcinomas in Japan. J Hum Genet 44:96–102, 1999.

282. Santoro M, Dathan NA, Berlingieri MT, et al: Molecular characterization of RET/PTC3; a novel rearranged version of the RET proto-oncogene in a human thyroid papillary carcinoma. Oncogene 9:509–516, 1994.

283. Lee CH, Hsu LS, Chi CW, et al: High frequency of rearrangement of the RET protooncogene (RET/PTC) in Chinese papillary thyroid carcinomas. J Clin Endocrinol Metab 83:1629–1632, 1998.

284. Bongarzone I, Butti MG, Coronelli S, et al: Frequent activation of ret protooncogene by fusion with a new activating gene in papillary thyroid carcinomas. Cancer Res 54:2979–2985, 1994.

285. Bongarzone I, Fugazzola L, Vigneri P, et al: Age-related activation of the tyrosine kinase receptor protooncogenes RET and NTRK1 in papillary thyroid carcinoma. J Clin Endocrinol Metab 81:2006–2009, 1996.

286. Zou M, Shi Y, Farid NR: Low rate of ret proto-oncogene activation (PTC/retTPC) in papillary thyroid carcinomas from Saudi Arabia. Cancer 73:176–180, 1994.

287. Tallini G, Ghossein RA, Emanuel J, et al: Detection of thyroglobulin, thyroid peroxidase, and RET/PTC1 mRNA transcripts in the peripheral blood of patients with thyroid disease. J Clin Oncol 16:1158–1166, 1998.

288. Mayr B, Potter E, Goretzki P, et al: Expression of Ret/PTC1, -2, -3, -delta3 and -4 in German papillary thyroid carcinoma. Br J Cancer 77:903–906, 1998.

289. Mayr B, Potter E, Goretzki P, et al: Expression of wild-type ret, ret/PTC and ret/PTC variants in papillary thyroid carcinoma in Germany. Langenbecks Arch Surg 384:54–59, 1999.

290. Soares P, Fonseca E, Wynford-Thomas D, Sobrinho-Simoes M: Sporadic ret-rearranged papillary carcinoma of the thyroid: a subset of slow growing, less aggressive thyroid neoplasms? J Pathol 185:71–78, 1998.

291. Nikiforov YE, Rowland JM, Bove KE, et al: Distinct pattern of ret oncogene rearrangements in morphological variants of radiation-induced and sporadic thyroid papillary carcinomas in children. Cancer Res 57:1690–1694, 1997.

292. Sugg SL, Ezzat S, Zheng L, et al: Oncogene profile of papillary thyroid carcinoma. Surgery 125:46–52, 1999.

293. Klugbauer S, Lengfelder E, Demidchik EP, Rabes HM: High prevalence of RET rearrangement in thyroid tumors of children from Belarus after the Chernobyl reactor accident. Oncogene 11:2459–2467, 1995.

294. Fugazzola L, Pilotti S, Pinchera A, et al: Oncogenic rearrangements of the RET proto-oncogene in papillary thyroid carcinomas from children exposed to the Chernobyl nuclear accident. Cancer Res 55:5617–5620, 1995.

295. Pisarchik AV, Ermak G, Demidchik EP, et al: Low prevalence of the ret/PTC3r1 rearrangement in a series of papillary thyroid carcinomas presenting in Belarus ten years post-Chernobyl. Thyroid 8:1003–1008, 1998.

296. Bounacer A, Wicker R, Schlumberger M, et al: Oncogenic rearrangements of the ret proto-oncogene in thyroid tumors induced after exposure to ionizing radiation. Biochimie 79:619–623, 1997.

297. Kopp P, Jameson JL: Thyroid disorders. In Jameson JL (ed): Principles of Molecular Medicine. Totowa, NJ, Humana Press, 1998, pp 459–473.

298. Bongarzone I, Vigneri P, Mariani L, et al: RET/NTRK1 rearrangements in thyroid gland tumors of the papillary carcinoma family: correlation with clinicopathological features. Clin Cancer Res 4:223–228, 1998.

299. Beimfohr C, Klugbauer S, Demidchik EP, et al: NTRK1 rearrangement in papillary thyroid carcinomas of children after

the Chernobyl reactor accident. Int J Cancer 80:842–847, 1999.

300. Chan JKC, Tsang WYW: Endocrine malignancies that may mimic benign lesions. Semin Diagn Pathol 12:45–63, 1995.

301. Cheifetz RE, Davis NL, Robinson BW, et al: Differentiation of thyroid neoplasms by evaluating epithelial membrane antigen, Leu-7 antigen, epidermal growth factor receptor, and DNA content. Am J Surg 167:531–534, 1994.

302. Viale G, Dell'Orto P, Coggi G, Gambacorta M: Coexpression of cytokeratins and vimentin in normal and diseased thyroid glands. Lack of diagnostic utility of vimentin immunostaining. Am J Surg Pathol 13:1034–1040, 1989.

303. Yamamoto Y, Izumi K, Otsuka H: An immunohistochemical study of epithelial membrane antigen, cytokeratin, and vimentin in papillary thyroid carcinoma. Recognition of lethal and favorable prognostic types [see comments]. Cancer 70:2326–2333, 1992.

304. Damiani S, Fratamico F, Lapertosa G, et al: Alcian blue and epithelial membrane antigen are useful markers in differentiating benign from malignant papillae in thyroid lesions. Virchows Arch A Pathol Anat Histopathol 419:131–135, 1991.

305. Lucas SD, Ek B, Rask L, et al: Aberrantly expressed cytokeratin 1, a tumor-associated autoantigen in papillary thyroid carcinoma. Int J Cancer 73:171–177, 1997.

306. Miettinen M, Kovatich AJ, Karkkainen P: Keratin subsets in papillary and follicular thyroid lesions. A paraffin section analysis with diagnostic implications. Virchows Arch 431:407–413, 1997.

307. Tanaka T, Umeki K, Yamamoto I, et al: Immunohistochemical loss of thyroid peroxidase in papillary thyroid carcinoma: strong suppression of peroxidase gene expression. J Pathol 179:89–94, 1996.

308. Umeki K, Tanaka T, Yamamoto I, et al: Differential expression of dipeptidyl peptidase IV (CD26) and thyroid peroxidase in neoplastic thyroid tissues. Endocr J 43:53–60, 1996.

309. Khan A, Baker SP, Patwardhan NA, Pullman JM: CD57 (Leu-7) expression is helpful in diagnosis of the follicular variant of papillary thyroid carcinoma. Virchows Arch 432:427–432, 1998.

310. Loy TS, Darkow GV, Spollen LE, Diaz-Arias AA: Immunostaining for Leu-7 in the diagnosis of thyroid carcinoma. Arch Pathol Lab Med 118:172–174, 1994.

311. Chhieng DC, Ross JS, McKenna BJ: CD44 immunostaining of thyroid fine-needle aspirates differentiates thyroid papillary carcinoma from other lesions with nuclear grooves and inclusions. Cancer 81:157–162, 1997.

312. Ross JS, del Rosario AD, Sanderson B, Bui HX: Selective expression of CD44 cell-adhesion molecule in thyroid papillary carcinoma fine-needle aspirates. Diagn Cytopathol 14:287–291, 1996.

313. van Hoeven KH, Kovatich AJ, Miettinen M: Immunocytochemical evaluation of HBME-1, CA 19-9, and CD-15 (Leu-M1) in fine-needle aspirates of thyroid nodules. Diagn Cytopathol 18:93–97, 1998.

314. Anwar F, Emond MJ, Schmidt RA, et al: Retinoblastoma expression in thyroid neoplasms. Mod Pathol 13:562–569, 2000.

315. Gimm O, Rath FW, Dralle H: Pattern of lymph node metastases in papillary thyroid carcinoma. Br J Surg 85:252–254, 1998.

316. Lindsay A: Papillary thyroid carcinoma revisited. In Hedinger CE (ed): Thyroid Cancer. Berlin, Springer-Verlag, 1969, pp 29–32.

317. Cady B, Rossi R: An expanded view of risk-group definition in differentiated thyroid carcinoma. Surgery 104:947–953, 1988.

318. Cady B: Papillary carcinoma of the thyroid gland: treatment based on risk group definition. Surg Oncol Clin North Am 7:633–644, 1998.

319. Hay ID, Bergstralh EJ, Goellner JR, et al: Predicting outcome in papillary thyroid carcinoma: development of a reliable prognostic scoring system in a cohort of 1779 patients surgically treated at one institution during 1940 through 1989. Surgery 114:1050–1057, discussion 1057–1058, 1993.

320. Sanders LE, Cady B: Differentiated thyroid cancer: reexami-

nation of risk groups and outcome of treatment. Arch Surg 133:419–425, 1998.

321. Woolner LB, Beahrs OH, Black BM, et al: Thyroid carcinoma: general considerations and follow-up data on 1181 cases. In Young S, Inman DR (eds): Thyroid Neoplasia. London, Academic Press, 1968, pp 51–76.

322. Tubiana M, Schlumberger M, Rougier P, et al: Long-term results and prognostic factors in patients with differentiated thyroid carcinoma. Cancer 55:794–804, 1985.

323. Mazzaferri EL: Papillary thyroid carcinoma: factors influencing prognosis and current therapy. Semin Oncol 14:315–332, 1987.

324. Beenken S, Guillamondegui O, Shallenberger R, et al: Prognostic factors in patients dying of well-differentiated thyroid cancer. Arch Otolaryngol Head Neck Surg 115:326–330, 1989.

325. Shaha AR, Shah JP, Loree TR: Risk group stratification and prognostic factors in papillary carcinoma of thyroid. Ann Surg Oncol 3:534–538, 1996.

326. Salvesen H, Njolstad PR, Akslen LA, et al: Papillary thyroid carcinoma: a multivariate analysis of prognostic factors including an evaluation of the p-TNM staging system. Eur J Surg 158:583–589, 1992.

327. Bellantone R, Lombardi CP, Boscherini M, et al: Prognostic factors in differentiated thyroid carcinoma: a multivariate analysis of 234 consecutive patients. J Surg Oncol 68:237–241, 1998.

328. Noguchi S, Murakami N, Kawamoto H: Classification of papillary cancer of the thyroid based on prognosis. World J Surg 18:552–557, discussion 558, 1994.

329. Kashima K, Yokoyama S, Noguchi S, et al: Chronic thyroiditis as a favorable prognostic factor in papillary thyroid carcinoma. Thyroid 8:197–202, 1998.

330. Frauenhoffer CM, Patchefsky AS, Cobanoglu A: Thyroid carcinoma: a clinical and pathologic study of 125 cases. Cancer 43:2414–2421, 1979.

331. Tennvall J, Biorklund A, Moller T, et al: Prognostic factors of papillary, follicular and medullary carcinomas of the thyroid gland. Retrospective multivariate analysis of 216 patients with a median follow-up of 11 years. Acta Radiol Oncol 24:17–24, 1985.

332. Tennvall J, Biorklund A, Moller T, et al: Is the EORTC prognostic index of thyroid cancer valid in differentiated thyroid carcinoma? Retrospective multivariate analysis of differentiated thyroid carcinoma with long follow-up. Cancer 57:1405–1414, 1986.

333. Rodriguez JM, Moreno A, Parrilla P, et al: Papillary thyroid microcarcinoma: clinical study and prognosis. Eur J Surg 163:255–259, 1997.

334. Vickery AL Jr, Wang CA, Walker AM: Treatment of intrathyroidal papillary carcinoma of the thyroid. Cancer 60:2587–2595, 1987.

335. McCaffrey TV, Bergstralh EJ, Hay ID: Locally invasive papillary thyroid carcinoma: 1940–1990 [see comments]. Head Neck 16:165–172, 1994.

336. Yasumoto K, Miyagi C, Nakashima T, et al: Papillary and follicular thyroid carcinoma: the treatment results of 357 patients at the National Kyushu Cancer Centre of Japan. J Laryngol Otol 110:657–662, 1996.

337. Hughes CJ, Shaha AR, Shah JP, Loree TR: Impact of lymph node metastasis in differentiated carcinoma of the thyroid: a matched-pair analysis. Head Neck 18:127–132, 1996.

338. Scheumann GF, Gimm O, Wegener G, et al: Prognostic significance and surgical management of locoregional lymph node metastases in papillary thyroid cancer. World J Surg 18:559–567, discussion 567–568, 1994.

339. Akslen LA, LiVolsi VA: Prognostic significance of histologic grading compared with subclassification of papillary thyroid carcinoma [see comments]. Cancer 88:1902–1908, 2000.

340. Pilotti S, Collini P, Manzari A, et al: Poorly differentiated forms of papillary thyroid carcinoma: distinctive entities or morphological patterns? Semin Diagn Pathol 12:249–255, 1995.

341. Andersen PE, Kinsella J, Loree TR, et al: Differentiated carcinoma of the thyroid with extrathyroidal extension. Am J Surg 170:467–470, 1995.

342. Sakamoto A, Kasai N, Sugano H: Poorly differentiated carcinoma of the thyroid. A clinicopathologic entity for a high-risk group of papillary and follicular carcinomas. Cancer 52:1849–1855, 1983.

343. Akslen LA: Prognostic importance of histologic grading in papillary thyroid carcinoma. Cancer 72:2680–2685, 1993.

344. Schroder S, Schwarz W, Rehpenning W, et al: Dendritic/Langerhans cells and prognosis in patients with papillary thyroid carcinomas. Immunocytochemical study of 106 thyroid neoplasms correlated to follow-up data. Am J Clin Pathol 89:295–300, 1988.

345. Schroder S, Schwarz W, Rehpenning W, et al: Prognostic significance of Leu-M1 immunostaining in papillary carcinomas of the thyroid gland. Virchows Arch A Pathol Anat Histopathol 411:435–439, 1987.

346. Goldenberg JD, Portugal LG, Wenig BL, et al: Well-differentiated thyroid carcinomas: p53 mutation status and microvessel density. Head Neck 20:152–158, 1998.

347. Godballe C, Asschenfeldt P, Jorgensen KE, et al: Prognostic factors in papillary and follicular thyroid carcinomas: p53 expression is a significant indicator of prognosis. Laryngoscope 108:243–249, 1998.

348. Omura K, Nagasato A, Kanehira E, et al: Retinoblastoma protein and proliferating-cell nuclear antigen expression as predictors of recurrence in well-differentiated papillary thyroid carcinoma. J Clin Oncol 15:3458–3463, 1997.

349. Dhar DK, Kubota H, Kotoh T, et al: Tumor vascularity predicts recurrence in differentiated thyroid carcinoma. Am J Surg 176:442–447, 1998.

350. Ishiwata T, Iino Y, Takei H, et al: Tumor angiogenesis as an independent prognostic indicator in human papillary thyroid carcinoma. Oncol Rep 5:1343–1348, 1998.

351. Akslen LA, Livolsi VA: Increased angiogenesis in papillary thyroid carcinoma but lack of prognostic importance [see comments]. Hum Pathol 31:439–442, 2000.

352. Hamming JF, Schelfhout LJ, Cornelisse CJ, et al: Prognostic value of nuclear DNA content in papillary and follicular thyroid cancer. World J Surg 12:503–508, 1988.

353. Hara H, Fulton N, Yashiro T, et al: N-ras mutation: an independent prognostic factor for aggressiveness of papillary thyroid carcinoma. Surgery 116:1010–1016, 1994.

354. Carcangiu ML, Zampi G, Rosai J: Poorly differentiated ("insular") thyroid carcinoma. A reinterpretation of Langhans' "wucherende Struma." Am J Surg Pathol 8:655–668, 1984.

355. Papotti M, Botto Micca F, Favero A, et al: Poorly differentiated thyroid carcinomas with primordial cell component. A group of aggressive lesions sharing insular, trabecular, and solid patterns. Am J Surg Pathol 17:291–301, 1993.

356. van den Brekel MW, Hekkenberg RJ, Asa SL, et al: Prognostic features in tall cell papillary carcinoma and insular thyroid carcinoma. Laryngoscope 107:254–259, 1997.

357. Tallini G, Garcia-Rostan G, Herrero A, et al: Downregulation of p27KIP1 and Ki67/Mib1 labeling index support the classification of thyroid carcinoma into prognostically relevant categories. Am J Surg Pathol 23:678–685, 1999.

358. Ringel MD, Burman KD, Shmookler BM: Clinical aspects of miscellaneous and unusual types of thyroid cancers. *In* Wartofsky L (ed): Thyroid Cancer, A Comprehensive Guide to Clinical Management. Totowa, NJ, Humana Press, 2000, pp 421–451.

359. Kapp DS, LiVolsi VA, Sanders MM: Anaplastic carcinoma following well-differentiated thyroid cancer: etiological considerations. Yale J Biol Med 55:521–528, 1982.

360. Flynn SD, Forman BH, Stewart AF, Kinder BK: Poorly differentiated ("insular") carcinoma of the thyroid gland: an aggressive subset of differentiated thyroid neoplasms. Surgery 104:963–970, 1988.

361. Pietribiasi F, Sapino A, Papotti M, Bussolati G: Cytologic features of poorly differentiated 'insular' carcinoma of the thyroid, as revealed by fine-needle aspiration biopsy. Am J Clin Pathol 94:687–692, 1990.

362. Resnick MB, Schacter P, Finkelstein Y, et al: Immunohistochemical analysis of p27/kip1 expression in thyroid carcinoma. Mod Pathol 11:735–739, 1998.

363. Pilotti S, Collini P, Del Bo R, et al: A novel panel of antibodies that segregates immunocytochemically poorly differentiated carcinoma from undifferentiated carcinoma of the thyroid gland. Am J Surg Pathol 18:1054–1064, 1994.

364. Dobashi Y, Sakamoto A, Sugimura H, et al: Overexpression of p53 as a possible prognostic factor in human thyroid carcinoma. Am J Surg Pathol 17:375–381, 1993.

365. Manenti G, Pilotti S, Re FC, et al: Selective activation of ras oncogenes in follicular and undifferentiated thyroid carcinomas. Eur J Cancer 7:987–993, 1994.

366. Lam KY, Lo CY, Chan KW, Wan KY: Insular and anaplastic carcinoma of the thyroid: a 45-year comparative study at a single institution and a review of the significance of p53 and p21. Ann Surg 231:329–338, 2000.

367. Johnson MW, Hunnicutt JW, Bilbao JE, et al: Poorly differentiated thyroid carcinoma with focal insular pattern: clinicopathologic correlation (abstract). Am J Clin Pathol 94:497–498, 1990.

368. Sasaki A, Daa T, Kashima K, et al: Insular component as a risk factor of thyroid carcinoma. Pathol Int 46:939–946, 1996.

369. Ashfaq R, Vuitch F, Delgado R, Albores-Saavedra J: Papillary and follicular thyroid carcinomas with an insular component. Cancer 73:416–423, 1994.

370. LiVolsi VA, Brooks JJ, Arendash-Durand B: Anaplastic thyroid tumors. Immunohistology. Am J Clin Pathol 87:434–442, 1987.

371. Nishiyama RH, Dunn EL, Thompson NW: Anaplastic spindle-cell and giant-cell tumors of the thyroid gland. Cancer 30:113–127, 1972.

372. Venkatesh YS, Ordonez NG, Schultz PN, et al: Anaplastic carcinoma of the thyroid. A clinicopathologic study of 121 cases. Cancer 66:321–330, 1990.

373. Rosai J, Saxen EA, Woolner L: Undifferentiated and poorly differentiated carcinoma. Semin Diagn Pathol 2:123–126, 1985.

374. Aldinger KA, Samaan NA, Ibanez M, Hill CS Jr: Anaplastic carcinoma of the thyroid: a review of 84 cases of spindle and giant cell carcinoma of the thyroid. Cancer 41:2267–2275, 1978.

375. Spires JR, Schwartz MR, Miller RH: Anaplastic thyroid carcinoma. Association with differentiated thyroid cancer. Arch Otolaryngol Head Neck Surg 114:40–44, 1988.

376. Galera-Davidson H, Bibbo M, Dytch HE, et al: Nuclear DNA in anaplastic thyroid carcinoma with a differentiated component. Histopathology 11:715–722, 1987.

377. Lo CY, Lam KY, Wan KY: Anaplastic carcinoma of the thyroid. Am J Surg 177:337–339, 1999.

378. Cibull ML, Gray GF: Ultrastructure of osteoclastoma-like giant cell tumor of thyroid. Am J Surg Pathol 2:401–405, 1978.

379. Silverberg SG, DeGiorgi LS: Osteoclastoma-like giant cell tumor of the thyroid. Report of a case with prolonged survival following partial excision and radiotherapy. Cancer 31:621–625, 1973.

380. Gaffey MJ, Lack EE, Christ ML, Weiss LM: Anaplastic thyroid carcinoma with osteoclast-like giant cells. A clinicopathologic, immunohistochemical, and ultrastructural study. Am J Surg Pathol 15:160–168, 1991.

381. Wan SK, Chan JK, Tang SK: Paucicellular variant of anaplastic thyroid carcinoma. A mimic of Reidel's thyroiditis. Am J Clin Pathol 105:388–393, 1996.

382. Blasius S, Edel G, Grunert J, et al: Anaplastic thyroid carcinoma with osteosarcomatous differentiation. Pathol Res Pract 190:507–510, discussion 511–512, 1994.

383. Bakri K, Shimaoka K, Rao U, Tsukada Y: Adenosquamous cell carcinoma of the thyroid after radiotherapy for Hodgkin's disease. Cancer 52:465–470, 1983.

384. Harada T, Katagiri M, Tsukayama C, et al: Squamous cell carcinoma with cyst of the thyroid. J Surg Oncol 42:136–143, 1989.

385. Huang TY, Assor D: Primary squamous cell carcinoma of the thyroid gland: a report of four cases. Am J Clin Pathol 55:93–98, 1971.

386. Huang TY, Lin SG: Primary squamous cell carcinoma of the thyroid. Indiana Med 79:763–764, 1986.

387. Sarda AK, Bal S, Arunabh, et al: Squamous cell carcinoma of the thyroid. J Surg Oncol 39:175–178, 1988.

388. Simpson WJ, Carruthers J: Squamous cell carcinoma of the thyroid gland. Am J Surg 156:44–46, 1988.
389. Shimaoka K, Tsukada Y: Squamous cell carcinomas and adenosquamous carcinomas originating from the thyroid gland. Cancer 46:1833–1842, 1980.
390. Theander C, Loden B, Berglund J, Seidal T: Primary squamous carcinoma of the thyroid—a case report. J Laryngol Otol 107:1155–1158, 1993.
391. Harada T, Shimaoka K, Katagiri M, et al: Rarity of squamous cell carcinoma of the thyroid: autopsy review. World J Surg 18:542–546, 1994.
392. Burt A, Goudie RB: Diagnosis of primary thyroid carcinoma by immunohistological demonstration of thyroglobulin. Histopathology 3:279–286, 1979.
393. Ralfkiaer N, Gatter KC, Alcock C, et al: The value of immunocytochemical methods in the differential diagnosis of anaplastic thyroid tumours. Br J Cancer 52:167–170, 1985.
394. Myskow MW, Krajewski AS, Dewar AE, et al: The role of immunoperoxidase techniques on paraffin embedded tissue in determining the histogenesis of undifferentiated thyroid neoplasms. Clin Endocrinol 24:335–341, 1986.
395. Eusebi V, Damiani S, Riva C, et al: Calcitonin free oat-cell carcinoma of the thyroid gland. Virchows Arch A Pathol Anat Histopathol 417:267–271, 1990.
396. Wolf BC, Sheahan K, DeCoste D, et al: Immunohistochemical analysis of small cell tumors of the thyroid gland: an Eastern Cooperative Oncology Group study. Hum Pathol 23:1252–1261, 1992.
397. Totsch M, Dobler G, Feichtinger H, et al: Malignant hemangioendothelioma of the thyroid. Its immunohistochemical discrimination from undifferentiated thyroid carcinoma [see comments]. Am J Surg Pathol 14:69–74, 1990.
398. Eckert F, Schmid U, Gloor F, Hedinger C: Evidence of vascular differentiation in anaplastic tumours of the thyroid—an immunohistological study. Virchows Arch A Pathol Anat Histopathol 410:203–215, 1986.
399. Albores-Saavedra J, Nadji M, Civantos F, Morales AR: Thyroglobulin in carcinoma of the thyroid: an immunohistochemical study. Hum Pathol 14:62–66, 1983.
400. Matias-Guiu X, Villanueva A, Cuatrecasas M, et al: p53 in a thyroid follicular carcinoma with foci of poorly differentiated and anaplastic carcinoma. Pathol Res Pract 192:1242–1249, discussion 1250–1251, 1996.
401. Holm R, Nesland JM: Retinoblastoma and p53 tumour suppressor gene protein expression in carcinomas of the thyroid gland. J Pathol 172:267–272, 1994.
402. Soares P, Cameselle-Teijeiro J, Sobrinho-Simoes M: Immunohistochemical detection of p53 in differentiated, poorly differentiated and undifferentiated carcinomas of the thyroid. Histopathology 24:205–210, 1994.
403. Dobashi Y, Sugimura H, Sakamoto A, et al: Stepwise participation of p53 gene mutation during dedifferentiation of human thyroid carcinomas. Diagn Mol Pathol 3:9–14, 1994.
404. Pollina L, Pacini F, Fontanini G, et al: bcl-2, p53 and proliferating cell nuclear antigen expression is related to the degree of differentiation in thyroid carcinomas. Br J Cancer 73:139–143, 1996.
405. Garcia-Rostan G, Tallini G, Herrero A, et al: Frequent mutation and nuclear localization of beta-catenin in anaplastic thyroid carcinoma. Cancer Res 59:1811–1815, 1999.
406. Sherman SI: Anaplastic carcinoma: prognosis. In Wartofsky L (ed): Thyroid Cancer, A Comprehensive Guide to Clinical Management. Totowa, NJ, Humana Press, 2000, pp 345–348.
407. Kobayashi T, Asakawa H, Umeshita K, et al: Treatment of 37 patients with anaplastic carcinoma of the thyroid. Head Neck 18:36–41, 1996.
408. Passler C, Scheuba C, Prager G, et al: Anaplastic (undifferentiated) thyroid carcinoma (ATC). A retrospective analysis. Langenbecks Arch Surg 384:284–293, 1999.
409. Lu WT, Lin JD, Huang HS, Chao TC: Does surgery improve the survival of patients with advanced anaplastic thyroid carcinoma? Otolaryngol Head Neck Surg 118:728–731, 1998.
410. Nel CJ, van Heerden JA, Goellner JR, et al: Anaplastic carcinoma of the thyroid: a clinicopathologic study of 82 cases. Mayo Clin Proc 60:51–58, 1985.
411. Tan RK, Finley RK 3rd, Driscoll D, et al: Anaplastic carcinoma of the thyroid: a 24-year experience. Head Neck 17:41–47, discussion 47–48, 1995.
412. Nilsson O, Lindeberg J, Zedenius J, et al: Anaplastic giant cell carcinoma of the thyroid gland: treatment and survival over a 25-year period. World J Surg 22:725–730, 1998.
413. Evans HL: Columnar-cell carcinoma of the thyroid. A report of two cases of an aggressive variant of thyroid carcinoma. Am J Clin Pathol 85:77–80, 1986.
414. Ferreiro JA, Hay ID, Lloyd RV: Columnar cell carcinoma of the thyroid: report of three additional cases. Hum Pathol 27:1156–1160, 1996.
415. Sobrinho-Simoes M, Nesland JM, Johannessen JV: Columnar-cell carcinoma. Another variant of poorly differentiated carcinoma of the thyroid. Am J Clin Pathol 89:264–267, 1988.
416. Mizukami Y, Nonomura A, Michigishi T, et al: Columnar cell carcinoma of the thyroid gland: a case report and review of the literature. Hum Pathol 25:1098–1101, 1994.
417. Berends D, Mouthaan PJ: Columnar-cell carcinoma of the thyroid. Histopathology 20:360–362, 1992.
418. Gaertner EM, Davidson M, Wenig BM: The columnar cell variant of thyroid papillary carcinoma. Case report and discussion of an unusually aggressive thyroid papillary carcinoma. Am J Surg Pathol 19:940–947, 1995.
419. Akslen LA, Varhaug JE: Thyroid carcinoma with mixed tall-cell and columnar-cell features. Am J Clin Pathol 94:442–445, 1990.
420. Genton CY, Dutoit M, Portmann L, et al: Pathologic fracture of the femur neck as first manifestation of a minute columnar cell carcinoma of the thyroid gland. Pathol Res Pract 194:861–863, 1998.
421. Shimizu M, Hirokawa M, Manabe T: Tall cell variant of papillary thyroid carcinoma with foci of columnar cell component. Virchows Arch 434:173–175, 1999.
422. Wenig BM, Thompson LD, Adair CF, et al: Thyroid papillary carcinoma of columnar cell type: a clinicopathologic study of 16 cases. Cancer 82:740–753, 1998.
423. Hui PK, Chan JK, Cheung PS, Gwi E: Columnar cell carcinoma of the thyroid. Fine needle aspiration findings in a case. Acta Cytol 34:355–358, 1990.
424. Evans HL: Encapsulated columnar-cell neoplasms of the thyroid. A report of four cases suggesting a favorable prognosis. Am J Surg Pathol 20:1205–1211, 1996.
425. Fukunaga M, Shinozaki S, Miyazawa Y, Ushigome S: Columnar cell carcinoma of the thyroid. Pathol Int 47:489–492, 1997.
426. Putti TC, Bhuiya TA, Wasserman PG: Fine needle aspiration cytology of mixed tall and columnar cell papillary carcinoma of the thyroid. A case report. Acta Cytol 42:387–390, 1998.
427. Smith AE, Couch M, Argani P: Pathologic quiz case 1. Papillary thyroid carcinoma (PTC), combined tall cell and columnar variants. Arch Otolaryngol Head Neck Surg 124:1170, 1172, 1998.
428. Franssila KO, Harach HR, Wasenius VM: Mucoepidermoid carcinoma of the thyroid. Histopathology 8:847–860, 1984.
429. Katoh R, Sugai T, Ono S, et al: Mucoepidermoid carcinoma of the thyroid gland. Cancer 65:2020–2027, 1990.
430. Rhatigan RM, Roque JL, Bucher RL: Mucoepidermoid carcinoma of the thyroid gland. Cancer 39:210–214, 1977.
431. Mizukami Y, Matsubara F, Hashimoto T, et al: Primary mucoepidermoid carcinoma in the thyroid gland. A case report including an ultrastructural and biochemical study. Cancer 53:1741–1745, 1984.
432. Harach HR, Day ES, de Strizic NA: Mucoepidermoid carcinoma of the thyroid. Report of a case with immunohistochemical studies. Medicina (B Aires) 46:213–216, 1986.
433. Tanda F, Massarelli G, Bosincu L, et al: Primary mucoepidermoid carcinoma of the thyroid gland. Surg Pathol 3:317–324, 1990.
434. Bondeson L, Bondeson AG, Thompson NW: Papillary carcinoma of the thyroid with mucoepidermoid features. Am J Clin Pathol 95:175–179, 1991.
435. Sambade C, Franssila K, Basilio-de-Oliveirz C: Mucoepidermoid carcinoma of the thyroid revisited. Surg Pathol 3:271–280, 1990.

436. Wenig BM, Adair CF, Heffess CS: Primary mucoepidermoid carcinoma of the thyroid gland: a report of six cases and a review of the literature of a follicular epithelial-derived tumor. Hum Pathol 26:1099–1108, 1995.

437. Arezzo A, Patetta R, Ceppa P, et al: Mucoepidermoid carcinoma of the thyroid gland arising from a papillary epithelial neoplasm. Am Surg 64:307–311, 1998.

438. Viciana MJ, Galera-Davidson H, Martin-Lacave I, et al: Papillary carcinoma of the thyroid with mucoepidermoid differentiation. Arch Pathol Lab Med 120:397–398, 1996.

439. Miranda RN, Myint MA, Gnepp DR: Composite follicular variant of papillary carcinoma and mucoepidermoid carcinoma of the thyroid. Report of a case and review of the literature. Am J Surg Pathol 19:1209–1215, 1995.

440. Cameselle-Teijeiro J, Febles-Perez C, Sobrinho-Simoes M: Papillary and mucoepidermoid carcinoma of the thyroid with anaplastic transformation: a case report with histologic and immunohistochemical findings that support a provocative histogenetic hypothesis. Pathol Res Pract 191:1214–1221, 1995.

441. Cameselle-Teijeiro J, Febles-Perez C, Sobrinho-Simoes M: Cytologic features of fine needle aspirates of papillary and mucoepidermoid carcinoma of the thyroid with anaplastic transformation. A case report. Acta Cytol 41:1356–1360, 1997.

441a. Baloch ZW, Solomon AC, LiVolsi VA: Primary mucoepidermoid carcinoma and sclerosing mucoepidermoid carcinoma with eosinophilia of the thyroid gland: a report of nine cases. Mod Pathol 13:802–807, 2000.

442. Harach HR: A study on the relationship between solid cell nests and mucoepidermoid carcinoma of the thyroid. Histopathology 9:195–207, 1985.

443. Chan JK, Albores-Saavedra J, Battifora H, et al: Sclerosing mucoepidermoid thyroid carcinoma with eosinophilia. A distinctive low-grade malignancy arising from the metaplastic follicles of Hashimoto's thyroiditis. Am J Surg Pathol 15:438–448, 1991.

444. Sim SJ, Ro JY, Ordonez NG, et al: Sclerosing mucoepidermoid carcinoma with eosinophilia of the thyroid: report of two patients, one with distant metastasis, and review of the literature. Hum Pathol 28:1091–1096, 1997.

445. Geisinger KR, Steffee CH, McGee RS, et al: The cytomorphologic features of sclerosing mucoepidermoid carcinoma of the thyroid gland with eosinophilia. Am J Clin Pathol 109:294–301, 1998.

446. Chung J, Lee SK, Gong G, et al: Sclerosing mucoepidermoid carcinoma with eosinophilia of the thyroid glands: a case report with clinical manifestation of recurrent neck mass. J Korean Med Sci 14:338–341, 1999.

447. Cavazza A, Toschi E, Valcavi R, et al: Sclerosing mucoepidermoid carcinoma with eosinophilia of the thyroid: description of a case. Pathologica 91:31–35, 1999.

448. Diaz-Perez R, Quiroz H, Nishiyama RH: Primary mucinous adenocarcinoma of thyroid gland. Cancer 38:1323–1325, 1976.

449. Sobrinho-Simoes M, Stenwig AE, Nesland JM, et al: A mucinous carcinoma of the thyroid. Pathol Res Pract 181:464–471, 1986.

450. Sobrinho-Simoes MA, Nesland JM, Johannessen JV: A mucin-producing tumor in the thyroid gland. Ultrastruct Pathol 9:277–281, 1985.

451. Cruz MC, Marques LP, Sambade CC, et al: Primary mucinous carcinoma of the thyroid gland. Surg Pathol 4:266–273, 1991.

452. Williams ED: Histogenesis of medullary carcinoma of the thyroid. J Clin Pathol 19:114–118, 1966.

453. Raue F, Kotzerke J, Reinwein D, et al: Prognostic factors in medullary thyroid carcinoma: evaluation of 741 patients from the German Medullary Thyroid Carcinoma Register. Clin Invest 71:7–12, 1993.

454. Williams ED: Medullary carcinoma of the thyroid. In DeGroot LJ (ed): Endocrinology. New York, Grune & Stratton, 1979, pp 777–792.

455. Saad MF, Ordonez NG, Rashid RK, et al: Medullary carcinoma of the thyroid. A study of the clinical features and prognostic factors in 161 patients. Medicine (Baltimore) 63:319–342, 1984.

456. Rosenberg-Bourgin M, Gardet P, de Sahb R, et al: Comparison of sporadic and hereditary forms of medullary thyroid carcinoma. Henry Ford Hospital J 37:141–143, 1989.

457. Donovan DT, Levy ML, Frust EJ: Familial cutaneous lichen amyloidosis in association with MEN2A: a new variant. Henry Ford Hospital J 37:147–150, 1989.

458. Sobol H, Narod SA, Schuffenecker I, et al: Hereditary medullary thyroid carcinoma: genetic analysis of three related syndromes. Henry Ford Hospital J 37:109–111, 1989.

459. Farndon JR, Leight GS, Dilley WG: Familial medullary thyroid carcinoma without associated endocrinopathies: a distinct clinical entity. Br J Surg 73:278–281, 1986.

460. Wolfe HJ, DeLellis RA: Familial medullary thyroid carcinoma and C cell hyperplasia. Clin Endocrinol Metab 10:351–365, 1981.

461. Carney JA, Sizemore GW, Hayles AV: C-cell disease of the thyroid gland in multiple endocrine neoplasia, type 2b. Cancer 44:2173–2183, 1979.

462. Mulligan LM, Kwok JB, Healey CS, et al: Germ-line mutations of the RET proto-oncogene in multiple endocrine neoplasia type 2A. Nature 363:458–460, 1993.

463. Mulligan LM, Eng C, Healey CS, et al: Specific mutations of the RET proto-oncogene are related to disease phenotype in MEN 2A and FMTC. Nat Genet 6:70–74, 1994.

464. Hofstra RM, Landsvater RM, Ceccherini I, et al: A mutation in the RET proto-oncogene associated with multiple endocrine neoplasia type 2B and sporadic medullary thyroid carcinoma [see comments]. Nature 367:375–376, 1994.

465. Chong GC, Beahrs OH, Sizemore GW, Woolner LH: Medullary carcinoma of the thyroid gland. Cancer 35:695–704, 1975.

466. Mure A, Gicquel C, Abdelmoumene N, et al: Cushing's syndrome in medullary thyroid carcinoma. J Endocrinol Invest 18:180–185, 1995.

467. Modigliani E: Medullary thyroid carcinoma. Curr Ther Endocrinol Metab 5:112–117, 1994.

468. Henry JF, Denizot A, Puccini M, et al: Latent subclinical medullary thyroid carcinoma: diagnosis and treatment. World J Surg 22:752–756, discussion 756–757, 1998.

469. Rieu M, Lame MC, Richard A, et al: Prevalence of sporadic medullary thyroid carcinoma: the importance of routine measurement of serum calcitonin in the diagnostic evaluation of thyroid nodules [see comments]. Clin Endocrinol (Oxf) 42:453–460, 1995.

470. Kaserer K, Scheuba C, Neuhold N, et al: C-cell hyperplasia and medullary thyroid carcinoma in patients routinely screened for serum calcitonin. Am J Surg Pathol 22:722–728, 1998.

471. Kakudo K, Carney JA, Sizemore GW: Medullary carcinoma of thyroid. Biologic behavior of the sporadic and familial neoplasm. Cancer 55:2818–2821, 1985.

472. Carney JA, Sizemore GW, Hayles AB: Multiple endocrine neoplasia, type 2b. Pathobiol Annu 8:105–153, 1978.

473. Kebebew E, Ituarte PH, Siperstein AE, et al: Medullary thyroid carcinoma: clinical characteristics, treatment, prognostic factors, and a comparison of staging systems. Cancer 88:1139–1148, 2000.

474. Bigner SH, Cox EB, Mendelsohn G, et al: Medullary carcinoma of the thyroid in the multiple endocrine neoplasia IIA syndrome. Am J Surg Pathol 5:459–472, 1981.

475. Ibanez ML: Medullary carcinoma of the thyroid gland. Pathol Annu 9:263–290, 1974.

476. Albores-Saavedra J, LiVolsi VA, Williams ED: Medullary carcinoma. Semin Diagn Pathol 2:137–146, 1985.

477. Hazard JB: The C cells (parafollicular cells) of the thyroid gland and medullary thyroid carcinoma. A review. Am J Pathol 88:213–250, 1977.

478. Uribe M, Fenoglio-Preiser CM, Grimes M, Feind C: Medullary carcinoma of the thyroid gland. Clinical, pathological, and immunohistochemical features with review of the literature. Am J Surg Pathol 9:577–594, 1985.

479. Zaatari GS, Saigo PE, Huvos AG: Mucin production in medullary carcinoma of the thyroid. Arch Pathol Lab Med 107:70–74, 1983.

480. Krueger JE, Maitra A, Albores-Saavedra J: Inherited medul-

lary microcarcinoma of the thyroid: a study of 11 cases. Am J Surg Pathol 24:853–858, 2000.

481. Harach HR, Williams ED: Glandular (tubular and follicular) variants of medullary carcinoma of the thyroid. Histopathology 7:83–97, 1983.

482. Sambade C, Baldaque-Faria A, Cardoso-Oliveira M, Sobrinho-Simoes M: Follicular and papillary variants of medullary carcinoma of the thyroid. Pathol Res Pract 184:98–107, 1988.

483. Dominguez-Malagon H, Delgado-Chavez R, Torres-Najera M, et al: Oxyphil and squamous variants of medullary thyroid carcinoma. Cancer 63:1183–1188, 1989.

484. Harach HR, Bergholm U: Medullary (C cell) carcinoma of the thyroid with features of follicular oxyphilic cell tumours. Histopathology 13:645–656, 1988.

485. Kakudo K, Miyauchi A, Ogihara T, et al: Medullary carcinoma of the thyroid. Giant cell type. Arch Pathol Lab Med 102:445–447, 1978.

486. Mendelsohn G, Baylin SB, Bigner SH, et al: Anaplastic variants of medullary thyroid carcinoma: a light-microscopic and immunohistochemical study. Am J Surg Pathol 4:333–341, 1980.

487. Bussolati G, Monga G: Medullary carcinoma of the thyroid with atypical patterns. Cancer 44:1769–1777, 1979.

488. Landon G, Ordonez NG: Clear cell variant of medullary carcinoma of the thyroid. Hum Pathol 16:844–847, 1985.

489. Holm R, Sobrinho-Simoes M, Nesland JM, et al: Medullary carcinoma of the thyroid gland: an immunocytochemical study. Ultrastruct Pathol 8:25–41, 1985.

490. Marcus JN, Dise CA, LiVolsi VA: Melanin production in a medullary thyroid carcinoma. Cancer 49:2518–2526, 1982.

491. Beerman H, Rigaud C, Bogomoletz WV, et al: Melanin production in black medullary thyroid carcinoma (MTC). Histopathology 16:227–233, 1990.

492. Ikeda T, Satoh M, Azuma K, et al: Medullary thyroid carcinoma with a paraganglioma-like pattern and melanin production: a case report with ultrastructural and immunohistochemical studies. Arch Pathol Lab Med 122:555–558, 1998.

493. Schroder S, Bocker W, Baisch H, et al: Prognostic factors in medullary thyroid carcinomas. Survival in relation to age, sex, stage, histology, immunocytochemistry, and DNA content. Cancer 61:806–816, 1988.

494. Kakudo K, Miyauchi A, Takai S, et al: C cell carcinoma of the thyroid—papillary type. Acta Pathol Jpn 29:653–659, 1979.

495. Harach HR, Bergholm U: Small cell variant of medullary carcinoma of the thyroid with neuroblastoma-like features. Histopathology 21:378–380, 1992.

496. Huss LJ, Mendelsohn G: Medullary carcinoma of the thyroid gland: an encapsulated variant resembling the hyalinizing trabecular (paraganglioma-like) adenoma of thyroid. Mod Pathol 3:581–585, 1990.

497. Harach HR, Bergholm U: Medullary carcinoma of the thyroid with carcinoid-like features. J Clin Pathol 46:113–117, 1993.

498. Butler M, Khan S: Immunoreactive calcitonin in amyloid fibrils of medullary carcinoma of the thyroid gland. An immunogold staining technique. Arch Pathol Lab Med 110:647–649, 1986.

499. Krisch K, Krisch I, Horvat G, et al: The value of immunohistochemistry in medullary thyroid carcinoma: a systematic study of 30 cases. Histopathology 9:1077–1089, 1985.

500. Schmid KW, Fischer-Colbrie R, Hagn C, et al: Chromogranin A and B and secretogranin II in medullary carcinomas of the thyroid. Am J Surg Pathol 11:551–556, 1987.

501. Lloyd RV, Sisson JC, Marangos PJ: Calcitonin, carcinoembryonic antigen and neuron-specific enolase in medullary thyroid carcinoma. Cancer 51:2234–2239, 1983.

502. Schroder S, Kloppel G: Carcinoembryonic antigen and nonspecific cross-reacting antigen in thyroid cancer. An immunocytochemical study using polyclonal and monoclonal antibodies. Am J Surg Pathol 11:100–108, 1987.

503. Matias-Guiu X, Machin P, Pons C, et al: Sustentacular cells occur frequently in the familial form of medullary thyroid carcinoma. J Pathol 184:420–423, 1998.

504. Emmertsen K, Ernø H, Henriques U, Schrøder HD: C-cells

505. Albores-Saavedra J, Monforte H, Nadji M, Morales AR: C-cell hyperplasia in thyroid tissue adjacent to follicular cell tumors. Hum Pathol 19:795–799, 1988.

506. Santensanio G, Iafrate E, Partenzi A, et al: A critical reassessment of the concept of C-cell hyperplasia of the thyroid—a quantitative immunohistochemical study. Appl Immunohistochem 5:160–172, 1997.

507. DeLellis RA, Wolfe HJ: The pathobiology of the human calcitonin (C)–cell: a review. Pathol Annu 16:25–52, 1981.

508. Chan JKC, Tse CCH: Solid cell nest-associated C-cells: another possible explanation for "C-cell hyperplasia" adjacent to follicular cell tumors (letter). Hum Pathol 10:498, 1989.

509. Baschieri L, Castagna M, Fierabracci A, et al: Distribution of calcitonin- and somatostatin-containing cells in thyroid lymphoma and in Hashimoto's thyroiditis. Appl Pathol 7:99–104, 1989.

510. Perry A, Molberg K, Albores-Saavedra J: Physiologic versus neoplastic C-cell hyperplasia of the thyroid: separation of distinct histologic and biologic entities. Cancer 77:750–756, 1996.

511. Komminoth P: The RET proto-oncogene in medullary and papillary thyroid carcinoma. Molecular features, pathophysiology and clinical implications. Virchows Arch 431:1–9, 1997.

512. Lloyd RV: RET proto-oncogene mutations and rearrangements in endocrine diseases. Am J Pathol 147:1539–1544, 1995.

513. Mulligan LM, Marsh DJ, Robinson BG, et al: Genotype-phenotype correlation in multiple endocrine neoplasia type 2: report of the International RET Mutation Consortium. J Intern Med 238:343–346, 1995.

514. Komminoth P, Kunz EK, Matias-Guiu X, et al: Analysis of RET protooncogene point mutations distinguishes heritable from nonheritable medullary thyroid carcinomas. Cancer 76:479–489, 1995.

515. Eng C, Mulligan LM: Mutations of the RET protooncogene in the multiple endocrine neoplasia type 2 syndromes, related sporadic tumors, and Hirschsprung disease. Hum Mutat 9:97–109, 1997.

516. Lallier M, St-Vil D, Giroux M, et al: Prophylactic thyroidectomy for medullary thyroid carcinoma in gene carriers of MEN2 syndrome. J Pediatr Surg 33:846–848, 1998.

517. Hinze R, Holzhausen HJ, Gimm O, et al: Primary hereditary medullary thyroid carcinoma—C-cell morphology and correlation with preoperative calcitonin levels. Virchows Arch 433:203–208, 1998.

518. Dralle H, Gimm O, Simon D, et al: Prophylactic thyroidectomy in 75 children and adolescents with hereditary medullary thyroid carcinoma: German and Austrian experience. World J Surg 22:744–750, discussion 750–751, 1998.

519. Eng C, Mulligan LM, Smith DP, et al: Mutation of the RET protooncogene in sporadic medullary thyroid carcinoma. Genes Chromosomes Cancer 12:209–212, 1995.

520. Bugalho MJ, Frade JP, Santos JR, et al: Molecular analysis of the RET proto-oncogene in patients with sporadic medullary thyroid carcinoma: a novel point mutation in the extracellular cysteine-rich domain. Eur J Endocrinol 136:423–426, 1997.

521. Romei C, Elisei R, Pinchera A, et al: Somatic mutations of the ret protooncogene in sporadic medullary thyroid carcinoma are not restricted to exon 16 and are associated with tumor recurrence. J Clin Endocrinol Metab 81:1619–1622, 1996.

522. Marsh DJ, Learoyd DL, Andrew SD, et al: Somatic mutations in the RET proto-oncogene in sporadic medullary thyroid carcinoma. Clin Endocrinol (Oxf) 44:249–257, 1996.

523. Matias-Guiu X, LaGuette J, Puras-Gil AM, Rosai J: Metastatic neuroendocrine tumors to the thyroid gland mimicking medullary carcinoma: a pathologic and immunohistochemical study of six cases. Am J Surg Pathol 21:754–762, 1997.

524. Girelli ME, Nacamulli D, Pelizzo MR, et al: Medullary thyroid carcinoma: clinical features and long-term follow-up of seventy-eight patients treated between 1969 and 1986. Thyroid 8:517–523, 1998.

for differentiation between familial and sporadic medullary thyroid carcinoma. Dan Med Bull 30:353–356, 1983.

525. Modigliani E, Cohen R, Campos JM, et al: Prognostic factors for survival and for biochemical cure in medullary thyroid carcinoma: results in 899 patients. The GETC Study Group. Groupe d'etude des tumeurs a calcitonine. Clin Endocrinol (Oxf) 48:265–273, 1998.

526. Scopsi L, Sampietro G, Boracchi P, et al: Multivariate analysis of prognostic factors in sporadic medullary carcinoma of the thyroid. A retrospective study of 109 consecutive patients. Cancer 78:2173–2183, 1996.

527. Bergholm U, Bergstrom R, Ekbom A: Long-term follow-up of patients with medullary carcinoma of the thyroid. Cancer 79:132–138, 1997.

528. Rossi RL, Cady B, Meissner WA, et al: Nonfamilial medullary thyroid carcinoma. Am J Surg 139:554–560, 1980.

529. Fuchshuber PR, Loree TR, Hicks WL Jr, et al: Medullary carcinoma of the thyroid: prognostic factors and treatment recommendations. Ann Surg Oncol 5:81–86, 1998.

530. Brierley J, Tsang R, Simpson WJ, et al: Medullary thyroid cancer: analyses of survival and prognostic factors and the role of radiation therapy in local control. Thyroid 6:305–310, 1996.

531. Norton JA, Froome LC, Farrell RE, et al: Multiple endocrine neoplasia type IIb: the most aggressive form of medullary thyroid carcinoma. Surg Clin North Am 59:109–118, 1979.

532. Guyetant S, Dupre F, Bigorgne JC, et al: Medullary thyroid microcarcinoma: a clinicopathologic retrospective study of 38 patients with no prior familial disease. Hum Pathol 30:957–963, 1999.

533. Williams ED, Brown CL, Doniach I: Pathological and clinical findings in a series of 67 cases of medullary carcinoma of the thyroid. J Clin Pathol 19:103–113, 1966.

534. Ruppert JM, Eggleston JC, deBustros A, Baylin SB: Disseminated calcitonin-poor medullary thyroid carcinoma in a patient with calcitonin-rich primary tumor. Am J Surg Pathol 10:513–518, 1986.

535. Saad MF, Ordonez NG, Guido JJ, Samaan NA: The prognostic value of calcitonin immunostaining in medullary carcinoma of the thyroid. J Clin Endocrinol Metab 59:850–856, 1984.

536. Mendelsohn G, Wells SA Jr, Baylin SB: Relationship of tissue carcinoembryonic antigen and calcitonin to tumor virulence in medullary thyroid carcinoma. An immunohistochemical study in early, localized, and virulent disseminated stages of disease. Cancer 54:657–662, 1984.

537. Schroder S, Schwarz W, Rehpenning W, et al: Leu-M1 immunoreactivity and prognosis in medullary carcinomas of the thyroid gland. J Cancer Res Clin Oncol 114:291–296, 1988.

538. Langle F, Soliman T, Neuhold N, et al: CD15 (LeuM1) immunoreactivity: prognostic factor for sporadic and hereditary medullary thyroid cancer? Study Group on Multiple Endocrine Neoplasia of Austria. World J Surg 18:583–587, 1994.

539. Viale G, Roncalli M, Grimelius L, et al: Prognostic value of bcl-2 immunoreactivity in medullary thyroid carcinoma. Hum Pathol 26:945–950, 1995.

540. Scopsi L, Sampietro G, Boracchi P, Collini P: Argyrophilia and chromogranin A and B immunostaining in patients with sporadic medullary thyroid carcinoma. A critical appraisal of their prognostic utility. J Pathol 184:414–419, 1998.

541. Roncalli M, Viale G, Grimelius L, et al: Prognostic value of N-myc immunoreactivity in medullary thyroid carcinoma. Cancer 74:134–141, 1994.

542. Fontanini G, Vignati S, Pacini F, et al: Microvessel count: an indicator of poor outcome in medullary thyroid carcinoma but not in other types of thyroid carcinoma. Mod Pathol 9:636–641, 1996.

543. el-Naggar AK, Ordonez NG, McLemore D, et al: Clinicopathologic and flow cytometric DNA study of medullary thyroid carcinoma. Surgery 108:981–985, 1990.

544. Ekman ET, Bergholm U, Backdahl M, et al: Nuclear DNA content and survival in medullary thyroid carcinoma. Swedish Medullary Thyroid Cancer Study Group. Cancer 65:511–517, 1990.

545. Gonzalez-Campora R, Lopez-Garrido J, Martin-Lacave I, et al: Concurrence of a symptomatic encapsulated follicular carcinoma, an occult papillary carcinoma and a medullary carcinoma in the same patient. Histopathology 21:380–382, 1992.

546. Sobrinho-Simoes M: Mixed medullary and follicular carcinoma of the thyroid. Histopathology 23:287–289, 1993.

547. Pfaltz M, Hedinger CE, Muhlethaler JP: Mixed medullary and follicular carcinoma of the thyroid. Virchows Arch A Pathol Anat Histopathol 400:53–59, 1983.

548. Parker LN, Kollin J, Wu SY, et al: Carcinoma of the thyroid with a mixed medullary, papillary, follicular, and undifferentiated pattern. Arch Intern Med 145:1507–1509, 1985.

549. Apel RL, Alpert LC, Rizzo A, et al: A metastasizing composite carcinoma of the thyroid with distinct medullary and papillary components. Arch Pathol Lab Med 118:1143–1147, 1994.

550. Lax SF, Beham A, Kronberger-Schonecker D, et al: Coexistence of papillary and medullary carcinoma of the thyroid gland—mixed or collision tumour? Clinicopathological analysis of three cases. Virchows Arch 424:441–447, 1994.

551. Albores-Saavedra J, Gorraez de la Mora T, de la Torre-Rendon F, Gould E: Mixed medullary-papillary carcinoma of the thyroid: a previously unrecognized variant of thyroid carcinoma. Hum Pathol 21:1151–1155, 1990.

552. Pastolero GC, Coire CI, Asa SL: Concurrent medullary and papillary carcinomas of thyroid with lymph node metastases. A collision phenomenon. Am J Surg Pathol 20:245–250, 1996.

553. Ljungberg O: Biopsy Pathology of the Thyroid and Parathyroid. London, Chapman & Hall, 1992.

554. Burt AD, MacGuire J, Lindop GB, et al: Mixed follicular-parafollicular carcinoma of the thyroid. Scott Med J 32:50–51, 1987.

555. Papotti M, Negro F, Carney JA, et al: Mixed medullary-follicular carcinoma of the thyroid. A morphological, immunohistochemical and in situ hybridization analysis of 11 cases. Virchows Arch 430:397–405, 1997.

556. Papotti M, Volante M, Komminoth P, et al: Thyroid carcinomas with mixed follicular and C-cell differentiation patterns. Semin Diagn Pathol 17:109–119, 2000.

557. Ljungberg O, Ericsson UB, Bondeson L, Thorell J: A compound follicular-parafollicular cell carcinoma of the thyroid: a new tumor entity? Cancer 52:1053–1061, 1983.

558. Ljungberg O, Bondeson L, Bondeson AG: Differentiated thyroid carcinoma, intermediate type: a new tumor entity with features of follicular and parafollicular cell carcinoma. Hum Pathol 15:218–228, 1984.

559. Mizukami Y, Nonomura A, Michigishi T, et al: Mixed medullary-follicular carcinoma of the thyroid gland: a clinicopathologic variant of medullary thyroid carcinoma. Mod Pathol 9:631–635, 1996.

560. Volante M, Papotti M, Roth J, et al: Mixed medullary-follicular thyroid carcinoma. Molecular evidence for a dual origin of tumor components. Am J Pathol 155:1499–1509, 1999.

561. Holm R, Sobrinho-Simoes M, Nesland JM, et al: Medullary thyroid carcinoma with thyroglobulin immunoreactivity. A special entity? Lab Invest 57:258–268, 1987.

562. Chan JK, Rosai J: Tumors of the neck showing thymic or related branchial pouch differentiation: a unifying concept. Hum Pathol 22:349–367, 1991.

563. Lewis JE, Wick MR, Scheithauer BW, et al: Thymoma, a clinicopathologic review. Cancer 60:2727–2743, 1987.

564. Murao T, Nakanishi M, Toda K, et al: Malignant teratoma of the thyroid gland in an adolescent female. Acta Pathol Jpn 29:109–117, 1979.

565. Levey M: An unusual thyroid tumor in a child. Laryngoscope 86:1864–1868, 1976.

566. Weigensberg C, Dalsley H, Asa SL, et al: Thyroid thymoma in childhood. Endocrinol Pathol 1:123–127, 1990.

567. Harach HR, Saravia Day E, Franssila KO: Thyroid spindle-cell tumor with mucous cysts. An intrathyroid thymoma? Am J Surg Pathol 9:525–530, 1985.

568. Kingsley DPE, Elton A, Bennett MH: Malignant teratoma of the thyroid, case report and a review of the literature. Br J Cancer 22:7–11, 1968.

569. Hofman P, Mainguene C, Michiels JF, et al: Thyroid spindle epithelial tumor with thymus-like differentiation (the "SET-

TLE" tumor). An immunohistochemical and electron microscopic study. Eur Arch Otorhinolaryngol 252:316–320, 1995.

570. Saw D, Wu D, Chess Q, Shemen L: Spindle epithelial tumor with thymus-like element (SETTLE), a primary thyroid tumor. Int J Surg Pathol 4:169–174, 1997.

571. Chetty R, Goetsch S, Nayler S, Cooper K: Spindle epithelial tumour with thymus-like element (SETTLE): the predominantly monophasic variant. Histopathology 33:71–74, 1998.

572. Kirby PA, Ellison WA, Thomas PA: Spindle epithelial tumor with thymus-like differentiation (SETTLE) of the thyroid with prominent mitotic activity and focal necrosis. Am J Surg Pathol 23:712–716, 1999.

573. Asa SL, Dardick I, Van Nostrand AW, et al: Primary thyroid thymoma: a distinct clinicopathologic entity. Hum Pathol 19:1463–1467, 1988.

574. Kakudo K, Mori I, Tamaoki N, Watanabe K: Carcinoma of possible thymic origin presenting as a thyroid mass: a new subgroup of squamous cell carcinoma of the thyroid. J Surg Oncol 38:187–192, 1988.

575. Miyauchi A, Kuma K, Matsuzuka F, et al: Intrathyroidal epithelial thymoma: an entity distinct from squamous cell carcinoma of the thyroid. World J Surg 9:128–135, 1985.

576. Miyauchi A, Ishikawa H, Maedea M: Intrathyroid epithelial thymoma: a report of six cases with immunohistochemical and ultrastructural studies [in Japanese]. Endocrinol Surg 6:289–295, 1989.

577. Mizukami Y, Kurumaya H, Yamada T, et al: Thymic carcinoma involving the thyroid gland: report of two cases. Hum Pathol 26:576–579, 1995.

578. Watanabe I, Tezuka F, Yamaguchi M, et al: Thymic carcinoma of the thyroid. Pathol Int 46:450–456, 1996.

579. Attaran SY, Omrani GH, Tavangar SM: Lymphoepithelial-like intrathyroidal thymic carcinoma with foci of squamous differentiation. Case report. APMIS 104:419–423, 1996.

580. Damiani S, Filotico M, Eusebi V: Carcinoma of the thyroid showing thymoma-like features. Virchows Arch A Pathol Anat Histopathol 418:463–466, 1991.

581. Cheuk W, Jacobson AA, Chan JKC: Spindle epithelial tumor with thymus-like element: a distinctive malignant thyroid tumor with significant metastatic potential. Mod Pathol 13:1150–1155, 2000.

582. Dorfman DM, Shahsafaei A, Miyauchi A: Intrathyroidal epithelial thymoma (ITET)/carcinoma showing thymus-like differentiation (CASTLE) exhibits CD5 immunoreactivity: new evidence for thymic differentiation. Histopathology 32:104–109, 1998.

583. Berezowski K, Grimes MM, Gal A, Kornstein MJ: CD5 immunoreactivity of epithelial cells in thymic carcinoma and CASTLE using paraffin-embedded tissue. Am J Clin Pathol 106:483–486, 1996.

584. Tse LLY, Shek TWH, Lam KY, et al: Carcinoma showing thymus-like differentiation (CASTLE) of the thyroid: an intrathyroid thymic carcinoma (abstract). Int J Surg Pathol (in press).

585. Choi P, To KF, Lai FM, et al: Follicular dendritic cell tumor of the neck: a report of two cases complicated by pulmonary metastasis. Cancer 89:664–672, 2000.

586. Sawady J, Mendelsohn G, Sirota RL, Taxy JB: The intrathyroidal hyperfunctioning parathyroid gland. Mod Pathol 2:652–657, 1989.

587. de la Cruz Vigo F, Ortega G, Gonzalez S, et al: Pathologic intrathyroidal parathyroid glands. Int Surg 82:87–90, 1997.

588. Freeman C, Berg JW, Cutler SJ: Occurrence and prognosis of extranodal lymphomas. Cancer 29:252–260, 1972.

589. Anscombe AM, Wright DH: Primary malignant lymphoma of the thyroid—a tumour of mucosa-associated lymphoid tissue: review of seventy-six cases. Histopathology 9:81–97, 1985.

590. Aozasa K, Inoue A, Tajima K, et al: Malignant lymphomas of the thyroid gland. Analysis of 79 patients with emphasis on histologic prognostic factors. Cancer 58:100–104, 1986.

591. Burke JS, Butler JJ, Fuller LM: Malignant lymphomas of the thyroid: a clinical pathologic study of 35 patients including ultrastructural observations. Cancer 39:1587–1602, 1977.

592. Compagno J, Oertel JE: Malignant lymphoma and other lymphoproliferative disorders of the thyroid gland. A clinicopathologic study of 245 cases. Am J Clin Pathol 74:1–11, 1980.

593. Devine RM, Edis AJ, Banks PM: Primary lymphoma of the thyroid: a review of the Mayo Clinic experience through 1978. World J Surg 5:33–38, 1981.

594. Rasbach DA, Mondschein MS, Harris NL, et al: Malignant lymphoma of the thyroid gland: a clinical and pathologic study of twenty cases. Surgery 98:1166–1170, 1985.

595. Woolner LB, McConahey WM, Beahrs OH, Black BM: Primary malignant lymphoma of the thyroid. Review of forty-six cases. Am J Surg 111:502–523, 1966.

596. Singer JA: Primary lymphoma of the thyroid. Am Surg 64:334–337, 1998.

597. Pledge S, Bessell EM, Leach IH, et al: Non-Hodgkin's lymphoma of the thyroid: a retrospective review of all patients diagnosed in Nottinghamshire from 1973 to 1992. Clin Oncol 8:371–375, 1996.

598. Hamburger JI, Miller JM, Kini SR: Lymphoma of the thyroid. Ann Intern Med 99:685–693, 1983.

599. Derringer GA, Thompson LD, Frommelt RA, et al: Malignant lymphoma of the thyroid gland: a clinicopathologic study of 108 cases. Am J Surg Pathol 24:623–639, 2000.

600. Thompson LD, Rosai J, Heffess CS: Primary thyroid teratomas: a clinicopathologic study of 30 cases. Cancer 88:1149–1158, 2000.

601. Luboshitzky R, Dharan M, Nachtigal D, et al: Syncytial variant of nodular sclerosing Hodgkin's disease presenting as a thyroid nodule. A case report. Acta Cytol 39:543–546, 1995.

602. Aozasa K, Inoue A, Yoshimura H, et al: Intermediate lymphocytic lymphoma of the thyroid. An immunologic and immunohistologic study. Cancer 57:1762–1767, 1986.

603. Coltrera MD: Primary T-cell lymphoma of the thyroid. Head Neck 21:160–163, 1999.

604. Abdul-Rahman ZH, Gogas HJ, Tooze JA, et al: T-cell lymphoma in Hashimoto's thyroiditis. Histopathology 29:455–459, 1996.

605. Yamaguchi M, Ohno T, Kita K: Gamma/delta T-cell lymphoma of the thyroid gland (letter). N Engl J Med 336:1391–1392, 1997.

606. Shanks JH, Harris M, Howat AJ, Freemont AJ: Angiotropic lymphoma with endocrine involvement. Histopathology 31:161–166, 1997.

607. Isaacson PG: Lymphomas of mucosa-associated lymphoid tissue (MALT). Histopathology 16:617–619, 1990.

608. Hyjek E, Isaacson PG: Primary B cell lymphoma of the thyroid and its relationship to Hashimoto's thyroiditis. Hum Pathol 19:1315–1326, 1988.

609. Isaacson PG, Androulakis-Papachristou A, Diss TC, et al: Follicular colonization in thyroid lymphoma. Am J Pathol 141:43–52, 1992.

610. Mizukami Y, Michigishi T, Nonomura A, et al: Primary lymphoma of the thyroid: a clinical, histological and immunohistochemical study of 20 cases. Histopathology 17:201–209, 1990.

611. Rosen IB, Sutcliffe SB, Gospodarowicz MK, et al: The role of surgery in the management of thyroid lymphoma. Surgery 104:1095–1099, 1988.

612. Maurer R, Taylor CR, Terry R, et al: Non-Hodgkin's lymphoma of the thyroid, a clinicopathological review of 29 cases applying the Lukes-Collins classification and an immunoperoxidase method. Virchows Arch A Pathol Anat Histopathol 383:293–317, 1979.

613. Bateman AC, Wright DH: Epitheliotropism in high-grade lymphomas of mucosa-associated lymphoid tissue. Histopathology 23:409–415, 1993.

614. Tennvall J, Cavallin-Stahl E, Akerman M: Primary localized non-Hodgkin's lymphoma of the thyroid: a retrospective clinicopathological review. Eur J Surg Oncol 13:297–302, 1987.

615. Stone CW, Slease RB, Brubaker D, et al: Thyroid lymphoma with gastrointestinal involvement: report of three cases. Am J Hematol 21:357–365, 1986.

616. Pedersen RK, Pedersen NT: Primary non-Hodgkin's lymphoma of the thyroid gland: a population based study. Histopathology 28:25–32, 1996.

617. Laing RW, Hoskin P, Hudson BV, et al: The significance of MALT histology in thyroid lymphoma: a review of patients from the BNLI and Royal Marsden Hospital. Clin Oncol (R Coll Radiol) 6:300–304, 1994.

618. Skacel M, Ross CW, Hsi ED: A reassessment of primary thyroid lymphoma: high-grade MALT-type lymphoma as a distinct subtype of diffuse large B-cell lymphoma. Histopathology 37:10–18, 2000.

619. Aozasa K, Inoue A, Yoshimura H, et al: Plasmacytoma of the thyroid gland. Cancer 58:105–110, 1986.

620. Hussong JW, Perkins SL, Schnitzer B, et al: Extramedullary plasmacytoma. A form of marginal zone cell lymphoma? Am J Clin Pathol 111:111–116, 1999.

621. Yapp R, Linder J, Schenken JR, Karrer FW: Plasma cell granuloma of the thyroid. Hum Pathol 16:848–850, 1985.

622. Mizukami Y, Nonomura A, Michigishi T, et al: Pseudolymphoma of the thyroid gland. A case report. Pathol Res Pract 192:166–169, discussion 170–171, 1996.

623. Thompson LD: Langerhans cell histiocytosis isolated to the thyroid gland. Eur Arch Otorhinolaryngol 253:62–65, 1996.

624. Thompson LDR, Wenig BM, Adair CF, Heffess CS: Peripheral nerve sheath tumors of the thyroid gland, a series of four cases and a review of the literature. Endocr Pathol 7:309–318, 1996.

625. Tsang WY, Lau MF, Chan JK: Incidental Langerhans' cell histiocytosis of the thyroid. Histopathology 24:397–399, 1994.

626. Coode PE, Shaikh MU: Histiocytosis X of the thyroid masquerading as thyroid carcinoma. Hum Pathol 19:239–241, 1988.

627. Wang WS, Liu JH, Chiou TJ, et al: Langerhans' cell histiocytosis with thyroid involvement masquerading as thyroid carcinoma. Jpn J Clin Oncol 27:180–184, 1997.

628. Kitahama S, Iitaka M, Shimizu T, et al: Thyroid involvement by malignant histiocytosis of Langerhans' cell type. Clin Endocrinol (Oxf) 45:357–363, 1996.

629. Egloff B: The hemangioendothelioma of the thyroid. Virchows Arch A Pathol Anat Histopathol 400:119–142, 1983.

630. Maiorana A, Collina G, Cesinaro AM, et al: Epithelioid angiosarcoma of the thyroid. Clinicopathological analysis of seven cases from non-Alpine areas. Virchows Arch 429:131–137, 1996.

631. Eusebi V, Carcangiu ML, Dina R, Rosai J: Keratin-positive epithelioid angiosarcoma of thyroid. A report of four cases. Am J Surg Pathol 14:737–747, 1990.

632. Lamovec J, Zidar A, Zidanik B: Epithelioid angiosarcoma of the thyroid gland. Report of two cases. Arch Pathol Lab Med 118:642–646, 1994.

633. Ritter JH, Mills SE, Nappi O, Wick MR: Angiosarcoma-like neoplasms of epithelial organs: true endothelial tumors or variants of carcinoma? Semin Diagn Pathol 12:270–282, 1995.

634. Mills SE, Stallings RG, Austin MB: Angiomatoid carcinoma of the thyroid gland. Anaplastic carcinoma with follicular and medullary features mimicking angiosarcoma. Am J Clin Pathol 86:674–678, 1986.

635. Mills SE, Gaffey MJ, Watts JC, et al: Angiomatoid carcinoma and 'angiosarcoma' of the thyroid gland. A spectrum of endothelial differentiation. Am J Clin Pathol 102:322–330, 1994.

636. Taccagni G, Sambade C, Nesland J, et al: Solitary fibrous tumour of the thyroid: clinicopathological, immunohistochemical and ultrastructural study of three cases. Virchows Arch A Pathol Anat Histopathol 422:491–497, 1993.

637. Cameselle-Teijeiro J, Varela-Duran J: CD34 and thyroid fibrous tumor (letter). Am J Surg Pathol 19:1096, 1995.

638. Cameselle-Teijeiro J, Varela-Duran J, Fonseca E, et al: Solitary fibrous tumor of the thyroid. Am J Clin Pathol 101:535–538, 1994.

639. Kie JH, Kim JY, Park YN, et al: Solitary fibrous tumour of the thyroid. Histopathology 30:365–368, 1997.

640. Thompson LD, Wenig BM, Adair CF, et al: Primary smooth muscle tumors of the thyroid gland. Cancer 79:579–587, 1997.

641. Kawahara E, Nakanishi I, Terahata S, Ikegaki S: Leiomyosarcoma of the thyroid gland. A case report with a comparative study of five cases of anaplastic carcinoma. Cancer 62:2558–2563, 1988.

642. Iida Y, Katoh R, Yoshioka M, et al: Primary leiomyosarcoma of the thyroid gland. Acta Pathol Jpn 43:71–75, 1993.

643. Chetty R, Clark SP, Dowling JP: Leiomyosarcoma of the thyroid: immunohistochemical and ultrastructural study. Pathology 25:203–205, 1993.

644. Ozaki O, Sugino K, Mimura T, et al: Primary leiomyosarcoma of the thyroid gland. Surg Today 27:177–180, 1997.

645. Tulbah A, Al-Dayel F, Fawaz I, Rosai J: Epstein-Barr virus–associated leiomyosarcoma of the thyroid in a child with congenital immunodeficiency: a case report. Am J Surg Pathol 23:473–476, 1999.

646. Andrion A, Bellis D, Delsedime L, et al: Leiomyoma and neurilemoma: report of two unusual non-epithelial tumours of the thyroid gland. Virchows Arch A Pathol Anat Histopathol 413:367–372, 1988.

647. Galati LT, Barnes EL, Myers EN: Dendritic cell sarcoma of the thyroid. Head Neck 21:273–275, 1999.

648. Pickleman JR, Lee JF, Straus FHd, Paloyan E: Thyroid hemangioma. Am J Surg 129:331–333, 1975.

649. Andrion A, Gaglio A, Dogliani N, et al: Liposarcoma of the thyroid gland. Fine-needle aspiration cytology, immunohistology, and ultrastructure. Am J Clin Pathol 95:675–679, 1991.

650. Nielsen VT, Knudsen N, Holm IE: Liposarcoma of the thyroid gland. Tumori 72:499–502, 1986.

651. Tseleni-Balafouta S, Arvanitis D, Kakaviatos N, Paraskevakou H: Primary myxoid chondrosarcoma of the thyroid gland. Arch Pathol Lab Med 112:94–96, 1988.

652. Nitzsche EU, Seeger LL, Klosa B, et al: Primary osteosarcoma of the thyroid gland. J Nucl Med 33:1399–1401, 1992.

653. Sichel JY, Wygoda M, Dano I, et al: Fibrosarcoma of the thyroid in a man exposed to fallout from the Chernobyl accident. Ann Otol Rhinol Laryngol 105:832–834, 1996.

654. Berthelsen A: Fibrosarcoma in the thyroid gland: recurrence treated with radiotherapy. J Laryngol Otol 92:933–936, 1978.

655. Heffess CS, Adair FF, Wenig BM: Paraganglioma of the thyroid gland (abstract). Int J Surg Pathol 2(suppl):188, 1995.

656. de Vries EJ, Watson CG: Paraganglioma of the thyroid. Head Neck 11:462–465, 1989.

657. Bale GF: Teratoma of the neck in the region of the thyroid gland, a review of the literature and report of four cases. Am J Pathol 26:565–580, 1950.

658. Fisher JE, Cooney DR, Voorhess ML, Jewett TC Jr: Teratoma of thyroid gland in infancy: review of the literature and two case reports. J Surg Oncol 21:135–140, 1982.

659. Kimler SC, Muth WF: Primary malignant teratoma of the thyroid: case report and literature review of cervical teratomas in adults. Cancer 42:311–317, 1978.

660. Hajdu SI, Hajdu EO: Malignant teratoma of the neck. Arch Pathol 83:567–570, 1967.

661. Bowker CM, Whittaker RS: Malignant teratoma of the thyroid: case report and literature review of thyroid teratoma in adults. Histopathology 21:81–83, 1992.

662. Buckley NJ, Burch WM, Leight GS: Malignant teratoma in the thyroid gland of an adult: a case report and a review of the literature. Surgery 100:932–937, 1986.

663. Ueno NT, Amato RJ, Ro JJ, Weber RS: Primary malignant teratoma of the thyroid gland: report and discussion of two cases. Head Neck 20:649–653, 1998.

664. Chen JS, Lai GM, Hsueh S: Malignant thyroid teratoma of an adult: a long-term survival after chemotherapy. Am J Clin Oncol 21:212–214, 1998.

665. Ivy HK: Cancer metastatic to the thyroid: a diagnostic problem. Mayo Clin Proc 59:856–859, 1984.

666. McCabe DP, Farrar WB, Petkov TM, et al: Clinical and pathologic correlations in disease metastatic to the thyroid gland. Am J Surg 150:519–523, 1985.

667. Lam KY, Lo CY: Metastatic tumors of the thyroid gland: a study of 79 cases in Chinese patients. Arch Pathol Lab Med 122:37–41, 1998.

668. Nakhjavani MK, Gharib H, Goellner JR, van Heerden JA: Metastasis to the thyroid gland. A report of 43 cases. Cancer 79:574–578, 1997.

tion, the specimen's condition and how it was identified, the type of procedure, and a clear description of the tumor. The description of the tumor includes orientation, size, weight, findings on external examination and representative cross-section, and appearance of the adrenal remnant. Weight should be obtained intact, but in some conditions (e.g., hyperplasia), precise weighing after the gland has been meticulously stripped of periadrenal fat and other connective tissue is essential. The diagnosis provides the histologic type, the grade, a descriptive diagnosis (if pertinent), descriptive features (if pertinent), the status of the margins, the status of regional lymph nodes, and the results of special studies.

## CONGENITAL ABNORMALITIES

Congenital abnormalities of the adrenal gland do not usually come to the attention of the surgical pathologist. Accessory adrenal tissues are usually found between the upper abdomen and the gonads, particularly in the area of the celiac axis, adjacent to the upper pole of the kidney, the broad ligament, or the spermatic cord. At histologic examination, the heterotopic tissues may be exclusively cortical or, as often seen in the celiac axis, composed of a mixture of cortex and medulla.

Congenital adrenal hyperplasia, also known as the adrenogenital syndrome, is an inborn error of metabolism that is inherited in an autosomal recessive fashion.[9, 10] It usually affects newborn infants, who often present with a salt-wasting syndrome or ambiguous genitalia in girls and precocious puberty in boys. Ninety-five percent of cases are secondary to a deficiency of the enzyme 21-hydroxylase; deficiency of the enzyme 11$\beta$-hydroxylase accounts for the majority of the remaining 5% of cases.[10] Gross evaluation shows that the adrenals are bilaterally enlarged and darker than usual, with their outer surfaces markedly convoluted. At histologic examination, the zona fasciculata and the zona reticularis layers are diffusely expanded and thickened, with lipid depletion.[11] The diagnosis is usually established before surgery; however, the weight of the gland should be documented and frozen tissue should be saved for possible biochemical or histochemical studies. Rarely, cases may be complicated by the occurrence of adrenocortical adenomas and carcinomas or even myelolipoma.[12] Many of these patients develop testicular lipid cell proliferations.

## ACQUIRED ADRENOCORTICAL HYPERPLASIA

Acquired adrenal gland hyperplasia usually results from either pituitary or nonpituitary oversecretion of corticotropin or, less commonly, corticotropin-releasing hormone.[13–16] In unusual cases, it may present without detectable hormone abnormalities outside of the adrenal gland. Patients usually present with

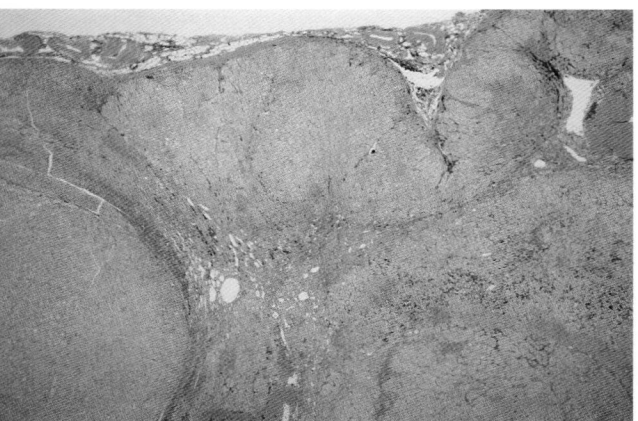

FIGURE 45–1. Acquired adrenocortical hyperplasia associated with Cushing's syndrome. Nodular and diffuse expansion of adrenocortical cells is seen.

Cushing's syndrome or, rarely, Conn's syndrome. It is almost always recognized clinically, obviating the need for a surgical procedure. Pathologic examination reveals that hyperplasia is almost always bilateral and may be diffuse or nodular; nodular glands are usually associated with a more advanced form of hyperplasia.

At gross evaluation, the glands have more rounded contours than normal. If resection is performed, it is important to weigh the glands and measure the cortical thickness. Normal glands weigh up to 6 g and usually have a cortical thickness of no more than 1 to 2 mm. Glands of cases associated with ectopic production of corticotropin or corticotropin-releasing hormone are usually larger than those seen in association with hyperplasia due to pituitary corticotropin overproduction. An expansion of the zona fasciculata or zona reticularis is seen at histologic examination in almost all cases, often with the formation of nodules up to 1 cm or larger (Fig. 45–1). Cases associated with Conn's syndrome show hyperplasia of the zona glomerulosa, with or without micronodules. There may be invaginations of the zona glomerulosa into the zona fasciculata. Problems may be encountered when macronodules greater than 0.5 to 1 cm and up to 5 cm are encountered, raising the differential diagnosis of adrenocortical adenoma. However, the remaining adrenal cortex is hyperplastic in adrenocortical hyperplasia but atrophic or normal with an adrenocortical adenoma. Congenital adrenocortical hyperplasia may be distinguished from acquired hyperplasia by its distinctive clinical features, notably virilization.

## PRIMARY PIGMENTED NODULAR ADRENOCORTICAL DISEASE

Primary pigmented nodular adrenocortical disease (micronodular dysplasia) is a rare disease of unknown etiology that may be either sporadic or asso-

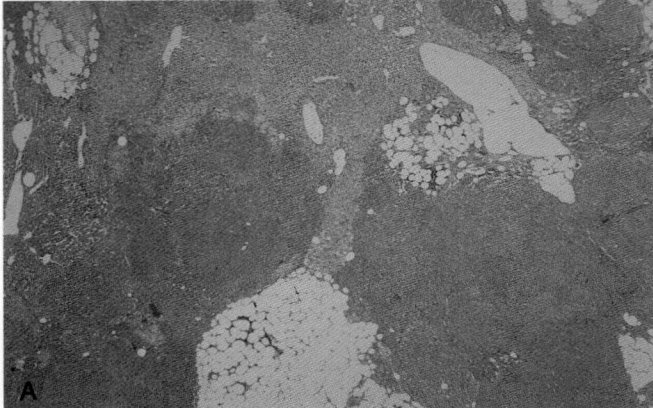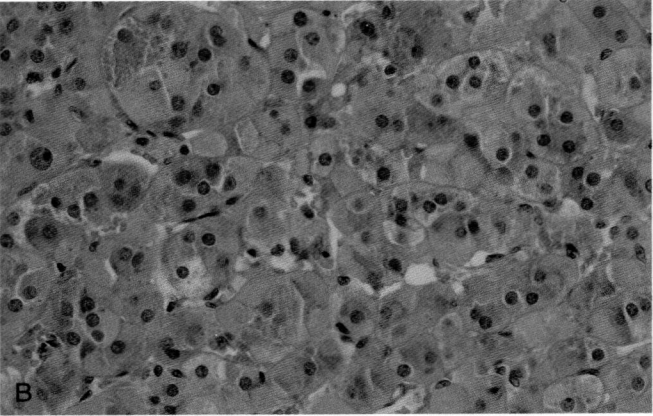

**FIGURE 45–2.** Primary pigmented nodular adrenocortical disease. *A,* At low magnification, a nodular appearance is seen. Note the focal myelolipomatous change. The intervening cortex is atrophic. *B,* At high magnification, a brown pigment can be seen in the cytoplasm of the cells.

ciated with an autosomal dominant familial syndrome, the most common being Carney's complex (cardiac myxomas, spotty pigmentation, neurofibromatosis, cerebral hemangiomas, and endocrine overactivity).[17] The familial disorder has been mapped to genomic loci on chromosomes 2p16 and 17q23–34.[18, 19] Patients are usually young, with a slight female predominance, and present with corticotropin-independent Cushing's syndrome. An autoimmune etiology may be due to adrenal-stimulating antibodies, which stimulate corticotropin receptor sites in the adrenal cortex.[20]

At gross evaluation, the normal-sized adrenal glands are studded with multiple small cortical nodules, 0.1 to 0.3 cm in diameter.[21–23] The nodules are pigmented, either brown or black.[14] The cortex between the nodules is not hyperplastic.[14] The nodules are histologically composed of cells with eosinophilic cytoplasm and abundant brown, granular pigment, representing lipofuscin[21–24] (Fig. 45–2). There may be foci of myelolipomatous change. The cell nuclei are vesicular and may contain prominent eosinophilic nucleoli; occasional binucleation and multinucleation may be present. The intervening cortical tissue is atrophic. Primary pigmented nodular adrenocortical disease is distinguished from adrenocortical hyperplasia by the normal size of the gland, the pigmentation and nuclear atypia in the nodules, and the lack of hyperplasia in the non-nodular cortex.

## INCIDENTAL ADRENOCORTICAL NODULES

Cortical nodules without clinical evidence of hyperfunction are detected in about 1% to 10% of cases at autopsy; an increased incidence is found in patients with systemic hypertension or diabetes mellitus.[25–27] With the use of sensitive radiologic imaging studies, cortical nodules are being detected more frequently

in vivo and becoming the target of surgical intervention.

At gross evaluation, incidental adrenocortical nodules are usually defined as less than 1 cm, whereas adenomas are defined as greater than 1 cm, although some consider all solitary nonfunctional nodules to represent adenomas, and still others consider all solitary nonfunctional nodules to represent nodules. They are often multiple and bilateral. Typically, they are yellow on cut section, although a subset of incidental adrenocortical nodules may be pigmented. The nodules generally arise in the cortex but may protrude into the medulla or into the surrounding adipose tissue, or they may even be found outside the boundaries of the adrenal gland, either attached to the capsule or free within the adipose tissue.[12, 18, 28, 29] The smaller nodules are not encapsulated, but the larger ones may show a pseudocapsule. The nodules are histologically well circumscribed but not encapsulated and are usually composed of cytologically normal cells of the zona fasciculata arranged in various architectural patterns. The pigmented nodules are composed of cells resembling the zona reticularis.

## ADRENOCORTICAL ADENOMA

Adrenocortical adenomas are benign neoplasms of the adrenal cortex, usually defined as greater than 1 cm in size. They occur in both adults and children, with a slight predilection for females. In children, most adenomas occur before 5 years of age.[30] Adults with adenomas usually present with symptoms and signs of endocrine dysfunction, most often Cushing's syndrome, but also primary hyperaldosteronism and, rarely, virilization or feminization.[31] Adults with adenomas may also be asymptomatic. In contrast, almost all children with adenomas present with mixed endocrine syndromes, most often Cushing's syndrome and virilization.[30] By radiologic studies, cortical adenomas are usually homogeneous, with a well-defined outline. Properly diagnosed, adrenocortical adenoma is a benign lesion, with no propensity for recurrence or metastasis.

Gross evaluation shows typical adenomas to be solitary, encapsulated, and relatively small. Adenomas are rarely larger than 50 g or 5 cm in diameter.[31–34] Adenomas found in patients with primary hyperaldosteronism are commonly smaller than usual, often no larger than 2 cm in diameter, and orange-yellow or yellow; they may be multiple or even bilateral.[35] Glucocorticoid-secreting neoplasms are larger, with a bright yellow or orange cut surface secondary to the presence of abundant lipid (Fig. 45–3). Adenomas associated with virilization or feminization are usually the largest. They are often tan to brown on cut section. Functional adenomas may suppress the uninvolved cortex, resulting in atrophy, although hyperplasia of the adjacent cortex may be seen in many adenomas associated with Conn's syndrome. A subset of adenomas are pigmented; these are usually nonfunctional, but they also occur with Cushing's syndrome or, more rarely, Conn's syndrome. On occasion, adenomas may be associated with extensive hemorrhage[36]; however, a more common phenomenon is the presence of myelolipomatous foci within the adenoma that mimics an area of hemorrhage.[37]

Mineralocorticoid-secreting tumors may show a fibrous pseudocapsule at histologic examination and are usually not well encapsulated. The tumor cells are organized in a variety of architectural patterns, from ball-like to trabecular. They are composed of cells that may resemble zona glomerulosa cells, but they may also resemble cells of the zona fasciculata or zona reticularis or cells with hybrid features of all three cell types. Nuclear atypia is infrequent, and mitotic figures are rare. Necrosis is usually absent. The adjacent adrenal cortex often contains nodules. In patients treated with spironolactone, spironolactone bodies may be found in the neoplastic cells as

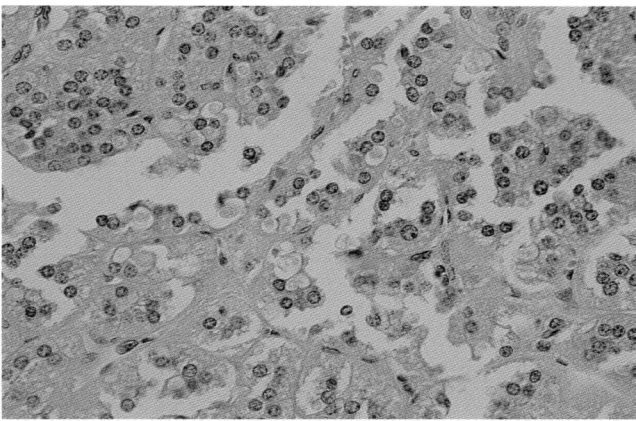

**FIGURE 45–4.** Adrenocortical adenoma associated with hyperaldosterone secretion and treated with spironolactone. Numerous spironolactone bodies are seen.

well as in the adjacent non-neoplastic zona glomerulosa (Fig. 45–4). These bodies are eosinophilic globules, 2 to 15 $\mu$m, in the tumor cell cytoplasm, often surrounded by clear spaces.[38, 39] Electron microscopic studies have shown these bodies to be composed of lamellar whorls of membranes thought to be derived from smooth endoplasmic reticulum.[38, 39] Glucocorticoid-secreting adenomas also have a pseudocapsule rather than a true capsule. Cystic change may be seen in larger tumors. They are composed of lipid-rich cortical cells that usually resemble those of the zona fasciculata or zona reticularis, or a mixture of these cell types, arranged in nests or cords (Fig. 45–5). Although these tumors may have nuclear atypia, including nucleomegaly and hyperchromasia, mitotic figures are extremely rare or absent[32, 34] (Fig. 45–6). Foci of lipomatous or myelolipomatous change or lymphocytic aggregates may be found. Rarely, a well-developed myelolipoma may coexist within an adenoma.[37] Virilizing or feminizing ade-

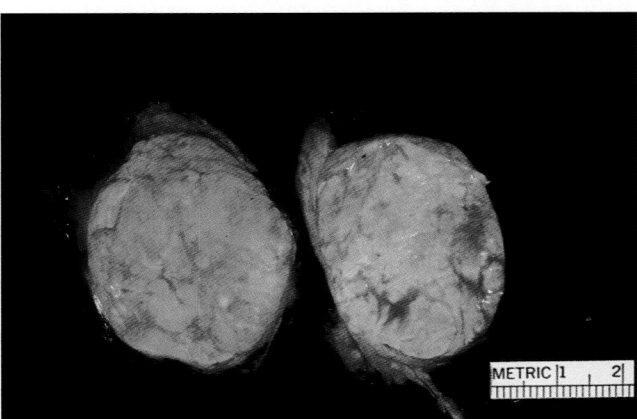

**FIGURE 45–3.** Adrenocortical adenoma associated with Cushing's syndrome. The yellow indicates a high lipid content.

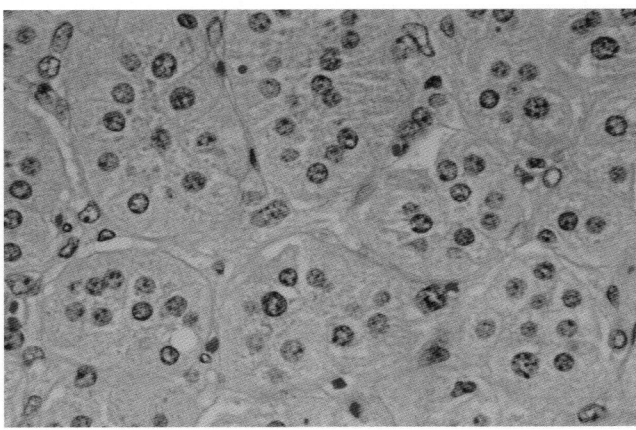

**FIGURE 45–5.** Adrenocortical adenoma associated with Cushing's syndrome. In this example, the nuclei are not pleomorphic, and the cytoplasm resembles that found in the normal zona reticularis.

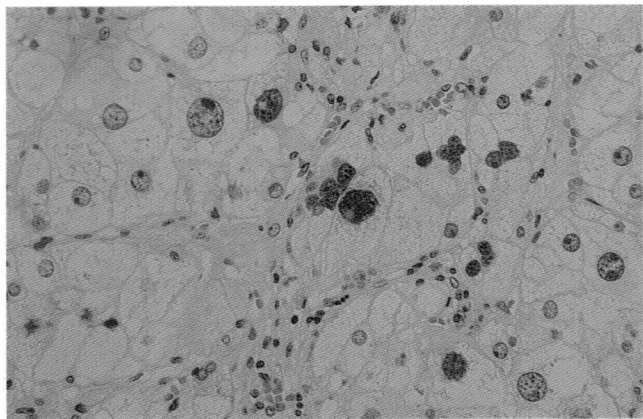

**FIGURE 45–6.** Adrenocortical adenoma. The cells are highly pleomorphic. Mitotic figures were absent.

nomas are rare; these symptoms are much more commonly found in cortical carcinomas. A mixture of cells resembling the zona fasciculata and the zona reticularis cells is usually seen, with the latter cells usually in the majority. Black adenomas are identical to other cortical adenomas, with the exception that the neoplastic cells have abundant cytoplasmic brown pigment.[40] Most investigators have concluded that the pigment is most consistent with lipofuscin, although Damron and colleagues[41] have suggested that it may be neuromelanin.

Immunohistochemical studies in adrenocortical adenoma reveal positivity for α-inhibin and Melan-A in most cases. Most cases are positive for vimentin, and a subset are positive for keratin. Occasional cases are positive for synaptophysin, although reactivity for chromogranin is consistently absent. A negative reaction is seen for S-100 protein, epithelial membrane antigen, and most other epithelial markers. Electron microscopic studies of adenomas have revealed findings similar to those for normal adrenal cortex.[42] The endoplasmic reticulum may be arranged in parallel arrays, referred to as lamellar or stacklike. Cell junctions, but not desmosomes, are found. Adenoma cells also have distinctive mitochondrial changes that correlate with the secretory activity of the neoplastic cells. In mineralocorticoid-secreting tumors, the mitochondria are relatively small and round or slightly elongated, with sacculo-tubular cristae. By contrast, in glucocorticoid-secreting tumors, the mitochondria are large and spherical and contain tubular or vesicular cristae.[43]

The differential diagnosis of adrenocortical adenoma includes adrenal pseudocyst, pheochromocytoma, and adrenocortical carcinoma. Rarely, adrenocortical adenomas may have extensive hemorrhage and secondary change, mimicking a pseudocyst.[36] Although pseudocysts may have a greater amount of adrenocortical tissue than one might expect, the amount of adrenocortical tissue in an adenoma with hemorrhage and secondary change will always be a great deal more. In addition, evidence of hormone overproduction is present in most cases of adenoma, whereas pseudocysts do not present with such symptoms. Pheochromocytoma may mimic an adrenocortical adenoma, particularly on frozen section. However, pheochromocytomas do not have the orange-yellow lipid color at gross examination. Although both neoplasms may be positive for synaptophysin, only pheochromocytoma has chromogranin expression, usually intense. The differential diagnosis of adrenocortical adenoma versus carcinoma is discussed in the section on adrenocortical carcinoma.

## ADRENOCORTICAL ONCOCYTIC NEOPLASMS

Rare cases of oncocytic adrenocortical neoplasms have been described.[36, 44, 45] All the reported cases occurred in adults; the mean age is about 45 years. There is a female predominance. Almost all patients lack clinical evidence of abnormal adrenal function; most of the tumors were discovered after radiologic examination of the patient was performed for a variety of reasons.

Gross evaluation indicates that the tumors range from 3 to 15 cm, with a median weight of about 200 g. On cut section, they typically have a mahogany brown color. Histologic examination reveals that these tumors are composed of lipid-depleted cells with intensely eosinophilic, granular cytoplasm, similar to oncocytes seen at other sites (Fig. 45–7). The tumor cell nuclei are vesicular, some of which may be enlarged with prominent nucleoli or hyperchromasia. Mitotic figures are usually rare or absent, but more than 1 mitosis per high-power field has been found in occasional cases. Immunohistochemical study has demonstrated positivity for vimentin, the mitochondrial antibody MES-13, neuron-specific enolase, synaptophysin, and keratin and negativity for epithelial membrane antigen, chromogranin A, and

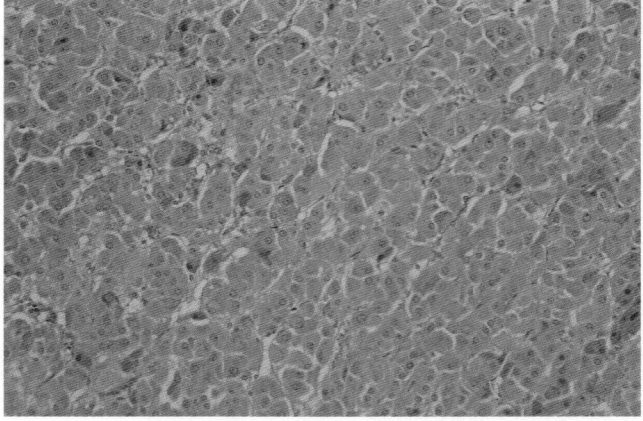

**FIGURE 45–7.** Adrenal oncocytoma. Like oncocytoma occurring in other organs, this neoplasm is characterized by a homogeneous population of cells with abundant eosinophilic cytoplasm. An MES-13 immunohistochemical stain for mitochondria was intensely positive.

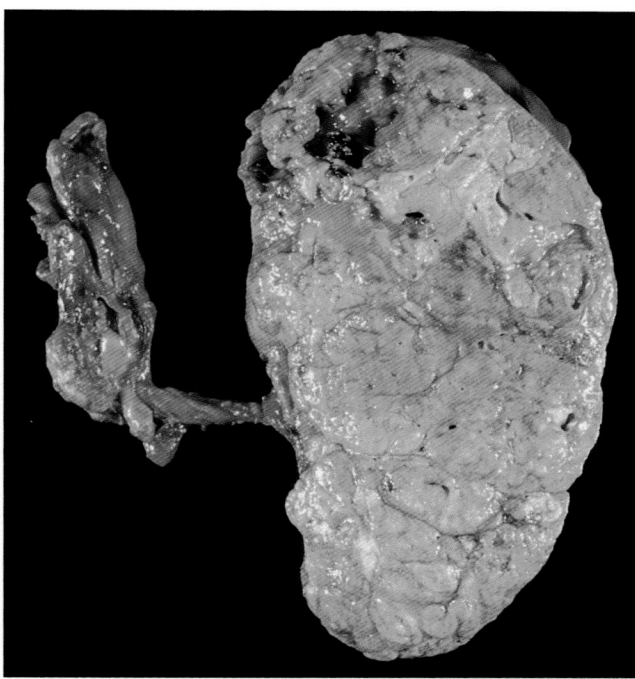

**FIGURE 45–8.** Adrenocortical carcinoma. This large neoplasm had a tumor thrombus in the adrenal vein (thrombus seen at left). Focal hemorrhage is near the top.

S-100 protein. Electron microscopic analysis has revealed abundant mitochondria as would be expected in oncocytoma, occasionally with electron-dense or crystalline inclusions.[46]

None of the tumors has shown clinical evidence of malignant behavior, although the follow-up times have been short in some patients. Most cases have been considered to represent benign neoplasms, although one has been diagnosed as carcinoma, and two have been diagnosed as oncocytic neoplasms of uncertain malignant potential. The differential diagnosis should also include pheochromocytoma, which may appear oncocytic on occasion. Pheochromocytomas are positive for chromogranin, whereas oncocytomas are negative.

## ADRENOCORTICAL CARCINOMA

Adrenocortical carcinoma, at a rate of two cases per million people, is rare.[47] It occurs in both children and adults, with a bimodal peak in age incidence. In adults, the median age is about 45 years; in children, the median age is about 4 years. In both children and adults, there is a slight female predilection. Adrenocortical carcinoma is associated with Li-Fraumeni syndrome, hemihypertrophy, and Beckwith-Wiedemann syndrome. Patients usually present with symptoms relating to the presence of a mass, and carcinomas are much more likely than adenomas to be nonfunctional, particularly when they occur in men.[48–50] Functional tumors in adults are most likely to be associated with Cushing's syndrome, with or without virilization, or rarely hyperaldosteronism.[51] In children, functional tumors are much more common, usually manifesting as mixed hypercortisolism and virilization.[30] Rare adults have had clinical symptoms and biochemical evidence of elevated catecholamine secretion in serum or urine.[52] Adrenocortical carcinomas are highly malignant neoplasms for which the best current therapy is radical surgical excision with en bloc resection of any local invasion, particularly in low-stage neoplasms.[53, 54] Unfortunately, most patients present with metastases at the time of diagnosis. The survival of patients with adrenocortical carcinoma is extremely poor; median survival time is about 1 to 2 years.[48, 55, 56] These tumors may recur locally or metastasize, most frequently to the liver, regional lymph nodes in the retroperitoneum, lungs, and bones.[48, 57, 58] Mitotane has been used to treat adrenocortical carcinoma but is generally ineffective in advanced stages.[56]

At gross evaluation, adrenocortical carcinomas are most often large (and occasionally enormous) neoplasms, usually greater than 5 cm and 100 g, with a median of about 15 cm and 500 g.[32–34] However, some carcinomas may be as small as 3 cm.[59, 60] On cut section, they are usually tan-yellow, with areas of hemorrhage and necrosis (Fig. 45–8). On histologic examination, adrenocortical carcinoma classically forms patternless sheets of cells interrupted by a fine sinusoidal network. However, there may also be broad or thin trabeculae or nests of varying size. Although there are commonly broad bands of fibrosis, single-cell infiltration of fibrous tissue is not usually seen. Venous or sinusoidal invasion is often present (Fig. 45–9). At high magnification, adrenocortical carcinoma is composed of either cells with eosinophilic cytoplasm resembling cells of the zona reticularis or cells with clear cytoplasm resembling cells of the zona fasciculata; the former usually predominate (Fig. 45–10). Atypia varies from mild to highly pleomorphic. Mitotic figures can be found and are frequently numerous; atypical mitotic figures are present. Rarely, these tumors may be spindled or contain abundant myxoid

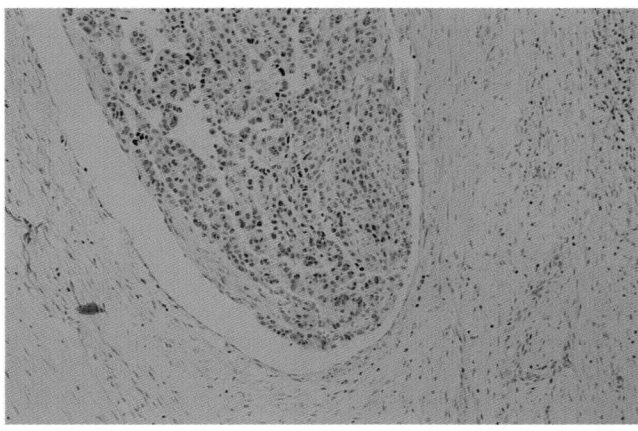

**FIGURE 45–9.** Adrenocortical carcinoma. Obvious vascular invasion is seen.

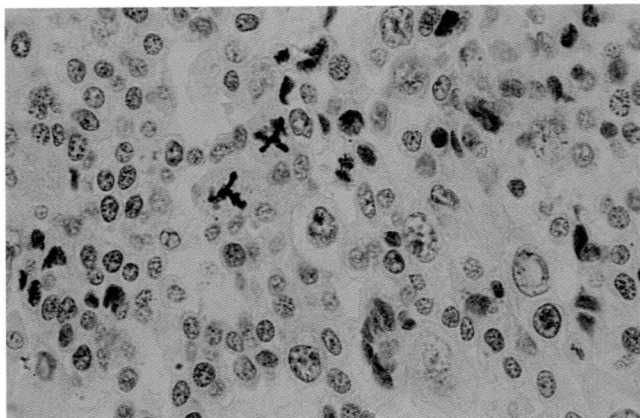

FIGURE 45–10. Adrenocortical carcinoma. This case showed highly atypical cells, with numerous mitotic figures, including atypical forms.

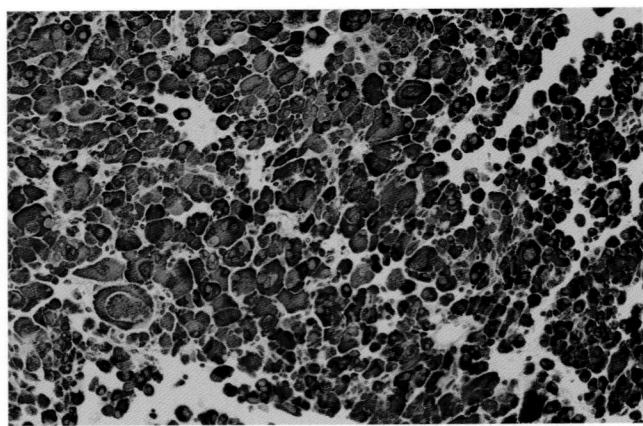

FIGURE 45–11. Adrenocortical carcinoma. This Melan-A stain shows intense positivity.

material.[61] Periodic acid–Schiff and mucin stains are generally negative, although rare cases have been described with focal cytoplasmic mucin.[62] Ultrastructural studies reveal features of steroid-producing cells with abundant rough and smooth endoplasmic reticulum that may be present in parallel arrays, numerous mitochondria with unusually shaped cristae, and cytoplasmic lipid.[42, 63] Dense-core granules may be identified in a subset of cases.[52, 64] Primitive intercellular junctions may be seen, but well-formed desmosomes are absent.

Although keratin has consistently been demonstrated by Western blotting, only a minority of adrenocortical carcinomas have demonstrable cytokeratin by paraffin section immunohistochemistry.[65] This keratin is usually recognized by the antibody CAM 5.2 (keratins 8 and 18) but is usually AE1 negative. Antibodies directed against α-inhibin and the A103 antibody directed against Melan-A are relatively sensitive markers for adrenocortical neoplasms, including carcinoma (Fig. 45–11). α-Inhibin is a peptide hormone expressed in sex cord–stromal neoplasms as well as in normal and neoplastic adrenocortical cells. It is expressed in almost all adrenocortical carcinomas, showing a diffuse cytoplasmic and granular staining pattern, and is not expressed in adrenomedullary cells and tumors or other carcinomas, including renal cell carcinomas.[66–68] There may be a greater intensity of staining for α-inhibin in tumors associated with hypercortisolism.[66] Melan-A was originally described as a melanocytic differentiation marker. However, the A103 anti–Melan-A antibody also stains sex cord–stromal tumors and normal and neoplastic adrenocortical cells.[69, 70] This staining is not seen with another Melan-A antibody (M2-7C10); thus, the staining is most likely due to cross-reactivity with a similar epitope of a different gene. Nonetheless, staining with A103 is seen in almost all adrenocortical neoplasms and is not seen in other carcinomas, including renal cell carcinoma. A subset of adrenocortical carcinomas may contain low-density neurofilaments, synaptophysin, and non-specific enolase[52, 64] (Fig. 45–12). However, chromogranin and three neuropeptides (calcitonin, gastrin, and somatostatin) are consistently absent.[64] Although normal adrenocortical cells are usually negative for vimentin, most adrenocortical carcinomas strongly express vimentin.

Vimentin expression in benign and malignant adrenocortical cells appears to have an inverse relationship with keratin expression.[65, 71–74] In non-neoplastic cortex, vimentin is usually not detected. By contrast, a subset of adenomas and the majority of adrenocortical carcinomas intensely express vimentin.[64, 65, 71, 72, 74] Epithelial membrane antigen, carcinoembryonic antigen, α-fetoprotein, anti–HMFG-2, and various blood group antigens are generally not expressed by normal or neoplastic adrenocortical cells.[65, 75] In addition, S-100 protein reactivity is usually negative.

Flow cytometric studies show aneuploidy in a majority of cases. Unfortunately, this does not have diagnostic significance, because aneuploidy may be seen in a significant subset of cortical adenomas.[76, 77]

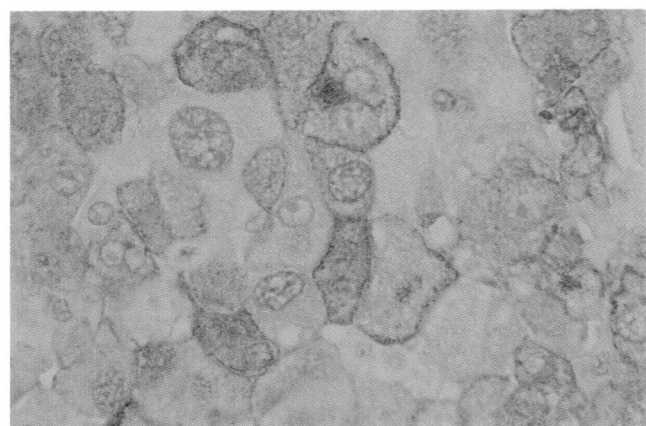

FIGURE 45–12. Adrenocortical carcinoma. A subset of cases may be positive for neuroendocrine markers, including synaptophysin.

Molecular studies have demonstrated somatic *TP53* mutations in about 30% to 50% of cases.[78] Comparative genomic hybridization has identified chromosome band 9p34 amplification in a subset of cases.[79] In addition, there are a number of other chromosome gains and losses, with gains more common than losses.[79, 80] In general, there is a correlation between the number of genetic aberrations detected and tumor size. Activating mutations of the *MEN1* gene probably do not play a prominent role in the tumorigenesis of adrenocortical carcinoma.[81]

Numerous prognostic factors have been proposed for adrenocortical carcinoma: stage, tumor size, mitotic count, presence of intratumoral hemorrhage, and markers of cell proliferation. One of the most commonly used staging systems is given in Table 45–2.[82] Patients with stage I and stage II disease generally have a fair prognosis, whereas those with stage III and stage IV disease usually have a dismal prognosis. Although the distinction between stage I and stage II is based on size greater than or less than 5 cm, another study has also shown that those patients with tumors greater than 12 cm have a worse prognosis than those with smaller tumors do.[83] Mitotic activity has been shown to be of prognostic significance in several studies.[83, 84] Patients with tumors with 20 or more mitoses per 50 high-power fields had a significantly worse prognosis.[84] Similarly, Ki-67, DNA topoisomerase IIα, and proliferating cell nuclear antigen antibodies have been used to assess prognosis.[85–88] In general, there is good correlation to the mitotic rate.[85] In one study, the number of nuclei positive for MIB-1 (an antibody against Ki-67) per 1000 tumor cells was 15 in adenomas and 208 in carcinomas.[88] None of the 20 benign lesions had more than 80 positive nuclei per 1000 tumor cells, compared with only 1 of 20 carcinomas having less than 80 positive nuclei per 1000 tumor cells. Staining for p53 has been reported in about half of carcinomas but not in adenomas.[88] Staining for p27 has also been found to be of use, with the labeling index significantly lower in carcinoma than in adenoma.[87] In contrast, antibodies to retinoblastoma protein have been found not to be of use, with similar staining of adenomas and carcinomas.[88]

By far, the most important differential diagnosis is the distinction of adrenocortical carcinoma from adrenocortical adenoma. Histologic features can be used to distinguish benign from malignant adrenocortical neoplasms. The mitotic count is the most reliable single determinant of malignancy, but it is best to use a multifactorial analysis to diagnose adrenocortical carcinoma. Three main systems are available[34, 84, 89, 90] (Tables 45–3 to 45–5); all three are reliable, although the Weiss system may be the simplest to use. However, in the Weiss system, it is critical to count mitoses with scrupulous care, counting 10 high-power fields in each of the five areas that have the highest mitotic rate. The distinction

**TABLE 45–3.** Histopathologic Criteria\* Proposed by Weiss for Distinguishing Benign from Malignant Adrenocortical Neoplasms

High nuclear grade (criteria of Fuhrman and coworkers†)
Mitotic rate >5 per 50 high-power fields
Atypical mitotic figures
Eosinophilic tumor cell cytoplasm (≥75% of tumor cells)
Diffuse architecture (≥33% of tumor)
Necrosis
Venous invasion (smooth muscle in wall)
Sinusoidal invasion (no smooth muscle in wall)
Capsular invasion

\* The presence of three or more criteria correlates highly with subsequent malignant behavior.
† Fuhrman SA, Lasky LC, Limas C: Prognostic significance of morphologic parameters in renal carcinoma. Am J Surg Pathol 6:655–663, 1982.
Data from Weiss LM: Comparative histologic study of 43 metastasizing and nonmetastasizing adrenocortical tumors. Am J Surg Pathol 8(3):163–169, 1984; and Weiss LM, Medeiros LJ, Vickery AL Jr: Pathologic features of prognostic significance in adrenocortical carcinoma. Am J Surg Pathol 13(3):202–206, 1989.

**TABLE 45–2.** Staging of Adrenocortical Carcinoma

**Staging Criteria**

| | |
|---|---|
| T1 | Tumor ≤5 cm, localized |
| T2 | Tumor >5 cm, localized |
| T3 | Tumor any size, locally invasive but not involving adjacent organs |
| T4 | Tumor any size, involving adjacent organs |
| N0 | Negative regional lymph nodes |
| N1 | Positive regional lymph nodes |
| M0 | No distant metastases |
| M1 | Distant metastases |

**Stage**

| | |
|---|---|
| I | T1N0M0 |
| II | T2N0M0 |
| III | T1 or T2N1M0 or T3N0M0 |
| IV | Any T and N with M1, T3N1, or T4 |

Modified from Henley DJ, Heerden JAV, Grant CS, et al: Adrenal cortical carcinoma—a continuing challenge. Surgery 94:926–931, 1983.

**TABLE 45–4.** System of Van Slooten and Colleagues for Distinguishing Benign from Malignant Adrenocortical Neoplasms

| Histologic Criteria\* | Weighted Value |
|---|---|
| Mitotic activity (2 per 10 high-power fields) | 9.0 |
| Extensive regressive changes (necrosis, hemorrhage, fibrosis, calcification) | 5.7 |
| Abnormal nucleoli | 4.1 |
| Vascular or capsular invasion | 3.3 |
| Nuclear hyperchromasia (moderate to marked) | 2.6 |
| Nuclear atypia (moderate to marked) | 2.1 |
| Loss of normal structure | 1.6 |

\* Histologic index greater than 8 correlates with subsequent malignant behavior.
Data from Van Slooten H, Schaberg A, Smeenk D, et al: Morphologic characteristics of benign and malignant adrenocortical tumors. Cancer 55:766–773, 1985.

**TABLE 45–5.** System of Hough and Colleagues for Distinguishing Benign from Malignant Adrenocortical Neoplasms

| Criteria* | Numeric Value |
|---|---|
| ***Histologic Criteria*** | |
| Broad fibrous bands | 1.00 |
| Diffuse growth pattern | 0.92 |
| Vascular invasion | 0.92 |
| Tumor cell necrosis | 0.69 |
| Mitotic index (1 per 10 high-power fields) | 0.60 |
| Pleomorphism (moderate to marked) | 0.39 |
| Capsular invasion | 0.37 |
| ***Nonhistologic Criteria*** | |
| Weight loss (10 lb/3 mo) | 2.00 |
| Tumor mass ($\geq$100 g) | 0.60 |
| Response to corticotropin (17-hydroxysteroids increased 2 times after intravenous administration of 50 $\mu$g of corticotropin) | 0.42 |
| Cushing's syndrome with virilism, virilism alone, or no clinical manifestations | 0.42 |
| Urinary 17-ketosteroids (10 mg/g creatinine/24 h) | 0.30 |

* In this system, both histologic and nonhistologic indices are derived. The mean histologic index of malignant tumors was 2.91; of indeterminate tumors, 1.00; and of benign tumors, 0.17.

Data from Hough AJ, Hollifield JW, Page DL, et al: Prognostic factors in adrenal cortical tumors: a mathematical analysis of clinical and morphologic data. Am J Clin Pathol 72:390–399, 1979.

between cortical adenoma and cortical carcinoma in children is a more controversial issue, because they constitute a small proportion of most series of adrenocortical neoplasms or are excluded entirely. Some believe, as I do, that they should be assessed like tumors occurring in adults, whereas others believe that size (and not histologic features) is the most (and perhaps only) reliable pathologic criterion of malignancy in children.[76, 91]

Adrenocortical carcinoma must also be distinguished from pheochromocytoma. At gross evaluation, adrenocortical neoplasms are yellow-orange; pheochromocytoma is tan-gray. At microscopic examination, pheochromocytoma shows a more distinct nesting pattern. A subset of adrenocortical carcinomas may be positive for synaptophysin; however, they are not positive for chromogranin, a consistent marker of pheochromocytoma.

Metastatic carcinoma is usually bilateral, whereas adrenocortical carcinoma is usually unilateral, but exceptions occur. Immunohistochemical studies help in distinguishing adrenocortical carcinoma from metastatic carcinoma. Metastatic carcinoma is consistently keratin positive and usually epithelial membrane antigen positive, whereas adrenocortical carcinoma is usually negative for these two markers; furthermore, adrenocortical carcinoma is usually positive for $\alpha$-inhibin and the A103 antibody to Melan-A. Although malignant melanoma is also keratin negative and A103 positive, it is almost always positive for S-100 protein; adrenocortical carcinomas are consistently negative.

# ADRENAL MEDULLARY HYPERPLASIA

Adrenal medullary hyperplasia is a pathologic increase in the number of chromaffin cells.[92–94] It is a rare disorder that almost always occurs in a familial setting but may also rarely occur as a sporadic disorder. It usually occurs in the setting of multiple endocrine neoplasia (MEN) 2 but may be associated with Beckwith-Wiedemann syndrome, cystic fibrosis, or sudden infant death syndrome. MEN 2 is an autosomal dominant disorder that occurs in two forms. MEN 2A, the most common form, usually consists of a triad of hyperplasia or neoplasia of the C cells of the thyroid, the chromaffin cells of the adrenal medulla, and the chief cells of the parathyroid. MEN 2A is caused by mutations of the *ret* proto-oncogene in one of five cysteine codons.[95] MEN 2B occurs in about 5% of cases of MEN and consists of hyperplasia or neoplasia of the C cells of the thyroid and the chromaffin cells of the adrenal medulla along with a variety of musculoskeletal abnormalities and neuromas and ganglioneuromas of the orodigestive tract and eye. MEN 2B is caused by a single-point mutation in the *ret* proto-oncogene at a locus distinct from those that cause MEN 2A.[95] Medullary hyperplasia occurs in the majority of cases of MEN 2A or 2B as well as in the Beckwith-Weidemann syndrome. Sporadic medullary hyperplasia may present with symptoms suggesting pheochromocytoma (pseudopheochromocytoma syndrome). Laboratory studies usually show abnormalities of catecholamine secretion.

The diagnosis of medullary hyperplasia may be obvious or subtle, requiring careful morphometric evaluation. Therefore, the adrenal gland should be carefully stripped of its periadrenal soft tissues, weighed precisely, and sectioned entirely at 3- to 4-mm intervals at right angles to the long axis of the gland, with all pieces submitted for histologic examination. Hyperplasia, when it is evident grossly, manifests as expansion of the tan-gray medulla or expansion of the medulla into both alae and the tail of the gland. It may be diffuse or nodular and may be complicated by pheochromocytoma. Microscopic examination may show compression of the adjacent cortex, but true encapsulation or invasion is not seen (Fig. 45–13). A nesting or trabecular pattern may be seen, or the architecture may be normal. The cells may be normal or may show spindling, vacuolation, granularity, hyperchromasia, or pleomorphism. Occasional mitotic figures may be present, and hyaline globules, usually minimal in number in a normal gland, may be numerous. The distinction between hyperplasia and normal adrenal medulla can be difficult, requiring morphometric evaluation. A simple morphometric evaluation requires use of a grid, attributing squares to the medulla or the rest of the gland (cortex, capsule, or blood vessels).[92] Using the weight of the gland (carefully determined, see earlier), one then calculates the weight of the medulla

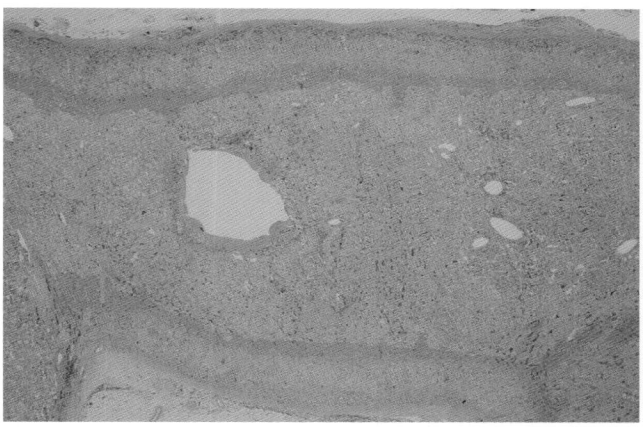

FIGURE 45-13. Adrenal medullary hyperplasia. There is marked expansion of the medulla. The cortex thickness is normal.

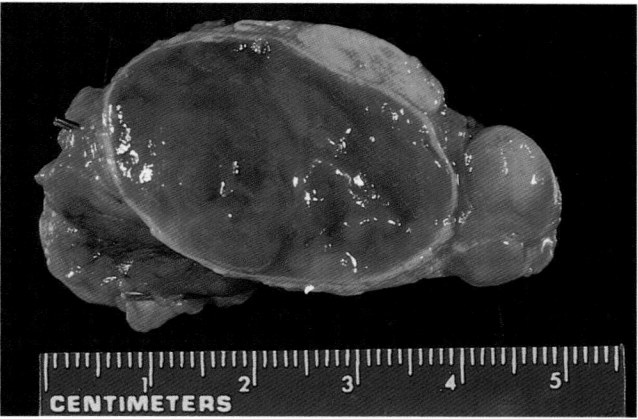

FIGURE 45-14. Adrenal pheochromocytoma. The cut section shows a hemorrhagic appearance. Note the rim of yellow cortex encircling the neoplasm.

by the ratio of the medullary area to the entire gland; a weight greater than 0.5 g (normal, 0.43 to 0.47 g) represents hyperplasia.

The distinction between hyperplasia and pheochromocytoma is definitional in the context of medullary hyperplasia; any nodules 1 cm or larger are arbitrarily regarded as pheochromocytoma.[93] However, flow cytometric studies reveal a diploid or euploid DNA content in medullary hyperplasia, in comparison to an aneuploid DNA content in the majority of cases of pheochromocytoma arising in this setting.[96]

## ADRENAL PHEOCHROMOCYTOMA

Adrenal pheochromocytoma (adrenal medullary paraganglioma) is a neoplasm that arises from the chromaffin cells of the adrenal medulla. It is rare, occurring in about 1 in 100,000 people in the United States. It affects patients of all ages, with a peak incidence in the fifth decade; 10% of cases occur in children. There is no striking sex predilection. About 10% of cases are familial, generally in a younger age group. Pheochromocytoma may be seen in the setting of MEN 2A and 2B (in about 40% of cases; see earlier), von Recklinghausen's disease (about 1% to 5% of cases), and von Hippel–Lindau disease (about 10% to 20% of cases) or as a familial syndrome unassociated with any other disease.[97, 98] Pheochromocytomas may present with myriad signs and symptoms, including intermittent, episodic, or sustained hypertension; sudden death; anxiety attacks; headaches; tachycardia, palpitations, reflex bradycardia, or postural hypotension; diaphoresis; weight loss; and tremor. Helpful laboratory tests include measurement of urinary catecholamines, vanillylmandelic acid, and metanephrines; analysis of plasma epinephrine and norepinephrine levels; and the clonidine suppression test. Rarely, pheochromocytomas may give rise to Cushing's syndrome.[99] Helpful localization studies include CT, magnetic resonance imaging, and nuclear scanning after the administration of labeled metaiodobenzylguanidine. About 10% of cases are malignant,[100] manifesting by metastasis—most commonly to liver, lymph node, lung, and bone—or extensive local invasion. The 5-year survival rate is about 50%.

The hallmark of the gross appearance of a pheochromocytoma is a gray-tan or hemorrhagic mass that is larger than 1 cm; however, there is wide variation in size (Fig. 45–14). Occasional cases may be pigmented because of melanin. Neoplasms average about 4 cm in diameter and weigh about 90 g. There may be adherence to or invasion of local structures, particularly large veins. On cut section, there may be cystic degeneration or dystrophic calcification. In pheochromocytomas occurring in a familial setting, the neoplasm is usually bilateral and is seen in the context of medullary hyperplasia.[97, 98, 101] At low magnification, pheochromocytomas typically show a distinct nesting pattern (*Zellballen*), a trabecular pattern, or a mixture of the two[102] (Fig. 45–15). Rarely, there may be spindle cell

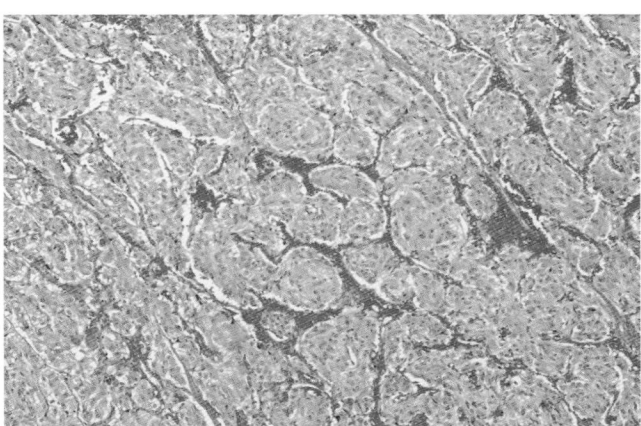

FIGURE 45-15. Adrenal pheochromocytoma. At low magnification, a *Zellballen* pattern is seen.

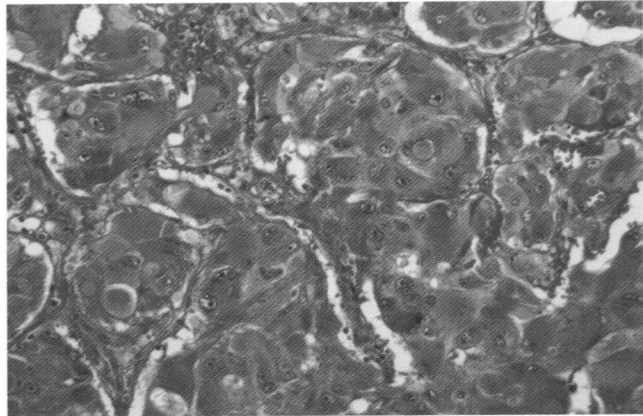

FIGURE 45–16. Adrenal pheochromocytoma. The cells have abundant eosinophilic cytoplasm. Note the cytoplasmic nuclear pseudoinclusion.

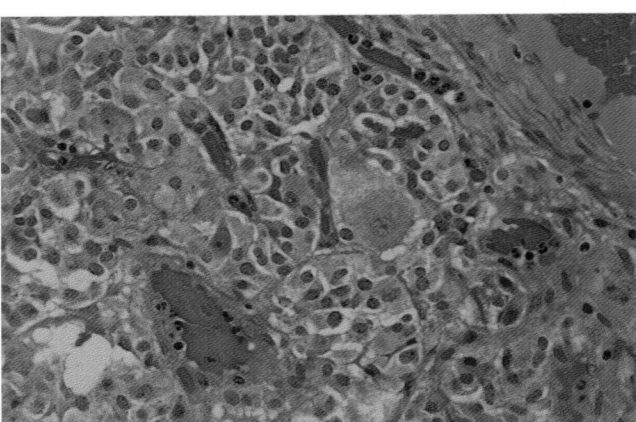

FIGURE 45–18. Adrenal pheochromocytoma. Note the admixed ganglion cells.

areas.[103] The border between the neoplasm and the adjacent non-neoplastic adrenal is usually indistinct, and there is no clear fibrous capsule. At high magnification, the cells typically have relatively abundant, finely granular cytoplasm that may be eosinophilic, amphophilic, or basophilic (Fig. 45–16). There may be hyaline globules (similar to those seen in the non-neoplastic medulla) or large vacuoles (Fig. 45–17). The nuclei vary from bland to highly pleomorphic. Scattered mitotic figures may be seen, and cytoplasmic nuclear pseudoinclusions may be present. Rarely, cells resembling mature ganglion cells may be present[103] (Fig. 45–18). Sustentacular cells are generally not evident by light microscopy. Stroma is usually scanty but contains a rich sinusoidal-capillary vascular network. Rarely, the vessels may be so prominent as to suggest a vascular neoplasm.[104] On occasion, there may be sclerosis or areas of amyloid deposition.[102, 105]

Ultrastructural studies demonstrate variable numbers of membrane-bound dense-core granules. Well-formed desmosomes are not seen. Immunohis-

tochemical studies show consistent positivity for chromogranin, synaptophysin, neuron-specific enolase, and neurofilament.[106–110] S-100 protein reactivity is negative in the tumor cells, but a population of spindled sustentacular cells is often labeled, usually at the periphery of nests of tumor cells. This S-100 protein positivity detects more sustentacular cells in familial pheochromocytomas than in sporadic tumors[106, 111] but probably does not (contrary to early reports) label cells more consistently in benign than in malignant pheochromocytomas.[112] Pheochromocytomas may also express a variety of neuropeptides, including leu-enkephalins and met-enkephalins, somatostatin, pancreatic polypeptide, vasoactive intestinal polypeptide, substance P, corticotropin, calcitonin, bombesin, and neurotensin (in descending order of frequency).[113, 114] Vasoactive intestinal polypeptide is expressed in rare ganglion cells in a subset of cases. Pheochromocytomas may also be positive for vimentin and even keratin in a subset of cases[115] but are negative for vascular markers and muscle markers. One study has reported expression of HMB-45 in one third of pheochromocytomas.[116]

Malignant pheochromocytomas are defined by the presence of distant metastases to parenchymal organs, lymph nodes, or other sites where normal sympathoadrenal tissue is not found.[117] There are no absolute clinical or pathologic features that distinguish benign from malignant pheochromocytoma. Clinically, malignant tumors are more likely to occur in males. Malignant tumors are significantly larger than benign tumors and more likely to have a coarse nodularity at gross evaluation. At microscopic examination, malignant tumors are significantly more likely to have confluent tumor necrosis and extensive local or vascular invasion and lack hyaline globules.[103] In addition, malignant tumors are somewhat more likely to have a higher mitotic rate, although the difference is not generally statistically significant. One study showed the tumor cell nuclei to be generally smaller with a narrow size

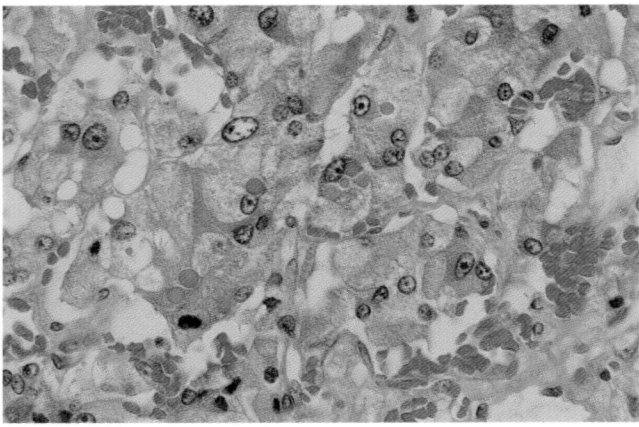

FIGURE 45–17. Adrenal pheochromocytoma. Numerous hyaline globules are present.

distribution in malignant tumors compared with benign neoplasms.[118] Tumor angiogenesis studies may be of potential use in determining the likelihood of malignant behavior, but their use in regular diagnostic pathology is still undergoing evaluation.[119] Immunohistochemical studies have revealed expression of fewer neuropeptides in malignant tumors than in benign ones.[113] Flow cytometric studies have yielded conflicting results, but aneuploid DNA content has been identified in both benign and malignant pheochromocytomas in several studies.[96, 120] Although groups have attempted to use statistical models of multiple factors to predict malignant behavior, it is nonetheless difficult to make an absolute distinction in a significant subset of cases.

The differential diagnosis of pheochromocytoma includes adrenocortical neoplasms and metastatic tumors. Adrenocortical neoplasms are generally yellow-orange on cut section, whereas pheochromocytomas are more often gray-tan. Although a subset of adrenocortical neoplasms may be positive for synaptophysin, they are not positive for chromogranin, a consistent marker of pheochromocytoma. Almost all metastatic carcinomas and malignant melanomas are keratin positive or S-100 protein positive, respectively, whereas the neoplastic cells of pheochromocytoma are usually negative for both markers.

## EXTRA-ADRENAL PARA-AORTIC SYMPATHOADRENAL PARAGANGLIOMA

Approximately 10% of pheochromocytomas arise in the extra-adrenal sympathoadrenal neuroendocrine system; approximately 80% of these cases arise in the para-aortic region.[121] These neoplasms are commonly termed paragangliomas. They occur in all age groups; the median age is about 35 years. There may be a slight male predominance. Patients usually present with signs and symptoms identical to those seen in adrenal pheochromocytoma, although some are identified as a result of abdominal pain; others are discovered as an abdominal mass or as an incidental finding. Tumors arise in the superior para-aortic area in about two thirds of cases and in the inferior para-aortic area (including the area of the organ of Zuckerkandl) in about one third of cases. Laboratory abnormalities and radiologic findings are similar to those seen in adrenal pheochromocytoma. The incidence of malignancy is higher than that seen in adrenal pheochromocytoma, about 25%. The pattern of spread is similar to that seen in adrenal pheochromocytoma, but the 5-year survival rate may be somewhat lower, about 35%.

Gross evaluation shows that most neoplasms are solitary, but approximately 20% of patients have multiple primary tumors, and rare patients may have 10 or more separate masses. There is a wide range in size, averaging about 10 cm. The cut section appearance is similar to that of adrenal pheo-chromocytoma; a gray-white color may be complicated by hemorrhage and cystic change. A subset of cases may show brown pigmentation from melanin.[122] The histologic appearance is identical to that of adrenal pheochromocytoma, and the localization of the tumor and the adrenal gland before or at the time of surgery is the best means of discriminating between an adrenal and an extra-adrenal primary. As with adrenal pheochromocytoma, there are no reliable means for distinguishing benign from malignant tumors.

## NEUROBLASTIC NEOPLASMS

Neuroblastic neoplasms arise from the primitive precursor cells of the sympathetic nervous system. The family of neuroblastic neoplasms includes the historical entities of neuroblastoma, ganglioneuroblastoma, and ganglioneuroma; each represents a point along the spectrum of neuroblastic maturation.[123–128] Neuroblastic neoplasms represent the third most common type of tumors in children of all ages (after leukemia-lymphoma and central nervous system neoplasms), and they are the most common solid tumor of children younger than 1 year.[129, 130] The median age is about 2 years, although rare cases may occur in adults.[130–132] There is no sex predilection. Some cases are familial, and there is an association with von Recklinghausen's disease. Interestingly, there is a low incidence of neuroblastic neoplasms in black persons, including those of equatorial Africa.[133]

Patients usually present with a mass in an area where the sympathetic nervous system can be found. Therefore, the most common sites are in the adrenal and the periadrenal retroperitoneum, which account for more than 50% of cases.[134] In adults, adrenal and periadrenal primaries are less common. Typically, the mass is large, firm, and irregular and often crosses the midline. In addition to the primary mass, patients may present with a variety of unusual syndromes; these include the "blueberry muffin baby" due to cutaneous masses, the opsoclonus-polymyoclonus syndrome, and intractable watery diarrhea due to secretion of vasoactive intestinal polypeptide. Common laboratory abnormalities include elevated urinary vanillylmandelic acid and homovanillic acid levels. CT is the most sensitive radiologic study and identifies calcifications in about 90% of patients. The staging system for neuroblastoma is given in Table 45–6.[135] Most patients present with evidence of metastases, which most commonly occur in lymph nodes, bone marrow, bone, liver, and skin (lung metastases are rare). The staging system recognizes a unique high-stage presentation with an excellent prognosis, stage IVS, in which there is localized primary tumor with dissemination limited to liver, skin, and bone marrow. These cases usually occur in infants.[136, 137] The treatment of neuroblastoma requires a multidisciplinary approach. Surgery and radiation therapy are gener-

**TABLE 45–6.** Staging System for Neuroblastoma Proposed by the International Staging System Working Party

| Stage | Criteria |
|-------|----------|
| I | Tumor confined to the organ or structure of origin with complete gross excision, with or without microscopic residual disease; lymph nodes negative |
| IIa | Unilateral tumor with incomplete gross excision; lymph nodes negative |
| IIb | Unilateral tumor with complete or incomplete gross excision; positive ipsilateral and negative contralateral lymph nodes |
| III | Tumor infiltrating across the midline (with or without lymph node involvement) or midline tumor with bilateral lymph nodes |
| IV | Remote disease involving skeleton, organs, soft tissues, or distant lymph node groups |
| IVS | Patients who would otherwise be assigned to stage I or II but who have remote disease confined to only one or more of the following sites: liver, skin, or bone marrow (without radiographic evidence of bone metastases on complete skeletal survey) |

Modified from Recommendations for reporting of tumors of the adrenal cortex and medulla. Association of Directors of Anatomic and Surgical Pathology. Hum Pathol 30:887–890, 1999.

ally used for low-stage disease; chemotherapy is used for unresectable or metastatic disease. Metastases usually occur in bone marrow, bone, lymph nodes, and liver, in descending frequency. Rarely, spontaneous regression has been reported for patients with stage IVS.[137] Another rare progression is maturation of neuroblastoma or ganglioneuroblastoma to ganglioneuroma. Adrenal masses with the histologic appearance of ganglioneuroma usually do not recur after excision.

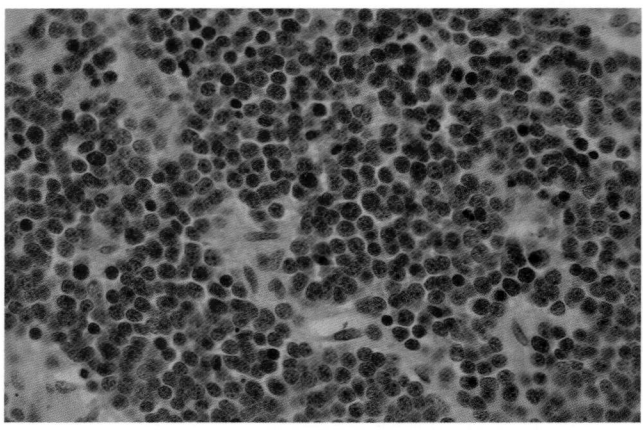

**FIGURE 45–20.** Undifferentiated type of adrenal neuroblastoma. Without special studies, this neoplasm is indistinguishable from other small round blue cell tumors.

Most gross tumors measure between 5 and 10 cm, although there may be wide variation in size (Fig. 45–19). On cut section, one may identify a rim of adrenal in primaries arising from that organ. The consistency of the tumor varies from fibrous and gray-white in patients with more differentiated tumors to soft and hemorrhagic in undifferentiated tumors. Calcification may also be identified. It is important to examine fibrous tumors carefully for evidence of a softer nodule, which may represent a less differentiated area of a nodular ganglioneuroblastoma. Neuroblastic neoplasms generally consist microscopically of two main cell populations, neuroblastic-ganglionic cells and Schwann cells, with a stroma that varies from nonexistent to fibrillary to schwannian stroma rich (Figs. 46–20 to 46–26). The Schwann cells most likely represent a reactive component recruited by tissue factors released by the neoplastic component, the neuroblastic-ganglionic

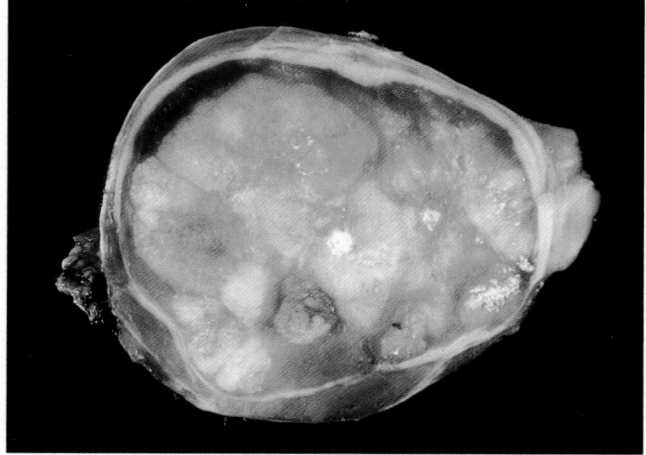

**FIGURE 45–19.** Adrenal neuroblastic tumor. This tumor is gray-tan, with flecks of calcification. (Courtesy of David Pinkhasov, Long Island Jewish Hospital, New York, NY.)

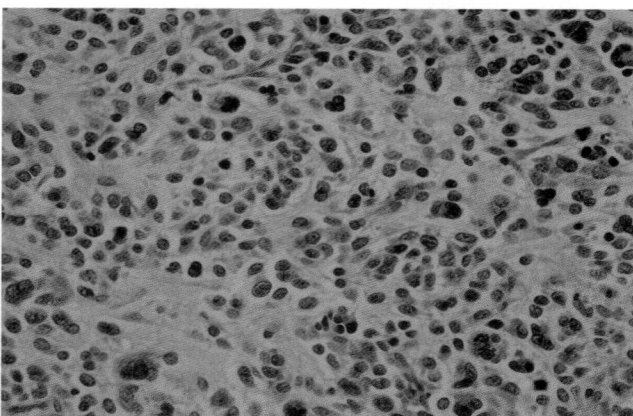

**FIGURE 45–21.** Poorly differentiated type of adrenal neuroblastoma. More than 5% but less than 50% of the cells show differentiation toward neuroblasts.

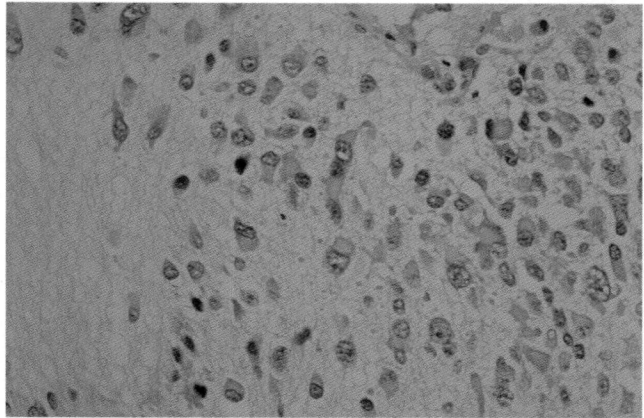

**FIGURE 45–22.** Differentiating type of adrenal neuroblastoma. More than 50% of the cells show differentiation toward neuroblasts, but the stroma is still neuropil.

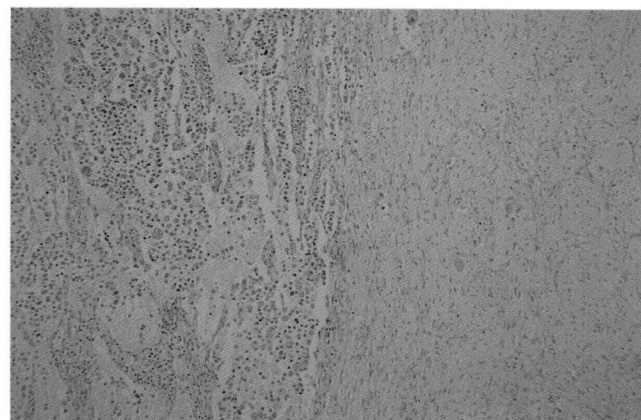

**FIGURE 45–24.** Nodular type of adrenal ganglioneuroblastoma. There is a gross nodule of neuroblastic tissue in a background of schwannian stroma.

cells. The neuroblastic-ganglionic cells may vary from small round blue cells with no differentiated features (aside from a dispersed salt-and-pepper chromatin pattern), to small blue cells with early ganglion cell differentiation as evidenced by an enlarged eccentric nucleus with a vesicular chromatin pattern and usually a single prominent nucleolus with a conspicuous rim of cytoplasm, to dysplastic-appearing ganglion cells, to perfectly formed mature ganglion cells. The amount and character of the stroma vary in direct proportion to the maturity of the neuroblasts. In the most undifferentiated cases, the stroma is nonexistent, although the tumor cells tend to be organized into packets by thin fibrovascular septa. Hemorrhage and necrosis may be prominent features, and there may be pseudoangiomatoid spaces. The first stroma to appear is a fine fibrillary neuropil, representing neuritic cell processes. On occasion, this stroma can be surrounded by a round rosette of neuroblasts—the Homer Wright rosette[123, 131, 138] (Fig. 45–27). With greater degrees of maturation, the stroma becomes fibrous, with large numbers of Schwann cells.

The degree of organization of the maturational process determines the specific classification of a neuroblastic tumor. The most recent classification of neuroblastic tumors is that of the International Neuroblastoma Pathology Committee (Table 45–7),[128] which represents a modification of that proposed by Shimada.[123] The International Neuroblastoma Pathology Committee classification recognizes four major types of neuroblastic tumors: neuroblastoma, intermixed ganglioneuroblastoma, nodular ganglioneuroblastoma, and ganglioneuroma. Neuroblastoma is a neuroblastic schwannian stroma–poor neoplasm. Although some tumors may have some degree of schwannian features, the proportion of tumor tissue with stroma-rich histology must not exceed 50% by

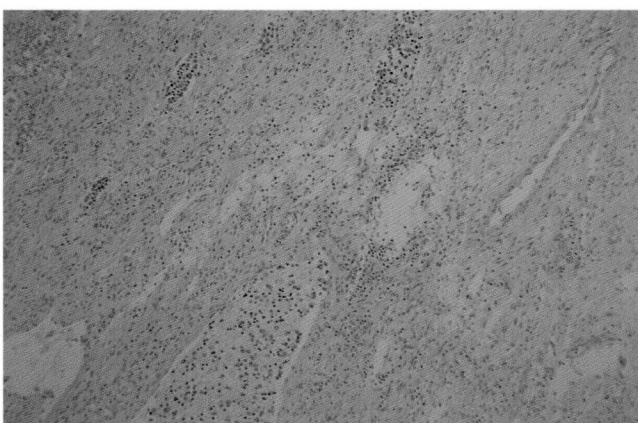

**FIGURE 45–23.** Intermixed type of adrenal ganglioneuroblastoma. There are nests of neuroblasts in a background that is more than 50% schwannian.

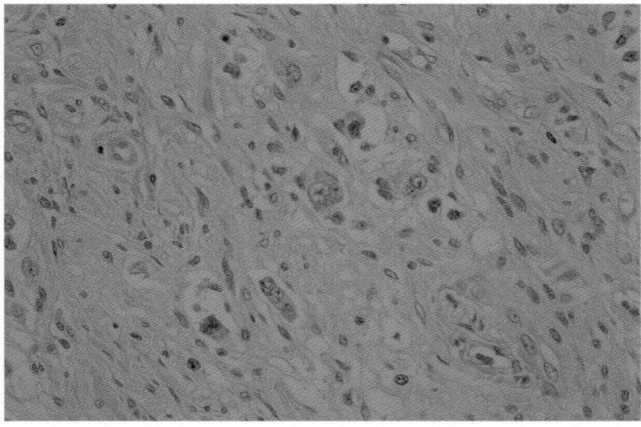

**FIGURE 45–25.** Maturing type of ganglioneuroma. There are scattered neuroblasts in an essentially schwannian stroma. The neuroblasts have some atypical features.

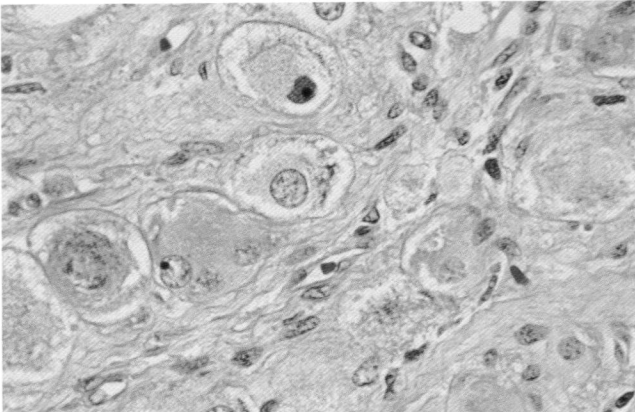

**FIGURE 45–26.** Mature subtype of ganglioneuroma. The neuroblasts are entirely mature; the stroma is exclusively schwannian.

definition. Neuroblastoma can be subdivided into undifferentiated, poorly differentiated, and differentiating subtypes. The undifferentiated subtype includes neoplasms for which special studies are required for distinction from other small round blue cell tumors (see Fig. 45–20). In the poorly differentiated subtype, neoplasms have a readily distinguishable background of neuropil; 5% or less of the tumor cell population shows definitive features of differentiation toward ganglion cells (see Fig. 45–21). In a differentiating neuroblastoma, more than 5% of the cells show differentiation toward ganglion cells (see Fig. 45–22). There is usually a greater degree of neuropil than in poorly differentiated neuroblastomas, but the degree of ganglionic differentiation is the defining feature. However, there may be significant schwannian stromal formation and ganglion cell differentiation, particularly at the periphery of the tumor, but the schwannian areas are less than 50% of the tumor.

There are two subtypes of ganglioneuroblastoma, intermixed and nodular. In the intermixed

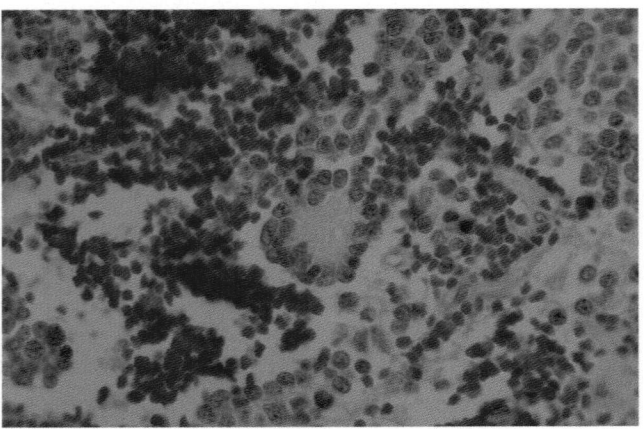

**FIGURE 45–27.** Homer Wright rosette. There is a central area of neuropil that is surrounded by a rosette of neuroblast nuclei.

**TABLE 45–7.** International Neuroblastoma Pathology Committee Classification of Neuroblastoma

| | |
|---|---|
| **Neuroblastoma** | |
| Undifferentiated | <50% stroma-rich No neuroblastic features seen histologically |
| Poorly differentiated | <5% of cells with differentiation toward ganglion cells |
| Differentiating | >5% of cells with differentiation toward ganglion cells |
| **Ganglioneuroblastoma** | |
| Intermixed | >50% stroma-rich; well-defined microscopic nests of neuroblastic cells |
| Nodular | Macroscopic nodules of neuroblastic tissue, with >50% stroma-rich in areas outside nodules |
| **Ganglioneuroma** | |
| Maturing | >50% stroma-rich with a minor component of scattered collections of neuroblastic areas, without discrete nests |
| Mature | Mature ganglion cells in an exclusively schwannian stroma |

Data from Shimada H, Ambros IM, Dehner LP, et al: Terminology and morphologic criteria of neuroblastic tumors. Recommendations by the International Neuroblastoma Pathology Committee. Cancer 86:349–363, 1999.

subtype, there are well-defined microscopic nests of neuroblastic cells intermixed or randomly distributed throughout the tumor (see Fig. 45–23). The nests are composed of neuroblastic cells in various stages of maturation, in a background of abundant neuropil. By definition, the schwannian component represents more than 50% of the tumor. The nodular subtype of ganglioneuroblastoma features macroscopic nodules of neuroblastic tissue. In about half of cases, there is a single nodule; two or more nodules are present in the remaining cases. Microscopic examination shows that there is often an abrupt transition at the edge of the nodule, which is composed of stroma-poor neuroblastic areas (see Fig. 45–24). In contrast, the tumor outside of the nodules has more than 50% schwannian areas.

There are two subtypes of ganglioneuroma, maturing and mature. The maturing subtype consists of more than 50% schwannian areas along with a minor component of scattered collections of neuroblastic areas (see Fig. 45–25). It is distinguished from the intermixed subtype of ganglioneuroblastoma by the lack of discrete nests of neuroblastic areas; in maturing ganglioneuromas, the neuroblasts blend into the schwannian areas. The mature subtype of ganglioneuroma is composed entirely of mature ganglion cells in an exclusively schwannian stroma (see Fig. 45–26). The stroma is usually organized into fascicles, and the ganglion cells are typically surrounded by satellite cells.

Tiny foci of neuroblastoma must be distinguished from neuroblastic nodules that may appear in the adrenal glands of newborns. These foci occur in about 1% of neonates and consist of clusters of immature neuroblasts, often with cystic degeneration. Because the incidence of neuroblastoma is much less than this, it is presumed that most undergo spontaneous regression. It has been suggested that a size of 2 mm be used as a cutoff; lesions smaller than this represent "normal" findings, whereas lesions larger than this represent neuroblastomas of uncertain biologic behavior.[139]

As mentioned earlier, immunohistochemical and electron microscopic studies are essential for diagnosis of undifferentiated neuroblastomas. Neuroblastomas are typically positive for neuron-specific enolase, synaptophysin, chromogranin, and neurofilament. The most immature neuroblastomas express only one type of neurofilament, whereas the more mature neoplasms express all three. In addition, neuroblastomas are usually positive for tyrosine hydroxylase, protein gene product 9.5, the ganglioside $GD_2$, and NB84.[140, 141] Significantly, neuroblastomas are negative for vimentin as well as for keratin, muscle markers, CD99, and leukocyte markers. S-100 protein is negative in the ganglion cells but highlights the Schwann cells and satellite cells, when they are present.[142] By electron microscopy, the neuroblastic cells show neuritic extensions of cell cytoplasm in which small dense-core neurosecretory granules may be found.[143–145] With increasing differentiation, these features are better developed. The molecular biology of neuroblastoma has been the subject of intensive study.[146] Amplification of the N-myc proto-oncogene is seen in about 20% to 25% of cases and correlates with high stage and aggressive behavior.[147–149] In addition, unbalanced translocations resulting in gain of genetic material from chromosome band 17q23-qter have been identified in more than 50% of cases. Other regions, including chromosome bands 1p36 and 11q23, show chromosome loss in a subset of cases. The loss of 1p36 is an adverse prognostic indicator.[150]

Numerous prognostic factors have been identified in neuroblastoma. The most important factors include age, stage, histologic subtype, mitosis-karyorrhexis index, presence of calcification, ploidy, N-myc amplification, and loss of 1p36. Age is an important factor; age older than 1 year identifies a group of patients with a poor prognosis.[123, 151] Among the three subtypes of neuroblastoma, the undifferentiated subtype has a significantly worse prognosis; the 3-year survival is about 30% for the undifferentiated subtype, in contrast to about 70% for the poorly differentiated and differentiating subtypes.[127] The nodular form of ganglioneuroblastoma has a worse prognosis than the intermixed subtype. The mitosis-karyorrhexis index is the number of mitotic or karyorrhectic cells based on a cell count of 5000 in random fields; a low index is regarded as less than 100, intermediate is 100 to 200, and high is more than 200.[123] The presence of calcification indicates a good prognosis. Diploidy or near-diploidy is an adverse prognostic indicator, as opposed to hyperdiploidy or near-triploidy.

Because of the multidisciplinary work-up of neuroblastoma, tissue needs to be obtained for more than light microscopy.[128] The tissue is obtained in a fresh state as soon as possible. At least two pieces are taken from the cut section. Multiple air-dried touch preparations are prepared for possible in situ hybridization studies (for N-myc and chromosome 1p). A portion of each piece is snap frozen at −70°C for possible molecular biology studies (N-myc). If available, tissue is placed in sterile culture medium for cytogenetics. Tiny pieces of tissue may also be saved in glutaraldehyde for electron microscopy. Histologic sections are taken for each 1 cm of tumor, with sampling of both central and peripheral areas of the tumor.

The surgical pathology report gives the histologic diagnosis, clearly stating the category of neuroblastic tumor, with subtyping, as described before.[127] The presence or absence of calcifications is clearly stated. The margin is assessed; cases with positive margins are identified as to whether there is microscopic or macroscopic residual tissue. The results of molecular studies are optimally incorporated into the surgical pathology report. The status of lymph nodes should, of course, also be reported. Regional ipsilateral and contralateral lymph nodes are always sampled whenever possible, and biopsy of other nodes is also done if they are greater than 2 cm.

## COMPOSITE PHEOCHROMOCYTOMA AND NEUROBLASTIC TUMOR

On occasion, mature ganglion-like cells can be found within otherwise unremarkable pheochromocytomas.[103] More rarely, complex tumors consisting of pheochromocytoma with foci of neuroblastoma, ganglioneuroblastoma, ganglioneuroma, or malignant peripheral nerve sheath sarcoma have been described.[152–158] In about 20% of cases, there is a his-

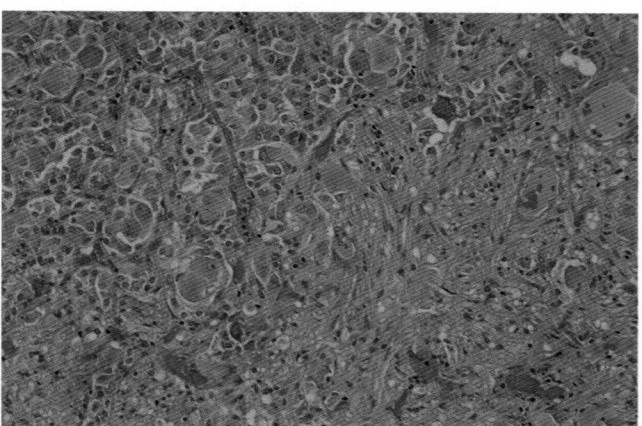

**FIGURE 45–28.** Composite pheochromocytoma and ganglioneuroma. The two components are intimately intermingled.

tory of neurofibromatosis, and rare cases have been associated with adrenocortical neoplasms. Patients usually present with symptoms of pheochromocytoma or, more rarely, symptoms of excess secretion of vasoactive intestinal polypeptide (watery diarrhea). Pheochromocytoma represents the predominant component, but definite foci of other tumors are also present at pathologic examination (Fig. 45–28). Immunohistochemical studies show typical staining patterns for each type of tumor present.

## COMPOSITE CORTICAL AND MEDULLARY TUMORS

Extremely rare cases of composite corticomedullary tumors have been described.[159] In one report of two cases, both patients suffered from Cushing's syndrome and paroxysmal hypertension. The tumors consist of cortical adenoma in a background of pheochromocytoma (Fig. 45–29). In one case, there was a complicating spindle cell sarcoma, apparently arising from the pheochromocytoma.

## PSEUDOCYSTS, INCLUDING "ENDOTHELIAL" CYSTS

Adrenal pseudocysts are uncommon but not rare lesions; about 500 cases have been reported in the literature.[160] Some divide these lesions into hemorrhagic and endothelial types, depending on whether endothelium-lined channels are present; there are no other significant clinical or pathologic differences. Because I consider the presence of endothelium-lined channels a stage in the repair of these lesions, both are discussed together here. Clinically, about 50% of cases have no signs or symptoms and are discovered incidentally; the rest present with abdominal pain, an abdominal mass, or hypertension and rarely in hemorrhagic shock. Radiologic studies

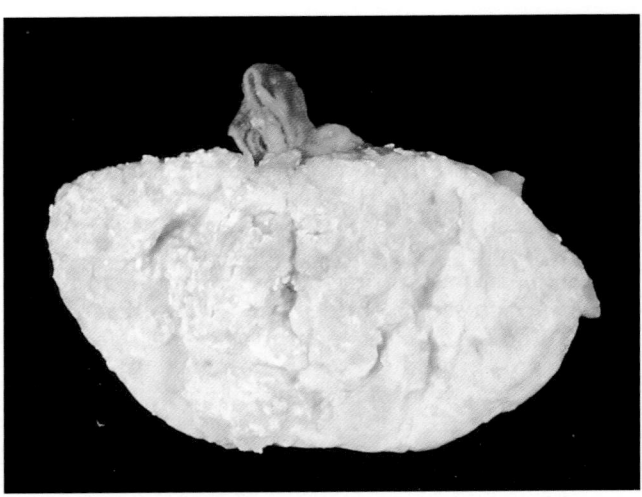

FIGURE 45–30. Adrenal pseudocyst. This example shows grumous, calcified material on its inner aspect. The pseudocyst was filled with a turbid fluid.

demonstrate a mass that is often calcified, occasionally showing a characteristic diffuse "eggshell" calcification.[161]

At gross evaluation, the lesions are usually large; the median size is about 10 cm[162–164] (Fig. 45–30). On cut section, the contents may be cystic, containing clear, brown, or bloody fluid, or they may be filled with necrotic material or thrombus. Microscopic examination shows a thick fibrous capsule that lacks a lining of epithelial cells; the wall may contain foci of macrophages, hemosiderin, elastic tissue, or smooth muscle in some cases. The center of the pseudocyst is composed of a variable mixture of necrotic debris, cholesterol clefts, thrombus, blood, lipid- or hemosiderin-laden macrophages, and endothelium-lined spaces (Fig. 45–31). On occasion, there may be adipose tissue or myelolipomatous metaplasia.[165] Nests of adrenocortical tissue may be seen, and these may be abundant, but no atypia of the adrenocortical cells is present. Immunohistochemical studies confirm the endothelial nature of the lining cells, with positivity for factor VIII–related antigen, CD34, and *Ulex europaeus.*

The most important differential diagnostic consideration is an adrenocortical neoplasm. Although abundant adrenocortical tissue may be present, the lesions do not present with hormone abnormalities, the necrotic areas lack the ghost outlines of tumor cells, and there is no cytologic atypia or mitotic activity in the adrenocortical cells. Both adrenocortical neoplasms and pheochromocytoma may undergo cystic change, but in both cases, the underlying neoplasm is usually obvious. Metastatic neoplasms may have widespread areas of necrosis. However, evidence of the underlying neoplasm is usually evident somewhere within the cavity. There has been one reported case of an adrenal pseudocyst with an apparently incidental metastasis from a breast carcinoma[165]; thus, thorough sampling of adrenal pseu-

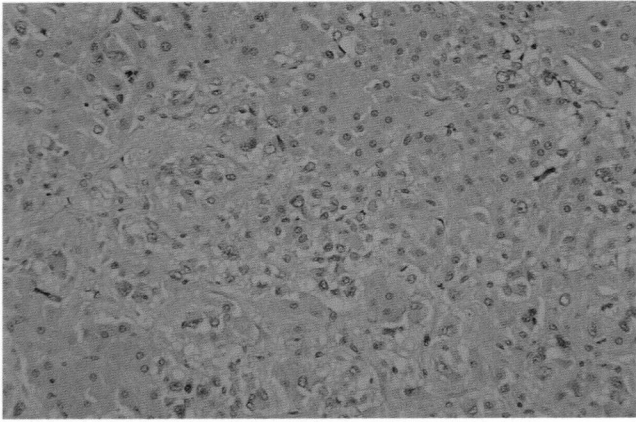

FIGURE 45–29. Composite adrenocortical adenoma and pheochromocytoma. The two components are classic for each neoplasm but are intermixed with one another.

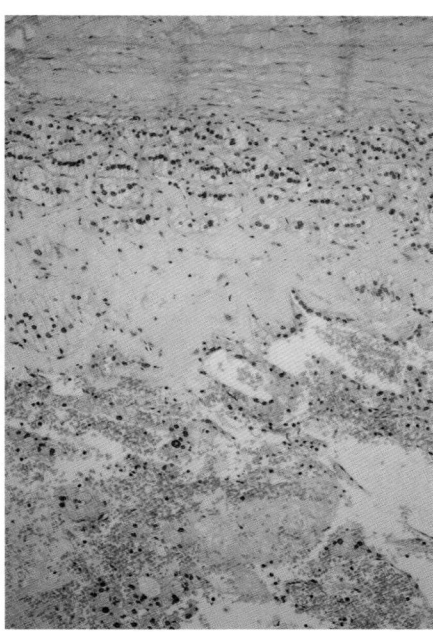

**FIGURE 45–31.** Adrenal pseudocyst. At the top is a fibrous wall that includes some normal adrenal cortex. The center of the cavity was filled with thrombus and hemorrhage; it is partially lined by endothelial cells, macrophages, and adrenocortical cells.

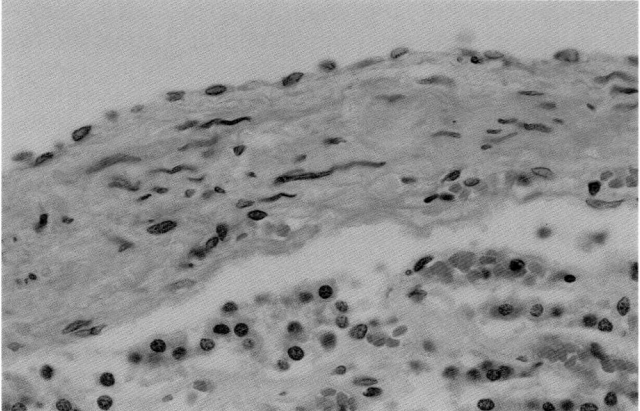

**FIGURE 45–32.** True adrenal cyst. There is a lining of epithelial cells (as demonstrated by a keratin stain).

docysts seems to be indicated. Infectious agents, such as fungi or mycobacteria, may cause widespread adrenal necrosis. These lesions are often bilateral; culture of the mass and special stains should be obtained in suspicious cases, particularly if epithelioid histiocytes and giant cells are seen. True hemangiomas of the adrenal are rare but have been reported (see later); they generally lack the degenerative changes seen in pseudocysts and do not reach a large size.

## TRUE ADRENAL CYSTS

True adrenal cysts consist of cystic spaces lined by a layer of true epithelium or mesothelium. They are extremely rare and are usually incidental findings.[166] They commonly measure between 1 and 5 cm and are usually filled with a clear serous fluid. The lining cells are usually flattened or cuboid (Fig. 45–32). Immunohistochemical stains demonstrate keratin positivity along with negativity for endothelial markers, consistent with epithelial or mesothelial derivation. Similar microscopic cysts smaller than 1 cm have been regarded as glandular retention cysts, embryonal cysts, or mesothelial inclusions.

## ADENOMATOID TUMOR

Adrenal adenomatoid tumor is a rare tumor that has been erroneously described as locally invasive lymphangioma.[167–169] The few reported cases have

been incidental findings, measuring up to 3 cm. The tumor is gray or pale white on cut section. There is a close histologic resemblance to adenomatoid tumors occurring in other organs, with nests and cords of relatively bland epithelial cells with cytoplasmic vacuoles and glandlike spaces (Fig. 45–33). There is no encapsulation, and the cells infiltrate between the adrenocortical cells, in one case extending into the periadrenal adipose tissue. Ultrastructural studies reveal desmosomes and long microvilli; immunohistochemical studies show positivity for keratin, consistent with a mesothelial derivation. The positivity for keratin, bland cytology, and characteristic infiltrating pattern make this tumor unlikely to be confused with anything else.

## MYELOLIPOMA

Adrenal myelolipoma is a benign, probably nonclonal, tumor. There is a wide age range; the median age is about 50 years. There is no sex predilection.

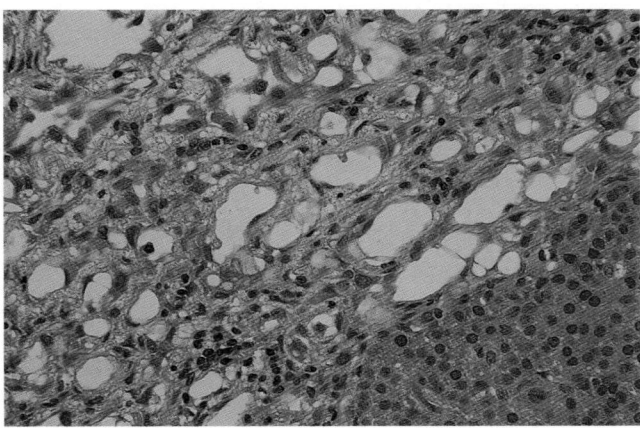

**FIGURE 45–33.** Adrenal adenomatoid tumor. Small pseudoglandular spaces lined by mesothelial cells are adjacent to and infiltrating normal adrenocortical cells.

The tumors occur more commonly in nodular adrenal glands and may be found within cortical adenomas (particularly those associated with Cushing's syndrome) or as a metaplastic phenomenon within a pseudocyst.[29, 37] They are not associated with extramedullary hematopoiesis in other organs. The tumor is usually discovered as an incidental finding, but larger lesions may present with abdominal pain, with an abdominal mass, or rarely as an acute abdomen due to rupture.[170, 171] The tumors are often distinctive on CT scan (nonenhancing mass with fat density), particularly when they have a high content of adipose tissue.

Myelolipomas are highly variable in size, from microscopic to enormous; most lesions are between 5 and 10 cm. On cut section, the tumor is usually yellow (because of the adipose tissue) with intermixed areas of red (reflecting hematopoiesis and hemorrhage) (Fig. 45–34). At microscopic examination, the lesions are usually not well encapsulated, with tumor elements directly apposed to adjacent adrenal parenchyma. The tumor consists of normal marrow containing adipocytes admixed with hematopoietic elements (Fig. 45–35). The hematopoietic elements contain myeloid, erythroid, and megakaryocytic lineages showing normal maturation. Rarely, foci of metaplastic ossification may be seen, and areas of infarction, hemorrhage, or thrombosis may occur. Myelolipoma is not likely to be confused with any other neoplasm, but one must ensure that the myelolipoma is not present within or coexisting with a cortical adenoma. The distinction between myelolipoma and myelolipomatous metaplasia associated with another lesion is arbitrary. Lipomas of the adrenal have been described (see later) but lack hematopoietic elements. Rarely, myelolipomas may occur in the retroperitoneum (or other sites).[172]

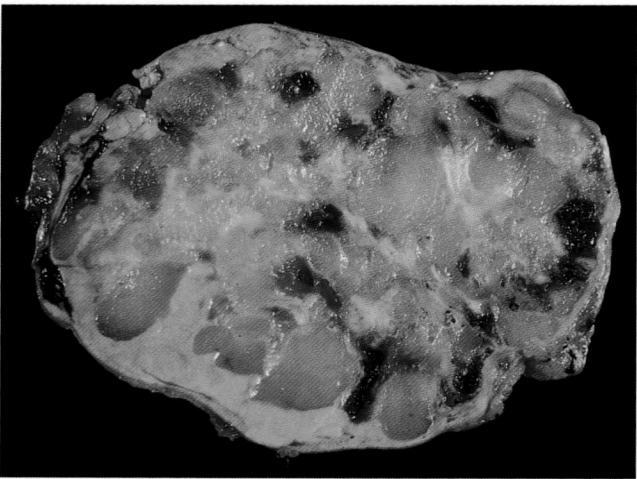

FIGURE 45–34. Adrenal myelolipoma. On cut section, a fatty appearance predominates, although there are focal areas of hemorrhage. (Courtesy of David Pinkhasov, Long Island Jewish Hospital, New York, NY.)

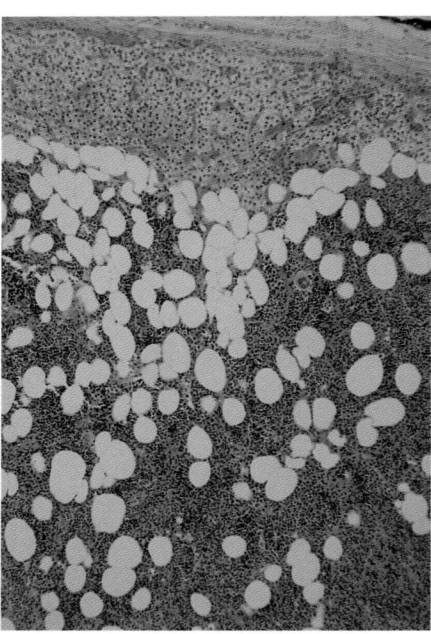

FIGURE 45–35. Adrenal myelolipoma. The lesion consists of marrow with normal hematopoiesis.

## RARE MESENCHYMAL NEOPLASMS

Primary mesenchymal neoplasms are rare in the adrenal gland but have been well described; this topic is better covered in specialized textbooks of adrenal pathology.[121] Rare cases of adrenal lipoma have been reported.[173, 174] They are usually incidental findings occurring in adults. They usually measure between 5 and 10 cm and consist histologically of mature adipose tissue. They should be distinguished from lipomatous metaplasia, which may occur in cortical adenoma and hyperplasia or in pseudocysts. A case of extensive lipomatous metaplasia in bilateral macronodular adrenocortical hyperplasia has been reported.[175] Lipomas should also be distinguished from myelolipoma, which contains hematopoietic elements admixed with the adipose tissue.

Hemangiomas of the adrenal have been reported but are rare.[176] Most present as incidental findings in adults, although hemangiomas may occur in infants as part of a larger syndrome. There may be a female predilection. Lymphangiomas have been reported, but they probably represent adenomatoid tumors. Primary adrenal angiosarcomas have been reported, particularly epithelioid angiosarcoma[177] (Fig. 45–36). In one series, the neoplasms were between 5 and 10 cm. Despite the epithelioid features, the neoplasm can be recognized by the formation of vascular-like spaces lined by cells that are positive for CD31, CD34, and other vascular markers. Epithelioid angiosarcomas may be positive for keratin.

Adrenal leiomyoma is usually an incidental finding at autopsy. Rare cases of adrenal leiomyosarcoma have been reported, most recently in an

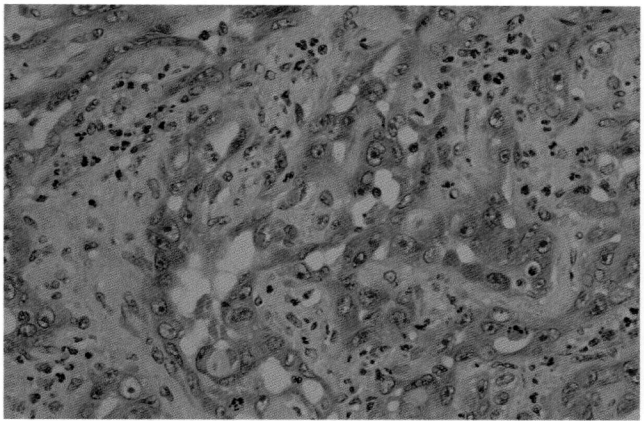

FIGURE 45–36. Adrenal epithelioid angiosarcoma. This neoplasm was keratin positive but also expressed several vascular markers.

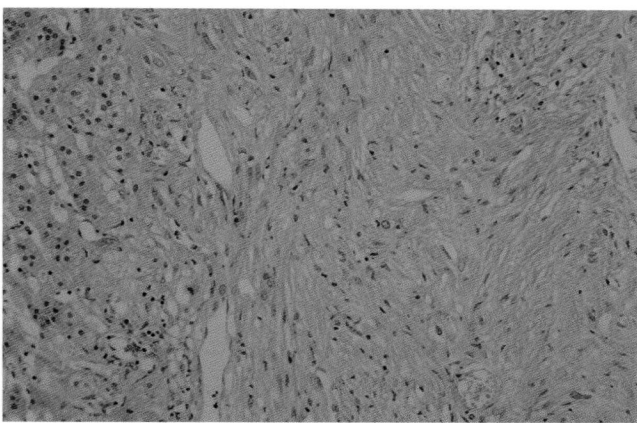

FIGURE 45–38. Adrenal neurofibroma. No ganglion cells are seen.

Epstein-Barr virus–positive tumor arising in association with the acquired immunodeficiency syndrome.[178, 179]

One case of solitary fibrous tumor of the adrenal has been reported.[180] The mass was discovered incidentally in a 42-year-old woman and remained unchanged for 5 years before surgical intervention. The histologic and immunohistochemical findings were identical to those of other solitary fibrous tumors. Microscopic areas of spindle cell proliferation may represent ovarian thecal metaplasia[181] (Fig. 45–37), and this lesion may rarely be responsible for the formation of a clinical mass.[182]

Schwannoma, neurofibroma, and malignant peripheral nerve sheath tumor of the adrenal have all been reported.[183–185] The absence of ganglion cells distinguishes neurofibroma from ganglioneuroma (Fig. 45–38). One must also distinguish neurofibroma involving a ganglion from ganglioneuroma; in the former, the ganglion cells are clustered in one area; in the latter, the ganglion cells are more dispersed. Occasional cases of malignant peripheral nerve sheath tumor occur as a composite tumor with pheochromocytoma.[158]

## MALIGNANT MELANOMA

Primary malignant melanoma is extremely rare in the adrenal gland but has been described.[121, 186] For a case to be accepted as primary, there must be no history of malignant melanoma or dysplastic melanocytic lesion at another site (including the eye or mucosa), and the lesion must be unilateral. Primary malignant melanoma must be distinguished from other neoplasms of the adrenal, including pheochromocytoma, neuroblastic neoplasms, and adrenocortical tumors, that may rarely contain pigment from melanin, lipofuscin, or the lipofuscin-like pigment neuromelanin. Adrenocortical neoplasms may stain

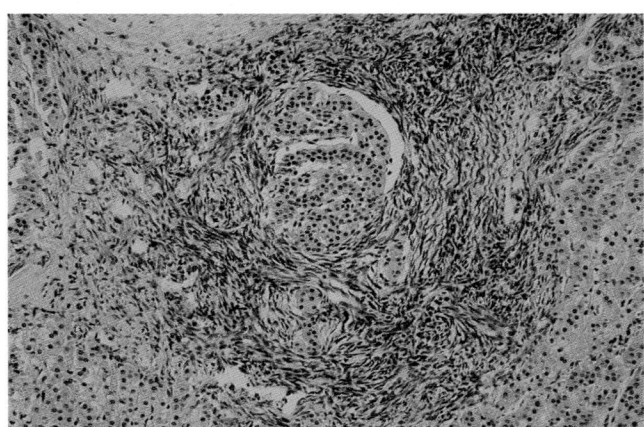

FIGURE 45–37. Thecal metaplasia of the adrenal. When microscopic, this lesion is not an uncommon finding. Note the clustered luteinized cells.

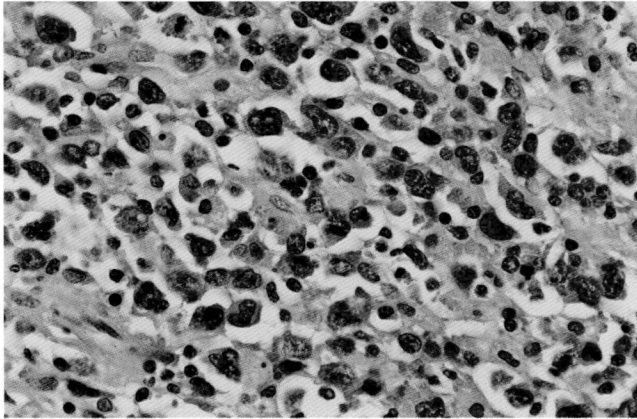

FIGURE 45–39. Adrenal lymphoma. This neoplasm showed a T cell lineage and was the only known site of lymphoma at presentation.

with the A107 antibody to Melan-A and a subset of pheochromocytomas may be positive for HMB-45, but neither of these neoplasms is positive for S-100 protein.

## HEMATOLYMPHOID NEOPLASMS

Secondary involvement of the adrenals by leukemia and lymphoma is a common occurrence at autopsy but only rarely presents as a clinical mass. Intravascular lymphomatosis has rarely presented as an adrenal mass, but it is usually shown to involve other sites on further investigation. Rare cases of primary B and T large cell lymphomas have been reported in the literature, including one case of bilateral primary involvement.[187, 188] In addition, I have seen two cases of peripheral T cell lymphoma that have presented as isolated adrenal masses (Fig. 45–39).

## METASTATIC CARCINOMA

The adrenal gland is commonly involved by metastatic carcinoma; metastatic disease is present at autopsy cases of carcinoma in about one quarter of cases.[189] Breast, lung, and kidney are the three most common primary sites of carcinoma to metastasize to the adrenal. Bilateral metastases occur in about 40% of cases.[190] In surgical pathology, the question of metastatic carcinoma to the adrenal arises in three main settings: 1) in the differentiation of the initial presentation of metastatic carcinoma from a primary adrenal neoplasm, 2) in the determination of whether an adrenal mass is a metastasis or a primary adrenal neoplasm in a patient with a history of carcinoma, and 3) in the determination of whether an adrenal nodule is metastatic carcinoma in a patient who has undergone adrenalectomy as part of cancer surgery or staging. Metastatic carcinomas are almost always keratin positive, whereas adrenocortical carcinoma is usually keratin negative. In contrast, adrenocortical carcinoma is usually positive for the A107 antibody to Melan-A and for $\alpha$-inhibin, whereas most carcinomas are negative for these markers. In regard to adrenalectomies performed at the time of nephrectomy for renal cell carcinoma, one study has shown a metastatic rate of less than 1.5% in the ipsilateral adrenal in unselected cases,[191] whereas another study has shown a metastatic rate of 11% when neoplasms larger than 5 cm were selected[192] (Fig. 45–40). In the first study, all but one of the positive cases was identified by preoperative abdominal CT. In the second study, tumors from the superior pole of the kidney occasionally showed direct extension to the adrenal gland but did not have a higher rate of metastasis.

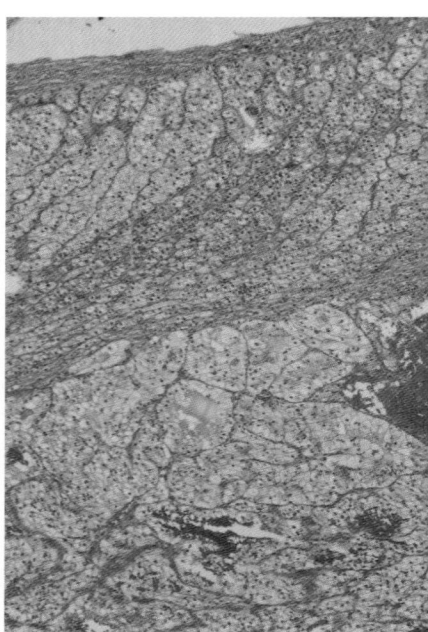

**FIGURE 45–40.** Metastasis of renal cell carcinoma to adrenal. Note the pseudoacinar spaces filled with hemorrhage characteristic of this neoplasm when it metastasizes.

## REFERENCES

1. Norton JA: Adrenal tumors. *In* DeVita VT Jr, Hellman S, Rosenberg SA (eds): Cancer. Principles and Practice of Oncology. 5th ed. Philadelphia, JB Lippincott, 1997, pp 1659–1677.
2. Bornstein SR, Stratakis CA, Chrousos GP: Adrenocortical tumors: recent advances in basic concepts and clinical management. Ann Intern Med 130:759–771, 1999.
3. Glazer HS, Weyman PJ, Sagel SS, et al: Nonfunctioning adrenal masses: incidental discovery on computed tomography. Am J Radiol 139:81–85, 1982.
4. Prinz RA, Brooks MH, Churchill R, et al: Incidental asymptomatic adrenal masses detected by computed tomographic screening: is operation required? JAMA 248:701–704, 1982.
5. Herrera MF, Grant CS, van Heerden JA, et al: Incidentally discovered adrenal tumors: an institutional perspective. Surgery 110:1014–1021, 1991.
6. Latronico AC, Chrousos GP: Extensive personal experience: adrenocortical tumors. J Clin Endocrinol Metab 82:1317–1324, 1997.
7. Korman JE, Ho T, Hiatt JR, et al: Comparison of laparoscopic and open adrenalectomy. Am Surg 63:908–912, 1997.
8. Recommendations for reporting of tumors of the adrenal cortex and medulla. Association of Directors of Anatomic and Surgical Pathology. Hum Pathol 30:887–890, 1999.
9. Mininberg DT, Levine LS, New MI: Current concepts in congenital hyperplasia. Pathol Annu 17:179–195, 1982.
10. White PC, New MI, Dupont C: Congenital adrenal hyperplasia. N Engl J Med 316:1519–1524, 1987.
11. Sasano H, Masuda T, Ojima M, et al: Congenital 17$\alpha$-hydroxylase deficiency: a clinicopathologic study. Hum Pathol 18:1002–1007, 1987.
12. Daeschner GL: Adrenal cortical adenoma arising in a girl with congenital adrenogenital syndrome. Pediatr Pathol 36:140–142, 1965.
13. Orth DN, Little GW: Results of treatment in 108 patients with Cushing's syndrome. N Engl J Med 285:243–247, 1971.
14. Gold EM: The Cushing syndromes: changing views of diagnosis and treatment. Ann Intern Med 90:829–844, 1979.
15. Jex RK, Heerden JAV, Carpenter PC, et al: Ectopic ACTH syndrome: diagnostic and therapeutic aspects. Am J Surg 149:276–282, 1985.
16. Jessop DS, Cunnah D, Millar JGB, et al: A pheochromocytoma presenting with Cushing's syndrome associated with

increased concentrations of circulating corticotrophin-releasing factor. J Endocrinol 113:133–138, 1987.

17. Carney JA, Hruska LS, Beauchamp GD, et al: Dominant inheritance of the complex of myxomas, spotty pigmentation and endocrine overactivity. Mayo Clin Proc 61:165–172, 1986.

18. Stratakis CA, Carney JA, Lin JP, et al: Carney complex, a familial multiple neoplasia with lentiginosis syndrome. Analysis of 11 kindreds and linkage to the short arm of chromosome 2. J Clin Invest 97:599–607, 1996.

19. Casey M, Mah C, Merliss AD, et al: Identification of a novel genetic locus for familial cardiac myxomas and Carney complex. Circulation 98:2560–2566, 1998.

20. Wulffraat NM, Drexhage HA, Wiersinga WM, et al: Immunoglobulins of patients with Cushing's syndrome due to pigmented adrenocortical micronodular dysplasia stimulate in vitro steroidogenesis. J Clin Endocrinol Metab 66:301–307, 1988.

21. Shenoy BV, Carpenter PC, Carney JA: Bilateral primary pigmented nodular adrenocortical disease: rare cause of Cushing's syndrome. Am J Surg Pathol 8:335–344, 1984.

22. Travis WD, Tsokos M, Doppman JL, et al: Primary pigmented nodular adrenocortical disease: a light and electron microscopic study of eight cases. Am J Surg Pathol 13:921–930, 1989.

23. Iseli BE, Hedinger CH: Histopathology and ultrastructure of primary adrenocortical nodular dysplasia with Cushing's syndrome. Histopathology 9:1171–1193, 1985.

24. Aiba M, Hirayama A, Iri H, et al: Primary adrenocortical micronodular dysplasia: enzyme histochemical and ultrastructural studies of two cases with a review of the literature. Hum Pathol 21:503–511, 1990.

25. Commons RR, Callaway CP: Adenomas of the adrenal cortex. Arch Intern Med 81:37–41, 1948.

26. Spain DM, Weinsaft P: Solitary adrenal cortical adenoma of elderly female: frequency. Arch Pathol Lab Med 78:231–233, 1964.

27. Robinson MJ, Pardo V, Rywlin AM: Pigmented nodules (black adenomas) of the adrenal: an autopsy study of incidence, morphology, and function. Hum Pathol 3:317–325, 1972.

28. Boggan JE, Tyrrell JB, Wilson CB: Transsphenoidal microsurgical management of Cushing's disease: report of 100 cases. J Neurosurg 59:195–200, 1983.

29. Dobbie JW: Adrenocortical nodular hyperplasia: the aging adrenal. J Pathol 99:1–18, 1969.

30. Hayles AB, Hahn HB, Sprague RG, et al: Hormone-secreting tumors of the adrenal cortex in children. Pediatrics 37:19–25, 1966.

31. Kay S: Hyperplasia and neoplasia of the adrenal gland. Pathol Annu 11:103–137, 1976.

32. Medeiros LJ, Weiss LM: New developments in the pathologic diagnosis of adrenal cortical neoplasms: a review. Am J Clin Pathol 97:73–83, 1992.

33. Tang CL, Gray GF: Adrenocortical neoplasms: prognosis and morphology. Urology 5:691–695, 1975.

34. Weiss LM: Comparative histologic study of 43 metastasizing and nonmetastasizing adrenocortical tumors. Am J Surg Pathol 8:163–169, 1984.

35. Neville AM, Symington T: The pathology of the adrenal gland in Cushing's syndrome. J Pathol Bacteriol 93:19–35, 1967.

36. Granger JK, Houn H-Y, Collins C: Massive hemorrhagic functional adrenal adenoma histologically mimicking angiosarcoma: report of a case with immunohistochemical study. Am J Surg Pathol 15:699–704, 1991.

37. Vyberg M, Sestoft L: Combined adrenal myelolipoma and adenoma associated with Cushing's syndrome. Am J Clin Pathol 86:541–545, 1986.

38. Shrago SS, Waisman J, Cooper PH: Spironolactone bodies in an adrenal adenoma. Arch Pathol Lab Med 99:416–420, 1975.

39. Davis DA, Medline NM: Spironolactone (aldactone) bodies: concentric lamellar formations in the adrenal cortices of patients treated with spironolactone. Am J Clin Pathol 54:22–32, 1970.

40. Macadam RF: Black adenoma of the human adrenal cortex. Cancer 27:116–119, 1971.

41. Damron TA, Schelper RL, Sorensen L: Cytochemical demonstration of neuromelanin in black pigmented adrenal nodules. Am J Clin Pathol 87:334–341, 1987.

42. Tannenbaum M: Ultrastructural pathology of the adrenal cortex. Pathol Annu 8:109–156, 1973.

43. Osanai T, Konta A, Chui D, et al: Electron microscopic findings in benign deoxycorticosterone and 11-deoxycortisol-producing adrenal tumor. Arch Pathol Lab Med 114:829–831, 1990.

44. Lin BT, Bonsib SM, Mierau GW, et al: Oncocytic adrenocortical neoplasms: a report of seven cases and review of the literature. Am J Surg Pathol 22:603–614, 1998.

45. Sasano H, Suzuki T, Sano T, et al: Adrenocortical oncocytoma: a true nonfunctioning adrenocortical tumor. Am J Surg Pathol 15:949–956, 1991.

46. El-Naggar AK, Evans DB, Mackay B: Oncocytic adrenal cortical carcinoma. Ultrastruct Pathol 15:549–556, 1991.

47. Third National Cancer Survey: Incidence Data. Bethesda, MD, National Cancer Institute, 1975. Publication (NIH)75–787.

48. Didolkar MS, Bescher RA, Elias EG, et al: Natural history of adrenal cortical carcinoma: a clinicopathologic study of 42 patients. Cancer 47:2153–2161, 1981.

49. Heinbecker P, O'Neal LW, Ackerman LV: Functioning and nonfunctioning adrenal cortical tumors. Surg Gynecol Obstet 105:21–33, 1957.

50. Wooten MD, King DK: Adrenal cortical carcinoma. Epidemiology and treatment with mitotane and a review of the literature. Cancer 72:3145–3155, 1993.

51. Alterman SL, Dominguez C, Lopez-Gomez A, et al: Primary adrenocortical carcinoma causing aldosteronism. Cancer 24:602–609, 1969.

52. Alsabeh R, Mazoujian G, Goates J, et al: Adrenal cortical tumors clinically mimicking pheochromocytoma. Am J Clin Pathol 104:382–390, 1995.

53. Pommier RF, Brennan MF: An eleven-year experience with adrenocortical carcinoma. Surgery 112:963–970, 1992.

54. Young WF Jr: Pheochromocytoma and primary aldosteronism: diagnostic approaches. Endocrinol Metab Clin North Am 26:801–827, 1997.

55. Greenberg PH, Marks C: Adrenal cortical carcinoma: a presentation of 22 cases with a review of the literature. Am J Surg 44:81–85, 1978.

56. Luton J-P, Cerdas S, Billaud L, et al: Clinical features of adrenocortical carcinoma, prognostic factors, and the effect of mitotane therapy. N Engl J Med 322:1195–1201, 1990.

57. Nader S, Hickey RC, Sellin RV, et al: Adrenal cortical carcinoma: a study of 77 cases. Cancer 52:707–711, 1983.

58. Nakano M: Adrenal cortical carcinoma: a clinicopathologic and immunohistochemical study of 91 autopsy cases. Acta Pathol Jpn 38:163–180, 1988.

59. Lewinsky BS, Grigor KM, Symington T, et al: The clinical and pathologic features of non-hormonal adrenocortical tumors. Report of twenty new cases and review of the literature. Cancer 33:778–790, 1974.

60. Gandour MJ, Grizzle WE: A small adrenocortical carcinoma with aggressive behavior: an evaluation of criteria for malignancy. Arch Pathol Lab Med 110:1076–1079, 1986.

61. Tang C-K, Harriman BB, Toker C: Myxoid adrenal cortical carcinoma. Arch Pathol Lab Med 103:635–638, 1979.

62. Tartour E, Caillou B, Tenenbaum F, et al: Immunohistochemical study of adrenocortical carcinoma. Predictive value of the D11 monoclonal antibody. Cancer 72:3296–3303, 1993.

63. Wiedemann HR: Tumors and hemihypertrophy associated with Wiedemann-Beckwith syndrome. Eur J Pediatr 141:129, 1983.

64. Miettinen M: Neuroendocrine differentiation in adrenocortical carcinoma: new immunohistochemical findings supported by electron microscopy. Lab Invest 66:169–174, 1992.

65. Gaffey MJ, Traweek ST, Mills SE, et al: Cytokeratin expression of adrenocortical neoplasia: an immunohistochemical and biochemical study with implications for the differential diagnosis of adrenocortical, hepatocellular, and renal cell carcinoma. Hum Pathol 23:144–153, 1992.

66. Munro LM, Kennedy A, McNicol AM: The expression of inhibin/activin subunits in the human adrenal cortex and its tumours. J Endocrinol 161:341–347, 1999.

67. McCluggage WG, Burton J, Maxwell P, et al: Immunohistochemical staining of normal, hyperplastic, and neoplastic adrenal cortex with a monoclonal antibody against alpha inhibin. J Clin Pathol 51:114–116, 1998.

68. Fetsch PA, Marincola FM, Abati A: The new melanoma markers: MART-1 and Melan-A (the NIH experience). Am J Surg Pathol 23:607–610, 1999.

69. Busam KJ, Iversen K, Coplan KA, et al: Immunoreactivity for A103, an antibody to Melan-A (MART-1), in adrenocortical and other steroid tumors. Am J Surg Pathol 22:57–63, 1998.

70. Busam KJ, Jungbluth AA: Melan-A, a new melanocytic differentiation marker. Adv Anat Pathol 6:12–18, 1999.

71. Cote RJ, Cordon-Cardo C, Reuter VE, et al: Immunopathology of adrenal and renal cortical tumors: coordinated change in antigen expression is associated with neoplastic conversion in the adrenal cortex. Am J Pathol 136:1077–1084, 1990.

72. Henzen-Logmans SC, Stel HV, Muijen GNPV, et al: Expression of intermediate filament proteins in adrenal cortex and related tumors. Histopathology 12:359–372, 1988.

73. Suzuki T, Sasano H, Nisikawa T, et al: Discerning malignancy in human adrenocortical neoplasms: utility of DNA flow cytometry and immunohistochemistry. Mod Pathol 5:224–231, 1992.

74. Miettinen M, Lehto V-P, Virtanen I: Immunofluorescence microscopic evaluation of the intermediate filament expression of the adrenal cortex and medulla and their tumors. Am J Pathol 118:360–366, 1985.

75. Wick MR, Cherwitz DL, McGlennen RC, et al: Adrenocortical carcinoma: an immunohistochemical comparison with renal cell carcinoma. Am J Pathol 122:343–352, 1986.

76. Zerbini C, Kozakewich HP, Weinberg DS, et al: Adrenocortical neoplasms in childhood and adolescence: analysis of prognostic factors including DNA content. Endocr Pathol 3:116–128, 1992.

77. Cibas ES, Medeiros LJ, Weinberg DS, et al: Cellular DNA profiles of benign and malignant adrenocortical tumors. Am J Surg Pathol 14:948–955, 1990.

78. Wagner J, Portwine C, Rabin K, et al: High frequency of germline p53 mutations in childhood adrenocortical cancer. J Natl Cancer Inst 86:1707–1710, 1994.

79. Figuereido BC, Stratakis CA, Sandrini R, et al: Comparative genomic hybridization (CGH) analysis of adrenocortical tumors in childhood. J Clin Endocrinol Metab 84:1116–1121, 1999.

80. Kjellman M, Kallioniemi OP, Karhu R, et al: Genetic aberrations in adrenocortical tumors detected using comparative genomic hybridization correlate with tumor size and malignancy. Cancer Res 56:4219–4223, 1996.

81. Gortz B, Roth J, Speel EJ, et al: MEN1 gene mutation analysis of sporadic adrenocortical lesions. Int J Cancer 80:373–379, 1999.

82. Henley DJ, Heerden JAV, Grant CS, et al: Adrenal cortical carcinoma—a continuing challenge. Surgery 94:926–931, 1983.

83. Harrison LE, Gaudin PB, Brennan MF: Pathologic features of prognostic significance for adrenocortical carcinoma after curative resection. Arch Pathol 134:181–185, 1999.

84. Weiss LM, Medeiros LJ, Vickery AL Jr: Pathologic features of prognostic significance in adrenocortical carcinoma. Am J Surg Pathol 13:202–206, 1989.

85. Goldblum JR, Shannon R, Kaldjian EP, et al: Immunohistochemical assessment of proliferative activity in adrenocortical neoplasms. Mod Pathol 6:663–668, 1993.

86. Iino K, Sasano H, Yabuki N, et al: DNA topoisomerase II alpha and Ki-67 in human adrenocortical neoplasms: a possible marker of differentiation between adenomas and carcinomas. Mod Pathol 10:901–907, 1997.

87. Nakazumi H, Sasano H, Iino K, et al: Expression of cell cycle inhibitor p27 and Ki-67 in human adrenocortical neoplasms. Mod Pathol 11:1165–1170, 1998.

88. Vargas MP, Vargas HI, Kleiner DE, et al: Adrenocortical neoplasms: role of prognostic markers MIB-1, P53, and RB. Am J Surg Pathol 21:556–562, 1997.

89. Hough AJ, Hollifield JW, Page DL, et al: Prognostic factors in adrenal cortical tumors: a mathematical analysis of clinical and morphologic data. Am J Clin Pathol 72:390–399, 1979.

90. Van Slooten H, Schaberg A, Smeenk D, et al: Morphologic characteristics of benign and malignant adrenocortical tumors. Cancer 55:766–773, 1985.

91. Cagle PT, Hough AJ, Pysher J, et al: Comparison of adrenal cortical tumors in children and adults. Cancer 57:2235–2237, 1986.

92. Visser JW, Axt R: Bilateral adrenal medullary hyperplasia: a clinicopathologic entity. J Clin Pathol 28:298–304, 1975.

93. Carney JA, Sizemore GW, Sheps SG: Adrenal medullary disease in multiple endocrine neoplasia, type 2: pheochromocytoma and its precursors. Am J Clin Pathol 66:279–290, 1976.

94. DeLellis RA, Wolfe HJ, Gagel RF, et al: Adrenal medullary hyperplasia: a morphometric analysis in patients with familial medullary carcinoma. Am J Pathol 83:177–196, 1976.

95. Eng C: RET proto-oncogene in the development of human cancer. J Clin Oncol 17:380–393, 1999.

96. Padberg BC, Garbe E, Achilles E, et al: Adrenomedullary hyperplasia and pheochromocytoma. DNA cytophotometric findings in 47 cases. Virchows Arch A Pathol Anat Histopathol 416:443–446, 1990.

97. Wilson RA, Ibanez ML: A comparative study of 14 cases with familial and nonfamilial pheochromocytomas. Hum Pathol 9:181–188, 1978.

98. Webb TA, Sheps SG, Carney JA: Differences betwen sporadic pheochromocytoma and pheochromocytoma in multiple endocrine neoplasia, type 2. Am J Surg Pathol 4:121–126, 1980.

99. Berenyi MR, Singh G, Gloster ES, et al: ACTH-producing pheochromocytoma. Arch Pathol Lab Med 101:31–35, 1977.

100. Gifford RW, Bravo EL, Manger WM: Diagnosis and management of pheochromocytoma. Cardiology 72(suppl 1):126–130, 1985.

101. Schimke RN: The multiple endocrine neoplasia syndromes. *In* Humphrey GB, Grindey GB, Dehner LP, et al (eds): Adrenal and Endocrine Tumors in Children. Boston, Martinus Nijhoff, 1983, pp 249–264.

102. Medeiros LJ, Wolf BC, Balogh K, et al: Adrenal pheochromocytoma: a clinicopathologic review of 60 cases. Hum Pathol 15:580–589, 1985.

103. Linnoila RI, Keiser HR, Steinberg SM, et al: Histopathology of benign versus malignant sympathoadrenal paragangliomas: clinicopathologic study of 120 cases including unusual histologic features. Hum Pathol 21:1168–1180, 1990.

104. Shin W-Y, Groman GS, Berkman JI: Pheochromocytoma with angiomatous features: a case report and ultrastructural study. Cancer 40:275–283, 1977.

105. Steinhoff MM, Wells SA, DeSchryver-Kecskemeti K: Stromal amyloid in pheochromocytomas. Hum Pathol 23:33–36, 1992.

106. Lloyd RV, Blaivas M, Wilson BS: Distribution of chromogranin and S100 protein in normal and abnormal adrenal medullary tissues. Arch Pathol Lab Med 109:633–635, 1985.

107. Lloyd RV, Shapiro B, Sisson JC, et al: An immunohistochemical study of pheochromocytomas. Arch Pathol Lab Med 108:541–544, 1984.

108. Gould VE, Wiedenmann B, Lee I, et al: Synaptophysin expression in neuroendocrine neoplasms as determined by immunocytochemistry. Am J Pathol 126:243–257, 1987.

109. Hartmann C-A, Gross U, Stein H: Cushing syndrome–associated pheochromocytoma and adrenal carcinoma: an immunohistological investigation. Pathol Res Pract 188:287–295, 1992.

110. Trojanowski JQ, Lee VM-Y: Expression of neurofilament antigens by normal and neoplastic human adrenal chromaffin cells. N Engl J Med 313:101–104, 1985.

111. Unger P, Hoffman K, Pertsemlidis D, et al: S100 protein–positive sustentacular cells in malignant and locally aggressive adrenal pheochromocytomas. Arch Pathol Lab Med 115:484–487, 1991.

112. Linnoila RI, Becker RL Jr, Steinberg SM, et al: The role of S-100 protein containing cells in the prognosis of sympathoadrenal paragangliomas. Mod Pathol 6:39A, 1993.

113. Linnoila RI, Lack EE, Steinberg SM, et al: Decreased expression of neuropeptides in malignant paragangliomas: an immunohistochemical study. Hum Pathol 19:41–50, 1988.

114. DeLellis RA, Tischler AS, Lee AK, et al: Leu-enkephalin–like immunoreactivity in proliferative lesions of the human adrenal medulla and extranodal paraganglia. Am J Surg Pathol 7:29–37, 1983.

115. Kimura N, Nakazato Y, Nagura H, et al: Expression of intermediate filaments in neuroendocrine tumors. Arch Pathol Lab Med 114:506–510, 1990.

116. Unger PD, Hoffman K, Thung SN, et al: HMB-45 reactivity in adrenal pheochromocytomas. Arch Pathol Lab Med 116:151–153, 1992.

117. Melicow MM: One hundred cases of pheochromocytoma (107 tumors) at the Columbia-Presbyterian Medical Center, 1926–1976: a clinicopathologic analysis. Cancer 40:1987–2004, 1977.

118. Hoffman K, Gil J, Barba J, et al: Morphometric analysis of benign and malignant adrenal pheochromocytomas. Arch Pathol Lab Med 117:244–247, 1993.

119. Liu Q, Djuricin G, Staren ED, et al: Tumor angiogenesis in pheochromocytomas and paragangliomas. Surgery 120:938–942, 1996.

120. Amberson JB, Vaughan ED, Gray GF, et al: Flow cytometric determination of nuclear DNA content in benign adrenal pheochromocytomas. Urology 30:102–104, 1987.

121. Lack EE: Tumors of the Adrenal Gland and Extra-adrenal Paraganglia. Atlas of Tumor Pathology. Third Series, Fascicle 19. Washington, DC, Armed Forces Institute of Pathology, 1997.

122. Moran CA, Albores-Saavedra J, Wenig BM, et al: Pigmented extraadrenal paragangliomas. A clinicopathologic and immunohistochemical study of 5 cases. Cancer 79:398–402, 1997.

123. Shimada H, Chatten J, Newton WA, et al: Histopathologic prognostic factors in neuroblastic tumors: definition of subtypes of ganglioneuroblastoma and an age-linked classification of neuroblastomas. J Natl Cancer Inst 73:405–416, 1984.

124. Joshi VV, Cantor AB, Altshuler G, et al: Recommendations for modification of terminology of neuroblastic tumors and prognostic significance of Shimada classification. A clinicopathologic study of 213 cases from the Pediatric Oncology Group. Cancer 69:2183–2196, 1992.

125. Joshi VV, Cantor AB, Altshuler G, et al: Age-linked prognostic categorization based on a new histologic grading system of neuroblastomas. A clinicopathologic study of 211 cases from the Pediatric Oncology Group. Cancer 69:2197–2211, 1992.

126. Joshi VV, Silverman JF, Altshuler G, et al: Systematization of primary histopathologic and fine-needle aspiration cytologic features and description of unusual histopathologic features of neuroblastic tumors: a report from the Pediatric Oncology Group. Hum Pathol 24:493–504, 1993.

127. Shimada H, Ambros IM, Dehner LP, et al: The International Neuroblastoma Pathology Classification (the Shimada system). Cancer 86:364–372, 1999.

128. Shimada H, Ambros IM, Dehner LP, et al: Terminology and morphologic criteria of neuroblastic tumors. Recommendations by the International Neuroblastoma Pathology Committee. Cancer 86:349–363, 1999.

129. Young JL, Miller RW: Incidence of malignant tumors in U.S. children. J Pediatr 86:254–258, 1975.

130. Rosen EM, Cassady JR, Frantz CN, et al: Neuroblastoma: the Joint Center for Radiation Therapy/Dana-Farber Cancer Institute/Children's Hospital experience. J Clin Oncol 2:719–732, 1984.

131. Kinnier Wilson LM, Draper GJ: Neuroblastoma, its natural history and prognosis: a study of 487 cases. Br Med J 3:301–307, 1974.

132. Allan SG, Cornbleet MA, Carmichael J, et al: Adult neuroblastoma: report of three cases and review of the literature. Cancer 57:2419–2421, 1986.

133. Miller RW: Ethnic differences in cancer occurrence: genetic and environmental influences with particular reference to neuroblastoma. In Mulvihill J, Miller RW, Fraumeni JF Jr (eds): Genetics of Human Cancer. New York, Raven, 1977, pp 1–14.

134. Jaffe N: Neuroblastoma: review of the literature and an examination of factors contributing to its enigmatic character. Cancer Treat Rev 3:61–82, 1976.

135. Grondal S, Cedermark B, Eriksson B, et al: Adrenocortical carcinoma. A retrospective study of a rare tumor with a poor prognosis. Eur J Surg Oncol 16:500–506, 1990.

136. Evans AE, Chatten J, D'Angio GJ, et al: A review of 17 IV-S neuroblastoma patients at the Children's Hospital of Philadelphia. Cancer 45:833–839, 1980.

137. Evans AE, Baum E, Chard R: Do infants with stage IV-S neuroblastoma need treatment? Arch Dis Child 56:271–274, 1981.

138. Dehner LP: Classic neuroblastoma: histopathologic grading as a prognostic indicator. The Shimada system and its progenitors. Am J Pediatr Hematol Oncol 10:143–154, 1988.

139. Bolande RP: Developmental pathology. Am J Pathol 97:623–683, 1979.

140. Brook FB, Raafat F, Eldeeb BB, et al: Histologic and immunohistochemical investigation of neuroblastomas and correlation with prognosis. Hum Pathol 19:879–888, 1988.

141. Tsokos M, Linnoila RI, Chandra RS, et al: Neuron-specific enolase in the diagnosis of neuroblastoma and other small, round-cell tumors in children. Hum Pathol 15:575–584, 1984.

142. Shimada H, Aoyama C, Chiba T, et al: Prognostic subgroups for undifferentiated neuroblastoma: immunohistochemical study with anti-S100 protein antibody. Hum Pathol 16:471–476, 1985.

143. Taxy JB: Electron microscopy in the differential diagnosis of neuroblastoma. Arch Pathol Lab Med 104:355–360, 1980.

144. Triche TJ, Askin FB: Neuroblastoma and the differential diagnosis of small-, round-, blue-cell tumors. Hum Pathol 14:569–595, 1983.

145. Misugi K, Misugi N, Newton WA: Fine structural study of neuroblastoma, ganglioneuroblastoma, and pheochromocytoma. Arch Pathol Lab Med 86:160–170, 1968.

146. Maris JM, Matthay KK: Molecular biology of neuroblastoma. J Clin Oncol 17:2264–2279, 1999.

147. Brodeur GM: Molecular pathology of human neuroblastomas. Semin Diagn Pathol 11:125, 1994.

148. Seeger RC, Brodeur GM, Sather H, et al: Association of multiple copies of the N-*myc* oncogene with rapid progression of neuroblastomas. N Engl J Med 313:1111–1116, 1985.

149. Brodeur GM, Seeger RC, Schwab M, et al: Amplification of N-*myc* in untreated human neuroblastomas correlates with advanced disease stage. Science 224:1121–1124, 1984.

150. Maris JM, Weiss MJ, Guo C, et al: Loss of heterozygosity at 1p36 independently predicts for disease progression but not decreased overall survival probability in neuroblastoma patients: A children's cancer group study. J Clin Oncol 18:1888–1899, 2000.

151. Carlsen NLT, Christensen IBJ, Schroeder H, et al: Prognostic factors in neuroblastoma treated in Denmark from 1943 to 1980. Cancer 58:2726–2735, 1986.

152. Tischler AS, Dayal Y, Balogh K, et al: The distribution of immunoreactive chromogranins, S-100 protein and vasoactive intestinal peptide in compound tumors of the adrenal medulla. Hum Pathol 18:909–917, 1987.

153. Schmid KW, Dockhorn-Dworniczak B, Fahrenkamp A, et al: Chromogranin A, secretogranin II and vasoactive intestinal peptide in phaeochromocytomas and ganglioneuromas. Histopathology 22:527–533, 1993.

154. Chetty R, Duhig JD: Bilateral pheochromocytoma-ganglioneuroma of the adrenal type I neurofibromatosis. Am J Surg Pathol 17:837–841, 1993.

155. Balazs M: Mixed pheochromocytoma and ganglioneuroma of the adrenal medulla: a case report with electron microscopic examination. Hum Pathol 19:1352–1355, 1988.

156. Nakagawara A, Ikeda K, Tsuneyoshi M, et al: Malignant pheochromocytoma with ganglioneuroblastomatous elements in a patient with von Recklinghausen's disease. Cancer 55:2794–2798, 1985.

157. Aiba M, Hirayama A, Fujimoto Y, et al: A compound adrenal medullary tumor (pheochromocytoma and ganglioneuroma) and a cortical adenoma in the ipsilateral adrenal gland: a case report with enzyme histochemical and immunohistochemical studies. Am J Surg Pathol 12:559–566, 1988.

158. Min K-W, Clemens A, Bell J, et al: Malignant peripheral nerve sheath tumor and pheochromocytoma: a composite tumor of the adrenal. Arch Pathol Lab Med 112:266–270, 1988.

159. Michal M, Havlicek F: Corticomedullary tumors of the adrenal glands. Report of two cases. Association of corticomedullary tumor with spindle cell sarcoma. Pathol Res Pract 192:1082–1089, 1996.

160. Bellantone R, Ferrante A, Raffaeli M, et al: Adrenal cystic lesions: report of 12 surgically treated cases and review of the literature. J Endocrinol Invest 21:109–114, 1998.

161. Costandi YT, Wendel RG, Inaba Y, et al: Calcified adrenal cysts. Urology 5:777–779, 1975.

162. Torres C, Ro JY, Batt MA, et al: Vascular adrenal cysts: a clinicopathologic and immunohistochemical study of six cases and a review of the literature. Mod Pathol 10:530–536, 1997.

163. Gaffey MJ, Mills SE, Fechner RE, et al: Vascular adrenal cysts: a clinicopathologic and immunohistochemical study of endothelial and hemorrhagic (pseudocystic) variants. Am J Surg Pathol 13:740–747, 1989.

164. Medeiros LJ, Lewandrowski KB, Vickery AL: Adrenal pseudocyst: a clinical and pathologic study of eight cases. Hum Pathol 20:660–665, 1989.

165. Gaffey MJ, Mills SE, Medeiros LJ, et al: Unusual variants of adrenal pseudocysts with intracystic fat, myelolipomatous metaplasia, and metastatic carcinoma. Am J Clin Pathol 94:706–713, 1990.

166. Medeiros LJ, Weiss LM, Vickery AL: Epithelial-lined (true) cyst of the adrenal gland: a case report. Hum Pathol 20:491–492, 1989.

167. Plaut A: Lymphangioma of the adrenal gland. Cancer 15:1165–1169, 1962.

168. Simpson PR: Adenomatoid tumor of the adrenal gland. Arch Pathol Lab Med 114:725–727, 1990.

169. Travis WT, Lack EE, Azumi N, et al: Adenomatoid tumor of the adrenal gland with ultrastructural and immunohistochemical demonstration of mesothelial origin. Arch Pathol Lab Med 114:722–724, 1990.

170. Medeiros LJ, Wolf BC: Traumatic rupture of an adrenal myelolipoma (letter). Arch Pathol Lab Med 107:500, 1983.

171. Sharma MC, Kashyap S, Sharoma R, et al: Symptomatic adrenal myelolipoma. Clinicopathological analysis of 7 cases and brief review of the literature. Urol Int 59:119–124, 1997.

172. Grignon DJ, Shkrum MJ, Smout MS: Extra-adrenal myelolipoma. Arch Pathol Lab Med 113:52–54, 1989.

173. Lam KY, Chan AC, Ng IO: Giant adrenal lipoma: a report of two cases and review of literature. Scand J Urol Nephrol 31:89–90, 1997.

174. Ghavamian R, Pullman JM, Menon M: Adrenal lipoma: an uncommon presentation of the incidental asymptomatic adrenal mass. Br J Urol 82:136–137, 1998.

175. Finch C, Davis R, Truong LD: Extensive lipomatous metaplasia in bilateral macronodular adrenocortical hyperplasia. Arch Pathol Lab Med 123:167–169, 1999.

176. Goren E, Bensal D, Reif RM, et al: Cavernous hemangioma of the adrenal gland. J Urol 135:341–342, 1986.

177. Wenig BM, Abbondanzo SL, Heffess CS: Epithelioid angiosarcoma of the adrenal glands. A clinicopathologic study of nine cases with a discussion of implications of finding epithelial-specific markers. Am J Surg Pathol 18:62–73, 1994.

178. Dugan MC: Primary adrenal leiomyosarcoma in acquired immunodeficiency syndrome. Arch Pathol Lab Med 120:797–798, 1996.

179. Zetler PJ, Filipenko JD, Bilbey JH, et al: Primary adrenal leiomyosarcoma in a man with acquired immunodeficiency syndrome (AIDS). Further evidence for an increase in smooth muscle tumors related to Epstein-Barr infection in AIDS. Arch Pathol Lab Med 119:1164–1167, 1985.

180. Prevot S, Penna C, Imbert JC, et al: Solitary fibrous tumor in the adrenal gland. Mod Pathol 9:1170–1174, 1996.

181. Fidler WJ: Ovarian thecal metaplasia in adrenal glands. Am J Clin Pathol 67:318–323, 1977.

182. Carney JA: Unusual tumefactive spindle-cell lesions in the adrenal glands. Hum Pathol 18:980–985, 1987.

183. Bedard YC, Horvath E, Kovacs K: Adrenal schwannoma with apparent uptake of immunoglobulins. Ultrastruct Pathol 1986:505–513, 1986.

184. Travis WD, Oertel JE, Lack EE: Miscellaneous tumors and tumefactive lesions of the adrenal gland. *In* Lack EE (ed): Pathology of the Adrenal Glands. New York, Churchill Livingstone, 1990, pp 351–378.

185. Ayala GE, Ettinghausen SE, Epstein AH, et al: Primary malignant peripheral nerve sheath tumor of the adrenal gland. Case report and literature review. J Urol Pathol 2:265–272, 1994.

186. Dao AH, Page DL, Reynolds VH, et al: Primary malignant melanoma of the adrenal gland. A report of two cases and review of the literature. Am Surg 56:199–203, 1990.

187. Schnitzer B, Smid D, Lloyd RV: Primary T-cell lymphoma of the adrenal glands with adrenal insufficiency. Hum Pathol 17:634–636, 1986.

188. Choi C-H, Durishin M, Garbadawala ST, et al: Non-Hodgkin's lymphoma of the adrenal gland. Arch Pathol Lab Med 114:883–885, 1990.

189. Abrams HL, Spiro R, Goldstein N: Metastases in carcinoma. Analysis of 1,000 autopsied cases. Cancer 3:74–85, 1950.

190. Sahagian-Edwards A, Holland JF: Metastatic carcinoma to the adrenal glands with cortical hypofunction. Cancer 7:1242–1245, 1954.

191. Wunderlich H, Schlichter A, Reichelt O, et al: Real indications for adrenalectomy in renal cell carcinoma. Eur Urol 35:272–276, 1999.

192. Li GR, Soulie M, Escourrou G, et al: Micrometastatic adrenal invasion by renal carcinoma in patients undergoing nephrectomy. Br J Urol 78:826–828, 1996.

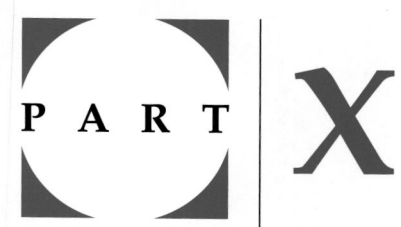
# Soft Tissue and Skeletal System

# 46

# Soft Tissues

Lawrence M. Weiss

Peripheral Neuroectodermal Tumor and Extraosseous
  Ewing's Sarcoma
Desmoplastic Small Round Cell Tumor
Malignant Melanoma of Soft Parts
**TUMORS AND TUMORLIKE PROLIFERATIONS SHOWING
CARTILAGINOUS OR CHORDOID DIFFERENTIATION**
Soft Tissue Chondroma
Parachordoma
Myxoid Chondrosarcoma (Chordoid Sarcoma)
Mesenchymal Chondrosarcoma

**TUMORS AND TUMORLIKE PROLIFERATIONS SHOWING
OSTEOGENIC DIFFERENTIATION**
Myositis Ossificans
Extraskeletal Osteosarcoma
**MALIGNANT MESENCHYMOMA**
**MALIGNANT LYMPHOMA**
**NON-NEOPLASTIC PROLIFERATIONS**
Infectious Disease
Noninfectious Histiocyte Proliferations

The soft tissues present a wide range of lesions to surgical pathologists. Although many lesions represent true neoplasms, a bewildering array of pseudoneoplastic proliferations are also frequently encountered. Even for the neoplasms, a wide range of clinical behaviors can be seen, from clearly benign to locally invasive through obviously malignant with a high risk of distant metastasis. In the soft tissues, it is not easy to classify tumors on the basis of their expected clinical behavior. Soft tissue lesions have classically been separated on the basis of their alleged histogenesis. However, because this is a concept that has proved to be a false one, this chapter presents a classification of soft tissue tumors based on their histodifferentiation, that is, documented tissue patterns as evidenced by light microscopy, immunohistochemistry, or other means. This classification is shown in Table 46–1. The reader should consult specialized textbooks on soft tissue tumors for discussion of rare entities not included in this chapter.[1, 2]

**TABLE 46–1.** Classification of Soft Tissue Tumors Utilized in This Chapter

*Tumors and Tumorlike Proliferations with Differentiation Toward Adipose Tissue*
Benign lipoma, including intramuscular lipoma
Angiolipoma
Myolipoma
Chondroid lipoma
Spindle cell and pleomorphic lipomas
Myelolipoma
Angiomyolipoma
Lipoblastoma-lipoblastomatosis
Hibernoma
Lipomatosis
Liposarcoma

*Tumors and Tumorlike Proliferations with Differentiation Toward Fibrous Tissue*
Ischemic fasciitis
Nodular fasciitis, including intravascular, ossifying, parosteal, and cranial variants
Proliferative fasciitis and proliferative myositis
Solitary fibrous tumor
Elastofibroma
Nuchal-type fibroma
Collagenous fibroma (desmoplastic fibroblastoma)
Fibroma of tendon sheath
Fibrous hamartoma of infancy
Infantile-type fibromatosis
Infantile digital fibromatosis
Calcifying aponeurotic fibromatosis
Fibromatosis colli
Superficial fibromatosis
Desmoid fibromatosis
Inflammatory myofibroblastic tumor or low-grade inflammatory fibrosarcoma
Low-grade fibromyxoid sarcoma
Fibrosarcoma

*Tumors and Tumorlike Proliferations with Predominantly Myxoid Differentiation*
Intramuscular myxoma
Aggressive angiomyxoma
Ossifying fibromyxoid tumor

*Tumors and Tumorlike Proliferations with Predominantly Fibrohistiocytic Differentiation*
Fibrous histiocytoma
Giant cell tumor of tendon sheath
Plexiform fibrohistiocytic tumor

**TABLE 46–1.** Classification of Soft Tissue Tumors Utilized in This Chapter *Continued*

Angiomatoid fibrous histiocytoma
Giant cell angiofibroma
Giant cell fibroblastoma
Dermatofibrosarcoma
Pleomorphic hyalinizing angiectatic tumor of soft parts
Acral myxoinflammatory fibroblastic sarcoma
Malignant fibrous histiocytoma

***Tumors and Tumorlike Proliferations with Vascular (Including Lymphatic and Perivascular) Differentiation***
Papillary endothelial hyperplasia
Capillary hemangioma
Cavernous hemangioma
Intramuscular hemangioma
Synovial hemangioma
Angiomatosis
Benign lymphangioma
Lymphangiomyomatosis
Glomus tumor
Hemangiopericytoma
Spindle cell hemangioendothelioma
Low-grade epithelioid angiosarcoma (epithelioid hemangioendothelioma)
Conventional angiosarcoma

***Tumors and Tumorlike Proliferations with Smooth Muscle Differentiation***
Benign leiomyoma
Angiomyoma (vascular leiomyoma, angioleiomyoma)
Leiomyosarcoma

***Tumors and Tumorlike Proliferations with Skeletal Muscle Differentiation***
Fetal rhabdomyoma
Adult rhabdomyoma
Rhabdomyosarcoma
Alveolar soft part sarcoma

***Tumors and Tumorlike Proliferations with Epithelial Differentiation***
Synovial sarcoma
Epithelioid sarcoma
Extrarenal rhabdoid tumor

***Tumors and Tumorlike Proliferations with Neural Differentiation***
Benign schwannoma
Neurofibroma
Perineurioma
Malignant peripheral nerve sheath sarcoma (malignant schwannoma, neurofibrosarcoma, neurogenic sarcoma)
Peripheral neuroectodermal tumor and extraosseous Ewing's sarcoma
Desmoplastic small round cell tumor
Malignant melanoma of soft parts (clear cell sarcoma)

***Tumors and Tumorlike Proliferations with Cartilaginous or Chordoid Differentiation***
Soft tissue chondroma
Parachordoma
Myxoid chondrosarcoma (chordoid sarcoma)
Mesenchymal chondrosarcoma

***Tumors and Tumorlike Proliferations with Osteogenic Differentiation***
Myositis ossificans
Extraskeletal osteosarcoma

***Malignant Mesenchymoma***

***Malignant Lymphoma***

## GENERAL CONSIDERATIONS

Lesions of the soft tissues are relatively common. Most benign lesions, such as lipomas, do not come to medical attention. Of those that do come to medical attention, benign lesions still greatly outnumber malignant ones, even though sarcomas attract the most attention from the surgical pathologist. However, sarcomas of the soft tissues, relatively uncommon neoplasms representing about 6600 cases a year in the United States, account for less than 0.5% of all malignant tumors.[3] Soft tissue sarcomas are more common in males than in females and more common in adults than in children, but individual types of sarcomas have specific age-incidence rates, and several (i.e., rhabdomyosarcoma) occur more commonly in children than in adults. There are no striking differences in the incidence of soft tissue sarcomas between different ethnic groups, by geographic regions, or over time. Soft tissue sarcomas occur more commonly at certain sites, such as the deep soft tissues of the extremities and the retroperitoneum, but individual types of sarcomas have specific site-incidence rates.

## Pathogenesis

Genetic factors are probably the most important known determinants in the development of soft tissue neoplasms, particularly those neoplasms occurring in childhood. Numerous types of soft tissue neoplasms occur on an inherited basis or follow a familial distribution. These range from syndromes that primarily manifest in the appearance of specific types of soft tissue neoplasms, such as neurofibromatosis type 1 and type 2,[4] to syndromes in which there is a wide variety of neoplasms including soft tissue neoplasms, such as Li-Fraumeni syndrome.[5, 6] These also include familial syndromes in which only one specific type of soft tissue tumor occurs, such as with multiple lipomas.[7]

Exposure to radiation is also a significant risk factor, but with modern radiation techniques, soft tissue neoplasms develop in less than 1% of patients. A sarcoma may be said to be a postirradiation sarcoma when the sarcoma occurred in the radiated field and there has been at least 3 years between the time of treatment and the development of the sarcoma.[8] Postirradiation sarcomas are most often high-grade malignant neoplasms, usually malignant fibrous histiocytomas, and occur primarily in adults. A herpesvirus (Kaposi's sarcoma–related herpesvirus or human herpesvirus 8) has been closely tied to the development of Kaposi's sarcoma.[9, 10] In addition, the Epstein-Barr virus has been identified in some smooth muscle neoplasms, particularly those occurring in immunocompromised patients.[11] However, there is little evidence for a viral etiology for the majority of soft tissue neoplasms. Prior injury has frequently been invoked as a cause of sarcomas, but aside from case reports, this must be unusual when the issue is carefully examined. One exception may be the development of vascular sarcomas in lymphedematous areas, such as in Stewart-Treves syndrome (lymphangiosarcomas occurring after radical mastectomy).[12] Various toxins, such as dioxin, have been investigated as a possible cause of sarcoma, but the evidence is still not strong.[13]

Regardless of the specific etiology of soft tissue tumors, great progress has been made in understanding the pathogenesis of many of these neoplasms. Classic cytogenetics has revealed that many soft tissue neoplasms, both benign and malignant, are associated with specific chromosome abnormalities, usually reciprocal translocations (see Table 7–2). Molecular characterization of many of these translocations has revealed that these often involve the formation of a novel chimeric gene, which represents the fusion of a gene with an RNA-binding domain that is ubiquitously expressed to a transcription factor encoding a gene with DNA-binding domains. Thus, the fusion product functions as an oncogene. In addition to translocations, ring chromosomes and giant marker chromosomes occur in certain sarcomas, usually low-grade sarcomas such as well-differentiated liposarcoma, and may allow amplification of selected DNA sequences. Finally, complex karyotypes without consistently recurring abnormalities are common in high-grade sarcomas and may represent a final common pathway of genetic derangements.[14] Overall, abnormal cell populations can be detected by either cytogenetics or DNA ploidy studies in about 85% of all soft tissue sarcomas.[15]

A variety of oncogenes and tumor suppressor genes have been found to be important in a large number of soft tissue sarcomas. *TP53* mutations, the most frequently detected genetic mutation in human tumors in general, have been identified in a significant proportion of soft tissue sarcomas.[16] Many although not all of these mutations can be detected by p53 immunohistochemistry.[17] In addition to *TP53* mutation, p53 overexpression with possible complexing to Mdm-2 protein has also been described in soft tissue sarcomas.[18–20] Altered patterns of retinoblastoma gene product expression are also frequently observed in sarcomas.[21] However, overexpression of the c-*erb*-b2 oncogene is rare or absent.[22] About 40% of soft tissue sarcomas show intrinsic expression of the *MDR1* gene before any chemotherapy with anticancer drugs.[23]

## Grading and Staging

Despite all of the attention given to the problem in the literature and the obvious clinical need for a practical solution, there is still no uniformly accepted grading system for soft tissue sarcomas. The two most clearly published systems are those of the French Federation of Cancer Centers and the National Cancer Institute[24, 25] (Tables 46–2 and 46–3). Neither has gained complete acceptance, although a comparative study of the two favored the French system because it was better able to predict the development of distant metastasis and tumor mortality.[26] It is clear that the type of histodifferentiation is important in determining prognosis, as are a variety of gross and histologic features, such as tumor size, necrosis, mitotic rate, and nuclear atypia. Some groups have also studied the possible use of other parameters, such as cell proliferation markers (e.g., Ki-67), oncogenes, and flow cytometric analysis; nonetheless, the most popular systems use a combination of gross and light microscopic features to give a three-tiered stratification. Enzinger and Weiss[2] advocated using the histologic type alone to assign a rough range for the neoplasm (e.g., malig-

**TABLE 46–2.** French Federation of Cancer Centers Sarcoma Group Grading System[26]

| | |
|---|---|
| Grade 1 | Score of 2–3 |
| Grade 2 | Score of 4–5 |
| Grade 3 | Score of 6–8 |

Score = sum of differentiation score + mitotic rate score + necrosis score

| | Differentiation Score |
|---|---|
| Well-differentiated liposarcoma | 1 |
| Well-differentiated fibrosarcoma | 1 |
| Well-differentiated malignant schwannoma | 1 |
| Well-differentiated leiomyosarcoma | 1 |
| Well-differentiated chondrosarcoma | 1 |
| Myxoid liposarcoma | 2 |
| Conventional fibrosarcoma | 2 |
| Conventional malignant schwannoma | 2 |
| Well-differentiated malignant hemangio-pericytoma | 2 |
| Myxoid or typical storiform-pleomorphic MFH* | 2 |
| Conventional leiomyosarcoma | 2 |
| Myxoid chondrosarcoma | 2 |
| Conventional angiosarcoma | 2 |
| Round cell, pleomorphic, or dedifferen-tiated liposarcoma | 3 |
| Poorly differentiated fibrosarcoma | 3 |
| Poorly differentiated or epithelioid malig-nant schwannoma | 3 |
| Malignant triton tumor | 3 |
| Conventional malignant hemangiopericy-toma | 3 |
| Giant cell and inflammatory MFH | 3 |
| Poorly differentiated, pleomorphic, or epi-thelioid leiomyosarcoma | 3 |
| All rhabdomyosarcoma | 3 |
| All synovial sarcoma | 3 |
| Mesenchymal chondrosarcoma | 3 |
| Poorly differentiated or epithelioid angio-sarcoma | 3 |
| Extraskeletal osteosarcoma | 3 |
| Ewing's sarcoma/peripheral neuroectoder-mal tumor | 3 |
| Alveolar soft part sarcoma | 3 |
| Malignant rhabdoid tumor | 3 |
| Clear cell sarcoma | 3 |
| Undifferentiated sarcoma | 3 |

| | Mitotic Rate Score |
|---|---|
| 0–9 per 10 HPF* | 1 |
| 10–19 per 10 HPF | 2 |
| More than 20 per 10 HPF | 3 |

| | Necrosis Score |
|---|---|
| No histologic necrosis | 0 |
| Less than 50% histologic necrosis | 1 |
| Greater than 50% histologic necrosis | 2 |

*MFH, Malignant fibrous histiocytoma; HPF, high-power field (0.174 mm²).

**TABLE 46–3.** National Cancer Institute Sarcoma Grading System[25, 380]

**Grade 1**
Well-differentiated and myxoid liposarcoma
Subcutaneous myxoid malignant fibrous histiocytoma
Well-differentiated malignant hemangiopericytoma
Well-differentiated fibrosarcoma
Well-differentiated leiomyosarcoma
Well-differentiated malignant schwannoma
Well-differentiated myxoid chondrosarcoma

**Grade 3**
Ewing's sarcoma/peripheral neuroectodermal tumor
Extraskeletal osteosarcoma
Mesenchymal chondrosarcoma
Malignant triton tumor
Other types of sarcoma with greater than 15% gross necrosis
Some types of pleomorphic liposarcoma, rhabdomyosarcoma, and synovial sarcoma

**Grade 2**
Other types of sarcoma with less than 15% gross necrosis
Some types of pleomorphic liposarcoma, rhabdomyosarcoma, and synovial sarcoma

system would take into account tumor site, depth (superficial or deep soft tissues), size, and spread (lymph node or distant metastasis). The American Joint Committee on Cancer staging system is given in Table 46–5.[28] Because of the lack of acceptance of

**TABLE 46–4.** Soft Tissue Sarcoma Grading System of Pediatric Oncology Group*

**Grade I**
Myxoid and well-differentiated liposarcoma
Deep-seated dermatofibrosarcoma protuberans
Well-differentiated or infantile (≤4 y old) fibrosarcoma or he-mangiopericytoma
Well-differentiated malignant peripheral nerve sheath tumor
Extraskeletal myxoid chondrosarcoma
Angiomatoid (malignant) fibrous histiocytoma

**Grade II**
Sarcomas not specifically included in grades I and III, and in which <15% of the surface area shows necrosis, and the mitotic count is ≤5 per 10 high-power fields using a ×40 objective. As secondary criteria, nuclear atypia is not marked, and the tumor is not markedly cellular.

**Grade III**
Pleomorphic or round cell liposarcoma
Mesenchymal chondrosarcoma
Extraskeletal osteosarcoma
Malignant triton tumor
Alveolar soft part sarcoma
Sarcomas not included in grade I and with >15% of surface area with necrosis, or with ≥5 mitoses per 10 high-power fields using a ×40 objective
Marked atypia or cellularity is less predictive but may assist in placing tumors in this category

Modified from Parham DM, Webber BL, Jenkins JJ III, et al: Non-rhabdomyosarcomatous soft tissue sarcomas of childhood: formulation of a simplified system of grading. Mod Pathol 8:705–710, 1995.
*See Table 46–7 for classification of pediatric rhabdomyosar-comas.

nant fibrous histiocytomas span grades 1 to 3, whereas epithelioid sarcomas span grades 2 and 3). For pediatric sarcomas, a separate grading system has been developed and appears to be of clinical use[27] (Table 46–4).

Similarly, there is no uniformly accepted staging system for soft tissue sarcomas. An optimal staging

**TABLE 46-5.** American Joint Committee on Cancer Staging of Soft Tissue Sarcomas[28]

| Stage IA | G1–2T1a–1bN0M0 |
|---|---|
| Stage IB | G1–2T2aN0M0 |
| Stage IIA | G1–2T2bN0M0 |
| Stage IIB | G3–4T1a–1bN0M0 |
| Stage IIC | G3–4T2aN0M0 |
| Stage III | G3–4T2bN0M0 |
| Stage IV | G1–4T1–2N1 or M1 |
| T | Primary tumor |
| T1 | ≤5 cm |
| | a. Superficial |
| | b. Deep |
| T2 | >5 cm |
| | a. Superficial |
| | b. Deep |
| N | Regional lymph nodes |
| N0 | No metastasis |
| N1 | Histologically verified metastasis |
| M | Distant metastasis |
| M0 | No metastasis |
| M1 | Distant metastasis |
| G | Histologic grade |
| G1 | Low (well-differentiated) |
| G2 | Moderate (moderately differentiated) |
| G3 | High (poorly differentiated) |
| G4 | Undifferentiated |

Modified from Fleming ID, Cooper JS, Henson DE, et al: AJCC Cancer Staging Manual. 5th ed. Philadelphia, JB Lippincott, 1997.

a single grading and staging system, close communication with clinical colleagues is needed in all cases of sarcoma.

## Prognostic Factors

The overall grade and stage (including size) of soft tissue sarcomas, however determined, have been found to be the most significant prognostic factors.[25–27] Age of the patient and assessment of the surgical margins have also been shown to be important.[29] Individual prognostic factors include specific type of histodifferentiation, mitotic rate, Ki-67 index, argyrophilic stain for nucleolar organizer regions (AgNOR counts), nuclear atypia, DNA aneuploidy or S phase fraction as determined by flow cytometry, p53 overexpression, Mdm-2 overexpression, mutations of the *TP53* gene, mutations or overexpression of the retinoblastoma gene, size of tumor, depth of tumor, presence of spread, and presence of gross necrosis.[19, 20, 23, 30–39] However, many factors are subordinate to other factors. Thus, the presence of DNA aneuploidy as determined by flow cytometry is probably merely reflective of the presence of nuclear atypia, and the Ki-67 index should correlate with the mitotic rate. In the future, nuclear magnetic resonance may be used to analyze the tissue lipid biochemistry in soft tissue tumors to provide another parameter in the development of a clinically relevant prognostic system.[40]

## Therapy[41]

A plethora of different therapies is used for soft tissue tumors, as might be expected from the myriad clinical behaviors exhibited by the different neoplasms. A multidisciplinary approach involving surgery, radiation therapy, and oncology is usually the best in dealing with soft tissue sarcomas. Simple excision, the complete removal of the gross lesion with a minimum of normal adjacent tissue, is adequate only for lesions that are clearly benign and for small and superficial tumors. Wide or radical excisions are usually employed for sarcomas. Wide excision entails excision of the neoplasm and adjacent normal tissues, but leaving in place some portion of the compartment; radical excisions involve excision of the entire compartment. In a radical muscle compartment excision, the entire muscle of that compartment, from origin to insertion, is excised. Neoplasms that are not limited to one distinct anatomic compartment or that abut bone or key neurovascular structures may require radical amputation for complete removal with a low risk of local recurrence, although a lesser procedure may be combined with another therapy, such as radiation therapy, to minimize the risk of recurrence.

Postoperative radiation therapy is often employed in cases with incomplete or suboptimal resection but may also be useful after an adequate wide surgical excision to minimize the risk of local recurrence, particularly in those patients with high-grade sarcomas. Preoperative radiation therapy may be employed to increase the chances of a complete surgical excision or to "downsize" the type of operation that must be performed to achieve complete excision. Adjuvant postoperative chemotherapy, usually including doxorubicin, for the treatment of soft tissue sarcomas is still somewhat controversial. Similarly, the efficacy of preoperative (neoadjuvant) chemotherapy to shrink sarcomas before surgical resection is also controversial. Isolated recurrences of soft tissue sarcomas should be considered for surgical reexcision. Patients with metastatic disease should be considered for surgical excision if the tumor is localized within one organ system. Systemic chemotherapy is generally employed if resection is no longer practical.

Certain pediatric sarcomas, such as Ewing's sarcoma/peripheral neuroectodermal tumor and rhabdomyosarcoma, are treated in a multidisciplinary fashion in which chemotherapy plays a much greater role than in the typical adult sarcoma. For these specialized neoplasms, referral to an institution with experience employing protocols for these specific neoplasms is often recommended.

## Content of Report[42]

A complete surgical pathology report for a benign soft tissue tumor includes the tumor's size, prefera-

**TABLE 46–6.** Contents of the Final Report[42]: Soft Tissue Sarcoma

*Gross*
Size (preferably in three dimensions)
Distance from margins (measured if less than 2 cm)
Character of border (circumscribed vs. infiltrating, satellite nodules, relationship to adjacent structures)
Depth (e.g., subcutaneous, deep fascia, intramuscular)
Necrosis (with approximate percentage)
Lymph nodes

*Microscopic*
Histodifferentiation or specific name
Indication of grade
Margins (measure if less than 2 cm)
*Mitotic rate
*Indication of degree of cytologic atypia
*Vascular invasion
*Character of margin
*Necrosis (with approximate percentage)

* Optional.

bly in three dimensions. For a soft tissue sarcoma (Table 46–6), the gross dictation includes the size of the tumor, its distance from margins (precisely measured if less than 2 cm), the character of its border (circumscribed versus infiltrating) and the presence of satellite nodules, its relationship to adjacent structures (particularly major blood vessels, nerve, and bone), an indication of the depth (e.g., related to skin, superficial to deep fascia, within deep fascia, within muscle), and the presence and amount of gross necrosis or calcification. The presence and location of any lymph nodes within the specimen should be given. In addition, mention should be made of a scar or previous biopsy site.

Microscopic sampling is documented by site in the gross dictation and includes at least all areas that appear different macroscopically. One section per centimeter of largest dimension is a good rule, although it may be relaxed in large neoplasms, particularly if initial sections document a high-grade neoplasm. Margins should be sampled, preferably by perpendicular sections, unless the neoplasm is obviously clear of the margin and is not the type (i.e., angiosarcoma) in which occult spread is common. The microscopic description includes the specific line of histodifferentiation, an indication of the histologic grade, and mention of any positive margins or the location and distance from the closest negative margin. If the specific line of histodifferentiation cannot be given, some qualifier as to the architecture (e.g., myxoid, round cell) should be given. Optional features to mention are the mitotic rate (usually given as the number of mitoses per 10 high-power fields), an indication of the degree of cytologic atypia (usually mild, moderate, marked), the presence or absence of vascular invasion, the character of the lesion margin, and the presence (give extent) or absence of microscopic evidence of necrosis.

## Tissue Procurement

The initial specimen of a soft tissue mass may be obtained by fine-needle aspiration biopsy, core needle biopsy, incisional biopsy, or excisional biopsy. Fine-needle aspiration biopsy usually has a limited role in the diagnosis of soft tissue lesions but should be considered in deep-seated tumors not easily amenable to other biopsy techniques. The primary role of fine-needle aspiration biopsy should be to determine the presence of malignant change and whether the process is mesenchymal. In many cases, a specific diagnosis can be given; however, even in experienced hands, it is often difficult to provide accurate typing and grading on such scant specimens. Grading, in particular, should be done with caution, because undergrading is common, given the constraints of the sampling. Similarly, core needle biopsies also usually have a limited role in diagnosis. Again, they are most useful in deep-seated tumors; they have the added advantage over fine-needle aspiration that a greater amount of tissue can usually be obtained, often sufficient for the performance of immunohistochemical and other special studies. As mentioned previously, excisional biopsy should be limited to lesions that are strongly suspected to be benign or to small and superficial tumors that can easily be re-resected, if necessary.

Incisional biopsy is usually the procedure of choice for the diagnosis of most soft tissue lesions. The exact site of the incision should be chosen to maximize the possibility of removing the entire biopsy site when the definitive resection is performed. At the time of surgery, frozen section may be performed to assess the adequacy of tissue obtained for diagnosis and the status of the margins. A specific diagnosis should be rendered only with great caution and great confidence at the time of frozen section, particularly because there is usually no clinical necessity for an immediate diagnosis. At the time of biopsy, consideration should be given to saving a small sample in glutaraldehyde for electron microscopy. Consideration should also be given to snap-freezing a sample for potential DNA and RNA studies. This is particularly important in pediatric tumors and other situations in which entities such as Ewing's sarcoma/peripheral neuroectodermal tumor, rhabdomyosarcoma, or desmoplastic small round cell tumor may be under consideration. In addition, sending tissue (sterilely) for classic cytogenetic analysis should also be considered; it may give diagnostic aid in a wide variety of soft tissue neoplasms, both benign and malignant. Unfortunately, the tissue must be sent to a cytogenetics laboratory with special experience in solid tissue cytogenetics because these studies are often difficult to perform on many soft tissue tumors. The role of flow cytometry is still controversial. Although several studies have shown that the identification of DNA aneuploidy has adverse prognostic significance, DNA aneuploidy often correlated with nuclear atypia. However, several studies have demonstrated some utility for analysis of DNA ploidy in high-grade soft tissue sarcoma.

## TUMORS AND TUMORLIKE PROLIFERATIONS WITH DIFFERENTIATION TOWARD ADIPOSE TISSUE

### Benign Lipoma, Including Intramuscular Lipoma[43, 44]

Benign lipomas are perhaps the most common of all soft tissue tumors, and biopsy is usually not done. They most often occur in adults of either sex and usually come to clinical attention as a slow-growing mass that has been present for many years. Most often presenting in the subcutaneous tissue of the trunk and proximal limbs, they may also occur intramuscularly or intermuscularly as well as rarely in unusual deep-seated locations, such as the mediastinum or the periosteum of bone. Intramuscular lipomas most commonly occur in the thigh; intermuscular lipomas most commonly occur in the anterior abdominal wall. Excised lipomas usually measure between 3 and 6 cm. Multiple lipomas may occur in about 5% of patients; a subset of these patients have a familial syndrome. Lipomas are usually cured by excision but may recur in about 1% of cases. Deep lipomas may have a higher recurrence rate; intramuscular lipomas may recur in 10% to 20% of cases, particularly in those cases with infiltrative edges.

In the ordinary subcutaneous lipoma, the histologic appearance is that of mature adipose tissue. Although a thin fibrous capsule is often present, sometimes it is not evident and one must render a diagnosis of mature adipose tissue consistent with lipoma. The intramuscular lipoma has the same histologic appearance as the subcutaneous lipoma but shows an infiltrating pattern between normal and atrophic skeletal muscle fibers (Fig. 46–1). Deep lipomas are often more irregular in appearance. A small subset of lipomas are associated with other histologic features, most often other mesenchymal elements. Fibrolipomas contain trabeculae or nodular aggregates of admixed fibrous tissue. Myxolipomas show foci of myxoid degeneration in an otherwise unremarkable lipoma. Like normal adipose tissue, lipomas are positive for S-100 protein. The majority of lipomas have cytogenetic abnormalities, most commonly 12q13–15 aberrations, 6p rearrangements, 13q rearrangements, 8q11–13 aberrations, and ring or giant marker chromosomes or both.[45] Interestingly, abnormal karyotypes are more common in patients older than 30 years, but there is no significant association between cytogenetic pattern and the patient's sex or age and the tumor's site, size, or depth.[45]

The clinical impression is important in differentiation of some mature lipomas from normal adipose tissue, particularly if the specimen is fragmented.

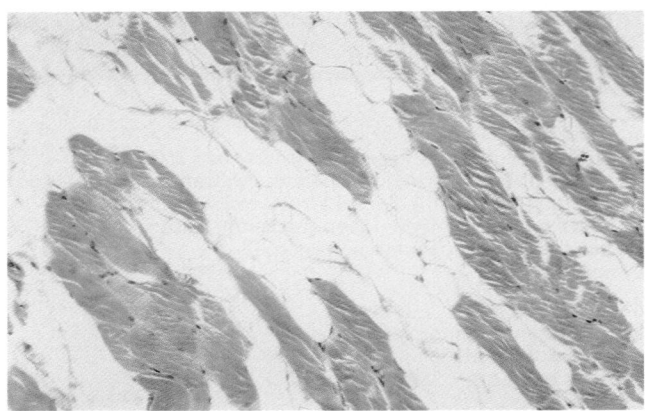

**FIGURE 46–1.** Intramuscular lipoma. Mature adipose tissue infiltrates between skeletal muscle fibers.

Although benign lesions of the synovium are termed synovial lipoma, particularly when they involve multiple synovial villi, they probably represent a reactive or metaplastic phenomenon, but rare circumscribed true synovial or tendon sheath lipomas have been reported. The complete lack of cytologic atypia distinguishes lipoma from atypical lipoma and well-differentiated liposarcoma (see later).

### Angiolipoma[46]

Angiolipomas occur primarily in males and present most often in young adulthood. They usually present as painful subcutaneous masses; multiple lesions (occasionally more than 10) outnumber solitary ones. A subset of cases are familial. The forearm is the most common site, followed by the upper arm and anterior abdominal wall. The lesions tend to be smaller than lipomas, possibly because they often present with pain. The prognosis of these tumors is excellent with essentially no recurrence; however, new lesions may appear. The gross tumors are firm and usually have a fleshy red-yellow cut surface.

The angiolipoma is distinguished from a typical subcutaneous lipoma by the presence of capillary-sized blood vessels, usually concentrated at the periphery (Fig. 46–2). It is said that the capillaries often contain fibrin thrombi, but this is rare in my experience. Although adipose tissue usually predominates, the vascular component is occasionally predominant. In some angiolipomas, secondary changes such as fibrosis and myxomatous change may also be present. The adipose component stains for S-100 protein, whereas the vascular component is positive for CD34 and other vascular markers. Cytogenetic studies have shown a normal karyotype, in contrast to many other types of lipomas, including ordinary lipomas and spindle cell and pleomorphic lipomas.[46]

The distinct vascular component distinguishes angiolipoma from lipoma. Angiolipomas do not oc-

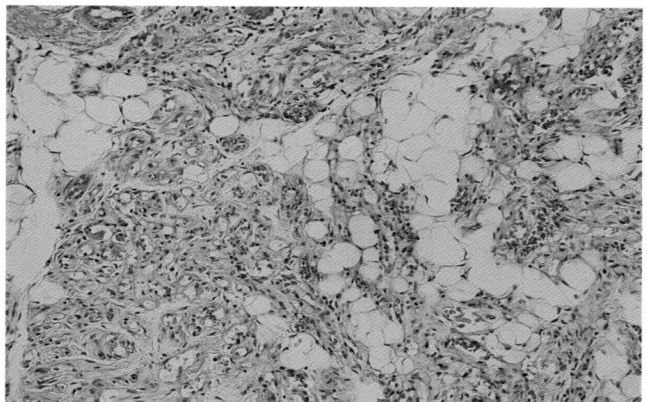

**FIGURE 46–2.** Angiolipoma. Capillary-sized blood vessels are interspersed within mature adipose tissue at the periphery of this lesion.

cur in an intramuscular location, so that a benign mesenchymal intramuscular lesion containing both adipocytic and vascular components probably represents an intramuscular hemangioma with fatty metaplasia.

## Myolipoma[47]

Myolipomas occur primarily in adults with a slight female predominance. They occur in subcutaneous tissue as well as in the abdominal wall and cavity, retroperitoneum, and pelvis. They tend to be larger than 10 cm. The clinical course appears to be benign. At gross evaluation, they are well circumscribed. They are composed histologically of mature adipose tissue and benign smooth muscle (Fig. 46–3); because the benign smooth muscle usually predominates, the tumors have also been called lipoleiomyoma. Attention to the bland cytologic features of both the adipocytic and smooth muscle components should lead to recognition as a benign neo-

plasm. Distinction from angiomyolipoma rests on the absence of abnormal vessels and immunonegativity for HMB-45.

## Chondroid Lipoma[48]

Chondroid lipomas occur in adults with a female predominance. They may be found in subcutaneous fat, muscle, or deep soft tissues. They occur in a variety of sites, most often the upper and lower limbs. They usually present when they are small (less than 5 cm). At gross evaluation, they are well circumscribed, with a rubbery, yellow cut surface. The neoplasm does not recur after complete excision.

Chondroid lipomas are composed histologically of mature adipocytes, multivacuolated lipoblasts, and eosinophilic vacuolated cells with irregular, hyperchromatic nuclei that resemble chondroblasts (Fig. 46–4). The last population is arranged in nests and cords in a chondroid matrix. Vascularity is usually increased. All three cell types are positive for S-100 protein.

The differential diagnosis includes soft tissue chondroma and a sarcoma, particularly extraskeletal myxoid chondrosarcoma. Soft tissue chondroma lacks cells resembling adipocytes and lipoblasts and is usually relatively avascular. Myxoid chondrosarcoma is usually more lobulated, with peripheral concentration of the tumor cells, and also lacks adipocytes and lipoblasts.

## Spindle Cell and Pleomorphic Lipomas[49, 50]

Although they were originally described as separate neoplasms, these lesions are discussed together because they probably represent two ends of the same clinicopathologic entity. These neoplasms present primarily in adults older than 45 years, with a

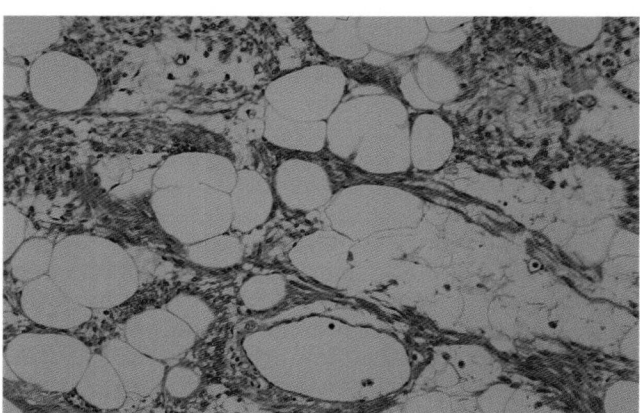

**FIGURE 46–3.** Myolipoma. A mixture of mature adipose tissue and benign smooth muscle is seen.

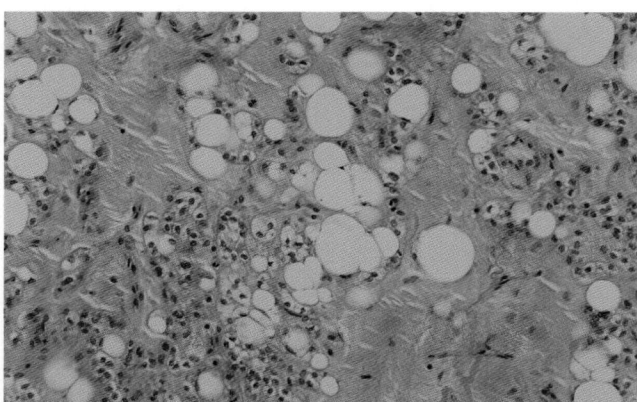

**FIGURE 46–4.** Chondroid lipoma. A mixture of mature adipose tissue and benign chondrocytes is embedded in a chondroid matrix.

strong male predominance. They occur in the subcutaneous tissue, most often in the posterior neck, shoulder region, upper back, and anterior neck. They are slow growing and painless, and they usually present at a somewhat smaller size than typical subcutaneous lipomas do. Rare cases may have multiple lesions. After adequate excision, there is almost never recurrence. In gross appearance, the lesions resemble lipomas with focal areas that are more gelatinous.

At histologic examination, the neoplasms are composed of a mixture of mature adipose tissue and fibromyxoid areas in varying proportions. The fibromyxoid areas contain bland spindled cells (spindle cell lipoma), highly pleomorphic cells (pleomorphic lipoma), or mixtures of the two in varying proportions (Figs. 46–5 and 46–6). The spindled cells have uniform nonatypical nuclei that may be aligned one to another. The pleomorphic cells are usually hyperchromatic and are often multinucleated, classically with a floretlike appearance. Neither the spindled nor the pleomorphic cells have mitotic activity. The fibromyxoid areas also contain varying amounts of collagen with varying degrees of vascularity. The spindled cells stain positively for CD34. Cytogenetic studies of spindle cell and pleomorphic lipomas have demonstrated 16q rearrangements in a large number of cases, a finding that may distinguish them from other lipomatous tumors.[51]

The presence of atypical cells raises the differential diagnosis of atypical lipoma or well-differentiated liposarcoma; however, the subcutaneous location and the circumscription of the lesion rule out these diagnoses. The presence of bland, CD34+ cells raises the possibility of solitary fibrous tumor, but the presence of admixed mature adipose tissue rules out that diagnosis. Occasional cases can have an extensive branching vascular pattern, and this feature, along with CD34 positivity, raises the possibility of hemangiopericytoma; again, the presence of mature adipose tissue rules out that diagnosis.

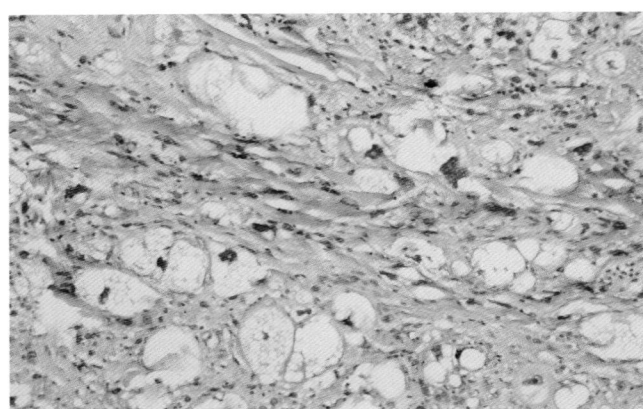

**FIGURE 46–6.** Pleomorphic lipoma. Markedly atypical cells are seen. Nonetheless, this lesion was a well-circumscribed subcutaneous mass.

## Myelolipoma[52]

Myelolipoma, which is much more common in the adrenal gland (see Chapter 45) and the liver, may rarely occur in the soft tissues. This soft tissue lesion occurs in adults with a marked female predilection. It has been reported most commonly in the retroperitoneal, pelvic, and presacral regions. Occasional cases have had multiple lesions. Patients usually present with an asymptomatic mass that may be large. The lesions are histologically identical to myelolipomas of the adrenal, with varying proportions of mature adipose tissue and normal marrow components.

Soft tissue myelolipoma must be distinguished from extramedullary hematopoiesis; the presence of mature adipose tissue rules out that possibility. If there is any question about the differential diagnosis, a bone marrow examination should resolve the issue.

## Angiomyolipoma[53]

This tumor, which is much more common in the kidney (see Chapter 30) and the liver than in the soft tissues, may extremely rarely occur in the retroperitoneum, pelvic soft tissue, spermatic cord, and mediastinum—in one case presenting as a 30-cm mass. As in the kidney, these neoplasms are almost always benign. The same histologic criteria used for diagnosis of this neoplasm in the kidney are applied to those in extrarenal sites. A combination of adipose tissue, abnormal blood vessels, and smooth muscle, often atypical in appearance and radiating from the blood vessels, should be sought by histologic examination. The muscle cells are positive for HMB-45 (and negative for S-100 protein), an unusual phenotype that is commonly seen in neoplasms that occur in the tuberous sclerosis complex.[54]

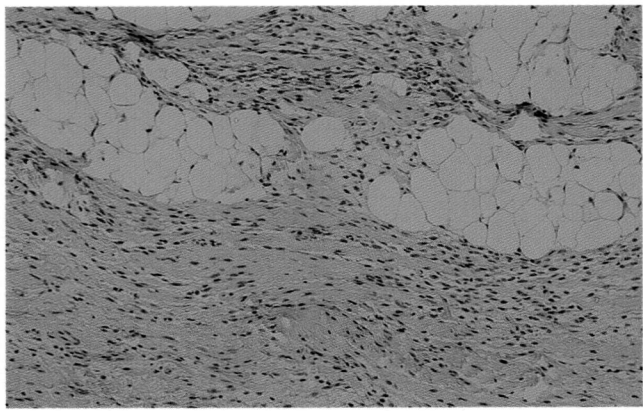

**FIGURE 46–5.** Spindle cell lipoma. In this typical example, a mixture of mature adipose tissue and bland spindled cells is seen.

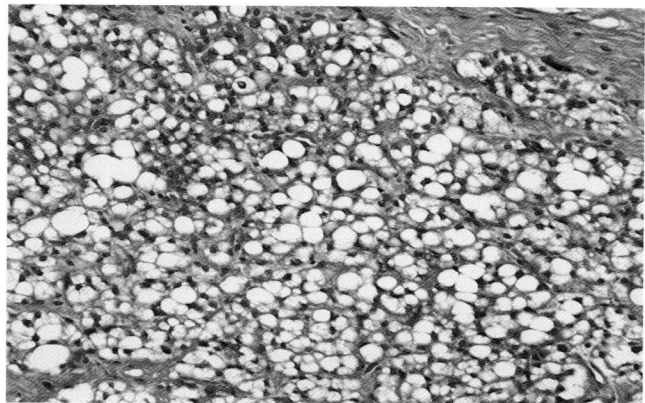

FIGURE 46–7. Lipoblastoma. A spectrum of lipoblasts and lipocytes is seen.

The differential diagnosis of a retroperitoneal angiomyolipoma includes a liposarcoma and a leiomyosarcoma. Liposarcoma lacks a component of smooth muscle and does not have the abnormal vessels of angiomyolipoma, whereas a leiomyosarcoma also lacks abnormal vessels and is negative for HMB-45.

## Lipoblastoma-Lipoblastomatosis[55, 56]

Lipoblastoma-lipoblastomatosis is restricted to childhood and usually occurs before the age of 5 years, affecting boys more than girls. It presents as a painless circumscribed subcutaneous mass (lipoblastoma) or as a diffuse lesion involving the subcutaneous tissue and underlying skeletal muscle (lipoblastomatosis). It may be associated with other benign soft tissue lesions. It usually occurs in the extremities, although it may affect any soft tissue site. Recurrence is uncommon in lipoblastoma, but lipoblastomatosis may recur. These gross lesions are usually less than 5 cm and are more gelatinous than a mature lipoma.

Histologically, the neoplasm has a distinct lobular appearance, separated by fibrous septa. The lobules are composed of nonatypical lipoblasts, mature adipocytes, cells showing intermediate differentiation, and stellate to spindled mesenchymal cells (Fig. 46–7). The lobules may show varying degrees of maturity, even within the same tumor. Mitotic figures are infrequent. The lipoblasts are associated with myxoid change of the stroma, and vascularity may be prominent. Cytogenetic studies of lipoblastoma have demonstrated 8q rearrangements, which may distinguish them from other lipomatous tumors.[51]

The most important differential diagnosis is with a myxoid liposarcoma. The clinical setting is perhaps the most important helpful feature; lipoblastoma-lipoblastomatosis rarely occurs after the age of 8 years, whereas liposarcomas are exceedingly rare in this age group (and are usually of low grade

anyway). The distinct lobularity, the range of maturation, the absence of cytologic atypia, and the relative absence of mitotic activity are helpful histologic features. Rarely, lipoblastomas may include cells resembling brown fat, raising consideration of a hibernoma, but this tumor is rare in children.

## Hibernoma[57]

Hibernoma occurs in adults with a median age of about 30 years; both sexes are affected equally. It usually occurs in the subcutaneous region, most commonly in axial locations such as the upper back, the back of the neck, the axilla, and the upper thorax. However, it may uncommonly occur in deep sites, such as the retroperitoneum or within muscle. It usually presents as a slow-growing, painless mass of 5 to 15 cm. At gross evaluation, it is a distinctive tan-brown.

Hibernomas are vaguely lobulated, although distinct fibrous septa are lacking. Several cell types are present. The most distinctive are small and large hibernoma cells—rounded cells with eosinophilic, granular cytoplasm, with multiple fine to coarse clear lipid vacuoles and a bland nonindented nucleus (Fig. 46–8). In addition, mature adipocytes as well as multivacuolated lipoblasts are present in varying proportions.

Several other neoplasms may have hibernoma-like cells, including lipoblastoma and well-differentiated liposarcoma, but the context should not lead to confusion. Cytogenetic studies of hibernomas have shown 11q abnormalities, which may distinguish them from other lipomatous tumors.[51]

## Lipomatosis[43, 58]

Lipomatosis is a term that encompasses numerous clinicopathologic syndromes, all of them rare. It in-

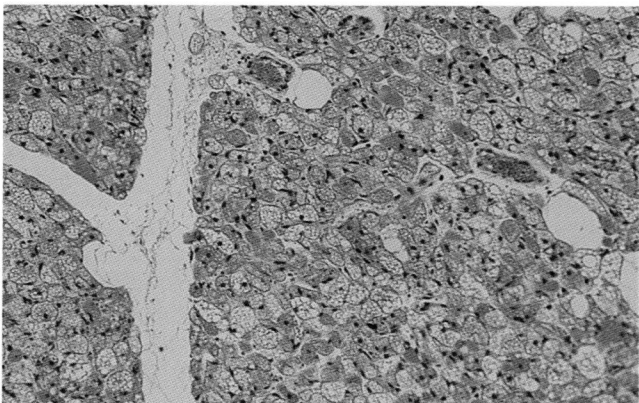

FIGURE 46–8. Hibernoma. Lobules composed of characteristic cells with granular cytoplasm and multiple lipid vacuoles are apparent.

cludes diffuse (asymmetric or congenital) lipomatosis, an overgrowth of adipose tissue affecting large portions of an extremity or the trunk; symmetric lipomatosis (Madelung's disease), a symmetric overgrowth of adipose tissue principally affecting the neck; pelvic lipomatosis, an overgrowth of adipose tissue around the rectum and bladder; steroid lipomatosis, a diffuse overgrowth of adipose tissue affecting axial areas associated with prolonged exposure to steroids; nevus lipomatosus cutaneus superficialis (including the Michelin tire baby syndrome), aggregates of adipose tissue occurring along skinfolds; and several other rare syndromes.

The histologic appearances of all the syndromes are similar, with an overgrowth of mature adipose tissue. In diffuse lipomatosis, the proliferation involves the subcutaneous tissue and adjacent muscle. In symmetric lipomatosis, the adipose tissue affects the subcutaneous tissue and deep soft tissue spaces, extending around and between muscles. In pelvic lipomatosis, abnormal deposits of adipose tissue are present in the perivesical and perirectal areas of the retroperitoneum. Steroid lipomatosis affects the sites of normal adipose tissue, particularly in axial regions. In nevus lipomatosus cutaneus superficialis, the adipose tissue is present in the middle to upper dermis.

## Liposarcoma[59–64]

Liposarcoma, one of the two most common soft tissue sarcomas (along with malignant fibrous histiocytoma), accounts for about 10% to 20% of cases. It occurs most commonly in adults with a median age of about 50 years. However, it can occur in all age groups, including pediatric patients (most often in their teens). Myxoid–round cell liposarcomas tend to occur at a younger age than well-differentiated or pleomorphic liposarcoma and are the exclusive type found in children. Men are affected slightly more than are women. Liposarcoma usually comes to attention as a long-standing mass. Pain and secondary symptoms such as weight loss and anorexia usually occur late. Recent growth of a long-standing mass may reflect progression to a higher grade. Liposarcomas almost always affect the deep soft tissues. The thigh is most commonly affected (about 30% of cases), followed by the retroperitoneum (20%) and inguinal region (10%). Liposarcoma is uncommon in the head and neck and the hands and feet. Well-differentiated and dedifferentiated liposarcomas have a predilection for the retroperitoneum; myxoid–round cell and pleomorphic liposarcomas have a predilection for the thigh. Pure low-grade liposarcomas virtually never metastasize without conversion to a high-grade liposarcoma but tend to recur, with a median time to recurrence of about 3 years. High-grade liposarcomas both recur and metastasize, at a relatively short interval. Low-grade liposarcomas have a 5-year survival of about 90% and a 10-year survival of about 50%; high-grade liposarcomas have a 5-year survival of about 10% and a 10-year survival of about 1%.

Liposarcomas generally measure between 5 and 15 cm, although some neoplasms may be enormous. They usually appear to be grossly encapsulated, although this is not generally confirmed by histologic examination. Satellite nodules may be present. Low-grade neoplasms tend to have a myxoid, gelatinous, or lipomatous appearance; high-grade neoplasms may look like a nondescript sarcoma, with areas of hemorrhage and necrosis.

Liposarcomas may be separated into three main groups histologically (and biologically): well-differentiated, myxoid–round cell, and pleomorphic. Well-differentiated liposarcomas represent approximately 50% of liposarcomas and may be divided into several subtypes: adipocytic (lipoma-like), sclerosing, spindle cell, inflammatory, and dedifferentiated. The lipoma-like subtype of well-differentiated liposarcoma has also been termed atypical lipoma, and this term is preferred by many when it occurs in the subcutaneous tissue or intramuscularly. These terms may be used synonymously because both may recur (although the more superficial lesions recur infrequently), both do not metastasize in pure form, and both have the capacity to dedifferentiate and then metastasize. The myxoid and round cell variants of liposarcoma are discussed together because it is now thought that they are two ends of a spectrum representing the same clinicopathologic entity. They make up 30% of cases, whereas pleomorphic liposarcomas make up about 10% of cases. In about 10% of cases, mixtures of the three major types are observed or the liposarcoma cannot be clearly categorized.

The lipoma-like subtype of well-differentiated liposarcoma is composed histologically of numerous adipocytes of various sizes and various degrees of nuclear atypia (Fig. 46–9). Occasional multivacuolar lipoblasts may also be present. Multivacuolar lipoblasts are mesenchymal cells with more than one optically clear, round vacuole; at least one of the

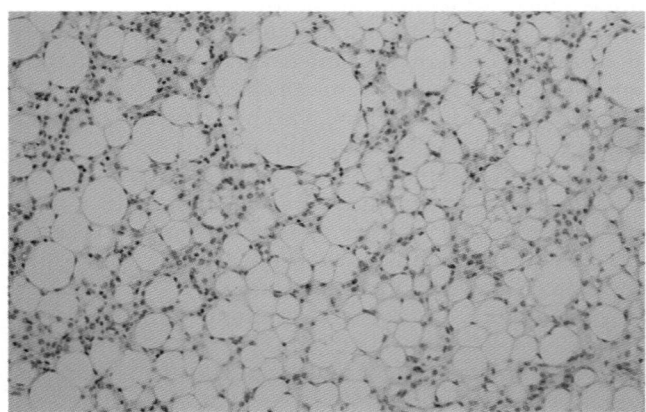

**FIGURE 46–9.** Well-differentiated liposarcoma, lipocytic type. A spectrum of lipocytes and lipoblasts is present. This neoplasm occurred in the retroperitoneum.

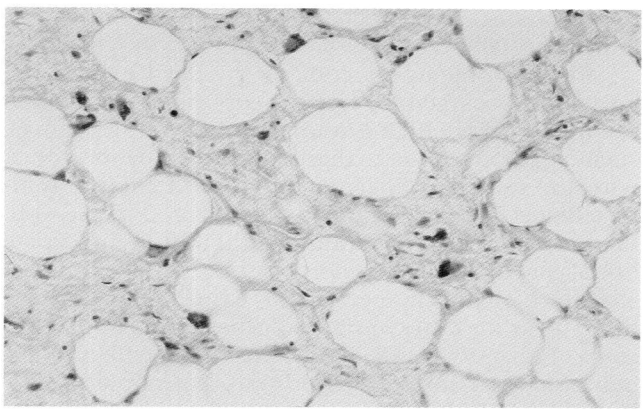

FIGURE 46–10. Well-differentiated liposarcoma, sclerosing type. Mature adipose tissue is admixed with fibrous tissue. Note the floretlike giant cells. This neoplasm also occurred in the retroperitoneum.

vacuoles indents the nucleus. In addition, there are often scattered spindle cells with atypia, sometimes within fibrous septa, as well as occasional floretlike multinucleated cells. The lipoma-like subtype of well-differentiated liposarcoma is particularly common in the retroperitoneum. The sclerosing subtype of well-differentiated liposarcoma is typically composed of predominantly mature adipose tissue admixed with varying amounts of collagenous fibrous tissue with a loose mucoid change (Fig. 46–10). The fibrous tissue contains spindled cells with varying degrees of nuclear atypia and multinucleated stromal cells; multinucleated lipoblasts may not always be present. Adipose tissue may be difficult to identify in some sections but should be present in at least some portion of the neoplasm. Sclerosing liposarcomas are particularly common in the inguinal region (spermatic cord and paratesticular). The inflammatory subtype of well-differentiated liposarcoma is a rare variant that has a prominent lymphoplasmacytic infiltrate within a background of lipoma-like liposarcoma that may be exceedingly bland; it is found almost exclusively in the retroperitoneum. The spindle cell variant is composed of relatively bland spindle cells arranged in short fascicles admixed with more typical areas of lipoma-like liposarcoma. The spindle cell area may show hyalinization or myxoid change. These rare neoplasms are often found in the subcutaneous tissue, most frequently in or near the upper extremities. Cytogenetic studies have shown that clonal chromosome abnormalities can be found in more than 90% of cases, with the most common abnormalities being supernumerary ring or giant marker chromosomes that have been found to contain amplified 12q sequences[65]; amplified 12q sequences may be critical to the pathogenesis of these neoplasms.[66]

Dedifferentiated liposarcoma is defined as a well-differentiated liposarcoma that contains a component of high-grade sarcoma (90% of cases) or recurs as high-grade sarcoma (10% of cases).[67, 68] The

high-grade sarcoma does not show adipocytic differentiation but usually has the histologic appearance of a malignant fibrous histiocytoma, an undifferentiated sarcoma, or a rhabdomyosarcoma (Fig. 46–11). The dedifferentiated area is usually obvious but may occasionally be either multifocal or focal; obviously, this phenomenon means that well-differentiated liposarcomas must be generously sampled to rule out this possibility. Dedifferentiated liposarcoma most commonly occurs in the retroperitoneum but may occur at any site in which well-differentiated liposarcoma occurs. The prognosis of dedifferentiated liposarcoma is poor but better than that of other pleomorphic sarcomas.

Myxoid–round cell liposarcoma represents two ends of a spectrum of a clinicopathologic type of liposarcoma. Myxoid liposarcoma may be regarded as a low-grade liposarcoma because it does not metastasize in its pure form, whereas round cell liposarcoma is a high-grade neoplasm, fully capable of metastatic behavior. Classic myxoid liposarcomas usually show a lobular low-magnification appearance and are composed of a myxoid matrix, a branching plexiform capillary vascular pattern, and a population of small mesenchymal cells, with or without recognizable multivacuolar lipoblasts (Fig. 46–12). The myxoid matrix consists of hyaluronic acid and may pool to form pseudocystic spaces. In addition, cellular elements may concentrate at the edges of the pools to create pseudoacinar patterns. The vascular pattern is highly characteristic, with a "chicken wire" appearance. The mesenchymal cells are spindled or stellate and have bland nuclei, without appreciable mitotic activity. Although some cases completely lack lipoblasts, the typical case contains scattered monovacuolar and multivacuolar lipoblasts, often concentrated along the periphery of lobules. Cells resembling hibernoma cells may also be present. Classic round cell liposarcomas are composed of numerous monovacuolar lipoblasts in a background otherwise acceptable for myxoid liposarcoma (Fig. 46–13). These cells may form cords

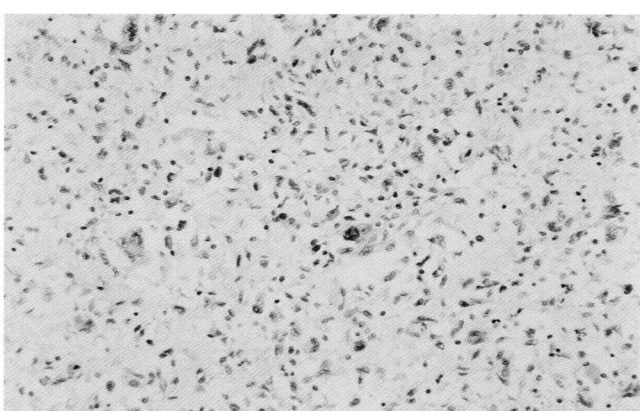

FIGURE 46–11. Dedifferentiated liposarcoma. Without the history of a preceding well-differentiated liposarcoma, this neoplasm would have been diagnosed as a malignant fibrous histiocytoma.

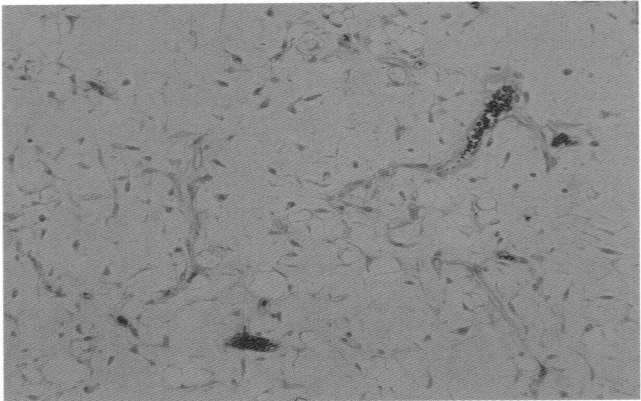

**FIGURE 46–12.** Myxoid liposarcoma. A myxoid stroma is seen in which occasional multivacuolar lipoblasts can be identified. Note the chicken wire arborization of capillary-like vessels.

and clusters and be so numerous as to mimic a small round blue cell tumor. Nonetheless, the mitotic rate is still usually low. When the percentage of round cell areas is above 75%, a diagnosis of pure round cell liposarcoma may be rendered. When the percentage of round cell areas is between 10% and 75%, a diagnosis of mixed myxoid and round cell sarcoma seems appropriate because the presence of greater than 10% round cell areas has been shown to be an adverse prognostic marker. Less than 10% round cell areas might still be regarded as a myxoid liposarcoma, although it may be prudent to mention the percentage of round cell area in the microscopic description. Occasional cases of myxoid liposarcoma are associated with a poorly differentiated spindle cell–type component. Myxoid–round cell liposarcoma most frequently occurs in the lower extremities. The natural history of myxoid–round cell liposarcoma is for progressive recurrences with greater proportions of round cell areas, although dedifferentiation (similar to the dedifferentiation of well-differentiated liposarcoma) may also rarely occur. Cytoge-

netic studies have revealed a t(12;16)(q13;p11) in more than 90% of cases.[69]

Pleomorphic liposarcoma is the third major category of liposarcoma. These neoplasms most often resemble other high-grade spindle cell sarcomas, such as pleomorphic malignant fibrous histiocytoma, with the exception that unequivocal diagnostic multivacuolar lipoblasts can be identified (Fig. 46–14). Frequently, there are numerous highly pleomorphic lipoblasts, including numerous abnormal multinucleated forms, but in occasional cases, they may be difficult to find. In contrast to other types of liposarcoma, the mitotic rate is usually high, with numerous abnormal forms. In addition, eosinophilic hyaline globules, although of no diagnostic significance, are usually easy to identify. Pleomorphic liposarcomas most commonly occur in the extremities.

The differential diagnosis of liposarcoma is wide and includes benign lipomatous proliferations, other benign lesions, and other sarcomas. A good deal of literature has been written on the distinction of lipoma from the lipoma-like variant of well-differentiated liposarcoma. As discussed earlier, the term *atypical lipoma* may be used to describe lesions with the histologic appearance of well-differentiated liposarcoma but that occur in the subcutaneous tissue or intramuscularly, because these neoplasms do not metastasize (when they occur in pure form) and have a lower incidence of recurrence than similar lesions occurring in deeper sites. However, as defined, atypical lipomas have the capacity to dedifferentiate and then metastasize (also similar to lesions occurring in deeper sites).

In distinguishing liposarcoma from other nonlipomatous lesions, both benign and malignant, much discussion has been spent on the definition of a lipoblast—a cell with one or (usually) more optically clear, round cytoplasmic inclusions, at least one of which indents a nucleus that shows at least some atypical features. However, just as it is hazardous to base a diagnosis of Hodgkin's disease on one "classic" Reed-Sternberg cell, it is best to diagnose liposarcoma on the basis of the entire constellation of

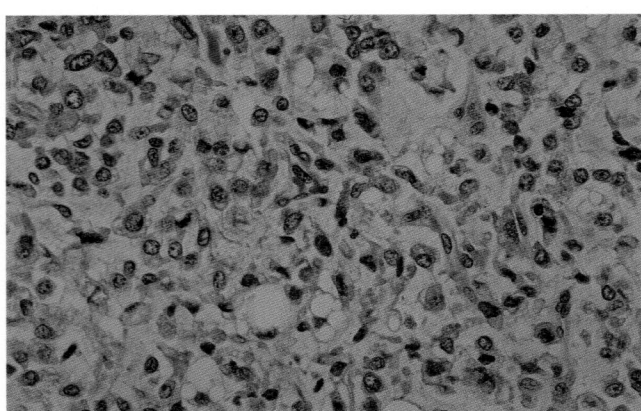

**FIGURE 46–13.** Round cell liposarcoma. Numerous lipoblasts are seen.

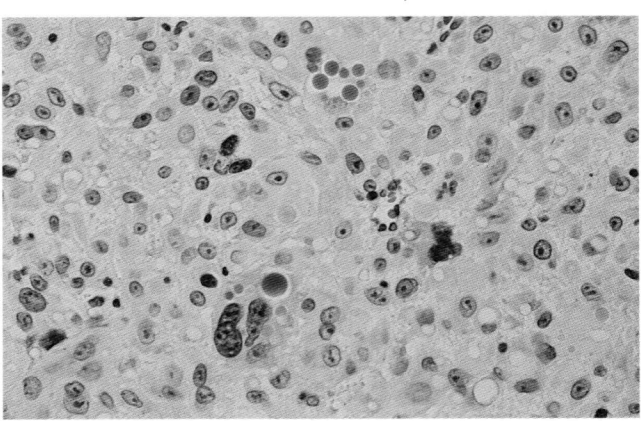

**FIGURE 46–14.** Pleomorphic liposarcoma. This highly pleomorphic sarcoma has identifiable lipoblasts.

cytologic and histologic findings (and if necessary, immunohistochemistry or other special studies). That having been said, the distinction of pleomorphic liposarcoma from other pleomorphic sarcomas does occasionally come down to the presence or absence of lipoblasts. However, in most cases, other features can be equally or more helpful. Myxoma or myxoid change in soft tissues lacks the characteristic rich vascular pattern of liposarcoma. Similarly, aggressive angiomyxoma, although more vascular than myxoma, lacks the fine capillary network of liposarcoma. Myxoid chondrosarcoma again lacks the rich capillary network of liposarcoma, is more multinodular at low magnification, and tends to feature cords of cells. Myxoid malignant fibrous histiocytoma has the closest resemblance to myxoid liposarcoma, but it usually has more cellular pleomorphism, has curved rather than chicken wire capillaries, and lacks S-100 protein positivity.

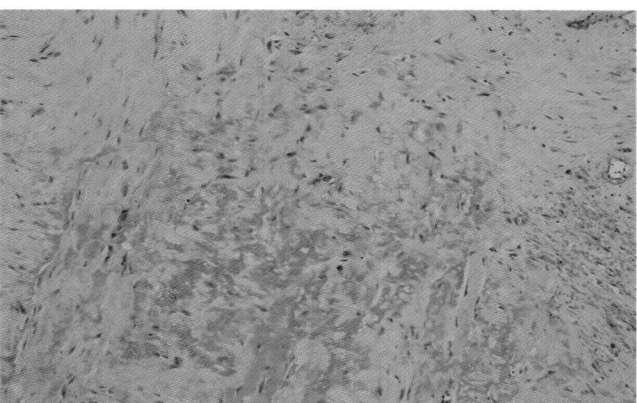

**FIGURE 46–15.** Ischemic fasciitis. Abundant fibrinoid necrosis is seen.

## TUMORS AND TUMORLIKE PROLIFERATIONS WITH DIFFERENTIATION TOWARD FIBROUS TISSUE

### Ischemic Fasciitis[70, 71]

Ischemic fasciitis, also known as atypical decubital fibroplasia, is a reactive as opposed to neoplastic lesion, probably representing ischemic changes with superimposed attempts at healing. It occurs in the subcutaneous tissue and muscle overlying bony prominences of the major limb girdles of immobilized patients, particularly elderly individuals. It presents as a painless mass that is poorly demarcated. Histologic examination often reveals a zone of fibrinoid necrosis and hemorrhage surrounded by exuberant granulation tissue in which there are abundant plump fibroblasts (Fig. 46–15). These fibroblasts may be mitotically active and have an "activated" although not pleomorphic nuclear chromatin. The uniformity of the fibroblasts, the zonation of the process at low magnification, and the clinical history should establish the diagnosis.

### Nodular Fasciitis, Including Intravascular, Parosteal, and Cranial Variants[72–78]

Fasciitis, a term technically denoting inflammation of the fascia, pathologically encompasses a wide array of different processes, including inflammatory and proliferative lesions. The lesions discussed in this section all have a similar histologic appearance and probably represent a similar disease process, although there are some distinctive clinical findings related to each specific entity. Parosteal fasciitis is also known as fibro-osseous pseudotumor and florid reactive periostitis.

Nodular fasciitis is an uncommon lesion, although it is the most common of the proliferative pseudosarcomas. It occurs in all age groups but has a peak of incidence around 30 years of age, and it has no sex predilection. It most commonly occurs at or near the superficial fascia, sometimes centered in the subcutaneous tissues and other times within skeletal muscle. About 50% of cases occur in the upper extremity, most often the volar aspect of the forearm or the upper arm, although the trunk, particularly the chest wall, and the lower extremities, particularly the thigh, are also relatively common sites. However, nodular fasciitis may occur at any site; the head and neck may be a particularly frequent site in infants and children. Patients usually present with a mass of less than 3 months' duration (often less than 1 month), and there is usually no history of preceding trauma. Rapid growth is commonly reported. Rare cases have more than one lesion. Nodular fasciitis does not recur after adequate excision, and even after incomplete excision, it recurs in less than 5% of cases. Most recurrences appear within several months of the initial surgery. With all recurrences, but particularly those that appear after 6 months or more, the original diagnostic material should be reviewed. Gross evaluation reveals that nodular fasciitis is usually about 2 cm (fitting on one slide) and is almost always less than 4 cm. The cut section may be myxoid or firm.

Intravascular fasciitis may affect a slightly younger population than nodular fasciitis does; again, there is no sex predilection. It differs from nodular fasciitis in having a greater proportion of cases involving deep soft tissues of the head and neck region, and the symptoms, although similar to those of nodular fasciitis, tend to be of longer duration before surgery. A multinodular appearance may be noted grossly. The ossifying variant of nodular fasciitis has the same clinical features as other types of nodular fasciitis. Parosteal fasciitis also has epidemiologic features similar to those of nodular fasciitis, but it has a female predominance. The lesion is usually centered at or near the periosteum. The tubular bones of the hands and feet are most commonly affected, but lesions involving the long bones have also been reported. Patients usually present with pain or swelling, generally of several months' duration. Soft tissue swelling, focal calcification, and a periosteal reaction are typical radiologic findings. Most lesions are about 2 cm. Recurrences are rare. Cranial fasciitis almost always occurs in the first 2 years of life and shows a male predominance. The lesion is usually centered at or near the periosteum of the skull. Patients usually present with a scalp mass of short duration, which often is fast growing. Soft tissue swelling and lytic changes in the outer table are typical radiologic findings. The lesion is usually 1 to 2 cm.

Nodular fasciitis and its closely related congeners show similar histologic features. Nodular fasciitis represents the prototypical type. Nodular fasciitis is usually relatively well circumscribed, although projecting tongues of the lesion may be present. It is composed of a loose proliferation of spindle cells. The spindle cells are generally patternless, with a flowing tissue culture appearance, although vague storiform formations may be present (Fig. 46–16). The background is usually loose, often with myxoid (and occasionally cystic) areas, but it may be somewhat fibrous. The lesion is usually vascular, with granulation tissue–like capillaries containing plump endothelial cells. There are often numerous extravasated red blood cells, and a scattering of inflammatory cells may be present. The individual spindle cells are cytologically bland and uniform from one to another. Mitotic figures are numerous, generally more than 1 mitosis per high-power field. Osteoclast-like giant cells are also present in a subset of cases.

In intravascular fasciitis, a similar proliferation is found within the lumina of small to medium-sized veins or arteries. However, there is usually a more fibrous matrix and a greater number of multinucleated giant cells. In ossifying fasciitis, foci of metaplastic osteoid rimmed by osteoblasts are present. In parosteal fasciitis, there are also foci of metaplastic osteoid as well as nests of immature cartilage, which in some cases may be more prominent than the underlying fasciitis. Some cases may show a zonal distribution, but these cases may be more closely related to myositis ossificans. Cranial fasciitis has a histologic appearance similar to that of parosteal fasciitis.

Immunohistochemical studies demonstrate that the spindle cells are reactive for vimentin, muscle-specific actin (usually weak), and smooth muscle–specific actin (usually strong). However, the cells lack envelopment by collagen IV, a common feature of smooth muscle. CD68 labels most of the osteoclast-like giant cells and may also label many of the spindle cells, although usually weakly. By electron microscopy, myofibroblastic features are seen, with abundant rough endoplasmic reticulum, microtubules, pinocytotic vesicles, and myofilaments. Diploid DNA content is identified by flow cytometric studies. Limited numbers of cytogenetic analyses have been reported. Some cases have demonstrated clonal cytogenetic abnormalities in a subset of cells; however, additional study is needed before any conclusions can be drawn.

The differential diagnosis of nodular fasciitis is broad. Obviously, it is most important to distinguish nodular fasciitis from a sarcoma. The short clinical history, small size, patternless architecture, and uniform nuclear features suggest nodular fasciitis rather than sarcoma. Paradoxically, nodular fasciitis usually has a higher mitotic rate than most sarcomas, and atypical mitoses are generally not seen. A sarcoma with a mitotic rate approximating that of nodular fasciitis usually has a greater degree of pleomorphism. Fibromatosis has a longer clinical history, is usually larger in size, has a much more infiltrative growth pattern, is more fibrous, and has a more consistent architectural pattern. Benign fibrous histiocytoma may be the most difficult to distinguish from nodular fasciitis, but fortunately the distinction is least important. Fibrous histiocytoma is usually less well circumscribed, has a more patterned storiform architecture, and is usually more fibrous. In addition, the cells of fibrous histiocytoma are generally actin negative.

Intravascular fasciitis must be distinguished from infantile myofibromatosis and a plexiform fibrohistiocytic tumor. Both of these lesions may be multifocal, but the proliferation is not within blood vessels. Ossifying fasciitis, parosteal fasciitis, and cranial fasciitis must be distinguished from myositis ossificans. Myositis ossificans is much less cellular and has a distinct zonation that is absent in fasciitis. Bizarre parosteal osteochondromatous proliferation is a lesion that shares many features with parosteal fasciitis. This lesion, however, is firmly attached to the cortex, generally has a greater amount of calcified matrix, and contains areas of mature cartilage. Cranial fasciitis may be difficult to distinguish from infantile myofibromatosis, both clinically and patho-

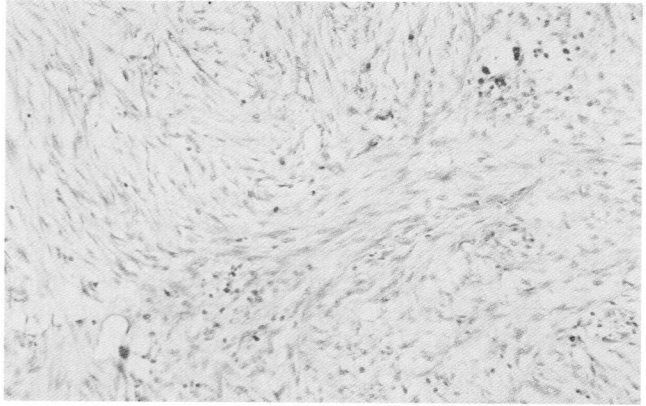

**FIGURE 46–16.** Nodular fasciitis. The loose proliferation of fibroblasts imparts a tissue culture appearance.

logically. Cranial fasciitis is more circumscribed and usually has a more prominent myxoid matrix, whereas infantile myofibromatosis often has a more hemangiopericytomatous appearance and lacks extravasated erythrocytes or metaplastic osteoid.

## Proliferative Fasciitis and Proliferative Myositis[79, 80]

Proliferative fasciitis and proliferative myositis are discussed together because they share many clinicopathologic features and probably represent variants of the same disease process. Both affect older adults with a median age of about 50 years (slightly older than the case for nodular fasciitis) but may occur in children. There is no sex preference. Proliferative fasciitis is usually centered in the superficial fascia; proliferative myositis involves skeletal muscle and the overlying fascia. The majority of cases of proliferative fasciitis occur in the upper and lower extremities; proliferative myositis is most common in the trunk, the shoulder girdle, and the upper extremities. As with nodular fasciitis, patients usually present with a rapidly growing mass of less than 3 months' duration (often less than 1 month). Recurrences are rare. At gross evaluation, both lesions are usually about 2 cm and almost always less than 5 to 6 cm. Both are usually poorly demarcated.

Proliferative fasciitis and proliferative myositis have a similar histologic appearance. At low magnification, the margins are poorly circumscribed, often extending in fingerlike projections along fascial planes. The stroma varies from loose to fibrous and rarely includes focal metaplastic osteoid. Similar to nodular fasciitis, a rich granulation tissue network of capillaries is usually present. Two distinctive cellular elements are present in various proportions. The first is a bland spindle cell, similar to that seen in nodular fasciitis. The second is a ganglion-like cell with a rounded outline, abundant amphophilic or basophilic cytoplasm, and one or several relatively prominent nuclei with a vesicular chromatin pattern and prominent nucleoli (Fig. 46–17). As in nodular fasciitis, the mitotic rate is usually high, although atypical mitoses are not generally seen. In proliferative myositis, the cellular proliferation is most prominent in the skeletal muscle septa but also insinuates around individual muscle fibers, imparting a checkerboard appearance. The muscle fibers may show atrophy but do not disappear. In proliferative fasciitis, the proliferation may entrap subcutaneous adipose tissue, simulating an adipocytic neoplasm. Proliferative fasciitis and proliferative myositis occurring in childhood are often more cellular and may contain foci of acute inflammation and necrosis.

Immunohistochemical studies demonstrate the proliferating cells, including the ganglion-like cells, to be positive for vimentin, muscle-specific actin, and smooth muscle–specific actin, although the last two reactions may be weak and variable. CD68

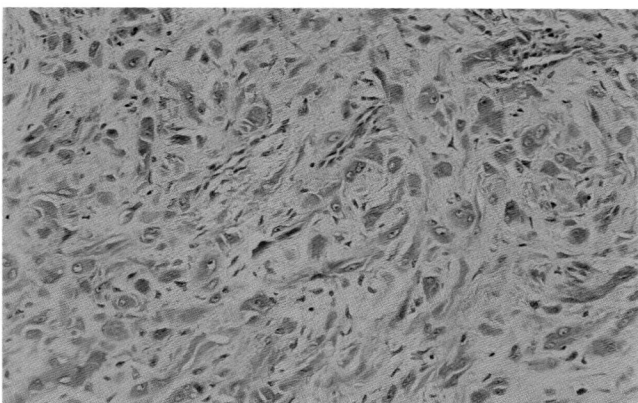

**FIGURE 46–17.** Proliferative fasciitis. Numerous ganglion-like cells are apparent.

staining may be variably positive. As in nodular fasciitis, the collagen IV stain is usually negative around the cells. Electron microscopy shows abundant rough endoplasmic reticulum, intracellular collagen, pinocytotic vesicles, and thin filaments, consistent with myofibroblastic differentiation. Flow cytometric studies show a nonaneuploid DNA content. One cytogenetic study reported trisomy 2 in a subset of cells in one case, a finding in need of confirmation.

In view of the presence of ganglion-like cells in proliferative fasciitis and proliferative myositis, the differential diagnosis includes ganglioneuroma (ganglion cells) and rhabdomyosarcoma (rhabdomyoblasts). The clinical setting goes a long way in distinguishing these lesions from proliferative fasciitis and proliferative myositis. Neither ganglioneuroma nor rhabdomyosarcoma occurs in skeletal muscle, and rhabdomyosarcoma always includes cytologically atypical cells in addition to rhabdomyoblasts. If any doubt exists, immunostains (neural and muscle markers) should be definitive.

## Solitary Fibrous Tumor[81–84]

Solitary fibrous tumor, a neoplasm that is much more common in the pleura (see Chapter 16) and other serosal cavities, also involves soft tissue. In the soft tissues, it generally occurs in adults with a peak in the fourth decade, with a female predilection. Patients present with a slow-growing, painless mass that may involve literally any site. Extrapleural tumors have had a good prognosis; they are generally cured after complete excision, although local recurrence and even metastasis have been described (usually but not always in association with atypical histologic features). The gross lesions range in size from 1 to 10 cm, are circumscribed, and are gray and firm on cut section.

The histologic appearance is similar to that of solitary fibrous tumor occurring in the pleura. There

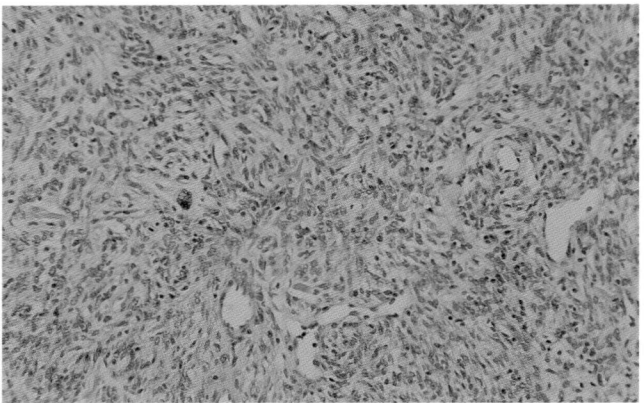

**FIGURE 46–18.** Solitary fibrous tumor. There is a bland fibrous proliferation. Note the occasional ropy collagen fibers.

is a proliferation of bland spindle cells alternating with ropy collagen. The spindle cells show variable cellularity, and there are often areas of dense hyalinization (Fig. 46–18). On occasion, the vascular pattern may show a staghorn hemangiopericytomatous arrangement. Cases with pleomorphism, extensive necrosis, and high mitotic rate are unusual outside of the pleura but have been described.[84] Immunohistochemical studies demonstrate CD34 positivity in most cases. Cytogenetic studies have not revealed consistent aberrations to date.[85]

The differential diagnosis includes a benign or malignant neural tumor (S-100 protein positive), a monophasic synovial sarcoma (keratin positive), fibrosarcoma (more cellular and CD34[-]), and a low-grade fibromyxoid sarcoma (CD34[-]). The most difficult distinction is with hemangiopericytoma, which shares the same immunophenotype and may share many histologic features. It is possible that some cases of hemangiopericytoma are closely related or actually represent solitary fibrous tumor involving the soft tissues.

## Elastofibroma[86]

Elastofibroma is a tumorlike lesion whose pathogenesis is still unknown; it may be a reactive, neoplastic, or possibly metabolic disorder. It occurs exclusively in older adults, sometimes with a long history of manual labor, and affects women more than men. Patients present with a slowly growing mass that is almost always located between the scapula and the seventh and eighth ribs. Less commonly, it may be bilateral, and it may rarely occur in other sites. The lesion is completely benign, and there is no recurrence after excision. The gross lesion averages between 5 and 10 cm and has a gray-yellow appearance on cut section.

At histologic examination, there is densely collagenous fibrous tissue in which thick eosinophilic elastic fibers are embedded, with residual adipose tissue (Fig. 46–19). The elastic fibers are highly abnormal, with fragmentation, beading, and serration. Once the elastic fibers are recognized, there is really nothing else to consider in the differential diagnosis.

## Nuchal-Type Fibroma[87–89]

Nuchal-type fibroma occurs in all age groups with a striking male predominance. There is a strong association with diabetes and previous neck injury, and it may also be associated with Gardner's syndrome. Patients present with a slow-growing mass that arises in the paraspinal area of the posterior neck region in about three quarters of cases. It is a benign lesion, but it can recur; the recurrences are usually easily controlled. The gross tumor averages about 3 cm and is poorly circumscribed, centered in the subcutaneous tissue. At microscopic examination, there is hypocellular, densely collagenized fibrous tissue with inconspicuous fibroblasts (Fig. 46–20). Entrapped adipose tissue is common, particularly at the periphery of the lesion.

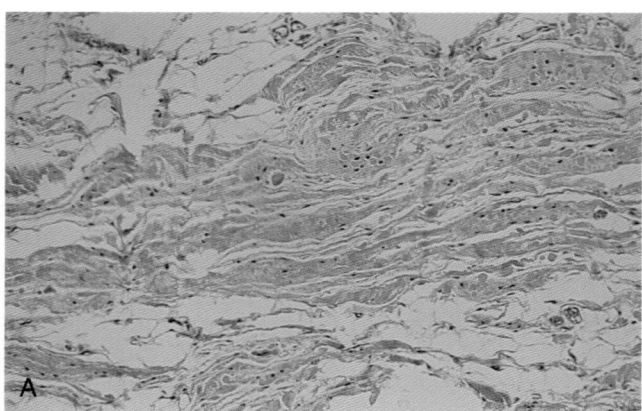
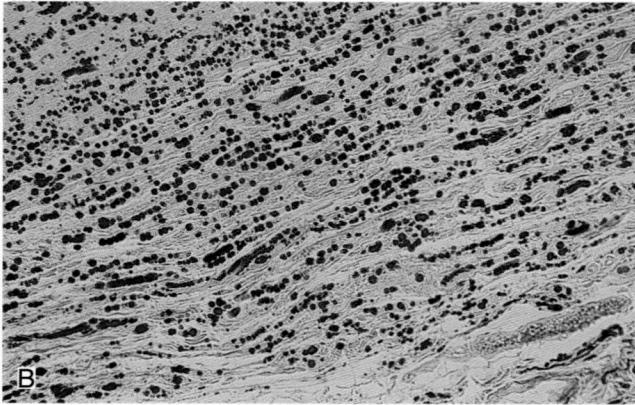

**FIGURE 46–19.** Elastofibroma. *A.* Dense fibrous tissue is seen. *B.* The elastin stain reveals numerous fragmented elastic fibers.

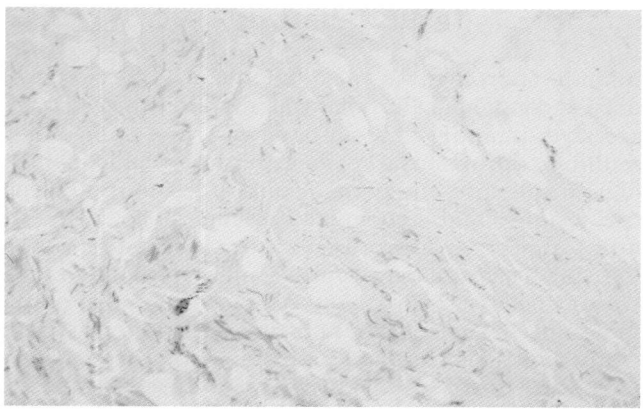

FIGURE 46–20. Nuchal-type fibroma. Hypocellular densely collagenized fibrous tissue is seen.

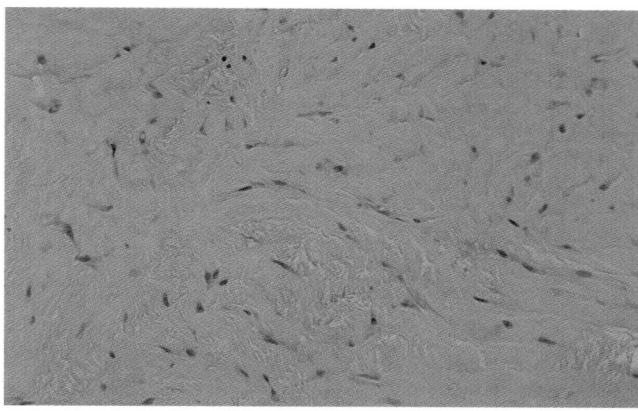

FIGURE 46–21. Collagenous fibroma. There is a hypocellular fibromyxoid stroma, with bland fibroblasts.

The differential diagnosis includes fibrolipoma and fibromatosis. Fibrolipoma is an encapsulated tumor that usually has a greater component of adipose tissue. Fibromatosis is much more cellular than nuchal-type fibroma.

### Collagenous Fibroma (Desmoplastic Fibroblastoma)[90]

Collagenous fibroma is a rare soft tissue tumor with a benign biologic behavior; it has also been reported under the name of desmoplastic fibroblastoma. It occurs primarily in adults with a mean age around 50 years; there is a female predilection. The tumor usually presents as a slowly growing solitary mass, although multiple lesions were present in one reported case. It occurs principally in the neck and shoulder region but may occur in a wide variety of sites. No tumor has recurred after excision. The gross tumor is a well-circumscribed, firm mass involving subcutaneous or deep soft tissue, usually about 5.0 cm in greatest diameter.

The tumors are histologically hypocellular with a collagenous or fibromyxoid stroma. There are widely separated spindle-shaped and stellate fibroblastic cells arranged haphazardly to one another (Fig. 46–21). Immunohistochemical studies demonstrate myofibroblastic features, with focal staining for muscle-specific actin, smooth muscle–specific actin, and desmin.

The differential diagnosis includes fibromatosis, nodular fasciitis, low-grade fibromyxoid sarcoma, and solitary fibrous tumor, all lesions that are more cellular than collagenous fibroma. The differential diagnosis also includes fibroma of tendon sheath, which has a lobular growth pattern and is more vascular; calcifying fibrous pseudotumor, which affects children and is associated with psammomatous and dystrophic calcifications; elastofibroma, which has characteristic elastic fibers; nuchal fibroma, which is more infiltrative; and neurofibroma, which is S-100 protein positive.

### Fibroma of Tendon Sheath[91–95]

Fibroma of tendon sheath most commonly occurs in young adults; it has a 2:1 male-to-female ratio. It occurs most often in the hands and feet, attached to a tendon sheath. Patients usually present with a small, painless mass. After excision, the lesion may recur, but there is usually little morbidity. The gross lesions are well-circumscribed and lobulated, usually measuring less than 2 cm in greatest diameter. On cut section, they are gray and firm. At low magnification, they are distinctly lobulated, with the lobules separated by narrow cleftlike vascular spaces. The individual lobules are composed of dense collagenous fibrous tissue containing slitlike vessels. The fibrous tissue contains bland spindle cells of variable cellularity ranging from hypocellular to moderately cellular (Fig. 46–22). Ultrastructural studies demon-

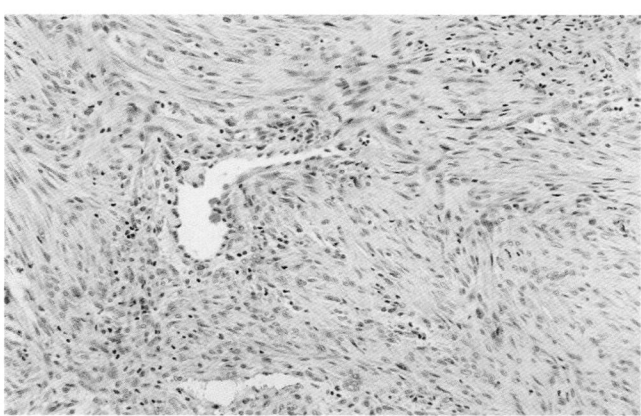

FIGURE 46–22. Fibroma of tendon sheath. There is a moderately cellular proliferation of bland fibroblasts. Note the slitlike vessels.

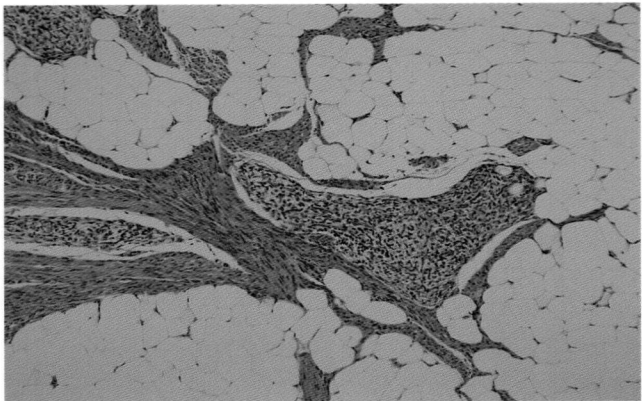

**FIGURE 46–23.** Fibrous hamartoma of infancy. There are areas of mature adipose tissue, cellular fibrous tissue, and cellular mesenchyme.

strate myofibroblastic differentiation. Immunohistochemical studies also show myofibroblastic features, with positivity for muscle-specific actin and smooth muscle–specific actin.

The differential diagnosis includes desmoplastic fibroma, which usually involves the head and neck, is less well circumscribed, and is less vascular. More cellular variants of fibroma of tendon sheath may resemble a late stage of nodular fasciitis or a fibrous histiocytoma. However, the localization to a tendon, the presence of hypocellular and hypercellular areas, and the circumscription favor fibroma of tendon sheath. The clinical presentation may resemble giant cell tumor of tendon sheath, but these lesions are pigmented on cut section and have a completely different histologic appearance.

## Fibrous Hamartoma of Infancy[96]

Fibrous hamartoma of infancy is a hamartomatous lesion that usually occurs in the first 2 years of life; it has a marked male predilection. The lesion usually presents as a painless enlarging subcutaneous mass in the region of the shoulder girdle or in the inguinal region. Complete excision is curative; incompletely excised lesions may recur. The gross lesions usually measure about 4 cm and show a variegated fatty and fibrous appearance on cut section.

The microscopic lesions consist of varying proportions of mature adipose tissue; irregularly disposed fascicles of mature fibrous tissue with bland fibroblasts, thick-walled blood vessels, and varying numbers of inflammatory cells; and nests and small sheets of undifferentiated spindled to stellate cells in a loose stroma (Fig. 46–23). Ultrastructural studies confirm the presence of a variety of cell types, and immunohistochemical studies demonstrate variable positivity for actin and desmin in the spindled cells.

## Infantile-Type Fibromatosis[97–100]

Infantile fibromatosis, also known as myofibroma, diffuse congenital fibromatosis, myofibromatosis, aggressive infantile myofibromatosis, and congenital multiple fibromatosis, comes in three clinicopathologic forms, presenting as a solitary lesion, multicentric lesions, and generalized lesions. The last two forms almost always present at or shortly after birth; the solitary form may present later, most often still within the first 2 years, but it may rarely also occur in adults.[101] The solitary and multicentric forms generally have an excellent outcome, but the generalized form leads to death in most cases. At gross evaluation, individual lesions tend to measure 1 to 3 cm and are firm on cut section.

A zonal microscopic pattern is often seen; more cellular areas are present in the center of the lesion, particularly around blood vessels (Fig. 46–24). These central areas have a close histologic resemblance to congenital hemangiopericytoma, and many now believe that congenital hemangiopericytoma is just a cellular example of infantile myofibromatosis. The mitotic rate is often high, but atypical forms are generally not seen. The periphery tends to be more collagenized, composed of spindled cells with bland nuclei. Polypoid projections into vascular spaces are common. Ultrastructural study shows myofibroblastic or smooth muscle differentiation, and there is reactivity for vimentin and smooth muscle actin on immunohistochemical analysis.

## Infantile Digital Fibromatosis[102, 103]

Infantile digital fibromatosis, also known as digital fibrous tumor and inclusion body fibromatosis, presents at birth or within the first year of life as a rapidly growing small nodule on the lateral or dorsal surfaces of the second through fifth fingers or, less commonly, the second through fifth toes. Rare cases have been reported in adults, usually in extra-

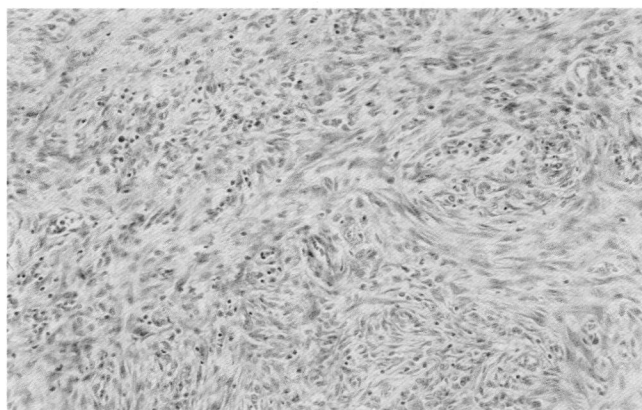

**FIGURE 46–24.** Infantile-type fibromatosis. There is a highly cellular but bland proliferation of fibroblast-like cells. This central area is less collagenized than the periphery of the lesion.

digital sites. Recurrences are frequent despite seemingly adequate excision.

Gross and microscopic examinations show that the lesions are centered in the dermis and extend into the subcutaneous tissue. They consist of a proliferation of bland fibroblasts in a dense collagenous stroma (Fig. 46–25). The most distinctive feature is the presence of small round eosinophilic cytoplasmic inclusions in the fibroblasts. Ultrastructural studies demonstrate the inclusions to consist of whorled bundles of cytoplasmic filaments. Immunohistochemical studies demonstrate positivity for actin and desmin in the spindled cells; the inclusions stain for actin.

## Calcifying Aponeurotic Fibromatosis[104, 105]

This extremely rare lesion occurs in children and adults with a male predilection. Patients present with a slow-growing, small mass usually involving the palm of the hand or the plantar aspect of the feet. Calcifications may be identified by radiologic examination. Complete excisions are difficult owing to infiltration of nerves and blood vessels; therefore, recurrences are common. Gross evaluation shows that most lesions are less than 3 cm and have a hard consistency.

At histologic examination, there is a proliferation of plump fibroblasts, with scattered hyaline, cartilaginous, or calcified foci (Fig. 46–26). The fibroblast nuclei tend to palisade—particularly around the foci of calcification—and may have a mild degree of atypia, although mitoses are rare. The differential diagnosis includes desmoid fibromatosis or Dupuytren's fibromatosis. Calcifying aponeurotic fibromatosis tends to occur in a younger age group and contains more plump fibroblasts; the presence of hyaline, cartilaginous, or calcified foci establishes the diagnosis.

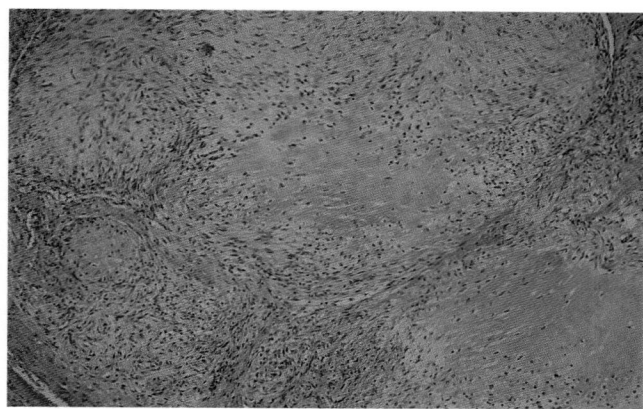

**FIGURE 46–26.** Calcifying aponeurotic fibromatosis. There is a cellular but bland spindle cell proliferation with occasional hyalinized areas.

## Fibromatosis Colli

Fibromatosis colli generally presents in the neonatal period as a hard, nontender mass at the lower end of the sternocleidomastoid muscle. It may be related to a difficult delivery. Left untreated, the mass resolves spontaneously in most cases. The gross lesions are usually less than 3 cm and are gray-white and firm on cut section. Histologic examination shows infiltration of the muscle fibers by hypocellular fibrous tissue with bland fibroblasts (Fig. 46–27).

## Superficial Fibromatosis[95, 106]

The superficial fibromatoses include palmar fibromatosis, knuckle pads, and plantar fibromatosis. Palmar fibromatosis (Dupuytren's contracture) almost always occurs in adults, increasing in incidence with age, with a marked preference for males. It is rare in blacks and Asians. Bilateral lesions occur in about 50% of cases, and a subset of cases are associated

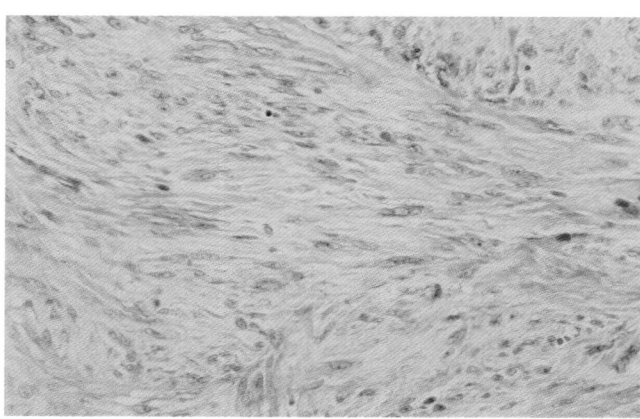

**FIGURE 46–25.** Infantile digital fibromatosis. There is a spindle cell proliferation. Note the several eosinophilic cytoplasmic inclusions.

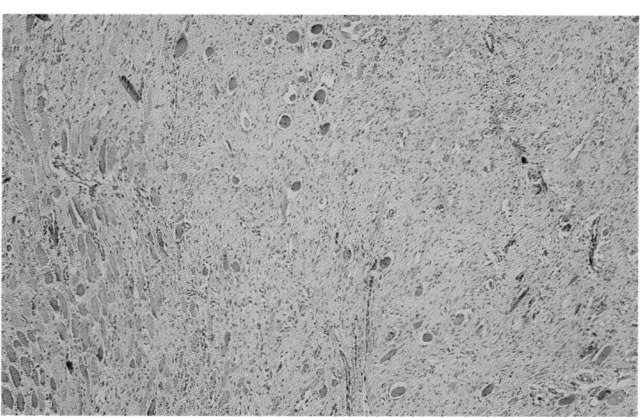

**FIGURE 46–27.** Fibromatosis colli. The dense hypocellular fibrous proliferation envelopes skeletal muscle.

with knuckle pads or plantar fibromatosis. Patients present with a nodule in the palmar surface of the hand that progresses to flexion contractures. Patients are treated by fasciectomy or aponeurectomy, but the lesion may still recur. Knuckle pads are thickenings on the dorsal aspect of the joints of the fingers; they do not lead to contractures. The epidemiologic features are similar to those of palmar fibromatosis, with which they are often associated. Treatment is not generally necessary. Plantar fibromatosis (Ledderhose's disease) has epidemiologic features similar to those of palmar fibromatosis but occurs in a wider age range. Lesions are bilateral in about 20% of cases and occur in approximately 10% of patients with palmar fibromatosis. Patients present with a nodule on the plantar aspect of the foot that causes discomfort on standing; contractures generally do not occur. Most cases do not require treatment. Fasciectomy is performed when discomfort is caused; however, recurrences are not uncommon.

The histologic appearances of all three lesions are similar. Early in the process, a uniform population of plump spindle cells with vesicular nuclei is present in loose fascicles. The mitotic rate is often high, but atypical forms are not generally seen. Later in the process, when specimens are most likely to be obtained, a population of thin spindle cells with slender nuclei is present in a dense collagenized fibrous tissue. Mitoses are usually not evident at this stage. Biopsy specimens may also show features intermediate between these two appearances. Plantar fibromatosis more often shows features of early lesions, probably because biopsy of these cases is performed at an earlier stage of the disease. Immunohistochemical studies show positivity for muscle-specific actin and the α-isoform of smooth muscle actin in early lesions; negativity for these markers is found in late lesions.

Early lesions may simulate fibrosarcoma, but attention to the clinical features should avoid misdiagnosis. Fibrosarcomas occurring in adults are rarely found in the hands or feet and generally involve deeper soft tissues.

## Desmoid Fibromatosis[106–111]

Desmoid fibromatosis is also known as deep or musculoaponeurotic fibromatosis. It occurs in all age groups but has a peak of incidence in the 20s; females are affected more than males. A subset of cases are associated with Gardner's syndrome (familial adenomatous polyposis with osteomas, cutaneous cysts, and other neoplasms and abnormalities), and about 1% of cases are familial outside of the setting of Gardner's syndrome.[112] Patients present with insidious masses that are deeply situated. Any site may be affected, but the abdominal wall, abdominal cavity, shoulder girdle, chest wall, and back are most commonly involved. Lesions that arise in childhood frequently occur in the head and

neck region. Some cases have a prior history of radiation, and other cases develop at the site of a previous scar. Mesenteric and retroperitoneal lesions are particularly common in patients with Gardner's syndrome who have undergone prior abdominal surgery; patients with abdominal fibromatosis are often women who have recently undergone childbirth, especially those who had a cesarean section. Multiple lesions are seen in about 5% of cases and are more common in familial cases; they tend to occur close to one another. Recurrences, usually multiple, are the rule even after seemingly complete resection. The surgical goal is to achieve as wide a margin as possible, without compromise of function or major morbidity. Postoperative radiation therapy is often employed when adequate margins cannot be achieved. Hormonal therapy is often used because there are usually no major side effects, and it may be useful. The gross lesion is poorly circumscribed and usually measures between 5 and 15 cm. On cut section, it is hard and tan-white. The lesion is poorly circumscribed and is centered in skeletal muscle and the adjacent fascia. There is often infiltration and obliteration of adjacent structures.

The histologic appearance is usually consistent within a given case as well as from case to case. At low magnification, there are broad fascicles of dense collagenous fibrous tissue. In between the collagen fibers are long spindle cells with slender, pointed nuclei (Fig. 46–28). The nuclei lack cytologic atypia and have a vesicular chromatin pattern and small nucleoli. The mitotic rate is low—less than 1 mitosis per high-power field. In some cases, there may be variation in the cellularity, and occasional cases may show a keloidal hyalinization. Fibromatosis occurring in childhood may have a uniformly high degree of cellularity. Electron microscopic studies demonstrate a prominent rough endoplasmic reticulum, pinocytotic vesicles, microtubules, and thin filaments consistent with myofibroblastic differentiation. Immunohistochemical studies generally show that the

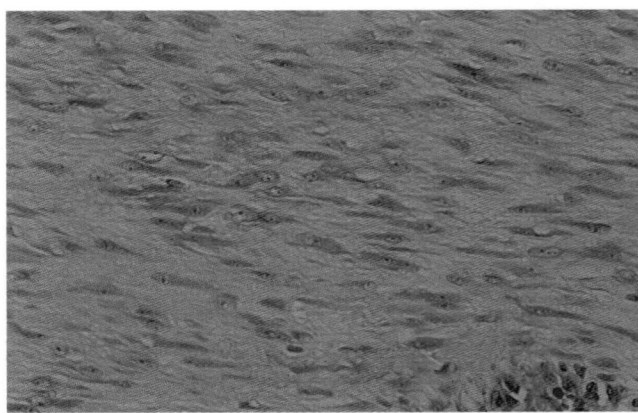

**FIGURE 46–28.** Desmoid fibromatosis. This spindle cell proliferation is composed of cells with identical flattened nuclei with a vesicular chromatin pattern and small but evident nucleoli.

spindle cells are positive for muscle-specific actin and $\alpha$-isoform smooth muscle actin, and many cases show positivity for estrogen and progesterone receptor.

The differential diagnosis includes nodular fasciitis and neurofibroma, on the one hand, and sarcoma (namely, fibrosarcoma or low-grade fibromyxoid sarcoma) on the other hand. Nodular fasciitis has a higher mitotic rate and a looser stroma, and it is usually much smaller than desmoid fibromatosis, whereas neurofibromas are S-100 protein positive. Fibrosarcomas have a higher mitotic rate and are less collagenous, whereas low-grade fibromyxoid sarcoma has a biphasic stroma consisting of both fibrous and loose areas; these latter areas are not a feature of fibromatosis.

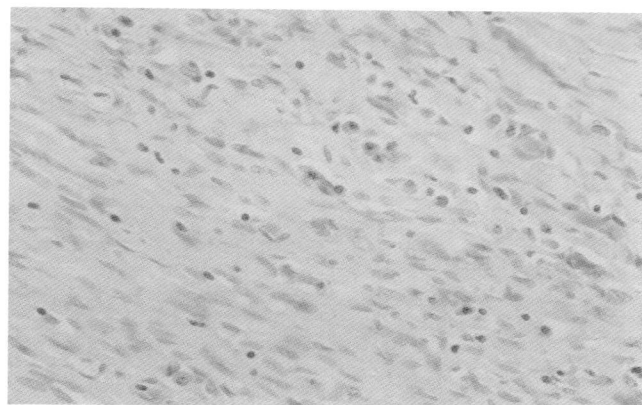

**FIGURE 46–29.** Inflammatory myofibroblastic tumor or low-grade inflammatory fibrosarcoma. There is a relatively hypocellular spindle cell proliferation with scattered inflammatory cells. There is a mild degree of nuclear atypia.

## Inflammatory Myofibroblastic Tumor or Low-Grade Inflammatory Fibrosarcoma[113, 114]

This lesion has been called inflammatory pseudotumor or plasma cell granuloma in the past. There is currently controversy as to whether inflammatory myofibroblastic tumor is inflammatory or neoplastic, benign or of uncertain behavior, and independent of or closely related to low-grade inflammatory fibrosarcoma. The majority of cases present in childhood through young adulthood, but a wide age range may be affected; there is no clear age predilection. Patients present with a mass accompanied by constitutional symptoms. Among soft tissue presentations, the lesion occurs most commonly in the abdominal cavity, the retroperitoneum, the mediastinum, and the head and neck. Although most lesions are solitary, presentation is occasionally multifocal, either within a single anatomic region or involving noncontiguous sites. Recurrences are relatively frequent, particularly in lesions from the abdominal cavity; rarely, the recurrences have had a histologic appearance more compatible with sarcoma. There are also rare cases in which secondary lesions have occurred in sites traditionally regarded as metastases (e.g., lung, bone, and brain).

At gross evaluation, inflammatory myofibroblastic tumors may be circumscribed or infiltrative and multinodular. They have a wide range in size; the largest lesions are found in the abdominal cavity and retroperitoneum. Microscopic examination reveals several histologic patterns: a myxoid-vascular pattern, with loosely arranged stellate or spindle-shaped cells in a myxoid edematous matrix; a compact pattern, with cellular fascicles or storiform bundles; and a hypocellular fibrous pattern, with dense collagen. Regardless of the pattern, the predominant cell type is a relatively bland spindle cell, with scattered lymphocytes, plasma cells, or eosinophils (Fig. 46–29). Ultrastructural studies show features of myofibroblasts. Immunohistochemical studies show positivity for smooth muscle actin and muscle-specific actin in most cases, also consistent with myofibroblastic differentiation. Flow cytometric studies have shown either diploid or aneuploid DNA content.[115] Cytogenetic studies performed in a small number of cases (arising in bone) have shown clonal abnormalities.[116]

The differential diagnosis includes myxoid lesions, such as nodular fasciitis; cellular spindle cell lesions, such as a follicular dendritic tumor; fibrous lesions, such as desmoid fibromatosis; and fibrosclerotic disorders. A key to the recognition of inflammatory fibroblastic tumor is the identification of more than one histologic pattern in a given tumor. There is as yet no good way to identify those cases that may metastasize from those that may not, although any significant degree of atypia should suggest a low-grade sarcoma.

## Low-Grade Fibromyxoid Sarcoma[117, 118]

Low-grade fibromyxoid sarcoma is a rare sarcoma that occurs most often in adults 25 to 45 years of age, without a sex predilection. Patients present with a long-standing deep-seated mass. Most cases have been reported in the thigh, inguinal region, and shoulder region. Although optimal treatment has not been decided, the neoplasms have been treated by excision. Most patients have experienced recurrences, and about half have developed metastases, although these may take years to manifest. One tumor underwent dedifferentiation over time. Gross tumors have been variable in size, with a median of about 10 cm.

At histologic examination, the neoplasms have characteristic biphasic fibrous and myxoid areas of various proportions, with bland spindle cells ar-

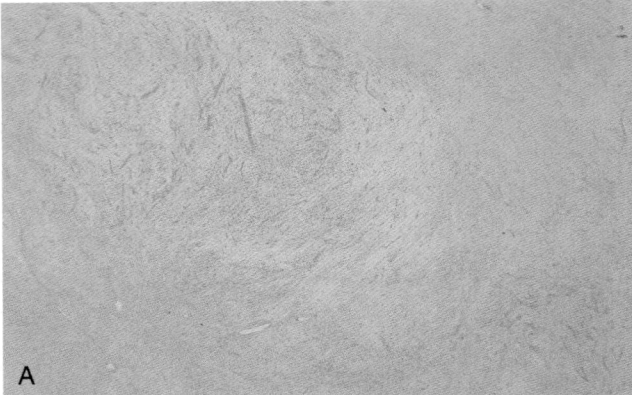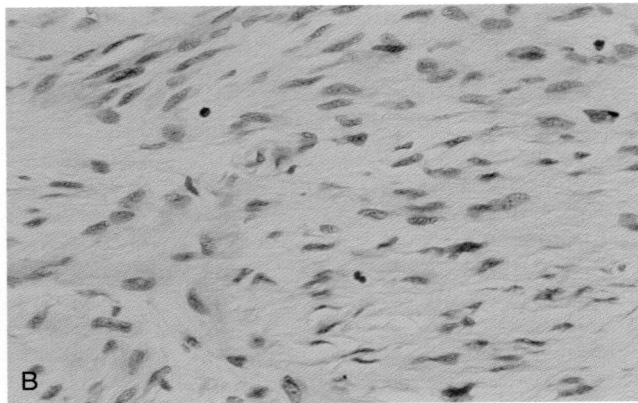

**FIGURE 46–30.** Low-grade fibromyxoid sarcoma. At low magnification *(A)*, a variably cellular proliferation is seen. At high magnification *(B)*, there is only mild nuclear pleomorphism.

ranged in a whorling pattern (Fig. 46–30). Cellularity is low to moderate but may be accentuated in perivascular areas. Vascularity is usually not prominent, but increased numbers of capillaries may be present in the myxoid areas. Nuclear pleomorphism is absent to slight, and mitotic figures are uncommon. Recurrences may show a greater degree of cellularity and pleomorphism than the primary tumor. Immunohistochemical studies have not been reported, but the tumors are negative for desmin, muscle-specific actin, CD34, and S-100 protein in my experience.

The differential diagnosis includes fibromatosis, neurofibroma, and a variety of low-grade sarcomas. Fibromatosis is more uniformly fibrous and lacks myxoid areas. Neurofibromas are usually much smaller and should be S-100 protein positive. Myxoid malignant fibrous histiocytoma shows a greater degree of pleomorphism and is usually much more vascular. Fibrosarcoma is much more cellular.

## Fibrosarcoma[119, 120]

Fibrosarcoma, a rare neoplasm, occurs as distinct clinicopathologic entities: infantile (congenital) fibrosarcoma and adult fibrosarcoma. Infantile fibrosarcoma usually occurs in the first year of life and in many cases is present at birth; there is a slight male predilection. Infants present with a fast-growing mass that usually involves one of the extremities in the subcutaneous tissue or the deeper soft tissues. Despite the ominous clinical and pathologic findings, the prognosis is excellent. Most cases are cured by wide local excision; metastasis occurs in less than 10%. Radiotherapy and chemotherapy are generally reserved for unresectable or recurrent and metastatic cases. At gross evaluation, there is a wide variation in size; the neoplasms may be well or poorly circumscribed and are firm and tan-white on cut section.

The adult type of fibrosarcoma has a peak incidence in the 40s but may affect any age group, including children; there is a slight predilection for men. A subset of cases arise after radiation, and rare cases occur at the sites of previous scars, particularly after burns, usually after an interval of decades. Adult fibrosarcoma usually presents as a deep-seated mass, most often involving the lower extremities, particularly the thigh, but it also commonly occurs in the upper extremities and the trunk. The prognosis for adult fibrosarcoma is much worse than that for the infantile variety, with 5-year survival rates of 40% to 50%. The neoplasms are usually treated by radical resection, often followed by radiation therapy, with chemotherapy also used in high-grade tumors. At gross evaluation, the tumors generally range from 5 to 10 cm; they may be well or poorly circumscribed and are firm and tan-white on cut section.

Infantile fibrosarcoma and adult fibrosarcoma show similar histologic features. At low magnification, there is a spindle cell proliferation that shows a fascicular arrangement, classically forming acute-angle or herringbone patterns (Fig. 46–31). The neoplasms are usually more cellular than collagenous. However, some well-differentiated examples may have abundant collagenation, and one variant of fi-

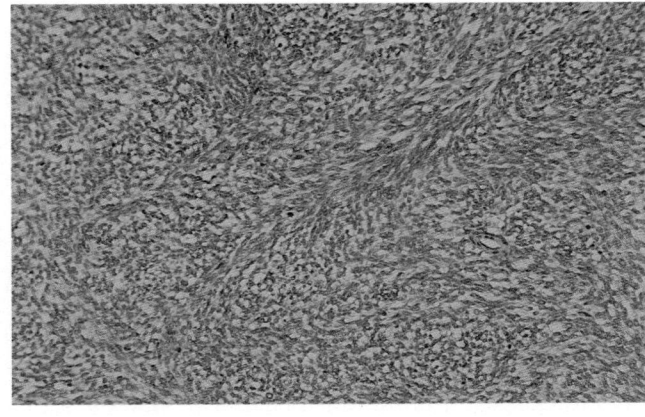

**FIGURE 46–31.** Fibrosarcoma. A herringbone pattern is seen.

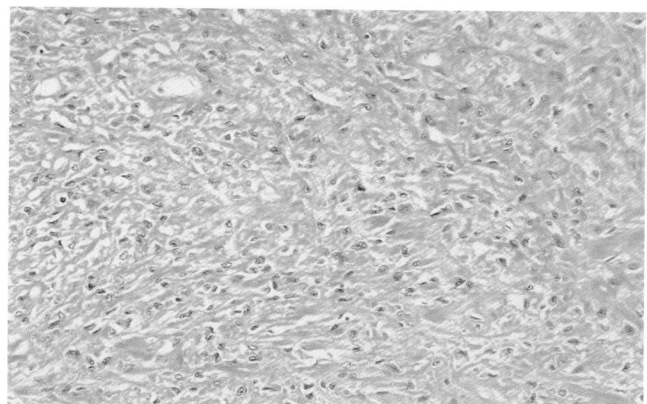

**FIGURE 46–32.** Sclerosing epithelioid fibrosarcoma. Dense collagenation is present; isolated cells take on an epithelioid appearance.

brosarcoma, the sclerosing epithelioid variant, has abundant hyalinizing collagen, which may isolate individual neoplastic cells (Fig. 46–32). The constituent cells are usually highly spindled and generally uniform from one to another (Fig. 46–33). However, in some infantile cases, the cells may be more oval than spindled, and in the sclerosing epithelioid variant, the cells may even be rounded. The nuclei range from mildly to markedly atypical. The mitotic rate is generally high and is always more than 1 mitosis per high-power field, and atypical forms may be seen. Electron microscopic studies show prominent rough endoplasmic reticulum and thin filaments, consistent with myofibroblastic differentiation. Immunohistochemical studies may demonstrate positivity for actin, particularly in the childhood cases. Cytogenetic studies of infantile fibrosarcoma have revealed several abnormalities, particularly a t(12;15)(p13;q25) and a nonrandom gain of extra chromosomes.[120, 121]

The differential diagnosis of fibrosarcoma includes both benign and malignant neoplasms. Nodular fasciitis is much smaller than fibrosarcoma and lacks the well-defined architecture of fibrosarcoma. Deep fibrous histiocytoma is also much smaller than fibrosarcoma, is usually more superficial (centered in the subcutaneous tissue), is more collagenized, and has a more variable cell population. Desmoid fibromatosis may be difficult to distinguish from fibrosarcoma. However, it is usually more collagenous and less cellular; the mitotic rate is lower (less than 1 mitosis versus more than 1 mitosis per high-power field), and the cells have less nuclear atypia. Inflammatory pseudotumor has a greater admixture of inflammatory cells, particularly lymphocytes and plasma cells, but some cases have been considered to be fibrosarcomas (inflammatory fibrosarcoma); this issue is discussed further in the section on inflammatory myofibroblastic tumor. Distinguishing cellular forms of infantile fibromatosis may be extremely difficult or even impossible. It is fortunate that there may not be distinct clinical differences at the borderline histologic appearances; one should probably err on the side of fibrosarcoma in such cases.

Dermatofibrosarcoma is a more superficial neoplasm than adult fibrosarcoma, being centered in the subcutaneous tissue, and is CD34⁺. Low-grade fibromyxoid sarcoma (which may be a variant of fibrosarcoma) usually has biphasic myxoid and fibrous areas; the myxoid areas should not be seen in fibrosarcoma. Monophasic synovial sarcoma and malignant schwannoma may be histologically indistinguishable from adult fibrosarcoma; immunostains are necessary for their distinction. A neoplasm with the histologic features of fibrosarcoma should be considered a monophasic synovial sarcoma if clusters of cells are positive for keratin or epithelial membrane antigen, and it should be considered a malignant schwannoma if the keratin and epithelial membrane antigen stains are negative but the S-100 protein stain is positive. Similarly, demonstration of desmin positivity is more in keeping with a spindle cell variant of a myosarcoma. The most controversial issue is the distinction of fibrous variants of malignant fibrous histiocytoma from fibrosarcoma. In my opinion, fibrosarcoma should consist of a relatively uniform population of spindle cells and should lack a significant component of histiocyte-like cells or multinucleated or pleomorphic giant cells.

The prognosis of adult fibrosarcoma has been closely related to the histologic grade as determined by the degree of cytologic atypia and the amount and character of the stroma. Two-, three-, and four-tiered systems exist. Given the rarity of fibrosarcoma, a two-grade approach is recommended. High-grade fibrosarcomas (with about 30% 5-year survival) feature significant cytologic atypia, increased cellularity, and little fibrosis, and they may show gross or microscopic foci of necrosis; low-grade fibrosarcomas (with about 60% 5-year survival) generally lack these features. Of course, treatment factors, such as adequacy of the excision and whether adjuvant radiation therapy was used, also have a major impact on prognosis.

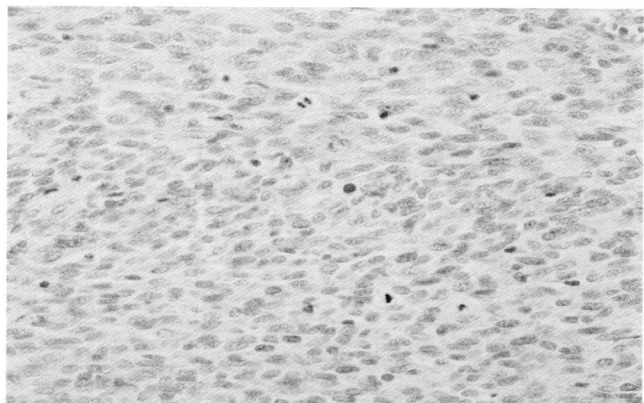

**FIGURE 46–33.** Fibrosarcoma. The cells are highly uniform, but the mitotic rate is high.

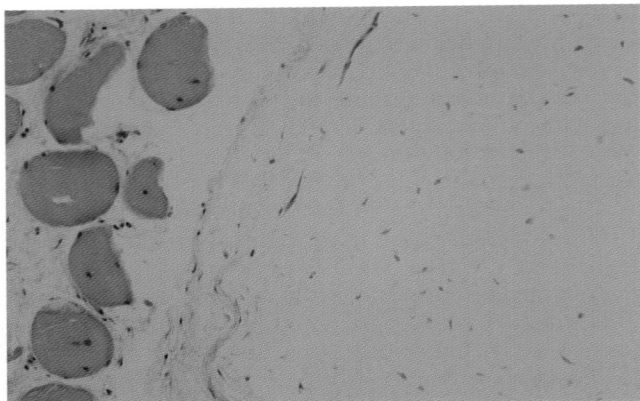

FIGURE 46–34. Intramuscular myxoma. The myxoid lesion is relatively avascular and acellular.

## TUMORS AND TUMORLIKE PROLIFERATIONS SHOWING PREDOMINANTLY MYXOID DIFFERENTIATION

### Intramuscular Myxoma[122–126]

Intramuscular myxoma occurs virtually always in adults, with a female predilection. It usually presents as a slow-growing, painless mass in the major muscle groups, such as the thigh, shoulder, and buttocks. Multiple lesions occur in about 5% of cases; these cases are usually associated with monostotic or polyostotic fibrous dysplasia, most often involving the adjacent underlying bone. Recurrence is uncommon after local excision. The gross lesions have infiltrative margins, are generally lobular and highly gelatinous on cut section, and vary widely in size, averaging between 3 and 10 cm.

The microscopic lesion is usually relatively avascular, nonfibrous, and cell poor, consisting of sparse stellate to spindled cells in a sea of myxoid, edematous stroma (Fig. 46–34). However, there may be focal areas with increased numbers of cells, more prominent vascularity, and often increased collagen content.[126] The stellate cells are uniformly bland, and mitotic figures are not present. There may be scattered macrophages, mast cells, and occasional multinucleated giant cells. At the edge of the lesion, there is often an infiltrative border with adjacent tissues. Immunohistochemical studies are negative for S-100 protein, muscle markers, and endothelial markers. Ultrastructural examination reveals myofibroblast-like cells.

The differential diagnosis includes myxoid sarcomas such as fibromyxoid sarcoma, myxoid liposarcoma, and the myxoid variant of malignant fibrous histiocytoma. The uniformly bland appearance of the cells and the absence of an extensive vascular network should distinguish intramuscular myxoma from myxoid sarcomas, even though myxomas may have focal areas of increased cellularity. Although intramuscular myxoma may have occasional macrophages with lipid vacuoles, these cells lack cytologic atypia, and the vacuoles do not indent the nuclei as seen in true lipoblasts.

### Aggressive Angiomyxoma[127, 128]

Aggressive angiomyxoma primarily affects young adults and is not a neoplasm of infants and children; there is a marked female predominance. Patients usually present with a slow-growing, painless mass. It usually occurs in the vulva and vagina but may occur in other pelvic and perineal sites. After excision, there is local recurrence in a high proportion of cases, although metastasis has not been reported. The gross tumor appears well circumscribed, is generally larger than 10 cm, and is gelatinous on cut section.

At histologic examination, aggressive angiomyxoma generally has infiltrative margins. The neoplasm consists of relatively bland stellate and spindled cells in a myxoid matrix (Fig. 46–35). The myxoid matrix usually contains scattered thick collagen fibers and focal areas of extravasation of erythrocytes. There is often condensation of the stroma into a thickened adventitial or periadventitial sheath around the blood vessels. The vasculature is distinctive and consists of numerous thin to thick, ectatic blood vessels. The stellate to spindled cells are extremely bland and generally lack mitotic activity. Scattered mast cells may also be present. Immunohistochemical studies demonstrate that the stellate and spindled cells are often positive for muscle-specific actin and smooth muscle–specific actin, but they are usually negative for desmin (except in one notable series), S-100 protein, and endothelial markers. Ultrastructural studies show features of myofibroblasts or fibroblasts.

The differential diagnosis of aggressive angiomyxoma includes myxoma, a variety of myxoid sarcomas, and angiofibroblastoma. Myxoma lacks the vascular pattern of aggressive angiomyxoma and does not usually occur in the sites most often affected by aggressive angiomyxoma. Myxoid sarcomas generally

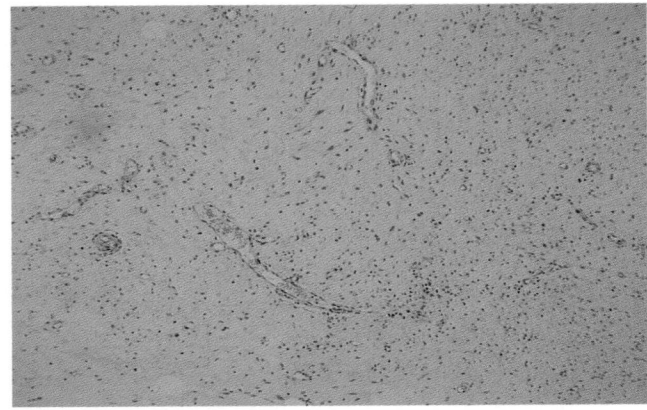

FIGURE 46–35. Aggressive angiomyxoma. This myxoid proliferation is relatively acellular but features prominent open blood vessels.

possess a greater degree of cellularity and cytologic atypia. Myxoid liposarcoma may show little cellularity or atypia, but it generally has a better developed network of small arborizing blood vessels, has lesional cells that are S-100 protein positive, and often contains diagnostic lipoblasts. Angiofibroblastoma occurs in sites similar to those in which aggressive angiomyxoma does, but it is usually more superficially situated, lacks an infiltrating border, has a more variable cellularity from area to area, and contains desmin-positive proliferating cells.

## Ossifying Fibromyxoid Tumor[129–132]

Ossifying fibromyxoid tumor is a rare tumor that affects adults with a median age of 50 years; there is a male predominance. Patients present with a slow-growing, painless mass. It most commonly occurs in the deep subcutaneous tissue in the extremities, although the head and neck region and the torso are also sites of involvement. Rare patients may have multiple sites of involvement. Approximately one third of patients develop recurrences after excision, and cases with metastases have been reported. The gross neoplasm is usually well circumscribed, usually measures less than 5 cm, and shows a lobulated appearance on cut section, often with a distinctive calcified peripheral shell.

The microscopic lesion has a lobulated low-magnification appearance. There is usually a thickened collagenized capsule that extends into the lesion to form septa that divide the lobules (Fig. 46–36). In about 90% of cases, the capsule contains lamellar bone, often rimmed by a thin stratum of bland osteoblasts. The lobules are composed of cords of uniform round to stellate cells embedded in a myxoid or fibromyxoid stroma. The cells usually have a monomorphic appearance with vesicular nuclei containing small nucleoli and a rim of eosinophilic cytoplasm. Mitotic activity is low. Immunohistochemical studies reveal positivity for S-100 protein in about 75% of cases, and collagen IV stains usually outline single cells. In some studies, staining for desmin and smooth muscle–specific actin has been reported. There is no staining for endothelial markers, HMB-45, or epithelial markers. Ultrastructural studies demonstrate a variety of findings, with no consistent lineage found. The cells have elongated cell processes, a partial or discontinuous basal lamina that may be reduplicated, and arrays of intermediate filaments.

A minority of cases of ossifying fibromyxoid tumor have an osseous component that appears to be produced by the tumor cells. Rare cases have a greater cellularity and mitotic rate. Some of these cases have behaved in an aggressive manner, suggesting that an overtly malignant form of this neoplasm exists.

The differential diagnosis of ossifying fibromyxoid tumor includes myxoid chondrosarcoma, chondroid syringoma, and nerve sheath tumor. Myxoid chondrosarcoma lacks lamellar bone and lacks collagen IV staining around single cells. Chondroid syringoma is keratin positive. Ossifying fibromyxoid tumor may represent a peculiar nerve sheath tumor, but it can be distinguished from nerve sheath myxoma by the presence of lamellar bone and its deeper localization (nerve sheath myxoma is usually a dermal-based tumor).

## TUMORS AND TUMORLIKE PROLIFERATIONS SHOWING FIBROHISTIOCYTIC DIFFERENTIATION

This section covers tumors and tumorlike lesions showing fibrohistiocytic differentiation. No one thinks any more that these tumors are actually derived from cells with the capacity to differentiate into both fibroblasts and true histiocytes—or even that these cells necessarily show histodifferentiation toward both fibroblasts and histiocytes. Rather, it is highly likely that the proliferating cells composing

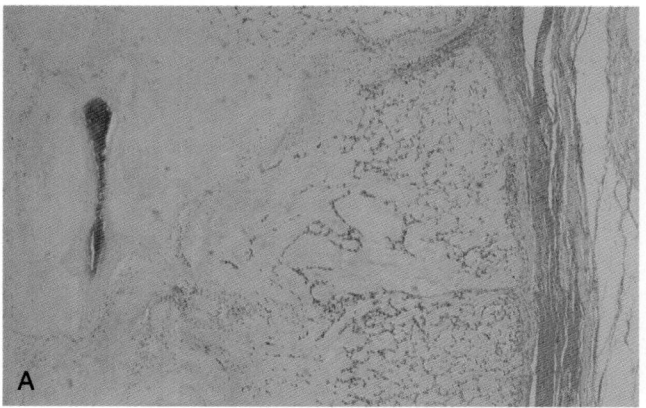
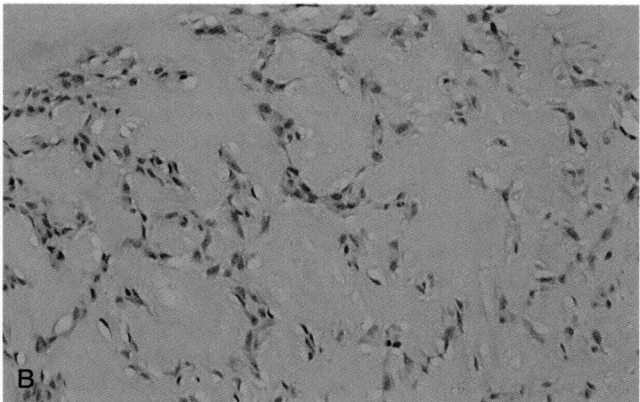

FIGURE 46–36. Ossifying fibromyxoid tumor. At low magnification (A), there is a dense capsule, and focal calcification is also evident. At high magnification (B), there are cords of relatively bland cells in a loosely collagenized stroma.

these tumors arise from undifferentiated cells committed to mesenchymal differentiation. Many of the cells that make up these tumors have some morphologic features reminiscent of fibroblasts or histiocytes, and they have conventionally been classified in this manner. If it can be demonstrated that a neoplasm has features suggesting definite differentiation toward any specific cell type, the neoplasm should probably be classified as a neoplasm of that type. Therefore, the category of tumor and tumorlike lesions showing fibrohistiocytic differentiation becomes defined by what it is (at least morphologically) as well as by what it is not.

## Fibrous Histiocytoma[133]

The overwhelming majority of cases of fibrous histiocytoma occur in the dermis (dermatofibroma). However, about 1% may occur in a deeper location, usually the subcutaneous tissue, or more rarely within skeletal muscle or the abdominal cavity. All ages are affected, with a median age of occurrence in young adulthood; there is a male predominance. The lesions usually present as painless masses, most often in the extremities, particularly the lower extremity, or in the head and neck. At gross evaluation, they are circumscribed, are generally greater than 4 cm in diameter, and may show hemorrhage on cut section. About 25% of these tumors recur, but none metastasizes.

The deep variant of fibrous histiocytoma has a histologic appearance similar to that of the more common cutaneous lesion. However, it tends to be less infiltrative at the edges, and there is usually more monomorphism of the proliferating cells. On occasion, there may be hemangiopericytomatous areas within the tumor. Mitoses may be present but should be less than 5 mitoses per 10 high-power fields. Immunohistochemical studies show positivity for factor XIIIa and negativity for CD34 and S-100 protein; CD68 shows variable staining. The factor XIIIa positivity has suggested differentiation toward dermal dendrocytes. Ultrastructural studies show a variety of cell types, from fibroblasts to histiocyte-like cells.

The differential diagnosis of deep fibrous histiocytoma includes angiomatoid fibrous histiocytoma, dermatofibrosarcoma, and malignant fibrous histiocytoma. Angiomatoid fibrous histiocytoma shows a more histiocytoid appearance, more consistently has cystic areas of hemorrhage, and is usually surrounded by a cuff of lymphoid tissue. Dermatofibrosarcoma is almost always CD34+, whereas malignant fibrous histiocytoma has a greater degree of cytologic atypia and mitotic activity.

## Giant Cell Tumor of Tendon Sheath[94, 134]

Giant cell tumor of tendon sheath encompasses several related clinicopathologic entities that involve the joint and bone as well as the soft tissues. It is still not resolved whether it represents a true neoplasm or a tumorlike reactive proliferation. In the soft tissues, the lesion occurs with a female predominance mainly in young adults. It usually presents clinically as a slow-growing, small nodule involving the soft tissues near joints. The digits, particularly the distal fingers, are most often affected, although the soft tissues around the knee and ankle are also commonly affected. Although the lesion may "recur" after excision, this is due to incomplete resection. The gross lesion is well circumscribed, generally measures between 1 and 2 cm, and is firm and gray-yellow on cut section.

Giant cell tumor of tendon sheath is composed histologically of sheets of histiocytoid mononuclear cells admixed with variable numbers of multinucleated osteoclast-like giant cells, foamy macrophages, and hemosiderin-laden macrophages. On occasion, a pure population of histiocytoid mononuclear cells is present (Fig. 46–37). The mitotic rate may be high, although atypical mitotic figures are not seen. Older lesions may show focal or extensive fibrosis. Immunohistochemical studies show the mononuclear cells to be positive for CD68 and other histiocyte markers.[135] Nonetheless, ultrastructural studies have shown features suggestive of synoviocytes.

Highly cellular examples of giant cell tumor of tendon sheath with a high mitotic rate may be confused with a malignant neoplasm (including a hematopoietic tumor or a small round cell sarcoma). However, the clinical presentation should remind the pathologist to consider the correct diagnosis; once it is considered a possibility, there really should be no problems in differential diagnosis.

## Plexiform Fibrohistiocytic Tumor[136–138]

The plexiform fibrohistiocytic tumor occurs primarily in children, adolescents, and young adults; there is a female predilection. Patients present with an ill-

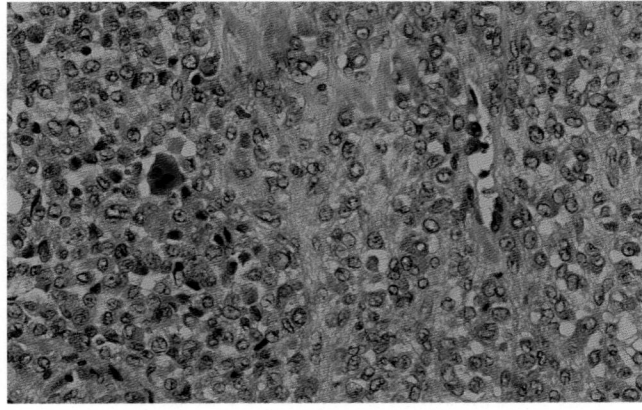

**FIGURE 46–37.** Giant cell tumor of tendon sheath. In this example, there was a large number of histiocytic cells with only rare giant cells.

defined, painless mass centered in the subcutaneous tissue, sometimes with extension into the dermis or skeletal muscle. Most cases occur in the extremities, particularly the fingers, hands, and wrist. Plexiform fibrohistiocytic tumor should be considered a low-grade malignant neoplasm. Recurrences are usually due to incomplete excision. Metastases may also occur, most commonly reported in regional lymph nodes or lungs. The gross tumor is poorly circumscribed, about 2.0 to 3.0 cm in diameter, and multinodular on cut section.

At histologic examination, a plexiform arrangement is seen at low magnification, with nodules of fibrohistiocytic and spindled cells in various proportions (Fig. 46–38). Rare cases may show vascular invasion. The fibrohistiocytic areas may have osteoclast-like giant cells or foamy macrophages; the spindled areas are composed of fascicles of bland fusiform cells that may resemble fibromatosis. Cytologic atypia is usually absent or minimal, but mitoses may be present, usually less than 3 mitoses per 10 high-power fields. Immunohistochemical studies may show positivity for smooth muscle actin, a feature that may suggest myofibroblastic differentiation, and many cells are CD68+, including the osteoclast-like giant cells. Staining for keratin, desmin, S-100 protein, factor XIIIa, and endothelial markers is negative. Ultrastructural studies have shown features of myofibroblastic and histiocytic differentiation. Flow cytometric studies have demonstrated a diploid population.

The differential diagnosis includes granulomatous inflammation, other plexiform tumors such as plexiform neurofibroma, fibrous hamartoma of infancy, and cellular neurothekeoma as well as nodular fasciitis or fibromatosis. Lesions with central necrosis or an accompanying inflammatory infiltrate should raise consideration of granulomatous inflammation. Plexiform neurofibroma is S-100 protein positive; fibrous hamartoma of infancy contains a hamartomatous proliferation of immature-appearing spindle cells. Cellular neurothekeoma is based more in the dermis and is more ill-defined at low magnifi-

cation. Nodular fasciitis and fibromatosis lack the low-power plexiform appearance of the plexiform fibrohistiocytic tumor.

## Angiomatoid Fibrous Histiocytoma[139–142]

Angiomatoid fibrous histiocytoma used to be considered one of the variants of malignant fibrous histiocytoma. However, the name has been changed to angiomatoid fibrous histiocytoma to reflect its unique clinicopathologic features that are more favorable than those of other types of malignant fibrous histiocytoma. The demonstration of features of muscle differentiation (see later) may warrant designation as a tumor showing features of muscle differentiation in future classifications of soft tissue tumors. Angiomatoid fibrous histiocytoma occurs primarily in children and adolescents with a mean age of about 15 years. However, it may occur in all age groups; there is no striking sex predilection. Patients generally present with a slow-growing tumor involving the subcutaneous tissue or nearby soft tissues, and systemic complaints are present in about 20% of cases. The extremities, particularly the upper extremity, are involved in most cases, but the trunk and, less commonly, the head and neck region may also be affected. With wide excision, recurrence appears in about 10% of cases, and metastases occur in less than 5% of cases. The gross tumor is usually well circumscribed, averaging about 4 cm in diameter, and contains cystic spaces or hemorrhagic areas on cut section.

Histologic examination shows multinodular masses of spindled to histiocytic cells interspersed with hemorrhagic, often cystic areas, with a peripheral lining of lymphoplasmacytic cells (Fig. 46–39). The cystic spaces are usually filled with erythrocytes but lack a true endothelial lining, being rimmed by the proliferating lesional cells. These cells are fibroblast-like or, more often, histiocyte-like and form sheets and nodules. Interspersed between the prolif-

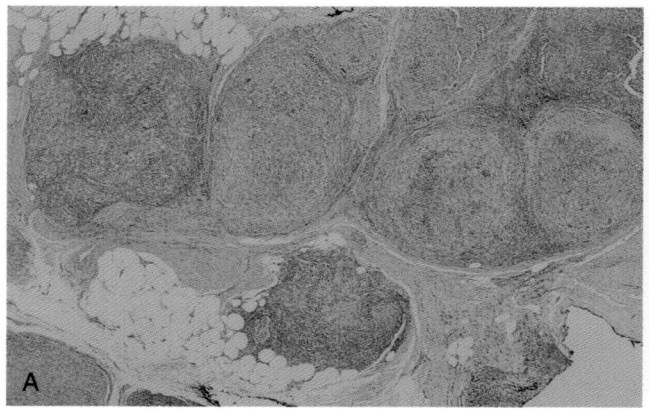
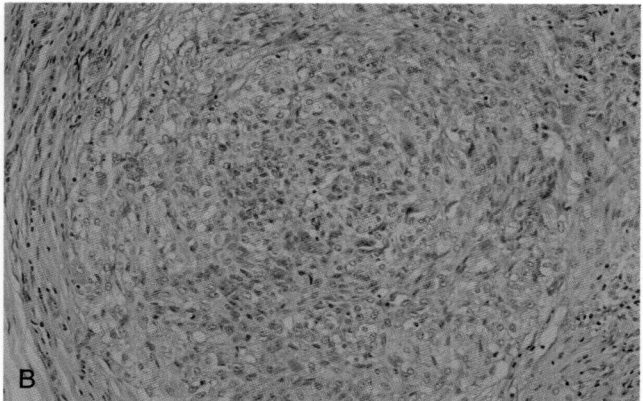

**FIGURE 46–38.** Plexiform fibrohistiocytic tumor. Low magnification *(A)* shows a plexiform arrangement. High magnification *(B)* shows a bland fibrohistiocytic proliferation. Note the occasional giant cells.

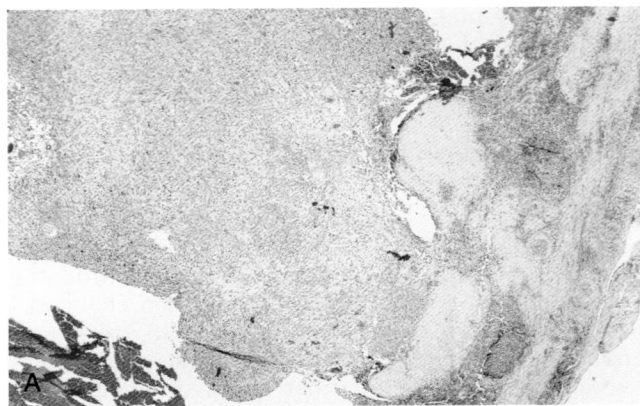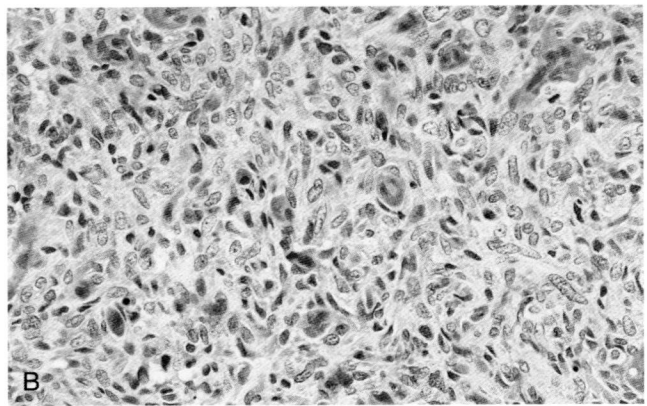

**FIGURE 46–39.** Angiomatoid fibrous histiocytoma. At low magnification (A), there is a fibrous pseudocapsule that contains aggregates of lymphoid cells. Note the hemorrhagic spaces. At high magnification (B), there is a relatively bland fibrohistiocytic proliferation.

erating cells are an intense vascularity, interstitial hemorrhage, and hemosiderin deposits. The periphery of the lesion contains numerous lymphocytes and plasma cells (which may include germinal centers), giving a superficial resemblance to the outer portion of a lymph node; however, a true lymph node capsule and subcapsular sinuses are absent. The most external portion of the lesion consists of dense, fibrocollagenous tissue. In some cases, infiltrating margins have been described.

Immunohistochemical studies have demonstrated the proliferating cells to be variably positive for muscle-specific actin and desmin and uniformly negative for smooth muscle–specific actin, myoglobin, vascular markers, and S-100 protein, suggesting myodifferentiation. Ultrastructural studies have not demonstrated features of muscle cells but have been interpreted as showing endothelial, histiocytic, fibroblastic, or myofibroblastic features in different cases and different studies.

Adverse prognostic features include incomplete resection, infiltrating margins, origin in the head and neck, and involvement of skeletal muscle. Other histologic features, including nuclear pleomorphism and mitotic rate, have no prognostic significance.

The differential diagnosis includes dermatofibroma, malignant fibrous histiocytoma, a primary vascular lesion, synovial sarcoma, or even a disorder of lymph nodes. Dermatofibroma may have abundant hemorrhagic areas (aneurysmal fibrous histiocytoma). However, the clinicopathologic setting is completely different and hemorrhage is found in the background of a storiform proliferation. Malignant fibrous histiocytoma possesses a greater degree of cytologic atypia. Immunohistochemical studies for vascular markers should distinguish angiomatoid fibrous histiocytoma from a primary vascular lesion, failing to demonstrate a lining of endothelial cells around the vascular spaces in angiomatoid fibrous histiocytoma. Synovial sarcoma should have at least some cells positive for keratin or epithelial membrane antigen. A disorder of lymph nodes should be ruled out on more than casual inspection of the lymphoid infiltrate; absence of a true lymph node capsule should be noted.

## Giant Cell Angiofibroma[143–145]

Giant cell angiofibroma is a rare neoplasm that usually presents as a soft tissue mass in the head and neck region of adults, most often occurring in the orbit. It has not yet been reported to metastasize, but the disease may persist or nondestructive local recurrences may appear.

At low magnification, giant cell angiofibroma is relatively well circumscribed and has a prominent network of small open blood vessels that occasionally show hyalinization. Between the blood vessels and pseudovessels is a patternless proliferation of round to plump spindled cells and multinucleated giant cells in a loose collagenous to myxoid matrix. The neoplastic cells may also line pseudovessels. The individual neoplastic cells have ill-defined cytoplasm and plump to round nuclei, often with irregular folding and pseudoinclusions. The neoplastic cells are positive for CD34 and are negative for S-100 protein and CD31.

The differential diagnosis includes solitary fibrous tumor and giant cell fibroblastoma, both of which are CD34+. Solitary fibrous tumor is more collagenous, lacks the open vascular pattern of giant cell angiofibroma, and has more bland and spindled proliferating cells. Giant cell fibroblastoma is more common in children, is more infiltrative, and lacks the prominent vascular pattern seen in giant cell angiofibroma.

## Giant Cell Fibroblastoma[146, 147]

Giant cell fibroblastoma is a rare soft tissue tumor that affects mostly children; there is a marked male predominance. Patients present with a painless, slowly growing mass centered in the subcutaneous tissue. There is a wide distribution, but the lesion most commonly occurs in the trunk or lower extremity. Local recurrence is due to incomplete resection in about 50% of cases. Rare cases have recurred as dermatofibrosarcoma. At gross evaluation, giant cell fibroblastoma is infiltrative, usually less than 5 cm in diameter, and firm or gelatinous on cut section.

At histologic examination, giant cell fibroblastoma is poorly circumscribed and has a variable low-magnification appearance, from collagenous to myxoid. The most characteristic feature is often the presence of ectatic pseudovascular spaces. The cells consist of spindle cells with varying degrees of hyperchromasia and giant cells with clustered or floret-like nuclei. Despite the presence of cytologic atypia, the mitotic rate is less than 1 mitosis per 10 high-power fields. Immunohistochemical studies show positivity for CD34 (similar to dermatofibrosarcoma) but negativity for S-100 protein, endothelial markers, and muscle markers. On ultrastructural study, the cells resemble fibroblasts. A t(17;22)(q22;q13) has been reported in giant cell fibroblastoma (similar to dermatofibrosarcoma).[148]

The differential diagnosis includes a variety of sarcomas as well as juvenile xanthogranuloma and giant cell angiofibroma. Giant cell angiofibroma is less infiltrative, occurs primarily in adults, and has a more prominent vascular pattern. Although the cells of giant cell fibroblastoma may have significant hyperchromasia, it generally lacks pleomorphism or significant mitotic activity and is more superficial than most sarcomas. Dermatofibrosarcoma may have a close relationship with giant cell fibroblastoma; both are CD34+, both share the same chromosome translocation, rare cases with features of both have been reported, and both neoplasms have been reported to recur as the other in rare cases.[149] Some have speculated that giant cell fibroblastoma represents a juvenile form of dermatofibrosarcoma.[146]

## Dermatofibrosarcoma[150, 151]

Dermatofibrosarcoma (dermatofibrosarcoma protuberans) occurs most often with a male predominance in young adults. Most patients present with a slow-growing plaque that progresses to a nodule. The deep dermis and subcutaneous tissue are affected, most frequently on the trunk and the proximal extremities, the groin, or the head and neck. The gross lesion is poorly circumscribed, averaging about 5 cm in diameter, and is gray-white on cut section. Even after wide local excision, recurrences are frequent, appearing in 20% to 50% of cases; metastases are fortunately rare, but they have been reported in 1% to 5% of cases.

At histologic examination, dermatofibrosarcoma usually demonstrates a monotonous storiform spindle cell proliferation involving the deep dermis and subcutaneous tissue. The overlying epidermis is often atrophic and not hyperplastic as seen in derma-

tofibroma. There is always a sparing Grenz zone between the neoplasm and the epidermis. The pattern of infiltration of the subcutaneous tissue is highly characteristic, with insinuation around single adipose cells and lobules of adipose tissue (Fig. 46–40). Stroma and vascularity are usually not prominent, but a myxoid pattern is occasionally a focal or prominent finding (myxoid variant of dermatofibrosarcoma).[152] The individual neoplastic cells usually have minimal pleomorphism and bland spindled nuclei. The mitotic rate is usually low, most often less than 1 mitosis per 10 high-power fields. Rarely, the cytoplasm is pigmented, a variant termed a Bednar tumor. In rare cases, there are areas resembling giant cell fibroblastoma or areas resembling a sarcoma, most often fibrosarcoma or malignant fibrous histiocytoma.[153] When there is a significant component of sarcoma, the prognosis is adversely affected.[154] Immunohistochemical studies demonstrate positivity for CD34 in about 90% of cases. Staining is negative for S-100 protein or muscle markers. Ultrastructural studies demonstrate cells resembling fibroblasts and other cells resembling histiocytes. Cytogenetic studies have reported a t(17;22)(q22;q13). Cases with fibrosarcomatous transformation have been associated with p53 overexpression or *TP53* mutation and may also have overexpression of Mdm-2 and p21[Waf1].[155]

The differential diagnosis of dermatofibrosarcoma includes neurofibroma, fibrous histiocytoma, nodular fasciitis, malignant fibrous histiocytoma, and fibrosarcoma. Neurofibroma generally lacks storiform areas and is S-100 protein positive. Fibrous histiocytoma usually shows more cellular polymorphism, fails to show spindle cell infiltration of individual adipose cells and lobules of adipose tissue, and is positive for factor XIIIa and negative for CD34. Nodular fasciitis generally shows a looser spindle cell proliferation with a higher mitotic rate, has a more polymorphic infiltrate, and is CD34−. Malignant fibrous histiocytoma shows a greater degree of cellular pleomorphism. Fibrosarcoma usually shows a more fascicular rather than storiform prolif-

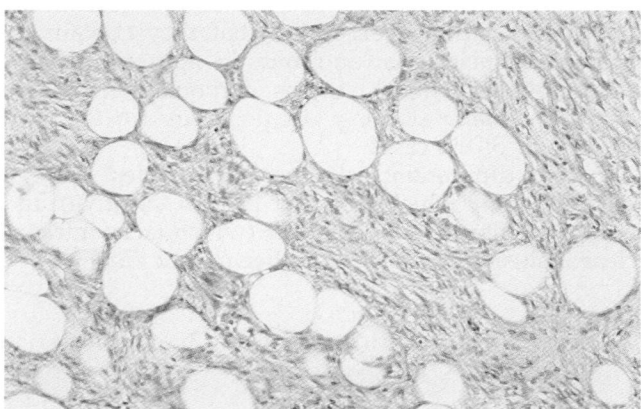

**FIGURE 46–40.** Dermatofibrosarcoma. The characteristic pattern of envelopment of subcutaneous adipose tissue is seen.

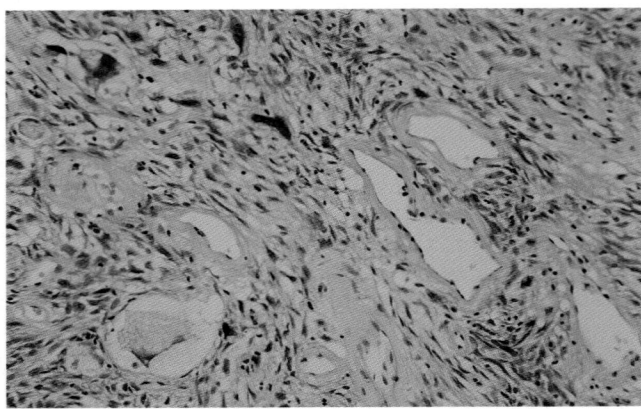

FIGURE 46–41. Pleomorphic hyalinizing angiectatic tumor of soft parts. There are hyalinized blood vessels, between which are pleomorphic tumor cells. The mitotic rate is low in this lesion.

eration, is more deeply seated, and usually has a higher mitotic rate.

## Pleomorphic Hyalinizing Angiectatic Tumor of Soft Parts[156]

This entity behaves like a low-grade sarcoma and has features of a fibrohistiocytic neoplasm with a distinctive vascular pattern. In the small number of cases reported to date, it has affected adults, both men and women. Patients present with a slowly enlarging mass in the subcutaneous tissue occurring mostly in the extremities, particularly the lower extremity. Follow-up in the small number of reported cases has demonstrated a high incidence of local recurrence, although no metastases have been reported. The gross lesions ranged from 2 to 8 cm and had a lobulated appearance.

The microscopic examination reveals clusters of thin-walled ectatic blood vessels scattered throughout the lesion (Fig. 46–41). These vessels are often surrounded by perivascular hyalinization composed of fibrin and collagen. The tumor cells consist of plump, spindled, and rounded pleomorphic cells usually resembling those of a malignant fibrous histiocytoma, with the exception that they contain intranuclear inclusions, and mitotic figures are rare. Immunohistochemical studies demonstrate absence of S-100 protein staining but positivity for CD34 in about half of the cases.

The differential diagnosis includes benign schwannoma (which is S-100 protein positive) and malignant fibrous histiocytoma (which lacks intranuclear inclusions and has a higher mitotic rate).

## Acral Myxoinflammatory Fibroblastic Sarcoma[157, 158]

Acral myxoinflammatory fibroblastic sarcoma, a low-grade sarcoma, is also known as inflammatory myxohyaline tumor of distal extremities with viro-

cyte or Reed-Sternberg–like cells. The neoplasm occurs in patients of all ages; there is no sex predilection. Patients present with a painless mass in the distal extremities, usually in the subcutaneous tissues. Recurrences have been common, and distal metastasis has been reported, although it is rare. The gross lesions are infiltrative, multinodular masses.

There is histologically a prominent myxoid matrix with numerous acute and chronic inflammatory cells (Fig. 46–42). Within the myxoid areas are scattered, large tumor cells with bizarre, vesicular nuclei and prominent nucleoli and abundant eosinophilic cytoplasm, resembling Reed-Sternberg cells. Mitotic activity is low. Ultrastructural study of the cells shows fibroblastic differentiation. Immunohistochemical studies demonstrate focal positivity for CD68 and CD34 in a subset of cases.

The differential diagnosis includes myxoid malignant fibrous histiocytoma (which usually has a higher mitotic rate), myxoid liposarcoma (which is rare in the distal extremities and lacks the bizarre atypical cells), an inflammatory disorder (which lacks the bizarre atypical cells), and even Hodgkin's disease (rare presenting in soft tissue and differentiated by immunohistochemical studies).

## Malignant Fibrous Histiocytoma[159–165]

As mentioned at the beginning of this section, the diagnosis of a tumor showing fibrohistiocytic differentiation is essentially one of exclusion, and this is certainly true of malignant fibrous histiocytoma. Malignant fibrous histiocytoma is no longer thought to show differentiation toward fibroblasts and true histiocytes but should be considered a diagnosis of exclusion; spindle cell sarcomas that show definite histologic, immunohistochemical, or ultrastructural features of specific cellular differentiation should be classified accordingly. Therefore, the incidence varies in different series, depending on how stringently one excludes other types of sarcomas. Nonetheless,

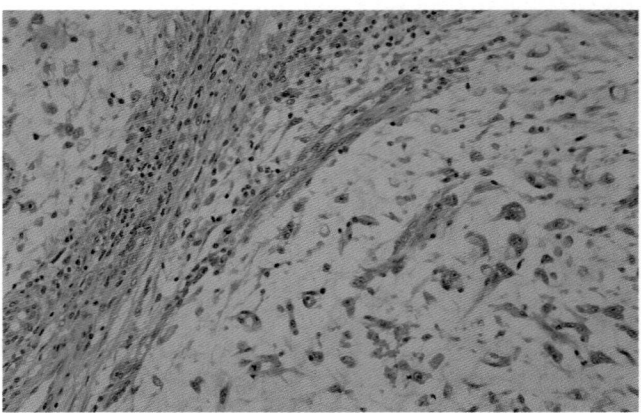

FIGURE 46–42. Acral myxoinflammatory fibroblastic sarcoma. Note the scattered cells with large nuclei and large prominent nucleoli in the myxoid foci.

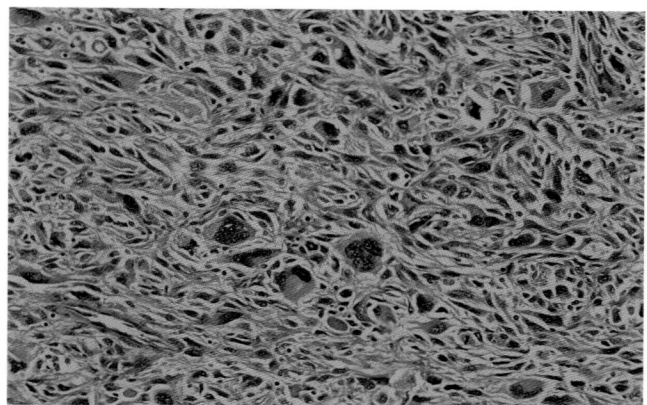

FIGURE 46–43. Malignant fibrous histiocytoma, storiform-pleomorphic type. The histologic appearance is that of a generic high-grade spindle cell sarcoma, without specific lineage-defining histologic or immunohistochemical features.

malignant fibrous histiocytoma is a common sarcoma, representing between 5% and 20% of adult sarcomas.

Malignant fibrous histiocytoma occurs in all age groups but is usually a neoplasm of late adulthood. There is a male preponderance of about 2:1, and whites are affected more than other racial groups. Patients present with a painless mass of months to years in duration. It is most often located on the extremities, particularly the thigh. The retroperitoneum is another common site of occurrence, particularly with the inflammatory variant. A small subset of cases, again of the inflammatory variant, are associated with systemic symptoms or increased white blood cell count. A minority of cases have been associated with previous radiation. The gross neoplasms are usually large, multinodular masses greater than 5 cm in diameter. On cut section, the tumors are usually gray but may have areas of hemorrhage or necrosis or appear xanthomatous. Malignant fibrous histiocytomas have a high recurrence rate of about 50% when they have been inadequately treated. There is also a high rate of metastasis, of about 30% to 40%. Metastases most commonly occur to the lung; regional lymph node metastasis is much less frequent.

Several variants have been recognized at histologic examination, including storiform-pleomorphic, myxoid, giant cell, and inflammatory types, but there may be overlap in individual cases. The storiform-pleomorphic type is most common, and it also represents the most classic type (Fig. 46–43). Although there is a wide variation from case to case as well as within a single case, the neoplasm usually consists, at least in part, of spindle cells with varying degrees of atypia arranged in a storiform pattern. The storiform areas often merge with areas of fascicle formation or areas of patternless growth. Vascularity is increased but is not a prominent feature. Areas of myxoid change may be found, but when this is a prominent feature, it is more characteristic of the myxoid variant (see later). The stroma

may also be densely collagenized in areas or may contain areas of metaplastic cartilage or bone; many (including me) believe that the diagnosis of extraosseous osteosarcoma is more appropriate when these features are present, especially when they represent a prominent finding. The proliferating cells vary widely, from bland to highly pleomorphic spindled cells to cells with a histiocytoid appearance to multinucleated giant cells, all with a wide range of cytologic atypia. The mitotic rate is often high and usually includes atypical forms. In addition, scattered inflammatory cells, including foamy macrophages, may be present.

In the myxoid variant of malignant fibrous histiocytoma, at least half the neoplasm shows prominent myxoid features (Fig. 46–44). The neoplasm can be myxoid throughout or, more commonly, contains other areas typical of the storiform-pleomorphic variant. These other areas usually blend between one another, but they may show an abrupt transition. The vascularity is usually more evident in the myxoid areas and shows curved arcs of thin capillaries and veins. Cytologic atypia varies in the myxoid variant, from cases with uniformly bland cells (which some term myxofibrosarcoma) to highly pleomorphic variants with cytologic atypia similar to the storiform-pleomorphic variant. The giant cell variant of malignant fibrous histiocytoma consists of a multinodular proliferation of histiocytes and fibroblasts, with numerous giant cells dispersed throughout the tumor. Although the histiocytes and fibroblasts may have widely varying degrees of atypia, the multinucleated giant cells have nuclei resembling benign osteoclasts. Metaplastic cartilage and bone are found in about 50% of cases, features that some regard as indicative of extraosseous osteosarcoma. The inflammatory variant of malignant fibrous histiocytoma contains numerous acute and chronic inflammatory cells (Fig. 46–45). Neutrophils, eosinophils, benign histiocytes, and foamy macrophages may dominate; the neoplastic spindle and histiocytoid cells, which are invariably present, may be difficult to discern.

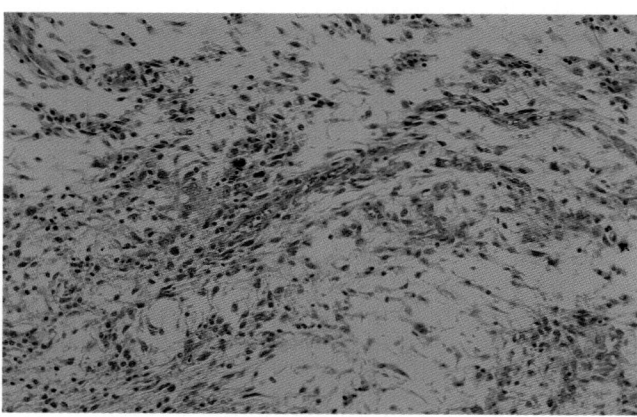

FIGURE 46–44. Malignant fibrous histiocytoma, myxoid type. Pleomorphic fibrohistiocytic cells are present in a myxoid background. Note the curved blood vessels, in contrast to the chicken wire vessels of myxoid liposarcoma.

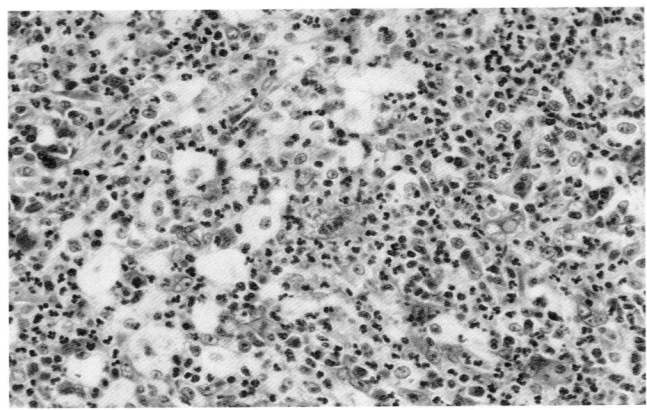

**FIGURE 46–45.** Malignant fibrous histiocytoma, inflammatory type. There is a prominent infiltrate of acute and chronic inflammatory cells, which almost obscures the neoplastic population.

Immunohistochemical studies, by definition, lack definitive evidence of differentiation toward specific cell types. Therefore, reactivity to stains for S-100 protein, endothelial markers, and definitive muscle markers is absent. Staining for muscle-specific actin may occur and may reflect myofibroblastic differentiation, and focal, particularly weak staining for keratin or desmin does not rule out the diagnosis. Although there may be staining for the lysosome marker CD68, malignant fibrous histiocytomas lack staining for CD45 (leukocyte common antigen) and other specific histiocyte-hematopoietic markers. Ultrastructural studies demonstrate features suggestive of fibroblastic or histiocytic differentiation.

The major prognostic factors include tumor size, depth of the lesion (superficial tumors do well), and histologic grade (nuclear pleomorphism and mitoses). In addition, vascular invasion, tumor necrosis, and aneuploidy adversely affect the patient's outcome. Myxoid variants of malignant fibrous histiocytoma tend to have a recurrence rate higher than that of other types; the giant cell variant may have the highest metastatic rate.

The differential diagnosis of malignant fibrous histiocytoma is enormous and includes benign and malignant neoplasms of numerous lineages, from mesenchymal to hematopoietic tumor. Clinically, it is most important to distinguish malignant fibrous histiocytoma from benign tumors and malignant neoplasms of nonmesenchymal lineage. Malignant fibrous histiocytoma is distinguished from atypical fibroxanthoma solely by location; if the lesion is centered in the dermis, it is an atypical fibroxanthoma, whereas if it is centered more deeply, it is a malignant fibrous histiocytoma. Malignant fibrous histiocytoma has a greater degree of atypia and a greater number of mitoses than does benign fibrous histiocytoma and, with the exception of the rare deep fibrous histiocytoma, is situated more deeply. The inflammatory type of malignant fibrous histiocytoma may be confused with xanthogranulomatous inflammation, but careful cytologic examination always

demonstrates highly atypical cells in malignant fibrous histiocytoma.

Malignant fibrous histiocytoma, particularly the inflammatory type, may be confused with hematopoietic neoplasms, including Hodgkin's disease and anaplastic large cell lymphoma. Inflammatory malignant fibrous histiocytoma should have at least some highly atypical cells showing definite spindled features; if there is any doubt, stains for leukocyte antigens should easily resolve the dilemma. Stains for keratin and S-100 protein may be of use if metastatic carcinoma and malignant melanoma are being considered; keratin staining, if present in malignant fibrous histiocytoma, should be weak and focal, in contrast to the strong, diffuse keratin staining seen in the large majority of cases of carcinoma.

It is less crucial but still worthwhile to distinguish malignant fibrous histiocytoma from other spindle cell sarcomas, particularly pleomorphic sarcomas of other types. Pleomorphic liposarcoma usually lacks a well-developed storiform architecture and should, by definition, contain at least some diagnostic lipoblasts. Pleomorphic myosarcomas should have more than weak, focal staining for desmin and other muscle markers. Some sarcomas of specific types may have large areas resembling malignant fibrous histiocytoma; rather than being considered composite tumors, these neoplasms should be classified by the specific type present.

The myxoid variant of malignant fibrous histiocytoma is most commonly confused with myxoid liposarcoma. Myxoid liposarcoma usually has a richer vasculature, more chicken wire in appearance, whereas the vessels of myxoid malignant fibrous histiocytoma are usually more irregular in spacing and arcing rather than chicken wire. Myxoid liposarcoma may contain round cell lipoblasts, whereas myxoid malignant fibrous histiocytoma usually contains at least some more pleomorphic cells. Myxomas are usually less vascular, are less cellular, and lack any degree of cytologic atypia. Nodular fasciitis usually has a more tissue culture appearance, and although it may have a high mitotic rate, it lacks atypical mitotic figures.

## TUMORS AND TUMORLIKE PROLIFERATIONS SHOWING VASCULAR (INCLUDING LYMPHATIC AND PERIVASCULAR) DIFFERENTIATION

### Papillary Endothelial Hyperplasia[166–168]

Papillary endothelial hyperplasia (vegetant intravascular hemangioendothelioma, Masson's lesion) is a pseudomalignant reactive process that probably represents an organizing thrombus. It occurs in all age groups, without sex predilection, and generally presents as a small mass; there is usually no history of trauma, but it may occur in a preexisting vascular lesion. It usually occurs in the head and neck or digits, in the skin, subcutaneous tissue, or deep soft tissue. The gross lesion consists of a multicystic mass containing blood and clot; a preexisting vessel may be evident at the periphery. If it is not detected by gross examination, a blood vessel wall, usually a vein, is often found at the periphery of the lesion at microscopic examination. The center of the lesion features papillae of bland endothelial cells surrounding fibrin (Fig. 46–46). The endothelial cells may be plump and mitotically active, but they are never pleomorphic and lack atypical mitotic figures. The papillary formations may simulate angiosarcoma, but intravascular location and the lack of cytologic atypia should establish the correct diagnosis.

## Capillary Hemangioma[169]

Capillary hemangioma is the most common type of vascular neoplasm and, after lipoma, probably the most common soft tissue neoplasm. There is a female predominance. The lesions usually present in the first decade of life and are often present at birth. The elevated, red lesion deepens to purple as it somewhat regresses over time. Multiple lesions may occur. In the soft tissue, the head and neck predominate, but the trunk and extremities are also commonly affected. At gross evaluation, a spongy appearance is noted.

The typical capillary hemangioma is composed of well-formed small vascular spaces lined by benign-appearing endothelial cells. Capillary hemangiomas vary in cellularity, including highly cellular lesions that typically occur in infants (infantile hemangioendothelioma, strawberry nevus, or juvenile hemangioma, hypertrophic angioma, nevus vasculosus). The most cellular lesions may show a high mitotic rate, although atypical mitoses are not seen. Lesions showing clinical signs of regression are often associated with thrombosis, calcification, fibrosis,

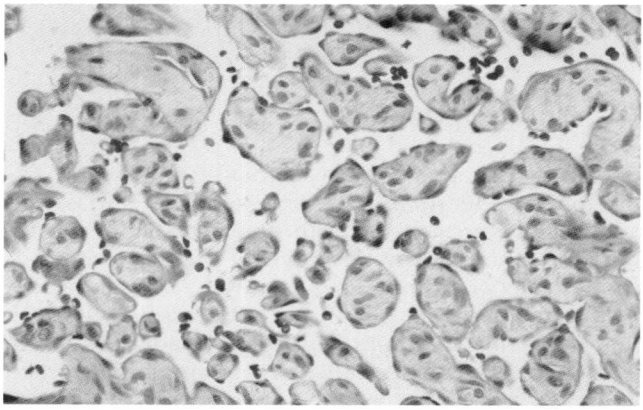

**FIGURE 46–46.** Papillary endothelial hyperplasia. Bland endothelial cells line and infiltrate pseudopapillae composed of fibrin.

or even fatty metaplasia. A distinct lobular appearance is often noted in capillary hemangioma, in which each lobule is organized around a larger vessel. Lobular capillary hemangioma (pyogenic granuloma) represents a highly lobular variant that occurs subjacent to skin and mucous membranes, often showing superficial ulceration. More rarely, it may occur in a subcutaneous or intravenous location. Lesions in the gingivae of pregnant women have been referred to as granuloma gravidarum. Special studies are not usually necessary for diagnosis of capillary hemangioma. Immunohistochemical studies show that the lining endothelial cells express CD34, CD31, factor VIII–related protein, and other vascular markers; interstitial cells may also show this staining pattern. Collagen IV stains often delineate clusters of cells, even in areas in which clear-cut vessels are not seen histologically. Electron microscopy shows evidence of endothelial differentiation in the lining cells, including Weibel-Palade bodies, sitting on a basal lamina surrounded by pericytes. These studies are most helpful in the histologically more mature-appearing areas.

Highly cellular capillary hemangiomas may be confused with malignant tumors, particularly if a high mitotic rate is seen. The most cellular lesions tend to occur in the youngest individuals, in whom a malignant vascular neoplasm would be most unusual. Reticulin or collagen IV stains demonstrate the well-formed vascular channels, and mitoses, if abundant, are never atypical.

## Cavernous Hemangioma[169]

Cavernous hemangiomas are less frequent than capillary hemangiomas and occur in a slightly older age group, with a peak in the second decade; there is no sex predominance. Occasional lesions occur as a part of clinical syndromes, including Maffucci's syndrome and blue rubber bleb nevus syndrome. Large cavernous hemangiomas may be associated with a coagulopathy (Kasabach-Merritt syndrome). Cavernous hemangiomas are usually larger, less circumscribed, and more deeply seated than capillary hemangiomas. They usually do not undergo regression over time. They occur in the extremities, trunk, and head and neck region. Gross lesions are usually spongy and may show calcification. If not completely resected, they may recur.

Cavernous hemangiomas consist histologically of large blood-filled spaces lined by flat, bland endothelial cells, often with an incomplete adventitial rimming. Areas resembling capillary hemangioma and areas transitional between capillary and cavernous hemangioma may also be present. Foci of regression, such as thrombosis, calcification, fibrosis, or fatty metaplasia, are often seen. Special studies demonstrate clear-cut evidence of vascular differentiation, although these studies are seldom required. There is usually no problem in differential diagnosis.

## Intramuscular Hemangioma[170, 171]

Intramuscular hemangioma (skeletal muscle hemangioma, infiltrating hemangioma, infiltrating angiolipoma) is a benign hemangioma involving skeletal muscle. It occurs in children and adults, with a predilection for young adults; there is an equal sex distribution. Patients present with a slowly enlarging, often painful soft tissue mass, with little indication of its vascular nature. Radiologic studies may be helpful, although atypical patterns are common. Intramuscular hemangioma occurs in the limbs, trunk, and head and neck area; the thigh represents the single most common site. Although the lesion does not metastasize, recurrence may commonly follow incomplete resections. The gross lesions appear circumscribed but not encapsulated and vary from pink and spongy to yellow-tan and firm, sometimes with calcification.

At histologic examination, there is infiltration of skeletal muscle by a bland vascular proliferation (Fig. 46–47). The lesions vary from the appearance of capillary hemangioma to cavernous hemangioma; most show mixed patterns. Pure capillary patterns are more common in head and neck tumors. Most lesions show signs of regression, including thrombosis, calcification, fibrosis, fatty metaplasia, and lymphocytic infiltrate. Immunohistochemical and ultrastructural studies show clear-cut evidence of vascular differentiation.

Differential diagnosis is usually not a problem, but pure capillary patterns may occasionally have areas in which the cellularity may suggest a malignant tumor. However, most cases have other areas showing more obvious vascular differentiation; angiosarcoma of the skeletal muscle is rare. Cases with fatty metaplasia may mimic liposarcoma, but assessment of the entire lesion usually obviates that problem. The overall clinical findings separate intramuscular hemangioma from angiomatosis (see later).

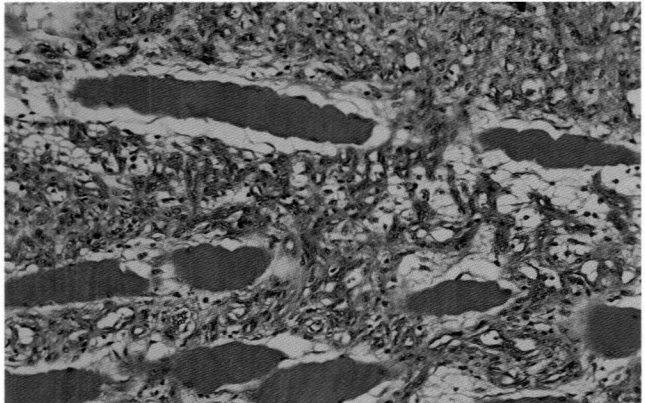

**FIGURE 46–47.** Intramuscular hemangioma. This lesion has the appearance of a capillary hemangioma.

## Synovial Hemangioma[172]

Synovial hemangioma is a rare variant of hemangioma that occurs in children or young adults, with a male predilection. Patients present with a long history of a painful, swollen joint. The knee is most commonly affected, followed by the elbow. The lesions generally do not recur after simple excision. Most lesions have the histologic appearance of cavernous hemangiomas, and the overlying synovium usually shows a villous hyperplasia.

## Angiomatosis[173, 174]

Angiomatosis (diffuse hemangioma, hemangiomatosis, infiltrating angiolipoma) is a hamartoma of blood vessels that is usually present in infancy and childhood. It occurs in a number of clinicopathologic syndromes—angiomatosis of soft tissue, skeletal-extraskeletal angiomatosis, diffuse neonatal hemangiomatosis, benign neonatal hemangiomatosis, and proliferative cutaneous angiomatosis. In the most common type, angiomatosis of soft tissue, patients usually present in childhood with diffuse persistent swelling sometimes associated with pain and discoloration. Two patterns of involvement are seen. In the more common pattern, there is extensive vertical involvement of multiple tissue planes; in the second, there is extensive involvement of tissue of the same type. Treatment is usually conservative, given the usually extensive nature of the process and the high rates of recurrence.

At histologic examination, most cases show a mixture of different types of vessels, including capillaries, veins (often with irregularly thick walls), and cavernous spaces, often with small vessels clustering adjacent to larger vessels. Some cases show a more uniform proliferation of capillaries. In either type, there is often a prominent component of adipose tissue.

The differential diagnosis is limited. Clinical features separate hemangiomatosis from intramuscular hemangioma. The presence of abundant adipose tissue raises consideration of a fatty tumor, which should be eliminated on examination of the whole lesion.

## Benign Lymphangioma[175, 176]

Benign lymphangioma may actually represent a hamartoma rather than a benign neoplasm. It is rare and usually presents at birth or somewhat less commonly within the first few years of life; there is a slight male predominance. A variety of syndromes, including Turner's syndrome, are associated with the occurrence of lymphangiomas. In addition, there is a rare syndrome called lymphangiomatosis in which lymphomas occur in a multifocal fashion, with widely different extents of disease varying from multiple bone lesions to soft tissue involvement to involvement of most parenchymal organs. Most patients with solitary lymphangioma present with a mass, although infection sometimes brings the lesion to medical attention. Lymphangiomas are most often located in the sites of the richest lymphatic drainage, such as the head and neck, the axilla, the abdominal cavity, and the skin (lymphangioma circumscriptum). When these lesions have the gross appearance of large cystic cavities, usually in loose areas such as the lower neck and axilla, cystic hygroma has often been the term applied. Although lymphangiomas do not recur in the usual sense, they are often difficult to completely resect without significant morbidity.

Histologic examination shows cysts and dilated thin-walled channels filled with proteinaceous fluid and lymphocytes (Fig. 46–48). The lining is that of thin endothelial cells, and smooth muscle or lymphoid aggregates are also sometimes present within the wall. On occasion, there is extravasation of blood in the spaces, and a long-standing lesion may contain significant areas of fibrosis. In lymphangiomatosis, extensive dissection of collagen may be seen. Immunohistochemical studies demonstrate the staining pattern of normal endothelial cells of lymphomas, with positivity for CD31 and factor VIII–associated protein and focal staining for CD34.

The differential diagnosis includes cavernous hemangioma, particularly when there are abundant intraluminal red blood cells. The distinction may be difficult, but the clinicopathologic setting or the identification of lymphoid follicles in the wall may help. Intra-abdominal lymphangiomas may be confused with benign cystic mesothelioma, but keratin stains should easily resolve this problem. Rare cases may be confused with angiosarcoma because of the presence of anastomosing vascular channels dissecting between collagen bundles, but there is a complete absence of cytologic atypia, and the clinicopathologic setting should again be useful. Cutaneous lesions may easily be confused with lymphangiectasis, an acquired lesion that results after long-standing lymphedema; the clinical history should suggest the correct diagnosis.

## Lymphangiomyomatosis[54]

This rare lesion is probably related to the tuberous sclerosis complex. It occurs only in female patients, usually of reproductive age, who generally present with dyspnea. The thoracic duct and mediastinal lymph nodes are most often involved, but involvement of lung and retroperitoneal lymph nodes may also occur. Patients with localized lesions may do well, but those with lung involvement generally do poorly; hormonal therapy has been tried with success in some cases. At gross evaluation, pink spongy masses are found along the sites of involvement; a chylous effusion is often present.

The microscopic lesions consist of lymphatic channels surrounded by bundles and short fascicles of smooth muscle cells, often arranged in a perithelial pattern around the lymphatics (Fig. 46–49). Immunohistochemical analysis reveals that the smooth muscle cells, in addition to possessing markers of smooth muscle differentiation, are positive for HMB-45, the melanosome-associated marker also found in the smooth muscle cells of angiomyolipoma. Ultrastructural studies demonstrate lamellated granules that may be related to premelanosomes.

The differential diagnosis of lymphangiomyomatosis includes metastatic leiomyosarcoma and benign metastasizing leiomyoma, but neither of these lesions contains a component of lymphangiomatous channels.

## Glomus Tumor[177, 178]

The glomus tumor is a rare tumor in which the proliferating cell has a striking resemblance to the

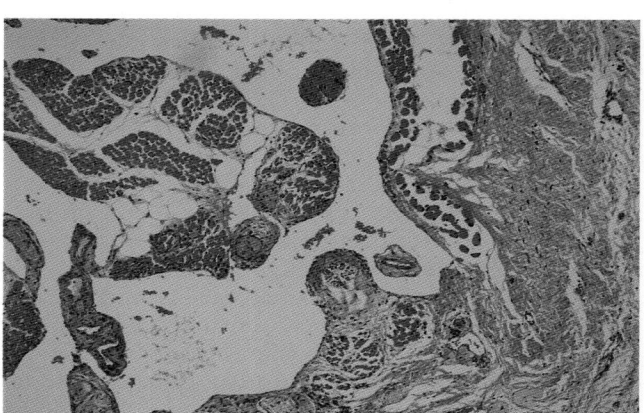

**FIGURE 46–48.** Lymphangioma. This intramuscular example shows the cavernous system with a few extravasated red blood cells lined by bland endothelial cells.

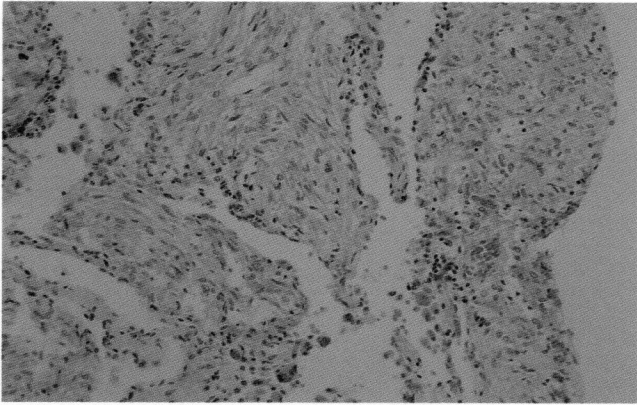

**FIGURE 46–49.** Lymphangiomyomatosis. Note the presence of smooth muscle cells in the wall of the endothelial-lined lymphatics.

cells of the normal glomus body involved in thermal regulation. It usually occurs in young adults; there is an equal sex distribution except for digital lesions, which have a 3:1 female predominance. A minority of cases occur in children, in which about 10% of cases are congenital, with an autosomal dominant pattern of inheritance. In adults, glomus tumors usually present as solitary, often highly painful blue-red nodules. The most common sites of occurrence are the subungual region of the fingers and other sites on the extremities. In children, a subungual presentation is unusual; the lesions are multiple in about 25% of cases. The lesions seldom recur after simple excision. The gross lesions usually measure less than 1 cm.

Most glomus tumors are histologically well circumscribed, although rare cases, most often occurring in childhood, may show infiltration of surrounding soft tissue. They are composed of varying proportions of glomus cells, vascular channels, and smooth muscle. Most tumors consist wholly or mostly of glomus cells (Fig. 46–50). Glomus cells are uniform round cells, usually with a round bland nucleus and pale cytoplasm. Rarely, the glomus cells may show cytologic atypia or oxyphilic cytoplasmic change. When vascular channels are prominent, it may be termed glomangioma, and when vascular channels and smooth muscle are prominent, it may be termed glomangiomyoma. The blood vessels resemble those of cavernous hemangiomas, and the glomus cells may be present in an attenuated lining or in perithelial clusters. Rarely, otherwise typical examples of glomus tumors may be associated with foci of sarcoma; these cases have been called glomangiosarcoma, although no case has yet been associated with metastasis. Even more rarely, malignant examples of glomus tumor have been reported; some of these have been associated with metastasis. Immunohistochemical studies demonstrate the glomus cells to be positive for muscle-specific actin and smooth muscle–specific actin; collagen IV stains usually show envelopment of single glomus cells.[179, 180] Interestingly, many cases have been re-

ported to be only focally positive or negative for desmin. Ultrastructural studies demonstrate features of smooth muscle cells.

The differential diagnosis of glomus tumor includes a skin adnexal tumor and nevus, distinguished by reactivity for keratin and S-100 protein expression, respectively. Glomangiomas may be mistaken for simple cavernous hemangiomas if a lining of glomus cells is not specifically sought.

## Hemangiopericytoma[179–184]

Hemangiopericytoma is a controversial neoplasm that shows differentiation toward the pericytes of blood vessels. Many cases previously regarded as hemangiopericytoma have been shown to actually represent examples of other neoplasms. Nonetheless, there are still cases in which a diagnosis of hemangiopericytoma is appropriate. Most cases occur in adults; there is no striking sex predominance. The most common sites of occurrence are soft tissue, nasal cavity and environs, meninges, and bone. In the soft tissues, it most often occurs in the lower extremity, pelvis, retroperitoneum, and orbit. Most patients with soft tissue hemangiopericytoma present with a slowly enlarging, painless mass. Hypoglycemia has been reported in rare cases. The gross neoplasm is well circumscribed, averaging between 5 and 10 cm, and has the cut section appearance of a typical sarcoma.

Infantile (congenital) hemangiopericytoma is a special clinicopathologic variant of hemangiopericytoma that occurs at birth or within the first year of life; it is thought to be closely related or identical to cellular forms of infantile myofibromatosis.[100] It typically presents as a rapidly growing mass (or multiple masses) in the subcutaneous tissues of the head and neck or extremities; it has a male predilection. Despite the alarming clinical presentation, most cases follow a benign clinical course, and spontaneous regression has been reported in some cases.

Hemangiopericytomas are histologically well circumscribed. The most distinctive appearance is the vascular pattern, composed of a monotonous network of endothelium-lined blood vessels forming a branching, staghorn pattern (Fig. 46–51). The vessels may vary from capillary-like to sinusoid-like in size, but the branching pattern is consistent throughout the tumor. The proliferating cells outside of the endothelial cells are more variable and range from thin spindled cells to plump spindled cells to rounded cells with epithelioid features. The proliferating cells generally form clusters to small sheets and do not show long fascicles. Areas of myxoid degeneration are not uncommon. The proliferating cells generally have uniform cytologic features, although some pleomorphism can be present. The mitotic rate is variable. Immunohistochemical studies demonstrate positivity for CD34. Staining is negative for the vascular markers CD31 and factor VIII–related antigen; the muscle markers desmin, muscle-specific actin,

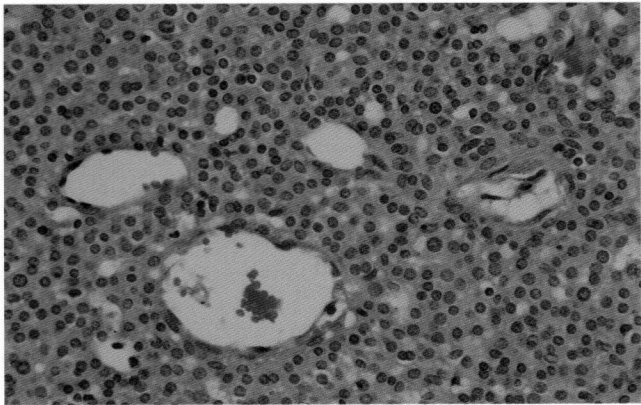

**FIGURE 46–50.** Glomus tumor. The glomus cells are composed of rounded cells with uniform round nuclei.

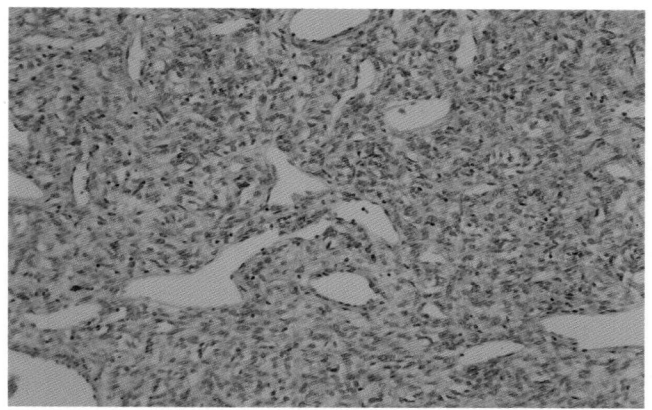

FIGURE 46–51. Hemangiopericytoma. There are ectatic branching blood vessels, and the intervening cells are ovoid to spindled.

and smooth muscle–specific actin; the epithelial markers keratin and epithelial membrane antigen; and S-100 protein. Collagen IV stains demonstrate positivity around single cells. Ultrastructural studies show evidence of pericytic differentiation; cells with numerous elongated cytoplasmic projections, numerous pinocytotic vesicles, and small bundles of myofilaments are separated from endothelial cells and from each other by basal lamina.

Infantile hemangiopericytoma generally resembles its adult counterpart but has several distinguishing features. The infantile neoplasm is often multinodular rather than well circumscribed and has intravascular and perivascular satellite nodules away from the main mass. The vascular pattern often shows a more irregular distribution than the repetitive staghorn pattern of adult tumors, and a fascicular pattern to the spindled cells can sometimes be seen. In addition, areas resembling infantile myofibromatosis or congenital fibrosarcoma may be seen, both neoplasms that overlap infantile hemangiopericytoma on clinical grounds as well.

The differential diagnosis of adult hemangiopericytoma from other neoplasms can be extremely difficult because many other neoplasms may show hemangiopericytomatous differentiation as a major component. These particularly include but are not limited to synovial sarcoma, mesenchymal chondrosarcoma, fibrous histiocytoma, and solitary fibrous tumor. Synovial sarcoma can be distinguished by the presence of epithelial membrane antigen or keratin positivity, even in monophasic examples. Mesenchymal chondrosarcoma should show at least some areas containing well-differentiated cartilage. Fibrous histiocytoma generally shows at least some areas besides the hemangiopericytomatous component, usually the more common storiform pattern, and is not CD43[+]. Solitary fibrous tumor may show great histologic similarities with benign forms of hemangiopericytoma; in addition, it shares the same immunohistochemical profile of CD34 positivity. Many pathologists have speculated that many cases previously reported as benign hemangiopericytoma are

in fact more accurately considered cases of solitary fibrous tumor.

The distinction of benign from malignant hemangiopericytoma is extremely difficult; some have advocated creating an intermediate or borderline category to handle equivocal cases. Increased numbers of mitoses, increased cellularity, and necrosis should raise concern for a malignant tumor. In general, 4 mitoses or more per 10 high-power fields indicate a malignant hemangiopericytoma. Proliferating cell nuclear antigen staining has also been reported to be of use in distinguishing benign from malignant neoplasms.[185]

## Spindle Cell Hemangioendothelioma[186–191]

Spindle cell hemangioendothelioma affects all age groups, although young adults are most commonly affected; there is no sex predilection. The extremities, most often the hands and feet, are most commonly involved. Patients usually present with a painless nodule in the superficial soft tissue. The clinical behavior is that of multiple recurrences after simple excision, and transformation to angiosarcoma has been reported. The gross spindle cell hemangioendothelioma is usually a hemorrhagic nodule that is small and spongy on cut section.

Spindle cell hemangioendothelioma is characterized histologically by a biphasic pattern, with cavernous endothelium-lined blood vessels and cellular areas. The cavernous blood vessels contain blood or thrombi. The cellular areas consist of uniform spindled to occasionally epithelioid cells forming slitlike vascular spaces with extravasated red blood cells (Fig. 46–52). The proliferating cells usually have bland nuclei with few or no mitoses. Immunohistochemical and ultrastructural studies show features of vascular differentiation. The histologic features of spindle cell hemangioendothelioma usually raise consideration of Kaposi's sarcoma. However, Kaposi's sarcoma usually occurs in patients affected

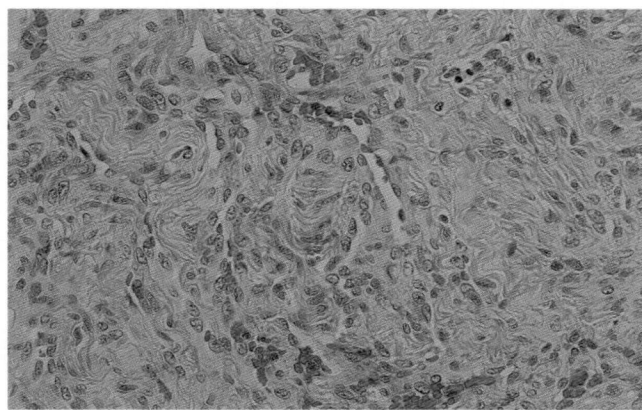

FIGURE 46–52. Spindle cell hemangioendothelioma. There are slitlike vessels, with spindled to epithelioid intervening cells.

with human immunodeficiency virus or in older adults. In addition, the cavernous spaces of spindle cell hemangioendothelioma are not present in Kaposi's sarcoma; the cytologic atypia, higher mitotic rate, and hyaline globules of Kaposi's sarcoma are not present in spindle cell hemangioendothelioma.

## Low-Grade Epithelioid Angiosarcoma (Epithelioid Hemangioendothelioma)[191–193]

Low-grade epithelioid angiosarcoma (epithelioid hemangioendothelioma, histiocytoid hemangioma) is a low-grade angiosarcoma that occurs uncommonly in the soft tissues, being more common in the lung (formerly known as intravascular bronchioloalveolar tumor), the bone, and the liver. In soft tissues, it occurs in all ages, but primarily in adults; there is a slight predilection for males. Clinically, it presents as a single, painful mass. All soft tissues may be involved; the lower extremity and head and neck are most commonly affected. The tumor usually arises in the subcutaneous tissue or skeletal muscle. Patients with low-grade epithelioid angiosarcoma of the soft tissues undergo recurrence in about 15% of cases and metastasis in about 30% of cases; even with metastasis, which most often involves regional lymph nodes, the patients usually do well. Gross evaluation shows that the tumors usually arise in association with a large vessel, commonly a vein, and are often gray or white-red.

Low-grade epithelioid angiosarcoma is composed histologically of relatively large, epithelioid to fusiform cells (Fig. 46–53). At low magnification, those cases arising from a vein tend to expand the vessel, maintaining its overall architecture. The individual cells tend to be distinct from one another or may form small vascular channels. Cytoplasm is usually abundant and eosinophilic, and there is occasional lumen formation, recapitulating vascular

differentiation. The tumor nuclei are usually bland, and the mitotic rate varies from none to brisk. Increased numbers of mitoses and areas of necrosis have been associated with increased clinical aggressiveness. Immunohistochemical studies demonstrate positivity for CD31, CD34, and factor VIII–related antigen, consistent with vascular differentiation. Collagen IV stains also help in demonstrating basal lamina that often encloses small clusters of cells. Staining for keratin is generally negative (but has been reported in similar neoplasms arising in different sites). Ultrastructural examination shows features of endothelial cells, including basal lamina, pinocytotic vesicles, junctional cell attachments, and occasionally Weibel-Palade bodies, along with abundant cytoplasmic intermediate filaments.

The differential diagnosis includes benign and more malignant vascular tumors as well as other malignant neoplasms. Epithelioid hemangioma has a more well developed vascular component, with well-formed blood vessels, and usually has a prominent inflammatory component that often includes eosinophils. Epithelioid examples of high-grade angiosarcomas have a greater degree of nuclear atypia and may contain areas of more conventional angiosarcoma. Epithelioid sarcoma and metastatic carcinoma are both keratin positive, lack positivity for vascular markers, and usually have a greater component of necrosis. Extraskeletal myxoid chondrosarcoma is usually larger and more myxoid, lacks vascular markers, and is usually positive for S-100 protein.

## Conventional Angiosarcoma[194, 195]

Conventional angiosarcoma is a relatively rare neoplasm. It most commonly occurs in skin, particularly in the scalp and forehead or in areas affected by chronic lymphedema. Outside of the skin, angiosarcoma most commonly occurs in the soft tissue, breast, liver, bone, spleen, and heart. Occasional cases occur as a long-term complication of radiation therapy or long-term lymphedema (Stewart-Treves syndrome); rare cases have been associated with foreign bodies.[12, 196, 197] When angiosarcoma occurs in the soft tissues, it occurs in all age groups with a 2:1 male predominance. The extremities are the most common site of occurrence, although the trunk and head and neck are not uncommon primary sites. Patients usually present with a mass that at gross examination shows prominent hemorrhage and necrosis. Conventional angiosarcoma is a high-grade neoplasm with a high rate of recurrence and metastasis.

At histologic examination, angiosarcoma typically shows anastomosing vascular channels lined by atypical endothelial cells (Fig. 46–54). The vascular channels do not respect normal architecture but tend to spread through normal structures, dissecting between individual collagen bundles and infiltrating through adipose tissue. The atypical endothelial cells

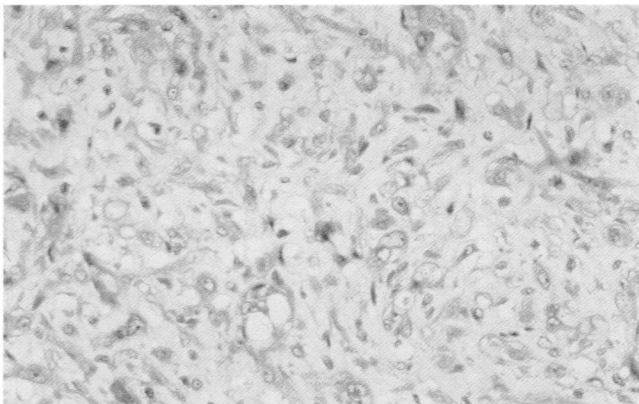

**FIGURE 46–53.** Low-grade epithelioid angiosarcoma (epithelioid hemangioendothelioma). The proliferating cells are ovoid to epithelioid; many contain intracellular lumina that represent abortive vascular channels.

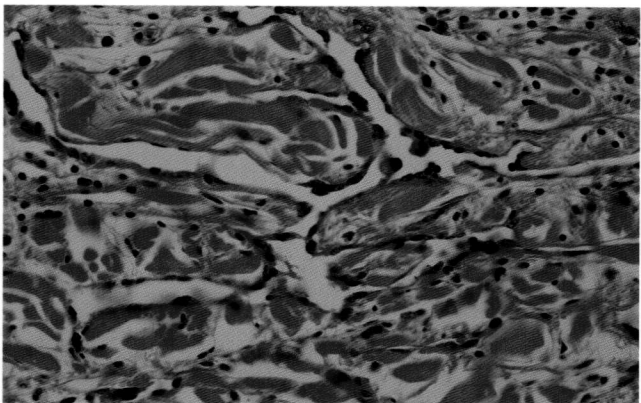

**FIGURE 46–54.** Angiosarcoma. Irregular vascular channels are lined by atypical endothelial cells.

vary from showing only slight differences from normal endothelial cells to highly pleomorphic cells with abundant mitoses. They may form a single lining along the vascular channels, but more often they pile up, forming micropapillary structures. In occasional cases, particularly in angiosarcoma occurring in the soft tissues, the endothelial cells may form sheets of cells having highly epithelioid features, with rounded, abundant eosinophilic cytoplasm, a variant referred to as epithelioid angiosarcoma.[198] Occasional epithelioid cells may have cytoplasmic vacuoles, which are rudimentary vascular channels, or may line channels, mimicking adenocarcinoma (Fig. 46–55). Ultrastructural studies of angiosarcoma demonstrate features of endothelial differentiation, including basal lamina, pinocytotic vesicles, desmosome-like junctions, and, in many cases, Weibel-Palade bodies. Epithelioid cases often have prominent aggregates of intermediate filaments. Immunohistochemical studies of angiosarcoma, including the epithelioid variant, demonstrate positivity for CD34, CD31, factor VIII–related antigen, and other vascular markers. Some cases of the epithelioid variant

have been keratin positive.[199] The collagen IV stain may be useful in demonstrating poorly formed vascular channels by outline of a basal lamina around these structures. Studies have demonstrated overexpression of Mdm-2, *TP53* gene mutation, and high vascular endothelial growth factor expression in a majority of cases.[200]

The differential diagnosis includes benign and low-grade vascular tumors in addition to other types of malignant neoplasms. Although some conventional angiosarcomas may have low-grade cytologic features, they usually exhibit abnormal infiltrating patterns through collagen and adipose tissue. However, even when the cytology is extremely low grade, there is usually at least some discernible cytologic atypia or piling up of cells along the vascular lumen. The epithelioid variant of angiosarcoma may easily be confused with other types of malignant neoplasms, including carcinoma, malignant melanoma, and other epithelioid sarcomas. Immunohistochemical demonstration of vascular markers such as CD34, CD31, and factor VIII–related antigen is of great use; some cases of epithelioid angiosarcoma may be keratin positive.

No histologic features correlate with clinical behavior. Conventional angiosarcoma, including the epithelioid variant, behaves like a uniformly high-grade neoplasm.

## TUMORS AND TUMORLIKE PROLIFERATIONS WITH DIFFERENTIATION TOWARD SMOOTH MUSCLE

### Benign Leiomyoma[201]

Benign leiomyomas occur in several clinicopathologic forms, including pilar leiomyoma, genital leiomyoma, and leiomyoma of deep soft tissue. Pilar leiomyomas arise from the arrector pili muscle of hair apparatuses and present as solitary or multiple painful papules to nodules that usually occur on the extremities or the trunk. Genital leiomyomas may be more common than pilar leiomyomas; they are more often single, painless nodules and usually involve the nipple, scrotum, or labium. Leiomyomas of the deep soft tissues usually occur in adults; there is no sex predilection. They usually present as an asymptomatic mass and occur most frequently in the extremities, the trunk, the abdominal cavity, and the retroperitoneum. At gross evaluation, they are well-circumscribed lesions, gray-white on cut section, and often show calcification. When properly diagnosed, they do not recur or metastasize after excision.

Benign leiomyomas of the soft tissues usually show obvious histologic features of smooth muscle differentiation, with fascicles of spindle cells with oblong, bland nuclei and no mitotic activity. The neoplasms commonly show degenerative features, including hyalinization, myxoid degeneration, and

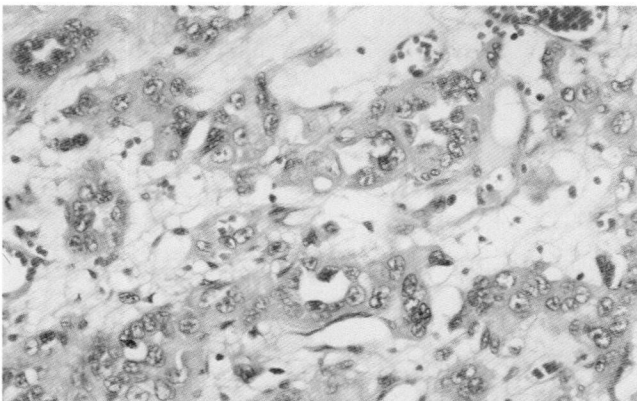

**FIGURE 46–55.** Epithelioid angiosarcoma. Highly atypical epithelioid cells form vascular channels, mimicking an adenocarcinoma.

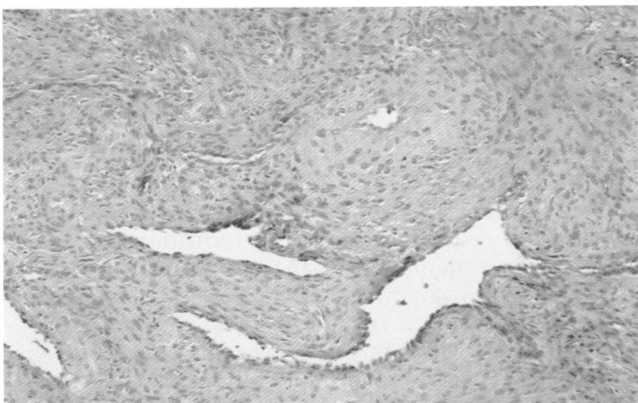

FIGURE 46–56. Angiomyoma. There are thick-walled blood vessels, with intervening smooth muscle cells.

calcification. In some cases, the nuclei may also show atypia, but mitoses should also be absent. The presence of any mitotic activity should raise concern for leiomyosarcoma. Rarely, the cytoplasm may show a clear cell change. Immunohistochemical studies show clear evidence of smooth muscle differentiation, with positivity for muscle-specific actin, smooth muscle–specific actin, and desmin. In addition, collagen IV stains demonstrate positivity around single cells. Ultrastructural studies also demonstrate clear evidence of smooth muscle differentiation, with basal lamina, pinocytotic vesicles, myofilaments, and dense bodies.

The differential diagnosis is usually not difficult. Any degree of mitotic activity in a possible soft tissue leiomyoma should probably raise consideration of at least borderline malignancy. In cases in which the histodifferentiation is not clear, immunohistochemical studies should easily resolve the problem.

## Angiomyoma (Vascular Leiomyoma, Angioleiomyoma)[202, 203]

Angiomyomas, which are benign neoplasms, usually occur in middle adulthood, with a female predominance. They usually present as a painful, slowly enlarging nodule arising in the subcutaneous region. Most occur in the extremities, particularly the lower extremity. At gross evaluation, they are well circumscribed and white-gray on cut section. They do not recur after simple excision.

Angiomyoma consists histologically of thick-walled blood vessels with radiating bundles and whorls of smooth muscle (Fig. 46–56). Areas of myxoid degeneration are often seen between the bundles of muscle, and other degenerative features may also be present.

## Leiomyosarcoma[204–211]

Leiomyosarcoma of the soft tissues occurs in several clinicopathologic settings. Most commonly, it arises in the retroperitoneal space and abdominal cavity, particularly the omentum and mesentery, of older adults; there is a female predilection. Patients present with an abdominal mass, similar to other abdominal or retroperitoneal tumors. The gross masses are usually greater than 10 cm and may be large, involving adjacent structures. On cut section, they have the appearance of a sarcoma, with foci of hemorrhage and necrosis. These neoplasms are often unresectable, and even when they are apparently resectable, they have a high recurrence and metastatic rate with a corresponding poor survival.

In the second most common clinicopathologic setting, leiomyosarcoma occurs in the extremities, most often the thigh. These cases affect adults and have no sex predilection. Patients present with a large mass, usually between 5 and 10 cm. Although the survival rate is better than that for abdominal leiomyosarcoma, recurrences and metastases are still relatively common. Cutaneous leiomyosarcoma occurs in the dermis or subcutaneous tissue of adults and predominates in men. It occurs most often in the extremities, particularly the lower leg, and has a predilection for the hair-bearing extensor surfaces. Patients usually present with a slowly growing mass that may be painful. Although local recurrence is common, metastases are rare, particularly in the dermal lesions.

Leiomyosarcoma arising from major blood vessels (vascular leiomyosarcoma) is the least common clinicopathologic setting. These leiomyosarcomas arise most frequently from the inferior vena cava, the pulmonary artery, and veins of the lower extremity. All usually occur in older adults. There is a striking predilection of inferior vena cava leiomyosarcoma for women, but interestingly, the others have an equal sex distribution. The symptoms vary, depending on the affected vein, and the morbidity and survival also usually depend on the particular presentation.

All clinicopathologic forms of leiomyosarcoma show a similar histologic appearance (Fig. 46–57). Most leiomyosarcomas show some areas in which

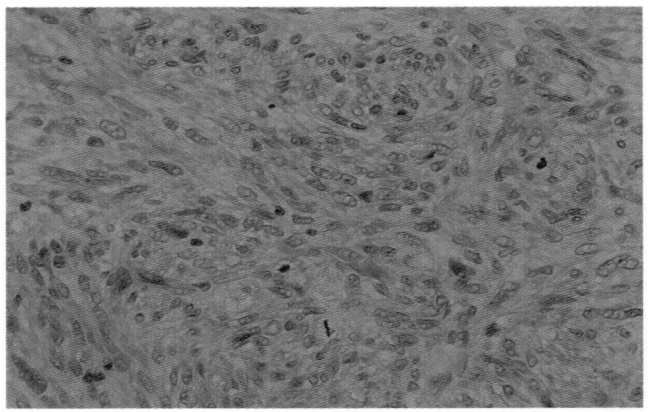

FIGURE 46–57. Leiomyosarcoma. Although this smooth muscle proliferation lacks atypical nuclei, several mitotic figures are present.

there are fascicles of spindle cells intersecting at 90° angles. Other areas, however, may show a more nondescript spindle cell proliferation; rarely, there may be myxoid change (Fig. 46–58). On occasion, there is palisading of nuclei, mimicking a neural tumor. The cells most often have discernible spindled eosinophilic cytoplasm. Often, there is an artifactual paranuclear vacuolization. In addition, the cytoplasm may occasionally show epithelioid features, with rounding of the cytoplasm and pale or clear cell change (although this is much less frequent than in smooth muscle tumors of the gastrointestinal tract), or granular cell change. The nuclei are usually oblong, with blunting of the edges. However, they may vary from extremely bland to highly pleomorphic; the mitotic rate may vary widely as well. Rarely, they may feature numerous osteoclast-like giant cells, mimicking the giant cell variant of malignant fibrous histiocytoma.[212] Histochemical studies often show a linear fuchsinophilia on a trichrome stain and positivity for glycogen on a periodic acid–Schiff (PAS) stain. Immunohistochemical studies on well-differentiated leiomyosarcomas usually show positivity for desmin, muscle-specific actin, and smooth muscle–specific actin. A dotlike paranuclear keratin positivity may be present.[213, 214] In addition, collagen IV stains demonstrate positivity around single cells. However, poorly differentiated examples may be desmin negative, the actin staining may be focal, and the characteristic collagen IV staining pattern may be lost. Similarly, ultrastructural studies are most helpful in the most differentiated tumors but may be equivocal in poorly differentiated examples.

The differential diagnosis of leiomyosarcoma includes benign leiomyoma and other spindle cell sarcomas. The presence of more than a rare mitotic figure in a smooth muscle neoplasm arising in the soft tissues should be enough for the designation uncertain or low malignant potential. Smooth muscle neoplasms of the soft tissues with more than 5 mitoses per 10 high-power fields should be considered malignant. The differentiation of poorly differentiated leiomyosarcoma from other poorly differentiated spindle cell sarcomas is controversial.

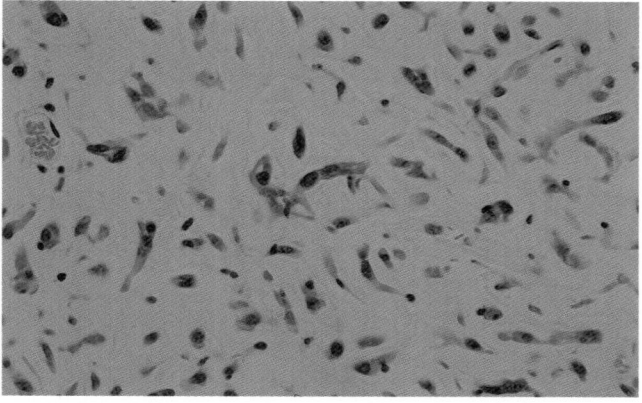

**FIGURE 46–58.** Myxoid leiomyosarcoma. This myxoid leiomyosarcoma was recognized by its immunohistochemical profile.

Cytologic studies show that leiomyosarcomas usually have blunt-ended nuclei, in contrast to the more pointed ends of the nuclei of fibrosarcoma or malignant schwannoma. I consider neoplasms that are positive on immunohistochemical analysis for desmin and smooth muscle–specific actin to most likely represent leiomyosarcomas, particularly if collagen IV surrounds single cells. Spindle cell neoplasms that are positive for smooth muscle–specific actin and muscle-specific actin but negative for desmin probably also represent leiomyosarcomas, particularly if the collagen IV staining is consistent with that diagnosis.

The prognosis of leiomyosarcoma is most determined by site. Retroperitoneal tumors have the worst prognosis, and cutaneous leiomyosarcomas virtually never metastasize if they are contained within the dermis.

## TUMORS AND TUMORLIKE PROLIFERATIONS SHOWING DIFFERENTIATION TOWARD SKELETAL MUSCLE

### Fetal Rhabdomyoma[215–217]

Fetal rhabdomyoma, an extremely rare neoplasm, occurs in all ages but has a predilection for the first 3 years of life; there is a 3:1 male predominance. This neoplasm may occur as a part of the nevoid basal cell carcinoma syndrome. The head and neck region, especially the postauricular region, is most commonly affected, but it may occur in a wide variety of sites. Patients with fetal rhabdomyomas usually present with an asymptomatic mass in the subcutaneous tissue. When it is properly excised, recurrence or metastasis does not occur. Fetal rhabdomyomas average about 4 cm in diameter and are typically pink or gray on cut section.

Fetal rhabdomyoma shows a spectrum of histologic appearances, mimicking the normal development of skeletal muscle. Most cases show primitive mesenchymal cells embedded in a myxoid matrix, within which immature rhabdomyoblasts can be identified; often, the most immature areas are seen centrally. Mitotic figures are usually few, and marked cellularity or nuclear atypia is generally absent. Other cases show a mature pattern, lacking a myxoid matrix and containing a large number of maturing myocytes with obvious differentiating features; these lesions have been called cellular fetal rhabdomyoma or juvenile rhabdomyoma. Immunohistochemical stains usually exhibit obvious evidence of skeletal muscle differentiation, including positivity for muscle-specific actin, desmin, and myoglobin. Gross circumscription, the histologic presence of zonal areas of maturation, and the absence of marked atypia favor the diagnosis of fetal rhabdomyoma over embryonal rhabdomyosarcoma. A minority of fetal rhabdomyomas may have significant mitotic activity.

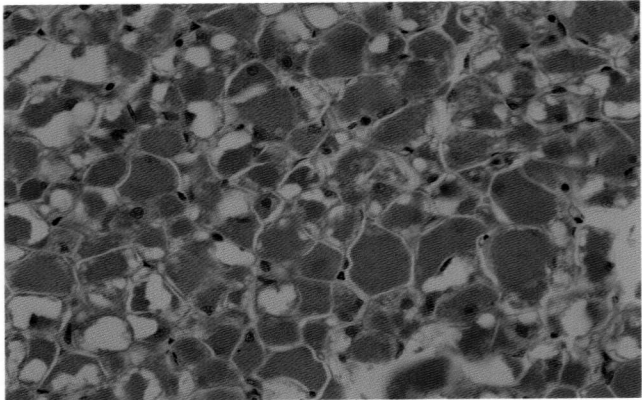

**FIGURE 46–59.** Adult rhabdomyoma. There is a resemblance to normal skeletal muscle, with peripherally located bland nuclei and abundant eosinophilic cytoplasm.

## Adult Rhabdomyoma[218]

Adult rhabdomyomas have a histologic appearance distinct from that of fetal rhabdomyomas and do not arise from them; thus, they should be considered a distinct entity. They may rarely occur in children, but they most commonly occur in middle-aged or older adults; similar to fetal rhabdomyoma, there is about a 3:1 male predominance. There is a marked predilection for the neck, particularly the oropharynx and the larynx; they do not occur in the limbs. Patients present with a mass that may be multifocal in about 10% to 20% of cases. The neoplasm may recur if it is incompletely excised. The gross lesions are well circumscribed, usually measure between 2 and 4 cm, and are yellow to brown on cut section.

The lesions consist histologically of variously sized rhabdomyocytes with abundant eosinophilic cytoplasm, occasional intracellular vacuoles (probably representing the traces of intracellular glycogen), and peripherally placed nuclei without mitotic activity (Fig. 46–59). Cross-striations and crystalline structures may be seen and can be highlighted with a phosphotungstic acid–hematoxylin stain. Electron microscopic and immunohistochemical studies show obvious evidence of muscle differentiation. Cytogenetic studies have identified clonal abnormalities. There is little diagnostic confusion if skeletal muscle differentiation is recognized.

## Rhabdomyosarcoma[219–237]

Rhabdomyosarcoma is a sarcoma showing skeletal muscle differentiation, without other prominent patterns of differentiation (mixed sarcomas). Rhabdomyosarcoma can be divided into at least three major types, with several variants: embryonal rhabdomyosarcoma, with botryoid and spindle cell variants; alveolar rhabdomyosarcoma, with a solid variant; and pleomorphic rhabdomyosarcoma. An international classification of rhabdomyosarcoma proposed for pediatric patients has been shown to be both reproducible and predictive of outcome[238] (Table 46–7). Rhabdomyosarcoma occurs most commonly in children, with peaks of incidence around the ages of 5 and 15 years and a median incidence about the age of 10 years. About 10% of all cases occur in adults. Embryonal rhabdomyosarcoma, the most common type, occurs predominantly in the youngest population; alveolar rhabdomyosarcoma has a peak of incidence in adolescents, and pleomorphic rhabdomyosarcoma occurs almost exclusively in adults. There is a slight male predominance in the embryonal and pleomorphic types but not in the alveolar type. Congenital cases occur in about 2% of patients; rhabdomyosarcoma may occur as a part of a variety of inherited disorders, including Li-Fraumeni syndrome and neurofibromatosis type 1.

Patients with rhabdomyosarcoma generally present with a painless mass or loss of function of affected structures. Rare neoplasms may present with widespread metastasis that may extensively involve the bone marrow, mimicking acute leukemia. Rhabdomyosarcomas occur most often in the head and neck region, the genitourinary tract, the extremities, and the trunk. The head and neck region is most often involved by rhabdomyosarcomas of the embryonal type, including the botryoid subtype. The periorbital region and parameningeal sites are most frequently involved. The genitourinary tract is also most often involved by rhabdomyosarcomas of the embryonal type; there is a particular predilection for the spindle cell variant to occur in paratesticular neoplasms. Extremity tumors are most likely alveolar rhabdomyosarcomas in adolescents and pleomorphic rhabdomyosarcomas in adults.

Optimally, rhabdomyosarcomas are completely resected; however, they so often occur adjacent to essential structures that only biopsy is performed. Radiation therapy has an important role for unresectable or incompletely resected tumors. Multidrug chemotherapy is part of the management of virtually all patients with rhabdomyosarcoma, and its implementation has led to markedly improved sur-

**TABLE 46–7.** International Classification of Rhabdomyosarcoma for Pediatric Patients

Superior prognosis
  Botryoid rhabdomyosarcoma
  Spindle cell rhabdomyosarcoma
Intermediate prognosis
  Embryonal rhabdomyosarcoma
Poor prognosis
  Alveolar rhabdomyosarcoma
  Undifferentiated sarcoma
Subtypes whose prognosis is not presently evaluable
  Rhabdomyosarcoma with rhabdoid features

Modified from Newton WA Jr, Gehan EA, Webber BL, et al: Classification of rhabdosarcomas and related sarcomas. Pathologic aspects and proposal for a new classification—an Intergroup Rhabdosarcoma Study. Cancer 76:1073–1085, 1995.

vival; overall survival is now about 50%. Local recurrence is common, including bone involvement. Metastases commonly occur in the lung, lymph nodes, and bone.

Rhabdomyosarcomas are variable in gross appearance. Although some may seem to be circumscribed, they are generally infiltrative when carefully examined. Tumors growing beneath mucosal surfaces tend to form a polypoid or grapelike configuration; these neoplasms constitute the botryoid variant of embryonal rhabdomyosarcoma. On cut section, rhabdomyosarcomas may be soft or firm. Pleomorphic rhabdomyosarcomas are grossly indistinguishable from other adult pleomorphic sarcomas. Nonextremity tumors tend to be small, averaging less than 2 to 4 cm; extremity neoplasms, particularly those arising in adults, are usually somewhat larger.

The histologic appearance of rhabdomyosarcoma varies with the different histologic subtypes. Typical embryonal rhabdomyosarcoma has a variably myxoid stroma infiltrated by undifferentiated round to spindled cells. Cellularity varies from neoplasm to neoplasm and also varies from area to area within a particular neoplasm. Although some cases may completely lack cells with discernible cytoplasm, most cases have a subset of cells with eosinophilic cytoplasm, often eccentrically exhibited (Fig. 46–60). These cells often take on characteristic shapes, the so-called strap or tadpole cells. Less commonly, the differentiated cells possess clearer evidence of skeletal muscle differentiation, with granular eosinophilic cytoplasmic material, concentrically arranged fibrils around the nucleus or the nuclear membrane, or definite cross-striations. The nuclei usually have a light chromatin pattern with inconspicuous nucleoli; they usually show some atypia and have a high mitotic rate. Some tumors, particularly in recurrences, show a uniform population of highly differentiated rhabdomyoblasts. Rare tumors may show uniformly highly anaplastic nuclei (so-called anaplastic rhabdomyosarcoma). Rare tumors may have cytoplasmic hyaline inclusions similar to those seen in rhabdoid tumors.

The botryoid variant of embryonal rhabdomyosarcoma has a similar histologic appearance, but the cellularity is accentuated beneath the intact overlying mucosal surface in a zone called the cambium layer. The cambium layer is at least several cells thick. Often, the most differentiated rhabdomyoblasts are present in this area. A thin hypocellular zone separates the cambium layer from the epithelium; it is usually discontinuous. The remainder of the neoplasm may also be hypocellular. The spindle cell variant of embryonal rhabdomyosarcoma is characterized by a relatively uniform population of eosinophilic spindle cells.[239–242] The cells are arranged in either a fascicular or a storiform pattern.

The alveolar type of rhabdomyosarcoma has a different histologic appearance more similar to small round blue cell tumors. There are usually characteristic fibrous septa, enclosing "alveolar" nests of neo-

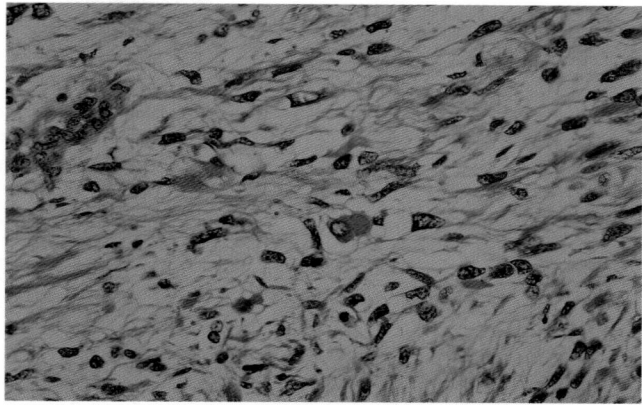

**FIGURE 46–60.** Embryonal rhabdomyosarcoma. There is an atypical spindle cell proliferation with occasional cells with abundant eosinophilic cytoplasm—rhabdomyoblasts.

plastic cells (Fig. 46–61). The neoplastic cells usually adhere to the edges of the septa, often clinging by cytoplasmic processes, simulating adenocarcinoma. Many neoplasms have solid areas in addition to areas with fibrous septa, whereas a minority of cases lack fibrous septa completely; these cases are regarded as the solid variant of alveolar rhabdomyosarcoma (Fig. 46–62). Alveolar rhabdomyosarcoma is defined by its cellular composition. In the lumen of the alveoli are sheets, clusters, and individual round cells, sometimes showing necrosis. Although most of the cells are undifferentiated and lack discernible cytoplasm, some cells may be larger and possess rounded, eosinophilic cytoplasm. The nuclei have dark chromatin, nuclear pleomorphism is usually marked, and the mitotic rate is high. Multinucleated giant cells may be present, often with the nuclei disposed in a wreathlike appearance, and have nuclear and cytoplasmic features similar to the larger differentiating cells. Some cases may show areas indistinguishable from embryonal rhabdomyosarcoma; these cases should be regarded as alveolar rhabdomyosarcoma, as long as there are at least fo-

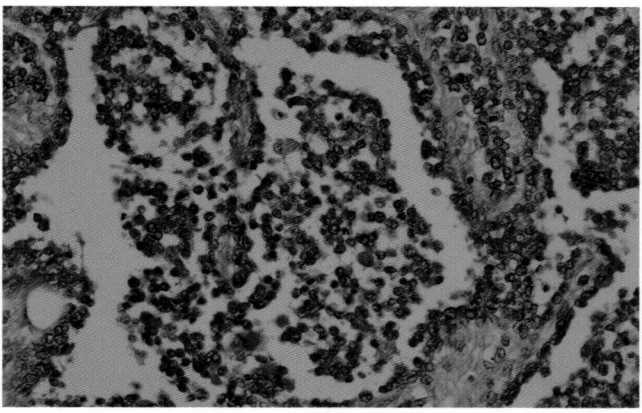

**FIGURE 46–61.** Classic alveolar rhabdomyosarcoma. Relatively undifferentiated round cells are seen in spaces and lining septa. Occasional rhabdomyoblasts may be seen.

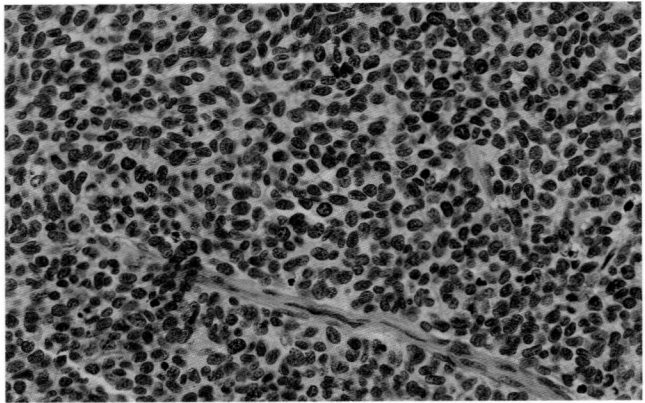

**FIGURE 46–62.** Solid variant of alveolar rhabdomyosarcoma. Patternless sheets of small blue cells are present. Immunohistochemical studies confirmed the presence of rhabdomyoblastic differentiation in this case.

cal clear-cut areas fitting the definition of alveolar rhabdomyosarcoma.

Pleomorphic rhabdomyosarcoma does not usually resemble the embryonal or alveolar types of rhabdomyosarcoma; it has a closer resemblance to other pleomorphic adult sarcomas, such as pleomorphic malignant fibrous histiocytoma or pleomorphic liposarcoma (Fig. 46–63). There is often a storiform or fascicular proliferation of highly pleomorphic cells in a variably fibrous background. There are frequently large cells with abundant eosinophilic cytoplasm with large nuclei frequently containing large nucleoli. Definite evidence of cytoplasmic cross-striations is rare, and electron microscopy or immunohistochemical stains are the most reliable way to establish the diagnosis.

Ultrastructural study of rhabdomyosarcomas may reveal a variety of findings, from nonspecific to definitive evidence of skeletal muscle differentiation. In general, a range of cellular differentiation is seen, from primitive cells with nonspecific filamentous material to cells with distinct sarcomeres. Features diagnostic of rhabdomyosarcoma include the identification of a mixture of thick (myosin) and thin (actin) filaments, the presence of thick filaments in association with ribosomes (ribosome and myosin complex), and definitive evidence of Z bands. On immunohistochemical analysis, rhabdomyosarcoma is typically positive for desmin and muscle-specific actin but negative for smooth muscle–specific actin (which is positive in leiomyosarcoma).[243] Antibodies to myoglobin and MyoD1 are relatively specific for rhabdomyosarcoma as opposed to leiomyosarcoma, but the antibody to myoglobin lacks great sensitivity, and MyoD1 antibody works reliably only in frozen sections. Occasional cells may be keratin positive. Rhabdomyosarcomas are negative for CD99.

Flow cytometric studies may show hyperdiploid, diploid or near-diploid, tetraploid, or hypertetraploid DNA content. Hyperdiploid tumors are more often of the embryonal subtype, whereas tetraploidy is associated with the alveolar subtype. Molecular studies have shown differences among the types of rhabdomyosarcomas. Embryonal rhabdomyosarcoma shows loss of heterozygosity at chromosome 11p15.5, close to but not at the *MYOD1* locus; deletions of chromosome 11 can be seen in other "blastomas" of childhood.[244] In addition, there are often gains of chromosomes 2q, 8, and 20. Alveolar rhabdomyosarcoma, including the classic and solid types, shows a characteristic translocation involving the *FKHR* gene on chromosome 13. In about two thirds of cases, there is a t(2;13)(q35;q14) involving the *PAX3* gene; in one third of cases, there is a t(1;13)(p36;q14) involving the *PAX7* gene.[244] Reverse transcription–polymerase chain reaction tests are available that can detect both in frozen or paraffin sections.[245] Patients with the t(2;13) may be older, have truncal tumors, and present with more advanced disease than patients with the t(1;13), who are more likely to have an extremity lesion and event-free survival.[246, 247] In both translocations, fusion proteins are formed that appear to act as transcriptional activators. There are other molecular

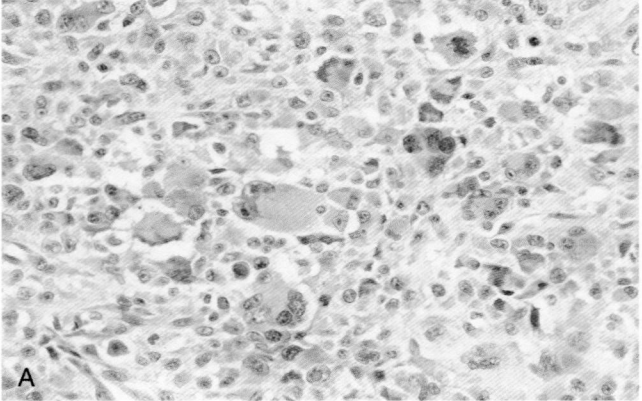
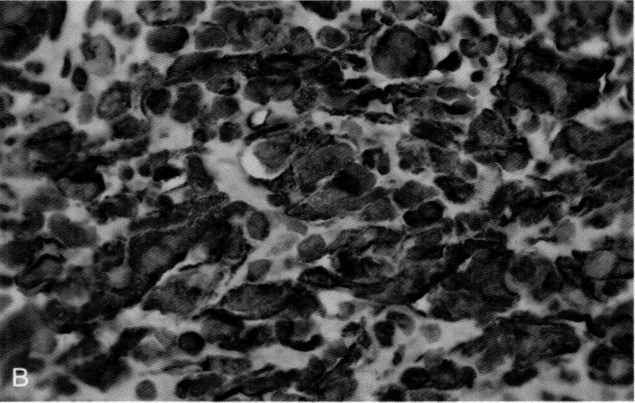

**FIGURE 46–63.** Pleomorphic rhabdomyosarcoma. There is a pleomorphic sarcoma with identifiable rhabdomyoblasts *(A)*, confirmed by the immunohistochemical study for desmin *(B)*.

lesions that distinguish alveolar from embryonal rhabdomyosarcoma; for example, the N-MYC gene is amplified in alveolar but not in embryonal rhabdomyosarcoma.[248] There are no distinctive molecular findings in pleomorphic rhabdomyosarcoma.

Embryonal, alveolar, and pleomorphic rhabdomyosarcomas are usually easy to distinguish from one another. The presence of any alveolar areas in a neoplasm that is otherwise an embryonal rhabdomyosarcoma warrants a diagnosis of alveolar rhabdomyosarcoma. One should diagnose pleomorphic rhabdomyosarcoma with the greatest caution in childhood, because most cases represent embryonal rhabdomyosarcoma with a high degree of pleomorphism (so-called anaplastic variant of embryonal rhabdomyosarcoma). Embryonal rhabdomyosarcoma may be mistaken for other spindle cell sarcomas of childhood; however, the presence of cells with eosinophilic cytoplasm should raise the possibility of the diagnosis. The diagnosis of embryonal rhabdomyosarcoma can be confirmed histologically with the identification of cells with definitive cross-striations or may require the use of immunohistochemical studies; rarely, electron microscopy may be necessary to establish the diagnosis. Similarly, the diagnosis of alveolar rhabdomyosarcoma can be suggested by the variation in cell size and the presence of cells with eccentric eosinophilic cytoplasm in a small round blue cell tumor. If the characteristic fibrous septa are not evident, immunostains usually provide confirmation of the diagnosis. Molecular biologic studies to detect the t(2;13) or the t(1;13) may also be of use. The distinction of pleomorphic rhabdomyosarcoma from other pleomorphic sarcomas such as pleomorphic malignant fibrous histiocytoma cannot usually be done in the absence of immunohistochemical studies. Extrarenal rhabdoid tumors may be difficult to distinguish from rhabdomyosarcoma, but these tumors do not express muscle markers. Rhabdomyosarcoma may occur as a component of mixed neoplasms. This may be seen in malignant peripheral nerve sheath tumors, as part of other blastic neoplasms of childhood, in malignant mixed müllerian tumor of the gynecologic tract, in spermatocytic seminomas, and in other neoplasms. Thus, it is always important to examine the entire neoplasm carefully to rule out components of other types of neoplasms.

The most important prognostic factors in rhabdomyosarcoma are stage, histologic type, age, and site of primary. The clinical staging system for patients with rhabdomyosarcoma used in the Intergroup Rhabdomyosarcoma Studies has helped in stratifying patients for studies and determining prognosis. Briefly, stage I represents localized disease that is completely resected, stage II represents microscopic residual disease, stage III represents macroscopic residual disease, and stage IV represents distant metastases. In the International Classification of Rhabdomyosarcoma, the different histologic types and variants are graded according to prognosis.[238] The botryoid and spindle cell variants

of embryonal rhabdomyosarcoma have a superior prognosis; other types of embryonal rhabdomyosarcoma have an intermediate prognosis, whereas alveolar rhabdomyosarcoma has a poor prognosis. Although not included in that classification, pleomorphic rhabdomyosarcoma should probably be considered a rhabdomyosarcoma of poor prognosis. Young age, orbital or nonbladder genitourinary location, and small size (less than 5 cm) are additional favorable prognostic factors. Finally, ploidy and S phase fraction have been found to identify selected groups of patients at high risk of treatment failure, even if the tumor's presentation is favorable according to standard criteria.[249] Specifically, patients with childhood rhabdomyosarcomas whose tumors are hyperdiploid have a much better overall survival than do those patients whose tumors are diploid or tetraploid.

## Alveolar Soft Part Sarcoma[250–256]

Alveolar soft part sarcoma is an extremely rare sarcoma that typically occurs in young adults with a median age of about 25 years; there is a marked female predominance. Patients generally present with a slow-growing, painless, deep-seated mass. It most frequently occurs in the lower extremity, with an unusual predilection for the anterior aspect of the right thigh. A head and neck presentation is next frequent, most commonly in children. These neoplasms are most often fatal, despite aggressive treatment; metastases to lung and brain are particularly common. Alveolar soft part sarcoma is the sarcoma most likely to present with a metastasis before discovery of the primary lesion. The gross neoplasms show a wide range in size, are poorly circumscribed, and often show evidence of hemorrhage on cut section.

The histologic appearance is remarkably uniform from case to case (Fig. 46–64). There are usually nests of neoplastic cells separated by dilated thin

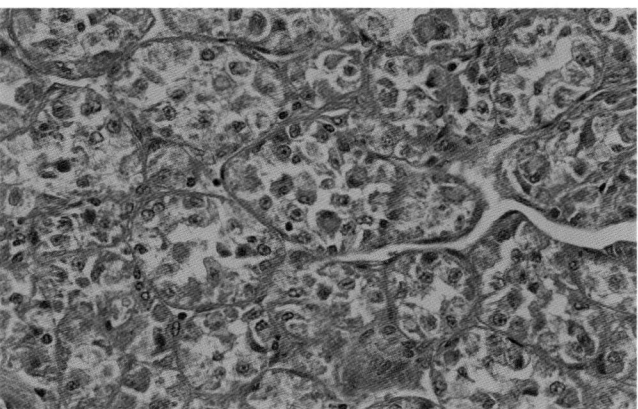

**FIGURE 46–64.** Alveolar soft part sarcoma. The classic appearance is seen with atypical cells with abundant eosinophilic cytoplasm lining and filling alveolar spaces.

vascular channels. Nests of tumor cells are often found within vessels at the edge of the tumor. In some nests, the centers may be filled with necrotic tumor; more commonly, the centers may have dropped out, leaving pseudoglandular formations. The individual tumor cells have abundant, strongly eosinophilic cytoplasm. PAS stains demonstrate characteristic crystalline inclusions. On occasion, the ghost outlines of these crystals can be seen on H&E-stained sections. The nuclei are eccentric and have a vesicular chromatin pattern with a prominent nucleolus. Paradoxically, the mitotic rate is usually not high. Ultrastructural studies demonstrate crystals and electron-dense secretory-like granules. Obvious evidence of muscle differentiation is not seen. Numerous immunohistochemical studies have been reported, not always with consistent results. However, it appears that the tumor cells are positive for desmin, muscle-specific actin, and MyoD1, consistent with differentiation toward skeletal muscle. Some cases are also positive for neuron-specific enolase and S-100 protein. Vimentin has been reported to be positive or negative.

Given the distinctive histologic features, the differential diagnosis is relatively limited. Renal cell adenocarcinoma may show a close resemblance to alveolar soft part sarcoma, but it is positive for keratin and epithelial membrane antigen. Paraganglioma may show a similar nesting pattern but does not occur in the extremities and is positive for endocrine markers such as chromogranin. Although alveolar soft part sarcoma shares some morphologic features as well as frequent S-100 protein positivity with malignant melanoma of soft parts, the latter neoplasm is consistently positive for HMB-45 and strongly positive for vimentin. Although alveolar soft part sarcoma is a rare neoplasm, it should be considered in the differential diagnosis of an undifferentiated epithelioid neoplasm that is negative for both keratin and vimentin.

## TUMORS AND TUMORLIKE PROLIFERATIONS SHOWING EPITHELIAL DIFFERENTIATION

### Synovial Sarcoma[257–264]

Synovial sarcoma is a relatively common sarcoma that occurs in a wide age range, including in children, but it has a broad peak of incidence between 10 and 30 years of age. There is a mild predilection for males. Patients generally present with a long history of a slow-growing, deep-seated mass that may be painful. It tends to occur in the extremities, although almost any soft tissue site, including the head and neck, may be involved. It generally occurs in the para-articular regions, although true involvement of the joint space is not typically seen. The knee and lower portion of the thigh are particularly frequent sites of occurrence, whereas the fingers and

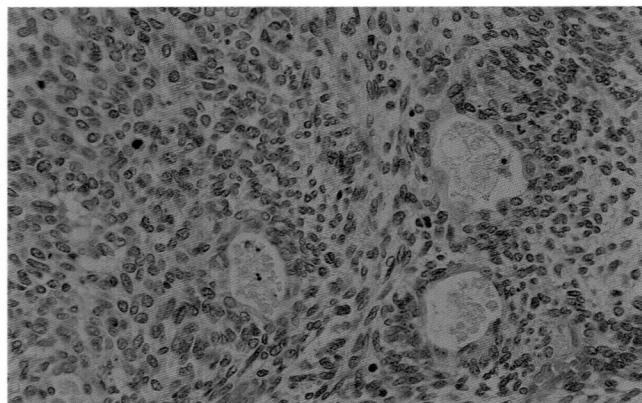

**FIGURE 46–65.** Biphasic synovial sarcoma. Glandular structures are formed, amid a spindle cell background.

toes are uncommon sites. Radical excision is the treatment of choice, usually followed by adjuvant radiotherapy and possibly chemotherapy. Recurrences are still common, even years after treatment, and metastases, which also occur early or late, may include spread to local lymph nodes. Synovial sarcomas may be suggested radiologically; about one fifth of cases have multiple calcifications, which in some cases may be striking. At gross evaluation, synovial sarcomas tend to be smaller than most sarcomas at presentation.

Synovial sarcomas may have either the classic biphasic or the more common monophasic histologic appearance. The biphasic variant features discrete epithelial and spindle cell areas (Fig. 46–65); the monophasic variant is exclusively spindle cell in appearance (Fig. 46–66). In both variants, the spindle cell area is usually similar to the appearance of fibrosarcoma, with sheets of long spindle cells with uniform elongated nuclei with tapered ends. The nuclei are usually only mildly to moderately atypical, and the mitotic rate is relatively low, often less than 1 or 2 mitoses per high-power field. There are

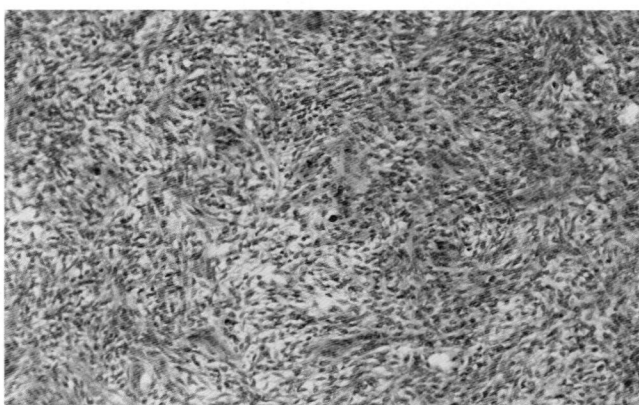

**FIGURE 46–66.** Monophasic synovial sarcoma. This appearance is indistinguishable from that of a fibrosarcoma. Immunohistochemical staining showed multifocal areas of keratin positivity.

often occasional foci in which the cells seem to cluster and have a more epithelioid appearance, suggesting incipient epithelial differentiation. However, some cases are more poorly differentiated, composed of less spindled to oval cells with a higher mitotic rate (more than 2 mitoses per high-power field). The degree of vascularity varies in the spindle cell areas, but it is not uncommon for there to be a staghorn hemangiopericytomatous arrangement of thin-walled vessel. Often, the stroma contains an abundant fine, ropy collagen, and there may be dense fibrosis in some cases. Scattered mast cells are usually present among the spindle cells. In about 25% of cases, calcifications, osteoid, or even bone formation is present, which rarely may be a prominent finding.[261, 265] Occasional cases may have myxoid areas, which may be a focal or extensive finding. The biphasic variant also contains discrete areas of epithelial differentiation in addition to the spindle cell areas. The epithelial areas are usually glandular but may also show squamous features. The glands are composed of cuboid to columnar cells bordering cleftlike spaces. Mucicarmine stains may be positive, particularly in the glandular spaces. Extremely rarely, the neoplasm may be composed entirely of these epithelial areas (monophasic epithelial type of synovial sarcoma). Immunohistochemical studies demonstrate the epithelial areas to be keratin and epithelial membrane antigen positive. In addition, multifocal clusters of keratin-positive and epithelial membrane antigen–positive cells can also be demonstrated in the spindle cell areas, particularly in those foci showing incipient epithelial differentiation. Collagen IV and reticulin stains usually show a discrete basement membrane separating the epithelial from spindle cell areas and may also highlight the incipient epithelial areas by outlining nests and clusters of cells. Vimentin stains are positive in the spindle cell areas but usually negative in the epithelial elements. Occasional cases may also be positive for S-100 protein in the spindle cell areas. Ultrastructural studies generally confirm the epithelial differentiation seen by light microscopy, complete with well-defined cell junctions and microvilli on the luminal cell membranes. Flow cytometric studies have found aneuploidy in approximately one third of synovial sarcomas. Cytogenetic studies have demonstrated that a t(X;18)(p11.2;q11.2) is a reproducible and specific marker for synovial sarcomas, of both biphasic and monophasic types.[85] A reverse transcription–polymerase chain reaction assay is also available to detect this translocation.[266]

The differential diagnosis of synovial sarcoma usually involves separation from other types of sarcomas. Immunoreactivity of small clusters of cells for keratin or epithelial membrane antigen effectively rules out fibrosarcoma and malignant schwannoma. The diagnosis of rare glandular variant of malignant schwannoma can be made most easily by demonstration of a clear origin from a nerve or a history of neurofibromatosis, because some cases of synovial sarcoma are S-100 protein positive. In addition, the glandular elements of that neoplasm are of the intestinal type with goblet cells. The presence of staghorn vessels raises the possibility of a hemangiopericytoma. Because synovial sarcomas are much more common than hemangiopericytomas, a spindle cell tumor with a hemangiopericytomatous vascular pattern is more likely to be a synovial sarcoma than a hemangiopericytoma; in cases of doubt, a CD34 stain (positive in hemangiopericytoma) along with epithelial markers should resolve the problem. The presence of cells positive for epithelial markers raises consideration of epithelioid sarcoma. However, in this tumor, the neoplastic cells do not form glands and are uniformly positive for epithelial markers (and also for vimentin); in synovial sarcoma, most spindled neoplastic cells are keratin negative. Finally, one should rule out the possibility of a primary adnexal tumor (superficial location) and metastatic carcinoma, particularly of pulmonary origin, in all cases in which the monophasic glandular variant of synovial sarcoma is being considered.

Prognostic factors have been intensively investigated in synovial sarcoma. The most important clinical factors indicating a worse prognosis are age of the patient (older than 20 years) and an inadequate excision. Unfavorable pathologic factors include size of the tumor (larger than 5 cm), extensive necrosis, vascular invasion, and demonstration of aneuploidy by flow cytometry. The presence of extensive calcification throughout the neoplasm is a favorable prognostic factor, as is localization to the distal extremities. The prognostic significance for monophasic versus biphasic tumors is controversial, but patients with monophasic neoplasms may fare worse.

## Epithelioid Sarcoma[267–271]

Epithelioid sarcoma most commonly occurs in young adults; the peak incidence occurs at about 30 years, although it may present in a wide age range. There is a predilection for males. Patients generally present with a long-standing history of one or several soft tissue masses that may be painful. It occurs most often in the distal extremities, the upper more than the lower, particularly the wrist, hands, fingers, and feet. However, there is a variant of epithelioid sarcoma called proximal-type epithelioid sarcoma, which occurs predominantly in the pelvis or perineal region.[271] Even after it is treated by radical excision, epithelioid sarcoma recurs in most patients, and the recurrences are often multiple. Metastases, when they occur, generally follow repeated recurrences; involvement of local lymph nodes generally occurs before lung metastases. Ultimately, most patients die of their disease, but this may take years. The proximal-type of epithelioid sarcoma may be more aggressive, with earlier metastasis than in conventional epithelioid sarcoma. At gross evaluation, epithelioid sarcoma may be superficial or deep and consist of a single mass or multiple masses. Superficial lesions may be centered in the dermis or subcutaneous tissue and may show ulceration of the overlying skin; deeper lesions are typically centered in the deep fascia, with infiltration of adjacent tendons. Tumor size is generally small, usually less than 5 cm.

A variety of histologic appearances may be seen. The tumors are usually poorly demarcated, with infiltration of adjacent structures, including tendons, blood vessels, and nerves. Often, separate nodules of tumor may be present at a distance from the primary mass. Classically, epithelioid sarcoma is described as consisting of multinodular masses of epithelioid cells with central necrosis, simulating granulomas (Fig. 46–67). Areas of extensive necrosis are seen in about 50% of cases. However, epithelioid sarcoma may also be composed of fascicles or may show a single cell pattern of infiltration. In most cases, the neoplastic cells have relatively abundant, eosinophilic cytoplasm and rounded, generally uniform nuclei. On occasion, the cytoplasm may be vacuolated or contain densely eosinophilic inclusions. However, in some cases, the tumor cells may be spindled, and in other cases, they may have a cuboid appearance, resembling lobular carcinoma of the breast. The nuclei tend to have a vesicular chromatin pattern with small nucleoli. The mitotic index is usually low, although atypical mitoses can be identified. In proximal-type epithelioid sarcoma, the neoplastic cells tend to have more prominent epithelioid or rhabdoid features, with marked cytologic atypia (Fig. 46–68).

Ultrastructural studies show aggregates of intermediate filaments and tonofilament-like structures. Although there is no basal lamina or basement membrane, most cases contain at least primitive cell junctions, and blunt filopodia or elongated microvilli, occasionally lining glandlike spaces, have also been noted. Cases of proximal-type epithelioid sarcoma often show prominent aggregates of cytoplasmic intermediate filaments, similar to those seen in extrarenal rhabdoid tumors. Although the electron microscopic studies are not conclusive in determin-

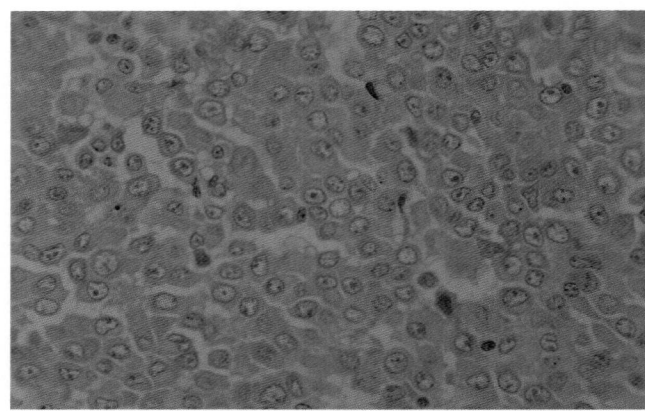

**FIGURE 46–68.** Proximal-type epithelioid sarcoma. The cells are more pleomorphic than is typically seen in epithelioid sarcoma.

ing the type of differentiation, the immunohistochemical studies unequivocally demonstrate an epithelial phenotype, with strong and consistent expression of keratin and epithelial membrane antigen by the majority of the neoplastic cells. Almost all cases are positive for keratin 8, the majority are positive for keratin 19, and only a minority are positive for keratin 7 or 34βE12.[272] Vimentin is another relatively consistent marker, although a minority of cases may be vimentin negative.[273] Other markers that may be positive in a significant number of cases include muscle-specific actin (about half), CD34 (about 40%), and *Ulex europaeus* I lectin; however, epithelioid sarcoma is negative for other vascular and muscle markers, including CD31, factor VIII–related antigen, and desmin.

The differential diagnosis of epithelioid sarcoma includes benign lesions, malignant melanoma, other sarcomas, and carcinoma. Because the cells may be bland and central necrosis may be seen, epithelioid sarcoma may be confused with granuloma annulare, necrobiosis lipoidica, rheumatoid nodules, and even necrotizing granulomatous inflammation; in cases of doubt, the demonstration of keratin positivity in the proliferating cells provides confirmation of epithelioid sarcoma. Malignant melanoma and clear cell sarcoma are generally positive for S-100 protein and HMB-45 and negative for keratin. An epithelioid angiosarcoma may be particularly difficult to distinguish histologically from epithelioid sarcoma and may express keratin, CD34, and *U. europaeus* I lectin; however, these neoplasms are positive for CD31 and factor VIII–related antigen. Synovial sarcoma may also mimic epithelioid sarcoma. Even though both neoplasms are keratin positive, the keratin stain is still useful because only clusters of cells are keratin positive in synovial sarcoma, whereas the majority of the neoplastic population is positive in epithelioid sarcoma. Carcinoma, including spread from both a skin primary tumor and a metastatic lesion, should be considered in the differential diagnosis. Evidence of dysplasia in the overlying skin and the presence

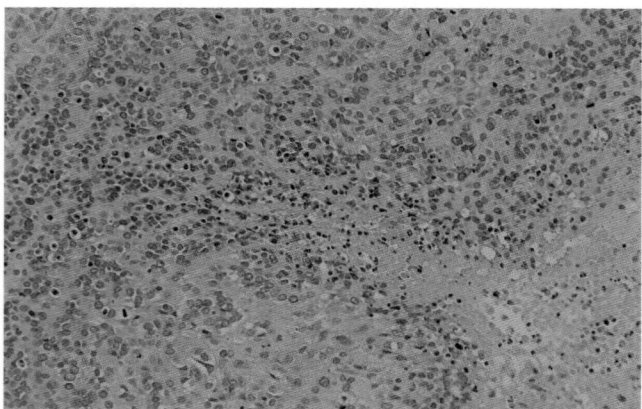

**FIGURE 46–67.** Epithelioid sarcoma. There are epithelioid masses of cells with central necrosis, showing a vague resemblance to a granuloma.

of marked pleomorphism might favor spread from a primary carcinoma. The possibility of a metastatic lesion should be ruled out clinically, especially if the vimentin stain is negative. Finally, an extrarenal rhabdoid tumor may be extremely difficult or impossible to distinguish from proximal-type epithelioid sarcoma; possibly, they represent the same or a similar entity.

## Extrarenal Rhabdoid Tumor[274–279]

Rhabdoid tumor was originally described in the kidney of infants as a rhabdomyosarcomatoid variant of Wilms' tumor. It has now been clearly separated from rhabdomyosarcoma and Wilms' tumor and is regarded as a unique neoplasm that may occur at many sites, including the soft tissues. Patients with extrarenal rhabdoid tumor presenting in the soft tissues have a median age of about 10 years (much older than with renal rhabdoid tumor), but the neoplasm occurs in a wide age range through old age. There is a slight male predilection. Rarely, familial cases have occurred. A wide variety of anatomic sites have been reported, including the chest wall and paraspinal areas, the extremities (particularly the lower extremity), the head and neck region, and the intra-abdominal soft tissues. It is a highly aggressive neoplasm; most patients are dead within 5 years. Gross evaluation shows that the neoplasm may be centered in the skin, subcutaneous tissue, or deep soft tissues. It tends to be between 5 and 10 cm at presentation, is poorly circumscribed, and is gray and fleshy on cut section, often with areas of necrosis and hemorrhage.

At microscopic examination, there are sheets and nests of highly anaplastic cells with abundant eosinophilic cytoplasm (Fig. 46–69). A proportion of the cells have a large cytoplasmic, glassy, eosinophilic inclusion-like mass. These structures are PAS positive and diastase resistant, and they also stand out on a Masson trichrome stain. The nuclei typi-

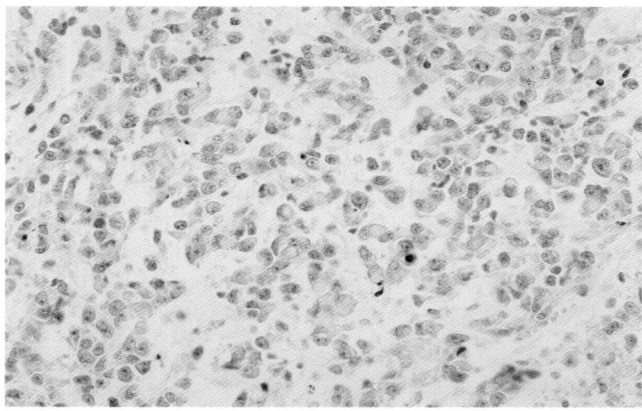

**FIGURE 46–69.** Extrarenal rhabdoid tumor. There are sheets of cells with pleomorphic nuclei and abundant, often inclusion-like, eosinophilic cytoplasm.

cally have a vesicular chromatin pattern with a central prominent nucleolus and thick nuclear membranes. Electron microscopy demonstrates that the cytoplasm contains numerous intermediate filaments that may show a variety of arrangements. The hyaline masses seen histologically also correspond to masses of these filaments. Immunohistochemical studies show strong expression of vimentin and, in most cases, expression of keratin and epithelial membrane antigen. Cytogenetics and fluorescent in situ hybridization studies of rhabdoid tumors have demonstrated a characteristic deletion at chromosome 22q11, supporting the hypothesis that extrarenal rhabdoid tumors represent a distinct clinicopathologic entity rather than merely a distinctive phenotype.[280] Deletion at this site leads to inactivation of the chromatin-remodeling *hSNF5/INI1* gene.[281]

The differential diagnosis of extrarenal rhabdoid tumor is large. Many neoplasms may show rhabdoid features, that is, cells with abundant eosinophilic cytoplasm; these neoplasms include epithelioid sarcoma (see earlier section), rhabdomyosarcoma, malignant melanoma, anaplastic carcinoma, synovial sarcoma, and angiosarcoma. The diagnosis of an extrarenal rhabdoid tumor becomes a diagnosis of exclusion; a large battery of immunohistochemical studies is required to rule out all other possible neoplasms.

## TUMORS AND TUMORLIKE PROLIFERATIONS SHOWING NEURAL DIFFERENTIATION

### Benign Schwannoma[282]

Schwannoma (neurilemoma) is a relatively common benign soft tissue tumor of all age groups but occurs predominantly in young adults; there is no age predilection. The tumors usually arise in association with a nerve. In most cases, they occur sporadically; but in 10% to 20% of cases, there is an association with a syndrome, either neurofibromatosis type 2 or a syndrome of multiple schwannomas, unassociated with neurofibromatosis, that may or may not be accompanied by central nervous system tumors. Neurofibromatosis type 2 is a rare autosomal dominant syndrome caused by abnormalities of the gene on chromosome 22 coding for merlin protein; the abnormality in the other syndrome has not yet been characterized. Schwannomas arise most frequently in the head and neck, particularly affecting cranial nerve 8 (especially in neurofibromatosis type 2). They also have a predilection for the flexor aspects of the extremities. Patients usually present with a slow-growing, painless, solitary mass in the subcutaneous tissue, although multiple masses may be seen in patients with a syndrome. Lesions are usually easily excised, without damage to the attached nerve, and recurrence or malignant transformation is rare, even in incompletely resected tumors. At gross evaluation, schwannomas are usually well-encapsulated, rubbery masses smaller than 5 cm, with a pink-tan cut section; larger tumors may have cystic change.

The typical microscopic schwannoma is well encapsulated and may contain small nerves with the capsule. Classically, a biphasic pattern, designated Antoni A and B, is found in varying proportions (Fig. 46–70). Antoni A areas consist of a cellular proliferation of bland spindle cells arranged in short bundles or fascicles. The cytoplasm is fibrillar or indistinct, and the nuclei are elongated and twisted with pointed ends. Occasional mitotic figures may be seen. Characteristically, the nuclei and cytoplasm line up with adjacent cells, with the formation of so-called Verocay bodies. Antoni B areas are relatively hypocellular areas with blood vessels showing thick hyaline walls. Cells similar to those seen in Antoni A areas are present but are much more loosely packed. Antoni B areas usually show degenerative changes such as myxoid change, cyst formation, stromal hemorrhage, and calcification.

Aside from the classic features of schwannoma, several histologic variants have been described, some of which have characteristic clinical features. Rarely, a plexiform architecture may be present (plexiform schwannoma); these tumors are commonly superficial and located on the trunk.[283, 284] In contrast to plexiform neurofibromas, they are usually not associated with neurofibromatosis and do not undergo malignant degeneration. Rare schwannomas may be composed of highly cellular Antoni A areas without Antoni B areas (Fig. 46–71). Mitotic figures may be numerous, up to 1 per high-power field.[285–287] These tumors commonly occur in deep-seated regions such as the retroperitoneum. On occasion, marked atypia can be seen in schwannomas. This is usually seen in Antoni B areas in cells that are not mitotically active and is associated with degenerative changes; thus, the designation ancient schwannoma has been applied to these variants.[288] Ancient schwannomas also occur in large tumors in

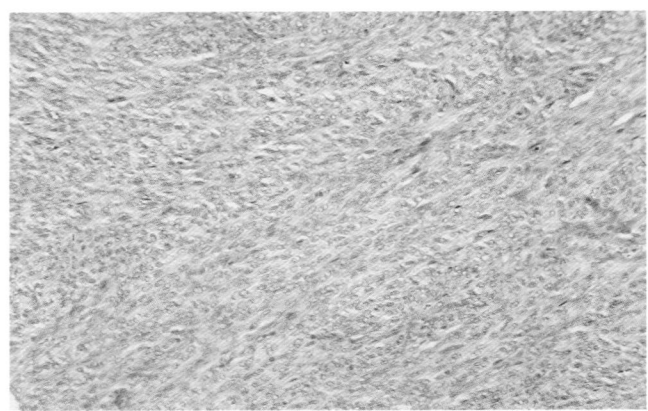

FIGURE 46–71. Benign cellular schwannoma. Although cellularity is markedly increased in this example, the lesion otherwise had typical features of schwannoma, including encapsulation.

deep-seated regions. Rarely, schwannomas may be associated with melanin formation.[289]

Ultrastructural studies of schwannomas show Schwann cells with abundant and redundant basal lamina. The Schwann cells have interdigitating cell processes. On immunohistochemical analysis, schwannomas have consistent expression of S-100 protein, present in all or nearly all the Schwann cells. The cells in Antoni A areas are more strongly labeled than are the cells in Antoni B areas, but the Antoni B areas are still consistently positive. In addition, collagen IV stains show a characteristic strong expression around individual cells. In addition, there may be variable expression of glial fibrillary acidic protein and CD57.

The differential diagnosis of schwannoma includes neurofibroma, malignant peripheral nerve sheath sarcoma, and other benign and malignant spindle cell tumors. In contrast to neurofibroma, schwannoma shows a true capsule, lacks true nerves within the mass, and has more consistent S-100 protein expression in the spindle cells. Malignant peripheral nerve sheath sarcoma is difficult to distinguish from cellular schwannoma. However, cellular schwannoma usually lacks atypia in the mitotically active areas, may have small Antoni B areas, and has more consistent S-100 protein expression. Both neoplasms may show foci of necrosis, but these areas are usually limited in cellular schwannoma and not rimmed by atypical cells. The consistent S-100 protein positivity should distinguish schwannoma from most non-neural benign and malignant spindle cell tumors. One should always seek out the presence of a true capsule and Antoni B areas to suggest the possibility of a schwannoma in the differential diagnosis of a spindle cell tumor.

## Neurofibroma[282]

Neurofibroma is another relatively common benign neural tumor. Neurofibromas occur in all age groups but are most common in young adults; there

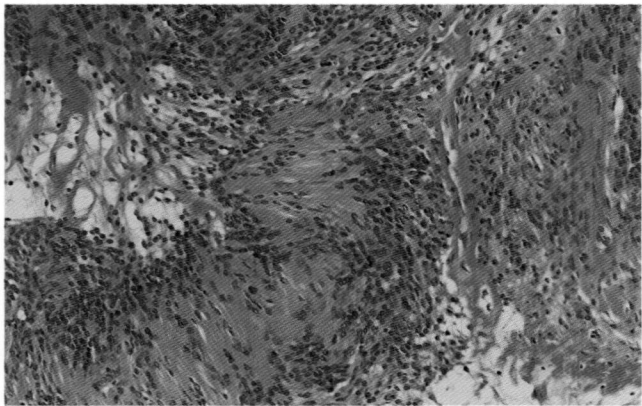

FIGURE 46–70. Benign schwannoma. Antoni A areas containing Verocay bodies predominate. Focal Antoni B areas, containing hyalinized vessels, are also present.

is no sex predilection. About 90% occur sporadically, whereas about 10% occur in the setting of neurofibromatosis type 1 or type 2. Neurofibromas occur much more commonly in neurofibromatosis type 1. Neurofibromatosis type 1 is 10 times more common than neurofibromatosis type 2 and is characterized by café au lait spots, neurofibromas, freckling, optic gliomas, iris hamartomas, and skeletal abnormalities. It is an autosomal dominant syndrome caused by abnormalities in the *NF1* gene, a tumor suppressor gene on chromosome 17. This gene encodes the protein neurofibromin, a microtubule-associated protein.

Neurofibromas arise within the nerve. They may occur in the skin or subcutaneous tissue (solitary neurofibroma) or the deep soft tissues, usually axial. Patients generally present with a painless skin lesion, a deep-seated mass, or other stigmata of neurofibromatosis type 1. Although these lesions do not recur after removal, the excision may have morbidity because the lesion arises within nerves. The gross lesion may be a small, rubbery, well-circumscribed superficial or deep nodule into which a nerve may occasionally be seen entering and exiting (localized neurofibroma); a poorly circumscribed, large subcutaneous mass (diffuse neurofibroma); or a large plexiform mass, which may be superficial or deep (plexiform neurofibroma). Localized and diffuse neurofibromas are usually not associated with neurofibromatosis type 1; diffuse neurofibromas tend to occur in children and young adults. The plexiform neurofibroma is diagnostic of neurofibromatosis type 1; it tends to occur in children and is often the first manifestation of the syndrome. It may be associated with abnormalities of the overlying skin and underlying bone (elephantiasis neuromatosa).

The localized neurofibroma is microscopically a circumscribed yet unencapsulated mass. The diffuse neurofibroma expands the subcutaneous tissue, spreading between individual fat cells and along fibrous septa. The plexiform neurofibroma is a mass of expanded nerves (Fig. 46–72). All three variants have similar proliferating elements, with a mixture of spindle cells, small nerves, and mast cells embed-

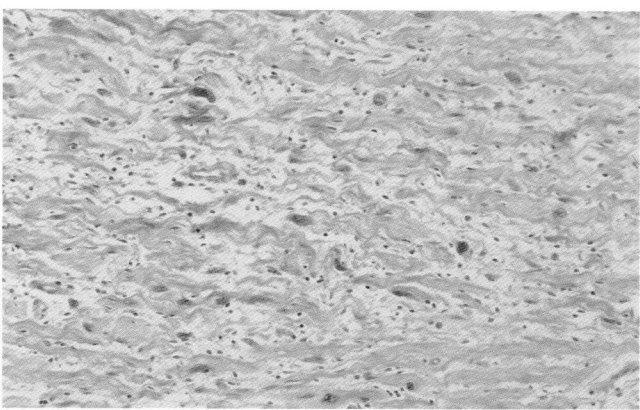

FIGURE 46–73. Benign neurofibroma with atypical cells. Mitotic activity was absent.

ded in a myxoid to collagenous stroma. The stroma is usually consistent within a single lesion and often contains ropy collagen fibers. Most of the spindle cells have wavy nuclei with pointed ends, similar to the cells of schwannoma. The cellularity is usually not high; however, a minority of neurofibromas may show mild to marked nuclear atypia (Fig. 46–73). Most lesions lack mitotic activity, but low mitotic activity may be seen in some. In a subset of lesions, structures resembling Pacini or Meissner corpuscles may be present; the latter are particularly common in the diffuse variant of neurofibroma. Rarely, neurofibromas may contain xanthoma cells, granular cells, melanin production, epithelioid cells, glandular structures, rosettelike structures, or cells showing rhabdomyosarcomatous differentiation.[290]

Ultrastructural studies demonstrate that the spindle cells of neurofibroma consist predominantly of Schwann cells, with an admixture of perineurial cells and fibroblasts. The Schwann cells are enveloped by a basal lamina. In virtually all cases, a significant subset (up to 50%) of the spindle cells stain for S-100 protein. In addition, there is usually staining for collagen IV around many of the spindle cells. Flow cytometric studies demonstrate a diploid DNA content.

The differential diagnosis of neurofibroma includes schwannoma, malignant peripheral nerve sheath sarcoma, and a variety of benign and malignant non-neural neoplasms. Schwannomas are encapsulated, lack nerves within the lesion, and have a greater proportion of cells expressing S-100 protein, and most schwannomas have a more variable appearance within a given lesion (with Antoni A and B areas). Rare schwannomas may have a plexiform appearance, but the proliferation within the nerve bundles is that of schwannoma rather than neurofibroma in those cases. Dermatofibrosarcoma may have a close resemblance to the diffuse variant of neurofibroma; both lesions infiltrate the subcutaneous tissue, leaving the adipose cells intact. However, dermatofibrosarcoma is CD34$^+$ and S-100 protein negative, whereas neurofibroma is CD34$^-$ and S-100 protein positive. The S-100 protein expression serves

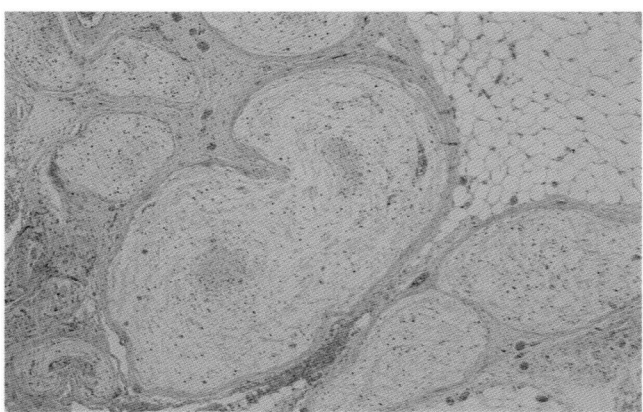

FIGURE 46–72. Benign neurofibroma. A plexiform pattern is illustrated.

to distinguish neurofibroma from most non-neural spindle cell tumors. The most important and the most difficult distinction is between neurofibroma and malignant peripheral nerve sheath sarcoma. This is complicated by the fact that about 2% of the neurofibromas arising in neurofibromatosis type 1 may show malignant degeneration; this is particularly true of plexiform neurofibromas. Typically, a preexisting neurofibroma undergoes rapid enlargement or begins to cause pain. Small (less than 5 cm) neurofibromas may have some cytologic atypia associated with low mitotic activity and areas of increased cellularity.[291] However, mitotic activity greater than 1 mitosis per 10 high-power fields, particularly when the lesion is large, should probably be regarded as malignant.

## Perineurioma[292-295]

Perineurioma is a rare tumor derived from the perineurium of nerves. It occurs predominantly in middle-aged adults and has a predilection for women. There is no association with neurofibromatosis. It occurs in subcutaneous or deep soft tissues, most often on the limbs or trunk. One variant, the sclerosing perineurioma, has a predilection for the fingers and palms of young adults. Patients with perineurioma usually present with a painless mass. The lesion is completely benign, with no reports of recurrence. At gross evaluation, the mass is well circumscribed and usually less than 5 cm in diameter.

There is a close microscopic resemblance to neurofibroma or meningioma. There is a proliferation of elongated spindle cells with loose storiform or short fascicular growth patterns (Fig. 46–74). Cellularity may vary. Cellular atypia and mitoses are generally absent. The sclerosing variant shows abundant dense collagen and variable numbers of small, epithelioid, and spindled cells with corded, trabecular, and whorled growth patterns. Ultrastructural studies

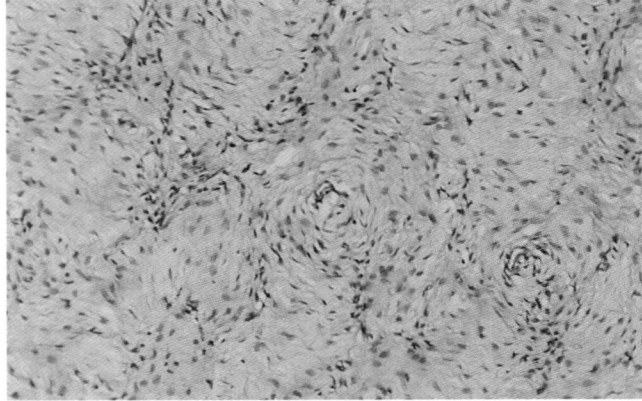

**FIGURE 46–74.** Perineurioma. There is a loose spindle cell proliferation, forming whorls. This lesion stained for epithelial membrane antigen.

show evidence of perineurial differentiation, with an elongated cell process with basal lamina and pinocytotic vesicles. Immunohistochemical studies show consistent reactivity for epithelial membrane antigen and negativity for S-100 protein.[296] Collagen IV stains show positivity around single cells. Sporadic positivity for keratin, muscle-specific actin, and smooth muscle–specific actin has also been reported.

The differential diagnosis includes neurofibroma, which may be histologically indistinguishable from perineurioma, and meningioma. The epithelial membrane antigen positivity distinguishes perineurioma from neurofibroma, and the S-100 protein negativity distinguishes it from most cases of meningioma. The sclerosing variant of perineurioma may be difficult to distinguish histologically from fibroma of tendon sheath; again, the immunohistochemical studies are of great use.

## Malignant Peripheral Nerve Sheath Sarcoma (Malignant Schwannoma, Neurofibrosarcoma, Neurogenic Sarcoma)[297-310]

Malignant peripheral nerve sheath sarcoma is one of the more common soft tissue sarcomas. About one third to one half of cases arise in the setting of neurofibromatosis type 1; approximately 2% of patients with neurofibromatosis develop a malignant peripheral nerve sheath sarcoma. Another 10% of cases of malignant peripheral nerve sheath sarcoma follow radiation. The sarcomas may occur de novo or in a preexistent neurofibroma; rarely, they may arise in a preexistent schwannoma or ganglioneuroma. They occur in a wide age range, with a predilection for young adults. Patients with a neurofibromatosis type 1 develop sarcomas about 10 years earlier in life than those without the syndrome do. There is an overall male predominance, accounted for by a marked predilection for the occurrence of malignant peripheral nerve sheath sarcoma in men with neurofibromatosis type 1.

Malignant peripheral nerve sheath sarcomas are usually deep-seated masses that arise in association with major nerve trunks. They most commonly occur in the proximal extremities and the trunk. Patients present with enlarging masses, often accompanied by pain. Rapid enlargement of a preexisting neurofibroma with the development of pain in a patient with neurofibromatosis type 1 is a common history. The 5-year survival is about 50%. Patients with neurofibromatosis type 1 tend to do worse, but this may be due to the fact that their neoplasms tend to be larger and more deeply seated. The worst survival is seen in patients with postirradiation sarcomas. At gross evaluation, malignant peripheral nerve sheath sarcomas are usually large, typically greater than 5 to 10 cm in diameter. There is often an attached major nerve, and a preexisting benign neoplasm may occasionally be identified grossly. On cut section, malignant peripheral nerve sheath sarcoma is tan and often shows areas of necrosis.

Malignant peripheral nerve sheath sarcomas usually have the histologic appearance of a nondescript spindle cell sarcoma, similar to the appearance of fibrosarcoma or a monophasic synovial sarcoma (Fig. 46–75). Low-magnification features that might favor the diagnosis of malignant peripheral nerve sheath sarcoma include the presence of densely cellular areas alternating with less cellular myxoid areas; a perivascular increase in cellularity, often with extension into the vessel walls; extensive perineural or intraneural spread of tumor (nerves should be specifically sampled when margins are assessed); plexiform areas; peculiar nodular whorled structures suggestive of tactile corpuscular differentiation; and extensive geographic areas of necrosis. Rarely, nuclear palisading may be seen, but this feature is actually more common in smooth muscle tumors. A high-magnification feature that might favor the diagnosis of malignant peripheral nerve sheath sarcoma is the presence of wavy nuclei with pointy ends. Pleomorphism and hyperchromatism are usually present, and mitotic figures are usually easy to find. Occasional epithelioid variants are seen.[311, 312] About 10% of cases contain heterologous elements, which may include chondrosarcoma, osteosarcoma, rhabdomyosarcoma (malignant triton tumor), angiosarcoma, liposarcoma, and even benign-appearing mucinous glands; heterologous elements may be more common in the malignant peripheral nerve sheath sarcomas arising in association with neurofibromatosis type 1.[297, 313]

Ultrastructural studies identify schwannian features in most cases, with long processes containing microtubules and neurofilaments, occasional junctional complexes, and variable amounts of basal lamina. Immunohistochemical studies show positivity for S-100 protein in about 75% of cases. In contrast to the benign neural tumors, the staining for S-100 protein is often only in a small percentage of the spindle cells. In addition, there is expression of myelin basic protein and CD57 in about 50% of cases and expression of glial fibrillary acidic protein, keratin, and muscle-specific actin in a small subset of cases. Collagen IV is variable but outlines individual neoplastic cells in well-differentiated examples. Cytogenetic studies have revealed a variety of abnormalities, including structural abnormalities of chromosomes 17 and 22 (the sites of the genes in neurofibromatosis type 1 and type 2, respectively).[85]

The differential diagnosis is broad and includes benign schwannoma (particularly cellular schwannoma), neurofibroma, and other sarcomas. Benign schwannoma may have mitotic activity but usually lacks atypia in the mitotically active areas, usually contains Antoni B areas, and has more consistent S-100 protein expression in all or virtually all spindle cells. Both neoplasms may show foci of necrosis, but these areas are usually limited in schwannoma and not rimmed by atypical cells. Neurofibroma may be extremely difficult to distinguish from malignant peripheral nerve sheath sarcoma, particularly when one is evaluating a neurofibroma for evidence of sarcomatous transformation. The presence of necrosis, mitotic activity greater than 1 mitosis per 10 high-power fields, and marked cytologic atypia favor the diagnosis of malignant peripheral nerve sheath sarcoma. Malignant peripheral nerve sheath sarcoma may be extremely difficult to distinguish from fibrosarcoma, monophasic synovial sarcoma, leiomyosarcoma, and even malignant fibrous histiocytoma. Within this differential diagnosis, the diagnosis of malignant peripheral nerve sheath sarcoma can be made with the identification of a major nerve in association with the tumor or the expression of S-100 protein in the absence of other markers characteristic of other types of sarcoma. S-100 protein may be expressed in synovial sarcoma, and keratin may be expressed in malignant peripheral nerve sheath sarcoma; the keratin positivity in monophasic synovial sarcoma is usually clustered, whereas the keratin positivity in malignant peripheral nerve sheath sarcoma is more randomly distributed. Malignant peripheral nerve sheath sarcomas may have heterologous glands, raising the differential with biphasic synovial sarcoma, but the glands in malignant peripheral nerve sheath sarcoma are often mucinous and have an abrupt transition to the spindle cell elements; those in synovial sarcoma usually lack mucinous features entirely and show transitions between the spindle cell areas and the glands.

Prognostic features in malignant peripheral nerve sheath sarcoma include histologic grade, tumor size, location (deep unfavorable), presence of necrosis, age, history of radiation exposure, plexiform features (favorable), and presence of rhabdomyosarcomatous areas (unfavorable). Although patients with neurofibromatosis type 1 have a poor prognosis, this may be related to the frequently deep location and large size of the neoplasms.

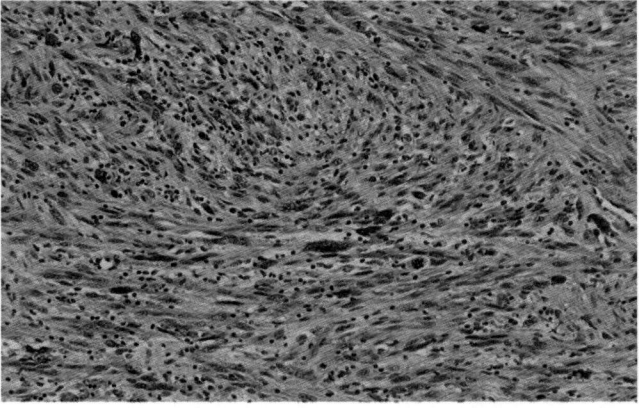

**FIGURE 46–75.** Malignant peripheral nerve sheath sarcoma. This example shows pleomorphism and high cellularity. This case arose in a patient with neurofibromatosis type 1.

## Peripheral Neuroectodermal Tumor and Extraosseous Ewing's Sarcoma[314–319]

These neoplasms are discussed together because they share many clinical, pathologic, and biologic similarities and probably represent essentially the same clinicopathologic entity. The neoplasm has also been referred to as primitive neuroectodermal tumor and Askin tumor. It occurs in a wide age range but primarily affects children and young adults; there is no sex predilection. Patients usually present with a rapidly growing, painful mass. A wide variety of sites may be involved, particularly the chest wall, paravertebral region, and lower extremity. Multidrug chemotherapy regimens represent the primary form of therapy, so that patients with these tumors may undergo only incisional biopsy. Modern intensive chemotherapy regimens have improved the formerly dismal survival of patients with these tumors to greater than 50%. Patients who do not survive generally succumb to disseminated disease. Consideration should be given to referral of patients with this neoplasm to a center that has experience with its treatment and participates in multi-institutional protocols. Cases with bone involvement seen radiologically should be considered primary bone tumors with secondary extension to soft tissue. The gross evaluation shows that the tumors are usually large (5 to 15 cm), are soft and fleshy on cut section, and often contain areas of hemorrhage and necrosis. In a minority of cases, attachment to nerves may be demonstrated.

At microscopic examination, most tumors involve the deep fascia or skeletal muscle. They consist of a small round cell proliferation that is present in sheets or packaged into ill-formed lobules and nests by a scanty cell-poor loose fibrovascular stroma (Fig. 46–76). The individual neoplastic cells range from small to intermediate (atypical large cell variant) and are usually uniform in size within a given case. Some have referred to dark and pale cell populations, but the dark cell population probably represents apoptotic cells. The neoplastic cells are usually round to oval but may occasionally show spindling. The cytoplasm ranges from scanty to moderate in amount. The nuclei are round to oval and generally have a fine chromatin pattern with small nucleoli. In cases in which larger cells are present, the nuclei tend to be larger and may possess a more prominent nucleolus. Mitotic figures are usually easy to identify. In occasional cases, Homer Wright–like rosettes are present, usually taken as evidence of neural differentiation consistent with peripheral neuroectodermal tumor rather than Ewing's sarcoma. The PAS stain is often positive.

Ultrastructural studies usually demonstrate abundant glycogen, perinuclear intermediate filaments, microtubules, variable numbers of dense-core granules, and cytoplasmic processes that interdigitate with one another. Cell junctions are usually present. The most consistent immunohistochemical findings are vimentin and CD99 (p30/32, MIC2) positivity.[320, 321] There is also variable expression of neural markers, including synaptophysin, chromogranin, neuron-specific enolase, S-100 protein, CD57, neurofilament, and neuron surface antigen. Some have proposed that the expression of two or more neural markers indicates peripheral neuroectodermal tumor rather than Ewing's sarcoma. Occasional cases may contain scattered keratin-positive cells, particularly when they are tested in frozen sections.

Cytogenetic studies have demonstrated a characteristic t(11;22)(q24;q12) (80% of cases) or t(21;22)(q22;q12) (10% of cases), in which the *FLI1* and *ERG* genes, respectively, are juxtaposed to the *EWS* gene to form a chimeric protein. A reverse transcription–polymerase chain reaction test is available that can detect both of the translocations in fresh or frozen tissue.[322] Those patients with fusion of *EWS* exon 7 to *FLI1* exon 6 may have a better prognosis[323]; this may be because this fusion product may encode a less active chimeric transcription factor.[324]

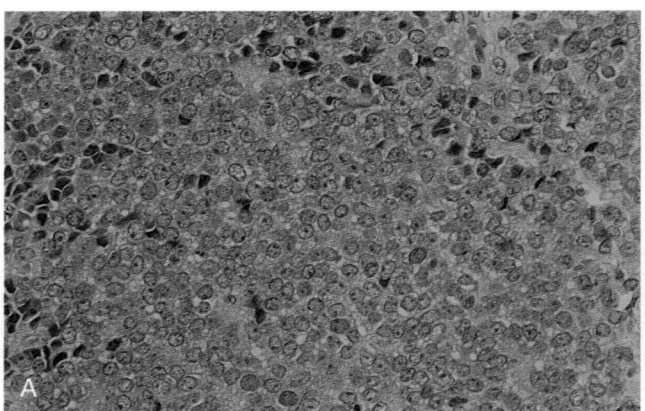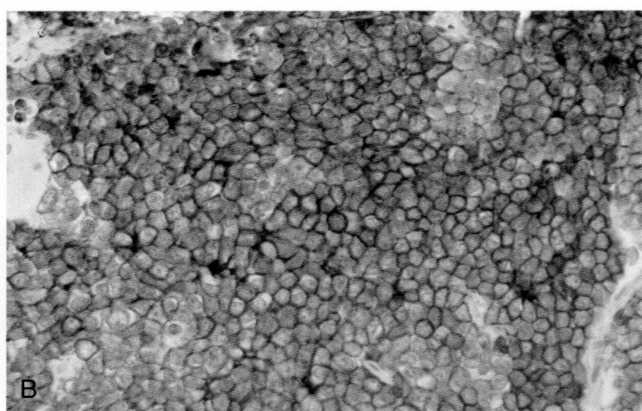

**FIGURE 46–76.** Peripheral neuroectodermal tumor/extraosseous Ewing's sarcoma. This case is a pure example of a small round blue cell tumor. There was strong diffuse staining for CD99.

The translocation may rarely involve similar genes on chromosomes 7, 2, or 17. Deletions of the *p16* tumor suppressor gene constitute the most frequent secondary molecular aberration.[325]

The differential diagnosis is that of a small round blue cell tumor. Malignant lymphoma, particularly lymphoblastic neoplasms, can histologically mimic peripheral neuroectodermal tumor/Ewing's sarcoma; furthermore, these tumors are also generally positive for CD99. However, they show nuclear positivity for terminal deoxyribonucleotidyl transferase and membrane positivity for other lymphoid markers such as CD45 and CD43. Rhabdomyosarcomas should show some reactivity for muscle markers such as desmin and muscle-specific actin. In contrast to peripheral neuroectodermal tumor/Ewing's sarcoma, neuroblastoma is a vimentin-negative and CD99⁻ neoplasm. It is impossible to distinguish extraosseous peripheral neuroectodermal tumor/Ewing's sarcoma from osseous examples unless radiologic studies have shown no involvement of adjacent bone.

Some but not most studies have claimed that peripheral neuroectodermal tumor, as defined by the presence of Homer Wright rosettes or the presence of two or more neuroendocrine immunohistochemical markers, has a worse prognosis than Ewing's sarcoma. If differences in prognosis exist, these are not terribly significant in this difficult to treat neoplasm.

## Desmoplastic Small Round Cell Tumor[326-330]

Desmoplastic small round cell tumor usually involves the abdominal or pelvic peritoneum of children or young adults. This neoplasm is more extensively discussed in Chapter 16. Only rare cases have been described in extraserosal locations.

## Malignant Melanoma of Soft Parts[331-337]

Malignant melanoma of soft parts is also known as clear cell sarcoma, because its behavior seems to be intermediate between a sarcoma and typical cutaneous malignant melanoma. It occurs primarily in young adults with a median age of 30 years; there is a predilection for women. Patients present with a long history of a deep-seated mass that is often painful. There should be no history of prior cutaneous malignant melanoma. The neoplasm occurs in the lower extremity in 75% of cases, particularly in the foot, ankle, and knee. The upper extremity, particularly the hand, is involved in about 20% of cases; the axial regions are a rare site of tumor. Malignant melanoma of soft parts treated with radical excision, which often requires amputation given its typi-

cal localization close to joints. Like cutaneous melanoma, malignant melanoma of soft parts spreads to regional lymph nodes, which should be incorporated into the surgical resection. Eventually, most patients develop recurrences and systemic metastases, although these may take a long time to manifest. Therefore, malignant melanoma of soft parts is often treated with adjuvant chemotherapy, radiotherapy, or both. Because of the rarity of the tumor, however, it is not clear whether these modalities are definitely beneficial. The gross neoplasm averages less than 5 cm and is usually intimately associated with tendons. Only a minority of cases show definite evidence of melanin pigment on cut section.

The histologic examination reveals the neoplasm centered around the deep fascia, often with infiltration of the overlying subcutaneous tissue and extension along nerves and tendons. Although it may extend to the deep dermis, there should not be any connection to or origin from the overlying epidermis. The neoplasm consists of loose fascicles and nests of neoplastic cells enclosed by delicate fibrous septa (Fig. 46–77). The individual cells, which typically have abundant clear or eosinophilic cytoplasm, may be round, oval, or spindled. The nuclei typically have a vesicular chromatin pattern and a prominent nucleolus. Many cases also contain osteoclast-like giant cells and multinucleated cells arranged in a wreath around the periphery of the cytoplasm (Touton giant cells), which are part of the neoplastic process. Only a minority of cases have histologically detectable melanin pigment, and this may require careful search. The mitotic rate is usually lower than expected for a melanoma, usually less than 1 mitosis per high-power field. PAS stains generally demonstrate abundant glycogen. Stains for melanin, such as the Fontana-Masson or Warthin-Starry stains, are positive in a majority of cases. Electron microscopic studies reveal melanosomes in varying stages of development. Immunohistochemical studies show strong positivity for vimentin and strong and consistent staining for HMB-45; the stain-

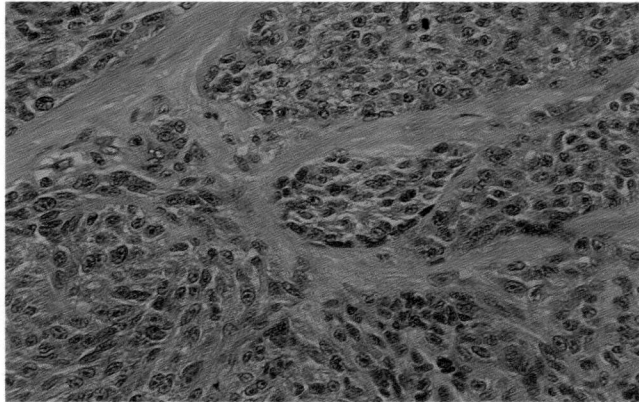

**FIGURE 46–77.** Malignant melanoma of soft parts (clear cell sarcoma). There are nests and fascicles of pale cells.

ing for HMB-45 is typically stronger and more consistent than is usually present in cutaneous melanoma. Interestingly, cytogenetic studies have demonstrated a characteristic t(12;22)(q13;q13) in most but not all cases; this is a specific marker for this neoplasm and is not present in cutaneous malignant melanoma.[338-340] In this translocation, the *EWS* on chromosome 12 (similar to Ewing's sarcoma/primitive neuroectodermal tumor) combines to a transcription factor called *ATF1*.[341, 342]

The differential diagnosis of malignant melanoma of soft parts includes cutaneous malignant melanoma as well as other sarcomas. To minimize the possibility of confusion with cutaneous malignant melanoma, there should be no history of cutaneous malignant melanoma, and there should be no evidence of involvement of the overlying epidermis; certainly, there must not be any evidence of junctional activity at the dermis-epidermis junction. Immunohistochemical studies for S-100 protein and HMB-45 should provide clear distinction from all other sarcomas. Malignant epithelioid schwannoma may have similar histologic findings and may be S-100 protein positive, but unless melanin pigment is present, a rare phenomenon in these neoplasms, malignant epithelioid schwannoma is HMB-45 negative, in contrast to the consistent and usually strong staining of HMB-45 in malignant melanoma of soft parts. Epithelioid sarcoma may resemble malignant melanoma of soft parts but is keratin positive and S-100 protein negative.

Clinical prognostic factors include age and adequacy of resection. Adverse pathologic prognostic factors are size of the lesion (greater than 5 cm), site of disease, depth, proliferation index, and demonstration of aneuploidy by flow cytometry.[336, 337, 343]

## TUMORS AND TUMORLIKE PROLIFERATIONS SHOWING CARTILAGINOUS OR CHORDOID DIFFERENTIATION

### Soft Tissue Chondroma[344, 345]

Soft tissue chondroma is a rare lesion that primarily affects middle-aged adults, although it may affect all age groups, including children. Patients usually present with a painless mass almost always in the hands or feet. The gross lesion is smaller than 3 cm, is lobulated and well demarcated, and may show areas of degeneration on cut section; it may be connected to adjacent tendon. Radiologic studies may demonstrate calcifications. Local recurrences may follow local excision, but metastasis or transformation to sarcoma should never occur.

The histologic examination reveals lobules of mature hyaline cartilage. Focal areas of increased cellularity, cytologic atypia, and even mitotic figures may be seen. Myxoid change may be seen and may even predominate, particularly in the center of the

lesion. Focal calcification or other degenerative changes may also be found. Immunohistochemical studies demonstrate positivity for S-100 protein, similar to normal cartilage.

The differential diagnosis includes chondromas of bone, synovial chondromatosis, and myxoid chondrosarcoma. The radiographic studies should help distinguish juxtacortical or periosteal chondroma from soft tissue chondroma. Synovial chondromatosis is similar histologically to soft tissue chondroma but may be distinguished clinically by its location adjacent to large joints. Myxoid chondrosarcoma is rare in the hands and feet and is almost always larger than 3 cm. The presence of mature cartilage at the periphery of the lesion strongly favors the diagnosis of chondroma.

### Parachordoma[346, 347]

Parachordoma is an extremely rare neoplasm that may occur in children or adults with a mean age of about 35 years. It presents as a slow-growing mass in the deep soft tissues, predominantly in the extremities. It generally behaves in a benign fashion, although recurrence is possible. At gross evaluation, it is usually a multinodular mass ranging from about 5 to 10 cm.

At microscopic examination, there are vague nodules of cords and nests of cells resembling those of chordoma in a myxoid or hyaline matrix (Fig. 46–78). The neoplastic cells are rounded and have large vesicular nuclei and vacuolated clear or eosinophilic cytoplasm. Occasional multivacuolated (physaliferous-like) cells are usually present in varying numbers. Parachordomas consistently express cytokeratins 8 and 18 but not other cytokeratins and are also positive for epithelial membrane antigen, S-100 protein, and vimentin. They have a linear pattern of type IV collagen immunoreactivity around nests of cells, which is distinct from chordoma or extraskeletal myxoid chondrosarcoma. Cytogenetic analysis in one case showed trisomy 15, without the

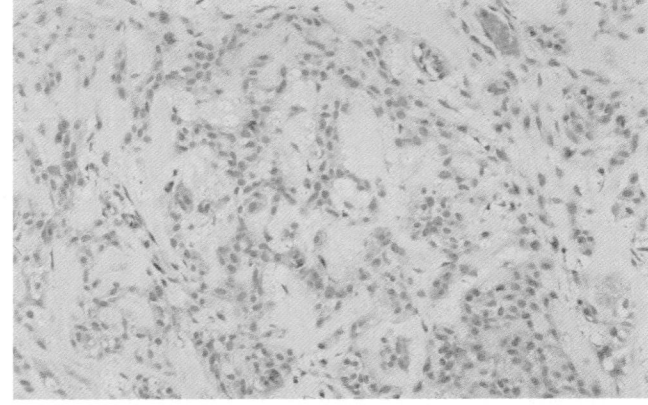

**FIGURE 46–78.** Parachordoma. There are cords of cells in a chondroid stroma. The cells of this case were positive for keratin.

t(9;22) characteristic of extraskeletal myxoid chondrosarcoma or the monosomies of various chromosomes that have been reported in chordoma. Parachordoma may be distinguished from a deeply situated adnexal tumor by the absence of myoepithelial markers (e.g., smooth muscle–specific actin).

## Myxoid Chondrosarcoma (Chordoid Sarcoma)[348-354]

Myxoid chondrosarcoma is a rare neoplasm that occurs predominantly in older adults; there is a male predominance. Patients usually present with a slow-growing mass that may be painful. The proximal extremities and the limb girdles are most often affected, particularly the thigh. Although the tumor is slow growing, recurrence or metastasis occurs in the majority of patients after wide local excision. Metastases most often occur in the lung and soft tissues, and patients may live for years with disease. The gross neoplasms are generally large, with a median size of around 5 to 10 cm, and are multilobular. On cut section, they are soft and fleshy and may show areas of cystic degeneration or hemorrhage.

A lobular histologic pattern is seen at low magnification, with intervening fibrous septa. The lobules are composed of myxoid stroma and polygonal to spindled cells. Foci of ill-formed chondroid areas are sometimes seen, but well-formed cartilage is rare. A prominent vascular network is not seen. The cells are often arranged in cords and strands, rings, and aggregates or are singly disposed (Fig. 46–79). They usually have a moderate rim of cytoplasm that may be vacuolated. Although the nuclei are frequently hyperchromatic, cytologic atypia is usually mild and mitotic activity is not abundant. On occasion, highly cellular areas are seen in which the cells may be round or spindled. Electron microscopic studies show prominent Golgi complex, abundant rough endoplasmic reticulum filled with dense granular material, and abundant glycogen; some cases

show bundles or parallel arrays of microtubules. Immunohistochemical studies demonstrate positivity for S-100 protein in many cases, and some cases are also positive for CD57 or neuron-specific enolase. Rare cases may be positive for keratin and other epithelial markers. Cytogenetic studies have revealed a t(9;22)(q22;12) in the majority of cases, in contrast to myxoid chondrosarcoma of bone.[355] The translocation involves the *EWS* gene on chromosome 22 (similar to several other malignant neoplasms, such as Ewing's sarcoma/primitive neuroectodermal tumor, desmoplastic small round cell tumor, and malignant melanoma of soft parts) and a novel gene on chromosome 9 designated *TEC*. Adverse prognostic factors include clinical features such as older age of the patient, larger tumor size, and tumor location in the proximal extremity or limb girdle; histologic features may not be predictive of survival.

The differential diagnosis includes soft tissue chondroma (discussed earlier), mixed tumor of salivary or sweat gland origin, chordoma, skeletal forms of myxoid chondrosarcoma, other myxoid sarcomas, and even cellular sarcomas such as Ewing's sarcoma/primitive neuroectodermal tumor or small cell variants of poorly differentiated synovial sarcoma. Salivary or sweat gland mixed tumors are positive for epithelial markers and occur in characteristic sites (salivary gland or skin). Chordoma is also consistently positive for keratin and other epithelial markers and usually occurs in an axial location. Skeletal forms of myxoid chondrosarcoma, including juxtacortical (parosteal) chondrosarcoma, usually show radiographic abnormalities and usually lack myxoid features. Myxoid malignant fibrous histiocytoma has a greater degree of nuclear pleomorphism, its cells are more uniformly spindled, and it generally lacks S-100 protein expression. Myxoid liposarcoma is generally S-100 protein positive but has a characteristic rich and plexiform capillary pattern. Ewing's sarcoma/primitive neuroectodermal tumor or small cell variants of poorly differentiated synovial sarcoma can be distinguished by their distinctive immunohistochemical and molecular profile.

## Mesenchymal Chondrosarcoma[356-358]

Mesenchymal chondrosarcoma, in contrast to myxoid chondrosarcoma, occurs predominantly in young adults and has a slight female predilection. It generally presents as a painless or painful slow-growing mass. It most often occurs in the soft tissue of the orbit or the proximal extremities, particularly the thigh. Again in contrast to myxoid chondrosarcoma, mesenchymal chondrosarcoma is a high-grade neoplasm, with a high metastatic rate—usually to lung—and poor survival. The gross tumors are generally much larger, often greater than 10 cm. They are fleshy on cut section but may have focal areas of cartilage or calcification.

At histologic examination, a distinct biphasic neoplasm is seen (Fig. 46–80). In one portion, there

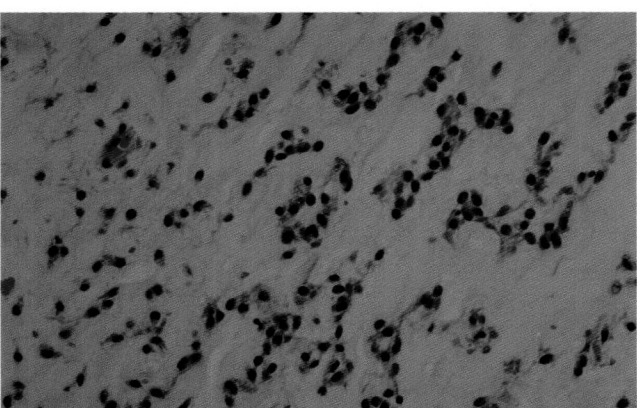

**FIGURE 46–79.** Myxoid chondrosarcoma. Strands of chondroid cells in a myxoid background are seen.

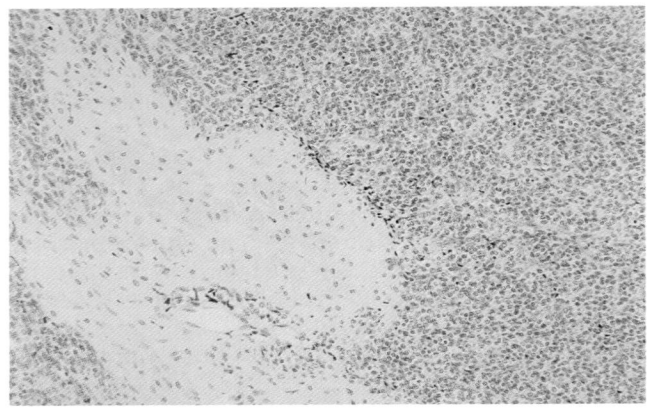

**FIGURE 46–80.** Mesenchymal chondrosarcoma. Most of the field shows an undifferentiated sarcoma, which is interrupted by distinct cartilaginous areas.

are well-formed hyaline cartilaginous nodules. These nodules have abrupt transition to areas of poorly differentiated sarcoma. The poorly differentiated sarcoma may be composed of undifferentiated round or oval cells, or it may be indistinguishable from hemangiopericytoma. Ultrastructural studies demonstrate features of cartilaginous differentiation in the cartilaginous areas and no clear differentiating features in the undifferentiated areas. The cartilaginous areas and scattered less differentiated cells are S-100 protein positive. The undifferentiated areas are generally negative for all markers, including CD99.

The differential diagnosis includes small round blue cell tumors such as Ewing's sarcoma/peripheral neuroectodermal tumor, hemangiopericytoma, and other sarcomas with a hemangiopericytoma-like pattern, and osteosarcoma. The identification of chondroid areas rules out both small round blue cell tumors and hemangiopericytoma, but of course, these areas may not be present in a small biopsy specimen. On rare occasions, sarcomas with a hemangiopericytomatous pattern may have metaplastic cartilage; other differentiated features should be sought. Osteosarcoma arises in the differential diagnosis; however, malignant osteoid, the defining feature of osteosarcoma, should be absent.

## TUMORS AND TUMORLIKE PROLIFERATIONS SHOWING OSTEOGENIC DIFFERENTIATION

### Myositis Ossificans[359–361]

Myositis ossificans is a rare lesion that primarily affects young adults, with a male predilection. However, it can affect all age groups. Patients present with a rapidly growing mass that is usually centered in skeletal muscle but may also occur in the subcutaneous tissue. Rarely, multiple lesions are seen; in children, this is an autosomal dominant hereditary syndrome, usually in association with skeletal abnormalities such as malformation or absence of one or more digits (fibrodysplasia ossificans progressiva). Myositis ossificans involves the extremities in most cases. The lesion usually resolves if it is left untreated (although it may continue to grow for a short time) and does not recur if it is completely excised. Radiographs generally demonstrate a well-circumscribed lesion with peripheral calcification. The gross lesions usually measure about 5 cm and are well circumscribed. On cut section, the center is soft; the periphery is gritty or shows obvious calcification.

At histologic examination, myositis ossificans shows a distinct zonal phenomenon. The center of the lesion resembles nodular fasciitis, with a loose spindle cell proliferation (Fig. 46–81). Mitotic figures may be numerous, but atypical forms are generally not seen. There is a transition zone that contains active bone formation, with osteoid often admixed with chondroid areas. External to this is a layer of mature lamellar bone, also rimmed by osteoblasts (Fig. 46–82). This is surrounded by a thin layer of compressed fibrous tissue.

The most important differential diagnosis is with extraskeletal osteosarcoma. Attention to the zoning phenomenon, the lack of cytologic atypia, and particularly the lack of atypical cells in between osteoid seams should distinguish myositis ossificans from osteosarcoma. Radiographs may be necessary to distinguish myositis ossificans from a primary bone lesion, such as a fracture callus.

### Extraskeletal Osteosarcoma[362–365]

Extraskeletal osteosarcoma is extremely rare, representing only 1% to 5% of all osteosarcoma. In contrast to conventional osteosarcoma, extraskeletal osteosarcoma most often affects older adults; there is a

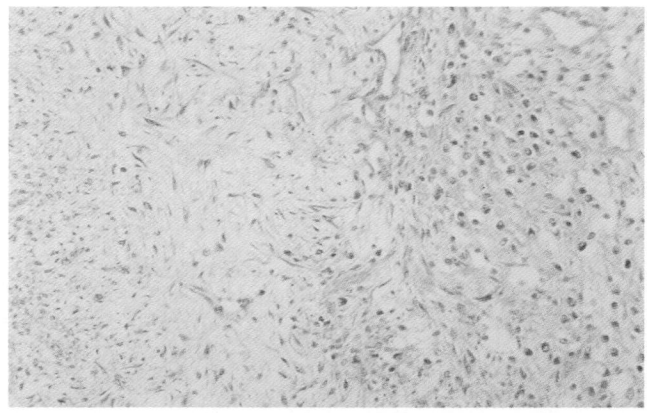

**FIGURE 46–81.** Myositis ossificans. At one end, an area indistinguishable from nodular fasciitis is seen; at the other end, immature but orderly osteoid is present.

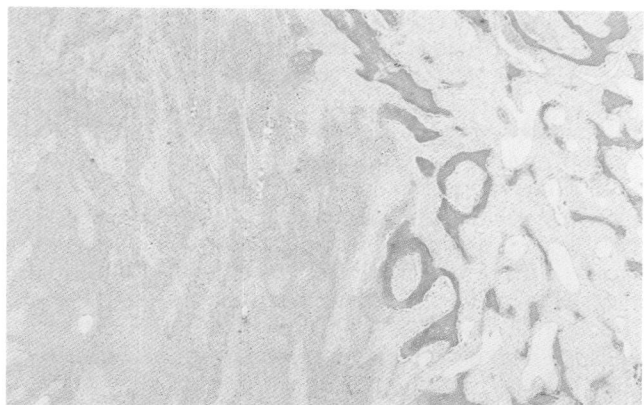

**FIGURE 46–82.** Myositis ossificans. At one side, there is osteoid formation; at the other end, there is mature bone.

slight male predilection. Patients present with a mass, which may be painful. A subset of cases are associated with radiation, occurring 3 years or more after radiation therapy. The neoplasm usually occurs in skeletal muscle, most often in or near the extremities, particularly the thigh, or the retroperitoneum. The prognosis is extremely poor, and patients should be treated with modern protocols used for conventional osteosarcoma. Radiologic studies are essential to exclude connection with the underlying bone. The gross lesion is usually larger than 5 cm, may or may not appear circumscribed, and may be either soft or firm and gritty.

The histologic appearance is similar to that of conventional osteosarcoma. The neoplasm usually shows a high degree of atypia associated with at least some osteoid formation. It may be predominantly osteoblastic, fibroblastic (simulating the giant cell variant of malignant fibrous histiocytoma), or chondroblastic (simulating chondrosarcoma), or it may contain a predominance of osteoclast-like giant cells (simulating the giant cell variant of malignant fibrous histiocytoma). However, in my opinion and like the situation in skeletal osteosarcoma, if the lesion contains at least focal clear-cut evidence of neoplastic osteoid formation, it should be considered an osteosarcoma. As stated before, extraskeletal osteosarcoma can be distinguished from myositis ossificans by the cellular atypia and the absence of a zoning phenomenon where more mature bone is seen at the periphery; in fact, in extraskeletal osteosarcoma, the areas appearing most osseous are often centrally located.

## MALIGNANT MESENCHYMOMA[366, 367]

Malignant mesenchymoma is defined as a spindle cell sarcoma showing two or more specific lines of frankly malignant mesenchymal differentiation as recognized histologically in addition to any undiffer-

entiated, fibrosarcomatous, or hemangiopericytomatous areas. However, by convention, malignant schwannoma with rhabdomyosarcoma (malignant triton tumor) is usually excluded. As defined, it is a rare neoplasm, with few large series. Patients are usually elderly and most often present with a large soft tissue mass, most commonly in the retroperitoneum or the thigh. Clinically, these neoplasms have generally been regarded as high grade, although one series has suggested less aggressive behavior.[367]

Malignant mesenchymoma most often microscopically contains components of rhabdomyosarcoma, liposarcoma, osteosarcoma or chondrosarcoma, or malignant schwannoma (Fig. 46–83). Either the two components coexist as major components within the same neoplasm, or one component predominates with foci—usually osteosarcomatous or chondrosarcomatous—of the second component. The predominant and least differentiated component should be used in determining the grade of the neoplasm. Carcinosarcomas (keratin positive) and malignant mixed mesodermal tumors (history of gynecologic tumor) should be considered in the differential diagnosis.

## MALIGNANT LYMPHOMA

Malignant lymphomas involving the soft tissues usually represent the sites of secondary spread from a local lymph node or the thymus. True primary lymphomas involving the soft tissues are rare but may most often involve the extremities.[368] Some cases are associated with a history of immunosuppression; rare lymphomas have been described arising at the site of injection of an immunosuppressant drug. The most common histologic appearance is large cell lymphoma (Fig. 46–84). The survival is similar to that of primary large cell lymphoma arising in other extranodal sites, unless there is a history of immunosuppression.

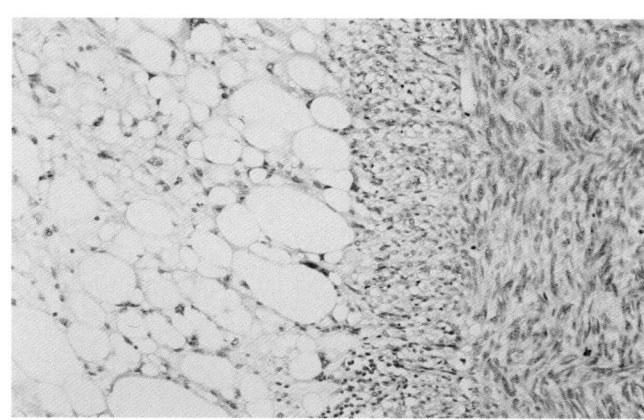

**FIGURE 46–83.** Malignant mesenchymoma. At one side is a liposarcoma, with an abrupt transition to a leiomyosarcoma.

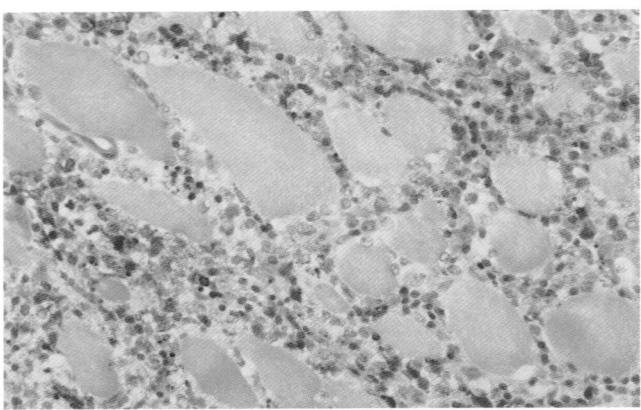

**FIGURE 46–84.** Diffuse large cell lymphoma. Lymphoma cells encircle skeletal muscle fibers.

## NON-NEOPLASTIC PROLIFERATIONS

### Infectious Disease

Necrotizing fasciitis is a disease that is rapidly increasing in incidence.[369] It is most commonly due to group A streptococcus but also may be caused by *Clostridium perfringens, Clostridium septicum,* or even mixed microorganisms. At histologic examination, one sees extensive necrosis, a comparably mild acute inflammatory infiltrate, and numerous bacteria (Fig. 46–85). Organisms including fungi and bacteria may cause the formation of abscesses, which may have thick fibrous capsules, simulating a neoplasm. In addition, organisms may induce a chronic inflammatory process with a high content of foamy macrophages, simulating inflammatory malignant fibrous histiocytoma; this lesion has a predilection for the retroperitoneum, where it has been termed retroperitoneal xanthogranuloma. In addition, acid-fast organisms or, even more rarely, other bacterial organisms can cause formation of fibrohistiocytic proliferations, again closely simulating fibrous histiocy-

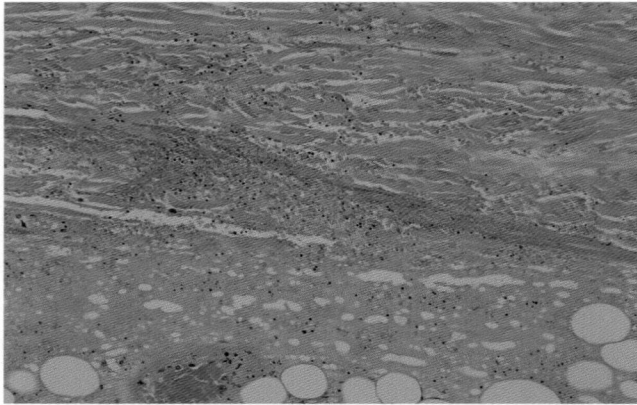

**FIGURE 46–85.** Necrotizing fasciitis. There is widespread necrosis. The blue haze represents numerous coccal organisms.

toma. This has been particularly well described for leprosy, in which it has been termed histoid leprosy, but in this era, it occurs more often in immunocompromised individuals, particularly from atypical mycobacteria. Another rare reaction to bacteria occurring primarily in immunocompromised individuals is bacillary angiomatosis.[370] In this disease, infection by *Bartonella henselae* or possibly other related species causes a vascular proliferation of small capillaries with an epithelioid endothelial lining, with numerous admixed acute inflammatory cells. In addition, there is often a fibrillar material in the extracellular matrix, which represents clumps of bacteria that may be identified with a Warthin-Starry stain.

Malacoplakia represents an unusual host reaction to a variety of bacterial antigens, usually those of gram-negative bacteria.[371, 372] Most often occurring in (but not limited to) soft tissues around the genitourinary tract or the colon, this host reaction consists of sheets of bland histiocytes along with acute and chronic inflammatory cells. The histiocytes contain iron- and calcium-positive cytoplasmic spherules termed Michaelis-Gutmann bodies as well as PAS-positive, diastase-resistant cytoplasmic granules. Although the lesions are usually sterile by stain and culture, electron microscopic studies may demonstrate scattered organisms within the histiocytes.

### Noninfectious Histiocyte Proliferations

A variety of histiocyte proliferations may occur in the soft tissues. Most result from a reaction to foreign materials. A histiocyte reaction to silica may be secondary to the now-discontinued practice of injection therapy for hernia.[373] These lesions present in the inguinal region or abdominal wall, many years after the injection of silica, and grossly are ill-defined masses. Histologic examination shows sheets of histiocytes, which may have various degrees of cytologic atypia, along with various amounts of fibrosis. Once the diagnosis is suspected, polarization demonstrates refractile intracellular and extracellular silica crystals. The sites of vaccination may also show similar reactions, possibly because of the inorganic vehicles in which the vaccine proteins are mixed; this is particularly common after tetanus vaccine.[374] Alternatively, the vaccination sites may show necrobiotic granulomas or may be more inflammatory in nature. In contrast to silica reaction, the interval between the injection and the clinical findings is usually short. In addition, a histiocytic reaction may result from exposure to polyvinylpyrrolidone, a material that has been used as a plasma expander or a vehicle in various intravenous preparations[375, 376] (Fig. 46–86). In this instance, there are collections of cytologically bland histiocytes and occasional multinucleated giant cells, without inflammatory cells or necrosis. The histiocytes contain a blue material in H&E-stained sections. The material is mucicarmine positive but does not stain for PAS or Giemsa. The

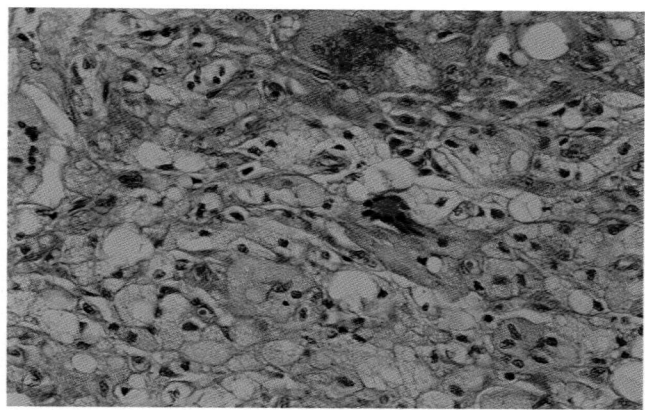

**FIGURE 46–86.** Histiocytic reaction due to polyvinylpyrrolidone. There are sheets of histiocytes, including foamy macrophages and multinucleated giant cells.

mucicarmine positivity may raise the differential of a metastatic carcinoma, but the nuclear features of the histiocytes are completely bland. A granular cell reaction may occur at the site of trauma, usually surgically induced. There is usually a central zone of amorphous debris or necrosis, with a peripheral accumulation of histiocytes with a granular cytoplasm. In contrast to a granular cell tumor, the granules are larger, more variable in size, and acid-fast positive.

Histiocyte reactions may also rarely be due to abnormal nonforeign materials. Crystal-storing histiocytosis represents a reaction to abnormally high amounts of immunoglobulins.[377] In this lesion, there is a proliferation of cytologically bland histiocytes with abundant polygonal cytoplasm containing crystalline inclusions. If the abnormal immunoglobulins are produced locally, there may be an accompanying infiltrate of lymphoplasmacytoid cells, occasionally with Dutcher bodies. The crystalline inclusions may mimic the cross-striations of rhabdomyoma or rhabdomyosarcoma, but these cells are negative for

muscle markers and strongly positive for the lysosomal marker CD68.

Rosai-Dorfman disease may rarely affect soft tissues, most often in the orbit.[378, 379] Patients may or may not have concomitant nodal disease; those with only extranodal disease tend to be older than those with nodal disease. Patients with soft tissue involvement tend to present with painless masses, unless compromise of vital structures is present. The histologic appearance in the soft tissues is similar to that seen in the lymph node, although there is often more extensive fibrosis and less prominent lymphophagocytosis (Fig. 46–87). Immunohistochemistry to demonstrate S-100 protein positivity in the proliferating histiocytes usually distinguishes soft tissue Rosai-Dorfman disease from morphologic simulants.

## REFERENCES

1. Coffin CM: Pediatric Soft Tissue Tumors. Baltimore, Williams & Wilkins, 1997.
2. Enzinger FM, Weiss SW: Soft Tissue Tumors. 2nd ed. St. Louis, CV Mosby, 1988.
3. Parker SL, Tong T, Bolden S, Wingo PA: Cancer statistics, 1997. CA Cancer J Clin 47:5–27, 1997.
4. Mulvihill JJ, Parry DM, Sherman JL, et al: Neurofibromatosis 1 (Recklinghausen disease) and neurofibromatosis 2 (bilateral acoustic neurofibromatosis). Ann Intern Med 113:39–52, 1990.
5. Malkin D, Li FP, Strong LC, et al: Germ line *p53* mutations in a familial syndrome of breast cancer, sarcomas, and other neoplasms. Science 250:1233–1238, 1990.
6. Malkin D, Jolly KW, Barbier N, et al: Germline mutations of the *p53* tumor-suppressor gene in children and young adults with second malignant neoplasms. N Engl J Med 326:1309–1315, 1992.
7. Shanks JA, Paranchych W, Tuba J: Familial multiple lipomatosis. Can Med Assoc J 77:881, 1957.
8. Arlen M, Higinbotham NL, Huvos AG, et al: Radiation-induced sarcoma of bone. Cancer 28:1087–1099, 1971.
9. Chang Y, Cesarman E, Pessin MS, et al: Identification of herpesvirus-like DNA sequences in AIDS-associated Kaposi's sarcoma. Science 266:1865–1869, 1994.
10. Moore PS, Chang Y: Detection of herpesvirus-like DNA sequence in AIDS-associated Kaposi's sarcoma lesions from persons with and without HIV infection. N Engl J Med 332:1181–1185, 1995.
11. McClain KL, Leach CT, Jenson HB, et al: Association of Epstein-Barr virus with leiomyosarcomas in children with AIDS. N Engl J Med 332:12–18, 1995.
12. Stewart FW, Treves N: Lymphangiosarcoma in postmastectomy lymphedema. Cancer 1:64–81, 1949.
13. Fingerhut MA, Halperin WE, Marlow DA: Cancer mortality in workers exposed to 2,3,7,8-tetrachlorodibenzo-*p*-dioxin. N Engl J Med 324:212–218, 1991.
14. Mertens F, Akerman M, Dal Cin P, et al: Cytogenetic analysis of 46 pleomorphic soft tissue sarcomas and correlation with morphologic and clinical features: a report of the CHAMP Study Group. Genes Chromosomes Cancer 22:16–25, 1998.
15. Mohamed AN, Zalupski MM, Ryan JR, et al: Cytogenetic aberrations and DNA ploidy in soft tissue sarcoma. A Southwest Oncology Group Study. Cancer Genet Cytogenet 99:45–53, 1997.
16. Latres E, Drobnjak M, Pollack D, et al: Chromosome 17 abnormalities and *TP53* mutation in adult soft tissue sarcomas. Am J Pathol 145:345–355, 1994.
17. Taubert H, Wurl P, Bache M, et al: The p53 gene in soft tissue sarcomas: prognostic value of DNA sequencing versus immunohistochemistry. Anticancer Res 18:183–187, 1998.
18. Cordon-Cardo C, Latres E, Drobnjak M, et al: Molecular

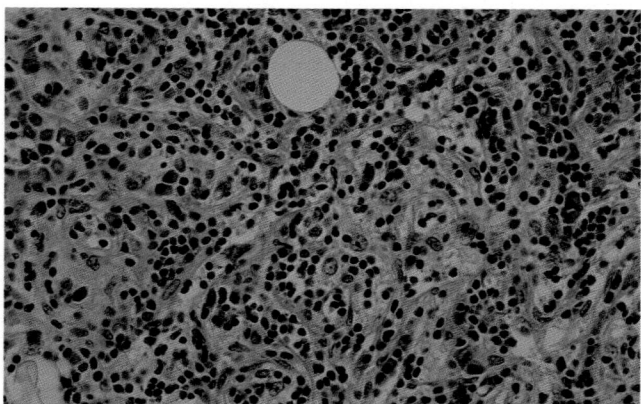

**FIGURE 46–87.** Rosai-Dorfman disease involving the soft tissues. The characteristic histiocytic cells with vesicular nuclei are seen, although the lesion is usually more fibrotic than the typical appearance in lymph nodes.

abnormalities of *mdm2* and *p53* genes in adult soft tissue sarcomas. Cancer Res 54:794–799, 1994.

19. Wurl P, Meye A, Berger D, et al: Prognostic relevance of C-terminal Mdm2 detection is enhanced by p53 positivity in soft tissue sarcomas. Diagn Mol Pathol 6:249–254, 1997.

20. Wurl P, Meye A, Berger D, et al: Significance of retinoblastoma and *mdm2* gene expression as prognostic markers for soft-tissue sarcoma. Langenbecks Arch Surg 383:99–103, 1998.

21. Karpeh MS, Brennan MF, Cance WG, et al: Altered patterns of retinoblastoma gene product expression in adult soft-tissue sarcomas. Br J Cancer 72:986–991, 1995.

22. George E, Niehans GA, Swanson PE, et al: Overexpression of the *c-erbB*-2 oncogene in sarcomas and small round-cell tumors of childhood. An immunohistochemical investigation. Arch Pathol Lab Med 116:1033–1035, 1992.

23. Stein U, Shoemaker RH, Schlag PM: *MDR1* gene expression: evaluation of its use as a molecular marker for prognosis and chemotherapy of bone and soft tissue sarcomas. Eur J Cancer 32A:86–92, 1996.

24. Coindre JM, Trojani M, Contesso G, et al: Reproducibility of a histopathologic grading system for adult soft tissue sarcoma. Cancer 58:306–309, 1986.

25. Costa J, Wesley RA, Glatstein E, Rosenberg SA: The grading of soft tissue sarcomas. Results of a clinicohistopathologic correlation in a series of 163 cases. Cancer 53:530–541, 1984.

26. Guillou L, Coindre J-M, Bonichon F, et al: Comparative study of the National Cancer Institute and French Federation of Cancer Centers Sarcoma Group Grading System in a population of 410 adult patients with soft tissue sarcomas. J Clin Oncol 15:350–362, 1997.

27. Parham DM, Webber BL, Jenkins JJ III, et al: Nonrhabdomyosarcomatous soft tissue sarcomas of childhood: formulation of a simplified system for grading. Mod Pathol 8:705–710, 1995.

28. Fleming ID, Cooper JS, Hensen DE, et al: AJCC Cancer Staging Manual. 5th ed. Philadelphia, JB Lippincott, 1997.

29. Li XQ, Parkekh SG, Rosenberg AE, Mankin HJ: Assessing prognosis for high-grade soft-tissue sarcomas: search for a marker. Ann Surg Oncol 3:550–557, 1996.

30. Schneider-Stock R, Radig K, Oda Y, et al: p53 mutations in soft-tissue sarcomas—correlations with p53 immunohistochemistry and DNA ploidy. J Cancer Res Clin Oncol 123: 211–218, 1997.

31. Collin F, Chassevent A, Bonichon F, et al: Flow cytometric DNA content analysis of 185 soft tissue neoplasms indicates that S-phase fraction is a prognostic factor for sarcomas. French Federation of Cancer Centers (FNCLCC) Sarcoma Group. Cancer 79:2371–2379, 1997.

32. Drobnjak M, Latres E, Pollack D, et al: Prognostic implications of p53 nuclear overexpression and high proliferation index of Ki-67 in adult soft-tissue sarcomas. J Natl Cancer Inst 86:549–554, 1994.

33. Golouh R, Bracko M, Novak J: Predictive value of proliferation-related markers, p53, and DNA ploidy for survival in patients with soft tissue spindle-cell sarcomas. Mod Pathol 9: 919–924, 1996.

34. Heslin MJ, Cordon-Cardo C, Lewis JJ, et al: Ki-67 detected by MIB-1 predicts distant metastasis and tumor mortality in primary, high grade extremity soft tissue sarcoma. Cancer 83:490–497, 1998.

35. Niezabitowski A, Rys J, Roessner A, et al: Assessment of proliferative activity, DNA values and some clinicopathologic parameters in mesenchymal tumors. Immunohistochemical and flow cytometric study. Gen Diagn Pathol 142: 327–333, 1997.

36. Plaat BE, Muntinghe FL, Molenaar WM, et al: Clinical outcome of patients with previously untreated soft tissue sarcomas in relation to tumor grade, DNA ploidy karyotype. Int J Cancer 74:396–402, 1997.

37. Rudolph P, Bonichon F, Gloeckner ZK, et al: Comparative analysis of prognostic indicators for sarcomas of the soft parts of the viscerae. Verh Dtsch Ges Pathol 82:246–252, 1998.

38. Stefanou DG, Nonni AV, Agnantis NJ, et al: p53/MDM-2 immunohistochemical expression correlated with proliferative activity in different subtypes of human sarcomas: a ten-year follow-up study. Anticancer Res 18:4673–4681, 1998.

39. Taubert H, Meye A, Wurl P: Prognosis is correlated with p53 mutation type for soft tissue sarcoma patients. Cancer Res 56:4134–4136, 1996.

40. Singer S: New diagnostic modalities in soft tissue sarcoma. Semin Surg Oncol 17:11–22, 1999.

41. Chang AE, Sondak VK: Clinical evaluation and treatment of soft tissue tumors. *In* Enzinger FM, Weiss SW (eds): Soft Tissue Tumors. St. Louis, Mosby–Year Book, 1995, pp 17–38.

42. Association of Directors of Anatomic and Surgical Pathology: Recommendations for reporting soft tissue sarcomas. Am J Clin Pathol 111:594–598, 1999.

43. Allen PW: Tumors and Proliferations of Adipose Tissue: A Clinicopathologic Approach. New York, Masson Publishing, 1981.

44. Fletcher CDM, Martin-Bates E: Intramuscular and intermuscular lipoma: neglected diagnoses. Histopathology 12:275–287, 1988.

45. Willen H, Akerman M, Da Cin P, et al: Comparison of chromosomal patterns with clinical features in 165 lipomas: a report of the CHAMP study group. Cancer Genet Cytogenet 102:46–49, 1998.

46. Sciot R, Akerman M, Da Cin P, et al: Cytogenetic analysis of subcutaneous angiolipoma: further evidence supporting its difference from ordinary pure lipomas: a report of the CHAMP study group. Am J Surg Pathol 21:441–444, 1997.

47. Meis JM, Enzinger FM: Myolipoma of soft tissue. Am J Surg Pathol 15:121–125, 1991.

48. Meis JM, Enzinger FM: Chondroid lipoma. A unique tumor simulating liposarcoma and myxoid chondrosarcoma. Am J Surg Pathol 17:1103–1112, 1993.

49. Fletcher CDM, Martin-Bates E: Spindle cell lipoma: a clinicopathological study with some original observations. Histopathology 11:803–817, 1987.

50. Shmookler BM, Enzinger FM: Pleomorphic lipoma: a benign tumor simulating liposarcoma. A clinicopathologic analysis of 48 cases. Cancer 47:126–133, 1981.

51. Fletcher CD, Akerman M, Dal Cin P, et al: Correlation between clinicopathological features and karyotype in lipomatous tumors. A report of 178 cases from the Chromosomes and Morphology (CHAMP) Collaborative Study Group. Am J Pathol 148:623–630, 1996.

52. Hunter SB, Schemakewitz EH, Patterson C, Varma VA: Extraadrenal myelolipoma. A report of two cases. Am J Clin Pathol 97:402–404, 1992.

53. Hruban RH, Bhagavan BS, Epstein JI: Massive retroperitoneal angiomyolipoma. A lesion that may be confused with well-differentiated liposarcoma. Am J Clin Pathol 92:445–455, 1989.

54. Chan JKC, Tsang WYW, Pau MY, et al: Lymphangiomyomatosis and angiomyolipoma: closely related entities characterized by hamartomatous proliferation of HMB-45 positive smooth muscle. Histopathology 22:445–455, 1993.

55. Collins MH, Chatten J: Lipoblastoma/lipoblastomatosis: a clinicopathologic study of 25 tumors. Am J Surg Pathol 21: 1131–1137, 1997.

56. Mentzel T, Calonje R, Fletcher CDM: Lipoblastoma and lipoblastomatosis: a clinicopathological study of 14 cases. Histopathology 23:527–533, 1993.

57. Gaffney EF, Hargreaves HK, Semple E, Vellios F: Hibernoma: distinctive light and electron microscopic features and relationship to brown adipose tissue. Hum Pathol 14:677–687, 1983.

58. Enzi G: Multiple symmetric lipomatosis: updated clinical report. Medicine (Baltimore) 63:56–64, 1984.

59. Evans HL, Soule EH, Winkelmann RK: Atypical lipoma, atypical intramuscular lipoma and well differentiated retroperitoneal liposarcoma. A reappraisal of 30 cases formerly classified as well differentiated liposarcoma. Cancer 43:574–584, 1979.

60. Evans HL: Liposarcomas and atypical lipomatous tumors: a study of 66 cases followed for a minimum of 10 years. Surg Pathol 1:41–54, 1988.

61. Azumi N, Curtis J, Kempson RL, Hendrickson MR: Atypical and malignant neoplasms showing lipomatous differentiation. A study of 111 cases. Am J Surg Pathol 11:161–183, 1987.
62. Shmookler BM, Enzinger FM: Liposarcoma occurring in children. An analysis of 17 cases and review of the literature. Cancer 52:567–574, 1993.
63. Smith TA, Easley KA, Goldblum JR: Myxoid/round cell liposarcoma of the extremities: a clinicopathologic study of 29 cases with particular attention to extent of round cell liposarcoma. Am J Surg Pathol 20:171–180, 1996.
64. Weiss SW, Rao VK: Well-differentiated liposarcoma (atypical lipoma) of deep soft tissue of the extremities, retroperitoneum and miscellaneous sites. A follow-up study of 92 cases with analysis of the incidence of "dedifferentiation." Am J Surg Pathol 16:1051–1058, 1992.
65. Rosai J, Akerman M, Cin PD, et al: Combined morphologic and karyotypic study of 59 atypical lipomatous tumors: evaluation of their relationship and differential diagnosis with other adipose tissue tumors (a report of the CHAMP study group). Am J Surg Pathol 20:1182–1189, 1996.
66. Mandahl N, Akerman M, Aman P, et al: Duplication of chromosome segment 12q15–35 is associated with atypical lipomatous tumors: a report of the CHAMP collaborative study group. Int J Cancer 67:632–635, 1996.
67. Henricks WH, Chu YC, Goldblum JR, Weiss SW: Dedifferentiated liposarcoma: a clinicopathological analysis of 155 cases with a proposal for an expanded definition of dedifferentiation. Am J Surg Pathol 21:271–287, 1997.
68. McCormick D, Mentzel T, Beham A, Fletcher CDM: Dedifferentiated liposarcoma: clinicopathologic analysis of 32 cases suggesting a better prognostic subgroup among pleomorphic sarcomas. Am J Surg Pathol 18:1213–1223, 1994.
69. Tallini G, Akerman M, Dal Cin P, et al: Combined morphologic and karyotypic study of 28 myxoid liposarcomas: implications for a revised morphologic typing (a report from the CHAMP Group). Am J Surg Pathol 20:1047–1055, 1996.
70. Perosio PM, Weiss SW: Ischemic fasciitis: a juxta-skeletal fibroblastic proliferation with a predilection for elderly patients. Mod Pathol 6:69–72, 1993.
71. Montgomery EA, Meis JM, Mitchell MS, Enzinger FM: Atypical decubital fibroplasia. A distinctive fibroblastic pseudotumor occurring in debilitated patients. Am J Surg Pathol 16:708–715, 1992.
72. Lauer DH, Enzinger FM: Cranial fasciitis of childhood. Cancer 45:401–406, 1980.
73. Konwaler BE, Keasbey L, Kaplan L: Subcutaneous pseudosarcomatous fibromatosis (fasciitis). Am J Clin Pathol 25:241–252, 1955.
74. Bernstein KE, Lattes R: Nodular (pseudosarcomatous) fasciitis, a non-recurrent lesion: clinicopathologic study of 134 cases. Cancer 49:1668–1678, 1982.
75. Meister P, Buckmann FW, Konrad E: Extent and level of fascial involvement in 100 cases with nodular fasciitis. Virchows Arch A Pathol Anat Histopathol 380:177–185, 1978.
76. Montgomery EA, Meis JM: Nodular fasciitis. Its morphologic spectrum and immunohistochemical profile. Am J Surg Pathol 15:942–948, 1991.
77. Patchefsky AS, Enzinger FM: Intravascular fasciitis. A report of 17 cases. Am J Surg Pathol 5:29–36, 1981.
78. Shimizu S, Hashimoto H, Enjoji M: Nodular fasciitis: an analysis of 250 patients. Pathology 16:161–166, 1984.
79. Meis JM, Enzinger FM: Proliferative fasciitis and myositis of childhood. Am J Surg Pathol 16:364–372, 1992.
80. Chung EB, Enzinger FM: Proliferative fasciitis. Cancer 36:1450–1458, 1975.
81. Goodlad JR, Fletcher CDM: Solitary fibrous tumour arising at unusual sites: analysis of a series. Histopathology 19:515–522, 1991.
82. Nascimento AG: Solitary fibrous tumor: a ubiquitous neoplasm of mesenchymal differentiation. Adv Anat Pathol 3:388–395, 1996.
83. Suster S, Nascimento AG, Miettinen M, et al: Solitary fibrous tumors of soft tissue: a clinicopathologic and immunohistochemical study of 12 cases. Am J Surg Pathol 19:1257–1266, 1995.
84. Vallat-Decouvelaere A-V, Dry SM, Fletcher CDM: Atypical and malignant solitary fibrous tumors in extrathoracic locations: evidence of their comparability to intra-thoracic tumors. Am J Surg Pathol 22:1501–1511, 1998.
85. Fletcher CD, Akerman M, Dal Cin P, et al: Correlation between clinicopathologic features and karyotype in spindle cell sarcomas: a report of 130 cases from the CHAMP study group. Am J Pathol 154:1841–1847, 1999.
86. Barr JR: Elastofibroma. Am J Clin Pathol 45:679–683, 1966.
87. Michal M, Fetsch JF, Hes O, Miettinen M: Nuchal-type fibroma: a clinicopathologic study of 52 cases. Cancer 85:156–163, 1999.
88. O'Connell JX: Nuchal fibrocartilaginous pseudotumor: a distinctive soft-tissue lesion associated with prior neck injury. Am J Surg Pathol 21:836–840, 1997.
89. Balachandran K, Allen PW, MacCormac LB: Nuchal fibroma: a clinicopathologic study of nine cases. Am J Surg Pathol 19:313–317, 1995.
90. Miettinen M, Fetsch JF: Collagenous fibroma (desmoplastic fibroblastoma): a clinicopathologic analysis of 63 cases of a distinctive soft tissue lesion with stellate-shaped fibroblasts. Hum Pathol 29:676–682, 1998.
91. Chung EB, Enzinger FM: Fibroma of tendon sheath. Cancer 44:1945–1954, 1979.
92. Humphreys S, McKee PH, Fletcher CDM: Fibroma of tendon sheath: a clinicopathologic study. J Cutan Pathol 13:331–338, 1986.
93. Pulitzer DR, Martin PC, Reed RJ: Fibroma of tendon sheath. A clinicopathologic study of 32 cases. Am J Surg Pathol 13:472–479, 1989.
94. Satti MB: Tendon sheath tumours: a pathological study of the relationship between giant cell tumour and fibroma of tendon sheath. Histopathology 20:213–220, 1992.
95. Ushijima M, Tsuneyoshi M, Enjoji M: Dupuytren type fibromatosis. A clinicopathologic study of 62 cases. Acta Pathol Jpn 34:991–1001, 1984.
96. Paller AS, Gonzalez-Crussi F, Sherman JO: Fibrous hamartoma of infancy. Eight additional cases and a review of the literature. Arch Dermatol 125:88–91, 1989.
97. Briselli MF, Soule EH, Gilchrist GS: Congenital fibromatosis. Report of 18 cases of solitary and 4 cases of multiple tumors. Mayo Clin Proc 55:554–562, 1980.
98. Chung EB, Enzinger FM: Infantile myofibromatosis. Cancer 48:1807–1818, 1981.
99. Fletcher CDM, Achu P, van Noorden S, McKee PH: Infantile myofibromatosis: a light microscopic, histochemical and immunohistochemical study suggesting true smooth muscle differentiation. Histopathology 11:245–258, 1987.
100. Mentzel T, Calonje E, Nascimento AG, Fletcher CD: Infantile haemangiopericytoma versus infantile myofibromatosis: a study of a series suggesting a spectrum of infantile myofibroblastic lesions. Am J Surg Pathol 18:922–930, 1994.
101. Daimaru Y, Hashimoto H, Enjoji M: Myofibromatosis in adults (adult counterpart of infantile myofibromatosis). Am J Surg Pathol 13:859–865, 1989.
102. Allen PW: Recurring digital fibrous tumours of childhood. Pathology 4:215–223, 1972.
103. Reye RDK: Recurring digital fibrous tumors in childhood. Arch Pathol 80:228–231, 1965.
104. Keasbey LE: Juvenile aponeurotic fibroma (calcifying fibroma). A distinctive tumor arising in the palms and soles of young children. Cancer 6:338–346, 1953.
105. Allen PW, Enzinger FM: Juvenile aponeurotic fibroma. Cancer 26:857–867, 1970.
106. Allen PW: The fibromatoses: a clinicopathologic classification based on 140 cases. Part I. Am J Surg Pathol 1:255–270, 1977.
107. Das Gupta TK, Brasfield RD, O'Hara J: Extra-abdominal desmoids: a clinicopathologic study. Ann Surg 170:109–121, 1969.
108. Burke AP, Sobin LH, Shekitka KM, et al: Intra-abdominal fibromatosis. A pathologic analysis of 130 tumors with comparison of clinical subgroups. Am J Surg Pathol 14:335–341, 1990.
109. Hayry P, Reitamo JJ, Totterman S, et al: The desmoid tumor.

II. Analysis of factors possibly contributing to the etiology and growth behavior. Am J Clin Pathol 77:674–680, 1982.

110. Yokoyama R, Tsuneyoshi M, Enjoji M: Extra-abdominal desmoid tumors: correlations between histologic features and biologic behavior. Surg Pathol 2:29–42, 1989.

111. Ayala AG, Ro JY, Goepfert H, et al: Desmoid fibromatosis: a clinicopathologic study of 25 children. Semin Diagn Pathol 3:138–150, 1986.

112. Jones IT, Jagelman DJ, Fazio VW, et al: Desmoid tumors in familial polyposis coli. Ann Surg 204:94–97, 1986.

113. Coffin CM, Watterson J, Priest JR, Dehner LP: Extrapulmonary inflammatory myofibroblastic tumor (inflammatory pseudotumor): a clinicopathologic and immunohistochemical study of 84 cases. Am J Surg Pathol 19:859–872, 1995.

114. Meis JM, Enzinger FM: Inflammatory fibrosarcoma of the mesentery and retroperitoneum. A tumor closely simulating inflammatory pseudotumor. Am J Surg Pathol 15:1146–1156, 1991.

115. Biselli R, Ferlini C, Fattorossi A, et al: Inflammatory myofibroblastic tumor (inflammatory pseudotumor): DNA flow cytometric analysis of nine pediatric cases. Cancer 77:778–784, 1996.

116. Sciot R, Dal Cin P, Fletcher CD, et al: Inflammatory myofibroblastic tumor of bone: report of two cases with evidence of clonal chromosomal changes. Am J Surg Pathol 21:1166–1172, 1997.

117. Evans HL: Low-grade fibromyxoid sarcoma. A report of 12 cases. Am J Surg Pathol 17:595–600, 1993.

118. Evans HL: Low-grade fibromyxoid sarcoma. A report of two metastasizing neoplasms having deceptively benign appearance. Am J Clin Pathol 88:615–619, 1987.

119. Scott SM, Reiman HM, Pritchard DJ, Ilstrup DM: Soft tissue fibrosarcoma. A clinicopathologic study of 132 cases. Cancer 64:925–931, 1989.

120. Schofield DE, Fletcher JA, Grier HE, Yunis EJ: Fibrosarcoma in infants and children. Application of new techniques. Am J Surg Pathol 18:14–24, 1994.

121. Knezevich SR, McFadden DE, Tao W, et al: A novel ETV6-NTRK3 gene fusion in congenital fibrosarcoma. Nat Genet 18:184–187, 1998.

122. Enzinger FM: Intramuscular myxoma. A review and follow-up study of 34 cases. Am J Clin Pathol 43:104–113, 1965.

123. Hashimoto H, Tsuneyoshi M, Daimaru Y, et al: Intramuscular myxoma. A clinicopathologic, immunohistochemical and electron microscopic study. Cancer 58:740–747, 1986.

124. Ireland DCR, Soule EH, Ivins JC: Myxoma of somatic soft tissues. A report of 58 patients, 3 with multiple tumors and fibrous dysplasia of bone. Mayo Clin Proc 48:401–410, 1973.

125. Kindblom L-G, Stener B, Angervall L: Intramuscular myxoma. Cancer 34:1737–1744, 1974.

126. Nielsen GP, O'Connell JX, Rosenberg AE: Intramuscular myxoma: a clinicopathologic study of 51 cases with emphasis on hypercellular and hypervascular varients. Am J Surg Pathol 22:1222–1227, 1998.

127. Skalova A, Michal M, Husek K, et al: Aggressive angiomyxoma of the pelvioperineal region. Immunohistological and ultrastructural study of seven cases. Am J Dermatopathol 15:446–451, 1993.

128. Steeper TA, Rosai J: Aggressive angiomyxoma of the female pelvis and perineum. Report of nine cases of a distinctive type of gynecologic soft tissue neoplasm. Am J Surg Pathol 7:463–475, 1983.

129. Enzinger FM, Weiss SW, Liang CY: Ossifying fibromyxoid tumor of soft parts. A clinicopathologic analysis of 59 cases. Am J Surg Pathol 13:817–827, 1989.

130. Kilpatrick SE, Ward WG, Mozes M, et al: Atypical and malignant variants of ossifying fibromyxoid tumor: clinicopathologic analysis of six cases. Am J Surg Pathol 19:1039–1046, 1995.

131. Miettinen M: Ossifying fibromyxoid tumor of soft parts. Additional observations of a distinctive soft tissue tumor. Am J Clin Pathol 95:142–149, 1991.

132. Schofield JB, Krausz T, Stamp GWH, et al: Ossifying fibromyxoid tumour of soft parts—immunohistochemical and ultrastructural analysis of a series. Histopathology 22:101–112, 1993.

133. Fletcher CDM: Benign fibrous histiocytoma of subcutaneous and deep soft tissue: a clinicopathologic analysis of 21 cases. Am J Surg Pathol 14:801–809, 1990.

134. Ushijima M, Hashimoto H, Tsuneyoshi M, Enjoji M: Giant cell tumor of the tendon sheath (nodular tenosynovitis). A study of 207 cases to compare the large joint group with the common digit group. Cancer 57:875–884, 1986.

135. Wood GS, Beckstead JH, Medeiros LG, et al: The cells of giant cell tumor of tendon sheath resemble osteoclasts. Am J Surg Pathol 12:444–452, 1988.

136. Hollowood K, Holley MP, Fletcher CDM: Plexiform fibrohistiocytic tumour: clinicopathological, immunohistochemical and ultrastructural analysis in favour of a myofibroblastic lesion. Histopathology 19:503–513, 1991.

137. Enzinger FM, Zhang RY: Plexiform fibrohistiocytic tumor presenting in children and young adults. An analysis of 65 cases. Am J Surg Pathol 12:818–826, 1988.

138. Remstein ED, Arndt CAS, Nascimento AG: Plexiform fibrohistiocytic tumor: clinicopathologic analysis of 22 cases. Am J Surg Pathol 23:662–670, 1999.

139. Costa MJ, Weiss SW: Angiomatoid malignant fibrous histiocytoma. A follow-up study of 108 cases with evaluation of possible histologic predictors of outcome. Am J Surg Pathol 14:1126–1132, 1990.

140. Enzinger FM: Angiomatoid malignant fibrous histiocytoma. A distinct fibrohistiocytic tumor of children and young adults simulating a vascular neoplasm. Cancer 44:2147–2157, 1979.

141. Fletcher CDM: Angiomatoid "malignant fibrous histiocytoma": an imunohistochemical study indicative of myoid differentiation. Hum Pathol 22:563–568, 1991.

142. Pettinato G, Manivel JC, Rosa GD, et al: Angiomatoid malignant fibrous histiocytoma: cytologic, immunohistochemical, ultrastructural and flow cytometric study of 20 cases. Mod Pathol 3:479–487, 1990.

143. Mentzel T, Fletcher CDM: Recent advances in soft tissue tumor diagnosis. Am J Clin Pathol 110:660–670, 1998.

144. Dei Tos AP, Seregard S, Calonje E, et al: Giant cell angiofibroma. A distinctive orbital tumor in adults. Am J Surg Pathol 19:1286–1293, 1995.

145. Mikami Y, Shimizu M, Hirokawa M, Manabe T: Extraorbital giant cell angiofibromas. Mod Pathol 10:1082–1087, 1997.

146. Shmookler BM, Enzinger FM, Weiss SW: Giant cell fibroblastoma. A juvenile form of dermatofibrosarcoma protuberans. Cancer 64:2154–2161, 1989.

147. Fletcher CDM: Giant cell fibroblastoma of soft tissue: a clinicopathological and immunohistochemical study. Histopathology 13:499–508, 1988.

148. Dei Tos AP, Dal Cin P: The role of cytogenetics in the classification of soft tissue tumours. Virchows Arch 431:83–94, 1997.

149. Alguacil-Garcia A: Giant cell fibroblastoma recurring as dermatofibrosarcoma protuberans. Am J Surg Pathol 15:798–801, 1991.

150. Taylor HB, Helwig EB: Dermatofibrosarcoma protuberans. Cancer 15:717–725, 1962.

151. Fletcher CD, Evans BJ, MacArtney JC, et al: Dermatofibrosarcoma protuberans: a clinicopathological and immunohistochemical study with a review of the literature. Histopathology 9:921–938, 1985.

152. Frierson HF, Cooper PH: Myxoid variant of dermatofibrosarcoma protuberans. Am J Surg Pathol 7:445–450, 1983.

153. Connelly JH, Evans HL: Dermatofibrosarcoma protuberans: a clinicopathologic review with emphasis on fibrosarcomatous areas. Am J Surg Pathol 16:921–925, 1992.

154. Mentzel T, Beham A, Katenkamp D, et al: Fibrosarcomatous ("high grade") dermatofibrosarcoma protuberans: clinicopathologic and immunohistochemical study of a review of 41 cases with emphasis on prognostic significance. Am J Surg Pathol 22:576–587, 1998.

155. Hisaoka M, Okamoto S, Morimitsu Y, et al: Dermatofibrosarcoma protuberans with fibrosarcomatous areas. Molecular abnormalities of the p53 pathway in fibrosarcomatous transformation of dermatofibrosarcoma protuberans. Virchows Arch 433:323–329, 1998.

156. Smith MEF, Fisher C, Weiss SW: Pleomorphic hyalinizing angiectatic tumor of soft parts. A low-grade neoplasm resembling neurilemoma. Am J Surg Pathol 20:21–29, 1996.
157. Meis-Kindblom JM, Kindblom LG: Acral myxoinflammatory fibroblastic sarcoma: a low-grade tumor of the hands and feet. Am J Surg Pathol 22:911–924, 1998.
158. Montgomery EA, Devaney KO, Giordano TJ, Weiss SW: Inflammatory myxohyaline tumor of distal extremities with virocyte or Reed-Sternberg–like cells: a distinctive lesion with features simulating inflammatory conditions, Hodgkin's disease, and various sarcomas. Mod Pathol 11:384–391, 1998.
159. Enzinger FM: Malignant fibrous histiocytoma 20 years after Stout. Am J Surg Pathol 10(suppl 1):43–53, 1986.
160. Fletcher CDM: Pleomorphic malignant fibrous histiocytoma: fact or fiction? A critical reappraisal based of 159 tumors diagnosed as pleomorphic sarcoma. Am J Surg Pathol 16:213–228, 1992.
161. Guccion JG, Enzinger FM: Malignant giant cell tumor of soft parts. An analysis of 32 cases. Cancer 29:1518–1529, 1972.
162. Kyriakos M, Kempson RL: Inflammatory fibrous histiocytoma. An aggressive and lethal lesion. Cancer 37:1584–1606, 1976.
163. Mentzel T, Calonje E, Wadden C, et al: Myxofibrosarcoma: clinicopathologic analysis of 75 cases with emphasis on the low-grade variant. Am J Surg Pathol 20:391–405, 1996.
164. Merck C, Angervall L, Kindblom L-G: Myxofibrosarcoma. A malignant soft tissue tumour of fibroblastic-histiocytic origin. A clinicopathologic and prognostic study of 110 cases using multivariate analysis. Acta Pathol Microbiol Immunol Scand Suppl 282:1–40, 1983.
165. Weiss SW, Enzinger FM: Myxoid variant of malignant fibrous histiocytoma. Cancer 39:1672–1685, 1977.
166. Hashimoto H, Daimaru Y, Enjoji M: Intravascular papillary endothelial hyperplasia. A clinicopathologic study of 91 cases. Am J Dermatopathol 5:539–545, 1983.
167. Kuo TT, Sayers CP, Rosai J: Masson's "vegetant intravascular hemangioendothelioma": a lesion often mistaken for angiosarcoma. Study of seventeen cases located in the skin and soft tissues. Cancer 38:1227–1236, 1976.
168. Pins MR, Rosenthal DI, Springfield DS, Rosenberg AE: Florid extravascular papillary endothelial hyperplasia (Masson's pseudoangiosarcoma) presenting as a soft tissue sarcoma. Arch Pathol Lab Med 117:259–263, 1993.
169. MacCollum DW, Martin LW: Hemangiomas in infancy and childhood. A report based on 6479 cases. Surg Clin North Am 36:1647–1663, 1956.
170. Allen PW, Enzinger FM: Hemangioma of skeletal muscle. An analysis of 89 cases. Cancer 29:8–22, 1972.
171. Beham A, Fletcher CDM: Intramuscular angioma: a clinicopathological analysis of 74 cases. Histopathology 18:53–59, 1991.
172. Lewis RC Jr, Coventry MB, Soule EH: Hemangioma of the synovial membrane. J Bone Joint Surg 41:264–271, 1959.
173. Howat AJ, Campbell PE: Angiomatosis: a vascular malformation of infancy and childhood. Report of 17 cases. Pathology 19:377–382, 1987.
174. Rao VK, Weiss SW: Angiomatosis of soft tissue. An analysis of the histologic features and clinical outcome in 51 cases. Am J Surg Pathol 16:764–771, 1992.
175. Whimster IW: The pathology of lymphangioma circumscriptum. Br J Dermatol 94:473–486, 1976.
176. Gomez CS, Calonje E, Ferrar DW, et al: Lymphangiomatosis of the limbs: clinicopathologic analysis of a series with a good prognosis. Am J Surg Pathol 19:125–133, 1995.
177. Gould EW, Manivel JC, Albores-Saavedra J, Monforte H: Locally infiltrative glomus tumors and glomangiosarcoma. A clinical ultrastructural and immunohistochemical study. Cancer 65:310–318, 1990.
178. Beham A, Fletcher CDM: Intravascular glomus tumour: a previously undescribed phenomenon. Virchows Arch A Pathol Anat Histopathol 418:175–177, 1991.
179. Schurch W, Skalli O, Lagace R, et al: Intermediate filament proteins and actin isoforms as markers for soft tissue tumor differentiation and origin. III. Hemangiopericytomas and glomus tumors. Am J Pathol 136:771–786, 1990.
180. Porter PL, Bigler SA, McNutt M, Gown AM: The immunophenotype of hemangiopericytomas and glomus tumors with special reference to muscle protein expression: an immunohistochemical study and review of the literature. Mod Pathol 4:46–52, 1991.
181. Enzinger FM, Smith BH: Hemangiopericytoma. An analysis of 106 cases. Hum Pathol 7:61–82, 1976.
182. Fletcher CDM: Haemangiopericytoma—a dying breed? Reappraisal of an "entity" and its variants. Curr Diagn Pathol 1:19–23, 1994.
183. Stout AP, Murran MR: Hemangiopericytoma: a vascular tumor featuring Zimmermann's pericytes. Ann Surg 116:26–33, 1942.
184. Tsuneyoshi M, Daimaru Y, Enjoji M: Malignant hemangiopericytoma and other sarcomas with hemangiopericytoma-like pattern. Pathol Res Pract 178:446–453, 1984.
185. Yu C-W, Hall PA, Fletcher CDM, et al: Haemangiopericytomas: the prognostic value of immunohistochemical staining with a monoclonal antibody to proliferating cell nuclear antigen (PCNA). Histopathology 19:29–33, 1991.
186. Fletcher CDM, Beham A, Schmid C: Spindle cell hemangioendothelioma: a clinicopathological and immunohistochemical study indicative of a non-neoplastic lesion. Histopathology 18:291–301, 1991.
187. Imayama S, Murakamai Y, Hashimoto H, Hori Y: Spindle cell hemangioendothelioma exhibits the ultrastructural features of a reactive vascular proliferation rather than of angiosarcoma. Am J Clin Pathol 97:279–287, 1992.
188. Perkins P, Weiss SW: Spindle cell hemangioendothelioma: an analysis of 78 cases with reassessment of its pathogenesis and biologic behavior. Am J Surg Pathol 20:1196–1204, 1996.
189. Scott GA, Rosai J: Spindle cell hemangioendothelioma. Report of seven additional cases of a recently described vascular neoplasm. Am J Dermatopathol 10:281–288, 1988.
190. Weiss SW, Enzinger FM: Spindle cell hemangioendothelioma, a low grade angiosarcoma resembling a cavernous hemangioma and Kaposi's sarcoma. Am J Surg Pathol 10:521–530, 1986.
191. Weiss SW, Ishak KG, Dail DH, et al: Epithelioid hemangioendothelioma and related lesions. Semin Diagn Pathol 3:259–287, 1986.
192. Weiss SW, Enzinger FM: Epithelioid hemangioendothelioma. A vascular tumor often mistaken for carcinoma. Cancer 50:970–981, 1982.
193. Mentzel T, Hull MT, Ulbright TM, et al: Epithelioid hemangioendothelioma of skin and soft tissues: clinicopathologic and immunohistochemical study of 30 cases. Am J Surg Pathol 21:363–374, 1997.
194. Meis-Kindblom JM, Kindblom L-G: Angiosarcoma of soft tissue: a study of 80 cases. Am J Surg Pathol 22:683–697, 1998.
195. Maddox JC, Evans HL: Angiosarcoma of skin and soft tissues: a study of forty-four cases. Cancer 48:1907–1921, 1981.
196. Jennings TA, Peterson L, Axiotis CA, et al: Angiosarcoma associated with foreign body material. Cancer 62:2436–2444, 1988.
197. Capo V, Ozzello L, Fenoglio CM, et al: Angiosarcomas arising in edematous extremities: immunostaining for factor VIII related antigen and ultrastructural features. Hum Pathol 16:144–150, 1985.
198. Fletcher CDM, Beham A, Bekir S, et al: Epithelioid angiosarcoma of deep soft tissue: a distinctive tumor readily mistaken for an epithelial neoplasm. Am J Surg Pathol 15:915–924, 1991.
199. Gray MF, Rosenberg AE, Dickersin GR, Bhan AK: Cytokeratin expression in epithelioid vascular neoplasms. Hum Pathol 21:212–217, 1990.
200. Zietz C, Rossle M, Haas C, et al: MDM-2 oncoprotein overexpression, p53 gene mutation, and VEGF upregulation in angiosarcomas. Am J Pathol 153:1425–1433, 1998.
201. Kilpatrick SE, Mentzel T, Fletcher CDM: Leiomyoma of deep soft tissue: clinicopathologic analysis of a series. Am J Surg Pathol 18:576–582, 1994.
202. Hachisuga T, Hashimoto H, Enjoji M: Angioleiomyoma. A clinicopathologic reappraisal of 562 cases. Cancer 54:126–130, 1984.

203. Fox SB, Heryet A, Khong TY: Angioleiomyomas: an immunohistological study. Histopathology 16:495–496, 1990.

204. Fletcher CDM, Kilpatrick SE, Mentzel T: The difficulty in predicting behavior of smooth muscle tumors in deep soft tissue. Am J Surg Pathol 19:116–117, 1995.

205. Gustafson P, Willen H, Baldertorp B, et al: Soft tissue leiomyosarcoma. A population-based epidemiologic and prognostic study of 48 patients, including cellular DNA content. Cancer 70:114–119, 1992.

206. Hashimoto H, Daimaru Y, Tsuneyoshi M, Enjoji M: Leiomyosarcoma of the external soft tissues. A clinicopathologic, immunohistochemical and electron microscopic study. Cancer 57:2077–2088, 1986.

207. Lack EE: Leiomyosarcomas in childhood: a clinical and pathologic study of 10 cases. Pediatr Pathol 6:181–197, 1986.

208. Oliver GF, Reiman HM, Gonchoroff NJ, et al: Cutaneous and subcutaneous leiomyosarcoma: a clinicopathological review of 14 cases with reference to antidesmin staining and nuclear DNA patterns studied by flow cytometry. Br J Dermatol 124:252–257, 1991.

209. Shmookler BM, Lauer DH: Retroperitoneal leiomyosarcoma. A clinicopathologic analysis of 36 cases. Am J Surg Pathol 7:269–280, 1983.

210. Swanson PE, Wick MR, Dehner LP: Leiomyosarcoma of somatic soft tissues in childhood: an immunohistochemical analysis of six cases with ultrastructural correlation. Hum Pathol 22:569–577, 1991.

211. Varela-Duran J, Oliva H, Rosai J: Vascular leiomyosarcoma. The malignant counterpart of vascular leiomyoma. Cancer 44:1684–1691, 1979.

212. Mentzel T, Calonje E, Fletcher CDM: Leiomyosarcoma with prominent osteoclast-like giant cells: analysis of eight cases closely mimicking the so-called giant cell variant of "MFH." Am J Surg Pathol 18:258–265, 1994.

213. Norton AJ, Thomas AJ, Isaacson PG: Cytokeratin-specific monoclonal antibodies are reactive with tumours of smooth muscle derivation. An immunocytochemical and biochemical study using antibodies to intermediate filament cytoskeletal proteins. Histopathology 11:487–499, 1987.

214. Brown DC, Theaker JM, Banks PM, et al: Cytokeratin expression in smooth muscle and smooth muscle tumours. Histopathology 11:477–486, 1987.

215. Dehner LP, Enzinger FM, Font RL: Fetal rhabdomyoma. An analysis of nine cases. Cancer 30:160–166, 1972.

216. Kodet R, Fajstavr J, Kabelka Z, et al: Is fetal cellular rhabdomyoma an entity or a differentiated rhabdomyosarcoma? A study of patients with rhabdomyoma of the tongue and sarcoma of the tongue enrolled in the Intergroup Rhabdomyosarcoma Studies I, II and III. Cancer 67:2907–2913, 1991.

217. Kapadia SB, Meis JM, Frisman DM, et al: Fetal rhabdomyoma of the head and neck. A clinicopathologic and immunophenotypic study of 24 cases. Hum Pathol 24:754–765, 1993.

218. Eusebi V, Ceccarelli C, Daniele E, et al: Extracardiac rhabdomyoma: an immunocytochemical study and a review of the literature. Appl Pathol 6:197–207, 1988.

219. Coffin CM: The new International Rhabdomyosarcoma Classification, its progenitors, and considerations beyond morphology. Adv Anat Pathol 4:1–16, 1997.

220. Bale PM, Parsons RE, Stevens MM: Diagnosis and behaviour of juvenile rhabdomyosarcoma. Hum Pathol 14:596–611, 1983.

221. Crist WM, Garnsey L, Beltangady M: Prognosis in children with rhabdomyosarcoma: a report of the Intergroup Rhabdomyosarcoma Studies I and II. J Clin Oncol 8:443–452, 1990.

222. Gaffney EF, Dervan PA, Fletcher CDM: Pleomorphic rhabdomyosarcoma in adulthood: analysis of 11 cases with definition of diagnostic criteria. Am J Surg Pathol 17:601–609, 1993.

223. Hollowood K, Fletcher CDM: Rhabdomyosarcoma in adults. Semin Diagn Pathol 11:47–57, 1994.

224. Kodet R, Newton WA, Hamoudi AB, Asmar L: Rhabdomyosarcomas with intermediate filament inclusions and features of rhabdoid tumors. Light microscopic and immunohistochemical study. Am J Surg Pathol 15:257–267, 1991.

225. Kodet R, Newton WA, Hamoudi AB, et al: Childhood rhabdomyosarcoma with anaplastic (pleomorphic) features. A report of the Intergroup Rhabdomyosarcoma Study. Am J Surg Pathol 17:443–453, 1993.

226. Lloyd RV, Hajdu SI, Knapper WH: Embryonal rhabdomyosarcoma in adults. Cancer 51:557–565, 1983.

227. Maurer HM, Beltangady M, Gehan E, et al: The Intergroup Rhabdomyosarcoma Study I. A final report. Cancer 61:209–220, 1988.

228. Maurer HM, Gehan EA, Beltangady M, et al: The Intergroup Rhabdomyosarcoma Study II. Cancer 71:1904–1922, 1993.

229. Parham DM: The molecular biology of childhood rhabdomyosarcoma. Semin Diagn Pathol 11:39–46, 1994.

230. Parham DM, Webber B, Holt H, et al: Immunohistochemical study of childhood rhabdomyosarcomas and related neoplasms. Cancer 67:3072–3080, 1991.

231. Parham DM: Immunohistochemistry of childhood sarcomas: old and new markers. Mod Pathol 6:133–138, 1993.

232. Schurch W, Begin LR, Seemayer TA, et al: Pleomorphic soft tissue myogenic sarcomas of adulthood: a reappraisal in the mid-1990's. Am J Surg Pathol 20:131–147, 1996.

233. Scrable H, Witte D, Shimada H, et al: Molecular differential pathology of rhabdomyosarcoma. Genes Chromosomes Cancer 1:23–35, 1989.

234. Seidal T, Kindblom L-G, Angervall L: Rhabdomyosarcoma in middle-aged and elderly individuals. APMIS 97:236–248, 1989.

235. Tsokos M: The role of immunocytochemistry in the diagnosis of rhabdomyosarcoma (editorial). Arch Pathol Lab Med 110:776–778, 1986.

236. Tsokos M, Webber BL, Parham DM, et al: Rhabdomyosarcoma. A new classification scheme related to prognosis. Arch Pathol Lab Med 116:847–855, 1992.

237. Tsokos M: The diagnosis and classification of childhood rhabdomyosarcoma. Semin Diagn Pathol 11:26–38, 1994.

238. Newton WA Jr, Gehan EA, Webber BL, et al: Classification of rhabdomyosarcomas and related sarcomas. Pathologic aspects and proposal for a new classification—an Intergoup Rhabdomyosarcoma Study. Cancer 76:1073–1085, 1995.

239. Cavazzana AO, Schmidt D, Ninfo V, et al: Spindle cell rhabdomyosarcoma. A prognostically favorable variant of rhabdomyosarcoma. Am J Surg Pathol 16:229–235, 1992.

240. Leuschner I, Newton WA, Schmidt D, et al: Spindle cell variants of embryonal rhabdomyosarcoma in the paratesticular region. A report of the Intergroup Rhabdomyosarcoma Study. Am J Surg Pathol 17:221–230, 1993.

241. Enterline HT, Horn RC: Alveolar rhabdomyosarcoma. A distinctive tumor type. Am J Clin Pathol 29:356–366, 1958.

242. Enzinger FM, Shiraki M: Alveolar rhabdomyosarcoma. An analysis of 110 cases. Cancer 24:18–31, 1969.

243. Carter RL, McCarthy KP, Machin LG, et al: Expression of desmin and myoglobin in rhabdomyosarcomas and in developing skeletal muscle. Histopathology 15:585–595, 1988.

244. Wang-Wuu S, Soukup S, Ballard E, et al: Chromosomal analysis of sixteen human rhabdomyosarcomas. Cancer Res 48:983–987, 1988.

245. Anderson J, Renshaw J, McManus A, et al: Amplification of the t(2;13) and t(1;13) translocations of alveolar rhabdomyosarcoma in small formalin-fixed biopsies using a modified reverse transcriptase polymerase chain reaction. Am J Pathol 150:477–482, 1997.

246. Douglass EC, Shapiro DM, Valentine M, et al: Alveolar rhabdomyosarcoma with the t(1;13): cytogenetic findings and clinicopathologic correlations. Med Pediatr Oncol 21:83–87, 1993.

247. Kelly KM, Womer RB, Sorensen PH, et al: Common and variant gene fusions predict distinct clinical phenotypes in rhabdomyosarcoma. J Clin Oncol 15:1831–1836, 1997.

248. Dias P, Kumar P, Marsden HB, et al: N-*myc* gene is amplified in alveolar rhabdomyosarcomas (RMS) but not in embryonal RMS. Int J Cancer 45:593–596, 1990.

249. De Zen L, Sommaggio A, d'Amore ES, et al: Clinical relevance of DNA ploidy and proliferative activity in childhood rhabdomyosarcoma: a retrospective analysis of patients enrolled onto the Italian Cooperative Rhabdomyosarcoma Study RMS88. J Clin Oncol 15:1198–1205, 1997.

250. Auerbach HE, Brooks JJ: Alveolar soft part sarcoma. A clinicopathologic and immunohistochemical study. Cancer 60:66–73, 1987.

251. Christopherson WM, Foote FW, Stewart FW: Alveolar soft-part sarcomas: structurally characteristic tumors of uncertain histogenesis. Cancer 5:100–111, 1952.

252. Cullinane C, Thorner PS, Greenberg ML, et al: Molecular, genetic, cytogenetic and immunohistochemical characterization of alveolar soft part sarcoma. Implications for cell of origin. Cancer 70:2444–2450, 1992.

253. Foschini MP, Eusebi V: Alveolar soft-part sarcoma: a new type of rhabdomyosarcoma? Semin Diagn Pathol 11:58–68, 1994.

254. Lieberman PH, Brennan MF, Kimmel M, et al: Alveolar soft-part sarcoma. A clinicopathologic study of half a century. Cancer 63:1–13, 1989.

255. Ordonez NG, Ro JY, Mackay B: Alveolar soft part sarcoma. An ultrastructural and immunocytochemical investigation of its histogenesis. Cancer 63:1721–1736, 1989.

256. Persson S, Willems JS, Kindblom L-G: Alveolar soft part sarcoma. An immunohistochemical, cytologic and electron microscopic study and a quantitative DNA analysis. Virchows Arch A Pathol Anat Histopathol 412:499–513, 1988.

257. Cadman NL, Soule EH, Kelly PJ: Synovial sarcoma. An analysis of 134 tumors. Cancer 18:613–627, 1965.

258. Cagle LA, Mirra JM, Storm K, et al: Histological features relating to prognosis in synovial sarcoma. Cancer 59:1810–1814, 1987.

259. Fisher C: Synovial sarcoma: ultrastructural and immunohistochemical features of epithelial differentiation in monophasic and biphasic tumors. Hum Pathol 17:996–1008, 1986.

260. Folpe AL, Schmidt RA, Chapman D, Gown AM: Poorly differentiated synovial sarcoma: immunohistochemical distinction from primitive neuroectodermal tumors and high-grade malignant peripheral nerve sheath tumors. Am J Surg Pathol 22:673–682, 1998.

261. Milchgrub S, Ghandur-Mnaymneh L, Dorfman HD, Albores-Saavedra J: Synovial sarcoma with extensive osteoid and bone formation. Am J Surg Pathol 17:357–363, 1993.

262. Ordonez NG, Mahfouz SM, Mackay B: Synovial sarcoma: an immunohistochemical and ultrastructural study. Hum Pathol 21:733–749, 1990.

263. Oda Y, Hashimoto H, Tsuneyoshi M, Takeshita S: Survival in synovial sarcoma. A multivariate study of prognostic factors with special emphasis on the comparison between early death and long-term survival. Am J Surg Pathol 17:35–44, 1993.

264. Schmidt D, Thun P, Med C, et al: Synovial sarcoma in children and adolescents. A report from the Kiel Pediatric Tumor Registry. Cancer 67:1667–1672, 1991.

265. Varela-Duran J, Enzinger FM: Calcifying synovial sarcoma. Cancer 50:345–352, 1982.

266. Argani P, Zakowski MF, Klimstra DS, et al: Detection of the SYT-SSX chimeric RNA of synovial sarcoma in paraffin-embedded tissue and its application in problematic cases. Mod Pathol 11:65–71, 1998.

267. Chase DR, Enzinger FM: Epithelioid sarcoma. Diagnosis, prognostic indicators and treatment. Am J Surg Pathol 9:241–263, 1985.

268. Dabska M, Koszarowski T: Clinical and pathologic study of aponeurotic (epithelioid) sarcoma. Pathol Annu 17:129–153, 1982.

269. Enzinger FM: Epithelioid sarcoma. A sarcoma simulating a granuloma or a carcinoma. Cancer 26:1029–1041, 1970.

270. Evans HL, Baer SC: Epithelioid sarcoma: a clinicopathologic and prognostic study of 26 cases. Semin Diagn Pathol 10:286–291, 1993.

271. Guillou L, Wadden C, Coindre J-M, et al: "Proximal-type" epithelioid sarcoma, a distinctive aggressive neoplasm showing rhabdoid features: clinicopathologic, immunohistochemical, and ultrastructural study of a series. Am J Surg Pathol 21:130–152, 1997.

272. Miettinen M, Fanburg-Smith JC, Virolainen M, et al: Epithelioid sarcoma: an immunohistochemical analysis of 112 classical and variant cases and a discussion of the differential diagnosis. Hum Pathol 30:934–942, 1999.

273. Arber DA, Kandalaft PL, Mehta P, Battifora H: Vimentin-negative epithelioid sarcoma. The value of an immunohistochemical panel that includes CD34. Am J Surg Pathol 17:302–307, 1993.

274. Kodet R, Newton WA, Sachs N, et al: Rhabdoid tumors of soft tissue: a clinicopathologic study of 26 cases enrolled on the Intergroup Rhabdomyosarcoma Study. Hum Pathol 22:674–681, 1991.

275. Parham DM, Weeks DA, Beckwith JB: The clinicopathologic spectrum of putative extrarenal rhabdoid tumors. An analysis of 42 cases studied with immunohistochemistry and/or electron microscopy. Am J Surg Pathol 18:1010–1029, 1994.

276. Tsuneyoshi M, Daimaru Y, Hashimoto H, Enjoji M: Malignant soft tissue neoplasms with the histologic features of renal rhabdoid tumors: an ultrastructural and immunohistochemical study. Hum Pathol 16:1235–1242, 1985.

277. Tsuneyoshi M, Daimaru Y, Hashimoto H: The existence of rhabdoid cells in specified soft tissue sarcomas. Histopathological, ultrastructural and immunohistochemical evidence. Virchows Arch A Pathol Anat Histopathol 411:509–514, 1987.

278. Sotelo-Avila C, Gonzalez-Crussi F, deMello D, et al: Renal and extrarenal rhabdoid tumors in children: a clinicopathologic study of 14 patients. Semin Diagn Pathol 3:151–163, 1986.

279. Weeks DA, Beckwith JB, Mierau GW: Rhabdoid tumor. An entity or phenotype? Arch Pathol Lab Med 113:113–114, 1989.

280. White FV, Dehner LP, Belchis DA, et al: Congenital disseminated malignant rhabdoid tumor: a distinct clinicopathologic entity demonstrating abnormalities of chromosome 22q11. Am J Surg Pathol 23:249–256, 1999.

281. Rousseau-Merck MF, Versteege I, Legrand I, et al: hSNF5/INI1 inactivation is mainly associated with homozygous deletions and mitotic recombinations in rhabdoid tumors. Cancer Res 59:3152–3156, 1999.

282. Harkin JC, Reed RJ: Tumors of the Peripheral Nervous System. Atlas of Tumor Pathology. Second Series, Fascicle 3. Washington, DC, Armed Forces Institute of Pathology, 1969.

283. Fletcher CDM, Davies SE: Benign plexiform (multinodular) schwannoma: a rare tumour unassociated with neurofibromatosis. Histopathology 10:971–980, 1986.

284. Iwashita T, Enjoji M: Plexiform neurilemmoma: a clinicopathological and immunohistochemical analysis of 23 tumours from 20 patients. Virchows Arch A Pathol Anat Histopathol 411:305–309, 1987.

285. Fletcher CDM, Davies SE, McKee PH: Cellular schwannoma: a distinct pseudosarcomatous entity. Histopathology 11:21–35, 1987.

286. White WM, Shiu MFH, Rosenblum MK, et al: Cellular schwannoma. A clinicopathologic study of 57 patients and 58 tumors. Cancer 66:1266–1275, 1990.

287. Woodruff JM, Godwin TA, Erlandson RA, et al: Cellular schwannoma. A variety of schwannoma sometimes mistaken for a malignant tumor. Am J Surg Pathol 5:733–744, 1981.

288. Dahl I: Ancient neurilemmoma (schwannoma). Acta Pathol Microbiol Scand A 85:812–818, 1977.

289. Mennemeyer RP, Hammar SP, Tytus JS, et al: Melanocytic schwannoma. Clinical and ultrastructural studies of three cases with evidence of intracellular melanin synthesis. Am J Surg Pathol 3:3–10, 1979.

290. Woodruff JM, Christensen WM: Glandular peripheral nerve sheath tumors. Cancer 72:3618–3628, 1993.

291. Lin BT, Weiss LM, Medeiros LJ: Neurofibroma and cellular neurofibroma with atypia: a report of 14 tumors. Am J Surg Pathol 21:1443–1449, 1997.

292. Fetsch JF, Miettinen M: Sclerosing perineurioma: a clinicopathologic study of 19 cases of a distinctive soft tissue lesion with a predilection for the fingers and palms of young adults. Am J Surg Pathol 21:1433–1442, 1997.

293. Giannini C, Scheithauer BW, Jenkins RB, et al: Soft-tissue perineurioma: evidence for an abnormality of chromosome 22, criteria for diagnosis, and review of the literature. Am J Surg Pathol 21:164–173, 1997.

294. Mentzel T, Tos APD, Fletcher CDM: Perineurioma (storiform

perineurial fibroma): clinicopathological analysis of four cases. Histopathology 25:261–267, 1994.

295. Tsang WYW, Chan JKC, Chow LTC, Tse CCH: Perineurioma: an uncommon soft tissue neoplasm distinct from localized hypertrophic neuropathy and neurofibroma. Am J Surg Pathol 14:756–763, 1992.

296. Ariza A, Bilbao JM, Rosai J: Immunohistochemical detection of epithelial membrane antigen in normal perineurial cells and perineurioma. Am J Surg Pathol 12:678–683, 1988.

297. Ducatman BS, Scheithauer BW: Malignant peripheral nerve sheath tumors showing divergent differentiation. Cancer 54:1049–1057, 1984.

298. Ducatman BS, Scheithauer BW, Piepgras DG, et al: Malignant peripheral nerve sheath tumors. A clinicopathologic study of 120 cases. Cancer 57:2006–2021, 1986.

299. Ghosh BC, Ghosh L, Huvos AG, Fortner JG: Malignant schwannoma. A clinicopathologic study. Cancer 31:184–190, 1973.

300. Hirose T, Hasegawa T, Kudo E, et al: Malignant peripheral nerve sheath tumors: an immunohistochemical study in relation to ultrastructural features. Hum Pathol 23:865–870, 1992.

301. Johnson TL, Lee MW, Meis JM: Immunohistochemical characterization of malignant peripheral nerve sheath tumors. Surg Pathol 4:121–135, 1991.

302. Meis JM, Enzinger FM, Martz KL, Neal JA: Malignant peripheral nerve sheath tumors (malignant schwannomas) in children. Am J Surg Pathol 16:694–707, 1992.

303. Meis-Kindblom JM, Enzinger FM: Plexiform malignant peripheral nerve sheath tumor of infancy and childhood. Am J Surg Pathol 18:479–485, 1994.

304. Wick MR, Swanson PE, Scheithauer BW, Manivel JC: Malignant peripheral nerve sheath tumor. An immunohistochemical study of 62 cases. Am J Clin Pathol 87:425–433, 1987.

305. Hruban RH, Shiu MH, Senie RT, Woodruff JM: Malignant peripheral nerve sheath tumors of the buttock and lower extremity. Cancer 66:1253–1265, 1990.

306. Sordillo PP, Helson L, Hajdu SI, et al: Malignant schwannoma: clinical characteristics, survival, and response to therapy. Cancer 47:2503–2509, 1981.

307. White HR: Survival in malignant schwannoma: an 18-year study. Cancer 27:720–729, 1971.

308. Sorensen SA, Mulvihill JJ, Nielsen A: Long-term follow-up of von Recklinghausen neurofibromatosis. Survival and malignant neoplasms. N Engl J Med 314:1010–1015, 1986.

309. Ducatman BS, Scheithauer BW: Postirradiation neurofibrosarcoma. Cancer 51:1028–1033, 1983.

310. Guccion JG, Enzinger FM: Malignant schwannoma associated with von Recklinghausen's neurofibromatosis. Virchows Arch A Pathol Anat Histopathol 383:43–57, 1979.

311. Lodding P, Kindblom L-G, Angervall L: Epithelioid malignant schwannoma. A study of 14 cases. Virchows Arch A Pathol Anat Histopathol 409:433–451, 1986.

312. DiCarlo EF, Woodruff JM, Bansal M, Erlandson RA: The purely epithelioid malignant peripheral nerve sheath tumor. Am J Surg Pathol 10:478–490, 1986.

313. Woodruff JM, Perino G: Non–germ-cell or teratomatous malignant tumors showing additional rhabdomyoblastic differentiation, with emphasis on the malignant Triton tumor. Semin Diagn Pathol 11:69–81, 1994.

314. Angervall L, Enzinger FM: Extraskeletal neoplasm resembling Ewing's sarcoma. Cancer 36:240–251, 1975.

315. Askin FB, Rosai J, Sibley RK, et al: Malignant small cell tumor of the thoracopulmonary region in childhood. A distinctive clinicopathologic entity of uncertain histogenesis. Cancer 43:2438–2451, 1979.

316. Contesso G, Llombart-Bosch A, Terrier P, et al: Does malignant small round cell tumor of the thoracopulmonary region (Askin tumor) constitute a clinicopathologic entity? An analysis of 30 cases with immunohistochemical and electron-microscopic support treated at the Institut Gustave Roussy. Cancer 69:1012–1020, 1992.

317. Dehner LP: Peripheral and central primitive neuroectodermal tumors. A nosologic concept seeking a consensus. Arch Pathol Lab Med 110:997–1005, 1986.

318. Dehner LP: Primitive neuroectodermal tumor and Ewing's sarcoma. Am J Surg Pathol 17:1–13, 1993.

319. Shimada H, Newton WA, Soule EH, et al: Pathologic features of extraosseous Ewing's sarcoma: a report from the Intergroup Rhabdomyosarcoma study. Hum Pathol 19:442–453, 1988.

320. Ambros IM, Ambros PF, Strehl S, et al: MIC2 is a specific marker for Ewing's sarcoma and peripheral primitive neuroectodermal tumors. Cancer 67:1886–1893, 1991.

321. Weidner N, Tjoe J: Immunohistochemical profile of monoclonal antibody O13: antibody that recognizes glycoprotein p30/32 MIC2 and is useful in diagnosing Ewing's sarcoma and peripheral neuroepithelioma. Am J Surg Pathol 18:486–494, 1994.

322. Meier VS, Kuhne T, Jundt G, Gudat F: Molecular diagnosis of Ewing tumors: improved detection of *EWS–FLI-1* and *EWS-ERG* chimeric transcripts and rapid determination of exon combinations. Diagn Mol Pathol 7:29–35, 1998.

323. De Alvara E, Kawai A, Healey JH, et al: *EWS–FLI1* fusion transcript structure is an independent determinant of prognosis in Ewing's sarcoma. J Clin Oncol 16:1248–1255, 1998.

324. Lin PP, Brody RI, Hamelin AC, et al: Differential transactivation by alternative EWS-FLI1 fusion proteins correlates with clinical heterogeneity in Ewings's sarcoma. Cancer Res 59:1428–1432, 1999.

325. Kovar H, Jug G, Aryee DN, et al: Among genes involved in the RB dependent cell cycle regulatory cascade, the *p16* tumor suppressor gene is frequently lost in the Ewing family of tumors. Oncogene 15:2225–2232, 1997.

326. Ordonez NG: Desmoplastic small round cell tumor: I: a histopathologic study of 39 cases with emphasis on unusual histological patterns. Am J Surg Pathol 22:1303–1313, 1998.

327. Ordonez NG: Desmoplastic small round cell tumor: II: an ultrastructural and immunohistochemical study with emphasis on new immunohistochemical markers. Am J Surg Pathol 22:1314–1327, 1998.

328. Gerald WL, Miller HK, Battifora H, et al: Intra-abdominal desmoplastic small round-cell tumor. Report of 19 cases of a distinctive type of high-grade polyphenotypic malignancy affecting young individuals. Am J Surg Pathol 15:499–513, 1991.

329. de Alvara E, Ladanyi M, Rosai J, Gerald WL: Detection of chimeric transcripts in desmoplastic small round cell tumor and related developmental tumors by reverse transcriptase polymerase chain reaction. A specific diagnostic assay. Am J Pathol 147:1584–1591, 1995.

330. Ladanyi M, Gerald WL: Fusion of the *EWS* and *WT1* genes in the desmoplastic small round cell tumor. Cancer Res 54:2837–2840, 1994.

331. Chung EB, Enzinger FM: Malignant melanoma of soft parts. A reassessment of clear cell sarcoma. Am J Surg Pathol 7:405–413, 1983.

332. Enzinger FM: Clear cell sarcoma of tendons and aponeuroses. An analysis of 21 cases. Cancer 18:1163–1174, 1965.

333. Hasegawa T, Hirose T, Kudo E, Hizawa K: Clear cell sarcoma. An immunohistochemical and ultrastructural study. Acta Pathol Jpn 39:321–327, 1985.

334. Kindblom L-G, Lodding P, Angervall L: Clear cell sarcoma of tendons and aponeuroses. An immunohistochemical and electron microscopic analysis indicating neural crest origin. Virchows Arch A Pathol Anat Histopathol 401:109–128, 1983.

335. Lucas DR, Nascimento AG, Sim FH: Clear cell sarcoma of soft tissues. Mayo Clinic experience with 35 cases. Am J Surg Pathol 16:1197–1204, 1992.

336. Montgomery EA, Meis JM, Ramos AG: Clear cell sarcoma of tendons and aponeuroses. A clinicopathologic study of 58 cases with analysis of prognostic factors. Int J Surg Pathol 1:89–100, 1993.

337. Sara AS, Evans HL, Benjamin RS: Malignant melanoma of soft parts (clear cell sarcoma). A study of 17 cases with emphasis on prognostic factors. Cancer 65:367–374, 1990.

338. Sreekantaiah C, Ladanyi M, Rodriguez E, Changanti RS: Chromosomal aberrations in soft tissue tumors. Relevance to diagnosis, classification and molecular mechanisms. Am J Pathol 144:1121–1134, 1994.

339. Reeves BR, Fletcher CDM, Gusterson BA: Translocation t(12;22)(q13;q13) is a nonrandom rearrangement in clear cell sarcoma. Cancer Genet Cytogenet 64:101–103, 1992.

340. Bridge JA, Sreekantaiah C, Neff JR, Sandberg AP: Cytogenetic findings in clear cell sarcoma of tendons and aponeuroses. Malignant melanoma of soft parts. Cancer Genet Cytogenet 52:101–106, 1991.

341. Fujimura Y, Ohno T, Siddique H, et al: The *EWS–ATF-1* gene involved in malignant melanoma of soft parts with t(12;22) chromosome translocation, encodes a constitutive transcriptional activator. Oncogene 12:159–167, 1996.

342. Zucman J, Delattre O, Desmaze C, et al: *EWS* and *ATF-1* gene fusion induced by t(12;22) translocation in malignant melanoma of soft parts. Nat Genet 4:341–345, 1993.

343. El-Naggar AK, Garcia GM: Epithelioid sarcoma. Flow cytometric study of DNA content and regional DNA heterogeneity. Cancer 69:1721–1728, 1992.

344. Dahlin C, Salvador H: Cartilaginous tumors of the soft tissues of the hands and feet. Mayo Clin Proc 49:721–726, 1974.

345. Chung EB, Enzinger FM: Benign chondromas of soft parts. Cancer 41:1414–1424, 1978.

346. Dabska M: Parachordoma. A new clinicopathologic entity. Cancer 40:1586–1592, 1977.

347. Folpe AL, Agoff SN, Willis J, Weiss SW: Parachordoma is immunohistochemically and cytogenetically distinct from axial chordoma and extraskeletal myxoid chondrosarcoma. Am J Surg Pathol 23:1059–1067, 1999.

348. Meis-Kindblom JM, Bergh P, Gunterberg B, Kindblom L-G: Extraskeletal myxoid chondrosarcoma. Am J Surg Pathol 23:636–650, 1999.

349. Dardick I, Lagace R, Carlier MR: Chordoid sarcoma (extraskeletal myxoid chondrosarcoma). A light and electron microscopic study. Virchows Arch 399:61–78, 1983.

350. Enzinger FM: Extraskeletal myxoid chondrosarcoma. An analysis of 34 cases. Hum Pathol 3:421–435, 1972.

351. Fletcher CDM, Powell G, McKee PH: Extraskeletal myxoid chondrosarcoma: a histochemical and immunohistochemical study. Histopathology 10:489–499, 1986.

352. Hachitanda Y, Tsuneyoshi M, Daimaru Y, et al: Extraskeletal myxoid chondrosarcoma in young children. Cancer 61:2521–2526, 1988.

353. Saleh G, Evans HL, Ro JY, Ayala AG: Extraskeletal myxoid chondrosarcoma. A clinicopathologic study of ten patients with long-term follow-up. Cancer 70:2827–2830, 1992.

354. Tsuneyoshi M, Enjoji M, Iwasaki H, Shinohara N: Extraskeletal myxoid chondrosarcoma. A clinicopathologic and electron microscopic study. Acta Pathol Jpn 31:439–447, 1981.

355. Sciot R, Dal Cin P, Fletcher C, et al: t(9;22)(q22–31;q11–12) is a consistent marker of extraskeletal myxoid chondrosarcoma: evaluation of three cases. Mod Pathol 8:765–768, 1995.

356. Lichtenstein L, Bernstein D: Unusual benign and malignant chondroid tumors of bone: a survey of some mesenchymal cartilage tumors and malignant chondroblastic tumors, including a few multicentric ones, as well as many atypical benign chondroblastomas and chondromyxoid fibromas. Cancer 12:1142–1157, 1959.

357. Nakashima Y, Unni KK, Shives TC, et al: Mesenchymal chondrosarcoma of bone and soft tissue: a review of 111 cases. Cancer 57:2444–2453, 1986.

358. Swanson PE, Lillemoe TJ, Manivel JC, Wick MR: Mesenchymal chondrosarcoma: an immunohistochemical study. Arch Pathol Lab Med 114:943–948, 1990.

359. Sumiyoshi K, Tsuneyoshi M, Enjoji M: Myositis ossificans. A clinicopathologic study of 21 cases. Acta Pathol Jpn 35:1109–1122, 1985.

360. Nuovo MA, Norman A, Chumas J, Ackerman LV: Myositis ossificans with atypical clinical and radiographic and pathologic findings: a review of 23 cases. Skeletal Radiol 21:87–101, 1992.

361. Ackerman LV: Extra-osseous localized non-neoplastic bone and cartilage formation (so-called myositis ossificans): clinical and pathological confusion with malignant neoplasms. J Bone Joint Surg Am 40:279–298, 1958.

362. Allan CJ, Soule EH: Osteogenic sarcoma of the somatic soft tissues. Clinicopathologic study of 26 cases and review of the literature. Cancer 27:1121–1133, 1971.

363. Chung EB, Enzinger FM: Extraskeletal osteosarcoma. Cancer 60:1132–1142, 1987.

364. Jensen ML, Schumacher B, Jensen OM, et al: Extraskeletal osteosarcomas: a clinicopathologic study of 25 cases. Am J Surg Pathol 22:588–594, 1998.

365. Sordillo PP, Hadju SI, Magill GB, Golbey RB: Extraosseous osteogenic sarcoma. A review of 48 patients. Cancer 51:727–734, 1983.

366. Brady MS, Perino G, Tallini G, et al: Malignant mesenchymoma. Cancer 77:467–473, 1996.

367. Newman PL, Fletcher CDM: Malignant mesenchymoma. Clinicopathologic analysis of a series with evidence of low-grade behavior. Am J Surg Pathol 15:607–614, 1991.

368. Travis WD, Banks PM, Reiman HM: Primary extranodal soft tissue lymphoma of the extremities. Am J Surg Pathol 11:359–366, 1987.

369. Kaul R, McGeer A, Low DE, et al: Population-based surveillance for group A streptococcal necrotizing fasciitis: clinical features, prognostic indicators, and microbiologic analysis of seventy-seven cases. Ontario Group A Streptococcal Study. Am J Med 103:18–24, 1997.

370. LeBoit PE, Berger TG, Egbert BM, et al: Bacillary angiomatosis. The histopathology and differential diagnosis of a pseudoneoplastic infection in patients with human immunodeficiency virus disease. Am J Surg Pathol 13:909–920, 1989.

371. Terner JY, Lattes R: Malakoplakia of the colon and retroperitoneum. Report of a case with histochemical study of the Michaelis-Guttmann inclusion bodies. Am J Clin Pathol 44:20–31, 1965.

372. Damjanov I, Katz SM: Malakoplakia. Pathol Annu 16:103–131, 1981.

373. Weiss SW, Enzinger FM, Johnson FB: Silica reaction simulating fibrous histiocytoma. Cancer 42:2738–2745, 1978.

374. Miliauskas JR, Mukherjee T, Dixon B: Postimmunization (vaccination) injection-site reactions. A report of four cases and review of the literature. Am J Surg Pathol 17:516–524, 1993.

375. Kuo T-T, Hsueh S: Mucicarcinophilic histiocytosis. A polyvinylpyrrolidone (PVP) storage disease simulating signet-ring cell carcinoma. Am J Surg Pathol 8:419–428, 1984.

376. Hizawa K, Inaba H, Nakanishi S, et al: Subcutaneous pseudosarcomatous polyvinylpyrrolidone granuloma. Am J Surg Pathol 8:393–398, 1984.

377. Kapadia SB, Enzinger FM, Heffner DK, et al: Crystal-storing histiocytosis associated with lymphoplasmacytic neoplasms. Report of three cases mimicking adult rhabdomyoma. Am J Surg Pathol 17:461–467, 1993.

378. Montgomery EA, Meis JM, Frizzera G: Rosai-Dorfman disease of soft tissue. Am J Surg Pathol 16:122–129, 1992.

379. Foucar E, Rosai J, Dorfman R: Sinus histiocytosis with massive lymphadenopathy (Rosai-Dorfman disease): review of the entity. Semin Diagn Pathol 7:19–73, 1990.

380. Costa J: The grading and staging of soft tissue sarcomas. *In* Fletcher CDM, McKee PH (eds): Pathobiology of Soft Tissue Tumours. Edinburgh, Churchill Livingstone, 1990, pp 221–238.

# 47

# *Bone and Joint Pathology*

Noel Weidner    Michael Kyriakos

## JOINTS

### Normal Anatomy

Bone joints (diarthroses) are covered by hyaline cartilage and enclosed by a joint capsule. The capsule is composed of an inner synovial layer and an outer fibrous layer that is continuous with the bone periosteum. The synovial layer (synovial membrane) contains fibroblast-like cells (synoviocytes or type B cells) and macrophage-like cells (type A cells).[13] Synoviocytes secrete collagen and proteoglycan and express vascular cell adhesion molecule-l and vimentin; they are negative for epithelial markers, such as cytokeratin.[13] A layer of loose connective tissue or adipose tissue may be present between the synovial and the fibrous layers, producing joint-space folds or villi. Tendons are made of densely packed type I collagen fibers that are surrounded by a connective tissue layer, the tendon sheath. In long tendons, this sheath is composed of an inner movable layer, adjacent to the collagen, and an outer layer that is bound loosely to the tissues surrounding the tendon; the result is a potential space similar to the joint cavity.[1–12] (see note)

### Ganglia, Baker's Cyst, and Carpal Tunnel Syndrome

Ganglion cysts (ganglia) occur near joints or around tendon sheaths, especially the dorsal carpal area of the hand or volar wrist. They are common tumefac-tive deformities that may cause local compression, leading to pain, weakness, joint disability, and secondary bony changes.[14–16] Intraosseous ganglia, either primary or as a result of extension from an extraosseous ganglion, occur. Ganglia are caused by myxoid degeneration, followed by cyst formation, within the connective tissue of the joint capsule or tendon sheath. Repeated bouts of trauma may be contributory because typists and pianists are prone to develop ganglia of the hand. As a result of compression by its mucoid content, pressure atrophy usually causes disappearance of the synovial lining cells of the ganglion cyst; however, at times these cells still may be found. Bursae, which occur where muscles, tendons, and skin glide over bony prominences, may develop diseases similar to those occurring in large joint spaces. Subdeltoid bursitis results from degeneration of a tendon or muscle in the rotator cuff of the shoulder followed by deposition of calcium in necrotic collagenous tissue (i.e., calcareous tendinitis).[17]

Baker's cyst is a form of ganglion cyst that occurs in the popliteal space from herniation of the synovial membrane through the posterior part of the joint capsule or from escape of joint fluid through normal anatomic connections of the knee joint with the semimembranous bursa. The cyst is lined by true synovium and may have cartilage in its wall. Any joint disease leading to increased intra-articular pressure, such as degenerative joint disease, neuropathic arthropathy, and rheumatoid arthritis, may result in the formation of Baker's cyst.[18]

The carpal tunnel lies between the flexor retinaculum or transverse carpal ligament and the carpal bones. The medial nerve travels through the carpal tunnel, and compression produces carpal tunnel syndrome.[19–21] The compression may be caused by bony deformity, masses within the tunnel (hemangiomas, lipomas, ganglia), arthritis, or amyloidosis;[22] often, however, no clear-cut cause is apparent.

---

Note: References 1–12 represent general references that can be used to document and elaborate the widely known general comments for each lesion. They will not be repeated throughout the text.

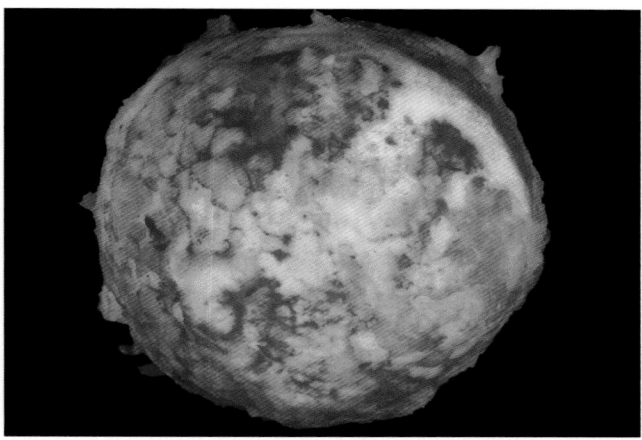

**FIGURE 47-1.** Osteoarthritis. Surface view of femoral head shows erosion of the articular cartilage.

## Arthritis

Degenerative joint disease (osteoarthritis) is caused by secondary degenerative changes (i.e., age related) that are exacerbated by repeated trauma[23-26] (Figs. 47-1 and 47-2). The process starts with fibrillation of the hyaline cartilaginous matrix at the articular surface after disappearance of the spindle cell perichondrium. Fibrillation develops at right angles to the articular surface, causing the smooth articular surface to become papillary or fibrillar. Eventually the cartilage develops clefts or fissures that extend through the cartilage to the underlying bone. The cartilage becomes attenuated, most pronounced on the surfaces directly exposed to weight bearing or movement, but also in areas of the joint not subject to these mechanical forces.[27] The loss of cartilage thickness leads to narrowing of the joint space and loss of stability of the chondro-osseous junction. Reactive changes in the residual joint cartilage produce an irregular, further dysfunctional joint surface that magnifies and accelerates the destruction. This pro-

cess ultimately results in exposure of variably sized areas of the underlying bone. With disappearance of the cartilage, the articulating bony surfaces are brought into direct contact, and the resulting friction between them produces polished, ivory-like, condensed bone (so-called eburnation). Altered joint shape leads to subluxations, reduced joint motion, and abnormal bone formation at the periphery of the joint where the cartilage and capsule meet (e.g., osteophytes or Heberden's nodes). Fibrous or bony ankylosis is rare. Often subchondral cysts develop that are located close to the articular surface. These cysts are surrounded by dense bone and contain mucinous fluid or loose connective tissue. Usually, there is no increase in the thickness of the joint capsule, but sometimes there is synovial membrane thickening producing papillary or pedunculated masses, which may show cartilaginous, bony, or fatty metaplasia. Detachment of these pedunculated masses may give rise to loose bodies or "joint mice." Some degree of synovial hyperplasia, hyperemia, and lymphocytic infiltration may develop in advanced stages of the disease. These changes should not be confused with rheumatoid arthritis. *Chondromalacia patellae* refers to softening, fibrillation, fissuring, and erosion of the articular cartilage of the patella.[28] The pathologic changes are those of degenerative joint disease.

Rheumatoid arthritis is a chronic-active polyarticular disease most commonly found in young women[29, 30] (Figs. 47-3 and 47-4). Although the exact cause of rheumatoid arthritis is unknown, human leukocyte antigen associations and essentially universal autoantibody production support an autoimmune process.[31, 32] The feet and hands nearly always are involved, but the elbows, knees, wrists, ankles, hips, spine, and temporomandibular joints also may develop rheumatoid arthritis. The disease begins with hyperemia of the synovium followed by proliferation (i.e., hyperplasia) of the synovial lining cells and infiltration by plasma cells and lymphocytes. Lymphoid follicles develop frequently.[32] This

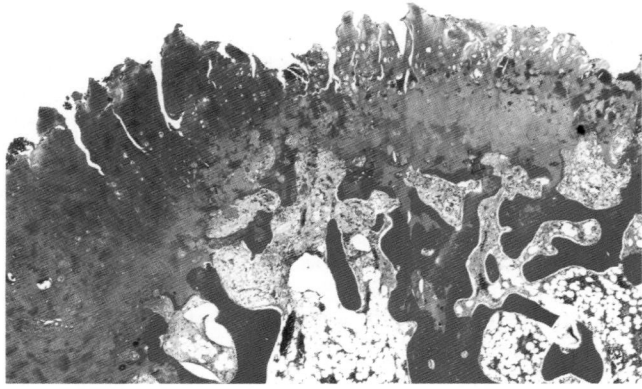

**FIGURE 47-2.** Osteoarthritis. View shows fibrillation and degeneration of the articular cartilage with cleftlike spaces that extend toward the subchondral bone.

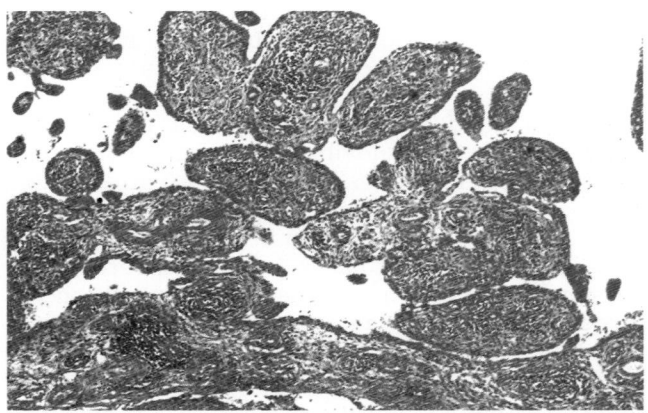

**FIGURE 47-3.** Rheumatoid arthritis. Villus proliferation of the synovium; some villi contain aggregates of lymphocytes.

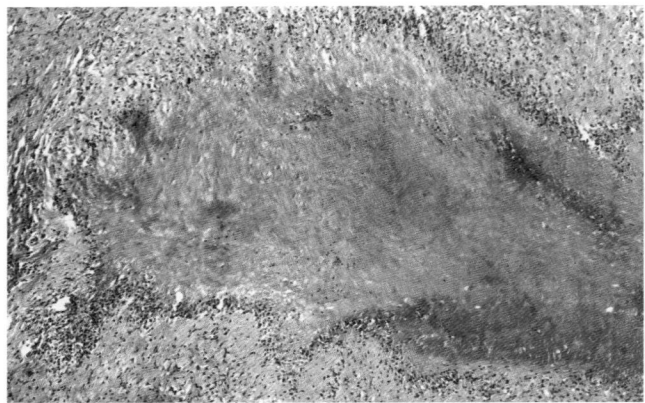

**FIGURE 47–4.** Rheumatoid nodule within the substance of the synovial membrane in a patient with rheumatoid arthritis. Central necrobiotic area is surrounded at its periphery by pallisading stromal and inflammatory cells.

histopathology, although supporting a diagnosis of rheumatoid arthritis, is not specific. Other microscopic features, which also are nonspecific, include the presence of synovial giant cells (approximately 33% of cases) and bone and cartilage fragments within the synovial membrane. Multinucleated plasma cells, foreign-body giant cells, and Touton giant cells also may occur in rheumatoid arthritis joints. The cartilage and bone fragments tend to occur in joints with advanced disease. They seem to arise as a result of the erosive destructive process of the articular surface (i.e., secondary osteoarthritis), which is common in prolonged rheumatoid arthritis. Prominent inflamed and hyperplastic synovial tissue (pannus) eventually grows over the articular cartilage; cartilage and bone may form in this pannus. Granulation tissue in the subchondral bone area and pannus within the joint cause degeneration and destruction of the articular cartilage,[33] contributing further to destabilization of the joint and secondary degenerative joint changes. Eventually, fibrous or bony ankylosis occurs. Increased articular pressure may cause acute joint rupture,[34] bone cysts ("rheumatoid geodes"),[35] or herniation of the capsule into the soft tissues.[36] The joint disease may lead to disuse osteoporosis and lead to fractures in the long bones (particularly the femoral neck) and the pelvis.[37]

Rheumatoid arthritis is a systemic disease, and extra-articular tenosynovitis and rheumatoid nodules are common expressions[38, 39] (Fig. 47–4). Rheumatoid nodules occur in approximately 20% of patients. The nodules are found most often in tendons and tendon sheaths and periarticular subcutaneous tissue, but they may occur in many sites, including the heart, large vessels, lung, pleura, kidney, meninges, breast, and synovial membrane.[40] Rheumatoid nodules contain a necrotic center with fibrin, surrounded by a distinctive border of palisaded fibrohistiocytic cells. Essentially identical nodules sometimes are found in rheumatic fever or systemic lupus erythematosus

and in otherwise asymptomatic children (i.e., subcutaneous granuloma annulare).[41–43] Non-necrotizing arteritis occurs in 10% of patients with rheumatoid arthritis,[44] but necrotizing arteritis and polyneuritis also may develop.[45, 46] The pulmonary manifestations of rheumatoid arthritis include chronic fibrosing interstitial lung disease, chronic inflammatory infiltrates, bronchiolitis obliterans, nodular fibrosis with pneumoconiosis (Caplan's syndrome), and rheumatoid nodule formation. Rheumatoid arthritis–associated pleuritis shows nonspecific inflammation but may have palisaded necrotizing changes suggestive of rheumatoid nodules. Lymphadenopathy is common in patients with rheumatoid arthritis; lymphadenopathy may precede the development of arthritis. Rheumatoid arthritis–associated lymphadenopathy shows diffuse follicular hyperplasia and striking plasma cellular infiltration. Vascular proliferation also is common and may mimic the plasma cell type of Castleman's disease. Amyloidosis complicates rheumatoid arthritis; in the United States, rheumatoid arthritis is the most common underlying disorder associated with amyloid deposition.

Infectious arthritis may be caused by bacteria, fungi, or parasites. These organisms enter joints by hematogenous spread or by extension from adjacent osteomyelitis. One important bacterial form of infectious arthritis is Lyme disease, caused by a tick-transmitted spirochete, *Borrelia burgdorferi*, which also involves the skin, heart, and nervous system.[47, 48] The ticks are encountered in the woods, where they normally infest deer and deer mice. The microscopic changes in the synovium are those of a nonspecific chronic synovitis, but the spirochete occasionally may be detected with the Dieterle stain.[49] It is important to recognize the possibility of Lyme disease because early therapy can result in cure, whereas delayed diagnosis may lead to chronic disease.

Gout may cause approximately 5% of chronic joint disease with the metatarsophalangeal joints being involved most frequently, but other joints of the hands and feet or long bones may develop disease.[50] In gout, urate deposits destroy the cartilage and subchondral bone. Deposits may extend from the joint into the adjacent soft tissues, causing destruction of ligaments and, eventually, skin erosion. Alcohol fixation is best for urate crystal preservation in tissue sections. The urate crystals appear as sheaves of needle-like, doubly refractile crystals. A granulomatous reaction develops around the deposits, composed of histiocytes and foreign-body giant cells, often with a palisaded appearance. Although rheumatoid nodules are in the differential diagnosis, they lack crystals by polarization. Polarization also is useful in excluding chondrocalcinosis or pseudogout, a common finding in routine pathology practice, in which there is deposition of calcium pyrophosphate crystals in the articular cartilage and ligaments.[51–53] Focal deposits of calcium pyrophosphate crystals also are frequent in specimens from patients with degenerative joint disease. They appear as rounded hematoxylinophilic pools or aggregates containing rhomboid crystals, which weakly polarize. Sometimes these deposits induce a granulomatous response similar to gout, but they lack the typical needle-like crystals characteristic of urate deposits. Whether the calcium pyrophosphate crystals are secondary to the degenerative joint changes or contributory is unclear sometimes from the clinical presentation.

Scleroderma (progressive systemic sclerosis)−related arthritis shows superficial deposition of fibrin along the synovial membrane, mild mononuclear infiltration of the synovial membrane, minimal hyperplasia of synovial lining cells, proliferation of collagen fibers, and focal obliteration of small vessels.[54] In systemic lupus erythematosus, the synovial pathology may be indistinguishable from that of rheumatoid arthritis. As a rule, however, there is a more intense surface fibrin deposition and a lesser degree of proliferation of synovial cells.[55]

Amyloid may occur in the synovium, articular cartilage, periarticular tissue, and intervertebral disk in old age, apparently unrelated to osteoarthritis and in the absence of systemic amyloidosis.[56–59] Larger amounts occur as an expression of primary amyloidosis or multiple myeloma. Amyloidosis is one of the causes of carpal tunnel syndrome.[60, 61]

## Tumors and Tumor Like Conditions

*Giant cell tumor of tendon sheath or synovium (nodular tenosynovitis)* is a common tumor that may present as either localized or diffuse disease. Other diagnostic terms used for this lesion include *nodular or diffuse pigmented villonodular tenosynovitis, giant cell tumor of tendon sheath, xanthogranuloma, benign synovioma,* and *fibrous histiocytoma of the tendon sheath or synovium.* This variable terminology has resulted from controversy over the nature of this disease. Some authors consider it a reactive process and prefer to designate it as *nodular or diffuse pigmented tenosynovitis*[62]; others regard it as neoplastic and a form of fibrous histiocytoma. Trisomy 7 has been documented in a diffuse case of *pigmented villonodular tenosynovitis,* suggesting that these lesions represent clonal, neoplastic proliferations.[63] Finally, ultrastructural and immunologic studies of giant cell tumor of tendon sheath have shown tumor cells with variable fibrohistiocytic differentiation, entirely consistent with a form of fibrous histiocytoma.[64–66]

The lesions may be classified into intra-articular and extra-articular types and further divided into localized and diffuse forms. On gross examination, the intra-articular localized form presents as a single nodular mass usually measuring 1 to 3 cm in diameter; the diffuse form grows as a papillary lesion that diffusely involves the synovium and may spread beyond the joint space into surrounding soft tissues. The localized extra-articular form, most commonly referred to as *giant cell tumor of tendon sheath or nodular tenosynovitis,* occurs more frequently in women than men, especially in young and middle-aged in-

dividuals. These localized extra-articular lesions are found in the fingers and toes, with the former being far more common. Localized giant cell tumor of tendon sheath has a fairly well-defined capsule, may be lobulated, and varies from whitish gray to yellow-brown. Histologic features include closely packed, medium-sized, polyhedral cells with a variable admixture of osteoclast-like giant cells. Mitotic activity may be brisk, but cytologic atypia is minimal. Hemosiderin is common, and patches or areas may show numerous xanthoma cells (foamy histiocytes). Areas of hyalinization may develop, and the whole tumor may become hypocellular and hyalinized; the so-called tendon sheath fibroma may be a closely related lesion.[67, 68] The great cellularity of this tumor, its variable pattern, and the presence of mitotic figures may lead to an erroneous diagnosis of sarcoma. These tumors almost always are benign, but they may simulate malignancy by eroding into contiguous bone. If incompletely removed, they may recur locally; new lesions may develop after excision.[69] A rare malignant counterpart of this lesion has been described.[70] Features that should suggest malignancy are numerous mitotic figures with atypical forms, marked nuclear hyperchromasia, clumped or coarse chromatin, and paucity of multinucleated giant cells.[70]

Diffuse forms of tenosynovitis (so-called pigmented villonodular synovitis or bursitis) occur primarily in young adults.[1–12, 71, 72] Although any joint may be involved, the knee joint is the usual site, with the hip, ankle, shoulder, and elbow joint frequent locations.[73, 74] The lesion is most often uniarticular, but bilateral disease may develop. Similar to the localized tumor, the adjacent bone can be penetrated or eroded, producing a destructive or lytic radiologic appearance that may simulate a bone malignancy.[75] This locally invasive character has been attributed to the production of metalloproteinases, such as collagenase and stromelysin (i.e., *biochemical pressure*).[76] Macroscopically, diffuse giant cell tumor of tendon sheath or synovium is made up of brownish yellow spongy, villous papillary tissue; the color is caused by its hemosiderin and lipid content. Over time, the villous projections fuse to form nodular areas that may become indistinguishable from the localized synovial forms. Except for the papillary character of the diffuse form, the histologic features of all of these lesions are similar. The diffuse intra-articular form is treated best by complete synovectomy, whereas the localized form may be treated by partial synovectomy.

*Synovial chondromatosis (synovial chondrometaplasia; synovial osteochondromatosis)* is an infrequent disease of unknown cause associated with the formation of cartilaginous or osteocartilaginous bodies in the synovial membranes[77] (Figs. 47−5 and 47−6). The condition is most often monarticular, usually affecting the knee or hip joints and communicating bursae. Rarely a similar condition may develop in the soft tissue adjacent to but not communicating with the joint.[78] The gross osteocartilaginous bodies

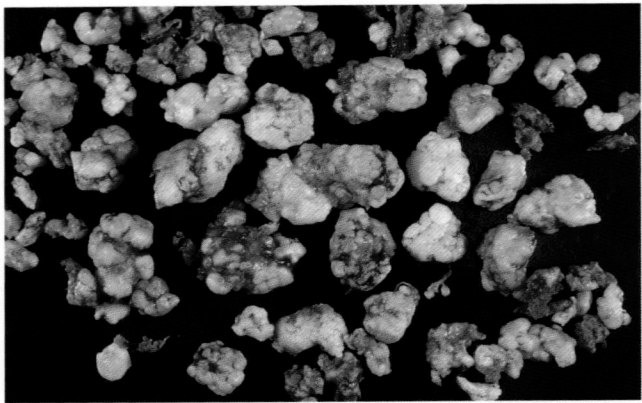

**FIGURE 47–5.** Synovial chondromatosis. Multiple nodules of cartilage and ossified cartilage removed from the knee of an adult. Nodules are irregular and cauliflower-like.

may remain confined to the synovium or be extruded into the joint cavity in large numbers.[79] For the histologic diagnosis, cartilaginous or osteocartilaginous bodies should be found within the synovial membrane, regardless of any such nodules free within the joint spaces, because such loose bodies may occur in degenerative joint disease, neuropathic arthropathy, and osteochondritis dissecans. The cartilage cells may show mild atypia, including binucleated forms, but this does not indicate malignancy in this context.[80] Treatment is surgical, but recurrences may develop.

*Synovial chondrosarcoma* is a rare primary joint tumor that may resemble synovial chondromatosis in its clinical presentation.[81, 82] Invasion beyond the joint capsule is strong evidence of the lesion's malignant character. Cytologically, high-grade morphology is required for diagnosis, because the cartilage in benign synovial chondromatosis may be atypical, resembling that found in low-grade chondrosarcoma.

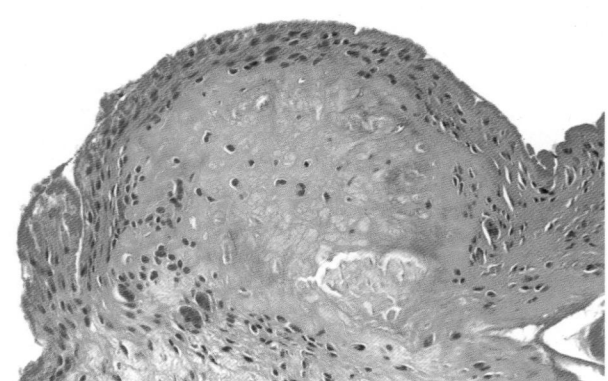

**FIGURE 47–6.** Synovial chondromatosis. Synovial lining is seen, beneath which is an ill-defined island of chondroid, at the periphery of which are a few osteoclast-type giant cells.

The only primary tumor of the synovium that is seen with any frequency, in addition to those already mentioned, is *synovial hemangioma*. Most patients are young adults, and there is a male predominance. The knee is the most common site, followed by the elbow and finger. In most cases, the tumor is confined to the intra-articular synovium, but sometimes it is located in a bursa adjacent to a joint. Cavernous hemangioma is the most common type, followed by lobular capillary hemangioma, arteriovenous hemangioma, and venous hemangioma.[83] Finally, rare cases of primary intra-articular hemangiopericytoma, synovial sarcoma, and epithelioid sarcoma have been observed.[84]

## BONE

### Normal Anatomy

Bones, including associated ligaments, cartilage, and tendons, are designed anatomically to withstand stresses of compression, tension, and shear forces. Active bone growth begins at the epiphyseal plate or disk (physis). Enchondral ossification occurs at the epiphyseal plate and articular cartilage, wherein longitudinal, regularly spaced columns of vascularized cartilage become calcified and converted to bone. At maturity and maximal adult length, bone growth stops, and the epiphyseal plate becomes ossified and disappears. The time of closure of the epiphysis differs in various bones and in the sexes (i.e., females earlier than males).

Mature bone has an outer cortex (*cortical bone* or *compact bone*) and a central medulla (*spongiosa* or *cancellous bone*).[1–12] The cortex contains two types of vascular channels: longitudinal (haversian canals) and transverse or oblique (Volkmann's canals). Except for that part of the bone covered by articular cartilage, the cortex is surrounded by a periosteum composed of an outer fibrous layer and an inner cellular (cambium) layer of fibroblasts and osteoblasts. The periosteum contains nerve fibers that may pass into the medullary canal along with the nutrient vessels. Bundles of collagen fibers penetrate the outer cortex from the outer layer of the periosteum; these are called *Sharpey's fibers* or *perforating fibers*. The periosteum may become detached and elevated from the bone as a result of trauma, infection, or tumors. New bone formation subsequently occurs between the elevated periosteum and the underlying bone. By radiographic examination, this new bone formation appears as fine spicules or layers that are perpendicular or parallel to the long axis of the bone. This periosteal reaction also may occur as a consequence of metastatic carcinoma or subperiosteal hemorrhage.

Osteoblasts synthesize the collagenous matrix of bone and regulate its mineralization. Osteoblasts may have a flat or variably plump appearance, sometimes with a perinuclear halo resulting from a prominent Golgi apparatus. Flat osteoblasts along a

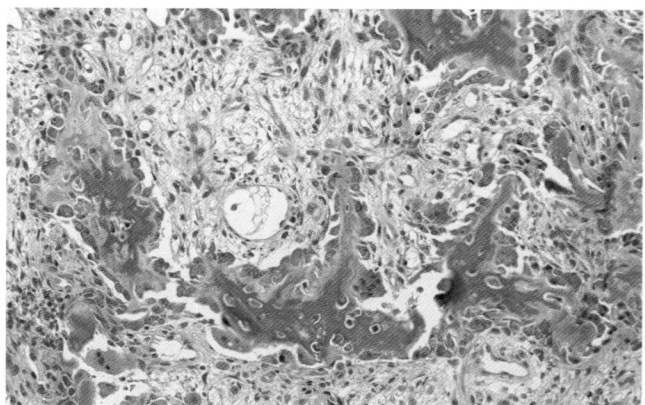

**FIGURE 47–7.** New bone formation. Trabeculae of bone produced by the active proliferation of plump osteoblasts that rim the trabeculae. Central cores of the trabeculae consist of osteoid that has become calcified, producing immature bone. Background stroma is vascular.

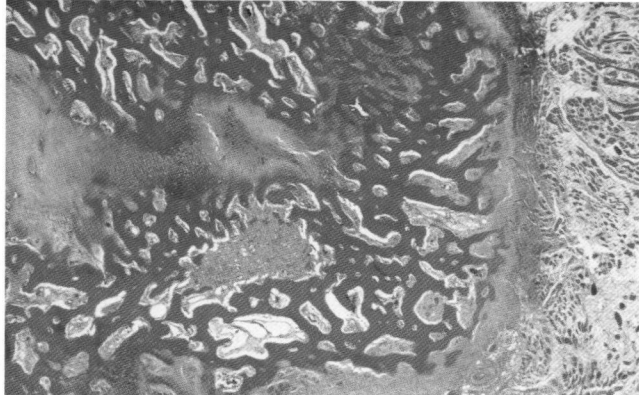

**FIGURE 47–8.** Fracture callus. Low-power view shows callus consisting of immature cartilage with active bone proliferation on either side of the fracture line.

bone surface are relatively inactive and may be difficult to see by light microscopy; plump or polygonal osteoblasts are metabolically active and usually indicate bone production (Fig. 47–7). Osteoblasts have a high cytoplasmic content of alkaline phosphatase, have abundant rough endoplasmic reticulum, and resemble fibroblasts. When osteoblasts become incorporated within the bone matrix, they reside within lacunae and are termed *osteocytes*. Osteocytes maintain contact with each other and with the bone surface through cellular processes that run through a network of canaliculi within the bone matrix to form a functional syncytium. This network likely plays a major role in mineral and structural homeostasis.

Osteoclasts are large, multinucleated cells important in bone resorption. Osteoclasts may be found in shallow concavities on the surface of bone (i.e., Howship's lacunae) and arise from monocyte-macrophage precursors.[85] An osteoclast is considered active by its mere presence on the bone surface. Osteoclasts contain abundant tartrate-resistant acid phosphatase and respond to various osteotropic hormones, such as calcitonin or parathyroid hormone. Osteoclast cytoplasm contains many mitochondria and scanty lysosomes; a ruffled edge is present in the area of the cell membrane that is in the process of bone resorption. Various matrix metalloproteinases have been detected by immunohistochemistry in osteoclasts.[86]

Osteoid, the unmineralized precursor matrix of bone, is composed of collagen (mainly type I); acid mucopolysaccharides; and noncollagen proteins,[87] including osteopontin, osteocalcin, and bone morphogenetic protein.[88–91] The last-mentioned is thought to play a crucial role in initiating the process that begins with cartilage formation and ends with bone formation.[92] Osteoid may be difficult to distinguish from hyalinized collagen, a problem when attempting to recognize osteosarcoma (see later).

Bone forms through mineralization of the osteoid by hydroxyapatite mineral deposition.[93, 94] Nor-

mal growth results from a balance between the processes of bone matrix synthesis and resorption. Among other growth factors, transforming growth factor-$\beta$ is particularly important for bone matrix production; vitamin D and parathyroid hormone make important contributions.[95–97] Increased physical activity and fluoride also have a positive trophic influence, whereas corticosteroid hormones and inactivity have a negative trophic influence.

In immature bone (woven or fiber bone), there is a haphazard arrangement of collagen fibers within the matrix, which is appreciated best with reticulin stains or under polarized light. Woven bone formation occurs preferentially in fibrous dysplasia, but it develops in any condition with accelerated bone turnover or deposition or both, such as the callus of a healing fracture (Figs. 47–8 and 47–9) or osteitis fibrosa cystica. Lamellar or mature bone shows concentric parallel lamellae under polarized light.

Bone necrosis (osteonecrosis) is recognized by the staining quality of the dead bone, which is a deeper blue than normal bone. Osteocytes are ab-

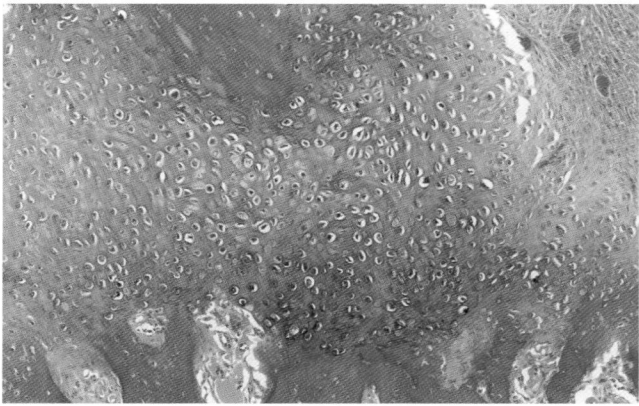

**FIGURE 47–9.** Close-up view of immature cartilage in a fracture callus. The organization and the ossification at the periphery of the cartilage distinguish it from low-grade chondrosarcoma, although the individual chondrocytes may appear atypical in the early phase of callus formation.

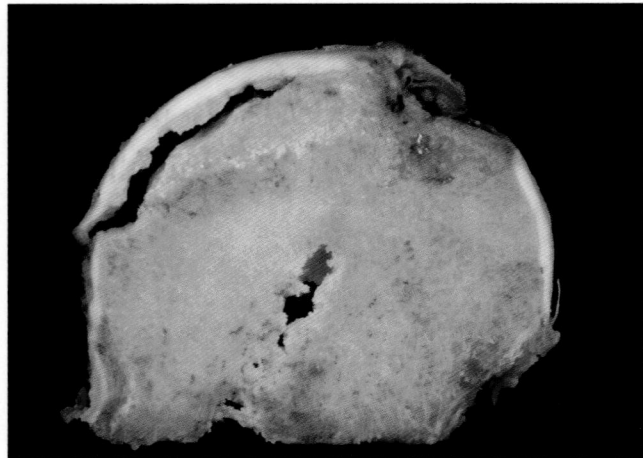

**FIGURE 47–10.** Hyperparathyroidism. Bone shows proliferation of osteoblasts with active osteoclastic reabsorption.

sent, the margins of the bone are ragged, and nearby fatty marrow elements are necrotic. Bone marrow necrosis (i.e., fat necrosis) is a more sensitive indicator of osteonecrosis because it may take a week or more for the osteocytes in necrotic bone to disappear but only a few days for fat necrosis to become evident on histologic examination.

## Metabolic Bone Disease

Complete and accurate evaluation of metabolic bone disease is a complex process using laboratory techniques often available only at specialized laboratories where undecalcified sections can be prepared and evaluated. Routinely stained sections of decalcified bone usually are not sufficient, but some metabolic lesions may be apparent if proper routine bone histologic sections are prepared.

*Osteoporosis* refers to a decreased amount of mineralized bone that develops when an individual is unable to repair and maintain the mass of bone that has been acquired throughout growth and maturation.[98–100] In osteoporosis, there is an increase in the amount of bone resorption, whereas bone formation is generally normal. It usually is a generalized and long-standing process, but transient regional osteoporosis also may occur. Histologic evaluation shows scant, disconnected, and thin bone trabeculae, and there may be increased surface osteoclastic activity. Osteoporosis may become severe enough to cause fracture, especially vertebral compression fractures resulting in loss of height in elderly people; hip fractures also are common. Osteoporosis occurs frequently in women after menopause, perhaps because of estrogen deficiency,[101] but the causes of osteoporosis are multiple.[102] Fluoride consumption and regular exercise may help prevent osteoporosis.[103, 104]

*Osteomalacia* (in adults with closed epiphyses) or *rickets* (in children with open epiphyses) refers to the accumulation of unmineralized bone matrix caused by a diminished rate of mineralization. It may result from a wide spectrum of congenital and acquired metabolic abnormalities that cause a decrease in serum calcium, phosphorus, or both to impair mineralization of the skeleton and epiphyseal growth.[105] This condition usually is due to vitamin D deficiency (either dietary or metabolic) or dietary calcium deficiency, or both. Bone and soft tissue neoplasms, collectively known as *phosphaturic mesenchymal tumors,* cause some cases. When these tumors are removed, the patients are cured of their oncogenic osteomalacia or rickets (see discussion under Miscellaneous Lesions). In osteomalacia, bone matrix is formed, but its calcification is incomplete, and this gives rise to noncalcified matrix at the periphery of the bone trabeculae. These changes can be shown in adequate biopsy tissue obtained from the long bones or the iliac crest with preparation of noncalcified specimens and examination with bright-field and phase-contrast microscopy and with the use of fluorescent tetracycline markers.

Another important metabolic bone disease is *osteogenesis imperfecta.*[1–12] Affected patients have short stature, a proclivity to fracture, poorly formed dentin, hearing loss, bluish sclerae, and swollen epiphyseal ends of long bones filled with nodules of cartilage. The last-mentioned appears as the "bag of popcorn" deformity on radiographs. In osteogenesis

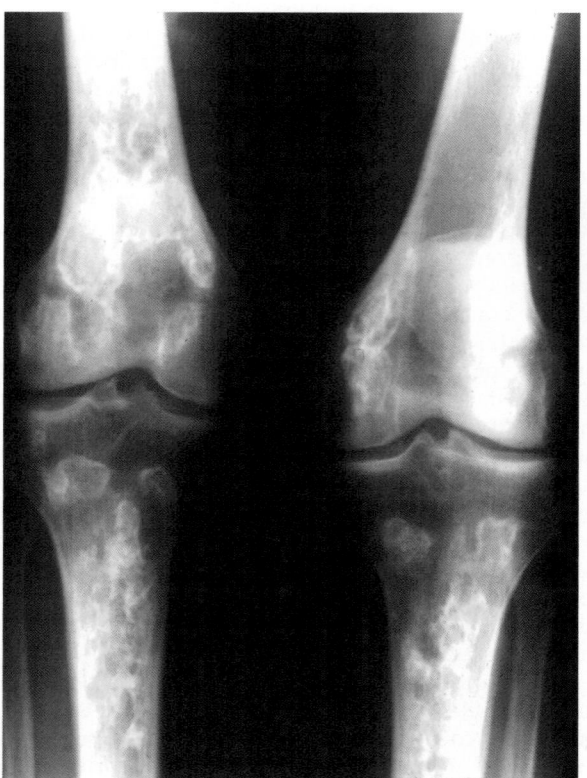

**FIGURE 47–11.** Roentgenograms of the lower extremities show irregular multiple infarcts in the distal femora and proximal tibiae. Each area of infarction shows irregular dense calcification, ossification, or both and is outlined by dense borders.

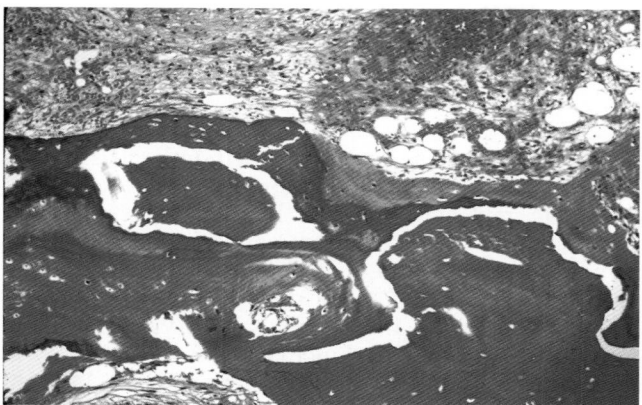

**FIGURE 47–12.** Ischemic necrosis of bone shows bone trabeculae with lacunae lacking osteocyte nuclei. The edge of the necrotic bone shows deposition on it of a pale seam of new bone.

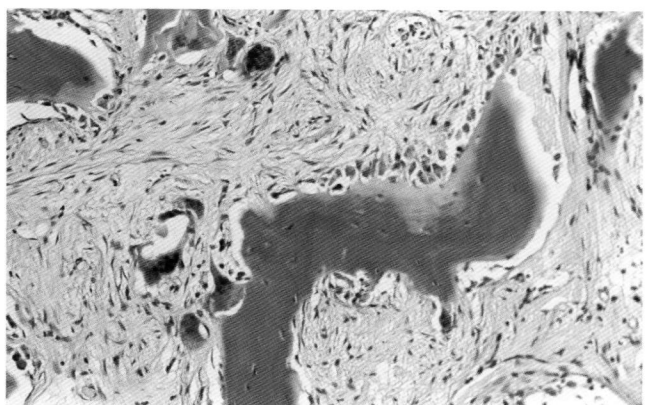

**FIGURE 47–14.** Hyperparathyroidism (Brown tumor). Aggregation of osteoclast-type giant cells in an area of extravasated red blood cells.

imperfecta, there is diminished collagen synthesis, crowded osteocytes and osteoblasts, no organized trabecular bone pattern, increased woven bone, and osteoporosis.

The pathologic features of *hyperparathyroidism*, either primary or secondary, are essentially similar (Figs. 47–10 and 47–11). There is diffuse osteopenia, especially of the hands with erosion of the distal phalanges and subperiosteal resorption of the radial side of the middle and proximal phalanges; loss of the dental lamina; and the presence of lytic bone lesions ("brown" tumors), increased osteoclastic activity with osteoclastic burrowing or tunneling into the bone matrix, increased bone formation, and peritrabecular fibrosis. The last-mentioned contrasts with the marrow fibrosis seen in myelofibrosis, in which marrow fibrosis is diffuse. The changes of hyperparathyroidism may be difficult to distinguish from those of giant cell reparative granuloma, which are similar to brown tumor, and the acute phase of

Paget's disease. Clinical and laboratory findings help resolve these problem cases.

*Osteopetrosis (Albers-Schönberg disease; marble bone disease)* is a rare congenital disorder characterized by a marked increase in the density of all bones. The bones are shortened and do not show the normal metaphyseal flare. Erlenmeyer flask deformity develops as a result. Despite the sclerotic appearance on radiographs, the bones are weak, resulting in many fractures, and there may be anemia, presumably owing to a diminished marrow space by excessive bone presence. In the adult form, there may be uniform bone opacity, or there may be alternating areas of variable involvement resulting in striped opacity. Osteopetrosis must be differentiated from widespread osteoblastic metastases and from myelosclerosis. Histologic evaluation shows irregular, thickened bone trabeculae containing cores of blue calcified cartilage filling the medullary space. Osteopetrosis is thought to represent a defect in bone remodeling secondary to a malfunction of osteoclasts resulting from a lysosomal defect. This disease is reversible by bone marrow transplantation or the use of recombinant human interferon-$\gamma$.[106]

## Paget's Disease

Paget's disease is common in northern Europeans but rare in blacks and Asians (Figs. 47–15 and 47–16). The highest incidence is in England, Australia, and Western Europe.[107] Among autopsies from England, approximately 3% of patients older than age 40 had Paget's disease.[108] Most patients with Paget's disease are older than age 55; the disease is rare before age 40.[109] It affects men slightly more often than women. Common sites are the lumbosacral spine, pelvis, and skull, but it may occur in any bone.[110] Paget's disease usually is polyostotic and accompanied by elevation of serum alkaline phosphatase levels; however, it also may appear as a monostotic process, wherein the serum alkaline phosphatase level may be normal. The usual com-

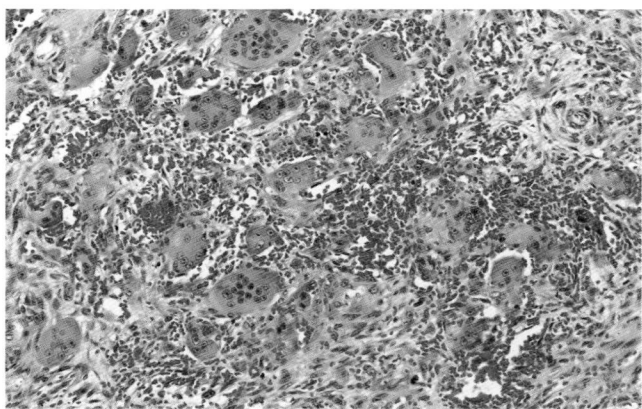

**FIGURE 47–13.** Ischemic necrosis of the proximal femoral head. Compact, deeply yellow area of necrosis is seen in the subchondral area. The overlying articular cartilage is intact but has separated from the underlying area of infarction.

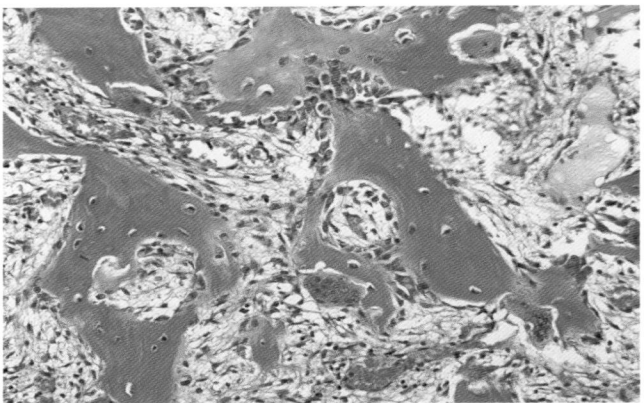

FIGURE 47–15. Paget's disease. Area of active Paget's disease shows osteoblastic proliferation with formation of new bone with simultaneous active osteoclastic resorption of the bone. Background stroma is edematous and highly vascular.

plaints include pain in the involved bone or signs and symptoms related to associated complications (i.e., fracture, arthritis, or secondary malignant degeneration). Fractures are of the transverse type, and patients who are immobilized because of long bone fractures may undergo rapid dissolution of bone substance.[111, 112] Early radiologic findings in Paget's disease vary from radiolucency in its early phases to radiopacity in the later stages; the normal distinction between cancellous and cortical bone may be lost. Rapid bone remodeling and repeated microfractures lead to bone deformity which, when near the joint, causes degenerative osteoarthritis. Tissue from active Paget's disease shows irregular and disorganized bone trabeculae, which are lined by plump osteoblasts and numerous multinucleated osteoclasts and a hypervascular stroma. The bone trabeculae may have a woven pattern. In the later or "burnt-out" phases, there is thickened trabecular bone that shows increased numbers of densely stained cement lines (mosaic pattern) and fibrosis of the marrow cavity. The irregular cement lines are caused by the abrupt interruptions and changes in direction of

bone lamellae and fibers resulting from rapid resorption and regeneration of masses of bone during the course of the disease.[113] Other pathologic processes that involve active reparative change accompanied by new bone formation also result in similar cement lines. These processes include irradiation effect, chronic osteomyelitis, and reactive bone surrounding metastatic cancer. In general, the cement lines seen in these conditions are more orderly and structurally better oriented than those of Paget's disease. The cause of Paget's disease is unknown, but some investigators have suggested a viral cause by the finding of nuclear inclusions resembling viral nucleocapsids of the measles type in the lesional osteoclasts.[114–116] The *virus* is thought to cause a massive localized increase in osteoclastic activity. The incidence of secondary bone sarcoma in Paget's disease is relatively low, especially given the relative frequency of Paget's disease in the general population.[108] Osteosarcoma is the most common type of sarcoma to develop, but chondrosarcoma, fibrosarcoma, and giant cell tumors are reported.[117–120]

## Fracture

Trauma causing breaks or fractures of the calcified bone matrix may cause tears of the periosteum, blood vessels, tendons, adjacent muscles, and skin. Bone fragments may become displaced, there may be many bone fragments (*comminuted fracture*), or the skin may be perforated (*compound fracture*). *Incomplete stress* or *fatigue fractures* occur when there is repeated stress to the bone, as sometimes develops with long-distance running and ballet dancing. Incomplete stress fractures often occur without a clear history of trauma. Repeated traumatic stress at ligamentous or tendinous insertions may result in *avulsion fractures* at the insertion points. Avulsion fractures are common along the inferior pubic ramus and lower femur where the adductor muscles originate and insert. Avulsion fractures of the tibial tubercle cause fragmentation (Osgood-Schlatter disease).

Fracture repair depends on patient age and nutrition, severity of the fracture, vascularity, treatment, and proper immobilization (Figs. 47–8 and 47–9). Delayed repair may result from bone devascularization, superimposed infection, and fibrous tissue interposition between the ends of the fragments. After a fracture, a hematoma forms between the ends of the broken bone, which acts as scaffolding for ingrowth of young capillaries. Within 3 to 5 days, devitalized bone fragments begin to be resorbed, and intramembranous bone growth appears from the inner layer of the periosteum proximal and distal to the fracture site. Cartilage and bone are formed.[121] This process on each side of the fracture meets at the fracture site to form the primary callus, which is resorbed later and replaced by mature lamellar bone. The new bone is laid down predominately along lines of stress. With early proper reduc-

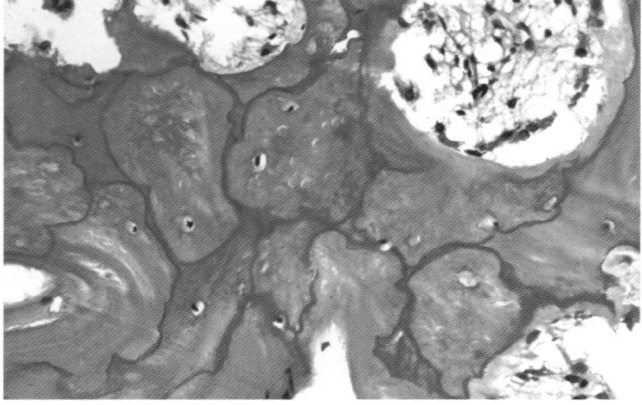

FIGURE 47–16. Mature phase of Paget's disease shows mosaic ("jigsaw") pagetic bone with intensely stained cement lines.

tion of the fracture, adequate blood supply, no infection, and normal metabolism, the fracture heals rapidly with little visible callus. Exuberant callus usually means slow fracture healing. In children, even with prominent angulation or deformity, the bone models itself to an astonishing degree.[122] The formation of exuberant cartilage and disorderly membranous bone in rapidly forming primary callus results in a microscopic pattern that potentially may be confused with osteosarcoma.

## Osteomyelitis

In developed countries, infections of bone and joints have declined as a result of modern preventive medicine, improved surgical techniques, and use of antibiotics. Currently, osteomyelitis is seen primarily in debilitated patients (i.e., elderly or young immunocompromised patients), as a complication of compound fractures, or after operation on the bone (Figs. 47–17 and 47–18). The source of the infectious agent may be from local contamination or hematogenous dissemination from a distant infected site.[123] Hematogenous seeding of the marrow cavity likely is related to its sluggish vascular flow, which is complicated by thrombosis and colonization by bacteria. Hematogenous osteomyelitis occurs most

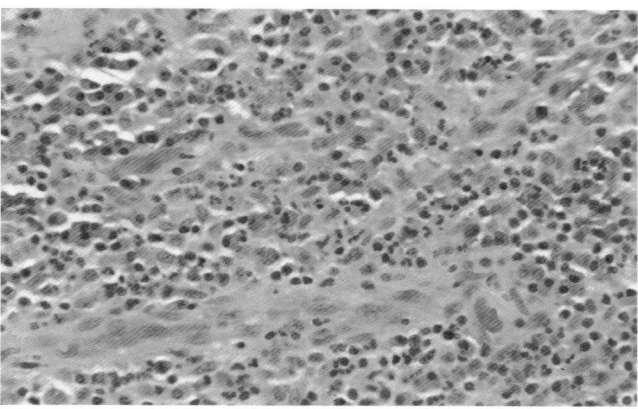

FIGURE 47–18. Acute and chronic osteomyelitis of bone. Numerous neutrophils are interspersed among plasma cells and occasional lymphocytes.

often in patients younger than age 20 years and involves the bones of the lower extremity in about 75% of cases. These young patients present with high fever and localized bone pain. In infants younger than 1 year old, epiphyseal damage and joint infection usually occur, but there is little damage to the metaphysis or diaphysis. In contrast, older children develop extensive metaphyseal cortical involvement, and damage to cartilage and joints is rare. Some young patients present with chronic recurrent multifocal osteomyelitis (sometimes with concomitant skin lesions), characterized by periods of exacerbation and improvement over several years and negative bacterial cultures.[124] In this condition, the most common histologic finding is subacute or chronic osteomyelitis characterized by a predominance of plasma cells.

Acute osteomyelitis is largely bacterial and caused by a variety of microorganisms. Approximately 90% are due to coagulase-positive staphylococci,[125] but *Klebsiella, Aerobacter, Proteus, Pseudomonas,* streptococcus, pneumococcus, gonococcus, meningococcus, *Brucella,* and *Salmonella* all may be the causative agent.[126, 127] Often, *Salmonella* causes osteomyelitis in patients with sickle cell disease.[128] Hematogenous pyogenic vertebral osteomyelitis frequently is underdiagnosed radiologically because of the subtle nature of the disease.[129] The more long-standing lesions of subacute and chronic osteomyelitis may simulate a malignant bone tumor radiologically, particularly Ewing's sarcoma, malignant lymphoma, and osteosarcoma.[130] A variant of osteomyelitis characterized by extensive regenerative bone changes is referred to as *Garré's osteomyelitis, sclerosing osteomyelitis,* or *periostitis ossificans.* This form is particularly common in the jaw bones.[131] Chronic osteomyelitis in a long bone (Brodie's abscess) may produce a radiologic pattern that simulates osteoid osteoma.

The pathologic change in osteomyelitis is determined by the age of the patient, bone involved, type of organism, and host factors.[132] From its origin in the metaphysis, the infection permeates the cortex

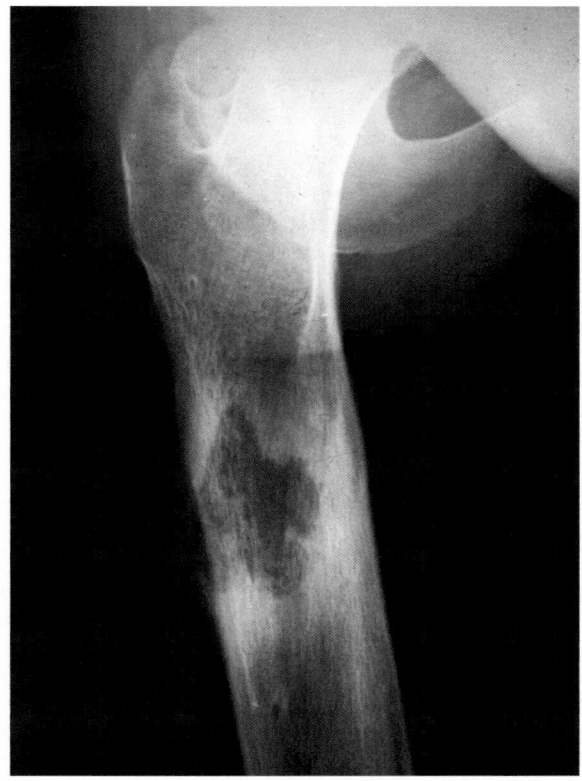

FIGURE 47–17. Osteomyelitis. Destructive lesion is present in the shaft of the proximal femur, with cortical erosion and peripheral bone sclerosis. Pattern resembles that of an aggressive tumor of bone.

through the Volkmann's canals and may spread along the medullary space to the rest of the bone. The infection causes focal bone necrosis. This dead bone (sequestrum) later is surrounded by new bone (involucrum) laid around the entire bone. Chronic osteomyelitis persists as long as infected dead bone remains. The dead bone is surrounded by granulation tissue that attacks the sequestrum, making it pitted on the surface next to the marrow cavity. The cortical surface remains smooth. Surgical removal of the sequestrum at the proper time usually allows the osteomyelitis to heal, but it may recur many years later if bacteria remain within the scar.

Osteomyelitis usually results in an admixture of inflammatory cells, including neutrophils, lymphocytes, and plasma cells, associated with variable marrow fibrosis, bone necrosis, and new bone formation.[1-12] When plasma cells are prominent, cases have been designated as *plasma cell osteomyelitis*[133]; when foamy macrophages are abundant, cases are termed *xanthogranulomatous osteomyelitis*.[134] Chronic osteomyelitis may be accompanied by prominent periosteal bone proliferation. In the adult, cutaneous sinuses may develop that become lined by squamous epithelium that extend deeply into the bone. Rarely, squamous cell carcinoma develops within these sinuses, a complication often heralded by a marked increase in pain and increasingly malodorous discharge.[135, 136]

Tuberculous osteomyelitis usually is seen in young adults or children, developing as a hematogenous infection. The vertebrae and bones of the hip, knee, ankle, elbow, and wrist are affected most often with involvement of the metaphysis, epiphysis, or synovium.[137] Fungal infections of bone include blastomycosis, actinomycosis, histoplasmosis, and coccidioidomycosis.[138, 139]

## Bone Infarcts and Necrosis

Bone infarcts have a propensity to develop in patients with sickle cell disease and Gaucher's disease but can result from many causes (Figs. 47–12 to 47–14), including trauma, corticosteroid therapy, pancreatic disease, occlusive vascular disease, thromboembolic disease, large vessel vasculitis, pheochromocytoma, osteomyelitis, decompression sickness (caisson disease), histiocytosis X, and sarcoidosis. An increased incidence of primary malignant bone tumors occurs in association with long-standing, large infarcts in the long bones. Such tumors (malignant fibrous histiocytoma, osteosarcoma, or fibrosarcoma) have usually developed in the medulla of the femur or tibia, often in men.[141-143]

During the first 1 or 2 weeks, no radiologic abnormality may be detected in a case of bone infarct, but resorption of the dead bone eventually results in decreased bone density. In time, new bone formation, growing in apposition to the dead bone trabeculae ("creeping apposition"), leads to increased bone density. This process is irregular, and the combination of incomplete resorption of dead bone and focal deposition of new bone produces a mottled, irregular roentgenographic appearance. Usually a moderately thick, radiopaque serpentine border is observed outlining an elongated area of central lucency ("coil of smoke" appearance). The pattern may resemble a calcified enchondroma or an osteosarcoma.[143]

Aseptic bone necrosis (avascular necrosis or osteonecrosis) has been reported in most secondary epiphyses and many primary epiphyses.[144] Some of these have been given eponyms, such as *Osgood-Schlatter disease* (necrosis of the tibial tuberosity) and *Legg-Calvé-Perthes disease* (necrosis of the upper femoral epiphysis). Aseptic necrosis is caused by interruption of blood flow induced by a mechanical disruption, such as fracture, dislocation, or thrombosis.[145, 146] Initial necrotic epiphyseal bone is surrounded by hyperemic tissue. Subsequently, dead bone is resorbed gradually (so-called creeping substitution) resulting, after months to years, in a dense radiologic lesion.[145] The newly formed bone, which is of soft consistency, may flatten because of pressure, resulting in degenerative joint disease. It is typical to see osteoclastic activity on one side of the dead trabeculae and osteoblastic activity on the other. The overlying cartilage is spared because its nutrition is supplied by the joint fluid.

Osteochondritis dissecans results from separation of the articular cartilage and subchondral bone from the underlying bone. This osteochondromatous fragment remains attached to the joint surface or synovium, and bone and cartilage remain viable. If it becomes detached completely, its osseous portion dies, but the cartilage remains viable from nutrients within the synovial fluid. The cause of osteochondritis dissecans is uncertain but possibly related to trauma.[148]

Bone necrosis may be a complication of radiation therapy.[149] Virtually any bone may be involved. In radiation necrosis of the pelvis and femoral neck, the changes of radiation osteonecrosis usually occur within 3 years of the therapy. On histologic evaluation, the new bone formed about the necrotic bone may show reactive prominent cement lines, simulating Paget's disease.

## Tumors

According to the World Health Organization, skeletal tumors may be classified as either benign or malignant.[149, 150] Intermediate or borderline tumors exist, however, such as giant cell tumor and some well-differentiated or low-grade cartilaginous tumors. Most malignant bone tumors arise de novo, but there are a few benign lesions that predispose the patient to the development of skeletal malignancies, including Paget's disease, enchondromatosis, osteochondromatosis, fibrous dysplasia, and bone infarcts.[151]

Each type of skeletal tumor or tumor-like lesion

has characteristic clinicopathologic features,[152] including patient age; bone involved; site of involvement within the bone (e.g., epiphysis, metaphysis, diaphysis, cortex, medulla, periosteum); and its radiologic, macroscopic, and microscopic appearance. Accurate pathologic diagnosis usually requires detailed knowledge of the clinical and radiologic features of the lesion.[153] No primary tumor of bone should be diagnosed by histologic evaluation without prior review of the radiologic studies with an expert bone radiologist.

## BONE-FORMING TUMORS

*Osteoma* is a benign lesion that probably is not a true neoplasm. It occurs in the flat bones of the skull and face as a hard bony protuberance, usually asymptomatic. Some osteomas may protrude into a paranasal sinus, most commonly the frontal sinus, and block the normal drainage from these sinuses.[154] The male-to-female ratio of occurrence is approximately 2:1, with most patients 40 to 50 years old. Patients with Gardner's syndrome may have multiple osteomas, most frequently in the mandible, that may become manifest several years before finding the intestinal polyps.[155] Occasionally, osteomas involve bones other than the skull and face. Most of these have a parosteal location and need to be distinguished from parosteal osteosarcoma.[156]

Radiologically, osteoma appears as a dense,

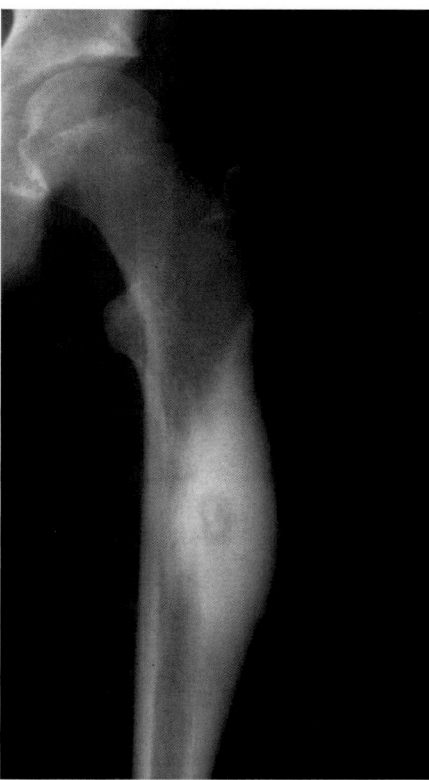

**FIGURE 47–19.** Osteoid osteoma. Roentgenogram shows highly sclerotic cortical bone with a partially lucent nidus with central ossification, creating a targetoid appearance.

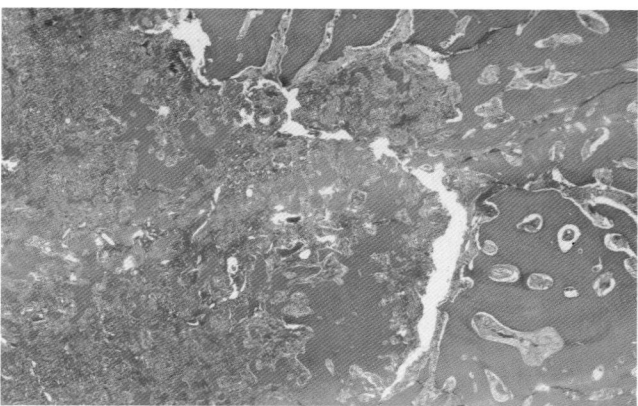

**FIGURE 47–20.** Low-power view of an osteoid osteoma nidus surrounded by dense bone.

opaque, well-defined mass measuring roughly from 1.0 to 9.0 cm. Most osteomas are composed of compact lamellar bone similar to cortical bone with haversian systems present; others are composed predominantly of mature lamellar bone with intervening fat and marrow elements.

Benign *osteoid osteoma* has been found in virtually every bone (Figs. 47–19 to 47–21), but the femur, tibia, humerus, bones of the hands and feet, and vertebrae are involved most often.[157] Long bone lesions usually are metaphyseal but may be epiphyseal, juxta-articular, or intra-articular.[158] Most osteoid osteomas arise in the bony cortex, but they may occur in the spongiosa or subperiosteal region.[159] Vertebral lesions usually affect the posterior elements.[160] The typical radiographic finding is that of a radiolucent central nidus (most often <1.5 cm) that is surrounded by a peripheral sclerotic reaction that may extend for several centimeters along both sides of the cortex. The central nidus consists of variably calcified trabeculae of osteoid, lined by plump osteoblasts that reside within a highly vascu-

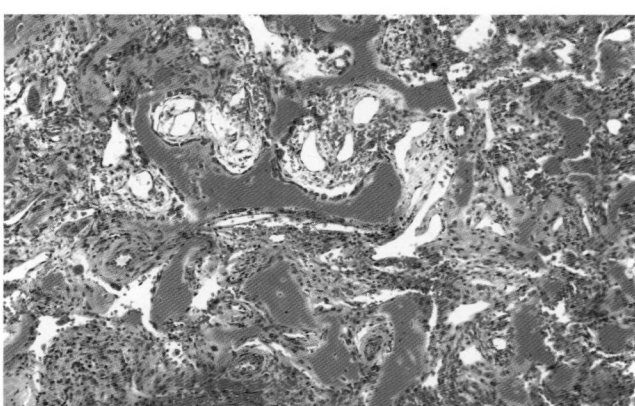

**FIGURE 47–21.** Higher magnification of osteoid osteoma nidus shows abundant new bone formation with trabeculae lined by enlarged osteoblasts. The trabeculae reside within a highly vascular stroma. Such a pattern is indistinguishable from the nidus of osteoblastoma.

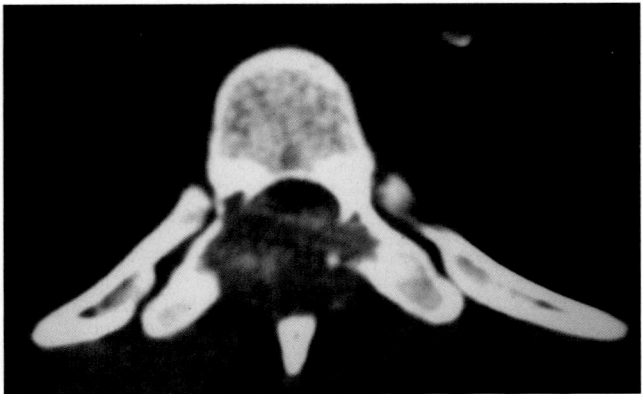

FIGURE 47–22. Osteoblastoma. Computed tomography scan shows an osteoblastoma involving the posterior vertebral elements in a 15-year-old girl. The lesion has destroyed the pedicles and involves the transverse processes and extends into the spinal canal.

larized stroma. When in a cortical location, a thick layer of dense bone surrounds the nidus. Osteoid osteoma usually occurs in patients 10 to 30 years old, exhibiting a 2:1 male-to-female ratio.[161, 162] Intense, sharply localized pain is almost universally present, only rarely being absent.[163] The pain is more intense at night and characteristically is relieved by nonsteroidal anti-inflammatory drugs (e.g., aspirin). Prostaglandin $E_2$, which is produced by os-

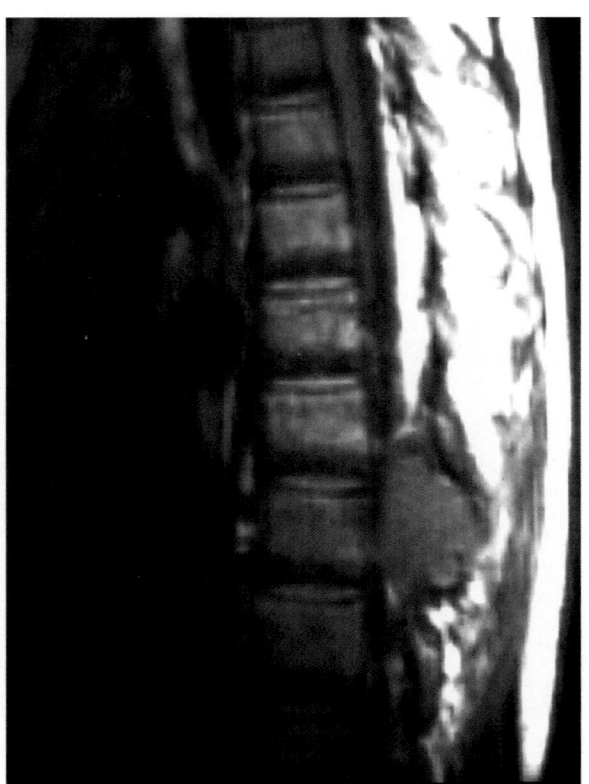

FIGURE 47–23. Osteoblastoma. Magnetic resonance image of the lesion in Figure 47–22.

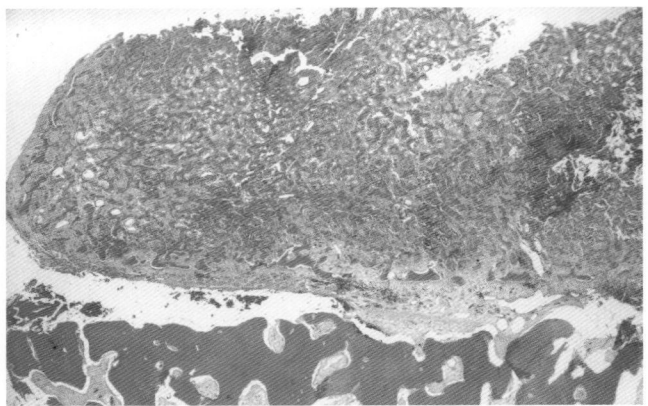

FIGURE 47–24. Nidus of osteoblastoma is sharply circumscribed, without permeation into the adjacent normal bone.

teoblasts, is present in increased amounts in osteoid osteoma and possibly contributes to the pain by stimulating nerve fibers within the lesion.[164, 165]

Surgical excision of osteoid osteoma is curative in almost all cases, provided that the nidus is removed completely. Failure to remove the nidus may result in local recurrence. Percutaneous needle ablation of the nidus has become an increasingly prevalent form of therapy for osteoid osteoma.

*Osteoblastoma* is similar clinically and pathologically to osteoid osteoma[166, 167] (Figs. 47–22 to 47–25); however, it is a larger lesion with a nidus greater than 1.5 cm, has no or minimal surrounding reactive bone, and may lack the intense nighttime pain of osteoid osteoma. In contrast to osteoid osteoma, which is more common in the long bones than in the vertebrae, the latter is the most common site for osteoblastoma, the long bones being involved less commonly. In the long bones, it usually arises within the spongiosa of the metaphysis, but cortical and subperiosteal forms occur.[159, 168, 169] Similar to osteoid osteoma, osteoblastoma usually occurs in pa-

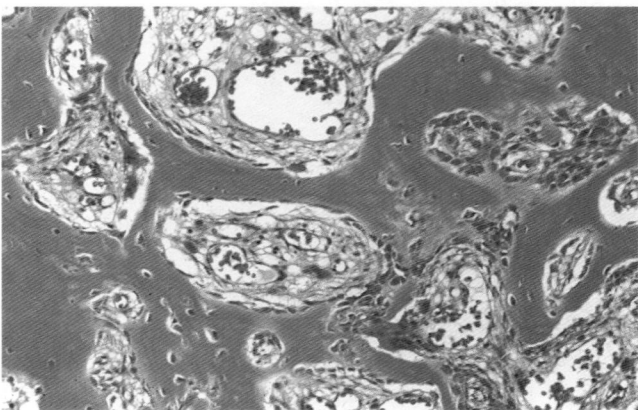

FIGURE 47–25. Higher magnification view of nidus of osteoblastoma shows netlike pattern of interconnecting bone trabeculae formed by active osteoblastic activity; osteoclasts are distributed randomly on the surface of the bone. The bone resides within a highly vascular edematous stroma.

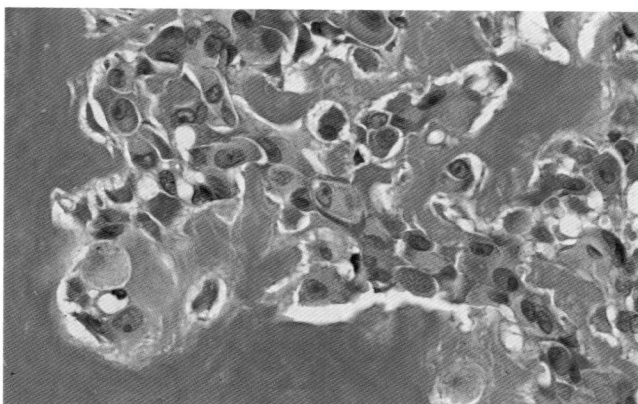

**FIGURE 47–26.** Aggressive osteoblastoma. High-power view shows plump epithelioid osteoblasts that have abundant eosinophilic cytoplasm, some with prominent nucleoli.

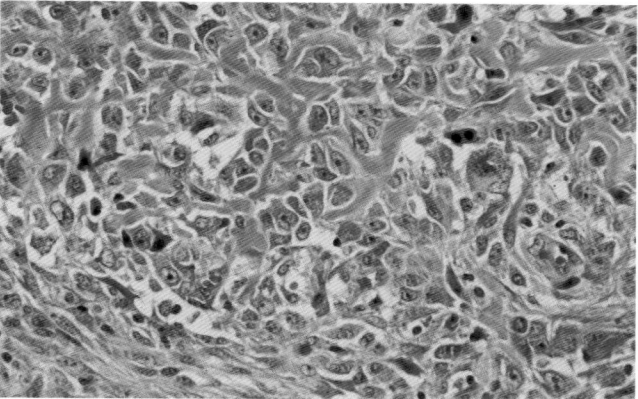

**FIGURE 47–28.** Osteosarcoma. Malignant stromal cells, with a high degree of cellular atypia, are present between which are ribbon-like strands of osteoid.

tients 10 to 30 years old, also exhibiting a 2:1 male-to-female ratio.[161, 162] Histologic evaluation shows the nidus of osteoblastoma is identical to that of osteoid osteoma, although in contrast to the latter, cartilaginous foci may rarely be found in osteoblastoma.[170] Distinguishing osteoblastoma from osteosarcoma may be difficult[168] because osteosarcoma contains numerous well-differentiated malignant osteoblasts, whereas osteoblastoma may contain scattered bizarre cells of *degenerative* nature.[171]

So-called *aggressive osteoblastoma* shows the radiologic and morphologic features of osteoblastoma but has atypical cytologic features and may have a greater local recurrence rate[1–12] (Fig. 47–26). Aggressive osteoblastoma characteristically contains epithelioid-appearing osteoblasts lining the osteoid trabeculae.[172] The osteoblasts are about twice the size of their conventional counterparts, having an abundant eosinophilic cytoplasm and large nuclei with promi-

nent nucleoli. In contrast to conventional osteosarcoma, aggressive osteoblastoma has a low mitotic rate without atypical mitoses, contains no lacelike osteoid, and lacks permeation of the surrounding trabecular bone. This form of aggressive osteoblastoma should not be confused with lesions reported as malignant osteoblastoma, osteosarcoma resembling osteoblastoma, osteoblastoma-like osteosarcoma, or osteoblastoma dedifferentiating to osteosarcoma.[171–175] The term should not be applied to conventional osteoblastomas that may have an aggressive-appearing radiologic pattern, sometimes simulating osteosarcoma, or that simply develop local recurrences after aggressive therapy.

Surgical therapy is the treatment of choice for osteoblastoma, with complete removal curative in all cases. Radiation therapy has been used to treat spinal cases that cannot be removed surgically because of their large size.

*Osteosarcoma* is the most frequent primary, malignant, bone-forming tumor (Figs. 47–27 to 47–43). It has a slight male predominance (3:2) and usually

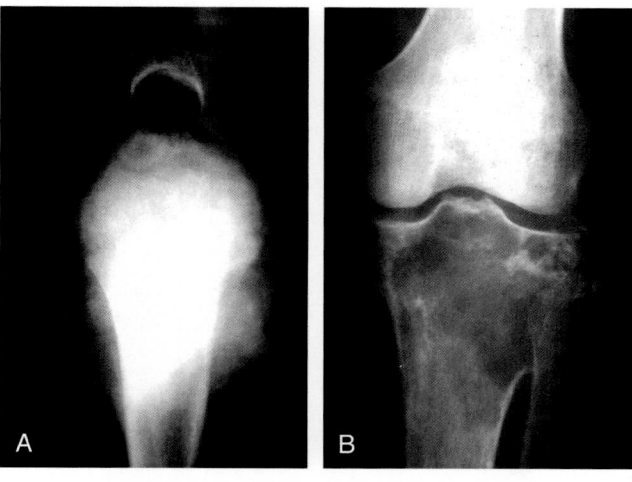

**FIGURE 47–27.** Osteosarcoma. Roentgenograms of osteosarcoma show proximal tibia (*A*) with highly dense tumor bone that extends into the soft tissues, and a predominately lytic destructive pattern (*B*) in a proximal tibia, with destruction of the cortex and extension to the subchondral area; matrix formation is minimal.

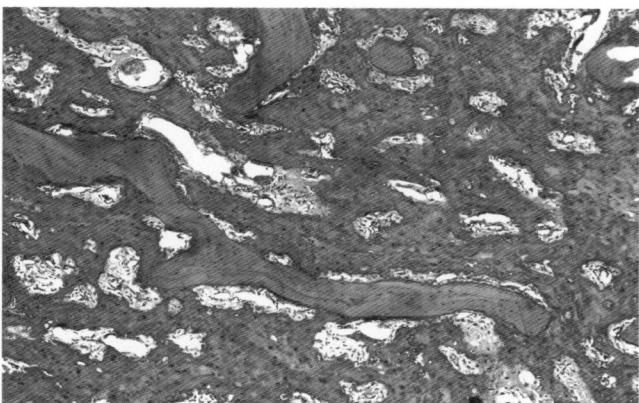

**FIGURE 47–29.** Osteoblastic osteosarcoma. Extensive tumor bone is seen deposited on a residual normal bone trabecula. Such dense tumor bone is diagnostic of osteosarcoma even in the absence of osteoid formation.

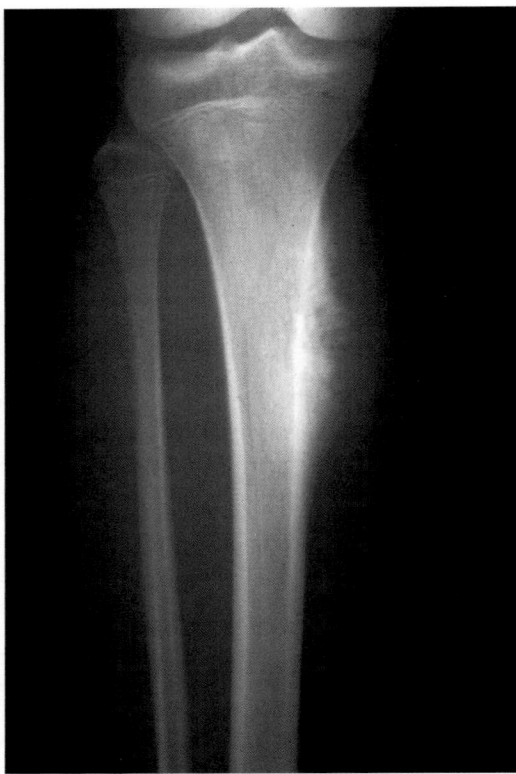

**FIGURE 47–30.** Periosteal osteosarcoma. Roentgenogram of proximal tibia shows surface-based lesion with radiating spicules at right angles to the long axis of the bone, and a soft tissue mass. Note the absence of any apparent medullary involvement.

arises in patients 10 to 30 years old.[176–178] A second peak age incidence occurs after age 40 years, most often in association with various preexisting bone conditions, including Paget's disease; prior radiation or chemotherapy or both; bone lesions such as fibrous dysplasia, osteochondromatosis, and enchondromatosis; bone infarcts; the *dedifferentiated* component of low-grade chondrosarcoma or chordoma; and, rarely, the site of a metallic foreign body.[179–187]

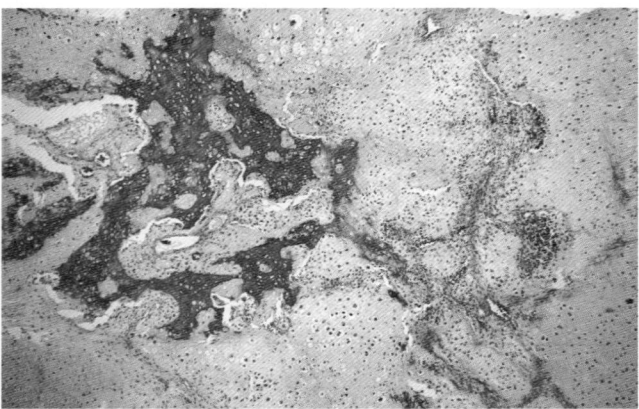

**FIGURE 47–31.** Periosteal osteosarcoma shows extensive high-grade malignant cartilage undergoing calcification and ossification.

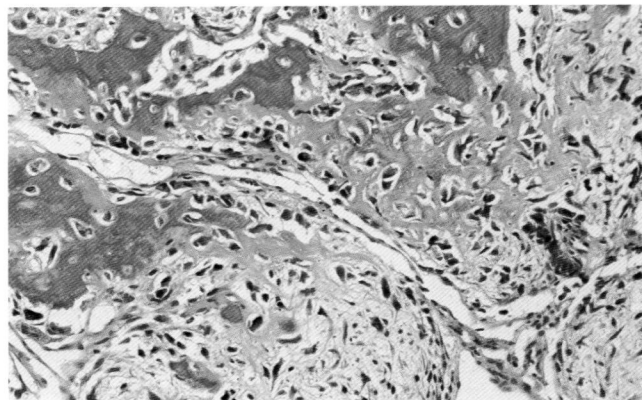

**FIGURE 47–32.** Small, focal region within a periosteal osteosarcoma shows osteoid formation with conversion to tumor bone. Such foci may be difficult to find within the mass of malignant cartilage that predominates in periosteal osteosarcoma.

Most de novo osteosarcomas occur in the metaphysis of the long bones, particularly about the knee and in the proximal humerus.[188] Uncommonly, it arises in the diaphysis or epiphysis of long bones; in the short bones of the distal extremities; or in the craniofacial or pelvic bones.[189, 190] The usual osteosarcoma initially involves the medullary cavity, later growing into and permeating the cortex; rarely, osteo-

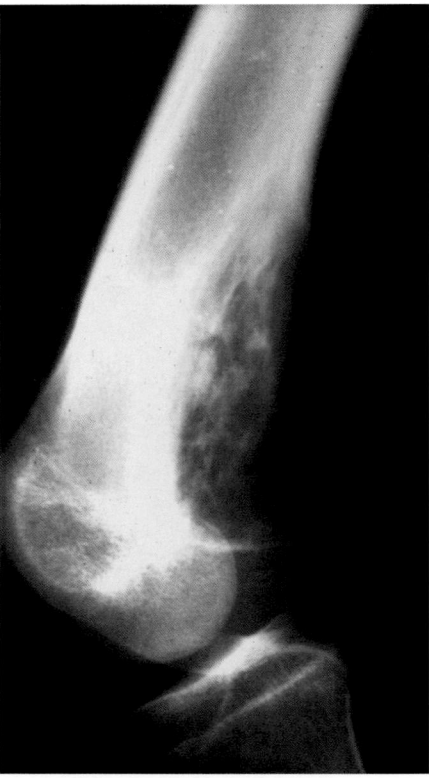

**FIGURE 47–33.** Well-differentiated osteosarcoma. Roentgenogram shows large, lytic, destructive lesion involving the posterior aspect of the distal femur in a 13-year-old girl. No soft tissue extension is apparent.

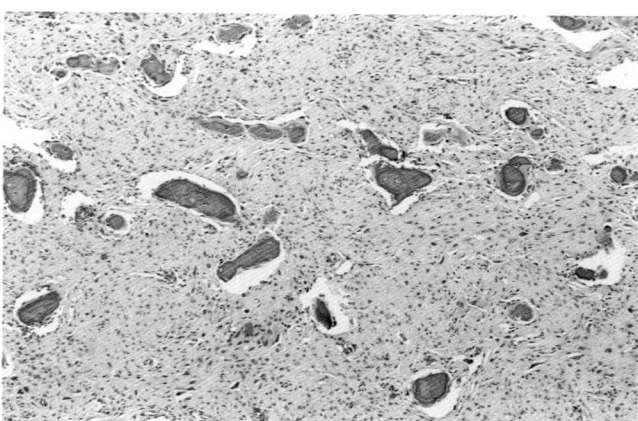

FIGURE 47–34. Well-differentiated osteosarcoma. Low-power view shows a pattern of bone formation that resembles fibrous dysplasia, consisting of irregular distribution of small bone trabeculae and ossicles within a fibrous stroma.

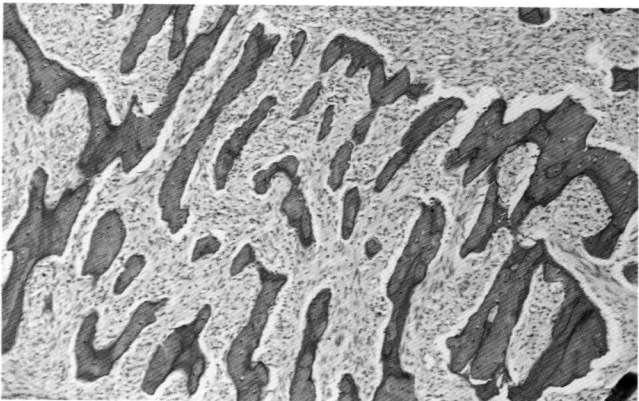

FIGURE 47–36. Well-differentiated osteosarcoma shows parallel arrangement of tumor bone trabeculae residing within a bland fibrous stroma. Such parallel arrangement of tumor bone is also found in parosteal osteosarcoma, the surface-based counterpart of well-differentiated osteosarcoma.

sarcomas arise within the cortex.[191] Osteosarcomas typically are unicentric, but multicentric examples occur, which may be synchronous or metachronous. Multicentric osteosarcoma tends to be aggressive and develop predominantly in children.[192, 193]

On roentgenographs, conventional osteosarcoma may appear totally opaque or lucent or, most commonly, have combined radiodense and lucent areas. Rarely the tumor may simulate a benign cyst of bone (*pseudocystic osteosarcoma*).[194] When osteosarcoma perforates the cortex, Codman's triangle may be evident as a result of elevation of the periosteum by the tumor with reactive new bone formation. Codman's triangle is not specific for osteosarcoma or for malignancy; any lesion that elevates the periosteum, including infection or hematoma, may produce it. At the time of diagnosis, osteosarcoma almost always is found to have extended into the soft tissues. It also may invade the epiphysis and joint space; form satellite nodules in the same bone or transarticularly (so-called skip metastases); and me-

tastasize through the bloodstream, especially to the lung, other bones, pleura, or heart.[195, 196] Metastases to lymph nodes are rare.

The gross tumor may be hard or cystic, friable, soft, necrotic, and hemorrhagic. Osteosarcoma cells may show variable anaplasia; they may be spindled, oval, or round (i.e., epithelioid), and their size may

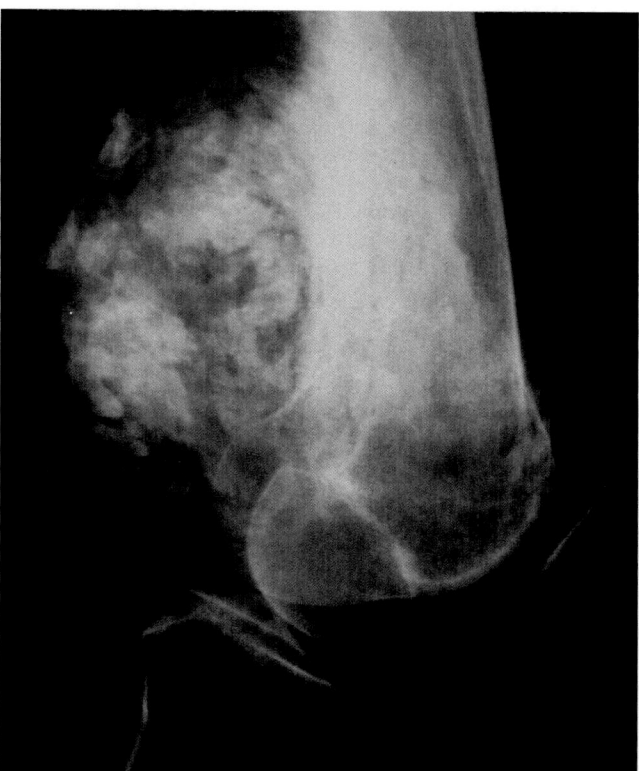

FIGURE 47–37. Parosteal osteosarcoma. Roentgenogram shows a large mass on the posterior surface of the distal femur in a 54-year-old woman. The mass, with abundant matrix formation, has extended anteriorly to the suprapatellar area.

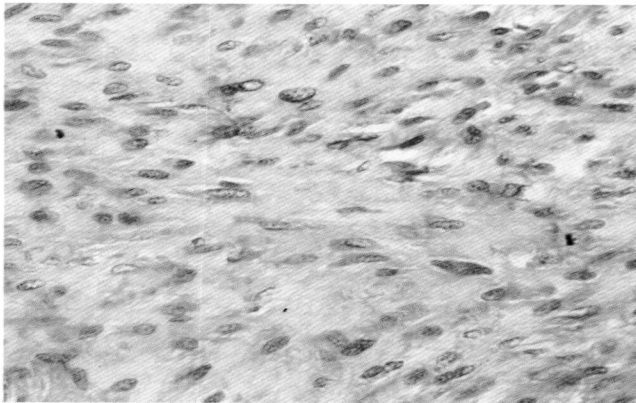

FIGURE 47–35. Higher magnification view of the spindle cell stroma in a well-differentiated osteosarcoma shows mild degree of atypia within some cells and mitotic activity. Such atypia would not be present in the stromal cells of fibrous dysplasia.

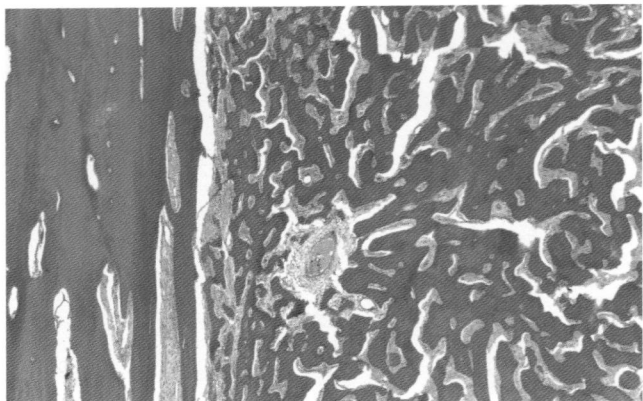

**FIGURE 47–38.** Low-power view of parosteal osteosarcoma shows normal cortical bone to the left of the field, juxtaposed to trabeculae of tumor bone.

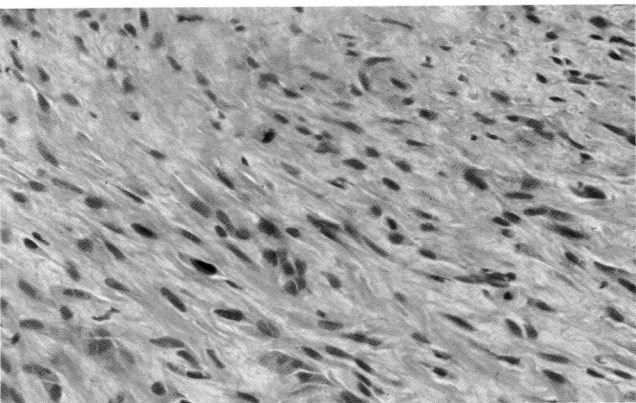

**FIGURE 47–40.** Stroma of parosteal osteosarcoma shows mostly bland-appearing spindle cells; however, occasional cells have dense, hyperchromatic atypical nuclei; some atypical mitotic figures are present.

range from small to giant.[197–200] Invasive tumor may destroy the preexisting bony trabeculae or grow or permeate around them in an appositional fashion. For the diagnosis of osteosarcoma, the pathologist must find, somewhere in the tumor, osteoid or tumor bone that is produced directly by malignant stromal cells, regardless of how much neoplastic cartilage (with or without endochondral ossification) or malignant-appearing fibrous tissue is present. Osteoid is recognized by its glassy eosinophilic-staining quality and irregular contours. In benign tumors, osteoid trabeculae often are surrounded by a rim of osteoblasts, but this osteoblastic rimming is absent or poorly developed in osteosarcoma. It may be difficult to distinguish osteoid from hyalinized collagen, but a glassy or homogeneous rather than fibrillary appearance, punctate calcification, and a plump appearance of the cells around it favor a diagnosis of osteoid. Most osteosarcomas are osteoblastic (Fig. 47–29), producing abundant osteoid and tumor bone, but they also frequently contain areas of malignant cartilage and malignant spindle cell fibrous regions. The relative proportion of these components varies from case to case;[201–203] depending on which

component predominates, osteosarcomas have been divided into osteoblastic, fibroblastic, and chondroblastic subtypes, but to date this classification is of little prognostic significance. The amount of osteoid may be sparse or abundant; usually in osteosarcoma one finds ribbon-like streamers of osteoid surrounded by obviously malignant stromal cells. As more osteoid accumulates, it may form large, sheet-like masses. On calcification and its conversion to tumor bone, the latter may become so extensive that it replaces and chokes off the stromal cells, resulting in acellular masses of tumor bone and osteoid.

Osteoclast-like multinucleated giant cells sometimes are numerous, producing a giant cell–rich osteosarcoma. These osteoclast-like giant cells are benign and apparently recruited into the tumor from monocyte/histiocyte precursors. Cartilaginous areas may be immature, mineralized, or myxoid but have obvious malignant features. The fibroblastic areas may have a fibrosarcomatous appearance. Osteosar-

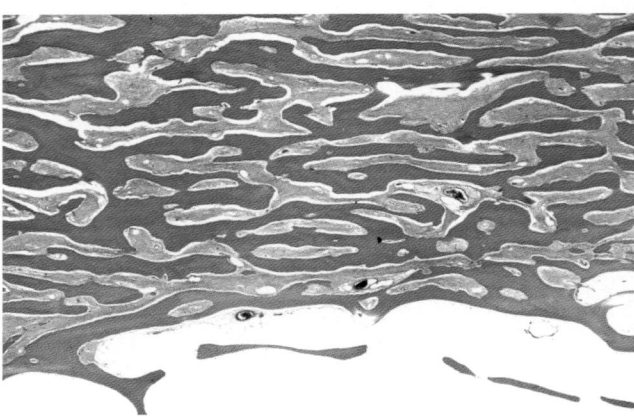

**FIGURE 47–39.** Parosteal osteosarcoma. In some areas, the tumor bone trabeculae are organized in parallel arrays.

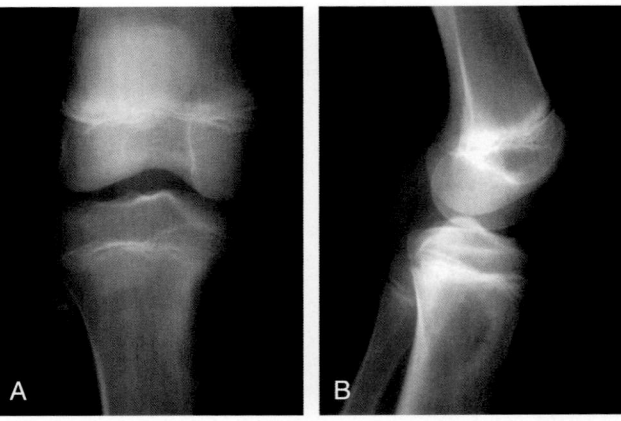

**FIGURE 47–41.** Telangiectatic osteosarcoma. Anterior and posterior roentgenograms of the proximal tibia of a 12-year-old girl. A destructive lesion is eccentrically present, with some degree of bone sclerosis about its inner margin. No apparent soft tissue mass is evident. The lesion is predominantly lytic.

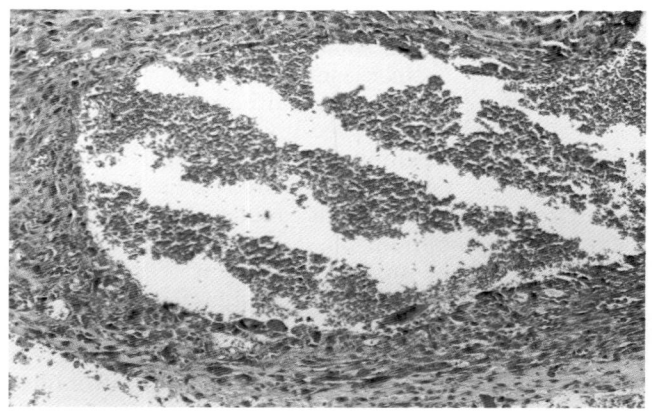

**FIGURE 47–42.** View of telangiectatic osteosarcoma shows dilated vascular space, similar to that found in an aneurysmal bone cyst; however, here the wall contains highly atypical and anaplastic tumor cells.

coma cells express vimentin and alkaline phosphatase; sometimes they contain smooth muscle actin and desmin. Immunoreactivity for keratin and epithelial membrane antigen is noted occasionally.[204–206] As expected, S-100 protein is found in cartilaginous areas, but it also may occur in osteoblastic areas.[204] Osteonectin and osteopontin are bone matrix proteins, antibodies to which have been used to help in the diagnosis of osteosarcoma; however, their presence in nonosteosarcomas has limited their diagnostic utility. The most common cytogenetic abnormalities detected in osteosarcoma involve chromosomes 1, 2, 6, 12, and 17; however, no specific chromosomal abnormality has been found.[207]

Osteosarcoma may also develop on the surface of the bone. These juxtacortical (surface-based) osteosarcomas are classified into parosteal, periosteal, and high-grade types. *Parosteal osteosarcoma* (Figs. 47–37 to 47–40), the most common form, occurs in patients older (mean age, approximately 40 years) than those with conventional, intramedullary osteo-

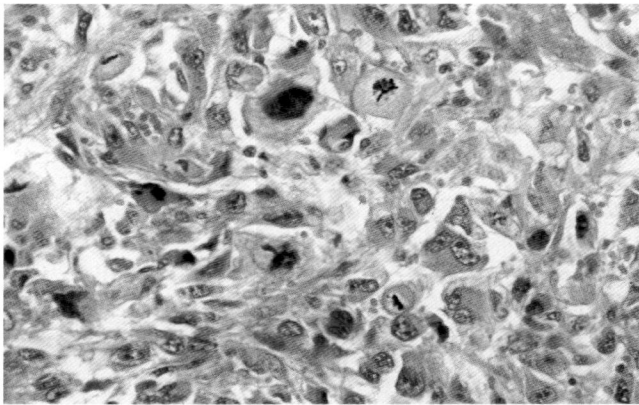

**FIGURE 47–43.** Higher magnification view of telangiectatic osteosarcoma shows highly atypical tumor cells with atypical mitotic figures. Other areas within this tumor had focal areas of osteoid formation. Osteoid may be scant and, at times, almost totally absent in telangiectatic osteosarcoma.

sarcoma. It most commonly affects the long bones, especially the metaphyseal region of the posterior distal femur, but may occur in other bones, including the jaw bones.[208] The tumor grows slowly; patients complain of mild pain or an enlarging mass sometimes for several years.[209–211] Radiologically, it appears as a dense, oval-to-spheroidal, lobulated mass that seems to be pasted onto the cortex. Over time, the mass encircles the bone and eventually may invade into the medullary space.[211–214] Mineralization of the tumor proceeds from the base, which rests on a thickened cortex, to the periphery. This activity is in contrast to what occurs in myositis ossificans (with which parosteal osteosarcoma may be confused),[215] in which mineralization develops initially at the periphery. Histologically, parosteal osteosarcoma is composed of varying proportions of a fibrous stroma and bone. The cells of the stroma are cytologically bland, and an extensive search for atypia or abnormal mitotic figures is frequently required. The bone appears to be metaplastic and to arise directly from the stroma. The bone trabeculae tend to be aligned in arrays that run parallel to the long axis of the parent bone. At its periphery, the tumor invades and incorporates the adjacent soft tissue; cartilaginous foci, having features of low-grade chondrosarcoma, are found in 50% to 80% of cases but, in contrast to periosteal osteosarcoma, are never a dominant feature. Foci of dedifferentiation may develop within parosteal osteosarcoma, most commonly after local recurrence but rarely also at the time of initial diagnosis. Treatment of parosteal osteosarcoma is purely surgical. In contrast to conventional osteosarcoma, the tumor has a relatively good prognosis after either wide en bloc excision for smaller lesions or amputation for larger tumors, with a 5-year survival rate of approximately 80%; 10-year survival rates decrease to 60% to 70% owing to the development of late metastases.[216] Patients with dedifferentiated tumors have a poor prognosis. Medullary extension does not seem to affect prognosis.

Periosteal osteosarcoma (Figs. 47–30 to 47–32) most frequently occurs in patients in their teens and young adults. In contrast to the metaphyseal location of parosteal osteosarcoma, periosteal osteosarcoma usually occurs on the medial or lateral aspect of the diaphysis or metaphysis of the proximal tibia or distal femur. The tumor tends to be smaller than parosteal osteosarcoma and radiologically shows a lucent concavity on the bone surface accompanied by a nonhomogeneous pattern of radiating spicules that extend outward from a thickened cortex into the soft tissue.[217, 218] The medullary cavity is involved only rarely and usually found only on microscopic examination. In contrast to its absence in parosteal osteosarcoma, Codman's triangle formation commonly is present in periosteal osteosarcoma. On gross and microscopic examination, periosteal osteosarcoma is predominantly a chondroblastic osteosarcoma with lobules of cartilage seen on macroscopic examination and intermediate-grade to high-grade malignant cartilage present microscopically.[211] Osteoid or tumor bone formation may be scarce. Reactive new bone formation and large areas of calcification are common. The histologic distinction between high-grade surface osteosarcoma and periosteal osteosarcoma may not be possible in all cases, but high-grade surface osteosarcoma tends to be osteoblastic rather than chondroblastic. Periosteal osteosarcoma has a prognosis that is better than that of conventional medullary osteosarcoma but worse than that of parosteal osteosarcoma.

High-grade osteosarcoma is the least common surface osteosarcoma.[219, 220] Most patients are teenagers or young adults. The tumor usually involves the metaphysis or metadiaphysis of a long bone, most typically the distal femur or proximal humerus. The tumor creates a radiologic pattern similar to that of periosteal osteosarcoma except for its denser, more irregular mineralization. Histologically the lesion is similar to conventional intramedullary osteosarcoma with osteoblastic predominance. The treatment and prognosis are similar to that of conventional osteosarcoma.

In *telangiectatic osteosarcoma*, blood-filled cavities are prominent, resulting in an appearance similar to that of aneurysmal bone cyst (Figs. 47–41 to 47–43). In contrast to aneurysmal bone cyst, malignant tumor cells exist in the septa (walls) of the cavities.[221] Osteoid in these tumors may be difficult to find.[221–223] In *small cell osteosarcoma*, the small size and uniformity of the tumor cells and their diffuse growth pattern mimics Ewing's sarcoma or malignant lymphoma.[224–227] Some of these small cell tumors also express the *MIC2* gene product (CD99) and have the t(11;22) translocation typically found in Ewing's sarcoma, and primitive neuroectodermal tumor (PNET). *Fibrohistiocytic osteosarcoma* contains areas indistinguishable from malignant fibrous histiocytoma, which may occur as a primary bone tumor in its own right. The distinction is based on finding tumor osteoid in fibrohistiocytic osteosarcoma. *Well-differentiated (low-grade) intraosseous osteosarcoma* is a cytologically bland spindle cell tumor that may be underdiagnosed as benign, particularly as fibrous dysplasia[228, 229] (Figs. 47–33 to 47–36). In contrast to fibrous dysplasia, however, there is cortical destruction and invasive growth.[230] Occasional atypical spindle cells are found, and a few atypical mitoses are seen among the metaplastic-appearing bone trabeculae. Some authors claim that these tumors are predominantly chondroblastic, whereas others have found no such pattern.

*Osteosarcoma of the jaw* occurs more commonly in the mandible than in the maxilla and accounts for approximately 5% of all osteosarcomas. These osteosarcomas tend to occur in patients with an older mean age than osteosarcomas elsewhere. Swelling, pain, and associated paresthesia are typical symptoms. There is a wide range of radiologic appearances, from radiolucent to radiopaque with a classic "sunburst" pattern. A uniformly widened periodontal membrane space is seen often when the tumor involves the alveolus.[231, 232] The histologic subtypes of jaw osteosarcomas include, in order of descending frequency, osteoblastic, chondroblastic, fibroblastic, and telangiectatic, although some series show a chondroblastic predominance. The histologic subtypes do not exhibit different clinical behaviors. The prognosis for jaw osteosarcoma is better than for extremity-based lesions; metastases from these lesions are uncommon.[233]

As a result of modern polyagent chemotherapy, the prognosis for conventional osteosarcoma has improved from only approximately 20% to an approximately 70% 5-year disease-free survival.[234–237] Osteosarcomas arising in the jaws or distal extremities seem to have a less aggressive course, whereas those arising from Paget's disease; after radiation therapy; in the craniofacial bones or vertebrae; or are multicentric have a significantly poorer prognosis. It has been shown that the amount of tumor necrosis after chemotherapy is related directly to the survival rate, with tumors showing greater than 90% necrosis being considered *good* responders with the best prognosis.[238, 239] This feature may be the most important prognostic parameter in patients with conventional osteosarcoma of extremities with no evidence of distant metastases at presentation.[240]

Traditional therapy for osteosarcoma of the extremities has consisted of amputation or disarticulation, depending on the location of the tumor. More recently, more limited forms of surgical therapy (limb-sparing procedures) have been coupled with preoperative and postoperative adjuvant chemotherapy.[241–245] Surgical removal of metastatic nodules of osteosarcoma in the lungs seems to prolong survival in selected patients.[246, 247]

## CARTILAGE-FORMING TUMORS

*Chondroma* is a benign cartilage-forming tumor usually occurring in the small bones of the hands and feet, especially the proximal phalanges (Figs. 47–44 to 47–47). Less commonly, it develops within the ribs and long bones. When in the long bones, massive "cloudy" calcification may occur.[248] Most chondromas develop within the spongiosa (enchondroma), where they grow and thin the cortex. They also may arise on the surface of the bone from the periosteal or parosteal tissue.[249, 250] These *juxtacortical chondromas* tend to erode and cause sclerosis of the underlying cortex. Enchondroma is multiple in approximately 30% of cases, and when having a predominantly unilateral distribution, the condition is referred to as *Ollier's disease*[251] (Fig. 47–45). When found in association with soft tissue hemangiomas, the condition is referred to as *Maffucci's syndrome*.[252] In both of these conditions, there is a significant risk of malignant transformation, usually to chondrosarcoma.[253–256] Ollier's disease may also be associated with ovarian sex cord tumors.[257]

Chondromas are composed of mature lobules of benign hyaline-like cartilage whose chondrocytes may be distributed diffusely or arranged in small nests of several cells. Their nuclei are usually small

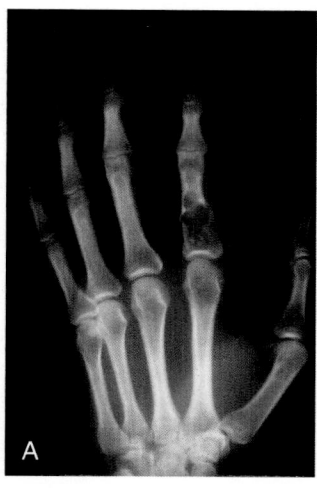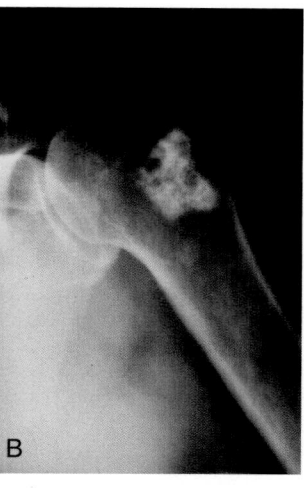

**FIGURE 47–44.** Enchondroma. *A,* Roentgenogram of the hand shows a fracture through an enchondroma of proximal phalanx. The lesion is largely lytic with punctate calcifications and endosteal scalloping of the adjacent bone cortex. *B,* Roentgenogram shows an incidental finding, in a 74-year-old man, of a densely calcified enchondroma in the proximal metaphysis of the humerus.

and hyperchromatic (ink-dot), with no visible chromatin pattern. Foci of myxoid degeneration, calcification, and enchondral ossification may be present. In enchondroma, the ossification tends to form a rim

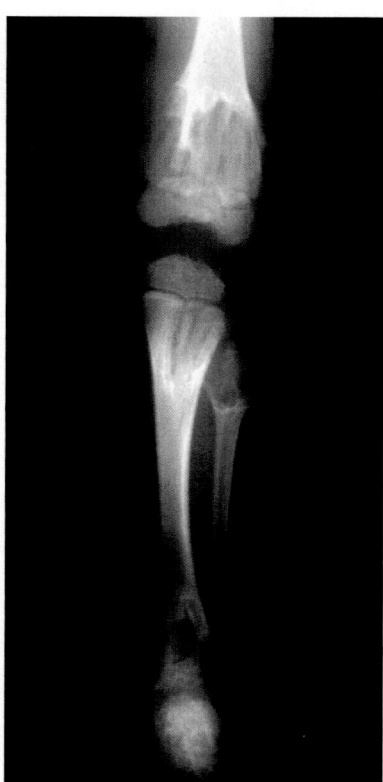

**FIGURE 47–45.** Ollier's disease. Roentgenogram shows multiple enchondromas involving the femur, tibia, and fibula. Note the expansion of the epiphysis and metaphysis; the striated appearance is caused by columns of uncalcified cartilage.

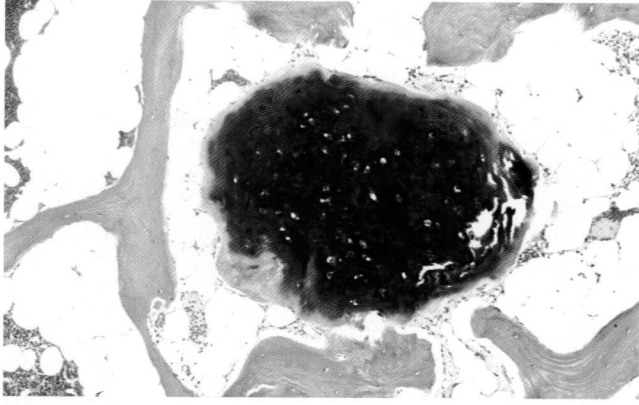

**FIGURE 47–46.** Enchondroma. Island of bland hyaline cartilage resides among bone trabeculae.

about the lobules of cartilage. This bony encasement pattern is a sign of slow growth and favors a benign diagnosis.[258] Juxtacortical chondroma tends to be more cellular than its medullary counterpart and may contain chondrocytes with occasional plump or double nuclei suggestive of low-grade chondrosarcoma. Surgical curettage of enchondroma or en-bloc excision of juxtacortical lesions is curative. A chest wall lesion in infancy, *mesenchymal hamartoma,* contains chondroma-like areas (often with enchondral ossification) that are admixed with areas having an aneurysmal bone cyst–like appearance. Most are present at birth and are benign.[259–261]

*Osteochondroma* is the most common benign bone tumor and is most likely the result of growth of aberrant foci of cartilage on the surface of the bone and thus is not a true neoplasm (Figs. 47–48 to 47–51). Although usually asymptomatic, osteochondroma may cause deformity or impair function of nearby structures. Common locations include the metaphyses of the lower femur, upper tibia, and upper humerus and the pelvic flat bones. When in a long bone, it extends in a mushroom-like or poly-

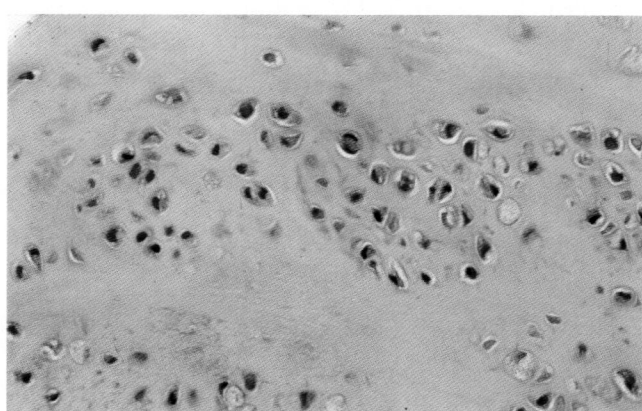

**FIGURE 47–47.** Enchondroma. Chondrocytes are arranged in loose clusters. The nuclei are small and dense (ink-dot appearance), in contrast to the large chondrocyte nuclei seen in chondrosarcoma whose chromatin pattern is frequently easily discernible.

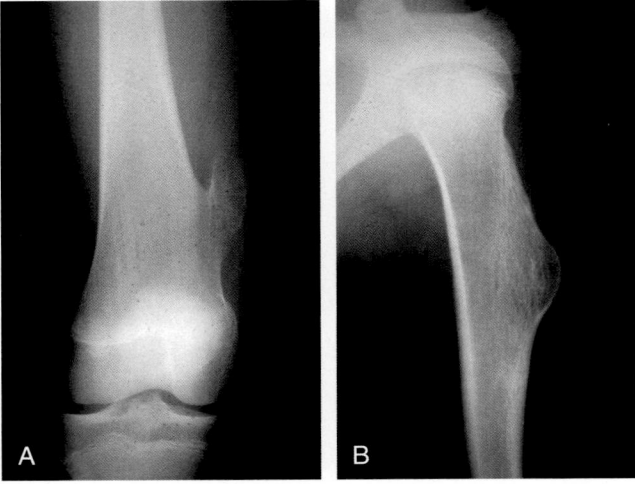

**FIGURE 47–48.** Osteochondroma. *A*, Roentgenogram shows polypoid osteochondroma, the central portion of which is continuous with the underlying medulla of the parent bone. *B*, Roentgenogram shows a sessile-type osteochondroma in which there is a less prominent polypoid projection.

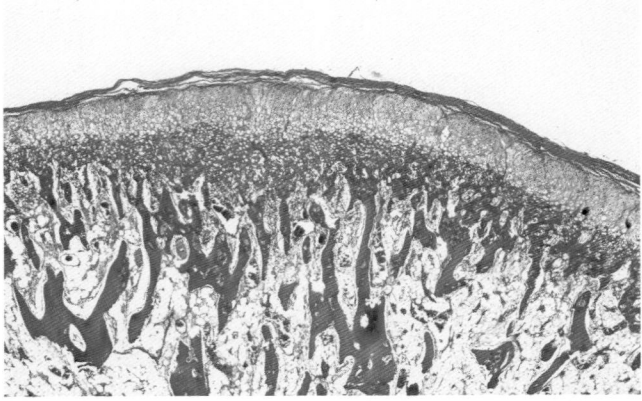

**FIGURE 47–50.** Osteochondroma. Low-power view shows hyaline cartilage cap covered by perichondrium; enchondral ossification is present.

poid fashion in a direction away from the adjacent joint. Osteochondroma usually develops in children and adolescents (<20 years old). Most are only a few centimeters in maximal dimension, but they may measure 10 cm. Radiologically the spongiosa of

the osteochondroma is in direct continuity with that of the underlying bone. Histologic characteristics include a peripheral cap of hyaline cartilage, of variable thickness, covered by a fibrous membrane (perichondrium) that joins with the periosteum of the adjacent bone. Typically the thickness of the cartilage cap in adults is approximately 0.5 cm and rarely greater than 1 cm.[262, 263] Often, it may be ab-

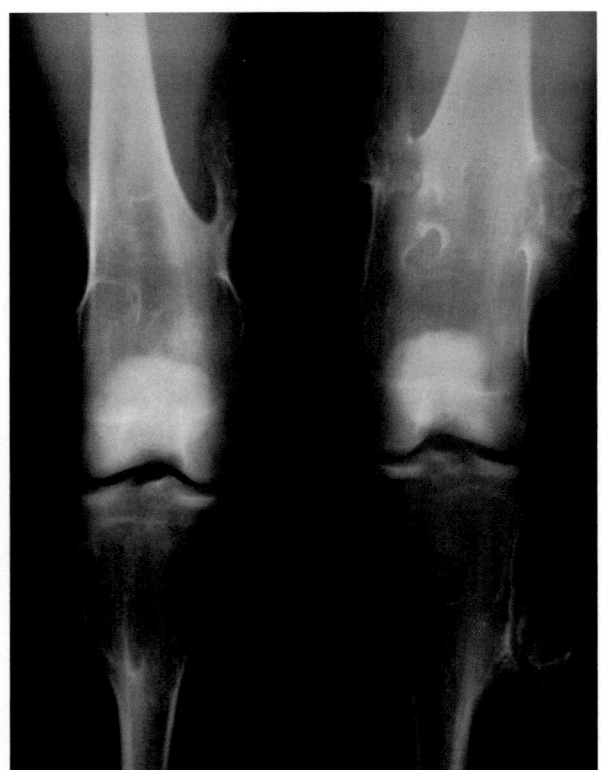

**FIGURE 47–49.** Osteochondromatosis. Multiple osteochondromas are seen in the femora and tibiae. There is widening of the metaphyses of both bones, and in one area there is column-like streaking similar to that found in Ollier's disease.

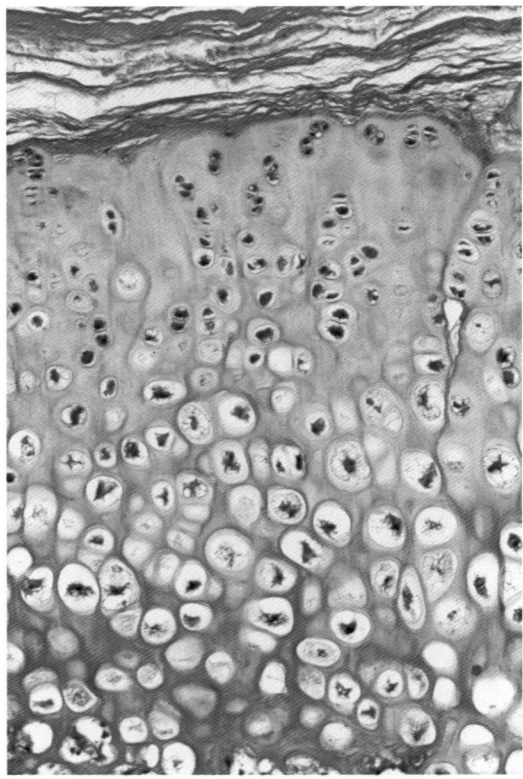

**FIGURE 47–51.** Higher magnification view of osteochondroma shows columnation of the chondrocytes in the cartilage cap. Such cartilage columnation is seen in actively growing individuals, in contrast to osteochondromas found after skeletal maturity in which there may be no evidence of enchondral ossification.

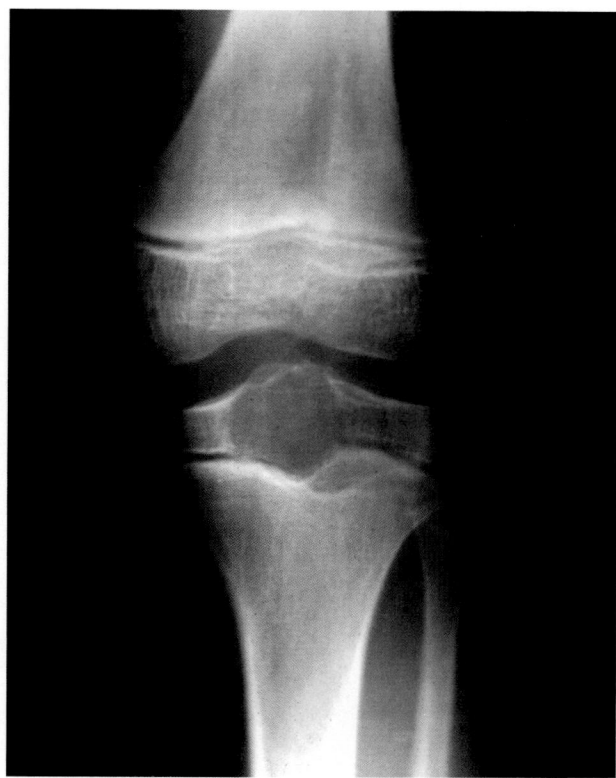

**FIGURE 47–52.** Chondroblastoma. Roentgenogram shows a well-defined, lytic lesion involving the epiphysis of the proximal tibia in a 9-year-old boy who had a painful knee.

sent owing to frictional erosion. In children, the cap may be several centimeters thick. Beneath the cap, there is mature bone trabeculae, containing normal bone marrow that is in continuity with the bone marrow of the underlying parent bone. From puberty until the cessation of skeletal growth, there is enchondral ossification present between the cartilage cap and the underlying bone. A bursa may develop about the head of an osteochondroma, which may develop osteocartilaginous loose bodies and synovial osteochondromatosis.[264] Osteochondromas may be multiple, a condition (autosomal dominant) known as osteochondromatosis or multiple cartilaginous exostoses[265, 266] (Fig. 47–49).

Complete surgical removal of osteochondroma is virtually always curative. However, a few (<1%) solitary osteochondromas develop into a chondrosarcoma (usually low-grade type), but the incidence of this change increases to approximately 10% in osteochondromatosis.[265, 267] This form of secondary chondrosarcoma in adults is suggested by an accelerated growth of the lesion during adolescence, large tumor size (i.e., >8 cm), a calcified center surrounded by a lesser dense periphery, and a thick cartilage cap (i.e., >2 to 3 cm).

It is important to distinguish osteochondroma from so-called bizarre parosteal osteochondromatous proliferation (*Nora's lesion*), which usually occurs in the bones of the hands and feet but may involve

long bones.[268] This parosteal proliferation simulates chondrosarcoma because it often contains cartilage with enlarged, bizarre, and binucleated chondrocytes.[268, 269] The cartilage has areas that mature into trabecular bone, however, which stains intensely with hematoxylin and is separated by a bland spindle cell proliferation. In contrast to osteochondroma, the lesion does not involve the underlying spongiosa of the affected bone. More than 50% of patients with these peculiar proliferations experience local recurrence after excision, but no malignant transformation has been reported.

Subungual exostosis (Dupuytren's exostosis) is usually located on the great toe, where it protrudes from beneath the toenail and may ulcerate through the skin. Although thought to represent a different entity from osteochondroma, it also is composed of a proliferating cartilaginous cap that merges into mature trabecular bone at its base. The lesion is benign but may recur after excision.[270, 271]

*Chondroblastoma* occurs in children and young adults in whom it most commonly arises in the epiphysis of a long bone (Figs. 47–52 to 47–54). Patients usually seek help because of pain. Chondroblastoma has a propensity for the distal end of the femur, proximal end of the humerus, and proximal end of the tibia.[272] Approximately 10% occur in the hands and feet, especially the calcaneus and talus. A metaphyseal origin is extremely rare. The lesion is almost completely lucent on roentgenograms but may show punctate calcification. The tumor is fairly well delineated but may extend into the metaphysis. Histologically, chondroblastoma is composed of polyhedral or epithelioid-appearing chondroblasts with well-defined cell borders and dense eosinophilic cytoplasm. Nuclei vary in shape from round to lobulated and sometimes, similar to Langerhans's cells, are clefted. Mitoses are rare, cytoplasmic glycogen granules often are present, and reticulin fibers surround individual cells. Scattered collections of osteoclast-type giant cells are evident. Chondroid islands

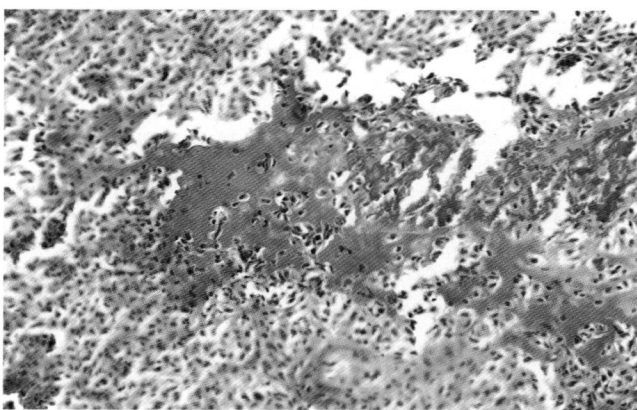

**FIGURE 47–53.** Area within chondroblastoma shows an island of pink chondroid material surrounded by chondroblasts. The finding of such chondroid is considered by some as necessary for the diagnosis of chondroblastoma.

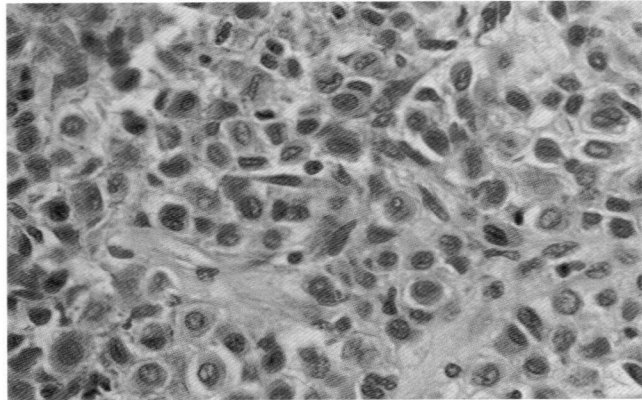

FIGURE 47–54. High-power view of chondroblastoma shows chondroblasts that have a relatively large amount of pink cytoplasm; some nuclei are clefted.

are present, and some authors insist on their presence for the diagnosis. Small zones of dystrophic calcification frequently are present that range from a network of thin lines about individual cells ("chicken wire pattern") to patternless aggregates. Aneurysmal bone cyst–like areas may occur (*cystic chondroblastoma*).[272] The cells of chondroblastoma express vimentin and S-100 protein, but they also may express neuron-specific enolase and low-molecular-weight cytokeratin.[273] Curettage with bone grafting provides initial local control in approximately 80% of cases. Rare cases of chondroblastoma have behaved aggressively, by invading the soft tissues, developing tumor thrombi in lymph channels, or spreading distantly (usually to lungs).[274–276]

*Chondromyxoid fibroma* is the least common of the benign cartilaginous lesions. It most frequently occurs in the long bones, especially of the lower extremities, in young adults (usually <30 years old). It also has occurred in the small bones of the hands and feet, pelvis, ribs, and vertebrae. In a long bone, the lesion is mainly metaphyseal but frequently extends into the epiphysis or diaphysis. In a short tubular bone, the entire bone may be expanded by the tumor. It is radiolucent, almost always lacking radiologic evidence of calcification. It may be eccentric with an inner sclerotic border or, at times, may have an aggressive appearance[277–279] (Figs. 47–55 to 47–57). Chondromyxoid fibroma is composed of hypocellular lobules that are separated by intersecting bands of relatively cellular tissue composed of fibroblast-like spindle cells and osteoclast-like giant cells and eosinophilic chondroblasts with dense eosinophilic cytoplasm.[280] The lobules themselves contain stellate-to-oval cells well separated by a myxochondroid matrix. The periphery of the lobules tends to be more cellular than the central zones. The cells may have atypical nuclei, leading to a misdiagnosis of chondrosarcoma. Mitotic figures are exceptional. Some tumors show a combination of chondroblastoma and chondromyxoid fibroma features.[281] The cells within the lobules and the eosinophilic chon-

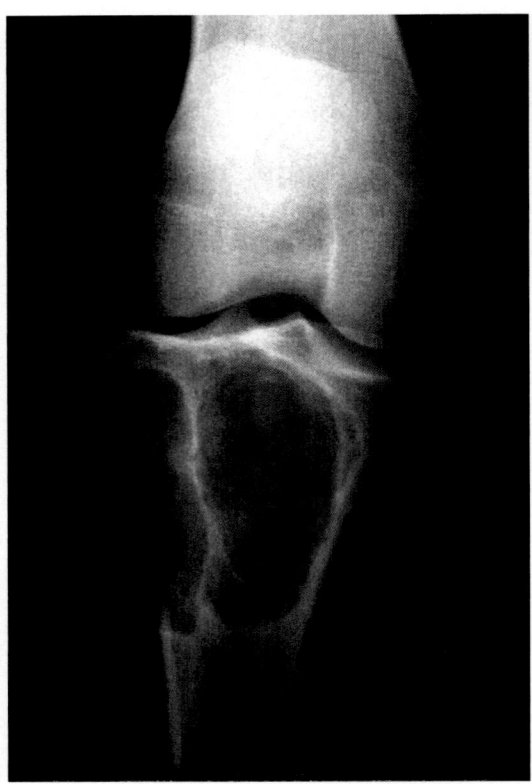

FIGURE 47–55. Chondromyxoid fibroma. Roentgenogram of proximal tibia shows a well-defined lytic lesion, with sclerotic borders and absence of any matrix formation.

droblasts are reactive for S-100 protein, supporting the presumed cartilaginous differentiation. The lobules may undergo progressive collagenation to form fibrocartilage. Local recurrence follows curettage of chondromyxoid fibroma in approximately 25% of cases; en-bloc excision is recommended. Soft tissue extension or implantation may occur, but distant metastases have not been reported. Fibromyxoma is

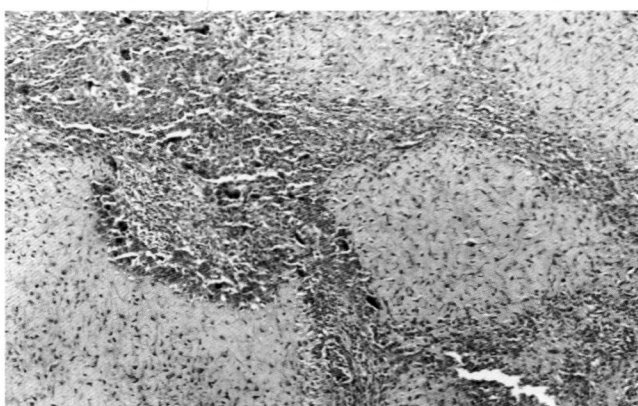

FIGURE 47–56. Nodules of chondromyxoid fibroma with peripheral hypercellular zones between the lobules in which are scattered chondroblasts and osteoclast-type giant cells. The cells within the nodules have a stellate appearance and are well separated by a myxoid matrix.

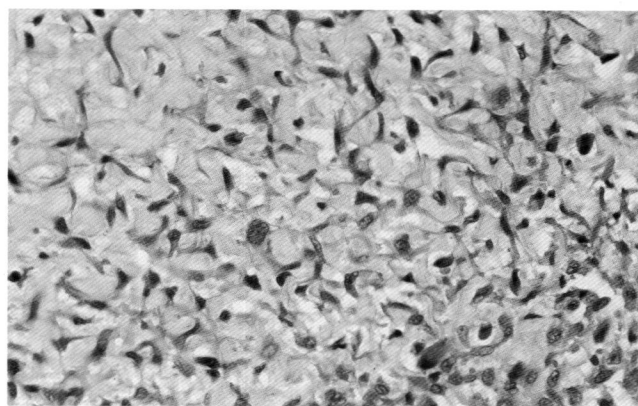

FIGURE 47–57. Close-up view of nodule of chondromyxoid fibroma. Stellate cells are scattered within a myxoid matrix. Some cell nuclei are enlarged and atypical, but this pattern should not be confused with low-grade chondrosarcoma.

similar to chondromyxoid fibroma, but it lacks cartilaginous areas and tends to occur in older individuals.

*Chondrosarcoma* is the most common malignant cartilage-forming tumor (Figs. 47–58 to 47–63). Most patients with conventional chondrosarcoma are 30 to 60 years old. The tumor is encountered in childhood rarely[282]; most malignant bone tumors in childhood showing cartilage formation prove to be chondroblastic osteosarcomas. Conventional chondrosarcomas may be classified according to location as central, peripheral, or juxtacortical (periosteal).[283, 284] Central chondrosarcoma develops in the medullary cavity, usually of a flat or long bone, and radiologically has an osteolytic pattern of bone destruction with splotchy, cloudy, or "popcorn" calcifications. It often shows irregular (i.e., permeative or infiltrative) margins, fusiform thickening of the

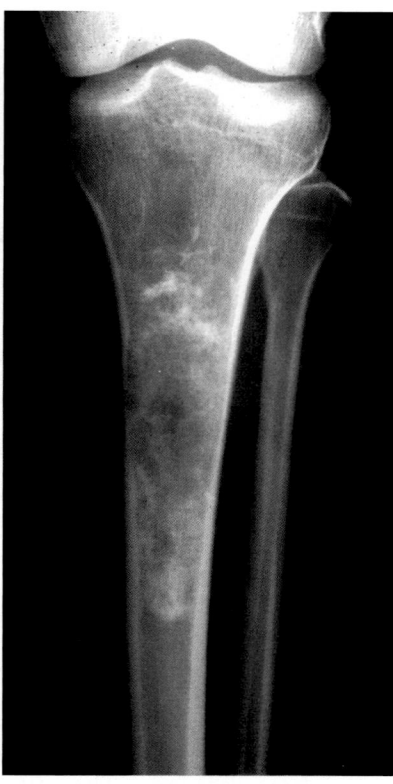

FIGURE 47–59. Chondrosarcoma involving the metadiaphysis of the tibia in a 45-year-old woman. The medial cortical bone is extensively thinned by a tumor that has well-defined borders and focal calcification.

shaft, endosteal scalloping of the cortex, and perforation of the cortex with soft tissue extension. The pelvic bones, ribs usually costochondral junction), and shoulder girdle are the common locations. Chondrosarcoma may develop in the bones of the skull, especially the temporal bone,[285] and, rarely, in the small bones of the hands and feet, especially the os calcis.[286, 287] Peripheral chondrosarcoma arises from the cartilaginous cap of a preexisting osteo-

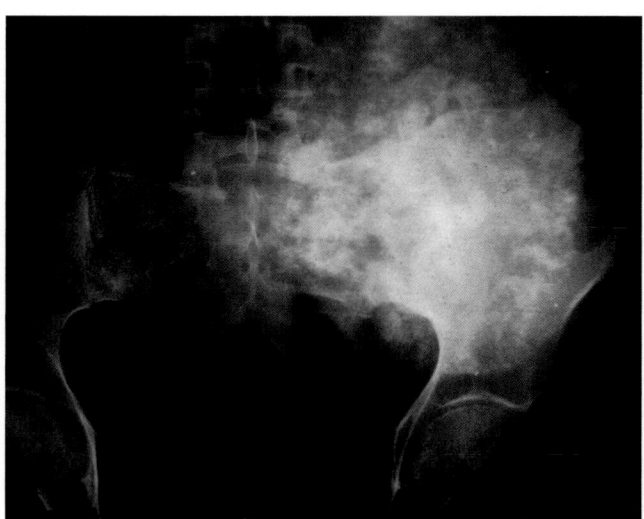

FIGURE 47–58. Chondrosarcoma. Roentgenogram shows massive chondrosarcoma involving the left side of the pelvis. "Popcorn" calcification is present throughout the tumor.

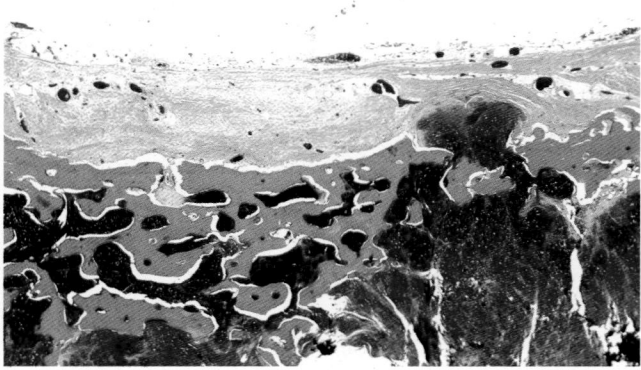

FIGURE 47–60. Low-grade chondrosarcoma shows tumor permeation and penetration through the cortex. Such haversian canal permeation by tumor is diagnostic of malignancy.

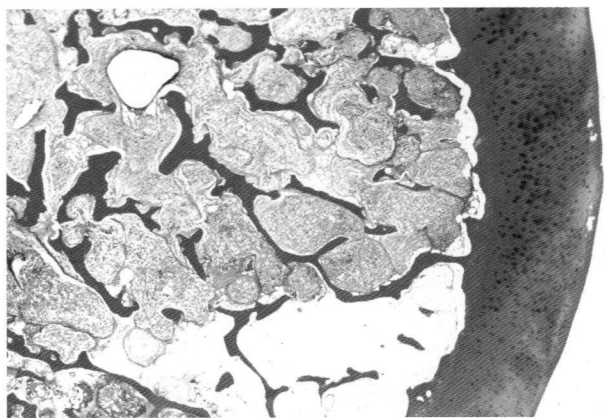

**FIGURE 47–61.** Low-power view of chondrosarcoma shows tumor permeating through and between existing normal bone trabeculae, without apparent destruction of the bone, filling the intratrabecular spaces and extending to the subarticular region.

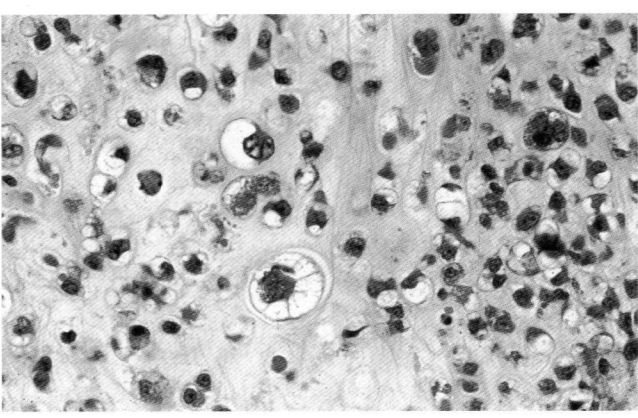

**FIGURE 47–63.** High-grade chondrosarcoma shows extreme degree of individual chondrocyte pleomorphism. Cells vary considerably in size and shape, with many appearing anaplastic.

chondroma. Juxtacortical (periosteal) chondrosarcoma develops on the surface of the bone, most often the shaft of a long bone (usually the femur).[283, 288] It has a cartilaginous lobular pattern with spotty calcification and enchondral ossification.[288] This form of chondrosarcoma may be difficult to distinguish from periosteal osteosarcoma. The diagnosis depends on the finding of osteoid production in the latter lesion. Also, in contrast to periosteal osteosarcoma, periosteal chondrosarcoma usually is well differentiated compared with the high-grade morphology of periosteal osteosarcoma.[283]

Conventional chondrosarcoma has a variable histopathology, but the common denominator is cartilaginous matrix production and the lack of direct bone or osteoid formation by the tumor cells. Bone may occur on chondrosarcoma, but this develops through a process of calcification and enchondral ossification of the malignant cartilage rather than by direct production of osteoid by the tumor cells as in

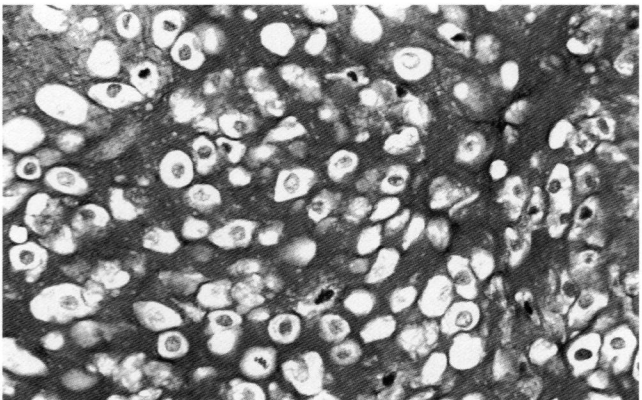

**FIGURE 47–62.** Low-grade chondrosarcoma shows hypercellularity with presence of abnormal chondrocytes that have enlarged nuclei whose chromatin pattern is easily seen. Mitotic figures, a rare finding in most chondrosarcomas, are also apparent.

osteosarcoma. Even in high-grade chondrosarcoma, the resulting bone may appear normal. Chondrosarcoma can be graded as well, moderately, or poorly differentiated, with most cases well to moderately differentiated.[1–12] Survival rates correlate with differentiation, with 5-year survival rates being 75% (well differentiated), 50% (moderately differentiated), and 25% (poorly differentiated).[289] The distinction between well-differentiated chondrosarcoma and an enchondroma is based on a combination of radiologic, clinical, and cytoarchitectural features, all of which should be evaluated thoroughly before a final diagnosis.[290, 291] In well-differentiated chondrosarcoma, the nuclei are large, with an open chromatin pattern; double nucleated cells may be numerous, and there may be single cell necrosis. The malignant cartilage permeates the bone marrow with trapping of the host lamellar bone on all sides by the tumor; such permeation is not found in chondroma. Haversian canal penetration and cortical penetration are good signs of malignancy. Large tumors of the long bones or ribs usually are malignant.[292, 293] Minor or moderate degrees of cell atypia in the chondrocytes in cartilaginous tumors of the hands and feet, osteochondromas, synovial osteochondromatosis, and soft tissue neoplasms are much less predictive of malignant behavior.[290] Myxoid change in an otherwise low-grade chondrosarcoma may be a sign of increased aggressiveness.

Cartilage lesions in children may appear cytologically atypical and, in an adult, would be diagnosed as a chondrosarcoma. However, in the absence of bone destruction, these lesions pursue a benign course. By electron microscopy, chondrosarcoma cells contain glycogen, lipid droplets, and dilated cisternae of granular endoplasmic reticulum similar to normal cartilage cells.[294] The tumor cells contain S-100 protein.[295, 296] Amplification of the *c-myc* proto-oncogene and expression of the *c-erbB-2* proto-oncogene have been detected in chondrosarcomas,[297, 298] and overexpression of *p53* seems limited to the high-grade (poorly differentiated) types.[301]

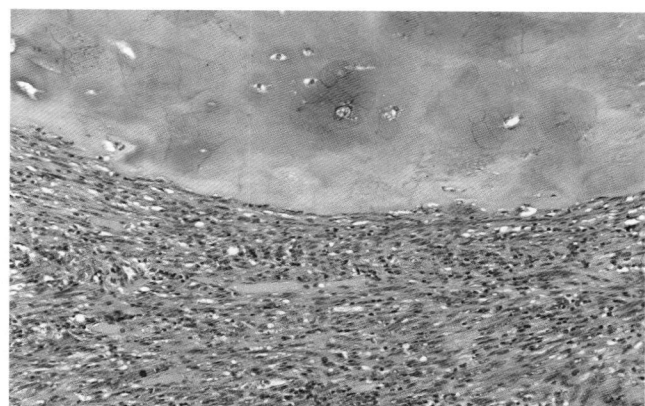

**FIGURE 47–64.** Dedifferentiated chondrosarcoma. Island of benign-appearing cartilage is juxtaposed to a spindle cell tumor.

Surgical excision is the treatment of choice for chondrosarcoma. The adequacy of the initial excision is crucial to prognosis. The biopsy site and skin incision point should be excised entirely in continuity, when definitive resection is performed. Chondrosarcoma of the rib should be excised en bloc along with the immediately adjacent uninvolved ribs and the underlying pleura.[300–302] Well-differentiated chondrosarcoma of the extremities is amenable to conservative therapy in the form of segmental resection[303], or complete curettage for low-grade tumors. Recurrences often are of a higher microscopic grade than the original tumor; metastases are usually to the lung.

Chondrosarcoma variants include clear cell chondrosarcoma, myxoid chondrosarcoma, dedifferentiated chondrosarcoma, and mesenchymal chondrosarcoma. The cells of clear cell chondrosarcoma have an abundant clear or ground-glass cytoplasm, sharply defined cell membranes, central round nuclei, and interspersed small trabeculae of woven bone. The tumor cells have features most consistent with cartilage cells in various stages of differentiation, and they express S-100 protein.[304–306] Osteoclast-like giant cells are often present, a rare finding in conventional chondrosarcoma. Lobulation usually is apparent, and in approximately 50% of cases, areas of conventional, well-differentiated chondrosarcoma are found. Clear cell chondrosarcoma is a radiolucent, well-defined lesion usually occurring in the epiphysis of a long bone, most frequently the proximal femur. Calcification is seen in approximately 30% of cases. This radiologic pattern is similar to that of chondroblastoma, such that clear cell chondrosarcoma may represent its malignant counterpart. Patients are generally older than those with chondroblastoma, however (usually in their 20s to 40s).[307, 308] The tumor is slow growing and has a better prognosis than conventional chondrosarcoma.

Myxoid chondrosarcoma occurs only rarely in bone, being found more commonly in the soft tissues of the extremities, usually in patients older than age 40 years. Histologic features include lob-

ules that contain an abundant myxoid stroma in which reside polygonal, spindle, or stellate cells that have small, bland nuclei. The cytoplasm frequently is vacuolated, creating an appearance similar to that of physaliphorous cells of chordoma. The cells may be arranged in radial formations at the periphery of the lobules.[309] The tumor cells express S-100 protein and vimentin, but not cytokeratin.[310]

Dedifferentiated chondrosarcoma (Figs. 47–64 and 47–65) is a biphasic tumor consisting of a poorly differentiated sarcomatous component juxtaposed to an otherwise typical low-grade chondrosarcoma.[311–313] This pattern of dedifferentiation may occur at the time of original presentation but more often develops in recurrent tumors. The dedifferentiated component most frequently resembles malignant fibrous histiocytoma or fibrosarcoma, but rhabdomyosarcoma, osteosarcoma, angiosarcoma, and undifferentiated spindle cell sarcomas also occur.[314–318] Cytogenetic and immunophenotyping studies indicate that the differentiated and the dedifferentiated components originate from a common primitive mesenchymal cell progenitor.[319] Dedifferentiated chondrosarcoma has an extremely poor prognosis (<10% 5-year survival), with frequent pulmonary metastases.[313, 320, 321]

*Mesenchymal chondrosarcoma* accounts for 1% to 2% of all chondrosarcomas[1–12, 315, 322–335](Figs. 47–66 to 47–69). Some mesenchymal chondrosarcomas have been reported as "hemangiopericytomas with cartilaginous differentiation," "primitive multipotential primary sarcomas of bone," and "polyhistioma." About two thirds of cases occur primarily in bone and one third in the soft tissues. Patients are usually young adults (mean age, 25 years), but there is a broad age range (5 to 74 years). The most frequently involved osseous sites are the femur, ribs, spine, and craniofacial bones. The cranial meninges and soft tissue of the lower extremities are common sites for the extraosseous lesions. Radiologically, mesenchymal chondrosarcoma shows a permeative pattern of bone destruction with features of conventional chon-

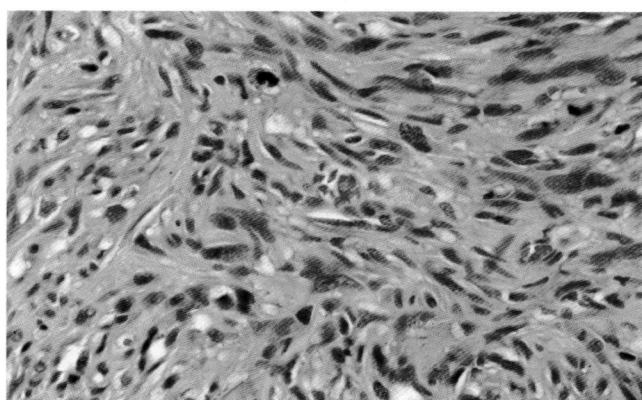

**FIGURE 47–65.** Spindle cell stroma in a dedifferentiated chondrosarcoma shows marked cellular atypia with numerous atypical mitotic figures.

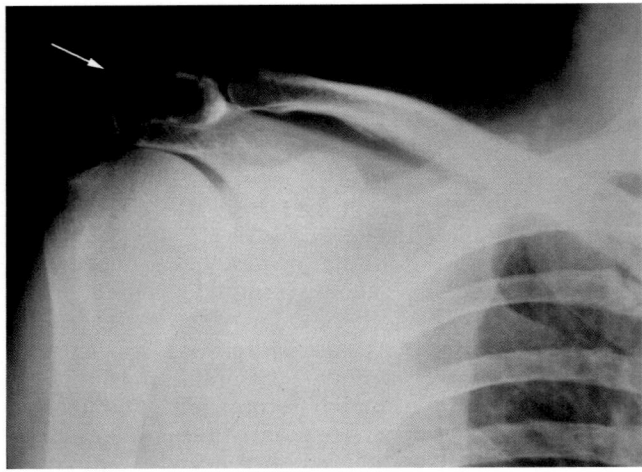

FIGURE 47–66. Mesenchymal chondrosarcoma. Roentgenogram shows a lytic lesion in the distal end of the acromion process in a 45-year-old man.

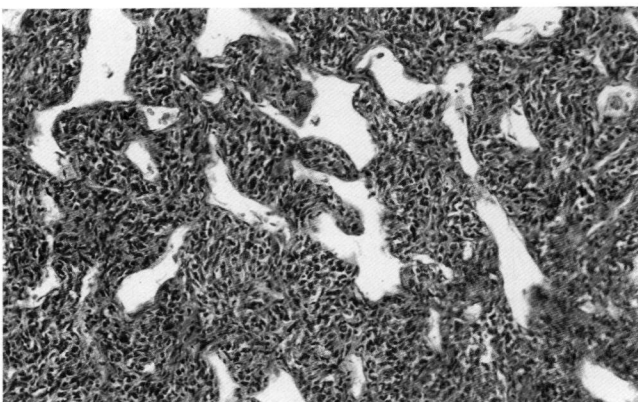

FIGURE 47–68. Mesenchymal chondrosarcoma shows proliferation of small cells in a background containing so-called staghorn-type vascular spaces, creating a hemangiopericytomatous pattern.

drosarcoma. Calcification, usually stippled, is seen in the osseous and extraosseous tumors. On gross examination, mesenchymal chondrosarcoma may be lobulated with distinct chondroid areas or predominately soft with a fleshy consistency. Gritty calcification commonly is found.

Bone and extraskeletal mesenchymal chondrosarcoma have the same histopathology, consisting of variable combinations of richly cellular areas of undifferentiated mesenchymal cells (i.e., small blue cells) and islands of well-differentiated hyaline cartilage. The small blue cells have uniform, small, round–to–spindle-shaped, hyperchromatic nuclei, with scant cytoplasm, and resemble the cells of Ewing's sarcoma. They may grow in either compact masses or diffuse sheets with a rich vascularity that creates hemangiopericytoma-like regions. At times, the cells assume spindle shapes, creating a herringbone pattern of fibrosarcoma (spindle-cell pattern). These patterns intermingle, and their prominence varies from region to region within the tumor. Cyto-

plasmic glycogen may be present. There is either a sudden or a gradual transition from the small blue cells to the islands of chondroid or well-formed cartilage. The cartilage cells tend to be well differentiated, appearing to be either normal or consistent with those of a low-grade chondrosarcoma. The cartilaginous islands may show enchondral-type ossification. The relative proportions of cartilage and small cells may vary considerably, with some tumors having abundant, easily found cartilage foci, whereas in others the cartilage is sparse and may take extensive sampling to find. Immunohistochemical studies have shown that the small blue cells fail to express S-100 protein, whereas the cartilaginous portions (i.e., lacunar cells) do stain for S-100 protein. The small blue cells and cartilaginous cells show reactivity for vimentin, leu-7, and neuron-specific enolase; they are nonreactive for synaptophysin, desmin, muscle-specific actin (HHF-35), cytokeratin (AE1/3, MAK 6, CAM 5.2), and epithelial membrane antigen. Strong immunoreactivity of the small blue cells for the *MIC2* gene product (CD99) using

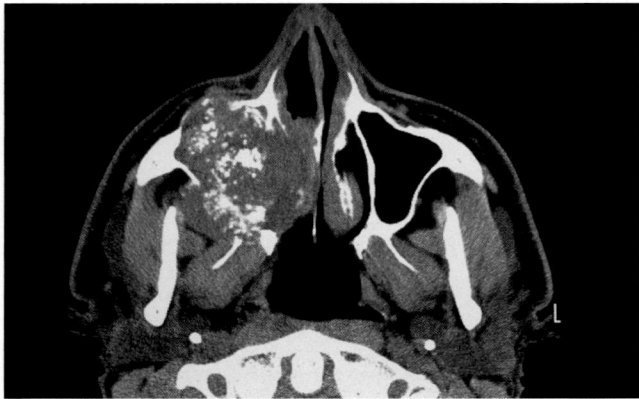

FIGURE 47–67. Mesenchymal chondrosarcoma. Computed tomography scan shows large, destructive mass, containing calcified matrix, involving the maxillary sinus in a 33-year-old man.

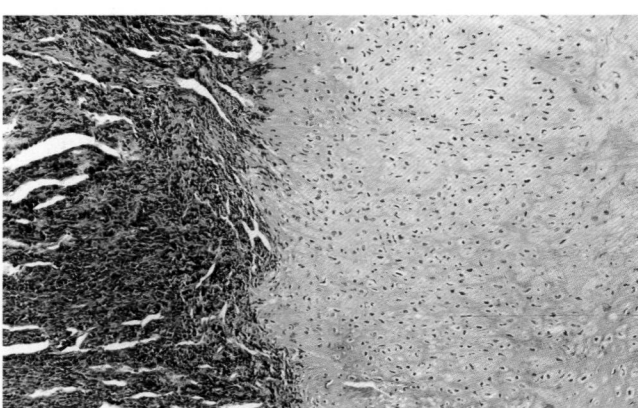

FIGURE 47–69. Mesenchymal chondrosarcoma. A well-differentiated cartilaginous nodule is seen juxtaposed to a small cell hemangiocytomatous area. These small cells may resemble the cells of Ewing's sarcoma.

the monoclonal antibody O13 has been found, consistent with the demonstration of the t(11;22)(q24; q12) translocation in cells cultured from a mesenchymal chondrosarcoma.[336]

Mesenchymal chondrosarcoma is an aggressive tumor whose clinical course is unpredictable. The overall 5-year survival is approximately 50%, with 10-year survival of 25%, despite radical surgical therapy, radiation therapy, and chemotherapy. Local recurrences and eventual metastases are typical events. This progression occurs rapidly in some patients, whereas in others the course may be prolonged, in terms of many years, even in the presence of pulmonary metastases.

## GIANT CELL TUMOR

Giant cell tumor, or osteoclastoma, usually develops in patients 20 to 50 years old.[337, 338] Cases occurring in younger patients are likely to be in skeletally mature girls (Figs. 47–70 to 47–72). Although any bone may be involved, the most common sites include the distal femur, proximal tibia, distal radius, sacrum, and proximal humerus.[337, 339–341] Location in the mobile spine is rare; true giant cell tumor of the craniofacial bones is extremely rare in the absence of Paget's disease in the area.[342] At the time of diagnosis, virtually all long bone giant cell tumors involve the epiphysis with extension to the end of the bone. The metaphysis also almost always is involved; in the rare lesions occurring in children, the metaphysis alone may be involved, suggesting that the actual site of origin of giant cell tumor is the metaphysis. A lesion in an adult that has the appearance of a giant cell tumor in an unusual location, such as the metaphysis or diaphysis of a long bone or in the short tubular bones or flat bones, should raise the suspicion of another lesion, such as aneurysmal

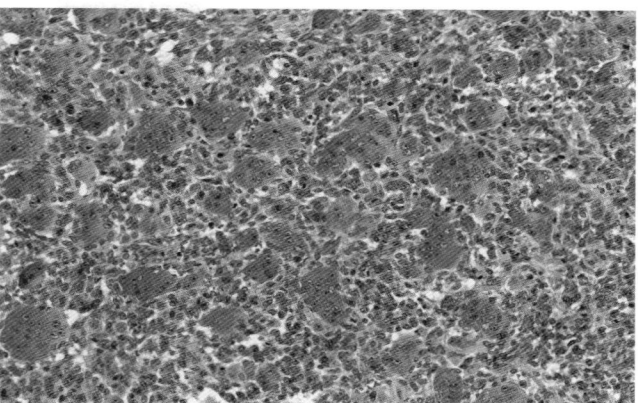

**FIGURE 47–71.** Low-power view of giant cell tumor shows diffuse proliferation of osteoclast-type giant cells, between which is a proliferation of smaller stromal cells.

bone cyst, osteosarcoma, giant cell reparative granuloma, or hyperparathyroidism.[343, 344] The typical giant cell tumor is an entirely lytic, expansile, frequently eccentric, and destructive lesion, usually without peripheral bone sclerosis or a periosteal reaction. Recurrent lesions that occur in the soft tissues, or in the rare instances of pulmonary metastases, may develop a peripheral shell of ossification. On gross inspection, the cut surface of a giant cell tumor is soft and tan or light brown, traversed by fibrous trabeculae, and often focally cystic and hemorrhagic.

The primary components of giant cell tumor are stromal cells and osteoclast-like giant cells. The giant cells usually are distributed diffusely and evenly, are relatively large, and often contain 20 to 30 nuclei. The giant cells are thought not to be neoplastic elements but rather the result of fusion of circulating monocytes or histiocytes that have been recruited into the lesion, possibly through an autocrine or paracrine mechanism mediated by various growth factors (e.g., transforming growth factor-$\beta$), which

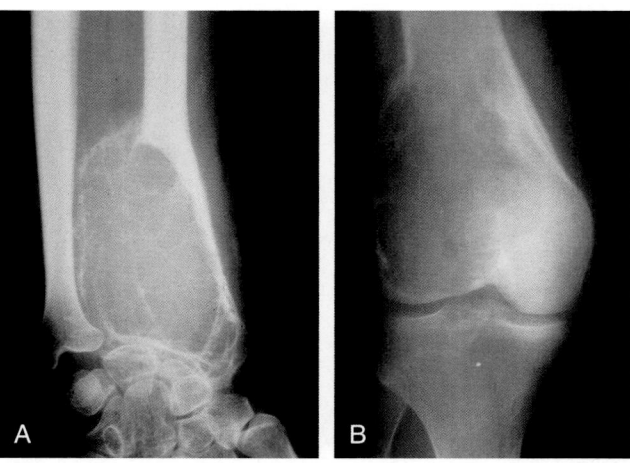

**FIGURE 47–70.** Giant cell tumor. *A,* Roentgenogram on the left shows a lesion within the distal radius having a "blown-out" appearance. Although appearing aggressive, the periphery of the lesion still has a thin rim of periosteal new bone formation, indicating its benign nature. *B,* The lesion on the right, located in the distal femur, shows a more ill-defined process (aggressive pattern), indicating rapidity of growth, with focal destruction of the bone cortex.

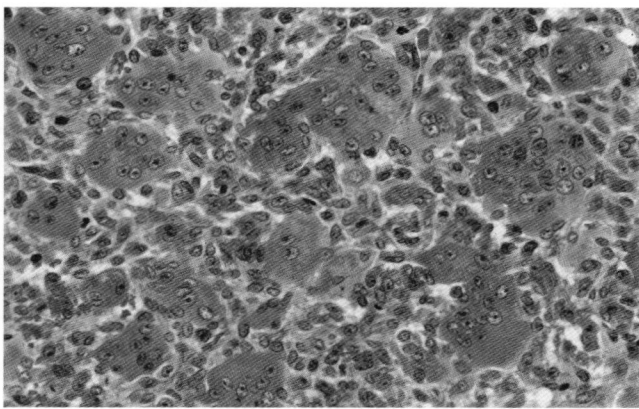

**FIGURE 47–72.** Higher magnification view of giant cell tumor shows the similarity between the nuclei of the smaller stromal cells and those of the osteoclast-type giant cells. Mitotic figures are present in some stromal cells but absent in the giant cells.

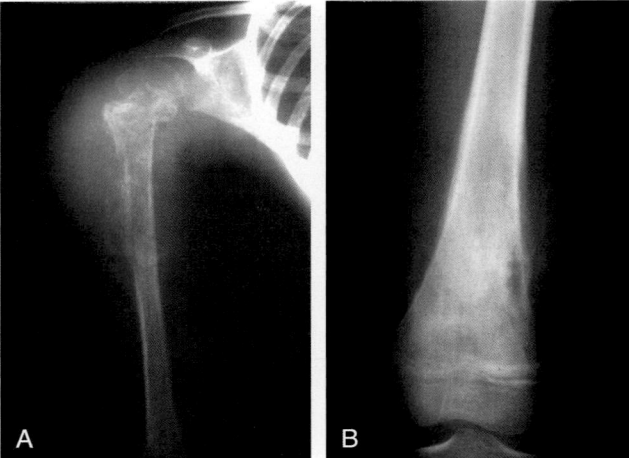

**FIGURE 47–73.** Ewing's sarcoma. Roentgenograms of affected bones (*A*, left humerus; *B*, right distal femur) show destructive permeative lesions, with soft tissue extension.

are released by the neoplastic mononuclear stromal cells or associated inflammatory cells.[345] The stromal cells are mononuclear cells whose nuclei are similar to the nuclei of the giant cells. These stromal cells are the only proliferating elements in the lesion[346] and the one cell type that exhibits atypia.[347, 348] The neoplastic stromal cells have fibroblastic or osteoblastic differentiation.[349–357] Although mitotic activity occurs in the stromal cells and may be brisk, atypical mitotic figures should not be seen in a true giant cell tumor. Variations in the classic appearance include areas of secondary aneurysmal bone cyst, collections of foam cells, spindle areas of stromal cells (sometimes with a storiform pattern), new bone formation, and necrosis; the necrosis sometimes is fairly extensive.[1–12] Histologic grading of conventional giant cell tumor has not been found to be reproducibly useful in managing patients.[358]

Conventional giant cell tumor may behave as an aggressive lesion with uncontrollable local recurrence; metastases are reported in approximately 10% of cases.[359, 360] The type of initial surgical removal is the most significant factor in local recurrence; in one large series, the recurrence rate was 34% after curettage and only 7% after wide resection.[361] The treatment of giant cell tumor should be complete surgical excision whenever feasible. It consists of curettage with bone grafting or fixation with methyl methacrylate cement, or en-bloc excision.[361–364] Special care should be taken to prevent implantation of the tumor into the adjoining soft tissues because this may lead to local recurrence. Radiation therapy should be reserved only for inoperable cases, given the number of reported cases of malignant transformation after use of radiation therapy.[343] Most, but not all, cases of metastasizing giant cell tumor have occurred after surgical therapy of the primary tumor. Some of these metastases have developed from tumors with an entirely benign microscopic appearance, and the metastases themselves may be cytolog-

ically bland.[365] The metastases are usually solitary, although multiple metastases may occur, and the patients have a good prognosis if the lesion is removed. Special techniques so far have not been found to help predict the clinical outcome of giant cell tumor.[366–369] Today, with the use of curettage, local recurrence rates are only approximately 5% to 10%.

So-called malignant giant cell tumor is a controversial issue.[3] Uncommon bone tumors develop that have the clinical, topographic, and general microscopic features of giant cell tumor but also show clear-cut evidence of malignancy in the mononuclear stromal component. Such tumors need to be distinguished from other giant cell–containing malignant tumors, particularly giant cell–rich osteosarcoma and malignant fibrous histiocytoma.[3] Occasionally a typical benign-appearing giant cell tumor is seen juxtaposed to high-grade sarcoma. This phenomenon has been referred to as *dedifferentiation*, in analogy to the situation occurring more commonly with chondrosarcoma and chordoma.[370] Most commonly, high-grade sarcomatous change in giant cell tumor develops after its treatment with radiation therapy; de novo malignant giant cell tumor is extremely rare.[342] The prognosis for malignant giant cell tumor is the same as for an equivalent high-grade primary spindle cell sarcoma.

### EWING'S SARCOMA

Ewing's sarcoma (Figs. 47–73 to 47–75) is an uncommon primary bone tumor that now is regarded by some as a member of a family of small round cell neoplasms of bone and soft tissue generically known as *primitive neuroectodermal tumor* (PNET). It is characterized by a cytogenetic abnormality involving a translocation between chromosomes 11 and 22 (i.e., t(11;22)).[371–375] Although some authors refer to the tumors of this family as *Ewing's sarcoma/PNET*, others retain the designation *Ewing's sarcoma* for bone and soft tissue tumors that do not exhibit evidence of neural differentiation and use *PNET* for

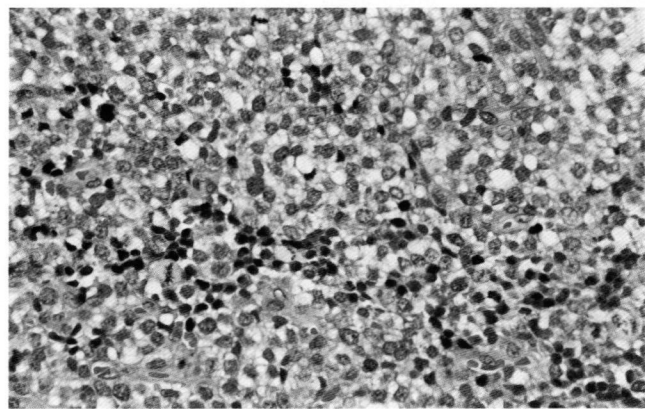

**FIGURE 47–74.** Ewing's sarcoma. Light and dark small tumor cells, many of which appear vacuolated because of their cytoplasmic glycogen content.

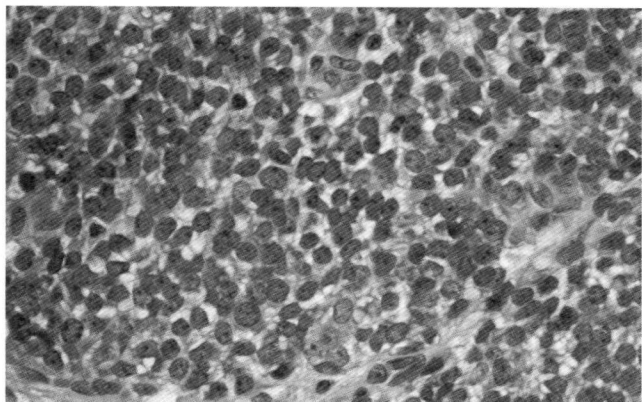

**FIGURE 47–75.** Higher magnification view of Ewing's sarcoma shows cells with fairly uniform nuclei, most of which have a fine chromatin pattern, and cytoplasmic borders that are ill defined.

tumors that show some neural differentiation by routine histology, immunohistochemistry, or electron microscopy. These small cell tumors may occur primarily in bone or soft tissue.[376-382] The *MIC2* gene product, CD99 or p30/32$^{MIC2}$, which can be detected by monoclonal antibodies such as 12E7, HBA71, or O13, is a cell membrane protein coded by a gene located on the short arms of the X and Y chromosomes that is expressed in a high percentage of cases by the cells of Ewing's sarcoma/PNET.[383, 384] Although sensitive, it is nonspecific because it may be found in a variety of other tumors, including acute lymphoblastic leukemia, lymphoblastic lymphoma, rhabdomyosarcoma, granulocytic sarcoma, sex cord–stromal tumors, synovial sarcoma, mesenchymal chondrosarcoma, and small cell osteosarcoma.[385-390] Some of these other *MIC2* product–expressing lesions are small cell tumors that are included in the histologic differential diagnosis with Ewing's sarcoma, and a panel of other antibodies must thus be employed in the immunohistochemical testing for Ewing's sarcoma/PNET.[390-392] Desmosome-associated proteins may be demonstrable immunohistochemically, and cytokeratin in some cases, but neural cell adhesion molecules are not.[393]

The tumors of the Ewing's sarcoma/PNET family show mainly the reciprocal translocation (11;22) (q24;q12), but other translocations also may occur, such as (21;22) (q22;q12), (7;22) (p22;q12), (17;22) (q12;q12), or (2;22) (q33;q12). These translocations result in the fusion of the *EWS* (Ewing's sarcoma) gene and the *FLI-1, ERG, ETV1, E1AF,* or *FEV* genes,[394-397] producing a variety of fusion genes (i.e., *EWS/FLI-1, EWS/ERG, EWS/ETV1, EWS/E1AF, EWS/FEV*) that can be detected by in situ hybridization or by reverse transcriptase–polymerase chain reaction (RT-PCR) reaction. These techniques can be used for the primary diagnosis and for the detection of metastatic or residual disease.[398-401]

Ewing's sarcoma of bone occurs most commonly in patients 5 to 20 years old.[402-404] It is rare before age 5 years, an age group in which metastatic neuroblastoma is more common. Black and Asian patients rarely are involved. The tumor often causes pain, swelling, weight loss, fever, leukocytosis, and an elevated erythrocyte sedimentation rate. The bones of the sacrum, pelvis, and lower extremity account for two thirds of all cases; the tumor rarely occurs in the craniofacial bones. In a tubular bone, the tumor is usually metaphyseal. Radiologic studies show a permeative and destructive process, which may be extensive and associated with pronounced layered periosteal new bone formation, producing the so-called onionskin appearance. However, the radiologic patterns in Ewing's sarcoma vary considerably from case to case and are not specific. At diagnosis, almost all patients have extraosseous soft tissue extension of the tumor. The metastatic spread of this tumor is to the lungs, other bones (particularly the skull), central nervous system, and (rarely) regional lymph nodes. About 25% of the patients have multiple bone or visceral lesions at the time of presentation.[405, 406]

On gross examination, Ewing's sarcoma has a fleshy, white appearance with a variable degree of necrosis. Histologically, the tumor cells are small, round, and uniform with relatively high nuclear-to-cytoplasmic ratios. The presence of clear-cut spindle cells should make one strongly consider a different diagnosis. The cytoplasm is scant, being indistinct to clear, the latter areas containing glycogen. Mitotic figures may be uncommon. With tumor necrosis, a perithelial pattern (i.e., viable-appearing tumor cells clustered around blood vessels with areas away from the vessel being necrotic) may be prominent. At times, the tumor cells are larger than usual, the tumor designated as an *atypical* or *large cell Ewing's sarcoma*. Ewing's sarcoma does not contain rosettes, the presence of which indicates neural differentiation. As indicated previously, the differential diagnosis includes such tumors as small cell osteosarcoma, mesenchymal chondrosarcoma, lymphoblastic lymphoma, and metastatic neuroblastoma. Neuroblastoma cells lack reactivity for CD 99.

Surgical excision alone results in 5-year survival rates of only about 10%; however, combining high-dose radiation therapy, polyagent chemotherapy, and surgical excision has been effective.[407-410] Currently, local control occurs in approximately 85% of cases, the actuarial 5-year disease-free survival being approximately 75%. Surgical excision of expendable bones, or amputation in the case of young children, in whom radiation therapy would cause severe growth retardation of the bones within the radiation field, yields better results than when excision is not done. All patients receive neoadjuvant chemotherapy, and similar to the situation in osteosarcoma, greater than 90% tumor necrosis is considered a good response; such a response usually indicates improved survival. DNA cell cycle analysis seems to correlate with prognosis in that patients with diploid tumors do better than those with aneuploid tumors.[411]

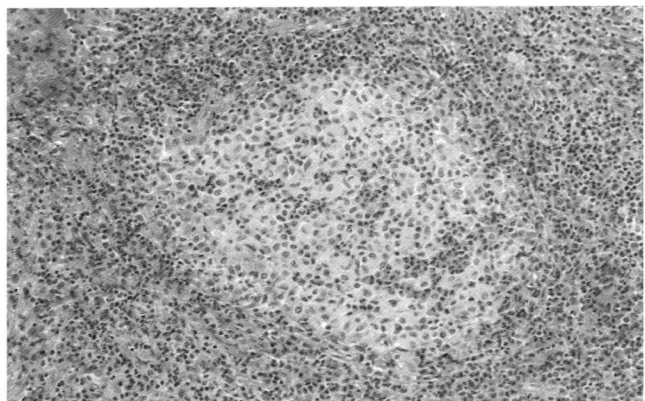

FIGURE 47–76. Eosinophilic granuloma. Pale zone in center of field consists of large histiocytes that are surrounded by an inflammatory infiltrate consisting of lymphocytes and eosinophils.

## MALIGNANT LYMPHOMA

Primary *large cell lymphoma* of bone is a tumor of adults, with approximately 60% of cases developing in patients older than age 30 years. Most of these tumors produce extensive, permeative bone destruction (i.e., mixed lytic and sclerotic), most commonly bones containing abundant red marrow (i.e., usually the diaphysis or metaphysis of long bones or the vertebrae), although any bone may be involved. Histologic features are similar to those of the known variants of large cell lymphomas at other anatomic sites, but in bone the cells may show marked spindling, with associated fibrosis, such that the tumor may be misdiagnosed as a sarcoma.[412-416] The cells are relatively large and contain nuclei with clumped chromatin and prominent nucleoli; cytoplasm is abundant, often is eosinophilic, and typically does not contain glycogen. These large cells may be mixed with a population of smaller lymphoid cells (i.e., a combination that helps eliminate Ewing's sarcoma in the differential diagnosis because the latter is composed of a uniform population of cells). In contrast to primary bone sarcomas, large cell lymphoma cells are positive for lymphocyte markers, such as CD45, CD20, or CD30 (Ki-1 or BerH2).[419, 420] Most of these tumors show B-cell differentiation. Treatment consists of a combination of irradiation and chemotherapy.[421] The 5-year survival rate for localized malignant lymphoma of bone has been reported to be approximately 60% in most series; pathologic stage seems to be the most important prognosticator, although cell type also may be important.[414, 422-426] African Burkitt's lymphoma typically presents with massive jaw bone involvement, but it can create tumor masses in the long bones and pelvis as well.[427] Rarely, Hodgkin's disease presents as a primary bone lesion.[428] Acute childhood leukemia frequently causes radiologic skeletal abnormalities (i.e., 90% of cases),[429, 430] but bone lesions are extremely rare in chronic leukemias.[431] Granulocytic sarcoma may present as a primary bone tumor; the tumor cells are positive for myelo-peroxidase, lysozyme, or CD43. Plasma cell myeloma and plasma cell dyscrasias are discussed in the chapters on the hematolymphatic system.

## LANGERHANS' CELL GRANULOMATOSIS (HISTIOCYTOSIS)

*Langerhans' cell granulomatosis (histiocytosis X; eosinophilic granuloma)* results from an abnormal infiltrate of Langerhans' cells (Langerhans histiocytes), which are cells of the accessory immune system[432] (Figs. 47–76 and 47–77). Characteristically, chronic inflammatory cells, especially eosinophils, are admixed with the Langerhans' cells. Osteoclast-like giant cells, neutrophils, foam cells, and areas of necrosis and fibrosis also may be found. Mitotic figures, sometimes atypical, are common. Langerhans' cell nuclei often are lobulated or indented (i.e., reniform), sometimes with a central longitudinal groove. By electron microscopy, their usually abundant acidophilic cytoplasm contains Birbeck's granules, which are specific to these cells. By immunohistochemistry, the cells are positive for CD1a and S-100 protein.

Langerhans' cell granulomatosis has been divided into three major categories based on the type and extent of organ involvement: 1) solitary bone involvement, 2) multiple bone involvement (with or without organ involvement), and 3) multiple organ involvement (bone, liver, spleen, and others). Cases with solitary bone involvement, which represent the most common variety, are referred to as *eosinophilic granuloma*. Young adults are affected most commonly; any bone may be involved, but bones of the hands and feet rarely are affected. The most common sites are the cranial vault, jaw, humerus, rib, and femur. Eosinophilic granuloma causes lytic lesions, often in the metaphysis of a long bone. There may be periosteal new bone proliferation or pathologic fracture. In some cases, the radiologic pattern may appear aggressive and simulate osteosarcoma or Ewing's sarcoma. In the skull, the lytic areas have a punched-out appearance. The lesions of eosino-

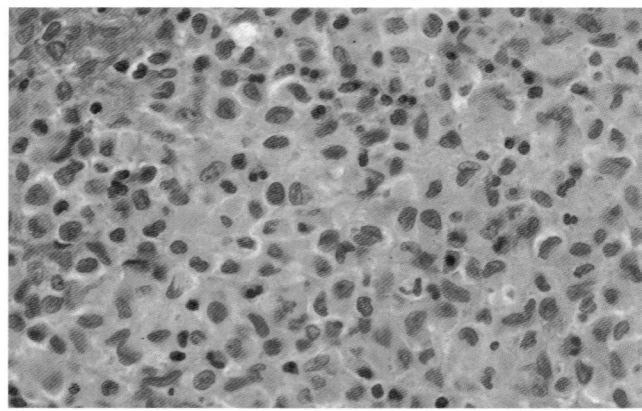

FIGURE 47–77. Higher magnification of eosinophilic granuloma shows epithelioid-type histiocytes, some of whose nuclei are seen to contain irregularly shaped, raisin-like, or clefted nuclei. Scattered eosinophils are present.

philic granuloma may regress spontaneously; they are extremely radiosensitive and may be cured with small amounts of radiation. The long-term prognosis is excellent.

Langerhans' cell granulomatosis with multiple bone involvement has been designated *multiple or polyostotic eosinophilic granuloma*, and the eponym *Hand-Schüller-Christian disease* has been applied to this subtype.[433, 434] The process may cause proptosis (exophthalmos), diabetes insipidus, chronic otitis media, or a combination of these conditions. This form of Langerhans' cell histiocytosis is characterized by a prolonged clinical course, often marked by alternating episodes of regressions and recrudescences, but eventually the outcome is favorable in most cases. This type of histiocytosis blends imperceptibly with the third form, in which there is bone and multisystem organ involvement. After the skeletal system, the skin and the lungs are the two most common sites affected. The outcome is variable and difficult to predict in the individual case, but unfavorable prognostic factors are young age (<18 months) at presentation, hepatosplenomegaly, anemia or thrombocytopenia or both, polyostotic bone involvement (three or more bones), and hemorrhagic skin lesions. Seborrhea-like skin lesions, diabetes insipidus, and pulmonary lesions are not associated with a poor prognosis. Histopathologically, it is dif-

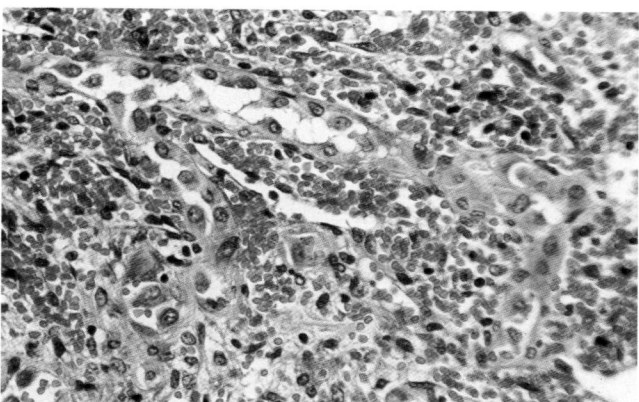

**FIGURE 47–79.** Epithelioid hemangioma with vessel formation. The vessels are lined by cells, with a relatively large amount of eosinophilic cytoplasm, that bulge into the lumina. The lumina are created by the coalescence of the clear cytoplasmic vacuoles in these cells.

ficult to separate the aggressive from the indolent forms; pathologic stage seems to be the best prognosticator. The differential diagnosis of Langerhans' cell granulomatosis of bone includes osteomyelitis, osseous manifestations of Rosai-Dorfman disease, metastatic tumor, lymphoma, osteomyelitis, and Ewing's sarcoma.

## VASCULAR TUMORS

*Benign hemangiomas* of vertebral bone have been detected in approximately 12% of autopsies, although this is controversial because some of these lesions may not be true tumors but represent malformations (Figs. 47–78 to 47–85). Symptomatic osseous hemangiomas are rare. The skull and vertebral column are the most common sites, with extremity lesions rare.[435] In the vertebral column, they may cause compression fracture or extend into the spinal canal to produce neurologic symptoms.[436, 437] Multiple cystic hemangiomas in children may be associated, in approximately 50% of the cases, with cutaneous, soft

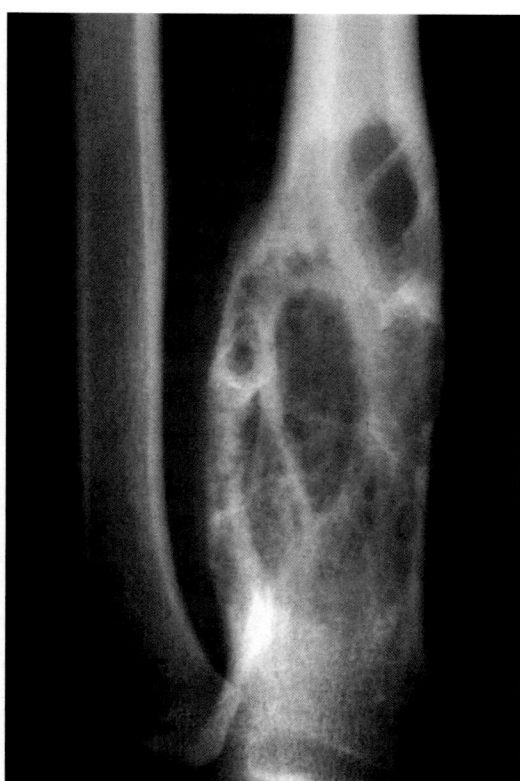

**FIGURE 47–78.** Epithelioid hemangioma. Roentgenogram of the distal end of the radius shows a cystic lesion with expansion of the bone and irregular periosteal reaction. The bone appears intact.

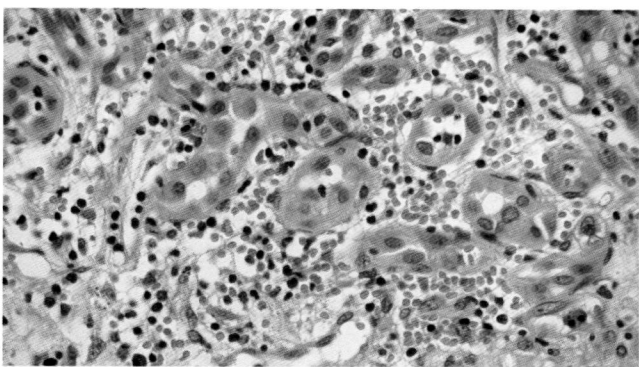

**FIGURE 47–80.** Cross-section of vessels in epithelioid hemangioma shows endothelial cell nuclei bulging into the lumina of the vessels, occasionally producing a tombstone-like appearance. The stroma contains a percolation of lymphocytes; eosinophils also may be prominent, although not shown in this field.

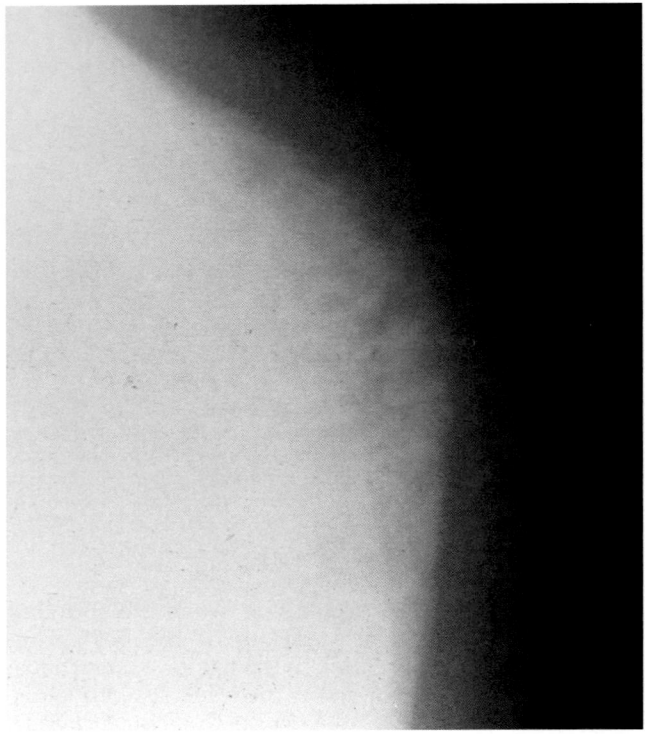

**FIGURE 47–81.** Hemangioma. Roentgenogram of the skull shows a hemangioma of the temporal bone in a 13-year-old boy. The lesion bulges into the outer table of the skull with some suggestion of radiating spicule-like formations throughout the lesion.

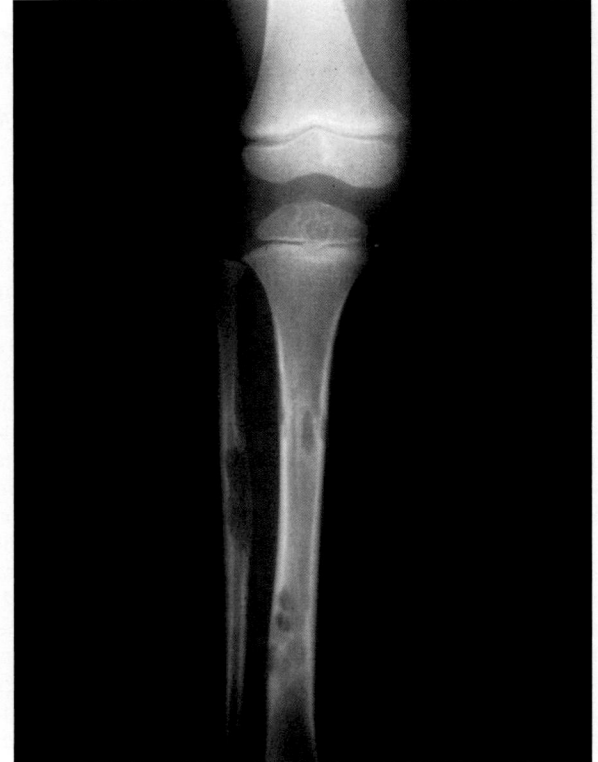

**FIGURE 47–83.** Angiomatosis. Roentgenogram shows multiple cystlike hemangiomas within the tibia and fibula.

tissue, or visceral hemangiomas.[438] Hemangiomas of the skull may produce lytic, punched-out areas on roentgenograms that may have radiating spicules of bone, producing the characteristic "sunburst" appearance. Vertebral body involvement creates a striped or corduroy pattern of vertical lines of vascular channels alternating with columns of thickened bone. On computed tomography scan, the pattern produces the so-called polka-dot appearance. He-

mangiomas of the long bones have a wide range of nonspecific radiologic appearances.[435] Most osseous hemangiomas consist of widely dilated cavernous spaces filled with blood (cavernous hemangioma); small vessel hemangiomas (capillary hemangioma) are uncommon. In hemangiomas, the endothelial cells are small and flat and show no atypia. A low-grade angiosarcoma may be difficult to separate from hemangioma, especially when in a small bi-

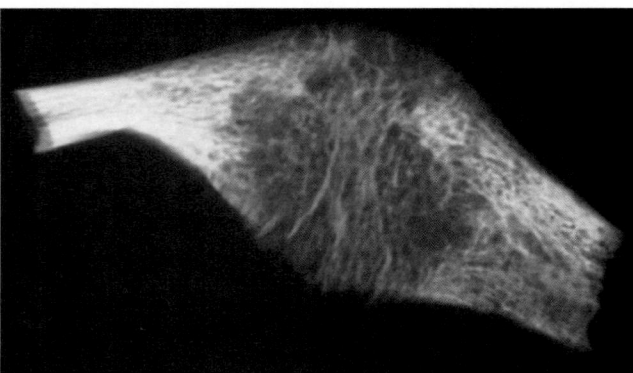

**FIGURE 47–82.** Specimen roentgenogram of the lesion in Figure 47–81 shows rarefied section of the skull table with coarse trabeculae, between which are microspaces representing the hemangiomatous process.

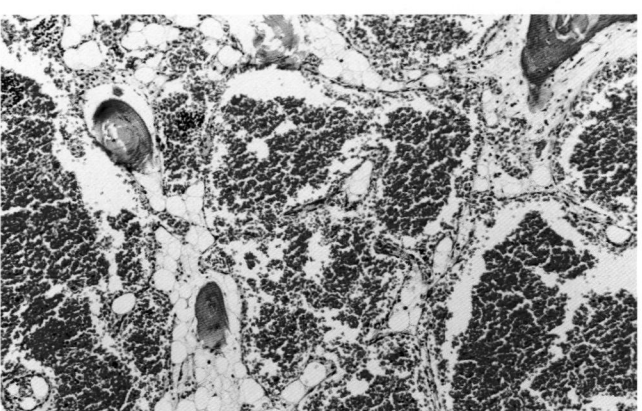

**FIGURE 47–84.** Cavernous hemangioma of bone consists of large, thin-walled, dilated vascular spaces interspersed between residual bone trabeculae.

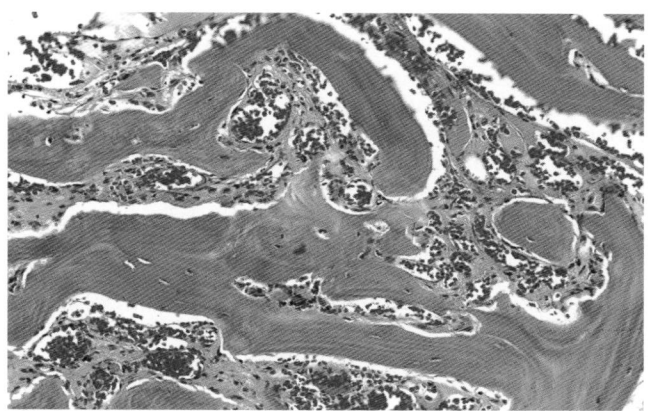

**FIGURE 47–85.** Capillary hemangioma of bone. Vessels are smaller than those in Figure 47–84 and not as dilated. There is a similar growth of the lesion between existing bone trabeculae without evident bone destruction.

opsy fragment. The distinction is made by finding endothelial cell cytologic atypia in low-grade angiosarcoma.

*Massive osteolysis* (Gorham's disease) is of unknown cause but has microscopic similarities with osseous hemangioma and lymphangioma. Gorham's disease is a destructive process that results in extensive reabsorption of one or several bones, with disappearance of the entire bone in some instances, and the filling of the residual spaces by a heavily vascularized fibrous tissue.[439, 440] *Lymphangiomas* of bone are rare, usually occurring with similar soft tissue lesions.[441] *Glomus tumors* develop within the terminal phalanx[442]; *hemangiopericytoma* may occur as a primary bone tumor; however, metastatic hemangiopericytoma to bone from another site must be excluded because this event is much more common than that of a primary osseous hemangiopericytoma.

*Epithelioid hemangioendothelioma* was described by Weiss and Enzinger[443] as a distinctive vascular tumor of soft tissue that mimicked carcinoma on histologic examination and showed clinical behavior intermediate between a benign hemangioma and a high-grade angiosarcoma.[443, 444] Intravascular bronchioloalveolar tumor of lung and so-called sclerosing cholangiocarcinoma of the liver are examples of epithelioid hemangioendothelioma.[444] Although epithelioid hemangioendothelioma most commonly occurs in the soft tissue of the extremities, it does occur within bone,[445–451] where some cases have been reported under the rubric of *myxoid angioblastoma* or *myxoid angioblastomatosis*[452, 453] or illustrated as individual cases under the heading of *hemangioendothelial sarcoma* or *angiosarcoma of bone*.[454–460]

Epithelioid hemangioendothelioma of bone is rare, with fewer than 100 cases reported in the English-language literature. Patients are usually children and young adults, but there is a broad age range. The long bones, especially those of the lower extremity, are involved most commonly, but any bone may be affected. In approximately 50% of cases, multiple bones are involved, or there are multiple sites within a single bone. In some cases, there is associated visceral organ involvement. Radiologically, epithelioid hemangioendothelioma is usually radiolucent, with sclerotic borders and expansion of the bone; cortical destruction with soft tissue extension may occur and suggests a malignant process.

An understanding of epithelioid hemangioendothelioma of bone is important because it may be mistaken for metastatic carcinoma on histologic evaluation. On microscopic examination, epithelioid hemangioendothelioma is composed of endothelial cells that are large, round, polygonal–to–slightly elongated or fusiform cells with an abundant eosinophilic cytoplasm.[443–478] The cells may be located about blood vessels, most often large veins. Cell nuclei are round, oval, and regular but may show folds or grooves and contain one or two small nucleoli. Overall, the cells have a distinct epithelioid appearance. They are frequently arranged in strands, cords, or small nests and characteristically embedded in a basophilic hyaline-to-myxoid stroma that may resemble chondroid tissue (myxochondroid stroma). Actual blood vessel formation by these epithelioid cells is uncommon; however, primitive vasoformation usually is present and characterized, at the cellular level, by the presence of cytoplasmic vacuoles that may become so large as to bulge eccentrically and distort the cell, creating a blister-like or signet ring–like effect.[443–478] Although these vacuolated or blister cells may resemble the signet ring cells of an adenocarcinoma, the vacuoles do not contain mucin, but they may contain red blood cells. The cells lack glycogen by periodic acid–Schiff stains. A lymphocytic or lymphoplasmacytic inflammatory component may be found at the periphery of the lesion, but this is not prominent. Examples of epithelioid hemangioendothelioma are reported in which numerous osteoclast-type giant cells are found. Mitotic figures are usually few in number or totally absent. By electron microscopy, the tumor cells have many of the features of normal endothelial cells, possessing basal lamina, numerous pinocytotic vesicles, junctional cell attachments (some desmosome-like), small amounts of rough endoplasmic reticulum, and mitochondria. Cytoplasmic vacuoles, at times containing flocculent amorphous material and surrounded by microvilli, also are found. Weibel-Palade bodies, characteristic of endothelial cells, may or may not be found. The feature that distinguishes normal endothelial cells from those of epithelioid hemangioendothelioma is the presence of abundant cytoplasmic intermediate filaments in the latter, which imparts to the cell its *epithelioid* quality when viewed by light microscopy.

Immunohistochemical studies have shown tumor cell reactivity for a variety of endothelial cell markers,[467, 479, 480] including factor VIII–related antigen, *Ulex europaeus-1* lectin, and CD34 antigen. Less consistently, CD31 may mark epithelioid hemangioendothelioma tumor cells, especially along the *endothelial luminal* margins. In some cases, cytokeratin reactivity also is present.[481, 482] Epithelioid hemangioendothelioma cells are strongly positive for vimentin and negative for S-100 protein and may show reactivity for muscle-specific actin (HHF-35).[462] The presence of signet ring–type or epithelioid-like cells raises the histologic possibility of metastatic carcinoma. The lack of significant cell atypia and mitotic activity in epithelioid hemangioendothelioma, the lack of epithelial mucin, and the presence of specific endothelial markers make the distinction between epithelioid hemangioendothelioma and carcinoma fairly straightforward in most cases. The basophilic myxoid and chondroid-like stroma of epithelioid hemangioendothelioma, with its content of sulfated acid mucopolysaccharide, and the dispersed pattern of the tumor cells may suggest a diagnosis of skeletal or extraskeletal myxoid chondrosarcoma. On gross inspection, myxoid chondrosarcoma is multilobular and characteristically gelatinous or myxoid, in contrast to the solitary, firm, gray-white–to–hemorrhagic appearance of epithelioid hemangioendothelioma. In common with the cells of epithelioid hemangioendothelioma, those of myxoid chondrosarcoma frequently are vacuolated, have an eosinophilic cytoplasm, and rarely may appear epithelioid. The cells of myxoid chondrosarcoma contain glycogen, in contrast to its absence in epithelioid hemangioendothelioma, and are reactive for S-100 protein and not for endothelial markers. By electron microscopy, the cells of myxoid chondrosarcoma show dilated rough endoplasmic reticulum, at times with microtubules, irregular cytoplasmic processes, lipid droplets, and long spacing collagen, all of which are absent in the cells of epithelioid hemangioendothelioma. Weibel-Palade bodies also are not present in chondrosarcoma.

The epithelioid character of the cells of epithelioid hemangioendothelioma with their cytoplasmic vasoformative vacuoles that contain red blood cells may suggest the possibility of an epithelioid angiosarcoma.[483–488] Both of these tumors share common immunohistochemical and electron microscopic features. In contrast to epithelioid hemangioendothelioma, epithelioid angiosarcoma is not angiocentric and usually grows as a solid sheet of cells that are far more pleomorphic than the cells of epithelioid hemangioendothelioma, with large prominent nucleoli. Epithelioid angiosarcoma also lacks the chondroid-like stroma of epithelioid hemangioendothelioma. Although primitive cytoplasmic vasoformative vacuoles are found in both tumors, they are more frequent in epithelioid hemangioendothelioma. Epithelioid angiosarcoma may contain areas of conventional angiosarcoma with well-formed intercommunicating vascular channels lined by atypical endothelial cells, a feature never found in epithelioid hemangioendothelioma.

The cytoplasmic vacuolization with signet ring features and the epithelioid character of the cells of epithelioid hemangioendothelioma may suggest the possibility of a chordoma. The presence of physaliphorous cells, mucin, glycogen, S-100 protein, cyto-

keratin, and epithelial membrane antigen in chordoma cells and their nonreactivity for endothelial markers should enable one to distinguish easily between these two lesions.[489, 490] Epithelioid hemangioendothelioma should be distinguished from epithelioid hemangioma, in which epithelioid endothelial cells also predominate and which also may occur within bone. Epithelioid hemangioendothelioma has a less definitive vascular pattern than occurs in epithelioid hemangioma, in which well-formed vascular channels are common. Epithelioid hemangioendothelioma contains a lesser degree of inflammation than found in epithelioid hemangioma, including significantly fewer eosinophils; tends to occur less often in the head and neck region; and is more angiocentric than epithelioid hemangioma. The small cords and strands of cells without extensive vascular channel formation in epithelioid hemangioendothelioma are not found in epithelioid hemangioma, and the cytoplasmic lumina are more distinct in epithelioid hemangioendothelioma than they are in epithelioid hemangioma. Finally, the myxoid hyaline stroma in which the cells of epithelioid hemangioendothelioma are embedded is not found in epithelioid hemangioma.

Most cases of osseous epithelioid hemangioendothelioma are indolent, with a benign course after resection. Local recurrences do occur, however, as do rare cases of metastases. Patients with multifocal involvement or with concomitant visceral organ involvement have a generally poorer prognosis than patients with solitary bone lesions.

*Angiosarcoma* (Figs. 47–86 to 47–89) is a rare bone tumor that usually occurs in patients in the third to fifth decades of life. The long bones are affected in approximately 60% of cases, with location in the metaphysis or diaphysis being typical. Multicentric disease, either synchronous or metachronous, occurs in 20% to 50% of cases in the form of multiple lesions within a single bone or in multiple bones. Angiosarcoma usually is a lucent lesion on roentgenograms but on rare occasions may be associated with sclerosis. It may involve the cortex or medulla as an ill-defined, destructive, permeative lesion or show multiple, sharply punched-out, oval-to-round lucencies throughout the bone. Cortical destruction with soft tissue tumor extension develops in the more poorly differentiated angiosarcomas. The gross tumor may have the appearance of currant jelly, with a soft or fleshy consistency. The tumor's histologic characteristics include blood vessel formation, with the vessels showing an intercommunicating, anastomotic pattern. These vessels are lined by endothelial cells that show mild-to-marked atypia. Vessels with a mild degree of atypia (low-grade angiosarcoma) may be difficult to distinguish from hemangioma, especially in small biopsy specimens. In high-grade lesions, these endothelial cells are crowded together and are larger with an abundant eosinophilic cytoplasm. They bulge into the vessel lumina, creating a "hobnail" pattern. The cells may crowd together, become spindle shaped, and

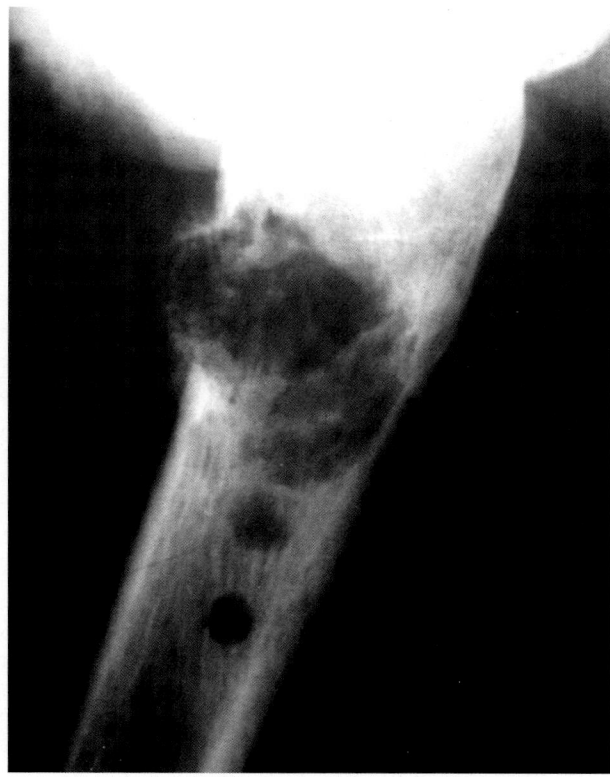

**FIGURE 47–86.** Angiosarcoma. Roentgenogram shows cystlike destructive lesions in the proximal femur of a 75-year-old man. There is extension of tumor beyond the confines of the cortex.

obliterate any evidence of vessel formation. At times, the cells have a distinct epithelioid appearance, and the lesion is misdiagnosed as a metastatic carcinoma. Immunohistochemical studies are helpful in establishing a diagnosis because the tumor cells are reactive for vimentin and endothelial markers, such as factor VIII–associated antigen, CD31, and CD34. True angiosarcoma of bone must be distin-

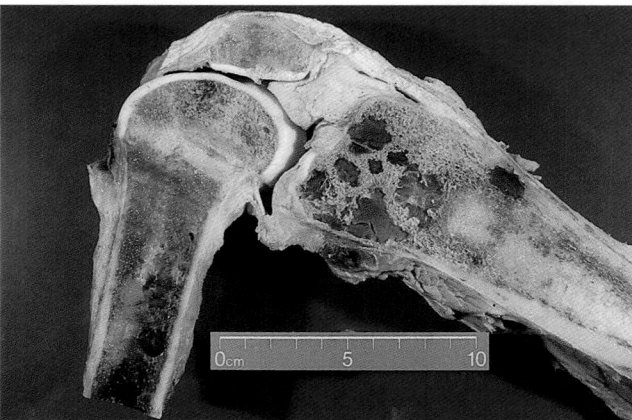

**FIGURE 47–87.** Cross-section of a knee joint from a patient with a multicentric angiosarcoma of bone. The dark gray–to–brown areas in the medulla of the femur and tibia represent sites of angiosarcoma.

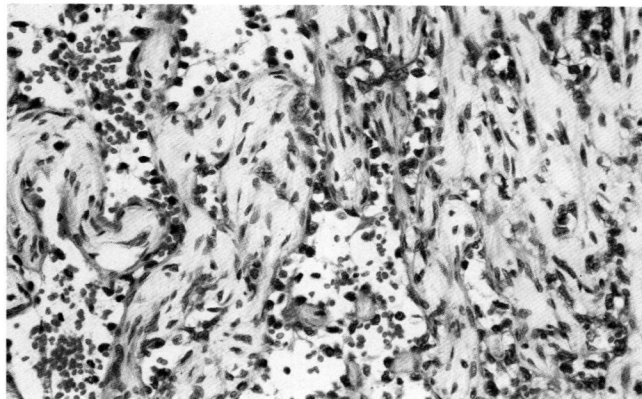

**FIGURE 47–88.** Low-grade angiosarcoma shows interconnecting vascular channels that are lined by small cells with little cytoplasm and nuclei that bulge into the lumina in a tombstone-like fashion. The intervening stroma is edematous.

guished from epithelioid hemangioma and epithelioid hemangioendothelioma. The prognosis of angiosarcoma depends on its differentiation, with low-grade lesions having a better prognosis than high-grade tumors, which have a poor outcome because of early metastases.

## FIBROGENIC TUMORS

*Desmoplastic fibroma* is a rare bone tumor composed of mature fibroblasts and myofibroblasts surrounded by well-developed collagen[491, 492] (Figs. 47–90 to 47–92). Occurring most often in the long bones, jaw, and pelvic bones, it represents the osseous counterpart of soft tissue fibromatosis or desmoid tumor. Most patients are men younger than age 30 years.[493] The lesion is radiologically lucent, with a trabeculated, soap-bubble or honeycomb pattern.[493] Most cases are well delimited, but at times the lesion may have an aggressive radiologic appearance with permeative bone destruction with soft tissue extension. Desmoblastic fibroma is a hypocellular spindle cell tumor lacking cytologic atypia with only rare nor-

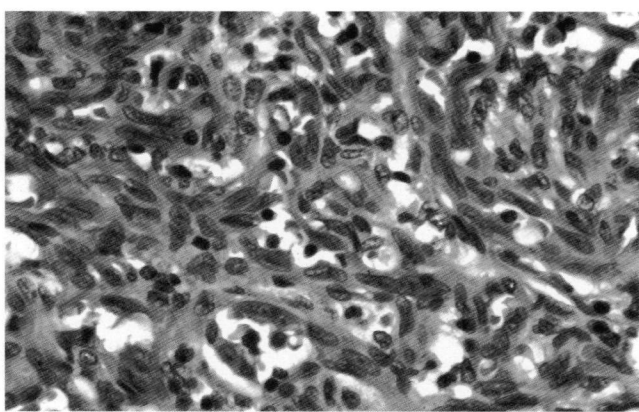

**FIGURE 47–89.** High-grade angiosarcoma shows vascular channels, lined by cells with more atypia than those present in the lesion in Figure 47–88.

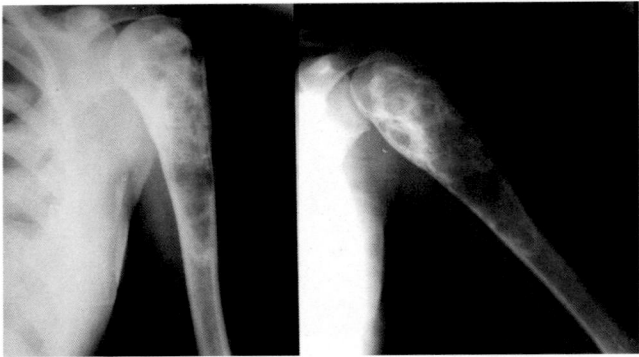

FIGURE 47–90. Desmoplastic fibroma. A 17-year-old girl with a painful proximal humerus. Roentgenograms show a multicystic lesion involving the epiphysis, metaphysis, and portion of the shaft; no extraosseous extension of the lesion is seen.

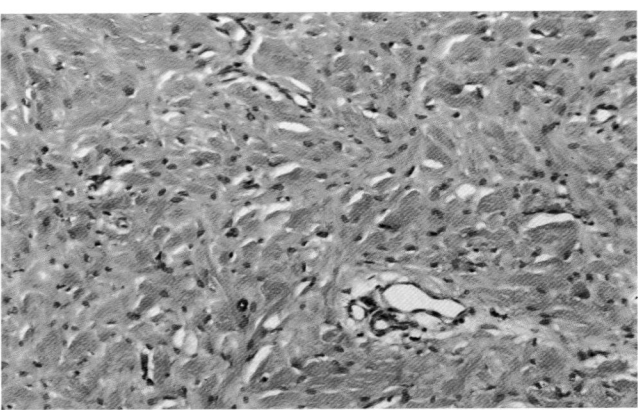

FIGURE 47–92. Higher magnification of desmoplastic fibroma shown in Figure 47–91 shows dense collagenation, a proliferation of small blood vessels, and a lack of cellular atypia or mitotic activity, distinguishing the lesion from a low-grade fibrosarcoma.

mal mitotic figures. It often recurs after incomplete excision but, in contrast to fibrosarcoma, it does not metastasize.[494, 495] *Infantile myofibromatosis*, histopathologically identical to the soft tissue counterpart, may occur as a solitary bone lesion, usually in infants younger than 2 years of age. Solitary fibrous tumor, which is reported in almost all body sites, has been described as a pedunculated periosteal mass.[496]

Primary osseous *fibrosarcoma* arises most commonly in the metaphysis of the long bones,[497–499] usually in the distal femur or proximal tibia,[500] although any bone may be involved (Figs. 47–93 to 47–95). Less commonly, it develops in the periosteum. Radiologically, osseous fibrosarcoma is osteolytic, with a variety of bone destruction patterns, including permeative destruction.[501] Fibrosarcoma does not produce tumor osteoid or chondroid matrix, being composed of relatively uniform spindle cells with relatively hyperchromatic nuclei, high nuclear-to-cytoplasmic ratios, and brisk mitotic activity. In the better differentiated tumors, the spindle cells are arranged in a herringbone pattern and lack sig-

nificant nuclear pleomorphism. The presence of extensive pleomorphism should suggest that the tumor is not a fibrosarcoma. Well-differentiated fibrosarcoma may be histologically misdiagnosed as a desmoplastic fibroma, but its destructive radiologic appearance usually suggests its malignant nature. Wide local excision and amputation are the main therapeutic choices for the treatment of fibrosar-

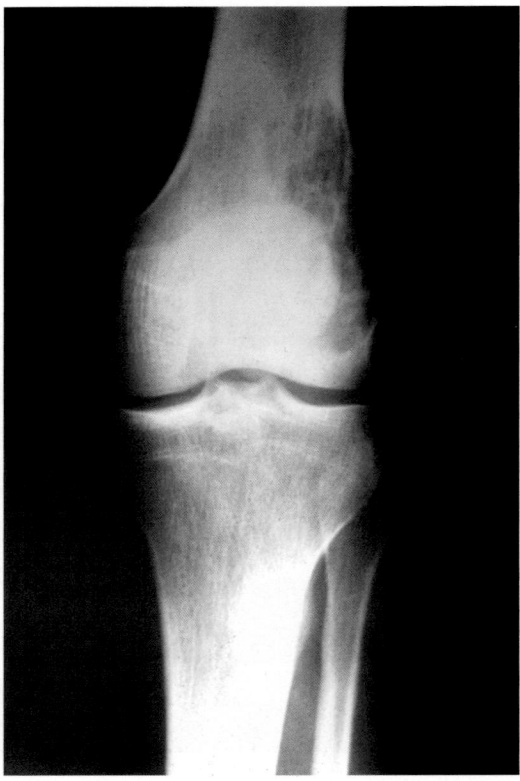

FIGURE 47–93. Fibrosarcoma. Roentgenogram shows destructive lytic lesion involving the distal end of the femur, with partial loss of the cortex, in a 45-year-old man.

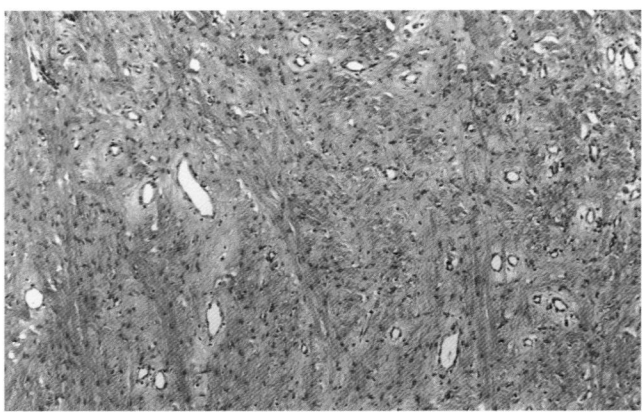

FIGURE 47–91. Desmoplastic fibroma. Low-power view shows a proliferation of small blood vessels within a bland-appearing fibrous stroma that resembles that of a desmoid tumor.

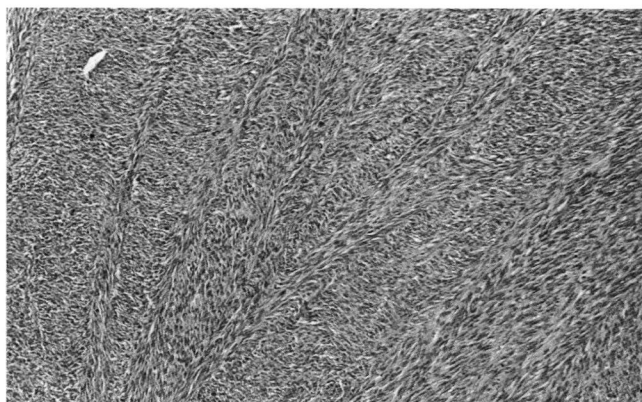

FIGURE 47–94. Low-power view of well-differentiated fibrosarcoma shows herringbone pattern formed by alternating fascicles of spindle cells.

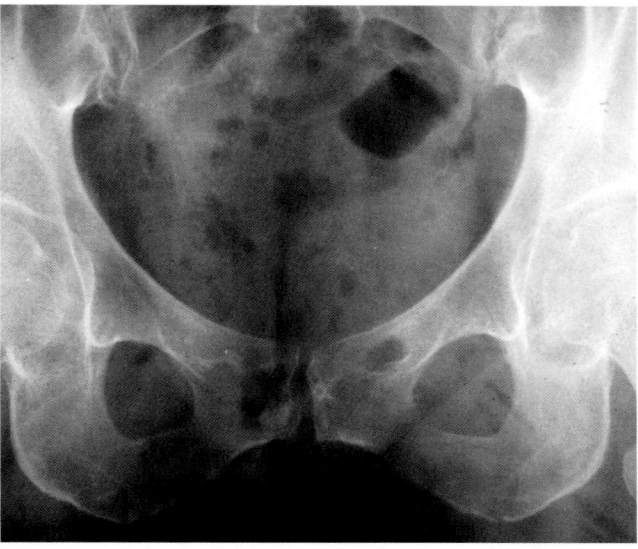

FIGURE 47–96. Chordoma. Roentgenogram of the sacrococcygeal area in a 57-year-old woman shows absence of the sacrum caused by a large destructive chordoma.

coma. The 10-year survival rate is approximately 80% for low-grade lesions and approximately 30% for high-grade tumors.[501, 502] Fibrosarcoma also may develop secondary to preexisting conditions, such as bone infarct, Paget's disease, low-grade cartilaginous tumor, or prior radiation exposure.

Intraosseous *malignant fibrous histiocytoma* is a high-grade, pleomorphic spindle cell sarcoma that occurs primarily in adults in the fifth to seventh decades of life. Its anatomic distribution is similar to that of osteosarcoma, with the metaphysis of a long bone the most common site. Radiologically, malignant fibrous histiocytoma has a destructive, osteolytic appearance. On histologic evaluation, it has the same morphologic features as its more common soft tissue counterpart[503–509] and does not produce tumor osteoid or chondroid matrix. Areas indistinguishable from those of malignant fibrous histiocytoma may be focally found in otherwise typical examples of osteosarcoma or chondrosarcoma.[510] A definitive diagnosis of primary malignant fibrous histiocytoma of bone cannot be made on biopsy tissue and must await examination of more abundant resection mate-

rial to rule out a malignant fibrous histiocytoma–like osteosarcoma with its osteoid formation. Malignant fibrous histiocytoma also has arisen in association with bone infarcts,[511, 512] foreign bodies,[513, 514] after irradiation therapy,[515] in Paget's disease, or as the spindle cell component of dedifferentiated chondrosarcoma and chordoma.[516, 517] The overall prognosis is poor.[509, 518, 519]

## CHORDOMA

*Chordoma* is a malignant bone tumor believed to arise from the remnants of the fetal notochord (Figs. 47–96 to 47–100). The notochord develops within the vertebral body but soon is displaced during vertebral development and comes to form the nucleus pulposus of the intervertebral disk.[531–534] In adults, even this vestige virtually always is no longer histologically identifiable. Despite this sequence, chordo-

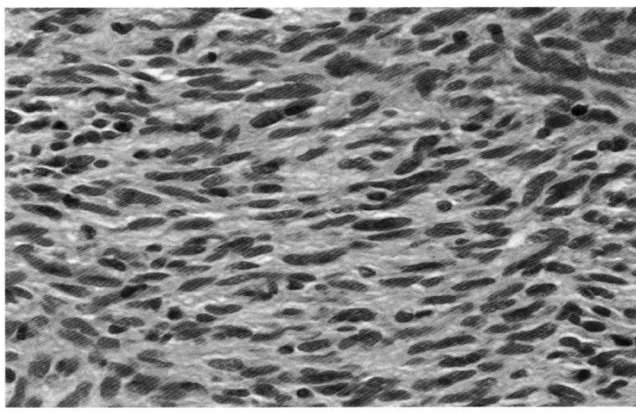

FIGURE 47–95. Well-differentiated fibrosarcoma shows fibroblasts with spindle-shaped nuclei lacking significant atypia. Mild collagen formation is present between the individual cells.

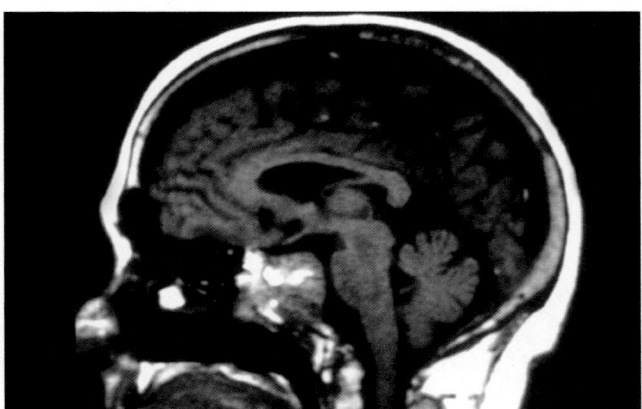

FIGURE 47–97. Magnetic resonance image shows a sphenooccipital chordoma arising in the clivus of a 73-year-old woman.

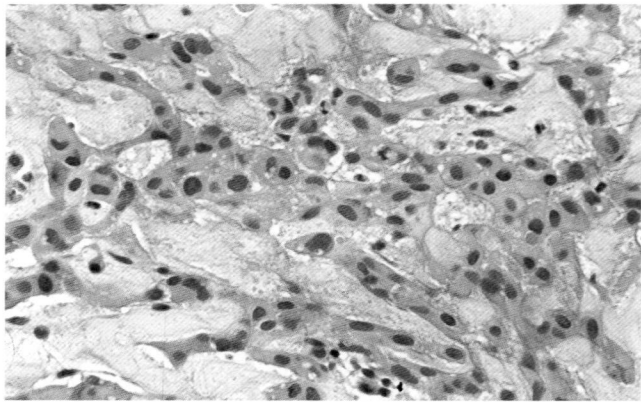

FIGURE 47–98. Chordoma shows large epithelioid-like cells with relatively abundant pink cytoplasm and nuclei that vary in size and shape. Background shows a loose, bluish, mucinous matrix.

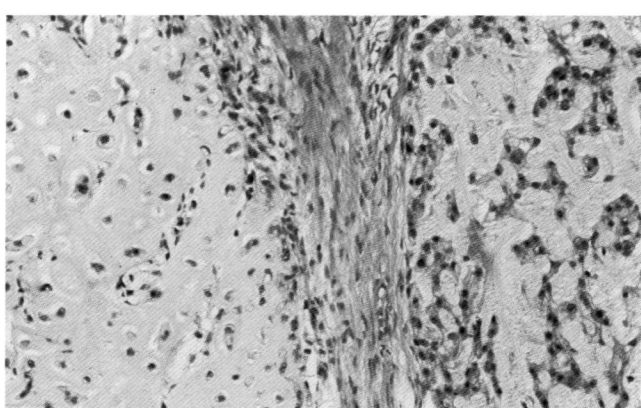

FIGURE 47–100. Chondroid chordoma. Area of conventional chordoma is seen to the right of the field, separated by a narrow band of fibrous tissue from a chondroid, cartilaginous-appearing area on the left.

mas seem to arise from the vertebral body and not from the disks. Virtually all these tumors are midline in origin, yet some apparent and controversial soft tissue examples have been reported away from the midline. Benign vestiges of the notochord, termed *ecchordosis physaliphora*, are found in the spheno-occipital region in 0.5% to 2.0% of autopsies. About 50% of chordomas arise in the sacrococcygeal area, approximately 35% in the spheno-occipital area, and the remainder within the mobile spine.[535, 536] These lesions usually occur in patients in their fifth to sixth decades of life, but may develop at all ages, although they are distinctly uncommon in patients younger than age 30 years. In children, spheno-occipital chordomas are more common than those at other sites.[537, 538] Chordoma grows slowly; the duration of symptoms before diagnosis often is longer than 5 years. Chordoma is an osteolytic tumor that destroys bone and that, by the time of diagnosis, almost always has extended beyond the confines of the bone to invade the soft tissues. Because of cra-

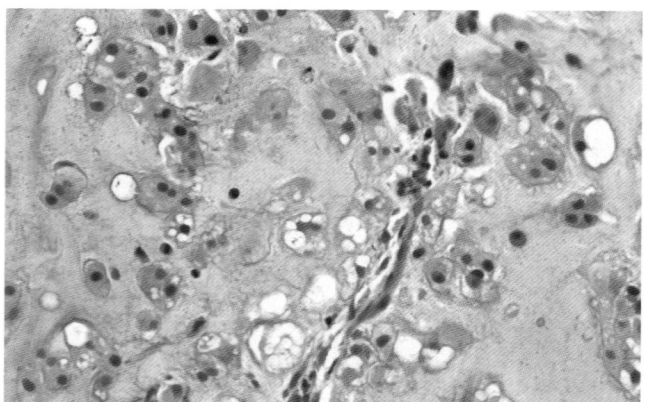

FIGURE 47–99. Another focus within the chordoma in Figure 47–98 shows physaliphorous cells produced by cytoplasmic vacuoles that distend the epithelioid-like cells.

nial nerve or spinal cord compression, neurologic symptoms and signs may dominate the clinical presentation. The skin or retroperitoneum or both may be involved by direct extension that is enough to compromise local structures.[539] Spheno-occipital chordoma may present as a nasal, paranasal, or nasopharyngeal mass causing compromised function of local organs and structures.[540, 541] Grossly chordoma is gelatinous and soft with areas of hemorrhage and composed of distinct lobules. This lobulated pattern is a useful diagnostic feature. The tumor cells vary in shape and have an abundant eosinophilic cytoplasm that often is vacuolated. As a result of mucin production, the cells may have an epithelioid appearance, and with increased accumulation of mucin, the vacuoles become more numerous and displace the nucleus to the periphery, creating signet ring cells. So-called physaliphorous cells are large tumor cells with a highly vacuolated or "bubbly" cytoplasm and a prominent vesicular nucleus.[542, 543] The tumor cells may exist as solid masses or be arranged in cords or strands within a mucinous matrix. Mitotic figures generally are scanty or absent; areas of cartilage and bone may be present.[544] The differential diagnosis includes metastatic carcinoma, myxoid chondrosarcoma, and myxopapillary ependymoma. Chordoma cells have strong reactivity for S-100 protein, cytokeratin, epithelial membrane antigen, and vimentin.[545–550] Glial fibrillary acidic protein is encountered with the use of polyclonal antibodies but less often with monoclonal antibodies.[551]

Surgical resection is the treatment for sacrococcygeal and vertebral chordoma. Spheno-occipital chordoma is less amenable to total resection, but use of proton-beam radiation therapy has improved the prognosis significantly.[533, 552, 553] Postoperative local recurrences may develop 10 or more years after initial therapy.[554] Distant metastases (occurring in approximately 40%) usually develop late in the evolution of the disease[555, 556]; most patients who die of chordoma do so because of local extension. Sometimes, pleomorphic, high-grade, spindle cell sarcoma occurs along with areas of typical chordoma (i.e., dedifferentiated chordoma), either in the primary tumor or in the recurrence.[557] This development portends a poor prognosis.[558, 559] Chondroid chordoma is a chordoma in which there is a cartilaginous component that may be so extensive that a misdiagnosis of chondrosarcoma is made. This form of chordoma occurs usually in the spheno-occipital region, but also may occur in the sacrococcygeal region[536, 560] (Fig. 47–100). Prognosis may be better than that of conventional chordoma,[561] although this is controversial. Chondroid chordoma cells are immunoreactive for S-100 protein and cytokeratin. The main differential diagnosis is with chondrosarcoma, whose cells react only for S-100 protein and not for cytokeratin.

## ADAMANTINOMA

*Adamantinoma* is a primary epithelial tumor[562–566] that occurs mainly in the tibia and less commonly in the fibula, femur, and ulna; it occurs usually in patients in the fourth to fifth decades of life.[567–570] (Figs. 47–101 to 47–104). The pathogenesis of adamantinoma is unclear but probably relates to neoplastic transformation of osseous epithelial rem-

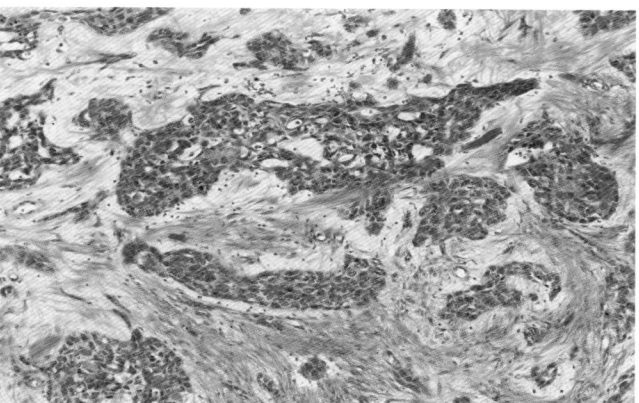

**FIGURE 47–102.** Adamantinoma with islands and nests of epithelial cells within a fibrous stroma.

nants.[571] It arises in the shaft or metaphysis,[572] producing single or multiple lytic areas in the cortex or medulla surrounded by marked sclerosis. The shaft of the tibia may show marked anterior bowing. The tumor is composed of solid nests of basaloid cells, with peripheral palisading; however, a variety of other histologic patterns may be found, including spindle cell, squamoid, and tubular, the last of which may simulate the channels of a vascular tumor.[572] Histologically adamantinoma sometimes is accompanied, especially at its periphery, by changes similar to osteofibrous dysplasia, and the relative proportions of these two components may vary greatly from case to case.[573–576] The tumor cells of adamantinoma show immunoreactivity for epithelial markers (cytokeratin, epithelial membrane antigen) and for vimentin.[577]

The main histologic differential diagnosis is metastatic carcinoma, but adamantinoma occurs in a younger patient group than does metastatic carcinoma, and the latter usually has a higher degree of cellular atypia than is found in adamantinoma. Adamantinoma is a slow-growing, low-grade malig-

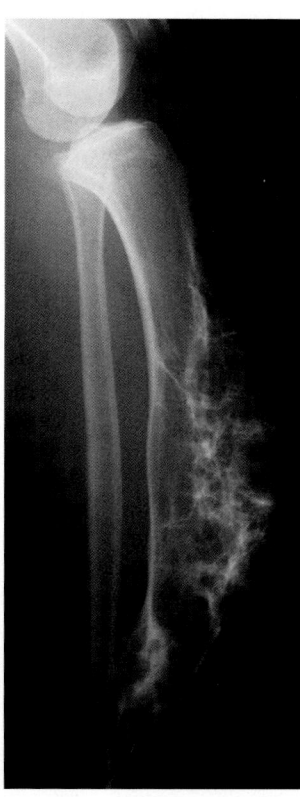

**FIGURE 47–101.** Adamantinoma. A 17-year-old girl with a several-year history of increasing size of her leg. Roentgenogram shows anterior bowing of the tibia caused by a cystic, multilocular lesion involving the diaphysis. The lesion involves the cortex and the medulla.

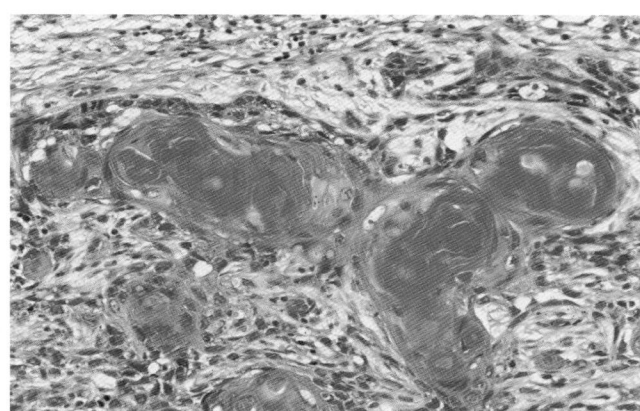

**FIGURE 47–103.** Area within adamantinoma shows keratinization within the islands of epithelial tumor cells. Keratohyalin granules are present in the cytoplasm of some cells.

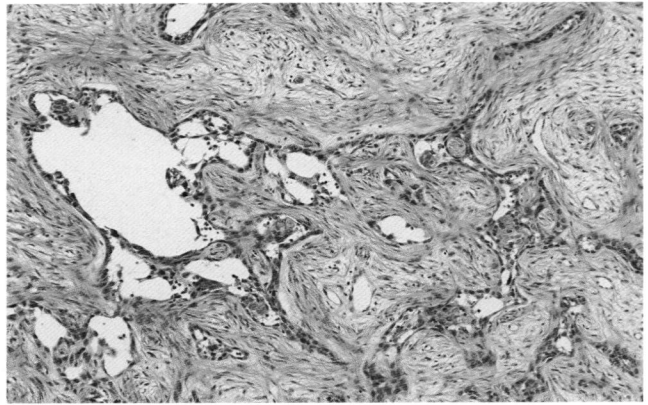

FIGURE 47–104. Pseudoangiomatous area within adamantinoma. Epithelial islands show central clearing, creating intercommunicating channels resembling vascular spaces; however, the cells lining these spaces are epithelial and not endothelial.

nancy with a tendency toward local recurrence and occasional development of lymph node or distant metastases, particularly to the lung. Complete excision or amputation is the usual therapeutic choice.

Studies have suggested that osteofibrous dysplasia may represent a regressing form of adamantinoma. In greater than 90% of cases of osteofibrous dysplasia, immunohistochemical studies show cytokeratin reactivity in the stromal cells, either in individual cells or in aggregates of several cells.[578] Some adamantinomas may show a predominant pattern of osteofibrous dysplasia, but careful search of routine sections shows small nests of epithelial cells, consistent with adamantinoma. These cases have been referred to as *differentiated* adamantinoma.[574]

### MISCELLANEOUS TUMORS

Although *intraosseous neurofibromas* occur, they are extremely rare, with two thirds arising in the mandible.[1–12] *Intraosseous schwannoma* occurs with greater frequency than osseous neurofibroma[579–581] and usually occurs in the mandible, but the sacrum, maxilla, and long bones also are sites of involvement.[582, 583] Both lesions show the typical histopathology of their soft tissue counterparts; however, the biphasic pattern of Antoni A and B areas may not be as distinct in osseous neurilemmoma as it is in the soft tissue lesion. Patients with von Recklinghausen's disease may have skeletal abnormalities, such as scoliosis, bowing, and pseudarthrosis.[584]

*Xanthoma* of bone is a rare lesion that usually presents in patients older than age 20 years.[585] It almost always is solitary, and the flat bones (pelvis, ribs, skull) are the most frequent sites. It shows an admixture of foamy cells, multinucleated giant cells, cholesterol clefts, and fibrosis.

*Fibrocartilaginous mesenchymoma* is a benign lesion that affects the metaphysis of the long bones, particularly the fibula. It is composed of an admixture of spindle cells, whose arrangement may simulate a fibrosarcoma; bone trabeculae; and islands of cartilage. Some of this cartilage is in the form of structures resembling epiphyseal plates, as is found in chest wall hamartoma and fibrocartilaginous dysplasia. Although local recurrence may occur in 40% of patients, to date no examples of metastasis have occurred.[586]

Rarely, *leiomyosarcoma* may occur primarily in bone, especially in the femur and tibia; however, before accepting this diagnosis, exclusion of a metastasis from a primary tumor in an extraosseous site is necessary.[520, 521] Typically, leiomyosarcoma cells contain smooth muscle actin and desmin, and they are enveloped by type IV collagen and laminin.[522] They also may show reactivity for cytokeratin and S-100 protein, which may cause diagnostic confusion.[523, 524]

Rare examples of primary *rhabdomyosarcoma* of bone are reported.[525, 526] *Lipoma* of bone is rare,[527, 528] whereas osseous *liposarcoma* is even more exceptional.[529, 530]

## Cystic Lesions

### SIMPLE SOLITARY BONE CYST

Most often, solitary bone cyst develops in long bones (90%), especially in the metaphysis of the humerus and femur[587, 588] (Figs. 47–105 to 47–108). Much less commonly, cysts occur in short bones, particularly the calcaneus.[589] Most develop in patients younger than age 20 years; in older patients, the lesion usually is found in sites other than the long bones. Most cases of solitary bone cyst are asymptomatic until the bone fractures after only minor trauma. Radiologic studies show a lucent, trabeculated lesion involving the metaphysis and extending to the epiphyseal plate; lesions so located are termed *active*. With growth of the bone, the cyst appears to move away from the epiphyseal plate

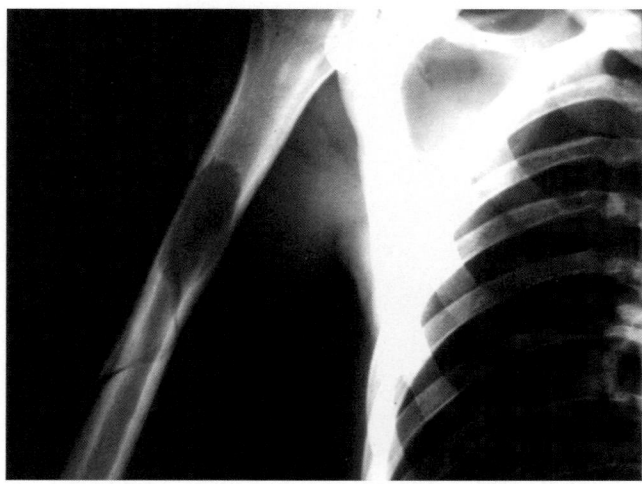

FIGURE 47–105. Solitary bone cyst. Well-circumscribed, lytic lesion in the diaphysis of the humerus. A spiral fracture through the lesion and portion of the shaft is present. Such cysts, located at a distance from the physis, have been termed *latent*.

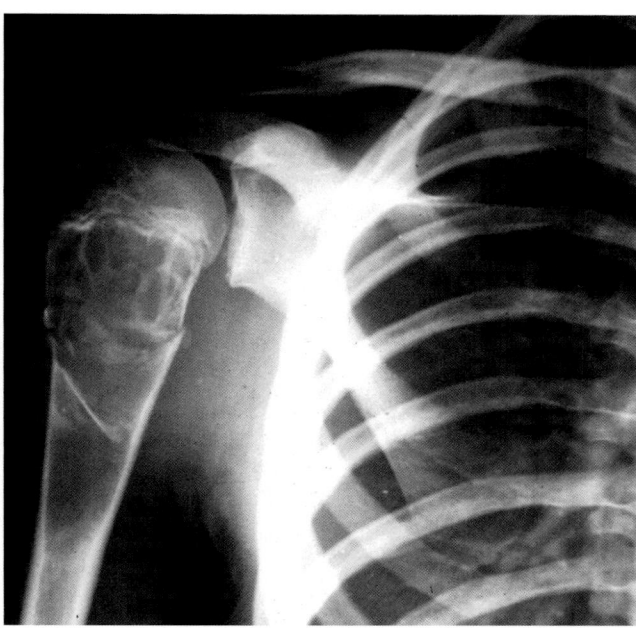

**FIGURE 47–106.** Solitary bone cyst with its base located juxta-posed to the epiphyseal plate. Such cysts have been termed *active*. Although the lesion appears to show multilocularity, this is caused by bony ridges on the endosteal surface, the lesion being unilocular.

owing to normal deposition of bone between it and the plate. Then the lesion may be found in the meta-diaphysis or diaphysis and in these locations is termed *latent*. Whatever the location, the long axis of the lesion is in the long axis of the bone and it causes uniform expansion of the bone. Magnetic resonance imaging (MRI) studies are useful in establishing the fluid content of the cyst. The cyst erodes and thins the cortex, but periosteal bone proliferation is not present, unless there is superimposed pathologic fracture.[587] At operation, the cyst is filled with serous or sanguineous fluid and is lined by a

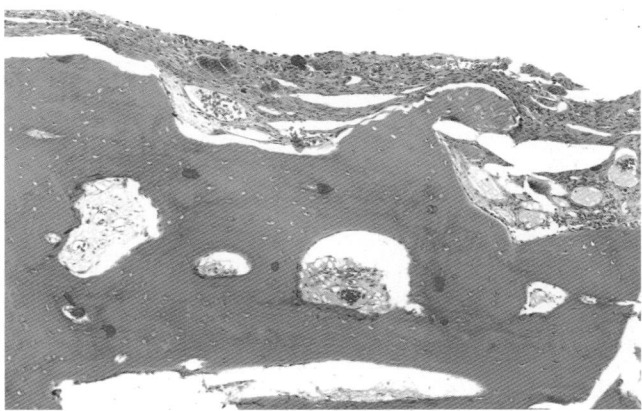

**FIGURE 47–107.** Solitary bone cyst. Thin membrane lining the cyst is adherent to the cortical bone and contains multinucleated osteoclast-like giant cells dispersed in a fibrous stroma.

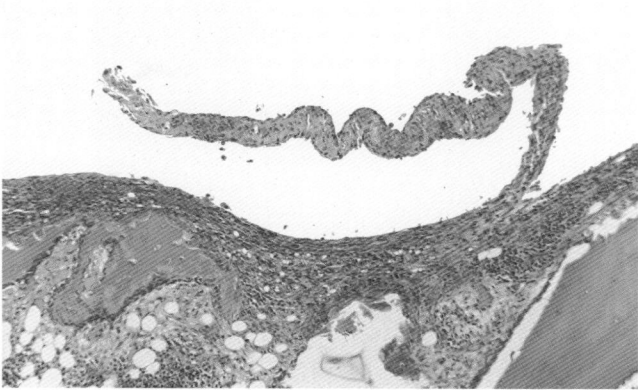

**FIGURE 47–108.** Solitary bone cyst membrane shows spindle cell stroma with bone formation. The membrane may be histologically similar to the walls of the vascular spaces in aneurysmal bone cyst.

smooth fibrous membrane. The membrane is composed of well-vascularized connective tissue; hemosiderin, often within macrophages; and scattered osteoclast-type giant cells. Bone adjacent to the cyst may be dense, with irregular cement lines.[590, 591] The presence within the membrane of flocculent, fibrin-like eosinophilic masses occurs in 10% to 15% of cases and has been thought incorrectly by some to represent cementum. This material may condense and be converted to osteoid and bone. The finding of this material is a strong indicator that the lesion is a solitary bone cyst. Treatment of solitary bone cyst is curettage and packing of the cyst with bone chips; the prognosis is excellent, although local recurrences may develop. The use of steroid injections into the cyst has been successful in healing the cyst in 70% to 95% of the cases, although repeated injections over time may be required before successful healing occurs.

## ANEURYSMAL BONE CYST

Aneurysmal bone cyst develops in patients 10 to 20 years old (80% of cases)[592–594] (Figs. 47–109 to 47–113). Favored sites of involvement include the long bones and the vertebrae, which together account for 65% of cases, but cysts also develop in the flat bones and small bones of the hands and feet.[595, 596] Aneurysmal bone cyst–like lesions may develop rarely in the soft tissue and within the walls of major arteries.[597] Aneurysmal bone cyst may be primary or develop secondarily in a preexisting bone lesion,[598–600] such as chondroblastoma, giant cell tumor, fibrous dysplasia, nonossifying fibroma, osteoblastoma, chondrosarcoma, osteosarcoma, and mesenchymal hamartoma of the chest wall in infants.

In a long bone, aneurysmal bone cyst is a radiologically lucent lesion centered on the metaphysis, but which may extend into the epiphysis if the physeal plate is closed. It expands the bone, usually causing erosion and destruction of the cortex with the eventual production of a peripheral rim of per-

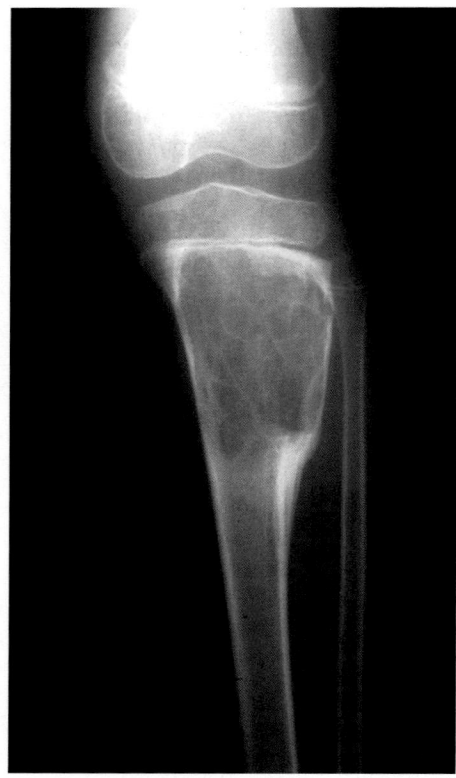

**FIGURE 47–109.** Aneurysmal bone cyst. Roentgenogram of the proximal tibia in a 5-year-old girl shows an expanded, lytic lesion within the metaphysis. Distal aspect of the lesion shows some periosteal new bone formation, but the lesion appears confined to the bone.

iosteal new bone formation. The bone expansion is typically, but not always, eccentric, producing the classic "blownout" appearance. When in a short tubular bone, the lesion may more commonly produce a fusiform expansion of the entire bone. In the vertebrae, the posterior elements are predominantly involved, but the lesion also may extend into the vertebral body; isolated vertebral body involvement is

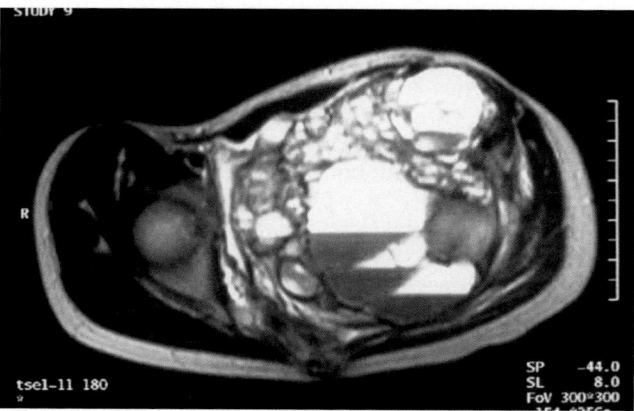

**FIGURE 47–110.** Magnetic resonance image of an aneurysmal bone cyst of the pelvis in a 12-year-old girl shows multiple fluid levels within the lesion.

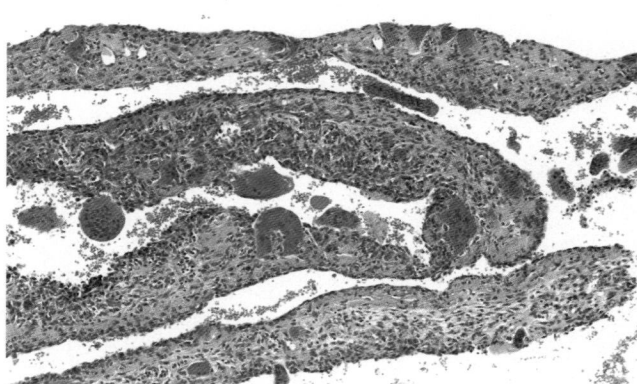

**FIGURE 47–111.** Walls of aneurysmal bone cyst have a serpentine appearance as a result of a curettage that has disrupted the vascular spaces. The lining of the spaces is composed of fibroblasts, some chronic inflammatory cells, and multinucleated osteoclast-type giant cells. Pink osteoid is noted in the walls of some of the fragments.

rare. Aneurysmal bone cyst also may extend across the intervertebral space, through the intervertebral disk, to involve an adjacent vertebra. Computed tomography and MRI studies may show fluid levels within the cysts, and MRI may show inhomogeneity of signal intensity with septations within the lesion.

On gross examination, aneurysmal bone cyst appears as a spongy, cystic hemorrhagic mass covered by a thin shell of reactive bone that may extend into the soft tissue. Histologically, aneurysmal bone cyst contains large spaces filled with blood. The walls (septa) of these spaces contain fibroblasts, myofibroblasts, histiocytes, and osteoclast-like giant cells, all of which also may line the spaces which lack endothelial cells.[601] Osteoid and plates of lamellar bone also are commonly present in the fibrous septa. Of diagnostic value is the presence of a peculiar calcified fibromyxoid tissue that is hematoxyphilic. This material is found in approximately 25% of aneurys-

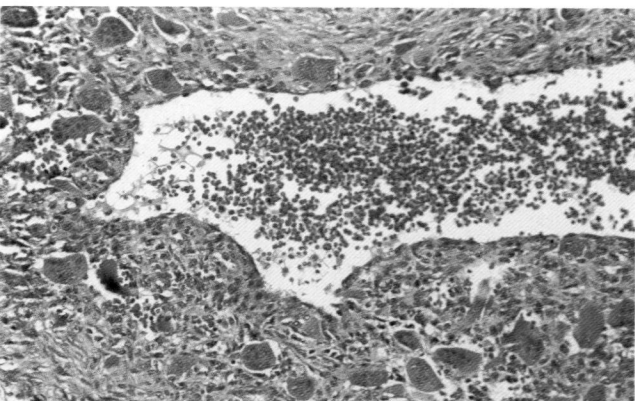

**FIGURE 47–112.** Close-up view of a typical vascular space in an aneurysmal bone cyst shows multiple, osteoclast-type giant cells within the walls that form the cystic spaces. Note the absence of stromal cell atypia as would be expected in a telangiectatic osteosarcoma.

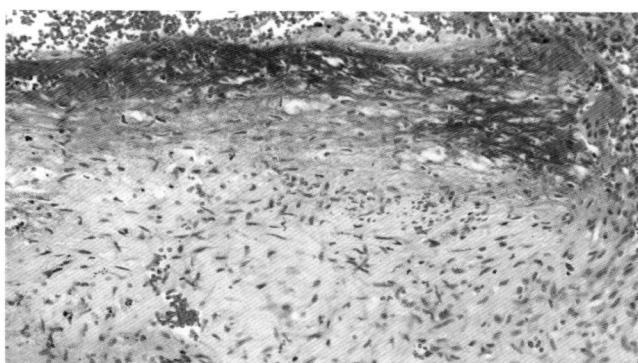

**FIGURE 47–113.** Focal area within an aneurysmal bone cyst shows highly hematoxyphilic fibrochondroid-like area. Such areas, although seen in a minority of aneurysmal bone cysts, are highly specific for this entity.

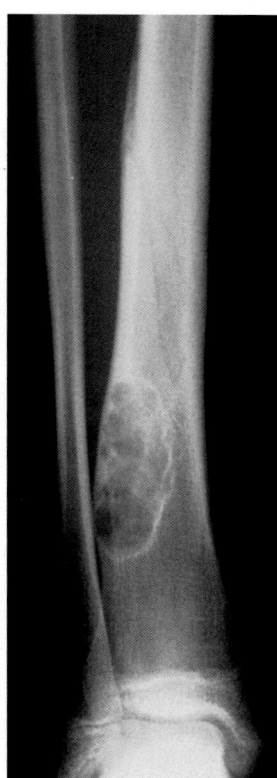

**FIGURE 47–114.** Nonossifying fibroma. A well-circumscribed, multiloculated lesion, with a sclerotic border, is seen within the distal metaphysis of the tibia in a 13-year-old girl.

mal bone cysts and seems to be specific to this lesion. At times, the multinucleated osteoclast-type giant cells are so numerous as to suggest a giant cell tumor, and recourse to the clinical and radiologic features of the lesion must be made to reach a correct diagnosis. This difficulty is compounded by the fact that true giant cell tumor is the most common primary bone lesion to contain areas of secondary aneurysmal bone cyst. Almost all aneurysmal bone cysts have areas that are more solid, wherein the stromal cells may show brisk mitotic activity but lack atypia. In these more solid areas, lacelike or trabecular osteoid also may be found. A solid variant of aneurysmal bone cyst has been described that has a minor, or even absent, cystic component; however, most, perhaps all, such lesions are probably examples of giant cell reparative granuloma.

Aneurysmal bone cyst recurs in approximately 20% of cases when treated by curettage alone, presumably because of incomplete excision.[594, 602] En-bloc resection or curettage with bone grafting affords better results.[603] Malignant transformation of aneurysmal bone cyst has been reported, but this possibility must be distinguished from the more likely event of telangiectatic osteosarcoma and osteosarcoma with aneurysmal bone cyst–like areas.[604]

### EPIDERMOID CYSTS

Epidermoid cysts most commonly occur in the skull bones and distal phalanges of the hand. They produce sharply defined radiolucent lesions. Histologically, the cyst wall consists of stratified squamous epithelium resting on a fibrous stroma. Exfoliated squames may fill the cyst. The cyst may rupture into the adjacent fibrous tissue and elicit an intense foreign-body reaction.

## Miscellaneous Lesions

Metaphyseal *fibrous cortical defect* and *nonossifying fibroma* are benign lesions that occur in adolescents. They occur almost exclusively in the metaphysis of

the long bones, especially the tibia and femur[605, 606] (Figs. 47–114 to 47–116). It is unclear whether these are neoplastic or developmental abnormalities.[607] Fibrous cortical defect is the smaller of the two lesions. Radiologically, it forms a focal, partially radiolucent oval-to-round lesion within or immediately adjacent to the cortex. Nonossifying fibroma is a large medullary lesion, usually involving one half or more of the width of the bone. It is characteristi-

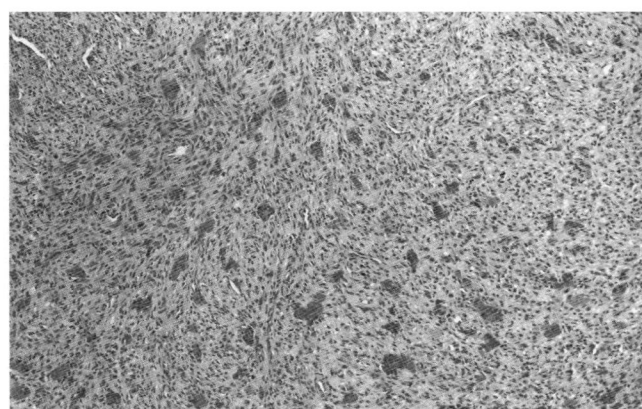

**FIGURE 47–115.** Nonossifying fibroma. Area shows a bland spindle cell stroma in which are scattered osteoclast-type giant cells.

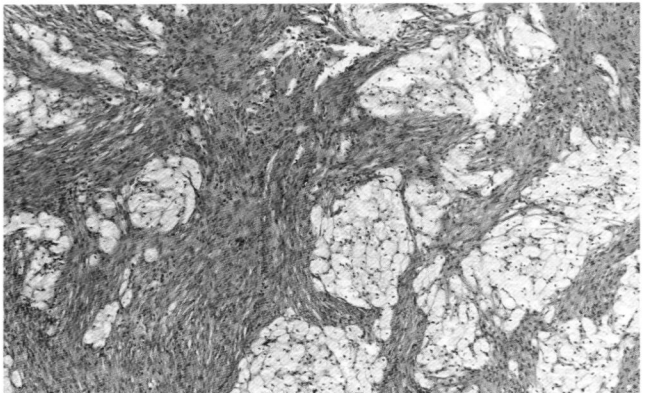

FIGURE 47–116. Area within nonossifying fibroma shows spindle cells interspersed with islands and nests of large foam cells.

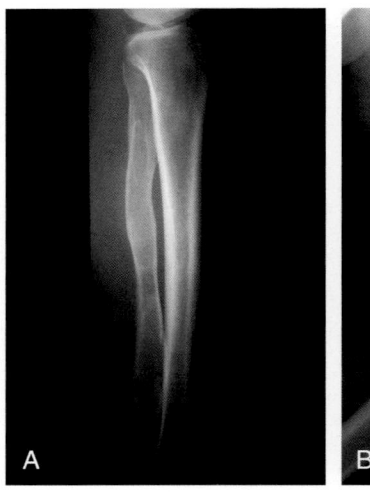
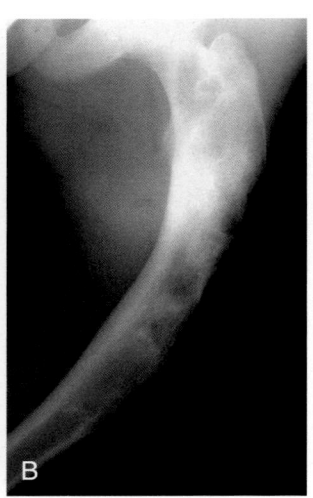

FIGURE 47–117. Fibrous dysplasia. *A,* Roentgenogram shows distortion of the fibula by a lesion having a ground-glass appearance. The distal and proximal margins of the lesion show slightly sclerotic borders. *B,* Roentgenogram shows the classic shepherd's crook deformity of the proximal femur.

cally radiolucent, with lobulated sclerotic borders and internal trabeculation. Fibrous cortical defect is an asymptomatic incidental lesion that occurs in approximately 40% of growing children and eventually involutes, becoming incorporated into the cortex; however, rare cases have continued to grow and develop into a nonossifying fibroma. Nonossifying fibroma is usually asymptomatic, pain developing usually after fracture of the lesion produced by minor trauma. Multiple nonossifying fibromas do occur, and in some cases, they are associated with extraskeletal anomalies (Jaffe-Campanacci syndrome) that include mental retardation, hypogonadism, ocular abnormalities, and cardiovascular malformations. Grossly, the bone lesions are brownish red to yellowish and composed of cellular fibrous tissue, growing in fascicular and storiform patterns, containing an admixture of osteoclast-like giant cells and islands of foamy or hemosiderin-laden macrophages. This is identical to the histologic pattern of benign fibrous histiocytoma of soft tissue; the latter term is used by some authors if the lesion occurs in an adult patient and in a site other than the metaphysis of a long bone.[608, 609] Fibrous cortical defect requires no therapy, whereas simple curettage usually is sufficient for the curative treatment of nonossifying fibroma.[610]

*Fibrous dysplasia* is a condition of unknown cause that results in the replacement of normal lamellar bone by fibrous connective tissue and structurally weak woven bone[611–613] (Figs. 47–117 to 47–119). It may be limited to one bone (monostotic type—80% of cases) or involve several bones (polyostotic type). The monostotic variant usually occurs in older children and young adults, frequently affecting the rib, femur, tibia, or skull.[611, 612] When the polyostotic type occurs in association with endocrine abnormalities, particularly precocious puberty associated with cutaneous pigmentation, it is referred to as *McCune-Albright syndrome.* The latter seems to result from a somatic mutation of the *c-fos* oncogene. Fibrous dysplasia is a self-limiting process that usually starts in childhood, but because of its slow growth, it may go

unnoticed until adulthood. The process usually stabilizes during puberty, persisting in a quiescent state indefinitely. As the name indicates, it is generally regarded as a dysplastic process rather than neoplastic. Radiologically, fibrous dysplasia is usually a radiolucent lesion that may have a hazy or ground-glass appearance depending on the amount of bone within it. It may expand the bone, at times in a fusiform fashion, and cause endosteal cortical scalloping and thinning, but it does not disrupt the cortex. The borders of the lesion tend to be sclerotic. The poor quality of the bone produced in fibrous dysplasia causes weakness in the affected bone that may result in bone deformities, especially in weight-bearing bones, most notably the "shepherd's crook" deformity produced by involvement of the proximal femur. Occasionally the lesion protrudes far beyond the normal bone contour (*fibrous dysplasia protuber-*

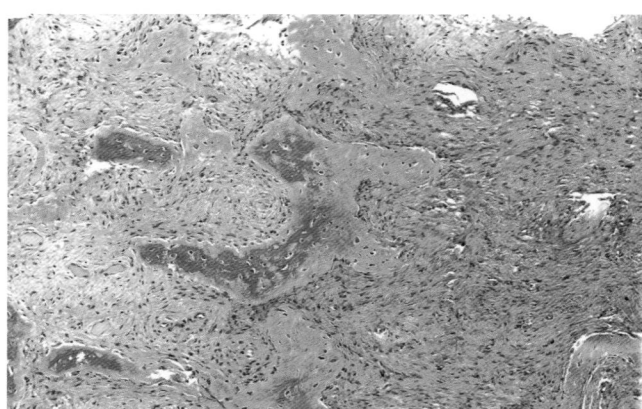

FIGURE 47–118. Fibrous dysplasia. Fibrous stroma contains irregular trabeculae of metaplastic bone arising directly from the stroma, without the presence of osteoblastic rimming.

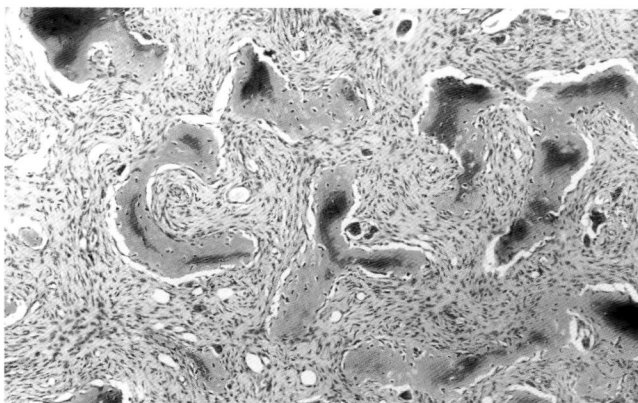

**FIGURE 47–119.** So-called Chinese character pattern of the bone trabeculae in fibrous dysplasia.

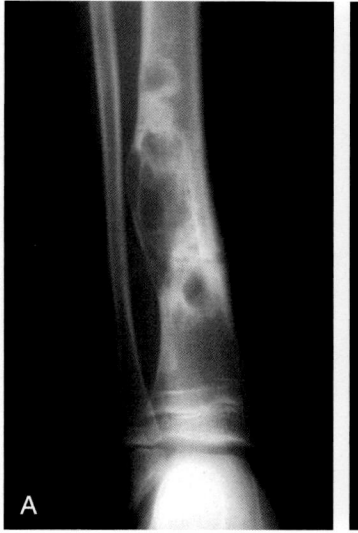
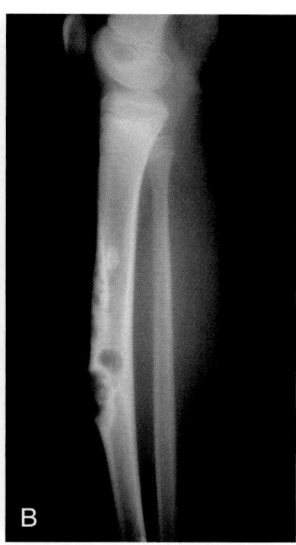

**FIGURE 47–120.** Osteofibrous dysplasia. *A,* Roentgenogram shows a lesion in the distal aspect of the tibia in a 9-year-old boy. The lesion consists of multiloculated cystlike spaces involving the cortex of the bone, although from this view one cannot rule out involvement of the medullary canal. A pathologic fracture is present in the distal portion of the lesion. *B,* Lateral roentgenogram of the tibia in a 9-year-old girl shows a thickened anterior cortex containing cystlike areas; a large, bitelike defect is present in the anterior cortex. There is anterior bowing of the bone, a feature characteristic of osteofibrous dysplasia and adamantinoma.

*ans*).[614] Grossly fibrous dysplasia is gritty and grayish white. Histologically, the lesion has a variably cellular fibrous stroma that contains scattered, irregularly shaped bone trabeculae, such as S or C shapes, likened to "Chinese figures." These trabeculae are composed of coarse fibers ("woven" bone) that do not mature to lamellar bone, suggesting that fibrous dysplasia is a maturation defect wherein bone formation is arrested at an early stage, resembling membranous ossification. Appositional osteoblasts do not appear on the surface of these trabeculae except as a pattern of reaction after fracture. Often, one sees the trabeculae arising directly from the fibrous stroma (metaplastic bone formation). Osteoclast-like giant cells and mitotic activity are typically inconspicuous. Variations on this theme include the presence of small calcified spherules similar to those seen in cementifying fibromas of the jaw bones,[615–617] highly cellular areas that may be diagnosed incorrectly as sarcoma, focal areas of hyaline cartilage, and cystic areas. The cartilaginous areas may dominate the microscopic picture and cause the mistaken diagnosis of a malignant transformation to chondrosarcoma.[618] Such cases have been designated as *fibrocartilaginous dysplasia*. The lack of nuclear atypia and abnormal mitoses helps separate fibrous dysplasia from low-grade osteosarcoma; lack of inflammatory cells helps separate it from osteomyelitis. If the affected bone previously has been biopsied or treated, the above-described classic histologic features may be lost, and a nonspecific picture be present.

Fibrous dysplasia may be accompanied by intramuscular myxoma of the same extremity[619]; the combination is referred to as *Mazabraud's syndrome*. Fibrous dysplasia of either monostotic or polyostotic type rarely may undergo malignant transformation to osteosarcoma, chondrosarcoma, or malignant fibrous histiocytoma.[620–622] Because of its postpubertal stability, the treatment of fibrous dysplasia is confined mostly to surgical correction of any bone deformity. Fibrous dysplasia must be distinguished from osteofibrous dysplasia (ossifying fibroma of

long bones). The latter is distinguished from fibrous dysplasia by the osteoblastic rimming of its bone trabeculae, the presence of maturation to lamellar bone, a cortical rather than a medullary location, and a greater tendency to recur[623, 624] (Figs. 47–120 to 47–122), in contrast to fibrous dysplasia, which involves many different bones while the tibia and fibula are affected almost exclusively in osteofibrous dysplasia. Clonal chromosomal abnormalities suggest that osteofibrous dysplasia is neoplastic.[625] Im-

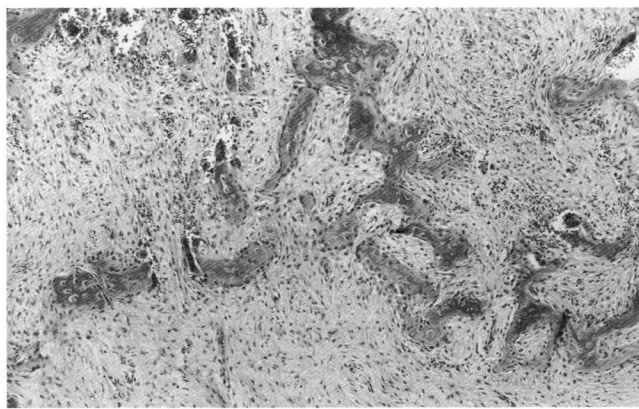

**FIGURE 47–121.** View of osteofibrous dysplasia shows edematous-appearing stroma in which there is active bone formation with the trabeculae of bone rimmed by osteoblasts. This is in contrast to fibrous dysplasia, in which such osteoblastic rimming is absent.

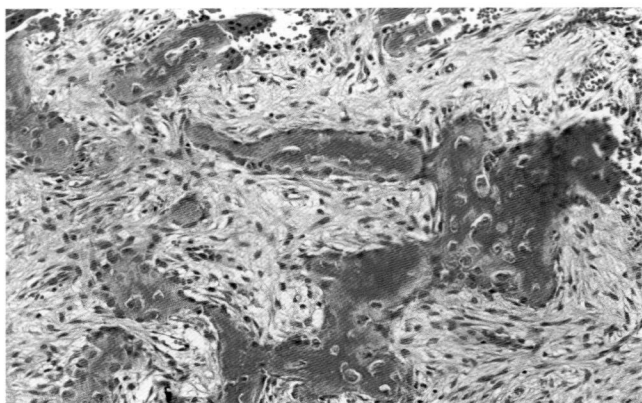

FIGURE 47–122. Higher magnification view of osteofibrous dysplasia shows the trabeculae to have centers of immature woven bone.

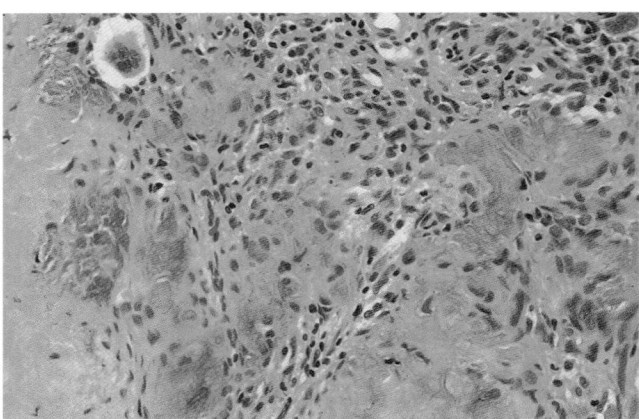

FIGURE 47–124. Phosphaturic mesenchymal tumor composed of lobules of peculiar cartilage-like matrix, which is calcified, spindle shaped, and has scattered osteoclast-like cells.

munoreactivity for cytokeratin may be found in the spindle cells of osteofibrous dysplasia and not in the cells of fibrous dysplasia.[623, 626] (See discussion of adamantinoma.)

*Oncogenic* or *tumor-induced osteomalacia or rickets* is a syndrome caused by tumors that secrete a phosphaturic substance that causes total-body phosphate depletion resulting in osteomalacia or rickets.[626–629] Most patients present with severe, often debilitating bone pain (sometimes with fractures), osteopenia, hypophosphatemia, hyperphosphaturia, normocalcemia, and decreased serum 1,25-dihydroxyvitamin $D_3$ levels. The tumors may occur in bone, skin, or soft tissue; may be small; and clinically may be quite difficult to find. Some patients have symptoms for years before discovery of the tumor. When a suspicious mass is found, it should be removed surgically with a clear margin. The morphologic features of the tumor may help confirm the diagnosis of oncogenic osteomalacia or rickets, especially if it has the unique morphologic features of a phospha-

turic mesenchymal tumor (see later) (Figs. 47–123 to 47–125). Postoperatively, serum phosphate and 1,25-dihydroxyvitamin $D_3$ should be measured because biochemical abnormalities may begin to resolve within hours. In other cases, it may take days to weeks before the abnormal serum values return to normal. If the chemical abnormalities resolve, the patient's symptoms disappear, and the tumor appears totally resected and benign, the diagnosis is confirmed and the prognosis is excellent. If this does not occur, however, and the tumor shows morphologic features not typical for a phosphaturic mesenchymal tumor, the clinician should continue the search for the right tumor or consider an alternative clinical diagnosis. If the patient's serum abnormalities and symptoms improve only partially, this may mean that there is residual or multifocal tumor present, especially if the tumor was resected only partially or shows malignant cytologic features. In the latter event, additional operative therapy, chemotherapy, or radiation therapy may be neces-

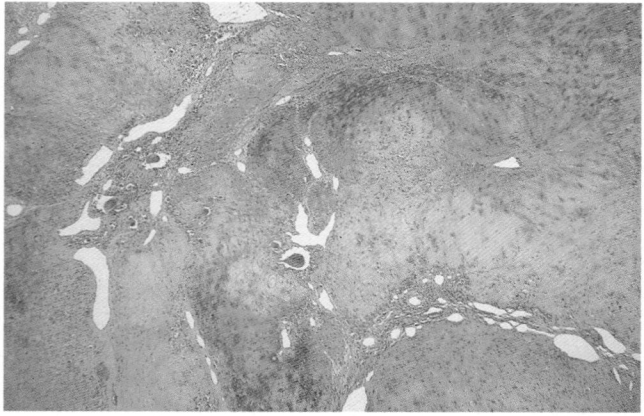

FIGURE 47–123. Phosphaturic mesenchymal tumor composed of lobules of peculiar cartilage-like matrix separated by dilated vascular channels, some of which contain osteoclast-like giant cells.

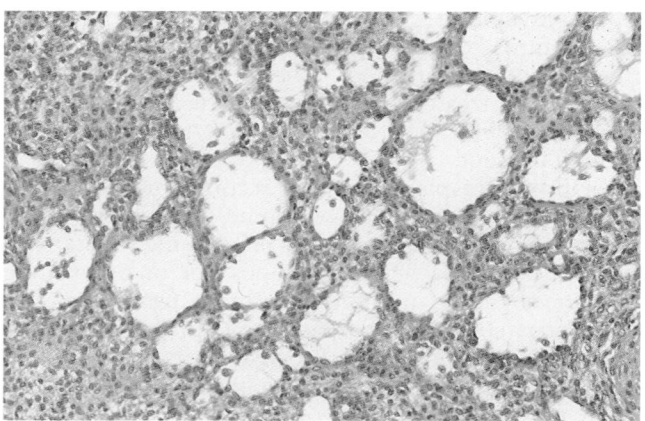

FIGURE 47–125. Phosphaturic mesenchymal tumor containing microcystic spaces.

sary to effect cure. If it is not possible to find or eradicate the tumor causing the osteomalacia or rickets, supplemental phosphorus and vitamin D therapy is indicated.

Although histologically polymorphous, personal (N.W.) review of 16 tumors documented to cause this syndrome revealed four tumor groups. The first group contained 10 connective tissue tumors having variably prominent vessels, osteoclast-like giant cells, focal microcystic changes, dystrophic calcification, osseous metaplasia, and poorly developed cartilage-like areas. With one exception, all tumors of this group occurred in the soft tissue and were benign. The single malignant tumor originated in bone, recurred locally, and metastasized to the lung. The remaining tumors occurred in bone and showed benign clinical behavior. They resembled osteoblastoma (three tumors), nonossifying fibroma (two tumors), and ossifying fibroma (one tumor). It is important to separate oncogenic osteomalacia or rickets from other tumor-associated osteomalacia or hypophosphatemic syndromes, such as tumor-induced malabsorption or diarrhea, ectopic parathyroid hormone production, or phosphorus uptake by leukemia/lymphoma cells. Oncogenic osteomalacia or rickets should be suspected in any patient who presents with hypophosphatemia and inappropriate phosphaturia. Serum 1,25-dihydroxyvitamin $D_3$ always is low, and the serum alkaline phosphatase is elevated. Because clinical osteomalacia or rickets may not be present when the biochemical abnormalities first develop, a bone biopsy might be helpful in securing the diagnosis. Tetracycline labeling should precede biopsy. The mesenchymal tumors may occur in almost any location. Approximately 50% have occurred in bone, 45% in soft tissues, and 3% in skin. About 45% have involved the lower extremities; 30%, the head-and-neck area; and 20%, the upper extremities. One phosphaturic mesenchymal tumor (mixed connective tissue variant) showed marked uptake of technetium-99m methylene diphosphonate, a property that, if present, may hasten tumor discovery. Finally, if a phosphaturic mesenchymal tumor is not found, one should consider other tumors that cause oncogenic osteomalacia or rickets. These include prostate cancer, breast cancer, oat cell carcinoma, fibrous dysplasia, and soft tissue tumors occurring in neurofibromatosis.

## Metastatic Bone Lesions

The most common malignant tumor to involve bone is a metastatic carcinoma.[629] Usually the clinical history (i.e., in the older patient) and multifocality make the diagnosis clear; however, multiple myeloma also presents in older patients with multiple bone lesions and must be considered in the differential diagnosis. Metastatic carcinoma almost always is positive on isotope bone scan, whereas myeloma frequently is negative (50% of cases); myeloma also often is associated with a serum paraprotein.

Greater than 80% of metastatic carcinomas to bone originate from breast, lung, prostate, thyroid, or kidney.[1-12, 630] In contrast, primary soft tissue sarcomas uncommonly metastasize to the skeletal system, but childhood embryonal rhabdomyosarcoma is an exception.[631] Sarcomatoid carcinomas may spread to the bone and cause diagnostic confusion with a primary bone sarcoma, especially when they arise from an occult renal primary. Metastases tend to develop in sites containing red marrow,[632] the axial skeleton (i.e., cranium, ribs, spine, and sacrum) being favored (approximately 70% of cases), but the long bones also may be involved, especially the proximal metaphyseal regions. Bone metastases distal to the knees or elbows are rare.[633-635] Bone metastases are usually osteolytic but may be osteoblastic or mixed. Osteoblastic metastases tend to develop from prostatic carcinoma, neuroendocrine tumors, and occasionally breast carcinoma.[636] Bone metastases, if extensive enough, may lead to hypercalcemia and elevation of serum acid phosphatase.[637] The microscopic recognition of a metastasis is usually simple, but some metastatic lesions may be populated by osteoclast-like giant cells, mimicking a primary giant cell tumor.[638] The primary source of the metastasis may be suggested microscopically, particularly in cases of carcinoma of the kidney, thyroid, or large bowel, and immunohistochemical evaluation can be useful. Most cases of metastatic squamous carcinoma derive from the lung. Metastatic bone lesions often cause pain and may produce pathologic fracture; treatment is for pain relief or to prevent or treat fracture. Radiation therapy is highly effective, inducing partial or complete relief of pain in more than 80% of cases. Symptoms of metastatic breast or prostate carcinoma often can be managed with hormonal manipulation. Sometimes a single metastatic focus, especially from the thyroid or kidney, may be excised with benefit.

## REFERENCES

1. Unni KK: Dahlin's Bone Tumors. General Aspects and Data on 11,087 Cases. 5th ed. Philadelphia, Lippincott-Raven, 1996.
2. Bullough PG, Vigorita VJ: Atlas of Orthopaedic Pathology with Clinical and Radiologic Correlations. 2nd ed. New York, Gower Medical Publishing, 1992.
3. Mirra JM: Bone Tumors. Clinical, Radiologic, and Pathologic Correlations. Philadelphia, Lea & Febiger, 1989.
4. Huvos AG: Bone Tumors. Diagnosis, Treatment, and Prognosis. 2nd ed. Philadelphia, WB Saunders, 1991.
5. Fechner RE, Mills SE: Tumors of the Bones and Joints. Third Series, Fascicle 8. Washington, DC, Armed Forces Institute of Pathology, 1993.
6. Dorfman HD, Czerniak B: Bone Tumors. St. Louis, MO, Mosby, 1998.
7. Schajowicz F: Tumors and Tumorlike Lesions of Bone: Pathology, Radiology and Treatment. New York, Springer-Verlag, 1994.
8. Mulder JD, Schütte HE, Kroon HM, Taconis WK: Radiologic Atlas of Bone Tumors. Amsterdam, Elsevier, 1993.
9. Forest M, Tomeno B, Vanel D: Orthopedic Surgical Pathology. Edinburgh, Churchill Livingstone, 1998.
10. Milgram JW: Radiologic and Histologic Pathology of Nontumorous Diseases of Bones and Joints. Northbrook, IL, Northbrook, 1990.

11. Resnick D: Diagnosis of Bone and Joint Disorders. 3rd ed. Philadelphia, WB Saunders, 1995.

12. Resnick D, Kyriakos M, Greenway GD: Tumors and tumor-like lesions of bone: Imaging and pathology of specific lesions. In Resnick D (ed): Diagnosis of Bone and Joint Disorders. 3rd ed. Philadelphia, WB Saunders, 1995, pp 3628–3938.

13. Wilkinson LS, Pitsillides AA, Worrall JG, Edwards JCW: Light microscopic characterization of the fibroblast-like synovial intimal cell (synoviocyte). Arthritis Rheum 35:1179–1184, 1992.

14. Lichtenstein L: Tumors of synovial joints, bursae, and tendon sheaths. Cancer 8:816–830, 1955.

15. McEvedy BY: Simple ganglia. Br J Surg 49:585–594, 1962.

16. Stack RE, Bianco AH Jr, MacCarthy CS: Compression of the common peroneal nerve by ganglion cyst. Report of nine cases. J Bone Joint Surg Am 47:773–778, 1965.

17. Pederson HE, Key JA: Pathology of calcareous tendinitis and subdeltoid bursitis. Arch Surg 62:50–63, 1951.

18. Wagner T, Abgarowicz T: Microscopic appearance of Baker's cyst in cases of rheumatoid arthritis. Rheumatologia 8:21–26, 1970.

19. Entin MA: Carpal tunnel syndrome and its variants. Surg Clin North Am 48:1097–1112, 1968.

20. Phalen GS: The carpal-tunnel syndrome. Seventeen years' experience in diagnosis and treatment of six hundred and fifty-four hands. J Bone Joint Surg Am 48:211–228, 1966.

21. Spinner RJ, Bachman JW, Amadio PC: The many faces of carpal tunnel syndrome. Mayo Clin Proc 64:829–836, 1989.

22. Bastian FO: Amyloidosis and the carpal tunnel syndrome. Am J Clin Pathol 61:711–717, 1974.

23. Bauer W, Bennett GA: Experimental and pathological studies in the degenerative type of arthritis. J Bone Joint Surg 18:1–18, 1936.

24. Silverberg M, Frank EL, Jarrett SR, Silberberg R: Aging and osteoarthritis of the human sternoclavicular joint. Am J Pathol 35:851–865, 1959.

25. Hamerman D: The biology of osteoarthritis. N Engl J Med 320:1322–1330, 1989.

26. Sokoloff L: Pathology and pathogenesis of osteoarthritis. In McCarty DJ (ed): Arthritis and Applied Conditions. 9th ed. Philadelphia, Lea & Febiger, 1979, pp 1135–1153.

27. Harrison MHM, Schajowicz F, Tureta J: Osteoarthritis of the hip. A study of the nature and evolution of the disease. J Bone Joint Surg Br 35:598–626, 1953.

28. Outerbridge RE: The etiology of chondromalacia patellae. J Bone Joint Surg Br 43:752–757, 1961.

29. Sokoloff L: Biopsy in rheumatic diseases. Med Clin North Am 45:1178–1180, 1961.

30. Sokoloff L: Pathology of rheumatoid arthritis and allied disorders. In McCarty DJ (ed): Arthritis and Applied Conditions. 9th ed. Philadelphia, Lea & Febiger, 1979, pp 429–447.

31. Winchester R: The molecular basis of susceptibility to rheumatoid arthritis. Adv Immunol 56:389–466, 1994.

32. Imai Y, Sato T, Yamakawa M, et al: A morphological and immunohistochemical study of lymphoid germinal center in synovial and lymph node tissue, from rheumatoid arthritis patients with special reference to complement components and their receptors. Acta Pathol Jpn 39:127–134, 1989.

33. Cooper NS: Pathology of rheumatoid arthritis. Med Clin North Am 52:607–621, 1968.

34. Dixon AStJ, Grant C: Acute synovial rupture in rheumatoid arthritis. Clinical and experimental observations. Lancet 1:742–745, 1964.

35. Palmer OO: Synovial cysts in rheumatoid disease. Ann Intern Med 70:61–68, 1969.

36. Jayson MI, Dixon AS, Kates A, et al: Popliteal and calf cysts in rheumatoid arthritis. Treatment by anterior synovectomy Ann Rheum Dis 31:9–15, 1972.

37. Taylor RT, Huskisson EC, Whitehouse GH, Hart FD: Spontaneous fractures of pelvis in rheumatoid arthritis. BMJ 4:663–664, 1971.

38. Hart FD: Rheumatoid arthritis. Extra-articular manifestations. Part I. BMJ 3:131–136, 1969.

39. Hart FD: Rheumatoid arthritis. Extra-articular manifestations. Part II. BMJ 2:747–752, 1970.

40. Roberts WC, Kehol JA, Carpenter DF, Golden A: Cardiac valvular lesions in rheumatoid arthritis. Arch Intern Med 122:141–146, 1968.

41. Beatty Jr EC: Rheumatic-like nodules occurring in nonrheumatic children. Arch Pathol 68:154–159, 1959.

42. Bennett GA, Zeller JW, Bauer W: Subcutaneous nodules of rheumatoid arthritis and rheumatic fever. Arch Pathol 30:70–89, 1940.

43. Hahn BH, Yardley JH, Stevens MB: "Rheumatoid" nodules in systemic lupus erythematosus. Ann Intern Med 72:49–58, 1970.

44. Sokoloff L, Wilens SL, Bunim JJ: Arteritis of striated muscle in rheumatoid arthritis. Am J Pathol 27:157–173. 1951.

45. Mongan ES, Cass RM, Jacox RF, Vaughan JH: A study of the relation of seronegative and seropositive rheumatoid arthritis to each other and to necrotizing vasculitis. Am J Med 47:23–25, 1969.

46. Schmid FR, Cooper NS, Ziff M, McEwen C: Arteritis in rheumatoid arthritis. Am J Med 30:56–83, 1961.

47. Meyerhoff J: Lyme disease. Am J Med 75:663–670, 1983.

48. Steere AC: Lyme disease. N Engl J Med 321:586–596, 1989.

49. Johnston YE, Duray PH, Steere AC, et al: Lyme arthritis. Spirochetes found in synovial microangiopathic lesions. Am J Pathol 18:26–34, 1985.

50. Lichtenstein L, Scott HW, Levin MH: Pathologic changes in gout-survey of eleven necropsied cases. Am J Pathol 32:871–895, 1956.

51. Chaplin AJ: Calcium pyrophosphate. Histological characterization of crystals in pseudogout. Arch Pathol Lab Med 100:12–15, 1976.

52. Ishida T, Dorfman HD, Bullough PG: Tophaceous pseudogout (tumoral calcium pyrophosphate dihydrate crystal deposition disease). Hum Pathol 26:587–593, 1995.

53. Moskowitz RW, Katz D: Chondrocalcinosis and chondrocalsynovitis (pseudo-gout syndrome). Analysis of 24 cases. Am J Med 43:322–334, 1967.

54. Rodnan GP, Medsger TA: The rheumatic manifestations of progressive systemic sclerosis (scleroderma). Clin Orthop 57:81–93, 1968.

55. Goldenberg DL, Cohen AS: Synovial membrane histopathology in the differential diagnosis of rheumatoid arthritis. Gout, pseudogout, systemic lupus erythematosus, infectious arthritis and degenerative joint disease. Medicine (Baltimore) 57:239–252, 1978.

56. Athanasou NA, Sallie B: Localized deposition of amyloid in articular cartilage. Histopathology 20:41–46, 1992.

57. Cary NRB: Clinicopathological importance of deposits of amyloid in the femoral head. J Clin Pathol 38:868–872, 1985.

58. Ladefoged C, Merrild U, Jorgensen B: Amyloid deposits in surgically removed articular and periarticular tissue. Histopathology 15:289–296, 1989.

59. Mihara S, Kawai S, Gondo T, Ishihara T: Intervertebral disc amyloidosis. Histochemical, immunohistochemical and ultrastructural observations. Histopathology 25:415–420, 1994.

60. Kyle RA, Eilers SG, Linscheid RL, Gaffey TA: Amyloid localized to tenosynovium at carpal tunnel release. Natural history of 124 cases. Am J Clin Pathol 91:393–397, 1989.

61. Kyle RA, Gertz MA, Linke RP: Amyloid localized to tenosynovium at carpal tunnel release. Immunohistochemical identification of amyloid type. Am J Clin Pathol 97:250–253, 1992.

62. Jaffe HL, Lichtenstein L, Sutro CJ: Pigmented villonodular synovitis, bursitis, and tenosynovitis. Arch Pathol 31:731–765, 1941.

63. Ray RA, Morton CC, Lipinski KK, et al: Cytogenetic evidence of clonality in a case of pigmented villonodular synovitis. Cancer 67: 121–125, 1991.

64. Alguacil-Garcia A, Unni KK, Goellner JR: Giant cell tumor of tendon sheath and pigmented villonodular synovitis. An ultrastructural study. Am J Clin Pathol 69:6–17, 1978.

65. O'Connell JX, Fanburg JC, Rosenberg AE: Giant cell tumor of tendon sheath and pigmented villonodular synovitis. Immunophenotype suggests a synovial cell origin. Hum Pathol 26:771–775, 1995.

66. Tashiro H, Iwasaki H, Kikuchi M, et al: Giant cell tumors of

tendon sheath. A single and multiple immunostaining analysis. Pathol Int 45:147–155, 1995.

67. Chung EB, Enzinger FM: Fibroma of tendon sheath. Cancer 44:1945–1954, 1979.

68. Maluf HM, DeYoung BR, Swanson PE, Wick MR: Fibroma and giant cell tumor of tendon sheath. A comparative histological and immunohistological study. Mod Pathol 8:155–159, 1995.

69. Wright CJE: Benign cell synovioma. An investigation of 85 cases. Br J Surg 38:257–271, 1951.

70. Ushijima M, Hashimoto H, Tsuneyoshi M, et al: Malignant giant cell tumor of tendon sheath. Report of a case. Acta Pathol Jpn 35:699–709, 1985.

71. Greenfield MM, Wallace KM: Pigmented villonodular synovitis. Radiology 54:350–356, 1950.

72. Nilsonne U, Moberger G: Pigmented villonodular synovitis of joints. Histological and clinical problems in diagnosis. Acta Orthop Scand 40:448–460, 1969.

73. Atmore WG, Dahlin DC, Ghormley RK: Pigmented villonodular synovitis. A clinical and pathologic study. Minn Med 39:196–202, 1956.

74. Rao AS, Vigorita VJ: Pigmented villonodular synovitis (giant-cell tumor of the tendon sheath and synovial membrane). A review of eighty-one cases. J Bone Joint Surg Am 66:76–94, 1984.

75. Scott FM: Bone lesions in pigmented villonodular synovitis. J Bone Joint Surg Br 50:306–311, 1968.

76. Darling JM, Glimcher LH, Shortkroff S, et al: Expression of metalloproteinases in pigmented villonodular synovitis. Hum Pathol 25:825–830, 1994.

77. Baunsgaard P, Nielsen BB: Primary synovial chondrometaplasia. Histologic variations in the structure of metaplastic nodules. Acta Pathol Microbiol Immunol Scand (A) 92:455–460, 1984.

78. Sviland L, Malcolm AJ: Synovial chondromatosis presenting as painless soft tissue mass. A report of 19 cases. Histopathology 27:275–279, 1995.

79. Milgram JW: Synovial osteochondromatosis. A histopathological study of thirty cases. J Bone Joint Surg Am 59:792–801, 1977.

80. Murphy FP, Dahlin DC, Sullivan CR: Articular synovial chondromatosis. J Bone Joint Surg Am 44:77–86, 1962.

81. Bertoni F, Unni KK, Beabout JW, Sim FH: Chondrosarcomas of the synovium. Cancer 67:155–162, 1991.

82. Goldman RL, Lichtenstein L: Synovial chondrosarcoma. Cancer 12:1233–1240, 1964.

83. Devaney K, Vinh TN, Sweet DE: Synovial hemangioma. A report of 20 cases with differential diagnostic considerations. Hum Pathol 24:737–745, 1993.

84. Ladefoged C, Jensen NK: Synovial haemangiopericytoma of the knee joint. Histopathology 15:635–637, 1989.

85. Udagawa N, Takahashi N, Akatsu T, et al: Origin of osteoclasts. Mature monocytes and macrophages are capable of differentiating into osteoclasts under a suitable microenvironment prepared by bone marrow-derived stromal cells. Proc Natl Acad Sci U S A 87:7260–7264, 1990.

86. Okada Y, Naka K, Kawamura K, et al: Localization of matrix metalloproteinase 9 (92-kilodalton gelatinase/type IV collagenase or gelatinase B) in osteoclasts. Implications for bone resorption. Lab Invest 72:311–322, 1995.

87. Heinegard D, Oldberg A: Structure and biology of cartilage and bone matrix noncollagenous macromolecules. FASEB J 3:2042–2051, 1989.

88. Noda M, Vogel RL, Craig AM, et al: Identification of a DNA sequence responsible for binding of the 1,25-dihydroxyvitamin $D_3$ receptor and 1,25-dihydroxyvitamin $D_3$ enhancement of mouse secreted phosphoprotein I (SPP-I or osteopontin) gene expression. Proc Natl Acad Sci U S A 87:9995–9999, 1990.

89. Owen TA, Bortell R, Yocum SA, et al: Coordinate occupancy of AP-I sites in the vitamin O-responsive and CCAAT box elements by Fos-Jun in the osteocalcin gene: Model for phenotype suppression of transcription. Proc Natl Acad Sci U S A 87:9990–9994, 1990.

90. Reinholt FP, Hultenby K, Oldberg A, Heinegard D: Osteo-

91. Wozney JM, Rosen V, Celeste AJ, et al: Novel regulators of bone formation: Molecular clones and activities. Science 242:1528–1534, 1988.

92. Zheng MH, Wood DJ, Papadimitriou JM: What's new in the role of cytokines on osteoblast proliferation and differentiation? Pathol Res Pract 188:1104–1121, 1992.

93. Anderson HC: Mechanism of mineral formation in bone. Lab Invest 60:320–330, 1989.

94. Glimcher MJ: Mechanism of calcification. Role of collagen fibrils and collagen-phosphoprotein complexes in vitro and in vivo. Anat Rec 224:139–153, 1989.

95. Centrella M, McCanhy TL, Canalis E: Skeletal tissue and transforming growth factor beta. FASEB J 2:3066–3073, 1988.

96. Huffer WE: Morphology and biochemistry of bone remodeling. Possible control by vitamin D, parathyroid hormone, and other substances. Lab Invest 59:418–442, 1988.

97. Marks Jr SJ, Popoff SN: Bone cell biology. The regulation of development, structure, and function in the skeleton. Am J Anat 83:1–44, 1988.

98. Riggs BL, Melton III U: Involutional osteoporosis. N Engl J Med 314:1676–1686, 1986.

99. Vigorita VJ: Osteoporosis. A diagnosable disorder? Pathol Annu 23(pt 2):185–212, 1988.

100. Jowsey J, Kelly PJ, Riggs BL, et al: Quantitative microradiographic studies of normal and osteoporotic bone. J Bone Joint Surg Am 47:785–806, 1965.

101. Davis ME, Slrandjord NM, Lanzl LH: Estrogens and the aging process. JAMA 196:219–224, 1966.

102. Raisz LO: Local and systemic factors in the pathogenesis of osteoporosis. N Engl J Med 318:818–828, 1988.

103. Bemstein DS, Sadowsky N, Hegsted DM, et al: Prevalence of osteoporosis in high- and low-fluoride areas in North Dakota. JAMA 198:499–504, 1966.

104. Riggs BL, Melton U: The prevention and treatment of osteoporosis. N Engl J Med 327:620–627, 1992.

105. Mankin HJ: Rickets, osteomalacia, and renal osteodystrophy. Part II. J Bone Joint Surg Am 56:352–386, 1974.

106. Key Jr LL, Radriguiz RM, Willi SM, et al: Long-term treatment of osteopetrosis with recombinant human interferon gamma. N Engl J Med 332:1594–1599, 1995.

107. Barry HC: Paget's disease of bone. Edinburgh, E & S Livingstone, 1969.

108. Collins DH: Paget's disease of bone. Incidence and subclinical forms. Lancet 2:51–57, 1956.

109. Greenspan A, Norman A, Sterling AP: Precocious onset of Paget's disease—a report of three cases and review of the literature. J Can Assoc Radiol 28:69–72, 1977.

110. Smith BJ, Eveson JW: Paget's disease of bone with particular reference to dentistry. J Oral Pathol 10:233–247, 1981.

111. Lake ME: The pathology of fracture in Paget's disease. Aust N Z J Surg 27:307–312, 1958.

112. Reifenstein Jr EC, Albright F: Paget's disease. Its pathologic physiology and the importance of this in the complications arising from fracture and immobilization. N Engl J Med 231:343–355, 1944.

113. Schmorl G: Ueber Ostitis deformans Paget. Virchows Arch [A] 283:694–751, 1931.

114. Fallon MD, Schwamm HA: Paget's disease of bone. An update on the pathogenesis, pathophysiology, and treatment of osteitis deformans. Pathol Annu 24(pt 1):115–159, 1989.

115. Mii Y, Miyauchi Y, Honoki K, et al: Electron microscopic evidence of a viral nature for osteoclast inclusions in Paget's disease of bone. Virchows Arch Pathol 424:99–104, 1994.

116. Mills BG, Singer FR: Nuclear inclusions in Paget's disease of bone. Science 194:201–202, 1976.

117. Hadjipavlou A, Lander P, Srolovitz H, Enker IP: Malignant transformation in Paget disease of bone. Cancer 70:2802–2808, 1992.

118. Price CHG, Goldie W: Paget's sarcoma of bone. A study of 80 cases from the Bristol and the Leeds bone tumour registries. J Bone Joint Surg Br 51:205–224, 1969.

119. Collins DH, Winn JM: Focal Paget's disease of the skull (osteoporosis circumscripta). J Pathol Bacteriol 69:1–9, 1955.

120. Eisman JA, Martin TJ: Osteolytic Paget's disease. Recognition and risks of biopsy. J Bone Joint Surg Am 68:112–117, 1986.
121. Ham AW, Harris WR: Repair and transplantation of bone. In Bourne GH (ed): The Biochemistry and Physiology of Bone. Vol 3. 2nd ed. New York, Academic Press, 1956, pp 338–379.
122. Odell RT, Leydig SM: The conservative treatment of fractures in children. Surg Gynecol Obstet 92:69–74, 1951.
123. Bohm E, Josten C: What's new in exogenous osteomyelitis? Pathol Res Pract 188:254–258, 1992.
124. Solheim LF, Paulus B, Liverud K: A new clinical-radiological syndrome. Acta Orthop Scand 51:37–41, 1980.
125. Waldvogel FA, Vasey H: Osteomyelitis. The past decade. N Engl J Med 300:360–370, 1980.
126. Lewis P, Sutler VL, Finegold M: Bone infections involving anaerobic bacteria. Medicine (Baltimore) 57:279–305, 1978.
127. Wu P-C, Khin N-M, Pang S-W: Salmonella osteomyelitis. An important differential diagnosis of granulomatous osteomyelitis. Am J Surg Pathol 9:531–537, 1985.
128. Silver HK, Simon JL, Clement DH: Salmonella osteomyelitis and abnormal hemoglobin disease. Pediatrics 20:439–447, 1957.
129. Garcia Jr A, Grantham SA: Hematogenous pyogenic vertebral osteomyelitis. J Bone Joint Surg Am 42:429–436, 1960.
130. Cabanela ME, Sim FH, Beabout JW, Dahlin DC: Osteomyelitis appearing as neoplasms. A diagnostic problem. Arch Surg 109:68–72, 1974.
131. Felsberg GJ, Gore RL, Schweitzer ME, Jui V: Sclerosing osteomyelitis of Garre (periostitis ossificans). Oral Surg Oral Med Oral Pathol 70:117–120, 1990.
132. Trueta J: The three types of acute haematogenous osteomyelitis. J Bone Joint Surg Br 41:671–680, 1959.
133. Yasuma T, Nakajima Y: Clinicopathological study on plasma cell osteomyelitis. Acta Pathol Jpn 31:835–844, 1981.
134. Cozzutlo C: Xanthogranulomatous osteomyelitis. Arch Pathol Lab Med 108:973–976, 1984.
135. Farrow R, Cureton RJR: Carcinomatous invasion of bone in osteomyelitis. Br J Surg 50:107–109, 1962.
136. Johnson LL, Kempson RL: Epidermoid carcinoma in chronic osteomyelitis. Diagnostic problems and management J Bone Joint Surg Am 47:133–145, 1965.
137. Bemey S, Goldstein M, Bishko F: Clinical and diagnostic features of tuberculous arthritis. Am J Med 53:36–42, 1972.
138. Moore RM, Green NE: Blastomycosis of bone. A report of six cases. J Bone Joint Surg Am 64:1097–1101, 1982.
139. Schwarz J: What's new in mycotic bone and joint diseases? Pathol Res Pract 178:617–634, 1984.
140. Galli SJ, Weintraub HP, Proppe KH: Malignant fibrous histiocytoma and pleomorphic sarcoma in association with medullary bone infarcts. Cancer 41:607–619, 1978.
141. Mirra JM, Bullough PG, Marcove RC, et al: Malignant fibrous histiocytoma and osteosarcoma in association with bone infarcts. Report of four cases, two in caisson workers. J Bone Joint Surg Am 56:932–940, 1974.
142. Torres FX, Kyriakos M: Bone infarct-associated osteosarcoma. Cancer 70:2418–2430, 1992.
143. Strecker W, Gilula LA, Kyriakos M: Case report 479. Idiopathic healing infarct of bone simulating osteosarcoma. Skeletal Radiol 17:220–225, 1988.
144. Mankin HJ: Nontraumatic necrosis of bone (osteonecrosis). N Engl J Med 326:1473–1479, 1992.
145. Bohr H, Larsen E: On necrosis of the femoral head after fracture of the neck of the femur. J Bone Joint Surg Br 47:330–338, 1965.
146. Golding JSR, Maciver JF, Went LN: The bone changes in sickle-cell anaemia and its genetic variants. J Bone Joint Surg Br 41:711–718, 1959.
147. Milgram JW: Radiological and pathological manifestations of osteochondritis of the distal femur. A study of 50 cases. Radiology 126:305–311, 1978.
148. Sengupta S, Prathap K: Radiation necrosis of the humerus. A report of three cases. Acta Radiol 12:313–320, 1973.
149. Schajowicz F, Ackernan LV, Sissons HA: Histologic Typing of Bone Tumours. International Histological Classification of Tumours, No. 6. Geneva, World Health Organization, 1972.
150. Schajowicz F, Sissons HA, Sobin LH: The World Health Organization's histologic classification of bone tumors. A commentary on the second edition. Cancer 75:1208–1214, 1995.
151. Dorfman HD: Malignant transformation of benign bone lesions. In Proceedings of the Seventh National Cancer Conference. Vol. 7. Philadelphia, JB Lippincott, 1973, pp 901–913.
152. Dorfman HD, Czemiak B: Bone cancers. Cancer 75:203–210, 1995.
153. Hudson TM: Radiologic-pathologic correlation of musculoskeletal lesions. Baltimore, Williams & Wilkins, 1987.
154. Hallberg OE, Begley Jr JW: Origin and treatment of osteomas of the paranasal sinuses. Arch Otolaryngol 51:750–760, 1950.
155. Chang CHJ, Piatt ED, Thomas KE, Watne AL: Bone abnormalities in Gardner's syndrome. Am J Roentgenol Radium Ther Nucl Med 103:645–652, 1968.
156. Bertoni F, Unni KK, Beabout JW, Sim FH: Parosteal osteoma of bones other than of the skull and face. Cancer 75:2466–2473, 1995.
157. Loizaga JM, Calvo M, Lopez Barea F, et al: Osteoblastoma and osteoid osteoma. Clinical and morphological features of 162 cases. Pathol Res Pract 189:33–41, 1993.
158. Bauer TW, Zehr RJ, Belhobek GH, Marks KE: Juxta-articular osteoid osteoma. Am J Surg Pathol 15:381–387, 1991.
159. Schajowicz F, Lemos C. Osteoid osteoma and osteoblastoma. Acta Orthop Scand 41:272–291, 1970.
160. MacLennan DI, Wilson FC Jr: Osteoid osteoma of the spine. A review of the literature and report of six new cases. J Bone Joint Surg Am 49:111–121, 1967.
161. Jaffe HL: Osteoid-osteoma of bone. Radiology 45:319–334, 1945.
162. Rigault P, Mouterde P, Padovani JP, et al: Osteomeosteoide chez l'enfant. A propos de 29 cas. Rev Chir Orthop 61:627–646, 1975.
163. McDermott MB, Kyriakos M, McEnery K: Painless osteoid osteoma of the rib in an adult. A case report and a review of the literature. Cancer 77:1442–1449, 1996.
164. Healey JH, Ghalman B: Osteoid osteoma and osteoblastoma. Current concepts and recent advances. Clin Orthop 204:76–85, 1986.
165. Wold LE, Pritchard DJ, Bergert J, Wilson DM: Prostaglandin synthesis by osteoid osteoma and osteoblastoma. Mod Pathol 1: 129–131, 1988.
166. Byers PD: Solitary benign osteoblastic lesions of bone: Osteoid osteoma and benign osteoblastoma. Cancer 22:43–57, 1968.
167. Sleiner GC: Ultrastructure of osteoid osteoma. Hum Pathol 7: 309–325, 1976.
168. Lucas DR, Unni KK, McLeod RA, et al: Osteoblastoma: Clinicopathologic study of 306 cases. Hum Pathol 25:117–134, 1994.
169. McLeod RA, Dahlin DC, Beabout JW: The spectrum of osteoblastoma. Am J Roentgenol AJR 126:321–335, 1976.
170. Bertoni F, Unni KK, Lucas DR, McLeod RA: Osteoblastoma with cartilaginous matrix. An unusual morphologic presentation in 18 cases. Am J Surg Pathol 17:69–74, 1993.
171. Bertoni F, Unni KK, McLeod RA, Dahlin DC: Osteosarcoma resembling osteoblastoma. Cancer 55:416–426, 1985.
172. Dorfman HD, Weiss SW: Borderline osteoblastic tumors. Problems in the differential diagnosis of aggressive osteoblastoma and low-grade osteosarcoma. Semin Diagn Pathol l: 215–234, 1984.
173. Bertoni F, Bacchini P, Donali D, et al: Osteoblastoma-like osteosarcoma. The Rizzoli Institute experience. Mod Pathol 6: 707–716, 1993.
174. Beyer WF, Kuhn H: Can an osteoblastoma become malignant? Virchows Arch [A] 408:297–305, 1985.
175. Schajowicz F, Lemos C: Malignant osteoblastoma. J Bone Joint Surg Br 58:202–211, 1976.
176. Atik OS, Caglar M, Bolukbasi S, et al: Osteogenic sarcoma of the distal femur in a young child. Hum Pathol 13:766, 1982.
177. Enneking WF (ed): Symposium Osteosarcoma. Clin Orthop 111:1–104, 1975.
178. Kozakewich H, Perez-Atayde AR, Goorin AM, et al: Osteosarcoma in young children. Cancer 67:638–642, 1991.
179. Manland HS, Humphries RE: Osteogenic sarcoma in dial painters using luminous paint. Arch Pathol 7:406–417, 1929.

180. Polednak AP: Bone cancer among female radium dial workers. Latency periods and incidence rates by time after exposure. Brief communication. J Natl Cancer Inst 60:77–82, 1978.
181. Sindelar WF, Costa J, Ketcham AS: Osteosarcoma associated with Thorotrast administration. Cancer 42:2604–2609, 1978.
182. Varela-Duran J, Dehner LP: Postirradiation osteosarcoma in childhood. A clinicopathologic study of three cases and review of the literature. Am J Pediatr Hematol Oncol 2:263–271, 1980.
183. Tucker MA, D'Angio GJ, Boice Jr JD, et al: Bone sarcomas linked to radiotherapy and chemotherapy in children. N Engl J Med 317:588–593, 1987.
184. Huvos AG, Woodard HQ, Cahan WG, et al: Postradiation osteosarcoma of bone and soft tissues. A clinicopathologic study of 66 patients. Cancer 55:1244–1255, 1985.
185. Weatherby RP, Dahlin DC, Ivins JC: Postradiation sarcoma of bone. Review of 78 Mayo Clinic cases. Mayo Clin Proc 56:294–306, 1981.
186. Smith GD, Chalmers J, McQueen MM: Osteosarcoma arising in relation to an enchondroma. A report of three cases. J Bone Joint Surg Br 68:315–319, 1986.
187. Penman HO, Ring PA: Osteosarcoma in association with total hip replacement J Bone Joint Surg Br 66:632–634, 1984.
188. Dahlin DC, Coventry MB: Osteogenic sarcoma. A study of 600 cases. J Bone Joint Surg Am 49:101–110, 1967.
189. Kellie SJ, Pratt CB, Parham DM, et al: Sarcomas (other than Ewing's) of flat bone in children and adolescents. A clinicopathologic study. Cancer 65:1011–1016, 1990.
190. Okada K, Wold LE, Beabout JW, Shives TC: Osteosarcoma of the hand. A clinicopathologic study of 12 cases. Cancer 72:719–725, 1993.
191. Kyriakos M: Intracortical osteosarcoma. Cancer 56:2525–2533, 1980.
192. Amstutz HC: Multiple osteogenic sarcomata-metastatic or multicentric? Report of two cases and review of literature. Cancer 24:923–931, 1969.
193. Parham DM, Prat CB, Parvey LS, et al: Childhood multifocal osteosarcoma. Clinicopathologic and radiologic correlates. Cancer 55:2653–2658, 1985.
194. Sundaram M, Totty WG, Kyriakos M, et al: Imaging findings in pseudocystic osteosarcoma. AJR Am J Roentgenol 176:783–788, 2001.
195. Uribe-Botero G, Russell WO, Sutow WW, Martin RG: Primary osteosarcoma of bone. A clinicopathologic investigation of 243 cases, with necropsy studies in 54. Am J Clin Pathol 67:427–435, 1977.
196. Wakasa K, Sakurai M, Uchida A, et al: Massive pulmonary tumor emboli in osteosarcoma. Occult and fatal complication. Cancer 66:583–586, 1990.
197. Dardick I, Schatz J, Colgan T: Osteogenic sarcoma with epithelial differentiation. Ultrastruct Pathol 16:463–474, 1992.
198. Hasegawa T, Shibata T, Hirose T, et al: Osteosarcoma with epithelioid features. An immunohistochemical study. Arch Pathol Lab Med 117:295–298, 1993.
199. Kramer K, Hicks DO, Palis J, et al: Epithelioid osteosarcoma of bone. Immunocytochemical evidence suggesting divergent epithelial and mesenchymal differentiation in a primary osseous neoplasm. Cancer 71:2977–2982, 1993.
200. Yoshida H, Yumoto T, Adachi H, et al: Osteosarcoma with prominent epithelioid features. Acta Pathol Jpn 39:439–445, 1989.
201. Dahlin DC, Unni KK: Osteosarcoma of bone and its important recognizable varieties. Am J Surg Pathol l:61–72, 1977.
202. Scranton PE, DeCicco FA, Totten RS, Yunis EJ: Prognostic factors in osteosarcoma. A review of 20 years' experience at the University of Pittsburgh Heath Center Hospitals. Cancer 36:2179–2191, 1975.
203. Yunis EL, Barnes L: The histologic diversity of osteosarcoma. Pathol Annu 21(pt 1):121–141, 1986.
204. Hasegawa T, Hirose T, Kudo E, et al: Immunophenotypic heterogeneity in osteosarcomas. Hum Pathol 22:583–590, 1991.
205. Jaffe N, Raymond AK, Ayala A, et al: Effect of cumulative courses of intraarterial cisdiamminedichloroplatin-11 on the primary tumor in osteosarcoma. Cancer 63:63–67, 1989.
206. Swanson PE, Dehner LP, Sirgi KE, Wick MR: Cytokeratin immunoreactivity in malignant tumors of bone and soft tissue. A reappraisal of cytokeratin as a reliable marker in diagnostic immunohistochemistry. Appl Immunohistochem 2:103–112, 1994.
207. Ozisik YY, Meloni AM, Peier A, et al: Cytogenetic findings in 19 malignant bone tumors. Cancer 74:2268–2275, 1994.
208. Millar B, Browne R, Flood T: Juxtacortical osteosarcoma of the jaws. Br J Oral Maxillofac Surg 28:73–79, 1990.
209. Scaglietti O, Calandriello B: Ossifying parosteal sarcoma. J Bone Joint Surg Am 44:635–647, 1962.
210. van der Wall JD, Ryan JF: Parosteal osteogenic sarcoma of the hand. Histopathology 16:75–78, 1990.
211. Unni KK, Dahlin DC, Beabout JW, Ivins JC: Perosteal osteogenic sarcoma. Cancer 37:2466–2475, 1976.
212. Campanacci M, Picci P, Gherlinzoni F, et al: Parosteal osteosarcoma. J Bone Joint Surg Br 66:313–321, 1984.
213. Ahuja SC, Yillacin AB, Smith J, et al: Juxtacortical (parosteal) osteogenic sarcoma. Histologic grading and prognosis. J Bone Joint Surg Am 59:632–647, 1977.
214. Wold LE, Unni KK, Beaboul JW, et al: Dedifferentiated parosteal osteosarcoma. J Bone Joint Surg Am 66:53–59, 1984.
215. Edeiken J, Farrell C, Ackerman LV, et al: Parosteal sarcoma. Am J Roentgenol Radium Ther Nucl Med 111:579–583, 1971.
216. Dwinnell LA, Dahlin DC, Ghormley RK: Parosteal (juxtacortical) osteogenic sarcoma. J Bone Joint Surg Am 36:732–744, 1954.
217. deSantos LA, Murray JA, Finklestein JB, et al: The radiographic spectrum of periosteal osteosarcoma. Radiology 127:123–129, 1978.
218. Hall RB, Robinson LH, Malawar MM, Dunham WK: Periosteal osteosarcoma. Cancer 55:165–171, 1985.
219. Farr GH, Huvos AG: Juxtacortical osteogenic sarcoma. J Bone Joint Surg Am 51:1205–1216, 1972.
220. Wold LE, Unni KK, Beabout JW, Pritchard DJ: High-grade surface osteosarcomas. Am J Surg Pathol 8:181–186, 1984.
221. Bertoni F, Pignatti G, Bachini P, et al: Telangiectatic or hemorrhagic osteosarcoma of bone. A clinicopathologic study of 41 patients at the Rizzoli Institute. Prog Surg Pathol 10:63–82, 1989.
222. Huvos AG, Rosen G, Bretsky SS, Butler A: Telangiectatic osteosarcoma. A clinicopathologic study of 124 patients. Cancer 49:1679–1689, 1982.
223. Matsuno T, Unni KK, McLeod RA, Dahlin DC: Telangiectatic osteogenic sarcoma. Cancer 38:2538–2547, 1976.
224. Bertoni F, Present D, Bacchini P, et al: The Istituto Rizzoli experience with small cell osteosarcoma. Cancer 64:2591–2599, 1989.
225. Ayala AG, Ro JY, Raymond AK, et al: Small cell osteosarcoma. A clinicopathologic study of 27 cases. Cancer 64:2162–2173, 1989.
226. Manin SE, Dwyer A, Kissane JM, Costa J: Small-cell osteosarcoma. Cancer 50:990–996, 1982.
227. Sim FH, Unni KK, Beabout JW, Dahlin DC: Osteosarcoma with small cells simulating Ewing's tumor. J Bone Joint Surg Am 61:207–215, 1979.
228. Unni KK, Dahlin DC, McLeod RA, Prtichard DJ: Intraosseous well-differentiated osteosarcoma. Cancer 40:1337–1347, 1977.
229. Bertoni F, Bacchii P, Fabbri N, et al: Osteosarcoma. Low-grade intraosseous-type osteosarcoma, histologically resembling parosteal osteosarcoma, fibrous dysplasia, and desmoplastic fibroma. Cancer 71:338–345, 1993.
230. Kun AM, Unni KK, McLeod RA, Pritchard DJ: Low-grade intraosseous osteosarcoma. Cancer 65:1418–1428, 1990.
231. Bertoni F, Dallera P, Bacchini P, et al: The Istituto Rizzoli-Beretta experience with osteosarcoma of the jaws. Cancer 68:1555–1563, 1991.
232. Tanzawa H, Uchiyama S, Sato K: Statistical observation of osteosarcoma of the maxillofacial region in Japan. Oral Surg Oral Med Oral Pathol 72:444–448, 1991.
233. Clark JL, Unni KK, Dahlin DC, Devine KD: Osteosarcoma of the jaw. Cancer 51:2311–2316, 1983.
234. Glasser DB, Lane JM, Huvos AG, et al: Survival, prognosis, and therapeutic response in osteogenic sarcoma. The Memorial Hospital experience. Cancer 69:698–708, 1992.

235. Harvei S, Solheim O: The prognosis in osteosarcoma. Norwegian national data. Cancer 48:1719–1723, 1981.
236. Lane JM, Hurson B, Boland PJ, et al: Osteogenic sarcoma. Clin Orthop Mar(204):93–110, 1986.
237. Rosen G, Marcove RC, Caparros B, et al: Primary osteogenic sarcoma. The rationale for preoperative chemotherapy and delayed surgery. Cancer 43:2163–2177, 1979.
238. Bjornsson J, Inwards CY, Wold LE, et al: Prognostic significance of spontaneous tumour necrosis in osteosarcoma. Virchows Arch [A] 423:195–199, 1993.
239. Raymond AK, Chawla SP, Carrasco CH, et al: Osteosarcoma chemotherapy effect. A prognostic factor. Semin Diagn Pathol 4:212–236, 1987.
240. Davis AM, Bell RS, Goodwin PJ: Prognostic factors in osteosarcoma. A critical review. J Clin Oncol 12:423–431, 1994.
241. Bacci G, Picci P, Ruggieri P, et al: Primary chemotherapy and delayed surgery (neoadjuvant chemotherapy) for osteosarcoma of the extremities. The Istituto Rizzoli experience in 127 patients treated preoperatively with intravenous methotrexate (high versus moderate doses) and intraarterial cisplatin. Cancer 65:2539–2553, 1990.
242. Burgers JM, van Glabbeke M, Busson A, et al: Osteosarcoma of the limbs. Report of the EORTC-SIOP 03 trial 20781 investigating the value of adjuvant treatment with chemotherapy and/or prophylactic lung irradiation. Cancer 61:1024–1031, 1988.
243. Campanacci M, Bacci G, Genoni F, et al: The treatment of osteosarcoma of the extremities. Twenty years' experience at the Istituto Ortopedico Rizzoli. Cancer 48:1569–1581, 1981.
244. Rao BN, Champion JE, Pratt CB, et al: Limb salvage procedures for children with osteosarcoma: An alternative to amputation. J Pediatr Surg 18:901–908, 1983.
245. Winkler K, Bielack S, Delling G, et al: Effect of intraarterial versus intravenous cisplatin in addition to systemic doxorubicin, high-dose methotrexate, and ifosfamide on histologic tumor response in osteosarcoma (study COSS-86). Cancer 66:1703–1710, 1990.
246. Belli L, Scholl S, Livartowski A, et al: Resection of pulmonary metastases in osteosarcoma. A retrospective analysis of 44 patients. Cancer 63:2546–2550, 1989.
247. Schaller Jr RT, Haas J, Schaller J, et al: Improved survival in children with osteosarcoma following resection of pulmonary metastases. J Pediatr Surg 17:546–550, 1982.
248. Laurence W, Franklin EL: Calcifying enchondroma of long bones. J Bone Joint Surg Br 35:224–228, 1953.
249. Boriani S, Bacchini P, Bertoni F, Campanacci M: Periosteal chondroma. A review of twenty cases. J Bone Joint Surg Am 65:205–212, 1983.
250. Nosanchuk JS, Kaufer H: Recurrent periosteal chondroma. Report of two cases and a review of the literature. J Bone Joint Surg Am 51:375–380, 1969.
251. Takigawa K: Chondroma of the bones of the hand. J Bone Joint Surg Am 53:1591–1600, 1971.
252. Lewis RJ, Kelcham AS: Maffucci's syndrome. Functional and neoplastic significance. Case report and review of the literature. J Bone Joint Surg Am 55:1465–1479, 1973.
253. Cannon SR, Sweelnam DR: Multiple chondrosarcomas in dyschondroplasia (Ollier's disease). Cancer 55:836–840, 1985.
254. Cowan WK: Malignant change and multiple metastases in Ollier's disease. J Clin Pathol 18:650–653, 1965.
255. Liu J, Hudkins PG, Swee RG, Unni KK: Bone sarcomas associated with Ollier's disease. Cancer 59:1376–1385, 1987.
256. Sun T-C, Swee RG, Shives TC, Unni KK: Chondrosarcoma in Maffucci's syndrome. J Bone Joint Surg Am 67:1214–1215, 1985.
257. Tamimi HK, Bolen JW: Enchondromatosis (Ollier's disease) and ovarian juvenile granulosa cell tumor. A case report and review of the literature. Cancer 53:1605–1608, 1984.
258. Mirra JM, Gold R, Downs J, Eckardt JJ: A new histologic approach to the differentiation of enchondroma and chondrosarcoma of the bones. A clinicopathologic analysis of 51 cases. Clin Orthop 201:214–237, 1985.
259. Brand T, Halch EI, Schaller RT, et al: Surgical management of the infant with mesenchymal hamartoma of the chest wall. J Pediatr Surg 21:556–558, 1986.
260. Campbell AN, Waggel J, Moll MG: Benign mesenchymoma of the chest wall in infancy. J Surg Oncol 21:267–270, 1982.
261. McCarthy EF, Dorfman HD: Vascular and cartilaginous hamartoma of the ribs in infancy with secondary aneurysmal bone cyst formation. Am J Surg Pathol 4:247–253, 1980.
262. del Rosario AD, Bui HX, Singh J, et al: Intracytoplasmic eosinophilic hyaline globules in cartilaginous neoplasms. A surgical, pathological, ultrastructural, and electron probe x-ray microanalytic study. Hum Pathol 25:1283–1289, 1994.
263. Hwang W-S, McQueen D, Monson RC, Reed MH: The significance of cytoplasmic chondrocyte inclusions in multiple osteochondromatosis, solitary osteochondromas, and chondrodysplasias. Am J Clin Pathol 78:89–91, 1982.
264. Josefczyk MA, Huvos AG, Smith J, Unnacher C: Bursa formation in secondary chondrosarcoma with intrabursal chondrosarcomatosis. Am J Surg Pathol 9:309–314, 1985.
265. Fairbank HAT: An Atlas of General Affictions of the Skeleton. Edinburgh, E & S Livingstone, 1951.
266. Unni KK, Dahlin DC: Premalignant tumors and conditions of bone. Am J Surg Pathol 3:47–60, 1979.
267. Ochsner PE: Zum problem der neoplastischen Entartung bei mulliplcn kartilaginaren Exostosen. Z Orthop 116:369–378, 1978.
268. Nora FE, Dahlin DC, Beabout JW: Bizarre parosteal osteochondromatous proliferations of the hands and feet. Am J Surg Pathol 7:245–250, 1983.
269. Meneses MF, Unni KK, Swee RG: Bizarre parosteal osteochondromatous proliferation of bone (Nora's lesion). Am J Surg Pathol 17:691–697, 1993.
270. Landon GC, Johnson KA, Dahlin DC: Subungual exostoses. J Bone Joint Surg Am 61:256–259, 1979.
271. Miller-Breslow A, Dorfman HD: Dupuytren's (subungual) exostosis. Am J Surg Pathol 12:368–378, 1988.
272. Springfield DS, Capanna R, Gherlinzoni F, et al: Chondroblastoma. A review of seventy cases. J Bone Joint Surg Am 67:748–754, 1985.
273. Semmclink HJ, Prusczynski M, Wiersma-van Tilburg A, et al: Cytokeratin expression in chondroblastomas. Histopathology 16:257–263, 1990.
274. Birch PJ, Buchanan R, Golding P, Pringle JAS: Chondroblastoma of the rib with widespread bone metastases. Histopathology 25:583–585, 1994.
275. Kahn LB, Wood FM, Ackerman LV: Malignant chondroblastoma. Report of two cases and review of the literature. Arch Pathol 88:371–376, 1969.
276. Kyriakos M, Land VJ, Penning HL, Parker SG: Metastatic chondroblastoma. Report of a fatal case with a review of the literature on atypical, aggressive, and malignant chondroblastoma. Cancer 55:1770–1789, 1985.
277. Jaffe HL, Lichtenstein L: Chondromyxoid fibroma of bone. A distinctive benign tumor likely to be mistaken especially for chondrosarcoma. Arch Pathol 45:541–551, 1948.
278. Kreicbergs A, Lonnquist PA, Willems J: Chondromyxoid fibroma. A review of the literature and a report on our own experience. Acta Pathol Microbiol Immunol Scand (A) 93:189–197, 1985.
279. Wilson AJ, Kyriakos M, Ackerman LV: Chondromyxoid fibroma. Radiologic appearance in 38 cases and in a review of the literature. Radiology 179:513–518, 1991.
280. Gherlinzoni F, Rock M, Picci P: Chondromyxoid fibroma. The experience at the Istituto Ortopedico Rizzoli. J Bone Joint Surg Am 65:198–204, 1983.
281. Dahlin DC: Chondromyxoid fibroma of bone, with emphasis on its morphological relationship to benign chondroblastoma. Cancer 9:195–203, 1956.
282. Young CL, Sim FH, Unni KK, McLeod RA: Chondrosarcoma of bone in children. Cancer 66:1641–1648, 1990.
283. Bertoni F, Boriani S, Laus M, Campanacci M: Periosteal chondrosarcoma and periosteal osteosarcoma. Two distinct entities. J Bone Joint Surg Br 64:370–376, 1982.
284. Campanacci M, Guemelli N, Leonessa C, Boni A: Chondrosarcoma. A study of 133 cases, 80 with long term follow up. Ital J Orthop Traumatol l:387–414, 1975.
285. Coltrerd MD, Googe PB, Harrist TJ, et al: Chondrosarcoma of the temporal bone. Diagnosis and treatment of 13 cases and review of the literature. Cancer 58:2689–2696, 1986.

286. Dahlin DC, Salvador AH: Chondrosarcomas of bones of the hands and feet. A study of 30 cases. Cancer 34:755–760, 1974.

287. Lansche WE, Spjut HL: Chondrosarcoma of the small bones of the hand. J Bone Joint Surg Am 40:1139–1145, 1958.

288. Schajowicz F: Juxtacortical chondrosarcoma. J Bone Joint Surg Br 59:473–480, 1977.

289. Sanerkin NG, Gallagher P: A review of the behaviour of chondrosarcoma of bone. J Bone Joint Surg Br 61:395–400, 1979.

290. Lichtenstein L, Jaffe HL: Chondrosarcoma of bone. Am J Pathol 19:553–589, 1943.

291. Schiller AL: Diagnosis of borderline cartilage lesions of bone. Semin Diagn Pathol 2:42–62, 1985.

292. Marcove RC, Huvos AG: Cartilaginous tumors of the ribs. Cancer 27:794–801, 1971.

293. Mirra JM, Gold R, Downs J, Eckardt JJ: A new histologic approach to the differentiation of enchondroma and chondrosarcoma of the bones. A clinicopathologic analysis of 51 cases. Clin Orthop 201:214–237, 1985.

294. Erlandson RA, Huvos AG: Chondrosarcoma: A light and electron microscopic study. Cancer 34:1642–1652, 1974.

295. Nakamura Y, Becker LE, Marks A: S-100 protein in tumors of cartilage and bone. An immunohistochemical study. Cancer 58:1820–1824, 1983.

296. Okajima K, Honda I, Kitagawa T: Immunohistochemical distribution of S-100 protein in tumors and tumorlike lesions of bone and cartilage. Cancer 61:792–799, 1988.

297. Castresana J, Barrios C, Gomez L, Kreicbergs A: Amplification of the c-myc proto-oncogene in human chondrosarcoma. Diagn Mol Pathol l:235–238, 1992.

298. Wrba F, Gullick WJ, Fertl H, et al: Immunohistochemical detection of the c-erbB-2 proto-oncogene product in normal, benign and malignant cartilage tissues. Histopathology 15:71–76, 1989.

299. Dobashi Y, Sugimura H, Sato A, et al: Possible association of p53 overexpression and mutation with high-grade chondrosarcoma. Diagn Mol Pathol 2:257–263, 1993.

300. McAfee MK, Pairolero PC, Bergstralh EJ, et al: Chondrosarcoma of the chest wall. Factors affecting survival. Ann Thorac Surg 40:535–541, 1985.

301. McKenna RJ, Schwinn CP, Soong KY, Higinbotham NL: Sarcomata of the osteogenic series (osteosarcoma, fibrosarcoma, chondrosarcoma, parosteal osteogenic sarcoma, and sarcomata arising in abnormal bone). J Bone Joint Surg Am 48:1–26, 1966.

302. O'Neal LW, Ackerman LV: Cartilaginous tumors of ribs and sternum. J Thorac Surg 21:71–108, 1951.

303. Smith WS, Simon MA: Segmental resection for chondrosarcoma. J Bone Joint Surg Am 57:1097–1103, 1975.

304. Faraggiana T, Sender B, Glicksman P: Light- and electron-microscopic study of clear cell chondrosarcoma. Am J Clin Pathol 75:117–121, 1981.

305. Wang LT, Liu TC: Clear cell chondrosarcoma of bone. A report of three cases with immunohistochemical and affinity histochemical observations. Pathol Res Pract 189:411–415, 1993.

306. Weiss AP, Dorfman HD: 5-100 protein in human cartilage lesions. J Bone Joint Surg Am 68:521–526, 1986.

307. Bjornsson J, Unni KK, Dahlin DC, et al: Clear cell chondrosarcoma of bone. Observations in 47 cases. Am J Surg Pathol 8:223–230, 1984.

308. Unni KK, Dahlin DC, Beabout JW, Sim FH: Chondrosarcoma. Clear-cell variant. A report of sixteen cases. J Bone Joint Surg Am 58:676–683, 1976.

309. Manin RF, Melnick PJ, Warner NE, et al: Chordoid sarcoma. Am J Clin Pathol 59:623–635, 1972.

310. Miettinen M, Lehto V-P, Dahl D, Virtanen I: Differential diagnosis of chordoma, chondroid, and ependymal tumors as aided by anti-intermediate filament antibodies. Am J Pathol 112:160–169, 1983.

311. Bertoni F, Present D, Bacchini P, et al: Dedifferentiated peripheral chondrosarcomas. A report of seven cases. Cancer 63:2054–2059, 1989.

312. Dahlin DC, Beabout JW: Dedifferentiation of low-grade chondrosarcomas. Cancer 28:461–466, 1971.

313. McFarland GB, McKinley LM, Reed RJ: Dedifferentiation of low-grade chondrosarcomas. Clin Orthop 122:157–164, 1977.

314. Dervan PA, O'Loughlin J, Hurson BJ: Dedifferentiated chondrosarcoma with muscle and cytokeratin differentiation in the anaplastic component. Histopathology 12:517–526, 1988.

315. Tetu B, Ordonez NG, Ayala AG, Mackay B: Chondrosarcoma with additional mesenchymal component (dedifferentiated chondrosarcoma). II. An immunohistochemical and electron microscopic study. Cancer 58:287–298, 1986.

316. Johnson S, Tetu B, Ayala AG, Chawla SP: Chondrosarcoma with additional mesenchymal component (dedifferentiated chondrosarcoma). I. A clinicopathologic study of 26 cases. Cancer 58:278–286, 1986.

317. Abernoza P, Neumann MP, Manivel JC, Wick MR: Dedifferentiated chondrosarcoma. An ultrastructural study of two cases, with immunocytochemical correlations. Ultrastruct Pathol 10:529–538, 1986.

318. Jaworski RC: Dedifferentiated chondrosarcoma. An ultrastructural study. Cancer 53:2674–2678, 1984.

319. Bridge JA, De Boer J, Travis J, et al: Simultaneous interphase cytogenetic analysis and fluorescence immunophenotyping of dedifferentiated chondrosarcoma. Implications for histopathogenesis. Am J Pathol 144:215–220, 1994.

320. Meis JM: "Dedifferentiation" in bone and soft-tissue tumors. A histological indicator of tumor progression. Pathol Annu 26(pt 1):37–62, 1991.

321. Mirra JM, Marcove RC: Fibrosarcomatous dedifferentiation of primary and secondary chondrosarcoma. Review of five cases. J Bone Joint Surg Am 56:285–296, 1974.

322. Devoe K, Weidner N: Immunohistochemistry of small round cell tumors. Semin Diagn Pathol 17:216–224, 2000.

323. Bertoni F, Picci P, Bacchini P, et al: Mesenchymal chondrosarcoma of bone and soft tissues. Cancer 52:533–541, 1983.

324. Dabska M, Huvos AG: Mesenchymal chondrosarcoma in the young. A clinicopathologic study of 19 patients with explanation of histogenesis. Virchows Arch (A) 399:89–104, 1983.

325. Dowling EA: Mesenchymal chondrosarcoma. J Bone Joint Surg Am 46:747–754, 1964.

326. Frydman CP, Klein MJ, Abdelwahab IF, Zwass A: Primitive multipotential primary sarcoma of bone. A case report and immunohistochemical study. Mod Pathol 4:768–772, 1991.

327. Goldman RL: "Mesenchymal" chondrosarcoma, a rare malignant chondroid tumor usually primary in bone. Report of a case arising in extraskeletal soft tissue. Cancer 20:1494–1498, 1967.

328. Guccion JG, Font RL, Enzinger PM, Zimmerman LE: Extraskeletal mesenchymal chondrosarcoma. Arch Pathol 95:336–340, 1973.

329. Huvos AG, Rosen G, Dabska M, Marcove RC: Mesenchymal chondrosarcoma. A clinicopathologic analysis of 35 patients with emphasis on treatment. Cancer 51:1230–1237, 1983.

330. Jacobson SA: Polyhistioma. A malignant tumor of bone and extraskeletal tissues. Cancer 40:2116–2130, 1977.

331. Ling LL, Steiner GC: Primary multipotential malignant neoplasm of bone. Chondrosarcoma associated with squamous cell carcinoma. Hum Pathol 17:317–320, 1986.

332. Nakashima Y, Unni KK, Shives TC, et al: Mesenchymal chondrosarcoma of bone and soft tissue. A review of 111 cases. Cancer 57:2444–2453, 1986.

333. Salvador AH, Beabout JW, Dahlin DC: Mesenchymal chondrosarcoma. Observations on 30 new cases. Cancer 28:605–615, 1971.

334. Steiner GC, Mirra JM, Bullough PG: Mesenchymal chondrosarcoma. A study of the ultrastructure. Cancer 32:926–939, 1973.

335. Swanson PE, Lillemoe TJ, Manivel JC, Wick MR: Mesenchymal chondrosarcoma. An immunohistochemical study. Arch Pathol Lab Med 114:943–948, 1990.

336. Sainati L, Scapinello A, Nontaldi A, et al: A mesenchymal chondrosarcoma of a child with the reciprocal translocation (11;22) (q24;q12). Cancer Genet Cytogenet 71:144–147, 1993.

337. Campanacci M, Giunti A, Olmi R: Giant-cell tumours of bone. A study of 209 cases with long-term follow-up in 130. Ital J Orthop Traumatol l:249–277, 1975.

338. Sung HW, Kuo DP, Shu WP, et al: Giant-cell tumor of bone.

Analysis of two hundred and eight cases in Chinese patients. J Bone Joint Surg Am 64:755–761, 1982.

339. Bertoni F, Unni KK, Beabout JW, Ebersold MJ: Giant cell tumor of the skull. Cancer 70:1124–1132, 1992.

340. Emley WE: Giant cell tumor of the sphenoid bone. A case report and review of literature. Arch Otolaryngol 94:369–374, 1971.

341. Wolfe JT III, Scheithauer BW, Dahlin OC: Giant-cell tumor of the sphenoid bone. Review of 10 cases. J Neurosurg 59:322–327, 1983.

342. Leonard J, Gökden M, Kyriakos M, et al: Malignant giant-cell tumor of the parietal bone. Case report and review of the literature. Neurosurgery 48:424–429, 2001.

343. Savini R, Gherlinzoni F, Morandi M, et al: Surgical treatment of giant-cell tumor of the spine. Istituto Ortopedico Rizzoli. J Bone Joint Surg Am 65:1283–1290, 1983.

344. Wold LE, Swee RG: Giant cell tumor of the small bones of the hands and feet. Semin Diagn Pathol l:173–184, 1984.

345. Zheng MH, Fan Y, Wysocki SJ, et al: Gene expression of transforming growth factor-beta 1 and its type II receptor in giant cell tumors of bone. Possible involvement in osteoclast-like cell migration. Am J Pathol 145:1095–1104, 1994.

346. Roessner A, Bassewitz DBV, Schlake W, et al: Biologic characterization of human bone tumors. III. Giant cell tumor of bone. A combined electron microscopical, histochemical, and autoradiographical study. Pathol Res Pract 178:431–440, 1984.

347. Kasahara K, Yamamuro T, Kasahara A: Giant-cell tumour of bone. Cytological studies. Br J Cancer 40:201–209, 1979.

348. Nascimento AG, Huvos AG, Marcove RC: Primary malignant giant cell tumor of bone. A study of eight cases and review of the literature. Cancer 44:1393–1402, 1979.

349. Aparisi T: Giant cell tumor of bone. Acta Orthop Scand 173(suppl):1–38, 1978.

350. Aparisi T, Arborgh B, Ericsson JLE: Giant cell tumor of bone. Virchows Arch [A] 381:159–178, 1979.

351. Aqel NM, Pringle JA, Honon MA: Cellular heterogeneity in giant cell tumour of bone (osteoclastoma). An immunohistological study of 16 cases. Histopathology 13:675–685, 1988.

352. Goldring SR, Schiller AL, Mankin HJ, et al: Characterization of cells from human giant cell tumors of bone. Clin Orthop 204:59–75, 1986.

353. Bouropoulou V, Kontogeorgos G, Manika Z: A histological and immunoenzymatic study on the histogenesis of "giant cell tumor of bones." Pathol Res Pract 180:61–67, 1985.

354. Emura I, Inoue Y, Ohnishi Y, et al: Histochemical, immunohistochemical and ultrastructural investigations of giant cell tumors of bone. Acta Pathol Jpn 36:691–702, 1986.

355. Fornasier VL, Flores L, Hastings D, Sharp T: Virus-like filamentous intranuclear inclusions in a giant-cell tumor, not associated with Paget's disease of bone. A case report. J Bone Joint Surg Am 67:333–336, 1985.

356. Negoescu A, Mandache E: The ultrastructure of nuclear inclusions in the giant-cell tumor of bone. Pathol Res Pract 184:410–417, 1989.

357. Schajowicz F, Ubios AM, Santini Araujo E, Cabrini RL: Virus-like intranuclear inclusions in giant cell tumor of bone. Clin Orthop 201:247–250, 1985.

358. Sanerkin NG: Malignancy, aggressiveness, and recurrence in giant cell tumor of bone. Cancer 46:1641–1649, 1980.

359. Dahlin DC, Cupps RE, Johnson EW Jr: Giant-cell tumor. A study of 195 cases. Cancer 25:1061–1070, 1970.

360. Murphy WR, Ackerman LV: Benign and malignant giant-cell tumors of bone. Cancer 9:317–339, 1956.

361. McDonald DJ, Sim FH, McLcod RA, Dahlin OC: Giant-cell tumor of bone. J Bone Joint Surg Am 68:235–242, 1986.

362. Eckardt JJ, Grogan TJ: Giant cell tumor of bone. Clin Orthop 204:45–58, 1986.

363. Mankin HJ, Fogelson FS, Thrashcr AZ, Jaffer F: Massive resection and allograft transplantation in the treatment of malignant bone tumors. N Engl J Med 294:1247–1255, 1976.

364. Parrish FF: Allograft replacement of all or part of the end of a long bone following excision of a tumor. Report of twenty-one cases. J Bone Joint Surg Am 55:1–22, 1973.

365. Rock MG, Pritchard DJ, Unni KK: Metastases from histologically benign giant-cell tumor of bone. J Bone Joint Surg Am 66:269–274, 1984.

366. Bridge JA, Neff JR, Bhatia PS, et al: Cytogenetic findings and biologic behavior of giant cell tumors of bone. Cancer 65:2697–2703, 1990.

367. Fukunaga M, Nikaido T, Shimoda T, et al: A new cytometric DNA analysis of giant cell tumors of bone including two cases with malignant transformation. Cancer 70:1886–1894, 1992.

368. Ladanyi M, Traganos F, Huvos AG: Benign metastasizing giant-cell tumors of bone. A DNA flow cytometric study. Cancer 64:1521–1526, 1989.

369. Sara AS, Ayala AG, El-Naggar A, et al: Giant cell tumor of bone. A clinicopathologic and DNA flow cytometric analysis. Cancer 66:2186–2190, 1990.

370. Meis JM, Dorfman HD, Nathanson SD, et al: Primary malignant giant cell tumor of bone. "Dedifferentiated" giant cell tumor. Mod Pathol 2:541–546, 1989.

371. Dehner LP: Primitive neuroectodermal tumor and Ewing's sarcoma. Am J Surg Pathol 17:1–13, 1993.

372. Ewing's sarcoma and its congeners. An interim appraisal (editorial). Lancet 339:99–100, 1992.

373. Ladanyi M, Heinemann FS, Huvos AG, et al: Neural differentiation in small round cell tumors of bone and soft tissue with the translocation t(11;22)(q24;q12). An immunohistochemical study of 11 cases. Hum Pathol 21:1245–1251, 1990.

374. Navarro S, Cavazzana AO, Llombart-Bosch A, Triche TL: Comparison of Ewing's sarcoma of bone and peripheral neuroepithelioma. An immunocytochemical and ultrastructural analysis of two primitive neuroectodermal neoplasms. Arch Pathol Lab Med 118:608–615, 1994.

375. Rellig WJ, Garin-Chesa P, Huvos AG: Ewing's sarcoma. New approaches to histogenesis and molecular plasticity. Lab Invest 66:133–137, 1992.

376. Roessner A, Jurgens H: Round cell tumours of bone. Pathol Res Pract 189:111–136, 1993.

377. Shishikura A, Ushigome S, Shimoda T: Primitive neuroectodermal tumors of bone and soft tissue. Histological subclassification and clinicopathologic correlations. Acta Pathol Jpn 43:176–186, 1993.

378. Cavazzana AO, Miser JS, Jefferson J, Triche TJ: Experimental evidence for a neural origin of Ewing's sarcoma of bone. Am J Pathol 127:507–518, 1987.

379. Hasegawa T, Hirose T, Kudo E, et al: Atypical primitive neuroectodermal tumors. Comparative light and electron microscopic and immunohistochemical studies on peripheral neuroepitheliomas and Ewing's sarcomas. Acta Pathol Jpn 41:444–454, 1991.

380. Schmidt D, Mackay B, Ayala AG: Ewing's sarcoma with neuroblastoma-like features. Ultrastruct Pathol 3:143–151, 1982.

381. Tsuneyoshi M, Yokoyama R, Hashimoto H, Enjoji M: Comparative study of neuroectodermal tumor and Ewing's sarcoma of the bone. Histopathologic, immunohistochemical and ultrastructural features. Acta Pathol Jpn 39:573–581, 1989.

382. Ushigome S, Shimoda T, Takaki K, et al: Immunocytochemical and ultrastructural studies of the histogenesis of Ewing's sarcoma and putatively related tumors. Cancer 64:52–62, 1989.

383. Ambros IM, Ambros PF, Strehl S, et al: MIC2 is a specific marker for Ewing's sarcoma and peripheral primitive neuroectodermal tumors. Evidence for a common histogenesis of Ewing's sarcoma and peripheral primitive neuroectodermal tumors from MIC2 expression and specific chromosome aberration. Cancer 67:1886–1893, 1991.

384. Ramani P, Rampling D, Link M: Immunocytochemical study of 12E7 in small round-cell tumours of childhood. An assessment of its sensitively and specificity. Histopathology 23:557–561, 1993.

385. Fellinger EJ, Garin-Chesa P, Glasser DB, et al: Comparison of cell surface antigen HBA71 (p30/32MIC2), neuron-specific enolase, and vimentin in the immunohistochemical analysis of Ewing's sarcoma of bone. Am J Surg Pathol 16:746–755, 1992.

386. Fellinger EJ, Garin-Chesa P, Su SL, et al: Biochemical and genetic characterization of the HBA 71 Ewing's sarcoma cell surface antigen. Cancer Res 51:336–340, 1991.

387. Fellinger EJ, Garin-Chesa P, Triche TJ, et al: Immunohistochemical analysis of Ewing's sarcoma cell surface antigen p30/32MIC2. Am J Pathol 139:317–325, 1991.

388. Perlman EJ, Dickman PS, Askin FB, et al: Ewing's sarcoma: Routine diagnostic utilization of MIC2 analysis. A Pediatric Oncology Group/Children's Cancer Group Intergroup Study. Hum Pathol 25:304–307, 1994.

389. Stevenson AJ, Chatteu J, Bertoni F, Miettinenm: CD99 (p30/32MIC2) neuroectodermal/Ewing's sarcoma antigen as an immunohistochemical marker. Review of more than 600 tumors and the literature experience. Appl Immunohistochem 2:231–240, 1994.

390. Weidner N, Tjoe J: Immunohistochemical profile of monoclonal antibody O13: An antibody that recognizes glycoprotein p30/32MIC2 and is useful in diagnosing Ewing's sarcoma and peripheral neuroepithelioma. Am J Surg Pathol 18:486–494, 1994.

391. Vartanian RK, Weidner N: MIC2 gene product (CD99) expression in lymphomas. Including lymphoblastic and non-lymphoblastic non-Hodgkin's lymphomas and Hodgkin's disease. Appl Immunohistochem 4:43–55, 1996.

392. Devoe K, Weidner N: Immunohistochemistry of small round-cell tumors. Semin Diagn Pathol 17:216–224, 2000.

393. Garin-Chesa P, Fellinger EJ, Huvos AG, et al: Immunohistochemical analysis of neural cell adhesion molecules. Differential expression in small round cell tumors of childhood and adolescence. Am J Pathol 139:275–286, 1991.

394. Delallre O, Zucman J, Melot T, et al: The Ewing family of tumors. A subgroup of small-round-cell tumors defined by specific chimeric transcripts. N Engl J Med 331:294–299, 1994.

395. Dockhom-Dwomiczak B, Schafer KL, Dantcheva R, et al: Diagnostic value of the molecular genetic detection of the t(11;22) translocation in Ewing's tumours. Virchows Arch 425:107–112, 1994.

396. Ladanyi M, Lewis R, Garin-Chesa P, et al: EWS rearrangement in Ewing's sarcoma and peripheral neuroectodermal tumor. Molecular detection and correlation with cytogenetic analysis and MIC2 expression. Diagn Mol Pathol 2:141–146, 1993.

397. Pfeifer JD, Hill DA, O'Sullivan MJ, Dehner LP: Diagnostic gold standard for soft tissue tumours. Morphology or molecular genetics. Histopathology 37:485–500, 2000.

398. Downing JR, Head DR, Parham DM, et al: Detection of the (11;22) (q24;qI2) translocation of Ewing's sarcoma and peripheral neuroectodermal tumor by reverse transcription polymerase chain reaction. Am J Pathol 143:1294–1300, 1993.

399. Selleri L, Hermanson GG, Eubanks JH, et al: Molecular localization of the t(11,22)(q24;q12) translocation of Ewing sarcoma by chromosomal in situ suppression hybridization. Proc Natl Acad Sci U S A 88:887–891, 1991.

400. Sorensen P, Liu X, Delattre O, et al: Reverse transcriptase PCR amplification of EWS/FL-I fusion transcripts as a diagnostic test for peripheral primitive neuroectodermal tumors of childhood. Diagn Mol Pathol 2:147–157, 1993.

401. Stephenson CF, Bridge JA, Sandberg AA: Cytogenetic and pathologic aspects of Ewing's sarcoma and neuroectodermal tumors. Hum Pathol 23:1270–1277, 1992.

402. Kissane JM, Askin FB, Nesbit M, et al: Sarcomas of bone in childhood. Pathologic aspects. J Natl Cancer Inst 56:29–41, 1981.

403. Spjut HJ, Ayala AG: Skeletal tumors in childhood and adolescence. In Finegold M (ed): Pathology of Neoplasia in Children and Adolescents. Vol 18. Major Series in Pathology. Philadelphia, WB Saunders, 1986.

404. Maygarden SL, Askin FB, Siegal GP, et al: Ewing sarcoma of bone in infants and toddlers. A clinicopathologic report from the Intergroup Ewing's Study. Cancer 71:2109–2118, 1993.

405. Cangir A, Vietti TJ, Gehan EA, et al: Ewing's sarcoma metastatic at diagnosis. Results and comparisons of two intergroup Ewing's sarcoma studies. Cancer 66:887–893, 1990.

406. Gasparini M, Bami S, Lalluada A, et al: Ten years experience with Ewing's sarcoma. Tumori 63:77–90, 1977.

407. Bacci G, Toni A, Avella M, et al: Long-term results in 144 localized Ewing's sarcoma patients treated with combined therapy. Cancer 63:1477–1486, 1989.

408. Neff JR: Nonmetastatic Ewing's sarcoma of bone. The role of surgical therapy. Clin Orthop 204:111–118, 1980.

409. Razek A, Perez CA, Tefft M, et al: Intergroup Ewing's sarcoma study. Local control related to radiation dose, volume, and site of primary lesion in Ewing's sarcoma. Cancer 46:516–521, 1980.

410. Rosen G, Caparros B, Nirenberg A, et al: Ewing's sarcoma. Ten-year experience with adjuvant chemotherapy. Cancer 47:2204–2213, 1981.

411. Dierick AM, Langlois M, Van Oostveldt P, Roels H: The prognostic significance of the DNA content in Ewing's sarcoma. A retrospective cytophotometric and flow cytometric study. Histopathology 23:333–339, 1993.

412. Boston HC, Dahlin DC, Ivins LC, Cupps RE: Malignant lymphoma (so-called reticulum cell sarcoma) of bone. Cancer 34:1131–1137, 1974.

413. Clayton F, Butler LL, Ayala AG, et al: Non-Hodgkin's lymphoma in bone. Pathologic and radiologic features with clinical correlates. Cancer 60:2494–2501, 1987.

414. Ivins IC: Reticulum-cell sarcoma of bone. J Bone Joint Surg Am 35:835–842, 1953.

415. Reimer RR, Chabner BA, Young RC, et al: Lymphoma presenting in bone. Results of histopathology, staging, and therapy. Ann Intern Med 87:50–55, 1977.

416. Vassallo J, Roessner A, Vollmer E, Grundmann E: Malignant lymphomas with primary bone manifestations. Pathol Res Pract 182:381–389, 1987.

417. Chan IK, Ng CS, Hui PK, et al: Anaplastic large cell Ki-1 lymphoma of bone. Cancer 68:2186–2191, 1991.

418. Falini B, Binazzi R, Pileri S, et al: Large cell lymphoma of bone. A report of three cases of B-cell origin. Histopathology 12:177–190, 1988.

419. Pettit CK, Zukerberg LR, Gray MH, et al: Primary lymphoma of bone. A B-cell neoplasm with a high frequency of multilobated cells. Am J Surg Pathol 4:329–334, 1990.

420. Radaszkiewicz T, Hansmann ML: Primary high-grade malignant lymphomas of bone. Virchows Arch [A] 413:269–274, 1988.

421. Baar L, Burkes RL, Bell R, et al: Primary non-Hodgkin's lymphoma of bone. A clinicopathologic study. Cancer 73:1194–1199, 1994.

422. Bacci G, Jaffe N, Emiliani E, et al: Therapy for primary non-Hodgkin's lymphoma of bone and a comparison of results with Ewing's sarcoma. Ten years' experience at the Istituto Ortopedico Rizzoli. Cancer 57:1468–1472, 1986.

423. Shoji H, Miller TR: Primary reticulum cell sarcoma of bone. Significance of clinical features upon the prognosis. Cancer 28:1234–1244, 1971.

424. Wang CC, Aeischli DJ: Primary reticulum cell sarcoma of bone with emphasis on radiation therapy. Cancer 22:994–998, 1968.

425. Ostrowskj ML, Unni KK, Banks PM, et al: Malignant lymphoma of bone. Cancer 58:2646–2655, 1986.

426. Dosoretz DE, Raymond AK, Murphy GF, et al: Primary lymphoma of bone. The relationship of morphologic diversity to clinical behavior. Cancer 50:1009–1014, 1982.

427. Fowles LV, Olweny CLM, Katongole-Bidde E, et al: Burkitt's lymphoma in the appendicular skeleton. J Bone Joint Surg Br 65:464–471, 1983.

428. Chan K-W, Rosen G, Miller DR, Tan CTC: Hodgkin's disease in adolescents presenting as a primary bone lesion. A report of four cases and review of literature. Am J Pediatr Hematol Oncol 4:11–17, 1982.

429. Marsh WL, Bylund DL, Heath VC, Anderson ML: Osteoarticular and pulmonary manifestations of acute leukemia. Case report and review of the literature. Cancer 57:385–390, 1986.

430. Thomas LB, Forkner CE, Frei E, Slabenau JR: The skeletal lesions of acute leukemia. Cancer 14:608–621, 1961.

431. Chabner BA, Haskell CM, Canellos GP: Destructive bone lesions in chronic granulocytic leukemia. Medicine (Baltimore) 48:401–410, 1969.

432. Nezelof C, Basset F, Rousseau MF: Histiocytosis X. Histoge-

netic arguments for a Langerhans cell origin. Biomed J 18: 365–371, 1973.

433. Daneshbod K, Kissane JM: Histiocytosis-X. The prognosis of polyostotic eosinophilic granuloma. Am J Clin Pathol 65: 601–611, 1976.

434. Lieberman PH, Jones CR, Dargeon HWK, Begg CF: A reappraisal of eosinophilic granuloma of bone. Hand-Schuller-Christian syndrome and Letterer-Siwe syndrome. Medicine (Baltimore) 48:375–400, 1969.

435. Kaleem Z, Kyriakos M, Totty WG: Solitary skeletal hemangioma of the extremities. Skeletal Radiol 29:502–513, 2000.

436. Unni KK, Ivins JC, Beabout JW, Dahlin DC: Hemangioma, hemangiopericytoma, and hemangioendothelioma (angiosarcoma) of bone. Cancer 27:1403–1414, 1971.

437. Wold LE, Swee RG, Sim FH: Vascular lesions of bone. Pathol Annu 20:101–137, 1985.

438. Spjut HJ, Lindbom A: Skeletal angiomatosis. Report of two cases. Acta Pathol Microbiol Scand 55:49–58, 1962.

439. Gorham LW, Stout AP: Massive osteolysis (acute spontaneous absorption of bone, phantom bone, and disappearing bone). Its relation to hemangiomatosis. J Bone Joint Surg Am 37:985–1004, 1955.

440. Halliday DR, Dahlin DC, Pugh OO, Young HH: Massive osteolysis and angiomatosis. Radiology 82:627–644, 1964.

441. Jumbelic M, Feuerstein IM, Dorfman HD: Solitary intraosseous lymphangioma. A case report. J Bone Joint Surg Am 66:1479–1480, 1984.

442. Mackenzie DH: Intraosseous glomus tumors. Report of two cases. J Bone Joint Surg Br 44:648–651, 1962.

443. Weiss SW, Enzinger FM: Epithelioid hemangioendothelioma. A vascular tumor often mistaken for carcinoma. Cancer 50: 970–981, 1982.

444. Weiss SW, Ishak KG, Dail DH, et al: Epithelioid hemangioendothelioma and related lesions. Semin Diagn Pathol 3: 259–287, 1986.

445. Tsuneyoshi M, Dorfman HD, Bauer TW: Epithelioid hemangioendothelioma of bone. A clinicopathologic, ultrastructural and immunohistochemical study. Am J Surg Pathol 10:754–764, 1986.

446. Maruyama N, Kumagai Y, Ishida Y, et al: Epithelioid hemangioendothelioma of the bone tissue. Virchows Arch A [Pathol Anat] 407:159–165, 1985.

447. Abrahams TG, Bula W, Jones M: Epithelioid hemangioendothelioma of bone. A report of two cases and review of the literature. Skeletal Radiol 21:509–513, 1992.

448. Krajca-Radcliffe JB, Nicholas RW, Lewis JM: Multifocal epithelioid hemangioendothelioma in bone. Orthop Rev 21:973–975, 1992.

449. Bollinger BK, Laskin WB, Knight CB: Epithelioid hemangioendothelioma with multiple site involvement. Literature review and observations. Cancer 73:610–615, 1994.

450. Pins MR, Mankin HJ, Xavier RJ, et al: Malignant epithelioid hemangioendothelioma of the tibia associated with a bone infarct in a patient who had Gaucher disease. A case report. J Bone Joint Surg Am 77:777–781, 1995.

451. Carmody E, Loftus B, Corrigan J, et al: Case report 759. Malignant epithelioid hemangioendothelioma of bone. Skeletal Radiol 21:538–541, 1992.

452. Reed RJ: Consultation case: Malignant myxoid angioblastoma of bone. Am J Surg Pathol 6:159–163, 1982.

453. Mirra JM, Kameda N: Myxoid angioblastomatosis of bones. A case report of a rare, multifocal entity with light, ultramicroscopic, and immunopathologic correlation. Am J Surg Pathol 9:459–458, 1985.

454. Wold LE, Unni KK, Beabout JW, et al: Hemangioendothelial sarcoma of bone. Am J Surg Pathol 6:59–70, 1982.

455. Volpe R, Mazabraud A: Hemangioendothelioma (angiosarcoma) of bone. A distinct clinicopathologic entity with an unpredictable course. Cancer 49:727–736, 1982.

456. Wu K, Guise ER: Malignant hemangioendothelioma of bone. A clinical analysis of 11 cases treated at the Henry Ford Hospital. Orthopedics 4:58–64, 1981.

457. Campanacci M, Boriani S, Giunti A: Hemangioendothelioma of bone. A study of 29 cases. Cancer 46:804–814, 1980.

458. Larsson S-E, Lorentzon R, Boquist L: Malignant hemangioendothelioma of bone. J Bone Joint Surg Am 57:84–89, 1975.

459. Otis J, Hutter RVP, Foote FW, et al: Hemangioendothelioma of bone. Surg Gynecol Obstet 127:295–305, 1968.

460. Hartman WH, Stewart FW: Hemangioendothelioma of bone. Unusual tumor characterized by indolent course. Cancer 15: 846–854, 1962.

461. Chow LT-C, Chow W-H, Fong DT-S: Epithelioid hemangioendothelioma of the brain. Am J Surg Pathol 16:619–625, 1992.

462. Weidner N: Atypical tumor of the mediastinum: Epithelioid hemangioendothelioma containing metaplastic bone and osteoclast giant cells. Ultrastruct Pathol 15:481–488, 1991.

463. Zagzag D, Yang G, Seidman L, Lusskin R: Malignant epithelioid hemangioendothelioma arising in an intramuscular lipoma. Cancer 71:764–768, 1993.

464. Kelleher MB, Iwatsuki S, Sheahan DB: Epithelioid hemangioendothelioma of liver. Am J Surg Pathol 13:999–1008, 1989.

465. Scoazec J-Y, Lamy P, Degott C, et al: Epithelioid hemangioendothelioma of liver. Gastroenterology 94:1447–1453, 1988.

466. Harris EJ, Taylor LM, Porter JM: Epithelioid hemangioendothelioma of the iliac vein. A primary vascular tumor presenting as traumatic venous obstruction. J Vasc Surg 10:693–699, 1989.

467. van Haelst UJGM, Pruszczynski M, Cate LN: Ultrastructural and immunohistochemical study of epithelioid hemangioendothelioma of bone. Coexpression of epithelial and endothelial markers. Ultrastruct Pathol 14:141–149, 1990.

468. Ellis GL, Kratochvil FJ: Epithelioid hemangioendothelioma of the head and neck: A clinicopathologic report of twelve cases. Oral Surg, Oral Med, Oral Pathol 61:61–68, 1986.

469. Marrogi AJ, Boyd D, El-Mofty SK, Waldron C: Epithelioid hemangioendothelioma of the oral cavity. J Oral Maxillofac Surg 49:633–638, 1991.

470. Kim CJ, Chi JG, Yoo CG, et al: Unusual endobronchial pulmonary epithelioid hemangioendothelioma. A case report. Int J Surg Pathol 3:59–64, 1995.

471. Battifora H: Epithelioid hemangioendothelioma imitating mesothelioma. Appl Immunohistochem 1:220–222, 1993.

472. Verbeken E, Beyls J, Moeran P, et al: Lung metastasis of malignant epithelioid hemangioendothelioma mimicking a primary intravascular bronchioloalveolar tumor. A histologic, ultrastructural, and immunohistochemical study. Cancer 55: 1741–1746, 1985.

473. Williams SB, Butler BC, Gilkey FW, et al: Epithelioid hemangioendothelioma with osteoclast-like giant cells. Arch Pathol Lab Med 117:315–318, 1993.

474. Toursarkissian B, O'Connor WN, Dillon ML: Mediastinal epithelioid hemangioendothelioma. Ann Thorac Surg 49:680–685, 1990.

475. Yousem SA, Hochholzer L: Unusual thoracic manifestations of epithelioid hemangioendothelioma. Arch Pathol Lab Med 111:459–463, 1987.

476. Lamovec J, Sobel HJ, Zidar A, Jerman J: Epithelioid hemangioendothelioma of the anterior mediastinum with osteoclast-like giant cells. Am J Clin Pathol 9:813–817, 1990.

477. Elhosseiny AA, Ramaswamy GR, Healy RO: Epithelioid hemangioendothelioma of the penis. Urology 28:243–245, 1986.

478. Strayer SA, Yum MN, Sutton GP: Epithelioid hemangioendothelioma of the clitoris: A case report with IHC and EM findings. Int J Gynecol Pathol 11:234–239, 1992.

479. Sirgi KE, Wick MR, Swanson PE: B72.3 and CD34 immunoreactivity in malignant epithelioid soft tissue tumors. Adjuncts in the recognition of endothelial neoplasms. Am J Surg Pathol 17:179–185, 1993.

480. Miettinen M, Lindemayer AE, Chaubal A: Endothelial cell markers CD31, CD34, and BNH9 antibody to H- and Y-antigens. Evaluation of their specificity and sensitivity in the diagnosis of vascular tumors and comparison with von Willebrand factor. Mod Pathol 7:82–90, 1994.

481. Gray MH, Rosenberg AE, Dickersin GR, Bhan AK: Cytokeratin expression in epithelioid vascular neoplasms. Hum Pathol 21:212–217, 1990.

482. Maiorana A, Fante R, Fano RA, Collina G: Epithelioid angiosarcoma of the buttock. Case report with immunohistochem-

ical study on expression of keratin polypeptides. Surg Pathol 4:325–332, 1991.

483. Freedman PD, Kerpel SM: Epithelioid angiosarcoma of the maxilla. Oral Surg Oral Med Oral Pathol 74:319–325, 1992.

484. Fletcher C, Behman A, Bekir S, et al: Epithelioid angiosarcoma of deep soft tissue. A distinctive tumor readily mistaken for an epithelial neoplasm. Am J Surg Pathol 15:915–924, 1991.

485. Wening B, Abbondanzo SL, Heffess C: Epithelioid angiosarcoma of the adrenal glands. A clinicopathological study of nine cases with a discussion of the implications of finding "epithelial-specific" markers. Am J Surg Pathol 18:62–73, 1994.

486. Prescott RJ, Banerjee SS, Eyden BP, Haboubi NY: Cutaneous epithelioid angiosarcoma. A clinicopathological study of four cases. Histopathology 25:421–429, 1994.

487. Byers RJ, McMahon RFT, Freemont AJ, et al: Epithelioid angiosarcoma arising in an arteriovenous fistula. Histopathology 21:87–89, 1992.

488. Perez-Atayde AR, Achenbach H, Lack EE: High-grade epithelioid angiosarcoma of the scalp. Am J Dermatopathol 8:411–418, 1986.

489. Rosai J: Angiolymphoid hyperplasia with eosinophilia of the skin. Its nosological position in the spectrum of histiocytoid hemangioma. Am J Dermatopathol 4:175–184, 1982.

490. Rosai J, Gold J, Landy R: Letter to the editor. Vascular disorder. Am J Surg Pathol 11:651–652, 1987.

491. Bertoni F, Calderoni P, Bacchini P, Campanacci M: Desmoplastic fibroma of bone. A report of six cases. J Bone Joint Surg Br 66:265–268, 1984.

492. Lagace R, Delage C, Bouchard HL, Seemayer TA: Desmoplastic fibroma of bone. An ultrastructural study. Am J Surg Pathol 3:423–430, 1979.

493. Inwards CY, Unni KK, Beabout JW, Sim FH: Desmoplastic fibroma of bone. Cancer 68:1978–1983, 1991.

494. Gebhardt MC, Campbell CJ, Schiller AL, Mankin HJ: Desmoplastic fibroma of bone. A report of eight cases and review of the literature. J Bone Joint Surg Am 67:732–747, 1985.

495. Rabham WN, Rosai J: Desmoplastic fibroma. Report of ten cases and review of the literature. J Bone Joint Surg Am 50:487–502, 1968.

496. O'Connell JX, Logan PM, Beauchamp CP: Solitary fibrous tumor of the periosteum. Hum Pathol 26:460–462, 1995.

497. Cunningham MP, Arlen M: Medullary fibrosarcoma of bone. Cancer 21:31–37, 1968.

498. Gilmer Jr WS, MacEwen GD: Central (medullary) fibrosarcoma of bone. J Bone Joint Surg Am 40:121–141, 1958.

499. Huvos AG, Higinbotham NL: Primary fibrosarcoma of bone. A clinicopathologic study of 130 patients. Cancer 35:837–847, 1975.

500. McLeod JJ, Dahlin DC, Ivins JC: Fibrosarcoma of bone. Am J Surg 94:431–437, 1957.

501. Bertoni F, Capanna R, Calderoni P, et al: Primary central (medullary) fibrosarcoma of bone. Semin Diagn Pathol 1:185–198, 1984.

502. Taconis WK, Van Rijssel THG: Fibrosarcoma of long bones. A study of the significance of areas of malignant fibrous histiocytoma. J Bone Joint Surg Br 67:111–116, 1985.

503. Huvos AG, Heilweil M, Bretsky SS: The pathology of malignant fibrous histiocytoma of bone. A study of 130 patients. Am J Surg Pathol 9:853–871, 1985.

504. Kahn LB, Webber B, Mills E, et al: Malignant fibrous histiocytoma (malignant fibrous xanthoma: xanthosarcoma) of bone. Cancer 42:640–651, 1978.

505. Katenkamp D, Stiller D: Malignant fibrous histiocytoma of bone. Light microscopic and electron microscopic examination of four cases. Virchows Arch [A] 391:323–335, 1981.

506. Kristensen IB, Jensen OM: Malignant fibrous histiocytoma of bone. A clinicopathologic study of 9 cases. Acta Pathol Microbiol Immunol Scand (A) 92:205–210, 1984.

507. McCarthy EF, Matsuno T, Dorfman HD: Malignant fibrous histiocytoma of bone. A study of 35 cases. Hum Pathol 10:57–70, 1979.

508. Nakashima Y, Morishita S, Kotoura Y, et al: Malignant fibrous histiocytoma of bone. A review of 13 cases and an ultrastructural study. Cancer 55:2804–2811, 1985.

509. Spanier SS, Enneking WF, Enriquez P: Primary malignant fibrous histiocytoma of bone. Cancer 36:2084–2098, 1975.

510. Dahlin DC, Unni KK, Matsuno T: Malignant (fibrous) histiocytoma of bone—fact or fancy? Cancer 39:1508–1516, 1977.

511. Fechner RE, Stallings RG, Wang G-J: Malignant fibrous histiocytoma in bone infarct. Association with sickle cell trait and alcohol abuse. Cancer 59:496–500, 1987.

512. Heselson NG, Price SK, Mills EED, et al: Two malignant fibrous histiocytomas in bone infarcts (case reports). J Bone Joint Surg Am 65:1166–1171, 1983.

513. Bago-Granell J, Aguirre-Canyadell M, Nardi J, Tallada N: Malignant fibrous histiocytoma of bone at the site of a total hip arthroplasty. A case report. J Bone Joint Surg Br 66:38–40, 1984.

514. Lee Y-S, Pho RWH, Nathder A: Malignant fibrous histiocytoma at site of metal implant. Cancer 54:2286–2289, 1984.

515. Huvos AG, Woodard HQ, Heilweil M: Postradiation malignant fibrous histiocytoma of bone. A clinicopathologic study of 20 patients. Am J Surg Pathol 10:9–18, 1986.

516. Belza MG, Urich H: Chordoma and malignant fibrous histiocytoma. Evidence for transformation. Cancer 58:1082–1087, 1986.

517. Miettinen M, Lehto Y-P, Yirtanen I: Malignant fibrous histiocytoma within a recurrent chordoma. A light microscopic, electron microscopic, and immunohistochemical study. Am J Clin Pathol 82:738–743, 1984.

518. Boland PJ, Huvos AG: Malignant fibrous histiocytoma of bone. Clin Orthop 204:130–134, 1986.

519. Yokoyama R, Tsuneyoshi M, Enjoji M, et al: Prognostic factors of malignant fibrous histiocytoma of bone. A clinical and histopathologic analysis of 34 cases. Cancer 72:1902–1908, 1993.

520. Angervall L, Berlin A, Kindblom L-G, Stener B: Primary leiomyosarcoma of bone. A study of five cases. Cancer 46:1270–1279, 1980.

521. von Hochstetter AR, Eberle H, Rittner JR: Primary leiomyosarcoma of extragnathic bones. Case report and review of literature. Cancer 53:2194–2200, 1984.

522. Kawai T, Suzuki M, Mukai M, et al: Primary leiomyosarcoma of bone. An immunohistochemical and ultrastructural study. Arch Pathol Lab Med 107:433–437, 1983.

523. Jundt G, Moll C, Nidecker A, et al: Primary leiomyosarcoma of bone. Report of eight cases. Hum Pathol 25:1205–1212, 1994.

524. Young MP, Freemont AJ: Primary leiomyosarcoma of bone. Histopathology 19:257–262, 1991.

525. Lamovec J, Zidar A, Bracko M, Golouh R: Primary bone sarcoma with rhabdomyosarcomatous component. Pathol Res Pract 190:51–60, 1994.

526. Oda Y, Tsuneyoshi M, Hashimoto H, et al: Primary rhabdomyosarcoma of the iliac bone in an adult. A case mimicking fibrosarcoma. Virchows Arch [A] 423:65–69, 1993.

527. Barcelo M, Pathria MN, Abdul-Karim FW: Intraosseous lipoma. A clinicopathologic study of four cases. Arch Pathol Lab Med 116:947–950, 1992.

528. Chow LT, Lee KC: Intra-osseous lipoma. A clinicopathologic study of nine cases. Am J Surg Pathol 16:401–410, 1992.

529. Mandard JC, Mandard AM, Le Gal Y: Les liposarcomes primitifs. A propos de 5 cas. Revue de la Littérature. Ann Anat Pathol (Paris) 18:329–346, 1973.

530. Pardo-Mindan FJ, Ayala H, Joly M, et al: Primary liposarcoma of bone. Light and electron microscopic study. Cancer 48:274–280, 1981.

531. Kaiser TE, Pritchard DJ, Unni KK: Clinicopathologic study of sacrococcygeal chordoma. Cancer 54:2574–2578, 1984.

532. Mindell ER: Chordoma. J Bone Joint Surg Am 63:501–505, 1981.

533. Rich TA, Schiller A, Suit HD, Mankin HJ: Clinical and pathologic review of 45 cases of chordoma. Cancer 56:182–187, 1985.

534. Sundaresan N: Chordomas. Clin Orthop 204:135–142, 1986.

535. Bjornsson J, Wold LE, Ebersold MJ, Laws ER: Chordoma of the mobile spine. A clinicopathologic analysis of 40 patients. Cancer 71:735–740, 1993.

536. Heffelfinger MJ, Dahlin DC, MacCarty CS, Beabout JW:

Chordomas and cartilaginous tumors at the skull base. Cancer 32:410–420, 1973.

537. Coffin CM, Swanson PE, Wick MR, Dehner LP: Chordoma in childhood and adolescence. A clinicopathologic analysis of 12 cases. Arch Pathol Lab Med 117:927–933, 1993.

538. Wold LE, Laws Jr ER: Cranial chordomas in children and young adults. J Neurosurg 59:1043–1047, 1983.

539. Gagne EJ, Su WP: Chordoma involving the skin. An immunohistochemical study of 11 cases. J Cutan Pathol 19:469–475, 1992.

540. Campbell WM, McDonald TJ, Unni KK, Laws Jr ER: Nasal and paranasal presentations of chordomas. Laryngoscope 90:612–618, 1980.

541. Richter HJ, Batsakis JG, Boles R: Chordomas. Nasopharyngeal presentation and atypical long survival. Ann Otol Rhinol Laryngol 84:327–332, 1975.

542. Crawford T: The staining reactions of chordoma. J Clin Pathol 11:110–113, 1958.

543. Lam R: The nature of cytoplasmic vacuoles in chordoma cells. A correlative enzyme and electron microscopic histochemical study. Pathol Res Pract 186:642–650, 1990.

544. Heaton JM, Turner DR: Reflections on notochordal differentiation arising from a study of chordomas. Histopathology 9:543–550, 1985.

545. Abenoza P, Sibley RK: Chordoma. An immunohistologic study. Hum Pathol 17:744–747, 1986.

546. Coffin CM, Swanson PE, Wick MR, Dehner LP: An immunohistochemical comparison of chordoma with renal cell carcinoma, colorectal adenocarcinoma, and myxopapillary ependymoma: A potential diagnostic dilemma in the diminutive biopsy. Mod Pathol 6:531–538, 1993.

547. Meis JM, Giraldo AA: Chordoma. An immunohistochemical study of 20 cases. Arch Pathol Lab Med 112:553–556, 1988.

548. Miettinen M: Chordoma. Antibodies to epithelial membrane antigen and carcinoembryonic antigen in differential diagnosis. Arch Pathol Lab Med 108:891–892, 1984.

549. Nakamura Y, Becker LE, Marks A: S100 protein in human chordoma and human and rabbit notochord. Arch Pathol Lab Med 107:118–120, 1983.

550. Salisbury JR, Isaacson PG: Demonstration of cytokeratins and an epithelial membrane antigen in chordomas and human fetal notochord. Am J Surg Pathol 9:791–797, 1985.

551. Witch R, Landaus SK: Glial fibrillary acidic protein expression in pleomorphic adenoma, chordoma, and astrocytoma. A comparison of three antibodies. Arch Pathol Lab Med 115:1030–1033, 1991.

552. O'Connell JX, Renard LG, Liebsch NJ, et al: Base of skull chordoma. A correlative study of histologic and clinical features of 62 cases. Cancer 74:2261–2267, 1994.

553. Pearlman AW, Friedman M.: Radical radiation therapy of chordoma. Am J Roentgenol Radium Ther Nucl Med 108:333–341, 1970.

554. Arial IM, Verdu C: Chordoma. An analysis of twenty cases treated over a twenty-year span. J Surg Oncol 7:27–44, 1975.

555. Chambers PW, Schwinn CP: Chordoma. A clinicopathologic study of metastasis. Am J Clin Pathol 72:765–776, 1979.

556. Higinbotham NL, Phillips RF, Farr HW, Hustu O: Chordoma. Thirty-five-year study at Memorial Hospital. Cancer 20:1841–1850, 1967.

557. Hruban RH, May M, Marcove RC, Huvos AG: Lumbo-sacral chordoma with high-grade malignant cartilaginous and spindle cell components. Am J Surg Pathol 14:384–389, 1990.

558. Meis JM, Raymond AK, Evans HL, et al: "Dedifferentiated" chordoma. A clinicopathologic and immunohistochemical study of three cases. Am J Surg Pathol 11:516–525, 1987.

559. Volpe R, Mazabraud A: A clinicopathologic review of 25 cases of chordoma (a pleomorphic and metastasizing neoplasm). Am J Surg Pathol 7:161–170, 1983.

560. Chu TA: Chondroid chordoma of the sacrococcygeal region. Arch Pathol Lab Med 111:861–864, 1987.

561. Mitchell A, Scheithauer BW, Unni KK, et al: Chordoma and chondroid neoplasms of the sphenooociput. An immunohistochemical study of 41 cases with prognostic and nosologic implications. Cancer 72:2943–2949, 1993.

562. Jundt G, Remberger K, Roessner A, et al: Adamantinoma of long bones. A histopathological and immunohistochemical study of 23 cases. Pathol Res Pract 191:112–120, 1995.

563. Perez-Atayde AR, Kozakewich HPW, Vawter GF: Adamantinoma of the tibia. An ultrastructural and immunohistochemical study. Cancer 55:1015–1023, 1985.

564. Rosai J: Adamantinoma of the tibia. Electron microscopic evidence of its epithelial origin. Am J Clin Pathol 51:786–792, 1969.

565. Rosai J, Pinkus GS: Immunohistochemical demonstration of epithelial differentiation in adamantinoma of the tibia. Am J Surg Pathol 6:427–434, 1982.

566. Yoneyama T, Winter WG, Milsow L: Tibial adamantinoma. Its histogenesis from ultrastructural studies. Cancer 40:1138–1142, 1977.

567. Baker PL, Dockerty MB, Coventry MB: Adamantinoma (so-called) of the long bones. J Bone Joint Surg 36:704–720, 1954.

568. Keeney GL, Unni KK, Beabout JW, Pritchard DR: Adamantinoma of long bones. A clinicopathologic study of 85 cases. Cancer 64:730–737, 1989.

569. Moon NF, Mori H: Adamantinoma of the appendicular skeleton. Clin Orthop 204:215–237, 1986.

570. Unni KK, Dahlin DC, Beabout JW, Ivins JC: Adamantinomas of long bones. Cancer 34:1796–1805, 1974.

571. Eisenstein W, Pitcock JA: Adamantinoma of the tibia. An eccrine carcinoma. Arch Pathol Lab Med 108:246–250, 1984.

572. Campanacci M, Giunti A, Bertoni F, et al: Adamantinoma of the long bones. The experience at the Istituto Ortopedico Rizzoli. Am J Surg Pathol 5:533–542, 1981.

573. Cohen DM, Dahlin DC, Pugh DG: Fibrous dysplasia associated with adamantinoma of the long bones. Cancer 15:515–521, 1961.

574. Czemiak B, Rojas-Corona RR, Dorfman HD: Morphologic diversity of long bone adamantinoma. The concept of differentiated (regressing) adamantinoma and its relationship to osteofibrous dysplasia. Cancer 64:2319–2334, 1989.

575. Ueda Y, Roessner A, Bosse A, et al: Juvenile intracortical adamantinoma of the tibia with predominant osteofibrous dysplasia-like features. Pathol Res Pract 187:1039–1034, 1991.

576. Weiss SW, Dorfman HD: Adamantinoma of long bone. An analysis of nine new cases with emphasis on metastasizing lesions and fibrous dysplasia-like changes. Hum Pathol 8:141–153, 1977.

577. Benassi MS, Campanacci L, Gamberi G, et al: Cytokeratin expression and distribution in adamantinoma of the long bones and osteofibrous dysplasia of tibia and fibula. An immunohistochemical study correlated to histogenesis. Histopathology 25:71–76, 1994.

578. Ruskin J, Cohen D, Davis L: Primary intraosseous carcinoma. Report of two cases. J Oral Maxillofac Surg 46:425–432, 1988.

579. Sweet DE, Vinh TN, Devaney K: Cortical osteofibrous dysplasia of long bone and its relationship to adamantinoma. A clinicopathologic study of 30 cases. Am J Surg Pathol 16:282–290, 1992.

580. De La Monte SM, Dorfman HD, Chandra R, Malawer M: Intraosseous schwannoma. Histologic features, ultrastructure, and review of the literature. Hum Pathol 15:551–558, 1984.

581. Fawcett KJ, Dahlin DC: Neurilemoma of bone. Am J Clin Pathol 47:759–766, 1967.

582. Turk PS, Peters N, Libbey NP, Wanebo HJ: Diagnosis and management of giant intrasacral schwannoma. Cancer 70:2650–2657, 1992.

583. Wirth WA, Bray CB: Intra-osseous neurilemoma. Case report and review of thirty-one cases from the literature. J Bone Joint Surg Am 59:252–255, 1977.

584. Hunt JC, Pugh OO: Skeletal lesions in neurofibromatosis. Radiology 76:1–19, 1961.

585. Bertoni F, Unni KK, McLeod RA, Sim FH: Xanthoma of bone. Am J Clin Pathol 90:377–384, 1988.

586. Bulychova IV, Unni KK, Bertoni F, Beabout JW: Fibrocartilaginous mesenchymoma of bone. Am J Surg Pathol 17:830–836, 1993.

587. Jaffe HL, Lichtenstein L: Solitary unicameral bone cyst. Arch Surg 44:1004–1025, 1942.

588. Stewart MJ, Hamel HA: Solitary bone cyst. South Med J 43:926–936, 1950.

589. Smith RW, Smith CF: Solitary unicameral bone cyst of the

calcaneus. A review of twenty cases. J Bone Joint Surg Am 56:49–56, 1974.

590. Amling M, Werner M, Posl M, et al: Calcifying solitary bone cyst: Morphological aspects and differential diagnosis of sclerotic bone tumours. Virchows Arch 426:235–242, 1995.

591. Mirra JM, Bernard AW, Bullough PO, et al: Cementum-like bone production in solitary bone cysts (so-called "cementoma" of long bones). Report of three cases. Electron microscopic observations support a synovial origin to the simple bone cyst. Clin Orthop 135:295–307, 1978.

592. Dabska M, Buraczewski J: Aneurysmal bone cyst. Pathology, clinical course and radiologic appearances. Cancer 23:371–389, 1969.

593. Lichtenstein L: Aneurysmal bone cyst. Observations on fifty cases. J Bone Joint Surg Am 39:873–882, 1957.

594. Vergel De Dios AM, Bond JR, Shives TC, et al: Aneurysmal bone cyst. A clinicopathologic study of 238 cases. Cancer 69:2921–2931, 1992.

595. Capanna R, Albisinni U, Picci P, et al: Aneurysmal bone cyst of the spine. J Bone Joint Surg Am 67:527–531, 1985.

596. Sabanathan S, Chen K, Robertson CS, Salama FD: Aneurysmal bone cyst of the rib. Thorax 39:125–130, 1984.

597. Rodriguez-Peralto JL, Lopez-Barea F, Sanchez-Herrera S, Atienza M: Primary aneurysmal cyst of soft tissues (extraosseous aneurysmal cyst). Am J Surg Pathol 18:632–636, 1994.

598. Buraczewski J, Dabska M: Pathogenesis of aneurysmal bone cyst. Relationship between the aneurysmal bone cyst and fibrous dysplasia of bone. Cancer 28:597–604, 1971.

599. Edging NP: Is the aneurysmal bone cyst a true entity? Cancer 18:1127–1130, 1965.

600. Levy WM, Miller AS, Bonakdarpour A, Aegerter E: Aneurysmal bone cyst secondary to other osseous lesions. Report of 57 cases. Am J Clin Pathol 63:1–8, 1975.

601. Alles JU, Schulz A: Immunocytochemical markers (endothelial and histiocytic) and ultrastructure of primary aneurysmal bone cysts. Hum Pathol 17:39–45, 1986.

602. Ruiter DJ, van Rijssel ThG, van der Velde EA: Aneurysmal bone cysts. A clinicopathological study of 105 cases. Cancer 39:2231–2239, 1977.

603. Koskinen EVS, Visuri TI, Holmstrom T, Roukkula MA: Aneurysmal bone cyst. Evaluation of resection and of curettage in 20 cases. Clin Orthop 118:136–146, 1976.

604. Kyriakos M, Hardy D: Malignant transformation of aneurysmal bone cyst, with an analysis of the literature. Cancer 68:1770–1780, 1991.

605. Cunningham JB, Ackerman LV: Metaphyseal fibrous defects. J Bone Joint Surg Am 38:797–808, 1956.

606. Jaffe HL, Lichtenstein L: Nonosteogenic fibroma of bone. Am J Pathol 18:205–221, 1942.

607. Hatcher CH: Pathogenesis of localized fibrous lesion in the metaphyses of long bones. Ann Surg 122:1016–1030, 1945.

608. Clarke BE, Xipell JM, Thomas DP: Benign fibrous histiocytoma of bone. Am J Surg Pathol 9:806–815, 1985.

609. Destouet JM, Kyriakos M, Gilula LA: Fibrous histiocytoma (fibroxanthoma) of a cervical vertebra. Skeletal Radiol 5:241–246, 1980.

610. Arata MA, Peterson HA, Dahlin DC: Pathological fractures through non-ossifying fibromas. Review of the Mayo Clinic experience. J Bone Joint Surg Am 63:980–988, 1981.

611. Dudley HR, Barry RJ: The natural history of fibrous dysplasia. J Bone Joint Surg Am 44:207–233, 1962.

612. Schlumberger HA: Fibrous dysplasia of single bones (monostotic fibrous dysplasia). Milit Surg 99:504–527, 1946.

613. Lichtenstein L, Jaffe HL: Fibrous dysplasia of bone. Arch Pathol 33:777–816, 1942.

614. Dorfman HD, Tsuneyoshi M: Exophytic variant of fibrous dysplasia (fibrous dysplasia protuberans). Hum Pathol 25:1234–1237, 1994.

615. Povysil C, Matejovsky Z: Fibro-osseous lesion with calcified spherules (cementifying fibromalike lesion) of the tibia. Ultrastruct Pathol 17:25–34, 1993.

616. Sissons HA, Steiner AC, Dorfman HD: Calcified spherules in fibro-osseous lesions of bone. Arch Pathol Lab Med 117:284–290, 1993.

617. Voytek TM, Ro JY, Edeiken J, Ayala AA: Fibrous dysplasia and cemento-ossifying fibroma. A histologic spectrum. Am J Surg Pathol 19:775–781, 1995.

618. Pelzmann KS, Nagel DZ, Salyer WR: Polyostotic fibrous dysplasia and fibrochondrodysplasia. Skeletal Radiol 5:116–118, 1980.

619. Aoki T, Kouho H, Hisaoka M, et al: Intramuscular myxoma with fibrous dysplasia. A report of two cases with a review of the literature. Pathol Int 45:165–171, 1995.

620. Huvos AG, Higinbotham NL, Miller TR: Bone sarcomas arising in fibrous dysplasia. J Bone Joint Surg Am 54:1047–1056, 1972.

621. Ishida T, Machinami R, Kojirna T, Kikuchi F: Malignant fibrous histiocytoma and osteosarcoma in association with fibrous dysplasia of bone. Report of three cases. Pathol Res Pract 188:757–763, 1992.

622. Ruggieri P, Sim FH, Bond JR, Unni KK: Malignancies in fibrous dysplasia. Cancer 73:1411–1424, 1994.

623. Park YK, Unni KK, McLeod RA: Osteofibrous dysplasia. Clinicopathologic study of 80 cases. Hum Pathol 24:1339–1347, 1993.

624. Campanacci M: Osteofibrous dysplasia of long bones: A new clinical entity. Ital J Orthop Traumatol 2:221–237, 1976.

625. Bridge JA, Dembinski A, De Boer J, et al: Clonal chromosomal abnormalities in osteofibrous dysplasia. Implications for histopathogenesis and its relationship with adamantinoma. Cancer 73:1746–1752, 1994.

626. Weidner N, Bar RS, Weiss D, Strottmann P: Neoplastic pathology of oncogenic osteomalacia-rickets. Cancer 55:1691–1695, 1985.

627. Weidner N, Santa Cruz D: Phosphaturic mesenchymal tumors, a polymorphous group causing osteomalacia-rickets. Cancer 59:1442–1454, 1987.

628. Weidner N: Review and update: Oncogenic osteomalacia-rickets. Ultrastruct Pathol 15:317–333, 1991.

629. Simon MA, Bartucci EJ: The search for the primary tumor in patients with skeletal metastases of unknown origin. Cancer 58:1088–1095, 1986.

630. Yamashita K, Ueda T, Komatsubara Y, et al: Breast cancer with bone-only metastases. Visceral metastases-frequency rate in relation to anatomic distribution of bone metastases. Cancer 68:634–637, 1991.

631. Caffey J, Andersen DH: Metastatic embryonal rhabdomyosarcoma in the growing skeleton. Clinical, radiographic, and microscopic features. Am J Dis Child 95:581–600, 1958.

632. Berrettoni HA, Carter JR: Mechanisms of cancer metastasis to bone. J Bone Joint Surg Am 68:308–312, 1986.

633. Healey JH, Tumbull ADM, Miedema B, Lane JM: Acrometastases. A study of twenty-nine patients with osseous involvement of the hands and feet. J Bone Joint Surg Am 68:743–746, 1986.

634. Morris DM, House HC: The significance of metastasis to the bones and soft tissues of the hand. J Surg Oncol 28:146–150, 1985.

635. Troncoso A, Ro JY, Han WS, et al: Renal cell carcinoma with acrometastasis. Report of two cases and review of the literature. Mod Pathol 4:66–69, 1991.

636. Thomas BM: Three unusual carcinoid tumours, with particular reference to osteoblastic bone metastases. Clin Radiol 19:221–225, 1968.

637. Quinn JM, Matsumura Y, Tarin D, Athanasou NA: Cellular and hormonal mechanisms associated with malignant bone resorption. Lab Invest 71:465–471, 1994.

638. Daroca Jr PJ, Reed RJ, Martin PC: Metastatic amelanotic melanoma simulating giant-cell tumor of bone. Hum Pathol 21:978–980, 1990.

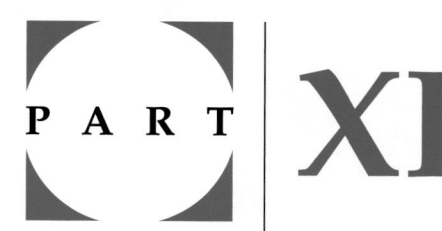

# PART XI

# Skin

# 48

# *Inflammatory Skin Conditions*

Scott R. Granter    Tai-Yuen Wong    Martin C. Mihm Jr.

DERMAL MUCINOSES
  Generalized Myxedema
  Pretibial Myxedema
  Lichen Myxedematosus and Scleromyxedema
  Scleredema

CUTANEOUS DEPOSITION DISORDERS
  Gout
  Calcinosis Cutis
  Xanthomas
  Amyloidosis
  Colloid Milium

Inflammatory skin pathology is perhaps one of the most complex and difficult areas in surgical pathology. This complexity may be attributed to several factors. First, accurate diagnoses are usually arrived at only after careful clinicopathologic correlation because many histologic patterns of inflammatory skin disease are not specific for a single disease. For example, lichen planus and lichenoid keratosis may show histologically identical patterns. A solitary lesion clinically resembling a basal cell carcinoma in a sun-exposed area would be consistent with lichenoid keratosis. On the other hand, multiple pruritic papules on the extremities would favor lichen planus. Second, many (if not most) inflammatory dermatoses evolve through acute, subacute, and chronic phases. These phases may have multiple histologic appearances. Familiarity with the histologic features of each of these phases is necessary for accurate diagnosis. Finally, the nomenclature and language of dermatopathology are complex and cumbersome, and many diagnostic terms are even misleading. This unfortunate aspect of dermatopathology often frustrates students of dermatopathology.

The goal of this chapter is to demonstrate a general approach to inflammatory skin diseases and exemplify this approach with a discussion of the more common and significant diseases encountered by the pathologist. For a more comprehensive study of inflammatory skin diseases, the reader is referred to several excellent dermatopathology textbooks.[1-4] In this chapter, disease processes are classified by the predominant reaction pattern of the various compartments of the skin or the dominant type of pathologic process displayed by the lesion. The following categories are addressed: skin conditions with predominantly epidermal (spongiotic, eczematous, psoriasiform, exfoliative, pustular) changes, interface dermatitis, bullous and acantholytic dermatoses, vasculitides, panniculitides, sclerosing disorders, granulomatous processes, dermal mucinoses, and deposition disorders. Some degree of overlap may be observed in the reaction patterns among these various conditions. However, they have been organized to illustrate the prototypical expression of disease that is most commonly exemplified by these conditions.

## ANATOMY OF NORMAL SKIN

The evaluation of inflammatory skin disease focuses on the three anatomic compartments of the skin: epidermis, dermis, and subcutaneous tissue. The epidermis is composed of stratified squamous epithelium. The lowermost layer of the epidermis, the basal cell layer, is composed of a single row of cuboid or columnar cells attached by hemidesmosomes to the basement membrane. In normal skin, mitoses are most commonly encountered in the basal cell layer, which is the germinative layer of the organ. The stratum spinosum or prickle cell layer composes the bulk of the epidermis and ranges in thickness according to anatomic site. As squamous cells within the stratum spinosum proceed toward the surface of the epidermis, these cells become flattened, and the cytoplasm becomes more densely eosinophilic. During pathologic processes that result in intercellular edema, the spinous cell-cell attachments may be more conspicuous. This finding is the hallmark of spongiotic dermatitides. In the superficial epidermis, flattened squamous cells accumulate keratohyalin granules. This layer, depending on the anatomic site, is composed of one to several cell layers and is referred to as the granular cell layer or stratum granulosum. The stratum corneum, or horny layer, is composed of flattened anucleated squamous cells and is arranged in a sievelike, basket weave pattern in nonacral sites. A thick compact stratum corneum characterizes skin in acral regions.

The dermis is separated into two major components, the papillary dermis and the reticular dermis. The papillary dermis is composed of delicate collagen fibers and is located immediately beneath the epidermis. In many sites, downward projections of the epidermis (rete ridges) alternate with upward projections of the papillary dermis (dermal papillae). In contrast to the papillary dermis, the reticular dermis is composed of dense thick bundles of collagen admixed with elastic fibrils. Subcutaneous adipose tissue lies deep to the reticular dermis. Thin fibrous septa divide the subcutaneous fat into lobules.

Within the dermis and subcutaneous adipose tissue are adnexal structures including eccrine sweat glands, apocrine glands, sebaceous glands, and hair follicles. Eccrine sweat coils are located within the deep dermis adjacent to the dermal-subcutaneous junction and extend to open onto the epidermis through a long slender duct. Eccrine sweat glands are particularly numerous in acral regions. Apocrine sweat glands are most numerous in the intertriginous regions. The secretory portion of the apocrine sweat gland is characterized by ectatic spaces lined by epithelial cells with abundant granular eosinophilic cytoplasm. The hair follicle is a complex structure. The deepest portion of the hair follicle, the hair bulb, comprises follicle and associated perifollicular connective tissue. The life cycle of a hair follicle may be divided into three different phases: the growing phase, referred to as the anagen follicle; the involutional phase, referred to as the catagen phase; and the resting phase, designated the telogen phase. Sebaceous glands may be found on most parts of the body (except the palms and soles) but are particularly numerous on the face and central chest regions. Sebaceous glands are multilobular and composed of epithelial cells with abundant, finely vacuolated cytoplasm. The oily sebaceous secretions are discharged into the associated hair follicle and then onto the surface of the skin.

## BIOPSY PREPARATION

The most common type of biopsy used to evaluate inflammatory conditions is the punch biopsy, a method that yields a cylindrical core of tissue that includes dermis and subcutaneous fat. A range of punch biopsy diameters is available. The punch biopsy is advantageous because it allows examination of the epidermis as well as the dermis. The shave biopsy is performed by a scalpel and usually yields a thin sliver of tissue that contains epidermis and superficial dermis only. The shave biopsy may be adequate for inflammatory dermatoses that predominantly affect the epidermis. Shave biopsies, however, are inadequate and often misleading in the evaluation of inflammatory dermatoses with a deep dermal and subcutaneous component. They may also be insufficient for diagnosis of tumors of the skin. When a deep dermal process or panniculitis is suspected, the excisional biopsy yields the most information. The excisional biopsy obtains an ellipse of skin, dermis, and adipose tissue. Fixation in 10% buffered formalin followed by routine H&E staining yields satisfactory nuclear and cytoplasmic detail.

## SKIN CONDITIONS WITH PREDOMINANTLY EPIDERMAL CHANGES

A variety of inflammatory skin conditions are characterized by changes that predominantly affect the epidermis. These include spongiotic-eczematous, psoriasiform, exfoliative, and pustular dermatitis.

### Spongiotic-Eczematous Dermatitis

Eczematous dermatitis represents a clinicopathologic spectrum of inflammatory skin disorders primarily involving the epidermis and, in most cases, the superficial dermis. Eczema can have many different causes, with overlapping but variable clinical and pathologic characteristics.[5] The clinical appearance of the rash depends greatly on the stage of the lesion's evolution and also on the presence of secondary changes produced by scratching, irritation, superimposed infection, and therapy. The timing, therefore, determines the character of the various components of the eczematous inflammation (such as erythema, scale, vesicles, and plaques). In the most simplified schema, eczema can be divided into three stages: acute, subacute, and chronic. Each stage represents a snapshot of a dynamic biologic process. In most situations, eczema can present at any stage, evolve or regress to another, or show a combination of different stages. The histopathologic appearance may vary and depends not only on the degree of inflammation but also on the stage at which the biopsy is performed. Furthermore, the histopathologic appearances may also be influenced by superimposed trauma, infection, or effects of previous treatment regimens.

In general, acute eczematous dermatitis is clinically characterized by erythema, microvesicles, sometimes vesicles and blisters, swelling, and oozing. Biopsy shows spongiosis or intercellular edema, which is evidenced by separation between keratinocytes within the stratum corneum, vesicles or bullae, lymphocyte exocytosis, dermal edema, and frequently a superficial perivascular, predominantly lymphoid infiltrate (Fig. 48–1). In general, subacute eczematous dermatitis is clinically characterized by erythema, scaling, and plaque formation with fissuring. Biopsy reveals variable psoriasiform hyperplasia, parakeratosis, hyperkeratosis, and frequently scale crust (Fig. 48–2). Chronic eczematous dermatitis is characterized by lichenification with thickened dry plaques, excoriation, and fissuring. Biopsy reveals psoriasiform hyperplasia that is frequently

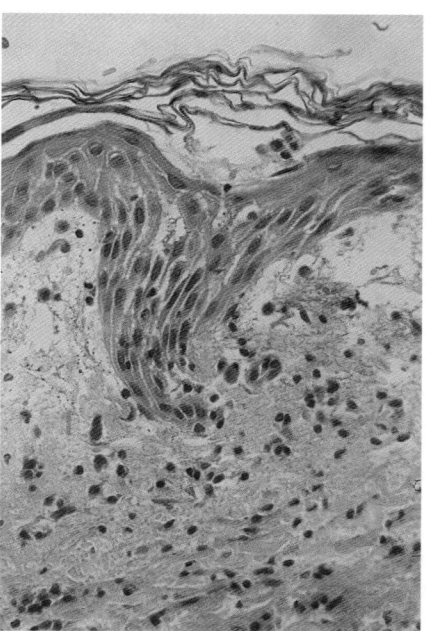

**FIGURE 48–1.** Acute spongiotic dermatitis. Early spongiosis is seen as separation between adjacent keratinocytes. Basket weave keratin overlying this lesion is evidence of the acute nature of this case.

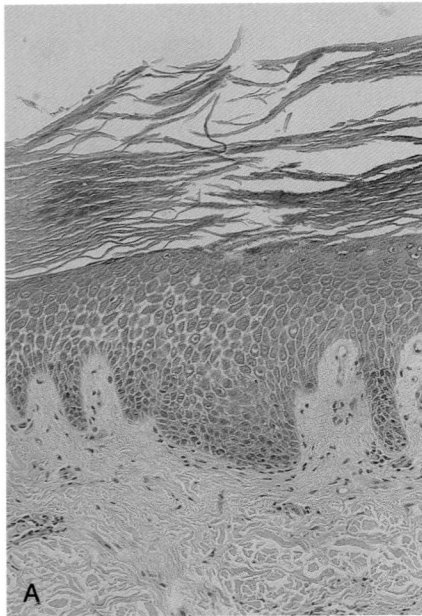
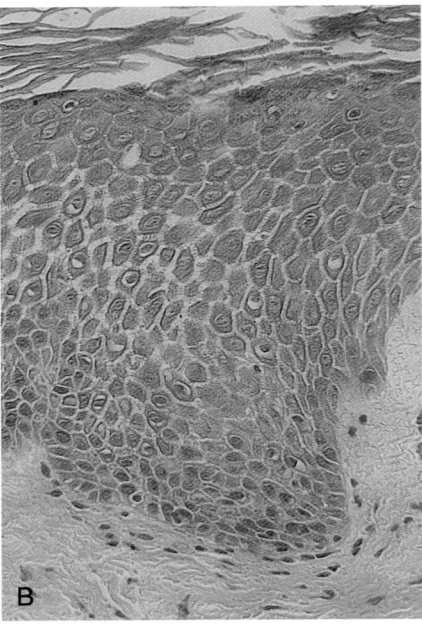

**FIGURE 48–2.** Subacute to chronic spongiotic dermatitis. *A.* Low-power magnification shows epidermal hyperplasia, with spongiosis, and overlying compact hyperkeratosis, features of chronicity. *B.* High-power magnification reveals diffuse spongiosis.

marked, hyperkeratosis, parakeratosis, hypergranulosis, focal spongiosis, fibrosis of the papillary dermis, and variable superficial perivascular inflammatory infiltrates. A single biopsy specimen may show different stages in the evolution of an eczematous dermatitis.

## Allergic Contact Dermatitis

Allergic contact dermatitis is a vesicular-bullous eruption resulting from contact with substances to which the patient is sensitized (e.g., nickel; poison ivy; organic chemicals, such as components commonly used in cosmetics, dyes, and deodorants, among others).[6] The location and distribution of lesions frequently provide clues to the etiology. Acute lesions may vary from erythematous papules and plaques to vesicles and, in severe cases, bullae formation. In situations with a less potent allergen or in chronic low-grade exposure, dry erythematous, scaly, and eczematous patches or plaques may be observed.

The histologic findings are similar to those described for eczematous dermatitides. As with other eczematous dermatitides, the histologic findings depend on the stage of the process when the biopsy specimen is taken. In the acute stage, the epidermis exhibits an acute reaction with exocytosis of mononuclear cells and occasional eosinophils, marked intercellular edema (spongiosis), and formation of microvesicles.[7] The presence of eosinophils admixed with intercellular edema is known as eosinophilic spongiosis. The papillary dermis is edematous and accompanied by a superficial perivascular lymphocytic infiltrate admixed with scattered eosinophils. A mild to moderate degree of psoriasiform epidermal hyperplasia with diffuse edema, exocytosis, micro-

vesicle formation, and parakeratotic scale formation is present in the subacute stage. Subacute allergic contact dermatitis shows epidermal changes similar to those of nummular eczema with spongiotic vesicle formation.

In the chronic stage, the epidermis shows irregular acanthosis, hyperkeratosis, confluent parakeratosis incorporated with scale crust, prominent granular cell layer, and minimal intercellular edema and exocytosis. The papillary dermis is no longer edematous and is thickened by coarse collagen arranged perpendicular to the epidermal surface. Scattered lymphocytes and rare eosinophils can still be found. The presence of scale crust containing neutrophils superimposed on features of spongiotic dermatitis suggests an impetiginized or superinfected lesion. The pathologic differential diagnosis encompasses other spongiotic dermatitides, including nummular dermatitis, dyshidrotic eczema, id reactions, and inflammatory pityriasis rosea. Eosinophilic spongiosis is observed in allergic contact dermatitis, but it can also be present in arthropod bites, bullous pemphigoid, herpes gestationis, incontinentia pigmenti, and the pemphigus group of disorders. Distinguishing among these differential diagnoses is frequently impossible without careful clinicopathologic correlation and often requires special stains such as immunofluorescence staining.

## Nummular Dermatitis

Nummular dermatitis is an eczematous eruption characterized clinically by round to oval coin-shaped lesions. They are intensely pruritic, minute, grouped papules and vesicles in discrete patches that evolve into plaques with abrupt distinct borders. Variable amounts of crusting, exudation, and scale formation are present. Lesions most commonly occur on the trunk and extensor surfaces of the extremities. The histologic appearance can be indistinguishable from allergic contact dermatitis.[8] The early lesions show acute spongiotic dermatitis with superficial dermal infiltrate and scattered eosinophils. The lesions most commonly examined by biopsy are from the well-developed coin-shaped plaques.

Histologic examination shows features of subacute spongiotic dermatitis with less pronounced intercellular edema and irregular elongation of rete ridges. Multifocal parakeratosis with scale crust is present over the acanthotic epidermis. The edema in the papillary dermis in the early phase is later replaced by a less remarkable dermal perivenular lymphocytic infiltrate with admixed eosinophils and focal fibrosis of the papillary dermis. Biopsy of subacute nummular dermatitis shows psoriasiform hyperplasia of the epidermis with overlying hyperkeratosis and parakeratosis admixed with scale crust. In contrast to psoriasis, the rete ridges are elongated but with a variable length, and there is no thinning of the suprapapillary plate. Spongiotic vesicles with surrounding intercellular edema can often be seen within the epidermis.[9] The dermal inflammatory infiltrate predominantly involves the superficial vascular plexus and is composed of perivenular lymphocytes and eosinophils. Careful clinicopathologic correlation is usually needed to distinguish nummular dermatitis from other forms of subacute spongiotic dermatitis, especially subacute allergic contact dermatitis.

## Id Reaction or Autosensitization

Id reaction or autosensitization is an acute eczematous eruption that results from an immunologic reaction to an active, but distant, inflammatory condition. It may be induced by such conditions as extensive fungal infection involving hair, feet, and nails; stasis dermatitis; or, less commonly, otitis media and otitis externa. The eruption usually occurs in patients with active localized dermatitis. An exacerbation of the primary localized skin lesion due to secondary infection, topical therapy, or rubbing usually precedes the allergic skin eruption. Generalized pruritus and increased sensitivity to irritation may follow. In the subsequent papulovesicular stage, the eruption is symmetric and composed of inflamed and impetiginized, eczematous, vesicular, or nummular eruptions with a predilection for the hands and flexor aspect of the forearm. In severe cases, the eruption results in confluent patches and plaques and, on rare occasions, in exfoliative erythroderma.

The histologic features depend on the type of id reaction. In the papillary stage, the lesion is characterized by the presence of perivenular lymphoid infiltrates within the dermis. In more diffuse eruptions, a picture of subacute spongiotic dermatitis similar to nummular eczema is observed. As with other spongiotic dermatitides, a specific pathologic diagnosis is difficult if not impossible, and careful clinicopathologic correlation is needed to establish the diagnosis.

## Dyshidrotic Dermatitis

Dyshidrotic dermatitis is an itchy, vesicular, and blistering disorder of unknown etiology primarily involving the palms and soles. It occasionally occurs in patients with atopy and may simulate superficial dermatophyte infection. Patients usually present with recurrent formation of vesicles or bullae involving the palms, soles, and characteristically the sides of the fingers. In chronic cases, eczematous changes including erythema, scaling, and lichenification are apparent.

An acute dermatitis is usually associated with vesicle and bullae formation within the acral epidermis (Fig. 48–3). Intercellular edema is prominent at the periphery and the base of the tense vesicle. The intravesicular inflammatory infiltrate is composed predominantly of mononuclear cells admixed with rare neutrophils. The dermal infiltrate is usually

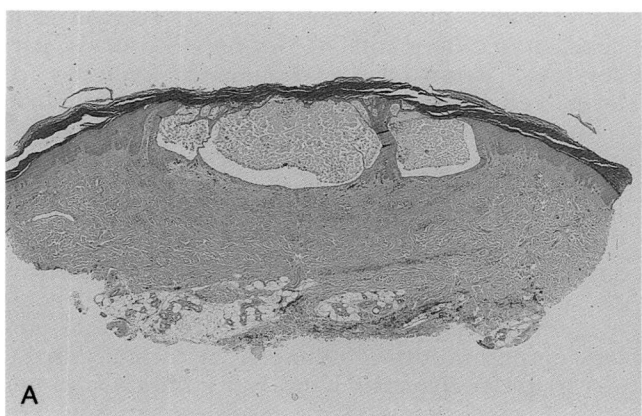
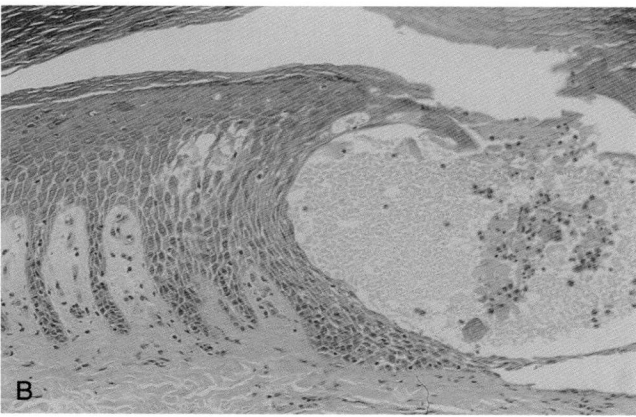

**FIGURE 48–3.** Dyshidrotic eczema. *A.* Low-power magnification shows acral skin with tense intraepidermal vesicles. *B.* At higher magnification, focal spongiosis is seen adjacent to a vesicle.

minimal. The histologic differential diagnosis encompasses other acute spongiotic dermatitides, including inflammatory dermatophytosis.

## Pityriasis Rosea

Pityriasis rosea is a common, self-limited, frequently pruritic, scaling eruption mostly presenting in young adults. The first sign of the disease is usually a solitary, oval, pink "herald" patch with fine surface scales. Lesions are most common on the trunk. Widespread secondary lesions appear within 1 to 2 weeks after formation of the herald patch. They appear as crops of oval, salmon-colored macules or minimally elevated plaques, each with a fine brown wrinkled central surface and a collarette of fine scale at the periphery. The trunk and proximal extremities are areas of predilection.[10] The distribution of lesions along the lines of cleavage at the back suggests a "pine tree" pattern. The face, hands, and feet are usually spared. A clinical variant with a more inflammatory presentation forms papules and vesicles. An atypical distribution involving intertriginous areas, face, arms, and legs (inverse pattern) can occur. Pruritus is variable but can be severe. Lesions usually resolve spontaneously after 6 to 8 weeks, without scarring.

Most established secondary plaques show mild subacute spongiotic dermatitis. There are spotty lens-shaped mounds of parakeratosis, focal intercellular edema occasionally with vesicle formation, and slight irregular acanthotic epidermis (Fig. 48–4). The parakeratotic scale is usually attached at one end to the stratum corneum and appears to lift off at an acute angle to the epidermis. In the papillary dermis, there are focal areas of extravasated red cells and edema associated with a focal perivascular lymphocytic infiltrate admixed with occasional eosinophils. A more severe spongiotic inflammatory pattern is present in the inflammatory variant of pityriasis rosea. The herald patch differs from the

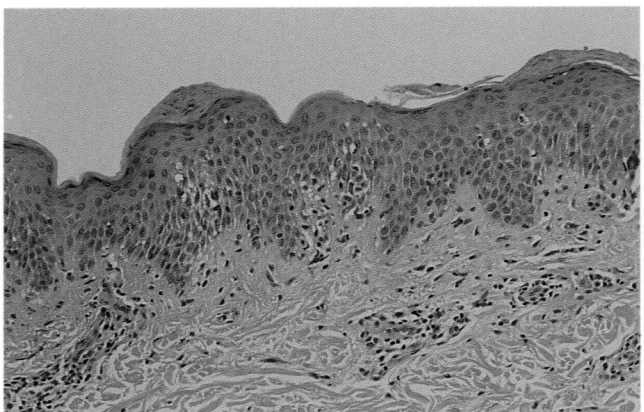

**FIGURE 48–4.** Pityriasis rosea. The biopsy specimen shows mild epidermal hyperplasia and focal mild spongiosis associated with a lens-shaped parakeratotic mound.

secondary lesions in exhibiting more acanthotic epidermis, less spongiosis, and a deep as well as a superficial infiltrate. In all types of pityriasis rosea, the red blood cells are confined to the papillary dermis without extravasation into the epidermis. The pathologic differential diagnosis encompasses other acute and subacute spongiotic dermatitides, including inflammatory dermatophytosis, erythema annulare centrifugum, and pityriasis lichenoides.[11]

## Atopic Dermatitis

Atopic dermatitis is an eczematous eruption often seen in association with a personal or family history of allergies, hay fever, or asthma.[12] It frequently occurs in early childhood and often resolves spontaneously during adolescence, but it occasionally recurs during adult life as dry, irritable skin. In the early months of life, the intensely pruritic eruption tends to involve the face, neck, upper trunk, and extensor surfaces and rarely becomes generalized. In late childhood and adolescence, the antecubital fossa and popliteal fossa are favored sites. During adulthood, a more widespread pattern can occur in the form of dry, itchy, scaling, irritable skin, especially affecting the hands and feet. Periorbital pruritus and scaling are characteristic. Exceptionally, severe cases may evolve into erythroderma. In the acute stage, the skin is moist, erythematous, and weeping in the form of exudative papules and plaques. Chronic eruption is characterized by dry scaling and lichenification, especially in the popliteal and antecubital fossae and periorbital areas. Weeping, crusting, and exudation may occur but usually result from superimposed trauma and infection. Adults are also susceptible to development of other dermatitides, including nummular eczema, dyshidrotic eczema, and hand eczema. There can be intermittent secondary infections with *Staphylococcus aureus*, group A β–hemolytic streptococci, and viruses, especially herpes simplex virus (eczema herpeticum) and vaccinia virus (eczema vaccinatum).

The histologic findings depend on the site of biopsy and stage of evolution of the disease.[8] In acute lesions such as those typically seen in childhood, atopic dermatitis shows hyperkeratosis, parakeratosis, abundant or diminished granular cell layer, and irregularly hyperplastic epidermis. Intercellular edema is mild, and vesiculation is uncommon. Occasional cases involve predominantly follicular epithelium. The dermal infiltrate is composed mostly of lymphocytes with sparse eosinophils. Chronic lichenoid lesions show features of lichen simplex chronicus. These lesions have increased hyperkeratosis, prominent granular cell layer, irregular epidermal hyperplasia, and vertical streaks of papillary dermal fibrosis resulting from chronic rubbing. A variable perivenular lymphoid infiltrate is present and is associated with mast cell hyperplasia. Perineural fibrosis associated with increased mast cells is often observed. On occasion, compact hyperkeratosis resembling ichthyosis vulgaris is present as well as hyperkeratotic follicular infundibula as noted in keratosis pilaris. Secondary changes in the form of exudation, erosion, and ulceration are evidence of excoriation.

## Seborrheic Dermatitis

Seborrheic dermatitis is a common, chronic, erythematous, greasy, scaling eruption involving the scalp, eyebrows, face, central chest, and intertriginous areas. It occurs most often in infancy and after puberty. It is also associated with severe stress and is seen in patients with neurologic disorders including Parkinson's disease and acquired immunodeficiency disorders. Scaling of the scalp is the most common feature and may evolve into plaques of yellow-red greasy scales that coalesce to involve the entire scalp. The rash usually presents as erythematous, greasy scaling patches but can vary from macular and papular erythematous lesions with dry scales on the trunk to moist, erythematous patches in the intertriginous areas. In rare instances, seborrheic dermatitis can present as generalized erythroderma. A chronic, recurrent diaper dermatitis that is frequently infected with *Candida* is common in infants. In seborrheic blepharitis, erythema and scaling involve the eyelid margins, often in association with mild conjunctivitis. Perioral dermatitis, considered by many a variant of seborrheic dermatitis (and by others to be a form of rosacea), is a papular erythematous eruption around the mouth.

In acute seborrheic dermatitis, the biopsy specimen may show subacute spongiotic dermatitis with a tendency to involve hair follicles, usually accompanied by scale crust with neutrophils aggregated around the edges of follicular ostia. Focal spongiosis and diffuse exocytosis of both mononuclear cells and neutrophils are noted. The papillary dermis is edematous, containing dilated vessels and a scattered lymphohistiocytic and neutrophilic infiltrate. Microabscesses and spongiform micropustules are occasionally found.[13] In chronic cases of seborrheic dermatitis, the epidermis exhibits mild to moderate psoriasiform hyperplasia and prominent parakeratosis concentrated especially around the follicular ostia and accompanied by follicular plugging with scales and neutrophils. Some cases of perioral dermatitis show features similar to those of acute seborrheic dermatitis. In patients with acquired immunodeficiency syndrome, the infiltrates are more extensive, consisting of admixed lymphocytes, histiocytes, and neutrophils involving both the superficial and deep perivascular plexuses. Eosinophils may also be found. Other frequently observed histologic characteristics are the presence of scattered apoptotic keratinocytes within the epidermis without associated acute inflammation and maturation disarray of keratinocytes.

## Incontinentia Pigmenti

Incontinentia pigmenti is an X-linked, dominantly inherited disorder with cutaneous and other associated neuroectodermal malformations.[14] The majority of patients are females who usually present during the neonatal period.[15] Three progressive stages of cutaneous involvement are recognized. The first stage features vesicles and bullae arranged in a linear fashion, with surrounding erythema, usually involving the extremities. In the second stage, verrucous papules and nodules are arranged in linear configuration on the extremities. Characteristic hyperpigmentation in an asymmetric, serpiginous pattern develops in the third stage, which (in contrast to lesions in the first and second stages) usually involves the trunk. Pigmentation tends to intensify at around the second year of life and involutes during a period of years. Other abnormalities of the eyes, teeth, bone, and central nervous system may be seen.

The histopathologic findings depend on the stage of the lesion. The earliest histologic expression of incontinentia pigmenti is spongiotic dermatitis with eosinophils (eosinophilic spongiosis). Vesicles in the first stage are filled with eosinophils (Fig. 48–5). Scattered dyskeratotic cells and whorls of keratinocytes are scattered within the epidermis (Fig. 48–6). Eosinophils frequently cluster around the dyskeratotic cells. Aggregates of eosinophils, forming eosinophilic microabscesses, are present within the epidermis and dermal papillae. Dermal edema with a mixed lymphocytic and eosinophilic infiltrate is present. In the second stage, the epidermis is acan-

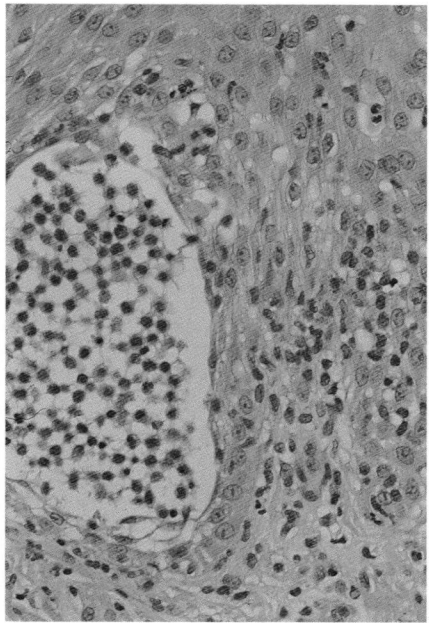

**FIGURE 48–5.** Incontinentia pigmenti. This early lesion shows eosinophilic spongiosis with intraepidermal eosinophilic pustules.

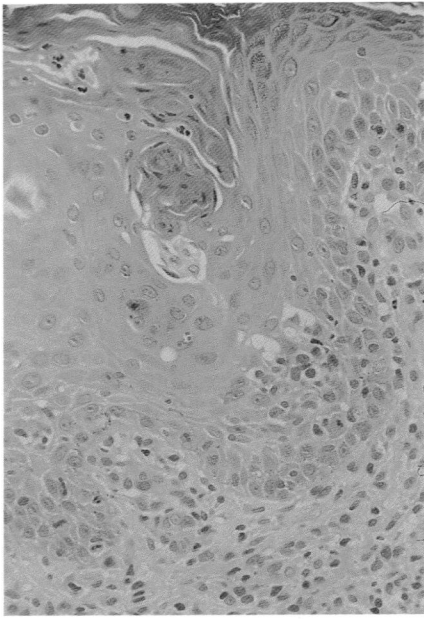

FIGURE 48-6. Incontinentia pigmenti. In this later lesion, spongiosis is minimal, and whorls of dyskeratotic squamous cells are scattered within the epidermis. Eosinophils may be seen in the epidermis and superficial papillary dermis along with melanophages.

thotic, accompanied by orthokeratosis and parakeratosis. Whorls of keratinocytes and dyskeratotic cells are more striking than in the first stage. The dermal infiltrate is predominantly lymphocytic, admixed with melanophages. Abundant melanophages are present in the dermis in the area of depigmentation in the third stage.

## Dermatophytosis

The dermatophytoses, or superficial fungal infections (usually called ringworm), are caused by a group of related fungal organisms involving the skin, nails, and hair.[16, 17] The terminology commonly used follows a classification according to the clinical pattern of disease rather than by offending organisms. These include tinea corporis (ringworm of the body), tinea pedis (athlete's foot), tinea manuum (tinea of the hands), tinea cruris (jock itch), tinea capitis (ringworm of the scalp), and tinea barbae (ringworm of the beard). The clinical appearance is variable and dependent on the involved body sites. Typical lesions are ring shaped, erythematous, and scaling. Lesions are most commonly located on the buttock, trunk, hands, and intertriginous areas. Areas with more intense inflammation are sometimes associated with vesicles or pustules. Tinea pedis is characterized by dry, hyperkeratotic scaling. Vesicles may occasionally appear in bullae formation. In tinea capitis, the clinical appearance is that of a pustular folliculitis that may result in scarring alopecia.

The histologic picture of dermatophytosis varies with the clinical features. In vesicular and bullous eruptions, spongiotic vesicles and tense bullae are noted in the epidermis, accompanied by exocytosis of a mixed infiltrate composed of lymphocytes, neutrophils, and occasionally eosinophils.[18] The dermal component is nonspecific and composed predominantly of lymphocytes centered around the superficial vascular plexus. The periodic acid–Schiff (PAS) stain should be performed on all biopsy specimens showing spongiotic dermatitis and eczematous plaques, particularly those refractory to topical steroid therapy (Fig. 48-7). In typical scaling lesions, the histologic examination reveals a hyperplastic epidermis with overlying hyperkeratosis and patchy parakeratosis admixed with neutrophils in the corneal layers. These features should always prompt examination with a PAS stain to search for fungal organisms. Elongated hyphae with septa formation and delicate parallel walls that stain brightly eosinophilic with a PAS stain confirm a diagnosis of superficial dermatophytosis.

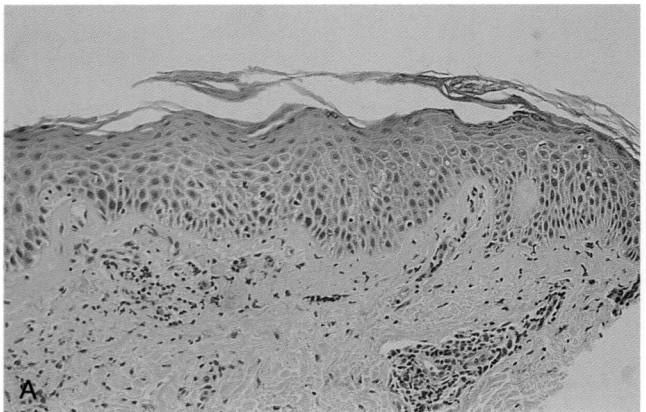 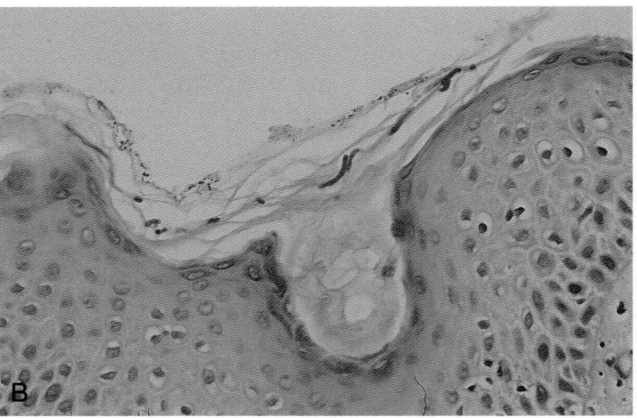

FIGURE 48-7. Dermatophytosis. *A.* This biopsy specimen shows mild spongiosis, slight epidermal hyperplasia, focal parakeratosis, and a superficial and interstitial mononuclear cell infiltrate. *B.* PAS stain reveals fungal forms. In some cases, the presence of neutrophils within parakecratosis is a histologic clue to diagnosis.

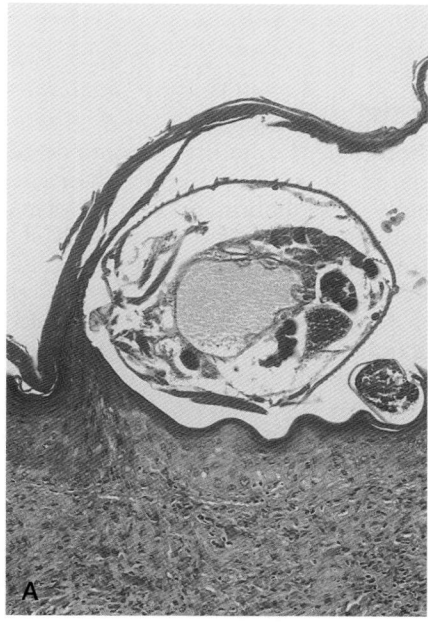

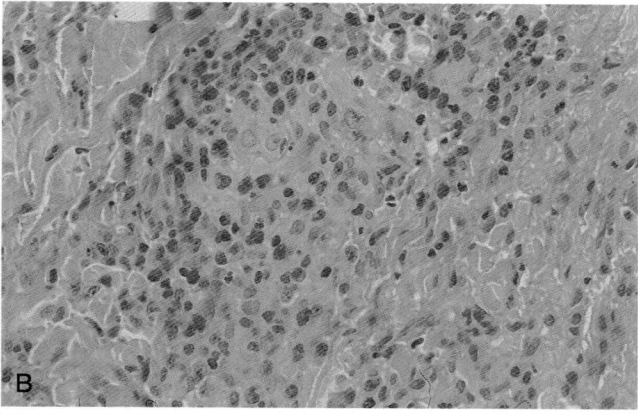

**FIGURE 48–8.** Scabies. *A.* Scabies infection was suspected clinically. Multiple levels revealed a single organism. An insect bite reaction could show similar histologic findings. *B.* The dermis of this biopsy specimen is remarkable for a perivascular and interstitial mononuclear cell infiltrate with numerous eosinophils. (Case courtesy of Dr. Margaret McGlaughlin, Boston, MA.)

## Arthropod Bite Reaction

Vesicles with spongiosis and occasionally eosinophilic exocytosis are commonly seen in cases of insect bite reactions. The dermis typically exhibits intense superficial and deep perivascular lymphocytic infiltrates, usually with eosinophils. Chronic bite reactions may be associated with a dense nodular lymphocytic infiltrate often accompanied by germinal center formation. Such patterns may be alarming and simulate a lymphoma (pseudolymphoma). In some cases, ancillary studies are needed to exclude this possibility.

The responses to arthropod bites and to mites vary and often represent an expression of delayed hypersensitivity. A spectrum of clinical lesions from urticaria to firm red nodules may be observed, depending on the response of the host. Some insect bites, especially those caused by fleas, mosquitoes, and bedbugs, result in clinical lesions called papular urticaria. These lesions are itchy, erythematous, urticarial papules distributed singly or multiply, depending on the number of bites on the body surface. Persistent lesions, which may be present for several weeks to even months, often result from the bites of mites or ticks. These lesions are large red nodules that are itchy and occasionally ulcerated.

The histology of arthropod bite reactions is highly variable. Urticarial lesions frequently show edema of the papillary dermis with sparse lymphocytes, extravasated red cells, and eosinophils scattered about the superficial vascular plexus. The epidermis may exhibit focal parakeratosis, spongiosis, and formation of vesicles.

In scabies, the organism is disposed in the subcorneal layer, and the epidermis exhibits psoriasiform hyperplasia. The superficial and deep dermis is involved by dense, perivascular to diffuse, nodular, polymorphous inflammatory infiltrates composed of lymphocytes, histiocytes, eosinophils, and plasma cells (Fig. 48–8).

In insect bite granulomas, or tick bite granulomas, the typical histology of the entry site of the insect is featured by psoriasiform epidermal hyperplasia with scale crust, neutrophilic exocytosis, or aggregation of neutrophils within the epidermis. Within the dermis, there is a dense, superficial and deep, perivascular lymphocytic infiltrate admixed with plasma cells and eosinophils. Endothelial proliferation is prominent. In some cases, extension of the inflammatory infiltrate into the subcutaneous fat and formation of lymphoid follicles with germinal centers mimicking a lymphomatous process may be observed.

Differentiation from a lymphoproliferative disorder is assisted by the presence of a polymorphous infiltrate composed of plasma cells and eosinophils in association with overlying pseudoepitheliomatous hyperplasia. In some cases, however, ancillary studies, such as immunohistochemical staining for $\kappa$ and $\lambda$ light chains, are needed for definitive diagnosis.

## Photoallergic Dermatitis

Photoallergic dermatitis is a form of allergic dermatitis that results from exposure of skin containing photosensitizing drugs or agents to ultraviolet light.[19] The eruption is an immunologically mediated delayed hypersensitivity response that is mounted after absorption of ultraviolet light. Most photoallergic eruptions are induced after topical contact with a sensitizing chemical; therefore, this form is also referred to as photocontact dermatitis. The drug or agent may also be administered orally or parenterally. Previous exposure to the agent is usually required. Early signs of eczematous eruption with erythema, papules, and occasional vesicles appear after an incubation period of 24 hours or more after exposure to ultraviolet light. The distribution of the rash predominantly involves sun-exposed areas but frequently extends to nonexposed areas. Cutaneous eruptions may continue to a subacute phase or even chronic phase, resulting in lichenification.

The histologic findings are variable and dependent on the stage of eruption. In the early phase, the epidermal changes are similar to those of acute allergic contact dermatitis with focal spongiosis, rare dyskeratosis, and exocytosis. The dermal infiltrate is composed of mononuclear cells and eosinophils predominantly involving the superficial vascular plexus, but they may extend to the midreticular or even deep vascular plexus. Endothelial cells may appear vacuolated and swollen. In the chronic phase, the epidermis shows acanthosis, hyperkeratosis, and hypergranulosis with fibrosis of the papillary dermis. Focal dyskeratosis and endothelial cell vacuolization may occur in any stage of the eruption and are helpful in making the diagnosis.

Actinic reticuloid is a chronic photosensitivity reaction predominantly affecting elderly men.[20] Both clinically and histologically, the involved skin may show many features similar to cutaneous T cell lymphoma. Patients initially present with erythema and edema only in sun-exposed areas. The skin becomes thickened with deep furrows as the disease progresses and also shows formation of papules, nodules, and plaques. In chronic cases, the lesions extend into unexposed areas and develop into generalized erythroderma. Localized and generalized lymphadenopathy may be present. Pruritus is characteristically severe. The eruption has been reported to resolve with complete skin protection from ultraviolet light.

The epidermis often shows psoriasiform hyperplasia with parakeratosis and hyperkeratosis. The dermal infiltrate is bandlike and predominantly involves the epidermis, but it may also diffusely involve the entire dermis or may be patchy and perivascular in distribution. The infiltrate is composed of lymphocytes, histiocytes, multinucleated giant cells, and eosinophils. The lymphoid cells may vary from normal to atypical, with hyperchromatic and hyperconvoluted nuclei. Small aggregates of atypical lymphocytes within the epidermis may resemble the Pautrier microabscesses seen in mycosis fungoides. One noticeable feature in any stage of the lesion, regardless of the degree of lymphocyte atypia, is the presence of histiocyte-like cells with stellate cytoplasmic processes oriented toward the epidermal surface. In facial lesions, a granulomatous component may be present within the infiltrate.

## Phototoxic Dermatitis

Phototoxic dermatitis results from an acute toxic exposure to ultraviolet light alone or in combination with a photosensitizing agent. The eruption usually occurs within a few hours of exposure. Common exogenous causative agents include sulfonamides, thiazides, phenothiazides, and griseofulvin. Topical agents, including psoralens and dyes, may also cause phototoxic dermatitis. Phototoxic reactions are characterized by sunburnlike erythema, edema, and occasionally vesiculation or bullae formation.[21] The rash involves sun-exposed areas with sharp demarcation from nonexposed areas. It usually presents less than 24 hours after exposure to light. Chronic exposure to topical agents, causing mild inflammatory reactions, may result in hyperpigmentation or hypopigmentation, atrophy, and telangiectasia.

Skin biopsy often shows prominent dyskeratosis and, in severe cases, necrosis and degeneration of the upper two thirds of the epidermis. Variable intercellular edema or vesicles are present. Vacuolization along the dermal-epidermal junction is characteristic. At times, keratinization of the basal layer may be observed. The papillary dermis is edematous and contains a variable perivascular mononuclear and neutrophilic infiltrate.

## Guttate (Small Plaque) Parapsoriasis

Parapsoriasis describes a group of several diverse dermatoses of unknown etiology, unresponsive to therapy, with a chronic clinical course. This group of disorders exhibits in common persistent, erythematous, scaling macules, papules, and plaques of various sizes. Guttate parapsoriasis, or small plaque parapsoriasis, represents one of the subtypes of parapsoriasis. Other variants are large plaque parapsoriasis and parapsoriasis variegata. Many authorities consider large plaque parapsoriasis to be a precursor lesion synonymous with early mycosis fungoides. Synonyms of guttate parapsoriasis include small plaque parapsoriasis, benign digitate dermatosis, and xanthoerythrodermia perstans.

Guttate parapsoriasis predominantly affects men and usually occurs after the age of 40 years. Clinical characteristics are multiple pink to yellow, slightly scaled, oval to elongated patches and ill-defined plaques occurring in parallel over the trunk or proximal thighs. The fine scale on the surface of the lesion often results in a wrinkled appearance resembling pityriasis rosea. The eruption is symmetric and infrequently involves the face, scalp, and distal extremities. The histologic changes are subtle and sometimes nonspecific. The epidermis is usually normal or slightly acanthotic with minimal to slight spongiosis and overlying mounds of parakeratosis and scale crust. The parakeratotic areas are elongated but discrete and described as lenticular in appearance. In the papillary dermis, there may be dilated lymphatics and a sparse perivascular lymphocytic infiltrate. The infiltrate focally extends into the epidermis. The lymphoid infiltrate is composed of CD4+ T cells. Clonal T cell populations have been demonstrated in some cases of guttate parapsoriasis.[22] Controversy still exists as to whether guttate parapsoriasis represents a precursor or an early stage of mycosis fungoides.[23, 24] The pathologic differential diagnosis includes pityriasis rosea, gyrate erythema, dermatophytosis, and mycosis fungoides.

## Psoriasis

Psoriasis, a common skin disorder, is characterized by erythematous papules with silvery white scales coalescing into sharply demarcated plaques.[25] The plaques characteristically involve the extensor surfaces, scalp, penis, and intertriginous areas. Scales become heaped up, and abrasive removal often exposes small bleeding points (Auspitz sign). At times, psoriasis may present in a generalized fashion or involve the total body surface in the form of an exfoliative dermatitis or so-called generalized erythroderma. Approximately 10% of the cases are associated with arthritis. A familial tendency has been documented.

A number of clinical variants have been described. Guttate psoriasis is often seen in children or young adults and is usually preceded by an upper respiratory tract infection. Lesions are characterized by small scaling papules that frequently resolve spontaneously. Inverse psoriasis predominantly involves the intertriginous areas and crural folds. Localized pustular psoriasis has a bilateral distribution and frequently affects the palms and soles. Generalized pustular psoriasis presents with widespread eruptions and is often associated with fever, generalized erythema, and toxicity. Psoriatic arthritis occurs in about 10% of cases. The patient is often seronegative for rheumatoid factor and presents with an asymmetric arthritis predominantly involving the interphalangeal joints and accompanied by severe nail changes, including onycholysis and punctate pitting of the nail plate.

The histologic picture of psoriasis is highly variable and dependent on the location, age of the lesion, and previous therapy.[26, 27] The early lesion, if biopsy is performed before 48 hours, shows slight irregular epidermal hyperplasia, patchy decrease in the granular cell layer, minimal hyperkeratosis, and sparse, irregularly parakeratotic scale (Fig. 48–9). The rete ridges appear plump, short, and irregularly spaced. Papillary dermal edema is present and may be associated with extravasated red blood cells. The epidermis shows spongiotic changes associated with lymphocytic and neutrophilic exocytosis. In subacute lesions, the rete ridges become markedly elongated and are regularly spaced (Fig. 48–10). Significant spongiosis associated with neutrophils is evident within the epidermis. The granular cell layer is decreased at sites of parakeratosis. The dermal papillae become bulbous secondary to edema, the presence of ectatic capillaries, and infiltration by neutrophils, lymphocytes, and histiocytes. In fully established lesions, the rete ridges are uniformly elongated and club shaped and may show fusion in their lower portions. The papillary dermis is markedly widened and contains ectatic, tortuous capillaries with a sparse mononuclear cell infiltrate. Thinning of the suprapapillary plate is noted. Microabscesses, composed of collections of neutrophils, form in the upper zone of the spinous layer and are referred to as spongiform pustules. The spongiform pustules, as they transgress the stratum corneum, are referred to as Munro microabscesses. The granular cell layer is decreased, especially in areas with overlying parakeratosis. Early lesions in guttate psoriasis show only minimal epidermal hyperplasia. The granular cell layer is preserved. Foci of spongiform pustules with neutrophils are present both below and within the stratum corneum, where they are admixed with the parakeratotic scales. The papillary dermis is edematous with ectatic capillaries, sparse dermal infiltrates, and extravasation of red blood cells.

The histologic differential diagnosis includes chronic eczematous dermatitis, seborrheic dermatitis, pityriasis rubra pilaris, cutaneous dermatophytosis, mycosis fungoides, and secondary syphilis. All cases showing psoriasiform dermatitis and parakeratosis associated with neutrophils should be carefully evaluated for fungal infection by use of a PAS stain. A definitive diagnosis of psoriasis should be rendered only after fungal infection has been excluded.

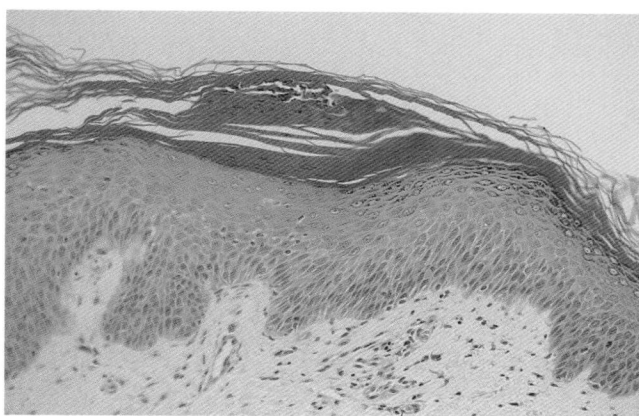

**FIGURE 48–9.** Early psoriasis. The biopsy specimen shows mild irregular epidermal hyperplasia with overlying hyperkeratosis associated with discrete areas of parakeratosis admixed with neutrophils.

## Lichen Simplex Chronicus and Prurigo Nodularis

Lichen simplex chronicus is characterized by pruritic, disklike or oval, well-circumscribed hyperkeratotic plaques secondary to repeated rubbing and scratching. The skin is markedly thickened. These lesions commonly occur on the back of the neck and on the shins, but they may occur in any area where patients scratch or rub their skin. The skin markings

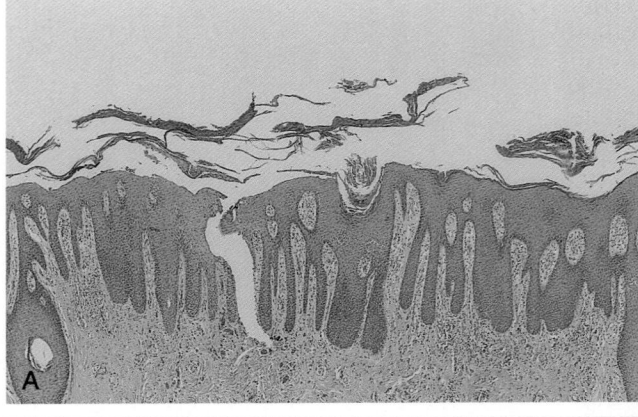

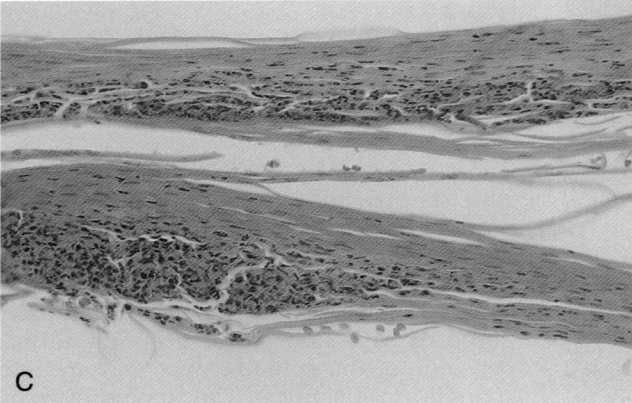

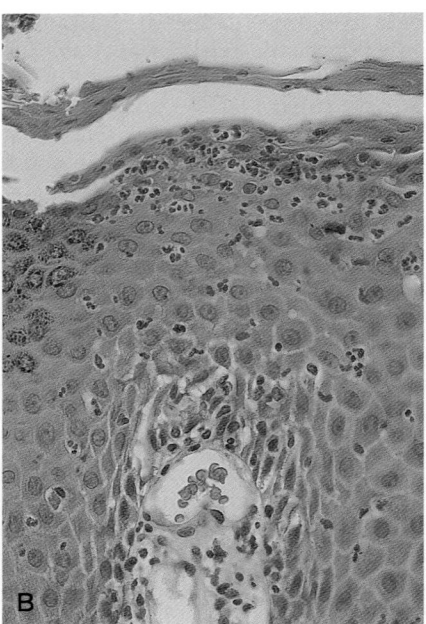

**FIGURE 48–10.** Psoriasis. *A.* Biopsy specimen of a well-developed psoriatic plaque shows regular psoriasiform epidermal hyperplasia. High magnification reveals spongiform intraepidermal pustules. *B,* so-called Munro microabscesses and parakeratosis with neutrophils (C).

are within the background of hyperkeratosis; this clinical finding is referred to as lichenification.

A localized hyperkeratotic nodule resulting from chronic irritation presenting predominantly on the extremities characterizes prurigo nodularis. Lesions of prurigo nodularis may be multiple and are firm, dome-shaped nodules ranging from 1 to 3 cm. The lesions are sometimes covered by a thickened keratotic scale.

The histologic picture of lichen simplex chronicus is that of chronic eczematous dermatitis. The findings include irregular psoriasiform epidermal hyperplasia characterized by hyperkeratosis and prominent hypergranulosis (Fig. 48–11). The rete ridges are irregular in length, size, and shape; some appear clublike and others are pointed. On occasion, residual spongiosis is noted, but vesicle formation is absent. The papillary dermis shows fibrosis with collagen bundles arranged in vertical streaks perpendicular to the epidermis. There are mild to moderate superficial perivascular dermal infiltrates composed predominantly of lymphoid cells with scattered eosinophils. Proliferation of cutaneous nerves with perineurial and endoneurial fibrosis has been described. These changes are especially prominent in lesions of atopic dermatitis. Superimposed epidermal changes, including ulceration, erosion, parakera-

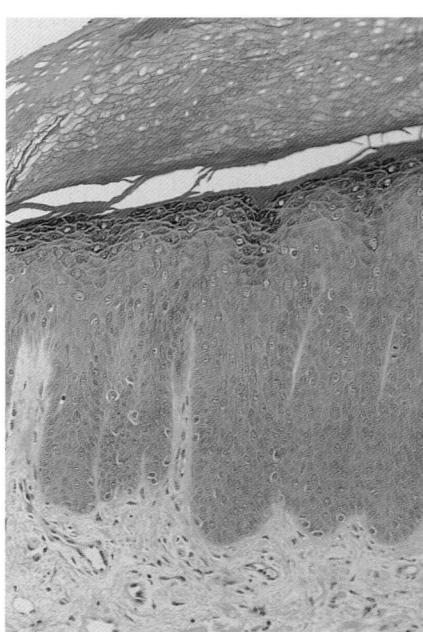

**FIGURE 48–11.** Lichen simplex chronicus. The biopsy specimen shows psoriasiform hyperplasia with hypergranulosis and dense hyperkeratosis. In contrast to psoriasis, the papillae are fibrotic and narrowed compared with the bulbous papillae of the psoriatic lesion.

tosis, and scale crust formation secondary to trauma and manipulation, are frequently seen in lichen simplex chronicus.

In prurigo nodularis, the degree of hyperkeratosis and epidermal hyperplasia with elongation of the rete ridges oriented toward the center of the lesion is more striking.[28] Lesions may be ulcerated. The papillary dermis is often fibrotic, and there may be associated neural proliferation and perineurial fibrosis. Increased numbers of eosinophils may be present within the dermal infiltrate.[29]

Lichen simplex chronicus and prurigo nodularis are reaction patterns to scratching and rubbing and do not represent discrete disease entities. Once a diagnosis of lichen simplex chronicus or prurigo nodularis has been rendered, the pathologist should search for clues to an underlying disorder. For example, careful scrutiny frequently reveals epidermal spongiosis, indicative of an associated eczematous dermatitis.

## Exfoliative Dermatitis (Erythroderma)

Exfoliative dermatitis is a generalized erythematous, scaling eruption that involves the entire cutaneous surface. It represents a secondary reactive process of the skin to an underlying systemic disease or is the result of progression of a skin disorder.[30] In approximately 25% of cases, the etiology is unknown. Examples of systemic diseases that may result in erythroderma are leukemia, mycosis fungoides, Sézary syndrome, and other lymphomas. Primary skin disorders that may be associated with erythroderma include psoriasis, seborrheic dermatitis, drug eruption, allergic contact dermatitis, stasis dermatitis, atopic dermatitis, pityriasis rubra pilaris, pemphigus foliaceus, sarcoidosis, and ichthyosiform erythroderma. The skin appears erythematous and scaly, accompanied by desquamation of fine to large sheets of keratinous scales. Distribution is generalized and includes palms and soles. Excess heat loss may result in chilliness and shivering. Patients may also have fever (especially if there is superimposed systemic and cutaneous infection), lymphadenopathy, alopecia, nail changes, or gynecomastia.

The histologic diagnosis of erythroderma may be challenging, and a definitive diagnosis cannot be rendered in a significant number of cases.[31] It is important to select a site of biopsy that includes a primary lesion that is not altered by secondary changes or at least a more palpable area in the midst of the reddish skin. In most cases, the biopsy specimen shows variable degrees of psoriasiform epidermal hyperplasia with diffuse epidermal edema.[32] Hyperkeratosis and irregular parakeratosis are usually detectable after erythema has been present for more than 2 weeks. The dermis is often edematous, containing large dilated capillaries and venules accompanied by a sparse to moderate inflammatory lymphoid infiltrate. The presence of bulbous papillae and small spongiform pustules leads to a diagnosis of psoriasis. In drug-induced erythroderma, eosinophils are frequently present within the edematous dermis. Atypical lymphoid cells in a bandlike distribution with significant epidermotropism and papillary dermal fibrosis suggests mycosis fungoides or Sézary syndrome. Thus, careful inspection of multiple levels is important.

Careful clinicopathologic correlation is needed to render a specific diagnosis. A complete medical evaluation with careful clinical history and physical examination, together with skin biopsy (and often other investigative procedures), are necessary to arrive at a specific diagnosis. Not uncommonly, multiple biopsies are needed to render a specific diagnosis. Sites of preexisting skin lesions are frequently most informative and should be sought for evaluation by biopsy. For example, biopsies of lesions on the extensor surfaces may reveal psoriasis; plaques in the antecubital and popliteal fossae may reveal changes of atopic eczema; and randomly scattered plaques may show mycosis fungoides. Furthermore, examination of several lesions with different clinical appearances may also be helpful.

## Pityriasis Rubra Pilaris

Pityriasis rubra pilaris is a rare cutaneous disorder characterized by a generalized erythematous scaling eruption, widespread follicular horny papules, and in most cases, hyperkeratosis of palms and soles.[33] Pityriasis rubra pilaris often starts on the scalp and face with diffuse erythema and scaling, simulating features of seborrheic dermatitis. The hallmark of this disease is the presence of fine, tapered, hyperkeratotic, follicular papules that usually begin on the dorsal aspects of the hands, especially over the fingers. The entire body may eventually become involved. Sharply demarcated, salmon-pink plaques with fine scales are characteristic. Coalescence of plaques in severe cases results in erythroderma, and the persistence of discrete areas of uninvolved skin on a background of erythroderma is characteristic of pityriasis rubra pilaris. The palms and soles are covered by thick hyperkeratotic scales and may be complicated by painful fissuring. Pruritus is often severe. In addition to the more common acquired type with adult onset, a familial variant with an early onset in infancy and childhood has been described.[34]

Early lesions show changes of psoriasiform epidermal hyperplasia with focal parakeratosis and hyperkeratosis (Fig. 48–12). Parakeratosis and hyperkeratosis alternate both vertically and horizontally within the stratum corneum. A collarette of parakeratosis around the follicular ostia is a common feature. Another helpful finding is the presence of a hyperkeratotic follicular plug containing remnants of hair shafts. Liquefactive degeneration of the basal cell layer is often noted. Acantholytic, dyskeratotic

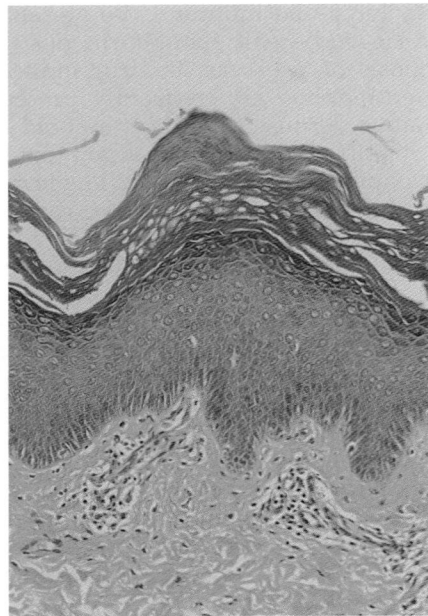

**FIGURE 48–12.** Pityriasis rubra pilaris. Mild irregular epidermal hyperplasia with alternating zones of vertical hyperkeratosis and linear parakeratosis is characteristic. Focal acantholysis of the granular cell layer is a characteristic finding when present.

foci are commonly found; they are usually less than 100 μm in thickness. In the dermis, the inflammatory infiltrate is typically minimal or sparse and is composed predominantly of lymphocytes with occasional eosinophils and neutrophils in a superficial perivascular distribution.[35]

The histologic differential diagnosis includes psoriasis, seborrheic dermatitis, subacute and chronic eczematous dermatitis, dermatophytosis, and keratosis pilaris. When the acantholytic, dyskeratotic foci are extensive, a bullous disorder may be considered. Immunofluorescence and clinical and pathologic correlation help in resolving the diagnosis.

## Lamellar Ichthyosis

Lamellar ichthyosis is a congenital disorder characterized by generalized, broad, grayish brown scales and variable background erythema.[36] Lamellar ichthyosis is usually present at birth or shortly thereafter. In some cases, the fetus is encased in a "collodion" membrane that sheds in several days. Later, the body is covered by large, white to brown scales that occasionally form thick, horny plaques. The flexural areas are most commonly affected. The palms and soles are always affected, varying from hyperkeratosis with increased skin markings to development of keratoderma.

The epidermis shows psoriasiform hyperplasia, variable papillomatosis, compact hyperkeratosis, and patchy parakeratosis. The granular cell layer is normal or increased in thickness (Fig. 48–13). A sparse chronic perivascular lymphocytic infiltrate is present

within the superficial dermis. The prominent granular cell layer and epidermal hyperplasia distinguish this entity from ichthyosis vulgaris that typically exhibits loss of the granular cell layer and often a thinned epidermis.[37] X-linked ichthyosis has a similar histologic appearance but usually exhibits focal parakeratosis and a more prominent perivascular infiltrate. The histologic differential diagnosis encompasses other forms of ichthyosis, including ichthyosis vulgaris, X-linked ichthyosis, and acanthosis nigricans.

## Necrolytic Migratory Erythema

Necrolytic migratory erythema is a cutaneous eruption associated with a glucagon-secreting α cell tumor of the pancreas. Characteristic clinical findings are weight loss, diabetes mellitus, anemia, and stomatitis.[38] The usual age of patients is between 40 and 70 years. The eruption is intensely pruritic and has a predilection for the lower extremities, lower abdomen, intertriginous areas, perioral areas, and face. The initial presentation is frequently an enlarging erythematous, often gyrate patch that may progress to plaques with erosions and blisters. Scale crust after rupture of blisters may be seen. The periphery has a characteristic double scale. Hyperpigmentation often remains after the lesion has resolved. Necrolytic migratory erythema may also be seen without the glucagonoma syndrome.[39]

The histologic picture varies with the age of the lesion. In early lesions, the epidermis shows abnormal maturation of the granular cell layer and the

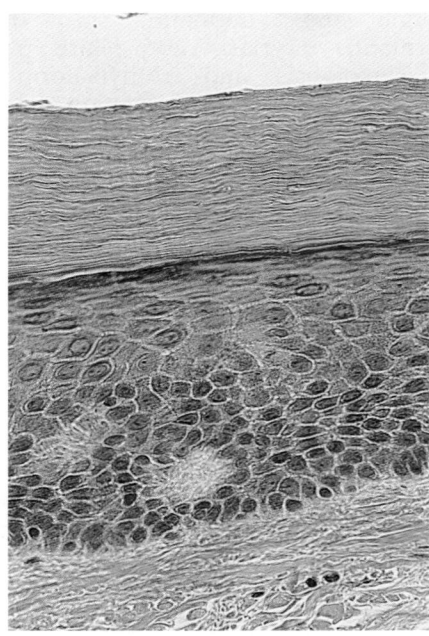

**FIGURE 48–13.** Lamellar ichthyosis. The findings are dense compact hyperkeratosis and increased granular cell layer with a normal to slightly hyperplastic epidermis. Variable parakeratosis may be observed, as in this case.

upper malpighian layer, resulting in dyskeratosis of keratinocytes in formation of subcorneal vesicles. The abrupt dyskeratosis within a subcorneal vesicle results in shedding of keratinocytes into the blister cavity. Other features include pallor of the upper epidermis due to intracellular edema and the presence of neutrophils within the epidermis and the superficial dermis.[40] In more established lesions, there is psoriasiform epidermal hyperplasia with hyperkeratosis and parakeratosis. The dermis shows a sparse neutrophilic and lymphocytic infiltrate around the superficial vascular plexus.

The histologic differential diagnosis includes psoriasis, impetiginized subacute spongiotic dermatitis, pellagra, acrodermatitis enteropathica, candidiasis, subcorneal pustular dermatosis, and staphylococcal scalded skin syndrome.

## Pellagra

Pellagra is a chronic generalized disorder secondary to niacin deficiency. It is characterized by dermatitis, dementia, and often diarrhea. The skin lesions are often the initial presentation of the disease. One theory postulates that the clinical manifestations of the disease are the result of increased extracellular matrix viscosity.[41] The rash begins as erythematous patches involving the sun-exposed areas of the body, such as the face, neck, forearm, and dorsal surface of the hands. It may progress to formation of blisters, ulceration, exudation, and superinfection. In chronic cases, the skin becomes thickened with hyperkeratosis, scaling, and hyperpigmentation.

Biopsy reveals psoriasiform epidermal hyperplasia associated with intracellular edema of the keratinocytes of the upper layer of the epidermis. Pallor is noted in the upper layers of the epidermis that abut the underlying, normal-appearing keratinocytes. The stratum corneum is thickened, with confluent parakeratosis. Vesicles and bullae, when present, are either intraepidermal or subepidermal in location. In the dermis, a superficial perivascular lymphocytic infiltrate is present. The histologic differential diagnosis includes necrolytic migratory erythema and acrodermatitis enteropathica.

## Acrodermatitis Enteropathica

Acrodermatitis enteropathica is a systemic disorder usually presenting in infants who have zinc deficiency.[42] Features of this entity are cutaneous eruptions, diarrhea, failure to thrive, irritability, photophobia, and ultimately death if it is untreated. The skin eruption frequently presents as an eczematous process with erosions and blistering affecting the hands, feet, neck, and perineal and facial areas. Alopecia often occurs. With time, the lesions evolve to form psoriasiform plaques.

Biopsy of early lesions reveals loss of the granular cell layer and focal distinct slight pallor of the

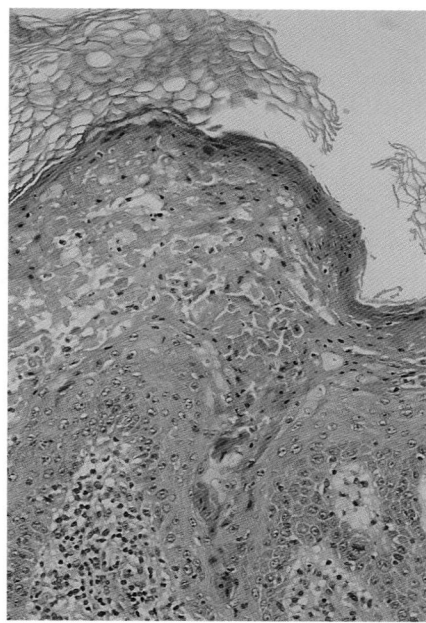

**FIGURE 48–14.** Acrodermatitis enteropathica. The biopsy specimen shows irregular psoriasiform and slightly papillomatous epidermal hyperplasia. A striking finding is epidermal pallor; necrosis (ballooning degeneration) spares the lower layers of the epidermis. Similar histologic findings may be seen in pellagra and glucagonoma syndrome.

upper layer of the epidermis (Fig. 48–14). In more advanced stages, the epidermis shows psoriasiform hyperplasia with confluent parakeratosis and hyperkeratosis. In addition, ballooning degeneration and necrosis of keratinocytes may be seen in established lesions. Bullous skin lesions have also been described.[43] The histologic differential diagnosis mainly includes necrolytic migratory erythema and pellagra.

## Inflammatory Linear Verrucous Epidermal Nevus

Inflammatory linear epidermal nevus is a hamartomatous overgrowth of skin, frequently in a linear and unilateral distribution.[44] The inflammatory linear verrucous epidermal nevus is a pruritic verrucous or excoriated plaque that often involves the lower extremities, buttock, or genitalia of females. The plaque is frequently linear and may extend along the entire length of an extremity, particularly the leg.

Biopsy shows psoriasiform hyperplasia of the epidermis, hyperkeratosis, and papillomatosis. A characteristic finding is confluent or patchy parakeratosis overlying areas of hypogranulosis, alternating with foci of orthokeratosis overlying zones of epidermis with an intact granular cell layer (Fig. 48–15). A mild perivascular lymphocytic infiltrate associated with ectatic vessels is present in the dermis. The histologic differential diagnosis includes psoriasis, lichen simplex chronicus, and porokeratosis.[45]

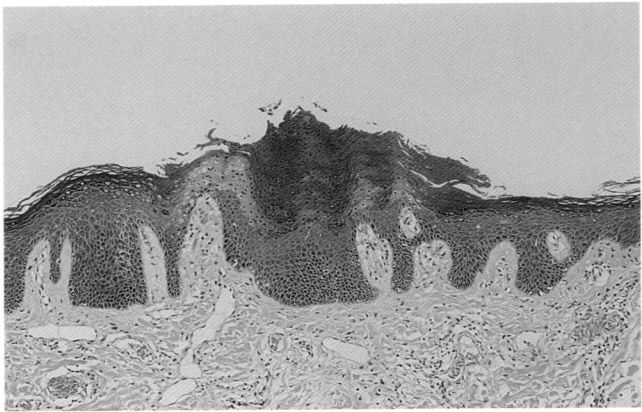

**FIGURE 48-15.** Inflammatory linear verrucous epidermal nevus. The biopsy specimen shows psoriasiform and papillomatous hyperplasia of the epidermis and hyperkeratosis alternating with parakeratosis. Variable inflammation accompanies these changes.

## Lichen Striatus

Lichen striatus is a unilateral, linear, self-limited skin eruption usually affecting the extremities in children. It is an eruption of acute onset and is characterized by erythematous, discrete, lichenoid papules coalescing into linear bands. The lesion often occurs unilaterally and most commonly affects the upper extremities of children. Spontaneous resolution is the usual clinical course.

The histopathologic features are highly variable.[46] The epidermis frequently shows hyperkeratosis, patchy parakeratosis, irregular psoriasiform epidermal hyperplasia, and focal spongiosis with exocytosis. There are scattered eosinophilic, dyskeratotic keratinocytes within the stratum malpighii. Focal vacuolar degeneration of the basal cell layer is present. The dermal perivascular lymphohistiocytic infiltrate predominantly involves the upper and midreticular dermis. The histologic differential diagnosis is mainly with inflammatory linear verrucous epidermal nevus and pityriasis lichenoides.

## Secondary Syphilis

Syphilis is a sexually transmitted disease caused by the spirochete *Treponema pallidum*. Untreated syphilis may progress through three stages. After an incubation period of 2 to 3 weeks, the primary stage is characterized by a painless ulcer (chancre) at the initial site of infection. The primary lesion may last 2 to 6 weeks or longer. The secondary stage is characterized by cutaneous involvement and lymphadenopathy lasting 6 weeks to 6 months. Late or tertiary syphilis develops in approximately one third of untreated patients and is characterized by cutaneous, cardiovascular, and central nervous system lesions.

The clinical appearance of secondary syphilis is notorious for mimicking other inflammatory skin conditions. In general, cutaneous lesions in secondary syphilis consist of scaling macules, papules, papulosquamous lesions, pustules, and nodules involving the trunk and the extremities symmetrically, including the palms and soles. Moist papules are present on the oral and genital mucosa. A characteristic "moth-eaten" pattern of alopecia may be seen. Other clinical variants include papular eruption in the anus producing condylomata, a diffuse erythematous exanthem (roseolar form), and in occasional cases, annular and circinate lesions. Late secondary lesions are scattered copper-colored or purple nodules.

Just as the clinical manifestations of syphilis may mimic other disorders, so too may syphilis mimic other diseases on histologic examination. The most typical histologic finding in secondary syphilis is a superficial and deep perivascular lymphohistiocytic infiltrate containing plasma cells surrounding prominent, hypertrophic endothelial cells.[47, 48] The epidermis shows psoriasiform hyperplasia with overlying parakeratosis, scale crust, and hyperkeratosis. Neutrophils are often present within the epidermis and may form small abscesses. Neutrophilic debris is common superficially. The dermal-epidermal junction is often obscured by the dermal infiltrate, which in some cases shows a lichenoid pattern. Silver stains may reveal spirochetes in the epidermis and around the blood vessels. Late secondary syphilis exhibits extensive infiltration of the dermis by lymphocytes, lymphoblastic cells, plasma cells, and eosinophils admixed with scattered epithelioid granulomas and may resemble a florid drug eruption or an insect bite granuloma.[49] The presence of plasma cells around vessels and endothelial cell swelling suggest a diagnosis of lues.

## Pustular Psoriasis

Pustular psoriasis generally occurs against the background of well-established psoriasis and presents as an eruption of pustules on erythematous skin, often originating in the hands and feet.[50] The eruptions are often associated with fever and chills. In the healing phase, the lesions resemble those of psoriasis. Acrodermatitis continua of Hallopeau and impetigo herpetiformis are probably variants of pustular psoriasis. Acrodermatitis continua is localized on the hands and feet but can occasionally disseminate. Impetigo herpetiformis is associated with hypocalcemia and may occur after removal of parathyroid glands or in the course of pregnancy.

In both localized and generalized pustular psoriasis, the characteristic features are spongiform pustules of Kogoj and neutrophilic exocytosis in the upper stratum malpighii.[51] The pustules vary in size from small micropustules to unilocular large, subcorneal, leukocyte-filled macropustules. Overlying the pustules is a hyperkeratotic stratum corneum with parakeratosis and collections of neutrophils. Elongation of the rete ridges is present but is often less pronounced than in psoriasis vulgaris. The dermis shows dilated blood vessels and an inflammatory infiltrate composed of both neutrophils and lymphocytes. The histologic differential diagnosis includes subcorneal pustular dermatosis, candidiasis, impetigo, and keratoderma blennorrhagicum.

## Keratoderma Blennorrhagicum (Reiter's Disease)

Reiter's disease consists of a classic triad of urethritis, arthritis, and conjunctivitis.[52] Characteristic lesions, usually on the soles of the feet and referred to as keratoderma blennorrhagicum, are thickened, crusted, scaling yellow papules and vesicles with an erythematous base. Other areas of the body, such as the fingers, toes, penis, and trunk, may also be involved. The urethritis is mucoid or mucopurulent. The arthritis is usually polyarticular, with some symmetric joint involvement. Sacroiliac joints are often affected. The conjunctivitis is mild, transient, and nonspecific. Approximately one third of patients will show painless oral lesions. Mild carditis, conduction defects, aortitis, and aortic insufficiency have been noted in approximately 10% of cases.

The distinctive histologic feature is the spongiform pustule, which may be seen in the oral, cutaneous, and penile lesions. On the penis, the lesion is referred to as balanitis circinata. The spongiform pustule is composed of a network of retained cell walls and damaged epidermal cells infiltrated by neutrophils. As micropustules enlarge with increased accumulation of neutrophils, they coalesce to form large subcorneal macropustules. The epidermis shows psoriasiform hyperplasia and overlying hyperkeratosis and parakeratosis.

The histologic differential diagnosis includes pustular psoriasis, subcorneal pustular dermatosis, candidiasis, and impetigo. Distinction between psoriasis and keratoderma blennorrhagicum may be impossible on the basis of histologic findings alone.[53] As with psoriasis, a diagnosis of keratoderma blennorrhagicum is made only after careful clinicopathologic correlation and the exclusion of fungal infection by special stains.

## Subcorneal Pustular Dermatosis (Sneddon-Wilkinson Disease)

Subcorneal pustular dermatosis is a chronic asymptomatic relapsing pustular eruption that affects the trunk, groin, and axilla and tends to spare the extremities and the face.[54] The pustules are sterile and tend to be grouped and flaccid; they are often arranged in an annular or serpiginous fashion. The oral mucosa is often spared.

The histologic picture shows significant overlap with pustular psoriasis, leading some authorities to propose that these conditions may be related. The epidermis shows mild irregular psoriasiform hyper-

plasia. Within the epidermis, there is neutrophilic exocytosis with collections of neutrophils in the subcorneal layer. In general, acantholysis, spongiform pustules, and underlying epidermal changes are absent. The dermal infiltrate is composed of neutrophils, eosinophils, and lymphocytes.

The histologic differential diagnosis includes pustular psoriasis, Reiter's syndrome, impetigo, candidiasis, pemphigus foliaceus, and pemphigus erythematosus. As with pustular psoriasis and Reiter's syndrome, fungal infection should be excluded before a diagnosis is rendered.

## INTERFACE DERMATITIS

Interface dermatitis refers to a group of disorders that share in common inflammation along the dermal-epidermal interface. There are two major categories of interface dermatitis, lichenoid interface dermatitis and vacuolar interface dermatitis. Lichenoid interface dermatitis is characterized by a dense band of lymphocytes in the superficial papillary dermis. Vacuolar interface dermatitis refers to a cell-poor interface dermatitis characterized by sparse inflammation at the dermal-epidermal junction associated with the development of vacuoles in the basal cell layer.

## Lichen Planus

Lichen planus is characterized by purple, pruritic, flat-topped papules and plaques. Lesions are most commonly seen on the flexor surfaces of the extremities. Careful examination of the papules and plaques reveals a white netlike pattern, referred to as Wickham striae. The mucous membranes of the mouth are frequently involved, and genitalia may also be involved.[55] Mucosal sites characteristically show a delicate white, lacelike pattern. Lichen planus may demonstrate the Koebner phenomenon, a phenomenon defined by the occurrence of new lesions at the site of minor trauma. A commonly encountered example is the development of a linear arrangement of lesions secondary to vigorous scratching. Lichen planus may preferentially involve hair follicles (lichen planopilaris) in some patients and is an important cause of alopecia. Rarely, a lichen planus–like picture (clinically and histologically) develops as a contact dermatitis to CD-2 color developer.

Biopsy of lichen planus reveals characteristic histologic features. The epidermis shows hyperkeratosis and variable atrophy or acanthosis. The basal cell layer is destroyed by a dense lichenoid (bandlike) infiltrate composed mainly of lymphocytes (Fig. 48–16). The epidermis typically shows hypergranulosis in a wedge-shaped pattern. The combination of destruction of the basal cell layer and the lichenoid tissue reaction creates a "sawtooth" silhouette of the epidermis. Separation between the epidermis and

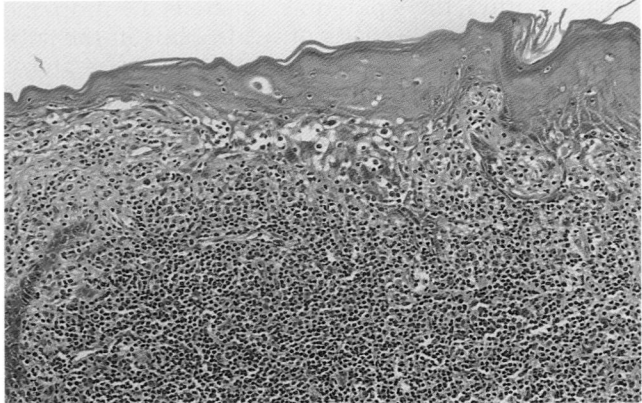

**FIGURE 48–16.** Lichen planus. This biopsy specimen of lichen planus reveals hyperkeratosis with an attenuated epidermis and ridges with a sawtooth pattern densely infiltrated by lymphocytes. The dense bandlike infiltrate is characteristic.

the underlying lichenoid infiltrate frequently produces clefts known as Max-Joseph spaces. A characteristic feature of lichen planus involving skin is the homogeneous lymphoid infiltrate. In general, plasma cells, neutrophils, and eosinophils are absent. When a mixed infiltrate is present, other causes of a lichenoid tissue reaction should be investigated, including lichenoid keratosis and lichenoid drug eruption. In addition, parakeratosis is rarely seen in lichen planus involving skin. Lichen planus involving mucosal sites may show parakeratosis and frequently shows a mixed inflammatory infiltrate, particularly including scattered plasma cells. Lichen planopilaris or lichen planus involving hair follicles shows changes similar to those seen in lichen planus involving the epidermis. Lichen planopilaris may involve the hair follicle alone, or it may involve the hair follicle in addition to the surrounding epidermis.[56] Lichen planus–like contact allergic reactions include eosinophils resembling a lichenoid drug eruption (see infra).

## Lichenoid Keratosis (Lichen Planus–like Keratosis)

Lichenoid keratosis typically occurs as a single lesion on the trunk or extremities of middle-aged to elderly adults. Lichenoid keratosis is more common in women than in men. The lesion is often an erythematous or pearly flat-topped papule and is frequently mistaken for basal cell carcinoma. On occasion, several lesions are present; however, usually only a single lesion appears. When multiple lesions are present, lichen planus must be excluded.

Like lichen planus, lichenoid keratosis is characterized by a lichenoid inflammatory response.[57] In contrast with lichen planus, however, a mixed inflammatory infiltrate with occasional eosinophils or plasma cells or parakeratosis may be seen. Careful inspection of the lateral aspect of the lesion fre-

quently reveals a subtle epidermal proliferation with features suggestive of early seborrheic keratosis. Lesions with significant squamous dysplasia arising in sun-damaged skin are often designated lichenoid actinic keratosis.

## Lichen Nitidus

Lichen nitidus is an uncommon lichenoid tissue reaction characterized by discrete 1- to 2-mm skin-colored to pink papules that are most commonly located on the genitalia and acral skin. Children are most commonly affected. This disease resolves spontaneously.

Low-power examination reveals a characteristic histologic pattern with a nodular superficial aggregate of mononuclear cells in the superficial papillary dermis, spanning only 1 or 2 mm (Fig. 48–17). Early lesions are composed predominantly of lymphocytes and occasional histiocytes. As lesions progress, histiocytes become more numerous. Late-stage lesions are composed predominantly of a granulomatous infiltrate. The epidermis frequently shows epidermal acanthosis at the edge of the inflammatory infiltrate, creating the so-called ball and claw effect. Compared with lichen planus, lichen nitidus demonstrates less vacuolization and necrosis of basal keratocytes. The clinical and pathologic features are distinctive; therefore, diagnosis is rarely difficult.[58]

## Lichenoid Drug Reaction

A lichenoid tissue reaction may be associated with exposure to various drugs and chemicals, such as gold, thiazide diuretics, antimalarials (chloroquine, quinidine), streptomycin, penicillamine, and arsenic.[59] Lichenoid drug eruptions frequently show papules and plaques that closely resemble lichen planus. Compared with other drug hypersensitivity

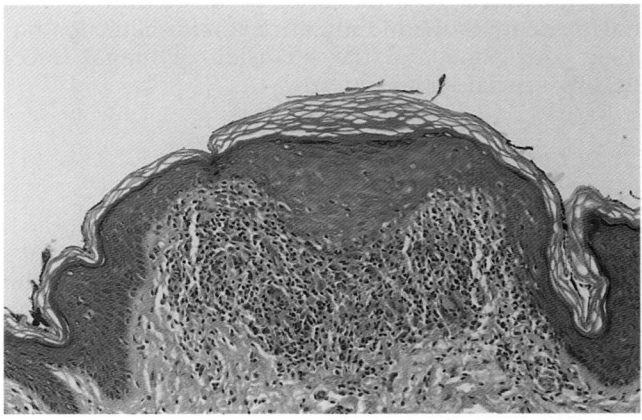

**FIGURE 48–17.** Lichen nitidus. The characteristic finding in lichen nitidus is a circumscribed lichenoid infiltrate that spans only one to a few rete ridges. Composite inflammation contains variable numbers of lymphocytes, mononuclear cells, giant cells, and even neutrophils.

reactions, lichenoid drug eruptions frequently occur many months after initiation of drug therapy. Lichenoid drug eruptions resemble lichen planus at low-power magnification. However, clues that a lichenoid tissue reaction represents a lichenoid drug eruption include parakeratosis; normal or diminished granular cell layer; and mixed inflammatory infiltrate including plasma cells, eosinophils, or neutrophils and infiltrate involving the mid to deep dermal vascular plexus. There is also a mid-dermal and sometimes a deep perivenular lymphoeosinophilic infiltrate. Nevertheless, careful clinicopathologic correlation and investigation for a history of drug ingestion are needed to establish a definitive diagnosis.

## Erythema Multiforme and Toxic Epidermal Necrolysis

Erythema multiforme is characterized by targetoid lesions, most often on the hands and feet, but they may be widespread. The targetoid pattern results from a dusky center surrounded by an outer erythematous ring. Central vesicle formation is common. Mucosal surfaces are frequently involved, and Stevens-Johnson syndrome is a term often applied to cases with extensive mucous membrane involvement with systemic symptoms.[60] Patients with Stevens-Johnson syndrome may also develop conjunctivitis. Some authorities consider toxic epidermal necrolysis to represent an extreme form of erythema multiforme characterized by widespread erythema, extensive blistering, and erosions.[61] It is controversial whether toxic epidermal necrolysis represents a separate entity or a form of erythema multiforme. They are considered together here because they often show histologic overlap.

Classic erythema multiforme is frequently associated with infection; the most common offending organisms are herpes simplex viruses or mycoplasmas, although other viral, fungal, and bacterial infections have also been documented. Drugs, most commonly sulfonamides, penicillin, barbiturates, contraceptives, and trimethoprim-sulfamethoxazole, may also be associated with erythema multiforme.[62] No etiology is identified in approximately half the cases.

Toxic epidermal necrolysis, in contrast to classic erythema multiforme, is nearly always associated with drug ingestion. Commonly associated drugs are sulfonamides, anticonvulsive agents, nonsteroidal anti-inflammatory agents, and allopurinol.[63-65]

Erythema multiforme is the prototypical vacuolar interface dermatitis. A sparse to moderate lymphocytic infiltrate around the superficial vascular plexuses and along the dermal-epidermal junction in association with vacuolar change and keratinocyte necrosis (dyskeratosis) is characteristic (Fig. 48-18). As the lesions progress, full-thickness epidermal necrosis becomes apparent. In well-developed lesions, extensive vacuolar degeneration leads to vesicle for-

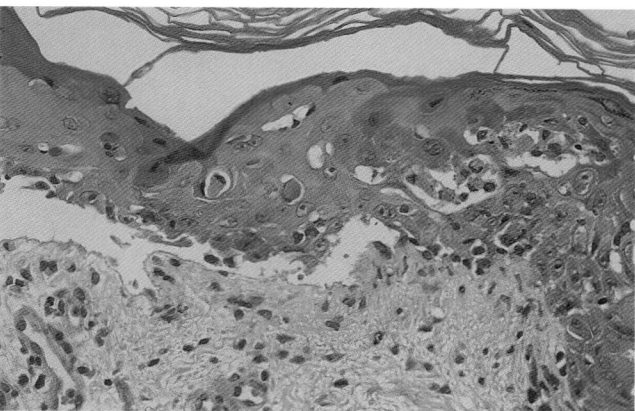

**FIGURE 48-18.** Erythema multiforme. Interface dermatitis with vacuolar change, dyskeratosis, and separation of the epidermis, resulting in subepidermal vesicle formation.

mation. Many cases that are clinically classified as toxic epidermal necrolysis show identical histologic findings; however, in general, toxic epidermal necrolysis is characterized by full-thickness epidermal necrosis associated with a sparser interface dermatitis.

## Graft-Versus-Host Disease

Approximately 50% to 70% of patients who have received HLA-matched allogeneic bone marrow transplants develop a widespread or localized macular erythematous rash due to donor T lymphocyte–mediated reactions to host tissue.[66-69] Immunocompromised patients may also develop graft-versus-host disease after transfusion of nonirradiated blood products or transplantation of solid tissue.[70] The clinical finding of a widespread macular erythematous rash, particularly involving the acral regions, in a bone transplant recipient is suggestive but not diagnostic of graft-versus-host disease. Graft-versus-host disease is most common between 10 days and 2 months after bone marrow transplantation.

The histopathologic findings of acute graft-versus-host disease are those of a vacuolar interface dermatitis. A minimal to moderately dense lymphocytic infiltrate along the dermal-epidermal junction is seen as "tagging" of lymphocytes (Fig. 48-19). Epidermal alteration, ranging from vacuolar degeneration to focal dyskeratosis associated with epidermal maturation disarray, is found. In extreme cases, extensive epidermal necrosis is seen. A characteristic but nonspecific finding is the presence of lymphocytes surrounding dyskeratotic squamous cells (so-called satellitosis or satellite cell necrosis). Furthermore, dermal appendage structures may be involved as well.

Two forms of chronic graft-versus-host disease have been described. Lichenoid chronic graft-versus-host disease is characterized by violaceous polygonal papules that closely resemble lichen planus

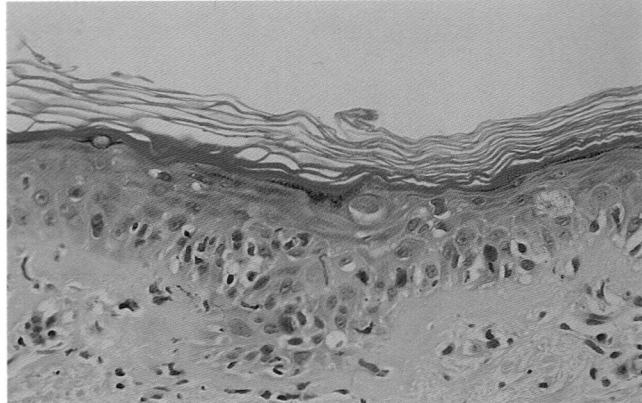

**FIGURE 48–19.** Graft-versus-host disease. This biopsy specimen shows a vacuolar interface dermatitis with maturation disarray, dyskeratosis, and satellitosis. These findings are characteristic but could be seen in erythema multiforme or a drug eruption.

clinically and pathologically. Biopsy of lichenoid graft-versus-host disease shows a dense lichenoid tissue reaction in the upper epidermis. Epidermal acanthosis with sawtoothing and hypergranulosis is present. Epidermal dysmaturation is also noted. Another form of chronic graft-versus-host disease, the sclerodermoid variant, resembles scleroderma both clinically and pathologically. Biopsy reveals dermal hyalinization and sclerosis.[71]

The diagnostic specificity of the histopathologic findings described for acute graft-versus-host disease is debatable. Drug eruptions may at times cause similar if not identical histologic changes. Therefore, careful clinicopathologic correlation is needed to establish a presumptive diagnosis of acute graft-versus-host disease. The finding of eosinophils or plasma cells in the setting of an interface dermatitis in a bone marrow transplant patient should prompt careful consideration of a drug etiology.

## Pityriasis Lichenoides

Pityriasis lichenoides has historically been separated into an acute form designated pityriasis lichenoides et varioliformis acuta (so-called PLEVA or Mucha-Habermann disease) and pityriasis lichenoides chronica (PLC). PLEVA is a papulovesicular eruption that usually occurs in children and young adults.[72] Lesions begin as erythematous papules that frequently develop central erosion, ulceration, or vesicle formation. The clinical course is variable; however, lesions usually resolve within weeks and frequently leave small residual scars. New crops of lesions often develop during a period of years. The lesions are widely distributed, usually affecting trunk and extremities. The chronic form of pityriasis lichenoides (PLC) is thought by some authorities to represent lesions that evolve more slowly than PLEVA.[73] The pathogenesis of pityriasis lichenoides is not understood.

Just as a clinical spectrum of lesions in pityriasis lichenoides is appreciated, the histopathologic features are also variable. Acute lesions (PLEVA) are characterized by a superficial and deep perivascular and interstitial infiltrate composed predominantly of lymphocytes (Fig. 48–20). At low-power examination, this infiltrate is wedge shaped, pointing toward the deep dermis. An interface dermatitis with extensive dyskeratosis and marked exocytosis is present. Some lesions demonstrate full-thickness epidermal necrosis or ulceration. Parakeratosis and associated scale crust may be seen. A characteristic feature is the presence of numerous extravasated red blood cells. Compared with PLEVA, PLC shows less inflammation and less epidermal necrosis. PLEVA and PLC seem to form a disease spectrum with overlapping clinical and pathologic findings.

## Fixed Drug Eruption

Fixed drug eruption is characterized by one or more well-defined, erythematous, dusky patches or plaques recurring in the same location and temporally related to repeated ingestion of medication. The most commonly associated medications are tetracycline, barbiturates, phenolphthalein, sulfonamides, and nonsteroidal anti-inflammatory agents. Genitalia and acral regions are the most common sites involved. New lesions may develop in different sites with repeated administration of offending agents.

Biopsy reveals an interface dermatitis associated

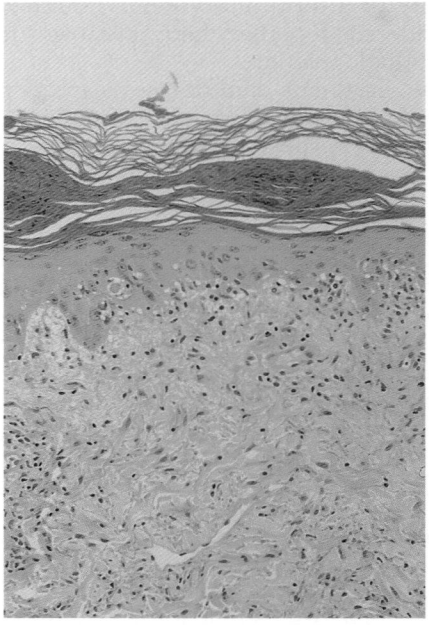

**FIGURE 48–20.** Pityriasis lichenoides. This acute lesion shows a superficial and deep perivascular and interstitial infiltrate in wedge-shaped distribution associated with an interface dermatitis, focal dyskeratosis, and extravasated red blood cells. Multifocal parakeratosis, often with scale crust, is characteristic.

with a mixed superficial and deep perivascular infiltrate composed of lymphocytes, neutrophils, and eosinophils. The overlying epidermis shows variable vacuolar degeneration of the dermal-epidermal junction with dyskeratosis and sometimes subepidermal vesiculation. Biopsy of late lesions shows melanophages within the superficial papillary dermis. The epidermal changes seen in fixed drug eruption greatly resemble erythema multiforme. In contrast to erythema multiforme, however, fixed drug eruption shows a superficial and deep, heavier inflammatory infiltrate that often contains neutrophils and eosinophils. Furthermore, the presence of melanophages aids in the differential diagnosis. In difficult cases, clinical correlation usually resolves this differential diagnosis.

## Lupus Erythematosus

Lupus erythematosus may be divided into three distinctive variants. Discoid lupus erythematosus (DLE), the most common variant, may be localized to one or several lesions, particularly involving the face, or it may be more generalized with widespread lesions. Systemic involvement is uncommon in patients who initially present with DLE; however, patients with systemic disease may develop discoid lesions. Typical lesions of DLE are erythematous plaques of varying size associated with scale. Examination of the undersurface of the scale removed from discoid lesions reveals keratinous follicular plugs ("carpet tack" sign). Lesions typically heal with scarring and hyperpigmentation or hypopigmentation.

Subacute cutaneous lupus erythematosus (SCLE) is characterized by widespread erythematous scaly lesions. In contrast to DLE, SCLE lesions are not associated with scarring. Approximately half of patients with SCLE have manifestations of systemic disease.[74] The lesions of SCLE often show a photosensitive distribution. The lesions are often annular in character. Psoriasiform and lichenoid lesions may also be observed.

Systemic lupus erythematosus is a complex disease with myriad manifestations. In addition to cutaneous disease, patients frequently manifest immunologic disease, hematologic disease, neurologic disease, renal disorders, serositis, arthritis, and oral ulcers. The most characteristic cutaneous manifestation is the malar ("butterfly") rash, an erythematous, scaly rash involving the central face. Multiple scaling, slightly atrophic papules may frequently affect sun-damaged skin. Patients with systemic lupus erythematosus may also develop discoid lesions and subacute cutaneous lesions.

Infants born to mothers with anti-Ro or La autoantibodies may develop erythematous scaly, usually annular plaques that resemble SCLE. This disorder is designated neonatal lupus erythematosus. The mothers of affected infants frequently do not have clinical manifestations of connective tissue disease; however, they may develop manifestations, particularly Sjögren's syndrome.[75] Most important, infants with neonatal lupus erythematosus may develop cardiac manifestations, usually congenital heart block.

It is debatable whether the variants of lupus described here can be separated on the basis of histology alone; therefore, their histologic features are considered together.[76, 77] It is our experience that there is overlap between subtypes, and they often cannot be reliably distinguished. However, some generalizations may be made. The morphologic common denominator for variants of lupus erythematosus is a vacuolar interface dermatitis (Fig. 48–21). A superficial papillary dermal perivascular and interstitial infiltrate, predominantly composed of lymphocytes, is characteristic. Variable vacuolization, dyskeratosis, follicular plugging, hyperkeratosis, epidermal atrophy, and basement membrane thickening may be seen. Early lesions frequently lack basement membrane thickening but show atrophy and a superficial neutrophilic infiltrate with nuclear debris. A dermal inflammatory infiltrate may involve both the superficial and deep vascular plexuses; in addition, it often shows a periadnexal distribution in subacute and chronic lesions (Fig. 48–22). The epidermal changes in DLE tend to be more marked than in SCLE or systemic lupus. Follicular plugging also tends to be more marked in DLE. Dermal mucin may be demonstrated in many cases, and mucin stains may be needed to demonstrate this finding. The edema of early lesions is a clue to mucin deposits. The so-called tumid form of lupus erythematosus shows minimal epidermal changes other than usual vasculopathy and is characterized by perivascular and periappendiceal mononuclear cell infiltrate and dermal mucin deposition.

Immunofluorescence staining of non–sun-exposed skin in patients with systemic lupus erythematosus usually demonstrates a combination of im-

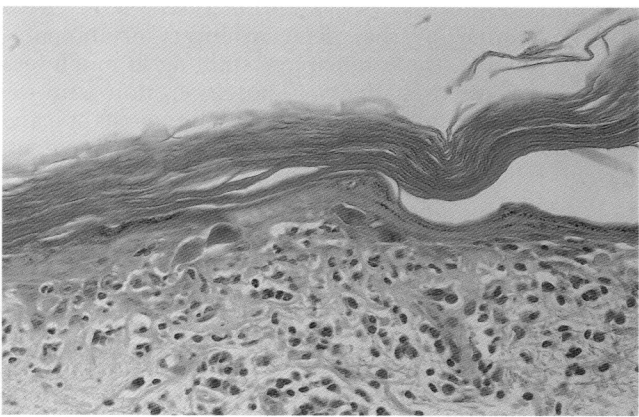

**FIGURE 48–21.** Lupus erythematosus. A vacuolar interface dermatitis with hyperkeratosis, dyskeratosis, and variable epidermal atrophy is characteristic. Marked vacuolopathy of the dermal-epidermal junction is present. All changes support a diagnosis of lupus erythematosus.

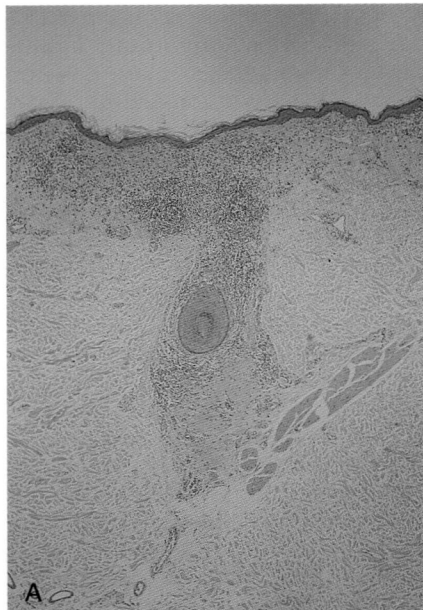 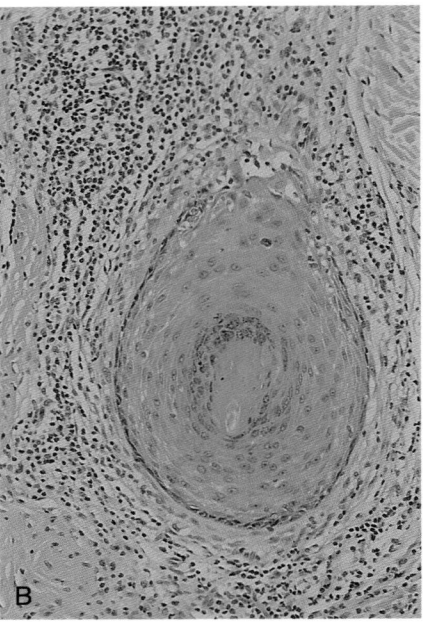

**FIGURE 48–22.** Lupus erythematosus. This biopsy specimen shows a dermal inflammatory infiltrate in a periadnexal and perivascular distribution involving both the superficial and deep vascular plexuses. (*A*, low power; *B*, high power.)

munoglobulins (IgG, IgA, IgM) and complement (C3) at the basement membrane. A positive lupus band test result, a pattern of multiple immunoreactants (so-called full house) at the dermal-epidermal junction of non–sun-damaged skin, is characteristic of lupus erythematosus. Strength of reactivity in a more or less continuous band and an increasing number of positive immunoreactants correlate with increased specificity. Most patients with discoid and systemic lupus erythematosus and approximately half of patients with SCLE show a positive lupus band test result with direct immunofluorescence testing of lesional skin. Most patients with active systemic lupus and a *minority* of patients with discoid lupus show a positive lupus band test result when sun-exposed nonlesional skin is tested. Immunoreactivity correlates with disease activity. Approximately 20% of nonaffected adults show immunoglobulin deposition in sun-damaged skin in a pattern similar to that seen in lupus erythematosus.[78] However, the intensity of staining is much less than in affected patients. Therefore, non–sun-exposed nonlesional skin provides the most specific substrate for immunofluorescence studies, even though false-negative results do occur.

### Dermatomyositis

Dermatomyositis is a connective tissue disease syndrome characterized by myositis and dermatitis. Skin manifestations include erythematous papules and plaques, periungual erythema, erythematous papules on the skin overlying knuckles (Gottron papules), and characteristic reddish purple periorbital swelling (heliotrope rash). Myositis results in severe proximal muscle weakness. Importantly, dermatomyositis may be associated with visceral malignant disease in adults.[79] In contrast, dermatomyositis in children is not associated with malignant disease.

The histologic findings in dermatomyositis show significant overlap with systemic lupus erythematosus. In general, however, changes tend to be more subtle in dermatomyositis. An interface vacuolar dermatitis, sometimes associated with sparse inflammation, is present. The papillary dermis exhibits an overall diminution in small vessels with some ectasia of the extant vessels. The inflammatory infiltrate is predominantly composed of lymphocytes and occasional plasma cells. Inflammation tends to be limited to the upper dermis. Dermal mucin deposition is a common and helpful finding but may require mucin stains for demonstration. As with lupus erythematosus, older lesions show basement membrane thickening. Immunofluorescence frequently demonstrates immunoglobulin and complement at the dermal-epidermal junction.[80, 81]

## BULLOUS AND ACANTHOLYTIC DERMATOSES

Bullous and acantholytic dermatoses encompass a large group of disorders produced by a variety of pathogenic mechanisms. Although definitive diagnosis may occasionally be rendered on the basis of biopsy alone, as with many inflammatory dermatoses, a definitive diagnosis should be rendered only after clinicopathologic correlation. In addition, definitive diagnosis of some of these diseases requires ancillary techniques such as immunofluorescence staining. In general, the differential diagnosis of a given bullous disorder is formulated on the basis of the plane of cleavage in vesicle formation and the nature of the inflammatory infiltrate.

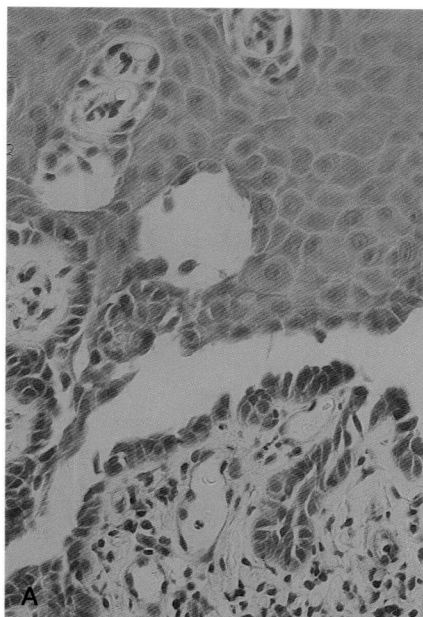
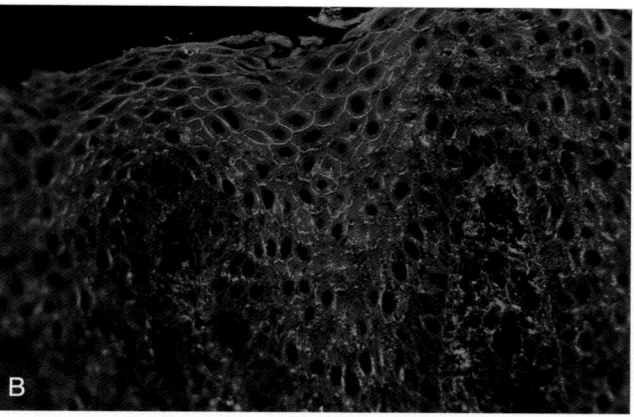

**FIGURE 48-23.** Pemphigus vulgaris. *A.* An intraepidermal vesicle caused by cleavage above the basal cell layer of the epidermis is seen. Note the suprabasilar acantholytic cells. *B.* Direct immunofluorescence reveals IgG and staining of the intercellular zones of epithelial keratinocytes. In some areas, at the periphery, a noncontinuous lacelike pattern of staining is seen around scattered individual cells. This finding is often seen in early lesions. (Courtesy of Christine Howard, Massachusetts General Hospital, Boston, MA.)

## Pemphigus Vulgaris

Pemphigus vulgaris is most commonly seen in middle-aged and elderly adults. Widespread vesicles, bullae, and erosions involve the oral mucosa, face, scalp, central chest, and intertriginous areas. Oral mucosal involvement is frequently the first manifestation of disease. The bullae vary in size and are typically flaccid and fragile. Pemphigus vegetans, considered a verrucous variant of pemphigus vulgaris, has a predilection for the intertriginous regions. Pemphigus vulgaris and its variants are believed to be caused by polyclonal IgG that binds to a component of desmosomes.[82, 83]

The classic histopathologic picture of pemphigus vulgaris is an intraepidermal vesicle caused by cleavage above the basal cell layer of the epidermis (Fig. 48-23). A variable superficial perivascular mixed inflammatory infiltrate, including occasional eosinophils, is often present. A characteristic feature is extension of the suprabasal cleft down the follicular epithelium. This feature is helpful in distinguishing pemphigus from Hailey-Hailey disease ("benign familial pemphigus"). Early lesions of pemphigus vulgaris, before development of the suprabasal intraepidermal cleft, are characterized by a nonspecific superficial perivascular infiltrate, usually composed of lymphocytes and variable numbers of eosinophils and eosinophilic spongiosis. In this prevesicular stage, distinction from bullous pemphigoid is not possible without assistance of ancillary studies such as immunofluorescence staining.

The histopathologic findings in early lesions are nonspecific, and a definitive diagnosis cannot be rendered without confirmatory immunofluorescence studies. Direct immunofluorescence reveals IgG and sometimes C3 in a lacelike pattern outlining the intercellular zones of epithelial keratinocytes. The plane of cleavage distinguishes pemphigus vulgaris from pemphigus erythematosus and pemphigus foliaceus. Positive immunofluorescence staining distinguishes pemphigus vulgaris from Hailey-Hailey disease and Grover's disease.

## Pemphigus Foliaceus and Pemphigus Erythematosus

Pemphigus foliaceus and pemphigus erythematosus are considered together because they share common histologic findings. Pemphigus foliaceus is a disease of adults characterized by widespread patches and fragile blisters, erosions, and scale crust. Because blisters are exceedingly fragile, a primary blistering disorder is frequently not considered in the clinical differential diagnosis. In contrast to pemphigus vulgaris, pemphigus foliaceus generally does not involve mucous membranes. Fogo selvagem is a poorly understood disease that is histologically and clinically similar to pemphigus foliaceus and is endemic in the rivers of Brazil.[84, 85] It has been proposed that the disease is mediated by an arthropod vector (*Simulium* species). Pemphigus erythematosus is characterized by an erythematous rash of the central face that resembles the butterfly rash of lupus erythematosus.

Pemphigus foliaceus, pemphigus erythematosus, and fogo selvagem are characterized by superficial vesicle formation with the plane of cleavage located within subcorneal keratinocytes near the level of the granular cell layer. A dyskeratotic acantholytic granular cell layer is characteristic. Because the vesicles are fragile, the roof of the blister is often not present, and biopsy reveals dyskeratotic cells on the

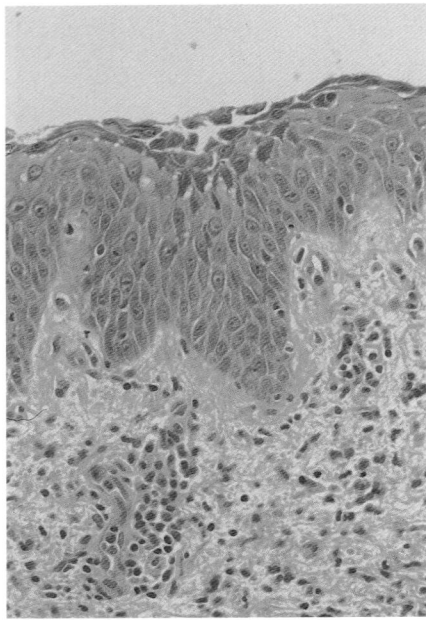

**FIGURE 48–24.** Pemphigus foliaceus. The findings are subtle and easily overlooked. A superficial vesicle formation with the plane of cleavage located within subcorneal keratinocytes near the level of the granular cell layer associated with dyskeratotic cells is seen.

surface of the epidermis and an absent granular cell layer and stratum corneum (Fig. 48–24). On occasion, bacterial superinfection is associated with a subcorneal vesicle containing numerous neutrophils admixed with acantholytic keratinocytes. Like pemphigus vulgaris, pemphigus foliaceus, pemphigus erythematosus, and fogo selvagem show staining of the intercellular region of the epidermis with IgG. Pemphigus erythematosus, in addition to intercellular staining with IgG, also shows staining with IgG along the basement membrane.[86]

## Drug-Induced Pemphigus

Drugs, most commonly penicillamine and captopril, may be associated with a pemphigus-like eruption.[87] Lesions frequently begin as a morbilliform rash or urticarial plaques that progress to blister formation. The blister may show a cleavage plane near the granular cell layer (similar to pemphigus foliaceus) or in the suprabasal plane (similar to pemphigus vulgaris). Direct immunofluorescence reveals intercellular staining with IgG and sometimes C3 in a pattern characteristic of the pemphigus group of disorders.

## Paraneoplastic Pemphigus

On occasion, patients with malignant disease develop papules, plaques, erosions, or vesicles. Oral lesions, frequently painful, are particularly common.

Hematopoietic malignant neoplasms are most commonly associated with paraneoplastic pemphigus; however, solid tumors have also been associated.[88, 89]

A combination of a vacuolar interface dermatitis and acantholysis above the basal cell layer is characteristic of paraneoplastic pemphigus. Lesions frequently also show spongiosis. Direct immunofluorescence usually reveals intercellular staining with IgG and sometimes C3. In addition, staining with IgG and C3 along the basement membrane is characteristic.

## Hailey-Hailey Disease

Hailey-Hailey disease, once referred to as benign familial chronic pemphigus, is an autosomal dominantly inherited genodermatosis that is now known not to be related to the pemphigus group of disorders. Hailey-Hailey disease, which most commonly presents in young adulthood, is characterized by grouped flaccid vesicles and erosions that most commonly involve the intertriginous regions. Because vesicles are extremely fragile, erosions and scale crust dominate the clinical picture. Mutations localized to chromosome 3q have been implicated in the pathogenesis of Hailey-Hailey disease.[90]

Well-developed lesions are characterized by a "dilapidated brick wall" appearance, secondary to extensive acantholysis (Fig. 48–25). Variable superficial perivascular lymphoid infiltrates are seen. Biopsy of early lesions occasionally shows a vesicle with a suprabasal cleft that closely mimics pemphigus vulgaris.[91] Unlike pemphigus vulgaris, Hailey-

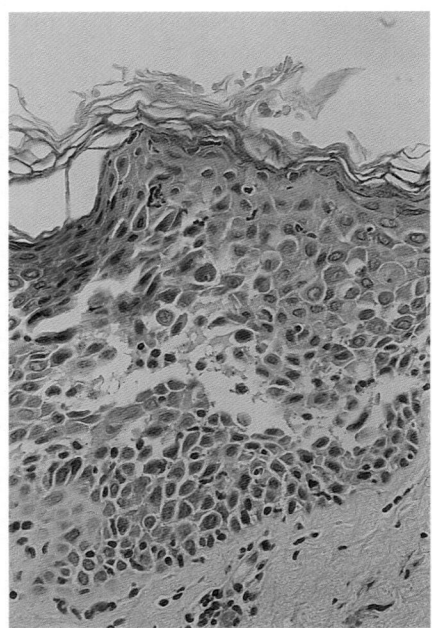

**FIGURE 48–25.** Hailey-Hailey disease. The lesions are characterized by a "dilapidated brick wall" appearance, secondary to extensive acantholysis.

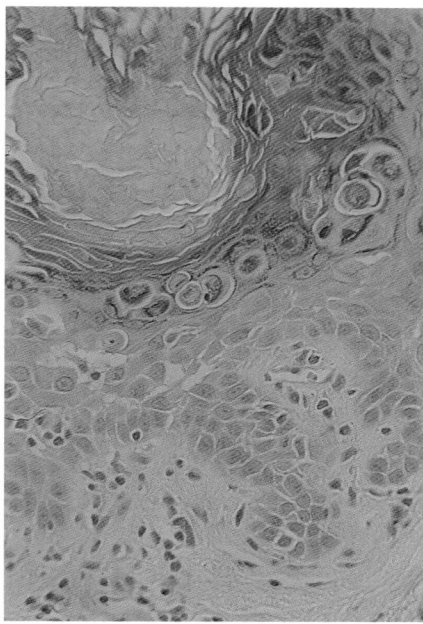

**FIGURE 48–26.** Darier's disease. Biopsy reveals variable acantholysis, dyskeratosis, and corps ronds, with overlying parakeratosis.

Hailey disease characteristically spares follicular epithelium. Hailey-Hailey disease should also be distinguished from Grover's disease, which tends to exhibit acantholysis in more discrete foci.

## Darier's Disease (Keratosis Follicularis)

Darier's disease is an autosomal dominantly inherited genodermatosis characterized by symmetric widespread keratotic papules and plaques that tend to involve the chest, back, neck, and scalp. Darier's disease presents most commonly during the first 2 decades of life.[92] Lesions are frequently distributed in the central chest in a so-called seborrheic distribution. Mucous membranes are occasionally involved. In addition, patients may show pitting of the palms; alternating white and red streaks on the fingernails with notches at the distal nail edge are characteristic.

Biopsy reveals variable acantholysis, dyskeratosis, and overlying parakeratosis (Fig. 48–26). Multiple corps ronds are found in the granular cell layer. These are squamous cells with a pyknotic nucleus and peripheral chromatin clumping that are surrounded by a halo. On occasion, suprabasal cleft formation mimics pemphigus vulgaris; however, the accompanying extensive dyskeratosis is a helpful diagnostic clue. Grover's disease may closely mimic Darier's disease but is characterized by smaller, more discrete foci of acantholysis and dyskeratosis. In difficult cases, clinical history usually allows distinction.

## Grover's Disease (Transient Acantholytic Dyskeratosis)

Grover's disease, predominantly a disease of middle-aged and elderly men, is characterized by scattered erythematous papules that tend to involve the trunk and sometimes the proximal extremities. Lesions frequently occur after sun exposure and sweating.[93–96] Patients often complain of intense pruritus. Lesions tend to be transient; however, recurrences are not uncommon, and they may persist in some patients.[97]

The histopathologic findings in Grover's disease are highly variable. In some cases, the dominant histologic finding is spongiosis, which may result in intraepidermal vesicle formation. A superficial perivascular lymphoeosinophilic infiltrate is characteristic. In many cases, the dominant histologic finding is the presence of discrete foci of acantholysis associated with dyskeratotic cells (Fig. 48–27). Grover's disease may closely mimic pemphigus vulgaris, Hailey-Hailey disease, and Darier's disease. Grover's disease tends to exhibit more discrete foci compared with these other diseases. Variants mimicking pemphigus foliaceus may also be seen. In difficult cases, immunofluorescence staining (which is negative in Grover's disease) aids in distinguishing it from the pemphigus family of vesiculobullous disorders. However, careful clinicopathologic correlation usually allows this distinction. Grover's disease may also closely mimic Darier's disease. The presence of foci mimicking more than one of the disorders in this differential diagnosis (Darier's disease, Hailey-Hailey disease, pemphigus) in a single lesion is suggestive of Grover's disease.

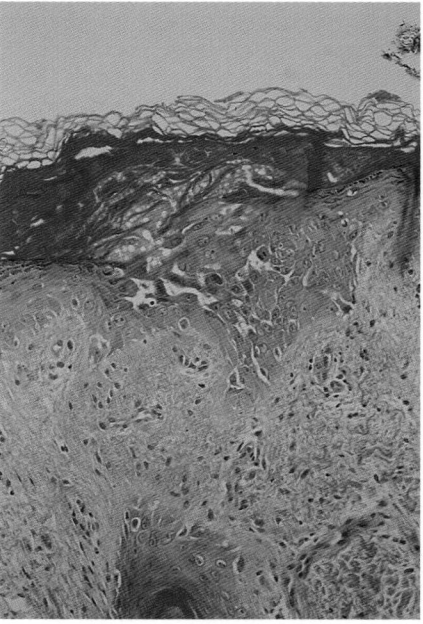

**FIGURE 48–27.** Grover's disease. Focal acantholysis with dyskeratosis is one of several appearances of Grover's disease.

## Impetigo

Impetigo is a superficial skin infection most commonly caused by *S. aureus* or group A streptococci. Papules, vesicles, and pustules erode and give rise to a characteristic honey-colored scale crust. Impetigo occurs most commonly in childhood. The face is the common site of infection. Bullous impetigo is most commonly caused by *S. aureus* (phage group II, type 71), which produces an epidermolytic toxin.[98]

Impetigo is characterized by subcorneal pustules. A superficial perivascular neutrophilic infiltrate within the edematous superficial dermis may be seen. Bullous impetigo is associated with a subcorneal blister with cleavage near the level of the granular cell layer. Early lesions may exhibit only rare neutrophils and occasional acantholytic keratinocytes. Established lesions may be associated with a denser collection of neutrophils within the vesiculopustule. Variable numbers of bacteria may be demonstrated with a Gram stain. In some cases, particularly in bullous impetigo, culture may be needed to definitively identify the infectious agent.

## Staphylococcal Scalded Skin Syndrome

Staphylococcal scalded skin syndrome, sometimes referred to as Ritter's disease, primarily affects infants with staphylococcal infection of the nasopharynx, inner ear, or conjunctiva. Like bullous impetigo, staphylococcal scalded skin syndrome is caused by *S. aureus* organisms that elaborate an epidermolytic exotoxin. Patients develop widespread erythematous patches, often originating on the face and intertriginous areas, which later become generalized.[99] Typically, large sheets of epidermis slough from flaccid bullae. The disease is self-limited, usually resolving within a 10-day period. However, in some patients (particularly adults), this disease may be fatal. This disorder occurs rarely in adults but usually only in the setting of compromised renal function.

Blister formation results from a subcorneal cleavage that is frequently centered near the granular cell layer. Acantholytic squamous cells may be noted. Early lesions are associated with minimal inflammation, whereas older lesions may give rise to a subcorneal pustule similar to that seen in impetigo.

The histologic differential diagnosis includes bullous impetigo, which may be histologically identical and requires clinical information for distinction. Pemphigus foliaceus and pemphigus erythematosus also show similar histologic findings. Clinical information and, when necessary, immunofluorescence studies distinguish these entities.

## Bullous Pemphigoid

Bullous pemphigoid is a blistering disorder that usually affects elderly patients; however, young adults may also be affected. Patients develop urticarial papules and plaques associated with tense vesicles and bullae. The characteristic distribution of lesions includes the intertriginous regions and the flexor surfaces of the extremities. Lesions may be arranged in serpiginous, annular, and occasionally herpetiform configurations. An uncommon variant, cicatricial pemphigoid, predominantly affects skin of the head and neck and mucosal surfaces. Involvement of ocular mucosa may lead to blindness. Some patients with cicatricial pemphigoid also have lesions characteristic of typical bullous pemphigoid.

Biopsy of urticarial lesions reveals a superficial perivascular mixed infiltrate composed of mononuclear cells and eosinophils. A helpful but not entirely specific clue to the diagnosis of urticarial lesions is the presence of tagging by eosinophils of the basal cell layer of the epidermis. Definitive diagnosis of urticarial lesions requires immunofluorescence studies. Biopsy of vesicles reveals a subepidermal cleavage plane associated with a variable mixed inflammatory infiltrate (Fig. 48–28). Eosinophils, lymphocytes, and neutrophils in variable numbers are present within the bullae. In the papillae adjacent to the bullae, eosinophils may often be observed at the dermal-epidermal junction. Variable eosinophilic spongiosis may be seen in urticarial lesions and at the edge of vesicles. Cicatricial pemphigoid shows, in addition to the features of bullous pemphigoid, a more prominent neutrophilic component and fibrosis of the superficial dermis. Immunofluorescence studies reveal linear deposition of C3 and IgG along the basement membrane.

## Herpes Gestationis

Herpes gestationis is a bullous eruption that occurs most commonly in the second or third trimester of pregnancy. Early lesions have a predilection for the periumbilical region. Lesions may become widespread and involve the trunk and extremities. Early lesions may be urticarial papules and plaques. Like bullous pemphigoid, the vesicles and bullae of herpes gestationis are tense and may be arranged in serpiginous, annular, or herpetiform configurations.

The histologic features of herpes gestationis are virtually identical to bullous pemphigoid. A subepidermal vesicle with variable mixed inflammatory infiltrate composed of lymphocytes, neutrophils, and eosinophils is noted. Early urticarial lesions may also be similar to bullous pemphigoid, with superficial perivascular infiltrate predominantly composed of lymphocytes and eosinophils. As with bullous pemphigoid, tagging of the dermal-epidermal junction by eosinophils is characteristic. Marked papil-

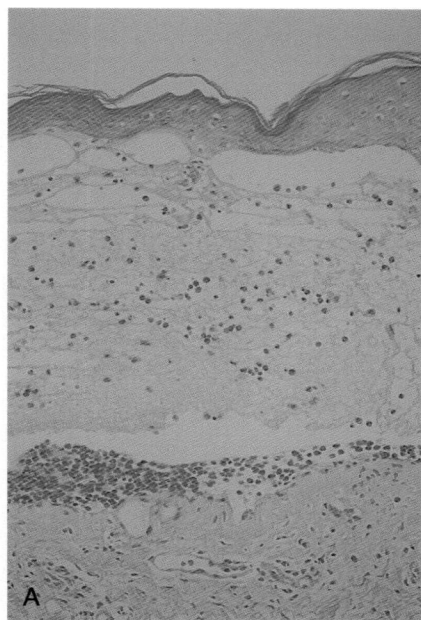
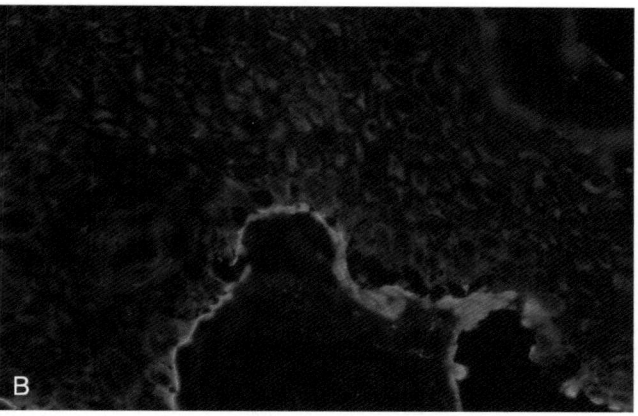

**FIGURE 48–28.** Bullous pemphigoid. *A.* A subepidermal vesicle with a variable mixed inflammatory infiltrate including numerous eosinophils is seen. *B.* Direct immunofluorescence shows staining with IgG along the dermal-epidermal junction in linear array.

lary dermal edema is frequently noted. The pathogenesis of herpes gestationis is similar to that of bullous pemphigoid. Both diseases appear to share the same target antigen within the hemidesmosome and lamina lucida.[100] Immunofluorescence studies reveal linear C3 and, less commonly, IgG at the dermal-epidermal junction.

## Dermatitis Herpetiformis

Dermatitis herpetiformis is an intensely pruritic eruption characterized by macules, papules, erosions, and occasionally vesicles distributed symmetrically over the extensor surfaces of the extremities, scalp, shoulders, back, and buttocks. Inherited as an autosomal dominant trait, this disease usually presents in early adulthood.[101] Because this eruption is so intensely pruritic, intact vesicles are often not present on physical examination. Dermatitis herpetiformis is frequently associated with a gluten-sensitive enteropathy, which is histologically similar to celiac disease. Skin lesions in some patients respond favorably to a gluten-free diet. However, dapsone therapy is usually needed to control the patient's symptoms.

Biopsy reveals a subepidermal blister with numerous neutrophils and variable numbers of eosinophils (Fig. 48–29). The superficial dermis shows a perivascular lymphocytic and neutrophilic infiltrate. The most characteristic feature is the presence of neutrophilic microabscesses associated with karyorrhexis (nuclear debris) within the dermal papillae. This feature is best appreciated just lateral to the blister. Immunofluorescence studies reveal granular deposits of IgA within the dermal papillae in the same distribution as the microabscesses.

The differential diagnosis of dermatitis herpetiformis includes linear IgA disease and bullous systemic lupus erythematosus. Clinical correlation and, when necessary, immunofluorescence studies aid in the distinction among these entities.

## Linear IgA Disease and Chronic Bullous Disease of Childhood

Linear IgA disease and chronic bullous disease of childhood have in common linear IgA deposition within the basement membrane zone and identical histopathologic features. In addition, the underlying pathogenesis appears to be IgA-mediated autoimmune disease.[102–105]

Linear IgA disease of adults is a rare disease that may mimic dermatitis herpetiformis or bullous pemphigoid clinically. Patients may develop excoriated pruritic lesions similar to those of dermatitis herpetiformis. Some patients develop annular vesicles that have been likened to a "string of beads."[106] Mucosal surfaces are frequently involved and may cause significant morbidity. Urticaria of the palms and soles, when present, is a helpful clinical feature. Occasional patients have associated gluten-sensitive enteropathy.

Linear IgA disease of childhood is characterized by vesicles and bullae with a predilection for perioral and genital regions. Like adult linear IgA disease, the childhood form may also be associated with blisters in an annular distribution that has been likened to a "cluster of jewels."[107] Like the adult form, childhood linear IgA disease is frequently associated with mucous membrane involvement.[108]

The histologic findings in childhood and adult linear IgA disease are identical to those of dermatitis

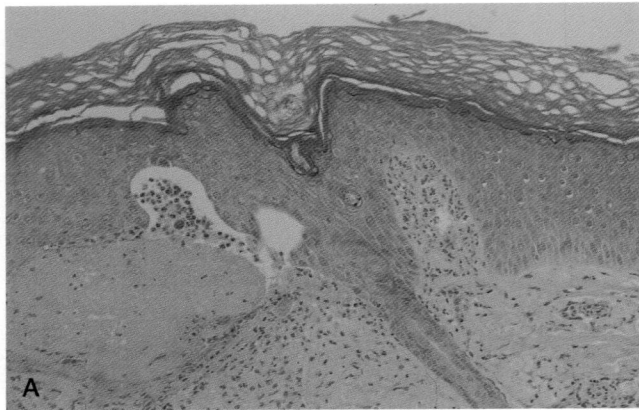
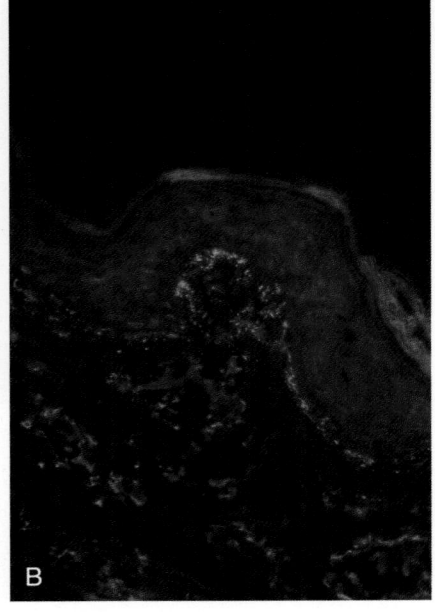

**FIGURE 48–29.** Dermatitis herpetiformis. *A.* The edge of the blister cavity shows neutrophilic microabscesses associated with karyorrhexis within the dermal papillae. *B.* Direct immunofluorescence shows granular deposits of IgA in the rete papillae.

herpetiformis. Subepidermal vesicles and bullae associated with a neutrophilic infiltrate and papillary dermal neutrophil microabscesses are seen. Immunofluorescence studies reveal linear IgA deposition along the basement membrane.

## Bullous Systemic Lupus Erythematosus

An unusual and rare variant of lupus erythematosus shows histologic findings similar to those of dermatitis herpetiformis and linear IgA disease. This form of lupus erythematosus, characterized by vesicles and bullae on sun-exposed sites, is most often seen in young black women.

Biopsy reveals subepidermal vesicles with numerous neutrophils and papillary dermal microabscesses similar to those seen in dermatitis herpetiformis. The presence of dermal mucin in some cases may provide a clue to the diagnosis. Other features typically seen in lupus erythematosus, including interface dermatitis, follicular plugging, and thickened basement membrane, are usually not seen in bullous systemic lupus erythematosus.[109] Granular or linear deposition of multiple immunoreactants, including IgG, IgA, IgM, and C3, helps distinguish bullous lupus erythematosus from dermatitis herpetiformis and linear IgA disease.

## Porphyria Cutanea Tarda

The porphyrias represent a heterogeneous group of diseases that have in common enzyme defects in the heme biosynthetic pathway. Porphyria cutanea tarda is the most common of the porphyrias, and discussion is limited to this variant.

Porphyria cutanea tarda is caused by a defect in uroporphyrinogen decarboxylase and is inherited as an autosomal dominant trait. The disease, most common in young and middle-aged adults, is characterized by vesicles and bullae on sun-damaged skin, particularly the dorsum of the hands. Vesicles frequently heal with scarring associated with miniaturized epidermal inclusion cysts called milia. Hypertrichosis and hyperpigmentation of the face are common findings. Risk factors include estrogen (oral contraceptives) and alcoholism.

Biopsy of vesicles reveals a subepidermal cleavage plane associated with minimal inflammatory infiltrate (Fig. 48–30). Solar elastosis is a frequent accompanying finding. A characteristic but nonspecific feature is the presence of rigid-appearing dermal papillae (festooning) projecting into the blister cavity. The vessels in the superficial papillary dermis demonstrate a homogeneous rim of eosinophilic hyalinized material that is best demonstrated with a PAS stain.

Pseudoporphyria is clinically and histologically similar to porphyria cutanea tarda but is not associated with defects in heme synthesis. Pseudoporphyria is associated with hemodialysis and ingestion of certain drugs, including furosemide, nalidixic acid, tetracycline, and naproxen as well as other nonsteroidal anti-inflammatory drugs.[110, 111] Distinction between porphyria and pseudoporphyria requires urine and fecal evaluation for abnormal porphyrins.

## Epidermolysis Bullosa (excluding epidermolysis bullosa acquisita)

Epidermolysis bullosa represents a complex group of inherited mechanobullous diseases with variable inheritance, clinical findings, and ultrastructural and

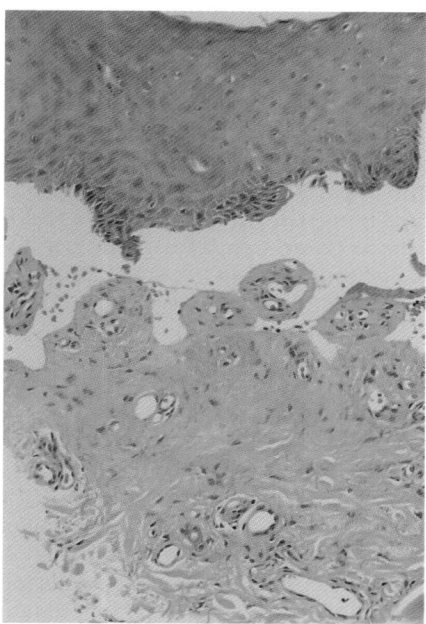

**FIGURE 48-30.** Porphyria cutanea tarda. This biopsy specimen shows a subepidermal vesicle without significant inflammatory infiltrate and festooning of dermal papillae. Note the prominent capillary-venular spaces associated with PAS-positive amorphous material within their walls.

molecular defects.[112] There are three major groups of epidermolysis bullosa and numerous complex subclassification schemes. For an excellent detailed review of the clinical and pathologic characteristics of this group of diseases, the reader is referred to more detailed discussions.[113]

Epidermolysis bullosa simplex is caused by an autosomal dominantly inherited defect in keratins that results in cytolysis and vesicle formation. Although the vesicle appears to be a subepidermal vesicle, in fact the cleavage plane occurs within the cytoplasm of the basal cell layer. The minute fragments of cytoplasm that adhere to the blister floor are usually appreciated only by use of ultrastructural techniques. However, one can often see vasculopathy of the basal cells in nonblistered skin. Furthermore, the roof of the bulla shows degenerative changes of the basal cells, a finding absent in other variants of epidermolysis bullosa.

Epidermolysis bullosa dystrophica may be inherited as either an autosomal dominant or autosomal recessive trait. This form of epidermolysis bullosa, which is typically more severe than epidermolysis bullosa simplex, is caused by a defect in anchoring fibrils, resulting in a subepidermal vesicle with a cleavage plane that forms below the lamina densa.

The third general category of epidermolysis bullosa, junctional epidermolysis bullosa, is inherited as an autosomal recessive trait associated with a defect in hemidesmosomes, which results in a vesicle with a cleavage plane within the lamina lucida. The clinical expression of junctional epidermolysis bullosa ranges from a fairly benign disease to a severe condition that resembles dystrophic epidermolysis bullosa.

All three forms of epidermolysis bullosa are characterized by subepidermal vesicles with minimal inflammatory infiltrates. Precise classification requires careful clinical correlation and ultrastructural studies or immunoelectron microscopy.

## Epidermolysis Bullosa Acquisita

Epidermolysis bullosa acquisita is a somewhat controversial entity with criteria that continue to undergo refinement. The disease is caused by antibodies directed against type VII collagen.[114] Epidermolysis bullosa acquisita mimics other blistering disorders both clinically and pathologically; therefore, ancillary techniques are needed to establish a definitive diagnosis.

The most common variant, the cell-poor variant, clinically resembles porphyria cutanea tarda. In this variant, hemorrhagic vesicles on the backs of the hands heal with scarring and milia and may be virtually indistinguishable from porphyria cutanea tarda. The inflammatory variant may mimic bullous pemphigoid, cicatricial pemphigoid, or dermatitis herpetiformis.[115, 116]

The cell-poor variant is characterized by a subepidermal vesicle associated with minimal inflammatory infiltrate and festooning of the dermal papillae in a pattern that mimics porphyria cutanea tarda. The inflammatory variant is characterized by a subepidermal vesicle associated with a variable inflammatory infiltrate composed of neutrophils, eosinophils, and lymphocytes. The inflammatory pattern may closely mimic dermatitis herpetiformis or bullous pemphigoid. As mentioned, immunofluorescence staining is required to distinguish epidermolysis bullosa from its mimics. Direct immunofluorescence reveals linear distribution of IgG and C3 lining the floor of the blister by use of the salt split skin method.[117] In contrast, split skin immunofluorescence studies of bullous pemphigoid reveal deposition of immunoreactants along the roof of the blister. This technique is also useful in evaluating lesions of bullous lupus erythematosus.

## Herpes Simplex, Herpesvirus, and Varicella Infections

After an incubation period of 11 to 20 days, varicella or chickenpox results in a widespread vesicular eruption on the face and trunk. Most patients are children, although infection is occasionally seen in adults in association with increased morbidity and even mortality. The vesicles tend to be grouped and have been likened to "dewdrops on a rose petal." Ruptured lesions develop scale crust and resolve in 1 to 2 weeks. Reactivation of latent varicella virus results in a painful vesicular eruption superimposed on an erythematous base with a dermatomal distri-

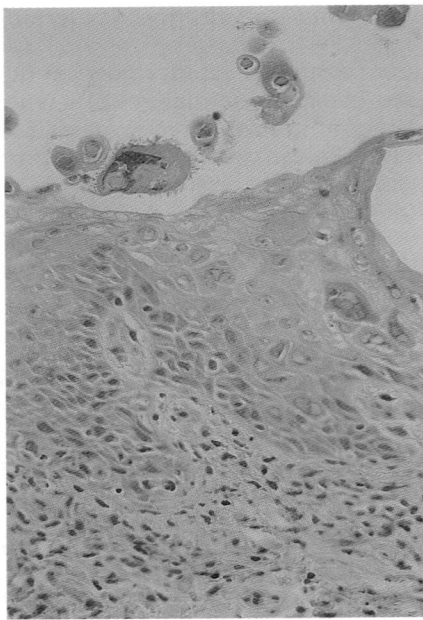

**FIGURE 48–31.** Herpesvirus infection. This biopsy specimen shows an intraepidermal vesicle with multinucleated keratinocytes with glassy intranuclear inclusions with a peripheral dark rim of chromatin.

bution. Multidermatomal lesions may occur in immunocompromised patients.

Herpes simplex virus infection is characterized by grouped vesicles superimposed on an erythematous base. Lesions occur most commonly in young adults. Herpes simplex virus type 1, colloquially known as a cold sore or fever blister, is characterized by clusters of vesicles and scale crust superimposed on an erythematous base in a perioral location. Herpes simplex virus type 2 infection causes herpetiform vesicles in the genitoanal region.

Biopsy of vesicles caused by herpesvirus infections show similar findings. Scanning magnification reveals extensive ballooning, degeneration, and acantholysis. High-power examination reveals multinucleated keratinocytes with glassy intranuclear inclusions with a peripheral dark rim of chromatin (Fig. 48–31). The intranuclear inclusions range from purple-blue to bright red. The classic Cowdry type A inclusion, an eosinophilic intranuclear inclusion surrounded by a clear halo, is often difficult to identify. It is nonviral and contains RNA and non–histone-containing protein. Nuclei with purple-blue or steel gray intranuclear inclusions are more common.

## VASCULITIDES

The term *vasculitis* refers to significant vascular injury associated with inflammation. Diseases associated with vasculitis are myriad and include disparate entities such as infection, connective tissue disorders, and paraneoplastic phenomena. In some circumstances, the vascular injury is secondary to a localized or systematized clinical phenomenon. In other cases, the vascular injury is the primary event. By definition, vasculitis is associated with inflammation and evidence of vessel wall injury. In general, vasculitides are classified by the character of the inflammatory infiltrate and type of vessel involved. Because most patterns of vasculitis are not specific for an underlying disorder, once a vasculitis is classified by these criteria, careful clinicopathologic correlation is needed to render a specific diagnosis.

### Leukocytoclastic Vasculitis

Leukocytoclastic vasculitis encompasses a heterogeneous group of vasculitides that share in common small vessel neutrophilic vasculitis associated with hypersensitivity to antigens. This form of vasculitis is sometimes referred to as hypersensitivity vasculitis. Leukocytoclastic vasculitis may be associated with infection, neoplasia, connective tissue disease, urticaria, cryoglobulinemia, paraproteinemia, and autoimmune diseases. Therefore, in patients with leukocytoclastic vasculitis, careful investigation should be made for signs and symptoms of visceral involvement. The most characteristic clinical manifestation is palpable purpura, evidenced by a purpuric rash, usually on the extremities, that does not blanch when pressure is applied.

Henoch-Schönlein purpura is a clinical syndrome that deserves special mention. Henoch-Schönlein purpura is a leukocytoclastic vasculitis most commonly encountered in children, but it may also be seen in adults. Palpable purpura of the buttocks and lower extremities may be clinically associated with abdominal pain, which tends to be exacerbated after meals. Henoch-Schönlein purpura is a self-limited disease and frequently follows an upper respiratory tract infection. In some cases, renal involvement is associated with morbidity and even mortality.

Biopsy of purpuric skin lesions is characterized by variable superficial and sometimes deep perivascular and interstitial neutrophilic infiltrates associated with karyorrhexis (Fig. 48–32). Fibrin deposition within the walls of small vessels (venules) is present. In early lesions and in urticarial vasculitis, careful examination may reveal only focal fibrin deposits. The histologic correlate of purpura is seen in the form of numerous extravasated erythrocytes. In fully developed lesions, the overlying epidermis may become necrotic, and erosions or ulcers may develop. The changes depend on the degree of skin involvement, which in turn reflects the basic etiologic disorder. Thus, postinfectious vasculitis is usually mild and superficial. The vasculitis secondary to systemic disorders such as polyarteritis nodosa results in extensive purpuric lesions.

The underlying cause of leukocytoclastic vasculitis cannot be determined on the basis of routine microscopic examination. Furthermore, biopsy does not aid in predicting systemic involvement. There-

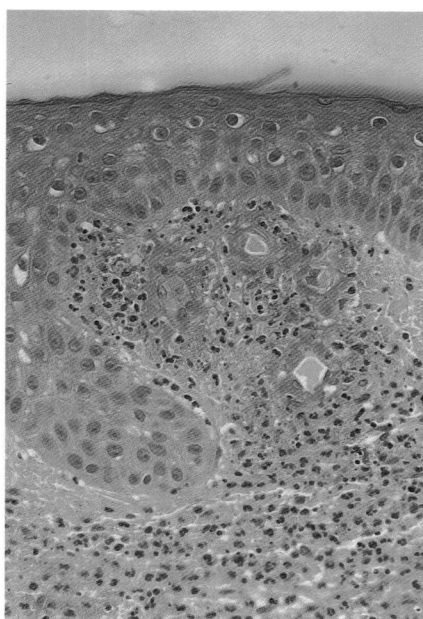

**FIGURE 48–32.** Leukocytoclastic vasculitis. The biopsy specimen shows superficial and deep perivascular and interstitial neutrophilic infiltrate associated with abundant karyorrhexis and perivascular fibrin deposition.

fore, careful clinicopathologic correlation in all patients with leukocytoclastic vasculitis is needed to evaluate for an associated underlying disorder.

## Granuloma Faciale

Granuloma faciale is considered a distinctive localized form of leukocytoclastic vasculitis. Clinically, granuloma faciale is characterized by one to several reddish brown or purple plaques, usually on the face. These lesions are usually asymptomatic and are only of cosmetic significance.

Granuloma faciale is characterized by a dense bandlike mixed infiltrate composed of neutrophils, eosinophils, lymphocytes, and plasma cells associated with karyorrhexis (Fig. 48–33). A grenz zone characteristically spares the papillary dermis between the inflammatory infiltrate and the overlying epidermis. In early lesions, careful examination reveals fibrinoid deposits surrounding vessels associated with karyorrhexis. With time, fibrosis appears, and the density of the inflammatory infiltrate diminishes. In chronic lesions, identification of unequivocal features of leukocytoclastic vasculitis may not be possible, but one may find brightly eosinophilic hyaline of the vessels in some cases.

## Erythema Elevatum Diutinum

Erythema elevatum diutinum, like granuloma faciale, is a rare disorder classified as a localized form of leukocytoclastic vasculitis. Erythema elevatum

diutinum occurs most commonly in young women, but it may occur in any age group. Papules, plaques, and nodules tend to cluster over joints, particularly the extensor surfaces of the hands, elbows, and ankles. Rarely, deep lesions mimic sarcoma clinically.[118] Erythema elevatum diutinum, like other forms of leukocytoclastic vasculitis, has been described in association with a number of different clinical disorders including cryoglobulinemia, multiple myeloma, hairy cell leukemia, polycythemia rubra vera, inflammatory bowel disease, rheumatoid arthritis, and systemic lupus erythematosus.[119–122]

Early lesions closely resemble granuloma faciale on biopsy examination, but with greater predominance of neutrophils and little if any grenz zone. Early lesions show a mixed inflammatory infiltrate with numerous neutrophils and associated karyorrhexis. Scattered eosinophils and lymphocytes are frequently present. Careful scrutiny of early lesions usually reveals fibrin deposition and fibrinoid necrosis within the walls of small vessels. As lesions progress, the density of the neutrophilic infiltrate declines, and lesions become increasingly fibrotic. Even in older lesions, neutrophils associated with nuclear debris may be identified. These cells are dispersed along collagen fibers and may be associated with lipid-laden histiocytes.

## Infectious Vasculitis

Infections should be considered in the differential diagnosis of any patient with leukocytoclastic vascu-

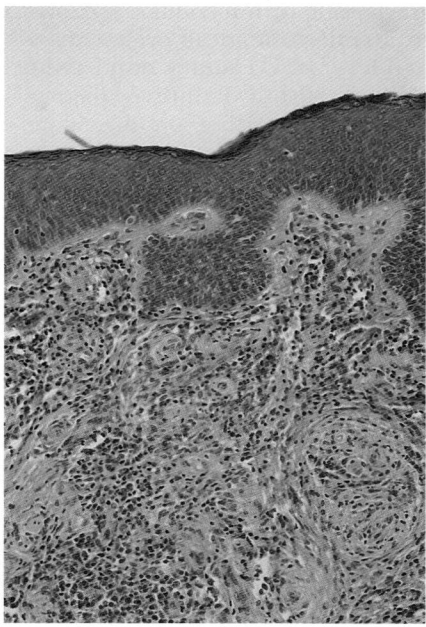

**FIGURE 48–33.** Granuloma faciale. Granuloma faciale is characterized by a dense bandlike mixed infiltrate composed of neutrophils, eosinophils, lymphocytes, and plasma cells associated with karyorrhexis. Note the grenz zone of sparing in the papillary dermis.

litis. Meningococcemia is caused by *Neisseria meningitidis,* a gram-negative coccus, which is transmitted person to person through nasopharyngeal secretions. Meningococcemia is most common in young children but rarely occurs in adults. Rapid onset of fever, chills, arthralgia, and myalgia eventually leading to stupor is characteristic. Severe hypotension may develop within a few hours of onset of symptoms.

Skin lesions are characterized by pink to purple macules or papules and purpura, which may progress to large confluent ecchymoses. The center of purpuric lesions may become necrotic. The lesions are most common on the trunk and extremities, and mucous membranes may be involved.

Disseminated gonococcal infection may also be associated with small vessel vasculitis. Disseminated gonococcal infection occurs in young, sexually active adults and is caused by the gram-negative diplococcus *Neisseria gonorrhoeae,* which is sexually transmitted. Fever, malaise, chills, arthralgia, and pustular skin lesions occur 7 to 30 days after infection. A countable number of skin lesions are characteristically present. The skin has a characteristic appearance; dusky, erythematous to purple-brown macules with a hemorrhagic or necrotic center are almost diagnostic. Other infectious organisms, including gram-positive bacteria, gram-negative bacteria, fungi, and rickettsiae, may also be associated with small vessel vasculitis.

Infectious vasculitis may involve small to large vessels and show variable degrees of perivascular and intravascular acute inflammation. Thrombus formation within the vessel lumen, a feature not often seen in noninfectious causes of small vessel vasculitis, is characteristic of infectious vasculitis. It may be difficult to identify offending organisms with special stains. Therefore, blood and wound culture may be necessary to establish a definitive diagnosis of infectious vasculitis. Depending on the stage of the lesion, variable dermal and epidermal necrosis may be present.

## Polyarteritis Nodosa

Polyarteritis nodosa is a primary form of vasculitis that may affect a range of vessel sizes. Patients frequently present with weight loss, fever, and other signs of systemic disease, such as neuritis, abdominal pain, melena, hypertension, arrhythmias, proteinuria, hematuria, and joint pain, in addition to skin lesions. Cutaneous involvement is characterized by livedo reticularis, a pattern of scattered hypererythematous macular lesions arranged in a netlike or mottled reticular configuration, or by extensive palpable purpura with ecchymoses. Epidermal infarction resulting in ulceration is also a common feature. The course of disease may be acute, subacute, or chronic and may be associated with symptom-free intervals. The disease is frequently fatal in untreated patients with systemic disease. Renal involvement,

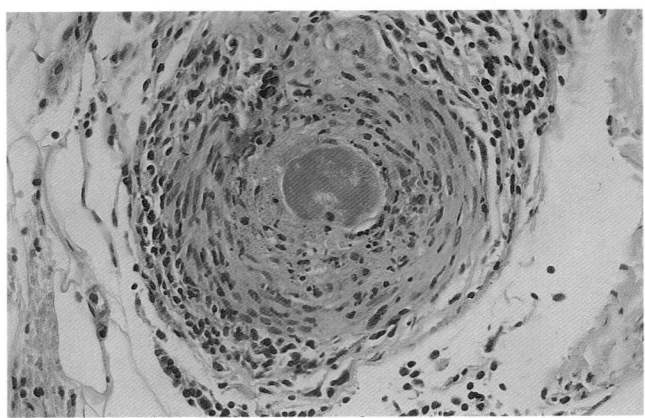

**FIGURE 48–34.** Polyarteritis nodosa. Vasculitis affecting medium-sized muscle arteries at the dermal-subcutaneous junction is seen. Thrombus formation within the vessel lumina is present.

which is present in most patients, is the most frequent cause of death.

Classic polyarteritis nodosa is characterized by vasculitis, usually affecting medium-sized muscle arteries in the deep dermis, dermal-subcutaneous junction, and subcutaneous fat (Fig. 48–34). In addition, vessels of other sizes are usually involved. The inflammatory infiltrate usually shows mixed neutrophils, lymphocytes, and eosinophils. Thrombus formation within the vessel lumina is also characteristic. As lesions age, a lymphohistiocytic infiltrate predominates over neutrophils.

Microscopic polyangiitis, considered by some to be a variant of polyarteritis nodosa, primarily affects arteriole- and capillary-sized vessels.[123] Cutaneous involvement with the microscopic polyangiitis is more common than in classic polyarteritis nodosa. Both classic polyarteritis nodosa and polyangiitis are associated with antineutrophil cytoplasmic antibodies that are specific for myeloperoxidase.[124–126]

## Allergic Granulomatosis (Churg-Strauss Syndrome)

Churg-Strauss syndrome is characterized by asthma, allergic rhinitis, pulmonary infiltrates, and tissue and blood eosinophilia. Churg-Strauss syndrome may show clinical and pathologic overlap with polyarteritis nodosa and Wegener's granulomatosis. Skin lesions include petechiae, ulcers, livedo reticularis, and subcutaneous nodules. The subcutaneous nodules typically affect the extensor surfaces of the extremities. Like polyarteritis nodosa, Churg-Strauss syndrome has been associated with antineutrophil cytoplasmic antibodies directed against myeloperoxidase.[127, 128]

The pathologic hallmark of Churg-Strauss syndrome is a combination of necrotizing vasculitis and extravascular granulomatous and eosinophilic inflammation. The Churg-Strauss granuloma, which is purported to be characteristic of Churg-Strauss syndrome, is composed of degenerated collagen surrounded by palisading histiocytes and multinucleated giant cells. The so-called Churg-Strauss granuloma may not be seen in all cases. Furthermore, this histologic finding is nonspecific and may be associated with a number of other disease processes.[129] Biopsy of lesions in some patients reveals a leukocytoclastic vasculitis accompanied by an eosinophil-rich infiltrate.

## Wegener's Granulomatosis

Wegener's granulomatosis, like polyarteritis nodosa and Churg-Strauss syndrome, is associated with antineutrophil cytoplasmic antibodies. In contrast, however, the antineutrophil cytoplasmic antibody in Wegener's disease reacts with proteinase 3 rather than with myeloperoxidase. Classic Wegener's granulomatosis is characterized by a clinicopathologic triad of necrotizing granulomatous lesions of the upper and lower respiratory tract, vasculitis, and glomerulonephritis.[130] More recently, a broader spectrum of disease has been accepted under the rubric of Wegener's granulomatosis. A less restrictive definition allows limited variants.[131] Skin lesions include palpable purpura, subcutaneous nodules, and necrosis that may be extensive.

A spectrum of histopathologic features may be seen. Skin biopsy in most patients reveals a nonspecific infiltrate.[132] In less than half of patients, a necrotizing small vessel vasculitis associated with extravascular, sometimes palisading granulomas is present. The most common finding is a leukocytoclastic vasculitis. Skin biopsies rarely reveal granulomatous vasculitis. Palisading granulomas that resemble those seen in the Churg-Strauss syndrome may also be identified. As can be seen, careful clinicopathologic correlation is needed to establish a diagnosis of Wegener's granulomatosis.

## Atheroembolism

Atheroembolism, a disease of adults with significant atherosclerosis, is caused when atheromatous plaque detaches and embolizes distally. Atheroembolism frequently follows vascular trauma associated with invasive medical procedures. Clinical manifestations include ulceration, livedo reticularis, and gangrene. Symptoms tend to localize to the distal lower extremities.

Biopsy reveals fibrin thrombi with or without intravascular atheromatous material, which is readily identified by needle-shaped clefts representing the outlines of dissolved crystals (Fig. 48–35). Not infrequently, examination of multiple step-sections from a deep biopsy specimen is needed to identify the embolus.

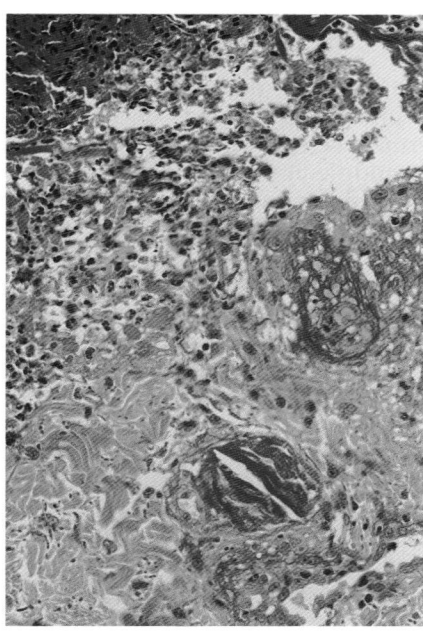

**FIGURE 48–35.** Atheroembolism. At the base of this ulcer is a vessel with a fibrin thrombus and central needle-shaped cleft.

## Erythema Nodosum Leprosum

Leprosy, an infectious disease caused by *Mycobacterium leprae*, can occasionally be accompanied by a vasculitic reaction (type II reaction) referred to as erythema nodosum leprosum. This occurs most often in lepromatous leprosy but may rarely also occur in borderline leprosy. The lesions are characterized clinically by tender red plaques and nodules together with areas of erythema. The eruption is generally widespread and accompanied by fever, malaise, and arthralgia. A type III reaction, known as Lucio's phenomenon, occurs exclusively in diffuse lepromatous leprosy, particularly in Mexico and Central America. It is usually seen in patients who have received inadequate treatment or no treatment. In contrast to erythema nodosum leprosum, there is no fever, tenderness, or arthralgia, and the lesions are limited to the lower extremities, buttocks, and forearms. The lesions consist of irregular plaques that develop into ulcers.

Erythema nodosum leprosum is characterized by leukocytoclastic vasculitis of dermal vessels admixed with scattered small, histiocytic granulomas containing bacilli. In Lucio's phenomenon, vascular changes are also prominent, but leukocytoclastic vasculitis is not featured. The lesions are characterized by endothelial proliferation leading to luminal obliteration with thrombosis of medium-sized vessels in the dermis and subcutis. Dense aggregates of acid-fast bacilli are found in the wall and the endothelium of normal-appearing vessels as well as within the vessels showing the proliferative changes. Ischemic necrosis secondary to vascular occlusion can lead to hemorrhagic infarcts and ulcers.

## Livedo Vasculitis

This condition, first described by the designation atrophie blanche, corresponds to a fibrinoid vasculitis of dermal vessels in the lower extremities of young to middle-aged women.[133] A familial form has also been described (the Georgian ulcers).[134] The lesions appear clinically as small purpuric macules and papules around the ankles and dorsa of the feet, accompanied by atrophic areas showing peripheral hypopigmentation. The lesions develop into small painful ulcers that have a tendency to recur. The ulcers tend to heal spontaneously, resulting in white atrophic scars that give the disease its name.

The histologic findings depend on the stage of the lesions. In the early lesions, eosinophilic fibrinoid material is present in the vessel walls of the dermis and in their lumina, producing partial occlusion. Infarction and hemorrhage of the dermis with necrosis of the epidermis are often noted. In atrophic lesions, the dermis is sclerotic, and the walls of dermal vessels show thickening and hyalinization of the intima with deposition of PAS-positive, diastase-resistant material. Direct immunofluorescence studies have demonstrated fibrin deposition in the vessel walls in early lesions and deposits of IgM, IgG, and C3 in late lesions.[135] Because inflammatory changes of the vessel walls are minimal, some authors believe that the process does not correspond to a true vasculitis and prefer to regard it as a vasculopathy. The histologic differential diagnosis includes stasis dermatitis. In stasis dermatitis, the capillary walls show only slight thickening without PAS-positive eosinophilic deposits, unlike the fibrinoid vasculitis of atrophie blanche.

## PANNICULITIDES

Panniculitis refers to a large and complex group of disorders that, by definition, are characterized by inflammation of subcutaneous adipose tissue. The panniculitides may also involve the dermis and soft tissue deep to subcutaneous adipose tissue. Classification of panniculitides is often difficult because many diseases show overlapping histologic and clinical features.

Panniculitis is classically divided into lobular and septal patterns. Although this is a logical starting point in any algorithmic approach to the diagnosis of panniculitis, both lobules and septa are frequently involved, and pure lobular or septal panniculitis is uncommon. A histologic differential is formulated by determination of the overall low-power pattern of fat involvement and evaluation of the composition of the inflammatory cells as well as by a search for concomitant epidermal and dermal alterations. As with other inflammatory conditions involving skin, only after careful clinicopathologic correlation is made should a definitive diagnosis be rendered. The timing of the biopsy is important. The diagnostic changes are frequently present early in the disease. Because the response of injury to fat involves fibrosis of the subcutaneous tissue, late lesions resulting from various causes often show similar changes, and definitive diagnosis may be difficult. Excisional biopsy specimens that contain abundant subcutaneous adipose tissue are more likely to yield a specific diagnosis. Punch biopsy specimens are generally inadequate for evaluation of a panniculitis.

## Erythema Nodosum

Erythema nodosum presents as multiple painful erythematous nodules most often on the lower extremity, particularly the anterior surface of the lower legs in women. Patients may experience multiple crops of lesions. The lesions are usually symmetric and bilateral.[136-138] Lesions resolve, leaving a bruiselike appearance. Ulceration and scarring are not seen.

Erythema nodosum represents the prototypical septal panniculitis (Fig. 48-36). Early lesions are characterized by predominantly septal inflammation, edema, and hemorrhage. The inflammatory components are composed of neutrophils, lymphocytes, histiocytes, and eosinophils. As the lesion ages, a lymphohistiocytic infiltrate with giant cells predominates. In addition, as the lesions evolve, there tends to be increased involvement of the lobule. Biopsy of resolving lesions reveals septal fibrosis and fibrosis of the paraseptal fat with a waning inflammatory response. The so-called Miescher granuloma is a septal aggregate of histiocytes that is said to be a

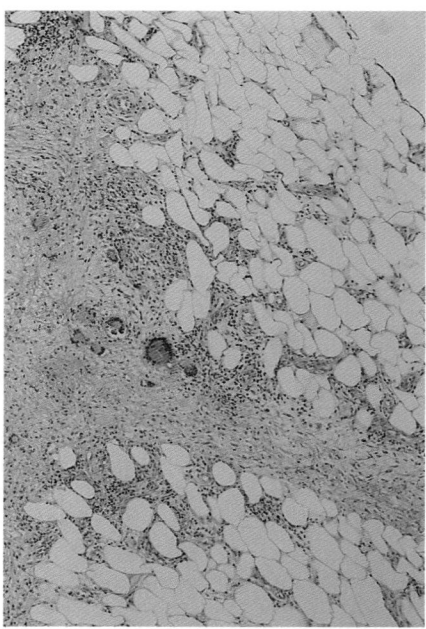

**FIGURE 48-36.** Erythema nodosum. A predominantly septal panniculitis with some lobular involvement composed of neutrophils, lymphocytes, histiocytes (including giant cells), and eosinophils is seen. A characteristic finding is the presence of paraseptal aggregates of mononuclear cells.

diagnostic clue but is probably not entirely specific for erythema nodosum. Furthermore, erythema nodosum must often be approached as a diagnosis of exclusion. In the presence of granulomas or abscesses, in particular, one should consider an infectious etiology and exclude this possibility with liberal use of culture and special stains for organisms. In addition, careful evaluation for necrotizing vasculitis is advised. Although low-grade vascular injury with extensive erythrocyte extravasation is characteristic of erythema nodosum, a frank necrotizing vasculitis should be carefully excluded. Vasculitides, in a manner similar to erythema nodosum, are characteristically associated with a septal pattern of panniculitis.

## Weber-Christian Disease

Many pathology texts still use the term Weber-Christian disease in reference to a form of lobular panniculitis that has been shown to be a nonspecific pattern that may be associated with a number of underlying clinical disorders.[139] Therefore, the most recent evidence supports the view that this term should be abandoned because it does not appear to represent a specific disorder.

## $\alpha_1$-Antitrypsin Deficiency

$\alpha_1$-Antitrypsin deficiency is a hereditary disorder associated with loss of a major inhibitor of a variety of proteases. The loss of protease inhibition results in unchecked consequences of inflammation. Patients develop recurrent erythematous nodules that frequently ulcerate and drain. Lesions most commonly involve the trunk and proximal extremities and frequently follow trauma. It now appears that patients with $\alpha_1$-antitrypsin deficiency were formerly classified under the rubric of Weber-Christian disease.[140-142]

Biopsy reveals a lobular panniculitis associated with extensive fat necrosis. Early lesions are dominated by neutrophilic inflammation with abscess formation. In some cases, a septal panniculitis may be seen. As with many other panniculitides, the histologic pattern in $\alpha_1$-antitrypsin deficiency is not diagnostic, and careful clinicopathologic correlation is needed to render a firm diagnosis. In particular, infection, trauma, and factitial disease should be excluded.

## Pancreatic Panniculitis

Patients with acute panniculitis may develop subcutaneous fat necrosis that is thought to be due to release of lipolytic enzymes from the pancreas into the systemic circulation.[143] Although pancreatic panniculitis is most commonly associated with acute alcohol-induced pancreatitis, other forms of inflamma-

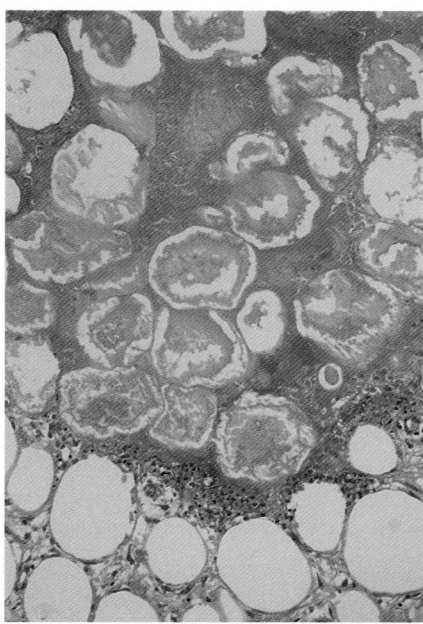

**FIGURE 48–37.** Pancreatic panniculitis. Extensive fat necrosis with basophilic degeneration and ghostlike cells surrounded by a palisade of neutrophils characteristic of saponification is seen in a patient with pancreatitis. (Case courtesy of Dr. P.H. McKee, Brigham and Women's Hospital, Boston, MA.)

tory pancreatic disease as well as pancreatic neoplasia may be associated with pancreatic panniculitis. Pancreatic panniculitis is usually manifested by painful erythematous nodules frequently associated with arthritis and polyserositis. Lesions tend to be tender and may occur at any site but show a predilection for the lower extremities. Ulceration of some lesions is associated with drainage of a hemorrhagic or oily fluid.

Biopsy usually reveals pathognomonic histologic features. Fat necrosis is seen in a pattern similar to that observed in the peripancreatic abdominal adipose tissue in patients with pancreatic fat necrosis (Fig. 48–37), namely, lobular panniculitis associated with necrosis and varying degrees of calcification. The zone of necrosis frequently abuts the septum. Granular basophilic degeneration of fat results in "ghost cells." The calcification is most prominent at the periphery of necrotic zones. Depending on the age of the lesion, variable acute, chronic, and granulomatous inflammation is associated with the fat necrosis.

## Nodular Vasculitis and Erythema Induratum

The existence of a distinctive vasculitis associated with *Mycobacterium tuberculosis* infection at a distant site (so-called tuberculoid reaction) is controversial. The term *erythema induratum* has been used to describe panniculitis associated with vasculitis in a setting of mycobacterial infection. The term *nodular vas-*

*culitis* has been used for a similar form of panniculitis in patients without evidence of mycobacterial infection.[144] By definition, special stains for tuberculosis are negative. Molecular evidence suggests that erythema induratum is due to a hypersensitivity reaction to fragments of mycobacterial organisms.[145, 146] Mycobacterial DNA has been detected in some cases of erythema induratum by polymerase chain reaction analysis.

Biopsy reveals a lobular panniculitis associated with vasculitis and ischemic and granular necrosis. Mixed inflammation including granulomas sometimes associated with caseous necrosis is seen. In addition, tuberculoid-type granulomas are frequently present. As mentioned, stains for mycobacteria are by definition negative. The vasculitis involves both arteries and veins, ranging from small to large vessels. Inflammation of vessels may be associated with acute, chronic, and granulomatous infiltrates.

## Subcutaneous Fat Necrosis of the Newborn

Subcutaneous fat necrosis of the newborn is a member of a distinctive group of crystalline panniculitides, a group of disorders characterized by panniculitis associated with crystal formation. Other members of this group of disorders are sclerema neonatorum and crystalline panniculitis associated with steroid withdrawal.

Subcutaneous fat necrosis of the newborn generally occurs in healthy neonates. Patients develop plaques and nodules that tend to be distributed over bone prominences, including cheeks, shoulders, back, buttocks, and thighs. The overlying skin is erythematous and may ulcerate. The lesions generally resolve during a period of several months.[147–149]

The pathogenesis of subcutaneous fat necrosis of the newborn is not understood.[150] Biopsy reveals a lobular panniculitis associated with a mixed inflammatory infiltrate composed of lymphocytes, neutrophils, histiocytes, and multinucleated giant cells.[151, 152] Both adipocytes and giant cells contain characteristic needle-shaped clefts that represent dissolved crystals (Fig. 48–38). Calcification of interlobular septa may also be a feature.

## Post-Steroid Panniculitis

Post-steroid panniculitis is rarely seen because of physicians' awareness of contraindications to rapid withdrawal of oral corticosteroids.[153, 154] Therefore, post-steroid panniculitis is of mostly historical interest.

The histologic features of post-steroid panniculitis are similar to those of subcutaneous fat necrosis of the newborn.

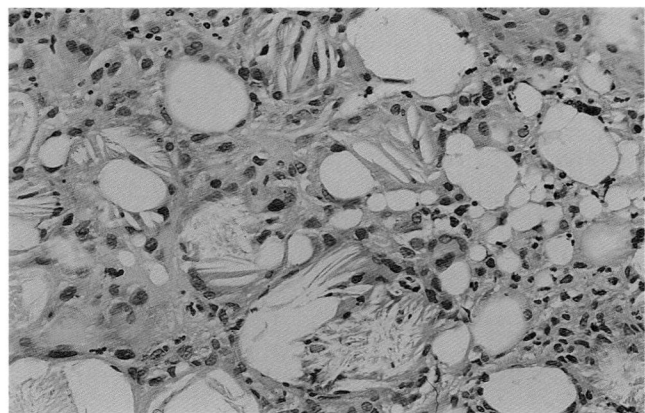

**FIGURE 48–38.** Subcutaneous fat necrosis of the newborn. Biopsy reveals a lobular panniculitis with mixed inflammatory infiltrate including multinucleated giant cells containing multiple needle-shaped clefts.

## Sclerema Neonatorum

In contrast to subcutaneous fat necrosis of the newborn, sclerema neonatorum is a crystalline panniculitis associated with serious neonatal illness. Neonates with sclerema neonatorum are frequently premature and commonly have other illnesses, such as infection and dehydration.[155] Sclerema neonatorum is characterized clinically by diffuse thickening and induration of a large percentage of the body surface. Palms, soles, and scrotum are characteristically spared. Sclerema neonatorum is associated with a high mortality rate.

Biopsy reveals adipocytes containing needle-shaped clefts in a radial arrangement. In contrast to subcutaneous fat necrosis of the newborn, inflammation is minimal or absent in sclerema neonatorum. Furthermore, the crystals are present within adipocytes. Giant cells containing crystals are absent.

## Lupus Panniculitis (Lupus Profundus)

Lupus panniculitis may be associated with discoid or systemic lupus erythematosus.[156–160] It is a rare disorder that most commonly occurs in adult women and presents as multiple nodules or plaques most often located on the face, trunk, buttocks, and proximal extremities. Associated discoid lupus may or may not be present, and ulceration may occur. Patients usually experience recurrent lesions that resolve, leaving areas of lipoatrophy and scarring.

Biopsy usually reveals characteristic findings. A mixed septal and lobular panniculitis associated with hyaline necrosis of fat lobules, karyorrhexis, and a lymphoplasmacytic infiltrate are characteristic of lupus panniculitis (Fig. 48–39). Blood vessels may

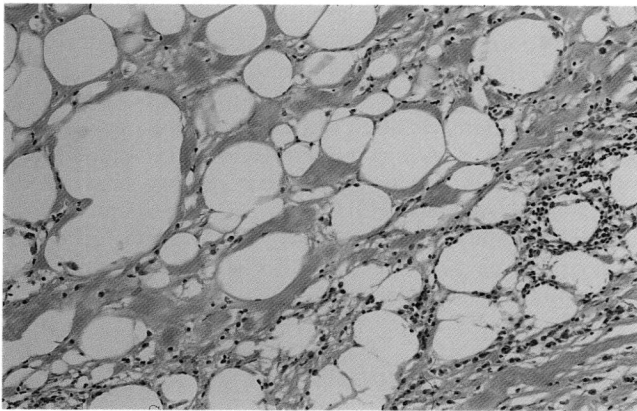

**FIGURE 48–39.** Lupus panniculitis. A mixed septal and lobular panniculitis associated with hyaline necrosis of fat lobules, karyorrhexis, and lymphoplasmacytic infiltrate is characteristic. A lymphocytic vasculitis frequently accompanies this picture.

demonstrate "onionskin" thickening, vasculopathy, and occasionally frank vasculitis. Dermal and subcutaneous mucin deposition is also a helpful diagnostic clue. The dermis and epidermis may show features of lupus erythematosus, such as basement membrane thickening, epidermal atrophy, follicular plugging, interface dermatitis, and perivascular and periadnexal chronic inflammatory infiltrate.

## SCLEROSING DISORDERS

Sclerosing disorders of the skin are those characterized by the deposition of increased amounts of collagenous matrix within the dermis.

### Scleroderma

Morphea, sometimes called localized scleroderma, is associated with a variety of clinical appearances. The most common lesions are single or multiple plaques with a white to ivory center and erythematous or violaceous border. In addition, lesions may be guttate, generalized, or linear. Young to middle-aged women are most commonly affected. The pansclerotic variant is more common in children. The etiology is unknown; however, rare cases are associated with *Borrelia burgdorferi* infection.[161]

Systemic scleroderma is a multiorgan disease commonly affecting the kidneys, lungs, and gastrointestinal tract in addition to the skin. Two clinical subtypes of systemic scleroderma are recognized. CREST syndrome is characterized by calcinosis cutis, Raynaud's phenomenon, esophageal dysfunction, sclerodactyly, and telangiectasia. Patients with CREST syndrome have a lower incidence of visceral involvement; hence, the prognosis is better compared with the progressive systemic sclerosis variant. The pathogenesis of systemic scleroderma is

poorly understood. Like localized scleroderma, systemic scleroderma is most common in young to middle-aged women. The most common skin lesions are nonpitting edema of the hands and feet and sclerosis with ulcerations of the fingers progressing to sclerodactyly. In some patients, progressive sclerosis of skin may result in flexion contractures.

The biopsy findings of sclerotic lesions in localized and systemic scleroderma show similar changes. The epidermis is usually not involved. The dominant finding is diffuse sclerosis of the dermis (Fig. 48–40). The mid and lower dermis are most strikingly affected. Dermal collagen bundles are sclerotic and swollen. The eccrine coil is compressed and distorted because of entrapment in the dermal sclerosis. A perivascular inflammatory infiltrate composed of lymphocytes and plasma cells, most marked in morphea, is seen around the superficial and deep dermal vasculature. A frequent finding in morphea is a nodular infiltrate of lymphocytes and plasma cells at the dermal-subcutaneous junction. Variable sclerosis often involves fibrous septa between fat lobules and fascia. A variant of morphea with extensive subcutaneous involvement has been termed morphea profunda. In addition, some cases may show sclerosis of the superficial reticular dermis and papillary dermis; such cases show morphologic overlap with lichen sclerosus.

### Lichen Sclerosus (et Atrophicus)

Lichen sclerosus is characterized by erythematous macules, papules, and plaques that resolve to leave an atrophic patch with a characteristic "cigarette-paper" appearance. Lichen sclerosus shows a marked female predominance and predilection for genitalia, but the trunk and limbs may also be involved. Lesions involving the genitalia tend to be particularly pruritic. Pruritic lesions, if rubbed, may

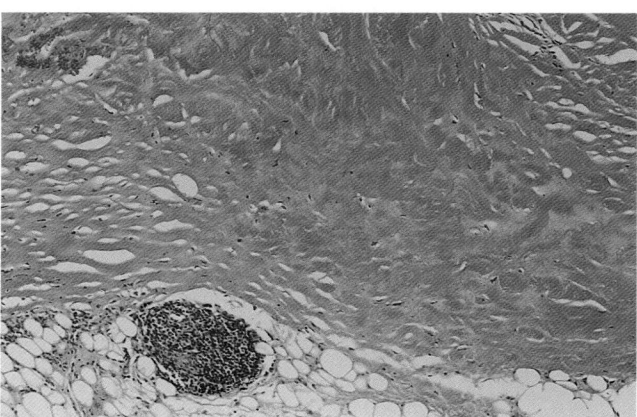

**FIGURE 48–40.** Morphea. This biopsy specimen shows deep dermal sclerosis with a pattern of linearity of the collagen fibers parallel to the epidermis. Note the nodular aggregate of lymphocytes and plasma cells.

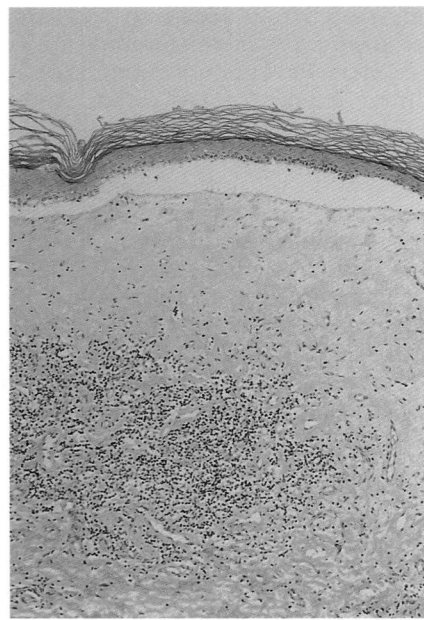

**FIGURE 48–41.** Lichen sclerosus. The papillary dermis and superficial reticular dermis are hyalinized. Below this zone of hyalinization, a perivascular and interstitial lymphoid infiltrate is seen. The epidermis is atrophic and separated from the underlying dermis, a common histologic artifact that is indicative of loss of integrity at the basement membrane.

develop superimposed lichenification. Lesions involving the penis are designated balanitis xerotica obliterans, a common cause of phimosis. An association between female genital involvement and development of squamous cell carcinoma has been described.[162, 163]

Early lesions are associated with a superficial perivascular and interstitial lymphoid infiltrate and vacuolar interface dermatitis. Edema of the papillary dermis is frequently present in early lesions and may be marked. As lesions age, the normal rete pattern is lost, and vacuolar alteration of the epidermis may become focal. The papillary dermis and superficial reticular dermis become hyalinized. Be-

low this zone of hyalinization, a variable perivascular and interstitial lymphoid infiltrate is present (Fig. 48–41). The epidermis frequently becomes atrophic, hence the designation lichen sclerosus et atrophicus. However, many lesions show epidermal acanthosis secondary to rubbing and superimposed lichen simplex chronicus. On occasion, cases show sclerosis of the deep dermis in addition to the superficial reticular dermis and papillary dermis. This has led some authorities to propose a relationship between lichen sclerosus and morphea.[164]

## Eosinophilic Fasciitis

Eosinophilic fasciitis is an inflammatory disorder showing significant clinical and pathologic overlap with morphea (localized scleroderma). However, there appear to be significant differences between these two disorders. Eosinophilic fasciitis is characterized by pain and thickening of the dermis and subcutaneous tissue, often in a ropelike fashion. Onset often follows strenuous exercise, and patients frequently have an associated peripheral eosinophilia.[165–167] Some patients develop a similar disorder after tryptophan ingestion (so-called tryptophan-related fasciitis or eosinophilia-myalgia syndrome).[168] *B. burgdorferi* has been indicated in occasional cases of eosinophilic fasciitis.[169, 170] Therefore, in endemic regions, we suggest serologic testing for spirochetal disease and tissue staining with silver stains to exclude borrelial infection.

An excisional biopsy is usually required to demonstrate the characteristic histopathologic features of eosinophilic fasciitis. In some cases, there is no significant change in the skin overlying the affected fascia. However, deep dermal sclerosis and fibrosis of septa between fat lobules associated with an inflamed, thickened fascia are characteristic when present. A mixed inflammatory infiltrate composed of lymphocytes, plasma cells, and variable numbers of eosinophils is present (Fig. 48–42). Extensive sclerosis results in obliteration of fat lobules. Inflamma-

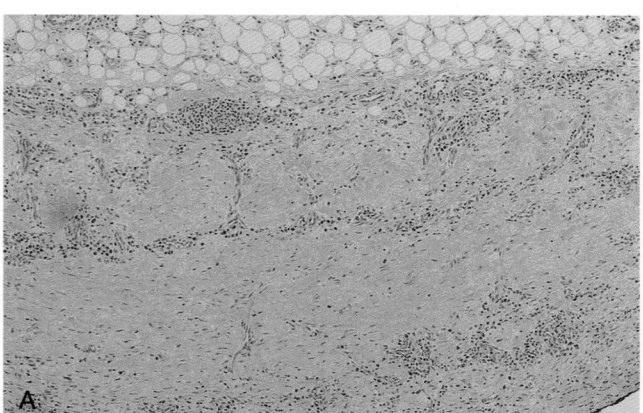 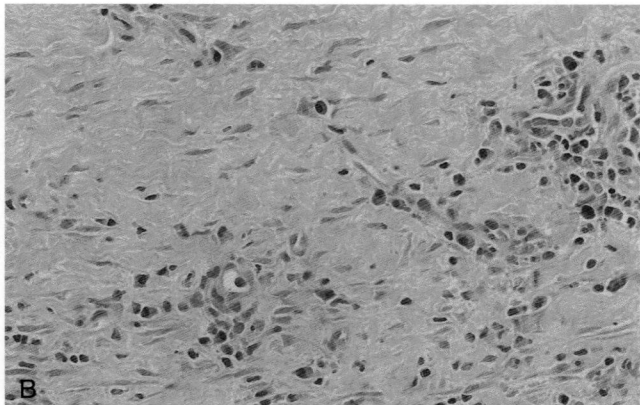

**FIGURE 48–42.** Eosinophilic fasciitis. *A.* Sclerosis and fibrosis of fascia is seen. *B.* High magnification shows a mixed inflammatory infiltrate composed of lymphocytes, plasma cells, mast cells, and eosinophils.

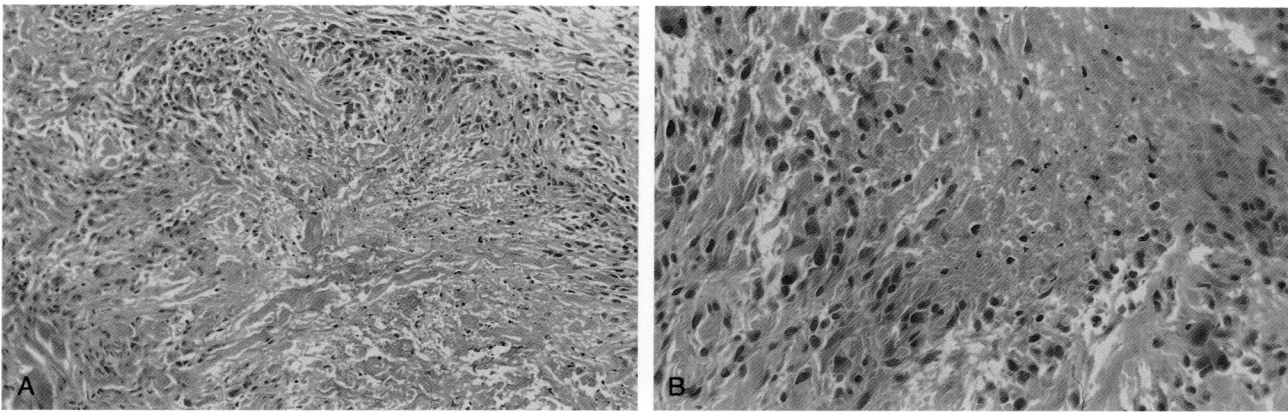

**FIGURE 48–43.** Granuloma annulare. Palisades of histiocytes arranged around necrobiotic collagen are present. (*A,* scanning magnification; *B,* high-power detail.)

tion is frequently most marked surrounding blood vessels.

## GRANULOMATOUS DERMATITIS

Granulomas are defined as focal collections of histiocytes. Granulomatous inflammation may be present in a wide range of conditions in the skin, from autoimmune responses to infectious agents to reactions to foreign material.

### Granuloma Annulare

Granuloma annulare is a benign skin disorder characterized clinically by papules and nodules, usually arranged in an annular configuration. Lesions typically involve the extensor surfaces of the extremities. A generalized form of granuloma annulare is characterized by pink to violaceous translucent lichenoid papules diffusely involving the trunk and flexor surfaces of the extremities. Deep dermal or subcutaneous granuloma annulare, sometimes referred to as pseudorheumatoid nodule, is characterized by firm, flesh-colored nodules usually seen on the extremities (frequently near joints) in young children. Perforating granuloma annulare is characterized by umbilicated papules most commonly located on the extremities of children.

The epidermis usually appears normal. In areas with collagen alteration, the upper and midreticular dermis are usually involved by well-demarcated areas of basophilic collagenous degeneration associated with deposition of mucin (acid mucopolysaccharides) and peripheral palisading of fibroblasts and histiocytes (Fig. 48–43). In lesions with incomplete collagen degeneration, the dermis shows an interstitial pattern of ill-defined basophilic areas of collagen alteration admixed with increased numbers of fibroblasts and histiocytes (Fig. 48–44). Perivascular lymphocytic infiltrates around both the superficial and deep vascular plexuses are often noted bordering areas of collagenous alteration. On occasion, fibrinoid alterations of venules are present. Giant cells and epithelioid granulomas simulating those seen in sarcoidosis are found infrequently in proximity to foci of collagenous degeneration. Generalized granuloma annulare shows a histologic pattern similar to classic granuloma annulare. In perforating granuloma annulare, transepidermal elimination of basophilic, mucinous material admixed with altered collagen is seen. Subcutaneous granuloma annulare is characterized by large areas of complete collagen degeneration with prominent peripheral palisading of histiocytes and abundant mucinous material present within the deep dermis or subcutaneous tissue.

### Necrobiosis Lipoidica

Necrobiosis lipoidica is a chronic necrobiotic dermatosis characterized by one or more discrete atrophic sclerotic plaques frequently located on the anterior tibial surface. Lesions begin as indurated erythematous macules or nodules with enlarging borders. Es-

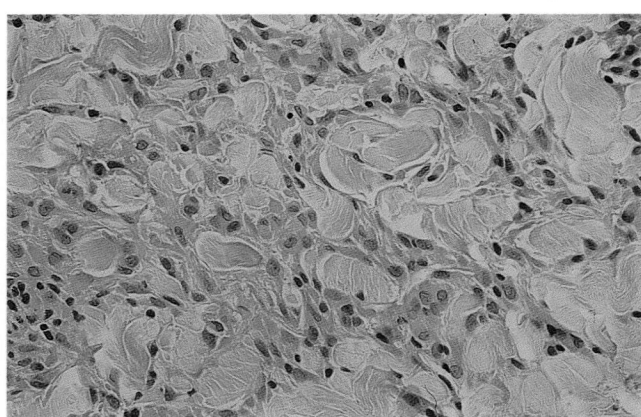

**FIGURE 48–44.** Granuloma annulare, interstitial variant. Necrobiotic collagen fibers are separated by interstitial histiocytes.

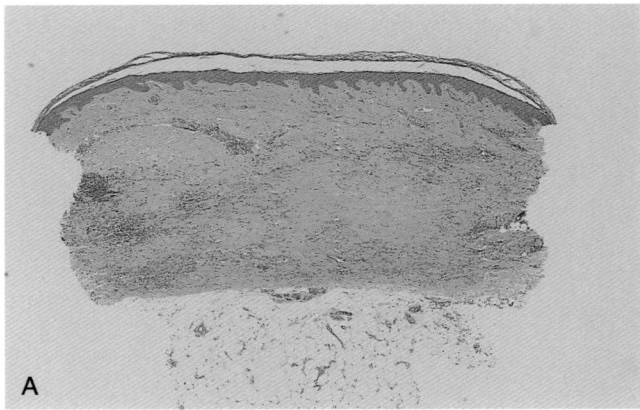
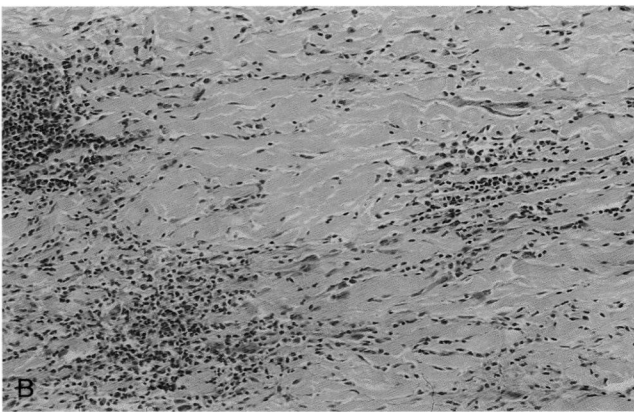

**FIGURE 48–45.** Necrobiosis lipoidica. *A.* Low-power magnification shows a typical square-shaped biopsy specimen indicating diffuse involvement of the dermis (in contrast to the focal lesions of granuloma annulare). *B.* Necrobiotic collagen identified as variable swollen structures with loss of refractility in often linear array is surrounded by chronic inflammation.

tablished lesions form a brown-yellow waxy, sclerotic surface with telangiectasia and a dark red outline. There may be ulceration and scarring from repeated ulcerations. Lesions are bilateral in more than half the cases. The lesions are usually asymptomatic, but pruritus and a burning sensation have been described by some patients. The patients frequently have diabetes mellitus, but not always.

The epidermis may be normal or atrophic and is occasionally ulcerated. Characteristic degeneration of collagen involves the reticular dermis, particularly the lower two thirds (Fig. 48–45). Large indistinct scattered areas of degenerated collagen appear eosinophilic and hyalinized and exhibit loss of refractility and normal architecture. These areas alternate with foci of spared, sclerotic dermal collagen surrounded by histiocytes, lymphocytes, and epithelioid cells. The alternating zones of "scarlike" tissue and necrobiotic collagen affecting the entire dermis form a characteristic picture. Lipid-filled multinucleated giant cells are present. Mucin deposition is usually minimal. Perivascular adventitial fibrosis and granulomatous inflammation may be present, resulting in a varying extent of luminal narrowing or obliteration. In 20% to 25% of cases, there is subcutaneous involvement, including septal necrobiosis, scarring, and mixed septal and paraseptal inflammation. Lipogranulomatous reaction and vascular changes may be present.

## Rheumatoid Nodule

Rheumatoid nodules are present in approximately 20% to 25% of patients with rheumatoid arthritis. Similar nodules may occur in patients with rheumatic fever and in rare cases of systemic lupus erythematosus. The nodules are firm, nontender, movable, subcutaneous masses. Lesions usually occur over bone prominences, especially the olecranon process, interphalangeal joints, and Achilles tendons.

Established lesions are often asymptomatic unless they are subjected to trauma or infection, which may result in complications such as ulceration, fistula track formation, osteomyelitis, and tendon rupture.

The nodule primarily involves the subcutaneous tissue or deep dermis. The epidermis and superficial dermis are usually normal. A central necrotic zone of amorphous, eosinophilic, fibrinoid material surrounded by palisading histiocytes and lymphocytes (Fig. 48–46) characterizes the established nodule. Peripherally, there is an outer zone of granulation tissue consisting of fibroblasts, inflammatory cells, and neovascularization. Mucin deposition is usually negligible.

## Rheumatic Fever Nodule

Rheumatic fever nodules are subcutaneous nodules found in approximately 30% of patients with rheumatic fever. Lesions are small (2 to 3 mm) and multiple, with a tendency to occur over bone prominences such as knuckles, olecranon process, and humoral epicondyles.

The established nodule exhibits lacelike fibrin deposition and focal alteration of collagen admixed with neutrophils and lymphocytes and surrounded by prominent blood vessels. Lesions are usually located in the deep dermis or subcutaneous tissue. Compared with other palisading granulomas, rheumatic fever nodules typically show a more acute inflammatory exudative reaction.

## Annular Elastolytic Granuloma

Annular elastolytic granuloma is a localized chronic dermal inflammatory process consisting of slowly enlarging annular plaques on sun-exposed areas. The lesions usually begin as small skin-colored or erythematous papules that gradually enlarge to form

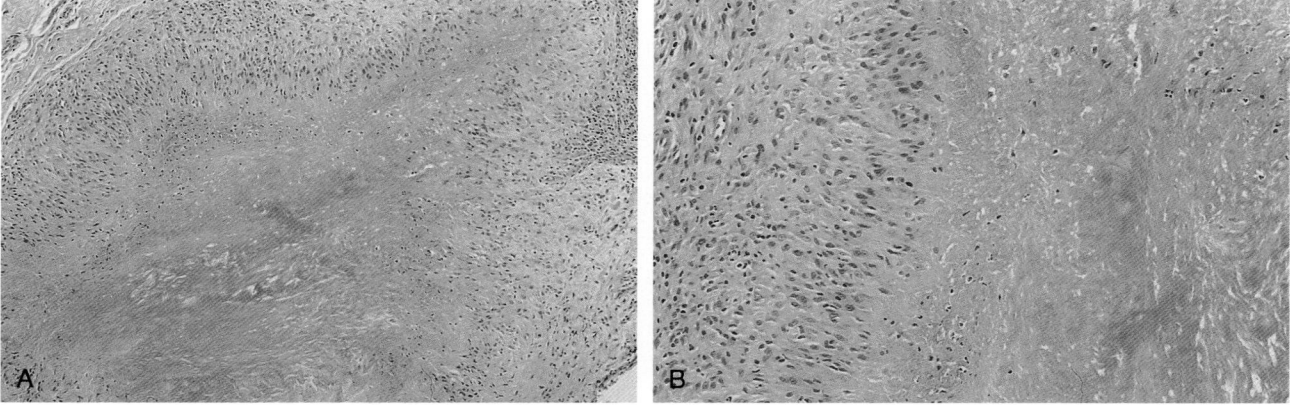

**FIGURE 48–46.** Rheumatoid nodule. *A.* Low-power magnification reveals a typical serpiginous zone of amorphous, eosinophilic, fibrinoid material surrounded by palisading histiocytes and lymphocytes. *B.* The histiocyte palisade is best developed in the rheumatoid nodule compared with other palisading granulomatous disorders.

a centrally hypopigmented 1- to 6-cm annular plaque. The most common sites are the face, scalp, neck, and arms. Most cases have occurred in white adults.

Biopsy of the annular border shows a granulomatous reaction within the mid dermis composed of epithelioid histiocytes, lymphocytes, and foreign body giant cells. A characteristic but nonspecific feature is the presence of multinucleated giant cells with intracytoplasmic elastic fibers. Asteroid bodies, which are believed to represent degenerative elastic fibers, have also been described. There is an associated perivascular lymphocytic and plasma cell infiltrate. Neither fibrinoid necrosis of collagen nor palisading of histiocytes is evident, and there is no mucin or lipid deposition. A biopsy specimen obtained from the central atrophic zone shows absence of elastotic material and absence of elastic fibers.

## Granulomatous Rosacea

Granulomatous rosacea is a histologic variant within the spectrum of acne rosacea that is characterized by epithelioid tubercle formation secondary to follicular damage and rupture. Synonyms include lupus miliaris disseminatus faciei, tuberculid-like rosacea, and rosacea-like tuberculid. Granulomatous rosacea is characterized by single or grouped discrete red-brown, firm, follicular and nonfollicular papules on the face. The papules are symmetrically distributed and may involve periorbital and perioral skin. The lesions usually involute spontaneously after a period of months to several years. Of the three variants, lupus miliaris disseminatus faciei has been observed in patients with tuberculosis. In these patients, it resolves with appropriate antibiotic therapy.

Epithelioid tubercles composed of epithelioid histiocytes, multinucleated giant cells, and lymphocytes surrounding areas of central granular necrosis are present within the dermis, usually in a perifollic-

ular pattern (Fig. 48–47). The granulomatous reaction is the result of a response to ruptured pilosebaceous units. By definition, mycobacteria are not identified.

## Infectious Granulomas

The development of immunodeficient states secondary to organ transplantation, immunosuppressive therapy, and infection with the human immunodeficiency virus has resulted in the increased incidence of unusual infections. A variety of cutaneous infections can present as palisading granulomas. These include juxta-articular nodes and gummatous lesions in syphilis, cutaneous tuberculosis, atypical mycobacterial infection, leprosy, cat-scratch disease, lymphogranuloma venereum, sporotrichosis, coccidioidomycosis, and other fungal infections.

Infectious granulomas usually exhibit more prominent central necrosis associated with a dense

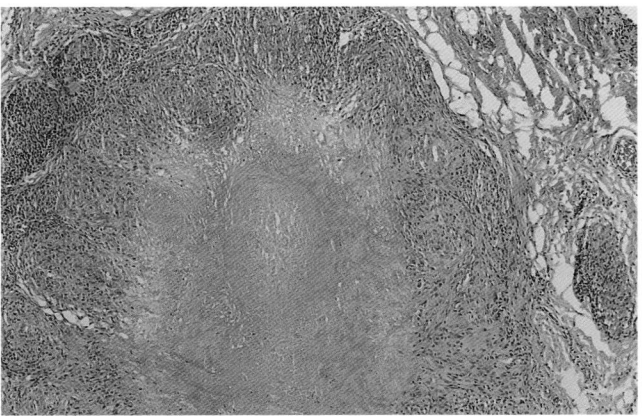

**FIGURE 48–47.** Granulomatous rosacea (lupus miliaris disseminatus faciei). Epithelioid histiocytes, multinucleated giant cells, and lymphocytes surround areas of central granular necrosis. The lesions are folliculocentric.

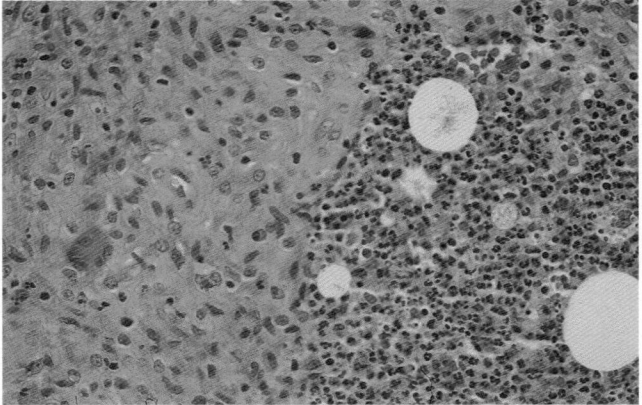

**FIGURE 48–48.** Infectious granuloma. Granulomatous inflammation with abscess formation containing bacteria-filled cystic spaces characterizes this atypical mycobacterial infection.

neutrophilic infiltration, especially in cat-scratch disease and in atypical mycobacterial infection (Fig. 48–48). Special stains for bacteria, fungi, and acid-fast bacilli are recommended to rule out an infectious etiology in palisading granulomas with central necrosis showing extensive inflammation, particularly when neutrophils are present. Immunocompromised patients may mount an unusual or atypical immune response to infection. In all patients, particularly in immunocompromised patients, the pathologist should have a low threshold for performing special stains for organisms. In addition, lesions that are suggestive of infection but fail to reveal organisms on special stains should be cultured when it is clinically appropriate.

## Palisading Granulomatous Dermatitis Associated with Systemic Disease

Palisading granulomatous dermatitis may be a manifestation of systemic disease or drug reaction.[171, 172] When the palisading dermal reaction occurs with a necrotizing vasculitis or granulomatous vasculitis, these changes may be associated with sarcoidosis, chronic bowel disease, rheumatoid arthritis, Behçet's disease, systemic lupus erythematosus, and certain endocrinopathies in addition to diabetes mellitus (such as thyroiditis). An interface dermatitis in association with the palisading granulomatous change may be observed in drug reactions, as with β-blockers, angiotensin-converting enzyme inhibitors, and calcium channel blockers. However, patients with these histologic reactions must be evaluated.

## DERMAL MUCINOSES

### Generalized Myxedema

Generalized myxedema results from chronic hypothyroidism, which causes accumulation of muco-polysaccharides within the dermis.[173, 174] Clinically, patients have symptoms of hypothyroidism including lethargy, cold intolerance, constipation, hair loss, and dry skin. The skin is pale and may demonstrate a "doughy" consistency, imparting an edematous appearance. However, in contrast to edema, pitting after pressure is not seen.

Biopsy reveals varying quantities of dermal mucin, ranging from only slight mucinosis to massive accumulation of dermal mucin. Frequently, dermal mucin is not readily apparent on routine H&E-stained sections. Histochemical stains, such as colloidal iron, toluidine blue, and alcian blue, are needed to demonstrate the dermal mucin, which exhibits metachromasia.

### Pretibial Myxedema

Pretibial myxedema is most often observed in patients with hyperthyroidism. Patients develop waxy plaques and nodules on the anterior shins and occasionally the dorsal aspect of the feet. On occasion, an extreme example mimics elephantiasis.

Biopsy reveals dermal expansion by large quantities of mucin, which splay apart collagen fibers. Distinction from dermal edema is easily demonstrated with histochemical stains for mucin. The location of the mucin is characteristically mid-dermal.

### Lichen Myxedematosus and Scleromyxedema

Lichen myxedematosus and scleromyxedema are thought to be related disorders. Lichen myxedematosus, sometimes referred to as papular mucinosis, is characterized by a papular eruption most commonly seen on the face and hands. A characteristic feature is the arrangement of papules in a linear pattern. Scleromyxedema is characterized by diffusely thickened skin in addition to papules similar to those seen in lichen myxedematosus. Patients characteristically have a circulating monoclonal gammopathy or paraprotein.[175] Biopsy reveals extensive dermal mucin. It is usually present in the upper third of the dermis, including the papillary dermis, and in contrast to the other dermal mucinoses, it shows increased fibroblasts and mast cells. Distinction from other forms of dermal mucinosis requires clinicopathologic correlation.

### Scleredema

Scleredema is characterized by nonpitting induration of the skin, particularly localized to the central upper back. Scleredema is often associated with upper respiratory tract infection or diabetes mellitus. Scleredema that follows an upper respiratory tract infection is associated with an abrupt and rapid onset (within several weeks of infection). Many infection-associated cases of scleredema resolve spontaneously during a period of months; however, some patients experience a prolonged course up to a period of years. Scleredema associated with diabetes mellitus has a prolonged course.[176]

Biopsy reveals a dermis that is expanded by thickened sclerotic collagen bundles widely separated from each other. The markedly thickened dermis may be recognized at low power by the abnormally placed eccrine glands within the superficial aspect of the dermis. Small quantities of mucin may be visualized on routine microscopy; however, special stains are usually needed to demonstrate dermal mucin. Scleredema is differentiated from scleroderma by the presence of mucin and the lack of scarring or sclerosis.

## CUTANEOUS DEPOSITION DISORDERS

A wide variety of exogenous and endogenous substances may form deposits within the dermis and subcutaneous tissue. In some cases, a wide variety of disorders may be associated with deposition of a single substance. For example, there are many causes of dermal mucin deposition.

### Gout

Cutaneous deposition of uric acid crystals occurs in patients with an abnormality in purine metabolism. Uric acid crystal deposits, sometimes referred to as gouty tophi, are typically deposited in small joints, particularly the great toe. The ear, although less commonly involved, is also a characteristic site of uric acid crystal deposition.

Uric acid crystals are dissolved during routine formalin fixation and processing for H&E-stained sections.[177] Nevertheless, the histopathologic features are diagnostic. Pale white, radially arranged amorphous material with a feathery or fibrillar border is surrounded by a granulomatous reaction.[178] Slender, slitlike clear spaces represent the outline of the dissolved crystals. Alcohol fixation preserves crystal structure. Polarization microscopy demonstrates bright birefringence in alcohol-fixed specimens.

### Calcinosis Cutis

There are several major causes of dermal calcium deposition. The underlying cause may not be discernible on light microscopic evaluation; therefore, careful clinical evaluation, such as for causes of hypercalcemia, should be instituted when it is appropriate. Dystrophic calcification refers to calcification of previously damaged tissue. Theoretically, this phenomenon may occur in any area of local tissue injury. By definition, patients have a normal serum calcium level. Extensive dystrophic calcification may

occur in the setting of connective tissue diseases, particularly dermatomyositis, scleroderma (especially CREST syndrome), and lupus erythematosus.

Calcification of neoplasms, both benign and malignant, may also be considered a form of dystrophic calcification. Idiopathic calcinosis cutis refers to calcification of dermis or subcutaneous tissue without apparent cause or association. Large tumor-like deposits may form in idiopathic calcinosis cutis. Calcified nodules frequently develop in scrotal skin and in many cases represent calcification of epidermal inclusion cysts.[179] Therefore, this form of calcification is probably best considered a form of dystrophic calcinosis cutis. "Metastatic" calcinosis cutis is an unsatisfactory term referring to cutaneous and subcutaneous calcification in the setting of defects in calcium metabolism. Most commonly, patients have hypercalcemia due to hyperparathyroidism, hyperphosphatemia, hypervitaminosis D, milk-alkali syndrome, and hyperphosphatemia associated with renal failure.[180, 181] In addition, diseases that destroy bone and raise serum calcium levels may also cause metastatic calcinosis cutis. Metastatic carcinoma to bone, multiple myeloma, and sarcoidosis are examples of diseases that may be associated with metastatic calcinosis cutis. Calciphylaxis is a rare, life-threatening condition most frequently seen in association with hyperparathyroidism in patients with chronic renal failure.[182, 183] Patients tend to develop widespread ulcers.

In H&E-stained sections, calcium stains deep blue to purple. Calcium is refractile and frequently demonstrates a "cracked" or fragmented appearance. Calcification is occasionally present as fine pale blue and gray granular material. When necessary, the von Kossa stain may be used to confirm the presence of calcification. Transepidermal elimination may be associated with calcinosis cutis. Calciphylaxis shows a distinctive histologic pattern; calcification within vessel walls associated with thrombosis is characteristic. The affected vessels are usually 100 $\mu$m in size and show intimal occlusion with fibrous and mural calcification. The surrounding dermis and soft tissue may also show focal calcification. The overlying dermis and epidermis are frequently infarcted.

### Xanthomas

Xanthomas are nodular dermal infiltrates composed mainly of foamy histiocytes. Their recognition is important because they may be associated with underlying defects in lipid metabolism or underlying disorders, including malignant neoplasia. Five distinctive clinical variants of xanthoma are recognized. Each variant tends to be associated with specific underlying clinical abnormalities.

Xanthelasmas occur most frequently around the eyes and are characterized by whitish yellow plaques that are frequently bilateral. Approximately half of patients have an underlying hyperlipidemia, most commonly hypercholesterolemia (type II-a) or dyslipoproteinemia (type III).

Plain xanthomas are characterized by yellowish macules with a predilection for the palmar creases. This form of xanthoma is associated with familial dysbetalipoproteinemia (type III). Plain xanthomas involving the intertriginous areas are associated with familial hypercholesterolemia.

Tendinous xanthomas typically involve the Achilles tendon or the extensor tendons of hands or feet. Tendinous xanthomas are associated with types II-a, III, and rarely II-b hyperlipidemia.

Tuberous xanthomas are characterized by macules, nodules, and occasionally large masses that typically involve pressure points such as elbows, knees, buttocks, and posterior thighs. Tuberous xanthomas are associated with types II-a, II-b, III, and IV hypercholesterolemia.

Eruptive xanthomas, which are associated with types I, II-b, III, IV, and V hypercholesterolemia, are characterized by sudden onset of numerous yellow papules that wax and wane with plasma triglyceride and lipid levels.[184]

It may be difficult to distinguish among the subtypes of xanthomas histologically. Therefore, careful clinicopathologic correlation is needed for precise classification. Xanthomas are characterized by dermal infiltrates composed of histiocytes with abundant foamy cytoplasm. A mixed inflammatory infiltrate is frequently present. Cholesterol clefts are frequently noted in tuberous and tendinous xanthomas. In addition, tuberous and tendinous xanthomas often demonstrate marked fibrosis. In chronic lesions, foamy histiocytes may be difficult to identify. Some patients with xanthomas lack hyperlipidemia owing to an inherited defect in lipid metabolism. Xanthomas in normal lipidemic patients may be associated with malignant neoplasia, particularly lymphoproliferative disorders.[185]

## Amyloidosis

Amyloid encompasses a group of similar-appearing proteins rather than a chemically distinct entity. On ultrastructural study, amyloid is composed of nonbranching fibrils that have a distinctive appearance despite the fact that a number of biochemically distinct forms of amyloid proteins have been described. All amyloid proteins have in common a $\beta$-pleated sheet pattern on examination with x-ray crystallography. The $\beta$-pleated sheet configuration confers birefringence with Congo red staining. Amyloid may be deposited in virtually any organ, under diverse clinical settings. Amyloid deposition may be limited to one organ (localized) or may be systemic, involving multiple organs.

Systemic amyloidosis may be divided into two distinct subtypes. Primary systemic amyloidosis is associated with immunocytic dyscrasia, particularly multiple myeloma. In these patients, the amyloid protein is composed of immunoglobulin light chains and the terminal fragments of light chains. Primary systemic amyloidosis occurs most commonly in older patients. Patients usually have symptoms of systemic involvement, including fatigue, weakness, weight loss, and carpal tunnel syndrome, and symptoms related to cardiac, renal, and hepatic dysfunction. Skin lesions are detected in approximately one third of patients with primary systemic amyloidosis. Because they may occur early in the disease course, their presence may be an important clue to an underlying B cell neoplasm.[186-188] The most common skin manifestation is hemorrhage due to vascular damage. A classic finding is the deposit of waxy purpuric macules and papules involving periorbital skin. Patients will often notice increased bruising after trauma.

The second form of systemic amyloidosis, secondary systemic amyloidosis, is associated with a number of chronic inflammatory diseases, including infections (such as tuberculosis, leprosy, osteomyelitis, and bronchiectasis) and inflammatory diseases (such as rheumatoid arthritis and familial Mediterranean fever). Skin lesions are rare in secondary systemic amyloidosis.

Biopsies of amyloid reveal dermal deposits of eosinophilic, amorphous hyaline material. The deposits form nodules or masses and also have a predilection for blood vessel walls and adnexal structures. Within the subcutaneous tissue, amyloid tends to be deposited around fat cells. Apple-green birefringence after Congo red staining is characteristic. However, the Congo red stain is not specific for amyloid. Immunohistochemical stains against the various chemical forms of amyloid may be helpful in precise chemical subclassification. As mentioned, skin lesions are uncommon in the setting of secondary systemic amyloidosis. However, biopsy of abdominal fat may reveal amyloid deposition in subcutaneous adipose tissue.[189-192]

Lichenoid amyloidosis and macular amyloidosis are two variants of localized amyloidosis; in contrast to systemic amyloidosis, they are localized to the skin and do not involve other organs. It has been postulated that the amyloid protein derives from lysosomal transformation from the $\alpha$-pleated sheet configuration of tonofilaments into a $\beta$-pleated sheet.[193] Immunostaining of this form of amyloid with antikeratin antibodies supports this hypothesis.[194] Lichenoid amyloidosis is characterized by discrete, pruritic, reddish brown papules that are most commonly seen on the shins and extensor surfaces of the forearms.[195, 196] Macular amyloidosis is characterized by pruritic gray-brown macular lesions that are most commonly seen on the upper back.

The histologic findings of papular and macular amyloidosis are subtle and easily overlooked. Both variants are characterized by small, amorphous eosinophilic deposits within the superficial papillary dermis. It is easy to overlook these small deposits of amyloid, and Congo red stain is helpful in highlighting amyloid deposits. In the lichenoid variant of localized amyloidosis, the histologic manifestations of chronic rubbing are seen, namely, acanthosis, hypergranulosis, and hyperkeratosis. Slight superficial dermal chronic inflammation and pigment incontinence are also appreciated.

Nodular amyloidosis is an uncommon form of localized amyloidosis that presents as nodules, often on the extremities or face.[197, 198] The amyloid in nodular amyloidosis is composed of immunoglobulin light chains. Some experts believe that this variant of amyloidosis represents a cutaneous plasmacytoma.[199] However, all patients with nodular deposits of amyloid should be carefully evaluated for systemic disease or progression of a lymphoproliferative disorder.

Biopsy of nodular amyloidosis reveals histologic findings similar to those in systemic amyloidosis. Large deposits of amorphous, eosinophilic material admixed with plasma cells are seen.

## Colloid Milium

Colloid milium is characterized by translucent papules and plaques on sun-damaged skin, most commonly on the face and dorsum of the hands. This disorder occurs most commonly in older men with a history of outdoor occupation with significant cumulative sun exposure. A juvenile variant, which is rare, has also been described. Juvenile and adult variants have a similar clinical appearance; however, juvenile colloid milium is usually limited to the face.

Histologic examination shows deposits of amorphous eosinophilic material with a characteristic cracked or fissured pattern (similar to that seen in amyloid). Often, a grenz zone of sparing in the superficial papillary dermis is identified. Colloid milium shows many histochemical features of amyloid. Colloid milium demonstrates apple-green birefringence with Congo red stain and stains with thioflavine T.

## REFERENCES

1. Barnhill RL (ed): Textbook of Dermatopathology. New York, McGraw-Hill, 1998.
2. Ackerman AB: Histologic Diagnosis of Inflammatory Skin Disease. 2nd ed. Baltimore, Williams & Wilkins, 1998.
3. McKee PH: Pathology of the Skin. 2nd ed. New York, Mosby-Wolfe, 1996.
4. Hood AF, Kwan TH, Mihm MC Jr, Horn TD: Primer of Dermatopathology. 2nd ed. Boston, Little, Brown, 1993.
5. Abell E: Spongiotic dermatitis. *In* Farmer ER, Hood AF (eds): Pathology of the Skin. Norwalk, CT, Appleton & Lange, 1990, pp 74–75.
6. Le TK, van der Valk PG, Schalwijk J, et al: Changes in epidermal proliferations and differentiation in allergic and irritant contact dermatitis reactions. Br J Dermatol 133:236–242, 1995.
7. Brand CU, Hunziker T, Schaffner T, et al: Activated immunocompetent cells in human skin lymph derived from irritant contact dermatitis: an immunomorphological study. Br J Dermatol 132:39–45, 1995.
8. Hurwitz RM, DeTrana C: The cutaneous pathology of atopic dermatitis. Am J Dermatopathol 12:544–551, 1990.
9. Braun-Falco O, Petry G: On the fine structure of the epider-
mis in chronic nummular eczema. II. Stratum spinosum. Arch Klin Exp Dermatol 224:63–80, 1966.
10. Bjornberg A, Hellgren L: Pityriasis rosea: a statistical, clinical and laboratory investigation of 826 patients and matched healthy controls. Acta Dermatol Venereol 42(suppl):1–36, 1962.
11. Jones HE: The atopic-chronic-dermatophytosis syndrome. Acta Dermatol Venereol 92(suppl):81–96, 1980.
12. Diepgen TL, Fartasch M: Recent epidemiological and genetic studies in atopic dermatitis. Acta Dermatol Venereol 176(suppl):13–18, 1992.
13. Pinkus H, Mehregan AH: The primary histologic lesions of seborrheic dermatitis and psoriasis. J Invest Dermatol 46:109–116, 1966.
14. Wicklund DA, Weston WL: Incontinentia pigmenti. A four-generation study. Arch Dermatol 116:701–703, 1980.
15. Carney RG Jr: Incontinentia pigmenti: a world statistical study. Arch Dermatol 112:535–542, 1976.
16. Weitzman I, Sumerbell RC: The dermatophytes. Clin Microbiol Rev 8:240–259, 1995.
17. Aly R: Ecology and epidemiology of dermatophyte infections. J Am Acad Dermatol 31:521–525, 1994.
18. Grossman ME, Silvers DN, Walther RR: Cutaneous manifestations of disseminated candidiasis. J Am Acad Dermatol 2:111–116, 1980.
19. Harber LC, Baer RL: Pathogenic mechanisms of drug-induced photosensitivity. J Invest Dermatol 58:327–342, 1972.
20. Norris PG, Hawk JL: Chronic actinic dermatitis. A unifying concept. Arch Dermatol 126:376–378, 1990.
21. Lim HW, Morison WL, Kamide R, et al: Chronic actinic dermatitis: an analysis of 51 patients evaluated in the United States and Japan. Arch Dermatol 130:1284–1289, 1994.
22. Haeffner AC, Smoller BR, Zepter K, Wood GS: Differentiation and clonality of lesional lymphocytes in small plaque parapsoriasis. Arch Dermatol 131:321–324, 1995.
23. Burg G, Dummer R: Small plaque (digitate) parapsoriasis is an "abortive cutaneous T-cell lymphoma" and is not mycosis fungoides. Arch Dermatol 131:336–338, 1995.
24. King ID, Ackerman AB: Guttate parapsoriasis/digitate dermatosis (small plaque parapsoriasis) is mycosis fungoides. Am J Dermatopathol 14:518–530, 1992.
25. Cram DL: Psoriasis: current advances in etiology and treatment. J Am Acad Dermatol 4:1–14, 1981.
26. Cox AJ, Watson H: Histologic variation in lesions of psoriasis. Arch Dermatol 106:503–507, 1972.
27. Ragaz A, Ackerman AB: Evolution, maturation and regression of lesions of psoriasis. Am J Dermatopathol 1:199–214, 1979.
28. Payne CMER, Wilkinson JD, McKee PH, et al: Nodular prurigo: a clinicopathological study of 46 patients. Br J Dermatol 113:431–439, 1985.
29. Feuerman EJ, Sandbank M: Prurigo nodularis: histological and electron microscopical study. Arch Dermatol 111:1472–1477, 1975.
30. Botella-Estrada R, San Martin O, Olivier V, et al: Erythroderma: a clinicopathological study of 56 cases. Arch Dermatol 130:1503–1507, 1994.
31. Zip C, Murray S, Walsh NM: The specificity of histopathology in erythroderma. J Cutan Pathol 20:393–398, 1993.
32. Walsh N, Prokopetz R, Tro V, et al: Histopathology in erythroderma: review of a series of cases by multiple observers. J Cutan Pathol 21:419–423, 1994.
33. Griffiths WAD: Pityriasis rubra pilaris. Clin Exp Dermatol 5:105–108, 1980.
34. Vanderhooft SL, Francis JS, Holbrook KA, et al: Familial pityriasis rubra pilaris. Arch Dermatol 131:448–453, 1995.
35. Soeprono FF: Histologic criteria for the diagnosis of pityriasis rubra pilaris. Am J Dermatopathol 8:277–283, 1986.
36. Traupe H: The Ichthyoses. A Guide to Clinical Diagnosis, Genetic Counseling, and Therapy. Berlin, Springer-Verlag, 1989.
37. Wells RS, Kerr CB: The histology of ichthyosis. J Invest Dermatol 46:530–535, 1966.
38. Mallinson CN, Bloom SR, Warin AP, et al: A glucagonoma syndrome. Lancet 2:1–5, 1974.
39. Marinkovich MP, Botella R, Datloff J, Sangueza OP: Necro-

lytic migratory erythema without glucagonoma in patients with liver disease. J Am Acad Dermatol 32:604–609, 1995.

40. Kahan RS, Perez-Figueredo RA, Neimanis A: Necrolytic migratory erythema. Arch Dermatol 113:792–797, 1977.

41. Stone OJ: Pellagra—increased viscosity of extracellular matrix. Med Hypotheses 40:355–359, 1993.

42. Lee MG: Transient symptomatic zinc deficiency in a full term breast fed infant. J Am Acad Dermatol 23:375–379, 1990.

43. Borroni G, Brazzelli V, Vignati G, et al: Bullous lesions in acrodermatitis enteropathica: histopathologic findings regarding two patients. Am J Dermatopathol 14:304–309, 1992.

44. Altman K, Mehregan AH: Inflammatory linear verrucose epidermal nevus. Arch Dermatol 104:385–389, 1971.

45. Golitz LE, Weston WL: Inflammatory linear verrucose epidermal nevus. Arch Dermatol 115:1208–1212, 1979.

46. Gianotti R, Restano L, Grimalt R, et al: Lichen striatus—a chameleon: a histopathological and immunohistological study of forty-one cases. J Cutan Pathol 22:18–23, 1995.

47. Jeerapaet P, Ackerman AB: Histologic pattern of secondary syphilis. Arch Dermatol 107:373–377, 1973.

48. Abell E, Marks R, Wilson Jones E: Secondary syphilis: a clinicopathological review. Br J Dermatol 93:251–254, 1976.

49. Cochran RIE, Thomson J, Fleming KA, et al: Histology simulating reticulosis in secondary syphilis. Br J Dermatol 95:251–254, 1976.

50. Baker H, Ryan TJ: Generalized pustular psoriasis: a clinical and epidemiological study of 104 cases. Br J Dermatol 80:771–782, 1968.

51. Zelickson B, Muller S: Generalized pustular psoriasis: a review of 63 cases. Arch Dermatol 127:1339–1345, 1991.

52. Huges R, Kear A: Reiter's syndrome and reactive arthritis: a current view. Semin Arthritis Rheum 24:190–210, 1994.

53. Wilkins RF: Reiter's syndrome: evaluation of preliminary criteria for definite diagnosis. Arthritis Rheum 24:844–848, 1981.

54. Burns RE, Fine G: Subcorneal pustular dermatosis. Arch Dermatol 80:72–74, 1959.

55. Eisenberg E, Krutchkoff D: Lichenoid lesions of oral mucosa. Oral Surg Oral Med Oral Pathol 73:699–704, 1992.

56. Mehregan DA, Van Hale HM, Muller SA: Lichen planopilaris: clinical and pathologic study of forty-five patients. J Am Acad Dermatol 27:935–942, 1992.

57. Prieto VG, Casals M, McNutt NS: Lichen planus–like keratosis: a clinical and histopathological reexamination. Am J Surg Pathol 17:259–263, 1993.

58. Smoller BR, Flynn T: Immunohistochemical examination of lichen nitidus suggests that it is not a localized papular variant of lichen planus. J Am Acad Dermatol 27:232–236, 1992.

59. Halvey S, Sahi A: Lichenoid drug eruptions. J Am Acad Dermatol 29:249–253, 1993.

60. Howland WW, Golitz LE, Weston WL, Huff JC: Erythema multiforme: clinical, histopathologic and immunologic study. J Am Acad Dermatol 10:438–446, 1984.

61. Wolkenstein P, Charue D, Laurent P, et al: Metabolic predisposition to cutaneous adverse drug reactions: role in toxic epidermal necrolysis caused by sulfonamides and anticonvulsants. Arch Dermatol 131:544–552, 1995.

62. Cote B, Wechsler J, Bastuji-Garin S, et al: Clinicopathologic correlation in erythema multiforme and Stevens-Johnson syndrome. Arch Dermatol 131:1268–1272, 1995.

63. Guillaume J-C, Roujeau J-C, Revuz J, et al: The culprit drugs in 87 cases of toxic epidermal necrolysis (Lyell's syndrome). Arch Dermatol 123:1166–1170, 1987.

64. Roujeau J-C, Chosidow O, Saiag P, Guillaume J-C: Toxic epidermal necrolysis. J Am Acad Dermatol 23:1039–1058, 1990.

65. Lyell A: A review of toxic epidermal necrolysis in Britain. Br J Dermatol 79:662–671, 1967.

66. Glucksberg J, Storb R, Fefer A, et al: Clinical manifestations of graft-versus-host disease in human recipients of marrow from HLA matched sibling donors. Transplantation 18:295–304, 1974.

67. James WD, Odom RB: Graft-versus-host disease. Arch Dermatol 119:683–689, 1983.

68. Saurat JH: Cutaneous manifestations of graft-versus-host disease. Int J Dermatol 20:249–251, 1981.

69. Tanaka K, Sullivan JM, Shulman HM, et al: A clinical review: cutaneous manifestation of acute and chronic graft-versus-host disease following bone marrow transplantation. J Dermatol 18:11–17, 1991.

70. Decoste SD, Boudreaux C, Dover JS: Transfusion-associated graft-vs-host disease in patients with malignancy. Arch Dermatol 26:1324–1329, 1990.

71. Chosidow O, Bagot M, Vernant JP, et al: Sclerodermatous chronic graft-versus-host disease: analysis of seven cases. J Am Acad Dermatol 26:49–55, 1992.

72. Gelmetti C, Rigoni C, Alessi E, et al: Pityriasis lichenoides in children: a long term follow-up of eighty-nine cases. J Am Acad Dermatol 23:473–478, 1990.

73. Ackerman AB: Histologic Diagnosis of Inflammatory Skin Diseases. 2nd ed. Baltimore, Williams & Wilkins, 1997, p 554.

74. Callen JP, Kelin J: Subacute cutaneous lupus erythematosus. Clinical, serologic, immunogenetic and therapeutic considerations in seventy-two patients. Arthritis Rheum 31:1007–1013, 1988.

75. Lee LA: Neonatal lupus erythematosus. J Invest Dermatol 100:9S–13S, 1993.

76. Bielsa I, Herrero C, Collada A, et al: Histopathologic findings in cutaneous lupus erythematosus. Arch Dermatol 130:54–58, 1994.

77. Jerdan MS, Hood AF, Moore GW, et al: Histologic comparison of the subsets of lupus erythematosus. Arch Dermatol 126:52–55, 1990.

78. Fabre VC, Lear S, Reichlin M, et al: Twenty percent of biopsy specimens from sun-exposed skin of normal young adults demonstrated positive immunofluorescence. Arch Dermatol 127:1006–1011, 1991.

79. Barnes BE: Dermatomyositis and malignancy. A review of the literature. Am Intern Med 84:68–76, 1976.

80. Chen Z, Maize JC, Silver RM, et al: Direct and indirect immunofluorescent findings in dermatomyositis. J Cutan Pathol 12:18–27, 1985.

81. Mascaro JM Jr, Hausmann G, Herrero C, et al: Membrane attack complex deposits in cutaneous lesions of dermatomyositis. Arch Dermatol 131:1386–1392, 1995.

82. Thivolet J: Pemphigus: past, present, and future. Dermatology 189(suppl):26–29, 1994.

83. Stanley JR, Koulu L, Thivolet C: Pemphigus vulgaris and pemphigus foliaceus autoantibodies bind different molecules (abstract). J Invest Dermatol 82:439, 1984.

84. Ahmed AR, Kurgi BS, Rogers RS III: Cicatricial pemphigoid. J Am Acad Dermatol 24:987–1001, 1991.

85. Sarrett Y, Hall R, Cobo M, et al: Salt–split skin substrate for the immunofluorescent screening of serum from patients with cicatricial pemphigoid and a new method of immunoprecipitation with IgA antibodies. J Am Acad Dermatol 24:952–958, 1991.

86. Chorzelski T, Jablonska S, Blaszcyk M: Immunopathological investigation in Senear-Usher syndrome (coexistence of pemphigus and lupus erythematosus). Br J Dermatol 80:211–217, 1968.

87. Ruocco V, Sacerdoti G: Pemphigus and bullous pemphigoid due to drugs. Int J Dermatol 30:307–312, 1991.

88. Ostezan LB, Fabre VC, Caughman W, et al: Paraneoplastic pemphigus in the absence of a known neoplasm. J Am Acad Dermatol 33:312–315, 1995.

89. Camisa C, Helm TN, Valenzuela R, et al: Paraneoplastic pemphigus: three new cases (abstract). J Invest Dermatol 98:590, 1992.

90. Ikeda S, Welsh EA, Peluso AM, et al: Localization of the gene whose mutations underlie Hailey-Hailey disease to chromosome 3q. Hum Mol Genet 3:1147–1150, 1994.

91. Michel B: Hailey-Hailey disease. Familial benign chronic pemphigus. Arch Dermatol 118:781–783, 1982.

92. Burge SM, Wilkinson JD: Darier-White disease: a review of the clinical features in 163 patients. J Am Acad Dermatol 27:40–50, 1992.

93. Hu CH, Michel B, Farber EM: Transient acantholytic dermatosis (Grover's disease). A skin disorder related to heat and sweating. Arch Dermatol 121:1439–1441, 1985.

94. Heaphy MR, Tucker SB, Winkelman RK: Benign papular acantholytic dermatosis. Arch Dermatol 112:814–821, 1976.

95. Manteaux AM, Rapini RP: Transient acantholytic dermatosis in patients with skin cancer. Cutis 46:488–490, 1990.

96. Grover RW: Transient acantholytic dermatosis. Arch Dermatol 101:426–434, 1970.

97. Chalet M, Grover R, Ackerman AB: Transient acantholytic dermatosis. Arch Dermatol 113:431–435, 1977.

98. Baker DH, Dimond RL, Wuepper KD: The epidermolytic toxin of *Staphylococcus aureus*: its failure to bind to cells and its detection in blister fluids of patients with bullous impetigo. J Invest Dermatol 71:274–275, 1978.

99. Elias PM, Fritsch P, Epstein EH Jr: Staphylococcal scalded skin syndrome. Arch Dermatol 113:207–219, 1977.

100. Eady RA: The hemidesmosome: a target in autoimmune bullous disease. Dermatology 189(suppl 1):38–41, 1994.

101. Hall RP: Dermatitis herpetiformis. J Invest Dermatol 99:873–881, 1992.

102. Wojnarowska F, Bhogal BS, Black MM: Chronic bullous disease of childhood and linear IgA disease of adults are IgA1-mediated diseases. Br J Dermatol 131:210–214, 1994.

103. Wojnarowska F, Allen J, Collier P: Linear IgA disease: a heterogeneous disease. Dermatology 189(suppl 1):52–56, 1994.

104. Collier PM, Wojnarowska F, Millard PR: Variation in the deposition of the antibodies at different anatomical sites in linear IgA disease of adults and chronic bullous disease of childhood. Br J Dermatol 127:482–484, 1992.

105. Kuechle MK, Stegemeir E, Maynard B, et al: Drug-induced linear IgA bullous dermatosis: report of six cases and review of the literature. J Am Acad Dermatol 30:187–192, 1994.

106. Wojnarowska F, Marsden RA, Bhogal B, Black MM: Chronic bullous disease of childhood, childhood cicatricial pemphigoid and linear IgA disease of adults. A comparative study demonstrating clinical and immunopathologic overlap. J Am Acad Dermatol 19:792–805, 1988.

107. Marsden RA, McKee PH, Bhogal B, et al: A study of benign chronic bullous dermatosis of childhood and comparison with dermatitis herpetiformis and bullous pemphigoid. Clin Exp Dermatol 5:159–176, 1980.

108. Wojnarowska F, Marsden RA, Bhogal B, Black MM: Chronic bullous disease of childhood, childhood cicatricial pemphigoid and linear IgA disease of adults. A comparative study demonstrating clinical and immunological overlap. J Am Acad Dermatol 9:792–805, 1988.

109. Burrows NP, Bhogal BS, Black MM, et al: Bullous eruption of systemic lupus erythematosus: a clinicopathological study of four cases. Br J Dermatol 128:332–338, 1993.

110. Gilchrest B, Roore JW, Mihm MC Jr: Bullous dermatosis in hemodialysis. Am Intern Med 83:480–483, 1975.

111. Judd LE, Hendersen DW, Hill DC: Naproxen-induced pseudoporphyria. Arch Dermatol 122:451–454, 1986.

112. Fine JD, Bauer EA, Briggaman RA, et al: Revised clinical and laboratory criteria for subtypes of inherited epidermolysis bullosa. J Am Acad Dermatol 24:119–135, 1991.

113. McKee PH: Pathology of the Skin. 2nd ed. New York, Mosby-Wolfe, 1996, Chapter 2.

114. Woodley DT, Briggaman RA, Gammon WR: Acquired epidermolysis bullosa: a bullous disease associated with autoimmunity to type VII (anchoring fibril) collagen. Dermatol Clin 8:717–726, 1990.

115. Stewart MI, Woodley DT, Briggaman RA: Epidermolysis bullosa acquisita and associated symptomatic esophageal webs. Arch Dermatol 127:373–377, 1991.

116. Gammon WR, Briggaman RA, Woodley DT, et al: Epidermolysis bullosa acquisita: a pemphigoid-like disease. J Am Acad Dermatol 11:820–832, 1984.

117. Gammon WR, Fine JD, Briggaman RA: Autoimmunity to type VII collagen: features and roles in basement membrane zone injury. *In* Fine JD (ed): Bullous Diseases. New York, Igaku Shoin, 1993, p 75.

118. Yiannias JA, El-Azhary RA, Gibson LE: Erythema elevatum diutinum: a clinical and histopathologic study of 13 patients. J Am Acad Dermatol 26:38–44, 1992.

119. Katz SI, Gallin JL, Hertz KC, et al: Erythema elevatum diutinum: skin and systemic manifestations, immunologic studies and successful treatment with dapsone. Medicine (Baltimore) 56:443–455, 1977.

120. Cream JJ, Leven GM, Calnan CD: Erythema elevatum diutinum: an unusual reaction to streptococcal antigen and response to dapsone. Br J Dermatol 84:393–399, 1971.

121. Morrison JGL, Hull PR, Fourie E: Erythema elevatum diutinum, cryoglobulinaemia, and fixed urticaria on cooling. Br J Dermatol 97:99–104, 1977.

122. Dorsey JK, Penick GD: The association of hairy cell leukemia with unusual immunologic disorder. Arch Intern Med 142:902–903, 1982.

123. DeShazo RD, Levinson AL, Lawless OJ, Weisbaum G: Systemic vasculitis with co-existent large and small vessel involvement: a classification dilemma. JAMA 238:1940–1942, 1977.

124. Jennette JC, Falk RJ: Diagnostic classification of antineutrophil cytoplasmic autoantibody–associated vasculitis. Am J Kidney Dis 18:184–187, 1991.

125. Jennette JC, Falk RJ: Antineutrophil cytoplasmic antibodies and associated diseases: a review. Am J Kidney Dis 15:517–529, 1990.

126. Goeken J: Antineutrophil cytoplasmic and anti–endothelial cell antibodies: new mechanisms for vasculitis. Curr Opin Dermatol 19:75, 1995.

127. Manger B, Krapf FE, Grmatzki M, et al: IgE-containing circulating immune complexes in Churg-Strauss vasculitis. Scand J Immunol 21:369–373, 1985.

128. Cohen Tervaert JW, Limburg PC, Elema JD, et al: Detection of auto-antibodies against myeloid lysosomal enzymes: a useful adjunct to classification of patients with biopsy-proven necrotizing arteries. Am J Med 91:59–66, 1991.

129. Finan MC, Winklemann RK: The cutaneous extravascular necrotizing granuloma (Churg-Strauss granuloma) and systemic disease: a review of 27 cases. Medicine (Baltimore) 62:142–158, 1983.

130. Goodman GC, Churg J: Wegener's granulomatosis: pathology and review of the literature. Arch Pathol 58:533, 1954.

131. Jennette JC, Falk RJ, Andrassy K, et al: Nomenclature of systemic vasculitides: proposal of an international consensus conference. Arthritis Rheum 37:187–192, 1994.

132. Barksdale SK, Hallahan CW, Kerr GS, et al: Cutaneous pathology in Wegener's granulomatosis. Am J Surg Pathol 19:161–172, 1995.

133. Schroeter AL, Diaz-Perez JL, Winkelmann RK, et al: Livedo vasculitis (the vasculitis of atrophie blanche). Arch Dermatol 111:188–193, 1976.

134. Suster S, Ronnen M, Bubis JJ, Schewach-Millet M: Familial atrophie blanche–like lesions with subcutaneous fibrinoid vasculitis: the Georgian ulcers. Am J Dermatopathol 8:386–391, 1986.

135. Shornick JK, Nichols BK, Bergstresser PR, et al: Idiopathic atrophie blanche. J Am Acad Dermatol 8:792–798, 1983.

136. Föström L, Winklemann RK: Acute panniculitis: a clinical and histopathologic study of 34 cases. Arch Dermatol 113:909–917, 1977.

137. Föström L, Winklemann RK: Granulomatous panniculitis in erythema nodosum. Arch Dermatol 111:335–340, 1975.

138. Hannuksela M: Erythema nodosum. Clin Dermatol 4:88–95, 1986.

139. White JW, Winklemann RK: Weber-Christian panniculitis: a review of 30 cases with this diagnosis. J Am Acad Dermatol 56–62, 1998.

140. Smith KC, Pittelkow MR, Su WPD: Panniculitis associated with severe $\alpha_1$-antitrypsin deficiency. Arch Dermatol 123:1655–1661, 1987.

141. Su WPD, Smith KC, Pittelkow MR, Winklemann RK: $\alpha_1$-Antitrypsin deficiency panniculitis: a histopathologic and immunopathologic study of four cases. Am J Dermatopathol 9:483–490, 1987.

142. Smith KC, Su WP, Pittelkow MR, Winklemann RK: Clinical and pathologic correlations in 96 patients with panniculitis. J Am Acad Dermatol 21:1192–1196, 1989.

143. Föström L, Winklemann RK: Acute, generalized panniculitis with amylase and lipase in skin. Arch Dermatol 111:497–502, 1975.

144. Montgomery H, O'Leary PA, Barker NW: Nodular vascular diseases of the legs: erythema induratum and allied conditions. JAMA 128:335, 1945.

145. Penneys NS, Leonardi CL, Cook S, et al: Identification of *Mycobacterium tuberculosis* DNA in five different types of cutaneous lesions by the polymerase chain reaction. Arch Dermatol 129:1594–1598, 1993.

146. Ollert MW, Thomas P, Korting HC, et al: Erythema induratum of Bazin: evidence of T-lymphocyte hyperresponsiveness to purified protein derivative of tuberculin. Report of two cases and treatment. Arch Dermatol 129:469–473, 1993.

147. Chen TH, Shewmake SQ, Hansen DD, Lacey HL: Subcutaneous fat necrosis of the newborn. Arch Dermatol 117:36–37, 1981.

148. Silverman AK: Panniculitis in infants (letter). Arch Dermatol 121:834, 1985.

149. Fretzin DF, Arias AM: Sclerema neonatorum and subcutaneous fat necrosis of the newborn. Pediatr Dermatol 4:112–122, 1987.

150. Sharata H, Postellon DC, Hashimoto K: Subcutaneous fat necrosis, hypercalcemia and prostaglandin E. Pediatr Dermatol 12:43–47, 1995.

151. Oswalt GC Jr, Montes LF, Cassady G: Subcutaneous fat necrosis of the newborn. J Cutan Pathol 5:193–199, 1978.

152. Friedman SJ, Winklemann RK: Subcutaneous fat necrosis of the newborn: light, ultrastructural and histochemical microscopic studies. J Cutan Pathol 16:99–105, 1989.

153. Roenigk HH, Haserick JR, Arundell FD: Poststeroid panniculitis. Arch Dermatol 90:387–391, 1965.

154. Silverman RA, Newman AJ, LeVine MJ, Kaplan B: Poststeroid panniculitis. A case report. Pediatr Dermatol 5:92–93, 1988.

155. Jardine D, Artherton DJ, Trompeter RS: Sclerema neonatorum and subcutaneous fat necrosis of the newborn in the same infant. Eur J Dermatol 150:125–126, 1986.

156. Winklemann RK: Panniculitis and systemic lupus erythematosus. JAMA 211:472–475, 1970.

157. Fountain RB: Lupus erythematosus profundus. Br J Dermatol 80:571–579, 1985.

158. Peters MS, Su WPD: Lupus erythematosus panniculitis. Med Clin North Am 73:1113–1127, 1989.

159. Peters MS, Su WPD: Panniculitis. Dermatol Clin 10:37–57, 1992.

160. Izumi AK, Takiguchi P: Lupus erythematosus panniculitis. Arch Dermatol 119:61–64, 1983.

161. Aberer E, Klade H, Stanek G, et al: *Borrelia burgdorferi* and different types of morphea. Dermatologica 182:145–154, 1991.

162. Hart WR, Norris JH, Helwig EB: Relation of lichen sclerosus et atrophicus of the vulva to the development of carcinoma. Obstet Gynecol 45:369–377, 1975.

163. Carlson A, Ambros R, Malfetano J, et al: Vulvar lichen sclerosus and squamous cell carcinoma: a cohort, case control, and investigational study with historical perspective; implications for chronic inflammation and sclerosis in the development of neoplasia. Hum Pathol 29:932–948, 1998.

164. Glockenberg A, Cohen-Sobel E, Caseli M, Chico G: Rare case of lichen sclerosus et atrophicus associated with morphea. J Am Podiatr Med Assoc 84:622–624, 1994.

165. Torres VM, George WM: Diffuse eosinophilic fasciitis. A new syndrome or variant of scleroderma? Arch Dermatol 113:1591–1593, 1977.

166. Krauser RE, Tuthill RJ: Eosinophilic fasciitis. Arch Dermatol 113:1092–1093, 1977.

167. Fleishmajer R, Jacotot AB, Shore S, Binick SA: Scleroderma, eosinophilia, and diffuse fasciitis. Arch Dermatol 114:1320–1325, 1978.

168. Connolly SM, Quimby SR, Griffing WL, Winklemann RK: Scleroderma and L-tryptophan: a possible explanation of the eosinophilia-myalgia syndrome. J Am Acad Dermatol 23:451–457, 1990.

169. Granter SR, Barnhill RL, Hewins ME, Duray PH: Identification of *Borrelia burgdorferi* in diffuse fasciitis with peripheral eosinophilia: borrelial fasciitis. JAMA 272:1283–1285, 1994.

170. Granter SE, Barnhill RL, Duray PH: Borrelial fasciitis: diffuse fasciitis and peripheral eosinophilia associated with *Borrelia* infection. Am J Dermatopathol 18:465–473, 1996.

171. Magro CM, Crowson AN, Regauer S: Granuloma annulare and necrobiosis lipoidica tissue reactions as a manifestation of systemic disease. Hum Pathol 27:50–56, 1996.

172. Magro CM, Crowson AN, Schapiro BC: Interstitial and palisading granulomatous drug reactions: a distinctive clinical and pathologic entity. J Cutan Pathol 25:72–78, 1998.

173. Heymann WR: Cutaneous manifestations of thyroid disease. J Am Acad Dermatol 26:885–902, 1992.

174. Truhan AP, Roenigk HH Jr: The cutaneous mucinoses. J Am Acad Dermatol 14:14–18, 1986.

175. Braun-Falco O, Weidner F: Skleromyxödem Arndt-Gottron mit Knochemarks-Plasmozytose und Myositis. Arch Belg Dermatol Syphiligr 26:193–217, 1970.

176. Fleishmajer R, Faludi G, Krol S: Scleredema and diabetes mellitus. Arch Dermatol 101:21–26, 1970.

177. King DF, King LA: The appropriate processing of tophi for microscopy. Am J Dermatopathol 4:239, 1982.

178. Lichenstein L, Scott HW, Levin MH: Pathologic changes in gout. Am J Pathol 32:871, 1956.

179. Swinehart JM, Golitz LE: Scrotal calcinosis dystrophic calcification in epidermoid cysts. Arch Dermatol 118:985–988, 1982.

180. Mehregan AH: Calcinosis cutis: a review of the clinical forms and report of 75 cases. Semin Dermatol 3:53, 1984.

181. Tezuka T: Cutaneous calculus: its pathogenesis. Dermatologica 161:191–199, 1980.

182. Fischer AH, Morris D: Pathogenesis of calciphylaxis: study of three cases with literature review. Hum Pathol 26:1055–1064, 1995.

183. Ivker RA, Woosley J, Briggaman RA: Calciphylaxis in three patients with end-stage renal disease. Arch Dermatol 131:63–68, 1995.

184. Crow MJ, Gross DJ: Eruptive xanthoma. Cutis 50:31–32, 1992.

185. Moschella SL: Plane xanthomatosis associated with myelomatosis. Arch Dermatol 101:683–687, 1970.

186. Alexanian R, Fraschini G, Smith L: Amyloidosis in multiple myeloma or without apparent cause. Arch Intern Med 114:2158–2160, 1984.

187. Kyle RA, Greipp PR: Amyloidosis (AL): clinical and laboratory features in 229 cases. Mayo Clin Proc 58:665–683, 1983.

188. Kyle RA, Bayrd ED: Amyloidosis: review of 236 cases. Medicine (Baltimore) 54:271–299, 1975.

189. Blumenfeld W, Hildebrandt RH: Fine needle aspiration of abdominal fat for the diagnosis of amyloidosis. Acta Cytol 37:170–174, 1993.

190. Libbey CA, Skinner M, Cohen AS: Use of abdominal fat tissue aspirate in the diagnosis of systemic amyloidosis. Arch Intern Med 143:1549–1552, 1983.

191. Westermark P: Occurrence of amyloid deposits in the skin in secondary systemic amyloidosis. Acta Pathol Microbiol Scand A 80:718–720, 1972.

192. Orfila C, Giraud P, Modesto A, et al: Abdominal fat tissue aspirate in human amyloidosis. Hum Pathol 17:366–369, 1986.

193. Glenner GG: Amyloid deposits and amyloidosis. N Engl J Med 302:1283–1292, 1980.

194. Masu S, Hosokawa M, Seiji M: Amyloid in localized cutaneous amyloiditis: immunofluorescence studies with anti-keratin antiserum. Acta Derm Venereol (Stockh) 61:381–384, 1981.

195. Wang WJ: Clinical features of cutaneous amyloidoses. Clin Dermatol 2:13–19, 1990.

196. Wong CK: Cutaneous amyloidoses. Int J Dermatol 26:273–277, 1987.

197. Potter BA, Johnson WC: Primary localized amyloidosis cutis. Arch Dermatol 103:448–451, 1971.

198. Goerttler E, Anton-Lamprecht I, Kotzur B: Amyloidosis cutis nodularis. Hautarzt 27:16–25, 1976.

199. Breathnach SM: Amyloid and amyloidosis. J Am Acad Dermatol 18:1–16, 1988.

# 49

# Tumors of the Skin

Saul Suster   Tai-Yuen Wong   Martin C. Mihm, Jr.

The skin can give rise to a wide variety of benign and malignant tumors that may originate from the various elements of the dermis and epidermis. Because the skin is an easily accessible organ, skin tumors are a frequent source of specimens for biopsy interpretation by general pathologists and dermatopathologists. Numerous classifications have been proposed in the past for tumors of the skin. For ease of presentation, they are classified here according to their putative or realized lines of differentiation into epidermal epithelial proliferations, cutaneous adnexal tumors, neuroendocrine neoplasms, mesenchymal and neural neoplasms, lymphoproliferative disorders, and melanocytic proliferations.

## EPIDERMAL EPITHELIAL PROLIFERATIONS

### Epidermal Nevi

Epidermal nevi represent congenital proliferations of the squamous epithelium of the epidermis that are present from birth but may not become clinically apparent until later in life. They often present clinically as linear keratotic plaques that may be either localized or disseminated. On occasion, such lesions may be associated with pathologic central nervous system manifestations (epilepsy, mental retardation), skeletal defects, and various ocular and oral cavity abnormalities; such cases have been referred to as the epidermal nevus syndrome.[1] Sharply demarcated areas of hyperkeratosis with papillomatosis characterize the lesions histologically. On cytologic examination, they are composed of a thickened layer of keratinocytes displaying normal maturation. Because of the epidermal hyperplasia and papillomatosis, they may often be confused histologically with seborrheic keratoses. When an epidermal nevus is associated with underlying malformed adnexal structures, such as abnormal development of sebaceous and apocrine glands, it is designated organoid nevus (nevus sebaceus of Jadassohn). Such cases are often associated with the development of basal cell carcinoma and adnexal carcinomas in adults.

## Verrucae

Verrucae are benign squamous proliferations of the epidermis induced by infection by human papillomavirus.[2, 3] Viral warts are characterized by predominantly exophytic growth with marked hyperkeratosis, papillomatosis, hypergranulosis, cytoplasmic clearing of keratinocytes in the granular cell layer (koilocytosis), and dilated, elongated small vessels within the papillary dermis. Variants of verrucae include verruca plana and verruca plantaris, characterized by a platelike or an invaginated endophytic growth pattern, respectively. Condyloma acuminatum refers to virus-induced epidermal growths in the anogenital and perineal region. Condylomas characteristically show both endophytic and exophytic growth of squamous epithelium and can generally be distinguished from other hyperplastic epidermal proliferations by the presence of koilocytotic changes. Late or involuting lesions may not show the cytopathic features distinctive of viral infection and may be appropriately designated "verrucous keratosis consistent with old wart." Most verrucae have a benign clinical course and may regress spontaneously without treatment.

Deep palmoplantar warts (myrmecia) due to human papillomavirus type 1 are characterized by their distinctive, dense cytoplasmic eosinophilic inclusions composed of keratohyalin. Molluscum contagiosum, a lesion caused by infection by a poxvirus, corresponds to a dome-shaped endophytic epidermal growth that is also characterized by the abundance of large, deeply eosinophilic intracytoplasmic inclusions (so-called molluscum bodies). Rarely, malignant transformation has been observed in viral warts, such as in epidermodysplasia verruciformis, in which patients are afflicted by multiple flat warts, some of which evolve into squamous cell carcinoma.[4]

## Acanthomas

### LARGE CELL AND CLEAR CELL ACANTHOMA

Large cell acanthoma is characterized by a well-demarcated area of hyperkeratosis within the epidermis that is composed of a proliferation of large keratinocytes devoid of cytologic atypia.[5] The proliferating cells are approximately twice the size of normal keratinocytes; the lesions generally arise in sun-exposed skin. Some have interpreted large cell acanthoma as a variant of seborrheic keratosis. Clear cell acanthoma, on the other hand, represents a distinctive lesion that usually occurs as a solitary plaque or nodule on the lower extremities characterized histologically by a sharply demarcated endophytic proliferation of squamous epidermal cells containing abundant clear cytoplasm.[6] The clear appearance of the cytoplasm is due to the accumulation of intracytoplasmic glycogen, as demonstrated by positive staining with periodic acid–Schiff (PAS). Another distinctive feature of these lesions is the presence of scattered neutrophils admixed with the clear squamoid cells within the epidermis.

### KERATOACANTHOMA

Keratoacanthoma is characterized by a rapidly growing (weeks to a few months), cup-shaped squamous epidermal proliferation that generally involves sun-exposed skin of elderly individuals.[7] The tumors generally follow an indolent clinical course and regress spontaneously if left untreated. Multiple keratoacanthomas may be seen in the Muir-Torre syndrome associated with sebaceous neoplasms and carcinomas of internal organs. On histologic examination, the tumors are composed of an endophytic-exophytic, cup-shaped squamous epidermal proliferation containing a craterlike central portion filled with laminated keratotic material (Fig. 49–1). The proliferating squamous cells in the early stages of the lesion may show mild to moderate cytologic atypia and frequent mitoses. Distinguishing features are the presence of abrupt keratinization (i.e., keratin formation without an intervening granular cell layer) and intense lichenoid inflammation with the formation of intraepidermal neutrophilic microabscesses. In its later stages, the lesion becomes flatter and more superficial, and the keratin plug may disappear. Regressing keratoacanthomas can assume the configuration of a keratinous cyst with attenuation of the squamous epithelial elements and an entirely intradermal cystic cavity filled with acellular keratin squames.

The differential diagnosis of keratoacanthoma is with squamous cell carcinoma. In many instances, it may be impossible to establish the diagnosis on the basis of histology alone, and a history of recent, rapid growth is necessary for making that distinction. Some authors currently believe that keratoacanthoma may not represent a distinct biologic entity but rather corresponds to an unusual, well-differen-

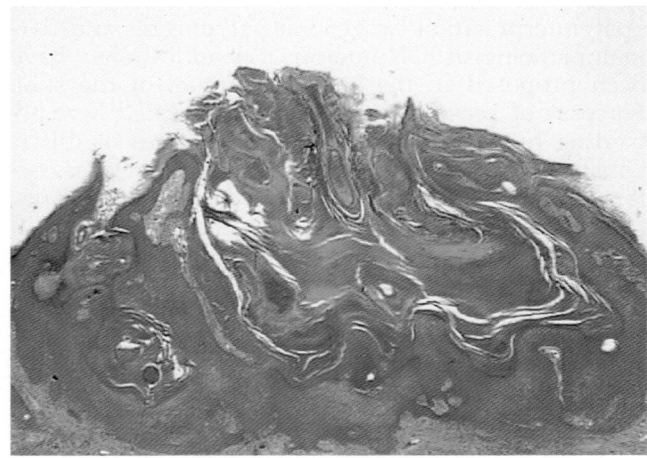

**FIGURE 49–1.** Keratoacanthoma. A cup-shaped endophytic proliferation of squamous epithelium characterizes the lesion.

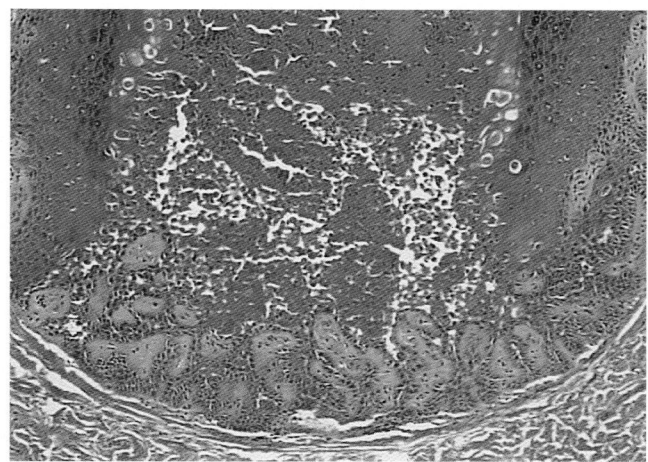

**FIGURE 49–2.** Warty dyskeratoma. An endophytic proliferation of squamous epithelium is seen containing a central, craterlike cavity filled with keratinous material; the suprabasal portion shows clefts with acantholysis and dyskeratosis.

tiated variant of squamous cell carcinoma (i.e., squamous cell carcinoma, keratoacanthoma type).[8] When in doubt, it is preferable to add a statement in the pathology report to the effect that a well-differentiated squamous cell carcinoma cannot be ruled out on the basis of histology.

## WARTY DYSKERATOMA

Warty dyskeratoma, a solitary, verrucous epidermal proliferation characterized by marked acantholysis and dyskeratosis of the proliferating tumor cells, usually involves hair follicles on sun-exposed areas.[9] On histologic examination, the lesions form well-circumscribed endophytic proliferations of squamous epithelium that appear to replace preexisting hair follicles and contain a central craterlike cavity filled with laminated keratinous material. The suprabasal portion of the squamous proliferation characteristically shows the formation of clefts with prominent acantholysis and dyskeratosis (Fig. 49–2). The lesions must be distinguished from Darier's disease, a genetically inherited disorder characterized by multiple keratotic papules displaying prominent acantholytic dyskeratosis.

## Keratoses

### SEBORRHEIC KERATOSIS

Seborrheic keratosis represents a benign localized epidermal proliferation of basaloid and squamoid cells most commonly present in elderly individuals. In rare instances, it may be associated with underlying malignancy (Leser-Trélat sign).[10] The most common histologic presentation is that of an exophytic epidermal growth with a dome-shaped configuration containing multiple cornified cysts. The proliferating cells have a generally rounded, basaloid ap-

pearance, and there may be varying degrees of melanin pigment deposition.

Several histologic variants have been described, including hyperkeratotic, adenoid, clonal, and inflamed or "irritated" seborrheic keratosis. Papillomatous or hyperkeratotic seborrheic keratosis is characterized by marked epidermal papillomatosis reminiscent of a verruca. A thinned epidermis with elongated, often anastomosing serpiginous cords of basaloid cells growing into the dermis characterizes adenoid seborrheic keratosis. Intraepidermal nests of basaloid squamous cells sharply demarcated from the surrounding keratinocytes characterize clonal seborrheic keratosis; this pattern has also been termed the Borst-Jadassohn phenomenon (Fig. 49–3, CD Fig. 49–1). The prominent intraepidermal nesting in these lesions should not be confused with a melanocytic process. A superficial dermal inflammatory infiltrate and prominent intraepidermal clusters of squamous cells (so-called squamous eddies) that adopt a characteristic whorling appearance characterize inflamed seborrheic keratosis.

When seborrheic keratosis involves the epithelium of hair follicles, it may proliferate in an endophytic manner and show features of squamous differentiation; such lesions have been termed inverted follicular keratosis. Another variant of seborrheic keratosis, melanoacanthoma, is characterized by the presence of multiple, dendritic benign melanocytes admixed with the basaloid epithelial proliferation at all levels of the epidermis. Dermatosis papulosis nigra refers to lesions showing the histologic features of pigmented seborrheic keratosis that are predominantly distributed on the face of black adolescents. Stucco keratosis refers to small hyperkeratotic seborrheic keratosis distributed symmetrically in the distal portion of the extremities.

### ACTINIC KERATOSIS

Actinic keratosis is an epidermal proliferation of atypical keratinocytes, generally induced by chronic

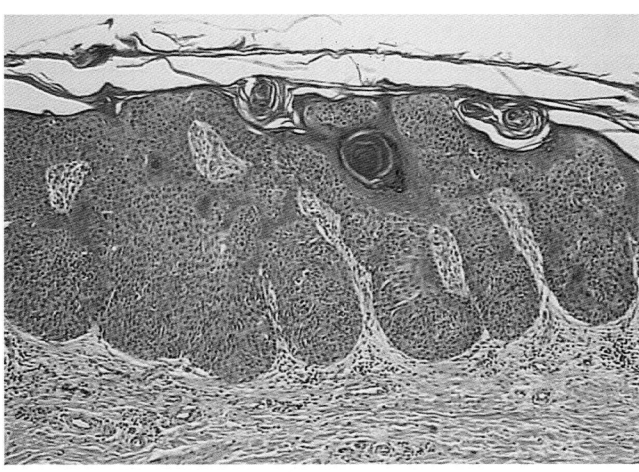

**FIGURE 49–3.** Clonal seborrheic keratosis showing prominent intraepidermal nesting (Borst-Jadassohn phenomenon).

sun exposure (solar keratosis).[11] Actinic keratosis is widely believed to represent a premalignant lesion that may progress to squamous cell carcinoma.[12] Exposure to ionizing radiation, carcinogenic hydrocarbons, and arsenicals may produce similar lesions. On histologic examination, actinic keratosis may show several distinctive growth patterns. All lesions share in common evidence of cytologic atypia of keratinocytes primarily involving the basal and suprabasal layer that may extend to involve the entire thickness of the epidermis. The cells usually show enlarged nuclei with clumping of chromatin and some mitotic activity. There are alternating zones of hyperkeratosis and parakeratosis with loss of the underlying granular layer. There is usually evidence of solar damage in the superficial dermis underlying the lesion.

The atrophic form of actinic keratosis is characterized by a thinned epidermis (three to four cell layers thick) in which the basal cells are replaced by a layer of atypical keratinocytes. The acantholytic form is characterized by the formation of frequent clefts containing large, rounded acantholytic cells. The lichenoid variant of actinic keratosis is characterized, in addition to the atypical epidermal changes, by a dense bandlike inflammatory infiltrate in the dermis. A pigmented variant is also recognized that is characterized by an admixture of pigmented dendritic melanocytes with the atypical keratinocytes; these lesions can easily be mistaken for a solar lentigo. The proliferative variant of actinic keratosis displays tongues of mildly atypical basaloid epithelium extending into the superficial dermis. In the hypertrophic form of actinic keratosis, the atypia of the basal keratinocytes may be minimal, and the epidermis is thickened and acanthotic. The bowenoid variant of actinic keratosis is characterized by full-thickness epidermal atypia resembling Bowen's disease. Actinic cheilitis designates similar lesions involving the oral squamous mucosa.[13]

## Bowen's Disease and Carcinoma In Situ

The concept of carcinoma in situ of the epidermis is still controversial. Carcinoma in situ has been defined as the presence of intraepithelial neoplasia involving the full thickness of the epidermis.[14, 15] Unfortunately, a wide variety of lesions of different etiology and with different biologic behavior may be classified as such under that definition. The most distinctive example of carcinoma in situ of the skin is Bowen's disease. The lesions may be associated with chronic solar damage, radiation therapy, or arsenical or paraquat exposure. Human papillomavirus types 2 and 16 have been found to be associated with extragenital and genital lesions, respectively.[16]

Bowen's disease generally presents clinically as a distinctive erythematous plaque that is often located on non–sun-exposed skin of the trunk or the lower extremities. The involved epidermis is charac-

terized histologically by psoriasiform hyperplasia and hyperkeratosis and parakeratosis with full-thickness atypia of keratinocytes (Fig. 49–4). The keratinocytes are generally enlarged and display atypical nuclei with abnormal mitotic figures as well as frequent dyskeratotic cells. The atypical keratinocytic proliferation may secondarily involve pilosebaceous structures and other adnexa. Solitary lesions indistinguishable histologically from Bowen's disease that are located on the glans penis have been termed erythroplasia of Queyrat. Such lesions are associated with a greater tendency for invasion and metastases. When the lesions are multiple and arise in the genital region (i.e., glans, penile shaft, vulva, and perineum), they are referred to as bowenoid papulosis. The lesions in bowenoid papulosis are distinguished clinically from Bowen's disease by their multiplicity, genital location, early age at onset, and tendency for spontaneous regression, and they are not associated with an increased incidence of invasive malignant behavior.[17]

## Squamous Cell Carcinoma

Squamous cell carcinoma most often arises in sun-damaged skin, although it may also occur as a complication of burn scars, chronic draining sinuses, or other types of ulcers (Marjolin's ulcers). It most commonly affects the head and neck region of elderly individuals. The tumor often presents clinically as a shallow ulcer with indurated borders. Histologic examination shows the tumor to be composed of a proliferation of atypical keratinocytes originating from the epidermis that infiltrate the underlying dermis, often showing horn pearl formation (Fig. 49–5A). The invasive component may show varying degrees of differentiation ranging from well-differentiated keratinocytes with clearly recognizable intercellular bridges and mild to moderate cytologic atypia to poorly differentiated cells with highly ana-

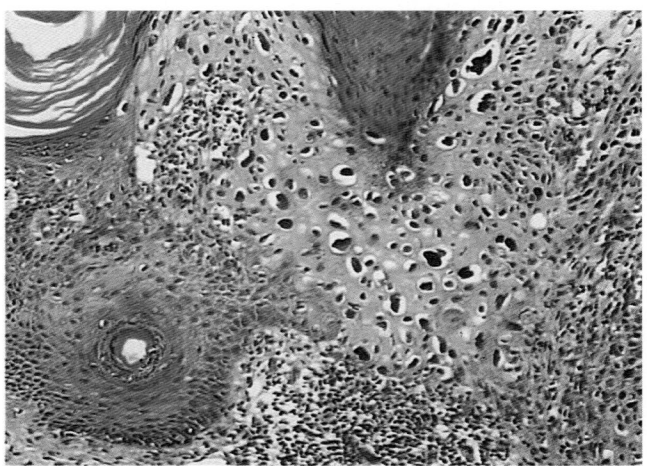

**FIGURE 49–4.** Bowen's disease. Notice full-thickness atypia of keratinocytes within the epidermis.

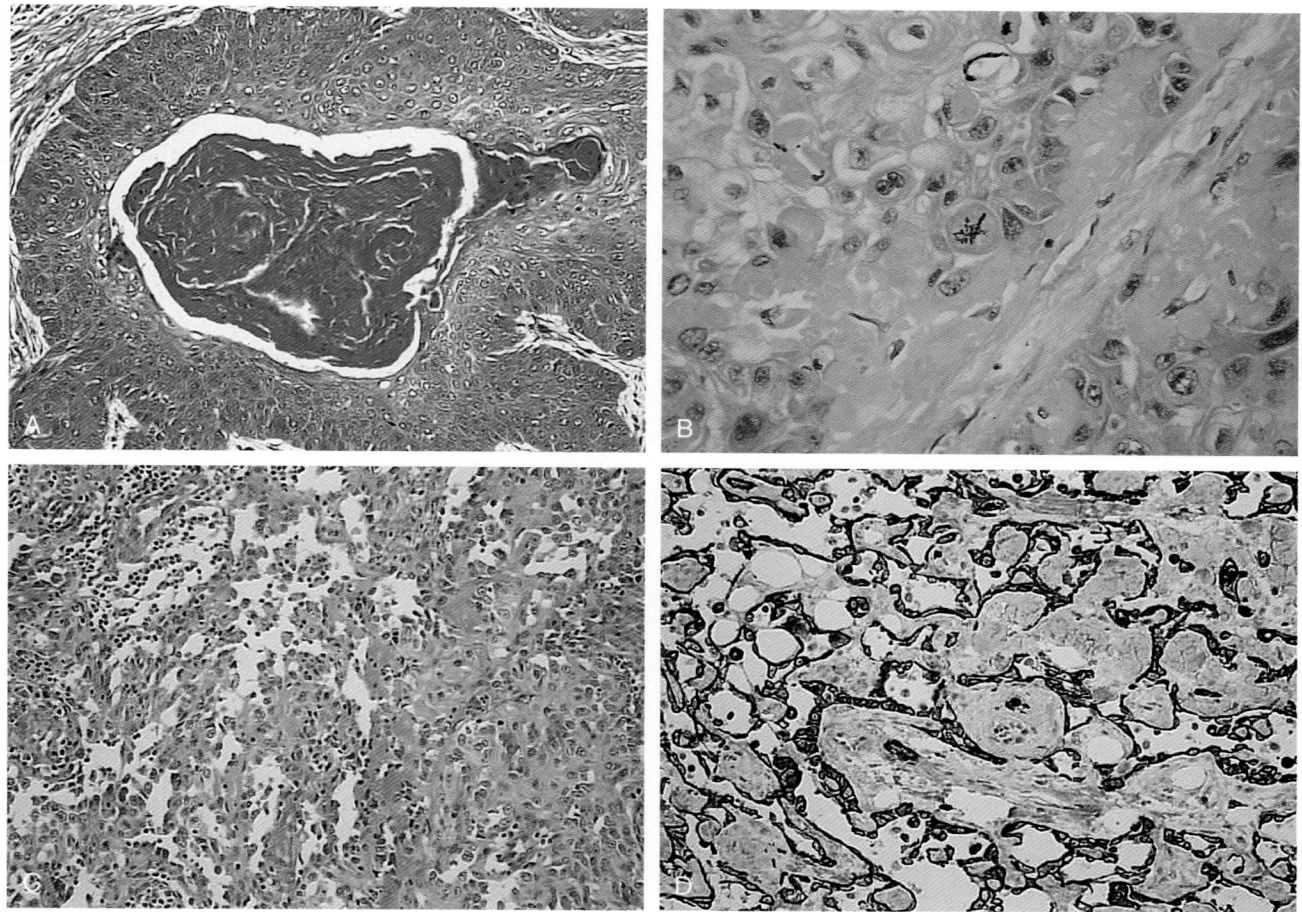

**FIGURE 49–5.** *A.* Squamous cell carcinoma. Notice islands of atypical squamous epithelium with central keratinization. *B.* Invasive, poorly differentiated squamous cell carcinoma showing marked cytologic atypia of keratinocytes. *C.* Pseudovascular squamous cell carcinoma. Cleftlike spaces are seen that resemble anastomosing vascular spaces. *D.* Pseudovascular spaces stain strongly positive for cytokeratin antibodies.

plastic nuclei, frequent mitotic figures, and only rare foci of single-cell keratinization (Fig. 49–5B). The tumors are often accompanied by a nonspecific inflammatory infiltrate in the dermis. Perineurial invasion by tumor cells is associated with a more aggressive behavior. Poor degree of differentiation, deep invasion, and immunosuppression are associated with a more aggressive clinical course. Metastases are rare but occur most often to lymph nodes and may also spread to distant organs such as lung, liver, bone, and brain.

Several unusual histologic variants of squamous cell carcinoma have been described. Spindle cell squamous carcinoma is characterized by oval or spindle-shaped atypical cells originating in the epidermis that infiltrate the dermis in a fascicular fashion closely resembling a sarcoma. The nuclei may be pleomorphic or vesicular with frequent mitoses. Areas of transition with well-differentiated squamous elements may or may not be identified. The diagnosis is supported by the demonstration of positivity for cytokeratin in the spindle cells by immunohisto-

chemistry or by the identification of tonofilaments in association with desmosomes in the tumor cells by electron microscopy.[18] Clear cell squamous carcinoma shows a proliferation of large, clear cells with empty cytoplasm that contains abundant glycogen as evidenced by strong PAS reaction that is abolished after digestion with diastase. Pseudovascular squamous cell carcinoma is characterized by a proliferation of tumor cells originating from the epidermis that form pseudoglandular and vessel-like spaces that may closely simulate an angiosarcoma (Fig. 49–5C). Demonstration of cytokeratin and epithelial membrane antigen positivity and absence of immunoreactivity for vascular endothelium–associated markers help support the diagnosis[19] (Fig. 49–5D). This variant is closely related to, and may in fact be indistinguishable from, acantholytic squamous cell carcinoma, a tumor characterized by a pseudoglandular growth pattern resulting from extensive acantholysis and dyskeratosis of tumor cells. A distinctive variant of poorly differentiated squamous cell carcinoma, the lymphoepithelioma-like carcinoma, has also been described in the skin. This tumor is composed of sheets of round cells with scant cytoplasm and large eosinophilic nucleoli surrounded by a dense lymphoid stroma, similar to its nasopharyngeal counterpart.[20]

Verrucous carcinoma, another variant of well-differentiated squamous cell carcinoma, characteristically presents as a large fungating, slow-growing tumor of the oral cavity. Identical lesions have been designated giant condyloma acuminatum of Buschke and Löwenstein in the anogenital region and epithelioma cuniculatum in the plantar region.[21] The lesions are characterized histologically by striking hyperkeratosis with parakeratosis and papillomatosis closely resembling a viral wart. The squamous cell proliferation is characteristically bland, with minimal cytologic atypia and paucity of mitotic figures. The tumors may show invasion of the dermis with pushing borders but do not display the irregular infiltration characteristic of conventional squamous cell carcinoma. Diagnosis requires strict clinicopathologic correlation and may not be possible on the basis of histology alone.

## Basal Cell Carcinoma

Basal cell carcinoma (BCC) is the most common malignant skin neoplasm. These tumors are traditionally thought to derive from the epidermis, in particular the basal cell layer and the outer root sheath of hair follicles, although current thinking favors origin from pluripotential stem cells capable of multiple lines of differentiation. They most commonly arise in sun-exposed skin of middle-aged to elderly individuals. The lesions may present as ulcers or plaques with raised, indurated borders or as flesh-colored firm nodules. Large tumors may infiltrate deeply and destroy adjacent structures (rodent ulcer). Metastases are extremely rare and most often occur in neglected lesions or immunosuppressed patients. Large tumor size is also associated with an increased risk for metastases.

On histologic examination, the hallmark of BCC is a uniform proliferation of small, round or oval hyperchromatic cells in the dermis that display prominent peripheral palisading of nuclei and are usually connected with the overlying epidermis (Fig. 49–6A). The tumors are often superficial and multicentric. More than 50% of BCC are of the nodular type.[22] These tumors grow as pearly nodules with rolled borders and telangiectasis. Histologic examination shows them to be composed of multiple solid tumor nodules within the dermis showing prominent peripheral palisading of nuclei and a distinctive "clefting" or retraction artifact from the surrounding stroma. The central portions of the nodules may contain abundant eosinophilic mucinous material that distends the nodule to create the impression of a cystic cavity. BCC can contain melanin within basaloid cells and melanophages, giving rise to a pigmented variant that may be confused clinically with a melanocytic lesion. The tumors may also occasionally show multiple cystic structures filled with keratin squames and parakeratotic material (keratotic BCC). Such cysts have been interpreted by some as attempts at hair shaft formation (Fig. 49–6B). BCC may also show foci of differentiation toward eccrine, pilosebaceous, infundibular, or follicular structures. Tumors showing light microscopic and immunohistochemical evidence of myoepithelial differentiation have also been described[23] (Fig. 49–6C).

A histologic variant associated with a more aggressive clinical behavior is the sclerosing (morphea) type. These tumors show islands of basaloid tumor cells in the dermis embedded within a sclerosing, desmoplastic stroma. The tumors are usually poorly circumscribed and deeply infiltrative; they are associated with an increased incidence of recurrence.[24] Metatypical BCC refers to a tumor that shows mixed features of BCC and squamous cell carcinoma. Islands of basaloid cells are seen that contain foci of keratinization, with occasional horn pearl formation and focal spindling of the tumor cells. The tumor overlaps with basosquamous carcinoma, in which clearly identifiable areas of BCC and squamous cell carcinoma are observed growing side by side within the same tumor mass; these lesions tend to be more aggressive than conventional BCC, with a greater incidence of perineurial and lymphatic invasion and, rarely, systemic metastasis after multiple recurrences.

A distinctive variant of BCC associated with a benign clinical course is the fibroepithelioma of Pinkus. This tumor is composed of branching strands of basaloid epithelial cells originating from the epidermis that surround islands of fibromucinous stroma (Fig. 49–6D). Other rare histologic variants of BCC include the clear cell variant, characterized by a predominantly clear cell population containing abundant cytoplasmic glycogen; signet ring cell BCC; adamantinoid BCC, which displays a close resemblance to odontogenic ameloblastomas; and adenoid BCC, characterized by serpiginous, lacelike formations and glandlike structures surrounded by a loose myxoid stroma.[25–27] Other unusual features occasionally seen in BCC are granular cell changes of the cytoplasm, anaplastic cytology, and amyloid deposition in the stroma.

The nevoid BCC syndrome is an autosomal dominant disorder in which hundreds of small nodules develop over the face and body between puberty and 35 years of age. During adulthood, many of the nodules may undergo malignant transformation and develop into invasive tumors. In addition to the nodules, the patients show multiple skeletal and central nervous system abnormalities.[28] The linear unilateral basal cell nevus is a rare condition in which closely clustered nodules of BCC grow since birth in a linear fashion following a zosteriform distribution. The Bazex syndrome is a dominantly inherited condition that consists of areas of follicular atrophoderma in the extremities and multiple, small BCC on the face.[29]

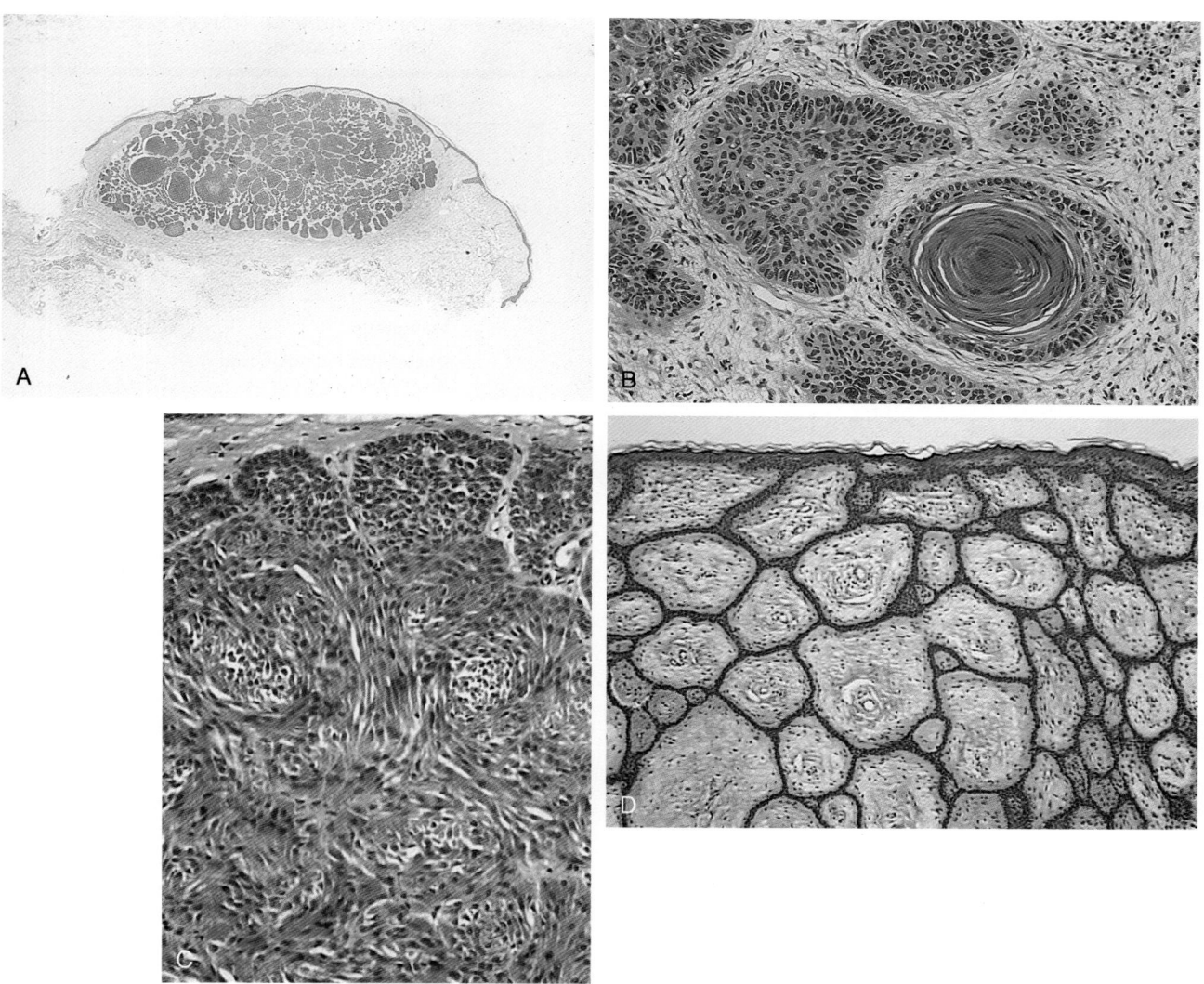

**FIGURE 49–6.** *A.* BCC. A nodular proliferation of basaloid cells is seen in the dermis. *B.* BCC with follicular differentiation. *C.* BCC with myoepithelial differentiation. The spindle cells depicted here were strongly positive for actin, keratin, and S-100 protein antibodies. *D.* Fibroepithelioma of Pinkus. Cords of epithelial cells extend into the dermis in a fibroepitheliomatous fashion.

## Paget's Disease

It is now well recognized that both mammary and extramammary Paget's disease most likely represents a primary intraepidermal neoplastic proliferation of atypical glandular cells showing apocrine differentiation.[30] In some cases, the tumors may develop as a result of epidermotropic spread from an underlying colorectal, genitourinary, or mammary ductal carcinoma. The last circumstance is most commonly observed with the mammary form of Paget's disease. Extramammary Paget's disease most often involves the skin of the anogenital and axillary regions, which are sites that normally contain a high density of apocrine cells.

Paget's disease is characterized histologically by a thickened epidermis containing a scattering of large cells with abundant clear cytoplasm admixed with the epidermal keratinocytes (Fig. 49–7). The tumor cells contain large nuclei with coarse chromatin pattern and occasional mitotic figures. The tumor cells are strongly positive for PAS and are diastase resistant; they also show a positive reaction with alcian blue at pH 2.5 and mucicarmine. The Paget cells can occasionally be identified within the epithelium of hair follicles or eccrine sweat ducts. Invasion from the epidermis into the dermis can also occasionally be observed, particularly in cases of extramammary Paget's disease, and is associated with aggressive behavior. Cases associated with an underlying carcinoma generally have a poor prognosis. Paget's disease unrelated to underlying carcinoma often recurs locally but is not associated with metastatic potential. Paget cells strongly immunoreact with carcinoembryonic antigen and with gross cystic disease fluid protein; the latter may be helpful in

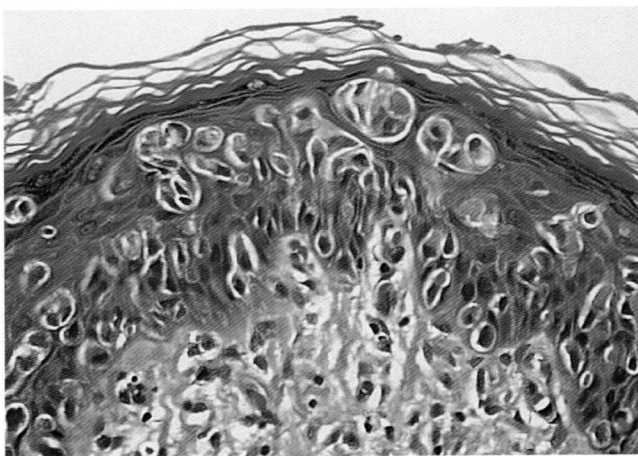

FIGURE 49–7. Paget's disease of the nipple epidermis. Numerous large cells with clear cytoplasmic halos are seen scattered throughout the epidermis.

TABLE 49–1. Dermal Adnexal Tumors with Eccrine Differentiation

| **Benign** |
| --- |
| Eccrine hidrocystoma |
| Syringoma |
| Chondroid syringoma |
| Eccrine poroma |
| Eccrine spiradenoma |
| Papillary eccrine adenoma |
| Eccrine hidradenoma |

| **Malignant** |
| --- |
| Ductal eccrine carcinoma |
| Microcystic carcinoma |
| Malignant chondroid syringoma |
| Malignant eccrine poroma |
| Malignant eccrine spiradenoma |
| Digital papillary carcinoma |
| Clear cell eccrine carcinoma |
| Mucinous carcinoma |
| Adenoid cystic carcinoma |
| Low-grade polymorphous carcinoma |

differential diagnosis, particularly for separating them from cases that closely resemble pagetoid malignant melanoma.[31]

## ADNEXAL NEOPLASMS

### Tumors with Eccrine Differentiation

Normal eccrine glands of the skin are composed of a secretory coil made up of cuboidal cells, a dermal duct segment composed of two layers of nonsecretory cuboidal epithelial cells lined by an acellular eosinophilic cuticle, and a coiled terminal portion (acrosyringium) that is lined by one layer of cuboidal epithelial cells surrounded by several layers of squamoid cells. Tumors with features reminiscent of these structures are regarded as showing evidence of eccrine differentiation.

BENIGN ADNEXAL TUMORS WITH ECCRINE DIFFERENTIATION. A variety of benign skin adnexal neoplasms showing features of eccrine differentiation have been described (Table 49–1).

*Eccrine Hidrocystoma.* Eccrine hidrocystoma is a non-neoplastic condition resulting from cystic dilatation of the dermal portion of the eccrine duct. The lesion is characterized by a large unilocular cyst in the dermis lined by two layers of cuboidal epithelium resembling the intradermal portion of the eccrine duct.

*Syringoma.* Syringoma represents another benign adnexal tumor characterized by a dermal proliferation of multiple small ductular structures lined by a double layer of flattened to cuboidal epithelial cells embedded in a dense collagenous stroma.[32] Many of the ductular structures adopt a distinctive tadpole or comma-shaped configuration. Some cases may contain dilated ductular structures filled with keratotic material. A clear cell variant of syringoma

composed of large cells containing abundant cytoplasmic glycogen has also been described.[33]

*Chondroid Syringoma.* Chondroid syringoma (also known as benign mixed tumor of the skin) is a benign adnexal neoplasm made up of a proliferation of tubular and ductal epithelium embedded within a chondromyxoid stroma. These tumors generally present as firm, skin-colored nodules distributed over the head and neck. The lesions are usually well circumscribed and composed of a proliferation of branching ducts lined by cuboidal cells and surrounded by a layer of myoepithelial cells. The surrounding stroma contains abundant connective tissue mucin rich in hyaluronic acid and variable amounts of immature to well-developed chondroid matrix (Fig. 49–8). Some of the ductular structures may show evidence of decapitation secretion indicative of apocrine differentiation.[34] Focal areas show-

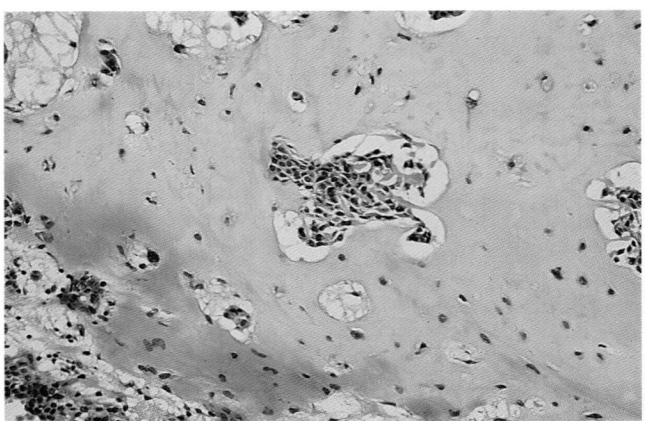

FIGURE 49–8. Chondroid syringoma. Glandular epithelial elements are seen embedded in mature cartilaginous matrix.

ing a solid proliferation of myoepithelial cells with plasmacytoid features can also be present occasionally. Epithelial cells with prominent nucleoli and rare mitotic figures may also be seen in some cases.

*Eccrine Poroma.* Eccrine poroma is the designation for a group of tumors that are thought to recapitulate the intraepidermal portion of the eccrine coil (acrosyringium). Three forms are recognized: an intraepidermal form (hidroacanthoma simplex), a dermal form (dermal duct tumor), and a combined dermal-epidermal form (eccrine poroma). The lesions generally present as slightly raised or nodular lesions on the distal extremities. In hidroacanthoma simplex, the epidermis is expanded by a monotonous population of small basaloid cells.[35] When the neoplastic proliferation predominantly involves the dermis, it tends to form ductlike spaces, hence the designation dermal duct tumor.[36] The majority of lesions, however, present with both an epidermal and a dermal component. The most distinguishing feature of eccrine poroma is a monotonous proliferation of bland-appearing, round to polygonal squamoid cells with abundant glycogen-rich cytoplasm (Fig. 49–9, CD Fig. 49–2). The cells have round, basophilic nuclei and inconspicuous intercellular bridges. Small ductlike structures lined by eosinophilic cuticles can occasionally be present.[37]

*Eccrine Spiradenoma.* Eccrine spiradenoma is a benign adnexal neoplasm showing features suggestive of differentiation along both the dermal duct and secretory segment of eccrine sweat glands. The tumors generally present as solitary, characteristically painful dermal nodules with no particular site predilection.[38] On histologic examination, the lesions are located deep in the dermis with no connection

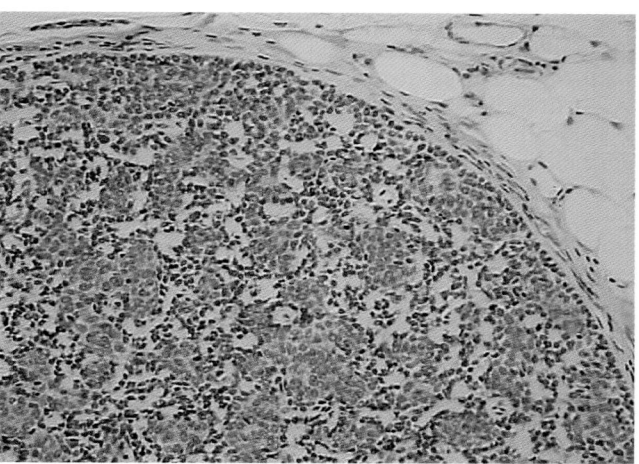

FIGURE 49–10. Eccrine spiradenoma. Notice dual cell population composed of small dark cells with scant cytoplasm and larger epithelial cells with pale cytoplasm disposed around small luminal structures.

to the epidermis and present as single or multiple well-circumscribed nodules. The nodules are composed of two distinct cell populations: cords of small round epithelial cells with dark nuclei and scant cytoplasm and larger epithelial cells with pale nuclei and scant cytoplasm disposed around small luminal structures (Fig. 49–10). Occasional ductular structures lined by an eosinophilic cuticle may also be present. Another distinctive feature is the presence of scattered small lymphocytes within the tumor stroma.

*Papillary Eccrine Adenoma.* Papillary eccrine adenoma generally presents as a dome-shaped nodular lesion on the extremities and is characterized histologically by an ill-defined proliferation of ductal structures in the dermis that contain numerous papillary projections within their lumina (Fig. 49–11). One or more layers of cuboidal epithelium line the

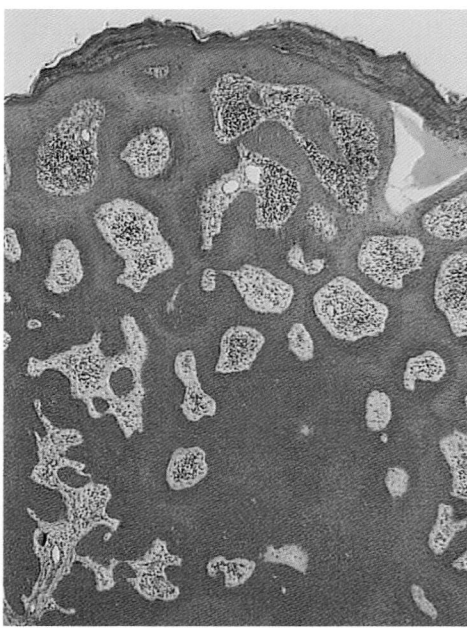

FIGURE 49–9. Eccrine poroma composed of monotonous proliferation of round to polygonal squamoid cells with abundant cytoplasm infiltrating the dermis.

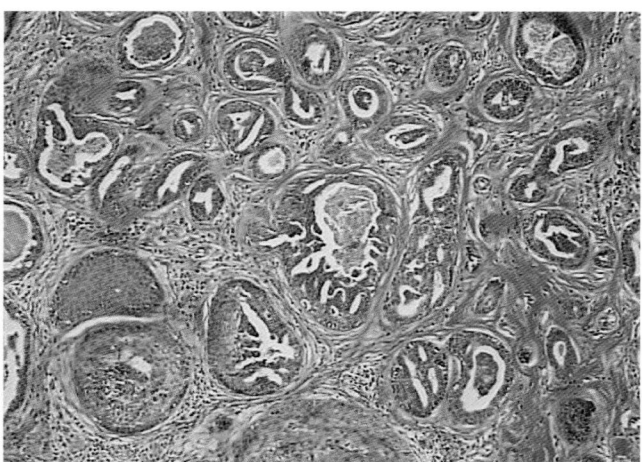

FIGURE 49–11. Papillary eccrine adenoma composed of proliferation of ductal structures in the dermis showing papillary projections into their lumina.

ductlike and glandular structures that compose the tumor. Keratin-filled cysts may often be admixed with the ductlike structures. The ductal and glandular structures show numerous slender papillary projections into the lumen arising from the lining epithelium.[39] On occasion, features of apocrine differentiation may be seen focally in these tumors. The cells lining the lumen and the papillae may occasionally display cytologic atypia with prominent nucleoli and mitoses. Widespread cytologic atypia, solid growth, high mitotic activity, and infiltrative growth pattern, however, should raise the consideration of eccrine papillary carcinoma.[40]

*Eccrine Hidradenoma.* Eccrine hidradenoma, also known as clear cell hidradenoma, nodular hidradenoma, or solid-cystic hidradenoma, is a benign adnexal tumor that generally presents as a solitary dermal nodule without any particular age or site distribution. The tumor is characterized histologically by well-circumscribed lobules located in the dermis that may show a connection with the epidermis and occasionally may extend into subcutaneous fat. The tumor lobules are surrounded by a distinctive densely eosinophilic, often hyalinized stroma that extends into the tumor, forming collagenous trabeculae. A monotonous population of large round to polygonal cells that contain abundant eosinophilic cytoplasm or that may display prominent cytoplasmic clearing characterizes the tumor lobules[41] (Fig. 49–12*A*). The cells may also focally adopt a fusiform appearance resembling myoepithelial cells (Fig. 49–12*B*). Mitoses and nuclear pleomorphism can be present but are usually inconspicuous. Branching tubular structures and large cysts are also a common feature of these tumors. Columnar secretory cells showing features of decapitation (apocrine) secretion may line the tubular structures. The cystic changes may sometimes be prominent, justifying the designation cystic hidradenoma. Small ductular spaces resembling sweat ducts lined by a dense eosinophilic cuticle may occasionally be observed. Foci of keratinization are frequently encountered, especially in cells lining the ductal lumina. Sharp circumscription and absence of irregular borders or infiltration beyond the surrounding layer of densely eosinophilic stroma on scanning magnification are predictive of a benign clinical course.

MALIGNANT ADNEXAL NEOPLASMS WITH ECCRINE DIFFERENTIATION. Malignant adnexal neoplasms with eccrine differentiation (see Table 49–1) represent a heterogeneous group of lesions that generally resemble, to some extent, their benign counterparts. For the most part, they are distinguished by increased nuclear pleomorphism, brisk mitotic activity, and infiltrative growth pattern. Thus, malignant forms of syringoma, eccrine spiradenoma, mixed tumor, eccrine poroma, and clear cell or nodular hidradenoma have been described.[42, 43] Areas displaying recognizable features of the benign counterpart must be identified to render such diagnoses. In addition to these, a group of primary eccrine carcinomas without benign counterparts has also been recognized, including ductal eccrine adenocarcinoma, mucinous carcinoma, adenoid cystic carcinoma, aggressive digital papillary adenocarcinoma, and low-grade polymorphous sweat gland carcinoma.

*Ductal Eccrine Adenocarcinoma.* Ductal eccrine adenocarcinoma probably represents the most common form of sweat gland carcinoma and is characterized by a proliferation of ductal structures lined by atypical cells with frequent mitoses displaying occasional cuticular lining. These tumors are highly aggressive with frequent spread to regional lymph nodes and internal organs. A distinctive variant of eccrine ductal carcinoma is the microcystic adnexal carcinoma, also known as syringoid carcinoma and sclerosing sweat duct carcinoma. The tumors have a tendency to occur in the face, particularly the lip and nasolabial fold, and generally present as indurated, plaquelike lesions. Histologic examination shows a monotonous proliferation of small nests

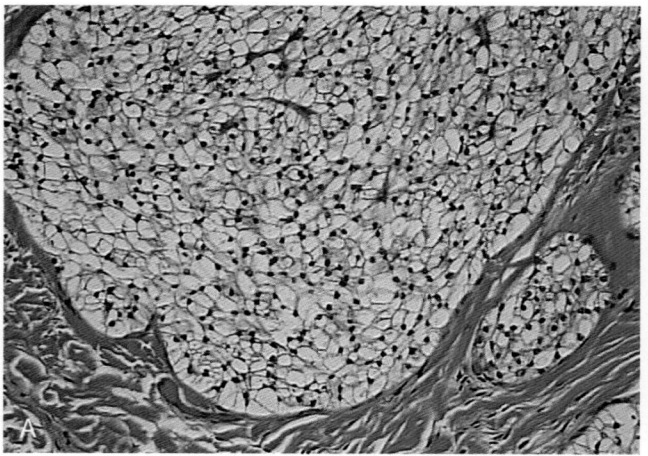 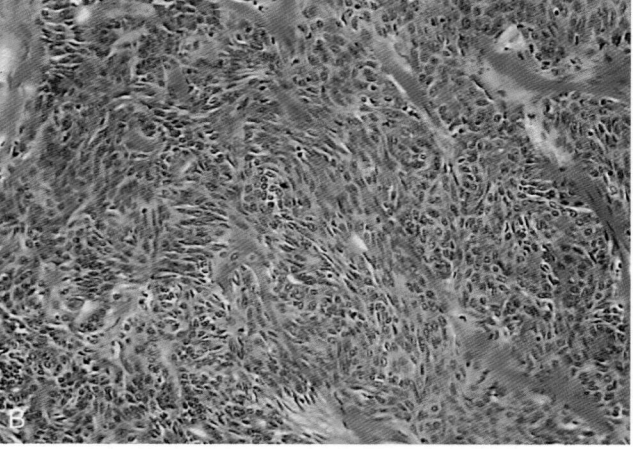

FIGURE 49–12. *A.* Eccrine hidradenoma showing lobular proliferation of monotonous large, clear cells in the dermis. *B.* Eccrine hidradenoma composed of monotonous oval to spindle cells with abundant cytoplasm that closely resemble myoepithelial cells.

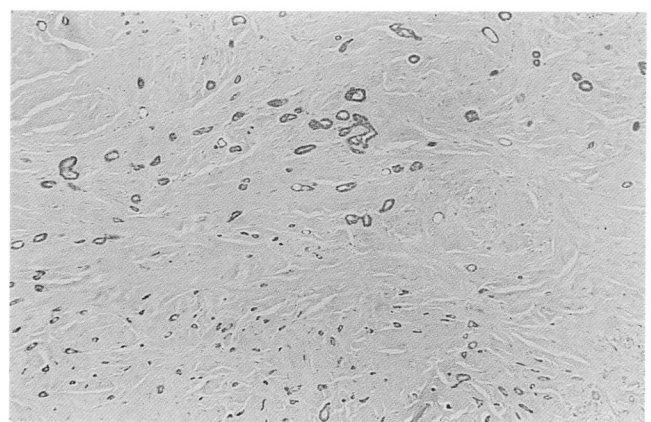

**FIGURE 49–13.** Microcystic adnexal sweat gland carcinoma. Notice small glandular structures diffusely infiltrating the dermis.

and cystlike structures made up of uniform squamoid cells diffusely infiltrating the dermis and surrounded by abundant collagenous stroma (Fig. 49–13).

*Mucinous Carcinoma.* Another distinctive type of sweat gland carcinoma, the mucinous carcinoma, is characterized by nests and cords of epithelial cells suspended in an abundant mucinous stroma.[42] These lesions must be distinguished from metastases of mucinous (so-called colloid) carcinoma of internal organs.

*Adenoid Cystic Carcinoma.* Adenoid cystic carcinoma of the skin is a rare form of eccrine carcinoma of low-grade malignant potential. It is characterized by a proliferation of basaloid epithelial islands in the dermis showing a prominent cribri-

form pattern of growth similar to that observed in adenoid cystic carcinoma of salivary glands.

*Digital Papillary Adenocarcinoma.* Digital papillary adenoma-adenocarcinoma encompasses a spectrum of lesions ranging from locally aggressive and destructive tumors with a tendency for local recurrence to metastasizing, fully malignant neoplasms. Most cases involve the distal extremities, particularly the fingers and toes. The tumor is composed of epithelium-lined cystic spaces in the dermis that contain numerous papillary infoldings. The papillae are lined by cuboidal epithelial cells showing varying degrees of nuclear atypia, mitotic activity, and occasionally multinucleation. The presence of more solid cellular areas, necrosis, and high mitotic activity is directly related to a higher metastatic potential.

*Low-Grade Polymorphous Sweat Gland Carcinoma.* Polymorphous sweat gland carcinoma is a variant of low-grade adnexal neoplasm with features of eccrine differentiation. The tumor is characterized by the admixture within the same lesion of various patterns of growth including solid, papillary, glandular, and cribriform areas reminiscent of low-grade polymorphous salivary gland carcinoma (Fig. 49–14). These tumors have a potential for local recurrence and regional lymph node metastases.[44]

## Tumors with Apocrine Differentiation

Apocrine secretory epithelium is characterized by polygonal to columnar cells that contain abundant, finely granular eosinophilic cytoplasm. These cells secrete their products by pinching off the apical por-

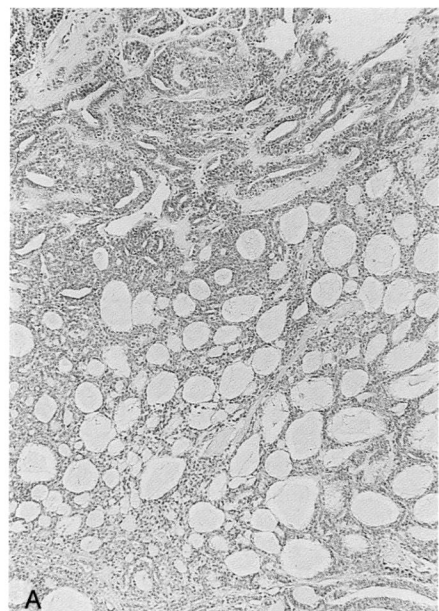 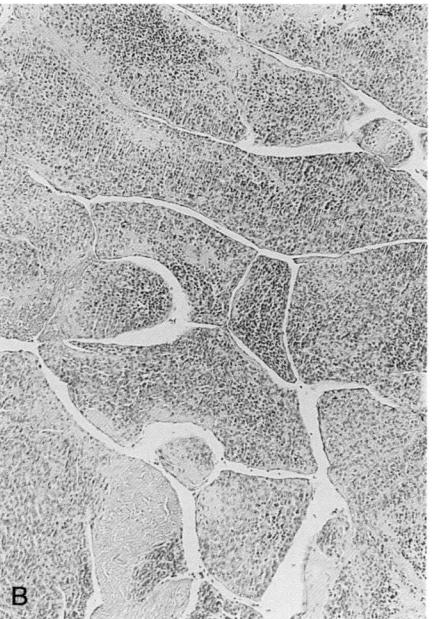

**FIGURE 49–14.** *A.* Low-grade polymorphous sweat gland carcinoma showing cribriform, adenoid cystic–like pattern of growth. *B.* Another area within the same tumor showing more solid, pseudopapillary growth pattern.

tion of the plasma membrane along with its secretory products and liberating them into the lumen, a process referred to as decapitation secretion.

BENIGN ADNEXAL TUMORS WITH APOCRINE DIFFERENTIATION. A number of benign tumors showing features of apocrine differentiation have been described (Table 49–2).

*Apocrine Cystadenoma.* Apocrine cystadenoma (or apocrine hidrocystoma) presents as small bluish nodules on the face, head, and neck or upper trunk that are often mistaken for a pigmented lesion. Similar lesions presenting in the penis are designated median raphe cysts. When located in the eyelids, they are referred to as Moll gland cysts. The lesion consists of a cystic cavity in the dermis lined by several layers of cuboidal to columnar apocrine-type secretory cells with abundant, finely granular eosinophilic cytoplasm and at least focal evidence of decapitation secretion.

*Hidradenoma Papilliferum.* Hidradenoma papilliferum is a cystic and papillary benign apocrine neoplasm that recapitulates the apocrine secretory coil and generally arises from the anogenital region in women. The tumor is composed of numerous complex papillary folds that project into a cystically dilated lumen (Fig. 49–15). The papillary projections are lined by two layers of cuboidal epithelium showing foci of decapitation secretion. The inner layer of the papillary structures is composed of myoepithelial cells.

*Syringocystadenoma Papilliferum.* Syringocystadenoma papilliferum is a distinctive lesion that most commonly occurs in the head and neck region, particularly the scalp, and presents as a solitary plaque or nodule predominantly in children. The lesion is composed of multiple papillary structures that project into a cystically dilated invagination of the epidermis. The papillary structures are lined by two rows of cells: a luminal row of cells composed of columnar cells displaying active decapitation secretion, similar to that seen in apocrine glands, and an outer row of cells composed of small, cuboidal cells. A distinctive feature is the presence of a dense plasma cell infiltrate in the fibrovascular stroma of the papillary structures. In approximately 30% of

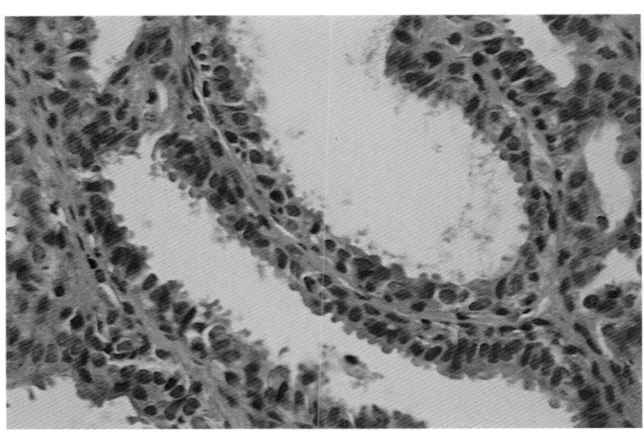

**FIGURE 49–15.** Hidradenoma papilliferum. The tumor shows numerous complex papillary projections within a dilated lumen.

cases, syringocystadenoma papilliferum is associated with a sebaceous nevus.

*Tubular Apocrine Adenoma.* Tubular apocrine adenoma is a rare benign lesion that usually presents as a well-defined nodule on the scalp. The tumor is distinguished histologically by a proliferation of numerous tubular structures lined by two rows of cells. Some of the tubules may contain small papillary projections into the lumen. Many of the cells lining the lumen show decapitation secretion. The lesion shows some similarities with, and, indeed, may be related to, papillary eccrine adenoma.[45]

*Apocrine Adenoma.* Apocrine adenoma is a term reserved for a variety of lesions showing a spectrum of histologic growth patterns that have as a common denominator the presence of columnar cells showing active decapitation secretion. The lesions most commonly arise in areas of the skin rich in apocrine glands, such as the axilla and perianal skin. Some lesions may demonstrate a solid growth pattern with focal glandular or tubular formations, others may be predominantly composed of branching tubular structures.[46] Cases showing prominent sclerotic stroma have been termed apocrine fibroadenomas. Lesions arising in the external or middle ear are termed ceruminous gland adenomas.

*Cylindroma.* Cylindroma is a benign adnexal tumor of disputed histogenesis generally thought to display features of apocrine differentiation. The lesions may be solitary but are more often multiple and commonly distributed along the scalp ("turban" lesion). When multiple, they tend to show a dominant pattern of inheritance. The tumor is characterized by a proliferation in the dermis of islands of basaloid cells surrounded by a thick layer of deeply eosinophilic collagenous material. The islands of tumor cells have irregular contours and appear to fit together like pieces of a jigsaw puzzle (Fig. 49–16).

APOCRINE CARCINOMA. Apocrine carcinoma is a rare malignant adnexal neoplasm that most commonly arises in areas with high apocrine gland density, such as the axilla. The tumors are characterized

**TABLE 49–2.** Dermal Adnexal Tumors with Apocrine Differentiation

| |
|---|
| **Benign** |
| Apocrine hidrocystoma |
| Hidradenoma papilliferum |
| Syringocystadenoma papilliferum |
| Tubular apocrine adenoma |
| Apocrine adenoma |
| Cylindroma |
| **Malignant** |
| Apocrine carcinoma |

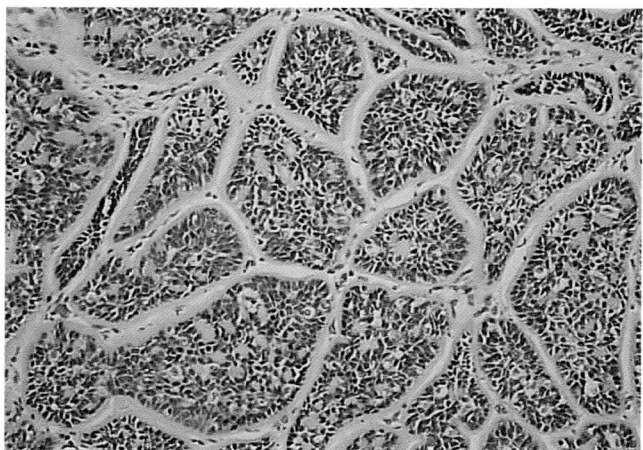

**FIGURE 49–16.** Dermal cylindroma showing irregular islands of dark tumor cells in the dermis that appear to interlock like pieces in a jigsaw puzzle.

**TABLE 49–3.** Dermal Adnexal Tumors with Follicular Differentiation

**Benign**

Tumors of the outer hair sheath and follicular infundibulum
  Tumor of the follicular infundibulum
  Pilar sheath acanthoma
  Dilated pore of Winer
  Trichoadenoma of Nikolowski
  Trichilemmoma
  Proliferating pilar tumor
  Infundibular cyst
  Trichilemmal cyst
  Steatocystoma multiplex
  Dermoid cyst
  Eruptive vellus hair cyst
Tumors of germinative follicular epithelium
  Trichofolliculoma
  Trichoepithelioma
  Immature trichoepithelioma
  Desmoplastic trichoepithelioma
  Pilomatricoma
  Trichoblastoma
  Trichodiscoma
  Perifollicular fibroma
  Fibrofolliculoma
Tumors with sebaceous differentiation
  Sebaceous hyperplasia
  Sebaceous adenoma

**Malignant**

Malignant folliculosebaceous neoplasms
  Trichilemmal carcinoma
  Pilomatrix carcinoma
  Sebaceous carcinoma

by a glandular or papillary proliferation composed of cells with abundant granular eosinophilic cytoplasm that exhibit nuclear atypia, atypical mitoses, and areas of necrosis. At least focally, some of the cells can exhibit decapitation secretion. The cytoplasm of the tumor cells contains PAS-positive, diastase-resistant material and often shows iron-positive granules. Areas of transition between benign-appearing apocrine glands and the neoplastic elements can often be found. The tumors are often locally invasive and may present with lymph node metastases in a high percentage of cases.[47] Up to one third of cases disseminate widely and lead to the death of the patient.

## Tumors with Pilosebaceous Differentiation

The normal hair follicle is composed of three segments: the lowermost segment or hair bulb, which is made up of basaloid matrix cells that harbor an invagination of the surrounding stroma known as the hair papilla; a middle segment or isthmus, which extends from the insertion of the arrector pili muscle to the entrance of the sebaceous duct and is characterized by "abrupt" (pilar) keratinization; and the upper portion, or infundibulum, which extends from the entrance of the sebaceous duct to the follicular orifice. The sebaceous gland is a specialized outgrowth of the hair follicle. In addition, free sebaceous glands unassociated with hair follicles are also present in certain areas such as the nipple and areola of the breast. A large number of benign and malignant proliferations displaying folliculosebaceous differentiation have been described[48] (Table 49–3).

TUMORS OF THE OUTER HAIR SHEATH AND FOLLICULAR INFUNDIBULUM. Tumors of the outer hair sheath and follicular infundibulum comprise a wide variety of lesions that share features of hair sheath and follicular infundibular differentiation.

*Tumor of the Follicular Infundibulum.* Tumor of the follicular infundibulum, also known as basal cell adenoma with follicular differentiation, is characterized by a platelike dermal growth originating from the epidermis and showing peripheral palisading of cells.

*Pilar Sheath Acanthoma.* Pilar sheath acanthoma is a growth typically occurring in the lip that forms a keratin-filled cyst extending from the epidermis into the dermis. The periphery of the cyst typically shows multiple short, elaborate anastomosing projections of epithelium resembling outer root sheath.

*Dilated Pore of Winer.* The dilated pore of Winer is essentially similar to pilar sheath acanthoma, except it displays a lesser degree of epithelial proliferation in the periphery.

*Trichoadenoma of Nikolowski.* Trichoadenoma of Nikolowski is a rare solitary tumor that usually occurs on the face and is composed of numerous cystlike structures in the dermis lined by pilar-type keratinizing epithelium with the occasional formation of centrally located horn cysts (CD Fig. 49–3). The cystic structures display a granular cell layer but do not contain any basaloid cells.

*Trichilemmoma.* Trichilemmoma is a relatively common verrucous lesion of the face and neck that may be associated with internal malignant disease in its multifocal, autosomal dominant form. The lesions are characterized by a lobular proliferation of monotonous polygonal cells with clear or pale, heavily glycogenated eosinophilic cytoplasm arising from the epidermis. The peripheral layer of the lobular growth shows basaloid cells with palisading and a thin layer of densely eosinophilic basement membrane material (CD Fig. 49–4).[49]

*Proliferating Pilar Tumor.* Proliferating pilar tumor (also known as proliferating trichilemmal cyst) is a distinctive lesion that typically arises in the scalp of elderly or middle-aged women. The lesions are centered in the deep dermis and slowly grow during the span of many years to reach a size of several centimeters. The most important diagnostic clue is the configuration of the lesion on scanning magnification. The tumor is characterized by sharp circumscription from the surrounding connective tissue and is composed of a proliferation of squamous cells with abundant "glassy" eosinophilic cytoplasm that appears to differentiate toward outer root sheath (trichilemmal) epithelium. The central portions of the lesion may display large areas of hemorrhage and necrosis, and mitotic figures and reactive nuclear atypia may be observed focally. Foreign body–type giant cell reaction to extruded keratinous material is a commonly observed feature (Fig. 49–17). The clue to the benign nature of the lesion lies in its smooth contours with sharp lateral circumscription. Lesions with irregular, infiltrating margins should be viewed with concern for the possibility of malignant behavior; some authors regard these as examples of malignant degeneration of a proliferating pilar tumor (malignant proliferating pilar tumor).[50]

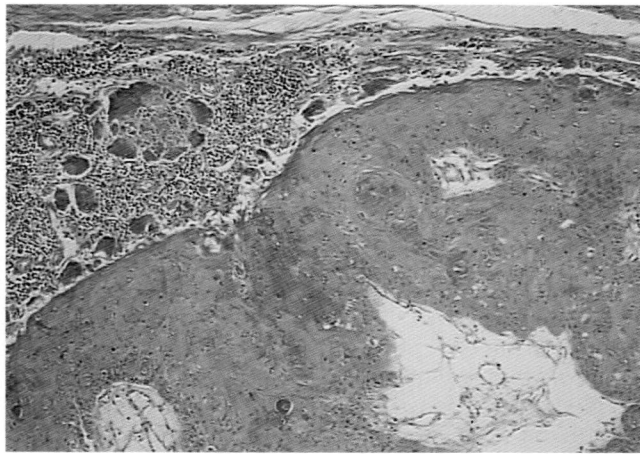

**FIGURE 49–17.** Proliferating trichilemmal cyst. A deeply invasive proliferation of squamous epithelium is present that is sharply demarcated from the surrounding stroma. Notice the prominent foreign body giant cell reaction in the surrounding stroma.

A variety of benign cysts may commonly arise from the various segments of the hair follicle.

*Infundibular Cyst.* Infundibular cyst, also known as epidermal inclusion cyst or epidermal cyst, results from progressive cystic dilatation of the infundibulum of the hair follicle. The cysts occupy the dermis and are characterized by a lining made up of keratinizing squamous epithelium with a well-developed granular cell layer.

*Trichilemmal Cyst.* Trichilemmal cyst, also known as pilar or sebaceous cyst, arises from the isthmus of the hair follicle and is characterized by a lining of squamous epithelium devoid of a granular cell layer (so-called trichilemmal keratinization).

*Steatocystoma Multiplex.* Steatocystoma multiplex is a disorder that often follows an autosomal dominant pattern of inheritance and presents as multiple small cystic nodules predominantly on the chest, upper arms, axilla, and scrotum. The squamoid cells that line the cyst form a thin layer of dense homogeneous material resembling an eosinophilic cuticle. This layer is generally referred to as a crenulated membrane owing to its characteristically undulated appearance. Another characteristic feature is the presence of mature sebaceous lobules in association with the outer portion of the cyst wall.

*Dermoid Cyst.* Dermoid cysts are congenital subcutaneous cysts that may superficially resemble infundibular cysts because of their squamous lining but also show adnexal structures, such as sebaceous or apocrine glands, associated with the cyst.

*Eruptive Vellus Hair Cyst.* Eruptive vellus hair cyst also resembles an infundibular cyst but is characterized by the accumulation of small vellus hairs within the cyst. Trichostasis spinulosa, a related condition, is characterized by multiple small vellus hair cysts affecting the skin of the back and is generally accompanied by pruritus.

TUMORS OF GERMINATIVE FOLLICULAR EPITHELIUM. Tumors of germinative follicular epithelium are those that show features of differentiation toward hair matrix cells, cortical cells, and cells of the inner root sheath.

*Trichofolliculoma.* Trichofolliculoma is a rare lesion most often arising in the head and neck. It is characterized by a dilated hair follicle that opens to the epidermal surface and is surrounded by numerous secondary follicles that bud out in a radial fashion around the main dilated follicle. The secondary follicles either differentiate toward germinative epithelium or form mature hairs.

*Trichoepithelioma.* Trichoepithelioma usually presents as a solitary nodule on the face arising during childhood. Multiple trichoepitheliomas can be seen in the Brooke-Fordyce syndrome that is transmitted as an autosomal dominant trait. The tumors are composed of lobules made up of basaloid cells in the dermis that closely resemble BCC (Fig. 49–18*A*). Within the lobules of basaloid cells are multiple keratinous cysts surrounded by cells showing infundibular or isthmic differentiation. The neoplastic proliferation appears to be embedded within its own

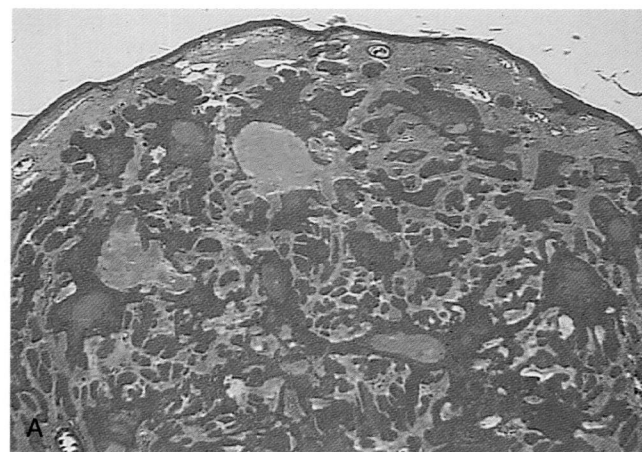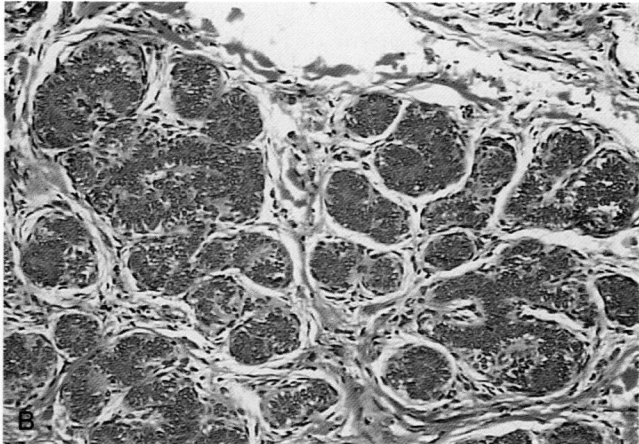

FIGURE 49–18. *A.* Trichoepithelioma shows lobules of basaloid cells in the dermis surrounded by a well-demarcated area of fibrotic stroma. *B.* Immature trichoepithelioma composed of small solid islands of basaloid cells showing invaginations that resemble the hair papilla.

fibrocollagenous stroma. The stroma often contains foci of dystrophic calcifications. Distinction from BCC with pilar differentiation may sometimes be difficult and in some instances even arbitrary.

An unusual variant designated immature trichoepithelioma has also been described that is characterized by a proliferation of small, solid islands of basaloid cells showing invaginations resembling the dermal hair papilla and lacking obvious keratinous cyst formation[51] (Fig. 49–18*B*). Another variant, desmoplastic trichoepithelioma, is composed of small nests and cords of basaloid cells embedded in a densely collagenized stroma that can closely resemble morpheaform BCC. The epithelial nests and cords can often be seen to connect with small keratin-filled cysts. Unlike BCC, desmoplastic trichoepithelioma is well circumscribed and appears to be contained within its own sclerotic stroma, a helpful feature for differential diagnosis.[52]

*Pilomatricoma.* Pilomatricoma, also known as calcifying epithelioma of Malherbe, is a distinctive tumor displaying features of matrix follicular differentiation. It frequently presents in children and adolescents as a deep-seated cystic or solid dermal nodule composed of a compact proliferation of small basaloid cells with small, round hyperchromatic nuclei characteristically displaying brisk mitotic activity (Fig. 49–19). The cells in the more central portions of the lesion show a tendency to exhibit a "washed out" appearance of the nuclei and more prominent eosinophilic cytoplasm, and these in turn eventually turn into "ghost" cells near the cyst lumen, in which only the cytoplasm of the cells can be discerned. Dystrophic calcifications are often encountered in the lumen of the cyst and can be prominent. Older lesions can show extensive replacement by ghost cells with abundant calcium deposits and extensive metaplastic bone formation. Extravasated keratin will often elicit a prominent foreign body–type reaction in the surrounding dermis. More superficially

located lesions can show transepidermal migration with extrusion of the ghost cells through the overlying epidermis.

*Trichoblastoma.* Trichoblastoma is a term originally proposed by Headington[53] to designate tumors exhibiting a relatively primitive appearance resembling that of embryonic hair that were accompanied by certain distinctive changes in the surrounding stroma. Although the terminology of these tumors has suffered numerous permutations since Headington's original description, trichoblastoma is still recognized as a useful designation for tumors exhibit-

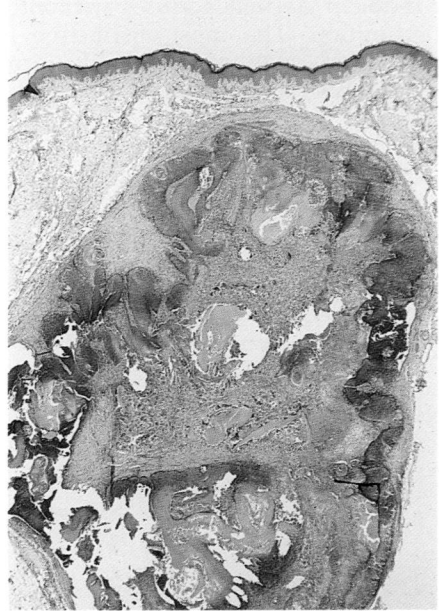

FIGURE 49–19. Pilomatricoma. A well-circumscribed dermal proliferation of small, dark basaloid cells is seen admixed with areas composed of "ghost" cells devoid of nuclei.

ing these features. Three distinctive variants or stages in the development of this tumor were originally recognized—trichogenic trichoblastoma, trichoblastic trichoblastoma, and trichoblastic fibroma—depending on the relative proportion and maturity of epithelium versus stroma. Because significant overlap can often be appreciated histologically between these different variants and the clinical evolution is the same regardless of the stage of the lesion, the unified terminology of "benign trichogenic tumor" has been proposed for these neoplasms.[54] The lesions generally present as firm, well-circumscribed nodules located anywhere within the dermis and can vary in size from 1 to 5 cm. They are characterized histologically by a proliferation of small basaloid cells arranged in cords, sheets, or discrete clusters that show prominent peripheral palisading. The cords of basaloid cells often grow as thin trabeculae that tend to branch out and often anastomose in a fibroepitheliomatous fashion (Fig. 49–20). The tumor cells are generally surrounded by a cellular stroma resembling perifollicular mesenchyme. Follicular differentiation may be observed in the form of foci resembling hair root structures or by the formation of rounded cellular clusters that contain focal indentations filled by a cellular stroma that closely resembles the primitive hair papilla and hair bulb (CD Fig. 49–5). Occasional mitoses may be present scattered throughout the lesion without this finding portending an aggressive behavior.

A variety of lesions showing purported features of differentiation toward follicle-related mesenchyme have also been described, including trichodiscoma, perifollicular fibroma, and fibrofolliculoma.

*Trichodiscoma.* Trichodiscoma, a tumor presumed to show differentiation toward the hair disk (haarscheibe), generally presents clinically as a group of indolent dermal nodules without any particular distribution. The most distinctive histologic feature is the presence of a platelike area in the superficial dermis composed of connective tissue with stromal mucin that contains microscopic nerve twigs, usually only demonstrable by silver stains.

*Perifollicular Fibroma.* Perifollicular fibroma is another fibroblastic proliferation with features similar to trichodiscoma, except that it generally surrounds hair follicles.

*Fibrofolliculoma.* Fibrofolliculoma refers to a perifollicular fibrous proliferation similar to that of perifollicular fibroma but in which the center of the hair follicle is dilated, and thin septa of proliferating epithelium and sebaceous lobules branch out into the perifollicular fibrous stroma.

TUMORS WITH SEBACEOUS DIFFERENTIATION. A variety of benign sebaceous proliferations have also been recorded.

*Sebaceous Hyperplasia.* Sebaceous hyperplasia is a benign, tumorlike condition that presents as tan-yellow, umbilicated papules in the face, areola, and genital skin of elderly individuals. Histologic examination shows a single dilated follicular canal that connects with the epidermal surface and contains four or more fully mature sebaceous lobules attached to the infundibulum of the pilosebaceous unit. The presence of ectopic sebaceous glands showing features of sebaceous hyperplasia on the vermilion border of the lip or oral mucosa is known as Fordyce's condition.

*Sebaceous Adenoma.* Sebaceous adenoma usually presents as a small yellowish nodule on the face of middle-aged patients. It is characterized histologically by a well-circumscribed proliferation of enlarged mature sebaceous lobules surrounded by a fibrous pseudocapsule. In the Muir-Torre syndrome, sebaceous adenomas have a tendency to show a less organized appearance, with less distinct lobulation and admixture of the mature lipidized sebocytes with smaller basaloid, nonlipidized cells in the periphery of the lobules. Tumors displaying these features have also been designated sebaceous epithelioma. When the small basaloid cells predominate, it may be difficult to distinguish the lesion from a BCC with sebaceous differentiation.

MALIGNANT FOLLICULOSEBACEOUS NEOPLASMS. Malignant folliculosebaceous neoplasms are quite rare.

*Trichilemmal Carcinoma.* Trichilemmal carcinoma is a distinctive neoplasm with follicular differentiation affecting hair-bearing areas of the skin in adult patients. The lesion shows sheets of large clear cells arising from the epidermis that infiltrate the underlying dermis in a nodular fashion (Fig. 49–21). The tumor cells contain abundant glycogen and show prominent peripheral palisading of nuclei. Subnuclear vacuolization and deposition of basement membrane material in the periphery of the tumor lobules are also often featured (CD Fig. 49–6). Foci of trichilemmal-type keratinization may be scattered throughout the lesion, and nuclear atypia and mitotic activity may also be present.[55]

*Pilomatrix Carcinoma.* Pilomatrix carcinoma is a tumor showing the same general features as con-

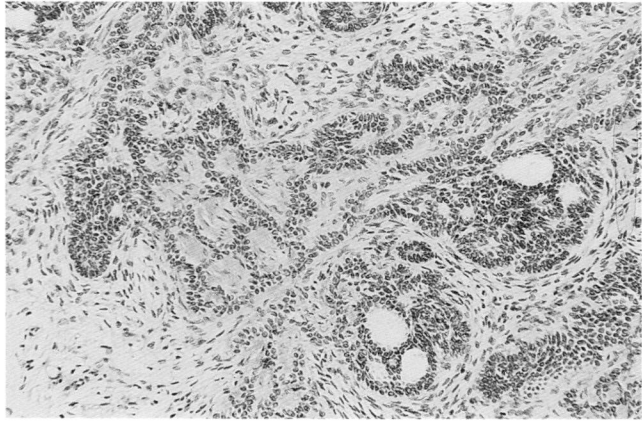

FIGURE 49–20. Trichogenic trichoblastoma. The tumor is characterized by branching cords of basaloid cells in the dermis surrounded by a cellular connective tissue stroma.

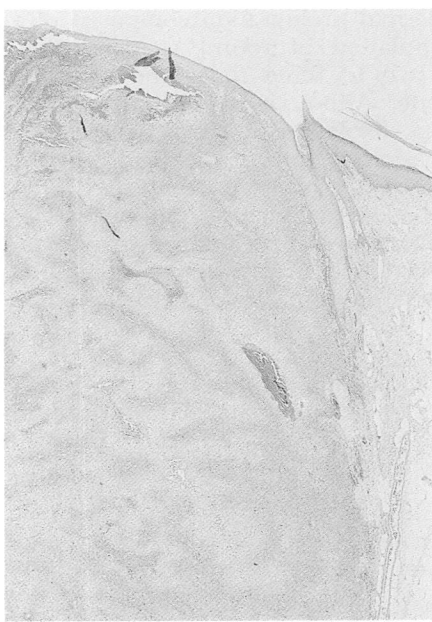

**FIGURE 49–21.** Trichilemmal carcinoma. A nodular proliferation of large clear cells with peripheral palisading of nuclei is seen invading the dermis.

ventional pilomatricoma, except that the tumor cells display more pronounced cytologic atypia, with increased nuclear-to-cytoplasmic ratios and large nucleoli, and display infiltrative growth and broad areas of necrosis.

*Sebaceous Carcinoma.* Sebaceous carcinoma is generally seen in middle-aged or elderly patients and shows a predilection for the ocular region, particularly the eyelids and the conjunctiva, where it arises in association with meibomian glands and the gland of Zeis, although extraocular lesions can also occur. The extraocular lesions are most often distributed in the head and neck but may also involve the trunk, genitalia, and extremities. Sebaceous carcinoma can also be seen as part of the Muir-Torre syndrome. On histologic examination, it is composed of lobules of polygonal tumor cells with sharp cell borders and abundant clear, multivacuolated cytoplasm. The tumor cells often have centrally placed nuclei with nucleoli and are characterized by prominent "scalloping" of the nuclei due to indentation by multiple lipid vacuoles (Fig. 49–22). Admixed in various proportions with the clear, obviously sebaceous cells are smaller, more primitive-appearing cells with high nuclear-to-cytoplasmic ratios, hyperchromatic nuclei with prominent nucleoli, and brisk mitotic activity. The tumors are often infiltrative and accompanied by vascular invasion and comedo-like areas of necrosis. Sebaceous carcinoma is an aggressive neoplasm with a high rate of local recurrence; up to 25% of cases present with distant metastases, and up to 20% of patients die of tumor-related causes. Ocular cases are thought to have a more aggressive behavior than that of tumors in extraocular locations.[56]

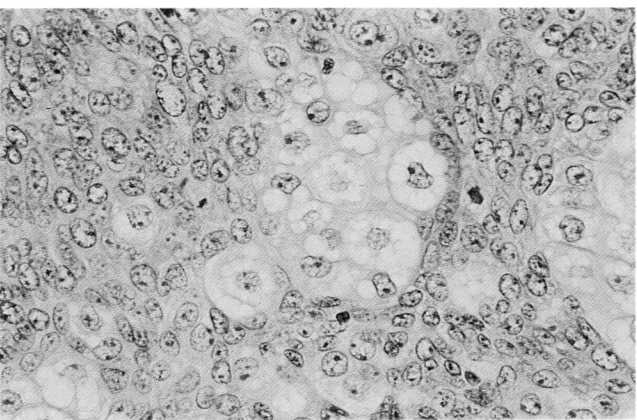

**FIGURE 49–22.** Sebaceous carcinoma. Atypical primitive cells are seen admixed with larger cells with abundant cytoplasm and scalloped nuclei.

## Tumors with Mixed Features of Adnexal Differentiation

Benign adnexal neoplasms may occasionally be encountered that show more than one type of adnexal epithelial differentiation. Thus, tumors exhibiting admixtures of eccrine and apocrine, sweat gland and pilar, sweat gland and sebaceous, or combinations of more than two of these features can occasionally be encountered. Such tumors are best regarded as examples of benign adnexal neoplasms with mixed or divergent differentiation.[57]

Malignant skin adnexal tumors showing mixed features of differentiation have also been described. Thus, tumors may on occasion show divergent lines of differentiation within the same neoplasm, including sebaceous, sweat gland, and pilar features. Such tumors are best characterized as adnexal carcinoma with mixed (or divergent) differentiation.[58]

## NEUROENDOCRINE NEOPLASMS

### Primary Neuroendocrine Carcinoma of the Skin (Toker Tumor)

Primary neuroendocrine carcinoma of the skin was first described by Toker[59] in 1972 under the designation "trabecular carcinoma of the skin" to emphasize one of its most distinctive morphologic attributes. The neuroendocrine nature of the lesion was first identified in 1978 by Tang and Toker,[60] who described on ultrastructural examination the presence of dense-core neurosecretory granules within the cytoplasm of the tumor cells and postulated that the tumors may be derived from Merkel cells in the skin. Since then, numerous studies on this condition appeared in the literature that further defined the clinicopathologic features of this neoplasm.[61–65] The tumor has since been known by a variety of designations, the most popular of which is Merkel cell carcinoma, although Merkel cell origin or differentiation has never been demonstrated to date. For this reason, the more generic designation of primary neuroendocrine carcinoma of the skin is still favored.[66]

Primary neuroendocrine carcinoma of the skin is most common in elderly patients with a slight female predilection; however, cases have been described over a broad range of age. The tumor involves mainly the head and neck area, followed by the extremities and the buttocks. On gross evaluation, the tumors are nodular masses with a pink-red or violaceous appearance. Rapid growth with early metastases and an aggressive clinical behavior with fatal outcome generally characterize the tumors. Histologic examination shows a poorly circumscribed,

diffuse dermal proliferation composed of a monotonous population of round to oval cells that are roughly two to three times the size of a mature lymphocyte. Although the tumor was initially described as displaying a characteristically trabecular growth pattern, a diffuse sheetlike growth pattern is more commonly observed that may often lead to confusion with malignant lymphoma (Fig. 49–23A). A trabecular growth pattern, however, can generally be appreciated at the edges of the tumor or may predominate in some lesions (Fig. 49–23B). The tumor cells contain large, often vesicular nuclei with dispersed chromatin and absent or inconspicuous nucleoli and scant cytoplasm (Fig. 49–23C). Extensive areas of necrosis, vascular and lymphatic invasion, high mitotic rate, and crush artifact in the tumor cells are also commonly found. Other features

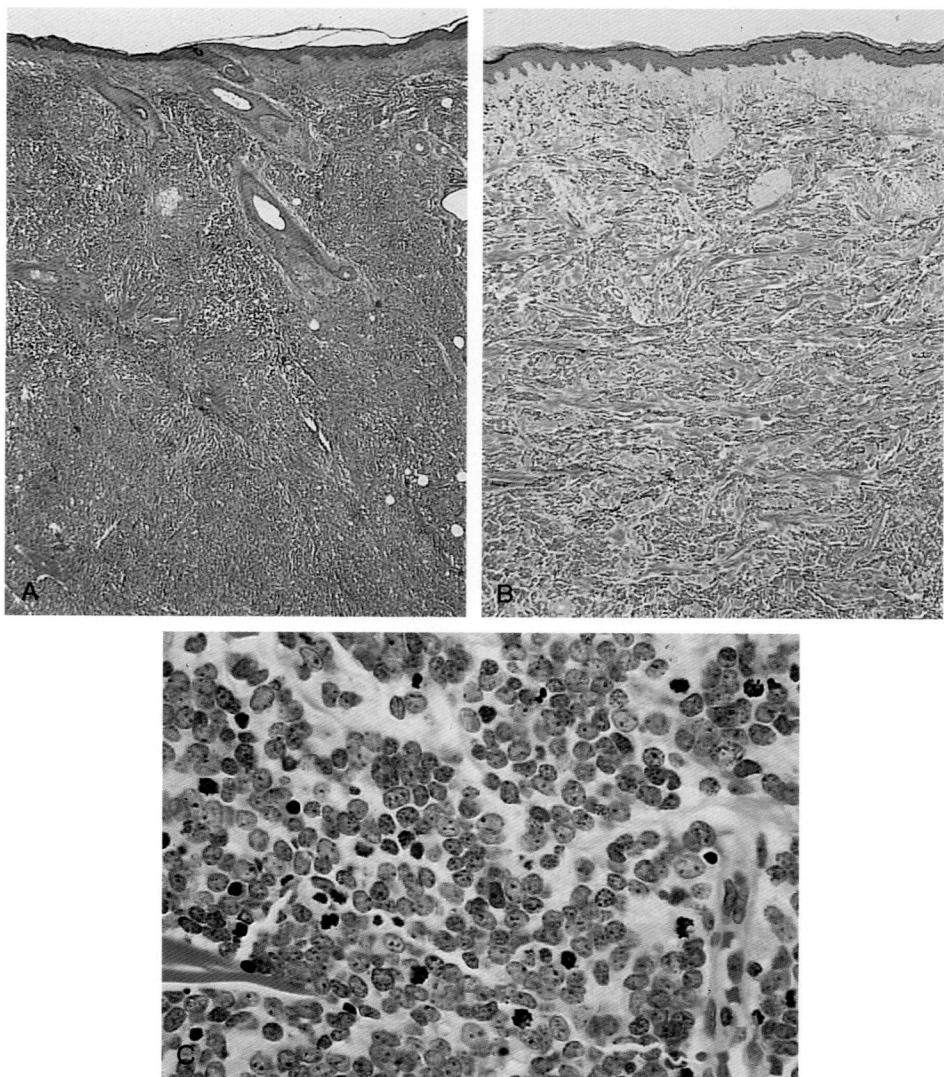

**FIGURE 49–23.** Neuroendocrine carcinoma of the skin (Toker tumor). *A.* Solid growth pattern of monotonous hyperchromatic tumor cells simulating a lymphoma. *B.* Trabecular growth pattern. *C.* Higher magnification shows round cells with characteristic evenly dispersed dense chromatin and scant rim of cytoplasm.

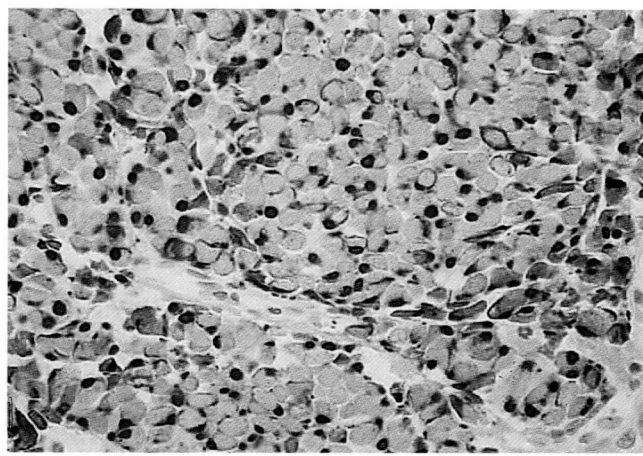

**FIGURE 49–24.** Neuroendocrine carcinoma of the skin showing distinctive dotlike paranuclear pattern of positivity with cytokeratin 20.

that can occasionally be encountered are the formation of rosettelike structures resembling Homer-Wright rosettes, pagetoid spread of tumor cells in the epidermis, and foci of squamous or eccrine glandular differentiation (CD Fig. 49–7).[67–69]

The tumors are characterized by strong immunoreactivity for neuroendocrine markers, including chromogranin, synaptophysin, neuron-specific enolase, somatostatin, calcitonin, and others.[70] The tumors also show a distinctive dotlike, perinuclear pattern of staining for low-molecular-weight cytokeratin and selectively stain for cytokeratin 20, a helpful feature for the differential diagnosis with a metastasis of small cell carcinoma of the lung[71] (Fig. 49–24). Other markers that have also been found to be expressed in these tumors are neurofilaments, Bcl-2, p53, and CD44.[72, 73] The differential diagnosis encompasses a variety of small round cell neoplasms including malignant lymphoma, metastatic neuroblastoma, Ewing's sarcoma/peripheral neural ectodermal tumor, embryonal rhabdomyosarcoma, poorly differentiated eccrine carcinoma, and malignant melanoma predominantly composed of small round cells. The most difficult and important differential diagnosis, however, is with a metastasis from a neuroendocrine carcinoma from internal organs.[74, 75] Differential staining for cytokeratin 7/20 may be of aid in defining the diagnosis under such circumstances.

## MESENCHYMAL AND NEURAL NEOPLASMS

A great variety of mesenchymal proliferations can involve the skin. Because of the similarity with their soft tissue counterparts detailed elsewhere in this text, only those showing distinctive features in the skin are dealt with in this chapter.

## Vascular Tumors of the Skin

A wide array of benign and malignant vascular proliferations, including vascular malformations, hyperplasias, and neoplasias, have been described in the skin.

VASCULAR MALFORMATIONS. Vascular malformations are congenital lesions characterized by disordered growth of normal vessel wall components. Several clinically distinctive forms of congenital vascular malformations have been described, including nevus flammeus (port-wine nevus), capillary hemangioma, cavernous hemangioma, angiokeratomas, lymphangiomas, and arteriovenous hemangiomas. All share features of vascular ectasia and proliferation of vessels devoid of cytologic features of malignancy.

VASCULAR HYPERPLASIA. Vascular hyperplasia is characterized by the proliferation of endothelial cells lining the vessels with increase in the number of vessels in the dermis.

*Acroangiodermatitis.* Acroangiodermatitis, also known as pseudo-Kaposi's sarcoma, is a form of vascular hyperplasia that essentially represents an exaggerated form of stasis dermatitis most often affecting the lower extremities of elderly individuals. It is characterized by a proliferation of superficial dermal vessels surrounded by increased fibroblastic proliferation in the surrounding stroma with hemosiderin deposition, edema, extravasated erythrocytes, and sparse inflammatory lymphoid infiltrate. Because the lesions may be hyperpigmented, purpuric, and indurated, they can be confused clinically with other conditions, such as Kaposi's sarcoma.

*Intravascular Papillary Endothelial Hyperplasia.* Intravascular papillary endothelial hyperplasia, also known as Masson's pseudoangiosarcoma, represents an exaggerated hyperplastic response of vascular endothelium to trauma within a vessel lumen. It presents clinically as a deep dermal or subcutaneous nodule in which numerous small pseudopapillary structures lined by a single layer of flattened endothelium appear to project into the lumen of a dilated, often thrombosed vessel. The pseudopapillary proliferation can closely resemble the endothelial tufting seen in angiosarcoma; however, it lacks frank nuclear atypia and is confined to the lumen of the involved vessel.

*Pyogenic Granuloma.* Pyogenic granuloma, also known as lobular capillary hemangioma, may represent a localized, exaggerated form of granulation tissue response to trauma. The lesion often shows an epidermal collarette surrounding a well-circumscribed proliferation of small dermal vessels against a stroma that contains abundant plasma cells admixed with small lymphocytes and neutrophils. Typical mitotic figures can often be identified; however, cytologic atypia is absent. Similar lesions may also be encountered in a subcutaneous or intravascular location or be located entirely within the dermis.

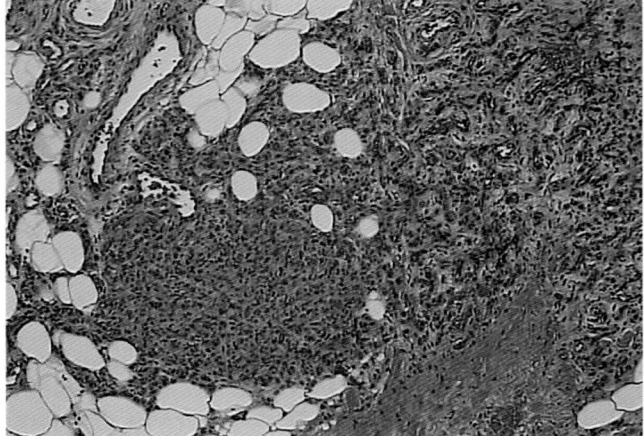

**FIGURE 49–25.** Acquired tufted hemangioma. Notice solid lobular proliferation of immature, small vessels scattered in the dermis.

VASCULAR NEOPLASIA. A wide variety of benign, borderline, and malignant vascular neoplasms are identified in the skin.[76] Hemangiomas in general show the same features as their soft tissue counterparts and are not discussed in detail. A few unusual variants, however, deserve special consideration.

*Acquired Tufted Hemangioma.* Acquired tufted hemangiomas, also known as progressive capillary hemangioma or angioblastoma of Nakagawa, present as slowly enlarging deep dermal plaques distributed on the neck and upper trunk of children and young adults. The lesions are characterized histologically by a lobular proliferation of small vessels scattered in a "cannonball" fashion throughout the dermis (Fig. 49–25). The capillary tufts may often project into dilated vascular lumina, imparting them with a crescentic appearance reminiscent of a glomerulus.[77, 78] The degree of cellularity within the vascular proliferation is often such that capillary lumina may not be readily apparent. Immunohistochemical stains for vascular endothelial markers may be of value for identifying vessel lumina in these lesions.

*Glomeruloid Hemangioma.* Glomeruloid hemangioma is a rare vascular proliferation characterized by multiple dilated vascular channels in the dermis containing a dense capillary proliferation that fill the lumina in a fashion vaguely reminiscent of renal glomeruli. PAS-positive eosinophilic globules may also be seen admixed with the vascular proliferation.[79] The lesions occur in the setting of the POEMS syndrome, a multisystem disorder consisting of polyneuropathy, organomegaly, endocrinopathy, M protein, and skin changes.[80]

*Microvenular Hemangioma.* Microvenular hemangioma is a rare vascular proliferation that preferentially involves the lower extremities of middle-aged adults. The lesions are composed of small, slitlike vessels that irregularly infiltrate the deep dermis (Fig. 49–26). Because of their deep infiltrative pattern, they may raise the possibility of a ma-

lignant vascular proliferation. Lack of cytologic atypia, necrosis, or mitotic activity helps distinguish them from other malignant vascular neoplasms.[81]

*Targetoid Hemosiderotic Hemangioma.* Targetoid hemosiderotic hemangioma is a benign vascular lesion that presents as a solitary, annular violaceous papule containing a pale ring surrounding the lesion and a more peripheral ecchymotic ring that grossly imparts the lesion with a targetlike appearance. On histologic examination, the lesion displays proliferation of widely dilated and irregular, thin-walled vascular lumina in the superficial dermis. Intraluminal papillary projections lined by a single layer of epithelioid endothelial cells displaying a "hobnail" appearance are present. The vessels in the deep portions of the lesion have a tendency to become angulated and irregular, appearing to dissect collagen bundles and surrounding adnexal structures.[82] The lesions may raise the possibility in the differential diagnosis of the patch stage of Kaposi's sarcoma.

*Epithelioid Hemangioma.* Epithelioid hemangioma is a benign vascular proliferation that incorporates several entities previously described as angiolymphoid hyperplasia with eosinophilia, Kimura's disease, atypical pyogenic granuloma, and histiocytoid hemangioma.[83-85] Its pathogenesis is still unsettled; some regard it as a reactive vascular proliferation, whereas others believe it represents a peculiar neoplastic vascular endothelial proliferation. The lesions generally present as multiple plaques or papules in the head and neck region of young to middle-aged adults with a female predilection, but they may also occur in other locations. Peripheral blood eosinophilia may be present in some cases. The lesions are characterized histologically by a vascular proliferation composed of large round to cuboidal, plump endothelial cells with abundant eosinophilic cytoplasm and large vesicular nuclei (Fig. 49–27). The endothelial proliferation usually lines vascular channels but may grow focally, forming sheets with a cohesive appearance within the vessel lumen that

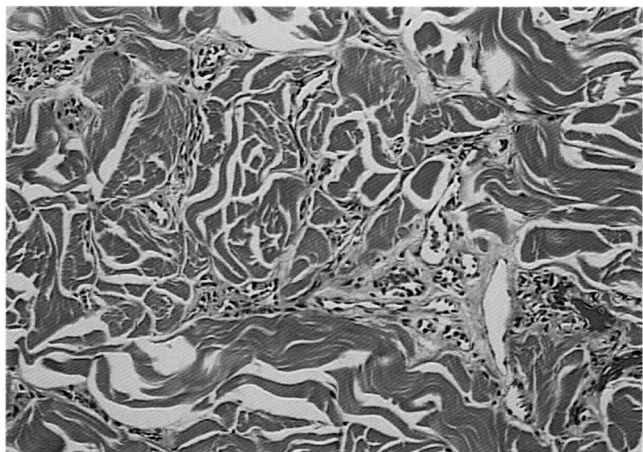

**FIGURE 49–26.** Microvenular hemangioma is characterized by multiple small, slitlike vessels that irregularly infiltrate the dermis.

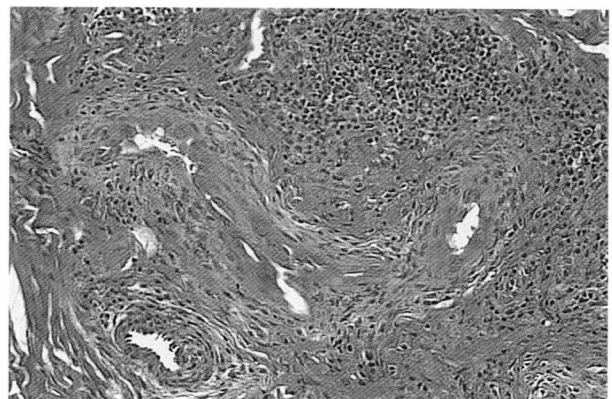

**FIGURE 49–27.** Epithelioid hemangioma (angiolymphoid hyperplasia with eosinophilia). A proliferation of vessels lined by large, prominent endothelial cells characterizes the lesions.

resemble epithelial cells. A characteristic feature is the presence of prominent cytoplasmic vacuoles; these vacuoles can sometimes contain single erythrocytes lying within their lumina. Some of the cells lining the vessel walls may adopt a hobnail configuration. A large "feeder" vessel is often identified within the vascular proliferation. A frequent accompanying feature in dermal lesions is the presence of an inflammatory lymphoid infiltrate containing germinal centers and abundant scattered eosinophils, the reason for the term *angiolymphoid hyperplasia with eosinophilia*. Late stages of the process may be devoid of an inflammatory infiltrate and can display significant regressive changes including prominent stromal fibrosis. Despite the often alarming epithelioid appearance of the cells, the process is benign.

*Glomus Tumor.* Glomus tumor is a benign neoplastic proliferation believed to recapitulate the normal myoarterial shunts concerned with temperature regulation that are located in the reticular dermis around the digits and distal extremities. Although, strictly speaking, glomus tumor represents a proliferation of tumor cells displaying a myoid phenotype without any evidence of vascular endothelial differentiation, it has been classed by convention among vascular endothelial neoplasms because of its close relationship with vessels. The tumors are most often solitary, although a multifocal type can be observed that is often familial and inherited as an autosomal dominant trait. The lesions present as deep dermal or subcutaneous nodules that typically produce a triad of symptoms including pain, tenderness, and temperature sensitivity. The tumors are characterized histologically by a monotonous proliferation of round to cuboidal cells that contain uniform round nuclei surrounded by a rim of amphophilic to eosinophilic cytoplasm (Fig. 49–28). The tumor cells may grow into sheets that form a solid, expansile nodule or may be distributed around ectatic blood vessels. An uncommon variant designated glomangiomyoma is characterized by an admixture of glomus cells with a population of spindle smooth muscle cells.

Immunohistochemical studies have shown strong positivity of the tumor cells in glomus tumors for actin and myosin stains but negative reaction for desmin, factor VIII–related antigen, and other vascular markers.

*Bacillary Angiomatosis.* Bacillary angiomatosis is a peculiar vascular endothelial proliferation identified in patients with the acquired immunodeficiency syndrome. The lesion shares features with epithelioid hemangioma and is characterized by a proliferation of vessels lined by large, epithelioid endothelial cells against a background of intense inflammation and stromal edema, often accompanied by a dense neutrophilic infiltrate with focal microabscesses. On silver impregnation, numerous rod-shaped bacilli are easily identified in the interstitium.[86] The aggregates of bacilli can sometimes be visualized on H&E examination as focal deposits of granular purplish material within the lesions. The bacilli are gram negative and acid-fast negative and are related to the cat-scratch bacillus. A closely related process caused by the organism *Bartonella bacilliformis* is seen in endemic areas of South America and gives rise to the lesions of verruga peruana, a disease with cutaneous lesions that clinically and histologically are indistinguishable from bacillary angiomatosis.

A variety of "borderline" vascular endothelial neoplasms have also been recognized that are believed to represent neoplastic vascular proliferations of low malignant potential, including spindle cell hemangioendothelioma, epithelioid hemangioendothelioma, retiform hemangioendothelioma, Kaposi's sarcoma, and endovascular papillary angioendothelioma (Dabska tumor).

*Spindle Cell Hemangioma.* This tumor was originally described as *spindle cell hemangioendothelioma* and thought to be a low-grade angiosarcoma with combined features of cavernous hemangioma and Kaposi's sarcoma.[87] The tumors are associated with a tendency for slow progression and multiple re-

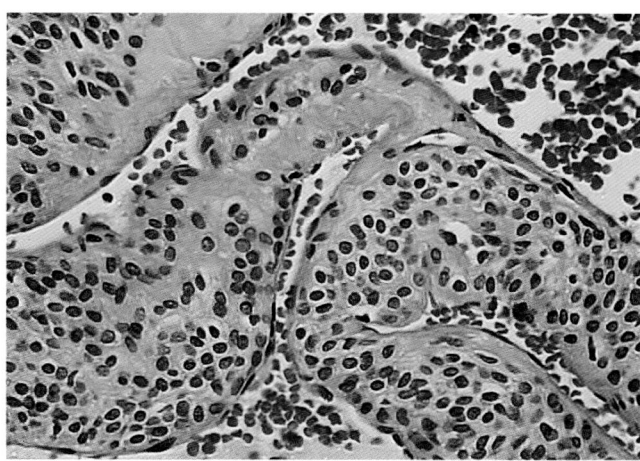

**FIGURE 49–28.** Glomus tumor composed of monotonous proliferation of round to polygonal tumor cells surrounded by a clear rim of cytoplasm.

currences but do not appear to display any capabilities for metastasis. Some authors have postulated that these lesions may not be neoplastic at all but rather represent a non-neoplastic, reactive vascular proliferation associated with malformed vessels and repeated cycles of thrombosis and recanalization. The lesions have a predilection for young adults and tend to affect the distal extremities. They usually manifest as either single or multiple asymptomatic nodules in the dermis or subcutaneous tissue. Local recurrence after simple excision is common; multiple recurrences with extensive local disease can also been observed. They are characterized histologically by two components, a proliferation of thin-walled cavernous vessels filled with blood and a dense spindle cell component that is generally admixed with the cavernous vessels. The spindle cells may form fascicles that contain slitlike spaces filled with extravasated erythrocytes reminiscent of Kaposi's sarcoma. Small clusters of plump epithelioid cells may also be seen admixed with the spindle cell elements. Cytologic atypia or mitotic activity is rarely present. Despite the close resemblance with Kaposi's sarcoma, the lack of significant mitotic activity and the conspicuous cavernous vessels seen throughout the tumor help to separate these two conditions.

*Epithelioid Hemangioendothelioma.* Epithelioid hemangioendothelioma is a distinctive low-grade vascular neoplasm believed to represent an intermediate stage between a benign hemangioma and an angiosarcoma.[88] The tumor is almost ubiquitous in distribution and can occasionally involve the skin as its primary manifestation. The lesions are often associated with local recurrence and lymph node metastases. The tumor cells are characterized histologically by their epithelioid appearance, with large vesicular nuclei surrounded by abundant eosinophilic cytoplasm. Intracytoplasmic vacuoles are a distinctive finding in the tumor cells (Fig. 49–29). Unlike epithelioid hemangioma, the tumor cells in epithelioid hemangioendothelioma are often not associated with the lumina of vessels and are seen growing as sheets or cords or are singly scattered within an extensively hyalinized and often myxoid stroma. The lesion often has an infiltrative appearance with irregular or ill-defined borders. Mitoses can vary from few to more than one per 10 high-power fields. Higher mitotic activity, presence of necrosis, and focal spindling of the cells have been associated with a more aggressive behavior.[89] Despite the close resemblance to metastatic carcinoma sometimes displayed by these tumors, the diagnosis can easily be accomplished with the use of immunohistochemical markers. The tumor cells stain strongly positive for factor VIII–related antigen and other vascular endothelial markers.

*Endovascular Papillary Angioendothelioma (Dabska Tumor).* Endovascular papillary angioendothelioma is a rare tumor originally described by Dabska[90] in 1969 as a distinctive vascular neoplasm of childhood. The tumor is often locally invasive with a potential for lymph node metastases; however, it is generally associated with a favorable prognosis. The most salient histologic feature of these tumors is the presence of intraluminal papillary structures expanding the vessel lumen. Endothelial cells displaying mild nuclear pleomorphism, hyperchromatism, and sparse mitotic activity line the papillary structures.

*Retiform Hemangioendothelioma.* Retiform hemangioendothelioma is a rare vascular tumor that is regarded as a low-grade form of angiosarcoma.[91] The tumor often presents in the extremities of young adults with a tendency for local recurrence; however, only one case of lymph node metastasis has been recorded to date. The tumor has a predominantly subcutaneous location and is composed of thin-walled arborizing blood vessels lined by a monotonous population of endothelial cells with a prominent hobnail appearance. The term *retiform* is derived from the branching appearance of the blood vessels that is reminiscent of the rete testis. Some authors regard retiform hemangioendothelioma as the adult counterpart of endovascular papillary angioendothelioma (Dabska tumor).

*Kaposi's Sarcoma.* Kaposi's sarcoma is a tumor of uncertain histogenesis that has been widely regarded to be of vascular endothelial origin, although this has not been proved. The isolation of human herpesvirus (HHV-8) in the lesions of Kaposi's sarcoma strongly suggests a role for this viral agent in its pathogenesis.[92] Before the advent of the acquired immunodeficiency syndrome (AIDS), Kaposi's sarcoma was a disease that more often affected the distal extremities of elderly individuals of Mediterranean or European descent or occurred in an endemic form in African children and young adults. With the advent of AIDS, a more aggressive, epidemic form in young adults, mostly homosexual or intravenous drug abusers, has become the most common form of the disease.

The clinical lesions of Kaposi's sarcoma typically evolve through stages as patches, plaques, and nodules. This is mirrored histopathologically by the changes observed in the skin. In the patch stage, the

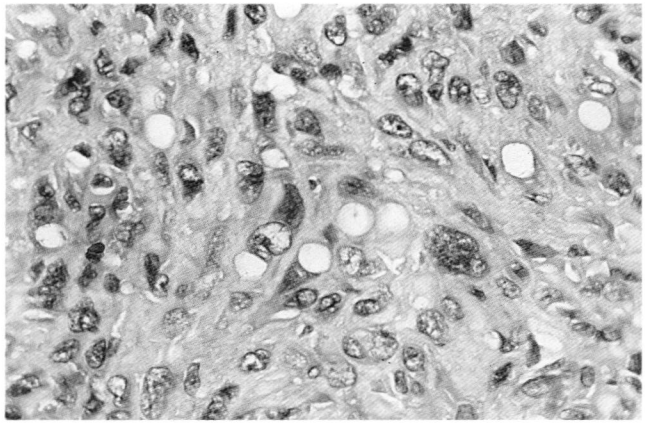

**FIGURE 49–29.** Epithelioid hemangioendothelioma. Cords and sheets of large epithelioid cells are seen containing abundant cytoplasm and frequent cytoplasmic vacuoles.

lesions can be subtle and consist of early vascular changes involving the reticular dermis. A proliferation of small vascular spaces is seen that is generally distributed around larger vessels or dermal adnexa (Fig. 49–30A, CD Fig. 49–9). The proliferating vessels are frequently angulated or branching, with open lumina. A distinctive feature is the protrusion of some of these small vessels into the lumina of larger vessels. The endothelium of these vessels is generally inconspicuous and devoid of cytologic atypia or mitotic activity. In the plaque stage, the vascular proliferation is denser and fills the entire dermis and may also involve the subcutis. The most distinctive feature of this stage is the emergence of a spindle cell proliferation surrounding the vascular proliferation. The spindle cells are generally devoid of significant cytologic atypia and are dispersed between dermal collagen bundles and around preexisting dermal vessels. Slitlike spaces containing extravasated erythrocytes can also be seen. Hemosiderin deposits and PAS-positive, round eosinophilic hyaline globules are also common features. The vascular and spindle proliferation is generally accompanied by an inflammatory infiltrate composed of small lymphocytes and plasma cells. The nodular lesions of Kaposi's sarcoma are characterized by an expansile, dense spindle cell proliferation forming fascicles that often cross each other at right angles (Fig. 49–30B). Interspersed with the spindle cells are numerous slitlike spaces filled with extravasated erythrocytes (Fig. 49–30C). The spindle cells show mild to moderate cytologic atypia with relatively frequent mitotic figures. There is frequently hemosiderin deposition and intracellular and extracellular clusters of PAS-positive, densely eosinophilic hyaline globules scattered throughout the lesion.

The immunohistochemical profile of Kaposi's sarcoma can be variable. Despite the obvious vascular features of these tumors, the spindle cells of Kaposi's sarcoma rarely react with factor VIII–related antigen (von Willebrand factor) and are only weakly positive for *Ulex europaeus* lectin 1. On the other hand, more recent studies have shown strong positivity of the tumor cells in a significant number of cases with CD34 and CD31, two vascular endothelium–related antigens.[93]

*Angiosarcoma.* Angiosarcoma is rare in the skin. Primary cutaneous angiosarcoma most often presents as lesions on the face and scalp of elderly individuals or in the setting of chronic lymphedema of the upper extremity as a late sequela of radical mastectomy for breast carcinoma (Stewart-Treves syndrome). Cases have also been described after radiation for breast cancer. The lesions are often multifocal and may present clinically as ill-defined plaques, patches, or nodules. On histologic examina-

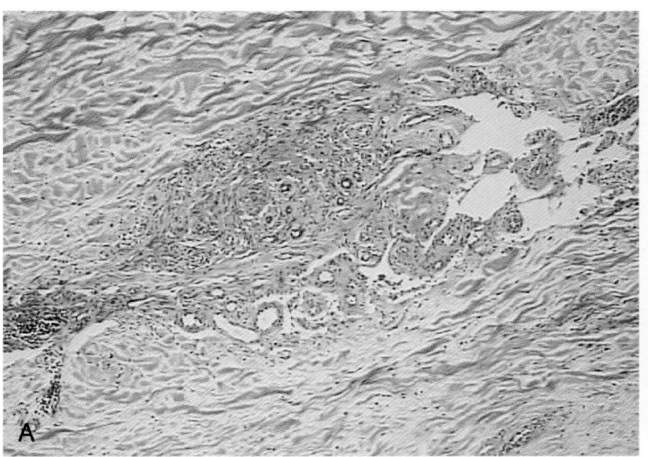

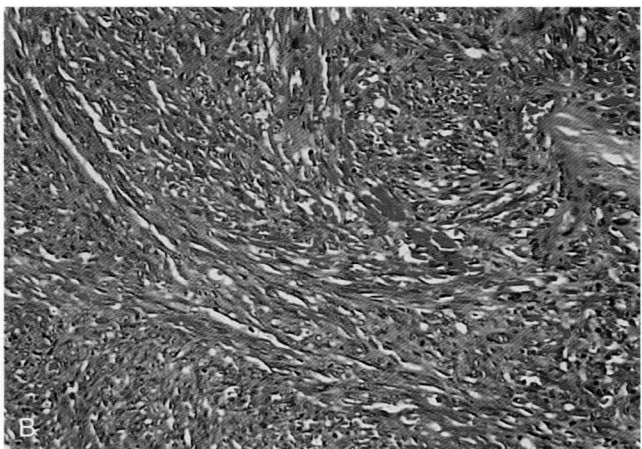

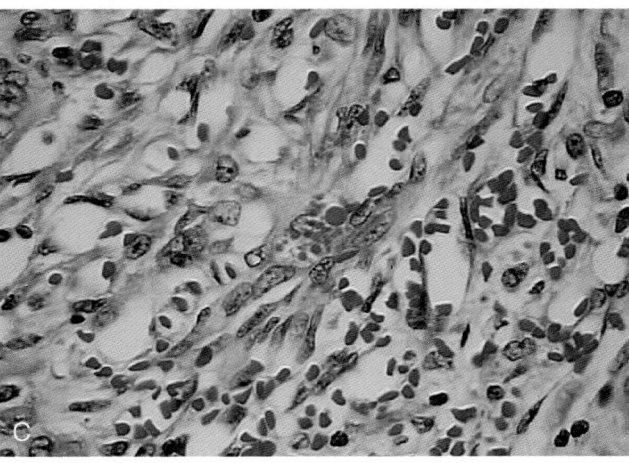

**FIGURE 49–30.** *A.* Kaposi's sarcoma. Patch stage showing discrete proliferation of small vascular spaces around larger vessels and dermal adnexa. *B.* Nodular stage of Kaposi's sarcoma showing fascicular spindle cell proliferation in the dermis. *C.* Nodular stage of Kaposi's sarcoma. Higher magnification shows atypical spindle cells with extravasated red blood cells.

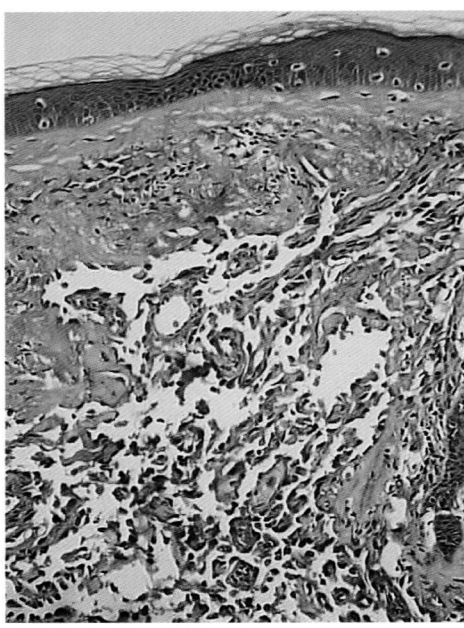

**FIGURE 49–31.** Well-differentiated angiosarcoma of the scalp. Notice anastomosing vascular proliferation lined by plump, hyperchromatic endothelial cells.

tion, the lesions tend to diffusely infiltrate the dermis and usually extend well beyond their grossly visible borders. The early lesions are characterized by a proliferation of small anastomosing vascular channels that are usually lined by a single layer of plump, hyperchromatic endothelial cells (Fig. 49–31). The vascular channels are seen to diffusely dissect among collagen bundles and infiltrate deep into the subcutis.[94] More advanced lesions often show highly cellular areas growing as sheets or nodules of atypical tumor cells with large, hyperchromatic nuclei and frequent atypical mitoses. These areas are usually closely associated with vascular channels lined by atypical endothelium in the periphery (CD Fig. 49–10). The tumor cells may adopt an epithelioid appearance, with abundant eosinophilic cytoplasm. In other lesions, the atypical cells may assume a spindled appearance, displaying large hyperchromatic nuclei and frequent atypical mitoses. Immunohistochemical markers of endothelial differentiation may not be helpful in the poorly differentiated variants because factor VIII–related antigen, CD34, and *Ulex europaeus* lectin 1 may not stain the tumor cells or may stain them only faintly.[95] The most reliable marker in this setting is CD31, which often identifies a number of the tumor cells.

## Fibroblastic, Myofibroblastic, and "Fibrohistiocytic" Tumors

Dermal proliferations predominantly composed of fibroblasts or myofibroblasts constitute a large group of lesions that can vary from benign, reactive, and non-neoplastic lesions to highly malignant neoplasms. The concept of "fibrohistiocytic" lesions, presumably derived from facultative fibroblasts capable of showing histiocytic differentiation, has largely been abandoned in recent years. It is now recognized that most of these lesions correspond to fibroblastic proliferations unrelated to histiocytic differentiation that often adopt a peculiar cartwheel or storiform pattern of growth. However, the term has become firmly entrenched in the literature and continues to be widely used.

BENIGN, REACTIVE, AND NON-NEOPLASTIC PROLIFERATIONS OF FIBROBLASTS. Benign, reactive, and non-neoplastic proliferations of fibroblasts include dermal scars and keloids, fibroepithelial polyps (acrochordon), acquired digital fibrokeratoma, periungual fibroma, fibroma molle (soft fibroma), nodular fasciitis, palmar and plantar fibromatosis, knuckle pads, and penile fibromatosis. All are characterized by a proliferation of mature fibroblasts-myofibroblasts surrounded by abundant intercellular collagen. Other unusual but distinctive benign dermal fibrous proliferations are dermatofibromas, atypical fibroxanthoma, infantile digital fibromatosis, and infantile myofibromatosis and solitary myofibroma.

***Dermatofibroma (Benign Fibrous Histiocytoma).*** Dermatofibroma (benign fibrous histiocytoma) is one of the most common skin neoplasms in adults. The tumors often present as flesh-colored nodules arising in the legs, arms, and trunks of young to middle-aged adults. The tumors are benign but may recur locally in up to 25% of cases when they are incompletely excised. On histologic examination, dermatofibroma may show a wide spectrum of features. The tumors may show wide variation, depending on the cellularity, shape of the cells, degree of sclerosis, hemosiderin deposition, and vascularity.[96] The hallmark of these tumors is their distinctive growth pattern under scanning magnification. Under low-power examination, the tumors grow as symmetric, well-circumscribed, unencapsulated dermal nodules that tend to infiltrate the dermis by wrapping their cells around collagen bundles, resulting in a characteristic pattern of entrapment of collagen at the periphery of the lesion (Fig. 49–32). The neoplastic cell population may be composed or monotonous round, epithelioid or histiocytoid cells with round nuclei and abundant cytoplasm, but it is more often made up of a proliferation of bland-appearing spindle cells that form tightly whorled fascicles arranged in a storiform or pinwheel pattern. Mitoses are extremely infrequent or absent. In addition to the spindle cells, lymphocytes, foamy macrophages, and osteoclast-type and Touton-type giant cells may be present. The overlying epidermis often displays changes such as acanthosis, basal cell hyperplasia, and basal hyperpigmentation. Cases containing a prominent central vascular component were designated sclerosing hemangiomas in the past. The vascular changes can sometimes adopt an aneurysmal appearance that can

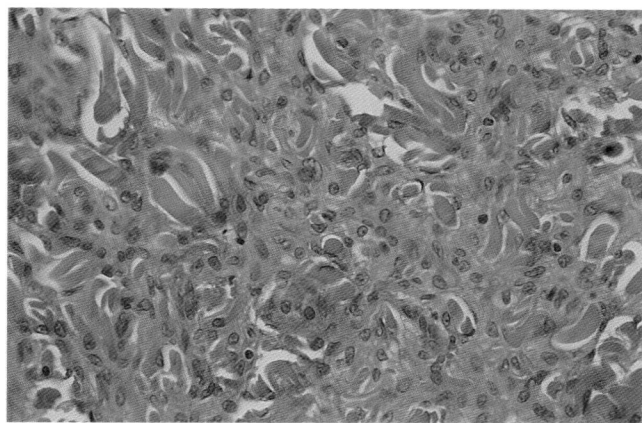

**FIGURE 49–32.** Dermatofibroma. Monotonous proliferation of bland-appearing round to oval cells with entrapment of collagen by the tumor cells.

lead to confusion with Kaposi's sarcoma or spindle cell hemangioendothelioma; however, the edges of the lesion display the characteristic features of dermatofibroma.

An unusual variant characterized by the presence of scattered bizarre giant cells interspersed with the spindle proliferation has been called dermatofibroma with monster cells.[97] Rare cases displaying prominent clearing of the cytoplasm have also been described under the designation clear cell dermatofibroma.[98] One of the most problematic variants described is the cellular variant of dermatofibroma, characterized by a more densely cellular fascicular growth pattern that may focally infiltrate the subcutaneous fat, causing confusion with dermatofibrosarcoma protuberans.[99] These lesions are associ-

ated with a higher propensity for local recurrence. On occasion, such lesions may attain a giant size (generally more than 5 cm) and are characterized by a storiform proliferation of spindle cells admixed with "lakes" of foamy macrophages that often infiltrate the subcutaneous fat and form large multinodular masses that can closely resemble dermatofibrosarcoma protuberans clinically. Unlike dermatofibrosarcoma protuberans, however, the lesions are devoid of significant cytologic atypia or mitotic activity.

Dermatofibromas are characterized by their immunoreactivity for factor XIIIa and vimentin but are negative for CD34 and Bcl-2, two markers often expressed in dermatofibrosarcoma protuberans.

*Atypical Fibroxanthoma.* Atypical fibroxanthoma represents a distinctive lesion characterized histologically by a highly atypical and pleomorphic cell population that is suggestive of a high-grade malignant neoplasm (Fig. 49–33). However, the lesions tend to be superficial, exophytic, well circumscribed, and often polypoid and are surrounded by an epidermal collarette. Despite their ominous cytologic appearances, the tumors behave in a completely benign fashion when they are completely excised.[100] These tumors tend to arise mostly in sun-damaged skin of elderly individuals. The tumor cells may vary from small, atypical spindle cells to large, multinucleated cells with bizarre nuclei and frequent abnormal mitotic figures reminiscent of malignant fibrous histiocytoma of soft tissue. Tumors showing areas of necrosis, vascular invasion, or invasion into the subcutis should be approached with caution and regarded as potentially malignant because similar cases have been known to recur and metastasize.[101] The diagnosis of atypical fibroxanthoma should be one of exclusion. Immunohistochemical stains may be of help to rule out alterna-

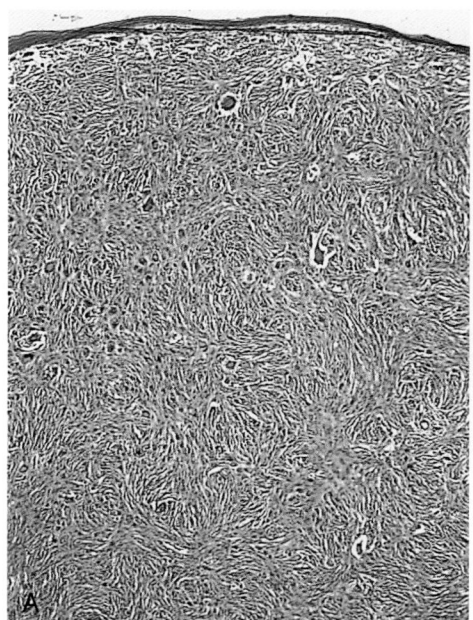
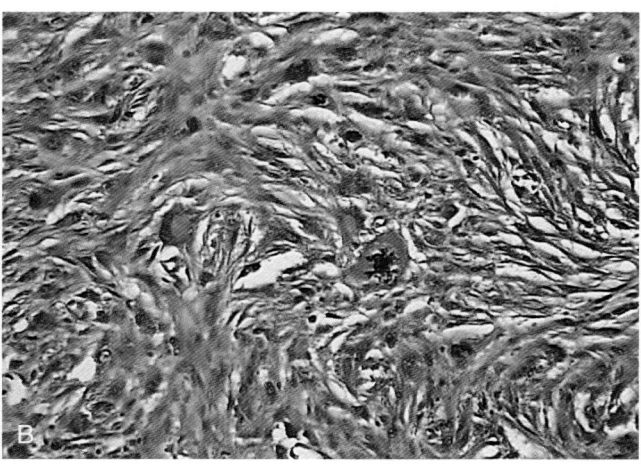

**FIGURE 49–33.** *A.* Atypical fibroxanthoma. A dense spindle cell proliferation admixed with tumor giant cells displaying a prominent storiform pattern is present in the dermis. *B.* Higher magnification shows marked nuclear pleomorphism and atypical mitotic figures in atypical fibroxanthoma.

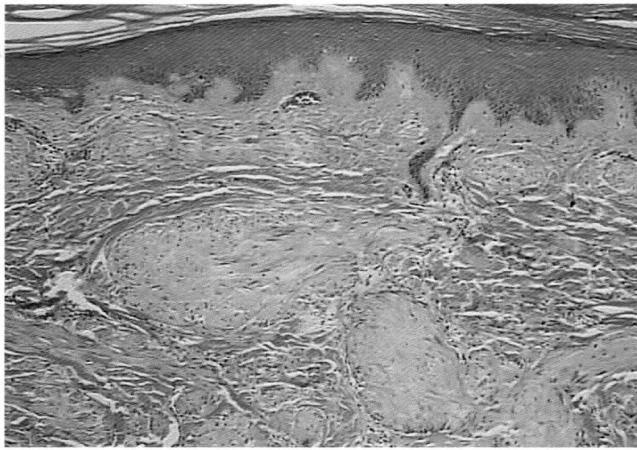

FIGURE 49–34. Solitary myofibroma of the adult. Well-circumscribed areas containing scant spindle cells predominantly concentrated in the periphery and with central areas of sclerosis are present in the dermis.

tive diagnoses, such as melanoma, leiomyosarcoma, and poorly differentiated carcinoma.

*Infantile Digital Fibromatosis.* Infantile digital fibromatosis is a distinctive benign dermal proliferation predominantly affecting the distal extremities (digits) of children and infants. The tumors are composed of interlacing bundles of benign-appearing fibroblasts and myofibroblasts embedded in a dense collagenous stroma. The most distinctive feature of these lesions is the presence of scattered intracytoplasmic eosinophilic inclusions that may range in size from that of a red blood cell to several times larger. The inclusions stain strongly with phosphotungstic acid–hematoxylin or trichrome stains and are composed of actin microfilaments.[102]

*Infantile Myofibromatosis and Solitary Myofibroma of the Adult.* Infantile myofibromatosis and solitary myofibroma of the adult represent proliferations of myofibroblasts involving mainly the deep

dermis and subcutis, but in the infantile form, they may often be multifocal and affect internal organs and bone.[103] The lesions in adults are more often cutaneous and solitary.[104] The cutaneous lesions are characterized by a biphasic pattern of growth. The central portions of the lesion are composed of a cellular proliferation of round to oval cells with scant cytoplasm that display a prominent hemangiopericytoma-like appearance, with numerous small, branching vessels with open lumina (CD Fig. 49–11). This central portion blends imperceptibly with more peripheral zones composed of fascicles of bland-appearing spindle cells with oval nuclei and abundant cytoplasm. These fascicles tend to be sharply delineated from the surrounding connective tissue stroma and often adopt a "wormlike" appearance within the dermis (Fig. 49–34). Necrosis, mitotic activity, and vascular invasion are not common features of these tumors; when present, they are not indicative of malignancy.[105] Although incompletely excised lesions can recur, their metastatic potential is low to none.

MALIGNANT FIBROBLASTIC OR FIBROHISTIOCYTIC LESIONS. Malignant fibroblastic or fibrohistiocytic lesions involving the skin, such as malignant fibrous histiocytoma and fibrosarcoma, are rare and more often the result of secondary infiltration from underlying soft tissue tumors.

*Dermatofibrosarcoma Protuberans.* Dermatofibrosarcoma protuberans is the most common malignant primary fibroblastic or "fibrohistiocytic" tumor of the skin. Dermatofibrosarcoma protuberans has a predilection for young or middle-aged adults and presents as an enlarging plaque or nodule that is frequently present for many years before diagnosis. The most common sites are the trunk and proximal extremities. The tumors are characterized histologically by a monotonous spindle cell proliferation that predominantly occupies the dermis and infiltrates the subcutaneous tissue (Fig. 49–35A). The spindle cells contain small oval nuclei with scant cytoplasm and have a tendency to adopt a prominent pinwheel

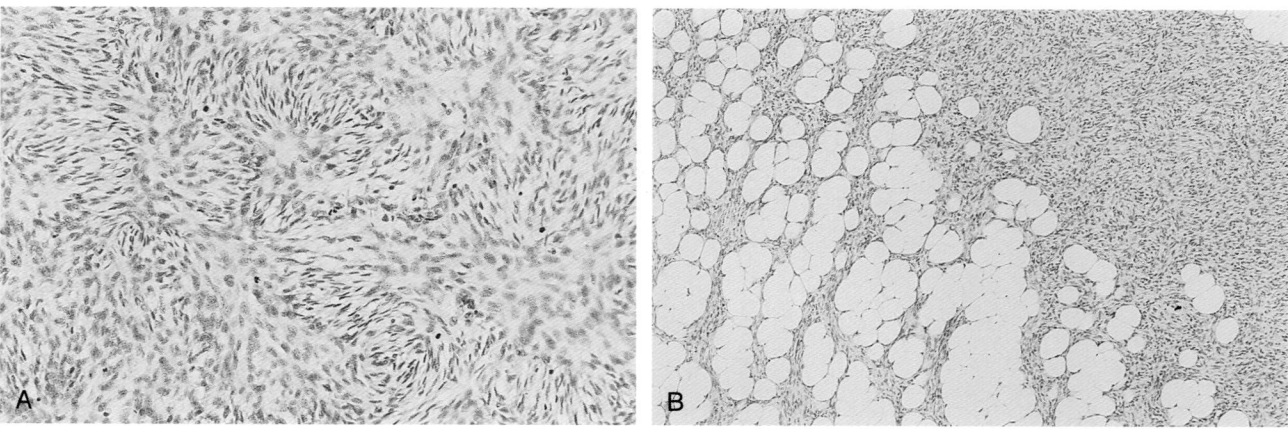

FIGURE 49–35. *A.* Dermatofibrosarcoma protuberans. A dense spindle cell proliferation is seen in the dermis displaying a prominent pinwheel or storiform pattern. *B.* Irregular, lacelike infiltration of the subcutaneous fat is seen in the deeper portions of the lesion.

or short storiform pattern of growth. The tumor may contain occasional mitotic figures. A characteristic feature is the pattern of infiltration of the subcutaneous fat. The tumor cells infiltrate the subcutaneous adipose tissue in a distinctive lacelike fashion, displacing and entrapping the fat without destroying it (Fig. 49–35B). Immunohistochemical analysis usually shows positivity of the tumor cells for vimentin, CD34, and Bcl-2 and negative staining for smooth muscle markers, S-100 protein, and factor XIIIa.[106, 107] A pigmented variant has been described under the designation of Bednar tumor. A myxoid variant characterized by abundant deposition of intercellular myxoid stroma has also been described.

Dermatofibrosarcoma protuberans is generally regarded as a clinically low-grade malignant neoplasm associated with a high tendency for local recurrence but with low metastatic potential. Metastases most often develop from recurrent tumors that show increased cellularity and atypia. Some cases can show areas of increased cellularity with marked cytologic atypia and increased mitotic activity that resemble a high-grade sarcoma. Such an event has been interpreted as the secondary development of fibrosarcoma superimposed on dermatofibrosarcoma protuberans. Fibrosarcomatous transformation in dermatofibrosarcoma protuberans is associated with a much more aggressive behavior and higher incidence of metastases (CD Fig. 49–12).[108]

***Giant Cell Fibroblastoma.*** A closely related condition, giant cell fibroblastoma, can also present as a solitary, slow-growing dermal or subcutaneous mass that is characterized by a proliferation of giant, pleomorphic, and spindle cells embedded in a myxoid stroma (CD Fig. 49–13). The giant cells show a tendency to line vessel-like channels and clefts. Recurrent lesions of dermatofibrosarcoma protuberans can occasionally display the features of giant cell fibroblastoma.[109]

## Skin Tumors with Myogenic Differentiation

Skin tumors with muscle differentiation are relatively rare. Most represent benign smooth muscle proliferations.

Smooth Muscle Tumors. Benign smooth muscle proliferations include leiomyoma, angioleiomyoma, and smooth muscle hamartoma.

***Leiomyoma.*** Leiomyoma can occur in any age group. Most cases arise from arrector pili muscles and tend to occur on the extensor surfaces of the extremities and on the trunk. The lesions are generally single and painful and usually present as small nodules. A subset of these tumors can arise from the skin of genital areas and the nipple. Genital leiomyomas arise from the dartos or vulvar smooth muscle and may grow to larger dimensions. The lesions are characterized histologically by fascicles of spindle cells with abundant eosinophilic cytoplasm

and oval nuclei with blunt ends and evenly distributed chromatin. Many of the cells may show perinuclear vacuoles. The tumors are unencapsulated and sometimes infiltrative, with common involvement of hair follicles and dermal adnexa. The tumors are generally devoid of mitotic activity. Presence of mitoses should raise the possibility of malignancy. Tumors containing a prominent vascular component are termed angioleiomyoma.

***Smooth Muscle Hamartoma.*** Smooth muscle hamartoma is a rare congenital lesion presenting in children most commonly on the torso. The lesions may measure up to 10 cm in diameter. Histologic examination shows them to be composed of fascicles of mature smooth muscle haphazardly arranged within the dermis and subcutis and intimately admixed with mature adipocytes and collagen fibers.[110]

***Leiomyosarcoma.*** Leiomyosarcoma can also arise in a superficial location as a primary skin neoplasm involving the dermis and subcutis. The lesions occur in all age groups and show a predilection for the extremities. They can exhibit a broad range of histologic features that vary from well-differentiated, low-grade lesions to poorly differentiated sarcomas. The well-differentiated lesions can closely resemble their benign counterparts, with fascicles of spindle cells with blunt-ended nuclei and abundant eosinophilic cytoplasm. Unlike leiomyomas, however, the tumor cells display mild nuclear pleomorphism, with conspicuous nucleoli and scattered mitotic figures. The poorly differentiated variants are characterized by marked nuclear pleomorphism, areas of necrosis, and high mitotic rates. Immunohistochemical studies show strong positivity of the tumor cells with smooth muscle markers, including smooth muscle actin and myosin, and desmin. Prognosis depends on the size of the lesion, tumor grade, depth of invasion, and completeness of the initial excision.[111] Up to 40% of dermal tumors recur, but metastases are extremely rare. In contrast, one third of subcutaneous lesions metastasize and have a fatal outcome.

Unusual histologic variants of cutaneous leiomyosarcomas include epithelioid leiomyosarcoma, myxoid leiomyosarcoma, and smooth muscle tumors with granular cell change. Epithelioid leiomyosarcomas are characterized by large, round to oval cells with abundant eosinophilic cytoplasm that may closely resemble an epithelial neoplasm. The tumors tend to arise in association with large dermal or subcutaneous vessels.[112] Granular cell leiomyosarcoma is characterized by the presence of abundant granular eosinophilic cytoplasm in the tumor cells. These neoplasms may be mistaken for other types of granular cell tumors of the skin. The granular cell change is believed to represent a secondary degenerative phenomenon.[113] Deposition of prominent myxoid matrix between the smooth muscle tumor cells is another unusual phenomenon that may lead to confusion with other myxoid skin neoplasms.

Skin Tumors with Features of Skeletal Muscle Differentiation. Skin tumors displaying features of skeletal muscle differentiation are extremely rare. Rare cases of embryonal rhabdomyosarcoma have been described in the skin, mainly of children and young adults. The tumors are composed of a proliferation of small, immature round to spindle cells often embedded in a myxoid stroma. The lesions show a tendency for recurrence and metastases. A case of malignant "triton" tumor showing a combination of embryonal rhabdomyosarcoma and malignant peripheral nerve sheath tumor has also been described.[114]

## Neural Tumors of the Skin

A wide variety of neural tumors may be encountered in the skin, ranging from hamartomatous processes and heterotopias to true benign and malignant nerve sheath neoplasms.

NEUROMAS. Neuromas are hamartomatous proliferations that attempt to recapitulate the normal structure of peripheral nerves. Neuromas can arise de novo or secondary to trauma (traumatic or amputation neuroma). Nontraumatic neuromas can be multiple or solitary. Multiple mucosal neuromas are part of the multiple endocrine neoplasia syndrome type 2A. Neuromas are characterized histologically by a fascicular proliferation of spindle cells that contain wavy nuclei and abundant eosinophilic cytoplasm. Solitary neuromas are generally encapsulated, whereas multiple neuromas are unencapsulated. The spindle cells in both types are strongly positive for S-100 protein. Silver impregnation demonstrates abundant axons in the tumor cells.

NEUROFIBROMAS. Neurofibromas are hamartomatous proliferations that recapitulate the various elements of neuromesenchyme, including Schwann cells, perineurial and endoneurial fibroblastic cells, and mast cells. Neurofibromas can occur as isolated, sporadic lesions involving the skin, but they are more often encountered in the setting of neurofibromatosis. The neurofibromas in neurofibromatosis are multiple and associated in nearly all cases with café au lait spots. The lesions can be superficial or deep and involve the subcutis. The superficial lesions are often polypoid and pedunculated. They are characterized histologically by a well-circumscribed, nonencapsulated proliferation of small oval to spindle cells embedded in the dermis (Fig. 49–36). The surrounding stroma may vary from densely fibrotic to hyalinized and myxomatous. Small aggregates of axons forming nerve twigs within the proliferating spindle cells can often be encountered. Mast cells are usually scattered in varying numbers throughout the lesion. Mitotic figures are absent. The tumor cells are usually positive for S-100 protein. Bundles and fascicles of markedly expanded nerves closely surrounded by a fibrous capsule or adjacent connective tissue characterize the plexiform variant.[115] A pigmented and a diffuse variant have also been described. The diffuse variant tends to be deep-seated

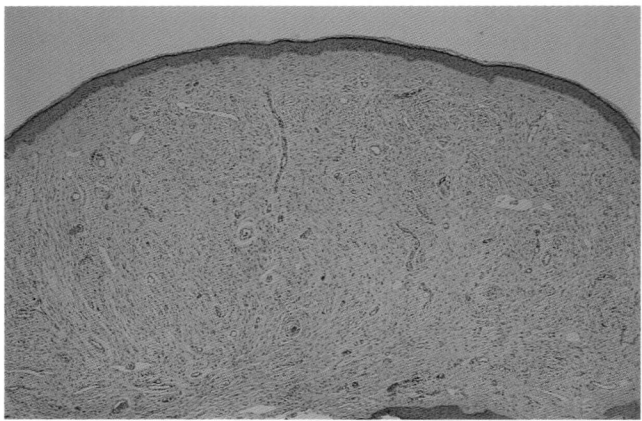

**FIGURE 49–36.** Neurofibroma. A uniform proliferation of small round to oval cells is seen occupying the dermis.

and is characterized by poorly circumscribed fascicles of bland, monotonous spindle cells that dissect among collagen fibers. The pigmented, diffuse, and plexiform variants are most frequently associated with neurofibromatosis. Deep infiltration of the dermis or subcutis, nuclear pleomorphism, and mitotic activity should raise the possibility of malignant transformation in neurofibroma, a relatively frequent occurrence in the setting of neurofibromatosis and in cases of desmoplastic melanoma with prominent neuroidal differentiation.

SCHWANNOMA. Schwannomas are benign peripheral nerve sheath neoplasms that are composed predominantly of cells displaying features of schwannian differentiation. They most often present as solitary dermal lesions with a predilection for the flexor aspect of the extremities and the head and neck. On histologic examination, the lesions are well encapsulated and may display two distinctive growth patterns referred to as Antoni type A and Antoni type B. The type A pattern refers to a fascicular proliferation of spindle cells that are often arranged in a parallel fashion resulting in a palisaded arrangement of the nuclei. A distinctive finding in the type A pattern is the presence of parallel rows of palisaded nuclei separated by an acellular matrix, the so-called Verocay bodies. The type B pattern is characterized by various degrees of cystic, edematous, or myxoid degeneration associated with thickened and hyalinized blood vessels and stromal fibrosis. The spindle cells in both patterns strongly label with S-100 protein. Degenerative changes involving the spindle cells resulting in marked cytologic atypia in the absence of mitoses have been designated "ancient" schwannoma.[116] Rare features in these tumors are melanotic pigmentation, glandular formations with mucus secretion, and plexiform growth pattern.

GRANULAR CELL NERVE SHEATH TUMOR. Granular cell nerve sheath tumor or granular cell tumor (myoblastoma) is still a tumor of disputed

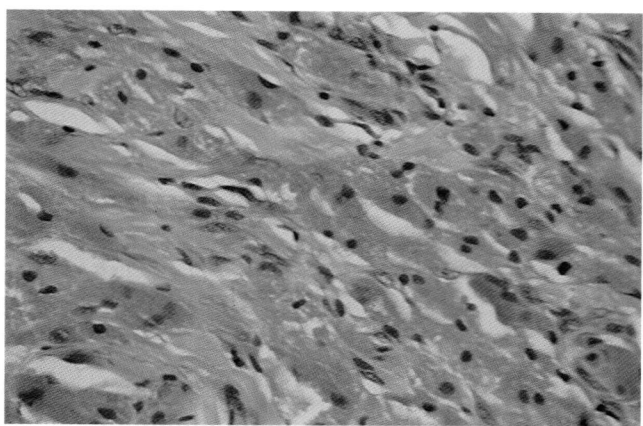

**FIGURE 49–37.** Granular cell nerve sheath tumor composed of large cells with small round nuclei surrounded by abundant granular, eosinophilic cytoplasm.

histogenesis, although most studies support a peripheral nerve sheath phenotype. The granular cells express S-100 protein, Leu-7 (CD57), and myelin basic protein, similar to normal peripheral nerves. The tumors are most often solitary, although multiple lesions can also occur. There is a female predilection, and the most commonly involved site is the tongue followed by the skin and internal organs. The skin lesions are characterized histologically by an ill-defined dermal proliferation of large cells with small, round, and centrally located nuclei surrounded by abundant granular, faintly eosinophilic cytoplasm (Fig. 49–37). The cytoplasmic granules are PAS positive and diastase resistant. The overlying epidermis is frequently hyperplastic and may show features of pseudocarcinomatous hyperplasia. The tumors can often attain a large size and infiltrate the subcutaneous fat. Tumors displaying rapid growth, ulceration of the overlying epidermis, marked nuclear pleomorphism and mitotic activity, and large size (>5 cm) should raise the suspicion of malignancy.

NERVE SHEATH MYXOMA (NEUROTHEKEOMA). Nerve sheath myxoma (neurothekeoma) is a benign cutaneous neoplasm composed of a proliferation of nerve sheath cells embedded in an abundant myxoid stroma. The lesions show a predilection for the head and upper extremities of middle-aged women; however, they can occur in any location at any age.[117] On histologic examination, the tumor shows a lobular growth pattern composed of fascicles of oval to spindle cells with slender cytoplasmic extensions embedded in a myxoid stroma (Fig. 49–38). The cells can occasionally adopt an epithelioid appearance or may be stellate or dendritic. The tumor cells stain strongly with S-100 protein and are also positive for collagen type IV and Leu-7 (CD57). A cellular variant has also been identified that is characterized by a paucity of myxoid stroma and an ill-defined, often infiltrative growth of epithelioid tumor cells in the dermis that often extend into the

subcutis.[118] The tumor cells in cellular neurothekeoma have large ovoid nuclei with prominent nucleoli surrounded by abundant eosinophilic cytoplasm with indistinct cell membranes. The tumor cells can adopt a fascicular, nodular, or plexiform growth pattern. Mitoses are frequent and may be associated with varying degrees of cytologic atypia. Unlike conventional neurothekeoma, the tumor cells in cellular neurothekeoma rarely react with S-100 protein or CD57 and have been referred to by some as immature nerve sheath myxoma.[119]

MALIGNANT PERIPHERAL NERVE SHEATH TUMOR. Malignant peripheral nerve sheath tumor, also known as malignant schwannoma, is usually a tumor of the deep soft tissue, mediastinum, and retroperitoneum that is commonly associated with neurofibromatosis. Cutaneous involvement is either the result of direct extension from a deep soft tissue lesion or the result of malignant transformation of a preexisting neurofibroma in a patient with neurofibromatosis. The lesions are characterized histologically by an atypical spindle cell proliferation disposed in fascicles that may often adopt a herringbone configuration or may show alternating hypercellular and hypocellular areas. The tumor cells can display varying degrees of cytologic atypia and mitotic activity.[120] Transitions with areas displaying the conventional features of neurofibroma are often present in patients with neurofibromatosis. Diagnosis is based on the history of neurofibromatosis, features of neural differentiation, or demonstration of close relationship with preexisting neurofibroma. S-100 protein has been claimed to stain approximately 50% of cases and can therefore be of limited value in poorly differentiated cases. Demonstration of features of schwannian differentiation by electron microscopy may be the only means of identifying such lesions. In addition to malignant peripheral nerve sheath tumor arising in the setting of neurofibromatosis, rare examples of sporadic cutaneous malignant peripheral nerve sheath tumor have

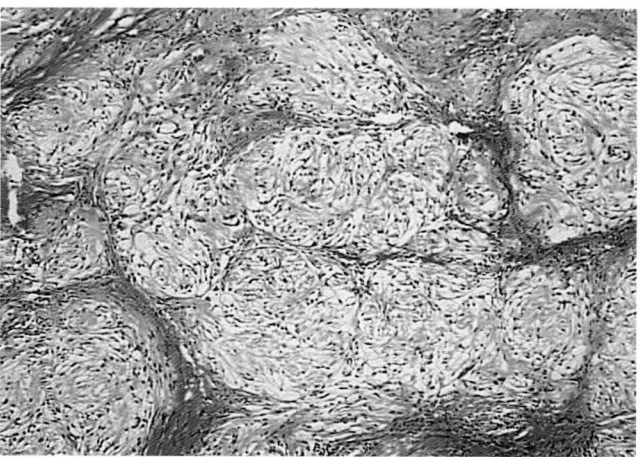

**FIGURE 49–38.** Nerve sheath myxoma showing lobular proliferation of spindle cells embedded in a myxoid stroma.

been described. Such tumors often adopt an epithelioid appearance that may closely resemble malignant melanoma.[121] Distinction from metastatic melanoma may be difficult and often impossible by routine histopathologic evaluation.

## LYMPHOPROLIFERATIVE DISORDERS

Cutaneous lymphoproliferations represent a relatively infrequent manifestation of skin disease that may span the range from benign, reactive, or hyperplastic conditions to indolent but atypical lymphoid proliferations to full-blown cutaneous lymphoma.

### Benign or Borderline Lymphoproliferations of the Skin

Cutaneous infiltrates predominantly composed of reactive B lymphocytes represent a frequent reaction pattern to a variety of stimuli, including insect bites, drug reactions, autoimmune disorders, and others. Their specific features are discussed elsewhere. Dense nodular lymphoid infiltrates were often categorized in the older literature as "pseudolymphoma cutis" or by other designations, such as lymphocytoma cutis and pseudolymphoma of Spiegler-Fendt. With the advent of modern immunologic techniques, it has become apparent that many of the "pseudolymphomas" represent clonal or low-grade malignant lymphoproliferations.[122, 123]

CUTANEOUS B CELL LYMPHOID HYPERPLASIA. Cutaneous B cell lymphoid hyperplasia is the term applied to cases in which a dense lymphoid infiltrate is present in the dermis, but special studies fail to reveal evidence of clonality or other aberrations in immunophenotype. The term should not be considered a specific diagnosis. Benign lymphoid hyperplasia is generally characterized by symmetric, well-circumscribed nodular aggregates in the dermis that are often wedge shaped and tend to involve the upper part of the dermis more than the deep dermis. They often contain a mixed cell infiltrate, with small lymphocytes, eosinophils, plasma cells, and histiocytes and can often show prominent germinal centers. The process generally spares adnexal structures and is devoid of atypia, necrosis, or mitotic activity. A combination of techniques, such as immunohistochemistry, flow cytometry, and molecular studies, may be necessary in such cases to rule out the possibility of early malignancy. Polyclonal immunoglobulin gene rearrangements favor a benign reactive process.

LYMPHOMATOID PAPULOSIS. Lymphomatoid papulosis is a clinical term that designates a chronic lymphoproliferative cutaneous disorder with a benign course often persisting for decades but with a malignant histologic appearance. The process is characterized clinically by a chronic, recurrent papu-

lar or nodular eruption that heals spontaneously, leaving hyperpigmented scars. The lesions preferentially affect women in their third and fourth decades and involve mainly the trunk, head, and proximal extremities. Although the process in the majority of instances behaves clinically like a benign disease, progression to malignant lymphoma has been observed in up to 10% of cases.

Molecular studies have suggested that this condition may belong in the spectrum of CD30+ lymphoproliferative disorders and may have a close histogenetic relationship with Hodgkin's disease and anaplastic large cell lymphoma.[124, 125] The characteristic, fully developed lesion consists of a superficial and deep nodular dermal infiltrate that may invade the subcutaneous fat and is composed of normal-appearing small lymphocytes admixed with loosely scattered medium- to large-sized pleomorphic lymphoid cells displaying atypical mitoses. Interphase lymphocytic exocytosis in association with epidermal necrosis is frequently observed. The proliferating cells label as activated helper T cells (CD3+, CD4+, CD5+, CD8−) and are also strongly positive for the CD30 antigen but do not express epithelial membrane antigen, CD15, or ALK-1. Clonal rearrangement of T cell receptor genes has been found in most cases studied so far.[125] The lesions are thus immunophenotypically indistinguishable from primary anaplastic large cell lymphoma of the skin. A diagnosis of lymphomatoid papulosis should thus be based on the characteristic clinical presentation and on the relative scarcity of the large anaplastic tumor cells in the infiltrate.

### Cutaneous T Cell Lymphoma

Cutaneous T cell lymphoma represents a heterogeneous group of lesions that share in common a clonal proliferation of T lymphocytes primarily originating from the papillary dermis. The clinical and histologic manifestations of cutaneous T cell lymphoma can be varied and range from chronic, indolent processes with subtle or minimal morphologic changes to rapidly growing, clinically aggressive lesions composed of highly atypical cells that may rapidly progress to disseminated disease.[126]

MYCOSIS FUNGOIDES. Mycosis fungoides represents the most common form of cutaneous T cell lymphoma. The disease is characterized by three well-defined clinical stages, the patch, plaque, and tumor stages. In the patch stage, the lesions present as slightly raised erythematous areas most often involving the trunk and the extremities that are often accompanied by scaling of the epidermis. The terms *parapsoriasis en plaque* and *large plaque parapsoriasis* were often used in the past to define the clinical appearance of the lesions in the patch stage.[127] In the plaque stage, the lesions are raised and indurated, often with a violaceous appearance, and show prominent scaling and pruritus. The patch and plaque stages of mycosis fungoides are relatively in-

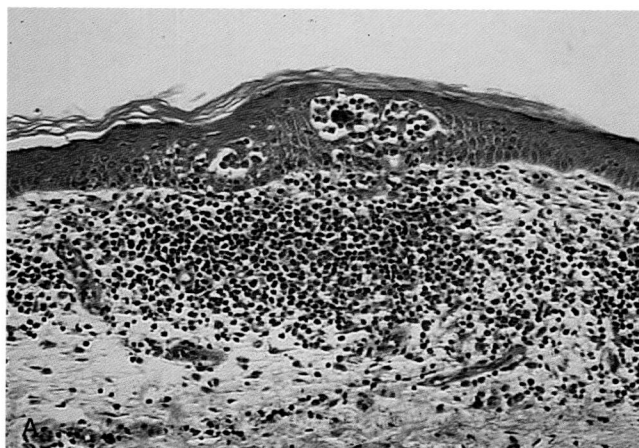
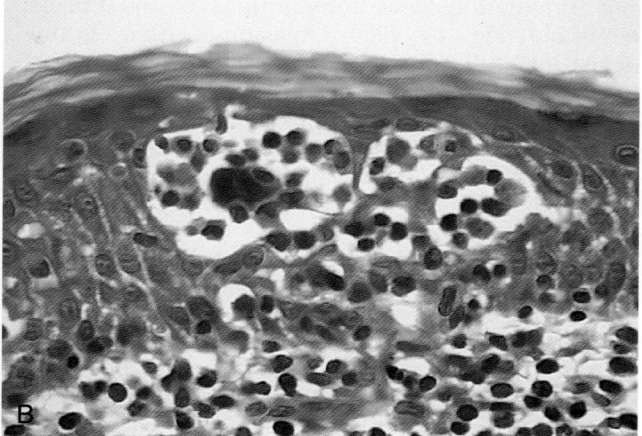

FIGURE 49–39. *A.* Mycosis fungoides, plaque stage, showing bandlike lymphoid infiltrate in the upper dermis. *B.* Mycosis fungoides, plaque stage, showing focal collections of atypical lymphocytes in the epidermis (Pautrier's microabscesses).

dolent and may progress slowly for many years without systemic disease. The tumor stage is characterized by the development of large, firm tumor nodules accompanied by erythroderma and scaling. The tumor stage often heralds systemic dissemination and portends a poor prognosis. When it is accompanied by high numbers of circulating tumor cells in the peripheral blood, the condition is referred to as Sézary syndrome.

The histologic findings in the patch stage can be subtle, with a scattering of perivascular small lymphocytes in the papillary dermis, superficial dermal fibroplasia, and rare lymphocytes within the epidermis. The sparse lymphoid infiltrate involving the epidermis may show mild nuclear atypia with convoluted nuclear contours in the absence of conspicuous spongiosis. In the plaque stage, the lymphoid infiltrate in the papillary and upper reticular dermis acquires a bandlike configuration and is composed of small to medium-sized lymphoid cells with hyperchromatic nuclei with irregular, convoluted nuclear membranes, admixed with plasma cells and eosinophils (Fig. 49–39A). The lymphoid elements may show a tendency to infiltrate the overlying epidermis, especially along the basal layer, and form discrete intraepidermal aggregates known as Pautrier microabscesses (Fig. 49–39B). The atypical lymphoid cells can also infiltrate dermal appendages, particularly hair follicles and eccrine duct epithelium, leading to mucinous degeneration that will result in hair loss (alopecia mucinosa). In the nodular stage, the papillary dermis and epidermis are generally spared, and there is massive dermal infiltration by sheets of enlarged atypical lymphoid cells with destruction of dermal skin adnexa (Fig. 49–40A). The atypical lymphocytes in these lesions demonstrate the same features as in the plaque stage, that is, large, irregular, and hyperchromatic nuclei with

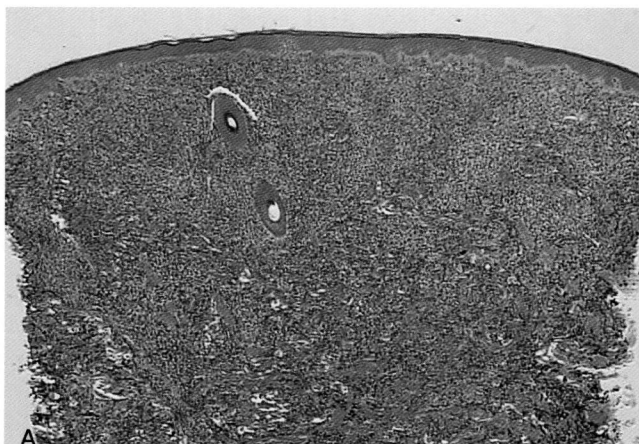
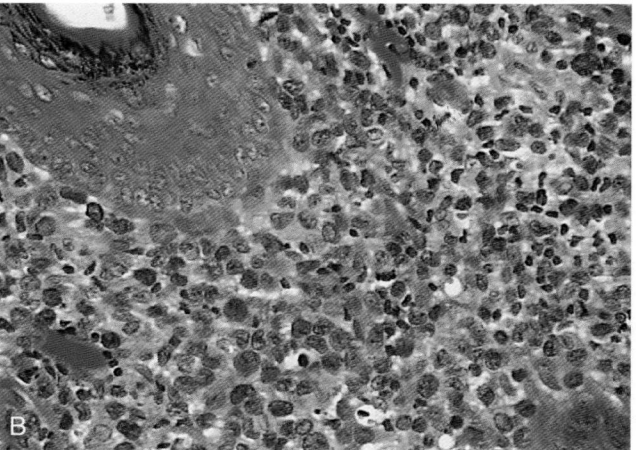

FIGURE 49–40. *A.* Mycosis fungoides, nodular stage, showing dense dermal infiltration by atypical lymphocytes with sparing of the epidermis. *B.* Mycosis fungoides, nodular stage. Higher magnification shows proliferation of atypical lymphocytes with nuclear convolutions.

deep indentations and convolutions of the nuclear membrane (Fig. 49–40*B*). Occasional larger, immunoblast-like cells are also often present.[128] The immunohistology of the lesions shows a CD1$^-$, CD2$^+$, CD3$^+$, CD4$^+$, CD5$^+$, CD7$^+$, CD8$^-$, and CD30$^-$ phenotype. In the tumor stage, an aberrant phenotype with loss of T cell antigens is a common finding. T cell receptor $\beta$-chain or $\gamma$-chain gene rearrangement is present in most cases.[129]

An unusual variant representing an abortive, localized form of the disease is known as pagetoid reticulosis (Woringer-Kolopp disease) (CD Fig. 49–14). Marked psoriasiform hyperplasia of the epidermis with parakeratosis and hyperkeratosis and a dense infiltrate of large atypical cells showing a pagetoid arrangement in the epidermis characterize this variant.[130] Another unusual and immunophenotypically closely related condition is known as granulomatous slack skin, which is characterized clinically by bulky folds of lax skin that hang from the flexural areas. On histologic examination, the lesions show a diffuse dermal infiltrate predominantly composed of small lymphocytes similar to those seen in mycosis fungoides. Admixed with the small lymphocytes are numerous large, multinucleated giant cells, many of which contain phagocytosed fragments of dermal elastic fibers.[131] Epidermotropism may not be readily apparent in these lesions. The lymphoid cells express the same immunophenotype as mycosis fungoides and also demonstrate clonal T cell receptor gene rearrangements.

ANAPLASTIC LARGE CELL LYMPHOMA. Anaplastic large cell lymphoma is a distinctive form of cutaneous T cell lymphoma characterized by single or multiple skin nodules that often show ulceration of the epidermis.[132, 133] Histologic examination shows the dermis to contain a mixed cell infiltrate composed of small lymphocytes admixed with plasma cells and histiocytes. Scattered throughout the dermal infiltrate are clusters and sheets of bizarre, atypical tumor cells with large, round, and irregular nuclei containing prominent eosinophilic nucleoli and surrounded by abundant cytoplasm. The tumor cells are often binucleated or multinucleated and may closely resemble the Reed-Sternberg cell and its variants[132] (Fig. 49–41). They also often adopt a kidney-shaped or "horseshoe" configuration.

The large anaplastic tumor cells show CD30 (Ki-1 antigen) positivity in a characteristic membranous and paranuclear (Golgi zone) pattern. They may also express T cell–associated antigens, such as CD45RO and CD43, with variable loss of pan–T cell antigens such as CD3 and CD5. Unlike their node-based counterpart, the tumor cells in primary cutaneous anaplastic large cell lymphoma are usually negative for epithelial membrane antigen and for the ALK-1 antigen.

The lesions have a tendency for spontaneous resolution, with multiple regressions and recurrences. In the past, many of these cases were regarded as a form of cutaneous malignant histiocyto-

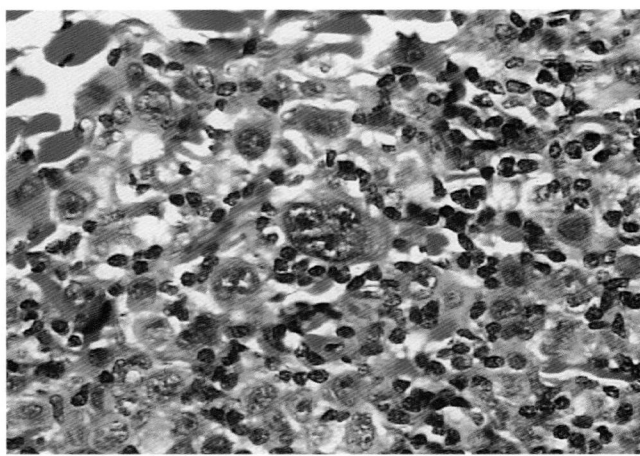

**FIGURE 49–41.** Cutaneous anaplastic large cell lymphoma with large, multinucleated tumor cells resembling Reed-Sternberg cells.

sis and designated regressing atypical histiocytosis. The term has now been abandoned because evidence has shown that the involved cells do not correspond to histiocytes but rather correspond to neoplastic T lymphocytes showing activation antigenic markers (i.e., CD30).

ANGIOCENTRIC T CELL LYMPHOMA. Angiocentric T cell lymphoma is a rare and aggressive form of cutaneous lymphoma that generally follows a rapidly progressive course with systemic dissemination. The lesions are composed of an atypical angiocentric lymphoid infiltrate admixed with variable numbers of immunoblasts, plasma cells, eosinophils, and histiocytes. The occlusion of vessels by the lymphoid infiltrate leads to extensive areas of ischemic necrosis. In the past, most of these cases fell under the rubric of lymphomatoid granulomatosis, a term referring to a systemic condition that frequently involved the lungs, skin, and central nervous system and was characterized by dense dermal infiltrates with prominent cuffing and transmural infiltration of the vessel walls by atypical lymphoid cells. More recently, similar cases have been described that are characterized by extensive infiltration and occlusion of vessel walls by CD56$^+$ lymphocytes. Infiltration and destruction of skeletal muscle is often present in these lesions. The tumor cells often show azurophilic granules in the cytoplasm and express the CD56 marker in conjunction with an aberrant T cell phenotype (CD4$^+$, CD2$^-$, CD3$^-$, CD8$^-$).[134] Despite the spurious expression of T cell markers, T cell receptor gene rearrangements have not been detected in these tumors. For this reason, these tumors have also been termed CD56$^+$ NK cell (null killer cell) lymphomas.

T CELL LYMPHOMATOUS PANNICULITIS. T cell lymphomatous panniculitis is another rare condition characterized by skin lesions that are deeply located in the subcutaneous fat and clinically resemble erythema nodosum. The lesions are distinguished histo-

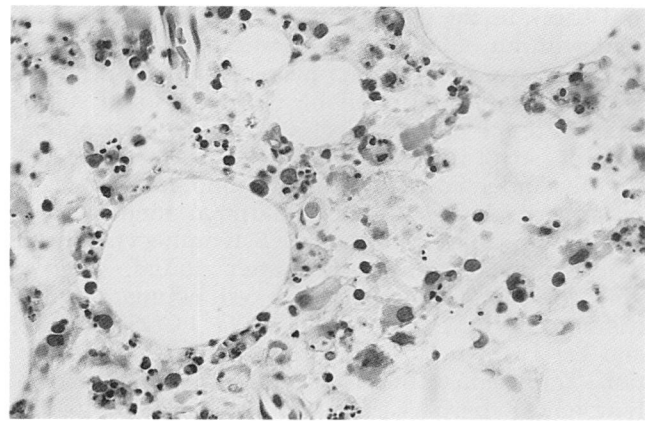

**FIGURE 49–42.** T cell lymphomatous panniculitis. Note large tumor cells within subcutaneous fat containing multiple ingested white blood cells ("beanbag cell").

logically by a proliferation of atypical lymphoid cells diffusely infiltrating the subcutaneous fat. Prominent hemophagocytosis and lymphophagocytosis accompany the neoplastic proliferation, with large, vesicular histiocytes often containing numerous cells within their cytoplasm[135] (Fig. 49–42). The tumor cells are positive for CD2, CD3, and CD5 and are negative for CD8 and CD4. T cell receptor gene rearrangements have been demonstrated in these tumors.

ADULT T CELL LYMPHOMA-LEUKEMIA. Adult T cell lymphoma-leukemia is a systemic lymphoproliferative disorder associated with the human T cell leukemia virus 1 (HTLV-1) that involves the skin in up to 49% of cases.[136] This form of leukemia-lymphoma is endemic in certain parts of Japan and the Caribbean islands but has also been observed sporadically in the southern United States and northern Europe. The disease may occur in an acute or a chronic form and courses with a leukemic blood picture with anemia, hypoalbuminemia, hypergammaglobulinemia, and hypercalcemia. The skin lesions may resemble those of mycosis fungoides and are characterized by a diffuse lichenoid infiltrate of medium to large atypical lymphoid cells that often show multilobated nuclei. Rare foci of epidermotropism may be present. The tumor cells often display a helper-inducer phenotype (CD4⁺ CD8⁻); however, other immunophenotypic profiles may be seen, such as CD4⁻ CD8⁺ or CD4⁻ CD8⁻.[137] HTLV-1 can be cultured from the lesions, and antibodies can also be found in the patient's serum for the virus.

## Cutaneous B Cell Lymphoma

Cutaneous B cell lymphomas are monoclonal B cell lymphoproliferations that can show a wide spectrum of clinical and histologic appearances.[138, 139] The neoplastic cell population is defined by the production of monoclonal immunoglobulins and is easily identi-

fied by the demonstration of light chain restriction. Cutaneous B cell lymphomas can be clinically divided into primary and secondary forms. Primary cutaneous B cell lymphoma is defined as cutaneous disease at presentation without evidence of extracutaneous manifestations for a period of at least 6 months; secondary cutaneous B cell lymphoma is defined by the concurrent presence of extracutaneous disease with secondary development of skin lesions. The lesions can be solitary or multiple and present as indurated plaques or nodules or as an erythematous macular-papular eruption. The nodular lesions frequently ulcerate; however, in contrast with cutaneous T cell lymphoma, there is usually no scaling or erythroderma. Preferred locations are the head and neck, the back, and the lower extremities. Primary cutaneous B cell lymphomas are associated with an excellent prognosis with a 5-year survival rate of more than 90%.

The histologic categorization of these tumors varies, depending on the proliferating cell type. In general, the majority of the histologic types encountered in lymph nodes have cutaneous counterparts. Terminology varies according to the classification scheme employed. The two most common forms of cutaneous B cell lymphoma are follicular lymphoma (follicle center cell lymphoma) and diffuse large cell lymphoma.

FOLLICULAR LYMPHOMA. Follicular lymphoma is characterized by the formation of large nodules reminiscent under scanning magnification of enlarged germinal centers that occupy the dermis and infiltrate deep into the subcutaneous fat[140, 141] (Fig. 49–43). Epidermotropism is usually not observed. The cell population within the follicles is usually monotonous and may be composed of small cleaved lymphocytes or large noncleaved lymphocytes. The interfollicular areas may contain a similar population of cells or may be composed of a mixture of small and large lymphocytes admixed with plasma cells and histiocytes. Areas in which the nodular

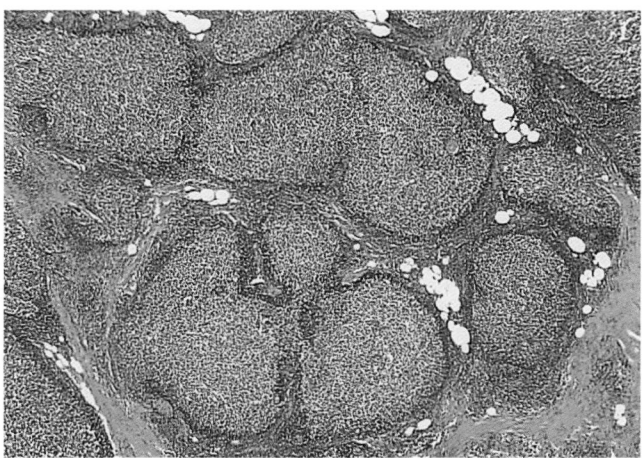

**FIGURE 49–43.** Follicular B cell lymphoma. The tumor is composed of large, monotonous lymphoid nodules within the dermis.

architecture is replaced by diffuse sheets of monotonous tumor cells are often found. The tumor cells express monotypic surface immunoglobulin and B cell–associated antigens such as CD20. Clonal immunoglobulin rearrangements by molecular techniques can also be demonstrated in these tumors. Tumor cells also strongly express Bcl-2 oncoprotein.[142]

DIFFUSE LARGE CELL LYMPHOMA. Diffuse large cell lymphoma is characterized by a diffuse dermal infiltrate of large, atypical lymphoid cells in the dermis and subcutis (Fig. 49–44). It shows a marked predilection for the lower extremities of elderly individuals. The tumor cells are positive for B cell markers such as CD20, CD79a, and Bcl-2.

SMALL LYMPHOCYTIC LYMPHOMA. Small lymphocytic lymphoma is another morphologic variant of cutaneous B cell lymphoma characterized by a monotonous proliferation of small lymphocytes or plasmacytoid cells. Reactive germinal centers may also be scattered among the lymphoid cell infiltrate. The tumors express monotypic cytoplasmic immunoglobulin and heavy and light chain gene rearrangements. The tumors can easily be confused with reactive lymphoid hyperplasia and may require molecular studies demonstrating clonality for their diagnosis. The lesions are clinically indolent and respond well to treatment.

MARGINAL ZONE B CELL LYMPHOMA. Marginal zone B cell lymphoma is a low-grade lymphoma thought to represent the cutaneous counterpart of lymphoma of the mucosa-associated lymphoid tissue of internal organs.[143, 144] The lesions present as plaques, papules, or nodules on the head

and trunk or the extremities. The tumors are associated with an indolent growth and excellent prognosis. They are characterized histologically by a diffuse lymphoid infiltrate involving the dermis and subcutaneous tissue composed of a monotonous proliferation of small to medium-sized lymphocytes with slightly indented nuclei and abundant pale cytoplasm that closely resemble marginal zone lymphocytes or so-called monocytoid B lymphocytes. Reactive lymphoid follicles are often found admixed with the neoplastic lymphoid cell population. The tumor cells have a CD20$^+$, CD79a$^+$, CD5$^-$, CD10$^-$, and Bcl-2$^+$ phenotype and exhibit light chain restriction. The lesions can easily be mistaken for reactive lymphoid hyperplasia and can be separated by identification of the monotonous interfollicular lymphoid proliferation and by demonstration of monoclonality.

INTRAVASCULAR-ANGIOTROPIC LYMPHOMATOSIS. Intravascular-angiotropic lymphomatosis corresponds to a predominantly B cell lymphoma characterized by systemic involvement with rapid dissemination in a variety of organs, particularly the central nervous system, in the absence of organomegaly or lymphadenopathy. Cutaneous involvement is common and an early manifestation of the disease. The lesions present as flat purpuric patches especially distributed over the lower extremities. The histology is characterized by marked angiotropism, with distention and occlusion of small venules, arterioles, and capillaries in the dermis by solid sheets of large, atypical mononuclear cells[145, 146] (Fig. 49–45). In the past, it was believed that the tumor cells represented vascular endothelial cells, hence the older designation of malignant angioendothelioma-

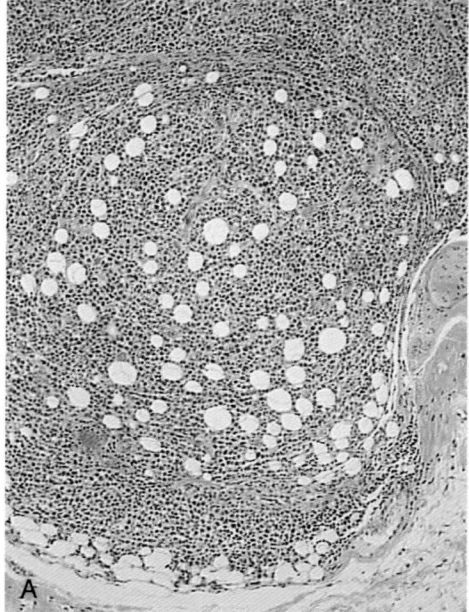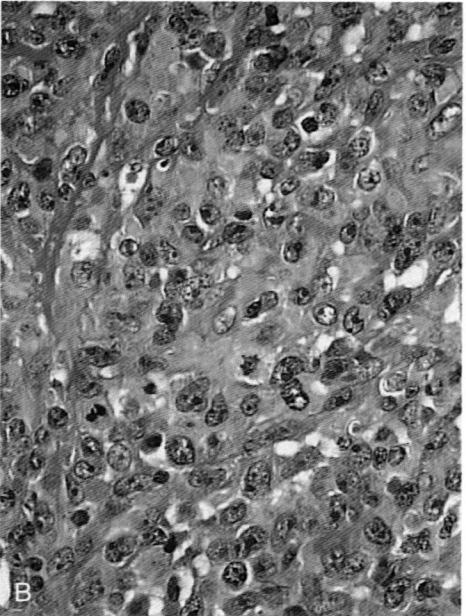

FIGURE 49–44. *A.* Diffuse large B cell lymphoma showing infiltration of deep dermis. Notice characteristic sparing of the fat by the lymphoma tumor cells. *B.* Diffuse large B cell lymphoma. Higher magnification shows a population of large atypical lymphoid cells.

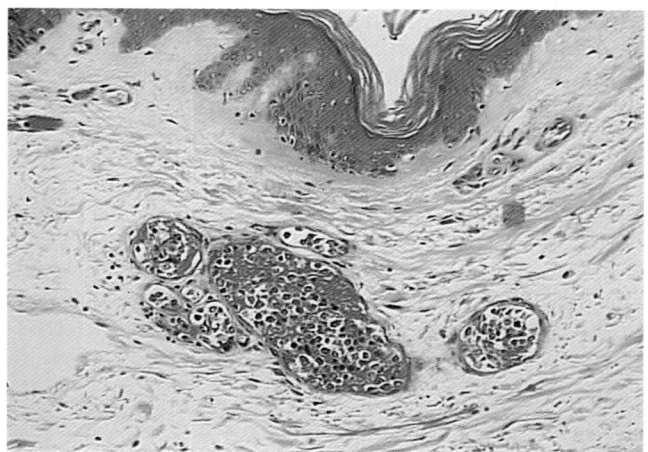

FIGURE 49–45. Angiotropic lymphoma. Dermal vessels show distention by a population of atypical lymphoid cells.

tosis proliferans. It is currently acknowledged that the proliferating cells filling the vessel lumen correspond to neoplastic B lymphocytes displaying a marked tendency for rapid and early dissemination through the peripheral circulation.

CUTANEOUS PLASMACYTOMA. Cutaneous plasmacytoma can rarely present as a primary skin tumor in the absence of systemic involvement by plasma cell myeloma (extramedullary plasmacytoma).[147] The lesions are characterized by a diffuse monoclonal proliferation of mature and immature plasma cells within the dermis and the subcutis.

## Cutaneous Leukemic Infiltrates

Cutaneous leukemic infiltrates may be the initial manifestation of an underlying systemic process or may be present concomitantly with or precede the development of leukemia.[148] The leukemic infiltrates may involve the epidermis, dermis, and subcutaneous tissue. Leukemia cutis has been used as a generic designation for this condition and is typically characterized by a dense perivascular and periadnexal infiltrate that is separated from the epidermis by a grenz zone. Diagnosis is dependent on the identification of the leukemic nature of the infiltrate by cytochemical and immunohistochemical studies and by close clinicopathologic correlation and hematologic evaluation. All types of leukemia can involve the skin; however, the types most commonly seen correspond to chronic lymphocytic leukemia, acute monocytic leukemia, and acute myelomonocytic leukemia. Chronic myeloid leukemia may also rarely involve the skin, giving rise to extramedullary myeloid tumors (granulocytic sarcoma, chloroma).

CHRONIC LYMPHOCYTIC LEUKEMIA. Chronic lymphocytic leukemia presents as red or violaceous macules, papules, or nodules that can often be large and ulcerated and are usually distributed on the face, scalp, trunk, and extremities. The lesions are composed of a dense perivascular and periadnexal infiltrate of small lymphocytes predominantly occupying the reticular dermis and separated from the epidermis by a grenz zone. The infiltrate may involve the subcutaneous tissue and dermal appendages.[150] Occasional lesions may initially become manifest as bullous lesions.[149] The lymphocytes show light chain restriction with monoclonal expression of κ or λ light chains. The lesions are indistinguishable from small lymphocytic lymphoma; clinical history is necessary to separate the two and establish the diagnosis of chronic lymphocytic leukemia.

CHRONIC MYELOID LEUKEMIA. Chronic myeloid leukemia is characterized by a dense infiltrate in the upper and deep dermis that extends into the subcutaneous tissue and is composed of immature myeloid cells with round or oval, vesicular nuclei that may closely resemble the immunoblastic cells seen in diffuse large cell lymphomas.[151] Mitoses can frequently be seen. Eosinophilic granules can sometimes be identified within the cytoplasm of the immature myelocytes. Some of the cells will stain positive with the chloroacetate esterase stain (Leder stain). The tumor cells stain strongly positive with CD43 and myeloperoxidase and may also react with lysozyme, CD15 (Leu-M1), and CD45. The cutaneous leukemic infiltrate in acute myeloid leukemia can be identical to that of chronic myeloid leukemia; clinical history is required to establish that distinction.[148]

ACUTE MONOCYTIC AND MYELOMONOCYTIC LEUKEMIA. Acute monocytic leukemia and acute myelomonocytic leukemia correspond to the most frequent skin manifestation of leukemia. The skin lesions may be widespread and are often accompanied by gingival hyperplasia. Rarely, the leukemic skin infiltrates may precede the development of bone marrow involvement by several months. A dense perivascular or diffuse dermal infiltrate characterizes the lesions histologically. The infiltrate is composed of a monotonous population of neoplastic cells with large folded or kidney-shaped nuclei and a thin rim of basophilic cytoplasm. The neoplastic cells often show the tendency to become arranged in a linear fashion resembling the "single-file" pattern of invasive lobular carcinoma of the breast[148, 152] (Fig. 49–46, CD Fig. 49–15). The leukemic cells generally stain positively with antilysozyme and CD43. They can also be positive for CD45 and CD15 and express other monocytic-granulocytic markers such as CD13, CD14, CD33, and CD68 on frozen section immunohistochemistry. Chloroacetate esterase is generally not found in these cells. Myelomonocytic leukemia (acute myelomonocytic leukemia) is characterized by showing the presence of both monocytic and granulocytic precursors. The dermal infiltrate is thus composed of an admixture of monocytoid and immature myeloid cells. The immunohistochemical staining pattern is similar to that of acute monocytic leukemia.

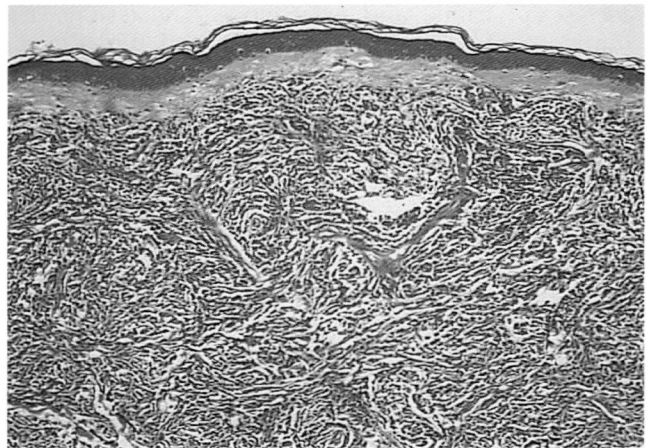

FIGURE 49–46. Acute myelomonocytic leukemia. Note single-file pattern of infiltration by the tumor cells.

## Other Related Conditions

A variety of other proliferative conditions involving the skin can enter into the differential diagnosis of hematolymphoid cutaneous proliferations.

LANGERHANS CELL HISTIOCYTOSIS. Langerhans cell histiocytosis (histiocytosis X) is a proliferative disorder of Langerhans cells, which are bone marrow–derived dendritic cells of monocytic-histiocytic lineage involved in immune-related activities. Langerhans cells are characterized by their distinctive morphologic features; the cells contain elongated and irregular nuclei with frequent infoldings or convolutions of the nuclear membrane, longitudinal nuclear grooves, small nucleoli, and indistinct eosino-

philic cytoplasm. These cells are characterized immunohistochemically by S-100 protein and CD1a positivity. At the ultrastructural level, the cells are distinguished by the presence of zipperlike and tennis racquet–like cytoplasmic structures called Birbeck granules. Cutaneous lesions may present as papules, nodules, plaques, vesicles, or ulcers and are usually distributed over the scalp, trunk, and intertriginous areas.[153] The dermal infiltrates also show a few scattered multinucleated histiocytes and eosinophils admixed with the Langerhans cells. The Langerhans cells often display marked epidermotropism. Extracutaneous involvement is often the rule in Langerhans cell histiocytosis; bone, liver, spleen, pituitary, and lung lesions often coexist with the skin lesions.

A closely related condition, congenital self-healing histiocytosis (Hashimoto-Pritzker disease, congenital self-healing reticulohistiocytosis), is characterized by identical histologic lesions that are limited exclusively to the skin.[154] The lesions are more frequent in neonates and infants and in the majority of cases show a tendency for spontaneous regression.

SINUS HISTIOCYTOSIS WITH MASSIVE LYMPHADENOPATHY. Sinus histiocytosis with massive lymphadenopathy (Rosai-Dorfman disease), a lymph node–based histiocytic proliferation, may involve the skin in up to 30% of cases.[155] The lesions may present as papules, nodules, or plaques composed of a diffuse dermal infiltrate of histiocytes admixed with small lymphocytes, plasma cells, and neutrophils. Lymphoid follicles with prominent germinal centers are often present (Fig. 49–47A). Large vesicular nuclei and abundant eosinophilic cytoplasm characterize the histiocytes. Emperipolesis (or phagocytosis) of inflammatory cells is a distinctive and significant finding (Fig. 49–47B). Cuffing of ves-

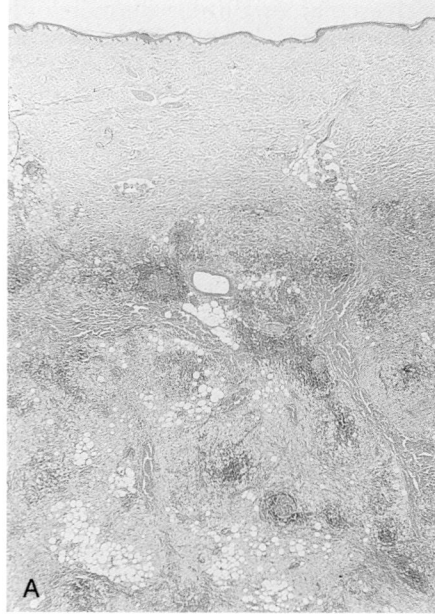

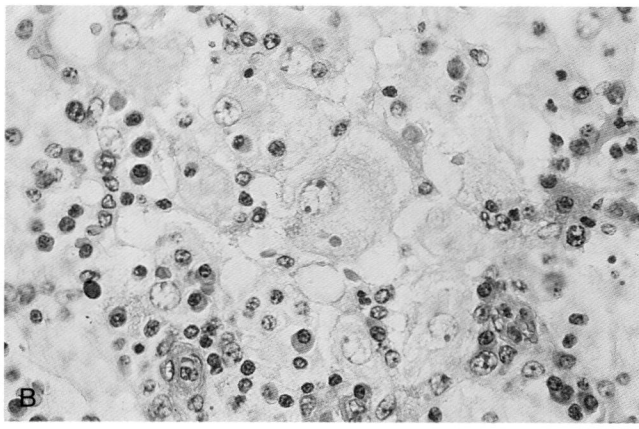

FIGURE 49–47. A. Cutaneous manifestation of sinus histiocytosis with massive lymphadenopathy. The deep dermis and subcutis are effaced by a dense histiocytic proliferation admixed with reactive germinal centers. B. Higher magnification of sinus histiocytosis with massive lymphadenopathy shows large histiocytes with phagocytosed lymphocytes (emperipolesis).

sels by sheets of plasma cells is another distinctive feature. The infiltrates can occasionally present as predominantly subcutaneous nodules simulating a panniculitis.[156] The histiocytes in Rosai-Dorfman disease are positive for S-100 protein and negative for CD1a. The cutaneous manifestations of Rosai-Dorfman disease generally follow an indolent course with spontaneous regression.

CUTANEOUS MASTOCYTOSIS. Cutaneous mastocytosis refers to the presence of excessive numbers of mast cells in the skin. The proliferating cells are characterized by pale-staining pink cytoplasm and centrally located, dark, densely basophilic round nuclei. The condition may become manifest in four clinical forms: solitary mastocytoma, urticaria pigmentosa, systemic mastocytosis, and telangiectasia eruptiva macularis perstans.[157] They are all characterized histologically by an increase in the number of mast cells in the dermis. Metachromatic stains such as toluidine blue and Giemsa easily highlight the mast cells. Lesions of solitary mastocytoma and urticaria pigmentosa are commonly seen in children. Urticaria pigmentosa may, over time, progress to systemic mastocytosis. Telangiectasia eruptiva macularis perstans is more often seen in adults and rarely progresses to systemic mastocytosis.

## MELANOCYTIC PROLIFERATIONS

Melanocytic proliferations constitute one of the main areas of difficulty in the histopathologic diagnosis of skin disorders. Melanocytic proliferations may present with a wide range of appearances that span benign to atypical and malignant neoplastic conditions. The cytologic characteristics of nevomelanocytes can also display a wide spectrum of appearances, often introducing difficulties for diagnosis. Accurate identification of the process is of critical importance for proper treatment and management of patients affected by these conditions.

### Lentigines and Dermal Melanocytoses

LENTIGINES. Lentigo simplex is thought to represent an abnormality in melanocyte migration of the skin that presents clinically as a small, well-circumscribed hyperpigmented macule. Elongated, club-shaped rete ridges showing basilar hyperpigmentation of the epidermis with increased frequency of basilar melanocytes characterize the process histologically. The lesions differ from a freckle (ephelis) because of the elongation of the rete ridges and the increased frequency of basilar melanocytes. They must also be distinguished from solar lentigo, which is characterized by a more pronounced elongation of rete ridges and increased basal pigmentation without increase in the number of melanocytes.

The café au lait spot refers to pale brown hypermelanotic macules resulting from hyperpigmentation of basal keratinocytes. These lesions may sporadically affect the general population but acquire their greatest significance in patients with neurofibromatosis, in whom they are generally present at birth. The presence of six or more café au lait macules in a patient should raise the possibility of neurofibromatosis.

Nevus spilus, a congenital lesion that may reach up to 20 cm in greatest diameter, is characterized clinically by slightly hyperpigmented macules and papules containing speckled, deeply hyperpigmented areas. The lesions may be histologically indistinguishable from a lentigo simplex, with lentiginous melanocytic hyperplasia associated with elongated rete ridges. The hyperpigmented macular foci may show lentiginous melanocytic hyperplasia or junctional nests of nevocytes.

DERMAL MELANOCYTOSES. Dermal melanocytoses are a series of conditions thought to be due to dermal arrest of cells migrating from the neural crest, resulting in skin hyperpigmentation. These include the Mongolian spot, nevus of Ota, nevus of Ito, acquired dermal melanocytosis, and dermal melanocytic hamartoma. They all present as bluish macular lesions characterized histologically by scattered dendritic melanocytes in the reticular dermis with little or no stromal alterations. Mongolian spots are usually large (up to 10 cm in diameter) macules present at birth that most often affect the lumbosacral region. Nevus of Ota is present at birth or during childhood as a bluish macule involving the face (periorbital, forehead, temple) along the distribution of the trigeminal nerve. Nevus of Ito is similar, except that it is distributed in the supraclavicular, scapular, or deltoid region. Acquired dermal melanocytosis of the face and extremities is similar to the nevus of Ota but also shows involvement of the extensor surfaces of the upper extremities. Dermal melanocyte hamartoma is characterized by scattered dermal melanocytes with prominent dendritic processes in the upper dermis that are unassociated with dermal fibrosis or other alterations of the stroma.

### Acquired Melanocytic Nevi

Acquired melanocytic nevi represent the most common dermal melanocytic lesions in humans. They generally present as small (<0.6 cm) hyperpigmented macules located virtually anywhere on the skin surface. Three variants have been classically recognized, depending on the location and distribution of the proliferating melanocytes: junctional nevi are proliferations of melanocytes confined to the dermal-epidermal junction; dermal nevus corresponds to those cases in which the melanocytes are exclusively present in the dermis; and compound nevi are those in which the tumor cells involve both the dermis and the epidermis (CD Fig. 49–16). The melanocytic proliferation in all cases is usually symmetric and well circumscribed. The lesions may be flat, dome shaped, polypoid, or verrucous-papillomatous. Junctional nevi show the formation of nests or theques of melanocytes within the epidermis, usually on the tips of elongated rete ridges rather than on the sides. Dermal nevi show similar nests of melanocytes within the dermis (Fig. 49–48). The melanocytes forming the theques are generally round to oval with round, centrally placed nuclei displaying evenly dispersed chromatin and abundant eosinophilic cytoplasm. Mitoses and anaplasia are not generally present. Long-standing lesions may undergo a process of neurotization, whereby the nevus cells acquire features of schwannian differentiation. A vertical gradient of cytologic maturation of nevocytes is another feature of benign acquired melanocytic nevi, whereby the cells tend to become smaller and cytologically bland as they go deeper into the dermis. Long-standing lesions tend to undergo involution that generally proceeds in a symmetric fashion from top to bottom of the lesion. Several unusual variants of benign acquired melanocytic nevi have been recognized.

BALLOON CELL NEVUS. Balloon cell nevus is a rare variant of melanocytic nevus characterized by cells that display abundant clear, foamy, or vacuolated cytoplasm. It has been postulated that the "balloon" features are the result of enlargement and lysis of melanosomes.[158]

HALO NEVUS. Halo nevus is characterized clinically by a white band or halo of hypopigmented skin surrounding the area of cutaneous hyperpigmentation. On histologic examination, the pale halo corresponds to infiltration of the papillary dermis by a dense mononuclear cell inflammatory infiltrate replacing the proliferating melanocytes at the periphery of the lesion.[159] On occasion, the melanocytes at the interphase zone in the periphery of the lesions may display nuclear enlargement and mild cytologic atypia, or they may appear to be undergoing degeneration. Despite these cytologic features of atypia, the lesions display normal maturation in depth, a helpful distinguishing feature from melanoma. It is believed that this process corresponds to a phenom-

enon of regression secondary to a humoral reaction to altered melanocytes.[160]

ATYPICAL NEVI OF VULVAR (GENITAL) SKIN. Atypical nevi of vulvar (genital) skin, pigmented lesions preferentially located on the vulva of premenopausal women but that can also occur on the scrotum or umbilicus, display worrisome histologic features not commonly observed in acquired benign melanocytic nevi.[161, 162] Such nevi are often slightly larger than ordinary acquired nevi (approximately 10 to 12 mm), are flat, and show variegation in color. They are usually well circumscribed and symmetric on histologic examination; however, they tend to display prominent lentiginous melanocytic proliferation with enlarged junctional nests, variation in the size and shape of the cellular theques with confluence and bridging of nests, and mild cytologic atypia of melanocytes. The dividing line between these lesions and dysplastic nevus is not clear, and some of the features displayed by both indeed show significant overlap.

RECURRENT MELANOCYTIC NEVUS. Recurrent melanocytic nevus (pseudomelanoma) represents a proliferation of residual melanocytes after incomplete removal of a melanocytic lesion.[163] The lesions are characterized by a circumscribed area of hyperpigmentation within scar tissue at the site of previous nevus removal. On histologic examination, there is an intraepidermal melanocytic proliferation overlying a dermal scar that may or may not display mild cytologic features of atypia and that may follow an irregular distribution. Residual nevus cells may also occasionally be observed beneath the dermal scar. Review of the previous biopsy is mandatory to rule out an atypical melanocytic proliferation or melanoma.[164]

DEEP PENETRATING NEVUS. Deep penetrating nevus is a term introduced to characterize a benign acquired melanocytic proliferation showing involvement of the deep reticular dermis and subcutis. The lesions are usually small (<1 cm) and symmetric and most commonly involve the face, upper trunk, and proximal extremities. They are characterized histologically by a symmetric, well-circumscribed, and wedge-shaped proliferation of melanocytes that extend into the deep dermis (Fig. 49–49). The superficial dermis shows a diffuse proliferation of pigmented spindle cells forming discrete fascicles or nests that display progressive maturation in depth. Junctional activity may occasionally be present. The spindle cell proliferation may grow in a polypoid or nodular pattern into the subcutaneous fat in a fashion reminiscent of cellular blue nevi. The spindle cells may occasionally show mild cytologic atypia; mitoses, however, are rare.[165]

## Congenital Melanocytic Nevi

Congenital melanocytic nevi represent pigmented lesions that are present since birth and generally achieve a larger size than acquired nevi. The lesions

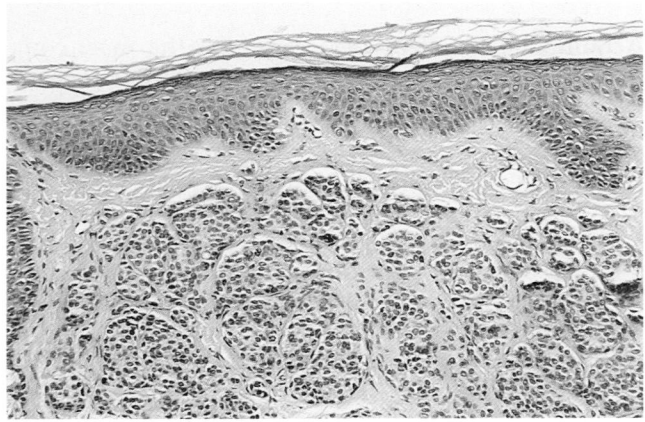

**FIGURE 49–48.** Dermal nevus showing nests of melanocytes in the dermis.

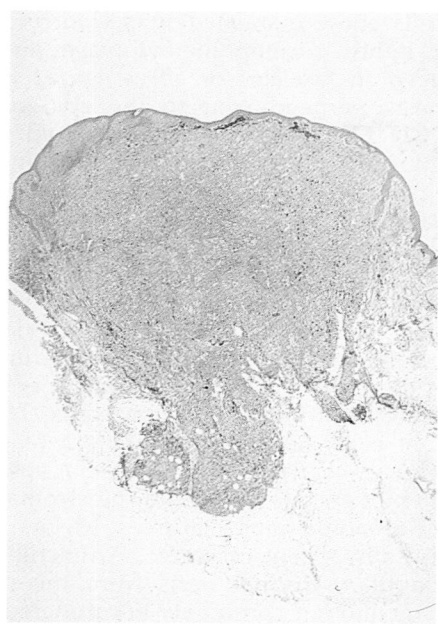

FIGURE 49–49. Deep penetrating nevus. A wedge-shaped melanocytic proliferation is seen that infiltrates deep into the subcutis.

Although some congenital nevi may be microscopically indistinguishable from acquired nevi, the majority of these lesions have distinctive histologic features that help to separate them from the acquired nevi. They are characterized histologically by a more extensive distribution of nevus cells throughout the dermis typically involving the lower two thirds of the reticular dermis and often infiltrating the subcutaneous fat. The nevus cells are often small, with scant cytoplasm and bland nuclear features. There is usually a grenz zone separating the epidermis from the dermal infiltrate; however, junctional nests may also be present. Another characteristic feature is the frequent involvement by nevus cells of dermal appendages and neurovascular structures (Fig. 49–50A). In contrast to acquired melanocytic nevi, the nevus cells in congenital nevi do not tend to form cellular theques and are characterized instead by their diffuse infiltration of dermal collagen, often arranged in a single-cell pattern or as cords of cells that appear to "fan out" into the dermis and splay the collagen fibers (Fig. 49–50B). Rarely, congenital nevi may show architectural or cytologic features of atypia involving both the intraepidermal and dermal component.

DERMAL NODULAR PROLIFERATIONS AND MELANOMA ARISING IN CONGENITAL NEVI. Giant congenital nevi may occasionally give rise to intradermal nodular proliferations displaying variable degrees of cytologic atypia, necrosis of melanocytes, and mitotic activity. Most such nodular proliferations, particularly during the neonatal period, are biologically benign, despite the features of atypia.[168] Conventional melanoma arising from congenital nevi more often develops from relatively small lesions and is usually of the pagetoid or nodular type. Malignant melanoma may also supervene in giant congenital nevi. Such tumors are often characterized by a small round cell proliferation of melanocytes that superficially may resemble a lymphoma or may be more rarely composed of epithelioid or spindle cells.[169] The majority of atypical epithelioid and

can range in size from 1.5 to 10 or 20 cm in diameter. They are generally well circumscribed with fairly uniform pigmentation and are often hair bearing. Giant forms often involve a large portion of the dorsal surface of the body and can have a papillary and verrucous surface. The significance of congenital melanocytic nevi, in particular the larger ones, is related to their risk for progression to malignant melanoma.[166] There is considerable controversy regarding the risk for subsequent development of melanoma in these lesions, but it has been estimated to be on the order of 5%.[167] This may be an overestimation, however, because giant congenital nevi are extremely rare (approximately 1 in every 20,000 births).

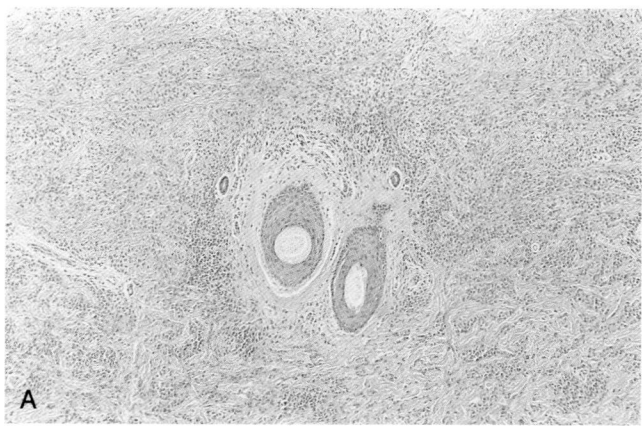
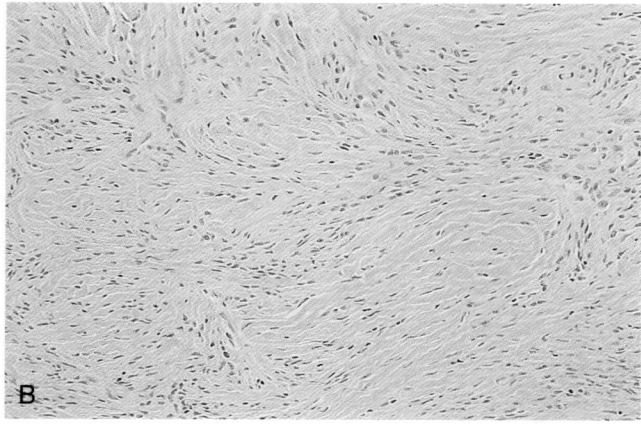

FIGURE 49–50. A. Congenital nevus. Monotonous population of small round nevus cells is seen in the deep dermis and around adnexal structures. B. Congenital nevus. Higher magnification shows "splaying" of collagen fibers in the dermis.

spindle cell proliferations arising in congenital nevi during infancy do not behave in a biologically aggressive fashion, unlike the small cell proliferations, which generally display full-blown clinical features of malignancy. A conservative approach, however, is recommended for any atypical proliferation originating in congenital nevi, including complete surgical removal of the lesion and close clinical follow-up of the patient.

## Spitz (Spindle and Epithelioid Cell) Nevus

This lesion, initially described as a juvenile form of melanoma by Spitz,[170] represents an acquired melanocytic proliferation characterized by a predominant proliferation of large epithelioid and spindle melanocytic cells. Spitz nevus represents one of the most important pitfalls for the diagnosis of cutaneous melanocytic lesions and is often misdiagnosed for malignant melanoma.

Spitz nevus most often presents clinically as a solitary, smooth, dome-shaped, flesh-colored nodule less than 1 cm in diameter. It may arise at any site but most commonly involves the face and extremities and shows a slight female predilection. The lesion may occur at any age, although it is more common in children and young adults. Rare cases may present as a focal cluster of lesions (agminated Spitz) or in a disseminated pattern involving numerous lesions distributed throughout the body.

On histologic examination, the lesions can adopt a junctional, compound, or dermal distribution.[171, 172] The most distinctive characteristic is the presence of large spindle and epithelioid melanocytes in various proportions showing a symmetric distribution. The

spindle cells show elongated nuclei surrounded by abundant, lightly eosinophilic cytoplasm and are often arranged in fascicles or as elongated teardrop-shaped nests perpendicular to the epidermis (Fig. 49–51A, CD Fig. 49–17). The epithelioid cells are large and round to polygonal, with round nuclei containing scattered chromatin with small nucleoli and surrounded by abundant eosinophilic cytoplasm. The epithelioid cells in Spitz nevus may occasionally adopt some degree of cellular pleomorphism, with large, irregular nuclei and prominent eosinophilic nucleoli, a feature that overlaps with some types of melanoma. A frequent finding associated with the epithelioid cell component is the presence of large, multinucleated giant cells. The nuclei in the giant cells, however, are devoid of cytologic atypia (Fig. 49–51B). Round, densely eosinophilic hyaline globules scattered within the stroma are also a frequent accompanying feature.[173] Melanin deposition is typically absent or scarce. Artifactual separation of papillary dermal nests from the overlying epidermis is another commonly encountered feature. Ectatic vessels in the stroma of the superficial dermis are often present and account for the pinkish gross appearance of the lesion. The two cell types may be admixed in varying proportions, although tumors composed of a predominantly spindle cell population are the most common type in adults. Regardless of the cell type, one of the hallmarks of Spitz nevus is the striking uniformity of the cells and nuclear features from side to side across the lesion. In addition to the symmetry and sharp lateral demarcation, other features necessary for the diagnosis are the lack of significant pagetoid spread in the epidermis, small size (<1 cm), lack of deep extension, and presence of maturation in depth. Mitotic activity may be present in Spitz nevus; how-

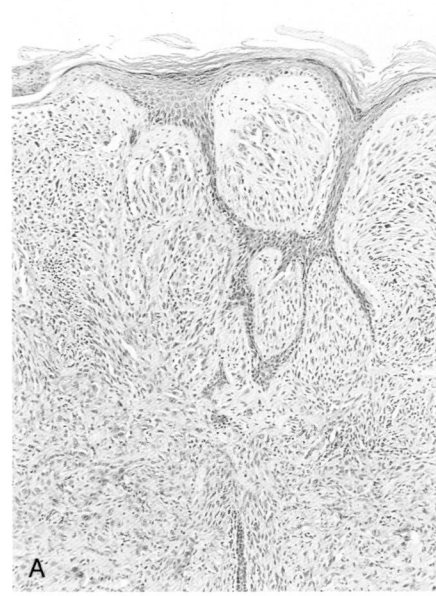

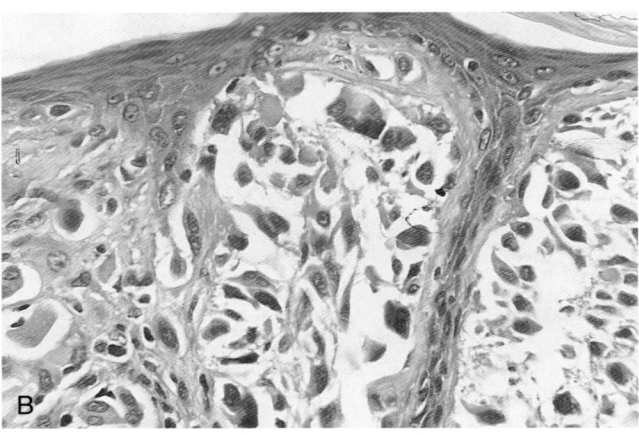

**FIGURE 49–51.** *A*. Spitz nevus. A spindle and epithelioid cell proliferation is seen in the dermis. *B*. Higher magnification of Spitz nevus shows large epithelioid melanocytes admixed with multinucleated giant cells.

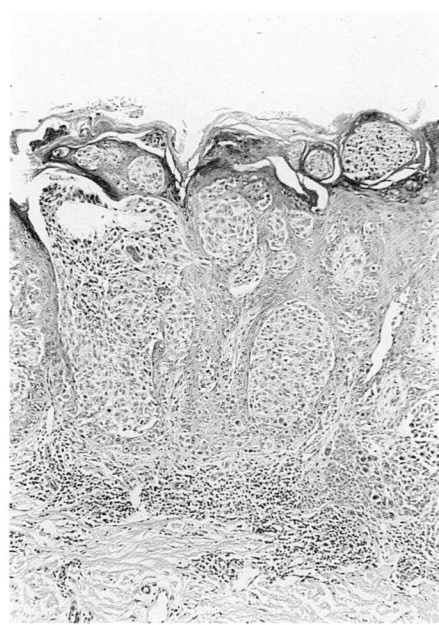

**FIGURE 49-52.** Spitz nevus showing transepidermal migration of theques of melanocytes.

ever, mitoses are most commonly seen in the upper portion of the lesion and are usually typical. Presence of mitoses in the deep component or abnormal (atypical) mitotic figures must raise the possibility of a nevoid melanoma.

Another feature of Spitz nevus that may lead to confusion with melanoma is the upward migration with transepidermal elimination of theques of melanocytes (Fig. 49-52). Unlike upward pagetoid spread in malignant melanoma, the migrating cells in Spitz nevus are focal and may form small, well-defined nests composed of more than three or four cells devoid of cytologic atypia. However, the presence of prominent pagetoid spread of atypical melanocytes in solitary units should raise the consideration of malignant melanoma transformation. Pseudocarcinomatous hyperplasia of the overlying epidermis is another feature that may occasionally be present in Spitz nevi and may lead to confusion with squamous cell carcinoma.

A few unusual variants of Spitz nevus have been described that deserve special consideration.

PIGMENTED SPINDLE CELL NEVUS. Pigmented spindle cell nevus is a distinctive variant of Spitz nevus that can often be confused with malignant melanoma.[174, 175] The lesion presents clinically as a small (<0.6 cm), well-circumscribed, plaquelike area of hyperpigmentation on the extremities or trunk. Women are affected more often than are men, and the peak incidence is in the third decade. The lesion is characterized histologically by a monotonous proliferation of heavily pigmented spindled melanocytes forming nests and fascicles that are distributed along the dermal-epidermal junction and within dermal papillae, in parallel to the long axis of the epi-

dermis (Fig. 49-53). The process may show a junctional or compound architecture. The base of the lesion, however, usually extends no deeper than the superficial reticular dermis. The spindled melanocytes usually show uniform oval nuclei that appear to be equal in size to those of adjacent keratinocytes. Nucleoli are usually inconspicuous, and mitoses are extremely rare. Occasional upward migration of nonatypical melanocytes or transepidermal migration of melanocytic theques can also be found. The papillary dermis may contain aggregates of melanophages. The small size, young age of the patients, and lack of invasion into the deep dermis serve to distinguish them from malignant melanoma.

DESMOPLASTIC SPITZ NEVUS. Desmoplastic Spitz nevus represents an unusual variant of Spitz nevus characterized histologically by its superficial resemblance to a fibrohistiocytic lesion.[176] The tumor is usually well circumscribed and small (<1 cm) and is composed of nests of epithelioid melanocytes surrounded by prominent connective tissue stroma containing spindled fibroblasts that may focally adopt a storiform distribution (Fig. 49-54A). The epithelioid melanocytes may show some mild degree of cytologic atypia but display maturation in depth and should be devoid of mitotic figures, except those rarely seen in the superficial dermal portion of the lesion.

HYALINIZING SPITZ NEVUS. Hyalinizing Spitz nevus represents another unusual variant of Spitz nevus that is characterized by a dyscohesive growth pattern of large epithelioid or plump spindled melanocytes that appear to be haphazardly scattered singly or in small groups throughout the dermis and embedded in abundant hyalinized, acellular collagen[177] (Fig. 49-54B). The melanocytic cells display nuclear enlargement with nucleolar prominence. Mitoses are extremely rare. Because of the unusual pattern of growth, the lesion can often be confused with metastatic carcinoma. The lesions are generally small and well circumscribed and show maturation

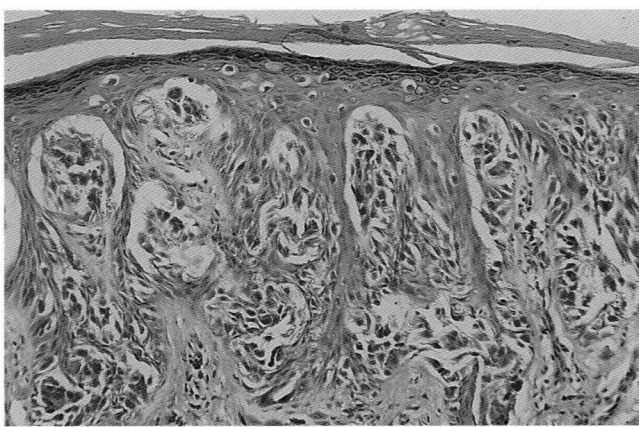

**FIGURE 49-53.** Pigmented spindle cell nevus. Nests of heavily pigmented epithelioid melanocytes are seen parallel to the long axis of the epidermis.

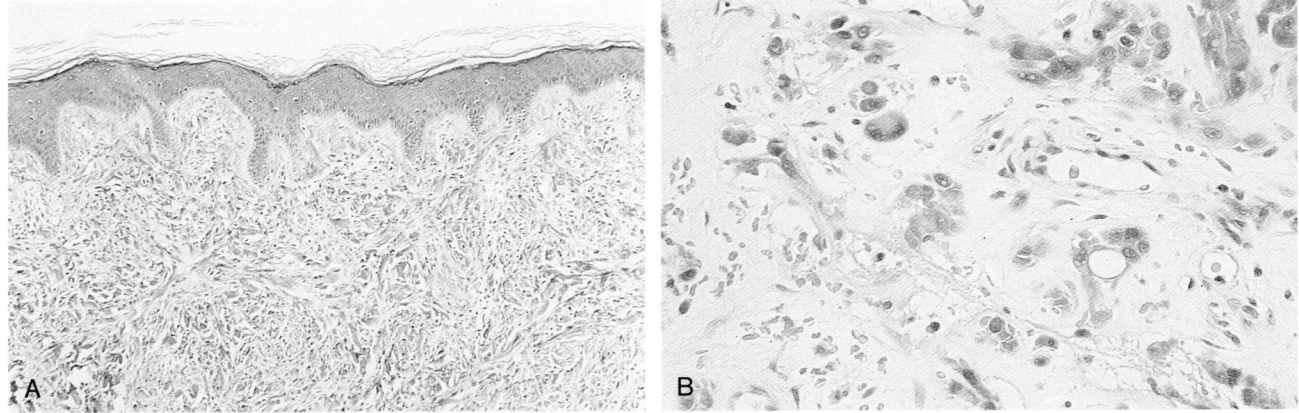

**FIGURE 49–54.** *A.* Desmoplastic Spitz nevus. A proliferation of epithelioid melanocytes is seen accompanied by a prominent spindled fibroblastic stromal proliferation in the dermis. *B.* Hyalinizing Spitz nevus. A dermal proliferation of epithelioid melanocytes is seen embedded in abundant hyalinized collagen.

in depth with progressive decrease in the size of the cells toward the base of the lesion. Immunohistochemical stains for S-100 protein and HMB-45 serve to highlight the melanocytic nature and distinguish it from metastatic carcinoma. The lack of marked cytologic atypia, neurotropism, vascular invasion, or superficial spreading component serves to distinguish it from desmoplastic-neurotropic variants of melanoma.

PLEXIFORM SPINDLE CELL NEVUS. Plexiform spindle cell nevus most likely represents an unusual variant of Spitz nevus composed predominantly of plump spindled melanocytes that is characterized by the striking plexiform arrangement of the tumor cells in the dermis.[178] The lesions are generally small, slightly raised, and symmetric and show a wedge-shaped configuration in the reticular dermis. The spindle cells contain abundant granular melanin and oval nuclei with delicate chromatin pattern and inconspicuous nucleoli. Occasional mild cytologic atypia and rare mitoses can be observed. Infiltration of cutaneous nerves, dermal adnexa, and arrector pili muscles in the dermis is a common feature. The most striking feature, however, is the plexiform arrangement of the tumor cells separated by collagenous bands, a feature best observed under scanning magnification. Another unusual and still controversial variant is the halo Spitz nevus.[179] These lesions may be extremely difficult to separate from melanoma, and this diagnosis should always be approached with extreme caution.

ATYPICAL AND METASTASIZING SPITZ NEVUS. The so-called atypical and metastasizing Spitz nevi are other manifestations of these tumors that may constitute a serious diagnostic problem. Although standardized criteria have not yet been established for the diagnosis of atypical Spitz nevus, a range of cytologic and architectural features of atypia may occasionally be encountered in these tumors. These include lentiginous melanocytic proliferation, asymmetry with lateral extension of epidermal melanocytes, significant variation in junctional nests with horizontal confluence and bridging, and cytologic atypia of melanocytes.[179, 180] Another unusual finding is the formation of well-defined, expansile nodules composed of a monotonous proliferation of epithelioid or spindled melanocytes occupying the dermis that may extend into the deep dermis and subcutaneous fat.[179] Because of the rarity of such lesions and the current lack of information regarding their clinical evolution, the significance of these various features has not yet been defined. It is possible that such cases may represent unusual variants of malignant melanoma with a nevuslike histologic appearance (see nevoid melanoma).

A similar consideration applies to those cases of Spitz nevus that are reported to spread to regional lymph nodes (metastasizing Spitz nevus).[181] Careful review of such lesions generally discloses subtle cytologic and architectural features of atypia and demonstrates that they tend to be larger and grow deeper than conventional Spitz nevi. Application of more stringent criteria for diagnosis and increased recognition of the Spitz-like nevoid variant of malignant melanoma may serve to avert underdiagnosis in such instances.

## Blue Nevus

Blue nevus is an acquired melanocytic lesion characterized by the proliferation within the reticular dermis of dendritic and spindled melanocytes, often accompanied by heavy melanin pigmentation (Fig. 49–55). The term derives from the characteristic blue color of the lesions observed clinically. This is the result of the Tyndall effect, which results in blue coloration of any deep-seated pigmented lesion of the skin because of the scattering of light by dermal

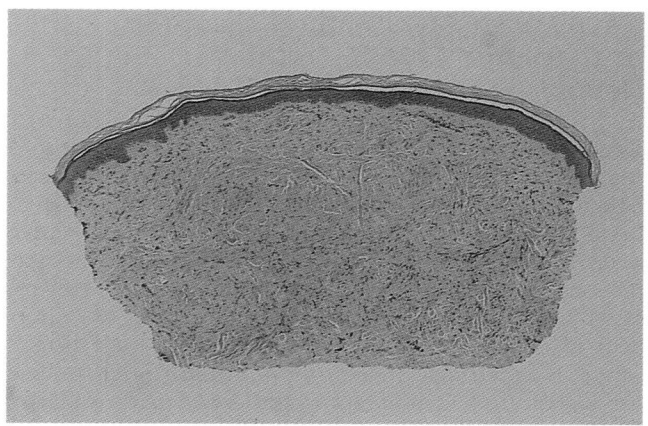

**FIGURE 49–55.** Blue nevus. A dendritic proliferation of pigmented melanocytes is seen in the reticular dermis.

collagen with preferential transmission of blue wavelengths. Blue nevi can show a wide spectrum of cellularity and atypia that ranges from the small, sparsely cellular common blue nevus, through cellular and atypical blue nevi, to the rare malignant blue nevus.[182-185]

COMMON BLUE NEVUS. Common blue nevus is a benign acquired melanocytic tumor composed of heavily pigmented, spindled or dendritic melanocytes located predominantly in the superficial reticular dermis. The lesions are usually dome shaped, well demarcated, and small (<1 cm). They are primarily distributed over the dorsal aspects of the hands and feet, face, and scalp. The dendritic melanocytes tend to infiltrate dermal appendages and neurovascular bundles. The nuclei are usually large and ovoid, with uniform chromatin pattern. The cells frequently have a stellate configuration and may show slender dendritic processes. Heavily pigmented melanophages are usually found admixed with the dendritic cell population. Variable degrees of fibrosis are generally also present. Features that allow distinction from metastatic melanoma are small size, lack of cytologic atypia, and absence of mitotic activity and necrosis.

SCLEROSING BLUE NEVUS. Sclerosing blue nevus is characterized by a prominent dermal fibrous component manifested clinically as a well-circumscribed fibrous nodule in the dermis. On histologic examination, the lesion shows a well-circumscribed expansion of the dermis composed of a sparse population of spindled and dendritic cells admixed with abundant fibroblasts (Fig. 49–56). Scattered melanin pigment can be observed in the dendritic cells as well as within melanophages (CD Fig. 49–18). The spindle and dendritic cells display little or no cytologic atypia and no mitoses. There may be infiltration of nerves and adnexal structures by spindle cells within the process.

COMBINED NEVUS. Combined nevus refers to a lesion displaying a combination of both the common

acquired melanocytic nevus or Spitz nevus and a blue nevus. The most common pattern is that of an ordinary nevus and blue nevus. The ordinary nevus component may be compound or dermal and is often seen overlying the blue nevus component. Because of the heavy pigmentation of the blue nevus component and the apparent invasion of the dermis by dendritic and spindled cells, these lesions may be mistakenly interpreted as malignant melanoma.[186] Features that help separate these lesions from melanoma are the orderly arrangement of the cells, good circumscription, and absence of cytologic atypia and mitotic activity.

CELLULAR BLUE NEVUS. Cellular blue nevus represents a distinctive variant of blue nevus characterized by a larger size (1 to 2 cm) and increased cellularity. The lesions frequently involve the buttocks, lumbosacral region, and scalp and are more frequent in children and young adults between the ages of 10 and 40 years. The lesions are benign and cured by conservative excision, although rare lesions have been reported to progress to malignancy. They are characterized histologically by a dense proliferation of large oval to spindle cells that occupy the reticular dermis and grow in an expansile, lobular fashion, often extending in a bulbous or dumbbell configuration into the subcutaneous fat (Fig. 49–57). Unlike the diffuse distribution of spindle cells in common blue nevus, the tumor cells in cellular blue nevi tend to organize in nests and fascicles sometimes separated by fibrous bands. The proliferating spindle cells are generally devoid of melanin pigment and show round to oval, slightly enlarged nuclei surrounded by abundant, lightly eosinophilic cytoplasm. Rare mitotic figures may occasionally be encountered. Clusters of heavily pigmented melanophages are often present, particularly surrounding the nests or fascicles of spindle cells. Multinucleated giant cells are occasionally noted in the cellular areas and may be associated with areas of cystic de-

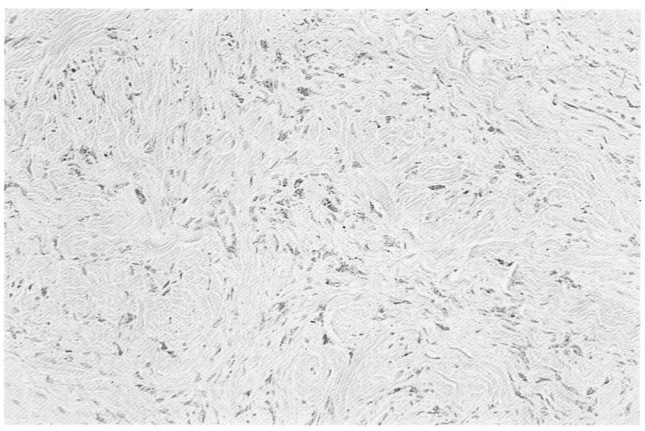

**FIGURE 49–56.** Collagenized blue nevus. A proliferation of heavily pigmented dendritic melanocytes is seen against a prominently collagenized stroma.

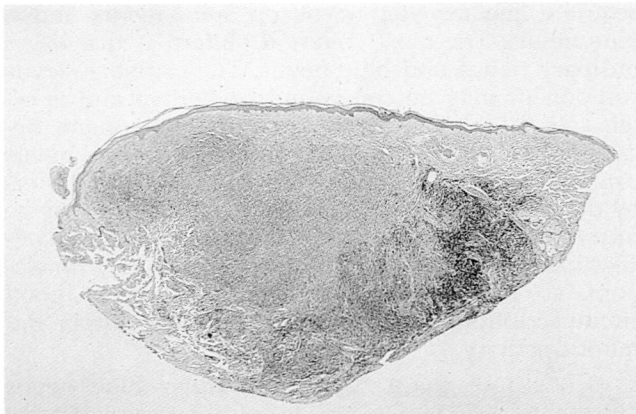

**FIGURE 49–57.** Cellular blue nevus. A dense population of dendritic and pigmented melanocytes is seen to infiltrate deeply into the subcutaneous fat.

generation of the stroma. A rare finding is the presence of focal balloon cell changes in the lesion.[187] Myxoid change of the stroma is another unusual histologic finding reported in these tumors.[188] Large telangiectatic vessels filled with pools of blood can sometimes be seen in the central portions of these tumors simulating a vascular neoplasm on scanning magnification. Combinations with areas displaying the features of more conventional blue nevus can also be seen. These areas are usually located in the superficial dermis overlying the lesion or at the periphery of the cellular lobules.

ATYPICAL CELLULAR BLUE NEVUS. Atypical cellular blue nevus is generally characterized by larger size, deep extension into the subcutis, and prominent cellularity with cytologic atypia and increased mitotic activity. Separation from a malignant blue nevus is often arbitrary because no well-defined criteria have been demonstrated to discriminate between the lesions that metastasize and those that do not.[184, 185] Atypical blue nevus should be treated by complete surgical excision, and the patients should be carefully monitored for the possibility of recurrence or metastases.

MALIGNANT BLUE NEVUS. Malignant blue nevus is thought to represent a process of malignant transformation in a cellular or atypical blue nevus.[189–191] Some authors prefer to designate this process as the development of a malignant melanoma in association with a cellular blue nevus. The main differential diagnosis is with a metastasis from malignant melanoma. The presence of a concomitant conventional blue nevus intimately associated with the lesion supports a diagnosis of malignant blue nevus. The tumors are characterized by an irregular, usually asymmetric dermal proliferation of pigmented and dendritic melanocytes showing significant nuclear anaplasia, frequent mitotic figures, and foci of necrosis. The absence of a junctional or epidermal component serves to distinguish them from conventional melanoma.

## Nevus with Architectural Disorder or Cytologic Atypia (Dysplastic Nevus)

Dysplastic nevus represents a variant of acquired melanocytic nevus that was first described in members of families in which at least two members had been affected by melanoma.[192] Such lesions have been shown to follow an autosomal dominant pattern of inheritance (dysplastic nevus syndrome) related to a single gene that is localized to the short arm of chromosome 1.[193] In addition to their occurrence in hereditary melanoma kindreds, such lesions are also found in melanoma patients with no family history of melanoma and in the general population.[194, 195] Their main significance lies in their role as markers of increased risk for melanoma. Because of the controversy surrounding these lesions, a National Institutes of Health Consensus Conference recommended that the term *dysplastic nevus* be abandoned in favor of the term *nevus with architectural disorder or cytologic atypia.*[196] Two types were identified by the National Institutes of Health Consensus Conference: (1) those associated with a low prospective risk for development of melanoma (<10% lifetime risk) and (2) those associated with a high prospective risk for melanoma development (up to 100% lifetime risk).[196, 197] The first type are those that occur in patients with no family or personal history of melanoma; the second type are those occurring in patients with a personal or family history of melanoma. Because the two groups are indistinguishable histologically, clinical history is indispensable for stratification of patients into these two categories.

Dysplastic nevi have been documented to occasionally progress to melanoma. These lesions are usually larger than common nevi (average, 4 to 12 mm) and show a propensity for the scalp, breast, buttocks, and dorsum of the feet. On gross evaluation, they are characterized by their variegation in color, asymmetry, and ill-defined borders.[198, 199] On histologic examination, they are defined by features of architectural disorder and cytologic atypia (Table 49–4). The most important architectural features of dysplastic nevus are the lateral extension with poor circumscription of the intraepidermal melanocytic component and the presence of a disordered intraepidermal melanocytic proliferation.[200] The lateral extension criterion involves extension of the melanocytes at the dermal-epidermal junction beyond the underlying papillary dermal nevus component (so-called shoulder phenomenon). The phenomenon of disordered intraepidermal melanocytic proliferation refers to the presence of a lentiginous (single-cell) melanocytic proliferation and the presence of irregular junctional nests. The lentiginous pattern of dysplastic nevus results in increase in number and confluence of single melanocytes along the basal layer of the epidermis, often focally replacing the basal keratinocytes completely. The architectural disorder of the nests of melanocytes is manifested by varia-

**TABLE 49–4.** Histologic Features of Dysplastic Nevi

Architectural features
    Lateral extension of melanocytes beyond dermal component ("shoulders")
    Disordered (single-cell) lentiginous proliferation of melanocytes in epidermis
    Irregular junctional nests often disposed at the sides of the rete ridges
    Confluence of theques with "bridging" of nests of melanocytes
Cytologic features
    Variability in the degree of cytologic atypia from cell to cell
    Nuclear enlargement, variation in chromatic pattern, and occasional prominent nucleoli
Stromal changes
    Lymphocytic infiltrate at the base of the lesion
    Concentric or lamellar fibroplasia

tion in the size and shape as well as in the placement of the junctional theques. The nests are often disposed at the sides of the rete ridges and tend to be localized perpendicular to the long axis of the rete, with confluence of adjacent theques often resulting in "bridging" between rete ridges (Fig. 49–58). In addition to the architectural features of disorganized growth, cytologic features of atypia are present in these lesions. This involves mainly the junctional and intraepidermal component and is characterized by great variability in the degree of atypicality from cell to cell. Gradual nuclear enlargement, pleomorphism, variation in the nuclear chromatin pattern, and occasional prominent nucleoli typify the nuclear atypia. The junctional nests may also contain epithelioid melanocytes with dusty melanin pigment. One characteristic feature of dysplastic nevus is the focal, spotty, and discontinuous character of the cytologically atypical melanocytes, as opposed to the uniform and monotonous evidence of cytologic atypia in melanoma. Another distinctive feature of dysplastic nevi is the presence of

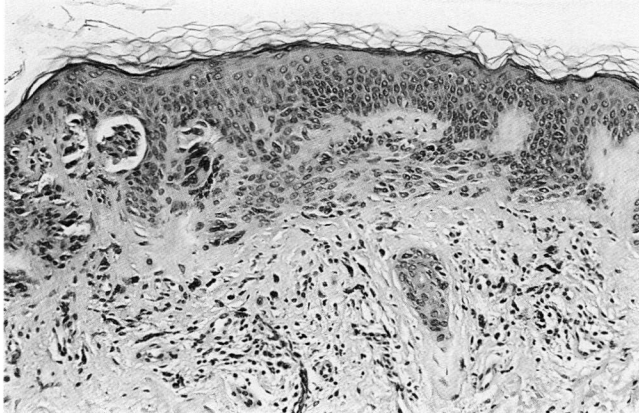

**FIGURE 49–58.** Dysplastic nevus. There is architectural disorder, with theques of melanocytes disposed at the sides of the rete ridges and "bridging" of rete ridges by elongated nests of melanocytes. A superficial inflammatory infiltrate and dermal fibroplasia are also present.

stromal changes surrounding the melanocytic proliferation. Lymphocytic infiltrates are often seen at the base of the lesion in dysplastic nevi. The inflammatory infiltrate may be sparse and perivascular or may be dense and bandlike and involve the papillary dermis. Compact concentric or lamellar fibroplasia is another frequent accompanying feature of these lesions.

Some authors have advocated grading of dysplastic nevi. High-grade lesions (i.e., those characterized by marked cytologic atypia and larger size) merit wider excision, particularly if the original lesion has been incompletely excised. Low-grade lesions (i.e., nevus with architectural disorder and only slight cytologic atypia) may not merit reexcision.[201] Close correlation with the clinical findings is recommended, however, to ascertain whether the histologic findings are representative of the entire lesion. If a residual lesion is present or if a clinical suspicion persists, complete excision with histologic examination is warranted.

## Malignant Melanoma

Malignant proliferations of melanocytes represent one of the most challenging and important problems in the field of cutaneous pathology. The increased awareness of the various clinical and epidemiologic features of melanoma during the past 20 to 30 years has resulted in a rapid rise in the incidence of this diagnosis in Western countries. Parallel to this process has been the evolution of the concept of melanoma over the years, with the recognition of the different stages of progression of melanocytic proliferations and their precursor lesions.[202, 203] These advances have resulted in increased understanding and further characterization of cutaneous melanocytic processes. The first classification of melanoma to take stock of the concept of tumor progression was that proposed in 1967 by Clark,[204] who recognized two basic stages in the development of these tumors. The "radial growth" phase was characterized by a proliferation confined to the epidermis of atypical melanocytes without the formation of a tumor nodule. The "vertical growth" phase was characterized by the subsequent invasion of the atypical melanocytes into the upper layers of the epidermis and into the dermis with the formation of an expansile nodular tumor growth. The radial growth phase in general terms was suggested to be associated with a lesser chance for metastasis, whereas the vertical growth phase was found to be associated with a higher risk of metastatic behavior. On the basis of these observations, Clark proposed a classification scheme that was based on the presence or absence of the radial growth phase. A similar proposal was made at about the same time by McGovern[205] and has been generally adopted since then for clinical practice (Table 49–5). Some authors, however, have contended that this classification has limited clinical application and poor correlation with prognosis and

**TABLE 49–5.** Classification of Malignant Melanoma Based on Radial or Vertical Growth Phase

| |
|---|
| With radial growth phase |
|    Superficial spreading melanoma |
|    Lentigo maligna melanoma |
|    Acral and mucosal lentiginous melanoma |
| Without radial growth phase |
|    Nodular melanoma |

have therefore questioned its utility.[206, 207] Moreover, the observation of great morphologic heterogeneity and overlap in the features of these tumors has led to the proposal that the different morphologic and clinical manifestations of melanoma represent part of a continuous spectrum rather than examples of distinct biologic entities.[207]

Another important concept to emerge from the study of malignant melanoma was the realization that the depth of invasion within the dermis might correlate with the clinical behavior of these lesions. Clark and associates[208] in 1969 divided the depth of invasion of malignant melanoma into five levels and demonstrated that the 5-year mortality increased with each level, from 8% in level II to 35% in level III, 46% in level IV, and 52% in level V. Breslow,[209] in 1970, introduced a method for objective measurement of tumor thickness using a micrometer in the evaluation of malignant melanoma (Table 49–6). Breslow demonstrated that malignant melanomas less than 0.76 mm thick did not metastasize and did not require regional lymph node dissection, whereas melanomas greater than 1.5 mm thick were associated with an increased risk of lymph node metastases. Currently, a combined approach for the prognostication of melanoma has been proposed in which tumors are assigned to three clinical risk categories according to a combination of the thickness and level of invasion of the lesions[210] (see Table 49–6).

Malignant melanoma predominantly affects white adults between the fourth and seventh decades of life with an equal sex distribution.[211] The most common sites are the back of the trunk, the upper and lower extremities, and the head and neck region. The lesions are more frequent in sun-ex-

posed areas. The gross appearance of melanoma varies considerably, depending on the stage and location. The lesions are generally greater than 1 cm in diameter and are characterized by irregular or notched borders, asymmetry, and marked variegation in color including shades of tan, brown, black, blue, gray, and white within the same lesion.[211, 212] Larger lesions can display ulceration and bleeding. Melanomas lacking pigment may be difficult to recognize clinically. Early lesions are usually flat, but more advanced lesions tend to become papular or nodular. Acral melanomas appear to be more common in blacks, Asians, and other ethnic groups. Subungual melanoma is a distinctive form of acral melanoma that most often involves the nail bed of the thumb or great toe and presents as an ulcerated tumor.[213] Another distinctive clinical form of malignant melanoma is the lentigo malignant melanoma. This form of melanoma occurs in sun-exposed areas of the skin of elderly patients and shows a more protracted clinical evolution during the course of many years.[214, 215] The lesion usually starts as a hyperpigmented macule that gradually spreads to attain a large size (lentigo maligna, Hutchinson's melanotic freckle). Progression to an invasive phase (lentigo maligna melanoma) may occur in up to 50% of cases of lentigo maligna. Invasion might not be recognizable clinically until after 10 to 15 years of evolution and after the lesion has attained a size of about 4 to 6 cm.[205] Malignant melanoma in children is extremely rare but when present displays behavior similar to that in adults.[216, 217]

The histologic diagnosis of malignant melanoma depends on the recognition of a constellation of features, and no single histologic feature can be regarded as a reliable marker for melanoma (CD Fig. 49–19).[218–220] The main criteria for the histologic diagnosis of malignant melanoma are detailed in Table 49–7.

**TABLE 49–6.** Combined Approach to Melanoma Prognostication Based on Level of Invasion (Clark) and Thickness (Breslow)[210]

| |
|---|
| Low-risk melanoma |
|   Tumors less than 0.76 mm thick and level II–III |
| Moderate-risk melanoma |
|   Tumors less than 0.76 mm thick and level IV |
|   Tumors between 0.76 mm and 1.5 mm thick |
|   Tumors more than 1.5 mm thick and level III |
| High-risk melanoma |
|   Tumors more than 1.5 mm thick and level IV or V |

**TABLE 49–7.** Histologic Criteria That Favor a Diagnosis of Malignant Melanoma

**Architectural**

Asymmetry
Poor lateral circumscription
Ulceration of overlying epidermis
Variation in size, shape, and location of nests of melanocytes or confluence of junctional melanocytic nests
Loss of cohesion of tumor cells with single-cell proliferation of melanocytes along dermal-epidermal junction
Upward migration of melanocytes (pagetoid spread) with predominance of single cells over nests of melanocytes
Infiltrative growth pattern with invasion of dermal adnexa, vessels, and nerves
Lack of maturation in deep dermal component

**Cytologic**

Marked nuclear atypia of melanocytes
Fine (dusty) melanin
Atypical mitoses, especially in deep dermal component
Necrosis of tumor cells

*Melanoma in situ* is the term currently used to designate a proliferation of atypical melanocytes entirely confined to the epidermis. Because the dividing line between morphologically atypical and frankly malignant melanocytes can often be arbitrary, Rywlin proposed the descriptive designation *atypical intraepidermal melanocytic proliferation* for this process.[221] Other proposed terms include atypical melanocytic hyperplasia, premalignant melanosis, melanocytic dysplasia, and pagetoid melanocytic proliferation.[208, 222, 223] Although inconsistencies and contradiction in use have been noted, malignant melanoma in situ continues to be the term employed by convention for the diagnosis of the radial growth phase of melanoma. The superficial spreading variant of melanoma in situ, also referred to as pagetoid melanoma in situ, is characterized by a proliferation of round, atypical melanocytes in a pagetoid fashion throughout all levels of the epidermis. *Superficial spreading melanoma* is characterized by a junctional proliferation of atypical melanocytes that invade from the epidermis into the dermis as well as by upward extension of atypical melanocytes into the upper layers of the epidermis (Fig. 49–59). *Nodular melanoma* is characterized by a nodular expansion of the dermis by an atypical proliferation of melanocytes. The overlying epidermis is usually thinned and may be ulcerated, and it shows pagetoid spread of atypical melanocytes. *Acral lentiginous melanoma* is characterized by a continuous proliferation of atypical melanocytes primarily along the basal layer of the epidermis, with invasion of the dermis in the form of round epithelioid or spindled melanocytes in aggregates or in single-cell fashion. *Lentigo maligna melanoma* is defined by the presence of dermal invasion by melanoma cells in a background lesion of lentigo maligna. The underlying dermis usually shows prominent features of solar damage. Dermal inflammatory infiltrates and histologic evidence of regression are usually present.

Melanomas can occasionally adopt a variety of unusual morphologic appearances that may introduce difficulties for histologic diagnosis.

## DESMOPLASTIC-NEUROTROPIC MELANOMAS.

Desmoplastic-neurotropic melanomas exhibit properties more consistent with neuroectodermal schwannian differentiation.[224–226] The tumors are often associated with a lentiginous melanocytic proliferation, but de novo forms of neurotropic melanoma originating from the dermis in the absence of a lentiginous component have also been recognized. The lesions usually present clinically as a raised, firm amelanotic nodule. Histologic examination shows an irregular proliferation of oval to spindle cells displacing the dermal collagen and infiltrating into the subcutaneous fat (Fig. 49–60A). The most common pattern is that of a desmoplastic tumor composed of individually scattered spindle cells that coalesce focally to form fascicles separated by abundant collagenous stroma.[224, 227, 228] The spindle cells generally show considerable pleomorphism with irregular nuclei and mitotic figures, although in some cases the cellular proliferation can be entirely banal and indistinguishable from conventional fibroblasts. Some cases may initially be mistaken for a dermal scar or fibromatosis. A prominent and diagnostic feature is the presence of neurotropism. Atypical spindle cells are seen to invade the endoneurium of cutaneous nerves as well as arrange themselves around the epineurium, forming a cuff of tumor cells around the nerve fibers[226, 228, 229] (Fig. 49–60B). Sheets and nests of plump, round or oval epithelioid cells that contain fine, dusty melanin pigment characterize another growth pattern. Sometimes the epithelioid cells may appear to blend with spindle cells as they extend from the papillary dermis into the upper reticular dermis, suggesting that the epithelioid cells with melanocytic differentiation may have the capability to differentiate into cells with fibroblastic as well as schwannian features. Neurotropism is also a prominent feature in the epithelioid cell variants of these tumors.[225–227]

Desmoplastic-neurotropic melanoma may be confused with a number of different lesions, including a variety of melanocytic and nonmelanocytic neoplasms composed of spindle cells infiltrating the

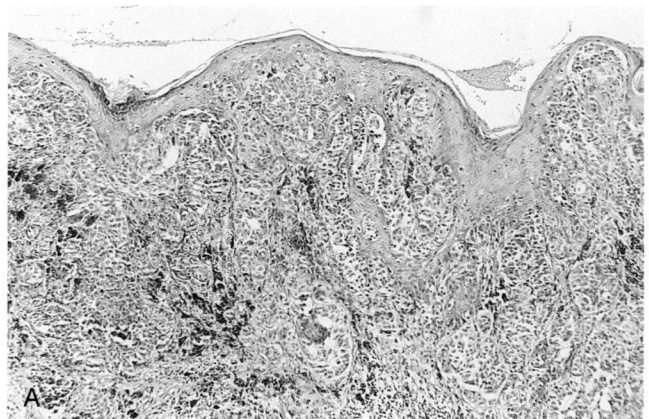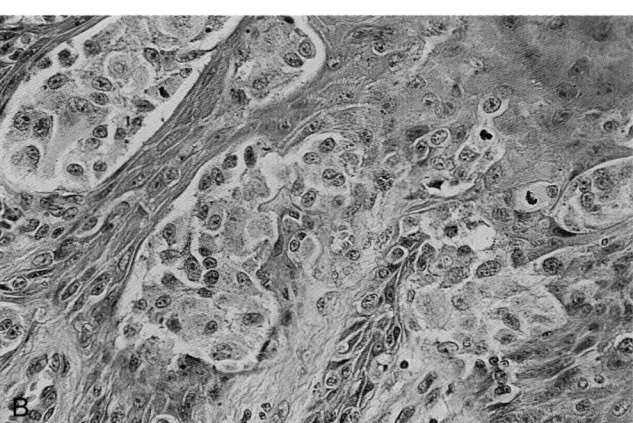

**FIGURE 49–59.** *A.* Superficial spreading malignant melanoma showing atypical proliferation of melanocytes that almost completely replace the epidermis and invade the underlying dermis. *B.* Superficial spreading malignant melanoma. Higher magnification shows marked atypia of melanocytes.

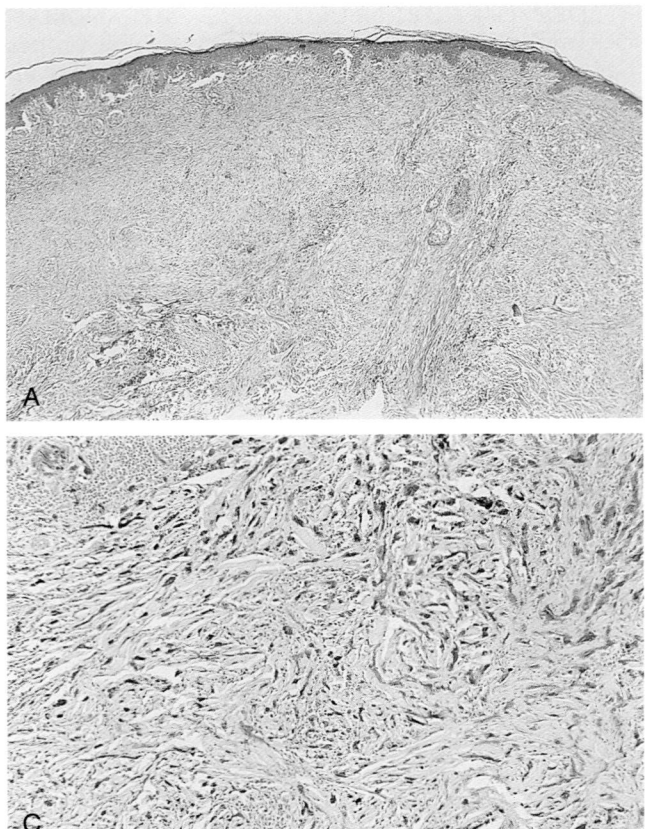
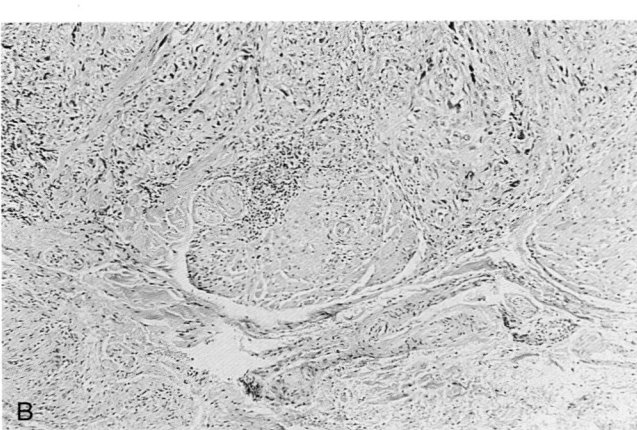

**FIGURE 49–60.** *A.* Desmoplastic melanoma. Diffuse infiltration and expansion of the dermis is noted by atypical spindled melanocytes. Note the atypical lentiginous melanocytic proliferation in the epidermis associated with the lesion *(top left). B.* Desmoplastic melanoma. Higher magnification of deep portion of the lesion shows atypical proliferation of spindled melanocytes wrapping around nerves. *C.* Desmoplastic melanoma. S-100 protein stain highlights atypical melanocytes.

dermis. Immunohistochemical stains for S-100 protein may be of help for diagnosis. Most desmoplastic-neurotropic melanomas show variable degrees of positivity for this marker in the atypical spindle cells[230] (Fig. 49–60C). Stains for the melanoma-associated marker HMB-45 are less commonly positive in such tumors.

The tumors are associated with aggressive behavior and frequent local recurrences, even after wide excision. The prognosis after local recurrence is usually poor. Although some authors make a distinction between desmoplastic and neurotropic melanoma, observing that fibroblast-like features and desmoplasia are more prominent in the former and epithelioid cell morphology more frequent in the latter, we believe that both probably represent different points in the spectrum of the same lesion (CD Figs. 49–20 and 49–21).

**BALLOON CELL MELANOMA.** Balloon cell melanoma is an unusual morphologic variant characterized by the presence of large cells with abundant clear cytoplasm and scalloped nuclei (Fig. 49–61). The balloon cell change has been considered a degenerative phenomenon.[231] Balloon cell melanoma may be confused with balloon cell nevus, xanthoma, granular cell tumors, sebaceous carcinoma, and metastatic clear cell tumors of internal organs such

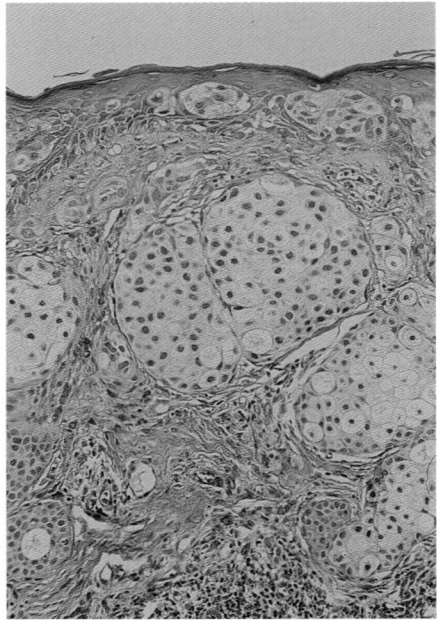

**FIGURE 49–61.** Balloon cell melanoma. The cells contain abundant clear cytoplasm and may superficially resemble sebaceous cells.

as renal cell carcinoma. The tumor cells are generally positive for S-100 protein and HMB-45.

**MINIMAL DEVIATION MELANOMA.** Minimal deviation melanoma is a term that was introduced to define lesions characterized by a proliferation of melanocytes with little cytologic atypia and a better prognosis than that of other conventional melanomas of the same thickness.[232, 233] The tumors often arise against the background of a common acquired nevus within which a nodular dermal expansion of monotonous tumor cells takes place. The proliferating cells within such nodules may resemble ordinary nevus cells or spindled melanocytes, or they may adopt the appearance of epithelioid cells similar to those of Spitz nevi, but without the full-blown cytologic features of conventional malignant melanoma or increase in mitotic activity. Because of the bland cytologic appearance of the proliferating cells in these tumors and the lack of well-defined criteria and objective markers for their diagnosis, minimal deviation melanoma is often a retrospective diagnosis that follows recurrence of a lesion.

**NEVOID MELANOMA.** Nevoid melanoma is a term applied to melanocytic lesions that closely resemble the growth pattern and architecture of a conventional or Spitz nevus.[234, 235] Good symmetry, minimal pagetoid spread, and a monotonous population of nevuslike cells in the dermis characterize the lesions (Fig. 49–62A). Some cases show a striking verrucous epidermal configuration with prominent papillomatosis, hyperkeratosis, and parakeratosis.[236] The lateral margins of the lesion are usually well demarcated, and there is generally absence of a host response. Despite the apparent banal appearance of the nevus cell population in the dermis, subtle features that identify the lesion as a melanoma are the absence of maturation in depth, presence of scattered mitotic figures throughout all levels of the lesion, and infiltrative growth of the cells into the deep dermis in cords and strands (Fig. 49–62B). Pa-

getoid extension of atypical melanocytes along dermal adnexa and replacement of the basal cell layer by singly dispersed atypical melanocytes lying side by side along the dermal-epidermal junction are two other features that distinguish these lesions. Many of these tumors are associated with recurrences and regional lymph node metastases, but their biologic behavior may appear to be less aggressive than that of conventional melanoma with comparable depth of invasion.[234] Additional studies are needed to better delineate the full clinical behavior of these lesions.

**OTHER VARIANTS OF MALIGNANT MELANOMA.** Other rare or unusual variants of malignant melanoma are amelanotic melanoma, spindle cell melanoma, melanoma with regression, melanoma with prominent myxoid stroma, melanoma with metaplastic bone formation, melanoma with signet ring cell features, and small cell melanoma that can closely resemble a lymphoma or other small round blue cell tumor.[217, 237–241]

## PROGNOSTIC FEATURES OF MELANOMA

During the past 20 years, intensive study has been devoted to identifying prognostic features of melanoma by use of large databases and multivariate analysis.[242–245] The two relatively more reliable predictors of survival that have emerged from such studies are the thickness of the primary lesion (as measured in millimeters from the granular layer of the epidermis to the deepest point of tumor invasion) and the stage of the disease at the time of diagnosis (tumor extent, nodal metastases, and distant metastases). A number of other factors, including ulceration, mitotic rate, lymphoid host response, regression, microscopic satellites, vascular-lymphatic invasion, tumor cell type, age, sex, and anatomic site, have also been reported to influence prognosis in patients with localized melanoma (Table 49–8). However, these various factors directly correlate

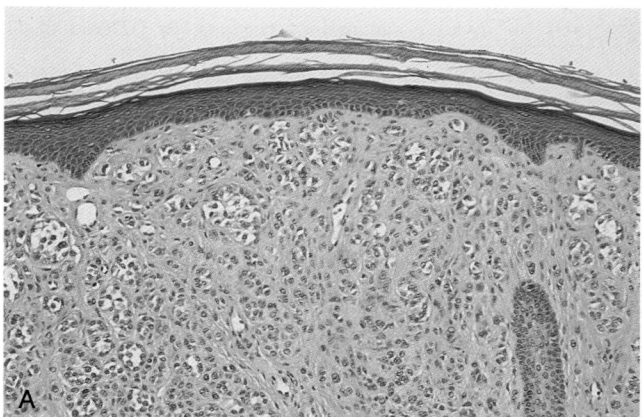
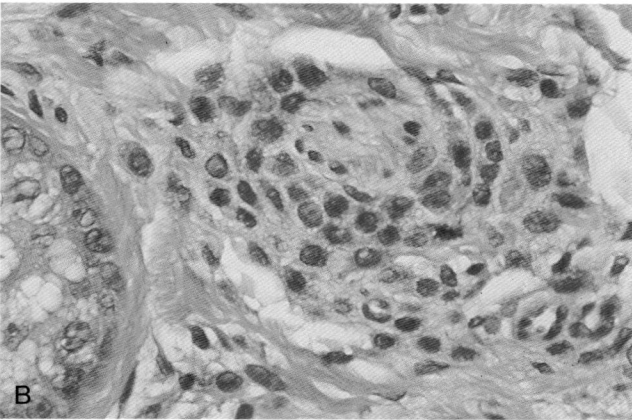

**FIGURE 49–62.** *A.* Nevoid melanoma. There is a symmetric, monotonous population of nevuslike cells in the dermis that closely resembles a Spitz nevus. *B.* Nevoid melanoma, higher magnification. Lack of maturation, perineural invasion, and occasional mitoses in depth characterize the lesion.

**TABLE 49–8.** Prognostic Features: Cutaneous Malignant Melanoma

Thickness of the lesion[209]
Staging (TNM)
Ulceration
Mitotic rate
Lymphoid host response
Evidence of regression
Microscopic satellites
Vascular-lymphatic invasion
Tumor cell type
Age
Sex
Anatomic site

**TABLE 49–9.** Contents of the Final Report: Cutaneous Malignant Melanoma

Minimal information necessary
  Location
  Size
  Histologic growth pattern
  Thickness[209]
  Depth of invasion[204]
  Status of margins
Additional valuable information
  Mitotic rate
  Ulceration
  Vascular-lymphatic invasion
  Neurotropism
  Microsatellites
  Regression

with melanoma thickness and generally fail to show statistical significance by multivariate analysis.[242]

Another area that has been the subject of study is the correlation between genetic changes and the development of melanoma. Mutations in *ras* have been found to play a role in the acquisition of aggressive metastatic properties by melanoma cells.[246] Cytogenetic and molecular studies have suggested that a tumor suppressor gene located on 9p21 (p16) has a pivotal role in the development of malignant melanoma.[247] Additional studies to elucidate the molecular pathogenesis of melanoma may lead to a better understanding of the underlying mechanisms associated with tumor progression and may serve to develop additional diagnostic and prognostic markers for these tumors.

Malignant melanoma is a highly aggressive neoplasm that is associated with a poor prognosis in its full-blown form. The median survival for patients with distant metastasis is approximately 6 months.[244] Factors influencing the time to death are the number of metastatic sites, the duration of remission, and the location of the metastases. Malignant melanoma is also notorious for its often unpredictable biologic behavior; large invasive lesions occasionally respond well to treatment, and small, relatively early lesions metastasize widely.

A report from the Association of Directors of Anatomic and Surgical Pathology issued the following recommendations for the reporting of malignant melanoma: site, type of procedure, histologic growth pattern, Clark level, Breslow thickness, mitotic rate, ulceration, features of regression, margins, vascular-lymphatic invasion, presence of microsatellites, neurotropism, and lymph node status.[248] We believe the pathology report should include the following minimal information (Table 49–9): location and size, histologic growth pattern, tumor thickness (Breslow), depth of invasion (Clarke), and status of the margins. Additional information of value that can be provided in the pathology report includes mitotic rate, ulceration, vascular-lymphatic invasion, neurotropism, microscopic satellites, and presence of features of regression.

## REFERENCES

1. Hodge JA, Ray MC, Flynn KJ: The epidermal nevus syndrome. Int J Dermatol 30:91–98, 1991.
2. Gross G, Pfister H, Hagedorn M, et al: Correlation between human papillomavirus (HPV) type and histology of warts. J Invest Dermatol 78:160–164, 1982.
3. Lutzner MA: The human papillomaviruses. A review. Arch Dermatol 119:631–635, 1983.
4. Lutzner MA, Blanchet-Bardon C, Orth G: Clinical observations, virologic studies, and treatment trials in patients with epidermodysplasia verruciformis, a disease induced by specific human papillomaviruses. J Invest Dermatol Suppl 83:18–25, 1984.
5. Sanchez Yus E, del Rio E, Requena L: Large cell acanthoma is a distinctive condition. Am J Dermatopathol 14:140–147, 1992.
6. Degos R, Civatte J: Clear-cell acanthoma. Br J Dermatol 83:248–254, 1970.
7. Schwartz RA: Keratoacanthoma. J Am Acad Dermatol 30:1–19, 1994.
8. LeBoit PE: Is keratoacanthoma a variant of squamous cell carcinoma: new insights into an old controversy . . . soon? Am J Dermatopathol 17:319–320, 1995.
9. Tanay A, Mehregan AH: Warty dyskeratoma. Dermatologica 138:155–164, 1969.
10. Schwartz RA: Sign of Leser-Trélat. J Am Acad Dermatol 35:88–95, 1996.
11. Frost CA, Green AC: Epidemiology of solar keratoses. Br J Dermatol 131:455–464, 1994.
12. Biesterfeld S, Pennings K, Gussendorf-Conen EI, et al: Aneuploidy in actinic keratosis and Bowen's disease: increased risk for invasive squamous carcinoma. Br J Dermatol 133:557–560, 1995.
13. Picascia DD, Robinson JK: Actinic cheilitis: a review of the etiology, differential diagnosis, and treatment. J Am Acad Dermatol 17:255–264, 1987.
14. Callen JD, Headington J: Bowen's and non-Bowen's squamous intraepithelial neoplasia of the skin: relationship to internal malignancy. Arch Dermatol 116:422–426, 1980.
15. Strayer DS, Santa Cruz DJ: Carcinoma in-situ of the skin: a review of histopathology. J Cutan Pathol 7:244–259, 1980.
16. Penneys NS, Mogollon RJ, Nadji M, et al: Papillomavirus common antigens. Papillomavirus antigen in verruca, benign papillomatous lesions, trichilemmoma, and bowenoid papulosis. An immunoperoxidase study. Arch Dermatol 120:859–861, 1984.
17. Wade TR, Kopf AW, Ackerman AB: Bowenoid papulosis of the genitalia. Arch Dermatol 115:306–308, 1979.
18. Smith KJ, Skelton HG, Morgan AM, et al: Spindle cell neoplasms coexpressing cytokeratin and vimentin (metaplastic squamous cell carcinoma). J Cutan Pathol 19:286–293, 1992.
19. Banerjee SS, Eyden BP, Wells S, et al: Pseudoangiosarcoma-

tous carcinoma: a clinicopathological study of seven cases. Histopathology 21:13–23, 1992.

20. Requena L, Sanchez Yus E, Jimenez E, et al: Lymphoepithelioma-like carcinoma of the skin: a light microscopic and immunohistochemical study. J Cutan Pathol 21:541–548, 1994.

21. McKee PH, Wilkinson JD, Black MM, et al: Carcinoma (epithelioma) cuniculatum: a clinicopathological study of nineteen cases and review of the literature. Histopathology 5: 425–436, 1981.

22. Betti R, Inselvini E, Carducci M, et al: Age and site prevalence of histologic subtypes of basal cell carcinomas. Int J Dermatol 34:174–176, 1995.

23. Suster S, Ramon y Cajal S: Myoepithelial differentiation in basal cell carcinoma. Am J Dermatopathol 13:350–357, 1991.

24. Salasche SJ, Amonette RA: Morpheaform basal-cell epithelioma. A study of subclinical extensions in a series of 51 patients. J Dermatol Surg Oncol 7:387–394, 1981.

25. Nishimura M, Hori Y: Adamantinoid basal cell carcinoma. Arch Pathol Lab Med 115:624–626, 1991.

26. Starink TM, Blomjous CEM, Stoof TJ, et al: Clear-cell basal cell carcinoma. Histopathology 17:401–405, 1990.

27. Seo IS, Warner TF, Priest JB: Basal cell carcinoma—signet ring type: ultrastructural study. J Cutan Pathol 6:101–107, 1979.

28. Shanley F, Ratcliffe J, Hockey A, et al: Nevoid basal cell carcinoma syndrome: review of 118 affected individuals. Am J Med Genet 50:282–290, 1994.

29. Bolognia JL: Bazex syndrome: acrokeratosis paraneoplastica. Semin Dermatol 14:84–89, 1995.

30. Jones RE, Ackerman AB: Extramammary Paget's disease: a critical reappraisal. Am J Dermatopathol 1:101–132, 1979.

31. Helm KF, Goellner JR, Peters MS: Immunohistochemical stains in extramammary Paget's disease. Am J Dermatopathol 14:402–407, 1992.

32. Hashimoto K, Gross BC, Lever WF: Syringoma: histochemical and electron microscopic studies. J Invest Dermatol 46: 150–166, 1966.

33. Feibelman CE, Maize JC: Clear cell syringoma: a study by conventional and electron microscopy. Am J Dermatopathol 6:139–150, 1984.

34. Hassab-El-Naby HM, Tam S, White WL, et al: Mixed tumor of the skin. A histological and immunohistochemical study. Am J Dermatopathol 11:413–428, 1989.

35. Mehregan AH, Levson DN: Hidroacanthoma simplex. Arch Dermatol 100:303–305, 1969.

36. Aloi FG, Pippione M: Dermal duct tumor. Appl Pathol 4: 175–178, 1986.

37. Pylyser K, DeWolf-Peeters C, Marien K: The histology of eccrine poroma. A study of 14 cases. Dermatologica 167:243–249, 1983.

38. Johnson BL Jr, Helwig EB: Eccrine acrospiroma. Cancer 23: 641–657, 1969.

39. Urmacher C, Liberman PH: Papillary eccrine adenoma: a light microscopic and immunohistochemical study. Am J Dermatopathol 9:243–249, 1987.

40. Kao GF, Helwig EB, Graham JH: Aggressive digital papillary adenoma and adenocarcinoma. J Cutan Pathol 14:129–146, 1987.

41. Suster S: Clear cell tumors of the skin. Semin Diagn Pathol 13:40–59, 1996.

42. Santa Cruz DJ: Sweat gland carcinomas: a comprehensive review. Semin Diagn Pathol 4:38–74, 1987.

43. Wong T-Y, Suster S, Nogita T, et al: Clear cell eccrine carcinomas of the skin. A clinicopathologic study of 9 cases. Cancer 73:1631–1643, 1994.

44. Suster S, Wong T-Y: Polymorphous sweat gland carcinoma. Histopathology 25:31–39, 1994.

45. Toribio J, Zulaica A, Peteiro C: Tubular apocrine adenoma. J Cutan Pathol 14:114–117, 1987.

46. Suster S: Tumors of the skin composed of large cells with abundant eosinophilic cytoplasm. Semin Diagn Pathol 16: 162–177, 1999.

47. Paties C, Taccagni GL, Papotti M, et al: Apocrine carcinoma of the skin: a clinicopathologic, immunocytochemical, and ultrastructural study, Cancer 71:375–381, 1993.

48. Wick MR, Swanson PE: Cutaneous Adnexal Tumors: A Guide to Pathologic Diagnosis. Chicago, ASCP Press, 1991.

49. Hidayat AA, Font RL: Trichilemmoma of the eyelid and eyebrow: a clinicopathologic study of 31 cases. Arch Ophthalmol 98:844–847, 1980.

50. Amaral A, Nascimento A, Goellner JR: Proliferating pilar (trichilemmal) cyst: report of 2 cases, one with carcinomatous transformation and one with distant metastases. Arch Pathol Lab Med 108:808–810, 1984.

51. Long SA, Hunt MA, Santa Cruz DJ: Immature trichoepithelioma: report of six cases. J Cutan Pathol 15:353–358, 1989.

52. Takei Y, Fukushiro S, Ackerman AB: Criteria for histologic differentiation of desmoplastic trichoepithelioma (sclerosing epithelial hamartoma) from morphea-like basal cell carcinoma. Am J Dermatopathol 7:207–211, 1985.

53. Headington JT: Tumors of the hair follicle. A review. Am J Pathol 85:480–505, 1976.

54. Wong T-Y, Reed JA, Suster S, Flynn S: Benign trichogenic tumors: a report of two cases supporting a simplified nomenclature. Histopathology 22:575–580, 1993.

55. Wong T-Y, Suster S: Tricholemmal carcinoma: a clinicopathologic study of 13 cases. Am J Dermatopathol 16:463–473, 1994.

56. Wolfe JT III, Wick MR, Campbell RJ: Sebaceous carcinomas of the oculocutaneous adnexa and extraocular skin. In Wick MR (ed): Pathology of Unusual Malignant Cutaneous Tumors. New York, Marcel Dekker, 1985, pp 77–106.

57. Wong T-Y, Suster S, Cheek RF, et al: Benign cutaneous adnexal tumors with combined folliculosebaceous, apocrine, and eccrine differentiation. Clinicopathologic and immunohistochemical study of 8 cases. Am J Dermatopathol 18:124–136, 1996.

58. Nahkleh RE, Swanson PE, Wick MR: Cutaneous adnexal carcinomas with mixed differentiation. Am J Dermatopathol 12: 325–334, 1990.

59. Toker C: Trabecular carcinoma of the skin. Arch Dermatol 105:107–110, 1972.

60. Tang CK, Toker C: Trabecular carcinoma of the skin: an ultrastructural study. Cancer 42:2311–2321, 1978.

61. Sibley RK, Dehner LP, Rosai J: Primary neuroendocrine (Merkel cell?) carcinoma of the skin: I. A clinicopathologic study of 46 cases with ultrastructural observations. Am J Surg Pathol 9:95–108, 1985.

62. Gould VE, Moll R, Moll I, et al: Neuroendocrine (Merkel) cells of the skin: hyperplasias, dysplasias, and neoplasms. Lab Invest 52:334–353, 1985.

63. Wick MR, Goellner JR, Scheithauer BW, et al: Primary neuroendocrine carcinomas of the skin (Merkel cell tumors). Am J Clin Pathol 79:6–13, 1983.

64. Pilotti S, Rilke F, Bartoli C, Grisotti A: Clinicopathologic correlations of cutaneous neuroendocrine Merkel cell carcinoma. J Clin Oncol 6:1863–1873, 1988.

65. Kroll MH, Toker C: Trabecular carcinoma of the skin. Further clinicopathologic and morphologic study. Arch Pathol Lab Med 106:404–408, 1982.

66. Wick MR, Scheithauer BW: Primary neuroendocrine carcinoma of the skin. In Wick MR (ed): Pathology of Unusual Malignant Cutaneous Tumors. New York, Marcel Dekker, 1985, p 107.

67. Toker C: Tumors: An Atlas of Differential Diagnosis. Baltimore, University Park Press, 1983, pp 1–36.

68. LeBoit PE, Crutcher WA, Shapiro PE: Pagetoid intraepidermal spread in Merkel cell (primary neuroendocrine) carcinoma of the skin. Am J Surg Pathol 16:584–593, 1992.

69. Gould ED, Albores-Saavedra J, Dubner B, et al: Eccrine and squamous differentiation in Merkel cell carcinoma. An immunohistochemical study. Am J Surg Pathol 12:768–772, 1989.

70. Layfield L, Ulich T, Liao S, et al: Neuroendocrine carcinoma of the skin: an immunohistochemical study of tumor markers and neuroendocrine products. J Cutan Pathol 13:268–274, 1986.

71. Chan JKC, Suster S, Wenig B, et al: Cytokeratin 20 immunoreactivity distinguishes Merkel cell (primary cutaneous neuroendocrine) carcinomas and salivary gland small cell carci-

nomas from small cell carcinomas of various sites. Am J Surg Pathol 21:226–234, 1997.

72. Visscher D, Cooper PH, Zarbo RJ, et al: Cutaneous neuroendocrine (Merkel cell) carcinoma: an immunophenotypic, clinicopathologic and flow cytometric study. Mod Pathol 2:331–336, 1989.

73. Penneys SA, Shapiro S: CD44 expression in Merkel cell carcinoma may correlate with risk of metastasis. J Cutan Pathol 21:22–26, 1994.

74. Silva EG, Mackay B, Goepfert H, et al: Endocrine carcinoma of the skin (Merkel cell carcinoma). Pathol Annu 19:1–30, 1984.

75. Suster S, Ronnen M, Lin E, Schewach MM: Trabecular carcinoma of the skin simulating metastatic disease. J Surg Oncol 32:73–75, 1986.

76. Hunt SJ, Santa Cruz DJ: Acquired benign and "borderline" vascular lesions. Dermatol Clin 10:97–112, 1992.

77. Padilla RS, Orkin M, Rosai J: Acquired "tufted" angioma (progressive capillary hemangioma): a distinctive clinicopathologic entity related to lobular capillary hemangioma. Am J Dermatopathol 9:292–300, 1987.

78. Wilson-Jones E, Orkin M: Tufted angioma (angioblastoma): a benign progressive angioma, not to be confused with Kaposi's sarcoma or low-grade angiosarcoma. J Am Acad Dermatol 20:214–225, 1989.

79. Chan JKC, Fletcher CDM, Hicklin GA, et al: Glomeruloid hemangioma: a distinctive cutaneous lesion of multicentric Castleman's disease associated with POEMS syndrome. Am J Surg Pathol 14:1036–1046, 1990.

80. Ishikawa O, Nihei Y, Ishikawa H: The skin changes of POEMS syndrome. Br J Dermatol 117:523–526, 1987.

81. Hunt SJ, Santa Cruz DJ, Barr RJ: Microvenular hemangioma. J Cutan Pathol 18:235–240, 1991.

82. Santa Cruz DJ, Aronberg J: Targetoid hemosiderotic hemangioma. J Am Acad Dermatol 19:550–558, 1988.

83. Olsen TG, Helwig EB: Angiolymphoid hyperplasia with eosinophilia: a clinicopathologic study of 116 patients. J Am Acad Dermatol 12:781–796, 1985.

84. Googe PB, Harris NL, Mihm MC Jr: Kimura's disease and angiolymphoid hyperplasia with eosinophilia: two distinct histopathologic entities. J Cutan Pathol 14:263–271, 1987.

85. Rosai J: Angiolymphoid hyperplasia with eosinophilia of the skin: its nosological position in the spectrum of histiocytoid hemangioma. Am J Dermatopathol 4:175–184, 1982.

86. Cockrell CJ, LeBoit PE: Bacillary angiomatosis: a newly characterized pseudoneoplastic, infectious, cutaneous vascular disorder. J Am Acad Dermatol 22:501–512, 1990.

87. Weiss SW, Enzinger FM: Spindle cell hemangioendothelioma: a low-grade angiosarcoma resembling a cavernous hemangioma and Kaposi's sarcoma. Am J Surg Pathol 10:521–530, 1986.

88. Weiss SW, Enzinger FM: Epithelioid hemangioendothelioma: a vascular tumor often mistaken for a carcinoma. Cancer 50:970–981, 1982.

89. Weiss SW, Ishak K, Dail DH, et al: Epithelioid hemangioendothelioma and related lesions. Semin Diagn Pathol 3:259–287, 1986.

90. Dabska M: Malignant endovascular papillary angioendothelioma of the skin in childhood. Cancer 24:503–510, 1969.

91. Calonje E, Fletcher CDM, Wilson-Jones E, Rosai J: Retiform hemangioendothelioma: a distinctive form of low-grade angiosarcoma delineated in a series of 15 cases. Am J Surg Pathol 18:115–125, 1994.

92. Chang Y, Cesarman E, Pessin MS, et al: Identification of herpesvirus-like DNA sequences in AIDS-associated Kaposi's sarcoma. Science 266:1865–1869, 1994.

93. Hoerl HD, Goldblum JR: Immunoreactivity patterns of CD31 and CD68 in 28 cases of Kaposi's sarcoma. Evidence supporting endothelial differentiation in the spindle cell component. Appl Immunohistochem 5:173–178, 1997.

94. Rosai J, Sumner HW, Kostianovsky M, Perez-Mesa C: Angiosarcoma of the skin: a clinicopathologic and fine structural study. Hum Pathol 7:83–109, 1976.

95. Suster S, Wong T-Y: On the discriminatory value of anti-HPCA-1 (CD34) in the differential diagnosis of benign and

96. Calonje E, Fletcher CDM: Cutaneous fibrohistiocytic tumors: an update. Adv Anat Pathol 1:2–15, 1994.

97. Tmada S, Ackeman AB: Dermatofibroma with monster cells. Am J Dermatopathol 9:380–387, 1987.

98. Zelger BW, Steiner H, Kutzner H: Clear cell dermatofibroma. Case report of an unusual fibrohistiocytic lesion. Am J Surg Pathol 18:668–676, 1994.

99. Calonje E, Mentzel T, Fletcher CDM: Cellular benign fibrous histiocytoma: clinicopathologic analysis of 74 cases with a distinctive variant of cutaneous fibrous histiocytoma with frequent recurrences. Am J Surg Pathol 18:668–676, 1994.

100. Fretzin DF, Helwig EB: Atypical fibroxanthoma of the skin. A clinicopathologic study of 140 cases. Cancer 31:1541–1552, 1973.

101. Helwig EB, May D: Atypical fibroxanthoma of the skin with metastases. Cancer 57:368–376, 1986.

102. Iwasaki H, Kikuchi M, Ohtsuki I, et al: Infantile digital fibromatosis. Identification of actin filaments in cytoplasmic inclusions by heavy meromyosin binding. Cancer 52:1653–1661, 1983.

103. Chung EB, Enzinger FM: Infantile myofibromatosis. Cancer 48:1807–1812, 1981.

104. Daimaru Y, Hashimoto H, Enjoji M: Myofibromatosis in adults (adult counterpart of infantile myofibromatosis). Am J Surg Pathol 13:859–865, 1989.

105. Beham A, Badve S, Suster S, Fletcher CDM: Solitary myofibroma in adults: clinicopathological analysis of a series. Histopathology 22:335–341, 1993.

106. Brathwaite C, Suster S: Dermatofibrosarcoma protuberans: a critical reappraisal of the role of immunohistochemical stains for diagnosis. Appl Immunohistochem 2:36–41, 1994.

107. Ma CK, Zarbo RJ, Gown AM: Immunohistochemical characterization of atypical fibroxanthoma and dermatofibrosarcoma protuberans. Am J Clin Pathol 97:478–483, 1992.

108. Wrotnowski U, Cooper PH, Shmookler BM: Fibrosarcomatous change in dermatofibrosarcoma protuberans. Am J Surg Pathol 12:287–293, 1988.

109. Beham A, Fletcher CDM: Dermatofibrosarcoma protuberans with areas resembling giant cell fibroblastoma: report of two cases. Histopathology 17:165–167, 1990.

110. Berger TG, Levin MW: Congenital smooth muscle hamartoma. J Am Acad Dermatol 11:709–712, 1984.

111. Fields JP, Helwig EB: Leiomyosarcoma of the skin and subcutaneous tissue. Cancer 47:156–169, 1981.

112. Suster S: Epithelioid leiomyosarcoma of the skin and subcutaneous tissue. Clinicopathologic, immunohistochemical and ultrastructural study of 5 cases. Am J Surg Pathol 18:232–240, 1994.

113. Suster S, Rosen LB, Sanchez J: Granular cell leiomyosarcoma of the skin. Am J Dermatopathol 10:234–239, 1988.

114. Wong T-Y, Suster S: Primary cutaneous sarcomas with rhabdomyoblastic differentiation. Histopathology 26:25–32, 1995.

115. Argenyi ZB, Cooper PH, Santa Cruz D: Plexiform and other unusual variants of palisaded encapsulated neuroma. J Cutan Pathol 17:329–333, 1990.

116. Argenyi ZB, Balogh K, Abraham AA: Degenerative ("ancient") changes in benign cutaneous schwannoma: a light microscopic, histochemical and immunohistochemical study. J Cutan Pathol 20:148–152, 1993.

117. Angervall L, Kindblom LG, Haglid K: Dermal nerve sheath myxoma: a light and electron microscopic, histochemical and immunohistochemical study. Cancer 53:1752–1759, 1984.

118. Argenyi ZB, LeBoit PE, Santa Cruz D, et al: Nerve sheath myxoma (neurothekeoma) of the skin: light microscopic and immunohistochemical reappraisal of the cellular variant. J Cutan Pathol 20:294–303, 1993.

119. Argenyi ZB: Neural and neuroendocrine tumors. In Barnhill RL (ed): Textbook of Dermatopathology. New York, McGraw-Hill, 1998, pp 747–762.

120. George E, Swanson PE, Wick MR: Malignant peripheral nerve sheath tumors of the skin. Am J Dermatopathol 11:213–220, 1989.

121. Suster S, Amazon K, Rosen LB, Ollague JM: Malignant epi-

thelioid schwannoma of the skin. A low-grade variant of neurotropic melanoma? Am J Dermatopathol 11:338–344, 1989.

122. Holbert JM Jr, Chesney TM: Malignant lymphoma of the skin: a review of recent advances in diagnosis and classification. J Cutan Pathol 9:133–168, 1982.

123. Braun-Falco O, Burg G, Schmoeckel C: Recent advances in the understanding of cutaneous lymphoma. Clin Exp Dermatol 6:89–109, 1981.

124. Kaudewitz P, Burg G, Stein H, et al: Atypical cells in lymphomatoid papulosis express the Hodgkin cell–associated antigen Ki-1. J Invest Dermatol 86:350–354, 1986.

125. Davis TH, Morton CC, Miller TR, et al: Hodgkin's disease, lymphomatoid papulosis, and cutaneous T-cell lymphoma derived from a common T-cell clone. N Engl J Med 315:475–479, 1986.

126. Burg G, Dummer R, Dommann S, et al: Pathology of cutaneous T-cell lymphoma. Hematol Oncol Clin North Am 9:961–995, 1995.

127. Altman J: Parapsoriasis: a histopathologic review and classification. Semin Dermatol 3:14–21, 1984.

128. Edelson RL: Cutaneous T cell lymphoma: mycosis fungoides, Sézary syndrome, and other variants. J Am Acad Dermatol 2:89–106, 1980.

129. LeBoit PE: Variants of mycosis fungoides and related cutaneous T-cell lymphomas. Semin Diagn Pathol 8:73–81, 1991.

130. Burns MK, Chan LS, Cooper KD: Woringer-Kolopp disease (localized pagetoid reticulosis) or unilesional mycosis fungoides: an analysis of eight cases with benign disease. Arch Dermatol 131:325–329, 1995.

131. LeBoit PE, Zackheim HS, White CR Jr: Granulomatous variants of cutaneous T-cell lymphoma: the histopathology of granulomatous mycosis fungoides and granulomatous slack skin. Am J Surg Pathol 12:83–95, 1988.

132. Willemze R, Beljaards RC: Spectrum of primary cutaneous CD30 (Ki-1)–positive lymphoproliferative disorders: a proposal for classification and guidelines for management and treatment. J Am Acad Dermatol 28:973–980, 1993.

133. Krishnan J, Tomaszewski MM, Kao GF: Primary cutaneous CD30-positive anaplastic large cell lymphoma: report of 27 cases. J Cutan Pathol 20:193–202, 1993.

134. Dummer R, Protoczna N, Haeffner AC, et al: A primary cutaneous non-T, non-B CD4+, CD56+ lymphoma. Arch Dermatol 132:550–553, 1996.

135. Wang CE, Su WPD, Kurtin P: Subcutaneous panniculitic T-cell lymphoma. Int J Dermatol 35:1–8, 1996.

136. Nagatani T, Miyazawa M, Matsuzaki T, et al: Adult T-cell leukemia/lymphoma (ATL): clinical, histopathological, immunological and immunohistochemical characteristics. Exp Dermatol 1:248–252, 1992.

137. Jaffe ES, Blattner WA, Blayney DW, et al: The pathologic spectrum of adult T-cell leukemia/lymphoma virus–associated lymphoid malignancies. Am J Surg Pathol 8:263–275, 1984.

138. Kerl H, Burg G: Histomorphology and cytomorphology of cutaneous B-cell lymphomas. J Dermatol Surg Oncol 10:266–270, 1984.

139. Sterry W, Kruger GR, Steigleder GK: Skin involvement of malignant B-cell lymphomas. J Dermatol Surg Oncol 10:291–295, 1984.

140. Garcia CF, Weiss LM, Warnke RA, Woods GS: Cutaneous follicular lymphoma. Am J Surg Pathol 10:454–462, 1986.

141. Pimpinelli N, Santucci M, Bosi A, et al: Primary cutaneous follicle center cell lymphoma: a lymphoproliferative disease with favorable prognosis. Clin Exp Dermatol 14:12–23, 1989.

142. Cerroni L, Volkenandt M, Rieger E, et al: bcl-2 protein expression and correlation with the interchromosomal 14;18 translocation in cutaneous lymphomas and pseudolymphomas. J Invest Dermatol 102:231–240, 1994.

143. LeBoit PE, McNutt NS, Reed JA, et al: Primary cutaneous immunocytoma. A B-cell lymphoma that can easily be mistaken for cutaneous lymphoid hyperplasia. Am J Surg Pathol 18:969–978, 1994.

144. Cerroni L, Signoretti S, Kutting B, et al: Marginal zone B-cell lymphoma of the skin. J Cutan Pathol 23:47–56, 1996.

145. Wick MR, Mills SE: Intravascular lymphomatosis: clinico-pathologic features and differential diagnosis. Semin Diagn Pathol 8:91–101, 1991.

146. Sleater JP, Segal GH, Scott MD, Masih AS: Intravascular (angiotropic) large cell lymphoma: determination of monoclonality by polymerase chain-reaction on paraffin-embedded tissues. Mod Pathol 7:593–598, 1994.

147. Wong KF, Chan JKC, Li LPK, et al: Primary cutaneous plasmacytoma. Report of two cases and review of the literature. Am J Dermatopathol 16:392–396, 1994.

148. Wong TY, Suster S, Bouffard D, et al: Histologic spectrum of cutaneous involvement in patients with myelogenous leukemia including the neutrophilic dermatoses. Int J Dermatol 34:323–329, 1995.

149. Bonvalet D, Foldes C, Civatte J: Cutaneous manifestations in chronic lymphocytic leukemia. J Dermatol Surg Oncol 10:278–284, 1984.

150. Rosen LB, Frank BL, Rywlin AM: A characteristic vesiculobullous eruption in patients with chronic lymphocytic leukemia. J Am Acad Dermatol 15:943–949, 1986.

151. Kaiserling E, Horny HP, Geerts ML, et al: Skin involvement in myelogenous leukemia. Morphologic and immunophenotypic heterogeneity of skin infiltrates. Mod Pathol 7:771–778, 1994.

152. Sepp N, Radaszkiewicz T, Meijer CJ, et al: Specific skin manifestations in acute leukemia with monocytic differentiation. A morphologic and immunohistochemical study of 11 cases. Cancer 71:124–127, 1993.

153. Burgdorf WH: Malignant histiocytic infiltrates. In Murphy GF, Mihm MC Jr (eds): Lymphoproliferative Disorders of the Skin. Boston, Butterworth, 1986, pp 217–255.

154. Hashimoto K, Bale GF, Hawkins HK, et al: Congenital self-healing reticulohistiocytosis (Hashimoto-Pritzker type). Int J Dermatol 25:516–520, 1986.

155. Chu P, LeBoit PE: Histologic features of cutaneous sinus histiocytosis (Rosai-Dorfman disease): study of cases both with and without systemic involvement. J Cutan Pathol 19:201–211, 1992.

156. Suster S, Cartagener N, Cabello-Inchausti B, et al: Histiocytic lymphophagocytic panniculitis: an unusual presentation of sinus histiocytosis with massive lymphadenopathy. Arch Dermatol 124:1246–1249, 1988.

157. Roupe G: Urticaria pigmentosa and systemic mastocytosis. Semin Dermatol 6:334–341, 1987.

158. Hashimoto K, Bale GF: An electron microscopic study of balloon cell nevus. Cancer 30:530–540, 1972.

159. Wayte DM, Helwig EB: Halo nevi. Cancer 22:69–90, 1968.

160. Bergmann W, Willemze R, de Graaff-Reitsma C, Ruiter DJ: Analysis of major histocompatibility antigens and the mononuclear cell infiltrate in halo nevi. J Invest Dermatol 85:25–29, 1985.

161. Friedman RJ, Ackerman AB: Difficulties in the histologic diagnosis of melanocytic nevi on the vulvae of premenopausal women. In Ackerman AB (ed): Pathology of Malignant Melanoma. New York, Masson, 1981, pp 119–127.

162. Christensen WN, Friedman KJ, Woodruff JD, Hood AF: Histologic characteristics of vulvar nevocellular nevi. J Cutan Pathol 14:87–91, 1987.

163. Kornberg R, Ackerman AB: Pseudomelanoma. Arch Dermatol 111:1588–1590, 1975.

164. Suster S: Pseudomelanoma. A pathologist's perspective. Int J Dermatol 25:506–507, 1986.

165. Seab JA Jr, Graham JH, Helwig EB: Deep penetrating nevus. Am J Surg Pathol 13:39–44, 1989.

166. Hendrickson MR, Ross JC: Neoplasms arising in congenital giant nevi: morphologic study of seven cases and a review of the literature. Am J Surg Pathol 5:109–135, 1981.

167. Rhodes AR: Neoplasms: benign neoplasias, hyperplasias, and dysplasias of melanocytes. In Fitzpatrick TB, Eisen AZ, Wolff K, et al (eds): Dermatology in General Medicine. 4th ed. New York, McGraw-Hill, 1993, pp 1026–1037.

168. Mancianti ML, Clark WH, Hayes FA, Herlyn M: Malignant melanoma simulants arising in congenital melanocytic nevi do not show experimental evidence for a malignant phenotype. Am J Pathol 136:817–827, 1990.

169. Rhodes AR, Sober AJ, Day CL, et al: The malignant potential of small congenital nevocellular nevi: an estimate of association based on a histologic study of 234 primary cutaneous melanomas. J Am Acad Dermatol 6:230–241, 1982.

170. Spitz S: Melanomas of childhood. Am J Pathol 24:591–609, 1948.

171. Paniago-Pereira C, Maize C, Ackerman A: Nevus of large spindle and/or epithelioid cells (Spitz's nevus). Arch Dermatol 114:1811–1823, 1978.

172. Busam KJ, Barnhill RL: The spectrum of Spitz tumors. In Kirkham N, Lemoine NR (eds): Progress in Pathology. Vol 2. Edinburgh, Churchill Livingstone, 1995, pp 31–46.

173. Kamino H, Misheloff E, Ackerman AB, et al: Eosinophilic globules in Spitz's nevi: new findings and a diagnostic sign. Am J Surg Pathol 1:319–324, 1979.

174. Smith N: The pigmented spindle cell tumor of Reed: an underdiagnosed lesion. Semin Diagn Pathol 4:75–87, 1987.

175. Barnhill RL, Mihm MC Jr: Pigmented spindle cell nevus and its variants: distinction from melanoma. Br J Dermatol 121:717–726, 1989.

176. Barr R, Morales R, Graham J: Desmoplastic nevus: a distinct histologic variant of mixed spindle and epithelioid cell nevus. Cancer 46:557–564, 1980.

177. Suster S: Hyalinizing spindle and epithelioid cell nevus. Study of five cases of a distinctive variant of Spitz's nevus. Am J Dermatopathol 16:593–598, 1994.

178. Barnhill RL, Mihm MC Jr, Magro CM: Plexiform spindle cell naevus: a distinctive variant of plexiform melanocytic nevus. Histopathology 18:243–247, 1991.

179. Barnhill RL: The pathology of melanocytic nevi and malignant melanoma. Boston, Butterworth-Heinemann, 1995, pp 1–76.

180. Barnhill RL, Barnhill MA, Berwick M, Mihm MC Jr: The histologic spectrum of pigmented spindle cell nevus: a review of 120 cases with emphasis on atypical variants. Hum Pathol 22:52–58, 1991.

181. Smith K, Skelton H, Lupton G, Graham J: Spindle cell and epithelioid cell nevi with atypia and metastasis (malignant Spitz nevus). Am J Surg Pathol 13:931–939, 1989.

182. Leopold JG, Richards DB: The interrelationship of blue and common nevi. J Pathol Bacteriol 95:37–46, 1968.

183. Rodriguez HA, Ackerman LV: Cellular blue nevus: clinicopathologic study of forty-five cases. Cancer 21:393–405, 1968.

184. Merkow LP, Burt RC, Hayeslip DW, et al: A cellular and malignant blue nevus: a light and electron microscopic study. Cancer 24:888–896, 1969.

185. Mishima Y: Cellular blue nevus: melanogenic activity and malignant transformation. Arch Dermatol 101:104–110, 1970.

186. Fletcher V, Sagebiel RW: The combined nevus: mixed patterns of benign melanocytic lesions must be differentiated from malignant melanomas. In Ackerman AB (ed): Pathology of Malignant Melanoma. New York, Masson, 1981, pp 273–283.

187. Perez M, Suster S: Balloon cell change in cellular blue nevus. Am J Dermatopathol 21:181–184, 1999.

188. Michal M, Bumruk K, Skalova A: Myxoid change within cellular blue nevi: a diagnostic pitfall. Histopathology 20:527–530, 1992.

189. Temple-Camp CRE, Saxe N, King H: Benign and malignant cellular blue nevus: a clinicopathological study of 30 cases. Am J Dermatopathol 10:289–296, 1988.

190. Goldenhersh MA, Savin RC, Barnhill RL, Stenn KS: Malignant blue nevus. J Am Acad Dermatol 19:712–722, 1988.

191. Connely J, Smith JL Jr: Malignant blue nevus. Cancer 67:2653–2657, 1991.

192. Clark WH Jr, Reimer RR, Green M, et al: Origin of familiar melanomas from heritable melanocytic lesions. "The B-K mole syndrome." Arch Dermatol 114:732–738, 1978.

193. Bale SJ, Dracopoli NC, Tucker MA, et al: Mapping the gene for hereditary cutaneous malignant melanoma–dysplastic nevus to chromosome 1p. N Engl J Med 320:1367–1372, 1989.

194. Elder DE, Goldman LI, Goldman SC, et al: Dysplastic nevus syndrome: a phenotypic association of sporadic cutaneous melanoma. Cancer 46:1787–1794, 1980.

195. Holly EA, Kelly JW, Shpall SN, Chiu S-H: Number of melanocytic nevi as a risk factor for malignant melanoma. J Am Acad Dermatol 17:459–468, 1987.

196. NIH Consensus Conference: Precursors to malignant melanoma. JAMA 251:1864–1866, 1984.

197. NIH Consensus Development Panel on Early Melanoma: Diagnosis and treatment of early melanoma. JAMA 268:1314–1319, 1992.

198. Roush GC, Barnhill RL: Correlation of clinical pigmentary characteristics with histopathologically-confirmed dysplastic nevi in nonfamilial melanoma patients. Studies of melanocytic nevi IX. Br J Cancer 64:943–947, 1991.

199. Kelly JW, Crutcher WA, Sagebiel RW: Clinical diagnosis of dysplastic melanocytic nevi: a clinicopathological correlation. J Am Acad Dermatol 14:1044–1052, 1986.

200. Rhodes AR, Mihm MC Jr, Weinstock MA: Dysplastic melanocytic nevi: a reproducible histologic definition emphasizing cellular morphology. Mod Pathol 2:306–319, 1989.

201. Barnhill RL: Tumors of melanocytes. In Barnhill RL (ed): Textbook of Dermatopathology. New York, McGraw-Hill, 1998, pp 537–591.

202. Mihm MC Jr, Clark WH Jr, From L: The clinical diagnosis, classification and histogenetic concepts of the early stages of cutaneous melanoma. N Engl J Med 284:1078–1082, 1971.

203. Clark WH Jr, Elder DE, Guerry D IV, et al: A study of tumor progression: the precursor lesions of superficial spreading and nodular melanoma. Hum Pathol 15:1147–1165, 1984.

204. Clark WH Jr. A classification of malignant melanoma in man correlated with histogenesis and biologic behavior. In Advances in the Biology of the Skin. Vol VIII. New York, Pergamon Press, 1967, pp 621–647.

205. McGovern VJ, Mihm MC Jr, Bailly C, et al: The classification of malignant melanoma and its histologic reporting. Cancer 32:1446–1457, 1973.

206. Ackerman AB: Malignant melanoma: a unifying concept. Hum Pathol 11:591–595, 1980.

207. Weyers W, Euler M, Diaz-Cascajo C, et al: Classification of cutaneous malignant melanoma. A reassessment of histopathologic criteria for the distinction of different types. Cancer 86:288–299, 1999.

208. Clark WH Jr, From L, Bernardino EH, et al: Histogenesis and biologic behavior of primary human malignant melanoma of the skin. Cancer Res 29:705–727, 1969.

209. Breslow A: Thickness, cross-sectional areas and depth of invasion in the prognosis of cutaneous melanoma. Ann Surg 172:902–908, 1970.

210. Bagley FH, Cady B, Lee A, Legg MA: Changes in clinical presentation and management of malignant melanoma. Cancer 47:2126–2134, 1981.

211. Barnhill RL, Mihm MC Jr, Fitzpatrick TB, Sober AJ: Neoplasms: malignant melanoma. In Fitzpatrick TB, Eisen AZ, Wolff K, et al (eds): Dermatology in General Medicine. Vol 1. New York, McGraw-Hill, 1993, pp 1078–1115.

212. Mihm MC Jr, Fitzpatrick TB, Brown MM, et al: Early detection of primary cutaneous malignant melanoma: a color atlas. N Engl J Med 289:989–996, 1973.

213. Patterson RH, Helwig EB: Subungual malignant melanoma: a clinical-pathologic study. Cancer 46:2074–2087, 1980.

214. Clark WH Jr, Mihm MC Jr: Lentigo maligna and lentigo maligna melanoma. Am J Pathol 55:39–67, 1969.

215. McGovern VJ, Shaw HM, Milton GW, Farago GA: Is malignant melanoma arising in Hutchinson's melanotic freckle a separate disease entity? Histopathology 4:235–242, 1980.

216. Barnhill RL, Flotte T, Fleischli M, Perez-Atayde AR: Cutaneous melanoma and atypical Spitz tumors in childhood. Cancer 76:1833–1845, 1995.

217. Handfield-Jones SE, Smith NP: Malignant melanoma in childhood. Br J Dermatol 134:607–613, 1996.

218. Price NM, Rywlin AM, Ackerman AB: Histologic criteria for the diagnosis of superficial spreading malignant melanoma: formulated on the basis of proven metastatic lesions. Cancer 38:2434–2441, 1976.

219. Cook MG, Clarke TJ, Humphreys S, et al: The evaluation of diagnostic and prognostic criteria and the terminology of

thin cutaneous malignant melanoma by the CRC Melanoma Pathology Panel. Histopathology 28:497–512, 1996.

220. Barnhill RL, Mihm MC Jr: The histopathology of cutaneous malignant melanoma. Semin Diagn Pathol 10:47–75, 1993.

221. Rywlin AM: Malignant melanoma in-situ, precancerous melanosis, or atypical intraepidermal melanocytic proliferation. Am J Dermatopathol 6(suppl):97–99, 1984.

222. Ten Seldam R, Helwig E, Sobin L, et al: Histological typing of skin tumors. *In* International Histological Classification of Tumors. No. 12. Geneva, World Health Organization, 1974, pp 1–136.

223. Clark H Jr, Evans HL, Everett MA, et al: Early melanoma: histologic terms. Am J Dermatopathol 13:579–582, 1991.

224. Connelly J, Lattes R, Orr W: Desmoplastic malignant melanoma (a rare variant of spindle cell melanoma). Cancer 28: 914–936, 1971.

225. Reed RJ, Leonard DD: Neurotropic melanoma: a variant of desmoplastic melanoma. Am J Surg Pathol 3:301–311, 1979.

226. Carlson JA, Dickersin GR, Sober AJ, Barnhill RL: Desmoplastic neurotropic malignant melanoma: a clinicopathologic analysis of 28 cases. Cancer 75:478–494, 1994.

227. Skelton HG, Smith KJ, Laskin WB, et al: Desmoplastic malignant melanoma. J Am Acad Dermatol 32:717–725, 1995.

228. Jain S, Allen PW: Desmoplastic malignant melanoma and its variants: a study of 45 cases. Am J Surg Pathol 13:358–373, 1989.

229. Smithers BM, McLeod GR, Little JH: Desmoplastic, neural transforming and neurotropic melanoma: review of 45 cases. Aust N Z J Surg 60:967–972, 1990.

230. Anstey A, Cerio R, Ramnarain N, et al: Desmoplastic malignant melanoma: an immunocytochemical study of 25 cases. Am J Dermatopathol 16:14–22, 1994.

231. Kao GF, Helwig EB, Graham JH: Balloon cell malignant melanoma of the skin: a clinicopathologic study of 34 cases with histochemical, immunohistochemical, and ultrastructural observations. Cancer 69:2942–2952, 1992.

232. Muhlbauer JE, Margolis RJ, Mihm MC Jr, Reed RJ: Minimal deviation melanoma: a histologic variant of cutaneous malignant melanoma in its vertical growth phase. J Invest Dermatol 80(suppl):63–65, 1983.

233. Reed RJ: Minimal deviation melanoma. *In* Mihm MC Jr, Murphy GK, Kaufman N (eds): Pathobiology and Recognition of Malignant Melanoma. Baltimore, Williams & Wilkins, 1988, pp 110–152.

234. Wong T-Y, Suster S, Duncan LM, Mihm MC Jr: Nevoid melanoma: a clinicopathological study of seven cases of malignant melanoma mimicking spindle and epithelioid cell nevus and verrucous dermal nevus. Hum Pathol 26:171–179, 1995.

235. McNutt NS, Urmacher C, Hakimian R, et al: Nevoid malignant melanoma: morphologic patterns and immunohistochemical reactivity. J Cutan Pathol 22:502–517, 1995.

236. Suster S, Ronnen M, Bubis JJ: Verrucous pseudonevoid melanoma. J Surg Oncol 36:134–137, 1987.

237. Nakhleh RE, Wick MR, Rocamora A, et al: Morphologic diversity in malignant melanoma. Am J Clin Pathol 93:731–740, 1990.

238. Prieto VJ, Kanik A, Salob S, McNutt NS: Primary cutaneous myxoid melanoma: immunohistologic clues to a difficult diagnosis. J Am Acad Dermatol 30:335–339, 1994.

239. Reed RJ, Martin P: Variants of melanoma. Semin Cutan Med Surg 16:137–158, 1997.

240. Sheibani K, Battifora H: Signet-ring cell melanoma. A rare morphologic variant of malignant melanoma. Am J Surg Pathol 12:28–34, 1988.

241. Kang S, Barnhill RL, Mihm MC Jr, Sober AJ: Regression in malignant melanoma: an interobserver concordance study. J Cutan Pathol 20:126–129, 1993.

242. Barnhill RL, Fine J, Roush GC, Berwick M: Predicting five-year outcome from cutaneous melanoma in a population-based study. Cancer 78:427–432, 1996.

243. Clark WH Jr, Elder DE, Guerry D IV, et al: Model predicting survival in stage I melanoma based on tumor progression. J Natl Cancer Inst 81:1893–1904, 1989.

244. Balch CM, Soong S-J, Shaw HM, et al: An analysis of prognostic factors in 8500 patients with cutaneous melanoma. *In* Balch CM, Houghton AN, Milton GW, et al (eds): Cutaneous Melanoma. 2nd ed. Philadelphia, JB Lippincott, 1992, pp 165–187.

245. Balch CM, Soong S-J, Murad TM, et al: A multifactorial analysis of melanoma: III. Prognostic factors in melanoma patients with lymph node metastases (stage II). Ann Surg 193:377–379, 1981.

246. Ball NJ, Yohn JJ, Meorelli JG, et al: Ras mutations in human melanoma: a marker of malignant progression. J Invest Dermatol 102:285–290, 1994.

247. Castellano M, Pollock PM, Walters MK, et al: CDKN2A/P16 is inactivated in most melanoma cell lines. Cancer Res 57: 4869–4875, 1997.

248. Recommendations for the reporting of tissues removed as part of the surgical treatment of cutaneous melanoma. Mod Pathol 10:387–390, 1997.

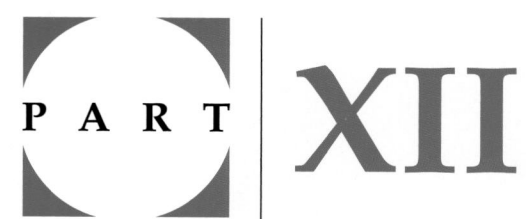

# PART XII

# Nervous System

# 50

# *Pituitary*

David R. Hinton   Sylvia L. Asa

## NEOPLASMS AND TUMORLIKE LESIONS

### Classification

Tumors of the pituitary region are common, accounting for about 15% of primary intracranial neoplasms that come to medical attention.[1, 2] The most frequent symptomatic tumor at this site is the pituitary adenoma; however, a wide spectrum of neoplastic and non-neoplastic lesions, including a variety of rare disorders, must be considered.[3, 4] Many of these lesions may clinically and radiologically mimic pituitary adenomas. The current World Health Organization (WHO) classification of central nervous system tumors recognizes under "Tumors of the Sellar Region" only tumors found primarily at this site, including pituitary adenoma, pituitary carcinoma, and craniopharyngioma and its variants.[5] The surgical pathologist who is confronted by a biopsy specimen from the sella requires a more complete differential of possible pathologic diagnoses; this is provided in the outline of this chapter. A detailed classification of pituitary adenomas is provided under that topic.

### Tissue Procurement

Transsphenoidal surgery has developed into an operation with relatively little morbidity and low mor-

tality; it is the route by which biopsy or excision of most sellar region lesions is done.[6] The specimens are often small and fragmented, providing, at times, a challenge to the skills of the surgical pathologist. Appropriate care in the processing of tissue must be taken to ensure the highest possible diagnostic yield. The value of pathologic intraoperative consultation for pituitary tumors has been the subject of a small number of reviews.[7–9] The indications (Table 50–1) vary from center to center, but intraoperative consultation is indicated to distinguish adenoma from other lesions, to identify an unexpected lesion, to determine whether margins are involved with tumor, and perhaps most important to ensure that tissue is appropriately divided and processed for accurate diagnosis.[3] When hormone hypersecretion is known and a pituitary tumor is identified on imaging studies, most surgeons do not believe it necessary to request intraoperative consultation. When hormone hypersecretion is present and no lesion is seen on imaging studies, as sometimes occurs in Cushing's disease, intraoperative touch or smear preparations by an experienced pathologist may help to identify the presence of a small microadenoma in one of several biopsy specimens; however, the lateralization of disease can be more reliably established by preoperative inferior petrosal sinus sampling.[10]

In general, the accuracy of frozen sections from the pituitary is lower than that from other sites,[7, 8] and because the damage to tissue caused by freezing

**TABLE 50–1.** Common Indications for Intraoperative Pathology Consultation in the Diagnosis of Pituitary Lesions

Appropriate division and processing of tissue for most accurate diagnosis
To confirm the presence of a pituitary adenoma
To distinguish pituitary adenoma from other lesions
To identify an unexpected lesion
To determine whether margins are involved with tumor

and thawing interferes with further analysis, frozen section analysis is not routinely recommended, especially when specimens are small. Cytologic smears and touch preparations stained with H&E are the methods of choice for the intraoperative assessment of most pituitary specimens.[9, 11] These methods provide a rapid and accurate means of identifying adenomatous tissue and most of the other lesions that enter the differential diagnosis and conserve tissue for paraffin embedding and electron microscopy. If the cytologic preparations are not adequate for diagnosis and the lesion is sufficiently large, frozen sections may occasionally be employed. This may be particularly useful when assessment of margins for tumor involvement has been requested.

# Tumors of Adenohypophysial Origin

## PITUITARY ADENOMA

### General Considerations

CLASSIFICATION. Endocrinologists, neurosurgeons, neuroradiologists, and pathologists have developed classification schemes to distinguish the various types of pituitary adenomas.

Functional classifications characterize tumors on the basis of in vivo hormone activity. Tumors may be divided into functional and nonfunctional categories. Functional tumors are classified with respect to clinical syndromes associated with excess prolactin (PRL), growth hormone (GH), thyroid-stimulating hormone (TSH), corticotropin, and rarely gonadotropins.[6]

Radiologic classifications rely on assessment of size and invasiveness. Originally proposed by Hardy,[12] this classification designates those tumors less than 10 mm as microadenomas and larger lesions as macroadenomas. The microadenomas are then divided into those that are intrasellar with a normal sellar appearance (grade 0) and those microadenomas that are noninvasive of bone but show focal sellar enlargement (grade I). The macroadenomas are divided into grades II to IV on the basis of the presence of diffuse sellar enlargement without bone erosion, focal erosion of the bony sella, and extensive erosion of skull base with involvement of extrasellar structures, respectively. The tumors are further classified according to the extent of suprasellar extension.

The histologic classification of pituitary adenomas based on the tinctorial characteristics of the tumor cells is no longer used; it has been replaced by classifications based on immunohistochemistry, which identifies hormone content, and electron microscopy, which identifies ultrastructural morphologic features. Classifying tumors on the basis of their major patterns of immunoreactivity is an approach that is easily accepted by most pathologists (Table 50–2). This approach may be augmented in the future by inclusion of other immunohistochemical markers as they become more widely available. For example, the family of tumors that shows major immunoreactivity with GH, PRL, or TSH also shows immunoreactivity with the pituitary-specific transcription factor Pit-1.[13] Similarly, those tumors with primary immunoreactivity for follicle-stimulating hormone (FSH)/luteinizing hormone (LH) react with antibodies against the transcription factor SF-1.[14] The addition of ultrastructural analysis provides another level of sophistication in classification schemes.[15] Electron microscopy allows definitive identification of the few tumor types that at present cannot be specifically identified by immunostaining.[3, 4]

Several attempts at formulating clinicopathologic classifications have been made. Thapar and Kovacs[4] divide pituitary adenomas into 17 distinct types on the basis of clinical presentations, immunohistochemical profile of major immunoreactivities, and ultrastructural characteristics. Kovacs and associates have further proposed a five-tier scheme including functional studies, imaging and surgical characteristics, histologic features (including invasiveness and concept of atypical adenoma), immunohistochemical features, and ultrastructural features; this scheme is under evaluation by the WHO.[16] Asa[3] has proposed a clinicopathologic classification that is practical, easily used, and consistent in organization with known cytodifferentiation pathways of adenohypophysial cells (Table 50–3). This classification is based primarily on clinical evidence of hormone hypersecre-

**TABLE 50–2.** Immunohistochemical Classification of Pituitary Adenomas

| Major Pattern of Immunoreactivity | Transcription Factors |
|---|---|
| GH cell adenoma (with and without cytokeratin-positive fibrous bodies) | Pit-1 |
| GH and PRL (mammosomatotroph adenoma) | Pit-1 |
| PRL cell adenoma | Pit-1 |
| PRL with GH reactivity (acidophil stem cell adenoma, confirm with electron microscopy) | Pit-1 |
| TSH cell adenoma (β-TSH and α-subunit) | Pit-1 |
| GH-, PRL-, and TSH-reactive adenomas | Pit-1 |
| FSH/LH cell adenoma (β-subunits and α-subunit) | SF-1 |
| Corticotropin cell adenoma | ? |
| Immunonegative tumors | ? |
| Unusual plurihormonal adenomas | ? |

tion and immunostaining profile, with selective ultrastructural analyses.

PATHOGENESIS. Pituitary adenomas are benign neoplasms that have been found to be monoclonal in virtually all cases that have been examined.[17] Because of the heterogeneity of adenoma subtypes, there is probably no single common etiologic event that defines the development of an adenoma.[18] Multiple molecular events are likely to be required that may vary according to the type of tumor formed. Early events are likely to be specific mutations, perhaps associated with oncogene activation or inactivation of tumor suppressor genes; however, most of these have yet to be defined. Mutations of the gene encoding the $\alpha$-subunit of the stimulatory guanosine triphosphate–binding protein $(G_s\alpha)$ result in the formation of the *gsp* oncogene and are found in some somatotroph[19] and nonfunctional adenomas.[20] Deletions of the multiple endocrine neoplasia gene (*MEN1*), a putative tumor suppressor gene, are found in pituitary adenomas in that disorder but in only about 5% of sporadic tumors,[21] and the gene is not downregulated by other mechanisms in these lesions.[22] Pituitary adenomas only rarely show mutations in *ras* and *p27/Kip1*,[23] and mutations are not seen in *TP53*,[24–26] *RB*,[27–29] or *c-erb*-B2/*neu*.[30] Subsequent dysregulated expression of hypothalamic trophic factors is probably critical in clonal expansion of the transformed cell.

Whereas the possibility that chronic stimulation of pituitary cells by hypothalamic hormones plays an initiating role in the development of certain adenomas has been argued, most evidence supports an important role of these hormones in tumor progression.[3, 18] Other growth factors and their receptors may also be dysregulated in adenomas, resulting in alterations in downstream signaling pathways regulating cell growth and differentiation. The factors implicated include insulin-like growth factor II, fi-

broblast growth factor (FGF) 4 (in lactotroph adenomas), basic FGF (FGF-2), FGF receptors, inhibins, activin and follistatin, and members of the epidermal growth factor family (transforming growth factor-$\alpha$, epidermal growth factor and its receptor).[31–37]

There has been interest in defining the genes regulating the aggressive behavior of invasive adenomas. The demonstration that increasing levels of invasive behavior are associated with increasing frequency of multiple allelic deletions suggests that invasive behavior is associated with progressive genetic changes.[38] Overexpression of p53 protein,[39] epidermal growth factor receptor,[37] FGF-2,[33] FGF-4,[32] a truncated form of FGF receptor-4,[224] and mutations in the $\alpha$-isozyme of protein kinase C[40] and a putative tumor suppressor gene at position 13q14[29] have been implicated. The genetic events involved in the rare progression of adenoma to carcinoma remain undetermined. Carcinomas may show prominent overexpression of p53 protein, and although transgenic mice with heterozygous deletions in *RB* gene develop pituitary carcinomas, loss of Rb expression is exceedingly rare in pituitary carcinoma.[29, 41] Point mutations in H-*ras* may be involved in the formation or growth of metastases in pituitary carcinoma.[42]

METHODS OF ASSESSMENT. In the routine assessment of pituitary adenoma, tissue should first be allocated appropriately. As indicated previously, touch or smear preparations are recommended in the intraoperative assessment to conserve the integrity of the small biopsy specimens.[9, 11] Fixation in neutral buffered formalin is recommended, with a small piece placed in 2.5% glutaraldehyde so that it is available for electron microscopy, if it is required. The H&E stain is used for routine histologic examination. Since the advent of immunocytochemistry, histochemical stains are not usually required except for the reticulin stain, which is essential in the analysis of tissue architecture, and the Congo red stain,

**TABLE 50–3.** Clinicopathologic Classification of Pituitary Adenomas

| Functioning Adenoma | Nonfunctioning Adenoma |
|---|---|
| **GH-PRL-TSH Family** | |
| Adenomas causing GH excess | Silent somatotroph adenoma |
|   Densely granulated somatotroph adenomas | |
|   Sparsely granulated somatotroph adenomas with fibrous bodies | |
|   Mammosomatotroph adenomas | |
| Adenomas causing hyperprolactinemia | Silent lactotroph adenoma |
|   Lactotroph adenomas | |
|   Lactotroph adenomas with GH reactivity (acidophil stem cell) | |
| Adenomas causing TSH excess | Silent thyrotroph adenoma |
|   Thyrotroph adenomas | |
| **Corticotropin Family** | |
| Adenomas causing corticotropin excess | Silent corticotroph adenomas |
|   Corticotroph adenoma | |
| **Gonadotropin Family** | |
| Adenomas causing gonadotropin excess | Silent gonadotroph adenoma |
|   Gonadotropin adenomas | Null cell adenoma |
| | Oncocytoma |
| **Unclassified Adenomas** | |
| Unusual plurihormonal adenomas | Hormone-negative adenomas |

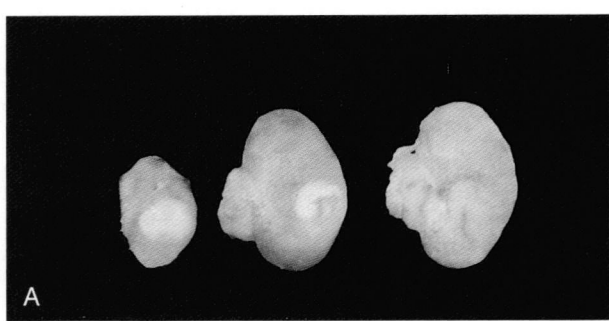

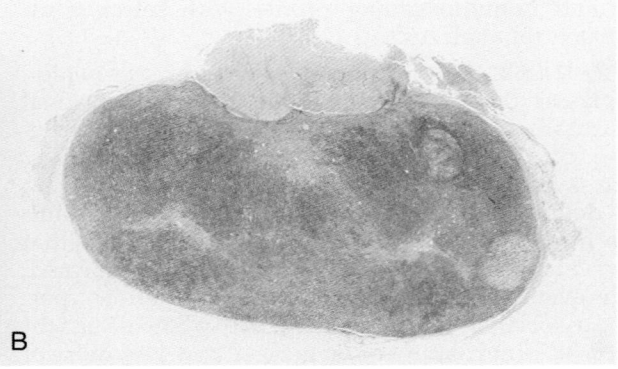

**Figure 50–1.** Microadenoma of the anterior pituitary gland. *A.* A gross photograph reveals a light-colored adenoma that contrasts with the yellow color of the adjacent anterior pituitary gland tissue. *B.* Horizontal section of a pituitary gland reveals the larger anterior lobe in apposition to the posterior lobe at the top of the figure; two small microadenomas are noted within the lateral lobe of the anterior pituitary. (Hematoxylin-phloxin-saffron.)

for the analysis of those rare tumors containing amyloid.

Immunohistochemistry for pituitary hormones is recommended in all primary pituitary adenomas.[3] This is required for appropriate classification of adenoma subtype. In particular, it allows the identification of endocrinologically silent but immunohistochemically positive adenomas. Such determinations may have prognostic importance by defining those adenoma subtypes with potential for aggressive behavior. Immunohistochemistry allows the pathologist to determine whether elevation of PRL in a patient with an adenoma is due to hormone secretion from the tumor or stalk compression with blockage of the normally inhibiting effect of dopamine.[43] It is also critical in the diagnosis of hyperplastic lesions, ectopic tumors, and the rare carcinoma. The availability of antisera against transcription factors adds a new dimension to the immunohistochemical analysis of these lesions. Staining for low-molecular-weight cytokeratins allows characterization of subtypes of adenomas and identification of Crooke's hyalinization that obviates the need for electron microscopy in most cases.

Electron microscopy has been a critical tool for the definition and classification of pituitary adenomas.[15] Although most adenomas do not require electron microscopy for appropriate classification and management, it does remain a necessary component in the analysis of a subset of tumors.[3] In particular, it is required for the accurate classification of the rare oncocytic tumors that have predominant PRL staining but may also contain GH, for the identification of many silent adenomas, and for the assessment of tumors in which the immunohistochemical pattern is unclear.

Molecular studies will most likely become an integral component of the analysis of pituitary tumors when the nature of the genes controlling pituitary tumorigenesis and growth is determined.[3] In situ hybridization studies may show evidence of hormone mRNA synthesis in rare tumors that are deficient in their ability to store detectable hormone. Immunohistochemical analysis of genes controlling cell growth (e.g., *TP53*) and analysis of growth fraction (e.g., MIB-1) and apoptosis have been reported in series of adenomas[39, 44, 45]; however, the practical value of applying these tools to the routine assessment of pituitary adenomas has not been established.

GENERAL CLINICAL FEATURES. Pituitary adenomas are common tumors. In selected autopsy series, up to 25% of pituitary glands will be found to harbor a small incidental microadenoma (Fig. 50–1).[46] The percentage of these tumors that become symptomatic is not known with certainty; increasing awareness probably accounts for the increase in annual incidence from 8.2 to 14.7 per 100,000 population during a period of 40 years.[47] Tumors of the pituitary usually become symptomatic because of overproduction of hypophysial hormones, decreased production of hypophysial hormones, local mass effect, or invasion of adjacent structures (Fig. 50–2 and Table 50–4). Symptomatic tumors are more fre-

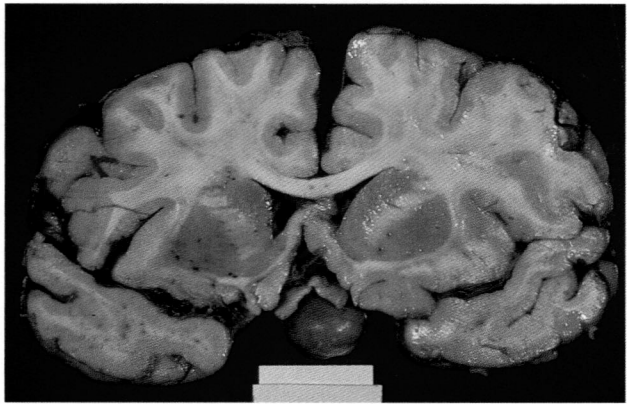

**Figure 50–2.** Coronal section of brain demonstrating suprasellar macroadenoma of pituitary compressing optic chiasm.

**TABLE 50–4.** Presentation of Pituitary Adenoma

**Hormone Excess**
| | |
|---|---|
| PRL | Amenorrhea-galactorrhea |
| GH | Acromegaly (adult) or gigantism (child) |
| Corticotropin | Cushing's disease |
| TSH | Secondary hyperthyroidism |

**Compression and Mass Effect**
| | |
|---|---|
| Pituitary stalk | Mild to moderate increase in PRL |
| Intrasellar | Hypopituitarism |
| Suprasellar | Optic chiasm: bitemporal hemianopia |
| | Hypothalamus: hypopituitarism; disruption of sleep, appetite |
| | Cerebrospinal fluid pathways: hydrocephalus |

**Invasion**
| | |
|---|---|
| Dura and bone | Cavernous sinus invasion with cranial nerve palsies |
| | Sphenoid sinus with local mass effect |
| | Skull base with local mass effect |

**Apoplexy**
| | |
|---|---|
| Acute infarction | Acute onset of headache, visual impairment, and ophthalmoplegia |
| | Alterations in consciousness |

quent in women, and they show an age-related incidence peak between the third and sixth decades; they are infrequent in childhood.[48] Prolactinomas (lactotroph adenoma) are the most common type of adenoma, making up about a third of surgical cases and half of incidental tumors. Next most common are the clinically nonfunctioning tumors, which together make up another third of symptomatic tumors. GH-secreting and corticotropin-secreting tumors each compose 10% to 15% of tumors; TSH-producing tumors are rare.[6]

GENERAL HISTOLOGIC FEATURES. In the histologic assessment of a pituitary tumor, one must first determine whether the appearance of the lesion is consistent with adenoma. In doing this, the lesion must be distinguished from normal structures of the sellar region, including anterior and posterior pituitary, as well as from other lesions that may mimic the appearance of these tumors, including hyperplasia. Distinguishing characteristics are shown in Table 50–5. The gross appearance of a pituitary adenoma is typically a soft pale or red-purple mass that contrasts with the firm yellow normal anterior pituitary (Fig. 50–1). On occasion, pituitary adenomas can also be firm or fibrotic. The major histologic features found in adenoma are loss of acinar architecture (best determined by use of reticulin stain), discohesiveness of cells (best seen on smear preparations), and cellular monomorphism (by H&E and immunostaining) (Figs. 50–3, 50–4, 50–5, and CD Fig. 50–1). The adenoma cells may grow in sheets, trabeculae, and papillae or form perivascular pseudorosettes. Cytologic examination reveals relatively uniform staining characteristics of the cytoplasm, variable pleomorphism and multinucleation (see Fig. 50–4) prominence of nucleoli, and occasionally mitotic activity. Some tumors contain microcalcifications or deposits of perivascular or stromal amyloid. Immunoperoxidase staining for pituitary hormones shows a distinctive pattern of predominant reactivity differing from the mixed population of adenohypophysial cells found in the normal gland. The distribution of cell types varies in the normal gland; corticotrophs are located primarily in median wedge, GH cells predominate in lateral lobe, PRL cells predominate in posterior lateral lobe, and gonadotrophs show diffuse distribution.[3, 4] Pituitary adenomas of different types show this same preferential pattern of intraglandular distribution, depending on their cell type of origin.

PROGNOSTIC FEATURES. There are currently no reliable histologic features that can distinguish a

**TABLE 50–5.** Features Distinguishing Normal Pituitary From Adenoma and Hyperplasia

| Method | Normal Pituitary | Adenoma | Hyperplasia |
|---|---|---|---|
| Gross appearance | Firm, yellow-tan gland | Soft pale tan-red mass (occasionally firm) | Nodular or diffuse enlargement of gland |
| Architecture and cytology | Acinar pattern with mixed population of cells | Lack of acinar structure; Sheetlike, papillary, or rosette pattern of growth; Monomorphic, discohesive, and variably pleomorphic cells; Mitotic figures rare | Expanded acini |
| Reticulin stain | Normal acini | Disrupted acinar structure | Expanded acini |
| Immunostains for pituitary hormones | Mixed population of adenohypophysial cell types (proportion varies with location in gland) | Distinctive patterns of predominant reactivity in monomorphic cells | Increased proportion of cells reactive for a specific cell type |
| Other features | Compression from adjacent adenoma; Crooke's hyaline in corticotrophs with hypercortisolemia | Microcalcifications in prolactinomas; Amyloid in some PRL- and GH-secreting tumors | |

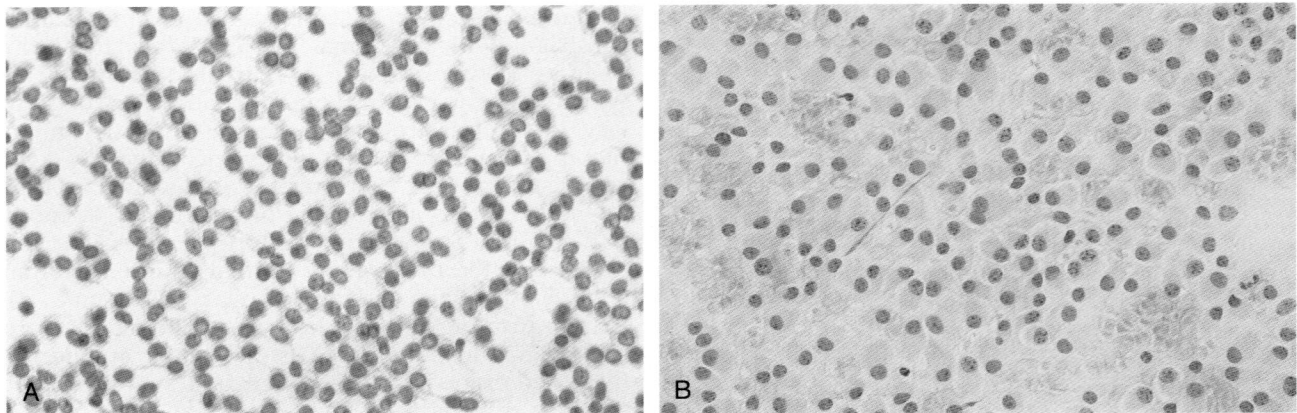

**Figure 50-3.** Smear preparations of fresh pituitary adenomas. Many tumors (*A*) are composed of discohesive, uniform nuclei, many of which have lost associated cytoplasm. In other adenomas (e.g., corticotroph adenoma shown in *B*), there is retention of cytoplasm with the nuclei. (H&E, magnification ×100.)

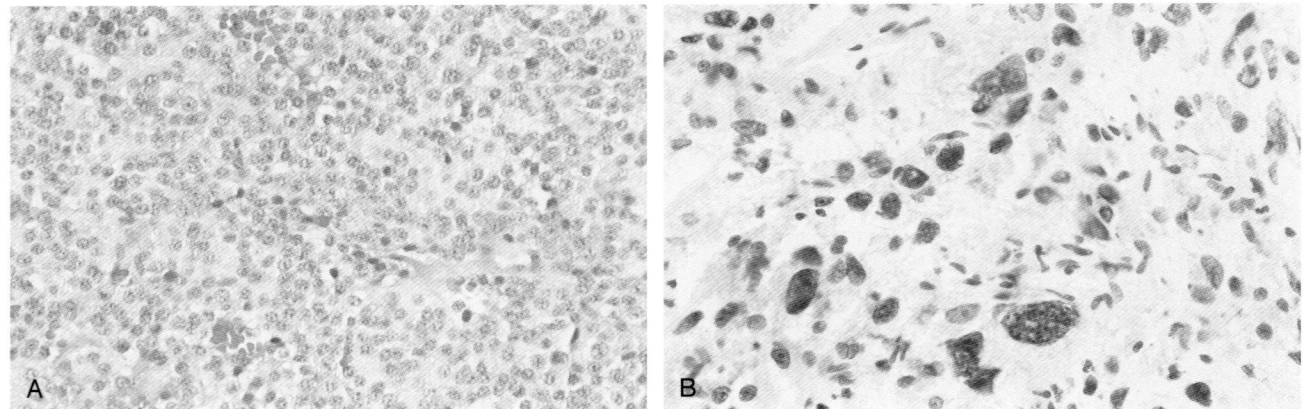

**Figure 50-4.** Nuclear pleomorphism in pituitary adenomas. Whereas many pituitary adenomas have uniform round to oval nuclei (*A*), other tumors show prominent nuclear pleomorphism (*B*). (H&E, magnification ×100.)

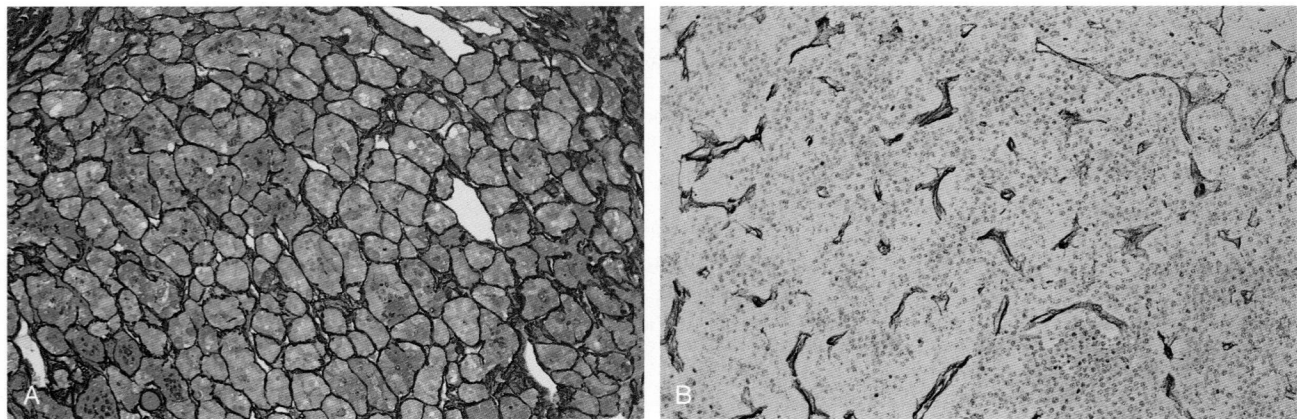

**Figure 50-5.** Reticulin stains in pituitary adenoma. *A.* In the normal anterior pituitary, reticulin clearly outlines the acini. *B.* In pituitary adenomas, there is loss of a reticulin framework. (Reticulin, magnification ×100.)

slowly growing pituitary adenoma from one that will have an aggressive and invasive course or even from one that will behave in a malignant manner. Invasive adenomas are defined by radiologic criteria or gross findings at surgery, whereas carcinoma is defined by the presence of metastasis. Microscopic invasion of dura is common, more frequent in macroadenomas, and is otherwise unrelated to prognosis.[49] Invasion of tumor into bone and adjacent sinuses indicates aggressive local disease but does not predict metastasis[50] (Fig. 50–6). Invasiveness is more common in macroadenomas than in microadenomas. It is also more common in some histologic subtypes, including silent corticotroph adenomas, thyrotroph adenomas, and acidophil stem cell adenomas.[3, 4] The presence of increased cellularity, nuclear pleomorphism, or atypia does not predict invasiveness.[11] Mitotic figures are infrequent in invasive tumors and are not typically valuable in predicting the behavior of a tumor.[11]

The possibility of predicting invasiveness or recurrence on the basis of immunohistochemical markers has been an area of investigation. The relationship between invasive growth of adenomas and an elevated growth fraction, as measured by labeling index for Ki-67 (MIB-1), is controversial.[11, 44, 51, 52] One study reported that although almost all noninvasive adenomas had a MIB-1 labeling index below 3%, there was a wide range of indices for invasive tumors, indicating that other factors must be involved.[44] The presence of nuclear p53 immunoreactivity has also been suggested to correlate with invasive growth,[39] but this has not been accepted by most investigators. Some authors have suggested that adenomas with elevated growth fraction and p53 labeling might be subclassified as atypical adenomas; however, the ability of these markers to independently predict increased invasiveness and recurrence in prospective studies has not yet been determined.

CONTENT OF REPORT FOR PITUITARY ADENOMA. For clinical correlation, the report for pituitary adenoma (Table 50–6) should state whether the current surgery is the original biopsy/resection or whether it is performed for recurrent disease. History of medical therapy for adenoma (e.g., dopamine agonists) should be obtained. Pituitary adenomas are classified in the context of clinical disease; therefore, it should be stated whether the tumor is functioning (producing excess pituitary hormone) or nonfunctioning. The endocrine syndrome associated with functioning tumors should be indicated. The size of tumor should be recorded on the basis of imaging studies. The presence and sites of radiologic or gross evidence of invasion should be noted.

The tumor samples are typically small and totally embedded in paraffin except for a small portion reserved for electron microscopy. Descriptions include the pattern of tumor growth, frequency of mitotic figures, and presence of features such as microcalcification or amyloid. The appearance of the reticulin pattern should be indicated. Indicate the presence of invaded, compressed, or normal adjacent anterior pituitary gland tissue and the presence or absence of Crooke's hyaline in corticotrophs. In-

 **TABLE 50–6. Contents of the Final Report: Pituitary Adenomas**

*Clinical Features*
Original biopsy or biopsy of recurrent lesion
Indicate whether patient is receiving medical therapy for inhibition of adenoma growth (e.g., dopamine or somatostatin agonists)
Nonfunctioning or functioning
  If functioning, indicate clinical syndrome (e.g., acromegaly)
Microadenoma (<10 mm) or macroadenoma (>10 mm on imaging study)
Radiologic or gross evidence of invasion
  If invasion, indicate structures invaded (e.g., cavernous sinus)

*Microscopic Features*
Pattern of growth
Reticulin pattern
Presence of microcalcification, amyloid, or frequent mitotic figures
Presence and appearance of adjacent pituitary gland tissue
Presence of Crooke's hyaline
Microscopic evidence of invasion including posterior pituitary, bone, nasal sinus
Oncocytic change

*Immunohistochemistry (all cases)*
Major and minor patterns of immunoreactivity for pituitary hormones
  Localization of immunoreactivity in cells (e.g., perinuclear)
Immunoreactivity for keratins and transcription factors
  Localization and patterns of keratin staining
(Labeling index for MIB-1, p53)—optional

*Electron Microscopy (in selected cases)*
Intracellular organelles (e.g., mitochondrial accumulation, oncocytic change)
Intracellular accumulation of filaments
Frequency, size and shape, and location (e.g., misplaced exocytosis) of secretory granules

*Diagnosis*
Classify tumor on basis of clinicopathologic features

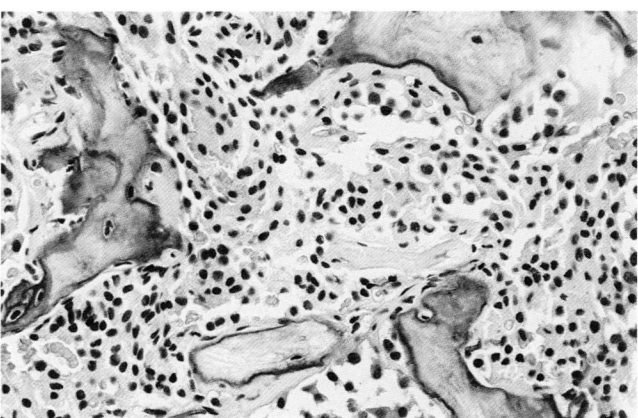
**Figure 50–6.** Invasive pituitary adenoma. This pituitary adenoma has invaded into and destroyed the bone of the adjacent sphenoid sinus. (H&E, magnification ×100.)

dicate whether microscopic evidence of invasion into bone or sinus tissues is present. If the patient was receiving medical therapy, the presence of associated histologic changes should be commented on. Immunoperoxidase studies should indicate the pattern and distribution of major and minor immunoreactivities of pituitary hormones as well as the pattern of cytokeratins. Electron microscopy is included in selected cases and should describe the cell's morphologic features, intracellular organelles, and secretory granules (abundance, morphologic features, and location).

### Adenomas Causing Excess Growth Hormone

CLINICAL CONSIDERATIONS. Chronic excess secretion of GH results in gigantism if epiphysial closure has not yet occurred or acromegaly after epiphysial closure. Acromegaly is phenotypically characterized by thickening of soft tissues of the face, prognathism, and acral enlargement; it may be complicated by diabetes mellitus, hypertension, carpal tunnel syndrome, and hypopituitarism.[53] Many of the biologic functions of GH are mediated by its stimulation of somatomedins, peptides also known as insulin-like growth factors. Patients with acromegaly, and particularly those with high post-treatment levels of GH, have increased incidence of colon cancer and higher mortality rate due to it.[54] Some patients have hyperprolactinemia and elevated blood levels of the $\alpha$-subunit of glycoprotein hormones, and occasional patients have clinical or subclinical TSH excess as a result of coexpression of these hormones by the tumor cells.[53]

DIAGNOSTIC AND IMMUNOHISTOCHEMICAL CONSIDERATIONS. GH-secreting adenomas are often detected when the tumor is small because of the prominent clinical effects of hormone excess. The microadenomas are typically located in the lateral wing of the gland. The clinical features are insidious, however, and the diagnosis is not infrequently delayed until the tumors present as macroadenomas with suprasellar extension or invasion.[53] GH-secreting tumors are derived from the mammosomatotroph line of differentiation and most contain immunoreactivity for Pit-1, the transcription factor that regulates differentiation of this line.[13] They may have trabecular, sinusoidal, or diffuse patterns of growth and may be acidophilic or chromophobic, depending on the density of secretory granules. They have been classified into three main groups on the basis of histologic, immunohistochemical, and ultrastructural characteristics.[3]

***Densely Granulated Somatotroph Adenoma.*** This is an acidophilic tumor that may grow in diffuse, sinusoidal, or trabecular patterns. Nuclear pleomorphism is mild to moderate. Most cells show strong immunoreactivity for GH in their cytoplasm (Fig. 50–7). Scattered cells may also show strong reactivity for glycoprotein hormone $\alpha$-subunit. Posi-

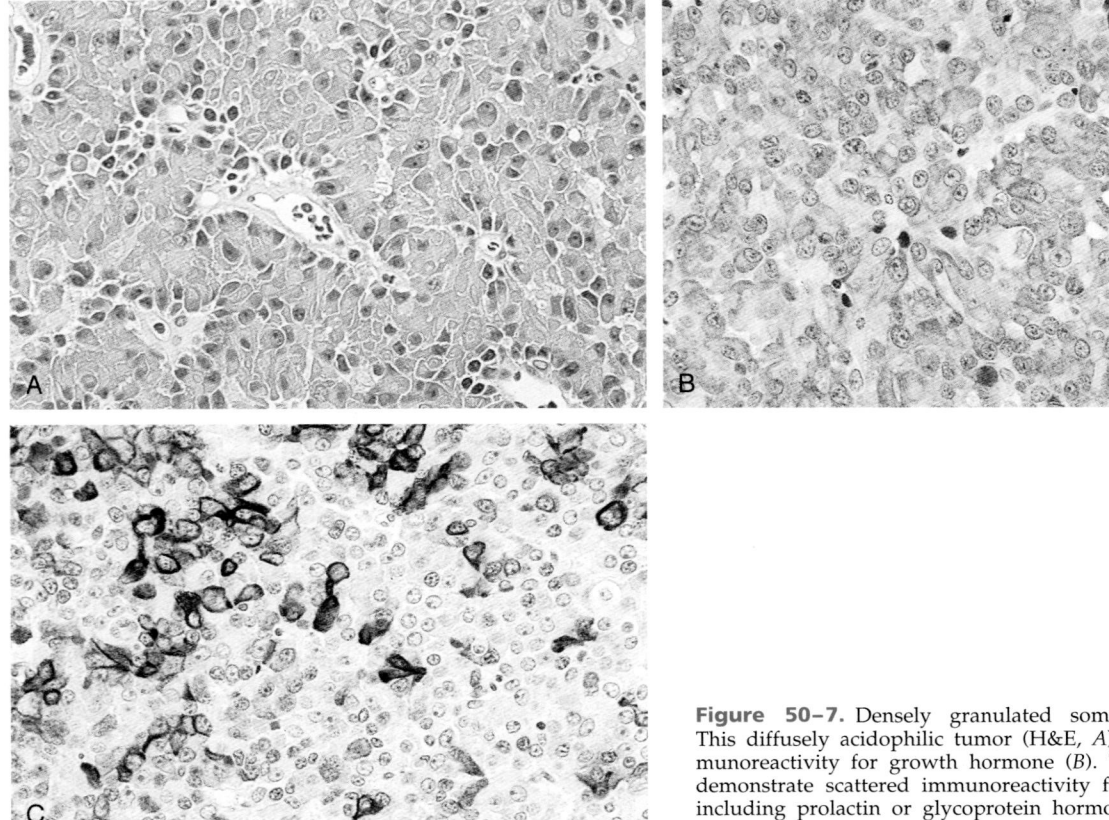

**Figure 50–7.** Densely granulated somatotroph adenoma. This diffusely acidophilic tumor (H&E, *A*) shows diffuse immunoreactivity for growth hormone (*B*). These tumors often demonstrate scattered immunoreactivity for other hormones, including prolactin or glycoprotein hormones such as $\alpha$-subunit shown here (*C*). (Magnification ×100.)

tivity for low-molecular-weight cytokeratins is often seen in a perinuclear location. Ultrastructural examination reveals well-developed endoplasmic reticulum, juxtanuclear Golgi complexes, and dense granulation (CD Fig. 50–2).

*Sparsely Granulated Somatotroph Adenoma.* This is a chromophobic tumor that grows in a diffuse pattern and typically is large at the time of presentation (Fig. 50–8). The tumor cells often show prominent nuclear pleomorphism, but this does not predict aggressive behavior. Immunoreactivity for GH is weak, focal, and often limited to the juxtanuclear region. These tumors demonstrate a characteristic cytoplasmic globular "fibrous body" that is strongly immunoreactive for low-molecular-weight cytokeratins. Ultrastructural examination reveals pleomorphic nuclei, variable prominence of endoplasmic reticulum, juxtanuclear accumulation of intermediate filaments (the fibrous body), and sparse small granules (CD Fig. 50–3).

*Mammosomatotroph Adenoma.* This acidophilic tumor contains interspersed chromophobic cells and grows in a solid or sinusoidal pattern. Cytoplasmic staining for GH is strong and diffuse; PRL staining is variable. Many tumors also show staining for α-subunit and on occasion staining for β-TSH. Perinuclear low-molecular-weight keratin staining is often seen. By electron microscopy, the tumors typically resemble densely granulated somatotroph adenomas but show increased and often striking pleomorphism in granule size, and the same cells also show "misplaced exocytosis," a feature characteristic of PRL secretion. On occasion, tumors composed of cells individually having features of GH and PRL secretion are identified.

DIFFERENTIAL DIAGNOSIS. The prominent nuclear pleomorphism found in sparsely granulated somatotroph adenomas may suggest the possibility of a pituitary carcinoma or metastatic tumor. Nuclear pleomorphism in an adenoma is not associated with increased aggressiveness, and pituitary carcinoma is diagnosed only by the presence of metastatic disease. Adenomas lack the increased mitotic rate and necrosis common in metastatic tumors and can easily be distinguished by immunohistochemistry. The rare hypothalamic gangliocytoma producing GH-releasing hormone (GRH) mixed with adenoma is identified by the presence of neuronal cells; they can be highlighted by immunostaining for neuronal markers (neurofilament, synaptophysin).[55, 56] Acro-

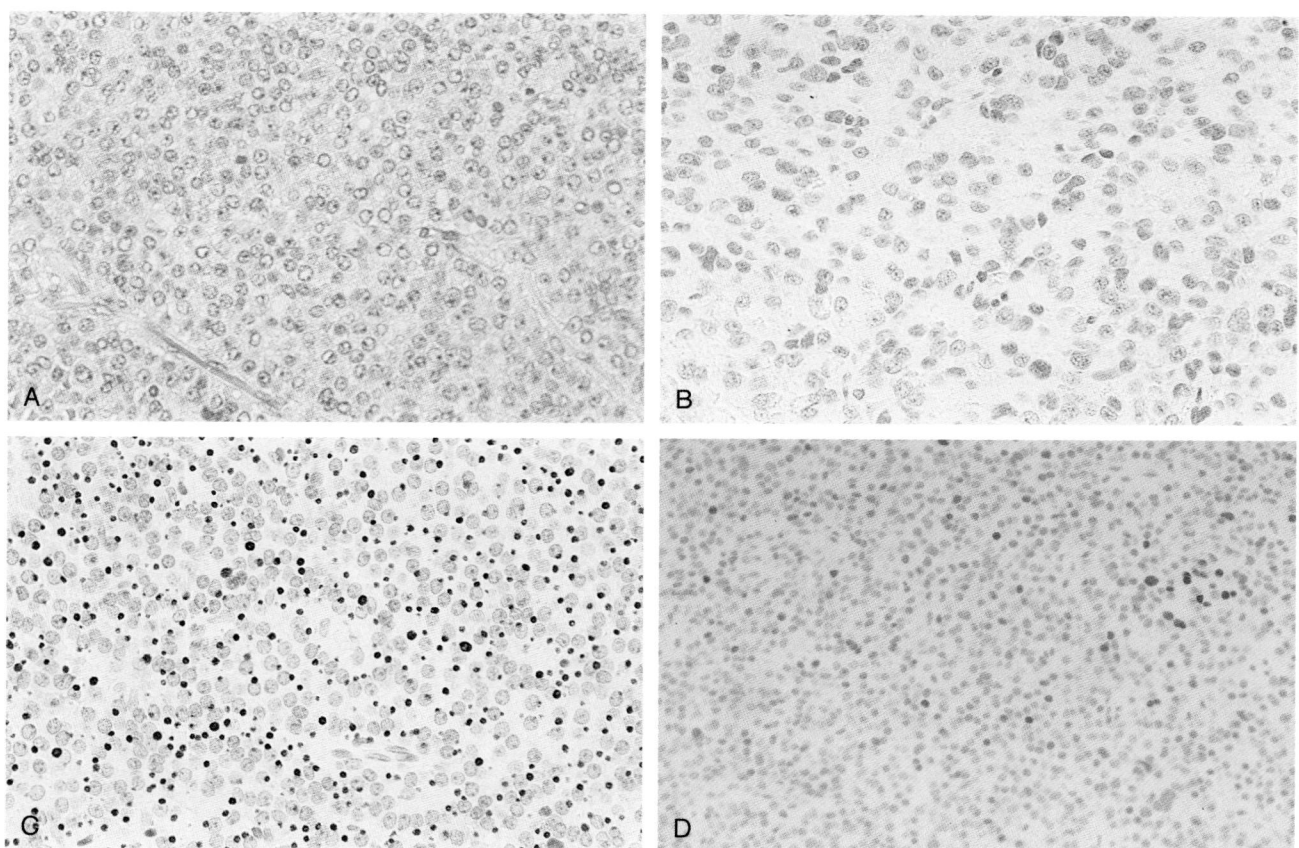

**Figure 50–8.** Sparsely granulated somatotroph adenoma. The tumor is often chromophobic (H&E, *A*). Immunoreactivity for growth hormone is usually scant (*B*). Fibrous bodies are clearly identified by their immunoreactivity for cytokeratin (*C*). Nuclear immunoreactivity for Pit-1 transcription factor is present (*D*). (Magnification ×100.)

megaly is rarely due to ectopic secretion of GRH; these patients usually have GH hyperplasia, but adenoma should be excluded.[57, 58]

### Adenomas Causing Excess Prolactin

CLINICAL CONSIDERATIONS. Secretion of excess PRL by lactotroph adenomas usually results in galactorrhea and ovulatory disorders in women and decreased libido and impotence in men. In the majority of patients who harbor well-differentiated sparsely granulated lactotroph adenomas, the tumor size correlates with serum level of PRL.[59] The primary mode of therapy for these tumors is medical (dopamine agonists); however, surgery is indicated for large tumors, for patients in whom medical therapy is ineffective or complicated by side effects, or by personal preference.[6, 59] Rarely, patients with PRL-secreting tumors will have a subtle form of acromegaly due to PRL and GH secretion from an unusual and particularly aggressive adenoma designated acidophil stem cell adenoma.[60]

DIAGNOSTIC AND IMMUNOHISTOCHEMICAL CONSIDERATIONS. PRL-secreting adenomas are often discovered as microadenomas in women and are more likely to be macroadenomas in men.[59] Microadenomas are more frequent in the posterolateral portion of the gland. Tumors may be gritty or calcified because of the presence of psammoma bodies.[61] These tumors may form amyloid; when this production is excessive, it may result in a caviar-like mass of amyloid spheres.[62] Adenomas with predominant excess secretion of PRL may be divided into three categories on the basis of light, immunostaining, and ultrastructural characteristics.[3, 4]

***Sparsely Granulated Lactotroph Adenoma.*** This is the most common form of lactotroph adenoma. It is composed of chromophobic cells with diffuse, papillary, or trabecular patterns of growth (Fig. 50–9). The stroma may be fibrotic, and the tumors occasionally contain calcified psammoma bodies. Some tumors produce endocrine amyloid that has been shown to be composed of a 4-kd proteolytic fragment of PRL.[62] The amyloid is identified by Congo red stain, and it may be focally deposited around vessels or form spherical masses (Fig. 50–10). Immunohistochemistry shows strong juxtanuclear, dot-like staining for PRL corresponding to the region of the Golgi complex. Nuclei stain for Pit-1[13] and may exhibit positivity for estrogen receptor.[63] On ultrastructural study, the tumor cells have prominent rough endoplasmic reticulum and well-developed Golgi complexes (CD Fig. 50–4). The sparse granules are spherical or occasionally pleomorphic; they are characteristically extruded into the extracellular space along the lateral cell borders, a feature known as misplaced exocytosis.[15]

***Densely Granulated Lactotroph Adenoma.*** This is a rare acidophilic tumor with strong, diffuse cytoplasmic immunoreactivity for PRL. On ultrastructural study, the tumor cells contain moderately well developed endoplasmic reticulum and Golgi complexes and numerous, spherical granules that may show misplaced exocytosis.

***Acidophil Stem Cell Adenoma.*** This rare tumor may manifest subtle clinical features of acromegaly along with typical features of PRL excess.[60] This oncocytic variant of PRL-producing adenoma is usually characterized by sheets of acidophilic cells. The acidophilia is due to mitochondrial accumulation; dilated mitochondria may also result in cytoplasmic vacuolization (Fig. 50–11). Immunohistochemistry reveals prominent PRL staining, which is variable in intensity but usually diffuse in nature. GH staining is weak or absent. Low-molecular-weight keratin focally accumulates to form globular fibrous bodies. Ultrastructural analysis may be needed to confirm the diagnosis.[15] The cells have moderately developed endoplasmic reticulum and Golgi regions and numerous, enlarged mitochondria (CD Fig. 50–5). Juxtanuclear accumulations of intermediate filaments (fibrous bodies) are present. The scant, small secretory granules show misplaced exocytosis.

DIFFERENTIAL DIAGNOSIS. There are numerous causes of an elevated PRL level, including stalk

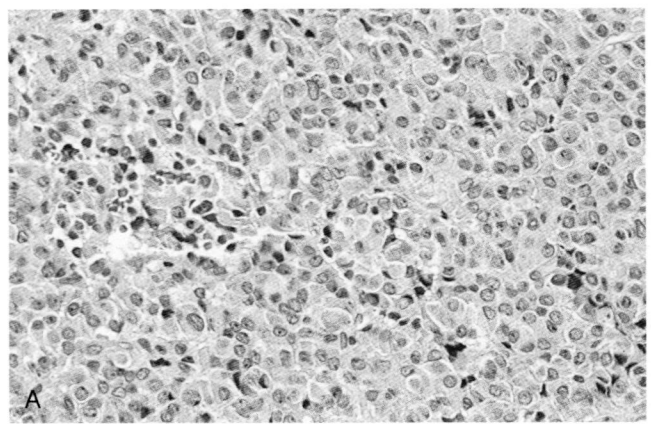 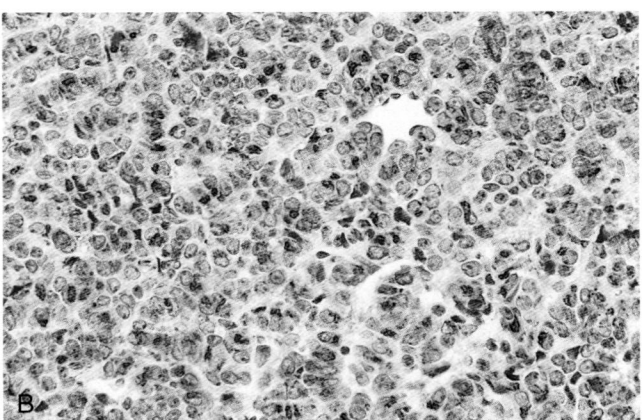

**Figure 50–9.** Sparsely granulated lactotroph adenoma. This typically chromophobic tumor (H&E, *A*) shows characteristic paranuclear immunoreactivity for prolactin (*B*). (Magnification × 100.)

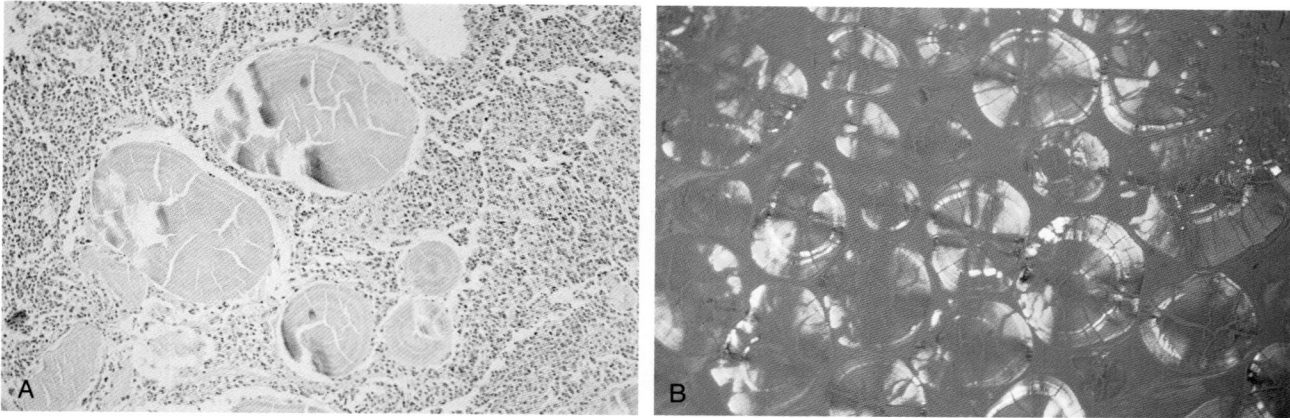

**Figure 50–10.** Amyloid deposited in a lactotroph adenoma. The extracellular, laminated bodies are strongly positive with Congo red stain (*A*). Characteristic birefringence is seen when the Congo red–stained section is viewed with polarized light (*B*). (Magnification ×100.)

compression by large adenomas or other lesions, drug therapy (e.g., phenothiazines, cimetidine), and hypothyroidism.[64] The elevated serum PRL level due to stalk effect from a non–PRL-secreting adenoma is usually relatively low and is not commensurate with the typically large size of the tumor.[43] Establishing that the resected tumor is causing the excess PRL requires proof that the lesion is an adenoma and is immunoreactive for PRL. Lactotroph or thyrotroph hyperplasia may also increase PRL and cause a pituitary mass lesion; distinction is by reticulin stain.[65, 66] PRL immunoreactivity may also be seen in some plurihormonal adenomas causing GH excess.

### Adenomas Causing Excess Thyrotropin

CLINICAL CONSIDERATIONS. This rare disorder represents less than 1% of pituitary adenomas.[6, 66] Chronic excess secretion of thyrotropin (TSH) from a pituitary adenoma results in hyperthyroidism, usually in association with a diffuse goiter; however, pituitary TSH-producing adenomas may be associated with euthyroidism or even hypothyroidism. In exceptional cases, TSH-producing adenomas may develop on the background of TSH cell hyperplasia in patients with long-standing primary hypothyroidism.[67]

DIAGNOSTIC AND IMMUNOHISTOCHEMICAL CONSIDERATIONS. These rare tumors are often large and invasive at the time of presentation. They are chromophobic tumors that grow in a diffuse or sinusoidal pattern and often show nuclear pleomorphism. Microcalcifications may be seen. Variable immunoreactivity for β-TSH and α-subunit is present.[3, 4] On ultrastructural analysis, the tumor cells are often elongated with eccentric nuclei. There is prominent rough endoplasmic reticulum and Golgi complexes and variable numbers of small, spherical granules that generally accumulate at the cell membrane and in the cell processes.[15]

DIFFERENTIAL DIAGNOSIS. It is crucial to distinguish TSH hyperplasia from adenoma; the role of reticulin staining cannot be overemphasized. Patients with mammosomatotroph adenomas may also develop hyperthyroidism and show weak immuno-

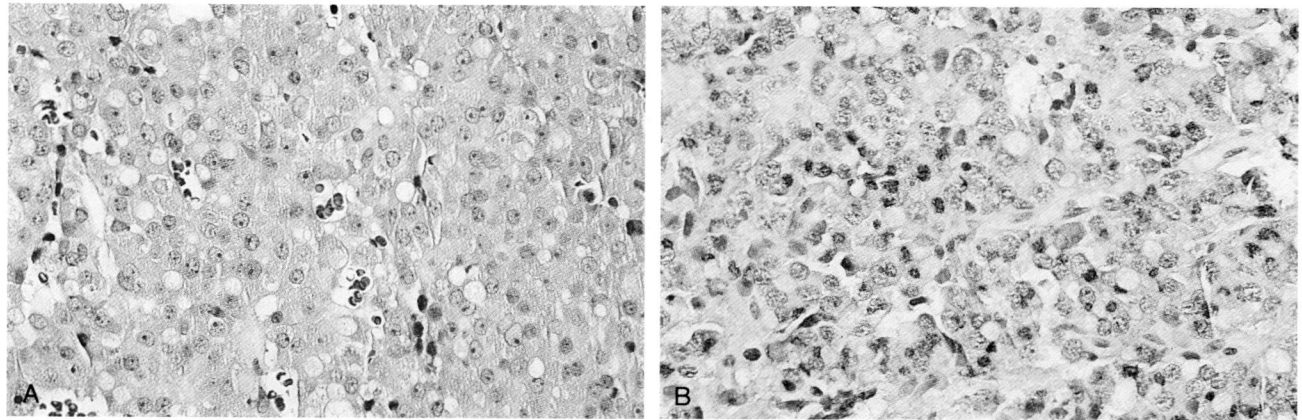

**Figure 50–11.** Acidophil stem cell adenoma. This usually chromophobic tumor often shows cytoplasmic vacuolization (H&E, *A*) and typically shows strong immunoreactivity for prolactin (*B*). (Magnification ×100.)

staining for TSH; however, these tumors also show positivity for GH and PRL.

### Adenomas Causing Excess Corticotropin

CLINICAL CONSIDERATIONS. Chronic excess secretion of cortisol results in Cushing's syndrome, a disorder characterized by central obesity, moon-shaped facies, hirsutism, acne, hypertension, muscle weakness, and mental disorders.[68] About two thirds of these cases are due to Cushing's disease, which represents hypercortisolism due to excess production of corticotropin by the pituitary. Patients with Cushing's disease have an elevated or high-normal corticotropin level in the context of cortisol excess. Nelson's syndrome occurs when a patient with a corticotropin-secreting pituitary adenoma is treated with bilateral adrenalectomy; the pituitary adenoma grows in the absence of hypercortisolemia, and the patient develops prominent hyperpigmentation of the skin because of associated secretion of melanocyte-stimulating hormone.[68] Most patients with Cushing's disease present when the tumors are small; in some cases, they may not be clearly detectable even by magnetic resonance imaging. Measurement of corticotropin in selective venous samples from the inferior petrosal sinus may then be used to determine the presence and laterality of a small microadenoma.[10]

DIAGNOSTIC AND IMMUNOHISTOCHEMICAL CONSIDERATIONS. Ninety percent of corticotropin-secreting adenomas are microadenomas. They can be localized in the median wedge of the gland but are usually lateralized to one side. Patients with Nelson's syndrome or sparsely granulated tumors may have macroadenomas.[68] Microscopic, immunohistochemical, and ultrastructural features divide these tumors into two types.[3, 4] If a biopsy specimen of the adjacent anterior pituitary gland is obtained in patients with Cushing's disease, the nontumorous corticotrophs exhibit massive perinuclear accumula-tion of low-molecular-weight cytokeratin in response to the hypercortisolemia, a phenomenon known as Crooke's hyaline change[69, 70] (Fig. 50–12). However, this is only an indication of glucocorticoid excess and is also seen with exogenous glucocorticoid administration, primary adrenal hypercortisolemia, and the ectopic corticotropin syndrome. A corticotroph adenoma may rarely develop prominent Crooke's change in the adenoma cells and is known as a Crooke's cell adenoma.[71]

***Densely Granulated Corticotroph Adenoma.*** Typically found as a cause of Cushing's disease, this basophilic tumor is usually a microadenoma with sinusoidal architecture (Fig. 50–13). The tumor cells stain positively with periodic acid–Schiff (PAS). Immunostaining reveals varying degrees of diffuse positivity for corticotropin, which is often accentuated in the periphery of the cell. There is also strong, diffuse positivity for low-molecular-weight cytokeratin; because keratins accumulate in corticotrophs in response to hypercortisolism, keratin staining is weak or undetectable in tumors from patients with Nelson's syndrome. Ultrastructural analysis reveals well-developed rough endoplasmic reticulum, prominent Golgi complexes, and numerous granules that vary considerably in size, shape, and electron density (CD Fig. 50–6). Some granules have a teardrop shape. Bundles of intermediate filaments are seen around the nucleus corresponding to the keratin identified by immunostaining.[15]

***Sparsely Granulated Corticotroph Adenoma.*** This rare, chromophobic, typically large tumor is composed of cells with a diffuse architecture. PAS stain is negative or weakly positive. Immunostaining for corticotropin is faint; however, keratin staining is strong. Electron microscopy reveals poorly developed organelles with scant, small, pleomorphic secretory granules and sparse accumulations of intermediate filaments.

DIFFERENTIAL DIAGNOSIS. The pathologist may be asked to determine whether a small microade-

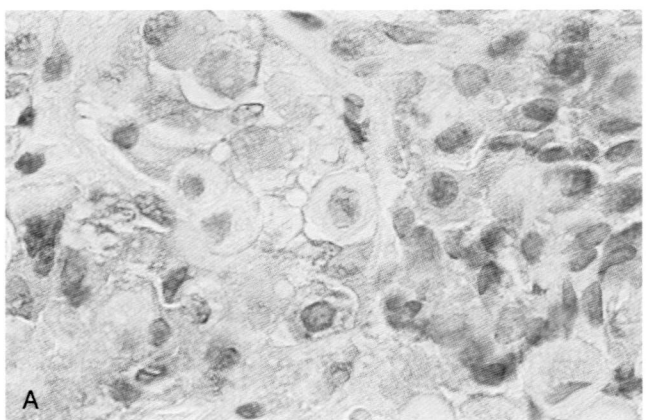
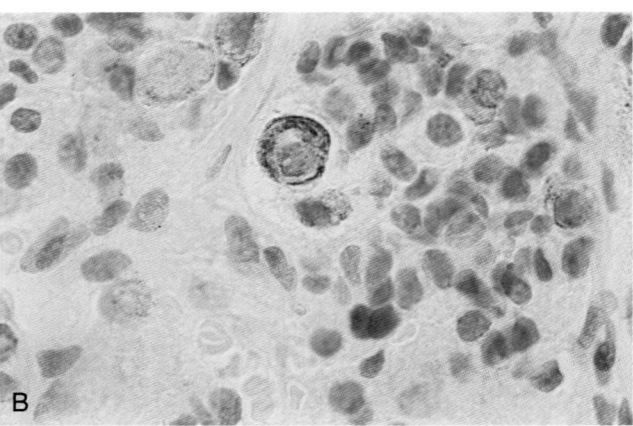

**Figure 50–12.** Crooke's hyaline change. Perinuclear hyaline material accumulates in nontumorous corticotrophs in the presence of hypercortisolemia (H&E, *A*). Immunoperoxidase staining reveals that Crooke's hyaline is composed of cytokeratin filaments (*B*). (Magnification ×100.)

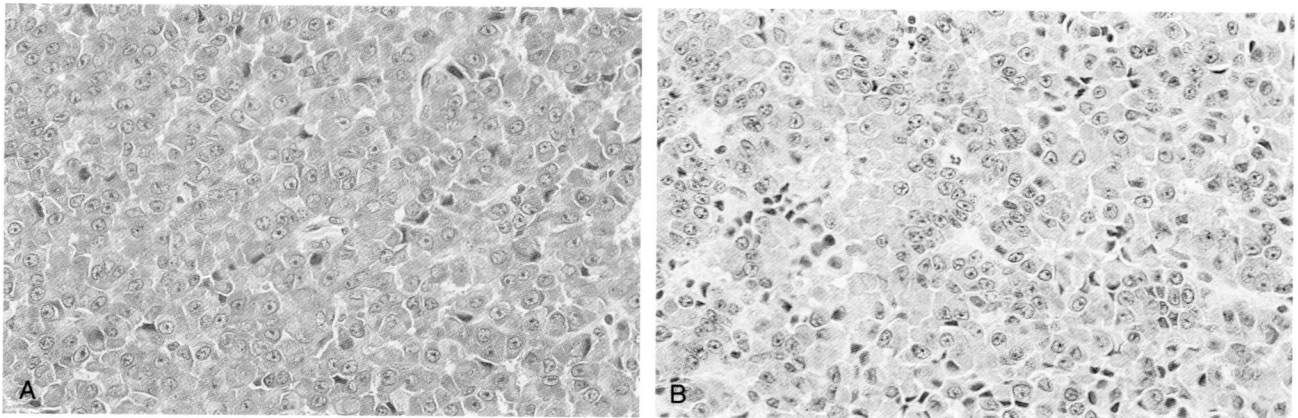

**Figure 50–13.** Densely granulated corticotroph adenoma. This tumor is typically basophilic (H&E, A) and shows diffuse immunoreactivity for corticotropin (B). (Magnification ×100.)

noma is present in one of several biopsy specimens from different regions of the gland when the neurosurgeon is unsure of the location of the tumor. Careful assessment of touch preparations may be essential so that the diagnosis can be made and tissue retained for reticulin staining and immunohistochemical studies. In a biopsy specimen from posterior pituitary, it is important not to misinterpret the presence of non-neoplastic corticotrophs that may normally be present in about 30% of pituitary glands at this site, a finding termed basophil invasion.[72] Primary corticotroph hyperplasia can cause Cushing's disease; the diagnosis relies on reticulin staining and prominence of corticotropin-immunoreactive cells. Ectopic sources of corticotropin-releasing hormone (CRH) may be associated with hyperplasia that can mimic adenoma. The development of prominent Crooke's change in a corticotroph adenoma can result in cells with hyperchromatic nuclei and a markedly atypical appearance that could suggest metastatic carcinoma or gangliocytoma. Immunostaining of a Crooke's cell adenoma shows strong positivity of tumor cells for keratin and weak corticotropin staining at the periphery of the tumor cells.[71]

### Adenomas Causing Excess Gonadotropin

CLINICAL CONSIDERATIONS. These patients typically present in middle age with mass effect due to large pituitary tumors, less frequently with gonadal dysfunction, and rarely with signs of gonadotropin excess. Suprasellar extension often leads to chiasmal compression with visual loss. The diagnosis in male patients is usually made when a nonfunctioning adenoma is suspected and biochemical studies reveal evidence of gonadotropin excess. The tumor is more difficult to diagnose in women because of physiologically elevated gonadotropins occurring in association with menopause. The diagnosis requires the demonstration of increased serum levels of FSH, LH, or both. Sometimes the $\alpha$- and $\beta$-subunits of these

glycoprotein hormones can circulate as free subunits.[73]

DIAGNOSTIC AND IMMUNOHISTOCHEMICAL CONSIDERATIONS. These tumors are usually large and vascular. The tumor cells grow in a sinusoidal, trabecular, or papillary pattern, and perivascular pseudorosette formation is often prominent (Fig. 50–14). Focal oncocytic change may be present. Immunostaining reveals focal positivity for $\beta$-FSH, $\beta$-LH, and $\alpha$-subunit.[3, 4] Nuclear staining for the steroidogenic transcription factor SF-1 is usually prominent.[14] Ultrastructural assessment reveals cellular heterogeneity with polar, round, and polygonal cells. Rough endoplasmic reticulum and Golgi complexes are often prominent, and secretory granules are variable in number, small, and localized at the end of the cell away from the nucleus (CD Fig. 50–7). Numerous dilated mitochondria correlate with the presence of oncocytic change.[15]

DIFFERENTIAL DIAGNOSIS. Immunostaining of densely granulated somatotroph, mammosomatotroph, and thyrotroph adenomas may also show $\alpha$-subunit, but staining for the FSH and LH $\beta$-subunits is lacking. Silent gonadotroph adenomas, which lack elevated serum levels of FSH and LH, may be morphologically indistinguishable from functional gonadotroph adenomas.[3]

### Clinically Nonfunctioning Adenomas

CLINICAL CONSIDERATIONS. These common adenomas are large because they usually do not present until they cause symptoms due to mass effect. Suprasellar extension with headache and chiasmal compression is common, and invasion into sphenoid sinus or cavernous sinus with local mass effect and cranial nerve palsies can occur. Some patients present suddenly with apoplexy due to acute tumor infarction. Biochemical evidence of hormone hypersecretion is not typically present except for mild hyperprolactinemia secondary to stalk com-

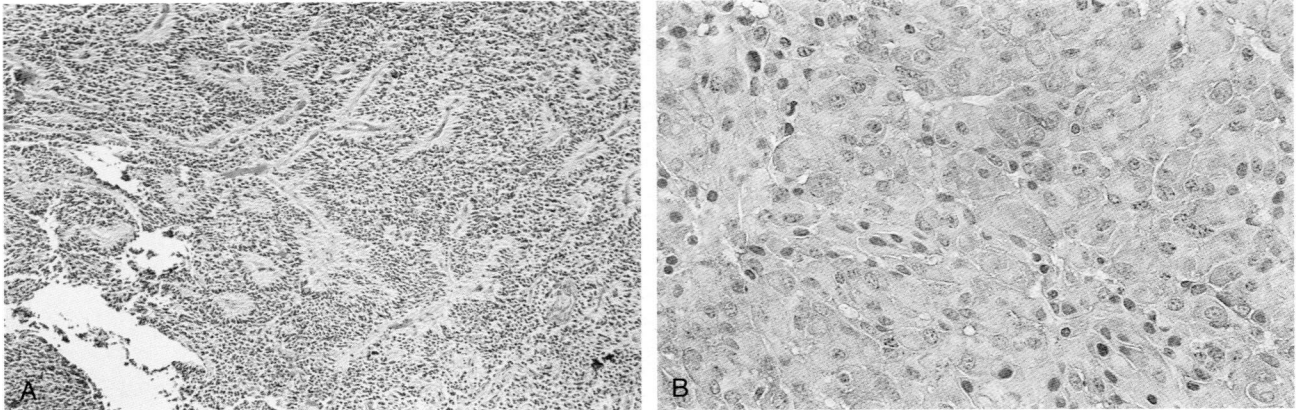

**Figure 50–14.** Gonadotroph adenoma. *A.* This chromophobic tumor often shows prominent perivascular pseudorosette formation. (H&E, magnification ×25.) *B.* Diffuse immunoreactivity for FSH is present. (Magnification ×100.)

pression, but hypopituitarism may occur. Some patients have elevated serum α-subunit.[3, 73]

DIAGNOSTIC AND IMMUNOHISTOCHEMICAL CONSIDERATIONS. These heterogeneous tumors have a wide range of morphologic appearances.

***Silent Somatotroph, Lactotroph, or Thyrotroph Adenomas.*** These rarely diagnosed tumors have the microscopic and ultrastructural appearance of their functional counterparts but are clinically silent. Some of these tumors may produce a biologically inactive hormone.[74, 75]

***Silent Corticotroph Adenoma.*** This tumor shows immunopositivity for corticotropin but is not associated with Cushing's syndrome. The clinical silence may be due to abnormal cleavage of the pro-opiomelanocortin molecule that is the precursor of corticotropin.[76] Type I adenomas are histologically and ultrastructurally indistinguishable from functional, densely granulated corticotroph adenomas with strong corticotropin and keratin immunoreactivity. They are important to recognize because they behave aggressively and tend to recur. A high percentage of these tumors (40%) present with hemorrhagic infarction.[4] Type II tumors are large macroadenomas that resemble the rare chromophobic corticotroph adenoma and stain for corticotropin. An unusual silent composite tumor has been described in a small number of young patients. This tumor is composed of pituitary adenoma cells strongly immunoreactive for corticotropin with interspersed cells showing ultrastructural and immunocytochemical features typical of adrenal cortical cells.[77]

***Silent Gonadotroph Adenoma.*** Many of these common tumors are indistinguishable from those that are diagnosed with clinical and biochemical findings. Others were previously categorized as null cell adenomas and oncocytomas. These chromophobic tumors usually show diffuse growth with focal trabecular or papillary patterning and perivascular pseudorosette formation. Oncocytic change is common, and when it is prominent, the tumor is called an oncocytoma (Fig. 50–15). Careful review of immunostains shows focal positivity for β-FSH, β-LH,

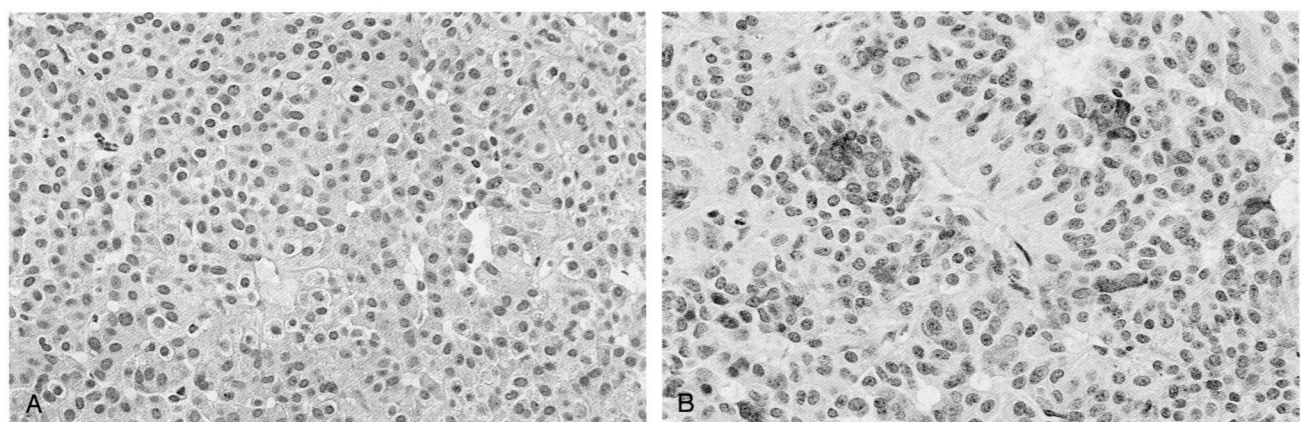

**Figure 50–15.** Oncocytoma. These weakly acidophilic tumors (H&E, *A*) have abundant cytoplasm and often show focal immunoreactivity for glycoprotein hormones such as FSH (*B*). (Magnification ×100.)

or α-subunit as well as for SF-1.[14, 73] Ultrastructural analysis reveals small cells with poorly developed organelles, sparse small secretory granules, and variable numbers of mitochondria (CD Fig. 50–8); in oncocytic tumors (CD Fig. 50–9), mitochondria may occupy up to 50% of cytoplasmic volume.[78] An unusual tumor that only rarely contains gonadotropins and may contain corticotropin-like material is the "female type of gonadotroph adenoma," a tumor that is reported to occur only in women. These tumors have a distinctive ultrastructural appearance with a honeycomb Golgi complex and sparse secretory granules.[3, 4]

DIFFERENTIAL DIAGNOSIS. Clinical information is required to appropriately separate these tumors from their clinically functional correlates. The differential diagnosis of clinically nonfunctioning pituitary adenoma includes various other hormonally inactive lesions that can occur in the sella, such as meningioma, and inflammatory lesions (see later).

### Plurihormonal Adenomas

Tumors coexpressing GH and PRL are well-recognized causes of acromegaly, gigantism, and hyperprolactinemia and are described in those sections of the chapter. α-Subunit and TSH are also coexpressed by some GH tumors. There are a number of tumors in which unusual combinations of hormones are found; these immunoreactivities are often silent and recognized only by immunohistochemistry.[3, 4, 79] One of these tumors has been designated the silent subtype III adenoma. In women, it may present with hyperprolactinemia, but it does not shrink in response to dopamine agonist therapy. In men, most tumors are macroadenomas. Rare tumors present with acromegaly. These tumors show diffuse growth and focal immunoreactivity for one or a number of pituitary hormones including GH, PRL, and corticotropin. Ultrastructural examination reveals characteristic nuclear inclusions, the sphaeridia, as well as sparse secretory granules in cell processes and interdigitating cell processes[15, 80] (CD Fig. 50–10).

### Ectopic Adenomas

Ectopic adenohypophysial tissue is commonly found within the sphenoid bone or adjacent structures along the path of the developing Rathke cleft.[81] Anterior lobe cells may also be seen in a suprasellar location attached to the supradiaphragmatic pituitary stalk.[82] These ectopic tissues may rarely be the site of origin of ectopic pituitary adenomas. The most common location for these tumors is the sphenoid sinus; less frequently, they may occur in a suprasellar location or even more rarely in petrous temporal bone, clivus, or third ventricle. Both functional and nonfunctional tumors have been described. Nonfunctional tumors may present with local mass effect. Careful immunohistochemical analysis and electron microscopy are often needed to determine the correct diagnosis.[81]

### Apoplexy in Pituitary Adenoma

CLINICAL CONSIDERATIONS. Pituitary apoplexy is defined by the sudden onset of headache, visual deficit, ophthalmoplegia, or altered mental status caused by hemorrhage or infarction of the pituitary gland. It occurs most frequently within large pituitary adenomas and only rarely in the nonadenomatous gland. In most patients, apoplexy is the first presentation of the adenoma. Approximately 1% to 2% of pituitary adenomas present in this manner.[83, 84]

DIAGNOSTIC CONSIDERATIONS. The mechanism of apoplexy has been considered by most authors to be acute hemorrhagic infarction. A study of 15 cases found that apoplexy may also be a consequence of nonhemorrhagic infarction and acute hemorrhage alone.[84] On histologic examination, the specimens removed during surgical decompression are composed of necrotic tumor, with or without acute hemorrhage (Fig. 50–16). The structure of the tumor is often retained and can be highlighted with the reticulin stain. On cytologic evaluation, only "ghosts" of the neoplastic cells remain, although focal clumps of apparently viable tumor are often seen. In cases in which surgery is delayed, biopsy specimens may show lymphocytic infiltration and replacement by granulation tissue.[84] Infarction of a pituitary adenoma has been proposed as one of the mechanisms for development of empty sella syndrome.[85]

IMMUNOHISTOCHEMISTRY. The presence of any viable tissue may allow immunohistochemical analysis of the tumor. The tumors most commonly represented are large nonfunctioning adenomas. Silent corticotroph adenomas are particularly likely to present in this manner.[4]

DIFFERENTIAL DIAGNOSIS. The characteristic clinical presentation of these patients alerts the pathologist to the correct diagnosis. The diagnosis can be made in the absence of viable tumor tissue by use of the reticulin stain to outline the typical adenoma pattern. The lymphocytic infiltration found in

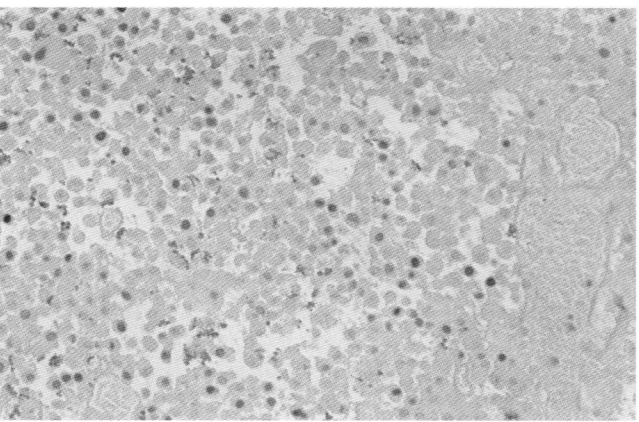

**Figure 50–16.** Pituitary apoplexy. Apoplexy is characterized by acute infarction of an adenoma. Although it is not shown here, many of these tumors are hemorrhagic. (H&E, magnification ×100.)

cases with delayed surgery does not approach that found in lymphocytic hypophysitis.

### Morphologic Effects of Medical Therapy for Adenoma

Dopamine agonists have become the primary therapeutic modality for most patients with prolactinomas.[86] Selective activation of $D_2$ receptors on the cell surface of lactotrophs by drugs such as bromocriptine leads to reversible, prominent inhibition of PRL transcription, synthesis, and secretion.[86] Responsive tumors shrink because of a marked decrease in tumor cell volume, leaving only a thin, perinuclear, cytoplasmic rim; these cells resemble lymphocytes. As a result, the density of tumor cells increases. Immunostaining for PRL becomes faint and often more focal. After long-term use, the tumors develop perivascular and stromal fibrosis and variable amounts of calcification.[87]

Somatostatin is a physiologic inhibitor of GH secretion. Somatostatin analogues, such as octreotide, are more stable and potent than the native molecule and have been used in the adjunctive treatment of somatotroph adenomas. There is good biochemical and symptomatic response to therapy but usually only a small decrease in tumor volume.[88] Microscopic changes are usually limited to mild perivascular and stromal fibrosis. Decreased number and size of secretory granules may be seen ultrastructurally.[88]

### Multiple Endocrine Neoplasia Type 1 Syndrome

Multiple endocrine neoplasia type 1 (MEN 1) is a variably penetrant, autosomal dominantly inherited disease caused by a mutation in one allele of the *MEN1* gene. Tumors of the parathyroids, enteropancreatic neuroendocrine system, anterior pituitary, and less commonly other tissues based on loss of heterozygosity involving the unaffected allele characterize it.[21] The reported prevalence of pituitary tumors in MEN 1 ranges from 16% to 65%. Prolactinomas are the most common pituitary tumors found in these patients; however, tumors of any hormone type including nonfunctional tumors may be seen. The age at onset of the pituitary adenomas in MEN 1 is indistinguishable from that found for sporadic tumors, with no morphologic differences in histologic features of the adenomas seen.[21] Multicentric tumors or double adenomas have been reported.[3, 89]

## PITUITARY CARCINOMA

CLINICAL CONSIDERATIONS. Pituitary carcinomas are rare primary adenohypophysial neoplasms that can be distinguished from locally invasive adenomas only by the presence of craniospinal or systemic metastases. More than 60 cases have been described in the English literature.[90, 91] The majority of patients have a protracted course in which the carcinoma is diagnosed as a result of metastasis, on average 6.5 years after an original diagnosis of adenoma is made. The longest intervals occur for patients with corticotroph adenomas and particularly those with Nelson's syndrome. Less frequently, patients present with invasive tumors that become metastatic soon after; a primary presentation with metastatic disease has not been reported. Most pituitary carcinomas are hormone secreting; PRL-secreting and corticotropin-secreting carcinomas are most common. Metastatic spread can involve the craniospinal axis or may be extraneural, involving liver, lung, bone, and lymph nodes. Extraneural metastatic spread is most common in corticotroph carcinomas. The immunophenotype of the metastasis is usually the same as that of the primary tumor. Blood hormone levels can be high in patients with extensive metastatic spread.[90]

DIAGNOSTIC CONSIDERATIONS. The diagnosis of pituitary carcinoma can be made only in a lesion with demonstrated metastases; it cannot at present be made on histologic analysis of the primary tumor alone. The histologic appearance of primary pituitary carcinomas is within the range found for adenoma with respect to pattern of growth, cellularity, and presence of necrosis, nuclear pleomorphism, or invasiveness of adjacent structures (Fig. 50–17). Mitotic figures are more frequently observed and are more abundant in carcinomas, but this feature cannot be used to predict the likelihood of an individual tumor's becoming malignant.

IMMUNOHISTOCHEMISTRY. Most pituitary carcinomas are functional and demonstrate appropriate patterns of immunoreactivity. Intensity of hormone immunoreactivity varies from case to case. Corticotropin-secreting tumors tend to show diffuse cytoplasmic staining for corticotropin; PRL-secreting carcinomas generally show juxtanuclear immunoreactivity for PRL. Studies of Ki-67–derived growth fraction using MIB-1 antibody have shown that carcinomas (primary and metastatic) have higher labeling indices than invasive adenomas do, although there is overlap between these categories.[44] Expression of p53 protein is rare in adenomas, may be seen in invasive adenomas, but is usually present in carcinomas.[39] In some cases, carcinomas show extensive p53 immunoreactivity.[41]

DIFFERENTIAL DIAGNOSIS. There is currently no way to identify carcinomas in the premetastatic phase or to accurately predict which tumors will become carcinomas. One group of authors has suggested the designation "adenoma of uncertain malignant potential" for tumors with increased mitotic activity and high (>3%) MIB-1 immunoreactivity; p53 expression may or may not be present.[16] The value of prospectively identifying such cases has not been established. Pituitary carcinoma must be distinguished from metastasis to the anterior pituitary or to a preexisting adenoma. Whereas metastatic carcinomas are usually easily differentiated from pituitary carcinoma by use of histologic and immunohistochemical criteria, a neuroendocrine carcinoma

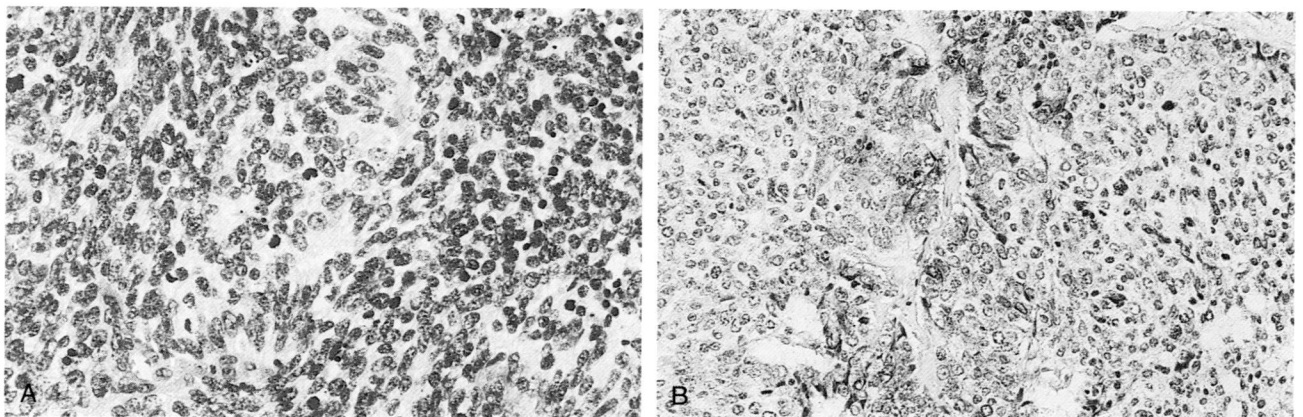

**Figure 50–17.** Pituitary carcinoma. This densely cellular, hyperchromatic and pleomorphic tumor has a high mitotic rate (H&E, *A*) and metastasized to the liver. Immunostaining reveals focal staining for corticotropin (*B*). (Magnification ×100.)

metastatic to pituitary could cause diagnostic confusion requiring careful clinical correlation.

## Tumors of the Hypothalamus and Neurohypophysis of Neuroepithelial Origin

### NEURONAL TUMORS (GANGLIOCYTOMA)

Symptomatic or asymptomatic masses in the hypothalamic region composed of mature neuronal elements have been designated gangliocytoma, hamartoma, or choristoma, depending on the location of the lesion and whether it is thought to be neoplastic or developmental in origin.[3, 55, 56] Individual cases may show morphologic features supporting one of these alternatives; however, there is no consensus on this issue, and distinction among these names may not be clinically important.

CLINICAL CONSIDERATIONS. Asymptomatic ectopic nodules containing neuronal elements may be identified in about 20% of random autopsies, commonly attached to the ventral hypothalamus.[55] They are usually of no clinical significance but may, on occasion, be of sufficient size to cause compressive symptoms. Symptomatic tumors are rare and may occur in the hypothalamus, in the suprasellar region, or rarely within the sella itself; a common location is behind the pituitary stalk.[4, 55] Lesions in the hypothalamus may lead to alterations in temperature and appetite control. Suprasellar masses can cause hypopituitarism with hyperprolactinemia or visual field deficits, and sellar lesions can cause hypopituitarism. Some neuronal tumors are hormonally active and may be associated with hyperplasias or adenomas of the pituitary gland, resulting in acromegaly,[56] precocious puberty, Cushing's disease, or amenorrhea-galactorrhea.[55]

DIAGNOSTIC CONSIDERATIONS. Symptomatic nodules may be nodular, pedunculated, solid, or cystic and may range in size from microscopic nodules to masses several centimeters in diameter. Microscopic examination reveals the presence of an abnormal arrangement of mature ganglion cells with abundant cytoplasm, Nissl granules, and large nuclei with prominent nucleoli (Fig. 50–18). In some cases, the neurons show abnormal morphology with binucleate or multinucleate forms. A glial stroma is usually present, sometimes showing fibrillary gliosis and calcification. In functional cases, the neuronal elements are often adjacent to or intimately admixed with an adenohypophysial hyperplastic lesion or adenoma.

IMMUNOHISTOCHEMISTRY. The ganglion cells within the lesion are positive for synaptophysin and neurofilament, supporting their neuronal phenotype.[55] The glial stroma may stain positively for glial fibrillary acidic protein and S-100 protein. The ganglion cells usually show immunoreactivity for a subset of hypothalamic peptides or hormones. Tumors from patients with acromegaly typically show immunoreactivity for GRH along with other peptides; associated pituitary adenomas in these patients stain positively for GH. Tumors from children with precocious puberty may show immunoreactivity for gonadotropin-releasing hormone; however, this is seen only in a subset of patients because precocious puberty may also be due to compressive effects. Tumors associated with Cushing's disease may be positive for CRH and other peptides, whereas tumors from patients with amenorrhea-galactorrhea may show positivity for vasoactive intestinal peptide and PRL. Nonfunctional tumors may also show positivity for peptides including vasoactive intestinal peptide, galanin, α-subunit, somatostatin, and serotonin.[3, 4, 55]

DIFFERENTIAL DIAGNOSIS. Hypothalamic neuronal tumors may be difficult to distinguish from normal tissues because of their cytologic maturity and low cellularity; the abnormal arrangement of cells, presence of binucleate cells, and propensity for

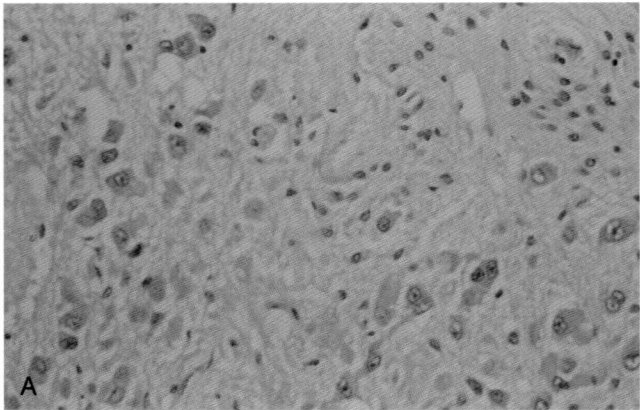
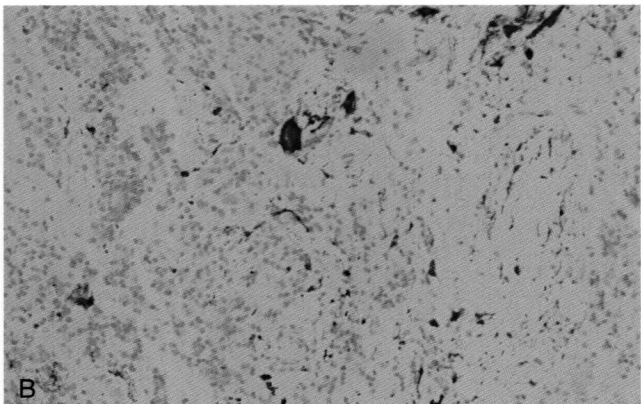

**Figure 50–18.** Gangliocytoma. This hypothalamic tumor is composed of abnormal ganglion cells with abundant cytoplasm, Nissl granules, and large nuclei with prominent nucleoli (H&E, *A*). Immunostaining for neurofilament reveals focal positivity in the neuronal cells (*B*). (Magnification ×100.)

calcification may be helpful in supporting a diagnosis of tumor. When intimate admixtures of ganglion cells and pituitary adenoma are present, it may be difficult to appreciate the ganglion cell elements. Neurofilament staining may be helpful in demonstrating the neuronal cell bodies in these tumors.

## GLIOMAS

CLINICAL CONSIDERATIONS. Glial neoplasms originating in the region of the hypothalamus compose about 15% of tumors in this site. They result in the diencephalic syndrome in children and visual disturbance and hydrocephalus in adults. Rare glial tumors are limited to the infundibulum and posterior pituitary and may cause diabetes insipidus.[92, 93] Malignant gliomas from other sites may infiltrate into the hypothalamic region but do not usually extend into the posterior pituitary.[92] Malignant gliomas may occur in the hypothalamic region 5 to 25 years after irradiation for pituitary adenoma, craniopharyngioma, or germinoma.[94, 95]

DIAGNOSTIC CONSIDERATIONS. The most common of the primary hypothalamic gliomas is the pilocytic astrocytoma, a circumscribed, WHO grade I tumor that is described in detail elsewhere (see Chapter 52). In this region, pilocytic astrocytomas have a propensity to involve optic nerves, the wall of the third ventricle, and the hypothalamus. Patterns of growth include more cellular areas of astrocytic cells with bipolar processes and Rosenthal fibers and looser areas in which the astrocytes are often associated with microcysts and granular bodies. Mitoses are usually not seen.[96]

Gangliogliomas may rarely be seen in the third ventricle or hypothalamic region and contain abnormal, often binucleate ganglion cells within the fibrillary or pilocytic astrocytic neoplasm.[97] Rarely, ependymomas involve the hypothalamic region or pituitary fossa.[98]

Little is known about primary gliomas of the posterior pituitary because of their rarity. They have been referred to as pituicytomas or infundibulomas by some authors because of some distinctive ultrastructural characteristics; however, they closely resemble pilocytic astrocytomas or, more rarely, fibrillary astrocytomas[99, 100] (Fig. 50–19).

IMMUNOHISTOCHEMISTRY. The tumor cells in pilocytic astrocytomas and the astrocytic component of gangliogliomas demonstrate positivity for glial fibrillary acidic protein.[96] In gangliogliomas, the ganglion cells demonstrate neuronal markers including synaptophysin and neurofilament protein.[97]

DIFFERENTIAL DIAGNOSIS. In some cases, the cellularity of these often low-grade astrocytic neoplasms can be low and difficult to distinguish from that of the vascular neurohypophysis. Reactive gliosis and particularly the atypical gliosis found surrounding some craniopharyngiomas and germinomas may be more difficult to distinguish until further sampling reveals the nature of the primary lesion. The rare ependymoma in the sellar region could be confused with pituitary adenoma showing

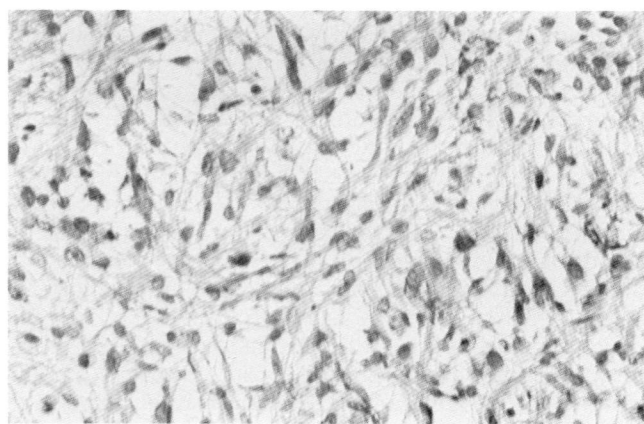

**Figure 50–19.** Pituicytoma. This tumor of the posterior pituitary is composed of astrocytic cells with elongated fibrillary processes. (H&E, magnification ×100.)

a prominent perivascular pseudorosette pattern; the strong immunoreactivity for glial fibrillary acidic protein in ependymoma should confirm the correct diagnosis.[98]

## MENINGIOMA

CLINICAL CONSIDERATIONS. Approximately 10% to 20% of intracranial meningiomas involve the sellar and parasellar region; they are found most commonly attached to dural structures of the sphenoid ridge, tuberculum sellae, diaphragma sellae, olfactory groove, or optic nerve sheath.[92, 101] Suprasellar tumors may secondarily invade the sella[102]; however, purely intrasellar meningiomas attached to the inferior surface of the diaphragma sellae are rare.[103] Meningiomas may occasionally arise in the irradiation field of patients treated for pituitary adenoma or craniopharyngioma.[104] Skull base meningiomas may compress brain structures such as optic chiasm or pituitary stalk and may erode, invade, or stimulate hyperostosis in adjacent bony structures. Suprasellar lesions are often associated with visual loss; less frequently, they cause hypopituitarism and hyperprolactinemia because of stalk compression.

DIAGNOSTIC CONSIDERATIONS. These histologically diverse tumors derived from arachnoidal cells have been classified into 11 types (WHO, 1993).[101] Separate categories are additionally included for the more aggressive atypical, papillary, and anaplastic variants. Detailed discussion of these tumors is provided in Chapter 52. All variants may be represented at this site. Benign meningiomas may invade the bony skull base or structures within the cavernous sinus, including cranial nerves. Growth of meningiomas into the sella may be associated with invasion of pituitary tissue.

IMMUNOHISTOCHEMISTRY. Meningiomas express both mesenchymal and epithelial markers. Vimentin is widely expressed in meningiomas and is the most abundant intermediate filament in these tumors. Many meningiomas react with cytokeratin antibodies, and virtually all meningiomas show some immunoreactivity to epithelial membrane antigen.[101] Meningothelial cells attach to one another by means of desmosomes, a feature reflected by immunoreactivity for the desmosomal protein desmoplakin.[105] Meningiomas frequently express progesterone receptors.[92]

DIFFERENTIAL DIAGNOSIS. An intrasellar meningioma may mimic a pituitary adenoma; recognition of the diverse histologic appearances of meningiomas is required for their differentiation. In general, whorls and indistinct cell borders in meningiomas may be helpful distinguishing features. A smear preparation at the time of intraoperative consultation demonstrates the more cohesive nature of meningothelial cells. Microcalcifications may be found in either meningiomas or pituitary adenomas, especially prolactinomas. Immunohistochemistry may be valuable in separating these entities. Meningiomas must be distinguished from the dural hemangiopericytoma. This malignant nonmeningothelial tumor can occur in the sellar region or may rarely arise within the sella itself.[106]

## GRANULAR CELL TUMORS

NOMENCLATURE. These distinctive benign tumors of the posterior lobe of the pituitary and infundibulum are of uncertain histogenesis.[107–111] Various authors have called them choristoma, myoblastoma, or pituicytoma; however, until the histogenesis is established, the more descriptive term *granular cell tumor* is most appropriate.[3] Although it is morphologically similar to granular cell tumor in extracranial sites, it is clear that the intracranial granular cell tumor is a distinct entity.

CLINICAL CONSIDERATIONS. Granular cell tumors are most commonly found as incidental, asymptomatic tumorlets at autopsy; they are identified as small groups of granular cells in the infundibulum or posterior lobe. In carefully studied cases, they are found in up to 17% of pituitaries.[107, 108] They are uncommon in individuals younger than 20 years, suggesting that they are acquired lesions. In contrast to these frequently observed tumorlets, only rarely do tumors enlarge to form symptomatic masses,[110, 111] usually in a suprasellar location in the fourth or fifth decade of life. The female-to-male ratio is 2:1. Suprasellar lesions cause chiasmal compression, hypopituitarism, and sometimes hydrocephalus or dementia. Less frequently, they become symptomatic while being confined to the posterior lobe of the pituitary; surprisingly, they are rarely associated with diabetes insipidus. The vascularity of the tumor stroma commonly leads to focal intraoperative hemorrhage.

DIAGNOSTIC CONSIDERATIONS. Symptomatic lesions are well circumscribed but unencapsulated firm nodular masses composed of large, polygonal cells with abundant, slightly eosinophilic, granular cytoplasm and uniformly regular, small nuclei (Fig. 50–20). The cytoplasm contains diastase-resistant

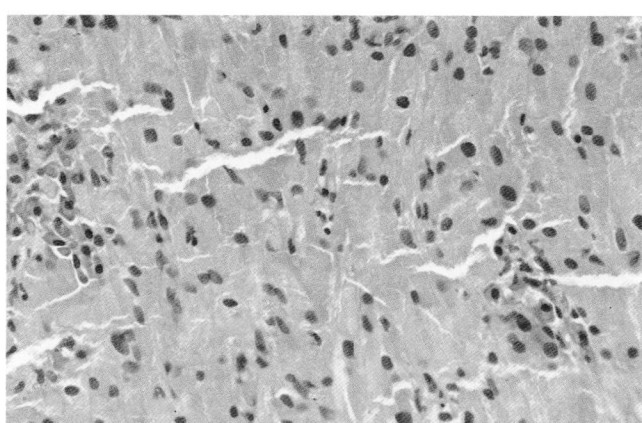

**Figure 50–20.** Granular cell tumor. This tumor is composed of large polygonal cells with finely granular cytoplasm. (H&E, magnification ×100.)

PAS positivity, and electron microscopy confirms that the granularity is due to accumulation of pleomorphic lysosomes (CD Fig. 50–11). Mitotic figures and other anaplastic histologic features are lacking in these uniformly benign tumors. The scant stroma contains a fine capillary network.

IMMUNOHISTOCHEMISTRY. The immunohistochemical profile of these tumors is distinct from that found in extracranial tumors.[111] They lack immunoreactivity for anterior pituitary hormones and are only occasionally positive for S-100 protein or glial fibrillary acidic protein. They may show positivity for histiocytic markers including CD68, $\alpha_1$-antitrypsin, $\alpha_1$-antichymotrypsin, and cathepsin B.[4, 92, 111]

DIFFERENTIAL DIAGNOSIS. The rarity of symptomatic granular cell tumors and their location means that they may be confused clinically with meningioma, craniopharyngioma, and pituitary adenoma. On gross evaluation, they lack the dural attachment of meningiomas, do not have cystic components typical of most craniopharyngiomas, and are generally firmer than pituitary adenomas. Their typical microscopic appearance then establishes the correct diagnosis.

## Primary Tumors of the Sellar Region Originating from Other Cell Types

### CRANIOPHARYNGIOMA

PATHOGENESIS. Craniopharyngiomas are histologically benign tumors thought to arise from epithelial rests. These rests may be left in place after involution of the craniopharyngeal duct formed by migration of Rathke pouch from the stomodeum to the uppermost part of the adenohypophysis.[112] An alternative view has been that the epithelial rests represent metaplastic adenohypophysial cells.[113] No genetic or environmental factors have been identified that contribute to the genesis or progression of craniopharyngiomas.

CLINICAL CONSIDERATIONS. Craniopharyngiomas inflict significant morbidity because of their location and inherent resistance to complete surgical excision. They represent approximately 3% of intracranial neoplasms but in children compose 10% of brain tumors. They can occur from infancy to old age, but peak incidence is from 5 to 20 years with a second smaller peak in the sixth decade.[92, 114] The majority of craniopharyngiomas are suprasellar (80%); however, they may also have an intrasellar component or arise in the sella itself. In childhood, patients present with endocrine disturbance (e.g., dwarfism), hypothalamic dysfunction, visual dysfunction, or elevated intracranial pressure. Adults frequently present with sexual dysfunction or visual problems. Biochemical studies may show hypogonadism due to destruction of hypothalamic tissue or mild elevation of PRL due to interruption of the pituitary stalk leading to loss of hypothalamic dopaminergic inhibition of PRL release in the anterior pituitary. Two patterns of craniopharyngioma growth have been described; the classic adamantinomatous tumor (90%) is found at any age, whereas the much less frequent papillary variant (10%) is found almost exclusively in adults.[92, 114]

DIAGNOSTIC CONSIDERATIONS. Craniopharyngiomas may be cystic (50%), solid (15%), or both. Tumors presenting in childhood tend to have cystic components; papillary craniopharyngiomas in adults are more likely to be solid. Although the tumor often appears to be well circumscribed, it does not have a capsule and may be tightly adherent to adjacent brain or vascular structures. The cystic components characteristically contain viscous oil-like fluid that often contains cholesterol crystals. Calcification may be prominent.

The adamantinomatous tumors are composed of cords and islands of epithelial cells within a loose fibrous stroma (Fig. 50–21). There is usually an

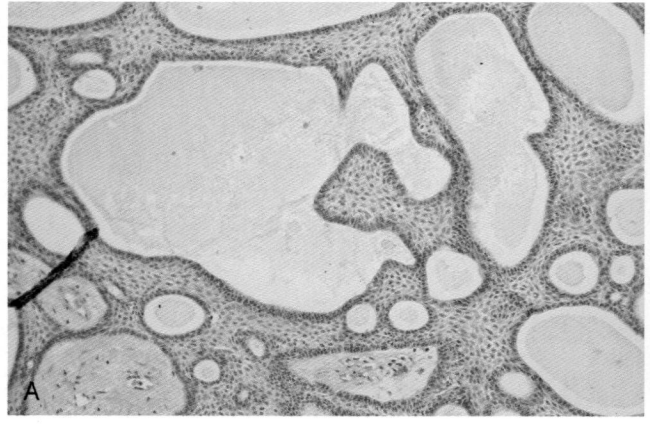
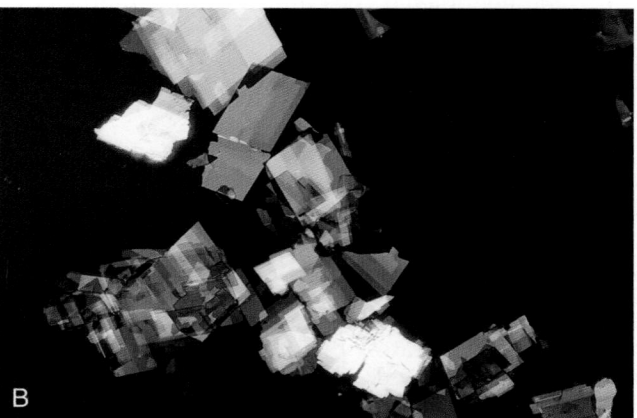

**Figure 50–21.** Craniopharyngioma. *A.* Adamantinomatous tumor composed of epithelial cells forming sheets and lining cystic spaces. (H&E, magnification ×25.) *B.* Tumor cyst fluid often contains cholesterol crystals exhibiting a characteristic shape when viewed under polarized light. (Magnification ×100.)

outer palisading layer, a middle zone of stellate epithelial cells, and a superficial keratinizing layer. A distinctive nodular keratinization ("wet keratin") is characteristic of this tumor and may be associated with calcification. The stroma often contains cholesterol clefts, chronic inflammatory cell infiltrates, and foam cells. Cystic degeneration is frequent. At the interface between tumor and brain, fingerlike projections of epithelium may be seen, often in association with a prominent gliotic response.

Papillary craniopharyngiomas are more circumscribed and lack the microcysts, calcifications, and palisading epithelium found in the adamantinomatous tumors. They are composed of stratified squamous papillary structures with fibrovascular cores. Malignant transformation in craniopharyngiomas is exceedingly rare; it has been described in only one previously irradiated case.[115]

IMMUNOHISTOCHEMISTRY. The epithelial component of craniopharyngiomas is positive for low- and high-molecular-weight keratins.[116] However, because of the distinctive histologic appearance of this tumor, immunohistochemical analysis is rarely required.

DIFFERENTIAL DIAGNOSIS. Craniopharyngiomas may be confused with Rathke cleft cysts or epidermoid cysts occurring in the sellar region. Craniopharyngiomas are more likely to show multiloculation, calcification, and nodular keratinization; epidermoid cysts are more likely to be unilocular, with orderly, stratified epithelium and sheets of keratin. Small sample size may make histologic distinction difficult; in those situations, the location and intraoperative appearance of the tumor may be of diagnostic value. The infiltrative nature of adamantinomatous craniopharyngiomas often results in surgical removal of adjacent brain tissue that may be highly gliotic. The presence of Rosenthal fibers in this tissue may lead to an erroneous diagnosis of pilocytic astrocytoma. The gliotic margin of craniopharyngioma lacks microcysts, is generally of lower cellularity than a pilocytic astrocytoma, and may show a gradient of cellularity decreasing with distance from the lesion. Further sampling may disclose the protruding fingers of epithelium of the adjacent craniopharyngioma.

## CHORDOMA

CLINICAL CONSIDERATIONS. Tumors derived from notochordal tissue are rare and occur most frequently in the sacrum and the clivus of adults; exceptional cases are intrasellar in location.[117–119] It is presumed that at least some of these cases derive from small ectopias of notochord, known as ecchordosis physaliphora, that are found over the clivus in about 2% of autopsies; however, most cases probably derive from notochordal remnants within the skull base.[117] Chordomas are expansile, erosive, intraosseous malignant tumors that show evidence of metastasis in 10% of patients at presentation, most commonly to lungs, lymph nodes, bones, and skin. They cause pain, local mass effect, and cranial nerve palsies; when present in a parasellar location, they may cause hypopituitarism.[92]

DIAGNOSTIC CONSIDERATIONS. The tumor is grossly mucoid and lobulated and often shows focal calcification. Lobules of tumor cells are typically arranged in cords and sheets within an abundant, mucinous, extracellular matrix. They often have abundant vacuolated, bubbly cytoplasm that has been termed physaliphorous. They are invasive of bone and may show microcalcification. Some chordomas contain distinct regions of malignant mesenchymal tissue resembling malignant fibrous histiocytoma, fibrosarcoma, or osteosarcoma.[120] A variant of chordoma in which cartilaginous differentiation is found has been described. These tumors have been called chondroid chordomas by some authors; however, most of these tumors are probably low-grade chondrosarcomas.[121]

IMMUNOHISTOCHEMISTRY. Chordomas are strongly positive for S-100 protein, epithelial membrane antigen, cytokeratin, and sometimes carcinoembryonic antigen. Chondroid chordomas are typically negative for cytokeratin and epithelial membrane antigen, providing support for the contention that many of these tumors are truly low-grade chondrosarcomas.[121]

DIFFERENTIAL DIAGNOSIS. The distinctive histologic appearance of this tumor does not usually cause diagnostic difficulty. The distinction between chordoma and chondrosarcoma is discussed before. Some meningiomas may show chondroid features; however, these tumors often show distinctive meningothelial areas and should not be strongly positive for cytokeratin and S-100 protein.[101] The presence of vacuolated cells may suggest a diagnosis of metastatic adenocarcinoma, although the presence of strong S-100 protein immunoreactivity and relative paucity of anaplasia support the diagnosis of chordoma.

## GERM CELL TUMORS

CLINICAL CONSIDERATIONS. The suprasellar region is the second most common site for intracranial germ cell tumors after the pineal[122]; in some cases, both of these sites are involved.[123] Most tumors occur in children younger than 20 years. Whereas germ cell tumors in the pineal region show a striking male predominance, those in the suprasellar region are more equally distributed between the sexes and in some series show a female predominance.[4] Growth in the suprasellar region can lead to hypopituitarism, diabetes insipidus, or chiasmal compression. Large tumors may cause obstructive hydrocephalus. Precocious puberty may be due to hypothalamic damage or result from production of human chorionic gonadotropin (hCG). Measurement of blood levels of hCG and $\alpha$-fetoprotein can be used diagnostically and to detect recurrences of syncytiotrophoblastic elements and endodermal sinus tumor, respectively. All tumor types with the exception of benign teratoma are capable of metastatic growth, most commonly in the craniospinal axis.

DIAGNOSTIC CONSIDERATIONS. The histologic appearance of suprasellar germ cell tumors is the same as for those found in the pineal and extracranial sites and is discussed in detail elsewhere. In the sellar region, germinomas are by far the most common lesion, although teratomas and mixed germ cell tumors are also represented (Fig. 50–22). Suprasellar germinomas are often widely infiltrative, making the exact site of origin often difficult to determine. Intrasellar extension may be present in up to 20% of cases, although isolated intrasellar tumors are rare.[124, 125]

IMMUNOHISTOCHEMISTRY. Intracranial germinomas may show immunohistochemical features that distinguish them from testicular seminomas and ovarian dysgerminomas.[126] Some intracranial germinomas exhibit cells that are positive for cytokeratin and epithelial membrane antigen and other cells positive for vimentin, whereas extracranial tumors lack these epithelial and mesenchymal markers. Germinomas are immunoreactive for placental alkaline phosphatase. Some germinomas contain isolated syncytiotrophoblastic cells reactive for hCG.[3, 4] The presence of isolated hCG-reactive syncytiotrophoblast cells in germinoma has been reported to predict a higher rate of recurrence; however, a study of germinomas with elevated hCG levels showed that prognosis does not appear to be different from that of pure germinomas when adequate radiation therapy is provided.[127] Embryonal carcinomas express α-fetoprotein and hCG, whereas endodermal sinus tumors express α-fetoprotein only.

DIFFERENTIAL DIAGNOSIS. The large malignant cells in germinomas can be hidden within an associated, often prominent, lymphocytic and granulomatous inflammatory infiltrate. Immunoperoxidase staining for placental alkaline phosphatase can help in the identification of the malignant cells. The infiltrating edge of a germinoma may show atypical reactive gliosis that could be misinterpreted as a glioma; however, adequate sampling of the lesion should demonstrate the neoplastic cells of the germinoma.

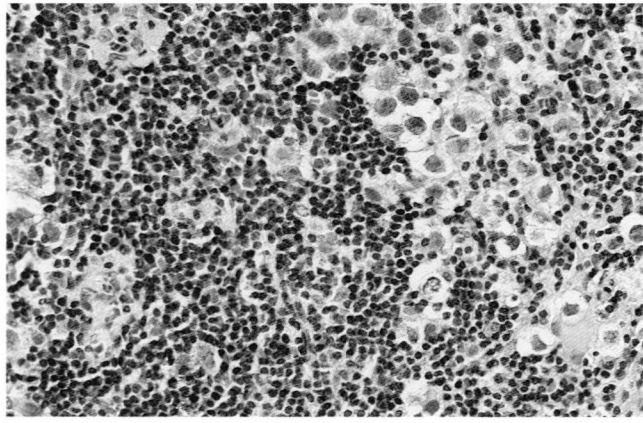

**Figure 50–22.** Germinoma. The large malignant cells with prominent nucleoli are mixed with a prominent lymphocytic infiltrate. (H&E, magnification ×100.)

## PRIMARY LYMPHOMA

CLINICAL CONSIDERATIONS. Involvement of the sellar region with primary central nervous system lymphoma is rare; when present, it is usually due to tumor originating in the hypothalamus or spreading directly from adjacent brain regions.[92] Primary lymphoma of the central nervous system is found most commonly in immunodeficient patients, such as those with acquired immunodeficiency syndrome, although it may also be seen in immunocompetent individuals. Hypothalamic involvement may lead to a hypothalamic syndrome including diabetes insipidus, somnolence, obesity, and hypopituitarism.[128] The tumor may rarely present as a suprasellar mass with chiasmal syndrome.[128-130]

DIAGNOSTIC CONSIDERATIONS. Primary lymphomas of the hypothalamus are similar to those found elsewhere in the central nervous system; most are high-grade B cell lymphomas. These tumors infiltrate hypothalamus and pituitary stalk and may extend to posterior pituitary.

DIFFERENTIAL DIAGNOSIS. Lymphoma in the sellar region is most commonly systemic and can often be differentiated from primary lymphoma by the pattern of spread; systemic lymphoma is usually subcapsular in location, whereas primary lymphoma involves the parenchyma directly. Histologic analysis can typically differentiate lymphoma from pituitary adenoma; however, immunohistochemical staining for leukocyte markers and pituitary hormones should resolve any difficult cases. Lymphocytic hypophysitis is distinguished from lymphoma by the identification of a polyclonal accumulation of mature lymphocytes.

## MISCELLANEOUS TUMORS OF THE SELLAR REGION

A number of tumors that characteristically occur elsewhere in the body or nervous system can occasionally occur in the sellar region and may clinically mimic pituitary adenoma or other common sellar tumors.

### Schwannoma

Schwannomas can rarely present in the intrasellar or parasellar regions and mimic pituitary adenoma.[131-135] Schwannomas in the cavernous sinus may originate in cranial nerves and extend medially into the sella. Purely intrasellar schwannomas are thought to derive from ectopic Schwann cells or Schwann cells ensheathing small nerve twigs innervating the dura. The schwannomas of the sellar region are histologically identical to those presenting elsewhere, with typical spindle cells arranged in compact Antoni A and loose Antoni B areas. In this location, they are most likely to be confused with meningioma. Schwannomas are strongly positive for S-100 protein and are negative for epithelial membrane antigen; meningiomas are usually positive for epithelial membrane antigen and show less frequent and less intense staining for S-100 protein.[101, 136]

### Hemangioblastoma

Hemangioblastomas have been reported as intrasellar or suprasellar lesions both in association with and in the absence of von Hippel–Lindau syndrome.[106, 137]

### Paraganglioma

Paragangliomas have rarely been reported as primary intrasellar tumors or as tumors extending from cavernous sinus. The cell of origin of the intrasellar tumors is unknown but may be from paraganglionic rests.[138, 139]

### Primary Sellar Melanoma

Primary sellar melanomas are rare but have been described; they are presumably derived from arachnoidal melanocytes. Most cases of melanoma in the sellar region are metastatic.[140, 141]

### Cavernous Angioma

Benign cavernous angiomas may rarely involve the pituitary and may be incidental findings at autopsy.[142, 143]

### Glomangioma

An intrasellar glomangioma has been reported that mimicked pituitary adenoma clinically and histologically. A derivation of this tumor from gomitoli, structures of the hypophysial portal system of the pituitary stalk with morphologic similarities to the glomus body, has been suggested.[144]

### Soft Tissue Tumors

Soft tissue tumors may involve the sellar region and include lipoma,[145] giant cell tumor,[146] chondromyxoid fibroma,[147] chondroma,[148] enchondroma,[149] chondrosarcoma,[150] alveolar soft part sarcoma,[151] and rhabdomyosarcoma.[152]

### Postirradiation Neoplasms

Irradiation of the sellar region for pituitary adenoma or craniopharyngioma has been associated with the development of postirradiation neoplasms, including sarcomas and gliomas; the average latency period is approximately 10 years. Sarcomas are most frequent and include osteosarcoma and fibrosarcoma.[153-155] Gliomas are usually astrocytic and invade the sellar region from adjacent diencephalic or neocortical regions.[94, 95]

## Metastatic Neoplasms of the Sellar Region

### METASTATIC CARCINOMA

CLINICAL CONSIDERATIONS. The sellar region is a common site for metastasis in the context of advanced systemic cancer. The most common primary sites of metastatic tumor are lung, breast, and gastrointestinal tract. Autopsy studies show that the pituitary is involved in 3% to 5% of cases[156] and,

when carefully looked for by microscopic examination, in up to 27% of cases.[157] The prominent vascularity of the pituitary gland has been suggested as a reason for the high rate of metastasis. Most of those who are found to have pituitary metastasis at autopsy were not known to be symptomatic for these pituitary tumors, presumably because they do not live long enough for symptoms to develop. Similarly, pituitary metastasis is only rarely the first manifestation of a cancer; however, it is much more commonly the presenting finding in patients who are symptomatic of their pituitary metastasis. Whereas all sites in the sellar region may be affected, the posterior pituitary appears to be most frequent. Tumors of the posterior pituitary, infundibulum, or hypothalamus may produce diabetes insipidus; only rarely do isolated tumors of the anterior pituitary result in hypopituitarism. Involvement of the cavernous sinus may result in headache and cranial nerve palsies.[158-160]

DIAGNOSTIC CONSIDERATIONS. Metastatic carcinoma is identified by recognition of the malignant features of the neoplasm and the differentiating characteristics of the primary tumor (Fig. 50–23). Immunohistochemical or ultrastructural studies may help in this characterization. On rare occasions, tumor may metastasize to a preexisting pituitary adenoma.[160]

DIFFERENTIAL DIAGNOSIS. A diagnosis of metastatic carcinoma is indicated, in most cases, by the history of cancer and correlation with histologic appearance of the primary lesion. In rare cases in which the patient presents with a metastatic pituitary mass, the lesion may be confused with pituitary adenoma or an inflammatory lesion. Biopsy of a highly anaplastic lesion raises the possibility of primary pituitary carcinoma. In less anaplastic tumors, the presence of mitotic activity and nuclear pleomorphism may be misleading because both features may also be present in some pituitary adenomas, such as the sparsely granulated somatotroph adenoma. In these situations, careful immunohistochemical and

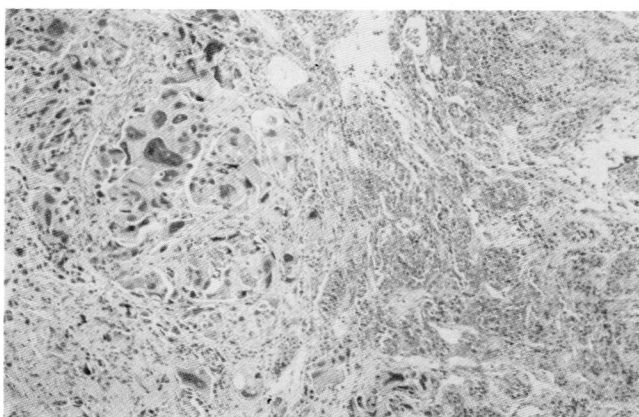

**Figure 50–23.** Metastatic carcinoma. An infiltrate of malignant cells originating from a primary tumor in the lung is present in the anterior pituitary. (H&E, magnification ×100.)

ultrastructural analysis looking for evidence of anterior pituitary hormone production is required.

### METASTATIC LYMPHOMA AND LEUKEMIA

CLINICAL CONSIDERATIONS. Most commonly, lymphoma or leukemia in the sellar region is metastatic and occurs in patients with systemic disease.[161] In one autopsy series, 23% of patients with hematopoietic neoplasms had microscopic evidence of hypophysial involvement.[162] The systemic tumors most frequently associated with involvement of the sellar region were non-Hodgkin's malignant lymphoma, lymphocytic leukemia, and myelogenous leukemia; Hodgkin's disease was unusual. Leukemic deposits are rarely symptomatic but may cause diabetes insipidus. Lymphoma can occasionally result in a sellar mass with mass effect and hypopituitarism.[163]

DIAGNOSTIC CONSIDERATIONS. Tumor metastatic to the pituitary usually infiltrates in the subcapsular region and only rarely infiltrates into the parenchyma. Tumor is often present in adjacent leptomeninges.

DIFFERENTIAL DIAGNOSIS. Metastatic lymphoma is distinguished from primary lymphoma by discerning the pattern of infiltration (subcapsular versus parenchymal) and determining whether systemic disease is present. Differentiation from pituitary adenoma is made by histologic analysis and immunohistochemistry for leukocyte antigens, if necessary.

### PLASMACYTOMA

CLINICAL CONSIDERATIONS. Patients with multiple myeloma may have involvement of the sella as part of their systemic disease. Rarely, a solitary intrasellar plasmacytoma may occur with or without an adjacent lytic lesion of the sella; such lesions may mimic pituitary adenoma clinically and radiologically.[164-166]

DIAGNOSTIC CONSIDERATIONS. Plasmacytomas are composed of a monomorphic population of cells, often with eccentric nuclei and basophilic cytoplasm with a pale Golgi zone. Immunohistochemistry confirms the diagnosis by demonstrating monoclonal immunoglobulin light or heavy chains.

DIFFERENTIAL DIAGNOSIS. The discohesive monomorphic cells of a plasmacytoma can mimic a chromophobic pituitary adenoma, especially at intraoperative frozen section. Whereas fibrous bodies may appear similar to the pale Golgi zone, they are not found in basophilic pituitary adenomas.[3] Immunohistochemical staining for immunoglobulin chains and pituitary hormones easily distinguishes these entities. Electron microscopy may be helpful in ruling out epithelial differentiation. Intrasellar plasmacytomas may also be mimicked by reactive plasma cell infiltrates. Plasma cell granuloma is a benign pseudotumor including plasma cells and lymphocytes; immunohistochemistry confirms the polyclonal nature of the infiltrate. Meningioma may occasionally be widely infiltrated by plasma cells; the infiltrate is polyclonal, and meningioma cells are identified within the infiltrate.

### LANGERHANS CELL HISTIOCYTOSIS

CLINICAL CONSIDERATIONS. Langerhans cell histiocytosis encompasses a group of disorders characterized by proliferation of epithelioid Langerhans cells, including histiocytosis X, Hand-Schüller-Christian disease, and Letterer-Siwe disease.[167] Central nervous system involvement occurs in about 25% of patients with systemic disease with a predilection for hypothalamus, pituitary stalk, and posterior pituitary. Adjacent bony structures may or may not be involved.[92] Isolated hypothalamic or neurohypophysial disease is rare and, when present, has historically been designated Gagel's granuloma.[168-171] Hypothalamic lesions may cause diabetes insipidus or less frequently hypopituitarism, often in association with increased PRL due to destruction of dopaminergic neurons or compression of the stalk. Direct destruction of anterior pituitary tissue is unusual and only rarely is the cause of hypopituitarism.

DIAGNOSTIC CONSIDERATIONS. Tissues are infiltrated by Langerhans cells admixed with lymphocytes, foamy macrophages, and eosinophils. The Langerhans cell is a large epithelioid histiocyte-like cell with a kidney-shaped nucleus and abundant cytoplasm. The ultrastructural demonstration of Birbeck granules (rod-shaped pentalaminar structures with a zipperlike central core and often a tennis racket–shaped dilated end) is pathognomonic for the disorder.[4]

IMMUNOHISTOCHEMISTRY. The Langerhans cell is positive for S-100 protein as well as for the leukocyte antigens HLA-DR and CD1.[172]

DIFFERENTIAL DIAGNOSIS. The clinical presentation may rarely mimic pituitary adenoma when the disease is localized to the sella; however, the lesions are easily separated histologically. Langerhans cell histiocytosis may be more difficult to differentiate from other polyclonal inflammatory proliferations, including lymphocytic hypophysitis, granulomatous inflammation, and the inflammation accompanying germinoma. The presence of eosinophils and the demonstration of Langerhans cells by S-100 protein staining or electron microscopy are helpful in establishing the correct diagnosis.

## NON-NEOPLASTIC TUMORLIKE CONDITIONS OF THE SELLAR REGION

### Hyperplasia of Adenohypophysial Cells

CLINICAL CONSIDERATIONS. Hyperplastic lesions of the anterior pituitary represent orderly proliferative responses of a class of anterior pituitary cells to physiologic or pathologic stimuli[173] (Table

**TABLE 50–7.** Underlying Conditions Associated with Hyperplasia of the Anterior Pituitary

| Cell Type | Underlying Conditions | |
| --- | --- | --- |
| | *Primary* | *Secondary* |
| Lactotroph | Idiopathic lactotroph hyperplasia | Pregnancy<br>Stalk compression<br>Primary hypothyroidism |
| Corticotroph | Primary corticotroph hyperplasia | Addison's disease<br>Ectopic CRH-secreting tumors |
| Somatotroph | Primary somatotroph hyperplasia | Ectopic GRH-secreting tumors (e.g., hypothalamic gangliocytoma, extracranial neuroendocrine tumor) |
| Mammosomatotroph | McCune-Albright syndrome | NA |
| Thyrotroph | NA | Primary hypothyroidism |
| Gonadotroph | NA | Primary hypogonadism (e.g., Klinefelter's) |

50–7). Hyperplasia of somatotrophs, lactotrophs, corticotrophs, or thyrotrophs may occasionally result in clinical syndromes indistinguishable from those caused by pituitary adenomas. Lactotroph hyperplasia occurs on a physiologic basis in pregnancy and results in enlargement of the gland up to twice the normal size.[174] Pathologic causes include stalk compression, which interrupts the normal inhibitory influence of dopamine on lactotrophs, and rare cases of idiopathic lactotroph hyperplasia.[3, 65] Somatotroph hyperplasia may occur in association with a hypothalamic gangliocytoma or other neuroendocrine tumors demonstrating ectopic production of GRH; some of these patients may have clinical acromegaly.[56–58] Primary somatotroph hyperplasia may be seen in some young patients with gigantism.[3] Mammosomatotroph hyperplasia has been described in patients with McCune-Albright syndrome.[175] Corticotroph hyperplasia may be present in rare patients with Cushing's disease or in those with untreated or inadequately treated Addison's disease.[176, 177] On occasion, ectopic secretion of CRH by tumors outside the pituitary induces corticotroph hyperplasia that can mimic an adenoma.[3] Thyrotroph hyperplasia may occur in the context of untreated primary hypothyroidism; these patients may present with hyperprolactinemia because of associated lactotroph hyperplasia.[66] Gonadotroph hyperplasia may occur after long-standing primary hypogonadism; however, it is rarely of sufficient size to cause symptoms.[3] Identification and treatment of the underlying hormone imbalance typically results in reversal of the hyperplasia; however, the pathologist will occasionally be presented with a hyperplastic lesion in which the underlying cause was not identified and adenoma is suspected.

DIAGNOSTIC CONSIDERATIONS. Hyperplasia must be distinguished from normal anterior pituitary and adenoma (see Table 50–5). Hyperplasia may result in diffuse enlargement of the gland or focal nodular changes that grossly may look like adenoma. Suprasellar extension of the hyperplastic lesion may even occur on occasion. Hyperplasia is recognized by the presence of expanded adenohypophysial acini identified by the reticulin stain (Fig. 50–24). In adenoma, the reticulin pattern is lost and fragmented; however, in hyperplasia, the reticulin pattern is maintained about the enlarged acini. In some rare cases, hyperplasia and adenoma may coexist in the same gland.

IMMUNOHISTOCHEMISTRY. The hyperplastic acini contain increased numbers of cells immunoreactive for the hyperplastic cell type. Interspersed cells within the acini are positive for other adenohypophysial hormones.

DIFFERENTIAL DIAGNOSIS. Hyperplasia is distinguished from normal gland by the presence of expanded acini. Focal, nodular hyperplasia is easier to detect than is diffuse hyperplasia because of the presence of normal adjacent tissue for comparison. Hyperplasia is distinguished from adenoma primarily by demonstrating the loss of the reticulin framework in adenoma; the presence of multiple hormone immunoreactivities should raise the suspicion of hyperplasia.

## Cysts

### RATHKE'S CLEFT CYST

CLINICAL CONSIDERATIONS. Rathke's cleft cysts originate from remnants of Rathke's pouch. In the human, the intermediate lobe of the pituitary is vestigial and often includes small cystic spaces derived from the cleft. These cysts are usually small and measure less than 5 mm in diameter.[178] When they enlarge, they may become symptomatic, causing hypopituitarism or more rarely diabetes insipidus. Symptomatic Rathke's cleft cysts usually present in adulthood, although childhood onset may occur. When lesions extend to become suprasellar, visual field defects or even hydrocephalus may occur.[179, 180]

DIAGNOSTIC CONSIDERATIONS. Gross examination reveals a unilocular, thin-walled, fluid-filled

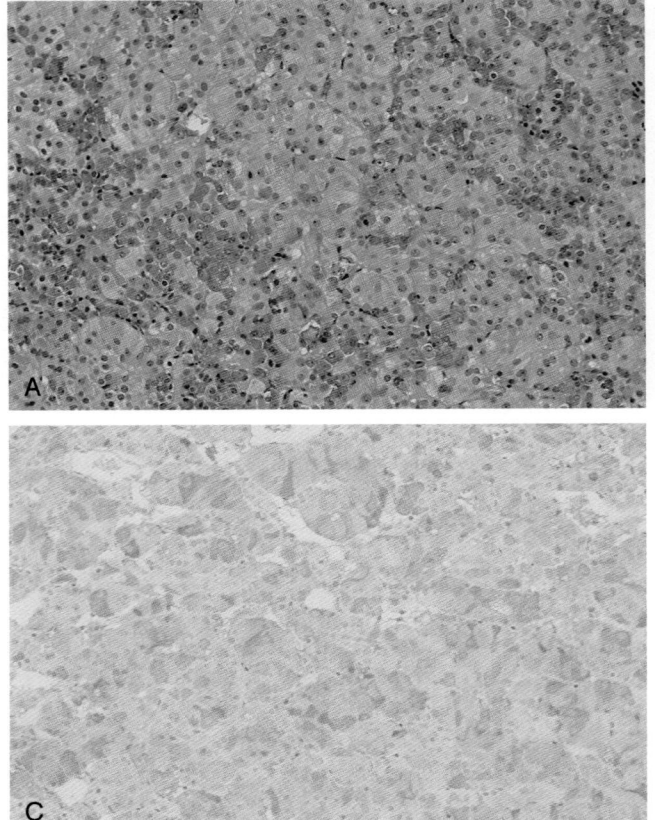

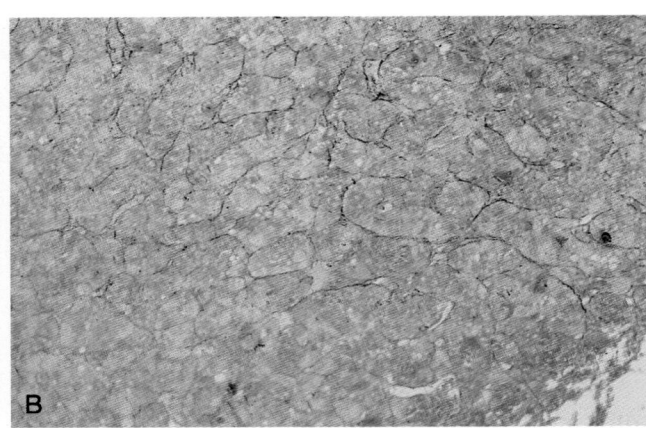

**Figure 50–24.** Hyperplasia. In this biopsy specimen from a patient with thyrotroph hyperplasia, there appears to be expansion of acini on H&E staining (*A*); however, reticulin stain is required to confirm the enlarged acini (*B*). Immunoperoxidase stains reveal the predominant reactivity for TSH in these expanded acini (*C*). (Magnification: ×100.)

cyst. The fluid may be watery to mucinous. The cyst is lined by a single layer of ciliated cuboidal or columnar epithelium with occasional goblet cells. Squamous metaplasia may occur. Nontumorous adenohypophysial parenchyma is found immediately adjacent to the epithelium in some specimens[181, 182] (Fig. 50–25).

IMMUNOHISTOCHEMISTRY. Identification of the typical cyst lining usually obviates the need for immunohistochemistry. The epithelial cells lining the cyst are positive for cytokeratins. Some of the cells may show positivity for glial fibrillary acidic protein.

DIFFERENTIAL DIAGNOSIS. Squamous metaplasia may lead to an erroneous diagnosis of papillary craniopharyngioma. Generous tissue sampling will generally lead to the finding of typical cuboidal or columnar epithelium in the Rathke's cleft cyst. Entirely suprasellar Rathke's cleft cysts may appear to be similar to colloid cysts of the roof of the third ventricle; the suprasellar location, greater degree of ciliation, and propensity for squamous metaplasia all support the diagnosis of Rathke's cleft cyst. Coexisting elements of Rathke's cleft cyst and pituitary adenoma in the same specimen probably represent sampling of coincidental lesions; however, the intimate association of these elements in some cases has suggested the presence of transitional tumors.[183]

## CYSTS OF OTHER ORIGIN

### Arachnoid Cysts

Arachnoid cysts of the sella or parasellar region may be congenital or acquired. When they arise in the sella, they may lead to hypopituitarism; when they form above the sella, they may lead to visual

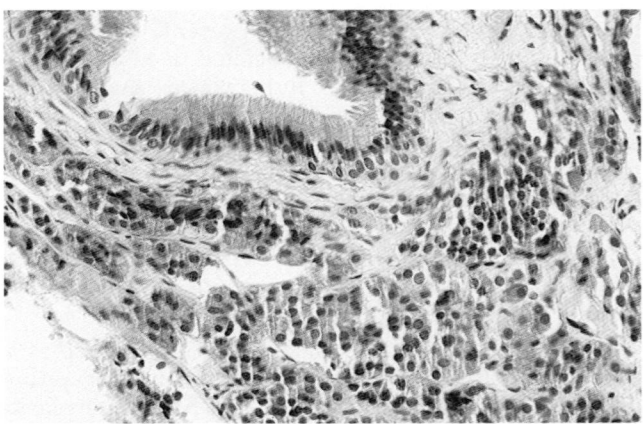

**Figure 50–25.** Rathke's cleft cyst. An epithelial cyst (top, left) lined by ciliated columnar cells rests on a fibrous stromal base containing residual adenophypophysial cells. (H&E, magnification ×100.)

or other neurologic deficits. The cysts are filled with clear, colorless fluid and are lined by a single layer of flattened arachnoidal cells.[184]

### Dermoid and Epidermoid Cysts

Dermoid and epidermoid cysts arise from epithelial cells misplaced during development. They may be seen in the suprasellar region, where they can cause hypopituitarism and elevated PRL as a result of stalk compression and visual field or other neurologic deficits.[91] Epidermoid cysts are lined by a thin squamous epithelium that shows abrupt keratinization forming sheets of keratin that fill the cyst[185, 186] (Fig. 50–26). In dermoid cysts, the epithelium also contains adnexal structures such as hair follicles or sweat glands.[92] Rupture of epidermoid cysts can lead to chemical meningitis. Development of a squamous carcinoma within an epidermoid cyst has been described.[187]

## Infections

Infections by bacteria, fungi, viruses, and protozoa may affect the sellar region.[188] In many cases, mass lesions may result, mimicking pituitary adenoma.

Acute bacterial infection with abscess formation may occur, particularly within preexisting cystic or neoplastic sellar lesions; the acute inflammatory infiltrate usually extends from an adjacent focus of acute infection, typically in the sphenoid or cavernous sinus. Less commonly, purulent pituitary abscesses may develop as a result of generalized sepsis or hematogenous dissemination from a distant septic source. Only rarely is transsphenoidal surgery complicated by abscess.[4, 188]

Chronic tuberculous meningitis may lead to functional compromise of the pituitary because of damage inflicted by plaques of basilar meningitis and secondary arteritis. Intrasellar tuberculomas may occur but are usually associated with active tuberculosis elsewhere.[189] Syphilitic granulomatous

infection may similarly affect the sella with destruction of pituitary tissue and hypopituitarism.[92] Whipple's disease involves the central nervous system in 10% to 20% of cases, and when it does, hypothalamic involvement is common. Infection with the rod-shaped bacillus *Tropheryma whippelii* results in strong PAS positivity of macrophages in the lesion. Definitive diagnosis is made by observing the organism by electron microscopy or by amplification of bacterial ribosomal RNA by the polymerase chain reaction.[190]

Infection with fungal organisms such as *Aspergillus* and *candida* or parasitic infection with *cysticercus* or *echinococcus* may produce mass lesions in this region.[191–194] Immunosuppressed patients, including those with acquired immunodeficiency syndrome, may have a variety of infections in the pituitary region, including *Pneumocystis carinii*, *Toxoplasma gondii*, and cytomegalovirus.[195]

## Inflammatory (Noninfectious) Disorders

### LYMPHOCYTIC HYPOPHYSITIS

CLINICAL CONSIDERATIONS. This chronic inflammatory disorder of the pituitary is thought to have an autoimmune basis. It occurs much more frequently in females than in males (8.5:1) with a particular predilection for women during pregnancy or in the postpartum period; 30% of the time, it coexists with another autoimmune disorder.[196–198] Recent data suggest that the precipitating antigen is alpha-enolase, a protein that is expressed by the placenta as well as pituitary, possibly explaining pregnancy as an initiating event.[225, 226] The inflamed pituitary gland may be diffusely enlarged and may even be associated with suprasellar extension, resulting in headaches and visual field impairment. Hypopituitarism is common; however, patients may rarely show

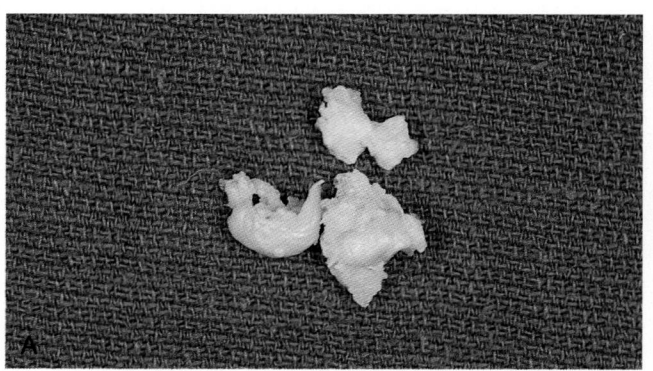 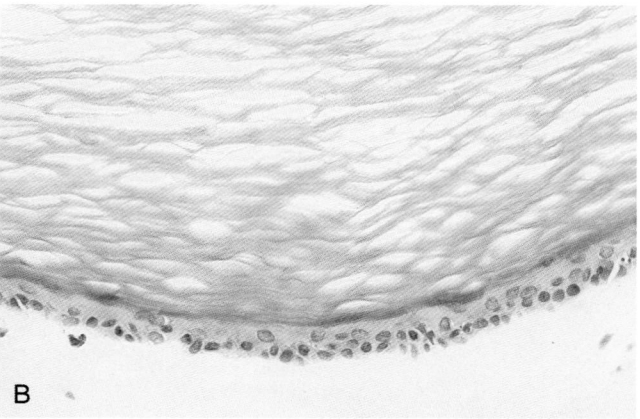

**Figure 50–26.** Epidermoid cyst. *A.* Gross fragments of excised epidermoid cyst reveal "pearly" appearance of the tissue. *B.* The fragments are composed of a thin squamous epithelium with numerous sheets of squames on the surface. (H&E, magnification ×100.)

isolated hormone insufficiency.[199] Hyperprolactinemia may be a result of an associated pregnancy, stalk compression by a suprasellar mass, or other alterations in local control of PRL release by inflammatory mediators. Because the diagnosis is established histologically in most patients, it is important that a correct frozen section diagnosis be rendered; surgery should then be limited to the biopsy specimen obtained for diagnosis.

DIAGNOSTIC CONSIDERATIONS. The adenohypophysial tissue is infiltrated by polyclonal lymphocytes and plasma cells accompanied by variable numbers of neutrophils, eosinophils, and macrophages (Fig. 50–27). Lymphoid follicles may be present. The adenohypophysis shows variable cell loss and fibrosis with residual islands of preserved acini, often with oncocytic change, separated by inflammatory cells. Inflammation may also involve the neurohypophysis.[196, 197] In rare cases, lymphocytic hypophysitis may overlap histologically with granulomatous hypophysitis.[200]

IMMUNOHISTOCHEMISTRY. The infiltrating lymphocytes may be labeled with common leukocyte antigen. Polyclonality can be established with antibodies against T and B cell markers and λ and κ light chains. Residual adenohypophysial cells can be identified with antibodies against pituitary hormones.

DIFFERENTIAL DIAGNOSIS. Lymphocytic hypophysitis can clinically mimic pituitary adenoma. Although inflammatory infiltrates may be present in some pituitary adenomas, they can easily be distinguished from hypophysitis by the greater degree of inflammation and presence of residual acini of normal gland in hypophysitis. Other inflammatory disorders, such as tuberculosis and sarcoidosis, are distinguished from hypophysitis by the finding of their characteristic granulomas. Giant cell granuloma is a disorder of unknown etiology that is characterized by granulomatous inflammation with aggregates of lymphocytes, epithelioid histiocytes, and multinucleated giant cells; infection must be excluded when this diagnosis is made.[200] Meningeal inflammatory pseudotumor may involve the sellar region; distinction is best made on clinical grounds because their histologic characteristics are similar.[201] Germinoma, lymphoma, and plasmacytoma all have inflammatory infiltrates and may involve the sellar region; however, they are identified by their defining neoplastic populations. Pregnant patients with complicated delivery may develop Sheehan's syndrome (postpartum pituitary necrosis), which may mimic lymphocytic hypophysitis because of the progressive postpartum hypopituitarism.[202]

## GRANULOMATOUS LESIONS

Granulomatous inflammation of noninfectious etiology can present in the sella as an isolated localized granulomatous process known as giant cell granuloma or granulomatous hypophysitis (Fig. 50–28) or rarely as the primary manifestation of sarcoidosis.[3, 203] The granulomas can enlarge the sella and mimic adenoma.[204] Granulomatous hypophysitis is considered by some authors to be part of the continuum of changes seen in the context of lymphocytic hypophysitis.[200] The infectious causes of granulomas including tuberculosis, syphilis, and fungal infection should always be ruled out when granulomas are identified. The granulomas are composed of epithelioid histiocytes, multinucleated giant cells, and lymphocytes.

## OTHER INFLAMMATORY LESIONS

*Neuroinfundibulohypophysitis* is a rare inflammatory condition that affects the infundibulum, the pituitary stalk, and the neurohypophysis. The inflammatory infiltrate resembles that of lymphocytic hypophysitis, and it is thought to be within the spectrum of autoimmune endocrine disorders that includes lymphocytic hypophysitis. Unlike, lymphocytic hypophysitis, infundibulohypophysitis shows no sexual predilection; it usually presents with diabetes insipidus and there is no direct involvement of the anterior lobe.[227]

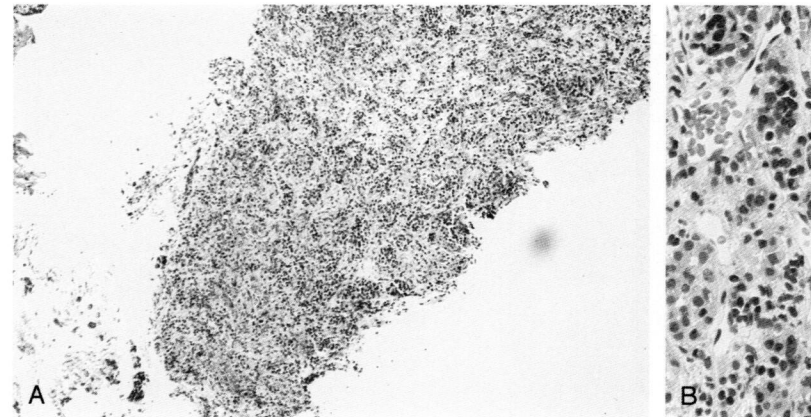
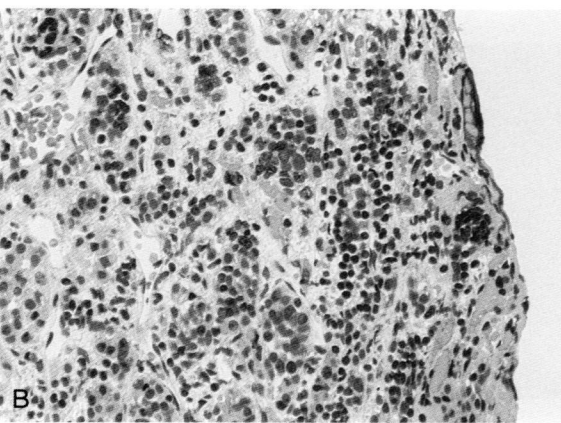

**Figure 50–27.** Lymphocytic hypophysitis. Biopsy specimen of anterior pituitary reveals prominent lymphocytic infiltrate within the anterior pituitary. (H&E; magnification: *A*, ×25; *B*, ×100.)

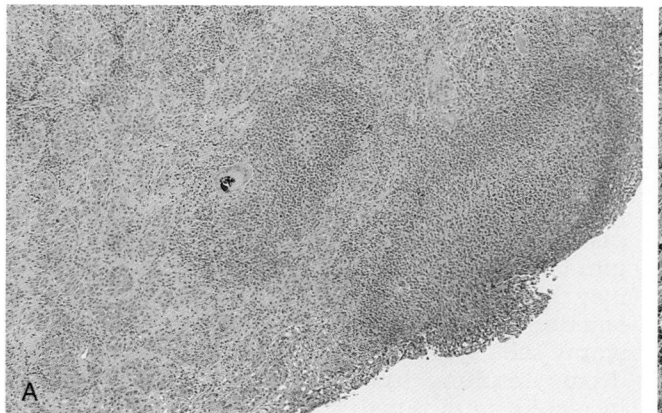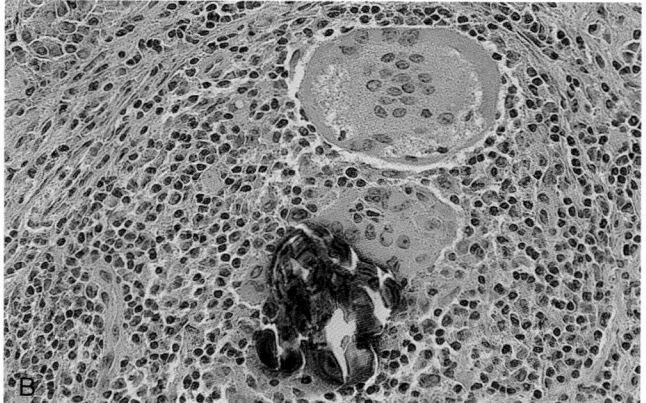

**Figure 50–28.** Granulomatous hypophysitis. *A.* Multiple granulomas in this patient are identified in the anterior pituitary enlarging the gland. (H&E, magnification ×25.) *B.* In this case, the granulomas are composed of epithelioid cells, giant cells with focal calcification, and lymphocytes. (H&E, magnification ×100.)

*Xanthomatous hypophysitis* is a rare form of primary hypophysitis that was first described in 1998 and has been occasionally reported since.[228, 229] It is characterized by an infiltrate of lipid-rich histiocytes with occasional lymphocytes, and resembles other xanthomatous inflammatory processes such as xanthomatous cholecystitis, endometritis or pyelonephritis. In other settings, this form of inflammation is attributed to cell debris of endogenous or infectious origin. Since these lesions have been reported to be cystic on radiologic or surgical evaluation, it may be that xanthomatous hypophysitis is a response to components of a ruptured cyst, however, this has not been proven.

## Arterial Intracranial Aneurysms

Aneurysm of the intracavernous or supraclinoid carotid artery, anterior communicating artery, or basilar tip may present as a suprasellar mass mimicking pituitary adenoma. If these lesions are not diagnosed before surgery, massive intraoperative bleeding may occur.[205] It is of interest that cerebral aneurysms may coexist with pituitary adenomas in approximately 7% of cases; this appears to be most frequently found with GH-secreting adenomas.[206]

Although rarely found in these locations, mucoceles of the sphenoid or ethmoid sinuses may erode into the sella to present as a sellar or suprasellar mass. Sellar involvement is usually not isolated but involves other areas of the skull base.[207]

## CONGENITAL AND DEVELOPMENTAL ABNORMALITIES

### Rathke's Pouch Remnants

Persistence of Rathke's pouch is common (20% to 30% of human pituitary glands). Small nests of squamous cells or small colloid-filled cysts are seen in the posterior lobe adjacent to the interface with the anterior pituitary; neither of these abnormalities has any clinical significance.[208]

## Hypoplasia or Aplasia

Defective formation of Rathke's pouch may lead to hypoplasia or aplasia of the anterior pituitary. The hypothalamus and posterior pituitary, which are of a different origin, develop normally. Survival of these infants is associated with hypopituitarism.[208] Mutations of the POU domain gene *PIT1* lead to selective loss of expression of GH, PRL, and TSH and hypoplasia of their respective cell types, and they have been described in two dwarf mouse strains.[209] *PIT1* mutations have been implicated in patients with cretinism and combined deficiency of the same three pituitary hormones.[210–212] Mutations of *PROP1*, a gene whose embryonic expression is required for Pit-1 expression, have been described in patients with deficiencies of GH, PRL, TSH, and gonadotropins.[213, 214] A number of other developmental defects have been causally associated with mutations of genes that encode proteins involved in development of the pituitary and the sellar region.[230–231] These include *septo-optic dysplasia* that is associated with inactivating mutations of HesX1, **Kallman's syndrome,** an X-linked developmental defect due to mutation of the KAL-1 gene that encodes an extracellular glycoprotein, **Prader-Willi syndrome** that has been linked with deletions of chromosome 15q11-q13; **Wolfram's syndrome (WS)** an autosomal recessive disorder characterized by diabetes insipidus, diabetes mellitus, optic atrophy and deafness that is due to compound heterozygous mutations of the WFS1 gene, a member of a novel gene family that encodes wolframin, an endoglycosidase H-sensitive membrane glycoprotein that localizes in the endoplasmic reticulum.

Anencephaly is a common malformation due to a major defect in closure of the cephalic neural tube.[215] This results in absence of the cranial vault and its associated soft tissues; defective brain development leads to absence of cerebral hemispheres, diencephalic structures, and posterior pituitary. The malformation results in intrauterine or early postnatal death. Although differentiation of adenohypophysial cells occurs, the hypothalamic abnormality leads to atrophy of the anterior pituitary and, after 32 weeks' gestation, reduced numbers of corticotrophs and virtual absence of gonadotrophs; somatotrophs, lactotrophs, and thyrotrophs are well represented.[216]

Encephaloceles, which also result from defective neural tube closure, can rarely extend into the sella, where they may form a mass lesion with hypopituitarism.[217]

## Salivary Gland Rests

Asymptomatic salivary gland rests can occur in the posterior lobe of the pituitary.[218] However, they may rarely be large enough to produce symptoms and may be the origin of rare salivary glandlike tumors of the sella.[219]

## MISCELLANEOUS DISORDERS

### Vascular Disorders of the Pituitary

Focal infarction of the anterior pituitary is not uncommon (1% to 6%) in unselected anterior pituitary glands at autopsy.[208] The small infarcts are usually not associated with known clinical abnormalities, although those cases with massive infarction (pituitary apoplexy) may develop hypopituitarism. Conditions associated with infarction include diabetes mellitus, traumatic head injury, stroke, increased intracranial pressure, and brain death of patients who are maintained on a respirator.[220]

Postpartum infarction of the pituitary (Sheehan's syndrome) is now rare in developed countries but may occur after severe blood loss causing shock around the time of delivery.[221] The resulting anterior hypopituitarism is characterized by headache, absence of lactation, persistent amenorrhea, and lethargy; diabetes insipidus is uncommon.

Rare cases of primary chronic intrasellar hematoma have been reported.[221]

### Empty Sella

Partial or complete filling of the sella by cerebrospinal fluid is referred to as empty sella; the sella itself may be of normal size or may be enlarged. An empty sella of normal size is common and represents a normal anatomic variant.[222] An enlarged empty sella, often termed empty sella syndrome, is

pathologic and may be primary, if there is no known cause, or secondary, if a definite cause for the condition is recognized. Primary empty sella syndrome is often found in obese, hypertensive females with headache and mild elevation of PRL. Some cases may be due to the effects of pulsatile cerebrospinal fluid transmitted through an incomplete diaphragma sellae. Others suggest that many cases are due to silent, spontaneous infarctions of pituitary adenomas.[85] Rarely, a pituitary adenoma may be found in association with the compressed anterior pituitary gland tissue of a patient with empty sella syndrome.[223] Secondary empty sella syndrome resulting from previous surgery, radiation, increased intracranial pressure, hydrocephalus, or clinically documented infarction of an adenoma has been described.

## Aging Changes in the Pituitary

A detailed analysis of the pituitary glands of 86 men and women older than 90 years showed that the pituitary has few morphologic changes with advanced age. The most significant difference is an increase in interstitial fibrosis, which occurs in men more than in women.[72]

## REFERENCES

1. Sutherland GR, Florell R, Louw D, et al: Epidemiology of primary intracranial neoplasms in Manitoba, Canada. Can J Neurol Sci 14:586–592, 1987.
2. Lovaste MG, Ferrari G, Rossi G: Epidemiology of primary intracranial neoplasms. Experiment in the province of Trento (Italy), 1977–1984. Neuroepidemiology 5:220–232, 1986.
3. Asa SL: Tumors of the Pituitary Gland. Atlas of Tumor Pathology. Third Series, Fascicle 22. Washington, DC, Armed Forces Institute of Pathology, 1998.
4. Thapar K, Kovacs K: Neoplasms of the sellar region. In Bigner DD, McLendon RE, Bruner JM (eds): Russel & Rubinstein's Pathology of Tumors of the Nervous System. Vol 2. 6th ed. New York, Oxford University Press, 1998, pp 561–677.
5. Kleihues P, Burger PC, Scheithauer BW: Histological Typing of Tumours of the Central Nervous System, World Health Organization, International Histological Classification of Tumours. Berlin, Springer-Verlag, 1993.
6. Wilson CB: Surgical management of pituitary tumors. Extensive personal experience. J Clin Endocrinol Metab 82:2381–2385, 1996.
7. Lloyd RV: Frozen sections in the diagnosis of pituitary lesions. In Lloyd RV (ed): Surgical Pathology of the Pituitary Gland. Philadelphia, WB Saunders, 1993, pp 22–24.
8. Lang HD, Saeger W, Ludecke DK, Muller D: Rapid frozen section diagnosis of pituitary tumors. Endocr Pathol 1:116–122, 1990.
9. Ng H-K: Smears in the diagnosis of pituitary adenoma. Acta Cytol 42:614–618, 1998.
10. Booth GL, Redelmeier DA, Grosman H, et al: Improved diagnostic accuracy of inferior petrosal sinus sampling over imaging for localizing pituitary pathology in patients with Cushing's disease. J Clin Endocrinol Metab 83:2291–2295, 1998.
11. Pegolo G, Buckwalter JG, Weiss MH, Hinton DR: Pituitary adenomas: correlation of the cytologic appearance with biologic behavior. Acta Cytol 39:887–891, 1995.
12. Hardy J, Verzina JL: Transsphenoidal microsurgery of intracranial neoplasms. In Thompson RA, Green JR (eds): Ad-

vances in Neurology. New York, Raven Press, 1976, pp 261–274.

13. Asa SL, Puy LA, Lew AM, et al: Cell type–specific expression of the pituitary transcription activator Pit-1 in the human pituitary and pituitary adenomas. J Clin Endocrinol Metab 77:1275–1280, 1993.
14. Asa SL, Bamberger AM, Cao B, et al: The transcription factor steroidogenic factor-1 is preferentially expressed in the human pituitary gonadotroph. J Clin Endocrinol Metab 81:2165–2170, 1996.
15. Horvath E, Kovacs K: Ultrastructural diagnosis of pituitary adenoma and hyperplasia. *In* Lloyd RV (ed): Surgical Pathology of the Pituitary Gland. Philadelphia, WB Saunders, 1993, pp 52–84.
16. Kovacs K, Scheithauer BW, Horvath E, Lloyd RV: The World Health Organization classification of adenohypophysial neoplasms. A proposed five-tier scheme. Cancer 78:502–510, 1996.
17. Herman V, Fagin J, Gonsky R, et al: Clonal origin of pituitary adenomas. J Clin Endocrinol Metab 71:1427–1433, 1990.
18. Asa SL, Ezzat S: The cytogenesis and pathogenesis of pituitary adenomas. Endocr Rev 19:798–827, 1998.
19. Vallar L, Spada A, Giannattasio G: Altered G_s and adenylate cyclase activity in human GH-secreting pituitary adenomas. Nature 330:566–568, 1987.
20. Tordjman K, Stern N, Ouaknine G, et al: Activating mutations of the G_s-gene in nonfunctioning pituitary tumors. J Clin Endocrinol Metab 77:765–769, 1993.
21. Zhuang Z, Ezzat SZ, Vortmeyer AO, et al: Mutations of the MEN1 tumor suppressor gene in pituitary tumors. Cancer Res 57:5446–5451, 1997.
22. Asa SL, Somers K, Ezzat S: The MEN-1 gene is rarely downregulated in pituitary adenomas. J Clin Endocrinol Metab 83:3210–3212, 1998.
23. Takeuchi S, Koeffler HP, Hinton DR, et al: Mutation and expression analysis of the cyclin-dependent kinase inhibitor gene p27/Kip1 in pituitary tumors. J Endocrinol 157:337–341, 1998.
24. Sumi T, Stefaneanu L, Kovacs K, et al: Immunohistochemical study of p53 protein in human and animal pituitary tumors. Endocr Pathol 4:95–99, 1993.
25. Levy A, Hall L, Yeundall WA, Lightman SL: P53 gene mutations in pituitary adenomas: rare events. Clin Endocrinol (Oxf) 41:809–814, 1994.
26. Buckley N, Bates AS, Broome JC, et al: P53 protein accumulation in Cushing's adenomas and invasive non-functional adenomas. J Clin Endocrinol Metab 79:1513–1516, 1994.
27. Cryns VL, Alexander JM, Klibanski A, Arnold A: The retinoblastoma gene in human pituitary tumors. J Clin Endocrinol Metab 77:644–646, 1993.
28. Zhu J, Leon SP, Beggs AH, et al: Human pituitary adenomas show no loss of heterozygosity at the retinoblastoma gene locus. J Clin Endocrinol Metab 78:922–927, 1994.
29. Pei L, Melmed S, Scheithauer B, et al: Frequent loss of heterozygosity at the retinoblastoma susceptibility gene (RB) locus in aggressive pituitary tumors: evidence for a chromosome 13 tumor suppressor gene other that RB. Cancer Res 55:1613–1616, 1995.
30. Ezzat S, Zheng L, Smyth HS, Asa SL: The c-erbB-2/neu proto-oncogene in human pituitary tumours. Clin Endocrinol 46:599–606, 1997.
31. Yokoyama S, Thapar K, Kovacs K, Stefeanu L: Localization of insulin-like growth factor-II mRNA in human pituitary adenomas. Virchows Arch 432:241–246, 1998.
32. Shimon I, Hinton DR, Weiss MH, Melmed S: Prolactinomas express human heparin-binding secretory transforming gene (hst) protein product: marker of tumor invasiveness. Clin Endocrinol 48:23–29, 1998.
33. Ezzat S, Smyth HS, Raymar L, Asa SL: Heterogeneous in vivo and in vitro expression of basic fibroblast growth factor by human pituitary adenomas. J Clin Endocrinol Metab 80:878–884, 1995.
34. Abbass SAA, Asa SL, Ezzat S: Altered expression of fibroblast growth factor receptors in human pituitary adenomas. J Clin Endocrinol Metab 82:1160–1166, 1997.
35. Alexander JM, Swearingen B, Tindall GT, Klibanski A: Human pituitary adenomas express endogenous inhibin subunit and follistatin messenger ribonucleic acids. J Clin Endocrinol Metab 80:147–152, 1995.
36. Penabad JL, Bashey HM, Asa SL, et al: Decreased follistatin gene expression in gonadotroph adenomas. J Clin Endocrinol Metab 81:3397–3403, 1996.
37. LeRiche VK, Asa SL, Ezzat S: Epidermal growth factor and its receptor (EGF-R) in human pituitary adenomas: EGF-R correlates with tumor aggressiveness. J Clin Endocrinol Metab 81:656–662, 1995.
38. Bates AS, Farrell WE, Bicjness EJ, et al: Allelic deletion in pituitary adenomas reflects aggressive biological activity and has potential value as a prognostic marker. J Clin Endocrinol Metab 82:818–824, 1997.
39. Thapar K, Scheithauer BW, Kovacs K, et al: p53 expression in pituitary adenomas and carcinomas: correlation with invasiveness and tumor growth factors. Neurosurgery 38:765–771, 1996.
40. Alvaro V, Touraine P, Raisman Vozari R, et al: Protein kinase C activity and expression in normal and adenomatous human pituitaries. Int J Cancer 50:724–730, 1992.
41. Hinton DR, Hahn JA, Weiss MH, Couldwell WT: Loss of RB expression in an ACTH-secreting pituitary carcinoma. Cancer Lett 126:209–214, 1998.
42. Pei L, Melmed B, Scheithauer B, et al: H-ras mutations in human pituitary carcinoma metastases. J Clin Endocrinol Metab 78:842–846, 1994.
43. Albuquerque FC, Hinton DR, Weiss MH: Excessively high prolactin level in a patient with a nonprolactin-secreting adenoma. J Neurosurg 89:1043–1046, 1998.
44. Thapar K, Kovacs K, Scheithauer BW, et al: Proliferative activity and invasiveness among pituitary adenomas and carcinomas: an analysis using the MIB-1 antibody. Neurosurgery 38:99–1071, 1996.
45. Kontogeorgos G, Sambaziotis D, Piaditis G, Karameris A: Apoptosis in human pituitary adenomas: a morphologic and in situ end-labeling study. Mod Pathol 10:921–926, 1997.
46. Burrow GN, Wortzman G, Rewcastle NB, et al: Microadenomas of the pituitary and abnormal sellar tomograms in an unselected autopsy series. N Engl J Med 304:156–158, 1981.
47. Annegers JF, Coulam CB, Abboud CF, et al: Pituitary adenoma in Olmstead County, Minnesota, 1935–1977. A report of an increasing incidence of diagnosis in women of childbearing age. Mayo Clin Proc 53:641–643, 1978.
48. Gold EB: Epidemiology of pituitary tumors. Epidemiol Rev 3:163–183, 1981.
49. Selman WR, Laws ER Jr, Scheithauer BW, Carpenter SM: The occurrence of dural invasion in pituitary adenomas. J Neurosurg 64:402–407, 1986.
50. Scheithauer BW, Kovacs KT, Laws ER Jr, Randall RV: Pathology of invasive pituitary tumors with special reference to functional classification. J Neurosurg 65:733–744, 1986.
51. Yonezawa K, Tamaki N, Kokunai T: Clinical features and growth fractions of pituitary adenomas. Surg Neurol 48:494–500, 1997.
52. Kawamoto H, Uozumi T, Kawamoto K, et al: Analysis of the growth rate and cavernous sinus invasion of pituitary adenomas. Acta Neurochir (Wien) 136:37–43, 1995.
53. Melmed S: Acromegaly. *In* Melmed S (ed): The Pituitary. Cambridge, MA, Blackwell Science, 1995, pp 413–442.
54. Orme SM, McNally RJ, Cartwright RA, Belchetz PE: Mortality and cancer incidence in acromegaly: a retrospective cohort study. United Kingdom Study Group. J Clin Endocrinol Metab 83:2730–2734, 1998.
55. Puchner MJ, Ludecke DK, Saeger W, et al: Gangliocytomas of the sellar region—a review. Exp Clin Endocrinol 103:129–149, 1995.
56. Asa SL, Scheithauer BW, Bilbao JM, et al: A case for hypothalamic acromegaly: a clinicopathologic study of six patients with hypothalamic gangliocytomas producing growth hormone–releasing factor. J Clin Endocrinol Metab 58:796–803, 1984.
57. Sano T, Asa SL, Kovacs K: Growth hormone–releasing hormone–producing tumors: clinical, biochemical and morphological manifestations. Endocr Rev 9:357–373, 1988.

58. Ezzat S, Asa SL, Stefaneanu L, et al: Somatotroph hyperplasia without pituitary adenoma associated with a long-standing growth hormone–releasing hormone–producing bronchial carcinoid. J Clin Endocrinol Metab 78:555–560, 1994.

59. Molitch ME: Prolactinoma. *In* Melmed S (ed): The Pituitary. Cambridge, MA, Blackwell Science, 1995, pp 443–477.

60. Horvath E, Kovacs K, Singer W, et al: Acidophil stem cell adenoma of the human pituitary: clinicopathologic analysis of 15 cases. Cancer 47:761–771, 1981.

61. Lipper S, Isenberg HD, Kahn LB: Calcospherites in pituitary prolactinomas. A hypothesis for their formation. Arch Pathol Lab Med 108:31–34, 1984.

62. Hinton DR, Polk RK, Linse KD, et al: Characterization of spherical amyloid protein from a prolactin-producing pituitary adenoma. Acta Neuropathol 93:43–49, 1997.

63. Zafar M, Ezzat S, Ramyar L, et al: Cell-specific expression of estrogen receptor in the human pituitary and its adenomas. J Clin Endocrinol Metab 80:3621–3627, 1995.

64. Ho KY, Evans WS, Thorner MO: Disorders of prolactin and growth hormone secretion. Clin Endocrinol Metab 14:1–32, 1985.

65. Jay V, Kovacs K, Horvath E, et al: Idiopathic prolactin cell hyperplasia of the pituitary mimicking prolactin cell adenoma: a morphological study including immunocytochemistry, electron microscopy, and in situ hybridization. Acta Neuropathol (Berl) 82:147–151, 1991.

66. Khalil A, Kovacs K, Sima AA, Burrow GN, Horvath E: Pituitary thyrotroph hyperplasia mimicking prolactin-secreting adenoma. J Endocrinol Invest 7:399–404, 1984.

67. Beck-Peccoz P, Brucker-Davis F, Persani L, et al: Thyrotropin-secreting pituitary tumors. Endocr Rev 17:610–638, 1996.

68. Bertagna X, Raux-Demay M-C, Guilhaume B, et al: Cushing's disease. *In* Melmed S (ed): The Pituitary. Cambridge, MA, Blackwell Science, 1995, pp 478–545.

69. Neumann PE, Horoupian DS, Goldman JE, Hess MA: Cytoplasmic filaments of Crooke's hyaline change belong to the cytokeratin class. An immunocytochemical and ultrastructural study. Am J Pathol 116:214–222, 1984.

70. Uei Y, Kanzaki M, Yabana T: Further immunohistochemical study of Crooke's hyalin. Pathol Res Pract 187:539–540, 1991.

71. Felix IA, Horvath E, Kovacs K: Massive Crooke's hyalinization in corticotroph cell adenomas of the human pituitary. A histological, immunocytological and electron microscopic study of three cases. Acta Neurochir (Wien) 58:235–243, 1981.

72. Sano T, Kovacs KT, Scheithauer BW, Young WF: Aging and the human pituitary gland. Mayo Clin Proc 68:971–977, 1993.

73. Snyder PJ: Gonadotroph adenoma. *In* Melmed S (ed): The Pituitary. Cambridge, MA, Blackwell Science, 1995, pp 559–575.

74. Kovacs K, Lloyd R, Horvath E, et al: Silent somatotroph adenomas of the human pituitary. A morphologic study of three cases including immunocytochemistry, electron microscopy, in vitro examination, and in situ hybridization. Am J Pathol 134:345–353, 1989.

75. Black PM, Hsu DW, Klibanski A, et al: Hormone production in clinically nonfunctioning pituitary adenomas. J Neurosurg 66:244–250, 1987.

76. Chabre O, Martinie M, Vivier J, et al: A clinically silent corticotroph adenoma (CSCPA) secreting a biologically inactive but immunoreactive assayable ACTH (abstract). J Endocrinol Invest 13(suppl 1):87, 1991.

77. Albuquerque FC, Weiss MH, Kovacs K, et al: A functioning composite "corticotroph" pituitary adenoma with interspersed adrenocortical cells. Pituitary 1:279–284, 1999.

78. Yamada S, Asa SL, Kovacs K: Oncocytomas and null cell adenomas of the human pituitary: morphometric and in vitro functional comparison. Virchows Arch A Pathol Anat Histopathol 413:333–339, 1988.

79. Kovacs K, Horvath E, Stefaneanu L, et al: Pituitary adenoma producing growth hormone and adrenocorticotropin: a histological, immunocytochemical, electron microscopic, and in situ hybridization study. Case report. J Neurosurg 88:1111–1115, 1998.

80. Horvath E, Kovacs K, Smyth HS, et al: A novel type of pituitary adenoma: morphological features and clinical correlations. J Clin Endocrinol Metab 66:1111–1118, 1988.

81. Coire CI, Horvath E, Kovacs K, et al: Cushing's syndrome from an ectopic pituitary adenoma with peliosis: a histological, immunohistochemical and ultrastructural study and review of the literature. Endocr Pathol 8:65–74, 1997.

82. Hori A: Suprasellar peri-infundibular ectopic adenohypophysis in fetal and adult brains. J Neurosurg 62:113–115, 1985.

83. Bills DG, Meyer FB, Laws ER Jr, et al: A retrospective analysis of pituitary apoplexy. Neurosurgery 33:602–609, 1993.

84. Kleinschmidt-Demasters BK, Lillehei KO: Pathological correlates of pituitary adenomas presenting with apoplexy. Hum Pathol 29:1255–1265, 1998.

85. Robinson DB, Michaels RD: Empty sella resulting from the spontaneous resolution of a pituitary macroadenoma. Arch Intern Med 152:1920–1923, 1992.

86. Shimon I, Melmed S: Management of pituitary tumors. Ann Intern Med 129:472–483, 1998.

87. Kovacs K, Stefaneanu L, Horvath E, et al: Effect of dopamine agonist medication on prolactin producing pituitary adenomas. A morphological study including immunohistochemistry, electron microscopy, and in situ hybridization. Virchows Arch A Pathol Anat Histopathol 418:439–446, 1991.

88. Ezzat S, Horvath E, Harris AG, Kovacs K: Morphological effects of octreotide on growth hormone–producing pituitary adenomas. J Clin Endocrinol Metab 79:113–118, 1994.

89. Kannuki S, Matsumoto K, Sano T, et al: Double pituitary adenomas—two case reports. Neurol Med Chir (Tokyo) 36:818–821, 1996.

90. Pernicone PJ, Scheithauer BW, Sebo TJ, et al: Pituitary carcinoma. A clinicopathologic study of 15 cases. Cancer 79:804–812, 1997.

91. Saeger W, Lubke D: Pituitary carcinoma. Endocr Pathol 7:21–35, 1996.

92. Scheithauer BW: The hypothalamus and neurohypophysis. *In* Kovacs K, Asa SL (eds): Functional Endocrine Pathology. 2nd ed. Malden, MA, Blackwell Science, 1998, pp 171–246.

93. Gillett GR, Symon L: Hypothalamic glioma. Surg Neurol 28:291–300, 1987.

94. Zampieri P, Zorat P, Mingrino S, Soattin G: Radiation-associated cerebral gliomas: a report of two cases and review of the literature. J Neurosurg Sci 33:271–279, 1989.

95. Tsang RW, Laperriere NJ, Simpson WJ, et al: Glioma arising after radiation therapy for pituitary adenoma. A report of four cases and estimation of risk. Cancer 72:2227–2233, 1993.

96. Forsythe PA, Shaw EG, Scheithauer BW, et al: Supratentorial pilocytic astrocytoma: a clinicopathologic prognostic and flow cytometric study of 51 cases. Cancer 72:1335–1342, 1993.

97. Johannsson JH, Rekate HL, Roessmann U: Gangliogliomas: pathological and clinical correlation. J Neurosurg 54:58–63, 1981.

98. Winer JB, Lidov H, Scaravilli F: An ependymoma involving the pituitary fossa. J Neurol Neurosurg Psychiatry 52:1443–1444, 1989.

99. Rossi ML, Bevan JS, Esiri MM, et al: Pituicytoma (pilocytic astrocytoma). J Neurosurg 67:768–772, 1987.

100. Posener L, Michener JW, Skwarok EW: Infundibuloma: a case report with a brief review of the literature. J Neurosurg 14:680–684, 1957.

101. Louis DN, Budka H, von Deimling A: Meningiomas. *In* Kleihues P, Cavanee WK (eds): Tumours of the Nervous System. Pathology and Genetics. Lyons, International Agency for Research on Cancer, 1997, pp 134–141.

102. Slavin MJ, Weintraub J: Suprasellar meningioma with intrasellar extension simulating pituitary adenoma. Case report. Arch Ophthalmol 105:1488–1489, 1987.

103. Grisoli F, Vincentelli F, Raybaud C, et al: Intrasellar meningioma. Surg Neurol 20:36–41, 1983.

104. Sridhar K, Ramamurthi B: Intracranial meningioma subsequent to radiation for a pituitary tumor: case report. Neurosurgery 25:643–645, 1989.

105. Parrish EP, Steart PV, Garrod DR, Weller RO: Antidesmosomal monoclonal antibody in the diagnosis of intracranial tumors. J Pathol 153:265–273, 1987.

106. Thapar K, Laws ER Jr: Vascular tumors: haemangioblasto-

mas, haemangiopericytomas and cavernous angiomas. *In* Sheaves R, Jenkins PT, Wass JAH (eds): Clinical Endocrine Oncology. Oxford, Blackwell Science, 1997, pp 264–272.

107. Luse S, Kernohan J: Granular cell tumors of the stalk and posterior lobe of the pituitary gland. Cancer 8:616–622, 1955.

108. Shanklin WM: The origin, histology and senescence of tumorettes in the human neurohypophysis. Acta Anat (Basel) 18:1–20, 1953.

109. Schaller B, Kirsch E, Tolnay M, Mindermann T: Symptomatic granular cell tumor of the pituitary gland: case report and review of the literature. Neurosurgery 42:166–171, 1998.

110. Parent A: Parasellar granular cell tumors. *In* Wilkins R, Rengachary S (eds): Neurosurgery. 2nd ed. New York, McGraw-Hill, 1996, pp 1415–1417.

111. Nishioka H, Li K, Llena JF, Hirano A: Immunohistochemical study of granular cell tumors of the neurohypophysis. Virchows Arch B Cell Pathol Incl Mol Pathol 60:413–417, 1991.

112. Erdheim J: Über Hypophysengangsgeshwulste und Hirnscholesteatome. Sitzungsbericht des Kaiselichen Akademie der Wissenchaften. Mathematisch-naturwissenschaftliche Classe 113:537–726, 1904.

113. Asa SL, Kovacs K, Bilbao JM: The pars tuberalis of the human pituitary. A histologic, immunohistochemical, ultrastructural and immunoelectron microscopic analysis. Virchows Arch A Pathol Anat Histopathol 399:49–59, 1983.

114. Petito CK, DeGirolami U, Earle KM: Craniopharyngiomas. A clinical and pathological review. Cancer 37:1944–1952, 1976.

115. Nelson GA, Bastian FO, Schlitt M, White RL: Malignant transformation in craniopharyngioma. Neurosurgery 12:427–429, 1988.

116. Asa SL, Kovacs K, Bilbao JM, Penz G: Immunohistochemical localization of keratin in craniopharyngiomas and squamous cell nests of the human pituitary. Acta Neuropathol 54:257–260, 1981.

117. Ho KL: Ecchordosis physaliphora and chordoma: a comparative ultrastructural study. Clin Neuropathol 4:77–85, 1985.

118. Heffelfinger MJ, Dahlin DC, MacCarty CS, Beabout JW: Chordomas and cartilaginous tumors at the skull base. Cancer 32:410–420, 1973.

119. Mathews W, Wilson CB: Ectopic intrasellar chordoma. J Neurosurg 39:260–263, 1974.

120. Tomlinson FH, Scheithauer BW, Forsythe PA, et al: Sarcomatous transformation in a cranial chordoma. Neurosurgery 31:13–18, 1992.

121. Brooks JJ, LiVolsi VA, Trojanowski JQ: Does chondroid chordoma exist? Acta Neuropathol 72:229–272, 1986.

122. Jennings MT, Gelman R, Hochberg T: Intracranial germ cell tumors: natural history and pathogenesis. J Neurosurg 63:155–167, 1985.

123. Ballesteros MD, Duran A, Arrazola J, et al: Primary intrasellar germinoma with synchronous pineal tumor. Neuroradiology 39:860–862, 1997.

124. Poon W, Ng HK, Wong K, South JR: Primary intrasellar germinoma presenting with cavernous sinus syndrome. Surg Neurol 30:402–405, 1988.

125. Kidooka M, Okada T, Nakajima M, Handa J: Intra- and suprasellar germinoma mimicking a pituitary adenoma—case report. Neurol Med Chir (Tokyo) 35:96–99, 1995.

126. Nakagawa Y, Perentes E, Ross GW, et al: Immunohistochemical differences between intracranial germinomas and their gonadal equivalents. An immunoperoxidase study of germ cell tumors with epithelial membrane antigen, cytokeratin, and vimentin. J Pathol 156:67–72, 1988.

127. Shibamoto Y, Takahashi M, Sasai K: Prognosis of intracranial germinoma with syncytiotrophoblastic giant cells treated by radiation therapy. Int J Radiat Oncol Biol Phys 37:505–510, 1997.

128. Maiuri F: Primary cerebral lymphoma presenting as a steroid responsive chiasmal syndrome. Br J Neurosurg 1:499–502, 1987.

129. Samaratunga H, Perry-Keane D, Apel RL: Primary lymphoma of pituitary gland: a neoplasm of acquired MALT? Endocr Pathol 8:335–341, 1997.

130. Singh VP, Mahapatra AK, Dinde AK: Sellar-suprasellar primary malignant lymphoma: case report. Indian J Cancer 30:88–91, 1993.

131. Sekhar L, Ross D, Sen C: Cavernous sinus and sphenocavernous neoplasms: anatomy and surgery. *In* Sekhar L, Janecka I (eds): Surgery of Cranial Base Tumors. New York, Raven Press, 1993, pp 521–604.

132. Ishege N, Ito C, Saeki N, Oka N: Neurinoma with intrasellar extension: a case report. Neurol Surg 13:79–84, 1985.

133. Perone TP, Robinson B, Holmes SM: Intrasellar schwannoma: case report. Neurosurgery 14:71–73, 1984.

134. Wilberger JE Jr: Primary intrasellar schwannoma: case report. Surg Neurol 32:156–158, 1989.

135. Civit T, Pinelli C, Klein M, et al: Intrasellar schwannoma. Acta Neurochir (Wien) 139:160–161, 1997.

136. Woodruff JM, Kourea HP, Louis DN: Schwannoma. *In* Kleihues P, Cavanee WK (eds): Tumours of the Nervous System. Pathology and Genetics. Lyons, International Agency for Research on Cancer, 1997, pp 126–128.

137. Dan NG, Smith DE: Pituitary hemangioblastoma in a patient with von Hippel–Lindau disease. J Neurosurg 42:232–235, 1975.

138. Steel TR, Dailey AT, Born D, et al: Paragangliomas of the sellar region: report of two cases. Neurosurgery 32:844–847, 1993.

139. Bilbao JM, Horvath E, Kovacs K, et al: Intrasellar paraganglioma associated with hypopituitarism. Arch Pathol Lab Med 102:95–98, 1978.

140. Neilson JM, Moffat AD: Hypopituitarism caused by a melanoma of the pituitary gland. J Clin Pathol 16:144–149, 1963.

141. Scholtz CL, Siu K: Melanoma of the pituitary. Case report. J Neurosurgery 45:101–103, 1976.

142. Chang WH, Khosla VK, Radotra BD, Kak VK: Large cavernous hemangioma of the pituitary fossa: a case report. Br J Neurosurg 5:627–629, 1991.

143. Sansone ME, Liwnicz BH, Mandybur TI: Giant pituitary cavernous hemangioma: case report. J Neurosurg 53:124–126, 1980.

144. Asa SL, Kovacs K, Horvath E, et al: Sellar glomangioma. Ultrastruct Pathol 7:49–54, 1984.

145. Esposito S, Nardi P: Lipoma of the infundibulum. Case report. J Neurosurg 67:304–306, 1987.

146. Watkins LD, Uttley D, Archer DJ, et al: Giant cell tumors of the sphenoid bone. Neurosurgery 30:576–581, 1992.

147. Viswanathan R, Jegathraman AR, Ganapathy K, et al: Parasellar chondromyxoid fibroma with ipsilateral total internal carotid artery occlusion. Surg Neurol 28:141–144, 1987.

148. Dutton J: Intracranial solitary chondroma. Case report. J Neurosurg 49:460–463, 1978.

149. Miki K, Kawamoto K, Kawamura Y, et al: A rare case of Maffucci's syndrome combined with tuberculum sellae enchondroma, pituitary adenoma and thyroid adenoma. Acta Neurochir (Wien) 87:79–85, 1987.

150. Sindou M, Daher A, Vighetto A, Goutelle A: Chondrosarcome parasellaire: report d'un cas opere par voie pterionotemporale et revue de la litterature. Neurochirurgie 35:186–190, 1989.

151. Bots GT, Tijssen CC, Wijnalda D, Teepen JL: Alveolar soft part sarcoma of the pituitary gland with secondary involvement of the right cerebral ventricle. Br J Neurosurg 2:101–107, 1988.

152. Jalalah S, Kovacs K, Horvath E, et al: Rhabdomyosarcoma in the region of the sella turcica. Acta Neurochir (Wien) 88:142–146, 1987.

153. Ahmad K, Fayos JV: Pituitary fibrosarcoma secondary to radiation therapy. Cancer 42:107–110, 1978.

154. Shi T, Farrell MA, Kaufmann JC: Fibrosarcoma complicating irradiated pituitary adenoma. Surg Neurol 22:277–284, 1984.

155. Amine AR, Sugar O: Suprasellar osteogenic sarcoma following radiation for pituitary adenoma. Case report. J Neurosurg 44:88–91, 1976.

156. Jin L, Lloyd RV: Metastatic neoplasms to the pituitary gland. *In* Lloyd RV (ed): Surgical Pathology of the Pituitary Gland. Philadelphia, WB Saunders, 1993, pp 137–140.

157. Roessmann U, Kaufman B, Friede RL: Metastatic lesions in the sella turcica and pituitary gland. Cancer 68:1673–1677, 1970.

158. Branch CL Jr, Laws ER Jr: Metastatic tumors of the sella

turcica masquerading as primary pituitary tumors. J Clin Endocrinol Metab 65:469–474, 1987.

159. Morita A, Meyer FB, Laws ER Jr: Symptomatic pituitary metastases. J Neurosurg 89:69–73, 1998.

160. Zager EL, Hedley-Whyte ET: Metastasis within a pituitary adenoma presenting with bilateral abducens palsies: case report and review of the literature. Neurosurgery 21:383–386, 1987.

161. Scheithauer BW: Pathology of the pituitary and sellar region: exclusive of pituitary adenoma. Pathol Annu 20:67–188, 1985.

162. Masse SR, Wolk RW, Conklin RH: Peripituitary gland involvement in acute leukemia in adults. Arch Pathol 96:141–142, 1973.

163. Sheehan T, Cuthbert RJ, Parker AC: Central nervous system involvement in haematological malignancies. Clin Lab Haematol 11:331–338, 1989.

164. Dhanani AN, Bilbao J, Kovacs K: Multiple myeloma presenting as a sellar plasmacytoma and mimicking a pituitary tumor: report of a case and review of the literature. Endocr Pathol 1:245–248, 1990.

165. Branch CL Jr, Laws ER Jr: Metastatic tumors of the sella turcica masquerading as primary pituitary tumors. J Clin Endocrinol Metab 65:469–474, 1987.

166. Mancardi GL, Mandybur TI: Solitary intracranial plasmacytoma. Cancer 51:2226–2233, 1983.

167. Lieberman PH, Jones CR, Dargeon HW, Begg CF: A reappraisal of eosinophilic granuloma of bone, Hand-Schüller-Christian syndrome and Letterer-Siwe syndrome. Medicine (Baltimore) 48:375–400, 1969.

168. Kepes JJ, Kepes M: Predominantly cerebral forms of histiocytosis-X. A reappraisal of "Gagel's hypothalamic granuloma," "granuloma infiltrans of the hypothalamus" and "Ayala's disease" with a report of four cases. Acta Neuropathol (Berl) 14:77–98, 1969.

169. Schmitt S, Wichmann W, Martin E, et al: Primary stalk thickening with diabetes insipidus preceding typical manifestations of Langerhans cell histiocytosis in children. Eur J Pediatr 152:399–401, 1993.

170. Nishio S, Mizuno J, Barrow DL, et al: Isolated histiocytosis X of the pituitary gland: case report. Neurosurgery 21:718–721, 1987.

171. Ober KP, Alexander E Jr, Challa VR, et al: Histiocytosis X of the hypothalamus. Neurosurgery 24:93–95, 1989.

172. Ornvold K, Ralfkiaer E, Carstensen H: Immunohistochemical study of the abnormal cells in Langerhans cell histiocytosis (histiocytosis X). Virchows Arch A Pathol Anat Histopathol 416:403–410, 1990.

173. Saeger W, Ludecke DK: Pituitary hyperplasia. Definition, light and electron microscopical structures and significance in surgical specimens. Virchows Arch A Pathol Anat Histopathol 399:277–287, 1983.

174. Stefaneanu L, Kovacs K, Lloyd RV, et al: Pituitary lactotrophs and somatotrophs in pregnancy: a correlative in situ hybridization and immunocytochemical study. Virchows Arch B Cell Pathol Incl Mol Pathol 62:291–296, 1992.

175. Kovacs K, Horvath E, Thorner MO, Rogol A: Mammosomatotroph hyperplasia associated with acromegaly and hyperprolactinemia in a patient with the McCune-Albright syndrome. A histologic, immunocytological, and ultrastructural study of surgically-removed adenohypophysis. Virchows Arch A Pathol Anat Histopathol 403:77–86, 1984.

176. Kubota T, Hayashi M, Kubuto M, et al: Corticotroph hyperplasia in a patient with Addison's disease: case report. Surg Neurol 37:441–447, 1992.

177. McKeever PE, Koppelman MC, Metcalf D, et al: Refractory Cushing's disease caused by multinodular ACTH-cell hyperplasia. J Neuropathol Exp Neurol 41:490–499, 1982.

178. McGrath P: Cysts of sellar and pharyngeal hypophyses. Pathology 3:123–131, 1971.

179. Yoshida J, Kobayashi T, Kageyama N, Kanzaki M: Symptomatic Rathke's cleft cyst. Morphologic study with light and electron microscopy and tissue culture. J Neurosurg 47:451–458, 1977.

180. Voelker JL, Campbell RL, Muller J: Clinical, radiographic, and pathological features of symptomatic Rathke's cleft cysts. J Neurosurg 74:535–544, 1991.

181. Nishio S, Mizuno J, Barrow DL, et al: Pituitary tumors composed of adenohypophyseal adenoma and Rathke's cleft cyst elements: a clinicopathologic study. Neurosurgery 21:371–377, 1987.

182. Keyaki A, Hirano A, Llena JF: Asymptomatic and symptomatic Rathke's cleft cysts: histologic study of 45 cases. Neurol Med Chir 29:88–93, 1989.

183. Kepes JJ: Transitional cell tumor of the pituitary gland developing from a Rathke's cleft cyst. Cancer 41:337–343, 1978.

184. Meyer FB, Carpenter SM, Laws ER Jr: Intrasellar arachnoid cysts. Surg Neurol 28:105–110, 1987.

185. Yamakawa K, Shitara N, Genka S, et al: Clinical course and surgical prognosis of 33 cases of intracranial epidermoid tumors. Neurosurgery 24:568–573, 1989.

186. Abramson RC, Morawetz RB, Schlitt M: Multiple complications from an intracranial epidermoid cyst: case report and literature review. Neurosurgery 24:574–578, 1989.

187. Lewis AJ, Cooper PW, Kassel EE, Schwartz ML: Squamous cell carcinoma arising in a suprasellar epidermoid cyst. Case report. J Neurosurg 59:538–541, 1983.

188. Berger SA, Edberg SC, David G: Infectious disease in the sella turcica. Rev Infect Dis 8:747–755, 1986.

189. Ranjan A, Chandy MJ: Intrasellar tuberculoma. Br J Neurosurg 8:179–185, 1994.

190. Mendel E, Khoo LT, Go JL, et al: Intracerebral Whipple's disease diagnosed by stereotactic biopsy: a case report and review of the literature. Neurosurgery 44:203–209, 1999.

191. Heary RF, Maniker AH, Wolansky LJ: Candidal pituitary abscess—case report. Neurosurgery 36:1009–1012, 1995.

192. Ramos-Gabatin A, Jordan RM: Primary pituitary aspergillosis responding to transsphenoidal surgery and combined therapy with amphotericin-B and 5-flurocytosine: case report. J Neurosurg 54:839–841, 1981.

193. Boecher-Schwaz HG, Hey O, Higer HP, Perneczky A: Intrasellar cysticercosis mimicking a pituitary adenoma. Br J Neurosurg 5:405–407, 1991.

194. Ozgen T, Bertan V, Kansu T, Akalin S: Intrasellar hydatid cyst. Case report. J Neurosurg 60:647–648, 1984.

195. Sano T, Kovacs K, Scheithauer BW, et al: Pituitary pathology in acquired immunodeficiency syndrome. Arch Pathol Lab Med 113:1066–1070, 1989.

196. Thodou E, Asa SL, Kontogeorgos G, et al: Clinical case seminar: lymphocytic hypophysitis: clinicopathological findings. J Clin Endocrinol Metab 80:2302–2311, 1995.

197. Asa SL, Bilbao JM, Kovacs K, et al: Lymphocytic hypophysitis of pregnancy resulting in hypopituitarism: a distinct clinicopathologic entity. Ann Intern Med 95:166–171, 1981.

198. Pestell RG, Best JD, Alford FP: Lymphocytic hypophysitis. The clinical spectrum of the disorder and evidence for an autoimmune pathogenesis. Clin Endocrinol (Oxf) 40:693–695, 1994.

199. Jensen MD, Handwerger BS, Scheithauer BW, et al: Lymphocytic hypophysitis with isolated corticotropin deficiency. Ann Intern Med 105:200–203, 1986.

200. Honegger J, Fahlbusch R, Bornemann A, et al: Lymphocytic and granulomatous hypophysitis: experience with nine cases. Neurosurgery 40:713–723, 1997.

201. Gartman JJ Jr, Powers SK, Fortune M: Pseudotumor of the sellar and parasellar areas. Neurosurgery 24:896–901, 1989.

202. Sheehan HL: Post-partum necrosis of the anterior pituitary. J Pathol Bacteriol 45:189–214, 1937.

203. Veseley DL, Maldonodo A, Levey GS: Partial hypopituitarism and possible hypothalamic involvement of sarcoidosis: report of a case and review of the literature. Am J Med 62:425–431, 1977.

204. Del Pozo JM, Roda JE, Montoya JG, et al: Intrasellar granuloma. Case report. J Neurosurg 53:717–719, 1980.

205. Dussault J, Plamondon C, Volpe R: Aneurysms of the internal carotid artery simulating pituitary tumors. Can Med Assoc J 101:51–56, 1969.

206. Weir B: Pituitary adenomas and aneurysms: case report and review of the literature. Neurosurgery 30:585–591, 1992.

207. Delfini R, Missori P, Iannetti G, et al: Mucoceles of the para-

nasal sinuses with intracranial and intraorbital extension: report of 28 cases. Neurosurgery 32:901–906, 1993.

208. Horvath E, Kovacs K: The adenohypophysis. *In* Kovacs K, Asa SL (eds): Functional Endocrine Pathology. 2nd ed. Malden, MA, Blackwell Science, 1998, pp 247–281.
209. Li S, Crenshaw EB III, Rawson EJ, et al: Dwarf locus mutants lacking three pituitary cell types result from mutations in the POU-domain gene *pit-1*. Nature 347:528–533, 1990.
210. Tatsumi K, Miyai K, Notomi T, et al: Cretinism with combined hormone deficiency caused by a mutation in the Pit-1 gene. Nat Genet 1:56–58, 1992.
211. Pfäffle RW, DiMattia GE, Parks JS,et al: Mutation of the POU-specific domain of Pit-1 and hypopituitarism without pituitary hypoplasia. Science 257:1118–1121, 1992.
212. Radovick S, Nations M, Du Y, et al: A mutation in the POU-homeodomain of Pit-1 responsible for combined pituitary hormone deficiency. Science 257:1115–1118, 1992.
213. Wu W, Cogan JD, Pfäffle RW, et al: Mutations in *PROP1* cause familial combined pituitary hormone deficiency. Nat Genet 18:147–149, 1998.
214. Fofanova O, Takamura N, Kinoshita E, et al: Compound heterozygous deletion of the prop-1 gene in children with combined pituitary hormone deficiency. J Clin Endocrinol Metab 83:2601–2604, 1998.
215. Norman MG, McGillivray, Kalousek DK, et al: Neural tube defect. Part 2. Anencephaly. *In* Congenital Malformations of the Brain. Pathological, Embryological, Clinical, Radiological and Genetic Aspects. New York, Oxford University Press, pp 17–129.
216. Pilavdzic D, Kovacs K, Asa SL: Pituitary morphology in anencephalic human fetuses. Neuroendocrinology 65:164–172, 1997.
217. Durham LH, Mackenzie IJ, Miles JB: Transsphenoidal meningohydroencephalocele. Br J Neurosurg 2:407–409, 1988.
218. Schochet SS Jr, McCormick WF, Halmi NS: Salivary gland rests in the human pituitary. Light and electron microscopical study. Arch Pathol 98:193–200, 1974.
219. Hampton TA, Scheithauer BW, Rojiani AM, et al: Salivary gland–like tumors of the sellar region. Am J Surg Pathol 21:424–434, 1997.

220. Reid RL, Quigley ME, Yen SSC: Pituitary apoplexy. A review. Arch Neurol 42:712–719, 1985.
221. Saito K, Takayasu M, Akabane A, et al: Primary chronic intrasellar haematoma: a case report. Acta Neurochir (Wien) 114:147–150, 1992.
222. Bjerre P: The empty sella. A reappraisal of etiology and pathogenesis. Acta Neurol Scand 82:1–24, 1990.
223. Benbow EW: Pituitary corticotroph adenoma in a primary enlarged empty sella turcica. Histopathology 32:186–187, 1998.
224. Ezzat S, Zhang L, Zhu XF, Wu GE, Asa SL: Targeted expression of a human pituitary tumor-derived isoform of FGF receptor-4 recapitulates pituitary tumorigenesis. J Clin Invest 109:69–78, 2002.
225. O'Dwyer DT, Smith AI, Matthew ML, Andronicos NM, Ranson M, Robinson PJ, Crock PA: Identification of the 49-kDa autoantigen associated with lymphocytic hypophysitis as alpha-enolase. J Clin Endocrinol Metab 87:752–757, 2002.
226. O'Dwyer DT, Clifton V, Hall A, Smith R, Robinson PJ, Crock PA: Pituitary Autoantibodies in Lymphocytic Hypophysitis Target Both gamma- and alpha-Enolase—A Link with Pregnancy? Arch Physiol Biochem 110:94–98, 2002.
227. Tubridy N, Saunders D, Thom M, Asa SL, Powell M, Plant GT, Howard R: Infundibulohypophysitis in a man presenting with diabetes insipidus and cavernous sinus involvement. Journal of Neurology, Neurosurgery and Psychiatry 71:798–801, 2001.
228. Folkerth RD, Price DL, Schwartz M, Black PM, De Girolami U: Xanthomatous hypophysitis. American Journal of Surgical Pathology 22:736–741, 1998.
229. Cheung CC, Ezzat S, Smyth HS, Asa SL: The spectrum and significance of primary hypophysitis. J Clin Endocrinol Metab 86:1048–1053, 2001.
230. Asa SL, Ezzat S: Molecular determinants of pituitary cytodifferentiation. Pituitary 1:159–168, 1999.
231. Scully KM, Rosenfeld MG: Pituitary development: regulatory codes in mammalian organogenesis. Science 295:2231–2235, 2002.

# Central Nervous System Tumors

M. Beatriz S. Lopes   Bruce C. Horten

## NEOPLASTIC LESIONS

### Classification

The classification system of central nervous system (CNS) tumors used in this chapter follows the now widely adopted format established by the World Health Organization (WHO).[1] This scheme wherever practical is based on the hypothesized cell of origin of the tumor and is modified and subclassified by associated histologic features (Table 51–1).

### General Considerations

#### PATHOGENESIS

The genesis of brain tumors remains largely a mystery, although many of the factors surrounding this puzzle have been clarified. As for environmental factors uncovered through epidemiologic investigations, only irradiation seems to play a reliably reproducible role.[2] Molecular biology and cytogenetic studies continue to reveal the genotypic heterogeneity of brain tumors.[3] To date, these studies point to endogenous genetic alterations at play in brain tumor evolution rather than exogenously induced mutations.[2]

#### GRADING AND STAGING

Many grading schemes have been employed since the 1950s, most of which concern principally or ex-clusively gliomas, especially astrocytomas. For the statistically significant astrocytomas, these grades have served to reflect clinical outcome and to guide therapy. The grading of all other gliomas and non-gliomatous CNS tumors to date has offered imperfect clinical correlation, however, and consequently has had less impact on patient care. Currently, most grading schemes for CNS tumors employ four grades.[4] Grade 1 is reserved for pilocytic astrocytoma and a few other glial, neuronal, or developmental lesions. Most well-differentiated tumors are graded 2, tumors with intermediate histologic features of malignancy are graded 3, and tumors with the greatest number of histologic features of malignancy are graded 4. The WHO designates these grades I through IV.[1] The precise histologic features distinguishing grades II from III and IV are a frequent subject of controversy. Nonetheless, it generally is accepted that necrosis or endothelial proliferation or both are features of grade IV tumors, significant mitotic activity is a feature of grade III and grade IV tumors, and neither necrosis nor significant mitotic activity is a feature of grade II tumors (Tables 51–2 and 51–3).

Staging generally is not employed in the evaluation of CNS tumors. Most CNS tumors spread to other regions of the body only after significant surgical intervention. Nonetheless, within the CNS compartment, the tendency of certain primary CNS tumors to spread to other CNS sites offers a significant guide to ultimate clinical outlook and appropriate therapy.

**TABLE 51–1.** Classification of Central Nervous System Tumors

I. Neoplastic lesions
   A. Glial tumors
      1. Astrocytic tumors
         a. Diffuse astrocytic tumors
            i. Low-grade astrocytoma
            ii. Anaplastic astrocytoma
            iii. Glioblastoma multiforme
            iv. Gliosarcoma
         b. Special subtypes of astrocytoma
            i. Pilocytic astrocytoma
            ii. Pleomorphic xanthoastrocytoma
            iii. Subependymal giant cell astrocytoma
            iv. Infantile desmoplastic astrocytoma
            v. Gliofibroma
      2. Oligodendroglial tumors
         a. Oligodendroglioma
         b. Mixed oligoastrocytoma
         c. Anaplastic oligodendroglioma
         d. Anaplastic oligoastrocytoma
      3. Ependymal tumors
         a. Ependymoma
         b. Anaplastic ependymoma
         c. Myxopapillary ependymoma
         d. Subependymoma
      4. Choroid plexus tumors
         a. Choroid plexus papilloma
         b. Choroid plexus carcinoma
      5. Neuroepithelial tumors of uncertain origin
         a. Astroblastoma
         b. Gliomatosis cerebri
   B. Neuronal and mixed neuronal-glial tumors
      1. Central neurocytoma and variants
      2. Gangliocytoma and dysplastic gangliocytoma of the cerebellum
      3. Ganglioglioma and malignant ganglioglioma
      4. Desmoplastic infantile ganglioglioma
      5. Dysembryoplastic neuroepithelial tumor
   C. Embryonal tumors
      1. Medulloblastoma and variants
      2. Central neuroblastoma and ganglioneuroblastoma
      3. Ependymoblastoma
      4. Medulloepithelioma
   D. Pineal parenchymal tumors
      1. Pineocytoma
      2. Pineoblastoma
      3. Mixed pineal parenchymal tumors
   E. Germ cell tumors
   F. Meningothelial tumors
      1. Meningioma and variants
      2. Atypical meningioma
      3. Papillary and clear cell meningiomas
      4. Malignant meningioma
   G. Tumors of cranial nerves
      1. Schwannoma and cellular schwannoma
      2. Neurofibroma
      3. Malignant peripheral nerve sheath tumor
   H. Primary central nervous system lymphomas and plasmacytomas
   I. Melanocytic tumors of the meninges
      1. Melanocytoma
      2. Melanoma
   J. Tumors of blood vessels and related tissues
      1. Vascular malformations
      2. Meningioangiomatosis
      3. Hemangiopericytoma
   K. Miscellaneous mesenchymal tumors
      1. Lipoma
      2. Solitary fibrous tumor
      3. Chordoma
      4. Mesenchymal chondrosarcoma
      5. Rhabdomyosarcoma
   L. Craniopharyngioma
   M. Paraganglioma
   N. Tumors of uncertain origin
      1. Capillary hemangioblastoma
      2. Atypical teratoid/rhabdoid tumor
   O. Benign cystic lesions of central nervous system
   P. Metastatic tumor to the central nervous system
      1. Metastatic carcinoma
      2. Lymphoma
      3. Leukemia

**TABLE 51–2.** Astrocytic Tumors and World Health Organization Grading

| Diffusely Infiltrating Astrocytomas | Grade |
| --- | --- |
| Astrocytoma | II |
| Anaplastic astrocytoma | III |
| Glioblastoma multiforme | IV |

| Special Subtypes of Astrocytomas | |
| --- | --- |
| Pilocytic astrocytoma | I |
| Pleomorphic xanthoastrocytoma | II–III |
| Subependymal giant cell astrocytoma | I |
| Desmoplastic cerebral astrocytoma of infancy | I |
| Gliofibroma | No grading |

From Kleihues P, Burger PC, Scheithauer BW: International Histological Classification of Tumours. Histological Typing of Tumours of the Central Nervous System, 2nd ed. Berlin, Springer Verlag, 1993.

## PROGNOSTIC FEATURES

In addition to the histologic features discussed previously, other techniques are available for establishing prognostic insights into CNS tumors (Table 51–4). Radiologic features[5] are crucial to the full interpretation of a CNS tumor. Margins of the tumor, the tumor-CNS interface, the extent of tumor, the vascular enhancement associated with the tumor, and other radiologic findings offer significant diagnostic and prognostic data. The immunohistochemical evaluation of tumor cell proliferation is becoming increasingly important for diagnostic and therapeutic accuracy in CNS tumors (see nuclear proliferation antigen Ki-67 data, Tables 51–3, 51–8, and 51–14). The cytogenetic and molecular features of CNS tumors are emerging as additional factors of significance in the complete evaluation of CNS tumors. In summary, prognostic evaluation of CNS tumors may include not only histologic features, but also radiologic, immunohistochemical, cytogenetic, and molec-

**TABLE 51–3.** Diffusely Infiltrating Astrocytoma

| Tumor Designation | WHO Grade | Histologic Features | Special Features | Ki-67 (Mean) |
|---|---|---|---|---|
| Astrocytoma | II | Nuclear atypia | Gemistocytic astrocytes >5% suggest shorter time to progression[11] | 2–4%[21, 23] |
| Anaplastic astrocytoma | III | Nuclear atypia<br>Mitotic activity | | 12–14%[21, 23] |
| Glioblastoma multiforme | IV | Nuclear atypia<br>Mitotic activity<br>Endothelial proliferation and/or necrosis | Gliosarcoma (mixed glioma-sarcoma) | 14–20%[20–23, 29–31] |

ular data, all of which contribute to as complete a picture as possible to guide therapy.

## THERAPY

The treatment of low-grade (see earlier) CNS tumors is confined to surgical biopsy and, if clinically feasible, surgical excision. Radiotherapy may be used with WHO grade II tumors. High-grade (WHO grades III and IV) CNS tumors traditionally are treated with supplemental radiotherapy and chemotherapy. This general treatment pattern has been employed for many years with innumerable variations in surgical therapy, radiotherapy, and especially chemotherapy protocols.[6] Gene-based therapy and antiangiogenesis have been introduced as two of several innovative therapeutic techniques to control CNS tumor proliferation.

## CONTENTS OF REPORT

The pathologist's report of a CNS tumor (Table 51–5) must include a discrete, crisp, clear-cut diagnosis with an accompanying tumor grade, preferably with an indication of the grading scheme employed (e.g., grade 2 [of 3] or grade 2 [of 4]). When appropriate, a microscopic description should be provided with comments concerning tumor growth pattern and invasion, immunohistochemical stains contributing to the diagnosis, and proliferation markers (generally Ki-67 [MIB-1]). Radiologic features affecting the diagnosis should be included in the textual description and any other clinical data that contributed significantly to the final diagnosis. Cytogenetics and molecular pathology, whenever available, should appear in the report with interpretation of the results an absolute requirement in this evolving supplement to tumor analysis. In summary a complete report ideally is subdivided into categories (clinical data, radiologic data, gross description, light microscopic description, important immunohistochemical results, prognostic markers, proliferation markers, cytogenetics, and molecular pathology) with a summary interpretive statement and a final diagnosis that includes the previously described tumor grade.

## CYTOLOGY

Smear preparations[5] in many centers have become the most important technique for intraoperative CNS tumor diagnosis, particularly when submitted specimens are minute as they often are if gathered stereotactically. Specifics regarding use of these smears are discussed in subsequent sections. Examination of cerebrospinal fluid[5] is a long-standing cy-

**TABLE 51–4.** Checklist of Prognostic Factors

Diagnosis
Histologic grade
Radiologic data
   Margins of tumor
   Extent of tumor
Histologic (mitotic count) and immunohistochemical (Ki-67 [MIB-1]) evaluation of tumor cell proliferation
Immunohistochemical predictive markers, in particular, p53 and EGFR
Additional cytogenetic and molecular factors (e.g., cytogenetic predictors of chemotherapy response in anaplastic oligodendroglioma[150])

**TABLE 51–5.** Contents of Final Report

1. Clinical data focusing on prior history of neoplasia and gross impressions of the present lesion
2. Radiologic data, preferably a brief summary of findings pertinent to the present diagnosis
3. Gross description, emphasizing necrosis, hemorrhage, cysts and their contents, and the number of blocks submitted
4. Light microscopic description, featuring criteria for benign versus malignant, primary versus metastatic, and tumor subtype
5. Immunohistochemical data, including particularly antibodies, both positive and negative, that contribute to the final diagnosis, such as GFAP, cytokeratins, and synaptophysin
6. Prognostic markers, in particular, p53, which may determine clinical outcome or guide therapy
7. Proliferation markers, principally MIB-1, reported as a specific percentage of tumor cell nuclei reactive
8. Cytogenetics and molecular pathology data particularly when of direct contribution to the final diagnosis and/or therapy, preferably with an explanation of the tests performed
9. A summary interpretive statement incorporating all of the previous 8 factors
10. Final diagnosis with a histologic grade, including the grading scheme employed (e.g., grade 2 [of 4])

tologic technique most effective in metastatic disease, in particular, adenocarcinoma and lymphoma, and in primary embryonal tumors of the brain, in particular, medulloblastoma.

## Glial Tumors

### ASTROCYTIC TUMORS

Astrocytic tumors are divided into two major groups according to their overall pattern of growth (see Table 51–2). The first group, diffuse astrocytic tumors, shows a capacity for diffuse infiltration of the adjacent brain regardless of histologic grade. In addition, these tumors have an intrinsic tendency to progress to more malignant phenotypes. This group includes *astrocytoma* (low grade or WHO grade II), *anaplastic astrocytoma* (WHO grade III), and *glioblastoma multiforme* (WHO grade IV) (see Table 51–3). The second group comprises relatively circumscribed astrocytic tumors that have a diminished malignant potential with infrequent anaplastic progression. These tumors include *pilocytic astrocytoma, pleomorphic xanthoastrocytoma, subependymal giant cell astrocytoma, desmoplastic cerebral astrocytoma of infancy,* and *gliofibroma.*

#### Diffuse Astrocytic Tumors

Diffuse astrocytomas represent 75% of cerebral astrocytic tumors and account for more than 60% of all primary brain tumors.[7] Low-grade astrocytomas commonly occur in patients in their 20s and 30s, whereas anaplastic tumors tend to arise in patients in their 30s to 50s. In general, men are affected more often than women. The location of the tumor is the most important factor in determining the nature of the symptoms and signs in diffuse astrocytomas. In low-grade astrocytomas, because of their usually slow growth, seizures may be the presenting clinical symptom and may precede the diagnosis by many years. Seizures are particularly likely to occur in lesions that involve the temporal lobe and the frontal lobe. Progressive lesions that expand to affect important areas of the brain may present with progressive neurologic deficits, such as hemiparesis, sensory changes, or difficulty with speech and language.

##### LOW-GRADE ASTROCYTOMA

*Synonyms.* Synonyms for low-grade astrocytoma are astrocytoma, fibrillary astrocytoma, and astrocytoma WHO grade II.

*Clinical Considerations.* Low-grade astrocytomas represent approximately 25% of all gliomas. Astrocytomas frequently involve the cerebral hemispheres of adults and the brain stem of children and adolescents. The peak incidence is in young adults between the ages of 30 and 40.[8]

*Diagnostic Considerations.* Macroscopically, low-grade astrocytomas often are difficult to distinguish from the adjacent brain. The tumors diffusely infiltrate the normal brain, causing an enlargement of preexisting anatomic structures (Fig. 51–1). They

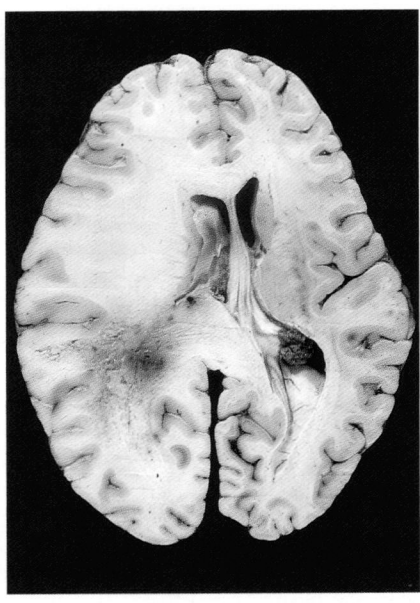

**FIGURE 51–1.** Astrocytoma (WHO grade II) diffusely infiltrating left parietotemporal lobes. Note absence of boundary between tumor and normal brain.

typically are firmer than the normal brain, however, because of the abundance of glial fibrils. The formation of small cysts with a delicate spongy appearance may be seen focally.

Astrocytomas classically have been divided into three major variants—*fibrillary, protoplasmic,* and *gemistocytic astrocytomas*—according to their resemblance to basic morphologic types of astrocytes in normal and reactive brain. Although the subclassification of astrocytomas by morphologic characteristics has significant limitations,[9] particular consideration should be given to the gemistocytic components of astrocytomas (see later). In practice, most tumors have a mixed population of the different subtypes.

Histologically, low-grade astrocytomas are characterized by low cellularity and minimal cellular and nuclear atypia (CD Fig. 51–1). Histologic features suggestive of anaplasia, including mitotic activity, endothelial (pericytic) proliferation, and necrosis, are not present in these tumors. Tumors with more fibrillary cellular components have prominent cytoplasmic processes that form a rich fibrillary matrix (Fig. 51–2). This matrix is particularly accentuated around blood vessels. In other instances, tumors may be composed of large numbers of protoplasmic astrocytes with stellate-shaped cells intermixed within an abundant eosinophilic matrix. Considerable microcystic formation and a loose matrix may be present.

Astrocytomas with a major component of gemistocytic cells are classified as *gemistocytic astrocytomas.* These tumors are rare as a pure histologic variant.[10] Gemistocytic astrocytomas are characterized by cells with abundant eosinophilic, round to slightly angulated cytoplasm and eccentric nuclei. The fibrillary

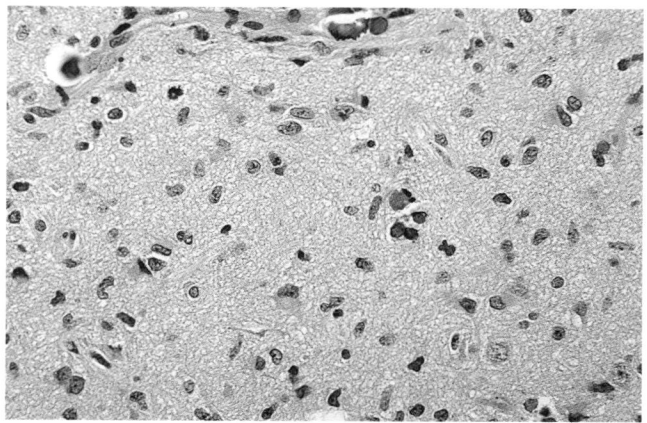

**FIGURE 51–2.** Astrocytoma grade II infiltrating cortex. Note the small gemistocytic astrocytes.

matrix, commonly seen in the more fibrillary tumors, is less conspicuous. Accumulated evidence has shown that the presence of gemistocytes is a sign of poor prognosis in low-grade astrocytomas.[10, 11] In a series of these tumors, low-grade astrocytomas containing more than 5% gemistocytes had a significantly shorter time to progression than tumors with less than 5% gemistocytes.[11]

Special stains are helpful to characterize the astrocytic nature of low-grade astrocytomas. Histochemical stains show high affinity of the glial fibrils for phosphotungstic acid–hematoxylin. As for immunohistochemical techniques, astrocytomas are conspicuously immunoreactive for glial fibrillary acidic protein (GFAP) (CD Fig. 51–2) and vimentin in cytoplasm and cellular processes. Tumor cells also show immunoreactivity to S-100 protein in the nucleus and in cell processes. Tumor astrocytes often are reactive with cytokeratin antibodies, especially those of higher molecular weight[12] (CD Fig. 51–3). In the differential diagnosis of glial versus metastatic tumor, poor reactivity with CAM 5.2 and focal-to-diffuse reactivity with GFAP strongly favor a primary glial tumor (Table 51–6).

Although these astrocytomas are considered *low grade,* natural history studies tend to show that they behave in an aggressive fashion, and the prognosis for many astrocytomas is guarded. For ordinary

**TABLE 51–6.** Immunoreactivity of Astrocytic Tumors

*Diagnostic*
GFAP
Vimentin
S-100
High-molecular-weight cytokeratin
Poor to no reactivity with CAM 5.2

*Prognostic*
p53—reactivity correlates with malignant progression
Ki67—reactivity correlates with malignant progression (see Table 51–3)

low-grade astrocytomas, the 5-year survival rate is approximately 50% with a tendency toward malignant progression over time. The incidence of progression within this group of astrocytomas may approach 80%.[8, 13–18] Studies indicate that the time interval for low-grade astrocytomas to progress to glioblastoma is shorter in low-grade astrocytomas carrying a *p53* mutation[11] (see later).

### ANAPLASTIC ASTROCYTOMA

*Synonyms.* Synonyms for anaplastic astrocytoma are malignant astrocytoma and astrocytoma WHO grade III.

*Clinical Considerations.* Anaplastic astrocytoma includes a heterogeneous group of tumors with the common features of cytologic anaplasia and proliferative activity. Anaplastic astrocytoma may arise de novo, without indication of a less malignant precursor tumor or, more commonly, may arise from low-grade astrocytoma. All types of diffuse astrocytomas are capable of undergoing progression to a more anaplastic form.

*Diagnostic Considerations.* When compared with low-grade astrocytomas, anaplastic astrocytomas tend to show increased cellularity and a variable degree of cytoplasmic pleomorphism or nuclear pleomorphism or both (Fig. 51–3). Gemistocytic elements are seen more commonly. Anaplastic astrocytomas typically display mitotic activity (CD Fig. 51–4), and markers for proliferative activity, such as Ki-67 (MIB-1), tend to show higher levels than in low-grade astrocytomas.[19–23] Mean values of the Ki-67 labeling index (LI) in anaplastic astrocytomas are 12% to 14%, whereas in low-grade astrocytomas, Ki-67 LI mean values are 2% to 4%.[21, 23] Endothelial (pericytic) proliferation and necrosis should not be present in accordance with the WHO classification.[1]

### GLIOBLASTOMA MULTIFORME

*Synonym.* A synonym for glioblastoma multiforme is astrocytoma WHO grade IV.

*Clinical Considerations.* Glioblastoma multiforme is the most malignant astrocytic tumor. It oc-

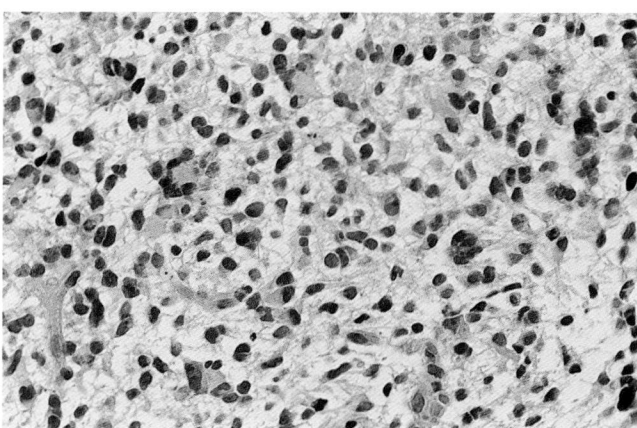

**FIGURE 51–3.** Anaplastic astrocytoma with moderate cellular atypia and increased cellularity in comparison to astrocytoma grade II.

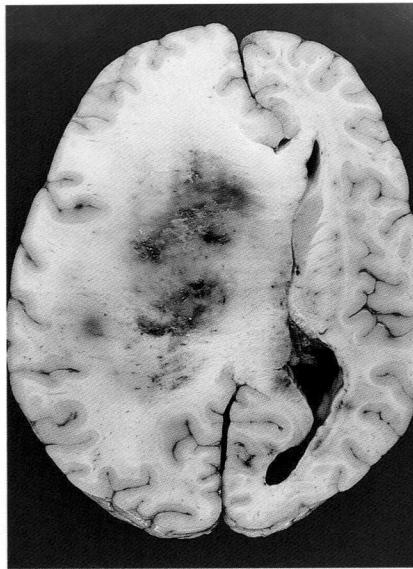

**FIGURE 51–4.** Glioblastoma multiforme involving the parietal-temporal region with massive edema and midline shift.

have a short clinical history. *Secondary glioblastomas* often develop from lower grade astrocytomas over months or years and typically occur in younger patients. Glioblastomas may occur rarely in children and adolescents.[7, 25]

Glioblastomas arise most frequently in the cerebral hemispheres, in particular the frontotemporal and parietal regions (Fig. 51–4). The tumors often present as expansive lesions, with ring enhancement on computed tomography (CT) scan and magnetic resonance imaging (MRI) giving an impression of well-delineated masses. Glioblastomas invariably infiltrate the adjacent brain in an aggressive manner, however, and may cross the midline infiltrating the opposite hemisphere. This latter pattern classically is described as the *butterfly* pattern. Less often, glioblastomas arise in the brain stem, spinal cord, and cerebellum (CD Fig. 51–5). In children, these tumors frequently are located in the brain stem and thalamus.[7, 25]

***Diagnostic Considerations.*** Macroscopically, glioblastomas are characterized by large areas of soft, gray-yellow tissue with extensive areas of necrosis and hemorrhage (CD Fig. 51–6). Tumors located in the cerebral hemispheres tend to infiltrate the cortical ribbon and white matter diffusely. The tumor infiltration of the adjacent brain, which gives an appearance of enlargement and distortion of the normal structures, sometimes is hard to distinguish from peritumoral edema.

Glioblastomas exhibit tremendous heterogeneity with multivariate histologic appearances. They are hypercellular and exhibit a high degree of cytoplasmic and nuclear pleomorphism. Most tumors contain populations with the obvious fibrillary astrocy-

curs predominantly in the cerebral hemispheres and has a peak incidence in patients in their 40s and 50s. In general, it represents approximately 15% to 20% of all intracranial tumors and 50% of all gliomas.[7] Glioblastomas may arise de novo, or they may develop from either low-grade astrocytomas or more often from anaplastic astrocytomas. These two types of glioblastomas are designated as *primary glioblastoma* and *secondary glioblastoma*.[24] *Primary glioblastomas* occur more commonly in older patients and

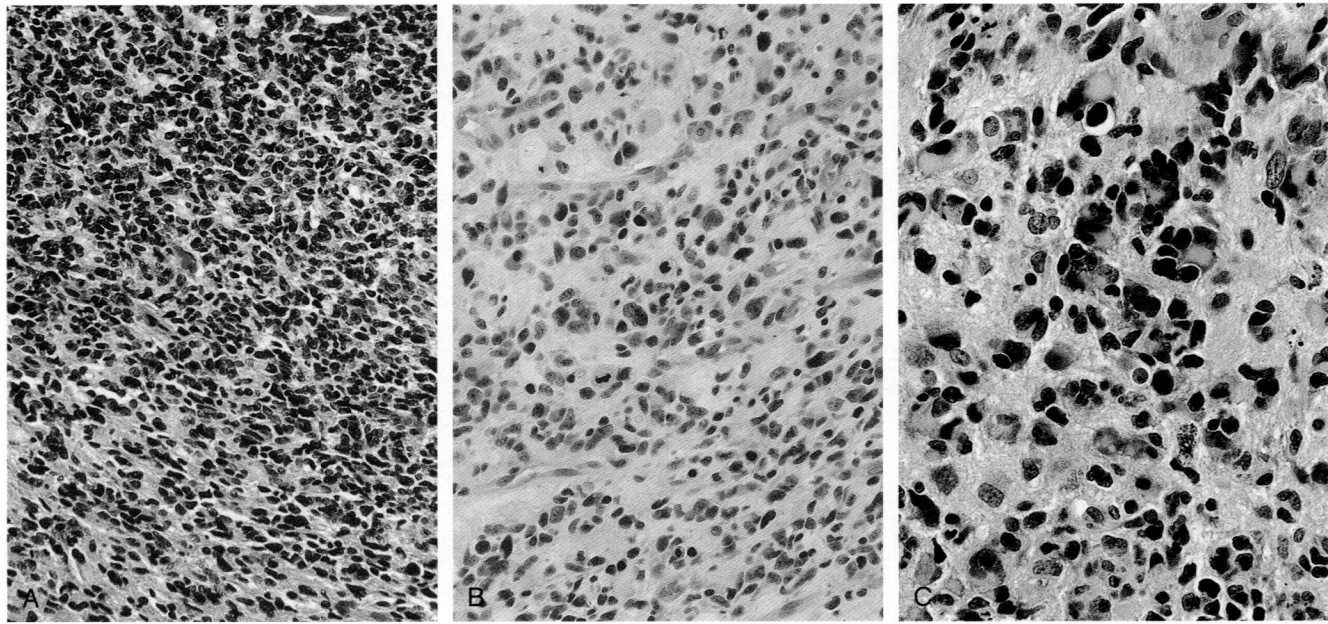

**FIGURE 51–5.** Glioblastomas have an abundance of cellular types and arrangements ranging from small cells *(A)*, to medium-size polygonal forms *(B)*, to multinucleated giant cells *(C)*.

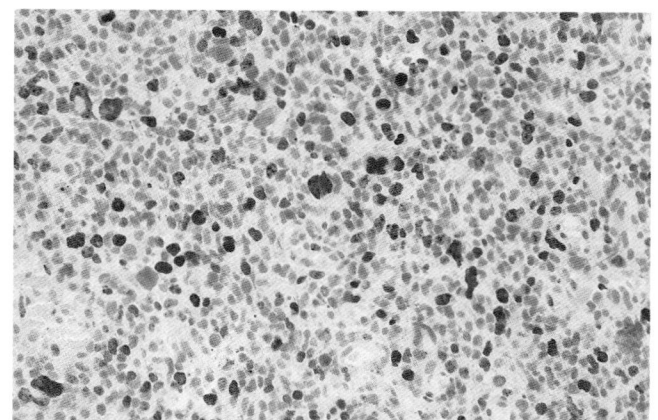

**FIGURE 51–6.** High Ki-67 labeling index is characteristic of glioblastoma.

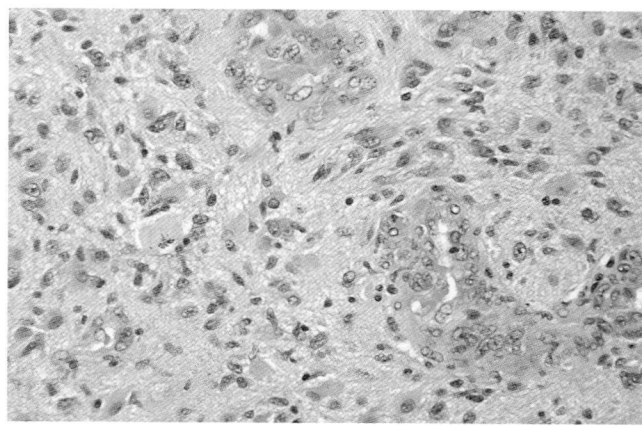

**FIGURE 51–7.** Vascular endothelial proliferation is typical of glioblastoma.

tic feature of delicate GFAP-immunoreactive processes. However, tumors may range from closely packed small cells with scant cytoplasm to larger cells with a gemistocytic appearance of ample cytoplasm (Fig. 51–5). Multinucleated giant cells are common. Cytoplasmic lipidization may be seen occasionally.[26] Foci of metaplastic change with squamous and adenomatous differentiation[27] or bone and cartilage formation[28] also may be present.

Mitotic figures are numerous, and studies with proliferative markers, mainly Ki-67, show high LIs (range of mean values, 14% to 20%) (Fig. 51–6), although these may vary significantly within an individual tumor.[20–23, 29–31] Microvascular proliferation with exuberant endothelial and pericytic proliferation, the so-called endothelial proliferation (Fig. 51–7), is seen throughout the tumor but is especially prominent in areas surrounding necrosis and at the tumor-brain interface. Geographic necrosis with pseudopalisading of the adjacent tumor cells is present in varying degrees (Fig. 51–8). Large areas of ischemic necrosis accompanied by thrombosed vessels also are observed.

***Giant Cell Glioblastoma.*** A variant of glioblastoma is important because of its distinctive histology. The giant cell glioblastoma is characterized by a predominance of bizarre, multinucleated giant cells (CD Fig. 51–7) and extensive areas of necrosis and hemorrhage. An increase of the stromal reticulin network also is seen, particularly related to blood vessels. Lymphocytic infiltration commonly is present.[32, 33] Giant cell glioblastomas, in contrast to ordinary glioblastomas, are well demarcated and arise in younger patients. These particular features of giant cell glioblastomas may account for their better prognosis as reported by some authors.[7, 32–34]

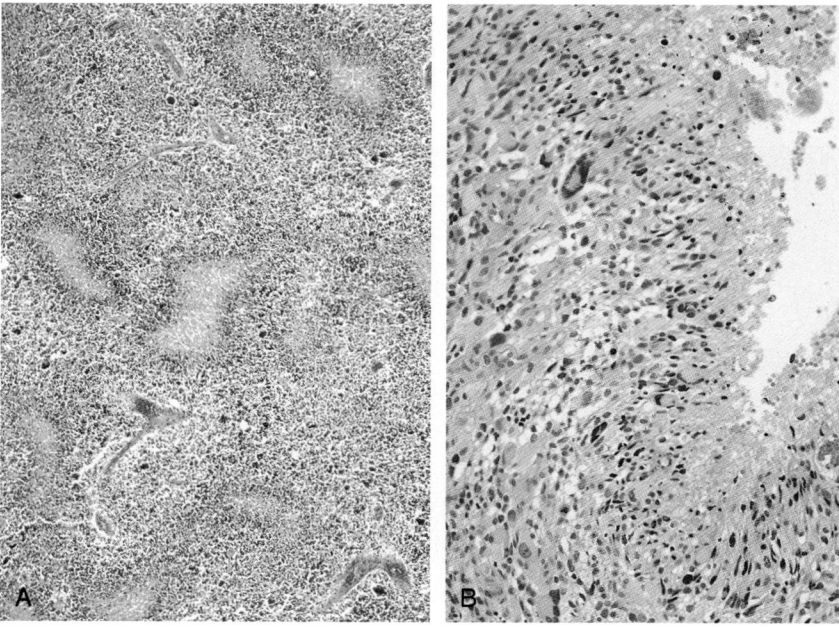

**FIGURE 51–8.** Areas of necrosis, particularly with pseudopalisading of tumor cells in glioblastoma (*A*). High magnification of the pseudo-palisading arrangement of tumor cells around a necrotic area (*B*).

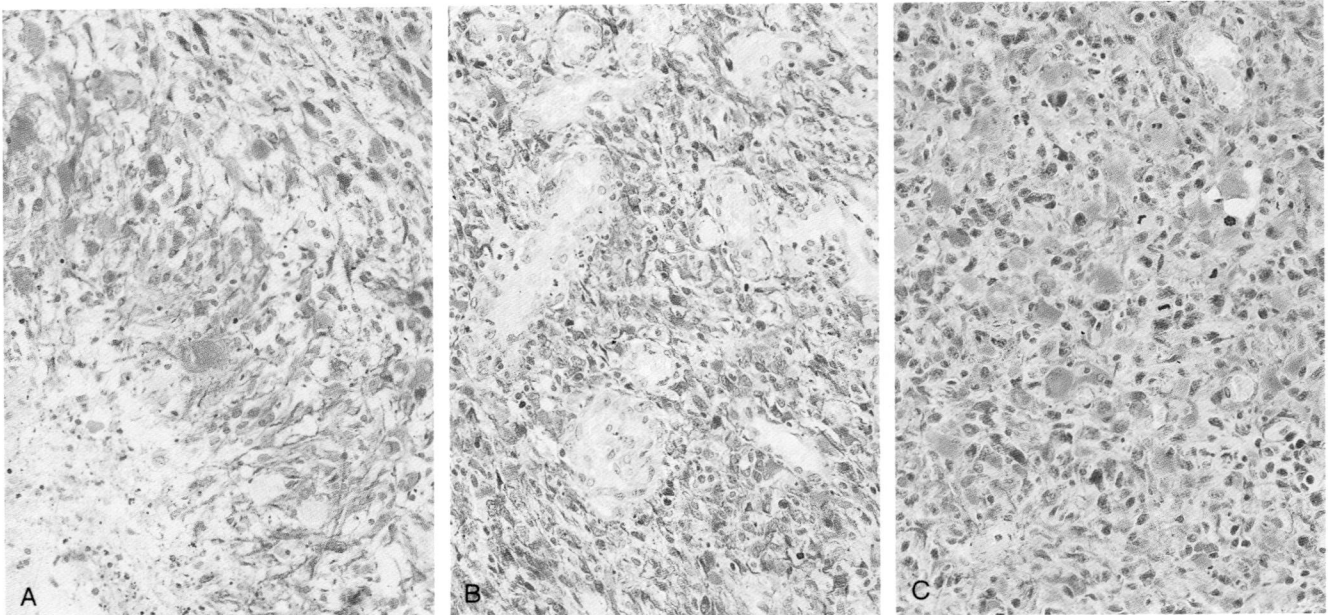

**FIGURE 51–9.** GFAP (*A* to *B*) and vimentin *(C)* immunohistochemistry accentuate the glial nature of glioblastoma cells. In contrast, vessels exhibiting endothelial proliferation are GFAP negative *(B)*.

Studies have shown that the molecular genetics of giant cell glioblastomas resembles *secondary glioblastomas* with *p53* gene mutations and rare *EGFR* gene amplification in most cases.[35, 36] These data are of particular interest because most giant cell glioblastomas develop de novo with a short preoperative history.[35]

Immunohistochemically, glioblastomas stain similarly to the low-grade diffuse astrocytomas with GFAP, vimentin, S-100, and cytokeratins (Fig. 51–9). As the degree of anaplasia increases, however, the intensity and percentage of GFAP reactivity tend to decrease.

### GLIOSARCOMA

***Synonym.*** A synonym for gliosarcoma is mixed glioblastoma/sarcoma.

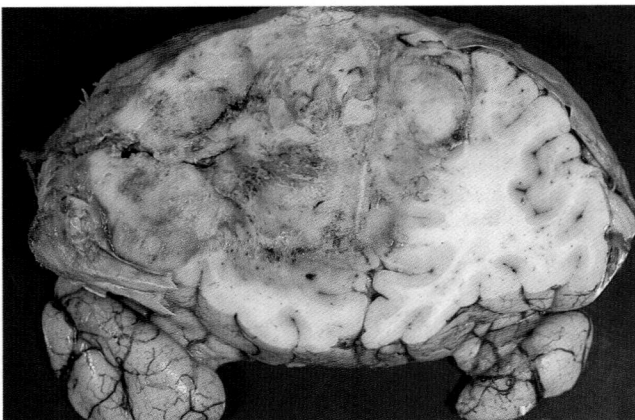

**FIGURE 51–10.** A gliosarcoma involving frontal lobes bilaterally with focal adherence to the dura matter.

***Clinical Considerations.*** The gliosarcoma (Fig. 51–10) is a variant of glioblastoma in which a biphasic tissue pattern with intermixed areas of glial and mesenchymal proliferation is present. The frequency of gliosarcomas ranges from approximately 2% to 8%.[37–39]

***Diagnostic Considerations.*** The glial component shows the typical features of a glioblastoma as previously described. The sarcomatous elements often show a diverse histologic appearance, most resembling fibrosarcoma, malignant fibrous histiocytoma, or angiosarcoma (CD Fig. 51–8) The proportions of glial and sarcomatous components are variable. GFAP immunohistochemistry and phosphotungstic acid–hematoxylin stain confirm the glial component, whereas the sarcomatous elements can be accentuated by vimentin or reticulin stains (Fig. 51–11). Gliosarcomas also may show mesenchymal metaplasia, including cartilaginous and bone formation.

Many immunohistochemical and ultrastructural studies had suggested in the past that the sarcomatous components probably were derived from an undifferentiated mesenchymal cell associated with the adventitia of tumor vessels.[40–43] Molecular genetic analyses have shown, however, that glial and mesenchymal elements of gliosarcomas share similar genetic alterations.[44–47] Identical *p53* gene mutations in gliomatous and sarcomatous elements have been identified,[46] suggesting that the sarcomatous areas may represent a phenotypic change of the glial cells.

***Molecular Genetics of Diffuse Astrocytomas.*** Molecular biologic studies have provided much insight into the mechanisms of diffuse astrocytoma tumorigenesis.[11, 35, 48–51] Molecular genetic analyses of astrocytomas have described specific genetic altera-

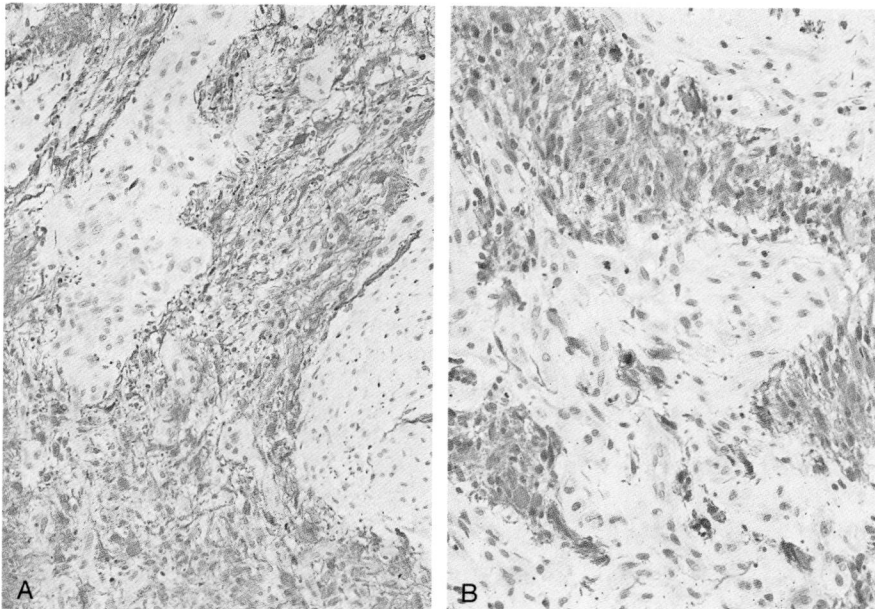

**FIGURE 51–11.** Glial (GFAP-positive) and mesenchymal (GFAP-negative) areas in gliosarcoma (A). A similar pattern is observed with S-100 protein immunostain (B).

tions that correlate with the different grades of tumor, from low-grade astrocytomas to glioblastomas.[50]

At least three mechanisms may be involved in the tumorigenesis of diffuse astrocytomas (Table 51–7). The molecular genetics of astrocytomas is complex, and a detailed discussion can be found elsewhere.[24, 49–50, 57]

Many other mechanisms have been associated with the progression of low-grade astrocytomas to glioblastomas (see Table 51–7). In glioblastoma, inactivation of putative tumor-suppressor genes on chromosome 10 is a principal genetic event. So far, the primary tumor-suppressor gene or genes on chromosome 10 have not been identified.

A large group of glioblastomas has exclusively

**TABLE 51–7.** Astrocytoma and Glioblastoma Molecular Genetics

I. Molecular genetics of diffuse astrocytoma tumorigenesis
  A. Inactivation of *p53* gene
    1. Most often mutation of one gene copy/loss of the other gene on short arm of chromosome 17
    2. Amplification of MDM2 oncogene inhibits *p53*[48,52]
    3. Up-regulation of *p21* causes *p53* accumulation[53]
  B. *EGFR* amplification/overexpression
  C. Alternate pathways
II. Molecular genetics of progression from low-grade to anaplastic astrocytoma
  A. Platelet-derived growth factor activation and ligand/receptor overexpression
  B. Chromosome 22q allelic loss
  C. Inactivation of tumor-suppressor genes[54,57] on:
    1. Chromosome 9p—*CDKN2/p16* gene
    2. Chromosome 11p
    3. Chromosome 13q—*RB* gene
    4. Chromosome 19q
III. Proposed molecular schemes of glioblastoma
  A. Primary glioblastoma
    1. Chromosome 10 tumor-suppressor gene inactivation or loss
    2. *EGFR* gene amplification
    3. Rare *p53* mutation
  B. Secondary glioblastoma
    1. *p53* mutation or loss of chromosome 17p
    2. Rare *EGFR* gene amplification
  C. Alternate scheme
    1. No *p53* mutation
    2. No *EGFR* gene amplification
IV. Clinical parameters of primary versus secondary glioblastoma

| | Origin | Age of patient | *p53* gene mutations | *EFGR* expression |
|---|---|---|---|---|
| **Primary** | De novo | Older | Rare | Common |
| **Secondary** | Slowly evolves from low-grade astrocytoma | Younger | Common | Rare |

either *p53* inactivation (Fig. 51–12) or *EGFR* gene amplification[50] (see Table 51–7). These genetic pathways denote not only different genetic trails of tumor formation, but also seem to reflect different clinical courses of glioblastomas (see Table 51–7). The clinical and epidemiologic data concerning these two sets of glioblastomas have been well characterized.[24] From the histologic viewpoint, however, these two types of glioblastomas are indistinguishable.

As previously mentioned, alternative pathways to those previously discussed have been described in the evolution of diffuse astrocytomas. One well-characterized pathway is that of giant cell glioblastoma, a histologically distinct variant of glioblastoma that occurs most frequently in younger patients and presents clinically as a *primary glioblastoma*. Most giant cell glioblastomas show *p53* gene mutation, a trait seen most commonly in *secondary glioblastomas*.[35, 36]

### Differential Diagnosis of Diffuse Astrocytomas.
Several conditions may mimic diffusely infiltrating astrocytomas (Table 51–8). Of particular importance is the pilocytic astrocytoma, a grade I neoplasm with a benign clinical course (see later) in contrast to the diffusely infiltrating astrocytoma which has a high propensity for malignant transformation. The differentiation of these tumors should be made not only on a histologic basis but also with the aid of clinical and radiographic data.

Anaplastic astrocytomas share many histologic features with anaplastic oligodendrogliomas. Their distinction (see Table 51–8) is of clinical relevance, however, because in contrast to anaplastic astrocytomas, anaplastic oligodendrogliomas are chemosensitive tumors.

The main differential diagnoses of glioblastoma include metastatic carcinoma, primary cerebral lymphoma, and abscess (see Table 51–8). All these conditions may present as contrast-enhancing ring lesions at neuroimaging.

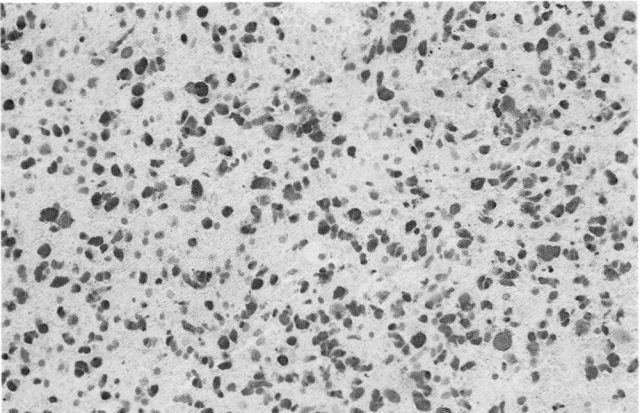

**FIGURE 51–12.** Immunohistochemistry for p53 protein (wild and mutated forms) in a secondary glioblastoma.

**TABLE 51–8.** Differential Diagnosis of Diffuse Astrocytoma

Low-grade astrocytoma
  Reactive gliosis—has less fibrillary background, less nuclear/cellular atypia
  Multiple sclerosis—has inflammatory cells and macrophages (CD68)
  Cerebral infarct—has inflammatory cells and macrophages (CD68)
  Pilocytic astrocytoma—has a biphasic pattern with Rosenthal and granular bodies
  Oligodendroglioma—has perinuclear halos, calcification, perineuronal satellitosis, no vimentin, and little GFAP reaction
  Fibrillary ependymoma—has perivascular pseudorosettes
Anaplastic astrocytoma
  Anaplastic oligodendroglioma—has a less fibrillary GFAP matrix
Glioblastoma
  Metastatic carcinoma—has only rare GFAP reactivity but marked CAM 5.2 and EMA reactivity
  Primary cerebral lymphoma—has perivascular tumor cells. Reactive with lymphoid markers (CD20)
  Abscess—has abundant macrophages (CD68) and a periphery of granulation tissue with reactive gliosis

### Intraoperative Diagnosis of Diffuse Astrocytomas.
Intraoperative diagnosis of astrocytic tumors can be performed by frozen sections (CD Fig. 51–9) and smear preparations. Smears and cytologic preparations are preferred by most neuropathology laboratories. Cytologic data from smear preparations are sufficient for intraoperative diagnosis and an important complement to the histopathologic data obtained from paraffin-embedded tissue sections. An additional advantage of smears is the fact that they eliminate the need to perform frozen sections on small specimens, mainly the ones originating from stereotactic biopsies, decreasing the incidence of freezing artifacts, which may lead to incorrect diagnosis.

Smears of astrocytomas show the typical fibrillary nature of these neoplasms better than frozen sections. The consistency of the tumor tissue depends on the predominant component of the tumor. Tumors with a high proportion of fibrillary astrocytes give a firmer consistency than tumors with more protoplasmic and gemistocytic components. Fibrillary astrocytic cells (CD Fig. 51–10) have a cytoplasmic geometry that ranges from a scant perinuclear rim with ill-defined borders to a more fusiform pattern with an elongate nucleus. Protoplasmic astrocytic populations have a more stellate shape with short, delicate processes. Tumors with more gemistocytic elements are characterized by cells with abundant eosinophilic, plump to slightly angulated cytoplasm and eccentric nuclei (CD Fig. 51–11). The matrix is conspicuously fibrillated but varies with the abundance of fibrillary astrocytes in the tumor.

Intraoperative differential diagnosis of low-grade astrocytomas and reactive astrocytosis usually is accomplished better by smears. Tumors show a fibrillary matrix, which usually is more ill-defined than the background accompanying a reactive astrocytosis. The tumor cells tend to produce only short, inconspicuous processes, a feature that distinguishes neoplastic from reactive astrocytes that tend to have long stellate-shaped processes. The nuclei of the tumor cells are slightly larger, more irregular, and hyperchromatic with coarser chromatin than reactive astrocytes.

Anaplastic astrocytomas show a higher degree of cellular atypia and nuclear pleomorphism than low-grade tumors. Although cellularity may be a subjective parameter, cytologic smears of higher grade astrocytomas in general show increased cellularity. The combination of vascular endothelial proliferation and necrosis is appreciated easily in smears that distinguish glioblastomas from anaplastic astrocytomas (CD Fig. 51–12).

***Prognostic Considerations of Diffuse Astrocytomas.*** The grading scheme for astrocytomas as adopted by the WHO employs four grades determined by cellularity, cytologic atypia, mitotic figures, endothelial proliferation, and necrosis (see earlier in text and see Table 51–3). Grades I and II for treatment purposes are considered benign or low grade, whereas grades III and IV are considered malignant. The arbitrary nature of this grading system has been discussed amply elsewhere, but as a functional guide for therapy it is serviceable.

The evaluation of proliferative activity in astrocytomas using Ki-67 (MIB-1) has found good correlation with WHO tumor grades[58–61] (see Table 51–3). Although proliferative indices are a valuable tool in the evaluation of individual cases, proliferation indices alone have not been shown to be a prognostic factor in astrocytomas.[61, 62] Molecular biology plays a significant role in the prognosis of diffuse astrocytomas as described previously (see "Molecular Genetics" and see Tables 51–6 and 51–7).

### Special Subtypes of Astrocytoma

#### PILOCYTIC ASTROCYTOMA

***Clinical Considerations.*** The pilocytic astrocytoma is a relatively well-circumscribed astrocytoma that occurs most frequently in children and young adults with a peak incidence in patients in their teens.[7] Pilocytic astrocytomas occur sporadically and in association with neurofibromatosis type 1 (NF1). The tumors arise throughout the neuraxis; however, they typically are located in midline structures, including the optic pathways, hypothalamus (Fig. 51–13) and third ventricular regions, cerebellum, brain stem, and less frequently spinal cord.[7] Cerebral hemispheric pilocytic astrocytomas also may occur and most frequently involve the frontoparietal lobes.[63] Of patients with NF1, 15% develop pilocytic astrocytoma of the optic nerve (also called *optic glioma*),[64] and about 70% of optic gliomas are associated with NF1.[65]

***Diagnostic Considerations.*** Most pilocytic astrocytomas are cystic lesions associated with a solid mural nodule. The nodule usually is soft and gray with variably sized cysts containing yellow fluid.

Pilocytic astrocytomas arising in the optic pathways are remarkable for infiltrating diffusely the optic nerve, producing a fusiform, expanded mass (CD Fig. 51–13). Microscopically, these tumors typically show a biphasic pattern of growth with compact areas intermixed with spongy areas displaying microcyst formations (Fig. 51–14). The compact component consists of bipolar, fibrillated or piloid cells arranged in fascicles. The spongy component is formed by smaller, stellate cells with short cellular processes arranged in loose, microcystic or spongy patterns.

Several distinctive structures are seen in pilocytic astrocytomas, including Rosenthal fibers and eosinophilic granular bodies. Rosenthal fibers (see Fig. 51–14*A*) are seen commonly in the compact areas, whereas eosinophilic granular bodies may be present in both tissues. Although these structures are not requisite for the diagnosis of pilocytic astrocytomas, they are helpful for establishing the diagnosis. Some degree of cellular atypia, including multinucleated cells, may be present in pilocytic astrocytomas. These features are considered degenerative features, however, not associated with anaplastic progression.

Pilocytic astrocytomas are highly vascular lesions. Hyalinized and telangiectatic vessels are seen often and may be accompanied by perivascular lymphocytic infiltrates. Microvascular proliferation may be present (CD Fig. 51–14), sometimes simulating the glomeruloid type of hyperplasia in glioblastomas, but this does not connote malignant transformation.

Immunohistochemically, compact and spongy cellular elements of the pilocytic astrocytoma are GFAP immunoreactive (Fig. 51–15). The bipolar cells are more strongly positive, however, than the stellate cells of the spongy areas. In contrast, vimentin immunoreactivity is equally conspicuous in both cellular patterns.[66] Mitotic activity is relatively low in pilocytic astrocytomas. Studies using proliferative markers, including Ki-67 (MIB-1), also have shown

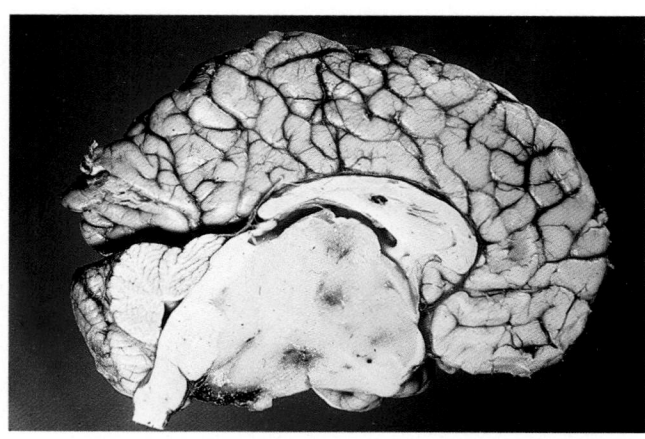

**FIGURE 51–13.** Sagittal view of a large hypothalamic pilocytic astrocytoma.

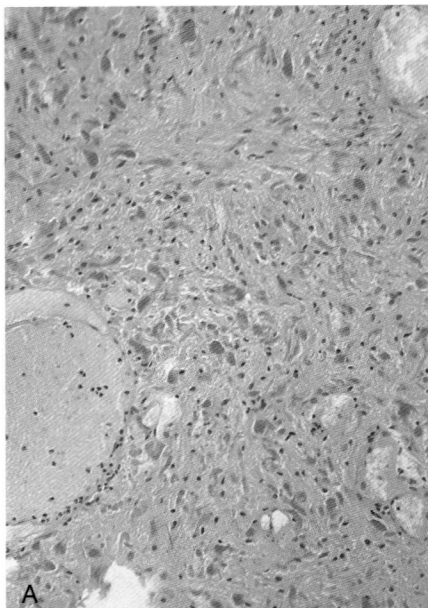 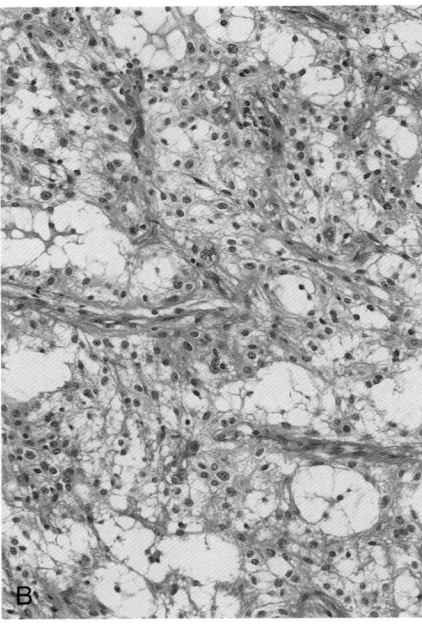

FIGURE 51–14. Pilocytic astrocytoma with a biphasic histologic arrangement of fusiform, fibrillated cells, with Rosenthal fibers *(A)* alternating with areas of looser stroma composed of stellate cells *(B)*.

low proliferative potential, although with some intratumoral variation.[61, 63, 67–69]

***Prognostic Considerations.*** Pilocytic astrocytomas are slowly growing masses and, compared with the diffuse infiltrating astrocytomas, are biologically less aggressive with a more favorable prognosis. They are a grade I neoplasm in the WHO classification.[1] Although the tumors often are macroscopically circumscribed, some degree of parenchymal infiltration and a significant propensity to invade the leptomeninges may occur.[70] Despite the indolent behavior of pilocytic astrocytomas, recurrence is possible, particularly after incomplete resections.[71] Anaplastic transformation is a rare phenomenon occurring in only 1% of cases.[70]

***Molecular Genetics.*** In contrast to diffuse astrocytomas, *p53* gene inactivation does not seem to play a role in the genesis and transformation of the pilocytic astrocytoma[50, 72–74] (Table 51–9). Allelic losses on chromosome 17 have been described in sporadic pilocytic astrocytomas, including the region encoding the *NF1* gene.[75] Nevertheless, the role for *NF1* as a tumor-suppressor gene in the genesis of pilocytic astrocytomas has not been confirmed.[75–77]

***Differential Diagnosis.*** In the differential diagnosis of pilocytic astrocytomas, two considerations are important. First, there has been a trend over many years to overcall diffuse fibrillary astrocytoma in the cerebral hemispheres of adults, whereas the actual diagnosis based largely on retrospective series is pilocytic astrocytoma. A lengthy discussion of this diagnostic challenge is found in an Armed Forces Institute of Pathology *Fascicle*.[78] Second, the histologic features of pilocytic astrocytoma may be mimicked at least in part by long-standing reactive gliosis, particularly in the brain tissue adjacent to a craniopharyngioma or a capillary hemangioblastoma. Review of preoperative and postoperative radiographic studies may assist in this latter dilemma.

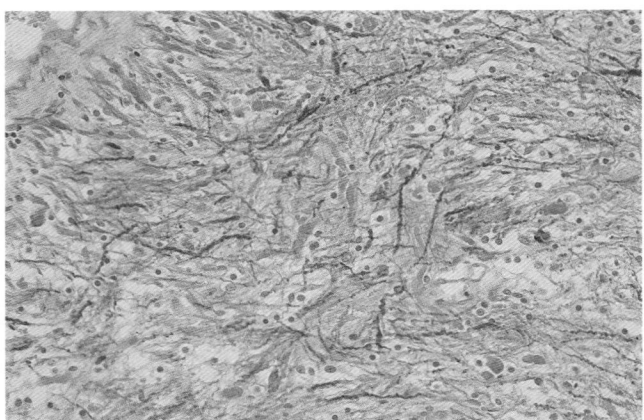

FIGURE 51–15. GFAP reactivity in pilocytic astrocytoma.

**TABLE 51–9.** Molecular Genetics of Special Subtypes of Astrocytoma

Pilocytic astrocytoma
  *p53*—no gene inactivation
  Chromosome 17—occasional allelic loss, region *NF1*
Pleomorphic xanthoastrocytoma
  *p53*—rare reports of gene mutation
  *EGFR*—rare reports of gene amplification
Subependymal giant cell astrocytoma
  16p13—*TSC2* gene region loss of heterozygosity with loss of gene product tuberin

## PLEOMORPHIC XANTHOASTROCYTOMA

***Clinical Considerations.*** The pleomorphic xanthoastrocytoma is a relatively rare glioma representing less than 1% of all astrocytomas. These tumors typically arise in children and young adults, without predilection for gender.[79] Tumors that occur in patients after their 30s are exceptional.[80-82] Typically, patients present with a long-standing history of seizures.

***Diagnostic Considerations.*** Pleomorphic xanthoastrocytomas arise most commonly in the cerebral hemispheres, in particular, the temporal lobe. They have a superficial location and commonly are attached to the meninges (CD Fig. 51–15). Dural invasion is uncommon, however. Grossly, these tumors are firm and well circumscribed with a conspicuous cystic component.

Three prominent histopathologic features are characteristic of these tumors. First is the high degree of cellular pleomorphism (Fig. 51–16). The second feature is cytoplasmic lipidization, especially conspicuous in polygonal and giant cells. The third feature, a prominent reticulin-positive stroma (CD Fig. 51–16), is most conspicuous in the areas adjacent to leptomeningeal involvement.[83] This last feature reflects the presence of a pericellular basement membrane–like deposition seen best at the ultrastructural level.[84, 85]

Immunohistochemically the tumor cells of the pleomorphic xanthoastrocytoma are reactive with GFAP (Fig. 51–17). The tumor cells and stroma also are reactive with vimentin.

Pleomorphic xanthoastrocytoma is rarely a component of a ganglioglioma.[86-88] The proportion of the neuronal and glial components varies considerably in these cases. The histogenic relationship between these rare cases and glioneuronal neoplasms is unclear.

***Molecular Genetics.*** No definitive molecular genetic events seem to play a role in the pathogenesis of pleomorphic xanthoastrocytoma. The genetic mutations seen in diffuse astrocytomas, mainly *p53* gene mutation and *EGFR* gene amplification, probably are not implicated in the pathogenesis of these tumors.[50] Mutations of *p53* have been described in a few pleomorphic xanthoastrocytomas, however, that later underwent malignant transformation.[89, 90] Amplification of the *EGFR* gene was observed in the recurrence of an ordinary pleomorphic xanthoastrocytoma that presented with anaplastic progression[90] (see Table 51–9).

***Prognostic Considerations.*** Most pleomorphic xanthoastrocytomas are classified as grade II neoplasms in the WHO classification.[1] Mitotic activity when present generally is low. Vascular endothelial proliferation and areas of necrosis commonly are not present. Anaplastic transformation has been reported in a few cases, however, with progression to anaplastic astrocytoma or glioblastoma or both.[84, 85, 91, 92]

***Differential Diagnosis.*** The differential diagnosis of pleomorphic xanthoastrocytoma involves the separation of this tumor from sarcoma and from a usual astrocytoma. Historically, this tumor was considered a sarcoma, and only with the use of GFAP antibody was its glial nature discerned. The distinctive clinical and gross features together with the vimentin-rich stroma distinguish this tumor from the usual astrocytoma.

## SUBEPENDYMAL GIANT CELL ASTROCYTOMA

***Clinical Considerations.*** Subependymal giant cell astrocytoma is the most common CNS neoplasm in association with the tuberous sclerosis complex (TSC).[93] Symptomatic tumors occur in about 6% of patients with TSC,[93] and in many TSC cases, symptoms referrable to the tumor may be the first manifestation of the disease.[94] In most cases, patients have a long-standing history of seizures resulting from cortical and white matter hamartomas. The subependymal giant cell astrocytoma also may occur without apparent signs of phakomatosis.[93, 95, 96] The tumor in any case usually presents in the first 2 decades of life.

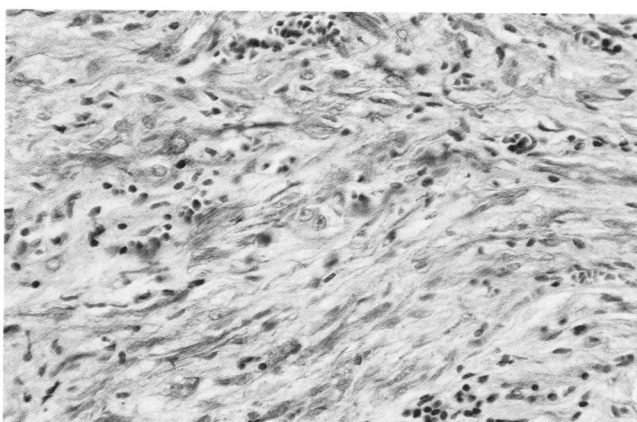

**FIGURE 51–17.** GFAP reactivity in both spindle and xanthomatous glial cells of pleomorphic xanthoastrocytoma.

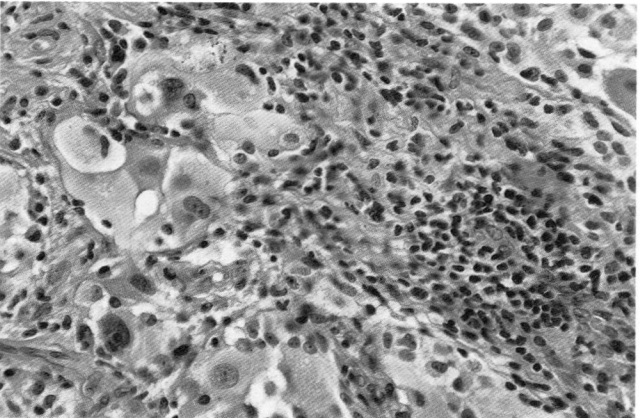

**FIGURE 51–16.** Pleomorphic xanthoastrocytoma with a variety of cell types.

*Diagnostic Considerations.* Subependymal giant cell astrocytomas are nodular, solid tumors arising from the wall of the lateral ventricle, often overlying the basal ganglia.[7] Less frequently, they arise in the third ventricle.

Microscopically, subependymal giant cell astrocytomas are heterogeneous tumors composed of spindle fibrillated cells admixed with more polygonal cells with abundant cytoplasm arranged in a fibrillated matrix. Large pyramidal cells with vesicular nuclei and prominent nucleoli, resembling ganglion cells, are common (CD Fig. 51–17). Some cellular pleomorphism and occasional multinucleate cells may be present. A conspicuous microvasculature features dilated vessels with hyalinized walls. These may hemorrhage, either spontaneously or after surgical manipulation. Calcifications often are seen. Mitotic activity may be present but is not indicative of anaplasia.[93] Similarly, foci of occasional vascular endothelial proliferation and necrosis do not indicate anaplastic progression. Subependymal giant cell astrocytomas are classified as a grade I neoplasm by the WHO classification,[1] and despite a few examples of recurrent tumor, no cases with malignant transformation have been described.[97]

Although subependymal giant cell astrocytomas are designated as a special type of astrocytoma,[1] these tumors have the capacity for divergent phenotypic expression of a mixed glioneuronal differentiation. Immunohistochemically, their primary astrocytic nature is confirmed by moderate GFAP and S-100 protein reactivity. Most tumors also express neuronal-associated proteins, however, including neurofilament proteins and neuronal-associated class III β-tubulin[98] (Fig. 51–18). Variable immunoreactivity for many neuropeptides also has been detected. These observations are confirmed by ultrastructural features suggestive of neuronal differentiation, including microtubules, rare dense-core granules, and occasional synapse formation.[99] Immunohistochemical and ultrastructural features are similar to those seen in the cortical tubers of the TSC. As a result, some authors have proposed that these tumors be designated *subependymal giant cell tumors.*[100]

*Molecular Genetics.* Loss of heterozygosity in the *TSC2* gene region (16p13) has been described in a few cases of subependymal giant cell astrocytoma.[101] Studies by immunohistochemistry for tuberin, the *TSC2* gene product, have shown loss of tuberin immunostaining in many subependymal giant cell astrocytomas, substantiating the presumed tumor-suppressor function of this gene[102, 103] (see Table 51–9).

*Differential Diagnosis.* The differential diagnosis of subependymal giant cell astrocytoma is principally the exclusion of a usual astrocytoma. The clinical setting, age of onset, and site of the tumor together with the characteristic giant cells expressing GFAP and neurofilament proteins are the basis of this important distinction.

### DESMOPLASTIC CEREBRAL ASTROCYTOMA OF INFANCY

*Clinical Considerations.* Desmoplastic cerebral astrocytoma of infancy is a rare astroglial tumor that arises in children during the first 2 years of life.[104, 105] These tumors have many clinical and histopathologic features similar to infantile desmoplastic ganglioglioma, which is discussed later in this chapter. The tumors typically are circumscribed and located in the superficial regions of the cerebral hemispheres, mainly the frontoparietal lobes.

*Diagnostic Considerations.* The tumors consist of a solid, firm nodule and a cystic component and often are adherent to the meninges.[105] The firmness of the tumors is due to the intense desmoplasia seen

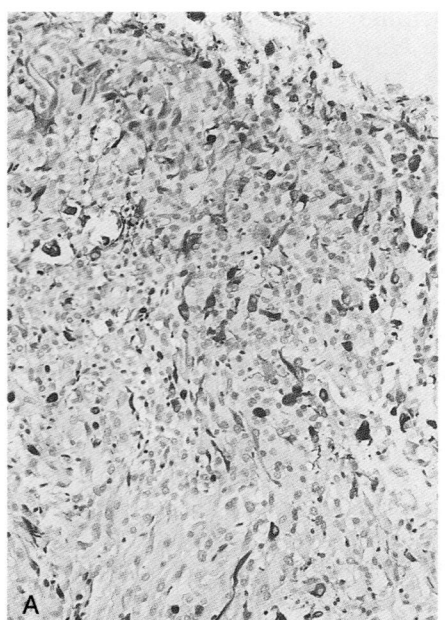
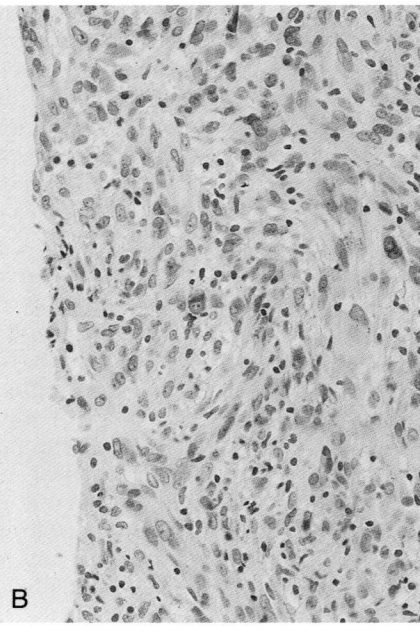

**FIGURE 51–18.** Giant cells in the subependymal astrocytoma may show glial (*A*, GFAP) and/or neuronal (*B*, neurofilament) markers by immunohistochemistry.

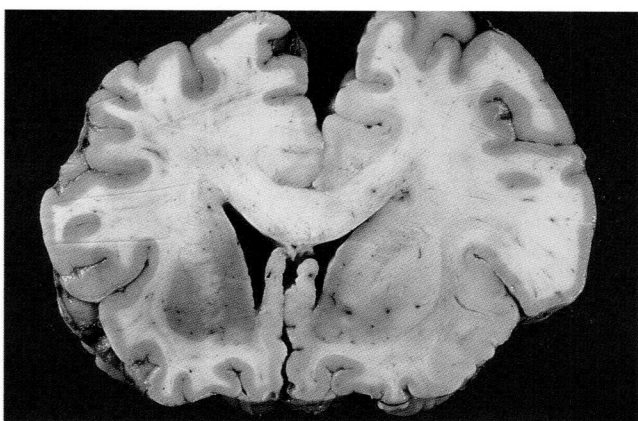

**FIGURE 51–19.** Oligodendroglioma infiltrating the right fronto-parietal region. Note the diffuse thickening of the cortical ribbon in the inferior portion of the frontal lobe.

intermixed with neoplastic elongated astroglial cells. In other areas, nodules or lobules of cells within a more obvious fibrillary matrix are seen. Immunohistochemically the glial tumor cells show intense immunoreactivity for GFAP. The origin of the desmoplastic stroma present in these tumors is still a matter of debate. True fibroblastic proliferation seems not to be present in these tumors. The reticulin-rich stroma is hypothesized to be elaborated by the neoplastic astrocytic cells themselves.[105, 106] Although some degree of cellular atypia and an elevated proliferative fraction may be present in these tumors, desmoplastic astrocytoma of infancy has a favorable prognosis.[104–106]

***Differential Diagnosis.*** The major differential diagnosis of desmoplastic cerebral astrocytoma is desmoplastic infantile ganglioglioma. The latter is a mixed glial-neuronal tumor in which neoplastic neuronal and astrocytic components are blended within a desmoplastic background.

### GLIOFIBROMA

***Clinical Considerations.*** Gliofibroma is a rare tumor that exhibits a prominent stromal component. In contrast to desmoplastic infantile astrocytoma previously discussed, these tumors have been described in children and adults[107–111] and may arise in the cerebrum, cerebellum, or spinal cord.[109–112]

***Diagnostic Considerations.*** Gliofibromas exhibit an admixture of two different cell types, astrocytes and fibroblasts, in variable degrees. The astroglial elements are spindle shaped and can be shown by GFAP and S-100 immunohistochemistry. The spindled fibroblasts are arranged in fascicles or dense hyaline zones that resemble fibromas. Prominent reticulin or vimentin stain is observed within the fibroblastic component of the tumor.

Tumors with low-grade histologic features and slow growth progression[111] and tumors with an anaplastic histologic appearance and aggressive behavior have been described.[107, 108, 112] The features of cellular pleomorphism and high mitotic activity are present in the tumors with a more aggressive clinical course.[107, 108, 112]

## OLIGODENDROGLIAL TUMORS

### *Oligodendroglioma*

CLINICAL CONSIDERATIONS. Oligodendrogliomas represent approximately 5% to 15% of intracranial gliomas.[113, 114] In a report from a single institution, oligodendrogliomas constituted 13% and 17% of all low-grade and high-grade gliomas.[115] Oligodendrogliomas most commonly arise in adults, with a peak incidence in the 30s and 40s.[113–116] About 6% to 12% of oligodendrogliomas occur in children and adolescents.[113, 115–118] Oligodendrogliomas affect both sexes with a 2:1 to 3:2 male-to-female ratio.[113, 115] Most tumors present with a slow clinical evolution, often associated with a history of seizures.[115, 118] The tumors occasionally may exhibit rapidly progressive symptoms, however, such as enlarging growths associated with enhancement on neuroimaging studies.[119]

Oligodendrogliomas can arise in any part of the neuraxis. Their incidence is proportional to the volume of white matter of the region.[120] The highest incidence of tumors is within the cerebral hemispheres, particularly the frontotemporal region. Bilateral involvement of cerebral hemispheres is noted in about 20% of cases,[113] and oligodendrogliomas commonly involve multiple lobes.[115, 116] The cerebellum, brain stem, and spinal cord are affected infrequently.

DIAGNOSTIC CONSIDERATIONS. Oligodendrogliomas are macroscopically soft, gelatinous masses, often relatively demarcated from the adjacent brain. The tumors tend to extend from the white to gray matter, obliterating the gray-white junction (Fig. 51–19). Oligodendrogliomas show a tendency to infiltrate leptomeninges focally. Areas of cystic degeneration are common in large tumors. Calcification is identified easily by neuroimaging in 70% of cases[121] (Fig. 51–20). Areas of hemorrhage are seen occasionally, but necrosis is limited to high-grade tumors.

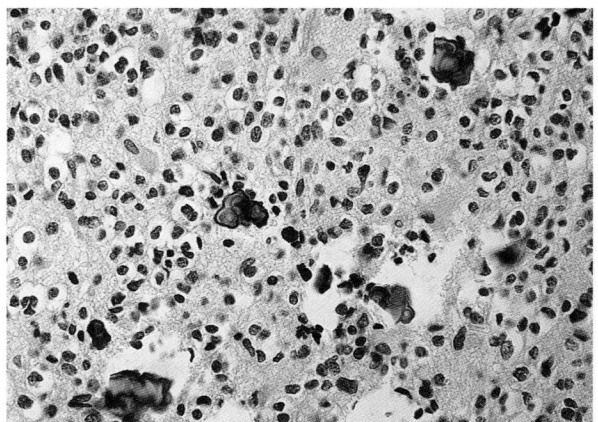

**FIGURE 51–20.** Small calcified concretions in oligodendroglioma.

**TABLE 51–10.** Oligodendroglial Tumors

| Tumor Designation | WHO Grade | Histologic Features | Ki-67 (mean) |
|---|---|---|---|
| Oligodendroglioma | II | Mild nuclear atypia<br>Low mitotic activity | <2% suggests longer survival[127]<br>>5% suggests shorter survival[127] |
| Anaplastic oligodendroglioma | III | Nuclear atypia<br>Increased mitotic activity<br>Endothelial proliferation (±)<br>Necrosis (±) | |
| Mixed oligoastrocytoma | II | Minor glial component >30%<br>Mild nuclear atypia<br>Low mitotic activity | |
| Anaplastic mixed oligoastrocytoma | III | Minor glial component >30%<br>Nuclear atypia<br>Increased mitotic activity<br>Endothelial proliferation (±)<br>Necrosis (±) | |

Smear preparations are helpful for the diagnosis of oligodendrogliomas during intraoperative consultations (CD Fig. 51–18). The tumors are typified by uniform discohesive tumor cells randomly distributed in an eosinophilic matrix composed of residual parenchyma. Nucleoli may be observed more readily than in astrocytomas, and multiple chromatin nodes are common. The lack of a conspicuous fibrillary matrix of cell processes helps to distinguish oligodendrogliomas from astrocytomas. Delicate branching microvasculature and calcifications also are helpful tools to make the diagnosis of oligodendrogliomas on smear preparations.

The microscopic appearance of most oligodendrogliomas is highly distinctive. Tumor cells commonly are arranged in a diffuse or pseudolobulated pattern, surrounded by delicate, geometric branching vessels. This characteristic vascular pattern often is referred to as a "chicken wire" pattern. On paraffin sections, a common artifact seen in oligodendrogliomas is the clearing of the cytoplasm, which gives the cell a characteristic "fried egg" appearance (CD Fig. 51–19A). The tumors also may show a wide variety of histologic patterns. Cellular arrangements include 1) nodular formation (CD Fig. 51–20); 2) palisades of cells with fusiform nuclear outlines mimicking those of polar spongioblastoma, a rare embryonal neuroepithelial tumor; 3) papillary-like structures surrounding blood vessels; and 4) microcystic formation with mucin deposition.

Frequently, oligodendrogliomas may display tumor cells with variable round-to-polygonal eosinophilic cytoplasm and eccentric nuclei termed *gliofibrillary oligodendrocytes* or *minigemistocytes*[122–124] (see CD Fig. 51–19B). Although these cellular elements have no prognostic value,[125] they must be distinguished from reactive astrocytes or neoplastic astrocytes or both within a true mixed oligoastrocytoma (see later), which has a less favorable prognosis than a pure oligodendroglioma.

Oligodendrogliomas frequently infiltrate the cerebral cortex diffusely, exhibiting perineuronal satellitosis (CD Fig. 51–21), and may spread along sub-pial zones. Reactive astrocytes often are found scattered throughout the tumor, particularly around blood vessels and in the areas of cortical infiltration.[126]

Oligodendrogliomas are a grade II neoplasm in the WHO classification (Table 51–10). Histopathologic features of anaplasia are not present in low-grade oligodendrogliomas. The cellular proliferative activity in oligodendrogliomas is low, but mitotic figures can be observed in low numbers without other evidence of malignant transformation. Although proliferative LIs may vary from laboratory to laboratory, a study has shown that the mean Ki-67 (MIB-1) LI in low-grade oligodendrogliomas is low (Ki-67 LI <2) (Fig. 51–21) and that tumors with Ki-67 LI greater than 5 are associated with shorter survival.[127]

No specific immunocytochemical marker of neoplastic oligodendrocytes is available for the purpose of diagnosis and tumor classification[128, 129] (Table 51–11). Major components of CNS myelin, including myelin basic protein, proteolipid protein, and myelin-associated glycoprotein, although present in oligodendrogliomas,[130–132] are variable and not specific

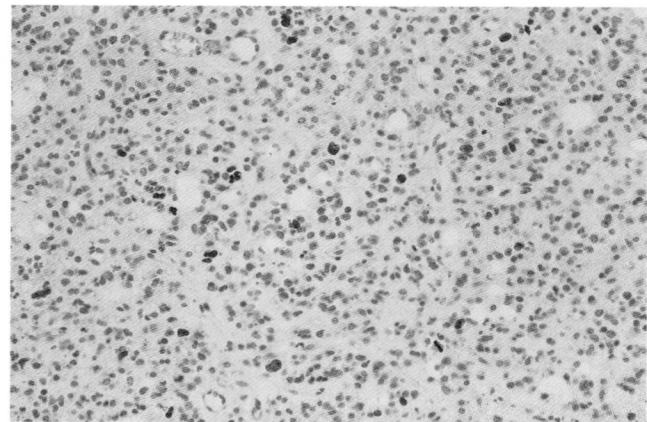

**FIGURE 51–21.** Low Ki-67 labeling index in an oligodendroglioma, grade II.

**TABLE 51–11.** Immunoreactivity, Diagnosis, and Molecular Genetics of Oligodendroglial Tumors

***Immunoreactivity***
No specific marker exists
Myelin and myelin-associated markers are not specific
Leu-7 (HNK-1) is not specific
Vimentin unreactive except in anaplastic oligodendroglioma
GFAP reactive, vimentin unreactive in minigemistocytes

***Diagnosis of Mixed Oligoastrocytoma***
No definitive criteria
Suggested criterion. The minor glial component, either astro-
 cytic or oligodendroglial, >30% of the tumor cells
Compact type. Two elements are distinct
Diffuse type. Two elements are intermixed

***Molecular Genetics***
Usual oligodendroglioma
 1p chromosomal loss
 19q chromosomal loss
 9p, 10q chromosomal losses with anaplastic change
 *p53* mutation with anaplastic change
Mixed oligoastrocytoma
 1p, 19q chromosomal loss. 30–70% of tumors especially if
  oligo predominant.
 *p53* mutation, 17p heterogeneity loss. 30% of tumors
  especially if astrocyte predominant

(e.g., myelin basic protein in neoplastic astrocytes).[130] Conflicting results also have been reported in studies analyzing galactocerebroside, a presumed oligodendrocyte-specific lipid.[128, 133] Leu-7, also designated *HNK-1*, a marker for natural killer cells,[134] identifies a carbohydrate epitope associated with myelin.[135, 136] Although present by immunohistochemical methods in most oligodendrogliomas, Leu-7 is not reliable in discriminating between oligo-

dendrogliomas and other gliomas, including astrocytomas and ependymomas.[132]

Among the intermediate filaments, vimentin is not expressed in most oligodendrogliomas[137] (CD Fig. 51–22). Because vimentin is expressed in neoplastic astrocytes and ependymal cells, the lack of vimentin may be useful in discriminating between oligodendrogliomas and astrocytomas and ependymomas. Anaplastic oligodendrogliomas are more likely to show vimentin expression.[138]

Gliofibrillary oligodendrocytes or minigemistocytes or both[122–124] commonly show intense GFAP immunoreactivity[124, 139–141] (Fig. 51–22) but are unreactive with vimentin, serving to distinguish these cells from reactive or neoplastic astrocytes. Ultrastructurally, gliofibrillary oligodendrocytes and minigemistocytes contain whorls of intermediate filaments within their cytoplasm, a pattern differing from the random distribution of short intermediate filaments noted in classic gemistocytes in astrocytic tumors.[124]

### Mixed Oligoastrocytoma

CLINICAL CONSIDERATIONS. Mixed oligoastrocytomas are composed of oligodendrocytes and a significant proportion of neoplastic astrocytes and are to be distinguished from oligodendrogliomas with reactive astrocytes or gliofibrillary neoplastic oligodendrocytes. Mixed oligoastrocytomas arise more commonly in the cerebral hemispheres, with the frontal lobes being affected most frequently, followed by the temporal lobes.[142, 143] Similar to low-grade oligodendrogliomas, the patients often present with a long-standing history of seizures.[143]

DIAGNOSTIC CONSIDERATIONS. Currently, there are no definitive histologic criteria to make the diagnosis of a mixed oligoastrocytoma (see Table 51–11).

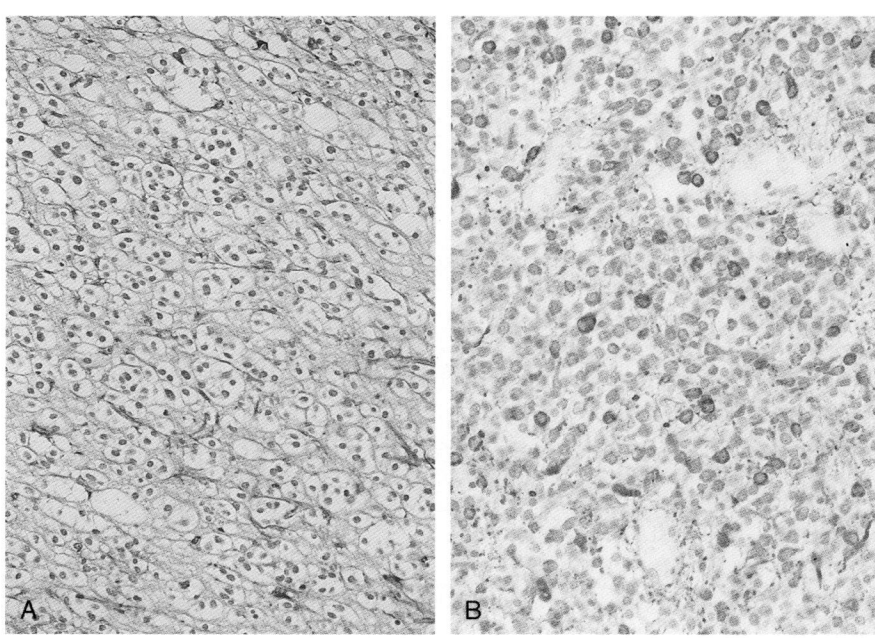

**FIGURE 51–22.** GFAP in two distinct cytologic areas of oligodendroglioma: fried egg region *(A)* and area with minigemistocytes *(B)*.

Frequently the predominant cell component is oligodendroglial.[126] Some investigators have defined a mixed glioma as a tumor in which a second minor glial component, either astrocytic or oligodendroglial, exceeds 30% of the cells.[144] More sophisticated methodology using cytometric image analysis may be an important adjunct to routine histopathology for the identification of mixed oligoastrocytomas.[145]

Mixed oligoastrocytomas have been subdivided into compact type or diffuse type, according to the distribution of the two cellular elements[142] (Fig. 51–23, CD Fig. 51–23). The compact type is characterized by distinct areas of each cytologic component, whereas the diffuse type has intermingled astrocytic and oligodendroglial cells. As in low-grade oligodendrogliomas, mixed oligoastrocytomas show a mild degree of pleomorphism and few mitotic figures. Endothelial proliferation and necrosis are absent. Mixed oligoastrocytomas correspond to WHO grade II (see Table 51–10).

The origin and histogenesis of these tumors are not completely understood. Theories have been postulated that the tumors may arise from *transitional* cells of mature oligodendrocytes and astrocytes.[122] The finding of bipotential O-2A progenitor cells associated with gliogenesis in the rodent may provide new advances in the understanding of these tumors.[140, 146, 147] As an alternative theory, the possibility that one glial component induces neoplastic transformation in the second cell population cannot be excluded completely in view of current concepts of tumorigenesis.

### Anaplastic Oligodendroglioma

CLINICAL CONSIDERATIONS. Only a few oligodendrogliomas are anaplastic, accounting for less than 5% of newly diagnosed malignant gliomas in one series.[119] Such tumors may evolve from a low-grade oligodendroglioma by a process of anaplastic transformation or appear de novo. Anaplastic oligodendrogliomas and anaplastic mixed oligoastrocyto-

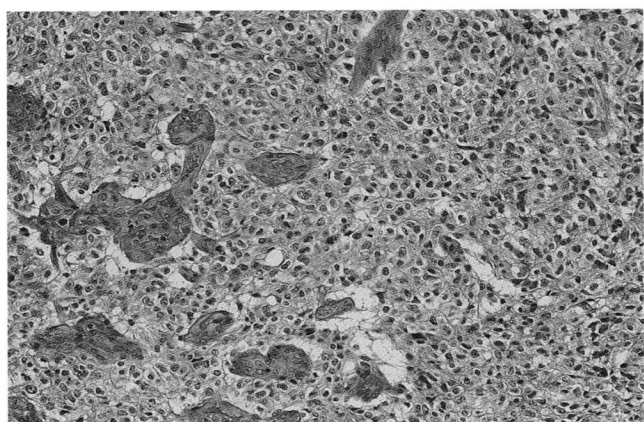

**FIGURE 51–24.** Anaplastic oligodendroglioma showing prominent endothelial proliferation.

mas, in contrast to other anaplastic gliomas, are highly chemosensitive tumors, particularly to the PCV (procarbazine, CCNU, and vincristine) regimen.[119, 148–150]

DIAGNOSTIC CONSIDERATIONS. Although there is no widely accepted grading system for oligodendrogliomas, the most significant morphologic criteria that indicate anaplasia include increased high nuclear-to-cytoplasmic ratios, nuclear pleomorphism, increased mitotic activity, and prominent endothelial proliferation[151] (Fig. 51–24, CD Fig. 51–24). Palisading necrosis also may be seen. Other investigators believe that proliferative activity assessed by proliferative markers, including Ki-67 (MIB-1) (Fig. 51–25) and proliferating cell nuclear antigen (PCNA), is associated more strongly with patient survival.[125, 127] Anaplastic oligodendrogliomas are a grade III neoplasm in the WHO classification (see Table 51–10).

As noted previously, GFAP-immunoreactive oligodendrocytes frequently are present in oligodendrogliomas and often increase in number with ana-

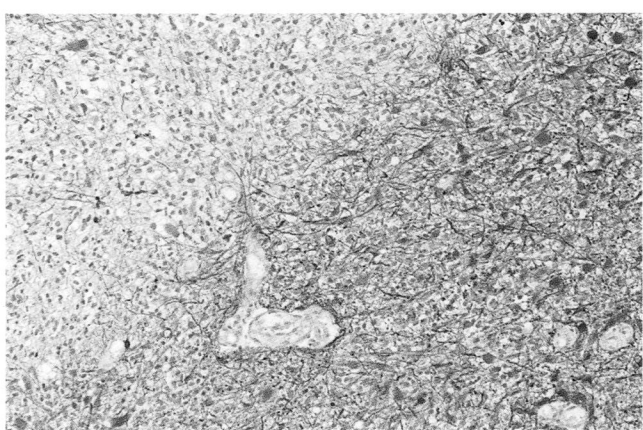

**FIGURE 51–23.** GFAP highlights the transitional zone of a mixed oligoastrocytoma with intense immunoreactivity in the astrocytic component *(right)* and an almost negative reaction in the oligodendrocytic component *(left).*

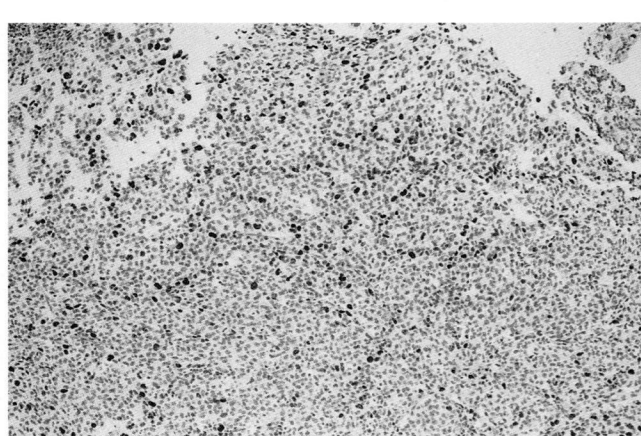

**FIGURE 51–25.** High Ki-67 labeling index in an anaplastic oligodendroglioma. Compare with the low labeling index of an oligodendroglioma grade II in Figure 51-21.

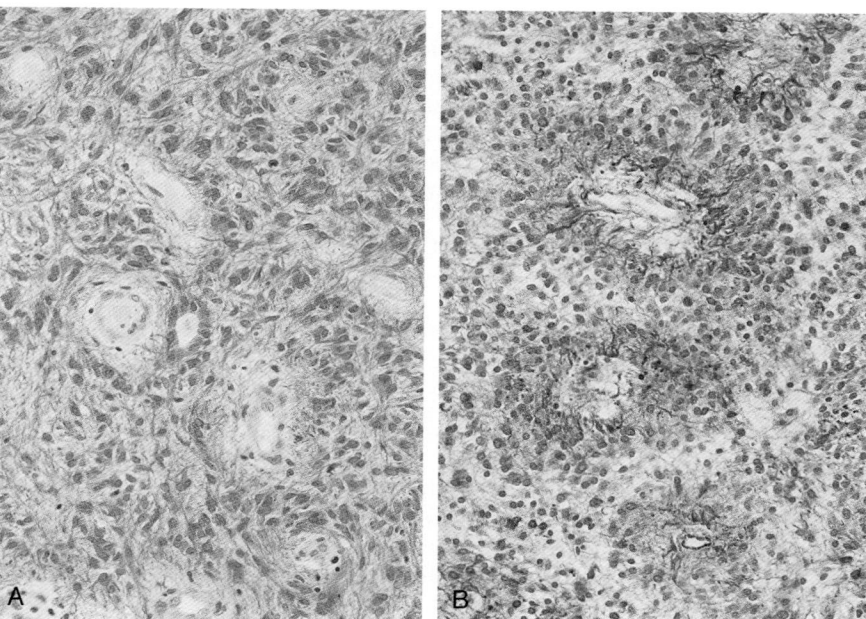

**FIGURE 51–27.** GFAP *(A)* and vimentin *(B)* immunohistochemistry highlight the fibrillary processes of an ependymoma.

(EMA) positive or both, particularly the papillary subtype (see later).[170–172] These epithelial markers are not as prominent in ependymomas, however, as in choroid plexus papillomas.

INTRAOPERATIVE DIAGNOSIS. Intraoperative smear preparations are helpful in showing the key features of ependymomas (CD Fig. 51–26). Tumor cells with well-defined cytoplasm, often arranged in thin processes, may form small pseudorosettes attached to blood vessels. The fibrillary background is the most significant finding to differentiate ependymomas from other papillary neoplasms, including choroid plexus papillomas. The nuclear chromatin usually is distributed irregularly in delicate nodes, producing an *open* pattern; this contrasts with the more coarse chromatin seen in astrocytomas and oligodendrogliomas.

EPENDYMOMA VARIANTS. Three histologic subtypes of ependymomas are recognized by the WHO classification: *cellular, papillary,* and *clear cell.* Although these tumor subtypes have the same clinical outcome as an ordinary ependymoma, their recognition as variants of ependymoma is important in distinguishing them from other gliomas.

*Cellular ependymomas* are characterized by prominent cellularity and only a few specialized ependymal formations, including perivascular pseudorosettes and ependymal rosettes. Indicators that aid in the correct diagnosis are the location of the tumors, the chromatin pattern of the tumor cells, and the fibrillary nature of the intercellular matrix.

*Papillary ependymomas* are distinguished by conspicuous formation of papillary and tubular structures, in a way similar to choroid plexus papillomas (see later). The ependymal nature of these tumors is confirmed easily, however, by immunoreactivity for GFAP and vimentin and variable cytokeratin immunoreactivity.[170]

*Clear cell ependymomas* are a rare subtype showing a distinctive appearance of perinuclear halo formation resembling that seen in oligodendroglial cells.[173] This appearance may present a problem in differential diagnosis with other neuroepithelial tumors, including oligodendrogliomas and central neurocytomas. The appropriate diagnosis is suggested by other clinicopathologic features, such as tumor location and distinct tumor demarcation. Ultrastructural analysis of the tumors is helpful for the identification of ependymal features, including the presence of cilia, microvilli, and junctional complexes.[173]

Histologic grading of ependymomas is controversial, and the value of each histologic feature suggestive of anaplasia as a prognostic factor is uncertain[164, 165, 174–177] (see Table 51–12). Tumor location and patient age are important factors in the prognosis of patients with ependymomas.[165, 178–180]

### Anaplastic Ependymoma

CLINICAL CONSIDERATIONS. Anaplastic progression of ependymomas is present in tumors at most sites but is rare in ependymomas of the spinal cord.[162] Anaplastic ependymomas (WHO grade III) have a high tendency to disseminate along the neuraxis with worsening of the patient's clinical course.[181]

DIAGNOSTIC CONSIDERATIONS. Anaplastic ependymomas are characterized histologically by their cellular density, cellular or nuclear atypia, mitotic activity, endothelial microvascular proliferation, and large areas of necrosis.[1, 177] Although these tumors are recognized by morphologic means, the correlation between the histopathology and the clinical outcome of patients with anaplastic ependymomas is not as direct as that seen in other gliomas.[175, 177]

The proliferative rate of ependymomas by means of mitotic index or proliferative LI or both seems to be the most important prognostic factor, particularly in supratentorial tumors.[182, 183] Immunohistochemistry for proliferative markers, mainly PCNA[183] and Ki-67 (MIB-1),[181, 184–186] shows that high LIs have a positive correlation with the histologic grade and early tumor recurrence (see Table 51–12). The presence of endothelial proliferation seems to be less relevant to the prognosis of these patients.[175, 182]

### Myxopapillary Ependymoma

CLINICAL CONSIDERATIONS. Myxopapillary ependymomas are a distinct variant of ependymoma that most commonly develops in the cauda equina and filum terminale of adults.[187] Less frequently, tumors may arise in the upper levels of the spinal cord[187] and lateral ventricles.[188] Ectopic tumors located in the extradural and presacral or retrosacral areas also have been reported.[167, 187, 189] The tumors are slow growing and usually have a favorable prognosis.

DIAGNOSTIC CONSIDERATIONS. Myxopapillary ependymomas are macroscopically discrete, encapsulated, sausage-shaped masses arising from the filum terminale and involving the spinal nerve roots of the cauda equina. Some tumors may disseminate locally along the spinal canal. On cut surface examination, the tumors are soft with a lobulated appearance.

Histologically, these tumors are characterized by papillary arrangements of columnar or cuboidal cells with fibrillary processes that radially extend to blood vessels (CD Fig. 51–27). The blood vessels have variable hyaline and mucinous degeneration that is typically periodic acid–Schiff positive. Mucin accumulation in the form of small *mucin lakes* also may accompany neoplastic cells not in contact with vessels. Although the papillary arrangements dominate the histologic picture, focal formation of ependymal tubules also can be seen. The glial nature of these tumors is verified by GFAP and vimentin immunoreactivity.[187] Ultrastructural analysis confirms ependymal differentiation with the demonstration of microvilli associated with cellular interdigitations and abundant basement membrane.[190, 191]

Most myxopapillary ependymomas are biologically benign and slow growing and correspond to WHO grade I. Local recurrences are common, however, and dissemination along the neuraxis occurs more frequently than with ordinary ependymomas of the spinal cord.[181] The prognosis of myxopapillary ependymoma seems to be related directly to successful total resection.[181, 187]

### Subependymoma

CLINICAL CONSIDERATIONS. Subependymomas are well-circumscribed, firm, generally asymptomatic masses of variable size located in the walls of the fourth and lateral ventricles[192–195] (CD Fig. 51–28). Most tumors are found incidentally at autopsy. Symptomatic subependymomas may present with either increased intracranial pressure owing to obstruction of cerebrospinal fluid flow or spontaneous tumor hemorrhage. Other tumor sites are the septum pellucidum, the foramen of Monro, and, less commonly, the spinal cord.[196–198] The tumors are found in both sexes and in all age groups, but most frequently symptomatic subependymomas affect middle-aged patients.[192, 195]

DIAGNOSTIC CONSIDERATIONS. Histologically, subependymomas exhibit ependymal and astrocytic differentiation, reflecting the probable lineage of these tumors.[162] The tumors are characterized by hypocellularity and a dense fibrillary matrix (CD Fig. 51–29). Ependymal differentiation is represented by perivascular pseudorosettes and, less frequently, true ependymal rosettes. Astrocytic differentiation is characterized by elongate, fibrillary-to-gemistocytic cells intermixed in a dense fibrillary matrix. The association of astrocytic and ependymal features has been confirmed by electron microscopic and tissue culture studies. Microcalcifications and microcystic degeneration are common. Hyalinized blood vessels and signs of prior subclinical hemorrhage, including hemosiderin deposition, often are present.

Subependymomas are WHO grade I tumors. Tumor location and surgical resection, particularly related to tumors situated on the floor of the fourth ventricle, are the most important prognostic factors.[193, 194]

MOLECULAR GENETICS OF EPENDYMAL TUMORS. Ependymomas have complex cytogenetic and molecular genetic alterations that are not observed in astrocytomas[199] (see Table 51–12). In contrast to astrocytomas, mutations of the *p53* tumor-suppressor gene have been shown only occasionally.[200, 201] About a third of ependymomas show abnormalities involving chromosome 22, and a tumor-suppressor gene on 22q may be present. Although some investigators have shown evidence of mutations of the *NF2* suppressor gene at 22q12,[202] others have been unable to identify such mutations in many ependymomas.[203–205]

DIFFERENTIAL DIAGNOSIS OF EPENDYMAL TUMORS. Classic ependymomas with prominent specialized structures, including perivascular pseudorosettes and especially ependymal rosettes, are easy to diagnose and are unlikely to be mistaken for any other glioma. Ependymomas may be a diagnostic problem, however, if these ependymal structures are less prominent. In fibrillary tumors without specialized ependymal arrangements, the possibility of a diffuse astrocytoma has to be excluded. In most of these tumors, even fibrillary ependymomas show foci of some perivascular pseudorosette formation. In addition to histology, the neuroradiologic finding of a circumscribed tumor with pushing borders is helpful in the diagnosis of ependymoma.

As previously described, the special variants of ependymoma, such as *cellular, papillary,* and *clear cell,* may resemble other gliomas, and it is important to distinguish them from anaplastic gliomas, choroid plexus tumors, and oligodendrogliomas, respectively.

Myxopapillary ependymomas may be mistaken for other tumors involving the cauda equina region, particularly paragangliomas and schwannomas. The presence of immunoreactivity for GFAP and vimentin verifying the presence of glial fibrils distinguishes this tumor from schwannoma and paraganglioma.[187] The lack of chromogranin helps to differentiate these tumors from paragangliomas.[206]

PROGNOSTIC CONSIDERATIONS. As described earlier, the histologic features generally associated with the grading of gliomas, such as high cellularity, mitotic activity, and especially endothelial proliferation, although pointing to a greater likelihood of recurrence, do not correlate with clinical outcome of ependymomas. Tumor location, patient age, and radiologic features of tumor delineation all contribute to the overall prognostic outlook. The immunohistochemical demonstration of high LI using Ki-67 (MIB-1) in general correlates with tumor recurrence. Molecular markers to date have not offered significant prognostic guidelines to ependymoma clinical outcome, however.

## CHOROID PLEXUS TUMORS

### Choroid Plexus Papilloma

CLINICAL CONSIDERATIONS. Choroid plexus papillomas are rare neuroepithelial tumors that account for less than 1% of all intracranial tumors.[207] Most involve children, producing 2% to 5% of CNS neoplasms in this age group,[208, 209] although papillomas also may arise in adults. Rare cases of prenatal choroid plexus papillomas have been cited in the literature.[210]

Papillomas may occur anywhere in the ventricular system, but in infants and children, the most frequent location is the lateral ventricles, and in adults, the most frequent location is the fourth ventricle. Multiple choroid plexus papillomas involving more than one ventricle also have been described.[211] Clinical symptoms are usually the result of hydrocephalus often resulting from either obstruction of the cerebrospinal fluid pathways or an overproduction of cerebrospinal fluid.[212]

Several observations suggest a possible role for simian virus 40 (SV40) in the pathogenesis of choroid plexus tumors.[213, 214] SV40 sequences have been shown in many choroid plexus papillomas and carcinomas and in ependymomas.[213, 214] These findings agree with experimental data showing that the expression of large T antigen of SV40 induces formation of choroid plexus papillomas and carcinomas in transgenic mice.[215]

Choroid plexus papillomas also have been described in association with Aicardi's syndrome.[216–219] However, choroid plexus cysts are considered the major diagnostic feature for this well-defined syndrome characterized by agenesis of the corpus callosum.[220]

DIAGNOSTIC CONSIDERATIONS. Choroid plexus papillomas are grossly well-demarcated, frequently calcified masses with a conspicuous papillary or cauliflower-like appearance. Although the tumors may be adherent to ventricular walls, brain invasion is infrequent. Areas of hemorrhage are seen commonly.

Histologically, choroid plexus papillomas are benign, papillary neoplasms composed of single or multiple layers of a cuboidal-to-columnar epithelium with a delicate fibrovascular core (CD Fig. 51–30). In contrast to normal choroid plexus, papillomas are hypercellular and exhibit cellular pleomorphism. Pseudostratification of the epithelium often is present, which contrasts with the ordered cell orientation that characterizes normal choroid plexus. The papillary appearance of these tumors is identified easily on intraoperative smear preparations.

Stromal metaplastic transformation of choroid plexus papillomas has been reported in a few cases, including chondroid and osseous metaplasia.[221–223] Xanthomatous and oncocytic changes also may be present. These morphologic changes are of no diagnostic significance, however.[224, 225]

The immunophenotype of choroid plexus tumors reflects the neuroepithelial nature of the normal choroid plexus. Epithelial antigens, such as cytokeratin or EMA, are expressed by most choroid plexus papillomas[226–229] (CD Fig. 51–31A). Although GFAP may be positive in a few papillomas,[226–228, 230] S-100 protein has been shown in most tumors.[226, 228, 230]

Transthyretin, formerly known as *prealbumin,* is a plasma protein involved in the transport of thyroxine and retinol and is secreted in great amounts by the choroid plexus epithelium. Transthyretin antibody is reactive in most choroid plexus papillomas,[228, 230, 231] and it has been considered a valuable marker for the identification of choroid plexus tumors[232] (CD Fig. 51–31B). Experience has shown, however, that transthyretin immunoreactivity is not restricted to choroid plexus tumors and that certain metastatic carcinomas also can express this protein.[233]

Recurrence of histologically benign papillomas has been associated with subarachnoid seeding.[236] Anaplastic transformation of papillomas should be suspected when increased mitotic activity and necrosis are present. These histologic features have been associated with a higher potential for tumor recurrence and spread.[209, 228, 234] Some authors refer to such tumors as *atypical choroid plexus papillomas.*[228, 235] The distinction between atypical tumors and true choroid plexus carcinomas has not been firmly established, however.

### Choroid Plexus Carcinomas

CLINICAL CONSIDERATIONS. Choroid plexus carcinomas are much rarer tumors than papillomas and tend to arise in young children.[212, 239, 240] Most of the carcinomas occur de novo; malignant transformation in choroid plexus papillomas is observed in less than 20% of cases.[208] Choroid plexus carcinomas have more aggressive behavior than papillomas, with a 5-year survival rate of 40% compared with a 100% rate of survival in papillomas.[212] In contrast to papillomas, choroid plexus carcinomas are frankly invasive lesions, and cerebrospinal fluid dissemination or subarachnoid spread or both commonly are seen.[212, 240] Metastases remote from the CNS have been reported in a few cases.[241, 242]

DIAGNOSTIC CONSIDERATIONS. Histologically, carcinomas have a less conspicuous papillary pattern, with tumor cells arranged in dense cellular sheets. Frank features of anaplasia, including nuclear atypia, cellular pleomorphism, increased mitotic activity, and necrosis, may be present focally or diffusely (CD Fig. 51–32). The possibility of a metastatic adenocarcinoma must be excluded, particularly in cases arising in adults. In children and adolescents, the differential diagnosis should include germ cell tumors with a papillary pattern, including embryonal carcinoma, choriocarcinoma, and yolk sac tumors.

Choroid plexus carcinomas have an immunohistochemical profile similar to the papillomas. Carcinomas stain only weakly for transthyretin, however.[228, 233] The value of transthyretin for differentiating choroid plexus carcinomas from other epithelial tumors, mainly metastatic carcinomas, is limited. It has been suggested, however, that the absence of transthyretin positivity may be associated with a poor prognosis in choroid plexus tumors.[228]

Studies with the proliferative marker MIB-1 have shown a mean labeling value of 1.0% to 3.7% for papillomas and a LI of 13% to 14% for carcinomas.[237, 238] These studies do not discriminate the so-called atypical papillomas, however.[238]

MOLECULAR GENETICS OF CHOROID PLEXUS TUMORS. The few cytogenetics reports have suggested that choroid plexus papillomas display hyperdiploidy, whereas choroid plexus carcinomas have a hyperhaploidy karyotype.[243–246] Duplication of chromosome 9p has been associated with abnormalities of choroid plexus, including hyperplasia and tumors.[247] A few cases of papilloma have been reported in families with Li-Fraumeni syndrome.[248, 249]

DIFFERENTIAL DIAGNOSIS OF CHOROID PLEXUS TUMORS. The papillary variant of ependymoma is the most important differential diagnosis of choroid plexus papilloma. In general, ependymomas lack the typical fibrovascular cores of choroid plexus papillomas but have a more obviously fibrillary neuroglial background. GFAP immunoreactivity is present in ependymomas and choroid plexus papillomas. Papillomas express strong reactivity for cytokeratin and transthyretin, however. Clinical and neuroradiologic data offer additional tools for precise diagnosis.

Distinction between choroid plexus carcinomas and metastatic carcinomas is essential in assessing an intraventricular epithelial tumor, particularly in cases affecting adults. The use of a wide immunohistochemical panel is necessary because choroid plexus carcinomas do not have a specific marker. The expression of GFAP or S-100 protein or both and positive cytokeratin and transthyretin immunohistochemistry are helpful clues to the diagnosis of a choroid plexus carcinoma. In children and adolescents, germ cell tumors, including embryonal carcinoma, choriocarcinoma, and yolk sac tumors, should be excluded.

PROGNOSTIC CONSIDERATIONS. The absence of transthyretin immunoreactivity has been associated with a poor prognosis in choroid plexus tumors.[228] Choroid plexus papillomas generally are associated with a good clinical outcome and are a WHO grade I neoplasm. Choroid plexus carcinomas are WHO grade III neoplasms with the histologic features of mitotic activity, necrosis, and brain invasion associated with recurrence and short survival time.

## NEUROEPITHELIAL TUMORS OF UNCERTAIN ORIGIN

### Astroblastoma

Astroblastoma is a rare glial neoplasm, usually occurring in older children and young adults.[250, 251] The histogenesis of astroblastoma is controversial. Although the tumor has a glial appearance and is GFAP immunoreactive, the ultrastructural features suggest a derivation from tanycytes,[252] specialized ependymal cells. Consequently, this tumor has been grouped in the category of neuroepithelial tumors of uncertain origin in the WHO classification.[1]

The astroblastoma usually is circumscribed and arises in the supratentorial compartment. Histologically, astroblastoma has a distinctive pattern of perivascular glial cells with broad, nontapering cytoplasmic processes radiating toward a central, often hyalinized blood vessel (CD Fig. 51–33). These perivascular pseudorosettes dominate the tumor with only a few intervening cells. Immunohistochemically the tumor is strongly positive for GFAP, vimentin, and S-100[253–255] (CD Fig. 51–34).

The WHO classification does not recommend a specific histologic grading for these tumors. Two histologic groups of astroblastomas have been proposed: low grade and high grade.[256] Low-grade tumors have a uniform architecture of perivascular pseudorosettes, minimal cellular atypia, low mitotic activity, and minimal or no proliferation of vascular endothelium. In contrast, high-grade astroblastomas show increased cellularity and cellular atypia, pseudorosettes with multiple cell layers, high mitotic activity, and microvascular endothelial proliferation. Necrosis may be a feature in low-grade and high-grade tumors. A report of seven cases has supported the initial impression that anaplastic histology is a prognostic factor in the behavior of astroblastomas.[251]

Astroblastoma should be differentiated from other tumors in which pseudorosette formation is present, particularly ependymomas. Astroblastoma pseudorosettes have thicker and shorter cytoplasmic processes than those of ependymal pseudorosettes. Occasional pseudorosette formation may occur in diffuse infiltrating astrocytoma (grades II through IV). The designation *astroblastoma* should be retained for tumors in which pseudorosetting dominates the lesion and foci of conventional fibrillary or gemistocytic astrocytoma are not present.

### Gliomatosis Cerebri

Gliomatosis cerebri is characterized by a diffuse growth of neoplastic glial cells throughout the cerebral hemispheres (CD Fig. 51–35). The lesion frequently is bilateral and may extend to infratentorial structures and the spinal cord. The diagnosis of gliomatosis cerebri is a neuroradiologic one. Imaging shows diffuse enlargement of cerebral structures causing little destruction of involved areas. Postmortem examination is necessary to confirm the diagnosis and the extent of tumor.

Histologically, gliomatosis cerebri resembles diffuse infiltrating astrocytoma[257] (CD Fig. 51–36), although a few cases showing an oligodendroglial pattern have been described.[258] The tumor cells vary in shape from oval to elongated and tend to invade along myelinated tracts, around blood vessels, and in the subpial and subependymal regions (CD Fig. 51–37). There is moderate cellular atypia and mitotic activity. GFAP and S-100 immunoreactivity is variable. Focal transformation to higher grade astrocytoma or glioblastoma or both may occur. Gliomatosis cerebri corresponds histologically to WHO grades III or IV.

## Neuronal and Mixed Neuronal-Glial Tumors

Table 51–13 presents the WHO grading system for neuronal and mixed neuronal-glial tumors.

### CENTRAL NEUROCYTOMA

CLINICAL CONSIDERATIONS. Central neurocytomas are rare benign neuronal tumors, most commonly found in the region of the lateral ventricles.[259] They usually occur in young patients; in one series, the age at surgery ranged from 6 to 52 years (mean age, 24 years).[260] Most present as well-demarcated, partially calcified masses in or adjacent to the lateral ventricles, typically in the region of the foramen of Monro. Massive tumors involving the lateral and the third ventricles also have been described. Neoplasms designated as *neurocytomas* have been reported in extraventricular sites.[261–265] It remains to be established whether these lesions are definitely neurocytomas that differ from the typical lesion only by their location.

**TABLE 51–13.** Neuronal and Mixed Neuronal-Glial Tumors World Health Organization Grading

| Neuronal | Grade |
|---|---|
| Central neurocytoma | I |
| Gangliocytoma | I |
| Dysplastic gangliocytoma of cerebellum | I |
| **Mixed Neuronal-Glial** | |
| Ganglioglioma | I–II |
| Anaplastic ganglioglioma | II–IV |
| Desmoplastic infantile ganglioglioma | I |
| Dysembryoplastic neuroepithelial tumor | I |

DIAGNOSTIC CONSIDERATIONS. Central neurocytomas are characterized by a homogeneous population of cells with round to slightly lobulated nuclei and finely speckled chromatin in a conspicuously fibrillated matrix (CD Fig. 51–38). A constant and distinctive histologic feature of these tumors is the presence of anuclear islands composed of a dense fibrillary matrix resembling neuropil (CD Fig. 51–39). Perinuclear halos may be prominent, and small concentric calcifications frequently are present. A delicate branching microvasculature, slightly reminiscent of oligodendrogliomas, typically is present. The uniform cell population, the finely fibrillated matrix, and the typical microvessels are recognized on smear preparations. Focal areas of necrosis rarely may be observed. Mitotic activity is low, and Ki-67 (MIB-1) LIs are generally low.[266–268] Endothelial proliferation is not present (see later). Mature ganglion cells have been reported infrequently in central neurocytomas,[269] and the term *ganglioneurocytoma* has been suggested for such cases.[262, 263, 267]

The histogenesis of central neurocytoma is controversial. Although most investigators regard this tumor as a neuronal neoplasm,[267] there has been speculation that the tumor may have a bipotential capacity for neuronal and glial differentiation.[269, 270] The neuronal nature of the tumor is confirmed by immunohistochemistry for synaptophysin (CD Fig. 51–40) and other neuronal-associated proteins, including neurofilament proteins and class III β-tubulin.[260, 267, 269] Ultrastructural features include clear and dense-core vesicles, cellular processes filled with parallel microtubular arrays, and mature synapses. GFAP immunoreactivity has been described in a few reported cases,[269] but in the authors' experience, it is restricted to reactive stromal astrocytes.[260]

DIFFERENTIAL DIAGNOSIS. The histologic features of central neurocytoma are reminiscent of ependymoma, oligodendroglioma, and neuroblastoma. Neuroblastoma is histologically less differentiated than neurocytoma with dense cellularity, hyperchromasia, and high mitotic activity. In ependymoma, perivascular pseudorosettes resemble the fibrillary anuclear areas of neurocytoma. The presence of these fibrillary zones helps to distinguish the neurocytoma from the oligodendroglioma. Immunohistochemistry for neuronal markers, especially synaptophysin, and the electron microscopic features of neurosecretory granules and synaptic junctions are important for the differential diagnosis of ependymoma and oligodendroglioma, in both of which these features are not seen. In addition, the expression of GFAP in ependymoma helps to distinguish it from the central neurocytoma.

PROGNOSTIC CONSIDERATIONS. Central neurocytomas are designated grade I in the WHO classification. Tumor recurrence has been reported,[268, 271-274] however, mainly in cases in which subtotal surgical resection was obtained at initial surgery. In a few cases, recurrence with ventricular and subarachnoid dissemination also has been noted.[274] Many tumors showing moderate mitotic activity, vascular proliferation, and focal necrosis also have been reported.[260, 261, 269-271, 273, 275] Some authors have advocated that the proliferative potential of central neurocytomas correlates with their clinical behavior[275] and that tumors with a MIB-1 LI of 2% have a higher chance of recurrence. In addition, their studies showed significant correlation between the presence of vascular endothelial proliferation and the MIB-1 LI. These authors suggested that tumors with high MIB-1 LI or vascular proliferation or both should be termed *atypical central neurocytoma* corresponding to a WHO grade II neoplasm.

## GANGLIOCYTOMA AND DYSPLASTIC GANGLIOCYTOMA OF THE CEREBELLUM

### Gangliocytoma

CLINICAL CONSIDERATIONS. Gangliocytomas are rare tumors composed of mature ganglionic neurons. The tumors generally are well circumscribed and most commonly arise in the temporal lobe and cervicothoracic spinal cord[276, 277] (CD Fig. 51–41). Other locations include the hypothalamus and pituitary region and the pineal gland.[276, 278, 279] Most lesions become clinically symptomatic within the first 3 decades, and in contrast to gangliogliomas (see later), clear association with a chronic seizure disorder is not observed. Tumors arising in the pituitary region have been associated with pituitary adenomas and clinical symptoms of endocrine disorders.[279] Hypothalamic neuronal hamartoma associated with gelastic seizures, mental retardation, or precocious puberty[280, 281] may be histologically difficult to separate from gangliocytoma. These clinically well-characterized lesions are regarded as hamartomas by the WHO classification.[1]

DIAGNOSTIC CONSIDERATIONS. Gangliocytomas are characterized by a proliferation of neoplastic ganglion cells in a poorly cellular glial-mesenchymal stroma (CD Fig. 51–42A). The ganglionic population is distributed irregularly and exhibits great cytologic pleomorphism, including bizarre and binucleate forms. Abnormal neuritic processes can be highlighted by silver impregnation techniques and immunohistochemical stains for neurofilament proteins (CD Fig. 51–42B). The inconspicuous glial elements of the tumor stroma are GFAP immunopositive.

Gangliocytomas are slow-growing tumors designated as grade I by the WHO. Because the scant glial elements of the lesion are not neoplastic in nature, these tumors have no potential for anaplastic progression.[276]

### Dysplastic Gangliocytoma of the Cerebellum

CLINICAL CONSIDERATIONS. The dysplastic gangliocytoma of the cerebellum, also known as *Lhermitte-Duclos disease*, is a rare form of gangliocytoma restricted to the cerebellum. The lesion usually becomes clinically apparent in patients during their 30s.[282] Patients with symptoms earlier in life have been reported, however, mainly as result of megencephaly and intracranial hypertension. Lhermitte-Duclos disease is associated with Cowden's syndrome in about 50% of the cases,[283] suggesting that this entity may have features of a hamartoma and a neoplasm. MRI of the thickened cerebellar folia is diagnostic.[284]

DIAGNOSTIC CONSIDERATIONS. The hypertrophic folia consist of abnormal ganglion cells and smaller neurons that occupy the normal granular and Purkinje cell layers (CD Fig. 51–43). Hypermyelinated parallel fibers and enlarged neurites replace the normal molecular layer. There usually is demyelination of the adjacent white matter. The histogenesis of these ganglionic and neuronal cells is still not well understood (CD Fig. 51–44). Some immunohistochemical studies have suggested a histogenetic relationship to Purkinje cell lineage,[285, 286] whereas other analyses have suggested an origin from granular cell neurons.[287, 288]

Dysplastic gangliocytoma of the cerebellum is a grade I neoplasm in the WHO classification. Most patients have a favorable postoperative course. Recurrences after a subtotal resection have been reported, however.[289-292]

## GANGLIOGLIOMA AND MALIGNANT GANGLIOGLIOMA

CLINICAL CONSIDERATIONS. Gangliogliomas are the most common mixed neuronal-glial tumors, but they represent only about 1% of all brain tumors[293] and 1% to 4% of all pediatric CNS tumors.[294, 295] Most arise within the first 3 decades of life,[296, 297] but they also may arise in adults.[298] Clinically, gangliogliomas present with seizure disorders,[293-295] in particular, complex partial seizures.[295]

Gangliogliomas may occur at any site in the neuraxis, but temporal lobes are most frequent, followed by parietal and frontal lobes.[293, 295-297, 299] Neuroimaging reveals a well-demarcated tumor with cystic and calcified components. Many cases are associated with cortical dysplasia in the vicinity of the tumor.[293, 299]

DIAGNOSTIC CONSIDERATIONS. Histologically, gangliogliomas are composed of clusters of neoplastic, abnormal ganglion cells and glial cells, most commonly fibrillary and pilocytic astrocytes (CD Fig. 51–45). An oligodendroglial component is considerably less common.[299, 300] The ganglionic elements may show considerable variation in size and density. Bizarre and binucleate forms may be present.[293, 301] A rich fibrocollagenous stroma with a significant deposition of collagen IV and laminin[302] often is accompanied by a variable angiomatosis and perivascular lymphocytic infiltrates. Tumor may involve leptomeninges.

Ganglionic elements are highlighted by silver stains and immunohistochemistry for neuronal-associated proteins. Neurofilament proteins, synaptophysin (CD Fig. 51–46A), and class III β-tubulin are shown in virtually all tumors.[293, 297] Chromogranin and many neuropeptides also may be present.[297] Dense synaptophysin perikaryal surface labeling has been promoted as a reliable indicator of neoplastic ganglion cells.[301, 303] This pattern of synaptophysin staining also may be observed in non-neoplastic neurons, however.[304, 305] The glial elements, usually astrocytic, are reactive with GFAP (CD Fig. 51–46B), vimentin, and S-100.

The ganglioglioma is a WHO grade I to II neoplasm. The glial component typically is responisble for recurrence and anaplastic progression as evidenced by MIB-1 labeling confined to the astrocytic elements.[293, 297] Although the MIB-1 LI is low in most gangliogliomas,[293, 297, 299] high labeling values may be indicative of more aggressive behavior.[297]

A report has described nine cases of a new variant of mixed neuronal-glial neoplasm.[306] These tumors show characteristic papillary formations containing astrocytic and neuronal elements. The neuronal elements vary from small neurocytes to ganglion cells. No histologic features of anaplasia are present.

Malignant transformation in gangliogliomas is reported to occur in about 10% of cases.[296] As previously mentioned, anaplastic progression invariably occurs in the glial component. The histopathologic picture resembles that of an anaplastic astrocytoma or a glioblastoma. The ganglionic elements may be difficult to detect in these more anaplastic tumors. Immunohistochemical stains for neuronal-associated markers are helpful in this context.

## DESMOPLASTIC INFANTILE GANGLIOGLIOMA

CLINICAL CONSIDERATIONS. Desmoplastic infantile ganglioglioma is a rare form of mixed neuronal-glial neoplasm that affects children younger than 2 years.[307, 308] The tumors typically are supratentorial, with a predilection for the frontal and parietal lobes. Characteristically, these tumors are massive with a prominent cystic component, dural attachment, and firm texture, particularly in superficial cortex.

DIAGNOSTIC CONSIDERATIONS. Histologically the tumors are composed of varied proportions of astrocytic and neuronal cells admixed in a variable mesenchymal stroma[307] (CD Fig. 51–47). The distribution of the astrocytic and neuronal elements within each tumor is relatively heterogeneous. The astrocytic cells are the most conspicuous, especially in more desmoplastic regions. The neuronal elements vary greatly, ranging from atypical ganglion-like cells to smaller polygonal cells. Typical ganglion cells similar to those seen in gangliogliomas are rarely present. A population of more primitive cells also is present. The desmoplastic stroma is marked by a conspicuous fibroblastic component and a dense deposition of reticulin and collagen fibrils intermixed within the neuroglial elements.

The mixed nature of the tumor cells is confirmed with special stains and immunohistochemistry. GFAP and vimentin highlight the glial elements, whereas neurofilament proteins, synaptophysin (CD Fig. 51–48), and silver impregnation facilitate identification of the neuronal cell populations. The reticulin stain and antibodies to collagen IV show the dense fibers of the desmoplastic stroma.

Mitotic activity and necrosis are uncommon but when present tend to occur in association with the most primitive cell populations. These features of anaplasia do not seem to indicate an anaplastic transformation. Microvascular endothelial proliferation is not evident.

PROGNOSTIC CONSIDERATIONS. Desmoplastic ganglioglioma of infancy has a favorable outcome with total or near-total surgical resection.[307] These tumors are grade I neoplasms in the WHO classification.

## DYSEMBRYOPLASTIC NEUROEPITHELIAL TUMOR

CLINICAL CONSIDERATIONS. DNT is a mixed neuronal-glial neoplasm[309] that was incorporated in the revised WHO classification of brain tumors in 1993.[1] It usually arises in children and young adults with long-standing complex partial seizures. DNTs are rare tumors and may represent less than 1% of all brain tumors.[310] In centers specializing in epilepsy surgery, the frequency may be 10%.[311] The tumors involve the supratentorial region, most frequently the temporal lobes.[309, 312] A few cases involving other sites also have been reported, including the caudate nucleus[313] and the cerebellum.[314] The lesions are predominantly intracortical and multinodular, but subcortical white matter involvement also is seen.[315, 316] A multicystic appearance frequently is appreciated on MRI.[316] A common radiographic sign is an overlying skull defect, suggesting a long-standing lesion.

DIAGNOSTIC CONSIDERATIONS. The characteristic histopathologic feature of DNT is the multinodular architecture of the tumor, best appreciated at low power (CD Fig. 51–49A). The nodules are composed of a mixture of small cells resembling oligodendroglia, astrocytes, and neuronal cells embedded within a mucinous and microcystic matrix (CD Fig. 51–49B). The neuronal component, which is composed mainly of large cells, may be inconspicuous, leading to the erroneous diagnosis of a mixed oligoastrocytoma. Neuronal-associated markers (synaptophysin, neurofilament proteins, class III β-tubulin) (CD Fig. 51–50A) confirm the distinct neuronal component, whereas GFAP (CD Fig. 51–50B), vimentin, and S-100 verify the glial elements.[317, 318] The small oligodendroglia-like cells seem to be a mixture of cells with early glial and neuronal differentiation.[317] Cellular atypia is not present. Mitotic activity may be observed, but proliferative indices are generally low (MIB-1, <1%).[318, 319] Tumor recurrence has been observed in cases with incomplete initial surgical resection.[319] Typically the brain surrounding a DNT has a variable degree of cortical dysplasia.[312]

DIFFERENTIAL DIAGNOSIS AND PROGNOSTIC CONSIDERATIONS. Considering the heterogeneity of these tumors, adequate sampling is important for the correct diagnosis of DNTs. The major differential diagnoses to be considered include oligodendroglioma and mixed oligoastrocytoma. The recognition of DNT is significant because surgical resection results in an extremely favorable prognosis. DNTs are grade I neoplasms in the WHO classification.

## Embryonal Tumors

The embryonal tumors are a group of clinically aggressive neoplasms that typically occur during the first decade of life. The embryonal designation of the tumors implies that these neoplasms are probably a result of transformation of immature or undifferentiated neuroepithelial cells.[320–323] Embryonal tumors have many common histologic features, including high cellularity, primitive-appearing small cell populations, and a usually high mitotic activity. These tumors exhibit a high tendency for cerebrospinal seeding. These features reflect the clinically aggressive behavior of embryonal tumors and their designation as grade IV neoplasms in the WHO classification (Table 51–14).

Despite the common properties shared by these neoplasms, many embryonal tumors are separated out on the basis of their distinctive histopathologic features and presumed histogenesis. The current WHO classification recognizes the central neuroblastoma and the ependymoblastoma as embryonal tumors showing differentiation toward neuronal and ependymal lineages. A rare embryonal neoplasm that has a characteristic cytomorphology and potential for expressing divergent neural cell types, the medulloepithelioma, is also a separate entity in the WHO classification. The designation of primitive neuroectodermal tumor is limited to medulloblastomas and neoplasms that are indistinguishable from medulloblastomas but located at other sites of the neuraxis.

### MEDULLOBLASTOMA

CLINICAL CONSIDERATIONS. Medulloblastomas by definition arise in cerebellum and are the most common and best characterized of the embryonal tumors. Most tumors arise in the cerebellar midline, although tumors involving the cerebellar hemispheres also may occur. Medulloblastomas occur mostly in children during the first decade of life with a mean age of 9 years.[324] Tumors also may arise in early adulthood and rarely in patients in their 40s and 50s.[325, 326] In children, medulloblastomas comprise approximately one quarter of all intracranial tumors.

DIAGNOSTIC CONSIDERATIONS. Grossly, medulloblastomas are soft, often friable gray masses distinct from the adjacent cerebellum (Fig. 51–28). Areas of necrosis and hemorrhage are frequent. Cyst formation, so common in the pilocytic astrocytoma of this region, is rare.

**TABLE 51–14.** Embryonal Tumors*

| Tumor Designation | Location | Special Histopathologic Features |
|---|---|---|
| Medulloblastoma | Cerebellum | Occasional neuroblastic (Homer Wright) rosettes<br>Neuronal and/or glial differentiation by immunohistochemistry<br>Variants: desmoplastic medulloblastoma, medullomyoblastoma, melanotic medulloblastoma |
| Other PNETs† | Supratentorial | Similar to medulloblastoma |
| Neuroblastoma | Supratentorial (fronto-parietal) | Occasional neuroblastic (Homer Wright) rosettes<br>Neuronal differentiation by immunohistochemistry |
| Ependymoblastoma | Supratentorial | Ependymoblastic rosettes; perivascular pseudorosettes<br>Glial differentiation by immunohistochemistry |
| Medulloepithelioma | Supratentorial<br>Cerebellum (less common) | Neural tube–like structures<br>Papillary, tubular, and trabecular arrangements<br>Focal neuronal and glial differentiation |

* All are WHO grade IV tumors.
† PNETs, Primitive neuroectodermal tumors.

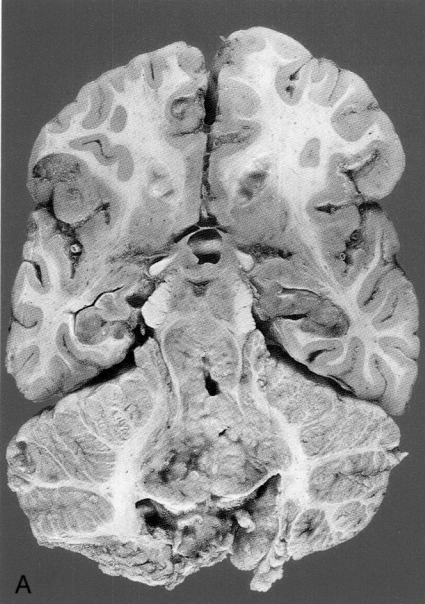
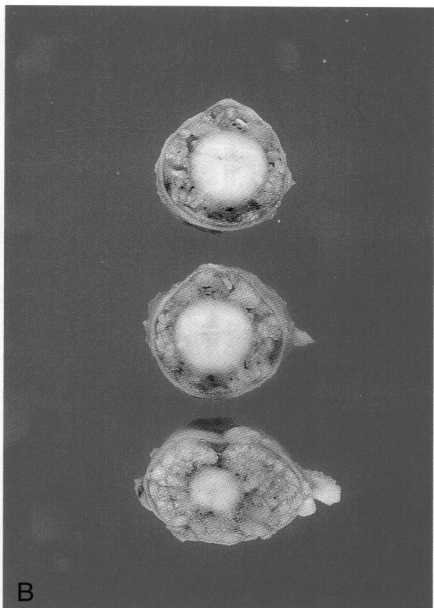

**FIGURE 51–28.** A large medulloblastoma occupying the cerebellar vermis and compressing the fourth ventricle *(A)*. Spinal cord encased by leptomeningeal dissemination of tumor through the CSF pathways *(B)*.

Medulloblastomas are hypercellular neoplasms composed of relatively small cells with hyperchromatic angular-to-ovoid nuclei and scant cytoplasm (Fig. 51–29*A*). The cells usually are arranged in sheets, although focal formation of rhythmic nuclear palisades can be seen. The tumor cells may infiltrate the cerebellar cortex diffusely with obliteration of the granular and molecular layers. Neuroblastic (Homer Wright) rosettes may be found in half of the cases[327] (Fig. 51–29*B*), and neoplastic ganglion-like cells are present in a few cases. Other signs of focal neuroblastic differentiation include a prominent intercellular fibrillated matrix and the proliferation of

cells with large and vesicular nuclei, similar to neurocytic cells. Mitoses are seen frequently. Focal or geographic necrosis is common, but endothelial vascular proliferation is rare.

Immunohistochemistry (Table 51–15) has shown that more than 50% of medulloblastomas show immunoreactivity for neuronal-associated markers, including synaptophysin, neurofilament proteins, class III β-tubulin, and microtubule-associated proteins[327–332] (Fig. 51–30). Astrocytic differentiation, as confirmed by GFAP reactivity, has been shown in nearly 10% of cases.[327, 333, 334] The distinction between reactive stromal astrocytes and a true neoplastic as-

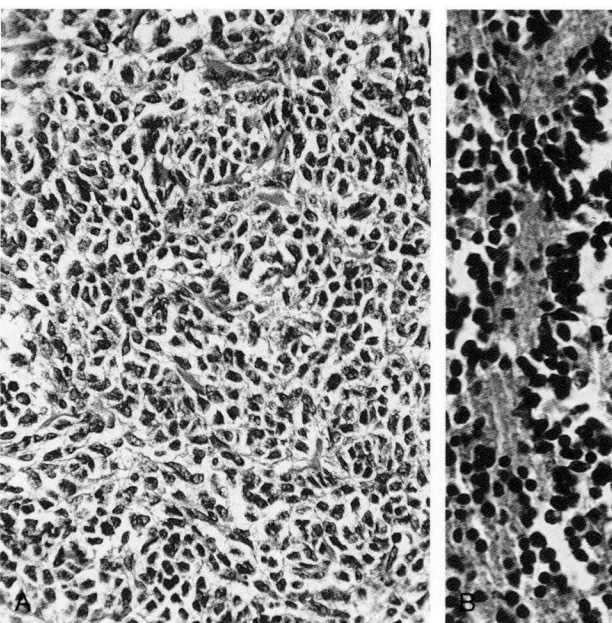
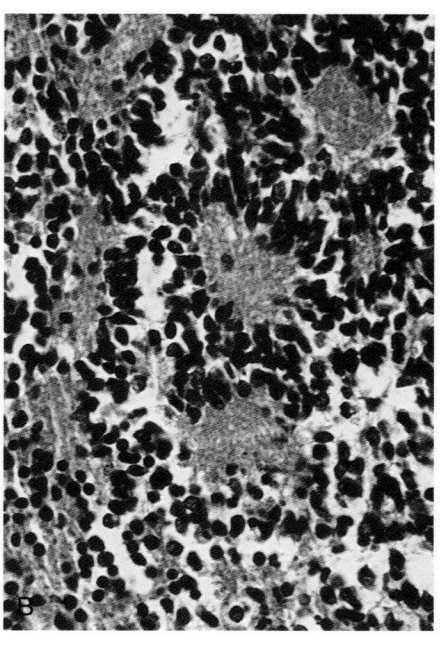

**FIGURE 51–29.** Small, poorly differentiated cells with a patternless arrangement in medulloblastoma *(A)*. Formation of neuroblastic Homer Wright rosettes *(B)*.

**TABLE 51–15.** Immunohistochemistry and Molecular Genetics of Medulloblastoma

*Immunohistochemistry*
Synaptophysin
Neurofilament proteins
β-tubulin, class III
Microtubule-associated proteins
GFAP—in 10% of cases, indicating glial differentiation
S-antigen and opsin—in photoreceptor differentiation

*Molecular Genetics*
Chromosome 17—isochromosome 17q. Loss of heterozygosity on 17p
Chromosome 1q—loss of heterozygosity
*p53*—no gene mutation

trocytic component is quite difficult, however. In addition, medulloblastomas may exhibit photoreceptor differentiation with S-antigen (S-Ag) and opsin immunoreactivity.[335, 336]

MEDULLOBLASTOMA VARIANTS. Many medulloblastoma variants are described. The most common is the *desmoplastic medulloblastoma*, which comprises about 10% to 20% of all medulloblastomas.[325, 327, 337, 338] These tumors are well-demarcated lesions with a firm consistency. They are more prevalent in the lateral portions of the cerebellar hemispheres, and leptomeningeal invasion commonly is seen. Microscopically the tumors have a biphasic arrangement with areas of hypercellularity alternating with nodular areas of hypocellularity (CD Fig. 51–51). The nodular or follicular areas feature cells with larger nuclei and a neuropil-like background intensely reactive with neuronal markers.[329] In contrast, the hypercellular areas are composed of small, primitive-appearing cells with increased mitotic ac-

tivity and proliferative LIs. The unique biphasic arrangement of this variant of medulloblastomas is most apparent on reticulin stain, wherein the nodules are markedly free of staining in contrast to rich intercellular deposition of reticulin in the hypercellular extranodular areas.

Other variants of medulloblastoma are extremely rare. *Medullomyoblastoma* exhibits striated muscle fibers admixed with the primitive neuroectodermal cells of an ordinary medulloblastoma. The myoblastic component is confirmed by myoglobin and desmin immunoreactivity. *Melanotic medulloblastoma* contains a population of pigmented cells in epithelial and papillary arrangements.

MOLECULAR GENETICS. Cytogenetics studies have shown a common and specific abnormality on chromosome 17, an isochromosome 17q, in about one third of medulloblastomas[339–341] (see Table 51–15). Molecular studies have confirmed this cytogenetic finding with the frequent loss of heterozygosity on chromosome 17p.[342–345] Although this is a region containing the *p53* gene locus, *p53* mutation generally is absent in medulloblastomas.[342, 345] Another gene located in the same region of the short arm of chromosome 17 is the lissencephaly gene 1 (*LIS-1*), which plays no role in the molecular pathogenesis of medulloblastomas.[344, 346] In addition, a third of the medulloblastomas show loss of heterozygosity on chromosome 1q.[344]

PROGNOSTIC CONSIDERATIONS. Medulloblastoma overall survival has improved significantly with 5-year survival rates 45% to 70%.[324, 347] The value of morphologic features in predicting the outcome of medulloblastoma is controversial, however. Although some reports have indicated that anaplastic features, including nuclear atypia, high mitotic index, necrosis, vascular endothelial proliferation,

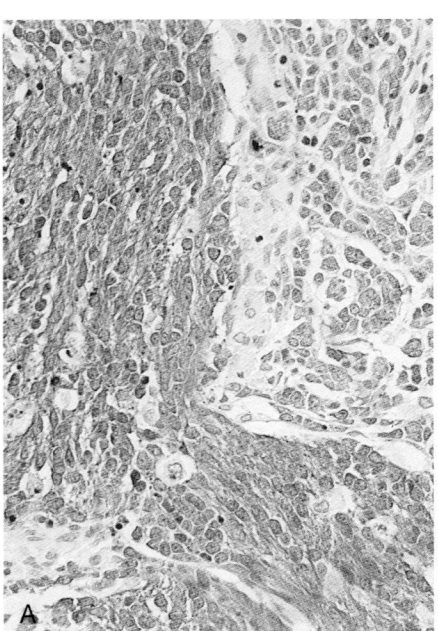
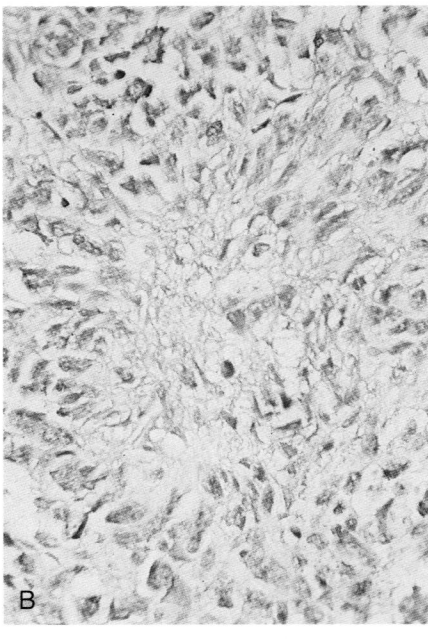

**FIGURE 51–30.** Neuronal differentiation in medulloblastoma confirmed by synaptophysin (*A*) and neurofilament (*B*) immunoreactivity.

and lack of neuronal differentiation, are important markers for a poorer prognosis, other authors have found no association with these parameters. An extensive discussion of these aspects is summarized by Giangaspero and colleagues.[347]

## NEUROBLASTOMA AND GANGLIONEUROBLASTOMA

CLINICAL CONSIDERATIONS. Central neuroblastomas are rare embryonal tumors that often affect children in the first decade of life.[348, 349] Most tumors are supratentorial with a predilection for the frontoparietal region (CD Fig. 51–52). They tend to be large and well demarcated by neuroimaging. Calcifications, cyst formation, and areas of hemorrhage are seen commonly.[350]

DIAGNOSTIC CONSIDERATIONS. Histologically, neuroblastomas are hypercellular tumors composed of small cells with round hyperchromatic nuclei and ill-defined cytoplasm. The cells are arranged in monotonous sheets alternating with areas of Homer Wright rosette formation (CD Fig. 51–53). In some tumors, larger polygonal cells with vesicular nuclei and abundant cytoplasm may be present. Ganglion-like cells are rare,[349, 351] however, and may indicate a ganglioneuroblastoma (see later). The exclusively neuroblastic differentiation of these embryonal tumors is confirmed by immunohistochemistry and ultrastructure. The tumor cells present processes containing microtubule arrays, neurosecretory granules, and synaptic junctions.[326] Immunohistochemistry reveals neuronal-associated cytoskeletal proteins, including neurofilaments, class III β-tubulin, and synaptophysin. Small neurites can be detected by silver stains, such as Bielschowsky.[348]

Ganglioneuroblastomas involving the CNS are extremely rare. Similar to the peripheral tumors, they are characterized by a variable number of ganglion-like cells intermingled within a neuroblastoma (CD Fig. 51–54). The prognosis and biologic behavior of central ganglioneuroblastoma seem similar to central neuroblastoma.

PROGNOSTIC CONSIDERATIONS. Cerebral neuroblastoma is a highly malignant tumor with poor prognosis because of local tumor recurrence and leptomeningeal extension. A report of 12 cases[350] described a mean survival of only 1.4 years (range, 2 days to 2.75 years).

## EPENDYMOBLASTOMA

CLINICAL CONSIDERATIONS. Ependymoblastomas are rare embryonal tumors with the capacity for ependymal differentiation. They affect young children with a median age of 3 years.[352, 353] Most tumors arise in the supratentorial compartment, and involvement of the ventricular cavities is frequent.[353]

DIAGNOSTIC CONSIDERATIONS. Ependymoblastomas have clear cytogenetic and histologic characteristics that permit their differentiation from medulloblastomas and other primitive neuroectodermal tumors. The tumors are macroscopically well-defined lesions, but leptomeningeal infiltration is common. Histologically the tumors are hypercellular and composed of poorly differentiated neuroepithelial cells forming either amorphous arrangements or characteristic ependymoblastic rosettes (CD Fig. 51–55). The latter consist of multilayered cellular arrangements surrounding a small lumen or a central canal (CD Fig. 51–56). Mitotic activity is frequent in the juxtaluminal areas. Perivascular rosettes, commonly seen in ependymomas, are rare in ependymoblastomas. Necrosis is seen commonly in the tumors. The cells composing the ependymoblastic rosettes and the amorphous groups of primitive cells are GFAP immunoreactive.[354, 355] Ultrastructural findings, including microvilli, 9+2 cilia, and juxtaluminal zonulae adherens, confirm the ependymal lineage of these tumors.[356]

Clear differentiation should be made between ependymoblastoma and malignant ependymoma (see "Ependymoma" section). Ependymoblastomas are separated from anaplastic ependymomas on the basis of their hypercellularity, the primitive nature of their tumor cells, the absence of pseudorosettes, and the lack of endothelial proliferation.

PROGNOSTIC CONSIDERATIONS. Ependymoblastomas are one of the most aggressive embryonal tumors. A review of 28 cases reported an average survival of 8.1 months.[353] Mortality often is related to tumor regrowth and seeding of the cerebrospinal fluid pathways.[352, 353] Extracranial metastases were described in one patient.[353]

## MEDULLOEPITHELIOMA

CLINICAL CONSIDERATIONS. Medulloepithelioma is a rare tumor that usually occurs early in the first decade of life.[326, 357, 358] The tumor involves most frequently the cerebral hemispheres with a tendency to arise in periventricular areas. A few cases arising in the posterior fossa have been reported.[358] Medulloepitheliomas also may occur in the eye.

DIAGNOSTIC CONSIDERATIONS. Histologically, medulloepithelioma consists of mitotically active, pseudostratified columnar epithelium resembling that of the primitive neural tube (CD Fig. 51–57). Cells are arranged in papillary, tubular, or trabecular arrangements outlined by external and internal limiting membranes, similar to the structure of the primitive neural tube. Most tumor cells, in the neural tube–like structures and the undifferentiated areas, are vimentin-positive as seen in the normal neuroepithelium.[357, 358] Neuronal and glial differentiation is present in only a few cells.[357, 358] Strong immunoreactivity for insulin-like growth factor I and basic fibroblastic growth factor also has been reported.[359] Mesenchymal differentiation may be seen occasionally with skeletal muscle formation or bone formation or both.

PROGNOSTIC CONSIDERATIONS. The prognosis of medulloepithelioma is poor. These tumors respond poorly to medical adjuvant therapy, and the overall survival in a series of eight cases was 20 months.[358]

## Pineal Parenchymal Tumors

Pineal parenchymal neoplasms comprise approximately 15% to 30% of pineal region tumors[360–363] and less than 1% of brain tumors.[364] These tumors are believed to originate from the intrinsic cell of the pineal gland, the pineocyte, a specialized neuroepithelial cell with neuroendocrine and photosensory properties.

### PINEOCYTOMA

Pineocytomas account for 25% to 30% of pineal parenchymal tumors[365, 366] and commonly arise in young adults in their teens and 20s.[362, 364, 367, 368] They are small, circumscribed lesions[365] that compress the surrounding brain with little tendency for brain parenchyma infiltration (CD Fig. 51–58). Pineocytomas have the most benign course of all pineal parenchymal tumors, with a 5-year patient survival rate of 86% in one large series.[366] Pineocytomas are classified as grade II tumors by the WHO.

Histologically, pineocytomas are moderately cellular and composed of cytologically mature cells arranged in sheets or in variable lobular formations that resemble the lobularity of the normal pineal gland. Most commonly, the cells are arranged in characteristic *pineocytomatous rosettes*[369] (CD Fig. 51–59). The presence of these specialized pineocytomatous rosettes has been associated with a more benign clinical course.[370]

Immunohistochemistry confirms the neurosecretory differentiation of pineal parenchymal tumors, especially pineocytomas. The tumors express neuronal-associated proteins, including class III β-tubulin, neurofilament proteins, and synaptophysin[368, 371–373] (CD Fig. 51–60). The neurosecretory differentiation of the tumor cells is confirmed by ultrastructure.[374] In addition, pineocytomas may express photosensory-associated protein retinal S-Ag.[375, 376] GFAP and S-100 highlight reactive stromal astrocytes.

### PINEOBLASTOMA

Pineoblastoma represents the other spectrum of pineal parenchymal tumors, the most primitive and malignant of these tumors. Pineoblastomas are more common than pineocytomas, accounting for 50% to 75% of all pineal parenchymal tumors.[362, 366, 377] They arise in young patients, mostly within the first 2 decades of life,[362, 377] with a male-to-female ratio of 2:1.[370] Cases involving adults also have been reported.[378] Pineoblastomas have a high potential for dissemination along the cerebrospinal fluid pathways and a poor response to therapy.[366]

Pineoblastomas are grossly soft, poorly demarcated tumors that tend to invade the surrounding brain and leptomeninges (CD Fig. 51–61). Calcification may be seen infrequently on MRI.[365] Microscopically, they display small, poorly differentiated cells containing round-to-oval hyperchromatic nuclei and scant cytoplasm arranged in densely cellular patternless sheets (CD Fig. 51–62). Homer Wright rosettes may be present and photosensory Flexner-Wintersteiner rosettes and fleurettes.[370, 379] Mitotic activity frequently is high, and areas of necrosis are evident.

Immunohistochemically the tumors express neuronal-associated proteins, including class III β-tubulin, neurofilament proteins, and synaptophysin, as seen in pineocytomas. Likewise, photosensory differentiation is documented in pineoblastomas with retinal S-Ag immunoreactivity.[375] Similar to other CNS embryonal tumors, pineoblastomas are regarded as grade IV tumors in the WHO classification.

### MIXED PINEOCYTOMA AND PINEOBLASTOMA

Many pineal parenchymal tumors have morphologic features of the well-differentiated pineocytoma and the poorly differentiated pineoblastoma. These tumors have a clinical course dependent on the mix of pineocytomatous and pineoblastomatous elements.[362] The potential for local infiltration and cerebrospinal fluid dissemination is significant, making these tumors usually more aggressive than pineocytoma.[362, 366]

MOLECULAR GENETICS OF PINEAL PARENCHYMAL TUMORS. Cytogenetic studies performed on a few tumors have found some concurrence, including abnormalities of chromosome 1p, deletions in chromosomes 11 and 12q, and monosomy or deletions in chromosome 22.[380, 381] Analysis of the *p53* tumor-suppressor gene failed to reveal *p53* gene mutations or overexpression of p53 protein by immunohistochemistry, suggesting that the *p53* gene pathway is not involved in pineal tumorigenesis.[382]

## Germ Cell Tumors

Primary CNS germ cell tumors are histologically indistinguishable from germ cell tumors of the gonads and other extragonadal sites (see Chapters 33 and 38). They occur primarily in the first 2 decades of life.[383–385] The incidence of primary germ cell tumors varies according to geographic regions of the globe.[386–390] In the brain, these tumors occur primarily in the pineal and suprasellar regions.[385, 391] Other less common intracranial locations are the basal ganglia and thalamus, the cerebral hemispheres, the posterior fossa, and lastly the spinal cord.[385, 390–400]

### GERMINOMA

Germinomas are the most common of the CNS germ cell tumors.[385, 387, 391] Grossly, they are soft, friable well-circumscribed masses with areas of hemorrhage and necrosis (Fig. 51–31) and are microscopically similar to germinoma (or dysgerminoma) of the gonads (CD Fig. 51–63).[401, 402] Most are immunoreactive for placental alkaline phosphatase[402–404] (Fig.

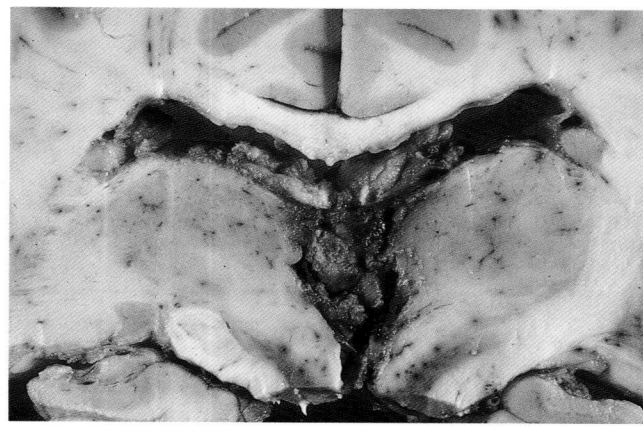

**FIGURE 51–31.** A germinoma of the supra-sellar region involving the 3rd ventricle.

51–32) but are generally unreactive for cytokeratin, although some have shown cytokeratin positivity in 30% of cases.[402, 404, 405]

## EMBRYONAL CARCINOMA

Embryonal carcinomas are rare, constituting only 5% of all intracranial germ cell tumors.[385, 399] Microscopically, epitheloid tumor cells may be arranged in cords, sheets, glands, or patternless groups of cells (CD Fig. 51–64). Embryonal carcinomas are diffusely positive for cytokeratin and placental alkaline phosphatase. Focal alpha fetoprotein–positive and β-human chorionic gonadotropin–positive cells also may be found[406–408] (CD Fig. 51–65).

## YOLK SAC TUMOR (ENDODERMAL SINUS TUMOR)

Yolk sac tumors as pure tumors are rare, representing about 7% of all intracranial germ cell tumors.[383, 387] Most are located in midline sites,[402, 409] but a few cases have been reported in the basal ganglia and posterior fossa.[393, 402] Histologically, CNS tumors resemble their gonadal counterparts.

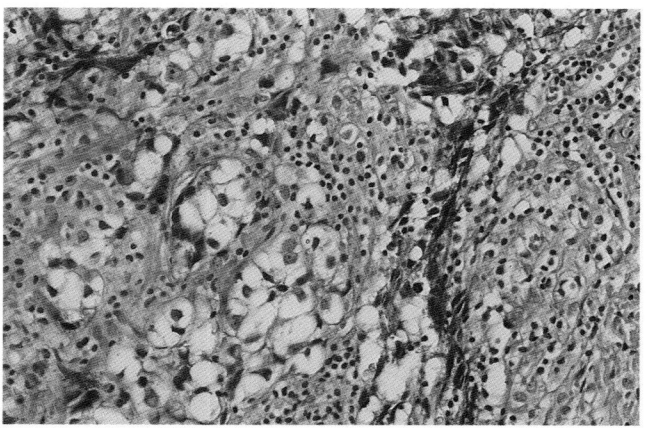

**FIGURE 51–32.** Placental alkaline phosphatase immunoreactivity in germinoma.

## CHORIOCARCINOMA

Pure primary choriocarcinomas are rare and constitute only 5% of all intracranial germ cell tumors.[383, 385–387, 402] The pineal region is the preferential site for these tumors, but the hypothalamus and sellar regions also are involved.[391]

## TERATOMA

Teratomas constitute only 0.5% of all intracranial neoplasms[386] but nearly 20% of all intracranial germ cell tumors.[383] The pineal region is the most common site, but other frequent locations are the sellar and suprasellar regions.[384, 391, 397, 410, 411]

Similar to their gonadal counterparts, CNS teratomas are divided into three categories: 1) mature teratoma, 2) immature teratoma, and 3) teratoma with malignant transformation. Mature teratomas are the least common (CD Fig. 51–66). Immature teratomas are the most common form.[385, 387] Although immature teratomas seem to have a less favorable clinical course compared with mature teratomas,[412] spontaneous maturation of the immature elements has been reported in residual or recurrent tumors with excellent postsurgical survival after successful removal.[413] Immature teratomas are likely to disseminate along cerebrospinal fluid pathways.[385, 414, 415] Teratomas with malignant transformation are teratomas (mature or immature) in which malignant components of epithelial or mesenchymal elements resembling ordinary carcinomas or sarcomas are present.[416]

## MIXED GERM CELL TUMORS

Of the various elements present in a CNS mixed germ cell tumor, the most common association is germinoma with teratoma, which has been estimated to occur in one fifth of all reported cases.[417]

# Meningothelial Tumors

## MENINGIOMA AND VARIANTS

CLINICAL CONSIDERATIONS. The term *meningioma* originally encompassed all tumors arising in the meninges[418] but now has been narrowed to designate tumors arising from meningothelial cells[419] (Table 51–16). Meningiomas constitute less than 20% of all primary brain tumors[420] and are most common in middle-aged women. Although meningiomas may occur virtually anywhere throughout the body, they are most frequent in the intracranial compartment, especially along the midline sagittal sinus, where meningothelial cells in arachnoid villi are especially abundant.[421] Meningiomas are typically firm, spherical, and discrete (Fig. 51–33). Even histologically benign meningiomas may invade overlying skull, eliciting a bony reactive hyperplasia.[422] Grossly the tumors in section are white to pale pink, whorled, and lobulated. Mineralized psammoma bodies and bony metaplasia may impart a gritty texture on sectioning.

**TABLE 51–16.** Meningothelial Tumors

| Tumor Designation | WHO Grade | Histologic Features | Ki-67 (Mean) |
|---|---|---|---|
| Meningioma | I | Meningothelial, transitional, psammomatous, fibroblastic, angiomatous, secretory variants | 4% |
| Atypical meningioma | II | Cellular with mitotic activity | 7% |
| Papillary meningioma | II–III | Cellular with perivascular tumor cell clusters | |
| Clear cell meningioma | II–III | Glycogen-rich clear cells. High recurrence rate | |
| Malignant meningioma | III | Necrosis, mitotic figures, brain invasion. Retained features of meningioma | 15% |

DIAGNOSTIC CONSIDERATIONS. Although meningiomas are notable for the extraordinary diversity of their histologic patterns (Fig. 51–34), the hallmark remains the cellular whorl—broad (meningothelial), tight (transitional), or mineralized (psammomatous). Certain subtypes may be difficult to identify as meningioma (e.g., the fibroblastic, angiomatous, or secretory variants). A careful examination of the slide usually discloses a rare telltale whorl or the distinctive cytologic features of nuclear clearing and nuclear inclusions (cytoplasmic invaginations).[421] Immunohistochemical reactivity (Fig. 51–35) includes EMA, nuclear progesterone receptor, and vimentin and variable reactivity (<50% of cases) for S-100. Cytokeratin and carcinoembryonic antigen reactivity are found in the secretory variant. There is no reactivity with GFAP and slight to no reactivity with nuclear estrogen receptor (Table 51–17).

The most common cytogenetic abnormality in meningiomas is deletion of chromosome 22[423] (see Table 51–17). This chromosome is also the site for the neurofibromatosis gene *NF2,* and it is not surprising that meningiomas are a feature of this familial disorder.[424] Numerous growth factors have been identified in meningiomas, including epidermal growth factor, insulin-like growth factor I and II, and fibroblast growth factor.[421] Meningiomas are benign tumors (WHO grade I) with a mean Ki-67 (MIB-1) LI of 3.8 ± 3.1%.[425]

The differential diagnosis of meningiomas occasionally is formidable because of their notorious histologic diversity. Confusion with glial tumors is resolved with GFAP and with nerve sheath tumors using the distinctive nuclear S100 reactivity characteristic of schwannomas and neurofibromas. Hemangiopericytoma (formerly angioblastic meningioma) and capillary hemangioblastoma are no longer regarded as meningiomas and are discussed in subsequent sections.

## ATYPICAL MENINGIOMA

The term *atypical meningioma* (WHO grade II) is a subjective diagnosis for meningiomas that exhibit increased cellularity and mitotic activity[430] (CD Fig. 51–67). Where the line is drawn to separate atypical from anaplastic or malignant meningiomas has not been established. Necrosis, anaplastic nuclei, and frank brain invasion are generally the mark of malignancy. Attempts to define atypical meningioma include mitotic figure counts (at least 4 or 5 mitotic figures per 10 high-powered fields)[426, 430] and Ki-67 (MIB-1) LI (mean, 7.2 ± 5.8%).[425, 431] There is clinical value in this designation because the atypical meningioma is known to exhibit a greater chance for recurrence compared with the usual meningioma.[427]

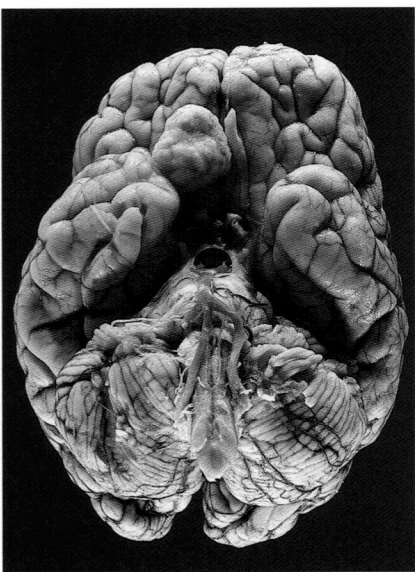

**FIGURE 51–33.** Olfactory groove meningioma, lobular and discrete, compressing adjacent frontal and temporal lobes of brain.

**TABLE 51–17.** Immunoreactivity and Molecular Genetics of Meningiomas

*Immunoreactivity*
EMA
Progesterone receptor
Vimentin
S-100—<50% of tumors
Cytokeratin/CEA—secretory variant
GFAP—unreactive
Estrogen receptor—slight to no reaction

*Molecular Genetics*
Chromosome 22—deletion. Also site for neurofibromatosis gene *NF2*

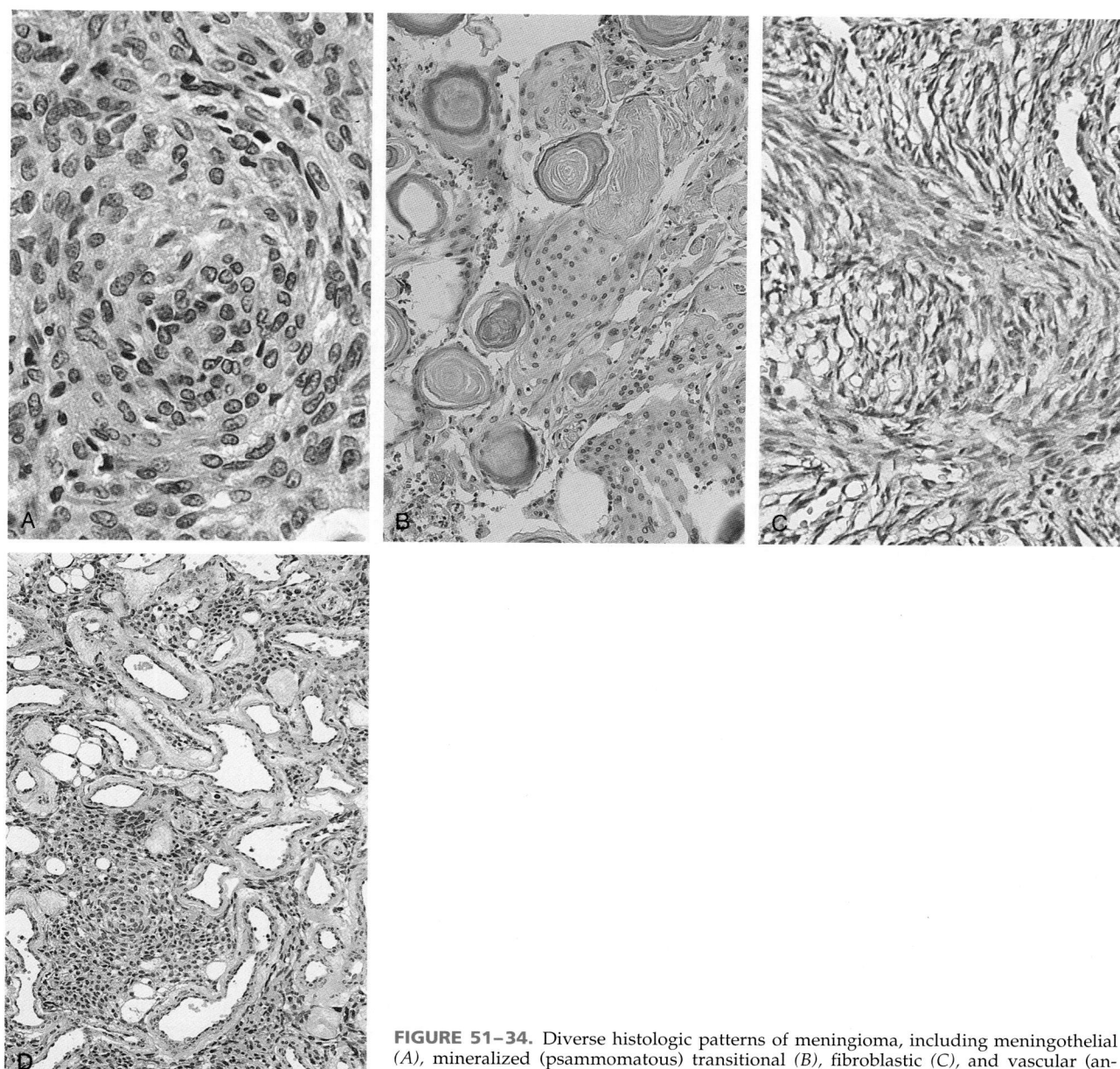

**FIGURE 51–34.** Diverse histologic patterns of meningioma, including meningothelial *(A)*, mineralized (psammomatous) transitional *(B)*, fibroblastic *(C)*, and vascular (angiomatous) *(D)*.

## PAPILLARY AND CLEAR CELL MENINGIOMAS

Two subtypes of meningioma bear special consideration because each has distinctive histologic features, and each is associated with an aggressive clinical course. Papillary meningioma (WHO grade II to III) has characteristic perivascular arrays of elongate tumor cells and usually is associated with more usual meningioma features (CD Fig. 51–68). This subtype is encountered most commonly in children and has a high mortality rate.[429] The clear cell meningioma[432] displays glycogen-rich clear cells arranged in broad sheets (CD Fig. 51–69) and is found in the lumbar spine and cerebellopontine angle. Despite a remark-

ably bland histologic appearance, this meningioma subtype exhibits a high recurrence rate (60%) with occasional local or widespread dissemination.

## MALIGNANT MENINGIOMA

Malignant (anaplastic WHO grade III) meningiomas, although displaying marked cellularity, nuclear anaplasia, necrosis, numerous mitotic figures, and brain invasion,[430] nonetheless retain histologic features of meningioma as described earlier (CD Fig. 51–70) and are to be distinguished from sarcomas, which may arise in meningial mesenchyme. Likewise, malignant meningioma is to be separated from the histologically usual meningioma that may invade bone

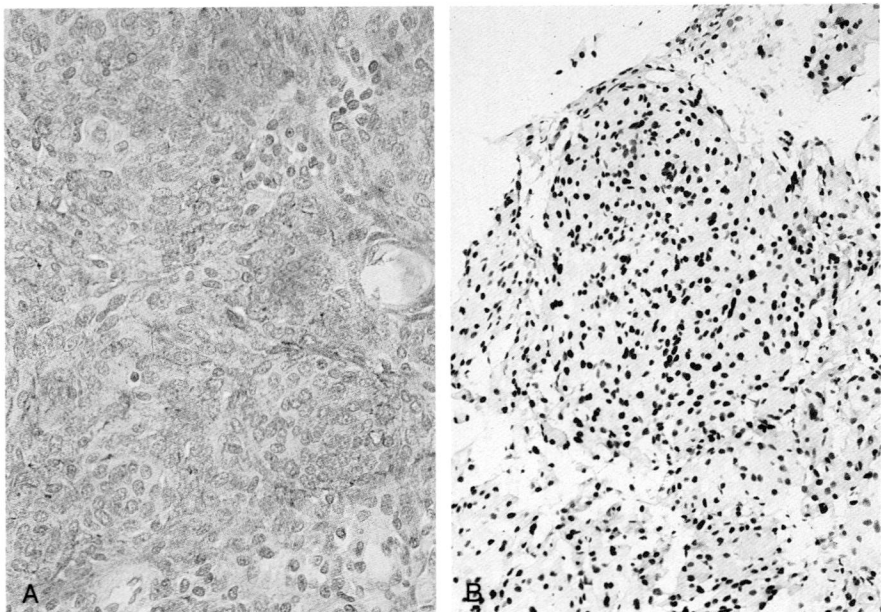

FIGURE 51–35. Meningioma immunore-activity for EMA *(A)* and progesterone receptor *(B)*.

(usually skull) and may spread (especially after surgical intervention) to distant organs, particularly lungs and pleura. Clinically, malignant meningiomas arise in the elderly with a virtual equal male-to-female ratio. Recurrence after surgery is 100% at 15 years versus 2% for usual meningiomas.[428]

Immunohistochemically, malignant meningiomas often display a decline or loss in reactivity for S-100, nuclear progesterone receptor, and on occasion EMA, while retaining vimentin reactivity. The proliferation marker Ki67 (MIB-1) is a valuable guide to malignancy in meningioma (Fig. 51–36). The LI for such tumors reveals a mean of $14.7 \pm 9.8\%$.[425]

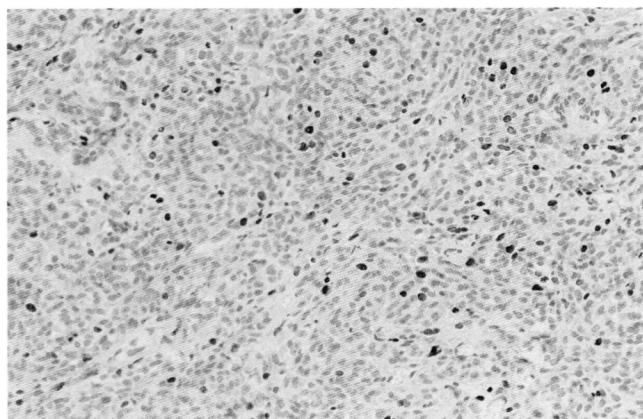

FIGURE 51–36. Proliferation marker Ki-67 (MIB-1) reactivity in malignant meningioma.

## Tumors of Cranial Nerves

A complete discussion of nerve sheath tumors is found in Chapter 46.

### SCHWANNOMA AND CELLULAR SCHWANNOMA

CLINICAL CONSIDERATIONS. The intracranial schwannoma comprises approximately 8% of all primary intracranial tumors,[433] and within this compartment 80% arise from the vestibular division of the eighth cranial (acoustic) nerve[434, 435] (Fig. 51–37). The rare (5%) bilateral acoustic schwannomas are a component of NF2. Spinal schwannomas arise from sensory nerve roots and in most series are the most common intraspinal tumor. Schwannomas rarely are intraparenchymal within cerebrum, brain stem, cerebellum, or spinal cord.[436, 437]

DIAGNOSTIC CONSIDERATIONS. Tables 51–18 and 51–19 delineate the histologic and immunohistochemical features of schwannoma (Fig. 51–38).[438] An important variant, the cellular schwannoma (CD Fig. 51–71), consists solely of the Antoni A cellular pattern and with its nuclear pleomorphism and mitotic activity (2 to 4 mitotic figures per 10 high-powered fields) may cause undue concern and diagnostic error.[439] Apart from the cellularity and mitoses, however, this tumor is in other histologic respects a schwannoma and behaves in a benign fashion.[440]

Deletion or mutation of selected loci on chromosome 22q, coinciding with the *NF2* gene of neurofibromatosis, is characteristic of schwannoma. The mutation is genomic in NF2, and the deletion is somatic in sporadic schwannoma[441] (see Table 51–19).

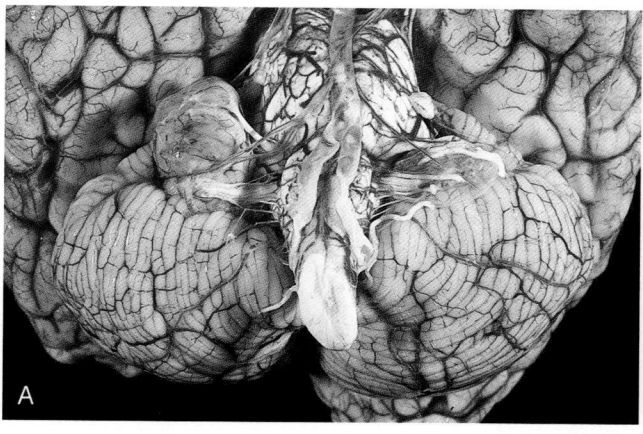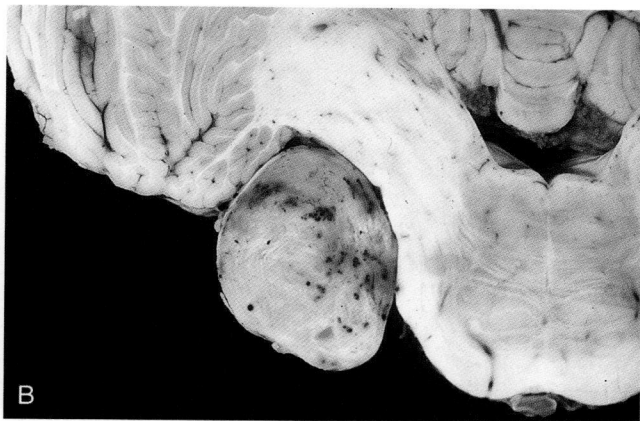

**FIGURE 51–37.** Cerebellopontine angle acoustic nerve schwannoma, lobular and discrete, compressing adjacent cerebellum and pons (A). Cross-section through the same tumor revealing the characteristic yellow hue, a result of hemosiderin deposits from focal hemorrhage (B).

## NEUROFIBROMA

Intracranial neurofibromas are vanishingly rare. Intraspinal neurofibromas arise from dorsal sensory nerve roots and are associated most frequently with NF1[442] (Fig. 51–39).

DIAGNOSTIC CONSIDERATIONS. Tables 51–18 and 51–19 delineate the histologic and immunohistochemical features of neurofibroma (Fig. 51–40). Although mitotic activity of mild-to-moderate degree is of only minor prognostic concern in schwannomas, even mild mitotic activity in a neurofibroma (1 to 2 mitotic figures per 10 high-powered fields) is cause for concern and when coupled with hypercellularity and nuclear atypia is grounds for a diagnosis of malignancy.

The *NF1* gene on the q arm of chromosome 17 is associated with neurofibromas occurring in the setting of neurofibromatosis. This gene probably is associated with sporadic neurofibromas as well[443] (see Table 51–19).

## MALIGNANT PERIPHERAL NERVE SHEATH TUMOR

Malignant transformation of a neurofibroma or de novo malignant nerve sheath tumor occurs frequently in the setting of neurofibromatosis (CD Fig. 51–72, Fig. 51–41). Malignant transformation of a schwannoma is exceedingly rare[444] (see Table 51–18).

Intracranial examples of such malignant tumors are rare, with the trigeminal (fifth) and the eighth cranial nerves most commonly involved, in that order.[443] Intraspinal involvement is most commonly the result of extension of tumor from an involved sciatic nerve or brachial plexus. Details of the diagnostic and prognostic considerations regarding ma-

## TABLE 51–18. Schwannoma Versus Neurofibroma

| | Schwannoma | Neurofibroma |
|---|---|---|
| Gross | Solitary. Displaces nerve | Multiple. Expands nerves |
| Cell(s) of origin | Schwann cells | Schwann cells, fibroblasts, perineurial cells |
| Tumor margin | Crisp and sharp | Diffuse and ill defined |
| Histologic pattern | Biphasic | Uniform sheets |
| | Cellular A/loosely cohesive B | |
| Foci of degeneration | Common | Uncommon in usual tumors |
| | Hemorrhage, histiocytes | |
| Cellularity | Cellular schwannoma | |
| Mitotic activity | Disturbing histology but benign | Even 1–2 mf/10 hpf* are cause for concern especially in association with cellularity and nuclear atypia |
| Malignant change | Exceedingly rare | Frequent in the setting of neurofibromatosis |
| Immunohistochemistry | S-100—marked nuclear and cytoplasmic | S-100—focal. Modestly nuclear |
| | EMA—unreactive | EMA—focally reactive |

* 1–2 mitotic figures per 10 high-powered fields.

**TABLE 51–19.** Immunohistochemistry and Molecular Genetics of Nerve Sheath Tumors

### Immunohistochemistry

S-100—nuclear and cytoplasmic reaction. Strong in schwannoma
Leu-7
CD 34—especially in myxoid areas
Vimentin
Myelin basic protein—of little to no diagnostic help
Neurofilament protein—of possible help in neurofibroma
EMA—focally reactive in neurofibroma

### Molecular Genetics

Schwannoma
   Chromosome 22q—somatic deletion in solitary tumors. Genomic mutation *(NF2)* in neurofibromatosis
Neurofibroma
   Chromosome 17q—*NF1* gene. Sporadic and in neurofibromatosis

lignant peripheral nerve sheath tumors are found in Chapter 46.

## Primary Central Nervous System Lymphomas and Plasmacytomas

### PRIMARY CENTRAL NERVOUS SYSTEM LYMPHOMA

Few CNS tumors have undergone such flux as have primary CNS lymphomas. In particular, long-standing confusion over the histogenesis of this tumor has been clarified with use of immunohistochemis-try. The historical rarity of this tumor (formerly 1% of primary CNS tumors) has given way in some series to an incidence approaching 7% of all primary CNS tumors.[445] Although much of this increase may be attributed to a comparable increase in immuno-compromised patients (congenital, transplant, and especially acquired immunodeficiency syndrome [AIDS] related), there also is at least in some series an increase in CNS lymphomas among the immunocompetent.[446] The most common patients with CNS lymphomas have been men in their 50s. With the advent of AIDS, however, age at onset in the 40s and in some series the 30s is now most common.[447] CNS lymphomas usually arise in deep white matter of the frontal lobe and, in contrast to most primary CNS intra-axial tumors, often are multiple and multifocal, simulating metastatic tumor. On gross examination, CNS lymphoma is often pale white and soft with ill-defined margins (Fig. 51–42). With therapy, now commonly employed especially in the setting of AIDS, tumor is often necrotic, hemorrhagic, and deceptively well defined.

DIAGNOSTIC CONSIDERATIONS. The periphery of a CNS lymphoma is ideal for diagnosis because it is here that the characteristic perivascular tumor deposits are most evident and where preservation is optimal (CD Fig. 51–73). Central tumor necrosis may hamper diagnosis, especially using stereotactic needle biopsies. Lymphomas arising as CNS primaries are typically of the diffuse, large cell, or immunoblastic variety[447] (Fig. 51–43A). Immunohistochemical evaluation reveals a B-cell histogenesis in more than 90% of cases (Fig. 51–43B), usually with IgM κ production. T-cell CNS lymphoma typically of peripheral T-cell type is exceedingly rare but when present often involves the leptomeningeal

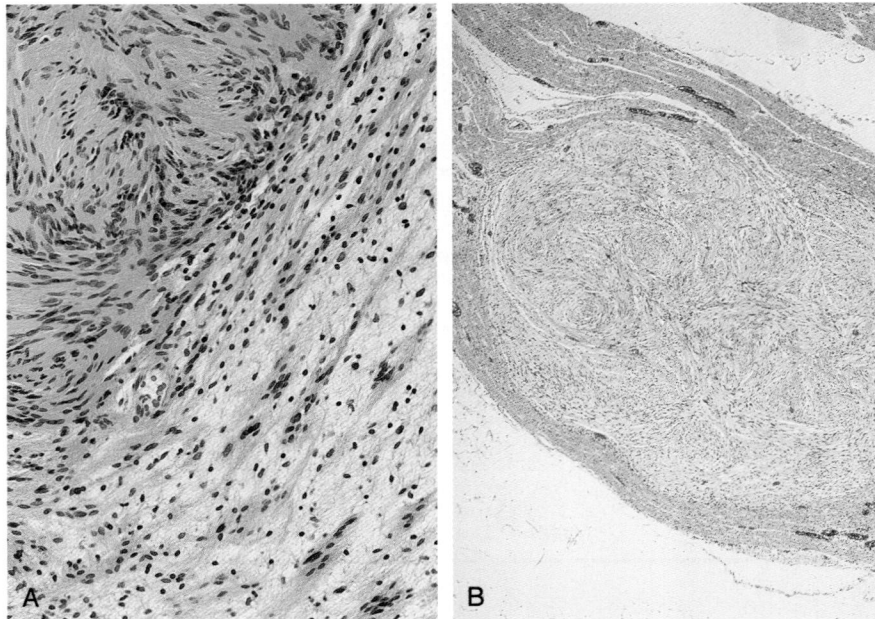

**FIGURE 51–38.** Histologic features of schwannoma, including Antoni A *(upper left)* and Antoni B *(lower right)* patterns *(A)*, and crisp tumor margins with compression of adjacent nerve *(B)*.

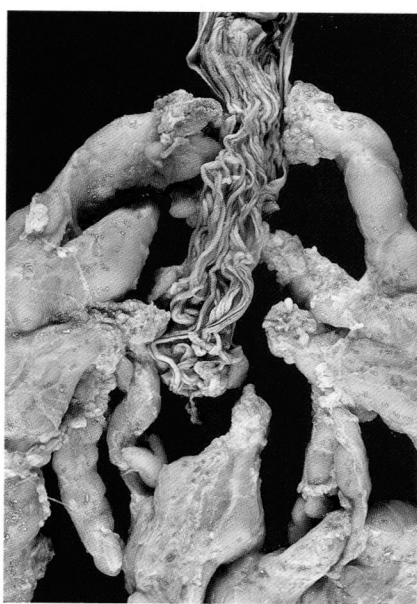

**FIGURE 51–39.** Cauda equina with associated peripheral nerve roots diffusely expanded by plexiform neurofibromas.

techniques in the tumor cells of most CNS lymphomas arising in immunocompromised individuals.[452] Epstein-Barr virus is not common in CNS lymphomas arising in immunocompetent patients.[453] In contrast, human herpesvirus 8 DNA has been identified in primary CNS lymphoma in patients with and without AIDS.[454]

The differential diagnosis of CNS lymphomas becomes a challenge when material is scanty or necrotic. Reactive gliosis may be marked in CNS lymphomas and cause confusion with glioma. A solid focus of lymphoma may resemble a primitive neuroepithelial tumor. In patients with AIDS, a *Toxoplasma* brain abscess may elicit a striking lymphocytic response. In each of these settings, immunohistochemical evaluation using L26 and CD3 clarifies the nature of the lymphoid infiltrate. A predominant infiltrate of large B cells in the brain is usually neoplastic and often is accompanied by a reactive infiltrate of small T cells.

PROGNOSTIC CONSIDERATIONS. CNS lymphomas are generally high-grade tumors with poor 5-year survival rates. Multifocal or leptomeningeal tumors offer a particularly grim prognosis, as do tumors arising in the setting of AIDS.[455] Proliferation studies using Ki-67 (MIB-1) have displayed high LIs (47% for high-grade lymphomas) but these results have not significantly predicted survival.[456]

### PLASMACYTOMA

A solitary proliferation of monoclonal plasma cells, plasmacytoma rarely arises in the CNS, most often in the skull or dura, mimicking a meningioma.[457] A few cases also have been reported within the brain.[458] Microscopically the tumor consists of sheets of mature plasma cells with monoclonality shown

compartment of immunocompetent individuals.[448] Still rarer is anaplastic lymphoma (Ki-1, often T-cell subtype).[449] Molecular studies, specifically of CNS lymphomas, are infrequent but have confirmed the gene rearrangements typical of a B-cell lymphoma.[450] A study of genetic alterations in immunocompetent individuals with primary CNS lymphoma showed frequent inactivation of the gene *CDKN2A* and only minor rare alterations of *p53* or *BCL2* genes.[451] Epstein-Barr virus has been identified by molecular

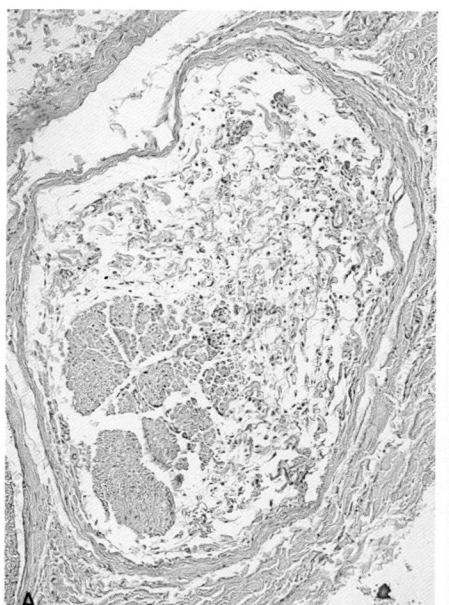
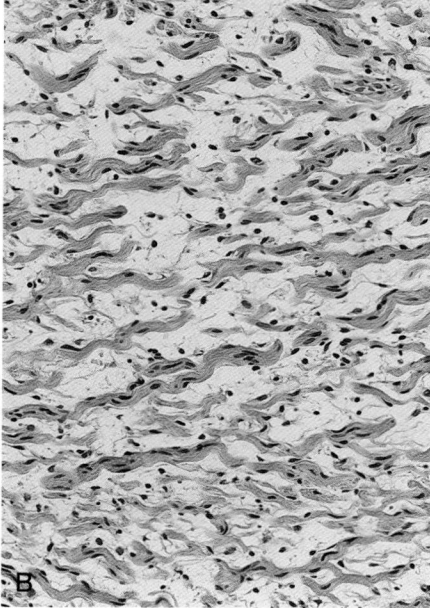

**FIGURE 51–40.** Peripheral nerve with surrounding epineurium and perineurium. Note focal replacement of nerve by neurofibroma composed of scattered spindle cells in an abundant myxoid stroma *(A)*. High magnification of neurofibroma displaying waving spindle cells with comma-shaped nuclei and a loose myxoid stroma *(B)*.

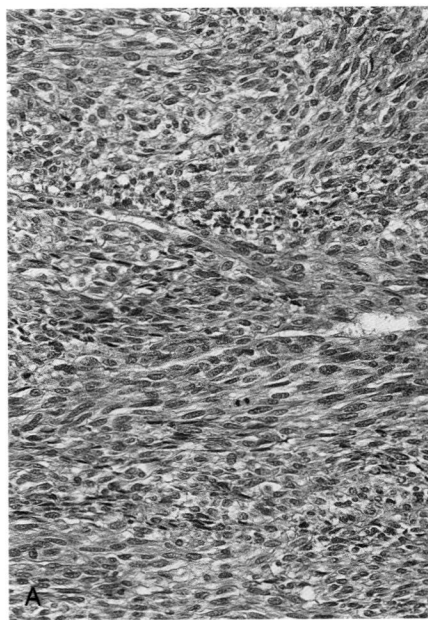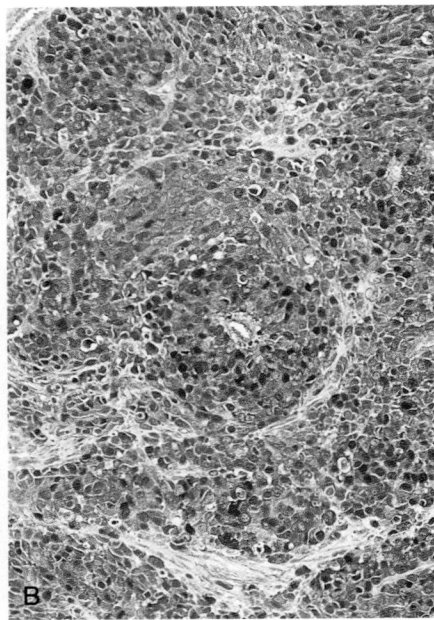

**FIGURE 51–41.** Malignant peripheral nerve sheath tumor displaying cellular streams of tumor with scattered mitotic figures (A). Nuclear and cytoplasmic S-100 reactivity, unusually strong, in a malignant nerve sheath tumor (B).

using immunohistochemistry for cytoplasmic κ or λ light chain production.

## Melanocytic Tumors of the Meninges

### MELANOCYTOMA

Melanocytoma is a rare benign tumor of melanocytes, usually solitary, spherical, and leptomeningeal lying often along the base of the posterior fossa. Although benign, they may recur, sometimes frequently.[459] Microscopically the tumor cells often are heavily pigmented with cytoplasmic melanin and cytologically vary from spindled to epithelioid. Mitoses are rare to absent. Whorled and insular patterns are common. Tumor cells are immunoreactive with S100, vimentin, and HMB-45.

The differential diagnosis is the greatest challenge regarding this rare entity. The overlap with melanoma is difficult to resolve. In general, melanocytoma is a solitary tumor with discrete margins, lack of mitoses, and low Ki67 (MIB-1) LI (<12%).[460] Pigmented schwannoma is another difficult differential diagnosis. The schwannoma has degenerative features (sclerotic vessels, hemosiderin, foamy histiocytes) and delicately spindled cells with small nuclei usually not apparent in melanocytoma. The pigmented meningioma is immunoreactive with EMA, again not a feature of melanocytoma.

### MELANOMA

Primary CNS melanoma exists principally in two forms. A third of these tumors are solid, often multiple masses, and the remaining two thirds are diffuse meningeal tumors spreading throughout the craniospinal axis (CD Fig. 51–74A). Primary CNS melanoma is associated in one fourth of cases with cutaneous pigmented nevi.[461]

DIAGNOSTIC CONSIDERATIONS. By light microscopy, primary CNS melanoma resembles in all respects extracranial melanoma with epithelioid to spindle pleomorphic cells displaying vesicular nuclei, prominent nucleoli, and frequent-to-abundant mitotic figures. Pigmentation may be abundant or slight (CD Fig. 51–74B). Immunohistochemical reactions include vimentin, HMB-45, and cytoplasmic and nuclear S-100. Cytokeratin also may be detected but usually the distribution is patchy and scant. The differential diagnosis of prime importance is metastatic melanoma, and this issue can be resolved only by a careful clinical and pathologic evaluation of the

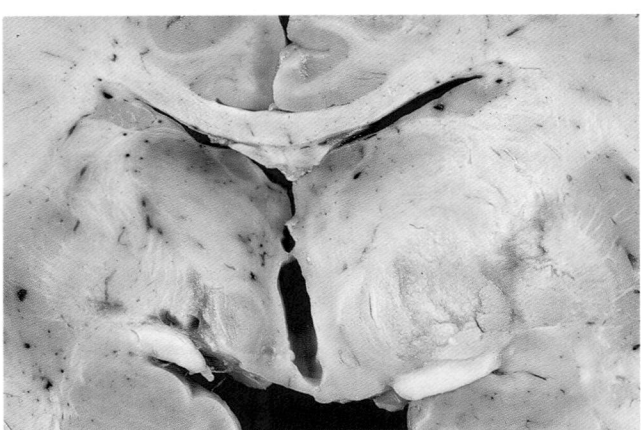

**FIGURE 51–42.** Primary cerebral lymphoma arising as an ill-defined white mass invading the right internal capsule and basal ganglia.

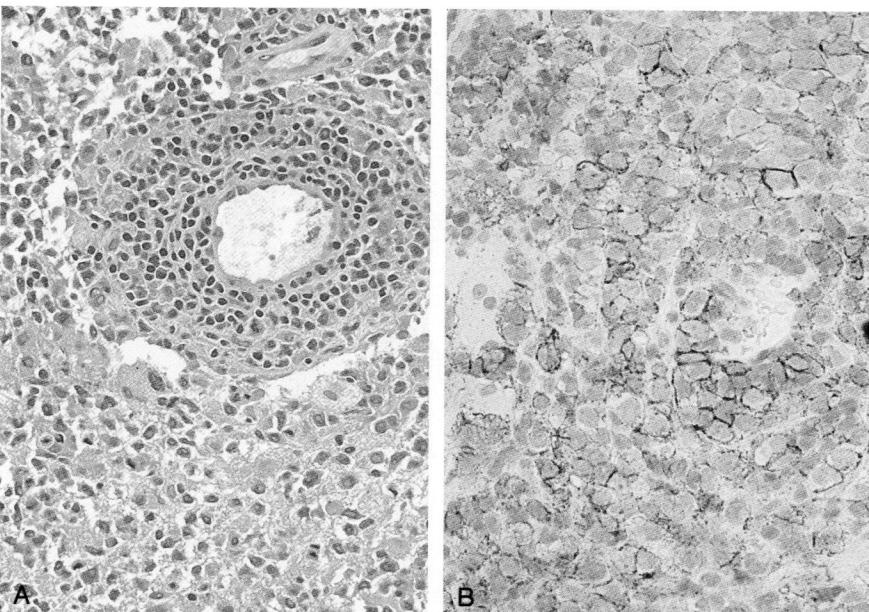

**FIGURE 51–43.** High power views of primary CNS lymphoma with H&E staining *(A)* and CD 20 immunoreactivity *(B)*.

patient's entire body. Neurocutaneous melanosis predisposes to primary CNS melanoma, but even in this setting the primary melanoma may arise initially outside the cranial compartment.

PROGNOSTIC CONSIDERATIONS. Primary CNS melanoma is a high-grade tumor with a poor prognosis and a tendency to spread throughout the craniospinal axis and extracranially.

## Tumors of Blood Vessels and Related Tissues

### VASCULAR MALFORMATIONS

The four subtypes of intracranial vascular malformations are described in Table 51–20. Capillary telangiectasis[462] is encountered most commonly in the midline pons as an incidental finding at autopsy (CD Fig. 51–75). Cavernous angioma[462] is found predominantly within the cerebral hemispheres, especially the region of the motor cortex of the frontal lobes, and creates symptoms either as a space-occu-

pying lesion or as a result of spontaneous hemorrhage (CD Fig. 51–76). Venous malformation is most commonly a varicosity found within the spinal cord and adjacent meninges, especially along the dorsal surface of the cord below the level of T6[462] (CD Fig. 51–77).

Arteriovenous malformation[463] may be minute (*cryptic*) or so large as virtually to replace a sizable portion of brain (Fig. 51–44). The distinctly abnormal vessels forming this lesion serve to distinguish it from the frequently submitted crush of vascular meninges and compressed but normally formed blood vessels often encountered by the pathologist and confused with a vascular malformation.

### MENINGIOANGIOMATOSIS

Meningioangiomatosis is a rare lesion presenting as a hamartomatous plaquelike thickening of leptomeninges and underlying cerebral cortex in young adults with seizures or in older individuals with NF2[465] (CD Fig. 51–78). The leptomeningeal component consists of hyperplastic meningothelial cells, psammoma bodies, and calcific deposits, giving the

**TABLE 51–20.** Vascular Malformations of Central Nervous System

| | Site | Symptoms | Histologic Features |
|---|---|---|---|
| Capillary telangiectasis | Midline pons | Incidental finding. Usually asymptomatic | Saccular capillaries with intervening brain tissue |
| Cavernous angioma | Cerebral hemispheres, especially frontal lobes | Mass lesion or source of spontaneous hemorrhage | Thin-walled, large vessels with no intervening brain tissue |
| Venous malformation | Spinal cord meninges | Ischemic damage to cord with paralysis | Large dilated veins in subarachnoid space |
| Arteriovenous malformation | Cerebral hemispheres in middle cerebral artery distribution | Seizures or massive hemorrhage | Malformed arteries and large veins with associated hemorrhage and thrombosis |

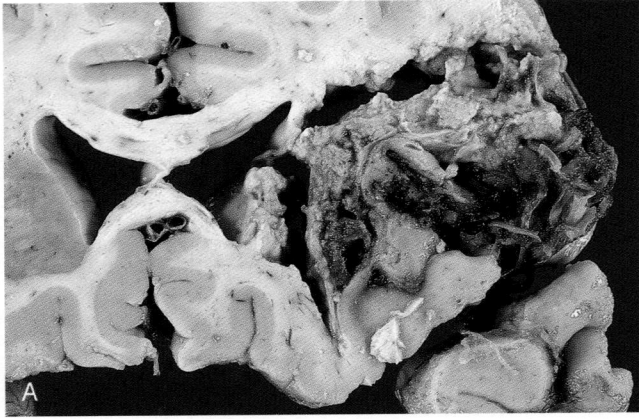
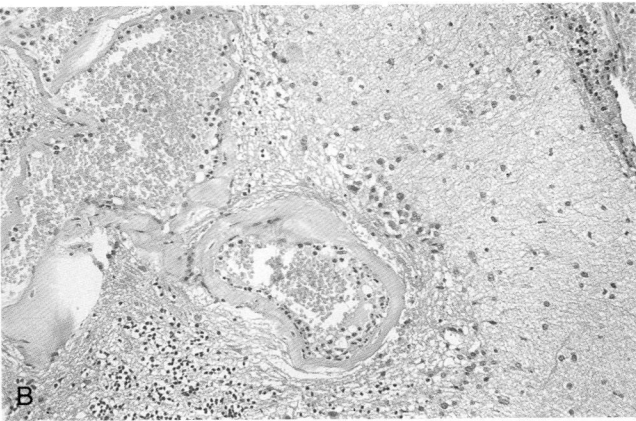

**FIGURE 51–44.** Arteriovenous malformation replacing the lateral inferior frontal lobe. There is adjacent subacute, hemosiderin-laden infarction of brain *(A)*. Microscopic view of malformed blood vessels with walls displaying alternating features of artery and vein *(B)*.

lesion a gritty texture. The cortical component is considerably more complex, including abundant capillaries accentuated by perivascular deposits of fibroblasts[464] and meningothelial cells, all accompanied by aberrant glial cell clusters[462] and neurons with cytoplasmic neurofibrillary tangles. The Ki67 (MIB-1) LI is low to absent, indicating the malformative nature of this lesion.[466]

## HEMANGIOPERICYTOMA

The primary CNS hemangiopericytoma[467] has pursued a nosologic route almost as circuitous as that of the primary CNS lymphoma. Once regarded as a particularly vascular (angioblastic) form of meningioma, it now is considered a soft tissue tumor, particularly because the term *meningioma* now is limited to tumors derived from meningothelial cells. It is

ironic that the new designation, *hemangiopericytoma*, links this tumor to one of the more controversial entities in soft tissue pathology.

Hemangiopericytoma (WHO grade II to III) arises from dura often in or about the tentorium and may compress or invade underlying brain tissue. It also may invade overlying skull but does not elicit the osteoblastic response typical of meningioma. The tumor comprises less than 1% of all primary CNS tumors and affects men slightly more often than women, in the 30 to 50 age range. Grossly, hemangiopericytoma usually is spherical, firm, and highly vascular, making surgical resection difficult.

DIAGNOSTIC CONSIDERATIONS. Microscopically the tumor consists of hypercellular sheets of oval-to-spindle tumor cells, interspersed by slitlike (staghorn) blood vessels (Fig. 51–45). Mitotic figures are

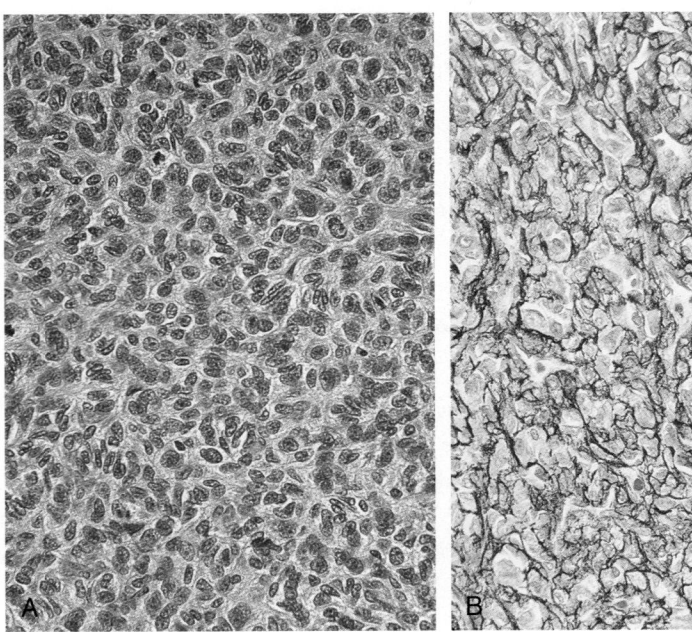

**FIGURE 51–45.** Meningeal hemangiopericytoma with sheets of oval cells interspersed by minute compressed capillaries *(A)*. A reticulin stain reveals the interlacing network of blood vessels *(B)*.

**TABLE 51–21.** Features of Meningeal Hemangiopericytoma

```
Immunohistochemistry
  Diagnostic
    Vimentin
    CD 34
    EMA—unreactive
    S100—unreactive
  Prognostic
    Ki67—LI (mean) 10%
WHO grade II–III
Molecular genetics
  Chromosome 12q13 rearrangement
  No chromosome 22 or NF2 abnormality
```

present but highly variable in number even within the same tumor. Immunohistochemical reactivity is seen with vimentin and CD34[468] (Table 51–21). The traditional meningioma reactivity to EMA and S100 is not present, however. In contrast to meningioma, there also is no evidence of a chromosome 22 abnormality. There is a frequent rearrangement of chromosome 12q13.[469] Hemangiopericytoma shows no NF2 familial gene mutation, which again is encountered often in meningioma. The differential diagnosis consists of meningioma and glioma. In each case, immunohistochemistry is a guide, with EMA distinguishing the meningioma and GFAP distinguishing the glioma.

PROGNOSTIC CONSIDERATIONS. Hemangiopericytoma of the meninges is best considered a low-grade (WHO grade II to III) dural sarcoma because of its virtually inevitable recurrence despite seemingly thorough surgical excision and high frequency of metastatic deposits in bone and lung.[470] The Ki67 (MIB-1) LI averages 10%,[471] and the mitotic rate averages fewer than 5 per 10 high-powered fields. Values above these levels together with evidence of nuclear pleomorphism and tumor necrosis may indicate a worse prognosis (higher tumor recurrence and rate of metastasis), but to date the value of these studies remains controversial.[470]

## Miscellaneous Mesenchymal Tumors

### LIPOMA

The lipoma[472] is a benign, hamartomatous, bright yellow tumor often lying in the midline of the brain or skull (CD Fig. 51–79). Location in the region of the corpus callosum frequently is associated with agenesis of that structure.

### SOLITARY FIBROUS TUMOR

The solitary fibrous tumor, once thought unique to pleura, now is identified throughout the body and also has been observed in meninges[473] (CD Fig. 51–80). Here this tumor may arise in cranial or spinal compartments and intrude on brain, spinal cord, or

nerves. The main differential diagnosis is meningioma, especially the fibroblastic subtype. Immunohistochemical stains offer diagnostic help because the solitary fibrous tumor is strongly reactive with CD34 but unreactive with EMA or progesterone receptor protein.

### CHORDOMA

The chordoma[474] arises from notochordal nests in the sacrococcygeal region (two thirds of cases) or skull base. Men are affected more often than women. The age of first symptoms varies from the late 30s for intracranial chordomas to the 40s for sacral tumors. Grossly the tumor is lobulated, soft, and gelatinous with ill-defined borders and an insinuating growth pattern making complete surgical excision difficult to impossible.

DIAGNOSTIC CONSIDERATIONS. The chordoma is formed of cuboidal-to-stellate cells with abundant intracytoplasmic and extracellular vacuoles and an often sizable intervening mucoid stroma (Fig. 51–46A). Immunohistochemistry is distinctive in that the tumor cells react with cytokeratin, EMA, S-100, vimentin, and HBME-1 (Fig. 51–46B–D). Distinguishing the tumor from carcinoma, especially renal cell carcinoma, depends on the immunoreactivity of chordoma for HBME-1.[475] Cartilaginous tumors are separated from chordomas immunohistochemically with the use of cytokeratin and EMA. The matter of chondroid chordoma is not yet resolved. Some authors[476] regard this entity as a cartilaginous neoplasm, whereas others[477] defend its independent status.

PROGNOSTIC CONSIDERATIONS. The chordoma, although histologically benign, behaves in a distinctly malignant fashion with multiple recurrences and metastatic dissemination after often radical surgical excision. Although mitotic counts may play a role in prognosis,[474] other studies suggest that only a young age at onset and ploidy[478] offer any valid prognostic insight.

### MESENCHYMAL CHONDROSARCOMA

In the craniospinal axis, mesenchymal chondrosarcoma[479] is found particularly in the skull base or upper spinal cord impinging on brain stem or spinal cord. Microscopically, in an ideal sample, there is a biphasic pattern of cartilagenous islands staining immunohistochemically with vimentin and S-100 (with no keratin or EMA reactivity) interspersed by stroma staining with vimentin and Leu 7 (with no S-100 reactivity).[480] If the sample is small and fails to contain a cartilagenous island, it is immunohistochemically impossible to distinguish this tumor from hemangiopericytoma. The best guide in this circumstance is the clinical history of an aggressive mass at the skull base or upper cervical cord.

### RHABDOMYOSARCOMA

Primary CNS rhabdomyosarcoma,[481] usually of embryonal subtype,[482, 483] is found typically in child-

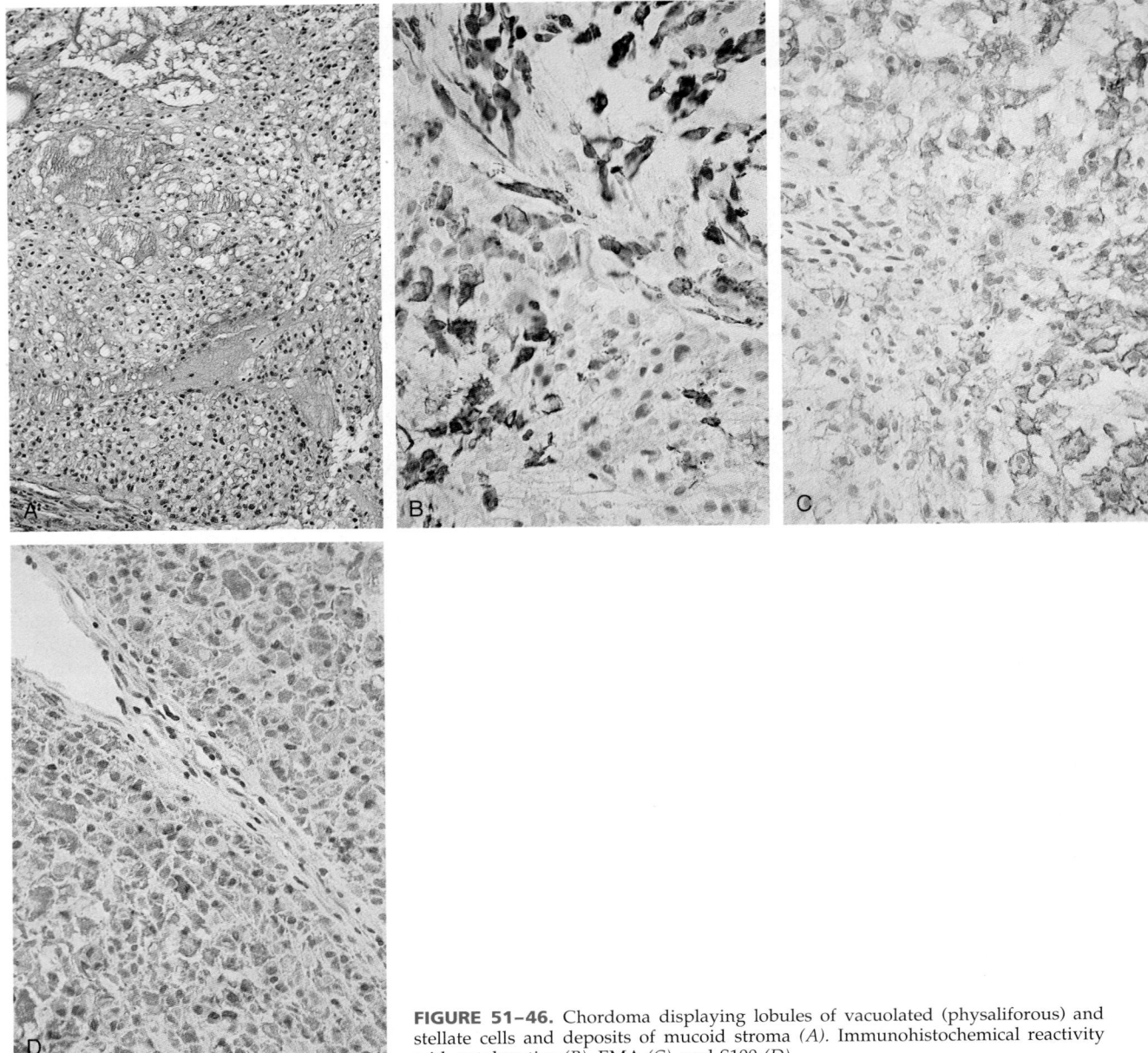

**FIGURE 51–46.** Chordoma displaying lobules of vacuolated (physaliforous) and stellate cells and deposits of mucoid stroma (A). Immunohistochemical reactivity with cytokeratins (B), EMA (C), and S100 (D).

hood as a midline mass in the posterior fossa either in meninges or within or adjacent to the fourth ventricle. Immunohistochemistry using desmin, myoglobin, myo D1, and myogenin is often essential to display the myoid origin of this tumor.

## Craniopharyngioma

CLINICAL CONSIDERATIONS. The craniopharyngioma has been separated into two subtypes.[484] The more common subtype, sometimes qualified as *adamantinomatous*, arises within and above the sella turcica, compresses the pituitary gland, and inserts itself into the overlying optic chiasm and brain of children and teenagers. The tumor grossly is cystic with distinctive cyst contents (viscous, dark brown-to-black liquid, likened to motor oil, in which float glistening flakes of cholesterol). Finger-like projections of tumor into overlying brain make complete resection of this tumor a neurosurgical challenge. The less common subtype, papillary craniopharyngioma,[485] arises within the third ventricle of adults (in their 40s). It is solid; well circumscribed; and free of calcification, cyst contents, or intracerebral tumor projections.

DIAGNOSTIC CONSIDERATIONS. Microscopically, adamantinomatous craniopharyngioma consists of squamous epithelium arranged in complex islands delimited by palisaded tumor cells, which give way to sheets of elongated-to-spindled squamous cells

(CD Fig. 51–81A). Brain tissue adjacent to tumor displays intense gliosis with focally abundant Rosenthal fibers (CD Fig. 51–81B). This remarkable gliosis may lead to confusion with pilocytic astrocytoma. The papillary subtype in contrast is formed of squamous epithelium arranged about blood vessels creating a partially artifactual papillary pattern (CD Fig. 51–82). There are no distinctive degenerative changes and no peripheral palisading of tumor cells.

Immunohistochemical reactivity includes cytokeratins and rare focal chromogranin.[486] Estrogen receptor activity has been shown by in situ hybridization.[487]

From a prognostic viewpoint, craniopharyngioma is histologically a benign tumor (WHO grade I). The deep central location of the tumor and the protrusions of tumor into brain tissue in the adamantinomatous subtype make complete surgical resection difficult, however, and recurrence of tumor a problem in 10% to 20% of cases. Tumors greater than 5 cm in diameter are particularly prone to a clinically poor outcome.[488] The differential diagnoses of craniopharyngioma include pilocytic astrocytoma (resulting, as described earlier, from biopsy of the gliotic brain tissue surrounding the tumor) and simple epidermoid cyst (which displays squamous maturation and keratohyaline granules but lacks palisading tumor cells and dystrophic calcification).[489]

## Paraganglioma

CLINICAL CONSIDERATIONS. Within the CNS, the paraganglioma arises most commonly in the cauda equina attached to the filum terminale or adjacent nerve roots.[490] The usual clinical setting is a middle-aged man with back pain.

DIAGNOSTIC CONSIDERATIONS. Distinctive for cauda equina paraganglioma is the frequency (50%) of ganglion cells within the cell nests, prompting the subclassification of gangliocytic paraganglioma.[491] Immunohistochemically, chief cells react with neuroendocrine markers, such as chromogranin (CD Fig. 51–83) and synaptophysin, whereas sustentacular cells react with S100. Cytokeratin reactivity, unusual in most paragangliomas, has been reported in chief cells in the cauda equina site.[492] GFAP may stain reactive astrocytes or occasionally sustentacular cells.[493] Cauda equina parganglioma is in general a benign neoplasm (WHO grade I), but if excision is incomplete, recurrence with craniospinal seeding may occur.[494]

## Tumors of Uncertain Origin

### CAPILLARY HEMANGIOBLASTOMA

CLINICAL CONSIDERATIONS. Capillary hemangioblastoma occurs either sporadically (15%) or in association with the autosomal dominant phakomatosis von Hippel–Lindau disease (CNS and retinal hemangioblastomas, pheochromocytoma, renal cell

carcinoma, and cysts of kidney and pancreas).[495] In the most common sporadic setting, a solitary hemangioblastoma arises in the cerebellum of a middle-aged man, whereas in the familial setting, tumors more often are multiple, sometimes supratentorial, and the patients are in their 20s or 30s. The capillary hemangioblastoma produces erythropoietin, and the resulting polycythemia serves as an indicator of tumor, particularly useful to survey tumor recurrence after surgical resection. Grossly the hemangioblastoma is characteristically cystic with the actual tumor often confined to a nodule projecting into the cyst, a setting similar to that of the cystic cerebellar astrocytoma (Fig. 51–47). The tumor nodule is intensely vascular, red to yellow, and although well delimited from adjacent brain is unencapsulated.

DIAGNOSTIC CONSIDERATIONS. Microscopically the capillary hemangioblastoma is composed of innumerable capillaries interspersed by foamy, lipid, and glycogen-laden stromal cells, the true neoplastic cells of this tumor (Fig. 51–48A). Stromal cells may be infrequent or abundant; small, cuboidal, or giant; and mononuclear or multinuclear. The compressed brain adjacent to the tumor typically is intensely gliotic with abundant astrocytic Rosenthal fibers reminiscent of the gliosis surrounding a craniopharyngioma (Fig. 51–48B). The origin of the stromal cells remains elusive despite a sizable battery of immunohistochemical and molecular biologic analyses. Stromal cells do not react immunohistochemically with endothelial or epithelial markers. They react instead with vimentin, neuron specific enolase (Fig. 51–48C), erythropoietin,[496] epidermal growth factor receptor,[497] and von Hippel–Lindau (VHL) gene product,[498] and they express vascular endothelial growth factor mRNA with in situ hybridization[499] (Table 51–22). The VHL gene is present on the short arm of chromosome 3, and mutations of this gene are observed in familial and sporadic capillary hemangioblastomas.[500] The differential diagnoses include metastatic renal cell carcinoma (both display clear cells) and pilocytic astrocytoma (the gliotic pe-

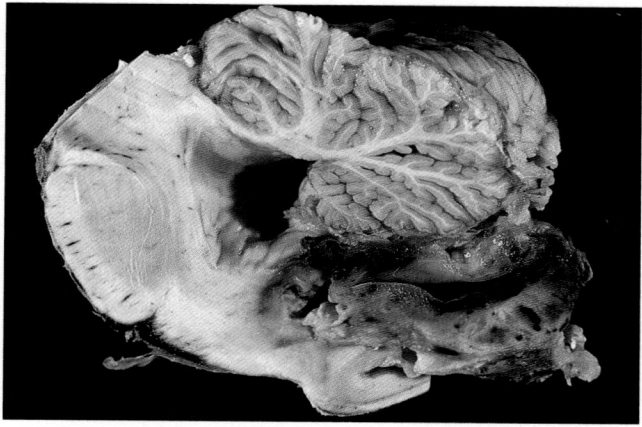

**FIGURE 51–47.** Cystic hemangioblastoma arising inferior to the cerebellum and compressing the underlying brain stem.

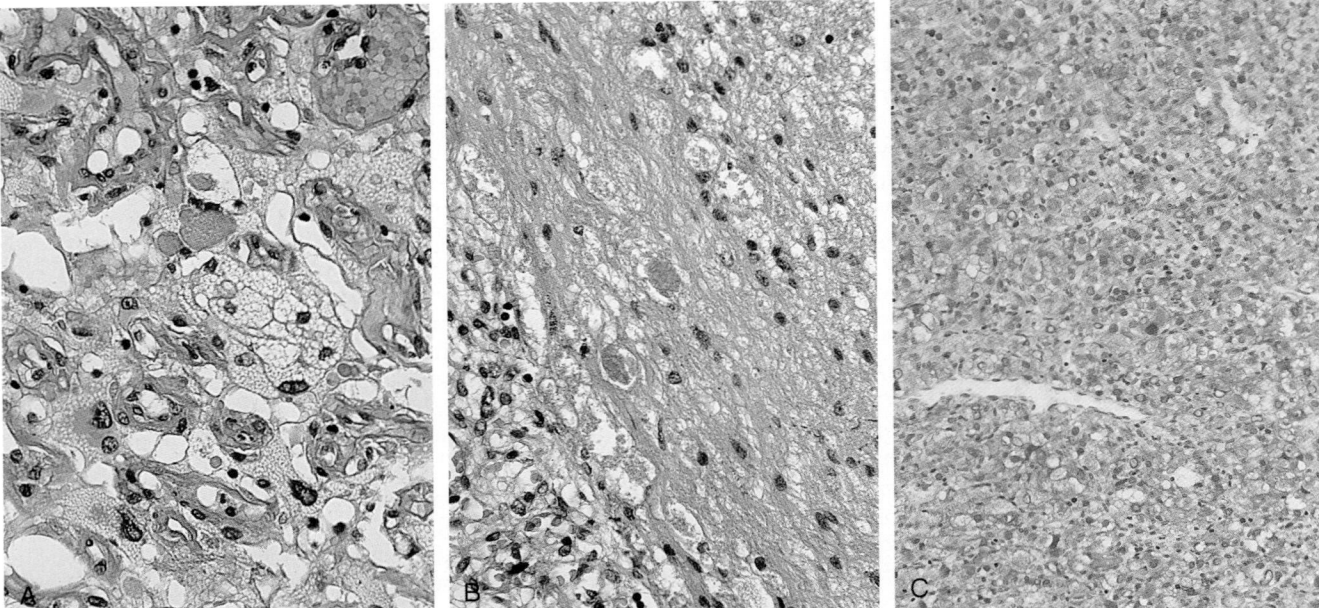

**FIGURE 51–48.** Microscopic view of hemangioblastoma with the foamy stromal cells interspersed by abundant capillaries *(A)*. Brain adjacent to the hemangioblastoma reveals gliosis and Rosenthal fibers *(B)*. Stromal cells immunoreactive with neuron specific enolase *(C)*.

riphery of the tumor). Immunohistochemical reactivity with cytokeratins and EMA distinguishes renal cell carcinoma from capillary hemangioblastoma. As for gliosis and presumed astrocytoma, the coordination of surgical biopsy with radiologic findings is crucial to guide proper sampling of tumor.

Capillary hemangioblastoma is a benign (WHO grade I) tumor. Complete surgical resection is difficult, however, and postsurgical recurrence is a problem in approximately 25% of cases. Factors that predispose to recurrence include association with von Hippel–Lindau syndrome (young age of onset, multiple tumors) and absence of cyst formation and diminished numbers of lipid-laden stromal cells.[501]

## ATYPICAL TERATOID AND RHABDOID TUMOR

CLINICAL CONSIDERATIONS. *Atypical teratoid and rhabdoid tumor* refers to a group of childhood brain tumors, all of which share the histologic feature of rhabdoid cells and some of which contain other tissue elements, including primitive neuroepithelium, mesenchyme, and mature epithelium.[502–505] These rare tumors arise most often in the posterior fossa, although supratentorial tumors and tumors involving multiple sites are common.[504, 505] Of patients, 75% are 3 years of age or younger with boys affected more commonly than girls. The tumors grossly are often large, soft, focally necrotic, and hemorrhagic.

DIAGNOSTIC CONSIDERATIONS. The distinctive rhabdoid cells, similar to those in the more common renal cell tumors, are large and polygonal with prominent nucleoli, eosinophilic cytoplasm, and spherical fibrillary intracytoplasmic inclusions (CD Fig. 51–84). These cells may be abundant or may be incorporated into a complex mix of primitive neuroepithelial tumor resembling medulloblastoma; mesenchymal spindle cells approaching the level of sarcoma; and glandular and epithelial elements consistent with adenocarcinoma, or squamous carcinoma, or both. Immunohistochemically the rhabdoid cells are variably reactive with EMA, vimentin, and smooth muscle actin and occasionally may react with GFAP, cytokeratin, and neurofilament protein (CD Fig. 51–85). Cytogenetic analysis reveals chromosome 22 abnormalities, either deletion (22q11) or translocation, which may[502] or may not[506] be distinctive for this tumor entity. Although this tumor entity is not part of the WHO CNS classification, the likely grading would be grade IV in view of the reported median survival of 6 months[502] and a proliferation rate approaching 80% of tumor cell nuclei[507] using Ki-67 (MIB-1).

**TABLE 51–22.** Features of Capillary Hemangioblastoma

Immunohistochemistry
  Vimentin
  Neuron specific enolase
  Erythropoietin
  Epidermal growth factor receptor
WHO grade I
Molecular genetics
  Chromosome 3—Mutations of *VHL* gene on short arm

# Benign Cystic Lesions of Central Nervous System

## COLLOID CYST

The colloid cyst is located within the third ventricle, where it may obstruct flow of cerebrospinal fluid and produce acute hydrocephalus (CD Fig. 51–86). The cyst usually presents in young to middle-aged adults with a slight male predominance.[508] Grossly the cyst is spherical and smooth with a delicate thin wall. Cyst contents are a distinctive glassy viscous liquid, which may present as a hyaline sphere after fixation. Cyst lining cells are reactive with cytokeratin (CD Fig. 51–87B), EMA, and focally CEA but are unreactive with GFAP. The presence of cilia and occasional goblet cells (CD Fig. 51–87A) suggests a link to respiratory epithelium rather than neuroepithelium.[509] The colloid cyst is benign, and after surgical resection there is generally no recurrence.

## ENDODERMAL CYST

The endodermal cyst is a rare cyst that usually is encountered in the spinal canal of young adults.[510] The lining is identical to that of the colloid cyst.

## RATHKE CLEFT CYST

The Rathke cleft cyst lies within and above the sella turcica and is lined by cells identical to the endodermal and colloid cysts.[511]

## EPIDERMOID CYST

The epidermoid cyst is found most often in the cerebellopontine angle of middle-aged adults and is lined by stratified squamous epithelium with keratohyaline granules.[512]

## DERMOID CYST

The dermoid cyst is a rare cyst that is found in the midline, especially in the posterior fossa adherent to cerebellar vermis or dura.[512] The lining consists of squamous epithelium and occasional dermal structures, such as hair follicles and sweat and sebaceous glands.

## ARACHNOID CYST

The arachnoid cyst is common in active neurosurgical services and compresses underlying brain. The sylvian sulcus is a favored site.[513] The cyst lining consists of delicate arachnoid cells adherent to a layer of collagen.

# Metastatic Tumor to the Central Nervous System

## METASTATIC CARCINOMA

CLINICAL CONSIDERATIONS. Although statistics vary widely with regard to CNS metastatic tumor, a reasonable estimate is that approximately 25% of intracranial tumors are metastatic.[514, 515] Lung carci-

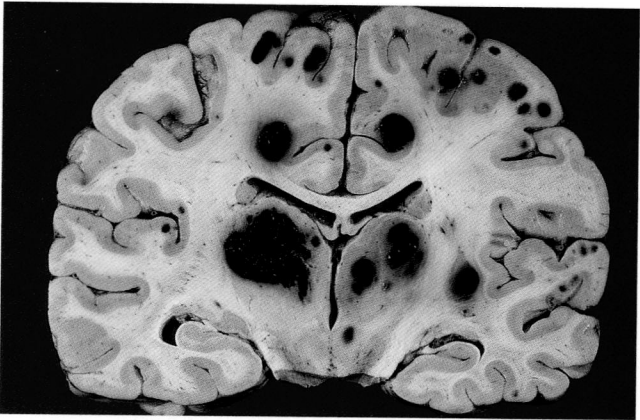

**FIGURE 51–49.** Metastatic melanoma in brain with multifocal hemorrhagic deposits virtually confined to gray matter, a distinctive feature of melanoma spread to CNS.

noma, breast carcinoma, and melanoma in that order are the most common primary sites for CNS metastatic tumor.[516] Certain tumors have a marked proclivity for spread to brain, including melanoma (Fig. 51–49), oat cell carcinoma, and choriocarcinoma.

Metastatic carcinoma in CNS is most often a hematogenous deposit at the junction of cortex with white matter, particularly in border zones of the arterial distribution, especially the zone between middle and posterior cerebral arteries[517] (CD Fig. 51–88).

Carcinoma also may deposit in dura, skull, or the leptomeningeal cerebrospinal fluid compartment (so-called carcinomatous meningitis) (CD Fig. 51–89). In the spine and spinal cord, carcinoma most often is present in the epidural space and vertebral body with consequent compression of the spinal cord (Fig. 51–50).

Grossly, intracerebral metastatic tumor is characteristically well circumscribed, spherical, and cen-

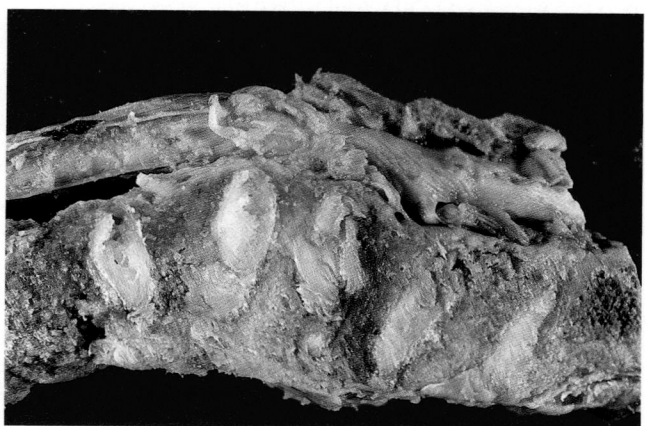

**FIGURE 51–50.** Metastatic lung carcinoma expanding and destroying vertebral bodies with compression of adjacent spinal cord.

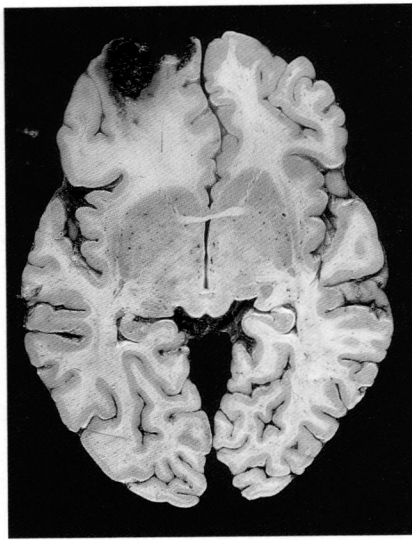

**FIGURE 51–51.** Horizontal section of brain with a solitary focus of hemorrhagic metastatic lung adenocarcinoma in the left frontal pole of brain and marked reactive edema in the subjacent white matter producing compression of the right frontal lobe.

trally necrotic (CD Fig. 51–90). Hemorrhagic metastases are common in tumor from melanoma, renal cell carcinoma, and choriocarcinoma. Peritumoral edema often is seen and may be disproportionate to the diameter of the actual tumor (Fig. 51–51).

The microscopic hallmark of metastatic CNS tumor is a sharp interface of tumor with adjacent brain tissue (CD Fig. 51–91). Exceptions do occur, however, most notably melanoma and oat cell carcinoma, both of which may display subtle single cell invasion of brain (CD Fig. 51–92). Metastatic tumor usually evokes a marked response from adjacent brain tissue, including astrogliosis, vascular edema, and vascular proliferation.

Immunohistochemistry is helpful in the diagnosis of metastatic brain tumor but must be used with caution (Fig. 51–52). Antibodies to cytokeratins and EMA, although strongly reactive with carcinoma, also focally react with glial, particularly astrocytic, tumors. To avoid error, it is crucial to supplement these antibodies with GFAP, which is only rarely and focally reactive with carcinoma.

In the differential diagnosis of metastatic CNS carcinoma, there are a few pitfalls to be avoided. Large cell carcinoma from lung may mimic a glioblastoma multiforme because both may have large anaplastic cells, a discrete margin with adjacent brain, and associated vascular proliferation. Melanoma and oat cell carcinoma through subtle invasion may resemble primary CNS glioma or medulloblastoma. These diagnostic issues generally are resolved by using appropriate immunohistochemical stains.

## LYMPHOMA

Systemic lymphoma of Hodgkin's (CD Fig. 51–93) and non-Hodgkin's types may involve the nervous system secondarily in 10% of patients.[518] Most common is subarachnoid invasion similar to carcinomatous meningitis. Tumor cells frequently extend along perivascular spaces to involve brain parenchyma and may invade cranial and spinal nerve roots. Systemic lymphomas most prone to such CNS extension include diffuse immunoblastic and large cell and small cell undifferentiated (Burkitt's and non-Burkitt's) lymphomas.[519] Lymphoma also may invade the spinal epidural space with resulting spinal cord compression.[519] Direct spread of lymphoma to brain parenchyma is exceedingly rare.[520]

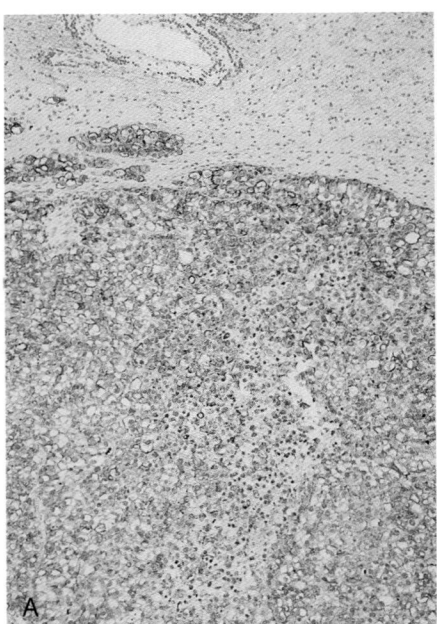
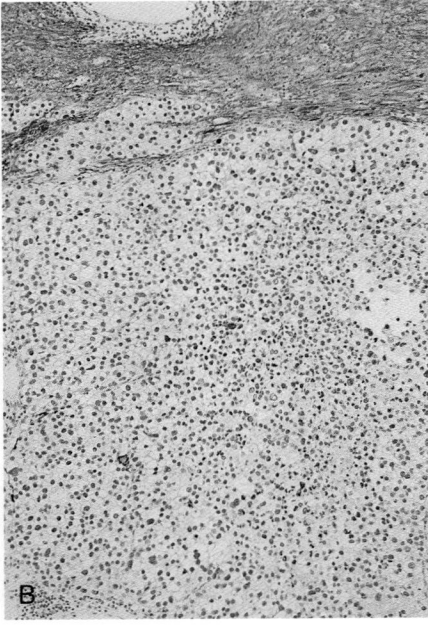

**FIGURE 51–52.** Immunohistochemical reactivity of metastatic carcinoma using high molecular weight cytokeratin to delineate tumor *(A)* and GFAP to highlight the adjacent gliotic brain *(B)*.

## LEUKEMIA

There are three principal manifestations of secondary CNS leukemia: 1) meningeal leukemia, 2) intraparenchymal intravascular leukostasis, and 3) nodular granulocytic sarcoma (chloroma).[521] Meningeal leukemia occurs most often in childhood acute lymphoblastic leukemia. In adults, secondary meningeal leukemia is less common but is associated with chronic lymphocytic leukemia and the monocytic or blastic phases of myeloid leukemia. Microscopic manifestations include subarachnoid, perivascular cellular deposits with extension into adjacent brain parenchyma and infiltration of nerve roots (CD Fig. 51–94). Current chemotherapy and radiation regimens have reduced the incidence of secondary childhood meningeal leukemia markedly[519] but have been accompanied by a rise in treatment-related tumors, especially gliomas.[522] Because systemic leukemia may produce a reactive meningeal leukocytosis, it is advisable to confirm the diagnosis of meningeal leukemia with immunohistochemical techniques.[519, 523]

Intraparenchymal intravascular leukostasis is a complication in 25% of patients with acute leukemia or the blast crisis of chronic leukemia[519] (CD Fig. 51–95A). Precipitate occlusion of cerebral vessels in uncontrolled acute leukemia may result in fatal intracerebral hemorrhage (CD Fig. 51–95B).

Granulocytic sarcoma, the solid tumor manifestation of acute myeloid leukemia, arises in skull, periosteum, or dural compartments with resulting compression of underlying brain or spinal cord. Histologic confusion with lymphoma is commonplace but may be avoided with use of immunohistochemistry.[524]

## NON-NEOPLASTIC LESIONS SIMULATING NEOPLASIA

### Cerebral Infarct

An acute cerebral infarct with space-occupying edema or a subacute infarct with its periphery of reactive, porous blood vessels producing ring enhancement may lead to an erroneous radiologic interpretation of brain tumor and consequent brain biopsy (CD Fig. 51–96A). A large tissue sample with an array of neurons undergoing eosinophilic necrosis generally causes little diagnostic difficulty. A small biopsy specimen, particularly a stereotactic or needle biopsy specimen, may cause confusion, however, especially if the infarct is subacute. In that stage, the tissue is hypercellular with reactive astrocytes and abundant lipid-laden macrophages engulfing disintegrating myelin (CD Fig. 51–96B). The presence of macrophages highlighted with CD68 (KP1) immunostaining is in general a warning to avoid a diagnosis of neoplasia, particularly if the accompanying astrocytes display uniform, vesicular nuclei and abundant fibrillary cytoplasm.

## Multiple Sclerosis

Solitary or multiple foci (plaques) of white matter demyelination, the hallmark of multiple sclerosis,[525] may be misinterpreted on radiologic (particularly MRI) examination as primary or metastatic brain tumor, leading to brain biopsy (Fig. 51–53A). The usual lesion of symptomatic multiple sclerosis at biopsy is the subacute plaque, an often intensely cellular mix of lipid-laden macrophages and reactive fibrillary astrocytes (Fig. 51–53B, C). To guard against a diagnosis of tumor, it is crucial as in infarct to recognize the macrophages with their vacuolated cytoplasm intensely reactive with CD68 (KP1) (Fig. 51–53D).

## Inflammatory and Infectious Lesions

### ABSCESS

The solitary or multifocal (CD Fig. 51–97A) brain abscess,[526] similar to the cerebral infarct, through its central cavitary necrosis and peripheral granulation tissue may simulate the ring enhancement of malignant glioma. Microscopically the necrotic debris and sheets of neutrophils within the abscess core present little diagnostic challenge (CD Fig. 51–97B). The periphery of the abscess with a mix of proliferating blood vessels (granulation tissue) and abundant reactive astrocytes (CD Fig. 51–97C) may create confusion. The orderly uniform astrocytes with their abundant cell processes intermixed with telltale lipid-laden macrophages should warn against a diagnosis of neoplasia, however.

### PROGRESSIVE MULTIFOCAL LEUKOENCEPHALOPATHY

Progressive multifocal leukoencephalopathy[527] presents as multiple, confluent, subcortical and white matter lesions produced by the JC papovavirus, which may simulate neoplasia with radiologic study (CD Fig. 51–98A). Biopsy reveals a cellular focus composed principally of lipid-laden macrophages (CD Fig. 51–98B). The diagnostic features include large, uniformly dense (and viral-laden) oligodendroglial nuclei and rare, large, highly atypical (transformed) astrocytes (CD Fig. 51–98C). To resolve questionable lesions, it is best to perform in situ hybridization for the JC virus using fixed, paraffin-embedded tissue sections.

### TOXOPLASMOSIS

*Toxoplasma* brain abscesses in cortex and basal ganglia are most common in immunocompromised patients[528] (CD Fig. 51–99A). Although radiologic examination often is sufficient for diagnosis, a questionable focus still may require biopsy. Most typical in such tissue is marked coagulative necrosis of all brain elements, accompanied by a variable cellularity ranging from scanty reactive glial cells to

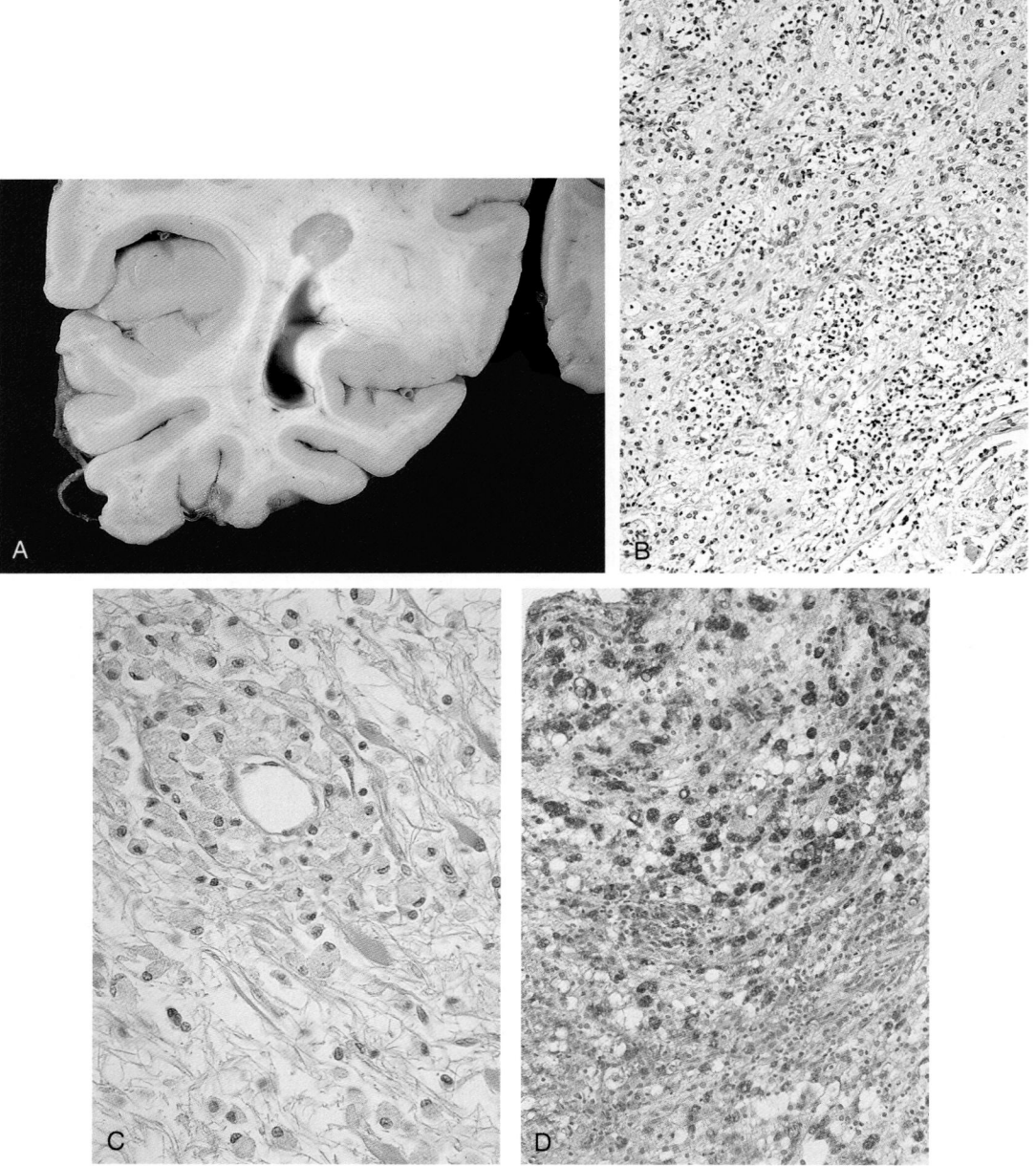

**FIGURE 51–53.** Chronic multiple sclerosis with a discrete spherical, demyelinated plaque at the upper edge of the ventricle *(A)*. Low power microscopic view of acute multiple sclerosis plaque with inflammatory cells, lipid-laden macrophages, and prominent blood vessels *(B)*. Closer view of perivascular macrophages and spindle-shaped adjacent reactive astrocytes *(C)*. CD68 immunostaining of macrophages in a plaque *(D)*.

numerous macrophages to abundant perivascular lymphocytes (CD Fig. 51–99B). Confusion may result with glioma or lymphoma. The diagnosis is confirmed with identification of *Toxoplasma* organisms as cysts or isolated endozoites in the intact brain just outside the zone of coagulative necrosis (CD Fig. 51–99C). Recognition of endozoites is enhanced using immunohistochemistry with antibody directed against *Toxoplasma* in fixed, paraffin-embedded tissues.

## Developmental and Syndrome-Related Lesions

### HYPOTHALAMIC HAMARTOMA

Lying at the base of the hypothalamus posterior to the pituitary stalk and attached or closely adjacent to the mammillary bodies or the tuber cinereum, the hypothalamic hamartoma, a mass of displaced neurons, nerve tracts, and glia, presents most commonly in young boys with precocious puberty.[529] Immunohistochemical evaluation of the neurons within the hamartoma reveals an array of releasing hormones native to the hypothalamus.[530]

## TUBEROUS SCLEROSIS

The complex genetic syndrome tuberous sclerosis, previously discussed in relation to subependymal giant cell astrocytoma, is associated with cerebral cortex developmental lesions, *tubers,* which give the syndrome its name.[531] The tuber is a firm, ill-defined, focally calcified mass replacing normal cortex and subjacent white matter, obscuring grossly the usually clear-cut gray-white junction (CD Fig. 51–100*A*). Histologically, it consists principally of gliosis particularly dense along the cortical surface, which imparts the sclerosis typical of the tuber. Intermixed in this glial meshwork is a disordered array of distinctive large cells with prominent nuclei and abundant cytoplasm exhibiting immunohistochemical features of neurons and astrocytes[532, 533] (CD Fig. 51–100*B*). The tuber is essentially a region of malformed brain tissue and as such is a fixed, nonexpansile mass, in contrast to the associated, deep-seated, subependymal giant cell astrocytoma, which may present as a true neoplasm extending into brain or more commonly into the lateral ventricle.

## Metabolic and Degenerative Lesions: Amyloidoma

One of the more unusual space-occupying lesions of the brain consists of an almost pure deposit of acellular amyloid protein within or adjacent to brain or spinal cord. Only rare lymphocytes or plasma cells may accompany the amyloidoma, and there is in general no association with myeloma or disseminated amyloidosis.[534, 535]

## REFERENCES

1. Kleihues P, Burger PC, Scheithauer BW: International Histological Classification of Tumours. Histological Typing of Tumours of the Central Nervous System, 2nd ed. Berlin, Springer Verlag, 1993.
2. Lantos PL, VandenBerg SR, Kleihues P: Tumours of the nervous system. *In* Graham DI, Lantos PL (eds): Greenfield's Neuropathology, 6th ed. London, Arnold, 1997, pp 586–588.
3. Bigner SH, Batra SK, Ahmed Rasheed BK: Mechanisms of altered growth control. Cytogenetics, oncogenes and suppressor genes. *In* Bigner DD, McLendon RE, Bruner JM (eds): Russell and Rubinstein's Pathology of Tumors of the Nervous System, 6th ed. London, Arnold, 1998, pp 47–82.
4. McLendon RE, Enterline DS, Tien RD, et al: Tumors of central neuroepithelial origin. *In* Bigner DD, McLendon RE, Bruner JM (eds): Russell and Rubinstein's Pathology of Tumors of the Nervous System, 6th ed. London, Arnold, 1998, pp 308–314.
5. Burger PC, Scheithauer BW: Atlas of Tumor Pathology. Tumors of the Central Nervous System. Third Series, Fascicle 10. Washington, DC, Armed Forces Institute of Pathology, 1994, pp 429–434.
6. Thapar K, Laws ER: Tumors of the central nervous system. *In* Murphy GP, Lawrence W, Lenhard RE (eds): ACS Textbook of Clinical Oncology, 2nd ed. Atlanta, ACS, 1995, pp 378–410.
7. Russell DS, Rubinstein LJ: Pathology of Tumours of the Nervous System, 5th ed. London, Edward Arnold, 1989, pp 95–161.
8. Piepmeier J, Christopher S, Spencer D, et al: Variations in the natural history of patients with supratentorial low-grade astrocytomas. Neurosurgery 38:872–878, 1996.
9. VandenBerg SR: Current diagnostic concepts of astrocytic tumors. J Neuropathol Exp Neurol 51:644–657, 1992.
10. Krouwer HG, Davis RL, Silver P, Prados M: Gemistocytic astrocytomas. A reappraisal. J Neurosurg 74:399–406, 1991.
11. Watanabe K, Osamu T, Yonekawa Y: Role of gemistocytes in astrocytoma progression. Lab Invest 76:277–284, 1997.
12. Hirato J, Nakazato Y, Ogawa A: Expression of non-glial intermediate filament proteins in gliomas. Clin Neuropathol 13:1–11, 1994.
13. Muller W, Afra D, Schroder R: Supratentorial recurrences of gliomas. Morphological studies in relation to time intervals with 544 astrocytomas. Acta Neurochir 37:75–91, 1977.
14. Afra D, Muller W, Benoist G, Schroder R: Supratentorial recurrences of gliomas. Results of reoperations on astrocytomas and oligodendrogliomas. Acta Neurochir 43:217–227, 1978.
15. Laws ER Jr, Taylor WF, Clifton MB, Okazaki H: Neurosurgical management of low-grade astrocytoma of the cerebral hemispheres. J Neurosurg 61:665–673, 1984.
16. Soffietti R, Chio A, Giordana MT, et al: Prognostic factors in well-differentiated cerebral astrocytomas in the adult. Neurosurgery 25:686–692, 1989.
17. Vertosick FT, Selker RG, Arena VL: Survival of patients with well-differentiated astrocytomas diagnosed in the era of computed tomography. Neurosurgery 28:496–501, 1991.
18. Weir B, Grace M: The relative significance of factors affecting survival in astrocytomas grades one and two. Can J Neurol Sci 3:47–50, 1976.
19. Raghavan R, Steart PV, Weller RO: Cell proliferation patterns in the diagnosis of astrocytomas, anaplastic astrocytomas and glioblastoma multiforme. A Ki-67 study. Neuropathol Appl Neurobiol 16:123–133, 1990.
20. Jaros E, Perry RH, Adam L, et al: Prognostic implications of p53, epidermal growth factor receptor, and Ki-67 labelling in brain tumours. Br J Cancer 66:373–385, 1992.
21. Karamitopoulu E, Perentes E, Diamantis I, Maraziotis T: Ki-67 immunoreactivity in human central nervous system tumors. A study with MIB 1 monoclonal antibody on archival material. Acta Neuropathol 87:47–54, 1994.
22. Coons SW, Johnson PC: Regional heterogeneity in the proliferative activity of human gliomas as measured by the Ki-67 labeling index. J Neuropathol Exp Neurol 52:609–618, 1993.
23. Montine TJ, Vandersteenhoven JJ, Aguzzi A, et al: Prognostic significance of Ki-67 proliferation index in supratentorial fibrillary astrocytic neoplasms. Neurosurgery 34:674–679, 1994.
24. Watanabe K, Tachibana O, Sato K, et al: Overexpression of the EGF receptor and p53 mutations are mutually exclusive in the evolution of primary and secondary glioblastomas. Brain Pathol 6:217–224, 1996.
25. Dohrmann GJ, Farwell JR, Flannery JT: Glioblastoma in children. J Neurosurg 44:442–448, 1975.
26. Kepes JJ, Rubinstein LJ: Malignant gliomas with heavily lipidized (foamy) tumor cells. A report of three cases with immunoperoxidase study. Cancer 47:2451–2459, 1981.
27. Mørk SJ, Rubinstein LJ, Kepes JJ, et al: Patterns of epithelial metaplasia in malignant gliomas. II. Squamous differentiation of epithelial-like formations in gliosarcomas and glioblastomas. J Neuropathol Exp Neurol 47:101–118, 1988.
28. Mathews T, Moossy J: Gliomas containing bone and cartilage. J Neuropathol Exp Neurol 33:456–471, 1974.
29. Burger PC, Shibata T, Kleihues P: The use of the monoclonal antibody Ki-67 in the identification of proliferating cells: Application to surgical neuropathology. Am J Surg Pathol 10:611–617, 1986.
30. Giangaspero F, Doglioni C, Rivano MT, et al: Growth fraction in human brain tumors defined by the monoclonal antibody Ki-67. Acta Neuropathol 74:179–182, 1987.
31. Deckert M, Reifenberger G, Wechsler W: Determination of

the proliferative potential of human brain tumors using the monoclonal antibody Ki-67. J Cancer Res Clin Oncol 115: 179–188, 1989.

32. Muller W, Slowik F, Firsching R, et al: Contribution to the problem of giant cell astrocytomas. Neurosurg Rev 10:213–219, 1987.

33. Palma L, Celli P, Maleci A, et al: Malignant monstrocellular brain tumours. A study of 42 surgically treated cases. Acta Neurochir 97:17–25, 1989.

34. Margetts JC, Kalyan-Raman UP: Giant-celled glioblastoma of brain. A clinico-pathological and radiological study of ten cases (including immunohistochemistry and ultrastructure). Cancer 63:524–531, 1989.

35. Peraud A, Watanabe K, Plate KH, et al: p53 mutations versus EGF receptor expression in giant cell glioblastomas. J Neuropathol Exp Neurol 56:1236–1241, 1997.

36. Meyer-Puttlitz B, Hayashi Y, Waha A, et al: Molecular genetic analysis of giant cell glioblastomas. Am J Pathol 151: 853–857, 1997.

37. Morantz RA, Feigin I, Ransohoff J III: Clinical and pathological study of 24 cases of gliosarcoma. J Neurosurg 45:398–408, 1976.

38. Meis JM, Martz KL, Nelson JS: Mixed glioblastoma multiforme and sarcoma. A clinicopathologic study of 26 Radiation Therapy Oncology Group cases. Cancer 67:2342–2349, 1991.

39. Galanis E, Buckner JC, Dinapoli RP, et al: Clinical outcome of gliosarcoma compared with glioblastoma multiforme. North Central Cancer Treatment Group results. J Neurosurgery 89:425–430, 1998.

40. Grant JW, Steart PV, Aguzzi A, et al: Gliosarcoma. An immunohistochemical study. Acta Neuropathol 79:305–309, 1989.

41. Ho K-L: Histogenesis of sarcomatous component of the gliosarcoma. An ultrastructural study. Acta Neuropathol 81:178–188, 1990.

42. Ng HK, Poon WS: Gliosarcoma of the posterior fossa with features of a malignant fibrous histiocytoma. Cancer 65: 1161–1166, 1990.

43. Haddad SF, Moore SA, Schelper RL, Goeken J: Smooth muscle cells can comprise the sarcomatous component of gliosarcomas. J Neuropathol Exp Neurol 51:493–498, 1992.

44. Albrecht S, Connelly JH, Bruner JM: Distribution of p53 protein expression in gliosarcomas. An immunohistochemical study. Acta Neuropathol 85:222–226, 1993.

45. Paulus W, Bayas A, Ott G, Roggendorf W: Interphase cytogenetics of glioblastoma and gliosarcoma. Acta Neuropathol 88:420–423, 1994.

46. Biernat W, Aguzzi A, Sure U, et al: Identical mutations of the p53 tumor suppressor gene in the glial and sarcomatous part of gliosarcomas suggest a common origin from glial cells. J Neuropathol Exp Neurol 54:651–656, 1995.

47. Boerman RH, Anderl K, Herath J, et al: The glial and mesenchymal elements of gliosarcoma share similar genetic alterations. J Neuropathol Exp Neurol 55:973–981, 1996.

48. Biernat W, Kleihues P, Yonekawa Y, Ohgaki H: Amplification and overexpression of MDM2 in primary (de novo) glioblastoma. J Neuropathol Exp Neurol 56:180–185, 1997.

49. Collins VP: Gene amplification in human gliomas. Glia 15: 289–296, 1995.

50. Louis DN: A molecular genetic model of astrocytoma histopathology. Brain Pathol 7:755–764, 1997.

51. Ohgaki H, Schaule B, zur Hausen A, et al: Genetic alterations associated with the evolution and progression of astrocytic brain tumours. Virchows Arch 427:113–118, 1995.

52. Reifenberger G, Ichimura K, Reifenberger J, et al: Refined mapping of 12q13–q15 amplicons in human malignant gliomas suggests CDK4/SAS and MDM2 as independent amplification targets. Cancer Res 56:5141–5145, 1996.

53. Ono Y, Tamiya T, Ichikawa T, et al: Accumulation of wild-type p53 in astrocytomas is associated with increased p21 expression. Acta Neuropathol 94:21–27, 1997.

54. Ichimura K, Schmidt EE, Goike HM, Collins VP: Human glioblastomas with no alterations of the CDKN2A (p16 INK4A, MTS1) and CDK4 genes have frequent mutations of the retinoblastoma gene. Oncogene 13:1065–1072, 1996.

55. Rollbrocker B, Waha A, Louis DN, et al: Amplification of the cyclin-dependent kinase 4 (CDK4) gene is associated with high cdk4 protein levels in glioblastoma multiforme. Acta Neuropathol 92:70–74, 1996.

56. Hayashi Y, Ueki K, Waha A, et al: Association of EGFR gene amplification and CDKN2 (p16/MTS1) gene deletion in glioblastoma multiforme. Brain Pathol 7:871–875, 1997.

57. Biernat W, Tohma Y, Yonekawa Y: Alterations of cell cycle regulatory genes in primary (de novo) and secondary glioblastomas. Acta Neuropathol 94:303–309, 1997.

58. Wakimoto H, Aoyagi M, Nakayama T, et al: Prognostic significance of Ki-67 labeling indices obtained using MIB-1 monoclonal antibody in patients with supratentorial astrocytomas. Cancer 77:373–380, 1996.

59. Ellison DW, Steart PV, Bateman AC, et al: Prognostic indicators in a range of astrocytic tumours. An immunohistochemical study with Ki-67 and p53 antibodies. J Neurol Neurosurg Psychiatry 59:413–419, 1995.

60. Sallinen PK, Haapasalo HK, Visakorpi T, et al: Prognostication of astrocytoma patient survival by Ki-67 (MIB-1), PCNA, and S-phase fraction using archival paraffin-embedded samples. J Pathol 174:275–282, 1994.

61. Giannini C, Scheithauer BW, Burger PC, et al: Cellular proliferation in pilocytic and diffuse astrocytomas. J Neuropathol Exp Neurol 58:46–53, 1999.

62. Stemmer-Rachaminov AO, Louis DN: Histopathologic and immunohistochemical prognostic factors in malignant gliomas. Curr Opin Oncol 9:230–234, 1997.

63. Forsyth PA, Shaw EG, Scheithauer BW, et al: Supratentorial pilocytic astrocytomas. A clinicopathologic, prognostic and flow cytometric study of 51 patients. Cancer 72:1335–1342, 1993.

64. Lewis RA, Gerson LP, Axelson KA, et al: von Recklinghausen neurofibromatosis. II. Incidence of optic gliomata. Ophthalmology 91:929–935, 1984.

65. Listernick R, Louis DN, Packer RJ, Gutmann DH: Optic pathway gliomas in children with neurofibromatosis 1. Consensus from the NF1 optic pathway glioma task force. Ann Neurol 41:143–149, 1997.

66. Schiffer D, Giordana MT, Mauro A, et al: Immunohistochemical demonstration of vimentin in human cerebral tumors. Acta Neuropathol 70:209–219, 1986.

67. Ito S, Hoshino T, Shibuya M, et al: Proliferative characteristics of juvenile pilocytic astrocytomas determined by bromodeoxyuridine labeling. Neurosurgery 31:413–418, 1992.

68. Kordek R, Biernat W, Debiec-Rychter M, et al: Comparative evaluation of p53-protein expression and the PCNA and Ki-67 proliferating cell indices in human astrocytomas. Pathol Res Pract 192:205–209, 1996.

69. Dirven CM, Koudstaal J, Mooji JJ, Molenaar WM: The proliferative potential of the pilocytic astrocytoma. The relation between MIB-1 labeling and clinical and neuro-radiological follow-up. J Neurooncol 37:9–16, 1998.

70. Tomlinson FH, Scheithauer BW, Hayostek CJ, et al: The significance of atypia and histologic malignancy in pilocytic astrocytoma of the cerebellum. A clinicopathologic and flow cytometric study. J Neurooncol 9:301–310, 1994.

71. Brown MT, Friedman HS, Oakes J, et al: Chemotherapy for pilocytic astrocytoma. Cancer 71:3165–3172, 1993.

72. Ohgaki H, Eibl RH, Schwab M, et al: Mutations of the p53 tumor suppressor gene in neoplasms of the human nervous system. Mol Carcinog 8:74–80, 1993.

73. Patt S, Gries H, Giraldo M, et al: p53 gene mutations in human astrocytic brain tumors including pilocytic astrocytomas. Hum Pathol 27:586–589, 1996.

74. Ishii N, Sawamura Y, Tada M, et al: Absence of p53 gene mutations in a tumor panel representative of pilocytic astrocytoma diversity using a p53 functional assay. Int J Cancer 76:797–800, 1998.

75. von Deimling A, Louis DN, Menon AG, et al: Deletions on the long arm of chromosome 17 in pilocytic astrocytoma. Acta Neuropathol 86:81–85, 1993.

76. Platten M, Giordano MJ, Dirven CM, et al: Up-regulation of specific NF1 gene transcripts in sporadic pilocytic astrocytomas. Am J Pathol 149:621–627, 1996.

77. Gutmann DH, Giordano MJ, Mahadeo DK, et al: Increased neurofibromatosis 1 gene expression in astrocytic tumors: Positive regulation by p21-ras. Oncogene 12:2121–2127, 1996.
78. Burger PC, Scheithauer BW: Tumors of the Central Nervous System. Atlas of Tumor Pathology. Third Series, Fascicle 10. Washington, DC, Armed Forces Institute of Pathology, 1994, pp 77–96.
79. Kepes JJ, Rubinstein LJ, Eng LF: Pleomorphic xanthoastrocytoma. A distinctive meningocerebral glioma of young subjects with relatively favorable prognosis. A study of 12 cases. Cancer 44:1839–1852, 1979.
80. Mackenzie JM: Pleomorphic xanthoastrocytoma in a 62 year-old male. Neuropathol Appl Neurobiol 13:481–487, 1987.
81. Nishio S, Takeshita I, Fujii K, et al: Supratentorial astrocytic tumours of childhood. A clinicopathologic study of 41 cases. Acta Neurochir 101:3–8, 1989.
82. Herpers MJ, Freling G, Beuls EA: Pleomorphic xanthoastrocytoma in the spinal cord. Case report. J Neurosurg 80:564–569, 1994.
83. Kawano N: Pleomorphic xanthoastrocytoma (PXA) in Japan. Its clinico-pathologic features and diagnostic clues. Brain Tumor Pathol 8:5–10, 1991.
84. Weldon-Linne CM, Victor TA, Groothuis DR, Vick NA: Pleomorphic xanthoastrocytoma. Ultrastructural and immunohistochemical study of a case with a rapidly fatal outcome following surgery. Cancer 52:2055–2063, 1983.
85. Kepes JJ, Rubinstein LJ, Ansbacher L, Schreiber DJ: Histopathological features of recurrent pleomorphic xanthoastrocytomas. Further corroboration of the glial nature of this neoplasm. A study of three cases. Acta Neuropathol 78:585–593, 1989.
86. Furuta A, Takahashi H, Ikuta F, et al: Temporal lobe tumor demonstrating ganglioglioma and pleomorphic xanthoastrocytoma components. Case report. J Neurosurg 77:143–147, 1992.
87. Lindboe C, Cappelen J, Kepes J: Pleomorphic xanthoastrocytoma as a component of a cerebellar ganglioglioma. Case report. Neurosurgery 31:353–355, 1992.
88. Kordek R, Biernat W, Sapieja W, et al: Pleomorphic xanthoastrocytoma with a gangliomatous component. An immunohistochemical and ultrastructural study. Acta Neuropathol 89:194–197, 1995.
89. Muñoz EL, Eberhard DA, Lopes MBS, et al: Proliferative activity and p53 mutation as prognostic indicators in pleomorphic xanthoastrocytoma. J Neuropathol Exp Neurol 55:606, 1996.
90. Paulus W, Lisle DK, Tonn JC, et al: Molecular genetic alterations in pleomorphic xanthoastrocytoma. Acta Neuropathol 91:293–297, 1996.
91. Whittle IR, Gordon A, Misra BK, et al: Pleomorphic xanthoastrocytoma. Report of four cases. J Neurosurg 70:463–468, 1989.
92. Daita G, Yonemasu Y, Muraoka S, et al: A case of anaplastic astrocytoma transformed from pleomorphic xanthoastrocytoma. Brain Tumor Pathol 8:63–66, 1991.
93. Shepherd CW, Scheithauer BW, Gomez MR, et al: Subependymal giant cell astrocytoma. A clinical, pathological, and flow cytometric study. Neurosurgery 28:864–868, 1991.
94. Kingsley DP, Kendall BE, Fitz CR: Tuberous sclerosis. A clinicoradiological evaluation of 110 cases with particular reference to atypical presentation. Neuroradiology 28:38–46, 1986.
95. Gomez MR: Phenotypes of the tuberous sclerosis complex with a revision of diagnostic criteria. Ann N Y Acad Sci 615:1–7, 1991.
96. Ahlsen G, Gillberg IC, Lindblom R, Gillberg C: Tuberous sclerosis in Western Sweden. A population study of cases with early childhood onset. Arch Neurol 51:76–81, 1994.
97. Halmagyi GM, Bignold LP, Allsop JL: Recurrent subependymal giant-cell astrocytoma in the absence of tuberous sclerosis. J Neurosurg 50:106–109, 1979.
98. Lopes MBS, Altermatt HJ, Scheithauer BW, et al: Immunohistochemical characterization of subependymal giant cell astrocytoma. Acta Neuropathol 91:368–375, 1996.
99. Hirose T, Scheithauer BW, Lopes MB, et al: Tuber and subependymal giant cell astrocytoma associated with tuberous sclerosis. An immunohistochemical, ultrastructural, and immunoelectron microscopic study. Acta Neuropathol 90:387–399, 1995.
100. Lantos PL, VandenBerg SR, Kleihues P: Tumours of the nervous system. In Graham DI, Lantos PL (eds): Greenfield's Neuropathology, 6th ed. London, Arnold, 1996, pp 625–627.
101. Henske EP, Scheithauer BW, Short MP, et al: Allelic loss is frequent in tuberous sclerosis kidney lesions but rare in brain lesions. Am J Hum Genet 59:400–406, 1996.
102. Henske EP, Wessner LL, Golden J, et al: Loss of tuberin in both subependymal giant cell astrocytomas and angiomyolipomas supports a two-hit model for the pathogenesis of tuberous sclerosis tumors. Am J Pathol 151:1639–1647, 1997.
103. Mizuguchi M, Kato M, Yamanouchi H, et al: Tuberin immunohistochemistry in brain, kidneys and heart with or without tuberous sclerosis. Acta Neuropathol 94:525–531, 1997.
104. Taratuto AL, Monges J, Lylyk P, Leiguarda R: Superficial cerebral astrocytoma attached to dura. Report of six cases in infants. Cancer 54:2502–2512, 1984.
105. VandenBerg SR: Desmoplastic infantile ganglioglioma and desmoplastic cerebral astrocytoma of infancy. Brain Pathol 3:275–281, 1993.
106. Louis DN, von Deimling A, Dickersin GR, et al: Desmoplastic cerebral astrocytomas of infancy. A histopathologic, immunohistochemical, ultrastructural, and molecular genetic study. Hum Pathol 23:1402–1409, 1992.
107. Snipes GJ, Steinberg GK, Lane B, Horoupian DS: Gliofibroma. Case report. J Neurosurg 75:642–646, 1991.
108. Schober R, Bayindir C, Canbolat A, et al: Gliofibroma. Immunohistochemical analysis. Acta Neuropathol 83:207–210, 1992.
109. Caldemeyer KS, Zimmerman RA, Azzarelli B, et al: Gliofibroma. CT and MRI. Neuroradiology 37:481–485, 1995.
110. Windisch TR, Naul LG, Bauserman SC: Intramedullary gliofibroma. MR, ultrasound, and pathologic correlation. J Comput Assist Tomogr 19:646–648, 1995.
111. Prayson RA: Gliofibroma. A distinct entity or a subtype of desmoplastic astrocytoma? Hum Pathol 27:610–613, 1996.
112. Friede RL: Gliofibroma. A peculiar neoplasia of collagen forming glia-like cells. J Neuropathol Exp Neurol 37:300–313, 1978.
113. Mørk SJ, Lindegaad K-F, Halvorsen TB, et al: Oligodendroglioma. Incidence and biological behavior in a defined population. J Neurosurg 63:881–889, 1985.
114. Zülch KJ: Brain Tumors. Their Biology and Pathology, 3rd ed. Berlin, Springer-Verlag, 1986.
115. Shaw EG, Scheithauer BW, O'Fallon JR, et al: Oligodendrogliomas. The Mayo Clinic experience. J Neurosurg 76:428–434, 1992.
116. Daumas-Duport C, Varlet P, Tucker M-L, et al: Oligodendrogliomas. Part I. Patterns of growth, histological diagnosis, clinical and imaging correlations. A study of 153 cases. J Neurooncol 34:37–59, 1997.
117. Dohrmann GJ, Farwell JR, Flannery JT: Oligodendrogliomas in children. Surg Neurol 10:21–25, 1978.
118. Rizk T, Mottolèse C, Bouffet E, et al: Cerebral oligodendrogliomas in children. An analysis of 15 cases. Childs Nerv Syst 12:527–529, 1996.
119. Cairncross JG, Macdonald DR, Ramsay DA: Aggressive oligodendroglioma. A chemosensitive tumor. Neurosurgery 31:78–82, 1992.
120. Fortuna A, Celli P, Palma L: Oligodendrogliomas of the spinal cord. Acta Neurochir 52:305–329, 1980.
121. Huk WJ, Gademann G, Friedmann G: Magnetic Resonance Imaging of the Central Nervous System Diseases. Berlin, Springer-Verlag, 1990, p 237.
122. Herpers MJHM, Budka H: Glial fibrillary acidic protein (GFAP) in oligodendroglial tumors. Gliofibrillary oligodendroglioma and transitional oligoastrocytoma as subtypes of oligodendroglioma. Acta Neuropathol 64:265–272, 1984.
123. Wondrusch E, Huemer M, Budka H: Production of glial fibrillary acidic protein (GFAP) by neoplastic oligodendrocytes. Gliofibrillary oligodendroglioma and transitional oligoastrocytoma revisited. Brain Tumor Pathol 8:11–15, 1991.

124. Kros JM, de Jong AA, van der Kwast ThH: Ultrastructural characterization of transitional cells in oligodendrogliomas. J Neuropathol Exp Neurol 51:186–193, 1992.

125. Schiffer D, Dutto A, Cavalla P, et al: Prognostic factors in oligodendrogliomas. Can J Neurol Sci 24:313–319, 1997.

126. Russell DS, Rubinstein LJ: Pathology of Tumours of the Nervous System, 5th ed. London, Edward Arnold, 1989, pp 172-187.

127. Coons SW, Johnson PC, Pearl DK: The prognostic significance of Ki-67 labeling indices for oligodendrogliomas. Neurosurgery 41:878–884, 1997.

128. Kennedy PGE, Watkins BA, Thomas DGT, Noble MD: Antigenic expression by cells derived from human gliomas does not correlate with morphological classification. Ann N Y Acad Sci 13:327–347, 1987.

129. Noble M, Ataliotis P, Barnett SC, et al: Development, regeneration and neoplasia of glial cells in the central nervous system. Ann N Y Acad Sci 633:35–47, 1991.

130. Figols J, Iglesias-Rozas JR, Kazner E: Myelin basic protein (MBP) in human gliomas. A study of twenty-five cases. Clin Neuropathol 4:116–120, 1985.

131. Nakagawa Y, Perentes E, Rubinstein LJ: Immunohistochemical characterization of oligodendrogliomas. An analysis of multiple markers. Acta Neuropathol 72:15–22, 1986.

132. Perentes E, Rubinstein LJ: Recent applications of immunoperoxidase histochemistry in human neuro-oncology. Arch Pathol Lab Med 111:796–812, 1987.

133. de la Monte SM: Uniform lineage of oligodendrogliomas. Am J Pathol 153:529–540, 1989.

134. Abo T, Balch TA: Differentiation antigen of human NK and K cells identified by a monoclonal antibody (HNK-1). J Immunol 127:1024–1029, 1981.

135. Sato S, Baba H, Tanaka M, et al: Antigenic determinant shared between myelin-associated glycoprotein from human brain and natural killer cells. Biomed Res 4:489–494, 1983.

136. McGarry RC, Helfand SL, Qaurles RH, et al: Recognition of myelin-associated glycoprotein by the monoclonal antibody HNK-1. Nature 306:376–378, 1983.

137. Jagadha V, Halliday WC, Becker LE: Glial fibrillary acidic protein (GFAP) in oligodendrogliomas. A reflection of transient GFAP expression by immature oligodendroglia. Can J Neurol Sci 13:307–311, 1986.

138. Cruz-Sanchez FF, Rossi ML, Buller JR, et al: Oligodendrogliomas. A clinical, histological, immunocytochemical and lectin-binding study. Histopathology 19:361–367, 1991.

139. Kros JM, Van Eden CG, Stefanko SZ, et al: Prognostic implications of glial fibrillary acidic protein containing cell types in oligodendrogliomas. Cancer 66:1204–1212, 1990.

140. Raff MC, Miller RH, Noble M: A glial progenitor cell that develops *in vitro* into an astrocyte or an oligodendrocyte depending on culture medium. Nature 303:390–396, 1983.

141. Bishop M, de la Monte SM: Dual lineage of astrocytomas. Am J Pathol 135:517–527, 1989.

142. Hart MN, Petito CK, Earle KM: Mixed gliomas. Cancer 33:134–140, 1974.

143. Shaw EG, Scheithauer BW, O'Fallon JR, Davis DH: Mixed oligoastrocytomas. A survival and prognostic factor analysis. Neurosurgery 34:577–582, 1994.

144. Hurtt MR, Moosy J, Donovan-Peluso M, Locker J: Amplification of epidermal growth factor receptor gene in gliomas. Histopathology and prognosis. J Neuropathol Exp Neurol 51:84–90, 1992.

145. Decaestecker C, Lopes MBS, Gordower L, et al: Quantitative chromatin pattern description in Feulgen-stained nuclei as a diagnostic tool to characterize the oligodendroglial and astroglial components in mixed oligo-astrocytomas. J Neuropathol Exp Neurol 56:391–402, 1997.

146. Miller RH, French-Constant C, Raff MC: The macroglial cells of the rat optic nerve. Ann Rev Neurosci 12:517–534, 1989.

147. Lillien LE, Raff MC: Differentiation signals in the CNS. Type-2 astrocyte development in vitro as a model system. Neuron 5:111–119, 1990.

148. Cairncross JG, Macdonald DR: Successful chemotherapy for recurrent malignant oligodendroglioma. Ann Neurol 23:360–364, 1988.

149. Cairncross JG, Macdonald DR, Ludwin S, et al: Chemotherapy for anaplastic oligodendroglioma. J Clin Oncol 12:2013–2021, 1994.

150. Cairncross JG, Ueki K, Zlatescu MC, et al: Specific genetic predictors of chemotherapeutic response and survival in patients with anaplastic oligodendrogliomas. J Natl Cancer Inst 90:1473–1479, 1998.

151. Burger PC: The grading of astrocytomas and oligodendrogliomas. *In* Fields WS (ed): Primary Brain Tumors. A Review of Histologic Classification. New York, Springer Verlag, 1989, pp 171–180.

152. Kim L, Hochberg FH, Thornton AF, et al: Procarbazine, lomustine, and vincristine (PCV) chemotherapy for grade III and IV oligoastrocytomas. J Neurosurg 85:602–607, 1996.

153. Jenkins RB, Kimmel DW, Moertel CA, et al: A cytogenetic study of 53 human gliomas. Cancer Genet Cytogenet 39:253–279, 1989.

154. Ransom DT, Ritland SR, Kimmel DW, et al: Cytogenetic and loss of heterozygosity studies in ependymomas, pilocytic astrocytomas, and oligodendrogliomas. Genes Chromosomes Cancer 5:348–356, 1992.

155. von Deimling A, Louis DN, von Ammon K, et al: Evidence for a tumor suppressor gene on chromosome 19q associated with human astrocytomas, oligodendrogliomas, and mixed gliomas. Cancer Res 52:4277–4279, 1992.

156. Maintz D, Fiedler K, Koopmann J, et al: Molecular genetic evidence for subtypes of oligoastrocytomas. J Neuropathol Exp Neurol 56:1098–1104, 1997.

157. Ohgaki H, Eibl RH, Wiestler OD, et al: *p53* mutations in nonastrocytic human brain tumors. Cancer Res 51:6202–6205, 1991.

158. Reifenberger J, Reifenberger G, Liu L, et al: Molecular genetic analysis of oligodendroglial tumors shows preferential allelic deletions on 19q and 1p. Am J Pathol 145:1175–1190, 1994.

159. Kraus JA, Koopmann J, Kaskel P, et al: Shared allelic losses on chromosomes 1p and 19q suggest a common origin of oligodendroglioma and oligo-astrocytoma. J Neuropathol Exp Neurol 54:91–95, 1995.

160. Zagzag D, Miller DC, Kleinman GM, et al: Demyelinating disease versus tumor in surgical neuropathology. Clues to a correct pathological diagnosis. Am J Surg Pathol 17:537–545, 1993.

161. Min K-W, Scheithauer BW: Clear cell ependymoma. A mimic of oligodendrogliomas. Clinicopathologic and ultrastructural considerations. Am J Surg Pathol 21:820–826, 1997.

162. Russell DS, Rubinstein LJ: Pathology of Tumours of the Nervous System, 5th ed. London, Edward Arnold, 1989, pp 187–219.

163. Yates AJ, Becker LE, Sachs LA: Brain tumors in childhood. Childs Brain 5:31–39, 1979.

164. Nazar GB, Hoffman HJ, Becker LE, et al: Infratentorial ependymomas in childhood. Prognostic factors and treatment. J Neurosurg 72:408–417, 1990.

165. Schiffer D, Chio A, Giordana MT, et al: Histologic prognostic factors in ependymoma. Childs Nerv Syst 7:177–182, 1991.

166. Salazar OM, Castro-Vita H, VanHoutte P, et al: Improved survival in cases of intracranial ependymoma after radiation therapy. Late report and recommendations. J Neurosurg 59:652–659, 1983.

167. Morantz RA, Kepes JJ, Batnitzky S, Materson BJ: Extraspinal ependymomas. Report of three cases. J Neurosurg 51:383–391, 1979.

168. Kline MJ, Kays DW, Rojiani AM: Extradural myxopapillary ependymoma. Report of two cases and review of the literature. Pediatr Pathol Lab Med 16:813–822, 1996.

169. Louis DN, Ramesh V, Gusella JF: Neuropathology and molecular genetics of neurofibromatosis 2 and related tumors. Brain Pathol 5:163–172, 1995.

170. Mannoji H, Becker LE: Ependymal and choroid plexus tumors. Cytokeratin and GFAP expression. Cancer 61:1377–1385, 1988.

171. Kaneko Y, Takeshita I, Matsushima T, et al: Immunohistochemical study of ependymal neoplasms. Histological subtypes and glial and epithelial characteristics. Virchows Arch A Pathol Anat Histopathol 417:97–103, 1990.

172. Hirato J, Nakazato Y, Ogawa A: Expression of non-glial intermediate filament proteins in gliomas. Clin Neuropathol 13:1–11, 1994.

173. Min KW, Scheithauer BW: Clear cell ependymoma. A mimic of oligodendroglioma. Clinicopathologic and ultrastructural considerations. Am J Surg Pathol 21:820–826, 1997.

174. Shaw EG, Evans RG, Scheithauer BW, et al: Radiotherapeutic management of adult intraspinal ependymomas. Int J Radiat Oncol Biol Phys 12:323–327, 1986.

175. Ross GW, Rubinstein LJ: Lack of histopathological correlation of malignant ependymomas with postoperative survival. J Neurosurg 70:31–36, 1989.

176. Ernestus RI, Wilcke O, Schoroder R: Supratentorial ependymomas in childhood. Clinicopathological findings and prognosis. Acta Neurochir 111:96–102, 1991.

177. Figarella-Branger D, Gambarelli D, Dollo C, et al: Infratentorial ependymomas of childhood. Correlation between histological features, immunohistochemical phenotype, silver nucleolar organizer region staining values and post-operative survival in 16 cases. Acta Neuropathol 82:208–216, 1991.

178. Bouffet E, Perilong G, Canete A, Massimino A: Intracranial ependymomas in children. A review of prognostic factors and a plea for cooperation. Med Pediatr Oncol 30:319–329, 1998.

179. Duffner PK, Krischer JP, Sanford RA, et al: Prognostic factors in infants and very young children with intracranial ependymomas. Pediatr Neurosurg 28:215–222, 1998.

180. Sala F, Talacchi A, Mazza C, et al: Prognostic factors in childhood intracranial ependymomas. The role of age and tumor location. Pediatr Neurosurg 28:135–142, 1998.

181. Rezai AR, Woo HH, Lee M, et al: Disseminated ependymomas of the central nervous system. J Neurosurg 85:618–624, 1996.

182. Schiffer D, Chio A, Cravioto H, et al: Ependymoma. Internal correlations among pathological signs. The anaplastic variant. Neurosurgery 29:206–210, 1991.

183. Schiffer D, Chio A, Giordana MT, et al: Proliferating cell nuclear antigen expression in brain tumors, and its prognostic role in ependymomas. An immunohistochemical study. Acta Neuropathol 85:495–502, 1993.

184. Rushing EJ, Yashima K, Brown DF, et al: Expression of telomerase RNA component correlates with the MIB-1 proliferation index in ependymomas. J Neuropathol Exp Neurol 56:1142–1146, 1997.

185. Rushing EJ, Brown DF, Hladik CL, et al: Correlation of bcl-2, p53, and MIB-1 expression with ependymoma grade and subtype. Mod Pathol 11:464–470, 1998.

186. Prayson RA: Clinicopathologic study of 61 patients with ependymoma including MIB-1 immunohistochemistry. Ann Diagn Pathol 3:11–18, 1999.

187. Sonneland PR, Scheithauer BW, Onofrio BM: Myxopapillary ependymoma. A clinicopathologic and immunocytochemical study of 77 cases. Cancer 56:883–893, 1985.

188. Sato H, Ohmura K, Mizushima M, et al: Myxopapillary ependymoma of the lateral ventricle. A study on the mechanism of its stromal myxoid change. Acta Pathol Jap 33:1017–1025, 1983.

189. Pulitzer DR, Martin PC, Collins PC, Ralph DR: Subcutaneous sacrococcygeal ("myxopapillary") ependymal rests. Am J Surg Pathol 12:672–677, 1988.

190. Rawlinson DG, Herman MM, Rubinstein LJ: The fine structure of a myxopapillary ependymoma of the filum terminale. Acta Neuropathol 25:1–13, 1973.

191. Specht CS, Smith TW, DeGirolami U, Price JM: Myxopapillary ependymoma of the filum terminale. A light and electron microscopic study. Cancer 58:310–317, 1986.

192. Scheithauer BW: Symptomatic subependymoma. Report of 21 cases with review of the literature. J Neurosurg 49:689–696, 1978.

193. Lombardi D, Scheithauer BW, Meyer FB, et al: Symptomatic subependymoma. A clinicopathological and flow cytometric study. J Neurosurg 75:583–588, 1991.

194. Ernestus RI, Schroder R: Clinical aspects and pathology of intracranial subependymoma—18 personal cases and review of the literature. Neurochirurgica 36:194–202, 1993.

195. Chiechi MV, Smirniotopoulus JG, Jones RV: Intracranial subependymomas. CT and MR imaging features in 24 cases. AJR Am J Roentgenol 165:1245–1250, 1995.

196. Pagni CA, Canavero S, Giordana MT, et al: Spinal intramedullary subependymomas. Case report and review of the literature. Neurosurgery 30:115–117, 1992.

197. Jallo GI, Zagzag D, Epstein F: Intramedullary subependymoma of the spinal cord. Neurosurgery 38:251–257, 1996.

198. Mineura K, Shioya H, Kowada M, et al: Subependymoma of the septum pellucidum. Characterization by PET. J Neurooncol 32:143–147, 1997.

199. Hamilton RL, Pollack IF: The molecular biology of ependymomas. Brain Pathol 7:807–822, 1997.

200. Ohgaki H, Eibl RH, Schwab M, et al: Mutations of the p53 tumor suppressor gene in neoplasms of the human nervous system. Mol Carcinog 8:74–80, 1993.

201. Fink KL, Rushing EJ, Schold SC Jr, Nisen PD: Infrequency of p53 gene mutations in ependymomas. J Neurooncol 27:111–115, 1996.

202. Birch BD, Johnson JP, Parsa A, et al: Frequent type 2 neurofibromatosis gene transcript mutations in sporadic intramedullary spinal cord ependymomas. Neurosurgery 39:135–140, 1996.

203. Rubio MP, Correa KM, Ramesh V, et al: Analysis of the neurofibromatosis 2 gene in human ependymomas and astrocytomas. Cancer Res 54:45–57, 1994.

204. Slavc I, MacCollin MM, Dunn M, et al: Exon scanning for mutations of the NF2 gene in pediatric ependymomas, rhabdoid tumors and meningiomas. Int J Cancer 64:243–247, 1995.

205. von Haken MS, White EC, Daneshvar Shyesther L, et al: Molecular genetic analysis of chromosome arm 17p and chromosome arm 22q DNA sequences in sporadic pediatric ependymomas. Genes Chromosomes Cancer 17:37–44, 1996.

206. Burger PC, Scheithauer BW: Tumors of the Central Nervous System. Atlas of Tumor Pathology. Third Series, Fascicle 10. Washington, DC, Armed Forces Institute of Pathology, 1994, pp 120–136.

207. Rubinstein LJ: Tumors of the Central Nervous System. Atlas of Tumor Pathology. Fascicle 6. Washington, DC, Armed Forces Institute of Pathology, 1972, pp 257–267.

208. Laurence KM: The biology of choroid plexus papilloma in infancy and childhood. Acta Neurochir 50:79–90, 1979.

209. Russell DS, Rubinstein LJ: Pathology of Tumours of the Nervous System, 5th ed. London, Edward Arnold, 1989, pp 394–404.

210. Romano F, Bratta FG, Caruso G, et al: Prenatal diagnosis of choroid plexus papillomas of the lateral ventricle. A report of two cases. Perinatal Diag 16:567–571, 1996.

211. Yoshino A, Katayama Y, Watanabe T, et al: Multiple choroid plexus papillomas of the lateral ventricle distinct from villous hypertrophy. J Neurosurg 88:581–585, 1998.

212. Pencalet P, Sainte-Rose C, Lellouch-Tubiana A, et al: Papillomas and carcinomas of the choroid plexus in children. J Neurosurg 88:521–528, 1998.

213. Bergsagel DJ, Finegold MJ, Butel JS, et al: DNA sequences similar to those of simian virus 40 in ependymomas and choroid plexus tumors of childhood. N Engl J Med 326:988–993, 1992.

214. Lednicky JA, Garcea RL, Bergsagel DJ, Butel JS: Natural simian virus 40 strains are present in human choroid plexus and ependymoma tumors. Virology 212:710–717, 1995.

215. Brinster RL, Chen HY, Messing A, et al: Transgenic mice harboring SV40 T-antigen genes develop characteristic brain tumors. Cell 37:367–379, 1984.

216. Hamano K, Matsubara T, Shibata S, et al: Aicardi syndrome accompanied by auditory disturbance and multiple brain tumors. Brain Dev 13:438–441, 1991.

217. Trifiletti RR, Incorpora G, Polizzi A, et al: Aicardi syndrome with multiple tumors. A case report with literature review. Brain Dev 17:283–285, 1995.

218. Aguiar MD, Cavalcanti M, Barbosa H, et al: Aicardi syndrome and choroid plexus papilloma. A rare association. Case report. Arq Neuropsiquiatr 54:313–317, 1996.

219. Uchiyama CM, Carey CM, Cherny WB, et al: Choroid plexus

papilloma and cysts in the Aicardi syndrome. Case reports. Pediatr Neurosurg 27:100–104, 1997.

220. Aicardi J, Chevrie J-J: The Aicardi syndrome. *In* Lassonde M, Jeeves MA (eds): Callosal Agenesis. A Natural Split Brain? New York, Plenum Press, 1994, pp 7–17.

221. Kawamata T, Kuco O, Kawamura H, et al: Ossified choroid plexus papilloma—case report. No Shinkei Geka (Neurol Surg) 16:989–994, 1988.

222. Doran SE, Blaivas M, Dauser RC: Bone formation within a choroid plexus papilloma. Case report. Pediatr Neurosurg 23:216–218, 1995.

223. Yap WM, Chuah KL, Tan PH: Choroid plexus papilloma with chondroid metaplasia. Histopathology 31:384–392, 1997.

224. Kepes JJ: Oncocytic transformation of choroid plexus epithelium. Acta Neuropathol 62:145–148, 1983.

225. Bonnin JM, Colon LE, Morawetz RB: Focal glial differentiation and oncocytic transformation in choroid plexus papilloma. Acta Neuropathol 72:277–280, 1987.

226. Doglioni C, Dell'Orto P, Coggi G, et al: Choroid plexus tumors. An immunocytochemical study with particular reference to the coexpression of intermediate filament proteins. Am J Pathol 127:519–529, 1987.

227. Lopes MBS, Rosemberg S, Cardoso de Almeida PC, Pestana CB: Glial fibrillary acidic protein and cytokeratin in choroid plexus tumors. An immunohistochemical study. Pathol Res Pract 185:339–341, 1989.

228. Paulus W, Jänisch W: Clinicopathologic correlations in epithelial choroid plexus neoplasms. A study of 52 cases. Acta Neuropathol 80:635–641, 1990.

229. Gottschalk J, Jautzke G, Paulus W, et al: The use of immunomorphology to differentiate choroid plexus tumors from metastatic carcinomas. Cancer 72:1343–1349, 1993.

230. Lach B, Scheithauer BW, Gregor A, Wick MR: Colloid cyst of the third ventricle. A comparative immunohistochemical study of neuraxis cysts and choroid plexus epithelium. J Neurosurg 78:101–111, 1993.

231. Megerian CA, Pilch BZ, Bhan AK, McKenna MJ: Differential expression of transthyretin in papillary tumors of the endolymphatic sac and choroid plexus. Laryngoscope 107:216–221, 1997.

232. Herbert J, Cavallaro T, Dwork AJ: A marker for primary choroid plexus neoplasms. Am J Pathol 136:1317–1325, 1990.

233. Albrecht S, Rouah E, Becker LE, Bruner J: Transthyretin immunoreactivity in choroid plexus neoplasms and brain metastases. Mod Pathol 4:610–614, 1991.

234. Masuzawa T, Shimabukuro H, Yoshimizu N, Sato F: Ultrastructure of disseminated choroid plexus papilloma. Acta Neuropathol 54:321–324, 1981.

235. Aguzzi A, Weber T, Paulus W: Choroid plexus tumours. *In* Kleihues P, Cavenee WK (eds): Pathology and Genetics of Tumours of the Nervous System. Lyon, International Agency for Research on Cancer (IARC), 1997, pp 58–60.

236. McGirr SJ, Ebersold MJ, Scheithauer BW: Choroid plexus papillomas. Long term follow-up of a surgically treated series. J Neurosurg 69:843–849, 1988.

237. Jay V, Parkinson D, Becker LE, Chan FW: Cell kinetic analysis in pediatric brain and spinal cord tumors. A study of 117 cases with Ki-67 quantitation and flow cytometry. Pediatr Pathol 14:253–276, 1994.

238. Vajtai I, Varga Z, Aguzzi A: MIB-1 immunoreactivity reveals different labelling in low-grade and in malignant epithelial neoplasms of the choroid plexus. Histopathology 29:147–151, 1996.

239. Newbould MJ, Kelsey AM, Arango JC, et al: The choroid plexus carcinomas of childhood. Histopathology, immunocytochemistry and clinicopathological correlations. Histopathology 26:137–143, 1995.

240. Berger C, Thiesse P, Lellouch-Tubiana A, et al: Choroid plexus carcinomas in childhood. Clinical features and prognostic factors. Neurosurgery 42:470–475, 1998.

241. Vraa-Jensen G: Papilloma of the choroid plexus with pulmonary metastases. Acta Psych Neurol 25:299–306, 1950.

242. Coffin CM, Wick MR, Braun JT, Dehner LP: Choroid plexus neoplasms. Clinicopathologic and immunohistochemical studies. Am J Surg Pathol 10:394–404, 1986.

243. Punnett HH, Tomczak EZ, de Chadaverian JP, Kanev PM: Cytogenetics analysis of a choroid plexus papilloma. Genes Chromosomes Cancer 10:282–285, 1994.

244. Rolando B, Pinto A: Hyperdiploid karyotype in a choroid plexus papilloma. Cancer Genet Cytogenet 90:130–131, 1996.

245. Li YS, Fan YS, Armstrong RF: Endoreduplication and telomeric association in a choroid plexus carcinoma. Cancer Genet Cytogenet 87:7–10, 1996.

246. Dobin SM, Donner LR: Pigmented choroid plexus carcinoma. A cytogenetic and ultrastructural study. Cancer Genet Cytogenet 96:37–41, 1997.

247. Norman MG, Harrison KJ, Poskitt KJ, Kalousek DK: Duplication of 9p and hyperplasia of the choroid plexus. A pathologic, radiologic, and molecular cytogenetics study. Pediatr Pathol Lab Med 15:109–120, 1995.

248. Yuasa H, Tokito S, Tokunaga M: Primary carcinoma of the choroid plexus in Li-Fraumeni syndrome. Case report. Neurosurgery 32:131–133, 1993.

249. Sedlacek Z, Kodet R, Seemanova E, et al: Two Li-Fraumeni syndrome families with novel germline p53 mutations. Loss of the wild-type p53 allele in only 50% of tumours. Br J Cancer 77:1034–1039, 1998.

250. Russell DS, Rubinstein LJ: Pathology of Tumours of the Nervous System, 5th ed. London, Edward Arnold, 1989, pp 161–169.

251. Thiessen B, Finlay J, Kulkarni R, Rosenblum MK: Astroblastoma. Does histology predict biologic behavior? J Neurooncol 40:59–65, 1998.

252. Rubinstein LJ, Herman MM: The astroblastoma and its possible cytogenetic relationship to the tanycyte. An electron microscopic, immunohistochemical, tissue- and organ-culture study. Acta Neuropathol 78:472–483, 1989.

253. Cabello A, Madero S, Castresana A, Diaz Lobato R: Astroblastoma. Electron microscopy and immunohistochemical findings. Case report. Surg Neurol 35:116–121, 1991.

254. Pizer BL, Moss T, Oakhill A, et al: Congenital astroblastoma. An immunohistochemical study. Case report. J Neurosurg 83:550–555, 1995.

255. Jay V, Edwards V, Squire J, Rutka J: Astroblastoma. Report of a case with ultrastructural, cell kinetic, and cytogenetic analysis. Pediatr Pathol 13:323–332, 1993.

256. Bonnin JM, Rubinstein LJ: Astroblastomas. A pathological study of 23 tumors, with a postoperative follow-up in 13 patients. Neurosurgery 25:6–13, 1989.

257. Lantos PL, Bruner JM: Gliomatosis cerebri. *In* Kleihues P, Cavenee WK (eds): Pathology and Genetics of Tumours of the Nervous System. Lyon, International Agency for Research on Cancer (IARC), 1997, pp 65–66.

258. Balko MG, Blisard KS, Samaha FJ: Oligodendroglial gliomatosis cerebri. Hum Pathol 23:706–707, 1992.

259. Hassoun J, Gambarelli D, Grisoli F, et al: Central neurocytoma. An electron-microscopic study of two cases. Acta Neuropathol 56:151–156, 1982.

260. Hessler RB, Lopes MBS, Frankfurter A, et al: Cytoskeletal immunohistochemistry of central neurocytomas. Am J Surg Pathol 16:1031–1038, 1991.

261. Louis DN, Swearingen B, Linggood RM, et al: Central nervous system neurocytoma and neuroblastoma in adults—report of eight cases. J Neurooncol 9:231–238, 1990.

262. Miller DC, Kim R, Zagzag D: Neurocytomas. Non-classical sites and mixed elements. J Neuropathol Exp Neurol 51:364, 1992.

263. Nishio S, Takeshita I, Fukui M: Primary cerebral ganglioneurocytoma in an adult. Cancer 66:358–362, 1990.

264. Coca S, Moreno M, Martos JA, et al: Neurocytoma of spinal cord. Acta Neuropathol 87:537–540, 1994.

265. Enam SA, Rosenblum ML, Ho K-L: Neurocytoma in the cerebellum. Case report. J Neurosurg 87:100–102, 1997.

266. Barbosa MD, Balsitis M, Jaspan T, Lowe J: Intraventricular neurocytoma. A clinical and pathological study of three cases and review of the literature. Neurosurgery 26:1045–1054, 1990.

267. Hassoun J, Söylemezoglu F, Gambarelli D, et al: Central neurocytoma. A synopsis of clinical and histological features. Brain Pathol 3:297–306, 1993.

268. Robbins P, Segal A, Narula S, et al: Central neurocytoma. A clinicopathological, immunohistochemical and ultrastructural study of 7 cases. Pathol Res Pract 191:100–111, 1995.

269. von Deimling A, Janzer R, Kleihues P, Wiestler OD: Patterns of differentiation potential in central neurocytoma. Acta Neuropathol 79:473–479, 1990.

270. von Deimling A, Kleihues P, Saremaslani P, et al: Histogenesis and differentiation potential of central neurocytomas. Lab Invest 64:585–591, 1991.

271. Yasargil MG, von Ammon K, von Deimling A, et al: Central neurocytoma. Histopathological variants and therapeutic approaches. J Neurosurg 76:32–37, 1992.

272. Sgouros S, Jackowski A, Carey MO: Central neurocytoma without intraventricular extension. Surg Neurol 42:335–339, 1994.

273. Kim DG, Kim JS, Chi JG, et al: Central neurocytoma: proliferative potential and biological behavior. J Neurosurg 84:742–747, 1996.

274. Eng DY, DeMonte F, Ginsberg L, et al: Craniospinal dissemination of central neurocytoma. J Neurosurg 86:547–552, 1997.

275. Söylemezoglu F, Scheithauer BW, Esteve J, Kleihues P: Atypical central neurocytoma. J Neuropathol Exp Neurol 56:551–556, 1997.

276. Russell DS, Rubinstein LJ: Pathology of Tumours of the Nervous System, 5th ed. London, Edward Arnold, 1989, pp 289–306.

277. Russo CP, Katz DS, Corona RJ, Winfield JA: Gangliocytoma of the cervicothoracic spinal cord. AJNR Am J Neuroradiol 16:889–891, 1995.

278. Beal MF, Kleinman GM, Pjemann RG, Hochberg FH: Gangliocytoma of third ventricle. Hyperphagia, somnolence, and dementia. Neurology 31:1224–1228, 1981.

279. Towfighi J, Salam MM, McLendon RE, et al: Ganglion cell-containing tumors of the pituitary gland. Arch Pathol Lab Med 120:369–377, 1996.

280. Zuniga OF, Tanner SM, Wild WO, Mosier HD Jr: Hamartoma of CNS associated with precocious puberty. Am J Dis Child 137:127–133, 1983.

281. Boyko OB, Curnes JT, Oakes WJ, Burger PC: Hamartomas of the tuber cinereum. CT, MR, and pathologic findings. AJNR Am J Neuroradiol 12:309–314, 1991.

282. Tuli S, Provias JP, Bernstein M: Lhermitte-Duclos disease. Literature review and novel treatment strategy. Can J Neurol Sci 24:155–160, 1997.

283. Vinchon M, Blond S, Lejeune JP, et al: Association of Lhermitte-Duclos and Cowden disease. Report of a new case and review of the literature. J Neurol Neurosurg Psychiatry 57:699–704, 1994.

284. Kulkantrakorn K, Awwas EE, Levy B, et al: MRI in Lhermitte-Duclos disease. Neurology 48:725–731, 1997.

285. Shiruba RA, Gessaga EC, Eng LF, et al: Lhermitte-Duclos disease. An immunohistochemical study of the cerebellar cortex. Acta Neuropathol 75:474–480, 1988.

286. Faillot T, Sichez J-P, Brault J-L, et al: Lhermitte-Duclos disease (dysplastic gangliocytoma of the cerebellum). Report of a case and review of the literature. Acta Neurochir 105:44–49, 1990.

287. Reznik M, Schoenen J: Lhermitte-Duclos disease. Acta Neuropathol 59:88–94, 1983.

288. Yachnis AT, Trojanowski JQ, Memmo M, Schlaepfer WW: Expression of neurofilament proteins in the hypertrophic granule cells of Lhermitte-Duclos disease. An explanation for the mass effect and the myelination of parallel fibers in the disease state. J Neuropathol Exp Neurol 47:206–216, 1988.

289. Marano SR, Johnson PC, Spetzler RF: Recurrent Lhermitte-Duclos disease in a child. J Neurosurg 69:599–603, 1988.

290. Williams DW 3d, Elster AD, Ginsberg LE, Stanton C: Recurrent Lhermitte-Duclos disease. Report of two cases and association with Cowden's disease. AJNR Am J Neuroradiol 13:287–290, 1992.

291. Stapleton SR, Wilkins PR, Bell BA: Recurrent dysplastic cerebellar gangliocytoma (Lhermitte-Duclos disease) presenting with subarachnoid haemorrhage. Br J Neurosurg 6:153–156, 1992.

292. Hashimoto H, Iida J, Masui K, et al: Recurrent Lhermitte-Duclos disease—case report. Neurol Med Chir 37:692–696, 1997.

293. Wolf HK, Muller MB, Spanle M, et al: Ganglioglioma. A detailed histopathological and immunohistochemical analysis of 61 cases. Acta Neuropathol 88:166–173, 1994.

294. Sutton LN, Packer RJ, Rorke LB, et al: Cerebral gangliogliomas during childhood. Neurosurgery 13:124–128, 1983.

295. Johnson JH Jr, Hariharan S, Berman J, et al: Clinical outcome of pediatric gangliogliomas. Ninety-nine cases over 20 years. Pediatr Neurosurg 27:203–207, 1997.

296. Russell DS, Rubinstein LJ: Pathology of Tumours of the Nervous System, 5th ed. London, Edward Arnold, 1989, pp 289–302.

297. Hirose T, Scheithauer BW, Lopes MB, et al: Ganglioglioma. An ultrastructural and immunohistochemical study. Cancer 79:989–1003, 1997.

298. Hakim R, Loeffler JS, Anthony DC, Black PM: Ganglioglioma in adults. Cancer 79:127–131, 1997.

299. Prayson RA, Khajavi K, Comair YG: Cortical architectural abnormalities and MIB1 immunoreactivity in gangliogliomas. A study of 60 patients with intracranial tumors. J Neuropathol Exp Neurol 54:513–520, 1995.

300. Allegranza A, Pileri S, Frank G, Ferracini R: Cerebral ganglioglioma with anaplastic oligodendroglial component. Histopathology 17:439–441, 1990.

301. Miller DC, Lang FF, Epstein FJ: Central nervous system gangliogliomas. Part 1. Pathology. J Neurosurg 79:859–866, 1993.

302. Jaffey PB, Mundt AJ, Baunoch DA, et al: The clinical significance of extracellular matrix in gangliogliomas. J Neuropathol Exp Neurol 55:1246–1252, 1996.

303. Miller DC, Koslow M, Budzilovich GN, Burstein DE: Synaptophysin. A sensitive and specific marker for ganglion cells in central nervous system neoplasms. Hum Pathol 21:271–276, 1990.

304. Zhang PJ, Rosenblum MK: Synaptophysin expression in the human spinal cord. Diagnostic implications of an immunohistochemcial study. Am J Surg Pathol 20:273–276, 1996.

305. Quinn B: Synaptophysin staining in normal brain. Importance for diagnosis of ganglioglioma. Am J Surg Pathol 22:550–556, 1998.

306. Komori T, Scheithauer BW, Anthony DC, et al: Papillary glioneuronal tumor. A new variant of mixed neuronal-glial neoplasm. Am J Surg Pathol 22:1171–1183, 1998.

307. VandenBerg SR, May EE, Rubinstein LJ, et al: Desmoplastic supratentorial neuroepithelial tumors of infancy with divergent differentiation ("desmoplastic infantile ganglioglioma"). Report on 11 cases of a distinctive embryonal tumor with favorable prognosis. J Neurosurg 66:58–71, 1987.

308. Taratuto AL, Rorke LB: Desmoplastic cerebral astrocytoma of infancy and desmoplastic infantile ganglioglioma. In Kleihues P, Cavenee WK (eds): Pathology and Genetics of Tumours of the Nervous System. Lyon, International Agency for Research on Cancer (IARC), 1997, pp 70–72.

309. Daumas-Duport C, Scheithauer BW, Chodkiewicz JP, et al: Dysembryoplastic neuroepithelial tumor. A surgically curable tumor of young patients with intractable partial seizures. Report of thirty-nine cases. Neurosurgery 23:545–556, 1988.

310. Rosemberg S, Vieira GS: Dysembryoplastic neuroepithelial tumor. An epidemiological study from a single institution. Arq Neuropsiquiatr 56:232–236, 1998.

311. Wolf HK, Campos MG, Zentner J, et al: Surgical pathology of temporal lobe epilepsy. Experience with 216 cases. J Neuropathol Exp Neurol 52:499–506, 1993.

312. Daumas-Duport C: Dysembryoplastic neuroepithelial tumours. Brain Pathol 3:283–295, 1993.

313. Cervera-Pierot P, Varlet P, Chodkiewicz JP, Daumas-Duport C: Dysembryoplastic neuroepithelial tumors located in the caudate nucleus area. Report of four cases. Neurosurgery 40:1065–1069, 1997.

314. Kuchelmeister K, Demirel T, Schlorer E, et al: Dysembryoplastic neuroepithelial tumour of the cerebellum. Acta Neuropathol 89:385–390, 1995.

315. Raymond AA, Halpin SF, Alsanjari N, et al: Dysembryoplas-

tic neuroepithelial tumor. Features in 16 patients. Brain 117: 461–475, 1994.

316. Ostertun B, Wolf HK, Campos MG, et al: Dysembryoplastic neuroepithelial tumors. MR and CT evaluation. AJNR Am J Neuroradiol 17:419–430, 1996.

317. Hirose T, Scheithauer BW, Lopes MBS, VandenBerg SR: Dysembryoplastic neuroepithelial tumor (DNT). An immunohistochemical and ultrastructural study. J Neuropathol Exp Neurol 53:184–195, 1994.

318. Taratuto AL, Pomata H, Sevlever G, et al: Dysembryoplastic neuroepithelial tumor. Morphological, immunocytochemical, and deoxyribonucleic acid analyses in a pediatric series. Neurosurgery 36:474–481, 1995.

319. Prayson RA, Morris HH, Estes ML, Comair YG: Dysembryoplastic neuroepithelial tumor. A clinicopathologic and immunohistochemical study of 11 tumors including MIB1 immunoreactivity. Clin Neuropathol 15:47–53, 1996.

320. Rorke LB: Primitive neuroectodermal tumor—a concept requiring an apologia? In Fields WS (ed): Primary Brain Tumors. A Review of Histologic Classification. New York, Springer Verlag, 1989, pp 5–15.

321. Rubinstein LJ: Justification for a cytogenetic scheme of embryonal central neuroepithelial tumors. In Fields WS (ed): Primary Brain Tumors. A Review of Histologic Classification. New York, Springer Verlag, 1989, pp 16–27.

322. Rubinstein LJ: Glioma cytology and differentiation viewed through the window of neoplastic vulnerability. In Salcman M (ed): Neurobiology of Brain Tumors. Baltimore, Williams & Wilkins, 1991, pp 35–51.

323. Lopes MBS, Scheithauer BW, VandenBerg SR: Ontogeny and classification of brain tumors. Neurooncology 23(part I):1–16, 1997.

324. Roberts RO, Lynch CF, Jones MP, Hart MN: Medulloblastoma. A population-based study of 532 cases. J Neuropathol Exp Neurol 50:134–144, 1991.

325. Hubbard JL, Scheithauer BW, Kispert DB, et al: Adult cerebellar medulloblastoma. The pathological, radiographic, and clinical disease spectrum. J Neurosurg 70:536–544, 1989.

326. Russell DS, Rubinstein LJ: Pathology of Tumours of the Nervous System, 5th ed. London, Edward Arnold, 1989, pp 247–289.

327. Kleihues P, Aguzzi A, Shibata T, Wiestler OD: Immunohistochemical assessment of differentiation and DNA replication in human brain tumors. In Fields WS (ed): Primary Brain Tumors. A Review of Histologic Classification. New York, Springer Verlag, 1989, pp 123–132.

328. Katsetos CD, Liu HM, Zacks SI: Immunohistochemical and ultrastructural observations on Homer Wright (neuroblastic) rosettes and the "pale islands" of human cerebellar medulloblastomas. Hum Pathol 19:1219–1227, 1988.

329. Katsetos CD, Herman MM, Frankfurter A, et al: Cerebellar desmoplastic medulloblastomas. A further immunohistochemical characterization of the reticulin-free pale islands. Arch Pathol Lab Med 113:1019–1029, 1989.

330. Molenaar WM, Jansson DS, Gould VE, et al: Molecular markers of primitive neuroectodermal tumors and other pediatric central nervous system tumors. Lab Invest 61:635–643, 1989.

331. Gould VE, Rorke LB, Jansson DS, et al: Primitive neuroectodermal tumors of the central nervous system express neuroendocrine markers and may express all classes of intermediate filaments. Hum Pathol 21:245–252, 1990.

332. Trojanowski JQ, Tohyama T, Lee VM-Y: Medulloblastomas and related primitive neuroectodermal brain tumors of childhood recapitulate molecular milestones in the maturation of neuroblasts. Mol Chem Neuropathol 17:121–135, 1992.

333. Schindler E, Gullotta F: Glial fibrillary acidic protein in medulloblastomas and other embryonic CNS tumours of children. Virchows Arch [A] 398:263–275, 1983.

334. Coffin CM, Mukai K, Dehner LP: Glial differentiation in medulloblastomas. Histogenetic insight, glial reaction, or invasion of brain? Am J Surg Pathol 7:555–565, 1983.

335. Korf HW, Czerwionka M, Reiner J, et al: Immunocytochemical evidence of molecular photoreceptor markers in cerebellar medulloblastomas. Cancer 60:1763–1766, 1987.

336. Bonnin JM, Perentes E: Retinal S-antigen immunoreactivity in medulloblastomas. Acta Neuropathol 76:204–207, 1988.

337. Burger PC, Grahmann FC, Bliestle A, Kleihues P: Differentiation in the medulloblastoma. A histological and immunohistochemical study. Acta Neuropathol 73:115–123, 1987.

338. Garton GR, Schomberg PJ, Scheithauer BW, et al: Medulloblastoma—prognostic factors and outcome of treatment. Review of the Mayo Clinic experience. Mayo Clin Proc 65: 1077–1086, 1990.

339. Biegel JA, Rorke LA, Packer RJ, et al: Isochromosome 17q in primitive neuroectodermal tumors of the central nervous system. Genes Chromosomes Cancer 1:139–147, 1989.

340. Karnes PS, Tran TN, Cui MY, et al: Cytogenetic analysis of 39 pediatric central nervous system tumors. Cancer Genet Cytogenet 59:12–19, 1992.

341. Giordana MT, Migheli A, Pavanelli E: Isochromosome 17q is a constant finding in medulloblastoma. An interphase cytogenetic study on tissue sections. Neuropathol Appl Neurobiol 24:233–238, 1998.

342. Saylors RL, Sidransky D, Friedman HS, et al: Infrequent p53 gene mutations in medulloblastoma. Cancer Res 51:4721–4723, 1991.

343. Biegel JA, Wentz E: No preferential parent of origin for the isochromosome 17q in childhood primitive neuroectodermal tumor (medulloblastoma). Genes Chromosomes Cancer 18: 143–146, 1997.

344. Pietsch T, Koch A, Wiestler OD: Molecular genetic studies in medulloblastomas. Evidence for tumor suppressor genes at the chromosomal regions 1q31-32 and 17p13. Klin Padiatr 209:150–155, 1997.

345. Steichen-Gersdorf E, Baumgartner M, Kreczy A, et al: Deletion mapping on chromosome 17p in medulloblastoma. Br J of Cancer 76:1284–1287, 1997.

346. Koch A, Tonn J, Kraus N, et al: Molecular analysis of the lissencephaly gene 1 (LIS-1) in medulloblastomas. Neuropathol Appl Neurobiol 22:233–242, 1996.

347. Giangaspero F, Bigner SH, Giordana MT, et al: Medulloblastoma. In Kleihues P, Cavenee WK (eds): Pathology and Genetics of Tumours of the Nervous System. Lyon, International Agency for Research on Cancer (IARC), 1997, pp 96–103.

348. Horten BC, Rubinstein LJ: Primary cerebral neuroblastoma. A clinicopathologic study of 35 cases. Brain 99:735–756, 1976.

349. Bennett JP Jr, Rubinstein LJ: The biologic behavior of primary cerebral neuroblastoma. A reappraisal of the clinical course in a series of 70 cases. Ann Neurol 16:21–27, 1984.

350. Davis PC, Wichman RD, Takei Y, Hoffman JC Jr: Primary cerebral neuroblastoma. CT and MR findings in 12 cases. AJNR Am J Neuroradiol 11:115–120, 1990.

351. Lantos PL, Kleihues P, VandenBerg SR: Tumours of the nervous system. In Graham DI, Lantos PL (eds): Greenfield's Neuropathology, 6th ed. London, Edward Arnold, 1996, pp 682–712.

352. Mørk SJ, Rubinstein LJ: Ependymoblastoma. A reappraisal of a rare embryonal tumor. Cancer 55:1536–1542, 1985.

353. Cervoni L, Celli P, Trillo G, Caruso R: Ependymoblastoma. A clinical review. Neurosurg Rev 18:189–192, 1995.

354. Cruz-Sanchez FF, Haustein J, Rossie ML, et al: Ependymoblastoma. A histological, immunohistochemical and ultrastructural study of five cases. Histopathology 12:17–27, 1988.

355. Pigott TJD, Punt JAG, Lowe JS, et al: The clinical, radiological and histopathological features of cerebral primitive neuroectodermal tumours. Br J Neurosurg 4:287–298, 1990.

356. Langford LA: The ultrastructure of the ependymoblastoma. Acta Neuropathol 71:136–141, 1986.

357. Caccamo DV, Herman MM, Rubinstein LJ: An immunohistochemical study of the primitive and maturing elements of human cerebral medulloepitheliomas. Acta Neuropathol 79: 248–254, 1989.

358. Molloy PT, Yachnis AT, Rorke LB, et al: Central nervous system medulloepithelioma. A series of eight cases including two arising in the pons. J Neurosurg 84:430–436, 1996.

359. Shiurba RA, Buffinger NS, Spencer EM, Urich H: Basic fibroblastic growth factor and somatomedin C in human medulloepithelioma. Cancer 68:798–808, 1991.

360. Herrick MK: Pathology of pineal tumors. *In* Neuwelt EA (ed): Diagnosis and Treatment of Pineal Region Tumors. Baltimore, Williams & Wilkins, 1984, pp 31–60.

361. Bruce JN, Stein BM: Pineal tumors. Neurosurg Clin N Am 1: 123–138, 1990.

362. Schild SE, Scheithauer BW, Schomberg PJ, et al: Pineal parenchymal tumors. Clinical, pathologic, and therapeutic aspects. Cancer 72:870–880, 1993.

363. Hoffman HJ, Yoshida M, Becker LE, et al: Pineal region tumors in childhood. Pediatr Neurosurg 21:91–104, 1994.

364. Vaquero J, Ramiro J, Martínez R, Bravo G: Neurosurgical experience with tumours of the pineal region at Clinica Puerta de Hierro. Acta Neurochir 116:23–32, 1992.

365. Chiechi MV, Smirniotopoulus JG, Mena H: Pineal parenchymal tumors. CT and MR features. J Comput Assist Tomogr 19:509–517, 1995.

366. Schild SE, Scheithauer BW, Haddock MG, et al: Histologically confirmed pineal tumors and other germ cell tumors of the brain. Cancer 78:2564–2571, 1996.

367. Herrick MK, Rubinstein LJ: The cytological differentiating potential of pineal parenchymal neoplasms (true pinealomas). A clinicopathologic study of 28 tumours. Brain 102: 289–320, 1979.

368. Mena H, Rushing EJ, Ribas JL, et al: Tumors of pineal parenchymal cells. A correlation of histological features, including nucleolar organizer regions, with survival in 35 cases. Hum Pathol 26:20–30, 1995.

369. Borit A, Blackwood W, Mair WGP: The separation of pineocytoma from pineoblastoma. Cancer 45:1408–1418, 1980.

370. Russell DS, Rubinstein LJ: Pathology of Tumours of the Nervous System, 5th ed. London, Edward Arnold, 1989, pp 380–394.

371. Coca S, Vaquero J, Escandon J, et al: Immunohistochemical characterization of pineocytomas. Clin Neuropathol 11:298–303, 1992.

372. Lopes MBS, Gonzalez-Fernandez F, Scheithauer BW, VandenBerg SR: Differential expression of retinal proteins in a pineal parenchymal tumor. J Neuropathol Exp Neurol 52: 516–524, 1993.

373. Fevre-Montange M, Jouvet A, Privat K, et al: Immunohistochemical, ultrastructural, biochemical and in vitro studies of a pineocytoma. Acta Neuropathol 95:532–539, 1998.

374. Min KW, Scheithauer BW, Bauserman SC: Pineal parenchymal tumors. An ultrastructural study with prognostic implications. Ultrastruct Pathol 18:69–85, 1994.

375. Perentes E, Rubinstein LJ, Herman MM, Donoso LA: S-antigen immunoreactivity in human pineal glands and pineal parenchymal tumors. A monoclonal antibody study. Acta Neuropathol 71:224–227, 1986.

376. Korf H-W, Klein DC, Zigler JS, et al: S-antigen-like immunoreactivity in a human pineocytoma. Acta Neuropathol 69: 165–167, 1986.

377. Hoffman HJ, Yoshida M, Becker LE, et al: Experience with pineal tumours in childhood. Neurol Res 6:107–112, 1984.

378. Chang SM, Lillis-Hearne PK, Larson DA, et al: Pineoblastoma in adults. Neurosurgery 37:383–390, 1995.

379. Stefanko SZ, Manschot WA: Pinealoblastoma with retinomatous differentiation. Brain 102:321–332, 1979.

380. Bello MJ, Rey JA, De Campos JM, Kusak ME: Chromosomal abnormalities in a pineocytoma. Cancer Genet Cytogenet 71: 185–186, 1993.

381. Sreekantaiah C, Jockin H, Brecher ML, Sandberg AA: Interstitial deletion of chromosome 11q in a pineoblastoma. Cancer Genet Cytogenet 39:125–131, 1989.

382. Tsumanuma I, Sato M, Okazaki H, et al: The analysis of p53 tumor suppressor gene in pineal parenchymal tumors. Noshuyo Byori 12:39–43, 1995.

383. Jennings MT, Gelman R, Hochberg F: Intracranial germ-cell tumors. Natural history and pathogenesis. J Neurosurg 63: 155–167, 1985.

384. Vaquero J, Ramiro J, Martinez R, Bravo G: Neurosurgical experience with tumors of the pineal region at Clinica Puerta de Hierro. Acta Neurochir 16:23–32, 1992.

385. Bjornsson J, Scheithauer BW, Okazaki H, Leech RW: Intracranial germ cell tumors. Pathobiological and immunohisto-

386. chemical aspects of 70 cases. J Neuropathol Exp Neurol 44: 32–46, 1985.

386. Zülch KJ: Brain Tumors. Their Biology and Pathology, 3rd ed. Berlin, Springer-Verlag, 1986.

387. Hoffman HJ, Otsubo H, Hendrick EB, et al: Intracranial germ-cell tumors in children. J Neurosurg 74:545–551, 1991.

388. Handa H, Yamashita J: Current treatment of pineal tumors. Neurol Med Chir (Tokyo) 21:147–154, 1981.

389. Takakura K: Intracranial germ cell tumors. Clin Neurosurg 32:429–444, 1985.

390. Tamaki N, Lin T, Shirataki K, et al: Germ cell tumors of the thalamus and the basal ganglia. Child Nerv Syst 6:3–7, 1990.

391. Russell DS, Rubinstein LJ: Pathology of Tumours of the Nervous System, 5th ed. London, Edward Arnold, 1989, pp 665–687.

392. Kobayashi T, Kageyama N, Kida Y, et al: Unilateral germinomas involving the basal ganglia and thalamus. J Neurosurg 55:55–62, 1981.

393. Masuzawa T, Shimabukuro H, Nakahara N, et al: Germ cell tumors (germinoma and yolk sac tumor) in unusual sites in the brain. Clin Neuropathol 5:190–202, 1986.

394. Ono N, Isobe I, Uki J, et al: Recurrence of primary intracranial germinomas after complete response with radiotherapy. Recurrence patterns and therapy. Neurosurgery 35:615–621, 1994.

395. Aguzzi A, Hedinger CE, Kleihues P, Yasargil MG: Intracranial mixed germ cell tumor with syncytiotrophoblastic giant cells and precocious puberty. Acta Neuropathol 75:427–431, 1988.

396. Komatsu Y, Narushima K, Kobayashi E, et al: CT and MR of germinoma in the basal ganglia. AJNR Am J Neuroradiol 10: S9–S11, 1989.

397. Ng HK, Poon WS, Chan YL: Basal ganglia teratomas. Report of three cases. Aust N Z J Surg 62:436–440, 1992.

398. Yasue M, Tanaka H, Nakajima M, et al: Germ cell tumors of the basal ganglia and thalamus. Pediatr Neurosurg 19:121–126, 1993.

399. Koeleveld RF, Cohen AR: Primary embryonal-cell carcinoma of the parietal lobe. J Neurosurg 75:468–471, 1991.

400. Higano S, Takahashi S, Ishii K, et al: Germinoma originating in the basal ganglia and thalamus. MR and CT evaluation. AJNR Am J Neuroradiol 5:1435–1441, 1994.

401. Wei Y-Q, Hang Z-B, Liu K-F: In situ observation of inflammatory cell-tumor cell interaction in human seminomas (germinomas). Light, electron microscopic, and immunohistochemical study. Hum Pathol 23:421–428, 1992.

402. Ho DM, Liu H-C: Primary intracranial germ cell tumor. Pathologic study of 51 patients. Cancer 70:1577–1584, 1992.

403. Shinoda J, Yamada H, Sakai N, et al: Placental alkaline phosphatase as a tumor marker for primary intracranial germinoma. J Neurosurg 68:710–720, 1988.

404. Felix I, Becker LE: Intracranial germ cell tumors in children. An immunohistochemical and electron microscopic study. Pediatr Neurosurg 16:156–162, 1990.

405. Nakagawa Y, Perentes E, Ross GW, et al: Immunohistochemical differences between intracranial germinomas and their gonadal equivalents. An immunoperoxidase study of germ cell tumours with epithelial membrane antigen, cytokeratin, and vimentin. J Pathol 156:67–72, 1988.

406. Yamagami T, Handa H, Yamashita J, et al: An immunohistochemical study of intracranial germ cell tumors. Acta Neurochir 86:33–41, 1987.

407. Niehans GA, Manivel C, Copland GT, et al: Immunohistochemistry of germ cell and trophoblastic neoplasms. Cancer 62:1113–1123, 1988.

408. Edwards MBS, Baumgartner JE: Pineal region tumors. *In* Cheek WR, Marlin AE, McLone DG, et al (eds): Pediatric Neurosurgery, 3rd ed. Philadelphia, WB Saunders, 1994, pp 429–436.

409. Kirkove CS, Brown AP, Symon L: Successful treatment of a pineal endodermal sinus tumor. J Neurosurg 74:832–836, 1991.

410. Bruce DA, Schut L, Sutton LN: Pineal region tumors. *In* McLaurin RL, Venes JL, Schut L, Epstein F (eds): Pediatric

Neurosurgery, 2nd ed. Philadelphia, WB Saunders, 1989, pp 409–416.

411. Dearnaley DP, A'Hern RP, Whittaker S, Bloom HJG: Pineal and CNS germ cell tumors. Royal Marsden Hospital experience 1962–1987. Int J Radiat Oncol Biol Phys 18:773–781, 1990.

412. Sano K, Matsutani M, Seto T: So-called intracranial germ cell tumours. Personal experiences and a theory of their pathogenesis. Neurol Res 11:118–126, 1989.

413. Shaffrey ME, Lanzino G, Lopes MBS, et al: Maturation of intracranial immature teratomas—report of two cases. J Neurosurg 85:672–676, 1966.

414. Kamiya M, Tateyama H, Fujiyoshi Y, et al: Cerebrospinal fluid cytology in immature teratoma of the central nervous system. A case report. Acta Cytol 35:757–760, 1991.

415. Smirniotopoulus JG, Rushing EJ, Mena H: Pineal region masses. Differential diagnosis. Radiographics 12:577–596, 1992.

416. Herrick MK: Pathology of pineal tumors. In Neuwelt EA (ed): Diagnosis and Treatment of Pineal Region Tumors. Baltimore, Williams & Wilkins, 1984, pp 31–60.

417. Dayan AD, Marshall AHE, Miller A, et al: Atypical teratomas of the pineal and hypothalamus. J Pathol Bacteriol 92:1–28, 1966.

418. Cushing H, Eisenhardt L: Meningiomas. Their Classification, Regional Behavior, Life History and Surgical End Results. Springfield, IL, Charles C Thomas, 1938.

419. Burger PC, Scheithauer BW: Tumors of the Central Nervous System. Atlas of Tumor Pathology. Third Series, Fascicle 10. Washington, DC, Armed Forces Institute of Pathology, 1994, pp 259–286.

420. Kepes JJ: Meningiomas. Biology, Pathology and Differential Diagnosis. New York, Masson, 1982.

421. Lantos PL, VandenBerg SR, Kleihues P: Tumours of the nervous system. Tumours of the meninges. In Graham DI, Lantos PL (eds): Greenfield's Neuropathology, 6th ed. London, Arnold, 1997, pp 727–752.

422. Bruner JM, Tien RD, Enterline DS: Tumors of the meninges and related tissues. In Bigner DD, McLendon RE, Bruner JM (eds): Russell and Rubinstein's Pathology of Tumors of the Nervous System, 6th ed. London, Arnold, 1998, pp 67–139.

423. Zang KD: Cytological and cytogenetical studies on human meningiomas. Cancer Genet Cytogenet 6:249–274, 1982.

424. Louis DN, Budka H, von Deimling A: Meningiomas. In Kleihues P, Cavenee WK (eds): Pathology and Genetics of Tumours of the Nervous System. Lyon, International Agency for Research on Cancer (IARC), 1997, pp 134–141.

425. Maier H, Wanschitz J, Sedivy R, et al: Proliferation and DNA fragmentation in meningioma subtypes. Neuropathol Appl Neurobiol 23:496–506, 1997.

426. Maier H, Ofner D, Hittmair A, et al: Classic, atypical, and anaplastic meningioma. Three histopathological subtypes of clinical relevence. J Neurosurg 77:616–623, 1992.

427. Chen WYK, Liu HC: Atypical (anaplastic) meningioma. Relationship between histological features and recurrence—a clinicopathologic study. Clin Neuropathol 9:74–81, 1990.

428. Mahmood A, Caccamo DV, Tomecak FJ, et al: Atypical and malignant meningiomas. A clinicopathological review. Neurosurgery 33:955–963, 1993.

429. Pasquier B, Gasnier F, Pasquier D, et al: Papillary meningioma. Clinicopathologic study of seven cases and review of the literature. Cancer 58:299–305, 1986.

430. Perry A, Stafford SL, Scheithauer BW, et al: Meningioma grading. An analysis of histologic parameters. Am J Surg Pathol 21:1455–1465, 1997.

431. Perry A, Stafford SL, Scheithauer BW, et al: The prognostic significance of MIB-1, p53, and DNA flow cytometry in completely resected primary meningiomas. Cancer 82:2262–2269, 1998.

432. Zorludemir S, Scheithauer BW, Hirose T, et al: Clear cell meningioma. A clinicopathologic study of a potentially aggressive variant of meningioma. Am J Surg Pathol 19:493–505, 1995.

433. Slooff JL: Pathological anatomical findings in the cerebellopontine angle. Adv Otorhinolaryngol 34:89–103, 1984.

434. Lantos PL, VandenBerg SR, Kleihues P: Tumours of the nervous system. Tumours of the peripheral nerves. In Graham DI, Lantos PL (eds): Greenfield's Neuropathology, 6th ed. London, Arnold, 1997, pp 713–723.

435. Consensus Development Panel: NIH Health Consensus Development Conference Statement on Acoustic Neuroma. Arch Neurol 51:201–207, 1991.

436. Beskonakli E, Cayli S, Turgut M, et al: Intraparenchymal schwannomas of the central nervous system. An additional case report and review. Neurosurg Rev 20:139–144, 1997.

437. Sharma MC, Karak AK, Gaikwad SB, et al: Intracranial intraparenchymal schwannomas. A series of eight cases. J Neurol Neurosurg Psychiatry 60:200–203, 1996.

438. Antoni N: Uber Ruchenmarkstumoren und Neurofibrome. Munich, Bergmann, 1920.

439. Woodruff JM: Cellular schwannoma and its necessary distinction from malignant peripheral nerve sheath tumor and sarcomas. Pathol Case Rev 3:118–122, 1998.

440. Casadei GP, Scheithauer BW, Hirose T, et al: Cellular schwannoma. A clinicopathologic, DNA flow cytometric, and proliferation marker study of 70 patients. Cancer 75:1109–1119, 1995.

441. Urich H, Tien RD: Tumors of cranial, spinal and peripheral nerve sheaths. In Bigner DD, McLendon RE, Bruner JM (eds): Russell and Rubinstein's Pathology of Tumors of the Nervous System, 6th ed. London, Arnold, 1998, pp 141–193.

442. Halliday AL, Sobel RA, Martuza RL: Benign spinal nerve sheath tumors. Their occurrence sporadically and in neurofibromatosis types 1 and 2. J Neurosurg 74:248–253, 1991.

443. Woodruff JM, Kourea HP, Louis DP: Tumours of cranial and peripheral nerves. In Kleihues P, Cavenee WK (eds): Pathology and Genetics of Tumours of the Nervous System. Lyon, International Agency for Research on Cancer (IARC), 1997, pp 125–132.

444. Woodruff JM, Selig AM, Crowley K, et al: Schwannoma (neurilemoma) with malignant transformation. Am J Surg Pathol 18:882–895, 1994.

445. Miller DC, Hochberg FH, Harris NL, et al: Pathology with clinical correlations of primary central nervous system non-Hodgkin's lymphoma. Cancer 74:1383–1397, 1994.

446. Eby NL, Grufferman S, Flannelly CM, et al: Increasing incidence of primary brain lymphomas in the U.S. Cancer 62:2461–2465, 1988.

447. Paulus W, Jellinger K, Morgello S: Malignant lymphomas In Kleihues P, Cavenee WK (eds): Pathology and Genetics of Tumours of the Nervous System. Lyon, International Agency for Research on Cancer (IARC), 1997, pp 154–159.

448. Grove A, Vyberg M: Primary leptomeningeal T-cell lymphoma. A case and a review of primary T-cell lymphoma of the central nervous system. Clin Neuropathol 12:7–12, 1993.

449. Paulus W, Ott MM, Strik H, et al: Large cell anaplastic (Ki-1) brain lymphoma of T-cell genotype. Hum Pathol 25:1253–1256, 1994.

450. Smith WJ, Garson JA, Bourne SP, et al: Immunoglobulin gene rearrangement and antigenic profile confirm B cell origin of primary cerebral lymphoma and indicate a mature phenotype. J Clin Pathol 41:128–132, 1988.

451. Cobbers JM, Wolter M, Reifenberger J, et al: Frequent inactivation of CDKN2A and rare mutation of TP53 in PCNSL. Brain Pathol 8:263–276, 1998.

452. Aboody-Guterman K, Hair L, Morgello S: Epstein-Barr virus and AIDS-related primary central nervous system lymphoma. Viral detection by immunohistochemistry, RNA in situ hybridization, and polymerase chain reaction. Clin Neuropathol 15:79–86, 1996.

453. Bignon YL, Clavelou P, Ramos F, et al: Detection of Epstein-Barr virus sequences in primary brain lymphoma without immunodeficiency. Neurology 41:1152–1153, 1991.

454. Cerboy JR, Garl PJ, Kleinschmidt-DeMasters BK: Human herpesvirus 8 DNA in CNS lymphomas from patients with and without AIDS. Neurology 50:335–340, 1998.

455. Tomlinson FH, Kurtin PJ, Suman VJ, et al: Primary intracerebral malignant lymphoma. A clinicopathological study of 89 patients. J Neurosurg 82:558–566, 1995.

456. Aho R, Haapasalo H, Alanen K, et al: Proliferative activity

and DNA index do not significantly predict survival in primary central nervous system lymphoma. J Neuropathol Exp Neurol 54:826–832, 1995.

457. Benli K, Inci S: Solitary dural plasmacytoma. Neurosurgery 36:1206–1209, 1995.

458. Wisniewski T, Sisti M, Inhirami G, et al: Intracerebral solitary plasmacytoma. Neurosurgery 27:826–829, 1990.

459. Litofsky NS, Zee C-S, Breeze RE, et al: Meningeal melanocytoma. Diagnostic criteria for a rare lesion. Neurosurgery 31: 945–948, 1992.

460. Jellinger KA, Bruner JM, Chou P, Paulus W: Melanocytic lesions. *In* Kleihues P, Cavenee K (eds): Pathology and Genetics of Tumours of the Nervous System. Lyon, International Agency for Research on Cancer (IARC), 1997, pp 149–151.

461. Bamborschke S, Ebhardt G, Szelies-Stock B, et al: Review and case report. Primary melanoblastosis of the leptomeninges. Clin Neuropathol 4:47–55, 1985.

462. Bruner JM, Tien RD, McLendon RE: Tumors of vascular origin. *In* Bigner DD, McLendon RE, Brunner JM (eds): Russell and Rubinstein's Pathology of Tumors of the Nervous System, 6th ed. London, Arnold, 1998, pp 239–293.

463. Stein BM, Kader A: Intracranial arteriovenous malformation. Clin Neurosurg 39:76–113, 1992.

464. Goates JJ, Dickson DW, Horoupian DS: Meningioangiomatosis. An immunocytochemical study. Acta Neuropathol 82: 527–532, 1991.

465. Stemmer-Rachamimov AO, Horgan MA, Taratuto AL, et al: Meningioangiomatosis is associated with neurofibromatosis 2 but not with somatic alterations of the NF2 gene. J Neuropathol Exp Neurol 56:485–489, 1997.

466. Prayson RA: Meningioangiomatosis. A clinicopathologic study including MIB1 immunoreactivity. Arch Pathol Lab Med 119:1061–1064, 1995.

467. Mena H, Ribas JL, Pezeshkour GH, et al: Hemangiopericytoma of the central nervous system. A review of 94 cases. Hum Pathol 22:84–91, 1991.

468. D'Amore ES, Manivel JC, Sung JH: Soft tissue and meningeal hemangiopericytomas. An immunohistochemical and ultrastructural study. Hum Pathol 21:414–423, 1990.

469. Herath SE, Stalboerger PG, Dahl RJ, et al: Cytogenetic studies of four hemangiopericytomas. Cancer Genet Cytogenet 72:137–140, 1994.

470. Vuorinen V, Salinen P, Haapasalo H, et al: Outcome of 31 intracranial hemangiopericytomas. Poor predictive value of cell proliferation indices. Acta Neurochir 138:1399–1408, 1996.

471. Jaaskelainen J, Louis DN, Paulus W, et al: Hemangiopericytoma. *In* Kleihues P, Cavenee WK (eds): Pathology and Genetics of Tumours of the Nervous System. Lyon, International Agency for Research on Cancer (IARC), 1997, pp 146–148.

472. Jellinger K, Paulus W: Mesenchymal, non-meningothelial tumors of the central nervous system. Brain Pathol 1:79–87, 1991.

473. Carneiro SS, Scheithauer BW, Nascimento AG, et al: Solitary fibrous tumor of the meninges. A lesion distinct from fibrous meningioma. A clinicopathologic and immunohistochemical study. Am J Clin Pathol 106:217–224, 1996.

474. Forsyth PA, Cascino TL, Shaw EG, et al: Intracranial chordomas. A clinicopathological and prognostic study of 51 cases. J Neurosurg 78:741–747, 1993.

475. O'Hara BJ, Paetau A, Miettinen M: Keratin subsets and monoclonal antibody HBME-1 in chordoma. Hum Pathol 29: 119–126, 1998.

476. Walker WP, Landas SK, Bromley CM, et al: Immunohistochemical distinction of classic and chondroid chordomas. Mod Pathol 4:661–666, 1991.

477. Wojno KJ, Hruban RH, Garin-Chesa P, et al: Chondroid chordomas and low-grade chondrosarcomas of the craniospinal axis. Am J Surg Pathol 16:1144–1152, 1992.

478. Schoedel KE, Martinez AJ, Mahoney TM, et al: Chordomas. Pathological features; ploidy and silver nucleolar organizing region analysis. A study of 36 cases. Acta Neuropathol 89: 139–143, 1995.

479. Rushing EJ, Armonda RA, Ansari Q, et al: Mesenchymal chondrosarcoma: a clinicopathologic and flow cytometric study of 13 cases presenting in the central nervous system. Cancer 77:1884–1891, 1996.

480. Swanson PE, Lillemoe TJ, Manivel JC, et al: Mesenchymal chondrosarcoma. An immunohistochemical study. Arch Pathol Lab Med 114:943–948, 1990.

481. Taratuto AL, Molina HA, Diez B, et al: Primary rhabdomyosarcoma of brain and cerebellum. Report of four cases in infants. An immunohistochemical study. Acta Neuropathol 66:98–104, 1985.

482. Kawamoto EH, Weidner N, Agostini RM, et al: Malignant ectomesenchymoma of soft tissue. Report of two cases and review of the literature. Cancer 59:1791–1802, 1987.

483. Stone JL, Zavala G, Bailey OT: Mixed malignant mesenchymal tumor of the cerebellar vermis. Cancer 44:2165–2172, 1979.

484. Sziefert GT, Sipos L, Horvath M, et al: Pathological characteristics of surgically removed craniopharyngiomas. Analysis of 131 cases. Acta Neurochir 124: 139–143, 1993.

485. Crotty TB, Scheithauer BW, Young WF, et al: Papillary craniopharyngioma. A clinico-pathologic study of 48 cases. J Neurosurg 83:206–214, 1995.

486. Yamada H, Haratake J, Narasaki T, et al: Embryonal craniopharyngioma. Case report of the morphogenesis of a craniopharyngioma. Cancer 75:2971–2977, 1995.

487. Thapar K, Stefaneanu L, Kovacs K, et al: Estrogen receptor gene expression in craniopharyngiomas—an in situ hybridization study. Neurosurgery 35:1012–1017, 1994.

488. Hetelekidis S, Barnes PD, Tao ML, et al: 20 year experience in childhood craniopharyngioma. Int J Radiat Oncol Biol Phys 27:189–195, 1993.

489. Burger PC, Scheithauer BW: Tumors of the Central Nervous System. Atlas of Tumor Pathology. Third Series, Fascicle 10. Washington, DC, Armed Forces Institute of Pathology, 1994, pp 349–354.

490. Raftopoulos C, Filament-Durand J, Brucher LM, et al: Paraganglioma of the cauda equina. Report of 2 cases and review of 59 cases from the literature. Clin Neurol Neurosurg 92: 263–270, 1990.

491. Sonneland PRL, Scheithauer BW, LeChago J, et al: Paraganglioma of the cauda equina region. Clinicopathologic study of 31 cases with special reference to immunocytology and ultrastructure. Cancer 58:1720–1735, 1986.

492. Orrell JM, Hales SA: Paragangliomas of the cauda equina have a distinct cytokeratin immunophenotype. Histopathology 21:479–481, 1992.

493. Achilles E, Padberg BC, Holl K, et al: Immunocytochemistry of paragangliomas—value of staining S-100 protein and glial fibrillary acidic protein in diagnosis and prognosis. Histopathology 18:453–458, 1991.

494. Roche PH, Figarella-Branger D, Regis J, et al: Cauda equina paraganglioma with subsequent intracranial and intraspinal metastases. Acta Neurochirurg 138:475–479, 1996.

495. Bohling T, Hatva E, Plate KH, et al: von Hippel–Lindau disease and capillary hemangioblastoma. *In* Kleihues P, Cavenee WK (eds): Pathology and Genetics of Tumours of the Nervous System. Lyon, International Agency for Research on Cancer (IARC), 1997, pp 179–181.

496. Tachibana O, Yamashima T, Yamashita J: Immunohistochemical study of erythropoietin in cerebellar hemangioblastomas associated with secondary polycythemia. Neurosurgery 28: 24–26, 1991.

497. Reifenberger G, Reifenberger J, Bilzer T, et al: Coexpression of transforming growth factor-alpha and epidermal growth factor receptor in capillary hemangioblastomas of the central nervous system. Am J Pathol 147:245–250, 1995.

498. Vortmeyer AO, Gnarra JR, Emmert-Buck MR, et al: von Hippel–Lindau gene deletion detected in the stromal cell component of a cerebellar hemangioblastoma associated with von Hippel–Lindau disease. Hum Pathol 28:540–543, 1997.

499. Wizigmann Voos S, Breier G, Risau W, et al: Up-regulation of vascular endothelial growth factor and its receptors in von Hippel–Lindau disease-associated and sporadic hemangioblastomas. Cancer Res 55:1358–1364, 1995.

500. Kanno H, Kondo K, Ito S, et al: Somatic mutations of the von Hippel–Lindau tumor suppressor gene in sporadic central nervous system hemangioblastomas. Cancer Res 54:4845–4847, 1994

501. de la Monte SM, Horowitz SA: Hemangioblastomas. Clinical and histopathological factors correlated with recurrence. Neurosurgery 25:695–698, 1989.

502. Rorke LB, Packer RJ, Biegel JA: Central nervous system atypical teratoid/rhabdoid tumors of infancy and childhood. J Neurosurg 85:56–65, 1996.

503. Burger PC, Yu IT, Tihan T, et al: Atypical teratoid/rhabdoid tumor of the central nervous system. A highly malignant tumor of infancy and childhood frequently mistaken for medulloblastoma. A Pediatric Oncology Group study. Am J Surg Pathol 22:1083–1092, 1998.

504. Chou SM, Anderson JS: Primary CNS malignant rhabdoid tumor (MRT). Report of two cases and review of literature. Clin Neuropathol 10:1–10, 1991.

505. Muller M, Hubbard SL, Fukuyama K, et al: Characterization of a pineal region malignant rhabdoid tumor. Toward understanding brain tumor cell invasion. Pediatr Neurosurg 22:204–209, 1995.

506. Bigner SH, McLendon RE, Fuchs H, et al: Chromosomal characteristics of childhood brain tumors. Cancer Genet Cytogenet 97:125–134, 1997.

507. Rorke LB: Atypical teratoid/rhabdoid tumours. In Kleihues P, Cavenee WK (eds): Pathology and Genetics of Tumours of the Nervous System. Lyon, International Agency for Research on Cancer (IARC), 1997, pp 110–111.

508. Nitta M, Symon L: Colloid cysts of the third ventricle. A review of 36 cases. Acta Neurochirurg 76:99–104, 1985.

509. Lach B, Scheithauer BW, Gregor A, et al: Colloid cyst of the third ventricle. A comparative immunohistochemical study of neuroaxis cysts and choroid plexus epithelium. J Neurosurg 78:101–111, 1993.

510. Agnoli AL, Laun A, Schonmayr R: Enterogenous intraspinal cysts. J Neurosurg 61:834–840, 1984.

511. Thapar K, Kovacs K: Neoplasms of the sellar region. In Bigner DD, McLendon RE, Bruner JM (eds): Russell and Rubinstein's Pathology of Tumours of the Nervous System, 6th ed. London, Arnold, 1998, pp 648–652.

512. Canley FK: Epidermoid and dermoid tumors. Clinical features and surgical management. In Wilkins RH, Rengachary SS (eds): Neurosurgery. Vol 1, 2nd ed. New York, McGraw-Hill, 1996, pp 971–976.

513. Rangachary SS, Watanabe T: Ultrastructure and pathogenesis of intracranial arachnoid cysts. J Neuropathol Exp Neurol 40:61–83, 1981.

514. Takahura K: Metastatic brain tumours. In Thomas DGT, Graham DI (eds): Malignant Brain Tumours. London, Springer Verlag, 1995, pp 203–220.

515. Posner JB: Management of brain metastases. Rev Neurol 148:477–487, 1992.

516. Routh A, Khansur T, Hickman BT, et al: Management of brain metastases. Past, present, and future. South Med J 87:1218–1226, 1994.

517. Delattre JY, Krol G, Thaler HT, et al: Distribution of brain metastases. Arch Neurol 45:741–744, 1988.

518. Mead GM, Kennedy P, Smith JL, et al: Involvement of the central nervous system by non-Hodgkin's lymphoma in adults. A review of 36 cases. QJM 60:699–714, 1986.

519. Traweek ST: Nervous system involvement by lymphomas, leukemia and other hematopoietic cell proliferations. In Bigner DD, McLendon RE, Bruner JM (eds): Russell and Rubinstein's Pathology of Tumors of the Nervous System, 6th ed. London, Arnold, 1998, pp 195–237.

520. Hair LS, Rogers JD, Chadburn A, et al: Intracerebral Hodgkin's disease in a human immunodeficiency virus-seropositive patient. Cancer 67:2931–2934, 1991.

521. Burger PC, Scheithauer BW: Tumors of the Central Nervous System. Atlas of Tumor Pathology. Third Series, Fascicle 10. Washington, DC, Armed Forces Institute of Pathology, 1994, p 423.

522. Salvati M, Puzzilli F, Bristot R, et al: Post-radiation gliomas. Tumori 80:220–223, 1994.

523. Homans AC, Barker BE, Forman EN, et al: Immunophenotypic characteristics of cerebrospinal fluid cells in children with acute lymphoblastic leukemia at diagnosis. Blood 76:1807–1811, 1990.

524. Traweek ST, Arber DA, Rappaport H, et al: Extramedullary myeloid cell tumors. An immunohistochemical and morphological study of 28 cases. Am J Surg Pathol 17:1011–1019, 1993.

525. McDonald WI: The pathological and clinical dynamics of multiple sclerosis. J Neuropathol Exp Neurol 53:338–343, 1994.

526. Wispelwey B, Dacey RE, Scheld WM: Brain abscess. In Scheld WM, Whitley RJ, Durack DT (eds): Infections of the Central Nervous System. New York, Raven Press, 1991, pp 457–486.

527. Major EO, Amemiya K, Tornatore CS, et al: Pathogenesis and molecular biology of progressive multifocal leukoencephalopathy, the JC virus-induced demyelinating disease of the human brain. Clin Microbiol Rev 5:49–73, 1992.

528. Wiley CA: Pathology of neurologic disease in AIDS. Psychiatr Clin North Am 17:1–15, 1994.

529. Albright AL, Lee PA: Neurosurgical treatment of hypothalamic hamartomas causing precocious puberty. J Neurosurg 78:77–82, 1993.

530. Asa SL, Scheithauer BW, Bilbao JM, et al: A case for hypothalamic acromegaly. A clinicopathologic study of six patients with hypothalamic gangliocytomas producing growth hormone-releasing factors. J Clin Endocrinol Metab 58:796–803, 1984.

531. Richardson EP: Pathology of tuberous sclerosis. Neuropathologic aspects. Ann N Y Acad Sci 615:128–139. 1991.

532. Hirose T, Scheithauer BW, Lopes MB, et al: Tuber and subependymal giant cell astrocytoma associated with tuberous sclerosis. An immunohistochemical, ultrastructural and immunoelectron microscopic study. Acta Neuropathol 90:387–399, 1995.

533. Crino PB, Trojanowski JQ, Dichter MA, et al: Embryonic neuronal markers in tuberous sclerosis. Single-cell molecular pathology. Proc Natl Acad Sci U S A 93:14152–14157, 1996.

534. Cohen M, Lanska D, Roessmann LL, et al: Amyloidoma of the CNS. I. Clinical and pathologic study. Neurology 42:2019–2023, 1992.

535. Vidal RG Ghiso J, Gallo G, et al: Amyloidoma of the CNS. II. Immunohistochemical and biochemical study. Neurology 42:2024–2028, 1992.

# 52

# The Molecular and Genetic Basis of Neurodegenerative Diseases

Stephen J. DeArmond   Jeffry P. Simko   David A. Gaskin

Two of the most fundamental and interrelated features of neurodegenerative diseases are that each disease targets a different set of neurons for degeneration (*selective vulnerability*) and that the morphologic characteristics of the degenerative process are unique for each disease (Table 52–1). The correlation of neuropathologic changes with the clinical presentation has been the mainstay for establishing a specific diagnosis; however, the final definitive diagnosis often requires examining the entire central nervous system, which is not possible until the patient dies. This is particularly true for the most common forms of neurodegenerative disorders, including Alzheimer's disease (AD), Lewy body disease variants, and the tauopathies, which together account for about 60% to 80% of all primary neurodegenerative disorders in patients older than age 55 years. It is also true for Creutzfeldt-Jakob disease (CJD). Even though CJD is rarer than AD, increasing evidence suggests that prion particles formed during the course of prion diseases in humans and in animals are responsible for the emergence of an increase of CJD acquired by medical procedures and by ingestion of prion-contaminated food products.[1–3] For these reasons, every suspected case of CJD requires a tissue diagnosis and genetic screening for

**TABLE 52–1.** Neuropathologic and Neurochemical Phenotypes of Common Neurodegenerative Diseases Including Genes Genetically Linked to Dominantly Inherited Forms

| Disease | Neuropathology | Peptide | Gene Mutation |
|---------|----------------|---------|---------------|
| AD | Neuritic plaques | A$\beta$ | |
| | Neurofibrillary tangles | tau | |
| Familial AD | Neuritic plaques | A$\beta$ | $\beta$APP (10%) |
| | Neurofibrillary tangles | tau | |
| | Neurofibrillary tangles | tau | PS-1 (40%) |
| | Neurofibrillary tangles | tau | PS-2 (10%) |
| | Neurofibrillary tangles | tau | ? (40%) |
| PD | Lewy body | $\alpha$-synuclein | $\alpha$-synuclein |
| Familial PD | Lewy body | $\alpha$-synuclein | |
| DLBD | Lewy body | $\alpha$-synuclein | |
| Prion disease | | | |
|   CJD | Vacuolation $\pm$ PrP amyloid | PrP$^{Sc}$ | |
|   Familial CJD | Vacuolation $\pm$ PrP amyloid | PrP$^{Sc}$ | PRNP |
|   FFI | Vacuolation $\pm$ PrP amyloid | PrP$^{Sc}$ | PRNP |
|   GSS | PrP amyloid | $^{tm}$PrP(?) | PRNP |
| ALS | Cytoplasmic inclusions | ? | |
| Familial ALS | Cytoplasmic inclusions | SOD-1 | SOD-1 (10%) |
| | Cytoplasmic inclusions | ? | ? (90%) |
| Pick's disease | Pick body | tau | |
| FTDPD-17 | Neurofibrillary tangles | tau | tau |

cases of familial prion disease to determine whether or not the incidence of CJD acquired by infection is increasing.

Since the 1970s, there has been a rapid shift from a purely cliniconeuropathologic classification of neurodegenerative diseases, which identified an often perplexing number of subtypes of a disorder (splitter approach), to the discovery of many of the genes and gene products causing or associating with each of the neurodegenerative diseases (see Table 52–1). Molecular genetics of these disorders indicate that there is a single gene or gene product abnormality that defines the disease and that the many subtypes of a disorder are due to biologic variations among humans, even within a family.

Two different strategies have been used to identify the genetic basis of neurodegenerative diseases—a biochemical approach and a molecular genetic approach. For the biochemical approach, pathologic products that accumulate in the brain are purified, partial amino acid sequences are determined, and a synthetic cDNA is constructed and used to probe a genomic library. This strategy was used to discover the $\beta$-amyloid precursor protein ($\beta$APP) gene on chromosome 21 in AD. A similar process was used to identify the human prion protein (*PrP*) gene[4] on chromosome 20[5] except that it began with the purification of the infectious agent that transmits scrapie from a hamster brain and with the discovery that it is a single protease-resistant protein designated *PrP$^{Sc}$*.[6]

The second discovery pathway has been through molecular genetic analysis of large pedigrees with familial forms of the neurodegenerative diseases. This approach, referred to as the *reverse genetic* or the *positional cloning* method, became possible in 1980 after the publication of a study by Botstein and colleagues[7] that described how to find any mutated gene by using polymorphic DNA markers. In essence, it is a protocol to identify a gene based on its "position" in the human genome without any prior knowledge of the gene product or its function. One of the first applications of this technique led to the discovery of the Huntington's disease (HD) gene. There are three criteria that must be fulfilled to apply this method[8]: 1) family pedigrees that segregate with the disease as a mendelian trait; 2) polymorphic markers that are distributed throughout the human genome; and 3) cosegregation of the disease gene with a genetic marker with the caveat that the closer the genetic marker is to the disease gene, the smaller the chance that a recombination event will occur between the marker and the gene, causing them to segregate independently. Polymorphisms are natural variations in the genome that distinguish two homologous chromosomes. Restriction fragment length polymorphisms (RFLPs) are differences in genomic DNA lengths generated by digestion with restriction enzymes.

This was the approach originally suggested by Botstein and colleagues[7] and was used in the first positional cloning studies. Southern hybridization is used to identify differences in restriction fragment sizes. Variations that are found can be caused by a mutation in a DNA sequence resulting in a loss or a creation of a restriction enzyme digestion site or an insertion or a deletion of DNA sequences, both of which can alter migration patterns of RFLPs on Southern transfers. Today, RFLP analysis is being replaced by microsatellite typing. Minisatellites and microsatellites are natural repeated sequences in the genome. Minisatellites are tandem repeats of DNA sequences that can show variations in numbers between homologous chromosome pairs and among different individuals. Microsatellites consist of dinucleotide, trinucleotide, or tetranucleotide repeats. These are used more frequently today because they are localized throughout the genome at small genetic intervals and are genotyped readily by polymerase chain reaction. Genotyping of microsatellites requires designing primers to the unique flanking sequences of the repeats for polymerase chain reaction. Polymorphisms of such repeats occur because of differences in the numbers of repeats. Positional cloning methods have been used to discover the genes and gene abnormalities genetically linked to most of the neurodegenerative diseases.

This chapter on molecular diagnostic procedures for neurodegenerative disorders briefly summarizes the history of discovery of mutations and relevant polymorphisms of disease genes. Many textbooks that discuss the molecular and genetic basis of neurologic diseases in great detail have been published and should be referred to for additional references to the many laboratories that have contributed to the advances in this field. The molecular biologic analysis of human neurodegenerative diseases has two goals. One is to secure a diagnosis that allows clinicians to advise the patient and the patient's family about prognosis, to establish an appropriate palliative treatment course, and to provide genetic counseling to the patient and family. The other goal is to learn more about the pathogenesis of nerve cell degeneration and to develop a rational basis for future pharmacologic intervention. For many neurodegenerative diseases, 85% to 90% present sporadically, with 10% to 15% dominantly inherited. Discovery of genetic linkage of a mutated gene to disease is helping clinicians understand how the wild-type gene might participate in pathogenesis. We cannot review all of the neurodegenerative diseases in this chapter; the major causes of neurodegeneration are described, and in the final section all of the inherited disorders of metabolism and protein dysfunction for which commercially available molecular genetic tests are available to the pathologist (neuropathologist) and neurologist are outlined.

## ALZHEIMER'S DISEASE

AD is the most common cause of dementia in patients older than age 55, with an annual incidence of 2.4 cases per 100,000 population 40 to 60 years old and 127 cases per 100,000 population older than age 60. It is estimated that 40% to 50% of cases of dementia in patients older than age 60 are caused by AD. The profound effect this disease has on family and national finances and on the ability of caregivers to support the patient is a function of the high incidence of the disease, the profound disability caused by the degeneration of cortical and subcortical neurons, and by the 10- to 20-year duration of the disease from onset of dementia to death. In 1907, Alzheimer[9] was the first to describe the association of neurofibrillary tangles (NFTs) and neuritic plaques (*miliary foci*) in the cerebral cortex (Fig. 52–1) with progressive dementia. The diagnosis of AD requires an estimate of the number of neuritic plaques and NFTs in multiple cerebral cortical regions,[10–12] a diagnostic procedure that currently can be performed only on autopsied brains.

## Molecular Pathogenesis of Neuritic Plaques and Amyloid Angiopathy

By electron microscopy, most of the plaque is composed of abnormal neuronal processes, mostly enlarged terminal axons and presynaptic boutons.[13] The dystrophic neurites contain NFTs identical to the NFTs in nerve cell bodies (see Fig. 52–1D and E).[14] The amyloid core of the plaque is an extracellular deposit of Aβ peptide (see Fig. 52–1B). For diffuse and primitive plaques, masses of abnormal neurites do not contain an identifiable amyloid core by light microscopy; however, extracellular amyloid fibrils often are identified among the dystrophic neurites (Fig. 52–1D).

The discovery of the amyloidogenic peptide comprising the core of neuritic plaques followed the development of methods to purify amyloid from AD and Down's syndrome patients in the 1970s. Brains of patients dying of Down's syndrome were used for this study because many patients older than age 40 with trisomy 21 develop a further dementing disease with neuritic plaques, NFTs, and amyloid angiopathy indistinguishable from AD. In 1984, Glenner and Wong[15] isolated and sequenced the major protein constituent from the amyloid angiopathy of AD and Down's syndrome. In 1985, Masters and coworkers[16] purified and sequenced the amyloidogenic peptide from the amyloid cores of neuritic plaques. Sequencing of the 4-kd amyloid peptide, designated the *amyloid β peptide* (Aβ), by both groups led to cloning the gene that encodes it and the discovery that Aβ peptide is derived from a larger precursor protein designated the βAPP.[17–20] Commercially available antibodies specific for the Aβ peptide strongly immunostain all types of neuritic plaques, including the amyloid core of mature plaques and the Aβ peptide dispersed diffusely among the dystrophic neurites comprising diffuse, primitive, and mature plaques (see Fig. 52–1A and C). The amyloid of amyloid angiopathy also immunostains strongly for Aβ peptide (see Fig. 52–1A).

## Molecular Pathogenesis of Neurofibrillary Tangles

NFTs accumulate in the cell bodies of medium and large neurons, displacing the nucleus and lipochrome. NFTs also accumulate in the dystrophic neurites of neuritic plaques and in neuropil threads (see Fig. 52–1D and E). Neuropil threads seem to be abnormal axons passing through the gray matter. In

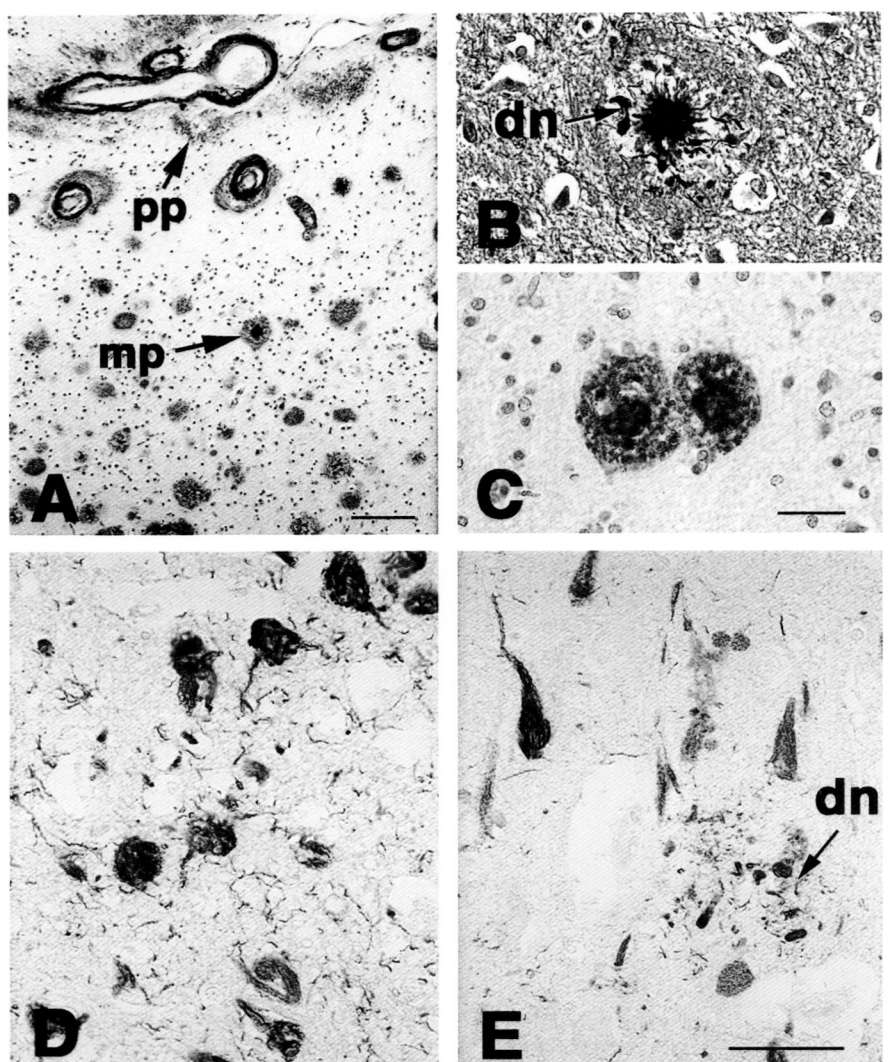

**FIGURE 52–1.** The neuropathologic features of Alzheimer's disease. *A.* A$\beta$ immunohistochemistry of the frontal cortex shows A$\beta$ peptide distributed to primitive neuritic plaques (pp), to mature neuritic plaques with an amyloid core (mp), and to blood vessel walls (amyloid angiopathy). B. Bielschowsky silver stain shows the amyloid core of a mature neuritic plaque and the halo of dystrophic neurites (dn) surrounding the core. C. Two mature neuritic plaques immunostained for A$\beta$ show intense reaction of the amyloid core and dispersion of A$\beta$ peptide among the dystrophic neurites. *D.* Globose neurofibrillary tangles in neurons of the subiculum immunostain strongly with phosphorylated tau antibodies, as do neuropil threads between the nerve cell bodies. E. Flame-shaped neurofibrillary tangles in pyramidal cells of the entorhinal cortex and dystrophic neurites of a neuritic plaque are immunopositive for phosphorylated tau protein. Bar in *A* is 100 $\mu$m. Bar in C also applies to *B* and is 50 $\mu$m. Bar in *E* also applies to *D* and is 50 $\mu$m.

larger pyramidal cells, NFTs are aligned in parallel, giving the aggregate a flame-shaped appearance (see Fig. 52–1E), whereas in other neurons they loop around each other, producing a globose pattern (see Fig. 52–1D). In addition to staining by the Bielschowsky silver technique, NFTs bind Congo red dye, which shows green birefringence with polarizing filters, arguing that they are an *intracellular amyloid*. Ultrastructurally, NFTs are composed of tightly packed paired helical filaments (PHFs)[21, 22] that can be isolated as tangle fragments[23, 24] or as dispersed filaments.[25] Chemical characterization of PHFs and molecular cloning have provided direct evidence that tau, a microtubule binding protein, is an integral structural component of PHFs.[23, 24, 26]

## Tau Physiology

The normal function of tau is to stabilize microtubules within the axons of neurons to facilitate ax-

onal transport and possibly to play a role in the elongation of axons during development.[27–29] Tau is located mainly in the axons, but also is present in neuronal cell bodies. Trace amounts are seen in other cell types. It is the product of a single gene that spans 6 kb of chromosome 17q21 and is composed of 11 coding exons.[30, 31] Sequencing of this gene in more than 200 white subjects identified two extended haplotypes without any recombination events, suggesting that it is located in a highly conserved region of the genome.[32] Six tau isoforms are produced from this gene by alternative mRNA splicing of exons 2, 3, and 10 to produce proteins ranging in size from 352 to 441 amino acids (45 to 65 kd).[30] These isoforms differ by the presence or absence of 58- or 29-amino acid inserts (correspond to exon-2 and exon-3 products) near the amino terminal of the protein and the presence or absence of a 31-amino acid insert (corresponding to exon 10) near the carboxyl terminal (Fig. 52–2).[30] The functions of the inserts near the amino terminal currently are

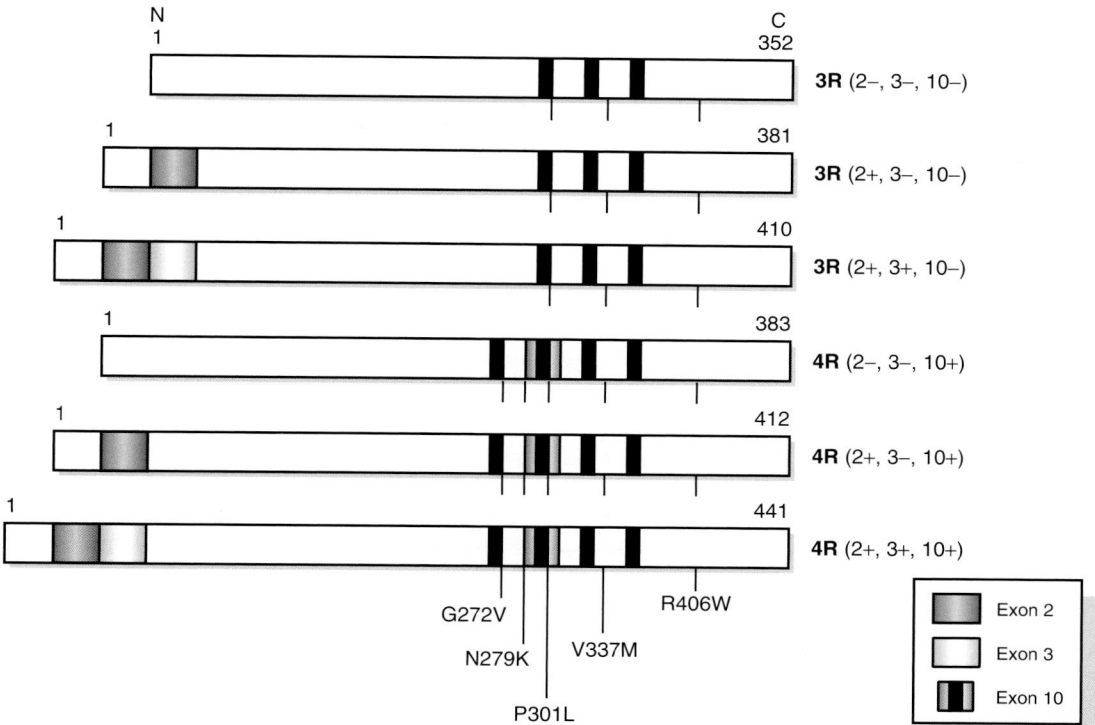

**FIGURE 52–2.** Schematic of the six human tau isoforms. Microtubule-binding domains are indicated in black. Only the shortest isoform is expressed in newborn brain, whereas all six isoforms are expressed in adult brain. The location of representative missense mutations responsible for tau pathology in familial tauopathies are shown in and around binding domains.

unknown. The insert encoded by exon 10 contains a microtubule binding domain.[33] Its absence results in three isoforms having only three microtubule binding domains each (designated *3R*), which are encoded by exons 9, 11, and 12. When the exon-10 encoded insert is present, it is the second binding domain from the amino end and yields three isoforms with four binding domains each (designated *4R*). These binding domains are composed of 18 amino acids and are highly conserved.[32, 34, 35]

Although the significance of these different isoforms is unknown, there is a shift in relative isoform concentrations through development, with only the shortest 3R isoform being present during fetal life and an equal representation of 3R and 4R isoforms present in the adult. The isoforms containing the 58-amino acid insert are expressed only weakly in the adult,[36] and 4R isoforms have been shown to have increased binding activity with microtubules relative to 3R isoforms.[37] Within the fetus, tau protein appears isolated at the ends of axons in developing neurons and is believed to participate in axonal elongation. In mice lacking the tau gene, normal development and life span are seen, with the only alterations being decreased microtubule stability in a subset of small-caliber axons and an increase in another microtubule-associated protein type.[38]

In vitro studies have shown that tau facilitates assembly and stabilization of tubulin into microtu-

bules through a phosphorylation-dephosphorylation modification of the tau protein, with phosphorylation leading to decreased tau-microtubule interaction and ultimate disassembly of the microtubule.[39, 40] More than 30 possible phosphorylation sites at serine and threonine residues have been identified on the tau protein that predominantly flank the microtubule binding domains (Fig. 52–3). Most of these sites are Ser-Pro and Thr-Pro motifs.[41] Only a few phosphorylation sites are reported to be within microtubule binding domains. In particular, phosphorylation at S262, which is present within the binding domain encoded by exon 9, has been shown to dramatically reduce microtubule binding in vitro.[42]

## Tau Pathology in Alzheimer's Disease

The NFTs seen in AD are composed predominantly of a pair of tau strands, each comprising six or seven tandem repeats (the microtubule binding region) bound together to form the core of a single strand (Fig. 52–4).[24] Each strand has a roughly rectangular cross-section. Commonly in AD, the two strands bind together along the shorter side of the rectangle; the resulting cross-sectional width of the paired filament is two to three times as long as its

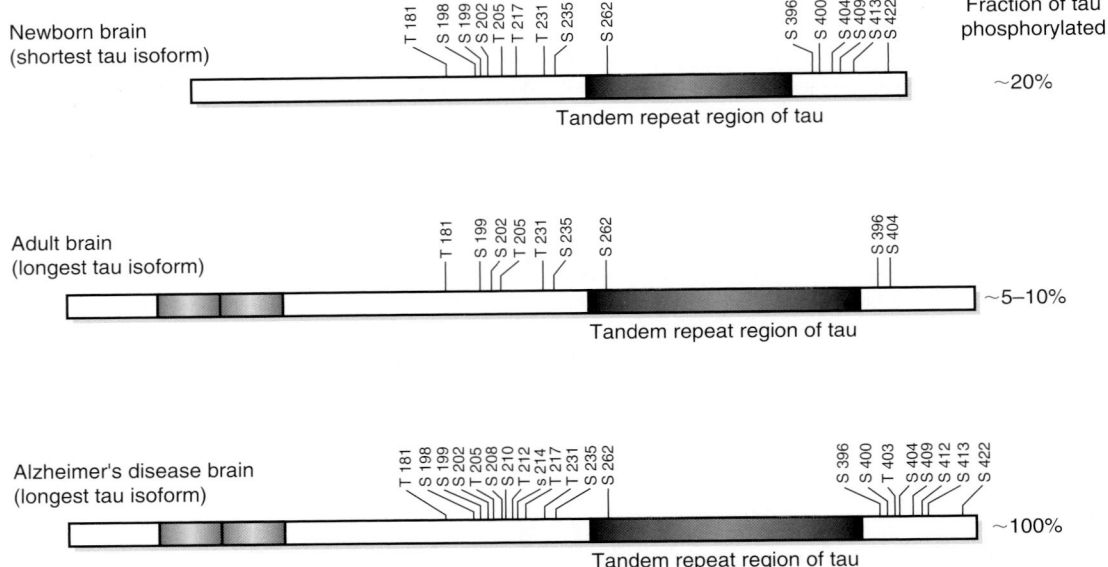

**FIGURE 52–3.** Known phosphorylation sites in tau in brains from a newborn, an adult, and a patient with Alzheimer's disease. Note that phosphorylation occurs at sites adjacent to the tandem repeat, microtubule binding domain. Note also, 100% of all six isoforms of tau in Alzheimer's disease are "hyperphosphorylated" relative to normal adult tau. (Courtesy of Michel Goedert.)

height. The relatively flat cross-section plus the natural twist of the two strands along the filament is visible by electron microscopy and has led to the term *paired helical filament* for the smallest unit NFT fiber.[43] When the broader sides of the two strands bind together to form a filament, the resulting cross-section has a roughly square profile. Although this filament has a natural twist along its length with a periodicity as in PHFs, because the cross-section is relatively symmetric, these paired filaments appear straight and without helical twists by standard electron microscopy. Tau in PHFs is hyperphosphorylated relative to normal tau (see Fig. 52–3). Western

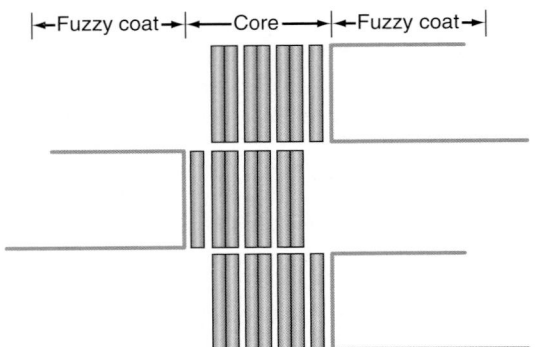

**FIGURE 52–4.** Model of one strand of the paired helical filament (PHF) structure. The core of the strand is composed exclusively of tau, in which six or seven tandem repeat domains bind as shown. The fuzzy coat of the PHF consists of the N- and C-terminal domains of tau. (Adapted from Wischik CM, Novak M, Thogersen HC, et al: Isolation of a fragment of tau derived from the core of the paired helical filament of Alzheimer disease. Proc Natl Acad Sci U S A 85:4506–4510, 1988.)

blot analysis indicates that PHFs are composed of approximately equal numbers of the hyperphosphorylated 3R and 4R tau isoforms in AD.[36, 44] In vitro studies have shown that hyperphosphorylated PHF-tau from AD patients causes normal tau to dissociate from microtubules and to form into insoluble filamentous tangles, suggesting that hyperphosphorylation is responsible for the tau pathology in AD.[45] Another report came to a different conclusion: It found that phosphorylation of certain sites in the shortest tau isoform, including the S262 site, prevents tau from forming filaments, even though it enhances the dissociation of tau from microtubules.[46] The authors concluded that hyperphosphorylation is a secondary phenomenon in PHF assembly.

Interactions of other proteins with tau have suggested other possible mechanisms for AD pathology. In particular, α-synuclein has been shown to bind to tau and to catalyze its phosphorylation at two serine residues (S262 and S356), indicating that it could play a role in PHF formation.[47] The mitotic regulatory protein Pin1, which is expressed in neurons, also has been shown to bind to phosphorylated tau in vitro.[48] Depletion of this key regulator of apoptosis by sequestration in abnormal tau deposits could be a possible mechanism for neuronal death.

## Pathogenic Mechanism of Dementia in Alzheimer's Disease

The definitive diagnosis of AD currently requires determining an age-adjusted semiquantitative estimate of the number of neuritic plaques and NFTs in a demented patient.[10-12] Plaques and NFTs must be counted because the combination provides the best correlation with the degree of dementia; however, it is the presence of neuritic plaques containing the Aβ peptide that is specific for AD because NFTs can be found in association with other neurodegenerative diseases, such as in postencephalitic parkinsonism, dementia pugilistica, amyotrophic lateral sclerosis (ALS)–Parkinson–dementia complex of Guam, subacute sclerosing panencephalitis, progressive supranuclear palsy,[49] and some familial forms of prion disease.[50] NFTs also are characteristic of the *tauopathies* (see later).

The histopathologic criteria for the diagnosis of AD are still evolving. There are three reasons for this ongoing evolution. First, there is a controversy regarding whether the number and distribution of senile plaques, NFTs, and neuropil threads or whether the Aβ and tau protein loads or both best correlate with the degree of dementia. Second, there are cases in which there are sufficient numbers of senile plaques distributed throughout the cerebral cortex to meet the morphologic criteria of AD, and yet the subject is cognitively normal.[51-56] Terry and colleagues[57] showed that the degree of generalized synapse loss in cortical and subcortical regions in AD correlates better with the degree of dementia than the number of plaques and NFTs, arguing that there are other mechanisms, in addition to Aβ peptide accumulation and NFT formation, that underlie dementia in AD. In this regard, it has been estimated that neuritic plaques account for about 10% to 20% of the synapse loss in AD. Third, there are cases in which there are insufficient numbers of amyloid plaques and NFTs to make a definitive morphologic diagnosis of AD, and yet the subject is demented. Some of these patients have coexisting vascular disease with infarcts, whereas others have widespread Lewy body degeneration of cerebral cortical and subcortical neurons.[58-60] It is possible that some of the cases of dementia without sufficient AD pathologic changes will be explained by the coexistence of a second form of neurodegeneration. It may be that etiologic factors that cause Lewy body degeneration and those that cause cerebrovascular disease also trigger neuritic plaque and NFT degeneration in some subjects.

## Formation of Aβ42 Peptide as a Result of Mismetabolism of βAPP Initiates the Events Leading to Alzheimer's Disease

Although alternative splicing during transcription of the βAPP gene results in six different mRNAs,[61-65] two do not contain the Aβ peptide domain (βAPP365 and βAPP563), and of the remaining four, APP714 is synthesized in only trace amounts. The βAPP695, βAPP751, and βAPP770 mRNAs differ by alternative splicing of exons 7 and 8. βAPP is a transmembrane protein with a portion of the C-terminal located intracellularly (Fig. 52–5). Of the 43 amino acids comprising the Aβ domain, 28 are on the outside of the cell membrane, whereas the remaining 15 are within the plasma membrane. Degradation of βAPP in the Aβ domain involves three enzymes designated *secretases*. α-Secretase cleaves at about 12 residues distal to the N-terminal end of the Aβ domain and divides it into two parts preventing Aβ peptide formation. β-Secretase cleaves the N-terminal end of the Aβ domain from the βAPP and is a potentially amyloidogenic cleavage. γ-Secretase also is potentially amyloidogenic because it cleaves the C-terminal Aβ domain, yielding mostly a non-amyloidogenic Aβ40 peptide, which is cleared from the central nervous system or, under conditions leading to AD, results in formation of more amyloidogenic Aβ42 than Aβ40. The former is not cleared from the central nervous system.

Selkoe[66, 67] has been a major proponent of the hypothesis that altered proteolytic cleavage of βAPP yielding the Aβ42 peptide is the key pathogenic event in AD. The main arguments include the following: 1) Aβ42 accumulation is an invariant feature of AD. 2) Some familial forms of AD are genetically linked to mutations of the βAPP gene, and the resulting neuropathologic phenotype is identical to that in sporadic AD. 3) A large proportion of patients with trisomy 21, who overexpress βAPP, develop AD. 4) Mutations of other genes genetically linked to familial AD also yield increased Aβ42 levels. Autosomal dominant AD has been linked to the presenilin-1 gene (*PS-1*, originally named *S182*) on chromosome 14 and the presenilin-2 gene (*PS-2*,

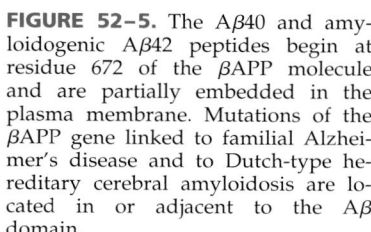

**FIGURE 52–5.** The Aβ40 and amyloidogenic Aβ42 peptides begin at residue 672 of the βAPP molecule and are partially embedded in the plasma membrane. Mutations of the βAPP gene linked to familial Alzheimer's disease and to Dutch-type hereditary cerebral amyloidosis are located in or adjacent to the Aβ domain.

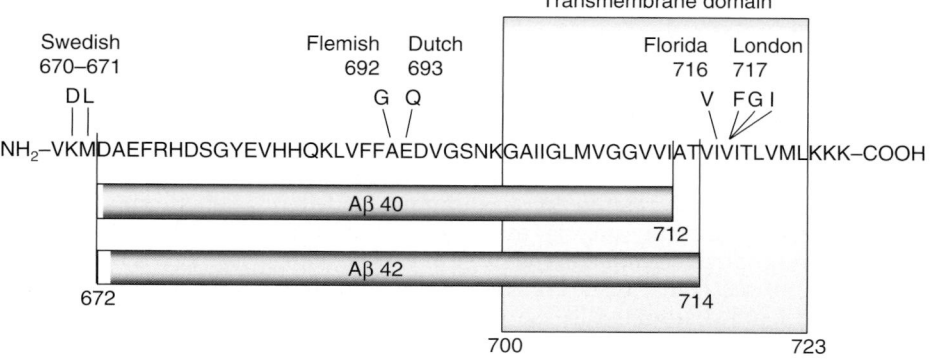

originally named *STM2*) on chromosome 1. 5) The ε4 allele of the apolipoprotein gene (*ApoE*) on chromosome 19, which is a risk factor for late-onset familial and sporadic AD, is associated with increased Aβ42 amyloid accumulation in the brain.

## Molecular Genetics of Familial Alzheimer's Disease

*Presenile dementia of the Alzheimer's type* is defined as AD occurring before the age of 55. Virtually all of these cases are dominantly inherited; however, not all forms of familial AD occur before age 55. Dominantly inherited forms of AD (familial AD) account for about 15% of all AD cases. Molecular genetic studies have revealed more about the cause and pathogenesis of sporadic AD and familial AD than they have provided diagnostic tools for the clinician during the life of the patient. Molecular genetics has shown that no single gene or gene product explains AD, in contrast to prion diseases and HD. To date, three genes have been linked genetically to different familial AD pedigrees; however, these account for only about 60% of familial AD families. The gene or genes causing 40% of familial AD cases remain to be found. All of the mutations result in increased formation of Aβ42.

## βAPP Mutations (Chromosome 21) in Familial Alzheimer's Disease

Three mutations of the *βAPP* gene have been linked to familial AD pedigrees (see Fig. 52–5). First, a double mutation has been linked to familial AD in a large Swedish kindred at codons 670 and 671 in exon 16. This mutation results in an asparagine-leucine substitution for lysine-methionine.[68] This mutation occurs immediately proximal to the N-terminal of the Aβ42 peptide, which begins at codon 673, at the β-secretase cut site. Transgenic mice expressing human 695 βAPP with the Swedish mutation show a 5-fold increase in Aβ40, a 13-fold increase in Aβ42, and deposition of Aβ amyloid plaques beginning at about 1 year of age.[69] Second, in Flemish pedigrees, two mutations have been identified near the α-secretase site within the Aβ domain. In pedigrees with a mutation at codon 692, there is an alanine-to-glycine substitution. Patients with this genotype present with presenile dementia with neuritic plaques and cerebral hemorrhage resulting from severe Aβ amyloid angiopathy.[70]

The second mutation site occurs at codon 693 (see Fig. 52–5) and results in a glutamic acid-to-glutamine substitution and is associated with the disease designated *hereditary cerebral hemorrhage with amyloidosis of the Dutch type* (HCHWA-D)[71, 72] to distinguish it from a similar disease that occurs among pedigrees in Iceland that is linked to mutations in the transthyretin gene and is designated *HCHWA-I*. HCHWA-D has been described in four families from two coastal villages in the Netherlands. It is characterized by extensive amyloid deposition in the walls of leptomeningeal and cerebral cortical vessels. Parenchymal amyloid deposits have been identified in some of these patients; however, these resemble immature plaques and preamyloid lesions and generally are not surrounded by dystrophic neurites. The disorder presents as strokes in otherwise healthy, nondemented, and normotensive individuals between the ages of 45 and 65.[73]

Third, multiple unrelated kindreds with familial AD have been identified on different continents with point mutations at codon 717 of exon 17 (see Fig. 52–5), which result in isoleucine, phenylalanine, or glycine for valine substitutions.[74–79] This mutation results in amino acid substitutions two residues distal to the γ-secretase cleavage site at the carboxy terminus of Aβ42, which ends at codon 714; this has been referred to as the *London mutation*. All of these mutations result in a "gain of function phenomenon" because they lead to greater levels of Aβ42 than normal and, in doing so, seem to foster amyloidogenesis. The Swedish mutation increases the rate of βAPP degradation through the β-secretase followed by the γ-secretase pathway.[80, 81] The London mutation, which is 3 amino acid residues distal to the 42nd residue of Aβ42, seems to alter the γ-secretase cleavage site leading to longer and less soluble Aβ42 and Aβ43.[82] In contrast, the Flemish mutation results in increased Aβ42 production by blocking the α-secretase pathway that cleaves within the Aβ domain.[83]

## PS-1 Mutations (Chromosome 14) in Familial Alzheimer's Disease

In 1992, a gene on chromosome 14 that cosegregates with early-onset AD was found.[84] In 1995, the gene was identified by Sherrington and colleagues[85] in St. George Hyslop's laboratory and originally was designated *S182* but is now designated *PS-1*. The *PS-1* gene contains 12 exons and codes for a protein with 467 amino acid residues.[85] The predicted sequence and hydrophobicity analysis indicated nine putative transmembrane domains,[85] although it is believed that eight exist in reality.[86, 87] In the eight-transmembrane model of PS-1, the N-terminal and C-terminal project into the cytoplasm (Fig. 52–6). In addition, there is a large hydrophilic loop between transmembrane six and transmembrane seven that also projects into the cytoplasm. Most of *PS-1* is believed to be localized to the smooth and rough endoplasmic reticulum. In the brain, little or no full-length *PS-1*, which is about 42 to 43 kd, is found. Most seems to be cleaved normally, yielding two peptides, a 27- to 28-kd N-terminal fragment and a 16- to 17-kd C-terminal fragment.[88] Cleavage normally occurs in the

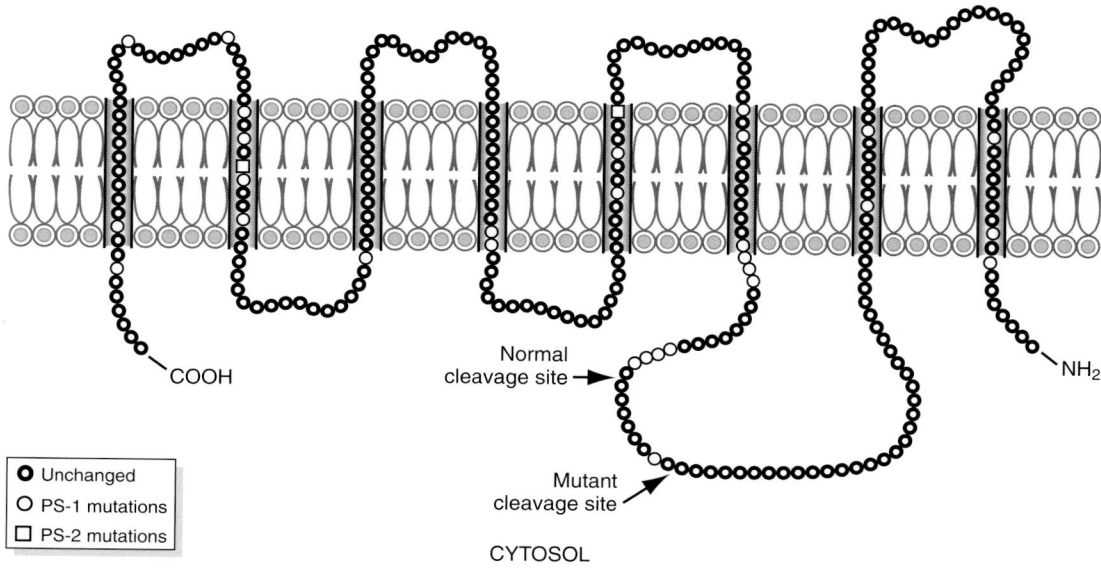

**FIGURE 52–6.** The eight-transmembrane model of presenilin-1 (PS-1) in the endoplasmic reticulum (ER). The N- and C-terminals as well as the large hydrophobic loop project into the cytosol. Normally, PS-1 is divided into two peptides at the cleavage site shown in the large hydrophobic loop.

large hydrophilic cytoplasmic loop, encoded by exon 9, near residue 299. A total of 45 different mutations of the *PS-1* gene have been linked to familial AD.[89] Greater than 50% of familial AD–linked *PS-1* mutations occur in exons 8 and 9 that code for the amino acids near the *PS-1* cleavage site in the large hydrophilic loop. The second most common cluster of *PS-1* mutations linked to familial AD occurs in exon 5, which codes for the transmembrane-2 domain. The average age of onset of familial AD linked to *PS-1* mutations is 40 years for exon 5 mutations and 43 years for exon 8 mutations compared with a mean age of onset of 47 years for all other *PS-1* mutations, which argues that these code for crucial functional or conformational domains.[89] Most mutations result in amino acid substitutions. One mutation occurs in the splice acceptor site for exon 9 and splices it out of *PS-1* mRNA (Δex9 mutation).[90]

How mutations of the *PS-1* and *PS-2* (see later) genes increase the formation of Aβ42 and lead to AD is being learned from *PS-1* knockout mice and transgenic mice expressing *PS-1*. Lack of *PS-1* in knockout mice markedly alters γ-secretase processing of βAPP, leading to defects in secretion of Aβ peptides and intracellular accumulation of Aβ containing C-terminal fragments, indicating that it may be necessary for the function of γ-secretase.[91] In contrast, patients with mutations of *PS-1* have significantly elevated Aβ42-to-Aβ40 ratios.[92] Double transgenic mice expressing human *PS-1* with an A246E mutation in the transmembrane-6 domain and human βAPP with the Swedish mutation develop Aβ plaques much earlier and in greater numbers than mice expressing human βAPP alone.[93] It has been

suggested that the presenilins modulate γ-secretase activity.[88]

## PS-2 Mutations (Chromosome 1) in Familial Alzheimer's Disease

Contemporaneous with the chromosome 14 linkage study, Levy-Lahad and associates[94] found that familial AD among the Volga German kindreds was not linked to chromosome 14 but to chromosome 1. Although the general rule for familial AD is early onset of disease (e.g., presenile dementia), Volga German familial AD cases were late onset. Based on the structure of *PS-1*, other groups simultaneously were searching for and found an isologous gene on chromosome 1 originally designated *STM2* because it potentially had seven transmembrane domains.[95, 96] Genetic linkage of two mutations with the Volga German familial AD samples (see Fig. 52–6) was established, and because of about 67% homology with *PS-1*, it was renamed *PS-2*.[95, 96]

## Genetic Predisposition to Late-Onset Alzheimer's Disease

The risk of sporadic AD correlates with getting older (>65 years), with gender (two to three times more prevalent in women than men), with Down's syndrome (trisomy 21), with level of education (inverse relationship), and with the expression of the ε4 allele of the *ApoE* gene.

## ApoE Genotype and Aβ Peptide Load in the Brain

It is not known whether AD is inevitable in all humans who live long enough or whether aging of the brain can take different pathways, including one without neuritic plaque and NFT formation. Workers who believe that AD is inevitable argue there are genetic factors that can accelerate or impede the development of AD and account for its variable presentation during life. Workers who believe the alternative hypothesis argue that AD is not inevitable; rather, it requires a combination of genetic and environmental factors to develop. These workers envision distinct pathways of aging and that AD is one possible pathway.

One of the most significant genetically determined risk factors that seems to influence which aging pathway is followed is the ApoE allotype.[97–105] The risks of late-onset familial AD and sporadic AD are associated with expression of the ApoE ε4 expression in dose-dependent and age-related manners. In contrast, the ε2 and ε3 alleles seem to be protective. ApoE is a 34-kd protein encoded by a 4-exon gene on the long arm of chromosome 19.[106] Three ApoE alleles, designated ε2, ε3, and ε4, result from Arg-Cys polymorphisms at residues 112 and 158. The most common allelic variants in the North American population are ε3/ε3 (60%) followed by ε3/ε4 (23%). The least common are ε2/ε2 (1%), ε2/ε4 (2%), and ε4/ε4 (2%). The ε2/ε3 (13%) occurs with an intermediate frequency. Similar frequencies have been found in the Framingham study.[107] With ε4/ε4, the odds of developing AD are about 19 times greater for senile dementia of the Alzheimer type and about 16 times greater for late-onset familial AD compared with ε3/ε3.[108] The ε3/ε4 population has a roughly 4 to 4.5 times increased incidence for late-onset familial and sporadic AD than ε3/ε3. Evidence for the protective effect of the ε2 allele was the finding that the ε2/ε3 population had about half the risk of late-onset familial and sporadic AD than the ε3/ε3 population. Also, when the ε2 allele is expressed with the ε4 allele (ε2/ε4 population), the incidence of AD was reduced by 25% to 35% compared with the ε3/ε4 population and about 90% compared with the ε4/ε4 population. The risk of AD as a function of the ApoE allele also varies greatly with age. The risk with the ε4 and the benefit of the ε2 alleles are highest for late-onset cases in patients aged 60 to 66. The ε4/ε4 genotype did not appear in patients after the age of 82, presumably because it confers an additional risk of death resulting from vascular disease. The ε2/ε3 genotype becomes more common with increasing age presumably because of decreased risk for common causes of death conferred by this genotype before the age of 70.

ApoE plays a major role in the mobilization and redistribution of cholesterol and phospholipid during reactive synaptic remodeling (note: the efficiency of tau reactive synaptogenesis may play a role in whether or not dementia occurs after deposition of Aβ peptide).[102, 109] ApoE also binds the Aβ peptide to its lipoprotein-binding domain, forming a stable complex.[110, 111] Binding seems to require oxidation of ApoE. ApoE-ε4 binds to Aβ within minutes in vitro, whereas ApoE-ε3 requires hours. ApoE-ε4 promotes Aβ polymerization into amyloid filaments.[112–114] ApoE-ε4 enhances fibrillogenesis of other amyloid-related peptides and has raised the hypothesis that it is a universal pathologic chaperone.[115] The amount of Aβ peptide that accumulates in the brain in subjects with sporadic AD is about 50% higher in ε4/ε4 subjects compared with ε3/ε3 subjects and 10% to 30% higher in ε3/ε4 subjects.[103, 116] The area of cortex occupied by Aβ peptide plaques also was greater for subjects carrying the ε4 allele. Immunohistochemistry with antibodies to ApoE has shown it localized to classic neuritic plaques, amyloid angiopathy, and neurofibrillary tangles in AD.[117]

## LEWY BODY DISORDERS: DISEASES ASSOCIATED WITH SYNUCLEIN ABNORMALITIES

Neurodegeneration with Lewy bodies occurs in three groups of diseases. First, idiopathic Parkinson's disease (PD) is characterized clinically by the triad of bradykinesia, rigidity, and tremor. The main neuropathologic features include greater than 70% loss of dopaminergic neurons of the pars compacta of the substantia nigra with Lewy bodies in some remaining nigral neurons (Fig. 52–7A) and variable numbers of Lewy bodies in other subcortical neuron populations, such as nucleus basalis of Meynert, locus coeruleus, dorsal efferent nucleus of the vagus nerve, and sympathetic chain ganglia.

The second disorder is named *diffuse Lewy body disease*, which is characterized by progressive waxing and waning psychiatric disturbances and dementia often in association with bradykinesia and rigidity. The disease is characterized neuropathologically by Lewy body inclusions in the neocortex, in limbic structures such as the cingulate gyrus, and in the substantia nigra with few or no neuritic plaques and NFTs. Analysis of the brain at postmortem from a patient suspected to have had diffuse Lewy body disease begins by examination of an H&E-stained section of the substantia nigra for classic Lewy bodies followed by immunohistochemical staining of the cingulate gyrus, amygdala, and hippocampus for neurons containing α-synuclein immunopositive Lewy bodies (Fig. 52–7B).[118] α-Synuclein immunohistochemistry frequently is required to identify cortical Lewy bodies because they often are obscure in the cerebral cortex with the routine H&E stain. α-Synuclein immunopositive neurites in the hippocampus are another diagnostic feature revealed by immunohistochemistry.

The third neurodegenerative disorder in which Lewy bodies feature is AD/Lewy body variant. The

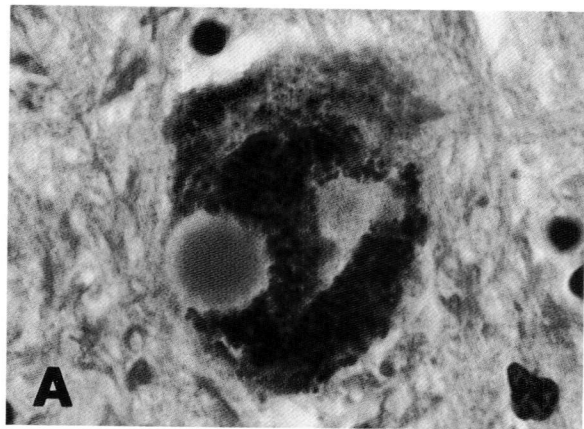

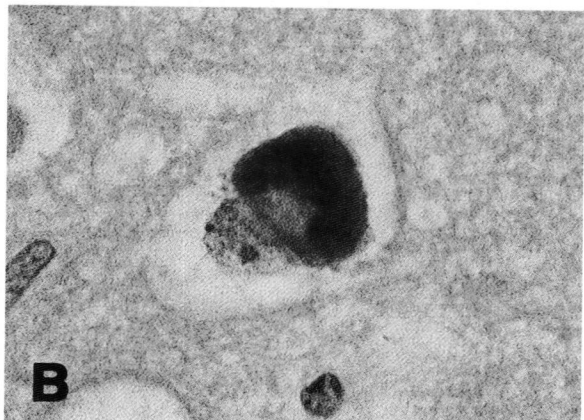

**FIGURE 52–7.** Lewy bodies. *A.* The classic Lewy body as seen in the cytoplasm of a substantia nigra neuron consists of a glassy spherical mass with a characteristic halo with the hematoxylin and eosin (H&E) stain. *B.* The cerebral cortical Lewy body is often more difficult to identify by a routine H&E stain but is easily recognized by α-synuclein immunohistochemistry. Note also that the neuropil surrounding the neuron has a granular immunopositivity as a result of α-synuclein staining of presynaptic boutons.

clinical features of this diagnostic category include dementia with or without parkinsonism. The neuropathologic features include neuritic plaques, NFTs, and nigral and cortical Lewy bodies. In some cases, there are sufficient neuritic plaques to meet the criteria for AD but no NFTs, whereas in other cases there are insufficient numbers of neuritic plaques and NFTs to qualify for AD. In these situations, if

the patient presented with dementia and little or no bradykinesia or tremor but has cortical Lewy bodies, we still apply the diagnosis of AD/Lewy body variant.

## α-Synuclein and Parkinson's Disease

Dominantly inherited Lewy body PD is rare. It was found, however, that genetic markers on chromosome 4 segregate with the PD phenotype in a large family of Italian descent.[119] Patients in this family presented with parkinsonism at a relatively early age (46 ± 13 years) compared with the mean onset of idiopathic parkinsonism of about 60 years. The chromosome 4 locus resolved to an A53T substitution in the α-synuclein gene open reading frame (Fig. 52–8). A year later, a second mutation, A30P, was reported that is linked genetically to a German pedigree.[120] Immunohistochemical localization of α-synuclein in Lewy bodies of idiopathic PD and diffuse Lewy body disease was published at about the same time as the first molecular genetic study.[121] These findings argue there is a causal relationship between mutated α-synuclein and familial Lewy body parkinsonism and implicate a primary abnormality of wild-type synuclein in idiopathic PD.

## Overlap of Alzheimer's Disease with Lewy Body Degeneration

The application of ubiquitin, then α-synuclein immunohistochemistry to identify cortical Lewy bodies has helped resolve the conundrum of how a patient could have insufficient numbers of plaques and NFTs for diagnosis of AD but still have dementia. Ubiquitin and α-synuclein immunohistochemistry indicate there is a more than coincidental overlap of AD changes with Lewy body degeneration. It has been estimated that 20% to 30% of patients with dementia with neuritic plaques and NFTs also have cortical and subcortical Lewy bodies.[60, 122–124] It is estimated that abnormal α-synuclein deposition as Lewy bodies in cortical neurons may be by themselves or in combination with AD changes the second most common form of neurodegeneration leading to dementia, accounting for 20% to 30% of cases in patients older than age 60.

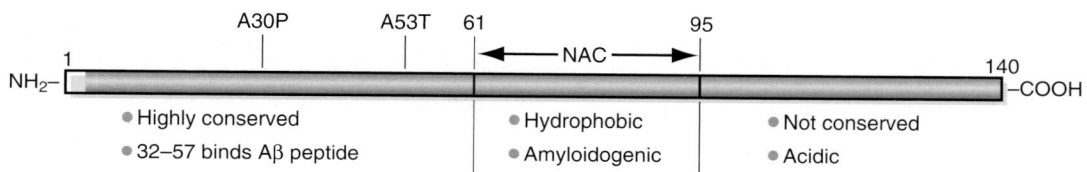

**FIGURE 52–8.** Schematic of the α-synuclein molecule showing the location of the NAC peptide found in amyloid plaques of Alzheimer's disease and the two mutations genetically linked to familial Parkinson's disease.

α-Synuclein is a 140-amino acid protein about 19 kd encoded by a gene on chromosome 4.[124] The molecule has three domains: 1) an N-terminal domain (residues 1 to 60) composed of incomplete KTKEGV repeats, 2) an extremely hydrophobic central domain (residues 61 to 95), and 3) an acidic C-terminal domain (residues 96 to 140) (see Fig. 52–8). α-Synuclein belongs to a family of proteins that include β-synuclein encoded on chromosome 5 and γ-synuclein encoded on chromosome 10. In humans, in addition to expression of full-length α-synuclein with 140 residues, two smaller 125- and 112-residue isoforms are expressed at lower levels. The isoforms result from deletions of codons encoding residues 41 to 54 and 103 to 130.

The overlap of α-synuclein abnormalities with AD first was discovered during purification of non-Aβ peptides from isolated amyloid plaques. An unknown hydrophobic, amyloidogenic peptide 35 residues in length, was found and named *NAC* for *non-Aβ component* of AD amyloid.[125, 126] Antisera raised to NAC immunostained neuritic plaques and vascular amyloid of AD. The precursor gene and protein were identified from cDNA libraries and designated the *NAC protein*. Immunohistochemistry localized NAC protein to presynaptic boutons (see Fig. 52–7B) often colocalizing with synaptophysin. NAC protein was found to be 95% homologous with α-synuclein, and the NAC domain was found to be the central hydrophobic region of the α-synuclein molecule (see Fig. 52–8).[126] Synuclein (NAC) antibodies react with 35% of the diffuse neuritic plaques and 55% of the mature neuritic plaques in AD but with no neuritic plaques in nondemented aged controls.[127] The numbers of synuclein immunopositive presynaptic bouton-like structures also were decreased 30% to 40% in AD but not in controls, providing further evidence that generalized cortical synapse loss is required for dementia in AD. The two mutations genetically linked to familial Lewy body PD, A30P and A53T, occur just proximal to the amyloidogenic NAC peptide domain, which extends from residues 61 to 95 (see Fig. 52–8). Residue 53 is predicted to be near the C-terminal end of a putative α-helical structure flanked on either side by β-sheet domains. These amino acid substitutions are predicted to extend the β-sheet structure of the molecule and to promote aggregation into Lewy bodies.

## α-Synuclein in Alzheimer's Disease

Whether abnormalities of α-synuclein play an active or passive role in the pathogenesis of AD is unknown. α-Synuclein expression is up-regulated only in the early stages of AD, in contrast to other synaptic proteins, including synaptophysin, which are decreased steadily throughout the course of the disease.[127, 128] Normally, α-synuclein is localized to presynaptic boutons (see Fig. 52–7B); immunogold-electron microscopy shows that it is associated with synaptic vesicles.[125] Given the aforementioned differences in synaptic bouton protein kinetics, it is of interest that the α-synuclein degradation product, NAC, becomes incorporated into neuritic plaques, whereas other synaptic proteins do not.[124] Aβ38 binds to α-synuclein, forming an SDS-insoluble complex in vitro.[129] The specific Aβ binding site in the NAC peptide seems to reside in residues 81 to 95. Given that NAC is highly hydrophobic and easily forms into amyloid fibrils[125] and given the absence of a linkage between α-synuclein polymorphisms and AD,[130] the possibility that α-synuclein is a bystander in AD, becoming incorporated in Aβ plaques when synapses degenerate, is raised. NAC peptides may contribute directly to the pathogenesis of AD dementia by α-synuclein-stimulated protein kinase A phosphorylation of tau, contributing to neurofibrillary tangle formation.[47]

## α-Synuclein in Other Neurodegenerative Diseases

The application of α-synuclein immunohistochemistry to other neurodegenerative diseases is revealing that disease-related abnormal accumulation of α-synuclein peptides may not be specific for Lewy body diseases and AD. Moreover, abnormal cytoplasmic α-synuclein deposits may not be confined

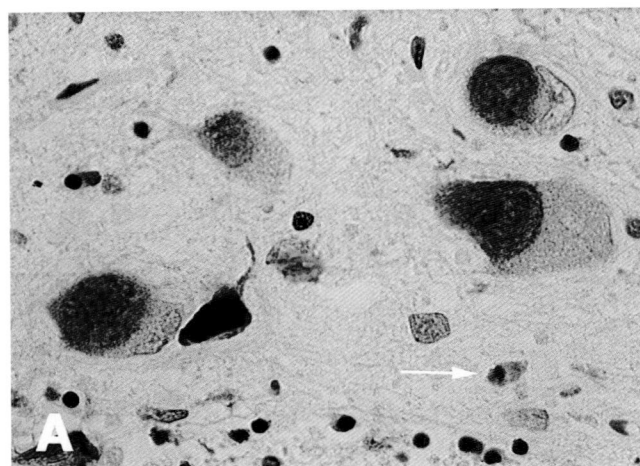

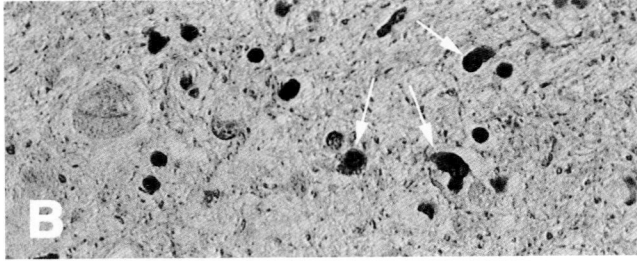

**FIGURE 52–9.** A case of olivopontocerebellar and striatonigral degeneration showing (*A*) abnormal α-synuclein immunopositive neurons in the base of the pons and (*B*) oligodendrocytes in the pontine white matter with cytoplasmic tau deposits (*arrows*). Note also, an oligodendrocyte in *A* has an α-synuclein immunopositive cell body (*arrow*).

exclusively to nerve cells. Two publications reported that α-synuclein peptides form cytoplasmic inclusions in neurons and oligodendrocytes of patients with multiple system atrophy.[131, 132] We have made the same observation in a case of the combined striatonigral-olivopontocerebellar degeneration form of multiple system atrophy (Fig. 52–9). The question raised by these findings is whether α-synuclein aggregates secondarily to abnormalities of axonal transport or whether it is a primary event leading to abnormal axonal transport. With regard to the presence of α-synuclein in glial cells, could it be that release of protease-resistant NAC peptide polymers into the extracellular space after the death of neurons leads to phagocytosis by glial populations? Or is there a general abnormality of α-synuclein that causes it to accumulate in any cell type in which it is synthesized?

## TAUOPATHIES INCLUDING THE FRONTOTEMPORAL DEMENTIAS

Although NFTs containing deposits of tau protein are a significant pathologic finding seen in the brains from AD patients (see Fig. 52–1D and E), there is a group of neurodegenerative disorders that are characterized by the presence of abnormal filamentous tau deposits without amyloid plaques or Lewy bodies. These disorders, collectively named *tauopathies*,[133] are a clinically, neuroanatomically, and ultrastructurally heterogeneous group (Table 52–2).[41, 134–141] In general, the pathologic findings in all of these disorders include neuronal loss; astrogliosis; and the presence of abnormal filamentous deposits of hyperphosphorylated tau protein within neurons or glial cells (or both) of the central nervous system, usually in a neuroanatomic distribution that correlates with the clinical findings of each individual entity. Ultrastructurally, different types of tau filaments are seen with each disorder.[41, 134–136, 142] Most of these disorders are familial with an autosomal dominant pattern of inheritance and presenile onset. Although AD, diffuse Lewy body disease, and anoxic brain injury are the main causes of dementia in individuals older than age 60, tauopathies are being recognized with greater frequency. Ten percent of all dementia cases[143, 144] and 10% to 20% of presenile dementias may be of this type.[145, 146] It has been estimated that 30% to 50% of these cases are familial.[143, 144]

Clinical and pathologic features of a few of these tauopathies are presented to highlight their heterogeneity. Progressive supranuclear palsy is characterized clinically by vertical gaze palsy and gait disturbances with progression to dementia and akinesia over an average course of 10 years with death around age 60.[147–151] Familial cases have been reported and suggest autosomal dominant transmission with incomplete penetrance.[152, 153] Pathologic findings include neuronal loss with astrocytic gliosis in the basal ganglia, subthalamic nucleus, cerebel-

lum, and prefrontal cortex.[148, 150] Filamentous tau deposits present within neurons and glial cells in the affected regions are composed of straight filaments.[134, 135, 154] Ballooned neurons similar to those seen in Pick's disease also may be present (Fig. 52–10).[135, 148, 150] Genetic analyses of familial forms have shown an overrepresentation of the most common wild-type tau genotype[32, 155]; as of yet, no tau gene mutations have been identified in progressive supranuclear palsy cases.[153]

Frontotemporal dementia presents with behavioral and personality changes including apathy, irritability, hyperorality, diminished speech output, and progressive dementia leading to death in patients usually in their 50s.[143, 156–158] Pathologic findings include severe neuronal loss and gliosis in the frontotemporal cortices that sometimes includes the basal ganglia and amygdala. In some cases, tau deposits are seen within these areas, but this has been an inconsistent finding.[156, 159] Balloon cells and Pick bodies (see Fig. 52–10) may be seen, arguing that such cases might be designated better as *Pick's disease* or *atypical Pick's disease*.[146, 158, 160–162] Other tauopathies, such as the ALS-parkinsonism-dementia complex of Guam and corticobasal degeneration,

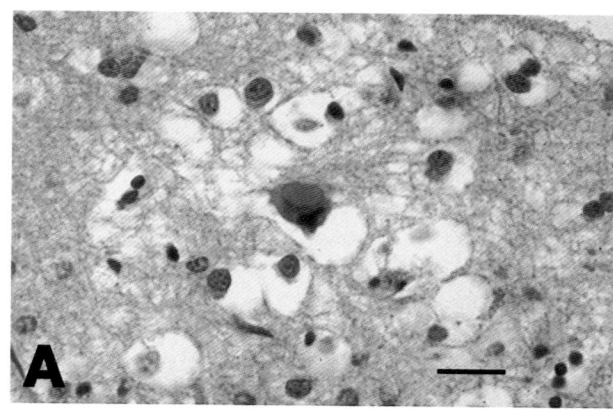

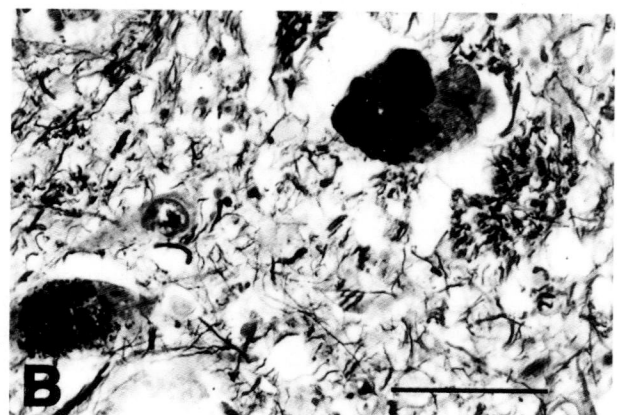

**FIGURE 52–10.** Pick's disease. *A.* A ballooned neuron in the cerebral cortex (H&E stain). *B.* Pick bodies, composed of filamentous tau deposits, are located in the cytoplasm of cortical neurons (Bielschowsky silver stain). Ballooned cells and Pick bodies are also seen in other Frontotemporal dementias as well as in Progressive supranuclear palsy. Bars in *(A)* and *(B)* are 25 µm.

**TABLE 52–2.** Neurodegenerative Disorders with Abnormal Tau Deposits

| Disorder | Glial Deposits | Familial Form? | Gene | Tau Pathology | Deposited Tau Isoforms | Comments |
|---|---|---|---|---|---|---|
| AD | No | Yes | APP<br>PS-1<br>PS-2 | PHF, SF* | All | Included as tauopathy by some<br>Familial forms ~5% of cases? |
| Down's syndrome | No | No | | PHF, SF | ? | Similar pathologic findings as AD |
| Dementia pugilistica | No | No | | | ? | *Punch drunk syndrome,* pathology owing to head trauma |
| Argyrophilic grain disease, dementia with grains | Yes, nonfilament tau deposits | ? | ? | Nonfilamentous tau deposits | ? | May be seen alone or with findings of other disorders (e.g., AD, Pick's disease) |
| Diffuse neurofibrillary tangles with calcification | ? | ? | ? | NFTs with calcification ? filament types | ? | Presenile dementia usually seen in women in Japan |
| Senile dementia with tangles | Yes, coiled and SF | No | | Coiled and SF | ? | Sporadic, late-onset dementia (age ~80s, F:M = 4:1, average 4-year course) |
| ALS-Parkinson's dementia complex of Guam | No | No | | PHF | All | Seems to be of environmental cause |
| Progressive supranuclear palsy | Yes, SF | Yes | ? | SF | 4R | Linkage disequilibrium with tau gene<br>No linkage to chromosome 17 shown |
| Corticobasal degeneration | Yes, TF* | ? | ? | TF | 4R | One report of tau gene mutation in one family |
| Pick's disease | Yes, coiled and SF | Yes | ? | Pick bodies (coiled and SF) | 3R | |
| Frontotemporal dementia | Not identified | Yes | Chromosome 3? | ? | ? | Some cases with no tau deposits |
| FTDP-17 | Yes, variable | Yes | Chromosome 17, tau gene | Variable | Variable | Includes multiple system tauopathy with presenile dementia, disinhibition-dementia-parkinsonism-amyotrophy complex, familial progressive subcortical gliosis, hereditary dysphasia dystonia dementia, pallidopontonigral degeneration |

* SF, straight filaments; TF, twisted filaments.

have different combinations of clinical features and distributions of pathologic findings.[163, 164]

Because of this confusing mix of different neuropathologic features in these disorders and marked variations in clinical presentations, many conventions and classification schemes[160, 165, 166] have been proposed to define this tauopathy group more accurately; nevertheless, there is still significant confusion and disagreement.[135, 167] Clinically suspicious cases of frontotemporal dementia sometimes show

the balloon cells of Pick's disease and may be classified as atypical Pick's disease, and other times cases do not show any distinctive inclusions or tau deposits. Some of the latter cases have been given other names, such as *dementia lacking distinctive histology* or *frontal lobe degeneration*.[145, 165, 166, 168, 169] It is hoped that molecular genetic analysis of sufficient numbers of these cases and families may help resolve the complexity. Genetic analysis of a family with an autosomal dominant pattern of inheritance for dementia lacking distinctive histology showed linkage to a pericentromeric region of chromosome 3[170]; however, no gene or mutation has been reported yet.

## Frontotemporal Dementia with Parkinsonism

One hopeful advance has been with another clinically heterogeneous subset of familial cases with an autosomal dominant pattern of inheritance and the clinical features of dementia and parkinsonism late in the disease course and filamentous tau deposits in the brain.[156, 157, 171] This group is so heterogeneous that individuals within the same family may present with the clinical picture of a different neurodegenerative syndrome. Linkage analysis performed on these families has shown segregation of disease to the long arm of chromosome 17 (ch17q21–22) where the tau gene is located.[156, 157, 171] Subsequent sequencing of the tau gene of affected family members has revealed mutations that are believed to be responsible for the pathology.[41, 156, 172–175] These disorders are listed in Table 52–2 with the disorder "frontotemporal dementia with parkinsonism linked to chromosome 17" (FTDP-17).[156] At least 17 different mutations of the tau gene have been identified in studies of more than 30 different affected families.[34, 35, 41, 172–183] Most have been shown to be present at highly conserved locations of the gene, have not been detected in unaffected individuals, and are present only in affected individuals or family members at a preonset age. Although not yet conclusive, this evidence strongly supports the hypothesis that tau mutations cause these disorders. A list of the known mutations, their associated clinical diagnosis, and their tau pathology is provided in Table 52–3.[184, 185] These mutations currently represent a small subset of familial frontotemporal dementia cases. Frontotemporal dementia families

without tau gene mutations already have been reported.[184, 185] Still, identification of genetic markers for various forms of these conditions is an extremely promising step in elucidating the pathogenesis of these disorders. The remainder of this section describes the pathophysiology of tau and the possible mechanism by which the genetic mutations in FTDP-17 patients may lead to tau pathology.

## Tau Pathology in the Tauopathies

Most of the studies of tau pathology have been in the context of AD (see earlier); nevertheless, these findings highlight the differences between AD NFTs and the tau filaments seen in tauopathies. Although all tau isoforms are present in the PHFs of AD, the filamentous tau deposits in tauopathies exhibit different isoform concentrations that sometimes are disease specific (see Table 52–2).[44, 186] The inclusions in Pick's disease contain only the 3R tau, which forms into tangles of coiled and straight filaments that are present in Pick bodies (see Fig. 52–10). Progressive supranuclear palsy and corticobasal degeneration deposits contain only 4R tau, but they aggregate differently: twisted filaments in corticobasal degeneration and straight filaments in progressive supranuclear palsy.[135, 136, 142] No disease-specific genetic mutations have been identified in familial cases of Pick's disease or progressive supranuclear palsy to date to help explain this pathology, as previously mentioned.[32, 153]

In FTDP-17, the isoforms detected in deposits are seen to be mutation specific. Most mutations involving exon 10 or its intron result in deposits containing predominantly the 4R isoforms, whereas other mutations yield pathology with all six isoforms present (see Table 52–2).[36, 172, 174, 180] It has been proposed that many of these mutations (S305N, E10+3, E10+12, E10+13, E10+14, E10+16)

**TABLE 52–3.** Reported Tau Gene Mutations in FTDP-17 and Related Disorders*

| Mutation | Exon | Disorder | Isoforms | Tau Pathology |
|---|---|---|---|---|
| G272V | 9 | FTDP-17 | All | ? |
| N279K | 10 | PPND | 4R >> 3R | ? |
| ΔK280 | 10 | Isolated case | ? 3R ? | ? |
| L284L | 10 | FTDP-17 | 4R >>> 3R | ? |
| P301L | 10 | FTDP-17 | 4R >> 3R | Narrow twisted filaments |
| P301S | 10 | FTDP-17 | ? | ? |
| S305N | 10 | FTDP-17 | 4R >> 3R | ? |
| Exon 10 + 3 | Intronic | MSTD† | 4R | Wide twisted filaments |
| Exon 10 + 12 | Intronic | FTDP-17 | 4R | ? |
| Exon 10 + 13 | Intronic | FTDP-17 | 4R | ? |
| Exon 10 + 14 | Intronic | FTDP-17 | 4R | ? |
| Exon 10 + 16 | Intronic | DDPAC,† FTDP-17 | 4R | ? |
| V337M | 12 | FTDP-17 | All | PHF, straight filaments |
| G389R | 13 | FTD | All | ? |
| R406W | 13 | FTDP-17 | All | PHF |

* Amino acids are numbered from amino to carboxyl end for the largest tau isoform 4R(2+,3+,10+) according to scheme of Goedert.[30]
† MSTD, multiple system tauopathy with presenile dementia; DDPAC, disinhibition-dementia-parkinsonism-amyotrophy complex.

interfere with an RNA stem loop structure at the 5' end of exon 10 that regulates its splicing (Fig. 52–11).[37, 172, 173] These mutations can destabilize this stem loop, allowing for increased splicing of exon 10 and higher levels of 4R isoforms.[180, 187, 188] Other mutations in exon 10 (N279K and L284L) have been shown to increase its splicing by an unknown mechanism, also leading to increased 4R isoforms. It has been proposed that they too interfere with a splicing regulatory element that has not been discovered yet.[180] Looking at these exon 10 mutations collectively, it is postulated that the 4R isoforms produced by these genes are normal but are out of proportion to 3R isoforms, and this excess promotes tau polymerization into filaments.[134] The 4R isoforms produced by genes with the N279K and S305N mutations show normal interaction with microtubules in vitro, supporting this hypothesis.[36, 180]

Tau products from other missense mutations (G272V, V337M, R405W), including the P301L of exon 10, contain all six isoforms and have been shown to have decreased affinity for microtubules.[36, 180, 189] For the P301L mutation, only the 4R isoforms are observed to have attenuated microtubule interaction; the 3R isoforms behave normally because they do not contain the mutation, indicating that the mutation is responsible for the decreased binding.[189] These results suggest that these mutations cause deleterious structural alterations in the protein that ultimately favor filament formation. Whether these structural alterations affect phosphorylation is unknown, but most mutations are within binding domains, favoring that it is an altered interaction with the microtubule that is the initiating step toward filament formation. Phosphorylation then is likely to occur secondarily.[90] Results from studies of tau gene mutations in FTDP-17 suggest various mechanisms for the development of pathology and highlight the genetic heterogeneity present in this disorder. The mechanisms can be generalized into two types—those that increase 4R isoforms and those that deleteriously alter tau-microtubule interactions. Both of these mechanisms seem quite different compared with how filaments are thought to form in AD. Although there is significant evidence that hyperphosphorylation plays some role in formation of PHFs in AD, the mechanism by which tau aggregates into filaments in AD is unknown. Likewise, the theories explaining tau pathology in FTDP-17 need further exploration, although data suggest that the presence of excess or nonbinding forms of tau leads to filament formation and pathology. Observations of abnormal forms of nonfilamentous tau in AD and results of recently described animal models also support this idea.[190–192] Mice transgenic for either the shortest or longest human tau isoforms showed axonal degeneration in brain and spinal cord with the formation of astrogliosis and accumulation of filamentous material in neurons that is immunoreactive with antibodies to tau. There is great promise that these newly developed transgenic models expressing mutated tau proteins will result in rapid progress in understanding of AD and other disorders in which abnormal tau deposits seem to foster neurodegeneration.

## PRION DISEASES

The neurodegenerative syndromes included among the human prion diseases are CJD, Gerstmann-Sträussler-Scheinker (GSS) disease, familial fatal insomnia (FFI), sporadic fatal insomnia, and kuru. The animal syndromes include scrapie of sheep and goats, transmissible mink encephalopathy, chronic wasting disease of mule deer and elk, feline spongiform encephalopathy, and bovine spongiform encephalopathy of Great Britain. Although prion diseases present sporadically 85% to 90% of the time in humans and by dominant inheritance 10% to 15% of the time similar to other neurodegenerative diseases, in contrast to other neurodegenerative diseases, prion diseases also are transmissible. Prion diseases are relatively rare compared to AD and Lewy body diseases, with an incidence of 3 to 5 per 1 million of the population older than age 50 and less than 1 per 10 million of the population younger than age 50. Nevertheless, prion diseases have acquired a far greater importance than their numbers would suggest because CJD has been transmitted among humans by medical procedures (iatrogenic CJD), such as through use of prion-contaminated intracerebral electroencephalogram electrodes, human growth hormone preparations, human pituitary gonadotropin preparations, human dura mater grafts, and corneas.[193–195] Since 1994, about 105 cases of new variant CJD in Great Britain were acquired from bovine spongiform encephalopathy–infected beef products, indicating that, under some circumstances, prion-contaminated food products can cause CJD.[3, 196] There is great fear that human blood and blood products have the potential to be a source of iatrogenic CJD.[197] The fear that CJD is an emerging infec-

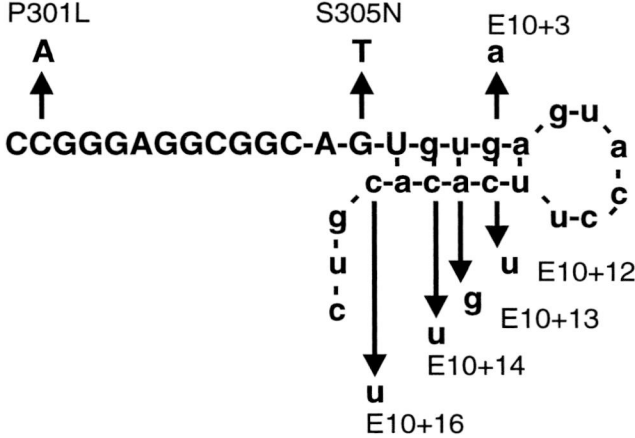

**FIGURE 52–11.** Schematic of the putative mRNA stem loop regulatory element at the 5' end of exon 10 of the tau gene. Known mutations in this region are also shown.

tious disease spreading among humans has led to a greater public awareness of prion diseases and the formation of new CJD surveillance programs led by the Centers for Disease Control in Atlanta, Georgia, and the American Association of Neuropathologists at the Institute of Pathology, Case Western Reserve University, Cleveland, Ohio. The goal is to determine whether or not there is an increased incidence of CJD in the United States, whether or not it is being transmitted by blood or blood products, and whether or not there are CJD cases caused by food products in the United States or acquired from food products by travelers to Great Britain or Europe.

In the past, these disorders were thought to be caused by "slow virus" because incubation times characteristically are several years in large animals and humans. The cause remained puzzling, however, because most cases of human prion disease could not be linked to infection and because the histologic features are not those of a typical infec-

tious process: No inflammatory infiltrates, no viral inclusions, no viral particles, and no viral antibodies can be shown. The vacuolation of the gray matter and PrP amyloid plaque formation that are characteristic of prion diseases are atypical for viral encephalitis (Fig. 52–12). An additionally puzzling characteristic of the human disorders is that about 15% of all human prion diseases are dominantly inherited, specifically, about 10% of CJD cases and, by definition, all cases of FFI and GSS disease. How these diseases could be sporadic, inherited, and infectious was resolved when Prusiner discovered that the infectious agent that transmits scrapie is composed of a single protease-resistant protein, designated $PrP^{Sc}$.[6] Prusiner introduced the term *prion* to designate the infectious particle to distinguish it from viruses and other conventional infectious agents. Subsequently, it was found that $PrP^{Sc}$ is derived from a normal cellular isoform expressed constitutively at particularly high levels in nerve cells,

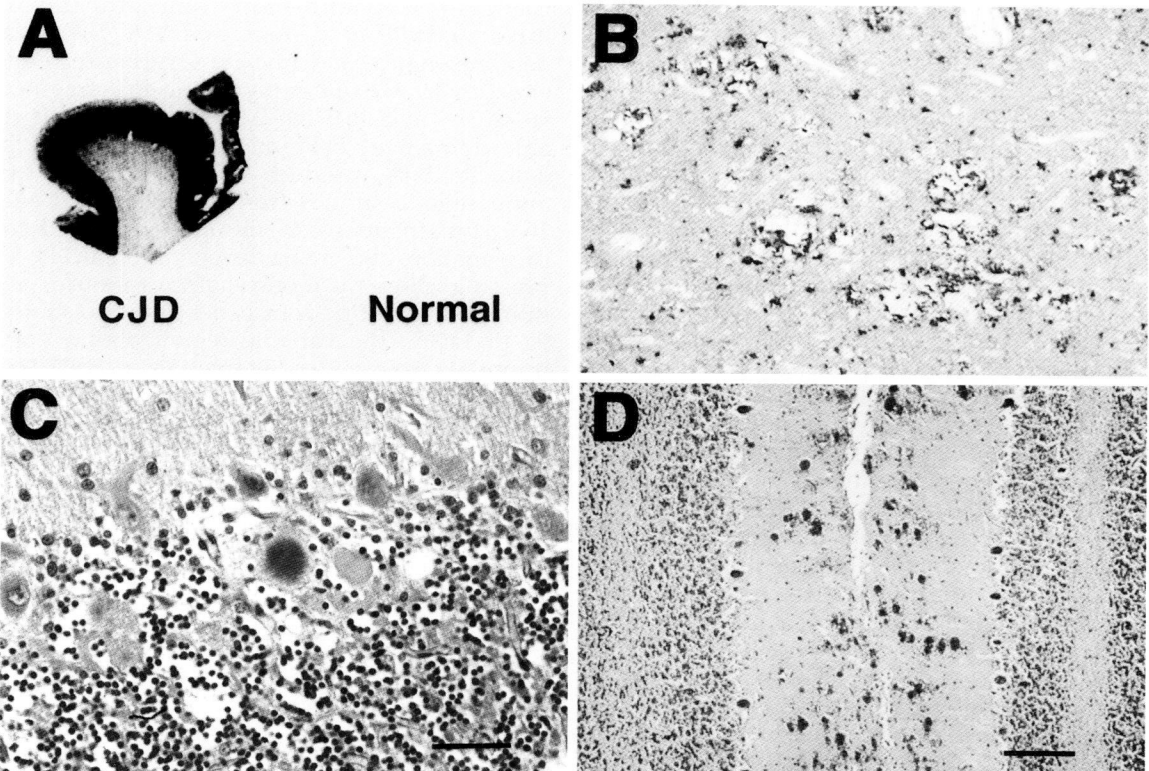

**FIGURE 52–12.** The definitive diagnosis of Creutzfeldt-Jakob disease (CJD) is made in tissue sections by demonstrating the presence of abnormal protease-resistant $PrP^{Sc}$ by one of two immunohistochemical techniques: *A.* With the histoblot technique, cryostat sections of unfixed frozen brain are mounted on nitrocellulose membranes and treated with proteinase K to eliminate $PrP^C$ and then with guanidinium to denature the protease-resistant $PrP^{Sc}$ so that PrP-specific antibodies will bind to it. $PrP^{Sc}$ is confined to the cerebral cortex in a case of CJD and is not found in normal cortex. *B.* The hydrolytic autoclaving method is used to detect $PrP^{Sc}$ in formalin-fixed, paraffin-embedded tissue sections. In this case, there are coarse deposits of $PrP^{Sc}$ surrounding vacuoles in the gray matter. *C.* PrP immunopositive amyloid plaques are found in only a small proportion of CJD cases. When present, they are usually found in small numbers in the cerebellar cortex (PAS histochemical stain). *D.* The diagnosis of Gerstmann-Sträussler-Scheinker (GSS) syndrome requires dominant inheritance and widespread PrP amyloid plaque deposition. In this case of GSS, innumerable amyloid plaques in the cerebellar molecular layer are stained blue-green by the sulfated alcian blue method. Bar in *C* also applies to *B* and is 50 $\mu$m. Bar in *D* is 200 $\mu$m.

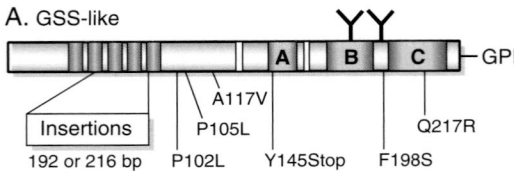

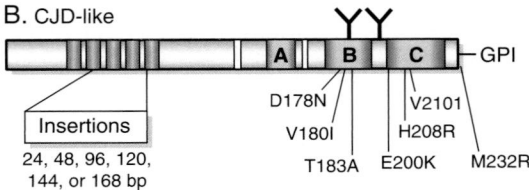

**FIGURE 52–13.** Mutations and insertions in the FRNP gene that segregate with dominantly inherited prion diseases. *A*. The Gerstmann-Sträussler-Scheinker syndrome, in which large amounts of PrP amyloid are deposited in the brain, is genetically linked to insertions of octarepeats of greater than 192 base pairs and to six nonconservative point mutations. Note, there is a tendency for the point mutations to be located between residues 90 and 150. *B*. Familial Creutzfeldt-Jakob disease is genetically linked to octapeptide insertions of 168 base pairs or less and to nonconservative point mutations primarily in the region of helices B and C.

designated *PrP^C*.[198, 199] The only difference between PrP^C and PrP^Sc is that the latter has a high proportion of β-sheet conformation accounting for its relative proteinase K resistance. Several groups have found that PrP^Sc is 43% β-sheet and 30% α-helix, whereas PrP^C is 3% β-sheet and 42% α-helix.[200, 201] PrP 27–30, the amyloidogenic and equally infectious proteinase K digestion product of PrP^Sc, has an even higher β-sheet content (54%) and lower α-helix content (21%) than PrP^Sc.[202, 203] Sequencing of the human prion protein gene, *PRNP*,[4] was followed rapidly by the discovery of its location in chromosome 20[5] and the discovery that all of the dominantly inherited prion diseases are genetically linked to mutations or insertions in the *PRNP* gene (Fig. 52–13). Today, many lines of evidence indicate that the cause and pathogenesis of sporadic forms, genetic forms, and forms acquired by infection (iatrogenic CJD and kuru) are due to abnormalities of a single plasma membrane glycolipid anchored protein, PrP (Fig. 52–14). The evidence that abnormal forms of PrP become transmissible particles (prions) and that their accumulation in the brain causes neuronal dysfunction and death has taken more than 25 years of intense laboratory investigation.[204, 205]

## Molecular Pathogenesis of Prion Diseases

There are two fundamental reasons why prion diseases exist and resemble conventional infectious diseases. First, the full-length PrP molecule can exist in two conformations, a constitutively expressed normal cellular conformer, PrP^C, and an abnormal pathogenic conformer found only in prion diseases,

PrP^Sc. Second, prion diseases resemble conventional infectious disorders because PrP^Sc can impose its conformation on PrP^C and initiate a self-perpetuating process, which results in the continuous conversion of PrP^C to nascent PrP^Sc and accumulation of PrP^Sc in the brain (i.e., increasing prion infectivity titer).

The PrP molecule has two domains that play different roles in the conversion of PrP^C to PrP^Sc (see Fig. 52–14). First, PrP^C has a "stable" or "ordered" core domain that contains two Asn-linked oligosaccharides; two α-helices, designated *helix-B* and *helix-C*, that are stabilized by a disulfide bridge between Cys^179 and Cys^214 (not shown in Fig. 52–14); a phosphatidylinositol glycolipid attached to the C-terminal at residue 231, which anchors PrP^C to the plasma membrane; and protein X binding sites, a putative cellular factor believed to lower the energy barrier for conversion of PrP^C to PrP^Sc when PrP^C binds to protein X.[206, 207] Second, PrP^C has a "variable" or "disordered" domain that contains the portion of the molecule that interacts with PrP^Sc and changes its conformation from primarily unstructured in PrP^C to β-sheet in PrP^Sc.[204] Nuclear magnetic resonance and nuclear Overhauser effect spectroscopy of two large synthetic PrP fragments, PrP 90–231[208] and PrP 29–231,[209] suggest that the variable domain of PrP^C contains a relatively short α-helix (helix-A, residues 144 to 156) and two short antiparallel β-strands (residues 129 to 131 and 161 to 163). Investigations of the steps required for prion propagation and neurodegeneration in Tg mice expressing chimeric mouse-hamster-mouse or mouse-human-mouse PrP transgenes indicate that residues 90 to 140 in the variable region play a particularly important role in the interaction of PrP^C with PrP^Sc leading to the conversion of the former to the latter.[207, 210] Residues 90 to 140 are largely unstructured or weakly helical in PrP^C[208, 209] but are predicted to be β-sheet in PrP^Sc.[204] In addition, helix-A may be converted to β-sheet along with other portions of the variable region during the conversion to PrP^Sc.

## Conversion of PrP^C to PrP^Sc and Accumulation of PrP^Sc Cause Neurodegeneration

PrP^Sc is derived from PrP^C, but in contrast to PrP^C, PrP^Sc is not degraded and accumulates in the cell. The PrP^C precursor pool from which PrP^Sc is formed must reach the cell surface before conversion occurs because blocking of PrP^C export from the endoplasmic reticulum–Golgi complex to the plasma membrane inhibits formation of PrP^Sc[211] and because exposure of scrapie-infected cells to phosphatidylinositol-specific phospholipase C, which releases PrP^C from the cell surface, also inhibits formation of PrP^Sc.[212] We found that greater than 90% of a cell's PrP^Sc and greater than 90% of a cell's PrP^C are localized to caveola-like, cholesterol-rich domains of the

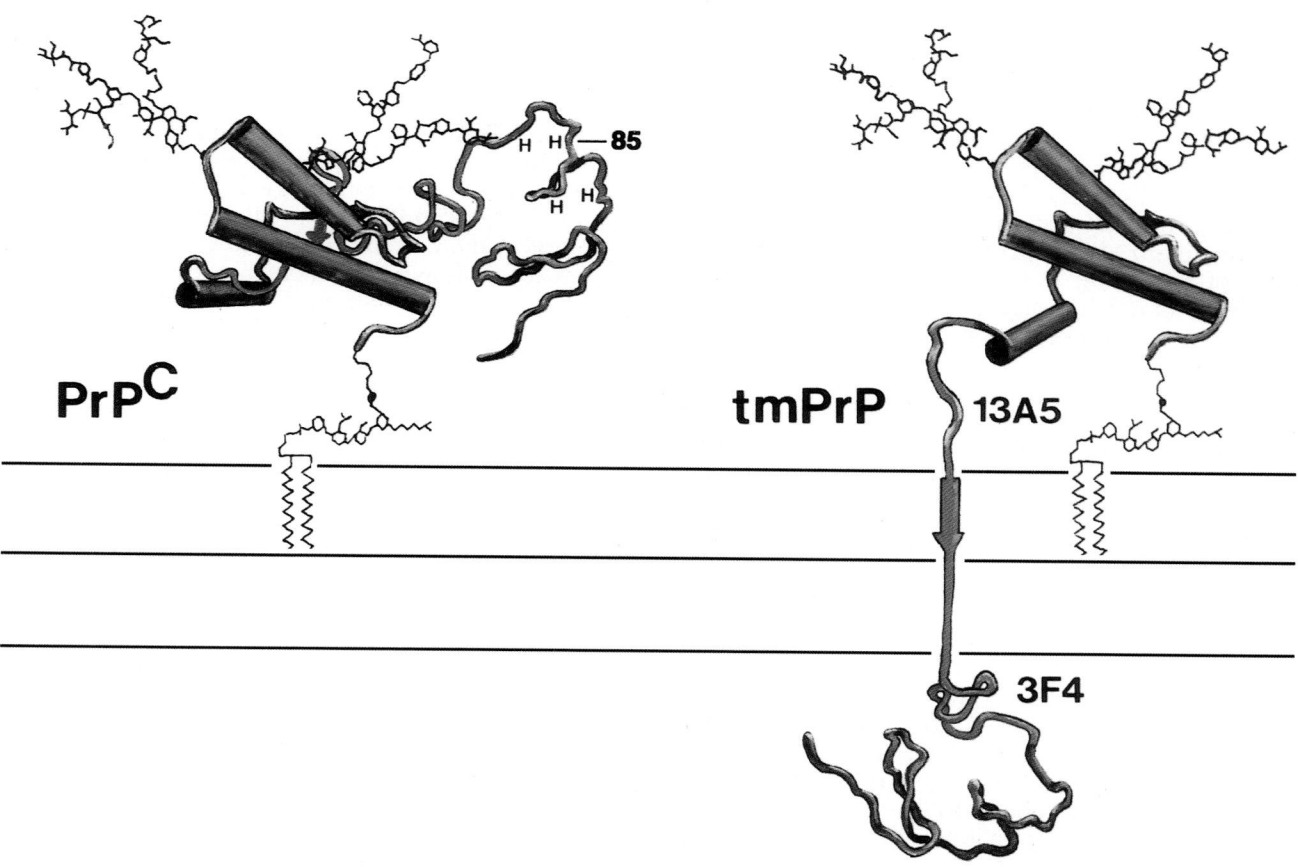

**FIGURE 52-14.** Models of the secretory form of PrP$^C$ (designated PrP$^C$) and the transmembrane form of PrP$^C$ (designated tmPrP). The secretory form is bound to the plasma membrane by a GPI anchor at the C-terminal (residue 231). The positions of the three helices are shown: Helix A, residues 144 to 157; Helix B, residues 172 to 193; and Helix C, residues 220 to 227. The four 'H's in the N-terminal domain are part of the four repeats that are believed to bind Cu$^{21}$. The most functionally important portion of the model, relative to conversion of PrP$^C$ to PrP$^{Sc}$, is the unstructured domain from residues 80 to 150. Vish Lingappa's laboratory has discovered that certain amino acid substitutions at residues 110, 111, and 117 cause PrP$^C$ to adopt a transmembrane topology (223). Whether or not tmPrP is also GPI anchored at its C-terminal is not known. The 3F4 monoclonal antibody epitope (residues 109 to 112) and the 13A5 epitope (residues 138 to 144) are indicated.

plasma membrane.[213] The site where exogenous PrP$^{Sc}$ comes into contact with PrP$^C$ and where PrP$^C$ is converted to nascent PrP$^{Sc}$ is not known with certainty; however, the colocalization of PrP$^{Sc}$ and PrP$^C$ in caveola-like, cholesterol-rich domains suggests that they may be the sites of conversion. Mice in which the *PrP* gene has been knocked out, Prnp$^{0/0}$ mice,[214] have yielded strong support for the concept that PrP$^{Sc}$ is derived from PrP$^C$ because no PrP$^{Sc}$ is formed, no prions are propagated, and no neuropathologic changes develop in these mice. Acute and chronic exposures of the brain in *PrP* knockout mice to PrP$^{Sc}$ have failed to propagate prions or to cause neuropathologic changes.[214–217] These findings indicate that exogenously derived PrP$^{Sc}$ by itself is not pathogenic; rather, for PrP$^{Sc}$ to cause neuronal degeneration, it must be derived from PrP$^C$. It is likely that, when nascent PrP$^{Sc}$ is derived from glycolipid-anchored PrP$^C$, it enters a

cellular compartment, where it can disrupt neuronal functions that PrP$^{Sc}$ in the extracellular space cannot. It is possible that PrP$^{Sc}$ must be anchored to membranes by a glycolipid anchor to be neuropathic and that it can do so only if it is derived from glycolipid-anchored PrP$^C$ (membrane hypothesis of neuronal degeneration in prion diseases[218]).

## Three Prion Disease Phenotypes

The previous discussion has focussed on conversion of PrP$^C$ to protease-resistant PrP$^{Sc}$. Hegde and colleagues[223] found that certain mutations of the *PrP* gene can cause PrP molecules to adopt a pathogenic transmembrane topography (tmPrP) (see Fig. 52–14). The latter finding is helping clinicians understand the basis of some of the differences in the prion disease phenotype.

Prion diseases in animals and humans can be divided into three broad categories based on their neurohistopatholgic features and the properties of nonamyloid abnormal PrP. The first category includes most prion diseases, including scrapie in sheep and rodents; bovine spongiform encephalopathy; kuru; sporadic, familial, and iatrogenic CJD; and sporadic fatal insomnia; and FFI. These diseases are characterized by vacuolar (spongiform) degeneration of the brain, little or no PrP amyloid plaque formation (amyloid plaques occur in only 5% of CJD cases in small numbers, as seen in Fig. 52–12C), and accumulation of protease-resistant PrP$^{Sc}$ that is derived from glycolipid-anchored PrP$^{C}$.

The second category occurs naturally only in humans, but has been reproduced in transgenic mice.[219, 220] The only prion diseases included in this category are the six dominantly inherited syndromes included in GSS disease. GSS syndromes are characterized by abundant amyloid plaque formation (see Fig. 52–12D), variable amounts of vacuolar degeneration, and abnormal PrP accumulation that is relatively protease-sensitive. The molecular mechanism causing GSS disease seems to be different from that causing CJD syndromes. Mutated PrP in GSS syndromes becomes highly truncated by cleavage of the N-terminal and C-terminal domains of the molecule, yielding PrP peptide fragments in each case spanning residues 80 to about 150.[221] In contrast to the protease-resistant PrP$^{Sc}$ that accumulates in the CJD/scrapie group, full-length mutated PrP found in the brain of human GSS cases and in GSS transgenic mice is relatively sensitive to protease digestion.[219, 222] Evidence suggests that the mutated PrP in GSS disease adopts a transmembrane topographic orientation that causes neuronal degeneration as the transmembrane form of mutated PrP accumulates with age (see Fig. 52–14).[223] The transmembrane form of PrP, $^{tm}$PrP, is more protease sensitive than PrP$^{Sc}$. The mechanism of amyloid formation in GSS disease seems to be due to the preservation of residues 80 to 150 during degradation of $^{tm}$PrP because of its transmembrane location. This PrP domain is converted to β-sheets and is highly amyloidogenic. The amyloid plaques formed during GSS disease are composed of this domain, providing further evidence of the great tendency of peptides 80 to 150 to adopt β-pleated structures and polymerize into amyloid filaments.

A third neurohistopathologic category of prion disease is the new variant CJD of Great Britain acquired from food products infected with bovine spongiform encephalopathy.[1, 3, 196] It has the histopathologic features of both CJD and GSS. It is characterized by widespread vacuolar degeneration of gray matter, accumulation of protease-resistant PrP$^{Sc}$ similar to other cases of CJD, and large numbers of PrP amyloid deposits throughout the brain similar to GSS cases. This similarity raises the possibility that PrP$^{Sc}$ and $^{tm}$PrP are formed in this unique prion disease acquired from bovine spongiform encephalopathy–infected cattle.

## Familial Prion Diseases

Almost 25 mutations of the *PRNP* gene are associated with familial prion diseases. Of these, there is sufficient genetic linkage to establish a causal relationship between five different *PRNP* mutations and central nervous system degeneration (see Fig. 52–13).[222, 224–227] Familial prion diseases are rarer than sporadic CJD, accounting for 10% to 15% of human prion diseases with an incidence of about 1 per 10 million of the population.

Neuropathologists have classified dominantly inherited prion diseases with abundant PrP amyloid accumulation as GSS diseases regardless of the *PRNP* mutation (see Fig. 52–12D). Three mutations associated with GSS disease occur in the putative PrP binding domain at codons 102, 105, and 117 (see Fig. 52–13). A fourth occurs at codon 145 and results in a stop codon and the synthesis of truncated PrP containing the amyloidogenic peptide.[228] Two other mutations associated with widely deposited PrP amyloid occur in the region of the third and fourth helical domains at codons 198 and 217.[224, 229] In both of these disorders, PrP amyloid plaque formation in the cerebral cortex is associated with neurofibrillary degeneration of neurons of the type seen in aging and AD. The codon 198 mutation, linked to a large pedigree in Indiana, is most remarkable because the PrP amyloid deposits in the cerebral cortex form the cores of neuritic plaques of the type characteristic of AD.[50] Transgenic mouse lines expressing a mutant mouse PrP that carries the codon 102 mutation linked to GSS(P102L) in humans have verified that this PrP amino acid sequence is amyloidogenic because the mice spontaneously develop a neurodegenerative disease that precisely duplicates the human disease in virtually every detail, including formation of large numbers of GSS-type PrP immunopositive amyloid plaques.[219, 230]

CJD-like clinicopathologic diseases have been found in patients with insertions of variable numbers of octapeptide repeats in the N-terminal domain of PrP and mutations at codons 178, 180, 200, 210, and 232. The mutation at codon 178 is of particular interest because it results in an Asn for Asp substitution and is linked to FFI and a CJD syndrome.[231–233] Subsequently, it was discovered that the *PRNP* allele carrying the 178 mutation in FFI also codes for a Met polymorphism at codon 129 (see Fig. 52–13), whereas the mutated allele in familial CJD (D178N) codes for Val at codon 129.[234] These findings show how a single amino acid difference in a mutated PrP molecule determines which population of neurons is vulnerable and the resulting clinical features. In FFI (D178N, M129), the neuropathology is confined largely to the mediodorsal and anterior ventral nuclei of the thalamus, whereas in familial CJD (D178N, V129), the neuropathology is widespread in the cerebral cortex and subcortical nuclei. Selective neuronal vulnerability is a feature of all forms of prion disease. In dominantly inherited prion diseases, differential neuronal targeting is attributed to the specific amino acid sequence of mutated PrP. Differential neuronal targeting for conversion of PrP$^C$ to PrP$^{Sc}$ in animals expressing wild-type PrP$^C$ infected with different prion strains seems to be due to neuron-specific differences in the carbohydrate structure of PrP$^C$.[235, 236]

The penetrance of some familial prion diseases is age dependent. The penetrance in pedigrees with CJD (E200K) is 1% for carriers of the mutation at age 40 and close to 100% for carriers at age 80.[237] Penetrance was found to be related to the expression levels of mutant PrP (E200K) mRNA and mutant PrP (E200K). They were lower than expression levels of the wild-type PrP mRNA and wild-type PrP$^C$ in healthy carriers, whereas most of the clinically ill E200K patients expressed equal levels of mutant and wild-type proteins.

## Homozygosity at Codon 129, a Risk Factor for Prion Disease

The most significant risk factor for sporadic CJD is age, with a mean incidence of about 62 years. In this regard, the age-related incidence of sporadic CJD is similar to that of AD. The second most significant risk factor is homozygosity at codon 129 of the *PRNP* gene (see Fig. 52–13), which influences expression of inherited, iatrogenic, and sporadic forms of prion disease.[238] Molecular genetic analysis of white patients with sporadic CJD has shown that 95% or more are homozygous for M or V at codon 129.[239, 240] This finding contrasts with the general population, in which frequencies for the codon 129 polymorphism in whites are 12% V/V, 37% M/M, and 51% M/V.[241] The frequency of the V allele in the Japanese population is much lower.[242] Heterozygosity at codon 129 (M/V) also is more frequent (18%) in Japanese CJD patients than in the general population, in which the polymorphism frequencies are 0% V/V, 92% M/M, and 8% M/V.[243] The risk factor for sporadic CJD associated with homozygosity at codon 129 is consistent with the dimer model of prion propagation in which interactions between PrP$^{Sc}$ and PrP$^C$ are favored when their amino acid sequences have a high degree of homology and an alternative PrP$^C$ allotype is not present to interfere with conversion of PrP$^C$ to PrP$^{Sc}$.[210, 244–246]

Susceptibility to iatrogenic or food-related infection with prions is influenced significantly by the *PRNP* codon 129 genotype.[241] In 16 patients (15 white, 1 African American) from the United Kingdom, United States, and France with iatrogenic CJD caused by contaminated human growth hormone extracts, 8 (50%) were V/V, 5 (31%) were M/M, and 3 (19%) were M/V.[195, 241, 247–251] Therefore, a disproportionate number of patients with iatrogenic CJD were homozygous at PrP codon 129. All of the patients who have acquired new variant CJD in Great Britain and Europe from bovine spongiform encephalopathy have been M/M at codon 129.[230] These data

suggest that heterozygosity at codon 129 may provide partial protection against acquiring CJD.

It is likely that homozygosity at codon 129 facilitates conversion of PrP$^C$ to PrP$^{Sc}$ by doubling the amount of PrP$^C$ with an identical amino acid sequence available to an infecting PrP$^{Sc}$. Conversely, heterozygous individuals express two PrP$^C$ allotypes that differ by one amino acid. A single amino acid difference in that region is sufficient to have a profound effect on scrapie incubation times in mice.[252, 253] Two PrP$^C$ allotypes can compete with each other for binding to PrP$^{Sc}$ and to protein X, both of which can have a profound effect on the rate of conversion of PrP$^C$ to nascent PrP$^{Sc}$.[254]

## Diagnostic Procedures for Prion Diseases

Consensus criteria for the diagnosis of prion diseases have been established.[255] A diagnosis of "probable CJD" can be made by biopsy or at autopsy if the quartet of clinical signs and symptoms are present and spongiform degeneration of gray matter is found in the absence of other confounding pathology. In the National Institutes of Health series, 52 of 55 autopsy-verified cases of CJD (95%) showed the characteristic spongiform degeneration of cerebral cortex in surgical biopsy specimens.[256] The definitive diagnosis of a human prion disease requires that one of the four following additional criteria be met: 1) presence of PrP amyloid plaques (see Fig. 52–12C), 2) transmission of spongiform encephalopathy to animals, 3) presence of PrP$^{Sc}$ (see Fig. 52–12A and B), or 4) presence of a pathogenic *PrP* gene mutation (see Fig. 52–13).

## AMYOTROPHIC LATERAL SCLEROSIS

The motor neuron diseases are important because they are relatively common and because they can present in adults as either a sporadic or a dominantly inherited form of ALS; in infants as Werdnig-Hoffmann disease (spinal muscular atrophy type I), which progresses rapidly to death in the first 2 years of life; in infants as a slowly progressive spinal muscular atrophy type II, which results in death in early adulthood; and as Kugelberg-Welander disease (spinal muscular atrophy type III), which is the mildest form and begins in childhood.

In this section, we focus on ALS and familial ALS primarily because of an interesting association made by Bredesen and colleagues.[257] ALS is a fatal motor neuron disease that is inherited in about 10% of cases and sporadic in about 90%. About 25% of familial ALS cases have been linked to mutations in the *sod1* gene, a gene that encodes copper/zinc superoxide dismutase (CuZnSOD). About 50 different *sod1* mutations have been identified in familial ALS families.[258] Most of the mutations lead to an amino acid substitution. They are located throughout the protein; however, most are clustered at the protein's $\beta$-barrel turns and at the dimerization interface. The mutations are predicted to result in a more open conformation of the CuZnSOD enzyme. Bredesen and colleagues[257] hypothesized that structural and functional effects similar to those of the familial ALS–associated CuZnSOD mutations may be achieved by age-associated post-translational modifications, such as glycation and carbonyl modification of CuZnSOD, and other modifications. Such changes are known to occur and alter CuZnSOD activity markedly. The known sites of these various age-associated modifications of CuZnSOD are in proximity to sites of familial ALS mutations, raising the possibility that this might be the link between the molecular mechanism of anterior horn cell degeneration in sporadic ALS and familial ALS. One could generalize the Bredesen hypothesis to other neurodegenerative diseases that present as sporadic and inherited disorders.

## HUNTINGTON'S DISEASE AND OTHER UNSTABLE TRIPLET REPEAT DISORDERS

The molecular genetic investigations of HD is one of the most remarkable sagas of neurology. The discovery of the genetic defect that causes HD was as much due to exceptional leadership as it was to advances in molecular genetic techniques. Martin, when he was the Head of Neurology at the Massachusetts General Hospital, had the foresight to bring together the team of molecular biologists and neurobiologists in 1980 for the task. The history of this triumph has been chronicled by Young.[259] Young related that it began in 1978 at a Hereditary Disease Foundation workshop in Los Angeles, where Botstein, Housman, and White suggested that the HD gene could be identified by genetic linkage analysis. At about the same time, Wexler, who was working at the National Institute of Neurological Disease, had identified and begun investigating a multigenerational Venezuelan pedigree of HD that was the largest in the world. This pedigree became the most important source of blood and skin samples for the linkage study. The samples were sent to Gusella's laboratory at the Massachusetts General Hospital for linkage analysis. Martin hired Gusella after his postdoctoral fellowship with Housman. In 1983, ahead of schedule, an anonymous marker on chromosome 4p was discovered that was linked genetically to HD.[260] That rapid success was followed by a laborious 10-year search for the HD gene. This search resulted in the discovery of an expanded unstable triplet CAG repeat in the N-terminal domain of the open reading frame of the HD gene that encodes the huntingtin protein.[261] In normal individuals, exon 1 of the huntingtin gene encodes 9 to 34 CAG repeats, whereas in patients with HD it encodes 37 to 120.[262–266]

Although HD was the first neurodegenerative disease for which genetic linkage analysis was undertaken, it was not the first in which a CAG triplet repeat expansion was found (Table 52–4). In 1991, X-linked spinobulbar muscular atrophy (Kennedy's disease) was the first CAG triplet repeat disorder to be identified.[267] Onset is in the 20s and is characterized by gynecomastia with slowly progressive lower motor neuron disease affecting facial muscles, tongue, and proximal limb muscles. Kennedy's disease was genetically linked to an expanded CAG repeat in the first exon of the androgen receptor gene on the X chromosome.[268] Normal subjects encode 11 to 33 CAG repeats, whereas patients with Kennedy's disease encode 40 to 62 CAG repeats.[269, 270]

The spinocerebellar ataxias (SCA) are a complex group of disorders that share in common degenera-

**TABLE 52–4.** Unstable Triplet Repeat Diseases

| Disease | Transmission | Expanded Repeats | Protein | Reference |
|---|---|---|---|---|
| Kennedy's disease | x-linked | CAG (exonic) | Androgen receptor | La Spada et al, 1991[268] |
| HD | 4 dominant | CAG (exonic) | Huntingtin | Huntington Group, 1993[298] |
| SCA-1 | 6 dominant | CAG (exonic) | Ataxin 1 | Orr et al, 1993[272] |
| SCA-2 | 12 dominant | CAG (exonic) | Ataxin 2 | Gispert et al, 1993[299] |
| SCA-3 | 14 dominant (allelic mutation) | CAG (exonic) | Ataxin 3 | Stevanin et al, 1994[300] |
| Machado-Joseph disease (SCA-3) | 14 dominant (allelic mutation) | CAG (exonic) | Ataxin 3 | Kawaguchi et al, 1994[301] |
| SCA-4 | 16 dominant | CAG (exonic) | Ataxin 4 | Flanigan et al, 1996[304] |
| SCA-5 | 11 dominant | CAG (exonic) | Ataxin 5 | Ranum et al, 1994[302] |
| SCA-6 | 19 dominant | CAG (exonic) | P/Q Ca$^{++}$ channel | Zhuchenko et al, 1997[303] |
| SCA-7 | 3 dominant | CAG (exonic) | Ataxin 7 | David et al, 1997[275] |
| Dentatorubral-pallidoluysial atrophy | 12 dominant | CAG (exonic) | Atrophin 1 | Koide et al, 1994[280]; Nagafuchi et al, 1994[282] |
| Friedreich's ataxia | 9 recessive | GAA (intronic) | Frataxin (loss of expression) | Campuzano et al, 1996[279] |

tion of cerebellar Purkinje cells and the dentate nucleus but also can involve afferent connections from the spinal cord (dorsal and ventral spinocerebellar tracts); the inferior olives; and nuclei of the base of the pons, efferent connection to red nucleus and thalamus, and the pyramidal and extrapyramidal systems. Consequently the final neuropathologic diagnosis often has remained descriptive and led to terms such as *cerebello-olivary degeneration, olivopontocerebellar degeneration,* or *dentatorubral degeneration.* When the ethnic background of the patient, dominant inheritance, age of onset, and clinical signs and symptoms were factored in, a specific disease might be suggested, such as Machado-Joseph disease. Classification of SCA types according to disease phenotype still is used frequently; however, if that classification does not incorporate molecular genetic correlates, it could be inappropriate and inaccurate and of little help for counseling the patient and the patient's family.[271] The limited way in which the spinocerebellar system responds to degeneration of its various components often makes phenotypic classification problematic. When viewed from the patient or pedigree genotype, at least 16 types of SCA can be identified.[271] Conner and Rosenberg[271] argued that molecular genetics and biochemical analysis would rewrite the classification of these diverse disorders as new mutations and genes are discovered.

Beginning in 1993, molecular genetic analysis of dominantly inherited SCA types led to a rapid determination of genotypic specificity that distinguished at least six SCAs with unstable CAG repeats that are numbered according to their appearance in the literature (see Table 52–4). Orr and associates[272] confirmed that SCA-1 with ataxia, ophthalmoplegia, and pyramidal and extrapyramidal findings maps to 6p22-p23 and consists of an expanded CAG repeat that results in an expanded polyglutamine repeat within the *SCA-1* gene product, ataxin-1. Although the *SCA-1* gene is expressed ubiquitously, only a subset of neurons are affected in the disease, including cerebellar Purkinje cells.[273] Similar to HD, normal subjects have 25 to 36 CAG repeats, whereas affected patients have more than 43 CAG repeats. There is an inverse relationship between the number of repeats and the age of onset of signs and symptoms similar to HD. Evidence for imprinting was the association of an increase in repeat number with paternal transmission.[274] A particularly interesting autosomal dominant cerebellar ataxia is SCA-7, which was found to be linked to unstable CAG repeats in exon 1 of the *SCA-7* gene on chromosome 3.[275-277] Although normal alleles have 4 to 35 repeats, Benton and coworkers[278] found that SCA-7 family members can vary from 37 repeats to the largest expansion recorded of 306.[278] The latter study verified the differential effect of paternal gender on the stability of the SCA-7 expansion and its association with anticipation. The largest expansion was transmitted paternally and resulted in infantile onset. SCA-7 is associated with a broad spectrum of abnormalities, including ataxia, maculopathy, dementia, motor and sensory abnormalities, and congenital heart defects and dysfunction. The authors proposed that large expansions of greater than 200 repeats may be responsible for the cardiac abnormalities. Other SCAs and the chromosome and gene to which they are linked are listed in Table 52–4.

Friedreich's ataxia is a recessively inherited disease with a prevalence of about 2 per 100,000 of the population. It accounts for about half of all hereditary ataxias.[271] It has been linked to a GAA triplet expansion in the first intron of the *FRDA* gene on chromosome 9q that results in loss of expression of the frataxin protein.[279] The main neuropathologic changes include degeneration of dorsal root ganglion cells with accompanying loss of large myelinated axons in the peripheral nervous system and in the dorsal columns of the spinal cord, severe neuron loss in Clarke's column of the spinal cord with accompanying degeneration of the dorsal spinocerebellar tract, secondary degeneration of the accessory cuneate and gracile nuclei, severe nerve cell loss in the dentate nucleus of the cerebellum, nerve cell loss in the vestibular and cochlear nuclei, and nerve cell loss in the globus pallidus and subthalamic nuclei. Also included in Table 52–4 is reference to dominantly inherited dentatorubral-pallidoluysial atrophy linked to unstable CAG repeats in the *DRPLA* gene.[280-282]

## Characteristics Shared by CAG Repeat Diseases

There are four characteristics of CAG repeat disorders that create problems for cliniconeuropathologic diagnosis and classification of a CAG disorder in an individual patient.[259]

1. *Variable age of onset:* A small percentage of individuals in a pedigree present with disease much earlier or much later than the mean.
2. *Anticipation:* In many pedigrees, age of onset of disease is younger with each succeeding generation. In HD, 80% to 90% of patients with the most marked anticipation leading to juvenile onset inherited the gene from their father.
3. *Phenotypic variation:* Marked variations in disease phenotype among pedigrees have led to clinical subclassifications of diseases such as HD. Phenotypic variation also can be seen among affected members of a single pedigree.
4. *New mutations:* Rare individuals with CAG repeat disorders can present with all the clinical and neuropathologic hallmarks of disease with no apparent family history. For these reasons, clinical and neuropathologic analysis must include a decision of whether or not to obtain molecular genetic analysis to arrive at a precise cause-based diagnosis to counsel the patient and the patient's family better.

## Molecular Consequence of Expanded Triplet Repeats

As described previously, HD, Kennedy's disease, SCA types 1 through 5, and dentatorubral-pallido-luysian atrophy all are linked genetically to abnormally expanded glutamine repeats near the N-terminal of the affected proteins. All four disease groups become more severe and begin earlier the longer the glutamine repeats. The repeats tend to lengthen in successive generations, especially with male transmission. Although no molecular function has been established for the repeats, Perutz and colleagues[283] have proposed that they act as polar zippers, joining protein molecules together similarly to the way leucine zippers join the transcription factors c-Jun and c-Fos. In their discussion of huntingtin with expanded repeats, Perutz and colleagues[283] began with the fact that the glutamine-rich segment starts at residue 18, which normally varies between 11 and 24 residues, but in HD it can vary between 37 and greater than 100 residues. The glutamine repeat is followed by an almost continuous stretch of 29 prolines, which forms a rigid helix; this indicates that the glutamine repeat is mounted at the end of a 90 Å long stalk. For spinobulbar muscular atrophy, the glutamine-rich expansion is in the N-terminal of the androgen receptor, which is a transcription factor with one C-terminal DNA-binding domain. Beginning at residue 58, normal individuals have 11 to 33 glutamine repeats, whereas in spinobulbar muscular atrophy patients, it is expanded to 40 to 62 repeats. Perutz and colleagues[283] reported that the androgen receptor with an expanded glutamine repeat transactivated an androgen-responsive reporter gene more weakly than a normal receptor.[284]

Through molecular modeling of polyglutamine repeats, Perutz and colleagues[283] proposed that they are capable of linking β-strands together into sheets or barrels with hydrogen bonds between their main chain amides and their polar side chains. They tested this experimentally and found that polyglutamine repeats, chemically modified for solubility, have the circular dichroism spectra of β-sheets independent of the solvent in which they are suspended, including trifluoroethanol, which normally induces α-helices. The precipitate formed by the β-sheeted polyglutamines consisted of 70 to 120 Å thick filaments of varying lengths that resemble amyloid filaments. More recently, huntingtin-encoded polyglutamine expansions were shown to form amyloid-like protein aggregates in vitro and in vivo.[285]

## Proteins with Expanded Polyglutamine Tracts Form Intracellular Inclusion Bodies

Aggregates of huntingtin[286, 287] and ataxin-1[288] with expanded polyglutamine repeats first were discovered to form intranuclear and sometimes intracyto-plasmic inclusion bodies in transgenic mice expressing these pathologic proteins.[289] Subsequently, these inclusion bodies were shown in the human cases of HD,[287] SCA-1,[288] SCA-3,[290] dentatorubral-pallidoluysian atrophy,[291] and spinobulbar muscular atrophy.[292] Klement and coworkers[289] commented that the two most striking characteristics of these inclusions are their selective limitation to nerve cells affected by the disease and their generally consistent nuclear location.

## Mechanisms of Nerve Cell Degeneration in CAG Repeat Diseases

The fundamental question is whether or not the subcellular accumulation of proteins with expanded glutamine tracts is important in pathogenesis. Sandou and associates[293] developed an in vitro model of HD by transfecting cultured striatal neurons with mutant huntingtin. They found that mutant huntingtin, not wild-type huntingtin, formed ubiquinated intranuclear inclusions and induced neurodegeneration by an apoptotic mechanism. Antiapoptotic agents or neurotrophic factors, such as brain-derived neurotrophic factor (BDNF) and ciliary neurotrophic factor (CNTF), protected the neurons against apoptosis and degeneration. To test whether or not nuclear localization was necessary for neurodegeneration, they added a small nuclear export signal to mutant huntingtin. Addition of the nuclear export signal completely blocked nuclear inclusion body formation and prevented neurodegeneration. Finally, Sandou and associates[293] asked whether or not neurodegeneration specifically was due to the presence of the ubiquinated intranuclear inclusions of mutated huntingtin. The fact that neurodegeneration could be prevented by exposing the cells to neurotrophic factors that did not prevent intranuclear inclusion formation suggested that the presence of intranuclear inclusions was not sufficient to cause nerve cell death. Sandou and associates[293] found that coexpression of a dominant negative ubiquitin-conjugating enzyme prevented the formation of intranuclear inclusions; it accelerated the neurodegeneration. They concluded that the formation of intranuclear inclusions by itself does not cause nerve cell death. The corollary is that smaller units of mutated huntingtin in the nucleus are pathogenic perhaps because they bind crucial nuclear proteins, transcription factors, or DNA promotor domains.

Klement and coworkers[289, 294] tested whether or not the subcellular location of mutant ataxin-1 is important in pathogenesis given that it is deposited in the nucleus and cytoplasm of Purkinje cells in the SCA-1 mouse model. With an in vitro model, they found that COS cells transfected with mutant ataxin-1 form inclusions in their nuclei similar to those in Purkinje cells. In a series of transfection experiments in which the mutated ataxin-1 molecule was dissected molecularly, they found an argine-rich and lysine-rich nuclear localization sequence near the C-terminal. A K772T mutation in the sequence completely eliminated activity of the nuclear localization sequence in COS cells and prevented formation of intranuclear inclusions. Similarly, transgenic mice expressing mutated ataxin-1$^{K772T}$ developed cytoplasmic inclusions only in Purkinje cells. These mice did not develop the characteristic histopathologic changes, arguing that nuclear localization of intact ataxin-1 was essential for SCA-1 pathogenesis. In the next series of experiments, 122 amino acids were deleted from a previously identified glutamine-rich self-aggregation domain within ataxin-1 between residues 495 and 605. Expression of this mutant ataxin-1 in transgenic mice resulted in sorting of this construct to the nucleus of Purkinje cells; however, no ubiquinated nuclear aggregates of ataxin-1 formed. Nevertheless, these mice developed Purkinje cell pathology and ataxia. These findings argue that although intranuclear ataxin-1 with expanded polyglutamine tracts is pathogenic, it does not have to be aggregated in the form of an inclusion to cause neurodegeneration.

## Other Dominantly Inherited Cerebellar Ataxias

The genetic basis of other forms of cerebellar ataxia remain to be found. Lowe and colleagues[295] summarized relatively current understanding of the clinico-neuropathologic types of autosomal dominant cerebellar ataxias (ADCA types I to IV).[296, 297] ADCA-I seems to encompass SCA-1 through SCA-5. ADCA-II presents with ataxia and retinal degeneration leading to blindness. No candidate gene has been identified. ADCA-III is a relatively pure cerebellar syndrome whose relationship to other SCAs is unclear. ADCA-IV is "almost certainly a manifestation of mitochondrial encephalopathy."[295]

## CONCLUSION

The molecular biology and genetics of neurodegenerative diseases have progressed extremely rapidly, so much so that it is impossible in a short chapter to capture the full scope of the discoveries. We have presented the basics of the most common and important neurodegenerative diseases of the central nervous system. In doing so, we hoped to outline the state of the art of techniques for making accurate diagnoses using the classic histologic and immunohistochemical tools of the neuropathologist and to give insight into when it is important to provide fine-tuning of the diagnosis with molecular genetic analysis. The latter is important for cases in which inheritance is suspected so that family and patient counseling can be initiated. Molecular genetic analysis also is important for cases for which there is no family history but the clinical and neuropathologic

**TABLE 52–5.** Partial List of Available Commercial and Research Laboratory Tests for Diseases of the Central Nervous System, Peripheral Nervous System, and Skeletal Muscle

| | |
|---|---|
| ***Alzheimer's Disease**** | |
| ApoE genotype | Blood; buccal swab |
| Tau/A$\beta$42 | Cerebrospinal fluid |
| *PS-1* | Blood |
| ***Movement Disorders**** | |
| Adrenoleukodystrophy Test (very long chain fatty acids) | Blood; plasma |
| Ataxia profiles (SCA 1, 2, 3, 6, 7, 8, and Friedreich's) | Blood |
| Dystonia (DYT1) DNA test | Blood |
| Huntington's disease DNA | Blood |
| ***Motor Neuron Disease**** | |
| Familial amyotrophic lateral sclerosis (sod1) | Blood |
| Kennedy's disease DNA test | Blood |
| Spinal muscular atrophy DNA test | Blood |
| ***Hereditary Peripheral Neuropathies**** | |
| Charcot-Marie-Tooth profile (CMT1A, CMT1X, CMT1B DNA tests) | Blood |
| Hereditary sensory motor neuropathies differential analysis | Blood |
| Congenital hypomyelination evaluation | Blood |
| Pressure palsy neuropathy (HNPP) DNA test | Blood |
| Refsum's disease test (phytanic acid) | Blood; plasma |
| Transthyretin Met 30 Amyloidosis test | Blood |
| ***Prion Disease (all Prion Diseases)***† | |
| Protease-resistant PrP$^{Sc}$ | Brain biopsy; autopsy |
| Familial prion diseases | Blood; brain biopsy |
| ***Mental Retardation**** | |
| Fragile X DNA test | Blood |
| Chromosome analysis with fragile X DNA | Blood |
| ***Neurogenetic Diagnosis (Neuromuscular Disorders)**** | |
| Myotonic dystrophy DNA test | Blood |
| Dystrophin test—males only (DMD and BMD)‡ | Frozen muscle |
| DMD/BMD DNA deletion test—males only | Blood |
| DMD/BMD carrier DNA test—females only | Blood |
| ***Metabolic Myopathy and Mitochondrial DNA (mtDNA) Mutation Profiles**** | |
| Individual (mtDNA) point mutation test | Blood; frozen muscle |
| Mitochondrial enzyme deficiency myopathies profile | Frozen muscle |
| Myoglobinuria profile | Frozen muscle |
| Glycogen storage myopathy A profile | Frozen muscle |
| Glycogen storage myopathy B profile | Frozen muscle |
| Lipid storage myopathy profile | Frozen muscle |

\* Commercial test.
† Research laboratory test.
‡ DMD, Duchenne muscular dystrophy; BMD, Becker muscular dystrophy.

features suggest a gene mutation. The latter is particularly true for the unstable trinucleotide repeat diseases in which anticipation is the rule. It is also true for individuals in whom a family history is not known, a situation which is common with the large migrations throughout the world. The final decision as to whether or not genetic testing will be done is in the hands of the attending physician, the patient, and the family. Although day-to-day patient care requirements for molecular genetic analysis must be based on practical and ethical considerations, research into the genes causing virtually all of the neurodegenerative diseases is involved actively in molecular analysis of every suspected familial form because many of the genes causing common diseases such as AD and familial ALS have not been found yet.

Finally, we did not discuss the large number of storage diseases, mitochondrial diseases, and metabolic disorders of the central and peripheral nervous systems in which molecular diagnostics plays perhaps an even more active role in clinical practice and in which great advances have been made. The same also can be said for skeletal muscle diseases. Table 52–5 outlines some of the more common tests available commercially and from research laboratories to aid the clinician faced with a neurologic disorder; this table emphasizes how many topics we did not cover.

*Acknowledgments*

*The authors thank Mrs. Helga Thordarson, for help in preparing the manuscript, and Juliana Cayetano-Balan and Cynthia Cowdrey, for neurohistologic and immunohistochemical stains of tissue sections. This work was supported by grants from the National Institutes of Health (AG02132, AG10770, and NS14069).*

## REFERENCES

1. Ironside JW: Creutzfeldt-Jakob disease. Brain Pathol 6:379–388, 1996.
2. Nathanson N, Wilesmith J, Wells GA, Griot C: Bovine spongiform encephalopathy and related diseases. *In* Prusiner SB (ed): Prion Biology and Diseases. Cold Spring Harbor, NY, Cold Spring Harbor Laboratory Press, 1999, pp 431–463.
3. Will RG, Ironside JW, Zeidler M, et al: A new variant of Creutzfeldt-Jakob disease in the UK. Lancet 347:921–925, 1996.
4. Kretzschmar HA, Stowring LE, Westaway D, et al: Molecular cloning of a human prion protein cDNA. DNA 5:315–324, 1986.
5. Sparkes RS, Simon M, Cohn VH, et al: Assignment of the human and mouse prion protein genes to homologous chromosomes. Proc Natl Acad Sci U S A 83:7358–7362, 1986.
6. Prusiner SB: Novel proteinaceous infectious particles cause scrapie. Science 216:136–144, 1982.
7. Botstein D, White RL, Skolnick M, Davis RW: Construction of a genetic linkage map in man using restriction fragment length polymorphisms. Am J Hum Genet 32:314–331, 1980.
8. Rosenberg RN, Prusiner SB, DiMauro S, Barchi RL: The Molecular and Genetic Basis of Neurological Disease, 2nd ed. Boston, Butterworth-Heinemann, 1997.
9. Alzheimer A: Ueber eine eigenartige Erkrankung der Hirnrinde. Cent Nervenheilk Psychiat 30:177–179, 1907.
10. Mirra SS, Heyman A, McKeel D, et al: The Consortium to Establish a Registry for Alzheimer's Disease (CERAD). Part II. Standardization of the neuropathologic assessment of Alzheimer's disease. Neurology 41:479–486, 1991.
11. Mirra SS, Gearing M, McKeel DJ, et al: Interlaboratory comparison of neuropathology assessments in Alzheimer's disease. A study of the Consortium to Establish a Registry for Alzheimer's Disease (CERAD) [published erratum appears in
12. Hyman BT, Trojanowski JQ: Consensus recommendations for the postmortem diagnosis of Alzheimer disease from the National Institute on Aging and the Reagan Institute Working Group on Diagnostic Criteria for the Neuropathological Assessment of Alzheimer disease (editorial). J Neuropathol Exp Neurol 56:1095–1097, 1997.
13. Gonatas NK, Anderson W, Evangelista I: The contribution of altered synapses in the senile plaque. An electron microscopic study in Alzheimer's dementia. J Neuropathol Exp Neurol 26:25–39, 1967.
14. Terry RD, Wisniewski H: The ultrastructure of the neurofibrillary tangle and the senile plaque. *In* Wolstenholme GEW, O'Connor M (eds): Ciba Foundation Symposium on Alzheimer's Disease and Related Disorders. New York, Churchill Livingstone, 1970, pp 145–168.
15. Glenner GG, Wong CW: Alzheimer's disease and Down's syndrome. Sharing of a unique cerebrovascular amyloid fibril protein. Biochem Biophys Res Commun 122:1131–1135, 1984.
16. Masters CL, Simms G, Weinman NA, et al: Amyloid plaque core protein in Alzheimer disease and Down syndrome. Proc Natl Acad Sci U S A 82:4245–4249, 1985.
17. Goldgaber D, Lerman MI, McBride OW, et al: Characterization and chromosomal localization of a cDNA encoding brain amyloid of Alzheimer's disease. Science 235:877–880, 1987.
18. Kang J, Lemaire H-G, Unterbeck A, et al: The precursor of Alzheimer's disease amyloid A4 protein resembles a cell-surface receptor. Nature 325:733–736, 1987.
19. Robakis N, Wisniewski HM, Jenkins EC, et al: Chromosome 21q21 sublocalisation of gene encoding beta-amyloid peptide in cerebral vessels and neuritic (senile) plaques of people with Alzheimer disease and Down syndrome. Lancet 1:384–385, 1987.
20. Tanzi RE, Gusella JF, Watkins PC, et al: Amyloid beta protein gene. cDNA, mRNA distribution, and genetic linkage near the Alzheimer locus. Science 235:880–884, 1987.
21. Kidd M: Paired helical filaments in electron microscopy in Alzheimer's disease. Nature 197:192–193, 1963.
22. Terry RD, Gonatas NK, Weiss M: Ultrastructural studies in Alzheimer's presenile dementia. Am J Pathol 44:269–297, 1964.
23. Kondo J, Honda T, Mori H, et al: The carboxyl third of tau is tightly bound to paired helical filaments. Neuron 1:827–834, 1988.
24. Wischik CM, Novak M, Thogersen HC, et al: Isolation of a fragment of tau derived from the core of the paired helical filament of Alzheimer disease. Proc Natl Acad Sci U S A 85: 4506–4510, 1988.
25. Lee VM, Balin BJ, Otvos LJ, Trojanowski JQ: A68. A major subunit of paired helical filaments and derivatized forms of normal Tau. Science 251:675–678, 1991.
26. Goedert M, Wischik CM, Crowther RA, et al: Cloning and sequencing of the cDNA encoding a core protein of the paired helical filament of Alzheimer disease. Identification as the microtubule-associated protein tau. Proc Natl Acad Sci U S A 85:4051–4055, 1988.
27. Kosik KS, Orecchio LD, Bakalis S, Neve RL: Developmentally regulated expression of specific tau sequences. Neuron 2:1389–1397, 1989.
28. Hirokawa N: Microtubule organization and dynamics dependent on microtubule-associated proteins. Curr Opin Cell Biol 6:74–81, 1994.
29. Goedert M, Jakes R, Spillantini MG, et al: Tau protein in Alzheimer's disease. Biochem Soc Trans 23:80–85, 1995.
30. Goedert M, Spillantini MG, Jakes R, et al: Multiple isoforms of human microtubule-associated protein tau. Sequences and localization in neurofibrillary tangles of Alzheimer's disease. Neuron 3:519–526, 1989.
31. Andreadis A, Brown WM, Kosik KS: Structure and novel exons of the human tau gene. Biochemistry 31:10626–10633, 1992.
32. Baker M, Litvan I, Houlden H, et al: Association of an extended haplotype in the tau gene with progressive supranuclear palsy. Hum Mol Genet 8:711–715, 1999.

J Neuropathol Exp Neurol 1994 Jul;53(4):425]. J Neuropathol Exp Neurol 53:303–315, 1994.

33. Goedert M, Spillantini MG, Potier MC, et al: Cloning and sequencing of the cDNA encoding an isoform of microtubule-associated protein tau containing four tandem repeats. Differential expression of tau protein mRNAs in human brain. EMBO J 8:393–399, 1989.

34. Rizzu P, Van Swieten JC, Joosse M, et al: High prevalence of mutations in the microtubule-associated protein tau in a population study of frontotemporal dementia in the Netherlands. Am J Hum Genet 64:414–421, 1999.

35. Iijima M, Tabira T, Poorkaj P, et al: A distinct familial presenile dementia with a novel missense mutation in the tau gene. Neuroreport 25:497–501, 1999.

36. Hong M, Zhukareva V, Vogelsberg-Ragaglia V, et al: Mutation-specific functional impairments in distinct tau isoforms of hereditary FTDP-17. Science 282:1914–1917, 1998.

37. Goode BL, Denis PE, Panda D, et al: Functional interactions between the proline-rich and repeat regions of tau enhance microtubule binding and assembly. Mol Biol Cell 8:353–365, 1997.

38. Harada A, Oguchi K, Okabe S, et al: Altered microtubule organization in small-calibre axons of mice lacking tau protein. Nature 369:488–491, 1994.

39. Drechsel DN, Hyman AA, Cobb MH, Kirschner MW: Modulation of the dynamic instability of tubulin assembly by the microtubule-associated protein tau. Mol Biol Cell 3:1141–1154, 1992.

40. Bramblett GT, Goedert M, Jakes R, et al: Abnormal tau phosphorylation at Ser396 in Alzheimer's disease recapitulates development and contributes to reduced microtubule binding. Neuron 10:1089–1099, 1993.

41. Buee L, Delacourte A: Comparative biochemistry of tau in progressive supranuclear palsy, corticobasal degeneration, FTP-17 and Pick's disease. Brain Pathol 9:681–693, 1999.

42. Biernat J, Gustke N, Drewes G, et al: Phosphorylation of Ser262 strongly reduces binding of tau to microtubules. Distinction between PHF-like immunoreactivity and microtubule binding. Neuron 11:153–163, 1993.

43. Goedert M, Jakes R, Spillantini MG, Crowther RA: Tau Protein and Alzheimer's Disease. New York, Wiley-Liss, 1994.

44. Sergeant N, Wattez A, Delacourte A: Neurofibrillary degeneration in progressive supranuclear palsy and corticobasal degeneration. Tau pathologies with exclusively "exon 10" isoforms. J Neurochem 72:1243–1249, 1999.

45. Alonso AC, Grundke-Iqbal I, Iqbal K: Alzheimer's disease hyperphosphorylated tau sequesters normal tau into tangles of filaments and disassembles microtubules. Nat Med 2:783–787, 1996.

46. Schneider A, Biernat J, von Bergen M, et al: Phosphorylation that detaches tau protein from microtubules (Ser262, Ser214) also protects it against aggregation into Alzheimer paired helical filaments. Biochemistry 38:3549–3558, 1999.

47. Jensen PH, Hager H, Nielsen M, et al: α-Synuclein binds to tau and stimulates the protein kinase A-catalyzed tau phosphorylation of serine residues. J Biol Chem 274:25481–25489, 1999.

48. Lu PJ, Wulf G, Zhou XZ, et al: The prolyl isomerase Pin1 restores the function of Alzheimer-associated phosphorylated tau protein. Nature 399:784–788, 1999.

49. Ghatak NR, Nochlin D, Hadfield MG: Neurofibrillary pathology in progressive supranuclear palsy. Acta Neuropathol (Berl) 52:73–76, 1980.

50. Ghetti B, Dlouhy SR, Giaccone G, et al: Gerstmann-Sträussler-Scheinker disease and the Indiana kindred. Brain Pathol 5:61–75, 1995.

51. Tomlinson BE, Blessed G, Roth M: Observations on the brains of non-demented old people. J Neurol Sci 7:331–356, 1968.

52. Wilcock GK, Esiri MM: Plaques, tangles and dementia. A quantitative study. J Neurol Sci 56:343–356, 1982.

53. Ulrich J: Alzheimer changes in nondemented patients younger than sixty-five. Possible early stages of Alzheimer's disease and senile dementia of Alzheimer type. Ann Neurol 17:273–277, 1985.

54. Katzman R, Terry R, DeTeresa R, et al: Clinical, pathological, and neurochemical changes in dementia. A subgroup with preserved mental status and numerous neocortical plaques. Ann Neurol 23:138–144, 1988.

55. Crystal H, Dickson D, Fuld P, et al: Clinico-pathologic studies in dementia. Nondemented subjects with pathologically confirmed Alzheimer's disease. Neurology 38:1682–1687, 1988.

56. de la Monte S, Wells SE, Hedley WT, Growdon JH: Neuropathological distinction between Parkinson's dementia and Parkinson's plus Alzheimer's disease. Ann Neurol 26:309–320, 1989.

57. Terry RD, Masliah E, Salmon DP, et al: Physical basis of cognitive alterations in Alzheimer's disease. Synapse loss is the major correlate of cognitive impairment. Ann Neurol 30:572–580, 1991.

58. Dickson DW, Crystal HA, Bevona C, et al: Correlations of synaptic and pathological markers with cognition of the elderly. Neurobiol Aging 16:285–298, discussion 298–304, 1995.

59. Gearing M, Mirra SS, Hedreen JC, et al: The Consortium to Establish a Registry for Alzheimer's Disease (CERAD). Part X. Neuropathology confirmation of the clinical diagnosis of Alzheimer's disease. Neurology 45:461–466, 1995.

60. Hansen L, Salmon D, Galasko D, et al: The Lewy body variant of Alzheimer's disease. A clinical and pathologic entity. Neurology 40:1–8, 1990.

61. De Sauvage F, Octave JN: A novel mRNA of the A4 amyloid precursor gene coding for a possibly secreted protein. Science 245:651–653, 1989.

62. Golde TE, Estus S, Usiak M, et al: Expression of beta amyloid protein precursor mRNAs. Recognition of a novel alternatively spliced form and quantitation in Alzheimer's disease using PCR. Neuron 4:253–267, 1990.

63. Jacobsen JS, Muenkel HA, Blume AJ, Vitek MP: A novel species-specific RNA related to alternatively spliced amyloid precursor protein mRNAs. Neurobiol Aging 12:575–583, 1991.

64. Ponte P, Gonzalez DP, Schilling J, et al: A new A4 amyloid mRNA contains a domain homologous to serine proteinase inhibitors. Nature 331:525–527, 1988.

65. Tanzi RE, McClatchey AI, Lamperti ED, et al: Protease inhibitor domain encoded by an amyloid protein precursor mRNA associated with Alzheimer's disease. Nature 331:528–530, 1988.

66. Selkoe DJ: Alzheimer's disease. A central role for amyloid. J Neuropathol Exp Neurol 53:438–447, 1994.

67. Selkoe DJ: Cellular and molecular biology of beta-amyloid precursor protein and Alzheimer's disease. *In* Rosenberg RN, Prusiner SB, DiMauro S, Barchi RL (eds): The Molecular and Genetic Basis of Neurological Disease. Boston, Butterworth-Heinemann, 1997, pp 601–611.

68. Mullan M, Houlden H, Windelspecht M, et al: A locus for familial early-onset Alzheimer's disease on the long arm of chromosome 14, proximal to the alpha 1-antichymotrypsin gene. Nat Genet 2:340–342, 1992.

69. Hsiao K, Chapman P, Nilsen S, et al: Correlative memory deficits, Aβ elevation, and amyloid plaques in transgenic mice. Science 274:99–102, 1996.

70. Hendriks L, van DC, Cras P, et al: Presenile dementia and cerebral haemorrhage linked to a mutation at codon 692 of the beta-amyloid precursor protein gene. Nat Genet 1:218–221, 1992.

71. Levy E, Carman MD, Fernandez-Madrid IJ, et al: Mutation of the Alzheimer's disease amyloid gene in hereditary cerebral hemorrhage, Dutch type. Science 248:1124–1126, 1990.

72. Fernandez MI, Levy E, Marder K, Frangione B: Codon 618 variant of Alzheimer amyloid gene associated with inherited cerebral hemorrhage. Ann Neurol 30:730–733, 1991.

73. Luyendijk W, Bots GT, Vegter van dVM, et al: Hereditary cerebral haemorrhage caused by cortical amyloid angiopathy. J Neurol Sci 85:267–280, 1988.

74. Goate A, Chartier HM, Mullan M, et al: Segregation of a missense mutation in the amyloid precursor protein gene with familial Alzheimer's disease. Nature 349:704–706, 1991.

75. Naruse S, Igarashi S, Kobayashi H, et al: Mis-sense mutation Val—-Ile in exon 17 of amyloid precursor protein gene in Japanese familial Alzheimer's disease (letter). Lancet 337:978–979, 1991.

76. Yoshioka K, Miki T, Katsuya T, et al: The 717Val—-Ile substitution in amyloid precursor protein is associated with familial Alzheimer's disease regardless of ethnic groups. Biochem Biophys Res Commun 178:1141–1146, 1991.

77. Hardy J, Group ASDR: Molecular characterization of Alzheimer's disease. Lancet 337:1342, 1991.

78. Murrell J, Farlow M, Ghetti B, Benson MD: A mutation in the amyloid precursor protein associated with hereditary Alzheimer's disease. Science 254:97–99, 1991.

79. Chartier HM, Crawford F, Houlden H, et al: Early-onset Alzheimer's disease caused by mutations at codon 717 of the beta-amyloid precursor protein gene. Nature 353:844–846, 1991.

80. Citron M, Oltersdorf T, Haass C, et al: Mutation of the beta-amyloid precursor protein in familial Alzheimer's disease increases beta-protein production. Nature 360:672–674, 1992.

81. Cai XD, Golde TE, Younkin SG: Release of excess amyloid beta protein from a mutant amyloid beta protein precursor. Science 259:514–516, 1993.

82. Suzuki N, Cheung TT, Cai XD, et al: An increased percentage of long amyloid beta protein secreted by familial amyloid beta protein precursor (beta APP717) mutants. Science 264:1336–1340, 1994.

83. Haass C, Schlossmacher MG, Hung AY, et al: Amyloid beta-peptide is produced by cultured cells during normal metabolism. Nature 359:322–325, 1992.

84. Schellenberg GD, Bird TD, Wijsman EM, et al: Genetic linkage evidence for a familial Alzheimer's disease locus on chromosome 14. Science 258:668–671, 1992.

85. Sherrington R, Rogaev EI, Liang Y, et al: Cloning of a gene bearing missense mutations in early-onset familial Alzheimer's disease. Nature 375:754–760, 1995.

86. Doan A, Thinakaran G, Borchelt DR, et al: Protein topology of presenilin 1. Neuron 17:1023–1030, 1996.

87. De Strooper B, Beullens M, Contreras B, et al: Phosphorylation, subcellular localization, and membrane orientation of the Alzheimer's disease–associated presenilins. J Biol Chem 272:3590–3598, 1997.

88. Sisodia SS, Thinakaran G, Borchelt DR, et al: Function and dysfunction of the presenilins. In Terry RD, Katzman R, Bick KL, Sisodia SS (eds): Alzheimer Disease, 2nd ed. Philadelphia, Lippincott Williams & Wilkins, 1999, pp 327–337.

89. Tanzi RE: The molecular genetics of Alzheimer's disease. In Martin JB (ed): Molecular Neurology. New York, Scientific American, 1998, pp 55–73.

90. Buee L, Permanne B, Perez TJ, et al: Alzheimer's disease. A beta or ApoE amyloidosis? (letter). Lancet 346:59, 1995.

91. De Strooper B, Saftig P, Craessaerts K: Deficiency of presenilin-1 inhibits the normal cleavage of amyloid precursor protein. Nature 391:387–390, 1998.

92. Scheuner D, Eckman C, Jensen M, et al: Secreted amyloid-protein similar to that in the senile plaques of Alzheimer's disease is increased in vivo by the presenilin 1 and 2 and APP mutations linked to familial Alzheimer's disease. Nature Med 2:864–870, 1996.

93. Borchelt DR, Ratovitski T, Van Lare J, et al: Accelerated amyloid deposition in the brains of transgenic mice co-expressing mutant presenilin-1 and amyloid precursor proteins. Neuron 19:939–945, 1997.

94. Levy-Lahad E, Wasco W, Poorkaj P, et al: Candidate gene for the chromosome 1 familial Alzheimer's disease locus. Science 269:973–977, 1995.

95. Levy-Lahad E, Wijsman EM, Nemens E, et al: A familial Alzheimer's disease locus on chromosome 1. Science 269:970–973, 1995.

96. Rogaeva EI, Sherrington R, Rogaeva EA, et al: Familial Alzheimer's disease in kindreds with missense mutations in a gene on chromosome 1 related to the Alzheimer's disease type 3 gene. Nature 376:775–778, 1995.

97. Borgaonkar DS, Schmidt LC, Martin SE, et al: Linkage of late-onset Alzheimer's disease with apolipoprotein E type 4 on chromosome 19 (letter). Lancet 342:625, 1993.

98. Chartier HM, Parfitt M, Legrain S, et al: Apolipoprotein E, epsilon 4 allele as a major risk factor for sporadic early and late-onset forms of Alzheimer's disease. Analysis of the 19q13.2 chromosomal region. Hum Mol Genet 3:569–574, 1994.

99. Corder EH, Saunders AM, Strittmatter WJ, et al: Gene dose of apolipoprotein E type 4 allele and the risk of Alzheimer's disease in late onset families. Science 261:921–923, 1993.

100. Corder EH, Saunders AM, Risch NJ, et al: Protective effect of apolipoprotein E type 2 allele for late onset Alzheimer disease. Nat Genet 7:180–184, 1994.

101. Liddell M, Williams J, Bayer A, et al: Confirmation of association between the e4 allele of apolipoprotein E and Alzheimer's disease. J Med Genet 31:197–200, 1994.

102. Poirier J, Davignon J, Bouthillier D, et al: Apolipoprotein E polymorphism and Alzheimer's disease. Lancet 342:697–699, 1993.

103. Rebeck GW, Reiter JS, Strickland DK, Hyman BT: Apolipoprotein E in sporadic Alzheimer's disease. Allelic variation and receptor interactions. Neuron 11:575–580, 1993.

104. Saunders AM, Strittmatter WJ, Schmechel D, et al: Association of apolipoprotein E allele ε4 with late-onset familial and sporadic Alzheimer's disease. Neurology 43:1467–1472, 1993.

105. Strittmatter WJ, Saunders AM, Schmechel D, et al: Apolipoprotein E, high-avidity binding to β-amyloid and increased frequency of type 4 allele in late-onset familial Alzheimer disease. Proc Natl Acad Sci U S A 90:1977–1981, 1993.

106. Das HK, McPherson J, Bruns GA, et al: Isolation, characterization, and mapping to chromosome 19 of the human apolipoprotein E gene. J Biol Chem 260:6240–6247, 1985.

107. Myers RH: Apolipoprotein E allele 4 is associated with dementia in the Framingham study. In Iqbal K, Mortimer J, Winblad B, Wisniewski H (eds): Research Advances in Alzheimer's Disease and Related Disorders. New York, John Wiley & Sons, 1995, pp 63–73.

108. Corder EH: Apolipoprotein E and the epidemiology of Alzheimer's disease. In Iqbal K, Mortimer J, Winblad B, Wisniewski H (eds): Research Advances in Alzheimer's Disease and Related Disorders. New York, John Wiley & Sons, 1995, pp 53–63.

109. Poirier J, Hess M, May PC, Finch CE: Astrocytic apolipoprotein E mRNA and GFAP mRNA in hippocampus after entorhinal cortex lesioning. Brain Res Mol Brain Res 11:97–106, 1991.

110. Strittmatter WJ, Weisgraber KH, Huang DY, et al: Binding of human apolipoprotein E to synthetic amyloid beta peptide. Isoform-specific effects and implications for late-onset Alzheimer disease. Proc Natl Acad Sci U S A 90:8098–8102, 1993.

111. Wisniewski T, Golabek A, Matsubara E, et al: Apolipoprotein E. Binding to soluble Alzheimer's beta-amyloid. Biochem Biophys Res Commun 192:359–365, 1993.

112. Ma J, Yee A, Brewer HB Jr, et al: Amyloid-associated proteins $\alpha_1$-antichymotrypsin and apolipoprotein E promote assembly of Alzheimer β-protein into filaments. Nature 372:92–94, 1994.

113. Wisniewski T, Castaño EM, Golabek A, et al: Acceleration of Alzheimer's fibril formation by apolipoprotein E in vitro. Am J Pathol 145:1030–1035, 1994.

114. Castano EM, Prelli F, Wisniewski T, et al: Fibrillogenesis in Alzheimer's disease of amyloid beta peptides and apolipoprotein E. Biochem J 306:599–604, 1995.

115. Soto C, Castano EM, Prelli F, et al: Apolipoprotein E increases the fibrillogenic potential of synthetic peptides derived from Alzheimer's, gelsolin and AA amyloids. FEBS Lett 371:110–114, 1995.

116. Schmechel DE, Saunders AM, Strittmatter WJ, et al: Increased amyloid beta-peptide deposition in cerebral cortex as a consequence of apolipoprotein E genotype in late-onset Alzheimer disease. Proc Natl Acad Sci U S A 90:9649–9653, 1993.

117. Namba Y, Tomonaga M, Kawasaki H, et al: Apolipoprotein E immunoreactivity in cerebral amyloid deposits and neurofibrillary in Alzheimer's disease and kuru plaque amyloid in Creutzfeldt-Jakob disease. Brain Res 541:163–166, 1991.

118. Dickson DW: Tau and synuclein and their roles in neuropathology. Brain Pathol 9:657–661, 1999.

119. Polymeropoulos MH, Lavedan C, Ide SE, et al: Mutation in the α-synuclein gene identified in families with Parkinson's disease. Science 276:2045–2047, 1997.

120. Kruger R, Kuhn W, Muller T, et al: Ala30Pro mutation in the gene encoding α-synuclein in Parkinson's disease. Nat Genet 18:106–108, 1998.
121. Sillantini MG, Schmidt ML, Lee VM-Y, et al: α-Synuclein in Lewy bodies. Nature 388:839–840, 1997.
122. Burkhardt CR, Filley CM, Kleinschmidt-DeMasters BK, et al: Diffuse Lewy body disease and progressive dementia. Neurology 38:1520–1528, 1988.
123. Hansen LA, Masliah E, Terry RD, Mirra SS: A neuropathological subset of Alzheimer's disease with concomitant Lewy body disease and spongiform change. Acta Neuropathol 78:194–201, 1989.
124. Hashimoto M, Masliah E: Alpha-synuclein in Lewy body disease and Alzheimer's disease. Brain Pathol 9:707–720, 1999.
125. Iwai A, Yoshimoto M, Masliah E, Saitoh T: Non-Aβ component of Alzheimer's disease amyloid (NAC) is amyloidogenic. Biochemistry 34:10139–10145, 1995.
126. Ueda K, Fukushima H, Masliah E, et al: Molecular cloning of a novel component of amyloid in Alzheimer's disease. Proc Natl Acad Sci U S A 90:11282–11286, 1993.
127. Masliah E, Iwai A, Mallory M, et al: Altered presynaptic protein NACP is associated with plaque formation and neurodegeneration in Alzheimer's disease. Am J Pathol 148:201–210, 1996.
128. Iwai A, Masliah E, Sundsmo MP, et al: The synaptic protein NACP is abnormally expressed during the progression of Alzheimer's disease. Brain Res 720:230–234, 1996.
129. Yoshimoto M, Iwai A, Kang D, et al: NACP, the precursor protein of non-amyloid β/A4 protein (Aβ) component of Alzheimer's disease amyloid, binds Aβ and stimulates Aβ aggregation. Proc Natl Acad Sci U S A 92:9141–9145, 1995.
130. Brookes AJ, St. Clair D: Synuclein proteins and Alzheimer's disease. Trends Neurosci 17:404–405, 1994.
131. Arima K, Ueda K, Sunohara N, et al: NACP/α-synuclein immunoreactivity in fibrillary components of neuronal and oligodendroglial cytoplasmic inclusions in the pontine nuclein in multiple system atrophy. Acta Neuropathol 96:439–444, 1998.
132. Wakabayashi K, Hayashi S, Kakita A, et al: Accumulation of α-synuclein/NACP is a cytopathological feature common to Lewy body disease and multiple system atrophy. Acta Neuropathol 96:445–452, 1998.
133. Goedert M, Trojanowski JQ, Lee VM-Y: The neurofibrillary pathology of Alzheimer's disease. In Rosenberg RN, Prusiner SB, DiMauro S, Barchi RL (eds): The Molecular and Genetic Basis of Neurological Disease. Boston, Butterworth-Heinemann, 1997, pp 613–627.
134. Yen SH, Hutton M, DeTure M, et al: Fibrillogenesis of tau. Insights from tau missense mutations in FTDP-17. Brain Pathol 9:695–705, 1999.
135. Komori T: Tau-positive glial inclusions in progressive supranuclear palsy, corticobasal degeneration and Pick's disease. Brain Pathol 9:663–679, 1999.
136. Goedert M, Spillantini MG, Davies SW: Filamentous nerve cell inclusions in neurodegenerative diseases. Curr Opin Neurobiol 8:619–632, 1998.
137. Jellinger KA: Dementia with grains (argyrophilic grain disease). Brain Pathol 8:377–386, 1998.
138. Jellinger KA, Bancher C: Senile dementia with tangles (tangle predominant form of senile dementia). Brain Pathol 8:367–376, 1998.
139. Guiroy DC, Miyazaki M, Multhaup G, et al: Amyloid of neurofibrillary tangles of Guamanian parkinsonism-dementia and Alzheimer disease share identical amino acid sequence. Proc Natl Acad Sci U S A 84:2073–2077, 1987.
140. McKenzie JE, Roberts GW, Royston MC: Comparative investigation of neurofibrillary damage in the temporal lobe in Alzheimer's disease, Down's syndrome and dementia pugilistica. Neurodegeneration 5:259–264, 1996.
141. Kosaka K: Diffuse neurofibrillary tangles with calcification. A new presenile dementia. J Neurol Neurosurg Psychiatry 57:594–596, 1994.
142. Ksiezak-Reding H, Morgan K, Mattiace L, et al: Ultrastructure and biochemical composition of paired helical filaments in corticobasal degeneration. Am J Pathol 145:1496–1508, 1994.
143. Gustafson L: Clinical picture of frontal lobe degeneration of non-Alzheimer type. Dementia 4:143–148, 1993.
144. Stevens M, van Duijn CM, Kamphorst W, et al: Familial aggregation in frontotemporal dementia. Neurology 50:1541–1545, 1998.
145. Knopman DS, Mastri AR, Frey WH 2, et al: Dementia lacking distinctive histologic features. A common non-Alzheimer degenerative dementia. Neurology 40:251–256, 1990.
146. Neary D, Snowden JS, Northen B, Goulding P: Dementia of frontal lobe type. J Neurol Neurosurg Psychiatry 51:353–361, 1988.
147. Litvan I, Mega MS, Cummings JL, Fairbanks L: Neuropsychiatric aspects of progressive supranuclear palsy. Neurology 47:1184–1189, 1996.
148. Verny M, Duyckaerts C, Agid Y, Hauw JJ: The significance of cortical pathology in progressive supranuclear palsy. Clinico-pathological data in 10 cases. Brain 119:1123–1136, 1996.
149. Steele JC, Richardson JC, Olszewski J: Progressive supranuclear palsy. A heterogeneous degeneration involving the brain stem, basal ganglia, and cerebellum with vertical gaze and pseudobulbar palsy, nuchal dystonia and dementia. Arch Neurol 2:473–486, 1964.
150. Bergeron C, Pollanen MS, Weyer L, Lang AE: Cortical degeneration in progressive supranuclear palsy. A comparison with cortical-basal ganglionic degeneration. J Neuropathol Exp Neurol 56:726–734, 1997.
151. Bergeron C, Davis A, Lang AE: Corticobasal ganglionic degeneration and progressive supranuclear palsy presenting with cognitive decline. Brain Pathol 8:355–365, 1998.
152. de Yébenes JG, Sarasa JL, Daniel SE, Lees AJ: Familial progressive supranuclear palsy. Description of a pedigree and review of the literature. Brain 118:1095–1103, 1995.
153. Rojo A, Pernaute RS, Fontán A, et al: Clinical genetics of familial progressive supranuclear palsy. Brain 122:1233–1245, 1999.
154. Nishimura M, Namba Y, Ikeda K, Oda M: Glial fibrillary tangles with straight tubules in the brains of patients with progressive supranuclear palsy. Neurosci Lett 143:35–38, 1992.
155. Conrad C, Andreadis A, Trojanowski JQ, et al: Genetic evidence for the involvement of tau in progressive supranuclear palsy. Ann Neurol 41:277–281, 1997.
156. Poorkaj P, Bird TD, Wijsman E, et al: Tau is a candidate gene for chromosome 17 frontotemporal dementia [published erratum appears in Ann Neurol 1998 Sep;44(3):428.]. Ann Neurol 43:815–825, 1998.
157. Foster NL, Wilhelmsen K, Sima AA, et al: Frontotemporal dementia and parkinsonism linked to chromosome 17. A consensus conference. Ann Neurol 41:706–715, 1997.
158. Brun A, Englund B, Gustafson L, et al: Clinical and neuropathological criteria for frontotemporal dementia, the Lund and Manchester Groups. J Neurol Neurosurg Psychiatry 57:416–418, 1994.
159. Jackson M, Lowe J: The new neuropathology of degenerative frontotemporal dementias. Acta Neuropathol 91:127–134, 1996.
160. Kertesz A, Hudson L, Mackenzie IR, Munoz DG: The pathology and nosology of primary progressive aphasia. Neurology 44:2065–2072, 1994.
161. Constantinidis J, Richard J, Tissot R: Pick's disease. Histological and clinical correlations. Eur Neurol 11:208–217, 1974.
162. Dickson DW: Pick's disease. A modern approach. Brain Pathol 8:339–354, 1998.
163. Rinne JO, Lee MS, Thompson PD, Marsden CD: Corticobasal degeneration. A clinical study of 36 cases. Brain 117:1183–1196, 1994.
164. Garruto RM, Gajdusek C, Chen KM: Amyotrophic lateral sclerosis among Chamorro migrants from Guam. Ann Neurol 8:612–619, 1980.
165. Brun A, Englund E: Regional pattern of degeneration in Alzheimer's disease. Neuronal loss and histopathological grading. Histopathology 5:549–564, 1981.
166. Mann DM: Dementia of frontal type and dementias with subcortical gliosis. Brain Pathol 8:325–338, 1998.
167. Hauw JJ, Duyckaerts C, Seilhean D, et al: The neuropatho-

logic diagnostic criteria of frontal lobe dementia revisited. A study of ten consecutive cases. J Neural Transm 47(suppl): 47–49, 1996.

168. Bergmann M, Kuchelmeister K, Schmid KW, et al: Different variants of frontotemporal dementia. A neuropathological and immunohistochemical study. Acta Neuropathol 92:170–179, 1996.
169. Kertesz A, Munoz DG: Pick's disease. Frontotemporal dementia. *In* Terry RD, Katzman R, Bick KL, Sisodia SS (eds): Alzheimer Disease, 2nd ed. Philadelphia, Lippincott Williams & Wilkins, 1999.
170. Brown J, Ashworth A, Gydesen S, et al: Familial non-specific dementia maps to chromosome 3. Hum Mol Genet 4:1625–1628, 1995.
171. Yamaoka LH, Welsh-Bohmer KA, Hulette CM, et al: Linkage of frontotemporal dementia to chromosome 17. Clinical and neuropathological characterization of phenotype. Am J Hum Genet 59:1306–1316, 1996.
172. Hutton M, Lendon CL, Rizzu P, et al: Association of missense and 5'-splice-site mutations in tau with the inherited dementia FTDP-17. Nature 393:702–705, 1998.
173. Spillantini MG, Murrell JR, Goedert M, et al: Mutation in the tau gene in familial multiple system tauopathy with presenile dementia. Proc Natl Acad Sci U S A 95:7737–7741, 1998.
174. Clark LPP, Wszolek Z, Geschwind DH, et al: Pathogenic implications of mutations in the tau gene in pallido-ponto nigral degeneration and related neurodegenerative disorders linked to chromosome 17. Proc Natl Acad Sci U S A 95:13103–13107, 1998.
175. Dumanchin C, Camuzat A, Campion D, et al: Segregation of a missense mutation in the microtubule-associated protein tau gene with familial frontotemporal dementia and parkinsonism. Hum Mol Genet 7:1825–1829, 1998.
176. Bugiani O, Murrell JR, Giaccone G, et al: Frontotemporal dementia and corticobasal degeneration in a family with a P301S mutation in tau. J Neuropathol Exp Neurol 58:667–677, 1999.
177. Delisle MB, Murrell JR, Richardson R, et al: A mutation at codon 279 (N279K) in exon 10 of the Tau gene causes a tauopathy with dementia and supranuclear palsy. Acta Neuropathol 98:62–77, 1999.
178. Mirra SS, Murrell JR, Gearing M, et al: Tau pathology in a family with dementia and a P301L mutation in tau. J Neuropathol Exp Neurol 58:335–345, 1999.
179. Nasreddine ZS, Loginov M, Clark LN, et al: From genotype to phenotype. A clinical pathological, and biochemical investigation of frontotemporal dementia and parkinsonism (FTDP-17) caused by the P301L tau mutation. Ann Neurol 45:704–715, 1999.
180. D'Souza I, Poorkaj P, Hong M, et al: Missense and silent tau gene mutations cause frontotemporal dementia with parkinsonism-chromosome 17 type, by affecting multiple alternative RNA splicing regulatory elements. Proc Natl Acad Sci U S A 96:5598–5603, 1999.
181. van Swieten JC, Stevens M, Rosso SM, et al: Phenotypic variation in hereditary frontotemporal dementia with tau mutations. Ann Neurol 46:617–626, 1999.
182. Goedert M, Spillantini MG, Crowther RA, et al: Tau gene mutation in familial progressive subcortical gliosis. Nat Med 5:454–457, 1999.
183. Bird TD, Nochlin D, Poorkaj P, et al: A clinical pathological comparison of three families with frontotemporal dementia and identical mutations in the tau gene (P301L) [published erratum appears in Brain 1999 Jul;122(pt 7):1398]. Brain 122:741–756, 1999.
184. Kertesz A, Kawarai T, Rogaeva E, et al: Familial frontotemporal dementia with ubiquitin-positive, tau negative inclusions. Neurology 54:818–827, 2000.
185. Savioz A, Kövari E, Anastasiu R, et al: Search for a mutation in the tau gene in a Swiss family with frontotemporal dementia. Exp Neurol 161:330–335, 2000.
186. Delacourte A, Sergeant N, Wattez A, et al: Vulnerable neuronal subsets in Alzheimer's and Pick's disease are distinguished by their tau isoform distribution and phosphorylation. Ann Neurol 43:193–204, 1998.

187. Grover A, Houlden H, Baker M, et al: 5' splice site mutations in tau associated with the inherited dementia FTDP-17 affect a stem-loop structure that regulates alternative splicing of exon 10. J Biol Chem 274:15134–15143, 1999.
188. Varani L, Hasegawa M, Spillantini MG, et al: Structure of tau exon 10 splicing regulatory element RNA and destabilization by mutations of frontotemporal dementia and parkinsonism linked to chromosome 17. Proc Natl Acad Sci U S A 96:8229–8234, 1999.
189. Hasegawa M, Smith MJ, Goedert M: Tau proteins with FTDP-17 mutations have a reduced ability to promote microtubule assembly. FEBS Lett 437:207–210, 1998.
190. Trojanowski JQ, Lee VM: Transgenic models of tauopathies and synucleinopathies. Brain Pathol 9:733–739, 1999.
191. Spittaels K, Van den Haute C, Van Dorpe J, et al: Prominent axonopathy in the brain and spinal cord of transgenic mice overexpressing four-repeat human tau protein. Am J Pathol 155:2153–2165, 1999.
192. Ishihara T, Hong M, Zhang B, et al: Age-dependent emergence and progression of a tauopathy in transgenic mice overexpressing the shortest human tau isoform. Neuron 24:751–762, 1999.
193. DeArmond SJ, Prusiner SB: Prions. *In* Purtilo DT, Damjanov I (eds): Anderson's Pathology. St. Louis, CV Mosby, 1996, pp 1042–1060.
194. DeArmond SJ, Prusiner SB: Prion diseases. *In* Graham DI, Lantos PL (ed): Greenfield's Neuropathology, 6th ed. Arnold, London, UK, 1997, pp 235–280.
195. Brown P, Preece MA, Will RG. "Friendly fire" in medicine. Hormones, homografts, and Creutzfeldt-Jakob disease. Lancet 340:24–27, 1992.
196. Scott MR, Will R, Ironside J, et al: Compelling transgenetic evidence for transmission of bovine spongiform encephalopathy prions to humans. Proc Natl Acad Sci U S A 96:15137–15142, 1999.
197. Evatt B, Austin H, Barnhart E, et al: Surveillance for Creutzfeldt-Jakob disease among persons with hemophilia. Transfusion 38:817–820, 1998.
198. Kretzschmar HA, Prusiner SB, Stowring LE, DeArmond SJ: Scrapie prion proteins are synthesized in neurons. Am J Pathol 122:1–5, 1986.
199. Oesch B, Westaway D, Wälchli M, et al: A cellular gene encodes scrapie PrP 27–30 protein. Cell 40:735–746, 1985.
200. Pan K-M, Baldwin M, Nguyen J, et al: Conversion of α-helices into β-sheets features in the formation of the scrapie prion proteins. Proc Natl Acad Sci U S A 90:10962–10966, 1993.
201. Safar J, Roller PP, Gajdusek DC, Gibbs CJ Jr: Conformational transitions, dissociation, and unfolding of scrapie amyloid (prion) protein. J Biol Chem 268:20276–20284, 1993.
202. Caughey BW, Dong A, Bhat KS, et al: Secondary structure analysis of the scrapie-associated protein PrP 27–30 in water by infrared spectroscopy. Biochemistry 30:7672–7680, 1991.
203. Gasset M, Baldwin MA, Fletterick RJ, Prusiner SB: Perturbation of the secondary structure of the scrapie prion protein under conditions associated with changes in infectivity. Proc Natl Acad Sci U S A 90:1–5, 1993.
204. Prusiner SB, Scott MR, DeArmond SJ, Cohen FE: Prion protein biology. Cell 93:337–348, 1998.
205. Prusiner SB: Prions. *In* Frängsmyr T (ed): Les Prix Nobel, The Nobel Prizes, 1997. Norstedts Tryckeri AB, Stockholm, Sweden, 1998, pp 268–323.
206. Kaneko K, Zulianello L, Scott M, et al: Evidence for protein X binding to a discontinuous epitope on the cellular prion protein during scrapie prion propagation. Proc Natl Acad Sci U S A 94:10069–10074, 1997.
207. Telling GC, Scott M, Mastrianni J, et al: Prion propagation in mice expressing human and chimeric PrP transgenes implicates the interaction of cellular PrP with another protein. Cell 83:79–90, 1995.
208. James TL, Liu H, Ulyanov NB, et al: Solution structure of a 142-residue recombinant prion protein corresponding to the infectious fragment of the scrapie isoform. Proc Natl Acad Sci U S A 94:10086–10091, 1997.
209. Donne DG, Viles JH, Groth D, et al: Structure of the recom-

binant full-length hamster prion protein PrP(29–231). The N terminus is highly flexible. Proc Natl Acad Sci U S A 94: 13452–13457, 1997.

210. Scott M, Groth D, Foster D, et al: Propagation of prions with artificial properties in transgenic mice expressing chimeric PrP genes. Cell 73:979–988, 1993.

211. Taraboulos A, Raeber AJ, Borchelt DR, et al: Synthesis and trafficking of prion proteins in cultured cells. Mol Biol Cell 3: 851–863, 1992.

212. Caughey B, Raymond GJ: The scrapie-associated form of PrP is made from a cell surface precursor that is both protease- and phospholipase-sensitive. J Biol Chem 266:18217–18223, 1991.

213. Vey M, Pilkuhn S, Wille H, et al: Subcellular colocalization of cellular and scrapie prion proteins in caveolae-like membranous domains. Proc Natl Acad Sci U S A 93:14945–14949, 1996.

214. Büeler H, Fischer M, Lang Y, et al: Normal development and behaviour of mice lacking the neuronal cell-surface PrP protein. Nature 356:577–582, 1992.

215. Büeler H, Aguzzi A, Sailer A, et al: Mice devoid of PrP are resistant to scrapie. Cell 73:1339–1347, 1993.

216. Prusiner SB, Groth D, Serban A, et al: Ablation of the prion protein (PrP) gene in mice prevents scrapie and facilitates production of anti-PrP antibodies. Proc Natl Acad Sci U S A 90:10608–10612, 1993.

217. Brandner S, Isenmann S, Raeber A, et al: Normal host prion protein necessary for scrapie-induced neurotoxicity. Nature 379:339–343, 1996.

218. DeArmond SJ, Qiu Y, Wong K, et al: Abnormal plasma membrane properties and functions in prion-infected cell lines. In: Function and Dysfunction in the Nervous System. Cold Spring Harbor, NY, Cold Spring Harbor Laboratory Press, 1996, pp 531–540.

219. Hsiao K, Scott M, Foster D, et al: Spontaneous neurodegeneration in transgenic mice with prion protein codon 101 prolineleucine substitution. Ann N Y Acad Sci 640:166–170, 1991.

220. Hsiao KK, Groth D, Scott M, et al: Serial transmission in rodents of neurodegeneration from transgenic mice expressing mutant prion protein. Proc Natl Acad Sci U S A 91:9126–9130, 1994.

221. Ghetti B, Piccardo P, Frangione B, et al: Prion protein amyloidosis. Brain Pathol 6:127–145, 1996.

222. Hsiao K, Baker HF, Crow TJ, et al: Linkage of a prion protein missense variant to Gerstmann-Sträussler syndrome. Nature 338:342–345, 1989.

223. Hegde RS, Mastrianni JA, Scott MR, et al: A transmembrane form of prion protein in neurodegenerative disease. Science 279:827–834, 1998.

224. Dlouhy SR, Hsiao K, Farlow MR, et al: Linkage of the Indiana kindred of Gerstmann-Sträussler-Scheinker disease to the prion protein gene. Nat Genet 1:64–67, 1992.

225. Gabizon R, Rosenmann H, Meiner Z, et al: Mutation and polymorphism of the prion protein gene in Libyan Jews with Creutzfeldt-Jakob disease. Am J Hum Genet 33:828–835, 1993.

226. Petersen RB, Tabaton M, Berg L, et al: Analysis of the prion protein gene in thalamic dementia. Neurology 42:1859–1863, 1992.

227. Poulter M, Baker HF, Frith CD, et al: Inherited prion disease with 144 base pair gene insertion. 1. Genealogical and molecular studies. Brain 115:675–685, 1992.

228. Kitamoto T, Iizuka R, Tateishi J: An amber mutation of prion protein in Gerstmann-Sträussler syndrome with mutant PrP plaques. Biochem Biophys Res Commun 192:525–531, 1993.

229. Hsiao K, Dlouhy S, Farlow MR, et al: Mutant prion proteins in Gerstmann-Sträussler-Scheinker disease with neurofibrillary tangles. Nat Genet 1:68–71, 1992.

230. DeArmond SJ, Ironside JW: Neuropathology of Prion diseases. In Prusiner SB (ed): Prion Biology and Diseases. Cold Spring Harbor, NY, Cold Spring Harbor Laboratory Press, 1999, pp 585–652.

231. Goldfarb LG, Brown P, Haltia M, et al: Creutzfeldt-Jakob disease cosegregates with the codon 178[Asn] PRNP mutation in families of European origin. Ann Neurol 31:274–281, 1992.

232. Medori R, Montagna P, Tritschler HJ, et al: Fatal familial insomnia. A second kindred with mutation of prion protein gene at codon 178. Neurology 42:669–670, 1992.

233. Medori R, Tritschler H-J, LeBlanc A, et al: Fatal familial insomnia, a prion disease with a mutation at codon 178 of the prion protein gene. N Engl J Med 326:444–449, 1992.

234. Goldfarb LG, Petersen RB, Tabaton M, et al: Fatal familial insomnia and familial Creutzfeldt-Jakob disease. Disease phenotype determined by a DNA polymorphism. Science 258:806–808, 1992.

235. DeArmond SJ, Sanchez H, Qiu Y, et al: Selective neuronal targeting in prion diseases. Neuron 19:1337–1348, 1997.

236. DeArmond SJ, Qiu Y, Sànchez H, et al: PrP$^C$ glycoform heterogeneity as a function of brain region. Implications for selective targeting of neurons by prion strains. J Neuropathol Exp Neurol 58:1000–1009, 1999.

237. Rosenmann H, Halimi M, Kahana I, et al: Differential allelic expression of PrP mRNA in carriers of the E200K mutation. Neurology 49:851–856, 1997.

238. Owen F, Poulter M, Collinge J, Crow TJ: Codon 129 changes in the prion protein gene in Caucasians. Am J Hum Genet 46:1215–1216, 1990.

239. Collinge J, Palmer M: Molecular genetics of inherited, sporadic and iatrogenic prion disease. In Prusiner S, Collinge J, Powell J, Anderton B (eds): Prion Diseases in Humans and Animals. New York, Ellis Horwood, 1992, pp 95–119.

240. Palmer MS, Dryden AJ, Hughes JT, Collinge J: Homozygous prion protein genotype predisposes to sporadic Creutzfeldt-Jakob disease. Nature 352:340–342, 1991.

241. Collinge J, Palmer MS, Dryden AJ: Genetic predisposition to iatrogenic Creutzfeldt-Jakob disease. Lancet 337:1441–1442, 1991.

242. Miyazono M, Kitamoto T, Doh-ura K, et al: Creutzfeldt-Jakob disease with codon 129 polymorphism (Valine). A comparative study of patients with codon 102 point mutation or without mutations. Acta Neuropathol 84:349–354, 1992.

243. Tateishi J, Kitamoto T: Developments in diagnosis for prion diseases. Br Med Bull 49:971–979, 1993.

244. Prusiner SB, Scott M, Foster D, et al: Transgenetic studies implicate interactions between homologous PrP isoforms in scrapie prion replication. Cell 63:673–686, 1990.

245. Prusiner SB: Molecular biology of prion diseases. Science 252:1515–1522, 1991.

246. Scott M, Foster D, Mirenda C, et al: Transgenic mice expressing hamster prion protein produce species-specific scrapie infectivity and amyloid plaques. Cell 59:847–857, 1989.

247. Brown P, Cervenáková L, Goldfarb LG, et al: Iatrogenic Creutzfeldt-Jakob disease. An example of the interplay between ancient genes and modern medicine. Neurology 44: 291–293, 1994.

248. Buchanan CR, Preece MA, Milner RDG: Mortality, neoplasia and Creutzfeldt-Jakob disease in patients treated with pituitary growth hormone in the United Kingdom. BMJ 302:824–828, 1991.

249. Deslys J-P, Marcé D, Dormont D: Similar genetic susceptibility in iatrogenic and sporadic Creutzfeldt-Jakob disease. J Gen Virol 75:23–27, 1994.

250. Fradkin JE, Schonberger LB, Mills JL, et al: Creutzfeldt-Jakob disease in pituitary growth hormone recipients in the United States. JAMA 265:880–884, 1991.

251. Goldfarb LG, Brown P, Gajdusek DC: The molecular genetics of human transmissible spongiform encephalopathy. In Prusiner SB, Collinge J, Powell J, Anderton B (eds): Prion Diseases of Humans and Animals. New York, Ellis Horwood, 1992, pp 139–153.

252. Carlson GA, Kingsbury DT, Goodman PA, et al: Linkage of prion protein and scrapie incubation time genes. Cell 46:503–511, 1986.

253. Carlson GA, Ebeling C, Yang S-L, et al: Prion isolate specified allotypic interactions between the cellular and scrapie prion proteins in congenic and transgenic mice. Proc Natl Acad Sci U S A 91:5690–5694, 1994.

254. Telling GC, Haga T, Torchia M, et al: Interactions between wild-type and mutant prion proteins modulate neurodegeneration in transgenic mice. Genes Dev 10:1736–1750, 1996.

255. Kretzschmar HA, Ironside JW, DeArmond SJ, Tateishi J: Diagnostic criteria for sporadic Creutzfeldt-Jakob disease. Arch Neurol 53:913–920, 1996.

256. Brown P, Gibbs CJ Jr, Rodgers-Johnson P, et al: Human spongiform encephalopathy. The National Institutes of Health series of 300 cases of experimentally transmitted disease. Ann Neurol 35:513–529, 1994.

257. Bredesen DE, Ellerby LM, Hart PJ, et al: Do posttranslational modifications of CuZnSOD lead to sporadic amyotrophic lateral sclerosis? Ann Neurol 42:135–137, 1997.

258. Siddique T, Deng H-X: Genetics of amyotrophic lateral sclerosis. Hum Mol Genet 5:1465–1470, 1996.

259. Young AB: Huntington's disease and other trinucleotide repeat disorders. *In* Martin JB (ed): Molecular Neurology. New York, Scientific American, 1998, pp 35–54.

260. Gusella JF, Wexler NS, Conneally PM, et al: A polymorphic DNA marker genetically linked to Huntington's disease. Nature 306:234–238, 1983.

261. Group HDCR: A novel gene containing a trinucleiotide repeat that is expanded and unstable on Huntington's disease chromosomes. Cell 72:971–983, 1993.

262. Andrew SE, Goldberg YP, Kremer B, et al: The relationship between trinucleotide (CAG) repeat length and clinical features of Huntington's disease. Nat Genet 4:398–403, 1993.

263. Duyao M, Ambrose C, Myers R, et al: Trinucleotide repeat length instability and age of onset in Huntington's disease. Nat Genet 4:387–392, 1993.

264. Gusella JF, MacDonald ME: Huntington's disease. Semin Cell Biol 6:21–28, 1995.

265. Snell RG, MacMillan JC, Cheadle JP, et al: Relationship between trinucleotide repeat expansion and phenotypic variation in Huntington's disease. Nat Genet 4:393–397, 1995.

266. Trottier Y, Devys D, Imbert G, et al: Cellular localization of the Huntington's disease protein and discrimination of the normal and mutated form. Nat Genet 10:104–110, 1995.

267. Kennedy WRAM, Sung JH: Progressive proximal spinal and bulbar muscular atrophy of late onset. A sex-linked recessive trait. Neurology 18:671–680, 1968.

268. La Spada AR, Wilson EM, Lubahn DB, et al: Androgen receptor gene mutations in X-linked spinal and bulbar muscular atrophy. Nature 352:77–79, 1991.

269. Belsham DD, Yee WC, Greenberg CR, Wrogemann K: Analysis of the CAG repeat region of the androgen receptor gene in a kindred with X-linked spinal and bulbar muscular atrophy. J Neurol Sci 112:133–138, 1992.

270. La Spada AR, Roling DB, Harding AE, et al: Meiotic stability and genotype-phenotype correlation of the trinucleotide repeat in X-linked spinal and bulbar muscular atrophy. Nat Genet 2:301–304, 1992.

271. Conner KE, Rosenberg RN: The genetic basis of ataxia. *In* Rosenberg RN, Prusiner SB, DiMauro S, Barchi RL (eds): The Molecular and Genetic Basis of Neurological Disease. Boston, Butterworth-Heinemann, 1997, pp 503–544.

272. Orr HT, Chung M-Y, Banfi S, et al: Expansion of an unstable trinucleotide CAG repeat in spinocerebellar ataxia type 1. Nat Genet 4:221–226, 1993.

273. Banfi S, Servadio A, Chung M-Y, et al: Identification and characterization of the gene causing type 1 spinocerebellar ataxia. Nat Genet 7:513–520, 1994.

274. Chung MY, Ranum LP, Duvick LA, et al: Evidence for a mechanism predisposing to intergenerational CAG repeat instability in spinocerebellar ataxia type I. Nat Genet 5:254–258, 1993.

275. David G, Abbas N, Stevanin G, et al: Cloning the SCA7 gene reveals a highly unstable CAG repeat expansion. Nat Genet 17:65–70, 1997.

276. Del-Favero J, Krols L, Michalik A, et al: Molecular genetic analysis of autosomal dominant cerebellar ataxia with retinal degeneration (ADCA type II) caused by CAG triplet repeat expansion. Hum Mol Genet 7:177–186, 1998.

277. Koob MD., Benzow KA, Bird TD, et al: Rapid cloning of expanded trinucleotide repeat sequences from genomic DNA. Nat Genet 18:72–75, 1998.

278. Benton CS, de Silva R, Rutledge SL, et al: Molecular and clinical studies in SCA-7 define a broad clinical spectrum and the infantile phenotype. Neurology 51:1081–1086, 1998.

279. Campuzano V, Montermini L, Moltò MD, et al: Friedreich's ataxia. Autosomal recessive disease caused by an intronic GAA triplet repeat expansion. Science 271:1423–1427, 1996.

280. Koide R, Ikeuchi T, Onodera O, et al: Unstable expansion of CAG repeat in hereditary dentatorubral-pallidoluysian atrophy (DRPLA). Nat Genet 6:9–13, 1994.

281. Nagafuchi S, Yanagisawa H, Sato K, et al: Dentatorubral and pallidoluysian atrophy expansion of an unstable CAG trinucleotide on chromosome 12p. Nat Genet 6:14–18, 1994.

282. Nagafuchi S, Yanagisawa H, Ohsaki E, et al: Structure and expression of the gene responsible for the triplet repeat disorder, dentatorubral and pallidoluysian atrophy (DRPLA). Nat Genet 8:177–182, 1994.

283. Perutz MF, Johnson T, Suzuki M, Finch JT: Glutamine repeats as polar zippers. Their possible role in inherited neurodegenerative diseases. Proc Natl Acad Sci U S A 91:5355–5358, 1994.

284. Mhatre AN, Trifiro MA, Kaufman M, et al: Reduced transcriptional regulatory competence of the androgen receptor in X-linked spinal and bulbar muscular atrophy [published erratum appears in Nat Genet 1994;6(2):214]. Nat Genet 5:184–188, 1993.

285. Scherzinger E, Lurz R, Turmaine M, et al: Huntingtin-encoded polyglutamine expansions form amyloid-like protein aggregates in vitro and in vivo. Cell 90:549–558, 1997.

286. Davies SW, Turmaine M, Cozens BA, et al: Formation of neuronal intranuclear inclusions underlies the neurological dysfunction in mice transgenic for the HD mutation. Cell 90:537–548, 1997.

287. DiFiglia M, Sapp E, Chase KO, et al: Aggregation of huntingtin in neuronal intranuclear inclusions and dystrophic neurites in brain. Science 277:1990–1993, 1997.

288. Skinner PJ, Koshy BT, Cummings CJ, et al: Ataxin-1 with an expanded glutamine tract alters nuclear matrix-associated structures. Nature 389:971–974, 1997.

289. Klement IA, Zoghbi HY, Orr HT: Pathogenesis of polyglutamine-induced disease. A model for SCA1. Mol Genet Metab 66:172–178, 1999.

290. Paulson HL, Perez MK, Trottier Y, et al: Intranuclear inclusions of expanded polyglutamine protein in spinocerebellar ataxia type 3. Neuron 19:333–244, 1997.

291. Becker MW, Rubinsztein DC, Leggo J, et al: Dentatorubral and pallidoluysian atrophy (DRPLA). Clinical and neuropathological findings in genetically confirmed North American and European pedigrees. Mov Disord 12:519–530, 1997.

292. Li M, Mina S, Kodayoshi Y, et al: Nuclear inclusion of the androgen receptor protein in spinal and bulbar muscular atrophy. Ann Neurol 44:249–254, 1998.

293. Sandou F, Finkbeiner S, Devys D, Greenberg ME: Huntingtin acts in the nucleus to induce apoptosis but death does not correlate with the formation of intranuclear inclusions. Cell 95:55–66, 1998.

294. Klement IA, Skinner PJ, Kaytor MD, et al: Ataxin-1 nuclear localization and aggregation. Role in polyglutamine-induced disease in SCA1 transgenic mice. Cell 95:41–53, 1998.

295. Lowe J, Lennox G, Leigh PN: Disorders of movement and system degenerations. *In* Graham DI, Lantos PL (eds): Greenfield's Neuropathology, 6th ed. Arnold, London, UK 1997, pp 281–366.

296. Harding A: The clinical features and classification of the late onset autosomal dominant cerebellar ataxias. A study of eleven families including descendants of the 'Drew family of Walworth.' Brain 105:1–28, 1982.

297. Harding A: Cerebellar and spinocerebellar disorders. *In* Bradley W, Daroff R, Fenichel F, Marsden C (eds): Neurology in Clinical Practice. Boston, Butterworth-Heinemann, 1996, pp 1773–1792.

298. Group THDCR: A novel gene containing a trinucleotide repeat that is expanded and unstable on Huntington's disease chromosomes. Cell 72:971–983, 1993.

299. Gispert S, Twells R, Orozco G, et al: Chromosomal assignment of the second locus for autosomal dominant cerebellar ataxia (SCA2) to chromosome 12q23–24.1. Nat Genet 4:295–299, 1993.

300. Stevanin G, Le Guern E, Ravisé N, et al: A third locus for autosomal dominant cerebellar ataxia type I maps to chromosome 14q24.3-qter. Evidence for the existence of a fourth locus. Am J Hum Genet 54:11–20, 1994.
301. Kawaguchi Y, Okamoto T, Taniwaki M, et al: CAG expansions in a novel gene for Machado-Joseph disease at chromosome 14q32.1. Nat Genet 8:221–228, 1994.
302. Ranum LP, Schut LJ, Lundgren JK, et al: Spinocerebellar ataxia type 5 in a family descended from the grandparents of President Lincoln maps to chromosome 11. Nat Genet 8: 280–284, 1994.
303. Zhuchenko O, Bailey J, Bonnen P, et al: Autosomal dominant cerebellar ataxia (SCA6) associated with small polyglutamine expansions in the alpha 1A-voltage-dependent calcium channel. Nat Genet 15:62–69, 1997.
304. Flanigan K, Gardner K, Alderson K, et al: Autosomal dominant spinocerebellar ataxia with sensory axonal neuropathy (SCA4): clinical description and genetic localization to chromosome 16q22.1. Am J Hum Genet 59:392–399, 1996.

# Muscle and Nerve Biopsy

James B. Atkinson    Mahlon D. Johnson
Thomas J. Montine    William O. Whetsell, Jr.

During earlier times, technology allowed examination of biopsy specimens of striated muscle and peripheral nerve by light microscopic methods only, but advanced techniques now permit study by specialized histochemical, immunohistochemical, ultrastructural, biochemical, and molecular biologic methods. These can provide precise information about the character and etiology of central nervous system dysfunction, peripheral nervous system dysfunction, dysfunction at the neuromuscular junction, and primary muscle dysfunction. The maximal value of these procedures depends on the cooperative efforts of the surgeon and the surgical pathologist to provide expert collection and preparation of specimens, because it is at these stages that most artifacts can be introduced or avoided in these delicate and capricious tissues. In this chapter, we provide detailed guidance in the technical aspects of collection and preparation of tissue and then discuss the interpretation of results of muscle biopsies and nerve biopsies in diagnosis of neuromuscular and peripheral nerve disorders.

## TECHNICAL CONSIDERATIONS AND APPROACHES

### Muscle Biopsies

Selection of the muscle to be examined is based on clinical evidence of specific muscle dysfunction. Because muscle diseases are often manifested to different extents in various muscles and muscle groups, both physical examination and electromyographic

evaluation influence the selection of the muscle to be removed at biopsy for diagnostic studies. The muscle to be sampled by the biopsy should not be the most involved muscle or a muscle that may have been traumatized by intramuscular injections or previous muscle biopsy. For open biopsy, the specimen is removed surgically through a skin incision of sufficient size (usually 3 to 4 cm long) to allow dissection of a portion of muscle approximately 1.0 by 0.5 by 0.5 cm in overall dimensions. On gentle removal of the biopsy specimen, the tissue should be kept cool and moist but should not be placed in isotonic solution or allowed to absorb fluid unnecessarily. It is recommended that the fresh muscle tissue specimen be laid directly onto a saline-moistened (not soaked) gauze pad that can be folded over the specimen to keep all sides of the tissue moist. In our experience, it is preferable that this specimen not be stretched, clamped, or tied; rather, it is simply laid on the moist pad in a way that maintains its longitudinal orientation. If a needle biopsy is preferable because of the patient's intolerance of an open biopsy, the specimen is handled in the same manner after it has been collected from the biopsy instrument needle. Once the specimen is collected and placed on the moist pad, it should be transported to the laboratory as quickly and safely as possible. If it is to be transported some distance or if there is some time delay in getting the specimen to the laboratory where it will be processed, the folded pad containing the fresh specimen should be placed in a plastic Petri dish in the operating room, and with lid secure, the dish should be cooled in a refrigerated container or on a water tight cooling pack for transport to the laboratory; the tissue should be carefully protected against any contact with the cooling liquid (e.g., water from melting ice) during transport.

In the laboratory, the orientation of the muscle specimen can be confirmed by direct observation or with a dissecting microscope; it is then divided appropriately for fixation or freezing. The oriented specimen is incised across its longitudinal axis to divide it first into two halves. One of the halves is further divided across its long axis into two more or less equal portions. The largest portion (the intact half) is set aside momentarily on the moist pad (for later freezing). One of the two smaller portions is gently cut into pieces approximating 0.5 cm³; these pieces are placed into a vial containing 2% glutaraldehyde and held for preparation for electron microscopy, if indicated. The other of the two smaller portions is placed into a vial containing 10% buffered formalin to be embedded in paraffin for routine histochemical studies. When these two smaller portions have been placed into the proper fixatives, the larger portion (the remaining half of the specimen) is snap-frozen—but only after certain precautions have been taken to minimize freezing artifacts. Specifically, an effective method found to avoid such artifacts is to cover this fresh tissue specimen completely with surgical talcum for 30 to 60 seconds immediately before freezing; this is done by sprinkling a heavy coating of dry talcum over all surfaces of the specimen. The tissue is then placed in a plastic freezing boat (Fisher Scientific, Pittsburgh, PA) in a thick slurry of talcum and mounting medium (OTC compound for frozen tissue specimens or a similar medium) and snap-frozen in liquid nitrogen. The tissue should be positioned in the boat so that the cross-sectional surface of the muscle will appear on the cutting face of the block formed by freezing. When this procedure is followed just before freezing, the talcum seems to absorb excess moisture that may have accumulated in the muscle tissue and thereby reduces or eliminates freeze artifacts in the tissue. With a previously frozen specimen in which freezing artifacts have already been introduced, the specimen is allowed to thaw completely, and if the procedure for coating in talcum and freezing (refreezing) is carried out, the initially observed artifacts can usually be eliminated. In this way, a poorly frozen specimen can be "rescued" and used effectively for histochemical or immunohistochemical studies requiring frozen sections. Because cross-sectional orientation is important for both frozen sections and paraffin sections, special attention must be given to proper orientation of the specimens at the outset.

Routine histochemical staining with H&E or other stains useful in formalin-fixed tissue is carried out with paraffin sections of standard thickness (5 to 6 μm). For special histochemical staining and immunohistochemical procedures, frozen sections of 8 μm are usually suitable. Histochemical stains recommended as a screening battery for frozen sections include H&E, modified Gomori trichrome, ATPase stain (pH 9.4), and NADH tetrazolium reductase (NADH-TR) stain. For immunohistochemical staining, frozen sections should be used according to protocols for such stains as dystrophins, sarcoglycans, and merosin (see later). Specimens for biochemical or molecular biologic analysis requiring frozen tissue can be prepared by the freezing techniques described before. In most instances, the same frozen specimen block from which frozen sections are cut for histochemical and immunohistochemical staining can also be submitted for biochemical and molecular biologic studies.

## Nerve Biopsies

The sural nerve is chosen for biopsy in most instances, but depending on the clinical indication and justification for selection, other nerves are occasionally submitted. In any case, it is of utmost importance that the nerve segment be removed without stretching, twisting, or other manipulation of the segment to be examined. This is achieved by stabilizing the nerve in situ before it is cut away and removed. Stabilization is best accomplished by use of a small clamping device. Once the nerve is isolated, a length of approximately 2 cm is secured with a muscle clamp. The nerve is then transected on either side of the clamp with care to leave a 1- to 2-mm stump extending from either side. The clamp containing the specimen is lifted away. If immunofluorescence studies are to be carried out, one or two thin cross-sections of the stump at either end of the clamp can be gently cut and placed immediately into Michel fixative. The clamp holding the remaining specimen is then placed into a vial of 2% glutaraldehyde for fixation for all additional studies. If no immunofluorescence studies are indicated, the entire specimen held in the clamp can be placed into the glutaraldehyde fixative as soon as it is removed. Both of these fixation procedures can be performed in the operating room, and they do not require the same kind of immediate transportation to the laboratory that the muscle biopsy specimen demands. Also, the clamping device described here is designated a muscle biopsy clamp. In our experience, such a clamp is ideal for nerve biopsies, but using such a clamp for muscle biopsies is not necessary if the procedures described for muscle biopsies are followed.

When the nerve biopsy specimen is placed into the glutaraldehyde solution, it should be allowed to fix for at least 12 hours. Cross-sections of the specimen excised from either end of the specimen after initial glutaraldehyde fixation can be carried through appropriate post-fixation and epoxy-embedding procedures and prepared for light and electron microscopic study.

For light microscopy, all nerve specimens are examined in 0.5-μm cross-sections stained with aqueous toluidine blue (0.5%), H&E, and Congo red stains. The central length of the specimen is prepared for the teasing procedure. Techniques for nerve teasing, although first described as early as the late 19th century,[1] have been considerably refined and are described in detail elsewhere.[2]

## DIAGNOSTIC CONSIDERATIONS AND APPROACHES FOR MUSCLE DISEASE

Various classifications of primary muscle diseases have been based on different defining features including clinical manifestations, mode of inheritance, etiology, and pathologic changes. A completely satisfactory classification of myopathies has yet to be devised, largely because of overlapping features. The muscle diseases described in this section are presented in a framework that should allow the pathologist to incorporate pathologic features into appropriate categories from which clinical criteria or results of ancillary testing (i.e., biochemical, genetic, and molecular studies) will provide a definitive diagnosis. Diseases affecting ion channels (i.e., periodic paralyses) and secondary muscle diseases (toxic, drug induced, endocrine, and trauma) are not discussed.

### Muscular Dystrophies

Muscular dystrophies are genetic diseases that cause progressive weakness and wasting of skeletal muscles because of a primary defect in the muscle cell. The diagnosis cannot be made solely on morphologic grounds but also depends on clinical features (including onset and distribution of weakness) as well as the mode of inheritance. In virtually no other area of medicine has molecular biology had as great an impact on diagnosis as in elucidating the nosology of the muscular dystrophies. Specifically, research during the last decade has shown that abnormalities in dystrophin and dystrophin-associated proteins located at the plasma membrane (sarcolemma) of individual muscle cells underlie various muscular dystrophies (dystrophinopathies). These findings have resulted in new approaches for the evaluation of patients who have proximal muscle weakness, elevated serum creatine kinase levels, and histopathologic evidence of a muscular dystrophy.

#### DUCHENNE'S AND BECKER'S MUSCULAR DYSTROPHIES

Duchenne's muscular dystrophy (DMD) affects 1 in 3300 live male births and is the second most common lethal genetic disorder in humans.[3] The disease is X linked and usually presents clinically in the first 5 years of life, progressing to wheelchair dependence during the second decade and death in the late teens or early 20s. Whereas DMD occurs almost exclusively in males, females may occasionally be affected as manifesting carriers. Proximal muscles are involved initially, resulting in a characteristic waddling gait and Gowers sign (in which patients use their hands and arms to raise the upper body on rising from a lying position).[4] Distal muscles become progressively involved, and muscles (particularly the calves) may exhibit pseudohypertrophy because of increased fat and connective tissue (see later). Serum creatine kinase levels are elevated until muscle mass becomes decreased.

Becker's muscular dystrophy (BMD), also an X-linked myopathy, has a less severe clinical course than that of DMD with a later and more unpredictable age at onset and a slower progression. Patients with BMD may not become wheelchair bound until their 20s or later, and life span may even be normal. The clinical features of BMD, although less severe, are essentially similar to those of DMD.

The cardinal histopathologic features of DMD and BMD are necrosis and degeneration of muscle fibers with gradual replacement of muscle by fat and fibrous connective tissue. Early in the disease, fiber diameters vary as a result of chronic myopathic degeneration, and fibers become smaller as disease progresses (CD Fig. 53–1A). Numerous hypercontracted, densely eosinophilic opaque hyaline fibers are seen in cross-sections, and although this finding is nonspecific, it can still be of diagnostic importance (Fig. 53–1A) (CD Fig. 53–1B). Internal nuclei are increased in number but usually not excessively. Hyaline fibers can become frankly necrotic with associated inflammation. As fibers undergo degeneration, attempts at regeneration result in proliferation and fusion of satellite cells, leading to formation of split fibers that represent two or more satellite cells developing within the same basement membrane. In DMD, muscle fiber necrosis reaches a peak at about 5 years of age, after which chronic myopathic degeneration becomes the prominent histopathologic feature with atrophic and occasional hypertrophic fibers. Progression of DMD is accompanied by a progressive increase in perimysial and endomysial fibrous connective tissue. Late stages are characterized by marked variation in fiber size, scattered necrotic fibers, increased fibrosis, and fatty infiltration such that ultimately these muscles consist almost entirely of fat and fibrous connective tissue (CD Fig. 53–1C). The diagnostic features are usually evident in H&E-stained sections but need confirmation by immunohistochemistry (see later). Gomori trichrome stain highlights the presence of fiber necrosis and increased connective tissue. ATPase staining shows that all fiber types are affected equally (although there may be some changes suggestive of denervation in BMD), and NADH-TR staining shows alteration in internal architecture. The histopathologic features of BMD are similar to those of DMD, although they are less severe at a given age and may be less predictable (CD Fig. 53–1D). In advanced cases, split fibers and internal nuclei may be more prominent in BMD than in DMD.

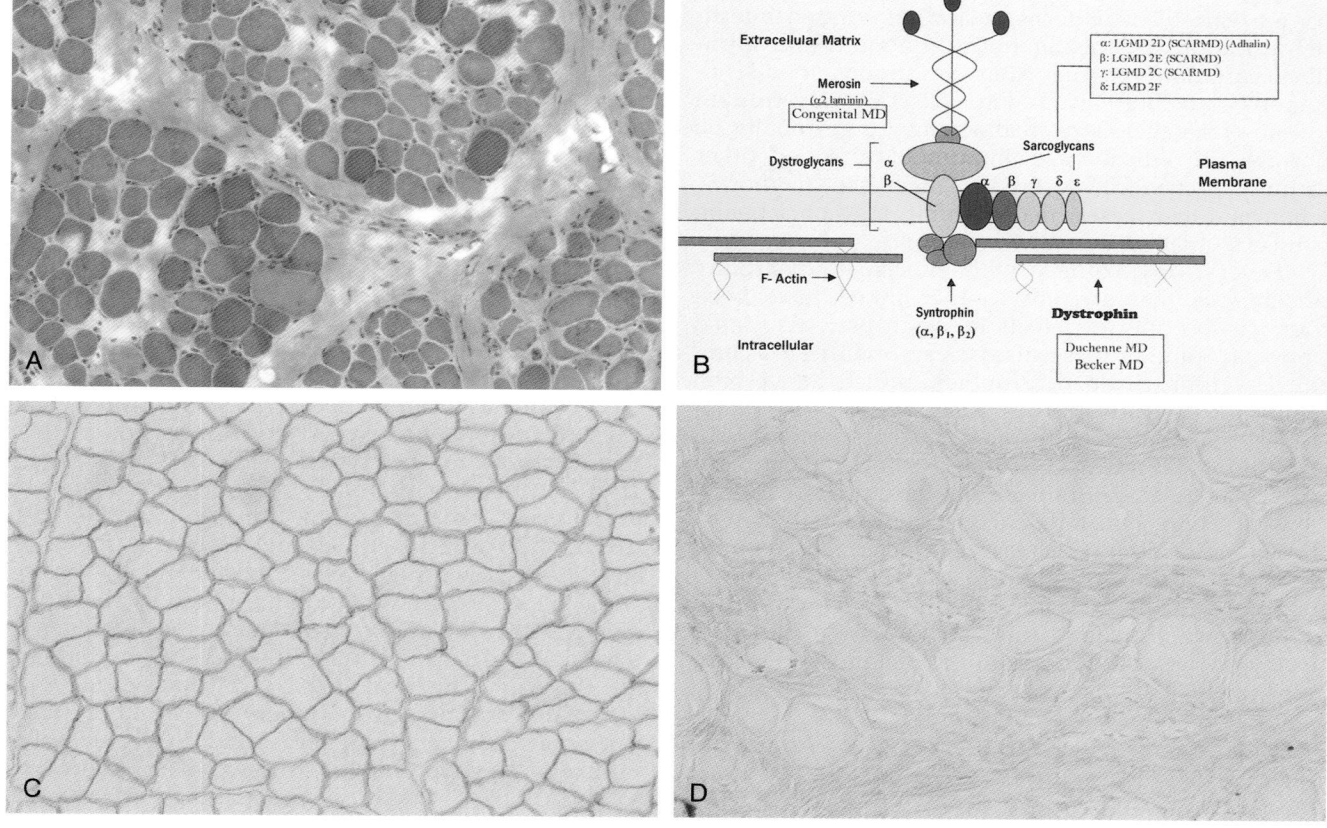

**FIGURE 53–1.** *A.* DMD. There is variation in fiber size and a striking increase in perimysial and endomysial fibrous connective tissue with focal fat deposition. Scattered hyalinized fibers are present. (Cryostat section, H&E.) *B.* Schematic diagram illustrates muscle plasma membrane (sarcolemma) and dystrophin and the dystrophin-associated proteins (merosin, dystroglycans, sarcoglycans, and syntrophin; merosin = $\alpha_2$-laminin; adhalin = $\alpha$-sarcoglycan). Muscle diseases with known defects are indicated in the boxes. LGMD, Limb-girdle muscular dystrophy; MD, muscular dystrophy; SCARMD, severe childhood autosomal recessive muscular dystrophy. *C.* Normal muscle. Immunostain for dystrophin demonstrates uniform labeling around the periphery of all fibers. *D.* DMD. Immunostain for dystrophin shows dystrophin-negative fibers.

## Dystrophin and Associated Proteins

DMD and BMD are caused by mutations in the gene for dystrophin. The locus that maps for dystrophin is at site Xp21.2 on the short arm of the X chromosome, and DMD and BMD represent the majority of cases of Xp21.2 myopathies. Dystrophin is a large protein (427 kd) encoded by a large, complex gene (2.4 million bases), which accounts for the high mutation rate.[5–7] Dystrophin is localized to the cytoplasmic surface of the sarcolemma in skeletal, cardiac, and smooth muscle and attaches intracellular actin to the extracellular basal lamina (Fig. 53–1B) (CD Fig. 53–1E). Dystrophin most likely provides structural support to the muscle sarcolemma, facilitates signal transduction between the sarcolemma and contractile apparatus, and regulates intracellular calcium.[5] Dystrophin-associated proteins also participate in those functions, and defects in the genes encoding many of these proteins result in other forms of muscular dystrophy[8] (see Fig. 53–1B and CD Fig. 53–1E). In DMD, dystrophin is completely

absent. In BMD, in-frame mutations result in expression of dystrophin with a reduced molecular weight (80% of cases), a reduced quantity (15% of cases), or an abnormally large molecule (5% of cases).[9]

Confirmation of the diagnosis of DMD and BMD now rests on analysis of dystrophin either at the messenger RNA level by analysis of DNA or at the protein level (immunohistochemistry, Western blot). Immunohistochemistry reveals continuous labeling around the periphery (sarcolemma) of normal muscle fibers (Fig. 53–1C) (CD Fig. 53–1F). In DMD, there is complete or nearly complete absence of immunolabeling, with isolated fibers (less than 1%) occasionally staining[10–12] (Fig. 53–1D) (CD Fig. 53–1G). Dystrophin immunostains should be interpreted only in non-necrotic fibers because necrosis is associated with loss of surface staining regardless of the etiology. In cases in which immunohistochemistry is equivocal, additional testing for DNA defects can be performed by multiplex polymerase chain reaction analysis with use of blood samples.

Dystrophin immunohistochemistry in BMD can have a variety of patterns, including marked interfiber variation in labeling (most common) and intrafiber variation ranging from continuous to discontinuous labeling[12] (CD Fig. 53–1H). Dystrophin immunohistochemistry in BMD may occasionally be normal (in which case immunoblotting or other techniques may be required to make the diagnosis), whereas other cases may exhibit loss of labeling similar to that seen in DMD.

Several myopathies with muscular dystrophy phenotypes that are not Xp21.2 linked have been found to be due to defects in dystrophin-associated proteins. Some of these diseases are manifested clinically as limb-girdle dystrophies, which affect both males and females and are inherited as either autosomal dominant or autosomal recessive traits.[8, 13] In addition to defects in dystrophin-associated proteins, molecular defects in other forms of muscular dystrophy are being elucidated (e.g., Emery-Dreifuss dystrophy, an X-linked disease characterized by mild proximal weakness and cardiac arrhythmias due to mutations in the gene for emerin, a nuclear protein of unknown function,[14] and a limb-girdle muscular dystrophy associated with mutations in the gene for calpain, a calcium-activated protease[15]).

## FASCIOSCAPULOHUMERAL MUSCULAR DYSTROPHY

Fascioscapulohumeral muscular dystrophy is an autosomal dominant disorder with onset from childhood to early adulthood. Weakness occurs in the facial and shoulder girdle muscles. The differential diagnosis may be difficult clinically because polymyositis, mitochondrial myopathies, and myasthenia gravis may have a similar distribution of weakness. The muscle biopsy specimen has moderate changes of myopathy with variation in fiber sizes and increased internal nuclei. Necrotic or hyalinized fibers are rare, but fibrosis can be pronounced. In addition to these changes, which are present in other muscular dystrophies, atrophic angulated fibers can be seen. Mononuclear inflammatory cell infiltrates may be prominent (CD Fig. 53–2A), and this feature can pose difficulties in making a distinction from inflammatory myopathies. The relative lack of overtly necrotic and regenerating fibers and the extent of fibrosis may be clues that help distinguish fascioscapulohumeral muscular dystrophy from inflammatory myopathies.

## MYOTONIC MUSCULAR DYSTROPHY

Myotonic muscular dystrophy, the most common inherited muscular dystrophy in adults, affects 1 of 7500 people.[16] It is autosomal dominant and characterized by facial and distal limb weakness and muscle atrophy and clinical and electromyographic evidence of myotonia (delayed muscle relaxation after contraction). Myotonic dystrophy is also a multisystem disease; other abnormalities include cataracts, cardiac conduction disturbances, testicular atrophy,

premature frontal alopecia, glucose intolerance, and in cases with early onset, mental retardation.[16] Although congenital (neonatal, infantile) myotonic dystrophy can be distinguished clinically from the adult form, the clinical expression can be variable, ranging from neonatal death to absence of symptoms. One of the interesting clinical features of myotonic dystrophy is the phenomenon of anticipation, in which a progressive decrease in the age at onset occurs through subsequent generations accompanied by a progressive increase in severity. The genetic defect in myotonic dystrophy is an expanded, noncoding CTG codon repeat at the 3' end of a gene thought to encode a ubiquitous protein kinase, myotonin protein kinase.[17, 18]

The muscle biopsy specimen in myotonic muscular dystrophy is characterized by variation in fiber sizes, with atrophy of type I fibers and hypertrophy of type II fibers. Muscle fiber necrosis and degeneration are less prominent than in other muscular dystrophies. A particularly striking feature is the presence of internal nuclei seen to form long chains when fibers are viewed in longitudinal sections (CD Fig. 53–2B). In later stages, ring fibers and sarcoplasmic masses can be seen. Ring fibers (ringbinden) are those in which myofibrils are wrapped circumferentially around the periphery of the fiber. They are nonspecific but may be found in considerable numbers in myotonic dystrophy. Ring fibers are frequently associated with sarcoplasmic masses, regions of disorganized and reduced myofibrils, usually subsarcolemmal in location. Although sarcoplasmic masses can be seen in other neuromuscular diseases, they are especially prominent and extensive in myotonic dystrophy. The muscle in later stages of myotonic dystrophy may also have interstitial fibrosis and extensive fiber hypertrophy.

## Inflammatory Myopathies

Inflammatory myopathies are a diverse group of muscle diseases that may constitute one of the most common indications for evaluation of myopathy by the surgical pathologist. They are responsive to therapy and therefore require precise diagnosis. Muscle fiber necrosis and regeneration with associated inflammatory cell infiltration characterize the inflammatory myopathies. Although inflammatory myopathies include infectious myopathies (bacterial, fungal, viral, and parasitic) and drug-induced myopathies, the idiopathic inflammatory myopathies (polymyositis, dermatomyositis, and inclusion body myositis [IBM]) are the focus of this section.

## POLYMYOSITIS

All three forms of idiopathic inflammatory myopathy are characterized by proximal (usually symmetric) weakness that develops during weeks to months, sometimes insidiously.[19, 20] Polymyositis occurs after the second decade, and remissions and exacerbations may characterize the clinical course.

Patients can have muscle pain and tenderness; other symptoms may include fever, malaise or fatigue, joint pain, and Raynaud phenomenon. Early in the disease, the erythrocyte sedimentation rate and serum creatine kinase values are elevated, and the electromyograph can be characteristic. Polymyositis is thought to be an autoimmune disease with a cell-mediated immune response directed toward muscle fibers, resulting in necrosis. In contrast to dermatomyositis, the incidence of malignant neoplasia is probably not increased in polymyositis.[19] Polymyositis can occur separately or in association with autoimmune or connective tissue disorders.

The cardinal pathologic features of polymyositis are muscle fiber necrosis and inflammation. These lesions are patchy, and therefore multiple tissue samples may be required if needle biopsies are used, or multiple tissue sections if an open biopsy is performed. The inflammatory infiltrates are predominantly mononuclear, composed of lymphocytes (T cells, 70%) and macrophages (30%). Inflammation can be located around individual necrotic muscle fibers or within the endomysial and perimysial connective tissue and sometimes (but not always) around blood vessels (Fig. 53–2A) (CD Fig. 53–3A). The distribution of fiber necrosis is diffuse and may vary from being virtually absent to so severe that the muscle, in rare cases, appears to have undergone infarction. A particularly prominent feature of polymyositis is regeneration of muscle fibers; regenerating fibers increase in number as the disease progresses and may even be present in the absence of necrotic fibers (Fig. 53–2B) (CD Fig. 53–3B). Regenerating muscle fibers are recognized by their basophilic sarcoplasm in H&E-stained sections and large, vesicular nuclei with prominent nucleoli.

## DERMATOMYOSITIS

Dermatomyositis is a distinct clinical entity characterized by a rash that often precedes muscle weakness. It occurs in both children and adults and is more common in females. The muscle weakness is similar to that of polymyositis in its presentation and course.[19, 20] Cutaneous lesions are variable and are manifest as dusky, erythematous eruptions in a butterfly distribution on the face, a heliotrope discoloration of the eyelids with periorbital edema, or erythema of the knuckles.[19] Although dermatomyositis usually occurs alone, it can be associated with mixed connective tissue diseases or other autoimmune disorders or malignant neoplasms in adults.[19, 20]

Dermatomyositis, like polymyositis, may be focal so that many muscle fascicles appear normal. The inflammatory infiltrates are predominantly perivascular or within interfascicular septa (perimysium), as opposed to polymyositis, in which they are predominantly found in the endomysium (the

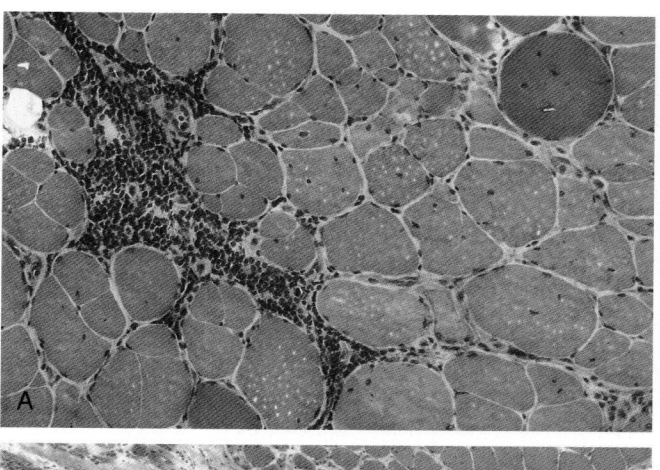

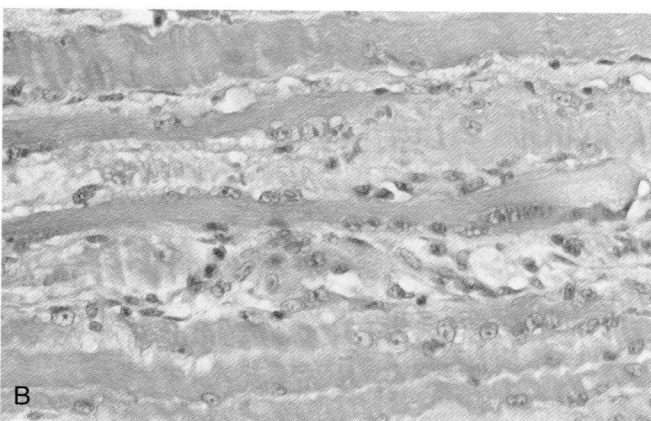

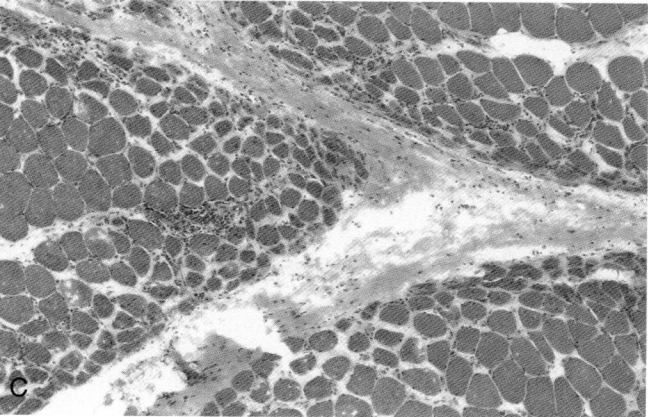

**FIGURE 53–2.** *A.* Polymyositis. Muscle biopsy specimen has myopathic features with fiber size variation, degenerating and split fibers, and internal nuclei. A focal mononuclear inflammatory cell infiltrate is present. (Cryostat section, H&E.) *B.* Polymyositis. Longitudinal section shows degenerating and regenerating fibers. Regenerating fibers are recognized by their basophilic sarcoplasm and large, vesicular nuclei with prominent nucleoli. (Paraffin section, H&E.) *C.* Dermatomyositis. This muscle exhibits striking perifascicular atrophy and focal lymphocytic infiltrates. (Cryostat section, H&E.)

connective tissue that surrounds individual muscle fibers). The most characteristic histopathologic feature of dermatomyositis is perifascicular atrophy, in which fibers around the periphery of the fascicle are atrophic (Fig. 53–2C) (CD Fig. 53–3C). Perifascicular atrophy occurs in about 90% of children and at least 50% of adults with dermatomyositis and is diagnostic even in the absence of inflammation. In occasional cases, the pattern of muscle injury is that of microinfarcts. Perifascicular atrophy and microinfarcts are evidence that the disease originates at the level of blood vessels. Restriction of atrophy to the edges of fascicles may be due to the vulnerability of that area to ischemia because of greater damage to blood vessels around the periphery of fascicles. Individual fiber necrosis is less common in dermatomyositis than in polymyositis; muscle fiber regeneration can be just as prominent. Surgical pathologists may also receive skin biopsy specimens from patients with suspected dermatomyositis; these are generally nonspecific, with mild superficial dermal chronic inflammation, unless there is an associated autoimmune or connective tissue disease.

## INCLUSION BODY MYOSITIS

IBM is a distinct clinical entity, and although its true incidence is not known, it may approach or equal that of polymyositis.[21] IBM is suspected when patients with presumed polymyositis do not respond to therapy. Early weakness of distal muscles (particularly foot extensors and finger flexors) may be a clue, however. Muscle involvement is painless and generalized in most patients, although it can be asymmetric and selective.[19–22] The serum creatine kinase level may be normal or only slightly elevated. IBM may be associated with a systemic autoimmune or connective tissue disorder in up to 15% of cases.[23] There are sporadic and familial forms. There is no effective therapy for IBM, and corticosteroids and intravenous administration of immunoglobulin produce only minor benefits.

IBM is characterized pathologically by muscle fiber necrosis and endomysial inflammation as well as by general myopathic features including internal nuclei, regenerating fibers, and mild fibrosis. In addition, there are several more distinctive histopathologic features. On cryostat sections, rimmed vacuoles are found usually around the periphery of the fiber (CD Fig. 53–3D). These are rounded or jagged spaces that exhibit basophilic material around their edges; in paraffin sections, they appear as empty vacuoles. By electron microscopy, rimmed vacuoles contain membranous whorls (lamella-like bodies). The frequency of muscle fibers containing rimmed vacuoles may be as great as 70%, or there may be so few that the diagnosis is difficult to make. They are not specific for IBM because they can also be found in chloroquine myopathy, acid maltase deficiency, and degenerating or necrotic muscle fibers. A characteristic ultrastructural feature from which the name of the disease is derived is the presence of 15- to 18-nm tubulofilaments by electron microscopy. These filaments are arranged in bundles and are present in small numbers in the sarcoplasm or nucleus (CD Fig. 53–3E). IBM filaments are found only in fibers that contain rimmed vacuoles but may be so rare as to be easily missed. The nature of these filaments has not been entirely elucidated, although some reports have indicated that they are congophilic and may represent amyloid. Some authors have suggested that Congo red stain helps in making the diagnosis of IBM.[24] The histopathologic diagnosis may be difficult because vacuolated fibers and tubulofilaments increase as disease progresses, and biopsy specimens obtained early in the course of the disease may not have sufficient diagnostic histologic features. In addition, the disease, like polymyositis, may be multifocal and therefore missed in any given biopsy specimen. The presence of more than one rimmed vacuole and more than one group of atrophic fibers per low-power field, with endomysial inflammation, is predictive of finding filamentous inclusions in more than 90% of cases.[25] The diagnosis may be missed if only paraffin-embedded sections are examined.

## GRANULOMATOUS AND OTHER INFLAMMATORY MYOPATHIES

In addition to muscle's involvement in the granulomatous inflammation that is associated with infectious diseases, muscle may be involved in sarcoidosis and in an idiopathic granulomatous myopathy. Sarcoid myopathy presents as a slowly progressive proximal myopathy of the extremities.[26] Muscle biopsy may have a low yield but can exhibit noncaseating granulomas near large blood vessels or in the perimysium[19] (CD Fig. 53–3F). An idiopathic granulomatous myopathy that has histologic features similar to those of sarcoidosis may occur in middle-aged and elderly patients, usually women.[27] This disease is slowly progressive and has a predilection for the lower extremities. The diagnosis is one of exclusion.[20]

Muscle biopsy may be performed to evaluate patients with presumed systemic connective tissue diseases, in which case they may be normal or have minimal nonspecific findings. The diagnostic yield is enhanced if the patient has muscle weakness or elevated serum creatine kinase levels.[20] Vasculitis may be found in muscle in systemic lupus erythematosus and polyarteritis nodosa. The muscle in rheumatoid arthritis shows nonspecific changes (usually type II fiber atrophy). Although polymyalgia rheumatica is associated with temporal arteritis and results in muscle stiffness and pain, it is not an inflammatory myopathy, and muscle biopsy findings usually do not show inflammation or atrophy with the exception of nonspecific type II fiber atrophy.[20, 28] A variety of drugs can produce an inflammatory myopathy and even mimic polymyositis. The best example is D-penicillamine, which is associated with interstitial and sometimes perivascular inflammation with eosinophils.[20] The eosinophilia-myalgia syndrome, described in patients receiving L-tryptophan, represents an adverse reaction to a contaminant and can produce an inflammatory infiltrate in muscle composed of lymphocytes and eosinophils.[29, 30]

## Congenital Myopathies

Congenital myopathies are nonprogressive or slowly progressive myopathies that present in the neonatal period with weakness and hypotonia. They are classified according to their pathologic features on cryostat sections. They make up a heterogeneous group of disorders that account, in part, for the floppy infant syndrome. In general, infants have decreased muscle tone, weakness, decreased spontaneous movement, and delayed motor milestones.[31] Severity and distribution vary, depending on the particular disease. Infants with congenital myopathies are distinguished from those with arthrogryposis multiplex congenita, in which joint contrac-

tures develop in utero and may be a component of congenital muscular dystrophy and denervating disorders.

### CONGENITAL FIBER-TYPE DISPROPORTION

Congenital fiber-type disproportion is defined histopathologically by type I fibers that are uniformly more than 15% smaller than type II fibers[31] (Fig. 53–3A) (CD Fig. 53–4A). In addition to being small, type I fibers are more variable in size than type II fibers (which are normal in size or slightly hypertrophic).

### CENTRONUCLEAR (MYOTUBULAR) MYOPATHY

In this group of disorders, the majority (80% or more) of muscle fibers contain internal nuclei in long rows (Fig. 53–3B) (CD Fig. 53–4B). There is often a clear "halo" around the internal nucleus, and in initial reports, these fibers were described as resembling myotubes, suggesting arrest of fetal development. The presence of central nuclei is wide-

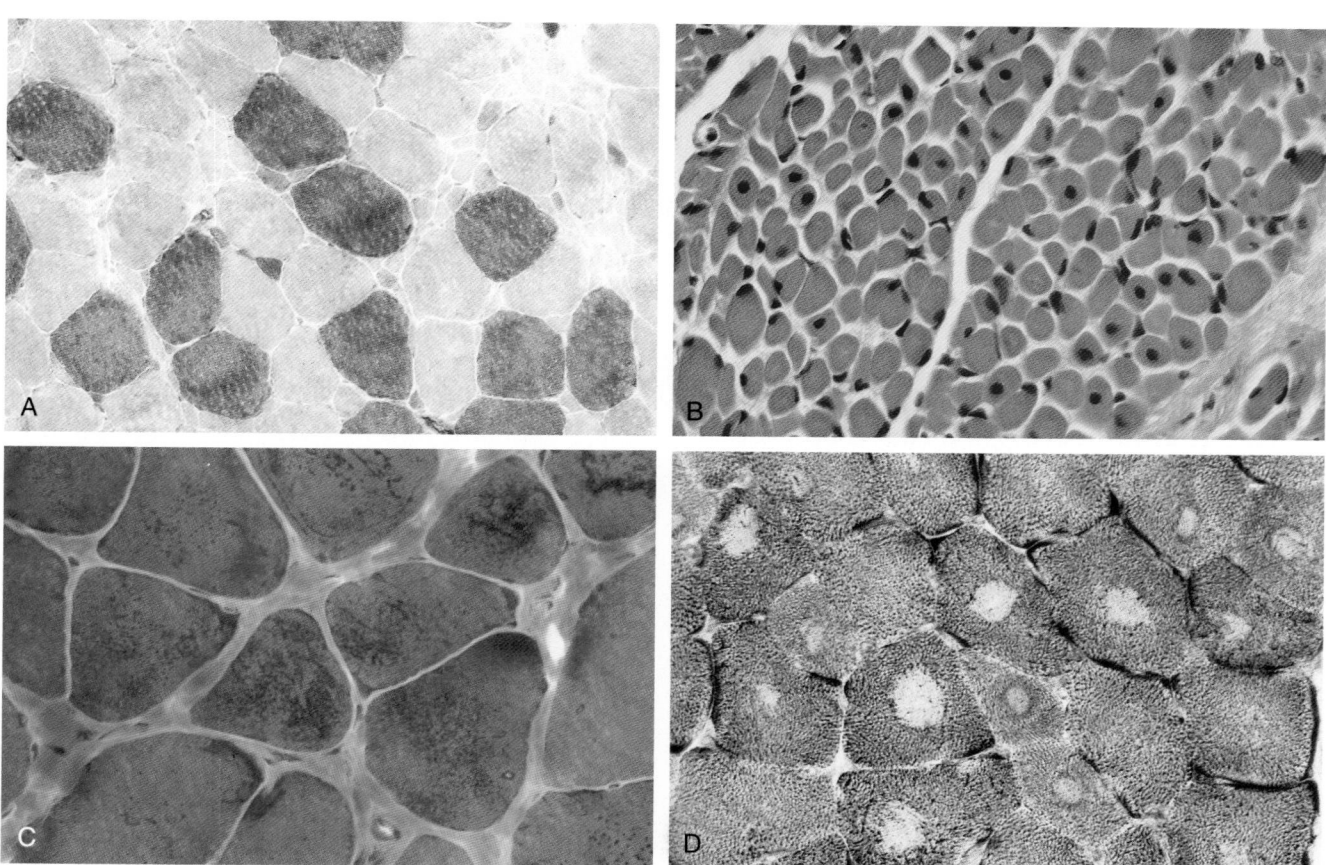

**FIGURE 53–3.** *A.* Congenital fiber-type disproportion. This muscle biopsy specimen has a predominance of type I fibers (lightly stained) that display marked variation in size and are generally smaller than type II fibers (darkly stained). (Cryostat section, ATPase, pH 9.4.) *B.* Centronuclear (myotubular) myopathy. These muscle fibers from a newborn infant contain large internal nuclei and have the appearance of fetal muscle (myotubes). (Paraffin section, H&E.) *C.* Nemaline myopathy. Muscle fibers contain particulate dark-staining nemaline rods. (Cryostat section, Gomori trichrome.) *D.* Central core disease. Muscle fibers have circular central areas of pallor that lack enzyme activity. (Cryostat section, NADH-TR.)

spread, affecting even the diaphragm and intercostal muscles, and type I fiber predominance is noted in most cases.[31]

## NEMALINE MYOPATHY

Two types of nemaline myopathy can be distinguished. The more common type is clinically evident at birth and has variable severity; a second form presents in adulthood. Although the disease is slowly progressive, death may occur early in life owing to respiratory failure. The adult form can present with cardiac involvement and only mild proximal weakness.

Nemaline myopathy is characterized histopathologically by dark red–staining material (rods) with Gomori trichrome stain that occurs almost exclusively in type I fibers (Fig. 53–3C) (CD Fig. 53–4C). Rods are not usually seen in H&E-stained sections, and they have a granular appearance on cross-section. Type I fiber predominance may also be present. By ultrastructural study, rods are 0.2 to 1.0 $\mu$m in diameter and have a density similar to that of Z lines (CD Fig. 53–4D). In cross-section, they have a tetragonal filamentous array. They are usually found in the sarcoplasm and occasionally in the nucleus. Rods appear to be composed of $\alpha$-actinin and actin, and it is thought that they are the result of abnormal activity of the protease dipeptidylpeptidase I.[32] They have also been described in a human immunodeficiency virus (HIV)–associated myopathy.[33]

## CENTRAL CORE DISEASE

Central core disease was the first specific myopathy found to be associated with infantile hypotonia. Clinical features include slowly progressive proximal muscle weakness, hypotonia, absent reflexes, and delayed motor milestones.[34] Muscle fibers in central core disease have well-circumscribed, circular areas in the center of most type I fibers that are devoid of mitochondria and sarcoplasmic reticulum and that lack oxidative enzymes and phosphorylase activity (Fig. 53–3D) (CD Fig. 53–4E). These fibers are best identified by NADH-TR histochemistry. There is also a predominance of type I fibers (which is generally true for most of the congenital myopathies). Two types of central cores are recognized ultrastructurally: structured cores, which have preserved myofibrillar architecture, and unstructured cores, in which the myofibrillar architecture is lost.

Other congenital myopathies have been described as multicore or minicore disease. These are nonprogressive myopathies that are usually sporadic.[31] The characteristic histopathologic feature is the presence of multiple foci with loss of cross-striations and decreased staining intensity. There may be several such zones within any given muscle fiber, and these areas have decreased oxidative enzyme and ATPase activities. Focal areas of sarcomere disintegration and Z band streaming as well as absent mitochondria are found by ultrastructural analysis. These changes are nonspecific because multiple foci of degeneration can be seen in a variety of diseases other than multicore and minicore disease.

## CENTRAL (INTRAUTERINE) MATURATIONAL DEFECT

Normal intrauterine development of skeletal muscle with regard to fiber type differentiation and morphologic features is complete by the 28th week of gestation. Some infants with hypotonia at birth do not manifest any of the pathologic features of the congenital myopathies, dystrophies, or neurogenic diseases. However, the muscle biopsy findings will show occasional large, hypereosinophilic fibers that appear to represent type II fibers.[35] An excessive number of these fibers (greater than 2%) can be associated with mild infantile hypotonia, which is thought to represent a delay in the normal intrauterine development of these fibers. The terms cerebral hypotonia and cerebral hypoplasia have also been applied to this disorder.

## Metabolic Myopathies

Three large groups of muscle diseases represent the metabolic myopathies: mitochondrial myopathies, disorders of lipid metabolism, and glycogen storage diseases. In general, patients with metabolic myopathies have gradually progressive limb-girdle myopathies or cramps induced by exercise or hypotonia (infants). These myopathies are diagnosed by the histochemical and ultrastructural features of muscle, the biochemical defects (specific enzyme deficiencies), and in some cases the results of molecular studies (analysis of mitochondrial DNA deletions).

### MITOCHONDRIAL MYOPATHIES

Mitochondrial myopathies are muscle diseases with structurally or numerically abnormal mitochondria and mitochondria with abnormal functions.[36] Mitochondrial myopathies can be classified biochemically as 1) defects of substrate transport (carnitine palmityltransferase [CPT] and carnitine deficiencies, which are discussed later), 2) defects of substrate utilization, 3) defects of the Krebs cycle, 4) defects of oxidative phosphorylation coupling, and 5) defects of the respiratory chain. A detailed description of the individual disorders that compose these groups, such as Kearns-Sayre syndrome, MERRF syndrome (myoclonus epilepsy with ragged red fibers), and MELAS syndrome (mitochondrial encephalopathy, myopathy, lactic acidosis, and strokelike episodes), is beyond the scope of this chapter; the reader is referred to more extensive sources.[37] The clinical presentation of mitochondrial myopathies may vary and can include progressive ophthalmoplegia, limb-girdle and fascioscapulohumeral myopathies, exercise-induced muscle cramps, and severe infantile hypotonia. Mitochondrial myopathies may also have cardiac involvement.

The histopathologic hallmark of mitochondrial

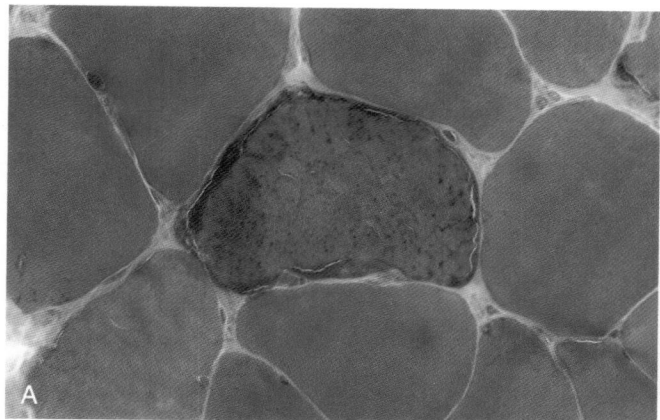 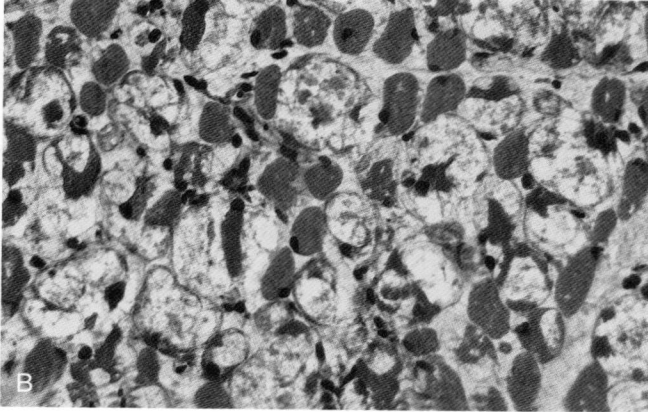

FIGURE 53–4. *A.* Mitochondrial myopathy. Ragged red fiber. (Cryostat section, Gomori trichrome.) *B.* Glycogen storage disease. Muscle biopsy specimen from a patient with type II glycogenosis (acid maltase deficiency, Pompe's disease) with marked vacuolization of virtually all muscle fibers. (Cryostat section, H&E.)

myopathies is the presence of ragged red fibers demonstrated in cryostat sections stained with the Gomori trichrome stain.[38] These appear as excessive amounts of coarse subsarcolemmal or intermyofibrillar red material that has slightly irregular shapes (Fig. 53–4*A*) (CD Fig. 53–5*A*). Ragged red fibers represent excessive abnormal mitochondria. NADH-TR shows dense subsarcolemmal accumulations of reaction product; when stained with succinic dehydrogenase or cytochrome *c* oxidase, these are indicative of mitochondria. They are randomly distributed but predominate in type I fibers. To be considered diagnostic, more than 2% of fibers should be ragged red fibers.[39] That ragged red fibers are present can initially be suggested in cryostat sections stained with H&E, in which punctate basophilic sarcoplasm is found next to the sarcolemma or within the fiber.

The Gomori trichrome and NADH-TR stains are useful in selecting samples for electron microscopy required for a morphologic diagnosis. At the ultrastructural level, mitochondria exhibit a variety of changes. They may be enlarged or have bizarre shapes (including ring shapes), and cristae may be abnormal (distorted, excessively branched, or concentrically arranged) (CD Fig. 53–5*B*); electron-dense material or granular material may replace the cristae. Various types of inclusions can be found, including paracrystalline structures (most commonly) and electron-dense bodies; paracrystalline inclusions are thought to be accumulated creatine kinase. Mitochondria may be increased in number, frequently as large subsarcolemmal aggregates (CD Fig. 53–5*C*). Mitochondria can be abnormal in one fiber but appear normal in neighboring fibers.

Morphologic criteria provide valuable information for the diagnosis of mitochondrial myopathies but cannot be used alone. Ragged red fibers can be found in nonmitochondrial disorders, such as DMD, myotonic dystrophy, and polymyositis,[40] or in patients who have received antiretroviral therapy with reverse transcriptase inhibitor.[41] Ragged red fi-

bers can be absent in some primary mitochondrial diseases (CPT deficiency or pyruvate dehydrogenase deficiency). Similarly, ultrastructural abnormalities of mitochondria have been described in several diseases, including muscular dystrophies, neurogenic atrophy, polymyositis, and acid maltase deficiency, and even in normal muscle.[39, 42] Therefore, determination of a precise etiology may require testing for specific enzyme deficiencies. Analysis of genetic defects in mitochondrial DNA has begun to provide additional diagnostic information because deletions of mitochondrial DNA are associated with Kearns-Sayre, MERRF, and MELAS syndromes.[39]

## LIPID METABOLISM DISORDERS (LIPID MYOPATHIES)

Disorders of lipid and glycogen metabolism can produce two syndromes, one characterized by progressive weakness and the other by exercise-induced cramps with or without myoglobinuria. Lipid myopathies are centered on defective metabolism of long-chain fatty acids, a crucial source of energy for muscle. Such defects can be at the level of substrate transport into the mitochondria (carnitine and CPT deficiencies) or at the level of β-oxidation, in which long-chain fatty acid derivatives are normally used as substrates for the Krebs cycle.[43]

### Carnitine Deficiency

Carnitine deficiency produces a slowly progressive limb-girdle myopathy and can be primary or associated with a large number of inborn metabolic errors (organic acidurias, disorders of β-oxidation, defects in the respiratory chain). There is a "myopathic" form of carnitine deficiency (in which serum carnitine levels are normal) and a systemic form. The muscle biopsy specimen contains small vacuoles within most fibers, and these vacuoles are oil red O positive. In some cases, vacuoles may obliterate most of the fiber architecture, and type I fibers are more severely affected. By electron microscopy, large lipid droplets are found either in a random distribution or in rows between myofibrils.

### Carnitine Palmityltransferase Deficiency

CPT deficiency is not associated with weakness; rather, exercise-induced muscle pain and cramps may occasionally be accompanied by myoglobinuria, and attacks are exacerbated by cold or by fasting. The extent of lipid seen in the biopsy specimen in CPT deficiency is not as great as that seen in carnitine deficiency, and it may even be mistaken for ice artifact on H&E-stained sections. Stains for lipid (oil red O) and electron microscopy confirm the presence of excess lipid in muscle. In some cases of CPT deficiency, the muscle biopsy findings may appear normal.

## GLYCOGEN STORAGE DISEASES

Skeletal muscle is involved in ten of the disorders that affect glycogen metabolism.[44] Like the disorders of lipid metabolism, glycogen storage diseases are associated with weakness or exercise-induced cramps with or without myoglobinuria; vacuolation of the muscle fibers is the histologic hallmark. Enzyme histochemistry in some of these myopathies can identify a specific enzyme defect, and additional biochemical testing using cultured fibroblasts can be confirmatory. Four types of glycogenosis affecting skeletal muscle, representing the most common forms and all transmitted as autosomal recessive traits, are discussed.

### Acid Maltase Deficiency

Acid maltase deficiency (type II glycogenosis, Pompe's disease) causes either a severe, generalized fatal disease in infancy or a myopathy that begins in childhood or adult life. Light microscopy of muscle shows a vacuolar myopathy that can be striking, particularly in the infantile form (Fig. 53–4B) (CD Fig. 53–5D). Muscle in the childhood and adult forms can be less striking and may even appear normal. Periodic acid–Schiff (PAS) stain demonstrates large amounts of glycogen (best seen in cryostat sections). Acid phosphatase, an enzyme not apparent in normal muscle but that indicates sites of lysosomal activity in abnormal muscle, is focally present in many fibers by histochemical staining and is indicative of abnormal lysosomes. At the ultrastructural level, massive amounts of glycogen are found, both membrane bound and free within the sarcoplasm, with displacement and loss of myofilaments (CD Fig. 53–5E).

### Branching Enzyme Deficiency

Branching enzyme deficiency (type IV glycogenosis, Andersen's disease) is characterized by liver disease and progressive cirrhosis; the myopathy is a minor component of the disease. Branching enzyme attaches short glucosyl chains with $\alpha$-1,6-glucosyl bonds to glycogen to start new chains that are subsequently lengthened by glycogen synthetase. A de-fect of branching enzyme therefore results in an abnormal polysaccharide similar to amylopectin, and this is reflected in the morphologic characteristics of the disease. Light microscopy of cryostat sections shows vacuoles that contain basophilic, PAS-positive material partially resistant to diastase digestion and that are alcian blue (at acid pH) positive. By electron microscopy, this material consists of filamentous and finely granular material often associated with normal glycogen particles.

### Myophosphorylase Deficiency

Myophosphorylase deficiency (type V glycogenosis, McArdle's disease) is characterized by exercise intolerance, myalgia, and cramps with exercise that are relieved by rest. Muscle biopsy shows subsarcolemmal and intermyofibrillar PAS-positive vacuoles that may be focal and mild in some cases. Histochemistry for myophosphorylase reveals absent activity. By electron microscopy, deposits of normal-appearing free glycogen are seen interspersed among myofibrils.

### Phosphofructokinase Deficiency

Phosphofructokinase deficiency (type VII glycogenosis, Tarui's disease) has a clinical presentation similar to that of McArdle's disease. In addition to PAS-positive material that is removed by diastase digestion, diastase-resistant material is present and represents an abnormal polysaccharide, ultrastructurally similar to that found in branching enzyme deficiency. The histochemical stain for phosphofructokinase can confirm the diagnosis.

## DIAGNOSTIC CONSIDERATIONS AND APPROACHES FOR PERIPHERAL NERVE DISEASE

A limited repertoire of pathologic reactions are observed in peripheral nerve, and these are shared by a number of primary and secondary disorders of the peripheral nervous system. Although it is essential to understand pathologic changes distinct to peripheral nerve, it is imperative to consider nerve biopsy specimens from the perspective of the general surgical pathologist. For example, angiotrophic lymphoma may produce a clinical pattern of mononeuritis multiplex and axonal degeneration developing in peripheral nerve secondary to ischemic damage. The goal in interpreting such a biopsy finding is not only to determine the characteristics of the peripheral neuropathy but also to identify the intravascular malignant lymphoma. Thus, the approach to nerve biopsy specimens requires clinical correlation as well as a sound foundation in general surgical pathology linked with specialized understanding of peripheral nerve diseases.

Two principal pathologic changes can occur in peripheral nerve: axonal degeneration and segmental demyelination (for more detailed discussions, see

Dyck and colleagues[2] and Richardson and De-Girolami[45]). Each is considered separately here, but they often occur together, and indeed, in some instances, one can induce the other. Thus, the surgical pathologist is commonly faced with a mixed peripheral neuropathy and must judge which process, axonal degeneration or demyelination, is more prominent. Axonal degeneration begins with disruption of the regular cytoskeletal architecture of axoplasm followed by accumulation of vesicular material in axoplasm (Fig. 53–5A) (CD Fig. 53–6A). In days, as the degeneration continues, it can be observed as structureless axoplasm within the disintegrating myelin sheath. Finally, scavenger cells engulf the degenerating axon and myelin debris (Fig. 53–5B) (CD Fig.

53–6B). Importantly, the basal lamina associated with the degenerating axon remains intact and, under the appropriate circumstances, may serve as a "tunnel" for proliferating Schwann cells (ultimately forming so-called bands of Büngner) that assist axonal regeneration. Regenerating axons are best identified by electron microscopy as multiple, small, and thinly myelinated neurites enclosed within a single basal lamina.

Axonal degeneration is typically of long standing by the time a biopsy is performed. Thus, in addition to these features, chronic axonal degeneration also displays reduction in axon density with increased endoneurial collagen deposition (Fig. 53–5C) (CD Fig. 53–6C). Methods for assessing axon

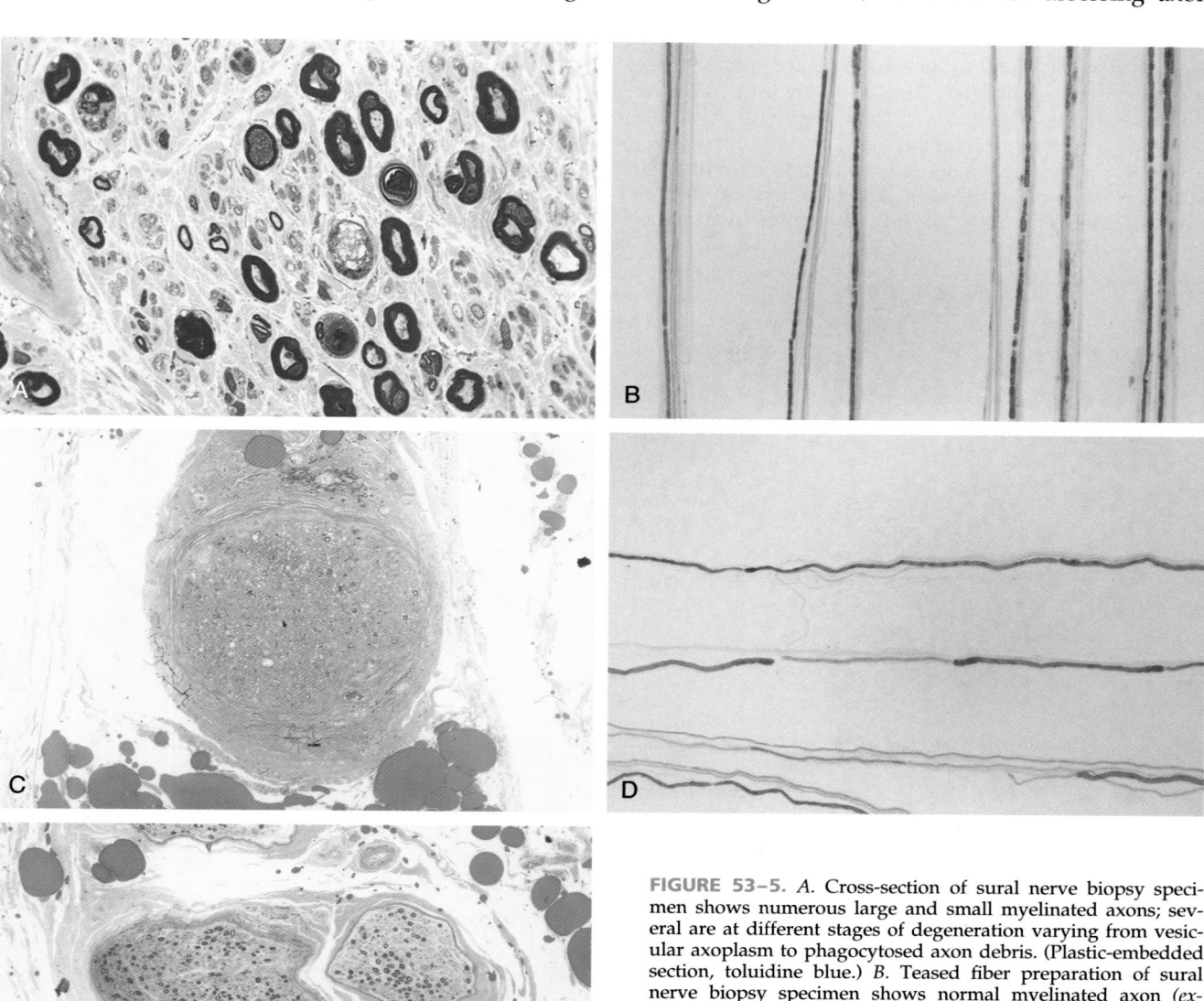

FIGURE 53–5. *A.* Cross-section of sural nerve biopsy specimen shows numerous large and small myelinated axons; several are at different stages of degeneration varying from vesicular axoplasm to phagocytosed axon debris. (Plastic-embedded section, toluidine blue.) *B.* Teased fiber preparation of sural nerve biopsy specimen shows normal myelinated axon (*extreme right*) and several degenerating axons (*left*) of different ages. *C.* Cross-section of sural nerve fascicle from a distal lower extremity amputation specimen shows chronic severe loss of axons secondary to long-standing peripheral vascular disease. (Toluidine blue.) *D.* Teased fiber preparation of sural nerve biopsy specimen shows segmental demyelination with remyelination. *E.* Cross-section of sural nerve biopsy specimen from a patient with rheumatoid arthritis and distal sensorimotor neuropathy shows focal axonal degeneration within the fascicle. (Toluidine blue.)

density vary from subjective interpretations based on experience to sophisticated enumeration of several different fiber types based on image analysis. We have adopted a semiquantitative method based on caricatures of a normal nerve fascicle (Fig. 53–6) (CD Fig. 53–7). With this system, one can approximate a mild (25%), moderate (50%), or severe (75%) reduction of large and small myelinated fibers. Caution must be exercised in the diagnosis of mild reduction in myelinated axon density because this change may be seen with increasing age in the absence of clinically apparent neurologic disease.

Segmental demyelination can occur after lesions to myelin itself or lesions to Schwann cells. Demyelination is rapidly attended by remyelination such that one rarely observes a large axon completely denuded of myelin. However, remyelination is inadequate, leaving myelin sheaths that are too thin and internodal segments that are too short and irregular. Because axonal diameter dictates myelin thickness, variation in myelin thickness among similarly sized axons strongly suggests segmental demyelination. In addition, repeated episodes of demyelination and remyelination may lead to layering of Schwann cell

processes around thinly myelinated axons or collagen fibers if the axon has degenerated. Despite these changes that may be seen in cross-sections of nerve biopsy specimens, teased fiber preparations are superior for the assessment of demyelinating disease. Here, internodal distances are irregularly shortened, myelin sheaths are abnormally thin, and perinodal myelin retraction may be present (Fig. 53–5D) (CD Fig. 53–6D). Irregularity of shortened and thinned internodal segments is a critical feature to determine because teased fiber preparations of regenerated axons show thinned and shortened internodal segments that are exquisitely regular in length.

As stated before, knowledge of histopathologic changes peculiar to peripheral nerve must be coupled with a comprehensive surgical pathology assessment of the nerve biopsy specimen, best accomplished with an H&E-stained cross-section of nerve. A central element of peripheral nerve biopsy evaluation is the vasculature, both epineurial and endoneurial, to determine evidence of thromboembolic disease, vasculitis, or diabetic vascular changes, among others. The culpable thromboembolism or vasculitic occlusion is typically focal and may be

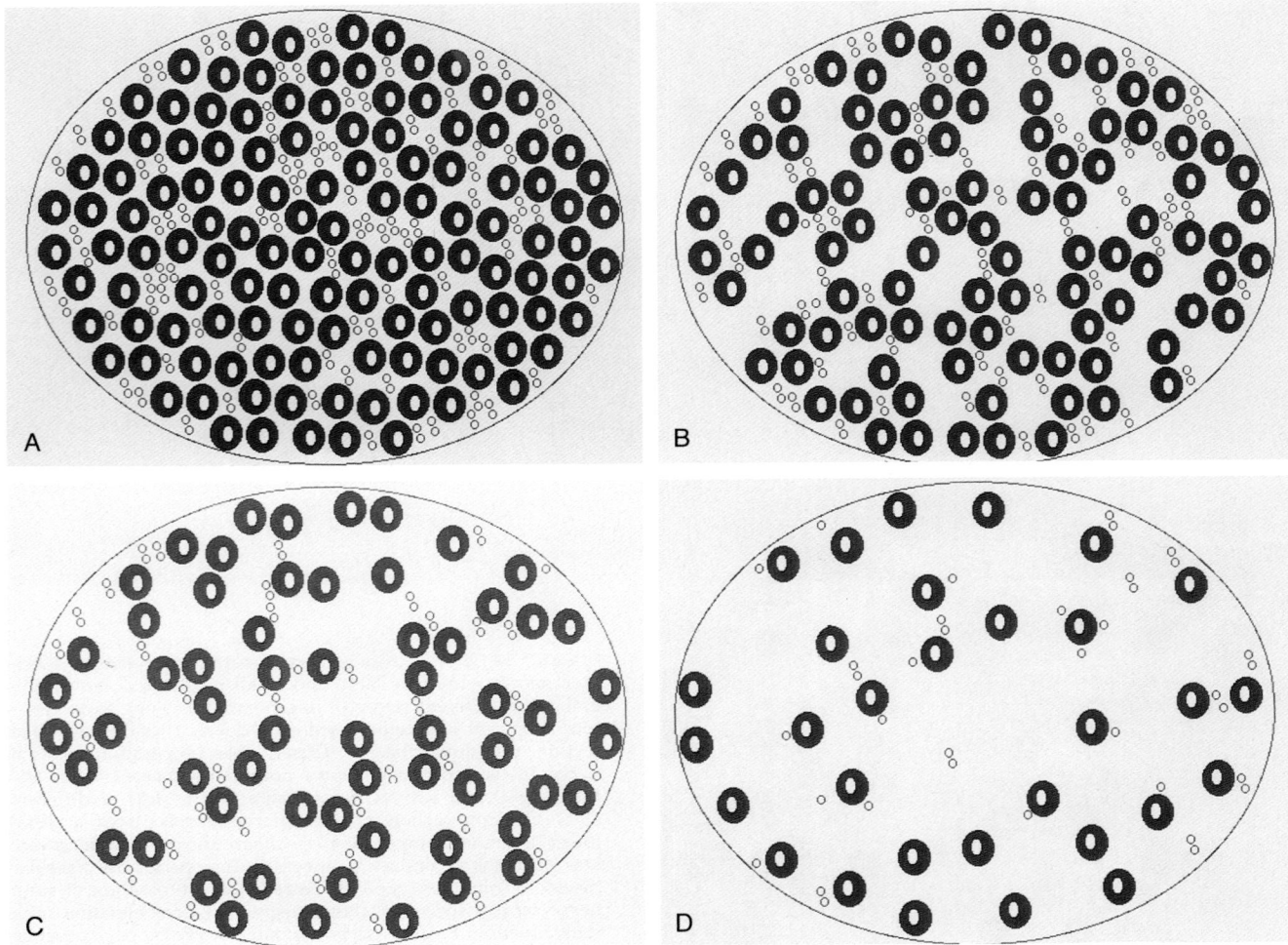

**FIGURE 53–6.** Caricatures of nerve fascicle cross-sections with normal complement of large and small myelinated axons (A) and reduction in axons of 25% (B), 50% (C), and 75% (D).

proximal to the segment of nerve removed at biopsy. Despite the absence of a demonstrable vascular lesion, focal axonal degeneration within nerve fascicles is highly suggestive of a proximal ischemic lesion (Fig. 53–5E) (CD Fig. 53–6E). In addition, routine Congo red staining of all nerve biopsy specimens provides screening for amyloid deposition, which may occur as focal collections, within vessel walls, or as diffuse accumulations in the endoneurium. Last, direct immunofluorescence for immunoglobulin deposition, especially immunoglobulin M in older patients with unexplained demyelinating disease, is becoming an important component in the evaluation of peripheral nerve biopsy specimens.

## DIAGNOSTIC CONSIDERATIONS AND APPROACHES FOR COMBINED NERVE AND MUSCLE DISEASE

Clinical features of denervation depend on the age of the patient and the site of motor unit injury. Whether the denervation is from loss of spinal mo-

tor neurons or peripheral nerves, the histologic changes in adults are largely the same. With denervation, there is loss of acetylcholine stimulation and trophic influences resulting in loss of thick and thin myofilaments and myofiber atrophy. Previously round or polygonal fibers collapse into elongated angular forms (Fig. 53–7A) (CD Fig. 53–8A), and such angulation of both type I and type II fibers (Fig. 53–7B) (CD Fig. 53–8B) distinguishes denervation from myopathic forms of myofiber atrophy that can produce atrophic fibers remaining round or polygonal. Because motor neurons innervate noncontiguous myofibers in a motor unit, initial atrophy from denervation is seen in individual myofibers scattered throughout a muscle fascicle; such atrophy, documented by myofibrillar ATPase staining, can involve both type I and type II fibers. With progressive denervation, groups of angular fibers may appear within one fascicle. Severely atrophic fibers with little remaining cytoplasm eventually appear as clusters of pyknotic nuclei sometimes resembling multinucleated giant cells or mononuclear cells. With prolonged denervation, muscle fascicles may also acquire myopathic features including round at-

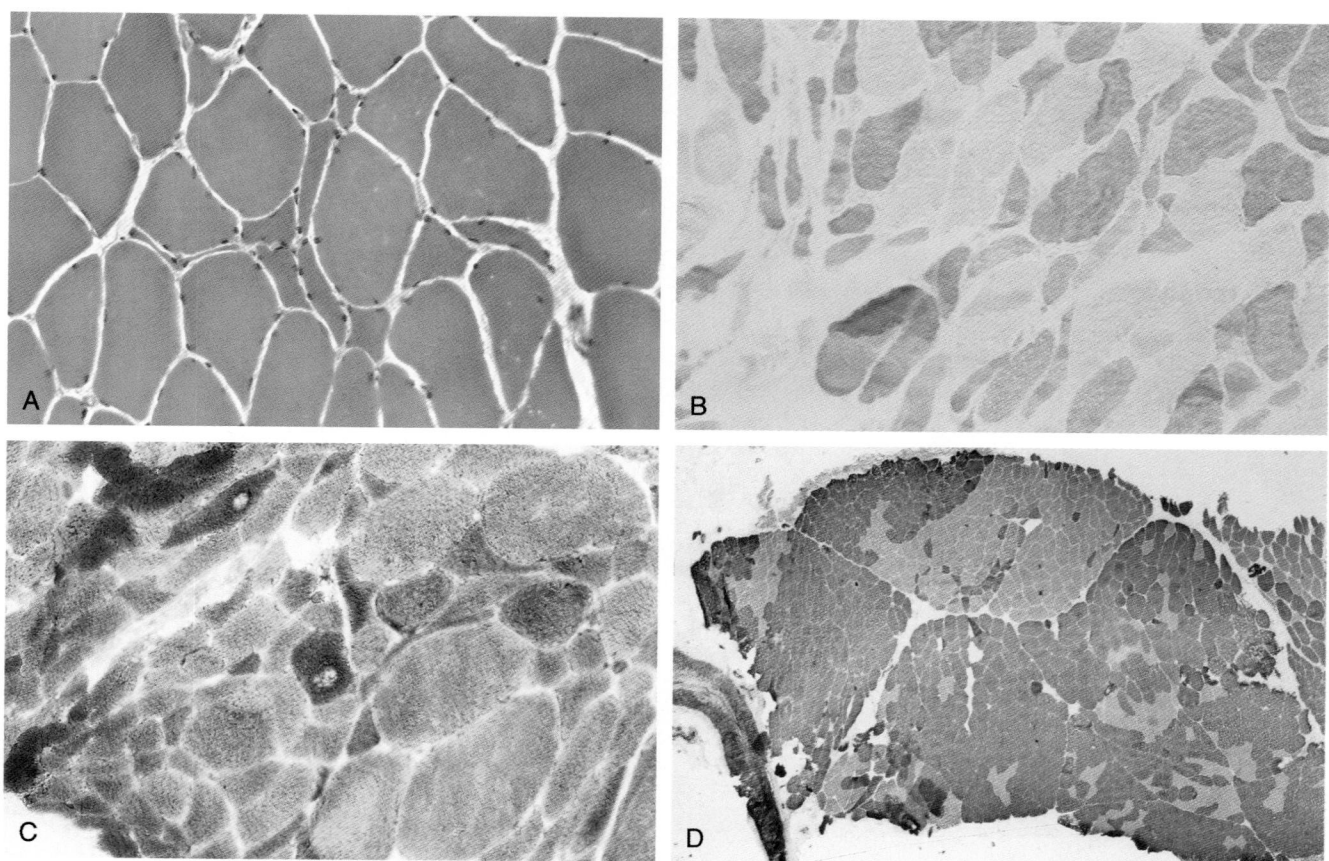

**FIGURE 53–7.** *A.* Neurogenic atrophy. Angular atrophy of type I and type II myofibers in the absence of myopathic features or inflammation. (Cryostat section, H&E.) *B.* Neurogenic atrophy of both type I fibers (lightly stained) and type II fibers (darkly stained) by ATPase reaction. (Cryostat section, pH 9.4.) *C.* Target fibers associated with reinnervation; usually seen in mildly atrophic type I fibers. (Cryostat section, NADH-TR stain.) *D.* Fiber-type grouping with 15 or more contiguous myofibers of one type; pathognomonic of chronic denervation and reinnervation. (Cryostat section, ATPase, pH 9.4.)

rophy of fibers, internal nuclei, split fibers, increased endomysial connective tissue, and occasionally even minimal focal inflammation.[46–48]

Reinnervation of individual myofibers results in changes in central myofibrillar organization producing target fibers. These represent one of the few changes of denervation and reinnervation demonstrable in formalin-fixed tissue and can be seen with trichrome, PAS, and phosphotungstic acid–hematoxylin stains. They are seen readily with NADH-TR staining (Fig. 53–7C) (CD Fig. 53–8C). Targets occur primarily in type I fibers and exhibit three zones: a central zone surrounded by a rim of increased staining encircled by a normal zone.[46–48] These must be distinguished from targetoid fibers, which lack the darkened rim and may be seen as a nonspecific change associated with denervation or myopathies. Although diagnostically helpful, target fibers are transient and may not be seen in small samples, particularly of chronically denervated muscle with extensive fiber-type grouping.[46–49]

With chronic denervation, nerve sprouts from remaining nerves reinnervate adjacent denervated myofibers, creating clusters of myofibers that, being innervated by a single motor nerve, acquire identical functional characteristics. Such structural change, called fiber-type grouping, is pathognomonic of denervation and reinnervation (Fig. 53–7D) (CD Fig. 53–8D). A minimum of 15 contiguous fibers of the same type and the presence of grouping of both type I and type II fibers are features considered diagnostic of fiber-type grouping.[46, 47, 50]

Neurogenic atrophy must be differentiated from artifact and other processes that produce angular atrophy of one or both fiber types. Type II atrophy is the most common process mimicking denervation (Fig. 53–8A) (CD Fig. 53–9A) and is associated with a number of diagnostic considerations including long-standing disuse, prolonged glucocorticoid administration, and chronic illnesses such as collagen-vascular disorders and endocrinopathies. H&E-stained sections reveal scattered angular fibers without grouping; myofibrillar ATPase reaction reveals involvement of only type II fibers; target fibers and

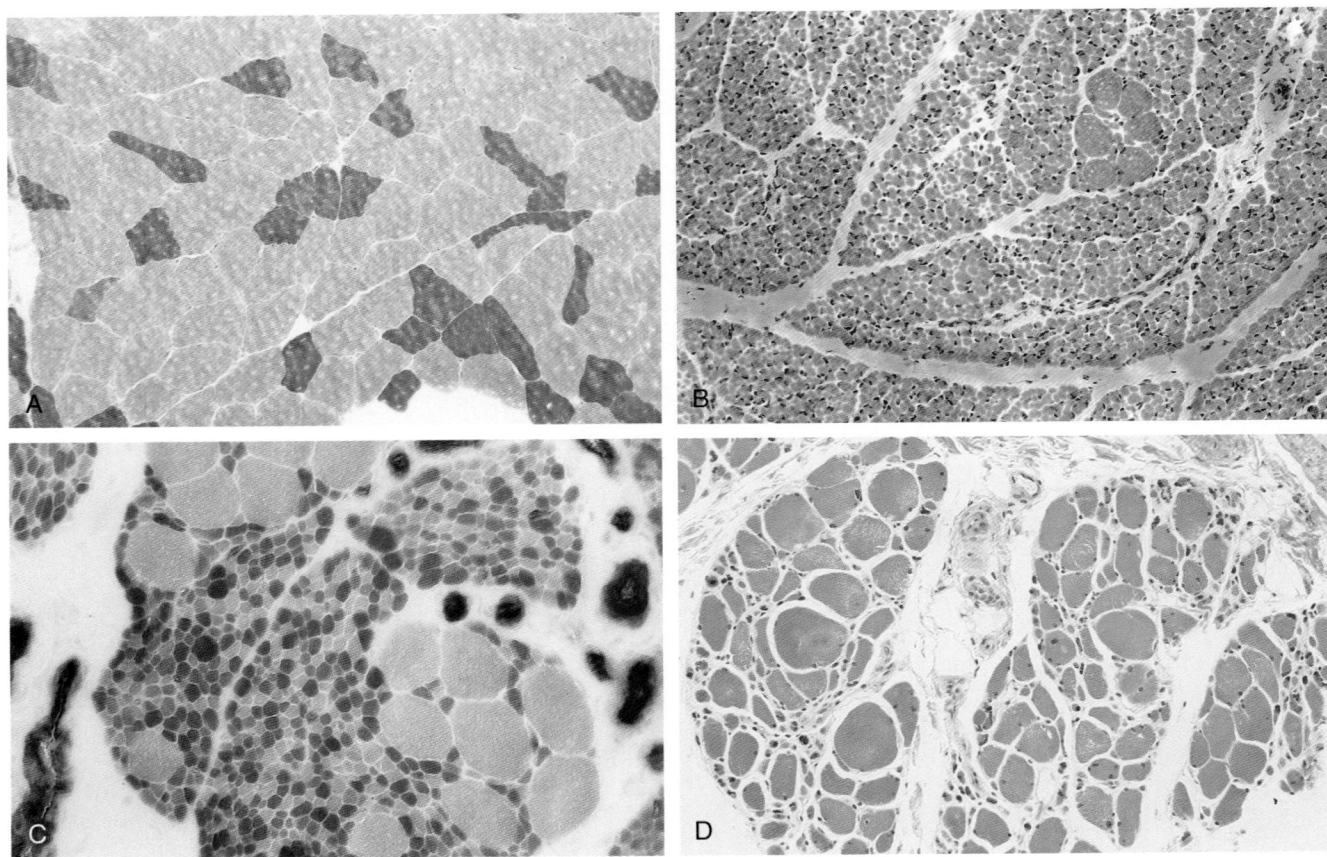

**FIGURE 53–8.** *A.* Type II fiber atrophy. Scattered angular fibers mimic denervation but are limited to type II fibers only. (Cryostat section, ATPase, pH 9.4.) *B.* SMA, type I. Denervated myofibers are rounded and often accompanied by clusters of hypertrophic fibers. (Cryostat section, H&E.) *C.* SMA, type I. Atrophic fibers are both type I and type II, whereas hypertrophic fibers are usually type I. (Cryostat section, ATPase, pH 9.4.) *D.* End-stage neurogenic atrophy, as is seen in amyotrophic lateral sclerosis, may be associated with myopathic changes such as atrophic round fibers, internal nuclei, and increased endomysial connective tissue. (Paraffin section, H&E.)

fiber-type grouping are absent. Muscular dystrophies, particularly fascioscapulohumeral, Becker's, and oculopharyngeal, may exhibit angular atrophy of scattered fibers. This can usually be distinguished from denervation by the absence of clinical features of denervation; the presence of dystrophic features, such as atrophic round fibers, regenerating fibers, and increased endomysial connective tissue; and the absence of other neurogenic changes.[46, 47]

## Primary Neurogenic Diseases

### SPINAL MUSCULAR ATROPHY

Spinal muscular atrophy (SMA) represents a spectrum of autosomal recessive diseases of anterior horn cells resulting in progressive symmetric atrophy of proximal muscles. Depending on the variant, symptoms may occur any time from in utero life to adolescence. Three variants reflecting different ages at onset and severity are recognized. SMA type I manifests before birth or in the first 3 months of life in 95% of cases, presenting as a floppy infant syndrome. SMA type II is clinically evident from 6 to 12 months of age, with leg weakness greater than arm weakness. Changes in skeletal muscle are similar to those in SMA type I but often less pronounced. SMA type III, usually presenting as proximal leg weakness in young adults, may be associated with some features of motor neuron disease in adults. The gene deletions associated with all three forms have been mapped to 5q11.2–13.3, which contains the survival motor neuron gene *(SMN)*. More than 95% of patients with SMA types I, II, and III have homozygous deletions in exon 7 of the *SMN* gene. Relative reductions of the SMN protein appear to influence the severity of the disease. Tests for *SMN* gene deletions are proving valuable in the diagnosis of atypical cases of SMA and genetic counseling.[51, 52]

In infantile forms of SMA, denervated myofibers undergo atrophy, resulting in collections of small, round (rather than angular) myofibers. These are usually substantially smaller than the mean myofiber diameter of 15 to 17 $\mu$m for this age (Fig. 53–8B) (CD Fig. 53–9B). Both type I and type II fibers are affected equally. Over time, the muscles exhibit fiber-type grouping involving large numbers of atrophic round fibers. Diagnostically important clusters of hypertrophic type I fibers are also seen in SMA type I and type II (Fig. 53–8C) (CD Fig. 53–9C). These changes are accompanied by increased perimysial connective tissue, although endomysial connective tissue is not changed. The infantile forms of SMA must be distinguished from cerebral hypotonia and normal immaturity of muscle. Randomly scattered hypertrophic type I and type II myofibers are seen in the developmentally delayed muscle of infants with cerebral hypotonia (see earlier). Early on, the diagnosis of SMA type I may be difficult because normal immature muscle fibers or those re-

flecting developmental delays are also round and exhibit mild variability in size. In SMA type III, muscle may exhibit angular atrophy typical of changes seen in adults as well as round atrophy that may be organized in broad fiber-type grouping. Type II fiber atrophy may also be present.[46, 47]

### AMYOTROPHIC LATERAL SCLEROSIS

Amyotrophic lateral sclerosis, also known as Lou Gehrig's disease and motor neuron disease, is the most common motor neuron disease in adults with an incidence of 1 to 3 per 100,000. In typical amyotrophic lateral sclerosis, muscle biopsy specimens obtained early in the course of the disease show characteristic features of denervation and reinnervation: angular atrophy of type I and type II fibers, target fibers, and hypertrophic type II fibers. In long-standing cases, fiber-type grouping is seen. Myopathic features, scattered regenerating fibers, and chronic inflammation may mimic muscular dystrophies[47, 53] (Fig. 53–8D) (CD Fig. 53–9D).

## Vascular-Based Combined Nerve and Muscle Diseases

Vasculitis accompanying a variety of diseases may produce a combination of neuropathy and myopathy. Although the pathogenesis varies, all afflict perineurial and epineurial or perimysial and endomysial arterioles, often producing fibrinoid necrosis and thrombosis of blood vessels, resulting in ischemic damage to both nerve and muscle (Fig. 53–9) (CD Fig. 53–10).

### POLYARTERITIS NODOSA

In contrast to systemic polyarteritis nodosa, nonsystemic or limited polyarteritis nodosa involving skin, nerves, and musculoskeletal system afflicts the peripheral nervous system in 50% to 75% of cases usu-

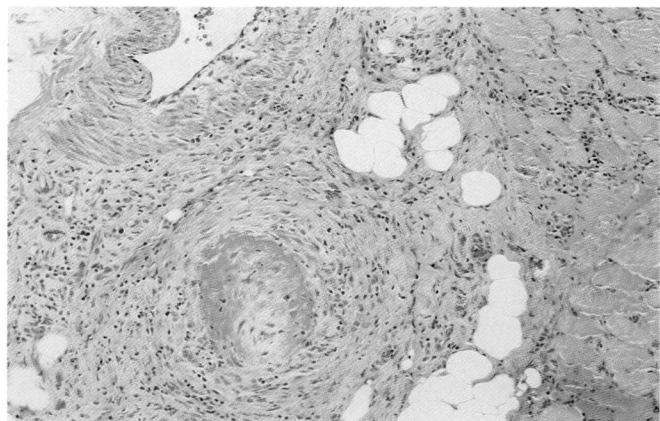

**FIGURE 53–9.** Necrotizing vasculitis. Necrotizing vasculitides typically involve epimysial and perimysial arterioles *(top)* but spare venules *(bottom)*. (Paraffin section, H&E.)

ally as a mononeuritis multiplex involving both motor and sensory nerves. Polyarteritis nodosa produces an acute necrotizing neutrophilic vasculitis of small epineurial arterioles of the vasa nervorum with fibrinoid necrosis of vascular walls. Acutely, limited numbers of eosinophils may be present; in older lesions, this acute infiltrate is replaced by lymphocytes, macrophages, and fibroblasts, producing medial fibrosis and narrowing of the lumen. The thrombotic occlusion produces ischemic damage to nerves, resulting in degeneration of axons in myelinated and unmyelinated nerves. Involvement of muscle is usually limited to endomysial and perimysial vasculitis.[46, 54]

## WEGENER'S GRANULOMATOSIS

Wegener's granulomatosis may produce a mononeuritis multiplex or symmetric polyneuropathy. Characteristically, this is a necrotizing arteritis of the vasa nervorum with T lymphocytes and plasmacytoid cells. Wegener's granulomatosis–associated myopathies may occasionally occur. The resultant denervation often produces muscle weakness. Diagnosis is based on evidence of Wegener's granulomatosis in other organs, characteristic histopathologic features, and antibodies to proteinase 3.[53, 56]

## RHEUMATOID ARTHRITIS

Patients with rheumatoid arthritis develop digital mononeuropathy or distal symmetric sensory or sensorimotor neuropathy associated with an arteritis primarily affecting the vasa nervorum. Chronic inflammation with fibrinoid necrosis and intimal hyperplasia of arterioles are thought to contribute to neuronal ischemia.[54, 57, 58] Skeletal muscle findings, predominantly type II atrophy, are described earlier.

## SYSTEMIC LUPUS ERYTHEMATOSUS

Peripheral neuropathies occur in about 10% of patients with systemic lupus erythematosus, most commonly a distal symmetric sensory or sensorimotor neuropathy, although mononeuritis multiplex can also occur. A T cell infiltrate and fibrinoid necrosis of epineurial vessels and a lymphocytic infiltrate of the adventitia are usually seen. As with other vasculitides, vascular fibrosis is seen in healed lesions.[59–61] As mentioned before, vasculitis, type II atrophy, and significant endomysial lymphocytic infiltrate may be seen in skeletal muscle.[60, 61]

## SJÖGREN'S SYNDROME

Sjögren's syndrome may be associated with symmetric sensory or sensorimotor neuropathy with perivascular lymphocytic infiltrates.[62] An asymptomatic lymphoplasmacytic infiltrate of muscle may be seen in 39% to 74% of patients. A symptomatic inflammatory myopathy with histopathologic features of polymyositis, dermatomyositis, or IBM develops in 2.5% to 10% of cases, usually involving proximal and rarely distal muscles.[62] A similar syndrome with a sensorimotor or motor axonal polyneuropathy

with CD8[+] suppressor T cells has been reported in association with HIV-1 diffuse infiltrative lymphocytosis syndrome.[63]

## ALLERGIC GRANULOMATOSIS (CHURG-STRAUSS SYNDROME)

Sixty-five percent to 80% of patients with allergic granulomatosis develop a symmetric polyneuropathy or mononeuritis multiplex. This is usually associated with the vasculitic phase of the disease, which may be accompanied by fatigue and significant weakness. The vascular lesions are seen as an eosinophilic necrotizing vasculitis of the vasa nervorum of peripheral nerves.[59]

## HIV-1–ASSOCIATED NEUROPATHY

At least 50% of patients with HIV-1 infection eventually develop peripheral neuropathies. The majority are segmental demyelinating inflammatory neuropathies with endoneurial and epineurial chronic inflammation and axonal degeneration. Early in HIV-1 infection, patients may develop an acute or chronic inflammatory demyelinating polyneuropathy. With immunosuppression, a distal symmetric polyneuropathy or mononeuritis multiplex becomes more common. Rarely, HIV-1 infections may be associated with a neutrophilic or mononuclear vasculitic neuropathy. Some vascular lesions resemble polyarteritis nodosa. Their pathogenesis may reflect immune complex–mediated or autoimmune-mediated vasculitides.[64] Polymyositis clinically identical to idiopathic polymyositis with endomysial infiltrates of CD8[+] suppressor T cells may also develop in immunosuppressed individuals. Rarely, nemaline myopathy is seen. Antiretroviral treatment with zidovudine (AZT) produces a reversible mitochondrial myopathy with myalgias, proximal weakness, and ragged red fibers in some patients.[65]

## PARANEOPLASTIC NEUROPATHY

Patients with occult neoplasms, particularly small cell carcinoma of the lung, may rarely develop a mononeuritis multiplex from a CD8[+]-sensitized cytotoxic-suppressor lymphocytic vasculitis involving epineurial and perimysial arterioles. This is associated with elevated anti-HU antibodies.[66] Muscle findings are described earlier.

## REFERENCES

1. Key A, Retzius G: Studien in der Anatomie de Nervensystems und des Bindegewebes. Vol II. Stockholm, PA Nordstedt & Soner, 1876.
2. Dyck PJ, Giannini C, Lais A: Pathologic alterations in nerves. *In* Dyck PJ, Thomas PK, Griffin JW, et al (eds): Peripheral Neuropathy. 3rd ed. Philadelphia, WB Saunders, 1993, pp 514–595.
3. Emery AE: Population frequencies of inherited neuromuscular diseases—a world survey. Neuromuscul Disord 1:19–29, 1991.
4. Iannaccone ST: Current status of Duchenne muscular dystrophy. Pediatr Neurol 39:879–894, 1992.
5. Campbell KP: Three muscular dystrophies: loss of cytoskeleton–extracellular matrix linkage. Cell 80:675–679, 1995.

6. Matsumara K, Campbell KP: Dystrophin-glycoprotein complex: its role in the molecular pathogenesis of muscular dystrophies. Muscle Nerve 17:2–15, 1994.
7. Hoffman EP, Wang J: Duchenne-Becker muscular dystrophy and the nondystrophic myotonias. Arch Neurol 50:1227–1237, 1993.
8. Brown RH: Dystrophin-associated proteins and the muscular dystrophies. Annu Rev Med 48:457–466, 1997.
9. Hoffman EP, Kunkel LM, Angelini C, et al: Improved diagnosis of Becker muscular dystrophy by dystrophin testing. Neurology 39:1011–1017, 1989.
10. Nicholson LVB, Davison K, Johnson MA, et al: Dystrophin in skeletal muscle II. Immunoreactivity in patients with Xp21 muscular dystrophy. J Neurol Sci 94:137–146, 1989.
11. Nicholson LVB, Johnson MA, Gardner-Medwin D, et al: Heterogeneity of dystrophin expression in patients with Duchenne and Becker muscular dystrophy. Acta Neuropathol 80: 239–250, 1990.
12. Muntoni F, Mateddu A, Cianchetti C, et al: Dystrophin analysis using a panel of anti-dystrophin antibodies in Duchenne and Becker muscular dystrophy. J Neurol Neurosurg Psychiatry 56:26–31, 1993.
13. Duggan DJ, Gorospe JR, Fanin M, et al: Mutations in the sarcoglycan genes in patients with myopathy. N Engl J Med 336:618–624, 1997.
14. Nagano A, Koga R, Ogawa M, et al: Emerin deficiency at the nuclear membrane in patients with Emery-Dreifuss muscular dystrophy. Nat Genet 12:255–259, 1996.
15. Richard I, Broux O, Allamand V, et al: Mutations in the proteolytic enzyme calpain 3 cause limb-girdle muscular dystrophy type 2a. Cell 81:27–40, 1995.
16. Harper PS: Myotonic Dystrophy. Philadelphia, WB Saunders, 1979.
17. Mahadevan M, Tsilfidis C, Sabourin L, et al: Myotonic dystrophy mutation: an unstable CTG repeat in the 3' untranslated region of the gene. Science 255:1253–1255, 1992.
18. Fischbeck KH: The mechanism of myotonic dystrophy. Ann Neurol 35:255–256, 1994.
19. Dalakas MC: Polymyositis, dermatomyositis, and inclusion-body myositis. N Engl J Med 325:1487–1498, 1991.
20. Heffner RR: Inflammatory myopathies. A review. J Neuropathol Exp Neurol 52:339–350, 1993.
21. Carpenter S: Inclusion body myositis, a review. J Neuropathol Exp Neurol 55:1105–1114, 1996.
22. Amato AA, Gronseth GS, Jackson CE, et al: Inclusion body myositis: clinical and pathological boundaries. Ann Neurol 40: 581–586, 1996.
23. Cole AJ, Kuzniecky R, Karpati G, et al: Familial myopathy with changes resembling inclusion body myositis and periventricular leucoencephalopathy. Brain 111:1025–1037, 1988.
24. Griggs RC, Askanas V, DiMauro S, et al: Inclusion body myositis and myopathies. Ann Neurol 38:705–713, 1995.
25. Lotz BP, Engel AG, Nishino H, et al: Inclusion body myositis. Brain 112:727–742, 1989.
26. Silverstein A, Siltzbach LE: Muscle involvement in sarcoidosis. Arch Neurol 21:235–241, 1969.
27. Lynch PG, Bansal DV: Granulomatous polymyositis. J Neurol Sci 18:1–9, 1973.
28. Brooke MH, Kaplan H: Muscle pathology in rheumatoid arthritis, polymyalgia rheumatica, and polymyositis. A histochemical study. Arch Pathol 94:101–118, 1972.
29. Winkelmann RK, Connolly SM, Quimby SR, et al: Histopathologic features of the L-tryptophan–related eoinophilia-myalgia (fasciitis) syndrome. Mayo Clin Proc 66:457–463, 1991.
30. Lin JD, Phelps RG, Gordon ML, et al: Pathologic manifestations of the eosinophilia myalgia syndrome: analysis of 11 cases. Hum Pathol 23:429–437, 1992.
31. Bodensteiner JB: Congenital myopathies. Muscle Nerve 17: 131–144, 1994.
32. Stauber WT, Riggs JE, Schochet SS, et al: Nemaline myopathy: evidence of dipeptidyl peptidase I deficiency. Arch Neurol 43: 39–41, 1986.
33. Dwyer BA, Mayer RF, Lee SC: Progressive nemaline (rod) myopathy as a presentation of human immunodeficiency virus infection (letter). Arch Neurol 49:440, 1992.
34. Goebel HH: Congenital myopathies. In Rowland LP, DiMauro S (eds): Handbook of Clinical Neurology, Myopathies. Vol 18. Amsterdam, Elsevier, 1992, pp 331–367.
35. Fenichel GM: Clinical Pediatric Neurology. 3rd ed. Philadelphia, WB Saunders, 1997, pp 153–175.
36. Sengers RC, Stadhouders AM, Trijbels JM: Mitochondrial myopathies. Clinical, morphological and biochemical aspects. Eur J Pediatr 141:192–207, 1984.
37. Morgan-Hughes JA: Mitochondrial myopathies. In Mastaglia FL, Walton JN (eds): Skeletal Muscle Pathology. 2nd ed. Edinburgh, Churchill Livingstone, 1992, pp 367–424.
38. Lindal S, Lund I: Mitochondrial diseases and myopathies: a series of muscle biopsy specimens with ultrastructural changes in the mitochondria. Ultrastruct Pathol 16:263–275, 1992.
39. Walker UA, Collins S, Byrne E: Respiratory chain encephalopathies: a diagnostic classification. Eur Neurol 36:260–267, 1996.
40. Rowland LP, Blake DM, Hirano M, et al: Clinical syndromes associated with ragged red fibres. Rev Neurol (Paris) 147:467–473, 1991.
41. Dalakas MC, Illa I, Pezeshkpour GH, et al: Mitochondrial myopathy caused by long-term zidovudine therapy. N Engl J Med 322:1098–1105, 1990.
42. DiMauro S, Bonilla E, Zeviani M, et al: Mitochondrial myopathies. Ann Neurol 17:521–538, 1985.
43. Brivet M, Boutron A, Slama A, et al: Defects in activation and transport of fatty acids. J Inherit Metab Dis 22:428–441, 1999.
44. DiMauro S, Bruno C: Glycogen storage diseases of muscle. Curr Opin Neurol 11:477–484, 1998.
45. Richardson EP, DeGirolami U: Pathology of the Peripheral Nerve. Major Problems in Pathology. Vol 32. Philadelphia, WB Saunders, 1995.
46. Schochet SS: Diagnostic Pathology of Skeletal Muscle and Nerve. New York, Appleton-Century-Crofts, 1986, pp 29–48.
47. Jennekens FGI: Neurogenic disorders of muscle. In Mastaglia FL, Walton JN (eds): Skeletal Muscle Pathology. 2nd ed. New York, Churchill Livingstone, 1992, pp 563–598.
48. Brooke MH, Engel WK: The histographic analysis of human muscle biopsies with regard to fiber types: 2. Diseases of the upper and lower motor neurons. Neurology 19:378–393, 1969.
49. De Reuck J, De Coster W, Van der Eecken H: The target phenomenon in rat muscle following tenotomy and neurotomy. Acta Neuropathol (Berl) 37:49–56, 1977.
50. Karpati G, Engel WK: "Type grouping" in skeletal muscles after experimental reinnervation. Neurology 18:447–455, 1968.
51. Crawford TO: From enigmatic to problematic: the new molecular genetics of childhood spinal muscular atrophy. Neurology 46:335–340, 1996.
52. Melki J: Spinal muscular atrophy. Curr Opin Neurol 10:381–385, 1997.
53. Iwasaki Y, Sugimoto H, Ikeda K, et al: Muscle morphometry in amyotrophic lateral sclerosis. Int J Neurosci 58:165–170, 1991.
54. Dyck PJ, Conn DL, Okazaki H: Necrotizing angiopathic neuropathy. Three dimensional morphology of fiber degeneration related to sites of occluded vessels. Mayo Clin Proc 47:461–475, 1972.
55. Hoffman GS, Kerr GS, Leavitt RY, et al: Wegener granulomatosis: an analysis of 158 patients. Ann Intern Med 116:488–498, 1992.
56. Nishino H, Rubino FA, DeRemee RA, et al: Neurological involvement in Wegener's granulomatosis: an analysis of 324 consecutive patients at Mayo Clinic. Ann Neurol 334:4–9, 1995.
57. Hart FD, Golding JR, Mackensie DH: Neuropathy in rheumatoid disease. Ann Rheum Dis 16:471–480, 1957.
58. Puechal X, Said G, Hilliquin P, et al: Peripheral neuropathy with necrotizing vasculitis in rheumatoid arthritis. Arthritis Rheum 38:1618–1629, 1995.
59. Hawke SHB, Davies L, Pamphlett R, et al: Vasculitic neuropathy. A clinical and pathological study. Brain 114:2175–2190, 1991.
60. Johnson, RT, Richardson EP: The neurological manifestations of systemic lupus erythematosus. A clinical-pathological study

of 24 cases and review of the literature. Medicine (Baltimore) 47:337–369, 1968.

61. McCombe PA, McLeod JG, Pollard JD, et al: Peripheral sensorimotor and autonomic neuropathy associated with systemic lupus erythematosus. Brain 110:533–549, 1987.

62. Alexander EL: Neurological disease in Sjögren's syndrome: mononuclear inflammatory vasculopathy affecting central/peripheral nervous system and muscle. Rheum Dis Clin North Am 19:869–905, 1993.

63. Moulignier A, Authier F-J, Baudrimont M, et al: Peripheral neuropathy in human immunodeficiency virus–infected pa-

tients with diffuse infiltrative lymphocytosis syndrome. Ann Neurol 41:438–445, 1997.

64. Gherardi R, Gelec L, Mhiri C, et al: The spectrum of vasculitis in human immunodeficiency virus–infected patients. Arthritis Rheum 36:1164–1174, 1993.

65. Chariot P, Gherardi R: Myopathy and HIV infection. Curr Opin Rheumatol 7:497–502, 1995.

66. Younger DS, Dalmau J, Ighirami G, et al: Anti-HU associated peripheral nerve and muscle microvasculitis. Neurology 44: 181–182, 1994.

# 54

# The Eye and Ocular Adnexa

Ian W. McLean   Lester O. Hosten

Ophthalmic pathology is limited to specimens that are generated by ophthalmologists. These include eyelid biopsy specimens, wedge (full-thickness) eyelid resections, conjunctival biopsy specimens, corneal buttons from penetrating keratoplasties, enucleated eyes, orbital tumor resections, optic nerve biopsy specimens, and orbital exenterations. Many of these specimens require special handling by the pathologist. Because many ophthalmic lesions are fairly comparable to their counterparts that occur elsewhere in the body, this chapter discusses only important lesions that do not occur elsewhere or are much more common in ophthalmic specimens than elsewhere.

## PROCESSING OPHTHALMIC SPECIMENS

Processing ophthalmic specimens is discussed in detail elsewhere,[1] but a brief overview should be helpful to pathologists who rarely handle these specimens. It is strongly recommended that a dissecting microscope be used to examine ophthalmic specimens because this provides the pathologist with similar magnification to that obtained by the ophthalmic surgeon with the operating microscope. In the gross laboratory, wedge resections of the eyelid should be cut sagittally, similar to a loaf of bread, so that each slice includes the palpebral conjunctiva and skin. The slices should be examined using a dissecting microscope for pathology. As a minimum, the medial (nasal)-most slice, the lateral (temporal)-most slice, and a central slice showing the pathology should be submitted for microscopic study. Excisional conjunctival biopsy specimens should be flattened on a piece of cardboard, then placed in fixative by the surgeon. The pathologist should inspect this specimen under a dissecting microscope for involvement of the margins of the lesion. The specimen should be sliced at approximately 2-mm intervals perpendicular to the margin that grossly appears closest to the lesion and embedded on edge. If the surgeon does not flatten the specimen, the conjunctiva tends to roll up, making identification of margins impossible.

Buttons from penetrating keratoplasties need to be examined with a dissecting microscope, looking for areas of vascularization or opacification. If these lesions are identified, the cornea should be bisected through them. If no lesion is identified, the specimen can be bisected in a random plane. Only half the cornea should be submitted, retaining the other half for special studies, if required. The technician embedding the corneal specimen should be instructed to embed all corneal specimens on edge.

Enucleated eyes need a careful gross examination because often the lesion of interest may be small compared with the whole eye and may not be included in the tissue submitted for histologic study. Based on the attachments for the extraocular muscles, the laterality usually can be identified. Transillumination to identify intraocular opacities is recom-

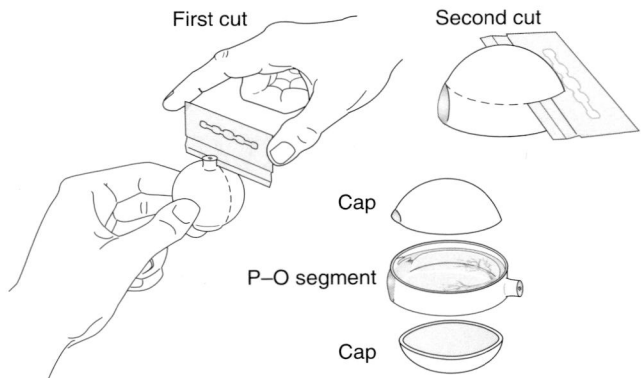

First cut · Second cut

Cap

P–O segment

Cap

**FIGURE 54–1.** Steps in gross examination of an eye for histologic processing.

mended. If no lesion is identified on external examination or transillumination, the eye should be opened in the horizontal plane so that a single section includes the pupil, optic nerve head, and macular area. It is worthwhile to get into the habit of always opening eyes the same way. When opening horizontally, we usually remove the superior cap first, and when opening vertically, we first remove the temporal cap. The caps are removed by slicing the globe from a point on the sclera adjacent to the optic nerve forward to exit the globe on the same side approximately halfway between the limbus and the center of the cornea (Fig. 54–1). This process allows viewing the specimen from a known direction, facilitating orientation. The following gross findings should be noted: dimensions of the eye; cornea and optic nerve length; character of the cornea; contents of anterior chamber; openness of the chamber angle; opacification of the lens; any mass in the vitreous, retina, subretinal space, or choroids; presence of subretinal exudates; cupping of the optic disk; and character of the cut section of optic nerve. After the internal examination, a second cap should be removed in the same way as the first by a cut parallel to the first cut starting on the other side of the optic nerve. The central disk of tissue should be submitted and embedded with instructions to the technician to "rough cut" until the histologic section contains the pupil and the optic nerve.

Orbital tumor resections need careful attention to margins as is true with optic nerve tumors. In the optic nerve, the dura mater provides a barrier to spread of the tumor, so the proximal and distal margins always should be examined histologically. After inspecting the dura mater for any defects, the remainder of the specimen can be examined with either multiple cross-sections or longitudinal sections.

Orbital exenteration specimens always require special handling. After examining the specimen to determine laterality and the character of the periosteum covering the orbital portion of the specimen and the conjunctiva and lids anteriorly, we recommend slicing the specimen sagittally in five or more 6- to 8-mm-thick pieces. Each slice should be examined for pathology. Often exenteration specimens are not completely fixed, and repeat formalin fixation of the slices may be necessary for preparation of good sections. If a tumor is suspected, the nasal and temporal margins should be examined in the end slices with multiple sections perpendicular to the original slices. We prefer to process the central slices that show the pathology in their entirety, but if the histology laboratory is unable to process such large blocks, they can be divided into smaller pieces. Attention must be given, however, to demonstration of the location of possible involvement of the margins.

## EYELID PATHOLOGY

In the eyelid, sebaceous carcinoma is the lesion that best fits the category of a unique or common lesion. Basal cell carcinoma is a more common eyelid malignancy, but basal cell carcinoma of the eyelid does not differ significantly from basal cell carcinoma elsewhere in the skin.[2] Sebaceous carcinoma arises much more often in the skin of the eyelid than elsewhere. Most sebaceous carcinomas of the eyelid arise in the meibomian (tarsal) glands. The second most common site of origin is the sebaceous glands of the lashes (glands of Zeis). Much less frequently, sebaceous carcinoma may originate from the sebaceous glands in the caruncle or the skin of the eyebrow. The upper eyelid is involved in about two thirds of cases, probably because the meibomian glands are more numerous in the upper tarsus than in the lower. Some tumors seem to originate from the meibomian glands and the glands of Zeis, whereas in others the exact site of origin cannot be determined. In advanced cases, the upper and lower eyelids may be involved.[3]

### Clinical Features

Sebaceous gland carcinomas affect elderly patients with a median age at diagnosis of 64 years. Except for one study of 40 cases,[4] all large series have shown a female preponderance. In a series of 104 patients from the Registry of Ophthalmic Pathology, 60% were female.[3] About two thirds of 156 cases reported from Shanghai were female.[5] Sebaceous gland carcinoma most commonly begins as a small, firm nodule resembling a chalazion. Frequently, it appears as an atypical or recurring chalazion, with a rubbery consistency. Patients with a more advanced meibomian gland carcinoma may have a diffuse, plaquelike thickening of the tarsus or a fungating or papillomatous growth involving the lid margin or palpebral conjunctiva. Lesions originating from the glands of Zeis appear as small, yellowish nodules located at the lid margin just in front of the gray line. A characteristic finding with sebaceous carcinoma arising in either meibomian or Zeis glands is loss of lashes caused by intraepithelial neoplastic invasion of the follicles. Carcinomas of the sebaceous

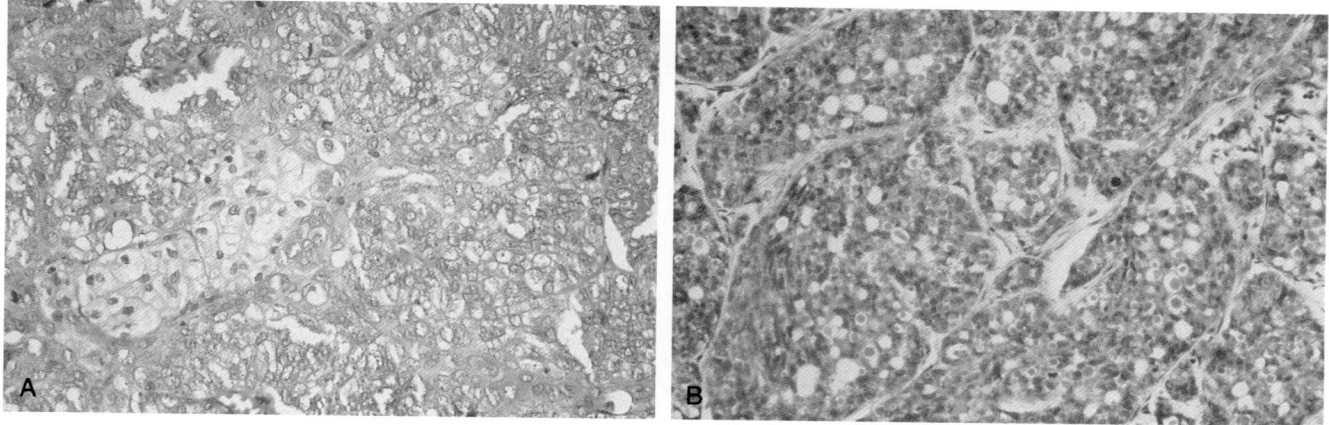

**FIGURE 54–2.** Sebaceous cell carcinoma. *A.* Undifferentiated sebaceous cells with pleomorphic nuclei and amphophilic cytoplasm surround well-differentiated neoplastic sebaceous cells with abundant vacuolated cytoplasm that has a foamy or frothy appearance. *B.* Oil red O stain for lipid with marked positivity within cytoplasmic vacuoles of neoplastic cells.

glands of the caruncle are usually grayish yellow masses covered by an intact epithelium.

A distinctive clinical feature of many sebaceous gland carcinomas is a persistent unilateral conjunctivitis, blepharitis, meibomianitis, or blepharoconjunctivitis. This clinical picture has been referred to as the *masquerade syndrome.*[6] This appearance is caused by invasion of sebaceous carcinoma cells into the conjunctival epithelium, which invokes an inflammatory response. Many patients with diffuse pagetoid invasion or carcinoma in situ–like changes involving the skin of the lids, the conjunctiva, and the cornea require orbital exenteration.

## Histologic Features

Sebaceous carcinoma can be classified by degree of differentiation into three groups. Well-differentiated tumors have a lobular pattern with cells in the center of the lobules exhibiting sebaceous differentiation

(Fig. 54–2*A*). These cells have an abundant, finely vacuolated cytoplasm that appears foamy or frothy. The nuclei are centrally placed. Moderately differentiated tumors show only a few areas of highly differentiated sebaceous cells. Most of the tumor is composed of anaplastic cells with hyperchromatic nuclei and prominent nucleoli and abundant amphophilic cytoplasm. In poorly differentiated tumors, most of the cells exhibit pleomorphic nuclei, with prominent nucleoli and amphophilic cytoplasm. These tumors often show moderate mitotic activity, and the mitotic figures may be atypical or bizarre. Frozen sections, which may be performed on formalin-fixed tissue, and oil red O stain for lipid may be necessary to establish an unequivocal diagnosis (Fig. 54–2*B*).

Sebaceous carcinoma can have a variety of histologic patterns.[3] The most common pattern is lobular (Fig. 54–3*A*). In the lobular pattern, the neoplastic cells form well-demarcated lobules of variable size. The lobules exhibit basaloid features but lack the

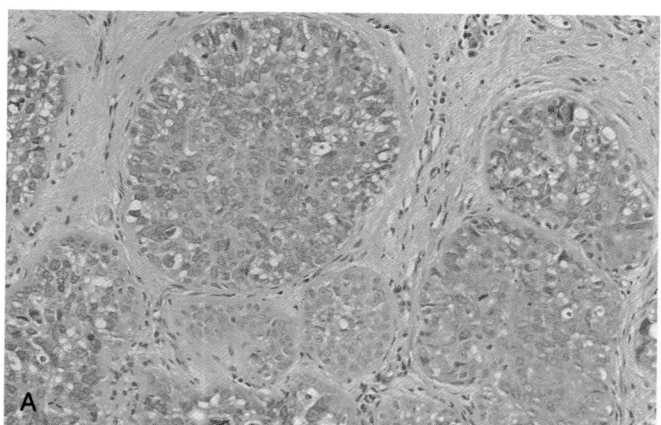
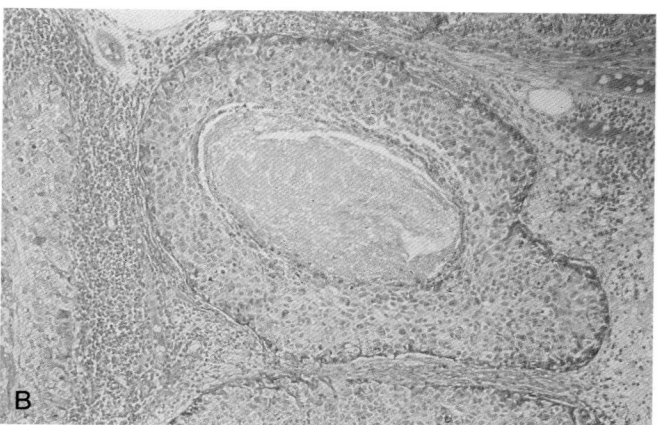

**FIGURE 54–3.** Sebaceous cell carcinoma. *A.* Lobular pattern with well defined lobules of neoplastic cells. *B.* Comedocarcinoma pattern with neoplastic cells arranged in large lobules with central necrosis.

peripheral palisading that is characteristic of a basal cell carcinoma. In better differentiated tumors, the cells in the centers of the lobules undergo sebaceous differentiation. Sebaceous tumors with the comedo-carcinoma pattern have larger lobules with prominent central foci of necrosis (Fig. 54–3B). The central necrotic tumor cells usually stain intensely for lipid. Tumors that erode from the tarsus to involve the conjunctival surface or less commonly the cutaneous surface may have a papillary pattern. These tumors resemble a squamous cell papilloma or carcinoma, but careful histologic examination usually reveals foci of sebaceous differentiation. Poorly differentiated tumors can have an infiltrative pattern that may be confused with a morphea-form basal cell carcinoma. Tumors often have mixed patterns. Most common is the mixture of lobular and comedocarcinoma-like areas, but any combination of patterns may be seen.

## Modes of Spread

Intraepithelial spread to the conjunctiva, cornea, or skin of the eyelids is observed frequently in sebaceous gland carcinoma. Intraepithelial spread can have two patterns: pagetoid and carcinoma in situ–like.[40, 41] The term *pagetoid* is used because it resembles the invasion of a ductal carcinoma of the breast into the epidermis of the nipple and surrounding areola in Paget's disease of the breast. The neoplastic cells in pagetoid spread invade the overlying epithelium as single cells or as small nests of cells that typically do not form intercellular bridges with the surrounding normal squamous epithelial cells. Pagetoid cells have hyperchromatic nuclei and abundant vacuolated cytoplasm that contains variable amounts of lipid (Fig. 54–4A).

The carcinoma in situ–like spread by sebaceous gland carcinoma cells is usually a diffuse process, with full-thickness replacement of surface epithelium by neoplastic cells (Fig. 54–4B). In the conjunctiva,

these changes frequently are misinterpreted as intra-epithelial (in situ) squamous cell carcinoma. Primary intraepithelial carcinoma of the palpebral conjunctiva is exceedingly rare, and in situ tumors in the palpebral conjunctiva should be considered secondary spread of sebaceous carcinoma from the eyelid until proved otherwise.[7]

Sebaceous carcinoma may spread by direct extension into the adjacent structures (lacrimal gland, orbit, paranasal sinuses, intracranial cavity).[3, 5, 8] Moderate to poorly differentiated tumors with infiltrative growth may have perineural infiltration and invasion of lymphatics. Among the 95 patients studied by Rao and colleagues,[9] 22 developed metastases to the preauricular and cervical lymph nodes. Some patients may present with a large preauricular mass and a relatively small primary eyelid tumor.

## Prognosis and Management

In the series of cases reported by Rao and colleagues,[9] the recurrence rate was 33%. Direct orbital invasion occurred in 19% of cases and metastases to preauricular or cervical lymph nodes or both in 23% of cases; 22 patients died as a result of the tumor. Distant metastases involving the lungs, liver, brain, and skull often were associated with previous or simultaneous regional lymph node metastases.

Rao and colleagues[3] analyzed the prognostic significance of the location and size of the sebaceous gland tumor, its site of origin, the duration of symptoms before excision, and the histologic pattern and degree of cellular differentiation. They concluded that a worse prognosis is indicated by origin of the tumor in the upper eyelid; size of 10 mm or more in maximal diameter; origin from the meibomian glands; duration of symptoms for more than 6 months; an infiltrative growth pattern; moderate-to-poor sebaceous differentiation; and invasion of lymphatic channels, vascular structures, and the orbit.

Early diagnosis and adequate treatment with

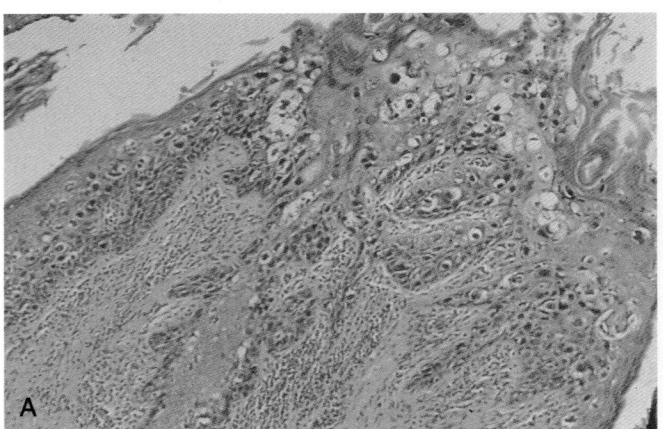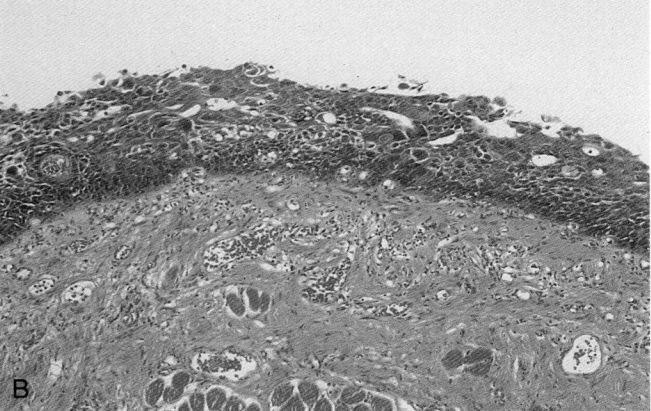

**FIGURE 54–4.** Sebaceous cell carcinoma. *A.* Skin: Pagetoid spread with invasion of overlying epithelium by cells with hyperchromatic nuclei and vacuolated cytoplasm. *B.* Conjunctiva: Carcinoma-in-situ spread with full thickness replacement of surface epithelium by neoplastic cells.

primary, wide surgical excision seem to improve the prognosis significantly. Because of the relatively high recurrence rate of incompletely excised sebaceous gland carcinoma, frozen section control is recommended to insure complete excision of the tumor. Because of the skip areas that occur with pagetoid invasion, Mohs' surgical technique has been less successful in the management of sebaceous carcinoma than basal cell carcinoma.[10] Sebaceous carcinoma is relatively radioresistant, and radiotherapy is unlikely to control the disease.[11] Radiation may be used for palliation in elderly patients with large tumors who are unable to tolerate extensive radical surgery.[9, 11] Removal of involved regional lymph nodes has resulted in long-term survival of some patients.[3]

## CORNEAL BUTTON PATHOLOGY

The subject of corneal pathology may be foreign to the general pathologist. In the cornea, the most common pathologic condition is loss of transparency. Understanding loss of corneal transparency requires knowing the physiologic processes that cause the cornea to be transparent. The cornea is composed mostly of collagen, and collagen is normally an opaque white tissue. Three features that are unique to corneal collagen make it transparent. First, the diameter of the bundles of collagen fibers in the cornea is much more uniform than elsewhere in the body. Second, the ground substance that surrounds the corneal collagen fibers has a greater concentration of keratan sulfate than elsewhere. Third, the corneal collagen fibers are less hydrated than elsewhere. Deturgescence is maintained in the cornea by its epithelium and endothelium. The corneal epithelium provides a barrier that prevents diffusion of water into the cornea from the tears, and the endothelium provides a pump that actively removes water from the corneal stroma. If any of these features of the cornea is altered, loss of transparency occurs.

## Loss of Corneal Transparency

With the exception of keratoconus, all corneal transplants are performed because of loss of transparency. In keratoconus, the shape of the cornea is abnormal resulting in a distorted visual image. Even in keratoconus, scarring resulting from contact lens use or complications of the disease, such as rupture of Descemet's membrane and hydrops, can cause loss of transparency.

A common reason for loss of corneal transparency is a scar resulting from an old infection or injury. In the scar, the collagen bundles are irregular in size, and keratan sulfate is replaced with dermatan sulfate resulting in opacification. Although the cornea is normally an avascular organ, many corneal scars become vascularized so that the presence of blood vessels in the cornea is an indication of scarring.

The most common cause of loss of corneal transparency requiring transplantation is damage to the corneal endothelium resulting from cataract extract. When this damage results in loss of a critical number of endothelial cells, the remaining cells no longer can pump a sufficient quantity of water out of the cornea to maintain the required dehydration, and the cornea becomes diffusely hazy. Water also collects between the corneal epithelium and Bowman's layer forming bullae. These subepithelial bullae are painful, and this condition is diagnosed as aphakic or pseudophakic bullous keratopathy, depending on whether a prosthetic intraocular lens (pseudophakos) was implanted during the cataract surgery (Fig. 54–5).

The histopathologic findings in aphakic or pseudophakic bullous keratopathy consist of subepithelial bullae, which can be distinguished from artifactitious separations of the corneal epithelium because in bullae the basal layer of the corneal epithelium is flattened; edema of the corneal stroma, which is characterized by swelling of the collagen bundles that obliterates the artifactitious spaces seen between the bundles in the normal cornea; normal or only slightly thickened Descemet's membrane; and a reduction in the number of and thinning of the remaining endothelial cells as they stretch to cover the posterior surface of the cornea. In an 8-$\mu$ histologic section from the center of a healthy adult cornea, there are at least 14 endothelial cell nuclei per 0.4-mm length (width of standard 40× field). In decompensated, hydrated corneas, the number of nuclei usually is reduced to less than 10 per 0.4-mm length. The finding of a normal Descemet's membrane is important because it rules out Fuchs' dystrophy. Fuchs' dystrophy is a chronic process in which the endothelial cells are lost over a long period. During this period, the sick endothelial cells lay down excessive amounts of basement membrane and collagen causing thickening, lamination, and ex-

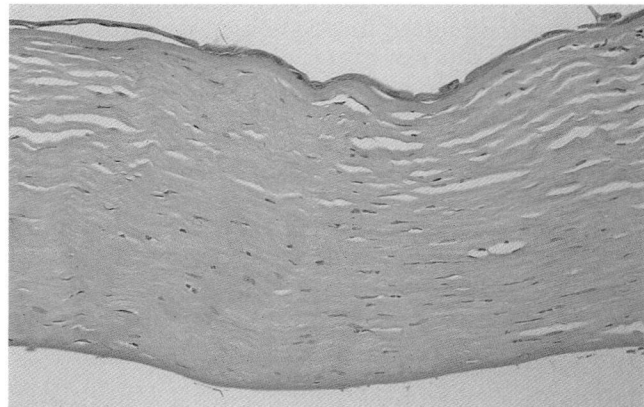

**FIGURE 54–5.** Bullous keratopathy. Corneal button with moderately edematous stroma, loss of endothelium and subepithelial bullae.

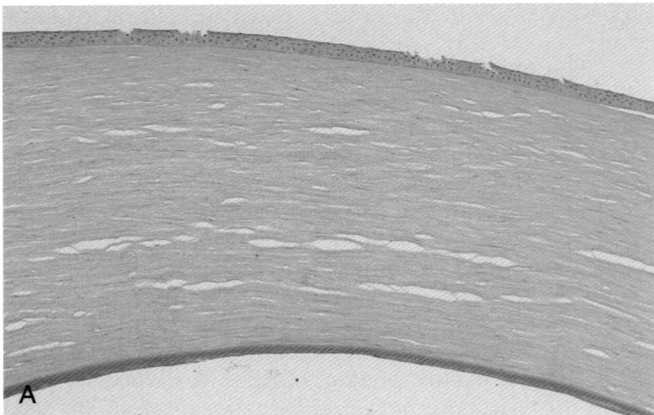 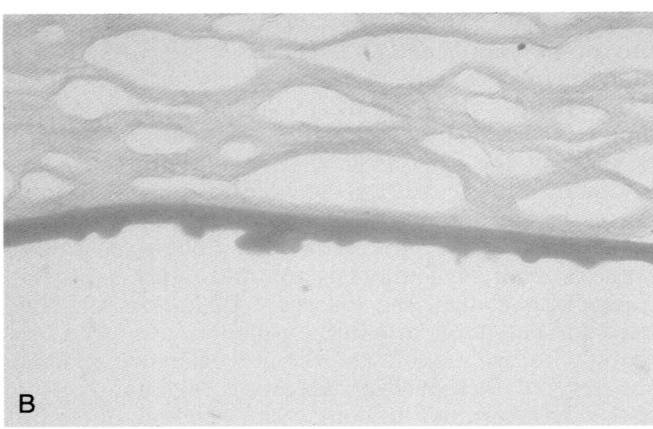

**FIGURE 54–6.** Fuchs' endothelial dystrophy. *A.* Corneal button with epithelial and stromal edema, thickened Descemet's membrane with embedded excrescences and loss of endothelial cells. *B.* Higher magnification of another specimen exhibiting thickened laminated Descemet's membrane with excrescences and absence of endothelial cells.

crescences of Descemet's membrane (Fig. 54–6). Because Fuchs' dystrophy and cataracts primarily affect elderly people, it is common to see cases in which cataract extraction exacerbates subclinical Fuchs' dystrophy to cause corneal decompensation. Because Fuchs' dystrophy is a bilateral disease, the fellow cornea may be predisposed to failure.

## PATHOLOGY OF ENUCLEATED EYES

Eyes are enucleated for only two reasons: 1) if they are blind and painful and 2) if they are suspected of containing a tumor. A pathologic description of all the entities in the differential diagnosis of the blind painful eye is beyond the scope of this chapter, but a few generalities are of interest. Retinal vascular disease is the leading cause of a blind painful eye, followed by trauma, endophthalmitis, and tumors. In all of these conditions, the final event causing pain in the blind eye is often secondary angle closure, which blocks the outflow of aqueous humor from the eye, resulting in elevated intraocular pressure and glaucoma. A variety of mechanisms lead to angle closure, but the most common is neovascularization of the anterior surface of the iris, referred to clinically as rubeosis iridis (Fig. 54–7). This fibrovascular membrane adheres to surrounding structures and undergoes contraction, causing an adhesion to form between the iris and cornea closing the anterior chamber angle. This condition is diagnosed as peripheral anterior synechia. The two most important intraocular tumors are retinoblastoma and uveal malignant melanoma.

## RETINOBLASTOMA AND RETINOCYTOMA

Retinoblastoma is a rare malignant tumor with a prevalence of about 1 in 20,000 live births. In 100

years, retinoblastoma has changed from an almost uniformly fatal disease to one in which 95% of patients are cured. The genetic cause of retinoblastoma is the loss of both alleles of a normal tumor-suppressor gene (the *RB1* gene) on the long arm of chromosome 13. This gene, classified as a recessive oncogene or antioncogene,[12] has been cloned.[13, 14] Researchers have discovered that mutations of the *RB1* gene play a role in the development of a wide variety of cancers in addition to retinoblastoma.[15, 16]

Retinoblastomas vary greatly in differentiation. Flexner-Wintersteiner rosettes were considered the highest degree of differentiation before 1969, when Tso and coworkers[17] described cytologically benign cells in retinoblastomas. They observed foci of benign-appearing cells that individually or in small bouquet-like clusters (fleurettes) exhibited photoreceptor differentiation.[18, 19] In most instances, such areas of benign-appearing tumor cells represented only a small component within an otherwise typical retinoblastoma, but rare tumors were composed en-

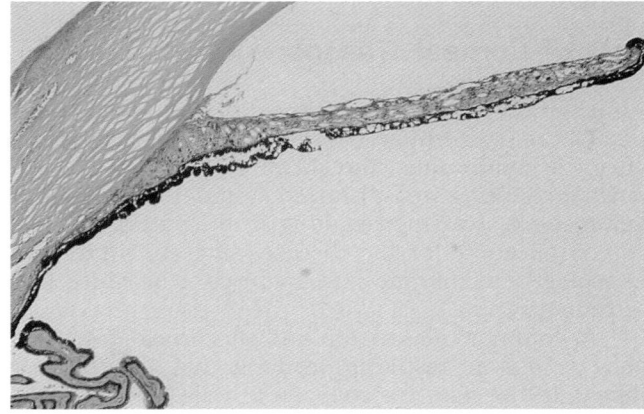

**FIGURE 54–7.** Diabetes mellitus. Anterior segment features including iris neovascularization (rubeosis iridis), ectropion uveae, vacuolization of iris pigment epithelium and peripheral anterior synechiae which cause secondary angle-closure glaucoma.

tirely of cells with benign cytologic features.[19] In 1983, Margo and associates[20] introduced the term *retinocytoma* for these tumors. This classification was patterned after neural tumors of the pineal: pineoblastoma for the malignant group and pineocytoma for the more highly differentiated and comparatively benign group.[21]

Based on long-term clinical observations, Gallie and coworkers[22] introduced a different name, *retinoma,* for small, often partially calcified retinal tumors exhibiting no growth. Although they studied 36 eyes with such lesions clinically, none was examined histologically. It seems clear, however, that the tumors they studied clinically are identical to the retinocytomas of Margo and associates.[20]

## Epidemiology and Genetics

Retinoblastoma is worldwide in distribution, affecting all racial groups without sex predilection. Analysis of data from the Netherlands,[23] Japan,[24] and United States[25] has shown that the incidence of retinoblastoma has been stable over periods of 10 to 20 years. Schipper[23] also showed that from 1920 through 1969, there was no change in the proportion of bilateral cases, which remained at about 33%. In Japan, 34% of the cases were bilateral.[24] In cases from the Registry of Ophthalmic Pathology obtained between 1922 and 1959, the prevalence of bilateral retinoblastoma was lower (21%)[26]. This lower prevalence is probably because of treatment or referral bias.

The incidence of retinoblastoma decreases with age, with most cases being diagnosed before age 3 years. Retinoblastoma has been observed in premature infants and term infants. In a series of 760 cases on file in the Registry of Ophthalmic Pathology, only five patients were older than 10 years of age,[27] and rarely the tumor does occur in adults.

Retinoblastoma can arise either as a germinal mutation or as a somatic mutation of the *RB1* gene. Multiple primary retinoblastomas, whether in one or both eyes, always result from a germinal mutation. Patients with a germinal mutation have the heritable type of retinoblastoma. Patients with a somatic mutation do not pass retinoblastoma to their children, which indicates that they have nonheritable retinoblastoma. The median age at the time of diagnosis of bilateral retinoblastoma is significantly less than for unilateral retinoblastoma.[26] Knudson[28] used age incidence data for patients with unilateral and bilateral retinoblastomas to formulate his *two-hit hypothesis.* He postulated that the development of any retinoblastoma requires two complementary tumor-inducing events to convert a normal retinal cell into a neoplastic cell. In cases of heritable retinoblastoma, the first mutation is in the germ cell, and every cell in the patient has the first hit. The second hit occurs in the somatic cell, which gives rise to the retinoblastoma. In nonheritable retinoblastoma, both hits must occur in the same somatic cell, which explains why patients with nonheritable retinoblastoma are older than patients with the heritable type.

With a germinal mutation, every cell of the body has one mutant allele of the RB-protein gene or one hit in Knudson's theory. Because there are at least 200 million cells in the developing retina, even though the probability of the second mutation occurring in any given cell is low, the chance of at least 1 of the 200 million cells developing the second hit is high. Only 5% to 10% of patients who are carriers of a mutation of the *RB* gene do not develop a retinoblastoma, 25% to 35% have unilateral retinoblastoma, and 60% to 75% have bilateral tumors. From these data, Knudson[28] estimated that the mean number of tumors in patients carrying the retinoblastoma mutation is between three and four. In Japan,[24] the average number of tumors in cases of bilateral retinoblastoma was 3.7, which is consistent with Knudson's estimate.

An additional major difference between patients with heritable and nonheritable retinoblastoma is that survivors of heritable retinoblastoma[16, 29–32] are highly susceptible to the development of other nonocular cancers. Based on data from the American Registry of Ophthalmic Pathology on patients with bilateral retinoblastoma, Roarty and coworkers[16] estimated that the 30-year cumulative incidence rate for nonocular tumors was 26%, which is in general agreement with data from large tumor registries from around the world.[30–32] For patients who received radiation, the 30-year incidence rate was 35%, and for patients who did not receive radiation therapy, it was 6%.[16] The most common tumors developing within and outside of the field of radiation were sarcomas, with osteogenic sarcomas being the most prevalent. It has been estimated that osteosarcoma of the lower extremities occurs 500-fold more frequently in survivors of bilateral retinoblastoma than in children who are not carriers of the mutant *RB* gene. Intracranial tumors, which resemble retinoblastoma closely, occur far more frequently in the pineal or in a parasellar location in patients with heritable retinoblastoma than in other patients.[33–35] The association of these intracranial tumors with bilateral retinoblastoma has been designated *trilateral retinoblastoma.*

Familial cases represent heritable retinoblastoma in which there is another family member affected. Less than 10% of cases of retinoblastomas are familial in the Registry of Ophthalmic Pathology, and in some underdeveloped countries where there are virtually no survivors, there are few familial cases. The remainder are sporadic, but this is a heterogeneous group: About one fourth of the sporadic group are heritable tumors arisen in patients with new germinal mutations; the remainder are nonheritable tumors derived from two somatic mutations in a retinal cell. Analysis of DNA polymorphism within the *RB* gene is being used to predict the risk of heritable retinoblastoma.[36]

Patients with chromosomal deletion retinoblastoma represent a subclass of patients with heritable retinoblastoma in which the germinal mutation affects more than the *RB* gene. These patients have an observable defect in one of the long arms of chromosome 13 involving the q14 band. In addition to retinoblastoma, these children typically have various somatic and mental developmental abnormalities.[37] When the q14 band is not included in the deleted segment, there is no retinoblastoma. This observation directed attention to the 13q14 band as the locus for the *RB* gene. This is the least common form of retinoblastoma. Deletions within the *RB* gene are much more frequent. Analysis of DNA in one series of 49 retinoblastomas revealed deletions within the *RB* gene in 12 tumors.[38]

## Clinical Features

The clinical manifestations of retinoblastoma vary with the stage of the disease. In the past and currently in underdeveloped regions, far advanced retinoblastoma with extraocular extension is still the rule. Common presenting symptoms in such cases are a fungating mass prolapsed through a corneal perforation, proptosis caused by massive posterior orbital invasion, buphthalmos from advanced secondary glaucoma, neurologic manifestations related to brain or leptomeningeal involvement, and enlarged preauricular or submandibular lymph nodes from metastasis. Before 1900, advanced retinoblastoma was observed commonly in Europe and North America. With improvement in the general medical education of the public, greater awareness on the part of physicians of the early signs of retinoblastoma, and increased availability of eye care, advanced cases now are seldom seen in Europe and the United States. In Shields and Shields'[39] review of 60 consecutive new cases seen between 1974 and 1978, none of the retinoblastomas had extraocular extension, buphthalmos, or manifestations of metastatic disease. In four cases, the tumor was asymptomatic, having been discovered on a routine examination.[39]

Today in most of North America, Japan, and Europe, most retinoblastomas are discovered when someone, usually a parent, notices the abnormal appearance of one or both pupils (Fig. 54–8). In Shields and Shields'[39] review of 60 consecutive cases, 90% had leukocoria. The pupil usually appeared white, pink, or grayish yellow. Strabismus was present in 35% of the cases. Other presenting signs observed in only a few cases included a dilated fixed pupil, hyphema, and heterochromia iridis. In the series from Japan,[24] the initial symptom was leukocoria in 60% of the patients and strabismus in 13%.

Leukocoria is most frequently the consequence of a retrolental mass, but a discrete intraretinal tumor situated at the posterior pole also may reflect light back, producing a white pupil. All leukocorias are not indicative of retinoblastoma because a broad spectrum of developmental, inflammatory, degenerative, and other pathologic conditions may be de-

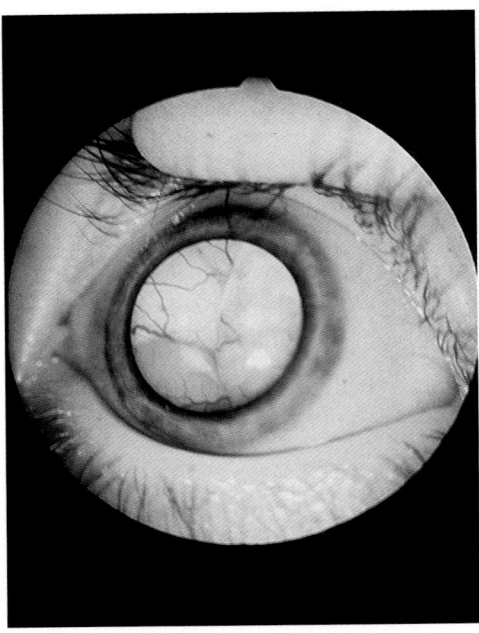

**FIGURE 54–8.** Leukocoria. Clinical appearance of leukocoria caused by retinal detachment as a result of a retinoblastoma exhibiting exophytic growth pattern into the subretinal space.

tected as a result of leukocoria. Computed tomography (CT) scanning of patients with retinoblastoma can aid in determining the size, location, and calcification of the tumor and can be used to detect macroscopic extraocular extension, but microscopic spread within the optic nerve beyond the lamina cribrosa is detected better with fat-suppressed magnetic resonance imaging than with CT.[40]

Small, often calcified tumors, typically found in eyes retaining useful vision, have been identified as retinocytomas.[20, 22, 41] These tumors have an ophthalmoscopic appearance that is similar to retinoblastomas that previously had been treated by radiation and undergone regression, and some authors consider retinocytomas to be spontaneously regressed retinoblastomas.[42, 43] This interpretation seems less likely because spontaneous regression usually occurs in a larger tumor and results in phthisis bulbi.[44] Gallie and coworkers[22] have described the clinical appearance of retinocytomas as a comparatively small homogeneous, translucent, gray, slightly elevated plaque shaped mass with functional retinal blood vessels looping into the mass in 90% of cases. Within the mass, there are opaque, white calcified flecks having the appearance of cottage cheese (78% of cases), and in areas underlying or adjacent to the tumor, there is atrophy, proliferation, and migration of retinal pigment epithelium (56% of cases).

Retinocytomas usually occur in a functional eye with clear media and no retinal detachment. Retinocytomas may be observed unilaterally in nongenetic or bilaterally in genetically determined cases of retinoblastoma.[22] Eagle and colleagues[45] reported a case of a retinocytoma that remained stationary for 3 years, then grew rapidly. Histologic examination revealed a typical retinocytoma except in the area where the growth occurred. In this location, the cytology was that of a poorly differentiated retinoblastoma, suggesting malignant transformation of the benign retinocytoma. This scenario may explain the rare cases of retinoblastoma that occur in adults.

## Pathologic Features

The gross features of intraocular retinoblastoma depend on the growth pattern of the tumor. Five growth patterns are recognized in retinoblastomas, which explain certain clinical variations and differences in intraocular and extraocular spread:

1. *Endophytic retinoblastomas* grow mainly from the inner surface of the retina into the vitreous. On ophthalmoscopic examination, the tumor is viewed directly. Retinal vessels typically are lost from view as they enter the tumor. As endophytic tumors grow large and become friable, tumor cells tend to be shed from the tumor into the vitreous, where they grow into separate tiny spheroidal masses that appear as fluff balls or cotton balls. The spheroidal masses of tumor can mimic inflammatory conditions, such as mycotic or nematodal endophthalmitis. Tumor cells in the vitreous may seed onto the inner surface of the retina, where they may invade into the retina. It is important to distinguish multicentric retinoblastoma from retinal seeding because the presence of multicentric tumors indicates a germinal mutation. Although this distinction is frequently difficult or impossible, some clues are helpful. If one can discern that the tumor lies mainly on the inner surface of the retina rather than within it or if one can see tumor cell clusters within the vitreous, such observations would suggest that retinal seeding has occurred. Tumor cells in the vitreous also may spread into the posterior chamber, then into the anterior chamber by aqueous flow. Secondary deposits on the lens, zonular fibers, ciliary epithelium, iris, corneal endothelium, and trabecular meshwork may be observed, and tumor cells may follow the aqueous outflow pathways out of the eye. In such cases, the anterior segment changes may be misinterpreted clinically as those of granulomatous iridocyclitis.

2. *Exophytic retinoblastomas* grow primarily from the outer retinal surface toward the choroid, producing first an elevation, then a detachment of the retina. On ophthalmoscopic examination, the tumor is viewed through the retina, and the retinal vessels course over the tumor. As the tumor grows larger, it may give rise to total retinal detachment, and tumor cells may escape into the subretinal exudate. Secondary implants may develop on the outer retinal surface, where they can invade into the retina or onto the inner surface of the retinal pigment epithelium. Then the implants may replace the pigment epithelium and eventually infiltrate through Bruch's membrane into the choroid. From the choroid, tumor cells may escape along ciliary vessels and nerves into the orbit and conjunctiva. From the orbit and conjunctiva, they can gain access to blood vessels and lymphatics and metastasize.

3. *Mixed endophytic-exophytic tumors* are probably more common than either purely endophytic or exophytic retinoblastomas, especially among the larger tumors. The combined features of endophytic and exophytic growth characterize these tumors.

4. *Diffuse infiltrating retinoblastomas* are the least common and often give rise to the greatest difficulty in clinical diagnosis.[46–48] The tumors grow diffusely within the periphery of the retina without greatly thickening it. Tumor cells are discharged into the vitreous often with seeding of the anterior chamber, producing a pseudohypopyon. Because of the absence of a mass, this type of retinoblastoma masquerades as a retinitis, vitritis, or *Toxocara* endophthalmitis. With anterior chamber involvement, hyperacute iritis with hypopyon, juvenile xanthogranuloma, or tuberculosis may be suspected.[48]

5. *Complete spontaneous regression* is believed to occur more frequently in retinoblastoma than in any other malignant neoplasm.[22] Typically, there is a severe inflammatory reaction followed by phthisis bulbi.[44] The mechanisms by which regression occurs are unknown. In several cases from the American Registry of Ophthalmic Pathology, bilateral retinoblastoma was observed in which there was total necrosis and phthisis bulbi on one side, whereas on the other side, a viable tumor massively filled the eye and invaded the orbit.[44] Such cases would seem to exclude the possibility of a systemic mechanism for tumor necrosis (e.g., production of antibodies against the tumor, a circulating toxin, or hypercalcemia). Occlusion of the central retinal artery has been observed in eyes with necrotic retinoblastomas, but whether this occurs before or after the tumor becomes necrotic cannot be established.

Histologically, retinoblastomas are malignant neuroblastic tumors that may arise in any of the nucleated retinal layers. The predominant cell has a large hyperchromatic basophilic nucleus of variable size and shape and scanty cytoplasm. Mitotic figures are typically numerous. The tumor cells have a striking tendency to outgrow their blood supply. Characteristically, especially in large tumors, sleeves of viable cells are present along dilated blood vessels. As the tumor cells become displaced more than 90 to 110$\mu$ away from the vessel, they undergo ischemic coagulative necrosis[23, 49] (Fig. 54–9). Although this is a relatively constant finding from one tumor to the next, Burnier and associates[49] showed an inverse relationship between the thickness of the cuff and the mitotic activity within the cuff. The cuff thickness of 100$\mu$ represents the approximate distance that oxygen can diffuse before it is consumed completely in a rapidly growing neoplasm.

When viable tumor cells are shed into the vitre-

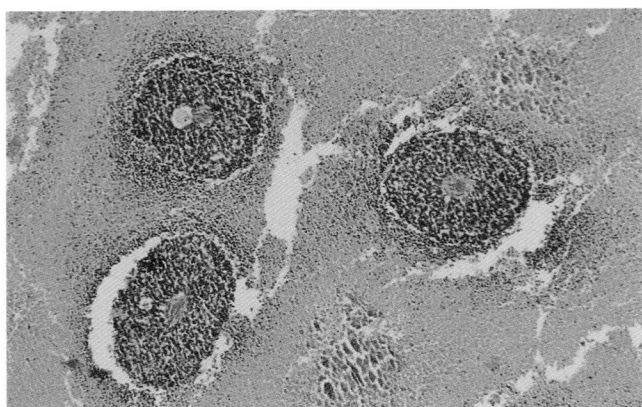

FIGURE 54–9. Retinoblastoma. Retinoblastoma displaying perivascular cuffs of viable tumor cells surrounded by necrotic (pink) cells, which are beyond the reach of oxygen diffusion from the vessels. The necrotic tissue has focal calcification.

ous or into subretinal fluid, they may grow into spheroidal aggregates with diameters that rarely exceed 1 mm.[23] Cells that are more peripherally situated derive their nutrition from the vitreous or subretinal fluid, and more central cells undergo necrosis. This represents the opposite situation from the cuffs of viable tumor cells that surround the vessels in retinoblastomas. If viable cells in the vitreous or subretinal space become attached to the retina, they may invade the retina. They gain oxygen from the retinal vasculature and release vascular growth factors that stimulate the proliferation of capillaries from the retina into the tumor. Similarly, tumor cells in the subretinal exudate may grow onto the inner surface of the retinal pigment epithelium, remaining viable by deriving nutrition from the choriocapillaris.

Almost without exception, the tumor's intrinsic blood vessels cannot keep pace with the prolifera-

tion of the neoplastic cells. The implication is that at this stage, the growth rate of the tumor is limited by the ability of the tumor to induce new vessel formation. Extensive areas of coagulative necrosis result. Foci of calcification occur frequently within the areas of necrosis. In most instances, the necrotic portions of retinoblastomas do not seem to provoke much of an inflammatory response. With marked necrosis, the DNA liberated from the tumor's nuclei may become absorbed preferentially in the walls of blood vessels and by the internal limiting membrane of the retina, giving hematoxylin and Feulgen staining to these tissues.[50] One also may observe similar basophilic staining of the lens capsule, vessels in the iris, or the tissues adjacent to Schlemm's canal, indicating that some of the disintegrated DNA escapes into the aqueous.

The formation of Flexner-Wintersteiner rosettes is highly characteristic of retinoblastomas. Pineoblastoma and medulloepithelioma are the only other neoplasms in which Flexner-Wintersteiner rosettes have been observed. The Flexner-Wintersteiner rosette represents differentiation by the tumor, but the cells of the rosettes are not benign. Characteristically, Flexner-Wintersteiner rosettes are found within areas of undifferentiated malignant cells exhibiting mitotic activity, and the cells that form rosettes may contain mitotic figures. Some rosettes are incompletely formed, and the cells blend with the surrounding undifferentiated cells.

The typical Flexner-Wintersteiner rosette (Fig. 54–10A) is lined by tall cuboidal cells that circumscribe an apical lumen. The basal ends of the cells that form the rosettes contain the nuclei. Terminal bars hold the apical ends of the cuboidal cells together, and the cells may have apical cytoplasmic projections into the lumen of the rosette. Electron microscopy has shown that these projections represent primitive inner and outer segments, and these cells represent an attempt by the tumor to form

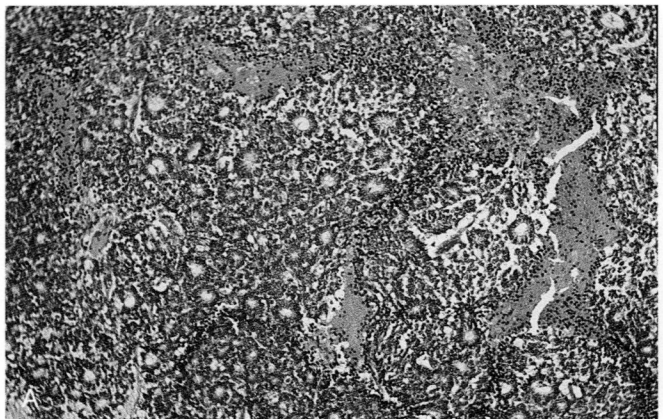
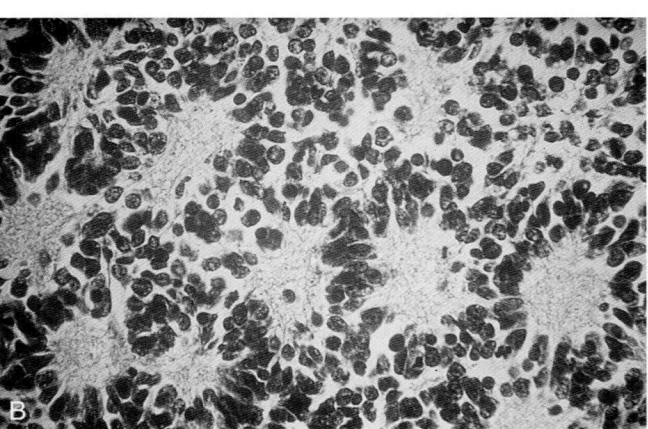

FIGURE 54–10. Retinoblastoma. *A.* Retinoblastoma cells arranged in characteristic Flexner-Wintersteiner rosettes where a central lumen is lined by cuboidal tumor cells with basally located nuclei. *B.* Homer-Wright rosettes, less commonly found in and less specific for retinoblastoma, are characterized by tumor cells arranged around a cobweb-like tangle of cytoplasmic processes in the center of the rosette.

photoreceptor cells.[51] Alcian blue and colloidal-iron stains reveal in the lumina of the rosettes a coating of hyaluronidase-resistant acid mucopolysaccharide that has similar staining characteristics to the glycosaminoglycan matrix that surrounds the rod and cones of the retina.[6] Tso and coworkers[51] described several additional ultrastructural features that the cells forming Flexner-Wintersteiner rosettes share with retinal photoreceptors: zonula occludens that form a luminal limiting membrane analogous to the cellular junctions that form the outer limiting membrane of the retina, cytoplasmic microtubules, cilia with the 9 + 0 pattern, and lamellated membranous structures resembling the disks of rod outer segments. Immunohistochemical and lectin histochemical studies also have supported the concept that retinoblastomas arise from undifferentiated retinal cells that may differentiate into photoreceptor-like cells.[52-54]

Homer-Wright rosettes (Fig. 54–10B) are seen much less commonly in retinoblastomas than Flexner-Wintersteiner rosettes. Because they are found in a variety of neuroblastic tumors, they are less specific for retinoblastoma. The Homer-Wright rosette first was described in sympathicoblastomas. They also are highly characteristic of cerebellar medulloblastomas.[55] In these rosettes, the cells are not arranged about a lumen but instead send out cytoplasmic processes that form a tangle within the center of the rosette.

In 1970, Tso and coworkers[19] reported that in 18 of 300 retinoblastomas (6%) treated by enucleation, there were foci of cytologically benign cells that had features of photoreceptors. In most of these 18 tumors, the areas exhibiting photoreceptor differentiation could be spotted easily at low magnification as discrete, comparatively eosinophilic islands standing out in contrast to the much more intensely basophilic portions of the tumor. The tumor cells that exhibited photoreceptor differentiation had more abundant cytoplasm and smaller, less basophilic nuclei that were much less densely packed. In these areas, mitotic figures were uncommon, necrosis was absent, and scattered deposits of calcium occasionally were present. Individual cells and clusters of cells had long cytoplasmic processes that stained brightly with eosin. The cytoplasmic processes that projected through a fenestrated membrane often fanned out like a bouquet of flowers (hence the name *fleurette*). Electron microscopy has revealed that the cells of the fleurettes resemble retinal cones.[18] The bulbous eosinophilic processes contain numerous mitochondria, which resemble cone inner segments.

In a subsequent study, Tso and colleagues[56] examined retinoblastomas in 54 eyes enucleated after having been irradiated. Only 42 eyes contained viable tumor cells, and 17 of these tumors (40%) exhibited photoreceptor differentiation. In seven cases, the residual tumor was composed entirely of cells showing photoreceptor differentiation. Consequently, Tso and colleagues[56] suggested that tumors containing

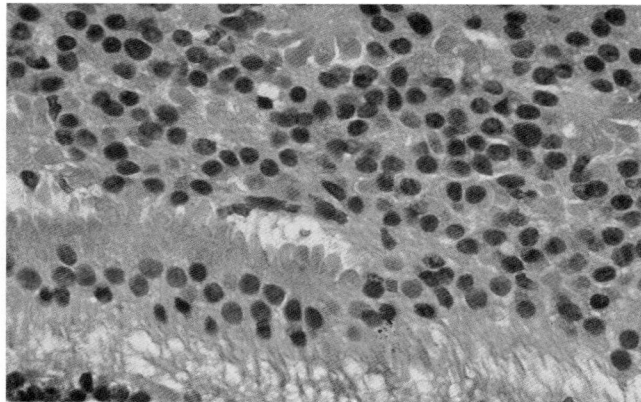

**FIGURE 54–11.** Retinocytoma. This uncommon variant of retinoblastoma is composed of benign-appearing cells exhibiting photoreceptor differentiation and formation of fleurettes.

such benign components might be incompletely radioresponsive because, as a general rule, benign and highly differentiated tumors are more radioresistant. Follow-up information was obtained in 13 of the 17 cases; there was only one tumor death. Despite uncontrolled tumor growth, the parents of the child refused to permit enucleation. The patient died of intracranial extension of the retinoblastoma. Histologic study revealed this tumor to be composed of areas of undifferentiated retinoblastoma and areas of benign-appearing cells that exhibited photoreceptor differentiation.

Tumors with benign-appearing histologic characteristics (Fig. 54–11) have been described in eyes that had not been irradiated before enucleation, and they have been designated *retinocytomas*.[20] Glial differentiation has been described in these benign variants of retinoblastoma,[20, 57] but it is difficult to be certain whether this represents reactive gliosis from the adjacent retina or glial differentiation of tumor cells.

In phthisical eyes with totally necrotic *regressed* retinoblastomas, it may be difficult to diagnose the retinoblastoma. Histologic examination reveals dense calcification in a tumor that exhibits complete coagulative necrosis (Fig. 54–12). Under high magnification, one usually can make out the ghostly outlines of fossilized tumor cells. Further confusion may be created by exuberant reactive proliferation of retinal pigment epithelial cells, ciliary epithelial cells, and glial cells and by ossification.

## Extraocular Extension and Metastasis

Most retinoblastomas exhibit the relentlessly progressive, rapidly invasive growth that is characteristic of blastic tumors of childhood. If left untreated, they usually fill the eye and completely destroy the internal architecture of the globe. The most common

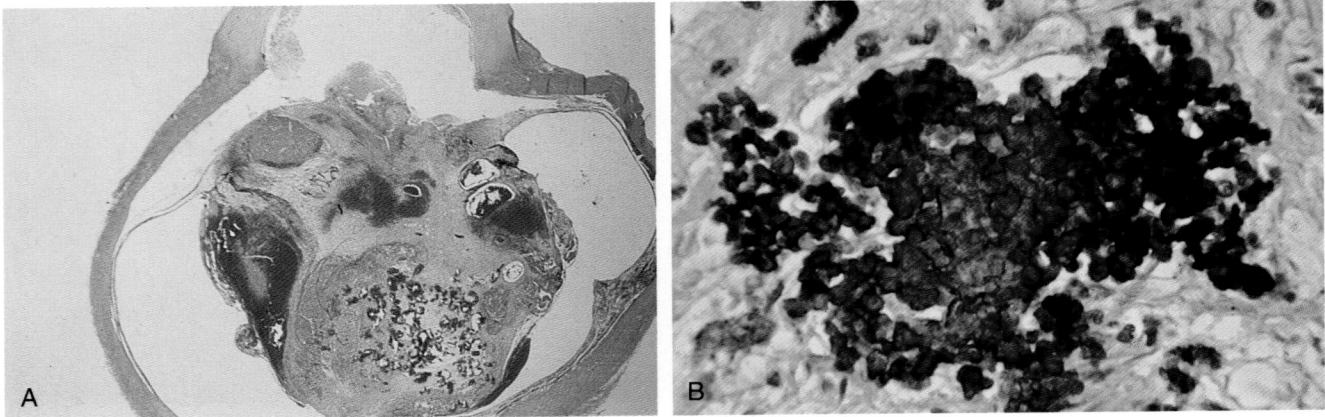

**FIGURE 54–12.** Retinoblastoma. *A.* Phthisical eye displaying partially regressed retinoblastoma composed of dark blue areas containing viable cells and calcification and light areas of necrotic cells all admixed with hemorrhage. *B.* Completely regressed retinoblastoma consisting of a shrunken scarred calcified mass.

method of spread is to the brain by invasion through the optic disk into the optic nerve (Fig. 54–13). When in the nerve, the tumor may spread directly along the nerve fiber bundles back toward the optic chiasm, or it may infiltrate through the pia mater into the subarachnoid space. From the subarachnoid space, tumor cells may be carried through the circulating cerebrospinal fluid to the brain and spinal cord. When the tumor has invaded the choroid, it may spread into the orbit through the scleral canals or by massively replacing the sclera. It has been estimated that approximately 6 months is required from when the retinoblastoma produces its first symptoms to when it invades outside the eye.[58] Orbital invasion dramatically increases the chances of hematogenous dissemination and permits access to conjunctival lymphatics and metastasis to regional lymph nodes.

Retinoblastomas exhibit metastatic potential in four ways:

1. Direct infiltrative spread may occur along the optic nerve from the eye to the brain. When the orbital soft tissues have been invaded, the tumor may spread directly into the orbital bones, through the sinuses into the nasopharynx, or through the various foramina into the cranium.
2. Dispersion of tumor cells may occur after cells in the optic nerve have invaded the leptomeninges and gained access to the circulating subarachnoid fluid. This dispersion may occur without involvement of cut end of the optic nerve. Flow of cerebrospinal fluid can carry tumor cells from the eye to the brain and spinal cord, and we have observed spread to the optic nerve on the opposite side.

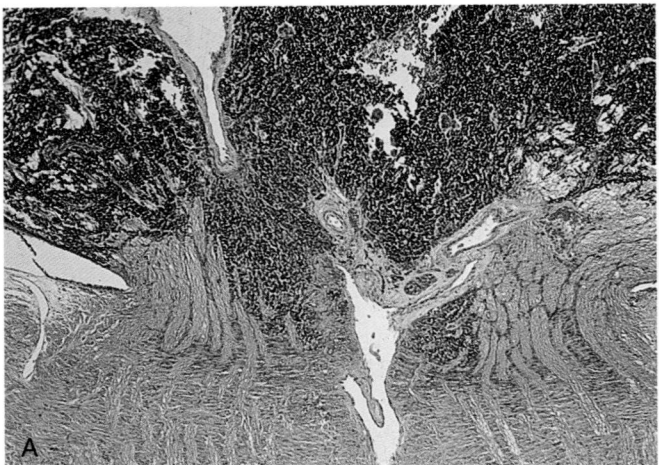
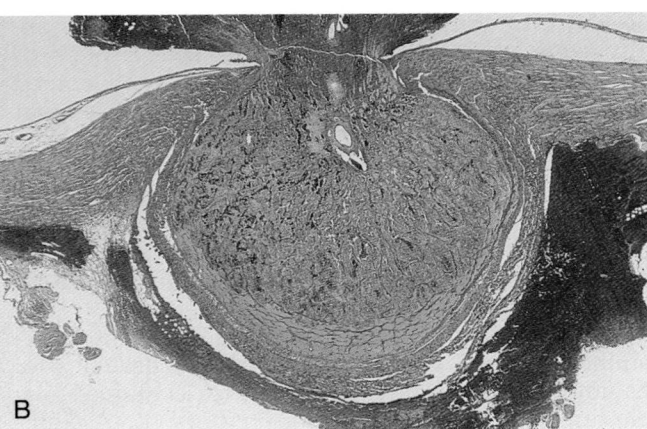

**FIGURE 54–13.** Retinoblastoma. *A.* Invasion of optic nerve by retinoblastoma tumor cells to the level of the lamina cribrosa, beyond which the optic nerve is spared. *B.* A different specimen displaying diffuse spread of retinoblastoma cells into the optic nerve but not to the level of transection.

3. Hematogenous dissemination leads to widespread metastasis to the lungs, bones, brain, and other viscera. Orbital invasion and to a lesser degree choroidal invasion increase the risk for hematogenous spread.

4. Lymphatic spread occurs in cases in which there has been anteriorly located or massive extraocular extension. There are no intraocular or orbital lymphatic channels, but the bulbar conjunctiva and lacrimal gland are richly supplied with lymphatic vessels.

When metastasis occurs, it is generally within the first year or two after treatment. Kopelman and associates[26] found that the median time to death in patients with fatal retinoblastoma was 6.4 months in unilateral cases and 14.2 months in bilateral cases. Late metastasis is so rare after treatment for retinoblastoma that when it is suspected, the question of an independent new primary tumor must be considered. Hematogenous metastasis from retinoblastoma is characteristically widespread, but in contrast to uveal melanoma, it frequently is preceded by spread to regional lymph nodes. The brain may be affected selectively when spread has occurred through the optic nerve. Invasion of leptomeninges of the optic nerve typically gives rise to a thick accumulation of tumor cells in the meninges along the basilar surface of the brain and in the ventricles, which can be detected by CT.[59]

Typically in metastatic lesions, retinoblastoma appears less differentiated than in the intraocular primary tumor. Rosettes, which may be numerous and highly organized in the primary tumors, are typically difficult to find and are poorly formed in metastatic lesions. Fleurettes are never observed in metastatic lesions.

The primary retinoblastomas observed in the pineal and in parasellar sites of patients with trilateral retinoblastoma[26, 33] have been confused with metastatic retinoblastoma, but in contrast to the latter, these tumors are solitary and not accompanied by other tumors, as one would expect with metastatic disease. They often appear several years after the successful treatment of intraocular tumors and may exhibit far greater differentiation with numerous rosettes, fleurettes, and individual cells exhibiting photoreceptor differentiation than one would expect to observe in a metastatic tumor. In addition to the primary retinoblastomas that occur intracranially, primitive neuroepithelial tumors have been observed in many locations in patients with heritable retinoblastoma. The sites of these tumors have included orbit, nasopharynx, trunk, and extremities.

Recurrence of retinoblastoma in the orbit after enucleation is almost always the result of tumor cells that were left untreated in the orbit. In some instances, this recurrence may be the result of subclinical orbital involvement that also may have escaped histopathologic recognition, but much more frequently it is a consequence of incomplete removal of the orbital component or invasion of the optic nerve beyond the plane of surgical transection. Rarely, orbital recurrence may be the result of lymphatic or hematogenous spread to the bony walls or soft tissues of the orbit to the lids.

## Prognosis

Many risk factors affect prognosis, but most important is the extent of invasion by the retinoblastoma. Kopelman and associates[26] in an analysis of cases from the Registry of Ophthalmic Pathology found that the extent of invasion into the optic nerve and through the ocular coats were the two most important predictors of patient outcome. The importance of extraocular invasion as the most important predictor of death is supported by many studies.[60–63] When the Registry data were evaluated by multivariate analysis, bilaterality was the only variable that proved to be more significantly associated with a fatal outcome than in univariate analysis, suggesting that bilaterality is related to death for reasons unrelated to the primary tumor. In some of these cases, the cause of death was attributed to spread of retinoblastoma to the brain, yet there was no optic nerve invasion. We believe that new intracranial primary tumors (trilateral retinoblastomas) are responsible for the deaths in these cases.

A problem with the study by Kopelman and associates[26] was that it was based on cases of retinoblastoma that were treated before 1962, and the possibility existed that more modern treatment could affect the results. Most of the more recent cases in the Registry of Ophthalmic Pathology are from less developed countries, where it is impossible to obtain follow-up data. Because of the lack of cases from the United States, McLean and coworkers[64] compared 514 cases of retinoblastoma from the Registry of Ophthalmic Pathology obtained between 1917 and 1962 (mean, 1945) with 460 cases from Germany obtained between 1963 and 1986 (mean, 1976). The cause-specific survival rate in which only deaths resulting from suspected spread or metastasis of the retinoblastoma were considered was lower in the older sample from the United States (66% at 5 years) than in the German sample (93% at 5 years). Invasion of the ocular coats and invasion into the optic nerve were the most significant prognostic factors in both samples. A multivariate logistic model using seven variables (post-1962 German versus pre-1963 American cases, unilateral versus bilateral, invasion of choroid, invasion of sclera, invasion of orbit, invasion of retrolaminar optic nerve, and invasion of the resected margin of the optic nerve) described the observed mortality patterns (Table 54–1). In the absence of other risk factors, there were no deaths in the German series and eight deaths in the series from the Registry of Ophthalmic Pathology. Because metastasis of retinoblastoma is unlikely in the absence of extraocular invasion, many oncologists no

**TABLE 54–1.** Relative Risk Associated with Prognostic Factors in Cases of Retinoblastoma

| Risk Factors Associated with Mortality | Odds Ratio* | Odds Ratio** |
|---|---|---|
| Invasion of ocular coats | | |
| Choroid | 1.8 | 2.9 |
| Sclera | 3.9 | 9.1 |
| Orbit | 21.6 | 37.6 |
| Invasion of optic nerve | | |
| Resected | 3.8 | 4.4 |
| Unresected | 8.6 | 13.3 |
| Bilaterality | 2.9 | 2.9 |
| Incorrect clinical diagnosis | 2.5 | |
| Pre 1963 case | | 4.1 |

* Kopelman JE, McLean IW, Rosenberg SH: Multivariate analysis of risk factors for metastasis in retinoblastoma treated by enucleation. Ophthalmology 94:371–377, 1987; ** McLean IW, Rosenberg SH, Messmer EP, et al: Prognostic factors in cases of retinoblastoma. Analysis of 974 patients from Germany and the United States treated by enucleation. In Bornfeld N, Gragoudas ES, Lommatzsch PK (eds): Tumors of the Eye. Proceedings of the International Symposium on Tumors of the Eye. Amsterdam, Kugler Publications, 1991, pp 151–154.

longer recommend lumbar punctures and bone marrow aspirates in patients with retinoblastoma confined within the eye.[65]

McLean and colleagues[66] reviewed 12 cases of fatal unilateral retinoblastoma from the Registry of Ophthalmic Pathology in which the tumor was confined to the eye without invasion into the optic nerve or sclera. In half of the 12 cases, there was choroidal invasion. In eight cases, four with choroidal invasion and four without choroidal invasion, there was an orbital recurrence, which preceded the development of distant metastasis. These histories suggest that there was probably microscopic extraocular spread that was not detected by histologic examination. This suggestion reemphasizes the importance of extraocular invasion as the pathway leading to metastasis of retinoblastoma and the great need for careful histologic examination aimed at detection of microscopic extraocular extension.

## Unsuspected Retinoblastoma

Stafford and coworkers,[67] in their analysis of 618 histologically proved cases in which adequate clinical data were available, found that almost 15% had been misdiagnosed initially. In 6.6% of the cases, the incorrect initial diagnosis had led to a delay in enucleation, while treatment was given for panophthalmitis, endophthalmitis, tuberculosis, or other forms of uveitis. In another 8.3%, a variety of noninflammatory, non-neoplastic conditions had been diagnosed. Shields and colleagues[68] described five patients with retinoblastoma who presented with orbital cellulitis, without extraocular extension of the tumor. In all five cases, the retinoblastoma had undergone extensive necrosis. Delays in enucleation were associated with a much greater mortality than in the cases in which a correct initial diagnosis had

been followed promptly by enucleation. Kopelman and associates[26] found that the odds of death were 2.5 times greater in patients with clinically undiagnosed retinoblastoma.

## Treatment

The management of retinoblastoma is complex, and the best treatment for each patient must be determined on an individual basis. The method of treatment should depend on the size and extent of the tumor, whether there is bilateral involvement, and the general health of the patient.[39] The age of the patient is an important consideration because younger patients are more likely to have a germinal mutation and are more likely to develop additional retinoblastomas. Enucleation is the most commonly employed treatment modality, but in the United States[69] and Great Britain,[70] the proportion of patients with retinoblastoma treated by enucleation is decreasing. The introduction of chemoreduction therapy for intraocular retinoblastomas should reduce further the number of retinoblastomas requiring enucleation.[71] For small tumors, photocoagulation and cryotherapy may be employed[72, 73]; for medium-sized tumors, there is plaque irradiation[74] or external-beam irradiation.[39] Large intraocular tumors usually can be managed with enucleation or chemoreduction.[71] For tumors with extraocular extension, there is enucleation combined with radiation and chemotherapy[75]; for orbital recurrence, radiation and chemotherapy[76, 77]; and for metastatic retinoblastoma, chemotherapy.[76, 77] Only with modern multidrug chemotherapy has there been survival of patients with retinoblastoma that has spread beyond the orbit.[76–78]

## MALIGNANT MELANOMA OF THE UVEAL TRACT

### Cause

The cause of uveal malignant melanoma is unknown, but several risk factors for the development of this tumor have been identified, including age, race, sex, predisposing lesions, genetic factors, and possibly environmental factors.[79]

#### AGE

The incidence of uveal malignant melanoma increases with age.[80] Median age at diagnosis is 53 in the cases on file in the Registry of Ophthalmic Pathology. Barr and associates[81] found that 1.6% of 6358 cases in the Registry of Ophthalmic Pathology were in patients younger than age 20. They noted that this prevalence probably is inflated because some of these cases were submitted to the Registry only because the patient was so young. Congenital uveal malignant melanoma is exceedingly rare.[81]

## RACIAL PIGMENTATION

The prevalence of uveal malignant melanoma in blacks is low in the Armed Forces Institute of Pathology (AFIP) Registry of Ophthalmic Pathology. Margo and McLean[82] reviewed 3876 cases of uveal malignant melanoma in which the race of the patient was known. Only 39 (1%) of these patients were black. Because the racial makeup of the population of patients whose cases are referred to the Registry of Ophthalmic Pathology is not known, the relative risk of uveal melanoma in blacks and whites cannot be calculated from these data. Scotto and coworkers[83] found that the incidence in whites (6 per 1 million per year) is 8.5 times greater than in blacks, which is consistent with Margo and McLean's data from the Registry of Ophthalmic Pathology, assuming that blacks make up 13% of their referral population. Comparing uveal malignant melanomas in blacks and whites, Margo and McLean[82] found that the tumors in blacks were larger, more heavily pigmented, and more extensively necrotic than the tumors in whites. Despite these differences, there was no difference in survival between the black and white patients.

In black Africans, there is suggestive evidence that the incidence of uveal malignant melanoma is lower than it is in American blacks, who often have some white ancestors. Asians have an incidence rate intermediate between American blacks and whites. Among whites, blue-eyed blondes have the highest incidence. These findings indicate an inverse correlation between skin pigmentation and the incidence of uveal malignant melanoma.

## SEX

Uveal malignant melanoma is more common in men than in women. In a survey of the cases in the Registry of Ophthalmic Pathology, there were 2764 men and 2231 women with choroidal and ciliary body melanomas. Gallagher and coworkers[79] reported a similar male predominance in cases from Canada, and the Third National Cancer Survey[80] from the United States found a higher incidence rate in men than women. The reason for the higher rate in men is unknown.

## GEOGRAPHIC FACTORS

There is great variation in the incidence of uveal malignant melanoma around the world, but these variations seem to reflect the skin pigmentation of the dominant racial groups in the different regions. The incidence is lowest in Africa, where the most heavily pigmented individuals predominate, and highest in the Scandinavian countries, where blond blue-eyed individuals predominate. There is suggestive data that actinic exposure is a pathogenetic factor in uveal malignant melanoma, but the relative risk is much lower than it is with cutaneous malignant melanoma.[84, 85] This finding is not surprising because most of the ultraviolet light that enters the eye is absorbed before it reaches the uveal melanocytes.

## PREDISPOSING LESIONS

Congenital melanosis[86, 87] and nevi[88–90] are the best-documented lesions that predispose to the development of uveal malignant melanoma. Ocular melanocytosis and oculodermal melanocytosis have been observed frequently to precede the development of a uveal malignant melanoma. Almost without exception malignant melanoma occurs in the more heavily pigmented eye. Congenital oculodermal melanocytosis (nevus of Ota) occurs more commonly in blacks and Asians than in whites. Patients of all races have been observed to develop uveal malignant melanoma in the eye involved by congenital melanosis, but the progression to uveal malignant melanoma has been observed most often in whites.

Uveal nevi progress to malignant melanoma less frequently than congenital melanosis. It has been estimated that the rate of transformation of nevi to malignant melanoma is 1 per 10,000 to 15,000 per year. Another reason for considering nevi a precursor of uveal malignant melanoma is that nevoid-appearing cells are observed at the periphery or along the scleral edge in about three quarters of the tumors. This frequency has been considered to be too high by some investigators, who believe that the nevoid appearance of cells along the sclera represents a compression artifact.

## GENETIC FACTORS

Although rare, the familial occurrence of uveal malignant melanoma has been recorded.[91, 92] Among the patients whose data are on file in the Registry of Ophthalmic Pathology, two families with uveal malignant melanoma in successive generations have been observed. The rarity of these cases suggests that family members of patients with uveal malignant melanoma have at most a low risk of developing this tumor, but this risk is probably greater than the low risk of the general population (7 per 1 million per year).

The role of specific gene alterations in the pathogenesis of uveal melanoma is less well defined than it is in retinoblastoma. Chromosomal analysis of many uveal melanomas has shown that abnormalities of chromosomes 3, 6, and 8 are observed most frequently.[93–95] In most tumors, there is loss of chromosome 3 alleles and multiplication of chromosome 6 and 8 alleles. These findings suggest that there is a tumor-suppressor gene (antioncogene) on chromosome 3 that is deleted and oncogenes on chromosomes 6 and 8 that are amplified in uveal melanomas. None of these genes have been identified. Detectable deletions of the long arm of chromosome 6 are probably less frequent in uveal melanomas than in cutaneous melanomas,[93–95] which suggests that the putative melanoma tumor-suppressor gene in this location[96] is altered less frequently in uveal melanomas than it is in cutaneous melanomas.

The tumor-suppressor gene *p53* located on the short arm of chromosome 17 is mutated in a variety of cancers, and it may play a role in the pathogenesis of uveal melanomas. The *p53* gene, similar to the *RB* gene, codes for a nucleoprotein that is involved in regulating the cell cycle. Point mutations in the *p53* gene alter the tumor-suppressor function of the protein product and increase its stability so that it accumulates in cells to levels that can be detected immunohistochemically. Immunohistochemical detection of p53 protein in cells can be used to screen for point mutations in the *p53* gene. In 12 of 18 uveal melanomas, Tobal and coworkers[97] measured increased expression of p53 protein. Polymerase chain reaction and sequencing of the *p53* gene in 2 of the 12 tumors revealed point mutations in both tumors. Neither of these mutations were cytosine-to-thymidine conversions, which are characteristic of ultraviolet light injury.[98]

Jay and McCartney[99] showed mutant *p53* gene product in a uveal malignant melanoma from a 150-year-old ocular specimen. This tumor was from a member of a family in which four generations had uveal melanoma associated with breast cancer. Parsons first described this family in 1905.[99]

## Associated Tumors

Although several authors have commented on the high rate of death resulting from other neoplasms in the follow-up of patients with uveal malignant melanoma, these authors failed to consider the expected mortality resulting from other cancers in their patients with uveal malignant melanoma. U.S. life tables indicate that approximately one fourth of the mortality in 55- to 75-year-old individuals is due to cancer. Using cases from the Registry of Ophthalmic Pathology, McLean and colleagues[100] compared the mortality resulting from cancers other than metastatic melanoma for patients treated for uveal melanoma with the expected mortality resulting from cancer of matched individuals obtained from U.S. life tables and found no difference. Holly and coworkers[101] found no increased risk of prior cancer in patients with uveal melanoma. These data suggest that there is not a strong association between uveal melanoma and other malignancies, but they do not exclude the possibility that there are small subgroups of uveal melanoma patients in which there is an association.

Ten cases of uveal malignant melanoma have been reported in patients with the dysplastic nevus syndrome.[102] McLean and colleagues[100] observed one case from the Registry of Ophthalmic Pathology in which a choroidal spindle cell nevus was associated with multiple cutaneous malignant melanomas. The association of uveal melanomas with dysplastic nevi seems to be weak because Taylor and associates[103] found the same prevalence of dysplastic nevi in patients with uveal melanoma as has been observed in the general population.

Bilaterality and multicentricity in one eye are rare in uveal melanoma, whereas in retinoblastoma multiple tumors are common and indicative of a genetic predisposition. There is a strong association with other cancers in a small subgroup of patients with bilateral uveal melanoma.[104] The subgroup of patients with associated tumors all had a unique constellation of findings: 1) rapid bilateral loss of vision in older patients (57 to 78 years old) who eventually died with carcinoma of bowel, ovary, gallbladder, pancreas, or lung; 2) a confusing clinical appearance that gave the impression of multiple choroidal tumors suggesting metastatic carcinoma or metastatic melanoma; and 3) bilateral diffuse melanocytic tumors in which most cells were cytologically benign.

## Clinical Features

Uveal malignant melanomas may arise in the iris, ciliary body, or choroid. Iris malignant melanomas are visible and usually noticed by the patient when relatively small. Choroidal and ciliary body malignant melanomas can be divided into stages based on clinical presentation. The first stage is asymptomatic and represents tumors discovered on a routine ophthalmoscopic examination. Use of the indirect ophthalmoscope has improved greatly the ability of ophthalmologists to detect and diagnose small choroidal tumors.[105] These tumors tend to be small lesions confined to the uvea without associated retinal detachment or involvement of the macular area. In the second stage, there is loss of vision, either a field defect or complete, which is usually due to associated retinal detachment. In the third stage, the patient develops ocular pain from glaucoma or inflammation. In the fourth stage, there are symptoms of extraocular extension, either proptosis or a visible subconjunctival mass. In 2627 cases of uveal melanoma from the Registry of Ophthalmic Pathology[106] that were obtained between 1936 and 1975, 2.8% had stage 1, 64% had stage 2, 32% had stage 3, and 1.4% had stage 4. Over the 40-year period in which these cases were collected, the proportion of patients who had stage 1 and 2 increased, and the proportion with more advanced disease decreased by 23%. Despite treatment at earlier stages, there was no significant improvement in survival rates.[106]

## Gross Pathology

The gross pathologic features of uveal malignant melanomas depend on the size and location of the tumors. Choroidal tumors are the most common. Although ophthalmologists use the diameter and the height of uveal malignant melanomas to classify them by size, most pathologists use a simpler classification based only on the largest dimension of the tumor. Uveal malignant melanomas are divided into three groups: small (largest dimension is ≤10 mm), medium (largest dimension is 11 to 15 mm), and large (largest dimension is >15 mm). Most small uveal malignant melanomas are discoid tumors that are confined to the choroid. The tough fibrous sclera prevents expansion of the tumor externally, but internally Bruch's membrane is relatively weak. As these tumors grow and produce a larger discoid mass, Bruch's membrane is stretched over the tumor and eventually ruptures. The tumor herniates through the rupture and grows into the subretinal space, giving the tumor a "collar button" configuration. The growth in the subretinal space is often greater than the growth in the choroids, and as the mass in the subretinal space becomes larger, the tumor develops a mushroom-like appearance. The collar button and mushroom configurations are typically seen in medium-sized tumors (Fig. 54–14). The retina overlying a uveal melanoma undergoes atrophy or cystoid degeneration, whereas the retina surrounding the tumor is detached by the accumulation of serous exudate between the retina and the retinal pigment epithelium. As the tumors become even larger, they invade and destroy the ocular tissues, eventually growing to fill the globe completely. Some tumors invade posteriorly through the sclera usually along the course of perforating nerves and vessels into the orbit or anteriorly into the conjunctiva.[107, 108]

The diffuse infiltrating type of choroidal melanoma is an uncommon variant on the usual growth pattern.[109] These tumors grow laterally in the choroid without producing much thickness. They are more likely to invade through the sclera than discoid uveal malignant melanomas, and these tumors may produce an orbital mass larger than the intraocular tumor (Fig. 54–15).

Malignant melanomas arising in the ciliary body are less common than tumors of the choroid. These

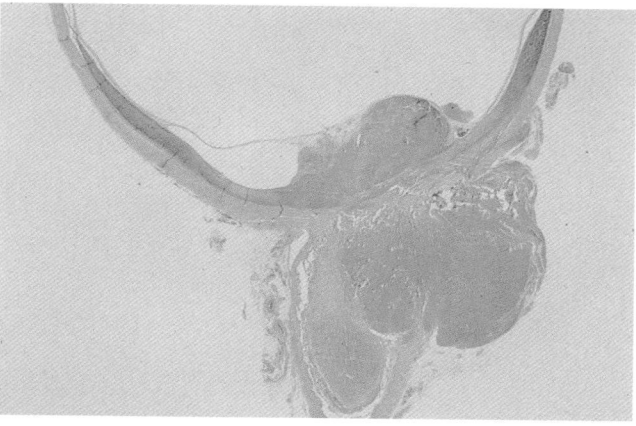

**FIGURE 54–15.** Uveal malignant melanoma. Diffuse infiltrating choroidal melanoma characterized by minimal choroidal thickening, extrascleral extension, and invasion of optic nerve.

tumors tend to be smaller and have a more spherical shape than choroidal tumors (Fig. 54–16). Anterior invasion to involve the iris root, angle structures, and anterior chamber is common. Clinically the anterior extension may be noticed by the patient, and what is thought to be a small iris tumor may represent only the tip of the iceberg. Bruch's membrane does not exist in the ciliary body, and the ciliary epithelium does not provide an effective barrier to inward growth. Ciliary body malignant melanomas commonly invade the posterior chamber and indent the lens, creating a lenticular notch or subluxation. The diffuse type of malignant melanoma also occurs in the ciliary body, where the tumor tends to grow in a ring configuration circumferentially within the ciliary body.[110] Similar to diffuse tumors of the choroids, these tumors frequently invade outside of the eye. The extraocular extension is usually along the aqueous outflow channels from

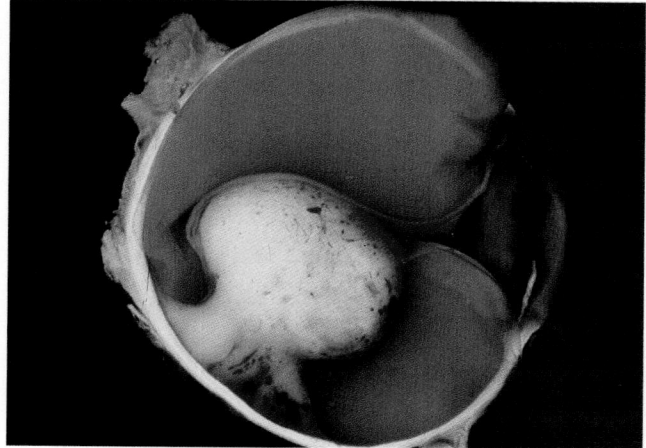

**FIGURE 54–14.** Uveal malignant melanoma. Choroidal melanoma exhibiting a mushroom-shaped appearance resulting from herniation of tumor through a rupture in Bruch's membrane with an associated serous retinal detachment. Passive venous congestion is present within the tumor mass.

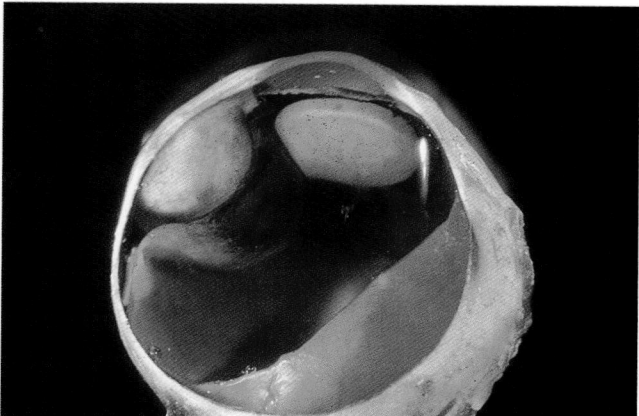

**FIGURE 54–16.** Uveal malignant melanoma. Ciliary body melanomas typically display a more spherical shape, with growth into the posterior chamber abutting the lens producing lenticular distortion.

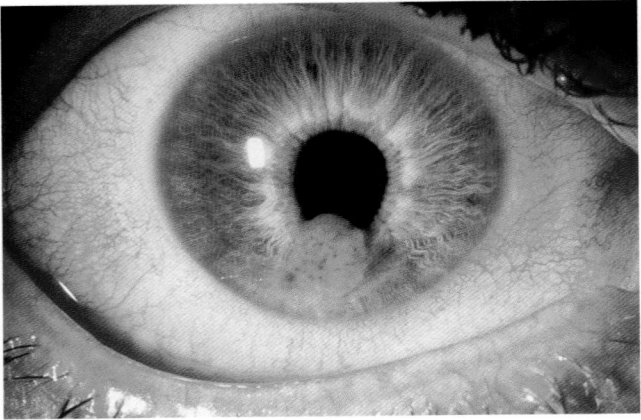

**FIGURE 54–17.** Uveal malignant melanoma. A malignant melanoma of the iris with prominent surface vasculature and distortion of the pupil.

the trabecular meshwork and Schlemm's canal. The extraocular extension may be mistaken for a primary malignant melanoma of the conjunctiva.

Tumors of the iris are the least common of the uveal malignant melanomas. Because the iris is visible to the patient, these tumors tend to be detected at relatively small sizes (Fig. 54–17) and in patients who are significantly younger. Tumors of the choroid measuring 10 mm are considered small, but a 10-mm tumor would fill the anterior chamber of the eye completely. Because iris tumors usually are detected earlier than ciliary body or choroidal tumors and because they are more surgically accessible, they usually are treated by local excision (iridectomy or iridocyclectomy). If the tumor is confined to the iris, a simple iridectomy is adequate; when the tumor extends into the ciliary body, a more extensive iridocyclectomy is required. These procedures enable the ophthalmologist to remove the tumor and preserve the eye, usually with useful vision. Because iris tumors are excised when relatively small, a large percentage of lesions removed for suspected malignant melanoma of the iris prove to be benign nevi.[111]

Iris nevi and melanomas may be associated with large dilated blood vessels. In some tumors, the tortuous enlarged blood vessels may be more prominent than the melanocytic component. Several of these tumors have been misdiagnosed clinically and pathologically as hemangioma of the iris. A true hemangioma of the iris is a rare lesion.

In the iris, there is no barrier between the stroma and the anterior chamber, and growth onto the anterior surface of the iris often is seen with nevi of the iris. Melanomas of epithelioid cell type are composed of cells that lack cohesion. With this type of tumor, it is common for malignant cells to be shed from the surface of the iris tumor and seed throughout the anterior chamber, clog the trabecular meshwork, and elevate the intraocular pressure. There also is a diffuse variant of malignant melanoma of the iris. These tumors spread through the

iris stroma and along the surface of the iris causing heterochromia but without producing a mass. These tumors tend to be of epithelioid cell type, and they usually seed the anterior chamber angle.

## Extraocular Extension

The sclera provides a barrier to egress of uveal malignant melanomas. Invasion outside of the eye usually is along the emissaries of the vortex veins and the ciliary arteries and nerves. Occasionally, neoplastic cells that have invaded into the lumen of the vortex veins can be observed, but vascular invasion within the tumor is a much more common source of hematogenous metastasis. Peripapillary uveal malignant melanomas frequently invade the optic nerve head, but in contrast to retinoblastomas, uveal malignant melanomas only rarely extend retrolaminarly within the optic nerve. Seeding of the cerebrospinal fluid has been reported,[112] but we have not observed this cause of death in other cases of uveal malignant melanoma.

## Cytology and Histopathology

In 1931, Callender[113] proposed a classification of uveal malignant melanomas based on cytologic and histopathologic features. Callender and coworkers,[114, 115] his successors at the AFIP,[116–119] and other investigators[120–124] have shown the prognostic value of this classification. Callender divided the cells of uveal malignant melanomas into two main cytologic types—spindle and epithelioid. Spindle-type cells of uveal malignant melanomas are fusiform in shape and usually are arranged in tightly cohesive bundles. Within the bundles by light microscopy, the plasma membranes of the cells are indistinct, giving the appearance of a syncytium. The cytoplasm has a fibrillar or finely granular character (Fig. 54–18A). Callender identified two subtypes of spindle cells based on nuclear features. Subtype A has a slender nucleus with fine chromatin and an indistinct nucleolus. Subtype A uveal malignant melanoma cells often have a longitudinal fold in the nuclear envelope giving the appearance of a chromatin streak. Subtype B cells have a plumper nucleus, coarser chromatin, and a more prominent and more eosinophilic nucleolus. Mitotic activity is rare in spindle A cells and infrequent in most spindle B cells.

Callender's epithelioid-type cells are larger and more pleomorphic than the spindle-type cells. Epithelioid cells usually have abundant glassy cytoplasm, giving the cell a polyhedral shape. The cells have a distinct cell border often with extracellular space between adjacent epithelioid-type cells. This loss of cohesion is characteristic of epithelioid-type cells, and it is one of the main features that distinguishes them from spindle-type cells. The nucleus of epithelioid-type cells is larger and rounder than that

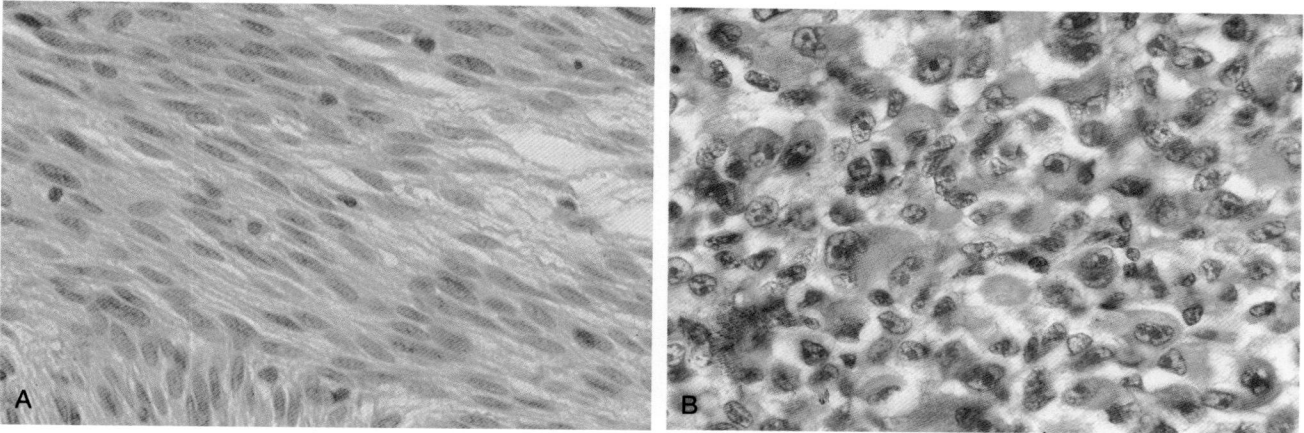

**FIGURE 54–18.** Uveal malignant melanoma. *A.* Spindle-type melanoma cells with tightly cohesive bundles of fusiform cells with indistinct plasma membranes and granular cytoplasm. *B.* Epithelioid-type melanoma cells with larger more pleomorphic cells with distinct plasma membranes and abundant glassy cytoplasm. Nuclei are larger and more round than in spindle-type cells and contain coarse marginated chromatin and prominent nucleoli.

of spindle-type cells. The nuclear envelope also is more angular with irregular indentations and outpouchings. The chromatin is coarse and marginated. A large eosinophilic nucleolus is one of the most important features of epithelioid cells (Fig. 54–18B). Occasional bizarre, multinucleated epithelioid cells may be seen. Mitotic activity usually is greater in epithelioid-type cells than in spindle-type cells.

Callender and coworkers[113, 114] classified uveal malignant melanomas into six groups. Four of these were based on the cytologic makeup of the tumor, and two were based on histologic features. The four groups based on cytology were tumors composed of spindle A cells, tumors composed of spindle B cells, tumors composed of epithelioid cells, and tumors composed of a mixture of epithelioid and spindle cells. The fifth group consisted of tumors with a fascicular pattern. Two fascicular patterns exist in uveal melanomas, vasocentric and Verocay-like. In tumors with the vasocentric pattern, the cells are predominantly of the spindle B type with their nuclei arranged in columns perpendicular to a central blood vessel. In tumors with the Verocay-like pattern, the cells, usually of the spindle A type, are arranged in bundles with palisading nuclei forming stripes across the bundle. The sixth group was composed of tumors that were too necrotic to classify into one of the other groups.

Changes have occurred in the use of Callender and coworkers' classification at the AFIP since Callender proposed his classification. The fascicular type was dropped because these tumors could be classified better by their cytologic makeup. In 1972, McLean and coworkers[125] reexamined 105 tumors classified as spindle A type by their predecessors at the AFIP. The purpose of this study was to investigate two problems with Callender and coworkers' classification. First, Callender provided no criteria for distinguishing spindle A malignant melanomas from nevi. Second, Callender provided no clear criteria for classifying tumors composed of a mixture of spindle A and B cells. In their study, McLean and coworkers[125] found that 15 of the 105 tumors originally classified as spindle A type were cytologically benign. These tumors were composed of spindle-shaped cells that had a lower nuclear-to-cytoplasmic ratio and finer, less hyperchromatic chromatin than the cytologically malignant spindle A cells. Because none of the 15 patients with these tumors died, McLean and coworkers[125] reclassified these tumors as spindle cell nevi. They documented several examples of tumors composed of cytologically malignant spindle A cells without the spindle B or epithelioid types of cells, which killed by metastasis. In one of these cases, examination of foci of metastatic melanoma in the liver revealed that the metastases were composed of a population of pure spindle A cells. Tumors classified as Callender's spindle A type included benign and malignant neoplasms. Because the prognosis with cytologically malignant spindle A tumors was similar to that with spindle B tumors, McLean and coworkers[125] recommended that Callender's spindle A and B types should be combined and designated *spindle cell melanomas*. This designation also eliminated the problem of how to classify tumors composed of a mixture of spindle A and B cells.

The major problem with Callender's classification is that it represents an oversimplification. Callender recognized only three types of cells in uveal malignant melanomas, but the cells of uveal malignant melanomas exist in a spectrum ranging from bland spindle A cells to anaplastic bizarre epithelioid cells. Within this spectrum, there are spindle-shaped cells that lack cohesion. These cells may have a relatively large eosinophilic nucleolus that is characteristic of epithelioid cells. There also are polyhedral cells that are cohesive with fibrillar cytoplasm and relatively small eosinophilic nucleoli that are characteristics of spindle B cells. Should these cells be classified purely on the basis of shape, or are the other features of these cells more important in their classification?

Callender's mixed cell type causes additional problems. There is no agreement among pathologists classifying uveal malignant melanomas as to what percentage of the cells have to be epithelioid to classify a tumor as mixed cell type. Does a diagnosis of a mixed cell type of tumor require fewer epithelioid cells if the epithelioid cells are large and anaplastic than if the epithelioid cells deviate only minimally from spindle B cells? Because of these complexities, there is poor agreement among pathologists in using Callender's classification. When five ophthalmic pathologists from different countries reviewed uveal melanomas for the World Health Organization, at least two of the five disagreed with the other pathologists' classification of cell type 60% of the time.

## Immunohistochemistry

Uveal melanocytic cells are of neural crest derivation, and these cells and tumors derived from them would be expected to contain S-100 protein.[126] HMB-45 is a monoclonal antibody against a protein obtained from cutaneous malignant melanoma, and it is a marker for cells derived from uveal melanocytes and cutaneous melanocytes. Neuron-specific enolase (NSE) is an enzyme found in neurons, but a variety of non-neuronal cells express NSE to varying degrees. Burnier and colleagues[127] compared the immunohistochemical reactivity of 13 uveal nevi and 20 uveal melanomas for HMB-45, S-100 protein, and NSE in formalin-fixed, paraffin-embedded sections. All 33 of the lesions were positive for HMB-45. The false-negative rates for S-100 protein and NSE were 21% and 18%. If only strongly positive reactions were considered, more than half of the tumors would be interpreted as negative for S-100 protein and NSE. Nevi stained with less intensity than melanomas using all three antibodies. The expression of HMB-45 seemed to be greater in active nevi than in inactive nevi.

## Recurrence and Metastasis

The relationship between extension outside of the eye, orbital recurrence, and metastasis is not as important in cases of uveal malignant melanoma as it is in cases of retinoblastoma. In cases of retinoblastoma, extraocular extension is the most important prognostic feature. In cases of uveal malignant melanoma, extraocular extension is of minor prognostic value. Most of the significance of extraocular extension is related to correlation with other features of the tumor. Tumors that are large and contain epithelioid cells are more likely to have extraocular extension. In almost all fatal cases with extraocular extension, the cause of death is hematogenous metastasis, most often to the liver.

Lorigan and colleagues[128] studied the location of metastases using imaging in 110 patients with uveal melanoma. Hepatic metastasis developed in 101 patients (92%). The liver was involved initially in 94 patients (85%), and it was the only initial metastatic site in 60 patients (55%). Only one patient had initially isolated lymph node metastases, which were located in the mediastinum. Abdominal and axillary lymph nodes were involved secondary to hepatic and pulmonary metastasis in 13 patients (12%). Only a few cases of uveal malignant melanoma have metastatic spread to regional lymph nodes, and in none of the cases in the AFIP Registry of Ophthalmic Pathology was the patient killed by local extension. These findings suggest that the biology of metastasis of uveal melanoma is different from cutaneous melanoma and retinoblastoma, which are more likely to invade locally and spread to regional lymph nodes. The high prevalence of hepatic metastasis with uveal melanoma cannot be explained by venous drainage and must indicate a selection process for the liver by the disseminated tumor cells.

## Prognosis and Prognostic Features

Uveal malignant melanoma kills in approximately 50% of the cases if the patient does not die of something else first. In contrast to retinoblastoma, uveal malignant melanoma kills slowly, with the median time to death being 6.5 years.[129] Callender's cell type, modified to two groups based on the presence of epithelioid-type cells, remains one of the most reliable prognosticators despite its lack of reproducibility. To improve on Callender's classification, Gamel and coworkers[130-133] in a series of articles found that measurements of nucleolar size were better predictors of outcome than measurements of nuclear size and that the standard deviations were better predictors than the means of the measurements. The most important prognostic feature in uveal malignant melanomas is not the shape of the cell but the size and variability in size of the nucleolus. McLean and associates[134] suggested that pathologists should place greater emphasis on nucleolar size and variability than on other cytologic features when using Callender's classification and have documented that this modification of Callender's classification results in excellent prediction of patient outcome.

The size of uveal malignant melanomas is as important a predictor of patient outcome as the cytologic features. The problem with using size as a prognostic feature has been related to measuring the size of an irregularly shaped object. McLean and coworkers[117] analyzed 217 cases of uveal malignant melanoma and found that simply measuring the largest tumor dimension was a better prognosticator than the maximal height or the product of the maximal length, width, and height.

Univariate and multivariate statistical analyses

have been employed in a variety of studies to investigate prognostic factors in uveal melanomas. Almost invariably these studies have reconfirmed the importance of size and cytology of the tumor.[116–118, 135, 136] Factors including invasion into the sclera, mitotic activity, necrosis, DNA aneuploidy, and neovascularization characterized by the presence of vascular loops have been found to be significant in most studies.[107, 116, 137–140] All of these studies have been based on malignant melanomas of the choroid and ciliary body. Because iris tumors are smaller, less likely to contain epithelioid-type cells, and less likely to metastasize than choroidal tumors, size and cell type are believed to be prognostic factors in malignant melanomas of the iris. Because of the rarity of metastasis of iris tumors, this belief has not been confirmed by direct analysis.[111, 141–143]

Most of the studies of prognostic factors in cases of uveal malignant melanoma have not examined host factors. McLean and coworkers[117] observed that even when multiple features of a uveal malignant melanoma were predictive of a fatal outcome, some patients survived for many years without developing metastasis. They suggested that a major reason for failure of predictions based on the features of the tumors was variations in host defenses. Most infiltrating lymphocytes in tumors including uveal malignant melanoma are cytotoxic/suppressor T lymphocytes.[144] These lymphocytes are believed to represent an important component of the host's immune response to tumors.[145] De la Cruz and associates[138] and Vit[146] have investigated the prognostic significance of infiltrating lymphocytes in uveal melanomas (Fig. 54–19). Both studies found that lymphocytic infiltration was associated with a worse prognosis.[138, 146] A possible explanation is suggested by the study of Kranda and colleagues.[147] They observed that an abnormal ganglioside profile on the surface of the melanoma cells was related to mixed cell type and lymphocytic infiltration, suggesting that more malignant uveal melanomas may be more antigenic.

## PATHOLOGY OF ORBITAL BIOPSY SPECIMENS AND ORBITAL EXENTERATION SPECIMENS

Orbital exenterations are performed more often for tumors of the lids, conjunctiva, eye, sinuses, nasopharynx, and brain that secondarily invade the orbit than for primary orbital tumors.[148] Life-threatening infections, such as mucormycosis, also are treated by exenteration (Fig. 54–20). Tumors of the lacrimal gland (Figs. 54–21 to 54–23) are similar to tumors of the salivary glands, and orbital soft tissue tumors are similar to soft tissue tumors elsewhere in the body. In the orbit, these tumors usually are discovered at a smaller size and because of this may have a better prognosis. Two soft tissue tumors that have a predilection for the orbit are embryonal rhabdomyosarcoma in children (Figs. 54–24 and 54–25) and fibrous histiocytomas in adults (Figs. 54–26 and 54–27). Lymphomas of the orbit and ocular adnexa (Fig. 54–28) are predominantly of the well-differentiated lymphocytic types and often have features of mucosa-associated lymphoid tumors that also may involve the gut, lungs, salivary glands, and thyroid.[149] One of the most common of the orbital tumors, idiopathic inflammation is the lesion most unique to ophthalmic pathology.

## IDIOPATHIC ORBITAL INFLAMMATION (PSEUDOTUMOR)

Idiopathic orbital inflammation or pseudotumor has no recognizable local or systemic cause in the orbit and is a diagnosis made by exclusion. Its differential

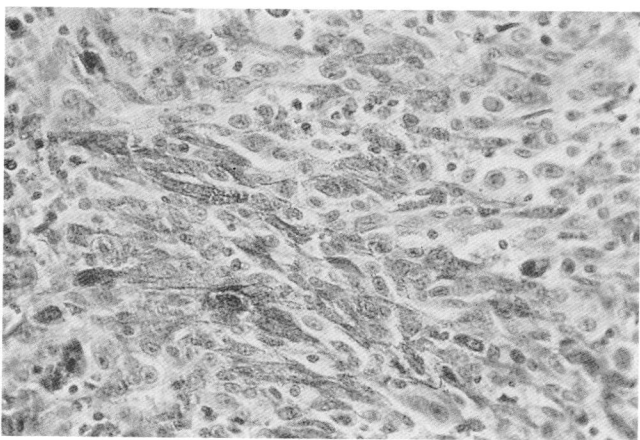

**FIGURE 54–19.** Uveal malignant melanoma. Epithelioid-type malignant uveal melanoma with tumor-infiltrating lymphocytes, which are associated with a worse survival rate.

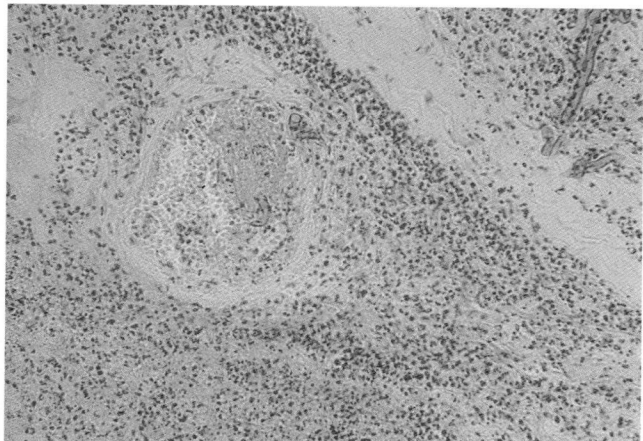

**FIGURE 54–20.** Mucormycosis. Broad, nonseptate, branching hyphae characteristic of *Mucor* and *Rhizopus* fungi may be associated with either granulomatous or nongranulomatous inflammation and typically invade blood vessels, causing thrombosis.

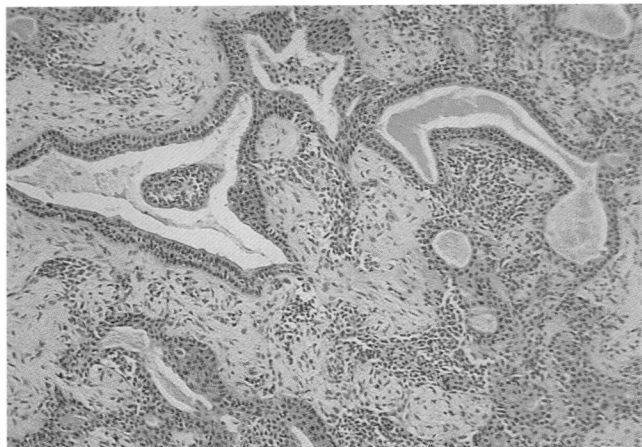

**FIGURE 54–21.** Lacrimal gland. Benign mixed tumor depicted by ducts lined with a double layer of epithelium arranged in an irregularly anastomosing pattern within a myxoid stroma.

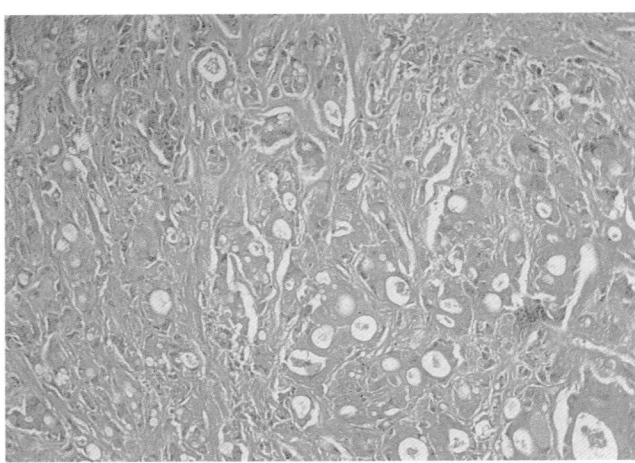

**FIGURE 54–23.** Lacrimal gland. Adenocarcinoma with irregularly anastomosing pattern of ducts within a fibrous stroma. The tumor arose in a pre-existing pleomorphic adenoma.

diagnosis includes infection; ruptured dermoid cyst; ectopic lacrimal gland[150, 151]; retained foreign body; hemorrhagic lymphangioma; Graves' disease; and systemic diseases such as autoimmune collagen diseases,[152] systemic vasculitis, Wegener's granulomatosis,[153] and Crohn's disease.[154] In several series based on orbital biopsy specimens,[155–157] strictly localized idiopathic orbital inflammation is one of the most common lesions. Because in most instances the diagnosis of orbital inflammation can be made clinically with ultrasonography and CT, the real incidence of inflammation may be far greater. It is probably the second most frequent cause of proptosis after Graves' disease.

## Clinical Findings

Patients with idiopathic orbital inflammation may be of any age, including childhood. The onset may be acute, subacute, or chronic. The disease may be recurrent in one orbit, may be bilateral, or may alternate from one orbit to the other. The inflammation can be classified further according to which orbital structure is predominantly involved: myositis (one or more extraocular muscles),[158] dacryoadenitis (lacrimal gland), periscleritis (epibulbar or tenon-level connective tissue and contiguous orbital fat), trochleitis (inflammation of the trochlear cartilage), and perineuritis (the outer dural sheath of the optic nerve and contiguous perioptic orbital fat). The lesions most often are diffuse, involving more than one structure, including the adipose tissue and extraocular muscles, but may be predominantly posterior or anterior.[159] Imaging studies are particularly valuable in determining the pattern and extent of orbital involvement.[160]

The acute form of the disease is the most striking and the easiest to distinguish from other orbital conditions, including Graves' disease and lymphoid

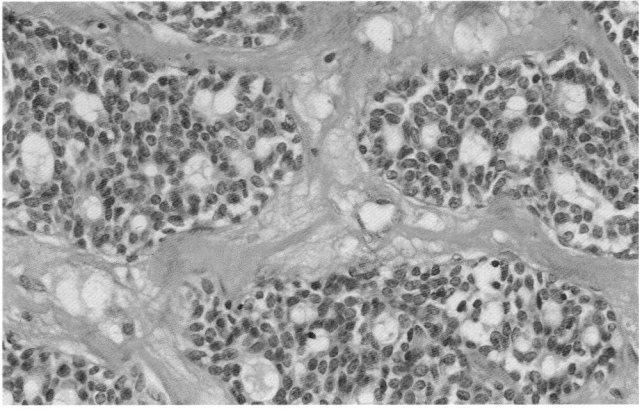

**FIGURE 54–22.** Lacrimal gland. Adenocystic carcinoma, whose low-power appearance resembles a swiss-cheese pattern, is composed of poorly differentiated epithelial cells arranged in islands containing mucin-filled cysts within a hyaline stroma.

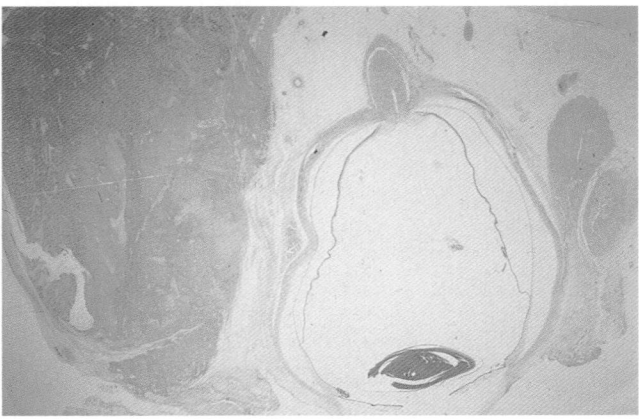

**FIGURE 54–24.** Rhabdomyosarcoma. Low-power photomicrograph of an orbital rhabdomyosarcoma commonly found in the superior orbit.

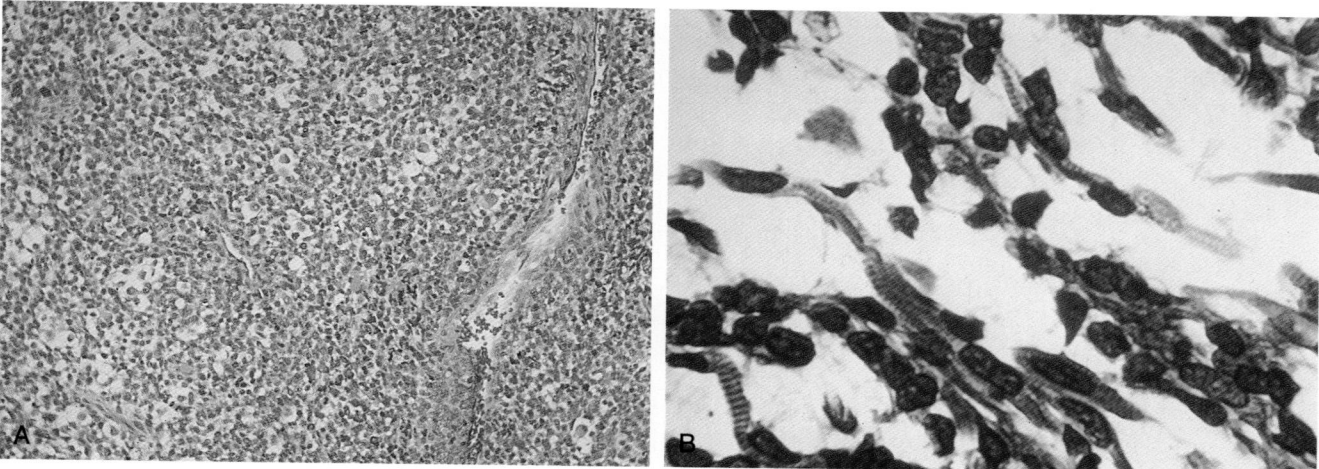

FIGURE 54–25. Rhabdomyosarcoma. *A.* Embryonic rhabdomyosarcoma, the most common histologic variant, is characterized by poorly differentiated cells with hyperchromatic nuclei. Scattered cells show rhabdomyoblastic differentiation. *B.* Masson trichrome stain effectively demonstrates spindle-shaped cells with cytoplasmic processes containing cross-striations of striated muscle differentiation.

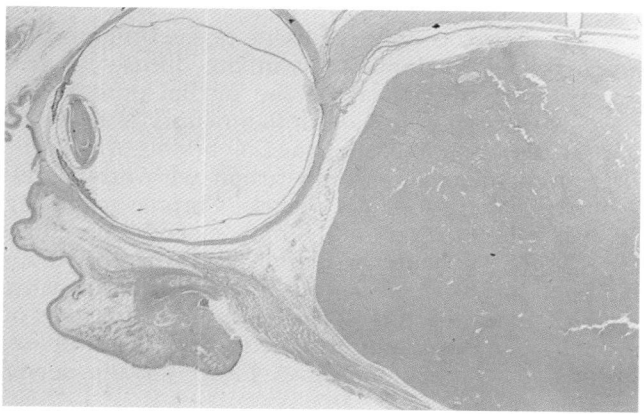

FIGURE 54–26. Fibrous histiocytoma. Low-power photomicrograph of an orbital mass with a pushing marginal displacement of the optic nerve.

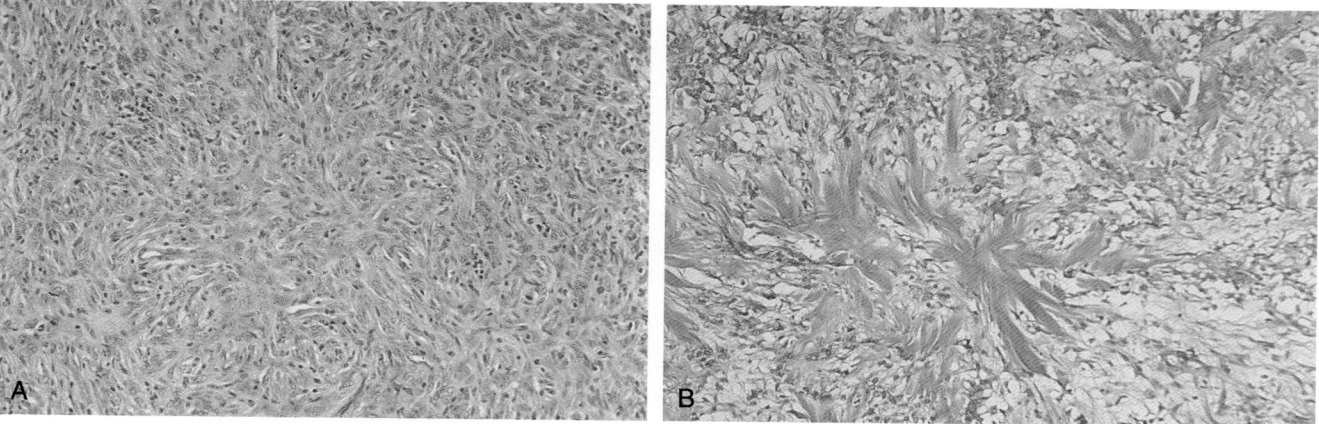

FIGURE 54–27. Fibrous histiocytoma. *A.* Mixture of spindle-shaped fibroblast-like cells and round-to-oval plump histiocyte-like cells, arranged in the characteristic storiform pattern, give fibrous histiocytoma its name. *B.* Higher-power photomicrograph of another lesion displays hyalinized bands of collagen, which make up stellate or cruciate scars within the tumor.

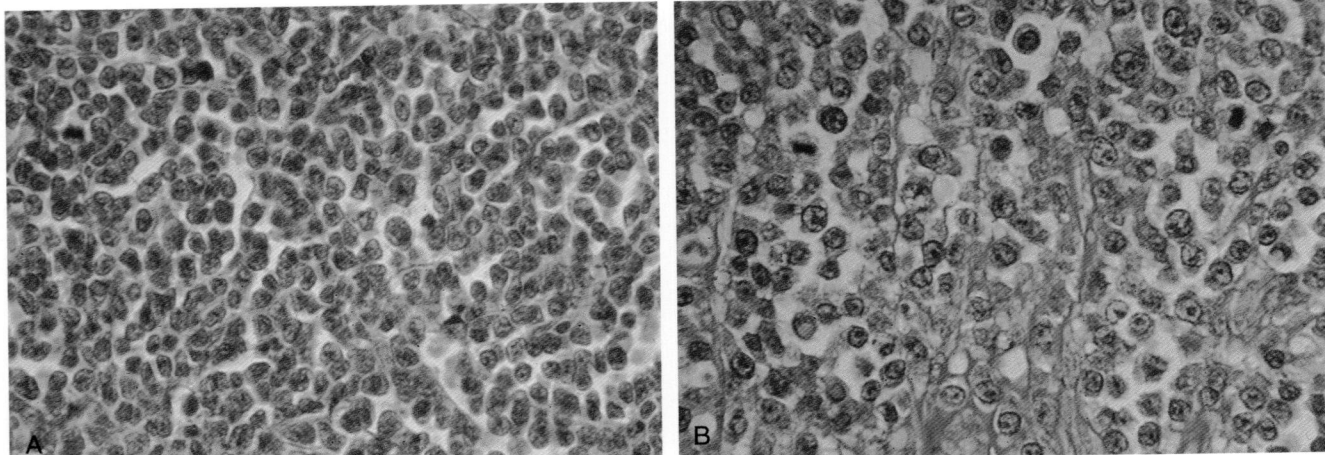

**FIGURE 54–28.** Malignant lymphoma. *A.* Orbital lymphoma exhibiting monomorphic round cells with an open chromatin pattern, distinct nucleoli, and occasional mitotic figures. *B.* Lymphoplasmacytoid variant whose cells have characteristics of both lymphocytes and plasma cells. The tumor displays monotonous immature lymphocytes, mitotic figures and intranuclear collections of finely granular immunoglobulin in cells referred to as Dutcher bodies. Delicate connective tissue septa are a distinctive feature of plasmacytic infiltrates, as are amorphous collections of eosinophilic material that are PAS positive, which is suggestive of immunoglobulin secretion.

tumors of the orbit. There is an abrupt onset of periocular pain accompanied by discomfort on movement of the globe, proptosis, chemosis, epibulbar injection, injection over the insertions of the rectus muscles, erythema of the lid skin, decreased visual acuity, or diplopia. Pronounced chemosis, lid swelling, and erythema may occur suggesting an orbital cellulitis, which generally can be ruled out by the absence of sinus disease on radiographic studies.

Subacute cases are characterized by less fulminant onset, with symptoms and signs developing more slowly over weeks to months. In the chronic variety, patients become symptomatic from proptosis, diplopia, or visual loss over months to years with few cutaneous or epibulbar signs of inflammation. If these lesions are situated anteriorly in the orbit and can be palpated through the lids, they offer a rock-hard feel that is mimicked only by metastatic scirrhous carcinomas.

In the myositis variant, the entire length of the involved extraocular muscle is enlarged, including the tendon; the latter feature helps distinguish idiopathic inflammation from Graves' disease. The inflammation may track along the intermuscular septa from one muscle to another and may spill over into the contiguous fat, which are findings not generally present in Graves' disease (Fig. 54–29).[158]

In the dacryoadenitis variant, the lacrimal gland is swollen, generally in an oblong fashion, with molding to the shape of adjacent structures, which differs from the rounded appearance of primary epithelial tumors in the lacrimal gland. In acute and chronic dacryoadenitides, there is generally no erosion of the contiguous orbital bone. Because of frequent involvement of the palpebral lobe and the orbital lobe, the gland may have a V shape (Fig. 54–30).

The fibrous connective tissue of the orbit and fat are involved predominantly in the diffuse variant. Rarely, inflammation along the medial orbital wall coexists with an ethmoidal inflammatory lesion with partial dissolution of the medial orbital wall. This inflammation may cause confusion with orbital cellulitis secondary to sinus disease. Chronic sclerosing orbital inflammation rarely may extend intracranially. In the subacute or chronic form of orbital inflammation, there is more uniform radiodensity, with confluence of the normally streaky infiltrates of orbital fat involvement observed in the acute phase, leading to solid radiodensities. Either the anterior or

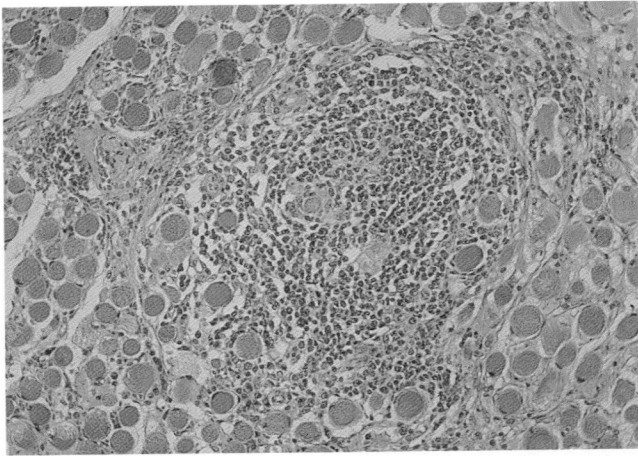

**FIGURE 54–29.** Pseudotumor. Involvement of the entire muscle including the tendon and involvement of the surrounding connective tissue is characteristic of myositis variant of pseudotumor and distinguishes it from thyroid related ophthalmopathy. Microscopically, muscle fibers are infiltrated with lymphocytes, plasma cells, and occasional eosinophils.

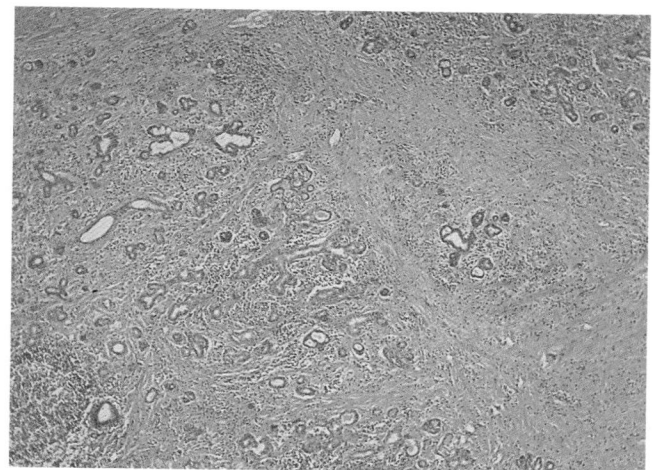

FIGURE 54–30. Pseudotumor. Dacryoadenitis with oblong molded appearance grossly differs from round appearance of primary epithelial tumors of the lacrimal gland. This moderately advanced case displays chronic inflammatory infiltrates as well as extensive fibrosis.

the posterior orbital fat may be selectively involved. Sclerosing orbital inflammation can lead to "wall-to-wall" radiodensity, in which the muscles, optic nerve, and globe are caught up entirely in a uniform ligneous mass (Fig. 54–31).

## Pathologic Features

Edema and a light polymorphic inflammatory infiltrate are highly characteristic in the early stages of inflammation. The infiltrating cells include lymphocytes, plasma cells, eosinophils, and less often polymorphonuclear leukocytes. Immunohistochemistry reveals that the lymphocytes are predominantly T

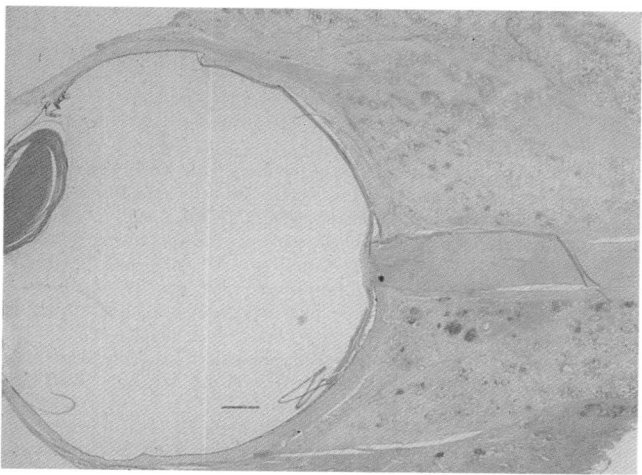

FIGURE 54–31. Pseudotumor. Sclerosing diffuse orbital variant showing lymphoid aggregates within extensive fibrosis, which has replaced the orbital fat and is firmly adherent to the sclera and optic nerve dural sheath.

cells. Eosinophilia may be especially evident in orbital biopsy specimens from children, and there may be an elevated absolute count of eosinophils in the peripheral blood.

As the disease progresses, collagen is laid down, and the inflammatory cells become more widely separated by fibrous tracts, which radiate outward from the tissue septa and blood vessels into the orbital fat. The connective tissues of the muscles thicken, and hyperplasia of the periacinar and periductal connective tissue of the lacrimal gland is observed. With progressive fibrosis, extraocular muscle degeneration occurs, and the secretory acinar units of the lacrimal gland are obliterated, leading to blind-duct proliferation or hyperplasia. When the acini of the lacrimal gland have been destroyed, they do not regenerate. In the inexorably sclerosing inflammation, all the orbital contents, including the optic nerve and sclera, are caught up in the strangulating fibrosis. There is only a light infiltrate of inflammatory cells, and necrosis is not featured, as in a true vasculitis or scleritis.

Frequently, perivascular lymphocytic cuffing is a prominent feature of idiopathic orbital inflammation, and occasionally eosinophils may be admixed. Such cuffing represents diapedesis of blood-borne cells into the adventitia of the capillaries and venules and does not constitute true vasculitis. In rare instances, a strictly localized idiopathic orbital inflammation seems to be caused by a true vasculitis of the orbital vessels, in which lymphocytes and polymorphonuclear leukocytes cause necrosis of the muscularis of orbital vessels. Henderson[155] pointed out that this subset frequently affects individuals younger than 30 years old. These lesions are less apt to be responsive to prednisone therapy and localized orbital radiotherapy and may require systemic administration of chemotherapeutic agents such as cyclophosphamide.

## Differential Diagnosis

The involvement of structures other than the extraocular muscles, combined with the presence of eosinophils, helps distinguish idiopathic orbital inflammation from Graves' disease. Compared with orbital lymphoid neoplasms, there is hypocellularity and far more cellular polymorphism, fibrosis, and edema. There is not the diffuse, sheetlike hyperplasia of lymphocytes that is characteristic of lymphoid tumors of the orbit. Lymphoid tumors of the orbit do not present acute inflammatory signs and generally are unifocal masses rather than the diffuse or multifocal processes represented by idiopathic orbital inflammations.[162] Locally invasive polymorphic orbital pseudotumors should be evaluated microscopically for cytologic atypia of fibrohistiocytic cells to exclude an inflamed malignant fibrous histiocytoma.

Idiopathic orbital inflammation can be indistinguishable clinically and histologically from systemic diseases, such as Wegener's granulomatosis, rheumatoid arthritis, Crohn's regional enteritis, systemic lupus erythematosus, and periarteritis nodosa. Although fewer than 10% of patients with orbital inflammation other than Graves' orbitopathy are found to have any underlying disease, it is probably wisest to have patients with inflammation studied for evidence of a multisystem autoimmune disease. Wegener's granulomatosis may produce only orbital signs and symptoms, but patients with this limited form of the disease often have antineutrophilic cytoplasmic antibodies in their serum.[153] Bilateral orbital lesions featuring many xanthoma cells should suggest the possibility of Erdheim-Chester disease.[163] Lesions with vascular endothelial proliferation and eosinophilia may represent angiolymphoid hyperplasia.[164, 165]

## Treatment

Therapy for acute fulminant cases of idiopathic orbital inflammation consisting of high doses of corticosteroids is generally curative. A less dramatic response to corticosteroids is found in subacute and chronic cases because of the heavy collagenization of the diseased tissues. Radiotherapy sometimes is administered in cases that are refractory to corticosteroids.[166] Many reports on radiotherapy for orbital inflammation actually dealt with lymphoid tumors rather than idiopathic inflammations, as defined and described in this chapter. Immunosuppressive therapy may be helpful in the small subset of patients who are refractory to corticosteroid therapy and radiotherapy.[167] Although idiopathic orbital inflammation generally is not a surgical disease, focal masses of hyalinized connective tissue in end-stage, burned-out cases may be surgically debulked to reduce proptosis or displacement of the eye. In extremely rare cases of refractory sclerosing orbital inflammation, there may be intractable pain, and vision may be lost from a compressive neuropathy as the fibrous tissue strangulates the optic nerve. Occasionally, when the patient has extraordinary pain and no vision, orbital exenteration may be indicated.

## REFERENCES

1. Eagle RC: Specimen handling in the ophthalmic pathology laboratory. Ophthalmol Clin N Am 8:1–15, 1995.
2. Bonner PK, Bregman BK, McLean IW, LaPiana FG: Mixed type basal cell carcinoma of the eyelid. Ophthalmic Plast Reconstr Surg 14:216–221, 1998.
3. Rao NA, Hidayat AA, McLean IW, Zimmerman LE: Sebaceous carcinomas of the ocular adnexa. A clinicopathologic study of 104 cases, with five-year follow-up data. Hum Pathol 13:113–122, 1982.
4. Doxanas MT, Green WR: Sebaceous gland carcinoma. Review of 40 cases. Arch Ophthalmol 102:245–249, 1984.
5. Ni C, Kuo PK: Meibomian gland carcinoma. A clinicopathological study of 156 cases with long-period follow-up of 100 cases. Jpn J Ophthalmol 23:388–401, 1979.
6. Brownstein S, Codere F, Jackson WB: Masquerade syndrome. Ophthalmology 87:259–262, 1980.
7. Margo CE, Lessner A, Stern GA: Intraepithelial sebaceous carcinoma of the conjunctiva and skin of the eyelid. Ophthalmology 99:227–231, 1992.
8. Bryant J: Meibomian gland carcinoma seeding intracranial soft tissues. Hum Pathol 8:455–457, 1977.
9. Rao NA, McLean IW, Zimmerman LE: Sebaceous carcinoma of the eyelid and caruncle. Correlation of clinical pathologic features with prognosis. In Jakobiec FA (ed): Ocular and Adnexal Tumors. Birmingham, Aesculapius Publishers, 1978, pp 289–342.
10. Folberg R, Whitaker DC, Tse DT, Nerad JA: Recurrent and residual sebaceous carcinoma after Mohs' excision of the primary lesion. Am J Ophthalmol 103:817–823, 1987.
11. Nunery WR, Welsh MG, McCord Jr CD: Recurrence of sebaceous carcinoma of the eyelid after radiation therapy. Am J Ophthalmol 96:10–15, 1983.
12. Benedict WF, Srivatsan ES, Mark C, et al: Complete or partial homozygosity of chromosome 13 in primary retinoblastoma. Cancer Res 47:4189–4191, 1987.
13. Friend SH, Bernards R, Rogelj S, et al: A human DNA segment with properties of the gene that predisposes to retinoblastoma and osteosarcoma. Nature 323:643–646, 1986.
14. Lee WH, Bookstein R, Hong F, et al: Human retinoblastoma susceptibility gene. Cloning, identification, and sequence. Science 235:1394–1399, 1987.
15. Benedict WF, Xu HJ, Takahashi R: The retinoblastoma gene. Its role in human malignancies. Cancer Invest 8:535–540, 1990.
16. Roarty JD, McLean IW, Zimmerman LE: Incidence of second neoplasms in patients with bilateral retinoblastoma. Ophthalmology 95:1583–1587, 1988.
17. Tso MOM, Fine BS, Zimmerman LE, et al: Photoreceptor elements in retinoblastoma. A preliminary report. Arch Ophthalmol 82:57–59, 1969.
18. Tso MOM, Fine BS, Zimmerman LE: The nature of retinoblastoma. II. Photoreceptor differentiation. An electron microscopic study. Am J Ophthalmol 69:350–359, 1970.
19. Tso MOM, Zimmerman LE, Fine BS: The nature of retinoblastoma. I. Photoreceptor differentiation. A clinical and histologic study. Am J Ophthalmol 69:339–359, 1970.
20. Margo C, Hidayat A, Kopelman J, et al: Retinocytoma. A benign variant of retinoblastoma. Arch Ophthalmol 101:1519–1531, 1983.
21. Rubinstein LJ: Tumors of the Central Nervous System. Atlas of Tumor Pathology. Second Series. Fascicle 6. Washington, DC, Armed Forces Institute of Pathology, 1982, pp 279–282.
22. Gallie BL, Phillips RA, Ellsworth RM, et al: Significance of retinoma and phthisis bulbi for retinoblastoma. Ophthalmology 89:1393–1399, 1982.
23. Schipper J: Retinoblastoma. A Medical and Experimental Study. Thesis. Utrecht, University of Utrecht, 1980.
24. Committee for the National Registry of Retinoblastoma: Survival rate and risk factors for patients with retinoblastoma in Japan. Jpn J Ophthalmol 36:121–131, 1992.
25. Tamboli A, Podgor MJ, Horm JW: The incidence of retinoblastoma in the United States. 1974 through 1985. Arch Ophthalmol 108:128–132, 1990.
26. Kopelman JE, McLean IW, Rosenberg SH: Multivariate analysis of risk factors for metastasis in retinoblastoma treated by enucleation. Ophthalmology 94:371–377, 1987.
27. Zimmerman LE: Retinoblastoma and retinocytoma. In Spencer WH (ed): Ophthalmic Pathology. An Atlas and Textbook. 3rd ed. Philadelphia, WB Saunders, 1985, pp 1292–1351.
28. Knudson Jr AG: Mutation and cancer. A statistical study of retinoblastoma. Proc Natl Acad Sci U S A 68:820–828, 1971.
29. Abramson DH, Ellsworth RM, Zimmerman LE: Nonocular cancer in retinoblastoma survivors. Trans Am Acad Ophthalmol Otolaryngol 81:454–456, 1976.
30. Derkinderen DJ, Koten JW, Wolterbeek R, et al: Non-ocular cancer in hereditary retinoblastoma survivors and relatives. Ophthalm Paediatr Genet 8:23–25, 1987.
31. Draper GJ, Sanders BM, Kingston JE: Second primary neoplasms in patients with retinoblastoma. Br J Cancer 53:661–671, 1986.
32. Lueder GT, Judisch GF, O'Gorman TW: Second nonocular

tumors in survivors of heritable retinoblastoma. Arch Ophthalmol 104:372–373, 1986.

33. Bader JL, Meadows AT, Zimmerman LE, et al: Bilateral retinoblastoma with ectopic intracranial retinoblastoma. Trilateral retinoblastoma. Cancer Genet Cytogenet 5:203–213, 1982.

34. Lueder GT, Judisch GF, Wen BC: Heritable retinoblastoma and pinealoma. Arch Ophthalmol 109:1707–1709, 1991.

35. Zimmerman LE, Burns RP, Wankum G, et al: Trilateral retinoblastoma. Ectopic intracranial retinoblastoma associated with bilateral retinoblastoma. J Pediatr Ophthalmol Strabismus 19:320–325, 1982.

36. Wiggs J, Nordenskjold M, Yandell D, et al: Prediction of the risk of hereditary retinoblastoma, using DNA polymorphisms within the retinoblastoma gene. N Engl J Med 318: 151–157, 1988.

37. Weichselbaum RR, Zakov ZN, Albert DM, et al: New findings in the chromosome 13 long-arm deletion syndrome and retinoblastoma. Trans Am Acad Ophthalmol Otolaryngol 86: 1191–1198, 1979.

38. Canning S, Dryja TP: Short, direct repeats at the breakpoints of deletions of the retinoblastoma gene. Proc Natl Acad Sci U S A 86:5044–5048, 1989.

39. Shields JA, Shields CL: Intraocular Tumors. A Text and Atlas. Philadelphia, WB Saunders, 1992.

40. John-Mikolajewski V, Messmer E, Sauerwein W, Freundlieb O: Orbital computed tomography. Does it help in diagnosing the infiltration of choroid, sclera and/or optic nerve in retinoblastoma? Ophthalmic Paediatr Genet 8:101–104, 1987.

41. Balmer A, Munier F, Gailloud C: Retinoma. Case studies. Ophthalmic Paediatr Genet 12:131–137, 1991.

42. Aaby AA, Price RL, Zakov ZN: Spontaneously regressing retinoblastomas, retinoma, or retinoblastoma group 0. Am J Ophthalmol 96:315–320, 1983.

43. Abramson DH, McCormick B, Fass D, et al: Retinoblastoma. The long-term appearance of radiated intraocular tumors. Cancer 67:2753–2755, 1991.

44. Boniuk M, Zimmerman LE: Spontaneous regression of retinoblastoma. Int Ophthalmol Clin 2:525–542, 1962.

45. Eagle Jr RC, Shields JA, Donoso L, Milner RS: Malignant transformation of spontaneously regressed retinoblastoma, retinoma/retinocytoma variant. Ophthalmology 96:1389–1395, 1989.

46. Mansour AM, Greenwald MJ, O'Grady R: Diffuse infiltrating retinoblastoma. J Pediatr Ophthalmol Strabismus 26:152–154, 1989.

47. Nicholson DH, Norton EW: Diffuse infiltrating retinoblastoma. Trans Am Ophthalmol Soc 78:265–289, 1980.

48. Shields JA, Shields CL, Eagle RC, Blair CJ: Spontaneous pseudohypopyon secondary to diffuse infiltrating retinoblastoma. Arch Ophthalmol 106:1301–1302, 1988.

49. Burnier MN, McLean IW, Zimmerman LE, Rosenberg SH: Retinoblastoma. The relationship of proliferating cells to blood vessels. Invest Ophthalmol Vis Sci 31:2037–2040, 1990.

50. Bunt AH, Tso MO: Feulgen-positive deposits in retinoblastoma. Incidence, composition, and ultrastructure. Arch Ophthalmol 99:144–150, 1981.

51. Tso MOM, Fine BS, Zimmerman LE: The Flexner-Wintersteiner rosettes in retinoblastoma. Arch Pathol 88:665–671, 1969.

52. Donoso LA, Shields CL, Lee EY: Immunohistochemistry of retinoblastoma. A review. Ophthalmic Paediatr Genet 10:3–32, 1989.

53. Kivelä T: Glycoconjugates in retinoblastoma. A lectin histochemical study of ten formalin-fixed and paraffin-embedded tumours. Virchows Arch [A] 410:471–479, 1987.

54. Vrabec T, Arbizo V, Adamus G, et al: Rod cell-specific antigens in retinoblastoma. Arch Ophthalmol 107:1061–1063, 1989.

55. Rubinstein LJ: Tumors of the Central Nervous System. Atlas of Tumor Pathology. Second Series, Fascicle 6. Washington, DC, Armed Forces Institute of Pathology, 1982.

56. Tso MOM, Zimmerman LE, Fine BS, et al: A cause of radioresistance in retinoblastoma. Photoreceptor differentiation. Trans Am Acad Ophthalmol Otolaryngol 74:959–969, 1970.

57. Smith JLS: Histology and spontaneous regression of retinoblastoma. Trans Ophthalmol Soc U K 94:953–967, 1974.

58. Erwenne CM, Franco EL: Age and lateness of referral as determinants of extra-ocular retinoblastoma. Ophthalmic Paediatr Genet 10:179–184, 1989.

59. Meli FJ, Boccaleri CA, Manzitti J, Lylyk P: Meningeal dissemination of retinoblastoma. CT findings in eight patients. AJNR Am J Neuroradiol 11:983–986, 1990.

60. Hungerford J, Kingston J, Plowman N: Orbital recurrence of retinoblastoma. Ophthalmic Paediatr Genet 8:63–68, 1987.

61. Magramm I, Abramson DH, Ellsworth RM: Optic nerve involvement in retinoblastoma. Ophthalmology 96:217–222, 1989.

62. Messmer EP, Heinrich T, Höpping W, et al: Risk factors for metastases in patients with retinoblastoma. Ophthalmology 98:136–141, 1991.

63. Stannard C, Lipper S, Sealy R, Sevel D: Retinoblastoma. Correlation of invasion of the optic nerve and choroid with prognosis and metastases. Br J Ophthalmol 63:560–570, 1979.

64. McLean IW, Rosenberg SH, Messmer EP, et al: Prognostic factors in cases of retinoblastoma. Analysis of 974 patients from Germany and the United States treated by enucleation. In Bornfeld N, Gragoudas ES, Lommatzsch PK (eds): Tumors of the Eye. Proceedings of the International Symposium on Tumors of the Eye. Amsterdam, Kugler Publications, 1991, pp 151–154.

65. Pratt CB, Meyer D, Chenaille P, Crom DB: The use of bone marrow aspirations and lumbar punctures at the time of diagnosis of retinoblastoma. J Clin Oncol 7:140–143, 1989.

66. McLean IW, Burnier MN, Zimmerman LE, Jokobiec FA: Tumor of the Eye and Ocular Adnexa. Atlas of Tumor Pathology. Third Series, Fascicle 12. Washington, DC, Armed Forces Institute of Pathology, 1994.

67. Stafford WR, Yanoff M, Parnell B: Retinoblastoma initially misdiagnosed as primary ocular inflammation. Arch Ophthalmol 82:771–773, 1969.

68. Shields JA, Shields CL, Suvarnamani C, et al: Retinoblastoma manifesting as orbital cellulitis. Am J Ophthalmol 112:442–449, 1991.

69. Shields JA, Shields CL, Sivalingam V: Decreasing frequency of enucleation in patients with retinoblastoma. Am J Ophthalmol 108:185–188, 1989.

70. Sanders BM, Draper GJ, Kingston JE: Retinoblastoma in Great Britain 1969–80. Incidence, treatment, and survival. Br J Ophthalmol 72:576–583, 1988.

71. Shields CL, Shields JA, Needle M, et al: Combined chemoreduction and adjuvant treatment for intraocular retinoblastoma. Ophthalmology 104:2101–2111, 1997.

72. Shields JA, Parsons H, Shields CL, Giblin ME: The role of cryotherapy in the management of retinoblastoma. Am J Ophthalmol 108:260–264, 1989.

73. Shields JA, Shields CL, Parsons H, Giblin ME: The role of photocoagulation in the management of retinoblastoma. Arch Ophthalmol 108:205–208, 1990.

74. Amendola BE, Markoe AM, Augsburger JJ, et al: Analysis of treatment results in 36 children with retinoblastoma treated by scleral plaque irradiation. Int J Radiat Oncol Biol Phys 17: 63–70, 1989.

75. Keith CG: Chemotherapy in retinoblastoma management. Ophthalmic Paediatr Genet 10:93–98, 1989.

76. Kingston JE, Hungerford JL, Plowman PN: Chemotherapy in metastatic retinoblastoma. Ophthalmic Paediatr Genet 8:69–72, 1987.

77. Grabowski EF, Abramson DH: Intraocular and extraocular retinoblastoma. Hematol Oncol Clin North Am 1:721–735, 1987.

78. White L: Chemotherapy for retinoblastoma. Where do we go from here? A review of published literature and meeting abstracts, including discussions during the Fifth International Symposium on Retinoblastoma, October 1990. Ophthalmic Paediatr Genet 12:115–130, 1991.

79. Gallagher RP, Elwood JM, Rootman J: Epidemiologic aspects of intraocular malignant melanoma. Cancer Treat Res 43:73–84, 1988.

80. Cutler SJ, Young JL: Third National Cancer Survey. Incidence data. Natl Cancer Inst Monogr Vol 41. Bethesda, MD, National Institutes of Health, 1975.

81. Barr CC, McLean IW, Zimmerman LE: Uveal melanoma in children and adolescents. Arch Ophthalmol 99:2133–2136, 1981.
82. Margo CE, McLean IW: Malignant melanoma of the choroid and ciliary body in black patients. Arch Ophthalmol 102:77–79, 1984.
83. Scotto J, Fraumenti JF, Lee JA: Melanomas of the eye and other noncutaneous sites. J Natl Cancer Inst 56:489–491, 1976.
84. Holly EA, Aston DA, Char DH, et al: Uveal melanoma in relation to ultraviolet light exposure and host factors. Cancer Res 50:5773–5777, 1990.
85. Seddon JM, Gragoudas ES, Glynn RJ, et al: Host factors, UV radiation, and risk of uveal melanoma. A case-control study. Arch Ophthalmol 108:1274–1280, 1990.
86. Gonder JR, Ezell PC, Shields JA, et al: Ocular melanocytosis. A study to determine the prevalence rate of ocular melanocytosis. Ophthalmology 89:950–952, 1982.
87. Gonder JR, Shields JA, Albert DM: Malignant melanoma of the choroid associated with oculodermal melanocytosis. Ophthalmology 88:372–376, 1981.
88. Gass JDM: Problems in the differential diagnosis of choroidal nevi and malignant melanomas. The XXXIII Edward Jackson Memorial Lecture. Am J Ophthalmol 83:299–323, 1977.
89. Naumann GOH, Yanoff M, Zimmerman LE: Histiogenesis of malignant melanomas of the uvea. I. Histopathologic characteristics of nevi of the choroid and ciliary body. Arch Ophthalmol 76:784–796, 1966.
90. Yanoff M, Zimmerman LE: Histogenesis of malignant melanomas of the uvea. II. Relationship of uveal nevi to malignant melanomas. Cancer 20:493–507, 1967.
91. Lynch HT, Anderson DE, Krush AJ: Heredity and intraocular malignant melanoma. Cancer 21:119–125, 1968.
92. Walker JP, Weiter JJ, Albert DM, et al: Uveal malignant melanoma in three generations of the same family. Am J Ophthalmol 88:723–726, 1979.
93. Prescher G, Bornfeld N, Becher R: Nonrandom chromosomal abnormalities in primary uveal melanoma. J Natl Cancer Inst 82:1765–1769, 1990.
94. Sisley K, Cottam DW, Rennie IG, et al: Non-random abnormalities of chromosomes 3, 6, and 8 associated with posterior uveal melanoma. Genes Chromosom Cancer 5:197–200, 1992.
95. Ghazvini S, Char DH, Kroll S, et al: Comparative genomic hybridization analysis of archival formalin-fixed paraffin-embedded uveal melanomas. Cancer Genet Cytogenet 90:96–101, 1996.
96. Copeman MC: The putative melanoma tumor-suppressor gene on human chromosome 6q. Pathology 24:307–309, 1992.
97. Tobal K, Warren W, Cooper CS, et al: Increased expression and mutation of p53 in choroidal melanoma. Br J Cancer 66:900–904, 1992.
98. Ziegler A, Leffell DJ, Kunala S, et al: Mutation hotspots due to sunlight in the p53 gene of nonmelanoma skin cancers. Proc Natl Acad Sci U S A 90:4216–4220, 1993.
99. Jay M, McCartney AC: Familial malignant melanoma of the uvea and p53. A Victorian detective story. Surv Ophthalmol 37:457–462, 1993.
100. McLean IW, Burnier MN, Zimmerman LE, Jokobiec FA: Tumor of the Eye and Ocular Adnexa. Atlas of Tumor Pathology. Third Series, Fascicle 12, Washington, DC, Armed Forces Institute of Pathology, 1994.
101. Holly EA, Aston DA, Ahn DK, et al: No excess prior cancer in patients with uveal melanoma. Ophthalmology 98:608–611, 1991.
102. Vink J, Crijns MB, Mooy CM, et al: Ocular melanoma in families with dysplastic nevus syndrome. J Am Acad Dermatol 23:858–862, 1990.
103. Taylor MR, Guerry D, Bondi EE, et al: Lack of association between intraocular melanomas and cutaneous dysplastic nevi. Am J Ophthalmol 98:478–482, 1984.
104. Barr CC, Zimmerman LE, Curtin VT, Font RL: Bilateral diffuse melanocytic uveal tumors associated with systemic malignant neoplasms. A recently recognized syndrome. Arch Ophthalmol 100:249–255, 1982.
105. Chang M, Zimmerman LE, McLean IW: The persisting pseudomelanoma problem. Arch Ophthalmol 102:726–727, 1984.
106. Zimmerman LE, McLean IW: Do growth and onset of symptoms of uveal melanomas indicate subclinical metastasis? Ophthalmology 91:685–691, 1984.
107. Affeldt JC, Minckler DS, Azen SP, Yeh L: Prognosis in uveal melanoma with extraocular extension. Arch Ophthalmol 98:1975–1979, 1980.
108. Shields JA, Shields CL: Massive orbital extension of posterior uveal melanomas. Ophthalmol Plast Reconstr Surg 7:238–251, 1991.
109. Font RL, Spaulding AG, Zimmerman LE: Diffuse malignant melanoma of the uveal tract. A clinicopathologic report of 54 cases. Trans Am Acad Ophthalmol Otolaryngol 72:877–894, 1968.
110. Manschot WA: Ring melanoma. Arch Ophthalmol 71:625–632, 1964.
111. Jakobiec FA, Silbert G: Are most iris "melanomas" really nevi? Arch Ophthalmol 99:2117–2132, 1981.
112. Sassani JW, Weinstein JM, Graham WP: Massively invasive diffuse choroidal melanoma. Arch Ophthalmol 103:945–948, 1985.
113. Callender GR: Malignant melanotic tumors of the eye. A study of histologic types in 111 cases. Trans Am Acad Ophthalmol Otolaryngol 36:131–142, 1931.
114. Callender GR, Wilder HC, Ash JE: Five hundred melanomas of the choroid and ciliary body. Followed five years or longer. Am J Ophthalmol 25:562–567, 1942.
115. Wilder HC, Paul EV: Malignant melanoma of the choroid and ciliary body. A study of 2,535 cases. Milit Surg 109:370–378, 1951.
116. Gamel JW, McCurdy JB, McLean IW: A comparison of prognostic covariates for uveal melanoma. Invest Ophthalmol Vis Sci 33:1919–1922, 1992.
117. McLean IW, Foster WD, Zimmerman LE: Prognostic factors in small malignant melanomas of choroid and ciliary body. Arch Ophthalmol 95:48–58, 1977.
118. McLean IW, Foster WD, Zimmerman LE: Uveal melanoma. Location, size, cell type, and enucleation as risk factors in metastasis. Hum Pathol 13:123–132, 1982.
119. Paul EV, Parnell BL, Fraker M: Prognosis of malignant melanomas of the choroid and ciliary body. Int Ophthalmol Clin 2:387–402, 1962.
120. Hayton S, Lafreniere R, Jerry LM, et al: Ocular melanoma in Alberta. A 38 year review pointing to the importance of tumor size and tumor histology as predictors of survival. J Surg Oncol 42:215–218, 1989.
121. Jensen OA: Malignant melanomas of the human uvea. Recent follow-up of cases in Denmark, 1943–1952. Acta Ophthalmol 48:1113–1128, 1970.
122. Rahi AHS, Agrawal PK: Prognostic parameters in choroidal melanomata. Trans Ophthalmol Soc U K 97:368–372, 1977.
123. Raivio IL: Uveal melanomas in Finland. An epidemiological, clinical, histological, and prognostic study. Acta Ophthalmol 133(suppl):1–64, 1977.
124. Shammas HF, Blodi FC: Prognostic factors in choroidal and ciliary body melanomas. Arch Ophthalmol 95:63–69, 1977.
125. McLean IW, Zimmerman LE, Evans RM: Reappraisal of Callender's spindle A type of malignant melanoma of choroid and ciliary body. Am J Ophthalmol 86:557–564, 1978.
126. Kan-Mitchell J, Rao N, Albert DM, et al: S100 immunophenotypes of uveal melanomas. Invest Ophthalmol Vis Sci 31:1492–1496, 1990.
127. Burnier MN Jr, McLean IW, Gamel JW: Immunohistochemical evaluation of uveal melanocytic tumors. Expression of HMB-45, S-100 protein, and neuron-specific enolase. Cancer 68:809–814, 1991.
128. Lorigan JG, Wallace S, Mavligit GM: The prevalence and location of metastases from ocular melanoma. Imaging study in 110 patients. AJR Am J Roentgenol 157:1279–1281, 1991.
129. McLean IW: The biology of haematogenous metastasis in human uveal malignant melanoma. Virchows Arch A Pathol Anat Histopathol 422:433–437, 1993.
130. Gamel JW, McLean IW: Computerized histopathologic assessment of malignant potential. II. A practical method for

predicting survival following enucleation for uveal melanoma. Cancer 52:1032–1038, 1983.

131. Gamel JW, McLean IW, Foster WD, Zimmerman LE: Uveal melanomas. Correlation of cytologic features with prognosis. Cancer 41:1897–1901, 1978.

132. Gamel JW, McLean IW, Greenberg RA, et al: Computerized histologic assessment of malignant potential. A method for determining the prognosis of uveal melanomas. Hum Pathol 13:893–897, 1982.

133. McCurdy J, Gamel J, McLean I: A simple, efficient, and reproducible method for estimating the malignant potential of uveal melanoma from routine H & E slides. Pathol Res Pract 187:1025–1027, 1991.

134. McLean IW, Foster WD, Zimmerman LE: Modifications of Callender's classification of uveal melanoma at the Armed Forces Institute of Pathology. Am J Ophthalmol 96:502–509, 1983.

135. Hayton S, Lafreniere R, Jerry LM, et al: Ocular melanoma in Alberta. A 38 year review pointing to the importance of tumor size and tumor histology as predictors of survival. J Surg Oncol 42:215–218, 1989.

136. Shammas HF, Blodi FC: Prognostic factors in choroidal and ciliary body melanomas. Arch Ophthalmol 95:63–69, 1977.

137. Augsburger JJ, Gamel JW: Clinical prognostic factors in patients with posterior uveal malignant melanoma. Cancer 66:1596–1600, 1990.

138. de la Cruz Jr PO, Specht CS, McLean IW: Lymphocytic infiltration in uveal malignant melanoma. Cancer 65:112–115, 1990.

139. Folberg R, Pe'er J, Gruman LM, et al: The morphologic characteristics of tumor blood vessels as a marker of tumor progression in primary human uveal melanoma. A matched case-control study. Hum Pathol 23:1298–1305, 1992.

140. McLean IW, Gamel JW: Prediction of metastasis of uveal melanoma. Comparison of morphometric determination of nucleolar size and spectrophotometric determination of DNA. Invest Ophthalmol Vis Sci 29:507–511, 1988.

141. Arentsen JJ, Green WR: Melanoma of the iris. Report of 72 cases treated surgically. Ophthalmic Surg 6:23–37, 1975.

143. Sunba MS, Rahi AHS, Morgan G: Tumors of the anterior uvea. I. Metastasizing malignant melanoma of the iris. Arch Ophthalmol 98:82–85, 1980.

144. Durie FH, George WD, Campbell AM, Damato BE: Analysis of clonality of tumour infiltrating lymphocytes in breast cancer and uveal melanoma. Immunol Lett 33:263–269, 1992.

145. Niederkorn JY: T cell subsets involved in the rejection of metastases arising from intraocular melanomas in mice. Invest Ophthalmol Vis Sci 28:1397–1403, 1987.

146. Vit VV: Prognostic role of morphologic characteristics of the immune response in uveal melanomas of various cellular types [ Russian]. Arkh Patol 45:25–30, 1983.

147. Kanda S, Cochran AJ, Lee WR, et al: Variations in the ganglioside profile of uveal melanoma correlate with cytologic heterogeneity. Int J Cancer 52:682–687, 1992.

148. Levin PS, Dutton JJ: A 20-year series of orbital exenteration. Am J Ophthalmol 112:496–501, 1991.

149. White WL, Ferry JA, Harris NL, Grove AS Jr: Ocular adnexal lymphoma. A clinicopathologic study with identification of lymphomas of mucosa-associated lymphoid tissue type. Ophthalmology 102:1994–2006, 1995.

150. Appel N, Som PM: Case report. Ectopic orbital lacrimal gland tissue. J Comput Assist Tomogr 6:1010–1012, 1982.

151. Green WR, Zimmerman LE: Ectopic lacrimal gland tissue. Report of 8 cases with orbital involvement. Arch Ophthalmol 78:318–327, 1967.

152. Grimson BS, Simona KB: Orbital inflammation, myositis and systemic lupus erythematosus. Arch Ophthalmol 101:736–738, 1983.

153. Kalina PH, Garrity JA, Herman DC, et al: Role of testing for anticytoplasmic autoantibodies in the differential diagnosis of scleritis and orbital pseudotumor. Mayo Clin Proc 65:1110–1117, 1990.

154. Weinstein JM, Koch K, Lane S: Orbital pseudotumor in Crohn's colitis. Ann Ophthalmol 16:275–278, 1984.

155. Henderson JW: Orbital Tumors. 2nd ed. New York, Brian C Decker, 1980.

156. Shields JA, Bakewell B, Augsburger JJ, Flanagan JC: Classification and incidence of space-occupying lesions of the orbit. A survey of 645 biopsies. Arch Ophthalmol 102:1606–1611, 1984.

157. McLean IW, Burnier MN, Zimmerman LE, Jokobiec FA: Tumor of the Eye and Ocular Adnexa. Atlas of Tumor Pathology. Third Series, Fascicle 12. Washington, DC, Armed Forces Institute of Pathology, 1994.

158. Ross WH: Myositic pseudotumor of the orbit. Can J Ophthalmol 18:199–201, 1983.

159. Kennerdell JS, Dresner SC: The nonspecific orbital inflammatory syndromes. Surv Ophthalmol 29:93–103, 1984.

160. Atlas SW, Grossman RI, Savino PJ, et al: Surface coil MR of orbital pseudotumor. AJR Am J Roentgenol 148:803–808, 1987.

161. Harr DL, Quencer RM, Abrams GW: Computed tomography and ultrasound in the evaluation of orbital infection and pseudotumor. Radiology 142:395–401, 1982.

162. Mauriello Jr JA, Flanagan JC: Pseudotumor and lymphoid tumor. Distinct clinicopathologic entities. Surv Ophthalmol 34:142–148, 1989.

163. Alper MG, Zimmerman LE, LaPiana FG: Orbital manifestations of Erdheim-Chester disease. Trans Am Ophthalmol Soc 81:64–85, 1983.

164. Hidayat AA, Cameron JD, Font RL, Zimmerman LE: Angiolymphoid hyperplasia with eosinophilia (Kimura's disease) of the orbit and ocular adnexa. Am J Ophthalmol 96:176–189, 1983.

165. Smith DL, Kincaid MC, Nicolitz E: Angiolymphoid hyperplasia with eosinophilia (Kimura's disease) of the orbit. Arch Ophthalmol 106:793–795, 1988.

166. Orcutt JC, Garner A, Henk JM, Wright JE: Treatment of idiopathic inflammatory orbital pseudotumours by radiotherapy. Br J Ophthalmol 67:570–574, 1983.

167. Paris GL, Waltuch GF, Egbert PR: Treatment of refractory orbital pseudotumors with pulsed chemotherapy. Ophthalmol Plast Reconstr Surg 6:96–101, 1990.

# Index

Note: Page numbers followed by the letter f refer to figures and those followed by t refer to tables.

Aβ peptide. *See* Amyloid β peptide (Aβ).
AAH (atypical adenomatous hyperplasia)
  prostatic, 1158–1159, 1158f–1159f, 1166, 1167
  pulmonary, 360, 383, 383f
AAT (α₁-antitrypsin), in yolk sac tumors
  ovarian, 1424, 1429, 1429t
  testicular, 1231
AAT deficiency. *See* α₁-Antitrypsin (AAT) deficiency.
Abdominal pregnancy, 1382
Abdominal trauma
  appendicitis caused by, 863
  splenic rupture caused by, 1578
    abscess and, 1576
    in infectious mononucleosis, 1577
Aberrant crypt foci, 756, 763
Abetalipoproteinemia, 741–742, 742f, 964
Abortion
  bleeding after, curettage for, 1337
  induced, 1466
    ectopic pregnancy subsequent to, 1382–1383
    mifepristone for, 1337
  spontaneous, 1452–1453, 1454, 1454f, 1466–1467, CD Figs. 40–1 and 40–2, CD Figs. 40–69 to 40–73
    causes of, 1466, 1467–1468, 1468f
    cytogenetics of, 1454, 1467–1468
    dating of, 1467, 1467t
    diethylstilbestrol and, 1277
    habitual, 1468
    in multiple gestation, 1468
    intrauterine infection and, 1468, CD Fig. 40–74
    leiomyoma causing, 1357
    retained fetal tissue following, 1338
    retained placenta following, 1470
    subchorionic hematomas in, 1459
  tubal, 1383–1384, 1385
Abrupt keratinization, 639, 640f
Abscess
  anal, 879
  appendiceal, 864
  bone, 1863
  breast, 545, 546, 548
  cerebral, 2107, CD Fig. 51–97
    in toxoplasmosis, 2107–2108, CD Fig. 51–99
  gallbladder-associated, 990
  hepatic, appendicitis causing, 864
  mediastinal, 496
  ovarian, 1434
  pancreatic
    acute pancreatitis causing, 907
    pseudocyst-associated, 908
  pelvic, appendicitis causing, 864
  pituitary, 2049
  prostatic, 1153

Abscess *(Continued)*
  pulmonary, in bronchogenic cyst, 495
  sellar region, 2049
  soft tissue, vs. neoplasm, 1844
  splenic, 1576
  testicular, 1246
  tubo-ovarian, 1380, 1381, 1434, CD Fig. 39–66
Acantholytic actinic keratosis, 1968
Acantholytic dyskeratosis, transient, 1941, 1941f
Acantholytic squamous cell carcinoma, 1969
  vulvar, 1265, 1265f, CD Figs. 35–30 and 35–31
Acanthoma(s), 1966–1967, 1966f–1967f
  pilar sheath, 1977
Acanthosis
  glycogenic, esophageal, 631–632
  overlying dermatofibroma, 1988
Acanthosis nigricans
  cutaneous, 1930
  esophageal, 656
Accessory tragus(i), 305, 305f
Accreditation of laboratories
  quality improvement and, 129, 130, 132
  turnaround time and, 135
ACE inhibitors, dermatitis caused by, 1958
Acetaminophen
  diverticulosis and, 818
  toxicity of, 948
Achalasia, 651, 651f
  Chagas' disease and, 654
  GERD secondary to, 657
  leiomyomatosis and, 635
  squamous carcinoma and, 636
Acid maltase deficiency, 84, 2160, 2163, 2164, CD Fig. 53–5
Acidophil stem cell adenoma, pituitary, 2029, 2032, 2033f, CD Fig. 50–5
Acidophilic bodies
  in acute hepatitis, 942, 942f
  in chronic hepatitis, 944, 945
Acinar cell carcinoma, pancreatic, 890–891, 890f
  vs. neuroendocrine neoplasms, 901–902
Acinar cell cystadenocarcinoma, pancreatic, 898
Acinic cell adenocarcinoma, salivary gland, 254–256, 254f–255f, CD Figs. 12–56 to 12–64
  mixed tumor transforming to, 258
  vs. cystadenocarcinoma, 263
  vs. epithelial-myoepithelial carcinoma, 262
  vs. salivary duct carcinoma, 263
Acinic cell carcinoma, bronchial gland, 357–358, 357f
Acne rosacea, granulomatous, 1957, 1957f

Acoustic schwannoma, 293, 2094, 2095f
Acquired immunodeficiency syndrome (AIDS). *See also* Human immunodeficiency virus (HIV) infection; Immunocompromised patient(s).
  adrenal leiomyosarcoma in, 1775
  appendiceal pathology in, 865
  bacillary angiomatosis in, 1985
    nodal, 1485
  bacillary peliosis hepatis in, 958
  BALT hyperplasia in, 375
  bronchiolitis in, follicular, 399
  cholangiopathy in, 994
  colitis in, adenovirus-induced, 830, 830f
  enterocolitis in, CMV-induced, 829
  enteropathy in, 734
    chronic bacterial, 826–827
  esophageal lesions in, 653
    in CMV infection, 651, 652, 653
    in HSV infection, 652
    in protozoal infection, 654
    in tuberculosis, 653
    inflammatory pseudotumor as, 634
  hairy leukoplakia in, 320, 321f
  hepatic infections in, 959, 960, CD Fig. 27–56
  herpes simplex infection in, anorectal, 830, 879
  Hodgkin's disease in, 1509
  iron overload in, 955
  Kaposi's sarcoma in, 1986
    esophageal, 648
    gallbladder, 986
    hepatic, 937–938, CD Fig. 27–26
    penile, 1206
    pulmonary, 371
    sinonasal, 187
  lymphadenopathy in, 1495
    Castleman's disease and, 1494
  microsporidial infection in, 85
  nephropathy in, 1009, 1010, 1011, 1011f, 1031
    TSRs in, 1011, 1021
  non-Hodgkin's lymphoma in, 1545
    anorectal, 800, 877
    Burkitt's, 693, 1534
    cardiac, 521
    CNS, 2044, 2096, 2097
    esophageal, 648
    gastric, 693
    hepatic, primary, 939
    oral, 317
    small intestine, 725
  pituitary infections in, 2049
  *Pneumocystis carinii* infection in
    otitis media seeded from, 299
    with granulomatous lymphadenitis, 1506
  prostatitis in, 1153

Breast *(Continued)*
  benign proliferative disease of. *See also*
      Adenoma; Duct hyperplasia, mam-
      mary, atypical; Fibroadenoma; Fi-
      brocystic breast disease.
    fibrocystic-related, 552–560, 553f–560f
  calcifications in
    in blunt-duct adenosis, 553
    in DCIS, 566, 566t, 568, 569
    in duct ectasia, 545
    in fibrocystic disease, 551, 552
    in sclerosing adenosis, 554
    mammography of, 564
    postmenopausal, 543
  carcinoma of. *See* Breast carcinoma.
  clear cell change in, 542–543, 543f
    in carcinoma, 574
    vs. LCIS, 573
  cystic hypersecretory hyperplasia of, 579
  development of, 539, 541–542
  duct ectasia in, 543, 544f, 545
    in cystic hypersecretory hyperplasia,
        579
    in fibrocystic disease, 551
  duct hyperplasia in. *See* Duct hyperpla-
      sia, mammary.
  ectopic tissue of, 539, 543
    lactating adenoma in, 550
  embryology of, 539
  fat necrosis in, 545–546
  fine-needle aspiration of, malpractice
      and, 140–141, 140t, 141t, 143, 146
  foreign body reaction in, 546, 590
  granular cell tumor of, 596
  gynecomastoid hyperplasia in, 545, 552
  hamartoma of, 596, 596f
  histology of, 540–543, 540f–544f
  infarct in, 548, 549
    with squamous metaplasia, 585
  inflammatory diseases of, 545–548,
      546f–548f
  lactational changes in, 542, 542f–543f
    in fibroadenoma, 549
  leiomyoma of, 595, 596
  lymphatic drainage of, 540, 541, 541f,
      611
  lymphoid tumors of, 547, 548f, 596–597
  male
    accessory tissue of, 543
    carcinoma in, 582, 589, 598–599
    diseases of, 545, 598–599
    estrogen-induced changes in, 542, 545
    fibroadenoma in, 591, 599
    gynecomastia of, 544–545, 545f, 598
      squamous metaplasia in, 585
    metastatic prostate carcinoma in, 597
    myofibroblastoma in, 593, 599
    phyllodes tumor in, 591, 599
    pubertal enlargement of, 539
  menopausal changes in, 539, 542, 543,
      543f
  menstrual changes in, 541–542
  mucocele-like tumor of, 579, 580f
  myoepithelial cells of, immunohisto-
      chemical markers in, 68
  pediatric diseases of, 597–598
  peripheral nerve tumors of, 596
  phyllodes tumor of. *See* Phyllodes tu-
      mor.
  pregnancy-like changes in, 542–543
  pregnancy-related changes in, 542, 544,
      548
  radiation-induced change(s) in, 590
    fat necrosis as, 545
    hypoplasia as, 543

Breast *(Continued)*
    lobular atypia as, 573, 574f
    vascular, 594
  skin tumors of, 594–595
  stromal tumors of, 590–593, 591f
  therapy-induced changes in, 590
  tissue specimen(s) from, 564–565, 565f
    from contralateral biopsy, 563–564
    frozen section of, 17, 19, 28, 29, 143,
        565
    malpractice claims involving, 140t,
        141–142, 141t, 143, 146
    pathology report on, 144t, 600, 600t
    specimen radiographs of, 564
    surgical margin evaluation of, 17, 28–
        29, 565
  vascular supply of, 539–540, 541, 541f
  vascular tumors of, 593–594, 593f–594f
Breast biopsy. *See* Breast, tissue speci-
    men(s) from.
Breast carcinoma, 563–590. *See also* Axil-
    lary lymph node metastases.
  arising in lymph node inclusions, 1484
  choriocarcinomatous features in, 589
  contralateral, 553–564
  detection of, 564–565, 565f
  diagnosis of, triple test strategy for, 140–
      141, 143, 144
  epidemiology of, 563
  genetic factors in, 118
    endometrial carcinoma and, 1345
    ovarian carcinoma and, 1413
  histologic grading of, 575–576, 599, 600,
      605–608, 610
  immunohistochemistry of, 17, 73, 575,
      597, 603, 604–605, 608, 609, 612
  in adolescence, 587, 587f, 598
  incidence of, 599
  intraoperative consultation on, 17, 19,
      28–29
  invasive type(s) of
    adenoid cystic, 587–589, 588f
    cribriform, 580–582, 581f
    cystic hypersecretory, 579
    inflammatory, 540, 589–590, 589f
    lobular, 576–578, 576f–578f
    medullary, 575–576, 585–586, 586f,
        607, 610
    metaplastic, 583–585, 584f
      vs. pleomorphic adenoma, 596
    miscellaneous variants of, 589
    mixed patterns in, 575
    mucinous, 578–580, 579f–580f
    not otherwise specified, 573–576,
        574f–575f, 578, 583, 586, 587
    occult, 590, 590r
    papillary, 560, 561f, 582–583, 582f–
        583f
    secretory (juvenile), 587, 587f, 598
    signet ring, intraductal, 588–589
    tubular, 580–582, 580f–581f
  locations of, 563
  lymph node metastases in. *See also* Axil-
      lary lymph node metastases.
    from lobular carcinoma, 578
    immunohistochemical studies of, 70
    PCR detection of, 114
  lymphatic-vascular invasion in, 574–575,
      599
  male, 598–599
    giant cell, 589
    papillary, 582
  metastases from, 597. *See also* Axillary
      lymph node metastases.
    from occult primary, 590, 590f

Breast carcinoma *(Continued)*
    in adenoid cystic carcinoma, 588
    in lobular carcinoma, 578
    in metaplastic carcinoma, 585
    malpractice claims involving, 140
    to bone marrow, 69, 69f, 597, 1639,
        1640f, CD Fig. 43–26
    to CNS, 2105
    to colon, 779
    to contralateral breast, 563
    to endometrium, 1350, CD Fig. 37–40
    to ovary, 578, 597, 1433, 1433f
    without invasion, 568
  metastatic, 597
  multicentric, 563, 564f
  multifocal, 563
  neural invasion in, 589
  neuroendocrine differentiation in, 575,
      589
  noninvasive, 566–573, 566t, 567f–573f.
      *See also* Carcinoma in situ (CIS),
      breast.
  osteoclast-like giant cells in, 589
  pathology report on, 144t, 600, 600t
  precursor lesion(s) of
    atypical lobular hyperplasia as, 570
    duct hyperplasia as, 561–562
    fibroadenoma as, 549
    fibrocystic disease as, 550, 552, 563,
        598
    LCIS as, 570
    microglandular adenosis as, 556
    sclerosing adenosis as, 553
  predictive tests in, 603
  prognostic factor(s) in, 599–613, 600t.
      *See also* Axillary lymph node metas-
      tases.
    adjuvant therapy and, 599, 600, 603
    for DCIS, 599–600
    histologic grading as, 575–576, 599,
        600, 605–608, 610
    ideal features of, 600
    local control and, 599
    molecular, 71–72, 74, 115t, 116–117,
        599, 600–605
    needed studies on, 601, 604
    proliferation markers as, 606, 608–611
    sentinel node biopsy as, 17, 70, 568,
        611–613, 1482
    traditionally accepted, 599
  risk factors for, 563
  sinus histiocytosis in, 1499
  staging of, 590, 599
  vs. adenomyoepithelioma, 557
  vs. duct adenoma, 559
  vs. fat necrosis, 545–546
  vs. granulomatous lobular mastitis, 546
  vs. intraductal papilloma, 559, 560
  vs. lymphoma, 547, 548f
  vs. microglandular adenosis, 556
  vs. radial scar, 557, 558
  vs. sclerosing adenosis, 553–555, 555f–
      556f
Breast implants, 590
Brenner tumor
  myometrial, 1368
  ovarian, 1410–1412, 1411f, CD Fig. 39–
      26
  paratesticular, 1244
Breslow thickness, 2010, 2010t, 2014
  vulvar melanomas and, 1269
Breus mole, 1459, CD Fig. 40–31
Bridging hepatic necrosis
  in acute hepatitis, 943, 943f
  in autoimmune hepatitis, 948

Cervical carcinoma *(Continued)*
in adenocarcinoma, 1298, 1299, 1305–1308, 1306f, 1311, CD Figs. 36–42 to 36–65
risk factors for, 1291–1292
squamous cell, 1308, 1308t
cytology of, 1299, 1299f, CD Fig. 36–16
epidemiology of, 1311–1312
in collision tumors, 1317, CD Fig. 36–108
invasive, 1312–1314, 1312f–1313f, CD Figs. 36–75 to 36–85
microinvasive, 1309–1310, 1309f–1310f, 1310t, CD Figs. 36–66 and 36–37
staging of, 1308–1309, 1308t
vascular involvement in
in invasive disease, 1313
in microinvasive disease, 1310, 1310f
Cervical cytology, 1295–1299, 1296f, 1298f–1299f, CD Figs. 36–1 to 36–15
computer-assisted, 1295
liquid-based, 1295, 1297
Cervical dysplasia, 1294, 1295, 1297, 1300, 1303
endocervical glandular, 1306
Cervical intraepithelial neoplasia (CIN)
basement membrane disruption in, 1310
cytology of, 1297, 1299
etiology of, 1292–1293
grading of, 1299–1300, 1300f, CD Figs. 36–17 to 36–23
CIN 1 in, 1300–1303, 1301f–1302f, CD Figs. 36–28 to 36–31
CIN 2 in, 1303–1304, 1303f–1304f, CD Figs. 36–32 to 36–37
CIN 3 in, 1304–1305, 1304f–1305f, CD Figs. 38–41
with microinvasive carcinoma, 1309, 1309f
HPV infection and, 1292–1293
cytology and, 1297
in CIN 1, 1301–1303, 1302f
in CIN 2, 1304
molecular detection of, 117, 1302–1303, 1302f, 1304
margin evaluation in, with LEEP, 1300, CD Figs. 36–24 to 36–27
terminology of, 1294–1295
with adenocarcinoma in situ (AIS), 1306
Cervical tumor(s)
epithelial
carcinoma as. *See* Cervical carcinoma.
miscellaneous, 1317–1319, 1318f, CD Figs. 36–107 to 36–117
mesenchymal, 1319–1320, 1319f–1320f
granulocytic sarcoma as, 1365
leiomyoma as, 1320, CD Figs. 36–119 and 36–120
lymphoma as, 1319, 1365
melanoma as, 1319, 1320
metastatic, 1320
mixed
adenofibroma as, 1354
adenomyoma as, 1354
adenosarcoma as, 1354
carcinosarcoma as, 1355
ovarian metastases from, 1434
Cervicitis, 1320
Cervicouterine junction, carcinoma of, 1315, CD Fig. 36–89
Cervix. *See also* Cervical carcinoma; Cervical tumor(s); Endocervical *entries.*
anatomy of, 1328
arteritis of, 1367, 1368

Cervix *(Continued)*
atrophic squamous epithelium in, 1304, 1305, CD Fig. 36–41
embryology of, 1291, 1327
endometriosis of, 1307, CD Figs. 36–60 and 36–61
epithelium of, 1291
extramedullary hematopoiesis in, 1357
functional role of, 1291
infectious or inflammatory conditions of, 1320
leukemic infiltration of, 1319
papillary endocervicitis of, 1307, CD Figs. 36–49 and 36–50
radiation-induced atypia in, 1307, CD Figs. 36–51 and 36–52
reactive squamous proliferations of, 1302, 1302f, 1303–1304, 1304f, CD Figs. 36–29, 36–34 and 36–35
CGCG (central giant cell granuloma), 164
of jaw, 331–332, 331f
Chagas' disease, esophageal motility disturbance in, 654
Chancroid, 1208
Charcot-Böttcher filaments, in Sertoli cell tumor, 1238
Charcot-Leyden crystals, in allergic fungal sinusitis, 191
Charcot-Marie-Tooth disease, hypertrophic, 84
Charge-coupled device, 49, 51f
Cheilitis, actinic, 1968
Chemical carcinogens
bladder cancer and, 1103–1104
non-Hodgkin's lymphoma and, 1518
renal cell carcinoma and, 1076
scrotal squamous cell carcinoma and, 1210
Chemical meningitis, ruptured epidermoid cyst causing, 2049
Chemotherapy
acute myeloid leukemia caused by, 1602, 1607–1608
bone marrow necrosis caused by, 1646
breast changes induced by, 590
cyclophosphamide, bladder cancer caused by, 1104
for oligodendroglioma, 2076, 2077
for osteosarcoma, 1872
for retinoblastoma, 2186
hepatic arterial, gallbladder injury by, 990
therapeutic response to
*p53* alterations and, 73, 1121
P-glycoprotein and, 73–74
veno-occlusive liver disease following, 956
Chernobyl accident–associated thyroid cancers, 1663, 1663t, 1683
Cherubism, 332, CD Figs. 14–4 and 14–5
Chiari syndrome. *See* Budd-Chiari syndrome.
Chiasmal syndrome, CNS lymphoma presenting as, 2044
Chief cell hyperplasia, 1734–1735. *See also* Parathyroid gland, hyperplasia of.
Chimeric proteins, 91
in soft tissue sarcomas, 1786
Chinese patient(s)
lymphoepithelial carcinoma in, salivary gland, 265
nasopharyngeal carcinoma in, 169
*Chlamydia pneumoniae,* in atherectomy specimens, 515

*Chlamydia trachomatis* infection. *See also* Lymphogranuloma venereum.
endometritis in, 1333
proctitis and colitis in, 830–831
salpingitis in, 1380
Chlorinated water, bladder cancer risk and, 1104
Chloroma. *See* Myeloid tumors, extramedullary.
Chloroquine
heart failure caused by, 511
lichenoid drug reaction to, 1934
myopathy caused by, 2160
Cholangiectasis(es), 994, CD Fig. 28–24
copper deposits in, 953, CD Fig. 27–42
Cholangiocarcinoma, 933–934, CD Figs. 27–16 and 27–17
Caroli's disease with, 933, 961
hepatocellular carcinoma combined with, 927, 929–930, CD Fig. 27–12
sclerosing, 930
hilar, 933, 934
primary biliary cirrhosis and, 950
primary sclerosing cholangitis and, 952
vs. inflammatory pseudotumor, 936
polycystic disease with, 961
primary biliary cirrhosis predisposing to, 950
primary sclerosing cholangitis and, 993–994
sclerosing, 930
staging of, 928t
trematode infections and, 933, 959
vs. hemangioendothelioma, epithelioid, 937
Cholangiohepatitis, Oriental, 954, CD Fig. 27–44
Cholangioles, 949, 950f
bile duct obstruction and, 950
in cystic fibrosis, 965
in primary biliary cirrhosis, 951
in sepsis, 950
Cholangiopathy
autoimmune, 952
ischemic, 994
Cholangitis
autoimmune, 952
choledochal cyst causing, 995
chronic, inflammatory pseudotumor and, 936
in Caroli's disease, 961
in congenital hepatic fibrosis, 961
in Kawasaki's disease, 962
in Langerhans cell histiocytosis, 962
in primary biliary cirrhosis, 952
in toxic shock syndrome, 954
post-transplantation, 968
primary recurrent pyogenic, 954, CD Fig. 27–44
primary sclerosing (PSC), 949, 951t, 952–953, 952f, CD Figs. 27–41 to 27–43
extrahepatic, 993–994, CD Figs. 28–22 to 28–26
in allograft, 969
with chronic cholecystitis, 991
with ulcerative colitis, 951t, 952
cholangiocarcinoma and, 933, 952
colorectal carcinoma and, 809
extrahepatic bile duct carcinoma and, 992
secondary sclerosing, 954, 994
simple obstructive, 954
suppurative, severe, 994
Cholangitis lenta, in sepsis, 950, 950f

Endometriosis, 433, 1366
  appendiceal, 801, 868
  bladder, 1134, CD Fig. 31–48
    vs. adenocarcinoma, 1127
  broad ligaments, 1391
  cervical, 1307, CD Figs. 36–60 and 36–61
  colorectal, 801–802
    germ cell tumor arising in, 800
  ectopic pregnancy and, 1382–1383, 1385
  fallopian tube, 1385, 1385f
  lymph node, 1483, 1487
  ovarian, 1436, 1436f
    clear cell adenocarcinoma with, 1409
    endometrioid adenocarcinoma with, 1407
    mixed cystadenoma with, 1412
    mucinous tumor with, 1406
    salpingitis associated with, 1385, 1385f
  paramesonephric duct cyst, 1391
  prostatic, 1134, 1160
  renal, 1134
  round ligaments, 1391
  serosal, 801
  small intestine, 739–740
  ureteral, 1134
  urethral, 1134
  uterine, 1366, 1368
  vaginal, vs. prolapsed fallopian tube, 1280
  with peritoneal leiomyomatosis, 434, 1361
Endometritis, 1332–1333, CD Fig. 37–8
  lymphoma-like lesions in, 1365
  metaplastic changes in, 1342
  syncytial, 1470, CD Fig. 40–88
Endometrium. See also Endometrial entries; Uterus.
  arteriovenous malformation of, 1368
  drug-related changes in, 1336–1337, CD Figs. 37–13 and 37–14
  ectopic pregnancy and, 1384, CD Fig. 38–10
  embryology of, 1327
  estrogen-related alterations in, 1334–1335, 1334f–1335f, CD Figs. 37–9 and 37–10
    exogenous hormone and, 1336, CD Fig. 37–13
  extramedullary hematopoiesis in, 1357, CD Fig. 37–63
  gestational changes in, 1455
  histology of, 1328–1329, 1328f–1329f
  in products of conception, 1453, CD Figs. 40–1 and 40–2
  inflammation of, 1332–1333, CD Fig. 37–8
    in tuberculosis, 1381
  lymphoma-like lesions of, 1365
  metaplasias of
    epithelial, 1341, 1342–1343, 1349–1350, CD Figs. 37–18 and 37–19
    nonepithelial, 1338, 1338f
  papillary syncytial change in, 1334, 1343, CD Fig. 37–10
  physiology of, 1328–1332, 1330f–1332f, CD Figs. 37–4 to 37–7
  primitive neuroectodermal tumor in, 1357
  progesterone-related alterations in, 1335–1336, CD Figs. 37–11 and 37–12
    exogenous hormone and, 1336, CD Fig. 37–13
  radiation-induced changes in, 1338

Endometrium (Continued)
  spindle cell nodule in, postoperative, 1368
  teratoma of, 1357
Endomyocardial biopsy, 505–515
  artifacts of, 506
  caveats related to, 506
  electron microscopy in, 84, 510
  in cardiac transplantation, 505, 511–515, 512f–514f, 512t
  in drug toxicity, 84, 505, 511, 511f, 511t
  in heart failure, 506–510, 507f, 508t, 509f–510f
  indications for, 505
  of neoplastic lesions, 506
  pathology report of, 505, 506t
  specimen processing in, 505
Endomyocardial fibrosis
  idiopathic, 508
  Löffler's. See Hypereosinophilic syndrome.
Endomyometrial junction, 1328, 1365
Endomyometritis, 1332, 1333
  after curettage, 1337
Endoneurial cells
  immunohistochemical markers of, 318
  in neurofibroma, 1992
Endophthalmitis, vs. retinoblastoma, 2181
Endoplasmic reticulum storage disorders, 963
Endosalpingiosis, 433–434, 434f, 1366, CD Figs. 37–84 and 37–85
  appendiceal, 868
  broad ligament, 1391
  fallopian tube, 1385, 1385f
  lymph node, 1483
  ovarian, 1435
  peritoneal, vs. ovarian tumor implants, 1403, CD Figs. 39–12 and 39–13
  with peritoneal leiomyomatosis, 434
Endoscopic retrograde cholangiopancreatography (ERCP)
  emphysematous cholecystitis secondary to, 990
  in primary sclerosing cholangitis, 952, 994
    vs. mastocytosis, systemic, 953
Endothelial cyst, adrenal, 1772
Endothelial hyperplasia, papillary, 1816–1817, 1817f
  cutaneous, 1983
  in atherectomy specimens, 515
Endothelial markers, 67
Endovascular papillary angioendothelioma, 1986
Enema solutions, intestinal mucosa and, 831–832
Enhancer, 91, 102f, 103
Entamoeba histolytica. See also Amebiasis.
  colitis caused by, 827–828, 828f
  hepatic lesions caused by, 959
Enteric cyst, mediastinal, 494, 495, 495f
Enterobius vermicularis infection
  appendiceal, 865, 865f, 866
  hepatic, 959
  tubal, 1381
Enterochromaffin cell tumors, pancreatic, 903
Enterochromaffin-like cells, 680
  hyperplasia of, 681
Enterocolitis. See also Colitis.
  Campylobacter causing, 822
  collagenous, 813
  Hirschsprung's-associated, 754
  necrotizing
    Hirschsprung's-associated, 754–755

Enterocolitis (Continued)
  in newborn, 826f
  neutropenic, 826, 826f
  pericrypt eosinophilic, 815
  Salmonella causing, 824
Enterocolitis lymphofollicularis, 725
Enteroendocrine system, 752
Enteropathy, autoimmune, 733
Enteropathy-associated T cell lymphoma, 728–729, 1538, 1539
  gastric involvement in, 693
Enucleated eye
  in retinoblastoma, 2185, 2186
  pathology in, 2178, 2178f
  processing of, 2173–2174
Enzymes, invasion-associated, 601
Eosinophilia, 1644
  growth factor administration and, 1645
  in Churg-Strauss syndrome, 1948
  orbital pseudotumor with, 2197
Eosinophilia-myalgia syndrome, 508, 1954, 2161
Eosinophilic cell metaplasia, endometrial, 1343
Eosinophilic cholecystitis, 991, CD Fig. 28–17
Eosinophilic cystitis, 1136
Eosinophilic enteritis, vs. subacute appendicitis, 864
Eosinophilic enterocolitis, pericrypt, 815
Eosinophilic esophagitis, idiopathic, 655, 655f
Eosinophilic fasciitis, 1954–1955, 1954f
Eosinophilic gastritis, 699, 700, 709, 709f
Eosinophilic gastroenteritis, 735–736
  vs. food hypersensitivity, 733
Eosinophilic granuloma, 304, 1546. See also Langerhans cell histiocytosis (histiocytosis X).
  appendiceal, Strongyloides and, 865
  gastric, 699
  jaw, 332, CD Fig. 14–6
  osseous, 1884–1885, 1884f
  pulmonary, 393t, 395, 397–398, 397f–398f
Eosinophilic leukemia, chronic, 1620
Eosinophilic microabscesses, in Langerhans cell histiocytosis, 1546
Eosinophilic pneumonia, 405–406, 406f
Eosinophilic spongiosis, 1920
  in bullous pemphigoid, 1942
  in incontinentia pigmenti, 1923, 1923f
  in pemphigus vulgaris, 1939
EPE (extraprostatic extension), 1176–1177, 1179, 1180
Ependymoblastoma, 2086, 2086t, 2089, CD Figs. 51–55 and 51–56
Ependymoma, 2078–2079, 2078f–2079f, 2078t, CD Figs. 51–25 and 51–26
  anaplastic, 2079–2080
    vs. ependymoblastoma, 2089
  clear cell, 2079
    electron microscopy of, 87
    vs. oligodendroglioma, 2077, 2081
  differential diagnosis of, 2080–2081
    vs. astroblastoma, 2083
  in hypothalamic region, 2040–2041
  molecular genetics of, 2080
  myxopapillary, 2080, 2081, CD Fig. 51–27
  papillary, 2079, 2081
    vs. choroid plexus papilloma, 2082
  prognostic features of, 2081
  simian virus 40 and, 2081
Ephelis (freckle), 2001
Epidermal cyst, 1978

Ewing's sarcoma *(Continued)*
  broad ligament, 1392
  mediastinal, 491
  sinonasal, 190
  in bone marrow, 1639, 1640
  molecular methods and, 1883
    for detecting extent of disease, 114
    for diagnosis, 103, 104t, 106–107, 106f
*EWS* gene, 103, 104t, 106–107, 108
  in desmoplastic small round cell tumor, 429
  in malignant melanoma of soft parts, 1840
  in myxoid chondrosarcoma, 1841
  in peripheral neuroectodermal tumor, 1838
Excisional skin biopsy, 1919
Exfoliative dermatitis, 1929
Exons, 91, 102
Exophytic endobronchial epidermoid carcinoma, 343
Exostosis
  cartilaginous, 1875
  of external auditory canal, 302
  subungual, 1875
Extrachorial placentation, 1457, CD Figs. 40–18 and 40–19
Extramedullary hematopoiesis
  in endometrium, 1357, CD Fig. 37–63
  in hepatic angiomyolipoma, 936, 936f
  in neonatal hepatitis, 943
  in tyrosinemia, 964
  soft tissue, vs. myelolipoma, 1792
  splenic, 1591, 1591f, 1592
  thyroid, 1725
Extranodal T cell lymphomas, 1538–1540, 1539f–1540f
Extraprostatic extension (EPE), 1176–1177, 1179, 1180
Extrinsic allergic alveolitis, 393t, 396–397, 397f
Eye. *See also* Conjunctiva; Cornea; Optic nerve; Orbit; Retinoblastoma; Uveal malignant melanoma.
  blind painful, 2178, 2198
  specimens from, processing of, 2173–2174, 2174f
Eyelid
  basal cell carcinoma of, 2174
  Moll gland cyst of, 1976
  sebaceous carcinoma of, 1981, 2174–2177, 2175f–2176f
  specimen from, processing of, 2173

Fabry's disease, 510, 964, 1049–1050, 1050f
  small intestine involvement in, 742
Facial nerve, chorda tympani of, 282
  adenoma and, 290
Facial palsy, in Wegener's granulomatosis, 307
Facioscapulohumeral muscular dystrophy, 2158, 2169, CD Fig. 53–2
Facioscapulohumeral myopathy, in mitochondrial disease, 2162
Factor VIII–related antigen, 67
Faggot cells, in acute promyelocytic leukemia, 1611
Fallopian tube(s), 1378–1391
  adenomatoid tumor of, 427, 1386, 1386f
  anatomy of, 1379
  arteritis of, 1367, 1368
  benign lesions of, 1385–1387, 1386f, CD Figs. 38–11 and 38–12
  congenital anomalies of, 1378, 1385

Fallopian tube(s) *(Continued)*
  diverticula in, 1382, 1382f
    tubal pregnancy and, 1383
  embryologic rests in, 1378, 1379f, CD Fig. 38–1
  embryology of, 1327, 1378
  endometriosis of, 1385, 1385f
  endosalpingiosis on, 1385
  foreign body or material in, 1381–1382
  histology of, 1379–1380
  hyperplastic epithelial changes in, 1387
  infection or inflammation of. *See* Salpingitis; Tubo-ovarian abscess.
  infertility and, 1385
  malignant lesions of, 1387–1388, 1390, CD Fig. 38–13
    checklist for, 1388t–1389t
    ovarian involvement by, 1434
    prognosis of, 1388, 1390, 1390t
  metaplastic epithelial changes in, 1386, 1386f, CD Fig. 38–12
  metastatic carcinoma of, 1390
  paratubal lesions associated with, 1390–1391
  physiology of, 1379–1380
  prolapsed, 1279–1280
  sterilization procedures on, 1385
  torsion of, 1390
  tubal pregnancy in, 1382–1385, 1383f–1384f, CD Figs. 38–5 to 38–10
  trophoblastic implants secondary to, 434
False vocal cord(s), 211, 212, 213. *See also* Vocal cord(s).
  amyloidosis of, 232
  rhabdomyoma of, 216
Familial adenomatous polyposis (FAP), 789–790, 790f. *See also* Gardner's syndrome.
  aberrant crypt foci and, 763
  hepatoblastoma in, 930
  nasopharyngeal angiofibroma and, 158
  small intestine adenomas in, 715
  small intestine carcinoma in, 717
  thyroid cancer in, 1664, 1695
  Turcot's syndrome and, 791
Familial breast-ovarian cancer syndromes, 1413
Familial enteropathy, 730, 733, 734f
Familial fatal insomnia (FFI), 2136, 2137, 2140
Familial juvenile polyposis. *See also* Juvenile polyps.
  gastric polyps in, 673, 698
Familial Mediterranean fevers, amyloid A protein in, 1027
Familial polyposis coli. *See* Familial adenomatous polyposis (FAP).
Fanconi's anemia, 1641
FAP. *See* Familial adenomatous polyposis (FAP).
Farmer's lung, 396, 397
Fasciitis
  cranial, 1798
  eosinophilic, 1954–1955, 1954f
  intravascular, 1797, 1798
  ischemic, 1797, 1797f
  necrotizing, 1844, 1844f
    perineal, 1209
  nodular, 1797–1799, 1798f
    vs. dermatofibrosarcoma, 1813
    vs. desmoid fibromatosis, 1805
    vs. fibroma of tendon sheath, 1802
    vs. malignant fibrous histiocytoma, 1816

Fasciitis *(Continued)*
  vs. plexiform fibrohistiocytic tumor, 1811
  parosteal, 1797–1798
  proliferative, 1799, 1799f
  tryptophan-related, 1954
Fat atrophy, serous, 1641, 1641f
Fat necrosis
  in $\alpha_1$-antitrypsin deficiency, 1951
  in bone marrow, 1860
  in breast, 545–546
  in lupus panniculitis, 1952, 1953f
  in pancreatic disease, 907, 907f, 1951, 1951f
  in scrotum, 1211
  of newborn, subcutaneous, 1952, 1952f
FATPWO (female adnexal tumor of probable wolffian origin), 1390–1391, 1392, 1392f, CD Fig. 38–14
  vs. endometrioid carcinoma, 1409
FCCL (follicular center cell lymphoma). *See* Follicular lymphoma.
Fecalith
  in appendix, 854, 862, 863
  in diverticulum, 819
Fechner's tumor, 357–358, 357f
Felty's syndrome, splenic pathology in, 1579
Female adnexal tumor of probable wolffian origin (FATPWO), 1390–1391, 1392, 1392f, CD Fig. 38–14
  vs. endometrioid carcinoma, 1409
Feminization, 1756
  adrenocortical adenoma causing, 1758, 1759–1760
Fenfluramine, valve disease associated with, 523, 524, 524f, 525
Ferritin, in iron overload, 954
Ferruginous bodies, 398–399
Fetal circulation
  chorioamnionitis and, 1463, 1463f
  thrombosis in, 1462, 1462f, CD Fig. 40–51
Fetal demise. *See also* Abortion.
  in multiple gestation, 1466, CD Fig. 40–68
  membrane coloration secondary to, 1457
  umbilical obstruction and, 1456, 1456f
  villus tissue alterations in, 1461–1462, 1462f, CD Figs. 40–48 and 40–49
Fetal hypoxia
  chorangiosis and, 1461
  chorioamnionitis and, 1463
  nucleated red blood cells and, 1462
Fetal membranes
  abnormalities of, 1457–1458, 1458f, CD Figs. 40–18 to 40–28
  examination of, 1452, 1453, 1454, 1454t
  in multiple gestation, 1465–1466, 1465f–1466f, CD Figs. 40–64 to 40–67
  infection of. *See* Chorioamnionitis.
Fetal rhabdomyoma, 1825
Fetal rhabdomyomatous nephroblastoma, 1068
Fetal tissue, retained, 1338
Fetal-type hepatoblastoma, 921t
Fetus
  examination of, 1452, 1453, 1454, 1466–1467, CD Figs. 40–69 to 40–70
  hydrops in, 1460, 1461f
  infection of, 1463, 1464
  tumors in, 1460
Fetus papyraceus, 1466, CD Fig. 40–68
FFI (familial fatal insomnia), 2136, 2137, 2140
FGF. *See* Fibroblast growth factor (FGF).

Hamartoma (*Continued*)
  gastric polypoid, 697f, 698
  hepatic, mesenchymal, 934, 934f
  hypothalamic, 2039, 2084, 2108–2109
  lymphangioma as, 1818
  melanocytic, dermal, 2001
  odontogenic, 328, 328f
  palatine tonsil, 198–199, 199f
  parathyroid, 1729t
  peribiliary gland, 931
  pulmonary, 380–381, 381f, CD Fig. 15–14
    genetic alterations in, 111
    vs. metastatic uterine leiomyosarcoma, 388
  sinonasal, 198–199, 199f
  smooth muscle, 1991
    of dartos, 1212
  splenic, 1582–1583, 1583f, CD Fig. 42–9
Hamartomatous polyp, colorectal, 764–765, 764f
Hamazaki-Wesenberg bodies, intranodal, in sarcoidosis, 1505
Hamman-Rich syndrome, 389, 390–391, 392t
Hand-Schüller-Christian syndrome, 304, 1546, 1885
Hard drive, 46
Hard metal pneumoconiosis, 391, 393t, 398, 398f
Hashimoto-Pritzker disease, 2000
Hashimoto's thyroiditis, 1716t, 1717, 1717f–1718f
  cysts associated with, 1714
  in sequestered thyroid tissue, 1714, 1715
  neoplasm(s) associated with
    lymphoma as, 1526, 1663, 1707–1708, 1717
    papillary carcinoma as, 1663
    sclerosing mucoepidermoid carcinoma with eosinophilia as, 1663, 1696
  vs. follicular carcinoma, 1677
  vs. lymphoma, 1708–1709
  vs. Riedel's thyroiditis, 1718
Hassall's corpuscles
  in mediastinal lymphoma, 481, 482
  in mediastinal seminoma, 466
  in multilocular thymic cyst, 493, 494, 494f
  in thymolipoma, 491
  in thymoma, 444, 447
  vs. atrophic follicles, in Castleman's disease, 492
HAV. *See* Hepatitis A virus (HAV) infection.
Haversian canals, 1858
HBV. *See* Hepatitis B virus (HBV) infection.
HC II assay, for high-risk HPV, 1297
HCC. *See* Hepatocellular carcinoma (HCC); Hepatocellular-cholangiolar carcinoma (HCC).
hCG. *See* Human chorionic gonadotropin (hCG).
HCV. *See* Hepatitis C virus (HCV) infection.
HD (Huntington's disease), 2122, 2142, 2142t, 2143, 2144
HDV. *See* Hepatitis D virus (HDV) infection.
H&E staining
  appropriate role of, 82, 90, 119
  mitotic figure counting and, 608
  of alcohol-fixed slides, 26
  of frozen sections, 24

Head and neck tumors. *See also* Sinonasal tract and nasopharynx.
  frozen sections of, 152–153
  metastatic to lung, 387
  prognostic markers in, molecular, 115t
  surgical margins of, 152
Health Level Seven (HL7) standard, 54, 55t
Heart. *See also* Cardiac *entries*.
  biopsy of. *See* Endomyocardial biopsy; Open heart biopsy.
  ischemic disease of, endomyocardial biopsy in, 510
  siderosis of, in neonatal hemochromatosis, 956
Heart block, in neonatal lupus, 1937
Heart failure. *See also* Cardiomyopathy.
  chronic
    Budd-Chiari syndrome associated with, 956
      hepatic centrilobular injury in, 956, 957
    drug-induced, 511
    endomyocardial biopsy in, 505, 506–510, 507f, 508t, 509f–510f
    in myocarditis, 506–508, 507f
    in primary amyloidosis, 1626
    lipomatous hypertrophy of atrial septum causing, 517
    unusual causes of, 508, 508t
Heat-induced epitope retrieval. *See* Antigen retrieval.
Heavy chain diseases, 726, 1626
Heavy chain restriction, immunostaining and, 66
Heberden's nodes, 1855
Heck's disease, 319
Heffner tumor, 294
*Helicobacter heilmannii*, 704
*Helicobacter pylori*
  detection of, 704
    immunohistochemical, 74
  duodenal effects of, gastric metaplasia as, 739
  esophageal effects of, in heterotopic gastric mucosa, 632
  gastric effects of, 668, 673
    in gastritis, 696, 701
      acute, 702, 703f
      chronic, 703–704, 704f–705f, 706, 707
    in lymphoid hyperplasia, 689, 690
    in lymphoma, 691, 695, 1526
  in gastric rests, in colon, 753
  phenotypic variation in, 703–704
Heliotrope rash, in dermatomyositis, 1938
HELLP syndrome, 959
Helper T lymphocytes
  in Hodgkin's disease, 1515
  in mycosis fungoides, 1538
  in peripheral T cell lymphoma, 1537
Hemangioblastoma
  capillary, 2103–2104, 2103f–2104f, 2104t
    vs. metastatic renal carcinoma, 1080, 2103, 2104
  of sellar region, 2045
Hemangioendothelioma
  epithelioid, 937, 938f, CD Fig. 27–25
    bone, 1887–1888
    cutaneous, 1986, 1986f
    mediastinal, 488–489, 488f–489f
    penile, 1206
    pulmonary, 371–372, 372f
    serosal, 430
    soft tissue, 1822, 1822f

Hemangioendothelioma (*Continued*)
  splenic, 1582
  infantile, 935, 935f, 1817, CD Fig. 27–20
    angiosarcoma arising in, 935, 936
  intranodal, 1486
  retiform, 1986
  spindle cell, 1821–1822, 1821f, 1985–1986
    vs. dermatofibroma, 1989
  thyroid, malignant, 1711–1712, 1711f
  vegetant intravascular. *See* Papillary endothelial hyperplasia.
Hemangioma
  adrenal, 1774
  appendiceal, 861
  arteriovenous, 1983
  bladder, 1130
  capillary, 1817
    cutaneous, 1983
    intramuscular, 1818, 1818f
    lobular, 157–158, 158f. *See also* Pyogenic granuloma.
    progressive, 1984
    scrotal, 1210
  cardiac, 517
  cavernous. *See* Cavernous hemangioma.
  chorionic, 1460, CD Figs. 40–41 to 40–43
  colorectal, 797–798
  cutaneous, 1983, 1984–1985, 1984f–1985f
    vs. epithelioid hemangioendothelioma and, 1986
  diffuse, 1818
  ear
    external, 301
    middle, 295
  epithelioid. *See also* Angiolymphoid hyperplasia with eosinophilia (ALHE).
    cutaneous, 1984–1985, 1985f
    intranodal, 1486, 1491
    temporal artery and, 529
    vs. epithelioid hemangioendothelioma, 1888, 1986
  fallopian tube, 1387
  gallbladder, 981
  gastric, 688, 688f
  glomeruloid, 1984
  hepatic, 934–935, CD Fig. 27–19
    focal nodular hyperplasia and, 922
    vs. hairy cell leukemia, 938
  histiocytoid, 517, 1822, 1984. *See also* Hemangioendothelioma, epithelioid.
  in Maffucci's syndrome, 1817, 1872
    colorectal, 797
  infantile hemangioendothelioma with, 935
  infiltrating, 1818, 1818f
  intramuscular, 1818, 1818f
  intranodal, 1486
  iris, 2190
  juvenile, 1817
  mediastinal, 488
  microvenular, 1984, 1984f
  nasopharyngeal, 157
  oral, congenital, 323
  osseous, 1885–1887, 1885f–1887f
  ovarian, 1431
  parotid, 267, 267f, CD Figs. 12–112 and 12–113
  penile, 1197
  renal, 1086–1087
  sclerosing, 1988
    pulmonary, 383–385, 384f, CD Fig. 15–16
  scrotal, 1210
  sinonasal, 157–158, 158f

Inguinal hernia
  carcinomatosis in, appendiceal adenocarcinoma causing, 857, 858, 858f, CD Fig. 24–4
  mobile cecum involved in, 753
  silica injection for, reaction to, 1844
  umbilical cord abnormalities and, 1456
Inguinal lymph nodes
  palisaded myofibroblastoma in, 1486
  para-amyloid in, 1487
  smooth muscle proliferation in, 1487
Inhibin
  in adrenocortical neoplasms, 1760, 1762
  in ovarian tumors, sex cord–stromal, 1422
  in pituitary adenoma, 2025
  in testicular tumor(s)
    gonadoblastoma as, 1240
    granulosa cell, 1239
    Leydig cell, 1237, 1237f
  in uterine stromal tumors, 1353
  spermatogenesis and, 1248
Inking of margins, 27, 27f, 28, 29. *See also* Surgical margin evaluation.
  documentation of, 31, 37
  of prostatectomy specimen, 1176
  of prostatic core biopsy, 1152
Inlet patch, in esophagus, 632
Insect bite reaction, 1925, 1925f
Insomnia, familial fatal (FFI), 2136, 2137, 2140
Instrument maintenance, 132
Insular carcinoma, 1689, 1689f–1690f, 1691
  vs. mixed carcinoma, 1705
  vs. nodular goiter, 1720
Insulin, β cells and, 883
  in transplanted pancreas, 910
Insulin-like growth factors
  growth hormone and, 2030
  in medulloepithelioma, 2089
  in meningioma, 2092
Insulinoma, 899, 900, 900t, 901, 902
  in MEN 1 syndrome, 904
*INT2* gene, in breast carcinoma, 601, 603
Intelligent reports, 52
Interdigitating dendritic cell sarcoma, 1548
Interdigitating dendritic cell tumor, 1547, 1548–1549
Interdigitating dendritic (reticular) cells, 87
Interface dermatitis, 1933–1938, 1934f–1938f
  with palisading granulomatous dermatitis, 1958
Interface engines, 54
Interface hepatitis, 945, 945f, 946
  autoimmune, 948
  in hypofibrinogenemia, 963
  in Wilson's disease, 962
Interface mucositis, 322, 322f, 322t
Interferon-α, for chronic myelogenous leukemia, 1618
Interferon-γ, for osteopetrosis, 1861
Interfollicular Hodgkin's disease, 1513, 1513f
Interlabial sulcus. *See* Labial sulcus.
Intermediate filaments, 63f, 64–65, 67
Intermediately differentiated lymphocytic lymphoma, 1529
International Classification of Diseases (ICD), 41, 55, 55t
Internet
  CAP reporting protocols on, 39–40, 40t
  for intraoperative consultation, 18
  for telepathology, 50
  resources for pathologists on, 36, 36t

Internet browser, for laboratory information system, 44, 45t
Interstitial cystitis, 1136
  vs. endometriosis, 1134
Interstitial fibrosis, pulmonary. *See also* Pulmonary fibrosis.
  after diffuse alveolar damage, 390
  asbestos-related, 393t, 398–399, 399f
  chronic, 391, 392t–393t, 394–396, 394f–396f, CD Figs. 15–20 and 15–21
  in acute interstitial pneumonia, 390
  vs. diffuse meningotheliomatosis, 377
Interstitial lung disease, respiratory bronchiolitis–associated, 395–396
Interstitial nephritis. *See* Tubulointerstitial disease (TID).
Interstitial pneumonia
  acute, 389, 390–391, 392t
  chronic fibrosing, 391, 392t–393t, 394–396, 394f–396f, CD Figs. 15–20 and 15–21
  definition of, 391
  idiopathic, 391
  lymphoid, 391
    vs. follicular bronchiolitis, 399
  open-lung biopsy of, 389
Interstitial pneumonitis, chronic fibrosing, 391, 392t–393t, 394–396, 394f–396f, CD Figs. 15–20 and 15–21
  in rheumatoid arthritis, 391, 394, 1856
Intervertebral disk, amyloid in, 1857
Intervillositis, 1460–1461, CD Figs. 40–45 and 40–46
  subchorionic, 1464
Intestinal metaplasia
  in bladder
    adenocarcinoma arising in, 1126, 1127
    vs. adenocarcinoma, 1136
  in cervix, 1307, CD Figs. 36–54 and 36–55
  in gallbladder, 982, CD Fig. 28–2
  in gastric mucosa
    carcinoma and, 673, 679, 706, 707
    chronic gastritis and, 703, 705f, 706, 707, 707f
    heterotopic in esophagus, 632
  incomplete
    in Barrett's esophagus, 642, 659, 660f
    in gastric cardia, 642
Intestinal mucosa, siderosis of, neonatal, 956, CD Fig. 27–45
Intestinal obstruction, by gallstone, 988
Intestinal T cell lymphoma, 1539
Intestine. *See* Large intestine; Small intestine.
Intimal fibroplasia, 1042, 1042t
Intracytoplasmic sperm injection (ICSI), 1246, 1247, 1248, 1249
Intraductal papillary mucinous neoplasm (IPMN), 884, 895–896, 896f
  vs. mucinous cystic neoplasms, 894, 895
Intraductal papilloma
  biliary, 934
  breast, 559–560, 560f, 562, 585
    in adolescence, 598
    in males, 599
    pleomorphic adenoma as, 595
  salivary gland, 250, 250f, CD Figs. 12–41 and 12–42
Intraoperative consultation, 17–32. *See also* Frozen section(s).
  accuracy of diagnosis in, 31–32, 132–133
  changing practices in, 17–18
  clinicopathologic correlation in, 19–21, 20f–21f, 30

Intraoperative consultation (Continued)
  communication of diagnosis in, 29–30
  costs of health care and, 17–18
  documentation of, 31, 37–38
  for pituitary tumors, 2023, 2024t
  in hyperparathyroidism, 1730–1731, 1730t
  indications for, 18–19
  laboratory design and, 5
  managerial decisions and, 29–30
  on brain tumor(s), 25, 26, 2061
    astrocytoma as, 21, 21f, 2068–2069, CD Figs. 51–10 to 51–12
    choroid plexus papilloma as, 2081
    ependymoma as, 2079, CD Fig. 51–26
    oligodendroglioma as, 2074, CD Fig. 51–18
  operating room visit during, 21, 30
  quality improvement in, 132–133
  recommendations to surgeon in, 30, 31
  techniques in, 21–26
    cytologic, 22, 24–26, 26f
    frozen section, 22–24, 23f
    gross examination, 22, 27, 29
    immunohistochemical, 17, 18
  turnaround time for diagnosis in, 31
Intratubular germ cell neoplasia. *See* Germ cell neoplasia, intratubular.
Intrauterine device (IUD)
  ectopic pregnancy and, 1383
  metaplastic changes caused by, 1342
  pelvic inflammatory disease caused by, 1333, 1381, 1434
Intrauterine infection. *See also* Chorioamnionitis; Villitis.
  spontaneous abortion and, 1468, CD Fig. 40–74
Intravascular fasciitis, 1797, 1798
Intravascular lymphomatosis
  as adrenal mass, 1776
  thyroid, 1708
Intravascular papillary endothelial hyperplasia. *See* Endothelial hyperplasia, papillary.
Intravascular-angiotropic lymphomatosis, cutaneous, 1998–1999, 1999f
Introns, 91, 102
Inuit (Eskimo) patient, lymphoepithelial carcinoma in, salivary gland, 265
Invasion-associated enzymes, 601
Invasive mole, 1469, 1470, CD Fig. 40–82
Inverse psoriasis, 1927
Inverted follicular keratosis, 1967
  of external ear, 285
Inverted papilloma
  bladder, 1132–1133, 1133f
    vs. invasive carcinoma, 1117, 1118f, 1126
  renal pelvis and ureter, 1092
  salivary gland, ductal, 249–250, 250f, CD Fig. 12–40
    vs. intraductal papilloma, 250
    vs. mucoepidermoid carcinoma, 250, 252–253
    vs. sialadenoma papilliferum, 251
  sinonasal, 154–155, 155f, 156
    vs. verrucous carcinoma, 172
Involucrin, 345
Iodine deficiency, thyroid cancers and, 1663
IPMN (intraductal papillary mucinous neoplasm), 884, 895–896, 896f
  vs. mucinous cystic neoplasms, 894, 895
IPSID (immunoproliferative small intestinal disease), 723, 725, 726–727, 726f

Microvilli *(Continued)*
  in mesothelioma, 85, 85f, 86, 422
  in renal cell carcinoma, 1080
Microvillus inclusion disease, 730, 733, 734f
Midline granuloma, oral lesions in, 320
Midmandibular cyst, 334
Midpalatine cyst, 334
Miescher granuloma, 1950–1951
Mifepristone, endometrial effects of, 1337
Migratory erythema, necrolytic, 1930–1931
Mikulicz cells, in *Klebsiella rhinoscleromatis* infection, 192, 192f
Miliary foci. *See* Neuritic plaques.
Milium(a)
  colloid, 1961
  in epidermolysis bullosa acquisita, 1945
  in porphyria cutanea tarda, 1944
Milk hypersensitivity
  proctocolitis in, 733
  small intestine abnormalities in, 733, 736
Milk lines, 539, 543
Milk-alkali syndrome, 1959
Milroy's syndrome, 741
Mineralocorticoids. *See* Conn's syndrome (primary hyperaldosteronism).
Minicore disease, 2162
Minigemistocytes, 2074, 2075, 2077, CD Fig. 51–19
Minimal change disease, 1008–1009, 1008f, 1010, 1011
  electron microscopy of, 83, 1008–1009, 1009f
  in HIV infection, 1031
  in sickle cell disease, 1030
Minimal deviation adenocarcinoma, cervical, 1312, 1316, 1316f–1317f, CD Figs. 36–96 to 36–98
Minisatellites, 2122–2123
Minocycline, black thyroid caused by, 1725, 1725f
Minor salivary glands
  esophageal submucosal, 631, 632f
    duct adenoma of, 634
  metaplastic change of. *See* Sialometaplasia.
  neoplasms of, 242
    staging of, 243
  of sinonasal tract and nasopharynx, 151
    benign neoplasms of, 156
    malignant neoplasms of, 181–182
  syringomatous tumor of, 595
Minute meningothelial nodules, 377, 377f
Miscarriage. *See* Abortion, spontaneous.
Mismatch repair. *See* DNA mismatch repair genes.
Misplaced exocytosis, in pituitary adenoma, 2031, 2032
Mitochondrial cytopathies, 965
Mitochondrial DNA, mutations in
  in cardiomyopathy, 510
  in metabolic myopathies, 2163
Mitochondrial encephalopathy, 2145
Mitochondrial myopathies, 84, 2162–2163, 2163f, CD Fig. 53–5
  zidovudine-associated, 2163, 2170
Mitotic indices, 608–610
Mitral insufficiency, 523, 524, 524f
Mitral stenosis, 524–525, 525f
  breast infarct and, 548
Mitral valve
  papillary fibroelastoma on, 516
  surgical excision of, specimen from, 523–524

Mitral valve prolapse, 524, 524f
  in Marfan's syndrome, 528
Mitrofanoff appendicovesicostomy, 868
Mixed cellularity Hodgkin's disease, 1510, 1510t, 1512, 1512f
  EBV and, 1509, 1515
  in AIDS patients, 1509
  vs. non-Hodgkin's lymphoma, 1517
Mixed follicular-parafollicular carcinoma, 1704–1705, 1705f, 1707
Mixed tumor. *See also* Müllerian tumor, mixed.
  bronchial gland, 357, 358, 358f, CD Fig. 15–7
  hepatic, malignant, 939
  lacrimal gland (pleomorphic adenoma), 2194f
  middle ear, in salivary ectopia, 305
  minor salivary gland (pleomorphic adenoma), 156
  salivary gland (pleomorphic adenoma), 244–245, 244f–245f, CD Figs. 12–1 to 12–10
    extending to auditory canal, 286
    genetic alterations in, 111
    GFAP in, 68
    malignant transformation of, 245, 258–259, 259f, CD Figs. 12–77 to 12–79
    metastasizing, 260, 260f
    oncocytic metaplasia in, 248
    vs. adenoid cystic carcinoma, 257
    vs. basal cell adenoma, 248
    vs. epithelial-myoepithelial carcinoma, 262
    vs. PLGA, 245, 257–258
  skin
    benign, 1972–1973, 1972f
    malignant, 1974
*MLL* gene abnormalities, 1602, 1612, 1615
Modem, 46, 46t
Mohs technique, 27–28, 28f–29f
  for sebaceous carcinoma, 2177
Mole
  Breus, 1459, CD Fig. 40–31
  hydatidiform, 1469–1470, 1469f, CD Figs. 40–76 to 40–81
  in ectopic pregnancy, 1385
  invasive, 1469, 1470, CD Fig. 40–82
Molecular studies, 90–119
  documentation of, 38, 39
  fixatives and, 37
  for determining extent of disease, 114–115
  for specimen identification, 118, 1182
  future prospects for, 118–119
  glossary of terms for, 91–92
  mutations in tumors and, 99
  of adrenocortical carcinoma, 1763
  of bladder cancer, 1119–1121
  of brain tumor(s), 113–114, 2059, 2061
    astrocytoma as
      diffuse, 2066–2068, 2067t, 2068f
      special types of, 2070, 2070t
    medulloblastoma as, 2088
    oligodendroglioma as, 2075t, 2077, 2078
  of breast cancer, 599, 600–605
  of endocrine tumors, 113
  of gastric carcinoma, 680
  of gastrointestinal tumors, 113
  of germ cell tumors, mediastinal, 468–469
  of gestational abnormalities, 1454

Molecular studies *(Continued)*
  of hematolymphoid malignancy, 103, 1481, 1602–1603
    ALL as, 1615
    AML as, 1609
    CML as, 1617–1618
    lymphoma as, 93, 103, 1481
      follicular center cell, 1635
      for identifying EBV, 117
      in residual disease, 1634
      mantle cell, 1635
      of CNS, 2097
  of hereditary cancers, 118
  of Hodgkin's disease, 1514–1515, 1517, 1518
  of infectious diseases, 117–118
  of lung cancer, 359–360, 360t
  of metabolic diseases, 118
  of muscular dystrophy, 2157, 2158
  of neuroblastoma, 1771
  of neurodegenerative diseases, 2122–2123. *See also specific disease.*
  of ovarian epithelial tumors, 1413–1414
  of pituitary adenoma, 2026
  of prostate cancer, 1173, 1181–1182
  of renal tumors, 111, 112t, 113
  of retinoblastoma, 2179
  of soft tissue sarcomas, 103, 104t–105t, 106–111, 106f, 110f, 1786
  of spinal muscular atrophy, 2169
  of thymic epithelial neoplasms, 452–453
  prognostic markers in, 115–117, 115t
  role of, 90
  specimen collection and handling in, 92, 96
  techniques in, 92–99, 94f–95f, 97f–98f
  transcription factors and, 99, 100t–101t, 102–103, 102f
    definition of, 92
    in lung cancer, 360
    in mesenchymal tumors, 103, 104t–105t, 106
Moll gland cyst, 1976
Molluscum contagiosum, 1966
  penile, 1208, CD Fig. 33–14
Mondor's disease, 548
Mongolian spot, 2001
Monoblastic leukemia, acute, 1611, 1611f, 1612, CD Fig. 43–6
  extramedullary presentation of, 1639
Monoclonal gammopathy
  in scleromyxedema, 1958
  of undetermined significance, 1625
Monocytic leukemia
  cutaneous infiltrate in, 1999, CD Fig. 49–15
  vs. dermatopathic lymphadenitis, 1499
Monocytoid B cell hyperplasia, 1499–1500, 1501f
  in cat-scratch disease, 1506
  vs. hemophagocytic syndrome, 1501
  vs. mastocytosis, 1551, 1551f
Monocytoid B cells, 1526
  in marginal zone lymphoma, 1526, 1527
Monocytosis, 1644
  growth factor administration and, 1645
Mononucleosis, infectious, 193
  appendiceal lymphoid hyperplasia in, 865
  liver manifestations of, 948–949, 949t
  paracortical hyperplasia in, 1497, 1498
  splenic involvement in, 1576–1577, 1576f
  vs. diffuse large B cell lymphoma, 1534
Monosomy 7 syndrome, infantile, 1622, 1623
Montgomery's tubercles, 540

O13 marker, 68
Oat cell carcinoma. *See also* Small cell carcinoma.
  bile duct extrahepatic, 993
  gallbladder, 985
  gastric, 683, 684
  laryngeal, 225
  metastatic to brain, 2105, 2106
  prostatic, 1169, 1170f
  pulmonary, 351t, 353, 354
    salivary gland metastasis from, 265
  small intestine, 719, 720, 720f
  thymic, 473–474, 474f
Obesity
  breast cancer risk and, 563
  endometrial hyperplasia in, 1340
  renal cell carcinoma and, 1076
  steatohepatitis in, 941
Obliterative bronchiolitis. *See* Bronchiolitis obliterans.
Obliterative endarteritis. *See* Endarteritis obliterans.
Obstructive colitis, 817
OC125 antibody, 71, 71f
Occult metastases, immunohistochemical detection of, 69–70, 69f
Occupational Safety and Health Administration (OSHA)
  formaldehyde exposure and, 13, 14
  gross room square footage and, 5
OCGT (osteoclast-like giant cell tumor), pancreatic, 891–892, 891f, CD Fig. 26–2
OCT (Optimal Cutting Temperature) compound, 23, 29f
  PCR inhibition by, 96
Octreotide, for somatotroph adenoma, 2038
Ocular melanocytosis, 2187
Ocular mucosa, cicatricial pemphigoid of, 1942
Ocular tumors. *See also* Orbit, tumor(s) of; Retinoblastoma; Uveal malignant melanoma.
  specimens from, 2174
Oculoauriculovertebral dysplasia, accessory tragi in, 305
Oculodermal melanocytosis, 2187
Odontogenic carcinoma, clear cell, 262
Odontogenic cyst(s), 332–333, 333f–334f, CD Figs. 14–7 to 14–11
  ameloblastoma arising from, 323
Odontogenic fibroma, central, 326, 326f
Odontogenic ghost cell tumor, 333, 334f
Odontogenic keratocyst, 333, 333f, CD Figs. 14–10 and 14–11
Odontogenic myxofibroma, 325–326, 326f
Odontogenic myxoma, 325–326, 326f
Odontogenic tumors. *See also* Ameloblastoma.
  epithelial, 323–325, 323f–326f
  mesenchymal, 325–328, 326f–328f
  mixed epithelial and mesenchymal, 328, 328f
Odontoma, 328, 328f
  in ameloblastic fibro-odontoma, 328
Oligoastrocytoma, mixed, 2074t, 2075–2076, 2075t, 2076f, CD Fig. 51–23
  anaplastic, 2074t, 2076, 2077
Oligodendroglioma, 2073–2075, 2073f–2075f, 2074t, 2075t, CD Figs. 51–18 to 51–22
  anaplastic, 2074t, 2076–2077, 2076f, CD Fig. 51–24
    vimentin expression in, 2075
  vs. anaplastic astrocytoma, 2068

Oligodendroglioma *(Continued)*
  arising in nasopharyngeal heterotopia, 198
  differential diagnosis of, 2077
  molecular genetics of, 114, 2075t, 2077, 2078
  prognostic features of, 2077–2078
  vs. clear cell ependymoma, 87
Oligohydramnios
  amnion nodosum in, 1457
  in transfusion syndrome, 1466
  renal anomalies and, 1002
  short umbilical cord in, 1456
Ollier's disease, 1872, 1873f
Omental cake, in mucinous peritoneal carcinomatosis, 857
Omentum(a)
  endosalpingiosis in, 433
  gastrointestinal-type stromal tumors of, 429–430
  in ovarian tumor specimen, 1397
  leiomyomatosis of, 1360
  serosal membranes of, 419
Oncocytic carcinoma
  breast, 589
  prostatic, 1171
  salivary gland, 267, CD Figs. 12–110 and 12–111
  vs. salivary duct carcinoma, 263
Oncocytic cystadenoma, salivary gland, 246
Oncocytic metaplasia
  endometrial, 1343
  thyroid, 1713
Oncocytoma
  adrenal, 1760–1761, 1760f
  electron microscopy of, 88
  laryngeal, vs. rhabdomyoma, 217
  minor salivary gland, 156
  pituitary, 2036, 2036f, 2037, CD Fig. 50–9
  pulmonary, 359
  renal, 1073–1074, 1073f–1074f, 1074t
    collecting duct origin of, 1083
    electron microscopy of, 88, CD Fig. 6–9
    genetic alterations in, 111, 112t
    vs. chromophobe cell carcinoma, 88
    with papillary adenomas, 1072
  salivary gland, 248–249, 248f, CD Figs. 12–28 to 12–31
Oncocytomatosis, renal, 1073
Oncocytosis, laryngeal, 231
Oncogene(s), 70, 71–72, 93, 99, 601, 602
  in bladder cancer, 1120–1121
  in breast cancer, 601–604
    c-*erb*-B2 *(HER2-neu)* as, 71–72, 74, 115t, 116, 601–603
  in colorectal carcinoma, 113, 768, 769t
  in lung cancer, 359, 360, 360t, 362–363, 364
  in non-Hodgkin's lymphomas, 1519, 1533
  in oral carcinogenesis, 313
  in ovarian carcinoma, 1413
  in pancreatic ductal adenocarcinoma, 886, 887, 888
  in pituitary adenoma, 2025
  in prostate cancer, 1181
  in soft tissue sarcomas, 1786
  in uveal malignant melanoma, 2187
Onion bulbs, electron microscopy of, 84
Oophoritis
  autoimmune, 1435
  cytomegalovirus, 1434, CD Fig. 39–67
  xanthogranulomatous, 1434

Open heart biopsy, 516–521
  of benign and low-grade neoplasms, 519. *See also* Myxoma, cardiac.
  of cardiac lymphoma, 520–521
  of cardiac sarcomas, 519–520, 520t
  of metastatic tumors, 520
  of non-neoplastic tumors and lesions, 516–518, 516f–517f
Open information systems, 54
Ophthalmic pathology. *See* Eye; Ocular tumors; Orbit.
*Opisthorchis*, 959
  cholangiocarcinoma and, 933
  extrahepetic bile duct carcinoma and, 992
Opsoclonus-polymyoclonus syndrome, 1767
Optic glioma, 2069, CD Fig. 51–13
Optic nerve
  pilocytic astrocytoma of, 2069, CD Fig. 51–13
  retinoblastoma invading into, 2180, 2184, 2184f, 2185, 2186
  specimen from, 2174
  uveal melanoma invading into, 2190
Optic nerve sheath
  inflammation of, 2194, 2197, 2197f, 2198
  meningioma of, 2041
Optical drives, 46, 49
Oral cavity. *See also* Oral mucosa; Salivary gland(s), neoplasm(s) of.
  fibromatosis of, 161
  frozen section from, 152
  leiomyoma of, 162
  lung metastases from, 387
  plasmablastic lymphoma of, 1545, 1545f
  teratoma of, 166
Oral contraceptives
  breast changes caused by, 542
    in granulomatous lobular mastitis, 546
  Budd-Chiari syndrome associated with, 956
  cervical cancer and, 1291, 1312
  cholestasis associated with, 954
  Crohn's disease and, 803
  endometrial changes caused by, 1336, CD Fig. 37–13
  hepatic lesion(s) and
    adenoma as, 921
    focal nodular hyperplasia as, 922
  lobular capillary hemangioma, 158
  peritoneal leiomyomatosis and, 434, 1360
  porphyria cutanea tarda and, 1944
  uterine leiomyoma and, hemorrhagic cellular, 1359, CD Figs. 37–65 and 37–66
  uterine leiomyosarcoma and, 1364
  vaginal *Candida* infection and, 1280
Oral mucosa. *See also* Oral cavity.
  neoplastic lesion(s) of, 313–319
    carcinoma in situ as, 313, 314f, 315
    Kaposi's sarcoma as, 317–318, 317f–318f, CD Figs. 14–1 and 14–2
    lymphoma as, 317
    melanoma as, 315–317, 316f
    neural, 318, 318f
    spindle cell tumors as, 318–319
    squamous cell carcinoma as, 313–315, 314f–315f, 1970
      papillary, 171, 315
      verrucous, 171
  non-neoplastic lesion(s) of, 319–323
    actinic cheilitis as, 1968
    congenital and hereditary, 322–323
    granulomatous, 320, 321f
    infectious, 319–320, 320f–321f
    interface mucositis as, 322, 322f, 322t

Promyelocytic leukemia, acute
(*Continued*)
  multidrug resistance in, 74
Promyelocytic leukemia, acute, 1602, 1610–
    1611, 1610f
Pronephros, 1002
Pro-opiomelanocortin, abnormal cleavage
    of, 2036
Prostaglandins
  in osteoid osteoma, 1866
  menstrual cycle and, 1331
Prostate
  abscess of, 1153
  adenocarcinoma of. *See* Prostate cancer.
  anatomy of, 1149–1150
  atrophy in, 1157, 1157f
    vs. atrophic adenocarcinoma, 1172
  benign processes of, miscellaneous, 1160
  bladder carcinoma extending to, 1113,
    1113t, 1119
  cysts of, 1160
  endometriosis of, 1134, 1160
  epithelium of, normal, 1151–1152,
    1151f–1152f
    basal cell immunohistochemistry in,
    68–69, 1151, 1152t, CD Fig. 5–3
  neuroendocrine cells in, 1151–1152,
    1151f, 1155–1156
  hyperplasia of, 1156–1160, 1157f–1160f.
    *See also* Benign prostatic hyperplasia
    (BPH).
  postatrophic (PAH), 1157, 1157f, 1166
    vs. phyllodes tumor, 1185t
    vs. pseudohyperplastic carcinoma,
    1171
  immunohistochemistry of
    of normal basal cells, 68–69, 1151,
    1152t, 1166, CD Fig. 5–3
    of normal neuroendocrine cells, 1152,
    1169
    of phyllodes tumor, 1184, 1185t
  infection or inflammation of, 1153–1155,
    1154f
    serum PSA level and, 1163
    with seminal vesiculitis, 1186
  melanin-like pigment in, 1152, 1152f
  metaplasia in, 1155–1156
  metastatic tumors in, 1185
  nodular hyperplasia of (BPH), 1156–
    1157
    bladder diverticula associated with,
    1138
    hyperthermia for, 1174–1175
    transition zone anatomy and, 1150
    vs. leiomyoma or fibroma, 1182
    with AAH, 1158
    with basal cell adenoma, 1158
  soft tissue tumors of, 1182–1184, 1183f
  tissue sampling of, 1152–1153. *See also*
    Core needle biopsy.
    Cowper's gland tissue in, 1150
    inflammation caused by, 1155, 1155f
    malpractice claims involving, 143, 145
    second opinion on, 133
    seminal vesicle epithelium in, 1150
    treatment-induced changes in, 1172–
    1175, 1172t, 1173f–1174f, 1173t,
    1174t
Prostate cancer, 1163–1182
  atypical adenomatous hyperplasia and,
    1158–1159
  clinical manifestations of, 1163
  collagenous micronodules in, 1165, 1165f
  crystalloids in, 1165, 1165f, 1167
  differential diagnosis of, 1164t

Prostate cancer (*Continued*)
    vs. atypical basal cell hyperplasia,
    1158
    vs. nephrogenic adenoma, 1133, 1134t
    vs. postatrophic hyperplasia, 1157
    vs. sclerosing adenosis, 1159
  epidemiology of, 1163
  estrogen therapy for
    breast tumors and, 598, 599
    endometriosis induced by, 1134
  genetic alterations in, 1181–1182
  grading of, 1164, 1164f–1165f, 1166–
    1168, 1167f
    after hormonal therapy, 1173
    after radiation, 1174
    DNA ploidy and, 1180
  gross pathology of, 1164, 1164f
  histologic variants of, 1168–1172, 1168f–
    1172f, 1168t
  immunohistochemistry of, 1166
    after treatment, 1173
    *BCL2* expression and, 1181–1182
    of lymph node micrometastases, 1177–
    1178
    vascular invasion and, 1180
  in cystoprostatectomy specimen, 1119,
    1172
  lymph node biopsy in, 1177–1178
  metastases from
    genetic alterations in, 1181, 1182
    to bladder, 1125
    to bone, 1170
    to breast, 597
    to lymph nodes, 1177–1178, 1180,
    1181
    to penis, 1206, CD Fig. 33–11
  microscopic features of, 1164–1166,
    1164f–1165f
  needle biopsy of. *See* Core needle bi-
    opsy.
  perineural invasion by, 1166, 1173f,
    1176, 1180
  preinvasive stage of. *See* Prostatic intra-
    epithelial neoplasia (PIN).
  prognostic factors in, 1176–1182, 1177t,
    1178t
  PSA levels in. *See* Prostate-specific anti-
    gen (PSA).
  radical prostatectomy specimens in,
    1175–1176, 1175t
  staging of, 1178, 1178t, 1180
  treatment-induced changes in, 1172–
    1175, 1172t, 1173f–1174f, 1173t,
    1174t
  urothelial, 1172
  vanishing cancer phenomenon in, 1173,
    1182
  vascular and lymphatic invasion by,
    1166, 1180
Prostatectomy, specimens from, 1175–
    1176, 1175t, 1179–1180
Prostate-specific antigen (PSA)
    immunohistochemical staining for
    in Cowper's glands, 1151
    in normal prostate epithelium, 1151,
    1156
    in prostate cancer, 1166, 1168, 1169,
    1170, 1171
    after therapy, 1173, 1174
    in prostatic intraepithelial neoplasia,
    1162
    in prostatic urethral polyp, 1187
    in sclerosing adenosis, 1159
  lymphoma and, 1184
  serum levels of, 1163–1164
    prognosis and, 1179, 1180

Prostate-specific antigen (PSA) (*Continued*)
    staging and, 1178
    soft tissue tumors and, 1182, 1183
Prostatic acid phosphatase (PAP)
    in normal prostate epithelium, 1151,
    1156
    in prostate cancer, 1166, 1168, 1169,
    1170, 1171
    after therapy, 1173, 1174
    in prostatic intraepithelial neoplasia,
    1162
    in prostatic urethral polyp, 1187
    in sclerosing adenosis, 1159
    soft tissue tumors and, 1183
Prostatic ducts, 1150
    adenocarcinoma arising in, 1168, 1168f
    bladder carcinoma extending to, 1110,
    1113, 1113t, 1119, 1138
    mucinous metaplasia in, 1155
Prostatic intraepithelial neoplasia (PIN),
    1160–1163, 1161f–1162f
    androgen deprivation therapy and, 1163,
    1172t
    aneuploidy in, 1180
    basal cell layer disruption in, 1166
    genetic alterations in, 1181
    radiation therapy and, 1163, 1173
Prostatic urethra. *See also* Urethra.
    anatomy of, 1150
    bladder carcinoma extending to, 1113,
    1138
    inflammation of, 1187
    metaplasia in, 1155, 1156, 1187
    neoplasms of, 1139, 1187
    polyps in, 1139, 1187
    stent-induced changes in, 1187
Prostatic utricle, 1150
Prostatitis, 1153–1155, 1154f
    serum PSA level and, 1163
    with seminal vesiculitis, 1186
Prosthesis, sinus histiocytosis associated
    with, 1499
Protein domains, 91
Proteinaceous lymphadenopathy, 1487,
    1487f
Protein-losing enteropathy, 744
    collagenous colitis causing, 812
    in Hirschsprung's disease, 755
    inflammatory polyps causing, 765
Proteinosis, alveolar, 404–405, 404f
Proteinuria. *See* Nephrotic syndrome.
Proton pump inhibitors, fundic gland
    changes caused by, 696, 697f, 698
Protoplasmic astrocytoma, 2062
    smears of, 2068
Protoporphyria, erythropoietic, 965
Protozoal infection, esophageal, 654
PrP amyloid plaques, 2137, 2137f–2138f,
    2138, 2140, 2141
PrP protein, 2122, 2137–2141, 2139f
Prune-belly syndrome, 1005, 1005f
    patent urachus in, 1138
Prurigo nodularis, 1928, 1929
Prussian blue stain, for iron, 1599
PSA. *See* Prostate-specific antigen (PSA).
Psammomatoid ossifying fibroma, 330–331
    sinonasal, 163–164, 163f
    vs. meningioma, 157
Psammomatous melanotic schwannoma,
    485–486, 487
PSC. *See* Primary sclerosing cholangitis
    (PSC).
Pseudoaneurysms, 532
    in Ehlers-Danlos syndrome, 528, 532
    of temporal artery, 529

Radial scar, 557–559, 558f
Radiation exposure. *See also* Radiation
    therapy, neoplasm(s) secondary to.
  brain tumors caused by, 2059
  lung cancer caused by, 340
  thyroid tumors caused by, 1663, 1663t,
    1683–1684
Radiation therapy
  breast change(s) caused by, 590
    fat necrosis as, 545
    hypoplasia as, 543
    lobular atypia as, 573, 574f
    vascular, 594
  cervical atypia caused by, 1307, CD Figs.
    36–51 and 36–52
  complication(s) of
    bone necrosis as, 1864
    colitis as, 832–833, 833f
      vs. collagenous colitis, 813
    cystitis as, 1137, 1137t, CD Fig. 31–55
      polypoid, 1137
    esophageal, 640, 656, 656f
    gastropathy as, 708–709
    in small intestine, 735, 741, 743
    liver disease as, veno-occlusive, 956
    marrow aplasia as, 1641
    nephropathy as, 1047–1048
  endometrial changes caused by, 1338
  for bone metastases, 1901
  for chordoma, 1892
  for CNS tumors, 2061
  for eosinophilic granuloma, 1885
  for Ewing's sarcoma, 1883
  for giant cell tumor of bone, malignant
    transformation and, 1882
  for orbital inflammation, idiopathic, 2198
  for retinoblastoma, 2179, 2183, 2186
  for sebaceous carcinoma, 2177
  for soft tissue sarcomas, 1788
  frozen section diagnosis subsequent to,
    152
  laryngeal changes caused by, 230f, 231
  neoplasm(s) secondary to
    after retinoblastoma therapy, 2179
    bladder cancer as, 1104
    colorectal cancer as, 767, 777, 779
    desmoid fibromatosis as, 1804
    esophageal, 636
    glioma as, 2107
    malignant peripheral nerve sheath tu-
      mor as, 486
    of middle ear, 295
    of salivary gland, 242
    osseous fibrosarcoma as, 1891
    osseous malignant fibrous histiocy-
      toma as, 1891
    osteosarcoma as, 1868, 1872, 2179
      of skull, 296
    parathyroid adenoma as, 1725
    prostate cancer as, adenosquamous,
      1170
    sarcoma as. *See* Soft tissue sarcoma(s),
      postirradiation.
    sellar, 2040, 2041, 2045
    thyroid cancer as, 1663
    uterine
      adenosarcoma as, 1355
      carcinosarcoma as, 1355
    vaginal carcinoma as, 1275
  prostatic effects of, 1173–1174, 1173t,
    1174f, 1174t
  in PIN, 1163, 1173
Radicular cyst, 332, CD Fig. 14–7
Radiographs, specimen
  equipment for, 11

Radiographs (*Continued*)
  scanning of, 49
  with breast specimens, 564
Ragged red fibers, 2163, 2163f, CD Fig.
  53–5
  zidovudine-associated, 2163, 2170
Random access memory (RAM), 46
Ranitidine, colonic intraepithelial lymphocytosis caused by, 814
Ranula, 268
Rapidly progressive glomerulonephritis,
  1018–1020, 1018f–1019f, 1018t
*RARA* gene, acute promyelocytic leukemias and, 1602
*ras* gene mutations
  in bladder cancer, 1120
  in breast cancer, 603
  in lung cancer, 360, 360t, 362, 363
  in melanoma, 2014
  in ovarian carcinoma, 1413, 1414
  in thyroid tumor(s)
    follicular adenoma as, 1669
    follicular carcinoma as, 1671t, 1677
    papillary carcinoma as, 1688
    poorly differentiated carcinoma as,
      1689, 1691
Ha-*ras* gene activation, in pancreatic endocrine neoplasms, 900
H-*ras* mutations, in pituitary carcinoma,
  2025
K-*ras* mutations
  in colorectal carcinoma, 113, 768, 769t,
    785
  in colorectal polyps, 756–757, 762
  in gastrointestinal tumors, 113
  in lung cancer, 360, 360t, 362, 363
  in mediastinal tumors, germ cell, 468,
    469
  pancreatic tumor(s) and, 113, 886, 887,
    888, 889, 891, 892
    endocrine, 899
    IPMN as, 896
    solid pseudopapillary tumor as, 897
  pseudomyxoma peritonei and, 432
Rathke's cleft cyst, 2047–2048, 2048f,
  2105
Rathke's pouch, remnants of, 2051
*RB* gene. *See* Retinoblastoma (*RB*) gene.
Rb protein. *See also* Retinoblastoma (*RB*)
  gene.
  human papillomavirus and, 172
  immunoreactivity of, 72
    in parathyroid carcinoma, 1733
    in soft tissue sarcomas, 1786, 1788
Records. *See* Medical records.
Rectal varices, 881
Rectum. *See also* Colorectal *entries*; Large
  intestine; Proctitis.
  ameboma in, 828
  amyloidosis in, 800
  anatomy of, 750, 751, 751f
    at anus, 871, 872f, CD Fig. 25–4
  carcinoid tumor of, 792
  carcinoma of. *See also* Colorectal carci-
    noma.
    anal involvement by, 875, 876, 877
    arising in squamous metaplasia, 779
    early, management of, 773
    grading of, 785
    in Crohn's disease, 809
    prognosis after resection of, 781, 783–
      784
    venous invasion by, 786
  Crohn's disease in, 806
  diversion colitis in, 815, 815f

Rectum (*Continued*)
  diverticula in, 818
  duplication cyst of, carcinoid tumor in,
    792
  endometriosis in, 801
  hemorrhage from, duplication cyst caus-
    ing, 753
  heterotopias in, 753
  leiomyoma of, 796
  lymphoid hyperplasia in, 766
  lymphoma of, 799, 800
  mucosa of, at anus, 871, CD Fig. 25–4
  prolapse of
    duplication cyst causing, 753
    polyp causing, 764, 766, 790
    solitary rectal ulcer and, 821
  salmonellosis in, 824
  spirochetosis in, 827
  ulcer of
    solitary, 820–821, 820f–821f
    stercoral, 819–820
  ulcerative colitis in, 804
Red blood cell disorders, splenomegaly in,
  1578–1579, CD Fig. 42–4
Red blood cell lakes, in splenic hairy cell
  leukemia, 1587, 1589f
Red blood cells
  nucleated
    in early gestation, 1454, 1455, 1455t,
      CD Fig. 40–6
    in term villi, 1462
    splenic removal of, 1572
Red cell aplasias, 1641–1642, 1642f
Red pulp, splenic, 1572, 1572f
  disease involving, 1573–1574, 1573f, 1574t
5α-Reductase, prostatic intraepithelial neoplasia and, 1163
Reed-Sternberg cells, 1511, 1511f–1514f,
  1512, 1513, 1514
  ancillary studies and, 1514
  immunophenotype of, 66, 67t, 1515,
    1515f, 1515t
  in mediastinal Hodgkin's disease, 477,
    477f, 478
  vs. binucleate immunoblasts, 1497, 1499
Reed-Sternberg–like cells
  in acral myxoinflammatory fibroblastic
    sarcoma, 1814
  in anaplastic large cell lymphoma, 692,
    1541, 1996, 1996f
  in immunoblastic lymphoma
    gastric, 692
    small intestine, 725
  in infectious mononucleosis, 193, 1576
  in lymphomatoid granulomatosis, 375
  in Mediterranean lymphoma, 726, 727
  in peripheral T cell lymphoma, 1536
  in small lymphocytic lymphoma, 1517
  in T cell–rich/histiocyte-rich B cell lym-
    phoma, 1517
Refrigerators, 11
Refsum's disease, 84
  infantile, 965
Regional alveolar damage, 390
Regressing atypical histiocytosis, 1550
Reichert cartilage, 281
Reinke crystalloids
  in Leydig cell tumor, 1237, 1237f
  in Leydig cells, 1248
Reiter's disease, 1933
  aortic insufficiency in, 523
Relapsing polychondritis, 306–307, 307f
  auricular cartilage in, 306
Remyelination, 2166
Renal. *See also* Glomerular disease; Kidney.

Seminoma *(Continued)*
    with early carcinomatous differentia-
      tion, 1225
Senile plaques. *See* Neuritic plaques.
Sentinel lymph node biopsy
    in breast cancer, 17, 70, 568, 611–613,
      1482
    in colorectal cancer, 785
    in melanoma, 1482
Sentinel pile, 880
Sepsis, cholestasis in, 950, 950f
Serosal membranes, 419–434
    anatomy of, 419
    embryology of, 419
    histology of, 419
    inflammation of, 433
    neoplasm(s) of, 420–432. *See also* Aden-
      omatoid tumor; Mesothelioma.
      desmoplastic small round cell tumor
        as, 428–429, 428f–429f
      gastrointestinal-type stromal tumors
        as, 429–430, 430f
      lymphoma as, 430–431, 431f
      metastatic carcinoma as, 431–432,
        431f–432f
        from breast, 578, 597
        from colon, 786
      primary serous peritoneal carcinoma
        as, 425–426, 426f
      sarcomas as, 430
      smooth muscle tumors as, 429–430
      solitary fibrous tumor as, 427–428,
        428f
      vascular, 430
    rare lesions of, 434, 434f
    reactive lesions of, 432–434, 432f–434f.
      *See also* Endocervicosis; Endome-
      triosis; Endosalpingiosis.
      vs. mesothelioma, 424
    sampling of, 419–420
Serotonin
    in carcinoid syndrome, 903
    in hypothalamic gangliocytoma, 2039
    valve disease associated with, 525
Serous adenocarcinoma
    broad ligament, 1392
    cervical, 1317, CD Figs. 36–101 and 36–
      102
    endometrial, 1343, 1343t, 1347–1348,
      1348f, 1349, CD Fig. 37–31
    ovarian, 1401, 1402f, 1403–1404, 1403f–
      1404f, 1415
    vs. mesothelioma, electron microscopy
      and, 85–86, 85f
Serous borderline tumor
    broad ligament, 1391
    fallopian tube, 1387
    ovarian. *See also* Serous LMP tumor,
      ovarian.
      tubal epithelium and, 1387
      vs. endosalpingiosis, 1366
    paratesticular, 1244, 1244f, CD Fig. 34–
      27
    peritoneal, 426, 426f, 1403
Serous carcinoma
    micropapillary, ovarian, 1403, 1403f
    papillary
      fallopian tube, 1387–1388, 1388f,
        1390t, CD Fig. 38–13
      ovarian, 1387
      peritoneal, 1404
      paratesticular, 1244
Serous carcinoma in situ, of fallopian tube,
    1387

Serous cystadenoma
    broad ligament, 1391
    fallopian tube, 1386
    hepatic, 932
    ovarian, 1401, 1401f–1402f, CD Fig.
      39–3
Serous fat atrophy, 1641, 1641f
Serous LMP tumor. *See also* Serous border-
    line tumor.
    ovarian, 1401–1403, 1401f–1402f, CD
      Fig. 39–6 to 39–8
      peritoneal implants from, 1403, CD
        Figs. 39–9 to 39–11
      trisomy 12 in, 1422
Serous ovarian tumors, 1401–1405, 1401f–
    1404f, 1422, CD Figs. 39–1 to 39–13
Serous psammocarcinoma
    of ovary and peritoneum, 1404
    of peritoneal cavity, 426
Serrated adenoma(s)
    appendiceal, 855, 855f
    colorectal, 762
    syndrome with, 791–792
Serres, rests of, 323
Sertoli cell nodules, 1238
Sertoli cell tumor
    ovarian, 1419–1420
    testicular, 1237–1238, 1238f, CD Fig. 34–
      20
      large cell calcifying, 1237, 1238–1239,
        1239f
      mixed tumors and, 1239
      vs. carcinoid tumor, 1234
      vs. seminoma, 1225, 1238
Sertoli cell–only syndrome, 1250–1251,
    1250f–1251f
Sertoli cells, 1247–1248
    infertility and, 1249, 1250, 1250f–1251f,
      1251
Sertoliform endometrial adenocarcinoma,
    1347, CD Fig. 37–30
Sertoli-Leydig cell tumor
    ovarian, 1419–1420, 1419f, CD Figs. 39–
      34 to 39–39
      vs. endometrioid adenocarcinoma,
        1409
      vs. mucinous adenocarcinoma, 1407
      vs. serous carcinoma, 1404
    testicular, 1239
SETTLE (spindle epithelial tumor with
    thymus-like element), 1706f–1707f,
    1706t, 1707
Severe combined immunodeficiency, 1544
    splenic lesions in, 1577
Sex cord–stromal tumors
    ovarian, 1415–1422
      cytogenetics of, 1422
      DNA ploidy of, 1422
      granulosa cell, 1415–1417, 1416f, CD
        Figs. 39–27 to 39–31
        DNA ploidy of, 1422
        trisomy 12 in, 1422
        vs. clear cell adenocarcinoma, 1410
        vs. small cell carcinoma, 1431
      immunohistochemistry of, 1422
      mixed with germ cell tumors, 1429–
        1430, CD Figs. 39–56 to 39–58
      Ollier's disease with, 1872
      Sertoli-Leydig cell, 1419–1420, 1419f,
        CD Figs. 39–34 to 39–39
        vs. endometrioid adenocarcinoma,
          1409
        vs. mucinous adenocarcinoma, 1407
        vs. serous carcinoma, 1404
      steroid cell, 1420–1422, 1421f–1422f

Sex cord–stromal tumors *(Continued)*
    thecoma-fibroma, 1417–1419, 1417f–
      1418f, CD Figs. 39–32 and 39–33
    unclassified, 1422
    with annular tubules, 1420, 1421f, CD
      Figs. 39–40 and 39–41
    testicular, 1236–1239, 1236f–1239f, CD
      Figs. 34–20 to 34–23
      clear cell, vs. seminoma, 1225, 1239
      immunohistochemistry of, 1221t, 1222
      mixed, 1239
      mixed with germ cell tumors, 1240,
        1240f, CD Fig. 34–24
      unclassified, 1239, 1240, CD Fig. 34–
        23
    uterine tumors resembling, 1347, 1353,
      1353f, CD Fig. 37–49
Sexually transmitted diseases. *See also* Cer-
    vical carcinoma.
    colitis in, 830–831
    penile lesions in, 1207–1208, 1207f–
      1208f, CD Figs. 33–13 and 33–14
Sézary cell leukemia, 1633
Sézary syndrome, 1538, 1633, 1633f, 1995
    exfoliative dermatitis in, 1929
Shaggy aorta syndrome, 816
Sharpey's fibers, 1858
Shave biopsy, 1919
Shave sections, 27
Sheehan's syndrome, 2050, 2052
Shiga toxin
    from enterohemorrhagic *E. coli*, 823, 824
    from *Shigella*, 823
Shigellosis, 822–823
Shock, hepatic centrilobular injury in, 956,
    957
Shock lung, 389–390, 389f, CD Fig. 15–18
Short intestine syndrome, 740
Shoulder, bursitis of, 1854
Shrapnell membrane, 303
Shwachman-Diamond syndrome, 1642
SIADH, neuroendocrine pulmonary carci-
    noma and, 341, 351, 353
Sialadenitis
    chronic
      in nicotine stomatitis, 321
      of minor salivary glands, in Sjögren's
        syndrome, 269–270
    chronic sclerosing, 268–269, 269f, CD
      Figs. 12–118 and 12–119
    myoepithelial. *See* Benign lymphoepithe-
      lial lesion (BLEL).
Sialadenoma papilliferum, 250–251, 251f,
    CD Figs. 12–43 and 12–44
    esophageal lesion resembling, 634
Sialoblastoma, 251, 251f, CD Figs. 12–45
    and 12–46
Sialolithiasis, 268, 269
Sialometaplasia
    necrotizing, 269, 269f, CD Fig. 12–120
      laryngeal, 220, 220f
      sinonasal, 199
Sicca syndrome, primary biliary cirrhosis
    with, 950
Sickle cell disease
    bone infarct in, 1864
    bone marrow necrosis in, 1646
    osteomyelitis in, 1863
    prenatal diagnosis of, 118
    renal complications of, 1030
    splenic involvement of, 1576, 1579
Sickle cell trait, medullary renal carcinoma
    and, 1083
Sideroblastic anemias, 1606, 1607, 1643

Suppressor T lymphocytes
  in peripheral myopathy and neuropathy, 2170
  in subcutaneous panniculitis–like T cell lymphoma, 1539–1540
Supraglottis, 211
  neoplasms of, 212t
Sural nerve biopsy. *See* Nerve biopsy.
Surface epithelial inclusion cyst, ovarian, 1435
Surfactant, pulmonary, 339, 340
Surfactant apoprotein
  in bronchioloalveolar carcinoma, 348
  in papillary adenoma, 382
  in pulmonary blastoma, 367
  in sclerosing hemangioma, 384
Surgical margin evaluation, 26–29, 27f–29f
  frozen section for, 22, 23, 23f, 27, 27f, 28, 29, 29f, 38
  inking for. *See* Inking of margins.
  Mohs technique for, 27–28, 28f–29f
  molecular methods for, 25
  of breast specimen, 28–29, 565
    from lumpectomy, 17
  of cervical electrosurgery specimen, 1300, CD Figs. 36–24 to 36–27
  of colorectal specimen, 775, 781, 783–784
  of cystectomy specimen, 1119
  of head and neck specimen, 152
  of liver resection specimen, 919
  of ophthalmic specimen, 2173, 2174
  of prostate specimen, 1176–1177, 1178–1179
Surgical pathology report. *See* Pathology report.
SVC. *See* Superior vena cava (SVC) syndrome.
Sweat gland carcinoma, 1974–1975, 1975f. *See also* Apocrine tumors; Eccrine tumors.
Swiss cheese disease, of breast, 598
Sympathetic nervous system tumors. *See also* Ganglioneuroblastoma; Ganglioneuroma; Neuroblastoma.
  mediastinal, 484–485, 484f
Synaptophysin, 67, 68
  Alzheimer's disease and, 2132
  in small cell carcinoma, cervical, 1318, 1318f
Syncytial endometritis, 1470, CD Fig. 40–88
Syncytial giant cell hepatitis, 944
Syncytial variant of nodular sclerosis Hodgkin's disease, 1513–1514, 1513f
  differential diagnosis of, 1516, 1517–1518
Syncytiotrophoblast, 1455, 1455t
Syncytiotrophoblastic tumor cells
  in choriocarcinoma
    mediastinal, 467
    ovarian, 1426
    testicular, 1220, 1231–1232, 1231f
  in dysgerminoma, 1423
  in embryonal carcinoma, ovarian, 1425
  in seminoma, 1223
  in suprasellar germ cell tumor, 2043, 2044
Synechia(e), peripheral anterior, 2178, 2178f
Synoptic reporting, 52
Synovial chondromatosis, 1857–1858, 1858f
  chondrosarcoma associated with, 1878
  of temporomandibular joint, 302–303
  osteochondroma associated with, 1857–1858, 1858f
  vs. soft tissue chondroma, 1840

Synovial chondrometaplasia. *See* Synovial chondromatosis.
Synovial chondrosarcoma, 1858
Synovial hemangioma, 1818, 1858
Synovial lipoma, 1790
Synovial membrane, 1854
  amyloid in, 1857
  giant cell tumor of, 1857. *See also* Giant cell tumor of tendon sheath.
  in rheumatoid arthritis, 1855–1856, 1855f–1856f
  in scleroderma-related arthritis, 1857
  in systemic lupus erythematosus, 1857
Synovial metaplasia, on breast implants, 590
Synovial osteochondromatosis. *See* Synovial chondromatosis.
Synovial sarcoma, 1830–1831, 1830f
  electron microscopy of, 86
  esophageal, 648
  intra-articular, 1858
  mediastinal, 491
  molecular methods and
    for diagnosis, 104t, 109
    for surgical margin evaluation, 114
  pleural, 430
    vs. mesothelioma, 423, 424
  prostatic, 1184
  pulmonary, 373–374, 373f–374f, CD Fig. 15–10
    vs. fibrosarcoma, 370
    vs. solitary fibrous tumor, 369
  sinonasal, 190
  vs. angiomatoid fibrous histiocytoma, 1812
  vs. epithelioid sarcoma, 1832
  vs. fibrosarcoma, 1807
  vs. hemangiopericytoma, 1821
  vs. malignant peripheral nerve sheath sarcoma, 1837
Synoviocytes, 1854
Synovioma. *See* Giant cell tumor of tendon sheath.
Synovitis, infectious, 1856
Synovium. *See* Synovial membrane.
α-Synuclein, 2126, 2130, 2131–2133, 2131f–2132f
Syphilis
  anorectal, 831, 879, 880
  aortitis in, 523, 526–527
  gastritis in, 710
  intrauterine infection in, 1464–1465
  laryngeal involvement in, 218, 231
  lymphadenitis in, 1491, 1492
    vs. Castleman's disease, 1494
  membranous glomerulopathy in, 1012, 1013
  otitis media in, 299
  penile, 1207
  pituitary involvement in, 2049, 2050
  secondary, 1932
Syringocystadenoma papilliferum, 1976
  of external ear, 285
Syringoid carcinoma, 1974
Syringoma, 1972
  chondroid, 1972–1973, 1972f
    vs. ossifying fibromyxoid tumor, 1809
  malignant, 1974
Syringomatous adenoma, infiltrating, of breast, 595
Syringomatous carcinoma, sweat duct, 595
Systematized Nomenclature of Medicine (SNOMED), 41, 55, 55t
Systemic sclerosis. *See* Scleroderma (systemic sclerosis).

T cell. *See* T lymphocytes.
T cell immunophenotyping, of thymic tumors, 451
T cell intracellular antigen 1 (TIA-1), 1539, 1540, 1542, 1587
T cell leukemia(s), 1630–1633, 1631f–1633f, CD Figs. 43–20 and 43–21. *See also* specific leukemia.
  acute lymphoblastic, 1614–1615, 1614f
  colorectal polyposis in, 799
T cell lymphocytosis, transient, 1644
T cell lymphoma(s), 1518, 1519. *See also* specific lymphoma.
  adrenal, 1775f, 1776
  anaplastic. *See* Anaplastic large cell lymphoma.
  classification of, 1519, 1520t
  CNS, 2096–2097
  colorectal, 799
  cutaneous, 1994–1997, 1995f–1997f, CD Fig. 49–14
    vs. actinic reticuloid, 1926
  gastric, 693, 694
  hemophagocytic syndrome in, 1500, 1576
  hepatosplenic γδ, 1538, 1540, 1587, 1587f, 1588t, 1589, CD Fig. 42–13
    hemophagocytic syndrome in, 1576
    vs. histiocytic lymphoma, 1550
  histiocytic medullary reticulosis as, 1550
  immunophenotype of, 1515t, 1537, 1537f
  in HIV-infected patients, 1545
  in organ transplant recipients, 1546
  intestinal, 728–729, 728f
    with celiac disease, 725, 1539
  lymphoblastic, 1542–1544, 1543f
    mediastinal, 483
    with myeloproliferative disorders, 1620
  mature (peripheral), 1535–1540
    extranodal, 1538–1540, 1539f–1540f
    in organ transplant recipients, 1546
    not otherwise characterized, 1536–1537, 1536f–1537f
    sinonasal, 183–184, 183f–184f
    subtypes of, 1538–1540, 1538f–1540f. *See also* specific subtype.
  transforming to anaplastic large cell lymphoma, 1540
  vs. B cell lymphomas, 1537
  vs. Hodgkin's disease, 1517
  vs. lymphoplasmacytic lymphoma, 1528–1529
  NK cells and. *See* T-NK cell lymphoma.
  splenic involvement in, 1574
  testicular, 1241
  thyroid, 1708
  uterine, 1365
T cell lymphomatous panniculitis, 1996–1997, 1997f
T cell receptor gene rearrangement, 1588t
  in lymphoblastic lymphoma, 483
  in peripheral T cell lymphoma, 1537, 1538, 1540
T cell–rich B cell lymphoma, 1533, 1533f, 1534
  bone marrow involvement by, 1636
  vs. Hodgkin's disease, 1517
T lymphocytes
  cytotoxic, in peripheral T cell lymphoma, 1537, 1539, 1540
  endometrial, 1329, 1331, CD Figs. 37–5 and 37–6
  helper
    in Hodgkin's disease, 1515
    in mycosis fungoides, 1538